WONG'S

Essentials
of Pediatric Nursing

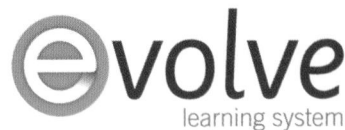 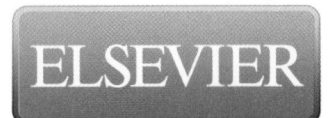
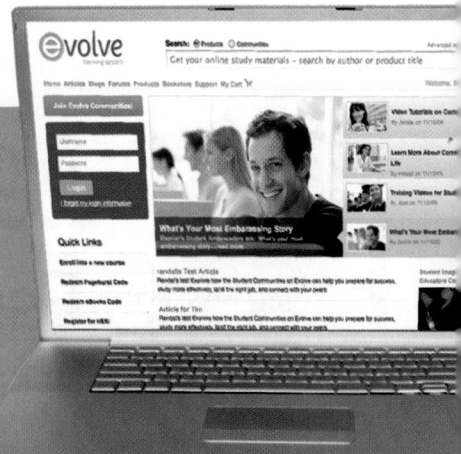

NINTH EDITION

WONG'S
Essentials
of Pediatric Nursing

Marilyn J. Hockenberry, PhD, RN, PNP-BC, FAAN
Professor, Duke School of Nursing;
Chair, Duke Institutional Research Board
Duke University
Durham, North Carolina

David Wilson, MS, RNC-NIC
Staff
Children's Hospital at Saint Francis
Tulsa, Oklahoma

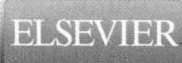

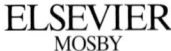

ELSEVIER
MOSBY

3251 Riverport Lane
St. Louis, Missouri 63043

WONG'S ESSENTIALS OF PEDIATRIC NURSING   ISBN: 978-0-323-08343-0
Copyright © 2013 by Mosby, an imprint of Elsevier Inc.

NCLEX®, NCLEX-RN®, and NCLEX-PN® are registered trademarks and service marks of the National Council of State Boards of Nursing, Inc.

Previous editions Copyright © 2009, 2005, 2001, 1997, 1993, 1989, 1985, 1982 by Mosby, Inc., an affiliate of Elsevier Inc.

Library of Congress Cataloging-in-Publication Data
Wong's essentials of pediatric nursing / [edited by] Marilyn J. Hockenberry, David Wilson.—9th ed.
    p. ; cm.
  Essentials of pediatric nursing
  Includes bibliographical references and index.
  ISBN 978-0-323-08343-0 (hardcover : alk. paper)
  I. Hockenberry, Marilyn J.   II. Wilson, David, 1950 Aug. 25–   III. Wong, Donna L., 1948–2008.
IV. Title: Essentials of pediatric nursing.
  [DNLM: 1. Pediatric Nursing.   WY 159]
  618.92′00231—dc23
                                                                    2012018414

Content Manager: Michele D. Hayden
Content Development Specialist: Heather Bays
Publishing Services Manager: Jeff Patterson
Project Manager: Megan Isenberg
Design Direction: Margaret Reid
Chapter Opener Art: © iStockphoto.com

Printed in the United States of America

Last digit is the print number: 9   8   7   6   5   4   3   2

CONTRIBUTORS

Annette L. Baker, RN, MSN, PNP
Pediatric Nurse Practitioner
Cardiovascular Program
Children's Hospital, Boston
Boston, Massachusetts

Rose Ann Urdiales Baker, PhD, PMHCNS-BC
Assistant Professor
University of Akron
College of Health Professionals
Akron, Ohio

Linda K. Ballard, CPNP, MSN
Pediatric Nurse Practitioner
Aflac Cancer Center and Blood Disorders
    Service
Children's Healthcare of Atlanta
Atlanta, Georgia

Ray Barfield, MD, PhD
Associate Professor of Pediatrics and
    Christian Philosophy;
Director, Pediatric Palliative Care
Duke University
Durham, North Carolina

Debra Brandon, PhD, RN, CCNS, FAAN
Associate Professor and Director PhD
    Program, Duke University School of
    Nursing;
Associate Professor, Department of
    Pediatrics;
Neonatal CNS, Duke Intensive Care Nursery
Durham, North Carolina

Christine A. Brosnan, DrPH, RN
Associate Professor of Nursing-Clinical
University of Texas Health Science Center
Houston School of Nursing
Houston, Texas

Terri L. Brown, MSN, RN, CPN
Clinical Specialist
Texas Children's Hospital
Houston, Texas

Rosalind Bryant, PhD, APRN-BC, PNP
Pediatric Nurse Practitioner
Texas Children's Hospital;
Instructor
Baylor College of Medicine
Houston, Texas

Patricia M. Conlon, RN, MS, CNS, CNP
Pediatric Clinical Nurse Specialist
Mayo Eugenio Litta Children's Hospital
Mayo Clinic Children's Center
Rochester, Minnesota

Martha Curry, MS, RN, CPNP
Pediatric Nurse Practitioner
Rheumatology Service
Texas Children's Hospital;
Instructor
Department of Pediatrics
Baylor College of Medicine
Houston, Texas

Amy E. Delaney, RN, MSN, CPNP-ACIP
Pediatric Nurse Practitioner
Hyde Park Pediatrics
Hyde Park, Massachusetts

Sharron L. Docherty, CPNP, PhD
Associate Professor, School of Nursing
Associate Professor, Department of
    Pediatrics, School of Medicine
Duke University
Durham, North Carolina

Quinn Franklin, MS, CCLS
Research Specialist Texas Children's Hospital
Adjunct Faculty University of Alabama
Adjunct Instructor San Jacinto Community
    College
Houston, Texas

Debbie Fraser, MN, RNC-NIC
Associate Professor
Advanced Nurse Practitioner Program
Centre for Nursing and Health Studies
Athabasca University
Athabasca, Alberta, Canada

Martina R. Gallagher, PhD, RN
Assistant Professor
University of Texas
Health Science Center at Houston
School of Nursing
Department of Nursing Systems
Houston, Texas

Valerie J. Groben, RN, MSN, APRN-BC
Pediatric Nurse Practitioner, Neuro
    Oncology
St. Jude Children's Research Hospital
Memphis, Tennessee

Sarah M. Gutknecht, DNP, RN, CPNP
Pediatric Nurse Practitioner
Pediatric Orthopaedics
Gillette Children's Specialty Healthcare
St. Paul, Minnesota

Eufemia Jacob, PhD, RN
Assistant Professor
University of California Los Angeles
Los Angeles, California

Kristine C. Jordan, PhD, MPH, RD
Assistant Professor
University of Utah
Salt Lake City, Utah

Linda M. Kollar, RN, MSN
Clinical Director
Surgical Weight Loss Program for Teens
Cincinnati Children's Hospital Medical
    Center
Cincinnati, Ohio

Deborah Suzanne Lammert, APRN-CNS, CCRN-P, MSN
Samaritans Purse International Relief
Boone, North Carolina;
Physician Support Services International
Tulsa, Oklahoma

Kathy McCarthy, BSN, RN
Senior Research Nurse
Baylor College of Medicine
Texas Children's Cancer and Hematology
    Centers
Houston, Texas

Patricia Barry McElfresh, MN, RN, PNP-BC
Pediatric Nurse Practitioner
Children's Healthcare of Atlanta
Aflac Cancer Center and Blood Disorders
    Service
Atlanta, Georgia

Tara Taneski Merck, MS, RN, CPNP
Pediatric Nurse Practitioner
Children's Healthcare of Atlanta
Aflac Cancer Center and Blood Disorders
    Service
Leukemia and Lymphoma Program
Atlanta, Georgia

Mary A. Mondozzi, MSN, PNP-BC
Burn Center Education/Outreach
    Coordinator
Akron Children's Hospital;
The Paul and Carol David Foundation Burn
    Institute
The Clifford R. Roeckman, MD Regional
    Burn Center
Akron, Ohio

Rebecca A. Monroe, MSN, RN, CPNP
Pediatric Nurse Practitioner
Pediatrics After Hours
Plano, Texas

Barbara Montagnino, MS, RN, CNS
Clinical Nurse Specialist
Progressive Care Unit
Texas Children's Hospital
Houston, Texas

Kim Mooney-Doyle, MSN, CPNP, CPON
PhD Student;
Instructor
University of Pennsylvania
School of Nursing
Philadelphia, Pennsylvania

Cynthia A. Prows, MSN, CNS, FAAN
Clinical Nurse Specialist, Genetics
Children's Hospital Medical Center
Cincinnati, Ohio

Elizabeth Record, BSN, MSN, DNP
Pediatric Nurse Practitioner
Hematology/Oncology Department
Children's Healthcare of Atlanta
Atlanta, Georgia

Robyn Rice, PhD, RN
Clinical Manager, SSM Hospice
St. Louis, Missouri;
Graduate Online Faculty
Department of Nursing
University of Phoenix
Phoenix, Arizona

Patricia A. Ring, MSN, RN, CPNP
Pediatric Nephrology
Children's Hospital of Wisconsin
Milwaukee, Wisconsin

**Cheryl C. Rodgers, RN, PhD, CPNP,
CPON**
Pediatric Nurse Practitioner
Texas Children's Cancer Center
Texas Children's Hospital;
Instructor
Department of Pediatrics
Baylor College of Medicine
Houston, Texas

**Margaret L. Schroeder, MSN, RN,
PNP-BC**
Cardiovascular Surgery Pediatric Nurse
    Practitioner
Children's Hospital Boston
Boston, Massachusetts

Jean C.K. Stansbury, RN, MSN, CNP
Pediatrics
Certified Pediatric Nurse Practitioner
Gillette Children's Specialty Healthcare
St. Paul, Minnesota

Cheryl Ann Thaxton, RN, MN, CPNP-PC
Certified Hospice and Palliative Pediatric
    Nurse;
Program Coordinator
Pediatric Quality of Life
Duke Children's Hospital and Health Center
Durham, North Carolina

Sandra L. Upchurch, PhD, RN,
Director of Curriculum
Review and Testing
Elsevier
Houston, Texas

**Barbara J. Wheeler, MN, RN,
IBCLC, RLC**
Neonatal Clinical Nurse Specialist
Lactation Consultant
St. Boniface General Hospital;
Professional Affiliate
Manitoba Centre for Nursing and Health
    Research
Winnipeg, Manitoba, Canada

Kristina D. Wilson, PhD, CCC-SLP
Senior Speech Language Pathologist and
    Clinical Researcher
Texas Children's Hospital;
Adjunct Assistant Professor
Department of Plastic Surgery
Baylor College of Medicine
Houston, Texas

Evidence-Based Practice Boxes
Olga A. Taylor, MPH
Senior Research Coordinator
Texas Children's Cancer and Hematology
    Centers
Quality Transformation Core
Houston, Texas

PowerPoint Lecture Slides
Brigit Carter, RN, PhD, CCRN
Assistant Professor
Duke University School of Nursing
Durham, North Carolina

Anne Derouin, RN, DNP, CPNP
Assistant Professor
Duke University School of Nursing
Durham, North Carolina

TEACH For Nurses
Case Studies
Lynne Tier, MSN, RN
Florida Hospital College of Health Sciences
School of Nursing
Orlando, Florida

**Teaching Strategies, Curriculum
Standards, and Teaching Focus**
**Cheryl C. Rodgers, RN, PhD, CPNP,
CPON**
Pediatric Nurse Practitioner
Texas Children's Cancer Center
Texas Children's Hospital;
Instructor
Department of Pediatrics
Baylor College of Medicine
Houston, Texas

Test Bank
Mary L. Dowell, PhD, RN, BC
Assistant Professor
Nursing Department
San Antonio College;
LVN-ADN Program Coordinator
Kerrville Distance Site
Kerrville, Texas

**The Authors Would Also Like
to Acknowledge the Following
Individuals for Contributing
to Earlier Editions**
**Terry Jean Brandt, RN, BSN,
CPON, CPN**
Education Coordinator
Inpatient Hematology Oncology Unit
Texas Children's Cancer Center and
    Hematology Service
Texas Children's Hospital
Houston, Texas

Carol Turnage Carrier, MSN, RN, CNS
Newborn Clinical Nurse Specialist
Texas Children's Hospital;
Clinical Faculty
The University of Texas Health Science
    Center at Houston
School of Nursing
Houston, Texas

Miguel F. Da Cunha, PhD
Former Professor
The University of Texas Health Science
    Center at Houston
School of Nursing
Houston, Texas

Janet DeJean, RN, CPON
Cancer Center and Hematology Service
Texas Children's Hospital
Houston, Texas

Jessica Hilburn, MT (ASCP), CIC
Director, Infection Control and Prevention
Eastern New Mexico Medical Center
Roswell, New Mexico

Brandi Horvath, RN, BSN, CPON
Cancer Center and Hematology Service
Texas Children's Hospital
Houston, Texas

Anh Mac, RN, BSN
Staff Nurse
Texas Children's Hospital
Houston, Texas

Angela C. Morgan, MS, RN, CCRN
Clinical Nurse Specialist, PICU
Texas Children's Hospital
Houston, Texas

Shelly Nalbone, MS, RN, CPNP
Assistant Director
Texas Children's Hospital
Houston, Texas

Theresa E. Reed, RN, BSN
Clinical Nurse Coordinator
Nutrition Support Nurses
Texas Children's Hospital
Houston, Texas

Curt Roberts, RN
Staff Nurse, PICU
Texas Children's Hospital
Houston, Texas

Danna Salinas, RN, BSN
Staff Nurse, PICU
Texas Children's Hospital
Houston, Texas

Angela Brocker, MS, RNC
Clinical Faculty
Georgetown University
Washington, DC

William T. Campbell, EdD, RN
Associate Professor
Department of Nursing
Salisbury University
Salisbury, Maryland

Claire M. Creamer, RN, MS, CPNP-BC
Assistant Professor
Rhode Island College
School of Nursing
Providence, Rhode Island

Nancy Crego, PHD-C, MSN, RN, CCRN
Faculty
Georgetown University
School of Nursing and Health Studies
Washington, DC

Nkonye Ezeobah, PhD, MSN, RN, FNP, CCDC
Associate Professor of Nursing
Los Angeles Southwest College
Los Angeles, California

Marian L. Farrell, PhD, PHM-NP, CRNP, CS
Professor of Nursing
University of Scranton
Scranton, Pennsylvania

Kathy Hodgson, RN, MSN
Nurse Educator
Lutheran School of Nursing
St. Louis, Missouri

Alan B. Jauregui, MD, APN, MSN
Lecturer
Scholarship Affairs Council Chairperson
University of Nevada Las Vegas, School of
Nursing
Las Vegas, Nevada

Katherine Moore, MS, RN-C (NICU)
Instructor
Langston University
Tulsa, Oklahoma

Kathleen Murphy-Ende, RN, PhD, AOCNP
Nurse Practitioner
Formally at the University of Wisconsin
Hospital and Clinics and School of
Nursing
Madison, Wisconsin;
Clinical Psychology Intern
Veterans Administration Hospital of Central
Iowa
Des Moines, Iowa

Katherine A. Roberts, MSN, RN
Assistant Professor of Nursing
Lamar University
Beaumont, Texas

Beverly J. Rossiter, MN, MSN, RN, CPNP
Assistant Professor
Indiana University of Pennsylvania
Indiana, Pennsylvania

Patricia L. Webb, DNP, APRN, CPNP-PC
Clinical Assistant Professor
Department of Nursing
Missouri State University
Springfield, Missouri

Kerstin West-Wilson, RNC, MS, IBCLC
Henry Zarrow Neonatal Intensive Care Unit
Children's Hospital at Saint Francis
Tulsa, Oklahoma

NCLEX-Style Review Questions and Student Case Studies

Colleen W. Bible, MSN, RN
Nursing Faculty
Division of Health Sciences, Nursing
Technical College of the Lowcountry
Beaufort, South Carolina

Test Bank

Alan B. Jauregui, MD, APN, MSN
Scholarship Affairs Committee Chairperson
University of Nevada, Las Vegas
School of Nursing
Las Vegas, Nevada

Christina Keller, RN, MSN
Instructor
Clinical Simulation Center
Radford University
Radford, Virginia

Wong's Essentials of Pediatric Nursing has been a leading book in pediatric nursing since it was first published more than three decades ago. This kind of support places a unique accountability and responsibility on us to earn your future endorsement with each new edition. So, with your encouragement and constructive comments, we offer this extensive revision, the ninth edition of *Wong's Essentials of Pediatric Nursing.*

To accomplish this, Marilyn J. Hockenberry, as editor-in-chief, along with David Wilson, co-editor, and many expert nurses and multidisciplinary specialists, have revised, rewritten, or authored portions of the text concerning areas that are undergoing rapid and complex change. These areas include community nursing, immunizations, genetics, home care, pain assessment and management, high-risk newborn care, adolescent health issues, end-of-life care, and numerous pediatric diseases. We have carefully preserved aspects of the book that have met with universal acceptance—its state-of-the-art research-based information; its strong, integrated focus on the family and community; its logical and user-friendly organization; and its easy-to-read style.

We have tried to meet the increasing demands of faculty and students to teach and to learn in an environment characterized by rapid change, enormous amounts of information, fewer traditional clinical facilities, and less time.

This text encourages students to *think critically.* This edition includes extensively revised nursing care plans that may be individualized according to the patient's needs. The nursing care plans include Nursing Interventions Classification and Nursing Outcomes Classification terminology as well as NANDA Defining Characteristics. The Critical Thinking Case Studies ask the nurse to examine the evidence, consider the assumptions, establish priorities, and evaluate alternative perspectives regarding each patient situation. The Critical Thinking Case Studies support our belief that the science of nursing and related health professions is not black and white. In many instances, it includes shades of gray, such as in the areas of genetic testing, resuscitation, cultural issues, end-of-life care, and quality of life. Revised evidence-based practice boxes include quality and safety competencies from the Quality and Safety Education for Nurses website. Competencies are designed specifically for prelicensed nurses.

This text also serves as a reference manual for practicing nurses. The latest recommendations have been included from authoritative organizations such as the American Academy of Pediatrics, the Centers for Disease Control and Prevention (CDC), the Institute of Medicine, the Agency for Healthcare Research and Quality, the American Pain Society, the American Nurses Association, and the National Association of Pediatric Nurse Associates and Practitioners. To expand the universe of available information, websites and e-mail addresses have been included for hundreds of organizations and other educational resources.

ORGANIZATION OF THE BOOK

The same general approach to the presentation of content has been preserved from the first edition, although some content has been added, condensed, and rearranged within this framework to improve the flow; minimize duplication; and emphasize health care trends, such as home and community care. The book is divided into two broad parts. The first part of the book, Chapters 1 through 17, follows what is sometimes called the "age and stage" approach, considering infancy, childhood, and adolescence from a developmental context. It emphasizes the importance of the nurse's role in health promotion and maintenance and in considering the family as the focus of care. From a developmental perspective, the care of common health problems is presented, giving readers a sense of the normal problems expected in otherwise healthy children and demonstrating when in the course of childhood these problems are most likely to occur. The remainder of the book, Chapters 18 through 32, presents the more serious health problems of infancy, childhood, and adolescence that are not specific to any particular age group and that frequently require hospitalization, major medical and nursing intervention, and home care.

UNIT ONE (Chapters 1 through 5) provides a longitudinal view of the child as an individual on a continuum of developmental changes from birth through adolescence and as a member of a family unit maturing within a culture and a community. Chapter 1 includes a discussion of morbidity and mortality in infancy and childhood and examines child health care from a historical perspective. Because unintentional injury is one of the leading causes of death in children, an overview of this topic is included. The nursing process, with emphasis on nursing diagnosis and outcomes and on the importance of developing critical thinking skills, is presented. In this edition, the critical components of evidence-based practice are added and provide the template for exploring the latest pediatric nursing research or practice guidelines throughout the book.

This book is about families with children, and the philosophy of family-centered care is emphasized. This book is also about providing atraumatic care—care that minimizes the psychologic and physical stress that health promotion and illness treatment can inflict. Features such as Evidence-Based Practice, Family-Centered Care, Community Focus, Research Focus, Drug Alert, and Atraumatic Care boxes bring these philosophies to life throughout the text. Finally, the philosophy of delivering nursing care is addressed. We believe strongly that children and families need consistent caregivers. The establishment of the therapeutic relationship with the child and family is explored as the essential foundation for providing quality nursing care.

Chapter 2 provides important information on community-based nursing care, with emphasis on epidemiology as it applies to the detection and identification of causes of morbidity and mortality in pediatrics. A community project presented in this chapter reflects the important components of the nursing process, such as completion of a community needs assessment, planning phase, implementation, and evaluation.

Chapter 3, devoted to the family, further emphasizes the importance of this social group in relation to the health and welfare of children. Family theories establish the tone of the chapter, which includes a variety of parenting situations that reflect contemporary society. Family strengths and vulnerabilities are addressed, and current findings on adoption, divorce, single-parenting, stepfamilies, and dual-earner families have been incorporated.

Chapter 4 provides the opportunity to expand the discussion of social, cultural, and religious influences on child development and health promotion, including socioeconomic factors, customs, and health beliefs and practices. The content more clearly describes the role of the nurse, with emphasis on cultural sensitivity and culturally competent care. Throughout this chapter, extensive revisions have been made to the tables, detailing cultural and religious factors to make the information more manageable and user friendly. The basic overview of child development in Chapter 5 remains up to date and expands on the theoretic approach to personality development and learning. Biologic systems development is not emphasized in this chapter but is discussed more fully in relation to major systems dysfunction in later chapters.

UNIT TWO (**Chapters 6 and 7**) is concerned with the principles of nursing assessment, including communication and interviewing skills, observation, physical and behavioral assessment, health guidance, and the latest information on preventive care guidelines. Chapter 6 contains guidelines for communicating with children, adolescents, and their families, as well as a detailed description of a health assessment, including discussion of family assessment, nutritional assessment, and a sexual history. Content on communication techniques is outlined to provide a concise format for reference. Chapter 6 continues by providing a comprehensive approach to physical examination and developmental assessment, with updated material on temperature measurement, body mass index–for-age guidelines, and the latest World Health Organization and CDC clinical growth charts. Chapter 7 is an important chapter, devoted to critical assessment and management of pain in children. Although the literature on pain assessment and management in children has grown considerably, this knowledge has not been widely applied in practice. Chapter 7 was added to address this concern by presenting detailed assessment and management strategies, including discussion of common pain states in children.

UNIT THREE (**Chapters 8 and 9**) stresses the importance of the neonatal period in relation to child survival during the first few months and the impact on health in later life. In Chapter 8, several areas have been revised to reflect current issues, especially in terms of the educational needs of the family during the infant's transition to extrauterine life as well as the recognition of newborn problems in the first few weeks of life. Current issues that have been updated include proactive measures to prevent infant abduction; hospital-based, baby-friendly breastfeeding initiatives; choices for circumcision analgesia; newborn atraumatic care; car safety seats; and newborn screening, including universal newborn hearing screening. Newborn skin care guidelines have also been updated, and choices for newborn umbilical cord care are discussed. Chapter 9 stresses the nurse's role in caring for the high-risk newborn and the importance of astute observations to the survival of this vulnerable group of infants. Modern advances in neonatal care have mandated extensive revision with a greater sensitivity to the diverse needs of infants, from those with extremely low birth weights, late-preterm infants, and those of normal gestational age who have difficulty making an effective transition to extrauterine life. Updates in Chapter 9 include information on late-preterm infant care; neonatal bilirubin monitoring and intervention guidelines; acid–base balance; therapeutic hypothermia; preterm infant nutrition; and neonatal exposure to maternal environmental conditions such as alcohol, tobacco, and recreational drugs, as well as exposure to viral infections, including human parvovirus and herpes. This chapter also includes the latest information regarding the detection and management of inborn errors of metabolism.

UNITS FOUR through SIX (**Chapters 10 through 17**) present the major developmental stages outlined in Unit One, which are expanded to provide a broader concept of these stages and the health problems most often associated with each age group. Special emphasis is placed on preventive aspects of care. The chapters on health promotion follow a standard approach that is used consistently for each age group.

Chapter 10 includes the latest information regarding childhood immunizations as well as a discussion regarding the association between childhood immunizations and autism. Chapter 11 has been streamlined in regard to vitamin and mineral imbalances yet continues to focus on the influence of nutrition in early childhood as it impacts health status in adulthood. The sections on colic, sudden infant death syndrome, and car seat safety in infancy have been updated as well. The influence of nutrition in preschool-age and school-age children (especially decreasing fat intake) in relation to later chronic diseases such as obesity and hypertension is also discussed. The potential negative effects of exposure to violence and terrorism are included as well.

The chapters on health problems in these units primarily reflect more typical and age-related concerns. The information on many disorders has been revised to reflect recent changes. Examples include sudden infant death syndrome, lead poisoning, wound healing, attention-deficit/hyperactivity disorder, contraception, teenage pregnancy, and substance abuse. The chapters on adolescence include the latest information regarding substance abuse, adolescent immunizations, and the impact of adolescent nutrition on cardiovascular health.

UNIT SEVEN (**Chapters 18 through 20**) deals with children who have the same developmental needs as growing children but who, because of congenital or acquired physical, cognitive, or sensory impairment, require alternative interventions to facilitate development. Chapter 18 reflects current trends in the care of families and children with chronic illness or disability such as providing home care, normalizing children's lives, focusing on developmental needs, enabling and empowering families, and promoting early intervention. Extensive revisions have been made to reflect increased awareness of the need for quality nursing care at the end of life. This section highlights common fears experienced by the child and family and includes discussion of symptom management and nurses' reactions to caring for dying children.

The content in Chapter 19 on cognitive or sensory impairment includes important updates on the definition and classification of cognitive impairment. Autism is discussed in this chapter to provide a cohesive overview of cognitive and sensory impairments. Chapter 20 has been completely revised by an expert in pediatric home health. This chapter provides an overview of home health in the context of the family as the expert in the care of the child with a chronic or acute illness requiring home care. This chapter presents important discussions related to the selection of a home health care agency, the role of the nurse in empowering the family, and case management in home health.

UNIT EIGHT (**Chapters 21 and 22**) is concerned with the impact of hospitalization on the child and family and presents a comprehensive overview of the stressors imposed by hospitalization and discusses nursing interventions to prevent or eliminate them. New research on short-stay or outpatient admissions addresses preparing children for these experiences. Chapter 21 provides updated information on the effects of illness and hospitalization on children at specific ages and the effects on their development. The increasing role of ambulatory and outpatient settings for surgical procedures is also discussed. Chapter 22 includes numerous revised Evidence-Based Practice boxes that include QSEN competencies and are designed to provide rationales for the interventions discussed in the chapter. A new focus in this chapter is the evidence related to preparation of the child for procedures commonly performed by nurses. Recommendations for practice are based on the evidence and concisely presented in Evidence-Based Practice boxes throughout the chapter.

UNITS NINE through TWELVE (**Chapters 23 through 32**) consider serious health problems of infants and children primarily from the biologic systems orientation, which has the practical organizational value of permitting health problems and nursing considerations to relate to specific pathophysiologic disturbances. Important revisions include discussions of hepatitis, cardiopulmonary resuscitation, all blood disorders, respiratory illnesses including influenza, acute lung injury and respiratory syncytial virus, tuberculosis, asthma, cystic fibrosis, effects of second-hand smoke exposure, seizures, chemotherapy, acquired immunodeficiency syndrome, diabetes mellitus, and burns. The information on orthopedic and muscular injuries in childhood as a result of sports participation or other injuries has been extensively revised to reflect current treatment modalities. Chapter 29 includes focused attention on type 2 diabetes and new information on insulin preparations and types of glucose meters.

Extensive **appendixes** are also included and contain information on growth measurements, pediatric laboratory values, and several foreign-language translations of the Wong-Baker FACES Pain Rating Scale. An appendix containing Spanish translations of common terms and phrases used in health care and pediatric nursing is included. All of the appendix material reflects the most current versions of forms, charts, and measurements.

UNIFYING PRINCIPLES

Several unifying principles have guided the organizational structure of this book since its inception. These principles continue to strengthen the book with each revision to produce a text that is consistent in approach throughout each chapter.

The Family as the Unit of Care

The child is an essential member of the family unit. Nursing care is most effective when it is delivered with the belief that *the family is the patient.* This belief permeates the book. When a child is healthy, the child's health is enhanced when the family is a fully functioning, health-promoting system. The family unit can be manifested in a myriad of structures; each has the potential to provide a caring, supportive environment in which the child can grow, mature, and maximize his or her human potential. In addition to the integration of family-centered care into every chapter, an entire chapter is devoted to understanding the family as the core focus in children's lives. Another chapter discusses the social, cultural, and religious influences that impact family beliefs. Separate sections in another chapter deal in depth with family communication and family assessment. The impact of illness and hospitalization, home care, community care, and the death of a child are covered extensively in four additional chapters. The needs of the family are emphasized throughout the text under Nursing Care Management in a separate section on family support. Numerous Family-Centered Care boxes are included to assist nurses in understanding and providing helpful information to families.

An Integrated Approach to Development

Children are not small adults but special individuals with unique minds, bodies, and needs. No book on pediatric nursing is complete without extensive coverage of communication, nutrition, play, safety, dental care, sexuality, sleep, self-esteem, and of course, parenting. Nurses promote the healthy expression of all these dimensions of personhood and need to understand how these functions are expressed by different children at different developmental ages and stages. Effective parenting depends on knowledge of development, and it is often the nurse's responsibility to provide parents with a developmental awareness of their children's needs. For these reasons, coverage of the many dimensions of childhood is integrated within the growth and development chapters rather than being presented in separate chapters. For example, safety concerns for a toddler are much different from those for an adolescent. Sleep needs change with age, as do nutritional needs. As a result, the units on each stage of childhood contain complete information on all these functions as they relate to the specific age. In the unit on school-age children, for instance, information is presented on nutritional needs, age-appropriate play and its significance, safety concerns characteristic of the age group, appropriate dental care, sleep characteristics, and means of promoting self-esteem—a particularly significant concern for school-age children. The challenges of being the parent of a school-age child are presented, and interventions are suggested that nurses can use to promote healthy parenting. Using the integrated approach, students gain an appreciation for the unique characteristics and needs of children at every age and stage of development.

Focus on Wellness and Illness: Child, Family, and Community

In a pediatric nursing text, a focus on illness is expected. Children become ill, and nurses typically are involved in helping children get well. However, it is not sufficient to prepare nursing students to care primarily for sick children. First, health is more than the absence of disease. Being healthy is being whole in mind, body, and spirit. Therefore, the majority of the first half of the book is devoted to discussions that promote physical, emotional, psychosocial, mental, and spiritual wellness. Much emphasis is placed on anticipatory guidance of parents to prevent injury or illness in their children. Second, health care is more than ever prevention focused. The objectives set forth in the *Healthy People 2020* report clearly establish a health care agenda in which solutions to medical and social problems lie in preventive strategies. Third, health care is moving from acute care settings to the community, the home, short-stay centers, and clinics. Nurses must be prepared to function in all settings. To be successful, they must understand the pathophysiology, diagnosis, and treatment of health conditions. Competent nursing care flows from this knowledge and is enhanced by an awareness of childhood development, family dynamics, and communication skills.

Nursing Care

Although the information in this text incorporates information from numerous disciplines (medicine, pathophysiology, pharmacology, nutrition, psychology, sociology), its primary purpose is to provide information on the nursing care of children and families. Discussions of all disorders conclude with a section on Nursing Care Management. In addition, 14 care plans are included. Taken together, they cover the nursing care for many childhood diseases, disorders, and conditions. The purposes of the care plans, like every other feature of the book, are to teach and to convey information. They include all current nursing diagnoses approved by NANDA International that have a potential bearing on the health problem. For every diagnosis, defining characteristics, appropriate patient outcomes, and select possible interventions with rationales are presented. The care plans are designed to stimulate critical thinking and encourage the student to individualize outcomes and interventions for the child rather than to provide an extensive picture of all nursing diagnoses, outcomes, and interventions for every given disease or condition.

Culturally Competent Care

Increasing cultural diversity in this country requires nurses caring for children and their families to develop expertise in the care of children from numerous backgrounds. Culturally competent nursing care requires more than acquiring knowledge about ethnic and cultural groups. It encompasses not only awareness of the influence of culture on the child and family but also the ability to intervene appropriately and effectively. The nurse must learn objective skills to focus on the child's, family's, and community's cultural characteristics. The nurse's self-awareness of unique personal cultural backgrounds must be acknowledged in order to understand how they contribute to cross-cultural communication. The importance of the environment of a cross-cultural care setting must be considered when providing clinical nursing care to culturally diverse families. This edition provides numerous learning experiences that examine cross-cultural communication, cultural assessment, cultural interpretation, and appropriate nursing interventions.

The Critical Role of Research and Evidence-Based Practice

This ninth edition is the product of an extensive review of the literature published since the book was last revised. Many readers and researchers have come to rely on the copious references that reflect significant contributions from a broad audience of professionals. To ensure that information is accurate and current, most citations are less than 5 years old, and almost every chapter has entries dated within 1 year of publication. This book reflects the art and science of pediatric nursing. A central goal in every revision is to base care on research rather than on tradition. Evidence-based practice produces measurable outcomes that nurses can use to validate their unique role in the health care system. Throughout the book, Evidence-Based Practice boxes reflect the importance of the science of nursing care.

CANADIAN CONTENT

The ninth edition of this text includes updated Canadian statistics regarding infant and child health in Chapter 1 and Canadian immunization schedules in Chapter 10. Numerous Canadian resource organizations are also provided throughout the text. These efforts are intended to make the text as valuable as possible to Canadian readers.

Much effort has been directed toward making this book easy to teach from and, more important, easy to learn from. In this edition, the following features have been included to benefit educators, students, and practitioners.

ATRAUMATIC CARE boxes emphasize the importance of providing competent care without creating undue physical and psychologic distress. Although many of the boxes provide suggestions for managing pain, atraumatic care also considers approaches to promoting self-esteem and preventing embarrassment.

COMMUNITY FOCUS boxes address issues that expand to the community, such as increasing immunization rates, preventing lead poisoning, and decreasing smoking among teens.

CRITICAL THINKING CASE STUDIES ask the nurse to examine the evidence, consider the assumptions, establish priorities, and evaluate alternative perspectives regarding each patient situation.

CULTURAL CONSIDERATIONS boxes integrate concepts of culturally sensitive care throughout the text. The emphasis is on the clinical application of the information, whether it focuses on toilet training or on male or female circumcision.

DRUG ALERTS highlight critical drug safety concerns for better therapeutic management.

EMERGENCY TREATMENT boxes are flagged by colored thumb tabs, enabling the reader to quickly locate interventions for crisis situations.

EVIDENCE-BASED PRACTICE boxes have been updated in this edition to focus the reader's attention on application of both research and critical thought processes to support and guide the outcomes of nursing care. The EBP boxes include QSEN competencies and provide measurable outcomes that nurses can use to validate their unique role in the health care system.

FAMILY-CENTERED CARE boxes present issues of special significance to families that have a child with a particular disorder. This feature is another method of highlighting the needs or concerns of families that should be addressed when family-centered care is provided.

NURSING ALERT features call the reader's attention to considerations that if ignored could lead to a deteriorating or emergency situation. Key assessment data, risk factors, and danger signs are among the kinds of information included.

NURSING CARE GUIDELINES summarize important nursing interventions for a variety of situations and conditions.

NURSING CARE PLANS include the latest NANDA nursing diagnoses and associated defining characteristics (signs and symptoms), which assist the nurse in the validation of the selected nursing diagnosis. The nursing care plans also include patient outcomes and Nursing Outcomes Classification terminology. Selected nursing interventions and Nursing Interventions Classification terminology are designed to guide the student to individualize the child's and family's care. The inclusion of the classification terminology, including NANDA diagnoses, Nursing Interventions Classification, and Nursing Outcomes Classification, provides a common language for the nurse to identify the unique needs of children and their families.

NURSING PROCESS boxes streamline the nursing process information on major diseases and conditions for easy identification.

NURSING TIPS notes present handy information of a nonemergency nature that makes patients more comfortable and the nurse's job easier.

PATHOPHYSIOLOGY REVIEWS have been added to this edition to provide the student with a visual representation of the effects of the disease process on the child. These illustrations provide knowledge required for the nurse to implement appropriate evidence-based nursing interventions and provide independent as well as collaborative care with other health care professionals.

QUALITY PATIENT OUTCOMES are added throughout the text to provide a framework for measuring nursing care performance. Nursing-sensitive outcome measures are integrated into the outcome indicators used throughout the book.

RESEARCH FOCUS boxes review new evidence on important topics in a concise way.

SAFETY ALERTS highlight patient safety as part of the QSEN initiative for better outcomes of nursing care.

Numerous pedagogic devices that enhance student learning have been retained from previous editions:

- **CHAPTER OUTLINES** with page numbers begin each chapter and allow readers to quickly locate topics of interest.
- A functional and attractive **FULL-COLOR DESIGN** visually enhances the organization of each chapter, as well as the special features.
- **EVOLVE** at the beginning of each chapter highlight additional resources and information included on the Evolve website. Marginal notes are included throughout the chapter to specify the location of the corresponding content.
- A detailed, cross-referenced **INDEX** allows readers to quickly access discussions.
- **KEY TERMS** are highlighted throughout each chapter to reinforce student learning.
- Hundreds of **TABLES** and **BOXES** highlight key concepts and nursing interventions.
- **KEY POINTS,** located at the end of each chapter, help the reader summarize major concepts, make connections, and synthesize information.
- **LEARNING OBJECTIVES** in each chapter provide the reader with a basic guideline for the major points presented in and learned from the chapter.
- Many of the **COLOR PHOTOGRAPHS** are new, and anatomic drawings are easy to follow, with color appropriately used to illustrate important aspects, such as saturated and desaturated blood. As an example, the full-color heart illustrations in Chapter 25 clearly depict congenital cardiac defects and associated hemodynamic changes.

ACKNOWLEDGMENTS

We are grateful to our mentor, **Donna Wong**, whose support made us better pediatric nurses. We still miss her greatly. We are also grateful to the many nursing faculty members, practitioners, and students who have offered their comments, recommendations, and suggestions. We are especially grateful to the contributors and the many reviewers who brought constructive criticism, suggestions, and clinical expertise to this edition. This edition could not have been completed without the dedication of these special people.

We are especially thankful to **Patrick Barrera** for his continued contributions. His commitment to excellence and attention to detail are essential to maintaining the quality of this book. Thanks go to **Olga Taylor** for her expert support in updating the evidence-based practice boxes throughout the book.

No book is ever a reality without the dedication and perseverance of the editorial staff. Although it is impossible to list every individual at Elsevier who has made exceptional efforts to produce this text, we are especially grateful to **Shelly Hayden, Heather Bays,** and **Megan Isenberg** for their support and commitment to excellence.

Finally, we thank our families and our children—for the unselfish love and endless patience that allows us to devote such a large part of our lives to our careers. Our children have given us the opportunity to directly observe the wonders of childhood.

Marilyn J. Hockenberry
David Wilson

CONTENTS

UNIT 1 CHILDREN, THEIR FAMILIES, AND THE NURSE, 1

1 Perspectives of Pediatric Nursing, 1
Marilyn J. Hockenberry and Patrick Barrera
  Health Care for Children, 2
    Health Promotion, 2
    Childhood Health Problems, 3
    Mortality and Morbidity, 6
  The Art of Pediatric Nursing, 8
    Philosophy of Care, 8
    Role of the Pediatric Nurse, 9
    Research and Evidence-Based Practice, 11
  Clinical Reasoning and the Process of Providing
    Nursing Care to Children and Families, 12
    Clinical Reasoning, 12
    Nursing Process, 12
  Quality Outcome Measures, 13

2 Community-Based Nursing Care of the Child and
  Family, 16
*Christine A. Brosnan, Sandra L. Upchurch, and
Martina R. Gallagher*
  Nursing in the Community, 16
  Community Concepts, 16
    Community, 16
    Demography, 18
    Epidemiology, 18
    Economics, 19
  Community Nursing Process, 19
    Community Needs Assessment and Diagnosis, 19
    Community Planning, 20
    Community Implementation, 20
    Community Evaluation, 20

3 Family Influences on Child Health Promotion, 23
Marilyn J. Hockenberry
  General Concepts, 24
    Definition of Family, 24
    Family Theories, 24
    Family Nursing Interventions, 25
  Family Structure and Function, 26
    Family Structure, 26
    Family Strengths and Functioning Style, 28
  Family Roles and Relationships, 28
    Parental Roles, 28
    Role Learning, 28
  Parenting, 31
    Motivation for Parenthood, 31
    Preparation for Parenthood, 31
    Transition to Parenthood, 31
    Parenting Behaviors, 33
    Limit Setting and Discipline, 33

  Special Parenting Situations, 35
    Parenting the Adopted Child, 35
    Parenting and Divorce, 37
    Single Parenting, 39
    Parenting in Reconstituted Families, 39
    Parenting in Dual-Earner Families, 39
    Foster Parenting, 41
    *Accommodating Contemporary Parenting
    Situations, 41*

4 Social, Cultural, and Religious Influences on Child
  Health Promotion, 43
Kim Mooney-Doyle
  Culture, 43
    The Child and Family in North America, 45
    Social Roles, 45
    Cultural Shock and Cultural Sensitivity, 46
  Subcultural Influences, 46
    Ethnicity, 47
    Minority-Group Membership, 47
    Socioeconomic Class, 47
    Schools, 48
    Communities, 48
    Peer Cultures, 48
    Biculture, 49
    Mass Media, 49
  Socioeconomic Influences, 50
    Poverty, 50
    Homelessness, 51
    Migrant Families, 51
  Cultural Influences, 52
    Cultural Relativity, 52
    Relationships with Health Care Providers, 52
    Communication, 53
    Food Customs, 54
  Health Beliefs and Practices, 54
    Health Beliefs, 55
    Health Practices, 55
    *Importance of Cultural Competence to
    Nurses, 56*
  Cultural Awareness, 57
    Religious Influences, 60
    Religious Beliefs, 60

5 Developmental and Genetic Influences on Child Health
  Promotion, 64
Quinn Franklin and Cynthia Prows
  Growth and Development, 65
    Foundations of Growth and Development, 65
    Biologic Growth and Physical Development, 67
    Physiologic Changes, 69
    Nutrition, 69
    Temperament, 70

Development of Personality and Mental Function, 71
  Theoretic Foundations of Personality Development, 71
  Theoretic Foundations of Mental Development, 72
  Development of Self-Concept, 74
Role of Play in Development, 75
  Classification of Play, 75
  Content of Play, 75
  Social Character of Play, 76
  Functions of Play, 77
  Toys, 78
Developmental Assessment, 78
  Denver II, 78
  Denver II Prescreening Developmental Questionnaire, 80
Genetic Factors That Influence Development, 80
  Overview of Genetics and Genomics, 80

UNIT 2 ASSESSMENT OF THE CHILD AND FAMILY, 86

6 Communication and Physical Assessment of the Child, 86
  Marilyn J. Hockenberry
  Guidelines for Communication and Interviewing, 87
    Establishing a Setting for Communication, 87
    Computer Privacy and Applications in Nursing, 88
    Telephone Triage and Counseling, 88
  Communicating with Families, 88
    Communicating with Parents, 88
    Communicating with Children, 90
    Communication Techniques, 92
  History Taking, 95
    Performing a Health History, 95
  Nutritional Assessment, 99
    Dietary Intake, 99
    Clinical Examination of Nutrition, 102
    Evaluation of Nutritional Assessment, 102
  General Approaches Toward Examining the Child, 102
    Sequence of the Examination, 102
    Preparation of the Child, 102
  Physical Examination, 106
    Growth Measurements, 106
    Physiologic Measurements, 111
    General Appearance, 118
    Skin, 119
    Lymph Nodes, 120
    Head and Neck, 120
    Eyes, 121
    Ears, 125
    Nose, 127
    Mouth and Throat, 128
    Chest, 129
    Lungs, 130
    Heart, 132
    Abdomen, 134
    Genitalia, 136
    Anus, 138
    Back and Extremities, 138
    Neurologic Assessment, 140
7 Pain Assessment and Management in Children, 144
  Eufemia Jacob
  Pain Assessment, 144
    Assessment of Acute Pain, 145
    Assessment of Chronic and Recurrent Pain, 151
    Multidimensional Measures, 151
  Assessment of Pain in Specific Populations, 152
    Pain in Neonates, 152
    Children with Communication and Cognitive Impairment, 153
    Cultural Differences, 156
    Children with Chronic Illness and Complex Pain, 156
  Pain Management, 156
    Nonpharmacologic Management, 159
    Pharmacologic Management, 162
    Consequences of Untreated Pain, 175
  Common Pain States in Children, 175
    Pain in Primary Care, 175
    Painful and Invasive Procedures, 176
    Postoperative Pain, 177
    Burn Pain, 177
    Recurrent Headaches, 177
    Recurrent Abdominal Pain, 178
    Pain with Sickle Cell Disease, 178
    Cancer Pain, 179
    Pain and Sedation in End-of-Life Care, 180

UNIT 3 FAMILY-CENTERED CARE OF THE NEWBORN, 185

8 Health Promotion of the Newborn and Family, 185
  Barbara J. Wheeler
  Adjustment to Extrauterine Life, 186
    Immediate Adjustments, 186
    Physiologic Status of Other Systems, 186
  Nursing Care of the Newborn and Family, 189
    Assessment, 189
    Maintain a Patent Airway, 206
    Maintain a Stable Body Temperature, 207
    Protect from Infection and Injury, 208
    Provide Optimal Nutrition, 214
    Promote Parent–Infant Bonding (Attachment), 219
    Prepare for Discharge and Home Care, 222

9 Health Problems of Newborns, 228
    Debbie Fraser
        Birth Injuries, 229
            Soft Tissue Injury, 229
            Head Trauma, 229
            Fractures, 230
            Paralysis, 231
        Common Problems in the Newborn, 232
            Erythema Toxicum Neonatorum, 232
            Candidiasis, 232
            Herpes Simplex Virus, 233
            Birthmarks, 234
        Nursing Care of the High-Risk Newborn and
            Family, 235
            Identification of High-Risk Newborns, 235
            Care of High-Risk Newborns, 235
        High Risk Related to Dysmaturity, 253
            Preterm Infants, 253
            Postterm Infants, 256
        High Risk Related to Physiologic Factors, 256
            Hyperbilirubinemia, 256
            Hemolytic Disease of the Newborn, 263
            Metabolic Complications, 266
            Respiratory Distress Syndrome, 267
            Respiratory Complications, 273
            Cardiovascular Complications, 279
            Neurologic Complications, 279
            Neonatal Seizures, 279
        High Risk Related to Infectious Processes, 282
            Sepsis, 282
            Necrotizing Enterocolitis, 284
        High Risk Related to Maternal Conditions, 285
            Infants of Diabetic Mothers, 285
            Drug-Exposed Infants, 286
            Maternal Infections, 290
        Congenital Anomalies, 293
            Genetic Etiology of Congenital Anomalies, 294
            Defects Caused by Chemical Agents, 294
        Inborn Errors of Metabolism, 295
            Congenital Hypothyroidism, 297
            Phenylketonuria, 298
            Galactosemia, 300
        Genetic Evaluation and Counseling, 301
            Psychologic Aspects of Genetic Disease, 302

**UNIT 4   FAMILY-CENTERED CARE OF THE
             INFANT, 308**

10 Health Promotion of the Infant and Family, 308
    David Wilson
        Promoting Optimal Growth and Development, 309
            Biologic Development, 309
            *Psychosocial Development: Developing a Sense of
                Trust (Erikson), 318*

            *Cognitive Development: Sensorimotor Phase
                (Piaget), 319*
            Development of Body Image, 320
            Social Development, 320
            Temperament, 322
            *Coping with Concerns Related to Normal Growth
                and Development, 323*
        Promoting Optimal Health During Infancy, 326
            Nutrition, 326
            Sleep and Activity, 330
            Dental Health, 330
            Immunizations, 330
            Safety Promotion and Injury Prevention, 344
            Anticipatory Guidance—Care of Families, 350

11 Health Problems of Infants, 354
    David Wilson
        Nutritional Disorders, 354
            Vitamin Imbalances, 355
            Mineral Imbalances, 355
            Nursing Care Management, 356
            *Protein-Energy Malnutrition (Severe Childhood
                Undernutrition), 356*
            Food Allergy, 358
            Growth Failure (Failure to Thrive), 362
            Sleep Problems, 364
        Positional Plagiocephaly, 366
            Therapeutic Management, 366
            Nursing Care Management, 367
        Disorders of Unknown Etiology, 367
            Colic (Paroxysmal Abdominal Pain), 367
            Sudden Infant Death Syndrome, 368
            Apparent Life-Threatening Event, 372

**UNIT 5   FAMILY-CENTERED CARE OF THE
             YOUNG CHILD, 378**

12 Health Promotion of the Toddler and Family, 378
    David Wilson
        Promoting Optimal Growth and Development, 379
            Biologic Development, 379
            Psychosocial Development, 380
            *Cognitive Development: Sensorimotor and
                Preoperational Phase (Piaget), 380*
            Spiritual Development, 382
            Development of Body Image, 383
            Development of Gender Identity, 383
            Social Development, 383
            *Coping with Concerns Related to Normal Growth
                and Development, 385*
        Promoting Optimal Health During
            Toddlerhood, 390
            Nutrition, 390
            Complementary and Alternative Medicine, 393
            Sleep and Activity, 393

Dental Health, 394
Safety Promotion and Injury Prevention, 396
Anticipatory Guidance—Care of Families, 403

13 Health Promotion of the Preschooler and Family, 407
Rebecca A. Monroe
Promoting Optimal Growth and Development, 408
Biologic Development, 408
Psychosocial Development, 408
Cognitive Development, 408
Moral Development, 409
Spiritual Development, 409
Development of Body Image, 409
Development of Sexuality, 410
Social Development, 410
Coping with Concerns Related to Normal Growth and Development, 412
Promoting Optimal Health During the Preschool Years, 417
Nutrition, 417
Sleep and Activity, 418
Dental Health, 419
Injury Prevention, 419
Anticipatory Guidance—Care of Families, 420

14 Health Problems of Toddlers and Preschoolers, 422
Kathy McCarthy
Infectious Disorders, 423
Communicable Diseases, 423
Conjunctivitis, 432
Stomatitis, 432
Intestinal Parasitic Diseases, 433
General Nursing Care Management, 433
Giardiasis, 434
Enterobiasis (Pinworms), 435
Ingestion of Injurious Agents, 436
Principles of Emergency Treatment, 437
Heavy Metal Poisoning, 441
Lead Poisoning, 441
Child Maltreatment, 445
Child Neglect, 445
Physical Abuse, 446
Sexual Abuse, 447
Nursing Care of the Maltreated Child, 448

UNIT 6   FAMILY-CENTERED CARE OF THE SCHOOL-AGE CHILD AND ADOLESCENT, 457

15 Health Promotion of the School-Age Child and Family, 457
Cheryl C. Rodgers
Promoting Optimal Growth and Development, 458
Biologic Development, 458
Psychosocial Development: Developing a Sense of Industry (Erikson), 459

Cognitive Development (Piaget), 460
Moral Development (Kohlberg), 460
Spiritual Development, 460
Social Development, 460
Developing a Self-Concept, 464
Coping with Concerns Related to Normal Growth and Development, 464
Promoting Optimal Health During the School Years, 468
Nutrition, 468
Sleep and Rest, 468
Exercise and Activity, 468
Dental Health, 469
Sex Education, 470
School Health, 471
Injury Prevention, 472
Anticipatory Guidance—Care of Families, 472

16 Health Promotion of the Adolescent and Family, 476
Linda M. Kollar
Promoting Optimal Growth and Development, 477
Biologic Development, 477
Psychosocial Development, 481
Cognitive Development (Piaget), 482
Moral Development (Kohlberg), 482
Spiritual Development, 482
Social Development, 483
Adolescent Sexuality, 485
Development of Self-Concept and Body Image, 486
Promoting Optimal Health During Adolescence, 487
Immunizations, 488
Nutrition, 489
Sleep and Rest, 490
Dental Health, 491
Personal Care, 491
Stress Reduction, 492
Sexuality Education and Guidance, 493
Safety Promotion and Injury Prevention, 493
Anticipatory Guidance—Care of Families, 495

17 Health Problems of School-Age Children and Adolescents, 498
Linda M. Kollar, Kristine Jordan, and David Wilson
Health Problems of School-Age Children, 499
Problems Related to Elimination, 499
School-Age Disorders with Behavioral Components, 501
Health Problems of Adolescents, 507
Altered Growth and Maturation, 507
Disorders Related to the Reproductive System, 508
Health Problems Related to Sexuality, 510
Nutrition and Eating Disorders, 517
Adolescent Disorders with a Behavioral Component, 527

UNIT 7   FAMILY-CENTERED CARE OF THE CHILD WITH SPECIAL NEEDS, 536

18 Quality of Life for Children Living with Chronic or Complex Diseases, 536
     Sharron L. Docherty, Raymond Barfield, Cheryl Thaxton, and Debra Brandon
          Perspectives on the Care of Children and Families Living with or Dying from Chronic or Complex Diseases, 537
               Scope of the Problem, 537
               Trends in Care, 538
          The Family of the Child with a Chronic or Complex Condition, 540
               Impact of the Child's Chronic Illness, 540
               Coping with Ongoing Stress and Periodic Crises, 542
               Assisting Family Members in Managing Their Feelings, 543
               Establishing a Support System, 544
          The Child with a Chronic or Complex Condition, 545
               Developmental Aspects, 545
               Coping Mechanisms, 545
               Responses to Parental Behavior, 547
               Type of Illness or Condition, 547
          Nursing Care of the Family and Child with a Chronic or Complex Condition, 548
               Assessment, 548
               Provide Support at the Time of Diagnosis, 548
               Support the Family's Coping Methods, 549
               Educate About the Disorder and General Health Care, 552
               Promote Normal Development, 552
               Establish Realistic Future Goals, 554
          Perspectives on the Care of Children at the End of Life, 555
               Principles of Palliative Care, 555
               Decision Making at the End of Life, 555
          Nursing Care of the Child and Family at the End of Life, 560
               Nursing Care Plan: The Child Who Is Terminally Ill or Dying, 560
               Fear of Pain and Suffering, 560
               Fear of Dying Alone or of Not Being Present When the Child Dies, 563
               Fear of Actual Death, 564
               Organ or Tissue Donation and Autopsy, 565
               Grief and Mourning, 565
               Nurses' Reactions to Caring for Dying Children, 566

19 Impact of Cognitive or Sensory Impairment on the Child and Family, 570
     Rosalind Bryant
          Cognitive Impairment, 571
               General Concepts, 571
               Nursing Care of Children with Impaired Cognitive Function, 572
               Down Syndrome, 576
               Fragile X Syndrome, 578
          Sensory Impairment, 579
               Hearing Impairment, 579
               Visual Impairment, 584
               Hearing–Visual Impairment, 589
               Retinoblastoma, 589
               Autism Spectrum Disorders, 590

20 Family-Centered Home Care, 596
     Robyn Rice
          General Concepts of Home Care, 596
               Home Care Trends, 597
               Effective Home Care, 598
               Discharge Planning and Selection of a Home Care Agency, 599
               Care Coordination (Case Management), 600
               Role of the Nurse, Training, and Standards of Care, 601
          Family-Centered Home Care, 603
               Diversity in Home Care, 603
               Parent–Professional Collaboration, 604
               The Nursing Process, 605
               Promotion of Optimum Development, Self-Care, and Education, 606
               Safety Issues in the Home, 608
               Family-to-Family Support, 609

UNIT 8   THE CHILD WHO IS HOSPITALIZED, 612

21 Family-Centered Care of the Child During Illness and Hospitalization, 612
     Tara Merck and Patricia McElfresh
          Stressors of Hospitalization and Children's Reactions, 613
               Separation Anxiety, 613
               Loss of Control, 615
               Effects of Hospitalization on the Child, 616
          Stressors and Reactions of the Family of the Child Who Is Hospitalized, 617
               Parental Reactions, 617
               Sibling Reactions, 617
          Nursing Care of the Child Who Is Hospitalized, 617
               Preparation for Hospitalization, 617
               Nursing Interventions, 621
          Nursing Care of the Family, 627
               Supporting Family Members, 627
               Providing Information, 628

Encouraging Parent Participation, 628
Preparing for Discharge and Home
   Care, 629
Care of the Child and Family in Special Hospital
   Situations, 629
   Ambulatory or Outpatient Setting, 629
   Isolation, 630
   Emergency Admission, 631
   Intensive Care Unit, 631

22 Pediatric Variations of Nursing Interventions, 635
   Terri L. Brown
   General Concepts Related to Pediatric
      Procedures, 636
      Informed Consent, 636
      Preparation for Diagnostic and Therapeutic
         Procedures, 637
      Surgical Procedures, 642
      Compliance, 646
   Skin Care and General Hygiene, 647
      Maintaining Healthy Skin, 647
      Bathing, 648
      Oral Hygiene, 649
      Hair Care, 649
      Feeding the Sick Child, 649
      Controlling Elevated Temperatures, 650
      Family Teaching and Home Care, 651
   Safety, 652
      Environmental Factors, 652
      Infection Control, 653
      Transporting Infants and Children, 654
      Restraining Methods and Therapeutic
         Holding, 655
   Positioning for Procedures, 657
      Femoral Venipuncture, 657
      Extremity Venipuncture or
         Injection, 657
      Lumbar Puncture, 657
      Bone Marrow Aspiration or Biopsy, 658
   Collection of Specimens, 658
      Fundamental Procedure Steps Common to All
         Procedures, 658
      Urine Specimens, 658
      Stool Specimens, 662
      Blood Specimens, 662
      Respiratory Secretion Specimens, 664
   Administration of Medication, 665
      Determination of Drug Dosage, 665
      Oral Administration, 665
      Intramuscular Administration, 667
      Subcutaneous and Intradermal
         Administration, 671
      Intravenous Administration, 671
      Nasogastric, Orogastric, and Gastrostomy
         Administration, 676
      Rectal Administration, 678
      Optic, Otic, and Nasal Administration, 679

Aerosol Therapy, 680
Family Teaching and Home Care, 680
Maintaining Fluid Balance, 681
   Measurement of Intake and Output, 681
   Parenteral Fluid Therapy, 681
Procedures for Maintaining Respiratory
   Function, 687
   Inhalation Therapy, 687
   End-Tidal Carbon Dioxide Monitoring, 689
   Bronchial (Postural) Drainage, 689
   Chest Physical Therapy, 689
   Intubation, 690
   Mechanical Ventilation, 690
   Chest Tube Procedures, 693
Alternative Feeding Techniques, 694
   Gavage Feeding, 695
   Gastrostomy Feeding, 698
   Nasoduodenal and Nasojejunal Tubes, 700
   Total Parenteral Nutrition, 701
   Family Teaching and Home Care, 701
Procedures Related to Elimination, 701
   Enema, 701
   Ostomies, 702
   Family Teaching and Home Care, 702

UNIT 9 THE CHILD WITH PROBLEMS RELATED TO THE TRANSFER OF OXYGEN AND NUTRIENTS, 706

23 The Child with Respiratory Dysfunction, 706
   Patricia M. Conlon
   Respiratory Infection, 707
      Nursing Care Plan: The Child with Acute
         Respiratory Tract Infection, 711
   Upper Respiratory Tract Infections, 710
      Acute Viral Nasopharyngitis, 710
      Acute Streptococcal Pharyngitis, 714
      Tonsillitis, 715
      Influenza, 716
      Otitis Media, 717
      Infectious Mononucleosis, 719
   Croup Syndromes, 720
      Acute Epiglottitis, 721
      Acute Laryngotracheobronchitis, 722
      Acute Spasmodic Laryngitis, 723
      Bacterial Tracheitis, 723
   Infections of the Lower Airways, 723
      Bronchitis, 723
      Respiratory Syncytial Virus and
         Bronchiolitis, 723
      Pneumonias, 725
   Other Infections of the Respiratory
      Tract, 728
      Pertussis (Whooping Cough), 728
      Tuberculosis, 729

Pulmonary Dysfunction Caused by Noninfectious
    Irritants, 731
    Foreign Body Aspiration, 731
    Aspiration Pneumonia, 732
    Pulmonary Edema, 733
    *Acute Respiratory Distress Syndrome and Acute
        Lung Injury, 733*
    Smoke Inhalation Injury, 734
    *Environmental Tobacco Smoke
        Exposure, 735*
Long-Term Respiratory Dysfunction, 736
    Asthma, 736
    *Nursing Care Plan: The Child with Acute
        Asthma Exacerbation, 742*
    *Nursing Care Plan: The Child with
        Asthma, 745*
    Cystic Fibrosis, 747
    *Obstructive Sleep-Disordered
        Breathing, 754*
Respiratory Emergency, 754
    Respiratory Failure, 754
    Cardiopulmonary Resuscitation, 755
    Airway Obstruction, 758
24 The Child with Gastrointestinal Dysfunction, 762
    *Debi S. Lammert, Kristina D. Wilson, and
    David Wilson*
    Distribution of Body Fluids, 763
        *Changes in Fluid Volume Related to
            Growth, 763*
        *Disturbances of Fluid and Electrolyte
            Balance, 764*
    Gastrointestinal Dysfunction, 771
        Disorders of Motility, 771
        *Recurrent and Functional Abdominal
            Pain, 784*
    Inflammatory Disorders, 785
        Acute Appendicitis, 785
        *Nursing Care Plan: The Child with
            Appendicitis, 787*
        Meckel Diverticulum, 786
        Inflammatory Bowel Disease, 789
        Peptic Ulcer Disease, 792
    Hepatic Disorders, 794
        Acute Hepatitis, 794
        Cirrhosis, 797
        Biliary Atresia, 798
    Structural Defects, 800
        Cleft Lip and Cleft Palate, 800
        *Esophageal Atresia and Tracheoesophageal
            Fistula, 803*
        Hernias, 805
    Obstructive Disorders, 805
        Hypertrophic Pyloric Stenosis, 805
        Intussusception, 809
        Malrotation and Volvulus, 810
        Anorectal Malformations, 810

Malabsorption Syndromes, 812
    *Celiac Disease (Gluten-Sensitive
        Enteropathy), 813*
    Short-Bowel Syndrome, 815

**UNIT 10   THE CHILD WITH PROBLEMS
             RELATED TO THE PRODUCTION
             AND CIRCULATION OF BLOOD, 819**

25 The Child with Cardiovascular Dysfunction, 819
    *Margaret L. Schroeder, Amy Delaney, and
    Annette L. Baker*
    Cardiovascular Dysfunction, 820
        History and Physical Examination, 820
    Congenital Heart Disease, 823
        Circulatory Changes at Birth, 823
        Altered Hemodynamics, 824
        Classification of Defects, 824
    Clinical Consequences of Congenital Heart
        Disease, 830
        Heart Failure, 830
        *Nursing Care Plan: The Child with Heart
            Failure, 837*
        Hypoxemia, 840
    Nursing Care of the Family and Child with
        Congenital Heart Disease, 843
        Help the Family Adjust to the Disorder, 843
        Educate the Family About the Disorder, 843
        *Help the Family Manage the Illness at
            Home, 844*
        *Prepare the Child and Family for Invasive
            Procedures, 845*
        Provide Postoperative Care, 845
        Plan for Discharge and Home Care, 847
    Acquired Cardiovascular Disorders, 848
        Bacterial (Infective) Endocarditis, 848
        Rheumatic Fever, 849
        Hyperlipidemia (Hypercholesterolemia), 850
        Cardiac Dysrhythmias, 853
        Pulmonary Artery Hypertension, 854
        Cardiomyopathy, 855
    Heart Transplantation, 856
    Vascular Dysfunction, 857
        Systemic Hypertension, 857
        *Kawasaki Disease (Mucocutaneous Lymph Node
            Syndrome), 858*
        Shock, 860
        Anaphylaxis, 862
        Septic Shock, 863
        Toxic Shock Syndrome, 864
26 The Child with Hematologic or Immunologic
    Dysfunction, 868
    Rosalind Bryant
    Hematologic and Immunologic
        Dysfunction, 869

Red Blood Cell Disorders, 869
  Anemia, 869
  Iron-Deficiency Anemia, 872
  Sickle Cell Anemia, 873
  Nursing Care Plan: The Child with Sickle Cell
    Anemia, 879
  β-Thalassemia (Cooley Anemia), 881
  Aplastic Anemia, 882
Defects in Hemostasis, 883
  Hemophilia, 883
  Immune Thrombocytopenia (Idiopathic
    Thrombocytopenic Purpura), 886
  Disseminated Intravascular Coagulation, 887
  Epistaxis (Nosebleeding), 888
Neoplastic Disorders, 888
  Leukemias, 888
  Lymphomas, 892
Immunologic Deficiency Disorders, 894
  Human Immunodeficiency Virus Infection
    and Acquired Immunodeficiency
    Syndrome, 894
  Severe Combined Immunodeficiency
    Disease, 897
  Wiskott-Aldrich Syndrome, 897
Technologic Management of Hematologic and
  Immunologic Disorders, 897
  Blood Transfusion Therapy, 897
  Hematopoietic Stem Cell Transplantation, 899
  Apheresis, 899

UNIT 11   THE CHILD WITH A DISTURBANCE OF REGULATORY MECHANISMS, 903

27 The Child with Genitourinary Dysfunction, 903
    Barbara A. Montagnino and Patricia A. Ring
    Genitourinary Dysfunction, 903
      Clinical Manifestations, 903
      Laboratory Tests, 904
      Nursing Care Management, 904
    Genitourinary Tract Disorders and
    Defects, 904
      Urinary Tract Infection, 904
      Obstructive Uropathy, 910
      External Defects, 911
    Glomerular Disease, 912
      Nephrotic Syndrome, 912
      Acute Glomerulonephritis, 915
    Miscellaneous Renal Disorders, 916
      Hemolytic Uremic Syndrome, 916
      Wilms Tumor, 917
    Renal Failure, 918
      Acute Renal Failure, 919
      Nursing Care Plan: The Child with Acute Renal
        Dysfunction, 920
      Chronic Renal Failure, 921

    Technologic Management of Renal Failure, 924
      Dialysis, 924
      Transplantation, 925
28 The Child with Cerebral Dysfunction, 927
    Cheryl C. Rodgers and Valerie J. Groben
    Cerebral Dysfunction, 928
      Increased Intracranial Pressure, 928
      Altered States of Consciousness, 928
      General Aspects, 929
      Neurologic Examination, 930
      Special Diagnostic Procedures, 932
    Nursing Care of the Unconscious Child, 934
      Respiratory Management, 935
      Intracranial Pressure Monitoring, 935
      Nutrition and Hydration, 937
      Medications, 937
      Thermoregulation, 937
      Elimination, 937
      Hygienic Care, 937
      Positioning and Exercise, 938
      Stimulation, 938
      Family Support, 938
    Cerebral Trauma, 938
      Head Injury, 938
      Submersion Injury, 945
    Nervous System Tumors, 946
      Brain Tumors, 946
      Neuroblastoma, 949
    Intracranial Infections, 949
      Bacterial Meningitis, 950
      Nonbacterial (Aseptic) Meningitis, 953
      Encephalitis, 954
      Rabies, 955
      Reye Syndrome, 956
    Seizure Disorders, 956
      Etiology, 956
      Pathophysiology, 956
      Seizure Classification and Clinical
        Manifestations, 957
      Nursing Care Plan: The Child with
        Seizures, 963
      Febrile Seizures, 966
    Cerebral Malformations, 966
      Cranial Deformities, 966
      Hydrocephalus, 967
29 The Child with Endocrine Dysfunction, 973
    Elizabeth Record and Linda K. Ballard
    The Endocrine System, 973
      Hormones, 976
    Disorders of Pituitary Function, 977
      Hypopituitarism, 977
      Pituitary Hyperfunction, 979
      Precocious Puberty, 979
      Diabetes Insipidus, 980
      Syndrome of Inappropriate Antidiuretic
        Hormone, 981

Disorders of Thyroid Function, 981
  Juvenile Hypothyroidism, 982
  Goiter, 982
  Lymphocytic Thyroiditis, 983
  Hyperthyroidism, 983
Disorders of Parathyroid Function, 985
  Hypoparathyroidism, 985
  Hyperparathyroidism, 986
Disorders of Adrenal Function, 987
  Acute Adrenocortical Insufficiency, 987
  Chronic Adrenocortical Insufficiency (Addison Disease), 988
  Cushing Syndrome, 989
  Congenital Adrenal Hyperplasia, 990
  Pheochromocytoma, 991
Disorders of Pancreatic Hormone Secretion, 992
  Diabetes Mellitus, 992
  Nursing Care Plan: The Child with Diabetes Mellitus, 1000

30 The Child with Integumentary Dysfunction, 1009
  Marilyn J. Hockenberry, Rose U. Baker, and Mary A. Mondozzi
  Integumentary Dysfunction, 1010
    Skin Lesions, 1010
    Wounds, 1010
    General Therapeutic Management, 1013
    Nursing Care Management, 1015
    Home Care and Family Support, 1016
  Infections of the Skin, 1017
    Bacterial Infections, 1017
    Viral Infections, 1017
    Dermatophytoses (Fungal Infections), 1017
    Systemic Mycotic (Fungal) Infections, 1020
  Skin Disorders Related to Chemical or Physical Contacts, 1022
    Contact Dermatitis, 1022
    Poison Ivy, Oak, and Sumac, 1022
    Drug Reactions, 1022
    Foreign Bodies, 1024
  Skin Disorders Related to Animal Contacts, 1024
    Arthropod Bites and Stings, 1024
    Scabies, 1024
    Pediculosis Capitis, 1027
  Rickettsial Diseases, 1028
    Lyme Disease, 1029
    Pet and Wild Animal Bites, 1029
    Human Bites, 1030
    Cat Scratch Disease, 1030
  Miscellaneous Skin Disorders, 1030
  Skin Disorders Associated with Specific Age Groups, 1030
    Diaper Dermatitis, 1030
    Atopic Dermatitis (Eczema), 1032

    Seborrheic Dermatitis, 1035
    Acne, 1035
  Thermal Injury, 1037
    Burns, 1037
    Sunburn, 1047
    Cold Injury, 1048

UNIT 12 THE CHILD WITH A PROBLEM THAT INTERFERES WITH PHYSICAL MOBILITY, 1050

31 The Child with Musculoskeletal or Articular Dysfunction, 1050
  Martha R. Curry, Sarah Gutknecht, and Linda Kollar
  The Immobilized Child, 1051
    Immobilization, 1051
  Traumatic Injury, 1055
    Soft-Tissue Injury, 1055
    Fractures, 1057
    The Child in a Cast, 1059
    The Child in Traction, 1062
    Distraction, 1065
    Amputation, 1066
  Sports Participation and Injury, 1066
    Overuse Syndromes, 1067
    Nurse's Role in Sports for Children and Adolescents, 1067
  Birth and Developmental Defects, 1068
    Developmental Dysplasia of the Hip, 1068
    Clubfoot, 1071
    Metatarsus Adductus (Varus), 1072
    Skeletal Limb Deficiency, 1072
    Osteogenesis Imperfecta, 1073
  Acquired Defects, 1074
    Legg-Calvé-Perthes Disease, 1074
    Slipped Capital Femoral Epiphysis, 1075
    Kyphosis and Lordosis, 1076
    Idiopathic Scoliosis, 1076
  Infections of Bones and Joints, 1079
    Osteomyelitis, 1079
    Septic Arthritis, 1080
    Skeletal Tuberculosis, 1081
  Bone and Soft-Tissue Tumors, 1081
    General Concepts: Bone Tumors, 1081
    Osteosarcoma, 1081
    Ewing Sarcoma (Primitive Neuroectodermal Tumor), 1082
    Rhabdomyosarcoma, 1083
  Disorders of Joints, 1084
    Juvenile Idiopathic Arthritis (Juvenile Rheumatoid Arthritis), 1084
    Systemic Lupus Erythematosus, 1086

32 The Child with Neuromuscular or Muscular Dysfunction, 1090
Jean Stansbury, Barbara Montagnino, and David Wilson
Congenital Neuromuscular or Muscular
    Disorders, 1090
    Cerebral Palsy, 1090
    Neural Tube Defects (Myelomeningocele), 1098
    *Spinal Muscular Atrophy, Type 1
        (Werdnig-Hoffmann Disease), 1105*
    *Spinal Muscular Atrophy, Type 3
        (Kugelberg-Welander Disease), 1106*
    Muscular Dystrophies, 1106
    *Duchenne (Pseudohypertrophic) Muscular
        Dystrophy, 1106*
Acquired Neuromuscular Disorders, 1109
    *Guillain-Barré Syndrome (Infectious
        Polyneuritis), 1109*

Tetanus, 1111
Botulism, 1113
Spinal Cord Injuries, 1114

APPENDIX, 1120

A Growth Measurements, 1120
B Common Laboratory Tests, 1129
C Translations of Wong-Baker FACES Pain Rating
    Scale, 1138
D Spanish–English Translations, 1140
E Blood Pressure Levels, 1143

ANSWERS TO CASE STUDIES, 1146

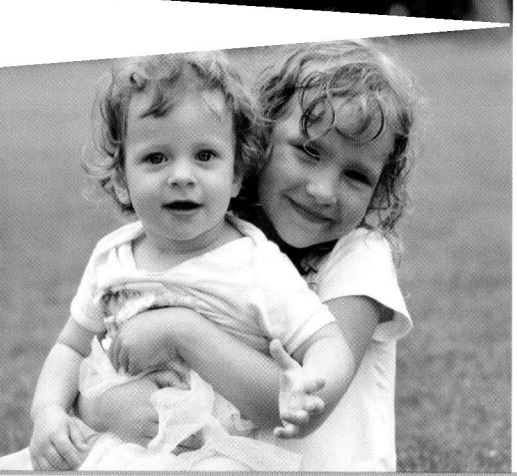

Perspectives of Pediatric Nursing

Marilyn J. Hockenberry and Patrick Barrera

evolve WEBSITE

http://evolve.elsevier.com/wong/essentials
Key Point Summaries
NCLEX-Style Review Questions

CHAPTER OUTLINE

Health Care for Children, 1
 Health Promotion, 2
  Nutrition, 2
  Dental Care, 2
  Immunizations, 3
 Childhood Health Problems, 3
  Obesity and Type 2 Diabetes, 3
  Childhood Injuries, 3
  Violence, 5
  Substance Abuse, 6
  Mental Health Problems, 6
 Mortality and Morbidity, 6
  Infant Mortality, 6
  Childhood Mortality, 7
  Childhood Morbidity, 8

The Art of Pediatric Nursing, 8
 Philosophy of Care, 8
  Family-Centered Care, 8
  Atraumatic Care, 8
 Role of the Pediatric Nurse, 9
  Therapeutic Relationship, 9
  Family Advocacy and Caring, 9
  *Disease Prevention and Health
   Promotion, 9*
  Health Teaching, 10
  Injury Prevention, 10
  Support and Counseling, 10
  Coordination and Collaboration, 11
  Ethical Decision Making, 11
 Research and Evidence-Based Practice, 11

Clinical Reasoning and the Process of
 Providing Nursing Care to Children and
 Families, 12
 Clinical Reasoning, 12
 Nursing Process, 12
  Assessment, 12
  Nursing Diagnosis, 12
  Planning, 13
  Implementation, 13
  Evaluation, 13
  Documentation, 13
 Quality Outcome Measures, 13

LEARNING OBJECTIVES

On completion of this chapter the reader will be able to:
- Define the terms *mortality* and *morbidity.*
- Identify two ways that knowledge of mortality and morbidity can improve child health.
- List three major causes of death during infancy, early childhood, later childhood, and adolescence.
- List two major causes of illness during childhood.
- Describe five broad functions of the pediatric nurse in promoting the health of children.

- Define *critical thinking.*
- Identify the five steps of the nursing process.
- Define *nursing diagnosis.*
- Define *evidence-based practice.*
- Identify the Institute of Medicine's six domains of patient care Quality Outcomes

HEALTH CARE FOR CHILDREN

The major goal for pediatric nursing is to improve the quality of health care for children and their families. In 2010, almost 75 million children 0 to 17 years of age lived in the United States, comprising 24% of the population (Federal Interagency Forum on Child and Family Statistics, 2011). The health status of children in the United States has improved in a number of areas, including increased immunization rates for all children, decreased adolescent birth rate, and improved child health outcomes. Unfortunately, millions of children and their families have no health insurance, which results in a lack of access to care and health promotion services. In addition, disparities in pediatric health care are related to race, ethnicity, socioeconomic status, and geographic factors (see Research Focus box). Patterns of child health are shaped by medical progress and societal trends (Starmer, Duby, Slaw, and others, 2010). Shifts in population demographics, family structure, income, education levels, and cultural norms directly affect the health of children (Leslie, Slaw, Edwards, and others, 2010). The Healthy People 2020 Leading Health Indicators (Box 1-1) provide a framework for identifying essential components for child health promotion programs designed to prevent future health problems among our nation's children.

HEALTH PROMOTION

Many leading causes of disease, disability, and death in children (i.e., prematurity, nutritional deficiencies, injuries, chronic lung disease, obesity, cardiovascular disease, depression, violence, substance abuse, and human immunodeficiency virus/acquired immunodeficiency syndrome [HIV/AIDS]) can be significantly reduced or prevented in children and adolescents by addressing six categories of behavior (World Health Organization, 2011):

1. Tobacco use
2. Behavior that results in injury and violence
3. Alcohol and substance use
4. Dietary and hygienic practices that cause disease
5. Sedentary lifestyle
6. Sexual behavior that causes unintended pregnancy and disease

Child health promotion provides opportunities to reduce differences in current health status among members of different groups and ensure equal opportunities and resources to enable all children to achieve their fullest health potential.

Nutrition

Nutrition is an essential component for healthy growth and development. Human milk is the preferred form of nutrition for all infants. Breastfeeding provides infants with micronutrients, immunologic properties, and several enzymes that enhance digestion and absorption of these nutrients. A recent resurgence in breastfeeding has occurred because of the education of mothers and fathers regarding its benefits and increased social support.

Children establish lifelong eating habits during the first 3 years of life, and nurses are instrumental in educating parents about the process of feeding and the importance of nutrition. Most eating preferences and attitudes related to food are established by family influences and culture. During adolescence, parental influence diminishes, and adolescents make food choices related to peer acceptability and sociability. Occasionally, these choices are detrimental to adolescents with chronic illnesses such as diabetes, obesity, chronic lung disease, hypertension, cardiovascular risk factors, and renal disease.

Families that struggle with lower incomes, homelessness, and migrant status generally lack the resources to provide their children with adequate food intake, nutritious foods such as fresh fruits and vegetables, and appropriate protein intake. The result is nutritional deficiencies with subsequent growth and developmental delays, depression, and behavior problems.

Dental Care

Dental caries is the single most common chronic disease of childhood (Cheng, Han, and Gansky, 2008; Heuer, 2007). Nearly one in five children between the ages of 2 and 4 years has visible cavities (Kagihara, Niederhauser, and Stark, 2009). The most common form of

---

BOX 1-1 HEALTHY PEOPLE 2020

Goals
- Attain high-quality, longer lives free of preventable disease, disability, injury, and premature death.
- Achieve health equity, eliminate disparities, and improve the health of all groups.
- Create social and physical environments that promote good health for all.
- Promote quality of life, healthy development, and healthy behaviors across all life stages.

Leading Health Indicators—Topics
- Access to Health Services
- Clinical Preventive Services
- Environmental Quality
- Injury and Violence
- Maternal, Infant, and Child Health
- Mental Health
- Nutrition, Physical Activity, and Obesity
- Oral Health
- Reproductive and Sexual Health
- Social Determinants
- Substance Abuse
- Tobacco

From U.S. Department of Health and Human Services, Office of Disease Prevention and Health Promotion: *Healthy people 2020*, Washington, DC, retrieved August 15, 2011, from http://www.healthypeople.gov/2020/about/default.aspx.

RESEARCH FOCUS
National Children's Study

The National Children's Study is the largest prospective, long-term study of children's health and development conducted in the United States. The study is designed to follow 100,000 children and their families from birth to age 21 years to understand the link between children's environments and their physical and emotional health and development (American Academy of Pediatrics, 2008). Researchers hope that a study of this magnitude will provide information on innovative interventions for families, children, and health care providers to eradicate unhealthy diets, dental caries, and childhood obesity and to bring a significant reduction in violence, injury, substance abuse, and mental health disorders among the nation's children. This study supports the *Healthy People 2020* primary goals to increase the quality and years of healthy life and eliminate health disparities related to race, ethnicity, and socioeconomic status (U.S. Department of Health and Human Services, 2009).

early dental disease is early childhood caries, which may begin before the first birthday and progress to pain and infection within the first 2 years of life (Kagihara, Niederhauser, and Stark, 2009). Preschoolers of low-income families are twice as likely to develop tooth decay and only half as likely to visit dentists as other children. Early childhood caries is a preventable disease, and nurses play an essential role in educating children and parents about practicing dental hygiene beginning with the first tooth eruption; drinking fluoridated water, including bottled water; and instituting early dental preventive care.

Immunizations

The two public health interventions that have had the greatest impact on world health are clean drinking water and childhood vaccination programs. Immunization rates can vary depending on a number of factors, including children's race and ethnicity, family income, geographic location, types of vaccinations, and the child's age. The nurse should review individual immunization records at every clinic visit, avoid missing opportunities to vaccinate, and encourage parents to keep immunizations current. Nurses are responsible for keeping up with changes in immunization schedules, recommendations, and research related to childhood vaccines.

CHILDHOOD HEALTH PROBLEMS

Changes in modern society, including advancing medical knowledge and technology, the proliferation of information systems, economically troubled times, and various changes and disruptive influences on the family, are leading to significant medical problems that affect the health of children (Leslie, Slaw, Edwards, and others, 2010). Recent concern has focused on groups of children who are at highest risk, such as children born prematurely or with very low birth weight (VLBW) or low birth weight (LBW), children attending child care centers, children who live in poverty or are homeless, children of immigrant families, and children with chronic medical and psychiatric illness and disabilities. In addition, these children and their families face multiple barriers to adequate health, dental, and psychiatric care. The new morbidity, also known as pediatric social illness, refers to the behavior, social, and educational problems that children face. Problems that can negatively impact a child's development include poverty, violence, aggression, noncompliance, school failure, and adjustment to parental separation and divorce. In addition, mental health issues cause challenges in childhood and adolescence.

Obesity and Type 2 Diabetes

Childhood obesity is the most common nutritional problem among American children, is increasing in epidemic proportions, and is associated with type 2 diabetes (Cali and Caprio, 2008; de Onis, Blössner, and Borghi, 2010; Matyka, 2008; Raj and Kumar, 2010). Obesity in children and adolescents is defined as a body mass index (BMI) at or greater than the 95th percentile for youth of the same age and gender (Schwartz and Chadha, 2008). The National Health and Nutrition Examination Survey reported that the prevalence of overweight children doubled and the prevalence of overweight adolescents tripled between 1980 and 2000 (American Dietetic Association, 2008).

Advancements in entertainment and technology such as television, computers, and video games have contributed to the growing childhood obesity problem in the United States. In the National Longitudinal Study of Adolescent Health, screen time (TV, video, computer use) interacts with genetic factors to influence BMI changes (Graff, North, Monda, and others, 2011). Lack of physical activity related to limited resources, unsafe environments, and inconvenient

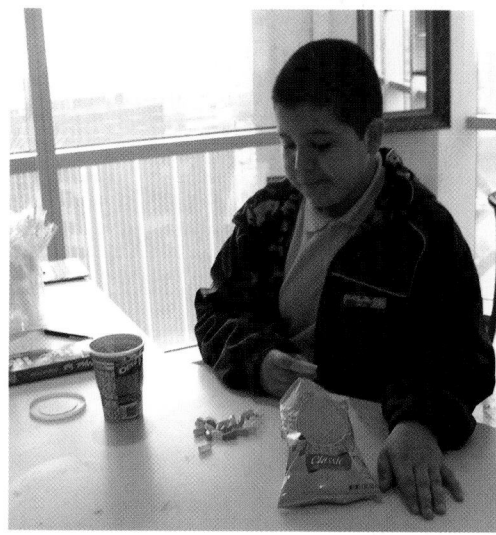

FIG 1-1 The American culture's intake of high-caloric fatty foods contributes to obesity in children.

play and exercise facilities combined with easy access to television and video games increases the incidence of obesity among low-income minority children. Overweight youth have increased risk for developing hypercholesterolemia, insulin resistance, diabetes, hypertension, and heart disease (Matyka, 2008; Schwartz and Chadha, 2008) (Fig. 1-1). The U.S. Department of Health and Human Services suggests that nurses focus on prevention strategies to reduce the incidence of overweight children in all ethnic groups from the current 20% to less than 6%.

Childhood Injuries

Injuries are the most common cause of death and disability to children in the United States (Schnitzer, 2006) (Table 1-1). Motor vehicle accidents (MVAs) continue to be the most common cause of death in children older than 1 year of age. Other unintentional injuries (head injuries, drowning, burns, and firearm accidents) take the lives of children every day. Many childhood injuries and fatalities could be prevented by implementing programs of accident prevention and health promotion.

The type of injury and the circumstances surrounding it are closely related to normal growth and development (Box 1-2). As children develop, their innate curiosity compels them to investigate the environment and to mimic the behavior of others. This is essential to acquire competency as an adult but can also predispose children to numerous hazards.

The child's developmental stage partially determines the types of injuries that are most likely to occur at a specific age and helps provide clues to preventive measures. For example, small infants are helpless in any environment. When they begin to roll over or propel themselves, they can fall from unprotected surfaces. Crawling infants, who have a natural tendency to place objects in their mouths, are at risk for aspiration or poisoning. Mobile toddlers, with the instinct to explore and investigate and the ability to run and climb, may experience falls, burns, and collisions with objects. As children grow older, their absorption with play makes them oblivious to environmental hazards such as street traffic and water. The need to conform and gain acceptance compels older children and adolescents to accept challenges and dares. Although the rate of injuries is high in children younger than 9 years of age, most fatal injuries occur in later childhood and adolescence.

TABLE 1-1   MORTALITY FROM LEADING TYPES OF UNINTENTIONAL INJURIES, UNITED STATES, 1997 (RATE PER 100,000 POPULATION IN EACH AGE GROUP)

TYPE OF ACCIDENT	AGE (YR)			
	<1	1–4	5–14	15–24
MALES				
All causes	818.0	39.8	24.0	124.4
Unintentional injuries (all types)	22.3	15.2	10.6	52.3
Motor vehicle accidents	4.4 (2)	5.3 (1)	5.8 (1)	38.3 (1)
Drowning	1.8 (4)	3.9 (2)	1.6 (2)	3.2 (2)
Fires and burns	1.5 (5)	2.5 (3)	0.8 (3)	—
Firearms	—	0.5 (4)	0.5 (4)	—
Ingestion of food or object	2.5 (3)	0.5 (5)	—	—
Falls	—	—	—	1.2 (5)
Mechanical suffocation	9.1 (1)	0.6 (4)	0.4 (5)	—
Poisoning	—	—	—	2.8 (3)
All other unintentional injuries	3.1	2.3	1.4	5.3
Accidents as a percentage of all deaths	2.7%	38.2%	44.3%	42.0%
FEMALES				
All causes	662.9	31.8	17.4	46.0
Unintentional injuries (all types)	18.1	10.9	6.7	20.0
Motor vehicle accidents	4.4 (2)	4.7 (1)	4.3 (1)	17.1 (1)
Drowning	1.4 (4)	2.0 (2)	0.6 (3)	0.4 (3)
Fires and burns	1.2 (5)	2.0 (2)	0.7 (2)	—
Firearms	—	—	0.1 (4)	0.1 (5)
Ingestion of food or object	1.5 (3)	0.4 (4)	—	—
Falls	—	—	—	0.2 (4)
Mechanical suffocation	6.9 (1)	0.3 (5)	0.1 (4)	—
Poisoning	—	—	—	0.8 (2)
All other unintentional injuries	2.7	1.5	0.9	1.5
Accidents as a percentage of all deaths	2.7%	34.2%	38.2%	43.4%

Modified from National Safety Council: *Injury facts*, Itaska, Ill, 2000, The Council. Data from National Center for Health Statistics.

BOX 1-2   CHILDHOOD INJURIES: RISK FACTORS

Sex—Preponderance of boys; difference mainly the result of behavioral characteristics, especially aggression

Temperament—Children with difficult temperament profile, especially persistence, high activity level, and negative reactions to new situations

Stress—Predisposes children to increased risk-taking and self-destructive behavior; general lack of self-protection

Alcohol and drug use—Associated with a higher incidence of motor vehicle injuries, drowning, homicides, and suicides

History of previous injury—Associated with an increased likelihood of another injury, especially if the initial injury required hospitalization

Developmental Characteristics
- Mismatch between child's developmental level and skill required for activity (e.g., all-terrain vehicles)
- Natural curiosity to explore the environment
- Desire to assert themselves and challenge rules
- In older children, desire for peer approval and acceptance

Cognitive Characteristics (Age Specific)
Infant—Sensorimotor: explores environment through taste and touch
Young child
- Object permanence—Actively searches for attractive object
- Cause and effect—Lacks awareness of consequential dangers
- Transductive reasoning—May fail to learn from experiences (e.g., perceives falling from a step as a different type of danger from climbing a tree)
- Magical and egocentric thinking—Is unable to comprehend danger to self or others

School-age child—Transitional cognitive processes: is unable to fully comprehend causal relationships; attempts dangerous acts without detailed planning regarding consequences

Adolescent—Formal operations: is preoccupied with abstract thinking and loses sight of reality; may lead to feeling of invulnerability

Anatomic Characteristics (Especially in Young Children)
- Large head—Predisposes to cranial injury
- Large spleen and liver with wide costal arch—Predisposes to direct trauma to these organs
- Small and light body—May be thrown easily, especially inside a moving vehicle

Other factors—Poverty, family stress (e.g., maternal illness, recent environmental change), substandard alternative child care, young maternal age, low maternal education, multiple siblings

The pattern of deaths caused by unintentional injuries, especially from MVAs, drowning, and burns, is remarkably consistent in most Western societies. The leading causes of death from injuries for each age group according to sex are presented in Table 1-1. The majority of deaths from injuries occur in boys. It is important to note that accidents continue to account for more than three times as many teen deaths as any other cause (Annie E. Casey Foundation, 2011). Fortunately, prevention strategies such as the use of car restraints, bicycle helmets, and smoke detectors have significantly decreased fatalities for children. Nevertheless, the overwhelming causes of death in children are MVAs, including occupant, pedestrian, bicycle, and motorcycle deaths; these account for more than half of all injury deaths (Centers for Disease Control and Prevention, 2006). Children younger than 1 year of age have the highest rate of death from MVAs, primarily from a failure to properly use car restraints (Fig. 1-2).

Pedestrian accidents involving children account for significant numbers of motor vehicle–related deaths. Most of these accidents occur at midblock, at intersections, in driveways, and in parking lots. Driveway injuries typically involve small children and large vehicles backing up.

Bicycle-associated injuries also cause a number childhood deaths. Children ages 5 to 9 years are at greatest risk of bicycling fatalities. The majority of bicycling deaths are from head injuries. Helmets greatly reduce the risk of head injury, but few children wear helmets (Castle, Burke, Arbogast, and others, 2010). Community-wide bicycle helmet campaigns and mandatory-use laws have resulted in significant increases in helmet use. Still, issues such as stylishness, comfort, and social acceptability remain important factors in noncompliance. Nurses can educate children and families about pedestrian and bicycle safety. In particular, school nurses can promote helmet wearing and encourage peer leaders to act as role models.

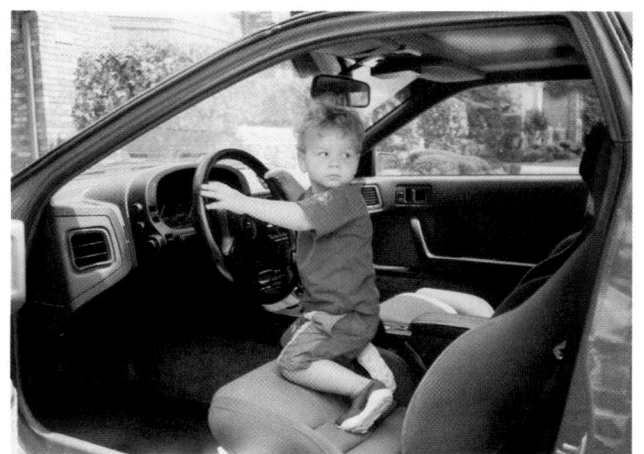

FIG 1-2 Motor vehicle injuries are the leading cause of death in children older than 1 year of age. The majority of fatalities involve occupants who are unrestrained.

Drowning and burns are among the top three leading causes of deaths for boys and girls throughout childhood (Fig. 1-3). In addition, improper use of firearms is the fourth leading cause of death from injury in children 5 to 14 years of age (Fig. 1-4). During infancy, more boys die from aspiration or suffocation than do girls (Fig. 1-5). Approximately 65% of all unintentional poisonings are reported in children younger than 5 years of age (Bronstein, Spyker, Cantilena, and others, 2010; Franklin and Rodgers, 2008) (Fig. 1-6). By ages 4 to 5 years, unintentional poisonings are uncommon. Intentional poisoning, associated with drug and alcohol abuse and suicide attempt, is the second leading cause of death in adolescent girls and third leading cause in adolescent boys.

Violence

Youth violence is a high-visibility, high-priority concern in every sector of U.S. society (U.S. Department of Health and Human Services, 2011). Strikingly higher homicide rates are found among minority populations, especially African-American children. The causes of violence

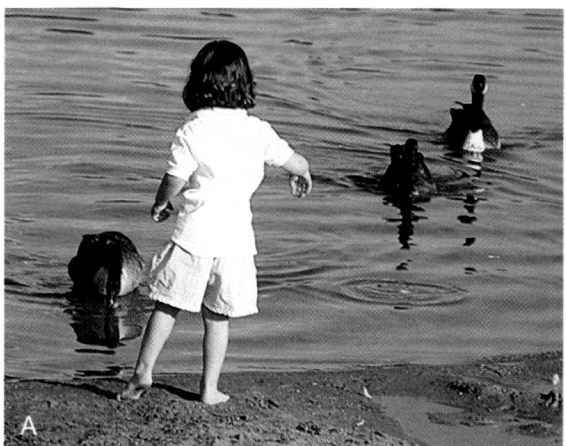 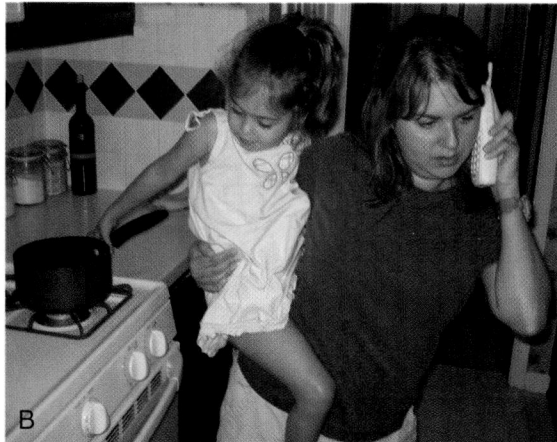

FIG 1-3 **A,** Drowning is one of the leading causes of death. Children left unattended are unsafe even in shallow water. **B,** Burns are among the top three leading causes of death from injury in children ages 1 to 14 years.

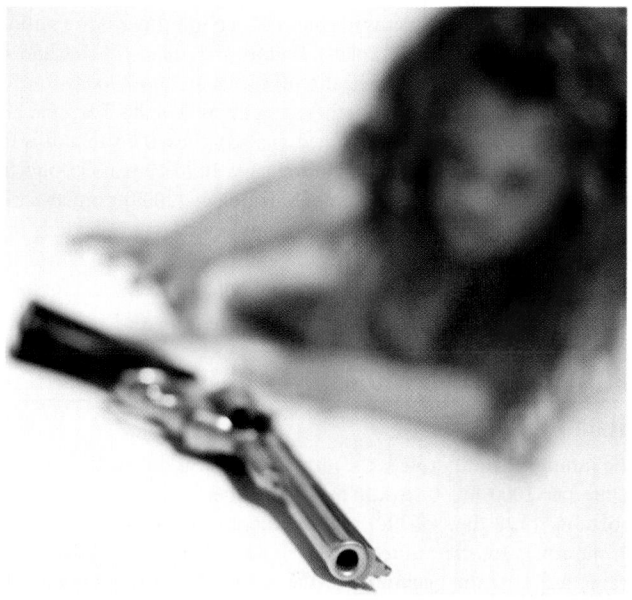

FIG 1-4 Improper use of firearms is the fourth leading cause of death from injury in children 5 to 14 years of age. (© 2012 Photos. com, a division of Getty Images. All rights reserved.)

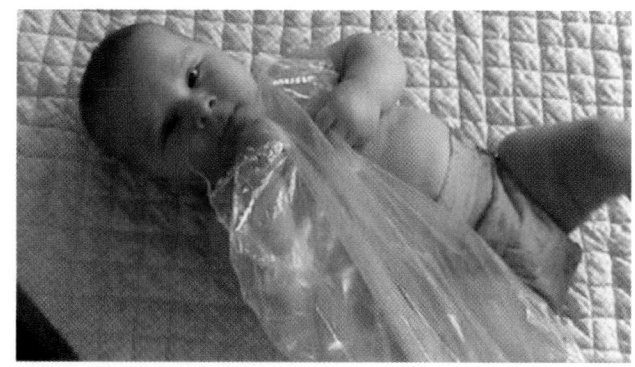

FIG 1-5 Mechanical suffocation is the leading cause of death from injury in infants.

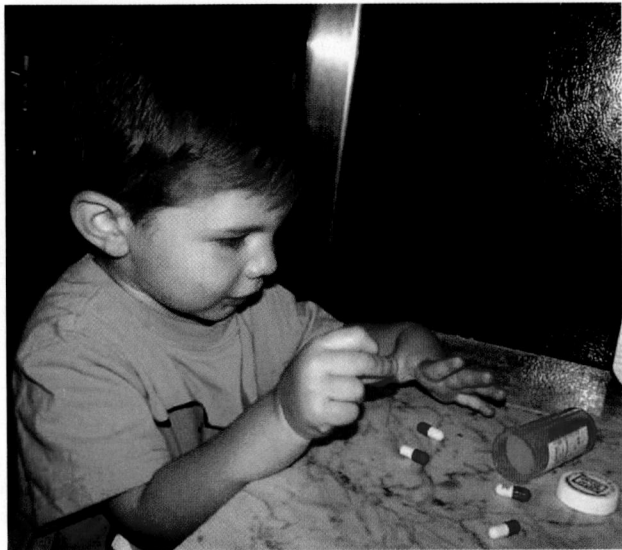

FIG 1-6 Poisoning causes a considerable number of injuries in children younger than 4 years of age. Medications should never be left where young children can reach them.

COMMUNITY FOCUS

Violence in Children

The serious problem of community violence affects the lives of many children and expands throughout the family, schools, and the workplace. Nurses working with children, adolescents, and families have a critical role in reducing violence through early identification and symptom recognition of the mental-emotional stress that can result from these experiences.

Violent crimes continue to be a significant health issue for children, with homicide being the second leading cause of death in 15- to 19-year-old teenagers (Annie E. Casey Foundation, 2011). The multifaceted origins of violence include developmental factors, gang involvement, access to firearms, drugs, the media, poverty, and family conflict. Often the silent and underrecognized victims are the children who witness acts of community violence. Studies suggest that chronic exposure to violence has a negative effect on children's cognitive, social, psychologic, and moral development. Also, multiple exposures to episodes of violence do not inoculate children against the negative effects; rather, continued exposure can result in lasting symptoms of stress. Children living with chronic violence may exhibit behaviors such as difficulty concentrating in school, memory impairment, aggressive play, uncaring behaviors, and constricted activities and thinking for fear of reliving the traumatic event.

National concern about the increasing prevalence of violent crimes has prompted nurses to actively participate in ensuring that children grow up in safe environments. Pediatric nurses are positioned to assess children and adolescents for signs of exposure to violence and well-known risk factors; nurses also can provide nonviolent problem-solving strategies, counseling, and referrals. These activities affect community practice and expand the nurse's role in the future health environment. Professional resources include:

National Domestic Violence Hotline
PO Box 161810
Austin, TX 78716
800-799-SAFE
www.ndvh.org

against children and self-inflicted violence are not fully understood. Violence seems to permeate American households through television programs, commercials, video games, and movies, all of which tend to desensitize the child toward violence. Violence also permeates the schools with the availability of guns, illicit drugs, and gangs. The problem of child homicide is extremely complex and involves numerous social, economic, and other influences. Prevention lies in better understanding of the social and psychologic factors that lead to the high rates of homicide and suicide. Nurses need to be especially aware of young people who harm animals or start fires, are depressed, are repeatedly in trouble with the criminal justice system, or are associated with groups known to be violent. Prevention requires early identification and rapid therapeutic intervention by qualified professionals.

Pediatric nurses can assess children and adolescents for risk factors related to violence. Families that own firearms must be educated about their safe use and storage. The presence of a gun in a household increases the risk of suicide by about fivefold and the risk of homicide by about threefold. Technologic changes such as childproof safety devices and loading indicators could improve the safety of firearms (see Community Focus box).

Substance Abuse

Risk-taking behaviors, particularly in boys, tend to begin in the first decade of life and continue into adolescence with drinking alcohol while driving, speeding, carrying a weapon, or using illicit drugs. Adolescent trends in cigarette smoking, alcohol use, and illicit drug abuse have declined since 2002. Approximately 9.8% of youth reported cigarette smoking, 15.9% reported alcohol use, and 9.5% reported illicit drug abuse within the past month (National Survey on Drug Use and Health, 2008). The slight decline in American youths' illicit drug use is attributed to education regarding the adverse effects of illicit drugs, parental disapproval, decreased availability of drugs, and consistent participation in church and organized activities such as scouts and sports.

Mental Health Problems

One in five adolescents has a mental health problem, and one in 10 has a serious emotional problem that affects daily functioning (Coury,

2006). Psychosocial problems in children seen in primary care settings in rural areas are common (Polaha, Dalton, and Allen, 2011). Children and adolescents with mental health problems are more likely to drop out of school than those with other disabilities (Porche, Fortuna, Lin, and others, 2011). **Suicide** is defined as a self-chosen death and is the third leading cause of death in children ages 10 to 19 years (Doucette, 2005). The American Association of Suicidology (2009) estimates that there are 11.5 youth suicides (15–24 years) every day. Suicide is preventable. Nurses should be alert to the symptoms of mental illness and potential suicidal ideation and be aware of potential resources for high-quality integrated mental health services.

MORTALITY AND MORBIDITY

Infant Mortality

The **infant mortality rate** is the number of deaths during the first year of life per 1000 live births. It may be further divided into **neonatal mortality** (<28 days of life) and **postneonatal mortality** (28 days–11 months). In the United States, infant mortality has decreased dramatically. At the beginning of the twentieth century, the rate was approximately 200 infant deaths per 1000 live births. In 2009, the infant mortality rate was 6.42 deaths per 1000 live births (Kochanek, Kirmeyer, Martin, and others, 2012).

From a worldwide perspective, however, the United States lags behind other nations in reducing infant mortality. In 2001, the United States ranked last among 27 nations that have a population of at least 2.5 million and had infant mortality rates equal to or lower than that of the United States in 2000. Hong Kong, Sweden, and Japan have the three lowest rates, with the United States ranked last behind Poland and Slovenia (Kochanek, Kirmeyer, Martin, and others, 2012).

Birth weight is considered the major determinant of neonatal death in technologically developed countries. There is a relationship between LBW and infant morbidity and mortality (Mathews, Miniño, Osterman, and others, 2011). The lower the birth weight, the higher the mortality. The relatively high incidence of LBW (<2500 g [5.5 lb]) in the United States is considered a key factor in its higher neonatal mortality rate compared with other countries. Access to and the use of high-quality prenatal care is a promising preventive strategy to decrease early delivery and infant mortality. Other factors that increase the risk of infant mortality include African-American race, male gender, short or long gestation, young or old maternal age, and lower level of maternal education (Martin, Kochanek, Strobino, and others, 2005).

As Table 1-2 demonstrates, many of the leading causes of death during infancy continue to occur during the perinatal period. The first four causes—congenital anomalies, disorders relating to short gestation and unspecified LBW, sudden infant death syndrome, and newborn affected by maternal complications of pregnancy—accounted for about half (51%) of all deaths of infants younger than 1 year of age (Kochanek, Kirmeyer, Martin, and others, 2012). LBW is a major indicator of infant health and a significant predictor of infant mortality (Mathews, Miniño, Osterman, and others, 2011). Many birth defects are associated with LBW, and reducing the incidence of LBW will help prevent congenital anomalies. Infant mortality resulting from HIV infection decreased significantly during the 1990s.

When infant death rates are categorized according to race, a disturbing difference is seen. Infant mortality for whites is considerably lower than for all other races in the United States, with African Americans having twice the rate of whites. Although the infant mortality of all racial groups increased slightly between 2001 and 2002, the gap has remained constant, with the infant mortality rate expressed as a ratio of deaths for African Americans to those for whites being relatively unchanged in the past decade (Kochanek, Kirmeyer, Martin, and others, 2012). The LBW rate is also much higher for African-American infants than for any other group. One encouraging note is that the gap in mortality rates between white and nonwhite races other than African Americans has narrowed in recent years. Infant mortality rates for Hispanics and Asian–Pacific Islanders have decreased dramatically during the past 2 decades (Mathews, Miniño, Osterman, and others, 2011).

Childhood Mortality

Death rates for children older than 1 year of age have always been lower than those for infants. Children ages 5 to 14 years have the lowest rate of death. However, a sharp rise occurs during later adolescence, primarily from injuries, homicide, and suicide (Table 1-3). In 2008, accidental injuries accounted for 38.8% of all deaths. The second leading cause of death was homicide, accounting for 12.4% of all deaths in 2008 (Mathews, Miniño, Osterman, and others, 2011). The trend in racial differences that occurs in infant mortality is also apparent in childhood deaths for all ages and for both sexes. Whites have fewer deaths for all ages, and male deaths outnumber female deaths.

TABLE 1-2	INFANT MORTALITY RATE AND PERCENTAGE OF TOTAL DEATHS FOR THE 10 LEADING CAUSES OF INFANT DEATH IN 2009 (RATE PER 1000 LIVE BIRTHS)		
RANK	**CAUSE OF DEATH (BASED ON 10th REVISION, INTERNATIONAL CLASSIFICATION OF DISEASES)**	**PERCENT**	**RATE**
	All races, all causes	100.0	642.1
1	Congenital anomalies	20.2	129.7
2	Disorders relating to short gestation and unspecified low birth weight	16.8	108.0
3	Sudden infant death syndrome	8.2	52.5
4	Newborn affected by maternal complications of pregnancy	6.0	38.4
5	Accidents (unintentional injuries)	4.4	28.0
6	Newborn affected by complications of the placenta, umbilical cord, and membranes	3.9	24.7
7	Bacterial sepsis of newborn	2.6	16.5
8	Respiratory distress of newborn	2.2	14.2
9	Diseases of circulatory system	2.1	13.7
10	Neonatal hemorrhage	2.0	13.0

Modified from Kochanek KD, Kirmeyer SE, Martin JA, and others: Annual summary of vital statistics: 2009, *Pediatrics* 129(2):338–348, 2012.

TABLE 1-3	FIVE LEADING CAUSES OF DEATH IN CHILDREN IN UNITED STATES: SELECTED AGE INTERVALS, 2009 (RATE PER 100,000 POPULATION)								
	AGES 1–4 YEARS		**AGES 5–9 YEARS**		**AGES 10–14 YEARS**		**AGES 15–19 YEARS**	
RANK	**CAUSE**	**RATE**	**CAUSE**	**RATE**	**CAUSE**	**RATE**	**CAUSE**	**RATE**
	All causes	26.1	All causes	12.2	All causes	15.6	All causes	53.2
1	Accidents	8.5	Accidents	3.8	Accidents	4.5	Accidents	22.1
2	Congenital anomalies	2.8	Cancer	2.3	Cancer	2.1	Homicide	8.8
3	Homicide	2.3	Congenital anomalies	0.9	Suicide	1.3	Suicide	7.7
4	Cancer	2.0	Homicide	0.6	Homicide	1.0	Cancer	3.0
5	Heart disease	0.9	Influenza and pneumonia	0.5	Congenital anomalies	0.8	Heart disease	1.5

Modified from Kochanek KD, Kirmeyer SE, Martin JA, and others: Annual summary of vital statistics: 2009, *Pediatrics* 129(2):338–348, 2012.

After 1 year of age, the cause of death changes dramatically, with unintentional injuries (accidents) being the leading cause from the youngest ages to the adolescent years. Violent deaths have been steadily increasing among young people ages 10 through 25 years, especially African Americans and males. Homicide is the second leading cause of death in the 15- to 19-year age group (see Table 1-3). Children 12 years of age and older tend to be killed by nonfamily members (acquaintances and gangs, typically of the same race) and most frequently by firearms. Suicide, a form of self-violence, is the third leading cause of death among children and adolescents 10 to 19 years of age.

Childhood Morbidity

Acute illness is defined as an illness with symptoms severe enough to limit activity or require medical attention. Respiratory illness accounts for approximately 50% of all acute conditions, 11% are caused by infections and parasitic disease, and 15% are caused by injuries. The chief illness of childhood is the common cold.

The types of diseases that children contract during childhood vary according to age. For example, upper respiratory tract infections and diarrhea decrease in frequency with age, but other disorders, such as acne and headaches, increase. Children who have had a particular type of problem are more likely to have that problem again. Morbidity is not distributed randomly in children. Recent concern has focused on groups of children who have increased morbidity: homeless children, children living in poverty, LBW children, children with chronic illnesses, foreign-born adopted children, and children in daycare centers. A number of factors place these groups at risk for poor health. A major cause is barriers to health care, especially for homeless people, poverty stricken individuals, and those with chronic health problems. Other factors include improved survival of children with chronic health problems, particularly infants of VLBW.

THE ART OF PEDIATRIC NURSING

PHILOSOPHY OF CARE

Nursing of infants, children, and adolescents is consistent with the definition of nursing as "the diagnosis and treatment of human responses to actual or potential health problems." This definition incorporates the four essential features of contemporary nursing practice (American Nurses Association, 2003):

1. Attention to the full range of human experiences and responses to health and illness without restriction to a problem-focused orientation
2. Integration of objective data with knowledge gained from an understanding of the patient or group's subjective experience
3. Application of scientific knowledge to the processes of diagnosis and treatment
4. Provision of a caring relationship that facilitates health and healing

Family-Centered Care

The philosophy of family-centered care recognizes the family as the constant in a child's life. Service systems and personnel must support, respect, encourage, and enhance the family's strength and competence by developing a partnership with parents (National Center for Cultural Competence, 2007). Nurses support families in their natural caregiving and decision-making roles by building on their unique strengths and acknowledging their expertise in caring for their children both within and outside the hospital setting (National Center for Cultural Competence, 2007). The nurse considers the needs of all family members in relation to the care of the child (Box 1-3). The philosophy

---

BOX 1-3   KEY ELEMENTS OF FAMILY-CENTERED CARE

Incorporating into policy and practice the recognition that the family is the constant in a child's life while the service systems and support personnel within those systems fluctuate

Facilitating family-professional collaboration at all levels of hospital, home, and community care:
- Care of an individual child
- Program development, implementation, and evaluation
- Policy formation

Exchanging complete and unbiased information between family members and professionals in a supportive manner at all times

Incorporating into policy and practice the recognition and honoring of cultural diversity, strengths, and individuality within and across all families, including ethnic, racial, spiritual, social, economic, educational, and geographic diversity

Recognizing and respecting different methods of coping and implementing comprehensive policies and programs that provide developmental, educational, emotional, environmental, and financial support to meet the diverse needs of families

Encouraging and facilitating family-to-family support and networking

Ensuring that home, hospital, and community service and support systems for children needing specialized health and developmental care and their families are flexible, accessible, and comprehensive in responding to diverse family-identified needs

Appreciating families as families and children as children, recognizing that they possess a wide range of strengths, concerns, emotions, and aspirations beyond their need for specialized health and developmental services and support

From Shelton TL, Stepanek JS: *Family-centered care for children needing specialized health and developmental services,* Bethesda, Md, 1994, Association for the Care of Children's Health.

---

acknowledges diversity among family structures and backgrounds; family goals, dreams, strategies, and actions; and family support, service, and information needs (Hooper, 2008).

Two basic concepts in family-centered care are enabling and empowerment. Professionals enable families by creating opportunities and means for all family members to display their current abilities and competencies and to acquire new ones to meet the needs of the child and family. Empowerment is the interaction of professionals with families in such a way that families maintain or acquire a sense of control over their family lives and acknowledge positive changes that result from helping behaviors that foster their own strengths, abilities, and actions.

Although caring for the family is strongly emphasized throughout this text, it is highlighted in features such as Cultural Considerations boxes (see p. 44) and Family-Centered Care boxes (see p. 13).

Atraumatic Care

Atraumatic care is the provision of therapeutic care in settings, by personnel, and through the use of interventions that eliminate or minimize the psychologic and physical distress experienced by children and their families in the health care system. Therapeutic care encompasses the prevention, diagnosis, treatment, or palliation of acute or chronic conditions. Setting refers to the place in which that care is given—the home, the hospital, or any other health care setting. Personnel include anyone directly involved in providing therapeutic care. Interventions range from psychologic approaches, such as preparing children for procedures, to physical interventions, such as providing space for a parent to room in with a child. Psychologic distress may include anxiety, fear, anger, disappointment, sadness, shame, or guilt. Physical distress may range from sleeplessness and immobilization to disturbances from sensory stimuli such as pain, temperature extremes, loud noises, bright lights, or darkness. Thus atraumatic care is concerned with the where, who, why, and how of any procedure performed on a child for the purpose of preventing or minimizing psychologic and physical stress (Wong, 1989).

The overriding goal in providing atraumatic care is first, do no harm. Three principles provide the framework for achieving this goal: (1) prevent or minimize the child's separation from the family, (2) promote a sense of control, and (3) prevent or minimize bodily injury and pain. Examples of providing atraumatic care include fostering the parent–child relationship during hospitalization, preparing the child before any unfamiliar treatment or procedure, controlling pain, allowing the child privacy, providing play activities for expression of fear and aggression, providing choices to children, and respecting cultural differences.

ROLE OF THE PEDIATRIC NURSE

The pediatric nurse is responsible for promoting the health and well-being of the child and family. Nursing functions vary according to regional job structures, individual education and experience, and personal career goals. Just as patients (children and their families) have unique backgrounds, each nurse brings an individual set of variables that affect the nurse–patient relationship. No matter where pediatric nurses practice, their primary concern is the welfare of the child and family.

Therapeutic Relationship

The establishment of a therapeutic relationship is the essential foundation for providing high-quality nursing care. Pediatric nurses need to have meaningful relationships with children and their families and yet remain separate enough to distinguish their own feelings and needs. In a therapeutic relationship, caring, well-defined boundaries separate the nurse from the child and family. These boundaries are positive and professional and promote the family's control over the child's health care. Both the nurse and the family are empowered and maintain open communication. In a nontherapeutic relationship, these boundaries are blurred, and many of the nurse's actions may serve personal needs, such as a need to feel wanted and involved, rather than the family's needs.

Exploring whether relationships with patients are therapeutic or nontherapeutic helps nurses identify problem areas early in their interactions with children and families (see Nursing Care Guidelines box). Although questions regarding the nurse's involvement may label certain actions negative or positive, no one action makes a relationship therapeutic or nontherapeutic. For example, a nurse may spend additional time with the family but still recognize his or her own needs and maintain professional separateness. An important clue to nontherapeutic relationships is the staff's concerns about their peer's actions with the family.

Family Advocacy and Caring

Although nurses are responsible to themselves, the profession, and the institution of employment, their primary responsibility is to the consumer of nursing services: the child and family. The nurse must work with family members, identify their goals and needs, and plan interventions that best address the defined problems. As an advocate, the

---

BOX 1-4 UNITED NATIONS' DECLARATION OF THE RIGHTS OF THE CHILD*

All children need:
- To be free from discrimination
- To develop physically and mentally in freedom and dignity
- To have a name and nationality
- To have adequate nutrition, housing, recreation, and medical services
- To receive special treatment if disabled
- To receive love, understanding, and material security
- To receive an education and develop his or her abilities
- To be the first to receive protection in disaster
- To be protected from neglect, cruelty, and exploitation
- To be brought up in a spirit of friendship among people

*Proclaimed by General Assembly Resolution 1386(XIV) of 20 November 1959.

---

nurse assists the child and family in making informed choices and acting in the child's best interest. Advocacy involves ensuring that families are aware of all available health services, adequately informed of treatments and procedures, involved in the child's care, and encouraged to change or support existing health care practices. The United Nations' Declaration of the Rights of the Child (Box 1-4) provides guidelines for nursing practice to ensure that every child receives optimum care.

As nurses care for children and families, they must demonstrate caring, compassion, and empathy for others. Aspects of caring embody the concept of atraumatic care and the development of a therapeutic relationship with patients. Parents perceive caring as a sign of quality in nursing care, which is often focused on the nontechnical needs of the child and family. Parents describe "personable" care as actions by the nurse that include acknowledging the parent's presence, listening, making the parent feel comfortable in the hospital environment, involving the parent and child in the nursing care, showing interest in and concern for their welfare, showing affection and sensitivity to the parent and child, communicating with them, and individualizing the nursing care. Parents perceive personable nursing care as being integral to establishing a positive relationship.

Disease Prevention and Health Promotion

Every nurse involved in caring for children must understand the importance of disease prevention and health promotion. A nursing care plan must include a thorough assessment of all aspects of child growth and development, including nutrition, immunizations, safety, dental care, socialization, discipline, and education. If problems are identified, the nurse intervenes directly or refers the family to other health care providers or agencies.

The best approach to prevention is education and anticipatory guidance. In this text each chapter on health promotion includes sections on anticipatory guidance. An appreciation of the hazards or conflicts of each developmental period enables the nurse to guide parents regarding childrearing practices aimed at preventing potential problems. One significant example is safety. Because each age group is at risk for special types of injuries, preventive teaching can significantly reduce injuries, lowering permanent disability and mortality rates.

Prevention also involves less obvious aspects of caring for children. The nurse is responsible for providing care that promotes mental well-being (e.g., enlisting the help of a child life specialist during a painful procedure such as an immunization).

NURSING CARE GUIDELINES

Exploring Your Relationships with Children and Families

To foster therapeutic relationships with children and families, you must first become aware of your caregiving style, including how effectively you take care of yourself. The following questions should help you understand the therapeutic quality of your professional relationships.

Negative Actions

Are you overinvolved with children and their families?
- Do you work overtime to care for the family?
- Do you spend off-duty time with children's families, either in or out of the hospital?
- Do you call frequently (either the hospital or home) to see how the family is doing?
- Do you show favoritism toward certain patients?
- Do you buy clothes, toys, food, or other items for the child and family?
- Do you compete with other staff members for the affection of certain patients and families?
- Do other staff members comment to you about your closeness to the family?
- Do you attempt to influence families' decisions rather than facilitate their informed decision making?

Are you underinvolved with children and families?
- Do you restrict parent or visitor access to children, using excuses such as the unit is too busy?
- Do you focus on the technical aspects of care and lose sight of the person who is the patient?

Are you overinvolved with the children and underinvolved with their parents?
- Do you become critical when the parents do not visit their children?
- Do you compete with the parents for their children's affection?

Positive Actions

Do you strive to empower families?
- Do you explore families' strengths and needs in an effort to increase family involvement?
- Have you developed teaching skills to instruct families rather than doing everything for them?
- Do you work with families to find ways to decrease their dependence on health care providers?
- Can you separate families' needs from your own needs?

Do you strive to empower yourself?
- Are you aware of your emotional responses to different people and situations?
- Do you seek to understand how your own family experiences influence reactions to patients and families, especially as they affect tendencies toward overinvolvement or underinvolvement?
- Do you have a calming influence, not one that will amplify emotionality?
- Have you developed interpersonal skills in addition to technical skills?
- Have you learned about ethnic and religious family patterns?
- Do you communicate directly with persons with whom you are upset or take issue?
- Are you able to "step back" and withdraw emotionally, if not physically, when emotional overload occurs, yet remain committed?
- Do you take care of yourself and your needs?
- Do you periodically interview family members to determine their current issues (e.g., feelings, attitudes, responses, wishes), communicate these findings to peers, and update records?
- Do you avoid relying on initial interview data, assumptions, or gossip regarding families?
- Do you ask questions if families are not participating in care?
- Do you assess families for feelings of anxiety, fear, intimidation, worry about making a mistake, a perceived lack of competence to care for their child, or fear of health care professionals overstepping their boundaries into family territory or vice versa?
- Do you explore these issues with family members and provide encouragement and support to enable families to help themselves?
- Do you keep communication channels open among yourself, family, physicians, and other care providers?
- Do you resolve conflicts and misunderstandings directly with those who are involved?
- Do you clarify information for families or seek the appropriate person to do so?

Do you recognize that from time to time a therapeutic relationship can change to a social relationship or an intimate friendship?
- Are you able to acknowledge the fact when it occurs and understand why it happened?
- Can you ensure that there is someone else who is more objective who can take your place in the therapeutic relationship?

Health Teaching

Health teaching is inseparable from family advocacy and prevention. Health teaching may be the nurse's direct goal, such as during parenting classes, or may be indirect, such as helping parents and children understand a diagnosis or medical treatment, encouraging children to ask questions about their bodies, referring families to health-related professional or lay groups, supplying patients with appropriate literature, and providing anticipatory guidance.

Health teaching is one area in which nurses often need preparation and practice with competent role models because it involves transmitting information at the child's and family's level of understanding and desire for information. As an effective educator, the nurse focuses on providing the appropriate health teaching with generous feedback and evaluation to promote learning.

Injury Prevention

Each year, injuries kill or disable more children older than 1 year than all childhood diseases combined. Nurses play an important role in preventing injuries by using a developmental approach to safety counseling for parents of children of all ages. Realizing that safety concerns for a young infant are completely different than injury risks of adolescents, nurses discuss appropriate injury preventions tips to parents and children as part of routine patient care.

Support and Counseling

Attention to emotional needs requires support and sometimes counseling. The role of a child advocate or health teacher is supportive by virtue of the individualized approach. The nurse can offer support by listening, touching, and being physically present. Touching and a physical presence are most helpful with children because they facilitate nonverbal communication. Counseling involves a mutual exchange of ideas and opinions that provides the basis for mutual problem solving. It involves support, teaching, techniques to foster the expression of feelings or thoughts, and approaches to help the family cope with stress. Optimally, counseling not only helps resolve a crisis or problem but also enables the family to attain a higher level of functioning, greater self-esteem, and closer relationships. Although counseling is often the role of nurses in specialized areas, counseling techniques are discussed in various sections of this text to help students and nurses cope with immediate crises and refer families for additional professional assistance.

Coordination and Collaboration

The nurse, as a member of the health care team, collaborates and coordinates nursing care with the care activities of other professionals. A nurse working in isolation rarely serves the child's best interests. The concept of holistic care can be realized through a unified, interdisciplinary approach by being aware of individual contributions and limitations and collaborating with other specialists to provide high-quality health services. Failure to recognize limitations can be nontherapeutic at best and destructive at worst. For example, a nurse who feels competent in counseling but who is really inadequate in this area may not only prevent the child from dealing with a crisis but also impede future success with a qualified professional.

Ethical Decision Making

Ethical dilemmas arise when competing moral considerations underlie various alternatives. Parents, nurses, physicians, and other health care team members may reach different but morally defensible decisions by assigning different weights to competing moral values. These competing moral values may include autonomy, the patient's right to be self-governing; nonmaleficence, the obligation to minimize or prevent harm; beneficence, the obligation to promote the patient's well-being; and justice, the concept of fairness. Nurses must determine the most beneficial or least harmful action within the framework of societal mores, professional practice standards, the law, institutional rules, the family's value system and religious traditions, and the nurse's personal values.

Nurses must prepare themselves systematically for collaborative ethical decision making. They can accomplish this through formal course work, continuing education, contemporary literature, and work to establish an environment conducive to ethical discourse. Moreover, nurses must be educated on the mechanisms for dispute resolution, case review by ethics committees, procedural safeguards, state statutes, and case law (Woods, 2005).

Nurses also use the professional code of ethics for guidance and as a means for professional self-regulation. The Code of Ethics for Nurses by the American Nurses Association focuses on the nurse's accountability and responsibility to patients and emphasizes the nursing role as an independent professional, one that upholds its own legal liability. Nurses may face ethical issues regarding patient care, such as the use of lifesaving measures for VLBW newborns or a terminally ill child's right to refuse treatment. They may struggle with questions regarding truthfulness, balancing their rights and responsibilities in caring for children with AIDS, whistle-blowing, or allocating resources. Conflicting ethical arguments are presented to help nurses clarify their value judgments when confronted with sensitive issues.

RESEARCH AND EVIDENCE-BASED PRACTICE

Nurses should contribute to research because they are the individuals observing human responses to health and illness. The current emphasis on measurable outcomes to determine the efficacy of interventions (often in relation to the cost) demands that nurses know whether clinical interventions result in positive outcomes for their patients. This demand has influenced the current trend toward evidence-based practice (EBP), which implies questioning why something is effective and whether a better approach exists. The concept of EBP also involves analyzing and translating published clinical research into the everyday practice of nursing. When nurses base their clinical practice on science and research and document their clinical outcomes, they are able to validate their contributions to health, wellness, and cure, not only to their patients, third-party payers, and institutions but also to the nursing profession. Evaluation is essential to the nursing process, and research is one of the best ways to accomplish this.

EBP is the collection, interpretation, and integration of valid, important, and applicable patient-reported, nurse-observed, and research-derived information. Evidence-based nursing practice combines knowledge with clinical experience and intuition. It provides a rational approach to decision making that facilitates best practice (Scott and McSherry, 2009; van Achterberg, Schoonhoven, and Grol, 2008). EBP is an important tool that complements the nursing process by using critical thinking skills to make decisions based on existing knowledge. The traditional nursing process approach to patient care can be used to conceptualize the essential components of EBP nursing. During the assessment and diagnostic phases of the nursing process, the nurse establishes important clinical questions and completes a critical review of existing knowledge. EBP also begins with identification of the problem. The nurse asks clinical questions in a concise, organized way that allows for clear answers. Good clinical questions should be asked in the PICOT (Population, Intervention, Control, Outcome, Time) format to assist with clarity and literature searching. PICOT questions assist with clarifying scope of the problem and clinical topic of interest. After the specific questions have been identified, extensive searching for the best information to answer the question begins. The nurse evaluates clinically relevant research, analyzes findings from the history and physical examinations, and reviews the specific pathophysiology of the defined problem. By integrating evidence with clinical expertise, the nurse focuses care on the patient's unique needs. The final step in EBP is consistent with the final phase of the nursing process: to evaluate the effectiveness of the care plan.

Searching for evidence in this modern era of technology can be overwhelming. For nurses to implement EBP, they must have access to appropriate, recent resources such as online search engines and journals. In many institutions, computer terminals are available on patient care units, with the Internet and online journals easily accessible. Another important resource for the implementation of EBP is time. The nursing shortage and ongoing changes in many institutions have compounded the issue of nursing time allocation for patient care, education, and training. In some institutions, nurses are given paid time away from performing patient care to participate in activities that promote EBP. This requires an organizational environment that values EBP and its potential impact on patient care. As knowledge is generated regarding the significant impact of EBP on patient care outcomes, it is hoped that the organizational culture will change to support the staff nurse's participation in EBP. As the amount of available evidence increases, so does our need to critically evaluate the evidence.

TABLE 1-4	THE GRADE CRITERIA TO EVALUATE THE QUALITY OF THE EVIDENCE
QUALITY	**TYPE OF EVIDENCE**
High	Consistent evidence from well-performed randomized clinical trials (RCTs) or exceptionally strong evidence from unbiased observational studies
Moderate	Evidence from RCTs with important limitations (inconsistent results, methodologic flaws, indirect evidence, or imprecise results) or unusually strong evidence from unbiased observational studies
Low	Evidence for at least one critical outcome from observational studies, from RCTs with serious flaws, or from indirect evidence
Very low	Evidence for at least one of the critical outcomes from unsystematic clinical observations or very indirect evidence
QUALITY	**RECOMMENDATION**
Strong	Desirable effects clearly outweigh undesirable effects or vice versa
Weak	Desirable effects closely balanced with undesirable effects

Adapted from Guyatt GH, Oxman AD, Visit GE, and others: GRADE: an emerging consensus on rating quality of evidence and strength of recommendations, *BMJ* 336:924–926, 2008.

Throughout this book, EBP boxes summarize the existing evidence that promotes excellence in clinical care. The GRADE criteria are used to evaluate the quality of research articles used to develop practice guidelines (Guyatt, Oxman, Vist, and others, 2008). Table 1-4 defines how nurses rate the quality of the evidence using the GRADE criteria and establish a strong versus a weak recommendation. Each EBP box rates the quality of existing evidence and the strength of the recommendation for practice change.

CLINICAL REASONING AND THE PROCESS OF PROVIDING NURSING CARE TO CHILDREN AND FAMILIES

CLINICAL REASONING

A systematic thought process is essential to a profession. It assists the professional in meeting the patient's needs. **Clinical reasoning** is a cognitive process that uses formal and informal thinking to gather and analyze patient data, evaluate the significance of the information, and consider alternative actions (Simmons, 2010). It is based on the scientific method of inquiry, which is also the basis for the nursing process. Clinical reasoning and the nursing process are considered crucial to professional nursing in that they constitute a holistic approach to problem solving.

Clinical reasoning is a complex developmental process based on rational and deliberate thought. Clinical reasoning provides a common denominator for knowledge that exemplifies disciplined and self-directed thinking. The knowledge is acquired, assessed, and organized by thinking through the clinical situation and developing an outcome focused on optimum patient care. Clinical reasoning transforms the way in which individuals view themselves, understand the world, and make decisions. In recognition of the importance of this skill, Critical

Thinking Case Studies included in this text demonstrate the importance of clinical reasoning. These exercises present a nursing practice situation that challenges the student to use the skills of clinical reasoning to come to the best conclusion. A series of questions leads students to explore the evidence, assumptions underlying the problem, nursing priorities, and support for nursing interventions that allow them to make rational and deliberate responses. These exercises are designed to enhance nursing performance in clinical reasoning.

NURSING PROCESS

The nursing process is a method of problem identification and problem solving that describes what the nurse actually does. The six-step nursing process model is assessment, diagnosis (problem identification), planning (with outcome development), implementation, evaluation, and documentation. The second step of the nursing process, nursing diagnosis, involves naming the child's or family's problem in standardized nursing language. In the American Nurses Association (2003) Standards of Practice, the nursing diagnosis phase of the nursing process is separated into two steps: nursing diagnosis and outcome identification.

Assessment

Assessment is a continuous process that operates at all phases of problem solving and is the foundation for decision making. Assessment involves multiple nursing skills and consists of the purposeful collection, classification, and analysis of data from a variety of sources. To provide an accurate and comprehensive assessment, the nurse must consider information about the patient's biophysical, psychologic, sociocultural, and spiritual background.

Nursing Diagnosis

The second step of the nursing process is problem identification and nursing diagnosis. At this point, the nurse must interpret and make decisions about the data gathered. The nurse organizes or clusters these data into categories to identify significant areas and makes one of the following decisions:

- No dysfunctional health problems are evident; no interventions are indicated.
- Risk for dysfunctional health problems exists; interventions are needed for health promotion.
- Actual dysfunctional health problems are evident; interventions are needed for health promotion.

The nursing diagnosis is the naming of the cue clusters that are obtained during the assessment phase. According to NANDA International (formerly the North American Nursing Diagnosis Association), the currently accepted definition of the term **nursing diagnosis** is that it is a clinical judgment about individual, family, or community responses to actual and potential health problems and life processes. The Nursing Care Plans in this text provide an understanding of the standardized language and how it relates to the individualized plan.

Not all children have actual health problems; some have a potential health problem, which is a risk state that requires nursing intervention to prevent the development of an actual problem. Potential health problems may be indicated by **risk factors**, or signs, that predispose a child and family to a dysfunctional health pattern and are limited to individuals at greater risk than the population as a whole. Nursing interventions are directed toward reducing risk factors. To differentiate actual from potential health problems, the word *risk* is included in the nursing diagnosis statement (e.g., Risk for Infection).

FAMILY-CENTERED CARE

Using Defining Characteristics to Select an Appropriate Nursing Diagnosis

An 18-month-old only child is admitted with respiratory distress and a presumptive diagnosis of epiglottitis. Initial nursing actions focus on the child's physiologic status. As the condition stabilizes, the nurse gathers family assessment data. The child's immunizations are current, he is clean and well nourished, and his developmental age is appropriate. The parents are both present at admission. The mother is distraught about the sudden onset of respiratory distress. She states that earlier her child had only a "runny nose," and she thought it was just a cold. When the child suddenly began to have difficulty breathing, she felt helpless and unable to relieve her child's discomfort. She states: "Nothing I did made him any better. If I had known this could happen, I would have brought him to the hospital sooner. I feel like a bad mother." In the hospital, after explanations by the nurses, the mother understands that epiglottitis is a sudden illness that typically follows symptoms of a cold. She is cooperative and asks what she can do to make her child more comfortable. She implements all of the suggestions of the health care team. The father supports both the child and the mother, although he assumes a more passive, "listening" role.

Three nursing diagnoses that relate to family and parent situations may be relevant. The first step is to review the diagnoses and the defining characteristics and decide which one is most appropriate:

1. Parenting, Impaired—Inability of the primary caretaker to create, maintain, or regain an environment that nurtures the child's growth and development
   Selected defining characteristics:
   - Insecure (or lack of) attachment to infant
   - Poor or inappropriate caretaking skills

2. Conflict, Parental Role—Parent experience of role confusion and conflict in response to crisis
   Selected defining characteristics:
   - Parent expressing concerns about changes in parental role
   - A demonstrated disruption in care or caretaking routines
   - Parent expressing concerns or feelings of inadequacy to provide for the child's physical and emotional needs during hospitalization or in home
   - Parent verbalizing or demonstrating feelings of guilt, anger, fear, anxiety, or frustration about effect of child's illness on family process

3. Family Processes, Interrupted—A change in family relationships or functioning
   Selected defining characteristics:
   - Expressions of conflict within the family
   - Changes in communication patterns among family members

Of these three diagnoses, the most relevant one is *Conflict, Parental Role.* The parents demonstrate attachment behavior to their child and are attentive to his needs. They appear to have appropriate parenting skills and are able to communicate effectively with each other. Neither parent expressed any conflict within the family. The sudden onset of this child's illness has interrupted the mother's usual role and caused her to feel inadequate, anxious, and guilty. However, the mother is able to adapt to this crisis. She demonstrates an ability to cope by learning and implementing new comforting skills for her child. The defining characteristics of the other two diagnoses require maladaptive characteristics that are clearly not demonstrated by these parents.

Signs and symptoms refer to a cluster of cues and defining characteristics that are derived from patient assessment and indicate actual health problems. When a defining characteristic is essential for the diagnosis to be made, it is considered critical. These critical defining characteristics help differentiate among diagnostic categories. For example, in deciding among the diagnostic categories related to family function and coping, the nurse uses defining characteristics to choose the most appropriate nursing diagnosis (see Family-Centered Care box).

Planning

After identifying the nursing diagnoses, the nurse develops a care plan and establishes outcomes or goals. The outcome is the projected or expected change in a patient's health status, clinical condition, or behavior that occurs after nursing interventions have been instituted. The ultimate goal of nursing care is to convert the nursing diagnoses into a desired health state. The care plan must be established before specific nursing interventions are developed and implemented.

Implementation

The implementation phase begins when the nurse puts the selected intervention into action and accumulates feedback data regarding its effects (or the patient's response to the intervention). The feedback returns in the form of observation and communication and provides a database on which to evaluate the outcome of the nursing intervention. It is imperative that continual assessment of the patient's status occurs throughout all phases of the nursing process, thus making the process a dynamic rather than static problem-solving method. Throughout the implementation stage, the main concerns are the patient's physical safety and psychologic comfort in terms of atraumatic care.

Evaluation

Evaluation is the last step in the decision-making process. The nurse gathers, sorts, and analyzes data to determine whether (1) the established outcome has been met, (2) the nursing interventions were appropriate, (3) the plan requires modification, or (4) other alternatives should be considered. The evaluation phase either completes the nursing process (outcome is met) or serves as the basis for selecting alternative interventions to solve the specific problem.

With the current focus on patient outcomes in health care, the patient's care is evaluated not only at discharge but thereafter as well to ensure that the outcomes are met and there is adequate care for resolving existing or potential health problems. One federal agency that has developed clinical guidelines containing outcome measures is the Agency for Healthcare Research and Quality.*

Documentation

Although documentation is not one of the five steps of the nursing process, it is essential for evaluation. The nurse can assess, diagnose and identify problems, plan, and implement without documentation; however, evaluation is best performed with written evidence of progress toward outcomes. The patient's medical record should include evidence of those elements listed in the Nursing Care Guidelines box.

QUALITY OUTCOME MEASURES

Quality of care refers to the degree to which health services for individuals and populations increase the likelihood of desired health outcomes and are consistent with current professional knowledge

---

*540 Gaither Road, Suite 2000, Rockville, MD 20850; 301-427-1364; info@ahrq.gov; http://www.ahrq.gov; http://guideline.gov.

NURSING CARE GUIDELINES

Documentation of Nursing Care

- Initial assessments and reassessments
- Nursing diagnoses, patient care needs, or both
- Interventions identified to meet the patient's nursing care needs
- Nursing care provided
- Patient's response to and the outcomes of the care provided
- Abilities of patient or, as appropriate, significant other(s) to manage continuing care needs after discharge

BOX 1-5 NATIONAL QUALITY FORUM: PATIENT-CENTERED OUTCOME MEASURES

Death among surgical inpatients with treatable serious complications (failure to rescue)—The percentage of major surgical inpatients who experience a hospital-acquired complication and die

Pressure ulcer prevalence—The percentage of inpatients who have a hospital-acquired pressure ulcer

Falls prevalence—The number of inpatient falls per inpatient days

Falls with injury—The number of inpatient falls with injuries per inpatient days

Restraint prevalence—The percentage of inpatients who have a vest or limb restraint

Urinary catheter–associated urinary tract infection for intensive care unit (ICU) patients—The rate of urinary tract infections associated with use of urinary catheters for ICU patients

Central line catheter–associated bloodstream infection rate for ICU and high-risk nursery patients—The rate of bloodstream infections associated with use of central line catheters for ICU and high-risk nursery patients

Ventilator-associated pneumonia for ICU and high-risk nursery patients—The rate of pneumonia associated with use of ventilators for ICU and high-risk nursery patients

Modified from National Quality Forum: *A status report, NQF Issue Brief No. 5, July 2007*, retrieved August 15, 2011, from http://www.qualityforum.org/Publications/2007/07/Nursing_Performance_Measurement_and_Reporting.aspx.

(Institute of Medicine, 2000). Because nurses are the principal caregivers within health care institutions, high-quality nursing outcomes are used as an indicator of the ability to provide excellence in patient care. Nurse-sensitive indicators are chosen by using specific evaluation criteria. Specific examples of patient-centered outcome measures established by the National Quality Forum are found in Box 1-5. A comprehensive resource, the Quality and Safety Education for Nurses (QSEN), is funded by the Robert Wood Johnson Foundation.* Each EBP box in this book ends with the QSEN competences related to knowledge, skills, and attitudes for evidence-based nursing practice.

Quality outcome evaluation criteria establish a framework for measuring nursing care performance. In addition to using the National Quality Forum's measurement evaluation criteria, nurses should evaluate each quality-nursing indicator to ensure it is an essential component of health care quality established by the Institute of Medicine (2000). These components include the following:

- Safe
- Effective
- Patient centered
- Timely
- Efficient
- Equitable

*University of North Carolina at Chapel Hill, School of Nursing, Carrington Hall, CB# 7460, Chapel Hill, NC 27599; 919-843-9985; fax: 919-843-3884; qsen@unc.edu; http://www.qsen.org

Throughout the chapters that focus on serious health problems, we have developed examples of quality outcome measures for specific diseases that reflect patient-centered outcomes. Quality outcome measures promote interdisciplinary teamwork, and the boxes throughout this book exemplify measures of effective collaboration to improve care. Quality Patient Outcomes boxes throughout this book are developed to assist health care professionals in identifying appropriate measures that evaluate the quality of patient care.

KEY POINTS

- Although the infant mortality rate in the United States has declined over the past few decades, the United States lags significantly behind most other major countries, such as Canada.
- LBW, which is closely related to early gestational age, is considered the leading cause of neonatal death in the United States.
- Injuries are the leading cause of death in children older than age 1 year, with the majority being MVA injuries.
- Childhood morbidity encompasses acute illness, chronic disease, and disability.
- Eighty percent of childhood illnesses are attributable to infections, with respiratory tract infections occurring two or three times more often than all other illnesses combined.
- The *new morbidity* refers to behavioral, social, and educational problems that can significantly alter a child's health.
- Developmental stage and environment are important determinants of the prevalence of injuries at a given age and thus help to direct preventive measures.
- The philosophy of family-centered care recognizes that the family is the constant in a child's life and that service systems and personnel must support, respect, and enhance the family's strength and competence.
- Atraumatic care is the provision of therapeutic care in settings, by personnel, and through the use of interventions that eliminate or minimize the psychologic and physical distress experienced by children and their families in the health care system.
- The pediatric nurse's roles include a therapeutic relationship, family advocacy, disease prevention and health promotion, health teaching, support and counseling, coordination and collaboration, ethical decision making, and research.
- EBP is the collection, interpretation, and integration of valid, important, and applicable patient-reported, nurse-observed, and research-derived information.
- The process of nursing children and families includes accurate and comprehensive assessment, analysis and synthesis of assessment data to arrive at a nursing diagnosis, planning of care, implementation of the plan, and evaluation of interventions.
- Because nurses are the principal caregivers within health care institutions, quality outcomes are used as a measure of the ability to provide excellence in patient care.

REFERENCES

Agency for Healthcare Research and Quality: *National healthcare disparities report*, Rockville, Md, 2008, U.S. Department of Health and Human Services.

American Academy of Pediatrics: *The national children's study*, 2008, retrieved January 2, 2011, from http://www.aap.org/family/natlchstudy.htm.

American Association of Suicidology: *Youth suicide fact sheet*, 2009, retrieved December 2, 2010, from http://www.suicidology.org.

American Dietetic Association: Position of the American Dietetic Association: nutrition guidance for healthy children ages 2 to 11 years, *J Am Dietetic Assoc* 108(6):1038–1047, 2008.

American Nurses Association: *Nursing: scope and standards of practice*, Washington, DC, 2003, Author.

Annie E. Casey Foundation: *2011 Kids count data book: state profiles of child well-being*, Baltimore, 2011, Author.

Bronstein AC, Spyker DA, Cantilena LR, and others: 2009 annual report of the American Association of Poison Control Centers' national poison data system: 27th annual report, *Clin Toxicol* 48(10):929–1178, 2010.

Cali AMG, Caprio S: Prediabetes and type 2 diabetes in youth: an emerging epidemic disease? *Curr Opin Endocrinol Diabetes Obes* 15:123–127, 2008.

Castle SL, Burke RV, Arbogast H, and others: Bicycle helmet legislation and injury patterns in trauma patients under age 18, *J Surg Res*, 2010.

Centers for Disease Control and Prevention: *CDC injury fact book*, Atlanta, 2006, National Center for Injury Prevention and Control.

Cheng NF, Han PZ, Gansky SA: Methods and software for estimating health disparities: the case of children's oral health, *Am J Epidemiol* 168(8):906–914, 2008.

Coury DL: Over the rainbow: advancing child health in the new millennium, *Ambul Pediatr* 6(3):134–137, 2006.

de Onis M, Blössner M, Borghi E: Global prevalence and trends of overweight and obesity among preschool children, *Am J Clin Nutr* 92(5):1257–1264, 2010.

Doucette A: Youth suicide. In Cosby AG, Greenberg RE, Southward LH, and others, editors: *About children: an authoritative resource on the state of childhood today*, Elk Grove Village, Ill, 2005, American Academy of Pediatrics.

Federal Interagency Forum on Child and Family Statistics: *America's children: key national indicators of well-being, 2011*. Washington, DC, 2011, U.S. Government Printing Office.

Franklin RL, Rodgers GB: Unintentional child poisoning treated in the United States hospital emergency departments: national estimates of incident cases, population-based poisoning rates, and product involvement, *Pediatrics* 122(6):1244–1251, 2008.

Graff M, North KE, Monda KL, and others: The combined influence of genetic factors and sedentary activity on body mass changes from adolescence to young adulthood: the National Longitudinal Adolescent Health Study, *Diabetes Metab Res Rev* 27(1):63–69, 2011.

Guyatt GH, Oxman AD, Vist GE, and others: GRADE: an emerging consensus on rating quality of evidence and strength of recommendations, *BMJ* 336:924–926, 2008.

Heuer S: Family-centered care, *J Spec Pediatr Nurs* 12(1):61–65, 2007.

Hooper VD: Patient-family centered care: are we there yet? *J Peri Anesthesia Nurs* 23(6):440–442, 2008.

Institute of Medicine: *Crossing the quality chasm*, Washington, DC, 2000, Author.

Kagihara LE, Niederhauser VP, Stark M: Assessment, management, and prevention of early childhood caries, *J Am Acad Nurse Pract* 21(1):1–10, 2009.

Kochanek KD, Xu J, Murphy SL, and others: Deaths: preliminary data for 2009, *Natl Vital Stat Rep* 59(4):1–57, 2011.

Leslie LK, Slaw KM, Edwards A, and others: Peering into the future: pediatrics in a changing world, *Pediatrics* 126(5):982–988, 2010.

Martin JA, Kochanek KD, Strobino DM, and others: Annual summary of vital statistics: 2003, *Pediatrics* 115(3):619–634, 2005.

Mathews TJ, Miniño AM, Osterman MJ, and others: Annual summary of vital statistics: 2008, *Pediatrics* 127(1):146–157, 2011.

Matyka KA: Type 2 diabetes in childhood: epidemiological and clinical aspects, *Br Med Bull* 86:59–75, 2008.

National Center for Cultural Competence: *A guide for advancing family-centered and culturally and linguistically competent care*, Washington, DC, 2007, Georgetown University Center for Child and Human Development.

National Survey on Drug Use and Health: *Trends in substance use, dependence or abuse, and treatment among adolescents: 2002–2007*, Rockville, Md, 2008, Office of Applied Studies.

Polaha J, Dalton WT 3rd, Allen S: The prevalence of emotional and behavior problems in pediatric primary care serving rural children, *J Pediatr Psychol* 36(6):652–660, 2011.

Porche MV, Fortuna LR, Lin J, and others: Childhood trauma and psychiatric disorders as correlates of school dropout in a national sample of young adults, *Child Dev* 82(3):982–998, 2011.

Raj M, Kumar RK: Obesity in children & adolescents, *Indian J Med Res* 132(5):598–607, 2010.

Schnitzer PG: Prevention of unintentional childhood injuries, *Am Fam Physician* 74(11):1864–1869, 2006.

Schwartz MS, Chadha A: Type 2 diabetes mellitus in childhood: obesity and insulin resistance, *J Am Osteopath Assoc* 108:518–524, 2008.

Scott K, McSherry R: Evidence-based nursing: clarifying the concepts for nurses in practice, *J Clin Nurs* 18(8):1085–1095, 2009.

Simmons B: Clinical reasoning: concept analysis, *J Adv Nurs* 66(5):1151–1158, 2010.

Starmer AJ, Duby JC, Slaw KM, and others: Pediatrics in the year 2020 and beyond: preparing for plausible futures, *Pediatrics* 126(5):971–981, 2010.

U.S. Department of Health and Human Services: *Youth violence: a report of the Surgeon General*, retrieved January 22, 2011, from http://www.surgeongeneral.gov/library/youthviolence.

van Achterberg T, Schoonhoven L, Grol R: Nursing implementation science: how evidence-based nursing requires evidence-based implementation, *J Nurs Scholar* 40(4):302–310, 2008.

Wong D: Principles of atraumatic care. In Feeg V, editor: *Pediatric nursing: forum on the future: looking toward the 21st century*, Pitman, NJ, 1989, Anthony J. Jannetti.

Woods M: Nursing ethics education: are we really delivering the good(s)? *Nurs Ethics* 12(1):5–18, 2005.

World Health Organization: *School health and youth health promotion, 2011*, retrieved January 21, 2011, from http://www.who.int/school_youth_health/en.

2

Community-Based Nursing Care of the Child and Family

*Christine A. Brosnan, Sandra L. Upchurch,
and Martina R. Gallagher*

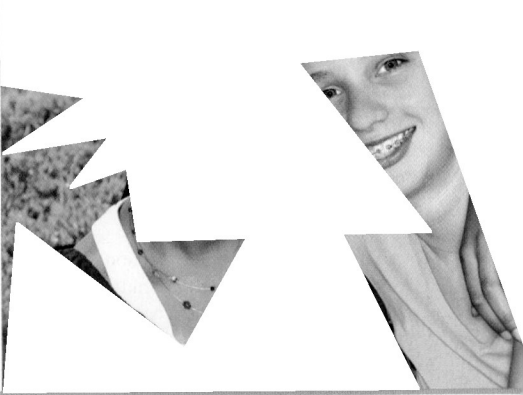

evolve WEBSITE

http://evolve.elsevier.com/wong/essentials
Key Point Summaries
NCLEX-Style Review Questions

CHAPTER OUTLINE

Nursing in the Community, 16
Community Concepts, 16
    Community, 16
        Community Health Nursing, 17
        Roles and Functions, 17
    Demography, 18
    Epidemiology, 18

*Distribution of Disease, Injury, or
    Illness, 18*
Epidemiologic Triangle, 18
Levels of Prevention, 19
Screening, 19
Economics, 19

Community Nursing Process, 19
    Community Needs Assessment and
        Diagnosis, 19
    Community Planning, 20
    Community Implementation, 20
    Community Evaluation, 20

LEARNING OBJECTIVES

On completion of this chapter the reader will be able to:
- Define a community.
- Describe community health nursing.
- Identify the roles and functions of the community health nurse.

- Discuss selected aspects of the epidemiologic process.
- Explain the purpose of an economic evaluation.
- Discuss the components of the community nursing process.

NURSING IN THE COMMUNITY

The health of children and their families is greatly influenced by their community, and nurses can make a significant contribution by working with the community to promote children's health. Nurses working with pediatric populations in the community need an understanding of the concepts and processes critical to address pediatric concerns from a community health perspective. Healthy communities provide not only excellent medical care but also a nurturing, safe place for children to live and grow. Healthy communities and cities address concerns through collaboration between and among citizens, health care providers, businesses, and governmental and private agencies (Riner, 2008).

This chapter discusses community health nursing as it relates to children. First, it identifies and defines the concepts and principles that serve as the basis of community health nursing. Then it describes the community health nursing process, step by step. It includes a box that demonstrates use of the process to address a very real child health concern: obesity.

COMMUNITY CONCEPTS

COMMUNITY

There are several ways to define a community. A community is a group of individuals with shared characteristics or interests who interact with each other (Rector, 2010). A community is a system that includes children and families, the physical environment, educational facilities, safety and transportation resources, political and governmental agencies, health and social services, communication resources, economic resources, and recreational facilities. The community is also the client of the community health nurse (Anderson and McFarland, 2010). Community health initiatives are directed either at the general health of the community as a whole or at specific populations within the community that have unique needs. In this context, populations can be described as groups of people who live in a community and have characteristics in common (e.g., school-age children). Target populations or subpopulations are more narrowly defined groups (e.g., non-immunized preschoolers, obese middle school children) toward whom nurses direct activities to improve the health status of individuals in the group. Common values often guide behaviors of populations and subpopulations in relation to health promotion and disease prevention (McEwen and Nies, 2011; Williams, 2010).

Community-oriented care involves a collaboration of individuals and groups, including health care providers, advocates, government, managed care organizations, businesses, children, and families, within a specific community. The goal of the collaborative effort is to provide services that promote the child health initiatives of *Healthy People 2020.** Community care is "without walls" in that the services of the health care system are frequently redesigned to meet the changing needs of the community. Those involved in community care partner with the community to identify, plan, intervene, and evaluate activities that improve the community's health (Anderson and McFarlane, 2010).

Community Health Nursing

Community health nursing focuses on promoting and maintaining the health of individuals, families, and groups in a community setting. Community health nursing is a synthesis of nursing and public health. It is population focused and involves collaboration with other disciplines to assess, plan, and implement care that emphasizes personal responsibility for health and self-care by community members (Warner, 2010; Williams, 2010). Community health nursing, at its best, empowers communities by enabling its members to gain the knowledge and skills needed to fulfill their own needs.

Although community health concepts can be used to address health concerns in any setting, traditional community health settings include home health agencies, schools, physician offices, ambulatory health clinics, emergency departments (EDs), triage call centers, insurance agencies, health departments, international relief agencies, health education agencies, juvenile detention facilities, camps, daycare centers, foster care facilities, hospice centers, and rehabilitation agencies. The American Nurses Association (1986) has established nine standards for community health nursing to guide practice across settings. They include the following categories: theory, data collection, diagnosis, planning, intervention, evaluation, quality assurance and professional development, interdisciplinary collaboration, and research. The revised scope and standards of public health nursing (American Nurses Association, 2007) describe the major components and measurement criteria for each standard.

Roles and Functions

The roles and functions of the community health nurse continue to evolve. In the future, more pediatric nurses will be working in community settings. The Health Resources and Services Administration (2004) reported that 14.9% of the total registered nurse workforce was employed in a community or public health setting and 11.5% in ambulatory care. Only 56.2% of registered nurses were employed in hospital settings. An example of the role evolution is the need for competent public health/community health nurses to work during times of natural disasters, public health threats, and terrorism attacks (Box 2-1).

BOX 2-1	**EVOLVING ROLE OF THE PEDIATRIC NURSE: NATURAL AND HUMAN-MADE DISASTERS**

Communities are affected by disasters, either natural disasters such as hurricanes and wildfires or human-made disasters such as terrorist attacks. During disasters, communities may not have the resources to respond and recover on their own. Pediatric nurses in all settings need to know disaster management stages, which include:

Prevention—Identification of disaster risks; education about what actions to take

Preparedness and planning
- For individuals and families—Training in first aid, an emergency disaster kit, a predetermined place to meet, and a communication plan
- For communities and agencies—Determination of the lines of authority and communication; coordination of personnel, supplies, and equipment; evacuation; rescue; and care of the dead

Response—Begins after the disaster; plans are implemented, which may include shelter in place for individuals, evacuation, or search and rescue. Calmness and patience are essential characteristics for all individuals involved

An important question for nurses to consider: Will nurses care for patients in the community during the disaster, or will they stay with their own families?

Modified from Mendias EP, Grimes DE: Preventing and managing community emergencies: disasters and infectious diseases. In Anderson ET, McFarlane J, editors: *Community as partner: theory and practice in nursing,* Philadelphia, 2010, Lippincott Williams & Wilkins; and Summerlin EB: Natural and man-made disasters. In Nies MA, McEwen M, editors: *Community/public health nursing: promoting the health of populations,* Philadelphia, 2011, Saunders.

Traditionally, the roles of community health nurses included caregiver, advocate, case manager, case finder, counselor, educator, epidemiologist, group process leader, health planner, and manager. For example, the nurse employed in a pediatric outpatient clinic functions in a number of roles to provide care to a child with type 2 diabetes. The nurse provides case management by coordinating care between the disciplines, counseling by supporting the child and family through developmental crisis, and case finding by identifying risk factors in the child's siblings.

The Institute of Medicine (1988) developed a list of core functions to guide the work of public health professionals, including nurses. The core functions are directed to population-wide services and to personal and home services for people at risk. The population-wide service is based on assessment of health status monitoring and disease surveillance, policy development, and assurance that policies are translated into service. The Council on Linkages Between Academia and Public Health Practice (2001), a group of university educators and public health professionals, further delineated the core functions and developed a list of skills to improve the ability of all public health workers, including nurses, to implement them. The eight categories of skills include analytic/assessment, policy development/program planning, communication, cultural competency, community dimensions of practice, basic public health sciences, financial planning and management, and leadership and systems thinking. Thus pediatric nurses employed in a managed care environment may be asked to develop a creative approach to teaching children from different cultures who have asthma about peak flow meters during ED visits. Included in the request may be a mechanism to evaluate the cost of the approach and the occurrence of repeated ED visits.

---

*http://www.healthypeople.gov.

DEMOGRAPHY

Demography is the study of population characteristics. Demographic characteristics include age, gender, race or ethnicity, socioeconomic status, and education. Individuals, families, and communities may have demographic characteristics that affect their health risks. Risk is an increased probability of developing a disease, injury, or illness. Age is one of the most important risk factors for disease prevention and certain health conditions. For example, infants are most likely to die as a result of congenital malformations, children and adolescents as a result of accidents, and middle-aged adults as a result of cancer (National Center for Health Statistics, 2011). Gender also plays an important role. Males are at much greater risk of hemophilia A and B than females. Race or ethnicity has long been associated with increased risk for disease and disability, but it is now thought that, aside from genetic predisposition, there is a complicated relationship between minority status and socioeconomic status that increases the risk for disease and disability (Smith, 2000). Low socioeconomic status predisposes children to a variety of problems. Poor children are more likely to be obese and to have untreated dental problems. They are more likely to have no regular site for medical care and to be treated in EDs (National Center for Health Statistics, 2011).

EPIDEMIOLOGY

Epidemiology is the science of population health applied to the detection of morbidity and mortality in a population. The epidemiologic process identifies the distribution and causes of disease or injury across a population (Cashaw, 2010). It also serves as an important component in developing health programs. For example, *Healthy People 2020* incorporates the process to develop a set of health objectives for the United States. Health professionals in community, state, and national health care organizations use the objectives as a guide to develop programs that have the greatest impact on the health of children.

Distribution of Disease, Injury, or Illness

Morbidity rates are used to measure disease and injury and, along with natality and mortality rates, present an objective picture of the health status of a community. There are two types of morbidity rates: incidence and prevalence. Incidence measures the occurrence of *new* events in a population during a time period. Prevalence measures *existing* events in a population during a time period (Hennekens and Buring, 1987). For example, the incidence of type 1 diabetes in a community is estimated by counting the new cases of type 1 diabetes in a population and dividing that figure by the population at risk. The prevalence of type 1 diabetes is estimated by counting the existing cases of type 1 diabetes in a population and dividing that figure by the population at risk. Both incidence and prevalence are usually given as rates per 1000, 10,000, or 100,000 population, depending on their frequency. Box 2-2 presents frequently used mortality and morbidity rates.

BOX 2-2   FREQUENTLY USED MORTALITY AND MORBIDITY RATES

$$\text{Crude birth rate} = \frac{\text{Number of births in a population within a time period} \times 1000}{\text{Total population}}$$

$$\text{Crude death rate} = \frac{\text{Number of deaths in a population within a time period} \times 1000}{\text{Total population}}$$

$$\text{Cause-specific death rate} = \frac{\text{Number of deaths in a population due to a certain disease within a time period} \times 1000}{\text{Total population}}$$

$$\text{Age-specific death rate} = \frac{\text{Number of deaths in a population in a certain age group within a time period} \times 1000}{\text{Total population in that age group}}$$

$$\text{Incidence of disease} = \frac{\text{Number of new events in a population within a time period} \times 1000}{\text{Total at-risk population}}$$

$$\text{Prevalence of disease} = \frac{\text{Number of existing events in a population within a time period} \times 1000}{\text{Total at-risk population}}$$

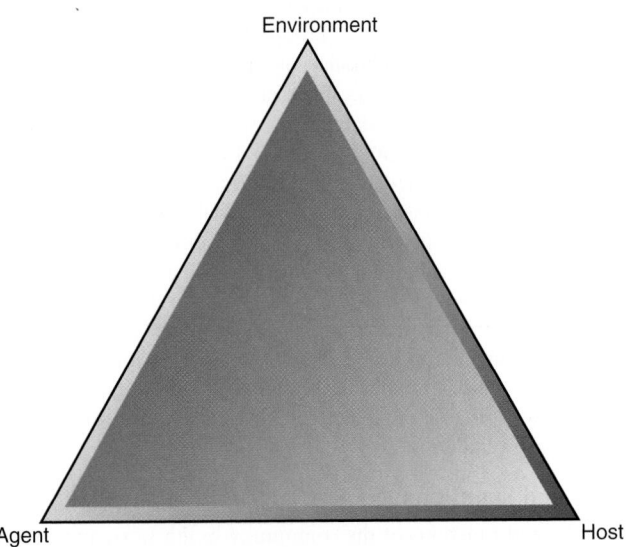

FIG 2-1 The epidemiologic triangle.

Epidemiologic Triangle

Three factors form the epidemiologic triangle, and their interrelationship alters the risk of acquiring a disease or condition (McKeown and Hilfinger, 2004). These factors are agent, host, and environment (Fig. 2-1).

An agent is responsible for causing a disease and may be an infectious agent such as *Mycobacterium tuberculosis,* a chemical agent such as lead in paint, or a physical agent such as fire. Host factors are those that are specific to an individual or group. These may be genetic factors that cannot be controlled, or they can be lifestyle factors (e.g., food selections or exercise patterns). **Environmental factors** provide a setting for the host and include the climatic conditions in which the host lives and factors related to the home, neighborhood, and school.

Levels of Prevention

Community health programs are based on three classic levels of prevention (Leavell and Clark, 1965). **Primary prevention** focuses on health promotion and prevention of disease or injury. Examples of primary prevention activities include well-child care clinics, immunization programs, safety programs (bike helmets, car seats, seat belts, childproof containers), nutrition programs, environmental efforts (clean air programs), sanitation measures (chlorinated water, garbage removal, sewage treatment), and community parenting classes. **Secondary prevention** focuses on screening and early diagnosis of disease. Examples of secondary interventions include tuberculosis and lead screening programs and mental health counseling for stressful events such as separation, divorce, death, or community natural disasters (e.g., earthquakes, floods, hurricanes). **Tertiary prevention** focuses on optimizing function for children with a disability or chronic disease. Tertiary interventions include rehabilitation and disease management programs for asthma, sickle cell disease, cancer, and anorexia and special education programs for children.

Screening

Community health nurses are frequently involved in **screening**, a secondary prevention activity. The purpose of screening is to detect and treat disease early in the period of pathogenesis to prevent the spread and progression of the disease (Wilson and Jungner, 1968). However, screening is not appropriate for every condition. Although screening may bring benefit, there is a certain amount of risk associated with any intervention. It is essential to determine the evidence for a proposed screening program before beginning the program so that the benefits of screening exceed the risks and cost. For example, acanthosis nigricans (AN) is a thickening and darkening of the skin that is commonly found on the neck and is associated with insulin resistance (Centers for Disease Control and Prevention, 2010). Some school health officials have recommended screening for AN as a way to identify early type 2 diabetes in children, but others have argued that screening may not be effective.

ECONOMICS

A basic understanding of the **economics** of health care is essential because it enables the nurse to participate in decision making about the worth of children's health programs. Economists theorize that individuals and societies view health as a basic utility, that is, something that is perceived as valuable (Gold, Patrick, Torrance, and others, 1996). Other basic utilities are food, shelter, and clothing. People are willing to trade resources, such as money and time, for a program or intervention that will improve their health. Economists measure the amount of resources individuals and communities are willing to pay for good health. They also examine how different groups prioritize health care needs and allocate health care dollars. Methods for defining and estimating cost have been well described, as has the need for a standardized approach to the measurement of cost and effects (Brosnan and Swint, 2001; Drummond, Sculpher, Torrance, and others, 2005).

Economic evaluation provides objective information to establish the value of a program to the community. An example is an evaluation of options designed to improve screening for colorectal cancer (Lairson, DiCarlo, Meyers, and others, 2008). There were four options: (1) usual

care; (2) mailed reminders and patient information; (3) mailed reminders and information applicable to the patients receiving them; and (4) mailed reminders, applicable information, and telephone calls. The authors concluded that mailed reminders and patient information (option 2) increased the number of patients screened at a reasonable cost.

BOX 2-3 THE COMMUNITY NURSING PROCESS

Assessment and diagnosis—The nurse collects subjective and objective information about a community and develops a diagnosis based on community needs and problems.

Planning—The nurse develops community-centered goals to address the identified needs and problems.

Implementation—The nurse implements a program that enables community members to reach their goals.

Evaluation—The nurse conducts a systematic evaluation to determine whether goals and program objectives were met.

COMMUNITY NURSING PROCESS

In community nursing, the focus of the nursing process shifts from the individual child and family to the community or target population (Box 2-3). The stages of the process (assessment, diagnosis, planning, implementation, and evaluation) are similar whether the client is one child or a population of children; only the type of interventions and indicators of wellness and illness differ (Anderson, 2010). **Assessment** is focused on collecting subjective and objective information about the target population to **diagnose** problems based on community needs. **Planning** involves the development of community-centered goals. During the **implementation** stage, the nurse works with the community to implement a program that enables members to reach their goals. Finally, the nurse **evaluates** whether the goals were met. Community nursing is collaborative, and the nurse is one member of a community team that includes other health professionals, educators, politicians, religious leaders, members of public and voluntary organizations, and consumers. The nurse's role depends on the scope of the project, the target population, and the expertise of team members.

Students may be introduced to community collaboration through service learning. The community partnership model is an example of a model that enables nursing students to become part of a collaborative team and to contribute directly to a community's well-being. In this model, the missions of nursing education, research, and practice are linked through three processes: evidence-based practice, service learning, and scholarly teaching (Brosnan, Upchurch, Meininger, and others, 2005).

COMMUNITY NEEDS ASSESSMENT AND DIAGNOSIS

The assessment phase of the community nursing process is called a **community needs assessment**. Assessment involves the collection of subjective and objective information about a community. **Subjective information** indicates what community members say are their most important needs and can be determined in a number of ways. One way is to distribute questionnaires to a sample of people living in the community. Another way is to interview community members directly, phoning or meeting with individuals (e.g., community leaders) who represent the group or who have a special role in the group.

Objective information is data that the nurse collects either by direct observation or through written sources. A windshield tour is one method of direct observation. Nurses drive through a neighborhood and take notes about the environment, including the appearance of houses, the presence of sidewalks and gutters, the number of public areas, and so on. Objective information about the community's health status can also be obtained from such sources as the Chamber of Commerce, Census Bureau, libraries, state health departments, and the Internet sites of voluntary health organizations or government agencies. Information about service agencies can be found in resource directories, including the local telephone book, community resource directories compiled by such organizations as the United Way, and population-specific books provided by public and voluntary agencies.

One way to organize an assessment is to use a guide that lists community systems that need to be examined. This process is similar to using a physical assessment guide to examine the different body systems in an individual patient. Anderson and McFarlane (2010) described eight community systems that the nurse should examine: health and social services, communication, recreation, physical environment, education, safety and transportation, politics and government, and economics. During the assessment, the nurse studies how well each component in the community functions and interacts to meet the health needs of children, identifies the strengths of the community, and determines whether any barriers disrupt the components and prevent access to care for children and their families.

After the assessment is completed, the community nurse collaborates with team members to analyze the results of surveys and questionnaires, determine whether the needs described by community members can be met by existing community agencies, and identify individuals at highest risk. During the analysis, the demographic characteristics, morbidity rates, and mortality rates in the community are compared with a standard. Comparisons can be made on the basis of time or place. In time comparisons, the nurse contrasts the rates in the current year with the rates during an earlier period. In comparisons of place, the nurse contrasts the rates in the community with those of a standard population. Standard rates may come from another community or from city, state, or national rates. For example, the rate of tuberculosis in a group of preschool children in the community in 2010 could be compared with the rate of tuberculosis in preschool children in the state in 2010.

A **community health diagnosis** is the reflection of health status, risks, or needs as determined by a causative agent. The format of a community diagnosis is similar to that of an individual nursing diagnosis, with a problem (need) and etiology related to that problem (causative agent). An example of a community nursing diagnosis is "Overweight among school age children related to decreased physical activity as demonstrated by the school nurse's report that 60% of children in the school have a BMI in the 85th to 95th percentile" (Cassells, 2010).

> **NURSING TIP** All communities have strengths and limitations. The community health nurse draws on the strengths of a community to solve problems.

COMMUNITY PLANNING

The nurse collaborates with community members in developing a plan that addresses the needs and problems of the target population. To maximize the use of community resources, problems should first be prioritized on the basis of their severity, the felt needs of the community, and the ability of the community nurse to bring about change. After prioritizing the problems, the nurse works with community members to develop at least one goal for each problem the members will address. **Goals** are outcomes that give direction to interventions and provide a measure of the change the interventions produced. Community interventions frequently take the form of **health programs** for improving the health status of the target population. Community health programs are based on the three levels of prevention: primary, secondary, and tertiary. For example, a goal for preventing bicycle injuries is "Within 1 year, all students in the first grade will wear bicycle helmets." The nurse and community members then plan a program that includes a health education program about bicycle safety for students and their parents (primary prevention).

The planning group considers the resources that are already available in the community and resources that will be needed to implement a health program, including personnel, supplies and equipment, office space, phones, and computers. Decisions are made about the timeline of the program, the budget, and strategies that can be used to obtain funding. The nurse may also contact health professionals who have implemented successful programs in other communities; they can provide valuable, time-saving tips and suggestions. Program descriptions are found through professional contacts, online resources, and reviews of the literature. An example of a community assessment and planning project is presented in Box 2-4.

COMMUNITY IMPLEMENTATION

During program implementation, the nurse and community members carry out the intervention. Whether the program is simple or complex, oversight is needed to ensure that everyone involved is communicating with one another, following the guidelines of the plan, keeping within the timeline, and documenting daily activities and expenses. The documentation will prove invaluable during the evaluation phase of the process.

COMMUNITY EVALUATION

Evaluation identifies whether the goals and program objectives were met. There are various models of program evaluation. The structure, process, and outcomes (evaluation) method is commonly used by health care organizations. Donabedian (1980) described this approach as:

Structure—Where and by whom is the care delivered in a program?

Process—Was the care delivered using operational standards and within the financial guidelines of the program?

Outcomes—What was the impact on health status? Was there any improvement?

Structure focuses on the qualifications of personnel; the adequacy of buildings, offices, supplies, and equipment; and the characteristics of the target population. Process focuses on the interaction of patients and providers. Process indicators include the number of people who attended a health education program, the number of pamphlets distributed, and the efficiency of the program. Outcome focuses on whether program objectives and community goals were met. Program evaluation should be ongoing so that performance improvement initiatives are monitored and so that an improvement in the way health care is delivered will affect the health status of the target population.

BOX 2-4 AN EXAMPLE OF COMMUNITY ASSESSMENT AND PLANNING

Lakewood is an elementary school with 500 prekindergarten to sixth grade children. The school nurse was asked to conduct a needs assessment of the school community and to develop a care plan. The schoolchildren and their families were the target population.

Community Needs Assessment

The school nurse formed a team of community members that included parents of students who attend Lakewood Elementary School, faculty and staff, health care professionals, local religious leaders, and politicians. The group met at regular intervals. Their first task was to complete the community assessment. Team members mailed questionnaires to a random sample of families who had children attending Lakewood. They held focus groups with community members to obtain subjective information about the needs of the school community. Team members obtained objective data from the local health department, school records, and the U.S. Census Bureau. The nurse also conducted a windshield tour of the neighborhood surrounding the school. The following information was collected:

People—Lakewood is located in an ethnically diverse area composed of 20% Hispanics, 40% African Americans, 30% non-Hispanic whites, and 10% Asians. The ethnicity of students in the school is representative of the surrounding area. Lakewood is located in a large southwestern city.

Safety and transportation—School bus service was rated excellent by a majority of those surveyed. The last school bus accident occurred 10 years ago. There were no fatalities, but a few children had minor injuries. Many children bicycle to school. Over the past 5 years, there were 10 bicycle accidents involving children from Lakewood. One of these accidents resulted in a fatality. In the 5 years before that, three bicycle accidents occurred, and none involved a fatality. Teachers noted that many of the children do not wear bicycle helmets and that the bicycles appear old and in need of repair. Parents complained that neighborhood streets are narrow, and few have curbs and sidewalks. In fact, most streets are bordered by ditches.

Economics—Although 94% of families had at least one fully employed member, 45% of the families lived below the poverty level. The number below poverty level had not changed in 10 years.

Education—Sixty percent of the adult population had a high school diploma, and 10% of this group had completed at least 1 year of college. School attendance at Lakewood was higher than overall state attendance rates.

Communication—Ninety-five percent of homes had telephones compared with 85% 10 years ago. An estimated 10% of the target population did not speak English; Spanish was the primary language spoken in this group.

Recreation—Few places were available for small children to play. The focus groups recommended more parks and playgrounds.

Politics and government—The school system was strongly centralized and headed by a school superintendent. The city had a mayor and city council.

Social—Of families living below the poverty level, 60% received some type of welfare assistance, including food stamps. The school lunch program served 95% of the children attending the school.

Health—Childhood immunization rates for all recommended diseases among kindergarten children in the community was 96%. This rate compared favorably with a report indicating that only 75% of states have attained the goal of having at least 95% of kindergarten children immunized. Vision and hearing screening programs at Lakewood resulted in the referral of 5% of the students for vision problems and 2% of the students for hearing problems. In focus groups, students and teachers noted that school breakfasts and lunches were high in carbohydrates and fats. They also observed that decreased recess time resulted in decreased student activity during school hours.

Based on the above assessment, the following community diagnoses were made:
- Increase in injuries related to bicycle accidents
- Increases in high intake of calories through school lunches and in sedentary lifestyle

Planning

Team members agreed that the increase in weight among the children should be closely monitored over the next 5 years. They also agreed that increased frequency of bicycle accidents among students was the highest priority problem, and the team developed the following goals: (1) within 6 months, all children will wear helmets when bicycling; (2) within 1 year, all students' bikes will be well maintained; and (3) within 2 years, no child going to or returning from school will be involved in a bicycle accident.

Team members reviewed the literature for examples of communities that had experienced similar problems, contacted school and health department officials in other areas of the country, examined the results of successful programs, and planned a health program that addressed the unique needs of the target population. The program was titled "Lakewood Bikes Safely." Program activities were the following:

1. Each September, the school nurse will address the school's parent association about the importance of bicycle safety, including the need to wear a helmet and to maintain bicycle equipment. As part of the presentation, a community police officer will discuss safety guidelines.
2. The school nurse will work with parents who have a financial need to help them obtain bicycle helmets for their children and funding for bike maintenance.
3. Within 6 months, school administrators and community members will petition the city to provide identified bicycle trails.

Team members determined the resources needed to implement the program, including personnel, supplies, and equipment. They estimated the total cost of setting up the program and maintaining it for 5 years and applied for funding to the school district and to the city and state health departments. The school nurse and other team members assumed responsibility for the timely implementation and evaluation of the Lakewood Bikes Safely program.

KEY POINTS

- Caring for children within a community requires a multidisciplinary approach.
- Healthy communities provide children with high-quality medical care and a nurturing, safe place in which to live and grow.
- Community health nursing focuses on promoting and maintaining the health of individuals, families, and groups in the community setting.
- Individual families and communities may have demographic characteristics that affect their risk for disease or injury.
- Epidemiology is the science of population health applied to the detection of morbidity and mortality in a population.
- Community health programs are based on three levels of intervention: primary, secondary, and tertiary.

- Economic evaluations provide objective information to establish the value of a program to society.
- A community needs assessment involves collection of subjective and objective information about the community.
- A community health diagnosis is a problem with a defined cause related to a community problem.

- Program planning and implementation in the community require collaboration between the nurse and community members who are in positions to promote change.
- Evaluation of effective community programs includes consideration of the structure, process, and outcomes related to the program.

REFERENCES

American Nurses Association: *Standards of community health nursing practice*, Kansas City, Mo, 1986, Author.

American Nurses Association: *Public health nursing scope and standards*, Washington, DC, 2007, Author.

Anderson ET: A model to guide practice. In Anderson ET, McFarlane J, editors: *Community as partner: theory and practice in nursing*, Philadelphia, 2010, Lippincott Williams & Wilkins.

Anderson ET, McFarlane J: Community assessment. In Anderson ET, McFarlane J, editors: *Community as partner: theory and practice in nursing*, Philadelphia, 2010, Lippincott Williams & Wilkins.

Brosnan CA, Swint JM: Cost analysis: concepts and application, *Public Health Nurs* 18(1):13–18, 2001.

Brosnan CA, Upchurch SL, Meininger JC, and others: Student nurses participate in public health research and practice through a school-based screening program, *Public Health Nurs* 22(3):260–266, 2005.

Cashaw SA: Epidemiology, demography and community health. In Anderson ET, McFarlane J, editors: *Community as partner: theory and practice in nursing*, Philadelphia, 2010, Lippincott Williams & Wilkins.

Cassells HB: Community assessment. In Nies MA, McEwen M, editors: *Community/public health: promoting the health of populations*, Philadelphia, 2010, Saunders.

Centers for Disease Control and Prevention: *CDC statement on screening children for acanthosis nigricans in schools and communities*, 2010, retrieved February 10, 2011, from http://www.cdc.gov/diabetes/news/docs/an.htm.

Council on Linkages Between Academia and Public Health Practice: *Core competencies for public health professionals*, 2001, retrieved January 4, 2008, from http://www.phf.org/competencies.htm.

Donabedian A: *The definition of quality and approaches to its assessment*, Ann Arbor, Mich, 1980, Health Administration Press.

Drummond MF, Sculpher MJ, Torrance GW, and others: *Methods for the economic evaluation of health care programmes*, ed 3, New York, 2005, Oxford University Press.

Gold MR, Patrick DL, Torrance GW, and others: Identifying and valuing outcomes. In Gold MR, Siegel JE, Russell LB, and others, editors: *Cost-effectiveness in health and medicine*, New York, 1996, Oxford University Press.

Health Resources and Services Administration: *The registered nurse population*, Rockville, Md, 2004, U.S. Department of Health and Human Services.

Hennekens CH, Buring JE: *Epidemiology in medicine*, Boston, 1987, Little, Brown.

Institute of Medicine: *The future of public health*, Washington, DC, 1988, National Academies Press.

Lairson DR, DiCarlo M, Meyers RE, and others: Cost-effectiveness of targeted and tailored interventions on colorectal cancer screening use, *Cancer* 112(4):779–788, 2008.

Leavell HR, Clark EG: *Preventive medicine for the doctor in his community: an epidemiologic approach*, New York, 1965, McGraw-Hill.

McEwen M, Nies MA: Health: a community view. In Nies MA, McEwen M, editors: *Community/public health: promoting the health of populations*, Philadelphia, 2011, Saunders.

McKeown RE, Hilfinger DK: Epidemiology. In Stanhope M, Lancaster J, editors: *Community and public health nursing*, St. Louis, 2004, Mosby.

National Center for Health Statistics: *Health, United States, 2010: with special feature on death and dying*, DHS Pub No 2011-1232, Hyattsville, Md, 2011, U.S. Department of Health and Human Services, retrieved February 2, 2011, from http://www.cdc.gov/nchs/data/hus/hus10.pdf.

Rector C: The journey begins: introduction to community health nursing. In Allender JA, Rector C, Warner K, editors: *Community health nursing: promoting and protecting the public's health*, Philadelphia, 2010, Lippincott Williams & Wilkins.

Riner ME: Health promotion through healthy communities. In Stanhope M, editor: *Public health nursing: population-centered care in the community*, St. Louis, 2008, Mosby.

Smith GD: Learning to live with complexity: ethnicity, socioeconomic position, and health in Britain and the United States, *Am J Public Health* 90:1694–1698, 2000.

Warner K: Setting the stage for community health nursing. In Allender JA, Rector C, Warner K, editors: *Community health nursing: promoting and protecting the public's health*, Philadelphia, 2010, Lippincott Williams & Wilkins.

Williams CA: Community-oriented nursing and community-based nursing. In Stanhope M, editor: *Foundations of nursing in the community: community oriented practice*, St. Louis, 2010, Mosby.

Wilson JMG, Jungner G: Principles and practice of screening for disease, *Public Health Papers*, no. 34, Geneva, 1968, World Health Organization.

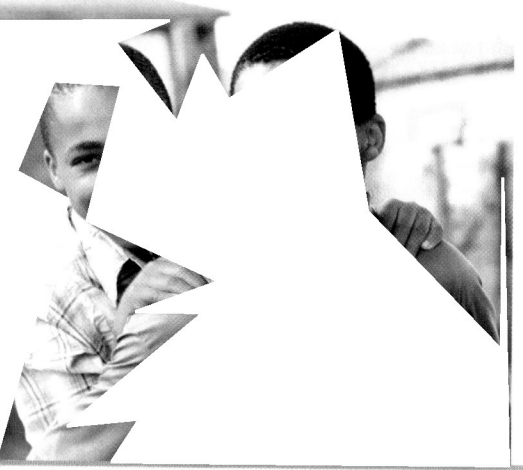

Family Influences on Child Health Promotion

Marilyn J. Hockenberry

evolve WEBSITE

http://evolve.elsevier.com/wong/essentials
Case Study—Family Functioning
Key Point Summaries
NCLEX-Style Review Questions

CHAPTER OUTLINE

General Concepts, 24
  Definition of Family, 24
  Family Theories, 24
    Family Systems Theory, 24
    Family Stress Theory, 24
    Developmental Theory, 25
  Family Nursing Interventions, 25
Family Structure and Function, 26
  Family Structure, 26
    Traditional Nuclear Family, 26
    Nuclear Family, 26
    Blended Family, 27
    Extended Family, 27
    Single-Parent Family, 27
    Binuclear Family, 27
    Polygamous Family, 27
    Communal Family, 27
    *Gay, Lesbian, Bisexual, and
      Transgender Families, 27*
  Family Strengths and Functioning
    Style, 28

Family Roles and Relationships, 28
  Parental Roles, 28
  Role Learning, 28
    Family Size and Configuration, 28
    Sibling Interactions, 29
    Ordinal Position, 29
    Multiple Births, 30
Parenting, 31
  Motivation for Parenthood, 31
  Preparation for Parenthood, 31
  Transition to Parenthood, 31
    *Parental Factors Affecting Transition to
      Parenthood, 31*
  Parenting Behaviors, 33
    Parental Styles of Control, 33
  Limit Setting and Discipline, 33
    Minimizing Misbehavior, 33
    *General Guidelines for Implementing
      Discipline, 33*
    Types of Discipline, 34

Special Parenting Situations, 35
  Parenting the Adopted Child, 35
    Issues of Origin, 36
    Adolescence, 36
    *Cross-Racial and International
      Adoption, 36*
  Parenting and Divorce, 37
    Impact of Divorce on Children, 37
    *Custody and Parenting
      Partnerships, 39*
  Single Parenting, 39
    Single Fathers, 39
  Parenting in Reconstituted
    Families, 39
  Parenting in Dual-Earner
    Families, 39
    Working Mothers, 40
  Foster Parenting, 41
  Accommodating Contemporary
    Parenting Situations, 41

LEARNING OBJECTIVES

On completion of this chapter the reader will be able to:
- Discuss definitions of family.
- Describe three major family theories.
- Identify different family structures found in the United States.
- Discuss the effect of family size and configuration on personality development.

- Discuss the role transition experienced by new parents.
- Explain various parenting behaviors such as parenting styles, disciplinary patterns, and communication skills.
- Demonstrate an understanding of special parenting situations such as adoption, divorce, single parenting, parenting in reconstituted families, and dual-earner families.

GENERAL CONCEPTS

DEFINITION OF FAMILY

The term family has been defined in many different ways according to the individual's own frame of reference, values, or discipline. There is no universal definition of family; a family is what an individual considers it to be. Biology describes the family as fulfilling the biologic function of perpetuation of the species. Psychology emphasizes the interpersonal aspects of the family and its responsibility for personality development. Economics views the family as a productive unit providing for material needs. Sociology depicts the family as a social unit interacting with the larger society, creating the context within which cultural values and identity are formed. Others define family in terms of the relationships of the persons who make up the family unit. The most common type of relationships are consanguineous (blood relationships), affinal (marital relationships), and family of origin (family unit a person is born into).

Earlier definitions of family emphasized that family members were related by legal ties or genetic relationships and lived in the same household with specific roles. Later definitions have been broadened to reflect both structural and functional changes. A family can be defined as an institution in which individuals, related through biology or enduring commitments, and representing similar or different generations and genders, participate in roles involving mutual socialization, nurturance, and emotional commitment (Coehlo, Kaakinen, Hanson, and others, 2009).

Considerable controversy has surrounded the newer concepts of family, such as communal families, single-parent families, and homosexual families. To accommodate these and other varieties of family styles, the descriptive term household is frequently used.

> **! NURSING ALERT**
>
> The nurse's knowledge and the sensitivity with which he or she assesses a household will determine the types of interventions that are appropriate to support family members.

Nursing care of infants and children is intimately involved with care of the child *and* the family. Family structure and dynamics can have an enduring influence on a child, affecting the child's health and well-being (American Academy of Pediatrics, 2003). Consequently, nurses must be aware of the functions of the family, various types of family structures, and theories that provide a foundation for understanding the changes within a family and for directing family-oriented interventions.

FAMILY THEORIES

A family theory can be used to describe families and how the family unit responds to events both within and outside the family. Each family theory makes assumptions about the family and has inherent strengths and limitations (Coehlo, Kaakinen, Hanson, and others, 2009). Most nurses use a combination of theories in their work with children and families. Commonly used theories are family systems theory, family stress theory, and developmental theory (Table 3-1).

Family Systems Theory

Family systems theory is derived from general systems theory, a science of "wholeness" that is characterized by interaction among the components of the system and between the system and the environment (Bomar, 2004). General systems theory expanded scientific thought from a simplistic view of direct cause and effect (A causes B) to a more complex and interrelated theory (A influences B, but B also affects A). In family systems theory, the family is viewed as a system that continually interacts with its members and the environment. The emphasis is on the interactions among the members; a change in one family member creates a change in other members, which in turn results in a new change in the original member. Consequently, a problem or dysfunction does not lie in any one member but rather in the type of interactions used by the family. Because the interactions, not the individual members, are viewed as the source of the problem, the family becomes the patient and the focus of care. Examples of the application of family systems theory to clinical problems are nonorganic failure to thrive and child abuse. According to family systems theory, the problem does not rest solely with the parent or child but with the type of interactions between the parent and the child and the factors that affect their relationship.

The family is viewed as a whole that is different from the sum of the individual members. For example, a household of parents and one child consists of not only three individuals but also four interactive units. These units include three dyads (the marital relationship, the mother–child relationship, and the father–child relationship) and a triangle (the mother–father–child relationship). In this ecologic model, the family system functions within a larger system, with the family dyads in the center of a circle surrounded by the extended family, the subculture, and the culture, with the larger society at the periphery.

Bowen's family systems theory (Coehlo, Kaakinen, Hanson, and others, 2009) emphasizes that the key to healthy family function is the members' ability to distinguish themselves from each other both emotionally and intellectually. The family unit has a high level of adaptability. When problems arise within the family, change occurs by altering the interaction or feedback messages that perpetuate disruptive behavior. Feedback refers to processes in the family that help identify strengths and needs and determine how well goals are accomplished. Positive feedback initiates change; negative feedback resists change (Goldenberg and Goldenberg, 2008). When the family system is disrupted, change can occur at any point in the system.

A major factor that influences a family's adaptability is its boundary, an imaginary line that exists between the family and its environment (Coehlo, Kaakinen, Hanson, and others, 2009).

Families have varying degrees of openness and closure in these boundaries. For example, whereas one family has the capacity to reach out for help, another considers help threatening. Knowledge of boundaries is critical when teaching or counseling families. Families with open boundaries may demonstrate a greater receptivity to interventions, but families demonstrating closed boundaries often require increased sensitivity and skill on the part of the nurse to gain their trust and acceptance. The nurse who uses family systems theory should assess the family's ability to accept new ideas, information, resources, and opportunities and to plan strategies.

Family Stress Theory

Family stress theory explains how families react to stressful events and suggests factors that promote adaptation to stress (Coehlo, Kaakinen, Hanson, and others, 2009). Families encounter stressors (events that cause stress and have the potential to effect a change in the family social system), including those that are predictable (e.g., parenthood) and those that are unpredictable (e.g., illness, unemployment). These stressors are cumulative, involving simultaneous demands from work, family, and community life. Too many stressful events occurring within a relatively short period (usually 1 year) can overwhelm the family's

TABLE 3-1 SUMMARY OF FAMILY THEORIES AND APPLICATIONS

ASSUMPTIONS	STRENGTHS	LIMITATIONS	APPLICATIONS
Family Systems Theory			
A change in any one part of a family system affects all other parts of the family system (circular causality). Family systems are characterized by periods of rapid growth and change and periods of relative stability. Both too little change and too much change are dysfunctional for the family system; therefore, a balance between morphogenesis (change) and morphostasis (no change) is necessary. Family systems can initiate change, as well as react to it.	Applicable for family in normal everyday life, as well as for family dysfunction and pathology Useful for families of varying structure and in various stages of the life cycle	More difficult to determine cause-and-effect relationships because of circular causality	Mate selection, courtship processes, family communication, boundary maintenance, power and control within family, parent–child relationships, teenage pregnancy and parenthood
Family Stress Theory			
Stress is an inevitable part of family life, and any event, even if positive, can be stressful for the family. Family encounters both normative expected stressors and unexpected situational stressors over its life cycle. Stress has a cumulative effect on family. Families cope with and respond to stressors with a wide range of responses and effectiveness.	Potential to explain and predict family behavior in response to stressors and to develop effective interventions to promote family adaptation Focuses on positive contribution of resources, coping, and social support to adaptive outcomes Can be used by many disciplines in the health field	Relationships among all variables in the framework not yet adequately described Not yet known if certain combinations of resources and coping strategies are applicable to all stressful events	Transition to parenthood and other normative transitions, single-parent families, families experiencing work-related stressors (dual-earner family, unemployment), acute or chronic childhood illness or disability, infertility, death of a child, divorce, teenage pregnancy and parenthood
Developmental Theory			
Families develop and change over time in similar and consistent ways. Family and its members must perform certain time-specific tasks set by themselves and by persons in the broader society. Family role performance at one stage of family life cycle influences family's behavioral options at next stage. Family tends to be in stage of disequilibrium when entering a new life-cycle stage and strives toward homeostasis within stages.	Provides a dynamic, rather than static, view of the family Addresses both changes within the family and changes in the family as a social system over its life history Anticipates potential stressors that normally accompany transitions to various stages and when problems may peak because of lack of resources	Traditional model more easily applied to two-parent families with children Use of age of oldest child and marital duration as marker of stage transition sometimes problematic (e.g., in stepfamilies, single-parent families)	Anticipatory guidance, educational strategies, and developing or strengthening family resources for management of transition to parenthood; family adjustment to children entering school, becoming adolescents, leaving home; management of "empty nest" years and retirement

ability to cope and place it at risk for breakdown or physical and emotional health problems among its members. When the family experiences too many stressors for it to cope adequately, a state of crisis ensues. For adaptation to occur, a change in family structure or interaction is necessary.

The resiliency model of family stress, adjustment, and adaptation emphasizes that the stressful situation is not necessarily pathologic or detrimental to the family but demonstrates that the family needs to make fundamental structural or systemic changes to adapt to the situation (McCubbin and McCubbin, 1994).

Developmental Theory

Developmental theory is an outgrowth of several theories of development. Duvall (1977) described eight developmental tasks of the family throughout its life span (Box 3-1). The family is described as a small group, a semiclosed system of personalities that interacts with the larger cultural social system. As an interrelated system, the family does not have changes in one part without a series of changes in other parts.

Developmental theory addresses family change over time using Duvall's family life cycle stages based on the predictable changes in the family's structure, function, and roles with the age of the oldest child

as the marker for stage transition. The arrival of the first child marks the transition from stage I to stage II. As the first child grows and develops, the family enters subsequent stages. In every stage, the family faces certain developmental tasks. At the same time, each family member must achieve individual developmental tasks as part of each family life cycle stage.

Developmental theory can be applied to nursing practice. For example, the nurse can assess how well new parents are accomplishing the individual and family developmental tasks associated with transition to parenthood. New applications should emerge as more is learned about developmental stages for nonnuclear and nontraditional families.

FAMILY NURSING INTERVENTIONS

In working with children, the nurse must include family members in their care plan. Research confirms parents' desire and expectation to participate in their child's care (Power and Franck, 2008). To discover family dynamics, strengths, and weaknesses, a thorough family assessment is necessary (see Chapter 6). The nurse's choice of interventions depends on the theoretic family model that is used (Box 3-2). For

BOX 3-1 DUVALL'S DEVELOPMENTAL STAGES OF THE FAMILY

Stage I—Marriage and an Independent Home: The Joining of Families
Reestablish couple identity.
Realign relationships with extended family.
Make decisions regarding parenthood.

Stage II—Families with Infants
Integrate infants into the family unit.
Accommodate to new parenting and grandparenting roles.
Maintain the marital bond.

Stage III—Families with Preschoolers
Socialize children.
Parents and children adjust to separation.

Stage IV—Families with Schoolchildren
Children develop peer relationships.
Parents adjust to their children's peer and school influences.

Stage V—Families with Teenagers
Adolescents develop increasing autonomy.
Parents refocus on midlife marital and career issues.
Parents begin a shift toward concern for the older generation.

Stage VI—Families as Launching Centers
Parents and young adults establish independent identities.
Parents renegotiate marital relationship.

Stage VII—Middle-Aged Families
Reinvest in couple identity with concurrent development of independent interests.
Realign relationships to include in-laws and grandchildren.
Deal with disabilities and the death of the older generation.

Stage VIII—Aging Families
Shift from a work role to leisure and semiretirement or full retirement.
Maintain couple and individual functioning while adapting to the aging process.
Prepare for own death and dealing with the loss of spouse, or siblings, and other peers.

Modified from Wright LM, Leahey M: *Nurses and families: a guide to family assessment and intervention*, Philadelphia, 1984, FA Davis.

BOX 3-2 FAMILY NURSING INTERVENTIONS

Behavior modification
Case management and coordination
Collaborative strategies
Contracting
Counseling, including support, cognitive reappraisal, and reframing
Empowering families through active participation
Environmental modification
Family advocacy
Family crisis intervention
Networking, including use of self-help groups and social support
Providing information and technical expertise
Role modeling
Role supplementation
Teaching strategies, including stress management, lifestyle modifications, and anticipatory guidance

From Friedman MM, Bowden VR, Jones EG: *Family nursing: research theory and practice,* ed 5, Upper Saddle River, NJ, 2003, Pearson Education.

FAMILY STRUCTURE AND FUNCTION

FAMILY STRUCTURE

The family structure, or family composition, consists of individuals, each with a socially recognized status and position, who interact with one another on a regular, recurring basis in socially sanctioned ways (Coehlo, Kaakinen, Hanson, and others, 2009). When members are gained or lost through events such as marriage, divorce, birth, death, abandonment, or incarceration, the family composition is altered, and roles must be redefined or redistributed.

Traditionally, the family structure was either a nuclear or extended family. In recent years, family composition has assumed new configurations, with the single-parent family and blended family becoming prominent forms. The predominant structural pattern in any society depends on the mobility of families as they pursue economic goals and as relationships change. It is common for children to belong to several different family groups during their lifetimes.

Nurses must be able to meet the needs of children from many diverse family structures and home situations. A family's particular structure affects the direction of nursing care. The U.S. Census Bureau uses four definitions for families: the traditional nuclear family, the nuclear family, the blended family or household, and the extended family or household.

Traditional Nuclear Family

A traditional nuclear family consists of a married couple and their biologic children. Children in this type of family live with both biologic parents and, if siblings are present, only full brothers and sisters (i.e., siblings who share the same two biologic parents). No other persons are present in the household (i.e., no steprelatives, foster or adopted children, half siblings, other relatives, or nonrelatives).

Nuclear Family

The nuclear family is composed of two parents and their children. The parent–child relationship may be biologic, step, adoptive, or foster. Sibling ties may be biologic, step, half, or adoptive. The parents are not necessarily married. No other relatives or nonrelatives are present in the household.

example, in family systems theory, the focus is on the interaction of family members within the larger environment (Goldenberg and Goldenberg, 2008). In this case, using group dynamics to involve all members in the intervention process and being a skillful communicator are essential. Systems theory also presents excellent opportunities for anticipatory guidance. Because each family member reacts to every stress experienced by that system, nurses can intervene to help the family prepare for and cope with changes. In family stress theory, the nurse uses crisis intervention strategies to help family members cope with the challenging event. In developmental theory, the nurse provides anticipatory guidance to prepare members for transition to the next family stage. Nurses who think family involvement plays a key role in the care of a child are more likely to include families in the child's daily care (Fisher, Lindhorst, Matthews, and others, 2008).

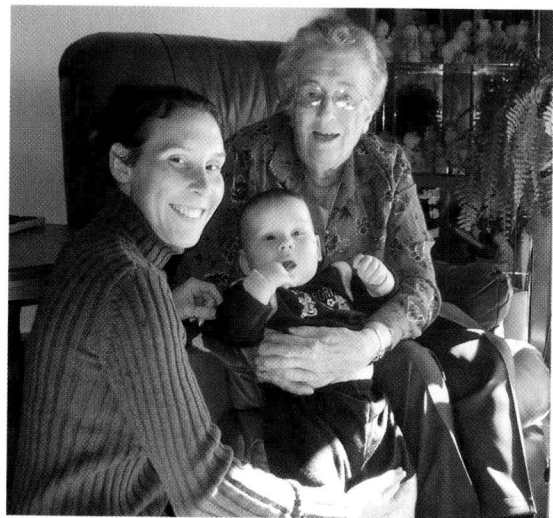

FIG 3-1 Children benefit from interaction with grandparents, who sometimes assume the parenting role.

Blended Family

A blended family or household, also called a reconstituted family, includes at least one stepparent, stepsibling, or half sibling. A stepparent is the spouse of a child's biologic parent but is not the child's biologic parent. Stepsiblings do not share a common biologic parent; the biologic parent of one child is the stepparent of the other. Half siblings share only one biologic parent.

Extended Family

An extended family or household includes at least one parent, one or more children, and one or more members (related or unrelated) other than a parent or sibling. Parent–child and sibling relationships may be biologic, step, adoptive, or foster.

In many nations and among many ethnic and cultural groups, households with extended families are common. Within the extended family, grandparents often find themselves rearing their grandchildren (Fig. 3-1). Young parents are often considered too young or too inexperienced to make decisions independently. Often, the older relative holds the authority and makes decisions in consultation with the young parents. Sharing residence with relatives also assists with the management of scarce resources and provides child care for working families. A resource for extended families is the Grandparent Information Center.*

Single-Parent Family

In the United States, an estimated 23.8 million children lived in single-parent families (Annie E. Casey Foundation, 2011). The contemporary single-parent family has emerged partially as a consequence of the women's rights movement and also as a result of more women (and men) establishing separate households because of divorce, death, desertion, or single parenthood. In addition, a more liberal attitude in the courts has made it possible for single people, both men and women, to adopt children. Although mothers usually head single-parent families, it is becoming more common for fathers to be awarded custody of dependent children in divorce settlements. With women's increased psychologic and financial independence and the increased

acceptability of single parents in society, more unmarried women are deliberately choosing mother–child families. Frequently, these mothers and children are absorbed into the extended family. The challenges of single-parent families are discussed on p. 39.

Binuclear Family

The term binuclear family refers to parents continuing the parenting role while terminating the spousal unit. The degree of cooperation between households and the time the child spends with each can vary. In joint custody, the court assigns divorcing parents equal rights and responsibilities concerning the minor child or children. These alternate family forms are efforts to view divorce as a process of reorganization and redefinition of a family rather than as a family dissolution. Joint custody and coparenting are discussed further on p. 39.

Polygamous Family

Although it is not legally sanctioned in the United States, the conjugal unit is sometimes extended by the addition of spouses in polygamous matings. Polygamy refers to either multiple wives (polygyny) or, rarely, multiple husbands (polyandry). Many societies practice polygyny that is further designated as sororal, in which the wives are sisters, or nonsororal, in which the wives are unrelated. Sororal polygyny is widespread throughout the world. Most often, mothers and their children share a husband and father, respectively, with each mother and her children living in the same or separate households.

Communal Family

The communal family emerged from disenchantment with most contemporary life choices. Although communal families may have divergent beliefs, practices, and organization, the basic impetus for formation is often dissatisfaction with the nuclear family structure, social systems, and goals of the larger community. Relatively uncommon today, communal groups share common ownership of property. In cooperatives, property ownership is private, but certain goods and services are shared and exchanged without monetary consideration. There is strong reliance on group members and material interdependence. Both provide collective security for nonproductive members, share homemaking and childrearing functions, and help overcome the problem of interpersonal isolation or loneliness.

Gay, Lesbian, Bisexual, and Transgender Families

A same-sex, homosexual, or gay/lesbian/bisexual/transgender (GLBT) family is one in which there is a legal or common-law tie between two persons of the same sex who have children (Blackwell, 2007). There are a growing number of families with same-sex parents in the United States, with an estimated one fourth of all same-sex couples raising children (Pawelski, Perrin, Foy, and others, 2006). Although some children in GLBT households are biologic from a former marriage or relationship, children may be present in other circumstances. They may be foster or adoptive parents, lesbian mothers may conceive through artificial fertilization, or a gay male couple may become parents through use of a surrogate mother.

When children are brought up in GLBT families, the relationships seem as natural to them as heterosexual parents do to their offspring. In other cases, however, disclosure of parental homosexuality ("coming out") to children can be a concern for families. A number of factors must be considered before disclosing this information to children. Parents should be comfortable with their own sexual orientation and should discuss it with their children as they become old enough to understand relationships. Discussions should be planned and take place in a quiet setting where interruptions are unlikely.

---

*For information, contact the local AARP representative or office; http://www.aarp.org/family/grandparenting.

BOX 3-3 **QUALITIES OF STRONG FAMILIES**

- A belief and sense of **commitment** toward promoting the well-being and growth of individual family members, as well as the family unit
- **Appreciation** for the small and large things that individual family members do well and **encouragement** to do better
- Concentrated effort to spend **time** and do things together, no matter how formal or informal the activity or event
- A sense of **purpose** that permeates the reasons and basis for "going on" in both bad and good times
- A sense of **congruence** among family members regarding the value and importance of assigning time and energy to meet needs
- The ability to **communicate** with one another in a way that emphasizes positive interactions
- A clear set of **family rules, values,** and **beliefs** that establishes expectations about acceptable and desired behavior
- A varied repertoire of **coping strategies** that promotes positive functioning in dealing with both normative and nonnormative life events
- The ability to engage in **problem-solving** activities designed to evaluate options for meeting needs and procuring resources
- The ability to be **positive** and see the positive in almost all aspects of their lives, including the ability to see crisis and problems as an opportunity to learn and grow
- **Flexibility** and **adaptability** in the roles necessary to procure resources to meet needs
- A **balance** between the use of internal and external family resources for coping and adapting to life events and planning for the future

From Dunst C, Trivette C, Deal A: Enabling and empowering families: principles and guidelines for practice, Cambridge, Mass, 1988, Brookline Books.

Nurses need to be nonjudgmental and to learn to accept differences rather than demonstrate prejudice that can have a detrimental effect on the nurse–child–family relationship (Blackwell, 2007). Moreover, the more nurses know about the child's family and lifestyle, the more they can help the parents and the child.

FAMILY STRENGTHS AND FUNCTIONING STYLE

Family function refers to the interactions of family members, especially the quality of those relationships and interactions (Bomar, 2004). Researchers are interested in family characteristics that help families function effectively. Knowledge of these factors guides the nurse throughout the nursing process and helps the nurse to predict ways that families may cope and respond to a stressful event, provide individualized support that builds on family strengths and unique functioning style, and assist family members in obtaining resources.

Family strengths and unique functioning styles (Box 3-3) are significant resources that nurses can use to meet family needs. Building on qualities that make a family work well and strengthening family resources make the family unit even stronger. All families have strengths as well as vulnerabilities.

FAMILY ROLES AND RELATIONSHIPS

Each individual has a position, or status, in the family structure and plays culturally and socially defined roles in interactions within the family. Each family also has its own traditions and values and sets its own standards for interaction within and outside the group. Each

determines the experiences the children should have, those they are to be shielded from, and how each of these experiences meets the needs of family members. When family ties are strong, social control is highly effective, and most members conform to their roles willingly and with commitment. Conflicts arise when people do not fulfill their roles in ways that meet other family members' expectations, either because they are unaware of the expectations or because they choose not to meet them.

PARENTAL ROLES

In all family groups, the socially recognized status of father and mother exists with socially sanctioned roles that prescribe appropriate sexual behavior and childrearing responsibilities. The guides for behavior in these roles serve to control sexual conflict in society and provide for prolonged care of children. The degree to which parents are committed and the way they play their roles are influenced by a number of variables and by the parents' unique socialization experience.

Parental role definitions have changed as a result of the changing economy and increased opportunities for women (Bomar, 2004). As women's role has changed, the complementary role of men has also changed. Many fathers are more active in childrearing and household tasks. As the redefinition of sex roles continues in American families, role conflicts may arise in many families because of a cultural lag of the persisting traditional role definitions.

ROLE LEARNING

Family Size and Configuration

Parenting practices differ between small and large families. Small families place more emphasis on the individual development of the children. Parenting is intensive rather than extensive, and there is constant pressure to measure up to family expectations. Children's development and achievement are measured against those of other children in the neighborhood and social class. In small families, children have more democratic participation than in larger families. Adolescents in small families identify more strongly with their parents and rely more on them for advice. They have well-developed, autonomous inner controls as contrasted with adolescents from larger families, who rely more on adult authority.

Children in a large family are able to adjust to a variety of changes and crises. There is more emphasis on the group and less on the individual (Fig. 3-2). Cooperation is essential, often because of economic necessity. The large number of people sharing a limited amount of space requires a greater degree of organization, administration, and authoritarian control. A dominant family member (a parent or older child) wields control. The number of children reduces the intimate, one-to-one contact between the parent and any individual child. Consequently, children turn to each other for what they cannot get from their parents. The reduced parent–child contact encourages individual children to adopt specialized roles to gain recognition in the family.

Older siblings in large families often administer discipline. Siblings are usually attuned to what constitutes misbehavior. Sibling disapproval or ostracism is frequently a more meaningful disciplinary measure than parental interventions. In situations such as the death or illness of a parent, an older sibling often assumes responsibility for the family at considerable personal sacrifice. Large families generate a sense of security in the children that is fostered by sibling support and cooperation. However, adolescents from large families are more peer oriented than family oriented.

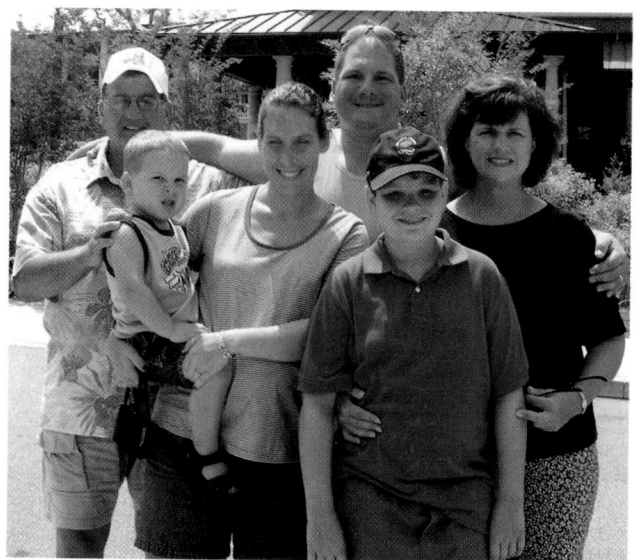

FIG 3-2 Family structure and function promotes strong relationships among its members.

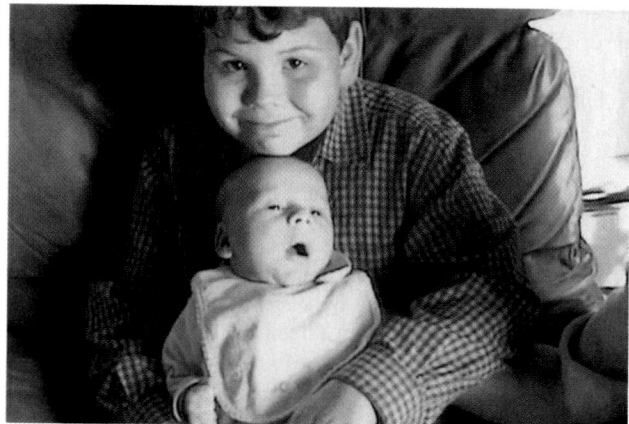

FIG 3-3 Older school-age children often enjoy taking responsibility for the care of a younger sibling.

Sibling Interactions
Spacing of Children

Age differences between siblings affect the childhood environment but to a lesser extent than does the gender of the sibling. The arrival of a sibling is difficult for toddlers and preschool children, especially between the ages of 2 and 3 years. At this age, they are still very attached to their parents and do not understand the concept of sharing. An older child is able to understand the situation and is less likely to see the newcomer as a threat, although the child does feel the loss of the only-child status (Coehlo, Kaakinen, Hanson, and others, 2009). In general, the narrower the spacing between siblings, the more the children influence one another, especially in emotional characteristics. The wider the spacing, the greater the influence of the parents.

Traditionally, sibling relationships were viewed from a Freudian perspective that emphasized the concept of sibling rivalry. Researchers have viewed siblings through developmental or ecologic frameworks that focus on interactions within family systems (Friedman, Bowden, and Jones, 2003). The results of these broader perspectives provide a picture of rich and varied sibling interactions (Fig. 3-3).

Sibling Functions

The sibling relationship's most unique feature is its duration. The longest relationship one will share with another human being is the sibling relationship, which lasts through a lifetime (often 50 to 80 years), compared with the child–parent relationship of approximately 30 to 50 years. Siblings spend long periods together and get to know each other at their best and worst.

Siblings exert power, exchange services, and express feelings in reciprocal ways that are often not revealed in the presence of the parents. They see themselves in their brothers and sisters, experience life vicariously through their siblings' behavior, and begin to expand on their own possibilities. Siblings can also be touchstones for what the other would *not* like to be, and they use each other as yardsticks for comparison. They provide a sounding board for each other and offer a safe forum for experimenting with new behaviors and roles. Brothers and sisters provide each other with tangible services (e.g., lending money, clothing, toys, or sports equipment; teaching a skill), help each other with childhood problems, provide support in dealing with parents or others outside the family, and provide introductions to new friendship groups. Children learn to negotiate and bargain, and sometimes to manipulate, from their siblings. Their interactions with each other provide opportunities for conflict and conflict resolution. They protect one another from parental-executive abuse of power and can form a coalition to deal with the issues of authority, power, and emotional support. Negotiating with parents is stronger when siblings act together rather than singly.

Tattling can be an important lever in sibling interactions. On the other hand, siblings often have a conspiracy of silence, leaving the parents feeling isolated and excluded. A willingness to maintain each other's privacy often forges a powerful bond of loyalty that distinguishes the relationship between siblings from that between friends.

More Active Sibling Relationships

Sibling relationships vary among cultures. Some factors may be giving the sibling relationship greater significance in American families than in the past. Shrinking family size, longer life spans, divorce and remarriage, geographic mobility, maternal employment, alternative sources of child care, competitive pressures, stress, and parental insufficiency may be propelling siblings into greater contact and emotional interdependence than ever before. Siblings often join forces to confront the trauma of divorce, and they frequently rely on each other for support when their parents remarry. The large number of working mothers means that young siblings today have significant amounts of time when a personally committed adult does not monitor their relationship. Often an older sibling is required to babysit, resulting in children spending more and more time together unsupervised. In a worried, mobile, small-family, high-stress, fast-paced, parent-absent society, children often turn to their brothers and sisters to meet their needs for contact, constancy, and permanency.

Ordinal Position

Researchers have observed that the birth position of children affects their personalities. Parents treat children differently, and sibling interactions are different, depending on the child's position within the family. Power is unequally distributed among siblings. Older siblings attempt to dominate younger ones. Therefore, younger siblings develop interpersonal skills, the ability to negotiate, and an ability to accept unfavorable outcomes to a greater extent than older siblings. Later-born children are obliged to interact with other siblings from birth and seem to be more outgoing and make friends more easily than first-borns. Children vary tremendously, and generalizations do not always

BOX 3-4   INFLUENCE OF ORDINAL POSITION ON CHILDREN

Firstborn Children

Are more achievement oriented

Are more dominant

Receive more physical punishment

Are allowed to show more aggression to siblings

Have stronger consciences; are more self-disciplined and inner directed

Are more socially anxious

Are prone to feelings of guilt

Identify more with parents than with peers

Are more conservative

Are subject to greater parental expectations

Begin to speak earlier in life

Demonstrate higher intellectual achievement

Plan better and experience fewer frustrations

Are likely to be most wanted

Middle Children

Have more demands made on them for household help

Are praised less often

Receive less of the parents' time

Learn to compromise and be adaptable

Are less stimulated toward achievement

Are more difficult to characterize because of a variety of positions in the family

Youngest Children

Are less dependent than firstborn children

Are less tense, more affectionate, and more good natured

Tend to identify more with peer group than with parents

Are more flexible in their thinking

Are popular with classmates

Have fewer demands placed on them for household help

Only Children

Have many of the same characteristics as firstborn children

Are more mature and cultivated

Experience greater parental pressure for mature behavior and achievement

Demonstrate superiority in language facility

Rarely develop into the stereotype of spoiled, selfish child

Often enjoy a rich fantasy life as a result of isolation

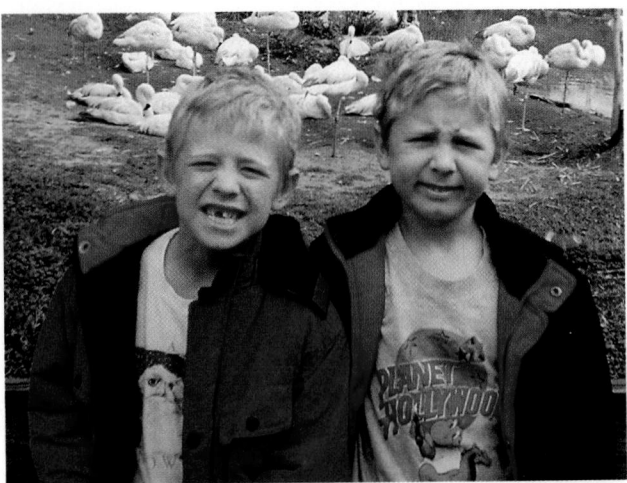

FIG 3-4 Fraternal twins.

apply to the individual. General characteristics of children in the various ordinal positions are presented in Box 3-4.

The Only Child

Being the only child in a family has traditionally been considered a disadvantage. Only children have been described as selfish, spoiled, dependent, and lonely. However, they do not demonstrate more evidence of maladjustment or self-centeredness than other children and tend to strongly resemble firstborn children in respects such as higher educational goals. Only children perform better on cognitive tests, are more mature, are more socially sensitive, and demonstrate superiority in language facility compared with other children.

Only children also enjoy the advantage of having parents who can devote more time to them, talk to them, and stimulate them in intellectual activities. However, parents also exert greater pressure for mature behavior at an early age and for achievement. Relative isolation from peers contributes to intellectual pursuits and encourages a rich fantasy life, independence, and originality.

Multiple Births

A deviation in early development that occurs with variable frequency is multiple births. Twins are common in the population, but triplets are rare, and quadruplets and quintuplets are extremely unusual. In any of these situations, the offspring can be of the like or unlike sex (i.e., derived from a single ovum; from multiple ova; or from a combination of the two, which can involve one or more cell divisions). The cause of twinning is unknown, but the increase in the number of larger multiples (quintuplets, sextuplets) in recent years has been associated with fertility treatments such as ovulation-inducing drugs and in vitro fertilization. Because women in their thirties are almost 2.5 times as likely as women in their twenties to have higher order plural births, increased childbearing among older women and the expanded use of fertility drugs have been associated with an increase in the multiple-birth ratio (Mathews, Minino, Osterman, and others, 2011).

Twins are of two distinct types: **identical**, or **monozygotic** (MZ), and **fraternal** (Fig. 3-4), or **dizygotic** (DZ) (Table 3-2). In 2007 in the United States, the overall rate of twin birth was 32.2 per 1000 births, a record high (Mathews, Minino, Osterman, and others, 2011); one third are MZ twins, and two thirds are DZ twins.

A special kind of sibling relationship is observed in twins, although getting along with each other and quarreling are not much different from these behaviors in any other two siblings, especially if they are different-sex fraternal twins. Twins tend to work out a relationship that is reasonably satisfactory to both and demonstrate early independence from parental attention. They develop a remarkable capacity for cooperative play and considerable loyalty and generosity toward each other. It is common for them to evolve a private language between themselves that may interfere with the development of the family language.

In a twinship, one member of the pair, to a greater or lesser extent, is more dominant, outgoing, and assertive than the other, often to the consternation of their parents. However, the seemingly more passive twin is able to accomplish as much and get his or her way as frequently as the more assertive twin.

Researchers have also observed a difference in behavior between identical and fraternal twins. There is near-unison in the actions of identical twins (although they alternate in assuming leadership), but fraternal twins, even of the same sex, do not display this quality. Sibling rivalry can be pronounced in fraternal twins, especially in different-sex twins.

TABLE 3-2	**CHARACTERISTICS OF TWINS**
MONOZYGOTIC OR IDENTICAL TWINS	**DIZYGOTIC OR FRATERNAL TWINS**
Characteristics	
Result of one fertilized ovum that became separated early in development	Result of fertilization of two ova
Alike physically and genetically	Differ physically and genetically
Same sex	May be same or opposite sex
Frequency	
Occurs uniformly in all populations	Varies among races (highest in African Americans, lowest in Asians, intermediate in whites)
Unaffected by maternal age	More common with advancing maternal age (maximum at ages 35 to 39 years; then decreases rapidly)
Tendency unaffected by heredity	Marked familial tendency
	Expressed only in the female
	Fathers appear to transmit disposition toward double ovulation to daughters
Similar behavior	Dissimilar behavior; more sibling rivalry

Identical twins also differ in their response to the tendency of some parents to treat twins exactly alike. The present philosophy is to determine the degree to which the children demonstrate an inclination toward togetherness. Some twins thrive best when they are constantly in each other's company; others prefer more individuality and separateness. Early years of togetherness are often the basis of the children's security, and separating them too early may produce unnecessary stresses. Fostering individual differences as they become evident could ease the process of separation when it becomes advisable.

Parental Adjustment

The entrance of any new member into a household creates stress, but with multiple births, two or more new members must be incorporated into the family at the same time. The problems are obvious. Two infants must be provided with physical care, including feeding, diapering, and all of the purchasing and preparation that accompany the care of any infant. Scheduling becomes crucial, and advancement in development brings new problems and adjustments (e.g., space and sleeping arrangements, selection of a stroller and other equipment). Care must be observed in selecting toys. As play becomes a serious business, some toys that would be safe and appropriate for a single child become weapons when two infants share a playpen. It is a good idea to select different toys for each child as they grow older and encourage sharing.

It is especially important for parents to maintain relationships with each other and other family members. Parents need to arrange time together as often as possible. The National Organization of Mothers of Twins Clubs, Inc.,* has local chapters throughout the United States to offer information and support to parents of twins and is highly recommended as a resource. *Twins Magazine* (http://www.twinsmagazine.com) is a place to seek and give advice about parenting multiples.

*NOMOTC Executive Office, 2000 Mallory Lane, Suite 130-600, Franklin, TN 37067; http://www.nomotc.org.

PARENTING

MOTIVATION FOR PARENTHOOD

A dominant characteristic in all societies is that adults are expected to become parents and to be gratified by the experience. Pressures of tradition, sentiment regarding the state of parenthood, and religious beliefs influence decision making because conformity to social-role expectations is a strong influence in family planning.

Factors that influence family size are social class, religion, race, financial stability, type of conjugal-role relationships, and the social-psychologic aspects of sexual relations (Coehlo, Kaakinen, Hanson, and others, 2009).

In the case of divorce and remarriage, an individual may decide to have more children with the new spouse.

PREPARATION FOR PARENTHOOD

The basic goals of parenting are to promote the physical survival and health of children, foster the skills and abilities necessary to be self-sustaining adults, and foster behavioral capabilities for optimizing cultural values and beliefs (Deave, Johnson, and Ingram, 2008). However, new parents often approach parenthood with limited experience and knowledge. Parents learn by trial and error, committing the same mistakes that have been committed by countless other parents, but they somehow manage to accomplish the task, becoming more skilled with each additional child.

Tradition, rather than rational planning, furnishes the chief norms for childrearing. Experience in having been nurtured as a child is an essential component of successful parenting. Their own parents are probably the only persons whom parents observe intimately in the parental role. This results in a generational continuity—parents rear their own children in much the same way that they themselves were reared. Other essential skills that parents need to feel comfortable in the parenting role include a basic understanding of childhood growth and development, bathing, feeding, use of play, and interpersonal communication skills.

TRANSITION TO PARENTHOOD

Although experts disagree as to whether the birth of the first child should be labeled a crisis, the early weeks of an infant's life call for parents to make drastic adjustments. A child's birth presents the challenge of providing total care 24 hours a day for a new member of the family (Deave, Johnson, and Ingram, 2008). A crisis may occur if the event is perceived as disturbing old habits and relationships and eliciting new responses. The birth requires role changes and significantly modifies former relationships. In addition to the roles of husband and wife, the couple must assume the roles of father and mother.

The advent of a new family member requires that the family cope with greater financial responsibilities, a possible loss of income, changes in sleeping habits, and less time for the parents to spend with each other (especially if the child is a firstborn) and with other children. If these events are perceived as aversive, they can disrupt the couple's bond and reduce their intimacy and affection.

Parental Factors Affecting Transition to Parenthood

No amount of preparation can fully prepare prospective parents for an infant's constant and immediate needs. The importance of early parent–infant interactions is addressed in the discussion of neonates, especially the attachment process (see Chapter 8). Factors affecting

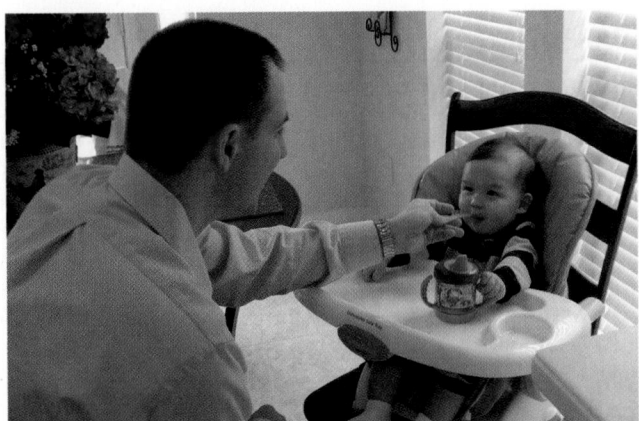

FIG 3-5 Fathers who assume care of their children may feel more comfortable and successful in their parenting role.

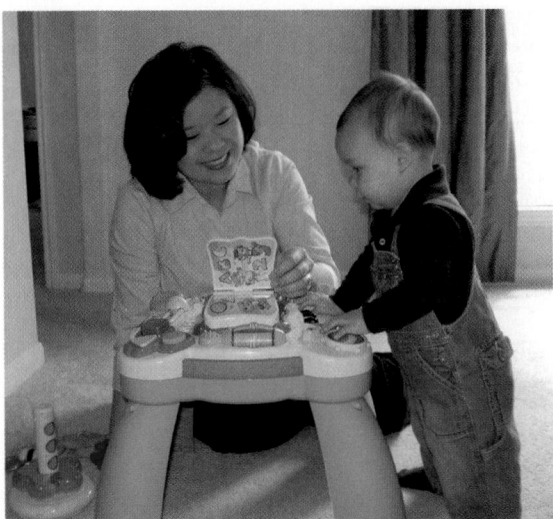

FIG 3-6 Quality time spent with a child is essential to a family's health and well-being.

parenting are the age of the parents, the quality of the parental relationship, the amount of previous experience with childrearing, parental support systems, and the effects of stress on parental behavior (Deave, Johnson, and Ingram, 2008).

Parental Age

From a physiologic health perspective, the most satisfactory ages for childbearing are between 18 and 35 years. During this time, parents are considered to be in optimum health, with a predicted life span that allows sufficient time and vigor to raise a family. However, the age at which parents begin their families has changed over the past few decades in the United States, with a substantial increase in the birth rate for women ages 30 to 44 years and a decline for women ages 20 to 29 years.

Father Involvement

Current practices that encourage early father–infant interaction indicate that fathers are as intrigued with their newborns as mothers are (see discussion on paternal engrossment under Promote Parent–Infant Bonding [Attachment], Chapter 8). Even fathers who have little initial contact with their newborns become involved with them over the next few months (Fig. 3-5), although the type of interaction is different from that of mothers. For example, whereas mothers are more likely to hold, soothe, care for, or play quietly with their infants, fathers are more boisterous and engage in more physically stimulating activities. However, fathers are more than just playmates. They are often successful at soothing distressed infants. A secure attachment to the father can help offset the consequences of an insecure attachment to the mother.

Parenting Education

First-time parents who have prepared themselves to be parents experience less stress adjusting to the birth of new baby than those who have not. Programs designed to take place near the time of birth or soon after can be more helpful in easing transitional stress than earlier programs (Deave, Johnson, and Ingram, 2008).

Many parents are looking for ways to be better parents. Nurses can offer a number of suggestions, including being an active listener, having an active role in education, keeping up with technology, keeping up with regular visits to the child's health care provider and vaccinations, ensuring safety in and out of the home, spending quality time with the child, and focusing on improving overall family communication (Fig. 3-6).

Other factors influencing the transition to the parental role include the following:
- Parents with previous experience, such as another child, appear to be more relaxed, have less conflict in disciplinary relationships, and are more aware of normal growth and development.
- The amount of stress experienced by one or both parents may interfere with their ability to be patient and understanding and to cope with their children's behavior.
- Special characteristics of the infant, such as being temperamentally difficult, can cause the parents to lose confidence and doubt their abilities. Infants with special care needs (e.g., those associated with a disability) can be a significant source of added stress.
- Stressed marital relationships can have a negative effect on parental transition because marital tension can alter caregiving routines and interfere with enjoyment of the infant. Conversely, parents' support and encouragement of one another serve as positive influences on establishing a satisfying parental role.

Support Systems

Successful adaptation to the stress of transition to parenthood involves at least two types of family resources (McCubbin and McCubbin, 1994). **Internal resources** such as adaptability and integration are the first type of resource. Changing from an orderly, predictable life to a relatively disordered, unpredictable one is a universal adaptation that families must make. Rigid schedules are impossible to maintain, and former activities must be curtailed or abandoned. **Adaptation** is reflected in learning to be patient, becoming better organized, and becoming more flexible. **Integration** refers to the couple's attempt to continue some activities they engaged in before they became parents. In this way, couples are able to maintain a sense of continuity and appreciate the importance of the husband–wife relationship (McCubbin and McCubbin, 1994).

The second resource is the use of **coping strategies** that strengthen the family's organization and functioning. These include the use of social support systems and community resources and the adoption of a future orientation. Interpersonal supports that provide information, advice, and caretaking can be derived from friends, relatives, and neighbors. Relationships with family, friends, and the community are essential. For parents, positive, supportive work relationships are important. Equally important is time spent with friends. Arranging

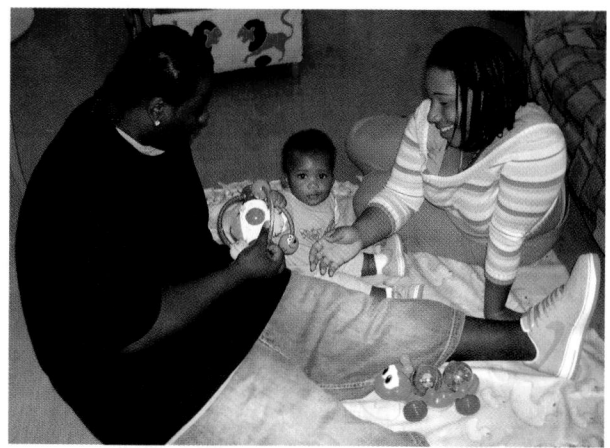

FIG 3-7 Learning new roles together as a mother and father can enhance parenting relationships.

for time away from the child or children is also beneficial. One parent can assume care of the family to allow the other parent some time to himself or herself. Adoption of a future orientation reassures parents that things will get better, that they will cope, and that it is realistic to plan for the time when they will be able to engage in self-fulfilling activities.

It is also reassuring to know that others experience ambivalent feelings toward parenthood and share the same difficulties and frustrations. Exchanging ideas and experiences with other parents and each other provides an opportunity to voice concerns and to learn new ways to cope with multiple childrearing problems (Fig. 3-7).

PARENTING BEHAVIORS

Parental Styles of Control

Parenting styles have been described in many different ways. Within a social interactional learning model, parenting can be positive or coercive (Liddle, Santisteban, Levant, and others, 2002). Whereas a positive approach to parenting encourages skill development, a coercive approach uses negative reinforcement and often causes a destructive effect on relationships.

Parenting styles are often classified as authoritarian, permissive, or authoritative (Hoeve, Dubas, Eichelsheim, and others, 2009; Hubbs-Tait, Kennedy, Page, and others, 2008). Authoritarian or dictatorial parents try to control their children's behavior and attitudes through unquestioned mandates. They establish rules and regulations or standards of conduct that they expect to be followed rigidly and unquestioningly. The message is: "Do it because I say so." Punishment need not be corporal but may be stern withdrawal of love and approval. Careful training often results in rigidly conforming behavior in the children, who tend to be sensitive, shy, self-conscious, retiring, and submissive. They are more likely to be courteous, loyal, honest, and dependable but docile. These behaviors are more typically observed when close supervision and affection accompany parental authority. If not, this style of parenting may be associated with both defiant and antisocial behavior.

Permissive parents exert little or no control over their children's actions. They avoid imposing their own standards of conduct and allow their children to regulate their own activity as much as possible. These parents consider themselves to be resources for the children, not role models. If rules do exist, the parents explain the underlying reason, elicit the children's opinions, and consult them in decision-making processes. They use lax, inconsistent discipline; do not set sensible limits; and do not prevent the children from upsetting the home routine. These parents rarely punish the children.

Authoritative or democratic parents combine practices from both of the previously described parenting styles. They direct their children's behavior and attitudes by emphasizing the reason for rules and negatively reinforcing deviations. They respect the individuality of each child and allow the child to voice objections to family standards or regulations. Parental control is firm and consistent but tempered with encouragement, understanding, and security. Control is focused on the issue, not on withdrawal of love or the fear of punishment. These parents foster "inner directedness," a conscience that regulates behavior based on feelings of guilt or shame for wrongdoing, not on fear of being caught or punished. Parents' realistic standards and reasonable expectations produce children with high self-esteem who are self-reliant, assertive, inquisitive, content, and highly interactive with other children.

There are differing philosophies in regard to parenting. Childrearing is a culturally bound phenomenon, and children are socialized to behave in ways that are important to their families. In the authoritative style, authority is shared, and children are included in discussions, fostering an independent and assertive style of participation in family life. When working with individual families, nurses should give these differing styles equal respect.

LIMIT SETTING AND DISCIPLINE

In its broadest sense, discipline means *to teach* or refers to a set of rules governing conduct. In a narrower sense, it refers to the action taken to enforce the rules after noncompliance. Limit setting refers to establishing the rules or guidelines for behavior. For example, parents can place limits on the amount of time children spend watching television or chatting online. The clearer the limits that are set and the more consistently they are enforced, the less need there is for disciplinary action.

Nurses can help parents establish realistic and concrete "rules." Limit setting and discipline are positive, necessary components of childrearing and serve several useful functions as they help children:
- Test their limits of control
- Achieve in areas appropriate for mastery at their level
- Channel undesirable feelings into constructive activity
- Protect themselves from danger
- Learn socially acceptable behavior

Children want and need limits. Unrestricted freedom is a threat to their security and safety. By testing the limits imposed on them, children learn the extent to which they can manipulate their environment and gain reassurance from knowing that others are there to protect them from potential harm.

Minimizing Misbehavior

The reasons for misbehavior may include attention, power, defiance, and a display of inadequacy (e.g., the child misses classes because of a fear that he or she is unable to do the work). Children may also misbehave because the rules are not clear or consistently applied. Acting-out behavior, such as temper tantrums, may represent uncontrolled frustration, anger, depression, or pain. The best approach is to structure interactions with children to prevent or minimize unacceptable behavior (see Family-Centered Care box).

General Guidelines for Implementing Discipline

Regardless of the type of discipline used, certain principles are essential to ensure the efficacy of the approach (see Family-Centered Care box). Many strategies, such as behavior modification, can only be

FAMILY-CENTERED CARE
Minimizing Misbehavior

- Set realistic goals for acceptable behavior and expected achievements.
- Structure opportunities for small successes to lessen feelings of inadequacy.
- Praise children for desirable behavior with attention and verbal approval.
- Structure the environment to prevent unnecessary difficulties (e.g., place fragile objects in an inaccessible area).
- Set clear and reasonable rules; expect the same behavior regardless of the circumstances; if exceptions are made, clarify that the change is for one time only.
- Teach desirable behavior through own example, such as using a quiet, calm voice rather than screaming.
- Review expected behavior before special or unusual events, such as visiting a relative or having dinner in a restaurant.
- Phrase requests for appropriate behavior positively, such as "Put the book down" rather than "Don't touch the book."
- Call attention to unacceptable behavior as soon as it begins; use distraction to change the behavior or offer alternatives to annoying actions, such as exchanging a quiet toy for one that is too noisy.
- Give advance notice or "friendly reminders," such as "When the TV program is over, it is time for dinner" or "I'll give you to the count of three, and then we have to go."
- Be attentive to situations that increase the likelihood of misbehaving, such as overexcitement or fatigue, or that decrease personal tolerance of minor infractions.
- Offer sympathetic explanations for not granting a request, such as "I am sorry I can't read you a story now, but I have to finish dinner. Then we can spend time together."
- Keep all promises made to children.
- Avoid outright conflicts; temper discussions with statements such as "Let's talk about it and see what we can decide together" or "I have to think about it first."
- Provide children with opportunities for power and control.

FAMILY-CENTERED CARE
Implementing Discipline

Consistency—Implement disciplinary action exactly as agreed on and for each infraction.

Timing—Initiate discipline as soon as the child misbehaves; if delays are necessary, such as to avoid embarrassment, verbally disapprove of the behavior and state that disciplinary action will be implemented.

Commitment—Follow through with the details of the discipline, such as timing of minutes; avoid distractions that may interfere with the plan, such as telephone calls.

Unity—Make certain that all caregivers agree on the plan and are familiar with the details to prevent confusion and alliances between the child and one parent.

Flexibility—Choose disciplinary strategies that are appropriate to the child's age and temperament and the severity of the misbehavior.

Planning—Plan disciplinary strategies in advance and prepare the child if feasible (e.g., explain the use of time-out); for unexpected misbehavior, try to discipline when you are calm.

Behavior orientation—Always disapprove of the behavior, not the child, with such statements as "That was a wrong thing to do. I am unhappy when I see behavior like that."

Privacy—Administer discipline in private, especially with older children, who may feel ashamed in front of others.

Termination—After the discipline is administered, consider the child as having a "clean slate" and avoid bringing up the incident or lecturing.

attention. When children use this technique, parents should end the explanation by stating, "This is the rule, and this is how I expect you to behave. I won't explain it any further."

Unfortunately, reasoning is often combined with **scolding**, which sometimes takes the form of shame or criticism. For example, the parent may state, "You are a bad boy for hitting your brother." Children take such remarks seriously and personally, believing that they *are* bad.

! NURSING ALERT

When reprimanding children, focus only on the misbehavior, not on the child. Use of "I" messages rather than "you" messages expresses personal feelings without accusation or ridicule. For example, an "I" message attacks the behavior—"I am upset when Johnny is punched; I don't like to see him hurt"—not the child who was misbehaving.

Positive and negative reinforcement is the basis of **behavior modification** theory—behavior that is rewarded will be repeated; behavior that is not rewarded will be extinguished. Using **rewards** is a positive approach. By encouraging children to behave in specified ways, the parents can decrease the tendency to misbehave. With young children, using paper stars is an effective method. For older children, the "token system" is appropriate, especially if a certain number of stars or tokens yields a special reward, such as a trip to the movies or a new book. In planning a reward system, the parents must explain expected behaviors to the child and establish rewards that are reinforcing. They should use a chart to record the stars or tokens and always give an earned reward promptly. Verbal approval should always accompany extrinsic rewards.

Consistently **ignoring** behavior will eventually extinguish or minimize the act. Although this approach sounds simple, it is difficult to implement consistently. Parents frequently "give in" and resort to previous patterns of discipline. Consequently, the behavior is actually reinforced because the child learns that persistence gains parental

implemented effectively when principles of consistency and timing are followed. A pattern of intermittent or occasional enforcement of limits actually prolongs the undesired behavior because children learn that if they are persistent, the behavior is permitted eventually. Delaying punishment weakens its intent, and practices such as telling the child "Wait until your father comes home," not only are ineffectual but also convey negative messages about the other parent.*

Types of Discipline

To deal with misbehavior, parents need to implement appropriate disciplinary action. Many approaches are available. **Reasoning** involves explaining why an act is wrong and is usually appropriate for older children, especially when moral issues are involved. However, young children cannot be expected to "see the other side" because of their egocentrism. Children in the preoperative stage of cognitive development (toddlers and preschoolers) have a limited ability to distinguish between their point of view and that of others. Sometimes children use "reasoning" as a way of gaining attention. For example, they may misbehave, thinking the parents will give them a lengthy explanation of the wrongdoing and knowing that negative attention is better than no

---

*For parenting of kindergarten through sixth-grade children, see http:// childparenting.about.com and http://www.kidshealth.org.

attention. For ignoring to be effective, parents should (1) understand the process, (2) record the undesired behavior before using ignoring to determine whether a problem exists and to compare results after ignoring is begun, (3) determine whether parental attention acts as a reinforcer, and (4) be aware of "response burst." Response burst is a phenomenon that occurs when the undesired behavior increases after ignoring is initiated because the child is "testing" the parents to see if they are serious about the plan.

The strategy of **consequences** involves allowing children to experience the results of their misbehavior. It includes three types:

1. Natural—Those that occur without any intervention, such as being late and having to clean up the dinner table
2. Logical—Those that are directly related to the rule, such as not being allowed to play with another toy until the used ones are put away
3. Unrelated—Those that are imposed deliberately, such as no playing until homework is completed or the use of time-out

Natural or logical consequences are preferred and effective if they are meaningful to children. For example, the natural consequence of living in a messy room may do little to encourage cleaning up, but allowing no friends over until the room is neat can be motivating! Withdrawing privileges is often an unrelated consequence. After the child experiences the consequence, the parent should refrain from any comment because the usual tendency is for the child to try to place blame for imposing the rule.

Time-out is a refinement of the common practice of sending the child to his or her room and is a type of unrelated consequence. It is based on the premise of removing the reinforcer (i.e., the satisfaction or attention the child is receiving from the activity). When placed in an unstimulating and isolated place, children become bored and consequently agree to behave in order to reenter the family group (Fig. 3-8). Time-out avoids many of the problems of other disciplinary approaches. No physical punishment is involved; no reasoning or scolding is given; and the parent does not need to be present for all of the time-out, thus facilitating consistent application of this type of discipline. Time-out offers both the child and the parent a "cooling off" time. To be effective, however, time-out must be planned in advance (see Family-Centered Care box).

Corporal or **physical punishment** most often takes the form of spanking (Larzelere, 2008). Based on the principles of aversive therapy,

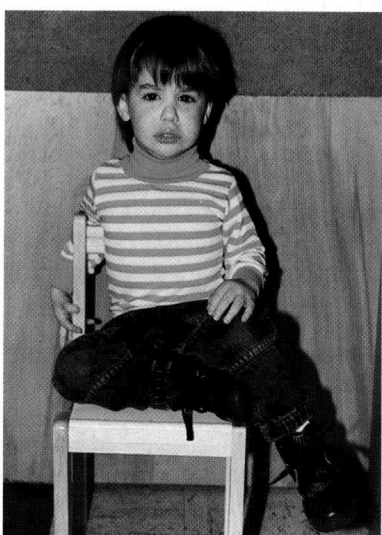

FIG 3-8 Time-out is an excellent disciplinary strategy for young children.

FAMILY-CENTERED CARE
Using Time-Out

Select an area for time-out that is safe, convenient, and unstimulating but where the child can be monitored, such as the bathroom, hallway, or laundry room.

Determine what behaviors warrant a time-out.

Make certain children understand the "rules" and how they are expected to behave.

Explain to children the process of time-out:
- When they misbehave, they will be given *one* warning.
- If they do not obey, they will be sent to the place designated for time-out.
- They are to sit there for a specified period.
- If they cry, refuse, or display any disruptive behavior, the time-out period will begin *after* they quiet down.
- When they are quiet for the duration of the time, they can then leave the room.

A rule for the length of time-out is *1 minute per year of age;* use a kitchen timer with an audible bell rather than a watch to record the time.

Implement time-out in a public place by selecting a suitable area or explain to children that time-out will be spent immediately on returning home.

inflicting pain through spanking causes a dramatic short-term decrease in the behavior. However, this approach has serious flaws: (1) it teaches children that violence is acceptable; (2) it may physically harm the child if it is the result of parental rage; and (3) children become "accustomed" to spanking, requiring more severe corporal punishment over time. Spanking can result in severe physical and psychologic injury, and it interferes with effective parent–child interaction (Cain, 2008). In addition, when the parents are not around, children are likely to misbehave because they have not learned to behave well for their own sake. Parental use of corporal punishment may also interfere with the child's development of moral reasoning.

SPECIAL PARENTING SITUATIONS

Parenting is a demanding task under ideal circumstances, but when parents and children face situations that deviate from "the norm," the potential for family disruption is increased. Situations that are encountered frequently are divorce, single parenthood, blended families, adoption, and dual-career families. In addition, as cultural diversity increases in our communities, many immigrants are making the transition to parenthood and a new country, culture, and language simultaneously. Other situations that create unique parenting challenges are parental alcoholism, homelessness, and incarceration. Although these topics are not addressed here, readers may wish to investigate them further.

PARENTING THE ADOPTED CHILD

Adoption establishes a legal relationship between a child and parents who are not related by birth but who have the same rights and obligations that exist between children and their biologic parents. In the past, biologic mothers alone made the decision to relinquish the rights to their children. In recent years, the courts have acknowledged the legal rights of biologic fathers regarding this decision. Concerned child advocates have questioned whether decisions that honor fathers' rights are in the best interests of their children. As children's rights have become recognized, older children have successfully dissolved their

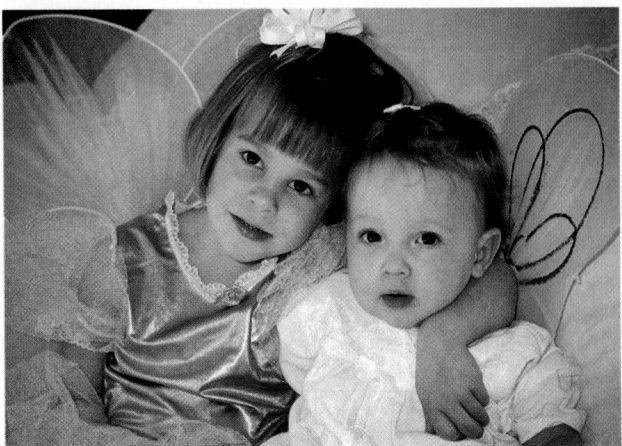

FIG 3-9 An older sister lovingly embraces her adopted sister.

? CRITICAL THINKING CASE STUDY
Parenting the Adopted Child

Twelve-month-old Justin was adopted at birth. His parents tell you that they wonder when they should tell Justin that he is adopted. As the nurse, what counseling and advice should you give Justin's parents?

Questions
1. Evidence—Is there sufficient information to draw any conclusions about this situation?
2. Assumptions—Describe some underlying assumptions about the following:
   a. The best time to tell children that they are adopted
   b. The manner in which parents should tell their child about adoption
   c. Children's reactions to being told they are adopted
3. What implications for nursing care can be drawn at this time?
4. Does the evidence support your conclusion?

---

legal bonds with their biologic parents to pursue adoption by adults of their choice. Furthermore, there is a growing interest and demand within the GLBT community to adopt.

Unlike biologic parents, who prepare for their child's birth with prenatal classes and the support of friends and relatives, adoptive parents have fewer sources of support and preparation for the new addition to their family. Nurses can provide the information, support, and reassurance needed to reduce parental anxiety regarding the adoptive process and refer adoptive parents to state parental support groups. Such sources can be contacted through a state or county welfare office.

The earlier infants enter their adoptive homes, the better the chances of parent–infant attachment. However, the more caregivers the infant had before adoption, the greater the risk for attachment problems. The infant must break the bond with the previous caregiver and form a new bond with the adoptive parents. Difficulties in forming an attachment depend on the amount of time the infant has spent with caregivers early in life as well as the number of caregivers (e.g., the birth mother, nurse, adoption agency personnel).

Siblings, adopted or biologic, who are old enough to understand should be included in decisions regarding the commitment to adopt with reassurance that they are not being replaced. Ways that the siblings can interact with the adopted child should be stressed (Fig. 3-9).

Issues of Origin

The task of telling children that they are adopted can be a cause of deep concern and anxiety. There are no clear-cut guidelines for parents to follow in determining when and at what age children are ready for the information. Parents are naturally reluctant to present such potentially unsettling news. However, it is important that parents not withhold the adoption from the child because it is an essential component of the child's identity (see Critical Thinking Case Study).

The timing arises naturally as parents become aware of the child's readiness. Most authorities believe that children should be informed at an age young enough so that, as they grow older, they do not remember a time when they did not know they were adopted. The time is highly individual but must be right for both the parents and the child. It may be when children ask where babies come from, at which time children can also be told the facts of their adoption. If they are told in a way that conveys the idea that they were active participants in the selection process, they will be less likely to feel that they were abandoned victims in a helpless situation. For example, parents can tell children that their personal qualities drew the parents to them. It is

wise for parents who have not previously discussed adoption to tell children that they are adopted before the children enter school to avoid having them learn it from third parties. Complete honesty between parents and children strengthens the relationship.

Parents should anticipate behavior changes after the disclosure, especially in older children. Children who are struggling with the revelation that they are adopted may benefit from individual and family counseling. Children may use the fact of their adoption as a weapon to manipulate and threaten parents. Statements such as "My real mother would not treat me like this" or "You don't love me as much because I'm adopted" hurt parents and increase their feelings of insecurity. Such statements may also cause parents to become overpermissive. Adopted children need the same undemanding love, combined with firm discipline and limit setting, as any other child.

Adolescence

Adolescence may be an especially trying time for parents of adopted children. The normal confrontations of adolescents and parents assume more painful aspects in adoptive families. Adolescents may use their adoption to defy parental authority or as a justification for aberrant behavior. As they attempt to master the task of identity formation, they may begin to have feelings of abandonment by their biologic parents. Gender differences in reacting to adoption may surface.

Adopted children fantasize about their biologic parents and may feel the need to discover their parents' identities to define themselves and their own identities. It is important for parents to keep the lines of communication open and to reassure their children that they understand the need to search for their identities. In some states, birth certificates are made legally available to adopted children when they come of age. Parents should be honest with questioning adolescents and tell them of this possibility (the parents themselves are unable to obtain the birth certificate; it is the children's responsibility if they desire it).

Cross-Racial and International Adoption

Adoption of children from racial backgrounds different from that of the family is commonplace. In addition to the problems faced by adopted children in general, children of a cross-racial adoption must deal with physical and sometimes cultural differences. It is advised that parents who adopt children with different ethnic background do everything to preserve the adopted children's racial heritage.

Although the children are full-fledged members of an adopting family and citizens of the adopted country, if they have a strikingly different appearance from other family members or exhibit distinct racial or ethnic characteristics, challenges may be encountered outside the family. Bigotry may appear among relatives and friends. Strangers may make thoughtless comments and talk about the children as though they are not members of the family. It is vital that family members declare to others that this is their child and a cherished member of the family.

In international adoptions, the medical information the parents receive may be incomplete or sketchy; weight, height, and head circumference are often the only objective information present in the child's medical record. Many internationally adopted children were born prematurely, and common health problems such as infant diarrhea and malnutrition delay growth and development. Some children have serious or multiple health problems that can be stressful for the parents.

PARENTING AND DIVORCE

Since the mid-1960s, a marked change in the stability of families has been reflected in increased rates of divorce, single parenthood, and remarriage. In 2009, the divorce rate for the United States was 3.4 per 1000 total population (Centers for Disease Control and Prevention, 2010). The divorce rate has changed little since 1987. In the decade before that, the rate increased yearly, with a peak in 1979. Although almost half of all divorcing couples are childless, it is estimated that more than 1 million children experience divorce each year.

The process of divorce begins with a period of marital conflict of varying length and intensity followed by a separation, the actual legal divorce, and the reestablishment of different living arrangements (Box 3-5). Because a function of parenthood is to provide for the security and emotional welfare of children, disruption of the family structure often engenders strong feelings of guilt in the divorcing parents.

During a divorce, parents' coping abilities may be compromised. The parents may be preoccupied with their own feelings, needs, and life changes and be unavailable to support their children. Newly employed parents, usually mothers, are likely to leave children with

---

BOX 3-5   STAGES OF THE DIVORCE PROCESS

Acute Phase

The married couple makes the decision to separate.

This phase includes the legal steps of filing for dissolution of the marriage and usually the departure of the father from the home.

This phase lasts from several months to more than 1 year and is accompanied by familial stress and a chaotic atmosphere.

Transitional Phase

The adults and children assume unfamiliar roles and relationships within a new family structure.

This phase is often accompanied by a change of residence, a reduced standard of living and altered lifestyle, a larger share of the economic responsibility being shouldered by the mother, and radically altered parent–child relationships.

Stabilizing Phase

The postdivorce family reestablishes a stable, functioning family unit.

Remarriage frequently occurs, with concomitant changes in all areas of family life.

Modified from Wallerstein JS: Children of divorce: stress and developmental tasks. In Garmezy N, Rutter M, editors: *Stress, coping, and development in children*, New York, 1988, McGraw-Hill.

---

new caregivers, in strange settings, or alone after school. The parent may also spend more time away from home, searching for or establishing new relationships. Sometimes, however, the adult feels frightened and alone and begins to depend on the child as a substitute for the absent parent. This dependence places an enormous burden on the child.

Common characteristics in the custodial household after separation and divorce include disorder, coercive types of control, inflammable tempers in both parents and children, reduced parental competence, a greater sense of parental helplessness, poorly enforced discipline, and diminished regularity in household routines. Noncustodial parents are seldom prepared for the role of visitor, may assume the role of recreational and "fun" parent, and may not have a residence suitable for children's visits. They may also be concerned about maintaining the arrangement over the years to follow.

Impact of Divorce on Children

Parental divorce is an additional childhood adversity that contributes to poor mental health outcomes, especially when combined with child abuse. Parental psychopathology may be one possible mechanism to explain the relationships between child abuse, parental divorce, and psychiatric disorders and suicide attempts (Afifi, Boman, Fleisher, and others, 2009). Even when a divorce is amicable and open, children recall parental separation with the same emotions felt by victims of a natural disaster, including loss, grief, and vulnerability to forces beyond their control. A recent study found that by increasing one of children's most important interpersonal resources, mother–child relationship quality, had a positive impact on coping with the adjustments surrounding divorce (Velez, Wolchik, Tein, and others, 2011).

The impact of divorce on children depends on several factors, including the ages and genders of the children, the outcome of the divorce, and the quality of the parent–child relationship and parental care during the years after the divorce. Family characteristics are more crucial to the child's well-being than specific child characteristics, such as age or gender. High levels of ongoing family conflict are related to problems of social development, emotional stability, and cognitive skills for the child.

A major problem occurs when children are "caught in the middle" between the divorced parents. They become the message bearer between the parents, are often quizzed about the other parent's activities, and have to listen to one parent criticize the other. A nurse may be able to help the child get out of the middle by stating "I messages" based on the formula of "I feel (state the feeling) when you (state the source). I would like it if you. . . ." An example of an "I message" is: "I do not feel comfortable when you ask me questions about Mom; maybe you could ask her yourself." This approach enables the child to feel in control.

Feelings of children toward divorce vary with age (Box 3-6). Previously, researchers believed that divorce had a greater impact on younger children, but recent observations indicate that divorce constitutes a major disruption for children of all ages. The feelings and behaviors of children may be different for various ages and gender, but all children experience stress second only to the stress produced by the death of a parent. Although considerable research has looked at gender differences in children's adjustments to divorce, the findings are not conclusive.

Some children feel a sense of shame and embarrassment concerning the family situation. Sometimes children see themselves as different, inferior, or unworthy of love, especially if they feel responsible for the family dissolution. Although the social stigma attached to divorce no longer produces the emotions it did in the past, such feelings may

BOX 3-6   FEELINGS AND BEHAVIORS OF CHILDREN RELATED TO DIVORCE

Infancy
Effects of reduced mothering or lack of mothering
Increased irritability
Disturbance in eating, sleeping, and elimination
Interference with attachment process

Early Preschool Children (Ages 2–3 Years)
Frightened and confused
Blame themselves for the divorce
Fear of abandonment
Increased irritability, whining, tantrums
Regressive behaviors (e.g., thumb sucking, loss of elimination control)
Separation anxiety

Later Preschool Children (Ages 3–5 Years)
Fear of abandonment
Blame themselves for the divorce; decreased self-esteem
Bewilderment regarding all human relationships
Become more aggressive in relationships with others (e.g., siblings, peers)
Engage in fantasy to seek understanding of the divorce

Early School-Age Children (Ages 5–6 Years)
Depression and immature behavior
Loss of appetite and sleep disorders
May be able to verbalize some feelings and understand some divorce-related changes
Increased anxiety and aggression
Feelings of abandonment by the departing parent

Middle School-Age Children (Ages 6–8 Years)
Panic reactions
Feelings of deprivation—loss of parent, attention, money, and secure future
Profound sadness, depression, fear, and insecurity
Feelings of abandonment and rejection

Fear regarding the future
Difficulty expressing anger at parents
Intense desire for reconciliation of parents
Impaired capacity to play and enjoy outside activities
Decline in school performance
Altered peer relationships—become bossy, irritable, demanding, and manipulative
Frequent crying, loss of appetite, sleep disorders
Disturbed routine, forgetfulness

Later School-Age Children (Ages 8–12 Years)
More realistic understanding of divorce
Intense anger directed at one or both parents
Divided loyalties
Ability to express feelings of anger
Ashamed of parental behavior
Desire for revenge; may wish to punish the parent they hold responsible
Feelings of loneliness, rejection, and abandonment
Altered peer relationships
Decline in school performance
May develop somatic complaints
May engage in aberrant behavior such as lying or stealing
Temper tantrums
Dictatorial attitude

Adolescents (Ages 12–18 Years)
Able to disengage themselves from parental conflict
Feelings of a profound sense of loss—of family, childhood
Feelings of anxiety
Worry about themselves, parents, siblings
Expression of anger, sadness, shame, embarrassment
May withdraw from family and friends
Disturbed concept of sexuality
May engage in acting-out behaviors

still exist in small towns or in some cultural groups and can reinforce children's negative self-image. The lasting effects of divorce depend on the children's and the parents' adjustment to the transition from an intact family to a single-parent family and, often, to a reconstituted family.

Although most studies have concentrated on the negative effects of divorce on youngsters, some positive outcomes of divorce have been reported. A successful postdivorce family, either a single-parent or a reconstituted family, can improve the quality of life for both adults and children. If conflict is resolved, a better relationship with one or both parents may result, and some children may have less contact with a disturbed parent. Greater stability in the home setting and the removal of arguing parents can be positive outcomes for the child's long-term well-being.

Telling the Children

Parents are understandably hesitant to tell children about their decision to divorce. Most parents neglect to discuss either the divorce or its inevitable changes with preschool children. Without preparation, even children who remain in the family home are confused by the parental separation. Frequently, children are already experiencing vague, uneasy feelings that are more difficult to cope with than being told the truth about the situation.

If possible, the initial disclosure should include both parents and siblings followed by individual discussions with each child. Sufficient time should be set aside for these discussions, and they should take place during a period of calm, not after an argument. Parents who physically hold or touch their children provide them with feelings of warmth and reassurance. The discussions should include the reason for the divorce, if age appropriate, and reassurance that the divorce is not the fault of the children.

Parents should not fear crying in front of the children because their crying gives the children permission to cry also. Children need to ventilate their feelings. Children may feel guilt, a sense of failure, or that they are being punished for misbehavior. They normally feel anger and resentment and should be allowed to communicate these feelings without punishment. They also have feelings of terror and abandonment. They need consistency and order in their lives. They want to know where they will live, who will take care of them, if they will be with their siblings, and if there will be enough money to live on. Children may also wonder what will happen on special days such as birthdays and holidays, whether both parents will come to school events, and whether they will still have the same friends. Children fear that if their parents stopped loving each other, they could stop loving them. Their need for love and reassurance is tremendous at this time.

Custody and Parenting Partnerships

In the past, when parents separated, the mother was given custody of the children with visitation agreements for the father. Now both parents and the courts are seeking alternatives. Current belief is that neither fathers nor mothers should be awarded custody automatically. Custody should be awarded to the parent who is best able to provide for the children's welfare. In some cases, children experience severe stress when living or spending time with a parent. Many fathers have demonstrated both their competence and their commitment to care for their children.

Often overlooked are the changes that may occur in the children's relationships with other relatives, especially grandparents. Grandparents are increasingly involved in the care of young children (Fergusson, Maughan, and Golding, 2008). Whereas grandparents on the noncustodial side are often kept from their grandchildren, those on the custodial side may be overwhelmed by their adult child's return to the household with grandchildren.

Two other types of custody arrangements are divided custody and joint custody. Divided, or split, custody means that each parent is awarded custody of one or more of the children, thereby separating siblings. For example, sons might live with the father and daughters with the mother.

Joint custody takes one of two forms. In joint physical custody, the parents alternate the physical care and control of the children on an agreed-on basis while maintaining shared parenting responsibilities legally. This custody arrangement works well for families who live close to each other and whose occupations permit an active role in the care and rearing of the children. In joint legal custody, the children reside with one parent, but both parents are the children's legal guardians, and both participate in childrearing.

Coparenting offers substantial benefits for the family: children can be close to both parents, and life with each parent can be more normal (as opposed to having a disciplinarian mother and a recreational father). To be successful, parents in these arrangements must be highly committed to providing normal parenting and to separating their marital conflicts from their parenting roles. No matter what type of custody arrangement is awarded, the primary consideration is the welfare of the children.

SINGLE PARENTING

An individual may acquire single-parent status as a result of divorce, separation, death of a spouse, or birth or adoption of a child. Although divorce rates have stabilized, the number of single-parent households continues to rise. In 2009, 34% of children younger than 18 years of age lived in single-parent families, and the majority of single parents were women (Annie E. Casey Foundation, 2011; Kreider and Elliott, 2009). Although some women are single parents by choice, most never planned on being single parents, and many feel pressure to marry or remarry.

Managing shortages of money, time, and energy is often a concern for single parents. Studies repeatedly confirm the financial difficulties of single-parent families, particularly single mothers. In 2009, only one third of mother-headed households reported having received any child support or alimony (Annie E. Casey Foundation, 2011). In fact, the stigma of poverty may be more keenly felt than the discrimination associated with being a single parent. These families are often forced by their financial status to live in communities with inadequate housing and personal safety concerns. Single parents often feel guilty about the time spent away from their children. Divorced mothers from marriages in which the father assumed the role of breadwinner and the mother assumed the household maintenance and parenting roles have

considerable difficulty adjusting to their new role of breadwinner. Many single parents have trouble arranging for adequate child care, particularly for a sick child.

Being a teenage parent adds to the financial burden of being a single parent and can have long-term consequences for the mother and child. Poverty is a well-known predictor of adverse effects on a child's health and well-being. Approximately 78% of children born to teenage mothers who did not marry or graduate high school live in poverty. In contrast, only 9% of children born to women over 20 years of age who marry and finish high school live in poverty (Annie E. Casey Foundation, 2009).

Social supports and community resources needed by single-parent families include health care services that are open on evenings and weekends; high-quality child care; respite child care to relieve parental exhaustion and prevent burnout; and parent enhancement centers for advancing education and job skills, providing recreational activities, and offering parenting education. Single parents need social contacts separate from their children for their own emotional growth and that of their children. Parents Without Partners, Inc.,* is an organization designed to meet the needs of single parents.

Single Fathers

Fathers who have custody of their children have many of the same problems as divorced mothers. They may feel overburdened by the responsibility; depressed; and concerned about their ability to cope with the emotional needs of the children, especially girls. Some fathers lack homemaking skills. They may find it difficult at first to coordinate household tasks, school visits, and other activities associated with managing a household alone.

PARENTING IN RECONSTITUTED FAMILIES

In the United States, many of the children living in homes where parents have divorced will experience another major change in their lives such as the addition of a stepparent or new siblings (Coehlo, Kaakinen, Hanson, and others, 2009). The entry of a stepparent into a ready-made family requires adjustments for all family members. Some obstacles to the role adjustments and family problem solving include disruption of previous lifestyles and interaction patterns, complexity in the formation of new ones, and lack of social supports. Despite these problems, most children from divorced families want to live in a two-parent home.

Cooperative parenting relationships can allow more time for each set of parents to be alone to establish their own relationship with the children. Under ideal circumstances, power conflicts between the two households can be reduced, and tension and anxiety can be lessened for all family members. In addition, the children's self-esteem can be increased, and there is a greater likelihood of continued contact with grandparents. Flexibility, mutual support, and open communication are critical in successful relationships in stepfamilies and stepparenting situations.

PARENTING IN DUAL-EARNER FAMILIES

No change in family lifestyle has had more impact than the large numbers of women moving away from the traditional homemaker role and entering the workplace (Coehlo, Kaakinen, Hanson, and others, 2009). The trend toward increased numbers of dual-earner families is unlikely to diminish significantly. As a result, families are subject to

---

*1650 South Dixie Hwy., Suite 402, Boca Raton, FL 33432; 800-637-7974; http://parentswithoutpartners.org.

considerable stress as members attempt to meet often competing demands of occupational needs and those regarded as necessary for a rich family life.

Role definitions are frequently altered to arrange a more equitable division of time and labor, as well as to resolve conflict, especially conflict related to traditional cultural norms. Overload is a common source of stress in a dual-earner family, and social activities are significantly curtailed. Time demands and scheduling are major problems for all individuals who work. When the individuals are parents, the demands can be even more intense. Dual-earner couples may increase the strain on themselves to avoid creating stress for their children. Although there is no evidence to indicate that the dual-earner lifestyle is stressful to children, the stress experienced by the parents may affect the children indirectly.

Working Mothers

Working mothers have become the norm in the United States. Maternal employment may have variable effects on preschool children's health (Mindlin, Jenkins, and Law, 2009). The quality of child care is a persistent concern for all working parents (see Evidence-Based Practice box). Determinants of child care quality are based on health and safety requirements, responsive and warm interaction among staff and children, developmentally appropriate activities, trained staff, limited group size, age-appropriate caregivers, adequate staff-to-child ratios, and adequate indoor and outdoor space. Nurses play an important role in helping families find suitable sources of child care and prepare children for this experience (see Alternate Child Care Arrangements, Chapter 10).

EVIDENCE-BASED PRACTICE

Daycare for Preschool Children

Ask the Question
PICOT Question
In preschool children, how does early daycare affect education, health, and welfare in the future?

Search for Evidence
Search Strategies
Search selection criteria included English language published within the past 5 years. Focus on research-based articles on daycare for preschool children.

Databases Used
PubMed, Cochrane Collaboration, MDConsult, Joanna Briggs Institute, AHRQ-National Guideline Clearinghouse, TRIP database Plus, PedsCCM, BestBETS

Critically Analyze the Evidence
A Cochrane Library systematic review found seven randomized control trials and one quasi-randomized study after examining 920 abstracts and 19 books (Zortich, Roberts, and Oakley, 2005). All of the eight studies were conducted in the United States. In these eight studies, a total of 2203 children were randomized to daycare or a control group. All subjects were younger than 4 years old at enrollment. Daycare ranged from 2 hr/wk for 8 months to 7 hr/day, 5 day/wk, for 7 years. All studies examined cognitive development, six studies examined school performance, four studies evaluated behavior, and one study assessed children's health. Studies found that daycare has beneficial effects on children's development, school achievement, and potential for future success.

The National Institute of Child Health and Human Development Early Child Care Research Network (Belsky, Vandell, Burchinal, and others, 2007) followed more than 1300 children receiving early child care and found that although parenting was a stronger and more consistent predictor of children's development than early child care experiences, higher quality care predicted higher vocabulary scores, and higher daycare exposure predicted more teacher-reported problem behaviors through sixth grade.

Bradley and Vandell (2007) evaluated studies of early child care with specific attention to the impact of the child's age, the time spent in child care, and quality and type of care facility on adaptive functioning. Children who were younger when child care began and were cared for 30 or more hours a week experienced stress-related behaviors. These children had higher language scores. The likelihood of communicable illness and ear infections was increased when six or more children were together.

Apply the Evidence: Nursing Implications
There is **strong evidence** with **strong recommendations** (Guyatt, Oxman, Vist, and others, 2008) to consider the following:
- Parenting remains a stronger and more consistent predictor of child development than the early child care experience.
- Out-of-home daycare has beneficial effects for children, enhancing cognitive development and preventing later school failures.
- Out-of-home daycare can have a positive effect on social outcomes for children and their families.

QSEN **Quality and Safety Competencies:**
Evidence-Based Practice*
Knowledge
Differentiate clinical opinion from research and evidence-based summaries.
Discuss current evidence on the influences of early child care on future development.

Skills
Base individualized care plan on patient values, clinical expertise, and evidence.
Integrate evidence into practice by considering the pros and cons of early out-of-home daycare and its influence on cognitive development and school success.

Attitudes
Value the concept of evidence-based practice as integral to determining best clinical practice.
Appreciate strengths and weakness of evidence on the influence of the early child care experience on a child's development.

References
Belsky J, Vandell DL, Burchinal M, and others: Are there long-term effects of early child care? *Child Development* 78(2):681–701, 2007.
Bradley RH, Vandell DL: Child care and the well-being of children, *Arch Pediatr Adolesc Med* 161(7):669–676, 2007.
Guyatt GH, Oxman AD, Vist GE, and others: GRADE: an emerging consensus on rating quality of evidence and strength of recommendations, *BMJ* 336:924–926, 2008.
Zortich B, Roberts I, Oakley A: Day care for pre-school children, *Cochrane Database Syst Rev* (2):CD000564, 2000. In *The Cochrane Library*, issue 3, 2005.

*Adapted from the QSEN at http://www.qsen.org.

FOSTER PARENTING

The term foster care is defined as 24-hour substitute care for children outside their own homes. The living situation may be nonrelative foster family homes, relative foster homes, group homes, emergency shelters, residential facilities, and preadoptive homes (Child Welfare Information Gateway, 2011). Each state provides a standard for the role of foster parent and a process by which to become one. These "parents" contract with the state to provide a home for children for a limited duration. Most states require about 27 hours of training before being on contract and at least 12 hours of continuing education a year. Foster parents may be required to attend a foster parent support group that is often separate from a state agency. Each state has guidelines regarding the relative health of the prospective foster parents and their families, background checks regarding legal issues for the adults, personal interviews, and a safety inspection of the residence and surroundings (Chamberlain, Price, Leve, and others, 2008).

Foster homes include both kinship and nonrelative placements. Since the 1980s, the proportion of children in out-of-home care placed with relatives has increased rapidly and been accompanied by a decrease in the number of foster families. As with their nonfoster counterparts, much of the child's adjustment depends on the family's stability and available resources. Even though foster homes are designed to provide short-term care, it is not unusual for children to stay for many years.

Nurses should be aware that 423,773 children spend time living in foster care in a given year, many of them facing developmental concerns (Annie E. Casey Foundation, 2011; Child Welfare Information Gateway, 2011). Children from lower income, single-mother, and mother–partner families are considerably more likely to be living in foster care (Berger and Waldfogel, 2004). Children in foster care tend to have a higher than normal incidence of acute and chronic health problems and may experience feelings of isolation or confusion (Annie E. Casey Foundation, 2009). Foster children are often at risk because of their previous caretaking environment. Nurses should strive to implement strategies to improve health care for this group of children. In particular, assessment and case management skills are required to involve other disciplines in meeting their needs.

ACCOMMODATING CONTEMPORARY PARENTING SITUATIONS

During recent years, both the private and government sectors have identified specific problems of contemporary families. Many of these issues involve working parents. One significant stressor for working single-parent and dual-earner families is when a child becomes ill. The frequency of childhood illness, exclusion practices of most licensed child care programs, and employers' limited sick-leave policies are other contributing factors. Most authorities agree that a familiar face and place are important components of sick-child care, and some argue that the only place for an ill child is at home with a parent or other relative.

Some employers have become more family focused and provide time off for parents to be with sick children. Increasing numbers are becoming more generous in the amount of time they allow parents (fathers as well as mothers) to remain at home after the birth or adoption of a child. Flexible work schedules and family-oriented legislation can ease the burden of managing family and work responsibilities. The passage of the Family and Medical Leave Act (FMLA) in 1993 set the stage for a greater focus on the issues of contemporary families. FMLA allows eligible employees to take up to 12 weeks of unpaid leave each year to care for newborn or newly adopted children, parents, or spouses who have serious health conditions or to recover from their own serious health condition.

KEY POINTS

- Because there is no agreement about the definition of family, a family is what an individual considers it to be.
- Three theories that have significant application to pediatric nursing are family systems theory, family stress theory, and developmental theory.
- Although the traditional family structure is nuclear or extended, in recent years, other forms, such as the single-parent family, have become more prominent.
- Family size and position within the family structure have a strong impact on children's development.
- Interpersonal skills and a basic understanding of childhood growth and development are two essential areas of focus for parents.

- Parental control tends to be predominantly one of three types: authoritarian, permissive, or authoritative.
- Three areas of special concern to adoptive families include the initial attachment process, the task of telling the children they are adopted, and identity formation during adolescence.
- Marital factors within the home significantly influence a child's development. The impact of divorce on a child depends on the child's age, the outcome, and the quality of the parent–child relationship and parental care after the divorce.
- Single parenting and stepparenting create adjustment difficulties and add stress to the already demanding parental role. Significant numbers of children will live in a single-parent or reconstituted family at some point.

REFERENCES

Afifi TO, Boman J, Fleisher W, and others: The relationship between child abuse, parental divorce, and lifetime mental disorders and suicidality in a nationally representative adult sample, *Child Abuse Negl* 33(3): 139–147, 2009.

American Academy of Pediatrics: Family pediatrics: report of the Task Force on the Family, *Pediatrics* 111(6): 1541–1571, 2003.

Annie E. Casey Foundation: *2009 Kids count data book: state profiles of child well-being*, Baltimore, 2009, Author.

Annie E. Casey Foundation: *2011 Kids count data book: state profiles of child well-being*, Baltimore, 2011, Author.

Berger L, Waldfogel J: Out-of-home placement of children and economic factors: an empirical analysis, *Rev Econo Household* 2(4):387–411, 2004.

Blackwell CW: Belief in the "free choice" model of homosexuality: a correlate of homophobia in registered nurses, *J LGBT Health Res* 3(3):31–40, 2007.

Bomar PJ: *Promoting health in families*, ed 3, Philadelphia, 2004, Saunders.

Cain DS: Parenting online and lay literature on infant spanking: information readily available to parents, *Soc Work Health Care* 47(2):174–184, 2008.

Centers for Disease Control and Prevention: Births marriages, divorces, and deaths: provisional data for 2009, *Natl Vital Stat Rep* 58(25):1–6, 2010.

Chamberlain P, Price J, Leve LD, and others: Prevention of behavior problems for children in foster care: outcomes and mediation effects, *Prev Sci* 9(1):17–27, 2008.

Child Welfare Information Gateway: *Foster care statistics 2009*, Washington, DC, 2011, U.S. Department of Health and Human Services, Children's Bureau.

Coehlo DP, Kaakinen JR, Hanson SMH, and others: *Family health care nursing*, ed 4, Philadelphia, 2009, FA Davis.

Deave T, Johnson D, Ingram J: Transition to parenthood: the needs of parents in pregnancy and early parenthood, *BMC Pregnancy Childbirth* 29(8):30, 2008.

Duvall ER: *Family development*, ed 5, Philadelphia, 1977, Lippincott.

Fergusson E, Maughan B, Golding J: Which children receive grandparental care and what effect does it have? *Child Psychol Psychiatry* 49(2):161–169, 2008.

Fisher C, Lindhorst H, Matthews T, and others: Nursing staff attitudes and behaviors regarding family presence in the hospital setting, *J Adv Nurs* 64(6):615–624, 2008.

Friedman MM, Bowden VR, Jones EG: *Family nursing: research theory and practice*, ed 5, Upper Saddle River, NJ, 2003, Prentice Hall.

Goldenberg I, Goldenberg H: *Family theory: an overview*, ed 7, Pacific Grove, Calif, 2008, Brooks-Cole Cengage Learning.

Hoeve M, Dubas JS, Eichelsheim VI, and others: The relationship between parenting and delinquency: a meta-analysis, *J Abnorm Child Psychol* 37(6):749–775, 2009.

Hubbs-Tait L, Kennedy TS, Page MC, and others: Parental feeding practices predict authoritative authoritarian, and permissive parenting styles, *J Am Diet Assoc* 108(7):1154–1161, 2008.

Kreider RM, Elliott DB: America's families and living arrangements: 2007, *Curr Pop Rep*, Washington, DC, 2009, U.S. Census Bureau.

Larzelere RE: Disciplinary spanking: the scientific evidence, *J Dev Behav Pediatr* 29(4):334–335, 2008.

Liddle HA, Santisteban DA, Levant RF, and others: *Family psychology*, Washington, DC, 2002, American Psychological Association.

Mathews TJ, Minino AM, Osterman MJ, and others: Annual summary of vital statistics: 2008, *Pediatrics* 127(1):146–157, 2011.

McCubbin MA, McCubbin HI: Families coping with illness: the resiliency model of family stress, adjustment, and adaptation. In Danielson CB, Bissel BH, Winstead-Fry P, editors: *Families, health, and illness*, St. Louis, 1994, Mosby.

Mindlin M, Jenkins R, Law C: Maternal employment and indicators of child health: a systemic review in pre-school children in OECD countries, *J Epidemiol Commun Health* 63(5):340–350, 2009.

Pawelski JG, Perrin EC, Foy JM, and others: The effects of marriage, civil union, and domestic partnership laws on the health and well-being of children, *Pediatrics* 118(1):349–364, 2006.

Power N, Franck L: Parent participation in the care of hospitalized children: a systematic review, *J Adv Nurs* 62(6):622–641, 2008.

Velez CE, Wolchik SA, Tein JY, and others: Protecting children from the consequences of divorce: a longitudinal study of the effects of parenting on children's coping processes, *Child Dev* 82(1):244–257, 2011.

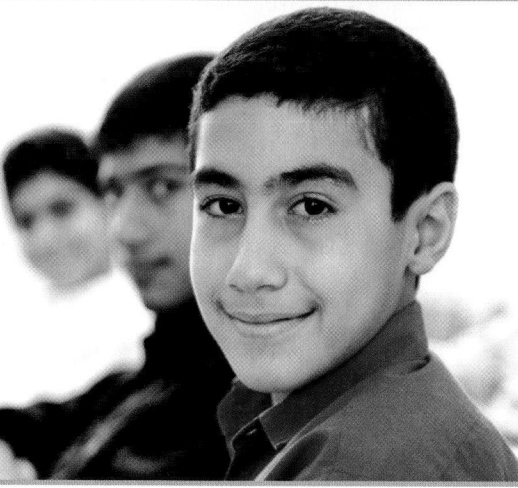

Social, Cultural, and Religious Influences on Child Health Promotion

Kim Mooney-Doyle

evolve WEBSITE

http://evolve.elsevier.com/wong/essentials
Case Study—Cultural Considerations
Key Point Summaries
NCLEX-Style Review Questions

CHAPTER OUTLINE

Culture, 43
    The Child and Family in North
        America, 45
    Social Roles, 45
        *Primary- and Secondary-Group
        Influences, 45*
        Self-Esteem and Culture, 45
    Cultural Shock and Cultural Sensitivity, 46
Subcultural Influences, 46
    Ethnicity, 47
    Minority-Group Membership, 47
    Socioeconomic Class, 47
        Communication Skills, 47
    Schools, 48
        Socialization, 48

Communities, 48
Peer Cultures, 48
Biculture, 49
Mass Media, 49
    Reading Materials, 49
    Television, 50
    New Technology, 50
Socioeconomic Influences, 50
    Poverty, 50
    Homelessness, 51
    Migrant Families, 51
Cultural Influences, 52
    Cultural Relativity, 52
    Relationships with Health Care
        Providers, 52

Communication, 53
    Food Customs, 54
Health Beliefs and Practices, 54
    Health Beliefs, 55
        Natural Forces, 55
        Supernatural Forces, 55
        Imbalance of Forces, 55
    Health Practices, 55
    Importance of Cultural Competence to
        Nurses, 56
Cultural Awareness, 57
    Religious Influences, 60
    Religious Beliefs, 60

LEARNING OBJECTIVES

On completion of this chapter the reader will be able to:
• Define *culture, cultural competence, ethnocentrism,* and *cultural relativity.*
• Describe the subcultural influences on child development.
• Discuss the population of minority children in the United States.

• Identify the impact of culture on health.
• Identify the impact socioeconomic influences have on health.
• Identify areas of potential conflict of values and customs for a nurse interacting with different cultural and ethnic groups.

❙CULTURE

Promoting the health of children requires a nurse to understand social, cultural, and religious influences on children and their families. This in turn depends on a purposeful awareness of the child's sociocultural context and also of oneself. The purpose of this chapter is to share with nursing students the significance of providing nursing care with a sense of cultural humility as a way to provide optimal care to all children and their families and to further understand the intersection of social, religious, and cultural forces that affect the health of children, their families, and their communities. Why is this important? The U.S. population is constantly evolving; patients experience negative health outcomes when social, cultural, and religious factors are not considered as influencing their health care; families may incorporate other health systems such as Eastern medicine or traditional healing into their lives; and it is required by legislative, regulatory, and credentialing bodies

(Tervalon, 2003). Educating health care providers is one way to reduce disparities in health care.

Cultural humility is a "commitment and active engagement in a lifelong process that individuals enter into on an ongoing basis with patients, communities, colleagues, and themselves" (Tervalon and Murray-Garcia, 1998, p. 118). It requires that health care providers participate in a continual process of self-reflection and self-critique that recognizes the power of the health care provider role, that views the patient and family as full members of the health care team, and that does not end after reading one chapter or attending one course but is an evolving aspect of being a health care provider. "Cultural competency is not an abdominal exam" (Kumagai and Lypson, 2009, p. 783). It is not a static endpoint to be checked off the list but an ongoing process that promotes deeper thinking and knowledge of oneself, others, and the world (Kumagai and Lypson, 2009).

Approaching nursing care from a position of cultural humility is important considering the ever-changing population. A sample of the demographic profile of the U.S. 2010 census includes 72.4% non-Hispanic white; 16.3% Hispanic/Latino; 12.6% Black/African American; and 3.6% Asian or American Indian/Alaskan Native (Humes, Jones, and Ramirez, 2011). Interestingly, the 2010 census data reveal that more than half of the population growth in the United States from 2000 to 2010 was attributable to increases in the Hispanic/Latino population. In addition, the population that defines their ethnicity as Asian grew faster than any other group, up 43% from the 2000 census. Children and adolescents 0 to 18 years of age comprised 24.3% of the U.S. population. The demographic profile includes white/non-Hispanic, 55.3%; Black/African American, 15.1%; Asian, 4.3%; Hispanic (any race), 22.5%; and all other, 4.7%. Traditionally, children younger than 5 years of age are highly underreported. This is problematic because the number and demographics of children determines the demand for schools, health care, and other services needed to meet the needs of families.

It is also important to understand nursing's contribution to culturally congruent care. A holistic view of care was first described by Madeleine Leininger, the recognized founder of transcultural nursing, in her culture care diversity and universality theory (Leininger, 2001; Munoz and Luckmann, 2005). The theory provides an intellectual framework and a research methodology for providing culturally congruent patient care. Nurses must remain aware that every family, child, and health care provider comes to a clinical encounter with a cultural lens through which they see and interpret the world.

Culture is a rich context through which people view and respond to their world (see Cultural Considerations box). It also provides the lens through which all facets of human behavior can be interpreted (Spector, 2009). Culture is composed of individuals who share a set of values, beliefs, practices (e.g., language, dress, diet, health care), social relationships, laws, politics, economics, and norms of behavior that are learned, integrative, social, and satisfying. Culture is an ingrained orientation to life that serves as a frame of reference for individual perception and judgment. Culture is, essentially, the way of life of a group of people that incorporates experiences of the past, influences thought and action in the present, and transmits these traditions to future group members. Families pass their culture on to children, and the children perceive the world through this cultural lens. Culture adapts to the ever-changing world as group members abandon, modify, or assume new patterns of living and behavior to meet the group's needs.

Material overt, or manifest, culture refers to the observable components of a culture, such as material objects (dress, art, utensils, and other artifacts) and actions. Nonmaterial covert culture refers to those aspects that cannot be observed directly, such as ideas, beliefs, customs,

---

🌐 CULTURAL CONSIDERATIONS

Cultural Definitions

Culture characterizes a particular group with its values, beliefs, norms, patterns, and practices that are learned, shared, and transmitted from one generation to another (Leininger, 2001). Culture differs from both race and ethnicity. *Race* is a term with roots in anthropology, distinguishing variety in humans by physical traits. *Ethnicity* is the affiliation of a set of persons who share a unique cultural, social, and linguistic heritage. *Gender* is an individual's self-identification as man or woman, and sex is the biological designation of male or female. *Social class* is a complex social construction that usually incorporates levels of education in the family, occupation, income, and access to resources. Socialization is the process by which society communicates its competencies, values, and expectations to children (Trawick-Smith, 2006). *Culture* is a complex whole in which each part is interrelated. It is an umbrella term that holds together many interrelated yet unique aspects of humanity, including beliefs, tradition, life ways, and heritage. It is much more than a country of origin or a demographic designation such as African American or white.

---

and feelings. Related to the large culture are many subcultures, each with an identity of its own. Children are socialized into a particular subculture rather than into the culture as a whole. Subcultural influences, such as ethnicity and social class, are discussed in more detail later in this chapter.

Cultures and subcultures contribute to the uniqueness of child members in such a subtle way and at such an early age that children grow up to think that their beliefs, attitudes, values, and practices are the "correct" or "normal" ones. By age 5 years, children can identify persons who belong to their cultural background. During later primary years, children can identify those from different cultures (Trawick-Smith, 2006). A set of values learned in childhood is likely to characterize children's attitudes and behavior for life, influencing their long-range goals and their short-range, impulsive inclinations. Thus, every ongoing society socializes each succeeding generation to its cultural heritage.

The manner and sequence of the growth and development phenomenon are universal and fundamental features of all children; however, children's varied behavioral responses to similar events are often determined by their culture. Culture plays a critical role in the parenting behaviors that facilitate children's development (Melendez, 2005). Children acquire the skills, knowledge, beliefs, and values important to their own family and culture. Cultural backgrounds can influence the pace of acquisition of cognitive and motor skills as well as the child's social and emotional development (Trawick-Smith, 2006).

Cultures may also differ in whether status in a group is based on age or on skill. Even children's play and their types of games are culturally determined. In some cultures, children play in groups composed of members of the same gender; in others, they play in mixed-gender groups. In some cultures, team games predominate; in others, most play is limited to individual games.

Standards and norms vary from culture to culture and from location to location; a practice that is accepted in one area may meet with disapproval or create tension in another. The extent to which cultures tolerate divergence from the established norm also varies among cultures and subcultural groups. Although conforming to cultural norms provides a degree of security, it is a decided deterrent to change.

THE CHILD AND FAMILY IN NORTH AMERICA

Context provides perspective for nursing care. The health and well-being of the child in the North American family is influenced by two distinct contexts: the context of family and the context of culture. Therefore, understanding these layers of influence on pediatric health is integral to developing a family-centered and culturally competent nursing practice (Thibodeaux and Deatrick, 2007). America's orientation toward homogenization—"the great melting pot"—is changing because of its increasingly diverse population.

The frontier background of the American culture has contributed to the overall orientation to life and childrearing. Americans have always had a basic optimistic view of the world, a belief that things can be better and that the children can and will be better off than their parents. With this hopeful outlook, a general future orientation, and the possibility of upward social mobility, American culture typically encourages development of self-confidence and autonomy in children. Children are generally permitted a greater degree of freedom than in more tradition-oriented cultures.

Family life in North America is characterized by increasing geographic and economic mobility. Families are less reliant on tradition, are fragmented, and have limited opportunity to transmit and acquire the traditional and accepted customs of a culture. Consequently, young adults rely to a greater extent on the professed experts, peers, and the mass media for acquisition of acceptable patterns of behavior, including childrearing practices. Conflicting information can be a source of confusion and frustration as parents attempt to determine the comparatively stable, essential components of the culture and transmit these to their children.

Children in North America grow up with a number of adults who differ from one another but who all provide input as role models, teachers, and standards for behavior. Most children live in some form of nuclear family located in sharply differentiated neighborhoods determined by income and ethnic status within a highly technical, largely urban society. Class differences in childrearing persist, but they are becoming less divergent.

Early in life, children in minority cultures become aware of their cultural context and the discriminatory attitudes of the majority culture toward their racial or ethnic group. The direct effects of discrimination are anger and low self-esteem, which manifest in a variety of behaviors. The most important influences on development of a positive self-image are warm, understanding parents who actively foster their children's growth. Parents who accept their children and react positively and constructively rather than in a negative manner will help their children develop feelings of self-worth, self-esteem, and self-acceptance. The more adequate children feel, the more positive their attitudes toward peers in both the majority and the minority groups and the greater their ability to withstand prejudice and intolerance and build lasting relationships.

SOCIAL ROLES

Much of children's self-concept comes from their ideas about their social roles. Roles are cultural creations; therefore, the culture prescribes patterns of behavior for persons in a variety of social positions. All persons who hold similar social positions have an obligation to behave in a particular manner. A role prohibits some behaviors and allows others. Because culture outlines and clarifies roles, it has a significant influence on the development of children's self-concept (i.e., attitudes and beliefs they have about themselves).

A social group consists of a system of roles carried out in both primary and secondary groups. A primary group has intimate, continued, face-to-face contact; mutual support of members; and the ability to order or constrain a considerable proportion of individual members' behavior. Two such groups are the family and the peer group, both of which have a great deal of influence on the child.

Secondary groups are groups that have limited, intermittent contact and generally less concern for members' behavior. These groups offer little in terms of support or pressure toward conformity except in rigidly limited areas. Examples of secondary groups are professional associations and social organizations such as church groups.

A concept of social role also depends largely on whether a child is reared in a primary- or secondary-group community. Children are subjected to perceptibly different forms of parental training in these two types of environments.

Primary- and Secondary-Group Influences

Children are raised within a primary-group environment and within a secondary-group environment. The influences, strengths, and limitations of both groups are significant. In a primary-group community (e.g., family; peer group; some contemporary rural, religious, or ethnic communities), all members know each other, most belong to the same subgroups, and all are concerned about each member's behavior. Community members have a high degree of material and psychologic support and one traditional set of values that the entire group agrees on and supports; thus, there is little conflict of values. In a stable community where the members remain within comparatively defined limits and relatives are likely to live close together, young members have ample opportunity to observe and absorb cultural practices and customs. Any member of the community feels justified in evaluating and censuring the conduct of another member.

Children reared in the relative isolation of secondary-group environmental influences tend to learn that there is only one acceptable way to respond to any given situation. The entire group agrees, and any tendency to deviate is met with collective disapproval. It is the parents' duty to see that the children learn and follow social roles and modes of behavior defined and strengthened by the views of the community.

The childrearing orientation in a secondary-group environment, such as urban communities, can differ considerably from that of a primary-group environment. The interaction between primary and secondary groups may reinforce values when both groups endorse that value or create confusion or conflict when one group rejects a value accepted by the other. An urban community is dynamic. Many of the traditional behaviors and values may not meet the needs of the changing society. Consequently, parents are often uncertain about what to teach their children. They may wish to rear their children with values consistent with their own, but the differences in experience between the generations are too great. As a result, they often grant their children autonomy in some areas of decision making early in the developmental process, and other secondary groups assume a greater influence. None of the groups is highly dominant in its influence; therefore, the children are exposed to an eclectic set of values and expectations, some in agreement and some in conflict. From these they must ultimately select those that they determine to be best for them and adopt them to form a consistent set of roles and behaviors to incorporate into the self-concept.

Self-Esteem and Culture

Culture influences a child's sense of self-esteem (Trawick-Smith, 2006). Some cultures are more collective in thought and action. A child from a collective culture will hold an inclusive view of him- or herself. Self-evaluation is related to the accomplishments or competencies of the entire family or community. School experiences that focus on personal achievement may promote positive self-esteem in some children but not in others who are more dependent on the success of a whole family or peer group. Their sense of control may not come from individual self-reliance but rather from a feeling of worth in their family or community (Trawick-Smith, 2006).

Families and culture also influence the criteria children use to evaluate their own abilities. Additionally, cultures vary in whether they instill an internal locus of control (a belief in the ability to regulate one's own life). Effects on self-esteem are minimal if these beliefs are directed by parents and are in accordance with cultural customs (Trawick-Smith, 2006). Ethnic pride can help children to maintain a positive self-image and counteract the effects of prejudice, which can have a negative impact on emotional health (Trawick-Smith, 2006).

CULTURAL SHOCK AND CULTURAL SENSITIVITY

Cultural shock is characterized by the inability to respond to or function within a new or strange situation. It can occur when the values and beliefs of a new cultural setting are radically different from those of the person's native culture (Munoz and Luckmann, 2005). This state of shock or uneasiness can happen to a patient in a hospital or to a nurse caring for patients with different cultural backgrounds. Immigrants to a new country and persons from a subcultural group experience the same cultural shock when they must adjust to the ways of an unfamiliar subgroup or setting.

Numerous factors influence reactions to a new environment. Language barriers, including dialects and jargon specific to a subcultural group, inhibit effective communication. Habits and customs, such as different role behaviors or etiquette, and differences in attitudes and beliefs are puzzling to newcomers in an unfamiliar environment. The child and family experiencing cultural shock can feel an intense sense of isolation, loneliness, and fear.

Nurses are challenged to overcome cultural shock and develop cultural sensitivity, an awareness of cultural similarities and differences. Doing so helps the nurse practice culturally competent care. This requires changing the way people think about, understand, and interact within the world around them (see Critical Thinking Case Study). The development of cultural competence is an ongoing, interactive process that involves six elements (Dunn, 2002):

1. Working on changing one's world view by examining one's own values and behaviors and working to reject racism and institutions that support it
2. Becoming familiar with core cultural issues by recognizing these issues and exploring them with patients
3. Becoming knowledgeable about the cultural groups one works with while learning about each individual patient's unique history
4. Becoming familiar with core cultural issues related to health and illness and communicating in a way that encourages patients to explain what an illness means to them
5. Developing a relationship of trust with patients and creating a welcoming atmosphere in the health care setting
6. Negotiating for mutually acceptable and understandable interventions of care

When minority groups immigrate from another country, a certain degree of cultural and ethnic blending occurs through the involuntary process of **acculturation**, gradual changes produced in a culture by the

? CRITICAL THINKING CASE STUDY
Reducing Cultural Shock

A woman from the Middle East is visiting her child who is hospitalized for a serious illness. Her husband left for home a short time ago to wash and change clothes. She speaks little English. You need to obtain her consent for an emergency procedure. She is hesitant and refuses to sign the consent form. What should you do?

1. Evidence—Are there sufficient data to draw any conclusions about this woman's actions?
2. Assumptions—Describe any underlying assumptions about each of the following:
   a. Arab culture
   b. Need for interpreter
   c. Approval for emergency procedures
   d. Documentation of the need for the emergency procedure
3. What priorities for nursing care should be established at this time?
4. Does the evidence support your nursing intervention(s)?

influence of another culture that cause one or both cultures to be more similar to each other. However, the changes occur to various degrees in different families and groups. Many groups continue to identify with their traditional heritage while adapting to the ill-defined concept of the "American way." Acculturation may be referred to as **assimilation**, which is the process of developing a new cultural identity (Spector, 2009).

SUBCULTURAL INFLUENCES

Except in rare situations, children grow and develop in a blend of cultures and subcultures. In a large, complex society such as the United States, different groups have their own set of standards, values, and expectations within the collective ways of the large culture. Most subcultures were formed when groups of people clustered together by preference, external pressures from the majority culture, or geographic isolation. Although many cultural differences are related to geographic boundaries, subcultures are not always restricted by location. Some subcultures are even related to the stages of development and have traditions, games, loyalties, and rules. The behavior of school-age children and adolescents demonstrates age-related subcultures. The culture is handed down by word of mouth from one "generation" to the next, and its rituals and behavior standards are highly resistant to outside influence.

Children's membership in a cultural subgroup is, for the most part, involuntary. They are each born into a family with a specific ethnic or racial heritage, socioeconomic level, and religious beliefs. Although the complex American society has countless subcultures and considerable variation in the way of life, the subcultures that seem to have the greatest influence on childrearing are ethnicity, social class, and occupational role. In addition, schools and peer-group subcultures are strong influences in the socialization of children.

! NURSING ALERT

American cultures and subcultures can be so diverse that it is essential that nurses be aware of and knowledgeable about the predominant groups in their work community and apply this knowledge in their practice.

ETHNICITY

Ethnicity is the classification of or affiliation with any of the basic groups or divisions of humankind or any heterogeneous population differentiated by customs, characteristics, language, or similar distinguishing factors. Ethnic differences extend to many areas and include such manifestations as family structure, language, food preferences, moral codes, and expression of emotion. Some standards of behavior (e.g., the traditional role of the father) result from the cultural heritage of the specific ethnic group. Others reflect the interaction between subcultures, most notably between members of the majority culture and a minority subculture. The term *ethnic* has aroused strong negative feelings, and the general population often rejects this term (Spector, 2009).

To establish their place in the group, children learn to follow a mode of behavior that is in accordance with standards distinctive to the group and learn how they can expect others to behave toward them. They take their cues by observing and imitating those to whom they are exposed. For example, children of a racial minority form a perception of their role as a group member by observing how role models within the subgroup respond to treatment by people outside the subgroup. When they see group members display an attitude of inferiority, they assume this to be the appropriate behavior and incorporate these perceptions into their own self-concept.

In the United States, the cross-cultural lines are becoming blurred as subcultures are assimilated and blended into the larger culture (Fig. 4-1). Although ethnic differences in childrearing are probably diminishing, they remain important. It is particularly difficult for

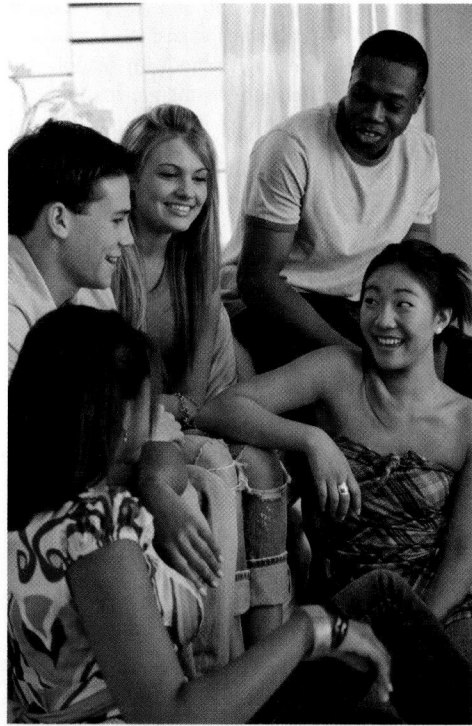

FIG 4-1 Youngsters from different cultural backgrounds interact within the larger culture. (© 2012 Photos.com, a division of Getty Images. All rights reserved.)

persons to attempt to maintain an identity within a subculture while living and conforming to the requirements of the larger culture.

Ethnocentrism is the emotional attitude that one's own ethnic group is superior to others; that one's values, beliefs, and perceptions are the correct ones; and that the group's ways of living and behaving are the best way (Spector, 2009). Ethnic stereotyping or labeling stems from ethnocentric views. Ethnocentrism implies that all other groups are inferior and that their ways are not in the best interests of the group. It is a common attitude among a dominant ethnic group and strongly influences a person's ability to evaluate objectively the beliefs and behaviors of others. Nurses must overcome the natural tendency to have ethnocentric attitudes when caring for people from different cultures. Culturally competent nurses have empathy for others, maintain an openness to feeling what others feel, and remain curious and willing to ask questions to gain a better understanding. In addition, nurses have a basic respect for themselves and others and acknowledge the intrinsic value of all humans.

MINORITY-GROUP MEMBERSHIP

The United States has more racial, ethnic, and religious minority groups than any other country. Ethnic minority groups are becoming increasingly important because these groups are producing children at a faster rate than the majority white population. Consequently, the minority population is increasing. The rapidly emerging U.S. minority population will present special needs and require resources beyond what is currently available (Murdock, 2005).

The U.S. 2010 census revealed more than 300 million people in the United States. The Hispanic population included 16.3% of the total population (Humes, Jones, and Ramirez, 2011). Currently, Hispanics are the fastest growing minority in the United States and have many health needs that are not being met (Murdock, 2005). In 2050, almost 30% of the U.S. population is expected to be Hispanic (Murdock, 2005).

SOCIOECONOMIC CLASS

Family relationships may be stronger in some ethnic or cultural groups than in others. However, the influence of socioeconomic class cannot be overlooked. This relates to the family's economic and educational levels. Strong family relationships exist among those of lower socioeconomic class who have few resources and must rely on the support of a family network to meet their physical and emotional needs. Middle- and upper-class people often have resources that reach beyond the extended family.

Communication Skills

Any concept that occurs to a person can be expressed in language. However, ease of communication and use of language codes vary among the social classes. Language is much more restricted in the lower classes, and grammar usage differs more than pronunciation. Persons in the middle classes use different grammar from those in the lower classes and are able to express more complicated ideas; persons in the lower classes use very simple grammar and are less likely to offer explanations.

These communication differences are highly significant in relation to school achievement. School is constructed around the elaborate language codes of the middle classes; therefore, children from the lower classes who lack an understanding of these language skills are placed at a decided disadvantage. This is particularly true for bilingual children and children from ethnic groups that have developed a unique dialect.

Historically, schools have participated in devaluing Native American languages, cultures, and traditional ways of learning and knowing.

Unfortunately, Native American children have been deficient in their preparation for school (Beaulieu, 2000). Also, children of Native American nations have been at risk for low achievement, overrepresentation in special education, and dropping out (Demmert, 2001). Many regional dialects and variations in language usage must be considered when communicating with persons from these groups. English words that sound like words in a foreign language can cause considerable misunderstanding.

SCHOOLS

When children enter school, their radius of relationships extends to include a wider variety of peers and a new focus of authority. Although parents continue to exert the major influence on children, in the school environment, teachers have the most significant psychologic impact on children's development and socialization. The teachers' function is primarily limited to teaching, but similar to parents, they are concerned about the children's emotional welfare. Both parents and teachers must constrain behavior and enforce standards of conduct.

Socialization

Next to the family, the schools exert the major force in providing continuity between generations by conveying a vast amount of culture from the older members to the young. This prepares children to carry out the traditional social roles they are expected to assume as adults in society. School is the center of cultural diffusion wherein the cultural standards of the larger group are disseminated to the local community. It governs what is taught and, to a large extent, how it is taught. School rules and regulations regarding attendance, authority relationships, and the system of penalties and rewards based on achievement transmit to children the behavioral expectations of the adult world of employment and relationships. School is often the only institution in which children systematically learn about the negative consequences of behaviors that depart from social expectations. In addition, the school provides an opportunity for some children to participate in the larger society in rewarding ways and often provides avenues for social mobility for both students and teachers. Individuals in the lower classes are offered the opportunity for further education and the capacity to move up in the social strata.

Teachers are responsible for transmitting the knowledge and values of the dominant culture (i.e., values on which there is broad consensus). They are expected to stimulate and guide children's intellectual development, sense of esthetics, and creative problem solving.

Traditionally the socialization process of school began when the child entered kindergarten or first grade. Today, with more than 60% of mothers of preschool children working outside the home, this socialization process begins much earlier for a significant number of children in a variety of child care settings.

Children of some cultural groups fare less well in school. They come from underrepresented groups, including African-American, Mexican American, Puerto Rican, and Native American children (Trawick-Smith, 2006). These cultural variations can be attributed to high rates of poverty, different cognitive styles, ineffective schools, and parents' views of schools as oppressive to cultural and traditional values (Trawick-Smith, 2006).

COMMUNITIES

Surveys of more than 1 million youth in the United States in grades 6 to 12 have shown that persons who experience a higher number of specific assets in their lives are more likely to make healthy choices and avoid high-risk behaviors. These assets offer a framework for positive child and adolescent development. The child or adolescent's community is made up of family, school, neighborhood, youth organization, and other members.

Four categories of external assets that youth receive from the community are (Search Institute, 2007):
1. **Support**—Young people need to feel support, care, and love from their families, neighbors, and others. They also need organizations and institutions that offer positive, supportive environments.
2. **Empowerment**—Young people need to feel valued by their community and be able to contribute to others. They need to feel safe and secure.
3. **Boundaries and expectations**—Young people need to know what is expected of them and what activities and behaviors are within the community boundaries and what are outside of them.
4. **Constructive use of time**—Young people need opportunities for growth through constructive, enriching opportunities and through quality time at home.

Internal assets must also be nurtured in the community's young members. These internal qualities guide choices and create a sense of centeredness, purpose, and focus. The four categories of internal assets are (Search Institute, 2007):
1. **Commitment to learning**—Young people need to develop a commitment to education and lifelong learning.
2. **Positive values**—Youth need to have a strong sense of values that direct their choices.
3. **Social competencies**—Young people need competencies that help them make positive choices and build relationships.
4. **Positive identity**—Young people need a sense of their own power, purpose, worth, and promise.

PEER CULTURES

Peer groups also have an impact on the socialization of children (Fig. 4-2). Peer relationships become increasingly important and influential as children proceed through school. In school, children have what can be regarded as a culture of their own. This is even more apparent in unsupervised playgroups because the culture in school is partly produced by adults.

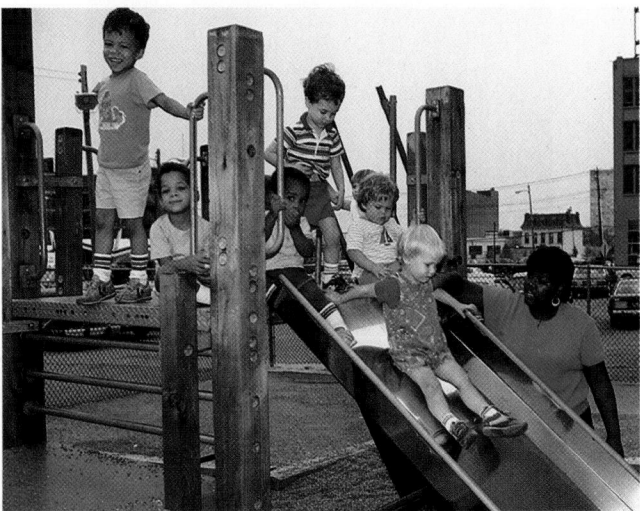

FIG 4-2 Children from a variety of cultural and ethnic backgrounds begin to socialize in the child care setting.

During their lives, children are exposed to value systems such as those of the family, ethnic group, and social class. In peer-group interactions, they confront a variety of these sets of values. The values imposed by the peer group are especially compelling because children must accept and conform to them to be accepted as members of the group. When the peer values are not too different from those of family and teachers, the mild conflict created by these small differences serves to separate children from the adults in their lives and to strengthen the feeling of belonging to the peer group.

The kind of socialization provided by the peer group depends on the subculture that develops from its members' background, interests, and capabilities. Some groups support school achievement, others focus on athletic prowess, and still others are decidedly against educative goals. Scholastic achievement is strongly related to the peer group's value system. Many conflicts between teachers and students and between parents and students can be attributed to fear of rejection by peers. What is expected from parents regarding academic achievement and what is expected from the peer culture often conflict, especially during high school. Chapter 19 discusses this in further detail.

Although the peer group has neither the traditional authority of the parents nor the legal authority of the schools for teaching information, it manages to convey a substantial amount of information to its members, especially on taboo subjects such as sex and drugs. Children's need for the friendship of their peers brings them into an increasingly complex social system. Through peer relationships, children learn to deal with dominance and hostility and to relate with persons in positions of leadership and authority. Other functions of the peer subculture are to relieve boredom and to provide recognition that individual members do not receive from teachers and other authority figures.

The peer-group culture has secrets, mores, and codes of ethics that promote group solidarity and detachment from adults. They have traditions and folkways, including age-related games and other activities, that are transferred from "generation to generation" of schoolchildren and that have a great influence over the behavior of all group members. As children move from one level to the next, they discard the folkways of the younger group as they adopt those of the new group. For example, a school-age child rides a bicycle to school; the high school student prefers a car. As they advance, children are forward oriented only—they look forward with anticipation but may look backward with contempt.

BICULTURE

Some children are exposed to the values, role relationships, and lifestyles of two or more cultures. This may occur because the child's parents are from two or more different cultures. In Hawaii, for example, it is common for children to be from four or more cultures. Other children straddle cultures as members of a minority culture within the dominant culture. This biculture is sometimes observed in the playgroup but usually is not a significant factor until children enter school. Then they must unlearn some of the established practices of one culture to become socialized in the other, especially in role relationships. For example, children from Hispanic and Asian cultures are taught to look away when scolded; in U.S. schools, the teacher expects direct eye contact—"Look at me when I speak to you." Children learn new roles and social behavior more rapidly than their adult counterparts.

This biculture is particularly marked in language differences. Bilingual children are said to be at a disadvantage in school situations of the dominant culture, in which there is controversy over bilingual education. Those supporting bilingual education adhere to the principle that children will understand more readily and perform more realistically (especially in testing situations) if learning is directed in their own language; others contend that children living in a dominant culture should adopt the ways of that culture, including its language. Children face less conflict when the school supports their language and culture even if the dominant language is used.

MASS MEDIA

The media provide children with a means for extending their knowledge about the world in which they live and have helped narrow the differences between groups. However, many people are concerned about the enormous influence the media can have on developing children and on health promotion behaviors. Children and adolescents in the United States spend more than 6 hours per day using entertainment media (Council on Communications and Media, 2009). Increased use of entertainment media has been associated with the epidemic of obesity in children and adolescents and increased aggression in children (Council on Communications and Media, 2009; Jordan, 2004). Anticipatory guidance around media utilization is among the most important a nurse can offer to a family. Because it can influence many areas of concern, such as aggression, sex, drugs, alcohol, obesity, eating disorders, and academic achievement (Strasburger, 2010), two important questions that nurses can ask to open the dialogue are "How much entertainment screen time does your child or teen spend each day?" and "Is there a TV, Internet connection, or wireless connection in the child or teen's bedroom?"

Researchers have established links between mass media and an increase in the use of tobacco, alcohol, and violent behavior in adolescents (Council on Communications and Media, 2009; Strasburger, 2010). The images of risky behavior presented by the media may serve to establish or reinforce teenagers' perceptions of their social environment. Also, media content may directly influence risk perception; media protagonists seldom experience the adverse consequences of their behaviors despite their grossly distorted experiences with violence, illness, or crime.

Children may identify closely with people or characters portrayed in reading materials, movies, and television programs and commercials. Pediatric nurses can educate and support parents on the effects of mass media on their children through the following recommendations (Jordan, 2004):

- Be aware of the content of the child's media and amount of time spent looking at a screen.
- Help young children watching television to find educational programs.
- Remove television, Internet-accessible computers, and video game systems from the bedroom to decrease the amount of time spent using these activities.
- Limit television viewing to 2 hours a day or less.
- Model good practices.
- Watch age-appropriate programs and play age-appropriate games with children.

Reading Materials

The oldest form of mass media—books, newspapers, and magazines—contributes to children's competence in almost every direction and provides enjoyment. Recognition of the impact that reading matter in schools has on value systems and the socialization process has prompted reevaluation of textbook content in several areas, such as stereotyped male and female role models, the sugar-coated view of life situations, and the biased history of minority groups.

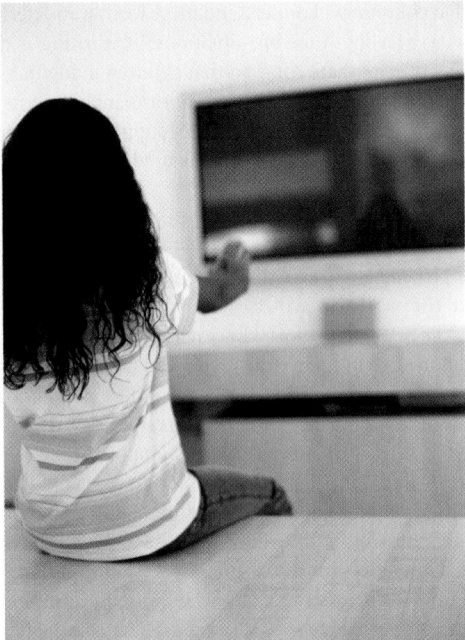

FIG 4-3 The average child in the United States spends more time watching television than in any other activity except sleeping. (© 2012 Photos.com, a division of Getty Images. All rights reserved.)

Reading aloud to children is a vital activity in promoting success in reading. It provides cognitive and language stimulation, is a forum for quality parent–child interaction, and may reduce parent stress (Klass, Needlman, and Zuckerman, 2002).

Television

The medium that has the most impact on children in the United States today is television; it has become one of the most significant socializing agents in the lives of young children. Its programs and commercials provide multiple sources for acquiring information, modeling behaviors, and observing value orientations. Besides producing a leveling effect on class differences in general information and vocabulary, TV exposes children to a wider variety of topics and events than they encounter in day-to-day life. Television always has time to talk to children and is a form of access to the adult world. Positive results occur only when viewing is relatively light, yet the average child in the United States older than the age of 8 years spends more time watching television or using a computer and video games (>6 hours/day) than in any other activity except sleeping (Fig. 4-3) (Council on Communications and Media, 2009).

Television can offer some beneficial effects on growing children by teaching healthy ideas and habits. Shows like *Sesame Street* promote school readiness by teaching letters and numbers, as well as teaching children about kindness and tolerance towards people who are different than them (Strasburger, 2010). Unfortunately, there is an imbalance in the availability of healthy and unhealthy media. Most researchers have concluded, however, that protracted television viewing can have negative effects on children. Increased verbal and physical aggressiveness, reduced persistence at problem solving, greater sex-role stereotyping, and reduced creativity have been reported repeatedly. In fairness, no one has yet defined the long-term effects of other electronic factors such as stereo headphones versus conversation, computer games or drills versus active social play, or DVDs versus books. However, clearly, children in the modern electronic environment are constantly stimulated from the outside, which allows them

little time to reflect and develop the inner speech that feeds brain development.

New Technology

Internet, cell phones, and social networking sites have added another layer to the mass media that influence children and adolescents. In many ways, this new technology is being used to access older forms of media (television, movies). It has also added a dimension to important social issues that affect children and teens, such as bullying; access to drugs, alcohol, and cigarettes; and partaking in other high-risk behaviors because of the popularity of social networking sites. Nurses must be familiar with potential risks and benefits and how to help families navigate this media. In addition, they must also offer families guidance in talking to their children and teens about proper use of this media.

Social Media

Social media and social networking sites serve as a community for adolescents and have potential to positively or negatively affect their health and well-being. Facebook is the most popular social networking site, with 130 million U.S. visitors (and counting) each year. Other avenues of social media, such as blogs and Twitter, may also be used readily by teens. Some benefits of social media are the sense of community it provides to children who may feel isolated or marginalized, such as children with chronic illnesses. There are important risks to consider, however. First are those mediated by the user themselves, such as what they display on their personal profiles, such as participation in high-risk behaviors or personal information (e.g., school). Second are those risks posed by other people accessing social networking sites, such as cyberbullying or sexual predation and solicitation (Moreno, 2010).

SOCIOECONOMIC INFLUENCES

POVERTY

A subcultural influence closely related to but different from social class is the condition known as **poverty**. It is a relative concept and is usually associated with the general standards of a population. The term *poverty* implies both visible and invisible impoverishment. It is a condition in which families live without adequate resources (Trawick-Smith, 2006). **Visible poverty** refers to lack of money or material resources, which includes poor nutrition, insufficient clothing, poor sanitation, and deteriorating housing. *Invisible poverty* refers to social and cultural deprivation such as limited employment opportunities, inferior educational opportunities, lack of or inferior medical services and health care facilities, and an absence of public services.

An **absolute standard** of poverty attempts to delimit a basic set of resources needed for adequate existence; a **relative standard** reflects the median standard of living in a society and is the term used in referring to childhood poverty in the United States; that is, what appears to be deprivation in one area may be a standard or norm in another.

An important development affecting American families since the end of World War II is the widening disparity in income status among generations. Children from families with a single mother comprise the largest group of children in poverty in the country (Wertheimer, 2005).

Growth in the number of poor children over the past decade has not been attributable to an increase in the number of welfare-dependent families but to growth in the ranks of the working poor. Approximately 20% of children in the United States live below the national poverty threshold, which is currently estimated at $22,350 for two adults and two children (Annie E. Casey Foundation, 2011). In addition,

| BOX 4-1 | INCOME, POVERTY, AND HEALTH INSURANCE COVERAGE IN THE UNITED STATES |

Children, 25% of the U.S. population, represent a disproportionate share of America's poor, making up 35% of those in poverty. Whereas approximately one-third of black and Hispanic children live in poverty, 10% to 15% of white (non-Hispanic) and Asian children in poverty.

A family is considered impoverished if a family with one adult and two children earned less than $18,530 in annual income. For a family of four (two adults and two children), this amount is $22,350.

Approximately 11 million children do not have health insurance, but more than 14 million are underinsured, meaning that their parents report spending a significant amount of money on out-of-pocket expenses related to their children's health.

More than 13 million children younger than 18 years, or approximately 18.5% of children, have specialized health care needs (campaign for children's health care).

From DeNavas-Walt C, Proctor BD, and Smith JC: U.S. Census Bureau, current population reports, P60-239, *Income, poverty, and health insurance coverage in the United States: 2010*, Washington, DC, 2011, U.S. Government Printing Office.

approximately 20% of children live in neighborhoods where more than 20% of the population currently lives below the federal poverty threshold. The official rate of poverty in 2009 was 14.3%, an increase in 1% since 2008. This is the second statistically significant rate of poverty in the United States since 2004. The poverty rate for children (younger than 18 years of age) increased from 19% to almost 21%. In addition, the poverty rate for individuals 18 to 64 years (the most likely ages of parents of children and adolescents) increased from 11.7% to almost 13%. Taken together, we can see that children and their families are particularly susceptible to negative economic forces across the nation and world (U.S. Census Bureau, 2010).

Such factors illustrate the growing inability of American families to provide economic essentials for their children. Approximately 11.6% (about 8.5 million) of all children in the United States were uninsured in 2002 (Szilagyi, 2005). Uninsured children are more likely to miss school, jeopardizing their education as well as their health (Box 4-1).

A high correlation between poverty and illness has long been observed. Impoverished families suffer from poor nutrition; without medical insurance, they have little if any preventive health care, inadequate health maintenance, and limited access to health services. One of the most significant health problems related to poverty is a high infant mortality rate. Although the rate of infant mortality has decreased in the United States, it still remains higher than that of most industrialized nations (Annie E. Casey Foundation, 2011). Day-to-day needs of food, clothing, and lodging take precedence over health care as long as the ailing person feels able to perform activities of daily living.

Poor families may be denied access to some institutions for emergency or other hospital care. Frequently, they must travel long distances to service centers that are willing to assume their care. In an emergency, they must find money for taxi fare, borrow an automobile, or seek other means of transportation. They must find care for dependents, such as other infants and small children, or take them along when taking the ill child for care. Families tend to delay preventive care indefinitely unless health services are relatively accessible. They are more likely to consult folk practitioners or other persons within their community.

Poor nutrition accounts for many health problems in the lower socioeconomic classes. Lack of funds, education, and readily available healthy foods results in a diet that may be seriously lacking in essential food substances, especially protein, vitamins, and iron. This inadequate diet often leads to nutritional deficiency disorders and growth retardation in children. On the other hand, these issues may contribute to pediatric overweight and type 2 diabetes because nonnourishing foods are less expensive and are easier to access in some neighborhoods.

Dental problems are more prevalent because of deficient preventive care. Lack of standard immunizations together with reduced resistance from poor nutrition renders children in poor segments of the population vulnerable to communicable diseases. Poor sanitation and crowded living conditions also contribute to the higher incidence and perpetuation of illness. In general, poor people become ill more frequently and remain ill for longer periods than those in the general population.

HOMELESSNESS

One of the most pressing problems in the United States is the growing number of homeless families. Homeless individuals are those persons who lack resources and community ties necessary to provide for their own adequate shelter. In the past the homeless population traditionally included single adults, mostly men. Families with children make up 40% of the homeless population, compared with single men, who make up about 41% of the group (Redlener, 2005). Homeless children have increased in numbers as poverty has become feminized, minorities have become poorer, and low-income housing has become less accessible. Estimates of the number of homeless children in the United States may be as high as 1 million; about 10% of the children living in poverty were homeless (Redlener, 2005). Many homeless children are younger than 5 years and are from minority groups.

Most homelessness is a direct result of an increasing number of people in poverty combined with a lack of decent, affordable housing. Other reasons include job layoffs, low incomes, parental mental illness, domestic conflict, and unexpected family or economic crises.

Another group of homeless children are the "runaway" and "throwaway" adolescents. Approximately 12% of the homeless population consists of adolescents (National Coalition to End Homelessness, 2009). Many runaways are victims of physical and sexual abuse and leave home because of long-term family or school problems. Poor parent–child relationships, extreme family conflict, feelings of alienation from parents, inconsistent supervision, and unpredictability in discipline are other often cited factors. These adolescents and young adults are at risk for violence, exploitation, substance abuse, and sexually transmitted infections (including HIV and AIDS).

Lack of a permanent housing deprives children of the most basic necessities for proper growth and development. Homelessness disrupts children's friendships and schooling. Homeless children experience physical and mental disorders more often than do poor children who have a permanent residence. Homeless children lack basic health care, including routine immunization and screening for routine problems, and they experience high rates of acute and chronic illnesses (Redlener, 2005).

MIGRANT FAMILIES

Children in migrant farm worker families are medically underserved. Their numbers are staggering; of the 2 million migrant farm workers who labor in the United States, 63% are accompanied by minor children (Gentry, Quandt, Davis, and others, 2007). These children face both acute and chronic health care issues as a result of poverty, parental occupation, and assimilation into American culture. They are often exposed to risks similar to those facing their parents because they may accompany them into the fields. These children frequently live in substandard housing conditions, which are subject to overcrowding and transmission of communicable diseases.

Migrant farm worker families face many obstacles when attempting to interface with the U.S. health care system. Three of every five families live below the federally designated poverty line and may lack insurance. The family's use of health care may be affected by parental work schedules and access to transportation. Their own limited English proficiency is further exacerbated by health care encounters that lack cultural sensitivity, translation services, and language capability. Cultural expectations of the health care system may differ between the farm worker families and health care providers. This may ultimately have a negative effect on families' utilization of the health care system. In fact, many families living on the United States–Mexico border seek the majority of care for their children in Mexico regardless of their insurance status. In addition, fewer than 20% of migrant farm worker families use the primary care and health promotion centers that are federally funded through the 1962 Migrant Health Act (Gentry, Quandt, Davis, and others, 2007).

Nurses and other health care providers should be mindful of the persistence of various forms of child labor in the United States (Hindman, 2006). Approximately 50% of 12- to 15-year-old children and teenagers participate in some sort of paid activity each year, and half of this population has jobs in which they are considered employees. Children, adolescents, and young adults may work in a variety of areas, including agriculture, construction, retail, or even street trades or scams. Youth who work on family farms often face the greatest risk of injury and death from handling dangerous or heavy machinery. Youth who work in street trades and scams or traveling sales crews may be subject to physical or verbal abuse or victimization (Hindman, 2006).

CULTURAL INFLUENCES

Nurses need to consider clients' cultural differences when providing health care. An understanding of the various beliefs regarding the causation of illness and disease, as well as traditional health practices, is essential to successful intervention. The more nurses know about the values, beliefs, and customs of other ethnic groups and how to elicit this information from families, the better they are able to meet the needs of these families and to gain their cooperation and compliance.

CULTURAL RELATIVITY

Although clinical characteristics of a disease or condition are essentially the same across cultures, how a child or family interprets or experiences the disease or condition varies. Culture as an influence is one obvious explanation for variance. Cultural relativity is the concept that any behavior must be judged first in the context of the culture in which it occurs. Cultural factors such as belief systems and view of the world influence the patient's and family's response to health care. These cultural beliefs and behaviors influence adherence to a treatment plan (Munoz and Luckmann, 2005). Some cultures, for example, may view a chronic illness or disability as affecting only particular aspects of a child's life, and the child as a whole is viewed as normal. In contrast, other families may describe the illness as having global effects on many aspects of the child's present and future life. These contrasting views may result in parents having different goals and expectations for their children.

Culture influences the assignment of gender roles, perception of disease, and perception of the side effects of the disease and the treatment the child should receive. For example, the family may expect the mother to be the primary caregiver. This places her at risk for caregiver strain when she is caring for a sick child.

Nurses can often recognize a family's health-related cultural perceptions and interpretations through discussion and observation. They should explore and consider implications of these perceptions when planning culturally appropriate interventions. Nurses must be comfortable having discussions with families about their cultural beliefs and practices. The conversations can begin easily as, "I want to take the best care of your child and family as possible. Is there anything in particular about your beliefs [cultural, religious, family] that you think I should know?"

RELATIONSHIPS WITH HEALTH CARE PROVIDERS

The manner of relating with health care providers differs considerably among cultural groups. For some nurses, one area of conflict is the attitude toward time and waiting that is part of some cultures. The time orientation of Hispanic and African-American ethnic groups is in the present. For example, African Americans are flexible in their time orientation; an African-American family may be late for or miss appointments because other issues take precedence, and they may not communicate this to the health agency. Hispanics, too, have a relaxed view of time. Whereas the dominant culture in the United States says that "time flies," the Hispanic says that "time walks."

The Japanese, on the other hand, consider time to be valuable and to be used wisely. They tend to be punctual for medical appointments and persistent in following prescribed regimens. A Vietnamese family will subordinate time to values considered to be more significant, such as propriety. They may be late for an appointment because of an overextended visit by a friend in their home. In general, Asian Americans view the American focus on time as offensive. They spend hours getting to know people and view predetermined, abrupt endings as rude. Introductory small talk is considered good manners.

Navajo Indians view time on a continuum with no beginning and no end. The present-time orientation may cause a Navajo to eat two meals a day today, four meals tomorrow, no meals the next day, and three meals the day after. This becomes an important nursing consideration if a Navajo is told to take medication with meals to ensure three doses per day.

In many cultural groups, the mother assumes the responsibility for health care; in others, both parents are involved equally in relationships with health workers. A somewhat different approach is apparent in some of the Asian cultures. For example, a Vietnamese or Filipino father, as unquestioned head of the family, is traditionally the one who interacts with persons, including health care providers, outside the family unit. In Hispanic families, the father, as head of the house, makes decisions regarding illness and treatment of adult family members, but the grandmother in the extended family is consulted regarding child care. Usually the family confers with other members before reaching a decision regarding treatment or hospitalization of a child. Arab families also rely on others to give advice and guidance in times of crisis. Japanese fathers may appear to be passive and uninvolved but actually are involved according to their own cultural standards.

Nurses should learn about any specific attitudes regarding the manner of approach to a child in a given culture. Navajo Indians do not like strangers near their infants. They fear that strangers may "witch" the child and cause the child harm. On the other hand, if a stranger, particularly a woman, lavishes attention on a Hispanic infant but fails to touch the child, some Hispanics believe the infant will develop symptoms of the "evil eye" (see p. 55). Vietnamese and Korean families may become upset if a newborn is admired at length for fear that evil spirits will overhear and desire the infant.

Some groups, such as the Amish, consider a child's admission to the hospital a family affair, with all members gathering to support and console the child and parents. In other groups, the family is willing to relinquish the care of the child to the hospital authority without interference. Their visits with the child are short but intense, and hospital staff may misinterpret this behavior as disinterest or abandonment.

All ethnic groups are entitled to be treated with dignity and respect. Family members should be addressed by their last names; many groups consider it an affront to be called by their first names. Stereotyping is to be condemned. People are individuals who are evaluated in relation to their cultural standards, needs, and preferences. For example, believing that fathers are never involved in the direct care of their children can result in wrong assumptions about a culture (Fig. 4-4).

Nurses who are members of a majority culture may encounter tension and distrust in a child from a minority culture as a result of the child's learned conceptions or relationships with other persons in the majority group. Based on these perceptions, minority children may suspect that nurses have hostile feelings toward them and fear ill treatment. When such children are hospitalized, this suspicion increases the feelings of loneliness and helplessness that accompany fearful events and separation from their families. The reverse situation may be encountered by a nurse from a minority culture attempting to meet the needs of a child who has been conditioned to view the nurse's cultural or ethnic group as inferior. Either situation is more likely to occur if the nurse or the child has had little or no personal contact with the other's culture. For example, a child from a minority culture from the inner city who lives in a neighborhood and attends school only with children from his or her minority culture may be more suspicious of a nurse from a different culture than would a child from the same minority group who lives in a culturally diverse neighborhood or attends an integrated school. Becoming familiar with cultures different from one's own and making an effort to know each other as individuals can shatter myths and, with time, build the trust needed to establish rewarding relationships among children, their families, and the nurse.

Communication

Communication is basic to all human relationships, but it may be a source of distress and misunderstanding between persons from different groups, such as speakers of different languages or even between the nurse and patient when the nurse only speaks in scientific, medical or nursing terms. Prejudice is one of the biggest barriers to cross-cultural communication. The Office of Minority Health and Health Disparities of the U.S. Department of Health and Human Services has established national standards on culturally and linguistically appropriate services in health care. Health care organizations must ensure the competence of language assistance provided to persons with limited English proficiency by interpreters and bilingual staff. Family and friends should not be used for interpretation services except on the patient's request (Shaw-Taylor, 2002). (See Communicating with Families Through an Interpreter, Chapter 6.)

Part of culturally sensitive communication is taking time to assess beliefs and values. In a study on childhood asthma, management researchers discovered that parents who believed asthma to be intermittent rather than a chronic condition provided suboptimal treatment to their children (Yoos, Kitzman, Henderson, and others, 2007). It is vital that the family members fully understand all implications of a child's care and management before they consent for special procedures or assume responsibility for the child's medication administration. Some persons with poor or limited language comprehension may simply smile and nod in agreement if they do not understand the questions or directives. It is common for an Asian family to indicate "yes" when in fact they mean "no" in order to avoid social disharmony. They tend to address issues indirectly rather than through confrontation and may become evasive when direct questioning makes them uncomfortable.

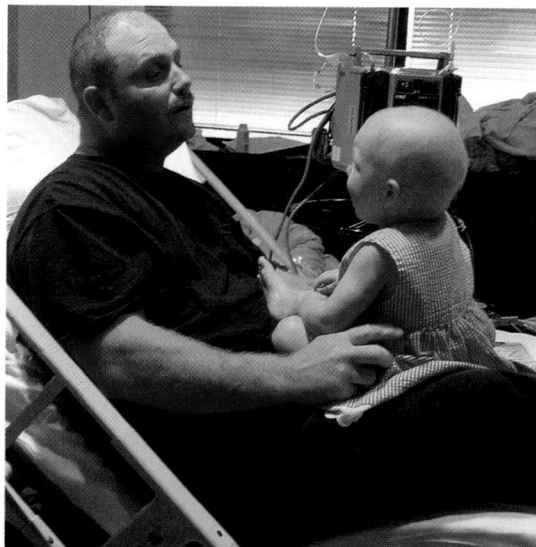

FIG 4-4 Many fathers assume an active parenting role. (Courtesy E. Jacob, Texas Children's Hospital, Houston.)

> **NURSING TIP** Helpful communication tools include:
> * Ask open-ended questions about cultural needs, health beliefs, and etiquette for communication.
> * If a live interpreter is not available, use a language line telephone interpreter.
> * Have legal consent forms and explanations of common diagnostic tests available in several languages.
> * Keep cards with common greetings, phrases, and names of body parts in the family's language with the patient's chart (e.g., *miseries* [pain] and *locked bowels* [constipation] for African Americans and *caida de la mollera* [fallen fontanel from dehydration]; *susto* [fright]; *dolor, duels,* or *lele* [pain]; and *la diarrhea* [diarrhea] for Hispanics).

Nonverbal communication is a practiced art in many Native American tribes, and the members are highly sensitive to body language. They emphasize periods of silence to formulate thoughts in preparation for speech and often remain silent after listening to others to properly assimilate what has been said. Interruption, interjection, or haste to arrive at a conclusion is perceived as immature behavior.

Different cultures view eye contact differently. European Americans are often advised to look people straight in the eye, but persons in other ethnic groups avoid eye contact and become uncomfortable when conversing with health care workers. In non-Western cultures, a patient may not look directly into the nurse's eyes as a sign of respect. Some Native Americans make eye contact during the initial greeting but consider continued, unwavering eye contact insulting and disrespectful. Asians may consider eye contact a sign of hostility or impoliteness.

The level of comfort with body space or distance from others varies among cultures. European Americans are generally comfortable at arm's length, Hispanics tend to get closer, and some Asians prefer a greater distance. Also, gestures may have different meanings. For example, some Asians consider pointing with a finger or foot disrespectful. Some Native Americans consider vigorous handshaking a sign of aggression, but for others, the gesture is a sign of goodwill and strong character.

Families may be reluctant to question or otherwise initiate contact with health professionals. In Asian cultures, for example, it is considered a sign of disrespect to question persons of authority. A Japanese family may wait silently rather than ask or question. They believe the health professionals know best and will meet their needs without being asked. They also think it is important to avoid criticism. Criticism can cause Japanese Americans to "lose face," or to feel ashamed, which is highly undesirable.

Many families have considered language the biggest barrier to the use of health care services. Often, families may have poor language comprehension, so it is necessary to speak slowly and carefully, not loudly, when conversing with them. Many persons are able to read and write English better than they can speak or understand it. Also, people usually revert to their dominant language in anxiety-provoking situations even if they are able to communicate satisfactorily under ordinary circumstances.

Terms of address and use of first and last names vary among cultures and can create confusion in institutions. For example, in Asian cultures, the family name is given first in respect for the family and the given names follow. Therefore, all siblings in a family have the same first name (or, in some families, the same middle name). The Mennonites refer to children as sons and daughters of a particular parent, such as "Josiah's son," rather than by the children's names.

Although all people share the basic emotions, there are decided ethnic variations in the ways emotions are expressed. People in some cultures (e.g., Italian, Latin, or Jewish background) express emotions openly and are accustomed to sharing their sorrows and joys with their family and friends. Conversely, Nordic and Asian groups are more restrained in expressing their emotions.

Health care providers generally ask questions and use handouts, booklets, and—particularly with children—dolls and pictures as communication aids. This is uncommon in some cultures. For example, Native American healers ask few questions and do not use forms. Nurses need to consider both verbal and nonverbal communication techniques to interact effectively with children and their families from different cultures.

FOOD CUSTOMS

Food customs and symbolism of various cultural, ethnic, and religious groups are an integral part of their lives. Although in a large country such as the United States most people have adopted the eclectic food habits that have evolved over generations, many still retain ethnic and geographic food traditions and preferences. Special holidays; ceremonies; and life experiences such as births, birthdays, weddings, and death are often marked by special food items or feasts. In many cultures, specific food practices are followed during pregnancy in the belief that certain foods damage or benefit developing fetuses. The distinctive food customs of ethnic groups are a product of their native environment, determined by availability.

A number of restrictions are related to food items. Some have a physiologic origin, such as lack of dairy foods in the diets of some persons of African or Asian ancestry with lactose intolerance. Others are religious restrictions, such as kosher foods and food preparation of the Orthodox Jewish faith and the vegetarian diet of Seventh Day Adventists. (See Vegetarian Diets, Chapter 13.)

Children in a strange environment, such as the hospital, feel much more comfortable when they are served familiar foods. Hospital food often tastes strange and bland, especially to children who enjoy the highly seasoned foods of their culture. Also, the family may be concerned that the child is not receiving foods appropriate to their culture and beliefs. When possible, provide the children's ethnic foods or allow families to bring favorite foods that are not on the hospital menu. Concern for differences in food habits and patterns projects an attitude of respect for the family's ethnic or religious heritage (Ohio State University Extension, 2005).

It is also important for nurses and other health care providers to be mindful of the meaning of food and eating within a family or community. Feeding and food preparation are ways in which families nurture and care for one another. This is especially true in the parent–child relationship. Parents and other family members may struggle with this desire to feed and nurture their child in circumstances when the child does not want to eat or cannot tolerate oral intake (i.e., a child receiving chemotherapy). Nurses can encourage families to nurture the sick child in other ways, such as touch, reading, or other enjoyable activities.

HEALTH BELIEFS AND PRACTICES

Nurses encounter people of many different racial and ethnic origins in the process of meeting the health needs of children and families. Some of these families have become so enculturated to the majority culture that their health beliefs and practices are consistent with those of the health care system. For many families, however, traditional practices and beliefs are an integral part of their daily lives. Health care workers should be aware that other people might live by different rules and priorities, which decisively influence their health-related behavior.

A model for learning about health traditions that differ from the Western, or modern, health care system is based on three dimensions:

1. What are the physical aspects of caring for the body (e.g., are there special clothes, foods, medicines)?
2. What are the mental parts of caring for health (e.g., feelings, attitudes, rituals, actions)?
3. What are the spiritual aspects of health (who I am, spiritual customs, prayers, healers)?

For each of these dimensions, one must consider the cultural traditions used to maintain health, protect health, and restore health (Spector, 2009).

HEALTH BELIEFS

The beliefs related to the cause of illness and the maintenance of health are integral parts of a family's cultural heritage. Often inseparable from religious beliefs, they influence the way families cope with health problems and respond to health care providers. Predominant among most cultures are beliefs related to natural forces, supernatural forces, and an imbalance between forces.

Natural Forces

The most common natural forces held responsible for ill health if the body is not adequately protected include cold air entering the body and impurities in the air. For example, a Chinese parent may overdress an infant in an effort to keep cold wind from entering the child's body. The Chinese believe that cold weather, rain, or wind is responsible for "cold" conditions. They also believe that an innate energy called *chi* enters and leaves the body through the mouth, nose, and ears and flows through the body in definite pathways, or meridians, at specific times and locations. The Chinese believe that a lack of chi and blood causes fatigue, low energy, and a variety of ailments.

Supernatural Forces

Some cultures view evil influences such as voodoo, witchcraft, or evil spirits as causes of illness, especially illnesses that cannot be explained by other means.

A health belief that is common among people from Latin American, Mediterranean, some Asian, and some African societies is the concept of the "evil eye" (Spector, 2009). It is part of the concept of health as a state of balance and illness as a state of imbalance (see following section). Strength and power are associated with the evil eye; therefore, as long as an individual's strength and weakness remain in balance, he or she is unlikely to become a victim of the evil eye. Weaknesses are not necessarily physical. For example, an excess of some emotion, such as envy, can create weakness. Infants and small children, because of immature development of their internal strength-weakness states, are especially vulnerable to the gaze of the evil eye. Consequently, the evil eye serves to rationalize an inexplicable onset of illness in children who display symptoms such as restlessness, crying, diarrhea, vomiting, and fever (see Complementary and Alternative Therapy box).

Imbalance of Forces

The concept of balance or equilibrium is widespread throughout the world. One of the most common imbalances is that which exists between "hot" and "cold." This belief derived from the ancient Greek concept of body humors (Andrews and Boyle, 2008), which states that illness is caused by an imbalance of the four humors: phlegm, blood, black bile, and yellow bile. These are balanced in healthy people and out of balance in those with illnesses. Such imbalance is thought to cause internal damage or altered function. Treatment of the illness is directed at restoring balance. The hot and cold understanding of disease is based in this concept. Diseases, areas of the body, foods, and illnesses are classified as either "hot" or "cold." Foods and beverages are designated hot or cold based on the effect they exert, not their actual temperature. In Chinese health belief, the forces are termed *yin* (cold) and *yang* (hot) (Spector, 2009).

Illness is treated by restoring normal balance through the application of appropriate "hot" or "cold" remedies. A "cold" condition such as a respiratory disease is believed to be caused by exposure to cold weather, rain, or cold wind entering the body; it is treated by administration of "hot" foods, herbs, or drugs. Menstruation is considered a "hot" condition; therefore, women are cautioned against ingesting "hot" foods, which might increase menstrual flow or produce cramping. Ingesting too much of either "hot" or "cold" foods can also be interpreted as a cause of illness.

Health care workers who are aware of this belief are better able to understand why some persons refuse to eat certain foods. It is often useful to discuss the diet with the family to determine their beliefs regarding food choices. It is possible to help families devise a diet that contains the necessary balance of basic food groups prescribed by the medical subculture while conforming to the beliefs of the ethnic subculture.

The "hot–cold" food classification may have adverse effects. For example, in some cultures, newborn infants are often started on evaporated milk formulas. Whereas evaporated milk is considered a "hot" food, whole milk is viewed as a "cold" food. Infants tend to develop rashes, which are believed to be caused by "hot" foods; in such cases, parents may decide to switch to whole milk. However, parents fear that it is dangerous to change too rapidly, so they often feed the child some type of neutralizing substance, which may create additional health problems. The nurse can help avoid such a problem by determining the family's preference before discharge from the hospital and prescribing a formula that is agreeable to both the family and the practitioner.

HEALTH PRACTICES

Cultures have numerous similarities regarding prevention and treatment of illness (see Complementary and Alternative Therapy box). The folk healers are powerful persons in their community and can

---

✿ COMPLEMENTARY AND ALTERNATIVE THERAPY
Cultural Health Influences

Cultural traditions used in the protection of health may include protective objects, which may be worn, carried, or hung in the home or room. For example, amulets are objects or charms that are worn on a string or chain to protect the wearer from the evil eye or evil spirits. It is important to allow people to wear these objects in the health care setting. Another cultural practice is the inclusion of substances in the diet that protect health. For example, the ginseng root is used to "build the blood" in the Chinese culture. Religious practices, such as burning candles or prayer, are also traditions used to protect health (Spector, 2009).

✿ COMPLEMENTARY AND ALTERNATIVE THERAPY
Spiritual Practices

All cultures have some types of home remedies that they apply before seeking help from other persons. Within various groups, folk healers who are endowed with the ability to "cure" maladies are sought for special situations and when home remedies are unsuccessful. The *curandero* (male) or *curandera* (female) of the Mexican-American community is believed to have healing powers that are a gift from God. The Asian family may consult an herbalist, knowledgeable in medicines, or perhaps a specialized practitioner of Asian therapies, including acupuncture (insertion of needles), acupressure (application of pressure), and moxibustion (application of heat). Native Americans consult a variety of healers with specific skills and knowledge. Specialized medicine persons diagnose illness, provide nonsacred treatments (usually by way of massage and herbs), and care for souls. Other specialists perform services or effect cures through the use of spiritual means. Native Hawaiians consult *kahunas* and practice *ho'oponopono* to heal family imbalance or disputes.

BOX 4-2   CULTURAL PRACTICES POSSIBLY CONSIDERED ABUSIVE BY THE DOMINANT CULTURE

Coining—A Vietnamese practice that may produce weltlike lesions on the child's back when the edge of a coin is repeatedly rubbed lengthwise on the oiled skin to rid the body of disease

Cupping—An Old World practice (also practiced by the Vietnamese) of placing a container (e.g., tumbler, bottle, jar) containing steam against the skin surface to "draw out the poison" or other evil element. When the heated air within the container cools, a vacuum is created that produces a bruiselike blemish on the skin directly beneath the mouth of the container.

Burning—A practice of some Southeast Asian groups whereby small areas of skin are burned to treat enuresis and temper tantrums

Female genital mutilation (female circumcision)—Removal of or injury to any part of the female genital organ; practiced in Africa, the Middle East, Latin America, India, Asia, North America, Australia, and Western Europe

Forced kneeling—A child discipline measure of some Caribbean groups in which a child is forced to kneel for a long time

Topical garlic application—A practice of Yemenite Jews in which crushed garlic cloves or garlic–petroleum jelly plaster is applied to the wrists to treat infectious disease. The practice can result in blisters or garlic burns.

Traditional remedies that contain lead—*Greta* and *azarcon* (Mexico; used for digestive problems), *paylooah* (Southeast Asia; used for rash or fever), and *surma* (India; used as a cosmetic to improve eyesight)

COMPLEMENTARY AND ALTERNATIVE THERAPY
Safety Topics

A health remedy that may be detrimental to a child's health is the mercury compound *azogue* (the Spanish name for quicksilver), which is commonly used in Mexico and sometimes sold illegally to low-income Hispanic families in the United States as a remedy for diarrhea. Alert health care workers know that the drug can cause permanent central nervous system damage. A careful history can reveal these practices, but it may require the collaboration of a folk healer to convince a user to stop.

FAMILY-CENTERED CARE
Cultural Awareness

A 15-month-old Bosnian girl in status epilepticus was carried in by her parents. They were frightened and spoke little English. I learned that the child had received a measles, mumps, and rubella (MMR) immunization the day before. As I proceeded to unwrap her from the blanket she was in, I quickly assessed the ABCs (airway, breathing, and circulation). I noticed that she was warm (probably a febrile seizure) and that a rag soaked in alcohol was tied around each thigh. Focusing on her potential airway compromise and trying to calm the parents, I proceeded to put an oxygen mask on her, undress her for a full assessment, and remove the alcohol rags. I spoke to the parents all the while in a calm, soothing voice. Once I had established an intravenous line and given her lorazepam (Ativan), the seizures stopped. So did the communication between her parents and me. I noticed that they would no longer give me eye contact, and the mother would not even speak to me after the seizures stopped. It wasn't until I was returning to the department from admitting her that I realized why they might have stopped communicating with me—I had removed the rags! Had I only thought to replace the rags or asked their permission to remove the rags, things may have been different.

Laura L. Kuensting, MSN(R), RN
Cardinal Glennon Children's Hospital
St. Louis, Missouri

---

acquire information about an illness without resorting to probing questions. They "speak the language" of the family who seeks help and often combine their rituals and potions with prayer and entreaties to God. They also are able to create an atmosphere conducive to successful management. Furthermore, they exhibit a sincere interest in the family and their problem.

Some folk remedies are compatible with the medical regimen and are useful to reinforce the treatment plan. For example, aspirin (a "hot" medication) is an appropriate therapy for "cold" diseases such as arthritis. It is common to discover that a folk prescription has a scientific basis. In any case, respect practices that do not harm patients.

In cultures that believe in the concept, overcoming the effect of the evil eye usually requires specialized rituals conducted by the appropriate practitioner. For example, the Latino *curandero* ascertains that the condition is truly the result of the evil eye by performing an assessment ritual and then performs a curative ritual. Sometimes faith in the folk practitioner delays obtaining needed medical treatment, although the practitioner usually suggests medical care if his or her efforts are unsuccessful.

Health practices of different cultures may also present problems of assessment and interpretation. For example, certain cultural practices or remedies can be mistakenly judged as evidence of child abuse by uninformed professionals (Box 4-2). It is important to keep the lines of communication open with families and approach the situation with a sense of cultural humility.

Faith healing and religious rituals are closely allied with many folk-healing practices. Wearing of amulets, medals, and other religious relics believed by the culture to protect the individual and facilitate healing is a common practice. It is important for health workers to recognize the value of this practice and keep the items where the family has placed them or nearby. It offers comfort and support and rarely impedes medical and nursing care. If an item must be removed during a procedure, it should be replaced, if possible, when the procedure is

completed. The nurse should explain the reason for its temporary removal to the family to reassure them their wishes will be respected (see Complementary and Alternative Therapy box and Family-Centered Care box).

IMPORTANCE OF CULTURAL COMPETENCE TO NURSES

Nurses are professionally, ethically, morally, and legally obligated to provide care that seeks to understand the varied and numerous cultural influences on the life of a child and family and that is consistent with their values and desires. The challenge for nurses is to gain knowledge about cultural care values, beliefs, and practices and to use this knowledge in the care they provide (Leininger, 2001). To understand and deal effectively with families in a multicultural community, nurses must be aware of their own attitudes and values. Nurses, too, are a product of their own cultural background and education. They are part of the "nursing culture." Nurses function within the framework of a professional culture with its own values and traditions and, as such, become socialized into that culture by educational programs and later by the work environment and professional associations.

Frequently, nurses and other health care workers are not aware of their own cultural values and how those values influence their thoughts

🌐 CULTURAL CONSIDERATIONS

Five Components of Cultural Competence

Cultural competence includes following five components (Munoz and Luckmann, 2005):

1. **Cultural awareness**—A cognitive process through which the nurse appreciates and is sensitive to the cultural values of the patient and family
2. **Cultural knowledge**—The foundation the nurse builds through formal and informal education that includes world views of different cultures, values, beliefs, and perceptions about health and illness
3. **Cultural skill**—The ability to include cultural data in the nursing assessment through the collection of cultural data in the health interview and observations
4. **Cultural encounter**—The process through which the nurse seeks opportunities to engage in cross-cultural interactions directly or indirectly
5. **Cultural desire**—The genuine and sincere motivation to work effectively with minority clients; can only be achieved if the individual wants to engage in the process of acquiring cultural competence

❗ NURSING ALERT

These generalizations are presented to help nurses learn the unique beliefs and practices of various groups and are not meant to be stereotypes of any group. It is critical to remember that no cultural group is homogeneous, every racial and ethnic group contains great diversity, and knowledge of a culture may not reflect an individual member's beliefs (Kleinman and Benson, 2006).

and actions. Nurses can practice self-reflection and critical reflection starting in the undergraduate nursing education. Self-reflection is integral to adjusting one's "frame of reference, which has been influenced by cultural assimilations and can serve to establish one's view of the world" (Boutin-Foster, Foster, and Konopasek, 2008, p. 108). A nurse can do this adjustment by thinking about his or her prior assumptions, considering the alternative perspective, and then shifting one's own perspective as he or she feels necessary. Critical reflection is another approach to self-reflection that encourages the nurse to understand how his or her perceptions of health, illness, and nursing have been formed over time (Boutin-Foster, and others, 2008). Cultural standards, values, and history; the family structure and function; and past experiences with health care influence a family's feelings and attitudes toward health, their children, and health care delivery systems. Relying only on one's own values and experiences for guidance can result in frustration and disappointment. It is one thing to know what is needed to deal with a health problem; it is often more difficult to implement a fruitful course of action unless nurses work within the cultural and socioeconomic framework of the family (see Critical Thinking Case Study, p. 46).

It is essential to make an effort to adapt health care practices to the family's health needs rather than attempt to change longstanding beliefs. Cultural humility is an active, dynamic, and lifelong process. The components of cultural competence outlined demonstrate not only the evolving nature of seeking the understanding of a child and family's culture but also how the nurse changes as a result (see Cultural Considerations box).

CULTURAL AWARENESS

Cultural and religious rituals are important practices among families from various cultures. An example is the Jewish upsherenish ceremony, which celebrates a boy's first haircut when he reaches 3 years of age. Any procedure requiring haircutting, such as placement of an intravenous line in a scalp vein, must be discussed with parents to obtain their permission.

Table 4-1 outlines some characteristics of selected cultures. Nurses must assess the cultural and religious practices of families to identify how these practices are similar to and different from those of their own cultural and religious backgrounds.

Concepts that come from medical anthropology can provide a framework for addressing health care issues. These concepts can have a direct impact on patient care. They lead the nurse away from an ethnocentric or medicocentric view of the health care encounter into the health care reality as constructed by the patient and family. This is relevant for addressing many of the problems that plague the American health care system, including patient dissatisfaction with the health care they receive, unequal distribution of high-quality health care, and excessive costs (Kleinman and Benson, 2006).

It is also important for nurses to recognize that disease and illness are distinct entities. Clinicians diagnose and treat diseases, abnormalities in the structure and function of body organs and systems. *Illness* and *disease* are not interchangeable; illness may occur even when disease is not present, and the course of a disease may vary substantially from the experience of illness.

Illness is culturally constructed; an individual's culture influences how a sickness is perceived, labeled, and explained. Culture also influences the meaning assigned to the illness, the role the individual with the sickness adopts, and the response of the family and community to the sickness.

Tension may arise when the perception of the illness and disease varies widely among the patient, family, and health care team. Failure of health care providers to recognize these disparities may be partially to blame in cases of noncompliance, delivery of inadequate care, and patient or family dissatisfaction. To begin addressing these issues, it is important for nurses to understand the various domains of health care in which individuals operate in American society, including professional (health care providers and institutions), popular (family, community, and lay literature), and folk (nonprofessional healers). Each domain possesses a method for defining and explaining the sickness and what should be done to address it. The challenge for nurses and other health care providers is to address this disconnect with families and develop mutually agreed on goals. Nurses are in a prime position to assume this role because understanding the human response to disease is central to their role. In addition, collaboration with the child and family is central to the role of the pediatric nurse.

Not all health care providers feel adequately prepared to care for culturally diverse populations. A study of 1700 resident physicians by Betancourt (2007) revealed that 25% to 30% of them did not feel prepared to deal with families who are mistrustful of the health care system, those with limited English proficiency, those whose health perspective differs from a Western-based model, adults who incorporate other family into the decision-making process, or those who bring their spirituality into the health care environment. Unfortunately, the numbers may not be too different for nursing and other health care professionals. Such statistics are a wake-up call for anyone who strives for high-quality patient care.

One method of addressing this disconnect with families and beginning collaboration is by understanding the family's explanatory model of illness. The questions in Box 4-3 (Kleinman and Benson, 2006) aim to elicit an individual's beliefs about the disease or illness, the meaning attached to it, goals, and expectations of the outcome and role of the

TABLE 4-1	BROAD CULTURAL CHARACTERISTICS RELATED TO THE HEALTH CARE OF CHILDREN AND FAMILIES		
HEALTH BELIEFS	**HEALTH PRACTICES**	**FAMILY RELATIONSHIPS**	**COMMUNICATION**
African			
Illness classified as:	Self-care and folk medicine prevalent	Strong kinship bonds in extended family; members come to aid of others in crisis	Alert to any evidence of discrimination
Natural—Affected by forces of nature without adequate protection (e.g., cold air, pollution, food and water)	Folk therapies usually religious in origin	Less likely to view illness as a burden	Place importance on nonverbal behavior
Unnatural—God's punishment for improper behavior	Folk therapies often not shared with the medical provider	Place strong emphasis on work and ambition	Affection shown by touching and hugging
May see illness as the "will of God"	Prayer as common means for prevention and treatment	Elders cared for and respected	Silence may indicate lack of trust
			Initial eye contact to show respect; maintaining eye contact can be viewed as aggressive
			Best to use direct but caring approach
Chinese			
A healthy body viewed as gift from parents and ancestors and must be cared for	Goal of therapy is to restore the balance of yin and yang	Extended family pattern common	Open expression of emotions unacceptable
Health seen as one of the results of balance between the forces of yin (cold) and yang (hot)—energy forces that rule the world	Acupuncturist needles applied to appropriate meridians identified in terms of yin and yang	Strong concept of loyalty of young to old	Often smile when they do not comprehend
Illness caused by an imbalance	Acupressure and tai chi replacing acupuncture in some areas	Respect for elders taught at early age—acceptance without questioning or talking back	Eye contact avoided as a sign of respect
Blood believed to be source of life and is not regenerated	Moxibustion—Application of heat to skin over specific meridians	Children's behavior a reflection on family	
Chi is innate energy	Wide use of medicinal herbs procured and applied in prescribed ways	Family and individual honor and "face" important	
	Meals may or may not be planned to balance hot and cold	Self-reliance and self-esteem highly valued; self-expression repressed	
Haitian			
Illness seen as a punishment	Health a personal responsibility	Maintenance of family reputation paramount	Recent immigrants and older persons may speak only Haitian Creole
Natural cause (*maladi bone die*—disease of the Lord) caused by environmental factors, movement of blood within the body, changes between hot and cold, and bone displacement	Foods have properties of "hot" or "cold" and "light" or "heavy" and must be in harmony with one's life cycle and bodily states	Lineal authority supreme; children in a subordinate position in family hierarchy	Often smile and nod in agreement when do not understand
Supernatural (*loa*—spirits' anger)	Natural illnesses treated by home and folk remedies first	Children valued for parental security in old age and expected to contribute to family welfare at an early age	Quiet and gentle communication style and lack of assertiveness lead health care providers to falsely believe they comprehend health teaching and are compliant
Good health seen as the maintenance of equilibrium	May use religious medallions, rosary beads, or figure of saint to pray with		May not ask questions if health care provider is busy or rushed
Prayer and good spiritual habits important			
Japanese			
Shinto religious influence	Energy restored by means of acupuncture, acupressure, massage, and moxibustion along affected meridians	Close intergenerational relationships	Make significant use of nonverbal communication with subtle gestures and facial expression
Human inherently good	*Kampō* medicine—Use of natural herbs	Generational categories:	Tend to suppress emotions
Evil caused by outside spirits		***Issei***—First generation to live in United States	Will often wait silently
Illness caused by contact with polluting agents (e.g., blood, corpses, skin diseases)	Believe in removal of diseased parts	***Nisei***—Second generation	
Health achieved through harmony and balance between self and society	Trend is to use both Western and Asian healing methods	***Sansei***—Third generation	
Disease caused by disharmony with society and not caring for body	Care for people with disabilities viewed as family's responsibility	***Yonsei***—Fourth generation	
	Take pride in child's good health	Family tends to keep problems to self	
	Seek preventive care and medical care for illness	Value self-control and self-sufficiency	
		Concept of *haji* (shame) imposes strong control; unacceptable behavior of children reflects on family	

TABLE 4-1	BROAD CULTURAL CHARACTERISTICS RELATED TO THE HEALTH CARE OF CHILDREN AND FAMILIES—cont'd		
HEALTH BELIEFS	**HEALTH PRACTICES**	**FAMILY RELATIONSHIPS**	**COMMUNICATION**
Mexican American			
Health controlled by environment, fate, and will of God Certain illnesses considered "hot" and "cold" states and are treated with food that complements those states Disease based on imbalance between individual and environment	Seek help from *curandero* or *curandera*, especially in rural areas *Curandero(a)* receives position by birth, apprenticeship, or a "calling" via dream or vision Treatments involve use of herbs, rituals, and religious artifacts Practice for severe illness—make promises, visit shrines, offer medals and candles, offer prayers Adhere to "hot" and "cold" food prescriptions and prohibitions for prevention and treatment of illness	Strong kinship—extended families include *compadres* (godparents) established by ritual kinship Children valued highly and desired, taken everywhere with family Elderly treated with respect	Spanish speaking or bilingual May have a strong preference for native language and revert to it in times of stress May shake hands or engage in introductory embrace Interpret prolonged eye contact as disrespectful Relaxed concept of time—may be late to appointments
Native American			
Believe health is state of harmony with nature and universe Respect bodies through proper management Depend on individual belief in traditional culture Traditional health beliefs holistic and wellness oriented	Distinction made between indigenous health problem requiring native healer or practice and Western disease requiring other medical care Health practices include self-sufficiency and harmonious living Participation in religious ceremonies and prayer promotes health	Cultures vary in kinship structure Extended family structure—usually includes relatives from both sides of family Elder members assume leadership roles	Use anecdotes or metaphors to discuss a situation Long pauses indicate careful consideration Nonverbal communication Respect indicated by avoiding eye contact Individuals usually speak for themselves
Puerto Rican			
Subscribe to the "hot–cold" theory of causation of illness Believe some illness caused by evil forces Destiny (*Si Dios quiere*—if God wants) is in control of health	Infrequent use of health care system Seek folk healers (*espiritistas*)—use of herbs, rituals Treatment classified as "hot" or "cold" Many varieties of herbal teas used to treat illness and promote healing	Family usually large and home centered—the core of existence Father has authority in family Great respect for elders Children valued—seen as a gift from God Children taught to obey and respect parents	Spanish speaking or bilingual Strong sense of family privacy—may view questions regarding family as impudent
Vietnamese			
Good health considered to be balance between yin and yang Concept of health based on harmony and balance Rituals used to prevent illness	Family uses all means possible before using outside agencies for health care Regard health as family responsibility; outside aid sought when resources run out Use herbal medicine, spiritual practices, and acupuncture May consider head sacred and feet profane; avoid touching head after feet May use cupping, coin rubbing, or pinching skin May inhale aromatic oils, take herbal teas, or wear strings tied on body	Family is revered institution Multigenerational families Family is chief social network Children highly valued Individual needs and interests subordinate to those of a family group Father is main decision maker Women taught submission to men Parents expect respect and obedience from children	May hesitate to ask questions Questioning authority is sign of disrespect; asking questions considered impolite May avoid eye contact with health professionals as a sign of respect

Data from Galanti G: *Caring for patients from different cultures*, ed 3, Philadelphia, 2004, University of Pennsylvania Press; Lipson JG, Dibble SL, Minarik PA: *Culture and clinical care: a pocket guide*, San Francisco, 2005, UCSF Nursing Press; Purnell LD, Paulanka BJ: *Transcultural health care: a culturally competent approach*, Philadelphia, 2003, FA Davis; and Spector RE: *Cultural diversity in health and illness*, ed 6, Upper Saddle River, NJ, 2004, Pearson Prentice Hall.

BOX 4-3   EXPLORING A FAMILY'S CULTURE, ILLNESS, AND CARE

What do you think caused your child's health problem?

Why do you think it started when it did?

How severe is your child's sickness? Will it have a short or long course?

How do you think your child's sickness affects your family?

What are the chief problems your child's sickness has caused?

What kind of treatment do you think your child should receive?

What are the most important results you hope to receive from your child's treatment?

What do you fear most about your child's sickness?

Adapted from Kleinman A, Eisenberg L, Good B: Culture, illness, and care: clinical lessons from anthropologic and cross-cultural research, *Ann Intern Med* 88:251-258, 1978.

health care provider. Nurses can use these questions to discern areas of discrepancy for further dialogue, negotiation, and collaboration. This discussion, when conducted with a genuine interest in the family and child's perspective, is a significant step in building trusting relationships, promoting adherence, decreasing disparities, and increasing health care satisfaction.

RELIGIOUS INFLUENCES

Religion and spirituality also exert a significant influence on the health of children and families and the decisions made around health and illness. Many immigrants came to the United States for religious freedom and established a religious and moral atmosphere that persists today. However, individual differences are part of the general culture.

The family's religious orientation dictates a code of behavior and influences the family's attitudes toward education, male and female role identity, and their ultimate destiny. It may also determine the school that the children attend, their companions, and often their mate selection. Religious beliefs are such an integral part of many cultures that it is difficult to distinguish the culture from the religion. In a few instances, such as in the Mennonite and Amish communities, religion is the basis for a common way of life that determines where the children are raised and their lifestyle. It is also important to remember that families that do not subscribe to a particular religion or that are atheist also have beliefs and convictions about family, the surrounding world, and life in general that influence children in these families.

RELIGIOUS BELIEFS

Religious and spiritual dimensions are among the most important influences in many people's lives (Fig. 4-5). The terms *religion* and *spirituality* are often used interchangeably, but this is a mistake. Spirituality is "concerned with the deepest levels of human experiencing, the places of deepest . . . meaning in and for our lives" (Mercer, 2006, p. 7). For children, in particular, spirituality possesses a relational consciousness; it concerns the child in relation to the source of power (God, Allah) that gives meaning to the relationship, other people, and the surrounding world, and within oneself (Mercer, 2006). Religion, on the other hand, is a particular and culturally influenced representation of human spirituality. Nurses promote holistic nursing care through an integration of spiritual and psychosocial care. The care focuses on activities that support a person's system of beliefs and worship, such as praying, reading religious materials, and performing religious rituals. In addition, it means being attentive and open to the

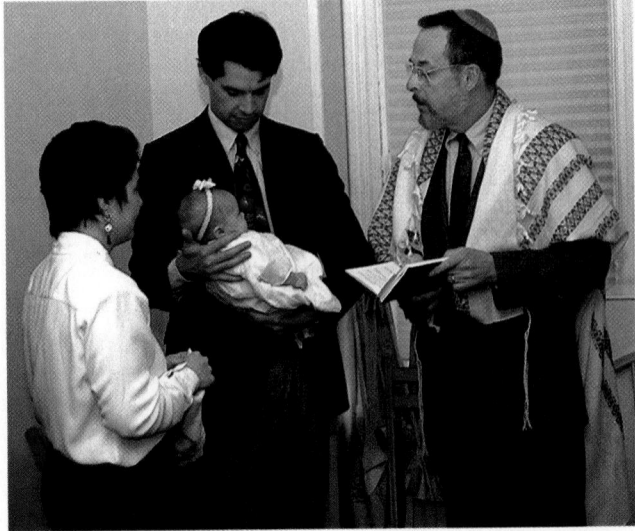

FIG 4-5 Soon after an infant is born, many families have special religious ceremonies.

BOX 4-4   GUIDELINES FOR INTEGRATING SPIRITUAL CARE INTO PEDIATRIC NURSING PRACTICE

- Respect the child and family's religious beliefs and practices.
- Consider the child's development when talking about spiritual concerns.
- Contact the institution's chaplaincy department for patients and families who have symptoms of spiritual distress or ask for specific religious rituals.
- Become knowledgeable about the religious world views of cultural groups found in the patients you care for.
- Encourage visitation with family members, members of the patient's spiritual community, and spiritual leaders.
- Allow children and families to teach you about the specifics of their religious beliefs.
- Develop awareness of your own spiritual perspective.
- Listen for understanding rather than agreement or disagreement.

Adapted from Brooks B: Spirituality. In Kline N, editor: *Essentials of pediatric oncology nursing: a core curriculum*, ed 2, Glenview, Ill, 2004, Association of Pediatric Oncology Nurses; Barnes LL, Plotnikoff GA, Fox K, and others: Spirituality, religion, and pediatrics: intersecting worlds of healing, *Pediatrics* 106(4 suppl):899–908, 2000.

unique spiritual experiences and insight of children. Unfortunately, "such insights may be dismissed as cute or the product of an overactive imagination" (Mercer, 2006, p. 8). Whereas meeting the spiritual needs of the child and family can provide strength, unmet spiritual needs can result in spiritual distress and debilitation. In practice, application of the nursing process for spiritual care (Box 4-4) can enhance the spiritual well-being of the child and family.

Religious beliefs that relate to health care and that may be a source of conflict between a family and the health care team remind us of the power of ordinary, daily life experience (e.g., childrearing and food preparation) to bring to life the concept of what is sacred (Mercer, 2006, p. 12). Religion and spirituality influence how individuals view an illness, a treatment regimen, and the role and utility of the health care provider. They also influence actions of food preparation and dietary restrictions and rituals surrounding birth and death (Table 4-2). A key role of nurses is to keep communication between the family and health care team open and ask about such influences.

TABLE 4-2 RELIGIOUS BELIEFS THAT MAY AFFECT NURSING CARE

BIRTH AND DEATH	DIET AND FOOD PRACTICES	MEDICAL CARE
Buddhist		
Birth—No baptism Infant presentation Death—Last rite chanting is often practiced at bedside soon after death; the deceased's family or Buddhist priest should be contacted Organ donation and transplantation—Organ donation is a matter of individual conscience	Restrictions on some food combinations; extremes must be avoided Some sects are strictly vegetarian Discourage use of alcohol and drugs	Illness is believed to be a trial to aid development of soul; illness results from Karmic causes Surgery is permitted, but extremes must be avoided Cleanliness is of great importance Family, community, and Buddhist priest are supportive visitors
Church of Christ, Scientist (Christian Science)		
Birth—No baptism Death—No last rites; autopsy is not permitted except in cases of sudden death; individuals can choose burial or cremation Organ donation and transplantation—Church takes no specific position on transplantation as distinct from other medical or surgical procedures Individuals decide on organ donation	Abstain from alcohol and some forms of tea and coffee	Oppose human intervention with drugs or other therapies; however, accept legally required immunizations Accept physical and moral healing Family, friends, and members of spiritual community may visit
Church of Jesus Christ of Latter-Day Saints (Mormon)		
Birth—No baptism Infant is blessed by church official at first opportunity after birth (in church) Baptism by immersion at 8 years Death—Believe that it is proper to bury the dead in the ground; cremation is discouraged Organ donation and transplantation—Individuals can choose whether to will organs to be used in transplants	Prohibit tea (except herbal), coffee, and alcohol Some individuals avoid chocolate and other products that contain caffeine Fasting for 24 hours each month	Devout adherents believe in divine healing Medical therapy is not prohibited Spiritual items—A "garment" (type of underwear) that is considered sacred; person may not want to remove it Family, friends, and church members are supportive visitors
Hindu		
Birth—No baptism Death—Certain prescribed rites are followed after death; priest may tie thread around neck or wrist to signify blessing; family will wash the body; are particular about who touches their dead; bodies are to be cremated Organ donation and transplantation—No religious laws prohibiting donation; individual decision	Many dietary restrictions Eating meat is forbidden	With an amputation, loss of a limb is believed to represent sins committed in previous life Accept most modern medical practices; some belief in faith healing Spiritual item—Person may wear a thread around wrist or body; do not remove it Family, community members, and priest are supportive visitors
Islam (Muslim/Moslem)		
Birth—At birth, the first words said to the infant in his or her right ear are *Allah-o-Akbar* (Allah is great), and the remainder of the Call for Prayer is recited; an *Aqeeqa* (party) to celebrate the birth of the child is arranged by the parents; male children are circumcised Death—At the time of death, specific rituals (e.g., bathing, wrapping the body in cloth) must be done by same-sex Muslim; before moving and handling the body, it is preferable to contact someone from the person's mosque or the local Islamic Society to perform these rituals Organ donation and transplantation—Individual decides	Prohibit all pork products and alcohol Fasting is practiced during the ninth month of the Islamic year (Ramadan)	Believers are encouraged in the Qu'ran to seek treatment; it is taught that only Allah cures; however, Muslims are taught not to refuse treatment in the belief that Allah will take care of them because he also chooses at times to work through the efforts of humans Other practices—Right hand is used for eating; left hand is for hygiene Family and friends are supportive visitors
Jehovah's Witnesses		
Birth—No baptism Death—No official last rites are practiced when death occurs Organ donation and transplantation—Organ donation is forbidden	No tobacco; moderate alcohol permissible	Blood or blood products are not allowed; volume expanders are permissible if not derived from blood

Continued

TABLE 4-2	RELIGIOUS BELIEFS THAT MAY AFFECT NURSING CARE—cont'd	
BIRTH AND DEATH	**DIET AND FOOD PRACTICES**	**MEDICAL CARE**
Judaism (Orthodox and Conservative) Birth—No baptism Ritual circumcision of male infants on eighth day; performed by *mohel* (ritual circumciser familiar with Jewish law and aseptic technique) Death—According to tradition, during last moments of life, relatives and close friends remain with the deceased Amputated limbs or surgically removed tissues should be made available to family for burial Cremation not allowed Organ donation and transplantation—A complex issue; sometimes they are practiced	Numerous dietary kosher laws exist; followers are allowed only meat from animals that are vegetable eaters and are ritually slaughtered; predatory fowl, shellfish, and pork are prohibited Milk products served first can be followed by meat in a few minutes, but milk may not be consumed for several hours after eating meat Fasting is part of Yom Kippur observance Matzo replaces leavened bread during Passover week	May resist surgical procedures during Sabbath, which extends from sundown Friday until sundown Saturday Illness is grounds for violating dietary laws Spiritual items—Men may wear prayer shawl, yarmulke (cap) while praying Family, friends, and rabbi are supportive visitors
Roman Catholic Birth—Infant baptism; especially urgent if poor prognosis, when it may be performed by anyone Death—Sacrament of the Sick is performed if prognosis is poor while patient is alive Organ donation and transplantation—Transplantation of organs is viewed by Catholics as ethically and morally acceptable to the Vatican; organ donation is viewed as an act of charity	Abstaining from meat is practiced on Ash Wednesday, Good Friday, and Fridays during Lent (as a rule)	Encourage anointing of the sick Spiritual items—Rosary beads, crucifix Traditional church teaching does not approve of contraceptives or abortion

Data from Galanti G: *Caring for patients from different cultures*, ed 3, Philadelphia, 2004, University of Pennsylvania Press; Lipson JG, Dibble SL, Minarik PA: *Culture and clinical care: a pocket guide*, San Francisco, 2005, UCSF Nursing Press; Purnell LD, Paulanka BJ: *Transcultural health care: a culturally competent approach*, Philadelphia, 2003, FA Davis; Spector RE: *Cultural diversity in health and illness*, ed 6, Upper Saddle River, NJ, 2004, Pearson Prentice Hall.

> **NURSING TIP** Children rarely voice a need for spiritual support. Listen closely for indirect references.

Respecting these rituals is especially important during a physical examination or preparation for surgery. An important role of the nurse is to be aware of families' spiritual needs and convey an attitude of concern for this important element of the child's care. Religion, which offers families understanding and spiritual support, is a valuable asset to health care. Table 4-2 outlines characteristics of selected religions with beliefs that affect health care.

In some instances, the rights of the family and the responsibility of the state may be in conflict. For example, Jehovah's Witnesses refuse blood transfusions for themselves and for their children. Parents, by law, have the primary obligation to care for and make decisions about their minor children. However, the legal principle of parens patriae says that the state has an overriding interest in the health and welfare of its citizens. Parents' refusal of medical treatment for their child that is deemed essential can be interpreted as neglect. In addition to advocating for the child and family, the nurse's role may include assuming the role of consultant to the staff and family regarding new, alternative methods of transfusion and, if necessary, coordinating with officials to petition juvenile or family court for temporary guardianship of the child.

▌ KEY POINTS

- Culture is the pattern of assumptions, beliefs, and practices encompassing other products of human work and thoughts specific to members of an intergenerational group, community, or population.
- Nurses have a responsibility to understand the influences of culture, race, and ethnicity on the development of social and emotional relationships, childrearing practices, and attitudes toward health.
- A child's self-concept evolves from ideas about his or her social roles.
- Primary groups are characterized by intimate contact, mutual support, and behavior constraint among members.
- Secondary groups have limited, intermittent contact; little mutual support; and no pressure for conformity.
- Culture influences a child's self-esteem.
- Important subcultural influences on children include ethnicity, social class, occupation, schools, peers, biculture, and mass media.
- A trend that has significantly influenced the American family is increasing geographic and economic mobility.
- The demographics of the U.S. population are shifting and demonstrate more racial and ethnic diversity. As of the 2010 census, the percentage of individuals who identify as Hispanic and African American has increased.

- Socioeconomic influences play a major role in opportunities for health promotion and wellness.
- Religious practices greatly influence health promotion beliefs in families.
- A child's physical characteristics and susceptibility to health problems are related to ethnic and cultural variations of hereditary and socioeconomic forces.
- Groups of children with greater physical and mental health problems are those living in poverty, those who are homeless, and those who have migrant families.
- Drug response, food sensitivity, disease resistance, physical characteristics, and disease states may demonstrate ethnic or cultural variations.

- Because verbal and nonverbal communication is an important cultural consideration, nurses need to acknowledge and respect their patients' practices for productive interaction to occur.
- Cultural beliefs related to cause of illness and maintenance of health may focus on natural forces, supernatural forces, or an imbalance of forces.
- The practice of cultural humility is continual and an important concept in the nursing process. Nurses can facilitate this process by recognizing cultural differences, integrating cultural knowledge, being aware of their own beliefs and practices, and acting in a culturally appropriate manner.
- No cultural group is homogeneous; every racial and ethnic group contains great diversity.

REFERENCES

Andrews MM, Boyle JS: *Transcultural concepts in nursing care*, ed 5, Philadelphia, 2008, Lippincott.

Annie E. Casey Foundation: *2011 kids count data book: state profiles of child well-being*, Baltimore, 2011, Author.

Beaulieu DL: Comprehensive reform and American Indian education. *J Am Indian Educ* 39(2): 29–38, 2000.

Betancourt J: Commentary on "Current approaches to integrating elements of cultural competence in nursing education," *J Transcult Nurs* 18(25 suppl):25S-27S, 2007.

Boutin-Foster C, Foster JC, Konopasek L: Physician, know thyself: the professional culture of medicine as a framework for teaching cultural competence, *Acad Med* 83:106–111, 2008.

Council on Communications and Media: Media violence—policy statement, *Pediatrics* 124(5): 1495–1503, 2009.

Demmert WG: *Improving academic performance among Native American students: a review of the research literature*, Charleston, WV, 2001, ERIC Clearinghouse on Rural Education and Small Schools, ED # 463 917.

Dunn AM: Culture competence and the primary care provider, *J Pediatr Health Care* 16(3):105–111, 2002.

Gentry K, Quandt SA, Davis SW, and others: Child healthcare in two farmworker populations, *J Commun Health* 32(6):419–431, 2007.

Hindman HD: Unfinished business: the persistence of child labor in the US, *Employee Responsibilities Rights J* 18(2): 125–131, 2006.

Humes KR, Jones NA, Ramirez RR: Overview of race and Hispanic origin: 2010, *U.S. Census Bureau 2010 Census Brief*, 2011, retrieved February 10, 2012 from http://www.census.gov/prod/cen2010/briefs/c2010br-02.pdf.

Jordan A: The role of media in children's development: an ecological perspective, *J Dev Behav Pediatr* 25(3):196–206, 2004.

Klass P, Needlman R, Zuckerman B: Reach out and get your patients to read, *Contemp Pediatr* 19(1):51–58, 2002.

Kleinman A, Benson P: Anthropology in the clinic: the problem of cultural competency

and how to fix it, *PLoS Med* 3(10):1673–1676, 2006.

Kumgari AK, Lypson ML: Beyond cultural competence: critical consciousness, social justice, and multicultural education, *Acad Med* 84(6):782–787, 2009.

Leininger MM: The theory of culture care diversity and universality. In Leininger MM, editor: *Culture care diversity and universality: a theory of nursing*, Sudbury, Mass, 2001, Jones & Bartlett.

Melendez L: Parental beliefs and practices around early self-regulation: the impact of culture and immigration, *Infants Young Child* 18(2):136–146, 2005.

Mercer JA: Children as mystics, sages, and holy fools: understanding the spirituality of children and its significance for clinical work, *Pastoral Psychology* 54(5):497–515, 2006.

Moreno M: Social networking sites and adolescents, *Pediatr Ann* 39(9):565–568, 2010.

Munoz CC, Luckmann J: *Transcultural communication in nursing*, Clifton Park, NY, 2005, Thomson Delmar Learning.

Murdock SH: Minority child population growth. In Cosby AG, Greenberg RE, Southward LH, and others, editors: *About children: an authoritative resource on the state of childhood today*, Elk Grove Village, Ill, 2005, American Academy of Pediatrics.

National Coalition to End Homelessness: *Youth*, 2009, retrieved March 28, 2009, from http://www.endhomelessness.org/section/policy/focusareas/youth.

Ohio State University Extension: *Cultural diversity: eating in America*, 2005, retrieved April 20, 2011, from http://www.nal.usda.gov/fnic/etext/000010.html.

Redlener I: Homelessness and its consequences. In Cosby AG, Greenberg RE, Southward LH, and others, editors: *About children: an authoritative resource on the state of childhood today*, Elk Grove Village, Ill, 2005, American Academy of Pediatrics.

Search Institute: *Developmental assets lists*, 2007, retrieved December 2, 2010, from http://www.search-institute.org/developmental-assets/lists.

Shaw-Taylor Y: Culturally and linguistically appropriate health care for racial or ethnic minorities: analysis of the US Office of Minority Health's recommended standards, *Health Policy* 62:211–221, 2002.

Spector RE: *Cultural diversity in health and illness*, ed 7, Upper Saddle River, NJ, 2009, Prentice-Hall.

Strasburger V: Children, adolescents, and the media: seven key issues, *Pediatr Ann* 39(9): 556–564, 2010.

Szilagyi PG: Health insurance. In Cosby AG, Greenberg RE, Southward LH, and others, editors: *About children: an authoritative resource on the state of childhood today*, Elk Grove Village, Ill, 2005, American Academy of Pediatrics.

Tervalon M: Components of culture in health for medical students' education. *Acad Med* 78(6):570–576, 2003.

Tervalon M, Murray-Garcia J: Cultural humility versus cultural competence: a critical distinction in defining physician training outcomes in multicultural education, *J Health Care Poor Underserved* 9(2):117–125, 1998.

Thibodeaux AG, Deatrick JA: Cultural influence on family management of children with cancer, *J Pediatr Oncol Nurs* 24(4):227–233, 2007.

Trawick-Smith J: *Early childhood development: a multicultural perspective*, ed 4, Upper Saddle River, NJ, 2006, Prentice-Hall.

U.S. Census Bureau: *Population distribution and change: 2000–2010*, retrieved May 7, 2011, from http://2010.census.gov/2010census.

U.S. Census Bureau: *Income, poverty, and health insurance in the United States: 2009*, Washington, DC, 2010, U.S. Government Printing Office.

Wertheimer R: Poverty. In Cosby AG, Greenberg RE, Southward LH, and others, editors: *About children: an authoritative resource on the state of childhood today*, Elk Grove Village, Ill, 2005, American Academy of Pediatrics.

Yoos HL, Kitzman H, Henderson C, and others: The impact of parental illness representation on disease management in childhood asthma, *Nurs Res* 56(3):167–174, 2007.

Developmental and Genetic Influences on Child Health Promotion

Quinn Franklin and Cynthia Prows

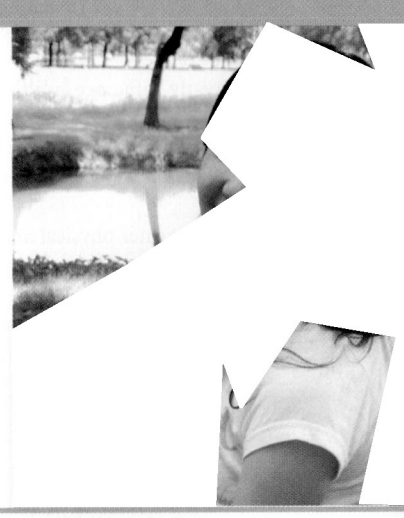

evolve WEBSITE

http://evolve.elsevier.com/wong/essentials
Key Point Summaries
NCLEX-Style Review Questions

CHAPTER OUTLINE

Growth and Development, 65
  Foundations of Growth and
    Development, 65
    Stages of Development, 65
    Patterns of Growth and
      Development, 65
    Individual Differences, 66
  Biologic Growth and Physical
    Development, 67
    External Proportions, 67
    Biologic Determinants of Growth and
      Development, 67
    Skeletal Growth and
      Maturation, 68
    Neurologic Maturation, 68
    Lymphoid Tissues, 68
    Development of Organ Systems, 69
  Physiologic Changes, 69
    Metabolism, 69
    Temperature, 69
    Sleep and Rest, 69
  Nutrition, 69
  Temperament, 70
    Significance of Temperament, 70

Development of Personality and Mental
  Function, 71
  Theoretic Foundations of Personality
    Development, 71
    Psychosexual Development (Freud), 71
    Psychosocial Development
      (Erikson), 71
  Theoretic Foundations of Mental
    Development, 72
    Cognitive Development (Piaget), 72
    Language Development, 73
    Moral Development (Kohlberg), 73
    Spiritual Development (Fowler), 74
  Development of Self-Concept, 74
    Body Image, 74
    Self-Esteem, 75
Role of Play in Development, 75
  Classification of Play, 75
  Content of Play, 75
  Social Character of Play, 76
  Functions of Play, 77
    Sensorimotor Development, 77
    Intellectual Development, 77
    Socialization, 77

    Creativity, 77
    Self-Awareness, 77
    Therapeutic Value, 77
    Morality, 78
  Toys, 78
Developmental Assessment, 78
  Denver II, 78
  Denver II Prescreening Developmental
    Questionnaire, 80
Genetic Factors that Influence
  Development, 80
  Overview of Genetics and Genomics, 80
    Genes, Genetics, and Genomics, 80
    Congenital Anomalies, 81
    Disorders of the Intrauterine
      Environment, 81
    Genetic Disorders, 81
    Role of Nurses in Genetics, 82
    Nursing Assessment: Applying and
      Integrating Genetic and Genomic
      Knowledge, 82
    Identification and Referral, 83
    Providing Education, Care, and
      Support, 83

LEARNING OBJECTIVES

On completion of this chapter the reader will be able to:
- Describe major trends in growth and development.
- Explain the alterations in the major body systems that take place during the process of growth and development.
- Discuss the development and relationships of personality, cognition, language, morality, spirituality, and self-concept.

- Describe the role of play in the growth and development of children.
- Demonstrate an understanding of the role of innate and environmental factors in the physical and emotional development of children.

GROWTH AND DEVELOPMENT

FOUNDATIONS OF GROWTH AND DEVELOPMENT

Growth and development, usually referred to as a unit, express the sum of the numerous changes that take place during the lifetime of an individual. The entire course is a dynamic process that encompasses several interrelated dimensions:

Growth—an increase in number and size of cells as they divide and synthesize new proteins; results in increased size and weight of the whole or any of its parts

Development—a gradual change and expansion; advancement from lower to more advanced stages of complexity; the emerging and expanding of the individual's capacities through growth, maturation, and learning

Maturation—an increase in competence and adaptability; aging; usually used to describe a qualitative change; a change in the complexity of a structure that makes it possible for that structure to begin functioning; to function at a higher level

Differentiation—processes by which early cells and structures are systematically modified and altered to achieve specific and characteristic physical and chemical properties; sometimes used to describe the trend of mass to specific; development from simple to more complex activities and functions

All of these processes are interrelated, simultaneous, and ongoing; none occurs apart from the others. The processes depend on a sequence of endocrine, genetic, constitutional, environmental, and nutritional influences (Seidel, Ball, Dains, and others, 2007). The child's body becomes larger and more complex; the personality simultaneously expands in scope and complexity. Very simply, growth can be viewed as a quantitative change and development as a qualitative change.

Stages of Development

Most authorities in the field of child development conveniently categorize child growth and behavior into approximate age stages or in terms that describe the features of a developmental age period. The age ranges of these stages are admittedly arbitrary and because they do not take into account individual differences, cannot be applied to all children with any degree of precision. However, categorization affords a convenient means to describe the characteristics associated with the majority of children at periods when distinctive developmental changes appear and specific developmental tasks must be accomplished. (A developmental task is a set of skills and competencies peculiar to each developmental stage that children must accomplish or master to deal effectively with their environment.) It is also significant for nurses to know that there are characteristic health problems peculiar to each major phase of development. The sequence of descriptive age periods and subperiods that are used here and elaborated in subsequent chapters is listed in Box 5-1.

Patterns of Growth and Development

There are definite and predictable patterns in growth and development that are continuous, orderly, and progressive. These patterns, or trends, are universal and basic to all human beings, but each human being accomplishes these in a manner and time unique to that individual.

Directional Trends

Growth and development proceed in regular, related directions or gradients and reflect the physical development and maturation of neuromuscular functions (Fig. 5-1). The first pattern is the cephalocaudal, or head-to-tail, direction. Whereas the head end of the organism develops first and is large and complex, the lower end is small and simple and takes shape at a later period. The physical evidence of this trend is most apparent during the period before birth, but it also applies to postnatal behavior development. Infants achieve structural control of the heads before they have control of their trunks and extremities, hold their backs erect before they stand, use their eyes

---

BOX 5-1   DEVELOPMENTAL AGE PERIODS

Prenatal Period—Conception to Birth
Germinal—Conception to ≈2 weeks
Embryonic—2 to 8 weeks
Fetal—8 to 40 weeks (birth)
A rapid growth rate and total dependency make this one of the most crucial periods in the developmental process. The relationship between maternal health and certain manifestations in the newborn emphasizes the importance of adequate prenatal care to the health and well-being of the infant.

Infancy Period—Birth to 12 Months
Neonatal—Birth to 27 or 28 days
Infancy—1 to ≈12 months
The infancy period is one of rapid motor, cognitive, and social development. Through mutuality with the caregiver (parent), the infant establishes a basic trust in the world and the foundation for future interpersonal relationships. The critical first month of life, although part of the infancy period, is often differentiated from the remainder because of the major physical adjustments to extrauterine existence and the psychologic adjustment of the parent.

Early Childhood—1 to 6 Years
Toddler—1 to 3 years
Preschool—3 to 6 years
This period, which extends from the time children attain upright locomotion until they enter school, is characterized by intense activity and discovery. It is a time of marked physical and personality development. Motor development advances steadily. Children at this age acquire language and wider social relationships, learn role standards, gain self-control and mastery, develop increasing awareness of dependence and independence, and begin to develop a self-concept.

Middle Childhood—6 to 11 or 12 Years
Frequently referred to as the *school age*, this period of development is one in which the child is directed away from the family group and centered around the wider world of peer relationships. There is steady advancement in physical, mental, and social development with emphasis on developing skill competencies. Social cooperation and early moral development take on more importance with relevance for later life stages. This is a critical period in the development of a self-concept.

Later Childhood—11 to 19 Years
Prepubertal—10 to 13 years
Adolescence—13 to ≈18 years
The tumultuous period of rapid maturation and change known as adolescence is considered to be a transitional period that begins at the onset of puberty and extends to the point of entry into the adult world—usually high school graduation. Biologic and personality maturation are accompanied by physical and emotional turmoil, and there is redefining of the self-concept. In the late adolescent period, the young person begins to internalize all previously learned values and to focus on an individual, rather than a group, identity.

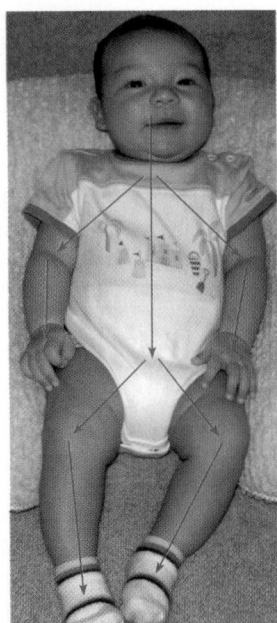

FIG 5-1 Directional trends in growth.

before their hands, and gain control of their hands before they have control of their feet.

Second, the **proximodistal**, or **near-to-far**, trend applies to the midline-to-peripheral concept. A conspicuous illustration is the early embryonic development of limb buds, which is followed by rudimentary fingers and toes. In infants, shoulder control precedes mastery of the hands, the whole hand is used as a unit before the fingers can be manipulated, and the central nervous system develops more rapidly than the peripheral nervous system.

These trends or patterns are bilateral and appear symmetric—each side develops in the same direction and at the same rate as the other. For some of the neurologic functions, this symmetry is only external because of unilateral differentiation of function at an early stage of postnatal development. For example, by the age of approximately 5 years, children have demonstrated a decided preference for the use of one hand over the other, although previously either one had been used.

The third trend, **differentiation**, describes development from simple operations to more complex activities and functions. From broad, global patterns of behavior, more specific, refined patterns emerge. All areas of development (physical, mental, social, and emotional) proceed in this direction. Through the process of development and differentiation, early embryonal cells with vague, undifferentiated functions progress to an immensely complex organism composed of highly specialized and diversified cells, tissues, and organs. Generalized development precedes specific or specialized development; gross, random muscle movements take place before fine muscle control.

Sequential Trends

In all dimensions of growth and development, there is a definite, predictable sequence, with each child normally passing through every stage. Children crawl before they creep, creep before they stand, and stand before they walk. Later facets of the personality are built on the early foundation of trust. The child babbles, then forms words, and finally sentences; writing emerges from scribbling.

Developmental Pace

Although development has a fixed, precise order, it does not progress at the same rate or pace. There are periods of accelerated growth and periods of decelerated growth in both total body growth and the growth of subsystems. Not all areas of development occur at the same pace. When a spurt occurs in one area such as gross motor, minimal advances may take place in language, fine motor, or social skills. After the gross motor skill has been achieved, development focus will shift to another area. The rapid growth before and after birth gradually levels off throughout early childhood. Growth is relatively slow during middle childhood, markedly increases at the beginning of adolescence, and levels off in early adulthood. Each child grows at his or her own pace. Distinct differences are observed among children as they reach developmental milestones.

> **NURSING TIP** Research suggests that normal growth, particularly height in infants, may occur in brief (possibly even 24-hour) bursts that punctuate long periods in which no measurable growth takes place. The researchers noted sex differences, with girls growing in length during the week they gained weight and boys growing in the week after a significant weight gain. Sex-specific growth hormone pulse patterns may coordinate body composition, weight gain, and linear growth (Lampl, Johnson, and Frongillo, 2001; Lampl, Thompson, and Frongillo, 2005). Furthermore, findings indicate a stuttering or saltatory pattern of growth that follows no regular cycle and can occur after "quiet" periods that last as long as 4 weeks. Mothers reported that their children were usually fussy and voraciously hungry a day or two before the growth spurt.

Sensitive Periods

There are limited times during the process of growth when the organism interacts with a particular environment in a specific manner. Periods termed **critical**, **sensitive**, **vulnerable**, and **optimal** are the times in the lifetime of an organism when it is more susceptible to positive or negative influences.

The quality of interactions during these sensitive periods determines whether the effects on the organism will be beneficial or harmful. For example, physiologic maturation of the central nervous system is influenced by the adequacy and timing of contributions from the environment such as stimulation and nutrition. The first 3 months of prenatal life are sensitive periods for physical growth of fetuses.

Psychologic development also appears to have sensitive periods when an environmental event has maximal influence on the developing personality. For example, primary socialization occurs during the first year when the infant makes the initial social attachments and establishes a basic trust in the world. A warm relationship with a parent figure is fundamental to a healthy personality. The same concept might be applied to readiness for learning skills such as toilet training or reading. In these instances, there appears to be an opportune time when the skill is best learned.

Individual Differences

Each child grows in his or her own unique and personal way. Great individual variation exists in the age at which developmental milestones are reached. The sequence is predictable; the exact timing is not. Rates of growth vary, and measurements are defined in terms of ranges to allow for individual differences. Some children are fast growers, others are moderate, and some are slower to reach maturity. Periods of fast growth, such as the pubescent growth spurt, may begin earlier or later in some children than in others. Children may grow fast or slowly during the spurt and may finish sooner or later than other children. Gender is an influential factor because girls seem to be more advanced in physiologic growth at all ages.

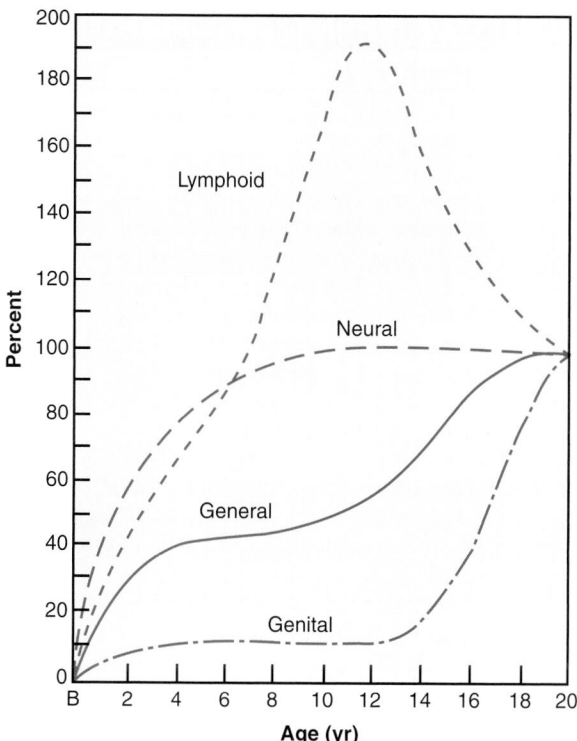

FIG 5-2 Growth rates for the body as a whole and three types of tissues. *Lymphoid:* thymus, lymph nodes, and intestinal lymph masses. *Neural:* brain, dura, spinal cord, optic apparatus, and head dimensions. *General:* body as a whole; external dimension; and respiratory, digestive, renal, circulatory, and musculoskeletal systems (Jackson, Patterson, and Harris, 1930).

BIOLOGIC GROWTH AND PHYSICAL DEVELOPMENT

As children grow, their external dimensions change. These changes are accompanied by corresponding alterations in structure and function of internal organs and tissues that reflect the gradual acquisition of physiologic competence. Each part has its own rate of growth, which may be directly related to alterations in the size of the child (e.g., the heart rate). Skeletal muscle growth approximates whole body growth; brain, lymphoid, adrenal, and reproductive tissues follow distinct and individual patterns (Fig. 5-2). When growth deficiency has a secondary cause, such as severe illness or acute malnutrition, recovery from the illness or the establishment of an adequate diet will produce a dramatic acceleration of the growth rate that usually continues until the child's individual growth pattern is resumed.

External Proportions

Variations in the growth rate of different tissues and organ systems produce significant changes in body proportions during childhood. The cephalocaudal trend of development is most evident in total body growth as indicated by these changes. During fetal development, the head is the fastest growing body part, and at 2 months of gestation, the head constitutes 50% of total body length. During infancy, growth of the trunk predominates; the legs are the most rapidly growing part during childhood; in adolescence, the trunk again elongates. In newborn infants, the lower limbs are one third the total body length but only 15% of the total body weight; in adults, the lower limbs constitute half of the total body height and 30% or more of the total body

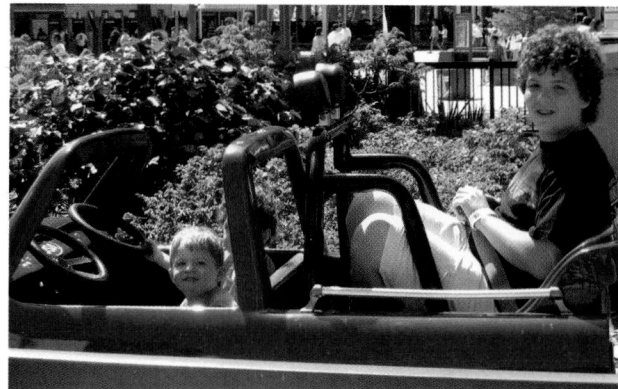

FIG 5-3 Changes in body proportions occur dramatically during childhood.

weight. As growth proceeds, the midpoint in head-to-toe measurements gradually descends from a level even with the umbilicus at birth to the level of the symphysis pubis at maturity.

Biologic Determinants of Growth and Development

The most prominent feature of childhood and adolescence is physical growth (Fig. 5-3). Throughout development, various tissues in the body undergo changes in growth, composition, and structure. In some tissues, the changes are continuous (e.g., bone growth and dentition); in others, significant alterations occur at specific stages (e.g., appearance of secondary sex characteristics). When these measurements are compared with standardized norms, a child's developmental progress can be determined with a high degree of confidence (Table 5-1). Growth in children with Down syndrome differs from that in other children. They have slower growth velocity between 6 months and 3 years and then again in adolescence. Puberty occurs earlier, and they achieve shorter stature. This population of patients is frequent users of the health care system, often with multiple providers, and benefit from the use of the Down syndrome growth chart to monitor their growth (Cronk, Crocker, Pueschel, and others, 1988; Myrelid, Gustafsson, Ollars, and others, 2002).

Linear growth, or height, occurs almost entirely as a result of skeletal growth and is considered a stable measurement of general growth. Growth in height is not uniform throughout life but ceases when maturation of the skeleton is complete. The maximum rate of growth in length occurs before birth, but newborns continue to grow at a rapid, although slower, rate.

> **NURSING TIP** Double the child's height at the age of 2 years to estimate how tall he or she may be as an adult.

At birth, weight is more variable than height and is, to a greater extent, a reflection of the intrauterine environment. The average newborn weighs from 3175 to 3400 g (7–7.5 pounds). In general, the birth weight doubles by 4 to 7 months of age and triples by the end of the first year. By the age of 2 to 2.5 years, the birth weight usually quadruples. After this point, the "normal" rate of weight gain, just as the growth in height, assumes a steady annual increase of approximately 2 to 2.75 kg (4.4–6 pounds) per year until the adolescent growth spurt.

Both bone age determinants and state of dentition are used as indicators of development. Because both are discussed elsewhere,

TABLE 5-1	GENERAL TRENDS IN HEIGHT AND WEIGHT GAIN DURING CHILDHOOD	
AGE GROUP	**WEIGHT***	**HEIGHT***
Infants		
Birth–6 months	Weekly gain—140–200 g (5–7 oz)	Monthly gain—2.5 cm (1 inch)
	Birth weight doubles by end of first 4–7 months†	
6–12 months	Weight gain—85–140 g (3–5 ounces)	Monthly gain—1.25 cm (0.5 inch)
	Birth weight triples by end of first year	Birth length increases by ≈50% by end of first year
Toddlers	Birth weight quadruples by age 2.5 years	Height at age 2 years is ≈50% of eventual adult height
		Gain during second year—about 12 cm (4.7 inches)
		Gain during third year—about 6–8 cm (2.4–3.1 inches)
Preschoolers	Yearly gain—2–3 kg (4.5–6.5 pounds)	Birth length doubles by age 4 years
		Yearly gain—5–7.5 cm (2–3 inches)
School-age children	Yearly gain—2–3 kg (4.5–6.5 pounds)	Yearly gain after age 7 years—5 cm (2 inches)
		Birth length triples by about age 13 years
Pubertal growth spurt		
Females—10–14 years	Weight gain—7–25 kg (15.5–55 pounds)	Height gain—5–25 cm (2–10 inches); ≈95% of mature height
	Mean—17.5 kg (38.5 pounds)	achieved by onset of menarche or skeletal age of 13 years
		Mean—20.5 cm (8 inches)
Males—11–16 years	Weight gain—7–30 kg (15.5–66 pounds)	Height gain—10–30 cm (4–12 inches); ≈95% of mature
	Mean—23.7 kg (52.2 pounds)	height achieved by skeletal age of 15 years
		Mean—27.5 cm (11 inches)

*Yearly height and weight gains for each age group represent averaged estimates from a variety of sources.
†Jung and Czajka-Narins, 1985.

neither is elaborated here (see next section for bone age; see also Chapters 10 and 12 for dentition).

Skeletal Growth and Maturation

The most accurate measure of general development is skeletal or bone age, the radiologic determination of osseous maturation. Skeletal age appears to correlate more closely with other measures of physiologic maturity (e.g., onset of menarche) than with chronologic age or height. Bone age is determined by comparing the mineralization of ossification centers and advancing bony form to age-related standards.

Bone formation begins during the second month of fetal life when calcium salts are deposited in the intercellular substance (matrix) to form calcified cartilage first and then true bone. Bone formation exhibits some differences. In small bones, the bone continues to form in the center, and cartilage continues to be laid down on the surfaces. In long bones, the ossification begins in the diaphysis (the long central portion of the bone) and continues in the epiphysis (the end portions of the bone). Between the diaphysis and the epiphysis, an epiphyseal cartilage plate (or growth plate) unites with the diaphysis by columns of spongy tissue, the metaphysis. Active growth in length takes place in the epiphyseal growth plate. Interference with this growth site by trauma or infection can result in deformity.

The first centers of ossification appear in 2-month-old embryos, and at birth, the number is approximately 400, about half the number at maturity. New centers appear at regular intervals during the growth period and provide the basis for assessment of bone age. Postnatally, the earliest centers to appear (at 5–6 months of age) are those of the capitate and hamate bones in the wrist. Therefore, radiographs of the hand and wrist provide the most useful areas for screening to determine skeletal age, especially before age 6 years. These centers appear earlier in girls than in boys.

Nurses must understand that the growing bones of children possess many unique characteristics. Bone fractures occurring at the growth plate may be difficult to discover and may significantly affect subsequent growth and development (Urbanski and Hanlon, 1996). Factors that may influence skeletal muscle injury rates and types in children and adolescents include (Caine, DiFiori, and Maffulli, 2006; Kaczander, 1997):

- Less protective sports equipment for children
- Less emphasis on conditioning, especially flexibility
- In adolescents, fractures that are more common than ligamentous ruptures because of the rapid growth rate of the physeal (segment of tubular bone that is concerned mainly with growth) zone of hypertrophy

Neurologic Maturation

In contrast to other body tissues, which grow rapidly after birth, the nervous system grows proportionately more rapidly before birth. Two periods of rapid brain cell growth occur during fetal life, a dramatic increase in the number of neurons between 15 and 20 weeks of gestation and another increase at 30 weeks, which extends to 1 year of age. The rapid growth of infancy continues during early childhood and then slows to a more gradual rate during later childhood and adolescence.

Postnatal growth consists of increasing the amount of cytoplasm around the nuclei of existing cells, increasing the number and intricacy of communications with other cells, and advancing their peripheral axons to keep pace with expanding body dimensions. This allows for increasingly complex movement and behavior. Neurophysiologic changes also provide the foundation for language, learning, and behavior development. Neurologic or electroencephalographic development is sometimes used as an indicator of maturational age in the early weeks of life.

Lymphoid Tissues

Lymphoid tissues contained in the lymph nodes, thymus, spleen, tonsils, adenoids, and blood lymphocytes follow a growth pattern unlike that of other body tissues. These tissues are small in relation to total body size, but they are well developed at birth. They increase rapidly to reach adult dimensions by 6 years of age and continue to grow. At about age 10 to 12 years, they reach a maximum development that is approximately twice their adult size. This is followed by a rapid decline to stable adult dimensions by the end of adolescence.

Development of Organ Systems

All tissues and organ systems undergo changes during development. Some are striking; others are subtle. Many have implications for assessment and care. Because the major importance of these changes relates to their dysfunction, the developmental characteristics of various systems and organs are discussed throughout the book as they relate to these areas. Physical characteristics and physiologic changes that vary with age are included in age-group descriptions.

PHYSIOLOGIC CHANGES

Physiologic changes that take place in all organs and systems are discussed as they relate to dysfunction. Other changes such as pulse and respiratory rates and blood pressure are an integral part of physical assessment (see Chapter 6). In addition, there are changes in basic functions, including metabolism, temperature, and patterns of sleep and rest.

Metabolism

The rate of metabolism when the body is at rest (**basal metabolic rate**, or **BMR**) demonstrates a distinctive change throughout childhood. Highest in newborn infants, the BMR closely relates to the proportion of surface area to body mass, which changes as the body increases in size. In both sexes, the proportion decreases progressively to maturity. The BMR is slightly higher in boys at all ages and further increases during pubescence over that in girls.

The rate of metabolism determines the caloric requirements of the child. The basal energy requirement of infants is about 108 kcal/kg of body weight and decreases to 40 to 45 kcal/kg at maturity. Water requirements throughout life remain at approximately 1.5 ml/calorie of energy expended. Children's energy needs vary considerably at different ages and with changing circumstances. The energy requirement to build tissue steadily decreases with age following the general growth curve; however, energy needs vary with the individual child and may be considerably higher. For short periods (e.g., during strenuous exercise) and more prolonged periods (e.g., illness), the needs can be very high.

> **NURSING TIP** Each degree of fever increases the basal metabolism 10%, with a correspondingly increased fluid requirement.

Temperature

Body temperature, reflecting metabolism, decreases over the course of development (see inside back cover). Thermoregulation is one of the most important adaptation responses of infants during the transition from intrauterine to extrauterine life. In healthy neonates, hypothermia can result in several negative metabolic consequences such as hypoglycemia, elevated bilirubin levels, and metabolic acidosis. Skin-to-skin care, also referred to as kangaroo care, is an effective way to prevent neonatal hypothermia in infants. Unclothed, diapered infants are placed on the parent's bare chest after birth, promoting thermoregulation and attachment (Galligan, 2006). After the unstable regulatory ability in the neonatal period, heat production steadily declines as the infant grows into childhood. Individual differences of 0.5° F to 1° F

are normal, and occasionally a child normally displays an unusually high or low temperature. Beginning at approximately 12 years of age, girls display a temperature that remains relatively stable, but the temperature in boys continues to fall for a few more years. Females maintain a temperature slightly above that of males throughout life.

Even with improved temperature regulation, infants and young children are highly susceptible to temperature fluctuations. Body temperature responds to changes in environmental temperature and is increased with active exercise, crying, and emotional stress. Infections can cause a higher and more rapid temperature increase in infants and young children than in older children. In relation to body weight, an infant produces more heat per unit than adolescents. Consequently, during active play or when heavily clothed, an infant or small child is likely to become overheated.

Sleep and Rest

Sleep, a protective function in all organisms, allows for repair and recovery of tissues after activity. As in most aspects of development, there is wide variation among individual children in the amount and distribution of sleep at various ages. As children mature, there is a change in the total time they spend in sleep and the amount of time they spend in deep sleep.

Newborn infants sleep much of the time that is not occupied with feeding and other aspects of their care. As infants grow older, the total time spent in sleep gradually decreases, they remain awake for longer periods, and they sleep longer at night. For example, the length of a sleep cycle increases from approximately 50 to 60 minutes in newborn infants to approximately 90 minutes in adolescents (Anders, Sadeh, and Appareddy, 2005). During the latter part of the first year, most children sleep through the night and take one or two naps during the day. By the time they are 12 to 18 months old, most children have eliminated the second nap. After age 3 years, children have usually given up daytime naps except in cultures in which an afternoon nap or siesta is customary. Sleep time declines slightly from ages 4 to 10 years and then increases somewhat during the pubertal growth spurt.

The quality of sleep changes as children mature. As children develop through adolescence, their need for sleep does not decline, but their opportunity for sleep may be affected by social, activity, and academic schedules. The time spent in deep, restful sleep increases from 50% in infancy to 80% in older children.

NUTRITION

Nutrition is probably the single most important influence on growth. Dietary factors regulate growth at all stages of development, and their effects are exerted in numerous and complex ways. During the rapid prenatal growth period, poor nutrition may influence development from the time of implantation of the ovum until birth. During infancy and childhood, the demand for calories is relatively great, as evidenced by the rapid increase in both height and weight. At this time, protein and caloric requirements are higher than at almost any period of postnatal development. As the growth rate slows, with its concomitant decrease in metabolism, there is a corresponding reduction in caloric and protein requirements.

Growth is uneven during the periods of childhood between infancy and adolescence, when there are plateaus and small growth spurts. Children's appetites fluctuate in response to these variations until the turbulent growth spurt of adolescence, when adequate nutrition is extremely important but may be subjected to numerous emotional influences. Adequate nutrition is closely related to good health throughout life, and an overall improvement in nourishment is

Healthy Food Choices

Current research indicates that new lower fat recipes in school lunch programs are well accepted by children (Matvienko, 2007). However, less-healthy foods are still more readily available than more-healthy foods in our nation's schools (Delva, O'Malley, and Johnston, 2007).

BOX 5-2 ATTRIBUTES OF TEMPERAMENT

Activity—Level of physical motion during activity such as sleep, eating, play, dressing, and bathing

Rhythmicity—Regularity in the timing of physiologic functions such as hunger, sleep, and elimination

Approach-withdrawal—Nature of initial responses to a new stimulus such as people, situations, places, foods, toys, and procedures. (**Approach** responses are positive and are displayed by activity or expression; **withdrawal** responses are negative expressions or behaviors.)

Adaptability—Ease or difficulty with which the child adapts or adjusts to new or altered situations

Threshold of responsiveness (sensory threshold)—Amount of stimulation, such as sounds or light, required to evoke a response in the child

Intensity of reaction—Energy level of the child's reactions regardless of quality or direction

Mood—Amount of pleasant, happy, friendly behavior compared with unpleasant, unhappy, crying, unfriendly behavior exhibited by the child in various situations

Distractibility—Ease with which a child's attention or direction of behavior can be diverted by external stimuli

Attention span and persistence—Length of time a child pursues a given activity (**attention**) and the continuation of an activity despite obstacles (**persistence**)

BOX 5-3 ACTIVITIES TO PROMOTE MASTERY MOTIVATION

- Encourage unobtrusive assistance during play.
- Share pleasure with infant in accomplishments.
- Don't give immediate assistance during tasks.
- Don't interrupt infant during tasks.
- Let infant initiate activities.
- Limit controlling feedback during play.
- Provide audio and visually responsive toys.
- Provide early kinesthetic stimulation (picking up, rocking).

From Morrow JD, Camp BW: Mastery motivation and temperament of 7-month-old infants, *Pediatr Nurs* 22(3):211–217, 1996.

---

evidenced by the gradual increase in size and early maturation of children in this century (see Community Focus box).

TEMPERAMENT

Temperament is defined as "the manner of thinking, behaving, or reacting characteristic of an individual" (Chess and Thomas, 1999) and refers to the way in which a person deals with life. From the time of birth, children exhibit marked individual differences in the way they respond to their environment and the way others, particularly the parents, respond to them and their needs. A genetic basis has been suggested for some differences in temperament. Nine characteristics of temperament have been identified through interviews with parents (Box 5-2). Temperament refers to behavioral tendencies, not to discrete behavioral acts. There are no implications of good or bad. Most children can be placed into one of three common categories based on their overall pattern of temperamental attributes:

The easy child—Easygoing children are even tempered, are regular and predictable in their habits, and have a positive approach to new stimuli. They are open and adaptable to change and display a mild to moderately intense mood that is typically positive. Approximately 40% of children fall into this category.

The difficult child—Difficult children are highly active, irritable, and irregular in their habits. Negative withdrawal responses are typical, and they require a more structured environment. These children adapt slowly to new routines, people, and situations. Mood expressions are usually intense and primarily negative. They exhibit frequent periods of crying, and frustration often produces violent tantrums. This group represents about 10% of children.

The slow-to-warm-up child—Slow-to-warm-up children typically react negatively and with mild intensity to new stimuli and, unless pressured, adapt slowly with repeated contact. They respond with only mild but passive resistance to novelty or changes in routine. They are inactive and moody but show only moderate irregularity in functions. Fifteen percent of children demonstrate this temperament pattern.

Thirty-five percent of children either have some, but not all, of the characteristics of one of the categories or are inconsistent in their behavioral responses. Many normal children demonstrate this wide range of behavioral patterns.

Significance of Temperament

Observations indicate that children who display the difficult or slow-to-warm-up patterns of behavior are more vulnerable to the development of behavior problems in early and middle childhood. Any child can develop behavior problems if there is dissonance between the child's temperament and the environment. Demands for change and adaptation that are in conflict with the child's capacities can become excessively stressful. However, authorities emphasize that it is not the temperament patterns of children that place them at risk; rather, it is the degree of fit between children and their environment, specifically their parents, that determines the degree of vulnerability. The potential for optimum development exists when environmental expectations and demands fit with the individual's style of behavior and the parents' ability to navigate this period (Chess and Thomas, 1999) (see Growth Failure [Failure to Thrive], Chapter 11).

Early identification of temperament provides a useful tool for caregivers in anticipating probable areas of difficulty or risk associated with development. For example, "difficult" children may be prone to colic in infancy, active children require more vigilance to prevent injury, and school entry requires different approaches for children with different temperaments.

Research indicates that irritable and unadaptable infants can raise doubts in mothers about their competence (Beck, 1996). Additional research indicates that a child's temperament can affect parent–child interactions and can influence the parents' self-esteem, marital harmony, mood, and overall satisfaction as parents (Carey, 1998). Studies on the relationship between temperament and the ability to perform a task successfully (mastery motivation) have found that infants with high mastery are more cooperative and less difficult (Morrow and Camp, 1996). Principles that can be used by nurses in direct patient care and in providing anticipatory guidance are listed in Box 5-3.

TABLE 5-2	SUMMARY OF PERSONALITY, COGNITIVE, AND MORAL DEVELOPMENT THEORIES			
PSYCHOSEXUAL (FREUD)	**PSYCHOSOCIAL (ERIKSON)**	**COGNITIVE (PIAGET)**	**MORAL JUDGMENT (KOHLBERG)**	**SPIRITUAL (FOWLER)**
I. Infancy—Birth–1 Year				
Oral	Trust vs mistrust	Sensorimotor (birth–2 years)		Undifferentiated
II. Toddlerhood—1–3 Years				
Anal	Autonomy vs shame and doubt	Preoperational thought, preconceptual phase (transductive reasoning [e.g., specific to specific]) (2–4 years)	Preconventional (premoral) level Punishment and obedience orientation	Intuitive-projective
III. Early Childhood—3–6 Years				
Phallic	Initiative vs guilt	Preoperational thought, intuitive phase (transductive reasoning) (4–7 years)	Preconventional (premoral) level Naive instrumental orientation	Mythical-literal
IV. Middle Childhood—6–12 Years				
Latency	Industry vs inferiority	Concrete operations (inductive reasoning and beginning logic) (7–11 years)	Conventional level Good-boy, nice-girl orientation Law-and-order orientation	Synthetic-convention
V. Adolescence—12–18 Years				
Genital	Identity vs role confusion	Formal operations (deductive and abstract reasoning) (11–15 years)	Postconventional or principled level Social-contract orientation	Individuating-reflexive

DEVELOPMENT OF PERSONALITY AND MENTAL FUNCTION

Personality and cognitive skills develop in much the same manner as biologic growth—new accomplishments build on previously mastered skills. Many aspects depend on physical growth and maturation. This is not a comprehensive account of the multiple facets of personality and behavior development. Many aspects are integrated with the child's emotional and social development in later discussion of various age groups. Table 5-2 summarizes some of the developmental theories.

THEORETIC FOUNDATIONS OF PERSONALITY DEVELOPMENT

Psychosexual Development (Freud)

According to Freud, all human behavior is energized by psychodynamic forces, and this psychic energy is divided among three components of personality: the id, ego, and superego (Freud, 1933). The id, the unconscious mind, is the inborn component that is driven by instincts. The id obeys the pleasure principle of immediate gratification of needs, regardless of whether the object or action can actually do so. The ego, the conscious mind, serves the reality principle. It functions as the conscious or controlling self that is able to find realistic means for gratifying the instincts while blocking the irrational thinking of the id. The superego, the conscience, functions as the moral arbitrator and represents the ideal. It is the mechanism that prevents individuals from expressing undesirable instincts that might threaten the social order.

Freud considered the sexual instincts to be significant in the development of the personality (Freud, 1964). However, he used the term *psychosexual* to describe any sensual pleasure. During childhood, certain regions of the body assume a prominent psychologic significance as the source of new pleasures and new conflicts gradually shifts from one part of the body to another at particular stages of development:

Oral stage (birth–1 year)—During infancy, the major source of pleasure seeking is centered on oral activities such as sucking, biting, chewing, and vocalizing. Children may prefer one of these over the others, and the preferred method of oral gratification can provide some indication of the personality they develop.

Anal stage (1–3 years)—Interest during the second year of life centers in the anal region as sphincter muscles develop and children are able to withhold or expel fecal material at will. At this stage, the climate surrounding toilet training can have lasting effects on children's personalities.

Phallic stage (3–6 years)—During the phallic stage, the genitalia become an interesting and sensitive area of the body. Children recognize differences between the sexes and become curious about the dissimilarities. This is the period around which the controversial issues of the Oedipus and Electra complexes, penis envy, and castration anxiety are centered.

Latency period (6–12 years)—During the latency period, children elaborate on previously acquired traits and skills. Physical and psychic energy are channeled into acquisition of knowledge and vigorous play.

Genital stage (age 12 years and older)—The last significant stage begins at puberty with maturation of the reproductive system and production of sex hormones. The genital organs become the major source of sexual tensions and pleasures, but energies are also invested in forming friendships and preparing for marriage.

Psychosocial Development (Erikson)

The most widely accepted theory of personality development is that advanced by Erikson (1963). Although built on Freudian theory, it is known as psychosocial development and emphasizes a healthy personality as opposed to a pathologic approach. Erikson also uses the biologic concepts of critical periods and epigenesis, describing key conflicts or core problems that the individual strives to master during critical periods in personality development. Successful completion or mastery of each of these core conflicts is built on the satisfactory completion or mastery of the previous stage.

Each psychosocial stage has two components—the favorable and the unfavorable aspects of the core conflict—and progress to the next stage depends on resolution of this conflict. No core conflict is ever mastered completely but remains a recurrent problem throughout life. No life situation is ever secure. Each new situation presents the conflict in a new form. For example, when children who have satisfactorily achieved a sense of trust encounter a new experience (e.g., hospitalization), they must again develop a sense of trust in those responsible for their care in order to master the situation. Erikson's life-span approach to personality development consists of eight stages; however, only the first five relating to childhood are included here:

Trust versus mistrust (birth–1 year)—The first and most important attribute to develop for a healthy personality is basic **trust**. Establishment of basic trust dominates the first year of life and describes all of the child's satisfying experiences at this age. Corresponding to Freud's oral stage, it is a time of "getting" and "taking in" through all the senses. It exists only in relation to something or someone; therefore, consistent, loving care by a mothering person is essential for development of trust. **Mistrust** develops when trust-promoting experiences are deficient or lacking or when basic needs are inconsistently or inadequately met. Although shreds of mistrust are sprinkled throughout the personality, from a basic trust in parents stems trust in the world, other people, and oneself. The result is **faith** and **optimism**.

Autonomy versus shame and doubt (1–3 years)—Corresponding to Freud's anal stage, the problem of autonomy can be symbolized by the holding on and letting go of the sphincter muscles. The development of autonomy during the toddler period is centered on children's increasing ability to control their bodies, themselves, and their environment. They want to do things for themselves using their newly acquired motor skills of walking, climbing, and manipulating and their mental powers of selecting and decision making. Much of their learning is acquired by imitating the activities and behavior of others. Negative feelings of doubt and shame arise when children are made to feel small and self-conscious, when their choices are disastrous, when others shame them, or when they are forced to be dependent in areas in which they are capable of assuming control. The favorable outcomes are self-control and willpower.

Initiative versus guilt (3–6 years)—The stage of initiative corresponds to Freud's phallic stage and is characterized by vigorous, intrusive behavior; enterprise; and a strong imagination. Children explore the physical world with all their senses and powers (Fig. 5-4). They develop a conscience. No longer guided only by outsiders, they have an inner voice that warns and threatens. Children sometimes undertake goals or activities that are in conflict with those of parents or others, and being made to feel that their activities or imaginings are bad produces a sense of guilt. Children must learn to retain a sense of initiative without impinging on the rights and privileges of others. The lasting outcomes are direction and purpose.

Industry versus inferiority (6–12 years)—The stage of industry is the latency period of Freud. Having achieved the more crucial stages in personality development, children are ready to be workers and producers. They want to engage in tasks and activities that they can carry through to completion; they need and want real achievement. Children learn to compete and cooperate with others, and they

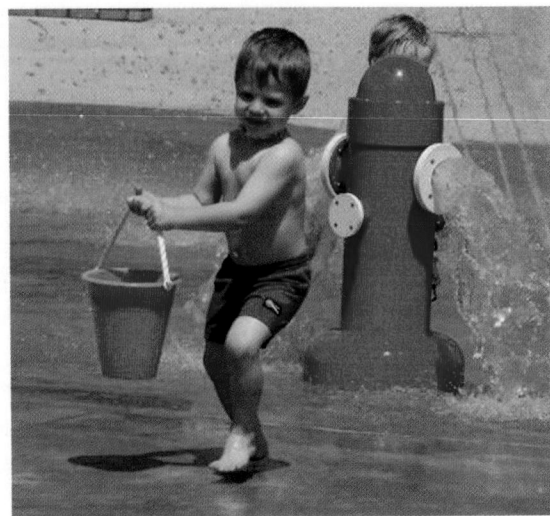

FIG 5-4 The stage of initiative is characterized by physical activity and imagination while children explore the physical world around them.

learn the rules. It is a decisive period in their social relationships with others. Feelings of inadequacy and inferiority may develop if too much is expected of them or if they believe that they cannot measure up to the standards set for them by others. The ego quality developed from a sense of industry is competence.

Identity versus role confusion (12–18 years)—Corresponding to Freud's genital period, the development of identity is characterized by rapid and marked physical changes. Previous trust in their bodies is shaken, and children become overly preoccupied with the way they appear in the eyes of others compared with their own self-concept. Adolescents struggle to fit the roles they have played and those they hope to play with the current roles and fashions adopted by their peers, to integrate their concepts and values with those of society, and to come to a decision regarding an occupation. An inability to solve the core conflict results in role confusion. The outcome of successful mastery is devotion and fidelity to others and to values and ideologies.

THEORETIC FOUNDATIONS OF INTELLECTUAL DEVELOPMENT

The term cognition refers to the process by which developing individuals become acquainted with the world and the objects it contains. Children are born with inherited potentials for intellectual growth, but they must develop that potential through interaction with the environment. By assimilating information through the senses, processing it, and acting on it, they come to understand relationships between objects and between themselves and their world. With cognitive development, children acquire the ability to reason abstractly, to think in a logical manner, and to organize intellectual functions or performances into higher order structures. Language, morals, and spiritual development emerge as cognitive abilities advance.

Cognitive Development (Piaget)

Cognitive development consists of age-related changes that occur in mental activities. The best-known theory regarding children's thinking, and a more comprehensive developmental theory than those already described, was developed by the Swiss psychologist Jean Piaget (1969). According to Piaget, intelligence enables individuals to make adaptations to the environment that increase the probability of survival, and through their behavior, individuals establish and maintain equilibrium with the environment.

Piaget (1969) proposed three stages of reasoning: (1) intuitive, (2) concrete operational, and (3) formal operational. When they enter the stage of concrete logical thought at about age 7 years, children are able to make logical inferences, classify, and deal with quantitative relationships about concrete things. Not until adolescence are they able to reason abstractly with any degree of competence. Each stage is derived from and builds on the accomplishments of the previous stage in a continuous, orderly process. The course of intellectual development is both maturational and invariant and is divided into the following stages (ages are approximate):

Sensorimotor (birth–2 years)—The sensorimotor stage of intellectual development consists of six substages (see pp. 319 and 380) that are governed by sensations in which simple learning takes place. Children progress from reflex activity through simple repetitive behaviors to imitative behavior. They develop a sense of cause and effect as they direct behavior toward objects. Problem solving is primarily by trial and error. They display a high level of curiosity, experimentation, and enjoyment of novelty and begin to develop a sense of self as they are able to differentiate themselves from their environment. They become aware that objects have **permanence**—that an object exists even though it is no longer visible. Toward the end of the sensorimotor period, children begin to use language and representational thought.

Preoperational (2–7 years)—The predominant characteristic of the preoperational stage of intellectual development is **egocentrism**, which in this sense does not mean selfishness or self-centeredness, but the inability to put oneself in the place of another. Children interpret objects and events not in terms of general properties but in terms of their relationships or their use to them. They are unable to see things from any perspective other than their own; they cannot see another's point of view, nor can they see any reason to do so (see Cognitive Development, Chapter 13).

Preoperational thinking is concrete and tangible. Children cannot reason beyond the observable, and they lack the ability to make deductions or generalizations. Thought is dominated by what they see, hear, or otherwise experience. However, they are increasingly able to use language and symbols to represent objects in their environment. Through imaginative play, questioning, and other interactions, they begin to elaborate concepts and to make simple associations between ideas. In the latter stage of this period, their reasoning is **intuitive** (e.g., the stars have to go to bed just as they do), and they are only beginning to deal with problems of weight, length, size, and time. Reasoning is also **transductive**—because two events occur together, they cause each other, or knowledge of one characteristic is transferred to another (e.g., all women with big bellies have babies).

Concrete operations (7–11 years)—At this age, thought becomes increasingly logical and coherent. Children are able to classify, sort, order, and otherwise organize facts about the world to use in problem solving. They develop a new concept of permanence—**conservation** (see Cognitive Development [Piaget], Chapter 16); that is, they realize that physical factors such as volume, weight, and number remain the same even though outward appearances are changed. They are able to deal with a number of different aspects of a situation simultaneously. They do not have the capacity to deal in abstraction; they solve problems in a concrete, systematic fashion based on what they can perceive. Reasoning is **inductive**. Through progressive changes in thought processes and

relationships with others, thought becomes less self-centered. They can consider points of view other than their own. Thinking has become socialized.

Formal operations (11–15 years)—Formal operational thought is characterized by adaptability and flexibility. Adolescents can think in abstract terms, use abstract symbols, and draw logical conclusions from a set of observations. For example, they can solve the following question: If A is larger than B and B is larger than C, which symbol is the largest? (The answer is A.) They can make hypotheses and test them; they can consider abstract, theoretic, and philosophic matters. Although they may confuse the ideal with the practical, most contradictions in the world can be dealt with and resolved.

Language Development

Children are born with the mechanism and capacity to develop speech and language skills. However, they do not speak spontaneously. The environment must provide a means for them to acquire these skills. Speech requires intact physiologic structure and function (including respiratory, auditory, and cerebral) plus intelligence, a need to communicate, and stimulation.

The rate of speech development varies from child to child and is directly related to neurologic competence and cognitive development. Gesture precedes speech, and in this way, a small child communicates satisfactorily. As speech develops, gesture recedes but never disappears entirely. Research suggests that infants can learn sign language before vocal language and that it may enhance the development of vocal language (Thompson, Cotner-Bichelman, McKerchar, and others, 2007). At all stages of language development, children's comprehension vocabulary (what they understand) is greater than their expressed vocabulary (what they can say), and this development reflects a continuing process of modification that involves both the acquisition of new words and the expanding and refining of word meanings previously learned. By the time they begin to walk, children are able to attach names to objects and persons.

The first parts of speech used are nouns, sometimes verbs (e.g., "go"), and combination words (e.g., "bye-bye"). Responses are usually structurally incomplete during the toddler period, although the meaning is clear. Next they begin to use adjectives and adverbs to qualify nouns followed by adverbs to qualify nouns and verbs. Later, pronouns and gender words are added (e.g., "he" and "she"). By the time children enter school, they are able to use simple, structurally complete sentences that average five to seven words.

Moral Development (Kohlberg)

Children also acquire moral reasoning in a developmental sequence. Moral development, as described by Kohlberg (1968), is based on cognitive developmental theory and consists of the following three major levels, each of which has two stages:

Preconventional level—The preconventional level of moral development parallels the preoperational level of cognitive development and intuitive thought. Culturally oriented to the labels of good/bad and right/wrong, children integrate these in terms of the physical or pleasurable consequences of their actions. At first, children determine the goodness or badness of an action in terms of its consequences. They avoid punishment and obey without question those who have the power to determine and enforce the rules and labels. They have no concept of the basic moral order that supports these consequences. Later, children determine that the right behavior consists of that which satisfies their own needs (and sometimes the needs of others). Although elements of fairness, give and take, and equal sharing are evident, they are interpreted in a practical, concrete manner without loyalty, gratitude, or justice.

Conventional level—At the conventional stage, children are concerned with conformity and loyalty. They value the maintenance of family, group, or national expectations regardless of consequences. Behavior that meets with approval and pleases or helps others is considered good. One earns approval by being "nice." Obeying the rules, doing one's duty, showing respect for authority, and maintaining the social order are the correct behaviors. This level is correlated with the stage of concrete operations in cognitive development.

Postconventional, autonomous, or **principled level**—At the postconventional level, the individual has reached the cognitive stage of formal operations. Correct behavior tends to be defined in terms of general individual rights and standards that have been examined and agreed on by the entire society. Although procedural rules for reaching consensus become important, with emphasis on the legal point of view, there is also emphasis on the possibility for changing law in terms of societal needs and rational considerations.

The most advanced level of moral development is one in which self-chosen ethical principles guide decisions of conscience. These are abstract and ethical but universal principles of justice and human rights with respect for the dignity of persons as individuals. It is believed that few persons reach this stage of moral reasoning.

Spiritual Development (Fowler)

Spiritual beliefs are closely related to the moral and ethical portion of the child's self-concept and, as such, must be considered as part of the child's basic needs assessment. Children need to have meaning, purpose, and hope in their lives. Also, the need for confession and forgiveness is present, even in very young children. Extending beyond religion (an organized set of beliefs and practices), spirituality affects the whole person, including the mind, body, and spirit. Fowler (1981) has identified seven stages in the development of faith, many of which are closely associated with and parallel cognitive and psychosocial development in childhood:

Stage 0: Undifferentiated—This stage of development encompasses the period of infancy during which children have no concept of right or wrong, no beliefs, and no convictions to guide their behavior. However, the beginnings of a faith are established with the development of basic trust through their relationships with the primary caregiver.

Stage 1: Intuitive-projective—Toddlerhood is primarily a time of imitating the behavior of others. Children imitate the religious gestures and behaviors of others without comprehending any meaning or significance to the activities. During the preschool years, children assimilate some of the values and beliefs of their parents. Parental attitudes toward moral codes and religious beliefs convey to children what they consider to be good and bad. Children still imitate behavior at this age and follow parental beliefs as part of their daily lives rather than through an understanding of their basic concepts.

Stage 2: Mythical-literal—Through the school-age years, spiritual development parallels cognitive development and is closely related to children's experiences and social interaction. Most children have a strong interest in religion during the school-age years. They accept the existence of a deity, and petitions to an omnipotent being are important and expected to be answered; good behavior is rewarded, and bad behavior is punished. Their developing conscience bothers them when they disobey. They have a reverence for thoughts and matters and are able to articulate their faith. They may even question the validity of their faith.

Stage 3: Synthetic-convention—As children approach adolescence, however, they become increasingly aware of spiritual disappointments. They recognize that prayers are not always answered (at least on their own terms) and may begin to abandon or modify some religious practices. They begin to reason, to question some of the established parental religious standards, and to drop or modify some religious practices.

Stage 4: Individuating-reflexive—Adolescents become more skeptical and begin to compare the religious standards of their parents with those of others. They attempt to determine which standards to adopt and incorporate into their own set of values. They also begin to compare religious standards with the scientific viewpoint. It is a time of searching rather than reaching. Adolescents are uncertain about many religious ideas but will not achieve profound insights until late adolescence or early adulthood.

DEVELOPMENT OF SELF-CONCEPT

Self-concept is how an individual describes him- or herself. The term self-concept includes all of the notions, beliefs, and convictions that constitute an individual's self-knowledge and that influence that individual's relationships with others. It is not present at birth but develops gradually as a result of unique experiences within the self, significant others, and the realities of the world. However, an individual's self-concept may or may not reflect reality.

In infancy, the self-concept is primarily an awareness of one's independent existence learned in part as a result of social contacts and experiences with others. The process becomes more active during toddlerhood as children explore the limits of their capacities and the nature of their impact on others. School-age children are more aware of differences among people, are more sensitive to social pressures, and become more preoccupied with issues of self-criticism and self-evaluation. During early adolescence, children focus more on physical and emotional changes taking place and on peer acceptance. Self-concept is crystallized during later adolescence as young people organize their self-concept around a set of values, goals, and competencies acquired throughout childhood.

Body Image

A vital component of self-concept, body image refers to the subjective concepts and attitudes that individuals have toward their own bodies. It consists of the physiologic (the perception of one's physical characteristics), psychologic (values and attitudes toward the body, abilities, and ideals), and social nature of one's image of self (the self in relation to others). All three of the components interrelate with one another. Body image is a complex phenomenon that evolves and changes during the process of growth and development. Any actual or perceived deviation from the "norm" (no matter how this is interpreted) is cause for concern. The extent to which a characteristic, defect, or disease affects children's body image is influenced by the attitudes and behavior of those around them.

The significant others in their lives exert the most important and meaningful impact on children's body image. Labels that are attached to them (e.g., "skinny," "pretty," or "fat") or body parts (e.g., "ugly mole," "bug eyes," or "yucky skin") are incorporated into the body image. Because they lack the understanding of deviations from the physical standard or norm, children notice prominent differences in others and unwittingly make rude or cruel remarks about such minor deviations as large or widely spaced front teeth, large or small eyes, moles, or extreme variations in height.

Infants receive input about their bodies through self-exploration and sensory stimulation from others. As they begin to manipulate their environment, they become aware of their bodies as separate from others. Toddlers learn to identify the various parts of their bodies and are able to use symbols to represent objects. Preschoolers become aware of the wholeness of their bodies and discover the genitalia. Exploration of the genitalia and the discovery of differences between the sexes become important. At this age, children have only a vague concept of internal organs and function (Stuart and Laraia, 2000).

School-age children begin to learn about internal body structure and function and become aware of differences in body size and configuration. They are highly influenced by the cultural norms of society and current fads. Children whose bodies deviate from the norm are often criticized or ridiculed. Adolescence is the age when children become most concerned about the physical self. The unfamiliar body changes, and the new physical self must be integrated into the self-concept. Adolescents face conflicts over what they see and what they visualize as the ideal body structure. Body image formation during adolescence is a crucial element in the shaping of identity, the psychosocial crisis of adolescence.

Self-Esteem

Self-esteem is the value that an individual places on oneself and refers to an overall evaluation of oneself (Willoughby, King, and Polatajko, 1996). Whereas self-esteem is described as the affective component of the self, self-concept is the cognitive component; however, the two terms are almost indistinguishable and are often used interchangeably.

The term self-esteem refers to a personal, subjective judgment of one's worthiness derived from and influenced by the social groups in the immediate environment and individuals' perceptions of how they are valued by others. Self-esteem changes with development. Highly egocentric toddlers are unaware of any difference between competence and social approval. On the other hand, preschool and early school-age children are increasingly aware of the discrepancy between their competencies and the abilities of more advanced children. Being accepted by adults and peers outside the family group becomes more important to them. Positive feedback enhances their self-esteem; they are vulnerable to feelings of worthlessness and are anxious about failure.

As children's competencies increase and they develop meaningful relationships, their self-esteem rises. Their self-esteem is again at risk during early adolescence when they are defining an identity and sense of self in the context of their peer group. Unless children are continually made to feel incompetent and of little worth, a decrease in self-esteem during vulnerable times is only temporary. Children assess the following aspects of themselves in forming an overall evaluation of their self-esteem (Sieving and Zirbel-Donisch, 1990):

Competence—How adequate are my cognitive, physical, and social skills?

Sense of control—How well can I complete tasks needed to produce desired actions? Is someone or something specific versus luck or chance responsible for my successes and failures?

Moral worth—How closely do my actions and behaviors meet moral standards that have been set?

Worthiness of love and acceptance—How worthy am I of love and acceptance from parents, other significant adults, siblings, and peers?

Factors that influence the formation of a child's self-esteem include (1) the child's temperament and personality, (2) abilities and opportunities available to accomplish age-appropriate developmental tasks, (3) how significant others interact with the child, and (4) social roles assumed and the expectations of these roles (see also Psychosocial History, Chapter 6).

ROLE OF PLAY IN DEVELOPMENT

Through the universal medium of play, children learn what no one can teach them. They learn about their world and how to deal with this environment of objects, time, space, structure, and people. They learn about themselves operating within that environment—what they can do, how to relate to things and situations, and how to adapt themselves to the demands society makes on them. Play is the work of children. In play, children continually practice the complicated, stressful processes of living, communicating, and achieving satisfactory relationships with other people.

CLASSIFICATION OF PLAY

From a developmental point of view, patterns of children's play can be categorized according to content and social character. In both there is an additive effect; each builds on past accomplishments, and some element of each is maintained throughout life. At each stage in development, the new predominates.

CONTENT OF PLAY

The content of play involves primarily the physical aspects of play, although social relationships cannot be ignored. The content of play follows the directional trend of the simple to the complex:

Social-affective play—Play begins with social-affective play, wherein infants take pleasure in relationships with people. As adults talk, touch, nuzzle, and in various ways elicit responses from an infant, the infant soon learns to provoke parental emotions and responses with such behaviors as smiling, cooing, or initiating games and activities. The type and intensity of the adult behavior with children vary among cultures.

Sense-pleasure play—Sense-pleasure play is a nonsocial stimulating experience that originates from without. Objects in the environment—light and color, tastes and odors, textures and consistencies—attract children's attention, stimulate their senses, and give pleasure. Pleasurable experiences are derived from handling raw materials (water, sand, food), body motion (swinging, bouncing, rocking), and other uses of senses and abilities (smelling, humming) (Fig. 5-5).

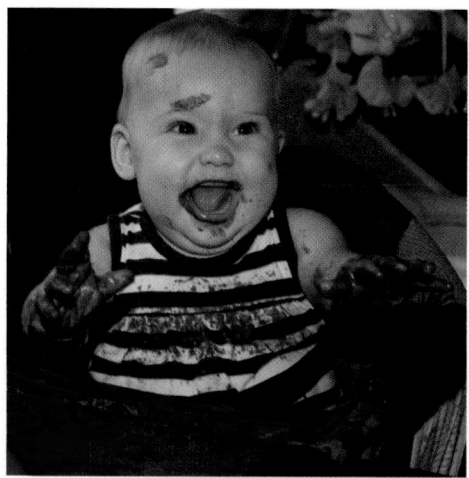

FIG 5-5 Children derive pleasure from handling raw materials. (Paints in this picture are nontoxic.)

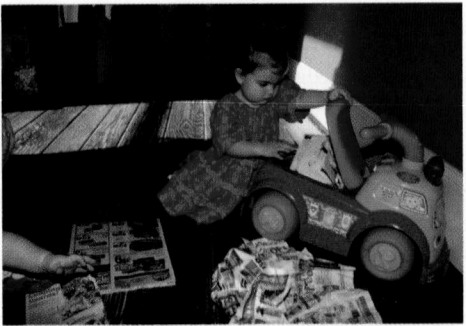

FIG 5-6 After infants develop new skills to grasp and manipulate, they begin to conquer new abilities such as putting paper in and taking it out of a toy car.

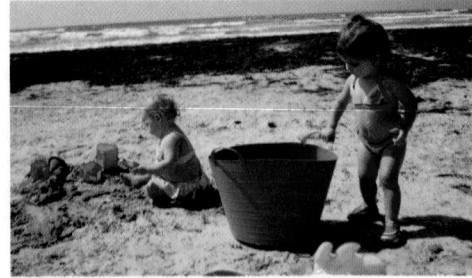

FIG 5-7 Parallel play at the beach.

Skill play—After infants have developed the ability to grasp and manipulate, they persistently demonstrate and exercise their newly acquired abilities through skill play, repeating an action over and over again. The element of sense-pleasure play is often evident in the practicing of a new ability, but all too frequently, the determination to conquer the elusive skill produces pain and frustration (e.g., putting paper in and taking it out of a toy car) (Fig. 5-6).

Unoccupied behavior—In unoccupied behavior, children are not playful but focusing their attention momentarily on anything that strikes their interest. Children daydream, fiddle with clothes or other objects, or walk aimlessly. This role differs from that of onlookers, who actively observe the activity of others.

Dramatic, or pretend, play—One of the vital elements in children's process of identification is dramatic play, also known as symbolic or pretend play. It begins in late infancy (11–13 months) and is the predominant form of play in preschool children. After children begin to invest situations and people with meanings and to attribute affective significance to the world, they can pretend and fantasize almost anything. By acting out events of daily life, children learn and practice the roles and identities modeled by the members of their family and society. Children's toys, replicas of the tools of society, provide a medium for learning about adult roles and activities that may be puzzling and frustrating to them. Interacting with the world is one way children get to know it. The simple, imitative, dramatic play of toddlers, such as using the telephone, driving a car, or rocking a doll, evolves into more complex, sustained dramas of preschoolers, which extend beyond common domestic matters to the wider aspects of the world and the society, such as playing police officer, storekeeper, teacher, or nurse. Older children work out elaborate themes, act out stories, and compose plays.

Games—Children in all cultures engage in games alone and with others. Solitary activity involving games begins as very small children participate in repetitive activities and progress to more complicated games that challenge their independent skills such as puzzles, solitaire, and computer or video games. Very young children participate in simple, **imitative games** such as pat-a-cake and peek-a-boo. Preschool children learn and enjoy **formal games**, beginning with ritualistic, self-sustaining games such as ring-around-a-rosy and London Bridge. With the exception of some simple board games, preschool children do not engage in **competitive games**. Preschoolers hate to lose and try to cheat, want to change rules, or demand exceptions and opportunities to change their moves. School-age children and adolescents enjoy competitive games, including cards, checkers, and chess, and physically active games such as baseball.

SOCIAL CHARACTER OF PLAY

The play interactions of infancy are between the child and an adult. Children continue to enjoy the company of adults but are increasingly able to play alone. As age advances, interaction with age-mates increases in importance and becomes an essential part of the socialization process. Through interaction, highly egocentric infants, unable to tolerate delay or interference, ultimately acquire concern for others and the ability to delay gratification or even to reject gratification at the expense of another. A pair of toddlers will engage in considerable combat because their personal needs cannot tolerate delay or compromise. By the time they reach age 5 or 6 years, children are able to arrive at compromises or make use of arbitration, usually after they have attempted but failed to gain their own way. Through continued interaction with peers and the growth of conceptual abilities and social skills, children are able to increase participation with others in the following types of play:

Onlooker play—During onlooker play, children watch what other children are doing but make no attempt to enter into the play activity. There is an active interest in observing the interaction of others but no movement toward participating. Watching an older sibling bounce a ball is a common example of the onlooker role.

Solitary play—During solitary play, children play alone with toys different from those used by other children in the same area. They enjoy the presence of other children but make no effort to get close to or speak to them. Their interest is centered on their own activity, which they pursue with no reference to the activities of the others.

Parallel play—During parallel activities, children play independently but among other children. They play with toys similar to those the children around them are using but as each child sees fit, neither influencing nor being influenced by the other children. Each plays beside, but not with, other children (Fig. 5-7). There is no group association. Parallel play is the characteristic play of toddlers, but it may also occur in other groups of any age. Individuals who are involved in a creative craft with each person separately working on an individual project are engaged in parallel play.

Associative play—In associative play, children play together and are engaged in a similar or even identical activity, but there is no organization, division of labor, leadership assignment, or mutual goal. Children borrow and lend play materials, follow each other with wagons and tricycles, and sometimes attempt to control who may or may not play in the group. Each child acts according to his or her own wishes; there is no group goal (Fig. 5-8). For example, two children play with dolls, borrowing articles of clothing from each other and engaging in similar conversation, but neither directs the other's actions or establishes rules regarding the limits of the play session. There is a great deal of behavioral contagion: when one child initiates an activity, the entire group follows the example.

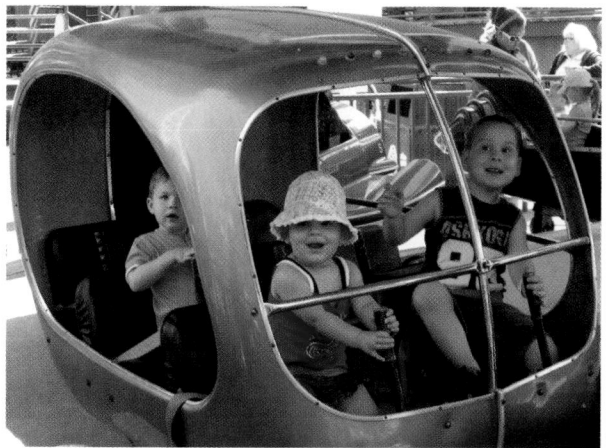

FIG 5-8 Associative play.

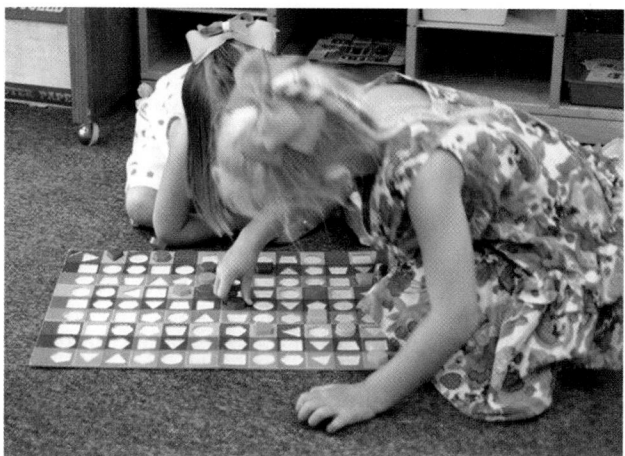

FIG 5-9 Cooperative play.

Cooperative play—Cooperative play is organized, and children play in a group with other children (Fig. 5-9). They discuss and plan activities for the purposes of accomplishing an end—to make something, attain a competitive goal, dramatize situations of adult or group life, or play formal games. The group is loosely formed, but there is a marked sense of belonging or not belonging. The goal and its attainment require organization of activities, division of labor, and role playing. The leader–follower relationship is definitely established, and the activity is controlled by one or two members who assign roles and direct the activity of the others. The activity is organized to allow one child to supplement another's function to complete the goal.

FUNCTIONS OF PLAY

Sensorimotor Development

Sensorimotor activity is a major component of play at all ages and is the predominant form of play in infancy. Active play is essential for muscle development and serves a useful purpose as a release for surplus energy. Through sensorimotor play, children explore the nature of the physical world. Infants gain impressions of themselves and their world through tactile, auditory, visual, and kinesthetic stimulation. Toddlers and preschoolers revel in body movement and exploration of objects in space. With increasing maturity, sensorimotor play becomes more differentiated and involved. Whereas very young children run for the sheer joy of body movement, older children incorporate or modify the motions into increasingly complex and coordinated activities such as races, games, roller skating, and bicycle riding.

Intellectual Development

Through exploration and manipulation, children learn colors, shapes, sizes, textures, and the significance of objects. They learn the significance of numbers and how to use them; they learn to associate words with objects; and they develop an understanding of abstract concepts and spatial relationships, such as *up*, *down*, *under*, and *over*. Activities such as puzzles and games help them develop problem-solving skills. Books, stories, films, and collections expand knowledge and provide enjoyment as well. Play provides a means to practice and expand language skills. Through play, children continually rehearse past experiences to assimilate them into new perceptions and relationships. Play helps children comprehend the world in which they live and distinguish between fantasy and reality.

Socialization

From very early infancy, children show interest and pleasure in the company of others. Their initial social contact is with the mothering person, but through play with other children, they learn to establish social relationships and solve the problems associated with these relationships. They learn to give and take, which is more readily learned from critical peers than from more tolerant adults. They learn the sex role that society expects them to fulfill, as well as approved patterns of behavior and deportment. Closely associated with socialization is development of moral values and ethics. Children learn right from wrong, the standards of the society, and to assume responsibility for their actions.

Creativity

In no other situation is there more opportunity to be creative than in play. Children can experiment and try out their ideas in play through every medium at their disposal, including raw materials, fantasy, and exploration. Creativity is stifled by pressure toward conformity; therefore, striving for peer approval may inhibit creative endeavors in school-age or adolescent children. Creativity is primarily a product of solitary activity, yet creative thinking is often enhanced in group settings where listening to others' ideas stimulates further exploration of one's own ideas. After children feel the satisfaction of creating something new and different, they transfer this creative interest to situations outside the world of play.

Self-Awareness

Beginning with active explorations of their bodies and awareness of themselves as separate from their mothers, the process of developing a self-identity is facilitated through play activities. Children learn who they are and their place in the world. They become increasingly able to regulate their own behavior, to learn what their abilities are, and to compare their abilities with those of others. Through play, children are able to test their abilities, assume and try out various roles, and learn the effects their behavior has on others. They learn the sex role that society expects them to fulfill, as well as approved patterns of behavior and deportment.

Therapeutic Value

Play is therapeutic at any age (Fig. 5-10). In play, children can express emotions and release unacceptable impulses in a socially acceptable fashion. Children are able to experiment and test fearful situations and can assume and vicariously master the roles and positions that they

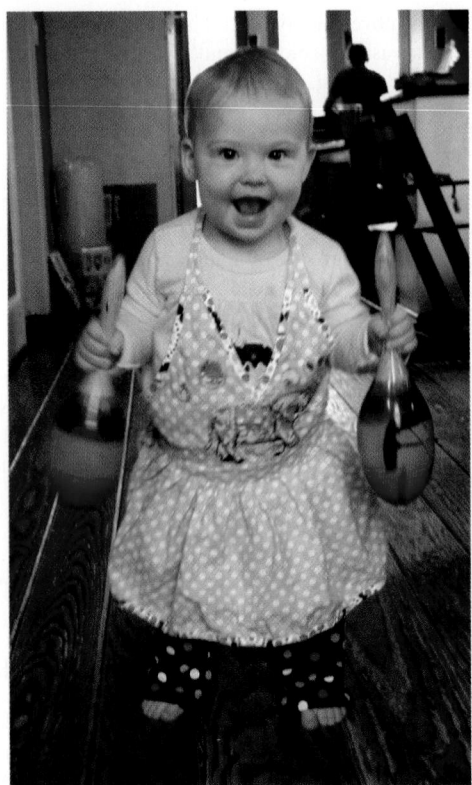

FIG 5-10 Play is therapeutic at any age and provides a means for release of tension and stress.

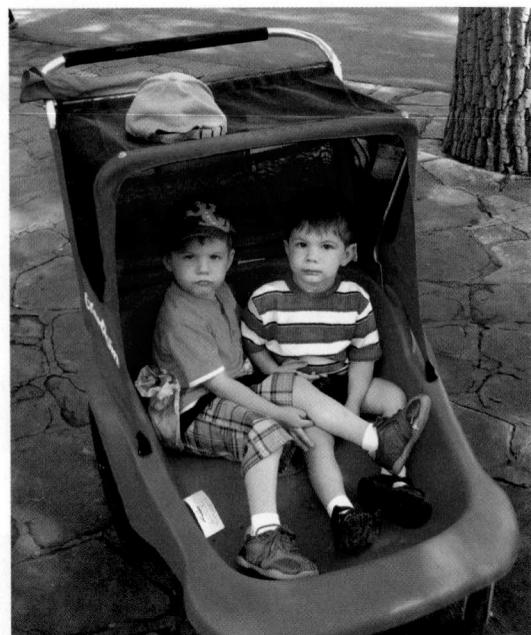

FIG 5-11 Peers become increasingly important as children develop friendships outside the family group.

are unable to perform in the world of reality. Children reveal much about themselves in play. Through play, children are able to communicate to the alert observer the needs, fears, and desires that they are unable to express with their limited language skills. Throughout their play, children need the acceptance of adults and their presence to help them control aggression and to channel their destructive tendencies.

Morality

Although children learn at home and at school those behaviors considered right and wrong in the culture, the interaction with peers during play contributes significantly to their moral training. Nowhere is the enforcement of moral standards as rigid as in the play situation. If they are to be acceptable members of the group, children must adhere to the accepted codes of behavior of the culture (e.g., fairness, honesty, self-control, consideration for others). Children soon learn that their peers are less tolerant of violations than are adults and that to maintain a place in the play group, they must conform to the standards of the group (Fig. 5-11).

TOYS

The type of toys chosen by or provided for children can support and enhance children's development in the areas just described. Although no scientific evidence shows that any toy is necessary for optimal learning, toys offer an opportunity to bring children and parents together. Research has indicated that a positive parent–child interaction can enhance early childhood brain development (American Academy of Pediatrics, 2003). Toys that are small replicas of the culture and its tools help children assimilate into their culture. Toys that require pushing, pulling, rolling, and manipulating teach them about physical properties of the items and help develop muscles and coordination. Rules and

the basic elements of cooperation and organization are learned through board games.

Because they can be used in a variety of ways, raw materials with which children can exercise their own creativity and imaginations are sometimes superior to ready-made items. For example, building blocks can be used to construct a variety of structures, count, and learn shapes and sizes.

DEVELOPMENTAL ASSESSMENT

One of the most essential components of a complete health appraisal is assessment of developmental function. Screening procedures are designed to identify quickly and reliably children whose developmental level is below normal for their age and who therefore require further investigation. They also provide a means of recording objective measurements of present developmental function for future reference. Since the passage of Public Law 99-457, the Education of the Handicapped Act Amendments of 1986, much greater emphasis is placed on developmental assessment of children with disabilities, and nurses can play a vital role in providing this service. It is estimated that 16% of children are affected by developmental disabilities, but fewer than 30% of these children are identified before kindergarten (Wagner, Jenkins, and Smith, 2006). All the procedures discussed in this section can be administered in a variety of settings: home, school, daycare center, hospital, practitioner's office, or clinic.

DENVER II

The most widely used developmental screening tests for young children are the series of tests developed by William Frankenburg and his colleagues (1994a). The oldest and best known—the **Denver Developmental Screening Test (DDST)** and its revision, the **DDST-R**—have been revised, restandardized, and renamed the **Denver II**. Before administering the Denver II, the examiner should be trained by and receive certification from a master instructor who has been trained by the Denver faculty.* The Denver II differs from the DDST in items, test form, interpretation, and referral. The previous total of 105 items has been increased to 125, including an increase from 21 DDST to 39 Denver II language items. Previous items that were difficult to administer or interpret have been either modified or eliminated. Many items that were previously tested by parental report now require observation by the examiner.

Each item was evaluated to determine whether significant differences exist on the basis of sex, ethnic group, maternal education, and place of residence. Items for which clinically significant differences exist were replaced or, if retained, are discussed in the technical manual. When evaluating children delayed on one of these items, the examiner can look up norms for the subpopulations to consider whether the delay may be caused by sociocultural or environmental differences.

The items on the test form are arranged in the same format as the DDST-R. The norms for the distribution bars were updated with the new standardization data but retain the 25th, 50th, 75th, and 90th percentile divisions. The test form contains a place to rate the child's behavioral characteristics (compliance, interest in surroundings, fearfulness, and attention span).

To determine relative areas of advancement and delay, enough items should be administered to establish the basal and ceiling levels in each sector. By scoring appropriate items as "pass," "fail," "refusal," or "no opportunity" and relating such scores to the child's age, the examiner can interpret each item as described in Box 5-4. To identify "cautions," all items intersected by the age line are administered. To screen solely for developmental delays, only the items located totally

to the left of the child's age line are administered. Criteria for referral are based on the availability of resources in the community.

Research on the Denver II's validity and accuracy continues. One study found that it identified most children with even subtle developmental problems. However, almost half the children without developmental problems received suspect scores, resulting in a high rate of overreferrals (Glascoe, Byrne, Ashford, and others, 1992). To minimize overreferrals, a decision for referral depends not only on the results of the Denver II but also on the practitioner's clinical judgment after considering the child's developmental history; general health status; and social, cultural, and emotional environment, as well as the availability of local resources for diagnosis and treatment (Frankenburg, 1994a, 1994b).

Although it is not the purpose of this discussion to detail the instruction manual, some points concerning preparation, administration, and interpretation of the Denver II are important to stress. Before beginning the screening, ask whether the child was born preterm and correctly calculate the adjusted age. Up to 24 months of age, allowances are made for preterm infants by subtracting the number of weeks of missed gestation from their present age and testing them at the adjusted age. For example, a 16-week-old infant who was born 4 weeks early is tested at a 12-week adjusted age level.

Explain to the parents and child, if appropriate, that the screenings are not intelligence tests but rather are a method of showing what the child can do at a particular age. Emphasize that the child is not expected to perform each item on the test. Tell the parent before the screening begins that the results of the child's performance will be explained after all of the items have been concluded. It is the nurse's responsibility to properly inform the parents of any testing or screening procedure before its administration so they are fully aware of its purpose and intent.

Prepare toddlers and preschoolers for the procedure by presenting it as a game. Frequently, the Denver II is an excellent way to begin a health appraisal because it is nonthreatening, requires no painful or unfamiliar procedures, and capitalizes on the child's natural activity of play. Because children are easily distracted, perform each item quickly and present only one toy from the kit at a time. After that toy's purpose is concluded, such as building a tower of blocks or identifying its color, replace the toy in the bag and take out another one. Temporary factors that may interfere with the child's performance include fatigue, illness, fear, hospitalization, separation from the parent, or general unwillingness to perform the activities. In addition, undiagnosed mental retardation, hearing loss, vision loss, or neurologic impairment or a familial pattern of slow development greatly influences the child's performance.

After completion of the Denver II, ask the parent whether the child's performance was typical of behavior at other times. If the parent replies affirmatively and the child's cooperation was satisfactory, explain the results, emphasizing all successful items first, then the items the child failed but was not expected to pass, and finally the items that represent delays. If the parent replies that the child's performance was not typical of usual behavior, it is best to defer any scoring or discussion of results, especially if the refusals yield a suspect score. In this situation, reschedule testing for a time when the child is more likely to cooperate.

In explaining a normal score, focus on how well the child performed and reinforce the parents' efforts in satisfactorily stimulating their child. In addition to assessing the child's present developmental level, the Denver II can be used to guide parents toward activities that are appropriate, although not necessarily expected, for the child's age. By testing for items to the right of the age line (ones the child is not

---

BOX 5-4   DENVER II SCORING

Interpretation of Denver II Scores

Advanced—Passed an item completely to the right of the age line (passed by less than 25% of children)

OK—Passed, failed, or refused an item intersected by the age line between the 25th and 75th percentiles

Caution—Failed or refused items intersected by the age line on or between the 75th and 90th percentiles

Delay—Failed an item completely to the left of the age line; refusals to the left of the age line may also be considered delays because the reason for the refusal may be inability to perform the task

Interpretation of Test

Normal—No delays and a maximum of one caution

Suspect—One or more delays or two or more cautions

Untestable—Refusals on one or more items completely to the left of the age line or on more than one item intersected by the age line in the 75th to 90th percentile area

Recommendations for Referral for Suspect and Untestable Results

Rescreen in 1 to 2 weeks to rule out temporary factors.

If rescreen is suspect or untestable, use clinical judgment based on the following: number of cautions and delays, which items are cautions and delays, rate of past development, clinical examination and history, and availability of referral resources.

---

*Forms and complete instructions are available from Denver Developmental Materials, PO Box 371075, Denver, CO 80237-5075; (800) 419-4729; http://www.denverii.com. The DDST and DDST-R are no longer available.

expected to perform), the examiner can identify children with advanced development, who may be gifted.

In explaining delays, carefully note the parent's response, especially casual acceptance such as "He'll catch up" or questions such as "Does this mean my child is retarded?" Be aware of personal anxieties during these situations and refrain from giving glib reassurances such as "I'm sure he will do better next time." Rather, respond honestly to parents' questions, yet with appropriate flexibility and concern, stressing the need for further developmental testing.

DENVER II PRESCREENING DEVELOPMENTAL QUESTIONNAIRE

The Prescreening Developmental Questionnaire (PDQ II) is a further revision of the PDQ and the R-PDQ. This version uses the norms (90th and 75th percentiles) from the Denver II. The PDQ II is a parent-answered prescreen consisting of 91 questions from the Denver II, although only a subset of questions is asked for each age group. The form may need to be read to parents and caregivers who are less educated.

Four different forms are available and are selected based on age: orange (0–9 months), purple (9–24 months), cream (2–4 years), and white (4–6 years). The caregiver answers questions until (1) three "nos" are circled (they do not have to be consecutive) or (2) all the questions on both sides of the form have been answered. Scoring is based on the number of delays or cautions (see Box 5-4). Children who have no delays or cautions are considered to be developing normally. If a child has one delay or two cautions, the caregiver is provided with age-appropriate developmental activities to pursue with the child, and a rescreen with the PDQ II is done 1 month later. If on rescreening the child has one or more delays, the Denver II is administered as soon as possible. If a child has two or more delays or three or more cautions on the first screening with the PDQ II, the Denver II is administered as soon as possible.

Several additional parent report developmental screening tools meet the standards for screening test accuracy. Some of the most common include the Ages and Stages Questionnaires (ASQ), Parents' Evaluation of Developmental Status (PEDS), Child Development Inventory, and the Pediatric Symptom Checklist. Although it is beyond the scope of this chapter to describe each screening tool, using a tool can aid the nurse in providing anticipatory guidance and appropriate referral (Wagner, Jenkins, and Smith, 2006).

GENETIC FACTORS THAT INFLUENCE DEVELOPMENT

OVERVIEW OF GENETICS AND GENOMICS

Nurses and other health care providers are increasingly faced with incorporating genetic and genomic information into their practice. In response to this need, the Consensus Panel on Genetic/Genomic Nursing Competencies was established in 2006. This independent panel of nurse leaders from clinical, research, and academic settings established essential minimal competencies necessary for nurses to deliver competent genetic- and genomic-focused nursing care. Subsequently, the American Association of Colleges of Nursing published the revised *The Essentials of Baccalaureate Education for Professional Nursing Practice* (2008, http://www.aacn.nche.edu/education/pdf/BaccEssentials08.pdf) and *The Essentials of Master's Education in Nursing* (2011, http://www.aacn.nche.edu/education/pdf/Master'sEssentials11.pdf) both of which identified genetics and genomics as strong forces influencing the role of nurses in patient care. This brief overview identifies key terms and concepts and highlights essential genetics and genomics competencies for all nurses (2008, http://www.genome.gov/Pages/Careers/HealthProfessionalEducation/geneticscompetency.pdf).

Genes, Genetics, and Genomics

Genes are segments of DNA that specify for proteins, segments of proteins or strands of RNA necessary to control physiologic functions or characteristics. These segments are often referred to as *sites* or *loci*, indicating a physical or "geographic" location on a chromosome. Variant forms of a gene commonly occur within a population. When referring to a particular form of a gene, the term *allele* is used. Specific differences within a gene are called *mutations* if they are rare within a population or are called *polymorphisms* if they are found within more than 1% of a particular population. Mutations and polymorphisms can be inherited or acquired. Variant alleles caused by mutations or polymorphisms may lead to no measureable or observable differences, may cause the person to be susceptible to clinically recognizable pathology within specific environmental contexts, may cause a clinically recognized disease or disorder, or may prove advantageous within a particular environmental context. Whereas genetics is the study of individual genes and the impact of their variant forms on relatively rare single gene disorders, genomics is the study of combinations of multiple genes, their interactions with each other, the environment, and other psychosocial and cultural factors (Guttmacher and Collins, 2002).

In earlier times, human diseases were thought to be either clearly genetic or typically environmental. However, the observation that some genetic disorders are congenital (present at birth) but others are expressed later in life has led scientists to conclude that many, if not most, diseases are caused by a genetic predisposition that can be activated by an environmental trigger. Examples of such interactions are found in single-gene disorders, such as phenylketonuria (PKU) and sickle cell disease, and **multifactorial conditions**, such as cancer and neural tube defects (NTDs). PKU is a disorder resulting from the (genetically determined) absence of an enzyme that metabolizes the amino acid phenylalanine. However, the deleterious effects in the infant are expressed only after sufficient ingestion of phenylalanine-containing substances, such as milk (environmental trigger). Even in the case of a "classic" genetic condition, such as sickle cell disease, its acute symptoms are precipitated by certain conditions such as lowered oxygen tension, infection, or dehydration.

Cancer is another example of genetic–environment interplay and explains the difference between inherited conditions and somatic cell genetic disorders. A normal **somatic cell** (any body cell other than the ova and sperm) may become a cancer cell after acquiring a series of gene changes. This process is the typical "genetic" cause of cancer. In a small subset of families, a mutation in a gene normally involved in regulation of cell growth, DNA repair, or cell death (**apoptosis**) is transmitted through the **germ cells** (ova and sperm). Children who inherit the genetic mutation will have it in all of their somatic cells, making them more susceptible to subsequent genetic changes in one or more cells that may transform into cancer cells. Beyond the genetic component of cancer, there is little dispute that environmental insult, such as tobacco smoking, sun exposure, and radiation, can be carcinogenic. Such environmental triggers are capable of spontaneously creating noninherited mutations in genes that regulate cell growth and cell response to cell abnormalities that can eventually lead to malignant transformation.

Evidence is growing that genes play an important role in human susceptibility and resistance to infection even in cases with a clear environmental cause of the infectious disease. Evidence for this genetic element in resistance gained heightened recognition during the first decade of the acquired immunodeficiency (AIDS) epidemic. Researchers discovered that adults with a specific deletion in both copies of their *CCR5* genes did not become infected with human immunodeficiency virus (HIV) despite repeated exposure. Later it was found that children exposed in utero to HIV typically had a significantly delayed onset of disease if at least one of their *CCR5* genes had the specific mutation (Romiti, Colognesi, Cancrini, and others, 2000). Understanding the mechanism of resistance associated with *CCR5* mutation led to a novel molecular therapy (Wilkin, Su, Kuritzkes, and others, 2007).

Congenital Anomalies

Embryogenesis and fetal development are an intricate and precisely timed series of events in which all parts must be properly integrated to ensure a coordinated whole. Insults during development or abnormalities in differentiation or in the proper timing of organogenesis may result in a variety of congenital anomalies. Congenital anomalies, or birth defects, occur in 2% to 4% of all live-born children and are often classified as deformations, disruptions, dysplasias, or malformations. Deformations are often caused by extrinsic mechanical forces on normally developing tissue. Club foot is an example of a deformation often caused by uterine constraint. Disruptions result from the breakdown of previously normal tissue. Congenital amputations caused by amniotic bands (fibrous strands of amnion that wrap around different body parts during development) are examples of disruption anomalies. Dysplasias result from abnormal organization of cells into a particular tissue type. Congenital abnormalities of the teeth, hair, nails, or sweat glands may be manifestations of one of the more than 100 different ectodermal dysplasia syndromes (National Foundation for Ectodermal Dysplasia, 2010). Malformations are abnormal formations of organs or body parts resulting from an abnormal developmental process. Most malformations occur before 12 weeks of gestation. Cleft lip, an example of a malformation, occurs at approximately 5 weeks of gestation when the developing embryo naturally has two clefts in the area. Normally, between 5 and 7 weeks, cells rapidly divide and migrate to fill in those clefts. If there is an abnormality in this developmental process, the embryo is left with either a unilateral or bilateral cleft lip that may also involve the palate.

The types of anomalies that can result from genetic or prenatal environmental causes can be major structural abnormalities with serious medical, surgical, or quality-of-life consequences, or they can be minor anomalies or normal variants with no serious consequences, such as a sacral dimple, an extra nipple, or a café-au-lait spot. Congenital anomalies can occur in isolation, such as congenital heart defect, or multiple anomalies may be present. A recognized pattern of anomalies resulting from a single specific cause is called a syndrome (e.g., Down syndrome, fetal alcohol syndrome). A nonrandom pattern of malformations for which a cause has not been determined is called an association (e.g., VACTERL [vertebral defects, anal atresia, cardiac defect, tracheoesophageal fistula, and renal and limb defects] association). When a single anomaly leads to a cascade of additional anomalies, the pattern of defects is referred to as a sequence. Pierre Robin sequence begins with the abnormal development of the mandible, resulting in abnormal placement of the tongue during development. The normal developmental process for the palate is prevented because the tongue obstructs the migration of the palatal shelves toward the midline, and a cleft palate remains. Consequently, infants born with Pierre Robin sequence have a recessed mandible and an abnormally placed tongue and are at risk for obstructive apnea. NTDs, cleft lip and palate, deafness, congenital heart defects, and cognitive impairment are examples of congenital malformations that can occur in isolation or as part of a syndrome, association, or sequence and can have different causes, such as single-gene or chromosome abnormalities, prenatal exposures, or multifactorial causes.

Disorders of the Intrauterine Environment

The intrauterine environment can have a profound and permanent effect on developing fetuses with or without chromosome or single-gene abnormalities. Intrauterine growth restriction, for example, can occur with many genetic syndromes, such as Down, Russell-Silver, Prader-Willi, and Turner syndromes (Rimoin, Connor, Pyeritz, and others, 2002), or it can be caused by nongenetic factors such as maternal alcohol ingestion. Placental abnormalities are increasingly being found to be the etiologic factor in neurodevelopmental disorders (e.g., cerebral palsy and cognitive impairment) that were previously attributed to asphyxia during delivery (Bos, Einspieler, Prechtl, and others, 2001).

Teratogens, agents that cause birth defects when present in the prenatal environment, account for the majority of adverse intrauterine effects not attributable to genetic factors. Types of teratogens include drugs (phenytoin [Dilantin], warfarin [Coumadin], isotretinoin [Accutane]), chemicals (ethyl alcohol, cocaine, lead), infectious agents (rubella, cytomegalovirus), physical agents (maternal ionizing radiation, hyperthermia), and metabolic agents (maternal PKU). Many of these teratogenic exposures and the resulting effects are completely preventable, such as ingestion of alcohol resulting in fetal alcohol syndrome or fetal alcohol effects, which causes severe birth defects, including cognitive impairment. The incidence of fetal alcohol syndrome is estimated at 5.2 per 10,000 live births (American Academy of Pediatrics, 2000).

Genetic Disorders

Genetic disorders can be caused by chromosome abnormalities as seen in Turner syndrome, Down syndrome, or velocardiofacial syndrome (VCFS); single-gene mutations as seen in sickle cell anemia, neurofibromatosis, or Duchenne muscular dystrophy; a combination of genetic and environmental factors as seen in NTDs or maturity-onset diabetes in the young; and mitochondrial DNA (mtDNA) mutations as seen in nonsyndromic deafness susceptibility caused by aminoglycoside sensitivity.

Both numeric and large structural abnormalities of autosomes (all chromosomes except the X and Y chromosomes) account for a variety of syndromes usually characterized by cognitive deficiencies. Nurses often note dysmorphic facial features, behavioral characteristics such as an unusual cry and poor feeding behavior, and other neurologic manifestations such as hypotonia or abnormal reflex responses, which may alert them to these and other chromosome abnormalities.

Somatic cells contain 44 autosomes (the 22 pairs of chromosomes that do not greatly influence sex determination at conception) and two sex chromosomes, XX in females and XY in males. For the purpose of cytogenetic studies, chromosomes are usually displayed in a karyotype, the laboratory-made arrangement of specially prepared chromosomes according to their size and centromere position. Numeric chromosome abnormalities occur whenever entire chromosomes are added or deleted. Down syndrome is an example of a condition caused by having an extra autosome, chromosome 21. Turner syndrome is the only example of a condition compatible with life that is caused by the absence of a chromosome. Children with Turner syndrome have one X chromosome. Chromosomes are subject to structural alterations resulting from breakage and rearrangement. A chromosome deletion occurs when chromosome breakage results in loss of the broken fragment at a chromosome's terminal end or within the chromosome.

Some structural chromosome abnormalities are too small to reliably visualize under a light microscope but are still clinically relevant. Fragile, or weak, sites associated with expanded triplet repeats have been identified on both the autosomes and the X chromosome. A classic example is fragile X syndrome. Contiguous gene syndromes are disorders characterized by a microdeletion or microduplication of smaller chromosome segments, which may require special analysis techniques or molecular testing to detect (Bar-Shira, Rosner, Rosner, and others, 2006).

Chromosome anomalies typically affect large numbers of genes; however, a single-gene disorder is caused by an abnormality within a gene or in a gene's regulatory region. Single-gene disorders can affect all body systems and may have mild to severe expressions. Single-gene disorders display a Mendelian pattern of dominant or recessive inheritance that was first delineated in the mid-nineteenth century by Gregor Mendel's experiments with plants.

Mendelian inheritance laws allow for risk prediction in single-gene disorders; however, phenotypic expression may be altered by incomplete penetrance or variable expressivity of the responsible allele. An allele is said to have reduced or incomplete penetrance in a population when a proportion of persons who possess that allele do not express the phenotype. An allele is said to have variable expressivity when individuals possessing that allele display the features of the syndrome in various degrees, from mild to severe. If a person expresses even the mildest possible phenotype, the allele is penetrant in that individual.

Role of Nurses in Genetics

All nurses need to be prepared to use genetic and genomic information and technology when providing care. Nearly 50 nursing organizations endorsed essential minimum competencies necessary for nurses to deliver competent genetic and genomic focused nursing care (Consensus Panel on Genetic/Genomic Nursing Competencies, 2006). The professional practice domains include applying and integrating genetic knowledge into nursing assessment; identifying and referring clients who may benefit from genetic information or services; identifying genetics resources and services to meet clients' needs; and providing care and support before, during, and after providing genetic information and services. Often a nurse is the first one to recognize the need for genetic evaluation by identifying an inherited disorder in a family history or by noting physical, cognitive, or behavioral abnormalities when performing a nursing assessment (Box 5-5).

Nursing Assessment: Applying and Integrating Genetic and Genomic Knowledge

Family health history is an important tool to identify individuals and families at increased risk for disease, risk factors for disease (e.g., obesity), and inheritance patterns of diseases. Because of its importance, all nurses need to be able to elicit family history information and document the collected information in pedigree format.

When eliciting a family health history, nurses should collect information about all family members within a minimum of three generations. This process usually takes 20 to 30 minutes. When possible, it is best to include both parents in the interview to elicit information about relatives on both sides of the family. Medical records, birth and death records, family Bibles, and photograph albums are helpful resources, and persons being interviewed should be instructed to bring such items if they are available. It may be necessary to consult other members of the family. The level of education and the degree of understanding vary widely among informants and influence their reliability. The informants may be reticent, particularly if they view the disorder as something to be ashamed of or in some way threatening. Sometimes

---

BOX 5-5   PEDIATRIC INDICATIONS FOR GENETIC CONSULTATION

Family History
- Family history of hereditary diseases, birth defects, or developmental problems
- Family history of sudden cardiac death or early-onset cancer
- Family history of mental illness

Medical History
- Abnormal newborn screen
- Abnormal genetic test result ordered by a nongenetics professional who lacks the knowledge and experience to discuss the implications of results
- Excessive bleeding or excessive clotting
- Progressive neurologic condition
- Recurrent infection or immunodeficiency

Developmental History
- Behavioral disorders
- Cognitive impairment or autism
- Development and speech delays or loss of developmental milestones

Physical Assessment
- Major congenital anomaly
- Minor anomalies and dysmorphic features
- Growth abnormalities
- Skeletal abnormalities
- Visual or hearing problems
- Metabolic disorder (unusual odor of breath, urine, or stool)
- Sexual development abnormalities or delayed puberty
- Skin disorders or abnormalities

Parental Requests That Child be Evaluated by a Genetics Professional

Adapted from Pletcher BA, Toriello HV, Noblin SJ, and others: Indications for genetic referral: a guide for healthcare providers, *Genet Med* 9(6):385-389, 2007.

---

true relationships may be concealed, such as adoption or misattributed paternity.

In addition to family history, nurses caring for children and families need to collect pregnancy, labor and delivery, perinatal, medical, and developmental histories. Although it is common for genetics nurses to obtain all of these histories before or during an initial genetics consultation, not all nurses are expected to obtain all of these assessment data from each patient during a pediatric visit. Electronic medical records are making it more practical to construct a comprehensive set of histories even when many health care professionals contribute only a portion of the total history.

All nurses are taught to perform physical assessments, but they are seldom taught to recognize minor anomalies and dysmorphology that may suggest a genetic disorder. Yet nurses are keen in recognizing delays in development, behavior differences, and global appearances that raise concern that a newborn, infant, child, or adolescent needs further evaluation. Although dysmorphology is beyond the scope of this chapter, readers are encouraged to review the January 2009 issue of *American Journal of Medical Genetics* (Carey, Cohen, Curry, and others, 2009). Drawings and photographs of normal and abnormal morphologic characteristics are provided for the head, face, and extremities together with accepted dysmorphology terminology. Nurses knowledgeable in dysmorphology are able to articulate specific concerns about a child's appearance rather than relying on the outdated and offensive phrase "funny looking kid." When a major anomaly is identified, nurses should raise suspicion that the child could have additional congenital anomalies. When three or more minor anomalies are identified, nurses should suspect the possibility of an underlying syndrome. However, it is important to consider the biologic parents' physical appearance, development, and behavior when considering the relevance of the child's combination of minor anomalies.

Identification and Referral

It is nurses' responsibility to learn basic genetic principles, to be alert to situations in which families could benefit from genetic evaluation and counseling, to know about special services that can help manage and support affected children, and to be familiar with facilities in their areas where these services are available. In this way, nurses are able to direct individuals and families to needed services and be active participants in the genetic evaluation and counseling process. A regularly updated resource for locating genetics clinics can be found at www.genetests.org (click on Clinic Directory tab). Contact information for specific genetics professionals can be found at the following websites: geneticists, www.acmg.net (click on Find a Geneticist); genetics nurses, www.isong.org (call or e-mail office); and genetic counselors, www.nsgc.org (click on Find a Counselor). In addition, state health departments either offer services or can help identify health professionals with specialty training in genetics.

Early identification of a genetic disorder allows anticipation of associated conditions and implementation of available preventive measures and therapy to avoid potential complications and to enhance the child's health. It may also prevent the unexpected birth of another affected child in the immediate or extended family. Nurses have an important role in identifying patients and families who have or are at risk for developing or transmitting a genetic condition (see Box 5-5). When facilitating genetics consultations, nurses should share with the genetics professional the findings in the histories they collected that triggered the consultation. Nurses can also help the referral process by determining and communicating the family's initial concerns, their state of knowledge about the reason for referral, and their attitudes and beliefs concerning genetics.

Genetic evaluation for diagnostic purposes may occur at any point in the life span. In the newborn period, birth defects and abnormal newborn screen results are obvious reasons for referral. Beyond the newborn period, indicators for referral include metabolic disorders, developmental delays, growth delays, behavioral problems, cognitive delays, abnormal or delayed sexual development, and medical problems known to be associated with genetic diseases. For example, a preschooler with hyperactivity and autistic-like behaviors may need evaluation for fragile X syndrome, and a 17-year-old girl with primary amenorrhea and short stature should be evaluated for Turner syndrome.

With so many recent advances in genetic testing, it is not unusual for a child or adult with longstanding medical problems, including cognitive impairment, to be referred for reevaluation of his or her condition as a possible genetic disorder that might not have been diagnosable a few years earlier, such as microdeletion disorders or single-gene mutations. If a genetic diagnosis is made, the patient is usually referred back to the primary care physician with recommendations for routine management.

Providing Education, Care, and Support

Maintaining contact with the family or making a referral to a health care practice or an agency that can provide a sustained relationship is

critical. It is becoming more common for genetics health care professionals to provide regular follow up and management, particularly for children with rare genetic disorders. However, some families choose not to have follow-up visits with genetic experts.

Regardless of whether families choose to receive continued care with a genetics center, clinic, or professional, nurses can help patients and families process and clarify the information they receive during a genetics visit. Misunderstanding of this information can have many causes, including cultural differences, the disparity of knowledge between the counselor and the family, and the heightened emotion surrounding genetic counseling. Family members have difficulty absorbing all of the information presented during a genetics evaluation and counseling session. Knowing this, genetics professionals write and send clinic summary letters to families. The nurse may need to help the family understand terminology in the letter, help them identify and articulate remaining questions or areas of clarification, and coach them through the process of accessing genetics health professionals to get remaining questions and concerns answered. Information often needs to be repeated several times before the family understands the content and its implications.

Nurses must assess for and address parents' feelings of guilt about carrying "bad genes" or having "made my child sick." Depending on the type of cytogenetic disorder, the nurse may be able to absolve the parents of guilt by explaining the random nature of segregation during both gamete formation and fertilization, and that those errors in cell division unique to the pregnancy in question are not likely to happen again and are not inherited. If the condition is a Mendelian-inherited or mitochondrial disorder, it is important to assess parents' understanding of recurrence risk, help them understand the chances that a subsequent pregnancy will not be affected, and ensure they have been given information about their options for future children (preimplantation diagnosis, use of donor egg or sperm, prenatal diagnosis, or adoption). Families often try to reason that some unrelated event caused the abnormality (e.g., a fall, a urinary tract infection, or "one glass of wine") before the mother was aware that she was pregnant. These misconceptions need to be assessed and dispelled.

After a genetics visit, and sometimes before the visit, parents often use the Internet to find answers to their questions. During the initial genetics evaluation, a diagnosis may not be possible. Instead, findings in medical, developmental, and family histories lead the professional to order genetic tests and other diagnostic procedures. Diagnoses under consideration are discussed briefly with the parents. Some parents are satisfied with the brief information and do not care to find out more until the actual diagnosis is established. Other parents go home and seek as much information as they can about the diagnoses under consideration. The information they find can be terrifying and overwhelming and inaccurate or misleading. Nurses can play an important role in helping parents identify reliable, accurate resources for information at whatever time they desire it. It is also important to stress that everything that is described for a genetic condition may not be relevant to their child. Before the follow-up genetics visit when test and procedure results are discussed, nurses can help parents identify and write down the questions and concerns they need addressed before leaving the clinic.

After a genetics diagnosis is made or a genetic predisposition to a delayed-onset disorder is identified, nurses need to have frequent contact with patients and families as they attempt to incorporate recommended therapies or disease-prevention strategies into their daily lives. For example, a disorder such as PKU requires conscientious diet management; therefore, it is important to make certain that the family understands and follows instructions and is able to navigate the health care system to access the essential formula and low-phenylalanine food products. An infant evaluated for cleft palate and cardiac defect and subsequently found to have VCFS requires surgical intervention for the congenital malformations. Such an infant also benefits from early intervention services and eventually an individualized education plan in school because developmental delays and eventual learning problems are common.

Initial and ongoing assessment of the family's coping abilities, resources, and support systems is vital to determine their need for additional assistance and support. As with any family who has a child with chronic health care needs, nurses must teach the family to become the child's advocate. Nurses can help families locate agencies and clinics specializing in a specific disorder or its consequences that can provide services (e.g., equipment, medication, and rehabilitation), educational programs, and parent support groups. Referral to local and national support groups or contact with a local family that has a child with the same condition can be helpful for new parents. Privacy and confidentiality are imperative, and both families must give permission before their contact information is given. Nurses can also be instrumental in helping parents start a support group when none is available.

Parental attachment and adjustment to the baby can be supported and facilitated by nursing interventions. Assessing the parents' understanding of the child's disorder and providing simple and truthful explanations can help them begin to understand their child's health issues. Guiding the parents in recognizing their child's cues, responses, and strengths can be helpful even for experienced parents. A caring attitude conveys the value of their child and, by extension, their value as parents. The nurse can help the parents identify their strengths as a family and identify support that is available to them.

Giving birth to and raising a child with a genetic disorder is not necessarily a lifetime burden. It is important for nurses to ask parents to describe their experience raising their child with a particular genetic condition. What has been the impact on their family? Although parents may initially experience negative outcomes, such as shock, emotional distress, and grief, families can adapt and thrive. Resources for managing stress and restoring balance in the lives of families affected by a genetic condition can help. Van Riper's (2007) research has identified nursing interventions that can promote resilience and adaptation in families of children with Down syndrome. Van Riper's recommendations are useful for families of children with any type of genetic disorder:

- Recognize multiple stressors, strains, and transitions in their lives (e.g., unmet family needs).
- Discuss and implement strategies for reducing family demands (e.g., setting priorities and reducing the number of outside activities family members are involved in).
- Identify and use individual, family, and community resources (e.g., humor, family flexibility, supportive extended family, respite care, local support groups, and Internet resources).
- Expand the range and efficacy of their coping strategies (e.g., increase the use of active strategies such as reframing, mobilize their ability to acquire and accept help, and decrease the use of passive appraisal).
- Encourage the use of an affirming style of family problem-solving communication (e.g., one that conveys support and caring and exerts a calming influence).

Some families do struggle after learning their child has a genetic disorder. Families may feel ashamed of a hereditary disorder and seek to blame their partner for transmitting a faulty gene or chromosome. Intrafamilial strife, hostility, and marital or couple disharmony, sometimes to the point of family disintegration, can occur. Nurses should be alert for evidence of risk factors that indicate poor adjustment (e.g., child abuse, divorce, or other maladaptive behaviors). Referral to psychosocial professionals for crisis intervention may be necessary.

KEY POINTS

- Growth is a change in quantity and occurs when cells divide and synthesize new proteins.
- Maturation, a qualitative change, is the aging process or an increase in competence and adaptability.
- Differentiation is a biologic description of the processes by which early cells and structures are modified and altered to achieve specific and characteristic physical and chemical properties.
- Development involves change from a lower to a more advanced stage of complexity.
- The five major developmental periods are prenatal, infancy, early childhood, middle childhood, and later childhood (pubescence and adolescence).
- Growth and development proceed in predictable patterns of direction, sequence, and pace.
- The directional trends in growth and development are cephalocaudal, proximodistal, and mass to specific.
- Physical development includes increase in height and weight and changes in body proportion, dentition, and some body tissues.
- The three broad classifications of child temperament are the easy child, the difficult child, and the slow-to-warm-up child.
- The developmental theories most widely used in explaining child growth and development are Freud's psychosexual stages, Erikson's stages of psychosocial development, Piaget's stages of cognitive development, Kohlberg's stages of moral development, and Fowler's stages of spiritual development.
- To develop a positive self-concept, children need recognition for their achievements and the approval of others.
- Through play, children learn about their world and how to relate to objects, people, and situations.
- Play provides a means of development in the areas of sensorimotor and intellectual progress, socialization, creativity, self-awareness, and moral behavior; it serves as a means for release of tension and expression of emotions.
- Growth and development are affected by a variety of conditions and circumstances, including heredity, physiologic function, gender, disease, physical environment, nutrition, and interpersonal relationships.
- Children's vulnerability and reaction to stress depend to a large extent on their age, coping behaviors, and support systems.
- Developmental screening tools are valuable in identifying infants and children who are at risk for developmental delays.
- Genetic mutations and polymorphisms can be inherited or acquired. Mutations are rare while polymorphisms occur in greater than 1% of a population.
- All nurses should be familiar with genetic or genomic information as it relates to the care of their patient.

REFERENCES

American Academy of Pediatrics, Committee on Early Childhood, Adoption, and Dependent Care: Selecting appropriate toys for young children: the pediatrician's role, *Pediatrics* 111(4):911–913, 2003.

American Academy of Pediatrics, Committee on Substance Abuse and Committee on Children With Disabilities: Fetal alcohol syndrome and alcohol-related neurodevelopmental disorders, *Pediatrics* 106(2 Pt 1):358–361, 2000.

Anders TF, Sadeh A, Appareddy V: Normal sleep in neonates and children. In Sheldon S, Ferber R, Kryger M, editors: *Principles and practice of sleep medicine in the child*, Philadelphia, 2005, Saunders.

Bar-Shira A, Rosner G, Rosner S, and others: Array-based comparative genome hybridization in clinical genetics, *Pediatr Res* 60(3):353–358, 2006.

Beck CT: A meta-analysis of the relationship between postpartum depression and infant temperament, *Nurs Res* 45(4):225–230, 1996.

Bos AF, Einspieler C, Prechtl HF, and others: Intrauterine growth retardation, general movements, and neurodevelopmental outcome: a review, *Dev Med Child Neurol* 43(1):61–68, 2001.

Caine D, DiFiori J, Maffulli N: Physeal injuries in children's and youth sports: reasons for concern? *Br J Sports Med* 40(9):749–760, 2006.

Carey JC, Cohen MM, Curry CJ, and others: Elements of morphology: standard terminology for the lips, mouth, and oral region, *Am J Med Genet A* 149A(1):77–92, 2009.

Carey WB: Teaching parents about infant temperament, *Pediatrics* 102(5 suppl E): 1311–1316, 1998.

Chess S, Thomas A: *Goodness of fit: clinical applications from infancy through adult life*, London, 1999, Routledge.

Consensus Panel on Genetic/Genomic Nursing Competencies: *Essential nursing competencies and curricula guidelines for genetics and genomics*, Silver Spring, Md, 2006, American Nurses Association.

Cronk C, Crocker AC, Pueschel SM, and others: Growth charts for children with Down syndrome: 1 month to 18 years of age, *Pediatrics* 81(1):102–110, 1988.

Delva J, O'Malley PM, Johnston LD: Availability of more-healthy and less-healthy food choices in American schools: a national study of grade, racial/ethnic, and socioeconomic differences, *Am J Prev Med* 33(4 suppl):S226-S239, 2007.

Erikson EH: *Childhood and society*, ed 2, New York, 1963, Norton.

Fowler J: *Stages of faith: the psychology of human development and the quest for meaning*, New York, 1981, HarperCollins.

Frankenburg WK: Preventing developmental delays: is developmental screening sufficient? I. Developmental screening and the Denver II, *Pediatrics* 93(4):586–589, 1994a.

Frankenburg WK: Preventing developmental delays: is developmental screening sufficient? II. Partners in health care, *Pediatrics* 93(4): 589–593, 1994b.

Freud S: *New introductory lectures in psychoanalysis*, New York, 1933, Norton.

Freud S: An outline of psychoanalysis. In Strachey J, editor and translator: *The standard edition of the complete psychological works of Sigmund Freud*, vol 23, London, 1964, Hogarth Press.

Galligan M: Proposed guidelines for skin to skin treatment of neonatal hypothermia, *MCN Am J Matern Child Nurs* 31(5):298–304, 2006.

Glascoe FP, Byrne KE, Ashford LG, and others: Accuracy of the Denver-II in developmental screening, *Pediatrics* 89(6 Pt 2):1221–1225, 1992.

Guttmacher AE, Collins FS: Genomic medicine—a primer, *N Engl J Med* 347(19):1512–1520, 2002.

Jackson JA, Patterson DG, Harris RE: *The measurement of man*, Minneapolis, 1930, University of Minnesota Press.

Jung FE, Czajka-Narins DM: Birth weight doubling and tripling times: an updated look at the effects of birth weight, sex, race, and type of feeding, *Am J Clin Nutr* 42:182–189, 1985.

Kaczander BI: Pediatric sports medicine: a unique perspective, *Podiatr Manage* 16(2):53–60, 1997.

Kohlberg L: Moral development. In Sills DL, editor: *International encyclopedia of the social sciences*, New York, 1968, Macmillan.

Lampl M, Johnson ML, Frongillo EA: Mixed distribution analysis identifies saltation and stasis growth, *Ann Hum Biol* 28(4):403–411, 2001.

Lampl M, Thompson A, Frongillo EA: Sex differences in the relationships among weight gain, subcutaneous skinfold tissue and salutatory length growth spurts in infancy, *Pediatr Res* 58(6):1238–1242, 2005.

Matvienko O: Impact of a nutrition education curriculum on snack choices of children ages six and seven years, *J Nutr Educ Behav* 39(5):281–285, 2007.

Morrow JD, Camp BW: Mastery motivation and temperament of 7-month-old infants, *Pediatr Nurs* 22(3):211–217, 1996.

Myrelid A, Gustafsson J, Ollars B, and others: Growth charts for Down's syndrome from birth to 18 years of age, *Arch Dis Child* 87(2):97–103, 2002.

National Foundation for Ectodermal Dysplasias: *Types of ectodermal dysplasias*, 2010. Retrieved June 29, 2011, from http://nfed.org/index.php/about_ed/types_of_ectodermal_dysplasias.

Piaget J: *The theory of stages in cognitive development*, New York, 1969, McGraw-Hill.

Rimoin DL, Connor MJ, Pyeritz RE, and others: *Emery and Rimoin's principles and practice of medical genetics*. London, Churchill Livingstone, 2002.

Romiti ML, Colognesi C, Cancrini C, and others: Prognostic value of a CCR5 defective allele in pediatric HIV-1 infection, *Mol Med* 6(1):28–36, 2000.

Seidel HM, Ball JW, Dains JE, and others: *Mosby's guide to physical examination*, ed 6, St. Louis, 2007, Mosby.

Sieving RE, Zirbel-Donisch ST: Development and enhancement of self-esteem in children, *J Pediatr Health Care* 4(6):290–296, 1990.

Stuart GW, Laraia MT: *Principles and practice of psychiatric nursing*, ed 7, St. Louis, 2000, Mosby.

Thompson R, Cotner-Bichelman N, McKerchar P, and others: Enhancing early communication through infant sign training, *J Appl Behav Anal* 40(1):15–23, 2007.

Urbanski LF, Hanlon DP: Pediatric orthopedics, *Top Emerg Med* 18(2):73–90, 1996.

Van Riper M: Families of children with Down syndrome: responding to "a change in plans" with resilience, *J Pediatr Nurs* 22(2):116–128, 2007.

Wagner J, Jenkins B, Smith J: Nurses' utilization of parent questionnaires for developmental screening, *Pediatr Nurs* 32(5):409–412, 2006.

Wilkin TJ, Su Z, Kuritzkes DR, and others: HIV type 1 chemokine coreceptor use among antiretroviral-experienced patients screened for a clinical trial of a CCR5 inhibitor: AIDS Clinical Trial Group A5211, *Clin Infect Dis* 44(4):591–595, 2007.

Willoughby C, King G, Polatajko H: A therapist's guide to children's self-esteem, *Am J Occup Ther* 50(2):124–132, 1996.

6

Communication and Physical Assessment of the Child

Marilyn J. Hockenberry

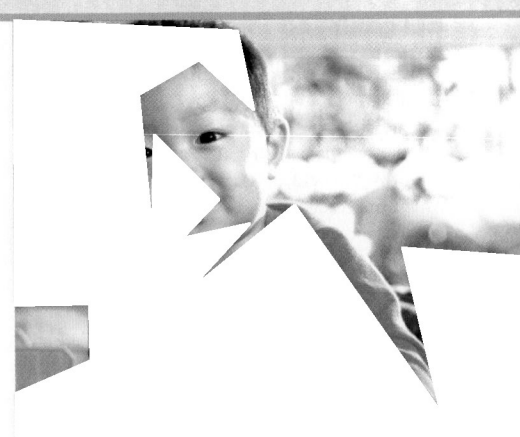

⊖volve WEBSITE

http://evolve.elsevier.com/wong/essentials

Animations—Abdominal Anatomy; Cranial Nerves; Organ Systems
  3-D Tour
Case Studies—Communicating with Adolescents; Pediatric
  Assessment
Key Point Summaries
NCLEX-Style Review Questions

CHAPTER OUTLINE

Guidelines for Communication and
  Interviewing, 87
  Establishing a Setting for
    Communication, 87
    Appropriate Introduction, 87
    *Assurance of Privacy and
      Confidentiality, 87*
  Computer Privacy and Applications in
    Nursing, 88
  Telephone Triage and Counseling, 88
Communicating with Families, 88
  Communicating with Parents, 88
    Encouraging the Parents to Talk, 88
    Directing the Focus, 88
    *Listening and Cultural
      Awareness, 89*
    Using Silence, 89
    Being Empathic, 89
    *Providing Anticipatory
      Guidance, 89*
    Avoiding Blocks to Communication, 89
    *Communicating with Families
      Through an Interpreter, 89*
  Communicating with Children, 90
    *Communication Related to
      Development of Thought
      Processes, 91*
  Communication Techniques, 92
    Play, 94

History Taking, 95
  Performing a Health History, 95
    Identifying Information, 95
    Chief Complaint, 95
    Present Illness, 96
    History, 96
    Sexual History, 98
    Family Medical History, 98
    Family Structure, 98
    Psychosocial History, 99
    Review of Systems, 99
Nutritional Assessment, 99
  Dietary Intake, 99
  Clinical Examination of Nutrition, 102
  Evaluation of Nutritional
    Assessment, 102
General Approaches Toward Examining
  the Child, 102
  Sequence of the Examination, 102
  Preparation of the Child, 102
Physical Examination, 106
  Growth Measurements, 106
    Growth Charts, 107
    Length, 109
    Height, 110
    Weight, 110
    *Skinfold Thickness and Arm
      Circumference, 111*
    Head Circumference, 111

Physiologic Measurements, 111
  Temperature, 111
  Pulse, 112
  Respiration, 112
  Blood Pressure, 115
General Appearance, 118
Skin, 119
  Accessory Structures, 119
Lymph Nodes, 120
Head and Neck, 120
Eyes, 121
  *Inspection of External
    Structures, 121*
  Inspection of Internal Structures, 121
  Vision Testing, 122
Ears, 125
  Inspection of External Structures, 125
  Inspection of Internal Structures, 125
  Auditory Testing, 127
Nose, 127
  Inspection of External Structures, 127
  Inspection of Internal Structures, 128
Mouth and Throat, 128
  Inspection of Internal Structures, 128
Chest, 129
Lungs, 130
  Auscultation, 131
Heart, 132
  Auscultation, 133

CHAPTER OUTLINE—cont'd

Abdomen, 134
  Inspection, 135
  Auscultation, 136
  Palpation, 136
Genitalia, 136
  Male Genitalia, 137
  Female Genitalia, 137

Anus, 138
Back and Extremities, 138
  Spine, 138
  Extremities, 139
  Joints, 139
  Muscles, 139

Neurologic Assessment, 140
  Cerebellar Function, 140
  Reflexes, 140
  Cranial Nerves, 140

LEARNING OBJECTIVES

On completion of this chapter the reader will be able to:

- Identify communication strategies for interviewing parents.
- Formulate guidelines for using an interpreter.
- Identify communication strategies for communicating with children of different age groups.
- Describe four communication techniques that are useful with children.
- State the components of a complete health history.
- List three areas that are evaluated as part of nutritional assessment.

- Prepare a child for a physical examination based on his or her developmental needs.
- Perform a comprehensive physical examination in a sequence appropriate to the child's age.
- Recognize expected normal findings for children at various ages.
- Record the physical examination according to the head-to-toe format.

GUIDELINES FOR COMMUNICATION AND INTERVIEWING

The most widely used method of communicating with parents on a professional basis is the interview process. Unlike social conversation, interviewing is a specific form of goal-directed communication. As nurses converse with children and adults, they focus on individuals to determine the kind of persons they are, their usual mode of handling problems, whether they need help, and the ways they react to counseling. Developing interviewing skills requires time and practice, but following some guiding principles can facilitate this process. An organized approach is most effective when using interviewing skills in patient teaching.

ESTABLISHING A SETTING FOR COMMUNICATION

Appropriate Introduction

Introduce yourself and ask the name of each family member who is present. Address parents or other adults by their appropriate titles, such as "Mr." and "Mrs.," unless they specify a preferred name. Record the preferred name on the medical record. Using formal address or their preferred names, rather than using first names or "mother" or "father," conveys respect and regard for the parents or other caregivers (Seidel, Ball, Dains, and others, 2011).

At the beginning of the visit, include children in the interaction by asking them their names, ages, and other information. Nurses often direct all questions to adults even when children are old enough to speak for themselves. This only terminates one extremely valuable source of information: the patient. When including the child, follow the general rules for communicating with children given in the Nursing Care Guidelines box on p. 91.

Assurance of Privacy and Confidentiality

The place where the nurse conducts the interview is almost as important as the interview itself. The physical environment should allow for as much privacy as possible with distractions, such as interruptions, noise, or other visible activity, kept to a minimum. At times, it is necessary to turn off a television, radio, or cellular telephone. The environment should also have some play provision for young children to keep them occupied during the parent–nurse interview (Fig. 6-1). Parents who are constantly interrupted by their children are unable to concentrate fully and tend to give brief answers to finish the interview as quickly as possible.

Confidentiality is another essential component of the initial phase of the interview. Because the interview is usually shared with other members of the health team care or the teacher (in the case of students), be certain to inform the family of the limits regarding confidentiality. If confidentiality is a concern in a particular situation, such as when talking to a parent suspected of child abuse or a teenager contemplating suicide, deal with this directly and inform the person

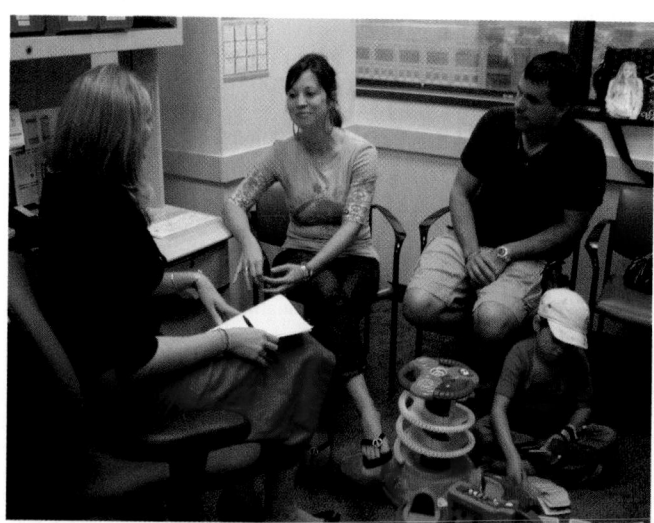

FIG 6-1 Child plays while nurse interviews parents.

that in such instances, confidentiality cannot be ensured. However, the nurse judiciously protects information of a confidential nature.

COMPUTER PRIVACY AND APPLICATIONS IN NURSING

The use of computer technology to store and retrieve health information has become widespread. The health care community is increasingly concerned about the privacy and security of this health information. Any person accessing confidential health information is charged with managing safeguards for disclosure because violations might incur civil damages.

Many institutions use computer and information applications in nursing (**nursing informatics**), such as electronic medical records, to record care and access information. Two important health care applications are record transmission, including facsimile (fax), electronic mail (e-mail), and telemedicine. The telemedicine application is capable of two-way video conferencing, transmission of radiographs, and clinical consultation between remote sites and centralized resources.*

TELEPHONE TRIAGE AND COUNSELING

Nurses are increasingly responsible for assessing children's symptoms and applying clinical judgment for further medical care (**triage**) via telephone report. Most often, health problems are assessed and prioritized according to urgency, and nurses provide treatment via telephone services. A well-designed telephone triage program is essential for safe, prompt, and consistent-quality health care (Beaulieu and Humphreys, 2008; Marklund, Ström, Månsson, and others, 2007). Telephone triage is more than "just a phone call" because a child's life is a high price to pay for poorly managed or incompetent telephone assessment skills. Typically, guidelines for telephone triage include asking screening questions; determining when to immediately refer to emergency medical services (dial 911); and determining when to refer to same-day appointments, appointments in 24 to 72 hours, appointments in 4 days or more, or home care (Box 6-1). Successful outcomes are based on the consistency and accuracy of the information provided. Telephone triage care management has increased access to high-quality health care services and empowered parents to participate in their children's medical care. Consequently, patient satisfaction has significantly improved. Unnecessary emergency department and clinic visits have decreased, saving medical costs and time (with less absence from work) for families in need of health care.

COMMUNICATING WITH FAMILIES

COMMUNICATING WITH PARENTS

Although the parent and the child are separate and distinct individuals, the nurse's relationship with the child is frequently mediated by the parent, particularly with younger children. For the most part, nurses acquire information about the child by direct observation or through communication with the parents. Usually it can be assumed that because of the close contact with the child, the parent gives reliable information. Assessing the child requires input from the child (verbal

---

*Resources: Nicoll LH: *Nurses' guide to the Internet*, ed 3, Philadelphia, 2001, Lippincott. Also available is a bimonthly publication, *CIN: Computers, Informatics, Nursing*. To order, call 800-638-3030; fax: 301-714-2300; e-mail: CustomerService@LWW.com; www.cinjournal.com.

BOX 6-1	TELEPHONE TRIAGE GUIDELINES

Date and time
Background
- Name, age, sex
- Chronic illness
- Allergies, current medications, treatments, or recent immunizations

Chief complaint
General symptoms
- Severity
- Duration
- Other symptoms
- Pain

Systems review
Steps taken
- Advised to call emergency medical services (911)
- Advised to see practitioner
- Advised regarding home care
- Advised to call back if symptoms worsen or fail to improve

Resources for Telephone Triage Protocols

Beaulieu R, Jumphreys J: Evaluation of a telephone advice nurse in a nursing faculty managed pediatric community clinic, *J Pediatr Health Care* 22(3):175–181, 2008.

Marklund B, Ström M, Månsson J, and others: Computer-supported telephone nurse triage: an evaluation of medical quality and costs, *J Nurs Manage* 15:180–187, 2007.

Simonsen SM: *Telephone assessment: guidelines for practice*, ed 2, St. Louis, 2001, Mosby.

---

and nonverbal), information from the parent, and the nurse's own observations of the child and interpretation of the relationship between the child and the parent. When children are old enough to be active participants in their own health maintenance, the parent becomes a collaborator in health care.

Encouraging the Parents to Talk

Interviewing parents not only offers the opportunity to determine the child's health and developmental status but also offers information about factors that influence the child's life. Whatever the parent sees as a problem should be a concern of the nurse. These problems are not always easy to identify. Nurses need to be alert for clues and signals by which a parent communicates worries and anxieties. Careful phrasing with broad, open-ended questions such as "What is Jimmy eating now?" provides more information than several single-answer questions, such as "Is Jimmy eating what the rest of the family eats?"

Sometimes the parent will take the lead without prompting. At other times, it may be necessary to direct another question on the basis of an observation, such as "Connie seems unhappy today" or "How do you feel when David cries?" If the parent appears to be tired or distraught, consider asking, "What do you do to relax?" or "What help do you have with the children?" A comment such as "You handle the baby very well. What kind of experience have you had with babies?" to new parents who appear comfortable with their first child gives positive reinforcement and provides an opening for questions they might have on the infant's care. Often all that is required to keep parents talking is a nod or saying "yes" or "uh-huh."

Directing the Focus

Directing the focus of the interview while allowing maximum freedom of expression is one of the most difficult goals in effective communication. One approach is the use of open-ended or broad questions followed by guiding statements. For example, if the parent proceeds to

CULTURAL CONSIDERATIONS

Interviewing Without Judgment

It is easy to inject one's own attitudes and feelings into an interview. Often nurses' own prejudices and assumptions, which may include racial, religious, and cultural stereotypes, influence their perceptions of a parent's behavior. What the nurse may interpret as a parent's passive hostility or lack of interest may be shyness or an expression of anxiety. For example, in Western cultures, eye contact and directness are signs of paying attention. However, in many non-Western cultures, including that of Native Americans, directness (e.g., looking someone in the eye) is considered rude. Children are taught to avert their gaze and to look down when being addressed by an adult, especially one with authority (Seidel, Ball, Dains, and others, 2011). Therefore, nurses must make judgments about "listening," as well as verbal interactions, with an appreciation of cultural differences.

list the other children by name, say, "Tell me their ages, too." If the parent continues to describe each child in depth, which is not the purpose of the interview, redirect the focus by stating, "Let's talk about the other children later. You were beginning to tell me about Paul's activities at school." This approach conveys interest in the other children but focuses the assessment on the patient.

Listening and Cultural Awareness

Listening is the most important component of effective communication. When the purpose of listening is to understand the person being interviewed, it is an active process that requires concentration and attention to all aspects of the conversation—verbal, nonverbal, and abstract. Major blocks to listening are environmental distraction and premature judgment.

Although it is necessary to make some preliminary judgments, listen with as much objectivity as possible by clarifying meanings and attempting to see the situation from the parent's point of view. Effective interviewers consciously control their reactions, responses, and the techniques they use (see Cultural Considerations box).

Careful listening relies on the use of clues, verbal leads, or signals from the interviewee to move along the interview. Frequent references to an area of concern, repetition of certain key words, or a special emphasis on something or someone serve as cues to the interviewer for the direction of inquiry. Concerns and anxieties are often mentioned in a casual, offhand manner. Even though they are casual, they are important and deserve careful scrutiny to identify problem areas. For example, a parent who is concerned about a child's habit of bedwetting may casually mention that the child's bed was "wet this morning."

Using Silence

Silence as a response is often one of the most difficult interviewing techniques to learn. The interviewer requires a sense of confidence and comfort to allow the interviewee space in which to think without interruptions. Silence permits the interviewee to sort out thoughts and feelings and search for responses to questions. Silence can also be a cue for the interviewer to go more slowly, reexamine the approach, and not push too hard (Seidel, Ball, Dains, and others, 2011).

Sometimes it is necessary to break the silence and reopen communication. Do this in a way that encourages the person to continue talking about what is considered important. Breaking a silence by introducing a new topic or by prolonged talking essentially terminates the interviewee's opportunity to use the silence. Suggestions for

breaking the silence include statements such as: "Is there anything else you wish to say?" "I see you find it difficult to continue; how may I help?" or "I don't know what this silence means. Perhaps there is something you would like to put into words but find difficult to say."

Being Empathic

Empathy is the capacity to understand what another person is experiencing from within that person's frame of reference; it is often described as the ability to put oneself in another's shoes. The essence of empathic interaction is accurate understanding of another's feelings (Mathiasen, 2006). Empathy differs from sympathy, which is *having* feelings or emotions similar to those of another person, rather than *understanding* those feelings (Mathiasen, 2006).

Providing Anticipatory Guidance

The ideal way to handle a situation is to deal with it *before* it becomes a problem. The best preventive measure is anticipatory guidance. Traditionally, anticipatory guidance focused on providing families information on normal growth and development and nurturing childrearing practices. For example, one of the most significant areas in pediatrics is injury prevention. Beginning prenatally, parents need specific instructions on home safety. Because of the child's maturing developmental skills, parents must implement home safety changes early to minimize risks to the child.

Unprepared parents can be disturbed by many normal developmental changes, such as a toddler's diminished appetite, negativism, altered sleeping patterns, and anxiety toward strangers. The chapters on health promotion provide nurses with information for counseling parents. However, anticipatory guidance should extend beyond giving general information during brief visits to empowering families to use the information as a means of building competence in their parenting abilities (Magar, Dabova-Missova, and Gjerdingen, 2006). To achieve this level of anticipatory guidance, the nurse should:

- Base interventions on needs identified by the family, not by the professional.
- View the family as competent or as having the ability to be competent.
- Provide opportunities for the family to achieve competence.

Avoiding Blocks to Communication

A number of blocks to communication can adversely affect the quality of the helping relationship. The interviewer introduces many of these blocks, such as giving unrestricted advice or forming prejudged conclusions. Another type of block occurs primarily with the interviewees and concerns information overload. When individuals receive too much information or information that is overwhelming, they often demonstrate signs of increasing anxiety or decreasing attention. Such signals should alert the interviewer to give less information or to clarify what has been said. Box 6-2 lists some of the more common blocks to communication, including signs of information overload.

The nurse can correct communication blocks by careful analysis of the interview process. One of the best methods for improving interviewing skills is audiotape or videotape feedback. With supervision and guidance, the interviewer can recognize the blocks and consciously avoid them.

Communicating with Families Through an Interpreter

Sometimes communication is impossible because two people speak different languages. In this case, it is necessary to obtain information through a third party, the interpreter. When using an interpreter, the nurse follows the same interviewing guidelines. Specific guidelines

BOX 6-2   BLOCKS TO COMMUNICATION

Communication Barriers (Nurse)
Socializing
Giving unrestricted and sometimes unasked for advice
Offering premature or inappropriate reassurance
Giving overready encouragement
Defending a situation or opinion
Using stereotyped comments or clichés
Limiting expression of emotion by asking directed, closed-ended questions
Interrupting and finishing the person's sentence
Talking more than the interviewee
Forming prejudged conclusions
Deliberately changing the focus

Signs of Information Overload (Patient)
Long periods of silence
Wide eyes and fixed facial expression
Constant fidgeting or attempting to move away
Nervous habits (e.g., tapping, playing with hair)
Sudden interruptions (e.g., asking to go to the bathroom)
Looking around
Yawning, eyes drooping
Frequently looking at a watch or clock
Attempting to change the topic of discussion

for using an adult interpreter are given in the Nursing Care Guidelines box.

Communicating with families through an interpreter requires sensitivity to cultural, legal, and ethical considerations (see Cultural Considerations box). For example, in some cultures, using a child as an interpreter is considered an insult to an adult because children are expected to show respect by not questioning their elders. In some cultures, class differences between the interpreter and the family may cause the family to feel intimidated and less inclined to offer information. Therefore, it is important to choose the translator carefully and provide time for the interpreter and family to establish rapport.

Legal and ethical concerns may also arise. For example, in obtaining informed consent through an interpreter, the nurse should fully inform the family of all aspects of the particular procedure to which they are consenting. Issues of confidentiality may arise when family members related to another patient are asked to interpret for the family, thus revealing sensitive information that may be shared with other families on the unit. With increased sensitivity toward patient rights and confidentiality, many institutions now require consent forms produced in the patient's primary language.

! NURSING ALERT

When using translated materials, such as a health history form, be certain the informant is literate in the foreign language.

COMMUNICATING WITH CHILDREN

Although the greatest amount of verbal communication is usually carried out with the parent, do not exclude the child during the interview. Pay attention to infants and younger children through play or by occasionally directing questions or remarks to them. Include older children as active participants.

NURSING CARE GUIDELINES

Using an Interpreter

- Explain to interpreter the reason for the interview and the type of questions that will be asked.
- Clarify whether a detailed or brief answer is required and whether the translated response can be general or literal.
- Introduce the interpreter to family and allow some time before the interview for them to become acquainted.
- Communicate directly with family members when asking questions to reinforce interest in them and to observe nonverbal expressions but do not ignore interpreter.
- Pose questions to elicit only one answer at a time, such as "Do you have pain?" rather than "Do you have any pain, tiredness, or loss of appetite?"
- Refrain from interrupting family members and the interpreter while they are conversing.
- Avoid commenting to the interpreter about family members because they may understand some English.
- Be aware that some medical words, such as *allergy,* may have no similar word in another language; avoid medical jargon whenever possible.
- Be aware that cultural differences may exist regarding views on sex, marriage, or pregnancy.
- Allow time after the interview for the interpreter to share something that he or she thought could not be said earlier; ask about the interpreter's impression of nonverbal clues to communication and family members' reliability or ease in revealing information.
- Arrange for the family to speak with the same interpreter on subsequent visits whenever possible.

🌐 CULTURAL CONSIDERATIONS

Using Children as Translators

When no one else is available to translate, children within the family are often asked to assume this role. In this situation, it is important to stress *literal* translation of parent responses. To ensure correct translations, it may be necessary to interrupt the parent and ask the child to translate every few sentences. When using children as interpreters, ask questions directed at specific answers and assess the interpreted translation in terms of nonverbal expressions of communication. Note that some institutions prohibit or discourage the use of children as interpreters; check institutional policy for compliance.

In communication with children of all ages, the nonverbal components of the communication process convey the most significant messages. It is difficult to disguise feelings, attitudes, and anxiety when relating to children. They are alert to their surroundings and attach meaning to every gesture and move that is made; this is particularly true of very young children.

Active attempts to make friends with children before they have had an opportunity to evaluate an unfamiliar person tend to increase their anxiety. Continue to talk to the child and parent but go about activities that do not involve the child directly, thus allowing the child to observe from a safe position. If the child has a special toy or doll, "talk" to the doll first. Ask simple questions, such as "Does your teddy bear have a name?" to ease the child into conversation. Other guidelines for communicating with children are in the Nursing Care Guidelines box. Specific guidelines for preparing children for procedures, a common nursing function, are provided in Chapter 22.

NURSING CARE GUIDELINES
Communicating with Children

- Allow children time to feel comfortable.
- Avoid sudden or rapid advances, broad smiles, extended eye contact, and other gestures that may be seen as threatening.
- Talk to the parent if the child is initially shy.
- Communicate through transition objects such as dolls, puppets, and stuffed animals before questioning a young child directly.
- Give older children the opportunity to talk without the parents present.
- Assume a position that is at eye level with the child (Fig. 6-2).
- Speak in a quiet, unhurried, and confident voice.
- Speak clearly, be specific, and use simple words and short sentences.
- State directions and suggestions positively.
- Offer a choice only when one exists.
- Be honest with children.
- Allow children to express their concerns and fears.
- Use a variety of communication techniques.

BOX 6-3 CHARACTERISTICS OF COMMUNICATIVE DEVELOPMENT IN YOUNG CHILDREN

Perlocutionary Stage (0 to 8–9 Months)
Child is reflexive to stimuli.
Child shows increasing purpose in action.

Emerging Illocutionary Stage (8–9 to 12–15 Months)
Child communicates intentionally with signals and gestures.

Conventional Illocutionary–Emerging Locutionary Stage (12–15 to 18–24 Months)
Child communicates intentionally with gestures, vocalizations, and verbalizations.

Modified from Hoge DR, Parette HP: Facilitating communicative development in young children with disabilities, *Transdisc J* 5(2):113–130, 1995.

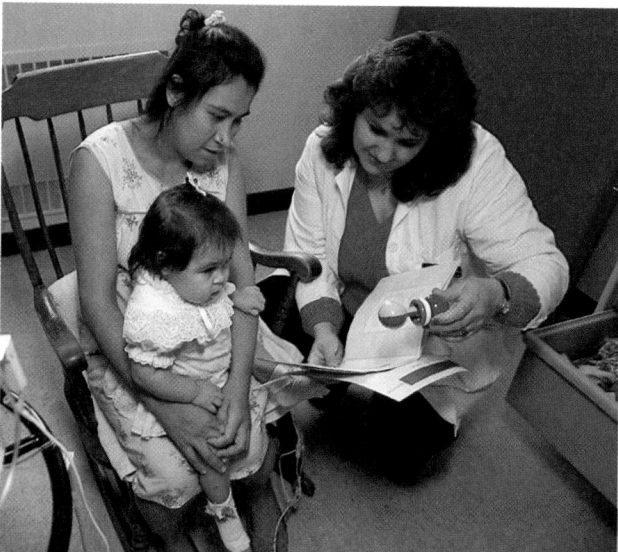

FIG 6-2 Nurse assumes position at child's level.

Communication Related to Development of Thought Processes

The normal development of language and thought offers a frame of reference for communicating with children. Thought processes progress from sensorimotor to perceptual to concrete and finally to abstract, formal operations. An understanding of the typical characteristics of these stages provides the nurse with a framework to facilitate social communication (Box 6-3).

Infancy

Because they are unable to use words, infants primarily use and understand nonverbal communication. Infants communicate their needs and feelings through nonverbal behaviors and vocalizations that can be interpreted by someone who is around them for a sufficient time. Infants smile and coo when content and cry when distressed. Crying is provoked by unpleasant stimuli from inside or outside, such as hunger, pain, body restraint, or loneliness. Adults interpret this to

mean that an infant needs something and consequently try to alleviate the discomfort and reduce tension. Crying (or the desire to cry) persists as a part of everyone's communication repertoire.

Infants respond to adults' nonverbal behaviors. They become quiet when they are cuddled, patted, or receive other forms of gentle physical contact. They receive comfort from the sound of a voice even though they do not understand the words that are spoken. Until infants reach the age at which they experience stranger anxiety, they readily respond to any firm, gentle handling and quiet, calm speech. Loud, harsh sounds and sudden movements are frightening.

Early Childhood

Children younger than 5 years of age are egocentric. They see things only in relation to themselves and from their point of view. Therefore, focus communication on them. Tell them what they can do or how they will feel. Experiences of others are of no interest to them. It is futile to use another child's experience in an attempt to gain the cooperation of small children. Allow them to touch and examine articles they will come in contact with. A stethoscope bell will feel cold; palpating a neck might tickle. Although they have not yet acquired sufficient language skills to express their feelings and wants, toddlers can effectively use their hands to communicate ideas without words. They push an unwanted object away, pull another person to show them something, point, and cover the mouth that is saying something they do not wish to hear.

Everything is direct and concrete to small children. They are unable to work with abstractions and interpret words literally. Analogies escape them because they are unable to separate fact from fantasy. For example, they attach literal meaning to such common phrases as "two-faced," "sticky fingers," and "coughing your head off." Children who are told they will get "a little stick in the arm" may not be able to envision an injection (Fig. 6-3). Therefore, avoid using a phrase that might be misinterpreted by a small child (see Table 22-1).

School-Age Years

Younger school-age children rely less on what they see and more on what they know when faced with new problems. They want explanations and reasons for everything but require no verification beyond that. They are interested in the functional aspect of all procedures, objects, and activities. They want to know why an object exists, why it

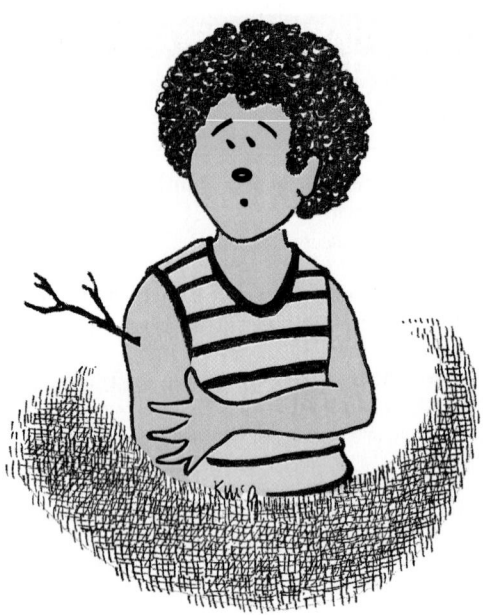

FIG 6-3 A young child may take the expression "a little stick in the arm" literally.

NURSING CARE GUIDELINES

Communicating with Adolescents

Build a Foundation
Spend time together.
Encourage expression of ideas and feelings.
Respect their views.
Tolerate differences.
Praise good points.
Respect their privacy.
Set a good example.

Communicate Effectively
Give undivided attention.
Listen, listen, listen.
Be courteous, calm, and open minded.
Try not to overreact. If you do, take a break.
Avoid judging or criticizing.
Avoid the "third degree" of continuous questioning.
Choose important issues when taking a stand.
After taking a stand:
- Think through all options.
- Make expectations clear.

is used, how it works, and the intent and purpose of its user. They need to know what is going to take place and why it is being done to them specifically. For example, to explain a procedure such as taking blood pressure (BP), show the child how squeezing the bulb pushes air into the cuff and makes the "silver" in the tube go up. Let the child operate the bulb. An explanation for the procedure might be as simple as, "I want to see how far the silver goes up when the cuff squeezes your arm." Consequently, the child becomes an enthusiastic participant.

School-age children have a heightened concern about body integrity. Because of the special importance they place on their body, they are sensitive to anything that constitutes a threat or suggestion of injury to it. This concern extends to their possessions, so they may appear to overreact to loss or threatened loss of treasured objects. Helping children voice their concerns enables the nurse to provide reassurance and to implement activities that reduce their anxiety. For example, if a shy child dislikes being the center of attention, ignore that particular child by talking and relating to other children in the family or group. When children feel more comfortable, they will usually interject personal ideas, feelings, and interpretations of events.

Adolescence

As children move into adolescence, they fluctuate between child and adult thinking and behavior. They are riding a current that is moving them rapidly toward a maturity that may be beyond their coping ability. Therefore, when tensions rise, they may seek the security of the more familiar and comfortable expectations of childhood. Anticipating these shifts in identity allows the nurse to adjust the course of interaction to meet the needs of the moment. No single approach can be relied on consistently, and encountering cooperation, hostility, anger, bravado, and a variety of other behaviors and attitudes is common. It is as much a mistake to regard an adolescent as an adult with an adult's wisdom and control as it is to assume that a teenager has the concerns and expectations of a child.

Interviewing an adolescent presents some special issues. The first may be whether to talk with the adolescent alone or with the adolescent and parents together. Of course, if the parent is not there, the only question is whether to suggest to the teenager that the parents

be interviewed at another time. If the parents and teenager are together, talking with the adolescent first has the advantage of immediately identifying with the young person, thus fostering the interpersonal relationship. However, talking with the parents initially may provide insight into the family relationship. In either case, give both parties an opportunity to be included in the interview. If time is limited, such as during history taking, clarify this at the onset to avoid appearing to "take sides" by talking more with one person than with the other.

Confidentiality is of great importance when interviewing adolescents. Explain to parents and teenagers the limits of confidentiality, specifically that young persons' disclosures will not be shared unless they indicate a need for intervention, as in the case of suicidal behavior.

Another dilemma in interviewing adolescents is that two views of a problem frequently exist—the teenager's and the parents'. Clarification of the problem is a major task. However, providing both parties an opportunity to discuss their perceptions in an open and unbiased atmosphere can, by itself, be therapeutic. Demonstrating positive communication skills can help families communicate more effectively (see Nursing Care Guidelines box).

COMMUNICATION TECHNIQUES

Nurses use a variety of verbal techniques to encourage communication. Some of these techniques are useful to pose questions or explore concerns in a less threatening manner. Others can be presented as word games, which are often well received by children. However, for many children and adults, talking about feelings is difficult, and verbal communication may be more stressful than supportive. In such instances, use several nonverbal techniques to encourage communication. Box 6-4 describes both verbal and nonverbal techniques.

Because of the importance of play in communicating with children, play is discussed more extensively below. Any of the verbal or nonverbal techniques can give rise to strong feelings that surface unexpectedly. Be prepared to handle them or to recognize when issues go beyond

BOX 6-4 CREATIVE COMMUNICATION TECHNIQUES WITH CHILDREN

Verbal Techniques
"I" Messages
Relate a feeling about a behavior in terms of "I."
Describe effect behavior had on the person.
Avoid use of "you."
"You" messages are judgmental and provoke defensiveness.
- **Example**—"You" message: "You are being uncooperative about doing your treatments."
- **Example**—"I" message: "I am concerned about how the treatments are going because I want to see you get better."

Third-Person Technique
Express a feeling in terms of a third person ("he," "she," "they"). This is less threatening than directly asking children how they feel because it gives them an opportunity to agree or disagree without being defensive.
- **Example**—"Sometimes when a person is sick a lot, he feels angry and sad because he cannot do what others can." Either wait silently for a response or encourage a reply with a statement such as "Did you ever feel that way?"

This approach allows children three choices: (1) to agree and, one hopes, express how they feel; (2) to disagree; or (3) to remain silent, which means they probably have such feelings but are unable to express them at this time.

Facilitative Response
Listen carefully and reflect back to patients the feelings and content of their statements.
Responses are empathic and nonjudgmental and legitimize the person's feelings.
Formula for facilitative responses: "You feel _____ because _____."
- **Example**—If child states, "I hate coming to the hospital and getting needles," a facilitative response is, "You feel unhappy because of all the things that are done to you."

Storytelling
Use the language of children to probe into areas of their thinking while bypassing conscious inhibitions or fears.
The simplest technique is asking children to relate a story about an event, such as "being in the hospital."
Other approaches:
- Show children a picture of a particular event, such as a child in a hospital with other people in the room, and ask them to describe the scene.
- Cut out comic strips, remove words, and have child add statements for scenes.

Mutual Storytelling
Reveal the child's thinking and attempt to change his or her perceptions or fears by retelling a somewhat different story (more therapeutic approach than storytelling).
Begin by asking the child to tell a story about something; then tell another story that is similar to child's tale but with differences that help the child in problem areas.
- **Example**—The child's story is about going to the hospital and never seeing his or her parents again. The nurse's story is also about a child (using different names but similar circumstances) in a hospital whose parents visit every day but in the evening after work until the child is better and goes home with them.

Bibliotherapy
Use books in a therapeutic and supportive process.
Provide children with an opportunity to explore an event that is similar to their own but sufficiently different to allow them to distance themselves from it and remain in control.
General guidelines for using bibliotherapy are:
1. Assess the child's emotional and cognitive development in terms of readiness to understand the book's message.
2. Be familiar with the book's content (intended message or purpose) and the age for which it is written.
3. Read the book to the child if child is unable to read.
4. Explore the meaning of the book with the child by having the child:
   - Retell the story.
   - Read a special section with the nurse or parent.
   - Draw a picture related to the story and discuss the drawing.
   - Talk about the characters.
   - Summarize the moral or meaning of the story.

Dreams
Dreams often reveal unconscious and repressed thoughts and feelings.
Ask the child to talk about a dream or nightmare.
Explore with the child what meaning the dream could have.

"What If" Questions
Encourage child to explore potential situations and to consider different problem-solving options.
- **Example**—"What if you got sick and had to go the hospital?" Children's responses reveal what they know already and what they are curious about, providing an opportunity for them to learn coping skills, especially in potentially dangerous situations.

Three Wishes
Ask, "If you could have any three things in the world, what would they be?"
If the child answers, "That all my wishes come true," ask the child for specific wishes.

Rating Game
Use some type of rating scale (numbers, sad to happy faces) to have the child rate an event or feeling.
- **Example**—Instead of asking youngsters how they feel, ask how their day has been "on a scale of 1 to 10, with 10 being the best."

Word Association Game
State key words and ask children to say the first word they think of when they hear the word.
Start with neutral words and then introduce more anxiety-producing words, such as "illness," "needles," "hospitals," and "operation."
Select key words that relate to some relevant event in the child's life.

Sentence Completion
Present a partial statement and have the child complete it. Some sample statements are:
- The thing I like best (least) about school is _____.
- The best (worst) age to be is _____.
- The most (least) fun thing I ever did was _____.
- The thing I like most (least) about my parents is _____.
- The one thing I would change about my family is _____.

Continued

BOX 6-4 CREATIVE COMMUNICATION TECHNIQUES WITH CHILDREN—cont'd

- If I could be anything I wanted, I would be _____.
- The thing I like most (least) about myself is _____.

Pros and Cons

Select a topic, such as "being in the hospital," and have the child list "five good things and five bad things" about it.

This is an exceptionally valuable technique when applied to relationships, such as things family members like and dislike about each other.

Nonverbal Techniques

Writing

Writing is an alternative communication approach for older children and adults. Specific suggestions include:

- Keep a journal or diary.
- Write down feelings or thoughts that are difficult to express.
- Write "letters" that are never mailed (a variation is making up a "pen pal" to write to).

Keep an account of the child's progress from both a physical and an emotional viewpoint.

Drawing

Drawing is one of the most valuable forms of communication—both nonverbal (from looking at the drawing) and verbal (from the child's story of the picture).

Children's drawings tell a great deal about them because they are projections of their inner selves.

Spontaneous drawing involves giving child a variety of art supplies and providing the opportunity to draw.

Directed drawing involves a more specific direction, such as "draw a person" or the "three themes" approach (state three things about child and ask the child to choose one and draw a picture).

Guidelines for Evaluating Drawings

Use spontaneous drawings and evaluate more than one drawing whenever possible.

Interpret the drawings in light of other available information about child and family, including the child's age and stage of development.

Interpret the drawings as a whole rather than focusing on specific details of the drawings.

Consider individual elements of the drawings that may be significant:

- Sex of figure drawn first—Usually relates to the child's perception of his or her own sex role
- Size of individual figures—Expresses importance, power, or authority
- Order in which figures are drawn—Expresses priority in terms of importance
- Child's position in relation to other family members—Expresses feelings of status or alliance
- Exclusion of a member—May denote feeling of not belonging or desire to eliminate
- Accentuated parts—Usually express concern for areas of special importance (e.g., large hands may be a sign of aggression)
- Absence of or rudimentary arms and hands—Suggest timidity, passivity, or intellectual immaturity; tiny, unstable feet may express insecurity, and hidden hands may mean guilt feelings
- Placement of drawing on the page and type of stroke—Whereas free use of paper and firm, continuous strokes express security, drawings restricted to a small area and lightly drawn in broken or wavering lines may be signs of insecurity
- Erasures, shading, or cross-hatching—Expresses ambivalence, concern, or anxiety with a particular area

Magic

Use simple magic tricks to help establish rapport with child, encourage compliance with health interventions, and provide effective distraction during painful procedures.

Although the "magician" talks, no verbal response from the child is required.

Play

Play is the universal language and "work" of children.

It tells a great deal about children because they project their inner selves through the activity.

Spontaneous play involves giving children a variety of play materials and providing the opportunity to play.

Directed play involves a more specific direction, such as providing medical equipment or a dollhouse for focused reasons, such as exploring children's fears of injections or exploring their family relationships.

---

your ability to deal with them. At that point, consider an appropriate referral.

Play

Play is a universal language of children. It is one of the most important forms of communication and can be an effective technique in relating to them. The nurse can often pick up on clues about physical, intellectual, and social developmental progress from the form and complexity of a child's play behaviors. Play requires minimum equipment or none at all. Many providers use therapeutic play to reduce the trauma of illness and hospitalization (see Chapter 22) and to prepare children for therapeutic procedures (see Chapter 22).

Because their ability to perceive precedes their ability to transmit, infants respond to activities that register on their physical senses. Patting, stroking, and other skin play convey messages. Repetitive actions, such as stretching infants' arms out to the side while they are lying on their back and then folding the arms across the chest or raising and revolving the legs in a bicycling motion, will elicit pleasurable sounds. Colorful items to catch the eye or interesting sounds, such as a ticking clock, chimes, bells, or singing, can be used to attract children's attention.

Older infants respond to simple games. The old game of peek-a-boo is an excellent means of initiating communication with infants while maintaining a "safe," nonthreatening distance. After this intermittent eye contact, the nurse is no longer viewed as a stranger but as a friend. This can be followed by touch games. Clapping an infant's hands together for pat-a-cake or wiggling the toes for "this little piggy" delights infants and small children. Talking to a foot or other part of the child's body is another effective tactic. Much of the nursing assessment can be carried out with the use of games and simple play equipment while the infant remains in the safety of the parent's arms or lap.

The nurse can capitalize on the natural curiosity of small children by playing games such as "Which hand do you take?" and "Guess what I have in my hand" or by manipulating items such as a flashlight or stethoscope. Finger games are useful. More elaborate materials, such as puppets and replicas of familiar or unfamiliar items, serve as excellent means of communicating with small children. The variety and extent are limited only by the nurse's imagination.

BOX 6-5 OUTLINE OF A PEDIATRIC HEALTH HISTORY

Identifying information
1. Name
2. Address
3. Telephone
4. Birth date and place
5. Race or ethnic group
6. Sex
7. Religion
8. Date of interview
9. Informant

Chief complaint (CC)—To establish the major specific reason for the child's and parents' seeking professional health attention

Present illness (PI)—To obtain all details related to the chief complaint

Past history (PH)—To elicit a profile of the child's previous illnesses, injuries, or operations
1. Birth history (pregnancy, labor and delivery, perinatal history)
2. Previous illnesses, injuries, or operations
3. Allergies
4. Current medications
5. Immunizations
6. Growth and development
7. Habits

Review of systems (ROS)—To elicit information concerning any potential health problem
1. General
2. Integument
3. Head
4. Eyes
5. Ears
6. Nose
7. Mouth
8. Throat
9. Neck
10. Chest
11. Respiratory
12. Cardiovascular
13. Gastrointestinal
14. Genitourinary
15. Gynecologic
16. Musculoskeletal
17. Neurologic
18. Endocrine

Family medical history—To identify genetic traits or diseases that have familial tendencies and to assess exposure to a communicable disease in a family member and family habits that may affect the child's health, such as smoking and chemical use

Psychosocial history—To elicit information about the child's self-concept

Sexual history—To elicit information concerning the child's sexual concerns or activities and any pertinent data regarding adults' sexual activity that influences the child

Family history—To develop an understanding of the child as an individual and as a member of a family and a community
1. Family composition
2. Home and community environment
3. Occupation and education of family members
4. Cultural and religious traditions
5. Family function and relationships

Nutritional assessment—To elicit information on the adequacy of the child's nutritional intake and needs
1. Dietary intake
2. Clinical examination

Through play, children reveal their perceptions of interpersonal relationships with their family, friends, or hospital personnel. Children may also reveal the wide scope of knowledge they have acquired from listening to others around them. For example, through needle play, children may reveal how carefully they have watched each procedure by precisely duplicating the technical skills. They may also reveal how well they remember those who performed procedures. In one example, a child painstakingly reenacted every detail of a tedious medical procedure, including the role of the physician who had repeatedly shouted at her to be still for the long ordeal. Her anger at him was most evident during the play session and revealed the cause for her abrupt withdrawal and passive hostility toward the medical and nursing staff after the test.

HISTORY TAKING

PERFORMING A HEALTH HISTORY

The format used for history taking may be (1) **direct**, in which the nurse asks for information via direct interview with the informant, or (2) **indirect**, in which the informant supplies the information by completing some type of questionnaire. The direct method is superior to the indirect approach or a combination of both. However, because time is limited, the direct approach is not always practical. If the nurse cannot use the direct approach, he or she should review the parents' written responses and question them regarding any unusual answers.

The categories listed in Box 6-5 encompass children's current and past health status and information about their psychosocial environment.

Identifying Information

Much of the identifying information may already be available from other recorded sources. However, if the parent and youngster seem anxious, use this opportunity to ask about such information to help them feel more comfortable.

Informant

One of the important elements of identifying information is the **informant**, the person(s) who furnishes the information. Record (1) who the person is (child, parent, or other), (2) an impression of reliability and willingness to communicate, and (3) any special circumstances such as the use of an interpreter or conflicting answers by more than one person.

Chief Complaint

The chief complaint is the specific reason for the child's visit to the clinic, office, or hospital. It may be the theme, with the present illness viewed as the description of the problem. Elicit the chief complaint by asking open-ended, neutral questions such as: "What seems to be the matter?" "How may I help you?" or "Why did you come here today?" Avoid labeling-type questions such as: "How are you sick?" or "What is the problem?" It is possible that the reason for the visit is not an illness or problem.

Occasionally, it is difficult to isolate one symptom or problem as the chief complaint because the parent may identify many. In this situation, be as specific as possible when asking questions. For example, asking informants to state which *one* problem or symptom prompted them to seek help now may help them focus on the most immediate concern.

Present Illness

The history of the present illness* is a narrative of the chief complaint from its earliest onset through its progression to the present. Its four major components are (1) the details of **onset,** (2) a complete **interval** history, (3) the **present** status, and (4) the reason for seeking help **now.** The focus of the present illness is on all factors relevant to the main problem even if they have disappeared or changed during the onset, interval, and present.

Analyzing a Symptom

Because pain is often the most characteristic symptom denoting the onset of a physical problem, it is used as an example for analysis of a symptom. Assessment includes (1) type, (2) location, (3) severity, (4) duration, and (5) influencing factors (see Nursing Care Guidelines box; see also Pain Assessment, Chapter 7).

History

The history contains information relating to all previous aspects of the child's health status and concentrates on several areas that are ordinarily passed over in the history of an adult, such as birth history, detailed feeding history, immunizations, and growth and development. Because this section includes a great deal of information, use a combination of open-ended and fact-finding questions. For example, begin interviewing for each section with an open-ended statement such as "Tell me about your child's birth" to provide the informants the opportunity to relate what they think is most important. Ask fact-finding questions related to specific details whenever necessary to focus the interview on certain topics.

Birth History

The birth history includes all data concerning (1) the mother's health during pregnancy, (2) the labor and delivery, and (3) the infant's condition immediately after birth. Because prenatal influences have significant effects on a child's physical and emotional development, a thorough investigation of the birth history is essential. Because parents may question what relevance pregnancy and birth have on the child's present condition, particularly if the child is past infancy, explain why such questions are included. An appropriate statement may be, "I will be asking you some questions about your pregnancy and _____'s [refer to child by name] birth. Your answers will give me a more complete picture of his [or her] overall health."

Because emotional factors also affect the outcome of pregnancy and the subsequent parent–child relationship, investigate (1) concurrent crises during pregnancy and (2) prenatal attitudes toward the fetus. It is best to approach the topic of parental acceptance of pregnancy through indirect questioning. Asking the parents if the pregnancy was planned is a leading statement because they may respond affirmatively for fear of criticism if the pregnancy was unexpected. Rather, encourage parents to state their true reactions by referring to specific facts relating to the pregnancy, such as the spacing between offspring, an

---

*The term *illness* is used in its broadest sense to denote any problem of a physical, emotional, or psychosocial nature. It is actually a history of the chief complaint.

NURSING CARE GUIDELINES

Analyzing the Symptom: Pain

Type

Be as specific as possible. With young children, asking the parents how they know the child is in pain may help describe its type, location, and severity. For example, a parent may state, "My child must have a severe earache because she pulls at her ears, rolls her head on the floor, and screams. Nothing seems to help." Help older children describe the "hurt" by asking them if it is sharp, throbbing, dull, or stabbing. Record whatever words they use in quotes.

Location

Be specific. "Stomach pains" is too general a description. Children can better localize the pain if they are asked to "point with one finger to where it hurts" or to "point to where Mommy or Daddy would put a Band-Aid." Determine if the pain radiates by asking, "Does the pain stay there or move? Show me with your finger where the pain goes."

Severity

Severity is best determined by finding out how it affects the child's usual behavior. Pain that prevents a child from playing, interacting with others, sleeping, and eating is most often severe. Assess pain intensity using a rating scale, such as a numeric or FACES scale (see Chapter 7).

Duration

Include the duration, onset, and frequency. Describe these in terms of activity and behavior, such as "pain reported to last all night; child refused to sleep and cried intermittently."

Influencing Factors

Include anything that causes a change in the type, location, severity, or duration of the pain: (1) precipitating events (those that cause or increase the pain), (2) relieving events (those that lessen the pain, such as medications), (3) temporal events (times when the pain is relieved or increased), (4) positional events (standing, sitting, lying down), and (5) associated events (meals, stress, coughing).

---

extended or short interval between marriage and conception, or a pregnancy during adolescence. The parent can choose to explore such statements with further explanations or, for the moment, may not be able to reveal such feelings. If the parent remains silent, return to this topic later in the interview.

Dietary History

Because parental concerns are common and nursing interventions are important in ensuring optimum nutrition, the dietary history is discussed in detail later in this chapter under Nutritional Assessment.

Previous Illnesses, Injuries, and Operations

When inquiring about past illnesses, begin with a general question such as "What other illnesses has your child had?" Because parents are most likely to recall serious health problems, ask specifically about colds; earaches; and childhood diseases such as measles, rubella (German measles), chickenpox, mumps, pertussis (whooping cough), diphtheria, tuberculosis, scarlet fever, strep throat, recurrent ear infections, gastroesophageal reflux, tonsillitis, or allergic manifestations.

In addition to illnesses, ask about injuries that required medical intervention, operations, and any other reason for hospitalization, including the dates of each incident. Focus on injuries such as accidental falls, poisoning, choking, or burns because these may be potential areas for parental guidance.

NURSING CARE GUIDELINES

Taking an Allergy History

- Has your child ever taken any drugs or tablets that have disagreed with him or her or caused an allergic reaction? If yes, can you remember the name(s) of these drugs?
- Can you describe the reaction?
- Was the drug taken by mouth (as a tablet or syrup), or was it an injection?
- How soon after starting the drug did the reaction happen?
- How long ago did this happen?
- Did anyone tell you it was an allergic reaction, or did you decide for yourself?
- Has your child ever taken this drug, or a similar one, again? If yes, did your child experience the same problems?
- Have you told the doctors or nurses about your child's reaction or allergy?

Allergies

Ask about commonly known allergic disorders such as hay fever and asthma; unusual reactions to drugs, food, or latex products; and reactions to other contact agents such as poisonous plants, animals, household products, or fabrics. If asked appropriate questions, most people can give reliable information about drug reactions (see Nursing Care Guidelines box).

 NURSING ALERT

Information about allergic reactions to drugs or other products is essential. Failure to document a serious reaction places the child at risk if the agent is given.

Current Medications

Inquire about current drug regimens, including vitamins, antipyretics (especially aspirin), antibiotics, antihistamines, decongestants, and herbs and homeopathic medications. List all medications, including their names, doses, schedules, durations, and reasons for administration. Often parents are unaware of a drug's actual name. Whenever possible, ask the parents to bring the containers with them to the next visit or ask for the name of the pharmacy and call for a list of all the child's recent prescription medications. However, this list will not include over-the-counter medications, which are important to know.

Immunizations

A record of all immunizations is essential. Because many parents are unaware of the exact name and date of each immunization, the most reliable source of information is a hospital, clinic, or private practitioner's record. All immunizations and "boosters" are listed, stating (1) the name of the specific disease, (2) the number of injections, (3) the dosage (sometimes lesser amounts are given if a reaction is anticipated), (4) the ages when administered, and (5) the occurrence of any reaction after the immunization.

 NURSING ALERT

Inquire about previous administration of any horse or other foreign serum. Inquire about recent administration of immune gamma globulin or blood transfusion because these necessitate a delay in giving live vaccines. And ask about anaphylactic reactions to neomycin, eggs, or any other component of a vaccine.

BOX 6-6   HABITS TO EXPLORE DURING A HEALTH INTERVIEW

- Behavior patterns such as nail biting, thumb sucking, pica (habitual ingestion of nonfood substances), rituals ("security" blanket or toy), and unusual movements (head banging, rocking, overt masturbation, walking on toes)
- Activities of daily living, such as hours of sleep and arising, duration of nighttime sleep and naps, type and duration of exercise, regularity of stools and urination, age of toilet training, and daytime or nighttime bedwetting
- Unusual disposition; response to frustration
- Use or abuse of alcohol, drugs, coffee, or tobacco

Growth and Development

The most important previous growth patterns to record are:
- Approximate weight at 6 months, 1 year, 2 years, and 5 years of age
- Approximate length at ages 1 and 4 years
- Dentition, including age of onset, number of teeth, and symptoms during teething

Developmental milestones include:
- Age of holding up head steadily
- Age of sitting alone without support
- Age of walking without assistance
- Age of saying first words with meaning
- Present grade in school
- Scholastic performance
- If the child has a best friend
- Interactions with other children, peers, and adults

Use specific and detailed questions when inquiring about each developmental milestone. For example, "sitting up" can mean many different activities, such as sitting propped up, sitting in someone's lap, sitting with support, sitting up alone but in a hyperflexed position for assisted balance, or sitting up unsupported with the back slightly rounded. A clue to misunderstanding of the requested activity may be an unusually early age of achievement (see Developmental Assessment, Chapter 5).

Habits

Habits are an important area to explore (Box 6-6). Parents frequently express concerns during this part of the history. Encourage their input by saying, "Please tell me any concerns you have about your child's habits, activities, or development." Investigate further any concerns that parents express.

One of the most common concerns relates to sleep. Many children develop a normal sleep pattern, and all that is required during the assessment is a general overview of nighttime sleep and nap schedules. However, a number of children develop sleep problems (see Sleep Problems, Chapters 10 and 13). When sleep problems occur, the nurse needs a more detailed sleep history to guide appropriate interventions.*

Habits related to use of chemicals apply primarily to older children and adolescents. If a youngster admits to smoking, drinking, or using drugs, ask about the quantity and frequency. Questions such as "Many kids your age are experimenting with drugs and alcohol; have you ever had any drugs or alcohol?" may give more reliable data than questions such as "How much do you drink?" or "How often do you drink or

---

*A sleep history and a sleep chart for the family to record the child's daily sleep and wake activities is available in Wilson D, Hockenberry M: *Wong's clinical manual of pediatric nursing,* ed 8, St. Louis, 2012, Mosby.

take drugs?" Clarify that "drinking" includes all types of alcohol, including beer and wine. When quantities such as a "glass" of wine or a "can" of beer are given, ask about the size of the container.

If older children deny use of chemical substances, inquire about past experimentation. Asking, "You mean you never tried to smoke or drink?" implies that the nurse expects some such activity, and the youngster may be more inclined to answer truthfully. Be aware of the confidential nature of such questioning, the adverse effect that the parents' presence may have on the adolescent's willingness to answer, and the fact that self-reporting may not be an accurate account of chemical abuse.

Sexual History

The sexual history is an essential component of adolescents' health assessment. The history uncovers areas of concern related to sexual activity; alerts the nurse to circumstances that may indicate screening for sexually transmitted infections or testing for pregnancy; and provides information related to the need for sexual counseling, such as safer sex practices. Box 6-7 gives guidelines for anticipatory guidance topics for parents and adolescents.

One approach to initiating a conversation about sexual concerns is to begin with a history of peer interactions. Open-ended statements and questions such as "Tell me about your social life" or "Who are your closest friends?" generally lead into a discussion of dating and sexual issues. To probe further, include questions about the adolescent's attitudes on such topics as sex education, "going steady," "living together," and premarital sex. Phrase questions to reflect concern rather than judgment or criticism of sexual practices.

In any conversation regarding sexual history, be aware of the language that is used in either eliciting or conveying sexual information. For example, avoid asking whether the adolescent is "sexually active" because this term is broadly defined. "Are you having sex with anyone?" is probably the most direct and best understood question. Because same-sex experimentation may occur, refer to all sexual contacts in nongender terms, such as "anyone" or "partners," rather than "girlfriends" or "boyfriends."

Family Medical History

The family medical history is used primarily to discover any hereditary or familial diseases in the parents and child. In general, it is confined to first-degree relatives (parents, siblings, grandparents, and immediate aunts and uncles). Information for each family member includes age; marital status; state of health if living; cause of death if deceased; and any evidence of conditions such as early heart disease, sudden death from unknown cause, hypercholesterolemia, hypertension, cancer, diabetes mellitus, obesity, congenital anomalies, allergies, asthma, seizures, tuberculosis, sickle cell disease, cognitive impairment, hearing or visual deficits, psychiatric disorders such as depression or psychosis, and emotional problems. Confirm the accuracy of the reported disorders by inquiring about the symptoms, course, treatment, and sequelae of each diagnosis.

Geographic Location

One of the important areas to explore when assessing the family health history is geographic location, including the birthplace and travel to different areas in or outside of the country, for identification of possible exposure to endemic diseases. Although the primary interest is the child's temporary residence in various localities, also inquire about close family members' travel, especially during tours of military service or business trips. Children are especially susceptible to parasitic infestation in areas of poor sanitary conditions and to vector-borne

diseases, such as those from mosquitoes or ticks in warm and humid or heavily wooded regions.

Family Structure

Assessment of the family, both its structure and function, is an important component of the history-taking process. Because the quality of the functional relationship between the child and family members is a major factor in emotional and physical health, family assessment is discussed separately and in greater detail apart from the more traditional health history.

Family assessment is the collection of data about the composition of the family and the relationships among its members. In its broadest sense, *family* refers to all those individuals who are considered by the family member to be significant to the nuclear unit, including relatives, friends, and social groups such as the school and church. Although family assessment is not family therapy, it can and frequently is therapeutic. Involving family members in discussing family

---

BOX 6-7 ANTICIPATORY GUIDANCE—SEXUALITY

Ages 12 to 14 Years

Have adolescent identify a supportive adult with whom to discuss sexuality issues and concerns.

Discuss the advantages of delaying sexual activity.

Discuss making responsible decisions regarding normal sexual feelings.

Discuss the roles of gender, peer pressure, and the media in sexual decision making.

Discuss contraceptive options (advantages and disadvantages).

Provide education regarding sexually transmitted infections (STIs), including human immunodeficiency virus (HIV) infection; clarify risks and discuss condoms.

Discuss abuse prevention, including avoiding dangerous situations, the role of drugs and alcohol, and the use of self-defense.

Have the adolescent clarify his or her values, needs, and ability to be assertive.

If the adolescent is sexually active, discuss limiting partners, use of condoms, and contraceptive options.

Have a confidential interview with the adolescent (including a sexual history).

Discuss the evolution of sexual identity and expression.

Discuss breast examination or testicular examination.

Ages 15 to 18 years

Support delaying sexual activity.

Discuss alternatives to intercourse.

Discuss "When are you ready for sex?"

Clarify values; encourage responsible decision making.

Discuss consequences of unprotected sex: early pregnancy; STIs, including HIV infection.

Discuss negotiating with partners and barriers to safer sex.

If the adolescent is sexually active, discuss limiting partners, use of condoms, and contraceptive options.

Emphasize that sex should be safe and pleasurable for both partners.

Have a confidential interview with the adolescent.

Discuss concerns about sexual expression and identity.

Data from Wright K: Anticipatory guidance: developing a healthy sexuality, *Pediatr Ann* 26(2 suppl):S142–S144, C3, 1997; and Fonseca H, Greydanus D: Sexuality in the child, teen and young adult: concepts for the clinician, *Prim Care Clin Office Pract* 34:275–292, 2007.

NURSING CARE GUIDELINES

Initiating a Comprehensive Family Assessment

Perform a comprehensive assessment on:
- Children receiving comprehensive well-child care
- Children experiencing major stressful life events (e.g., chronic illness, disability, parental divorce, death of a family member)
- Children requiring extensive home care
- Children with developmental delays
- Children with repeated accidental injuries and those with suspected child abuse
- Children with behavioral or physical problems that could be caused by family dysfunction

characteristics and activities can provide insight into family dynamics and relationships.

Because of the time involved in performing an in-depth family assessment as presented here, be selective in deciding when knowledge of family function may facilitate nursing care (see Nursing Care Guidelines box). During brief contacts with families, a full assessment is not appropriate, and screening with one or two questions from each category may reflect the health of the family system or the need for additional assessment.

The most common method of eliciting information on the family structure is to interview family members. The principal areas of concern are (1) family composition, (2) home and community environment, (3) occupation and education of family members, and (4) cultural and religious traditions (Box 6-8).

Psychosocial History

The traditional medical history includes a personal and social section that concentrates on children's personal status, such as school adjustment and any unusual habits, and the family and home environment. Because several personal aspects are covered under development and habits, only those issues related to children's ability to cope and their self-concept are presented here.

Through observation, obtain a general idea of how children handle themselves in terms of confidence in dealing with others, answering questions, and coping with new situations. Observe the parent–child relationship for the types of messages sent to children about their coping skills and self-worth. Do the parents treat the child with respect, focusing on strengths, or is the interaction one of constant reprimands with emphasis on weaknesses and faults? Do the parents help the child learn new coping strategies or support the ones the child uses?

Parent–child interactions also convey messages about body image. Do the parents label the child and body parts, such as "bad boy," "skinny legs," or "ugly scar?" Do the parents handle the child gently, using soothing touch to calm an anxious child, or do they treat the child roughly, using slaps or restraint to make the child obey? If the child touches certain parts of the body, such as the genitalia, do the parents make comments that suggest a negative connotation?

With older children, many of the communication strategies discussed earlier in the chapter are useful in eliciting more definitive information about their coping and self-concept. Children can write down five things they like and dislike about themselves. The nurse can use sentence completion statements, such as: "The thing I like best (or worst) about myself is _____"; "If I could change one thing about myself, it would be _____"; or "When I am scared, I _____."

Review of Systems

The review of systems is a specific review of each body system following an order similar to that of the physical examination (see Nursing Care Guidelines box). Often the history of the present illness provides a complete review of the system involved in the chief complaint. Because asking questions about other body systems may appear irrelevant to the parents or child, precede the questioning with an explanation of why the data are necessary (similar to the explanation concerning the relevance of the birth history) and reassure the parents that the child's main problem has not been forgotten.

Begin the review of a specific system with a broad statement such as "How has your child's general health been?" or "Has your child had any problems with his eyes?" If the parent states that the child has had problems with some body function, pursue this with an encouraging statement such as "Tell me more about that." If the parent denies any problems, query for specific symptoms (e.g., "No headaches, bumping into objects, or squinting?"). If the parent reconfirms the absence of such symptoms, record positive statements in the history, such as "Mother denies headaches, bumping into objects, and squinting." In this way, anyone who reviews the health history is aware of exactly what symptoms were investigated.

NUTRITIONAL ASSESSMENT

DIETARY INTAKE

Knowledge of the child's dietary intake is an essential component of a nutritional assessment. However, it is also one of the most difficult factors to assess. Individuals' recall of food consumption, especially amounts eaten, is frequently unreliable. The food intake history of children and adolescents is prone to reporting error, mostly in the form of underreporting. People from different cultures may have difficulty adequately describing the types of food they eat. Despite these obstacles, a dietary evaluation is an important component of the child's assessment.

The Dietary Reference Intakes (DRIs) are a set of four nutrient-based reference values that provide quantitative estimates of nutrient intake for use in assessing and planning dietary intake (American Academy of Pediatrics, 2009). The specific DRIs are:

Estimated Average Requirement (EAR)—Nutrient intake estimated to meet the requirement of half the healthy individuals (50%) for a specific age and gender group

Recommended Dietary Allowance (RDA)—Average daily dietary intake sufficient to meet the nutrient requirement of nearly all (97%–98%) healthy individuals for a specific age and gender group

Adequate Intake (AI)—Recommended intake level based on estimates of nutrient intake by healthy groups of individuals

Tolerable Upper Intake Level (UL)—Highest average daily nutrient intake level likely to pose no risk of adverse health effects; as intake increases above the UL, risk of adverse effects increases

Figure 6-4 contains MyPlate, which describes the recommended dietary intake. Specific questions used to conduct a nutritional assessment are given in Box 6-9. Every nutritional assessment should begin with a dietary history. The exact questions used to elicit a dietary history vary with the child's age. In general, the younger the child, the more specific and detailed the history should be. The overview elicited from the dietary history can be helpful in evaluating food frequency records. The history is also concerned with financial and cultural factors that influence food selection and preparation (see Cultural Considerations box).

BOX 6-8 FAMILY ASSESSMENT INTERVIEW

General Guidelines

Schedule the interview with the family at a time that is most convenient for all parties; include as many family members as possible; clearly state the purpose of the interview.

Begin the interview by asking each person's name and their relationships to one another.

Restate the purpose of the interview and the objective.

Keep the initial conversation general to put members at ease and to learn the "big picture" of the family.

Identify major concerns and reflect these back to the family to be certain that all parties receive the same message.

Terminate the interview with a summary of what was discussed and a plan for additional sessions if needed.

Structural Assessment Areas

Family Composition

Immediate members of the household (names, ages, and relationships)

Significant extended family members

Previous marriages, separations, death of spouses, or divorces

Home and Community Environment

Type of dwelling, number of rooms, occupants

Sleeping arrangements

Number of floors, accessibility of stairs and elevators

Adequacy of utilities

Safety features (fire escape, smoke and carbon monoxide detectors, guardrails on windows, use of car restraint)

Environmental hazards (e.g., chipped paint, poor sanitation, pollution, heavy street traffic)

Availability and location of health care facilities, schools, play areas

Relationship with neighbors

Recent crises or changes in home

Child's reaction and adjustment to recent stresses

Occupation and Education of Family Members

Types of employment

Work schedules

Work satisfaction

Exposure to environmental or industrial hazards

Sources of income and adequacy

Effect of illness on financial status

Highest degree or grade level attained

Cultural and Religious Traditions

Religious beliefs and practices

Cultural and ethnic beliefs and practices

Language spoken in home

Assessment questions include:

- Does the family identify with a particular religious or ethnic group? Are both parents from that group?
- How is religious or ethnic background part of family life?
- What special religious or cultural traditions are practiced in the home (e.g., food choices and preparation)?
- Where were family members born, and how long have they lived in this country?
- What language does the family speak most frequently?
- Do they speak and understand English?
- What do they believe causes health or illness?

- What religious or ethnic beliefs influence the family's perception of illness and its treatment?
- What methods are used to prevent or treat illness?
- How does the family know when a health problem needs medical attention?
- Who does the family contact when a member is ill?
- Does the family rely on cultural or religious healers or remedies? If so, ask them to describe the type of healer or remedy.
- Who does the family go to for support (clergy, medical healer, relatives)?
- Does the family experience discrimination because of their race, beliefs, or practices? Ask them to describe.

Functional Assessment Areas

Family Interactions and Roles

Interactions refer to ways family members relate to each other. The chief concern is the amount of intimacy and closeness among the members, especially spouses.

Roles refer to behaviors of people as they assume a different status or position.

Observations include:

- Family members' responses to each other (cordial, hostile, cool, loving, patient, short tempered)
- Obvious roles of leadership versus submission
- Support and attention shown to various members

Assessment questions include:

- What activities does the family perform together?
- Who do family members talk to when something is bothering them?
- What are members' household chores?
- Who usually oversees what is happening with the children, such as at school or health care?
- How easy or difficult is it for the family to change or accept new responsibilities for household tasks?

Power, Decision Making, and Problem Solving

Power refers to individual member's control over others in family; it is manifested through family decision making and problem solving.

Chief concern is clarity of boundaries of power between parents and children.

One method of assessment involves offering a hypothetical conflict or problem, such as a child failing school, and asking family how they would handle this situation.

Assessment questions include:

- Who usually makes the decisions in the family?
- If one parent makes a decision, can the child appeal to the other parent to change it?
- What input do children have in making decisions or discussing rules?
- Who makes and enforces the rules?
- What happens when a rule is broken?

Communication

Communication is concerned with clarity and directness of communication patterns.

Further assessment includes periodically asking family members if they understood what was just said and to repeat the message.

Observations include:

- Who speaks to whom
- If one person speaks for another or interrupts

BOX 6-8 FAMILY ASSESSMENT INTERVIEW—cont'd

- If members appear uninterested when certain individuals speak
- If there is agreement between verbal and nonverbal messages

Assessment questions include:
- How often do family members wait until others are through talking before "having their say"?
- Do parents or older siblings tend to lecture and preach?
- Do parents tend to "talk down" to the children?

Expression of Feelings and Individuality

Expressions are concerned with personal space and freedom to grow, with limits and structure needed for guidance.

Observing patterns of communication offers clues to how freely feelings are expressed.

Assessment questions include:
- Is it OK for family members to get angry or sad?
- Who gets angry most of the time? What do they do?
- If someone is upset, how do other family members try to comfort this person?
- Who comforts specific family members?
- When someone wants to do something, such as try out for a new sport or get a job, what is the family's response (offer assistance, discouragement, or no advice)?

NURSING CARE GUIDELINES

Review of Systems

General—Overall state of health, fatigue, recent or unexplained weight gain or loss (period of time for either), contributing factors (change of diet, illness, altered appetite), exercise tolerance, fevers (time of day), chills, night sweats (unrelated to climatic conditions), frequent infections, general ability to carry out activities of daily living

Integument—Pruritus, pigment or other color changes, acne, eruptions, rashes (location), tendency for bruising, petechiae, excessive dryness, general texture, disorders or deformities of nails, hair growth or loss, hair color change (for adolescents, use of hair dyes or other potentially toxic substances, such as hair straighteners)

Head—Headaches, dizziness, injury (specific details)

Eyes—Visual problems (behaviors indicative of blurred vision, such as bumping into objects, clumsiness, sitting close to television, holding a book close to face, writing with head near desk, squinting, rubbing the eyes, bending head in an awkward position), cross eyes (strabismus), eye infections, edema of the eyelids, excessive tearing, use of glasses or contact lenses, date of last optic examination

Ears—Earaches, discharge, evidence of hearing loss (ask about behaviors, such as the need to repeat requests, loud speech, inattentive behavior), results of any previous auditory testing

Nose—Nosebleeds (epistaxis), constant or frequent runny or stuffy nose, nasal obstruction (difficulty breathing), alteration or loss of sense of smell

Mouth—Mouth breathing, gum bleeding, toothaches, toothbrushing, use of fluoride, difficulty with teething (symptoms), last visit to dentist (especially if temporary dentition is complete), response to dentist

Throat—Sore throats, difficulty swallowing, choking (especially when chewing food; may be from poor chewing habits), hoarseness or other voice irregularities

Neck—Pain, limitation of movement, stiffness, difficulty holding head straight (torticollis), thyroid enlargement, enlarged nodes or other masses

Chest—Breast enlargement, discharge, masses, enlarged axillary nodes (for adolescent girls, ask about breast self-examination)

Respiratory—Chronic cough, frequent colds (number per year), wheezing, shortness of breath at rest or on exertion, difficulty breathing, sputum production, infections (pneumonia, tuberculosis), date of last chest x-ray examination, skin reaction from tuberculin testing

Cardiovascular—Cyanosis or fatigue on exertion, history of heart murmur or rheumatic fever, anemia, date of last blood count, blood type, recent transfusion

Gastrointestinal (questions in regard to appetite, food tolerance, and elimination habits are asked elsewhere)—Nausea, vomiting (not associated with eating; may be indicative of brain tumor or increased intracranial pressure), jaundice or yellowing skin or sclera, belching, flatulence, recent change in bowel habits (blood in stools, change of color, diarrhea or constipation)

Genitourinary—Pain on urination, frequency, hesitancy, urgency, hematuria, nocturia, polyuria, unpleasant odor to urine, force of stream, discharge, change in size of scrotum, date of last urinalysis (for adolescents, sexually transmitted infection, type of treatment; for male adolescents, ask about testicular self-examination)

Gynecologic—Menarche, date of last menstrual period, regularity or problems with menstruation, vaginal discharge, pruritus, date and result of last Papanicolaou (Pap) smear (include obstetric history, as discussed under birth history, when applicable); if sexually active, type of contraception, sexually transmitted infection and type of treatment

Musculoskeletal—Weakness, clumsiness, lack of coordination, unusual movements, back or joint stiffness, muscle pains or cramps, abnormal gait, deformity, fractures, serious sprains, activity level

Neurologic—Seizures, tremors, dizziness, loss of memory, general affect, fears, nightmares, speech problems, any unusual habits

Endocrine—Intolerance to weather changes, excessive thirst or urination, excessive sweating, salty taste to skin, signs of early puberty

The most common and probably easiest method of assessing daily intake is the 24-hour recall. The child or parent recalls every item eaten in the past 24 hours and the approximate amounts. The 24-hour recall is most beneficial when it represents a typical day's intake. Some of the difficulties with a daily recall are the family's inability to remember exactly what was eaten and inaccurate estimation of portion size. To increase accuracy of reporting portion sizes, the use of food models and additional questions are recommended. In general, this method is most useful in providing *qualitative* information about the child's diet.

To improve the reliability of the daily recall, the family can complete a **food diary** by recording every food and liquid consumed for a certain number of days. A 3-day record consisting of 2 weekdays and 1 weekend day is representative for most people. Providing specific charts to record intake can improve compliance. The family should record items immediately after eating.

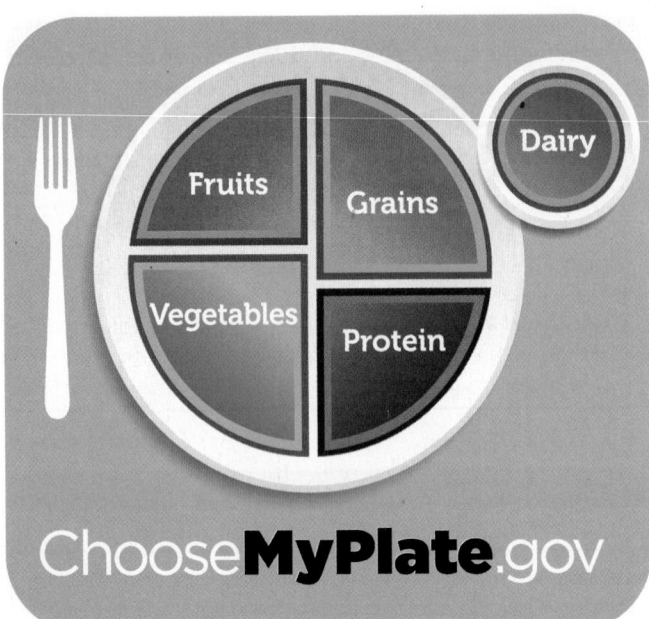

FIG 6-4 MyPlate. MyPlate advocates building a healthy plate by making half of your plate fruits and vegetables and the other half grains and protein. Avoiding oversized portions, making half your grains whole grains, and drinking fat-free or low-fat (1%) milk are additional recommendations for a healthy diet. (From U.S. Department of Agriculture: *MyPlate*, Washington, DC, June 2011, Author, retrieved from http://www.choosemyplate.gov.)

🌐 CULTURAL CONSIDERATIONS
Food Practices

Because cultural practices are prevalent in food preparation, consider carefully the kinds of questions that are asked and the judgments made during counseling. For example, some cultures, such as Hispanic, African American, and Native American, include many vegetables, legumes, and starches in their diet that together provide sufficient essential amino acids even though the actual amount of meat or dairy protein is low (see Food Customs, Chapter 4).

CLINICAL EXAMINATION OF NUTRITION

A significant amount of information regarding nutritional deficiencies comes from a clinical examination, especially from assessing the skin, hair, teeth, gums, lips, tongue, and eyes. Hair, skin, and mouth are vulnerable because of the rapid turnover of epithelial and mucosal tissue. Table 6-1 summarizes clinical signs of possible nutritional deficiency or excess. Few are diagnostic for a specific nutrient, and if suspicious signs are found, they must be confirmed with dietary and biochemical data. Generally, the clinical examination does not reveal children *at risk* for a deficiency or excess.

Anthropometry, an essential parameter of nutritional status, is the measurement of height, weight, head circumference, proportions, skinfold thickness, and arm circumference in young children. Height and head circumference reflect past nutrition, and weight, skinfold thickness, and arm circumference reflect present nutritional status, especially of protein and fat reserves. Skinfold thickness is a measurement of the body's fat content because approximately half the body's total fat stores are directly beneath the skin. The upper arm muscle circumference is correlated with measurements of total muscle mass. Because muscle serves as the body's major protein reserve, this measurement is considered an index of the body's protein stores. Ideally, growth measurements are recorded over time, and comparisons are made regarding the *velocity* of growth based on previous and present values.

Numerous **biochemical tests** are available for assessing nutritional status and include analysis of plasma; blood cells; urine; and tissues from liver, bone, hair, and fingernails. Many of these tests are complicated and are not performed routinely. Common laboratory procedures for nutritional status include measurement of hemoglobin, hematocrit, transferrin, albumin, creatinine, and nitrogen. Appendix B provides laboratory values for these tests and more specific nutrient measurements.

EVALUATION OF NUTRITIONAL ASSESSMENT

After collecting the data needed for a thorough nutritional assessment, evaluate the findings to plan appropriate counseling. From the data, assess whether the child is (1) malnourished, (2) at risk for becoming malnourished, (3) well nourished with adequate reserves, or (4) overweight or obese.

Analyze the daily food diary for the variety and amounts of foods suggested in MyPlate (see Fig. 6-4). For example, if the list includes no vegetables, inquire about this rather than assuming that the child dislikes vegetables because it is possible that none were served that day. Also, evaluate the information in terms of the family's ethnic practices and financial resources. Encouraging increased protein intake with additional meat is not always feasible for families on a limited budget and may conflict with food practices that use meat sparingly, such as in Asian meal preparation.

GENERAL APPROACHES TOWARD EXAMINING THE CHILD

SEQUENCE OF THE EXAMINATION

Ordinarily, the sequence for examining patients follows a head-to-toe direction. The main function of such a systematic approach is to provide a general guideline for assessment of each body area to avoid omitting segments of the examination. The standard recording of data also facilitates exchange of information among different professionals. The typical organization of a physical examination is in the chapter outline. In examining children, this orderly sequence is frequently altered to accommodate the child's developmental needs, although the examination is recorded following the head-to-toe model. Using developmental and chronologic age as the main criteria for assessing each body system accomplishes several goals:
- Minimizes stress and anxiety associated with assessment of various body parts
- Fosters a trusting nurse–child–parent relationship
- Allows for maximum preparation of the child
- Preserves the essential security of the parent–child relationship, especially with young children
- Maximizes the accuracy and reliability of assessment findings

PREPARATION OF THE CHILD

Although the physical examination consists of painless procedures, for some children the use of a tight arm cuff, probes in the ears and mouth, pressure on the abdomen, and a cold piece of metal to listen to the chest are stressful. Therefore, the nurse should use the same considerations discussed in Chapter 27 for preparing children for procedures.

BOX 6-9   DIETARY REFERENCE INTAKES FOR AN INDIVIDUAL

Estimated Average Requirement (EAR)—Used to examine the possibility of inadequacy.

Recommended Dietary Allowance (RDA)—Dietary intake at or above this level usually has a low probability of inadequacy.

Adequate Intake (AI)—Dietary intake at or above this level usually has a low probability of inadequacy.

Tolerable Upper Intake Level (UL)—Dietary intake above this level usually places an individual at risk of adverse effects from excessive nutrient intake.

Dietary History

What are the family's usual mealtimes?

Do family members eat together or at separate times?

Who does the family grocery shopping and meal preparation?

How much money is spent to buy food each week?

How are most foods prepared—baked, broiled, fried, other?

How often does the family or your child eat out?
- What kinds of restaurants do you go to?
- What kinds of food does your child typically eat at restaurants?

Does your child eat breakfast regularly?

Where does your child eat lunch?

What are your child's favorite foods, beverages, and snacks?
- What are the average amounts eaten per day?
- What foods are artificially sweetened?
- What are your child's snacking habits?
- When are sweet foods usually eaten?
- What are your child's toothbrushing habits?

What special cultural practices are followed? What ethnic foods are eaten?

What foods and beverages does your child dislike?

How would you describe your child's usual appetite (hearty eater, picky eater)?

What are your child's feeding habits (breast, bottle, cup, spoon, eats by self, needs assistance, any special devices)?

Does your child take vitamins or other supplements? Do they contain iron or fluoride?

Does your child have any known or suspected food allergies? Is your child on a special diet?

Has your child lost or gained weight recently?

Are there any feeding problems (excessive fussiness, spitting up, colic, difficulty sucking or swallowing)? Are there any dental problems or appliances, such as braces, that affect eating?

What types of exercise does your child do regularly?

Is there a family history of cancer, diabetes, heart disease, high blood pressure, or obesity?

Additional Questions for Infants

What was the infant's birth weight? When did it double? Triple?

Was the infant premature?

Are you breastfeeding or have you breastfed your infant? For how long?

If you use a formula, what is the brand?
- How long has the infant been taking it?
- How many ounces does the infant drink a day?

Are you giving the infant cow's milk (whole, low fat, skim)?
- When did you start?
- How many ounces does the infant drink a day?

Do you give your infant extra fluids (water, juice)?

If the infant takes a bottle to bed at nap or nighttime, what is in the bottle?

At what age did the child start on cereal, vegetables, meat or other protein sources, fruit or juice, finger food, table food?

Do you make your own baby food or use commercial foods, such as infant cereal?

Does the infant take a vitamin or mineral supplement? If so, what type?

Has the infant had an allergic reaction to any food(s)? If so, list the foods and describe the reaction.

Does the infant spit up frequently; have unusually loose stools; or have hard, dry stools? If so, how often?

How often do you feed your infant?

How would you describe your infant's appetite?

Modified from Murphy SP, Poos MI: Dietary reference intakes: summary of applications in dietary assessment, *Pub Health Nutr* 5(suppl 6A):843–849, 2002.

In addition to that discussion, general guidelines related to the examining process are given in the Nursing Care Guidelines box.

The physical examination should be as pleasant as possible, as well as educational. The paper-doll technique is a useful approach to teaching children about the body part that is being examined (Fig. 6-5). At the conclusion of the visit, the child can bring home the paper doll as a memento.

Table 6-2 summarizes guidelines for positioning, preparing, and examining children at various ages. Because no child fits precisely into one age category, it may be necessary to vary the approach after a preliminary assessment of the child's developmental achievements and needs. Even with the best approach, many toddlers are uncooperative and inconsolable for much of the physical examination. However, some seem intrigued by the new surroundings and unusual equipment and respond more like preschoolers than toddlers. Likewise, some early preschoolers may require more of the "security measures" used with younger children, such as continued parent–child contact, and less of the preparatory measures used with preschoolers, such as playing with the equipment before and during the actual examination (Fig. 6-6).

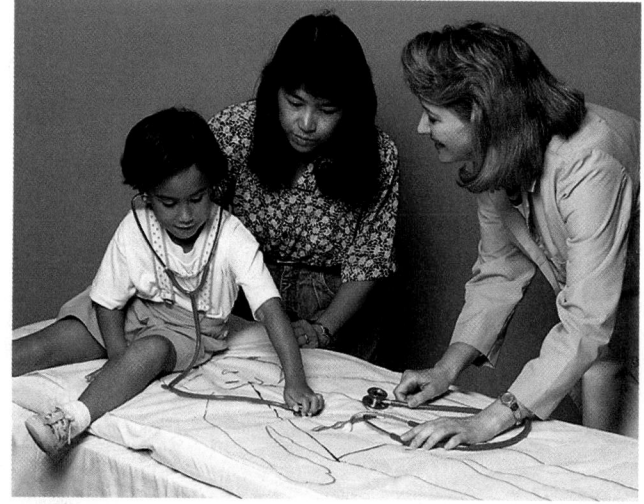

FIG 6-5 Using the paper-doll technique to prepare a child for physical examination.

TABLE 6-1 CLINICAL ASSESSMENT OF NUTRITIONAL STATUS

EVIDENCE OF ADEQUATE NUTRITION	EVIDENCE OF DEFICIENT OR EXCESS NUTRITION	DEFICIENCY OR EXCESS*
General Growth		
Between 5th and 95th percentiles for height, weight, and head circumference	<5th or >95th percentile for growth	Protein, calories, fats, and other essential nutrients, especially vitamin A, pyridoxine, niacin, calcium, iodine, manganese, zinc
Steady gain with expected growth spurts during infancy and adolescence	Absence of or delayed growth spurts; poor weight gain	
Sexual development appropriate for age	Delayed sexual development	Excess vitamins A, D
Skin		
Smooth, slightly dry to touch	Hardening and scaling	Vitamin A
Elastic and firm	Seborrheic dermatitis	Excess niacin
Absence of lesions	Dry, rough, petechiae	Riboflavin
Color appropriate to genetic background	Delayed wound healing	Vitamin C
	Scaly dermatitis on exposed surfaces	Riboflavin, vitamin C, zinc
	Wrinkled, flabby	Niacin
	Crusted lesions around orifices, especially nares	Protein, calories, zinc
	Pruritus	Excess vitamin A, riboflavin, niacin
	Poor turgor	Water, sodium
	Edema	Protein, thiamine
		Excess sodium
	Yellow tinge (jaundice)	Vitamin B$_{12}$
		Excess vitamin A, niacin
	Depigmentation	Protein, calories
	Pallor (anemia)	Pyridoxine, folic acid, vitamins B$_{12}$, C, E (in premature infants), iron
		Excess vitamin C, zinc
	Paresthesia	Excess riboflavin
Hair		
Lustrous, silky, strong, elastic	Stringy, friable, dull, dry, thin	Protein, calories
	Alopecia	Protein, calories, zinc
	Depigmentation	Protein, calories, copper
	Raised areas around hair follicles	Vitamin C
Head		
Even molding, occipital prominence, symmetric facial features	Softening of cranial bones, prominence of frontal bones, skull flat and depressed toward middle	Vitamin D
Fused sutures after 18 months	Delayed fusion of sutures	Vitamin D
	Hard, tender lumps in occiput	Excess vitamin A
	Headache	Excess thiamine
Neck		
Thyroid not visible, palpable in midline	Thyroid enlarged, may be grossly visible	Iodine
Eyes		
Clear, bright	Hardening and scaling of cornea and conjunctiva	Vitamin A
Good night vision	Night blindness	Vitamin A
Conjunctiva—Pink, glossy	Burning, itching, photophobia, cataracts, corneal vascularization	Riboflavin
Ears		
Tympanic membrane—Pliable	Calcified (hearing loss)	Excess vitamin D
Nose		
Smooth, intact nasal angle	Irritation and cracks at nasal angle	Riboflavin
		Excess vitamin A
Mouth		
Lips—Smooth, moist, darker color than skin	Fissures and inflammation at corners	Riboflavin
		Excess vitamin A
Gums—Firm, coral pink, stippled	Spongy, friable, swollen, bluish red or black, bleed easily	Vitamin C
Mucous membranes—Bright pink, smooth, moist	Stomatitis	Niacin

TABLE 6-1   CLINICAL ASSESSMENT OF NUTRITIONAL STATUS—cont'd

EVIDENCE OF ADEQUATE NUTRITION	EVIDENCE OF DEFICIENT OR EXCESS NUTRITION	DEFICIENCY OR EXCESS*
Tongue—Rough texture, no lesions, taste sensation	Glossitis	Niacin, riboflavin, folic acid
	Diminished taste sensation	Zinc
Teeth—Uniform white color, smooth, intact	Brown mottling, pits, fissures	Excess fluoride
	Defective enamel	Vitamins A, C, D; calcium; phosphorus
	Caries	Excess carbohydrates
Chest		
In infants, shape almost circular	Depressed lower portion of rib cage	Vitamin D
In children, lateral diameter increased in proportion to anteroposterior diameter	Sharp protrusion of sternum	Vitamin D
Smooth costochondral junctions	Enlarged costochondral junctions	Vitamins C, D
Breast development—Normal for age	Delayed development	See under General Growth; especially zinc
Cardiovascular System		
Pulse and blood pressure (BP) within normal limits	Palpitations	Thiamine
	Rapid pulse	Potassium
		Excess thiamine
	Arrhythmias	Magnesium, potassium
		Excess niacin, potassium
	Increased BP	Excess sodium
	Decreased BP	Thiamine
		Excess niacin
Abdomen		
In young children, cylindric and prominent	Distended, flabby, poor musculature	Protein, calories
	Prominent, large	Excess calories
In older children, flat	Potbelly, constipation	Vitamin D
Normal bowel habits	Diarrhea	Niacin
		Excess vitamin C
	Constipation	Excess calcium, potassium
Musculoskeletal System		
Muscles—Firm, well-developed, equal strength bilaterally	Flabby, weak, generalized wasting	Protein, calories
	Weakness, pain, cramps	Thiamine, sodium, chloride, potassium, phosphorus, magnesium
		Excess thiamine
	Muscle twitching, tremors	Magnesium
	Muscular paralysis	Excess potassium
Spine—Cervical and lumbar curves (double S curve)	Kyphosis, lordosis, scoliosis	Vitamin D
Extremities—Symmetric; legs straight with minimum bowing	Bowing of extremities, knock knees	Vitamin D, calcium, phosphorus
	Epiphyseal enlargement	Vitamins A, D
	Bleeding into joints and muscles, joint swelling, pain	Vitamin C
Joints—Flexible, full range of motion, no pain or stiffness	Thickening of cortex of long bones with pain and fragility, hard tender lumps in extremities	Excess vitamin A
	Osteoporosis of long bones	Calcium
		Excess vitamin D
Neurologic System		
Behavior—Alert, responsive, emotionally stable	Listless, irritable, lethargic, apathetic (sometimes apprehensive, anxious, drowsy, mentally slow, confused)	Thiamine, niacin, pyridoxine, vitamin C, potassium, magnesium, iron, protein, calories
		Excess vitamins A, D, thiamine, folic acid, calcium
Absence of tetany, convulsions	Masklike facial expression, blurred speech, involuntary laughing	Excess manganese
	Convulsions	Thiamine, pyridoxine, vitamin D, calcium, magnesium
		Excess phosphorus (in relation to calcium)
Intact peripheral nervous system	Peripheral nervous system toxicity (unsteady gait, numb feet and hands, fine motor clumsiness)	Excess pyridoxine
Intact reflexes	Diminished or absent tendon reflexes	Thiamine, vitamin E

*Nutrients listed are deficient unless specified as excess.

NURSING CARE GUIDELINES

Performing Pediatric Physical Examination

Perform the examination in an appropriate, nonthreatening area:

- Have the room well lit and decorated with neutral colors.
- Have room temperature comfortably warm.
- Place all strange and potentially frightening equipment out of sight.
- Have some toys, dolls, stuffed animals, and games available for children.
- If possible, have rooms decorated and equipped for different-age children.
- Provide privacy, especially for school-age children and adolescents.
- Provide time for play and becoming acquainted.

Observe behaviors that signal the child's readiness to cooperate:

- Talking to the nurse
- Making eye contact
- Accepting the offered equipment
- Allowing physical touching
- Choosing to sit on the examining table rather than the parent's lap

If signs of readiness are not observed, use the following techniques:

- Talk to the parent while essentially "ignoring" the child; gradually focus on the child or a favorite object, such as a doll.
- Make complimentary remarks about the child, such as about his or her appearance, dress, or a favorite object.
- Tell a funny story or play a simple magic trick.
- Have a nonthreatening "friend" available, such as a hand puppet, to "talk" to child for the nurse (see Fig. 6-26, *A*).

If the child refuses to cooperate, use the following techniques:

- Assess the reason for uncooperative behavior; consider that a child who is unduly afraid may have had a traumatic experience.
- Try to involve the child and parent in process.
- Avoid prolonged explanations about the examining procedure.
- Use a firm, direct approach regarding expected behavior.
- Perform the examination as quickly as possible.
- Have an attendant gently restrain child.
- Minimize any disruptions and stimulation.
- Limit the number of people in room.
- Use an isolated room.
- Use a quiet, calm, confident voice.

Begin the examination in a nonthreatening manner for young children or children who are fearful:

- Use activities that can be presented as games, such as test for cranial nerves (see Table 6-13) or parts of developmental screening tests (see Chapter 5).
- Use approaches such as Simon Says to encourage the child to make a face, squeeze a hand, stand on one foot, and so on.
- Use the paper-doll technique:
  1. Lay the child supine on an examining table or floor that is covered with a large sheet of paper.
  2. Trace around the child's body outline.
  3. Use the body outline to demonstrate what will be examined, such as drawing a heart and listening with a stethoscope before performing an activity on the child.

If several children in the family will be examined, begin with the most cooperative child to model desired behavior.

Involve the child in the examination process:

- Provide choices, such as sitting on the table or in the parent's lap.
- Allow the child to handle or hold the equipment.
- Encourage the child to use equipment on a doll, family member, or examiner.
- Explain each step of the procedure in simple language.

Examine the child in a comfortable and secure position:

- Sitting in the parent's lap
- Sitting upright if in respiratory distress

Proceed to examine the body in an organized sequence (usually head to toe) with the following exceptions:

- Alter the sequence to accommodate needs of different-age children (see Table 6-2).
- Examine painful areas last.
- In an emergency situation, examine vital functions (airway, breathing, and circulation) and the injured area first.

Reassure the child throughout the examination, especially about bodily concerns that arise during puberty.

Discuss findings with the family at the end of the examination.

Praise the child for cooperation during the examination; give a reward such as a small toy or sticker.

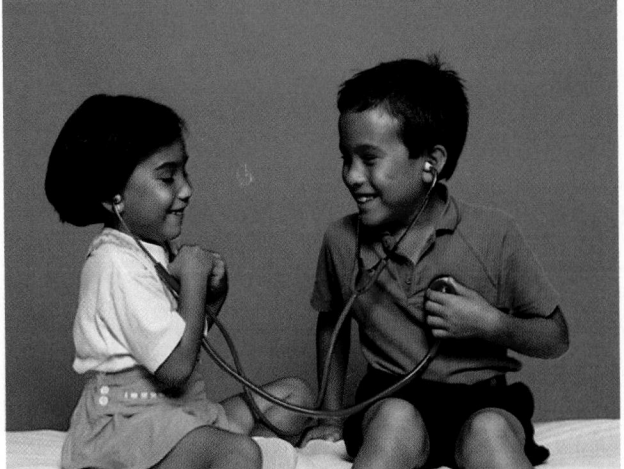

FIG 6-6 Preparing children for physical examination.

PHYSICAL EXAMINATION

Although the approach to and sequence of the physical examination differ according to the child's age, the following discussion outlines the traditional model for physical assessment. The focus includes all pediatric age groups; however, see Chapter 8 for a detailed discussion of a newborn assessment. Because the physical examination is a vital part of preventive pediatric care, Figure 6-7 gives a schedule for periodic health visits.

GROWTH MEASUREMENTS

Measurement of physical growth in children is a key element in evaluating their health status. Physical growth parameters include weight, height (length), skinfold thickness, arm circumference, and head circumference. Values for these growth parameters are plotted on percentile charts, and the child's measurements in percentiles are compared with those of the general population.

TABLE 6-2   AGE-SPECIFIC APPROACHES TO PHYSICAL EXAMINATION DURING CHILDHOOD

POSITION	SEQUENCE	PREPARATION
Infant		
Before able to sit alone—Supine or prone, preferably in parent's lap; before 4–6 months, can place on examining table	If quiet, auscultate heart, lungs, abdomen.	Completely undress if room temperature permits.
	Record heart and respiratory rates.	Leave diaper on male infant.
	Palpate and percuss same areas.	Gain cooperation with distraction, bright objects, rattles, talking.
	Proceed in usual head-to-toe direction.	Smile at infant; use soft, gentle voice.
After able to sit alone—Sitting in parent's lap whenever possible; if on table, place with parent in full view	Perform traumatic procedures last (eyes, ears, mouth [while crying]).	Pacify with bottle of sugar water or feeding.
	Elicit reflexes as body part is examined.	Enlist parent's aid for restraining to examine ears, mouth.
	Elicit Moro reflex last.	Avoid abrupt, jerky movements.
Toddler		
Sitting or standing on or by parent	Inspect body area through play: "count fingers," "tickle toes."	Have parent remove outer clothing.
Prone or supine in parent's lap		Remove underwear as body part is examined.
	Use minimum physical contact initially.	Allow to inspect equipment; demonstrating use of equipment is usually ineffective.
	Introduce equipment slowly.	
	Auscultate, percuss, palpate whenever quiet.	If uncooperative, perform procedures quickly.
		Use restraint when appropriate; request parent's assistance.
	Perform traumatic procedures last (same as for infant).	Talk about examination if cooperative; use short phrases.
		Praise for cooperative behavior.
Preschool Child		
Prefer standing or sitting	If cooperative, proceed in head-to-toe direction.	Request self-undressing.
Usually cooperative prone or supine		Allow to wear underpants if shy.
Prefer parent's closeness	If uncooperative, proceed as with toddler.	Offer equipment for inspection; briefly demonstrate use.
		Make up story about procedure (e.g., "I'm seeing how strong your muscles are" [blood pressure]).
		Use paper-doll technique.
		Give choices when possible.
		Expect cooperation; use positive statements (e.g., "Open your mouth").
School-Age Child		
Prefer sitting	Proceed in head-to-toe direction.	Respect need for privacy.
Cooperative in most positions	May examine genitalia last in older child.	Request self-undressing.
Younger child prefers parent's presence		Allow to wear underpants.
		Give gown to wear.
Older child may prefer privacy		Explain purpose of equipment and significance of procedure, such as otoscope to see eardrum, which is necessary for hearing.
		Teach about body function and care.
Adolescent		
Same as for school-age child	Same as older school-age child.	Allow to undress in private.
Offer option of parent's presence	May examine genitalia last.	Give gown.
		Expose only area to be examined.
		Respect need for privacy.
		Explain findings during examination: "Your muscles are firm and strong."
		Matter of factly comment about sexual development: "Your breasts are developing as they should be."
		Emphasize normalcy of development.
		Examine genitalia as any other body part; may leave to end.

Growth Charts

The most commonly used growth charts in the United States are from the National Center for Health Statistics (NCHS). The growth charts have been revised to include the body mass index–for-age (BMI-for-age) charts, 3rd and 97th smoothed percentiles for all charts, and the 85th percentile for the weight-for-stature and BMI-for-age charts. The data were collected from five national surveys between 1963 and 1994.

The revised charts have eliminated the disjunctions between the curves for infants and other children and have been extended for children and adolescents to age 20 years.

The weight-for-age percentile distributions are now continuous between the infant and the older child charts at 24 to 36 months. The length-for-age to stature-for-age and weight-for-length to weight-for-stature curves are parallel in the overlapping ages of 24 to 36 months.

Clinical Preventive Services for Normal-Risk Children*

Age	Infancy							Early Childhood							Middle Childhood						Adolescence							
	Newborn	3-5 d	By1mo	2 mo	4 mo	6 mo	9 mo	12mo	15mo	18mo	24mo	30mo	3 y	4 y	5 y	6 y	7 y	8 y	9 y	10 y	11 y	12 y	13 y	14 y	15 y	16 y	17 y	18 y
History Initial/Interval	●	●	●	●	●	●	●	●	●	●	●	●	●	●	●	●	●	●	●	●	●	●	●	●	●	●	●	●
Measurements																												
Length/Height and Weight	●	●	●	●	●	●	●	●	●	●	●	●	●	●	●	●	●	●	●	●	●	●	●	●	●	●	●	●
Head Circumference	●	●	●	●	●	●	●	●	●	●	●																	
Weight for Length	●	●	●	●	●	●	●	●	●	●																		
Body Mass Index											●	●	●	●	●	●	●	●	●	●	●	●	●	●	●	●	●	●
Blood Pressure	★	★	★	★	★	★	★	★	★	★	★	★	●	●	●	●	●	●	●	●	●	●	●	●	●	●	●	●
Sensory Screening																												
Vision	★	★	★	★	★	★	★	★	★	★	★	★	●	●	●	★	●	★	●	●	★	★	★	★	●	★	★	●
Hearing	●	★	★	★	★	★	★	★	★	★	★	★	★	●	●	●	★	●	★	●	★	★	★	★	★	★	★	★
Developmental/ Behavioral Assessment																												
Developmental Screening							●			●		●																
Autism Screening										●	●																	
Developmental Surveillance	●		●	●	●	●		●	●		●		●	●	●	●	●	●	●	●	●	●	●	●	●	●	●	●
Psychosocial/ Behavioral Assessment	●	●	●	●	●	●	●	●	●	●	●	●	●	●	●	●	●	●	●	●	●	●	●	●	●	●	●	●
Alcohol and Drug Use Assessment																					★	★	★	★	★	★	★	★
Physical Examination	●	●	●	●	●	●	●	●	●	●	●	●	●	●	●	●	●	●	●	●	●	●	●	●	●	●	●	●
Procedures																												
Newborn Metabolic/ Hemoglobin Screening	◄——	●	——►																									
Immunization	●	●	●	●	●	●	●	●	●	●	●	●	●	●	●	●	●	●	●	●	●	●	●	●	●	●	●	●
Hematocrit or Hemoglobin					★			●					★	★	★	★	★	★	★	★	★	★	★	★	★	★	★	★
Lead Screening						★	★	● or ★		★	● or ★		★	★	★	★												
Tuberculin Test			★			★		★		★	★		★	★	★	★	★	★	★	★	★	★	★	★	★	★	★	★
Dyslipidemia Screening											★			★		★		★		★	★	★	★	★	★	★	★	★
STI Screening																					★	★	★	★	★	★	★	★
Cervical Dysplasia Screening																					★	★	★	★	★	★	★	★
Oral Health						★	★	● or ★		● or ★	● or ★	● or ★	●			●												
Anticipatory Guidance	●	●	●	●	●	●	●	●	●	●	●	●	●	●	●	●	●	●	●	●	●	●	●	●	●	●	●	●

Key: ● = To be performed; ★ = risk assessment to be performed, with appropriate action to follow, if positive; ◄—●—► = range during which a service may be provided, with the symbol indicating the preferred age.

*For current immunization schedules, see Chapter 10.

FIG 6-7 Preventive health care chart. *STI,* Sexually transmitted infection. (Modified from American Academy of Pediatrics Committee on Practice and Ambulatory Medicine and Bright Futures Steering Committee: Recommendations for preventive pediatric health care, *Pediatrics* 120(6):1376, 2007.)

The revised weight-for-stature charts provide a smoother transition from the weight-for-length charts for preschool-age children.

The most prominent change to the complement of growth charts for older children and adolescents is the addition of the BMI-for-age growth curves. The BMI-for-age charts were developed with national survey data (1963 to 1994), excluding data from the 1988 to 1994 National Health and Nutrition Examination Surveys III (NHANES III) for children older than 6 years because an increase in body weight and BMI occurred between NHANES III and previous national surveys. Without this exclusion, the 85th and 95th percentile curves would have been higher, and fewer children and adolescents would have been classified as at risk of or overweight. Therefore, the BMI-for-age growth curves do not represent the current population of children older than 6 years of age.

> **! NURSING ALERT**
>
> The sex-specific BMI-for-age charts for ages 2 to 20 years replace the 1977 NCHS weight-for-stature charts that were limited to prepubescent boys younger than 11.5 years and with statures less than 145 cm (4 feet, 9 inches) and to prepubescent girls younger than 19 years and with statures less than 137 cm (4 feet, 6 inches).

Breast- and Formula-Fed Infants

The national survey data better represent the combined size and growth patterns of the general U.S. population (1971–1994). Over the past 30 years in the United States, approximately half of all infants were reported to have been breastfed, and approximately one third were breastfed for 3 months or more. Therefore, compared with the 1977 NCHS growth charts, the nationally representative data on which the revised infant growth charts are based better represent the combined growth patterns of breastfed and formula-fed infants in the U.S. population.

Special Groups

Although differences in size and growth occur among the major racial and ethnic groups in the United States, these appear to be small and inconsistent. Therefore, the revised growth charts include all infants and children whatever their race or ethnicity. Because the growth patterns of preterm, very low–birth-weight (VLBW) (<1500 g [3.3 lb]) infants are considerably different from those of higher birth-weight, full-term infants and specialized growth charts exist to track the growth of VLBW infants, data for VLBW infants were excluded from the revised charts.

Versions of the Growth Charts

Three different versions of the charts are available (www.cdc.gov/growthcharts). The first set contains all nine smoothed percentile lines (3rd, 5th, 10th, 25th, 50th, 75th, 90th, 95th, 97th), and the second and third sets contain seven smoothed percentile lines. The second set contains the 5th and 95th percentile lines, and the third set contains the 3rd and 97th percentile lines at the extreme ends of the distribution. In addition, the charts for weight-for-stature and BMI-for-age contain the 85th percentile. In all of the growth charts, age is truncated to the nearest full month, for example, 1 month (1.0–1.9 months), 11 months (11.0–11.9 months), and 23 months (23.0–23.9 months).

The three sets of charts are provided to meet the needs of various users. Set 1 shows all of the major percentile curves but may have limitations when the curves are close together, especially at the youngest ages. Most users in the United States may wish to use the format shown in set 2 for the majority of routine clinical applications. Pediatric endocrinologists and others dealing with special populations, such as children with failure to thrive, may wish to use the format in set 3.

Nurses are often responsible for measuring growth in children, so it is essential that they understand the revised growth charts. Several important differences exist between the 1977 and the revised charts with significant implications for classifying children as underweight or overweight. Nurses need to become familiar with determining BMI, which only requires information about the child's weight and height.* With the increasing number of overweight children in the United States, the BMI charts are a critical component of children's physical assessment.

> ### ! NURSING ALERT
>
> The Centers for Disease Control and Prevention (CDC, 2010) now recommends the World Health Organization (WHO) growth charts be used for children younger than 24 months of age instead of the CDC growth charts. The basis for this recommendation is that healthy breastfed infants are the standard against which all other infants of this age are compared in the WHO growth charts. The CDC growth charts continue to be recommended for children older than 24 months of age.

Centers for Disease Control and Prevention: Use of World Health Organization and CDC growth charts for children aged 0–59 months in the United States, *MMWR Recomm Rep* 59(rr09):1–15, 2010.

> ### ! NURSING ALERT
>
> BMI for age may be used to identify children and adolescents at the upper end of the distribution who are either overweight (≥95th percentile) or at risk for being overweight (≥85th and <95th percentile) (Ogden, Carroll, and Flegal, 2008). Formulas for determining BMI are available at http://www.cdc.gov/nccdphp/dnpa/bmi and in Appendix B.

Children whose growth may be questionable include:
- Children whose height and weight percentiles are widely disparate (e.g., height in the 10th percentile and weight in the 90th percentile, especially with above-average skinfold thickness)
- Children who fail to follow the expected growth velocity in height and weight, especially during the rapid growth periods of infancy and adolescence

---

*BMI = [Weight in pounds ÷ (Height in inches × Height in inches)] × 703. NOTE: This formula is the BMI calculation for adults used in some pediatric settings; for child and adolescent BMI table and plotting, see Appendix B.

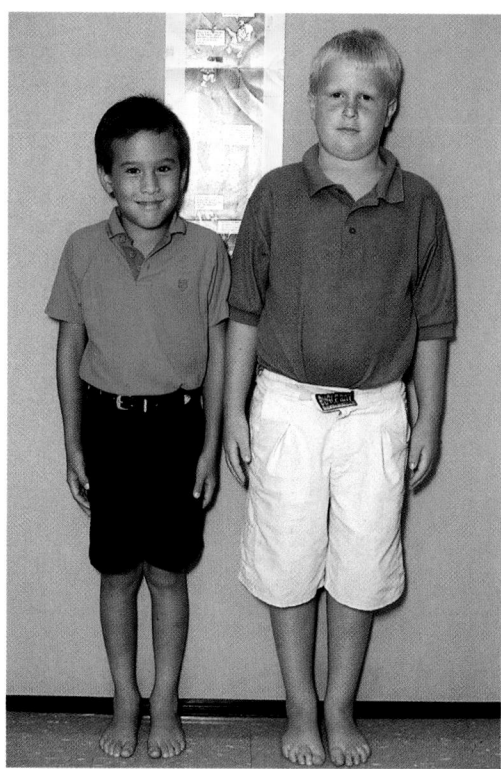

FIG 6-8 These children of identical age (8 years) are markedly different in size. The child on the left, of Asian descent, is at the 5th percentile for height and weight. The child on the right is above 95th percentile for height and weight. However, both children demonstrate normal growth patterns.

- Children who show a sudden increase (except during puberty), decrease, or no change in a previously steady growth pattern

Because growth is a continuous but uneven process, the most reliable evaluation lies in comparing growth measurements over time. It is important to remember that normal growth patterns vary among children the same age (Fig. 6-8).

Length

The term **length** refers to measurements taken when children are supine (also referred to as **recumbent length**). Until children are 24 months old (or 36 months if using the chart for birth to 36 months), measure recumbent length. Because of the normally flexed position during infancy, fully extend the body by (1) holding the head in midline, (2) grasping the knees together gently, and (3) pushing down on the knees until the legs are fully extended and flat against the table. If using a measuring board, place the head firmly at the top of the board and the heels of the feet firmly against the footboard.

If such a measuring device is not available, measure length by placing the child on a paper-covered surface, marking the end points of the top of the head and the heels of the feet, and measuring between these two points (Fig. 6-9). For accurate measurement, hold the writing utensil at a right angle to the table when marking the cephalic point; position the feet with the toes pointing directly to the ceiling when marking the heel point. Regardless of the method used, have someone assist in holding the child's head in midline while you extend the legs and take the measurements.

Height

The term **height** (or **stature**) refers to the measurement taken when a child is standing upright. Measure height by having the child, with the shoes removed, stand as tall and straight as possible with the head in midline and the line of vision parallel to the ceiling and floor. Be certain the child's back is to the wall or other vertical flat surface with the heels, buttocks, and back of the shoulders touching the wall and the medial malleoli touching if possible (Fig. 6-10). Check for and correct bending of the knees, slumping of the shoulders, or raising of the heels.

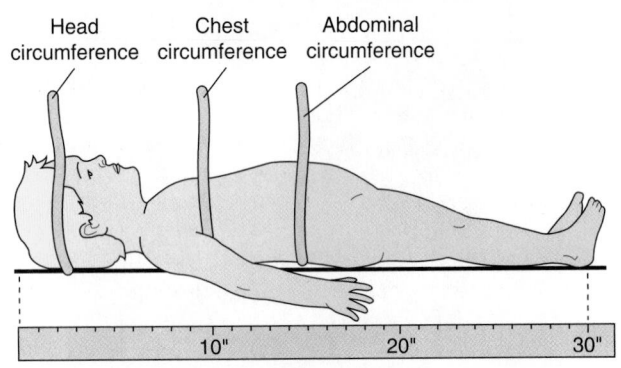

FIG 6-9 Measurement of head, chest, and abdominal circumference and crown-to-heel (recumbent) length. (From Price DL: *Pediatric nursing: an introductory text*, ed 10, St. Louis, 2007, Saunders.)

> **NURSING TIP** Normally, height is less if measured in the afternoon than in the morning. To minimize this variation, apply modest upward pressure under the jaw or the mastoid processes behind the ears.

For the most accurate measurement, use a wall-mounted unit (**stadiometer**; see Fig. 6-10). The movable measuring rod of platform scales is accurate only if it remains parallel to the floor and rests securely on the topmost part of the head. To improvise a flat surface for measuring length, attach a paper or metal tape or yardstick to the wall, position the child adjacent to the tape, and place a three-dimensional object, such as a thick book or box, on top of the head. Rest the side of the object firmly against the wall to form a right angle. Measure length or stature to the nearest 1 mm or 1/8 inch.

Weight

Weight is measured with an appropriately sized balance beam scale, which measures weight to the nearest 10 g (0.35 oz) for infants and 100 g (0.22 lb) for children. Before weighing the child, balance the scale by setting it at 0 and noting if the balance registers exactly in the middle of the mark. If the end of the balance beam rises to the top or bottom of the mark, more or less weight, respectively, is needed. Some scales are designed to self-correct, but others need to be recalibrated by the manufacturer. Scales vary in their accuracy; infant scales tend to be more accurate than adult platform scales, and newer scales tend to be more accurate than older ones, especially at the upper levels of weight measurement. When precise measurements are necessary, two nurses should take the weight independently; if there is a discrepancy, take a third reading.

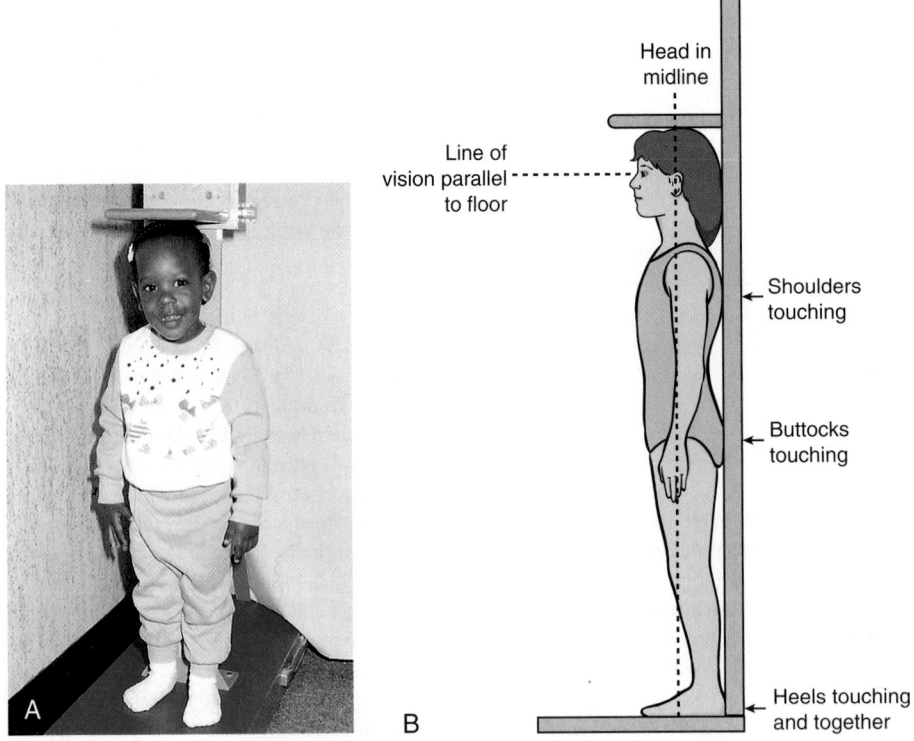

FIG 6-10 A and **B,** Measurement of height. (**A,** From Seidel HM, Ball JW, Dains JE, and others: *Mosby's guide to physical examination*, ed 6, St. Louis, 2007, Mosby. **B,** From Wilson S: *Health assessment for nursing practice*, ed 4, St. Louis, 2009, Mosby.)

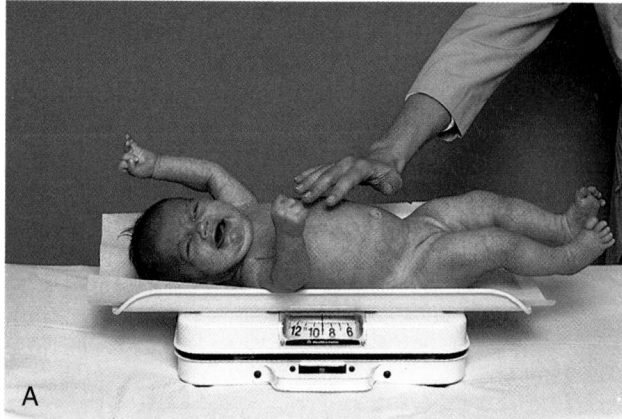

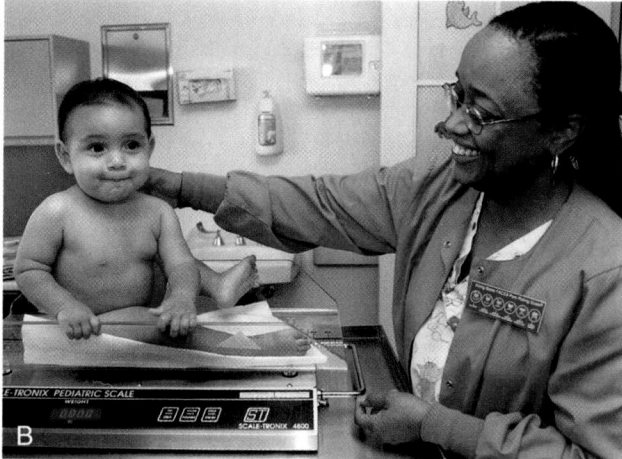

FIG 6-11 **A,** Infant on scale. **B,** Toddler on scale. Note the presence of the nurse to prevent falls. (**B,** Courtesy Paul Vincent Kuntz, Texas Children's Hospital, Houston.)

Take measurements in a comfortably warm room. When the birth to 36-month growth charts are used, children should be weighed nude. Older children are usually weighed while wearing their underpants or a light gown. However, always respect the privacy of all children. If the child must be weighed wearing some article of clothing or some type of special device, such as a prosthesis or an armboard for an intravenous device, note this when recording the weight. Children who are measured for recumbent length are usually weighed on an infant platform scale and placed in a lying or sitting position. When weighing a child, place your hand lightly above the infant to prevent him or her from accidentally falling off the scale (Fig. 6-11, *A*) or stand close to the toddler, ready to prevent a fall (Fig. 6-11, *B*). For maximum asepsis, cover the scale with a clean sheet of paper between each child's measurement.

Skinfold Thickness and Arm Circumference

Measures of relative weight and stature cannot distinguish between adipose (fat) tissue and muscle. One convenient measure of body fat is skinfold thickness, which is increasingly recommended as a routine measurement. Measure skinfold thickness with special calipers, such as the Lange calipers. The most common sites for measuring skinfold thickness are the triceps (most practical for routine clinical use), subscapula, suprailiac, abdomen, and upper thigh. For greatest reliability, follow the exact procedure for measurement and record the average of at least two measurements of one site.

Arm circumference is an indirect measure of muscle mass. Measurement of arm circumference follows the same procedure as for skinfold thickness except the midpoint is measured with a paper or steel tape. Place the tape vertically along the posterior aspect of the upper arm to the acromial process and to the olecranon process; half of the measured length is the midpoint. Percentiles for triceps skinfold and arm circumference in children are provided in Appendix B and may be used as reference data. However, the percentiles are not standards or norms because values between the 5th and 95th percentiles are not ranges of normal.

Head Circumference

Measure head circumference in children up to 36 months of age and in any child whose head size is questionable. Measure the head at its greatest circumference, usually slightly above the eyebrows and pinna of the ears and around the occipital prominence at the back of the skull (see Fig. 6-9). Because head shape can affect the location of the maximum circumference, more than one measurement at points above the eyebrows is necessary to obtain the most accurate measure. Use a paper or metal tape because a cloth tape can stretch and give a falsely small measurement. For greatest accuracy, use devices marked with tenths of a centimeter because the percentile charts have only 0.5-cm increments.

Plot the head size on the appropriate growth chart under head circumference. Generally, head and chest circumferences are equal at about 1 to 2 years of age. During childhood, chest circumference exceeds head size by about 5 to 7 cm (2–2.75 inches). (For newborns, see Physical Assessment, Chapter 8.)

PHYSIOLOGIC MEASUREMENTS

Physiologic measurements, key elements in evaluating physical status of vital functions, include temperature, pulse, respiration, and BP. Compare each physiologic recording with normal values for that age group (see Appendix E and inside back cover). In addition, compare the values taken on preceding health visits with present recordings. For example, a falsely elevated BP reading may not indicate hypertension if previous recent readings have been within normal limits. The isolated recording may indicate some stressful event in the child's life.

As in most procedures carried out with children, treat older children and adolescents much the same as adults. However, give special consideration to preschool children (see Atraumatic Care box). For best results in taking vital signs of infants, count respirations first (before the infant is disturbed), take the pulse next, and measure temperature last. If vital signs cannot be taken without disturbing the child, record the child's behavior (e.g., crying) along with the measurement.

ATRAUMATIC CARE
Reducing Young Children's Fears

Young children, especially preschoolers, fear intrusive procedures because of their poorly defined body boundaries. Therefore, avoid invasive procedures, such as measuring rectal temperature, whenever possible. Also, avoid using the word "take" when measuring vital signs because young children interpret words literally and may think that their temperature or other function will be taken away. Instead, say, "I want to know how warm you are."

BOX 6-10 RECOMMENDED TEMPERATURE SCREENING ROUTES IN INFANTS AND CHILDREN

Birth to 2 Years
Axillary
Rectal—If definitive temperature reading is needed for infants older than 1 month of age

2 to 5 Years
Axillary
Tympanic
Oral—When child can hold thermometer under tongue
Rectal—If definitive temperature reading is needed

Older Than 5 Years
Oral
Axillary
Tympanic

BOX 6-11 ALTERNATIVE TEMPERATURE MEASUREMENT SITES FOR ILL CHILDREN

Skin
A probe is placed on the skin to determine heat output in response to changes in the patient's skin temperature.
Skin temperature sensors are most often used for neonates and infants placed in radiant heat warmers or isolettes (using servocontrol feature of the apparatus). In turn, the heater unit warms to a set point to maintain the infant's temperature within a specified range.
ThermoSpot is an example of a device allowing continuous thermal monitoring in neonates.

Urinary Bladder
A thermistor or thermocouple is placed within the indwelling bladder catheter. The catheter tip immersed in the bladder provides a continuous temperature read-out on the bedside monitor.
This is not a true measure of core temperature but responds better than rectal and skin temperatures to core body changes.
Because of thermistor sizes, this method is unusable with neonates and small infants.

Pulmonary Artery
A catheter is placed into the heart to obtain a reading in the pulmonary artery.
It is used in critical care settings or operating rooms only in patients requiring aggressive monitoring.
Catheters are not available in sizes for neonates or small infants.

Esophageal Site
A probe is inserted into the lower third of the esophagus at the level of the heart.
This is used in critical care settings or operating rooms.
Several companies have esophageal stethoscopes with temperature probe monitors for patients in the operating room that show a continuous temperature reading.

Nasopharyngeal Site
A probe is inserted into the nasopharynx, posterior to the soft palate, and provides an estimate of hypothalamic temperature.
This is used in critical care settings or operating rooms.

Data from Kumar PR, Nisarga R, Gowda B: Temperature monitoring in newborns using ThermoSpot, *Indian J Pediatr* 71(9):795–796, 2004; Martin SA, Kline AM: Can there be a standard for temperature measurement in the pediatric intensive care unit? *AACN Clin Issues* 15(2):254–266, 2004; and Maxton FJC, Justin L, Gilles D: Estimating core temperature in infants and children after cardiac surgery: a comparison of six methods, *J Adv Nurs* 45(2):214–222, 2004.

Temperature

Temperature is the measure of heat content within an individual's body. The core temperature most closely reflects the temperature of the blood flow through the carotid arteries to the hypothalamus. Core temperature is relatively constant despite wide fluctuations in the external environment. When a child's temperature is altered, receptors in the skin, spinal cord, and brain respond in an attempt to achieve normothermia, a normal temperature state. In pediatrics, there is a lack of consensus regarding what temperature constitutes normothermia for every child. For rectal temperatures in children, a value of 37° to 37.5° C (98.6°–99.5° F) is an acceptable range, where heat loss and heat production are balanced. For neonates, a core body temperature between 36.5° and 37.6° C (97.7° and 99.7° F) is a desirable range. In neonates, obtain temperature measurements for monitoring adequacy of thermoregulation, not fever; therefore, temperature measurements in each infant should be carefully considered in the context of the *purpose* and the environment.

The nurse can measure temperature in healthy children at several body sites via oral, rectal, axillary, ear canal, tympanic membrane, temporal artery, or skin route (Box 6-10). For ill children, other sites for temperature measurement that have been investigated include the urinary bladder, pulmonary artery, and esophageal and nasopharyngeal sites (El-Radhi and Barry, 2006; Mains, Coxall, and Lloyd, 2008) (Box 6-11). One of the most important influences on the accuracy of temperature is improper temperature-taking technique. Detailed discussion of temperature-taking methods and visual examples of proper techniques are given in Table 6-3. For a critical review of the evidence on temperature taking methods, see the Evidence-Based Practice box.

The most frequently used temperature measurement devices in infants and children include:

Electronic intermittent thermometers—Measure the patient's temperature at oral, rectal, and axillary sites; these are used as primary diagnostic indicators

Infrared thermometers—Measure the patient's temperature by collecting emitted thermal radiation from a particular site (e.g., ear canal)

Electronic continuous thermometers—Measure the patient's temperature during the administration of general anesthesia, treatment of hypothermia or hyperthermia, and other situations that require continuous monitoring

Box 6-12 provides a detailed description of these devices.

! NURSING ALERT

The belief that core temperature can be estimated by adding 1° C to the temperature taken in the axilla is incorrect. Do not add a degree to the finding obtained by taking a temperature by the axillary route (Craig, Lancaster, Williamson, and others, 2000).

TABLE 6-3   TEMPERATURE MEASUREMENT LOCATIONS FOR INFANTS AND CHILDREN

TEMPERATURE SITE

Oral

Place tip under tongue in right or left posterior sublingual pocket, not in front of tongue. Have child keep mouth closed without biting on thermometer.

Pacifier thermometers measure intraoral or supralingual temperature and are available but lack support in the literature.

Several factors affect mouth temperature: eating and mastication, hot or cold beverages, open-mouth breathing, ambient temperature.

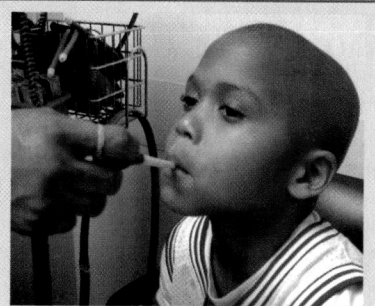

Axillary

Place tip under arm in center of axilla and keep close to skin, not clothing. Hold child's arm firmly against side. Temperature may be affected by poor peripheral perfusion (results in lower value), clothing or swaddling, use of radiant warmer, or amount of brown fat in cold-stressed neonate (results in higher value).

Advantage—Avoids intrusive procedure and eliminates risk of rectal perforation.

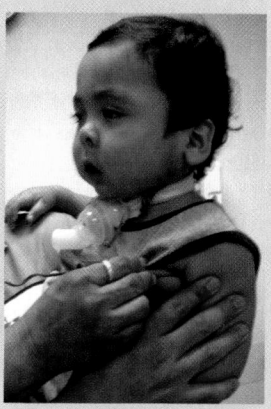

Ear Based (Aural)

Insert small infrared probe deeply into canal to allow sensor to obtain measurement. Size of probe (most are 8 mm) may influence accuracy of result. In young children, this may be a problem because of small diameter of canal. Proper placement of ear is controversial related to whether the pinna should be pulled in manner similar to that used during otoscopy (see p. 126).

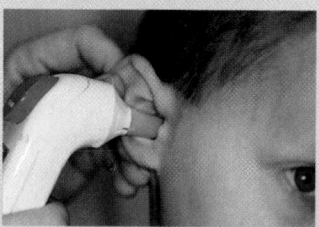

Rectal

Place well-lubricated tip at maximum 2.5 cm (1 inch) into rectum for children and 1.5 cm (0.6 inch) for infants; securely hold thermometer close to anus.

Child may be placed in side-lying, supine, or prone position (i.e., supine with knees flexed toward abdomen); cover penis because procedure may stimulate urination. A small child may be placed prone across parent's lap.

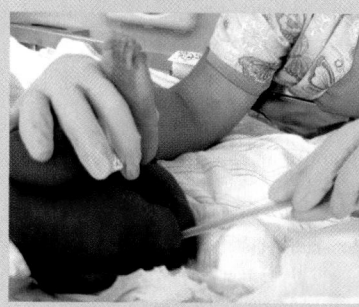

Temporal Artery

An infrared sensor probe scans across forehead, capturing heat from arterial blood flow. Temporal artery is only artery close enough to skin's surface to provide access for accurate temperature measurement.

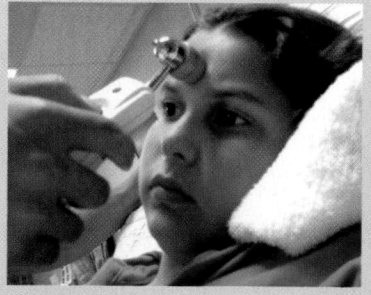

Data from Martin SA, Kline AM: Can there be a standard for temperature measurement in the pediatric intensive care unit? *AACN Clin Issues* 15(2):254–266, 2004; and Falzon A, Grech V, Caruana B, and others: How reliable is axillary temperature measurement? *Acta Paediatr* 92(3):309–313, 2003. Oral, axillary, rectal, and temporal artery images courtesy Paul Vincent Kuntz, Texas Children's Hospital, Houston.

EVIDENCE-BASED PRACTICE

Temperature Measurement in Pediatrics

Ask the Question
Picot Question
In infants and children, what is the most accurate method for measuring temperature in febrile children?

Search for the Evidence
Search Strategies
Clinical research studies related to this issue were identified by searching for English publications within past 10 years for infant and child populations; comparisons with gold standard: rectal thermometry.

Databases Used
PubMed, Cochrane Collaboration, MD Consult, Joanna Briggs Institute, National Guideline Clearinghouse (AHRQ), TRIP Database Plus, PedsCCM, BestBETs

Critically Analyze the Evidence
Rectal temperature—Rectal measurement remains the clinical gold standard for the precise diagnosis of fever in infants and children compared with other methods (Fortuna, Carney, Macy, and others, 2010; Greenes and Fleisher, 2004; Holzhauer, Reith, Sawin, and others, 2009; Riddell and Eppich, 2003; University of Michigan, 2003). However, this procedure is more invasive and is contraindicated for infants younger than 1 month old, children with recent rectal surgery, children with diarrhea or anorectal lesions, and children receiving chemotherapy (cancer treatment usually affects the mucosa and causes neutropenia).

Oral temperature (OT)—OT indicates rapid changes in core body temperature, but accuracy may be an issue compared with the rectal site (Jensen, Jensen, Madsen, and others, 2000). OTs are considered the standard for temperature measurement (Gilbert, Barton, and Counsell, 2002) but are contraindicated in children who have an altered level of consciousness, are receiving oxygen, are mouth breathing, are experiencing mucositis, had recent oral surgery or trauma, or are younger than 5 years of age (Carroll, 2000; El-Radhi and Barry, 2006). Limitations of OTs include the effects of ambient room temperature and recent oral intake (Carroll, 2000; Martin and Kline, 2004).

Axillary temperature—This is inconsistent and insensitive in infants and children older than 1 month old (Falzon, Grech, Caruana, and others, 2003; Jean-Mary, Dicanzio, Shaw, and others, 2002). In neonates with fever the axillary temperature cannot be used interchangeably with rectal measurement (Muller, van Berkel, and de Beaufort, 2008).

Ear (aural) temperature—This is not a precise measurement of body temperature. Meta-analysis of 101 studies comparing tympanic membrane temperatures with rectal temperatures in children concluded that the tympanic method demonstrated a wide range of variability, limiting its application in a pediatric setting (Craig, Lancaster, Taylor, and others, 2002). More recently published reviews continue to find poor sensitivity using infrared ear thermometry (Devrim, Ates, Ceyhan, and others, 2007; Dodd, Lancaster, Craig, and others, 2006). Diagnosis of fever without a focus should not be made based on tympanic thermometry because it is not an accurate measure of core temperature (Craig, Lancaster, Taylor, and others, 2002; Devrim, Ates, Ceyhan, and others, 2007; Dodd, Lancaster, Craig, and others, 2006; Riddell and Eppich, 2003).

Temporal artery temperature (TAT)—TAT is not predictable for fever in young children but can be used as a screening tool for detecting fever less than 38° C (100.4° F) in children 3 months to 4 years of age (Al-Mukhaizeem, Allen, Komar, and others, 2004; Callanan, 2003; Fortuna, Carney, Macy, and others, 2010; Greenes and Fleisher, 2001; Hebbar, Fortenberry, Rogers, and others,

2005; Holzhauer, Reith, Sawin, and others, 2009; Schuh, Komar, Stephens, and others, 2004; Siberry, Diener-West, Schappell, and others, 2002; Titus, Hulsey, Heckman, and others, 2009).

Apply the Evidence: Nursing Implications
There is **good** evidence with **strong** recommendations for the following (Guyatt, Oxman, Vist, and others 2008):
- No single site used for temperature assessment provides unequivocal estimates of core body temperature.
- Studies show that the axillary and tympanic measures demonstrate poor agreement when these modes are compared with more accurate core temperature methods. The differences are more evident as temperature increases, regardless of age.
- TAT is not predictable for fever and should be only used as a screening tool in young children.
- When an accurate method for obtaining a correct reflection of core temperature is needed, the rectal temperature is recommended in younger children and the oral route in older children.

QSEN Quality and Safety Competencies:
Evidence-Based Practice*
Knowledge
Differentiate clinical opinion from research and evidence-based summaries.
Demonstrate understanding of thermometry selection based on the developmental age of the child.

Skills
Base individualized care plan on patient values, clinical expertise, and evidence.
Integrate evidence into practice by using the correct type of thermometry to screen for fever compared with measures used for accurate determination of the degree of fever.

Attitudes
Value the concept of evidence-based practice as integral to determining best clinical practice.
Recognize strengths and weakness of evidence for the most accurate method for measuring fever in infants and children.

References
Al-Mukhaizeem F, Allen U, Komar L, and others: Comparison of temporal artery, rectal and esophageal core temperatures in children: results of a pilot study, *Paediatr Child Health* 9(7):461–465, 2004.
Callanan D: Detecting fever in young infants: reliability of perceived, pacifier, and temporal artery temperatures in infants younger than 3 months of age, *Pediatr Emerg Care* 19(4):240–243, 2003.
Carroll M: An evaluation of temperature measurement, *Nurs Stand* 14(44):39–43, 2000.
Craig JV, Lancaster GA, Taylor S, and others: Infrared ear thermometry compared with rectal thermometry in children: a systemic review, *Lancet* 360:603–609, 2002.
Devrim I, Kara A, Ceyhan M, and others: Measurement accuracy of fever by tympanic and axillary thermometry, *Pediatr Emerg Care* 23(1):16–19, 2007.
Dodd SR, Lancaster GA, Craig JV, and others: In a systematic review, infrared ear thermometry for fever diagnosis in children finds poor sensitivity, *J Clin Epidemiol* 59:354–357, 2006.
El-Radhi AS, Barry W: Thermometry in paediatric practice, *Arch Dis Child* 91(4):351–356, 2006.
Falzon A, Grech V, Caruana B, and others: How reliable is axillary temperature measurement? *Acta Paediatr* 92(3):309–313, 2003.
Fortuna EL, Carney MM, Macy M, and others: Accuracy of non-contact infrared thermometry versus rectal thermometry in young children evaluated in the emergency department for fever, *J Emerg Nurs* 36(2):101–104, 2010.
Gilbert M, Barton AJ, Counsell CM: Comparison of oral and tympanic temperatures in adult surgical patients, *Appl Nurs Res* 15(1):42–47, 2002.

*Adapted from the QSEN at http://www.qsen.org.

EVIDENCE-BASED PRACTICE

Temperature Measurement in Pediatrics—cont'd

Greenes DS, Fleisher GR: Accuracy of a noninvasive temporal artery thermometer for use in infants, *Arch Pediatr Adolesc Med* 155(3):376–381, 2001.

Greenes DS, Fleisher GR: When body temperature changes, does rectal temperature lag? *J Pediatr* 144(6):824–826, 2004.

Guyatt GH, Oxman AD, Vist GE, and others: GRADE: an emerging consensus on rating quality of evidence and strength of recommendations, *BMJ* 336:924–926, 2008.

Hebbar K, Fortenberry JD, Rogers K, and others: Comparison of temporal artery thermometer to standard temperature measurement in pediatric intensive care unit patients, *Pediatr Crit Care Med* 6(5):557–561, 2005.

Holzhauer JK, Reith V, Sawin K, and others: Evaluation of temporal artery thermometry in children 3–36 months old, *J Spec Pediatr Nurs* 14(4):239–244, 2009.

Jean-Mary MB, Dicanzio J, Shaw J, and others: Limited accuracy and reliability of infrared axillary and aural thermometers in a pediatric outpatient population, *J Pediatr* 141(5):671–676, 2002.

Jensen BN, Jensen FS, Madsen SN, and others: Accuracy of digital tympanic, oral, axillary, and rectal thermometers compared with standard rectal mercury thermometers, *Eur J Surg* 166(11):848–851, 2000.

Martin SA, Kline AM: Can there be a standard for temperature measurement in the pediatric intensive care unit? *AACN Clin Issues* 15(2):254–266, 2004.

Muller PCE, van Berkel LH, de Beaufort AJ: Axillary and rectal temperature measurements poorly agree in newborn infants, *Neonatology* 94:31–34, 2008.

Riddell A, Eppich W: Should tympanic temperature measurement be trusted? BestBETs, 2003, retrieved April 2005, from http://www.bestbets.org/cgi-bin/bets.pl?record=00340.

Schuh S, Komar L, Stephens D, and others: Comparison of the temporal artery and rectal thermometry in children in the emergency department, *Pediatr Emerg Care* 20(11):736–741, 2004.

Siberry GK, Diener-West M, Schappell E, and others: Comparison of temple temperatures with rectal temperatures in children under 2 years of age, *Clin Pediatr* 41(6):405–414, 2002.

Titus MO, Huley T, Heckman J, and others: Temporal artery thermometry utilization in pediatric emergency care, *Clin Pediatr* 48(2):190–193, 2009.

University of Michigan: Rectal temperature is still the gold standard for determining the presence or absence of fever, *Evidence-Based Pediatrics Web Site*, 2003, retrieved April 2005, from http://www.med.umich.edu/pediatrics/ebm/cats/fever.htm.

TABLE 6-4	GRADING OF PULSES
GRADE	**DESCRIPTION**
0	Not palpable
+1	Difficult to palpate, thready, weak, easily obliterated with pressure
+2	Difficult to palpate, may be obliterated with pressure
+3	Easy to palpate, not easily obliterated with pressure (normal)
+4	Strong, bounding, not obliterated with pressure

TABLE 6-5 — NORMATIVE DINAMAP BLOOD PRESSURE VALUES (SYSTOLIC/DIASTOLIC; MEAN ARTERIAL PRESSURE IN PARENTHESES)

AGE GROUP	MEAN	90TH PERCENTILE	95TH PERCENTILE
Newborn (1–3 days)	65/41 (50)	75/49 (59)	78/52 (62)
1 month–2 years	95/58 (72)	106/68 (83)	110/71 (86)
2–5 years	101/57 (74)	112/66 (82)	115/68 (85)

From Park M, Menard S: Normative oscillometric blood pressure values in the first 5 years in an office setting, *Am J Dis Child* 143(7):860–864, 1989.

Pulse

A satisfactory pulse can be taken radially in children older than 2 years of age. However, in infants and young children, the apical impulse (heard through a stethoscope held to the chest at the apex of the heart) is more reliable (see Fig. 6-33 for location of pulses). Count the pulse for 1 full minute in infants and young children because of possible irregularities in rhythm. However, when frequent apical rates are necessary, use shorter counting times (e.g., 15- or 30-second intervals). For greater accuracy, measure the apical rate while the child is asleep; record the child's behavior along with the rate. Grade pulses according to the criteria in Table 6-4. Compare radial and femoral pulses at least once during infancy to detect the presence of circulatory impairment, such as coarctation of the aorta. (See inside back cover for normal rates for pediatric age groups.)

Respiration

Count the respiratory rate in children in the same manner as for adult patients. However, in infants, observe abdominal movements because respirations are primarily diaphragmatic. Because the movements are irregular, count them for 1 full minute for accuracy (see also p. 130). (See inside back cover for normal respiratory rates in children.)

Blood Pressure

Blood pressure measurement by noninvasive methods is part of a routine vital sign determination. Measure BP annually in children 3 years of age through adolescence and in children with symptoms of hypertension, children in emergency departments and intensive care units, and high-risk infants (National High Blood Pressure Education Program Working Group on High Blood Pressure in Children and Adolescents, 2004).

Measurement Devices

Ambulatory BP monitoring in children and adolescents is a valuable method for assessing and managing suspected hypertension. Also measure BP using electronic devices that use oscillometric or Doppler techniques. In oscillometry, pressure changes are transmitted through the arterial wall to the pressure cuff, and the oscillations are detected by a pressure-sensitive indicator. Oscillometers have digital read-outs for systolic, diastolic, and mean arterial pressures (MAPs) and for pulse. The MAP is not the same as the mean BP (arithmetic average of systolic and diastolic pressures). Rather, it is a value somewhat lower than the arithmetic mean. BP readings using oscillometry, such as Dinamap, are generally higher (10 mm Hg higher) than measurements using auscultation (Park, Menard, and Schoolfield, 2005) (Table 6-5). Differences between Dinamap and auscultatory readings prevent the interchange of the readings by the two methods (Midgley, Wardhaugh, Macfarlane, and others, 2009).

Doppler ultrasonography translates changes in ultrasound frequency caused by blood movement within the artery to audible sound by means of a transducer in the cuff. This technique is useful for systolic pressure measurement but is unreliable for diastolic pressure measurement. Oscillometric and Doppler instruments are useful in measuring BP in infants and have largely replaced the flush method, which reflects only the mean BP, and the auscultatory method.

BOX 6-12 TYPES OF THERMOMETERS USED TO MEASURE TEMPERATURE IN INFANTS AND CHILDREN

Electronic Thermometer

Temperature is sensed with an electronic component called thermistor mounted at the tip of a plastic and stainless steel probe, which is connected to an electronic recorder. A disposable plastic cover is used for infection control.

Temperature measurement appears on digital display within 60 seconds.

The probe can be placed in the mouth, axilla, or rectum.

Infrared Thermometer

Thermal radiation is measured from the axilla, ear canal, or tympanic membrane.

Temperature measurement appears on the digital display in approximately 1 second.

Three types are available for ear-based use: tympanic, ear canal, and arterial heat balance via the ear canal (AHBE).

Often these devices are all inappropriately referred to as *tympanic thermometers*.

Temperatures measured in this way reflect arterial (bloodstream) temperature.

Ear-Based Temperature Sensor

Although this is frequently used in pediatric settings (especially ambulatory clinics), debate continues on the reliability of ear-based thermometry in screening febrile children.

Most models use "offsets" for internal calculations that transform ear temperature into supposedly equivalent oral or rectal temperatures.

Ear Sensor (LighTouch LTX)

This measures the infrared heat energy radiating from canal opening, scans canal for highest temperature reading, and then calculates arterial temperature (correlates highly with core or internal body temperature).

It is available in two sizes; the smaller size of LighTouch Pedi-Q is for infants and toddlers.

Axillary Sensor (LighTouch LTN)

This measures the infrared heat energy radiating from the axilla.

It can be used on wet skin; in incubators; or under radiant heaters, warming pads, or other heat sources.

Digital Thermometer

A probe is connected to a microprocessor chip, which translates signals into degrees and sends temperature measurement to digital display.

It is used like an oral electronic thermometer and can be used for measuring oral, rectal, and axillary temperature.

It is more accurate and easier to read but somewhat more expensive than a plastic strip thermometer.

Liquid Crystal Skin Contact Thermometer (Chemical Dot Thermometer)

This single-use, disposable, flexible thermometer has a specific chemical mixture in each circle that changes color to measure temperature increments of $\frac{2}{10}$ of a degree.

There are two types:

1. Kept in mouth (1 minute), axilla (3 minutes), or rectum (3 minutes); color change is read 10 to 15 seconds after removing the thermometer

2. Wearable, continuous-use thermometer, which is placed under axilla; may be read within 2 to 3 minutes after placement and continuously thereafter; discard and replace every 48 hours

---

RESEARCH FOCUS

Selection of a Blood Pressure Cuff

Researchers have found that selection of a cuff with a bladder width equal to 40% of the upper arm circumference most accurately reflects directly measured radial arterial pressure (Clark, Kieh-Lai, Sarnaik, and others, 2002).

Selection of Cuff

No matter what type of noninvasive technique is used, the most important factor in accurately measuring BP is the use of an appropriately sized cuff (**cuff size** refers only to the inner inflatable bladder, not the cloth covering). A technique to establish an appropriate cuff size is to choose a cuff with a bladder width that is approximately 40% of the arm circumference midway between the olecranon and the acromion (see Research Focus box). This will usually be a cuff bladder that covers 80% to 100% of the circumference of the arm (Fig. 6-12) (Beevers, Lip, and O'Brien, 2001). Cuffs that are either too narrow or too wide affect the accuracy of BP measurements. If the cuff size is too small, the reading on the device is falsely high. If the cuff size is too large, the reading is falsely low (Clark, Kieh-Lai, Sarnaik, and others, 2002).

Using limb circumference for selecting cuff width more accurately reflects direct arterial BP than using limb length because this method takes into account variations in arm thickness and the amount of pressure required to compress the artery. For measurement on sites other than the upper arms, use the limb circumference, although the

TABLE 6-6 RECOMMENDED DIMENSIONS FOR BLOOD PRESSURE CUFF BLADDERS

AGE	WIDTH (CM)	LENGTH (CM)	MAXIMUM ARM CIRCUMFERENCE (CM)*
Newborn	4	8	10
Infant	6	12	15
Child	9	18	22
Small adult	10	24	26
Adult	13	30	34
Large adult	16	38	44
Thigh	20	42	52

From National High Blood Pressure Education Program Working Group on High Blood Pressure in Children and Adolescents: The fourth report on the diagnosis, evaluation, and treatment of high blood pressure in children and adolescents, *Pediatrics* 114(2 suppl 4th Rep):555–576, 2004.

*Calculated so that largest arm would still allow bladder to encircle arm by at least 80%.

shape of the limb (e.g., conical shape of the thigh) may prevent appropriate placement of the cuff and inaccurately reflect intraarterial BP (Table 6-6).

When using a site other than the arm, BP measurements using noninvasive techniques may differ. Generally, systolic pressure in the

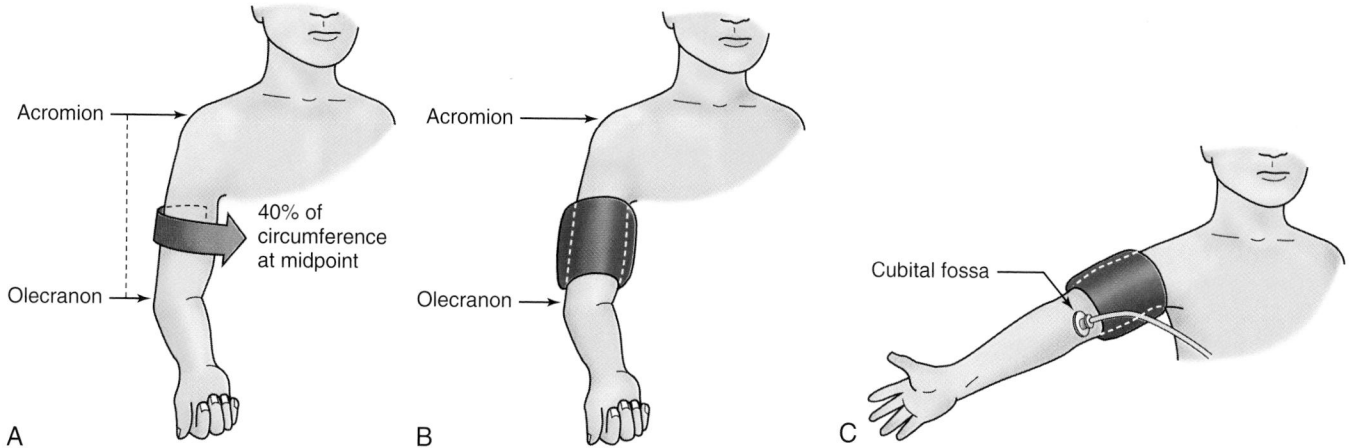

FIG 6-12 Determination of proper cuff size. **A,** Cuff bladder width should be approximately 40% of circumference of arm measured at a point midway between olecranon and acromion. **B,** Cuff bladder length should cover 80% to 100% of arm circumference. **C,** Blood pressure should be measured with the cubital fossa at the heart level. The arm should be supported. The stethoscope bell is placed over the brachial artery pulse proximal and medial to the cubital fossa and below the bottom edge of the cuff. (From National Institutes of Health, National Heart, Lung, and Blood Institute: *Update on the Task Force Report [1987] on high blood pressure in children and adolescents: a working group report from the National High Blood Pressure Education Program*, NIH Pub No 96-3790, Bethesda, Md, September 1996, Author.)

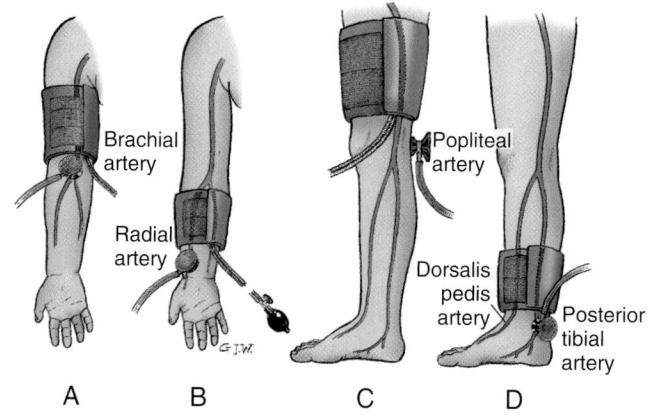

FIG 6-13 Sites for measuring blood pressure. **A,** Upper arm. **B,** Lower arm or forearm. **C,** Thigh. **D,** Calf or ankle.

TABLE 6-7	DIFFERENCES IN OSCILLOMETRIC SYSTOLIC BLOOD PRESSURE BETWEEN ARM AND LOWER EXTREMITY SITES IN NORMAL CHILDREN	
	SYSTOLIC BLOOD PRESSURE × (MEAN ± SD)	
AGE GROUP (YR)	**ARM-THIGH**	**ARM-CALF**
4–8	−7.1 ± 6.8	−9.3 ± 7.4
9–16	−2.4 ± 7.7	−5.0 ± 26.9

From Park M, Lee D, Johnson GA: Oscillometric blood pressures in the arm, thigh, and calf in healthy children and those with aortic coarctation, *Pediatrics* 91(4):761–765, 1993.

lower extremities (thigh or calf) is greater than pressure in the upper extremities, and systolic BP in the calf is higher than that in the thigh (Fig. 6-13). Table 6-7 lists these differences that are applied to oscillometric measurements taken on the right extremities with the child supine and the cuff size based on the circumference method.

Measurement and Interpretation

Measuring and interpreting BP in infants and children require attention to correct procedure because (1) limb sizes vary, and cuff selection must accommodate the circumference; (2) excessive pressure on the antecubital fossa affects the Korotkoff sounds; (3) children easily

! NURSING ALERT

Compare BP in the upper and lower extremities to detect abnormalities, such as coarctation of the aorta, in which the lower extremity pressure is less than the upper extremity pressure.

! NURSING ALERT

When taking BP, use an appropriately sized cuff. When the correct size is not available, use an oversized cuff rather than an undersized one or use another site that more appropriately fits the cuff size. Do not choose a cuff based on the name of the cuff (e.g., an "infant" cuff may be too small for some infants).

become anxious, which can elevate BP; and (4) BP values change with age and growth. In children and adolescents, determine the normal range of BP by body size and age. BP standards that are based on gender, age, and height provide a more precise classification of BP according to body size. This approach avoids misclassifying children who are very tall or very short. The revised BP tables now include the 50th, 90th, 95th, and 99th percentiles (with standard deviations) by gender, age, and height (see Appendix E).

To use the tables in a clinical setting, determine the height percentile by using the newly revised Centers for Disease Control and Prevention growth charts (www.cdc.gov/growthcharts). The child's measured systolic BP and diastolic BP are compared with the numbers provided in the table (boys or girls) according to the child's age and height percentile. The child is normotensive if the BP is below the 90th percentile. If the BP is at or above the 90th percentile, repeat the BP measurement at that visit to verify an elevated BP. BP measurements between the 90th and 95th percentiles indicate prehypertension and necessitate reassessment and consideration of other risk factors. In addition, if an adolescent's BP is more than 120/80 mm Hg, consider the patient prehypertensive even if this value is below the 90th percentile. This BP level typically occurs for systolic BP at 12 years old and for diastolic BP at 16 years old. If the child's BP (systolic or diastolic) is at or above the 95th percentile, the child may be hypertensive, and the measurement must be repeated on at least two occasions to confirm diagnosis (National High Blood Pressure Education Program Working Group on High Blood Pressure in Children and Adolescents, 2004) (see Nursing Care Guidelines box).

Orthostatic Hypotension

Orthostatic hypotension (OH), also called postural hypotension or orthostatic intolerance, often manifests as syncope (fainting), vertigo (dizziness), or lightheadedness and is caused by decreased blood flow to the brain (cerebral hypoperfusion). Normally, blood flow to the brain is maintained at a constant level by a number of compensating mechanisms that regulate systemic BP. When one assumes a sitting or standing position from a supine or recumbent position, peripheral capillary vasoconstriction occurs, and blood that was pooling in the lower vasculature is returned to the heart for redistribution to the head and remainder of the body. When this mechanism fails or is slow to respond, the person may experience vertigo or syncope. One of the most common causes of OH is hypovolemia, which may be induced by medications such as diuretics or vasodilator medications and by prolonged immobility or bed rest. Other causes of OH include dehydration, diarrhea, emesis, fluid loss from sweating and exertion, alcohol intake, dysrhythmias, diabetes mellitus, sepsis, and hemorrhage.

Blood pressure measurements taken with the child supine then standing (at least 2 minutes in each position) may demonstrate variability and assist in the diagnosis of OH. A child with a sustained drop in systolic pressure of more than 20 mm Hg or in diastolic pressure of more than 10 mm Hg after standing for 2 minutes without an increase in heart rate of more than 15 beats/min most likely has an autonomic deficit. Nonneurogenic causes of OH have a compensatory increase in pulse of more than 15 beats/min as well as a drop in BP, as noted previously. For children and adolescents with vertigo, lightheadedness, nausea, syncope, diaphoresis, and pallor, it is important to monitor BP and heart rate to determine the original cause. BP is an important diagnostic measurement in children and adolescents and must be a part of the routine monitoring of vital signs.

NURSING CARE GUIDELINES
Using the Blood Pressure Tables

1. Use the standard height charts to determine the height percentile.
2. Measure and record the child's systolic blood pressure (SBP) and diastolic blood pressure (DBP).
3. Use the correct gender table for SBP and DBP.
4. Find the child's age on the left side of the table. Follow the age row horizontally across the table to the intersection of the line for the height percentile (vertical column).
5. There, find the 50th, 90th, 95th, and 99th percentiles for SBP in the left columns and for DBP in the right columns.
   - BP less than 90th percentile is normal.
   - BP between the 90th and 95th percentiles is prehypertension. In adolescents, BP of 120/80 mm Hg or greater is prehypertension even if this figure is less than the 90th percentile.
   - BP over the 95th percentile may be hypertension.
6. If the BP is over the 90th percentile, the BP should be repeated twice at the same office visit, and an average SBP and DBP should be used.
7. If the BP is over the 95th percentile, BP should be staged. If BP is stage 1 (95th to 99th percentile plus 5 mm Hg), BP measurements should be repeated on two more occasions. If hypertension is confirmed, evaluation should proceed. If BP is stage 2 (>99th percentile plus 5 mm Hg), prompt referral should be made for evaluation and therapy. If the patient is symptomatic, immediate referral and treatment are indicated.

From National High Blood Pressure Education Program Working Group on High Blood Pressure in Children and Adolescents: The fourth report on the diagnosis, evaluation, and treatment of high blood pressure in children and adolescents, *Pediatrics* 114(2 suppl 4th Rep):555–576, 2004.

! NURSING ALERT

Published norms for BP, such as those in Appendix E, are valid only if you use the same method of measurement (auscultation and cuff size determination) in clinical practice.

GENERAL APPEARANCE

The child's general appearance is a cumulative, subjective impression of the child's physical appearance, state of nutrition, behavior, personality, interactions with parents and nurse (also siblings if present), posture, development, and speech. Although the nurse records the patient's general appearance at the beginning of the physical examination, it encompasses all the observations of the child during the interview and physical assessment.

Note the facies, the child's facial expression and appearance. For example, the facies may give clues to children who are in pain; have difficulty breathing; feel frightened, discontented, or unhappy; are mentally delayed; or are acutely ill.

Observe the posture, position, and types of body movement. A child with hearing or vision loss may characteristically tilt the head in an awkward position to hear or see better. A child in pain may favor a body part. A child with low self-esteem or a feeling of rejection may assume a slumped, careless, and apathetic pose. Likewise, a child with confidence, a feeling of self-worth, and a sense of security usually demonstrates a tall, straight, well-balanced posture. While observing such body language, do not interpret too freely but rather record objectively.

Note the child's hygiene in terms of cleanliness; unusual body odor; the condition of the hair, neck, nails, teeth, and feet; and the condition of the clothing. Such observations are excellent clues to possible instances of neglect, inadequate financial resources, housing difficulties (e.g., no running water), or lack of knowledge concerning children's needs.

Behavior includes the child's personality, activity level, reaction to stress, requests, frustration, interactions with others (primarily the parent and nurse), degree of alertness, and response to stimuli. Some mental questions that serve as reminders for observing behavior include the following: What is the child's overall personality? Does the child have a long attention span, or is he or she easily distracted? Can the child follow two or three commands in succession without the need for repetition? What is the youngster's response to delayed gratification or frustration? Does the child use eye contact during conversation? What is the child's reaction to the nurse and family members? Is the child quick or slow to grasp explanations?

SKIN

Assess skin for color, texture, temperature, moisture, turgor, lesions, and rashes. Examination of the skin and its accessory organs primarily involves inspection and palpation. Touch allows the nurse to assess the texture, turgor, and temperature of the skin. The normal color in light-skinned children varies from a milky white and rose to a deeply hued pink. Dark-skinned children, such as those of Native American, Hispanic, or African descent, have inherited various brown, red, yellow, olive green, and bluish tones in their skin. Asian persons have skin that is normally of a yellow tone. Several variations in skin color can occur, some of which warrant further investigation. The types of color change and their appearance in children with light or dark skin are summarized in Table 6-8.

Normally, the skin texture of young children is smooth, slightly dry, and not oily or clammy. Evaluate skin temperature by symmetrically feeling each part of the body and comparing upper areas with lower ones. Note any difference in temperature.

Determine tissue turgor, or elasticity in the skin, by grasping the skin on the abdomen between the thumb and index finger, pulling it taut, and quickly releasing it. Elastic tissue immediately resumes its normal position without residual marks or creases. In children with poor skin turgor, the skin remains suspended or tented for a few seconds before slowly falling back on the abdomen. Skin turgor is one of the best estimates of adequate hydration and nutrition.

Accessory Structures

Inspection of the accessory structures of the skin may be performed while examining the skin, scalp, or extremities.

Inspect the hair for color, texture, quality, distribution, and elasticity. Children's scalp hair is usually lustrous, silky, strong, and elastic. Genetic factors affect the appearance of hair. For example, the hair of African-American children is usually curlier and coarser than that of white children. Hair that is stringy, dull, brittle, dry, friable, and depigmented may suggest poor nutrition. Record any bald or thinning spots. Loss of hair in infants may indicate lying in the same position and may be a cue to counsel parents concerning the child's stimulation needs.

Inspect the hair and scalp for general cleanliness. Persons in some ethnic groups condition their hair with oils or lubricants that, if not thoroughly washed from the scalp, clog the sebaceous glands, causing scalp infections. Also examine the area for lesions; scaliness; evidence of infestation, such as lice or ticks; and signs of trauma, such as ecchymosis, masses, or scars.

In children who are approaching puberty, look for growth of secondary hair as a sign of normally progressing pubertal changes. Note precocious or delayed appearance of hair growth because, although not always suggestive of hormonal dysfunction, it may be of great concern to early- or late-maturing adolescents.

Inspect the nails for color, shape, texture, and quality. Normally, the nails are pink, convex, smooth, and hard but flexible (not brittle). The edges, which are usually white, should extend over the fingers. Dark-skinned individuals may have more deeply pigmented nail beds.

TABLE 6-8	DIFFERENCES IN COLOR CHANGES OF RACIAL GROUPS	
DESCRIPTION	**APPEARANCE IN LIGHT SKIN**	**APPEARANCE IN DARK SKIN**
Cyanosis—Bluish tone through skin; reflects reduced (deoxygenated) hemoglobin	Bluish tinge, especially in palpebral conjunctiva (lower eyelid), nail beds, earlobes, lips, oral membranes, soles, and palms	Ashen gray lips and tongue
Pallor—Paleness; may be sign of anemia, chronic disease, edema, or shock	Loss of rosy glow in skin, especially face	Ashen gray appearance in black skin More yellowish brown color in brown skin
Erythema—Redness; may be result of increased blood flow from climatic conditions, local inflammation, infection, skin irritation, allergy, or other dermatoses or may be caused by increased numbers of red blood cells as compensatory response to chronic hypoxia	Redness easily seen anywhere on body	Much more difficult to assess; rely on palpation for warmth or edema
Ecchymosis—Large, diffuse areas, usually black and blue, caused by hemorrhage of blood into skin; typically result of injuries	Purplish to yellow-green areas; may be seen anywhere on skin	Very difficult to see unless in mouth or conjunctiva
Petechiae—Same as ecchymosis except for size: small, distinct, pinpoint hemorrhages ≤2 mm in size; can denote some type of blood disorder, such as leukemia	Purplish pinpoints most easily seen on buttocks, abdomen, and inner surfaces of arms or legs	Usually invisible except in oral mucosa, conjunctiva of eyelids, and conjunctiva covering eyeball
Jaundice—Yellow staining of skin usually caused by bile pigments	Yellow staining seen in sclerae of eyes, skin, fingernails, soles, palms, and oral mucosa	Most reliably assessed in sclerae, hard palate, palms, and soles

Short, ragged nails are typical of habitual biting. Uncut, dirty nails are a sign of poor hygiene.

The palm normally shows three flexion creases (Fig. 6-14, *A*). In some situations such as Down syndrome, the two distal horizontal creases are fused to form a single horizontal crease (the **single palmar crease,** or **transpalmar crease**) (Fig. 6-14, *B*). If grossly abnormal lines or folds are observed, sketch a picture to describe them and refer the finding to a specialist for further investigation.

LYMPH NODES

Lymph nodes are usually assessed during examination of the part of the body in which they are located. The body's lymphatic drainage system is extensive. Figure 6-15 shows the usual sites for palpating accessible lymph nodes.

Palpate nodes using the distal portion of the fingers and gently but firmly pressing in a circular motion along the regions where nodes are normally present. During assessment of the nodes in the head and neck, tilt the child's head upward slightly but without tensing the sternocleidomastoid or trapezius muscles. This position facilitates palpation of the **submental, submandibular, tonsillar,** and **cervical nodes.** Palpate the axillary nodes with the child's arms relaxed at the sides but slightly abducted. Assess the inguinal nodes with the child in the supine position. Note size, mobility, temperature, and tenderness, as well as reports by the parents regarding any visible change of enlarged nodes. In children, small, nontender, movable nodes are usually normal. Tender, enlarged, warm, erythematous lymph nodes generally indicate infection or inflammation close to their location. Report such findings for further investigation.

HEAD AND NECK

Observe the head for general **shape** and **symmetry.** A flattening of one part of the head, such as the occiput, may indicate that the child continually lies in this position. Marked asymmetry is usually abnormal and may indicate premature closure of the sutures (craniosynostosis).

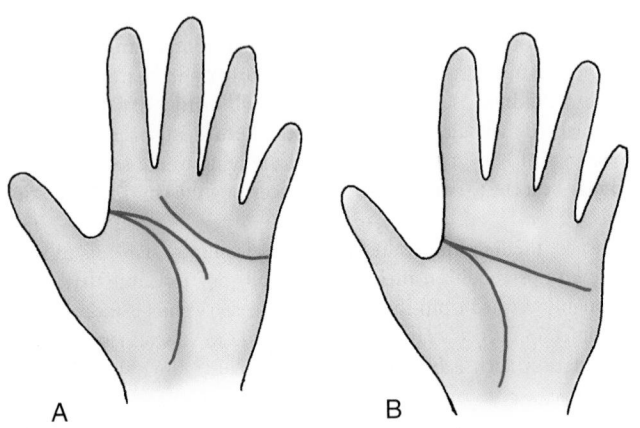

FIG 6-14 Examples of flexion creases on palm. **A,** Normal. **B,** Transpalmar crease.

> ### ! NURSING ALERT
>
> Significant head lag after 6 months of age strongly indicates cerebral injury and is referred for further evaluation.

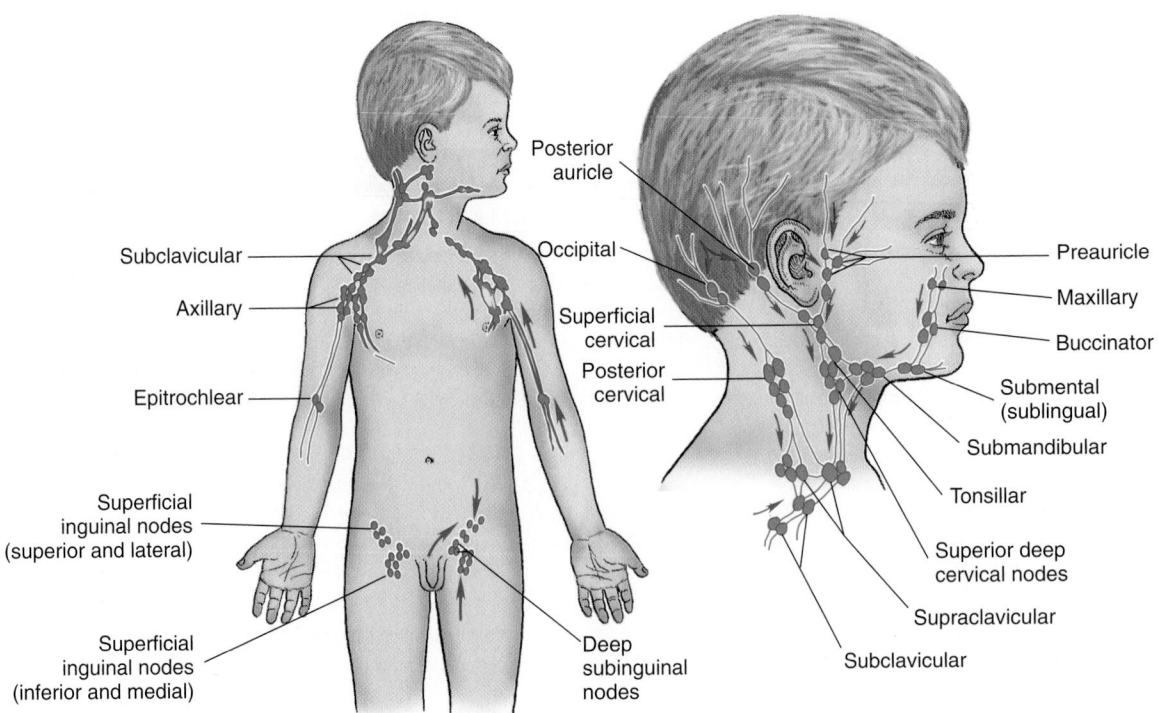

FIG 6-15 Location of the superficial lymph nodes. *Arrows* indicate directional flow of lymph.

Note **head control** in infants and **head posture** in older children. By 4 months of age, most infants should be able to hold the head erect and in midline when in a vertical position.

Evaluate **range of motion** by asking the older child to look in each direction (to either side, up, and down) or by manually putting the younger child through each position. Limited range of motion may indicate **wryneck**, or **torticollis**, in which the child holds the head to one side with the chin pointing toward the opposite side a result of injury to the sternocleidomastoid muscle.

> ### ! NURSING ALERT
>
> Hyperextension of the head (**opisthotonos**) with pain on flexion is a serious indication of meningeal irritation and is referred for immediate medical evaluation.

Palpate the **skull** for patent sutures, fontanels, fractures, and swellings. Normally, the posterior fontanel closes by the second month of life, and the anterior fontanel fuses between 12 and 18 months. Early or late closure is noted because either may be a sign of a pathologic condition. (For a more detailed discussion of the cranial bones, see Chapter 8.)

While examining the head, observe the face for symmetry, movement, and general appearance. Ask the child to "make a face" to assess symmetric movement and disclose any degree of paralysis. Note any unusual facial proportion, such as an unusually high or low forehead; wide- or close-set eyes; or a small, receding chin.

In addition to assessment of the head and neck for movement, inspect the neck for size and palpate its associated structures. The neck is normally short, with skinfolds between the head and shoulders during infancy; however, it lengthens during the next 3 to 4 years.

> ### ! NURSING ALERT
>
> If any masses are detected in the neck, report them for further investigation. Large masses can block the airway.

EYES

Inspection of External Structures

Inspect the **eyelids** for proper placement on the eye. When the eye is open, the upper eyelid should fall near the upper iris. When the eyes are closed, the eyelids should completely cover the cornea and sclera (Fig. 6-16).

Determine the general slant of the **palpebral fissures** or eyelids by drawing an imaginary line through the two points of the medial canthus and across the outer orbit of the eyes and aligning each eye on the line. Usually, the palpebral fissures lie horizontally. However, in Asians, the slant is normally upward.

Also inspect the inside lining of the eyelids, the **palpebral conjunctivae**. To examine the lower conjunctival sac, pull down the eyelid while the patient looks up. To evert the upper eyelid, hold the upper eyelashes and gently pull *down* and *forward* as the child looks down. Normally, the conjunctiva appears pink and glossy. Vertical yellow striations along the edge are the **meibomian glands**, or **sebaceous glands**, near the hair follicle. Located in the inner or medial canthus and situated on the inner edge of the upper and lower eyelids is a tiny opening, the **lacrimal punctum**. Note any excessive tearing, discharge, or inflammation of the lacrimal apparatus.

The **bulbar conjunctiva**, which covers the eye up to the limbus, or junction of the cornea and sclera, should be transparent. The sclera,

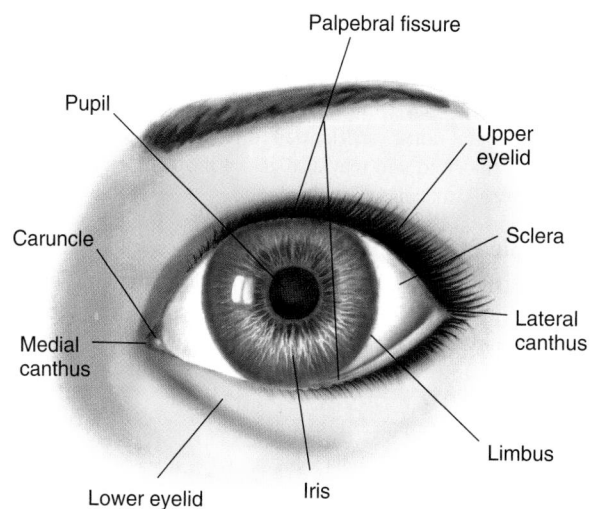

FIG 6-16 External structures of the eye.

or white covering of the eyeball, should be clear. Tiny black marks in the sclera of heavily pigmented individuals are normal.

The **cornea**, or covering of the iris and pupil, should be clear and transparent. Record opacities because they can be signs of scarring or ulceration, which can interfere with vision. The best way to test for opacities is to illuminate the eyeball by shining a light at an angle (**obliquely**) toward the cornea.

Compare the **pupils** for size, shape, and movement. They should be round, clear, and equal. Test their **reaction to light** by quickly shining a light toward the eye and removing it. As the light approaches, the pupils should constrict; as the light fades, the pupils should dilate. Test the pupil for any response of **accommodation** by having the child look at a bright, shiny object at a distance and quickly moving the object toward the face. The pupils should constrict as the object is brought near the eye. Record normal findings on examination of the pupils as **PERRLA**, which stands for "*p*upils *e*qual, *r*ound, *r*eact to *l*ight, and *a*ccommodation."

Inspect the iris and pupil for color, size, shape, and clarity. Permanent eye color is usually established by 6 to 12 months of age. While inspecting the iris and pupil, look for the lens. Normally, the lens is not visible through the pupil.

Inspection of Internal Structures

The ophthalmoscope permits visualization of the interior of the eyeball with a system of lenses and a high-intensity light. The lenses permit clear visualization of eye structures at different distances from the nurse's eye and correct visual acuity differences in the examiner and child. Use of the ophthalmoscope requires practice to know which lens setting produces the clearest image.

The ophthalmic and otic heads are usually interchangeable on one "body" or handle, which encloses the power source, either disposable or rechargeable batteries. The nurse should practice changing the heads, which snap on and are secured with a quarter turn, and replacing the batteries and light bulbs. Nurses who are not directly involved in physical assessment are often responsible for ensuring that the equipment functions properly.

Preparing the Child

The nurse can prepare the child for the ophthalmoscopic examination by showing the child the instrument, demonstrating the light source and how it shines in the eye, and explaining the reason for darkening the room. For infants and young children who do not respond to such explanations, it is best to use distraction to encourage them to keep their eyes open. Forcibly parting the eyelids results in an uncooperative, watery eyed child and a frustrated nurse. Usually, with some practice, the nurse can elicit a red reflex almost instantly while approaching the child and may also gain a momentary inspection of the blood vessels, macula, or optic disc.

Funduscopic Examination

Figure 6-17 shows the structures of the back of the eyeball, or the fundus. The fundus is immediately apparent as the red reflex. The intensity of the color increases in darkly pigmented individuals.

> **! NURSING ALERT**
>
> A brilliant, uniform red reflex is an important sign because it rules out many serious defects of the cornea, aqueous chamber, lens, and vitreous chamber. Any dark shadows or opacities are recorded because they indicate some abnormality in any of these structures.

As the ophthalmoscope is brought closer to the eye, the most conspicuous feature of the fundus is the optic disc, the area where the blood vessels and optic nerve fibers enter and exit the eye. The disc is

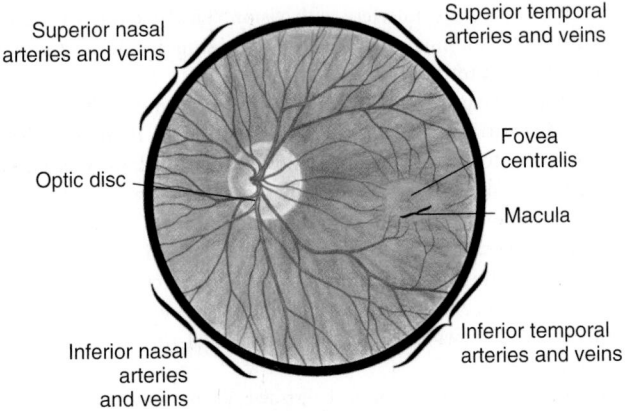

FIG 6-17 Structures of the fundus. (From Seidel HM, Ball JW, Dains JE, and others: *Mosby's guide to physical examination*, ed 6, St. Louis, 2007, Mosby.)

creamy pink and lighter in color than the surrounding fundus. Normally, it is round or vertically oval.

After locating the optic disc, inspect the area for blood vessels. The central retinal artery and vein appear in the depths of the disc and emanate outward with visible branching. The veins are darker and about one fourth larger than the arteries. Normally, the branches of the arteries and veins cross each other.

Other structures that are common are the macula, the area of the fundus with the greatest concentration of visual receptors, and in the center of the macula, a minute glistening spot of reflected light called the fovea centralis; this is the area of most perfect vision.

Vision Testing

Several tests are available for assessing vision. This discussion focuses on four areas: (1) ocular alignment, (2) visual acuity, (3) peripheral vision, and (4) color vision. Vision screening should be performed by age 3 years and annually after that or more often if there are concerns (American Academy of Pediatrics, 2003a; Wall, Marsh-Tootle, Evans, and others, 2002). Chapter 24 discusses behavioral and physical signs of visual impairment.

Ocular Alignment

Normally, by the age of 3 to 4 months, children are able to fixate on one visual field with both eyes simultaneously (binocularity). One of the most important tests for binocularity is alignment of the eyes to detect nonbinocular vision, or strabismus (Halle, 2002). In strabismus, or cross-eye, one eye deviates from the point of fixation. If the misalignment is constant, the weak eye becomes "lazy," and the brain eventually suppresses the image produced by that eye. If strabismus is not detected and corrected by ages 4 to 6 years, blindness from disuse, known as amblyopia, may result.

Tests commonly used to detect misalignment are the corneal light reflex and the cover tests. To perform the corneal light reflex test, or Hirschberg test, shine a flashlight or the light of the ophthalmoscope directly into the patient's eyes from a distance of about 40.5 cm (16 inches). If the eyes are orthophoric, or normal, the light falls symmetrically within each pupil (Fig. 6-18, *A*). If the light falls off center in one eye, the eyes are misaligned. Epicanthal folds, excess folds of skin that extend from the roof of the nose to the inner termination of the eyebrow and that partially or completely overlap the inner canthus of the eye, may give a false impression of misalignment

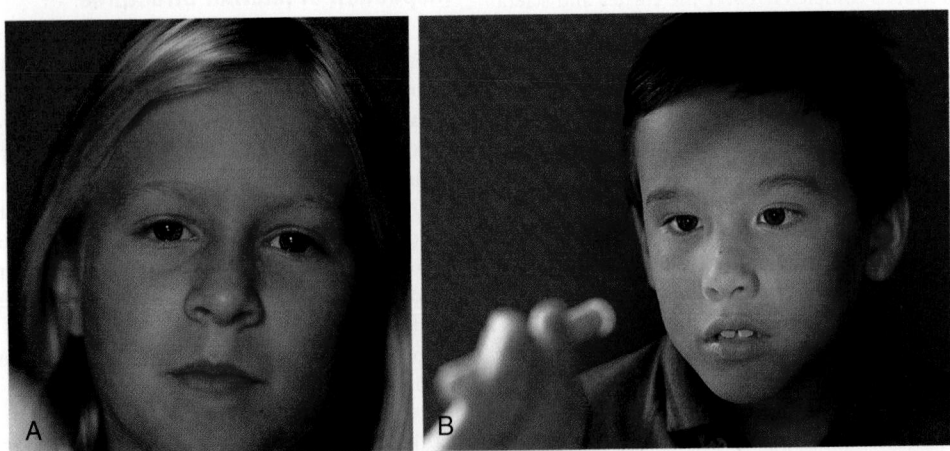

FIG 6-18 A, Corneal light reflex test demonstrating orthophoric eyes. **B,** Pseudostrabismus. Inner epicanthal folds cause the eyes to appear misaligned; however, the corneal light reflexes fall perfectly symmetrically.

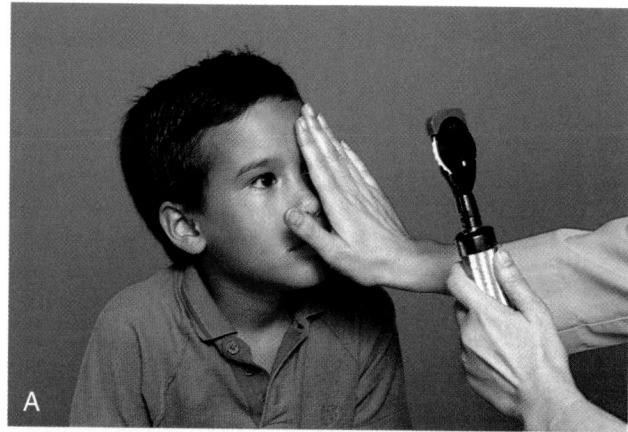

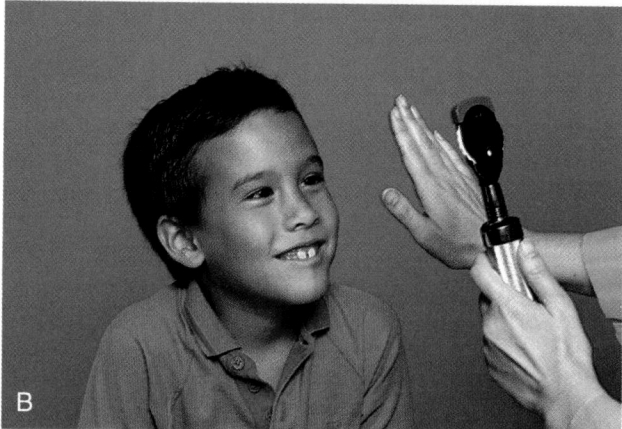

FIG 6-19 Alternate cover test to detect amblyopia in a patient with strabismus. **A,** The eye is occluded, and the child is fixating on light source. **B,** If the eye does not move when uncovered, the eyes are aligned.

(pseudostrabismus) (Fig. 6-18, *B*). Epicanthal folds are often found in Asian children.

In the cover test, one eye is covered, and the movement of the *uncovered* eye is observed while the child looks at a near (33 cm [13 inches]) or distant (6 m [20 feet]) object. If the uncovered eye does not move, it is aligned. If the uncovered eye moves, a misalignment is present because, when the stronger eye is temporarily covered, the misaligned eye attempts to fixate on the object.

In the alternate cover test, occlusion shifts back and forth from one eye to the other, and movement of the eye that was *covered* is observed as soon as the occluder is removed while the child focuses on a point in front of him or her (Fig. 6-19). If normal alignment is present, shifting the cover from one eye to the other will not cause the eye to move. If misalignment is present, eye movement will occur when the cover is moved. This test takes more practice than the other cover test because the occluder must be moved back and forth quickly and accurately to see the eye move. Because deviations can occur at different ranges, it is important to perform the cover tests at both close and far distances.

! NURSING ALERT

The cover test is usually easier to perform if the examiner uses his or her hand rather than a card-type occluder (see Fig. 6-19). Attractive occluders fashioned like an ice cream cone or happy-face lollipop cut from cardboard are also well received by young children.

Photoscreening is a technique used to screen for amblyopia, refractive disorders, and media opacities (American Academy of Pediatrics, 2003a). Using a camera, the nurse obtains images of the pupillary reflexes (reflections) and red reflexes (Bruckner test) (American Academy of Pediatrics, 2003a). Photoscreening offers an effective way to screen infants, preverbal children, and those with developmental delays who are difficult to screen.

Visual Acuity Testing in Children Beyond Infancy

The most common test for measuring visual acuity is the Snellen letter chart, which consists of lines of letters of decreasing size. The American Academy of Pediatrics (2003a) recommends that children stand 10 feet from the chart with their heels at the 10-foot line during testing. When screening for visual acuity in children, the nurse tests the child's right eye first by covering the left. Children who wear glasses should be screened with them on. Tell the child to keep both eyes open during the examination. If the child fails to read the current line, move up the chart to the next larger line. Continue up the chart until a line is found that the child can pass. Then begin moving down the chart again until the child fails to read the line. To pass each line, the child must correctly identify four of six symbols on the line. Repeat the procedure, covering the right eye. Table 6-9 provides a list of visual screening tests for children and guidelines for referral recommended by the American Academy of Pediatrics (2003a).

For children unable to read letters and numbers, the tumbling E or HOTV test is useful (Coats and Jenkins, 1997). The tumbling E test uses the capital letter E pointing in four different directions. The child is asked to point in the direction the E is facing. The HOTV test consists of a wall chart composed of the letters H, O, T, and V. The child is given a board containing a large H, O, T, and V. The examiner points to a letter on the wall chart, and the child matches the correct letter on the board held in his or her hand. The tumbling E and HOTV are excellent tests for preschool-age children.

Visual Acuity Testing in Infants and Difficult-to-Test Children

In newborns, vision is tested mainly by checking for light perception by shining a light into the eyes and noting responses such as pupillary constriction, blinking, following the light to midline, increased alertness, or refusal to open the eyes after exposure to the light. Although the simple maneuver of checking light perception and eliciting the pupillary light reflex indicates that the anterior half of the visual apparatus is intact, it does not confirm that the infant can see. In other words, this test does not assess whether the brain receives the visual message and interprets the signals.

Another test of visual acuity is the infant's ability to fix on and follow a target. Although any brightly colored or patterned object can be used, the human face is excellent. Hold the infant upright while moving your face slowly from side to side.

! NURSING ALERT

If visual fixation and following are not present by 3 to 4 months of age, further ophthalmologic evaluation is necessary.

Other signs that may indicate visual loss or other serious eye problems include fixed pupils, strabismus, constant nystagmus, the setting-sun sign, and slow lateral movements. Unfortunately, it is difficult to test each eye separately; the presence of such signs in one eye could indicate unilateral blindness.

TABLE 6-9	EYE EXAMINATION GUIDELINES*		
FUNCTION	**RECOMMENDED TESTS**	**REFERRAL CRITERIA**	**COMMENTS**
Ages 3 to 5 Years			
Distance visual acuity	Snellen letters Snellen numbers Tumbling E HOTV Picture test: • Allen figures • LEA symbols	1. <4 of 6 correct on 20-foot (6-m) line with either eye tested at 10 feet (3 m) monocularly (i.e., <10/20 or 20/40) or 2. Two-line difference between eyes, even within passing range (i.e., 10/12.5 and 10/20 or 20/25 and 20/40)	1. Tests are listed in decreasing order of cognitive difficulty; highest test that child is capable of performing should be used; in general, tumbling E or HOTV test should be used for children 3 to 5 years of age and Snellen letters or numbers for children 6 years of age and older. 2. Testing distance of 10 feet (3 m) is recommended for all visual acuity tests. 3. Line of figures is preferred over single figures. 4. Nontested eye should be covered by occluder held by examiner or by adhesive occluder patch applied to eye; examiner must ensure that it is not possible to peek with nontested eye.
Ocular alignment	Cross cover test at 10 feet (3 m) Random dot E stereo test at 18 inches (40 cm) Simultaneous red reflex test (Bruckner test)	Any eye movement <4 of 6 correct Any asymmetry of pupil color, size, brightness	Child must be fixing on a target while cross cover test is performed. Use direct ophthalmoscope to view both red reflexes simultaneously in a darkened room from 2 to 3 feet (0.6–0.9 m) away; detects asymmetric refractive errors as well.
Ocular media clarity (cataracts, tumors, etc.)	Red reflex	White pupil, dark spots, absent reflex	Use direct ophthalmoscope in a darkened room. View eyes separately at 12 to 18 inches (30–45 cm); white reflex indicates possible retinoblastoma.
Ages 6 Years and Older			
Distance visual acuity	Snellen letters Snellen numbers Tumbling E HOTV Picture test: • Allen figures • LEA symbols	1. <4 of 6 correct on 15-foot (4.5-m) line with either eye tested at 10 feet (3 m) monocularly (i.e., <10/15 or 20/30) or 2. Two-line difference between eyes, even within the passing range (i.e., 10/10 and 10/15 or 20/20 and 20/30)	1. Tests are listed in decreasing order of cognitive difficulty; highest test that child is capable of performing should be used; in general, tumbling E or HOTV test should be used for children 3 to 5 years of age and Snellen letters or numbers for children 6 years of age and older. 2. Testing distance of 10 feet (3 m) is recommended for all visual acuity tests. 3. Line of figures is preferred over single figures. 4. Nontested eye should be covered by occluder held by examiner or by adhesive occluder patch applied to eye; examiner must ensure that it is not possible to peek with nontested eye.
Ocular alignment	Cross cover test at 10 feet (3 m) Random dot E stereo test at 18 inches (40 cm) Simultaneous red reflex test (Bruckner test)	Any eye movement <4 of 6 correct Any asymmetry of pupil color, size, brightness	Child must be fixing on target while cross cover test is performed. Use direct ophthalmoscope to view both red reflexes simultaneously in a darkened room from 2 to 3 feet (0.6–0.9 m) away; detects asymmetric refractive errors as well.
Ocular media clarity (e.g., cataracts, tumors)	Red reflex	White pupil, dark spots, absent reflex	Use direct ophthalmoscope in a darkened room. View eyes separately at 12 to 18 inches (30–45 cm); white reflex indicates possible retinoblastoma.

From American Academy of Pediatrics, Committee on Practice and Ambulatory Medicine, Section on Ophthalmology: Eye examination in infants, children, and young adults by pediatricians, *Pediatrics* 111(4):902–907, 2003.
*Assessing visual acuity (vision screening) is one of the most sensitive techniques for detection of eye abnormalities in children. The American Academy of Pediatrics Section on Ophthalmology, in cooperation with American Association for Pediatric Ophthalmology and Strabismus and American Academy of Ophthalmology, has developed these guidelines to be used by physicians, nurses, educational institutions, public health departments, and other professionals who perform vision evaluation services.

Special tests are available for testing infants and other difficult-to-test children to assess acuity or confirm blindness. For example, in visually evoked potentials, the eyes are stimulated with a bright light or pattern, and electrical activity to the visual cortex is recorded through scalp electrodes. Acuity is assessed by using progressively smaller patterns.

Peripheral Vision

In children who are old enough to cooperate, estimate peripheral vision, or the visual field of each eye, by having the children fixate on a specific point directly in front of them while an object, such as a finger or a pencil, is moved from beyond the field of vision into the range of peripheral vision. As soon as children see the object, have them say "stop." At that point, measure the angle from the anteroposterior axis of the eye (straight line of vision) to the peripheral axis (point at which the object is first seen). Check each eye separately and for each quadrant of vision. Normally, children see about 50 degrees upward, 70 degrees downward, 60 degrees nasalward, and 90 degrees temporally. Limitations in peripheral vision may indicate blindness from damage to structures within the eye or to any of the visual pathways.

Color Vision

The tests available for color vision include the Ishihara test and the Hardy-Rand-Rittler test. Each consists of a series of cards (pseudoisochromatic) containing a color field composed of spots of a certain "confusion" color. Against the field is a number or symbol similarly printed in dots but of a color likely to be confused with the field color by a person with a color vision deficit. As a result, the figure or letter is invisible to an affected individual but is clearly seen by a person with normal vision.

EARS

Inspection of External Structures

The entire external earlobe is called the pinna, or auricle; one is located on each side of the head. Measure the height alignment of the pinna by drawing an imaginary line from the outer orbit of the eye to the occiput, or most prominent protuberance of the skull. The top of the pinna should meet or cross this line. Low-set ears are commonly associated with renal anomalies or cognitive impairment. Measure the angle of the pinna by drawing a perpendicular line from the imaginary horizontal line and aligning the pinna next to this mark. Normally, the pinna lies within a 10-degree angle of the vertical line (Fig. 6-20). If it falls outside this area, record the deviation and look for other anomalies.

Normally, the pinna extends slightly outward from the skull. Except in newborn infants, ears that are flat against the head or protruding away from the scalp may indicate problems. Flattened ears in an infant may suggest a frequent side-lying position and, just as with isolated areas of hair loss, may be a clue to investigate parents' understanding of the child's stimulation needs.

Inspect the skin surface around the ear for small openings, extra tags of skin, or sinuses. If a sinus is found, note this because it may

represent a fistula that drains into some area of the neck or ear. Cutaneous tags represent no pathologic process but may cause parents concern in terms of the child's appearance.

Also assess the ears for hygiene. An otoscope is not necessary for looking into the external canal to note the presence of cerumen, a waxy substance produced by the ceruminous glands in the outer portion of the canal. Cerumen is usually yellow-brown and soft. If an otoscope is used and any discharge is visible, note its color and odor. Avoid transmitting potentially infectious material to the other ear or to another child through handwashing and using disposable specula or sterilizing reusable specula between each examination.

Inspection of Internal Structures

The head of the otoscope permits visualization of the tympanic membrane by use of a bright light, a magnifying glass, and a speculum. Some otoscopes have an attachment for a pneumonic device to insert air into the canal to determine membrane compliance (movement). The speculum, which is inserted into the external canal, comes in a variety of sizes to accommodate different canal widths. The largest speculum that fits comfortably into the ear is used to achieve the greatest area of visualization. The lens, or magnifying glass, is movable, allowing the examiner to insert an object, such as a curette, into the ear canal through the speculum while still viewing the structures through the lens.

Positioning the Child

Before beginning the otoscopic examination, position the child properly and gently restrain (have the child sit on parent's lap and hold parent's hands) if necessary. Older children usually cooperate and do not need restraint. However, prepare them for the procedure by allowing them to play with the instrument, demonstrating how it works, and stressing the importance of remaining still. A helpful suggestion is to let them observe you examining the parent's ear. Restraint is needed for younger children because the ear examination upsets them (see Atraumatic Care box).

As you insert the speculum into the meatus, move it around the outer rim to accustom the child to the feel of something entering the ear. If examining a painful ear, touch a nonpainful part of the affected ear, then examine the unaffected ear, and finally return to the painful ear. By this time, the child is usually less fearful of anything causing discomfort to the ear and will cooperate more.

For their protection and safety, restrain infants and toddlers for the otoscopic examination. There are two general positions of restraint. In one, the child is seated sideways in the parent's lap with one arm hugging the parent and the other arm at the side. The ear to be examined is toward the nurse. With one arm, the parent holds the child's head firmly against his or her chest and with the other arm hugs the child, thereby securing the child's free arm (Fig. 6-21, *A*). Examine

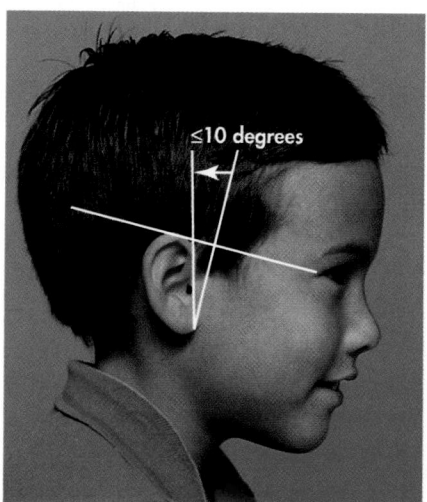

FIG 6-20 Ear alignment.

≤10 degrees

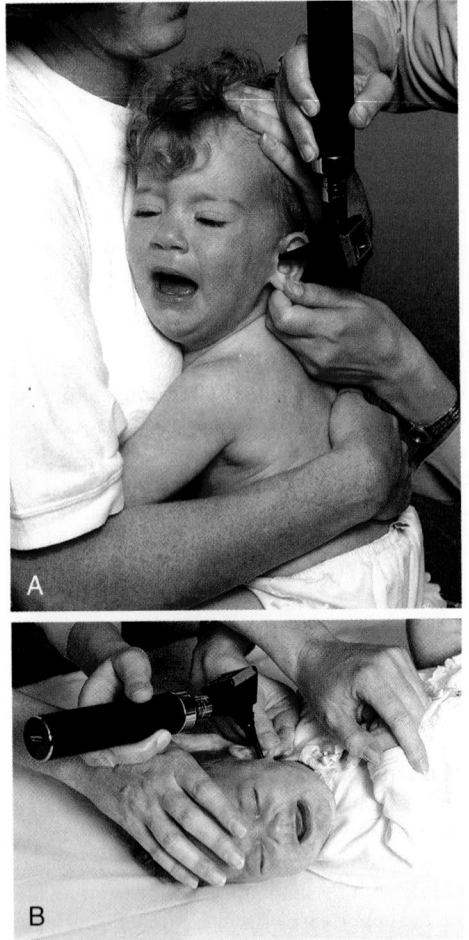

FIG 6-21 Position for restraining a child (**A**) and an infant (**B**) during otoscopic examination.

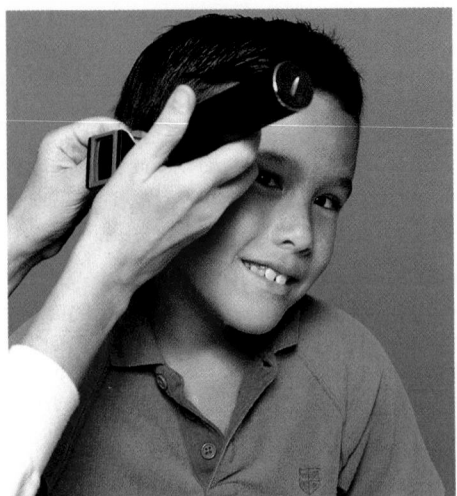

FIG 6-22 Positioning the head by tilting it toward opposite shoulder for full view of the tympanic membrane.

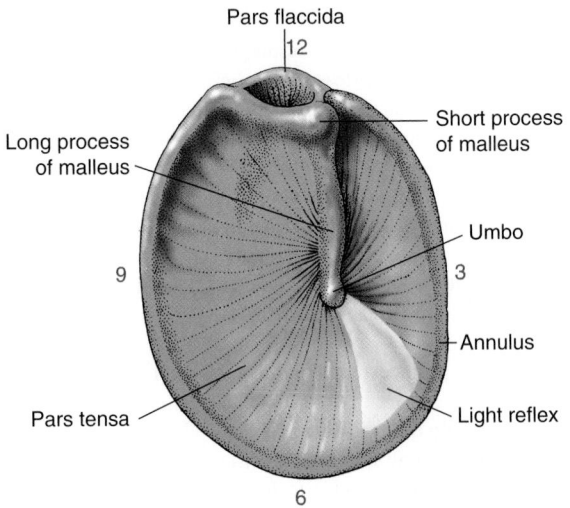

FIG 6-23 Landmarks of the tympanic membrane. (From Rothrock JC: *Alexander's care of the patient in surgery*, ed 13, St. Louis, 2006, Mosby.)

the ear using the same procedure for holding the otoscope as described later.

The other position involves placing the child on the side, back, or abdomen with the arms at the side and the head turned so the ear to be examined points toward the ceiling. Lean over the child, use the upper part of the body to restrain the arms and upper trunk movements, and use the examining hand to stabilize the head. This position is practical for young infants and for older children who need minimum restraint, but it may not be feasible for other children who protest vigorously. For safety, enlist the parent's or an assistant's help in immobilizing the head by firmly placing one hand above the ear and the other on the child's side, abdomen, or back (Fig. 6-21, *B*).

With cooperative children, examine the ear with the child in a side-lying, sitting, or standing position. One disadvantage to standing is that the child may "walk away" as the otoscope enters the canal. If the child is standing or sitting, tilt the head slightly toward the child's opposite shoulder to achieve a better view of the eardrum (Fig. 6-22).

With the thumb and forefinger of the free (usually nondominant) hand, grasp the auricle. For the two positions of restraint, hold the otoscope upside down at the junction of its head and handle with the thumb and index finger. Place the other fingers against the skull to allow the otoscope to move with the child in case of sudden movement. In examining a cooperative child, hold the handle with the otic head upright or upside down. Use the dominant hand to examine both ears or reverse hands for each ear, whichever is more comfortable.

Before using the otoscope, visualize the external ear and the tympanic membrane as being superimposed on a clock (Fig. 6-23). The numbers are important geographic landmarks. Introduce the speculum into the meatus between the 3 and 9 o'clock positions in a *downward* and *forward* position. Because the canal is curved, the speculum does not permit a panoramic view of the tympanic membrane unless the canal is straightened. In infants, the canal curves upward. Therefore, pull the pinna *down* and *back* to the 6 to 9 o'clock range to straighten the canal (Fig. 6-24, *A*). With older children, usually those older than 3 years of age, the canal curves downward and forward. Therefore, pull the pinna *up* and *back* toward a 10 o'clock position (Fig. 6-24, *B*). If you have difficulty visualizing the membrane, try repositioning the head, introducing the speculum at a different angle, and pulling the pinna in a slightly different direction. Do not insert the speculum past the cartilaginous (outermost) portion of the canal, usually a distance of 0.60 to 1.25 cm (0.23–0.5 inch) in older children. Insertion of the speculum into the posterior or bony portion of the canal causes pain.

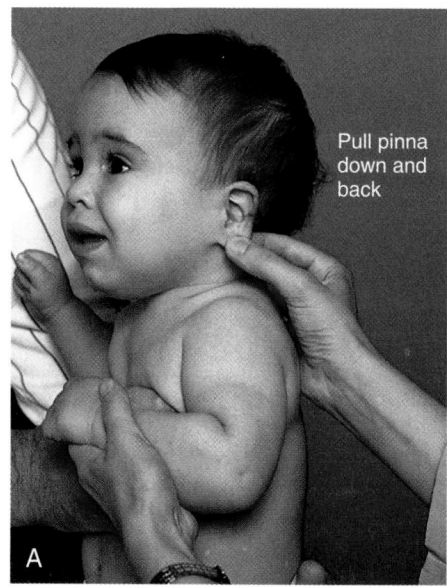
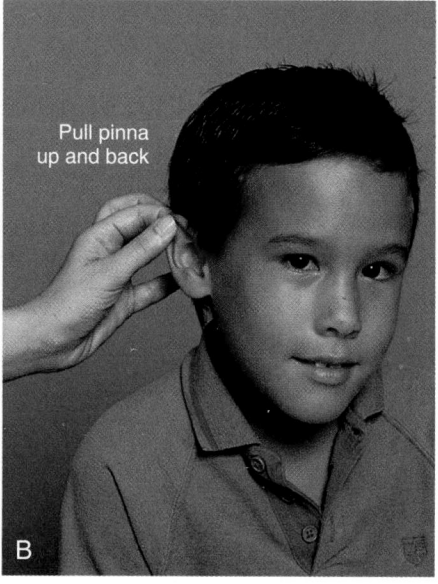

Pull pinna down and back

Pull pinna up and back

FIG 6-24 Positioning for visualizing the eardrum in an infant **(A)** and in a child older than 3 years of age **(B)**.

In neonates and young infants, the walls of the canal are pliable and floppy because of the underdeveloped cartilaginous and bony structures. Therefore, the very small 2-mm speculum usually needs to be inserted deeper into the canal than in older children. Exercise great care not to damage the walls or eardrum. For this reason, only an experienced examiner should insert an otoscope into the ears of very young infants.

Otoscopic Examination

As you introduce the speculum into the external canal, inspect the walls of the canal, the color of the tympanic membrane, the light reflex, and the usual landmarks of the bony prominences of the middle ear. The walls of the external auditory canal are pink, although they are more pigmented in dark-skinned children. Minute hairs are evident in the outermost portion, where cerumen is produced. Note signs of irritation, foreign bodies, or infection.

Foreign bodies in the ear are common in children and range from erasers to beans. Symptoms may include pain, discharge, and affected hearing. Remove soft objects, such as paper or insects, with forceps. Remove small, hard objects, such as pebbles, with a suction tip, a hook, or irrigation. However, irrigation is contraindicated if the object is vegetative matter, such as beans or pasta, which swells when in contact with fluid.

> ### ⚠ NURSING ALERT
>
> If there is any doubt about the type of object in the ear and the appropriate method to remove it, refer the child to the appropriate practitioner.

The tympanic membrane is a translucent, light pearly pink or gray. Note marked erythema (which may indicate suppurative otitis media); a dull, nontransparent grayish color (sometimes suggestive of serous otitis media); or ashen gray areas (signs of scarring from a previous perforation). A black area usually suggests a perforation of the membrane that has not healed.

The characteristic tenseness and slope of the tympanic membrane cause the light of the otoscope to reflect at about the 5 or 7 o'clock position. The light reflex is a fairly well-defined, cone-shaped reflection, which normally points away from the face.

The bony landmarks of the eardrum are formed by the umbo, or tip of the malleus. It appears as a small, round, opaque, concave spot near the center of the eardrum. The manubrium (long process or handle) of the malleus appears to be a whitish line extending from the umbo upward to the margin of the membrane. At the upper end of the long process near the 1 o'clock position (in the right ear) is a sharp, knoblike protuberance, representing the short process of the malleus. Note the absence of the light reflex or loss or abnormal prominence of any of these landmarks.

Auditory Testing

Several types of hearing tests are available and recommended for screening in infants and children (American Academy of Pediatrics, 2003b) (Table 6-10). Universal newborn hearing screening is available in almost every state in the United States. The nurse must operate under a high index of suspicion for those children who may have conditions associated with hearing loss, whose parents are concerned about hearing loss, and who may have developed behaviors that indicate auditory impairment (Cunningham and Cox, 2003). Chapter 24 discusses types of hearing loss, causes, clinical manifestations, and appropriate treatment.

NOSE

Inspection of External Structures

The nose is located in the middle of the face just below the eyes and above the lips. Compare its placement and alignment by drawing an imaginary vertical line from the center point between the eyes down to the notch of the upper lip. The nose should lie exactly vertical to this line, with each side exactly symmetric. Note its location, any deviation to one side, and asymmetry in overall size and in diameter of the nares (nostrils). The bridge of the nose is sometimes flat in Asian and African-American children. Observe the alae nasi for any sign of flaring, which indicates respiratory difficulty. Always report any flaring of the alae nasi. Fig. 6-25 illustrates the landmarks used in describing the external structures of the nose.

TABLE 6-10	AUDITORY TESTS FOR INFANTS AND CHILDREN		
AGE	AUDITORY TEST AND AVERAGE TIME	TYPE OF MEASUREMENT	PROCEDURE
All ages	Evoked otoacoustic emissions, 10-min test	Physiologic test specifically measuring cochlear (outer hair cell) response to presentation of stimulus	Small probe containing sensitive microphone is placed in ear canal for stimulus delivery and response detection.
Birth–9 months	Auditory brainstem response, 15-min test	Electrophysiologic measurement of activity in auditory nerve and brainstem pathways	Placement of electrodes on child's head detects auditory stimuli presented though earphones one ear at a time.
9 months–2.5 yr	Conditioned oriented responses or visual reinforced audiometry, 30-min test	Behavioral tests measuring child's responses to speech and frequency-specific stimuli presented through speakers	Both techniques condition child to associate speech or frequency-specific sound with reinforcement stimulus, such as lighted toy.

Modified with permission from Bachmann KR, Arvedson JC: Early identification and intervention for children who are hearing impaired, *Pediatr Rev* 19:155–165, 1998.

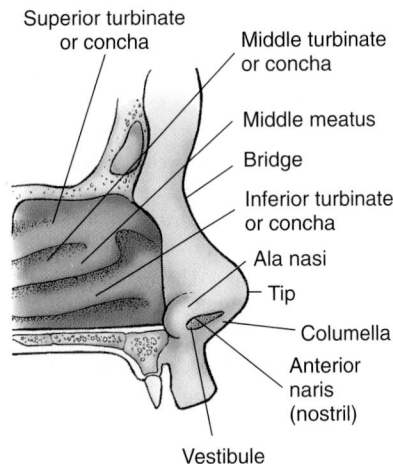

Superior turbinate or concha

Middle turbinate or concha

Middle meatus

Bridge

Inferior turbinate or concha

Ala nasi

Tip

Columella

Anterior naris (nostril)

Vestibule

FIG 6-25 External landmarks and internal structures of the nose.

Inspection of Internal Structures

Inspect the **anterior vestibule** of the nose by pushing the tip upward, tilting the head backward, and illuminating the cavity with a flashlight or otoscope without the attached ear speculum. Note the **color** of the **mucosal lining**, which is normally redder than the oral membranes, as well as any swelling, discharge, dryness, or bleeding. There should be no discharge from the nose.

On looking deeper into the nose, inspect the **turbinates**, or **concha**, plates of bone that jut into the nasal cavity and are enveloped by the mucous membranes. The turbinates greatly increase the surface area of the nasal cavity as air is inhaled. The spaces or channels between the turbinates are called the **meatus** and correspond to each of the three turbinates. Normally, the front end of the inferior and middle turbinate and the middle meatus are seen. They should be the same color as the lining of the vestibule.

Inspect the **septum**, which should divide the vestibules equally. Note any deviation, especially if it causes an occlusion of one side of the nose. A perforation may be evident within the septum. If this is suspected, shine the light of the otoscope into one naris and look for admittance of light to the other. Because olfaction is an important function of the nose, testing for smell may be done at this point or as part of cranial nerve assessment (see Table 6-13).

MOUTH AND THROAT

With a cooperative child, the nurse can accomplish almost the entire examination of the mouth and throat without the use of a tongue blade. Ask the child to open the mouth wide; to move the tongue in different directions for full visualization; and to say "ahh," which depresses the tongue for full view of the back of the mouth (tonsils, uvula, and oropharynx). For a closer look at the buccal mucosa, or lining of the cheeks, ask children to use their fingers to move the outer lip and cheek to one side (see Atraumatic Care box).

Infants and toddlers usually resist attempts to keep the mouth open. Because inspecting the mouth is upsetting, leave it for the end of the physical examination (along with examination of the ears) or do it during episodes of crying. However, the use of a tongue blade (preferably flavored) to depress the tongue may be needed. Place the tongue blade along the *side* of the tongue, not in the center back area where the gag reflex is elicited. Fig. 6-26, *B*, illustrates proper positioning of the child for the oral examination.

The major structure of the exterior of the mouth is the **lips**. The lips should be moist, soft, smooth, and pink or a deeper hue than the surrounding skin. The lips should be symmetric when relaxed or tensed. Assess symmetry when the child talks or cries.

Inspection of Internal Structures

The major structures that are visible within the oral cavity and oropharynx are the mucosal lining of the lips and cheeks, gums (or gingiva), teeth, tongue, palate, uvula, tonsils, and posterior oropharynx (Fig. 6-27). Inspect all areas lined with **mucous membranes** (inside the lips and cheeks, gingiva, underside of the tongue, palate, and back

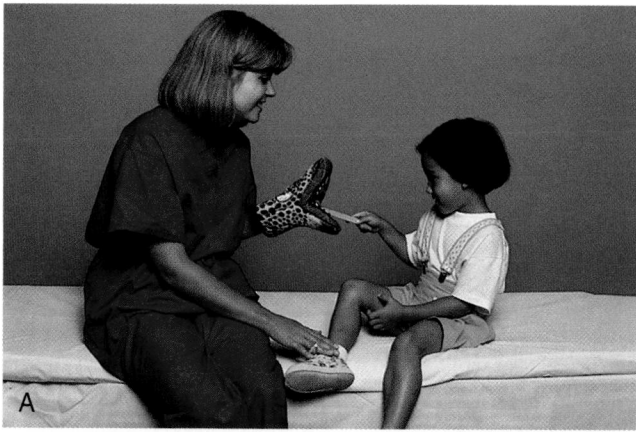

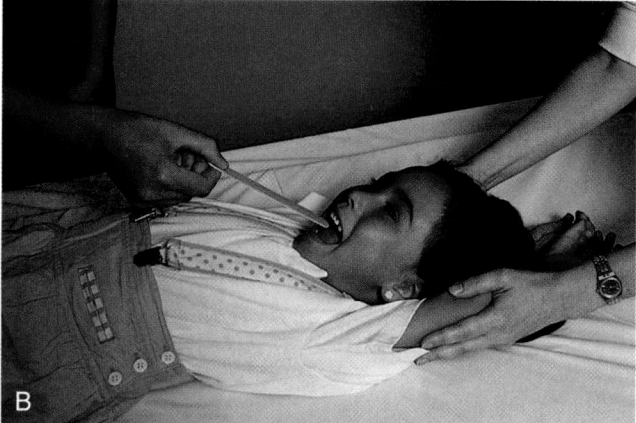

FIG 6-26 A, Encouraging a child to cooperate. **B,** Positioning a child for examination of the mouth.

tooth enamel with obvious plaque (whitish coating on the surface of the teeth) is a sign of poor dental hygiene and indicates a need for counseling. Brown spots in the crevices of the crown of the tooth or between the teeth may be caries (cavities). Chalky white to yellow or brown areas on the enamel may indicate fluorosis (excessive fluoride ingestion). Teeth that appear greenish black may be stained temporarily from ingestion of supplemental iron.

Examine the gums (gingiva) surrounding the teeth. The color is normally coral pink, and the surface texture is stippled, similar to the appearance of an orange peel. In dark-skinned children, the gums are more deeply colored, and a brownish area is often observed along the gum line.

Inspect the tongue for papillae, small projections that contain several taste buds and give the tongue its characteristic rough appearance. Note the size and mobility of the tongue. Normally, the tip of the tongue should extend to the lips or beyond.

The roof of the mouth consists of the hard palate, which is located near the front of the oral cavity, and the soft palate, which is located toward the back of the pharynx and has a small midline protrusion called the uvula. Carefully inspect the palates to ensure they are intact. The arch of the palate should be dome shaped. A narrow, flat roof or a high, arched palate affects the placement of the tongue and can cause feeding and speech problems. Test movement of the uvula by eliciting a gag reflex. It should move upward to close off the nasopharynx from the oropharynx.

Examine the oropharynx and note the size and color of the palatine tonsils. They are normally the same color as the surrounding mucosa; glandular, rather than smooth in appearance; and barely visible over the edge of the palatoglossal arches. The size of the tonsils varies considerably during childhood. However, report any swelling, redness, or white areas on the tonsils.

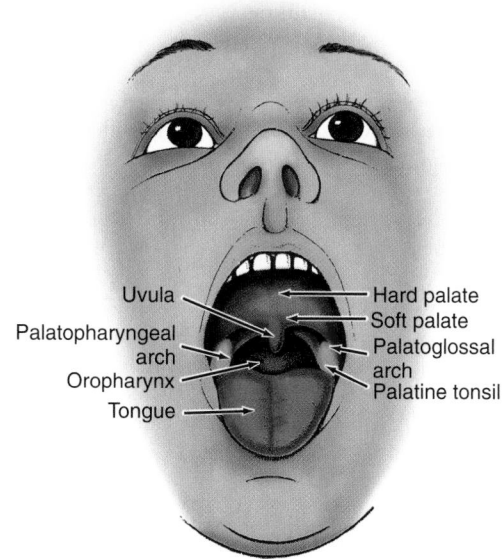

FIG 6-27 Interior structures of the mouth.

of the pharynx) for color, any areas of white patches or ulceration, bleeding, sensitivity, and moisture. The membranes should be bright pink, smooth, glistening, uniform, and moist.

Inspect the teeth for number in each dental arch, for hygiene, and for occlusion or bite (see also Teething, Chapter 12). Discoloration of

CHEST

Inspect the chest for size, shape, symmetry, movement, breast development, and the bony landmarks formed by the ribs and sternum. The rib cage consists of 12 ribs on each side and the sternum, or breast bone, located in the midline of the trunk (Fig. 6-28). The sternum is composed of three main parts. The manubrium, the uppermost portion, can be felt at the base of the neck at the suprasternal notch. The largest segment of the sternum is the body, which forms the sternal angle (angle of Louis) as it articulates with the manubrium. At the end of the body is a small, movable process called the xiphoid. The angle of the costal margin as it attaches to the sternum is called the costal angle and is normally about 45 to 50 degrees. These bony structures are important landmarks in the location of ribs and intercostal spaces (ICSs), which are the spaces between the ribs. They are numbered according to the rib directly *above* the space. For example, the space immediately below the second rib is the second ICS.

The thoracic cavity is also divided into segments by drawing imaginary lines on the chest and back. Fig. 6-29 illustrates the anterior, lateral, and posterior divisions.

Measure the size of the chest by placing the measuring tape around the rib cage at the nipple line (see Fig. 6-9). For greatest accuracy, take two measurements—one during inspiration and the other during expiration—and record the average. Chest size is important mainly in relation to head circumference (see p. 111). Always report marked disproportions because most are caused by abnormal head growth, although some may be a result of altered chest shape, such as barrel chest (chest is round) or pigeon chest (sternum protrudes outward).

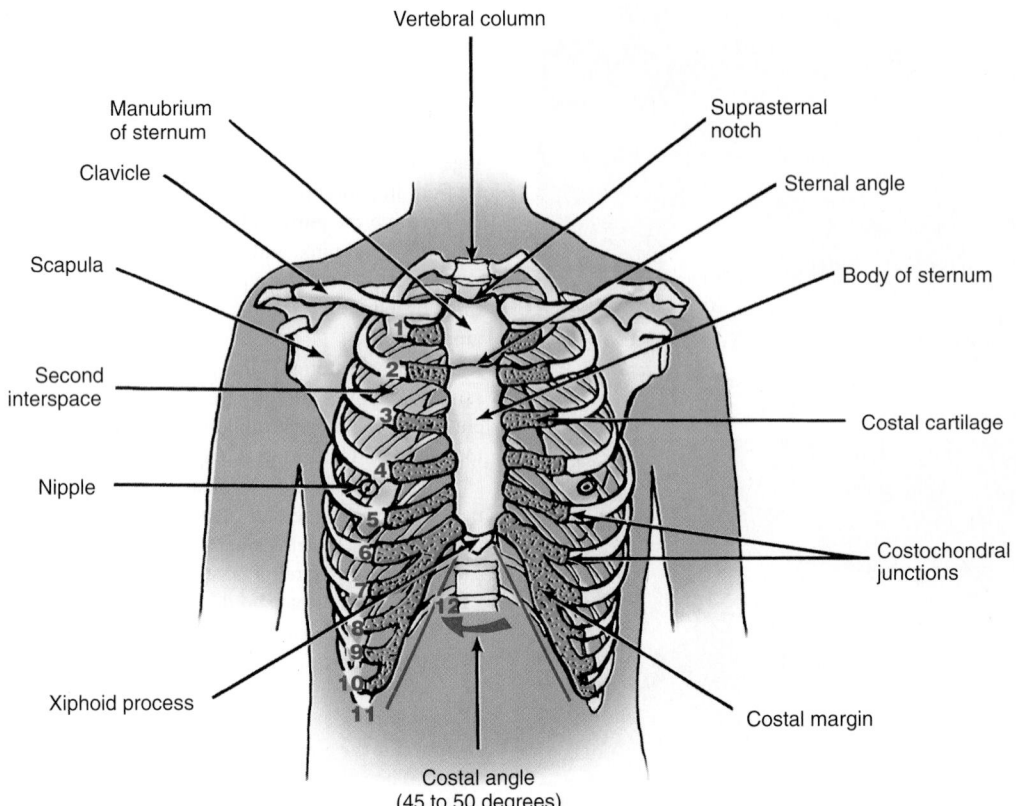

FIG 6-28 The rib cage.

During infancy, the chest's **shape** is almost circular, with the antero-posterior (front-to-back) diameter equaling the transverse, or lateral (side-to-side), diameter. As the child grows, the chest normally increases in the transverse direction, causing the anteroposterior diameter to be less than the lateral diameter. Note the **angle** made by the lower costal margin and the sternum and palpate the junction of the ribs with the costal cartilage (costochondral junction) and sternum, which should be fairly smooth.

Movement of the chest wall should be symmetric bilaterally and coordinated with breathing. During inspiration, the chest rises and expands, the diaphragm descends, and the costal angle increases. During expiration, the chest falls and decreases in size, the diaphragm rises, and the costal angle narrows (Fig. 6-30). In children younger than 6 or 7 years of age, respiratory movement is principally abdominal or diaphragmatic. In older children, particularly girls, respirations are chiefly thoracic. In either case, the chest and abdomen should rise and fall together. Always report any asymmetry of movement.

While inspecting the skin surface of the chest, observe the position of the **nipples** and any evidence of **breast development**. Normally, the nipples are located slightly lateral to the midclavicular line between the fourth and fifth ribs. Note symmetry of nipple placement and normal configuration of darker pigmented areolas surrounding flat nipples in prepubertal children.

Pubertal breast development usually begins in girls between 10 and 14 years of age (see Chapter 19). Record early (precocious) or delayed breast development, as well as evidence of any other secondary sexual characteristics. In males, **breast enlargement (gynecomastia)** may be caused by hormonal or systemic disorders, but more commonly is a result of adipose tissue from obesity or a transitory body change during early puberty. In either situation, investigate the child's feelings regarding breast enlargement.

In adolescent girls who have achieved sexual maturity, palpate the breasts for evidence of any masses or hard nodules. Use this opportunity to discuss the importance of routine breast self-examination. To decrease any fear or concern that results when a mass is felt, emphasize that most palpable masses are benign.

LUNGS

The lungs are situated inside the thoracic cavity, with one lung on each side of the sternum. Each lung is divided into an apex, which is slightly pointed and rises above the first rib; a base, which is wide and concave and rides on the dome-shaped diaphragm; and a **body**, which is divided into lobes. The right lung has three lobes: the upper, middle, and lower. The left lung has only two lobes, the upper and lower, because of the space occupied by the heart (Fig. 6-31).

Inspection of the lungs primarily involves observation of respiratory movements. Evaluate respirations for (1) **rate** (number per minute), (2) **rhythm** (regular, irregular, or periodic), (3) **depth** (deep or shallow), and (4) **quality** (effortless, automatic, difficult, or labored). Note the character of **breath sounds**, such as noisy, grunting, snoring, or heavy.

Evaluate respiratory movements by placing each hand flat against the back or chest with the thumbs in midline along the lower costal margin of the lungs. The child should be sitting during this procedure and, if cooperative, should take several deep breaths. During respiration, your hands will move with the chest wall. Assess the amount and speed of respiratory excursion and note any asymmetry of movement.

Experienced examiners may percuss the lungs. Percuss the anterior lung from apex to base, usually with the child in the supine or sitting position. Percuss each side of the chest in sequence to compare

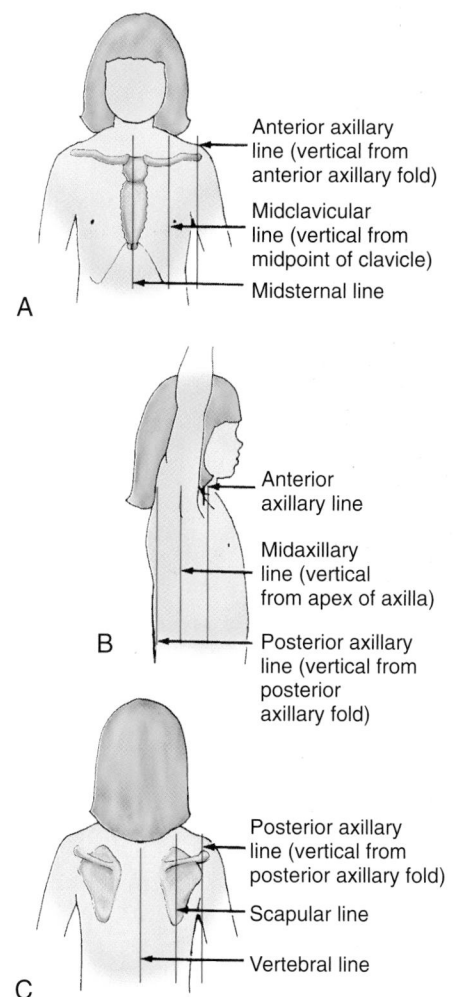

FIG 6-29 Imaginary landmarks of the chest. **A,** Anterior. **B,** Right lateral. **C,** Posterior.

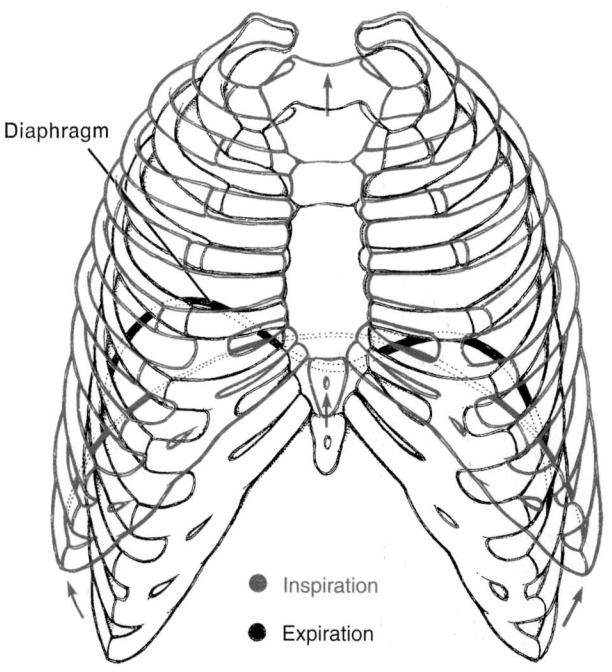

FIG 6-30 Movement of the chest during respiration.

NURSING CARE GUIDELINES
Effective Auscultation

- Make certain the child is relaxed and not crying, talking, or laughing. Record if the child is crying.
- Check that the room is comfortable and quiet.
- Warm the stethoscope before placing it against the skin.
- Apply firm pressure on the chest piece but not enough to prevent vibrations and transmission of sound.
- Avoid placing the stethoscope over hair or clothing, moving it against the skin, breathing on the tubing, or sliding the fingers over the chest piece, which may cause sounds that falsely resemble pathologic findings.
- Use a symmetric and orderly approach to compare sounds.

ATRAUMATIC CARE
Encouraging Deep Breaths

- Ask the child to "blow out" the light on an otoscope or pocket flashlight; discreetly turn off the light on the last try so the child feels successful.
- Place a cotton ball in the child's palm; ask the child to blow the ball into the air and have the parent catch it.
- Place a small tissue on the top of a pencil and ask the child to blow off the tissue.
- Have the child blow a pinwheel, a party horn, or bubbles.

BOX 6-13 CLASSIFICATION OF NORMAL BREATH SOUNDS

Vesicular Breath Sounds
Heard over the entire surface of the lungs with the exception of the upper intrascapular area and area beneath the manubrium.
Inspiration is louder, longer, and higher pitched than expiration.
The sound is a soft, swishing noise.

Bronchovesicular Breath Sounds
Heard over the manubrium and in the upper intrascapular regions where the trachea and bronchi bifurcate.
Inspiration is louder and higher pitched than in vesicular breathing.

Bronchial Breath Sounds
Heard only over trachea near suprasternal notch.
The inspiratory phase is short, and the expiratory phase is long.

---

the sounds. When percussing the posterior lung, the procedure and sequence are the same, although the child should be sitting. Resonance is heard over all the lobes of the lungs that are not adjacent to other organs. Record and report any deviation from the expected sound.

Auscultation

Auscultation involves using the stethoscope to evaluate breath sounds (see Nursing Care Guidelines box). Breath sounds are best heard if the child inspires deeply (see Atraumatic Care box). In the lungs breath sounds are classified as vesicular, bronchovesicular, or bronchial (Box 6-13).

Absent or diminished breath sounds are always an abnormal finding warranting investigation. Fluid, air, or solid masses in the pleural space interfere with the conduction of breath sounds. Diminished breath sounds in certain segments of the lung can alert the nurse to pulmonary areas that may benefit from chest physiotherapy.

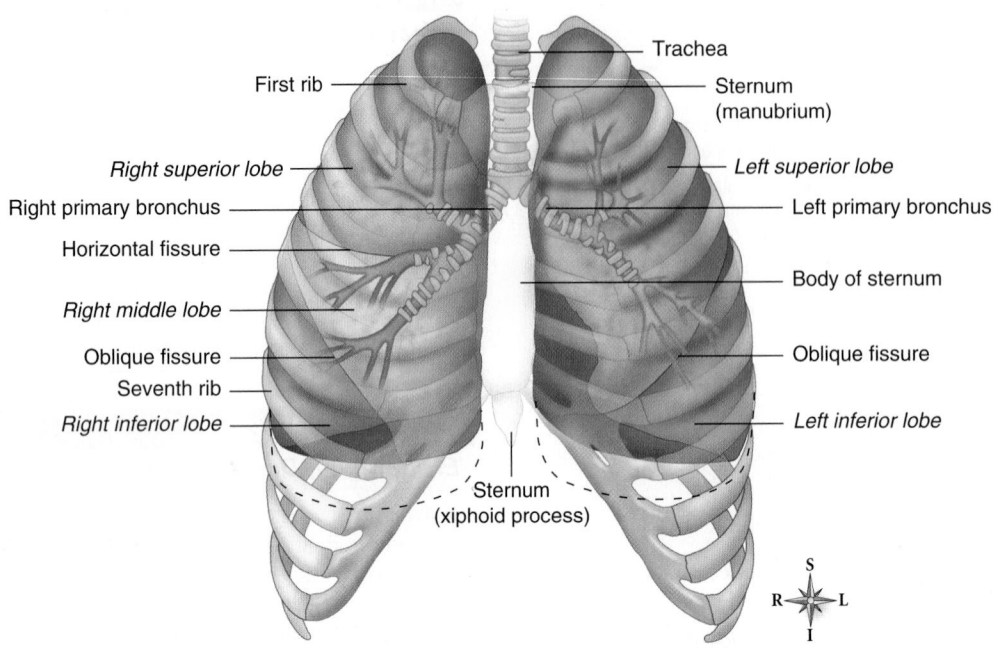

FIG 6-31 Location of the lobes of the lungs within the thoracic cavity. (From Patton KT, Thibodeau GA: *Anatomy and physiology,* ed 8, St. Louis, 2013, Mosby.)

BOX 6-14 VARIOUS PATTERNS OF RESPIRATION

Tachypnea—Increased rate
Bradypnea—Decreased rate
Dyspnea—Distress during breathing
Apnea—Cessation of breathing
Hyperpnea—Increased depth
Hypoventilation—Decreased depth (shallow) and irregular rhythm
Hyperventilation—Increased rate and depth
Kussmaul respiration—Hyperventilation, gasping and labored respiration; usually seen in diabetic coma or other states of respiratory acidosis
Cheyne-Stokes respiration—Gradually increasing rate and depth with periods of apnea
Biot respiration—Periods of hyperpnea alternating with apnea (similar to Cheyne-Stokes except that depth remains constant)
Seesaw (paradoxic) respirations—Chest falls on inspiration and rises on expiration
Agonal—Last gasping breaths before death

Increased breath sounds after pulmonary therapy indicate improved passage of air through the respiratory tract. Box 6-14 lists terms used to describe various respiration patterns.

Various pulmonary abnormalities produce **adventitious sounds** that are not normally heard over the chest. These sounds occur in addition to normal or abnormal breath sounds. They are classified into two main groups: **crackles**, which result from the passage of air through fluid or moisture, and **wheezes**, which are produced as air passes through narrowed passageways, regardless of the cause, such as exudate, inflammation, spasm, or tumor. Considerable practice with an experienced tutor is necessary to differentiate the various types of lung sounds. Often it is best to describe the type of sound heard in the lungs rather than trying to label it. Always report any abnormal sounds for further medical evaluation.

HEART

The heart is situated in the thoracic cavity between the lungs in the mediastinum and above the diaphragm (Fig. 6-32). About two thirds of the heart lies within the left side of the rib cage, with the other third on the right side as it crosses the sternum. The heart is positioned in the thorax like a trapezoid:

Vertically along the right sternal border (RSB) from the second to the fifth rib

Horizontally (long side) from the lower right sternum to the fifth rib at the left midclavicular line (LMCL)

Diagonally from the left sternal border (LSB) at the second rib to the LMCL at the fifth rib

Horizontally (short side) from the RSB and LSB at the second ICS—base of the heart

Inspection is easiest when the child is sitting in a semi-Fowler position. Look at the anterior chest wall from an angle, comparing both sides of the rib cage with each other. Normally, they should be symmetric. In children with thin chest walls, a pulsation may be visible. Because comprehensive evaluation of cardiac function is not limited to the heart, also consider other findings such as the presence of all pulses (especially the femoral pulses) (Fig. 6-33), distended neck veins, clubbing of the fingers, peripheral cyanosis, edema, BP, and respiratory status.

Use palpation to determine the location of the **apical impulse** (AI), the most lateral cardiac impulse that may correspond to the apex. The AI is found:

- Just lateral to the LMCL and fourth ICS in children older than 7 years of age
- At the LMCL and fifth ICS in children younger than 7 years of age

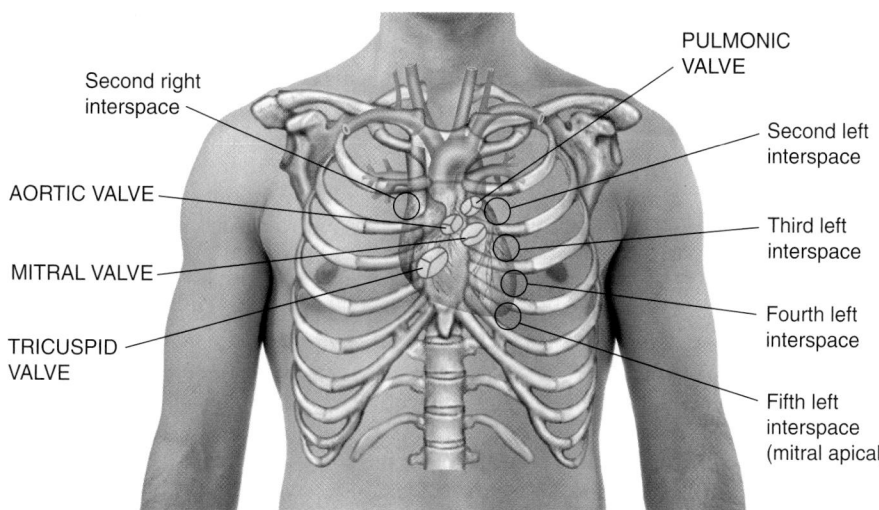

Second right
interspace

PULMONIC
VALVE

AORTIC VALVE

MITRAL VALVE

TRICUSPID
VALVE

Second left
interspace

Third left
interspace

Fourth left
interspace

Fifth left
interspace
(mitral apical)

FIG 6-32 Position of the heart within the thorax. (From Seidel HM: *Mosby's guide to physical examination*, ed 5, St. Louis, 2003, Mosby.)

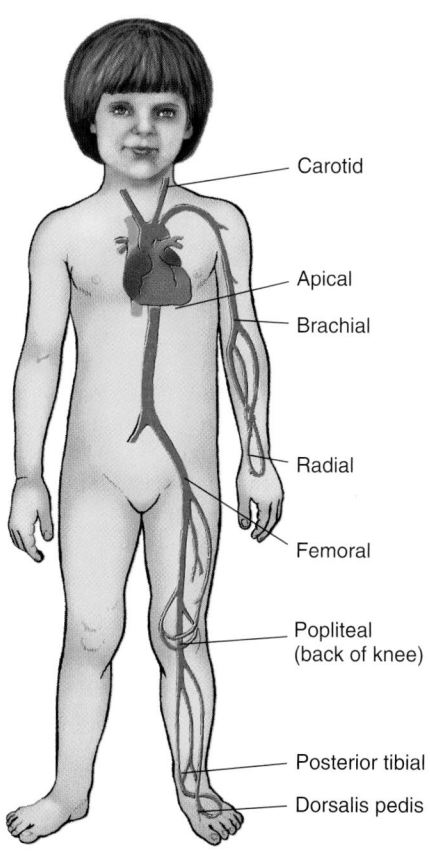

Carotid

Apical

Brachial

Radial

Femoral

Popliteal
(back of knee)

Posterior tibial

Dorsalis pedis

FIG 6-33 Location of pulses.

Although the AI gives a general idea of the size of the heart (with enlargement, the apex is lower and more lateral), its normal location is variable, making it an unreliable indicator of heart size.

The **point of maximum intensity** (PMI), as the name implies, is the area of most intense pulsation. Usually the PMI is located at the same site as the AI, but it can occur elsewhere. For this reason, the two terms should not be used synonymously.

Assess the **capillary refill time**, an important test for circulation and hydration, by pressing the skin lightly on a central site, such as the forehead, or a peripheral site, such as the top of the hand, to produce

a slight blanching. The time it takes for the blanched area to return to its original color is the **capillary refill time**.

> **! NURSING ALERT**
>
> Capillary refill should be brisk—less than 2 seconds. Prolonged refill may be associated with poor systemic perfusion or a cool ambient temperature.

Auscultation
Origin of Heart Sounds

The heart sounds are produced by the opening and closing of the valves and the vibration of blood against the walls of the heart and vessels. Normally, two sounds—S_1 and S_2—are heard, which correspond, respectively, to the familiar "lub dub" often used to describe the sounds. S_1 is caused by closure of the **tricuspid** and **mitral valves** (sometimes called the **atrioventricular valves**). S_2 is the result of closure of the **pulmonic** and **aortic valves** (sometimes called **semilunar valves**). Normally, the split of the two sounds in S_2 is distinguishable and widens during inspiration. **Physiologic splitting** is a significant normal finding.

> **! NURSING ALERT**
>
> Fixed splitting, in which the split in S_2 does not change during inspiration, is an important diagnostic sign of atrial septal defect.

Two other heart sounds, S_3 and S_4, may be produced. S_3 is normally heard in some children; S_4 is rarely heard as a normal heart sound; it usually indicates the need for further cardiac evaluation.

Differentiating Normal Heart Sounds

Figure 6-34 illustrates the approximate anatomic position of the valves within the heart chambers. Note that the anatomic location of valves does not correspond to the area where the sounds are heard best. The auscultatory sites are located in the direction of the blood flow through the valves.

Normally, S_1 is louder at the apex of the heart in the mitral and tricuspid area, and S_2 is louder near the base of the heart in the pulmonic and aortic area (Table 6-11). Listen to each sound by inching down the chest. Auscultate the following areas for sounds, such as murmurs that may radiate to these sites: sternoclavicular area above the clavicles and manubrium, area along the sternal border, area along the left midaxillary line, and area below the scapulae.

> **NURSING TIP** To distinguish between S_1 and S_2 heart sounds, simultaneously palpate the carotid pulse with the index and middle fingers and listen to the heart sounds; S_1 is synchronous with the carotid pulse.

Auscultate the heart with the child in at least two positions: sitting and reclining. If adventitious sounds are detected, further evaluate them with the child standing, sitting and leaning forward, and lying on the left side. For example, atrial sounds such as S_4 are heard best with the person in a recumbent position and usually fade if the person sits or stands.

Evaluate heart sounds for (1) **quality** (they should be clear and distinct, not muffled, diffuse, or distant); (2) **intensity**, especially in relation to the location or auscultatory site (they should not be weak or pounding); (3) **rate** (they should have the same rate as the radial pulse); and (4) **rhythm** (they should be regular and even). A particular arrhythmia that occurs normally in many children is sinus arrhythmia, in which the heart rate increases with inspiration and decreases with expiration. Differentiate this rhythm from a truly abnormal arrhythmia by having children hold their breath. In **sinus arrhythmia**, cessation of breathing causes the heart rate to remain steady.

Heart Murmurs

Another important category of the heart sounds is **murmurs**, which are produced by vibrations within the heart chambers or in the major arteries from the back-and-forth flow of blood. (For a more detailed discussion, see Cardiovascular Dysfunction, Chapter 25.) Murmurs are classified as:

Innocent—No anatomic or physiologic abnormality exists.
Functional—No anatomic cardiac defect exists, but a physiologic abnormality such as anemia is present.
Organic—A cardiac defect with or without a physiologic abnormality exists.

The description and classification of murmurs are skills that require considerable practice and training. In general, recognize murmurs as distinct swishing sounds that occur in addition to the normal heart sounds and record the (1) **location**, or the area of the heart in which the murmur is heard best; (2) **time** of the occurrence of the murmur within the S_1–S_2 cycle; (3) **intensity** (evaluate in relationship to the child's position); and (4) **loudness**. Table 6-12 lists the usual subjective method of grading the loudness or intensity of a murmur.

ABDOMEN

Examination of the abdomen involves inspection followed by auscultation and then palpation. Perform palpation last because it may distort the normal abdominal sounds. Knowledge of the anatomic placement of the abdominal organs is essential to differentiate normal, expected findings from abnormal ones (Fig. 6-35).

For descriptive purposes, the abdominal cavity is divided into four quadrants by drawing a vertical line midway from the sternum to the

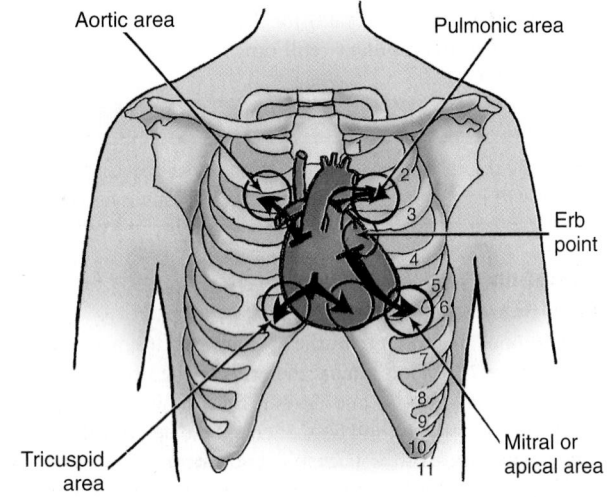

FIG 6-34 Direction of heart sounds for anatomic valve sites and areas *(circled)* for auscultation.

TABLE 6-11	SEQUENCE OF AUSCULTATING HEART SOUNDS*	
AUSCULTATORY SITE	**CHEST LOCATION**	**CHARACTERISTICS OF HEART SOUNDS**
Aortic area	Second right intercostal space close to sternum	S_2 heard louder than S_1; aortic closure heard loudest
Pulmonic area	Second left intercostal space close to sternum	Splitting of S_2 heard best, normally widens on inspiration; pulmonic closure heard best
Erb point	Second and third left intercostal spaces close to sternum	Frequent site of innocent murmurs and those of aortic or pulmonic origin
Tricuspid area	Fifth right and left intercostal spaces close to sternum	S_1 heard as louder sound preceding S_2 (S_1 synchronous with carotid pulse)
Mitral or apical area	Fifth intercostal space, left midclavicular line (third to fourth intercostal space and lateral to left midclavicular line in infants)	S_1 heard loudest; splitting of S_1 may be audible because mitral closure is louder than tricuspid closure
		S_3 heard best at beginning of expiration with child in recumbent or left side-lying position; occurs immediately after S_2; sounds like word $S_1 S_2 S_3$: "Ken-tuck-y"
		S_4 heard best during expiration with child in recumbent position (left side-lying position decreases sound); occurs immediately before S_1; sounds like word $S_4 S_1 S_2$: "Ten-nes-see"

*Use both diaphragm and bell chest pieces when auscultating heart sounds. Bell chest piece is necessary for low-pitched sounds of murmurs, S_3, and S_4.

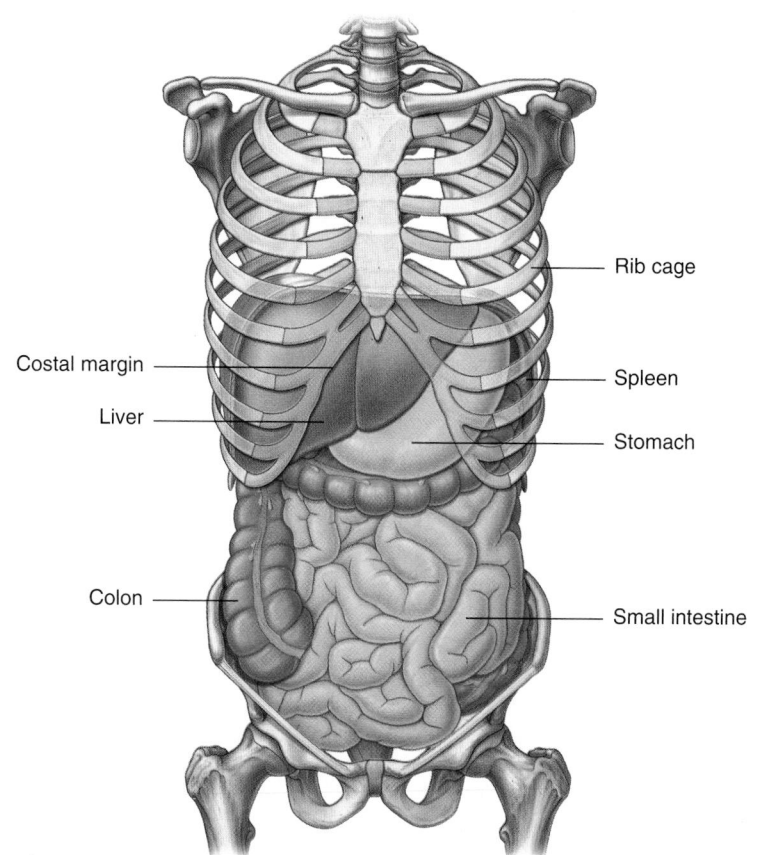

FIG 6-35 Location of structures in the abdomen. (From Drake RL, Vogl W, Mitchell AWM: *Gray's anatomy for students*, New York, 2005, Churchill Livingstone.)

Labels: Rib cage, Costal margin, Liver, Spleen, Stomach, Colon, Small intestine

TABLE 6-12	GRADING THE INTENSITY OF HEART MURMURS
GRADE	**DESCRIPTION**
I	Very faint; often not heard if child sits up
II	Usually readily heard; slightly louder than grade I; audible in all positions
III	Loud but not accompanied by a thrill
IV	Loud accompanied by a thrill
V	Loud enough to be heard with a stethoscope barely touching the chest; accompanied by a thrill
VI	Loud enough to be heard with the stethoscope not touching the chest; often heard with the human ear close to the chest; accompanied by a thrill

symphysis pubis and a horizontal line across the abdomen through the umbilicus. The sections are named:
- Left upper quadrant
- Left lower quadrant
- Right upper quadrant
- Right lower quadrant

Inspection

Inspect the **contour** of the abdomen with the child erect and supine. Normally, the abdomen of infants and young children is cylindric and, in the erect position, fairly prominent because of the physiologic lordosis of the spine. In the supine position, the abdomen appears flat. A midline protrusion from the xiphoid to the umbilicus or symphysis

pubis is usually **diastasis recti**, or failure of the rectus abdominis muscles to join in utero. In a healthy child, a midline protrusion is usually a variation of normal muscular development.

> **! NURSING ALERT**
>
> A tense, boardlike abdomen is a serious sign of paralytic ileus and intestinal obstruction.

The **skin** covering the abdomen should be uniformly taut without wrinkles or creases. Sometimes silvery, whitish striae ("stretch marks") are seen, especially if the skin has been stretched as in obesity. Superficial veins are usually visible in light-skinned, thin infants, but distended veins are an abnormal finding.

Observe **movement** of the abdomen. Normally, chest and abdominal movements are synchronous. In infants and thin children, **peristaltic waves** may be visible through the abdominal wall; they are best observed by standing at eye level to and across from the abdomen. Always report this finding.

Examine the **umbilicus** for size, hygiene, and evidence of any abnormalities, such as hernias. The umbilicus should be flat or only slightly protruding. If a herniation is present, palpate the sac for abdominal contents and estimate the approximate size of the opening. **Umbilical hernias** are common in infants, especially in African-American children.

Hernias may exist elsewhere on the abdominal wall (Fig. 6-36). An **inguinal hernia** is a protrusion of peritoneum through the abdominal wall in the inguinal canal. It occurs mostly in boys, is frequently bilateral, and may be visible as a mass in the scrotum. To locate a hernia,

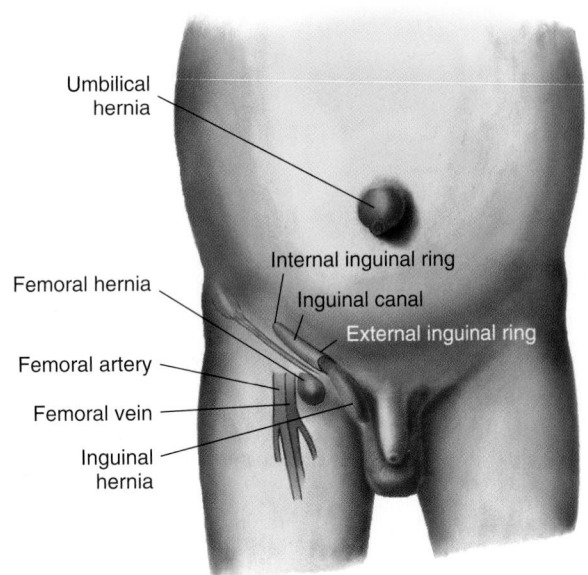

Umbilical hernia

Internal inguinal ring

Inguinal canal

External inguinal ring

Femoral hernia

Femoral artery

Femoral vein

Inguinal hernia

FIG 6-36 Location of hernias.

slide the little finger into the external inguinal ring at the base of the scrotum and ask the child to cough. If a hernia is present, it will hit the tip of the finger.

> **NURSING TIP** If the child is too young to cough, have the child blow up a balloon or laugh to raise the intraabdominal pressure sufficiently to demonstrate the presence of an inguinal hernia.

A **femoral hernia**, which occurs more frequently in girls, is felt or seen as a small mass on the anterior surface of the thigh just below the inguinal ligament in the femoral canal (a potential space medial to the femoral artery). Feel for a hernia by placing the index finger of your right hand on the child's right femoral pulse (left hand for left pulse) and the middle finger flat against the skin toward the midline. The ring finger lies over the femoral canal, where the herniation occurs. Palpation of hernias in the pelvic region is often part of the genital examination.

Auscultation

The most important finding to listen for is **peristalsis**, or **bowel sounds**, which sound like short metallic clicks and gurgles. Record their frequency per minute (e.g., 5 sounds/min). Stimulate bowel sounds by stroking the abdominal surface with a fingernail. Report absence of bowel sounds or hyperperistalsis because either usually denotes an abdominal disorder.

Palpation

There are two types of palpation: superficial and deep. For **superficial palpation**, lightly place your hand against the skin and feel each quadrant, noting any areas of tenderness, muscle tone, and superficial lesions such as cysts. Because superficial palpation is often perceived as tickling, use several techniques to minimize this sensation and relax the child (see Atraumatic Care box). Admonishing the child to stop laughing only draws attention to the sensation and decreases cooperation.

Deep palpation is for palpating organs and large blood vessels and for detecting masses and tenderness that were not discovered during

superficial palpation. Palpation usually begins in the lower quadrants and proceeds upward to avoid missing the edge of an enlarged liver or spleen. Except for palpating the liver, successful identification of other organs, such as the spleen, kidneys, and part of the colon, requires considerable practice with tutored supervision. Report any questionable mass. The lower edge of the liver is sometimes felt in infants and young children as a superficial mass 1 to 2 cm (0.4–0.8 inch) below the right costal margin (the distance is sometimes measured in fingerbreadths). Normally, the liver descends during inspiration as the diaphragm moves downward. Do not mistake this downward displacement as a sign of liver enlargement.

> **! NURSING ALERT**
>
> If the liver is palpable 3 cm (1.2 inch) below the right costal margin or the spleen is palpable more than 2 cm (0.8 inch) below the left costal margin, these organs are enlarged—a finding that is always reported for further medical investigation.

Palpate the **femoral pulses** by placing the tips of two or three fingers (index, middle, or ring) along the inguinal ligament about midway between the iliac crest and symphysis pubis. Feel both pulses simultaneously to make certain that they are equal and strong (Fig. 6-37).

> **! NURSING ALERT**
>
> Absence of femoral pulses is a significant sign of coarctation of the aorta and is referred for medical evaluation.

GENITALIA

Examination of the genitalia conveniently follows assessment of the abdomen while the child is still supine. In adolescents, inspection of the genitalia may be left to the end of the examination. The best approach is to examine the genitalia matter of factly, placing no more emphasis on this part of the assessment than on any other segment. It helps to relieve children's and parents' anxiety by telling them the

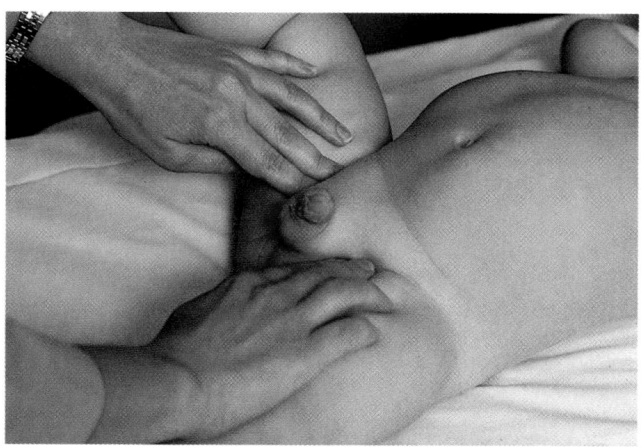

FIG 6-37 Palpating for femoral pulses.

results of the findings; for example, the nurse might say, "Everything looks fine here."

If it is necessary to ask questions, such as about discharge or difficulty urinating, respect the child's privacy by covering the lower abdomen with the gown or underpants. To prevent embarrassing interruptions, keep the door or curtain closed and post a "do not disturb" sign. Have a drape ready to cover the genitalia if someone enters the room.

In examining the genitalia, wear gloves when touching body substances. It might be helpful for the adolescent to know that wearing gloves also prevents skin-to-skin contact.

The genital examination is an excellent time for eliciting questions or concern about body function or sexual activity. Also use this opportunity to increase or reinforce the child's knowledge of reproductive anatomy by naming each body part and explaining its function. This part of the health assessment is an opportune time to teach testicular self-examination to boys.

Male Genitalia

Note the external appearance of the glans and shaft of the penis, the prepuce, the urethral meatus, and the scrotum (Fig. 6-38). The **penis** is generally small in infants and young boys until puberty, when it begins to increase in both length and width. In an obese child, the penis often looks abnormally small because of the folds of skin partially covering it at the base. Be familiar with normal pubertal growth of the external male genitalia to compare the findings with the expected sequence of maturation (see Chapter 16).

Examine the **glans** (head of the penis) and **shaft** (portion between the perineum and prepuce) for signs of swelling, skin lesions, inflammation, or other irregularities. Any of these signs may indicate underlying disorders, especially sexually transmitted infections.

Carefully inspect the **urethral meatus** for location and evidence of discharge. Normally, it is centered at the tip of the glans. Also note **hair distribution**. Normally, before puberty, no pubic hair is present. Soft, downy hair at the base of the penis is an early sign of pubertal maturation. In older adolescents, hair distribution is diamond shaped from the umbilicus to the anus.

Note the location and size of the **scrotum**. The scrota hang freely from the perineum behind the penis, and the left scrotum normally hangs lower than the right. In infants, the scrota appear large in relation to the rest of the genitalia. The skin of the scrotum is loose and highly rugated (wrinkled). During early adolescence, the skin normally becomes redder and coarser. In dark-skinned boys, the scrota are usually more deeply pigmented.

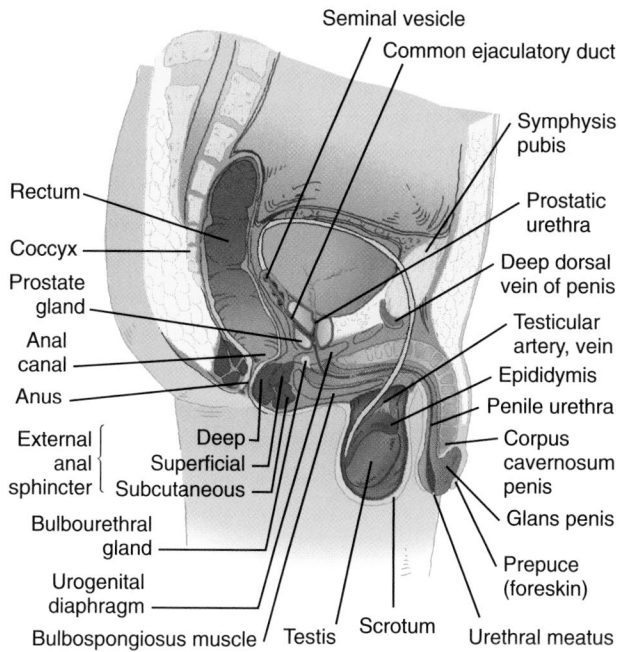

FIG 6-38 Major structures of genitalia in an uncircumcised postpubertal male. (From Black JM: *Medical-surgical nursing: clinical management for positive outcomes*, ed 8, St. Louis, 2008, Saunders.)

Palpation of the scrotum includes identification of the testes, epididymis, and, if present, inguinal hernias. The two **testes** are felt as small, ovoid bodies about 1.5 to 2 cm (0.6–0.8 inch) long—one in each scrotal sac. They do not enlarge until puberty, when they approximately double in size.

When palpating for the presence of the testes, avoid stimulating the **cremasteric reflex**, which is stimulated by cold, touch, emotional excitement, or exercise. This reflex pulls the testes higher into the pelvic cavity. Several measures are useful in preventing the cremasteric reflex during palpation of the scrotum. First, warm the hands. Second, if the child is old enough, examine him in a tailor or "Indian" position, which stretches the muscle, preventing its contraction (Fig. 6-39, *A*). Third, block the normal pathway of ascent of the testes by placing the thumb and index finger over the upper part of the scrotal sac along the inguinal canal (Fig. 6-39, *B*). If there is any question concerning the existence of two testes, place the index and middle fingers in a scissors fashion to separate the right and left scrota. If, after using these techniques, you have not palpated the testes, feel along the inguinal canal and perineum to locate masses that may be undescended testes. Although undescended testes may descend at any time during childhood and are checked at each visit, report any failure to palpate the testes.

Female Genitalia

The examination of female genitalia is limited to inspection and palpation of external structures. If a vaginal examination is required, the nurse should make an appropriate referral unless he or she is qualified to perform the procedure.

A convenient position for examination of the genitalia involves placing the young girl supine on the examining table or in a semireclining position on the parent's lap with the feet supported on your knees as you sit facing the child. Divert the child's attention from the examination by instructing her to try to keep the soles of her feet pressed against each other. Separate the labia majora with the thumb and index

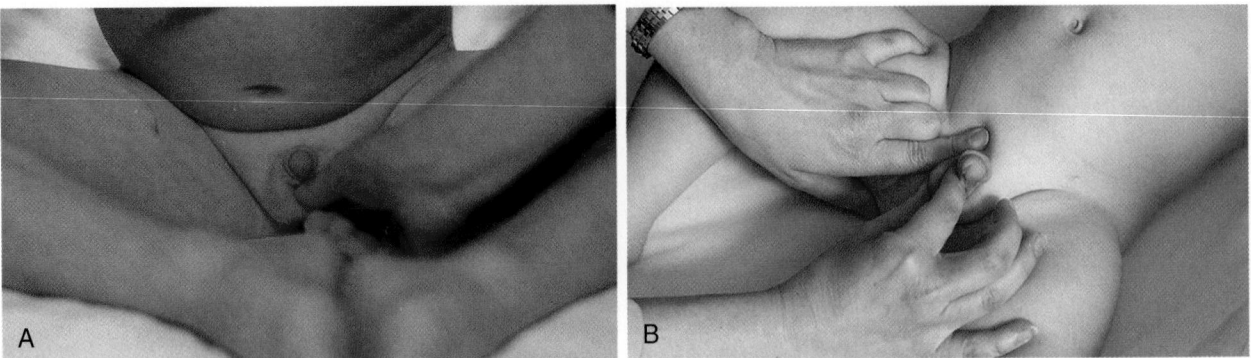

FIG 6-39 A, Preventing the cremasteric reflex by having the child sit in the tailor position. **B,** Blocking the inguinal canal during palpation of the scrotum for descended testes.

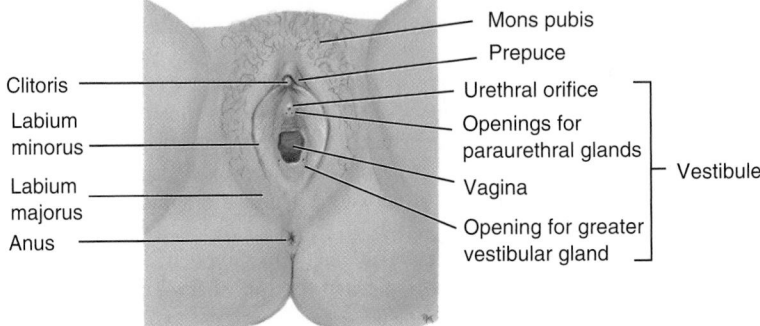

FIG 6-40 External structures of the genitalia in a postpubertal female. The labia are spread to reveal deeper structures. (From Applegate E: *The anatomy and physiology learning system,* ed 3, St. Louis, 2006, Saunders.)

finger and retract outward to expose the labia minora, urethral meatus, and vaginal orifice.

Examine the female genitalia for size and location of the structures of the **vulva,** or **pudendum** (Fig. 6-40). The **mons pubis** is a pad of adipose tissue over the symphysis pubis. At puberty, the mons is covered with hair, which extends along the labia. The usual pattern of female **hair distribution** is an inverted triangle. The appearance of soft, downy hair along the labia majora is an early sign of sexual maturation. Note the size and location of the **clitoris,** a small, erectile organ located at the anterior end of the labia minora. It is covered by a small flap of skin, the **prepuce.**

The **labia majora** are two thick folds of skin running posteriorly from the mons to the posterior commissure of the vagina. Internal to the labia majora are two folds of skin called the **labia minora.** Although the labia minora are usually prominent in newborns, they gradually atrophy, which makes them almost invisible until their enlargement during puberty. The inner surface of the labia should be pink and moist. Note the size of the labia and any evidence of fusion, which may suggest male scrota. Normally, no masses are palpable within the labia.

The **urethral meatus** is located posterior to the clitoris and is surrounded by the Skene glands and ducts. Although not a prominent structure, the meatus appears as a small V-shaped slit. Note its location, especially if it opens from the clitoris or inside the vagina. Gently palpate the glands, which are common sites of cysts and sexually transmitted lesions.

The **vaginal orifice** is located posterior to the urethral meatus. Its appearance varies depending on individual anatomy and sexual activity. Ordinarily, examination of the vagina is limited to inspection. In virgins, a thin crescent-shaped or circular membrane, called the **hymen,** may cover part of the vaginal opening. In some instances, it completely occludes the orifice. After rupture, small rounded pieces

of tissue called caruncles remain. Although an imperforate hymen denotes lack of penile intercourse, a perforate one does not necessarily indicate sexual activity (see also Sexual Abuse, Chapter 14).

> **! NURSING ALERT**
>
> In girls who have been circumcised, the genitalia will appear different. Do not show surprise or disgust but note the appearance and discuss the procedure with the young woman.

Surrounding the vaginal opening are **Bartholin glands,** which secrete a clear, mucoid fluid into the vagina for lubrication during intercourse. Palpate the ducts for cysts. Also note the discharge from the vagina, which is usually clear or white.

ANUS

After examination of the genitalia, it is easy to identify the anal area, although the child should be placed on the abdomen. Note the general firmness of the **buttocks** and symmetry of the **gluteal folds.** Assess the tone of the anal sphincter by eliciting the **anal reflex** (anal wink). Gently scratching the anal area results in an obvious quick contraction of the external anal sphincter.

BACK AND EXTREMITIES

Spine

Note the general **curvature** of the spine. Normally, the back of a newborn is rounded or C-shaped from the thoracic and pelvic curves. The development of the cervical and lumbar curves approximates development of various motor skills, such as cervical curvature with head control, and gives older children the typical double S curve.

Marked curvatures in posture are abnormal. Scoliosis, lateral curvature of the spine, is an important childhood problem, especially in girls. Although scoliosis may be identified by observing and palpating the spine and noting a sideways displacement, more objective tests include:

- With the child standing erect, clothed only in underpants (and bra if an older girl), observe from behind, noting asymmetry of the shoulders and hips.
- With the child bending forward so the back is parallel to the floor, observe from the side, noting asymmetry or prominence of the rib cage.

A slight limp, a crooked hemline, or complaints of a sore back are other signs and symptoms of scoliosis.

Inspect the back, especially along the spine, for any tufts of hair, dimples, or discoloration. Mobility of the vertebral column is easy to assess in most children because of their tendency to be in constant motion during the examination. However, you can test mobility by asking the child to sit up from a prone position or to do a modified sit-up exercise.

Movement of the cervical spine is an important diagnostic sign of neurologic problems, such as meningitis. Normally, movement of the head in all directions is effortless.

> **! NURSING ALERT**
>
> Hyperextension of the neck and spine, or opisthotonos, which is accompanied by pain when the head is flexed, is always referred for immediate medical evaluation.

Extremities

Inspect each extremity for symmetry of length and size; refer any deviation for orthopedic evaluation. Count the fingers and toes to be certain of the normal number. This is so often taken for granted that an extra digit (polydactyly) or fusion of digits (syndactyly) may go unnoticed.

Inspect the arms and legs for temperature and color, which should be equal in each extremity, although the feet may normally be colder than the hands.

Assess the shape of bones. There are several variations of bone shape in children. Although many of them cause parents concern, most are benign and require no treatment. Bowleg, or genu varum, is lateral bowing of the tibia. It is clinically present when the child stands with an outward bowing of the legs, giving the appearance of a bow. Usually, there is an outward curvature of both femur and tibia (Fig. 6-41, A). Toddlers are usually bowlegged after beginning to walk until all of their lower back and leg muscles are well developed. Unilateral or asymmetric bowlegs that are present beyond the age of 2 to 3 years, particularly in African-American children, may represent pathologic conditions requiring further investigation.

Knock knee, or genu valgum, appears as the opposite of bowleg, in that the knees are close together but the feet are spread apart. It is determined clinically by using the same method as for genu varum but by measuring the distance between the malleoli, which normally should be less than 7.5 cm (3 inches) (Fig. 6-41, B). Knock knee is normally present in children from about 2 to 7 years of age. Knock knee that is excessive, asymmetric, accompanied by short stature, or evident in a child nearing puberty requires further evaluation.

Next inspect the feet. Infants' and toddlers' feet appear flat because the feet are normally wide and the arches are covered by fat pads.

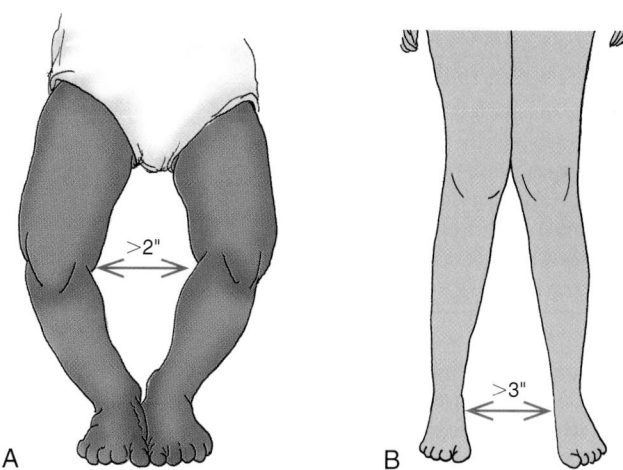

FIG 6-41 A, Bowleg. **B,** Knock knee.

Development of the arch occurs naturally from the action of walking. Normally, at birth the feet are held in a valgus (outward) or varus (inward) position. To determine whether a foot deformity at birth is a result of intrauterine position or development, scratch the outer and then the inner side of the sole. If the foot position is self-correctable, it will assume a right angle to the leg. As the child begins to walk, the feet turn outward less than 30 degrees and inward less than 10 degrees.

Toddlers have a "toddling" or broad-based gait, which facilitates walking by lowering the center of gravity. As the child reaches preschool age, the legs are brought closer together. By school age, the walking posture is much more graceful and balanced.

The most common gait problem in young children is pigeon toe, or toeing in, which usually results from torsional deformities, such as internal tibial torsion (abnormal rotation or bowing of the tibia). Tests for tibial torsion include measuring the thigh–foot angle, which requires considerable practice for accuracy.

Elicit the plantar or grasp reflex by exerting firm but gentle pressure with the tip of the thumb against the lateral sole of the foot from the heel upward to the little toe and then across to the big toe. The normal response in children who are walking is flexion of the toes. Babinski sign, dorsiflexion of the big toe and fanning of the other toes, is normal during infancy but abnormal after about 1 year of age or when locomotion begins (see Fig. 10-6).

Joints

Evaluate the joints for range of motion. Normally, this requires no specific testing if you have observed the child's movements during the examination. However, routinely investigate the hips in infants for congenital dislocation. Report any evidence of joint immobility or hyperflexibility. Palpate the joints for heat, tenderness, and swelling. These signs, as well as redness over the joint, warrant further investigation.

Muscles

Note symmetry and quality of muscle development, tone, and strength. Observe development by looking at the shape and contour of the body in both a relaxed and a tensed state. Estimate tone by grasping the muscle and feeling its firmness when it is relaxed and contracted. A common site for testing tone is the biceps muscle of the arm. Children are usually willing to "make a muscle" by clenching their fists.

BOX 6-15 TESTS FOR CEREBELLAR FUNCTION

Finger-to-nose test—With the child's arm extended, ask the child to touch the nose with the index finger with the eyes open and then closed.

Heel-to-shin test—Have the child stand and run the heel of one foot down the shin or anterior aspect of the tibia of the other leg, both with the eyes opened and then closed.

Romberg test—Have the child stand with the eyes closed and heels together; falling or leaning to one side is abnormal and is called the Romberg sign.

Estimate strength by having the child use an extremity to push or pull against resistance, as in the following examples:

Arm strength—The child holds the arms outstretched in front of the body and tries to raise the arms while downward pressure is applied.

Hand strength—The child shakes hands with the nurse and squeezes one or two fingers of the nurse's hand.

Leg strength—The child sits on a table or chair with the legs dangling and tries to raise the legs while downward pressure is applied.

Note symmetry of strength in the extremities, hands, and fingers, and report evidence of paresis, or weakness.

NEUROLOGIC ASSESSMENT

The assessment of the nervous system is the broadest and most diverse part of the examination process, since every human function, both physical and emotional, is controlled by neurologic impulses. Much of the neurologic examination has already been discussed, such as assessment of behavior, sensory testing, and motor function. The following focuses on a general appraisal of cerebellar function, deep tendon reflexes, and the cranial nerves.

Cerebellar Function

The cerebellum controls balance and coordination. Much of the assessment of cerebellar function is included in observing the child's posture, body movements, gait, and development of fine and gross motor skills. Tests such as balancing on one foot and the heel-to-toe walk assess balance. Test coordination by asking the child to reach for a toy, button clothes, tie shoes, or draw a straight line on a piece of paper (provided the child is old enough to do these activities). Coordination can also be tested by any sequence of rapid, successive movements, such as quickly touching each finger with the thumb of the same hand.

Several tests for cerebellar function can be performed as games (Box 6-15). When a Romberg test is done, stay beside the child if there is a possibility that he or she might fall. School-age children should be able to perform these tests, although in the finger-to-nose test, preschoolers normally can only bring the finger within 5 to 7.5 cm (2–3 inches) of the nose. Difficulty in performing these exercises indicates a poor sense of position (especially with the eyes closed) and incoordination (especially with the eyes open).

Reflexes

Testing reflexes is an important part of the neurologic examination. Persistence of primitive reflexes (see Chapter 8), loss of reflexes, or hyperactivity of deep tendon reflexes is usually a result of a cerebral insult.

Elicit reflexes by using the rubber head of the reflex hammer, flat of the finger, or side of the hand. If the child is easily frightened by equipment, use your hand or finger. Although testing reflexes is a

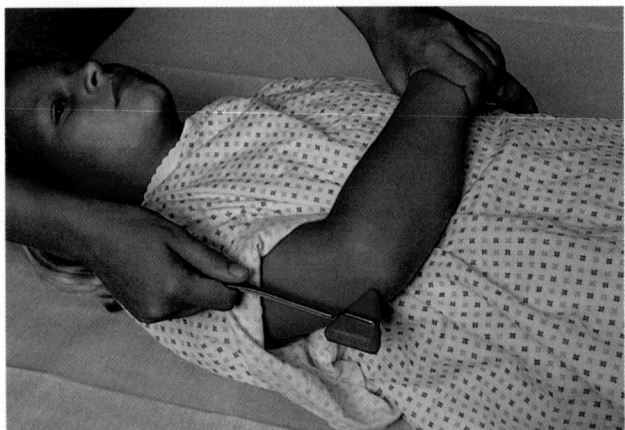

FIG 6-42 Testing for the triceps reflex. The child is placed supine, with the forearm resting over the chest, and the triceps tendon is struck. Alternate procedure: the child's arm is abducted with the upper arm supported and the forearm allowed to hang freely. The triceps tendon is struck. Normal response is partial extension of the forearm.

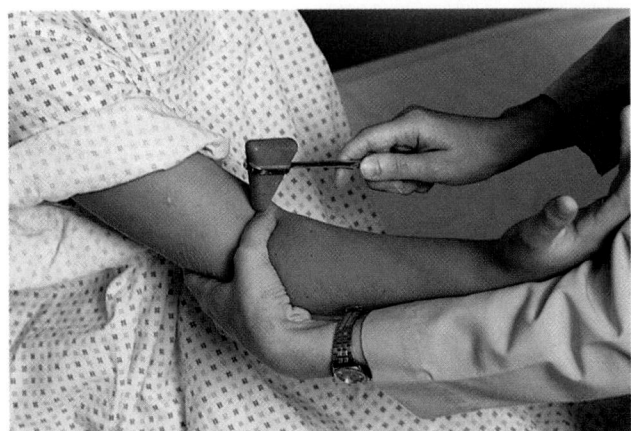

FIG 6-43 Testing for the biceps reflex. The child's arm is held by placing the partially flexed elbow in the examiner's hand with the thumb over the antecubital space. The examiner's thumbnail is struck with a hammer. Normal response is partial flexion of the forearm.

simple procedure, the child may inhibit the reflex by unconsciously tensing the muscle. To avoid tensing, distract younger children with toys or talk to them. Older children can concentrate on the exercise of grasping their two hands in front of them and trying to pull them apart. This diverts their attention from the testing and causes involuntary relaxation of the muscles.

Deep tendon reflexes are stretch reflexes of a muscle. The most common deep tendon reflex is the knee jerk reflex, or patellar reflex (sometimes called the quadriceps reflex). Figs. 6-42 to 6-45 illustrate the reflexes normally elicited. Report any diminished or hyperreflexive response for further evaluation.

Cranial Nerves

Assessment of the cranial nerves is an important area of neurologic assessment (Fig. 6-46; Table 6-13). With young children, present the tests as games to foster trust and security at the beginning of the examination. Also include the cranial nerve test when examining each system, such as tongue movement and strength, gag reflex, swallowing, cardinal positions of gaze (Fig. 6-47), and position of the uvula during examination of the mouth.

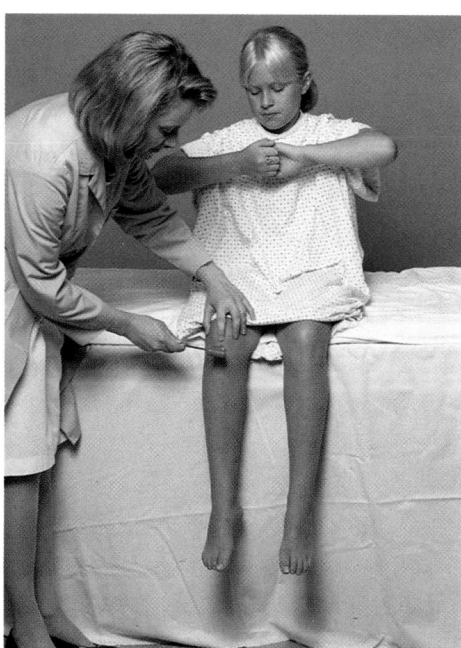

FIG 6-44 Testing for the patellar, or knee-jerk, reflex, using distraction. The child sits on the edge of the examining table (or on the parent's lap) with the lower legs flexed at the knee and dangling freely. The patellar tendon is tapped just below the kneecap. Normal response is partial extension of the lower leg.

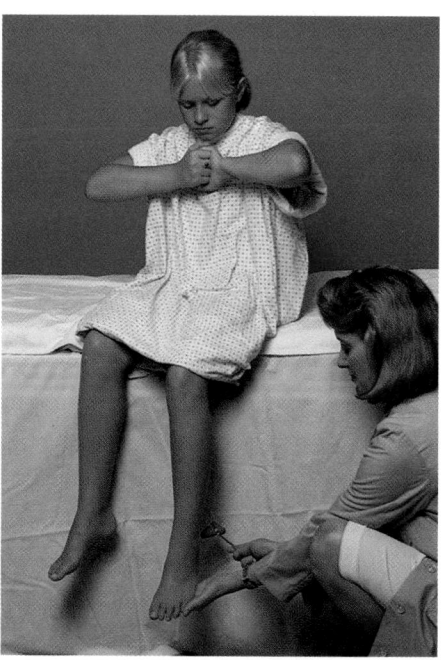

FIG 6-45 Testing for the Achilles reflex. The child should be in the same position as for the knee-jerk reflex. The foot is supported lightly in the examiner's hand, and the Achilles tendon is struck. Normal response is plantar flexion of the foot (the foot pointing downward).

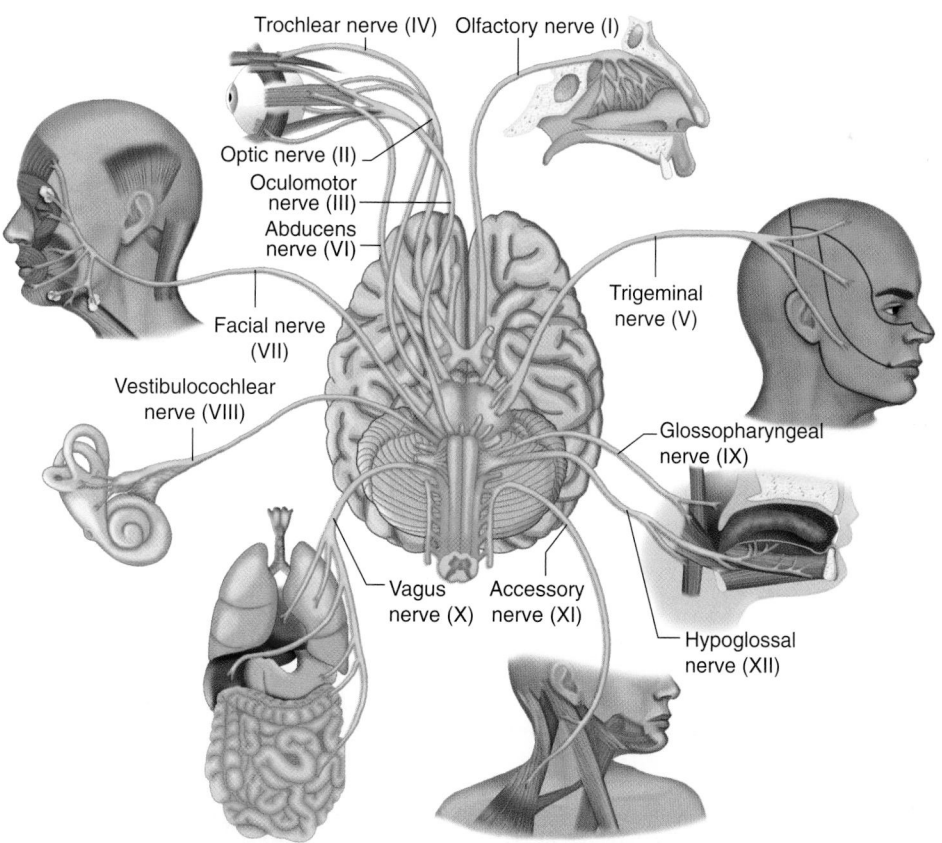

FIG 6-46 Cranial nerves. (From Patton KT, Thibodeau GA: *Anatomy and physiology,* ed 8, St. Louis, 2013, Mosby.)

TABLE 6-13　ASSESSMENT OF CRANIAL NERVES

DESCRIPTION AND FUNCTION	TESTS
I—Olfactory Nerve Olfactory mucosa of nasal cavity Smell	With eyes closed, have child identify odors such as coffee, alcohol from a swab, or other smells; test each nostril separately.
II—Optic Nerve Rods and cones of retina, optic nerve Vision	Check for perception of light, visual acuity, peripheral vision, color vision, and normal optic disc.
III—Oculomotor Nerve Extraocular muscles of eye: • Superior rectus—Moves eyeball up and in • Inferior rectus—Moves eyeball down and in • Medial rectus—Moves eyeball nasally • Inferior oblique—Moves eyeball up and out Pupil constriction and accommodation Eyelid closing	Have child follow an object (toy) or light in six cardinal positions of gaze (see Fig. 6-47). Perform PERRLA (*p*upils *e*qual, *r*ound, *r*eact to *l*ight, and *a*ccommodation). Check for proper placement of eyelid.
IV—Trochlear Nerve Superior oblique muscle (SO)—Moves eye down and out	Have child look down and in (see Fig. 6-47).
V—Trigeminal Nerve Muscles of mastication Sensory—Face, scalp, nasal and buccal mucosa	Have child bite down hard and open jaw; test symmetry and strength. With child's eyes closed, see if child can detect light touch in mandibular and maxillary regions. Test corneal and blink reflex by touching cornea lightly (approach from side so the child does not blink before cornea is touched).
VI—Abducens Nerve Lateral rectus (LR) muscle—Moves eye temporally	Have child look toward temporal side (see Fig. 6-47).
VII—Facial Nerve Muscles for facial expression Anterior two thirds of tongue (sensory)	Have child smile, make funny face, or show teeth to see symmetry of expression. Have child identify sweet or salty solution; place each taste on anterior section and sides of protruding tongue; if child retracts tongue, solution will dissolve toward posterior part of tongue.
VIII—Auditory, Acoustic, or Vestibulocochlear Nerve Internal ear Hearing and balance	Test hearing; note any loss of equilibrium or presence of vertigo.
IX—Glossopharyngeal Nerve Pharynx, tongue Posterior third of tongue Sensory	Stimulate posterior pharynx with a tongue blade; child should gag. Test sense of sour or bitter taste on posterior segment of tongue.
X—Vagus Nerve Muscles of larynx, pharynx, some organs of gastrointestinal system, sensory fibers of root of tongue, heart, and lung	Note hoarseness of voice, gag reflex, and ability to swallow. Check that uvula is in midline; when stimulated with tongue blade, it should deviate upward and to stimulated side.
XI—Accessory Nerve Sternocleidomastoid and trapezius muscles of shoulder	Have child shrug shoulders while applying mild pressure; with examiner's hands placed on shoulders, have child turn head against opposing pressure on either side; note symmetry and strength.
XII—Hypoglossal Nerve Muscles of tongue	Have child move tongue in all directions; have child protrude tongue as far as possible; note any midline deviation. Test strength by placing tongue blade on one side of tongue and having child move it away.

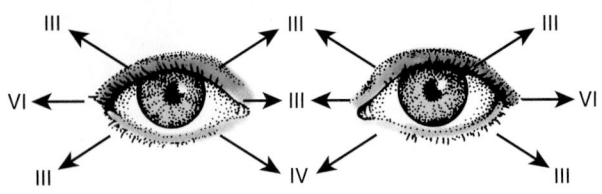

FIG 6-47 Checking extraocular movements in the six cardinal positions indicates the functioning of cranial nerves III, IV, and VI. (From Ignatavicius DD: *Medical-surgical nursing: patient-centered collaborative care*, ed 6, St. Louis, 2009, Saunders.)

KEY POINTS

- To effectively establish a setting for communication, nurses must make an appropriate introduction and ensure privacy and confidentiality.
- When communicating with parents, nurses need to encourage parental involvement, listen carefully, use silence, and be empathic.
- Communication with children must reflect their developmental stage.
- Nonverbal communication with children may take the form of writing, drawing, and play.
- The objectives of performing a health history are to identify pertinent information, determine the chief complaint, analyze the present illness, secure the patient's health history, review biologic systems, and record a family medical history and child psychosocial and sexual history.
- Family assessment is the collection of data about family composition and relationships among its members; it also focuses on home and community environment, parents' occupation and education, and cultural and religious traditions.
- The family function interview examines interaction and roles, power, decision making, problem solving, communication, and expression of feelings and individuality.
- Nutritional assessment is performed by determination of dietary intake, clinical examination, and biochemical analysis.
- Growth measurements during the physical examination focus on length or height, weight, skinfold thickness, and arm and head circumference. Assessment of growth is measured against standard growth charts to determine a child's status in comparison with other children of the same age.
- Measurements of temperature, pulse, respiration, and BP constitute the physiologic approach to assessment.
- The child's general appearance is a cumulative, subjective impression of physical appearance, state of nutrition, behavior, personality, interactions with parents and nurse, posture, development, and speech.
- Assessment of the skin, which primarily involves inspection and palpation, focuses on color, texture, temperature, moisture, and turgor. The nurse needs to be aware of both physiologic and ethnic factors that may affect these areas.
- In assessment of the lymph nodes, the nurse examines, by palpation, the part of the body in which the glands are located.
- The head is inspected for shape, symmetry, mobility, and muscle control.
- Examination of the eyes includes placement and alignment, inspection of external and internal structures, and vision testing.
- The ear examination encompasses placement and alignment, external and internal structures, and auditory testing.
- The lungs are examined by inspection, palpation, percussion, and auscultation.
- Auscultation is the most important procedure for examining the heart.
- Abdominal assessment follows an orderly sequence of inspection, auscultation, and palpation because palpation may distort normal abdominal sounds.
- Examination of the genitalia may provoke anxiety in the child, and the nurse must avoid any transference of anxiety.
- Neurologic assessment addresses behavior; motor, sensory, and cerebellar function; reflexes; and cranial nerves.

REFERENCES

American Academy of Pediatrics: *Pediatric nutrition handbook*, ed. 6, Elk Grove Village, Ill, 2009, Author.

American Academy of Pediatrics, Committee on Practice and Ambulatory Medicine, Section on Ophthalmology: Eye examination in infants, children, and young adults by pediatricians, *Pediatrics* 111(4):902–907, 2003a.

American Academy of Pediatrics, Committee on Practice and Ambulatory Medicine, Section on Otolaryngology and Bronchoesophagology: Hearing assessment in infants and children: recommendations beyond neonatal screening, *Pediatrics* 111(2):436–440, 2003b.

Beaulieu R, Humphreys J: Evaluation of a telephone advice nurse in a nursing faculty managed pediatric community clinic, *J Pediatr Health Care* 22(3):175–181, 2008.

Beevers G, Lip GYH, O'Brien E: ABC of hypertension blood pressure measurement, part I, Sphygmomanometry: factors common to all techniques, *BMJ* 322(7292):981–985, 2001.

Clark JA, Kieh-Lai MW, Sarnaik A, and others: Discrepancies between direct and indirect blood pressure measurements using various recommendations for arm cuff selection, *Pediatrics* 110(5):920–923, 2002.

Coats DK, Jenkins RH: Vision assessment of the pediatric patient: refinements, *Am Acad Ophthalmol* 1(1):1–12, 1997.

Craig JV, Lancaster GA, Williamson PR, and others: Temperature measured at the axilla compared with rectum in children and young people: systematic review, *BMJ* 320(7243):1174–1178, 2000.

Cunningham M, Cox EO: Hearing assessment in infants and children: recommendations beyond neonatal screening, *Pediatrics* 111(2):436–440, 2003.

Dodd SR, Lancaster GA, Craig JV, and others: In a systematic review, infrared ear thermometry for fever diagnosis in children finds poor sensitivity, *J Clin Epidemiol* 59(4):354–357, 2006.

El-Radhi AS, Barry W: Thermometry in paediatric practice, *Arch Dis Child* 91(4):351–356, 2006.

Halle C: Achieve new vision screening objectives, *Nurse Pract* 27(3):15–35, 2002.

Magar NA, Dabova-Missova S, Gjerdingen DK: Effectiveness of targeted anticipatory guidance during well-child visits: a pilot trial, *J Am Board Fam Med* 19(5):450–458, 2006.

Mains JA, Coxall K, Lloyd H: Measuring temperature, *Nurs Stand* 22(39):44–47, 2008.

Marklund B, Ström M, Månsson J, and others: Computer-supported telephone nurse triage: an evaluation of medical quality and costs, *J Nurs Manage* 15(2):180–187, 2007.

Mathiasen H: Empathy and sympathy: voices from literature, *Am J Cardiol* 97(12):1789–1790, 2006.

Midgley PC, Wardhaugh B, Macfarlane C, and others: Blood pressure in children aged 4–8 years: comparison of Omron HEM 711 and sphygmomanometer blood pressure measurements, *Arch Dis Child* 94(12):955–958, 2009.

National High Blood Pressure Education Program Working Group on High Blood Pressure in Children and Adolescents: The fourth report on the diagnosis, evaluation, and treatment of high blood pressure in children and adolescents, *Pediatrics* 114(2 suppl 4th rep):555–576, 2004.

Ogden CL, Carroll MD, Flegal KM: High body mass index for age among US children and adolescents, 2003–2006, *JAMA* 299(20):2401–2405, 2008.

Park MK, Menard SW, Schoolfield J: Oscillometric blood pressure standards for children, *Pediatr Cardiol* 26(5):601–607, 2005.

Seidel HM, Ball JW, Dains JE, and others: *Mosby's guide to physical examination*, ed 7, St. Louis, 2011, Mosby.

Wall TC, Marsh-Tootle W, Evans HH, and others: Compliance with vision-screening guidelines among a national sample of pediatricians, *Ambul Pediatr* 2(6):449–455, 2002.

Pain Assessment and Management in Children

Eufemia Jacob

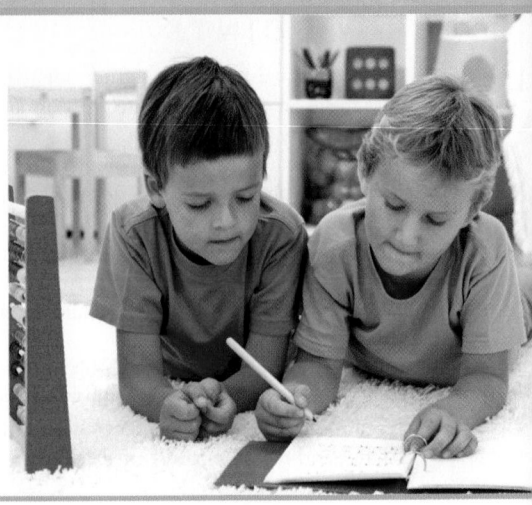

CHAPTER OUTLINE

Pain Assessment, 144
  Assessment of Acute Pain, 145
    Pain Intensity, 145
    *Global Judgment of Improvement and
      of Satisfaction With Treatment, 150*
    Adverse Events and Symptoms, 150
    Physical Recovery, 150
    Emotional Response, 151
  Assessment of Chronic and Recurrent
    Pain, 151
  Multidimensional Measures, 151
**Assessment of Pain in Specific
  Populations, 152**
  Pain in Neonates, 152

  Children with Communication
    and Cognitive Impairment, 153
  Cultural Differences, 156
  Children with Chronic Illness and
    Complex Pain, 156
Pain Management, 156
  Nonpharmacologic
    Management, 159
  Pharmacologic Management, 162
    Patient-Controlled Analgesia, 163
    Epidural Analgesia, 168
    *Transmucosal and Transdermal
      Analgesia, 168*
    Monitoring Side Effects, 169

  *Evaluation of the Effectiveness of Pain
    Regimens, 175*
  Consequences of Untreated Pain, 175
Common Pain States in Children, 175
  Pain in Primary Care, 175
  Painful and Invasive Procedures, 176
  Postoperative Pain, 177
  Burn Pain, 177
  Recurrent Headaches, 177
  Recurrent Abdominal Pain, 178
  Pain with Sickle Cell Disease, 178
  Cancer Pain, 179
  Pain and Sedation in End-of-Life
    Care, 180

LEARNING OBJECTIVES

On completion of this chapter the reader will be able to:
- Identify measures to assess pain in children.
- List various types of pain assessment tools for use with children.
- Outline essential pain management strategies to reduce pain in children.

- Review common types of pain experienced by children.
- Discuss evidence to support specific pain management strategies.

PAIN ASSESSMENT

Many children and adolescents continue to suffer from inadequately treated pain of all types (Perquin, Hazebroek-Kampschreur, Hunfeld, and others, 2000a, 2000b). Several research studies suggest that the undertreatment of pain in children is related to inconsistent practice in pain assessment, administration of analgesics at subtherapeutic levels, prolonged intervals in between medications (Jacob and Puntillo, 2000), and lack of systematic monitoring and evaluation of relief (Jacob, Miaskowski, Savedra, and others, 2003a, 2003b; Jacob and Mueller, 2008). Optimal pain management begins with thorough assessment, which will guide the selection of treatments. Acute pain

---

BOX 7-1 DEVELOPMENTAL CHARACTERISTICS OF CHILDREN'S RESPONSES TO PAIN

Young Infant
- Generalized body response of rigidity or thrashing, possibly with local reflex withdrawal of stimulated area
- Loud crying
- Facial expression of pain (eyebrows lowered and drawn together, eyes tightly closed, and mouth open and squarish)
- No association demonstrated between approaching stimulus and subsequent pain

Older Infant
- Localized body response with deliberate withdrawal of stimulated area
- Loud crying
- Facial expression of pain or anger
- Physical resistance, especially pushing the stimulus away after it is applied

Young Child
- Loud crying, screaming
- Verbal expressions such as "Ow," "Ouch," "It hurts"
- Thrashing of arms and legs
- Attempts to push away stimulus before it is applied

- Lack of cooperation; need for physical restraint
- Requests termination of procedure
- Clings to parent, nurse, or other significant person
- Requests emotional support, such as hugs or other forms of physical comfort
- May become restless and irritable with continuing pain
- Behaviors occurring in anticipation of actual painful procedure

School-Age Child
- May see all the behaviors of a young child, especially during actual painful procedure but less in the anticipatory period
- Stalling behavior, such as "Wait a minute" or "I'm not ready"
- Muscular rigidity, such as clenched fists, white knuckles, gritted teeth, contracted limbs, body stiffness, closed eyes, wrinkled forehead

Adolescent
- Less vocal protest
- Less motor activity
- More verbal expressions, such as "It hurts" or "You're hurting me"
- Increased muscle tension and body control

Data from Craig KD, McMahon RJ, Morison JD, and others: Developmental changes in infant pain expression during immunization injections, *Soc Sci Med* 19(12):1331-1337, 1984; and Katz ER, Kellerman J, Siegel SE: Behavioral distress in children with cancer undergoing medical procedures: developmental considerations, *J Consult Clin Psychol* 48(3):356–365, 1980.

---

assessment is easier to perform than complex pain that may be chronic, recurrent, or persistent.

The assessment of pain needs to reflect the variations in children's cognitive, emotional, and physical capabilities (Box 7-1). Six core domains and specific measures to assess and measure pain in children are recommended: (1) pain intensity, (2) global judgment of satisfaction with treatment, (3) symptoms and adverse events, (4) physical recovery, (5) emotional response, and (6) economic factors (McGrath, Walco, Turk, and others, 2008). These domains will be discussed as they relate to assessment of acute, chronic, and recurrent pain.

ASSESSMENT OF ACUTE PAIN

Acute pain in children may be attributable to several causes such as medical procedures (immunization, venipuncture for blood draw or intravenous [IV] therapy, lumbar puncture for diagnosis or treatment, bone marrow aspiration, skin debridement for severe burns), surgical (appendectomy, tonsillectomy) and orthopedic (spinal fusion) procedures, medical treatments (chemotherapy-induced mucositis or peripheral neuropathy), injury (falls, burns, motor vehicle crashes, other traumatic injuries), infection, and exacerbation of disease-related pain (arthritis, sickle cell disease, cancer).

Pain Intensity

Traditionally, assessment measures are defined as behavioral measures, physiologic measures, and measures of self-reports. These measures predominantly address the domain of pain intensity. The behavioral measures of pain (for infants and children younger than 4 years; Table 7-1) and self-reports of pain (for children 4 years and older; Table 7-2) have been developed, validated, and widely used. Self-report measures are not sufficiently valid for children younger than 3 years of age because many are not able to accurately self-report their pain. Distress behaviors, such as vocalization, facial expression, and body movement, have been associated with pain (Figs. 7-1 and 7-2). These behaviors are helpful in evaluating pain in infants and children with

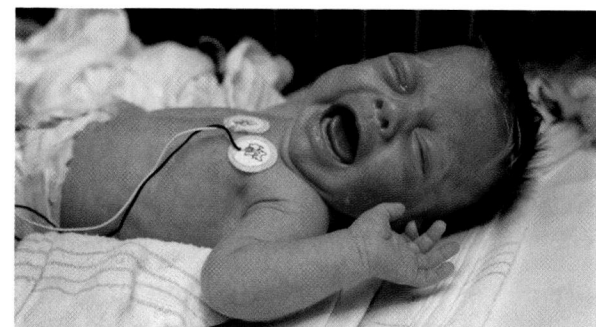

FIG 7-1 Full, robust crying of preterm infant after a heel stick. (Courtesy Halbouty Premature Nursery, Texas Children's Hospital, Houston; photo by Paul Vincent Kuntz.)

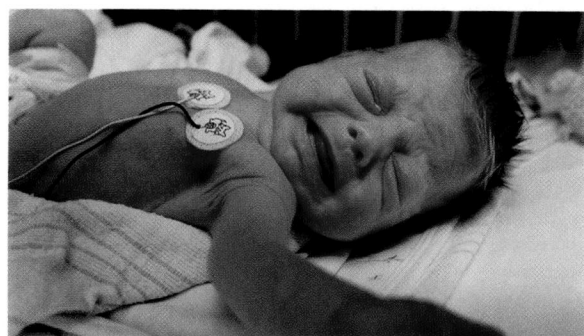

FIG 7-2 The face of pain after a heel stick. Note the eye squeeze, brow bulge, nasolabial furrow, and wide-spread mouth. (Courtesy Halbouty Premature Nursery, Texas Children's Hospital, Houston; photo by Paul Vincent Kuntz.)

TABLE 7-1	SUMMARY OF SELECTED BEHAVIORAL PAIN ASSESSMENT SCALES FOR YOUNG CHILDREN		
AGES OF USE	**RELIABILITY AND VALIDITY**	**VARIABLES**	**SCORING RANGE**
Objective Pain Score (OPS) (Hannallah, Broadman, Belman, and Others, 1987)			
4 mo–18 yr	Concurrent validity with linear analog pain scale, Spearman's r: 0.721 with scores ≥6 and 0.419 with scores <6 Interrater agreement, coefficient alpha: 0.986 for one rater and 0.983 for the other Concurrent validity with CHEOPS, Pearson correlation coefficient: 0.88 and 0.94	Blood pressure (0–2) Crying (0–2) Moving (0–2) Agitation (0–2) Verbal evaluation or body language (0–2)	0 = no pain; 10 = worst pain
Children's Hospital of Eastern Ontario Pain Scale (CHEOPS) (McGrath, Johnson, Goodman, and Others, 1985)			
1–5 yr	Interrater reliability: 90%–99.5% Internal correlation: significant correlations between pairs of items Concurrent validity between CHEOPS and visual analog scale (VAS): 0.91; between individual and total scores of CHEOPS and VAS: 0.50–0.86 Construct validity with preanalgesia and postanalgesia scores: 9.9–6.3	Cry (1–3) Facial (0–2) Child verbal (0–2) Torso (1–2) Touch (1–2) Legs (1–2)	4 = no pain; 13 = worst pain
Nurses Assessment of Pain Inventory (NAPI) (Stevens, 1990)			
Newborn–16 yr	Not tested by original author; later tested by Joyce, Schade, Keck, and others (1994) Interrater agreement: weighted kappa 0.37–0.80 Discriminant validity: statistically significant differences between preanalgesia and postanalgesia scores ($p <0.0001$) Reliability: Cronbach alpha: 0.35–0.69	Body movement (0–2) Facial (0–3) Touching (0–2)	0 = no pain; 7 = worst pain
Behavioral Pain Score (BPS) (Robieux, Kumar, Radhakrishnan, and Others, 1991)			
3–36 mo	Original article stated, "reliability of the VAS and BPS scores was tested by a k test"; no further testing of reliability or validity mentioned	Facial expression (0–2) Cry (0–3) Movements (0–3)	0 = no pain; 8 = worst pain
Modified Behavioral Pain Scale (MBPS) (Taddio, Nulman, Koren, and Others, 1995)			
4–6 mo	Concurrent validity between MBPS and VAS scores: correlation coefficient 0.68 ($p <0.001$) and 0.74 ($p <0.001$) Construct validity using prevaccination and postvaccination scores with EMLA vs. placebo: significantly lower scores with EMLA ($p <0.01$) Internal consistency of items: significant correlations between items Interrater agreement ICC: 0.95, $p <0.001$ Test–retest reliability: 0.95, $p <0.001$	Facial expression (0–3) Cry (0–4) Movements (0, 2, 3)	0 = no pain; 10 = worst pain
Riley Infant Pain Scale (RIPS) (Schade, Joyce, Gerkensmeyer, and Others, 1996)			
<36 mo and for children with cerebral palsy	Interrater agreement using intraclass correlation coefficient: 0.53–0.83, $p <0.0001$ Discriminant validity using Mann-Whitney U test with preanalgesia and postanalgesia scores: statistically significant ($p <0.001$) Sensitivity: 0.31–0.23 Specificity: 0.86–0.90 Interrater reliability using two-way cross-tabulations and kappa statistics (r[87] = 0.94; $p <0.001$) and kappa values above 0.50 for each category	0: Neutral face/smiling, calm, sleeping quietly, no cry, consolable, moves easily 1: Frowning/grimace, restless body movements, restless sleep, whimpering, winces with touch 2: Clenched teeth, moderate agitation, sleeps intermittently, difficult to console, cries with touch 3: Full cry expression, thrashing/flailing, sleeping prolonged periods interrupted by jerking or no sleep, screaming/high-pitched cry, inconsolable, screams when touched/moved	0 = no pain; 3 = worst pain

TABLE 7-1	**SUMMARY OF SELECTED BEHAVIORAL PAIN ASSESSMENT SCALES FOR YOUNG CHILDREN—cont'd**		

AGES OF USE	RELIABILITY AND VALIDITY	VARIABLES	SCORING RANGE
FLACC Postoperative Pain Tool (Merkel, Voepel-Lewis, Shayevitz, and Others, 1997)			
2 mo–7 yr	Validity using analysis of variance for repeated measures to compare FLACC scores before and after analgesia; preanalgesia FLACC scores significantly higher than postanalgesia scores at 10, 30, and 60 min (p <0.001 for each time) Correlation coefficients used to compare FLACC pain scores and OPS pain scores; significant positive correlation between FLACC and OPS scores (r = 0.80; p <0.001); positive correlation also found between FLACC scores and nurses' global ratings of pain (r[47] = 0.41; p <0.005)	Face (0–2) Legs (0–2) Activity (0–2) Cry (0–2) Consolability (0–2)	0 = no pain; 10 = worst pain

FLACC SCALE*			
	0	1	2
Face	No particular expression or smile	Occasional grimace or frown, withdrawn, disinterested	Frequent to constant frown, clenched jaw, quivering chin
Legs	Normal position or relaxed	Uneasy, restless, tense	Kicking or legs drawn up
Activity	Lying quietly, normal position, moves easily	Squirming, shifting back and forth, tense	Arched, rigid, or jerking
Cry	No cry (awake or asleep)	Moans or whimpers, occasional complaint	Crying steadily, screams or sobs, frequent complaints
Consolability	Content, relaxed	Reassured by occasional touching, hugging, or talking to; distractible	Difficult to console or comfort

*From Merkel SI, Voepel-Lewis T, Shayevitz JR, and others: The FLACC: a behavioral scale for scoring postoperative pain in young children, *Pediatr Nurs* 23(3):293–297, 1997. Used with permission of Jannetti Publications, Inc., and the University of Michigan Health System. Can be reproduced for clinical and research use.

limited communication skills. However, discriminating between pain behaviors and reactions from other sources of distress, such as hunger, anxiety, or other types of discomfort, is not always easy. These factors decrease the specificity and sensitivity of behavioral measures (see Table 7-1).

Behavioral assessment is useful for measuring pain in infants and preverbal children who do not have the language skills to communicate that they are in pain and in children with mental clouding and confusion that limit their ability to communicate meaningfully. Behavior provides important information that cannot be obtained from self-report. Behavioral assessment may provide a more complete picture of the total pain experience when administered in conjunction with a subjective self-report measure. However, behavioral pain scales may be more time consuming than self-reports. These measures depend on a trained observer to watch and record children's behaviors such as vocalization, facial expression, and body movements that suggest discomfort. Behaviors are assigned numbers from 0 to 4 to represent different intensities of distress. Scores are added to determine the child's pain rating.

Behavioral measures are most reliable when measuring short, sharp procedural pain, such as during injections or lumbar punctures, and in infants. They are less reliable when measuring longer-lasting pain and in older children, in whom pain scores on behavioral measures do not always correlate with the children's own reports of pain intensity. Behavioral pain measures have been developed and validated on short, sharp pain or on pain in the recovery room immediately after arousal from anesthesia.

The most commonly used behavioral pain measure is the FLACC. The FLACC Pain Assessment Tool (Manworren and Hynan, 2003;

Merkel, Voepel-Lewis, Shayevitz, and others, 1997) is an interval scale that includes five categories of behavior: facial expression (F), leg movement (L), activity (A), cry (C), and consolability (C). It measures pain by quantifying pain behaviors with scores ranging from 0 (no pain behaviors) to 10 (most possible pain behaviors). Other behavioral measures (see Table 7-1) include the Children's Hospital of Eastern Ontario Pain Scale (CHEOPS), which was developed in collaboration with experienced recovery room nurses who were queried as to what behaviors they most frequently observed to determine whether a child is in pain (McGrath, Vair, McGrath, and others, 1985; Suraseranivongse, Montapaneewat, Manon, and others 2005); the Toddler-Preschooler Postoperative Pain Scale (TPPPS), which is an observational scale developed for measuring postoperative pain in children ages 1 to 5 years (Suraseranivongse, Montapaneewat, Manon, and others, 2005; Tarbell, Cohen, and Marsh, 1992); the Parent's Postoperative Pain Rating Scale (PPPRS), which is a scale that parents may use to rate their children's pain by noting changes in the frequency of a number of behaviors (Chambers, 2003; Chambers and Craig, 1998; Finley, Chambers, McGrath, and others, 2003); and the Parents' Postoperative Pain Measure (PPPM), which was developed based on cues parents reported observing in their children after surgery (e.g., changes in appetite, activity level).

In critical care settings, the COMFORT scale (Ambuel, Hamlett, Marx, and others, 1992) is recommended. The COMFORT scale is a behavioral, unobtrusive method of measuring distress in unconscious and ventilated patients. It has eight indicators: alertness, calmness/agitation, respiratory response, physical movement, blood pressure, heart rate, muscle tone, and facial tension. Each indicator is scored between 1 and 5 based on the behaviors exhibited by the patient.

TABLE 7-2   PAIN RATING SCALES FOR CHILDREN

PAIN SCALE, DESCRIPTION	INSTRUCTIONS	RECOMMENDED AGE AND COMMENTS
FACES Pain Rating Scale* Consists of six cartoon faces ranging from smiling face for "no hurt" to tearful face for "hurts worst"	*Original instructions:* Explain to child that each face is for a person who feels happy because there is no pain (hurt) or sad because there is some or a lot of pain. FACE 0 is very happy because there is no hurt. FACE 1 hurts just a little bit. FACE 2 hurts a little more. FACE 3 hurts even more. FACE 4 hurts a whole lot, but FACE 5 hurts as much as you can imagine, although you don't have to be crying to feel this bad. Ask child to choose face that best describes own pain. Record number under chosen face on pain assessment record. *Brief word instructions:* Point to each face using the words to describe the pain intensity. Ask child to choose face that best describes own pain and record appropriate number.	Children as young as 3 yr Using original instructions without affect words, such as happy or sad, or brief words resulted in same range of pain rating, probably reflecting child's rating of pain intensity. For coding purposes, numbers 0, 2, 4, 6, 8, 10 can be substituted for 0–5 system to accommodate 0–10 system. The FACES provides three scales in one: facial expressions, numbers, and words. Research supports cultural sensitivity of FACES for white, African-American, Hispanic, Thai, Chinese, and Japanese children.

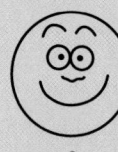 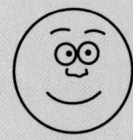 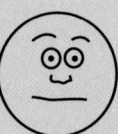 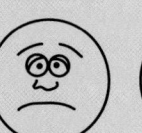 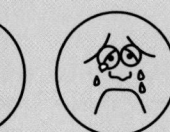

0 No hurt	1 or 2 Hurts little bit	2 or 4 Hurts little more	3 or 6 Hurts even more	4 or 8 Hurts whole lot	5 or 10 Hurts worst

Oucher (Beyer, Denyes, and Villarruel, 1992) Consists of six photographs of a white child's face representing "no hurt" to "biggest hurt you could ever have"; also includes vertical scale with numbers from 0 to 100; scales for African-American and Hispanic children have been developed (Villarruel and Denyes, 1991)	*Numeric scale:* Point to each section of scale to explain variations in pain intensity: "0 means no hurt." "This means little hurts" (pointing to lower part of scale, 1–29). "This means middle hurts" (pointing to middle part of scale, 30–69). "This means big hurts" (pointing to upper part of scale, 70–99). "100 means the biggest hurt you could ever have." Score is actual number stated by child. *Photographic scale:* Point to each photograph and explain variations in pain intensity using following language: first picture from the bottom is "no hurt," second is "a little hurt," third is "a little more hurt," fourth is "even more hurt than that," fifth is "pretty much or a lot of hurt," and sixth is "biggest hurt you could ever have." Score pictures from 0 to 5, with bottom picture scored as 0. *General:* Practice using Oucher by recalling and rating previous pain experiences (e.g., falling off bike). Child points to number or photograph that describes pain intensity associated with experience. Obtain current pain score from child by asking, "How much hurt do you have right now?"	Children 3–13 yr Use numeric scale if child can count off any two numbers or by tens (Jordan-Marsh, Yoder, Hall, and others, 1994). Determine whether child has cognitive ability to use photographic scale; child should be able to rate six geometric shapes from largest to smallest. Determine which ethnic version of Oucher to use. Allow child to select version of Oucher or use version that most closely matches physical characteristics of child. NOTE: Ethnically similar scale may not be preferred by child when given choice of ethnically neutral cartoon scale (Luffy and Grove, 2003).
Poker Chip Tool (Hester, Foster, Jordan-Marsh, and Others, 1998) Uses four red poker chips placed horizontally in front of child	Say to child: "I want to talk with you about the hurt you may be having right now." Align chips horizontally in front of child on bedside table, clipboard, or other firm surface. Tell child, "These are pieces of hurt." Beginning at chip nearest child's left side and ending at one nearest right side, point to chips and say, "This (first chip) is a little bit of hurt and this (fourth chip) is the most hurt you could ever have." For a young child or for any child who may not fully comprehend the instructions, clarify by saying, "That means this (1) is just a little hurt, this (2) is a little more hurt, this (3) is more yet, and this (4) is the most hurt you could ever have."	Children as young as 4 yr Determine whether child has cognitive ability to use numbers by identifying larger of any two numbers.

TABLE 7-2 PAIN RATING SCALES FOR CHILDREN—cont'd

PAIN SCALE, DESCRIPTION	INSTRUCTIONS	RECOMMENDED AGE AND COMMENTS
	Do not give children an option for 0 hurt. Research with Poker Chip Tool has verified that children without pain will so indicate by responses such as, "I don't have any." Ask child, "How many pieces of hurt do you have right now?" After initial use of Poker Chip Tool, some children internalize the concept "pieces of hurt." If child gives response such as "I have one right now," before you ask or before you lay out poker chips, record number of chips on Pain Flow Sheet. Clarify child's answer by statements such as "Oh, you have a little hurt? Tell me about the hurt."	
Word-Graphic Rating Scale[1] **(Tesler, Savedra, Holzemer, and Others, 1991)**		
Uses descriptive words (may vary in other scales) to denote varying intensities of pain	Explain to child, "This is a line with words to describe how much pain you may have. This side of the line means no pain, and over here the line means worst possible pain." (Point with your finger where "no pain" is, and run your finger along the line to "worst possible pain" as you say it.) "If you have no pain, you would mark like this." (Show example.) "If you have some pain, you would mark somewhere along the line, depending on how much pain you have." (Show example.) "The more pain you have, the closer to worst pain you would mark. The worst pain possible is marked like this." (Show example.) "Show me how much pain you have right now by marking with a straight, up-and-down line anywhere along the line to show how much pain you have right now." With millimeter rule, measure from the "no pain" end to mark and record this measurement as pain score.	Children 4–17 yr

No pain   Little pain   Medium pain   Large pain   Worst possible pain

| **Numeric Scale** | | |
| Uses straight line with end points identified as "no pain" and "worst pain" and sometimes "medium pain" in the middle; divisions along line marked in units from 0–10 (high number may vary) | Explain to child that at one end of line is 0, which means that person feels no pain (hurt). At other end is usually 5 or 10, which means the person feels worst pain imaginable. The numbers 1–5 or 1–10 are for very little pain to a whole lot of pain. Ask child to choose number that best describes own pain. | Children as young as 5 yr as long as they can count and have some concept of numbers and their values in relation to other numbers. Scale may be used horizontally or vertically. Number coding should be same as other scales used in facility. |

No pain   Worst pain
0 1 2 3 4 5 6 7 8 9 10

| **Visual Analog Scale (VAS) (Cline, Herman, Shaw, and Others, 1992)** | | |
| Defined as vertical or horizontal line that is drawn to certain length, such as 10 cm (4 in) and anchored by items that represent extremes of the subjective phenomenon, such as pain, that is measured | Ask child to place mark on line that best describes amount of own pain. With centimeter ruler, measure from "no pain" end to the mark and record this measurement as the pain score. | Children as young as 4.5 yr, preferably 7 yr Vertical or horizontal scale may be used. Research shows that children ages 3–18 yr least prefer VAS compared with other scales (Luffy and Grove, 2003; Wong and Baker, 1988). |

No pain   Worst pain

Continued

TABLE 7-2	PAIN RATING SCALES FOR CHILDREN—cont'd	
PAIN SCALE, DESCRIPTION	**INSTRUCTIONS**	**RECOMMENDED AGE AND COMMENTS**
Color Tool (Eland and Banner, 1999)		
Uses markers for child to construct own scale that is used with body outline	Present eight markers to child in random order. Ask child, "Of these colors, which color is like _____?" (the event identified by child as having hurt the most). Place the marker (represents severe pain) away from other markers. Ask child, "Which color is like a hurt but not quite as much as _____?" (the event identified by child as having hurt the most). Place this marker with the marker chosen to represent severe pain. Ask child, "Which color is like something that hurts just a little?" Place the marker with the other colors. Ask child, "Which color is like no hurt at all?" Show the four marker choices to the child in order from worst to no-hurt color. Ask child to show on body outlines where he or she hurts using markers chosen. After child has colored hurts, ask if they are current hurts or hurts from the past. Ask if child knows why the area hurts if it is not clear to you why it does.	Children as young as 4 yr, provided they know the colors, are not color blind, and are able to construct the scale if in pain

*Wong-Baker FACES Pain Rating Scale reference manual describing development and research of the scale is available from City of Hope Pain/Palliative Care Resource Center, 1500 East Duarte Road, Duarte, CA 91010; 626-359-8111, ext. 3829; fax 626-301-8941; http://www1.us.elsevierhealth.com/FACES/.

†Instructions for Word-Graphic Rating Scale from Acute Pain Management Guideline Panel: *Acute pain management in infants, children, and adolescents: operative and medical procedures; quick reference guide for clinicians,* ACHPR Pub No 92-0020, Rockville, Md, 1992, Agency for Health Care Research and Quality, U.S. Department of Health and Human Services. Word-Graphic Rating Scale is part of the Adolescent Pediatric Pain Tool and is available from Pediatric Pain Study, University of California, School of Nursing, Department of Family Health Care Nursing, San Francisco, CA 94143-0606; 415-476-4040.

Patients are observed unobtrusively for 2 minutes, and the total score is derived by adding the scores of each indicator. The total scores can range between 8 and 40. A score of 17 to 26 generally indicates adequate sedation and pain control. Because of the complexity of measuring blood pressure and heart rate, this scale is used primarily for patients in critical care settings.

For children ages 3 to 4 years, the most frequently used measure of pain intensity is a pictorial faces pain scale. There are many different "faces" scales. Faces pain scales provide a series of facial expressions depicting gradations of pain. They are appealing to children and easy to use because children can simply point to the face that represents how they feel. Two faces scales, the Bieri Faces Pain Scale–Revised (Hicks, von Baeyer, Spafford, and others, 2001) and the Wong-Baker FACES Pain Scale (Wong and Baker, 1988), are the most widely used. The Bieri scale is made up of six faces depicting increasing gradation of pain severity from 0 = "no pain" on the left face to 5 = "most pain possible" on the right face. In developing this scale, the authors did not include a smiling face at the "no pain" end or tears at the "most pain" end and validated it so that it is equivalent to a 0 to 10 metric system. The Wong-Baker FACES Pain Scale consists of six cartoon faces ranging from a smiling face for "no pain" to a tearful face for "worst pain." The child is asked to choose a face that describes his or her pain.

For children 8 years and older, the numerical rating scale (NRS), specifically the 0 to 10 scale, is most widely used in clinical practice because it is easy to use and document. However, there is little research to support the reliability and validity of the NRS, except in the context of the Oucher Pain Scale (see Table 7-2; Beyer, Turner, Jones, and others, 2005). The visual analog scale (VAS), a 10-cm line anchored by numbers or the words "no pain" on the left and "worst pain" on the right, is another measure of pain intensity with established reliability and validity (Tesler, Savedra, Holzemer, and others, 1991). It requires a higher degree of abstraction than the NRS, but it cannot be used in telephone follow-up.

Global Judgment of Improvement and of Satisfaction With Treatment

Although pain intensity is the dimension that is most commonly assessed, patients or patient surrogates should also be asked to rate a global judgment of satisfaction with pain treatment. The ratings will mean something different from one patient or surrogate to another. Whereas some may focus on the relief of pain, others may consider side effects of the treatment. The global question should be posed with indications of what should be considered in the answer, such as "Considering pain relief, side effects, physical recovery, and emotional recovery, how satisfied are you with the treatments your child is receiving for pain?"

Adverse Events and Symptoms

After pain medications are initiated, not only should pain intensity be reassessed, but treatment-emergent adverse events should also be evaluated. Adverse events refer to newly emerging signs, symptoms, laboratory findings, or diseases that occur after medications for pain are initiated. Constipation is the most frequent symptom and is often not assessed, particularly for patients on prolonged opioid treatments. There is no particular strategy to measure either the occurrence or the severity of the events. Children older than age 10 years may be able to provide this information. In younger children, parents or caregivers should be asked about adverse events and symptoms.

Physical Recovery

Another domain is physical recovery, which includes aspects of physical functioning that are influenced by the procedure or injury causing acute pain. For example, swallowing 50 ml of water is important after tonsillectomy. Possible assessments of the physical recovery domain include time to ambulation, time to resume swallowing, time to normal spirometry, oral intake, and time out of bed. However, measures such as tolerance of physical therapy may be inconsistent. One child may be intolerant of physical therapy because he or she did not want to go when asked, but another might be said to be intolerant of physiotherapy only if he or she cried and refused to continue with physical therapy. These measures of physical recovery should be systematically assessed for the purposes of evaluating interventions to control pain after procedures and injuries that have specific effects on physical functioning.

Emotional Response

The domain of emotional response includes all aspects of negative affect or distress secondary to pain, such as anxiety, depression, fear, distress, dysphoria, or unhappiness. Behaviors indicating avoidance, withdrawal, or resistance need to be assessed. In children 8 years of age and older, the PedIMMPACT group recommends the use of the Adolescent Pediatric Pain Tool (Savedra, Holzemer, Tesler, and others, 1993), which allows children to describe the quality of the pain using a word list. The 56 words are grouped according to sensory, affective, and evaluative qualities of pain; has been validated; and can be used for children 8 years of age and older.

ASSESSMENT OF CHRONIC AND RECURRENT PAIN

Pain that persists for 3 months or more or beyond the expected period of healing is defined as chronic pain (Merskey and Bogduk, 1994). Complex regional pain syndrome and chronic daily headache are most common chronic pain conditions in children. Pain that is episodic and reoccurs is defined as recurrent pain. The time frame within which episodes of pain recur is at least 3 months. Recurrent pain in children includes migraine headache, episodic sickle cell pain, recurrent abdominal pain (RAP), and recurrent limb pain. Van Dijk and colleagues (2006) reported that 57% of school-age children were having at least one recurrent pain (headaches, stomach pains, growing pains), and at least 6% had one or more chronic pain (disease related, back pain). Chronic and recurrent pain adversely affects the psychosocial and physical well-being of children. The domains for the assessment of chronic or recurrent pain are the same for acute pain (pain intensity, global judgment of satisfaction with treatment, symptoms and adverse events, physical functioning, emotional functioning, economic factors) and two additional domains (role functioning and sleep). Because the time course of chronic and recurrent pain is different from that of acute pain, measures used to assess chronic and recurrent pain must consider timing and duration as key factors.

Pain diaries are commonly used to assess pain symptoms and response to treatment in children and adolescents with recurrent and chronic pain (Dampier, Ely, Brodecki, and others, 2002a, 2002b; Ely, Dampier, Gilday, and others, 2002; Palermo and Valenzuela, 2003; Palermo, Valenzuela, and Stork, 2004; Stinson, Stevens, Feldman, and others, 2008; Stone, Broderick, Schwartz, and others, 2003). Most pain diaries use NRS or VAS with varying anchors such as faces scales or words. Children as young as 6 years have been included in diary studies. Conventional paper-and-pencil measures have been associated with several limitations such as poor compliance, missing data, hoarding of responses, and back and forward filling (Palermo and Valenzuela, 2003; Stone, Broderick, Schwartz, and others, 2003). An increasing number of studies are converting paper diaries into electronic diaries for use

in school-age children and adolescents with recurrent or chronic pain (Palermo, Valenzuela, and Stork, 2004; Stinson, Stevens, Feldman, and others, 2008; Stone, Broderick, Schwartz, and others, 2003). Electronic diaries were found to show higher accuracy of children's diary responses and higher compliance rates compared with the paper format. However, electronic diaries are more expensive and may have a number of logistical issues that must be resolved.

The PedIMMPACT group recommends the same approach for measuring global judgment of satisfaction with treatment and symptoms and adverse events. The physical functioning domain in chronic and recurrent pain is focused on activities of everyday life, such as sitting or walking, or on more vigorous activities such as running and other sports. The recommendation is to use a measure such as the Functional Disability Inventory (Walker and Greene, 1991) for assessing physical functioning in school-age children and adolescents. The Functional Disability Inventory assesses the child's ability to perform everyday physical activities and has established psychometric properties with different populations (Claar and Walker, 2006; Reid, Lang, and McGrath, 1997; Vervoort, Goubert, Eccleston, and others, 2006). For younger children (younger than 7 years of age), the PedsQL developed by Varni and colleagues (Varni, Seid, and Rode, 1999) is recommended for assessing the physical functioning domain as it relates to pain. The PedsQL is a multidimensional scale with both parent and child report versions. It assesses physical, emotional, social, and school functioning.

The emotional functioning domain most often refers to depression and anxiety because they are elevated in children with chronic and recurrent pain (Palermo, 2000). However, most children with chronic or recurrent pain do not have clinical levels of anxiety or depression. The Children's Depression Inventory (Kovacs, 1981) and the Revised Child Anxiety and Depression Scale (Chorpita, Yim, Moffitt, and others, 2000) have been used to assess anxiety and depression in children and adolescents with chronic or recurrent pain.

Chronic and recurrent pain can significantly interfere with the roles that children and adolescents perform, such as being a student, friend, and family member. School attendance is used as a measure of role functioning in school-age children with chronic or recurrent pain. Absence from school is an important measure of fulfillment of the role of student. Other measures such as the PedsQL (Varni, Seid, and Rode, 1999) and PedMIDAS (Hershey, Powers, Vockell, and others, 2001, 2004) have been validated for measurement of role functioning in children with chronic or recurrent pain.

Sleep disruption is also common in chronic and recurrent pain. More than half of children with pain-related conditions (headache, juvenile idiopathic arthritis, or sickle cell disease) report difficulties with sleeping (Palermo and Kiska, 2005; Walters and Williamson, 1999). Sleep diaries in which the child (or parent) keeps a record of the time to go to bed, fall asleep, and wake up are useful for assessment of pain interference with sleep. The sleep diary was validated using sleep actigraphy in healthy children ages 13 and 14 years (Gaina, Sekine, Chin, and others, 2004). In addition, the Sleep Habits Questionnaire (Owens, Spirito, and McGuinn, 2000) may be useful for assessing sleep behaviors in school-age children with chronic or recurrent pain.

MULTIDIMENSIONAL MEASURES

Several cognitive skills, such as measurement, classification, and seriation (the ability to accurately place in ascending or descending order), become explicit between approximately 7 and 10 years of age. Older children are able to use the 0 to 10 numeric rating scale that is currently used by adolescents and adults. However, the use of the 0 to 10 numeric

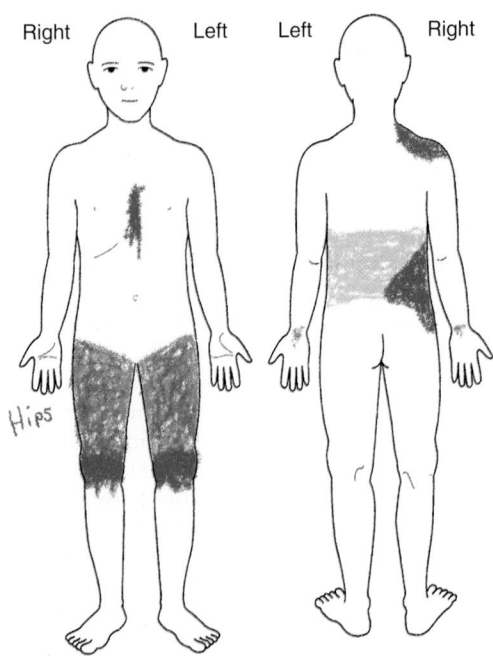

FIG 7-3 Adolescent Pediatric Pain Tool: body outlines for pain assessment. Instructions: "Color in the areas on these drawings to show where you have pain. Make the marks as big or as small as the place where the pain is." The tool has been completed by a child with sickle cell disease. (From Savedra MC, Tesler MD, Holzemer WL, Ward JA, School of Nursing, University of California–San Francisco; copyright 1989, 1992.)

rating scale is only an assessment of pain intensity, which may not change in some pain states (Jacob, Miaskowski, Savedra, and others, 2003a, 2003b). Other dimensions, such as pain quality, pain location, and spatial distribution of pain, may change without a change in pain intensity.

Two multidimensional assessment tools have been well validated in children ages 8 years and older that assess not only pain intensity but also pain location and pain quality. Modeled after the McGill Pain Questionnaire (Melzack, 1975), the **Adolescent Pediatric Pain Tool (APPT)** is a multidimensional pain instrument for children and adolescents that is used to assess three dimension of pain: location, intensity, and quality (Fig. 7-3). The APPT is a one-page, two-sided instrument with a front and back body outline on one side (Savedra, Tesler, Holzemer, and others, 1989, 1993). On the back side is a 100-mm word-graphic rating scale (Tesler, Savedra, Holzemer, and others, 1991) and a pain descriptor list (Wilkie, Holzemer, Tesler, and others, 1990). Each of the three components of the APPT is scored separately. The body outline is scored by placing a clear plastic template overlay with 43 body areas on the body outline diagram. An estimate of the pervasiveness of the pain is made by counting the number of body areas marked. A ruler or micrometer preprinted on the APPT is used to score the word-graphic rating scale. The number of millimeters from the left side of the scale to the point marked by the child is measured, and the numeric value provides an overall evaluation of the amount of pain the child is experiencing. The total number of words on the descriptor list is counted, and scores range from 0 to 56. The clinician then counts the number of words selected in each of three categories—evaluative (0–8), sensory (0–37), and affective (0–11)—and calculates a percentage score for each one (Savedra, Holzemer, Tesler, and others, 1993).

An advantage to using the APPT is that in some pain states, pain intensity ratings do not change, but pain location and spatial distribution of pain may decrease over time (Jacob, Miaskowski, Savedra, and others, 2003a, 2003b). The total surface area may decrease, but some children may perceive the remaining sites as equal in pain intensity. In addition to pain location, assessments of pain quality may be able to distinguish the presence of the different dimensions of pain (temporal, affective, evaluative, and sensory). Words may not be quantifiable on numeric rating scales yet represent the pain experience, such as *horrible* and *terrible* from the evaluative dimension, *screaming* and *terrifying* from the affective dimension, or *sharp* and *stabbing* from the sensory dimension. The different qualities of pain may also represent whether pain is of an ischemic and inflammatory nature in the cutaneous, subcutaneous, and musculoskeletal tissues as opposed to pain that is more neuropathic, which may be described using words such as *shooting, burning,* or *shocklike* (McCaffery and Pasero, 1999).

The Pediatric Pain Questionnaire (PPQ) is a multidimensional pain instrument used to assess patient and parental perceptions of the pain experience in a manner appropriate for the cognitive-developmental level of children and adolescents. The PPQ represents an attempt to assess the complexities of pediatric chronic, recurrent pain and targeted chronic musculoskeletal pain in children with juvenile rheumatoid arthritis. It consists of eight questions: (1) the pain history, (2) pain language, (3) the colors children associate with pain, (4) the emotions they experience, (5) their worst pain experiences, (6) the ways they cope with pain, (7) the positive aspects of pain, and (8) the location of their current pain. The PPQ includes three components: (1) VAS, (2) color-coded rating scales, and (3) verbal descriptors to provide information about the sensory, affective, and evaluative dimensions of chronic pain (Varni, Thompson, and Hanson, 1987). It also has information about the child's and family's pain history, symptoms, pain relief interventions, and socioenvironmental situations that may influence pain. The child, parent, and physician complete the form separately.

The number of pain measures available for use in infants and young children has increased dramatically and adds a layer of complexity to the assessment of pain in children. The current trend supports a common metric for measurement of pain in children (von Baeyer and Hicks, 2000). Most instruments consist of 0 for no pain to a range of 4 to 160 for the top anchors in pain measures. A pain score of 5 may mean a lot of pain (if a 0 to 5 scale is used) or very little (if a 0 to 100 scale is used), and it may not be clearly specified which score corresponds to which scale. Other health care providers who do not specialize in pediatric pain may be confused by the available instruments and scoring methods and may not be able to determine the effectiveness of interventions by the pain score documented. An advantage to using a common metric is that a certain score may be considered as the point at which an intervention is required or a point at which relief may be considered adequate (von Baeyer and Hicks, 2000). The 0 to 10 system was reported to be preferred by health care providers and would make pain scores easier to read, interpret, and integrate into research and practice.

ASSESSMENT OF PAIN IN SPECIFIC POPULATIONS

PAIN IN NEONATES

Assessment of pain in preverbal children is difficult, especially in neonates, because the most reliable indicator of pain, self-report, is not possible. Therefore, evaluation must be based on physiologic changes and behavioral observations (Box 7-2). Although behaviors such as vocalizations, facial expressions, body movements, and general

BOX 7-2 MANIFESTATIONS OF ACUTE PAIN IN NEONATES

Physiologic Responses

Vital signs: observe for variations
- Increased heart rate
- Increased blood pressure
- Rapid, shallow respirations

Oxygenation
- Decreased transcutaneous oxygen saturation ($tcPO_2$)
- Decreased arterial oxygen saturation (SaO_2)

Skin: observe color and character
- Pallor or flushing
- Diaphoresis
- Palmar sweating

Other observations
- Increased muscle tone
- Dilated pupils
- Decreased vagal nerve tone
- Increased intracranial pressure
- Laboratory evidence of metabolic or endocrine changes:
  - Hyperglycemia
  - Lowered pH
  - Elevated corticosteroids

Behavioral Responses

Vocalizations: observe quality, timing, and duration
- Crying
- Whimpering
- Groaning

Facial expression: observe characteristics, timing, orientation of eyes and mouth
- Grimaces
- Brow furrowed
- Chin quivering
- Eyes tightly closed
- Mouth open and squarish

Body movements and posture: observe type, quality, and amount of movement or lack of movement; relationship to other factors
- Limb withdrawal
- Thrashing
- Rigidity
- Flaccidity
- Fist clenching

Changes in state: observe sleep, appetite, activity level
- Changes in sleep–wake cycles
- Changes in feeding behavior
- Changes in activity level
- Fussiness, irritability
- Listlessness

relaxation state are common to all infants, they vary with different situations. Crying associated with pain is more intense and sustained (see Fig. 7-1). Facial expression is the most consistent and specific characteristic; scales are available to systematically evaluate facial features, such as eye squeeze, brow bulge, open mouth, and taut tongue (Hadjistavropoulos, Craig, Grunau, and others, 1997) (see Fig. 7-2). Most infants respond with increased body movements, but the infant may be experiencing pain even when lying quietly with the eyes closed. The preterm infant's response to pain may be behaviorally blunted

or absent; however, ample evidence indicates that such infants are neurologically capable of feeling pain. In addition, infants in awake or alert states demonstrate a more robust reaction to painful stimuli than infants in sleep states. Also, infants receiving muscle-paralyzing agents (e.g., vecuronium) are incapable of behavioral or visible pain responses.

Although regular use of pain assessment tools can better assist caregivers in determining whether the infant is in pain, caregivers must consider the infant's maturity, behavioral state, energy resources available to respond, and risk factors for pain. In infants with diminished ability to respond robustly to pain, it is imperative to presume that pain exists in all situations that are usually considered painful for adults and children even in the absence of behavioral or physiologic signs (Sweet and McGrath, 1998).

Several pain assessment tools have been developed for the assessment of pain in neonates (Table 7-3). One pain assessment tool used by nurses who work with premature and full-term infants in the neonatal intensive care setting is called CRIES, which is an acronym for the tool's physiologic and behavioral indicators of pain: crying, requiring increased oxygen, increased vital signs, expression, and sleeplessness. Each indicator is scored from 0 to 2—similar to the Apgar score for neonates. The total possible pain score, representing the worst pain, is 10. A pain score greater than 4 should be considered significant. This tool has been tested for reliability and validity for postoperative pain in infants between the ages of 32 weeks of gestation up to 20 weeks postterm (60 weeks) (Sweet and McGrath, 1998).

The Premature Infant Pain Profile (PIPP) is unique because it has been developed specifically for preterm infants (Sweet and McGrath, 1998). The category "gestational age at time of observation" gives a higher pain score to infants with lower gestational age. Infants who are asleep 15 seconds before the painful procedure also receive additional points for their blunted behavioral responses to painful stimuli.

The Neonatal Pain, Agitation, and Sedation Scale (NPASS) was originally developed to measure pain or sedation in preterm infants after surgery. It measures five criteria (see Table 7-3) in two dimensions (pain and sedation) and may be used in neonates as young as 23 weeks of gestation up to infants who are 100 days old. Extra points are added in the pain scale dimension for preterm infants based on gestational age.

CHILDREN WITH COMMUNICATION AND COGNITIVE IMPAIRMENT

The assessment of pain in children with communication and cognitive impairment can be challenging. Children who have significant difficulties in communicating with others about their pain include those with significant neurologic impairments (e.g., cerebral palsy), mental retardation, metabolic disorders, autism, severe brain injury, and communication barriers (e.g., critically ill children who are on ventilators or heavily sedated or have neuromuscular disorders, loss of hearing, or loss of vision). These children are at greater risk than other children for undertreatment of pain because they have medical problems that may cause pain and undergo painful procedures. Their behaviors include moaning, inconsistent patterns of play and sleep, changes in facial expression, and other physical problems that may mask expression of pain and be difficult to interpret (Hadden and von Baeyer, 2002). These children often experience spasticity, contractures, and orthopedic surgical treatment that may be painful.

The mother or primary caregiver is an important source of information during assessment (Breau, MacLaren, McGrath, and others, 2003). Up to 60% of parents of children with severe

TABLE 7-3	SUMMARY OF PAIN ASSESSMENT SCALES FOR INFANTS		
AGES OF USE	RELIABILITY AND VALIDITY	VARIABLES	SCORING RANGE
Postoperative Pain Score (POPS) (Barrier, Attia, Mayer, and Others, 1987)			
1–7 mo	Not tested by original authors; later tested by Joyce, Schade, Keck, and others (1994) High interrater agreement (reliability); discriminant validity (p <0.0001); reliability with high Cronbach alpha ranging from 0.79–0.88	Sleep (0–2) Flexion fingers/toes (0–2) Facial expression (0–2) Sucking (0–2) Quality of cry (0–2) Tone (0–2) Spontaneous motor activity (0–2) Consolability (0–2) Spontaneous excitability (0–2) Sociability (0–2)	0 = worst pain; 20 = no pain
Neonatal Infant Pain Scale (NIPS) (Lawrence, Alcock, Mcgrath, and Others, 1993)			
Average gestational age, 33.5 wk	Interrater reliability: 0.92 and 0.97 Construct validity using analysis of variance between before, during, and after procedure scores: F = 18.97, df = 2.42, p <0.001 Concurrent validity between NIPS and visual analog scale (VAS) using Pearson correlations: 0.53–0.84 Internal consistency using Cronbach alpha: 0.95, 0.87, and 0.88 for before, during, and after procedure scores	Facial expression (0–1) Arms (0–1) Cry (0–2) Legs (0–1) Breathing patterns (0–1) State of arousal (0–1)	0 = no pain; 7 = worst pain
Pain Assessment Tool (PAT) (Hodgkinson, Bear, Thorn, and Others, 1994)			
27 wk gestational age–full term	No reliability or validity discussed by original authors	Posture/tone (1–2) Respirations (1–2) Sleep pattern (0–2) Heart rate (1–2) Expression (1–2) Saturations (0–2) Color (0–2) Blood pressure (0–2) Cry (0–2) Nurse's perception (0–2)	4 = no pain; 20 = worst pain
Pain Rating Scale (PRS) (Joyce, Schade, Keck, and Others, 1994)			
1–36 mo	Interrater agreement: r = 0.65–0.84, p <0.0001 Discriminant validity: statistically significant t-tests (p <0.0001)	0: Smiling, sleeping, no change when moved/touched 1: Takes small amount orally, restless, moving, cries 2: Not drinking/eating, short periods of cries, distracted with rocking or pacifier 3: Change in behavior, irritable, arms/legs shake/jerk, facial grimace 4: Flailing, high-pitched wailing, parents request pain medication, unable to distract 5: Sleeping prolonged periods interrupted by jerking, continuous crying, rapid and shallow respirations	0 = no pain; 5 = worst pain
CRIES (Krechel and Bildner, 1995)			
32–60 wk of gestational age	Concurrent validity between CRIES and POPS: 0.73 (p <0.0001, n = 1382); Spearman correlation between subjective report and POPS and CRIES: 0.49 (p <0.0001, n = 1300) Discriminant validity using before and after analgesia scores: Wilcoxon sign rank test: mean decline of 3.0 units (p <0.0001, n = 74) Interrater reliability using Spearman correlation coefficient: r = 0.72 (p <0.0001, n = 680)	Crying (0–2) Requires increased oxygen (0–2) Increased vital signs (0–2) Expression (0–2) Sleepless (0–2)	0 = no pain; 10 = worst pain

TABLE 7-3 SUMMARY OF PAIN ASSESSMENT SCALES FOR INFANTS—cont'd

AGES OF USE	RELIABILITY AND VALIDITY	VARIABLES	SCORING RANGE
Premature Infant Pain Profile (PIPP) (Stevens, Johnston, Petryshen, and Others, 1996)			
28–40 wk of gestational age	Internal consistency using Cronbach alpha: 0.75–0.59; standardized item alpha for six items: 0.71 Construct validity using handling vs. painful situations: statistically significant differences (paired $t = 12.24$, two-tailed $p <0.0001$, and Mann-Whitney U = 765.5, $p <0.00001$) and using real versus sham heel stick procedures with infants ages 28–30 wk of gestational age ($t = 2.4$, two-tailed $p <0.02$, and Mann-Whitney U = 132, $p <0.016$) and with full-term boys undergoing circumcision with topical anesthetic versus placebo ($t = 2.6$, two-tailed $p <0.02$, or nonparametric equivalent Mann-Whitney U test, U = 145.7, two-tailed $p <0.02$)	Gestational age (0–3) Eye squeeze (0–3) Behavioral state (0–3) Nasolabial furrow (0–3) Heart rate (0–3) Oxygen saturation (0–3) Brow bulge (0–3)	0 = no pain; 21 = worst pain
Scale for Use in Newborns (SUN) (Blauer and Gerstmann, 1998)			
0–28 days	No reliability; face validity, content validity, construct validity using extreme groups	Central nervous system state (0–4) Movement (0–4) Breathing (0–4) Tone (0–4) Heart rate (0–4) Face (0–4) Mean blood pressure (0–4)	0 = no pain; 28 = worst pain Average baseline score 10–14 A 2 represents normal or baseline value
Neonatal Pain, Agitation, and Sedation Scale (NPASS) (Puchalski and Hummel, 2002)			
Birth (23 wk of gestational age) and full-term newborns ≤100 days	Interrater reliability using ICC: 0.95 confidence interval (CI) for preintervention and postintervention pain scale; 0.95 CI for preintervention and postintervention sedation scale Internal consistency (Cronbach alpha): Preintervention pain scale, 0.75 and 0.71 raters 1 and 2 Postintervention pain scale, 0.25 and 0.27 raters 1 and 2 Preintervention sedation scale, 0.88 and 0.81 raters 1 and 2 Postintervention sedation scale, 0.86 and 0.89 raters 1 and 2	Cry/irritability (0–2) Behavior/state (0–2) Facial expression (0–2) Extremities/tone (0–2) Vital signs—heart rate, respiratory rate, blood pressure, SaO_2 (0–2)	Pain score: 0 = no pain; 10 = intense pain Sedation score: 0 = no sedation; 10 = deep sedation

CRIES NEONATAL POSTOPERATIVE PAIN SCALE

	0	1	2
Crying	No	High pitched	Inconsolable
Requires oxygen for saturation >95%	No	<30%	>30%
Increased vital signs	Heart rate and blood pressure less than or equal to preoperative state	Heart rate and blood pressure increase <20% of preoperative state	Heart rate and blood pressure increase >20% of preoperative state
Expression	None	Grimace	Grimace/grunt
Sleepless	No	Wakes at frequent intervals	Constantly awake

cognitive impairments reported that their child experienced pain or severe discomfort that was not being effectively managed (Lenton, Stallard, Lewis, and others, 2001; Stallard, Williams, Velleman, and others, 2002). The most frequently reported pain behaviors are crying; being less active; seeking comfort; moaning; not cooperating; being irritable; being stiff, spastic, tense, or rigid; sleeping less; being difficult to satisfy or pacify; flinching or moving a body part away; and being agitated or fidgety (Hadden and von Baeyer, 2002). Parents also reported that some daily living activities, such as assisted stretching

and walking, independent standing, toileting, putting on splints, occupational therapy, range of motion, and physical therapy, were painful.

Stallard, Williams, Lenton, and others (2001) asked the parents of cognitively impaired and noncommunicative children to assess the presence, severity, and duration of their pain during a 2-week observation period. Parents reported that 84% experienced pain on 5 or more separate days, with 32% experiencing pain on 12 or more days. Of the 74 episodes that lasted longer than 30 minutes, 33.8% occurred at night. Most pain episodes were judged to last longer than 10 minutes, with 48% of the children having episodes lasting longer than 10 minutes on 5 or more days. Although the experience of pain was common among this group of children, none was receiving treatment for relief or management of pain.

The Non-communicating Children's Pain Checklist is a pain measurement tool specifically designed for children with cognitive impairments (Breau, McGrath, Camfield, and others, 2002). The scale discriminates between periods of pain and calm and can predict behavior during subsequent episodes of pain (Fig. 7-4). The scale consists of six subscales (vocal, social, facial, activity, body and limbs, physiological signs), which are scored based on the number of times the items are observed over a 10-minute period (0 = not at all, 1 = just a little, 2 = fairly often, 3 = very often).

Another tool, the Pain Indicator for Communicatively Impaired Children (PICIC), distinguishes between pain and nonpain in communicatively impaired children with life-threatening illnesses (Stallard, Williams, Velleman, and others, 2002). The PICIC has six core pain cues: (1) crying with or without tears; (2) screaming, yelling, groaning, or moaning; (3) a screwed up or distressed looking face; (4) body appearing stiff or tense; (5) difficulty in comforting or consoling; and (6) flinching or moving away if touched. The items are rated using a 4-point Likert scale (1 = not at all, 2 = a little, 3 = often, 4 = all the time).

CULTURAL DIFFERENCES

Several barriers to effective pain treatment in non–English-speaking patients have been documented and include inadequate assessment of pain, concern about side effects of and tolerance to analgesics, patient and family reluctance to report pain, fear that pain means worse disease, reluctance to take pain medications, and lack of adherence to prescribed analgesics (Abbe, Simon, Angiolilo, and others, 2006; Bruera, Willey, Ewert-Flannagan, and others, 2005; Flores, Abreu, Olivar, and others, 1998; Flores and Vega, 1998). Non–English-speaking patients pose additional language and cultural barriers that make pain assessment and treatments more challenging.

A major challenge in the assessment and management of pain in children is the cultural appropriateness of pain assessment tools that has been validated only in white and English-speaking children. Observational scales and interview questionnaires for pain may not be as reliable for pain assessment as self-report scales in Hispanic children. In Chinese children who learned to read Chinese characters vertically downward and from right to left, the use of vertically oriented VAS resulted in less error than horizontally oriented scales. Cultural background may therefore influence the reliability of pain assessment tools developed in a single cultural context (Bernstein and Pachter, 2003).

The Oucher Pain Scale (see Table 7-2), originally developed and validated as a self-report of pain intensity for white children 3 to 12 years old, now features culturally specific photographs with pictures of children who more closely match the physical characteristics of children (Beyer and Knott, 1998). The Oucher consists of a 0 to 10 numeric scale for older children and a six-picture photographic scale for younger children. The five versions of the Oucher are (1) White or Caucasian, (2) Black or African-American, (3) Hispanic, (4) First Nations (boy and girl), and (5) Asian (boy and girl). They can be downloaded free of charge at http://www.oucher.org and include instructions as well as information related to validity and reliability.

The Adolescent Pediatric Pain Tool also has a Spanish version (Van Cleve, Munoz, Bossert, and others, 2001) that has been used in children and adolescents with cancer (Jacob and Mueller, 2008; Van Cleve, Bossert, Beecroft, and others, 2004). Jacob and Mueller (2008) examined the pain experience of Spanish-speaking children with cancer who

were asked about their pain during the week before a scheduled oncology clinic appointment. They found that 41% of the patients were experiencing pain. Some were experiencing moderate to severe pain and did not receive medications because they were not reporting their pain. The APPT has a body outline that may be useful for non–English-speaking children to communicate the location and extensiveness of the pain. To minimize the risk of undertreatment of pain, non–English-speaking children and adolescents may be given the body outline diagram of the APPT, and clinicians may encourage them to use the body outline diagram for communicating their pain (Jacob and Mueller, 2008).

CHILDREN WITH CHRONIC ILLNESS AND COMPLEX PAIN

Questionnaires and pain assessment scales do not always provide the most meaningful means of assessing pain in children, particularly for those with complex pain. Some children cannot relate to a face or a number that describes their pain and may not be able to isolate pain from other concurrent symptoms they are experiencing. In children with cancer, experiencing multiple symptoms makes the task of having to isolate the pain symptom from other symptoms difficult. Rating the pain does not always accurately convey to others how they really feel (Woodgate and Yanofsky, 2004).

In children with chronic illness, particularly those with complex pain, the most important aspect of the assessment is the relationship developed between the child and the family, and it is in developing this relationship that the pain team gets the sense of what the pain experience is like for the child and family. The pain experience may interfere with the child's ability to eat, sleep, and perform daily activities and routines (Miaskowski and Lee, 1999; Morin, Gibson, and Wade, 1998). The pain experience may also be complicated by pain processes that occur in the central nervous system (CNS) (e.g., hyperalgesia, central sensitization, windup), by other symptoms (e.g., fatigue, nausea, vomiting, diarrhea, constipation) that accompany medical treatments, and by complications (e.g., infections, unexpected development of fistulas, typhlitis) from disease or treatments.

Other important questions to ask the family center around the onset of pain (Was the onset sudden, unexpected, off and on, or ongoing?); pain duration or pattern (When did the pain start? How long does pain last?); the effectiveness of the current treatment (What medications and doses help? What other strategies have you tried that work?); factors that aggravate or relieve the pain (What situations, positions, events, or activities make the pain worse? What makes the pain better?); other symptoms (e.g., nausea) and complications (e.g., fever, difficulty with breathing) that occur concurrently; and interference with the child's sleep, mood, function, and interactions with family (McCaffery and Pasero, 1999). Variations and rhythms of pain can also be assessed by asking if the pain is better or worse at certain times during the day or night. Other aspects warranting careful assessment that may pose barriers to effective management include family issues and relationships, fears and concerns about addictions (see Community Focus box, p. 175), the clinician's and family's lack of knowledge about pain, inappropriate use of pain medications, ineffective management of adverse effects from medications, and the use of different modalities (McCaffery and Pasero, 1999).

PAIN MANAGEMENT

Unrelieved pain may lead to potential long-term physiologic, psychosocial, and behavioral consequences (Goldschneider and Anand, 2003;

Non-communicating Children's Pain Checklist — Postoperative Version (NCCPC-PV)

NAME:_____ UNIT/FILE #: _____ DATE:_____ (dd/mm/yy)

OBSERVER:_____ START TIME:_____ AM/PM STOP TIME:_____ AM/PM

How often has this child shown these behaviours in the last 10 minutes? Please circle a number for each behaviour. If an item does not apply to this child (for example, this child cannot reach with his/her hands), then indicate "not applicable" for that item.

0 = NOT AT ALL	1 = JUST A LITTLE	2 = FAIRLY OFTEN	3 = VERY OFTEN	NA = NOT APPLICABLE

I. Vocal

	0	1	2	3	NA
1. Moaning, whining, whimpering (fairly soft)	0	1	2	3	NA
2. Crying (moderately loud)	0	1	2	3	NA
3. Screaming/yelling (very loud)	0	1	2	3	NA
4. A specific sound or word for pain (e.g., a word, cry, or type of laugh)	0	1	2	3	NA

II. Social

	0	1	2	3	NA
5. Not cooperating, cranky, irritable, unhappy	0	1	2	3	NA
6. Less interaction with others, withdrawn	0	1	2	3	NA
7. Seeking comfort or physical closeness	0	1	2	3	NA
8. Being difficult to distract, not able to satisfy or pacify	0	1	2	3	NA

III. Facial

	0	1	2	3	NA
9. A furrowed brow	0	1	2	3	NA
10. A change in eyes, including: squinching of eyes, eyes opened wide, eyes frowning	0	1	2	3	NA
11. Turning down of mouth, not smiling	0	1	2	3	NA
12. Lips puckering up, tight, pouting, or quivering	0	1	2	3	NA
13. Clenching or grinding teeth, chewing, or thrusting tongue out	0	1	2	3	NA

IV. Activity

	0	1	2	3	NA
14. Not moving, less active, quiet	0	1	2	3	NA
15. Jumping around, agitated, fidgety	0	1	2	3	NA

V. Body and Limbs

	0	1	2	3	NA
16. Floppy	0	1	2	3	NA
17. Stiff, spastic, tense, rigid	0	1	2	3	NA
18. Gesturing to or touching part of the body that hurts	0	1	2	3	NA
19. Protecting, favoring, or guarding part of the body that hurts	0	1	2	3	NA
20. Flinching or moving the body part away, being sensitive to touch	0	1	2	3	NA
21. Moving the body in a specific way to show pain (e.g., head back, arms down, curls up, etc.)	0	1	2	3	NA

VI. Physiological

	0	1	2	3	NA
22. Shivering	0	1	2	3	NA
23. Change in color, pallor	0	1	2	3	NA
24. Sweating, perspiring	0	1	2	3	NA
25. Tears	0	1	2	3	NA
26. Sharp intake of breath, gasping	0	1	2	3	NA
27. Breath holding	0	1	2	3	NA

Score Summary

Category	I	II	III	IV	V	VI	TOTAL
Score							

FIG 7-4 Non-communicating Children's Pain Checklist. (Copyright 2004, Lynn Breau, Patrick McGrath, Allen Finley, and Carol Camfield. Reprinted with permission.)

Continued

USING THE NCCPC-PV

The NCCPC-PV was designed to be used for children, aged 3 to 18 years, who are unable to speak because of cognitive (mental/intellectual) impairments or disabilities. It can be used *whether or not* a child has physical impairments or disabilities. Descriptions of the types of children used to validate the NCCPC-PV can be found in: Breau, L.M., Finley, G.A., McGrath, P.J. & Camfield, C.S. (2002). Validation of the Non-communicating Children's Pain Checklist — Postoperative Version. *Anesthesiology, 96* (3), 528-535. The NCCPC-PV was designed to be used without training by parents and caregivers (carers), or by other adults who are not familiar with a specific child (do not know them well).

The NCCPC-PV may be freely copied for clinical use or use in research funded by not-for-profit agencies. For-profit agencies should contact Lynn Breau: Pediatric Pain Research, IWK Health Centre, 5850 University Avenue, Halifax, Nova Scotia, Canada, B3J 3G9 (lbreau@ns.sympatico.ca).

The NCCPC-PV was intended for use for pain after surgery or due to other procedures conducted in hospital. If short- or long-term pain is suspected for a child at home or in a long-term residential setting, the **Non-communicating Children's Pain Checklist — Revised** may be used. It can be obtained by contacting Lynn Breau. Information regarding the NCCPC-R can be found in: Breau, L.M., McGrath, P.J., Camfield, C.S. & Finley, G.A. (2002). Psychometric Properties of the Non-communicating Children's Pain Checklist—Revised. *Pain, 99,* 349-357.

ADMINISTRATION

To complete the NCCPC-R, base your observations on the child's behavior over **10 minutes**. *It is not necessary to watch the child continuously for this period.* However, it is recommended that the observer be in the child's presence for the majority of this time (e.g., be in the same room with the child). Although shorter observation periods may be used, the cut-off scores described below may not apply.

At the end of the observation time, indicate how frequently (how often) each item was seen or heard. This should not be based on the child's typical behavior or in relation to what he or she usually does. A guide for deciding the frequency of items is below:

> 0 = Not present at all during the observation period. (Note: If the item is not present because the child is not capable of performing that act, it should be scored as "NA").
> 1 = Seen or heard rarely (hardly at all), but is present.
> 2 = Seen or heard a number of times, but not continuous (not all the time).
> 3 = Seen or heard often, almost continuous (almost all the time); anyone would easily notice this if they saw the child for a few moments during the observation time.
> NA = Not applicable. This child is not capable of performing this action.

SCORING

1. Add up the scores for each subscale and enter below that subscale number in the Score Summary at the bottom of the sheet. Items marked "NA" are scored as "0" (zero).
2. Add up all subscale scores for Total Score.
3. Check whether the child's score is greater than the cut-off score.

CUT-OFF SCORE

Based on the scores of 24 children aged 3 to 18 (Breau, Finley, McGrath & Camfield, 2002), a **Total Score of 11 or more** indicates a child has **moderate to severe pain**. Based on unpublished data from this same sample, a *Total score of 6-10* indicates a child has **mild pain**. When parents and caregivers completed the NCCPC-PV in hospital for the study group, this was accurate 88% of the time. When other observers completed the NCCPC-PV, this was accurate 75% of the time. A Total Score of 10 or less indicates less than moderate/severe pain. This was correct in the study group for parents and caregivers 81% of the time, and for other observers 63% of the time.

USE OF CUT-OFF SCORES

As with all observational tools, caution should be taken in using cut-off scores, because they may not be 100% accurate. They should not be used as the only basis for deciding whether a child should be treated for pain. In some cases children may have lower scores when pain is present. For more detailed instructions for use of the NCCPC-PV in such situations, please refer to the full manual, available from Lynn Breau: Pediatric Pain Research, IWK Health Centre, 5850 University Avenue, Halifax, Nova Scotia, Canada, B3J 3G9 (lbreau@ns.sympatico.ca).

FIG 7-4, cont'd

Weisman, Bernstein, and Schechter, 1998). Management of pain should be a priority for all clinicians.

NONPHARMACOLOGIC MANAGEMENT

Pain is often associated with fear, anxiety, and stress. A number of nonpharmacologic techniques (see Nursing Care Guidelines box), such as distraction, relaxation, guided imagery, and cutaneous stimulation, provide coping strategies that may help reduce pain perception, make pain more tolerable, decrease anxiety, and enhance the effectiveness of analgesics or reduce the dosage required (Rusy and Weisman, 2000). In addition, these techniques decrease the perceived threat of pain, provide a sense of control, enhance comfort, and promote rest and sleep (McCaffery and Pasero, 1999). Although there is a paucity of research on the effectiveness of many of these interventions, the strategies are safe, noninvasive, and inexpensive, and most are independent nursing functions. Environmental and psychologic factors may exert a powerful influence on children's pain perceptions and may be modified by using psychosocial strategies, education, parental support, and cognitive-behavioral interventions. For children undergoing repeated painful procedures, cognitive-behavioral interventions are effective for decreasing anxiety and distress (McGrath and Hillier, 2003).

If the child cannot identify a familiar coping technique, the nurse can describe several strategies and let the child select the most appealing one. Experimentation with several strategies that are suitable to the child's age, pain intensity, and abilities is often necessary to determine the most effective approach. Parents should be involved in the selection process; they may be familiar with the child's usual coping skills and can help identify potentially successful strategies. Involving the parents also encourages their participation in learning the skill with the child and acting as coach. If the parent cannot assist the child, other appropriate persons may include a grandparent, older sibling, nurse, or child-life specialist (McGrath and Hillier, 2003).

Children should learn to use a specific strategy before pain occurs or before it becomes severe. To reduce the child's effort, instructions for a strategy, such as distraction or relaxation, can be audiotaped and played during a period of comfort. However, even after they have learned an intervention, children often need help using it during a painful procedure. The intervention can also be used after the procedure. This gives the child a chance to recover, feel mastery, and cope more effectively (McGrath and Hillier, 2003).

Several studies have documented the effectiveness of nonpharmacologic analgesia, such as containment, positioning, nonnutritive sucking (Fig. 7-5), and kangaroo holding in neonates during painful

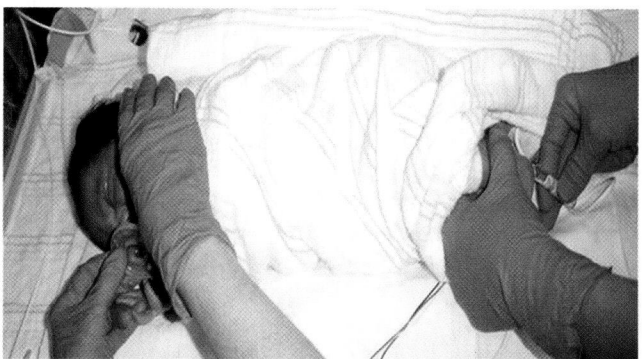

FIG 7-5 Sucking following oral sucrose can enhance analgesia before a heel stick in a preterm infant.

procedures. Containment is achieved through positioning and blanket rolls (Cole and Jorgensen, 1997). It provides a "nest" that enhances the infant's feelings of security and decreases stress. Comforting measures and swaddling have been demonstrated to reduce crying and heart rate after procedures such as heel punctures and injections. In infants between 27 and 34 weeks of gestational age, infants who were swaddled after a routine heel stick procedure were able to calm crying immediately, decrease their heart rate, and return to a sleep state; in comparison, infants who were not swaddled took a minimum of 10 minutes to return to baseline physiologic and behavioral levels (Fearon, Kisilevsky, Hains, and others, 1997). Proper positioning with the infant held in a midline orientation, hand-to-mouth activity, and proper flexion can promote self-soothing behaviors. "Facilitated tucking," which is holding the infant's extremities flexed and contained close to the trunk, during heel lance procedures has been demonstrated to decrease the heart rate, decrease crying time, and promote stability in the sleep–wake cycles after the lance.

Nonnutritive sucking (pacifier) attenuates behavioral, physiologic, and hormonal responses to pain from procedures such as heel punctures, venipuncture, and immunization injections. The administration of concentrated sucrose with and without nonnutritive sucking has been demonstrated to have calming and pain-relieving effects for invasive procedures in neonates (see Evidence-Based Practice box). The amount of time crying was decreased with 0.24 to 0.48 g (0.008–0.17 oz; 2 ml of a 12% to 24% sucrose solution) administered orally 2 minutes before a heel lance or venipuncture (Stevens, Yamada, and Ohlsson, 2005).

Kangaroo care is skin-to-skin holding of infants dressed only in diapers against their mother's or father's chest (Gray, Watt, and Blass, 2000; Johnston, Stevens, Pinelli, and others, 2003). Infants who spent 1 to 3 hours in kangaroo care showed increased frequency in quiet sleep, longer duration of quiet sleep, and decreased crying in the neonatal intensive care unit (NICU), and they cried less at the age of 6 months compared with neonates who did not receive skin-to-skin contact. Significant differences were found in pain responses during heel lancing between infants who were kangaroo held and those who were not. In the study by Gray, Watt, and Blass (2000), heart rate increased by 8 to 10 beats/min in the kangaroo care group versus 36 to 38 beats/min in the control group of neonates who were swaddled in bassinets; grimacing was 64% less, and crying was 82% less. In another study, infant responses to pain during heel lance procedures were compared using kangaroo holding (Fig. 7-6) with the neonate held upright at a 60-degree angle between the mother's breasts for maximal skin-to-skin contact (Johnston, Stevens, Pinelli, and others, 2003). A blanket was placed over the neonate's back, and the mother's clothes were wrapped around the neonate for 30 minutes before the lancing procedure, during, and at least 30 minutes after the heel stick. Another group remained in the isolette in a prone position, swaddled with a blanket and the heel accessible, for 30 minutes before the heel lancing procedure. Pain scores were significantly lower in kangaroo-held infants.

Many terms are used to describe approaches to health care that are outside the realm of conventional medicine as practiced in the United States. Complementary and alternative medicine (CAM), as defined by the National Center for Complementary and Alternative Medicine, is a group of diverse medical and health care systems, practices, and products that are not currently considered part of conventional medicine (Myers, Stuber, Bonamer-Rheingans, and others, 2005). Although some scientific evidence exists regarding some CAM therapies, for most, key questions are yet to be answered through well-designed scientific studies—questions such as whether these therapies are safe

NURSING CARE GUIDELINES

Nonpharmacologic Strategies for Pain Management

General Strategies

- Prepare the child before potentially painful procedures but avoid "planting" the idea of pain.
  - For example, instead of saying, "This is going to (or may) hurt," say, "Sometimes this feels like pushing, sticking, or pinching, and sometimes it doesn't bother people. Tell me what it feels like to you."
  - Use "nonpain" descriptors when possible (e.g., "It feels like heat" rather than "It's a burning pain"). This allows for variation in sensory perception, avoids suggesting pain, and gives the child control in describing reactions.
  - Avoid evaluative statements or descriptions (e.g., "This is a terrible procedure" or "It really will hurt a lot").
- Stay with child during a painful procedure.
  - Allow parents to stay with child if child and parent desire; encourage the parent to talk softly to child and to remain near the child's head.
- Educate the child about the pain, especially when explanation may lessen anxiety (e.g., that pain may occur after surgery and does not indicate something is wrong); reassure the child that he or she is not responsible for the pain.
- For long-term pain control, give child a doll, which represents "the patient" and allow the child to do everything to the doll that is done to the child; pain control can be emphasized through the doll by stating, "Dolly feels better after the medicine."

Specific Strategies

Distraction

- Involve the child in play; use a radio, tape recorder, CD player, or computer game; have the child sing or use rhythmic breathing.
- Have the child take a deep breath and blow it out until told to stop.
- Have the child blow bubbles to "blow the hurt away."
- Have the child concentrate on yelling or saying "ouch" with instructions to "yell as loud or soft as you feel it hurt; that way I know what's happening."
- Have the child look through a kaleidoscope (the type with glitter suspended in a fluid-filled tube) and encourage him or her to concentrate by asking, "Do you see the different designs?"
- Use humor, such as watching cartoons, telling jokes or funny stories, or acting silly with child.
- Have the child read, play games, or visit with friends.

Relaxation

- With an infant or young child:
  - Hold the child in a comfortable, well-supported position, such as vertically against the chest and shoulder.
  - Rock in a wide, rhythmic arc in a rocking chair or sway back and forth rather than bouncing the child.
  - Repeat one or two words softly, such as "Mommy's here."
- With a slightly older child:
  - Ask the child to take a deep breath and "go limp as a rag doll" while exhaling slowly; then ask the child to yawn (demonstrate if needed).
  - Help the child assume a comfortable position (e.g., a pillow under the neck and knees).

- Begin progressive relaxation: starting with the toes, systematically instruct the child to let each body part "go limp" or "feel heavy"; if child has difficulty relaxing, instruct the child to tense or tighten each body part and then relax it.
- Allow the child to keep the eyes open because children may respond better if their eyes are open rather than closed during relaxation.

Guided Imagery

- Have the child identify some highly pleasurable real or imaginary experience.
- Have the child describe details of the event, including as many senses as possible (e.g., "feel the cool breezes," "see the beautiful colors," "hear the pleasant music").
- Have the child write down or tape record a script.
- Encourage the child to concentrate only on the pleasurable event during the painful time; enhance the image by recalling specific details through reading the script or playing the tape.
- Combine with relaxation and rhythmic breathing.

Positive Self-Talk

- Teach the child positive statements to say when in pain (e.g., "I will be feeling better soon," "When I go home, I will feel better, and we will eat ice cream").

Thought Stopping

- Identify positive facts about the painful event (e.g., "It does not last long").
- Identify reassuring information (e.g., "If I think about something else, it does not hurt as much").
- Condense positive and reassuring facts into a set of brief statements and have the child memorize them (e.g., "Short procedure, good veins, little hurt, nice nurse, go home").
- Have the child repeat the memorized statements whenever thinking about or experiencing the painful event.

Behavioral Contracting

- Informal—May be used with children as young as 4 or 5 years of age:
  - Use stars, tokens, or cartoon character stickers as rewards.
  - Give a child who is uncooperative or procrastinating during a procedure a limited time (measured by a visible timer) to complete the procedure.
  - Proceed as needed if the child is unable to comply.
  - Reinforce cooperation with a reward if the procedure is accomplished within the specified time.
- Formal—Use a written contract, which includes:
  - A realistic (seems possible) goal or desired behavior
  - Measurable behavior (e.g., agrees not to hit anyone during procedures)
  - A contract written, dated, and signed by all persons involved in any of the agreements
  - Identified rewards or consequences that are reinforcing
  - Goals that can be evaluated
  - Commitment and compromise requirements for both parties (e.g., while the timer is used, the nurse will not nag or prod the child to complete the procedure)

Carol Turnage Carrier; Updated by Olga A. Taylor

EVIDENCE-BASED PRACTICE
Reduction of Minor Procedural Pain in Infants*

Ask the Question
PICOT Question
In newborns and infants, does sucrose provide adequate analgesia during minor painful procedures? Are the effects age dependent?

Search for the Evidence
Search Strategies
Search selection criteria included English publications within past 10 years, research-based articles (level 1 or lower) on neonates or infants undergoing venipuncture or immunizations.

Databases Used
PubMed, Cochrane Collaboration, MD Consult, Joanna Briggs Institute, National Guideline Clearinghouse (AHQR), TRIP Database Plus, PedsCCM, BestBETs

Critically Analyze the Evidence
Studies evaluated whether sucrose provides adequate analgesia for minor painful procedures.

Venipuncture versus heel lance for blood sampling
- Venipuncture performed by skilled phlebotomists results in less pain than heel stick for blood sampling (Shah and Ohlsson, 2004).
- Decreased pain scores, cry duration, and mother's rating of infant's pain demonstrated venipuncture as the preferred method of blood collection (Shah and Ohlsson, 2004).
- Infants receiving heel stick may also require more than one stick to get enough for the sample; venipuncture reduces the risk of additional sticks (Shah and Ohlsson, 2004).

Glucose versus EMLA cream for venipuncture in neonates
- 30% oral glucose and placebo on the skin group had significantly lower Premature Infant Pain Profile (PIPP) scores and duration of crying than the EMLA (lidocaine and prilocaine) and oral placebo group (Gradin, Lenclen, Gajdos, and others, 2002).
- Fewer patients in the glucose group were scored on the PIPP as having pain or a score above 6 (19.3% compared with 41.7%) (Gradin, Lenclen, Gajdos, and others, 2002).

Glucose compared with EMLA for venipuncture pain
- Combination of EMLA and 1 ml oral glucose (300 mg/ml) significantly reduced pain response associated with diphtheria–pertussis–tetanus immunizations in 3-month-old infants (Lindh, Wiklund, Blomquist, and others, 2003).

Sucrose for minor painful procedures (heel lance and venipuncture)
- A total of 150 full-term newborns were randomly assigned to one of six treatment groups: (1) no treatment, (2) 2 ml of sterile water placebo, (3) 2 ml of 30% glucose, (4) 2 ml of 30% sucrose, (5) 2 ml of 30% sucrose with pacifier, and (6) pacifier alone. The pacifier alone was more effective than sweet solutions, sweet solutions and the pacifier were significantly more effective than the placebo, and sucrose and glucose were equally effective in lowering pain scores (Carbajal, Chauvet, Couderc, and others, 1999).
- Behavioral state, difficulty, and duration of venipuncture were not significantly different between 2 ml of a placebo of sterile water or 25% sucrose slowly over 2 minutes into the mouth by syringe 4 minutes before

venipunctures. Heart rate, crying times, and neonatal facial coding system scores were significantly lower in the treatment group (25% sucrose) (Acharya, Annamali, Taub, and others, 2004).
- 2 ml of 24% sucrose solution alone was the most effective analgesic compared with placebo (spring water), EMLA, or EMLA combined with 2 ml of sucrose. The combination of EMLA and sucrose did not enhance the analgesic effects (Abad, Diaz-Gomez, Domenech, and others, 2001).
- Sucrose in a wide variety of dosages delivered by syringe or pacifier was found to decrease crying time, heart rate, facial action, and composite pain scores during venipuncture and heel lance (Stevens, Yamada, and Ohlsson, 2005).
- Use of sucrose in a range of 0.012 to 0.12 g (0.05 to 0.5 ml) of a 24% solution 2 minutes before a single heel lance or venipuncture is safe and effective for pain relief (Stevens, Yamada, and Ohlsson, 2005).
- Concomitant use of other methods of pain relief, including use of pacifier, rocking, kangaroo care, or holding along with sucrose intervention, is recommended (Stevens, Yamada, and Ohlsson, 2005).

Apply the Evidence: Nursing Implications
There is **good evidence** with **strong recommendation** (Guyatt, Oxman, Vist, and others, 2008) for using sucrose to provide adequate analgesia during minor painful procedures. Sucrose is effective in reducing pain response in infants 6 months of age and younger undergoing minor acute painful procedures. The most effective dose has been 24% solution given at least 2 minutes before a procedure. Doses of 50% to 75% have been effective for relieving pain during immunizations in infants up to 6 months of age, suggesting that higher concentrations may be required for older infants. Effective dose volumes range from 0.05 to 2 ml, with lower volumes used for low-birth-weight infants and larger volumes used for older infants. Sucrose in combination with nonpharmacologic support during a procedure may increase the analgesic response for older infants (2 months) even with lower concentrations of sucrose. Interventions include using a pacifier, holding, swaddling, skin-to-skin contact, and rocking. Administration can be by a labeled oral syringe, dipped pacifier, or bottle, depending on the infant's ability and age. Comparisons between sucrose and glucose have been inconclusive.

QSEN Quality and Safety Competencies:
Evidence-Based Practice*
Knowledge
Differentiate clinical opinion from research and evidence-based summaries.
Describe the use of sucrose to provide analgesia during minor painful procedures.

Skills
Base the individualized care plan on patient values, clinical expertise, and evidence.
Integrate evidence into practice by using sucrose for analgesia during minor painful procedures.

Attitudes
Value the concept of evidence-based practice (EBP) as integral to determining best clinical practice.
Appreciate strengths and weakness of evidence for sucrose use during minor painful procedures.

*Adapted from the QSEN at http://www.qsen.org.

Continued

EVIDENCE-BASED PRACTICE

Reduction of Minor Procedural Pain in Infants—cont'd

References

Abad F, Diaz-Gomez NM, Domenech E, and others: Oral sucrose compares favorably with lidocaine-prilocaine cream for pain relief during venepuncture in neonates, *Acta Paediatr* 90:160–165, 2001.

Acharya AB, Annamali S, Taub NA, and others: Oral sucrose analgesia for preterm infant venepuncture, *Arch Dis Child Fetal Neonatal Educ* 89:F17–F18, 2004.

Carbajal R, Chauvet X, Couderc S, and others: Randomised trial of analgesic effects of sucrose, glucose, and pacifiers in term neonates, *BMJ* 319(7222):1393–1397, 1999.

Gradin M, Lenclen R, Gajdos V, and others: Crossover trial of analgesic efficacy of glucose and pacifier in very preterm neonates during subcutaneous injections, *Pediatrics* 110(6):1053–1057, 2002.

Guyatt GH, Oxman AD, Vist GE, and others: GRADE: an emerging consensus on rating quality of evidence and strength of recommendations, *BMJ* 336:924–926, 2008.

Lindh V, Wiklund U, Blomquist HK, and others: EMLA cream and oral glucose for immunization pain in 3-month old infants, *Pain* 104(1–2):381–388, 2003.

Shah V, Ohlsson A: Venipuncture versus heel lance for blood sampling in term neonates, *Cochrane Database Syst Rev* (4):CD001452.pub2; DOI: 10.1002/14651858.CD001452.pub2, 2004.

Stevens B, Yamada J, Ohlsson A: *Sucrose for analgesia in newborn infants undergoing painful procedures* [review], 2005. In Cochrane Neonatal Collaboration, retrieved April 16, 2009, from http://www.thecochranelibrary.com.

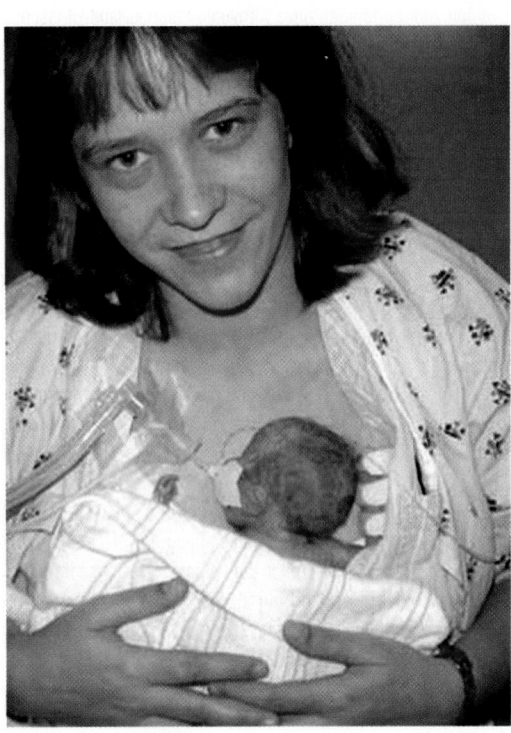

FIG 7-6 Mother using kangaroo hold with her newborn infant. Note the placement of the infant directly on the mother's skin.

and whether they work for the diseases or medical conditions for which they are used.

Complementary and alternative medicine therapies may be grouped into five classes: (1) biologically based (foods, special diets, herbal or plant preparations, vitamins, other supplements), (2) manipulative treatments (chiropractic, osteopathy, massage), (3) energy based (Reiki, bioelectric or magnetic treatments, pulsed fields, alternating and direct currents), (4) mind–body techniques (mental healing, expressive treatments, spiritual healing, hypnosis, relaxation), and (5) alternative medical systems (homeopathy, naturopathy, ayurvedic, traditional Chinese medicine that includes acupuncture and moxibustion).

Current estimates of pediatric CAM use range from 10% to 15%, derived from children sampled at health care facilities with chronic conditions or from countries other than the United States. For the U.S. population, pediatric CAM use was estimated to be 31% to 84% (Myers, Stuber, Bonamer-Rheingans, and others, 2005; Rusy and Weisman, 2000). Those who used CAM were found in each age group,

and the mean age was 10.3 years. The majority used unconventional therapy for chronic, as opposed to life-threatening, medical conditions. The therapies that are increasingly used include herbal medicine, massage, megavitamins, self-help groups, folk remedies, energy healing, and homeopathy (Myers, Stuber, Bonamer-Rheingans, and others, 2005; Rusy and Weisman, 2000).

PHARMACOLOGIC MANAGEMENT

For mild pain (<3 on 0 to 10 scale) or moderate pain (4 to 6 on 0 to 10 scale), acetaminophen (Tylenol, paracetamol) and nonsteroidal antiinflammatory drugs (NSAIDs) are suitable (Table 7-4). For moderate (5 to 6) to severe pain (7 to 10 on 0 to 10 scale), opioids are needed (Table 7-5). A combination (acetaminophen with codeine) works better in some cases because **nonopioids** act at the peripheral nervous system, and **opioids** act at the CNS (Table 7-6). Oxycodone is available without a nonopioid in an immediate release and controlled release preparation (OxyContin). Morphine is considered the gold standard for the management of severe pain. When morphine is not a suitable opioid, drugs such as hydromorphone (Dilaudid) and fentanyl (Sublimaze) are effective substitutes. Although fentanyl is used as an anesthetic in the operating room, it is classified as an analgesic. It can be safely administered by nurses by the IV, intramuscular (IM), transmucosal, and transdermal routes (Algren, Gursoy, Johnson, and others, 1998; Golianu, Krane, Galloway, and others, 2000).

> **! NURSING ALERT**
>
> The optimum dosage of an analgesic is one that controls pain without causing severe side effects. This usually requires titration, the gradual adjustment of drug dosage (usually by increasing the dose) until optimum pain relief without excessive sedation is achieved. Dosage recommendations are only safe initial dosages (see Tables 7-5 and 7-6), not optimum dosages.

Several drugs, known as **coanalgesics** or **adjuvant analgesics**, may be used alone or with opioids to control pain symptoms and opioid side effects. Drugs frequently used to relieve anxiety, cause sedation, and provide amnesia are diazepam (Valium) and midazolam (Versed). However, these drugs are not analgesics and should be used to enhance the effects of analgesics and not as a substitute for analgesics. Other adjuvants include tricyclic antidepressants (TCAs, e.g., amitriptyline, imipramine) and antiepileptics (e.g., gabapentin, carbamazepine, clonazepam) for neuropathic pain, stool softeners and laxatives for constipation, antiemetics for nausea and vomiting, diphenhydramine for itching, steroids for inflammation and bone pain, and

TABLE 7-4	NONSTEROIDAL ANTIINFLAMMATORY DRUGS (NSAIDS) APPROVED FOR CHILDREN*†	
DRUG	**DOSAGE**	**COMMENTS**
Acetaminophen (Tylenol)	10–15 mg/kg/dose every 4–6 hr not to exceed five doses in 24 hr or 75 mg/kg/day, orally	Available in numerous preparations Nonprescription Higher dosage range may provide increased analgesia
Choline magnesium trisalicylate (Trilisate)	Children <37 kg (81.5 lb): 50 mg/kg/day divided into two doses Children >37 kg (81.5 lb): 2250 mg/day divided into two doses	Available in suspension, 500 mg/5 ml Prescription
Ibuprofen (children's Motrin, children's Advil)	Children >6 mo: 5–10 mg/kg/dose every 6–8 hr not to exceed 40 mg/kg/day	Available in numerous preparations Available in suspension, 100 mg/5 ml, and drops, 100 mg/2.5 ml Nonprescription
Naproxen (Naprosyn)	Children >2 yr: 10 mg/kg/day divided into two doses	Available in suspension, 125 mg/5 ml, and several different dosages for tablets Prescription
Tolmetin (Tolectin)	Children >2 yr: 20 g/kg/day divided into three or four doses	Available in 200-mg, 400-mg, and 600-mg tablets Prescription

Data from Olin BR and others: *Drug facts and comparisons*, St. Louis, 2002, Facts and Comparisons.
*Newer formulations of NSAIDs selectively inhibit one of the enzymes of cyclooxygenase-2 (COX-2, which is responsible for pain transmission) but do not inhibit the other (COX-1). Inhibition of COX-1 decreases prostaglandin production, which is necessary for normal organ function. For example, prostaglandins help maintain gastric mucosal blood flow and barrier protection, regulate blood flow to the liver and kidneys, and facilitate platelet aggregation and clot formation. Theoretically, the COX-2 NSAIDs provide similar analgesic and antiinflammatory benefits with fewer gastric and platelet side effects than the nonselective agents. COX-2 NSAIDs are approved for use in patients older than 18 years of age.
†All NSAIDs in this table (except acetaminophen) have significant antiinflammatory, antipyretic, and analgesic actions. Acetaminophen has a weak antiinflammatory action, and its classification as an NSAID is controversial. Patients respond differently to various NSAIDs; therefore, changing from one drug to another may be necessary for maximum benefit. Acetylsalicylic acid (aspirin) is also an NSAID but is not recommended for children because of its possible association with Reye syndrome. The NSAIDs in this table have no known association with Reye syndrome. However, caution should be exercised in prescribing any salicylate-containing drug (e.g., Trilisate) for children with known or suspected viral infection. Side effects of ibuprofen, naproxen, and tolmetin include nausea, vomiting, diarrhea, constipation, gastric ulceration, bleeding nephritis, and fluid retention. Acetaminophen and choline magnesium trisalicylate are well tolerated in the gastrointestinal tract and do not interfere with platelet function. NSAIDs (except acetaminophen) should not be given to patients with allergic reactions to salicylates. All of the NSAIDs should be used cautiously in patients with renal impairment.

dextroamphetamine and caffeine for possible increased analgesia and decreased sedation (see Table 7-6) (McCaffery and Pasero, 1999).

Children (except infants younger than about 3 to 6 months) metabolize drugs more rapidly than adults; younger children may require higher doses of opioids to achieve the same analgesic effect. Therefore, the therapeutic effect and duration of analgesia vary. Children's dosages are usually calculated according to body weight, except in children with a weight greater than 50 kg (110 pounds), in whom the weight formula may exceed the average adult dose. In this case, the adult dose is used. Conversion factors for selected opioids must be used when a change is made from the IV (preferred) or IM to the oral route. Immediate conversion from IM or IV to the suggested equianalgesic oral dose may result in a substantial error. For example, the dose may be significantly more or less than what the child requires. Small changes ensure small errors. Several routes of analgesic administration can be used (Box 7-3), and the most effective and least traumatic route of administration should be selected.

Patient-Controlled Analgesia

A significant advance in the administration of IV, epidural, or subcutaneous analgesics is the use of patient-controlled analgesia (PCA). As the name implies, the patient controls the amount and frequency of the analgesic, which is typically delivered through a special infusion device. Children who are physically able to "push a button" (i.e., 5–6 years of age) and who can understand the concept of pushing a button to obtain pain relief can use PCA (Maxwell and Yaster, 2000). Although

it is controversial, parents and nurses have used the IV PCA system for the child. Nurses can efficiently use the infusion device on a child of any age to administer analgesics to avoid signing for and preparing opioid injections every time one is needed (Fig. 7-7). When PCA is used as "nurse- or parent-controlled" analgesia, the concept of patient control is negated, and the inherent safety of PCA needs to be monitored. Research has reported safe and effective analgesia in children when the patient, parent, or nurse controlled the PCA (Algren, Gursoy, Johnson, and others, 1998; Maxwell and Yaster, 2000).

Patient-controlled analgesia infusion devices typically allow for three methods or modes of drug administration to be used alone or in combination:

1. Patient-administered boluses that can be infused only according to the preset amount and lockout interval (time between doses). More frequent attempts at self-administration may mean the patient needs the dose and time adjusted for better pain control.

2. Nurse-administered boluses that are typically used to give an initial loading dose to increase blood levels rapidly and to relieve breakthrough pain (pain not relieved with the usual programmed dose).

3. Continuous basal rate infusion that delivers a constant amount of analgesic and prevents pain from returning during those times, such as sleep, when the patient cannot control the infusion.

As with any type of analgesic management plan, continued assessment of the child's pain relief is essential for the greatest benefit from

TABLE 7-5   DOSAGE OF SELECTED OPIOIDS FOR CHILDREN[*][†]

DRUG	APPROPRIATE EQUIANALGESIC	APPROXIMATE EQUIANALGESIC PARENTERAL DOSE	RECOMMENDED STARTING DOSE (CHILDREN <50 KG (110 LB) BODY WEIGHT)[‡]	
			ORAL	PARENTERAL[‡]
Morphine	30 mg every 3–4 hr	10 mg every 3–4 hr	0.2–0.4 mg/kg every 3–4 hr 0.3–0.6 mg/kg time released every 12 hr	0.1–0.2 mg/kg IM every 3–4 hr 0.02–0.1 mg/kg IV bolus every 2 hr 0.015 mg/kg every 8 min PCA 0.01–0.02 mg/kg/hr IV infusion (neonates) 0.01–0.06 mg/kg/hr IV infusion (child)
Fentanyl (Sublimaze) (oral mucosal form [Actiq])[§]	Not available	0.1 mg IV	5–15 mcg/kg; maximum dose 400 mcg	0.5–1.5 mcg/kg IV bolus every 30 min 1–2 mcg/hr IV infusion
Codeine[‖]	200 mg every 3–4 hr	130 mg every 3–4 hr	1 mg/kg every 3–4 hr	Not recommended
Hydromorphone[¶] (Dilaudid)	7.5 mg every 3–4 hr	1.5 mg every 3–4 hr	0.04–0.1 mg/kg every 3–4 hr	0.02–0.1 mg/kg every 3–4 hr 0.005–0.2 mg/kg IV bolus every 2 hr
Hydrocodone and acetaminophen (Lorcet, Lortab, Vicodin, others)	30 mg every 3–4 hr	Not available	0.2 mg/kg every 3–4 hr	Not available
Levorphanol (Levo-Dromoran)	4 mg every 6–8 hr	2 mg every 6–8 hr	0.04 mg/kg every 6–8 hr	0.02 mg/kg every 6–8 hr
Meperidine (Demerol)[#]	300 mg every 2–3 hr	100 mg every 3 hr	Not recommended	0.75 mg/kg every 2–3 hr
Methadone (Dolophine, others)[**]	20 mg every 6–8 hr	10 mg every 6–8 hr	0.2 mg/kg every 6–8 hr	0.1 mg/kg every 6–8 hr
Oxycodone (Roxicodone, OxyContin; also in Percocet, Percodan, Tylox, others)	20 mg every 3–4 hr	Not available	2 mg/kg every 3–4 hr[††]	Not available

Data from Acute Pain Management Guideline Panel: *Acute pain management: operative or medical procedures and trauma: clinical practice guideline,* AHCPR Pub No 92-0032, Rockville, Md, 1992, Agency for Health Care Policy and Research, Public Health Service, U.S. Department of Health and Human Services; Berde C, Ablin A, Glazer J, and others: American Academy of Pediatrics Report of the Subcommittee on Disease-Related Pain in Childhood Cancer, *Pediatrics* 86(5 pt 2):820, 1990.

IM, Intramuscular; *IV,* intravenous; *PCA,* patient-controlled analgesia.

[*]NOTE: Published tables vary in suggested doses that are equianalgesic to morphine. Clinical response is criterion that must be applied for each patient; titration to clinical response is necessary. Because there is not complete cross-tolerance among these drugs, it is usually necessary to use a lower than equianalgesic dose when changing drugs and to retitrate to response.

[†]CAUTION: Recommended doses do not apply to patients with renal or hepatic insufficiency or other conditions affecting drug metabolism and kinetics.

[‡]CAUTION: Doses listed for patients with body weight less than 50 kg (110 lb) cannot be used as initial starting doses in infants younger than 6 months of age. For nonventilated infants younger than 6 months, the initial opioid dose should be about ¼ to ⅓ of the dose recommended for older infants and children. For example, morphine could be used at a dose of 0.03 mg/kg instead of the traditional 0.1 mg/kg.

[§]Actiq is indicated only for management of breakthrough cancer pain in patients with malignancies who are already receiving and are tolerant to opioid therapy, but it can be used for preoperative or preprocedural sedation/analgesia.

[‖]CAUTION: Codeine doses above 65 mg often are not appropriate because of diminishing incremental analgesia with increasing doses but continually increasing constipation and other side effects. Dosages are from McCaffery M, Pasero C: *Pain: a clinical manual,* ed 2, St. Louis, 1999, Mosby.

[¶]For morphine, hydromorphone, and oxymorphone, rectal administration is an alternate route for patients unable to take oral medications, but equianalgesic doses may differ from oral and parenteral doses because of pharmacokinetic differences.

[#]Meperidine is not recommended for continuous pain control (i.e., postoperatively) because of risk of normeperidine toxicity.

[**]Initial dose is 10%–25% of equianalgesic morphine dose. Parenteral Dolophine is no longer available in the United States.

[††]CAUTION: Doses of aspirin and acetaminophen in combination with opioid or nonsteroidal antiinflammatory drug preparations must also be adjusted to patient's body weight. Daily dose of acetaminophen should not exceed 75 mg/kg, or 4000 mg.

PCA. Typical uses of PCA are for controlling pain from surgery, sickle cell crisis, trauma, and cancer. Morphine is the drug of choice for PCA and usually comes in a concentration of 1 mg/ml. Other options are hydromorphone (0.2 mg/ml) and fentanyl (0.01 mg/ml).

Hydromorphone is often used when patients are not able to tolerate side effects such as pruritus and nausea from the morphine PCA (Algren, Gursoy, Johnson, and others, 1998; Maxwell and Yaster, 2000). Some physicians may still prescribe meperidine. However, meperidine is the least potent and shortest acting of the synthetic opioids and the least effective in providing analgesia for severe pain. More important, it may increase the risk of seizures when administered chronically because of the excitatory effects on the nervous system of its metabolite, normeperidine. Some authors (Nadvi, Sarnaik, and Ravindranath, 1999) have argued that the incidence of meperidine-associated seizures is extremely small (0.4% of patients; 0.06% of admissions) and the risk of seizures should not dissuade clinicians from using this drug. However, the American Pain Society recommends that meperidine be reserved for brief treatment courses for patients who have reported and demonstrated its effectiveness or who have allergies or uncorrectable intolerances to other opioids. Meperidine should not be used for longer than 48 hours or in dosages greater than 600 mg/24 hr (Max, Payne, Edwards, and others, 1999).

TABLE 7-6 MANAGEMENT OF OPIOID SIDE EFFECTS

SIDE EFFECT	ADJUVANT DRUGS	NONPHARMACOLOGIC TECHNIQUES
Constipation	**Senna and docusate sodium** *Tablet:* 　2–6 yr: Start with ½ tablet once a day; maximum: 1 tablet twice a day 　6–12 yr: Start with 1 tablet once a day; maximum: 2 tablets twice a day 　>12 yr: Start with 2 tablets once a day; maximum: 4 tablets twice a day *Liquid:* 　1 mo–1 yr: 1.25–5 ml q hs 　1–5 yr: 2.5–5 ml q hs 　5–15 yr: 5–10 ml q hs 　>15 yr: 10–25 ml q hs **Casanthranol and docusate sodium** 　*Liquid:* 5–15 ml q hs 　*Capsules:* 1 cap PO q hs **Bisacodyl:** PO or PR 　3–12 yr: 5 mg/dose/day 　>12 yr: 10–15 mg/dose/day **Lactulose** 7.5 ml/day after breakfast Adult: 15–30 ml/day PO **Mineral oil:** 1–2 tsp/day PO **Magnesium citrate** 　<6 yr: 2–4 ml/kg PO once 　6–12 yr: 100–150 ml PO once 　>12 yr: 150–300 ml PO once **Milk of Magnesia** 　<2 yr: 0.5 ml/kg/dose PO once 　2–5 yr: 5–15 ml/day PO 　6–12 yr: 15–30 ml PO once 　>12 yr: 30–60 ml PO once	Increase water intake Prune juice, bran cereal, vegetables
Sedation	**Caffeine:** single dose of 1–1.5 mg PO **Dextroamphetamine:** 2.5–5 mg PO in AM and early afternoon **Methylphenidate:** 2.5–5 mg PO in AM and early afternoon Consider opioid switch if sedation is persistent	Caffeinated drinks (e.g., Mountain Dew, cola drinks)
Nausea, vomiting	**Promethazine:** 0.5 mg/kg q 4–6 hr; maximum: 25 mg/dose **Ondansetron:** 0.1–0.15 mg/kg IV or PO q 4 hr; maximum: 8 mg/dose **Granisetron:** 10–40 mcg/kg q 2–4 hr; maximum: 1 mg/dose **Droperidol:** 0.05–0.06 mg/kg IV q 4–6 hr; can be very sedating	Imagery, relaxation Deep, slow breathing
Pruritus	**Diphenhydramine:** 1 mg/kg IV or PO q 4–6 hr prn; maximum: 25 mg/dose **Hydroxyzine:** 0.6 mg/kg/dose PO q 6 hr; maximum: 50 mg/dose **Naloxone:** 0.5 mcg/kg q 2 min until pruritus improves (diluted in solution of 0.1 mg of naloxone per 10 ml of saline) **Butorphanol:** 0.3–0.5 mg/kg IV (use cautiously in opioid-tolerant children; may cause withdrawal symptoms); maximum: 2 mg/dose because mixed agonist-antagonist	Oatmeal baths, good hygiene Exclude other causes of itching Change opioids
Respiratory depression: mild to moderate	Hold dose of opioid Reduce subsequent doses by 25%	Arouse gently, give oxygen, encourage to deep breathe
Respiratory depression: severe	**Naloxone** *During disease pain management:* 　0.5 mcg/kg in 2-min increments until breathing improves (American Pain Society, 1999; McCaffery and Pasero, 1999) 　Reduce opioid dose if possible 　Consider opioid switch *During sedation for procedures:* 　5–10 mcg/kg until breathing improves (Yaster, Krance, Kaplan, and others, 1997) 　Reduce opioid dose if possible 　Consider opioid switch	Oxygen, bag and mask if indicated

Continued

TABLE 7-6 MANAGEMENT OF OPIOID SIDE EFFECTS—cont'd

SIDE EFFECT	ADJUVANT DRUGS	NONPHARMACOLOGIC TECHNIQUES
Dysphoria, confusion, hallucinations	Evaluate medications, eliminate adjuvant medications with central nervous system effects as symptoms allow Consider opioid switch if possible **Haloperidol** (Haldol): 0.05–0.15 mg/kg/day divided in 2–3 doses; maximum: 2–4 mg/day	Rule out other physiologic causes
Urinary retention	Evaluate medications, eliminate adjuvant medications with anticholinergic effects (e.g., antihistamines, tricyclic antidepressants) Occurs more frequently with spinal analgesia than with systemic opioid use **Oxybutynin** 1 yr: 1 mg tid 1–2 yr: 2 mg tid 2–3 yr: 3 mg tid 4–5 yr: 4 mg tid >5 yr: 5 mg tid	Rule out other physiologic causes In/out or indwelling urinary catheter

cap, Capsule; *hs,* at bedtime; *IV,* intravenous; *PO,* by mouth; *PR,* by rectum; *prn,* as needed; *q,* every; *tid,* three times a day.

BOX 7-3 ROUTES AND METHODS OF ANALGESIC DRUG ADMINISTRATION

Oral
- Preferred because of convenience, cost, and relatively steady blood levels
- Higher dosages of oral form of opioids required for equivalent parenteral analgesia
- Peak drug effect occurs after 1 to 2 hours for most analgesics
- Delay in onset a disadvantage when rapid control of severe pain or of fluctuating pain is desired

Sublingual, Buccal, or Transmucosal
- Tablet or liquid placed between cheek and gum (buccal) or under tongue (sublingual)
- Highly desirable because more rapid onset than oral route
- Produced less first-pass effect through liver than oral route, which normally reduces analgesia from oral opioids (unless sublingual or buccal form is swallowed, which occurs often in children)
- Few drugs commercially available in this form
- Many drugs can be compounded into sublingual troche or lozenge.*
- Actiq—Oral transmucosal fentanyl citrate in hard confection base on a plastic holder; indicated only for management of breakthrough cancer pain in patients with malignancies who are already receiving and are tolerant to opioid therapy but can also be used for preoperative or preprocedural sedation and analgesia

Intravenous (IV) (Bolus)
- Preferred for rapid control of severe pain
- Provides most rapid onset of effect, usually in about 5 minutes
- Advantage for acute pain, procedural pain, and breakthrough pain
- Needs to be repeated hourly for continuous pain control
- Drugs with short half-lives (morphine, fentanyl, hydromorphone) preferable to avoid toxic accumulation of drug

Intravenous (Continuous)
- Preferred over bolus and intramuscular (IM) injection for maintaining control of pain
- Provides steady blood levels
- Easy to titrate dosage

Subcutaneous (SC) (Continuous)
- Used when oral and IV routes not available
- Provides equivalent blood levels to continuous IV infusion
- Suggested initial bolus dose to equal 2-hour IV dose; total 24-hour dose usually requires concentrated opioid solution to minimize infused volume; use smallest gauge needle that accommodates infusion rate

Patient-Controlled Analgesia (PCA)
- Generally refers to self-administration of drugs regardless of route
- Typically uses programmable infusion pump (IV, epidural, SC) that permits self-administration of boluses of medication at preset dose and time interval (lockout interval is time between doses)
- PCA bolus administration often combined with initial bolus and continuous (basal or background) infusion of opioid
- Optimum lockout interval not known but must be at least as long as time needed for onset of drug
- Should effectively control pain during movement and procedures
- Longer lockout provides larger dose

Family-Controlled Analgesia
- One family member (usually a parent) or other caregiver designated as child's primary pain manager with responsibility for pressing PCA button
- Guidelines for selecting a primary pain manager for family-controlled analgesia:
  - Spends a significant amount of time with patient
  - Is willing to assume responsibility of being primary pain manager
  - Is willing to accept and respect patient's reports of pain (if able to provide) as best indicator of how much pain the patient is experiencing; knows how to use and interpret a pain rating scale
  - Understands the purpose and goals of patient's pain management plan
  - Understands the concept of maintaining a steady analgesic blood level
  - Recognizes signs of pain and side effects and adverse reactions to opioid

Nurse-Activated Analgesia
- Child's primary nurse designated as primary pain manager and is the only person who presses PCA button during that nurse's shift

BOX 7-3   ROUTES AND METHODS OF ANALGESIC DRUG ADMINISTRATION—cont'd

- Guidelines for selecting primary pain manager for family-controlled analgesia also applicable to nurse-activated analgesia
- May be used in addition to basal rate to treat breakthrough pain with bolus doses; patient assessed every 30 minutes for need for bolus dose
- May be used without a basal rate as a means of maintaining analgesia with around-the-clock bolus doses

Intramuscular

NOTE: Not recommended for pain control; not current standard of care

- Painful administration (hated by children)
- Some drugs can cause tissue and nerve damage
- Wide fluctuation in absorption of drug from muscle
- Faster absorption from deltoid than from gluteal sites
- Shorter duration and more expensive than oral drugs
- Time consuming for staff and unnecessary delay for child

Intranasal

- Available commercially as butorphanol (Stadol NS); approved for those older than 18 years of age
- Should not be used in patient receiving morphine-like drugs because butorphanol is partial antagonist that will reduce analgesia and may cause withdrawal

Intradermal

- Used primarily for skin anesthesia (e.g., before lumbar puncture, bone marrow aspiration, arterial puncture, skin biopsy)
- Local anesthetics (e.g., lidocaine) cause stinging, burning sensation
- Duration of stinging dependent on type of "caine" used
- To avoid stinging sensation associated with lidocaine:
  - Buffer the solution by adding 1 part sodium bicarbonate (1 mEq/ml) to 9 to 10 parts 1% or 2% lidocaine with or without epinephrine (see Evidence-Based Practice box, p. 171)
- Normal saline with preservative, benzyl alcohol, anesthetizes venipuncture site
- Use same dose as for buffered lidocaine (see Evidence-Based Practice box, p. 171)

Topical or Transdermal

- EMLA (eutectic mixture of local anesthetics [lidocaine and prilocaine]) cream and anesthetic disk or LMX4 (4% lidocaine cream)
  - Eliminates or reduces pain from most procedures involving skin puncture
  - Must be placed on intact skin over puncture site and covered by occlusive dressing or applied as anesthetic disc for 1 hour or more before procedure
- Synera, S-Caine (lidocaine/tetracaine)
  - Apply for 20 to 30 minutes
  - Do not apply to broken skin
- LAT (lidocaine–adrenaline–tetracaine), tetracaine–phenylephrine (tetraphen)
  - Provides skin anesthesia about 15 minutes after application on nonintact skin
  - Gel (preferable) or liquid placed on wounds for suturing
  - Adrenaline not for use on end arterioles (fingers, toes, tip of nose, penis, earlobes) because of vasoconstriction
- Transdermal fentanyl (Duragesic)
  - Available as patch for continuous pain control
  - Safety and efficacy not established in children younger than 12 years of age

- Not appropriate for initial relief of acute pain because of long interval to peak effect (12–24 hours); for rapid onset of pain relief, give an immediate-release opioid
- Orders for "rescue doses" of an immediate-release opioid recommended for breakthrough pain, a flare of severe pain that breaks through the medication being administered at regular intervals for persistent pain
- Has duration of up to 72 hours for prolonged pain relief
- If respiratory depression occurs, possible need for several doses of naloxone
- Vapocoolant
  - Use of prescription spray coolant, such as Fluori-Methane or ethyl chloride (Pain-Ease); applied to the skin for 10 to 15 seconds immediately before the needle puncture; anesthesia lasts about 15 seconds
  - Some children dislike cold; may be less uncomfortable to spray coolant on a cotton ball and then apply it to the skin
  - Application of ice to the skin for 30 seconds has been found to be ineffective

Rectal

- Alternative to oral or parenteral routes
- Variable absorption rate
- Generally disliked by children
- Many drugs able to be compounded into rectal suppositories*

Regional Nerve Block

- Use of long-acting local anesthetic (bupivacaine or ropivacaine) injected into nerves to block pain at site
- Provides prolonged analgesia postoperatively, such as after inguinal herniorrhaphy
- May be used to provide local anesthesia for surgery, such as dorsal penile nerve block for circumcision or for reduction of fractures

Inhalation

- Use of anesthetics, such as nitrous oxide, to produce partial or complete analgesia for painful procedures
- Side effects (e.g., headache) possible from occupational exposure to high levels of nitrous oxide

Epidural or Intrathecal

- Involves catheter placed into epidural, caudal, or intrathecal space for continuous infusion or single or intermittent administration of opioid with or without a long-acting local anesthetic (e.g., bupivacaine, ropivacaine)
- Analgesia primarily from drug's direct effect on opioid receptors in spinal cord
- Respiratory depression rare but may have slow and delayed onset; can be prevented by checking level of sedation and respiratory rate and depth hourly for initial 24 hours and decreasing dose when excessive sedation is detected
- Nausea, itching, and urinary retention are common dose-related side effects from the epidural opioid
- Mild hypotension, urinary retention, and temporary motor or sensory deficits are common unwanted effects of epidural local anesthetic
- Catheter for urinary retention inserted during surgery to decrease trauma to child; if inserted when child is awake, anesthetize urethra with lidocaine

Data primarily from American Pain Society: *Principles of analgesic use in the treatment of acute pain and chronic cancer pain,* ed 4, Glenview, Ill, 1999, Author; and McCaffery M, Pasero C: *Pain: a clinical manual,* ed 2, St. Louis, 1999, Mosby.
*For further information about compounding drugs in troche or suppository form, contact Professional Compounding Centers of America (PCCA), 9901 S. Wilcrest Drive, Houston, TX 77009; 800-331-2498; http://www.pccarx.com.

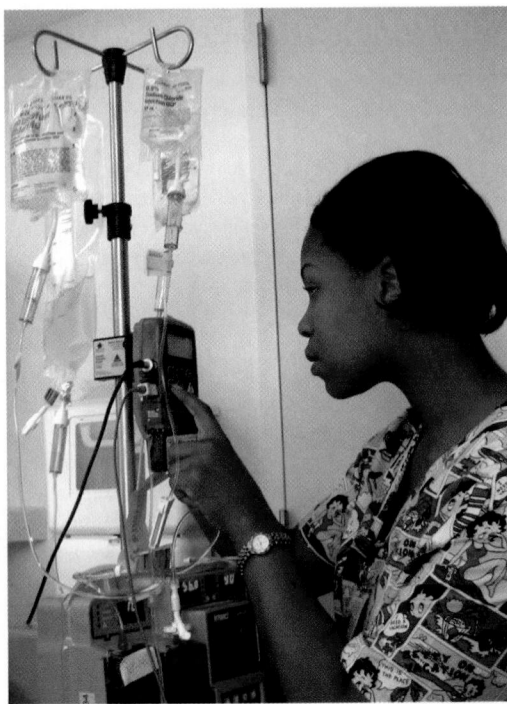

FIG 7-7 Nurse programming a patient-controlled analgesia pump to administer analgesia.

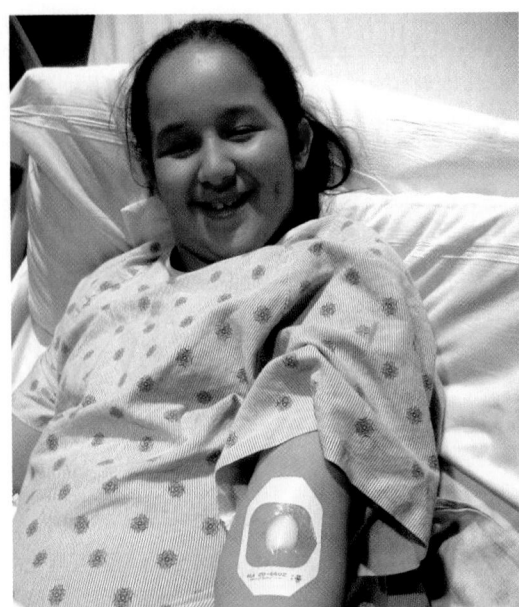

FIG 7-8 LMX (a 4% liposomal lidocaine cream) is an effective analgesic before intravenous insertion or blood draw.

Epidural Analgesia

Epidural analgesia is used to manage pain in selected cases. Although an epidural catheter can be inserted at any vertebral level, it is usually placed into the epidural space of the spinal column at the lumbar or caudal level. The thoracic level is usually reserved for older children or adolescents who have had an upper abdominal or thoracic procedure, such as a lung transplant. An opioid (usually fentanyl, hydromorphone, or preservative-free morphine, which is often combined with a long-acting local anesthetic such as bupivacaine or ropivacaine) is instilled via single or intermittent bolus, continuous infusion, or patient-controlled epidural analgesia. Analgesia results from the drug's effect on opiate receptors in the dorsal horn of the spinal cord rather than the brain. As a result, respiratory depression is rare, but if it occurs, it develops slowly, typically 6 to 8 hours after administration (Golianu, Krane, Galloway, and others, 2000). Properly securing the epidural catheter with an occlusive dressing decreases the possibility of soiling or inadvertently displacing the catheter. Careful monitoring of sedation level and respiratory status is critical to prevent opioid-induced respiratory depression. Assessment of pain and the skin condition around the catheter site are important aspects of nursing care (Golianu, Krane, Galloway, and others, 2000).

Transmucosal and Transdermal Analgesia

Oral transmucosal fentanyl (Oralet) provides nontraumatic preoperative and preprocedural analgesia and sedation (Golianu, Krane, Galloway, and others, 2000). Fentanyl is also available as a transdermal patch (Duragesic). Although contraindicated for acute pain management, it may be used for older children and adolescents who have cancer pain or sickle cell pain and for patients who are opioid tolerant.

One of the most significant improvements in the ability to provide atraumatic care to children is the anesthetic cream LMX (a 4% liposomal lidocaine cream) or EMLA (a eutectic mixture of local anesthetics) (Abdelkefi, Abdennebi, Mellouli, and others, 2004; Choi, Irwin, Hui, and others, 2003; Egekvist and Bjerring, 2000; Gad, Olsen, Lysgaard, and others, 2005; Rogers and Ostrow, 2004; Santiago, Abad, Fernandez, and others, 2000; Uziel, Berkovitch, Gazarian, and others, 2003). The eutectic mixture (lidocaine 2.5% and prilocaine 2.5%), whose melting point is lower than that of the two anesthetics alone, permits effective concentrations of the drug to penetrate intact skin (see Evidence-Based Practice boxes and Fig. 7-8).

In some situations, there is not ample time for topical preparations such as LMX or EMLA to take effect, and refrigerant sprays such as ethyl chloride and fluorimethane can be used (Reis and Holubkov, 1997). When sprayed on the skin, these sprays vaporize, rapidly cool the area, and provide superficial anesthesia. Hospital formularies may have other products with lidocaine, prilocaine, or amethocaine topical preparations that require less time for application. A randomized controlled trial compared the efficacy and safety of amethocaine gel (which is applied for 30 minutes) and EMLA cream (which is applied for 60 minutes) before a port-a-cath puncture. Children rated the pain after the puncture using the FACES scale (coded 0 to 5). Both groups had low pain scores, less than or equal to 2, and it did not make a significant difference whether the amethocaine or the EMLA cream was used. The researchers concluded that the amethocaine was clinically equivalent to EMLA, but the amethocaine gel required less time for anesthesia (Bishai, Taddio, Bar-Oz, and others, 1999).

Monitoring Side Effects

Although both nonopioids and opioids have side effects, the major concern is with side effects from opioids (Box 7-4). Respiratory depression is the most serious complication and is most likely to occur in sedated patients. The respiratory rate may decrease gradually, or

Analgesic Patches: Synera to Decrease Pain During Painful Procedures

Terri L. Brown; Updated by Olga A. Taylor

Ask the Question
PICOT Question

Do topical analgesic patches (e.g., lidocaine-tetracaine [Synera, S-Caine]) offer additional advantages (less time, ease of use, lower cost, higher effectiveness, decreased anxiety) in relieving pain during peripheral intravenous (PIV) cannulation in children compared with LMX (lidocaine) cream and buffered lidocaine via injection?

Search for the Evidence
Search Strategies

English research-based publications on lidocaine–tetracaine patches for venipuncture without time limitation were included. Exclusions included epidural use, dermatologic procedures, and S-Caine Peel.

Databases Used

Cochrane Collaboration Database, Joanna Briggs Institute, National Guideline Clearinghouse (AHRQ), PubMed, SUMSearch, CINAHL, Scopus, Micromedex, UpToDate, BestBETs, manufacturer's websites (Endo Pharmaceuticals, ZARS Pharma)

Critically Analyze the Evidence

Studies evaluated effectiveness of Synera patch in decreasing pain during painful procedures.

- Synera is as effective as EMLA in a much shorter time frame with fewer adverse reactions in adults (Sawyer, Febbraro, Masud, and others, 2009).
- Synera reduced PIV cannulation pain and did not alter the success rate in children 3 to 17 years old (Singer, Taira, Chisena, and others, 2008).
- Median self-reported pain using a visual analog scale or Wong-Baker FACES scale was significantly lower when the Synera patch was placed over the antecubital or hand vein versus the placebo patch ($p = 0.04$) (Singer, Taira, Chisena, and others, 2008).
- A 20-minute application of the S-Caine Patch (Synera) was effective in lessening pain in children scheduled for vascular access (Sethna, Verghese, Hannallah, and others, 2005).
- Synera pain patch significantly reduced pain compared with placebo (median Oucher scores of 0 versus 60; $p < 0.001$); 59% of children in the pain patch group reported no pain compared with 20% in the placebo group (Sethna, Verghese, Hannallah, and others, 2005).
- Mild skin erythema (<38%) and edema (<2%) occurred with similar frequencies between the groups (Sethna, Verghese, Hannallah, and others, 2005).

Apply the Evidence: Nursing Implications

There is **good evidence** with **strong recommendation** for using Synera patches to decrease pain during painful procedures (Guyatt, Oxman, Vist, and others, 2008). Synera use during PIV cannulation in children 3 years and older decreases pain. Synera should not be used in children with sensitivity to lidocaine, tetracaine, para-aminobenzoic acid (PABA), or amide- or ester-type anesthetics. Use with caution in patients with hepatic impairment and those receiving class I antiarrhythmic drugs (e.g., tocainide and mexiletine) and do not apply to broken skin. Use the patch immediately after opening the pouch, do not cut or remove any layers of the patch, and ensure that the holes on the patch are not covered by clothing. Do not keep the patch on longer than 20 to 30 minutes. As with all transdermal patches containing medication, after use, fold the adhesive together and dispose of used patches in a location out of the reach of children. Do not use in a magnetic resonance imaging suite.

QSEN **Quality and Safety Competencies:**
Evidence-Based Practice*
Knowledge

Differentiate clinical opinion from research and evidence-based summaries.

Describe the use of Synera to decrease pain during painful procedures.

Skills

Base individualized care plan on patient values, clinical expertise, and evidence.

Integrate evidence into practice by using Synera patches to decrease pain during painful procedures.

Attitudes

Value the concept of EBP as integral to determining best clinical practice.

Appreciate strengths and weakness of evidence for use of Synera patches to decrease pain during painful procedures.

References

Guyatt GH, Oxman AD, Vist GE, and others: GRADE: an emerging consensus on rating quality of evidence and strength of recommendations, *BMJ* 336:924–926, 2008.

Sawyer J, Febbraro S, Masud S, and others: Heated lidocaine/tetracaine patch (Synera™, Rapydan™) compared with lidocaine/prilocaine cream (EMLA®) for topical anaesthesia before vascular access, *Br J Anaesthesia* 102(2):210–215, 2009.

Sethna NF, Verghese ST, Hannallah RS, and others: A randomized controlled trial to evaluate S-Caine Patch™ for reducing pain associated with vascular access in children, *Anesthesiology* 102(2):403–408, 2005.

Singer AJ, Taira BR, Chisena EN, and others: Warm lidocaine/tetracaine patch versus placebo before pediatric intravenous cannulation: a randomized controlled trial, *Ann Emerg Med* 52(1):41–47, 2008.

*Adapted from the QSEN at http://www.qsen.org.

respirations may cease abruptly. Lower limits of normal are not established for children, but any significant change from a previous rate calls for increased vigilance. A slower respiratory rate does not necessarily reflect decreased arterial oxygenation; an increased depth of ventilation may compensate for the altered rate. If respiratory depression or arrest occurs, the nurse must be prepared to intervene quickly (see Nursing Care Guidelines box).

Although respiratory depression is the most feared side effect, constipation is a common, and sometimes serious, side effect of opioids.

Opioids decrease peristalsis and increase anal sphincter tone. If prolonged use of opioids is expected, prevention of constipation with stool softeners and laxatives is more effective than treatment after constipation occurs. Dietary treatment, such as increased fiber, is usually not sufficient to promote regular bowel evacuation. However, dietary measures, such as increased fluid and fruit intake, and physical activity are encouraged. Another common side effect is pruritus from epidural or IV infusion. Pruritus can be treated with low doses of IV naloxone, nalbuphine, or diphenhydramine. Children may also experience

EVIDENCE-BASED PRACTICE

Needle-Free Injection System: J-Tip to Administer Buffered Lidocaine

Terri Brown; Updated by Olga A. Taylor

Ask the Question
PICOT Question
In pediatrics, are needle-free injection systems (e.g., J-Tip) effective and safe in relieving pain during peripheral intravenous (PIV) cannulation?

Search for the Evidence
Search Strategies
English-language research-based publications on jet injectors for delivery of lidocaine during PIV cannulation without time limitation were included. Exclusions included dental products, insulin, growth factor, and medications other than lidocaine.

Databases Used
Cochrane Collaboration Database, Joanna Briggs Institute, National Guideline Clearinghouse (AHRQ), PubMed, SUMSearch, CINAHL, Scopus, UpToDate, Best-BETs, manufacturers' or distributors' websites (National Medical Products, Bioject, and Injex)

Critically Analyze the Evidence
- J-Tip is superior in pain prevention compared with LMX (lidocaine cream) or EMLA (a eutectic mix of lidocaine and prilocaine) (Jimenez, Bradford, Seidel, and others, 2006; Spanos, Booth, Koenig, and others, 2008).
- J-Tip with 0.2 ml of 1% buffered lidocaine provided greater anesthesia than a 30-minute application of LMX in children ages 8 to 15 years undergoing 22- or 24-gauge PIV catheter insertion (Spanos, Booth, Koenig, and others, 2008).
- Visual analog scale (VAS) scores were significantly different immediately after PIV catheter insertion (17.3 for J-Tip vs. 44.6 for LMX; $p < 0.001$). Blinded reviewer VAS scores were not statistically significant (21.7 for J-Tip vs. 31.9 for LMX; $p = 0.23$) (Spanos, Booth, Koenig, and others, 2008).
- J-Tip did not alter the insertion site or affect the success of PIV access on the first attempt; multiple injections could be performed if necessary without causing lidocaine toxicity (Spanos, Booth, Koenig, and others, 2008).
- J-Tip with 0.25 ml of 1% buffered lidocaine provided greater anesthesia than application of 2.5 g of EMLA in a study of 116 children ages 7 to 19 years undergoing PIV catheter insertion (Jimenez, Bradford, Seidel, and others, 2006).
- Subjects' self-report median pain ratings of PIV cannulation using a 0 to 10 VAS were 0 for J-Tip and 3 for EMLA ($p = 0.0001$ for patients receiving EMLA ≥ 60 minutes before cannulation and $p = 0.0013$ for those receiving EMLA <60 minutes before) (Jimenez, Bradford, Seidel, and others, 2006).
- More pain scores were favorable for the J-Tip application (84% reported no pain at the time of injection) compared with EMLA application (61% reported pain at time of Tegaderm dressing removal; $p = 0.004$) (Jimenez, Bradford, Seidel, and others, 2006).
- J-Tip with 0.2 ml of 1% buffered lidocaine was no more effective than jet-delivered placebo (preservative-free normal saline) during PIV cannulation but may provide superior analgesia compared with no local anesthetic pretreatment (Auerbach, Tunik, and Mojica, 2009).

- Children 5 to 18 years of age received either J-Tip (0.2 ml of buffered 1% lidocaine) or jet-delivered placebo (0.2 ml of preservative-free normal saline) 60 seconds before PIV cannulation in an emergency department. Subjects reported pain on injection and on PIV cannulation using a 100-mm color analog scale (Auerbach, Tunik, and Mojica, 2009).
- Mean needle insertion pain score for jet lidocaine, 28 mm, was similar to the mean score for placebo, 34 mm, and lower than the no device group, 52 mm; most patients reported that they would request this device for future PIV access (Auerbach, Tunik, and Mojica, 2009).

Apply the Evidence: Nursing Implications
There is **good evidence** with a **strong recommendation** for using J-Tip to administer buffered lidocaine (Guyatt, Oxman, Vist, and others, 2008). J-Tip with 0.2 ml of buffered lidocaine 1% decreases pain during PIV insertion. It is recommended to wait 1 minute after administration before attempting PIV insertion. J-Tip should not be used to administer buffered lidocaine in children with a known hypersensitivity to lidocaine or other amide-type local anesthetics such as prilocaine, mepivacaine, bupivacaine, or etidocaine.

QSEN Quality and Safety Competencies: Evidence-Based Practice*
Knowledge
Differentiate clinical opinion from research and evidence-based summaries.
Describe the use of J-Tip to administer buffered lidocaine.

Skills
Base individualized care plan on patient values, clinical expertise, and evidence.
Integrate evidence into practice by using J-Tip to administer buffered lidocaine.

Attitudes
Value the concept of EBP as integral to determining best clinical practice.
Appreciate strengths and weakness of evidence for using J-Tip to administer buffered lidocaine.

References
Auerbach M, Tunik M, Mojica M: A randomized, double-blind controlled study of jet lidocaine compared to jet placebo for pain relief in children undergoing needle insertion in the emergency department, *Acad Emerg Med* 16(1):1–6, 2009.
Guyatt GH, Oxman AD, Vist GE, and others: GRADE: an emerging consensus on rating quality of evidence and strength of recommendations, *BMJ* 336:924–926, 2008.
Jimenez N, Bradford H, Seidel KD, and others: A comparison of a needle-free injection system for local anesthesia versus EMLA® for intravenous catheter insertion in the pediatric patient, *Anesth Analg* 102(2):411–414, 2006.
Spanos S, Booth R, Koenig H, and others: Jet injection of 1% buffered lidocaine versus topical ELA-Max for anesthesia before peripheral intravenous catheterization in children: a randomized controlled trial, *Pediatr Emerg Care* 24(8):511–515, 2008.

*Adapted from the QSEN at http://www.qsen.org.

Buffered Lidocaine for Pain Reduction During Peripheral Intravenous Access in Children

Angela Morgan; Updated by Olga Taylor

Ask the Question
PICOT Question

In children, is buffered lidocaine an appropriate anesthetic for reducing pain during peripheral intravenous (PIV) access?

Search for the Evidence
Search Strategies

Search criteria included English-language publications within the past 5 years, research-based articles (level 3 or lower) on children undergoing PIV access. Two of the articles reviewed were more than 5 years old but were included based on the limited literature in this area.

Databases Used

PubMed, Cochrane Collaboration, MD Consult, Joanna Briggs Institute, National Guideline Clearinghouse (AHQR), TRIP Database, PedsCCM, BestBETs

Critically Analyze the Evidence

- Patients' comfort and satisfaction were improved when the pH of lidocaine solution was increased; it is recommended to increase pH of lidocaine solution using bicarbonate immediately before administration (Cepeda, Tzortzopoulou, Thackrey, and others, 2010).
- Buffered lidocaine versus LMX (liposomal lidocaine cream) was evaluated before PIV access in children (4–17 years of age; 61% female). Both interventions decreased pain; no significant differences in pain levels between buffered lidocaine and LMX groups were noted. The LMX group stated that the pain came with the removal of the occlusive dressing from the site (Luhmann, Hurt, Shootman, and others, 2004).
- PIV access without buffered lidocaine was significantly more painful than PIV access with buffered lidocaine in children (Fein, Boardman, Stevenson, and others, 1998).
- Subcutaneous lidocaine versus no pain control measures was evaluated in children younger than 2 years of age before PIV access in the emergency department; no significant differences in pain levels were found (Sacchetti and Carraccio, 1996).
- PIV access without lidocaine was significantly more painful than PIV access with lidocaine regardless of catheter size (Klein, Shugerman, Leigh-Taylor, and others, 1995).

Apply the Evidence: Nursing Implications

There is **good evidence** with a **strong recommendation** (Guyatt, Oxman, Vist, and others, 2008) for using buffered lidocaine as a pain reduction measure in children before PIV access. Buffered lidocaine should be used in children older than 2 years of age. Buffered lidocaine has an immediate time of onset and a duration of about 1 hour and can be injected at multiple sites. The following dosage is recommended: 0.1 to 0.5 ml buffered 1% lidocaine to a maximum of 0.45 ml/kg/dose; can repeat dose after 2 hours. Buffered lidocaine should not be used within 2 hours before vesicants or with abraded skin. There is a possibility of some vasoconstriction with use of buffered lidocaine, which may increase the difficulty of PIV access. An "extra stick" and ineffective buffered lidocaine administration may result in pain during both local administration and PIV access. Expertise in administering buffered lidocaine is an important factor related to its effectiveness.

QSEN Quality and Safety Competencies:
Evidence-Based Practice*
Knowledge

Differentiate clinical opinion from research and evidence-based summaries.

Describe the use of buffered lidocaine for pain reduction during PIV access in children.

Skills

Base individualized care plan on patient values, clinical expertise, and evidence.

Integrate evidence into practice by using buffered lidocaine for pain reduction during PIV access in children.

Attitudes

Value the concept of EBP as integral to determining best clinical practice.

Appreciate the strengths and weakness of the evidence for using buffered lidocaine for pain reduction during PIV access in children.

References

Cepeda MS, Tzortzopoulou A, Thackrey M, and others: Adjusting the pH of lidocaine for reducing pain on injection, *The Cochrane Collaboration* 12:1–64, 2010.

Fein JA, Boardman CR, Stevenson S, and others: Saline with benzyl alcohol as intradermal anesthesia for intravenous line placement in children, *Pediatr Emerg Care* 14(2):119–122, 1998.

Guyatt GH, Oxman AD, Vist GE, and others: GRADE: an emerging consensus on rating quality of evidence and strength of recommendations, *BMJ* 336:924–926, 2008.

Klein EJ, Shugerman RP, Leigh-Taylor K, and others: Buffered lidocaine: analgesia for intravenous line placement in children, *Pediatrics* 95(5):709–712, 1995.

Luhmann J, Hurt S, Shootman M, and others: A comparison of buffered lidocaine versus ELA-Max before peripheral intravenous catheter insertions in children, *Pediatrics* 113(3 Pt 1):217–220, 2004.

Sacchetti AD, Carraccio C: Subcutaneous lidocaine does not affect the success rate of intravenous access in children less than 24 months of age, *Acad Emerg Med* 3(11):1016–1019, 1996.

*Adapted from the QSEN at http://www.qsen.org.

---

nausea and vomiting; however, these subside after 2 days of opioid administration. Oral or rectal antiemetics may be necessary to minimize nausea and vomiting.

Both tolerance and physical dependence can occur with prolonged use of opioids (see Community Focus box). **Physical dependence** is a normal, natural, physiologic state of "neuroadaptation." When opioids are abruptly discontinued without weaning, **withdrawal symptoms** occur. Symptoms of withdrawal occur at 24 hours after abrupt discontinuation and reach a peak within 72 hours. Symptoms of withdrawal include signs of neurologic excitability (irritability, tremors, seizures, increased motor tone, insomnia), gastrointestinal dysfunction (nausea, vomiting, diarrhea, abdominal cramps), and autonomic dysfunction (sweating, fever, chills, tachypnea, nasal congestion, rhinitis). Withdrawal symptoms can be anticipated and prevented by weaning patients from opioids that were administered for more than 5 to 10 days. Adherence to a weaning protocol to prevent or minimize withdrawal symptoms from opioids will be required. A weaning flowsheet (Fig. 7-9, *A*) may be used to assess the efficacy of opioid weaning in neonates (Franck and Vilardi, 1995; Franck, Vilardi, Durand, and others, 1998). In older infants and young children (7 months to

BOX 7-4   SIDE EFFECTS OF OPIOIDS

General
- Constipation (possibly severe)
- Respiratory depression
- Sedation
- Nausea and vomiting
- Agitation, euphoria
- Mental clouding
- Hallucinations
- Orthostatic hypotension
- Pruritus
- Urticaria
- Sweating
- Miosis (may be sign of toxicity)
- Anaphylaxis (rare)

Signs of Tolerance
- Decreasing pain relief
- Decreasing duration of pain relief

Signs of Withdrawal Syndrome in Patients with Physical Dependence
Initial Signs of Withdrawal
- Lacrimation
- Rhinorrhea
- Yawning
- Sweating

Later Signs of Withdrawal
- Restlessness
- Irritability
- Tremors
- Anorexia
- Dilated pupils
- Gooseflesh
- Nausea, vomiting

NURSING CARE GUIDELINES
Managing Opioid-Induced Respiratory Depression

If Respirations Are Depressed
- Assess sedation level.
- Reduce the infusion by 25% when possible.
- Stimulate the patient (shake his or her shoulder gently, call by name, ask to breathe).

If the Patient Cannot Be Aroused or Is Apneic
- Administer naloxone (Narcan):
  - For children weighing less than 40 kg (88 pounds), dilute 0.1 mg of naloxone in 10 ml of sterile saline to make 10 mcg/ml solution and give 0.5 mcg/kg.
  - For children weighing more than 40 kg (88 pounds), dilute a 0.4-mg ampule in 10 ml of sterile saline and give 0.5 ml.
- Administer the bolus by slow intravenous push every 2 minutes until effect is obtained.
- Closely monitor patient. Naloxone's duration of antagonist action may be shorter than that of the opioid, requiring repeated doses of naloxone

NOTE: Respiratory depression caused by benzodiazepines (e.g., diazepam [Valium] or midazolam [Versed]) can be reversed with flumazenil (Romazicon). Pediatric dosing experience suggests 0.01 mg/kg (0.1 ml/kg); if there is no (or inadequate) response after 1 to 2 minutes, administer the same dose and repeat as needed at 60-second intervals for a maximum dose of 1 mg (10 ml) (Yaster, Krance, Kaplan, and others, 1997).

10 years) the Withdrawal Assessment Tool–1 (Fig. 7-9, *B*) may be used to assess and monitor withdrawal symptoms in pediatric critically ill children who are exposed to opioids and benzodiazepines for prolonged periods (Franck, Harris, Soetenga, and others, 2008).

Tolerance occurs when the dose of an opioid needs to be increased to achieve the same analgesic effects that was previously achieved at a lower dose (see Community Focus box). Tolerance may develop after 10 to 21 days of morphine administration. Treatment of tolerance involves increasing the dose or decreasing the duration between doses. Treatment of physical dependence involves gradually reducing the dose over several days to prevent withdrawal symptoms. Following are guidelines for treating physical dependence from morphine (Max, Payne, Edwards, and others, 1999):
- Gradually reduce the dose (similar to tapering of steroids).
- Give half of the previous daily dose every 6 hours for the first 2 days.
- Then reduce the dose by 25% every 2 days. Continue this schedule until the total daily dose of 0.6 mg/kg/day of morphine (or equivalent) is reached. After 2 days on this dose, discontinue the opioid.
- You may also switch to oral methadone, using one fourth of equianalgesic dose as the initial weaning dose and proceeding as described above.

Parents and older children may fear addiction when opioids are prescribed. The nurse should address these concerns with assurance that any such risk is extremely low. It may be helpful to ask the question, "If you did not have this pain, would you want to take this medicine?" The answer is invariably no, which reinforces the solely therapeutic nature of the drug. It is also important to avoid making statements to the family such as: "We don't want you to get used to this medicine," or "By now you shouldn't need this medicine," which may reinforce the fear of becoming addicted. Whereas both physical dependence and tolerance are physiologic states, addiction or psychologic dependence is a psychologic state and implies a "cause–effect" mode of thinking, such as "I need the drug because it makes me feel better." Infants and children do not have the cognitive ability to make the cause–effect association and therefore cannot become addicted. The use of opioid analgesics early in life has not been demonstrated to increase the risk for addiction later in life. Nurses need to explain to parents the differences among physical dependence, tolerance, and addiction and allow them to express their concerns about the use and duration of use of opioids. Infants and children, when treated appropriately with opioids, may be at risk for physical tolerance and physical dependence but not psychologic dependence or addiction (McCaffery and Pasero, 1999).

Unfortunately, individuals who have severe, unrelieved pain may become intensely focused on finding relief. Sometimes behaviors such as "clock watching" make patients appear to others to be preoccupied with obtaining opioids. However, this preoccupation focuses on finding relief of pain, not on using opioids for reasons other than pain control. This phenomenon has been termed *pseudoaddiction* and must not be confused with real addiction.

Evaluation of the Effectiveness of Pain Regimens

The effectiveness of analgesics can be enhanced by a supportive attitude toward the child. By reinforcing the cause and effect of the

Children's Hospital Oakland Opioid Weaning Flowsheet and Guidelines for Use of the Form
Analgesia/sedation orders (drug/dose/frequency)

Date			
Drug			
Administration time			
Dose ↑ or ↓ or freq change			

		Time:		
Choose one: Crying/agitated 25%-50% of interval Crying/agitated >50% of interval	2 3			
Choose one: Sleeps ≤25% of interval Sleeps 26%-75% of interval Sleeps >75% of interval	3 2 1			
Choose one: Hyperactive Moro Markedly hyperactive Moro	2 3			
Choose one: Mild tremors, disturbed Moderate/severe tremors, disturbed	1 2			
Increased muscle tone	2			
Temperature 37.2°-38.4°C	1			
Temperature >38.4°C	2			
Respiratory rate >60 (extubated)	2			
Suction >twice/interval (intubated)	2			
Sweating	1			
Frequent yawning (>3-4/interval)	1			
Sneezing (>3-4/interval)	1			
Nasal stuffiness	1			
Emesis	2			
Projectile vomiting	3			
Loose stools	2			
Watery stools	3			
TOTAL SCORE				
ADJUSTED SCORE				
INITIALS OF PERSON SCORING				

Directions: Score every 2-4 hours per guideline
Score greater than 8-12 may indicate withdrawal

Guidelines for use of the flow sheet

Use of form

Use the flowsheet for all infants who have received continuous or around-the-clock opioid medication for 3 days or more, or more than 3 doses per day for more than 5 days. This patient population will most often include postoperative patients, agitated intubated infants, and all post-ECMO patients.

Instructions
1. Write drug, dose, and frequency of analgesics and sedatives ordered.
2. Enter date, name of drug (abbreviated MS=morphine sulfate or FENT=fentanyl), and administration time of drugs given in the appropriate boxes; indicate if dose frequency given is an increase or decrease from the ordered dose.
3. Scoring must be performed every 4 hours during weaning of opioids, every 2 hours if score is 8 or greater. The score for each item indicates the presence of the sign during the previous 2-4 hours (depending on the scoring interval). Every 4-hour scoring should continue until the patient is off all opioids for 48-72 hours. Place a "0" in the column after the sign if it is not seen during the scoring period.

Central nervous system
Crying behavior: Score 2 points if patient exhibits crying or cry behavior for a duration of ≤50% of the scoring interval. Score 3 points if cumulative crying behavior totals >50% of the scoring interval.
NOTE: Crying behavior is accompanied by the facial expressions associated with crying, but without audible sounds because of endotracheal intubation.
Sleeping: Score 3 points if patient sleeps for ≤25% of the scoring interval. Score 2 points if patient sleeps for 26%-75% of the scoring interval. Score 1 point if patient sleeps for >75% of the scoring interval.
Moro (startle) reflex: Score 2 points if patient has some arm and/or leg extension when touched or when disturbed by loud noises. Score 3 points if patient has marked arm and/or leg extension that is accompanied by crying behavior, hyperalert state, or continued arm and/or leg tremors after being startled.
Tremors—disturbed: Score 1 point if patient has mild tremors when disturbed. Score 2 points if patient has moderate to severe tremors when disturbed. NOTE: Tremors are alternating movements that are rhythmic, of equal rate and amplitude, and can usually be stopped by flexion of the limb.
Increased muscle tone: Score 2 points if patient exhibits fisting or tight flexion of extremities that are difficult to extend.

Metabolic
Temperature: Score 1 point if patient's temperature is 37.2°-38.4°C. Score 2 points if patient's temperature is >38.4°C.
Respiratory rate: Score 1 point if patient's spontaneous respiratory rate is >60/minute. Score 2 points if patient's spontaneous respiratory rate is >60/minute and accompanied by retractions.
Suction: Score 2 points if patient is suctioned more than twice during a 4-hour period.
Sweating: Score 1 point if patient exhibits any type of sweating, including beads of sweat, or if skin is moist to touch.
Yawning: Score 1 point if patient yawns >3-4 times in succession or yawns 1-2 times often during a 4-hour period.
Sneezing: Score 1 point if patient sneezes >3-4 times in succession or sneezes 1-2 times during a 4-hour period.
Nasal stuffiness: Score 1 point for nasal stuffiness.

Gastrointestinal
Emesis of formula/stomach contents: Score 2 points if patient has 1 or more episodes of emesis during a 4-hour period.
Projectile vomiting: Score 3 points if patient has 1 or more episodes of projectile vomiting.
Loose stools: Score 2 points if patient has loose stools characterized by a water ring around some solid stool. The stools will often be frequent. NOTE: Do not score for "breast milk" stools: frequent, small, seedy, yellow stools.
Watery stools: Score 3 points if patient has stools that consist of only liquid. The stools will often be frequent.

Total score: Add up all the scores in the column and place the total score in this box. Clinical signs that appear continuously, such as respiratory rate >60 or regular poor feeding, should be included in the total score.
Adjusted score: The adjusted score is used when a sign is detected that is expected to occur independently of withdrawal, due to a preexisting condition (high respiratory rate in infant with bronchopulmonary dysplasia). The decision to adjust the score should be made after discussion with the healthcare team during rounds, and the rationale should be recorded in a problem-oriented note. Circle the signs to be excluded and deduct the points from the total score to obtain the adjusted score.
Initials of person scoring: The person scoring should write his/her initials in this space.

A

FIG 7-9 A, Weaning flowsheet to monitor opioid weaning in neonates. *ECMO,* Extracorporeal membrane oxygenation.
Continued

medication and analgesia, the nurse can condition the child to expect pain relief, provided the regimen is likely to be effective. A pain relief scale or periodic ratings of pain intensity should be used for evaluation of the effectiveness of pain regimens.

The response to therapy should be evaluated 15 to 30 minutes after each dose, and titration should continue to the highest achievable amount of relief (Max, Payne, Edwards, and others, 1999). In a retrospective study that examined the pain experience of children with sickle cell disease, evidence of pain relief from medications was documented for fewer than half (44.8%) of the patients in the emergency department (ED) (Jacob and Mueller, 2008). Even though The Joint Commission required documentation of pain assessments with vital signs, evidence of pain relief was not documented in 41.4% of the episodes. Titration methods in the ED or during the course of hospitalization, if used, were not reflected in the amount of medications received by the children (Jacob and Mueller, 2008; Jacob, Miaskowski, Savedra, and others, 2003a, 2003b).

Several harmful effects occur with unrelieved pain, particularly when pain is prolonged. A number of physiologic stress responses in the body are triggered during pain, and they lead to negative consequences that involve multiple systems. Unrelieved pain may prolong the stress response and adversely affect an infant's or child's recovery, whether it is from trauma, surgery, or disease. In a landmark study by Anand and Hickey (1992), 30 neonates received deep intraoperative

WITHDRAWAL ASSESSMENT TOOL – 1 (WAT – 1)

Patient Identifier														
	Date:													
	Time:													
Information from patient record, previous 12 hours														
Any loose /watery stools	No = 0 Yes = 1													
Any vomiting/wretching/gagging	No = 0 Yes = 1													
Temperature > 37.8°C	No = 0 Yes = 1													
2 minute pre-stimulus observation														
State	SBS* ≤ 0 or asleep/awake/calm = 0 SBS* ≥ +1 or awake/distressed = 1													
Tremor	None/mild = 0 Moderate/severe = 1													
Any sweating	No = 0 Yes = 1													
Uncoordinated/repetitive movement	None/mild = 0 Moderate/severe = 1													
Yawning or sneezing	None or 1 = 0 ≥2 = 1													
1 minute stimulus observation														
Startle to touch	None/mild = 0 Moderate/severe = 1													
Muscle tone	Normal = 0 Increased = 1													
Post-stimulus recovery														
Time to gain calm state (SBS* ≤ 0)	< 2min = 0 2 - 5min = 1 > 5 min = 2													
Total Score (0-12)														

WITHDRAWAL ASSESSMENT TOOL (WAT – 1) INSTRUCTIONS

- Start WAT-1 scoring from the **first day of weaning** in patients who have received opioids +/or benzodiazepines by infusion or regular dosing for prolonged periods (e.g., > 5 days). Continue twice daily scoring until 72 hours after the last dose.
- The Withdrawal Assessment Tool (WAT-1) should be completed along with the SBS[1] at least once per 12 hour shift (e.g., at 08:00 and 20:00 ± 2 hours). The progressive stimulus used in the SBS[1] assessment provides a standard stimulus for observing signs of withdrawal.

Obtain information from patient record (this can be done before or after the stimulus):
  ✓ **Loose/watery stools**: Score 1 if any loose or watery stools were documented in the past 12 hours; score 0 if none were noted.
  ✓ **Vomiting/wretching/gagging**: Score 1 if any vomiting or spontaneous wretching or gagging were documented in the past 12 hours; score 0 if none were noted
  ✓ **Temperature > 37.8°C**: Score 1 if the modal (most frequently occurring) temperature documented was greater than 37.8 °C in the past 12 hours; score 0 if this was not the case.

2 minute pre-stimulus observation:
  ✓ **State**: Score 1 if awake and distress (SBS[1]: ≥ +1) observed during the 2 minutes prior to the stimulus; score 0 if asleep or awake and calm/cooperative (SBS[1] ≤ 0).
  ✓ **Tremor**: Score 1 if moderate to severe tremor observed during the 2 minutes prior to the stimulus; score 0 if no tremor (or only minor, intermittent tremor).
  ✓ **Sweating**: Score 1 if any sweating during the 2 minutes prior to the stimulus; score 0 if no sweating noted.
  ✓ **Uncoordinated/repetitive movements**: Score 1 if moderate to severe uncoordinated or repetitive movements such as head turning, leg or arm flailing or torso arching observed during the 2 minutes prior to the stimulus; score 0 if no (or only mild) uncoordinated or repetitive movements.
  ✓ **Yawning or sneezing** > 1: Score 1 if more than 1 yawn or sneeze observed during the 2 minutes prior to the stimulus; score 0 if 0 to 1 yawn or sneeze.

1 minute stimulus observation:
  ✓ **Startle to touch**: Score 1 if moderate to severe startle occurs when touched during the stimulus; score 0 if none (or mild).
  ✓ **Muscle tone**: Score 1 if tone increased during the stimulus; score 0 if normal.

Post-stimulus recovery:
  ✓ **Time to gain calm state** (SBS[1] ≤ 0): Score 2 if it takes greater than 5 minutes following stimulus; score 1 if achieved within 2 to 5 minutes; score 0 if achieved in less than 2 minutes.
Sum the 11 numbers in the column for the total WAT-1 score (0-12).

B

FIG 7-9, cont'd B, Withdrawal assessment tool for infants and children. *SBS,* State behavioral scale. (**A,** Modified from Franck L, Vilardi J: Assessment and management of opioid withdrawal in ill neonates, *Neonatal Netw* 14[2]:39–48, 1995; **B,** © 2007 LS Franck and MAQ Curley. All rights reserved. Reprinted in Franck LS, Harris SK, Soetenga DJ, and others: The Withdrawal Assessment Tool–1 [WAT–1]: an assessment instrument for monitoring opioid and benzodiazepine withdrawal symptoms in pediatric patients, *Pediatr Crit Care Med* 9[6]:577, 2008.)
*From Curley MQ, Harris SK, Fraser KA, and others: State behavioral scale: a sedation assessment instrument for infants and young children supported on mechanical ventilation, *Pediatr Crit Care Med* 7(2):107–114, 2006.

Fear of Opioid Addiction

One of the reasons for the unfounded but prevalent fear of addiction from opioids used to relieve pain is a misunderstanding of the differences among physical dependence, tolerance, and addiction. Health care professionals and the community often confuse addiction with the physiologic effects of opioids when in reality these three events are unrelated.

The American Society of Addiction Medicine defines these three terms as follows:

- *Physical dependence* on an opioid is a physiologic state in which abrupt cessation of the opioid, or administration of an opioid antagonist, results in a withdrawal syndrome. Physical dependence on opioids is an expected occurrence in all individuals in the presence of continuous use of opioids for therapeutic or nontherapeutic purposes. It does not, in and of itself, imply addiction.

- *Tolerance* is a form of neuroadaptation to the effects of chronically administered opioids (or other medications) that is indicated by the need for increasing or more frequent doses of the medication to achieve the initial effects of the drug. A person may develop tolerance both to the analgesic effects of opioids and to some of the unwanted side effects, such as respiratory depression, sedation, or nausea. Tolerance is variable in occurrence, but it does not, in and of itself, imply addiction.

- *Addiction* in the context of pain treatment with opioids is characterized by a persistent pattern of dysfunctional opioid use that may involve any or all of the following:
  - Adverse consequences associated with the use of opioids
  - Loss of control over the use of opioids
  - Preoccupation with obtaining opioids, despite the presence of adequate analgesia

Nurses must educate older children, parents, and health professionals about the extremely low risk of real addiction (less than 1%) from the use of opioids to treat pain. Infants, young children, and comatose or terminally ill children simply cannot become addicted because they are incapable of a consistent pattern of drug-seeking behavior, such as stealing, drug dealing, prostitution, and use of family income, to obtain opioids for nonanalgesic reasons.

Data from American Society of Addiction Medicine: *Public policy statement on definitions related to the use of opioids for pain treatment*, February 2001, retrieved from http://www.asam.org.

anesthesia with high doses of the opioid sufentanil followed postoperatively with an infusion of opioids for 24 hours, and 15 neonates received lighter anesthesia with halothane and morphine followed postoperatively by intermittent morphine and diazepam. The 15 neonates who received the lighter anesthesia and intermittent postoperative opioids had more severe hyperglycemia and lactic acidemia, and four postoperative deaths occurred in the group. The 30 neonates who received deep anesthesia had a lower incidence of complications (sepsis, metabolic acidosis, disseminated intravascular coagulation) and no deaths.

Poorly controlled acute pain can predispose patients to **chronic pain syndromes**. A guiding principle in pain management is that prevention of pain is always better than treatment (Benjamin, Swinson, and Nagel, 2000). Pain that is established and severe is often more difficult to control. When pain is unrelieved, sensory input from injured tissues reaches spinal cord neurons and may enhance subsequent responses. Long-lasting changes in cells within spinal cord pain pathways may occur after a brief painful stimulus and may lead to the development of chronic pain conditions. Basbaum (1999a, 1999b)

reported a series of studies that emphasize a distinct neurochemistry of acute and persistent pain and concluded that persistent pain is not merely a prolonged acute pain symptom of some other disease. Underlying physiologic mechanisms lead to the persistence of pain (Marx, 2004; Woolf and Salter, 2000).

In a study of nursing practice related to pain assessment and management in different pediatric specialty units (Jacob and Puntillo, 2000), complaints of pain were noted, but specific pain scores or notations about responses to analgesics after administration were seldom documented. Pain scores were not available before and after analgesics, and it was therefore not possible to conclude whether analgesics were effective. Nurses therefore need to evaluate and monitor pain in a timely fashion after administration of analgesics; titrate dosage to effect; or make recommendations for an alternate analgesic, for addition of another analgesic, or for a combination of analgesics, adjuvants, and nonpharmacologic strategies, if pain persists.

CONSEQUENCES OF UNTREATED PAIN

Despite current research on neonates' experience of pain, infants' pain often remains inadequately managed. The mismanagement of infants' pain is partially the result of misconceptions regarding the effects of pain on neonates and the lack of knowledge of immediate and long-term consequences of untreated pain. Infants respond to noxious stimuli through physiologic indicators (increased heart rate and blood pressure, variability in heart rate and intracranial pressure [ICP]), decreases in SaO_2 and skin blood flow, and behavioral indicators (muscle rigidity, facial expression, crying, withdrawal, and sleeplessness) (Anand, Grunau, and Oberlander, 1997; Bildner and Krechel, 1996). The physiologic and behavioral changes, as well as a variety of neurophysiologic responses to noxious stimulation, are responsible for the acute and long-term consequences of pain.

Anand and Hickey (1987) described responses of infants to painful stimuli. Chemical and hormonal responses were observed after noxious stimuli without the use of an anesthetic or analgesic. Such responses included increases in β-endorphin (an endogenous opioid) secretion, plasma renin activity, plasma epinephrine and norepinephrine, catecholamines, growth hormone, glucagon, aldosterone, and other corticosteroids. The result of these chemical and hormonal increases includes the breakdown of fat and carbohydrate stores; prolonged hyperglycemia; and increased serum lactate, pyruvate, total ketone bodies, and nonesterified fatty acids. Such consequences can be attributed to a greater morbidity for neonates in the NICU. Several experimental studies revealed a significant decrease in these responses when adequate analgesia was used before the painful procedure. One study showed that the standardization of postoperative pain management strategies for infants in the NICU led to the following improvements: (1) decreased length of time to extubation, (2) decreased length of stay, (3) better fluid management, and (4) reduced side effects of opioids. The authors also noted improved pain management documentation, decreased cost, and decreased nursing time (Furdon, Eastman, Benjamin, and others, 1998). (See Atraumatic Care box.)

COMMON PAIN STATES IN CHILDREN

PAIN IN PRIMARY CARE

In normative problems such as teething; during immunizations and vaccinations; and in common childhood illnesses such as otitis media, pharyngitis, and viral infections, pain is the presenting symptom that can be distressing (Schechter, 2003). The inflammation or irritation of the gingiva as the tooth erupts is responsible for discomfort during teething. Teething infants show more mouthing and drooling than nonteething infants. A topical anesthetic such as benzocaine, cold or frozen teething rings, and hard crackers or bread can alleviate pain during teething.

Injections from immunizations, IM antibiotics in the emergency care department or physician's office, and blood draws are common sources of pain in children (Schechter, 2003). The immunization schedule for infants and young children requires at least 19 injections in the first 6 years of childhood; children receive four or five injections at multiple visits. Potential complications to needlesticks include fibrosis, contracture, abscess, and nerve injury. Factors that affect the incidence of complication are the injection site, the injectate itself (lower pH causing more burning and stinging), needle length, and the frequency of injection. Warming the injectate, using lidocaine as a diluent, and applying ice and pressure to the site immediately before the procedure may reduce the discomfort associated with IM injections. Topical analgesia such as EMLA, LMX, amethocaine, and cold sprays, and cognitive-behavioral techniques (distraction, bubbles, parental presence, age-appropriate explanations, kaleidoscopes, music, stories) have been used to minimize pain, stress, fear, distress, and anxiety during injections. If multiple injections are required, parents have reported that simultaneous administration rather than sequential administration is less painful and less traumatic for their children.

In patients with otitis media, the incidence of pain is lower in those who received ibuprofen three times a day when compared with children who received acetaminophen or who did not receive either ibuprofen or acetaminophen (Bertin, Pons, d'Athis, and others, 1996). Warm compresses using oatmeal or warm stones have also been found to be effective for otitis media. Local anesthetic combinations such as Auralgan (antipyrine, benzocaine, and oxyquinoline sulfate dissolved in dehydrated glycerine) have been demonstrated to provide relief, better than olive oil drops to the ear (Hoberman, Paradise, Reynolds, and others, 1997).

In children with pharyngitis, spontaneous pain resolved in 80% of children who received ibuprofen during the first 48 hours, 70% of children who received acetaminophen, and 55% of children who received neither ibuprofen nor acetaminophen (Bertin, Pons, d'Athis, and others, 1996). In patients who had culture-positive streptococcal pharyngitis, those who received IM injection of a steroid such as dexamethasone or betamethasone were able to achieve pain relief within

6 hours compared with those who did not receive either one (Marvez-Valls, Ernst, Gray, and others, 1998). Parents have also reported using salt water gargles, lozenges, and local anesthetic sprays for alleviation of their child's pain in acute pharyngitis.

Viral infections of the mouth such as primary herpetic gingivostomatitis (herpes simplex virus 1) and herpangina ulcers (coxsackievirus A) are extremely painful; if inadequately treated, the pain can inhibit oral intake in children. Viscous lidocaine can be swished and spit by children older than 3 years of age or applied with cotton-tipped applicator in children younger than 3 years. A 2% viscous lidocaine solution contains 100 mg/5 ml lidocaine hydrochloride, and dosages of more than 5 mg/kg every 3 hours can be potentially toxic in small children (Gonzales-Del-Rey, Wason, and Druckenbrod, 1994). Parents need careful instructions to place an accurate amount of lidocaine in the child's mouth. Benzocaine has also been used, and methemoglobinemia has been reported as a rare side effect associated with its administration in younger children. "Magic mouthwash" preparation has ingredients that adhere to the lesion and provide pain relief. It usually consists of equal parts of diphenhydramine, viscous lidocaine, and aluminum and magnesium hydroxide (Maalox); equal parts of diphenhydramine and attapulgite suspension (Kaopectate); or a sucralfate suspension plus diphenhydramine and attapulgite suspension solutions that coat the lesions.

PAINFUL AND INVASIVE PROCEDURES

Several painful and invasive procedures require the administration of anesthetics and analgesics. For circumcision pain, caudal or penile blocks are used before the procedure. Then the patient's parents are instructed how to apply lidocaine gels for the first 24 to 36 hours after the circumcision. For open wounds, bupivacaine may be instilled with or without epinephrine onto the dressing applied to skin to minimize pain for up to 48 hours after the procedure. For graft donor sites, analgesia is maintained by using a foam dressing soaked with bupivacaine (0.25%, 2 mg/kg; 0.8 ml/kg) applied to the donor surface. A continuous infusion of 0.25% bupivacaine at 1 to 3 ml/hr via a standard 18-gauge epidural catheter is then curled on the outer or inner surface of the foam (Cousins and Power, 2003). Wound perfusion of bupivacaine is useful for iliac crest bone graft donor sites (used for alveolar bone grafting in some techniques of cleft palate repair). A standard 18-gauge epidural catheter is also used with a very low infusion rate (1–3 ml/hr) of bupivacaine. For minor and some intermediate procedures, the local anesthetic infiltration with bupivacaine is commonly used. Some examples of these procedures include surface wounds and tunneling procedures in the anesthetized child requiring inguinal surgery; insertion of ventriculoperitoneal shunts, central venous lines, or central venous catheter-reservoir systems; and similar procedures.

Nitrous oxide, which is taken up rapidly and eliminated by the lungs, is highly insoluble in the blood and is delivered quickly to the brain to produce an analgesic effect equivalent to that of IV morphine. After approximately 2 minutes of inhalation, maximum pain relief can be achieved. The child breathes via face mask, nasal mask, or mouthpiece. It is not suitable for children younger than 3 years old and works best for children older than 5 years of age. Nitrous oxide inhalations are used frequently for a wide variety of procedures that require potent analgesia for a short time, such as suture insertion or removal, dressing removal or changes (including burns), drain or catheter removal, venipuncture or cannulation, lumbar puncture, physical therapy, and biopsies (skin, muscle, renal, or bone marrow). However, the use of nitrous oxide is contraindicated in children with pneumothorax, bowel obstruction, abnormal airway, recent head injury (especially with an intracranial air pocket), chronic respiratory disease with air trapping or bullous changes in the lung, and some types of uncorrected congenital heart disease (e.g., pulmonary hypertension). Nitrous oxide may lead to expansion of air pockets in confined spaces (chest, cranial cavities, bowel lumens) and create an increased pressure and tension effect. Tension pneumothorax, ischemia or shift of intracranial contents, and bowel distention with risk of perforation could occur. In addition, because nitrous oxide produces a degree of sedation and potentiates the sedative effects of other CNS depressants, caution is required when concurrently giving opioids, benzodiazepines, antihistamines, and similar drugs. Inspired concentrations of up to 50% nitrous oxide used for less than 30 minutes do not affect airway reflexes. Only trained personnel may administer nitrous oxide and monitor the child (Cousins and Power, 2003).

POSTOPERATIVE PAIN

Pain associated with surgery to the chest (e.g., repair of congenital heart defects, chest trauma) or abdominal regions (e.g., appendectomy, cholecystectomy, splenectomy) may result in pulmonary complications. Pain leads to decreased muscle movement in the thorax and abdominal area and leads to decreased tidal volume, vital capacity, functional residual capacity, and alveolar ventilation. The patient is unable to cough and clear secretions, and the risk for complications such as pneumonia and atelectasis is high. Severe postoperative pain also results in sympathetic overactivity, which leads to increases in heart rate, peripheral resistance, blood pressure, and cardiac output. The patient eventually experiences an increase in cardiac demand and myocardial oxygen consumption and a decrease in oxygen delivery to the tissues.

The basis for good postoperative pain control in children is preemptive analgesia. Preemptive analgesia involves administration of medications (e.g., local and regional anesthetics, analgesics) before the child experience the pain or before surgery is performed so that the sensory activation and changes in the pain pathways of the peripheral and CNS can be controlled. Preemptive analgesia has been demonstrated to lower postoperative pain, lower analgesic requirement, lower hospital stay, lower complications after surgery, and minimize the risks for peripheral and CNS sensitization that can lead to persistent pain (Cousins and Power, 2003).

A combination of medications (multimodal or balanced analgesia) is used for postoperative pain and may include NSAIDs, local anesthetics, nonopioids, and opioid analgesics to achieve optimum relief and minimize side effects. Opioids (see Table 7-5) administered around the clock during the first 48 hours or administered via PCA are commonly prescribed postoperatively. The duration of use is frequently limited to days because the cause of pain usually resolves. The combination of the IV NSAID ketorolac and morphine using a PCA device is frequently prescribed after thoracic surgery. Morphine delivered by PCA leads to a lower total dosage of opioid analgesia compared with the administration of intermittent doses of analgesic as required. After bowel surgery, a mixture of local anesthetics (bupivacaine) and a low-dose opioid (fentanyl) delivered by epidural route improves the rate of recovery and minimizes the gastrointestinal effects (e.g., bowel stasis, nausea, vomiting). After bowel function has been restored, oral opioids such as immediate-release and controlled-release preparations are preferred in older children. Controlled-release opioids facilitate ATC dosing and improve sleep. They are also associated with lower incidence of nausea, sedation, and breakthrough pain.

BURN PAIN

Because burn pain has multiple components, involves repeated manipulations over the injured painful sites, and has changing pattern over time, it is difficult and challenging to control. Burn pain includes a constant background pain that is felt at the wound sites and surrounding areas and can be exacerbated (breakthrough pain) by movements such as changing position, turning in bed, walking, or even breathing. Areas of normal skin that have been harvested for skin grafts (donor sites) also elicit pain. Pain is commonly experienced with intense tingling or itching sensations when skin grafting is required. During the healing process, when the tissue and nerve regenerate, the necrotic tissue (eschar) is excised until viable tissue is reached. The healing process may last for months to years. Pain or paresthetic sensations (e.g., itching, tingling, cold sensations) may persist. In addition, discomfort may be associated with immobilization of limbs in splints or garments, as well as multiple surgical interventions such as skin grafting and reconstructive surgery (Choiniere, 2003).

Multiple therapeutic procedures are carried out during the course of treatment. These procedures (dressing changes, wound débridement and cleansing, physical therapy sessions) occur daily or even several times a day. Providing proper analgesia without interfering with the patient's awareness during and after the procedure is the biggest challenge in the management of burn pain. Fentanyl or alfentanil has a major advantage over morphine because of its short duration. Fentanyl can prevent oversedation after the procedure. For less painful procedures, premedication with oral morphine, oral ketamine, or milder opioids 15 minutes before the procedure may be sufficient. Depending on the patient's anxiety level, a benzodiazepine (e.g., lorazepam) before the procedure may be beneficial. For longer procedures, morphine is the mainstay of treatment. Some patients may require moderate to deep sedation and analgesia. Oral oxycodone with midazolam and acetaminophen, in addition to nitrous oxide, may be needed. IV ketamine administered at subtherapeutic doses has been one of the most extensively used anesthetics for burn patients. The dysphoria and unpleasant reactions associated with ketamine administration may be minimized with premedication with a benzodiazepine. If ketamine is used with either morphine or fentanyl, the regimen could have opioid-sparing actions and reduce the opioid-related side effects.

Psychologic interventions can also be helpful in the treatment of burn pain. These interventions include hypnosis, relaxation training (breathing exercises, progressive muscle relaxation), biofeedback, stress inoculation training, cognitive-behavioral strategies (guided imagery, distraction, coping skills), and group and individual psychotherapy. They can be used alone or in combination. All of these techniques can help the patient relax and maintain a sense of control (Choiniere, 2003). A major disadvantage of these interventions is that they require time and discipline, and often patients are too stressed, fatigued, disoriented, or sick to engage in them.

RECURRENT HEADACHES

Recurrent headaches in children can be caused by several factors, including tension; dental braces; imbalance or weakness of eye muscles, causing deviation in alignment and refractive errors; and sequelae to accidents, sinusitis and other cranial infection or inflammation, increased ICP, epileptic attacks, drugs, obstructive sleep apnea, and rarely hypertension. Other causes may include arteriovenous malformations, disturbances in cerebrospinal fluid (CSF) flow or absorption, intracranial hemorrhages, ocular and dental diseases, bacterial infections, and brain tumors. Severe pain is the most disturbing symptom in migraine. Tension-type headache is usually mild or moderate, often producing a pressing feeling in the temples similar to a "tight band around the head." Continuous, daily, or near-daily headache with no specific cause occurs in a small subgroup of children. In epilepsy, headaches commonly occur immediately before, during, or after a seizure attack.

Treatment of recurrent headaches requires an understanding of the antecedents and consequences of headache pain. A headache diary can allow the child to record the time of onset, activities before the onset, any worries or concerns as far back as 24 hours before the onset, the severity and duration of pain, pain medications taken, and the activity pattern during headache episodes. The headache diary allows ongoing monitoring of headache activity, indicates the effects of interventions, and guides treatment planning.

There are two main approaches to management of headache using behavioral approaches: (1) teaching patients self-control skills to prevent headache (biofeedback techniques and relaxation training) and (2) modifying behavior patterns that increase the risk of headache occurrence or reinforce headache activity (cognitive-behavioral stress management techniques). Biofeedback is a technology-based form of relaxation therapy and can be useful in assessing and reinforcing learning of relaxation skills such as progressive muscle relaxation, deep breathing, and imagery. Children as young as 7 years of age have been taught these skills and with 2 to 3 weeks of practice are able to decrease the time needed to achieve relaxation.

To modify behavior patterns that increase the risk of headache occurrence or reinforce headache activity, the nurse instructs the parents to avoid giving excessive attention to their child's headache and to respond matter of factly to pain behavior and requests for special attention (Holden, Deichmann, and Levy, 1999). Parents are taught to assess whether school or social performance demands are being avoided because of headache. Parents are taught to focus attention on adaptive coping such as the use of relaxation techniques and maintenance of normal activity patterns. When using cognitive-behavioral stress management techniques, the parents identify negative thoughts and situations that may be associated with an increased risk for headache. The child is then taught to activate positive thoughts and engage in adaptive behavior appropriate to the situation.

RECURRENT ABDOMINAL PAIN

Recurrent abdominal pain or functional abdominal pain is defined as pain that occurs at least once per month for 3 consecutive months accompanied by pain-free periods and is severe enough that it interferes with a child's normal activities. Management of RAP is highly individualized to reflect the causes of the pain and the psychosocial needs of the child and family. A clear understanding of the child's characteristics (anxiety, physical health, temperament, coping skills, experience, learned response, depression), child's disability (school attendance, activities with family, social interactions, pain behaviors), environmental factors (family attitudes and behavioral patterns, school environment, community, friendships), and the pain stimulus (disease, injury, stress) is important in planning management strategies (Collins and Weisman, 2003).

Before any workup of the pain, the nurse informs the family that RAP is common in children and only 10% of children with RAP have an identifiable organic cause for their pain symptom. Medical workup is dictated by the child's symptoms and signs in combination with knowledge about common organic causes of RAP. If an organic cause is found, it is treated appropriately. Even if no organic cause is found, the nurse needs to communicate to the child and family a belief that the pain is real. Usually the abdominal pain goes away, but even if problems are identified, they may not be the actual cause and pain may persist, may be replaced by another symptom, or may go away on its own. The management plan includes regular follow-up at a 3- to 4-month intervals, a list of symptoms that call for earlier contact, and biobehavioral pain management techniques. The goal is to minimize the impact the pain has on the child's activities and the family's life (Collins and Weisman, 2003).

Case reports have demonstrated the effectiveness of implementing a time-out procedure, token systems, and positive reinforcement based on operant theory treatment modalities. Stress management and cognitive-behavioral strategies have also been reported to be successful. Parent training in how to avoid positive reinforcement of sick behaviors and focus on rewarding healthy behaviors is important. Over the course of several sessions, parents are educated about RAP, how to distinguish between sick and well behaviors, a reward system for well behaviors, and the importance of reinforcing relaxation and stressing coping skills taught to children for pain management. Treatment may consist of a varying number of sessions over 1 to 6 months and may include various components such as monitoring of symptoms, limited parent attention, relaxation training, increased dietary fiber, and requirements of school attendance. Response rates are 25% without abdominal pain and 56% to 75% improvements in symptoms (Collins and Weisman, 2003). The use of cognitive-behavioral therapy has been documented to reduce or eliminate pain in children with RAP and highlights the involvement of parents in supporting their child's self-management behavior. No negative side effects of symptom substitution occurred with the interventions. One study demonstrated that the combination of self-regulation and cognitive-behavioral interventions along with fiber intervention is more effective for treating RAP than using fiber alone (Weydert, Ball, and Davis, 2003).

PAIN WITH SICKLE CELL DISEASE

A painful episode is the most frequent cause for ED visits and hospital admissions among children with sickle cell disease. The acute painful episode in sickle cell disease is the only pain syndrome in which opioids are considered the major therapy and are started in early childhood and continued throughout adult life. A source of frustration for patients and clinicians is that the most current analgesic regimens are inadequate in controlling some of the most severe painful episodes. A multidisciplinary approach that involves both pharmacologic and nonpharmacologic modalities (cognitive-behavioral intervention, heat, massage, physical therapy) is needed but is not often implemented. The goals of treatment of the acute episode may not be to take all the pain away, which is usually impossible, but to make the pain tolerable to the patient until the episode resolves and to increase function and patient participation in activities of daily living (Benjamin, Dampier, Jacox, and others, 1999; Max, Payne, Edwards, and others, 1999).

Individuals coming to an ED for acute painful episodes usually have exhausted all home care options or outpatient therapy (Benjamin, Dampier, Jacox, and others, 1999; Max, Payne, Edwards, and others, 1999). The nurse should ask patients what the usual medication, dosage, and side effects were in the past; the usual medication taken at home; and medication taken since the onset of present pain. The patient may be on long-term opioid therapy at home and therefore may have developed some degree of tolerance. A different potent opioid or a larger dose of the same medication may be indicated. Because mixed opioid–agonist–antagonists (e.g., pentazozine, nalbuphine, butorphanol) may precipitate withdrawal syndromes, these should be avoided if patients were taking long-term opioids at home. A "passport" card with patient information about the diagnosis, previous complications, suggested pain management regimen, and name and contact information of the primary hematologist is helpful for parents and facilitates management of pain in the ED.

The patient is admitted for inpatient management of severe pain if adequate relief is not achieved in the ED (Benjamin, Dampier, Jacox, and others, 1999; Max, Payne, Edwards, and others, 1999). For severe pain, IV administration with bolus dosing and continuous infusion using a PCA device may be necessary. Patients requiring more than 5 to 7 days of opioids should have tapering doses to avoid the physiologic symptoms of withdrawal (dysphoria, nasal congestion, diarrhea, nausea and vomiting, sweating, and seizures). Appropriate weaning of the PCA schedules starts with reduction of the continuous infusion rate before discontinuation, while the patient can continue to use demand doses for analgesia. Morphine-equivalent equianalgesic conversions may be used to convert continuous infusion rates to equivalent oral analgesics. Doses of long-acting oral analgesics, such as sustained-release oral morphine, may also be used to replace continuous infusion dosing. The demand doses can be subsequently reduced if analgesia remains adequate.

Some patients whose pain is managed poorly will try to persuade medical staff to give them more analgesic, engage in clock watching, and request specific medications or dosages. These patients are often perceived as manipulative and demanding. Because patients with sickle cell disease have lifelong experiences with pain, they are knowledgeable about the medications and doses that are effective (Benjamin, Dampier, Jacox, and others, 1999; Max, Payne, Edwards, and others, 1999). Therefore the nurse should respect their requests for specific medications and doses and not interpret this as indications of drug-seeking behavior.

Patients who are administered doses of opioids that are inadequate to relieve their pain or whose doses are not tapered after a course of treatment may develop iatrogenic pseudoaddiction (Elander, Lusher, Bevan, and others, 2004), which resembles addiction. Pseudoaddiction or clock-watching behavior may be resolved by communicating with patients to ensure accurate assessment, involving them in decisions about their pain management, and administering adequate opioid doses (Elander, Lusher, Bevan, and others, 2004).

CANCER PAIN

Pain is the most prevalent symptom (84.4%) and was rated as moderate to severe (86.6%) and highly distressing (52.8%) in children with cancer (Collins, Byrnes, Dunkel, and others, 2000). Pain is present before diagnosis and treatment and may resolve after initiation of anticancer therapy. However, treatment-related pain is a common occurrence. Pain may be related to an operation; mucositis; a phantom limb; infection; chemotherapy; and procedures such as bone marrow aspiration, needle puncture, or lumbar puncture (Collins, Byrnes, Dunkel, and others, 2000). Tumor-related pain frequently occurs when the child relapses or when tumors become resistant to treatment. Intractable pain may occur in patients with solid tumors that metastasize to the central or peripheral nervous system. In young adult survivors of childhood cancer, chronic pain conditions may develop, including complex regional pain syndrome of the lower extremity, phantom limb pain, avascular necrosis, mechanical pain related to bone that failed to unite after tumor resection, and postherpetic neuralgia.

Oral mucositis (ulceration of the oral cavity and throat) may occur in 40% of patients undergoing chemotherapy or radiotherapy and in 76% of patients undergoing bone marrow transplant (Berger, Henderson, Nadoolman, and others, 1995). No present therapy adequately relieves the pain of these lesions. Antihistamines, local anesthetics, and opioids provide only temporary relief, may block taste perception, or may produce additional side effects such as lethargy and constipation. Initial treatment includes single agents (saline, opioids, sodium bicarbonate, hydrogen peroxide, sucralfate suspension, clotrimazole, nystatin, viscous lidocaine, amphotericin B, dyclonine) or mouthwash mixtures using a combination of agents (lidocaine, diphenhydramine, Maalox or Mylanta, nystatin). The mucositis after bone marrow transplantation may be prolonged, continuously intense, exacerbated by mouth care and swallowing, or worse during waking hours. The patient may be unable to eat or swallow. Morphine administered as a continuous infusion or delivered by a PCA device may be required until mucositis is resolved (Collins and Weisman, 2003).

Other treatment-related pain includes (1) abdominal pain after allogeneic bone marrow transplantation, which may be associated with acute graft-versus-host disease; (2) abdominal pain associated with typhlitis (infection of the cecum), which occurs when the patient is immunocompromised; (3) phantom sensations and phantom limb pain after an amputation; (4) peripheral neuropathy after administration of vincristine; and (5) medullary bone pain, which may be associated with administration of granulocyte colony–stimulating factor (Collins and Weisman, 2003).

Almost 40% of all pain episodes in children with cancer may be attributed to procedures (Ljungman, Gordh, Sorensen, and others, 1999, 2000, 2001; Ljungman, Kreuger, Andreasson, and others, 2000). Survivors of childhood cancer describe vivid memories of their experience with repeated painful procedures during treatment. These procedures include needle puncture for IM chemotherapy (L-asparaginase), IV lines, port access and blood draws, lumbar puncture, bone marrow aspiration and biopsy, removal of central venous catheters, and other invasive diagnostic procedures. Fear and anxiety related to these procedures may be minimized with parent and child preparation. The preparation starts with obtaining information from the parent about the child's coping styles, explaining the procedure, and enlisting their support followed by an age-appropriate explanation to the child. Topical analgesics (cold sprays, EMLA, amethocaine gels), as discussed previously, have been effective in providing analgesia before needle procedures.

Lumbar puncture for administration of chemotherapy (cytarabine, methotrexate) and collection of CSF may lead to a leak at the puncture site and low ICP (Collins and Weisman, 2003). Some children may experience postdural puncture headache, which may be treated by administering nonopioid analgesics and placing the patient in the supine position for 1 hour after the procedure. The pain related to bone marrow aspiration is caused by the insertion of a large needle into the posterior iliac space and the unpleasant sensation experienced at the time of marrow aspiration. Nonpharmacologic strategies such as cognitive-behavioral therapy, guided imagery, relaxation, music therapy, and hypnosis, as well as conscious sedation and general anesthesia, have been proven effective in decreasing pain and distress during the procedure.

Morphine is the most widely used opioid for moderate to severe pain and may be administered via the oral (including sustained-release formulations such as MS [Contin and Kadian], IV, subcutaneous, epidural, and intrathecal routes. When dose-limiting side effects of morphine develop, hydromorphone has been reported to be effective in several studies of children with cancer (Drake, Longworth, and Collins, 2004). In a study of children and adolescents with mucositis after bone marrow transplantation, which compared morphine with hydromorphone using PCA, hydromorphone was well tolerated and had a potency ratio of approximately 6:1 relative to morphine (Drake, Longworth, and Collins, 2004).

The most common clinical syndrome of neuropathic pain is painful peripheral neuropathy caused by chemotherapeutic agents, particularly vincristine and cisplatin and rarely cytarabine (Collins and Weisman, 2003). Withdrawal of the chemotherapy may resolve the neuropathy over weeks to months, or it may persist even after withdrawal. Neuropathic pain is associated with at least one of the following: (1) pain that is described as electric or shocklike, stabbing, or burning; (2) signs of neurologic involvement (paralysis, neuralgia, pain hypersensitivity) other than those associated with the progression of the tumor; and (3) the location of the solid organ cancer consistent with neurologic damage that could give rise to neuropathic pain. Dying children with cancer who experience neuropathic pain have higher baseline requirements of morphine and require rapid increases of morphine than dying children without neuropathic pain (Dougherty and DeBaun, 2003). Children with neuropathic pain often require massive opioid infusion (3 mg/kg/hr of IV morphine dose equivalent or approximately 100-fold greater than standard starting infusion rates). An epidural or subarachnoid infusion may be initiated if the patient experiences dose-limiting side effects of opioids or if pain was resistant to opioids.

Tricyclic antidepressants (amitriptyline, desipramine) and anticonvulsants (gabapentin, carbamazepine) have demonstrated effectiveness in neuropathic cancer pain. Randomized controlled trials showed that 60% to 70% of patients with neuropathic pain achieve relief with TCAs (Sindrup, Otto, Finnerup, and others, 2005). The TCAs have many actions that could be involved in their pain-relieving effect and have been considered the mainstay of therapy for neuropathic pain (Sindrup, Otto, Finnerup, and others, 2005).

Klepstad, Borchgrevink, Hval, and others (2001) reported the pain experience of a 12-year-old girl with severe neuropathic pain caused by a cervical spinal tumor. Two weeks after resection of the tumor, the child experienced increased pain in her neck, which was superficial and distributed in the dermatomes below the cervical medullary lesion. Pain was provoked by touch and did not decrease in intensity despite a subcutaneous infusion of morphine at 160 mg/24 hr. The child screamed from increased pain when her parents or siblings tried to comfort her with bodily contact. Pain was relieved after administration of 7.5 to 10 mg IV ketamine. Ketamine is an *N*-methyl-D-aspartate (NMDA) antagonist, which has undesirable side effects (sedation, nausea, dissociative reactions, muteness, dizziness, and visual distortions) and short duration of action (Sang, 2000). After administration of ketamine, the child was able to tolerate touch without pain paroxysms. A continuous IV infusion was eventually initiated for convenience, and benzodiazepines were added to avoid the psychomimetic effects associated with ketamine. More recently, Finkel, Pestieau, and Queszado (2007) used subanesthetic doses of ketamine to treat 11 children and adolescents who were taking high doses of opioids and had uncontrolled cancer pain. Ketamine appeared to improve pain control and to have an opioid-sparing effect. Members of a pain management consulting service directed and titrated the ketamine to address symptoms. The ketamine dose range used (0.1–1 mg/kg/hr) was low dose and is lower than that used for anesthetic purposes. Lorazepam (0.025 mg/kg every 12 hr) was administered concurrently during ketamine treatment. Continuous monitoring included heart rate, noninvasive blood pressure, respiratory rate, and oxygen saturation.

Although ketamine is frequently used to ensure analgesia and sedation during painful procedures in children, its long-term use for the treatment of neuropathic pain in children has not been systematically studied and is not of clinical benefit for all patients (Klepstad, Borchgrevink, Hval, and others, 2001). In randomized studies of patients with chronic neuropathic pain, only some patients had a beneficial response to ketamine (Haines and Gaines, 1999; Max, Byas-Smith, Gracely, and others, 1995; Mitchell, 2001). Other NMDA antagonists (dextromethorphan, memantine) are available for clinical use, but no reports on their use in children with neuropathic pain related to cancer have been documented.

PAIN AND SEDATION IN END-OF-LIFE CARE

Many patients require doses of opioids that make them sedated but arousable as their disease progresses (cancer, human immunodeficiency virus, cystic fibrosis, neurodegenerative disease) at the end of life. Comfort can be achieved with a combination of opioids and adjuvant analgesics in most situations. Parents need reassurance that the opioids are treating pain but not causing the child's death and that the child's advancing disease is the cause of death.

A small group of patients have intolerable side effects or inadequate analgesia despite extremely aggressive use of medications to relieve pain and side effects. Continuous sedation may be a means of relieving suffering when there is no feasible or acceptable means of providing analgesia that preserves alertness. A continuing high-dose infusion of opioids along with sedation is prescribed to reduce the possibility that a child might experience unrelieved pain but be too sedated to report it. Sedation in these situations is widely regarded as providing comfort, not euthanasia. Clinicians and ethicists have a range of views regarding assisted suicide and euthanasia, but they all agree that no child or parent should choose death because of inadequate efforts to relieve pain and suffering (Berde and Collins, 2003).

▌ KEY POINTS

- Although the ability to measure pain in children has improved dramatically in recent years, assessment of pain in children continues to be complex and challenging.
- Behavioral assessment is useful for measuring pain in infants and preverbal children who do not have the language skills to communicate that they are in pain or when mental clouding and confusion limit a child's ability to communicate.
- Physiologic measures are not able to distinguish between physical responses to pain and other forms of stress to the body.

- The number of pain measurement tools that are available for use in infants and young children has increased dramatically and adds a layer of complexity to the assessment of pain in children.
- Important components of assessment include the onset of pain; pain duration or pattern; effectiveness of the current treatment; factors that aggravate or relieve the pain; other symptoms and complications concurrently felt; and interference with the child's mood, function, and interactions with family.

- The administration of sucrose with and without nonnutritive sucking has a calming and pain-relieving effects for invasive procedures in neonates.
- One of the most significant improvements in the ability to provide atraumatic care to children is the anesthetic creams LMX or EMLA.
- Nonopioids, including acetaminophen (Tylenol, paracetamol) and NSAIDs, are suitable for mild to moderate pain; opioids are needed for moderate to severe pain.
- Several drugs, known as coanalgesics or adjuvant analgesics, may be used alone or with opioids to control pain symptoms and opioid side effects.
- A significant advance in the administration of IV, epidural, or subcutaneous analgesics is the use of PCA.
- Although respiratory depression is the most feared side effect of opioids, constipation is a common and sometimes serious side effect that decreases peristalsis and increases anal sphincter tone.
- Several harmful effects occur with unrelieved pain, particularly when pain is prolonged.
- Surgery and traumatic injuries (fractures, dislocations, strains, sprains, lacerations, burns) generate a catabolic state as a result of increased secretion of catabolic hormones and lead to alterations in blood flow, coagulation, fibrinolysis, substrate metabolism, and water and electrolyte balance and increase the demands on the cardiovascular and respiratory systems.
- Because burn pain has multiple components, involves repeated manipulations over the injured painful sites, and has changing pattern over time, it is difficult and challenging to control.
- Treatment of recurrent headaches requires an understanding of the antecedents and consequences of headache pain.
- RAP or functional abdominal pain is defined as pain that occurs at least once per month for 3 consecutive months accompanied by pain-free periods and is severe enough that it interferes with a child's normal activities.
- A painful episode is the most frequent cause for ED visits and hospital admissions among children with sickle cell disease.
- Pain is the most prevalent symptom reported by children with cancer.
- Injections from immunizations, IM antibiotics in the ED or physician's office, and blood draws are common sources of pain in children.
- For nonpainful procedures such as radiologic imaging studies, several medications are used to sedate, minimize anxiety, and induce amnesia.
- Several painful and invasive procedures require the administration of anesthetics and analgesics.

REFERENCES

Abbe M, Simon C, Angiolilo A, and others: A survey of language barriers from the perspective of pediatric oncologists, interpreters, and parents, *Pediatr Blood Cancer* 47(6):819–824, 2006.

Abdelkefi A, Abdennebi YB, Mellouli F, and others: Effectiveness of fixed 50% nitrous oxide oxygen mixture and EMLA cream for insertion of central venous catheters in children, *Pediatr Blood Cancer* 43(7):777–779, 2004.

Algren JT, Gursoy F, Johnson TD, and others: The effect of nitrous oxide diffusion on laryngeal mask airway cuff inflation in children, *Paediatr Anaesth* 8(1):31–36, 1998.

Ambuel B, Hamlett KW, Marx CM, and others: Assessing distress in pediatric intensive care environments: the COMFORT scale, *J Pediatr Psychol* 17(1):95–109, 1992.

American Pain Society: *Principles of analgesic use in the treatment of acute pain and chronic cancer pain*, ed 4, Glenview, Ill, 1999, Author.

Anand KJ, Grunau RE, Oberlander TF: Developmental character and long-term consequences of pain in infants and children, *Child Adolesc Psychiatr Clin North Am* 6(4):703–724, 1997.

Anand KJ, Hickey PR: Halothane-morphine compared with high-dose sufentanil for anesthesia and postoperative analgesia in neonatal cardiac surgery, *N Engl J Med* 326(1):1–9, 1992.

Anand KJ, Hickey P: Pain and its effects in the human neonate and fetus, *N Engl J Med* 317(21):1321–1329, 1987.

Barrier G, Attia J, Mayer MN, and others: Measurement of postoperative pain and narcotic administration in infants using a new clinical scoring system, *Anesthesiology* 67(3A):A532, 1987.

Basbaum AI: Distinct neurochemical features of acute and persistent pain, *Proc Natl Acad Sci USA* 96(14):7739–7743, 1999a.

Basbaum AI: Spinal mechanisms of acute and persistent pain, *Reg Anesth Pain Med* 24(1):59–67, 1999b.

Benjamin L, Swinson G, Nagel R: Sickle cell anemia day hospital: an approach for the management of uncomplicated painful crises, *Blood* 95:1130–1137, 2000.

Benjamin LJ, Dampier CD, Jacox AK, and others: *Guideline for the management of acute and chronic pain in sickle cell disease*, Glenview, Ill, 1999, American Pain Society.

Berde C, Collins J: Cancer pain and palliative care in children. In Melzack R, Wall P, editors: *Handbook of pain management*, St. Louis, 2003, Churchill Livingstone.

Berger A, Henderson M, Nadoolman W, and others: Oral capsaicin provides temporary relief for oral mucositis pain secondary to chemotherapy/radiation therapy, *J Pain Symptom Manage* 10(3):243–248, 1995.

Bernstein B, Pachter L: Cultural considerations in children's pain. In Schechter N, Berde C, Yaster M, editors: *Pain in infants, children, and adolescents*, Philadelphia, 2003, Lippincott Williams & Wilkins.

Bertin L, Pons G, d'Athis P, and others: A randomized double blind multicentre controlled trial of ibuprofen versus acetaminophen and placebo for symptoms of acute otitis media in children, *Fundam Clin Pharmacol* 10:387–392, 1996.

Beyer JE, Denyes MJ, Villarruel AM: The creation, validation and continuing development of the Oucher: a measure of pain intensity in children, *J Pediatr Nurs* 7(5):335–346, 1992.

Beyer JE, Knott CB: Construct validity estimation for the African-American and Hispanic versions of the Oucher scale, *J Pediatr Nurs* 13(1):20–31, 1998.

Beyer JE, Turner SB, Jones L, and others: The alternate forms reliability of the Oucher pain scale, *Pain Manag Nurs* 6(1):10–17, 2005.

Bildner J, Krechel SW: Increasing staff nurse awareness of postoperative pain management in the NICU, *Neonat Netw* 15(1):11–16, 1996.

Bishai R, Taddio A, Bar-Oz B, and others: Relative efficacy of amethocaine gel and lidocaine–prilocaine cream for port-a-cath puncture in children, *Pediatrics* 104(3):e31, 1999.

Blauer T, Gerstmann D: A simultaneous comparison of three neonatal pain scales during common NICU procedures, *Clin J Pain* 14(1):39–47, 1998.

Breau LM, MacLaren J, McGrath PJ, and others: Caregivers' beliefs regarding pain in children with cognitive impairment: relation between pain sensation and reaction increases with severity of impairment, *Clin J Pain* 19(6):335–344, 2003.

Breau LM, McGrath PJ, Camfield CS, and others: Psychometric properties of the Non-communicating Children's Pain Checklist–Revised, *Pain* 99:349–357, 2002.

Bruera E, Willey JS, Ewert-Flannagan PA, and others: Pain intensity assessment by bedside nurses and palliative care consultants: a retrospective study, *Support Care Cancer* 13(4):228–231, 2005.

Chambers C: The role of family factors in pediatric pain. In Finley G, McGrath PJ, editors: *Pediatric pain: biological and social context*, Seattle, 2003, IASP Press.

Chambers C, Craig K: An intrusive impact of anchors in children's faces pain scales, *Pain* 78:27–37, 1998.

Choi WY, Irwin MG, Hui TW, and others: EMLA cream versus dorsal penile nerve block for postcircumcision analgesia in children, *Anesth Analg* 96(2):396–399, 2003.

Choiniere M: Pain of burns. In Melzack R, Wall P, editors: *Handbook of pain management*, St. Louis, 2003, Churchill Livingstone.

Chorpita BF, Yim L, Moffitt C, and others: Assessment of symptoms of DSM-IV anxiety and depression in children: a revised child anxiety and depression scale, *Behav Res Ther* 38(8):835–855, 2000.

Claar RL, Walker LS: Functional assessment of pediatric pain patients: psychometric properties of the functional disability inventory, *Pain* 121(1–2):77–84, 2006.

Cline ME, Herman J, Shaw ER, and others: Standardization of the visual analogue scale, *Nurs Res* 41(6):378–380, 1992.

Cole J, Jorgensen K: Medical, developmental, and pharmacologic intervention: the essence of collaboration, *Neonat Netw* 16:56–58, 1997.

Collins J, Weisman S: Management of pain in childhood cancer. In Schechter N, Berde C, Yaster M, editors: *Pain in infants, children, and adolescents*, Philadelphia, 2003, Lippincott Williams & Wilkins.

Collins JJ, Byrnes ME, Dunkel IJ, and others: The measurement of symptoms in children with cancer, *J Pain Symptom Manage* 19(5):363–377, 2000.

Cousins M, Power I: Acute and postoperative pain. In Melzack R, Wall P, editors: *Handbook of pain management*, St. Louis, 2003, Churchill Livingstone.

Dampier C, Ely B, Brodecki D, and others: Characteristics of pain managed at home in children and adolescents with sickle cell disease by using diary self-reports, *J Pain* 3(6):461–470, 2002a.

Dampier C, Ely E, Brodecki D, and others: Home management of pain in sickle cell disease: a daily diary study in children and adolescents, *J Pediatr Hematol Oncol* 24(8):643–647, 2002b.

Dougherty M, DeBaun MR: Rapid increase of morphine and benzodiazepine usage in the last 3 days of life in children with cancer is related to neuropathic pain, *J Pediatr* 142(4):373–376, 2003.

Drake R, Longworth J, Collins JJ: Opioid rotation in children with cancer, *J Palliat Med* 7(3):419–422, 2004.

Egekvist H, Bjerring P: Effect of EMLA cream on skin thickness and subcutaneous venous diameter: a randomized, placebo-controlled study in children, *Acta Dermatol Venereol* 80(5):340–343, 2000.

Eland JA, Banner W: Analgesia, sedation, and neuromuscular blockage in pediatric critical care. In Hazinski ME, editor: *Manual of pediatric critical care*, St. Louis, 1999, Mosby.

Elander J, Lusher J, Bevan D, and others: Understanding the causes of problematic pain management in sickle cell disease: evidence that pseudoaddiction plays a more important role than genuine analgesic dependence, *J Pain Symptom Manage* 27(2):156–169, 2004.

Ely B, Dampier C, Gilday M, and others: Caregiver report of pain in infants and toddlers with sickle cell disease: reliability and validity of a daily diary, *J Pain* 3(1):50–57, 2002.

Fearon I, Kisilevsky BS, Hains SM, and others: Swaddling after heel lance: age-specific effects on behavioral recovery in preterm infants, *Develop Behav Pediatr* 18:222–232, 1997.

Finkel JC, Pestieau SR, Queszado ZM: Ketamine as an adjuvant for treatment of cancer pain in children and adolescents, *J Pain* 8(6):515–521, 2007.

Finley GA, Chambers CT, McGrath PJ, and others: Construct validity of the parents' postoperative pain measure, *Clin J Pain* 19(5):329–334, 2003.

Flores G, Abreu M, Olivar MA, and others: Access barriers to health care for Latino children, *Arch Pediatr Adolesc Med* 152(11):1119–1125, 1998.

Flores G, Vega LR: Barriers to health care access for Latino children: a review, *Fam Med* 30(3):196–205, 1998.

Franck LS, Harris SK, Soetenga DJ, and others: The Withdrawal Assessment Tool-1 (WAT-1): an assessment instrument for monitoring opioid and benzodiazepine withdrawal symptoms in pediatric patients, *Pediatr Crit Care Med* 9(6):573–580, 2008.

Franck L, Vilardi J: Assessment and management of opioid withdrawal in ill neonates, *Neonat Netw* 14(2):39–48, 1995.

Franck LS, Vilardi J, Durand D, and others: Opioid withdrawal in neonates after continuous infusions of morphine or fentanyl during extracorporeal membrane oxygenation, *Am J Crit Care* 7(5):364–369, 1998.

Furdon SA, Eastman M, Benjamin K, and others: Outcome measures after standardized pain management strategies in postoperative patients in the neonatal intensive care unit, *J Perinat Neonatal Nurs* 12(1):58–69, 1998.

Gad LN, Olsen KS, Lysgaard AB, and others: Optimized use of EMLA cream in children—secondary publication: a randomized, prospective, controlled comparison of two application regimes, *Ugeskr Laeger* 167(4):404–407, 2005.

Gaina A, Sekine M, Chen X, and others: Validity of child sleep diary questionnaire among junior high school children, *J Epidemiol* 14(1):1–4, 2004.

Goldschneider K, Anand K: Long-term consequences of pain in neonates. In Schechter N, Berde C, Yaster M, editors: *Pain in infants, children, and adolescents*, Philadelphia, 2003, Lippincott Williams & Wilkins.

Golianu B, Krane EJ, Galloway KS, and others: Pediatric acute pain management, *Pediatr Clin North Am* 47(3):559–587, 2000.

Gonzales-Del-Rey J, Wason S, Druckenbrod R: Lidocaine overdose: another preventable case? *Pediatr Emerg Care* 10:344–346, 1994.

Gray L, Watt L, Blass E: Skin-to-skin contact is analgesic in healthy newborns, *Pediatrics* 105(1):110–111, 2000.

Hadden KL, von Baeyer CL: Pain in children with cerebral palsy: common triggers and expressive behaviors, *Pain* 99(1–2):281–288, 2002.

Hadjistavropoulos HD, Craig KD, Grunau RE, and others: Judging pain in infants: behavioural, contextual, and developmental determinants, *Pain* 73(3):319–324, 1997.

Haines DR, Gaines SP: N of 1 randomised controlled trials of oral ketamine in patients with chronic pain, *Pain* 83(2):283–287, 1999.

Hannallah RS, Broadman LM, Belman AB, and others: Comparison of caudal and ilioinguinal/iliohypogastric nerve blocks for control of post-orchiopexy pain in pediatric ambulatory surgery, *Anesthesiology* 66:832–834, 1987.

Hershey AD, Powers SW, Vockell AL, and others: PedMIDAS: Development of a questionnaire to assess disability of migraines in children, *Neurology* 57(11):2034–2039, 2001.

Hershey AD, Powers SW, Vockell AL, and others: Development of a patient-based grading scale for PedMIDAS, *Cephalalgia* 24(10):844–849, 2004.

Hester NO, Foster RL, Jordan-Marsh M, and others: Putting pain measurement into clinical practice. In Finley GA, McGrath PJ, editors: *Measurement of pain in infants and children*, vol 10, Seattle, 1998, International Association for the Study of Pain Press.

Hicks CL, von Baeyer CL, Spafford PA, and others: The Faces Pain Scale–Revised: toward a common metric in pediatric pain measurement, *Pain* 93(2):173–183, 2001.

Hoberman A, Paradise JL, Reynolds EA, and others: Efficacy of Auralgan for treating ear pain in children with acute otitis media, *Arch Pediatr Adolesc Med* 151:675–678, 1997.

Hodgkinson K, Bear M, Thorn J, and others: Measuring pain in neonates: evaluating an instrument and developing a common language, *Aust J Adv Nurs* 12(1):17–22, 1994.

Holden E, Deichmann M, Levy J: Empirically supported treatments in pediatric psychology: recurrent pediatric headache, *J Pediatr Psychol* 24:91–100, 1999.

Jacob E, Miaskowski C, Savedra M, and others: Management of vaso-occlusive pain in children with sickle cell disease, *J Pediatr Hematol Oncol* 25(4):307–311, 2003a.

Jacob E, Miaskowski C, Savedra M, and others: Changes in intensity, location, and quality of vaso-occlusive pain in children with sickle cell disease, *Pain* 102(1-2):187–193, 2003b.

Jacob E, Mueller BU: Pain experience of children with sickle cell disease who had prolonged hospitalizations for acute painful episodes, *Pain Med* 9(1):13–21, 2008.

Jacob E, Puntillo KA: Variability of analgesic practices for hospitalized children on different pediatric specialty units, *J Pain Symptom Manage* 20(1):59–67, 2000.

Johnston CC, Stevens B, Pinelli J, and others: Kangaroo care is effective in diminishing pain response in preterm neonates, *Arch Pediatr Adolesc Med* 157(11):1084–1088, 2003.

Jordan-Marsh M, Yoder L, Hall D, and others: Alternate Oucher form testing gender ethnicity and age variations, *Res Nurs Health* 17:111–118, 1994.

Joyce BA, Schade JG, Keck JF, and others: Reliability and validity of preverbal pain assessment tools, *Issues Comp Pediatr Nurs* 17:121–135, 1994.

Klepstad P, Borchgrevink P, Hval B, and others: Long-term treatment with ketamine in a 12-year-old girl with severe neuropathic pain caused by a cervical spinal tumor, *J Pediatr Hematol Oncol* 23(9):616–619, 2001.

Kovacs M: Rating scales to assess depression in school-aged children, *Acta Paedopsychiatr* 46(5–6):305–315, 1981.

Krechel SW, Bildner J: CRIES: a new neonatal postoperative pain measurement score: initial testing of validity and reliability, *Pediatr Anaesth* 5:53–61, 1995.

Lawrence J, Alcock D, McGrath P, and others: The development of a tool to assess neonatal pain, *Neonat Netw* 12(6):59–66, 1993.

Lenton S, Stallard P, Lewis M, and others: Prevalence and morbidity associated with nonmalignant, life-threatening conditions in childhood, *Child Care Health Dev* 27(5):389–398, 2001.

Ljungman G, Gordh T, Sorensen S, and others: Pain in paediatric oncology: interviews with children, adolescents and their parents, *Acta Paediatr* 88(6):623–630, 1999.

Ljungman G, Gordh T, Sorensen S, and others: Pain variations during cancer treatment in children: a descriptive survey, *Pediatr Hematol Oncol* 17(3):211–221, 2000.

Ljungman G, Gordh T, Sorensen S, and others: Lumbar puncture in pediatric oncology: conscious sedation vs. general anesthesia, *Med Pediatr Oncol* 36(3):372–379, 2001.

Ljungman G, Kreuger A, Andreasson S, and others: Midazolam nasal spray reduces procedural anxiety in children. *Pediatrics* 105(1 Pt 1):73–78, 2000.

Luffy R, Grove SK: Examining the validity, reliability, and preference of three pediatric pain measurement tools in African-American children, *Pediatr Nurs* 29(1):54–60, 2003.

Manworren R, Hynan L: Clinical validation of FLACC: Preverbal Patient Pain Scale, *Pediatr Nurs* 29(2):140–146, 2003.

Marvez-Valls EG, Ernst AA, Gray J, and others: The role of betamethasone in the treatment of acute exudative pharyngitis, *Acad Emerg Med* 5:567–572, 1998.

Marx J: Pain research: prolonging the agony, *Science* 305(5682):326–329, 2004.

Max MB, Byas-Smith MG, Gracely RH, and others: Intravenous infusion of the NMDA antagonist, ketamine, in chronic posttraumatic pain with allodynia: a double-blind comparison to alfentanil and placebo, *Clin Neuropharmacol* 18(4):360–368, 1995.

Max MB, Payne R, Edwards WT, and others: *Principles of analgesic use in the treatment of acute pain and cancer pain*, Glenview, Ill, 1999, American Pain Society.

Maxwell L, Yaster M: Perioperative management issues in pediatric patients, *Anesthesiol Clin North Am* 18(3):601–632, 2000.

McCaffery M, Pasero C: *Pain clinical manual*, St. Louis, 1999, Mosby.

McGrath P, Hillier L, editors: *Modifying the psychologic factors that intensify children's pain and prolong disability*, Philadelphia, 2003, Lippincott Williams & Wilkins.

McGrath PJ, Johnson G, Goodman JT, and others: The CHEOPS: a behavioral scale to measure postoperative pain in children. In Fields H, Dubner R, Cervero F, editors: *Advances in pain research and therapy*, New York, 1985, Raven Press.

McGrath PJ, Walco GA, Turk DC, and others: Core outcome domains and measures for pediatric acute and chronic/recurrent pain clinical trials: PedIMMPACT recommendations, *J Pain* 9(9):771–783, 2008.

Melzack R: The McGill pain questionnaire: major properties and scoring methods, *Pain* 1:277–299, 1975.

Merkel SI, Voepel-Lewis T, Shayevitz JR, and others: The FLACC: a behavioral scale for scoring postoperative pain in young children, *Pediatr Nurs* 23(3):293–297, 1997.

Merskey H, Bogduk N, editors: *Classification of chronic pain: descriptions of chronic pain syndromes and definitions of pain terms*, ed 2, Seattle, 1994, IASP Press.

Miaskowski C, Lee K: Pain, fatigue, and sleep disturbances in oncology outpatients receiving radiation therapy for bone metastasis: a pilot study, *J Pain Symptom Manage* 17(5):320–332, 1999.

Mitchell AC: An unusual case of chronic neuropathic pain responds to an optimum frequency of intravenous ketamine infusions, *J Pain Symptom Manage* 21(5):443–446, 2001.

Morin C, Gibson D, Wade J: Self-reported sleep and mood disturbance in chronic pain patients, *Clin J Pain* 14(4):311–314, 1998.

Myers C, Stuber ML, Bonamer-Rheingans JI, and others: Complementary therapies and childhood cancer, *Cancer Control* 12(3):172–180, 2005.

Nadvi SZ, Sarnaik S, Ravindranath Y: Low frequency of meperidine-associated seizures in sickle cell disease, *Clin Pediatr (Phila)* 38(8):459–462, 1999.

Owens JA, Spirito A, McGuinn M: The Children's Sleep Habits Questionnaire (CSHQ): psychometric properties of a survey instrument for school-aged children, *Sleep* 23(8):1043–1051, 2000.

Palermo T, Valenzuela D: Use of pain diaries to assess recurrent and chronic pain in children, *Suffer Child* 3:1–14, 2003.

Palermo TM: Impact of recurrent and chronic pain on child and family daily functioning: a critical review of the literature, *J Dev Behav Pediatr* 21(1):58–69, 2000.

Palermo TM, Kiska R: Subjective sleep disturbances in adolescents with chronic pain: relationship to daily functioning and quality of life, *J Pain* 6(3):201–207, 2005.

Palermo TM, Valenzuela D, Stork P: A randomized trial of electronic versus paper pain diaries in children: impact on compliance, accuracy, and acceptability, *Pain* 107(3):213–219, 2004.

Perquin CW, Hazebroek-Kampschreur AA, Hunfeld JA, and others: Chronic pain among children and adolescents: physician consultation and medication use, *Clin J Pain* 16(3):229–235, 2000a.

Perquin CW, Hazebroek-Kampschreur AA, Hunfeld JA, and others: Pain in children and adolescents: a common experience, *Pain* 87(1):51–58, 2000b.

Puchalski M, Hummel P: The reality of neonatal pain, *Adv Neonatal Care* 2(5):233–244, 2002.

Reid GJ, Lang BA, McGrath P: Primary juvenile fibromyalgia: psychological adjustment, family

functioning, coping, and functional disability, *Arthritis Rheum* 40(4):752–760, 1997.

Reis E, Holubkov R: Vapocoolant spray is equally effective as EMLA cream in reducing immunization pain in school-aged children, *Pediatrics* 100(6):e5, 1997.

Robieux I, Kumar R, Radhakrishnan S, and others: Assessing pain and analgesia with a lidocaine-prilocaine emulsion in infants and toddlers during venipuncture, *J Pediatr* 118(6):971–973, 1991.

Rogers TL, Ostrow CL: The use of EMLA cream to decrease venipuncture pain in children, *J Pediatr Nurs* 19(1):33–39, 2004.

Rusy L, Weisman S: Complementary therapies for acute pediatric pain management, *Pediatr Clin North Am* 47(3):589–599, 2000.

Sang CN: NMDA-receptor antagonists in neuropathic pain: experimental methods to clinical trials, *J Pain Symptom Manage* 19(1 suppl):S21–S25, 2000.

Santiago A, Abad P, Fernandez C, and others: Premedication with EMLA cream for ambulatory surgery in children, *Ambu Surg* 8(3):157, 2000.

Savedra MC, Holzemer WL, Tesler MD, and others: Assessment of postoperation pain in children and adolescents using the adolescent pediatric pain tool, *Nurs Res* 42(1):5–9, 1993.

Savedra MC, Tesler MD, Holzemer WL, and others: Pain location: validity and reliability of body outline markings by hospitalized children and adolescents, *Res Nurs Health* 12:307–314, 1989.

Schade JG, Joyce BA, Gerkensmeyer J, and others: Comparison of three preverbal scales for postoperative pain assessment in a diverse pediatric sample, *J Pain Symptom Manage* 12(6):348–359, 1996.

Schechter N: Management of common pain problems in the primary care pediatric setting. In Schechter N, Berde C, Yaster M, editors: *Pain in infants, children, and adolescents*, Philadelphia, 2003, Lippincott Williams & Wilkins.

Sindrup SH, Otto M, Finnerup NB, and others: Antidepressants in the treatment of neuropathic pain, *Basic Clin Pharmacol Toxicol* 96(6):399–409, 2005.

Stallard P, Williams L, Lenton S, and others: Pain in cognitively impaired, non-communicating children, *Arch Dis Child* 85(6):460–462, 2001.

Stallard P, Williams L, Velleman R, and others: The development and evaluation of the pain indicator for communicatively impaired children (PICIC), *Pain* 98(1–2):145–149, 2002.

Stevens B: Development and testing of a pediatric pain management sheet, *Pediatr Nurs* 16(6):543–548, 1990.

Stevens B, Johnston C, Petryshen P, and others: Premature Infant Pain Profile: development and initial validation, *Clin J Pain* 12:13–22, 1996.

Stevens B, Yamada J, Ohlsson A: *Sucrose for analgesia in newborn infants undergoing painful procedures* (review), 2005. In Cochrane Neonatal Collaboration, retrieved from http://www.thecochranelibrary.com.

Stinson JN, Stevens BJ, Feldman BM, and others: Construct validity of a multidimensional electronic pain diary for adolescents with arthritis, *Pain* 136(3):281–292, 2008.

Stone AA, Broderick E, Schwartz JE, and others: Intensive momentary reporting of pain with an electronic diary: reactivity, compliance, and patient satisfaction, *Pain* 104(1–2):343–351, 2003.

Suraseranivongse S, Montapaneewat T, Manon J, and others: Cross-validation of a self-report scale for postoperative pain in school-aged children, *J Med Assoc Thai* 88:412–418, 2005.

Sweet S, McGrath P: Physiological measures of pain. In Finley G, McGrath P, editors: *Measurement of pain in infants and children*, Seattle, 1998, IASP Press.

Taddio A, Nulman I, Koren BS, and others: A revised measure of acute pain in infants, *J Pain Symptom Manage* 10(6):456–463, 1995.

Tarbell SE, Cohen IT, Marsh JL: The Toddler-Preschooler Postoperative Pain Scale: an observational scale for measuring postoperative pain in children aged 1–5: preliminary report, *Pain* 50(3):273–280, 1992.

Tesler MD, Savedra MC, Holzemer WL, and others: The word-graphic rating scale as a measure of children's and adolescents' pain intensity, *Res Nurs Health* 14:361–371, 1991.

Uziel Y, Berkovitch M, Gazarian M, and others: Evaluation of eutectic lidocaine/prilocaine cream (EMLA) for steroid joint injection in children with juvenile rheumatoid arthritis: a double blind, randomized, placebo controlled trial, *J Rheumatol* 30(3):594–596, 2003.

Van Cleve L, Bossert E, Beecroft P, and others: The pain experience of children with leukemia during the first year after diagnosis, *Nurs Res* 53(1):1–10, 2004.

Van Cleve L, Munoz C, Bossert EA, and others: Children's and adolescents' pain language in Spanish: translation of a measure, *Pain Manag Nurs* 2(3):110–118, 2001.

van Dijk A, McGrath PA, Pickett W, and others: Pain prevalence in nine- to 13-year-old schoolchildren, *Pain Res Manag* 11(4):234–240, 2006.

Varni JW, Seid M, Rode CA: The PedsQL: measurement model for the pediatric quality of life inventory, *Med Care* 37(2):126–139, 1999.

Varni JW, Thompson KL, Hanson V: The Varni/Thompson Pediatric Pain Questionnaire, Part I, Chronic musculoskeletal pain in juvenile rheumatoid arthritis, *Pain* 28:27–38, 1987.

Vervoort T, Goubert L, Eccleston C, and others: Catastrophic thinking about pain is independently associated with pain severity, disability, and somatic complaints in school children and children with chronic pain, *J Pediatr Psychol* 31(7):674–683, 2006.

Villarruel AM, Denyes MJ: Pain assessment in children: theoretical and empirical validity, *Adv Nurs Sci* 14(2):32–41, 1991.

von Baeyer C, Hicks C: Support for a common metric for pediatric pain intensity scales, *Pain Res Manage* 4(2):157–160, 2000.

Walker LS, Greene JW: The functional disability inventory: measuring a neglected dimension of child health status, *J Pediatr Psychol* 16(1):39–58, 1991.

Walters A, Williamson G: The role of activity restriction in the association between pain and depression: a study of pediatric patients with chronic pain, *Child Health Care* 28:33–50, 1999.

Weisman S, Bernstein B, Schechter N: Consequences of inadequate analgesia during painful procedures in children, *Arch Pediatr Adolesc Med* 152:147–149, 1998.

Weydert J, Ball T, Davis M: Systematic review of treatments for recurrent abdominal pain, *Pediatrics* 111(1):1–3, 2003.

Wilkie DJ, Holzemer WL, Tesler MD, and others: Measuring pain quality: validity and reliability of children's and adolescents' pain language, *Pain* 41(2):151–159, 1990.

Wong DL, Baker CM: Pain in children: comparison of assessment scales, *Pediatr Nurs* 14(1):917, 1988.

Woodgate R, Yanofsky R: A different perspective to approaching cancer symptoms in children, *J Pain Symptom Manage* 26(3):800–817, 2004.

Woolf CJ, Salter MW: Neuronal plasticity: increasing the gain in pain, *Science* 288(5472):1765–1769, 2000.

Yaster M, Krance EJ, Kaplan RF, and others: *Pediatric pain management and sedation handbook*, St. Louis, 1997, Mosby.

Health Promotion of the Newborn and Family

Barbara J. Wheeler

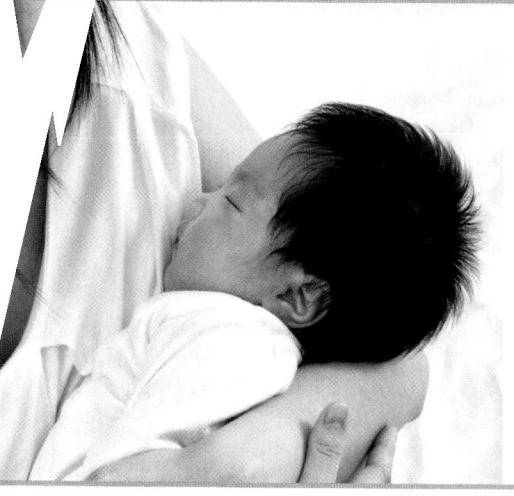

⊖volve WEBSITE

http://evolve.elsevier.com/wong/essentials
Animations—Bradycardia; Fetal Circulation
Case Studies—Breastfeeding; The Normal Newborn

Key Point Summaries
NCLEX-Style Review Questions

CHAPTER OUTLINE

Adjustment to Extrauterine Life, 186
Immediate Adjustments, 186
Respiratory System, 186
Circulatory System, 186
Physiologic Status of Other
Systems, 186
Thermoregulation, 186
Hematopoietic System, 186
Fluid and Electrolyte Balance, 187
Gastrointestinal System, 187
Renal System, 187
Integumentary System, 187
Musculoskeletal System, 188
Defenses Against Infection, 188
Endocrine System, 188
Neurologic System, 188
Sensory Functions, 188
**Nursing Care of the Newborn and
Family, 189**
Assessment, 189
Initial Assessment: Apgar Scoring, 189

*Clinical Assessment of Gestational
Age, 189*
*Transitional Assessment: Periods of
Reactivity, 201*
Behavioral Assessment, 201
*Assessment of Attachment
Behaviors, 202*
Physical Assessment, 202
Maintain a Patent Airway, 206
Maintain a Stable Body
Temperature, 207
Protect from Infection and Injury, 208
Identification, 208
Eye Care, 208
Vitamin K Administration, 208
*Hepatitis B Vaccine
Administration, 209*
Newborn Screening for Disease, 209
*Universal Newborn Hearing
Screening, 209*
Bathing, 209

Care of the Umbilicus, 211
Circumcision, 211
Provide Optimal Nutrition, 214
Human Milk, 214
Breastfeeding, 215
Bottle Feeding, 217
Commercially Prepared Formulas, 217
Preparation of Formula, 218
Alternate Milk Products, 218
Feeding Schedules, 218
Feeding Behavior, 218
Promote Parent–Infant Bonding
(Attachment), 219
Infant Behavior, 219
Maternal Attachment, 219
Paternal Engrossment, 220
Siblings, 221
*Multiple Births and Subsequent
Children, 221*
Prepare for Discharge and Home
Care, 222

LEARNING OBJECTIVES

On completion of this chapter the reader will be able to:
- Identify the principal cardiorespiratory changes that occur during the transition to extrauterine life.
- Identify the immature physiologic functioning of each body system and its significance to nursing care of the newborn.
- Perform an initial and transitional assessment of a newborn, including the Apgar score and gestational age assessment.

- Perform a newborn physical assessment based on recognition of expected normal findings.
- Outline a nursing plan of care for a well newborn.
- Assess and promote parent–infant attachment behaviors.

ADJUSTMENT TO EXTRAUTERINE LIFE

The most profound physiologic change required of neonates is transition from fetal or placental circulation to independent respiration. The loss of the placental connection means the loss of complete metabolic support, especially the supply of oxygen and the removal of carbon dioxide. The normal stresses of labor and delivery produce alterations of placental gas exchange patterns, acid–base balance in the blood, and cardiovascular activity in the infant. Factors that interfere with this normal transition or that interfere with fetal oxygenation (including conditions such as hypoxemia, hypercapnia, and acidosis) affect the fetus's adjustment to extrauterine life.

IMMEDIATE ADJUSTMENTS

Respiratory System

The most critical and immediate physiologic change required of newborns is the onset of breathing. The stimuli that help initiate the first breath are primarily chemical and thermal. Chemical factors in the blood (low oxygen, high carbon dioxide, and low pH) initiate impulses that excite the respiratory center in the medulla. The primary thermal stimulus is the sudden chilling of the infant, who leaves a warm environment and enters a relatively cooler atmosphere. This abrupt change in temperature excites sensory impulses in the skin that are transmitted to the respiratory center.

Tactile stimulation may assist in initiating respiration. Descent through the birth canal and normal handling during delivery help stimulate respiration in uncompromised infants. Acceptable methods of tactile stimulation include tapping or flicking the soles of the feet or gently rubbing the newborn's back, trunk, or extremities. Slapping the newborn's buttocks or back is a harmful technique and should not be done. Prolonged tactile stimulation, beyond one or two taps or flicks to the soles of the feet or rubbing the back once or twice, can waste precious time in the event of respiratory difficulty and can cause additional damage in infants who have become hypoxemic before or during the birth process.

The initial entry of air into the lungs is opposed by the surface tension of the fluid that filled the fetal lungs and the alveoli. Some lung fluid is removed during the normal forces of labor and delivery. As the chest emerges from the birth canal, fluid is squeezed from the lungs through the nose and mouth. After complete delivery of the chest, brisk recoil of the thorax occurs, and air enters the upper airway to replace the lost fluid. Remaining lung fluid is absorbed by the pulmonary capillaries and lymphatic vessels.

In the alveoli, the surface tension of the fluid is reduced by surfactant, a substance produced by the alveolar epithelium that coats the alveolar surface. The effect of surfactant in facilitating breathing is discussed in relation to respiratory distress syndrome (see Chapter 9).

Circulatory System

As important as the initiation of respiration are the circulatory changes that allow blood to flow through the lungs. These changes, which occur more gradually, are the result of pressure changes in the lungs, heart, and major vessels. The transition from fetal to postnatal circulation involves the functional closure of the fetal shunts: the foramen ovale, the ductus arteriosus, and eventually the ductus venosus. (For a review of fetal circulation, see Chapter 25.) Increased blood flow dilates the pulmonary vessels, pulmonary vascular resistance decreases, and systemic resistance increases, thus maintaining blood pressure (BP). As the pulmonary vessels receive blood, the pressure in the right atrium, right ventricle, and pulmonary arteries

decreases. Left atrial pressure increases above right atrial pressure, with subsequent foramen ovale closure. With the increase in pulmonary blood flow and dramatic reduction of pulmonary vascular resistance, the ductus arteriosus begins to close.

The most important factors controlling ductal closure are the increased oxygen concentration of the blood and the fall in endogenous prostaglandins. The foramen ovale closes functionally at or soon after birth. The ductus arteriosus is closed functionally by the fourth day. Anatomic closure takes considerably longer. Failure of the ductus arteriosus or foramen ovale to close results in persistence of fetal shunting of blood away from the lungs (see Chapter 25).

Because of the reversible flow of blood through the ductus during the early neonatal period, a functional murmur occasionally may be heard. In conditions such as crying or straining, the increased pressure shunts unoxygenated blood from the right side of the heart across the ductal opening, which may cause transient cyanosis.

PHYSIOLOGIC STATUS OF OTHER SYSTEMS

Thermoregulation

Next to establishing respiration, heat regulation is most critical to the newborn's survival. Although the newborn's capacity for heat production is adequate, three factors predispose newborns to excessive heat loss:

- The newborn's large surface area facilitates heat loss to the environment, although this is partially compensated for by the newborn's usual position of flexion, which decreases the amount of surface area exposed to the environment.
- The newborn's thin layer of subcutaneous fat provides poor insulation for conservation of heat.
- The newborn's mechanism for producing heat is different from that of the adult, who can increase heat production through shivering. A chilled neonate cannot shiver but produces heat through nonshivering thermogenesis (NST), which involves increased metabolism and oxygen consumption.

The principal thermogenic sources are the heart, liver, and brain. An additional source, once believed to be unique to newborns (Zingaretti, Crosta, Vitali, and others, 2009), is known as brown adipose tissue, or brown fat. Brown fat, which owes its name to its larger content of mitochondrial cytochromes, has a greater capacity for heat production through intensified metabolic activity than does ordinary adipose tissue. Heat generated in brown fat is distributed to other parts of the body by the blood, which is warmed as it flows through the layers of this tissue. Superficial deposits of brown fat are located between the scapulae, around the neck, in the axillae, and behind the sternum. Deeper layers surround the kidneys, trachea, esophagus, some major arteries, and adrenals. The location of brown fat may explain why the nape of the neck often feels warmer than the rest of the infant's body.

Because of these factors predisposing infants to loss of body heat, it is essential that newly born infants are quickly dried and either placed skin to skin with their mothers or provided with warm, dry blankets after delivery.

Although newborns' ability to conserve heat is usually a matter of concern, they may also have difficulty dissipating heat in an overheated environment, which increases the risk of hyperthermia.

Hematopoietic System

The blood volume of the newborn depends on the amount of placental transfer of blood. The blood volume of a full-term infant is about 80 to 85 ml/kg of body weight. Immediately after birth, the total blood volume averages 300 ml, but depending on how long umbilical cord clamping is delayed or if the umbilical cord is milked, as much as 100 ml can be added to the blood volume (Rabe, Jewison, Alvarez, and others, 2011). Blood values for the newborn are listed in Appendix C.

Fluid and Electrolyte Balance

Changes occur in the total body water volume, extracellular fluid volume, and intracellular fluid volume during the transition from fetal to postnatal life. At birth, the total weight of an infant is 73% fluid compared with 58% in an adult. Infants have a proportionately higher ratio of extracellular fluid than adults.

An important aspect of fluid balance is its relationship to other systems. An infant's rate of metabolism is twice that of an adult in relation to body weight. As a result, twice as much acid is formed, leading to more rapid development of acidosis. In addition, immature kidneys cannot sufficiently concentrate urine to conserve body water. These three factors make infants more prone to dehydration, acidosis, and possible overhydration or water intoxication.

Gastrointestinal System

The ability of newborns to digest, absorb, and metabolize foodstuff is adequate but limited in certain functions. Enzymes are adequate to handle proteins and simple carbohydrates (monosaccharides and disaccharides), but deficient production of pancreatic amylase impairs use of complex carbohydrates (polysaccharides). Deficiency of pancreatic lipase limits absorption of fats, especially with ingestion of foods with high saturated fatty acid content such as cow's milk. Human milk, despite its high fat content, is easily digested because the milk itself contains enzymes such as lipase, which assist in digestion.

The liver is the most immature of the gastrointestinal organs. The activity of the enzyme glucuronyl transferase is reduced, which affects the conjugation of bilirubin with glucuronic acid and contributes to physiologic jaundice of newborns. The liver is also deficient in forming plasma proteins. The decreased plasma protein concentration probably plays a role in the edema usually seen at birth. Prothrombin and other coagulation factors are also low. The liver stores less glycogen at birth than later in life. Consequently, newborns are prone to hypoglycemia, which may be prevented by early and effective feeding, ideally breastfeeding.

Some salivary glands are functioning at birth, but the majority do not begin to secrete saliva until about age 2 to 3 months, when drooling is frequent. Stomach capacity varies in the first few days of life, from about 5 ml on day 1 to about 60 ml on day 3 (Spangler, Randenberg, Brenner, and others, 2008); thus, infants require frequent small feedings. The colon also has a small volume; newborns may have a bowel movement after each feeding. Newborns who breastfeed usually have more frequent feedings and more frequent stools than infants who receive formula.

An infant's intestine is longer in relation to body size than that of the adult. Therefore, there are a larger number of secretory glands and a larger surface area for absorption compared with an adult's intestine. Infants have rapid peristaltic waves and simultaneous nonperistaltic waves along the entire esophagus, which propel nutrients forward. The relative immaturity of the peristaltic waves combined with decreased lower esophageal sphincter (LES) pressure, inappropriate relaxation of the LES, and delayed gastric emptying make regurgitation a common occurrence. Progressive changes in the stooling pattern indicate a properly functioning gastrointestinal tract (Box 8-1).

The neonatal gastrointestinal mucosa may perform an important function as a barrier to foreign antigens. Both immune and nonimmune factors may play a vital role in decreasing the absorption of antigens capable of causing serious neonatal illness; however, the

---

BOX 8-1 CHANGE IN STOOLING PATTERNS OF NEWBORNS

Meconium

Infant's first stool; composed of amniotic fluid and its constituents, intestinal secretions, shed mucosal cells, and possibly blood (ingested maternal blood or minor bleeding of alimentary tract vessels)

Passage of meconium should occur within the first 24 to 48 hours, although it may be delayed up to 7 days in very low–birth-weight infants.

Transitional Stools

Usually appear by third day after initiation of feeding; greenish brown to yellowish brown, thin, and less sticky than meconium; may contain some milk curds

Milk Stool

Usually appears by fourth day

In **breastfed infants** stools are yellow to golden, are pasty in consistency, and have an odor similar to that of sour milk.

In **formula-fed infants** stools are pale yellow to light brown, are firmer in consistency, and have a more offensive odor.

---

functional capacity of this system may be immature or altered. Feeding an infant human milk increases the effectiveness of this defense mechanism (Le Huërou-Luron, Blat, and Boudry, 2010).

Renal System

All structural components are present in the renal system, but there is a functional deficiency in the kidneys' ability to concentrate urine and to cope with conditions of fluid and electrolyte stress such as dehydration or a concentrated solute load.

Total volume of urine per 24 hours is about 200 to 300 ml by the end of the first week. However, the bladder voluntarily empties when stretched by a volume of 15 ml, resulting in as many as 20 voidings per day. The first voiding should occur within 24 hours. The urine is colorless and odorless and has a specific gravity of about 1.020.

Integumentary System

At birth, all of the structures within the skin are present, but many of the functions of the integument are immature. The outer two layers of the skin, the epidermis and dermis, are loosely bound to each other and very thin. Rete pegs, which later in life anchor the epidermis to the dermis, are not developed. Slight friction across the epidermis, such as from rapid removal of adhesive tape, can cause separation of these layers and blister formation. The transitional zone between the cornified and living layers of the epidermis is effective in preventing fluid from reaching the skin surface.

The sebaceous glands are very active late in fetal life and in early infancy because of the high levels of maternal androgens. They are most densely located on the scalp, face, and genitalia and produce the greasy vernix caseosa that covers infants at birth. Plugging of the sebaceous glands causes milia.

The eccrine glands, which produce sweat in response to heat or emotional stimuli, are functional at birth, and palmar sweating on crying reaches levels equivalent to those of anxious adults by 3 weeks of age. The eccrine glands produce sweat in response to higher temperatures than those required in adults, and the retention of sweat may result in miliaria. The apocrine glands remain small and nonfunctional until puberty.

The growth phases of hair follicles usually occur simultaneously at birth. During the first few months, the synchrony between hair loss and regrowth is disrupted, and there may be overgrowth of hair or temporary alopecia.

Because the amount of melanin is low at birth, newborns are lighter skinned than they will be as children. Consequently, they are more susceptible to the harmful effects of the sun.

Musculoskeletal System

At birth, the skeletal system contains more cartilage than ossified bone, although the process of ossification is fairly rapid during the first year. The nose, for example, is predominantly cartilage at birth and may be temporarily flattened or asymmetric because of the force of delivery. The six skull bones are relatively soft and are separated only by membranous seams. The sinuses are incompletely formed in newborns.

Unlike the skeletal system, the muscular system is almost completely formed at birth. Growth in size of muscular tissue is caused by hypertrophy, rather than hyperplasia, of cells.

Defenses Against Infection

Infants are born with several defenses against infection. The first line of defense is the skin and mucous membranes, which protect the body from invading organisms. The mature neonatal intestinal mucosal (gut) barrier also plays a vital role as an important defense mechanism against antigens. The second line of defense is the macrophage system, which produces several types of cells capable of attacking a pathogen. The neutrophils and monocytes are phagocytes, which means they can engulf, ingest, and destroy foreign agents. Eosinophils also probably have a phagocytic property because they increase in number in the presence of foreign protein. The lymphocytes (T cells and B cells) are capable of being converted to other cell types, such as monocytes and antibodies. Although the phagocytic properties of the blood are present in infants, the inflammatory response of the tissues to localize an infection is immature.

The third line of defense is the formation of specific antibodies to an antigen. Exposure to various foreign agents is necessary for antibody production to occur. Infants are generally not capable of producing their own immunoglobulin (Ig) until the beginning of the second month of life, but they receive considerable passive immunity in the form of IgG from the maternal circulation and from human milk (see p. 214). They are protected against most major childhood diseases, including diphtheria, measles, poliomyelitis, and rubella, for about 3 months, provided the mother has developed antibodies to these illnesses.

Endocrine System

Ordinarily, the endocrine system of newborns is adequately developed, but its functions are immature. For example, the posterior lobe of the pituitary gland produces limited quantities of antidiuretic hormone, or vasopressin, which inhibits diuresis. This renders young infants highly susceptible to dehydration.

The effect of maternal sex hormones is particularly evident in newborns. The labia are hypertrophied, and the breasts of both genders may be engorged and secrete milk from the first few days of life to as long as 2 months of age. Female newborns may have pseudomenstruation (more often seen as a milky secretion than actual blood) from a sudden drop in progesterone and estrogen levels.

Neurologic System

At birth, the nervous system is incompletely integrated but sufficiently developed to sustain extrauterine life. Most neurologic functions are primitive reflexes. The autonomic nervous system is crucial during transition because it stimulates initial respirations, helps maintain acid–base balance, and partially regulates temperature control.

Myelination of the nervous system follows cephalocaudal–proximodistal (head-to-toe–center-to-periphery) laws of development and is closely related to observed mastery of fine and gross motor skills. Myelin is necessary for rapid and efficient transmission of some, but not all, nerve impulses along the neural pathway. The tracts that develop myelin earliest are the sensory, cerebellar, and extrapyramidal tracts. This accounts for the acute senses of taste, smell, and hearing in newborns, as well as the perception of pain. All cranial nerves are present and myelinated except for the optic and olfactory nerves.

Sensory Functions

Newborns' sensory functions are remarkably well developed and have a significant effect on growth and development, including the attachment process.

Vision

At birth, the eye is structurally incomplete. The fovea centralis is not yet completely differentiated from the macula. The ciliary muscles are also immature, limiting the eyes' ability to accommodate and focus on an object for any length of time. The infant can track and follow objects. The pupils react to light, the blink reflex is responsive to minimal stimulus, and the corneal reflex is activated by a light touch. Tear glands usually do not begin to function until 2 to 4 weeks of age.

Newborns have the ability to focus momentarily on a bright or moving object that is within 20 cm (8 inches) and in the midline of the visual field. In fact, infants' ability to fixate on coordinated movement is greater during the first hour of life than during the succeeding several days. Visual acuity is reported to be between 20/100 and 20/400, depending on the vision measurement techniques.

Infants also demonstrate visual preferences: medium colors (yellow, green, pink) over bright (red, orange, blue) or dim colors; black-and-white contrasting patterns, especially geometric shapes and checkerboards; large objects with medium complexity rather than small, complex objects; and reflecting objects over dull ones.

Hearing

After the amniotic fluid has drained from the ears, infants probably have auditory acuity similar to that of adults. Neonates react to loud sounds of about 90 decibels with a startle reflex. Newborns' response to sounds of low frequency versus those of high frequency differs; whereas the former, such as the sound of a heartbeat, metronome, or lullaby, tends to decrease an infant's motor activity and crying, the latter elicits an alerting reaction. There is also an early sensitivity to the sound of human voices, although not specifically speech sounds. For example, infants younger than 3 days of age can discriminate the mother's voice from that of other women. As early as age 5 days, newborns can differentiate between stories repeated to them during the last trimester of pregnancy by their mother and the same stories recited after birth by a different woman.

The internal and middle ear is large at birth, but the external canal is small. The mastoid process and the bony part of the external canal have not yet developed. Consequently, the tympanic membrane and facial nerve are very close to the surface and can be easily damaged.

Smell

Newborns react to strong odors such as alcohol and vinegar by turning their heads away. Breastfed infants are able to smell breast milk and will cry for their mothers when they smell leaking milk. Infants are also able to differentiate the breast milk of their mothers from the breast milk of other women by smell. Maternal odors are believed to influence the attachment process and successful breastfeeding. Unnecessary routine washing of the breast may interfere with establishment of early breastfeeding.

Taste

The newborn has the ability to distinguish among tastes. Various types of solutions elicit differing gustofacial reflexes. A tasteless solution elicits no facial expression; a sweet solution elicits an eager suck and a look of satisfaction; a sour solution causes the usual puckering of the lips; and a bitter liquid produces an angry, upset expression. Newborns demonstrate preferential taste for glucose water to sterile water. During early childhood, the taste buds are distributed mostly on the tip of the tongue.

Touch

At birth, infants are able to perceive tactile sensation in any part of the body, although the face (especially the mouth), hands, and soles of the feet seem to be most sensitive. There is increasing documentation that touch and motion are essential to normal growth and development. Gentle patting of the back or rubbing of the abdomen usually elicits a calming response from infants. In turn, painful stimuli, such as a pinprick, elicit an upset response.

NURSING CARE OF THE NEWBORN AND FAMILY

ASSESSMENT

Newborns require thorough, skilled observation to ensure a satisfactory adjustment to extrauterine life. Physical assessment after delivery can be divided into four phases:
1. The initial assessment, which includes the Apgar scoring system
2. Transitional assessment during the periods of reactivity
3. Assessment of gestational age
4. Systematic physical examination

In addition, the nurse must be aware of behaviors that signal successful reciprocal attachment between the infant and parents. Awareness of the expected normal findings during each assessment process helps the nurse recognize any deviation that may prevent the infant from progressing uneventfully through the early postnatal period. With shorter hospitalizations, the accomplishment of thorough newborn assessment and parent teaching has become a challenge.

Initial Assessment: Apgar Scoring

The most frequently used method to assess newborns' immediate adjustment to extrauterine life is the Apgar scoring system, which is based on newborn heart rate, respiratory effort, muscle tone, reflex irritability, and color (Table 8-1). Each item is given a score of 0, 1, or 2. Evaluations of all five categories are made at 1 and 5 minutes after birth and repeated until the infant's condition stabilizes. Total scores of 0 to 3 represent severe distress, scores of 4 to 6 signify moderate difficulty, and scores of 7 to 10 indicate absence of difficulty in adjusting to extrauterine life. The Apgar score is affected by the degree of physiologic immaturity, infection, congenital malformations, maternal sedation or analgesia, and neuromuscular disorders.

The Apgar score reflects the general condition of the infant at 1 and 5 minutes based on the five parameters described previously. The Apgar score is not a tool, however, that stands on its own to interpret past events, determine need for newborn resuscitation, or predict

TABLE 8-1	INFANT EVALUATION AT BIRTH—APGAR SCORING SYSTEM		
SIGN	**0**	**1**	**2**
Heart rate	Absent	Slow, <100 beats/min	>100 beats/min
Respiratory effort	Absent	Irregular, slow, weak cry	Good, strong cry
Muscle tone	Limp	Some flexion of extremities	Well flexed
Reflex irritability	No response	Grimace	Cry, sneeze
Color	Blue, pale	Body pink, extremities blue	Completely pink

future events linked to the infant's eventual neurologic or physical status. Considerable discussion and controversy have centered on Apgar scoring because of its misuse as an indicator for the presence or absence of perinatal asphyxia in the medicolegal field (American Academy of Pediatrics [AAP] Committee on Fetus and Newborn, and American College of Obstetricians and Gynecologists [ACOG], Committee on Obstetric Practice, 2006, reaffirmed 2008).

Clinical Assessment of Gestational Age

Assessment of gestational age is an important criterion because perinatal morbidity and mortality are related to gestational age and birth weight. A frequently used method of determining gestational age is the New Ballard Scale (NBS) by Ballard, Khoury, Wedig, and others (1991) (Fig. 8-1, A). This scale, an abbreviated version of the Dubowitz scale, assesses six external physical and six neuromuscular signs. Each sign has a number score, and the cumulative score correlates with a maturity rating of 20 to 44 weeks of gestation.

The NBS includes −1 and −2 scores that reflect signs of extremely preterm infants, such as fused eyelids; imperceptible breast tissue; sticky, friable, transparent skin; no lanugo; and square-window (flexion of wrist) angle of greater than 90 degrees (see Fig. 8-1, A, and the description of the tests in Box 8-2). For infants with a gestational age of at least 26 weeks, the examination may be performed up to 96 hours after birth; however, it is recommended that the initial examination be performed within the first 48 hours of life. In a study of preterm infants ranging from 29 to 35 weeks at birth, Ballard scores completed after 7 days after birth were found to either overestimate or underestimate gestational age by up to 2 weeks (Sasidharan, Dutta, and Narang, 2009). In a blinded Spanish study, Marín, Martín, Lliteras, and others (2006) compared estimations of gestational age using NBS versus ultrasonography or the mother's last menstrual period. Researchers found general agreement between NBS and ultrasonography or last menstrual period; however, they noted that NBS tends to overestimate gestational age in very preterm newborns and in infants whose mothers had received prenatal corticosteroid therapy.

Weight Related to Gestational Age

The weight of the infant at birth also correlates with the incidence of perinatal morbidity and mortality. However, birth weight alone is a poor indicator of gestational age and fetal maturity. Maturity implies functional capacity—the degree to which the neonate's organ systems are able to adapt to the requirements of extrauterine life. Therefore, gestational age is more closely related to fetal maturity than is birth weight. Because heredity influences a newborn's size, noting the size of other family members is part of the assessment process.

ESTIMATION OF GESTATIONAL AGE BY MATURITY RATING

NEUROMUSCULAR MATURITY

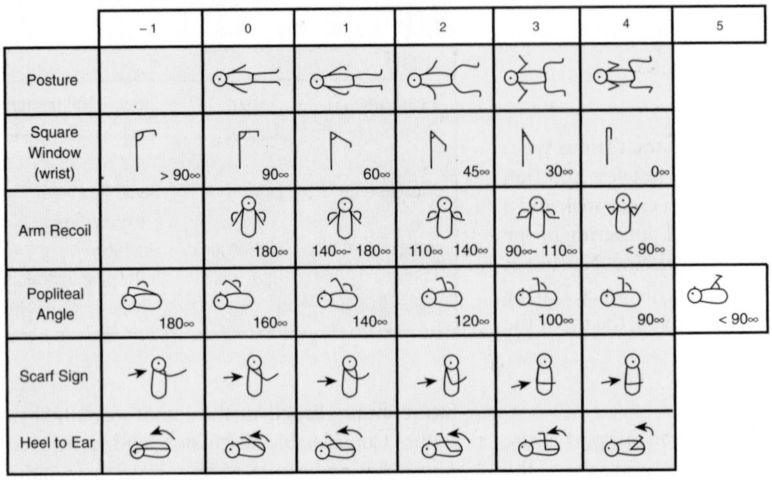

	−1	0	1	2	3	4	5
Posture							
Square Window (wrist)	>90∞	90∞	60∞	45∞	30∞	0∞	
Arm Recoil		180∞	140∞–180∞	110∞ 140∞	90∞–110∞	<90∞	
Popliteal Angle	180∞	160∞	140∞	120∞	100∞	90∞	<90∞
Scarf Sign							
Heel to Ear							

PHYSICAL MATURITY

Skin	sticky friable transparent	gelatinous red, translucent	smooth pink, visible veins	superficial peeling &/or rash, few veins	cracking pale areas rare veins	parchment deep cracking no vessels	leathery cracked wrinkled
Lanugo	none	sparse	abundant	thinning	bald areas	mostly bald	
Plantar Surface	heel-toe 40-50 mm: -1 <40 mm: -2	>50 mm no crease	faint red marks	anterior transverse crease only	creases ant. 2/3	creases over entire sole	
Breast	imperceptible	barely perceptible	flat areola no bud	stippled areola 1-2 mm bud	raised areola 3-4 mm bud	full areola 5-10 mm bud	
Eye/Ear	lids fused loosely: -1 tightly: -2	lids open pinna flat stays folded	slightly curved pinna; soft; slow recoil	well-curved pinna; soft but ready recoil	formed & firm instant recoil	thick cartilage ear stiff	
Genitals (male)	scrotum flat, smooth	scrotum empty faint rugae	testes in upper canal rare rugae	testes descending few rugae	testes down good rugae	testes pendulous deep rugae	
Genitals (female)	clitoris prominent labia flat	prominent clitoris small labia minora	prominent clitoris enlarging minora	majora & minora equally prominent	majora large minora small	majora cover clitoris & minora	

MATURITY RATING

score	weeks
-10	20
-5	22
0	24
5	26
10	28
15	30
20	32
25	34
30	36
35	38
40	40
45	42
50	44

A

FIG 8-1 A, New Ballard Scale for newborn maturity rating. Expanded scale includes extremely preterm infants and has been refined to improve accuracy in more mature infants.

BOX 8-2   TESTS USED IN ASSESSING GESTATIONAL AGE

Posture—With infant quiet and in a supine position, observe degree of flexion in arms and legs. Muscle tone and degree of flexion increase with maturity.
Full flexion of the arms and legs—4*

Square window—With thumb supporting back of arm below wrist, apply gentle pressure with index and third fingers on dorsum of hand without rotating infant's wrist. Measure angle between base of thumb and forearm.
Full flexion (hand lies flat on ventral surface of forearm)—4

Arm recoil—With infant supine, fully flex both forearms on upper arms, hold for 5 seconds; pull down on hands to fully extend and rapidly release arms. Observe rapidity and intensity of recoil to a state of flexion.
A brisk return to full flexion—4

Popliteal angle—With infant supine and pelvis flat on a firm surface, flex lower leg on thigh and then flex thigh on abdomen. While holding knee with thumb and index finger, extend lower leg with index finger of other hand. Measure degree of angle behind knee (popliteal angle).
An angle of less than 90 degrees—5

Scarf sign—With infant supine, support head in midline with one hand; use other hand to pull infant's arm across the shoulder so that infant's hand touches shoulder. Determine location of elbow in relation to midline.
Elbow does not reach midline—4

Heel to ear—With infant supine and pelvis flat on a firm surface, pull foot as far as possible up toward ear on same side. Measure degree of knee flexion (same as popliteal angle).
Knees flexed with a popliteal angle of less than 90 degrees—4

*Numeric ratings correspond with Fig. 8-1, *A.*

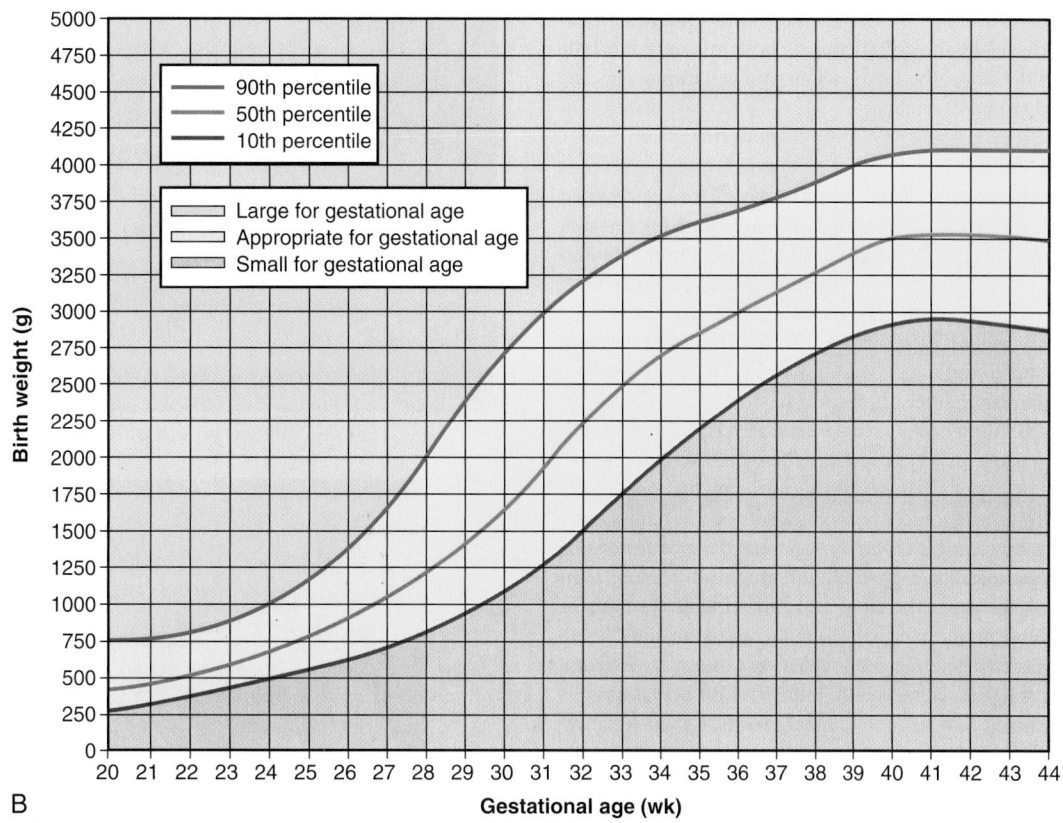

B

FIG 8-1, cont'd **B,** Intrauterine growth: birth weight percentiles based on live single births at gestational ages 20 to 44 weeks. (**A,** From Ballard JL, Khoury JC, Wedig K, and others: New Ballard Score, expanded to include extremely premature infants, *J Pediatr* 119[3]:418, 1991. **B,** Data from Alexander GR, Himes JH, Kaufman RB, and others: A United States national reference for fetal growth, *Obstet Gynecol* 87[2]:163–168, 1996.)

Intrauterine growth curves are used to classify infants according to birth weight and gestational age. The primary intrauterine growth charts that provide national reference data include the work of Alexander, Himes, Kaufman, and others (1996), which is representative of more than 3.1 million live births in the United States, and Thomas, Peabody, Turnier, and others (2000). Olsen, Groveman, Lawson, and others (2010) published new intrauterine growth curves based on more than 257,000 infants in the United States, noting that use of a contemporary, large, and racially diverse U.S. sample has produced intrauterine growth curves that differ from those produced earlier. Thomas, Peabody, Turnier, and others (2000) concluded that intrauterine growth measured by head circumference, birth weight, and length varies according to race and gender. These researchers also found that altitude did not seem to significantly affect birth weight, as has been suggested by other authors. It is recommended that readers access and use the most current intrauterine growth chart specific to the referent population being evaluated.

Classification of infants at birth by both **birth weight** and **gestational age** provides a more satisfactory method for predicting mortality risks and providing guidelines for management of the neonate than estimating gestational age or birth weight alone. The infant's birth weight, length, and head circumference are plotted on standardized graphs that identify normal values for gestational age (for birth weight see Fig. 8-1, *B*). Infants whose weight is **appropriate for gestational age (AGA)** (between the 10th and 90th percentiles) can be presumed to have grown at a normal rate regardless of the time of birth—preterm, term, or postterm. Infants who are **large for gestational age**

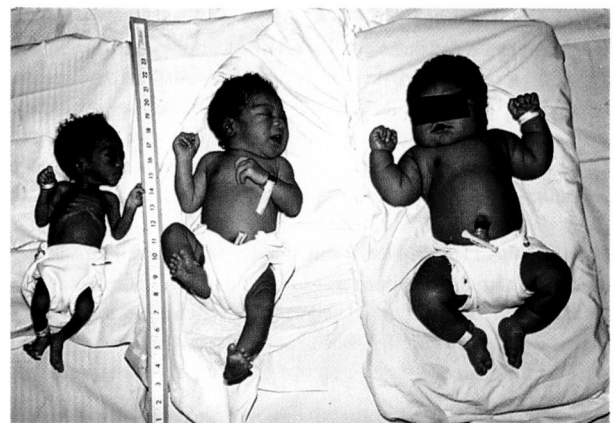

FIG 8-2 Three infants, same gestational age, weight 600, 1400, and 2750 g, respectively, from left to right. (From *Perinatal assessment of maturation*, National Audiovisual Center, Washington, DC.)

(LGA) (above the 90th percentile) can be presumed to have grown at an accelerated rate during fetal life; **small-for-gestational-age (SGA)** infants (below the 10th percentile) can be assumed to have intrauterine growth restriction or delay.

When gestational age is determined according to a standardized gestational age scale such as the NBS, the newborn will fall into one of the following nine possible categories for birth weight and gestational age: AGA—term, preterm, postterm; SGA—term, preterm, postterm; LGA—term, preterm, postterm. Figure 8-2 illustrates the disparity between birth weights of three preterm infants of the same gestational age, 32 weeks. Birth weight and gestational age both influence morbidity and mortality; the lower the birth weight and gestational age, the higher the morbidity and mortality.

General Measurements

Several important measurements of newborns have significance when compared with each other and when recorded over time on a graph. For full-term infants, average **head circumference** is between 33 and 35.5 cm (13 and 14 inches). Head circumference may be somewhat less immediately after birth because of the molding process that occurs during vaginal deliveries. Usually by the second or third day, the skull is normal in size and contour.

Chest circumference is 30.5 to 33 cm (12–13 inches) but is not routinely performed in the healthy term infant. Head circumference is usually about 2 to 3 cm (≈1 inch) greater than chest circumference. Because of the molding of the head during delivery, these measurements may initially appear equal. However, if the head is significantly smaller than the chest, **microcephaly** or premature closure of the sutures (**craniosynostosis**) is a possibility. If the head is more than 4 cm (1.6 inches) larger than the chest and this remains constant or increases over several days, then hydrocephalus must be considered. Other causes of increased head circumferences are caput succedaneum, cephalhematoma, subgaleal hemorrhage, and subdural hematoma.

Head circumference may also be compared with crown-to-rump length, or sitting height. **Crown-to-rump** measurements are usually 31 to 35 cm (12.2–13.8 inches) and are approximately equal to head circumference. The relationship of the head and crown-to-rump measurements is more reliable than that of the head and chest. Neonatal head circumference and crown-to-rump length may provide a more accurate means for identifying infants at risk; head circumference has been shown to be equal to or up to 1 cm more than crown-to-rump length in 62% of the infants examined and determined to be normocephalic.

Abdominal circumference need not be routinely measured in newborns but should be done in the event of abdominal distention to determine changes in girth over time. Abdominal circumference is measured just above the level of the umbilicus because the umbilical cord is still attached, making measurements across the umbilicus too variable in newborns. Measuring the abdominal circumference below the umbilical region is unsuitable because bladder status may affect the reading.

Head-to-heel length is also measured. Because of the usual flexed position of infants, it is important to extend the legs completely when measuring total body length. The average length of newborns is 48 to 53 cm (19–21 inches) (Fig. 8-3). Foote and colleagues (2011) have developed an evidence-based practice guideline for measuring length in infants and children.

Body weight should be measured soon after birth because weight loss occurs fairly rapidly. Normally, neonates lose about 10% of their birth weight by 3 to 4 days of age because of loss of extracellular fluid and meconium, as well as limited food intake, especially in breastfed infants. The birth weight is usually regained by the tenth to fourteenth day of life. Most newborns weigh 2700 to 4000 g (6–9 pounds), the average weight being about 3400 g (7.5 pounds). Accurate birth weights and lengths are important because they provide a baseline for assessment of future growth.

Another category of measurements is vital signs. **Axillary temperatures** are taken because insertion of a thermometer into the rectum can potentially cause perforation of the mucosa if performed incorrectly (see Table 6-3 and Fig. 8-4). Core body temperature varies

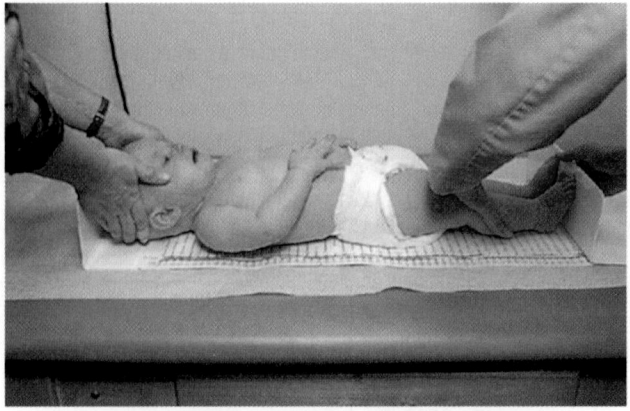

FIG 8-3 Measurement of infant length.

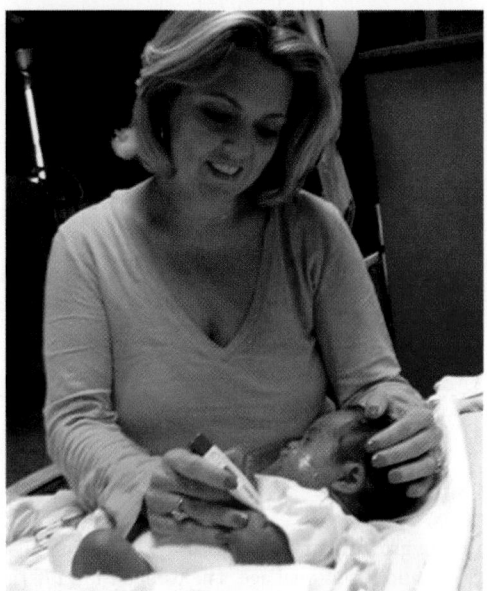

FIG 8-4 Mother taking axillary temperature with digital thermometer.

according to the periods of reactivity but is usually 36.5° to 37.6° C (97.7°–99.7° F). Skin temperature is slightly lower than core body temperature. Therefore axillary temperature is generally less than rectal temperature, measuring about 0.2° C lower (Hussink, van Berkel, and de Beaufort, 2008). Because brown adipose tissue is located in the axillary pocket, axillary readings may be elevated whenever NST occurs. However, axillary readings may be normal in cold-stressed infants when NST is not triggered or is overwhelmed.

The single best method for determining a newborn infant's temperature remains elusive when considering the available studies. Despite their usefulness in older children and adults, the accuracy of tympanic membrane sensors is problematic in infants. A meta-analysis of 101 studies comparing tympanic membrane temperatures with rectal temperatures in children concluded that the tympanic method demonstrated a wide range of variability, limiting its application in a pediatric setting (Craig, Lancaster, Taylor, and others, 2002). Dodd, Lancaster, Craig, and colleagues (2006) concur with this finding, stating that after a systematic review of studies involving almost 4100 children, they found that infrared ear thermometry would fail to diagnose fever in three or four of every 10 febrile children.

The Canadian Paediatric Society (CPS), Community Paediatrics Committee (2010) outlines concerns regarding the safety and accuracy of tympanic temperature measurement in newborns because of the size of a newborn's external ear canal relative to the size of the thermometer probe. To ensure accuracy, the probe, which may be up to 8 mm (0.3 inch) in diameter, must be deeply inserted into the ear canal to allow orientation of the sensor near or against the tympanic membrane. At birth, the average diameter of the canal is just 4 mm (0.16 inch); at 2 years of age, it is just 5 mm (0.2 inch). The CPS concludes that current infrared tympanic thermometry lacks sufficient safety and precision to meet clinical needs for use in newborn infants and children younger than 2 years of age.

Infrared axillary and digital thermometers are used in many neonatal units because they give rapid readings and are easy to clean; studies demonstrate their usefulness in well, full-term newborns (Sganga, Wallace, Kiehl, and others, 2000). Jones, Kleber, Eckert, and others (2003) compared rectal temperatures of infants younger than 2 months of age with calibrated digital thermometers and mercury glass thermometers; this study of 120 infants found that the digital thermometers measured a higher temperature (mean average of 0.7° F; range, 0°–1.6° F) than the mercury glass thermometers. The researchers concluded that the error in measurement was attributable to the digital thermometer used. Advantages of digital thermometers in neonatal care include relatively easy readability by parents and caretakers in the home, improvement of discharge planning effectiveness, and decreased risk of breakage and associated complications compared with glass thermometers.

Temporal artery thermometers (TATs) are available for use in the general pediatric population, and parents often report ease of use and less discomfort with such methods. Greenes and Fleisher (2001) concluded that the TAT had limited sensitivity in infants for detecting rectal fever, yet the TAT was more accurate than the tympanic thermometer. Siberry, Diener-West, Schappell, and others (2002) compared the infrared TAT (using an infrared device) with the rectal temperature measurement (digital thermometer) and found poor predictability for fever in children 0 to 3 months old. The authors concluded that the TAT could be used as a rapid assessment screening tool to identify rectal fever in children 3 to 24 months old, but TAT was unreliable as a screening tool for infants younger than 3 months. Schuh, Komar, Stephens, and others (2004) compared rectal temperatures with TAT measurements in an emergency department population of children younger than 24 months and concluded that the TAT was not reliable for detecting rectal fever in children younger than 3 months but could be used as a screening tool for detecting fever of at least 38.3°C (100.9° F) in children 3 to 24 months of age. Holzhauer, Reith, Sawin and colleagues (2009) determined that TAT did not accurately detect rectal fever in infants and children ages 3 to 36 months; the researchers did find that TAT was less traumatic for small children than rectal temperature measurement. Carr, Wilmoth, Eliades and colleagues (2011) found that TAT measurements (vs. rectal temperature measurements) in children 1 to 24 months with a fever of 38° C or more, resulted in saving nursing time and less child discomfort. In this small study there was an 87.4% level of agreement between TAT and rectal temperatures and 94.7% of the measurements differed by 1° C or less.

In most studies regarding newborn temperature, the glass mercury thermometer is the gold standard against which other methods are compared. There is no universal agreement on placement times for glass thermometers, although 3 minutes for rectal temperature and 5 minutes for axillary temperature are considered to be adequate. In 2007, the AAP, Committee on Environmental Health (2001, reaffirmed 2007) reaffirmed its statement recommending that mercury thermometers no longer be used in clinics and homes to decrease mercury exposure hazard.

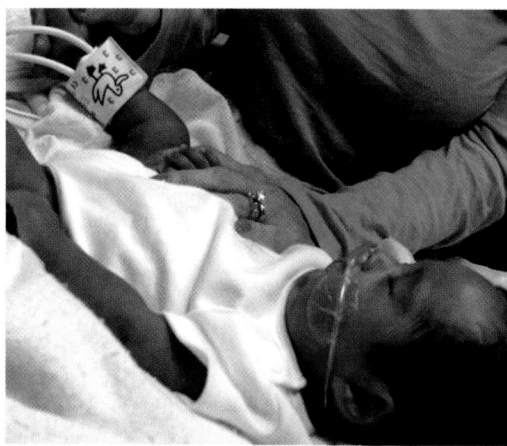

FIG 8-5 Measurement of blood pressure using oscillometry.

Nurses must be cognizant of the many variables involved:
Site—axillary, rectal, tympanic, skin
Environment—radiant warmer, open crib, incubator, clothing, or nesting
Purpose—fever, possible sepsis (in which case the temperature may be lower than normal in newborns), and thermoregulation in the transition phase
Instrument—electronic, digital, infrared

Nurses must also be able to make clear clinical decisions based on accurate and objective data. Further research is needed to perfect thermometers that accurately reflect infants' core temperature to effectively plan nursing care and maintain a stable temperature.

Pulse and respirations also vary according to the periods of reactivity and the infant's behaviors but are usually in the range of 120 to 140 beats/min and 30 to 60 breaths/min. Both are counted for a full 60 seconds to detect irregularities in rate or rhythm. The heart rate is taken apically with a stethoscope, and the femoral arteries are palpated for equality of strength or fullness.

Measurement of blood pressure (BP) provides baseline data and may indicate cardiovascular problems. BP is most easily and accurately assessed using oscillometry (Dinamap) when the newborn is in a quiet or sleep state using an appropriate cuff width–to-arm ratio of 0.45 to 0.70 (approximately half to three quarters) (Nuntnarumit, Yand, and Bada-Ellzey, 1999) (Fig. 8-5). For healthy term infants, the average oscillometric systolic/diastolic BP is 65/45 mm Hg on day 1 of life, changing to 69.5/44.5 mm Hg by day 3 (Kent, Kecskes, Shadbolt, and others, 2007). Blood pressure values in infants are higher in the awake state than in the sleep state. Mean BP values increase over the first month of life and are positively correlated with increasing gestational age and birth weight (Pejovic, Peco-Antic, and Marinkovic-Eric, 2007). Compare BP in the upper and lower extremities, which should be equal.

! NURSING ALERT

Although uncommon, the presence of neonatal hypertension may be a sign of a significant underlying problem such as renal, cardiac, or thromboembolic pathologic condition, or it may be associated with a medication treatment regimen. Neonatal hypertension is brought to the primary practitioner's attention for further evaluation.

The role of pulse oximetry in the early newborn period (after 24 hours of age) is now recommended as a screening tool to detect hypoxemia (SPO$_2$ ≤95%) in newborns with undiagnosed congenital heart disease (Mahle, Martin, Beekman, and others, 2012). Guidelines for newborn pulse oximetry screening are published elsewhere (Kemper, Mahle, Martin, and others, 2011) (see Evidence-Based Practice box).

A suggested schedule for monitoring heart rate, respiratory rate, and temperature is on admission to the nursery, once every 30 minutes until the newborn has been stable for 2 hours (AAP and ACOG, 2007), and then once every 8 hours until discharge. However, this schedule may vary according to institutional policy. Any change in the infant, such as color, breathing, muscle tone, or behavior, necessitates more frequent monitoring.

General Appearance

Before each body system is assessed, it is important to describe the general posture and behavior of the newborn. The overall appearance yields valuable clues to the infant's physical status.

In full-term neonates, the posture is one of complete flexion as a result of in utero position. Most infants are born in a vertex presentation with the head flexed and the chin resting on the upper chest, the arms flexed with the hands clenched, the legs flexed at the knees and hips, and the feet dorsiflexed. The vertebral column is also flexed. It is important to recognize any deviation from this characteristic fetal position.

The infant's behavior is carefully noted, especially the degree of alertness, drowsiness, and irritability; the latter two factors may reflect common signs of neurologic problems. Some questions to mentally ask when assessing behavior include:

- Is the infant awakened easily by a loud noise?
- Is the infant comforted by rocking, sucking, or cuddling?
- Do there seem to be periods of deep and light sleep?
- When awake, does the infant seem satisfied after a feeding?
- What stimuli elicit responses from the infant?
- When disturbed, how much does the infant protest?

Skin

The texture of the newborn's skin is velvety smooth and puffy, especially about the eyes, the legs, the dorsal aspect of the hands and the feet, and the scrotum or labia. Skin color depends on racial and familial background and varies greatly among newborns. In general, white infants are usually pink to red. African-American newborns may appear a pinkish or yellowish brown. Infants of Hispanic descent may have an olive tint or a slight yellow cast to the skin. Infants of Asian descent may be a rosy or yellowish tan. The color of American Indian newborns varies from a light pink to a dark, reddish brown. By the second or third day of life, the skin turns to its more natural tone and is drier and flakier. Several other color changes that may be noted on the skin are described later in this chapter (see Table 8-4).

At birth, the skin may be partially covered with a grayish white, cheeselike substance called vernix caseosa, a mixture of sebum and desquamating cells. It is absorbed by 24 to 28 hours. A fine, downy hair called lanugo may be present on the skin, especially on the forehead, cheeks, shoulders, and back.

Head

General observation of the contour of the head is important because molding occurs in almost all vaginal deliveries. In a vertex delivery, the head is usually flattened at the forehead, with the apex rising and forming a point at the end of the parietal bones and the posterior skull or occiput dropping abruptly. The usual, more oval contour of the head is apparent by 1 to 2 days after birth. The change in shape occurs

---

EVIDENCE-BASED PRACTICE

Role of Pulse Oximetry in Screening Newborns for Congenital Heart Disease

Olga A. Taylor

Ask the Question
PICOT Question
Is pulse oximetry useful in screening newborns for congenital heart disease?

Search for Evidence
Search Strategies
Search selection included English-language publications within the past 3 years on the role of pulse oximetry in screening newborns for congenital heart disease.

Database Used
PubMed

Critically Analyze the Evidence
- Current oximeters have a very low false-positive rate and are stable and reliable in screening newborns for congenital heart defects (de-Wahl Granelli, Wennergren, Sandberg, and others, 2009; Hoffman, 2011; Mahle, Newburger, Matherne, and others, 2009; Meberg, Brugmann-Pieper, Due, and others, 2008; Riede, Wornder, Dahnert, and others, 2010).
- Pulse oximetry screening in newborns had a sensitivity of 62.07% to 77.78%, specificity of 99.82% to 99.90%, positive predictive value of 20.69% to 25.93%, and negative predictive value of 99.97% to 99.99% (de-Wahl Granelli, Wennergren, Sandberg, and others, 2009; Riede, Wornder, Dahnert, and others, 2010).

- Estimated positive predictive value and sensitivity of pulse oximetry for detecting congenital heart disease from multiple studies was 47.0% and 69.6%, respectively; sensitivity varied drastically from 0% to 100% (Mahle, Newburger, Matherne, and others, 2009).
- When pulse oximetry is used in conjunction with physical examination, prenatal diagnosis, and clinical observation, delayed diagnosis of congenital heart disease was seen in only 4.4% of newborns (Riede, Wornder, Dahnert, and others, 2010).
- Duct-dependent lung circulation was detected in 100% of cases when pulse oximetry screening was used along with physical examination. Overall detection rate for duct-dependent circulation was increased to 92% with the use of pulse oximetry screening (de-Wahl Granelli, Wennergren, Sandberg, and others, 2009).
- Pulse oximetry screening detected cardiac heart disease in 88% of newborns. Use of pulse oximetry in addition to physical examination (vs. physical examination alone) increased detection rate by 14% (Meberg, Andreassen, Brunvand, and others, 2009).
- Pulse oximetry screening combined with physical examination detected congenital heart disease in 98% of newborns (Walsh, 2011).
- Pulse oximetry screens have low cost and risk of harm (de-Wahl Granelli, Wennergren, Sandberg, and others, 2009; Mahle, Newburger, Matherne, and others, 2009).

EVIDENCE-BASED PRACTICE

Role of Pulse Oximetry in Screening Newborns for Congenital Heart Disease—cont'd

- Of the 1045 pediatric cardiologists surveyed, 55% supported required pulse oximetry screening in newborns (Chang, Rodriguez, and Klitzner, 2009).
- Reliability of pulse oximetry is greatly impacted by factors such as probe placement time, training, and nursing degree (Reich, Connolly, Bradley, and others, 2008).
- Pulse oximetry screening can miss some cardiac anomalies such as coarctation of the aorta, interrupted arch, and hypoplastic left heart syndrome (Shastri, Clarke, and Roy, 2011).
- Pulse oximetry did not detect any congenital heart disease in newborns (Sendelbach, Jackson, Lai, and others, 2008).

Apply the Evidence: Nursing Implications

There is **good evidence** with **strong recommendations** for using pulse oximetry screening to detect cardiac heart disease in newborns (Guyatt, Oxman, Vist, and others, 2008). Pulse oximetry has a very low false-positive rate, high sensitivity, and very high specificity. Use of pulse oximetry in conjunction with other tests increases detection rates of cardiac anomalies in newborns. However, some factors such as user training and degree influence the reliability of pulse oximetry.

QSEN Quality and Safety Competencies:

Evidence-Based Practice*

Knowledge

Differentiate clinical opinion from research and evidence-based summaries.

Describe use of pulse oximetry screening for detection of cardiac heart disease in newborns.

Skills

Base individualized care plan on patient values, clinical expertise, and evidence.

Integrate evidence into practice for using pulse oximetry screening to detect cardiac heart disease in newborns.

Attitudes

Value the concept of evidence-based practice as integral to determining best clinical practice.

Appreciate strengths and weakness of evidence for using pulse oximetry screening to detect cardiac heart disease in newborns.

References

Chang RKR, Rodriguez S, Klitzner TS: Screening newborns for congenital heart disease with pulse oximetry: survey of pediatric cardiologists, *Pediatr Cardiol* 30:20–25, 2009.

de-Wahl Granelli A, Wennergren M, Sandberg K, and others: Impact of pulse oximetry screening on the detection of duct dependent congenital heart disease: a Swedish prospective screening study in 39 821 newborns, *BMJ* 338:a3037–a3049, 2009.

Guyatt GH, Oxman AD, Vist GE, and others: GRADE: an emerging consensus on rating quality of evidence and strength of recommendations, *BMJ*, 336:924–926, 2008.

Hoffman JIE: It is time for routine neonatal screening by pulse oximetry, *Neonatology* 99:1–9, 2011.

Mahle WT, Newburger JW, Matherne GP, and others: Role of pulse oximetry in examining newborns for congenital heart disease, *Circulation* 120:447–458, 2009.

Meberg A, Andreassen A, Brunvand L, and others: Pulse oximetry screening as a complementary strategy to detect critical congenital heart defects, *Acta Paediatrica* 98:682–686, 2009.

Meberg A, Brugmann-Pieper S, Due R, and others: First day of life pulse oximetry screening to detect congenital heart defects, *J Pediatr* 152:761–765, 2008.

Reich JD, Connolly B, Bradley G, and others: The reliability of a single pulse oximetry reading as a screening test for congenital heart disease in otherwise asymptomatic newborn infants, *Pediatr Cardiol* 29:885–889, 2008.

Riede FT, Wornder C, Dahnert I, and others: Effectiveness of neonatal pulse oximetry screening for detection of critical congenital heart disease in daily clinical routine: results from a prospective multicenter study, *Eur J Pediatr* 169:975–981, 2010.

Sendelbach DM, Jackson GL, Lai SS, and others: Pulse oximetry screening at 4 hours of age to detect critical congenital heart defects, *Pediatrics* 122:e815–e820, 2008.

Shastri AT, Clarke P, Roy R: Pulse oximetry screening for detection of critical congenital heart disease in newborns: a survey of current practices in the United Kingdom, *Acta Paediatrica* 100:636–637, 2011.

Walsh W: Evaluation of pulse oximetry screening in Middle Tennessee: cases for consideration before universal screening, *J Perinatol* 31:125–129, 2011.

*Adapted from the QSEN at http://www.qsen.org.

---

because the bones of the cranium are not fused, allowing for overlapping of the edges of these bones to accommodate to the size of the birth canal during delivery. Such molding usually does not occur in infants born by elective cesarean section.

Six bones—the frontal, occipital, two parietals, and two temporals—make up the cranium. Between the junction of these bones are bands of connective tissue called sutures. At the junction of the sutures are wider spaces of unossified membranous tissue called fontanels. The two most prominent fontanels in infants are the anterior fontanel formed by the junction of the sagittal, coronal, and frontal sutures and the posterior fontanel formed by the junction of the sagittal and lambdoid sutures (Fig. 8-6, *A*).

NURSING TIP The location of the suture is easily remembered because the coronal suture "crowns" the head, and the sagittal suture "separates" the head.

The skull is palpated for all patent sutures and fontanels, noting size, shape, molding, or abnormal closure. The sutures feel like cracks between the skull bones, and the fontanels feel like wider soft spots at the junction of the sutures. These are palpated by using the tip of the index finger and running it along the ends of the bones (Fig. 8-6, *B*).

The anterior fontanel is diamond shaped and measures anywhere from barely palpable to 4 to 5 cm (≈2 inches) at its widest point (from bone to bone rather than from suture to suture). The posterior fontanel is easily located by following the sagittal suture toward the occiput. The posterior fontanel is triangular, usually measuring between 0.5 and 1 cm (<0.5 inch) at its widest part. The fontanels should feel flat, firm, and well demarcated against the bony edges of the skull. Frequently, pulsations are visible at the anterior fontanel. Coughing, crying, or lying down may temporarily cause the fontanels to bulge and become more taut.

Palpate the skull for any unusual masses or prominences, particularly those resulting from birth trauma, such as caput succedaneum or cephalhematoma (see Chapter 9). Because of the pliability of the skull,

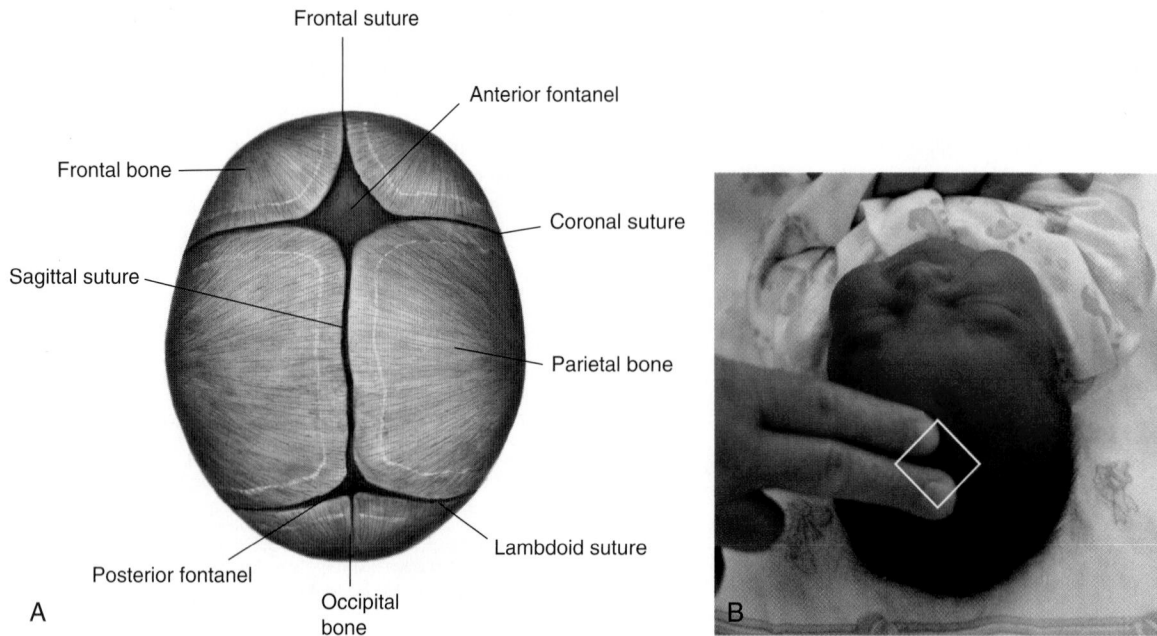

FIG 8-6 **A,** Location of sutures and fontanels. **B,** Palpating the anterior fontanel.

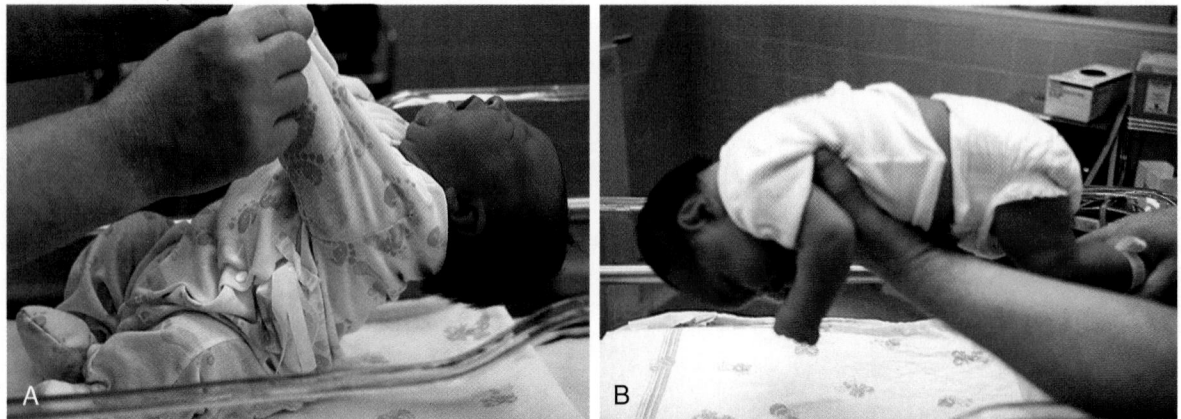

FIG 8-7 Head control in an infant. **A,** Inability to hold the head erect when pulled to sitting position. **B,** Ability to hold the head erect when placed in ventral suspension.

exerting pressure at the margin of the parietal and occipital bones along the lambdoid suture may produce a snapping sensation similar to the indentation of a ping-pong ball. This phenomenon, known as **physiologic craniotabes**, may be found normally, especially in newborns of breech birth, but also may indicate hydrocephalus, congenital syphilis, or rickets.

Assess the degree of **head control**. Although **head lag** is normal in newborns, the degree of ability to control the head in certain positions should be recognized. If a supine infant is pulled from the arms into a semi-Fowler position, marked head lag and hyperextension are noted (Fig. 8-7, *A*). However, as the infant is brought forward into a sitting position, the infant will attempt to control the head in an upright position. As the head falls forward onto the chest, many infants will attempt to right it into the erect position. Also, if the infant is held in ventral suspension (i.e., held prone above and parallel to the examining surface), the infant will hold the head in a straight line with the spinal column (Fig. 8-7, *B*). When lying on the abdomen, newborns have the ability to lift the head slightly, turning it from side to side. Marked head lag is seen in neonates with Down syndrome, prematurity, hypoxia, and neuromuscular compromise.

Eyes

Because newborns tend to have their eyes tightly closed, it is best to begin the examination of the eyes by observing the eyelids for edema, which is normally present for the first 2 days after delivery. The eyes are observed for symmetry. **Tears** may be present at birth, but purulent discharge from the eyes shortly after birth is abnormal. To visualize the surface structures of the eyes, the infant is held supine, and the head is gently lowered. The eyes will usually open, similar to the mechanism of a doll's eyes. The **sclera** should be white and clear.

The cornea is examined for the presence of any opacities or haziness. The corneal reflex is normally present at birth but may not be elicited unless neurologic or eye damage is suspected. The pupil will usually respond to light by constricting. The pupils are normally malaligned. A searching nystagmus is common. Strabismus is a normal finding because of the lack of binocularity. The color of the iris is noted. Most light-skinned newborns have slate gray or dark blue eyes, and dark-skinned infants have brown eyes.

A funduscopic examination may be difficult to perform because of the infant's tendency to keep the eyes tightly closed. However, a red reflex should be elicited. The absence of a red reflex in a newborn may indicate a cataract, glaucoma, retinal abnormalities, or retinoblastoma (see Chapter 6).

> **NURSING TIP** To elicit a red reflex, place the infant in a dark room. In an alert state, many newborns open their eyes in a supported sitting position.

Ears

The ears are examined for position, structure, and auditory function. The top of the pinna should lie in a horizontal plane to the outer canthus of the eye (see Fig. 6-20). The pinna is often flattened against the side of the head from pressure in utero. An otoscopic examination ordinarily may not be performed because the canals are filled with vernix caseosa and amniotic fluid, making visualization of the tympanic membrane difficult.

Auditory ability is tested by a number of objective hearing tests (see Table 6-10). Making a loud noise close to the infant's head may or may not elicit a response; the lack of a response, however, is not a definite indication of hearing loss. The startle reflex (Table 8-2) may be observed when there is a sudden loud noise near the infant or the bassinet is accidentally bumped, but this often depends on the infant's state at the time.

Nose

The nose is usually flattened after birth, and bruises are common. Patency of the nasal canals can be assessed by holding a hand over the infant's mouth and one canal and noting the passage of air through the unobstructed opening. If nasal patency is questionable, it is reported because most newborns are obligatory nose breathers. Sneezing and thin white mucus are common up to several hours after birth.

Mouth and Throat

An external defect of the mouth such as cleft lip is readily apparent; however, the internal structures require careful inspection. The palate is normally highly arched and somewhat narrow. Rarely, teeth may be present. A common finding is Epstein pearls, small, white, epithelial cysts along both sides of the midline of the hard palate. They are insignificant and disappear in several weeks.

The frenulum of the upper lip is a band of thick pink tissue that lies under the inner surface of the upper lip and extends to the maxillary alveolar ridge. It is particularly evident when the infant yawns or smiles. It disappears as the maxilla grows.

The lingual frenulum attaches the underside of the tongue to the lower palate midway between the ventral surface of the tongue and the tip. In some cases, a tight lingual frenulum, formerly referred to as tongue-tie, may restrict adequate sucking. Further evaluation may be required to ascertain adequate sucking, particularly in breastfed infants. The treatment for a tight lingual frenulum advocated by the

AAP is frenotomy, a safe and effective surgical procedure that improves comfort, effectiveness, and ease of breastfeeding for the mother and infant (Coryllos, Genna, and Salloum, 2004; Forlenza, Paradise Black, McNamara, and others, 2010; Segal, Stephenson, Dawes, and others, 2007).

Elicit the sucking reflex by placing a nipple or nonlatex gloved finger in the infant's mouth. The infant should exhibit a strong, vigorous suck. The rooting reflex is elicited by stroking the cheek and noting the infant's response of turning toward the stimulated side and sucking.

The uvula can be inspected while the infant is crying and the chin is depressed. However, it may be retracted upward and backward during crying. Tonsillar tissue is generally not seen in newborns. Natal teeth, teeth present at birth, as opposed to neonatal teeth, which erupt during the first month of life, are seen infrequently and erupt chiefly at the position of the lower incisors. Teeth are reported because they are frequently found with developmental abnormalities and syndromes, including cleft lip and palate. Most natal teeth are loosely attached. However, current thinking suggests preserving them until they exfoliate naturally (Leung and Robson, 2006) unless the tooth is attached loosely or breastfeeding is impaired by the neonate's biting the breast.

Neck

Because the newborn's neck is short and covered with folds of tissue, adequate assessment of the neck requires allowing the head to fall gently backward in hyperextension while the back is supported in a slightly raised position. Observe for range of motion, shape, and any abnormal masses and palpate each clavicle for possible fractures.

Chest

The shape of the newborn's chest is almost circular because the anteroposterior and lateral diameters are equal. The ribs are flexible, and slight intercostal retractions are normally seen on inspiration. The xiphoid process is commonly visible as a small protrusion at the end of the sternum. The sternum is generally raised and slightly curved.

Inspect the breasts for size; shape; and nipple formation, location, and number. Breast enlargement appears in many newborns of both genders by the second or third day and is caused by maternal hormones. Occasionally, a milky substance, sometimes called witch's milk, is secreted by the infant's breasts by the end of the first week. Supernumerary nipples may be found on the chest, on the abdomen, or in the axilla.

Lungs

The normal respirations of newborns are irregular and abdominal, and the rate is between 30 and 60 breaths/min. Pauses in respiration of less than 20 seconds' duration are considered normal. After the initial forceful breaths required to initiate respiration, subsequent breaths should be nonlabored and fairly regular in rhythm. Periodic breathing is commonly seen in full-term newborns and consists of rapid nonlabored respirations followed by pauses of less than 20 seconds; periodic breathing may be more prominent during sleep and is not accompanied by status changes such as cyanosis or bradycardia. Occasional irregularities occur in relation to crying, sleeping, stooling, and feeding.

Perform auscultation when the infant is quiet. Bronchial breath sounds should be equal bilaterally. Any differences in auscultatory findings between symmetric sites are reported. Crackles soon after birth indicate the presence of fluid, which represents the normal transition of the lungs to extrauterine life. However, wheezes, persistence

TABLE 8-2	ASSESSMENT OF REFLEXES IN THE NEWBORN
REFLEXES	**EXPECTED BEHAVIORAL RESPONSES**
Localized	
Eyes	
Blinking or corneal	Infant blinks at sudden appearance of a bright light or at approach of an object toward cornea; persists throughout life.
Pupillary	Pupil constricts when a bright light shines toward it; persists throughout life.
Doll's eye	As head is moved slowly to right or left, eyes lag behind and do not immediately adjust to new position of head; disappears as fixation develops; if persists, indicates neurologic damage.
Nose	
Sneeze	Sneezing is a spontaneous response of nasal passages to irritation or obstruction; persists throughout life.
Glabellar	Tapping briskly on glabella (bridge of nose) causes eyes to close tightly.
Mouth and Throat	
Sucking	Infant begins strong sucking movements of circumoral area in response to stimulation; persists throughout infancy even without stimulation, such as during sleep.
Gag	Stimulation of posterior pharynx by food, suction, or passage of a tube causes infant to gag; persists throughout life.
Rooting	Touching or stroking the cheek along side of mouth causes infant to turn head toward that side and begin to suck; should disappear at about age 3–4 mo but may persist for up to 12 mo.
Extrusion	When tongue is touched or depressed, infant responds by forcing it outward; disappears by age 4 mo.
Yawn	Yawning is a spontaneous response to decreased oxygen by increasing amount of inspired air; persists throughout life.
Cough	Irritation of mucous membranes of larynx or tracheobronchial tree causes coughing; persists throughout life; usually present after first day of birth.
Extremities	
Grasp	Touching palms of hands or soles of feet near base of digits causes flexion of fingers and toes (see Fig. 8-8, *A*); palmar grasp lessens after age 3 mo to be replaced by voluntary movement; plantar grasp lessens by 8 mo of age.
Babinski	Stroking outer sole of foot upward from heel and across ball of foot causes toes to hyperextend and hallux to dorsiflex (see Fig. 8-8, *B*); disappears after age 1 yr.
Ankle clonus	Briskly dorsiflexing foot while supporting knee in partially flexed position results in one or two oscillating movements ("beats"); eventually, no beats should be felt.
Mass	
Moro	Sudden jarring or change in equilibrium causes sudden extension and abduction of extremities and fanning of fingers, with index finger and thumb forming a C shape followed by flexion and adduction of extremities; legs may weakly flex; infant may cry (see Fig. 8-9, *A*); disappears after age 3–4 mo, usually strongest during first 2 mo.
Startle	A sudden loud noise causes abduction of the arms with flexion of elbows; hands remain clenched; disappears by age 4 mo.
Perez	While infant is prone on a firm surface, thumb is pressed along spine from sacrum to neck; infant responds by crying, flexing extremities, and elevating pelvis and head; lordosis of the spine, as well as defecation and urination, may occur; disappears by age 4–6 mo.
Tonic neck	When infant's head is turned to one side, arm and leg extend on that side, and opposite arm and leg flex (see Fig. 8-9, *B*); disappears by age 3–4 mo to be replaced by symmetric positioning of both sides of body.
Trunk incurvation (Galant)	Stroking infant's back alongside spine causes hips to move toward stimulated side; disappears by age 4 wk.
Dance or step	If infant is held so that sole of foot touches a hard surface, there is a reciprocal flexion and extension of the leg, simulating walking (see Fig. 8-9, *C*); disappears after age 3–4 wk to be replaced by deliberate movement.
Crawl	When placed on abdomen, infant makes crawling movements with arms and legs (see Fig. 8-9, *D*); disappears at about age 6 wk.
Placing	When infant is held upright under arms and dorsal side of foot is briskly placed against hard object, such as table, leg lifts as if foot is stepping on table; age of disappearance varies.

of medium or coarse crackles after the first few hours of life, and stridor should be reported for further investigation.

Heart

Heart rate is auscultated and may range from 100 to 180 beats/min shortly after birth and, when the infant's condition has stabilized, from 120 to 140 beats/min. The **point of maximum impulse (PMI)** may be palpated and is usually found at the fourth to fifth intercostal space, medial to the left midclavicular line. The PMI gives some indication of the location of the heart, which may be displaced in conditions such as congenital diaphragmatic hernia or pneumothorax. **Dextrocardia**, an anomaly wherein the heart is on the right side of the body, is reported because the abdominal organs may also be reversed, with associated circulatory abnormalities.

Auscultation of the specific components of the **heart sounds** is difficult because of the rapid rate and effective transmission of respiratory sounds. However, the **first (S_1)** and **second (S_2)** sounds should be clear and well defined; the second sound is somewhat higher in pitch and sharper than the first. A **murmur** is frequently heard in newborns, especially over the base of the heart or at the left sternal border at the third or fourth interspace. In newborns a murmur is not associated with specific cardiac defects but frequently represents the incomplete functional closure of fetal shunts. (See Chapter 6 for other characteristics of murmurs.) However, always record and report all murmurs and other unusual heart sounds.

Abdomen

The normal contour of the abdomen is cylindric and usually prominent with few visible veins. Bowel sounds are heard within the first 15 to 20 minutes after birth. Visible peristaltic waves may be observed in some newborns. Diastasis recti is a gap in the rectus muscles; this usually benign condition is visible as a raised and palpable bulge at midline, especially in crying infants.

Inspect the umbilical cord to determine the presence of two arteries, which look like papular structures, and one vein, which has a larger lumen than the arteries and a thinner vessel wall. At birth, the umbilical cord appears bluish white and moist. After clamping, it begins to dry and appears a dull, yellowish brown. It progressively shrivels in size and turns greenish black.

If the umbilical cord appears unusually large in diameter at the base, inspect for the presence of a hematoma or small omphalocele. If the cord is clamped over an existing omphalocele, part of the intestine will be clamped, causing tissue necrosis. One practical rule of thumb is to cut the cord distally 4 to 5 inches from a questionable enlargement until further examination is carried out by a practitioner. The extra length can later be cut if no pathologic condition has been identified.

> **! NURSING ALERT**
>
> An umbilical cord that is draining and erythematous at the base should be investigated by the primary practitioner. The cord undergoes a process of dry gangrene decay, which has an odor; therefore, odor alone may not be a reliable index of suspicion for omphalitis.

Palpate after inspecting the abdomen. The liver is normally palpable 1 to 3 cm ($\approx$0.5–1 inch) below the right costal margin. The tip of the spleen can sometimes be felt, but a palpable spleen more than 1 cm below the left costal margin suggests enlargement and warrants further investigation. Although both kidneys should be palpated, this maneuver requires considerable practice. When felt, the lower half of the right kidney and the tip of the left kidney are 1 to 2 cm above the umbilicus.

During examination of the lower abdomen, palpate for femoral pulses, which should be strong and equal bilaterally.

Female Genitalia

Normally, the labia minora, labia majora, and clitoris are edematous, especially after a breech delivery. However, the labia and clitoris must be carefully inspected to identify any evidence of ambiguous genitalia or other abnormalities. Normally, in a girl, the urethral opening is located behind and below the clitoris.

A hymenal tag is occasionally visible from the posterior opening of the vagina. It is composed of tissue from the hymen and the labia minora. It usually disappears in several weeks. Generally, the vaginal vault is not inspected.

Vaginal discharge may be noted during the first week of life. This pseudomenstruation is a manifestation of the abrupt decrease of maternal hormones and usually disappears by 2 to 4 weeks of age. Fecal discharge from the vaginal opening indicates a rectovaginal fistula and is always reported. Vernix caseosa may be present in large amounts between the labia.

Male Genitalia

The penis is inspected for the urethral opening, which is located at the tip. However, the opening may be totally covered by the prepuce, or foreskin, which covers the glans penis. A tight prepuce is a common finding in newborns. It should not be forcefully retracted; locating the urinary meatus is usually possible without retracting the foreskin. Smegma, a white cheesy substance, is commonly found around the glans penis under the foreskin. Small, white, firm lesions called epithelial pearls may be seen at the tip of the prepuce. An erection is common in newborns.

The scrotum may be large, edematous, and pendulous in full-term neonates, especially in infants born in breech position. It is more deeply pigmented in dark-skinned infants. A noncommunicating hydrocele commonly occurs unilaterally and disappears within a few months. Always palpate the scrotum for the presence of testes (see Chapter 6). In small newborns, particularly preterm infants, the undescended testes may be palpable within the inguinal canal. Absence of the testes may also be a sign of ambiguous genitalia (disorders of sex development), especially when accompanied by a small scrotum and penis. Inguinal hernias may or may not be manifested immediately after birth. A hernia is more easily detected when the infant is crying. Palpable lymph nodes are most commonly found in the inguinal area.

Back and Rectum

Inspect the spine with the infant prone. The shape of the spine is gently rounded, with none of the characteristic S-shaped curves seen later in life. Any abnormal openings, masses, dimples, or soft areas are noted. A protruding sac anywhere along the spine, but most commonly in the sacral area, indicates some type of spina bifida. A small sinus, which may or may not be communicating with the spine, is a pilonidal sinus. It is frequently covered with a tuft of hair. Although it may have no pathologic significance, a pilonidal cyst may indicate the existence of spina bifida occulta or be a portal of entry into the spinal column. With the infant still prone, note symmetry of the gluteal folds. Report any evidence of asymmetry; tests for developmental dysplasia of the hip are performed by trained (or skilled) examiners (see Chapter 31).

The presence of an anal orifice and passage of meconium from the anal orifice during the first 24 to 48 hours of life indicates anal patency. If an imperforate anus is suspected, report this to the primary practitioner for further evaluation.

> **! NURSING ALERT**
>
> The presence of meconium or stool in the rectal area is not an indication of rectal patency; a fistula may exist wherein stool is evacuated via the vagina, scrotum, or raphe. Therefore, it is imperative that anal patency be checked with a small rubber catheter if doubt regarding patency exists.

Extremities

Examine the extremities for symmetry, range of motion, and signs of malformation. Count the fingers and toes and note any supernumerary digits (polydactyly) or fusion of digits (syndactyly). A partial syndactyly between the second and third toes is a common variation seen in otherwise normal infants. The nail beds should be pink, although slight blueness is evident in acrocyanosis.

The palms of the hands should have the usual creases (see Fig. 6-14). Full-term newborns usually have creases covering the entire sole of the foot. The soles of the feet are flat with prominent fat pads.

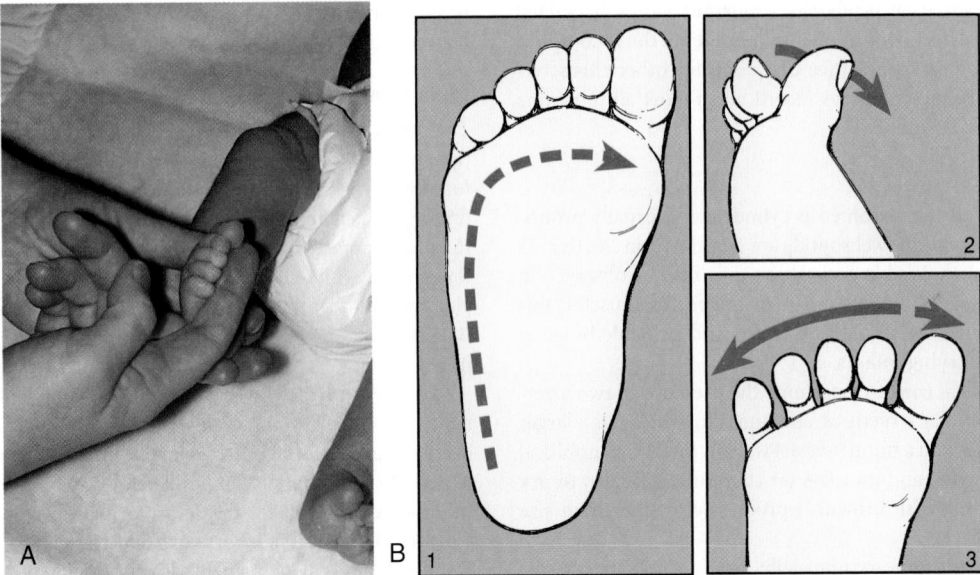

FIG 8-8 **A,** Plantar or grasp reflex. **B,** Babinski reflex. 1, Direction of stroke. 2, Dorsiflexion of big toe. 3, Fanning of toes. (**A,** From Zitelli BJ, McIntire SC, Nowalk AJ: *Zitelli and Davis' atlas of pediatric physical diagnosis*, ed 6, St. Louis, 2012, Saunders.)

Observe range of motion of the extremities throughout the entire examination. The absence of arm movement signals a potential birth injury paralysis such as Klumpke or Erb-Duchenne palsy. An asymmetric or partial Moro reflex should alert the practitioner to further evaluate upper extremity mobility. Examine the lower extremities for limb length, symmetry, and hip abduction and flexion. Newborns demonstrate full range of motion in the elbow, hip, shoulder, and knee joints. Movements should be symmetric, smooth, and unrestricted.

Also assess muscle tone. By attempting to extend a flexed extremity, determine if tone is equal bilaterally. Extension of any extremity is usually met with resistance, and when released, the extremity returns to its previous flexed position. Hypotonia suggests some degree of hypoxia or neurologic disorder and is common in an infant with Down syndrome. Asymmetry of muscle tone may indicate a degree of paralysis from brain damage or nerve damage. Failure to move the lower limbs suggests a spinal cord lesion or injury. Sustained rhythmic tremors, twitches, and myoclonic jerks characterize neonatal seizures or may indicate neonatal abstinence syndrome. (See Neonatal Seizures and Drug-Exposed Infants, Chapter 9.) Sudden asynchronous jerking movements, quivering, or momentary tremors are usually normal.

Neurologic System

Assessing neurologic status is a critical part of the physical examination of newborns. Much of the neurologic testing takes place during evaluation of body systems, such as eliciting localized reflexes and observing posture, muscle tone, head control, and movement. However, several important mass (total body) reflexes also need to be elicited. These should be tested at the end of the examination because they may disturb the infant and interfere with auscultation. Two common newborn reflexes are elicited. The first is the grasp reflex. Touching the palms of the hands or soles of the feet near the base of the digits causes flexion or grasping (Fig. 8-8, A). The other is the Babinski reflex. Stroking the outer sole of the foot upward from the heel across the ball of the foot causes the big toe to dorsiflex and the other toes to hyperextend (Fig. 8-8, B).

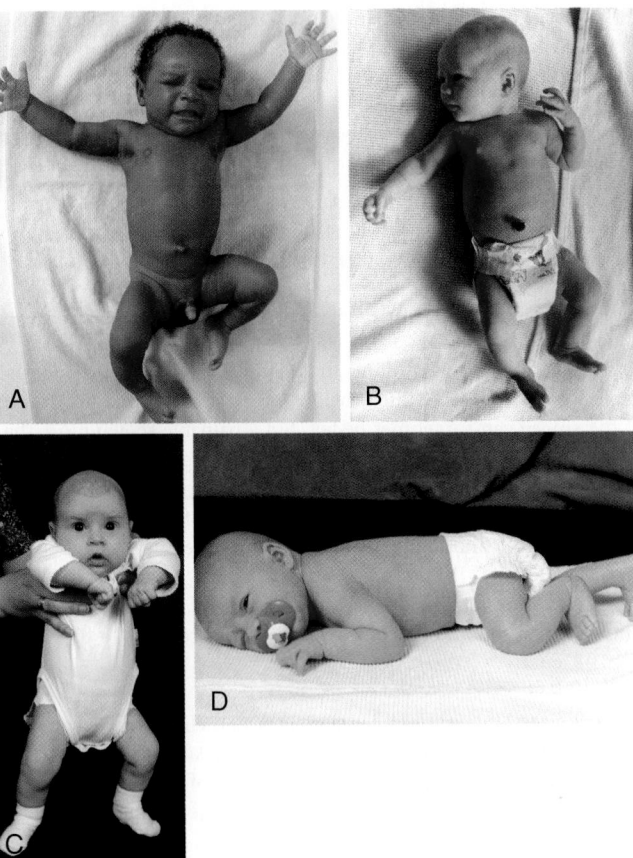

FIG 8-9 **A,** Moro reflex. **B,** Tonic neck reflex. **C,** Dance reflex. **D,** Crawl reflex. (Courtesy Paul Vincent Kuntz, Texas Children's Hospital, Houston.)

These reflexes, as well as several local reflexes, are described in Table 8-2. Record and report the absence, asymmetry, persistence, or weakness of a reflex.

Transitional Assessment: Periods of Reactivity

Newborns exhibit behavioral and physiologic characteristics that may at first appear to be signs of stress. However, during the initial 24 hours, changes in heart rate, respiration, motor activity, color, mucus production, and bowel activity occur in an orderly, predictable sequence that is normal and indicates lack of stress.

For 6 to 8 hours after birth, the newborn is in the **first period of reactivity**. During the first 30 minutes, the infant is very alert, cries vigorously, may suck his or her fingers or fist, and appears very interested in the environment. At this time, the newborn's eyes are usually open, making this an excellent opportunity for the mother, father, and child to see each other. Because the newborn has a vigorous suck, this is also an opportune time to begin breastfeeding. The infant will usually grasp the nipple quickly, satisfying both the mother and the infant. This is particularly important to point out to the parents because after this initially highly active state, the infant may be sleepy and uninterested in sucking. Physiologically, the respiratory rate during this period is as high as 80 breaths/min, crackles may be heard, heart rate reaches 180 beats/min, bowel sounds are active, mucus secretions are increased, and temperature may decrease. Maintaining appropriate temperature for newborns is best accomplished by practicing skin-to-skin care whereby only a diaper is worn to allow majority of skin surface to be in contact with the mother's skin. A light blanket is used to cover the mother and newborn. Research has shown that the mother's skin temperature will increase to ensure the newborn does not become hypothermic (Kimura and Matsuoka, 2007).

After this initial stage of alertness and activity, the infant enters the **second stage** of the first reactive period, which generally lasts 2 to 4 hours. Heart and respiratory rates decrease, temperature continues to fall, mucus production decreases, and urine and stool are usually not passed. The infant is in a state of sleep and relative calm. Any attempt at stimulation usually elicits minimal response. Because of the continued decline in body temperature, undressing or bathing is avoided during this time.

The **second period of reactivity** begins when the infant awakens from this deep sleep; it lasts about 2 to 5 hours and provides another excellent opportunity for child and parents to interact. The infant is again alert and responsive, heart and respiratory rates increase, the gag reflex is active, gastric and respiratory secretions are increased, and passage of meconium frequently occurs. This period is usually over when the amount of respiratory mucus has decreased. After this stage is a period of stabilization of physiologic systems and a vacillating pattern of sleep and activity.

Behavioral Assessment

Another important area of assessment is observation of behavior. Infants' behavior helps shape their environment, and their ability to react to various stimuli affects how others relate to them. The principal areas of behavior for newborns are sleep; wakefulness; and activity, such as crying.

One method of systematically assessing the infant's behavior is the use of the **Brazelton Neonatal Behavioral Assessment Scale (BNBAS)** (Brazelton and Nugent, 1996). The BNBAS is an interactive examination that assesses the infant's response to 28 items organized according to the clusters in Box 8-3. It is generally used as a research or diagnostic tool and requires special training.

BOX 8-3   CLUSTERS OF NEONATAL BEHAVIORS IN BRAZELTON NEONATAL BEHAVIORAL ASSESSMENT SCALE

Habituation—Ability to respond to and then inhibit response to discrete stimulus (light, rattle, bell, pinprick) while asleep

Orientation—Quality of alert states and ability to attend to visual and auditory stimuli while alert

Motor performance—Quality of movement and tone

Range of state—Measure of general arousal level or arousability of infant

Regulation of state—How infant responds when aroused

Autonomic stability—Signs of stress (tremors, startles, skin color) related to homeostatic (self-regulating) adjustment of the nervous system

Reflexes—Assessment of several neonatal reflexes

In addition to its use as an initial and ongoing tool to assess neurologic and behavioral responses, the scale can be used in assessment of initial parent–child relationships, as a preventive instrument that identifies a caregiver who may benefit from a role model, and as a guide to help parents focus on their infant's individuality and develop a deeper attachment to their child (Bruschweiler-Stern, 2009). Studies have demonstrated that showing parents the unique characteristics of their infant causes a more positive perception of the infant to develop, with increased interaction between infant and parent.

Patterns of Sleep and Activity

Newborns begin life with a systematic schedule of sleep and wakefulness that is initially evident during the periods of reactivity. After this initial period, it is not unusual for the infant to sleep almost constantly for the next 2 to 3 days to recover from the exhausting birth process.

Infants have six distinct sleep–wake states, which represent a particular form of neural control (Table 8-3). As maturity increases, each state becomes more precisely defined according to the behaviors observed. **State** is defined as a "group of characteristics that regularly occur together" (Blackburn, 2003) and includes body activity, eye and facial movements, respiratory pattern, and response to internal and external stimuli. The six sleep–wake states are quiet (deep) sleep, active (light) sleep, drowsy, quiet alert, active alert, and crying. Infants respond to internal and external environmental factors by controlling sensory input and regulating the sleep–wake states; the ability to make smooth transitions between states is called **state modulation**. The ability to regulate sleep–wake states is essential in infants' neurobehavioral development. The more immature the infant, the less able he or she is to cope with external and internal factors that affect the sleep–wake patterns.

Recognition and knowledge of sleep–wake states is important in the planning of nursing care. It is also important for nurses to help parents and caregivers understand the significance of the infant's behavioral responses to daily caregiving and how these states can be altered. A classic example is a newborn who feeds vigorously in the active alert state but poorly when he or she progresses to the crying state. The neurologic assessment of a newborn in the active alert state will differ significantly from that performed during the deep sleep state.

Newborns typically spend as much as 16 to 18 hours sleeping and do not necessarily follow a pattern of light–dark diurnal rhythm. With increasing age, sleep–wake states change, with increasing amounts of time spent in awake alert states and decreasing amounts of sleep time. Approximately 50% of total sleep time is spent in irregular or rapid eye movement sleep.

TABLE 8-3 STATES OF SLEEP AND ACTIVITY

STATE AND BEHAVIOR	IMPLICATIONS FOR PARENTING
Deep Sleep (Quiet)	
Closed eyes	Continue usual house noises because external stimuli do not arouse infant.
Regular breathing	
No movement except for occasional sudden bodily twitch	Leave infant alone if sudden loud noise awakens infant and he or she cries.
No eye movement	Do not attempt to feed.
Light Sleep (Active)	
Closed eyes	External stimuli that did not arouse infant during deep sleep may minimally arouse child.
Irregular breathing	
Slight muscular twitching of body	
Rapid eye movement (REM) under closed eyelids	Periodic groaning or crying is usual; do not interpret as an indication of pain or discomfort.
May smile	
Drowsy	
Eyes may be open	Most stimuli arouse infant but may return to sleep state.
Irregular breathing	
Active body movement variable with occasional mild startles	Pick infant up during this time rather than leaving in crib.
	Provide mild stimulus to awaken.
	Infant may enjoy nonnutritive sucking.
Quiet Alert	
Eyes wide open and bright	Satisfy infant's needs such as hunger or nonnutritive sucking.
Responds to environment by active body movement and staring at close-range objects	Place infant in area of home where activity is continuous.
Minimal body activity	Place a toy in crib or play yard.
Regular breathing	Place objects within 17.5–20 cm (7–8 in) of infant's view.
Focuses attention on stimuli	Intervene to console.
Active Alert	
May begin with whimpering and slight body movement	Remove intense internal or external stimuli because infant has increased sensitivity to stimuli.
Eyes open	
Irregular breathing	
Crying	
Progresses to strong, angry crying and uncoordinated thrashing of extremities	Comforting measures that were effective during alert state are usually ineffective.
Eyes open or tightly closed	Rock and swaddle to decrease crying.
Grimaces	Intervene to reduce fatigue, hunger, or discomfort.
Irregular breathing	

Portions adapted from Blackburn S, Loper DL: *Maternal, fetal, and neonatal physiology: a clinical perspective*, Philadelphia, 1992, Saunders.

Cry

Newborns should begin extrauterine life with a strong, lusty cry. The sounds produced by crying can be described as hunger, anger, pain, and "bid for attention" cries. Discomfort (pain) sounds initially consist of gasps and cries in which the consonant H is clearly distinguishable. The duration of crying is as variable in each infant as the duration of sleep patterns. Newborns may cry as little as 5 minutes or as much as

◻ NURSING CARE GUIDELINES

Assessing Attachment Behavior

- When the infant is brought to the parents, do they reach out for the child and call the child by name?
- Do the parents speak about the child in terms of identification—who the infant looks like; what appears special about their child compared with other infants?
- When parents are holding the infant, what kind of body contact is there? Do they feel at ease in changing the infant's position; are fingertips or whole hands used; are there parts of the body they avoid touching or parts of the body they investigate and scrutinize?
- When the infant is awake, what kinds of stimulation do the parents provide? Do they talk to the infant, to each other, or to no one? How do they look at the infant—direct visual contact, avoidance of eye contact, or looking at other people or objects?
- How comfortable do the parents appear in terms of caring for the infant? Do they express any concern regarding their ability or disgust for certain activities, such as changing diapers?
- What type of affection do they demonstrate to the newborn, such as smiling, stroking, kissing, or rocking?
- If the infant is fussy, what kinds of comforting techniques do the parents use, such as rocking, swaddling, talking, or stroking?

2 hours or more per day. Feeding usually terminates the state of crying when hunger is the cause. Holding the infant skin to skin or swaddling or wrapping an infant snugly in a blanket promotes sleep and maintains body temperature. Rocking the infant may reduce crying and induce quiet alertness or sleep. Variations in the initial cry can indicate abnormalities. A weak, groaning cry or grunting during expiration usually indicates respiratory disturbance. Absent, weak, or constant crying requires further investigation for possible drug withdrawal or a neurologic problem.

Assessment of Attachment Behaviors

One of the most important areas of assessment is careful observation of behaviors that are thought to indicate the formation of emotional bonds between the newborn and family, especially the mother. Such behaviors include the en face position; undressing and touching the infant; smiling, kissing, and talking to the infant; and holding, rocking, and cradling the child close to the body (see Nursing Care Guidelines box). Because assessment is closely related to interventions that promote attachment (e.g., encouraging these behaviors in parents), assessing attachment behaviors is further discussed on pp. 219–222.

Physical Assessment

An essential aspect of the care of the newborn is a thorough physical assessment that includes estimation of gestational age and physical examination to identify normal characteristics and existing abnormalities. These initial and ongoing assessments are critical to establishing baseline data for planning, implementing, and evaluating care and are a nursing priority in caring for the newborn. The discussion of physical examination focuses on normal findings and variations from the norm that require little or no intervention. Readers are encouraged to review Chapter 6 for further discussion of examination techniques. General guidelines for conducting a physical examination are presented in the Nursing Care Guidelines box. Table 8-4 summarizes physical examination of newborns.

The nursing care of newborns is discussed on the following pages. The nursing process in the care of newborns is outlined in the Nursing Process box.

TABLE 8-4   PHYSICAL ASSESSMENT OF THE NEWBORN

USUAL FINDINGS	COMMON VARIATIONS OR MINOR ABNORMALITIES	POTENTIAL SIGNS OF DISTRESS OR MAJOR ABNORMALITIES
General Appearance		
Posture—Flexion of head and extremities, which rest on chest and abdomen	**Frank breech**—Extended legs, abducted and fully rotated thighs, flattened occiput, extended neck	Limp posture, extension of extremities
Skin		
At birth, bright red, puffy, smooth	Neonatal jaundice after first 24 hours	Jaundice appearing in first 24 hr
Second to third day, pink, flaky, dry	Ecchymoses or petechiae caused by birth trauma	Generalized cyanosis
Vernix caseosa	**Milia**—Distended sebaceous glands that appear as	Pallor
Lanugo	tiny white papules on cheeks, chin, and nose	Mottling
Edema around eyes, face, legs, dorsa of	**Miliaria** or **sudamina**—Distended sweat (eccrine)	Grayness
hands, feet, and scrotum or labia	glands that appear as minute vesicles, especially	Plethora
Acrocyanosis—Cyanosis of hands and feet	on face	Hemorrhage, ecchymoses, or petechiae that persist
Cutis marmorata—Transient mottling when	**Erythema toxicum**—Pink papular rash with	**Sclerema**—Hard and stiff skin
infant is exposed to decreased	vesicles superimposed on thorax, back, buttocks,	Poor skin turgor
temperature	and abdomen; may appear in 24–48 hours and	Rashes, pustules, or blisters
	resolve after several days	**Café-au-lait spots**—Light brown spots
	Harlequin color change—Clearly outlined color	**Nevus flammeus**—Port-wine stain
	change as infant lies on side; lower half of body	
	becomes pink, and upper half is pale	
	Mongolian spots—Irregular areas of deep blue	
	pigmentation, usually in sacral and gluteal	
	regions; seen predominantly in newborns of	
	African, American Indian, Asian, or Hispanic	
	descent	
	Telangiectatic nevi ("stork bites")—Flat, deep	
	pink localized areas usually seen on back of neck	
Head		
Fontanels flat, soft, and firm	Molding after vaginal delivery	Fused sutures
Widest part of fontanel measured from bone	Third sagittal (parietal) fontanel	Bulging or depressed fontanels when quiet
to bone, not suture to suture	Bulging fontanel because of crying or coughing	Widened sutures and fontanels
	Caput succedaneum—Edema of soft scalp tissue	**Craniotabes**—Snapping sensation along lambdoid
	Cephalhematoma (uncomplicated)—Hematoma	suture that resembles indentation of ping-pong ball
	between periosteum and skull bone	
Eyes		
Eyelids usually edematous	Epicanthal folds in Asian infants	Pink color of iris
Color—Slate gray, dark blue, brown	Searching nystagmus or strabismus	Purulent discharge
Absence of tears	**Subconjunctival (scleral) hemorrhages**—	Upward slant in non-Asians
Presence of red retinal reflex	Ruptured capillaries, usually at limbus	Hypertelorism (3 cm)
Corneal reflex in response to touch		Hypotelorism
Pupillary reflex in response to light		Congenital cataract(s)
Blink reflex in response to light or touch		Constricted or dilated fixed pupil
Rudimentary fixation on objects and ability to		Absence of red retinal reflex
follow to midline		White reflex (leukocoria)
		Absence of pupillary or corneal reflex
		Inability to follow object or bright light to midline
		Yellow sclera
Ears		
Position—Top of pinna on horizontal line	Inability to visualize tympanic membrane because of	Low placement of ears
with outer canthus of eye	filled aural canals	Absence of startle reflex in response to loud noise should
Startle reflex elicited by a loud, sudden noise	Pinna flat against head	be evaluated but is not diagnostic
Pinna flexible, cartilage present	Irregular shape or size	Minor abnormalities may be signs of various syndromes,
	Pits or skin tags	especially renal
	Preauricular sinus	

Continued

TABLE 8-4	PHYSICAL ASSESSMENT OF THE NEWBORN—cont'd	
USUAL FINDINGS	COMMON VARIATIONS OR MINOR ABNORMALITIES	POTENTIAL SIGNS OF DISTRESS OR MAJOR ABNORMALITIES
Nose Nasal patency **Nasal discharge**—Thin white mucus (transient) Sneezing	Flattened and bruised	Nonpatent canals Thick, bloody nasal discharge Flaring of nares (alae nasi) Copious nasal secretions or stuffiness (may be minor)
Mouth and Throat Intact, high-arched palate Uvula in midline Frenulum of tongue Frenulum of upper lip **Sucking reflex**—Strong and coordinated Rooting reflex Gag reflex Extrusion reflex Absent or minimal salivation Vigorous cry	**Natal teeth**—Teeth present at birth; benign but may be associated with congenital defects **Epstein pearls**—Small, white epithelial cysts along midline of hard palate	Cleft lip Cleft palate Large, protruding tongue or posterior displacement of tongue Receding chin (lower jaw): micrognathia Profuse salivation or drooling **Candidiasis (thrush)**—White, adherent patches on tongue, palate, and buccal surfaces Inability to pass nasogastric tube Hoarse, high-pitched, weak, absent, or other abnormal cry
Neck Short, thick, usually surrounded by skinfolds Tonic neck reflex	**Torticollis (wry neck)**—Head held to one side with chin pointing to opposite side	Excessive skinfolds Resistance to flexion Absence of tonic neck reflex Fractured clavicle; crepitus
Chest Anteroposterior and lateral diameters equal Slight sternal retractions evident during inspiration Xiphoid process evident Breast enlargement	Funnel chest (pectus excavatum) Pigeon chest (pectus carinatum) Supernumerary nipples Secretion of milky substance from breasts	Depressed sternum Marked retractions of chest and intercostal spaces during respiration Asymmetric chest expansion Redness and firmness around nipples Wide-spaced nipples
Lungs Respirations chiefly abdominal Cough reflex absent at birth; may be present by 1–2 wk Bilateral equal bronchial breath sounds	Irregular rate and depth of respirations, periodic breathing Crackles shortly after birth	Inspiratory stridor Expiratory grunt Intercostal, substernal, or suprasternal retractions Persistent irregular breathing Periodic breathing with repeated apneic spells lasting >20 sec Seesaw respirations (paradoxic) Unequal breath sounds Persistent fine, medium, or coarse crackles Wheezing Cough Diminished breath sounds Peristaltic bowel sounds on one side with diminished breath sounds on same side
Heart **Apex**—Fourth to fifth intercostal space, lateral to left sternal border S_2 slightly sharper and higher in pitch than S_1	**Sinus arrhythmia**—Heart rate increasing with inspiration and decreasing with expiration Transient cyanosis on crying or straining	**Dextrocardia**—Heart on right side Displacement of apex, muffled or distant Cardiomegaly Abdominal bruit Murmur Thrill Persistent central cyanosis Hyperactive precordium

Animation—Bradycardia

TABLE 8-4   PHYSICAL ASSESSMENT OF THE NEWBORN—cont'd

USUAL FINDINGS	COMMON VARIATIONS OR MINOR ABNORMALITIES	POTENTIAL SIGNS OF DISTRESS OR MAJOR ABNORMALITIES
Abdomen Cylindric **Liver**—Palpable 2–3 cm below right costal margin **Spleen**—Tip palpable at end of first week of age **Kidneys**—Palpable 1–2 cm above umbilicus **Umbilical cord**—Bluish white at birth with two arteries and one vein **Femoral pulses**—Equal bilaterally	Umbilical hernia **Diastasis recti**—Midline gap between recti muscles **Wharton jelly**—unusually thick umbilical cord	Abdominal distention Localized bulging Distended veins Absent bowel sounds Enlarged liver and spleen Ascites Visible peristaltic waves Scaphoid or concave abdomen Moist umbilical cord Presence of only one artery in umbilical cord Urine, stool, or pus leaking from umbilical cord or cord insertion site Periumbilical erythema Palpable bladder distention after scanty voiding Absent femoral pulses Cord bleeding or hematoma **Omphalocele** or **gastroschisis**—Protrusion of abdominal contents through abdominal wall or cord
Female Genitalia Labia and clitoris usually edematous Urethral meatus behind clitoris Vernix caseosa between labia Urination within 24 hours	**Pseudomenstruation**—Blood-tinged or mucoid discharge Hymenal tag	Enlarged clitoris with urethral meatus at tip Fused labia Absence of vaginal opening Meconium from vaginal opening No urination within 24 hr Mass in labia Ambiguous genitalia Bladder exstrophy
Male Genitalia Urethral opening at tip of glans penis Testes palpable in each scrotum Scrotum usually large, edematous, pendulous, and covered with rugae; usually deeply pigmented in dark-skinned ethnic groups Smegma Urination within 24 hours	Urethral opening covered by prepuce Inability to retract foreskin **Epithelial pearls**—Small, firm, white lesions at tip of prepuce Erection or priapism Testes palpable in inguinal canal Scrotum small	**Hypospadias**—Urethral opening on ventral surface of penis **Epispadias**—Urethral opening on dorsal surface of penis **Chordee**—Ventral curvature of penis Testes not palpable in scrotum or inguinal canal No urination within 24 hr Inguinal hernia Hypoplastic scrotum **Hydrocele**—Fluid in scrotum Masses in scrotum Meconium from scrotum Discoloration of testes Ambiguous genitalia Bladder exstrophy
Back and Rectum Spine intact; no openings, masses, or prominent curves Trunk incurvation reflex Anal reflex Patent anal opening Passage of meconium within 48 hr	Green liquid stools in infant under phototherapy Delayed passage of meconium in very low–birth-weight neonates	Anal fissures or fistulas Imperforate anus Absence of anal reflex No meconium within 36–48 hr Missing vertebrae Pilonidal cyst or sinus Tuft of hair along spine Spina bifida cystica

Continued

TABLE 8-4	PHYSICAL ASSESSMENT OF THE NEWBORN—cont'd	
USUAL FINDINGS	**COMMON VARIATIONS OR MINOR ABNORMALITIES**	**POTENTIAL SIGNS OF DISTRESS OR MAJOR ABNORMALITIES**
Extremities		
Ten fingers and toes	Partial syndactyly between second and third toes	**Polydactyly**—Extra digits
Full range of motion	Second toe overlapping third toe	**Syndactyly**—Fused or webbed digits
Nail beds pink with transient cyanosis immediately after birth	Wide gap between first (hallux) and second toes	**Phocomelia**—Hands or feet attached close to trunk
Creases on anterior two thirds of sole	Deep crease on plantar surface of foot between first and second toes	**Hemimelia**—Absence of distal part of extremity
Sole usually flat	Asymmetric length of toes	Hyperflexibility of joints
Symmetry of extremities	Dorsiflexion and shortness of hallux	Persistent cyanosis of nail beds
Equal muscle tone bilaterally, especially resistance to opposing flexion		Yellowing of nail beds
Equal bilateral brachial pulses		Sole covered with creases
		Transverse palmar (simian) crease
		Fractures
		Decreased or absent range of motion
		Dislocated or subluxated hip
		Limitation in hip abduction
		Unequal gluteal or leg folds
		Unequal knee height
		Audible clunk on abduction of hip
		Asymmetry of extremities
		Unequal muscle tone or range of motion
Neuromuscular System		
Extremities usually in some degree of flexion	Quivering or momentary tremors	**Hypotonia**—Floppy, poor head control, extremities limp
Extension of an extremity followed by previous position of flexion		**Hypertonia**—Jittery, arms and hands tightly flexed, legs stiffly extended, startles easily
Head lag while sitting but momentary ability to hold head erect		Asymmetric posturing (except tonic neck reflex)
Ability to turn head from side to side when prone		Opisthotonic posturing—Arched back
Ability to hold head in horizontal line with back when held prone		Signs of paralysis
		Tremors, twitches, and myoclonic jerks
		Marked head lag in all positions

 NURSING CARE GUIDELINES

Physical Examination of the Newborn

1. Provide a normothermic and nonstimulating examination area.
2. Check that equipment and supplies are working properly and are accessible.
3. Undress only the body area examined to prevent heat loss.
4. Proceed in an orderly sequence (usually head to toe) with the following exceptions:
   - Observe the infant's attitude and position of flexion first to avoid disturbing him or her.
   - Perform all procedures that require quiet next, such as auscultating the lungs, heart, and abdomen.
   - Perform disturbing procedures, such as testing reflexes, last.
   - Measure head and length at same time to compare results.
5. Proceed quickly to avoid stressing the infant.
6. Comfort the infant during and after the examination.
   - Talk softly.
   - Hold the infant's hands against his or her chest.
   - Swaddle and hold the infant.
   - Offer a pacifier or nonlatex gloved finger to suck.
   - Use containment and positioning to maximize developmental state regulation.

MAINTAIN A PATENT AIRWAY

Establishing a patent airway is a primary objective in the delivery room and is the responsibility of the attending nurses and practitioners. However, maintaining a patent airway continues to be a priority goal in the nursery, with attention to proper positioning of infants to facilitate drainage of secretions, especially after feeding. The AAP, Section on Breastfeeding (2005) recommends the supine position during sleep for healthy newborns. This recommendation is based on the association between sleeping prone and sudden infant death syndrome (see Chapter 11). Since the initial recommendation in 1992 that all infants be placed in the supine position to sleep, there has been no evidence of an increased number of complications, such as choking or vomiting, when infants are placed in this position (Krous, Masoumi, Haas, and others, 2007; Malloy, 2002). There has, however, been an increase in the number of infants with cranial asymmetry, particularly unilateral flattening of the occiput (AAP, Task Force on Sudden Infant Death Syndrome, 2005, reaffirmed 2009). Health care professionals must educate parents on prevention of positional plagiocephaly by encouraging alternate positions when infants are awake (Laughlin, Luerssen, Dias, and others, 2011).

A bulb syringe is kept near the infant and is used if suctioning is required. If more forceful removal of secretions is required, mechanical suction is used. The use of the properly sized catheter and correct suctioning technique is essential to prevent mucosal damage and

◎ NURSING PROCESS

The Healthy Newborn and Family

Assessment

Assess the newborn according to the guidelines on pp. 202–206.

Diagnosis (Problem Identification)

After a thorough assessment, several nursing diagnoses for healthy newborns include:

- Readiness for Enhanced Parenting
- Risk for Injury
- Effective Breastfeeding
- Risk for Imbalanced Body Temperature
- Readiness for Enhanced Nutrition
- Ineffective Breathing Pattern
- Risk for Infection
- Risk for Neonatal Jaundice

Planning

Numerous outcomes for healthy newborns are discussed on pp. 206–223. Expected patient outcomes include:

- Newborn airway will remain patent.
- Effective breathing pattern will be established.
- Thermoregulation will be maintained.
- Parent–infant attachment behaviors will be observed.
- Breastfeeding or bottle feeding will be established.
- Infant will exhibit no evidence of infection; immune status will be maintained.
- Newborn will remain free of injury.

- Family will demonstrate ability to care for the infant's basic needs.
- Newborn jaundice will be detected and monitored effectively.

Implementation

Intervention strategies for healthy newborns and family are discussed on pp. 206–223.

Evaluation

The effectiveness of nursing interventions for the newborn and family is determined by continual assessment and evaluation of care based on the following guidelines:

- Observe infant's color and respiratory pattern.
- Monitor axillary temperature regularly; observe for signs of temperature instability such as respiratory distress.
- Observe for any evidence of infection, especially at the umbilicus or site of circumcision; check identification; and verify administration of prophylactic eye treatment, vitamin K injection, hepatitis B vaccine, and hearing and newborn screening tests, including bilirubin screening.
- Monitor infant's feeding ability and oral intake.
- Monitor daily weight.
- Observe interactions between infant and family members; interview family regarding their feelings about the newborn.
- Observe parents' ability to provide care for infant; interview parents regarding any concerns about infant's care at home.
- Observe parents' correct use of car safety seat restraint on discharge.

---

edema. Gentle suctioning is necessary to prevent reflex bradycardia, laryngospasm, and cardiac arrhythmias from vagal stimulation. Oropharyngeal suctioning is performed for 5 seconds, with sufficient time between suctioning to allow the infant to recuperate and reoxygenate.

> **❗ NURSING ALERT**
>
> To avoid aspiration of amniotic fluid or mucus, clear the pharynx first and then the nasal passages using a bulb syringe: remember, **m**outh before **n**ose. Vital signs are closely monitored, and any indication of respiratory distress is immediately reported.

> **❗ NURSING ALERT**
>
> The cardinal signs of respiratory distress in a newborn include tachypnea, nasal flaring, grunting, intercostal retractions, and cyanosis.

MAINTAIN A STABLE BODY TEMPERATURE

Conserving the newborn's body heat is an essential nursing goal. At birth, a major cause of heat loss is **evaporation**, the loss of heat through moisture. The amniotic fluid that bathes the infant's skin favors evaporation, especially when combined with the cool atmosphere of the delivery room. Heat loss through evaporation is minimized by rapidly drying the skin and hair with a warmed towel and placing the infant in a heated environment or skin-to-skin contact with the mother.

Another major cause of heat loss is **radiation**, the loss of heat to cooler solid objects in the environment that are not in direct contact with the infant. Loss of heat through radiation increases as these solid objects become colder and closer to the infant. The temperature of

ambient or surrounding air in the incubator essentially has no effect on loss of heat through radiation. This is a critical point to remember when attempting to maintain a constant temperature for the infant because even though the temperature of the ambient air is optimal, the infant can become hypothermic.

An example of radiant heat loss is the placement of the incubator close to a cold window, drafty doorway, or air-conditioning unit. The cold from any of these sources will cool the walls of the incubator and, subsequently, the body of the neonate. To prevent this, the infant is placed as far away as possible from exterior walls, windows, and ventilating units. If heat loss continues to be a problem, a radiant warmer or heat lamp may be used to maintain the infant's temperature.

The use of radiant heating devices or phototherapy lights with an incubator may cause overheating of the infant because infants cannot effectively dissipate radiant heat through the Plexiglas wall of the incubator. For this same reason, an incubator should not be exposed to direct sunlight.

Heat loss can also occur through conduction and convection. Conduction involves loss of heat from the body because of direct contact of skin with a cooler solid object. This can be minimized by placing the infant on a padded, covered surface and providing insulation through clothes and blankets rather than by placing the infant directly on a hard table. Placing the newborn skin to skin with the mother on her chest or abdomen immediately after delivery is physically beneficial in terms of conserving heat, as well as fostering maternal attachment.

Convection is similar to conduction except that heat loss is aided by surrounding air currents. For example, placing the infant in the direct flow of air from a fan or air-conditioner vent will cause rapid heat loss through convection. Transporting the neonate in a crib with solid sides reduces airflow around the infant.

PROTECT FROM INFECTION AND INJURY

The most important practice for preventing cross-infection is thorough hand washing of all individuals involved in the infant's care. Other procedures to prevent infection include eye care, umbilical care, bathing, and care of the circumcision. Artificial nails are prohibited (World Health Organization [WHO], 2009a), and long fingernails are discouraged for health care providers because the former have been implicated in the transmission of sepsis. Vitamin K is administered to protect against hemorrhage. In addition, several safety measures are practiced, particularly in terms of proper identification, and screening tests are used to detect various disorders.

Identification

Proper identification of the newborn is absolutely essential. The nurse must verify that identifying bands are securely fastened and verify the information (name, gender, mother's admission number, date, and time of birth) against the birth records and the child's actual gender. This identification process should take place optimally in the delivery room. Some institutions use methods of infant identification such as a color photograph kept in the medical record, storage of blood for DNA genotyping, or electronic surveillance systems for infant security. Footprinting or fingerprinting alone is not currently recommended for newborn identification (AAP and ACOG, 2007); however, the National Center for Missing and Exploited Children (NCMEC) does recommend the use of footprints as a form of identification in addition to a cord blood sample, which is stored until the day after discharge (NCMEC, 2009). Electronic tags that give off a radio frequency may also be used to prevent newborn abductions (Vincent, 2009). A tag is placed on the newborn and removed at the time of discharge by hospital personnel.

A proactive hospital emergency plan should be implemented to prevent infant abduction and to respond promptly and effectively in the event one happens. A mock newborn abduction drill is an effective method that can be used to evaluate staff competence and response to the incident (Shogan, 2002). All hospital personnel should be educated regarding newborn abduction, preventive aspects, and methods to identify the potential risk of such an occurrence.

The nurse should discuss safety issues with the mother the first time the infant is brought to her. The NCMEC* has reported that 58% of infant abductions occur in the mother's room (NCMEC, 2011). A written copy of the safety instructions should also be given to the parent. Parents are instructed to look at identification badges of nurses and hospital personnel who come to take infants and not to relinquish their infants to anyone without proper identification. Mothers are also advised not to leave the infant alone in the crib while they shower or use the bathroom; rather, they should ask to have the infant observed by a health care worker if a family member is not present in the room. Parents and staff are encouraged to use a password system when the newborn is taken from the room as a routine security measure. The nurse should document in the chart that these instructions were given and that appropriate identification band checks are routinely made throughout each shift. Nursing staff are also educated regarding the "typical" abductor profile and to be constantly aware of visitors with unusual behavior.

The typical profile of an abductor is a woman between the ages of 15 and 44 years who is often overweight and has low self-esteem; she may be emotionally disturbed because of the loss of her own child or an inability to conceive and may have a strained relationship with her husband or partner. The typical abductor may also be seen visiting the newborn nursery or neonatal intensive care unit area before the abduction and may ask questions about the care of or the health of a specific newborn. The abductor may familiarize herself with the hospital routine and may also impersonate a health care worker. Parents are made aware of the fact that infant safety measures must be implemented in the home as well. Measures to prevent and decrease infant abduction after discharge to the home include avoiding the publication of birth announcements in the local newspaper and avoiding using yard decorations to announce a newborn's arrival (Shogan, 2002).

Eye Care

Prophylactic eye treatment against ophthalmia neonatorum, infectious conjunctivitis of the newborn, includes the use of (1) silver nitrate (1%) solution, (2) erythromycin (0.5%) ophthalmic ointment or drops, or (3) tetracycline (1%) ophthalmic ointment or drops (preferably in single-dose ampules or tubes). *Chlamydia trachomatis* is the major cause of ophthalmia neonatorum in the United States. Silver nitrate is effective against gonococcal conjunctivitis.

Topical antibiotics such as tetracycline and erythromycin, silver nitrate, and a 2.5% povidone–iodine solution (currently unavailable in commercial form in the United States) have not proved to be effective in the treatment of chlamydial conjunctivitis.

A 14-day course of oral erythromycin or an oral sulfonamide may be given for chlamydial conjunctivitis (AAP, Committee on Infectious Diseases, 2009). Administration of oral erythromycin in infants younger than 6 weeks old has been associated with infantile hypertrophic pyloric stenosis; therefore, parents should be informed of the potential risks and signs of the illness (AAP, Committee on Infectious Diseases, 2009). Herpes simplex virus may also cause neonatal conjunctivitis; treatment in such cases involves the use of topical and systemic antiviral medications.

Because studies on maternal attachment emphasize that in the first hour of life a newborn has a greater ability to focus on coordinated movement than at any other time during the next several days and because eye contact is very important in the development of maternal–infant bonding, the routine administration of silver nitrate or topical ophthalmic antibiotics can be postponed for up to 1 hour after birth. However, practitioners must ensure that the drug is given by 1 hour of age. A chemical conjunctivitis may occur within 24 hours of instillation of ophthalmic prophylaxis. The clinical features include mild eyelid edema and a sterile, nonpurulent eye discharge (Fuloria and Kreiter, 2002). Purulent eye discharge should be reported to the primary practitioner for further investigation.

Vitamin K Administration

Shortly after birth, vitamin K is administered as a single intramuscular dose of 0.5 to 1 mg to prevent hemorrhagic disease of the newborn, also called vitamin K deficiency bleeding (VKDB). Normally, vitamin K is synthesized by the intestinal flora. However, because infants' intestines are relatively sterile at birth and because breast milk contains low levels of vitamin K, the supply is inadequate for at least the first 3 or 4 days. The major function of vitamin K is to catalyze the synthesis of prothrombin in the liver, which is needed for blood clotting. The vastus lateralis muscle is the traditionally recommended injection site, but the ventrogluteal (not the dorsogluteal) muscle can be used.

Several countries have noted a resurgence in later onset of VKDB after practicing orally administered prophylaxis (AAP, 2003). Current

---

*NCMEC has a variety of resources for parents and health professionals for the prevention of child abduction. Contact 800-THE-LOST (800-843-5678); http://www.missingkids.com.

recommendations are that vitamin K be given to all newborns as a single intramuscular dose of 0.5 to 1.0 mg (AAP, 2003). Additional study is needed on the efficacy, safety, and bioavailability of oral preparations and on the most effective dosing regimens to prevent VKDB.

Hepatitis B Vaccine Administration

To decrease the incidence of hepatitis B virus in children and its serious consequences (cirrhosis and liver cancer) in adulthood, the first of three doses of hepatitis B vaccine are recommended soon after birth and before hospital discharge for all newborns in the United States (AAP, Committee on Infectious Diseases, 2011). The injection is given in the vastus lateralis muscle because this site is associated with a better immune response than is the dorsogluteal area (a muscle typically not used in infants in the United States) (see also Immunizations, Chapter 10). Giving the infant concentrated oral sucrose can reduce the pain of the injection (Stevens, Yamada, and Ohlsson, 2010).

Preterm infants who weigh less than 2000 g (4.4 pounds) and are born to HBsAg-negative women may be vaccinated at a chronologic age of 1 month if medically stable or at hospital discharge if discharged before the infant reaches 1 month chronologic age (AAP, Committee on Infectious Diseases, 2009). Infants born to HBsAg-positive mothers should be immunized within 12 hours after birth with hepatitis B vaccine and hepatitis B immune globulin (HBIg) at separate sites, regardless of gestational age or birth weight; the birth dose in such infants should not be counted in the series of three hepatitis B vaccines, and the full three-dose series should be administered starting at age 1 month (AAP, Committee on Infectious Diseases, 2009). An infant who weighs less than 2000 g and whose mother's HBsAg status is unknown should receive the hepatitis B vaccine within 12 hours of birth; maternal status should be determined readily and, if unavailable, the infant should receive the dose of HBIg as soon as possible but within 7 days of birth. In Canada, hepatitis B vaccine is given to newborns only if their mothers are HBsAg positive at birth (see Immunizations, Chapter 10).

Newborn Screening for Disease

A number of genetic disorders can be detected in the newborn period. There is no national policy for such detection in the United States; therefore, the extent of neonatal screening is determined by state laws and voluntary guidelines. Most states require screening for phenylketonuria (PKU), congenital hypothyroidism, galactosemia, and hemoglobin defects such as sickle cell disease (see Chapters 9 and 26); screening for congenital hearing loss is recommended at the same time as disease screening. Because concern has been voiced regarding the inconsistency among states in screening for genetic disorders based on cost, population demographics, resource availability, and political environment, the Task Force on Newborn Screening was formed by the AAP and other federal health care agencies to address this issue. A number of resolutions and policies have been developed to better address the issue of newborn screening (see AAP, Committee on Genetics, 2006, reaffirmed 2011).

The nurse's responsibility is to educate parents regarding the importance of screening and to collect appropriate specimens at the recommended time (after 24 hours of age). With early newborn discharge before 24 hours, some authorities recommend a repeat screening for PKU within 2 weeks (AAP, Committee on Genetics, 2006). Accurate screening depends on high-quality blood spots on approved filter paper forms. The blood should completely saturate the filter paper spot on one side only. The paper should not be handled, placed on wet surfaces, or contaminated with any substance. (See Atraumatic Care box.)

The AAP and ACOG (2007) also recommend routine prenatal and perinatal human immunodeficiency virus (HIV) counseling and testing for all pregnant women and their newborns. Benefits of early identification of HIV-infected infants are early antiretroviral therapy and aggressive nutritional supplementation; appropriate changes in their immunization schedule; monitoring and evaluation of immunologic, neurologic, and neuropsychologic functions for possible changes caused by antiretroviral therapy; initiation of interventions for special educational needs; evaluation for the need of other therapies, such as immunoglobulin for the prevention of bacterial infections; tuberculosis screening and treatment; and management of communicable disease exposures. In addition, vertical transmission of HIV from the mother to the newborn may be reduced to 2% with a cesarean section before the rupture of membranes and onset of labor (AAP and ACOG, 2007). As a result of virologic diagnostic techniques such as HIV culture, polymerase chain reaction, and immune complex–dissociated p24 antigen, diagnosis of HIV infection can be made in 30% to 50% of infants at birth and in 100% of infants by 4 to 6 months of age. For information on additional diseases that may be screened in the newborn period, see Newborn Screening Fact Sheets (Kaye and AAP Committee on Genetics, 2006).

Universal Newborn Hearing Screening

Approximately one to six per 1000 newborns may have significant hearing loss, which may go undetected until later in life. Such deficits may lead to subsequent speech and language delays, which could be treated with early detection. The Joint Committee on Infant Hearing, AAP (2007), recommends that all birthing hospitals establish programs to screen all newborn infants before discharge for hearing loss by automated auditory brainstem response or transient evoked otoacoustic emissions. Newborns who fail the initial screening require documentation and referral for further testing by 1 month of age; newborns who do not receive initial screening before discharge should also be tested by 1 month. It is estimated that screening by high-risk factors alone fails to identify approximately 50% of all newborns with congenital hearing loss. Guidelines for screening infants and older children for hearing loss have been published by the Joint Committee on Infant Hearing Screening, AAP (2007). A subsequent audiologic assessment should be performed at least once by 24 to 36 months of age if the infant has any hearing risk factors despite passing the newborn hearing screening (AAP, 2009).

Bathing

Bath time is an opportunity for the nurse to accomplish much more than general hygiene. It is an excellent time for observing the infant's behavior, state of arousal, alertness, and muscular activity. Bathing is usually performed after the vital signs have stabilized, especially the temperature.

With the possibility of transmission of viruses such as hepatitis B virus and HIV via maternal blood and blood-stained amniotic fluid, the traditional timing of the newborn's bath has been questioned. Newborns must be considered a potential contamination source until proved otherwise. As part of standard precautions, nurses should wear gloves when handling newborns until blood and amniotic fluid are removed by bathing.

Studies indicate that healthy full-term newborns with a stable body temperature can be bathed as early as 1 hour of age without experiencing problems, provided that effective thermoregulation measures are taken after the bath (Behring, Vezeau, and Fink, 2003; Medves and O'Brien, 2004; Varda and Behnke, 2000). Nurses are cautioned, however, to avoid instituting routine newborn bathing according to a

ATRAUMATIC CARE

Heel Punctures

Repeated heel lancing is often necessary to obtain sufficient blood for a number of newborn blood tests, including newborn screening. It has been anecdotally observed that newborns appear to withdraw the heel when touched for subsequent heel punctures. Taddio, Shah, Gilbert-MacLeod, and others (2002) found that infants of diabetic mothers exposed to multiple heel punctures in the first 24 to 36 hours of life learned to anticipate pain and exhibited more intense pain responses. Additional studies have shown that venipuncture performed by an experienced phlebotomist elicited fewer pain responses (as measured by the Premature Infant Pain Profile [PIPP] from full-term newborns than did heel punctures (Shah and Ohlsson, 2001). Furthermore, the need for additional skin punctures was reduced with venipuncture. Although maternal anxiety was initially higher in the venipuncture group, mothers who observed the venipuncture reported observing less pain response than mothers who observed heel punctures.

Oral sucrose and nonnutritive sucking have proved effective in decreasing the pain associated with heel punctures in preterm and full-term infants during the first week of life (Gibbins, Stevens, Hodnett, and others, 2002; Harrison, Johnston, and Loughnan, 2003; Stevens, Yamada, and Ohlsson, 2010); however, the exact dose range that proves effective varies among several studies (Stevens, Yamada, and Ohlsson, 2010). In one study, infants experiencing venipuncture were either given oral sucrose (30%) and a skin placebo or the eutectic mixture of local anesthetic (EMLA). Pain scores were measured with the PIPP, and infants receiving the oral sucrose solution exhibited fewer pain symptoms than those in the EMLA group (Gradin, Eriksson, Holmqvist, and others, 2002). Newborns given 2 ml of concentrated oral sucrose solution showed a significant reduction in crying time and heart rate compared with control subjects (given sterile water) during heel stick sampling and other painful stimuli (Stevens, Yamada, and Ohlsson, 2010).

Evidence indicates that as little as 2 ml of a 24% oral sucrose solution is effective in decreasing pain in full-term and preterm infants. In addition, the best analgesic effect is achieved when sucrose is administered 2 minutes before the painful procedure with a pacifier or syringe. In one study protocol in which oral sucrose was effective, 0.5 ml of 24% oral sucrose solution was administered 2 minutes before, during, and 5 minutes after the heel puncture (Gibbins, Stevens, Hodnett, and others, 2002). Eriksson and Finnstrom (2004) found that repeated administration of a 30% sucrose solution before heel lance in healthy full-term infants did not decrease the pain-relieving effect of the sucrose solution; the study's aim was to determine whether multiple oral sucrose administrations would cause tolerance to sucrose. Monitoring for adverse effects must accompany each administration (Noerr, 2001).

The mother's holding the infant in skin-to-skin contact has also been shown to significantly reduce the child's distress during the procedure (Gray, Watt, and Blass, 2000; Johnston, Filion, Campbell-Yeo, and others, 2009; Johnston, Stevens, Pinelli, and others, 2003). Breastfeeding during heel puncture in full-term newborns has been shown to be effective in decreasing pain scores compared with placebo or an oral sucrose solution (Carbajal, Veerapen, Couderc, and others, 2003; Codipietro, Ceccarelli, and Ponzone, 2008).

After a review of several published studies examining the benefit of applying the topical anesthetic EMLA to reduce the pain of heel lance in full-term and preterm infants, Weise and Nahata (2005) report no differences in pain response between the use of EMLA versus placebo. Thus, this product appears to confer no benefit on newborns undergoing heel lance procedures.

Music was found to decrease the pain response to heel stick in a small group of preterm infants (Butt and Kisilevsky, 2000). A study comparing the effects of swaddling and containment on preterm infants undergoing heel stick failed to demonstrate significant differences between the two interventions (Huang, Tung, Kuo, and others, 2004).

These studies provide evidence of a number of effective ways to decrease the pain associated with heel puncture in full-term and preterm newborns. It is essential that nurses use *all* available resources to advocate for the prevention and management of neonatal pain during such procedures. Because the overall goal is to decrease the effect of painful interventions such as heel stick on infants, a combination of pharmacologic and nonpharmacologic interventions is recommended. (See also Atraumatic Care box, pp. 212–213.)

A number of commercially available oral sucrose solutions now exist, including TootSweet* and Sweet-Ease[†]; both are 24% sucrose solutions. When these are not available, the pharmacy may mix an oral sucrose solution to ensure a clean product. An approximate 25% sucrose solution may be made by mixing 1 tsp of granulated (table) sugar with 4 tsp of sterile water or by diluting simple syrup, a commonly used medication flavoring. However, these methods are the least desirable in terms of prevention of contamination of the solution.

*Natus Medical Incorporated, 1501 Industrial Road, San Carlos, Calif.
[†]Children's Medical Ventures, Norwell, Mass.

rigid schedule; nursing interventions such as bathing should instead be based on individualized assessment and family interaction needs.

The bath time provides an opportunity for the nurse to involve the parents in the care of their child, to teach correct hygiene procedures, and to learn about their infant's individual characteristics (Fig. 8-10). The appropriate types of bathing supplies and the need for safety in terms of water temperature and supervision of the infant at all times during the bath are stressed.

Parents are encouraged to examine their infant closely during bathing. Frequently, normal variations such as Epstein pearls, mongolian spots, or "stork bites" cause parents much distress if they are unaware of the significance of such findings. Minor birth injuries may appear as major defects to them. Explaining how these occurred and when they will disappear reassures parents of their infant's normalcy. Common variations are discussed further in Chapter 9.

One of the most important considerations in skin cleansing is preservation of the skin's acid mantle, which is formed from the uppermost horny layer of the epidermis; sweat; superficial fat; metabolic products; and external substances such as amniotic fluid, microorganisms, and chemicals. Infants' skin surface has a pH of about 5 soon after birth, and the bacteriostatic effects of this pH are significant. Consequently, only plain warm water or soap with appropriate pH should be used for the bath. Alkaline soaps, oils, powder, and lotions are not used because they alter the acid mantle, thus providing a medium for bacterial growth. Talcum powder has the added risk of aspiration if it is applied too close to the infant's face. A safer alternative is a cornstarch-based powder (see also Diaper Dermatitis, Chapter 30).

Parents should be involved in a discussion regarding the newborn's bath at home. It is recommended that for the first 2 weeks the infant be bathed no more than two or three times per week with a plain warm sponge bath. This practice helps maintain the integrity of the newborn's skin and allows time for the umbilical cord to completely dry. Routine daily soap bathing for newborns is no longer recommended (Association of Women's Health, Obstetric and Neonatal Nursing, 2007).

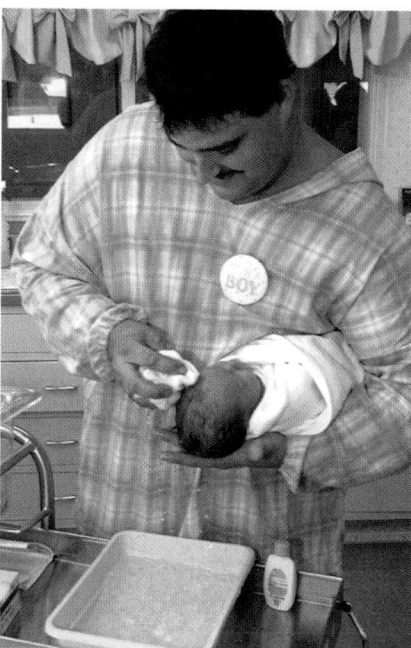

FIG 8-10 Bath time is an excellent opportunity for parents to learn about their newborn.

Care of the Umbilicus

Because the umbilical stump is an excellent medium for bacterial growth, various methods of cord care have been practiced to prevent infection. Some methods popular in the past include the use of an antimicrobial agent such as bacitracin or triple dye and agents such as alcohol or povidone–iodine. The use of antiseptic agents has been shown to prolong cord drying and separation (Zupan, Garner, and Omari, 2004). Studies regarding bacterial growth and colonization according to the cleansing method used have produced varied results (Dore, Buchan, Coulas, and others, 1998; Golombek, Brill, and Salice, 2002; Janssen, Selwood, Dobson, and others, 2003). A Cochrane review of 21 studies found no significant difference between cords treated with antiseptics compared with dry cord care or placebo; there were no reported systemic infections or deaths, and a trend toward reduced colonization was found in cords treated with antiseptics (Zupan, Garner, and Omari, 2004). Recommendations for cord care by the Association of Women's Health, Obstetric and Neonatal Nursing (2007) include cleaning the umbilical cord initially with sterile water or a neutral pH cleanser and then subsequently cleaning the cord with water.

Nurses working in neonatal care must carefully evaluate the available studies and compare the risks and benefits regarding the method of cord care within their own population of newborns and families. Regardless of the method used, nurses must include cord care teaching in the discharge planning because it has been demonstrated to be a concern for parents after discharge to the home. Particularly in the developing world, infants may encounter increased risk of potentially life-threatening sepsis; thus, antimicrobial treatment may be appropriate in some settings (Mullany, Darmstadt, Katz, and others, 2009).

The diaper is folded in front below the cord to avoid irritation and wetness on the site. The area is kept free of urine and stool and cleansed daily with water if needed. Parents are instructed regarding stump deterioration and proper umbilical care. The stump deteriorates through the process of dry gangrene. Cord separation time is influenced by a number of factors, including the type of cord care, type

---

BOX 8-4   RISKS AND BENEFITS OF NEONATAL CIRCUMCISION

Risks

Complications:
- Hemorrhage
- Infection
- Meatitis (from loss of protective foreskin)
- Adhesions
- Concealed penis
- Urethral fistula
- Meatal stenosis
- Necrosis or amputation

Pain in unanesthetized infants (long-term consequences unknown, but short-term stresses include increased heart rate, behavior changes, prolonged crying, increased cortisol levels, and decreased blood oxygenation)

Benefits*

Prevention of penile cancer and posthitis (inflammation of prepuce)

Decreased incidence of balanitis (inflammation of glans), urinary tract infections in male infants, and some sexually transmitted infections later in life (herpes, syphilis, gonorrhea)

Decreased incidence of human immunodeficiency virus (HIV) infection, human papillomavirus (HPV), and cervical cancer (in female partner)

Prevention of complications associated with later circumcision

Preservation of male's body image that is consistent with peers (only in countries or cultures where procedure is common)

*Although there is risk reduction for these conditions with circumcision, the absolute risk of conditions such as penile cancer and infant urinary tract infections is so low that neither the American Academy of Pediatrics nor the American Medical Association recommends circumcision for prevention. Recent evidence regarding circumcision and transmission of sexually transmitted infections has led some authorities to recommend that the American Academy of Pediatrics revisit its policy statement (Tobian, Gray, and Quinn, 2010); the Joint United Nations Programme on HIV/AIDS (2010) suggests long-term HIV prevention strategy is likely to include the provision of neonatal circumcision.

---

of delivery, and other perinatal events. The average cord separation time is 5 to 15 days. It takes a few more weeks for the cord base to heal completely after cord separation. During this time, care consists of keeping the base clean and dry and observing for any signs of infection.

Circumcision

Circumcision, the surgical removal of the foreskin on the glans penis, is usually done in the hospital, although it is not a common practice in most countries. In the United States, however, between 60% and 90% of newborn boys are circumcised, depending on the region (United Nations Programme on HIV/AIDS, 2010). Despite the frequency of the procedure in the United States, there is still controversy regarding the benefits and risks (Box 8-4). The AAP, Task Force on Circumcision (1999, reaffirmed 2005) issued a circumcision policy statement stating that the medical benefits of male newborn circumcision are not sufficiently significant to recommend it as a routine procedure. Recent research has explored the link between circumcision and reduced transmission of communicable illnesses such as HIV in later life (Bailey, Moses, Parker, and others, 2007; Gray, Kigozi, Serwadda, and others, 2007), and some authors advocate a need to revisit the Academy's policy statement based on potential risk reduction (Tobian, Gray, and Quinn, 2010).

The current AAP statement (1999, reaffirmed 2005) emphasizes parental autonomy to determine what is in the best interest of their male newborn. The policy encourages physicians to ensure that parents have been given accurate and unbiased information about the risks, benefits, and alternatives before making an informed choice and that they understand that circumcision is an elective procedure. In addition to examining the medical benefits of male newborn circumcision, the AAP recommends that procedural analgesia be provided if parents decide to have their male infant circumcised.

Nurses are in a unique position to educate parents regarding the care of their newborns, and they must take responsibility for ensuring that each parent has accurate and unbiased information with which to make an informed decision regarding the appropriateness of the circumcision procedure for their newborn. Parents need to know the options for pain control, especially the choice of topical or injected anesthesia, and their option of observing the procedure. Nurses should be proactive in advocating for circumcision analgesia.

Nurses should use nonpharmacologic interventions that can reduce the pain of this operative procedure (see Atraumatic Care box). Despite adequate scientific evidence that newborns feel and respond to pain, circumcisions may still be performed in the United States with either insufficient analgesia or no analgesia at all. Nurses can use the AAP's policy statement (1999, reaffirmed 2005) to advocate more effectively for the use of optimal pain relief for circumcision.

Four types of anesthesia and analgesia are used in newborns undergoing circumcision: ring block, dorsal penile nerve block (DPNB), topical anesthetic such as EMLA (prilocaine–lidocaine) or LMX4 (4% lidocaine), and concentrated oral sucrose. Oral acetaminophen and comfort measures such as music, sucking on a pacifier, and soothing voices have not proved to be effective in reducing the pain of circumcision when used alone (Williamson, 1997); however, these may be used in addition to analgesia and anesthesia to decrease procedural pain.

The Cochrane group exploring pain relief for neonatal circumcision (Brady-Fryer, Wiebe, and Lander, 2007) found that DPNB was the most effective intervention for decreasing the pain of circumcision. Studies exploring the use of several strategies concurrently, such as that conducted by Razmus, Dalton, and Wilson (2004), which included groups receiving both sucrose and ring block compared with ring block alone, have the most potential to clarify optimum strategies.

Circumcision should not be performed immediately after delivery because of neonates' unstable physiologic status and increased susceptibility to stress. Preoperative nursing care usually includes allowing

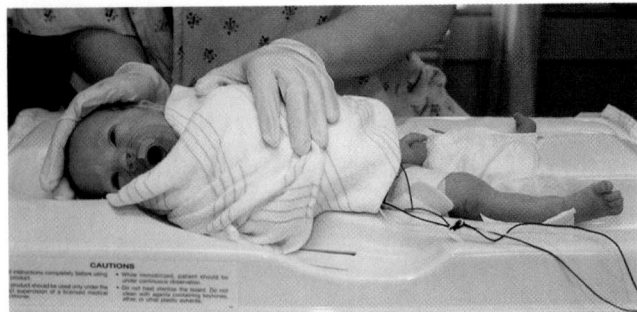

FIG 8-11 Proper positioning of infant in Circumstraint. (Photo by Paul Vincent Kuntz, Texas Children's Hospital, Houston.)

the infant nothing by mouth before the procedure to prevent aspiration of vomitus (≈2 hours); however, the necessity of this practice has been questioned (Kraft, 2003). Additional measures include the surgical time-out, checking for a signed consent form and adequately restraining the infant, usually on a special board (Fig. 8-11) or physiologic circumcision restraint chair. All of the equipment used for the procedure, such as gloves, instruments, dressings, and draping towels, must be sterile.

The procedure involves freeing the foreskin from the glans penis by using a scalpel, Gomco or Mogen clamp (see Cultural Considerations box), or Plastibell. In the Gomco technique, the foreskin is clamped, cut with a scalpel, and removed; the clamp crushes the nerve endings and blood vessels, promoting hemostasis. In the Plastibell procedure, the foreskin is removed using a plastic ring and a string tied around the foreskin like a tourniquet. The excess foreskin is trimmed. In about 5 to 8 days, the plastic ring separates and falls off.

After the procedure is completed, the infant is released from the restraints and comforted. If the parents were not present during the procedure, they are informed of the infant's status and reunited with their son.

Care of the circumcised penis depends on the type of procedure performed. If a clamp (Gomco or Mogen) was used, a petrolatum gauze dressing may be applied loosely to prevent adherence to the diaper. If the Plastibell was applied, no special dressing is required. Because the area is tender, the diaper is applied loosely to prevent friction against the penis. The penis is evaluated for excessive bleeding in the first few hours after the procedure, and the first void is recorded. A recommended standard is to evaluate the site every 30 minutes for at least 2 hours and then at least every 2 hours thereafter (Williamson, 1997).

ATRAUMATIC CARE

Guidelines for Pain Management During Neonatal Circumcision*

Pharmacologic Interventions

Use of Topical Anesthetic Only

One hour before the procedure, administer **acetaminophen** as ordered.

Place a thick layer (1 g) of **EMLA**† (lidocaine–prilocaine) cream around the penis where the prepuce (foreskin) attaches to the glans. Avoid placing cream on the tip of the penis where EMLA may come in contact with the urethral opening.

Cover the penis with a "finger cot" that is cut from a vinyl glove or a piece of plastic wrap and secure the bottom of the covering with tape. Avoid using

Tegaderm or large amounts of tape on the skin because removing the adhesive causes pain and can irritate or remove the fragile skin.

If the infant urinates during the time EMLA is applied (1 hr) and a significant amount of EMLA is removed, reapply the cream and covering. The total application of EMLA should not exceed a surface area of 10 cm² (1.25 × 1.25 inches).

Remove the cream with a clean cloth or tissue. Blanching of the skin is an expected reaction to EMLA's application under an occlusive dressing; erythema and some edema may also occur.

ATRAUMATIC CARE

Guidelines for Pain Management During Neonatal Circumcision—cont'd

Two minutes before starting the procedure, give the infant a **concentrated sucrose solution** (24%). Use this solution to coat the pacifier (recoat several times before and during the procedure) or administer 2 ml to the tongue. Allow the infant to suck on the pacifier dipped in oral sucrose during the procedure.

After the procedure, apply **petrolatum or A&D ointment** on a 2 × 2 dressing before diapering the infant to prevent the wound from adhering to the dressing or diaper. Topical anesthetic alone is not recommended for pain management of circumcision.

Administer **acetaminophen** as ordered by the practitioner 4 hours after the initial dose; give additional doses as needed but not to exceed five doses in 24 hours or a maximum dosage of 75 mg/kg/day.

Use of Dorsal Penile Nerve Block (DPNB) or Ring Block

One hour before the procedure, administer **acetaminophen**.

One hour before the procedure, apply **EMLA**. For the DPNB, apply EMLA to the prepuce as described previously and at the penile base. For the ring block, apply EMLA to the prepuce as described previously and to the shaft of the penis. A topical anesthetic should be used in conjunction with the DPNB or ring block to avoid the pain of injecting the anesthetic.

Two minutes before starting the procedure, give the infant a **concentrated sucrose solution** (24%). Use this solution to coat the pacifier (recoat several times before and during the procedure) or administer 2 ml to the tongue. Allow the infant to suck on the pacifier dipped in oral sucrose during the procedure.

DPNB and ring block are accomplished using a small-gauge needle to administer **lidocaine** in several areas at the base or shaft of the penis. Using buffered lidocaine (with sodium bicarbonate) and warming the solution may further decrease pain. (Lidocaine with epinephrine is not used in neonates.)

For maximum anesthesia, wait 5 minutes after the injection of lidocaine. An alternative anesthetic is chloroprocaine, which is as effective as lidocaine after 3 minutes.

Apply **A&D ointment or petrolatum** as described previously.

Administer **acetaminophen** as ordered by the practitioner (10–15 mg/kg) every 4 to 6 hours for 24 hours not to exceed five doses in 24 hours or a maximum dosage of 75 mg/kg/day.

Nonpharmacologic Interventions (To Accompany the Preceding Pharmacologic Interventions)

If a Circumstraint board is used, pad it with blankets or other thick, soft material such as "lamb's wool."

Provide the parents, caregiver, or another staff member with the option of holding the infant during the procedure or of being present during the circumcision.

Swaddle the upper body and legs during the procedure to provide warmth and containment and to reduce movement (see Fig. 8-11).

If the patient is not swaddled and is unclothed, use a radiant warmer to prevent hypothermia. Shield the infant's eyes from overhead lights as needed.

Prewarm any topical solutions to be used in sterile preparation of the surgical site by placing them in a warm blanket or towel.

Play infant relaxation music before, during, and after the procedure; allow the parents or other caregiver the option of providing the music of choice.[‡]

After the procedure, remove restraints and swaddle. Immediately have the parent, other caregiver, or nursing staff hold the infant. Continue to have the infant suck on the pacifier or offer feeding.

Combination analgesia is recommended: oral sucrose, acetaminophen, and topical anesthetic; or oral sucrose, acetaminophen, topical anesthetic, and DPNB or ring block in addition to nonpharmacologic comfort measures such as containment, positioning, nonnutritive sucking, and breastfeeding.

References

Anand KJS, International Evidence-Based Group for Neonatal Pain: Consensus statement for the prevention and management of pain in the newborn, *Arch Pediatr Adolesc Med* 155(2):173–180, 2001.

Cyna AM, Middleton P: Caudal epidural block versus other methods of postoperative pain relief for circumcision in boys, *Cochrane Database Syst Rev* 8(4):CD003005, 2008.

Geyer J, Ellsbury D, Kleiber C, and others: An evidence-based multidisciplinary protocol for neonatal circumcision pain management, *J Obstet Gynecol Neonatal Nurs* 31(4):403–410, 2002.

Howard CR, Howard FM, Weitzman ML: Acetaminophen analgesia in neonatal circumcision: the effect on pain, *Pediatrics* 93(4):641–646, 1994.

Joint United Nations Programme on HIV/AIDS: Neonatal and child male circumcision: a global review, Geneva, 2010, UNAIDS, retrieved March 23, 2011, from http://www.who.int/hiv/pub/malecircumcision/neonatal_child_MC_UNAIDS.pdf.

Kraft NL: A pictorial and video guide to circumcision without pain, *Adv Neonatal Care* 3(2):50–64, 2003.

Lehr VT, Cepeda E, Frattarelli DA, and others: Lidocaine 4% cream compared with lidocaine 2.5% and prilocaine 2.5% or dorsal penile block for circumcision, *Am J Perinatol* 22(5):231–237, 2005.

Razmus I, Dalton M, Wilson D: Pain management for newborn circumcision, *Pediatr Nurs* 20(5):414–417, 427, 2004.

Stevens B, Yamada J, Ohlsson A: Sucrose for analgesia in newborn infants undergoing painful procedures, *Cochrane Database Syst Rev* (1):CD001069, 2010.

Taddio A: Pain management for neonatal circumcision, *Paediatr Drugs* 3(2):101–111, 2001.

Taddio A, Ohlsson K, Ohlsson A: Lidocaine-prilocaine cream for analgesia during circumcision in newborn boys, *Cochrane Database Syst Rev* (1):CD000496, 2003.

Yamada J, Stinson J, Lamba J, and others: A review of systematic reviews on pain interventions in hospitalized infants, *Pain Res Manage* 13(5):413–420, 2008.

*Modified from Taddio A, Pollock N, Gilbert-MacLeod C, and others: Combined analgesia and local anesthesia to minimize pain during circumcision, *Arch Pediatr Adolesc Med* 154(6):620–623, 2000.

[†]EMLA is approved for use in infants age 37 or more weeks of gestation, provided practitioners follow recommendations regarding maximal dose and limits for exposure time to the medication. In addition, practitioners are advised not to use EMLA with infants who are receiving potentially methemoglobinemia-inducing medications such as acetaminophen or phenobarbital. Although the package insert warns that patients taking acetaminophen are at greater risk for developing methemoglobinemia, there have been no reported cases of this complication occurring in children taking acetaminophen and using EMLA.

[‡]Suggested infant relaxation music: *Heartbeat Lullabies* by Terry Woodford. Available from Baby-Go-To-Sleep Center, Audio Therapy Innovations, Inc., PO Box 550, Colorado Springs, CO 80901; 800-537-7714; http://www.babygotosleep.com.

⊕ CULTURAL CONSIDERATIONS

Circumcision

In the Jewish culture, circumcision is performed during a ceremony called a **berith**, or **brit**, which takes place on the eighth day of life. A specially trained professional known as a **mohel** stretches the prepuce over the glans, pulling it though a slit in a shield (usually a Mogen clamp) and cutting it with a knife. The traditional technique is not sterile, and bleeding is controlled by tight bandaging around the penis (Cohen, Drucker, Vainer, and others, 1992). The infant may be given some sweet wine before the procedure. Blankets instead of straps are usually used to restrain the infant on a board, and the parents are present (Trochtenberg, 1990).

Female circumcision (mutilation), or female genital mutilation (FGM), is also practiced in some countries, particularly in Africa, the Middle East, and Southeast Asia, and among immigrants from these countries to the United States, Australia, Canada, and Europe. In the most extensive operation (excision or infibulation), the clitoris, labia minora, and medial aspects of the labia majora are removed. The remaining labia majora are sewn closed except for a small opening for urine and menses (Abubakar, Iliyasu, Kabir, and others, 2004; McCleary, 1994). Anesthesia is used rarely. In African and Asian cultures, female circumcision is used to prove virginity and to reduce sexual pleasure, thus promoting fidelity. The World Health Organization (2010) condemns all forms of FGM. FGM is associated with an increased risk for adverse obstetric outcomes and numerous physical problems, which often may not receive medical care (Morrone, Hercogova, and Lotti, 2002; World Health Organization, 2006, 2010).

Normally, on the second day, a yellowish white exudate forms as part of the granulation process. This is not a sign of infection and is not forcibly removed. As healing progresses, the exudate disappears. Parents are educated to report any evidence of bleeding, unusual swelling, or absence of voiding to the practitioner.

PROVIDE OPTIMAL NUTRITION

Selection of a feeding method is one of the major decisions faced by parents. In general, there are two primary choices: human milk and commercially prepared whole cow's milk formula. These two methods have significant nutritional, economic, and psychologic advantages and differences. Nurses should be at the forefront in providing parent(s) with accurate and unbiased information needed to make a conscientious informed decision regarding the feeding method.

Human Milk

Human milk is the best option for infant nutrition up to 1 year of age. Breast milk consists of a number of micronutrients that are called bioavailable, meaning these nutrients are available in quantities and qualities that make them easily digestible by the newborn's intestine and absorbed for energy and growth. Breast milk offers a variety of immunologic properties that are found exclusively in human milk. Human milk has been shown to be effective in protecting newborns against respiratory tract infections, gastrointestinal infections, otitis media, numerous allergies, type 2 diabetes, and atopy.

The fat content of human milk is composed of lipids, triglycerides, and cholesterol; cholesterol is an essential element for brain growth. The function of these lipids is to allow optimal intestinal absorption of essential fatty acids and polyunsaturated fatty acids (PUFAs). Furthermore, lipids contribute approximately 50% of the total calories in human milk (Lawrence and Lawrence, 2011). Although the overall fat content in human milk is higher than in cow's milk, it is used more efficiently by infants.

The primary source of carbohydrate in human milk is lactose, which is present in higher concentrations (6.8 g/dl) than in cow's milk–based formula (4.9 g/dl). The carbohydrates not only serve as a large portion of total calories in human milk, but also have protective functions; the oligosaccharides (prebiotic) in human milk stimulate the growth of *Lactobacillus bifidus* (a probiotic) and prevent bacteria from adhering to epithelial surfaces. Additional carbohydrates found in human milk include glucose, galactose, and glucosamine.

Human milk also contains two proteins, whey (lactalbumin) and casein (curd), in a ratio of approximately 60:40 (vs. 80:20 in most cow's milk–based formula). This ratio in human milk makes it more digestible and produces the soft stools seen in breastfed infants. Thus, human milk has a laxative effect, and constipation is uncommon. The whey protein lactoferrin in human milk has iron-binding characteristics with bacteriostatic capabilities, particularly against gram-positive and gram-negative aerobes, anaerobes, and yeasts (Lawrence and Lawrence, 2011).

Lysozyme is found in large quantities in human milk and has bacteriostatic functions against gram-positive bacteria and *Enterobacteriaceae* organisms. Human milk also contains numerous other host defense factors such as macrophages, granulocytes, and T and B lymphocytes. Casein in human milk greatly enhances the absorption of iron, thus preventing iron-dependent bacteria from proliferating in the gastrointestinal tract (Biancuzzo, 2003). Secretory immunoglobulin A (IgA) is found in high levels in colostrum, but levels gradually decline over the first 14 days of life. Secretory IgA prevents bacteria and viruses from invading the intestinal mucosa in breastfed newborns, thus protecting from infection (Newburg and Walker, 2007). The whey protein is also believed to play an important role in preventing the development of certain allergies.

Several digestive enzymes also present in human milk include amylases, lipases, proteases, and ribonucleases, which enhance the digestion and absorption of various nutrients. The amounts of lipid- and water-soluble vitamins, electrolytes, minerals, and trace elements in human milk are sufficient for growth, development, and energy needs during the first 6 months of life. The one possible exception is vitamin D, which is found in varying amounts depending on the mother's intake of vitamin D–fortified food and exposure to ultraviolet light. Therefore, to prevent vitamin D–deficiency rickets, the AAP, Section on Breastfeeding (2008) now recommends that infants who are exclusively breastfed or who are ingesting less than 1000 ml/day of vitamin D–fortified formula be supplemented with 400 IU vitamin D (oral) per day. The CPS, First Nations, Inuit, and Métis Health Committee (2007) suggests that for children living in its northernmost climates, it may be reasonable to double this recommendation to 800 IU per day to compensate for extremely limited exposure to sunlight.

Additional beneficial components of human milk include prostaglandins; epidermal growth factor; desoxyhexanoic acid (DHA); arachidonic acid (AA); taurine; cystine; carnitine; cytokine; interleukins; and natural hormones such as thyroid-releasing hormone, gonadotropin-releasing hormone, and prolactin. Studies have demonstrated that breastfeeding is associated with a decrease in the incidence of type 2 diabetes (Kue Young, Chateau, and Zhang, 2002; Le Huërou-Luron, Blat, and Boudry, 2010; Young, Martens, Taback, and others, 2002), a decrease in the incidence of hospital admissions for respiratory tract illnesses in generally healthy infants (Bachrach, Schwarz, and Bachrach, 2003), and higher intelligence scores compared with cow's milk–based formula–fed infants (Michaelsen, Lauritzen, and

Mortensen, 2009). Some studies have demonstrated that breastfeeding has an analgesic effect on newborns during painful procedures such as heel puncture (Carbajal, Veerapen, Couderc, and others, 2003; Gray, Miller, Phillips, and others, 2002; Shah, Aliwalas, and Shah, 2006).

Breastfeeding

Human milk is the preferred form of nutrition for all infants. *Healthy People 2020* has a goal to increase breastfeeding rates in the United States to 81.9% in early postpartum and to 61% for mothers who continue to breastfeed for at least 6 months (U.S. Department of Health and Human Services, 2011). Some have voiced concern that early discharge of new mothers from hospitals, more aggressive marketing of infant formulas to the public, and more employed mothers contributed to the decline of breastfeeding in the 1990s. In addition, some hospital practices intended to provide optimal maternal–newborn health may instead undermine breastfeeding. Early separation of the mother and newborn, delays in initiating breastfeeding, provision of formula in the hospital and in discharge packs, conflicting information by health care workers, and formula coupons given at discharge have been implicated in the decline of breastfeeding after discharge. Rooming-in has correlated positively with successful breastfeeding, but the use of pacifiers has sometimes been associated with earlier weaning from breast to bottle.

Studies exploring breastfeeding mothers' reasons for early cessation of breastfeeding suggest several factors contribute to this decision, such as history of depression, obesity, and lower maternal education (Kehler, Chaput, and Tough, 2009). Modifiable factors associated with a decreased risk of early cessation of breastfeeding include professional and social support (Meedya, Fahy, and Kable, 2010; Thulier and Mercer, 2009). These findings have important implications for nurses in education and discussion regarding breastfeeding before, during, and after pregnancy. Teaching families about the importance of breastfeeding and their critical role in supporting the mother is imperative.

The AAP, Section on Breastfeeding (2005) has reaffirmed its position exclusively recommending breastfeeding until at least 1 year of age as the best form of infant nutrition. The Academy also supports programs that enable women to continue breastfeeding after returning to work. In its support of breastfeeding practices, the Academy further discourages the advertisement of infant formula to breastfeeding mothers and distribution of formula discharge packs without the advice of a health care provider.

The Baby-Friendly Hospital Initiative (BFHI) is a joint effort of the WHO and the United Nations Children's Fund (UNICEF) to encourage, promote, and support breastfeeding as the model for optimum infant nutrition. Ten research-supported practices were developed by the BFHI as a guideline for maternity facilities worldwide to promote breastfeeding (WHO, UNICEF, and Wellstart International, 2009) (Box 8-5). Research indicates that Baby-Friendly designated hospitals have higher rates for breastfeeding initiation and exclusivity than hospitals that are not Baby-Friendly designates (Abrahams and Labbok, 2009; Merewood, Mehta, Chamberlain, and others, 2005).

In addition to the physiologic qualities of human milk, the most outstanding psychologic benefit of breastfeeding is the close maternal–child relationship. The infant is nestled close to the mother's skin, can hear the rhythm of her heartbeat, can feel the warmth of her body, and has a sense of peaceful security. The mother has a close feeling of union with her child and feels a sense of accomplishment and satisfaction as the infant sucks milk from her.

Human milk is the most economical form of feeding. It is always available, ready to serve at room temperature, and free of contamination. Although human milk is not sterile, healthy full-term infants can

---

> ## BOX 8-5 TEN STEPS TO SUCCESSFUL BREASTFEEDING
>
> Every facility providing maternity services and care for newborn infants should:
> 1. Have a written breastfeeding policy that is routinely communicated to all health care staff.
> 2. Train all health care staff in skills necessary to implement this policy.
> 3. Inform all pregnant women about the benefits and management of breastfeeding.
> 4. Help mothers initiate breastfeeding within a half hour of birth.
> 5. Show mothers how to breastfeed and how to maintain lactation even if they should be separated from their infants.
> 6. Give newborn infants no food or drink other than breast milk unless medically indicated.
> 7. Practice rooming-in—allowing mothers and infants to remain together—24 hours a day.
> 8. Encourage breastfeeding on demand.
> 9. Give no artificial teats or pacifiers (also called dummies or soothers) to breastfeeding infants.
> 10. Foster the establishment of breastfeeding support groups, and refer mothers to them on discharge from the hospital or clinic.

Data from WHO, UNICEF, and Wellstart International: *Baby-friendly hospital initiative: revised, updated and expanded for integrated care,* Geneva, 2009, WHO, retrieved March 28, 2011, from http://whqlibdoc.who.int/publications/2009/9789241594967_eng.pdf.

---

tolerate varying amounts of nonpathogenic and pathogenic organisms. The protection against infection can provide additional cost savings in terms of fewer medical visits and less time lost from work for the employed mother.

Breastfed infants, especially beyond 2 to 3 months of age, tend to grow at a satisfactory but slower rate than bottle-fed infants.

Contraindications to breastfeeding include (Lawrence and Lawrence, 2011; AAP, Section on Breastfeeding, 2005):
- Maternal chemotherapy antimetabolites and certain antineoplastic drugs
- Active tuberculosis not under treatment in the mother
- HIV in the mother
- Galactosemia in the infant
- Maternal herpes simplex lesion on a breast
- Cytomegalovirus (CMV)—primary risk for preterm infants receiving CMV-infected donor milk, not for infected mother's infant (who already has CMV)
- Maternal substance abuse (e.g., cocaine, methamphetamine, and marijuana) (NOTE: Maternal methadone treatment for substance abuse is *not* a contraindication to breastfeeding.)
- Human T-cell leukemia virus types I and II
- Mothers who are receiving diagnostic or radioactive isotopes or who have had exposure to radioactive materials (for as long as there is radioactivity in milk)

Mastitis is usually not a contraindication if the discomfort is tolerable.

A small number of medications are contraindicated for breastfeeding mothers. Consult a reference text such as Hale (2010). Some herbal products are presented as safe and effective alternatives to prescription or over-the-counter medications; certain herbal agents, called **galactogogues**, are reported to increase breast milk production. However, insufficient data are available to confirm or deny the assertion of increased milk production using herbal galactogogues, and mothers

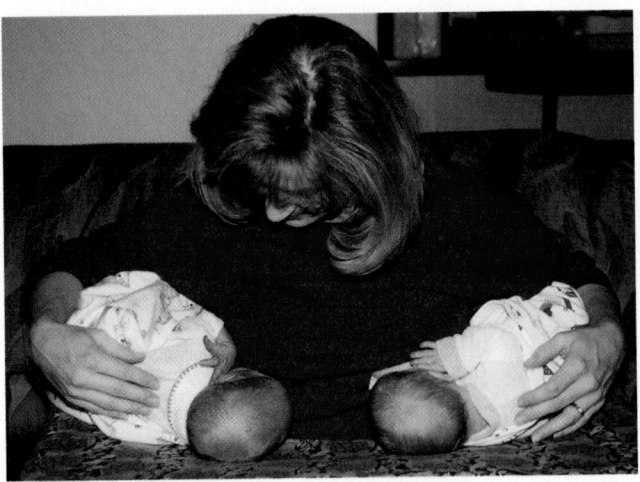

FIG 8-12 Simultaneous breastfeeding of twins.

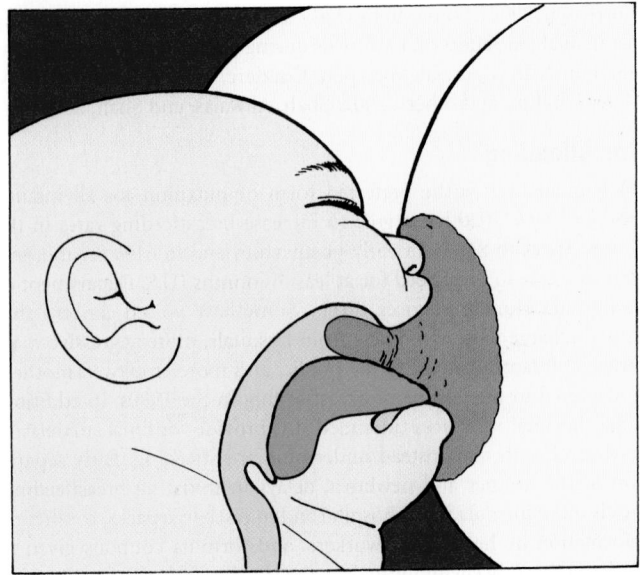

FIG 8-13 The tongue is under the areola with the tip of the nipple at the back of the wide-open mouth.

are cautioned to seek advice from a practitioner to ensure that the herbal preparations will not harm breastfeeding infants (Conover and Buehler, 2004; Jackson, 2010).

Breastfeeding with twins and other multiples requires specialized professional support. If both twins are full term, they can begin feeding immediately after birth (Fig. 8-12); late preterm infants should be evaluated individually but may be breastfed if stable. Simultaneous feeding promotes the rapid production of milk needed for both infants and makes the milk that would normally be lost in the letdown reflex available to one of the twins. When only one infant is hungry, the mother should feed singly. She should also alternate breasts when feeding each infant and avoid favoring one breast for one infant. The suckling patterns of infants vary, and each infant needs the visual stimulation and exercise that alternating breasts provides.

A concern mothers may have is the perceived inconvenience or loss of freedom and independence if they chose to breastfeed. Being committed to feeding the infant every 2 to 3 hours can seem overwhelming, especially to women with multiple responsibilities. Many women resume their careers shortly after their pregnancy and may believe bottle feeding is less work than breastfeeding. The preparation, storage, and heating of formula are important considerations for the family when comparing the effort required for bottle feeding versus breastfeeding. Combining breastfeeding and employment is possible, and many employers now provide space for mothers to pump and store their milk. This is likely an acknowledgement of the demonstrated health benefits of breastfeeding—a breastfed infant is far less likely to have infections of any sort; thus, the infant's mother is far less likely to need time away from work to care for an ill infant. Suggestions for breastfeeding mothers returning to work are discussed in Chapter 10. Although breastfeeding is the preferred form of infant feeding, mothers' decisions regarding their preferences must be supported and respected.

Successful breastfeeding probably depends more on the mother's desire to breastfeed, satisfaction with breastfeeding, and available support systems than on any other factors. Mothers need support, encouragement, and assistance during their postpartum hospital stays and at home to enhance their opportunities for success and satisfaction.

Three main criteria have been proposed as essential in promoting positive breastfeeding: absence of a rigid feeding schedule, correct positioning of the infant at the breast to achieve latch-on, and correct suckling technique. Correct suckling for breastfeeding is defined as a wide-open mouth, tongue under the areola, and expression of milk by effective alveolar compression (Fig. 8-13).

The following interventions promote breastfeeding:
- Frequent and early breastfeeding, especially during the first hour of life; immediate skin-to-skin contact; rooming-in; and feeding on demand
- Direct modeling of the importance of breastfeeding by health care providers, such as implementing demand nursing with no formula supplementation and decreased emphasis on infant formula products
- Increased information and support to mothers after discharge, including phone follow-up
- Early breast pumping every 2 to 3 hours for 10 to 15 minutes bilaterally if the newborn is unable to nurse immediately (increases oxytocin production and thus milk production)

Nurses play a significant role in the breastfeeding decision and must make themselves available to families for guidance and support. Several excellent books and organizations, such as La Leche League International,* are available as resources for professionals and breastfeeding mothers.

> ### ! NURSING ALERT
>
> Do not use microwaves to defrost frozen human milk. High-temperature microwaving (72°–98° C [162°–208° F]) significantly destroys the antiinfective factors and vitamin C content (Quan, Yang, Rubinstein, and others, 1992). The safety of low-temperature microwaving (20°–53° C [68°–127° F]) remains questionable. One of the best ways to thaw frozen human milk is to place it under a warm flow of tap water. Another option is to let the frozen milk thaw overnight in the refrigerator to maintain high levels of secretory IgA (Biancuzzo, 2003). Test the temperature of the milk before feeding.

*957 N. Plum Grove Road, Schaumburg, IL 60173; 847-519-7730; http://www.llli.org. In Canada: PO Box 700, Winchester, ON, KOC 2KO; 800-665-4324; http://www.lllc.ca.

Bottle Feeding

Bottle feeding generally refers to the use of bottles for feeding commercial or evaporated milk formula rather than using the breast, although human milk may be expressed and fed with a bottle when necessary. Bottle feeding is an acceptable method of feeding. Nurses should not assume that new parents automatically know how to bottle feed their infants. One study noted 77% of formula-feeding mothers did not receive instruction on formula preparation from a health professional; consequently, hands, bottles, and nipples were not washed properly, and storage and heating practices were unsafe in many instances (Labiner-Wolfe, Fein, and Shealy, 2008). Parents who choose bottle feeding also need support and assistance in meeting their infants' needs.

Providing newborns with nutrition is only one aspect of feeding. Holding them close to the body while rocking or cuddling them helps to ensure the emotional component of feeding. Similar to breastfed infants, bottle-fed infants need to be held on alternate sides of the lap to expose them to different stimuli. The feeding should not be hurried. Even though they may suck vigorously for the first 5 minutes and seem to be satisfied, they should be allowed to continue sucking. Infants need at least 2 hours of sucking a day. If there are six feedings per day, then about 20 minutes of sucking at each feeding provides for oral gratification.

Propping the bottle during infant feeding is discouraged for the following reasons:

- It denies the infant the important component of close human contact.
- The infant may aspirate formula into the trachea and lungs while sleeping.
- It may facilitate the development of middle ear infections. If the infant lies flat and sucks, milk that has pooled in the pharynx becomes a suitable medium for bacterial growth. Bacteria then enters the eustachian tube, which leads to the middle ear, causing acute otitis media.
- It encourages continuous pooling of formula in the mouth, which can lead to nursing caries when the teeth erupt (see Chapter 12).

Commercially Prepared Formulas

The analysis of human and whole cow's milk indicates that the latter is unsuitable for infant nutrition. Whole cow's milk has a high protein content and low fat and lipid content, and evidence indicates that it may cause intestinal bleeding and lead to iron-deficiency anemia in infants. Questions have also been raised regarding the unmodified protein content of whole cow's milk, which may trigger an undesired immune response and thus increase the incidence of allergies in children at an early age.

Commercially prepared formulas are cow's milk based and have been modified to resemble the nutritional content of human milk. These formulas are altered from cow's milk by removing butterfat, decreasing the protein content, and adding vegetable oil and carbohydrate. Some cow's milk–based formulas have demineralized whey added to yield a whey-to-casein ratio of 60 to 40. The standard cow's milk–based formulas, regardless of the commercial brand, have essentially the same compositions of vitamins, minerals, protein, carbohydrates, and essential amino acids, with minor variations such as the source of carbohydrate (Akers and Groh-Wargo, 2005); nucleotides to enhance immune function; and long-chain polyunsaturated fatty acids (LCPUFAs), DHA and AA, which have been reported to improve brain function (Georgieff, 2001). DHA and AA are both found in large quantities in human milk but until recently were not present in most infant formulas. Studies in full-term infants receiving supplements with LCPUFAs have produced mixed results regarding brain function and visual acuity (Simmer, Patole, and Rao, 2008). Many studies report a variety of sources for LCPUFAs, including egg yolk lipid, phospholipids, and triglycerides. The evidence for supplementation of formula for preterm infants with LCPUFAs, however, has been more convincing, producing some transient improvement in visual acuity and general development (AAP, Committee on Nutrition, 2009). There do not appear to be any adverse effects associated with LCPUFA supplementation in preterm infants with respect to the incidence of bronchopulmonary disease, necrotizing enterocolitis, or other conditions of prematurity (AAP, Committee on Nutrition, 2009). The Food and Drug Administration (FDA) regulates the manufacture of infant formula in the United States to ensure product safety. Standard cow's milk–based formulas are sold as low iron and iron fortified; however, only the iron-fortified formulas meet the requirements of infants (AAP, Committee on Nutrition, 2009).

There are four main categories of commercially prepared infant formulas: (1) cow's milk–based formulas, available in 20 kcal/fl oz as liquid (ready to feed), powder (requires reconstitution with water), or a concentrated liquid (requires dilution with water); (2) soy-based formulas, available commercially in ready-to-feed 20 kcal/fl oz powder and concentrated liquid forms, commonly used for children who are lactose or cow's milk protein intolerant; (3) casein- or whey-hydrolysate formulas, commercially available in ready-to-feed and powder forms and used primarily for children who cannot tolerate or digest cow's milk– or soy-based formulas; and (4) amino acid formulas.

The AAP (Bhatia, Greer, and Committee on Nutrition, 2008) recommends the use of soy protein–based formulas for infants with galactosemia and hereditary lactase deficiency and when a vegetarian diet is preferred. For infants with documented allergies caused by cow's milk, extensively hydrolyzed protein formula should be considered because up to 14% of these infants also have a soy protein allergy. Some researchers have speculated that exclusive use of soy formula in infants may adversely affect their endocrine, reproductive, and immune systems. This concern is related to isoflavones in soy and possible alteration in sexual maturity, immune response, and thyroid function (Chen and Rogan, 2004; Greim, 2004). Others report no long-term untoward effects from the ingestion of isoflavones in soy formula (Giampietro, Bruno, Furcolo, and others, 2004; Merritt and Jenks, 2004). There is currently no conclusive evidence that dietary soy products adversely affect human development, reproduction, or endocrine function (Bhatia, Greer, and Committee on Nutrition, 2008).

The casein- or whey-hydrolysate formulas are considered to be less antigenic than either cow's milk–based or soy-based formulas. The protein hydrolysate formulas (casein and whey) are derived from cow's milk–based formulas by a process of heat, filtration, and enzyme treatment designed to break the peptide chains into more digestible and hypoallergenic proteins. The hydrolysate formulas have the disadvantage of tasting bad; however, these may be made more palatable by adding a hypoallergenic flavoring. Neocate and EleCare are extensively hydrolyzed amino acid formulas designed for infants who are sensitive to cow's milk–based, soy-based, and partially hydrolyzed casein- and whey-based formulas. Both products are available in powder form. A wide variety of formulas are manufactured for infants and children with special needs; it is not within the scope of this text to discuss each one, but a formula company representative can provide product books that describe the purpose and content of each formula.

Follow-up formulas are marketed as a transitional formula for infants older than 6 months of age who are also eating solid foods.

These generally contain a higher percentage of calories from protein and carbohydrate sources, a higher amount of iron and vitamins, and a lower amount of fat than standard cow's milk–based formulas. Many nutrition experts (AAP, Committee on Nutrition, 2009), however, dispute the necessity of follow-up formulas if the infant is receiving an adequate amount of solid foods containing sufficient iron, vitamins, and minerals.

Preparation of Formula

Persons preparing infant formula must wash their hands well and then wash all of the equipment used to prepare the formula (including the cans of formula) with soap and water. Sterilizing bottles and nipples 5 minutes in boiling water may be required when a hot-water dishwasher is not available. It is generally recommended that the tap water used to reconstitute powdered infant formula or to dilute concentrated liquid be brought to a rolling boil for 1 minute and then allowed to cool before use (AAP, Committee on Nutrition, 2009). Bottled water should not be considered sterile unless otherwise indicated; bottled water without fluoride should be avoided for mixing infant formula (Morin, 2007). Following the manufacturer's instructions for preparing the formula is essential to ensure the infant receives adequate calories and fluid for adequate growth. Parents are cautioned not to alter the reconstitution or dilution of infant formula except under the specific directions of the primary practitioner. Powdered formula and concentrated formula are prepared and bottled and refrigerated if not used for feeding immediately. Warming the formula is optional, although many parents prefer to warm it before feeding. Any milk remaining in the bottle after the feeding is discarded because it is an excellent medium for bacterial growth. Opened cans of ready-to-feed or concentrated formula are covered and refrigerated immediately until the next feeding. Because of incidents involving contamination of powdered formula with *Enterobacter sakazakii* and subsequent infant death in a neonatal unit, it is now recommended that hospital formula preparation for newborns follow separate guidelines; these are discussed in Chapter 9.

Laws governing the labeling of infant formulas require that the directions for preparation and use of the formula include pictures and symbols for nonreading individuals. In addition, manufacturers are translating the directions into foreign languages, such as Spanish and Vietnamese, to prevent misunderstanding and errors in formula preparation.

> ### ! NURSING ALERT
>
> Stress to families that the proportions must not be altered—neither diluted with extra water to extend the amount of formula nor concentrated to provide more calories.

Alternate Milk Products

In the United States, few infants are fed **evaporated milk formula**, and its use is not recommended by the AAP, Committee on Nutrition (2009). However, it has advantages over whole milk. It is readily available in cans; needs no refrigeration if unopened; is less expensive than commercial formula; provides a softer, more digestible curd; and contains more lactalbumin and a higher calcium-to-phosphorus ratio. Disadvantages of evaporated milk for infant nutrition include low iron and vitamin C concentrations, excessive sodium and phosphorus, decreased vitamin A and D (except in fortified forms), and poorly digested fat. A common rule for preparing evaporated milk formula is diluting the 13-oz can of milk with 19.5 ounces of water and adding 3 Tbsp of sugar or commercially processed corn syrup.

Evaporated milk must not be confused with condensed milk, which is a form of evaporated milk with 45% more sugar. Because of its high carbohydrate concentration and disproportionately low fat and protein content, condensed milk is not used for infant feeding. Likewise, skim and low-fat milk must not be used for infant milk because they are deficient in caloric concentration, significantly increase the renal solute load and water demands, and deprive the body of essential fatty acids.

Goat's milk is a poor source of iron and folic acid. It has an excessively high renal solute load as a result of its high protein content, making it unsuitable for infant nutrition (AAP, Committee on Nutrition, 2009). Some believe that goat's milk is less allergenic than other available milk sources and may feed it to their infants to reduce allergic milk reactions. However, infants allergic to cow's milk are just as likely to be allergic to goat's milk; other complications such as hypernatremia and metabolic acidosis may ensue as a result of the high sodium and protein concentration found in goat's milk compared with human milk (Basnet, Schneider, Gazit, and others, 2010). Raw, unpasteurized milk from any animal source is unacceptable for infant nutrition.

Feeding Schedules

Ideally, feeding schedules should be determined by the infant's hunger. **Demand feedings** involve feeding infants when they signal readiness. **Scheduled feedings** are arranged at predetermined intervals. Some hospitals routinely feed infants every 3 to 4 hours. Although this may be satisfactory for bottle-fed infants, it hinders the breastfeeding process. Breastfed infants tend to be hungry every 2 to 3 hours because of the easy digestibility of the milk; therefore, they should be fed on demand.

Supplemental feedings should *not* be offered to breastfed infants before lactation is well established because they may satiate the infant and may cause nipple preference. Supplemental water is not needed in breastfed infants even in hot climates (AAP, Committee on Nutrition, 2009). Satiated infants suck less vigorously at the breast, and milk production depends on the breast being emptied at each feeding. If milk is allowed to accumulate in the ducts, causing breast engorgement, ischemia results, suppressing the activity of the acini, or milk-secreting cells. Consequently, milk production is reduced. In addition, the process of sucking from a bottle is different from breast nipple compression. The relatively inflexible rubber nipple prevents the tongue from its usual rhythmic action. Infants learn to put the tongue against the nipple holes to slow down the more rapid flow of fluid. When infants use these same tongue movements during breastfeeding, they may push the human nipple out of the mouth and may not grasp the areola properly.

Usually by 3 weeks of age, lactation is well established. Bottle-fed infants consume about 2 to 3 oz of formula at each feeding and are fed approximately six times a day. The quantity of formula consumed is based on the caloric need of 108 kcal/kg/day; therefore, a newborn who weighs 3 kg requires 324 kcal/day. Because commercial formula has 20 kcal/oz, approximately 16 oz (480 ml) provides the daily caloric requirement. Breastfed infants may feed as frequently as 10 to 12 times a day.

Feeding Behavior

Five behavioral stages occur during successful feeding. Recognizing these steps can assist nurses in identifying potential feeding problems caused by improper feeding techniques. **Prefeeding behavior**, such as crying or fussing, demonstrates the infant's level of arousal and degree of hunger. To encourage the infant to grasp the breast properly, it is preferable to begin feeding during the quiet alert state before the infant becomes upset. **Approach behavior** is indicated by sucking movements or the rooting reflex. **Attachment behavior** includes activities that occur from the time the infant receives the nipple and sucks (sometimes more pronounced during initial attempts at breastfeeding). **Consummatory behavior** consists of coordinated sucking and swallowing. Persistent gagging might indicate unsuccessful consummatory behavior. **Satiety behavior** is observed when infants let the parent know that they are satisfied, usually by falling asleep.

PROMOTE PARENT–INFANT BONDING (ATTACHMENT)

The process of parenting is based on a relationship between the parent and infant. As more is learned of the complexity of neonates and of their potential for influencing and shaping their environments, particularly their interaction with significant others, it is apparent that promoting positive parent–child relationships necessitates an understanding of behavioral steps in attachment, variables that enhance or hinder this process, and methods of teaching parents to develop a stronger relationship with their children, especially by recognizing potential problems. (See also Assessment of Attachment Behaviors, p. 202.)

Infant Behavior

Nurses must appreciate the individuality and uniqueness of each infant. According to the individual temperament, infants change and shape the environment, which influences their future development. (See Patterns of Sleep and Activity, p. 201.) An infant who sleeps 20 hours a day will be exposed to fewer stimuli than one who sleeps 16 hours a day. In turn, each infant will likely elicit a different response from parents. An infant who is quiet, undemanding, and passive may receive much less attention than one who is responsive, alert, and active. Behavioral characteristics such as irritability and consolability can influence the ease of transition to parenthood and the parents' perception of the infant.

Nurses can positively influence the attachment of the parent and child. The first step is recognizing individual differences and explaining to the parents that such characteristics are normal. For example, some people believe that infants sleep throughout the day except for feedings. For some newborns, this may be true, but for many, it is not. Understanding that the infant's wakefulness is part of a biologic rhythm and not a reflection of inadequate parenting can be crucial in promoting healthy parent–child relationships. Another aspect of helping parents' concerns includes supplying guidelines on how to enhance the infant's development during awake periods. Placing the child in a crib to stare at the same mobile every day is not exciting, but carrying the infant into each room as one does daily chores can be fascinating. Likewise, placing the infant in front of a television is not likely to provide appropriate stimulation. Infants enjoy human contact and often respond to visual and auditory stimuli in different ways depending on their sleep–wake state and the type of stimuli provided. Infants prefer black and white objects, geometric patterns and shapes, and reflective surfaces such as mirrors and eyeglasses. However, evidence indicates that infants prefer contact with human faces and enjoy interactions with others more than objects or television images.

Maternal Attachment

Research has suggested that there is a **maternal sensitive period** immediately and for a short time after birth when parents have a unique ability to attach to their infants (Klaus, Kennell, and Klaus, 1995). Mothers may demonstrate a predictable and orderly pattern of

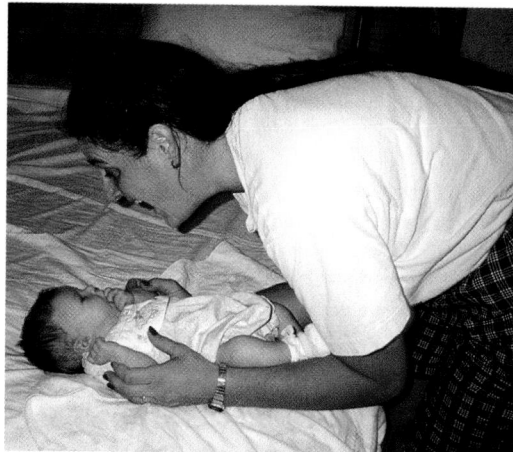

FIG 8-14 En face position between the parent and infant can be significant in attachment process.

behavior during the development of the attachment process. When mothers are presented with their nude infants, they begin to examine the infant with their fingertips, concentrating on touching the extremities, and then proceed to massage and encompass the trunk with their entire hands. Assuming the **en face position**, in which the mother's and infant's eyes meet in visual contact in the same vertical plane, is significant in the formation of affectional ties (Fig. 8-14). Although similar patterns of touching have been observed, additional studies demonstrate different patterns for mothers, as well as the same pattern for nonmaternal persons, such as male and female nurses. Some authors have suggested that mothers experiencing depression, as well as adolescent mothers, may have lower rates of secure attachment with their infants (Flaherty and Sadler, 2011), necessitating the need for caregivers to monitor such mothers closely and to model attachment behaviors. Nurses must observe for maternal attachment behaviors and exercise caution in interpreting such behaviors.

Several studies have attempted to substantiate the long-term benefits of providing parents with opportunities to optimally bond with their infants during the initial postpartum period. Although there has been some evidence that increased parent–child contact encourages prolonged breastfeeding and may minimize the risks of parenting disorders, conclusions about the long-term effects of such early intervention on parenting and child development must be viewed cautiously. In addition, some authorities claim that the emphasis on bonding has been unjustified and may lead to guilt and fear in parents who did not have early contact with their infants. There is concern that the literal interpretation of "sensitive" or "critical" might imply that without early contact, optimum bonding cannot occur or, conversely, that early contact alone is sufficient to ensure competent parenting.

The nurse should stress to parents that although early bonding is valuable, it does not represent an "all or none" phenomenon. Throughout the child's life, there will be multiple opportunities for development of parent–child attachment. Bonding is a complex process that develops gradually and is influenced by numerous factors, only one of which is the type of initial contact between the newborn and parent.

In a concept analysis of parent–infant attachment, Goulet, Bell, St-Cyr, and others (1998) describe attributes of parent–infant attachment as **proximity, reciprocity,** and **commitment.** Within these attributes are further dimensions, which include contact, emotional state, individualization, complementarity, sensitivity, centrality, and parent role exploration. The researchers describe the parent–infant attachment process as one that is complex and therefore cannot be evaluated simply by the observations of attitudes and behaviors of parents toward their infants (Goulet, Bell, St-Cyr, and others, 1998). Further research into the reciprocal relationships between infants and parents and the situational factors that influence such relationships is recommended.

One component of successful maternal attachment is the concept of reciprocity (Brazelton, 1974). As the mother responds to the infant, the infant must respond to the mother by some signal, such as sucking, cooing, eye contact, grasping, or molding (conforming to other's body during close physical contact). The first step is initiation in which interaction between infant and parent begins. Next is orientation, which establishes the partners' expectations of each other during the interaction. After orientation is acceleration of the attention cycle to a peak of excitement. The infant reaches out and coos, both arms jerk forward, the head moves backward, the eyes dilate, and the face brightens. After a short time, deceleration of the excitement and turning away occur in which the infant's eyes shift away from the parent's and the child grasps his or her shirt. During this cycle of nonattention, repeated verbal or visual attempts to reinitiate the infant's attention are ineffective. This deceleration and turning away probably prevents the infant from being overwhelmed by excessive stimuli. In a good interaction, both partners have synchronized their attention–nonattention cycles. Parents or other caregivers who do not allow the infant to turn away and who continually attempt to maintain visual contact encourage the infant to turn off the attention cycle and thus prolong the nonattention phase.

Although this description of reciprocal interacting behavior is usually observed in infants by 2 to 3 weeks of age, nurses can use this information to teach parents how to interact with their newborns. Recognizing the attention versus nonattention cycles and understanding that the latter is not a rejection of the parent helps parents develop competence in parenting.

Paternal Engrossment

Fathers also show specific attachment behaviors to their newborns. This process of paternal engrossment, forming a sense of absorption, preoccupation, and interest in the infant, includes (1) visual awareness of the newborn, especially focusing on the beauty of the child; (2) tactile awareness, often expressed in a desire to hold the infant; (3) awareness of distinct characteristics with emphasis on those features of the infant that resemble the father; (4) perception of the infant as perfect; (5) development of a strong feeling of attraction to the child that leads to intense focusing of attention on the infant; (6) experiencing a feeling of extreme elation; and (7) feeling a sense of deep self-esteem and satisfaction. These responses are greatest during the early contacts with the infant and are intensified by the neonate's normal reflex activity, especially the grasp reflex and visual alertness. In addition to behavioral reactions, fathers also demonstrate physiologic responses such as increased heart rate and BP during interactions with their newborns.

The process of engrossment has significant implications for nurses. It is imperative to recognize the importance of early father–infant contact in releasing these behaviors. Fathers need to be encouraged to express their positive feelings, especially if such emotions are contrary to any popular belief that fathers should remain stoic. If this is not clarified, fathers may feel confused and attempt to suppress the natural sensations of absorption, preoccupation, and interest in order to conform with societal expectations.

Mothers also need to be aware of the responses of the father toward the newborn, especially because one of the consequences of paternal preoccupation with the infant is less overt attention toward the mother.

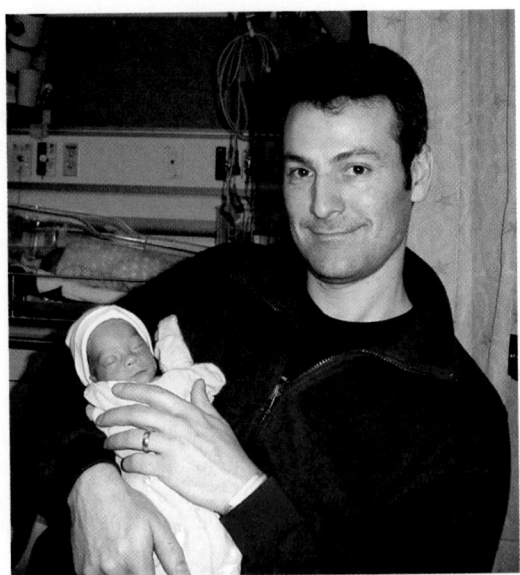

FIG 8-15 A desire to hold the infant and participate in caregiving activities is an indication of paternal engrossment.

If both parents are able to share their feelings, each can appreciate the process of attachment toward their child and will avoid the unfortunate conflict of being insensitive and unaware of the other's needs. In addition, a father who is encouraged to form a relationship with his newborn is less likely to feel excluded and abandoned after the family returns home and the mother directs her attention toward caring for the infant.

Ideally, the process of engrossment should be discussed with parents before the delivery, such as in prenatal classes, to reinforce the father's awareness of his natural feelings toward the expected child. Focusing on the future experience of seeing, touching, and holding one's newborn may also help expectant fathers become more comfortable in accepting their paternal feelings. This in turn can assist them in being more supportive toward the mother, especially as the labor and delivery draw near.

At the infant's birth, the nurse can play a vital role in helping the father express engrossment by assessing the neonate in front of the couple; pointing out normal characteristics; encouraging identification through consistent referral to the child by name; encouraging the father to cuddle, hold, talk to, or feed the infant; and demonstrating whenever necessary the soothing powers of caressing, stroking, and rocking the child (Fig. 8-15). Fathers are encouraged to be with the mother during labor and delivery, to spend time alone with the mother and newborn after delivery, and to room-in with the mother and infant. Many birthing centers have adopted a family-centered focus, including sleeping accommodations that more closely resemble the home environment for the new mother and father.

Fathers, like mothers, may demonstrate attachment not only after the infant's birth but during fetal life as well. Paternal attachment may proceed at a different pace than maternal attachment. Paternal preoccupation with events of labor and delivery and the spouse's health may detract from paternal attachment (Anderson, 1996). Research has noted that, although fathers spend similar amounts of time in interaction with their newborns as do mothers, the nature of their interaction is different. Mothers and infants focus on face-to-face exchange and mutual gazing, co-vocalization, and affectionate touch. Fathers' time with their infants includes quick peaks of high positive emotionality, including joint laughter and open exuberance. Interactions with

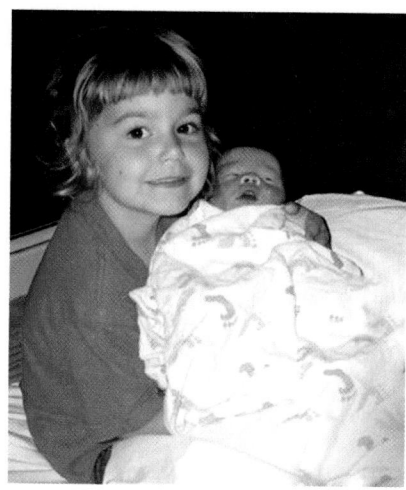

FIG 8-16 Sibling visitation shortly after birth can facilitate the attachment process.

fathers tend to center on physical games or games with an object focus rather than on face-to-face signals (Feldman, 2007).

The nurse observes for the same indications of affection from the father as those expected in the mother, such as making visual contact in the en face position and embracing the infant close to the body. When present, such behaviors are reinforced. If such responses are not obvious, the nurse needs to assess the father's feelings regarding this birth, cultural beliefs that may affect his expression of emotions, and other factors that influence his perception of the infant and the mother in order to facilitate a positive attachment during this critical period.

Siblings

Although the attachment process has been discussed almost exclusively in terms of the parents and infants, it is essential that nurses be aware of other family members, such as siblings and members of the extended family, who need preparation for the acceptance of this new child. Young children in particular need sensitive preparation for the birth to minimize sibling jealousy.

In support of family-centered care, the current trend is to allow siblings to visit the mother on the postpartum unit and to hold the newborn (Fig. 8-16). Another trend has been the presence of siblings at childbirth. Unlike sibling visitation, the evidence supporting this practice has been controversial, yet the nature of truly providing family-centered care encompasses siblings, grandparents, and other significant persons who comprise the extended family unit (Tomlinson, Bryan, and Esau, 1996). The AAP and ACOG (2007) support the presence of siblings at childbirth and visitation of the newborn and mother; basic guidelines for infection control and adult supervision are also recommended.

Children exhibit different degrees of involvement in the birth process. Some reported benefits include children's increased knowledge of the birth process, less regressive behavior after the birth, and more mothering and caregiving behavior toward the infant. Some practitioners add facilitated family bonding and assimilation of the newborn into the family as positive outcomes. Parents whose children attended the birth have echoed these same benefits and have expressed their desire to repeat the experience should another pregnancy occur. Despite these positive findings, opponents believe that allowing children to observe a delivery could lead to emotional difficulties, although there is no research to support this contention. As research mounts, birthing centers that allow siblings at the birth are developing more

definitive guidelines, such as an age requirement of at least 4 to 5 years, the presence of a supportive person for the sibling only, and an adequate sequence of preparation in which parents explore all options for preparing their other children.

From observations during sibling visitation, there is evidence that sibling attachment occurs. However, the en face position is assumed much less often among the newborn and siblings than between mother and newborn, and when this position is used, it is brief. Siblings focus more on the head or face than on touching or talking to the infant. The siblings' verbalizations are often focused less on attracting the infant's attention and more on addressing the mother about the newborn. Children who have established a prenatal relationship with the fetus have demonstrated more attachment behaviors, supporting the suggestion of encouraging prenatal acquaintance. Additional research is needed to establish theories on sibling bonding as have been constructed for parental bonding.

Multiple Births and Subsequent Children

A component of attachment that has special meaning for families with multiple births, monotropy refers to the principle that a person can become optimally attached to only one individual at a time. If a parent can form only one attachment at a time, how can all of the siblings of a multiple birth receive optimum emotional care? Research on bonding and multiple births is still lacking despite the recent increase in multiple births, and even less is known about paternal engrossment and sibling attachment. In regard to mother–twin bonding, the conclusions of different authors vary. Some report that mothers bond equally to each twin at the time of birth even if one twin is ill. Others suggest that mothers of twins may take months or years to form individual attachments to each child or even longer if the twins are identical.

Nurses can be instrumental in promoting bonding of multiple births. The most important principle is to assist the parents in recognizing the individuality of the children, especially in monozygotic (identical) twins. The mother should visit with each newborn, including a sick infant, as much as possible after birth. Rooming-in and breastfeeding are encouraged. Any characteristics that are unique to each child are emphasized, and each infant is called by name rather than referring to "the twins." Asking the family questions such as "How do you tell Ashley and Amy apart?" and "In what ways are Ashley and Amy different and similar?" helps point out their individual characteristics. Behaviors on the BNBAS can be used to illustrate these differences and to stress effective strategies for dealing with multiple personalities at the same time.

Cobedding (bed sharing) of twins or other multiples may be done in the hospital with the goal of maintaining the bond between siblings that was formed in utero (Fig. 8-17). Much research is focused on exploring the safety and benefits of the practice of cobedding (Hayward, Campbell-Yeo, Price, and others, 2007) (see also Sudden Infant Death Syndrome, Chapter 11); however, the AAP (2005, reaffirmed 2009) has recommended against families cobedding with infants at home. Because neither the safety nor the benefits of cobedding for newborns has been documented in the literature, the Academy recommends families be counseled to follow safe sleeping practices, which currently dictate that infants sleep alone for optimal safety.

Another area of attachment that has received minimal attention is maternal bonding of multiparous mothers. Research suggests that there are several additional tasks to "taking on" a second child. These include:

- Promoting acceptance and approval of the second child
- Grieving and resolving the loss of an exclusive dyadic relationship with the first child

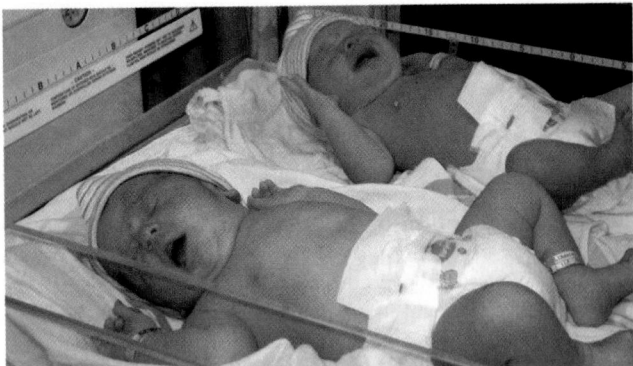

FIG 8-17 Newborn twins are placed in same bed during the newborn transition period.

- Planning and coordinating family life to include a second child
- Reformulating a relationship with the first child
- Identifying with the second child by comparing this child with the first child in terms of physical and psychologic characteristics
- Assessing one's affective capabilities in providing sufficient emotional support and nurturance simultaneously to two children

Employed mothers who have a second child report fewer concerns than with the first child regarding general aspects of separation from their child and the effect of separation on the child, but they have similar concerns regarding separation because of employment. It appears that although experience may decrease some concerns, it may not minimize others.

PREPARE FOR DISCHARGE AND HOME CARE

With short postpartum hospital stays as well as a trend toward mother–infant care, also called dyad or couplet care, discharge planning, referral, and home visits have become increasingly important components of comprehensive newborn care. First-time, as well as experienced, parents benefit from guidance and assistance with the infant's care, such as breastfeeding or bottle feeding, and with the family's integration of a new member, particularly sibling adjustment.

To assess and meet these needs, teaching must begin early, ideally before the birth. Not only is the postpartum stay sometimes very short (as little as 12–24 hours), but mothers are also in the taking-in phase during which they may demonstrate passive and dependent behaviors. On the first postpartum day, as a result of fatigue and excitement about the newborn, mothers may not be able to absorb large amounts of information. This time may need to be spent highlighting essential aspects of care, such as infant safety and feeding. Parents may also be given a list of mother and infant care topics as part of the nursing admission history to choose issues they wish to review. Teaching before discharge should focus on newborn feeding patterns, monitoring diapers for voiding and stooling, jaundice, and infant crying.

The AAP, Committee on Fetus and Newborn (2010) has established guidelines for postpartum discharge (see Family-Centered Care box). The Academy emphasizes that each mother–infant dyad should be evaluated individually to determine the optimal time of discharge.

Although some mothers and newborns may be safely discharged within 12 to 24 hours without detriment to their health, others require a longer stay. Follow-up home care within days (or even hours after discharge when minor problems are anticipated) appears to be the emerging trend in an effort to curtail hospital costs and provide adequate mother–newborn care with minimal complications. (See Community Focus boxes.)

Despite the changing spectrum of well-newborn health care, the nurse's role continues to be that of providing ongoing assessments of each mother–newborn dyad to ensure a safe transition to home and a successful adaptation into the family unit. The ultimate safety and success of early newborn discharge from hospital are contingent on using clear discharge criteria and having a high-quality early follow-up program (Radmacher, Massey, and Adamkin, 2002).

With family structures changing, it is essential that nurses identify the primary caregiver, which may not always be the mother but may be a father, grandparent, or babysitter. Depending on the family composition, the mother's primary support system in the care of the newborn may not always be the traditional husband or male companion.

Nurses should not assume that terminology associated with mother–infant care is understood. Words relating to the anatomy (e.g., *meconium*, *labia*, *edema*, and *genitalia*) and to breastfeeding (e.g., *areola*, *colostrum*, and *let-down reflex*) may be unfamiliar to mothers. Mothers with other children do not necessarily understand more words, and younger, less educated mothers may be at particular risk for not understanding teaching.

An essential area of discharge counseling is the safe transportation of the newborn home from the hospital. Ideally, this information should also be provided before delivery to allow parents an opportunity to purchase a suitable infant car safety seat. When purchasing a car safety seat, parents should consider cost and convenience. The convertible-type seats are more expensive initially but cost less than two separate systems (infant-only model and infant-toddler convertible model). Convenience is a major factor because a cumbersome restraint may be used less often or used improperly. Before buying a car safety seat, it is best to look carefully at different models. For example, some types are too large for subcompact cars. Asking friends about the advantages and disadvantages of their restraints is helpful,

🏠 COMMUNITY FOCUS

Early Newborn Discharge Checklist

Feeding—Adequate latch-on demonstrated for breastfeeding newborn; successfully feeding 1.5 to 2 oz of formula every 3 to 4 hours with minimum spitting up and no vomiting

Elimination—Voiding every 4 to 6 hours or more often; one stool passed in first 24 to 28 hours

Circumcision—Evidence of voiding; nonbleeding circumcision (does not require pressure); no excess edema at site

Color—Pink centrally and buccal mucosa moist; no evidence of jaundice in first 24 hours

Cord—No signs or symptoms of infection; if used, drying agent applied per institution protocol (see Care of the Umbilicus, p. 211)

Newborn screening—Completed phenylketonuria and other screenings per state law

Vital signs—Stable heart rate, respiratory rate, and temperature for at least 12 hours before discharge; no apnea

Activity—Wakeful periods before feedings; moves all extremities

Home visit or primary practitioner visit—Follow-up appointment within 48 hours after discharge

🏠 COMMUNITY FOCUS

Newborn Home Care After Early Discharge*

Wet diapers—Minimum of one for each day of life (day 2 = 2 wets; day 3 = 3 wets) until fifth or sixth day, at which time 5 or 6 per day to 14 days, then 6 to 10 per day

Breastfeeding—Successful latch-on and feeding every 1.5 to 3 hours daily; audible swallowing

Formula feeding—Successfully taking at least 1 to 2 oz every 3 to 4 hours; voiding as above

Circumcision—Wash with warm water only; yellow exudate forming, with no bleeding; Plastibell intact for 48 hours

Stools—At least one every 48 to 72 hours (bottle feeding), or two or three per day (breastfeeding)

Color—Pink to ruddy when crying; pink centrally when at rest or asleep

Activity—Has four or five wakeful periods per day and alerts to environmental sounds and voices

Jaundice—Physiologic jaundice (i.e., jaundice not appearing in the first 24 hours); feeding, voiding, and stooling as noted above or practitioner notification for suspicion of pathologic jaundice (appears within 24 hours of birth; hemolysis and ABO/Rh problem suspected), decreased activity, poor feeding, or dark orange skin color persisting on the fifth day in light-skinned newborn; obtain transcutaneous (or serum) bilirubin before discharge and identify risk with an hour-specific nomogram (see Hyperbilirubinemia, Chapter 9)

Umbilical cord—Kept above diaper line; drying, no drainage; periumbilical area nonerythematous

Vital signs—Heart rate, 120 to 140 beats/min at rest; respiratory rate, 30 to 55 breaths/min at rest without evidence of sternal retractions, grunting, or nasal flaring; temperature, 36.3° to 37° C (97.3°–98.6° F) axillary

Position of sleep—On back

*Any deviation from the above or suspicion of poor newborn adaptation should be immediately reported to the practitioner.

but borrowing a car seat or purchasing a used one can be dangerous. Parents should use only a restraint that has directions for use and a certification label stating that it complies with federal motor vehicle safety standards (both should be on the seat). They should not use a restraint that has been involved in a crash. Some service clubs and hospitals have loan programs for restraints. Information about approved models and other aspects of car safety seat restraints is available from several organizations and sources.*

Parents are cautioned against placing an infant in the front seat of a car with a passenger-side air bag. It is now recommended that infants and toddlers ride rear facing in a child safety seat in the back seat of the car until the age of 2 years or until they reach the maximum height and weight recommended by the car seat manufacturer (AAP, Committee on Injury, Violence, and Poison Prevention, 2011). Studies indicate that toddlers (up to 24 months of age) are safer riding in convertible seats in the rear-facing position (Bull and Durbin, 2008). A convertible safety seat is positioned semireclined and facing the rear of the car. After the child has outgrown the rear-facing seat, a forward-facing seat with a harness is recommended.

❗ NURSING ALERT

In a car seat, padding is never placed underneath or behind the infant because it creates slackness in the harness, leading to the possibility of the child's ejection from the seat in the event of a crash. In vehicles with front passenger-side air bags, the rear-facing safety seat must be placed in the back seat to avoid injury to the infant from the released air bag forcing the safety seat against the vehicle seat or passenger door.

Although federal safety standards do not specify the minimum weight of an infant and the appropriate type of restraint, newborns

---

*American Academy of Pediatrics, 141 Northwest Point Blvd., Elk Grove Village, IL 60007-1098; 847-434-4000; http://www.aap.org and http://www.HealthyChildren.org; and local division of traffic safety or National Highway Traffic Safety Administration Auto Safety Hotline, 888-327-4236. For children with disabilities, contact the Easter Seals, 800-221-6827, and ask about Special KARS (Kids Are Riding Safe).

weighing 2 kg (4.4 pounds) receive relatively good support in convertible seats with a seat back–to-crotch strap height of 14 cm (5.7 inches) or less. Rolled blankets or towels may be needed between the crotch and legs to prevent slouching and can be placed along the sides to minimize lateral movements. Placing the infant in a safety seat at a 45-degree angle will prevent slumping and airway obstruction (AAP, Committee on Injury, Violence, and Poison Prevention, 2011). Seats with shields (large padded surfaces in front of the child) and armrests (found on some other models) are unacceptable because of their proximity to the infant's face and neck. (For a discussion of appropriate car restraints for preterm infants, see Community Focus box, Chapter 9; and for infants, see Motor Vehicle Injuries in Chapters 10 and 12.)

In the United States and Canada, all states and provinces have mandated the use of child restraints. Therefore, hospitals and birthing centers should have policies regarding the safe discharge of newborns in car safety seats and provisions for parents to learn to use the devices correctly. In addition, hospital personnel should ensure that infants born before 37 weeks of gestation have a period of observation in the selected car seat to monitor for possible apnea, bradycardia, and oxygen desaturation (AAP, Committee on Injury, Violence, and Poison Prevention and the Committee on Fetus and Newborn, 2009). Parents are more likely to use a restraint correctly and consistently if the proper use of one is demonstrated and its necessity is stressed. Infants and children continue to be hurt and killed because car seat restraints are not installed properly.

KEY POINTS

- Transition from fetal or placental circulation to independent respiration is the most important physiologic change required of newborns.
- Chemical and thermal factors help initiate a neonate's first respiration.
- Circulatory changes in neonates result from shifts in pressure in the heart and major vessels and from functional closures of the fetal shunts.
- Newborns' large surface area, thin layer of subcutaneous fat, and unique mechanism for producing heat predispose them to excessive heat loss.
- Infants' high rate of metabolism is closely correlated with the rate of fluid exchange, which is much higher in infants than in adults.
- The skin and mucous membranes, the macrophage system, and antibodies are the first, second, and third lines, respectively, of defense against infection.
- The Apgar score, the initial assessment of newborns, focuses on heart rate, respiratory effort, muscle tone, reflex irritability, and color.

- Physical assessment of newborns includes clinical assessment of gestational age, general measurements, general appearance, head-to-toe assessment, and parent–infant attachment or bonding.
- Neurologic assessment focuses on localized reflexes and posture, muscle tone, head control, and movement and is best accomplished during the general physical examination.
- Behavioral assessment of newborns with the BNBAS examines responses to seven categories: habituation, orientation, motor performance, range of state, regulation of state, autonomic stability, and reflexes.
- Physical care for newborns includes maintaining a patent airway, maintaining a stable body temperature, protecting from infection and injury, and providing optimal nutrition.
- Although the attachment, or bonding, process primarily affects infants and parents, siblings also play an important role.
- An essential aspect of discharge teaching is ensuring newborns' safe transportation home in federally approved, backward-facing car safety seats.

REFERENCES

Abrahams SW, Labbok MH: Exploring the impact of the baby-friendly hospital initiative on trends in exclusive breastfeeding, *Int Breastfeed J* 29:4–11, 2009.

Abubakar I, Iliyasu Z, Kabir M, and others: Knowledge, attitude and practice of female genital cutting among antenatal patients in Aminu Kano Teaching Hospital, *Nigerian J Med* 13(3):254–258, 2004.

Akers SM, Groh-Wargo SL: Normal nutrition during infancy. In Samour PQ, Helm KK, Lang CE, editors: *Handbook of pediatric nutrition*, ed 3, Sudbury, Mass, 2005, Jones & Bartlett.

Alexander GR, Himes JH, Kaufman RB, and others: A United States national reference for fetal growth, *Obstet Gynecol* 87(2):163–168, 1996.

American Academy of Pediatrics: Controversies concerning vitamin K and the newborn (policy statement), *Pediatrics* 112(1):191–192, 2003, reaffirmed 2009.

American Academy of Pediatrics: Hearing assessment in infants and children: recommendations beyond neonatal screening, *Pediatrics* 124(4):1252–1263, 2009.

American Academy of Pediatrics, Committee on Environmental Health: Mercury in the environment: implications for pediatricians (technical report), *Pediatrics* 108(1):197–205, 2001, reaffirmed 2007.

American Academy of Pediatrics, Committee on Fetus and Newborn: Policy statement: hospital stay for healthy term newborns, *Pediatrics* 125(20):405–409, 2010.

American Academy of Pediatrics, Committee on Fetus and Newborn, American College of Obstetricians and Gynecologists, Committee on Obstetric Practice: The Apgar score, *Pediatrics* 117(4):1444–1447, 2006, reaffirmed 2008.

American Academy of Pediatrics, Committee on Genetics: Introduction to the newborn

screening fact sheets, *Pediatrics* 118(3):1304–1312, 2006, reaffirmed 2011.

American Academy of Pediatrics, Committee on Genetics: Newborn screening fact sheets, *Pediatrics* 118(3):e935–e963, 2006, reaffirmed 2011.

American Academy of Pediatrics, Committee on Infectious Diseases: Policy statement—recommended childhood and adolescent immunization schedules—United States 2011, *Pediatrics* 127(2):387–391, 2011.

American Academy of Pediatrics, Committee on Infectious Diseases: *Red book: 2009 report of the Committee on Infectious Diseases*, ed 28, Elk Grove Village, Ill, 2009, Author.

American Academy of Pediatrics, Committee on Injury, Violence, and Poison Prevention: Policy statement: child passenger safety, *Pediatrics* 127(4):788–793, 2011.

American Academy of Pediatrics, Committee on Injury, Violence, and Poison Prevention and the Committee on Fetus and Newborn: Safe transportation of preterm and low birth weight infants at hospital discharge, *Pediatrics* 123(5):1424–1429, 2009.

American Academy of Pediatrics, Committee on Nutrition: *Pediatric nutrition handbook*, ed 6, Elk Grove Village, Ill, 2009, Author.

American Academy of Pediatrics, Joint Committee on Infant Hearing: Year 2007 position statement: principle and guidelines for early hearing detection and intervention, *Pediatrics* 120(4):898–921, 2007.

American Academy of Pediatrics, Section on Breastfeeding: Breastfeeding and the use of human milk (policy statement), *Pediatrics* 115(2):496–506, 2005.

American Academy of Pediatrics, Section on Breastfeeding: Prevention of rickets and vitamin D deficiency in infants, children, and adolescents, *Pediatrics* 122(5):1142–1150, 2008.

American Academy of Pediatrics, Task Force on Circumcision: Circumcision policy statement, *Pediatrics* 103(3):686–693, 1999, reaffirmed 2005.

American Academy of Pediatrics, Task Force on Sudden Infant Death Syndrome: The changing concept of sudden infant death syndrome: diagnostic coding shifts, controversies regarding the sleeping environment, and new variables to consider in reducing risk, *Pediatrics* 116(5):1245–1255, 2005, reaffirmed 2009.

American Academy of Pediatrics, American College of Obstetricians and Gynecologists: *Guidelines for perinatal care*, ed 6, Elk Grove Village, Ill, 2007, Author.

Anderson AM: The father–infant relationship: becoming connected, *J Soc Pediatr Nurs* 1(2):83–92, 1996.

Association of Women's Health, Obstetric and Neonatal Nursing: *Evidence-based clinical practice guideline: neonatal skin care*, Washington, DC, 2007, Author.

Bachrach VR, Schwarz E, Bachrach LR: Breastfeeding and the risk of hospitalization for respiratory disease in infancy, *Arch Pediatr Adolesc Med* 157(3):237–243, 2003.

Bailey RC, Moses S, Parker CB, and others: Male circumcision for HIV prevention in young men in Kisumu, Kenya: a randomized controlled trial, *Lancet* 369(9562):643–656, 2007.

Ballard JL, Khoury JC, Wedig K, and others: New Ballard Score, expanded to include extremely premature infants, *J Pediatr* 119(3):417–423, 1991.

Basnet S, Schneider M, Gazit A, and others: Fresh goat's milk for infants: myths and realities—a review, *Pediatrics* 125(4):e973–e977, 2010.

Behring A, Vezeau TM, Fink R: Timing of the newborn first bath: a replication, *Neonat Netw* 22(1):39–46, 2003.

Bhatia J, Greer F, Committee on Nutrition: Use of soy protein–based formulas in infant feeding, *Pediatrics* 121(5):1062–1068, 2008.

Biancuzzo M: *Breastfeeding the newborn: clinical strategies for nurses*, ed 2, St. Louis, 2003, Mosby.

Blackburn ST: *Maternal, fetal, and neonatal physiology: a clinical perspective*, St. Louis, 2003, Saunders.

Brady-Fryer B, Wiebe N, Lander JA: Pain relief for neonatal circumcision, *Cochrane Database Syst Rev* 18(4):CD004217, 2007.

Brazelton TB: Mother–infant reciprocity. In Klaus M, Leger T, Trause MA, editors: *Maternal attachment and mothering disorders*, New Brunswick, NJ, 1974, Johnson & Johnson Baby Products.

Brazelton TB, Nugent JK: *Neonatal behavioural assessment scale*, London, 1996, MacKeith Press.

Bruschweiler-Stern, N: The neonatal moment of meeting—building the dialogue, strengthening the bond, *Child Adolesc Psychiatric Clin North Am* 18(3):533–544, 2009.

Bull MJ, Durbin DR: Rear-facing car safety seats: getting the message right, *Pediatrics* 121(3):619–620, 2008.

Butt ML, Kisilevsky BS: Music modulates behaviour of premature infants following heel lance, *Can J Nurs Res* 31(4):17–39, 2000.

Canadian Paediatric Society, Community Paediatrics Committee: Temperature measurement in paediatrics, reaffirmed 2010, retrieved March 31, 2011, from http://www.cps.ca/english/statements/cp/cp00-01.htm.

Canadian Paediatric Society, First Nations, Inuit, and Métis Health Committee: Vitamin D supplementation: recommendations for Canadian mothers and infants, *Paediatr Child Health* 12(7):583–589, 2007.

Carbajal R, Veerapen S, Couderc S, and others: Analgesic effect of breast feeding in term neonates: randomized controlled trial, *BMJ* 326(7379):13, 2003.

Carr EA, Wilmoth ML, Eliades AB, and others: Comparison of temporal artery to rectal temperature measurements in children up to 24 months, *J Pediatr Nurs* 26(3):179–185, 2011.

Chen A, Rogan W: Isoflavones in soy infant formula: a review of evidence for endocrine and other activity in infants, *Ann Rev Nutr* 24:33–54, 2004.

Codipietro L, Ceccarelli M, Ponzone A: Breastfeeding or oral sucrose solution in term neonates receiving heel lance: a randomized, controlled trial, *Pediatrics* 122(3):e716–e721, 2008.

Cohen HA, Drucker MM, Vainer S, and others: Postcircumcision urinary tract infection, *Clin Pediatr* 31(6):322–324, 1992.

Conover E, Buehler BA: Use of herbal agents by breastfeeding women may affect infants, *Pediatr Ann* 33(4):235–240, 2004.

Coryllos A, Genna C, Salloum A: Congenital tongue-tie and its impact on breastfeeding. In American Academy of Pediatrics, Section on Breastfeeding: *Breastfeeding: best for baby and mother*, Elk Grove Village, Ill, 2004, Author.

Craig JV, Lancaster GA, Taylor S, and others: Infrared ear thermometry compared with rectal thermometry in children: a systematic review, *Lancet* 360(9333):603–609, 2002.

Dodd SR, Lancaster GA, Craig JV, and others: In a systematic review, infrared ear thermometry for fever diagnosis in children finds poor sensitivity, *J Clin Endocrinol* 59(4):354–357, 2006.

Dore S, Buchan D, Coulas S, and others: Alcohol versus natural drying for newborn cord care, *J Obstet Gynecol Neonat Nurs* 27(6):621–627, 1998.

Eriksson M, Finnstrom O: Can daily repeated doses of orally administered glucose induce tolerance when given for neonatal pain relief? *Acta Paediatr* 93(2):246–249, 2004.

Feldman R: Parent–infant synchrony and the construction of shared timing: physiological precursors, developmental outcomes, and risk conditions, *J Child Psychol Psychiatry* 48(3):329–354, 2007.

Flaherty SC, Sadler LS: A review of attachment theory in the context of adolescent parenting, *J Pediatr Health Care* 25(2):114–121, 2011.

Foote JM, Brady LH, Burke AL, and others: Development of an evidence-based clinical practice guideline on linear growth measurement of children, *J Pediatr Nurs* 26(4):312–324, 2011.

Forlenza GP, Paradise Black NM, McNamara EG, and others: Ankyloglossia, exclusive breastfeeding, and failure to thrive, *Pediatrics* 125(6):e1500–e1504, 2010.

Fuloria M, Kreiter S: The newborn examination, part I, Emergencies and common abnormalities involving the skin, head, neck, chest, and respiratory and cardiovascular systems, *Am Fam Physician* 65(1):61–68, 2002.

Georgieff MK: Taking a rational approach to the choice of formula, *Contemp Pediatr* 18(8):112–130, 2001.

Giampietro PG, Bruno G, Furcolo G, and others: Soy protein formulas in children: no hormonal effects in long-term feeding, *J Pediatr Endocrinol Metab* 17(2):191–196, 2004.

Gibbins S, Stevens B, Hodnett E, and others: Efficacy and safety of sucrose for procedural pain relief in preterm and term neonates, *Nurs Res* 51(6):375–382, 2002.

Golombek SG, Brill PE, Salice AL: Randomized trial of alcohol versus triple dye for umbilical cord care, *Clin Pediatr* 41(6):419–423, 2002.

Goulet C, Bell L, St-Cyr D, and others: A concept analysis of parent–infant attachment, *J Adv Nurs* 28(5):1071–1081, 1998.

Gradin M, Eriksson M, Holmqvist G, and others: Pain reduction at venipuncture in newborns: oral glucose compared with local anesthetic cream, *Pediatrics* 110(6):1053–1057, 2002.

Gray L, Miller LW, Phillips BL, and others: Breastfeeding is analgesic in healthy newborns, *Pediatrics* 109(4):590–593, 2002.

Gray L, Watt L, Blass EM: Skin-to-skin contact is analgesic in healthy newborns, *Pediatrics* 105(1):110–111, 2000; retrieved July 20, 2007, from http://www.pediatrics.org/cgi/content/full/105/1/e14.

Gray RH, Kigozi G, Serwadda D, and others: Male circumcision for HIV prevention in men in Rakai, Uganda: a randomized controlled trial, *Lancet* 369(9562):657–666, 2007.

Greenes DS, Fleisher GR: Accuracy of a noninvasive temporal artery thermometer for use in infants, *Arch Pediatr Adolesc Med* 155(3):376–381, 2001.

Greim HA: The endocrine and reproductive system: adverse effects of hormonally active substances? *Pediatrics* 113(4):1070–1075, 2004.

Hale T: *Medications and mothers' milk*, ed 14, Amarillo, Tex, 2010, Hale Publishing.

Harrison D, Johnston L, Loughnan P: Oral sucrose for procedural pain in sick hospitalized infants: a randomized-controlled trial, *J Paediatr Child Health* 39(8):591–597, 2003.

Hayward K, Campbell-Yeo M, Price S, and others: Co-bedding twins: how pilot study findings guided improvements in planning a larger multicenter trial, *Nurs Res* 56(2):137–143, 2007.

Holzhauer JK, Reith V, Sawin KJ, and others: Evaluation of temporal artery thermometry in children 3–36 months old, *J Soc Pediatr Nurs* 14(4):239–244, 2009.

Huang CM, Tung WS, Kuo LL, and others: Comparison of pain responses of premature infants to the heelstick between containment and swaddling, *J Nurs Res* 12(1):31–40, 2004.

Hussink Muller PC, van Berkel LH, de Beaufort AF: Axillary and rectal temperature measurements poorly agree in newborn infants, *Neonatology* 94(1):31–34, 2008.

Jackson PC: Complementary and alternative methods of increasing breast milk supply for lactating mothers of infants in the NICU, *Neonatal Network* 29(4):225–230, 2010.

Janssen PA, Selwood BL, Dobson SR, and others: To dye or not to dye: a randomized, clinical trial of a triple dye/alcohol regime versus dry cord care, *Pediatrics* 111(1):15–20, 2003.

Johnston CC, Filion F, Campbell-Yeo M, and others: Enhanced kangaroo mother care for heel lance in preterm infants: a crossover trial, *J Perinatol* 29(1):51–56, 2009.

Johnston CC, Stevens B, Pinelli J, and others: Kangaroo care is effective in diminishing pain response in preterm neonates, *Arch Pediatr Adolesc Med* 157(11):1084–1088, 2003.

Joint United Nations Programme on HIV/AIDS: *Neonatal and child male circumcision: a global review*, Geneva, 2010, UNAIDS, retrieved March 23, 2011, from http://www.who.int/hiv/pub/malecircumcision/neonatal_child_MC_UNAIDS.pdf.

Jones HL, Kleber CB, Eckert GJ, and others: Comparison of rectal temperature measured by digital vs. mercury glass thermometer in infants under 2 months old, *Clin Pediatr* 42(4):357–359, 2003.

Kaye CI, American Association of Pediatrics Committee on Genetics: Newborn screening fact sheets, *Pediatrics* 118(3):e934–e963, 2006.

Kehler HL, Chaput KH, Tough SC: Risk factors for cessation of breastfeeding prior to six months postpartum among a community sample of women in Calgary, Alberta, *Can J Public Health* 100(5):376–380, 2009.

Kemper AR, Mahle WT, Martin GR, and others: Strategies for implementing screening for critical congenital heart disease, *Pediatrics* 128(5):e1259–e1267, 2011.

Kent AL, Kecskes Z, Shadbolt B, and others: Blood pressure in the first year of life in healthy infants born at term, *Pediatr Nephrol* 22(10):1743–1749, 2007.

Kimura C, Matsuoka M: Changes in breast skin temperature during the course of breastfeeding, *J Hum Lact* 23(1):60–69, 2007.

Klaus MH, Kennell JH, Klaus PH: *Bonding: building the foundations of secure attachment and independence*, Menlo Park, Calif, 1995, Addison-Wesley.

Kraft NL: A pictorial and video guide to circumcision without pain, *Adv Neonatal Care* 3(2):50–64, 2003.

Krous HF, Masoumi H, Haas EA, and others: Aspiration of gastric contents in sudden infant death syndrome without cardiopulmonary resuscitation, *J Pediatr* 150(3):241–246, 2007.

Kue Young T, Chateau D, Zhang M: Type 2 diabetes mellitus in children: prenatal and early infancy risk factors among native Canadians, *Arch Pediatr Adolesc Med* 156(7):651–655, 2002.

Labiner-Wolfe J, Fein SB, Shealy KR: Infant formula-handling education and safety, *Pediatrics* 122(suppl 2):S85–S90, 2008.

Laughlin J, Luerssen TG, Dias MS, and others: Prevention and management of positional skull deformities in infants, *Pediatrics* 128(6):1236–1241, 2011.

Lawrence RA, Lawrence RM: *Breastfeeding: a guide for the medical profession*, ed 7, St. Louis, 2011, Mosby.

Le Huërou-Luron I, Blat S, Boudry G: Breast- vs. formula-feeding: impacts on the digestive tract and immediate and long-term health effects, *Nutr Res Rev* 23(1):23–36, 2010.

Leung AKC, Robson WLM: Natal teeth: a review, *J Natl Med Assoc* 98(2):226–228, 2006.

Mahle WT, Martin GR, Beekman RH, and others: Endorsement of Health and Human Services recommendation for pulse oximetry screening for critical congenital heart disease, *Pediatrics* 129(1):190–192, 2012.

Malloy MH: Trends in postneonatal aspiration deaths and reclassification of sudden infant death syndrome: impact of the "Back to Sleep" program, *Pediatrics* 109(4):661–665, 2002.

Marín Gabriel MA, Martín Moreiras J, Lliteras Fleixas G, and others: Assessment of the New Ballard Score to estimate gestational age, *An Pediatr (Barc)* 64(2):140–145, 2006.

McCleary PH: Female genital mutilation and childbirth: a case report, *Birth* 21(4):221–223, 1994.

Medves M, O'Brien B: The effect of bather and location of first bath on maintaining thermal stability in newborns, *J Obstet Gynecol Neonat Nurs* 33(2):175–182, 2004.

Meedya S, Fahy K, Kable A: Factors that positively influence breastfeeding duration to 6 months: a literature review, *Women Birth* 23(4):135–145, 2010.

Merewood A, Mehta SD, Chamberlain LB, and others: Breastfeeding rates in U.S. Baby-Friendly hospitals: results of a national survey, *Pediatrics* 116(3):628–634, 2005.

Merritt RJ, Jenks BH: Safety of soy-based formulas containing isoflavones: the clinical evidence, *J Nutr* 134(5):1220S–1224S, 2004.

Michaelsen KF, Lauritzen L, Mortensen EL: Effects of breast-feeding on cognitive function, *Adv Exp Med Biol* 639:199–215, 2009.

Morin KH: Infant nutrition: what about water softeners and bottled water for babies? *MCN Am J Matern Child Nurs* 32(1):57, 2007.

Morrone A, Hercogova J, Lotti T: Stop female genital mutilation: appeal to the international dermatologic community, *Int J Dermatol* 41(5):253–263, 2002.

Mullany LC, Darmstadt GL, Katz J, and others: Risk of mortality subsequent to umbilical cord infection among newborns of southern Nepal: cord infection and mortality, *Pediatr Infect Dis J* 28(1):17–20, 2009.

National Center for Missing and Exploited Children: *Self assessment for healthcare facilities*, Alexandria, Va, 2009, Author, retrieved March 10, 2011, from http://www.missingkids.com/missingkids/servlet/ProxySearchServlet?sitenbr=152657769&k=newborn.

National Center for Missing and Exploited Children: *Newborn/infant abductions*, Alexandria, Va, 2011, Author, retrieved March 10, 2011, from http://www.missingkids.com/en_US/documents/InfantAbductionStats.pdf.

Newburg DS, Walker DA: Protection of the neonate by the innate immune system of developing gut and of human milk, *Pediatr Res* 61(1):2–8, 2007.

Noerr B: Sucrose for neonatal procedural pain, *Neonat Netw* 20(7):63–67, 2001.

Nuntnarumit P, Yang W, Bada-Ellzey HS: Blood pressure measurements in the newborn, *Clin Perinatol* 26(4):981–996, 1999.

Olsen IE, Groveman SA, Lawson ML, and others: New intrauterine growth curves based on United States data, *Pediatrics* 125(2):e215–e224, 2010.

Pejovic B, Peco-Antic A, Marinkovic-Eric J: Blood pressure in non-critically ill preterm and full-term neonates, *Pediatr Nephrol* 22(2):249–257, 2007.

Quan R, Yang C, Rubinstein S, and others: Effects of microwave radiation on anti-infective factors in human milk, *Pediatrics* 89(4 Pt 1):667–669, 1992.

Rabe H, Jewison A, Alvarez RF, and others: Milking compared with delayed cord clamping to increase placental transfusion in preterm neonates, a randomized controlled trial, *Obstet Gynecol* 117(2 Pt 1):205–211, 2011.

Radmacher P, Massey C, Adamkin D: Hidden morbidity with "successful" early discharge, *J Perinatol* 22(1):15–20, 2002.

Razmus I, Dalton M, Wilson D: Pain management for newborn circumcision, *Pediatr Nurs* 20(5):414–417, 427, 2004.

Sasidharan K, Dutta S, Narang A: Validity of New Ballard Score until 7th day of postnatal life in moderately preterm neonates, *Arch Dis Child Fetal Neonatal Ed* 94(1):F39–F44, 2009.

Schuh S, Komar L, Stephens D, and others: Comparison of the temporal artery and rectal thermometry in children in the emergency department, *Pediatr Emerg Care* 20(11):736–741, 2004.

Segal LM, Stephenson R, Dawes M, and others: Prevalence, diagnosis, and treatment of ankyloglossia: methodologic review. *Can Fam Physician* 53(6):1027–1033, 2007.

Sganga A, Wallace R, Kiehl E, and others: A comparison of four methods of normal newborn temperature measurement, *MCN Am J Matern Child Nurs* 25(2):76–79, 2000.

Shah PS, Aliwalas LI, Shah V: Breastfeeding or breast milk for procedural pain in neonates, *Cochrane Database Syst Rev* (3):CD004950, 2006.

Shah V, Ohlsson A: Venepuncture versus heel lance for blood sampling in term neonates, *Cochrane Database Syst Rev* (2):CD001452, 2001.

Shogan MG: Emergency management plan for newborn abduction, *J Obstet Gynecol Neonat Nurs* 31(3):340–346, 2002.

Siberry GK, Diener-West M, Schappell E, and others: Comparison of temple temperatures with rectal temperatures in children under 2 years of age, *Clin Pediatr* 41(6):405–414, 2002.

Simmer K, Patole SK, Rao SC: Longchain polyunsaturated fatty acid supplementation in infants born at term, *Cochrane Database Syst Rev* (1):CD000376, 2008.

Spangler AK, Randenberg AL, Brenner MG, and others: Belly models as teaching tools: what is their utility? *J Hum Lact* 24(2):199–205, 2008.

Stevens B, Yamada J, Ohlsson A: Sucrose for analgesia in newborn infants undergoing painful procedures, *Cochrane Database Syst Rev* (1):CD001069, 2010.

Taddio A, Shah V, Gilbert-MacLeod C, and others: Conditioning and hyperalgesia in newborns exposed to repeated heel lances, *JAMA* 288(7):857–861, 2002.

Thomas P, Peabody J, Turnier V, and others: A new look at intrauterine growth and the impact of race, altitude, and gender, *Pediatrics* 106(2):e21, 2000.

Thulier D, Mercer J: Variables associated with breastfeeding duration, *J Obstet Gynecol Neonatal Nurs* 38(3):259–268, 2009.

Tobian AAR, Gray RH, Quinn TC: Male circumcision for the prevention of acquisition and transmission of sexually transmitted infections, *Arch Pediatr Adolesc Med* 164(1):78–84, 2010.

Tomlinson PS, Bryan AA, Esau AL: Family centered intrapartum care: revisiting an old concept, *J Obstet Gynecol Neonat Nurs* 25(4):331–337, 1996.

Trochtenberg DS: Neonatal circumcision, *N Engl J Med* 323(17):1206, 1990 (letter to the editor).

United Nations Programme on HIV/AIDS: *Neonatal and child male circumcision: a global review*, Geneva, 2010, UNAIDS/WHO.

U.S. Department of Health and Human Services: *Healthy people 2020: about healthy people*, Washington, DC, 2011, Author, retrieved June 1, 2011, from http://www.healthypeople.gov/2020/topicsobjectives2020/objectiveslist.aspx?topicId=26.

Varda KE, Behnke RS: The effect of timing the initial bath on newborn's temperature, *J Obstet Gynecol Neonat Nurs* 29(1):27–32, 2000.

Vincent JL: Infant hospital abduction: security measures to aid in prevention, *MCN Am J Matern Child Nurs* 34(3):179–183, 2009.

Weiss ME, Nahata MC: EMLA for painful procedures in infants, *J Pediatr Health Care* 19(1):42–47, 2005.

Williamson ML: Circumcision anesthesia: a study of nursing implications for dorsal penile nerve block, *Pediatr Nurs* 23(10):59–63, 1997.

World Health Organization: *Global strategy to stop health-care providers from performing female genital mutilation*, Geneva, 2010, Author, retrieved March 23, 2011, from http://www.who.int/hiv/pub/malecircumcision/neonatal_child_MC_UNAIDS.pdf.

World Health Organization: *WHO guidelines on hand hygiene in health care, 2009*, Geneva, 2009, Author, retrieved March 10, 2011, from http://whqlibdoc.who.int/publications/2009/9789241597906_eng.pdf.

World Health Organization Study Group on Female Genital Mutilation and Obstetric Outcome: Female genital mutilation and obstetric outcome: WHO collaborative prospective study in six African countries, *Lancet* 367(9525):1835–1841, 2006.

World Health Organization, UNICEF, and Wellstart International: *Baby-friendly hospital initiative: revised, updated and expanded for integrated care*, Geneva, 2009, World Health Organization, retrieved March 28, 2011, from http://whqlibdoc.who.int/publications/2009/9789241594967_eng.pdf.

Young TK, Martens PJ, Taback SP, and others: Type 2 diabetes mellitus in children: prenatal and early infancy risk factors among native Canadians, *Arch Pediatr Adolesc Med* 156(7):651–655, 2002.

Zingaretti MC, Crosta F, Vitali A, and others: The presence of UCP1 demonstrates that metabolically active adipose tissue in the neck of adult humans truly represents brown adipose tissue, *FASEB J* 23(9):3113–3120, 2009.

Zupan J, Garner P, Omari AA: Topical umbilical cord care at birth, *Cochrane Database Syst Rev* (3):CD001057, 2004.

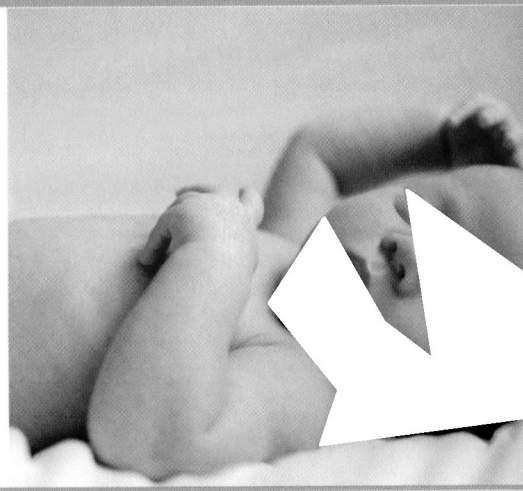

evolve WEBSITE

http://evolve.elsevier.com/wong/essentials

Animations—Erb Palsy; Paralyzed Diaphragm; Shoulder Dystocia

Case Studies—Health Problems of the Newborn; Hyperbilirubinemia

Key Point Summaries

Nursing Care Plans—The High-Risk Infant with Respiratory Distress Syndrome; The Infant with Bronchopulmonary Dysplasia; The Newborn with Jaundice

NCLEX-Style Review Questions

CHAPTER OUTLINE

Birth Injuries, 229
  Soft Tissue Injury, 229
  Head Trauma, 229
    Caput Succedaneum, 229
    Cephalhematoma, 229
    Subgaleal Hemorrhage, 229
  Fractures, 230
  Paralysis, 231
    Facial Paralysis, 231
    Brachial Palsy, 231
    Phrenic Nerve Paralysis, 232
Common Problems in the Newborn, 232
  Erythema Toxicum Neonatorum, 232
  Candidiasis, 232
    Oral Candidiasis, 232
  Herpes Simplex Virus, 233
  Birthmarks, 234
Nursing Care of the High-Risk Newborn and Family, 235
  Identification of High-Risk Newborns, 235
    Classification of High-Risk Newborns, 235
  Care of High-Risk Newborns, 235
    Systematic Assessment, 235
    Monitoring Physiologic Data, 235
    Respiratory Support, 236
    Thermoregulation, 236
    Protection from Infection, 239

Hydration, 239
Nutrition, 240
Feeding Resistance, 243
Energy Conservation, 243
Skin Care, 244
Administration of Medications, 244
Developmental Outcome, 246
Family Support and Involvement, 248
Facilitating Parent–Infant Relationships, 249
Discharge Planning and Home Care, 251
Neonatal Loss, 252
High Risk Related to Dysmaturity, 253
  Preterm Infants, 253
  Postterm Infants, 256
High Risk Related to Physiologic Factors, 256
  Hyperbilirubinemia, 256
  Hemolytic Disease of the Newborn, 263
    Blood Incompatibility, 263
  Metabolic Complications, 266
  Respiratory Distress Syndrome, 267
  Respiratory Complications, 273
    Acid–Base Imbalance, 277
  Cardiovascular Complications, 279
  Neurologic Complications, 279
  Neonatal Seizures, 279

High Risk Related to Infectious Processes, 282
  Sepsis, 282
  Necrotizing Enterocolitis, 284
High Risk Related to Maternal Conditions, 285
  Infants of Diabetic Mothers, 285
  Drug-Exposed Infants, 286
    Alcohol Exposure, 289
    Cocaine Exposure, 289
    Methamphetamine Exposure, 289
    Marijuana Exposure, 290
    Selective Serotonin Reuptake Inhibitors, 290
  Maternal Infections, 290
Congenital Anomalies, 293
  Genetic Etiology of Congenital Anomalies, 294
    Chromosomal Abnormalities, 294
    Single-Gene Defects, 294
    Multifactorial Inheritance, 294
  Defects Caused by Chemical Agents, 294
Inborn Errors of Metabolism, 295
  Congenital Hypothyroidism, 297
  Phenylketonuria, 298
  Galactosemia, 300
Genetic Evaluation and Counseling, 301
  Psychologic Aspects of Genetic Disease, 302

LEARNING OBJECTIVES

On completion of this chapter the reader will be able to:

- Recognize common deviations from normal characteristics in the newborn.
- Perform a systematic assessment of a high-risk newborn.
- Outline a general care plan for a high-risk infant.
- Recognize physiologic factors that compromise the preterm infant's health status.
- Discuss the role of the nurse in facilitating positive parent–infant relationships.

- Contrast the physical characteristics of preterm and full-term infants.
- Discuss the basis for screening newborns for health problems.
- Discuss the rationale for performing newborn screening and genetic counseling when a newborn has a hereditary condition.
- Modify a general care plan to meet the needs of an infant with specific high-risk health needs.

BIRTH INJURIES

Several factors predispose an infant to birth injuries (Mangurten and Puppala, 2011; Verklan and Lopez, 2011). Maternal factors include uterine dysfunction that leads to prolonged or precipitous labor, preterm or postterm labor, and cephalopelvic disproportion. Injury may result from dystocia caused by fetal macrosomia, multifetal gestation, abnormal or difficult presentation (not caused by maternal uterine or pelvic conditions), and congenital anomalies. Intrapartum events that can result in scalp injury include the use of intrapartum monitoring of fetal heart rate and collection of fetal scalp blood for acid–base assessment. Obstetric birth techniques can cause injury. Forceps birth, vacuum extraction, version and extraction, and cesarean birth are potential contributory factors. Often more than one factor is present, and multiple predisposing factors may be related to a single maternal condition.

SOFT TISSUE INJURY

Various types of soft tissue injury may be sustained during the process of birth, primarily in the form of bruises or abrasions secondary to dystocia. Soft tissue injury usually occurs when there is some degree of disproportion between the presenting part and the maternal pelvis (**cephalopelvic disproportion**). The use of forceps to facilitate a difficult vertex delivery may produce bruising or abrasion on the sides of the neonate's face. Petechiae or ecchymoses may be observed on the presenting part after a breech or brow delivery. After a difficult or precipitous delivery, the sudden release of pressure on the head can produce scleral hemorrhages or generalized petechiae over the face and head. Petechiae and ecchymoses may also appear on the head, neck, and face of an infant born with a nuchal cord, giving the infant's face a cyanotic appearance. A well-defined circle of petechiae and ecchymoses or abrasions may also be seen on the occipital region of the newborn's head when a vacuum suction cup is applied during delivery. Rarely, lacerations occur during cesarean section.

These traumatic lesions generally fade spontaneously within a few days without treatment. However, petechiae may be a manifestation of an underlying bleeding disorder or a systemic illness such as an infection and should be further evaluated as to their origin. Nursing care is primarily directed toward assessing the injury and providing an explanation and reassurance to the parents.

HEAD TRAUMA

Trauma to the head and scalp that occurs during the birth process is usually benign but occasionally results in more serious injury. The injuries that produce serious trauma, such as intracranial hemorrhage and subdural hematoma, are discussed in relation to neurologic disorders in the newborn (see Table 9-9). Skull fractures are discussed in association with other fractures sustained during the birth process. The three most common types of extracranial hemorrhagic injury are caput succedaneum, cephalhematoma, and subgaleal hemorrhage.

Caput Succedaneum

The most commonly observed scalp lesion is caput succedaneum, a vaguely outlined area of edematous tissue situated over the portion of the scalp that presents in a vertex delivery (Fig. 9-1, *A*). The swelling consists of serum, blood, or both accumulated in the tissues above the bone, and it often extends beyond the bone margins. The swelling may be associated with overlying petechiae or ecchymoses. No specific treatment is needed, and the swelling subsides within a few days.

Cephalhematoma

Infrequently, a cephalhematoma is formed when blood vessels rupture during labor or delivery to produce bleeding into the area between the bone and its periosteum. The injury occurs most often with primiparous delivery and is often associated with forceps delivery and vacuum extraction. Unlike caput succedaneum, the boundaries of the cephalhematoma are sharply demarcated and do not extend beyond the limits of the bone (suture lines) (Fig. 9-1, *B*). The cephalhematoma may involve one or both parietal bones. The occipital bones are less commonly affected, and the frontal bones are rarely affected. The swelling is usually minimal or absent at birth and increases in size on the second or third day. Blood loss is usually not significant.

No treatment is indicated for uncomplicated cephalhematoma. Most lesions are absorbed within 2 weeks to 3 months. Lesions that result in severe blood loss to the area or that involve an underlying fracture require further evaluation. Hyperbilirubinemia may result during resolution of the hematoma. A local infection can develop and is suspected when a sudden increase in swelling occurs. Parents should be counseled that, in some cases, a small area of calcification may develop and persist.

Subgaleal Hemorrhage

Subgaleal hemorrhage is bleeding into the subgaleal compartment (Fig. 9-1, *C*). The subgaleal compartment is a potential space that contains loosely arranged connective tissue; it is located beneath the galea aponeurosis, the tendinous sheath that connects the frontal and occipital muscles and forms the inner surface of the scalp. The injury occurs as a result of forces that compress and then drag the head through the pelvic outlet (Verklan and Lopez, 2011). Instrumented delivery, particularly vacuum extraction and forceps delivery, increase

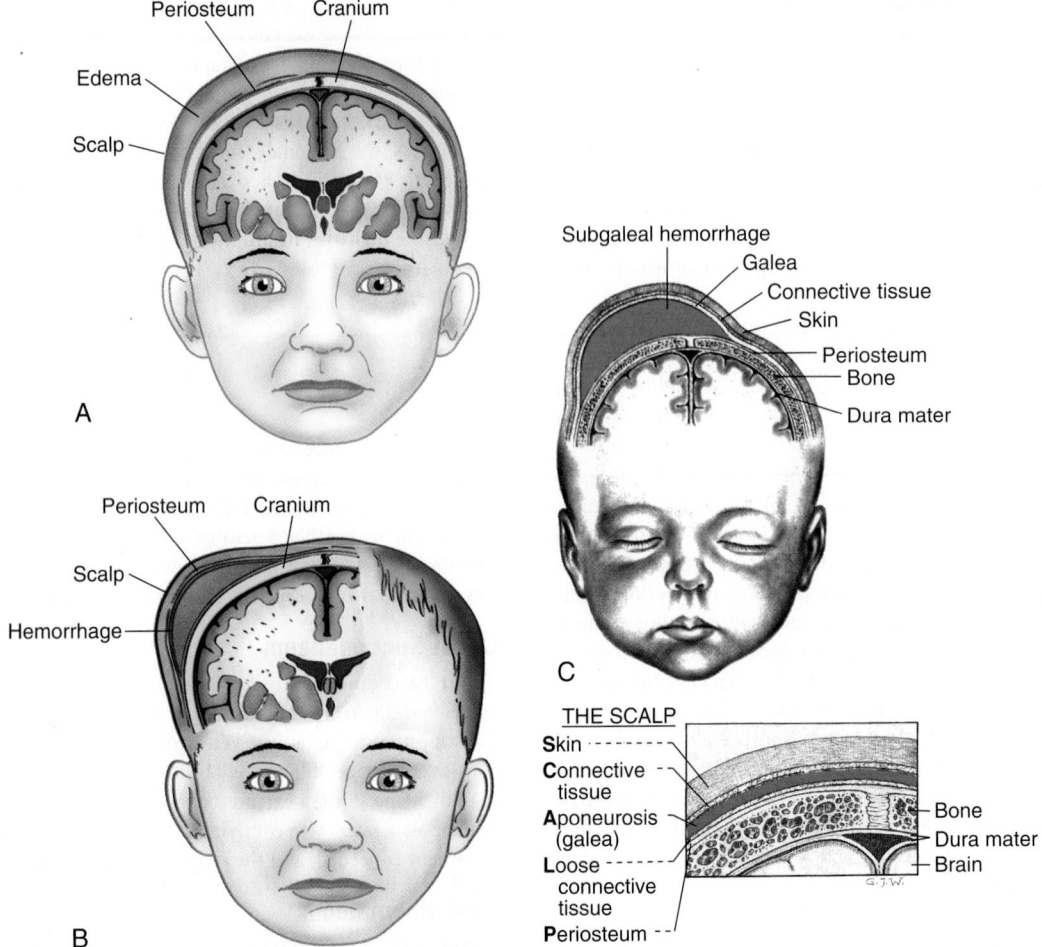

FIG 9-1 **A,** Caput succedaneum. **B,** Cephalhematoma. **C,** Subgaleal hemorrhage. (**A** and **B,** From Seidel HM, Ball JM, Davis JE, and others: *Mosby's guide to physical examination,* ed 6, St. Louis, 2006, Mosby.)

the risk of subgaleal hemorrhage. Additional risk factors include prolonged second stage of labor, fetal distress, macrosomia, failed vacuum extraction, and maternal primiparity (Doumouchtsis and Arulkumaran, 2006). The bleeding extends beyond bone, often posteriorly into the neck, and continues after birth, with the potential for serious complications such as anemia or hypovolemic shock.

Early detection of the hemorrhage is vital; serial head circumference measurements and inspection of the back of the neck for increasing edema and a firm mass are essential. A boggy fluctuant mass over the scalp that crosses the suture line and moves as the baby is repositioned is an early sign of subgaleal hemorrhage (Doumouchtsis and Arulkumaran, 2006). Other signs include pallor, tachycardia, and increasing head circumference (Reid, 2007). An early sign of subgaleal hemorrhage is a forward and lateral positioning of the newborn's ears because the hematoma extends posteriorly. Disseminated intravascular coagulation (DIC) has also been reported in association with subgaleal hemorrhage (Schierholz and Walker, 2010). Computed tomography (CT) or magnetic resonance imaging (MRI) is useful in confirming the diagnosis. Replacement of lost blood and clotting factors is required in acute cases of hemorrhage. Monitoring the infant for changes in level of consciousness and a decrease in the hematocrit are also key to early recognition and management. An increase in serum bilirubin levels may be seen as a result of the degradation of red blood cells (RBCs) within the hematoma.

Nursing Care Management

Nursing care is directed toward assessment and observation of the common scalp injuries and vigilance in observing for possible associated complications such as infection or, as in the case of subgaleal hemorrhage, acute blood loss and hypovolemia. Nursing care of a newborn with a subgaleal hemorrhage includes careful monitoring for signs of hemodynamic instability and shock (Schierholz and Walker, 2010). Because caput succedaneum and cephalhematoma usually resolve spontaneously, parents need reassurance of their usual benign nature.

FRACTURES

The clavicle, or collarbone, is the bone most frequently fractured during the birth process. It is often associated with shoulder dystocia or a difficult vertex or breech delivery of infants who are large for gestational age. Crepitus (the coarse crackling sensation produced by the rubbing together of fractured bone fragments) may be felt or heard on examination. A palpable, spongy mass, representing localized edema and hematoma, may also be a sign of a fractured clavicle. The infant may be reluctant to move the arm on the affected side, and the Moro reflex may be asymmetric. Radiographs usually reveal a complete fracture with overriding of the fragments.

Fractures of long bones, such as the femur or the humerus, are sometimes difficult to detect by radiographic examination in infants. Although osteogenesis imperfecta is a rare finding, a newborn infant with a fracture should be assessed for other evidence of this congenital disorder.

Fractures of the neonatal skull are uncommon. The bones, which are less mineralized and more compressible than bones in older infants and children, are separated by membranous seams that allow sufficient alteration in the head contour so that it adjusts to the birth canal during delivery. Skull fractures usually follow a prolonged, difficult delivery or forceps extraction. Most fractures are linear, but some may be visible as depressed indentations that compress or decompress like a ping-pong ball. Management of depressed skull fractures is controversial; many resolve without intervention. Nonsurgical elevation of the indentation using a hand breast pump or vacuum extractor has been reported (Mangurten and Puppala, 2011). Surgery may be required in the presence of bone fragments or signs of increased intracranial pressure (ICP) (Hill, 2008). A similar finding in neonates is craniotabes, which is usually benign or may be associated with prematurity or hydrocephalus (Johnson, 2009). In this condition, the cranial bone(s) move freely on palpation and may easily compress.

> **! NURSING ALERT**
>
> A newborn with a fractured clavicle may have no symptoms, but suspect a fracture if an infant has limited use of the affected arm, malpositioning of the arm, asymmetric Moro reflex, or focal swelling or tenderness or if he or she cries in pain when the arm is moved.

> **! NURSING ALERT**
>
> Any newborn who is large for gestational age or weighs more than 3855 g (8.5 pounds) and is delivered vaginally should be evaluated for a fractured clavicle.

Nursing Care Management

Often, no intervention is needed other than maintaining proper body alignment, careful dressing and undressing of the infant, and handling and carrying that support the affected bone. For example, if the infant has a fractured clavicle, it is important to support the upper and lower back rather than pulling the infant up from under the arms. Placing the infant in a side-lying position with the affected side down should also be avoided. Linear skull fractures usually require no treatment. A ping-pong ball–type skull fracture may require decompression by surgical intervention. The infant is carefully observed for signs of neurologic complications. The parents of infants with a fracture of any bone should be involved in caring for the infant during hospitalization as part of discharge planning for care at home.

PARALYSIS

Facial Paralysis

Pressure on the facial nerve (cranial nerve VII) during delivery may result in injury to that nerve. The primary clinical manifestations are loss of movement on the affected side, such as an inability to completely close the eye, drooping of the corner of the mouth, and absence of wrinkling of the forehead and nasolabial fold (Fig. 9-2). The paralysis is most noticeable when the infant cries. The mouth is drawn to the unaffected side, the wrinkles are deeper on the normal side, and the eye on the involved side remains open.

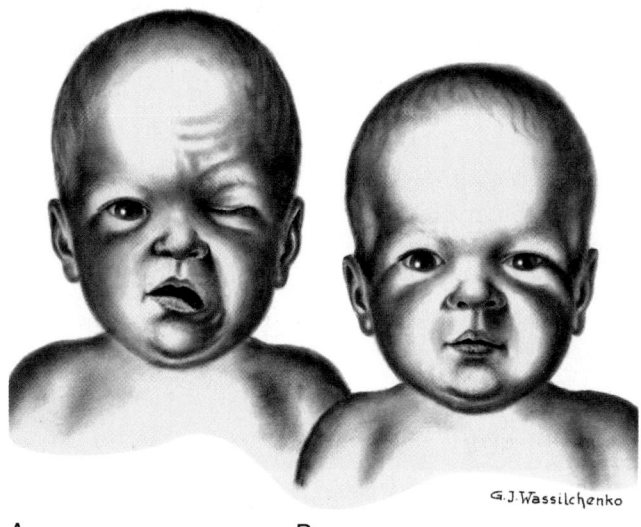

G.J.Wassilchenko

A   B

FIG 9-2 A, Paralysis of right side of face 15 minutes after forceps delivery. Absence of movement on the affected side is especially noticeable when the infant cries. **B,** The same infant 24 hours later.

No medical intervention is necessary. The paralysis usually disappears spontaneously in a few days but may take as long as several months.

Brachial Palsy

Plexus injury results from forces that alter the normal position and relationship of the arm, shoulder, and neck. **Erb palsy (Erb-Duchenne paralysis)** is caused by damage to the upper plexus and usually results from stretching or pulling away of the shoulder from the head, as might occur with shoulder dystocia or with a difficult vertex or breech delivery. Other identified risk factors include an infant with birth weight of more than 4000 g (8.8 pounds), a second stage of labor of less than 15 minutes, maternal body mass index greater than 29, a vacuum-assisted extraction, prolonged labor, and a previous history of brachial plexus injury (Hale, Bae, and Waters, 2009; Hudic, Fatusic, Sinanovic, and others, 2006). The less common lower plexus palsy, or **Klumpke palsy**, results from severe stretching of the upper extremity while the trunk is relatively less mobile.

The clinical manifestations of Erb palsy are related to the paralysis of the affected extremity and muscles. The arm hangs limp alongside the body while the shoulder and arm are adducted and internally rotated. The elbow is extended, and the forearm is pronated, with the wrist and fingers flexed; a grasp reflex may be present because finger and wrist movement remain normal (Tappero, 2009) (Fig. 9-3). In lower plexus palsy, the muscles of the hand are paralyzed, with consequent wrist drop and relaxed fingers. In a third and more severe form of brachial palsy, the entire arm is paralyzed and hangs limp and motionless at the side. The Moro reflex is absent on the affected side for all forms of brachial palsy.

Treatment of the affected arm is aimed at preventing contractures of the paralyzed muscles and maintaining correct placement of the humeral head within the glenoid fossa of the scapula. Complete recovery from stretched nerves usually takes 3 to 6 months. Full recovery is expected in 88% to 92% of infants (Verklan and Lopez, 2011). However, avulsion of the nerves (complete disconnection of the ganglia from the spinal cord that involves both anterior and posterior roots) results in permanent damage. For injuries that do not improve spontaneously

Animation—Erb Palsy

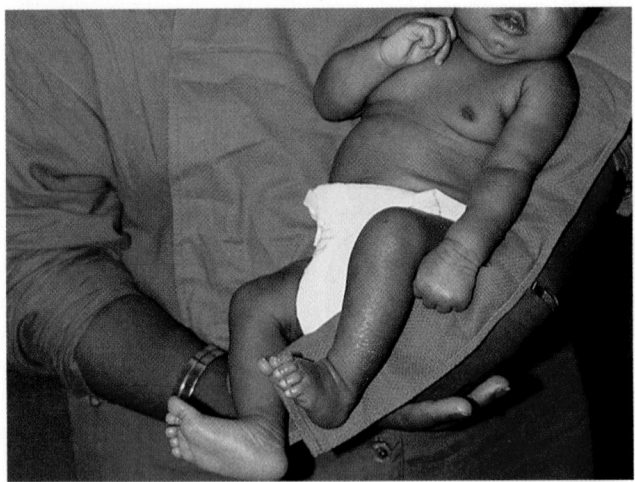

FIG 9-3 Left-sided brachial plexus (Erb) palsy. Note the extended, internally rotated arm and pronated wrist on the affected side.

by 3 months, surgical intervention may be needed to relieve pressure on the nerves or to repair the nerves with grafting (Joyner, Soto, and Adam, 2006). In some cases, injection of botulinum toxin A into the pectoralis major muscle may be effective in reducing muscle contractures after birth-related brachial plexus injuries (Price, Ditaranto, Yaylali, and others, 2007).

Phrenic Nerve Paralysis

Phrenic nerve paralysis results in diaphragmatic paralysis as demonstrated by ultrasonography, which shows paradoxic chest movement and an elevated diaphragm. Initially, radiography may not demonstrate an elevated diaphragm if the neonate is receiving positive-pressure ventilation (Volpe, 2008). The injury sometimes occurs in conjunction with brachial palsy. Respiratory distress is the most common and important sign of injury. Because injury to the phrenic nerve is usually unilateral, the lung on the affected side does not expand, and respiratory efforts are ineffectual. Breathing is primarily thoracic, and cyanosis, tachypnea, or complete respiratory failure may be seen. Pneumonia and atelectasis on the affected side may also occur.

Nursing Care Management

Nursing care of an infant with facial nerve paralysis involves aiding the infant in sucking and helping the mother with feeding techniques. Because part of the mouth cannot close tightly around the nipple, the use of a soft rubber nipple with a large hole may be helpful. The infant may require gavage feeding to prevent aspiration. Breastfeeding is not contraindicated, but the mother will need additional assistance in helping the infant grasp and compress the areolar area.

If the eyelid of the eye on the affected side does not close completely, artificial tears can be instilled daily to prevent drying of the conjunctiva, sclera, and cornea. The eyelid is often taped shut to prevent accidental injury. If eye care is needed at home, the parents are taught the procedure for administering eye drops before the infant is discharged from the nursery (see Chapter 22).

Nursing care of the newborn with brachial palsy is concerned primarily with proper positioning of the affected arm. The affected arm should be gently immobilized on the upper abdomen; passive range-of-motion exercises of the shoulder, wrist, elbow, and fingers are initiated at 7 to 10 days of age (Joyner, Soto, and Adam, 2006). Wrist flexion contractures may be prevented with the use of supportive splints. In dressing the infant, preference is given to the affected arm. Undressing

begins with the unaffected arm, and redressing begins with the affected arm to prevent unnecessary manipulation and stress on the paralyzed muscles. Teach parents to use the "football" position when holding the infant and to avoid picking up the child from under the axillae or by pulling on the arms.

The infant with phrenic nerve paralysis requires the same nursing care as any infant with respiratory distress. Mechanical ventilation may be required to prevent further respiratory compromise.

The family's emotional needs are also an important part of nursing care; the family will need reassurance regarding the neonate's progress toward an optimal outcome.

Follow-up is also essential because of the extended length of recovery. Parents may wish to contact the Brachial Plexus Palsy Foundation* and visit the website for further information.

COMMON PROBLEMS IN THE NEWBORN
ERYTHEMA TOXICUM NEONATORUM

Erythema toxicum neonatorum, also known as flea-bite dermatitis or newborn rash, is a benign, self-limiting eruption of unknown cause that usually appears within the first 2 days of life. The lesions are firm, 1- to 3-mm, pale yellow or white papules or pustules on an erythematous base; they resemble flea bites. The rash appears most commonly on the face, proximal extremities, trunk, and buttocks, but it may be located anywhere on the body except the palms and soles. The rash is more obvious during crying episodes. There are no systemic manifestations, and successive crops of lesions heal without pigmentation changes. The rash usually lasts about 5 to 7 days. The etiology is unknown. However, a smear of the pustule will show numerous eosinophils and a relative absence of neutrophils. When the diagnosis is questionable, bacterial, fungal, or viral cultures should be obtained. Although no treatment is necessary, parents are usually concerned about the rash and need to be reassured of its benign and transient nature.

CANDIDIASIS

Candidiasis, also known as moniliasis, is not uncommon in newborns. Candida albicans, the usual organism responsible, may cause disease in any organ system. It is a yeastlike fungus (it produces yeast cells and spores) that can be acquired from a maternal vaginal infection during delivery; from person-to-person transmission (especially from poor hand-washing technique); or from contaminated hands, bottles, nipples, or other articles. Mucocutaneous, cutaneous, and disseminated candidal infections are all observed in this age group. Candidiasis is usually a benign disorder in neonates, often confined to the oral and diaper regions. Diaper dermatitis caused by Candida organisms manifests as a moist, erythematous eruption with small white or yellow pebbly pustules. Small areas of skin erosion may also be seen (see Diaper Dermatitis, Chapter 30).

Oral Candidiasis

Oral candidiasis (thrush) is characterized by white, adherent patches on the tongue, palate, and inner aspects of the cheeks (Fig. 9-4). It is often difficult to distinguish from coagulated milk. The infant may refuse to suck because of pain in the mouth.

---

*210 Spring Haven Circle, Royersford, PA 19468; http://www.brachialplexus palsyfoundation.org.

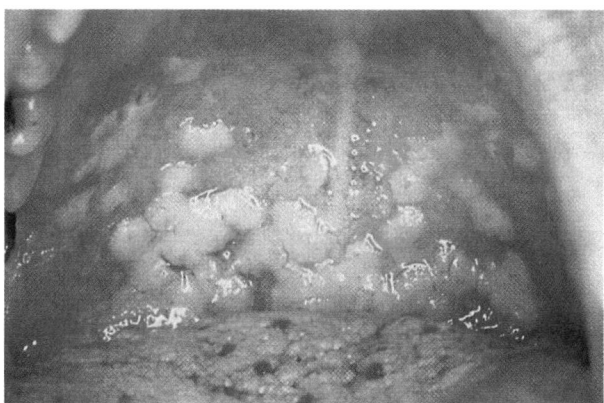

FIG 9-4 Oral candidiasis (thrush). (Courtesy J.A. Innes. In Goering RV, Dockrell HM, Wakelin D, and others: *Mims' medical microbiology*, ed 4, London, 2008, Mosby.)

This condition tends to be acute in newborns and chronic in infants and young children. Thrush appears when the oral flora is altered as a result of antibiotic therapy or poor hand washing by the infant's caregiver. Although the disorder is usually self-limiting, spontaneous resolution may take as long as 2 months, during which time lesions may spread to the larynx, trachea, bronchi, and lungs and along the gastrointestinal tract. The disease is treated with good hygiene, application of a fungicide, and correction of any underlying disturbance. The source of infection should be treated to prevent reinfection.

Topical application of 1 ml nystatin (Mycostatin) over the surfaces of the oral cavity 4 times a day, or every 6 hours, is usually sufficient to prevent spread of the disease or prolongation of its course. Several other drugs may be used, including amphotericin B (Fungizone), clotrimazole (Lotrimin, Mycelex), fluconazole (Diflucan), or miconazole (Monistat, Micatin) given intravenously, orally, or topically. To prevent relapse, therapy should be continued for at least 2 days after the lesions disappear (Lawrence and Lawrence, 2011). Gentian violet solution may be used in addition to one of the antifungal drugs in chronic cases of oral thrush; however, the former does not treat gastrointestinal *Candida* infection and may be irritating to the oral mucosa. Some practitioners avoid its use because it is messy, easily stains clothing, and may be irritating to the oral mucosa. Fluconazole is reportedly more effective than nystatin but it does not have Food and Drug Administration approval for use in infants (Su, Gaskie, and Jamieson, 2008).

> **! NURSING ALERT**
>
> Oral candidiasis can be distinguished from coagulated milk when attempts to remove the patches with a tongue blade are unsuccessful. The primary caregiver may also report that the infant does not nurse well or bottle feed as previously.

Nursing Care Management

Nursing care is directed toward preventing spread of the infection and correctly applying the prescribed topical medication. For candidiasis in the diaper area, the caregiver is taught to keep the diaper area clean and to apply the medication to affected areas as prescribed (see also Diaper Dermatitis, Chapter 30). Older infants with candidal diaper dermatitis can introduce the yeast into the mouth from contaminated hands. Placing clothes over the diaper can prevent this cycle of self-infection.

In cases of oral thrush, nystatin is administered after feedings. Distribute the medication over the surface of the oral mucosa and tongue with an applicator or syringe; the remainder of the dose is deposited in the mouth to be swallowed by the infant to treat any gastrointestinal lesions.

In addition to good hygienic care, other measures to control thrush include rinsing the infant's mouth with plain water after each feeding before applying the medication and boiling reusable nipples and bottles for at least 20 minutes after a thorough washing (spores are heat resistant). If used, pacifiers should be boiled for at least 20 minutes once daily. If the mother is breastfeeding, it is recommended that simultaneous treatment of the infant and mother occur if either is infected (Lawrence and Lawrence, 2011).

HERPES SIMPLEX VIRUS

Neonatal herpes is one of the most serious viral infections in newborns, with a mortality rate of up to 60% in infants with disseminated disease. Approximately 86% to 90% of herpes simplex transmission occurs during passage through the birth canal (Shet, 2011). The risk of transmission of genital herpes during vaginal birth is estimated to be between 30% and 50% with active primary infection at term (Gardella and Brown, 2011). However, in up to 80% of cases of neonatal herpes simplex virus (HSV) infection, the mother has no history or symptoms of infection at the time of birth, but serologic testing reveals evidence of the herpes virus (Gardella and Brown, 2011).

Neonatal herpes manifests in one of three ways: (1) with skin, eye, and mouth involvement (SEM); (2) as localized central nervous system (CNS) disease; or (3) as disseminated disease involving multiple organs. In skin and eye disease, a rash appears as vesicles or pustules on an erythematous base. Clusters of lesions are common. The lesions ulcerate and crust over rapidly. Most infants with neonatal herpes eventually develop this characteristic rash, but up to 20% of neonates with disseminated disease do not develop a skin rash (Kimberlin, 2007). Ophthalmologic clinical findings include chorioretinitis and microphthalmia; neurologic involvement such as microcephaly and encephalomalacia may also develop (James, Kimberlin, and Whitley, 2009). Disseminated infections may involve virtually every organ system, but the liver, adrenal glands, and lungs are most commonly affected. In HSV meningitis, infants develop multiple lesions of cortical hemorrhagic necrosis. It can occur alone or with oral, eye, or skin lesions. The presenting symptoms, which may occur in the second to fourth weeks of life, include lethargy, poor feeding, irritability, and local or generalized seizures.

Nursing Care Management

Neonates with herpesvirus or suspected infection (as a result of exposure) should be carefully evaluated for clinical manifestations. The absence of skin lesions in the neonate exposed to maternal herpesvirus does not indicate absence of disease. Contact precautions (in addition to standard precautions) should be instituted according to the American Academy of Pediatrics (AAP) and American College of Obstetricians and Gynecologists (ACOG) (2007) guidelines or hospital protocol. It is recommended that swabs of the mouth, nasopharynx, conjunctivae, rectum, and any skin vesicles be obtained from the exposed neonate; in addition, urine, stool, blood, and cerebrospinal fluid (CSF) specimens should be obtained for culture. Therapy with acyclovir and vidarabine is initiated if the culture results are positive or if there is strong suspicion of herpesvirus infection (AAP, Committee on Infectious Diseases, 2009; James, Kimberlin, and Whitley, 2009).

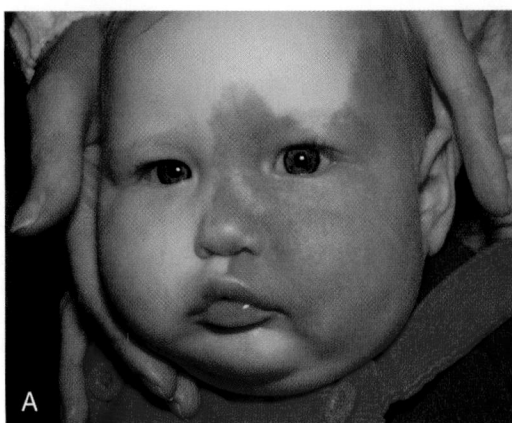 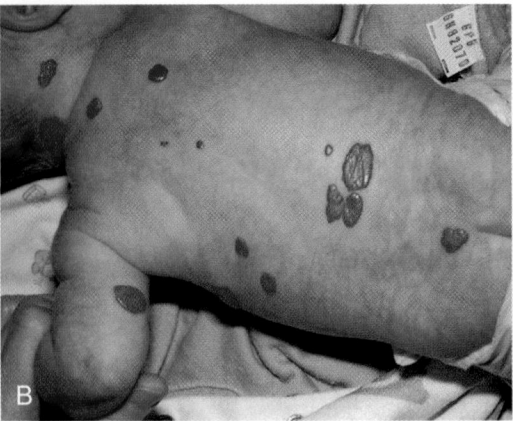

FIG 9-5 A, Port-wine stain. **B,** Strawberry hemangioma. (From Zitelli BJ, McIntire SC, Nowalk AJ: *Zitelli and Davis' atlas of pediatric physical diagnosis,* ed 6, St. Louis, 2012, Saunders.)

High-dose acyclovir (60 mg/kg/day) has been shown to decrease mortality rates in infants with disseminated HSV (James, Kimberlin, and Whitley, 2009).

BIRTHMARKS

Discolorations of the skin are common findings in newborn infants (see discussion on skin assessment of newborns, Chapter 8). Most, such as mongolian spots or telangiectatic nevi, involve no therapy other than reassurance to parents of the benign nature of these discolorations. However, some can be a manifestation of a disease that suggests further examination of the child and other family members (e.g., the multiple light brown café-au-lait spots that often characterize the autosomal dominant hereditary disorder neurofibromatosis and are common findings in Albright syndrome).

Darker or more extensive lesions demand further scrutiny, and excision of the lesion is recommended when feasible. Such lesions include a reddish brown solitary nodule that appears on the face or upper arm and usually represents a spindle and epithelioid cell nevus (juvenile melanoma); a giant pigmented nevus (or bathing trunk nevus), a dark brown to black, irregular plaque that is at risk of transformation to malignant melanoma; and the dark brown or black macules that become more numerous with age (junctional or compound nevi).

Vascular birthmarks may be divided into the following categories: vascular malformations, capillary hemangiomas, and mixed hemangiomas. Vascular stains (malformations) are permanent lesions that are present at birth and are initially flat and erythematous. Any vascular structure, capillary, vein, artery, or lymphatic may be involved. The two most common vascular stains are the transient macular stain (stork bite, salmon patch, or angel kiss) and the port-wine stain, or nevus flammeus. The port-wine lesions are pink, red, or, rarely, purple stains of the skin that thicken, darken, and proportionately enlarge as the child grows (Fig. 9-5, *A*). The macular stain is most often located on the eyelids, glabella, or nape of the neck and usually fades over several months but may be prominent with crying or environmental temperature changes (Morelli, 2011).

Port-wine stains may also be associated with structural malformations, such as glaucoma or leptomeningeal angiomatosis (tumor of blood or lymph vessels in the pia-arachnoid) (Sturge-Weber syndrome) or bony or muscular overgrowth (Klippel-Trenaunay-Weber syndrome). Children with port-wine stains on the eyelids, forehead, or cheeks should be monitored for these syndromes with periodic

ophthalmologic examination, neurologic imaging, and measurement of extremities.

The treatment of choice for port-wine stains is the use of the flashlamp-pumped pulsed-dye laser. A series of treatments is usually needed. The treatments can significantly lighten or completely clear the lesions with almost no scarring or pigment change.

Capillary hemangiomas, sometimes referred to as strawberry hemangiomas, are benign cutaneous tumors that involve only capillaries. These hemangiomas are bright red, rubbery nodules with a rough surface and a well-defined margin (Fig. 9-5, *B*). Strawberry hemangiomas may not be apparent at birth but may appear within a few weeks and enlarge considerably during the first year of life and then begin to involute spontaneously. It may take 5 to 12 years for complete resolution. As many as 50% of patients may be left with residual findings such as telangiectasia, redundant fatty tissue, or skin atrophy (Alster and Railan, 2006). Cavernous venous hemangiomas involve deeper vessels in the dermis and have a bluish red color and poorly defined margins. These latter forms may be associated with the trapping of platelets (Kasabach-Merritt syndrome) and subsequent thrombocytopenia (Kelly, 2010; Witt, 2009).

Hemangiomas may also occur as part of the PHACE syndrome (Sidbury, 2010):

P—Posterior fossa brain malformation
H—Hemangiomas (segmental cervicofacial)
A—Arterial anomalies
C—Cardiac defects, including coarctation of the aorta
E—Eye anomalies

Although most hemangiomas require no treatment because of their high rate of spontaneous involution, some vision and airway obstruction may necessitate therapy. Systemic propranolol or prednisone may deter further growth. Subcutaneous injections of interferon or vincristine may be required if prednisone therapy and the pulsed-dye laser fail to control a problematic hemangioma; however, the associated side effects may outweigh the benefits of therapy in some cases (Holland and Drolet, 2010).

Nursing Care Management

Birthmarks, especially those on the face, are upsetting to parents. Families need an explanation of the type of lesion, its significance, and possible treatment.* They can benefit from seeing photographs of

---

*Information is available from Vascular Birthmarks Foundation, http://www.birthmark.org.

other infants before and after treatment for port-wine stains or after the passage of time for hemangiomas. Pictures taken to follow the involution process may further help parents gain confidence that progress is taking place.

If laser therapy is performed, the lesion will have a purplish black appearance for 7 to 10 days, after which the blackness fades and gives way to redness with an eventual lightening of the treated area. During the treatment phase, parents are cautioned to avoid any trauma to the lesion or picking at the scab. The child's fingernails are trimmed as an added precaution. Washing the area gently with water and dabbing it dry is adequate, although in some cases, a topical antibiotic ointment may be used. No salicylates should be taken during the treatment phase because they decrease the effects of the therapy. The child should be kept out of the sun for several weeks and then protected with a sunscreen of at least SPF 25. Complications associated with laser treatment include redness and bruising and, less commonly, hyperpigmentation, hypopigmentation, and atrophic scarring (Alster and Railan, 2006).

NURSING CARE OF THE HIGH-RISK NEWBORN AND FAMILY

IDENTIFICATION OF HIGH-RISK NEWBORNS

A high-risk neonate can be defined as a newborn, regardless of gestational age or birth weight, who has a greater than average chance of morbidity or mortality because of conditions or circumstances associated with birth and the adjustment to extrauterine existence. The high-risk period encompasses human growth and development from the time of viability (the gestational age at which survival outside the uterus is believed to be possible, or as early as 23 weeks of gestation) up to 28 days after birth; thus, it includes threats to life and health that occur during the prenatal, perinatal, and postnatal periods.

There has been increased interest in late-preterm infants of 34 to 36⁶⁄₇ weeks of gestation who may receive the same treatment as term infants. Late-preterm infants often experience similar morbidities to preterm infants, including respiratory distress, hypoglycemia requiring treatment, temperature instability, poor feeding, jaundice, and discharge delays, as a result of illness. Therefore, assessment and prompt intervention in life-threatening perinatal emergencies often make the difference between a favorable outcome and a lifetime of disability. It is estimated that late-preterm infants represent 70% of the total preterm infant population and that the mortality rate for this group is significantly higher than that of term infants (7.9 vs. 2.4 per 1000 live births, respectively) (Tomashek, Shapiro-Mendoza, Davidoff, and others, 2007). Because late-preterm infants' birth weights often range from 2000 to 2500 g (4.4-5.5 pounds) and they appear relatively mature compared with smaller preterm infants, they may be cared for in the same manner as healthy term infants while risk factors for late-preterm infants are overlooked. Late-preterm infants are often discharged early from the birth institution and have a significantly higher rate of rehospitalization than term infants (Escobar, Clark, and Greene, 2006). Discussions regarding high-risk infants in this chapter also refer to late-preterm infants who are experiencing a delayed transition to extrauterine life. Nurses in newborn nurseries should be familiar with the characteristics of neonates and recognize the significance of serious deviations from expected observations. When providers can anticipate the need for specialized care and plan for it, the probability of successful outcome is increased.

The Association of Women's Health, Obstetric and Neonatal Nurses has published the *Late Preterm Infant Assessment Guide* (Askin, Bakewell-Sachs, Medoff-Cooper, and others, 2007) for the education of perinatal nurses regarding the late-preterm infant's risk factors and appropriate care and follow-up care.

Classification of High-Risk Newborns

High-risk infants are most often classified according to birth weight, gestational age, and predominant pathophysiologic problems. The more common problems related to physiologic status are closely associated with the state of maturity of the infant and usually involve chemical disturbances (e.g., hypoglycemia, hypocalcemia) or consequences of immature organs and systems (e.g., hyperbilirubinemia, respiratory distress, hypothermia). Because high-risk factors are common to several specialty areas—particularly obstetrics, pediatrics, and neonatology—specific terminology is needed to describe the developmental status of the newborn (Box 9-1).

Formerly, weight at birth was considered to reflect a reasonably accurate estimation of gestational age; that is, if an infant's birth weight exceeded 2500 g (5.5 pounds), the infant was considered to be mature. However, accumulated data have shown that intrauterine growth rates are not the same for all infants and that other factors (e.g., heredity, placental insufficiency, maternal disease) influence intrauterine growth and birth weight. From these data, a more definitive and meaningful classification system that encompasses birth weight, gestational age, and neonatal outcome has been developed. (See Fig. 8-2 for size comparison of newborn infants.)

CARE OF HIGH-RISK NEWBORNS

Systematic Assessment

A thorough systematic physical assessment is an essential component in the care of high-risk infants (see Nursing Care Guidelines box). Subtle changes in feeding behavior, activity, color, oxygen saturation (SaO_2), or vital signs often indicate an underlying problem. Low-birth-weight (LBW) preterm infants, especially very low–birth-weight (VLBW) or extremely low–birth-weight (ELBW) infants, are ill equipped to withstand prolonged physiologic stress and may die within minutes of exhibiting abnormal symptoms if the underlying pathologic process is not corrected. Alert nurses are aware of subtle changes and react promptly to implement interventions that promote optimum functioning in high-risk neonates. Changes in the infant's status are noted through ongoing observations of the infant's adaptation to the extrauterine environment.

Observational assessments of high-risk infants are made according to each infant's acuity; critically ill infants require close observation and assessment of respiratory function, including continuous pulse oximetry, electrolytes, and evaluation of blood gases. Accurate documentation of the infant's status is an integral component of nursing care. With the aid of continuous, sophisticated cardiopulmonary monitoring, nursing assessments and daily care may be coordinated to allow for minimal handling of the infant (especially VLBW or ELBW infants) to decrease the effects of environmental stress.

Monitoring Physiologic Data

Most neonates under intensive observation are placed in a controlled thermal environment and monitored for heart rate, respiratory activity, and temperature. The monitoring devices are equipped with an alarm system that indicates when the vital signs are above or below preset limits. However, it is essential to check the apical heart rate and compare it with the monitor reading.

Blood pressure (BP) is monitored routinely in sick neonates by either internal or external means. Direct recording with arterial catheters is often used but carries the risks inherent in any procedure in

BOX 9-1 CLASSIFICATION OF HIGH-RISK INFANTS

Classification According to Size

Low-birth-weight (LBW) infant—An infant whose birth weight is less than 2500 g (5.5 pounds) regardless of gestational age

Very low–birth-weight (VLBW) infant—An infant whose birth weight is less than 1500 g (3.3 pounds)

Extremely low–birth-weight (ELBW) infant—An infant whose birth weight is less than 1000 g (2.2 pounds)

Appropriate-for-gestational-age (AGA) infant—An infant whose weight falls between the 10th and 90th percentiles on intrauterine growth curves

Small-for-date (SFD) or small-for-gestational-age (SGA) infant—An infant whose rate of intrauterine growth was slowed and whose birth weight falls below the 10th percentile on intrauterine growth curves (see also Fig. 8-1, *B*)

Intrauterine growth restriction (IUGR)—Found in infants whose intrauterine growth is restricted (sometimes used as a more descriptive term for SGA infants)

Symmetric IUGR—Growth restriction in which the weight, length, and head circumference are all affected

Asymmetric IUGR—Growth restriction in which the head circumference remains within normal parameters while the birth weight falls below the 10th percentile

Large-for-gestational-age (LGA) infant—An infant whose birth weight falls above the 90th percentile on intrauterine growth charts

Classification According to Gestational Age

Preterm (premature) infant—An infant born before completion of 37 weeks of gestation regardless of birth weight

Full-term infant—An infant born between the beginning of the 38 weeks and the completion of the 42 weeks of gestation regardless of birth weight

Late-preterm infant—An infant born between 34 5/7 and 36 6/7 weeks of gestation regardless of birth weight*

Postterm (postmature) infant—An infant born after 42 weeks of gestational age regardless of birth weight

Classification According to Mortality

Live birth—Birth in which the neonate manifests any heartbeat, breathes, or displays voluntary movement regardless of gestational age

Fetal death—Death of the fetus after 20 weeks of gestation and before delivery with absence of any signs of life after birth

Neonatal death—Death that occurs in the first 27 days of life; early neonatal death occurs in the first week of life; late neonatal death occurs at 7 to 27 days

Perinatal mortality—Total number of fetal and early neonatal deaths per 1000 live births

*Definitions of *late-preterm infants* vary among experts, but Engle (2006) suggests the above (which corresponds to 239th day to 259th day from the first day of the last menstrual period).

which a catheter is introduced into an artery. BP values gradually increase over the first month of life in preterm and term infants. BP norms vary by gestational age and weight, medications such as corticosteroids, and disease process. One of the primary considerations in the preterm infant is the relationship between systemic BP and the determination of adequate cerebral blood flow. In the neonatal intensive care unit (NICU), frequent laboratory examinations and their interpretation are integral parts of the ongoing assessment of infants' progress. Accurate intake and output records are kept on all acutely ill infants. An accurate output can be obtained by collecting urine in a plastic urine collection bag specifically made for preterm infants (see Urine Specimens, Chapter 22) or by weighing the diapers, which is the simplest and least traumatic means of measuring urinary output. The preweighed wet diaper is weighed on a gram scale, and the gram weight of the urine is converted directly to milliliters (e.g., 25 g = 25 ml).

Blood examinations are a necessary part of the ongoing assessment and monitoring of the high-risk newborn's progress. The tests most often performed are blood glucose, bilirubin, calcium, hematocrit, serum electrolytes, and blood gases. Samples may be obtained from the heel; by venipuncture; by arterial puncture; or by an indwelling catheter in an umbilical vein, an umbilical artery, or a peripheral artery (see Atraumatic Care box, p. 210, and Collection of Specimens, Chapter 22).

When numerous blood samples must be drawn, it is important to maintain an accurate record of the amount of blood being removed, especially in ELBW and VLBW infants, who can ill afford to have their blood supply depleted during the acute phase of their illness. There is an increased emphasis on drawing as little blood as possible from high-risk neonates to minimize the depletion of blood volume and avoid blood transfusions and associated complications. To avoid the need for repeated arterial punctures, pulse oximetry, which measures the saturation or percentage of oxygen in the hemoglobin, is typically used. Although used less frequently than pulse oximetry, transcutaneous carbon dioxide ($tcPCO_2$) is monitored in some situations. The nurse notes changes in oxygenation (or other aspects being monitored) associated with handling and adjusts the infant's care accordingly. The frequency of vital signs is determined by the infant's acuity level (seriousness of condition) and response to handling.

The nursing process in the care of high-risk newborns and their families is described in the Nursing Process box.

Respiratory Support

The primary objective in the care of high-risk infants is to establish and maintain respiration. Many infants require supplemental oxygen and assisted ventilation. All infants require appropriate positioning to maximize oxygenation and ventilation. Oxygen therapy is provided on the basis of the infant's requirements and illness (see Respiratory Distress Syndrome, p. 267).

Thermoregulation

After or concurrent with the establishment of respiration, the most crucial need of LBW infants is application of external warmth. Prevention of heat loss in distressed infants is absolutely essential for survival, and maintaining a neutral thermal environment is a challenging aspect of neonatal intensive nursing care. Heat production is a complicated process that involves the cardiovascular, neurologic, and metabolic systems, and immature neonates have all of the problems related to heat production that are faced by full-term infants (see Thermoregulation, Chapter 8). However, LBW infants are placed at further disadvantage by a number of additional problems. They have an even smaller muscle mass and fewer deposits of brown fat for producing heat, lack insulating subcutaneous fat, and have poor reflex control of skin capillaries.

NURSING CARE GUIDELINES
Physical Assessment

General Assessment

Using an electronic scale, weigh daily, or more often if indicated.

Measure length and head circumference at birth.

Describe general body shape and size, posture at rest, ease of breathing, presence and location of edema.

Describe any apparent deformities.

Describe any signs of distress—poor color, hypotonia, lethargy, apnea.

Respiratory Assessment

Describe shape of chest (barrel, concave), symmetry, presence of incisions, chest tubes, or other deviations.

Describe use of accessory muscles—nasal flaring or substernal, intercostal, or suprasternal retractions.

Determine respiratory rate and regularity.

Auscultate and describe breath sounds—crackles, wheezing, wet or diminished sounds, grunting, diminished air movement, stridor, equality of breath sounds.

Describe cry if not intubated.

Describe ambient oxygen and method of delivery; if intubated, describe size and position of tube, type of ventilator, and settings.

Determine oxygen saturation by pulse oximetry and partial pressure of oxygen, and describe carbon dioxide by transcutaneous carbon dioxide ($tcPCO_2$).

Cardiovascular Assessment

Determine heart rate and rhythm.

Describe heart sounds, including any murmurs.

Determine the point of maximum impulse (PMI), the point at which the heartbeat sounds and palpates loudest (a change in the PMI may indicate a mediastinal shift).

Describe infant's color: cyanosis (may be of cardiac, respiratory, or hematopoietic origin), pallor, plethora, jaundice, mottling.

Assess color of mucous membranes, lips.

Determine blood pressure as indicated. Indicate extremity used and cuff size.

Describe peripheral pulses, capillary refill, and peripheral perfusion (mottling).

Describe monitors, their parameters, and whether alarms are in the "on" position.

Gastrointestinal Assessment

Determine presence of abdominal distention—increase in circumference, shiny skin, evidence of abdominal wall erythema, visible peristalsis, visible loops of bowel, status of umbilicus.

Determine any signs of regurgitation and time related to feeding; describe character and amount of residual if gavage fed; if nasogastric tube is in place, describe type of suction and drainage (color, consistency, pH).

Describe amount, color, consistency, and odor of any emesis.

Palpate liver margin (1–3 cm below right costal margin).

Describe amount, color, and consistency of stools.

Describe bowel sounds—presence or absence (must be present if feeding).

Genitourinary Assessment

Describe any abnormalities of genitalia.

Describe amount (as determined by weight), color, pH, labstick findings, and specific gravity of urine.

Check weight.

Neurologic–Musculoskeletal Assessment

Describe infant's movements—random, purposeful, jittery, twitching, spontaneous, elicited; describe level of activity with stimulation; evaluate based on gestational age.

Describe infant's position or attitude—flexed, extended.

Describe reflexes observed—Moro, sucking, Babinski, plantar, and other expected reflexes.

Determine level of response and consolability.

Determine changes in head circumference (if indicated), size and tension of fontanels, suture lines.

Determine pupillary responses in infant older than 32 weeks of gestation.

Check hip alignment (only experienced practitioner should perform).

Temperature

Determine axillary temperature.

Determine relationship to environmental temperature.

Skin Assessment

Note any skin lesions or birthmarks.

Describe any discoloration, reddened area, signs of irritation, blisters, abrasions, or denuded areas, especially where monitoring equipment, infusions, or other apparatus come in contact with skin; also check and note any skin preparation used (e.g., skin disinfectants).

Determine texture and turgor of skin—dry, smooth, flaky, peeling, and so on.

Describe any rash, skin lesion, or birthmarks.

Determine whether intravenous infusion catheter is in place and observe for signs of infiltration.

Describe parenteral infusion lines—location, type (arterial, venous, peripheral, umbilical, central, peripheral central venous), type of infusion (medication, saline, dextrose, electrolyte, lipids, total parenteral nutrition), type of infusion pump and rate of flow, type of catheter, and appearance of insertion site.

To delay or prevent the effects of cold stress, at-risk newborns are placed in a heated environment immediately after birth, where they remain until they are able to maintain thermal stability—the capacity to balance heat production and conservation with heat dissipation. Because overheating produces an increase in oxygen and calorie consumption, infants are also jeopardized in a hyperthermic environment. A neutral thermal environment is one that permits the infant to maintain a normal core temperature with minimum oxygen consumption and calorie expenditure (Bissinger and Annibale, 2010). Studies indicate that optimum thermoneutrality cannot be predicted for every high-risk infant's needs. In healthy term infants, it is recommended that axillary temperatures be maintained at 36.5° to 37.5° C (97.7°–99.5° F); in preterm infants, axillary temperatures of 36.3° and 36.9° C

(97.3° and 98.4° F) are considered appropriate (Brown and Landers, 2011).

Very low–birth-weight and ELBW infants, with thin skin and almost no subcutaneous fat, can control body heat loss or gain only within a limited range of environmental temperatures. In these infants, heat loss from radiation, evaporation, and transepidermal water loss is three to five times greater than in larger infants, and a decrease in body temperature is associated with an increase in mortality. Further research is needed to define a neutral thermal environment for ELBW infants.

The consequences of cold stress that produce additional hazards to neonates are (1) hypoxia, (2) metabolic acidosis, and (3) hypoglycemia. Increased metabolism in response to chilling creates a

◎ NURSING PROCESS

The High-Risk Newborn and Family

Assessment

At birth, the newborn is given a rapid yet thorough assessment to determine any apparent problems and identify those that demand immediate attention. This examination is primarily concerned with evaluation of cardiopulmonary and neurologic functions. The assessment includes assignment of an Apgar score (see Chapter 8) and evaluation for any obvious congenital anomalies or evidence of neonatal distress. A systematic assessment (see p. 235) is carried out after the high-risk newborn is stable. (See also Clinical Assessment of Gestational Age, Chapter 8.)

Diagnosis (Problem Identification)

Many nursing diagnoses may be evident after a careful assessment of the infant at risk. Some apply to all infants; others vary according to the needs and characteristics of individual infants and their families. Because a number of health problems accompany high-risk infants, the nurse is also alert to other conditions and complications discussed later in this chapter and elsewhere in the book. The nursing diagnoses that represent general guides for nursing intervention are:
- Ineffective Breathing Pattern related to pulmonary and neuromuscular immaturity
- Ineffective Thermoregulation related to immature temperature control and decreased subcutaneous fat
- Risk for Infection (risk factors include deficient immunologic defenses, exposure to environmental pathogens, required invasive procedures and invasive equipment)
- Imbalanced Nutrition: Less Than Body Requirements related to inability to ingest nutrients
- Risk for Impaired Skin Integrity (risk factors include immature skin structure, physical immobility, decreased fluid intake, and invasive procedures)
- Risk for Imbalanced Fluid Volume (risk factors include immature skin structure; extra fluid losses via skin, lungs, and urine; decreased ability to take in required amount of fluid to sustain hydration)
- Delayed Growth and Development related to preterm birth, immature physiologic capabilities at birth, neonatal intensive care unit environment, separation from parents, effects of concomitant illnesses
- Interrupted Family Processes related to preterm birth, situational crisis, interruption of parent–infant interaction
- Anticipatory Grieving related to unexpected birth of high-risk infant, knowledge deficit regarding infant's prognosis and eventual outcome

Planning

The nursing care plan for the high-risk infant depends to a large extent on the diagnosis of the health problem(s) that place the infant at risk. However, the following expected outcomes are appropriate for many high-risk infants and their families:
- Infant will exhibit adequate oxygenation.
- Infant will maintain stable body temperature.
- Infant will exhibit no evidence of nosocomial infection.
- Infant will receive adequate hydration and nutrition.
- Infant will maintain skin integrity.
- Infant will receive appropriate developmental support and care.
- Parents will experience positive parent–infant interactions.
- Parents will exhibit positive caretaking abilities with high-risk infant.
- Family will receive appropriate support, including preparation for home care or for infant's death.

Implementation

Intervention strategies for high-risk infants and their families are discussed on pp. 235 to 253.

Evaluation

The effectiveness of nursing interventions is determined by continual reassessment and evaluation of care based on the following observational guidelines:
- Take vital signs and perform respiratory assessments at time intervals based on infant's condition and needs; observe infant's respiratory efforts and response to therapy; check functioning of equipment; review laboratory test results.
- Measure body temperature at specified intervals.
- Observe infant's behavior and appearance for evidence of sepsis; monitor lab values for sepsis.
- Assess for hydration; assess and measure fluid intake; observe infant during feeding; measure amount of human milk, formula, or parenteral intake; weigh daily.
- Observe infant's skin for signs of irritation, excoriation, and breakdown.
- Observe infant's response to developmental care.
- Observe parental interaction with infant; interview family regarding their feelings, concerns, and readiness for home care.
- Assess family and observe their behaviors during and after the death of their infant.

---

compensatory increase in oxygen and calorie consumption. If available oxygen is not increased to accommodate this need, arterial oxygen tension is decreased. This is further complicated by a smaller lung volume in relation to the metabolic rate, which creates diminished oxygen in the blood and concurrent pulmonary disorders. A small advantage is gained by the presence of fetal hemoglobin because its increased capacity to carry oxygen allows the infant to exist for longer periods in conditions of lowered oxygen tension.

The three primary methods for maintaining a neutral thermal environment are the use of an incubator, a radiant warming panel (Fig. 9-6), and an open bassinet with cotton blankets. A dressed infant under blankets can maintain a certain temperature within a wider range of environmental temperatures; however, the close observations required with a high-risk infant are best accomplished if the infant remains partially unclothed. The incubator should always be

prewarmed before placing an infant in it. The use of double-walled incubators significantly improves the infant's ability to maintain a desirable temperature and reduce energy expenditure related to heat regulation. Inside or outside the incubator, head coverings are effective in preventing heat loss. A fabric-insulated or wool cap is more effective than one fashioned from stockinette. The use of a heated gel mattress with radiant heat has been shown to significantly decrease the incidence of radiation heat loss and preserve an adequate neutral thermal environment for the VLBW neonate (Lewis, Sanders, and Brockopp, 2011; Soll, 2008). An effective means for maintaining the desired range of temperature in the infant is the use of a manually adjusted or automatically controlled (servo-controlled) incubator. The latter mechanism, when set at the upper and lower limits of the desired circulating air temperature range, adjusts automatically in response to signals from a thermal sensor attached to the abdominal skin. If the

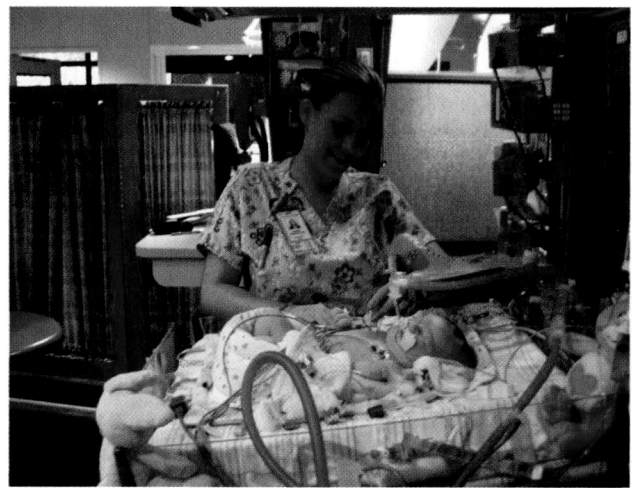

FIG 9-6 Nurse caring for an infant in a radiant warmer. (Photo courtesy E. Jacobs, Texas Children's Hospital, Houston.)

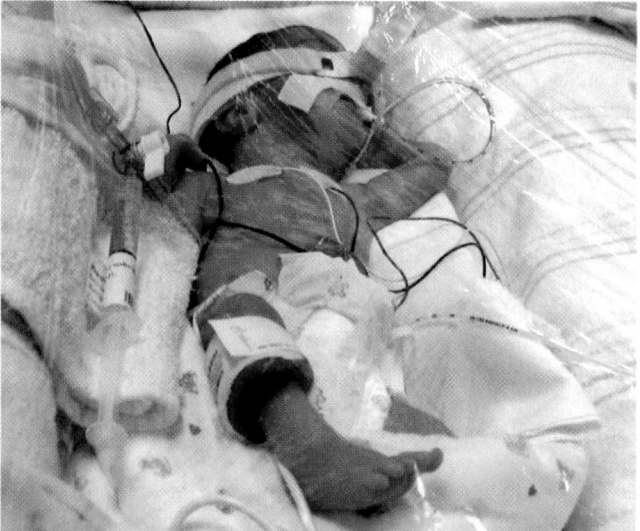

FIG 9-7 Infant under plastic wrap, which produces a draft-free environment. (Photo courtesy E. Jacobs, Texas Children's Hospital, Houston.)

infant's temperature drops, the warming device is triggered to increase heat output. The servo control is usually set to a desired skin temperature between 36° and 36.5° C (96.8° and 97.7° F) (Brown and Landers, 2011).

A high-humidity atmosphere contributes to body temperature maintenance by reducing evaporative heat loss. A number of "microenvironments" may be used with VLBW and ELBW infants to minimize evaporative and insensible water losses. These include items such as food-grade plastic bags or plastic wrap, humidified reservoirs for incubators, and humidified plastic heat shields covered with plastic wrap (Fig. 9-7). When such environments are used, special care must be taken to avoid bacterial contamination of the warm and humid environment by organisms such as *Pseudomonas* and *Serratia*, which have an affinity for moist environments; postnatally acquired pneumonia from such organisms may be fatal, particularly in VLBW infants. A systematic review of practices to decrease hypothermia at birth in LBW infants found that plastic wraps (polyethylene) or bags kept preterm infants warmer, leading to higher temperatures on admission to neonatal units and less hypothermia (Lewis, Sanders, and Brockopp,

2011; McCall, Alderdice, Halliday, and others, 2010). This practice is now recommended in the Neonatal Resuscitation Program guidelines published by the American Heart Association (Kattwinkel, Perlman, Aziz, and others, 2010).

Skin-to-skin (kangaroo) contact between a stable preterm infant and parent is also a viable option for interaction because of the maintenance of appropriate body temperature by the infant. Other benefits of skin-to-skin contact are discussed later in this chapter.

Protection from Infection

Protection from infection is an integral part of all newborn care, but preterm and sick neonates are particularly susceptible. The protective environment of a regularly cleaned and changed incubator provides effective isolation from airborne infective agents. However, thorough, meticulous, and frequent hand washing is the foundation of a preventive program. This includes *all* persons who come in contact with infants and their equipment. After handling another infant or equipment, no one should ever touch an infant without first washing their hands.

Personnel with infectious disorders are either barred from the unit until they are no longer infectious or are required to wear suitable shields, such as masks or gloves, to reduce the likelihood of contamination. An annual influenza vaccination is recommended for NICU personnel. Standard precautions as a method of infection control are instituted in all nursery areas to protect the infants and staff (see Chapter 22). The benefit of "gowning" by visitors and hospital staff to control infection is not supported by research. Sibling visitation in the NICU has not been shown to increase nosocomial infections (AAP and ACOG, 2007); however, appropriate screening for upper respiratory illness in siblings is often recommended.

The sources of infection rise in direct relationship to the number of persons and pieces of equipment coming in contact with the infants. Equipment used in the care of infants is cleaned on a regular basis in accordance with the manufacturer's recommendations or institutional protocol; this includes cleaning of cribs, mattresses, incubators, radiant warmers, cardiorespiratory monitors, pulse oximeters, and vital sign–monitoring equipment after usage with one infant and before usage with another. Because organisms thrive best in water, plumbing fixtures and humidifying equipment are particularly hazardous. Disposable equipment used for water-related therapies, such as nebulizers and plastic tubing, is changed regularly.

Hydration

High-risk infants often receive supplemental parenteral fluids to supply additional calories, electrolytes, and water. Adequate hydration is particularly important in preterm infants because their extracellular water content is higher (70% in full-term infants and up to 90% in preterm infants), their body surface is larger, and the capacity for handling fluid shifts is limited in preterm infants' underdeveloped kidneys. Therefore, these infants are highly vulnerable to fluid depletion.

Parenteral fluids may be given to the high-risk neonate via several routes depending on the nature of the illness, the duration and type of fluid therapy, and unit preference. Common routes of fluid infusion include peripheral, peripherally inserted central venous (or percutaneous central venous), surgically inserted central venous, and umbilical venous catheters. The preferred sites for peripheral intravenous (IV) infusions in neonates are the peripheral veins on the dorsal surfaces of the hands or feet. Alternative sites are scalp veins and antecubital veins. Special precautions and frequent observations must accompany the use of peripheral lines (Beauman and Swanson, 2006). In many neonatal centers the percutaneous central venous catheter is used for parenteral therapy and medication administration because of less expense and decreased neonatal trauma.

In most facilities, NICU nurses insert peripheral IV catheters and maintain the infusions. IV fluids must always be delivered by continuous infusion pumps that deliver minute volumes at a preset flow rate. The catheter is secured to the skin with a transparent dressing or minimum amount of tape (see Skin Care, p. 244) with care taken not to cause undue pressure from the catheter hub and tubing. Because all infants, especially those who are ELBW and VLBW, are highly vulnerable to any fluid shifts, infusion rates are carefully regulated and checked hourly to prevent tissue damage from extravasation, fluid overload, or dehydration. Pulmonary edema, congestive heart failure, patent ductus arteriosus, and intraventricular hemorrhage may occur with fluid overload. Dehydration may cause electrolyte disturbances with potentially serious CNS effects.

Infants who are ELBW, tachypneic, receiving phototherapy, or in a radiant warmer have increased insensible water losses that require appropriate fluid adjustments. Nurses must monitor fluid status by daily (or more frequent) weights and accurate intake and output of all fluids, including medications and blood products. Bedside urine-specific gravity and serum electrolytes are monitored per unit protocol, and urine electrolytes are obtained as warranted by the infant's condition. ELBW infants often require more frequent monitoring of these parameters because of their inordinate transepidermal fluid loss, immature renal function, and propensity to dehydration or overhydration. Intolerance of even dextrose 5% is not uncommon in ELBW infants, with subsequent glycosuria and osmotic diuresis. Alterations in behavior, alertness, or activity level in these infants receiving IV fluids may signal an electrolyte imbalance, hypoglycemia, or hyperglycemia. Nurses should also be observant for tremors or seizures in VLBW or ELBW infants because these may be a sign of hyponatremia or hypernatremia.

> ## ! NURSING ALERT
>
> Nurses should be constantly alert for signs of IV infiltration (e.g., erythema, edema, color change of tissue, blanching at site) and for signs of overhydration (weight gain of >30 g [1 oz] in 24 hr, periorbital edema, tachypnea, and crackles on lung auscultation).

A common problem observed in infants who have an umbilical artery catheter in place is vasoconstriction of peripheral vessels, which can seriously impair circulation. The response is triggered by arterial vasospasm caused by the presence of the catheter, the infusion of fluids, or injection of medication. Blanching of the buttocks, genitalia, or legs or feet is an indication of vasospasm. The problem is recognized promptly and reported to the practitioner. The nurse must also observe for signs of thrombi in infants with umbilical venous or arterial lines. The precipitation of microthrombi in the vascular bed with the use of such catheters is commonly manifested by a sudden bluish discoloration seen in the toes, called catheter toes. The problem is promptly reported to the practitioner because failure to alleviate the existing pathologic condition may result in the loss of toes or even a foot or leg.

Infants with umbilical venous or arterial catheters should also be observed closely for catheter dislodging and subsequent bleeding or hemorrhage; urinary output, renal function, and gastrointestinal function are also evaluated in these infants. Although the intent of such catheters is to effectively deliver IV fluids (and sometimes medications) and to obtain arterial blood gas samples, they are not without inherent complications.

Nutrition

Optimum nutrition is critical in the management of LBW and preterm infants, but there are difficulties in providing for their nutritional needs. The various mechanisms for ingestion and digestion of foods are not fully developed; the more immature the infant, the greater the problem. In addition, the nutritional requirements for this group of infants are not known with certainty. It is known that all preterm infants are at risk because of poor nutritional stores and several physical and developmental characteristics.

An infant's nutritional needs for rapid growth and daily maintenance must be met in the presence of several anatomic and physiologic disabilities. Although some sucking and swallowing activities are demonstrated before birth and in preterm infants, coordination of these mechanisms does not occur until approximately 32 to 34 weeks of gestation, and they are not fully synchronized until 36 to 37 weeks. Initial sucking is not accompanied by swallowing, and esophageal contractions are uncoordinated. Consequently, infants are highly prone to aspiration and its attendant dangers. As infants mature, the suck–swallow pattern develops but is slow and ineffectual, and these reflexes may also become easily exhausted.

The amount and method of feeding are determined by the infant's size and condition. Nutrition can be provided by either the parenteral or the enteral route or by a combination of the two. Infants who are ELBW, VLBW, or critically ill often obtain the majority of their nutrients by the parenteral route because of their inability to digest and absorb enteral nutrition. Illness factors resulting in hypoxia and major organ immaturity further preclude the use of enteral feeding until the infant's condition has stabilized; necrotizing enterocolitis (NEC) has previously been associated with enteral feedings in acutely ill or distressed infants (see Necrotizing Enterocolitis, p. 284). Total parenteral nutritional support of acutely ill infants may be accomplished successfully with commercially available IV solutions specifically designed to meet the infant's nutritional needs, including protein, amino acids, trace minerals, vitamins, carbohydrates (dextrose), and fat (lipid emulsion).

Studies have shown that there are benefits to the early introduction of small amounts of enteral feedings in metabolically stable preterm infants. These minimal enteral (trophic gastrointestinal priming) feedings have been shown to stimulate the infant's gastrointestinal tract, preventing mucosal atrophy and subsequent enteral feeding difficulties. Minimal enteral feedings with as little as 0.1 to 4 ml/kg of breast milk or preterm formula may be given by gavage as soon as the infant is medically stable. Parenteral hydration and nutrition are continued until the infant is able to tolerate an amount of enteral feeding sufficient to sustain growth. An increased incidence of NEC in VLBW infants receiving minimal enteral nutrition has not been substantiated (Reynolds and Thureen, 2007; Terrin, Passariello, Canani, and others, 2009). Minimal enteral feedings have been proved to increase mineral absorption, increase serum calcium and alkaline phosphatase activity, and substantially decrease the incidence of bilious gastric residuals and feeding intolerance in preterm infants (Schanler, Shulman, Lau, and others, 1999). Minimal enteral feedings are recommended as the standard of care for feeding VLBW infants (Hay, 2008).

Although the timing of the first feeding has been a matter of controversy, most authorities now believe that early feeding (provided that the infant is medically stable) reduces the incidence of complicating factors, such as hypoglycemia and dehydration, and the degree of hyperbilirubinemia. The feeding regimen used varies in different units.

Breastfeeding

Ample evidence indicates that human milk is the best source of nutrition for term and preterm infants. Studies indicate that small preterm infants are able to breastfeed if they have adequate sucking and swallowing reflexes and there are no other contraindications, such as respiratory complications or concurrent illness (Dougherty and Luther, 2008). Mothers who wish to breastfeed their preterm infants are encouraged to pump their breasts until their infants are sufficiently stable to tolerate breastfeeding. Appropriate guidelines for the storage of expressed mother's milk should be followed to decrease the risk of milk contamination and destruction of its beneficial properties.

Milk produced by mothers whose infants are born before term contains higher concentrations of protein, sodium, chloride, and immunoglobulin A (IgA). Growth factors, hormones, prolactin, calcitonin, thyroxine, steroids, and taurine (an essential amino acid) are also present in human milk. Secretory IgA concentration is higher in the milk from mothers of preterm infants than in the milk from mothers of full-term infants. IgA is important in the control of bacteria in the intestinal tract, where it inhibits adherence and proliferation of bacteria on epithelial surfaces. Additional protection from infection is provided by leukocytes, lactoferrin, and lysozyme, all of which are present in human milk. The milk produced by mothers for their infants changes in content over the first 30 days postnatally, at which time it is similar to full-term human milk. Despite its benefits, LBW infants (<1500 g [3.3 pounds]) who are exclusively fed unfortified human milk demonstrate decreased growth rates and nutritional deficiencies even beyond the hospitalization period. These infants often have inadequacies of calcium, phosphorus, protein, sodium, vitamins, and energy. Specially designed supplements for human milk have been developed to address these deficits. Fortifiers are commercially available, usually as a liquid or powder containing protein; carbohydrate; calcium; phosphorus; magnesium; sodium; and varied amounts of zinc, copper, and vitamins. Because fortifiers do not contain sufficient iron, an exogenous source must be administered after enteral feeding.

A number of studies regarding the effects of long-chain polyunsaturated fatty acids on cognitive development, visual acuity, and physical growth in full-term and preterm infants have prompted formula companies to add docosahexaenoic acid (DHA) and arachidonic acid (AA) to their infant formulas. AA and DHA are present in human milk, and their presence has been reported to lead to an increase in cognitive development in human milk–fed infants compared with infants fed a formula without these fatty acids. However, one meta-analysis of four clinical trials demonstrated no clinically significant developmental benefits to supplementation of formula with AA and DHA in term and preterm infants at 18 months of age (Beyerlein, Hadders-Algra, Kennedy, and others, 2010).

Preterm infants may be able to successfully breastfeed earlier than previously believed (28–36 weeks); in addition, preterm infants who are breastfed rather than bottle fed demonstrate fewer incidences of oxygen desaturation; absence of bradycardia; warmer skin temperature; and better coordination of breathing, sucking, and swallowing (Gardner and Lawrence, 2011). Preterm infants should be carefully evaluated for readiness to breastfeed, including assessment of behavioral state, ability to maintain body temperature outside an artificial heat source, respiratory status, and readiness to suckle at the mother's breast. The latter may be accomplished with nonnutritive suckling at the breast during skin-to-skin (kangaroo) contact so the mother and newborn may become accustomed to each other (Gardner and Lawrence, 2011). Nasal cannula oxygen may also be provided during preterm breastfeeding on the basis of the infant's assessed requirements.

Time, patience, and dedication on the part of the mother and the nursing staff are needed to help infants with breastfeeding. The process is begun slowly—beginning with one feeding daily and gradually increasing the feedings as the infant tolerates them. Supplementary bottle feeding is inefficient because the infant expends energy and calories to feed twice. Supplementing by gavage feeding or using a training nipple is more energy and calorie efficient. Breastfeeding preterm infants often requires additional guidance by a lactation consultant; continued support and encouragement by the nursing staff and family members are essential. In addition, postdischarge breastfeeding often requires further guidance, counseling, and support by nursing staff (Ahmed and Sands, 2010).

For infants who cannot be breastfed but who also cannot survive except on human milk, banked donor milk is important. Because of the antiinfective and growth-promoting properties of human milk, as well as its superior nutrition, donor milk is used in many NICUs for preterm or sick infants when the mother's milk is not available (AAP, 2005). Donor milk is also used therapeutically for medical purposes, such as in transplant recipients who are immunocompromised. Unprocessed human milk from unscreened donors is not recommended because of the risk of transmission of infectious agents (AAP, 2005).

The Human Milk Banking Association of North America* has established guidelines for the operation of donor human milk banks (Human Milk Banking Association, 2011). Donor milk banks collect, screen, process (pasteurize), and distribute milk donated by breastfeeding mothers who are feeding their own infants and pumping a few extra ounces each day for the milk bank.

Nipple Feeding

Vigorous infants can be fed from a nipple with little difficulty, but compromised preterm infants require alternative methods. The amount to be fed is determined largely by the infant's weight gain and tolerance of previous feeding and is increased by small increments until a satisfactory caloric intake is ensured.

The rate of increase that is well tolerated varies from one infant to another, and determining this rate is often a nursing responsibility. Preterm infants require more time and patience to feed compared with full-term infants, and the oropharyngeal mechanism may be stressed by an attempt to feed too rapidly. It is important not to tire the infants or overtax their capacity to retain the feedings. When infants require a prolonged time (arbitrarily, more than 30 minutes) to complete a feeding, gavage feeding may be considered for the next time.

A developmental approach to feeding considers the individual infant's readiness rather than initiating feedings based on weight and age or a predetermined time schedule. Feeding readiness is determined by each infant's medical status, energy level, ability to sustain a brief quiet alert state, gag reflex (demonstrated with a gavage tube insertion), spontaneous rooting and sucking behaviors, and hand-to-mouth behaviors (Nye, 2008). A preterm infant may experience difficulty coordinating sucking, swallowing, and breathing, with resultant apnea, bradycardia, and decreased oxygen saturation. The infant's ability to suck on a pacifier does not indicate complete readiness for nipple feeding or ability to coordinate the above-mentioned activities without some degree of stress; a gradual introduction of nippling in preterm infants is based on careful evaluation of their ability to maintain adequate cardiopulmonary functions while feeding. When infants are unable to tolerate bottle feedings, intermittent feedings by gavage

---

*http://www.hmbana.org.

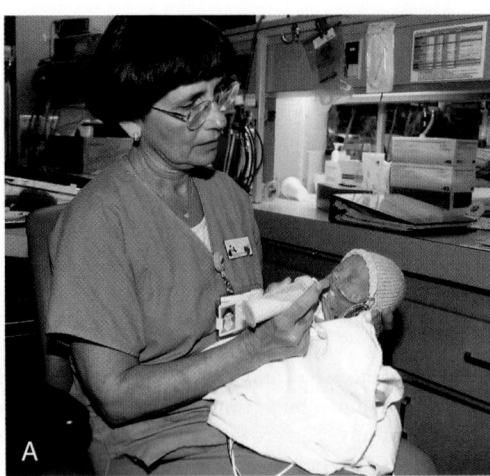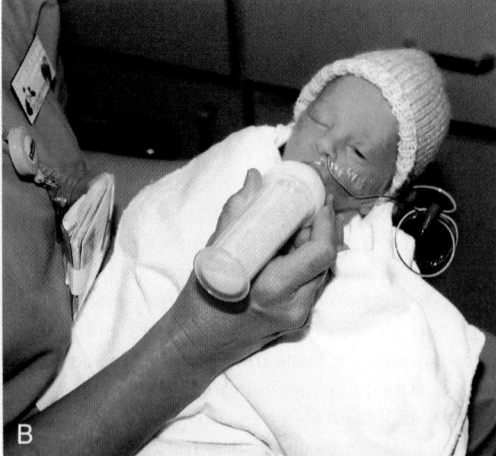

FIG 9-8 Nipple feeding the preterm infant. **A,** The infant is first brought to a quiet alert state in preparation for feeding. **B,** After readiness is demonstrated, the infant is nipple fed. (Courtesy Jeff Barnes, Education and Eastern Oklahoma Perinatal Center, St. Francis Hospital, Tulsa, Okla.)

> ⚠ **NURSING ALERT**
>
> Poor feeding behaviors such as apnea, bradycardia, cyanosis, pallor, and decreased oxygen saturation in any infant who has previously fed well may indicate an underlying illness.

are instituted until they gain enough strength and coordination to use the nipple.

The nipple used should be relatively firm and stable. Although a high-flow, pliable nipple requires less energy to use, it may provide a flow rate that is too rapid for some preterm infants to manage without a risk of aspiration. A firmer nipple facilitates a more "cupped" tongue configuration and allows for a more controlled, manageable flow rate.

The infant is positioned in the feeder's arms or placed semiupright in the lap (Fig. 9-8) and is held with the back curved slightly to simulate the position assumed naturally by most full-term newborns. The use of gentle cheek and jaw support for preterm infants has been shown to facilitate feedings. Stroking the infant's lips, cheeks, and tongue before feeding helps promote oral sensitivity. Inward and upward support to the infant's cheeks and a slightly upward lift to the chin are provided by the fingers to assist nipple compression during feeding.

Bottle feedings are continued if infants are able to tolerate the feedings and take the required amount. Some preterm infants respond more slowly than full-term infants; therefore, the feeding interval and the amount of the feeding are individualized. Preterm infants are often slow feeders and require patience, frequent rest periods, and burping (or bubbling).

Gavage Feeding

Gavage feeding is a safe means of meeting the nutritional requirements of infants who are unable to feed orally. These infants are usually too weak to suck effectively, are unable to coordinate swallowing, and lack a gag reflex. Gavage feedings may be provided by continuous drip regulated via infusion pump or by intermittent bolus feedings. Studies have demonstrated an overall decrease in total milk fat concentration delivery when continuous gavage infusions are administered, which

suggests that intermittent or bolus gavage of expressed mother's milk be administered when possible (Premji, Paes, Jacobson, and others, 2002). Intermittent gavage feeding is used as an energy-conserving technique for infants learning to nipple feed who become excessively tired, listless, or cyanotic.

A size 3.5-, 5-, 6-, or 8-Fr feeding tube is used to instill the feeding, and the usual methods for determining correct placement are used (see Chapter 22 for technique). Although the more relaxed lower esophageal sphincter makes passage of the tube easier, there may be changes in heart rate and BP in response to vagal stimulation.

When an indwelling tube is required, consideration should be given to using a product made of Silastic rather than polyvinyl chloride (PVC) because PVC becomes stiff when exposed to body fluids.

The stomach is aspirated, the contents measured, and the aspirate returned as part of the feeding. However, this practice may vary depending on circumstances and individual unit protocol. The amount of aspirate depends on the time since the previous feeding or concurrent illness. Some advocate deducting the amount aspirated to avoid overdistending the stomach.

The milk or formula is allowed to flow by gravity, and the length of time varies. This procedure is not used as a timesaving method for the nurse. Complications of indwelling tubes include aspiration, obstructed nares, mucous plugs, purulent rhinitis, epistaxis, infection, and possible stomach perforation. Current practice dictates a radiograph as the only certain way to determine nasogastric (NG) tube placement. Methods such as auscultation of an air bubble, and neck-ear-xiphoid (NEX) measurements for insertion depth, and pH measurements are considered imprecise when used as the only method for determination of placement (de Boer, Smit, and Mainous, 2009; Ellett, Croffie, Cohen, and others, 2005; Farrington, Lang, Cullen, and others, 2009; Quandt, Schraner, Ulrich Bucher, and others, 2009; Renner, 2010). One study found that age-related, height-based gastric tube insertion length was more precise than either nose–ear–xiohoid or nose–ear–mid-umbilicus measurements in placing nasogatric tubes in neonates under 1 month of age; the researchers recommend that nose–ear–xiphoid measurements for insertion depth be abandoned because of their unreliability in accurately placing feeding tubes in neonates (Cirgin-Ellett, Cohen, Perkins, and others, 2011). Further research is needed to determine optimal positioning of feeding tubes in high-risk infants on intermittent bolus or continuous gavage feedings.

> **! NURSING ALERT**
>
> The nurse must observe preterm infants closely for behaviors that indicate readiness for oral feedings. These include:
> - A strong, vigorous suck
> - Coordination of sucking and swallowing
> - A gag reflex
> - Sucking on the gavage tube, hands, or a pacifier
> - Rooting and wakefulness before and sleeping after feedings
>
> When these behaviors are noted, infants can be challenged with oral feedings that are introduced slowly.

The infant may be held during gavage feedings by the caregiver or parent. If necessary, oxygen may be supplied via nasal cannula to facilitate handling. It is not recommended that the infant be removed from a primary source of oxygen for feedings because doing so decreases oxygen availability. Nonnutritive sucking (NNS) on a pacifier may help bring the infant to a quiet alert state in preparation for feeding. Proposed benefits of NNS include improved weight gain, improved milk intake, more stable heart rate and oxygen saturation, earlier age at full oral feeds, and improved behavioral state. A systematic review of NNS found that infants receiving NNS were discharged significantly earlier than non-NNS infants and that they experienced a more rapid transition from tube to bottle feedings and better bottle-feeding performance. Additional research suggests that NNS may provide relief of mild to moderate pain associated with procedures such as heel sticks (Liaw, Yang, Blackburn, and others, 2010).

> **! NURSING ALERT**
>
> An increase in gastric residuals, abdominal distention, bilious vomiting, temperature instability, apneic episodes, and bradycardia may be indicative of early NEC and should be reported to the practitioner.

Feeding Resistance

Any feeding technique that bypasses the mouth precludes the opportunity for the infant to practice sucking and swallowing or to experience normal hunger and satiation cycles. Infants may demonstrate aversion to oral feedings by such behaviors as averting the head to the presentation of the nipple, extruding the nipple by tongue thrust, gagging, or even vomiting.

Other observations include disinterest in or active resistance to oral play, diminished spontaneity and motivation, and shallow interpersonal relationships, probably related to the absence of some early incorporative patterns of normal oral experiences. The longer the period of nonoral feeding, the more severe the feeding problems, especially if this period occurs during a time when the infant progresses from reflexive to learned and voluntary feeding actions. Infancy is the period during which the mouth is the primary instrument for reception of stimulation and pleasure.

Infants identified as being at risk for feeding resistance should be provided with regular oral stimulation such as stroking the oral area from the cheeks to the lips, touching the tongue, placing some of the feeding on the lips and tongue, and associating feeding with pleasurable activities (holding, talking, making eye contact) based on the child's developmental level. Those who exhibit feeding aversion should begin a stimulation program to overcome resistance and acquire the ability to take nourishment by the oral route. Because management requires long-term commitment, successful implementation of a plan

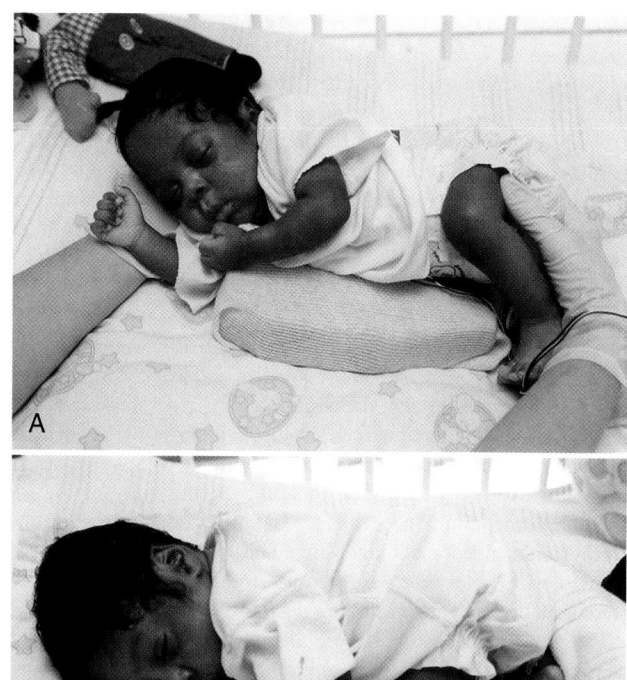

FIG 9-9 A, Preterm infant slowly transitioned to the prone position on a prone roll. **B,** Preterm infant positioned on a prone roll. (Courtesy Halbouty Premature Nursery, Texas Children's Hospital, Houston; photos by Paul Vincent Kuntz.)

for oral stimulation depends on maximum parental involvement and a multidisciplinary team approach.

Energy Conservation

One of the major goals of care for the high-risk infant is conservation of energy. Much of the care described in this section is directed toward this end (e.g., disturbing the infant as little as possible, maintaining a neutral thermal environment, gavage feeding as appropriate, promoting oxygenation, judiciously implementing any caregiving activities that increase oxygen intake and caloric consumption). An infant who is not required to expend excess energy to breathe, eat, or alter body temperature can use this energy for growth and development. Diminishing environmental noise levels and shading the infant from bright lights also promote rest (see Developmental Outcome, p. 246).

Early in hospitalization, the prone position is best for most preterm infants and results in improved oxygenation, better-tolerated feedings, and more organized sleep–rest patterns. Infants exhibit less physical activity and energy expenditure when placed in the prone position (Fig. 9-9). Prolonged supine positioning for preterm infants is not desirable because they appear to lose their sense of equilibrium when supine and use vital energy in attempts to recover balance by postural changes. In addition, prolonged supine positioning is associated with long-term problems such as decreased flexion of the limbs, pelvis, and trunk; widely abducted hips (frog-leg position); retracted and abducted shoulders; ankle and foot eversion; increased neck extension;

and increased trunk extension with neck and back arching (Altimier, 2007). The AAP, Task Force on Sudden Infant Death Syndrome (2005b) continues to affirm its position that healthy infants be placed to sleep in a supine position.* When medically stable, preterm infants should also be placed in a supine position to sleep unless conditions such as gastroesophageal reflux or upper airway anomalies make this impractical (see also Sudden Infant Death Syndrome, Chapter 11). Prone positioning for play should be provided in the nursery and encouraged after discharge.

Skin Care

The skin of preterm infants is characteristically immature relative to that of full-term infants. In most preterm infants, the skin barrier properties resemble those of the term infant by 2 to 4 weeks' postnatal age, regardless of gestational age at birth. Because of its increased sensitivity and fragility, no alkaline-based soap that might destroy the skin's acid mantle is used. The increased permeability of the skin facilitates absorption of ingredients. All skin products (e.g., alcohol, chlorhexidine, povidone–iodine) should be used with caution; the skin is rinsed with water afterward because these substances may cause severe irritation and chemical burns in VLBW and ELBW infants.

The skin is easily excoriated and denuded; therefore, care must be taken to avoid damage to the delicate structure. The total skin is thinner than that of full-term infants and lacks rete pegs, appendages that anchor the epidermis to the dermis. Therefore, there is less cohesion between the thinner skin layers. The use of adhesive tape or bandages may excoriate the skin or adhere to the skin surface so well that the epidermis can be separated from the dermis and pulled away with the tape. The use of pectin barriers and hydrocolloid adhesives may be useful because these products mold well to skin contours and adhere in moist conditions. Recommendations for protecting the

---

*Information is available from the National Institute of Child Health and Human Development's SIDS: "Back to Sleep" Campaign, http://www.nichd.nih.gov/sids.

integrity of the skin of preterm infants include using minimal adhesive tape, backing the tape with cotton, and delaying adhesive and pectin barrier removal until adherence is reduced (Lund and Kuller, 2007). Emollients such as Eucerin or Aquaphor have been used to promote skin integrity and prevent dry, cracking, and peeling skin in infants at risk for skin breakdown; however, the use of such agents has been shown to increase the risk for coagulase-negative infections in preterm infants and therefore should not be routinely used (Afsar, 2009).

It is unsafe to use scissors to remove dressings or tape from the extremities of very small and immature infants because it is easy to snip off tiny extremities or nick loosely attached skin. Solvents used to remove tape are avoided because they tend to dry and burn the delicate skin. Guidelines for skin care are listed in the Nursing Care Guidelines box.

During skin assessment of preterm infants, nurses are alert to the subtle signs that indicate zinc deficiency, a problem sometimes seen in infants who have inadequate intake or abnormal losses of zinc. Breakdown usually occurs in the areas around the mouth, buttocks, fingers, and toes. In preterm and VLBW infants, it may also occur in the creases of the neck, wrists, and ankles and around wounds. Zinc deficiency is most likely to appear in preterm infants with inadequate zinc intake, an ileostomy, short-bowel syndrome, or chronic diarrhea. Suspicious lesions are reported to the practitioner so that zinc supplements can be prescribed. Skin injuries have been reported during the use of phototherapy blankets. Caution is warranted in using these products in ELBW infants and infants who are at risk for skin breakdown.

Administration of Medications

Administration of therapeutic agents such as drugs, ointments, IV infusions, and oxygen requires judicious handling and meticulous attention to detail. The computation, preparation, and administration of drugs in minute amounts often require collaboration among members of the health care team to reduce the chance for error. In addition, the immaturity of an infant's detoxification mechanisms and

---

 NURSING CARE GUIDELINES

Neonatal Skin Care

General Skin Care
Assessment
Assess skin every day or more often as needed for redness, dryness, flaking, scaling, rashes, lesions, excoriation, and breakdown.
Identify risk factors for skin injury: gestational age ≤30 weeks, adhesive use, nutritional compromise high-frequency ventilation, extracorporeal membrane oxygenation, hypotension requiring vasopressors.
Use a valid assessment tool to provide reliable and objective measurement of skin condition.
Evaluate and report abnormal skin findings and analyze for possible causes.
Intervene according to interpretation of findings or physician order.

Bathing
Initial Bath
Assess to ensure that the infant has a stable temperature for a minimum of 2 to 4 hours before first bath.
Use cleansing agents with neutral pH or minimal dyes or perfume in water.
Use standard precautions; wear gloves.
Do not completely remove vernix; allow vernix to wear off with normal care and handling.

Bathe preterm infant younger than 32 weeks in warm water only for the first week.

Routine
Decrease frequency of baths to every second or third day by daily cleansing of eye, oral, and diaper areas and pressure points.
Use pH neutral cleanser or soaps no more than two or three times a week.
Avoid rubbing skin during bathing or drying.
Immerse stable infants fully (except head) in an appropriate-size tub.
Use swaddled immersion bathing technique: slowly unwrap after gently lowering into water for sensitive but stable infants needing assistance with motor system reactivity.

Emollients
Apply sparingly to dry, flaking, fissured areas as needed.
Choose petrolatum-based products that are free of preservatives, dyes, and perfumes.
Observe neonates ≤750 g receiving emollient therapy for increased risk of coagulase-negative *Staphylococcus* infections.
Consider dispensing emollients from hospital pharmacy, unit dose, or patient-specific container.

NURSING CARE GUIDELINES

Neonatal Skin Care—cont'd

Adhesives

Decrease use as much as possible.

Use semipermeable dressings to secure intravenous lines (IVs), nasogastric or orogastric tubes, silicone catheters, and central lines.

Use hydrogel or limb electrodes.

Consider pectin barriers beneath adhesives to protect skin.

Secure pulse oximeter probe or electrodes with elasticized dressing material (carefully avoid restricting blood flow).

Do not use adhesive remover, solvents, or bonding agents.

Avoid removing adhesives for at least 24 hours after application.

Adhesive removal can be facilitated using water, mineral oil, or petrolatum.

Remove adhesives or skin barriers slowly, supporting the skin underneath with one hand and gently peeling away the product from the skin with the other hand.

Antiseptic Agents

Apply before invasive procedures.

Consider the potential for skin breakdown or irritation with disinfectant.

No specific disinfectant is recommended over another for all neonates; remove completely with water or saline after use.

Avoid use of isopropyl alcohol for skin prep or removal of other disinfectants.

Transepidermal Water Loss (TEWL)

Minimize TEWL and heat loss in small preterm infants at <30 weeks of gestation by:

- Measuring ambient humidity during first weeks of life.
- Applying occlusive polyethylene body bag immediately at delivery and removing after infant is stabilized in the neonatal intensive care unit.
- Considering increasing humidity to 70% to 90% by using a humidified incubator for first 7 days; decrease to 50% until 28 days of age.
- Using supplemental conductive heat and reduce radiant heat source.
- Applying semipermeable transparent dressings to skin surfaces on infant's chest, abdomen, and back.

Skin Breakdown

Prevention

Decrease pressure from externally applied forces using water, air, or gel mattresses; sheepskin; or cotton bedding.

Provide adequate nutrition, including protein, fat, and zinc.

Apply transparent adhesive dressings to protect arms, elbows, and knees from friction injury.

Use tracheostomy and gastrostomy dressings (Hydrasorb or Lyofoam) for drainage and relief of pressure from tracheostomy or gastrostomy tube.

Use emollient in the diaper area (groin and thighs) to reduce urine irritation.

Treating Skin Breakdown

Irrigate wound every 4 to 8 hours with warm half-strength normal saline using a 20-ml or larger syringe and 20-gauge Teflon catheter.

Culture wound and treat if signs of infection are present (excessive redness, swelling, pain on touch, heat, or resistance to healing).

Use transparent adhesive dressing for uninfected wounds.

Apply hydrogel with or without antibacterial or antifungal ointments (as ordered) for infected wounds (may need to moisten before removal).

Use hydrocolloid for deep, uninfected wounds (leave in place for 5–7 days) or as an ostomy barrier and to improve appliance adhesion; warm barrier in hand for several minutes to soften before applying to skin.

Avoid use of antiseptic solutions for wound cleansing (use for intact skin only).

Treating Diaper Dermatitis

Maintain clean, dry skin; use absorbent diapers and change often.

If mild irritation occurs, use petrolatum barrier.

For developing dermatitis, apply a generous quantity of zinc-oxide barrier.

For severe dermatitis, identify cause and treat (frequent stooling from spina bifida, severe opiate withdrawal, or malabsorption syndrome).

Treat *Candida albicans* with antifungal ointment or cream.

Avoid powders and antibiotic ointments. (See Care of the Umbilicus and Circumcision, Chapter 8.)

Other Skin Care Concerns

Use of Substances on Skin

Evaluate all substances that come in contact with infant's skin.

Before using any topical agent, analyze components of preparation and:

- Use sparingly and only when necessary.
- Confine use to smallest possible area.
- Whenever possible and appropriate, wash off with water.
- Monitor infant carefully for signs of toxicity and systemic effects.

Use of Thermal Devices

Avoid heat lamps because of increased potential for burns. If needed, measure actual temperature of exposed skin every 15 minutes.

When using preheated transcutaneous electrodes:

- Avoid use on extremely low–birth-weight infants.
- Set at lowest possible temperature.
- Use pulse oximetry rather than transcutaneous monitoring whenever possible.

When prewarming heels before phlebotomy, avoid temperatures over 40° C.

Provide warm ambient humidity, directed away from infant; use aerosolized sterile water and maintain ambient temperature so as to not exceed 40° C.

Document use of all heating devices.

Use of Fluid Therapy and Hemodynamic Monitoring

Be certain fingers or toes are visible whenever extremity is used for peripheral IV or arterial line.

Secure catheter or needle with transparent dressing and tape to promote easy visualization of site.

Assess site hourly for signs of ischemia, infiltration, and inadequate perfusion (check capillary refill, pulses, color).

Avoid use of restraints (e.g., arm boards); if used, check that they are secured safely and not restricting circulation or movement (check for pressure areas).

Use commercial IV protector (e.g., I.V. House) with minimal tape.

Data from Johnson FE, Maikler VE: Nurses' adoption of the AWHONN/NANN Neonatal Skin Care Project, *NINR* 1(1):59–67, 2001; Kuller JM: Skin breakdown: risk factors, prevention, and treatment, *Newborn Infant Nurs Rev* 1(1):33–42, 2001; Lund CH, Kuller J, Lott JW: Neonatal skin care: clinical outcomes of the AWHONN/NANN evidence-based clinical practice guideline, *J Obstet Gynecol Neonatal Nurs* 30(1):41–51, 2001; Lund CH, Kuller J, Raines DA, and others: *Neonatal skin care: evidence-based clinical practice guideline,* ed 2, Washington, DC, 2007, AWHONN; Lund C, Lane A, Raines DA: Neonatal skin care: the scientific basis for practice, *J Obstet Gynecol Neonatal Nurs* 28(3):241–254, 1999; Taquino LT: Promoting wound healing in the neonatal setting: process versus protocol, *J Perinat Neonatal Nurs* 14(1):108–118, 2000.

inability to demonstrate symptoms of toxicity (e.g., signs of auditory nerve involvement from ototoxic drugs such as gentamicin) complicate drug therapy and require that nurses be particularly alert for signs of adverse reaction (see Administration of Medication, Chapter 22).

Nurses should be aware of the hazards of administering bacteriostatic and hyperosmolar solutions to infants. Benzyl alcohol, a common preservative in bacteriostatic water and saline, has been shown to be toxic to newborns, and products containing this preservative should not be used to flush IV catheters, to dilute or reconstitute medications, or as an anesthetic to start IVs. It is recommended that medications with preservative such as benzyl alcohol be avoided whenever possible. *Nurses must read labels carefully to detect the presence of preservatives in any medication to be administered to an infant.*

Hyperosmolar solutions present a potential danger to preterm infants. Hyperosmolar solutions given orally to infants can produce clinical, physiologic, and morphologic alterations, the most serious of which is NEC. Oral and parenteral medications should be sufficiently diluted to prevent complications related to hyperosmolality.

There has been heightened awareness of the impact of medication errors and subsequent poor outcomes for high-risk neonates. Nurses, physicians, and pharmacists must work in cooperation to implement strategies in the NICU environment to eradicate medication errors. Technology alone has not proved to be the solution; therefore, nurses must be extremely vigilant when administering medications to preterm and high-risk infants.

Developmental Outcome

Much attention has been focused on the effects of early developmental intervention on both normal and preterm infants. Infants respond to a great variety of stimuli, and the atmosphere and activities of the NICU are overstimulating. Consequently, infants in NICUs are subjected to inappropriate stimulation that can be harmful. For example, the noise level that results from monitoring equipment, alarms, and general unit activity has been correlated with the incidence of intracranial hemorrhage, especially in ELBW and VLBW infants. Personnel should reduce noise-generating activities, such as closing doors (including incubator portholes), listening to loud radios, talking loudly, and handling equipment (e.g., trash containers). Byers, Waugh, and Lowman (2006) suggest monitoring sound levels in the NICU to address problem areas. Nursing care activities, such as taking vital signs, changing the infant's position, weighing, and changing diapers, are associated with frequent periods of hypoxia, oxygen desaturation, and elevated ICP. The more immature the infant, the less able he or she is to habituate to a single procedure, such as taking an oscillometric BP, without becoming overstimulated.

Twenty-four-hour surveillance of sick infants implies maximum visibility and often bright lights. Units should establish a night-day sleep pattern by darkening the room, covering cribs with blankets, or placing eye patches over the infant's eyes at night. Infants need scheduled rest periods during which the lights are dimmed, the incubators are covered with blankets, and the infants are not disturbed for handling of any kind (Altimier, 2007). Sleep periods should be undisturbed for at least 50 minutes to allow complete sleep cycles.

Infants' eyes should be shielded from bright procedure lights to prevent potential harm. Many experts suggest that the human face, especially the parent's, is the best visual stimulus and that visual stimuli be kept to a minimum early in development. Developmental care, accentuating the infant's unique ability to achieve behavioral state organization, is tailored to the developmental level and tolerance of each infant based on a comprehensive behavioral assessment. During the early stages of development (especially before 33 weeks of gestation), external stimulation produces uncoordinated, random activity, such as jerky limb extension, hyperflexion, and irregular vital signs. At this stage, infants need to have minimum environmental stimulation. Using the developmental model of supportive care, the nurse closely monitors physiologic and behavioral signs to promote organization and well-being of the high-risk infant during handling. Softly calling the infant by name and then gently placing a hand on the body signal care is beginning and alleviate the abrupt interruption that precedes caregiving. Infants are handled with slow, controlled movements (some infants are unstable if moved abruptly), and their random movements are controlled with limbs held flexed close to their bodies during turning or other position changes. This containment or facilitated tucking may also be used before invasive procedures such as heel stick to alleviate distress. Blanket swaddling and nesting or containment have been shown to decrease physiologic and behavioral stress during routine care procedures such as bathing, weighing, and heel stick. A nest constructed by placing blanket rolls underneath the bed sheet helps infants maintain an attitude of flexion when prone or side lying.

Although it must be individually adjusted, skin-to-skin contact (kangaroo care) and short periods of gentle massage can help reduce stress in preterm infants. Regular passive skin-to-skin contact between parents (mother or father) and LBW infants has been shown to alleviate stress. The parent wears a loose-fitting, open-front top, and the undressed (except for diaper) infant is placed in a vertical position on the parent's bare chest, which permits direct eye contact, skin-to-skin sensations, and close proximity (Fig. 9-10). Skin-to-skin contact between the parent and infant, in addition to being a safe and effective method for VLBW infant–parent acquaintance, can have a positive healing effect for the mother with a high-risk pregnancy. Mothers may experience psychologic healing related to preterm delivery and regain

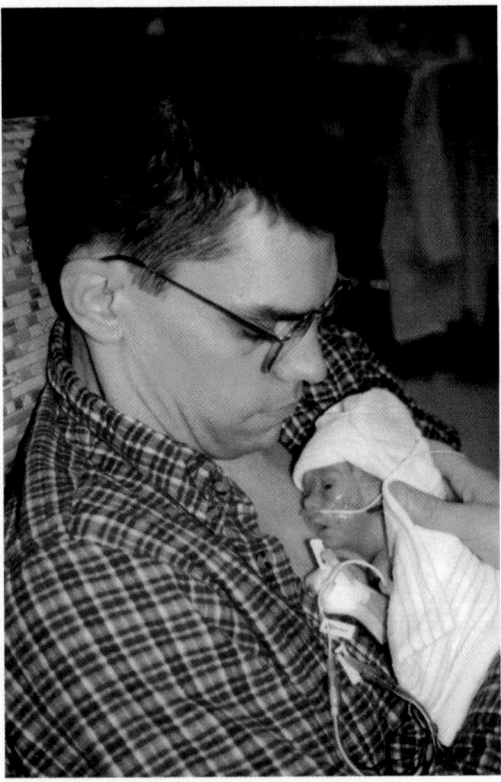

FIG 9-10 Father providing skin-to-skin (kangaroo) care. (Courtesy Judy Meyr, St. Louis.)

TABLE 9-1	SIGNS OF STRESS OR FATIGUE IN NEONATES
SUBSYSTEM	**SIGNS OF STRESS**
Autonomic	Physiologic instability
Respiratory	Tachypnea, pauses, gasping, sighing
Color	Mottled, flushed, dusky, pale or gray
Visceral	Hiccups, gagging, choking, spitting up, grunting and straining as if having a bowel movement, coughing, sneezing, yawning
Autonomic	Tremors, startles, twitches
Motor	Fluctuating tone; lack of control over movement, activity, and posture
Flaccidity	Low tone in trunk; limp, floppy upper and lower extremities; limp, drooping jaw (gape face)
Hypertonicity	Arm or leg extensions, arm(s) outstretched with fingers splayed in salute gesture, fingers stiffly outstretched, trunk arching, neck hyperextended
Hyperflexion	Trunk, extremities, fisting
Activity	Squirming; frantic, diffuse activity or little or no activity or responsiveness
State	Disorganized quality to state behaviors, including available states, maintenance of state control, and transition from one state to another
Sleep	Whimpering sounds, facial twitching, irregular respirations, fussing, grimacing, restless appearance
Awake	Glazed, unfocused look; staring; worried or pained expression; hyperalert or panicked appearance; eye roving; crying; cry-face; actively averting gaze or closing eyes; irritability; prolonged awake periods; inconsolability; frenzy
	Abrupt or rapid state changes
Other state-related behaviors and attention interaction	Efforts to attend to and interact with environmental stimulation eliciting signs of stress and disorganized subsystem functioning
Autonomic	Physiologic instability of varying degrees with autonomic, respiratory, color, and visceral responses
Motor	Fluctuating tone, increased motor activity, progressively frantic diffuse activity if stimulation continues
State	Roving eyes; gaze averting; glazed, unfocused look or worried, panicked expression; weak cry; cry-face; irritability
	Closed eyes and sleeplike withdrawal
	Abrupt state changes
	Signs of stress when presented with more than one type of stimulus at a time

Data from Als H: A synactive model of neonatal behavior organization: framework for the assessment of neurobehavioral development in the premature infant and for support of infants and parents in the neonatal intensive care environment, *Phys Occup Ther Pediatr* 6:3–55, 1986; Als H: Toward a synactive theory of development: promise for the assessment and support of infant individuality, *Infant Mental Health J* 3(4):229–243, 1982; Hunter JG: The neonatal intensive care unit. In Case-Smith J, Allen AS, Pratt PN, editors: *Occupational therapy for children*, ed 4, St. Louis, 2001, Mosby.

the mothering role through early skin-to-skin contact with their VLBW infants. Major neonatal benefits of skin-to-skin care include a reduced risk of mortality, fewer nosocomial infections, decreased length of hospital stay, maintenance of neonatal thermal stability and oxygen saturation, increased feeding vigor, and improved growth (Conde-Agudelo, Belizan, and Diaz-Rossello, 2011; Dodd, 2005). In full-term newborns, skin-to-skin contact has a strong analgesic effect during procedures such as heel lance (Cong, Ludington-Hoe, McCain, and others, 2009). LBW infants receiving skin-to-skin contact with breastfeeding mothers maintained higher oxygen saturation and were less likely to have desaturations below 90%, and their mothers were more likely to continue breastfeeding both in the hospital and for 1 month after discharge. Kangaroo care of preterm infants fosters appropriate neurobehavioral development by promoting stability of heart and respiratory function, minimizes purposeless movements, offers maternal proximity for attention, improves the infant's behavioral state, and permits self-regulating behaviors (McCain, Ludington-Hoe, Swinth, and others, 2005).

Additional research studies have confirmed the beneficial effects of developmental care with preterm infants. In addition to requiring fewer days of mechanical ventilation, preterm infants who received individualized developmental care had shorter hospital stays; a significant decrease in complications such as intraventricular hemorrhage and bronchopulmonary dysplasia; less need for sedation when critically ill; improved neurodevelopmental scores at 9, 18, and 36 months

of life; and a decrease in feeding intolerance (Symington and Pinelli, 2003; Westrup, Sizun, and Lagercrantz, 2007).

The arena of developmental care for preterm infants has expanded to include a wide variety of interventions such as infant massage, soothing soft music, recordings of parents reading stories, positioning to enhance self-regulatory abilities, enhancement of hand-to-mouth activities, uninterrupted sleep periods, decreased environmental light and noise, and even the use of stuffed animals to facilitate infant positioning. As a result of such interventions, parents may perceive the NICU environment as less threatening. Active participation in providing such an environment for their special infant also involves the parents in the provision of daily care when the newborn is critically ill and cannot be fed or held.

When infants have reached sufficient developmental organization and stability, interventions are designed and implemented to support their growing abilities. Nurses and parents become adept at learning to read infants' behavioral cues and supplying appropriate interventions (Table 9-1). Clues include both approach and avoidance behaviors. Approach behaviors that are supported and enhanced include tongue extension, hand clasp, hand-to-mouth movements, sucking, looking, and cooing. Signs of stress or fatigue that signal the infant's need for "time-out" are described in Table 9-1.

When infants are recovering and are free of support systems, medically stable, and on room air or smaller amounts of oxygen, they are assessed to document behavioral state organization and ability to

NURSING CARE GUIDELINES
Developmental Interventions

General Guidelines

Individualize interventions for each infant.

Offer stimulus only during periods of alertness.

Begin one type of stimulus at a time.

Provide intervention for short periods.

Space periods according to infant's tolerance.

Continually assess infant's response to developmental interventions.

Titrate interventions according to infant's cues.

Terminate stimulation if infant displays evidence of overstimulation (see Table 9-1).

Provide 50-minute uninterrupted sleep periods.

Handle to promote or maintain behavioral organization, providing for flexion, containment, firm pressure, grasp, and nonnutritive sucking (NNS).

Tactile

Stroke skin slowly and gently in head-to-toe direction (assess tolerance first).

Provide alternate textures (e.g., satin, velvet).

Provide firm boundaries: foot bracing, blankets, "nesting."

Encourage skin-to-skin (kangaroo) holding by parents and siblings as tolerated.

Provide containment holding in cupped palms of hand for nesting and comfort.

Auditory

Reduce noise levels.

Mother's voice is the best.

Maintain 50 dB with maximum 55 dB for only 10 minutes per hour.

Play tape of parents' and siblings' voices.

Softly play simple, soothing music, recording of womb sounds, or music box for short periods only.*

Call infant by name at each interaction.

Vestibular

Position with limbs and trunk in flexion with hands to face at midline.

Slowly change position during handling; avoid quick position changes.

Side-to-side slow movement is preferred over rocking.

Place in sling (hammock) and rock.

Close infant's fist around cloth toy.

Lift head to upright position, tip to right and then to left, stopping at midline (only with stable, more mature infants).

Avoid rapid horizontal to vertical movements in ill infant to minimize intracranial pressure and autonomic consequences (desaturation, apnea, bradycardia).

Olfactory

Pass open container or a cotton gauze dipped in breast milk or formula under nose.

Place cloth doll that has been in close contact with mother's skin in the infant's bed; avoid perfumes, scented soaps, and powders.

Use a pacifier dipped in mother's breast milk during gavage feeding for NNS.

Gustatory

Place infant's hand or a pacifier in mouth when sucking movements are observed or during gavage feeding.

Place one or two drops of milk in infant's mouth with each tube feeding.

Provide nonnutritive suckling at mother's breast.

Visual

Reduce light levels and protect eyes from direct lights such as examination or procedure lights.

Place photographs of parents and siblings in visual range (19–22 cm [7.5–8.5 in]) in en face position (maintain for short periods when awake and alert; constant picture in close proximity may be too much stimulus).

Initiate eye contact; repeat as tolerated once the infant reaches equivalent of 30 weeks of gestation. Monitor carefully for stress responses.

*Suggested infant relaxation music: *Heartbeat Lullabies* by Terry Woodford. Available from Baby-Go-To-Sleep Center, Audio Therapy Innovations, Inc., PO Box 550, Colorado Springs, CO 80901; 800-537-7748; http://www.babygotosleep.com.

self-regulate. When the infant is stable and mature enough to begin developmental intervention, activities are individualized according to each infant's cues, temperament, state, behavioral organization, and particular needs. Intervention periods are short (e.g., 2 to 3 minutes of voices, 5 minutes of quiet music). Hearing and vestibular interventions are initiated earlier than visual stimulation. One type of intervention at a time is applied to document the infant's tolerance and response (see Nursing Care Guidelines box). An intervention program for convalescing infants includes parents and siblings early in the infant's hospitalization; teaching parents to be responsive to the infant's individual cues is an important function of the NICU nurse. Parents, siblings, and health care providers are encouraged to adhere to the established developmental care plan to avoid disruption in sleep–wake cycles and minimize inappropriate stimuli.

Developmental care of preterm neonates is an ongoing process in the NICU and is incorporated into the daily care given to each infant. The nurse is cognizant of the preterm infant's developmental needs, temperament, and newborn state, as well as environmental conditions that adversely affect the infant; nursing care is planned accordingly to enhance optimum physical, psychosocial, and neurologic development. This task is often difficult to accomplish when invasive treatments or interventions are required to stabilize the critically ill neonate.

Family Support and Involvement

Professional health workers often are so absorbed in the lifesaving physical aspects of care that they ignore the emotional needs of infants and their families. The significance of early parent–child interaction and infant stimulation has been documented by reliable research. Nurses, aware of these infant and family needs, must incorporate activities that facilitate family interaction into the nursing care plan.

The birth of a preterm infant is an unexpected and stressful event for which families are emotionally unprepared. They find themselves simultaneously coping with their own needs, the needs of their infant, and the needs of their family (especially when they have other children). To compound the situation, their infant's precarious condition engenders an atmosphere of apprehension and uncertainty. They are faced with multiple crises and overwhelming feelings of responsibility, helplessness, and frustration.

All parents have some anxieties about the outcome of a pregnancy, but after a preterm birth, the concern is heightened regarding both the viability and the normalcy of their infant. Mothers may see their infant only briefly before the newborn is removed to the intensive care unit or even to another hospital, leaving them with just the recollection of the infant's very small size and unusual appearance. They often feel alone or lost on the mother–baby unit, belonging neither with mothers who have lost their infants nor with those who have delivered healthy, full-term infants. The staff and physicians are often guarded in discussing the infant's condition; mothers are continually expecting to hear that their infant has died, and they are sensitive to the anxieties of other mothers and staff members. Going home without their infant only compounds their feelings of disappointment, failure, and deprivation.

When an infant is to be transported from the hospital, the parents need a description of the facility where the infant is going. They need to know the location, reputation, and nature of the facility and the care that the infant is expected to receive. The name of the infant's physician and the telephone number of the nursery should be given to them, and unfamiliar terms such as *neonatologist, ventilator, infusion,* and *incubator* should be explained. Explanations should be kept simple, and parents are given the opportunity to ask questions. If booklets are available that describe the facility, they are given to the family.

Perhaps most important, the parents should have some contact with the infant before the transport. Being able to see, touch, and (if possible) hold their infant may help decrease the parents' anxiety. Often a photograph or even a videotape of their infant can serve as tangible evidence of the newborn's existence until the parents are able to travel to the regional facility. When possible, it is often advisable to transfer the mother to the same institution as her infant.

Parents need to be informed of their infant's progress and reassured that the infant is receiving proper care. They need to understand the smallest aspects of the infant's condition and treatment. Parents need a realistic, honest, and direct assessment of the situation. Using non-medical terminology, moving at a pace that is comfortable for parents to assimilate the information, and avoiding lengthy technical explanations facilitate communication with family members. Psychologic tasks that must be accomplished by parents during their infant's care are presented in Box 9-2.

Facilitating Parent–Infant Relationships

Because of their physiologic instability, infants are separated from their mothers immediately and surrounded by a complex, impenetrable barrier of glass windows, mechanical equipment, and special

---

BOX 9-2 PSYCHOLOGIC TASKS OF PARENTS OF A HIGH-RISK INFANT

- Work through the events surrounding labor and delivery.
- Acknowledge that the infant's life is endangered and begin the anticipatory grieving process.
- Confront and recognize feelings of inadequacy and guilt in not delivering a healthy child.
- Adapt to the neonatal intensive care environment.
- Resume parental relationships with the sick infant and initiate the caregiving role.
- Prepare to take the infant home.

Modified from Siegel R, Gardner SL, Dickey LA: Families in crisis: theoretical and practical considerations. In Gardner SL, Carter BS, Enzman-Hines M, and others, editors: *Merenstein and Gardner's handbook of neonatal intensive care,* ed 7, St. Louis, 2011, Mosby Elsevier.

---

caregivers. There is some evidence indicating that the emotional separation that accompanies the physical separation of mothers and infants may interfere with the normal mother–infant attachment process discussed in Chapter 8. Maternal attachment is a cumulative process that begins before conception, strengthens by significant events during pregnancy, and matures through mother–infant contact during the neonatal period and infancy.

When an infant is sick, the necessary physical separation appears to be accompanied by an emotional estrangement by the parents, which may seriously damage the capacity for parenting their infant. This detachment is further hampered by the tenuous nature of the infant's condition. When survival is in doubt, parents may be reluctant to establish a relationship with their infant. They prepare themselves for the infant's death while continuing to hope for recovery. This anticipatory grief (see Chapter 18) and hesitancy to embark on a relationship are evidenced by behaviors such as delay in giving the infant a name, reluctance in visiting the nursery (or when they do visit, focusing on equipment and treatments rather than on their infant), and hesitancy to touch or handle the infant when given the opportunity.

Family-centered care of high-risk newborns includes encouraging and facilitating parental involvement rather than isolating parents from their infant and associated care. This is particularly important in relation to mothers; to reduce the effects of physical separation, mothers are united with their newborn at the earliest opportunity.

Preparing the parents to see their infant for the first time is an important nursing responsibility. The nurse prepares parents for their infant's appearance, the equipment attached to the child, and the general atmosphere of the unit. The initial encounter with the intensive care unit is a stressful experience, and the frightening array of people, equipment, and activity is likely to be overwhelming. A book of photographs or pamphlets describing the NICU environment (infants in incubators or under radiant warmers, monitors, mechanical ventilators, and IV equipment) provides a useful and nonthreatening introduction to the NICU.

Parents are encouraged to visit their infant as soon as possible. Even if they saw the infant at the time of transport or shortly after birth, the infant may have changed considerably, especially if a number of medical and equipment requirements are associated with the infant's hospitalization. At the bedside, the nurse should explain the function of each piece of equipment and the role it plays in facilitating recovery. Explanations may often need to be patiently repeated because parents' anxiety over the infant's condition and the surroundings may prevent them from really "hearing" what is being said. When possible, some items related to therapy can be removed; for example, phototherapy can be temporarily discontinued and eye patches removed to permit eye-to-eye contact.

Parents appreciate the support of a nurse during the initial visit with their infant, but they may also appreciate some time alone with the infant for a short while. It is important during the early visits to emphasize the positive aspects of their infant's behavior and development so the parents can focus on their infant as an individual rather than on the equipment that surrounds the child. For example, the nurse may describe the infant's spontaneous behaviors during care, such as the grasp reflex and spontaneous movement, or make comments about the infant's biologic functions. Most institutions have open visiting policies so that parents and siblings may visit their infant as often as they wish.

Parents vary greatly in the degree to which they are able to interact with their infant. Some may wish to touch or hold their infant during the first visit, but others may not feel comfortable enough to even enter

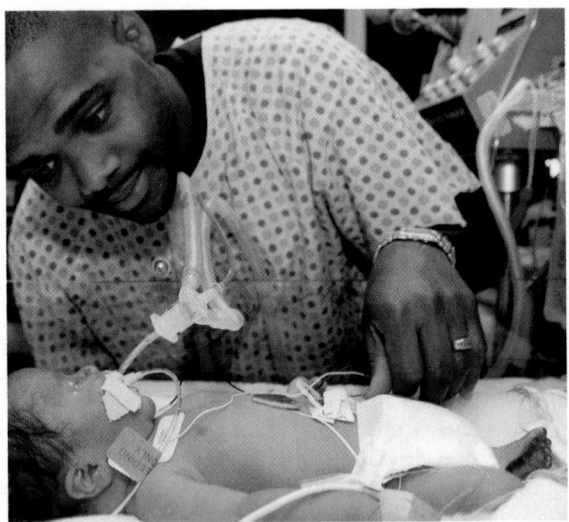

FIG 9-11 Father interacting with newborn receiving intensive care.

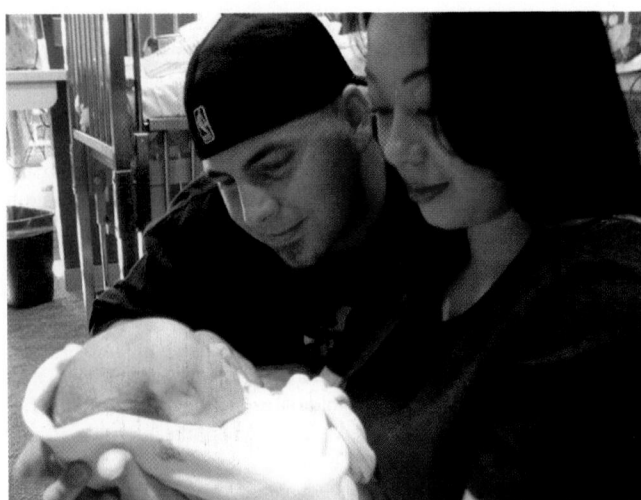

FIG 9-12 Mother and father interacting with their preterm infant. (Photo courtesy E. Jacobs, Texas Children's Hospital, Houston.)

the nursery. These reactions depend on a variety of prenatal and post-natal factors, such as the parity of the mother and her preparation before birth; the infant's size, condition, and physical appearance; and the type of treatment the infant is receiving. It is essential to recognize that the individualized pacing and quality of the interactions are more important than an early onset of these interactions. Parents may not be receptive to early and extended infant contact because they need time to adjust to the impact of an infant with birth problems and must be helped to grieve before they can accept their infant.

The parents' inability to focus on their infant is a clue for the nurse to assist the parents in expressing feelings of guilt, anxiety, helplessness, inadequacy, anger, and ambivalence. Nurses can help parents deal with these distressing feelings and recognize that they are normal responses shared by other parents. It is important to point out and reinforce the positive aspects of parents' behavior and interactions with their infant.

Most parents feel shaky and insecure about initiating interaction with their infant. Nurses can sense parents' level of readiness and offer encouragement in these initial efforts. Parents of preterm infants follow the same acquaintance process as do parents of term infants. They may quickly proceed through the process or may require several days or even weeks to complete the process. Parents begin by touching their infant's extremities with their fingertips and poking the infant tenderly and then proceed to caresses and fondling (Figs. 9-11 and 9-12). Touching is the first act of communication between parents and child. Parents need to be prepared for their infant's exaggerated and generalized startle responses to touch so they will not interpret these as negative reactions to their overtures. It may be necessary to limit tactile stimuli when the infant is critically ill and labile, but the nurse can offer other options such as speaking softly or sitting at the bedside.

Parents of acutely ill preterm infants may express feelings of help-lessness and lack of control. Involving the parent in some type of caregiving activity, no matter how minor it may seem to the nurse, enables the parent to "take on" a more active role. Examples of such caregiving for an acutely ill infant who cannot be held and is seemingly not responding positively include moistening the infant's lips with a small amount of sterile water on a cotton-tipped swab or slipping the diaper from under the infant when it is wet or soiled.

Eventually, parents begin to endow their infant with an identity—as part of the family. When an infant no longer appears as a foreign object and begins to take on aspects of family members, such as the father's

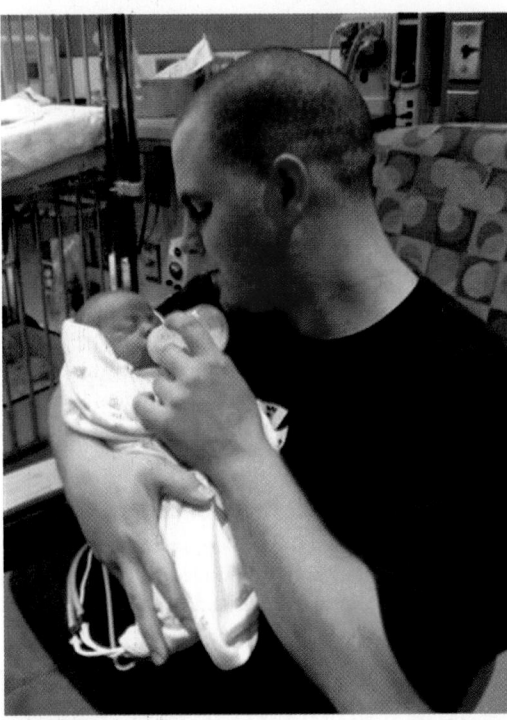

FIG 9-13 Father feeding preterm infant. (Photo courtesy E. Jacobs, Texas Children's Hospital, Houston.)

chin or the sister's nose, nurses can facilitate this incorporation. Parents are encouraged to bring in clothes, a toy, a stuffed animal, or a family snapshot for their infant, and the nurse can help parents set goals for themselves and for the infant. Parents may become involved by reading a children's storybook or nursery rhymes in a soft, soothing voice. Some families tape record the parents' voices telling or reading stories and play the tapes when the infant is able to cope with such stimuli. Feeding schedules are discussed, and parents are encouraged to visit at times when they can become involved in the care of their infant (Fig. 9-13).

Throughout the parent–infant acquaintance process, the nurse listens carefully to what the parents say to assess their concerns and their progress toward incorporating their infant into their lives. The manner in which parents refer to their infant and the questions they ask reveal their worries and feelings and can serve as valuable clues to future relationships with the infant. The alert nurse is attuned to these subtle indications of parents' needs, which provide guidelines for nursing intervention. Often all that the parents need is reassurance that they will have the support of the nurse during caregiving activities and that the behaviors about which they are concerned are normal reactions and will disappear as the infant matures.

Parents need guidance in their relationships with their infant and assistance in their efforts to meet their infant's physical and developmental needs. The nursing staff must help parents understand that their preterm infant offers few behavioral rewards and show them how to accept small rewards from their infant. The infant's reactions and behaviors are explained to parents, who take their infant's jerky, rejective behavior personally. They need reassurance that these behaviors are not a reflection on their parenting skills. Parents are taught to recognize their infant's cues regarding stimulation, handling, and other interaction, especially aversive behaviors that indicate a need for rest. Nurses need to include parents in planning their infant's care and sensory stimulation materials, such as a music box or recording.

Above all, nurses must encourage and reinforce parents during their caregiving activities and interactions with their infant to promote healthy parent–child relationships. It is also helpful for the parents to have contact and communication with a consistent group of nurses. This decreases the different information given to parents and often instills confidence that although the parents cannot be at their infant's bedside 24 hours a day, there are competent and caring nurses whom they may call to inquire about the infant's status. Periodic parent conferences involving the staff caring for the child serve to clarify misunderstandings or problems related to the infant's condition.

Siblings

In the past, concerns about sibling visitation in the NICU focused on fears of infection and disruption of nursing routines. These fears have not been substantiated, and sibling visits should be a part of the normal operation of NICUs (Fig. 9-14). Clearly defined policies and procedures should be developed to facilitate sibling visitation (AAP and ACOG, 2007; Griffin, 2006).

The birth of a preterm infant is a difficult time for siblings, who rely on the support of understanding parents. When the happy anticipation is changed to sadness, worry, and altered routines, siblings are bewildered and deprived of their parents' attention. They know something is wrong, but they have only a dim understanding of what

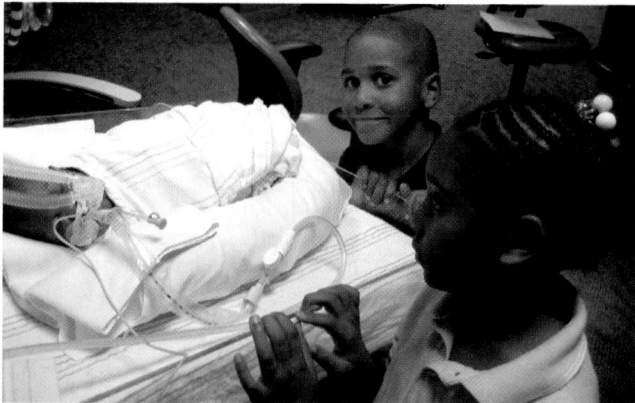

FIG 9-14 Siblings visiting in the neonatal intensive care unit. (Photo courtesy E. Jacobs, Texas Children's Hospital, Houston.)

it is. Concern about the negative effects on visiting siblings of seeing the ill newborn has not been confirmed. Children have not hesitated to approach or touch the infant, and children younger than 5 years of age have been less reluctant than older children; in addition, there have been no measurable differences between previsit and postvisit behaviors.

The potential benefits of sibling visits must be weighed against exposure of the child to the environment of the NICU. Children must be prepared for the unfamiliar NICU atmosphere, but contact with the infant appears to have a positive effect on siblings by helping them deal with the reality rather than the bizarre fantasies that are characteristic of young children. Such visits also help to bond the family as a unit.

Support Groups

Parents need to feel that they are not alone. Parent support groups have been of immeasurable value to families of infants in the NICU. Some groups consist of parents who have infants in the hospital and share the same anxieties and concerns. Other groups include parents who have had infants in the NICU and who have dealt with the crisis effectively. The groups are usually under the leadership of a staff person and involve physicians, nurses, and social workers, but the parents can offer other parents something that no one else can provide.

An excellent resource for parents of preterm infants is the book by J. Zaichkin, *Newborn Intensive Care: What Every Parent Needs to Know* (ed 3, pub. by AAP, 2010). This resource has technical and anecdotal information regarding different problems facing preterm infants, common treatments and therapies, preparation for home discharge, and home care for the preterm infant.

Discharge Planning and Home Care

Parents become apprehensive and excited as the time for discharge approaches. They have many concerns and insecurities regarding the care of their infant. They fear that the child may still be in danger, that they will be unable to recognize signs of distress or illness in their infant, and that the infant may not yet be ready for discharge. Nurses need to begin early to assist parents in acquiring or increasing their skills in the care of their infant. Appropriate instruction must be provided and sufficient time allowed for the family to assimilate the information and learn the continuing special care requirements. Where rooming-in or other live-in arrangements are available, parents can stay for a few days and nights and assume the care of their infant under the supervision and support of the nursery staff.

There should be appropriate medical and nursing follow-up and referrals to services that can benefit the family, including developmental follow-up. Parents of preterm infants should also be given adequate information about immunizations with other discharge planning information. With the trend toward earlier discharge, many hospital-based home health care agencies become involved in the follow-up and care of NICU "graduates" in the home. For the parents of an infant being discharged with equipment such as an oxygen tank, apnea monitor, or even a ventilator, discharge planning requires multidisciplinary collaborative practice to ensure that the family has not only the appropriate resources but also the available assistance for dealing with the infant's needs. Many communities have organized support groups, including those discussed previously, those designed for parents of infants who require special care because of specific defects or disabilities, and those for parents of multiple births.

Car seat safety is an essential aspect of discharge planning, and infants younger than 37 weeks of gestation should have a period of observation in an appropriate car seat to monitor for possible apnea, bradycardia, and decreased SaO$_2$ (Bull, Engle, and AAP, Committee on

Injury, Violence, and Poison Prevention and the Committee on Fetus and Newborn, 2009) (see Community Focus box). Several models can be adapted for small infants with the placement of blanket rolls on each side of the infant to support the head and trunk. For adequate support without slumping, the seat back–to-crotch strap distance must be 14 cm (5.5 inches) or less; a small rolled blanket may be placed between the crotch strap and the infant to reduce slouching. The distance from the lower harness strap to the seat bottom should be 25.5 cm (10 inches) or less to decrease the potential for the harness straps to cross the infant's ears (Howard-Salsman, 2006). The rear-facing position provides support for the head, neck, and back, thereby reducing the stress to the neck and spinal cord in a vehicle crash. Car seat manufacturers must specify recommended minimum and maximum weights for the occupant; therefore, it is important to check the manufacturer's recommendations before purchasing a car seat for a smaller infant. Additional guidelines are available from the AAP (Durbin and AAP, Committee on Injury, Violence, and Poison Prevention, 2011). (See Chapter 10 for a discussion of infant car restraints and the AAP's website* for a complete list of appropriate car seats for infants.)

An important part of discharge planning and care of preterm infants is nutrition for continued growth; thus, the choice of feeding must be carefully addressed. Human milk should be fortified according to the infant's corrected age and physiologic needs. In a Cochrane review, fortification of human milk with a multinutrient supplement for at least 12 weeks after hospital discharge was found to result in higher rates of growth (McCormick, Henderson, Fahey, and others, 2010). Full-term infant formulas are not considered adequate for proper growth in preterm infants.

Knowing that staff members are available for telephone or personal contact when the parents take the infant home provides a measure of security to anxious parents. Many NICU facilities maintain a policy of open communication between staff and parents both during the infant's hospitalization and after discharge. It is the responsibility of the NICU staff to make certain that parents are prepared to care for their infant, both emotionally and physically. At the same time, it is important that parents establish a trusting relationship with the infant's primary care provider in the community before discharge from the acute care facility.

Neonatal Loss

The precarious nature of many high-risk infants makes death a real and ever-present possibility. Although infant mortality has been reduced sharply with improved technology, the mortality rate is still greatest during the neonatal period. Nurses in the NICU are the persons who must prepare the parents for an inevitable death, provide end-of-life care for the infant and family, and facilitate a family's grieving process after an expected or unexpected death.

The loss of an infant has special meaning for the grieving parents. It represents a loss of a part of themselves (especially for mothers), a loss of the potential for immortality that offspring represent, and the loss of the dream child that has been fantasized about throughout the pregnancy. There is often a sense of emptiness and failure. In addition, when an infant has lived for such a short time, there may be few, if any, pleasant memories to serve as a basis for the identification and idealization that are part of the resolution of a loss.

To help parents understand that the death is a reality, it is important that they be encouraged to hold their infant before death and, if

possible, be present at the time of death so their infant can die in their arms if they choose. Many who deny the need to hold their infant may later regret the decision.

Parents are given the opportunity to actually "parent" the infant in any manner they wish or are able to do before and after the death. This

---

🏠 **COMMUNITY FOCUS**

Preterm and Near-Term Infant Car Seat Evaluation

The American Academy of Pediatrics (AAP) (Bull, Engle, and Committee on Injury, Violence, and Poison Prevention and the Committee on Fetus and Newborn, 2009) recommends that infants born before 37 weeks of gestation be evaluated for apnea, bradycardia, and oxygen desaturation episodes before hospital discharge.* The AAP suggests that facilities develop policies for the implementation of a program of evaluation; however, few evidence-based practice recommendations have been published to date delineating specific requirements for such a program. Based on the available literature, suggestions for providing a car seat evaluation of infants born before 37 weeks of gestation include:

- Use the parents' car seat for the evaluation.
- Perform the evaluation 1 to 7 days before the infant's anticipated discharge.
- Secure the infant in the car seat per guidelines using blanket rolls on the side.
- Set the pulse oximeter low alarm at 88% (or per unit protocol).
- Set the heart rate low alarm limit at 80 beats/min and apnea alarm at 20 seconds (cardiorespiratory monitor).
- Leave the infant undisturbed semiupright in the car seat for a minimum of 90 to 120 minutes or for the time period parents state it takes (whichever is longer) to arrive at their home.
- Document the infant's tolerance to the car seat evaluation.
- An episode of desaturation, bradycardia, or apnea (20 seconds or more) constitutes a failure, and evaluation by the practitioner must occur before discharge. If the infant experiences this in a semiupright position, a car bed with the infant supine should be considered, and similar testing should be undertaken in the car bed.
- Repeat the test after 24 hours after modifications have been made to the car seat, car bed, or infant's position in either restraint system.
- It is recommended that a certified car seat technician place the infant in the car seat (or bed) if a failure occurs (see National Highway Traffic Safety Administration website† for car seat inspection station).
- If the infant is being discharged on an apnea or cardiorespiratory monitor, this equipment should be used during the trip home.
- The technician will demonstrate appropriate positioning of the infant in the restraint device to the parents and have the parents do a return demonstration.
- Document the interventions, the infant's tolerance, and the parents' return demonstration.

Modified from American Academy of Pediatrics: Safe transportation of premature and low birth weight infants, *Pediatrics* 97(5):758–760, 1996; American Academy of Pediatrics: Transporting children with special health care needs, *Pediatrics* 104(4):988–992, 1999; Bull MJ, Engle WA, and Committee on Injury, Violence, and Poison Prevention and the Committee on Fetus and Newborn: Safe transportation of preterm and low birth weight infants at hospital discharge, *Pediatrics* 123(5):1424–1429, 2009.

*Infants at risk for obstructive apnea (e.g., Pierre Robin sequence or congenital neuromuscular disorders such as spinal muscular atrophy) may also need to be evaluated in a semiupright car seat or car bed before discharge.

†http://www.nhtsa.gov.

---

*http://www.aap.org/healthtopics/carseatsafety.cfm.

may include seeing, touching, holding, caressing, and talking to their infant privately; the parents may also wish to bathe and dress the infant. If parents are hesitant about seeing their dead infant, it is advisable to keep the body in the unit for a few hours because many parents change their minds after the initial shock of the death.

Parents may need to see and hold the infant more than once—the first time to say "hello" and the last time to say "good-bye." If parents wish to see the infant after the body has been taken to the morgue, the infant should be retrieved, wrapped in a blanket, rewarmed in a radiant warmer, and taken to the mother's room or other private place. The nurse should stay with the parents and provide them an opportunity for private time alone with their dead infant. Individual grief responses of the mother and father should be recognized and handled appropriately; gender differences and cultural and religious beliefs will affect the parents' grief responses.

A hospice approach for families with infants for whom the decision has been made to not prolong life and who are receiving only palliative care may be implemented in such cases. Another approach is to send the family home with the infant and allow them to spend time together until the eventual death; hospice services may be available, and supportive care is provided in the home setting. Some families find this option less restrictive and more family oriented than being in the hospital setting. (See Chapter 18 for further discussion of hospice care.)

A photograph of the infant taken before or after death is highly desirable. Parents may wish to have a special family portrait taken with the infant and other family members; this often helps personalize and make the experience more tangible. The parents may not wish to see the photograph at the time of death, but the chance to refer to it later will help make their infant seem more real, which is a part of the normal grief process. A photograph of their infant being held by the hand or touched by an adult offers a more positive image than a morgue type of photograph. A bereavement or memory packet can be given to the grieving parents and family; it may include the infant's handprints and footprints; a lock of hair; the bedside name card; the ID bracelet or armbands; and, as appropriate to the family's religious beliefs, a certificate of baptism.

Naming the deceased infant is an important step in the grieving process. Some parents may hesitate to give the newborn a name that had been chosen during the pregnancy for their "special baby." However, having a tangible person for whom to grieve is an important component of the grieving process.

A nurse who is familiar to the family should be present during the discussion about the dead or dying infant. The nurse should talk with parents openly and honestly about funeral arrangements because few parents have had experience with this aspect of death. Many funeral homes now offer inexpensive arrangements for these special cases. Someone from the NICU should take the responsibility for acquiring this type of information. It is often helpful to parents for the NICU to have a list of local funeral homes, services offered, and prices. Families need to be informed of the options available, but a funeral is preferable because the ritual provides an opportunity for parents to feel the support of friends and relatives. A member of the clergy of the appropriate faith may be notified if the parents wish. Issues regarding an autopsy or organ donation (when appropriate) are approached in a multidisciplinary fashion (primary practitioner and primary nurse) with respect, sensitivity to cultural and religious beliefs, tact, and consideration of the family's wishes. (For additional suggestions for helping families who experience neonatal loss, see Grief and Perinatal Loss by Gardner and Dickey, 2011, and Jansen, 2003.)

Before the parents leave the hospital, they are given the telephone number of the unit (if they do not have it) and invited to call any time

they have any further questions. Many intensive care units make a point to contact the parents several weeks after a neonatal death to assess the parents' coping mechanisms, evaluate the grieving process, and provide support as needed. Several organizations are available to offer support and understanding to families who have lost a newborn; these organization include the Compassionate Friends,* Aiding Mothers and Fathers Experiencing Neonatal Death (AMEND),† and Share Pregnancy and Infant Loss Support, Inc.‡ (See also Chapter 18 for further discussion of the family and the grief process.)

Nurses who care for critically ill infants also experience grief; NICU nurses may feel helpless and sorrowful. It is important that such grief be allowed and that nurses attend the funeral or memorial service as a part of working through the grief process. Nurses may fear that showing emotion is unprofessional and that the expression of grief indicates "loss of control." These fears are unfounded. Studies have demonstrated that to continue to be effective managers and providers of care, nurses must be allowed to grieve and support each other through the process (Gardner and Dickey, 2011).

Baptism

Because many Christian parents wish to have their child baptized if death is anticipated or is a decided possibility, this may become a nursing responsibility. Whenever possible, it is most desirable that a representative of the parents' faith (e.g., a Roman Catholic priest or a Protestant minister) perform such a ritual. When death is imminent, a nurse or a physician can perform the baptism by simply pouring water on the infant's forehead (a medicine dropper is a convenient means) while repeating the words, "I baptize you in the name of the Father and of the Son and of the Holy Spirit." This includes a birth of any gestational age, particularly when the parents are Roman Catholic.

When the parents' faith is uncertain, a conditional baptism can be carried out by saying, "If you are capable of receiving baptism, I baptize you in the name of the Father and of the Son and of the Holy Spirit." The baptism is recorded in the infant's chart, and a notice is placed on the crib or incubator. Parents are informed at the first opportunity.

▌HIGH RISK RELATED TO DYSMATURITY

PRETERM INFANTS

Prematurity accounts for the largest number of admissions to NICUs. Immaturity of most organ systems places infants at risk for a variety of neonatal complications (e.g., hyperbilirubinemia, respiratory distress syndrome [RDS], intellectual and motor delays). Low birth weight and prematurity were the second leading cause of infant mortality in the United States in 2006 (Heron, Hoyert, Murphy, and others, 2009). The actual cause of prematurity is not known in most instances. Factors such as poverty, maternal infections, previous preterm delivery, multiple pregnancies, pregnancy-induced hypertension, and placental problems that interrupt the normal course of gestation before completion of fetal development are responsible for a large number of preterm births. Additional factors are listed in Box 9-3.

---

*PO Box 3696, Oakbrook, IL 60522-3696; 630-990-0010, 877-969-0010; http://www.compassionatefriends.org/home.aspx.
†Contact Maureen Connelly, 4324 Berrywick Terrace, St. Louis, MO 63128; 314-487-7582; or Martha Eise, Martha@amendgroup.com; http://www.amendgroup.com.
‡National Share Office, 402 Jackson Street, St. Charles, MO, 63301; 800-821-6819.

BOX 9-3   ETIOLOGY OF PRETERM BIRTH

Maternal Factors

Socioeconomic
- Malnutrition
- Age
- Race

Chronic medical conditions
- Heart disease
- Renal disease
- Diabetes
- Hypertension

Behavioral
- Substance abuse
- Smoking
- Poor or absent prenatal care

Factors Related to Pregnancy

Multiple pregnancy

Low body mass index (<19.8 kg/m²) (Fanaroff, 2011)

Abruptio placentae or placenta previa

Incompetent cervix

Premature rupture of membranes or chorioamnionitis

Polyhydramnios or oligohydramnios

Infection

Trauma

Fetal Factors

Chromosomal abnormalities

Congenital anomalies

Nonimmune hydrops

Erythroblastosis

Unknown Factors

The outlook for preterm infants is largely, but not entirely, related to the state of physiologic and anatomic immaturity of the various organs and systems at the time of birth. Infants at term have advanced to a state of maturity sufficient to allow a successful transition to the extrauterine environment. Preterm infants must make the same adjustments but with functional immaturity proportional to the stage of development reached at the time of birth. These adjustments, however, may be limited or even hindered by the external environment to which the preterm infant is exposed. Exposure to excessive stimuli, bacteria, and viruses make the environment less conducive for preterm infants to grow and develop. The degree to which infants are prepared for extrauterine life can be predicted to some extent by birth weight and estimated gestational age (see Clinical Assessment of Gestational Age, Chapter 8).

Within the past decade, increasing attention has been given to late preterm infants, that is, infants born between 34 and 36⅞ weeks' gestation. Such infants have some of the same risk factors as those born before 34 weeks' gestation, but physical characteristics and adaptation to extrauterine life are variable. Late preterm infants have metabolic and physical immaturity that places them at risk for greater mortality and morbidity than term infants (Engle, Tomashek, Wallman, and others, 2007). Studies have demonstrated decreased cognitive and motor function in late preterm infants at 24 months compared with term infants (Woythaler, McCormick, and Smith, 2011). In the following sections, the discussion of preterm infants continues to apply to all infants who are born before a completed gestational age of 37 weeks.

Because prematurity now encompasses a wider age, weight, and physiologic maturity range, physical characteristics described may also vary; such descriptions are generalized for description purposes.

Diagnostic Evaluation

Preterm infants have a number of distinct characteristics at various stages of development. Identification of these characteristics provides valuable clues to the gestational age and hence to the infant's physiologic capabilities. The general, outward physical appearance changes as the infant progresses to maturity. Characteristics of skin, general attitude (or posture) when supine, appearance of hair, and amount of subcutaneous fat provide cues to a newborn's physical development. Observation of spontaneous, active movements and response to stimulation and passive movement contributes to the assessment of neurologic status. The appraisal is made as soon as possible after admission to the nursery because much of the observation and management of infants depends on this information.

On inspection, preterm infants are very small and appear scrawny because they have only minimal subcutaneous fat deposits (or none in some cases) and have a proportionately large head in relation to the body, which reflects the cephalocaudal direction of growth. The skin is bright pink (often translucent, depending on the degree of immaturity), smooth, and shiny, with small blood vessels clearly visible underneath the thin epidermis. The fine lanugo hair is abundant over the body (depending on gestational age) but is sparse, fine, and fuzzy on the head. The ear cartilage is soft and pliable, and the soles and palms have minimal creases, resulting in a smooth appearance. The bones of the skull and the ribs feel soft, and the eyes may be closed. Male infants have few scrotal rugae, and the testes are undescended; in girls, the labia and clitoris are prominent. Figure 9-15 compares the features of full-term and preterm infants.

In contrast to full-term infants' overall attitude of flexion and continuous activity, preterm infants may be inactive and listless. The extremities maintain an attitude of extension and remain in any position in which they are placed. Reflex activity is only partially developed—sucking is absent, weak, or ineffectual; swallow, gag, and cough reflexes are absent or weak; and other neurologic signs are absent or diminished. Physiologically immature, preterm infants are unable to maintain body temperature, have limited ability to excrete solutes in the urine, and have increased susceptibility to infection. A pliable thorax, immature lung tissue, and an immature regulatory center lead to periodic breathing, hypoventilation, and frequent periods of apnea. They are more susceptible to biochemical alterations such as hyperbilirubinemia and hypoglycemia, and they have a higher extracellular water content that renders them more vulnerable to fluid and electrolyte derangements. Preterm infants exchange fully half of their extracellular fluid volume every 24 hours compared with one seventh of the volume in adults.

The soft cranium is subject to characteristic unintentional deformation caused by positioning from one side to the other on a mattress. The head looks disproportionately longer from front to back, is flattened on both sides, and lacks the usual convexity seen at the temporal and parietal areas. This positional molding is often a concern to parents and may influence the parents' perception of the infant's attractiveness and their responsiveness to the infant. Positioning the infant on a waterbed or gel mattress can reduce or minimize cranial molding.

Neurologic impairment (e.g., intraventricular hemorrhage) and serious sequelae correlate with the size and gestational age of infants at birth and with the severity of neonatal complications. The greater the degree of immaturity, the greater the degree of potential disability. A greater incidence of cerebral palsy, attention-deficit/hyperactivity

PRETERM   TERM

Posture—The preterm infant lies in a "relaxed attitude," limbs more extended; the body size is small, and the head may appear somewhat larger in proportion to the body size. The term infant has more subcutaneous fat tissue and rests in a more flexed attitude.

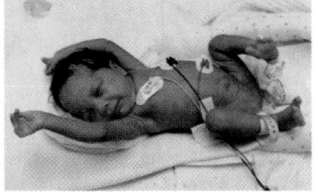 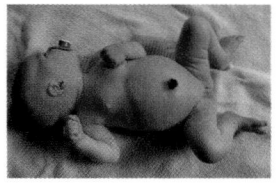

Ear—The preterm infant's ear cartilages are poorly developed, and the ear may fold easily; the hair is fine and feathery, and lanugo may cover the back and face. The mature infant's ear cartilages are well formed, and the hair is more likely to form firm, separate strands.

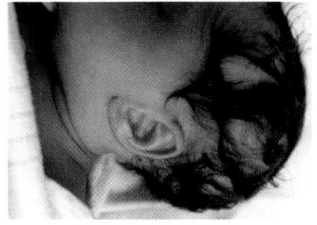 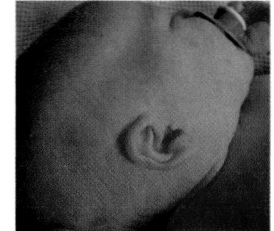

Sole—The sole of the foot of the preterm infant appears more turgid and may have only fine wrinkles. The mature infant's sole (foot) is well and deeply creased.

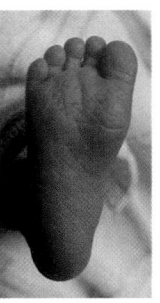 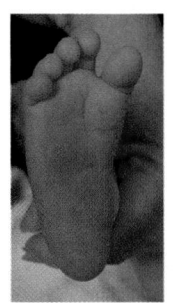

Female genitalia—The preterm female infant's clitoris is prominent, and labia majora are poorly developed and gaping. The mature female infant's labia majora are fully developed, and the clitoris is not as prominent.

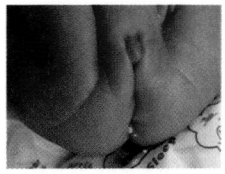 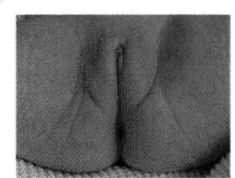

Male genitalia—The preterm male infant's scrotum is undeveloped and not pendulous; minimal rugae are present, and the testes may be in the inguinal canals or in the abdominal cavity. The term male infant's scrotum is well developed, pendulous, and rugated, and the testes are well down in the scrotal sac.

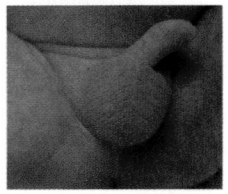 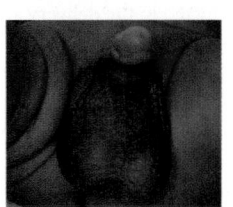

Scarf sign—The preterm infant's elbow may be easily brought across the chest with little or no resistance. The mature infant's elbow may be brought to the midline of the chest, resisting attempts to bring the elbow past the midline.

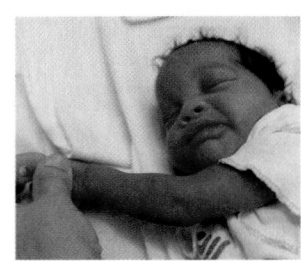 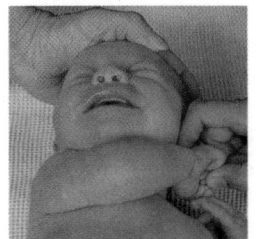

FIG 9-15 Clinical and neurologic examinations comparing preterm and full-term infants. (Data from Pierog SH, Ferrara A: *Medical care of the sick newborn*, ed 2, St. Louis, 1976, Mosby.)

Continued

NEUROLOGIC EVALUATION

PRETERM	TERM

Grasp reflex—The preterm infant's grasp is weak; the term infant's grasp is strong, allowing the infant to be lifted up from the mattress.

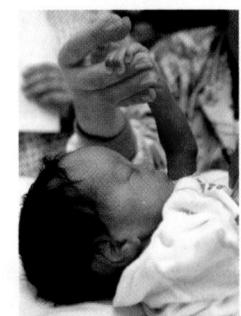 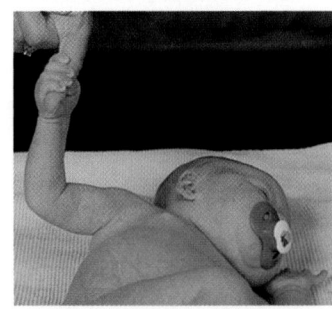

Heel-to-ear maneuver—The preterm infant's heel is easily brought to the ear, meeting with no resistance. This maneuver is not possible in the term infant, since there is considerable resistance at the knee.

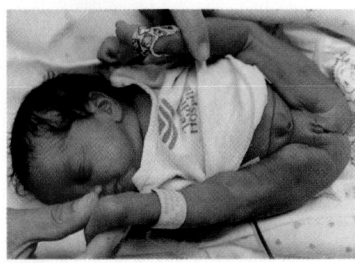 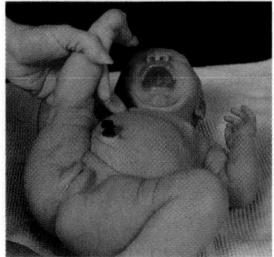

FIG 9-15, cont'd

disorder (ADHD), visual-motor deficits, and altered intellectual functioning is observed in preterm than in full-term infants. However, behavioral development can be enhanced when families are provided with support and infants are referred to appropriate services for neurologic and developmental interventions. Parental interest and involvement are important variables in the developmental progress of infants.

Therapeutic Management

When delivery of a preterm infant is anticipated, the intensive care nursery is alerted and a team approach implemented. Ideally, a neonatologist, an advanced practice nurse, a staff nurse, and a respiratory therapist are present for the delivery. Infants who do not require resuscitation are immediately transferred in a heated incubator to the NICU, where they are weighed and where IV lines, oxygen therapy, and other therapeutic interventions are initiated as needed. Resuscitation is conducted in the delivery area until infants can be safely transported to the NICU.

Subsequent care is determined by the infant's status. The general care of preterm infants differs from that of full-term infants primarily in the areas of respiratory support, temperature regulation, nutrition, susceptibility to infection, activity intolerance, neurodevelopmental care, and other consequences of physical immaturity.

Nursing Care Management

The nursing care, similar to the therapeutic management, is individualized for each infant. See appropriate discussions under Nursing Care of the High-Risk Newborn and Family for additional details of care.

POSTTERM INFANTS

Infants born of a gestation that extends beyond 42 weeks as calculated from the mother's last menstrual period (or by gestational age assessment) are considered to be postterm, or postmature, regardless of birth weight. This constitutes 3.5% to 15% of all pregnancies. The cause of delayed birth is unknown. Some infants are appropriate for gestational age but show the characteristics of progressive placental dysfunction. These infants display characteristics such as absence of lanugo, little if any vernix caseosa, abundant scalp hair, and long fingernails. The skin is often cracked, parchment-like, and desquamating. A common finding in postterm infants is a wasted physical appearance that reflects intrauterine deprivation. Depletion of subcutaneous fat gives them a thin, elongated appearance. The little vernix caseosa that remains in the skinfolds may be stained a deep yellow or green, which is usually an indication of meconium in the amniotic fluid.

There is a significant increase in fetal and neonatal mortality in postterm infants compared with those born at term. They are especially prone to fetal distress associated with the decreasing efficiency of the placenta, macrosomia, and meconium aspiration syndrome. The greatest risk occurs during the stresses of labor and delivery, particularly in infants of **primigravidas**, or women delivering their first child. Close surveillance with fetal assessment and induction of labor is usually recommended when infants are significantly overdue.

HIGH RISK RELATED TO PHYSIOLOGIC FACTORS

HYPERBILIRUBINEMIA

The term **hyperbilirubinemia** refers to an excessive level of accumulated bilirubin in the blood and is characterized by **jaundice**, or **icterus**, a yellowish discoloration of the skin, sclerae, and nails. Hyperbilirubinemia is a common finding in newborns and in most instances is relatively benign. However, in extreme cases, it can indicate a pathologic state.

Hyperbilirubinemia may result from increased unconjugated or conjugated bilirubin. The unconjugated form or indirect hyperbilirubinemia (Table 9-2) is the type most commonly seen in newborns. The following discussion of hyperbilirubinemia is limited to unconjugated hyperbilirubinemia.

TABLE 9-2	COMPARISON OF MAJOR TYPES OF UNCONJUGATED HYPERBILIRUBINEMIA*		
PHYSIOLOGIC JAUNDICE	BREASTFEEDING-ASSOCIATED JAUNDICE (EARLY ONSET)	BREAST MILK JAUNDICE (LATE ONSET)	HEMOLYTIC DISEASE
Cause			
Immature hepatic function plus increased bilirubin load from red blood cell (RBC) hemolysis	Decreased milk intake related to fewer calories consumed by infant before mother's milk is well established; enterohepatic shunting	Possible factors in breast milk that prevent bilirubin conjugation Less frequent stooling	Blood antigen incompatibility causing hemolysis of large numbers of RBCs Liver's inability to conjugate and excrete excess bilirubin from hemolysis
Onset			
After 24 hr (preterm infants, prolonged)	2nd–4th day	4th–8th day	During first 24 hr (levels increase >5 mg/dl/day)
Peak			
3rd–4th day	3rd–5th day	10th–15th day	Variable
Duration			
Declines on 5th–7th day	Variable	May remain jaundiced for 3–12 wk or more	Depends on severity and treatment
Therapy			
Increase frequency of feedings and avoid supplements. Evaluate stooling pattern. Monitor transcutaneous bilirubin (TcB) or total serum bilirubin (TSB) level. Perform risk assessment (see Fig. 9-16, *A*). Use phototherapy if bilirubin levels increase significantly or significant hemolysis is present	Breastfeed frequently (10–12 times/day); avoid supplements such as water, dextrose water, and formula. Evaluate stooling pattern; stimulate as needed. Perform risk assessment (see Fig. 9-16, *A*). Use phototherapy if bilirubin levels increase significantly or significant hemolysis is present. If phototherapy is instituted, evaluate benefits and harm of temporarily discontinuing breastfeeding; additional assessments may be required. Assist mother with maintaining milk supply; feed expressed milk as appropriate. After discharge, follow up according to hour of discharge (see pp. 258–259).	Increase frequency of breastfeeding; use no supplementation such as glucose water; cessation of breastfeeding is not recommended. Perform risk assessment (see Fig. 9-16, *A*). Consider performing additional evaluations: glucose-6-phosphate dehydrogenase, direct and indirect serum bilirubin, family history, and others as necessary. May include home phototherapy with a temporary (10–12 hr) discontinuation of breastfeeding; a subsequent TSB may be drawn to evaluate a drop in serum levels. Assist mother with maintenance of milk supply and reassurance regarding her milk supply and therapy. Use formula supplements only at practitioner's discretion.	Monitor TcB or TSB level. Perform risk assessment (see Fig. 9-16, *A*). Postnatal—Use phototherapy; administer intravenous immunoglobulin per protocol; if severe, perform exchange transfusion. Prenatal—Perform transfusion (fetus). Prevent sensitization (Rh incompatibility) of Rh-negative mother with Rh_0(D) immune globulin (RhIg). If mother is breastfeeding, assist with maintenance and storage of milk; may bottle feed expressed milk as appropriate to therapy. Minimize maternal–infant separation and encourage contact as appropriate.

*Table depicts patterns of jaundice in term infants; patterns in preterm infants vary according to factors such as gestational age, birth weight, and illness.

Pathophysiology

Bilirubin is one of the breakdown products of the hemoglobin that results from RBC destruction. When RBCs are destroyed, the breakdown products are released into the circulation, where the hemoglobin splits into two fractions: heme and globin. The globin (protein) portion is used by the body, and the heme portion is converted to unconjugated bilirubin, an insoluble substance bound to albumin.

In the liver, the bilirubin is detached from the albumin molecule and, in the presence of the enzyme glucuronyl transferase, is conjugated with glucuronic acid to produce a highly soluble substance, conjugated bilirubin, which is then excreted into the bile. In the intestine, bacterial action reduces the conjugated bilirubin to urobilinogen, the pigment that gives stool its characteristic color. Most of the reduced bilirubin is excreted through the feces; a small amount is eliminated in the urine.

Normally, the body is able to maintain a balance between the destruction of RBCs and the use or excretion of byproducts. However, when developmental limitations or a pathologic process interferes with this balance, bilirubin accumulates in the tissues to produce jaundice. Possible causes of hyperbilirubinemia in newborns are:

- Physiologic (developmental) factors (prematurity)
- An association with breastfeeding or breast milk
- Excess production of bilirubin (e.g., hemolytic disease, biochemical defects, bruises)
- Disturbed capacity of the liver to secrete conjugated bilirubin (e.g., enzyme deficiency, bile duct obstruction)
- Combined overproduction and undersecretion (e.g., sepsis)
- Some disease states (e.g., hypothyroidism, galactosemia, infant of a diabetic mother)
- Genetic predisposition to increased production (American Indians, Asians)

The most common cause of hyperbilirubinemia is the relatively mild and self-limited physiologic jaundice, or icterus neonatorum. Unlike hemolytic disease of the newborn (HDN) (see p. 263), physiologic jaundice is not associated with any pathologic process. Although almost all newborns experience elevated bilirubin levels, only about 50% to 60% demonstrate observable signs of jaundice (Blackburn, 2011).

Two phases of physiologic jaundice have been identified in full-term infants. In the first phase, bilirubin levels of formula-fed white and African-American infants gradually increase to approximately 5 to 6 mg/dl by 3 to 4 days of life and then decrease to a plateau of 2 to 3 mg/dl by the fifth day (Blackburn, 2011). Bilirubin levels maintain a steady plateau state in the second phase without increasing or decreasing until approximately 12 to 14 days, at which time levels decrease to the normal value of 1 mg/dl (Blackburn, 2011). This pattern varies according to racial group, method of feeding (breast vs. bottle), and gestational age. In preterm formula-fed infants, serum bilirubin levels may peak as high as 10 to 12 mg/dl at 5 or 6 days of life and decrease slowly over a period of 2 to 4 weeks (Blackburn, 2011).

As noted above, infants of Asian descent (as well as American Indians) have mean bilirubin levels almost twice those seen in whites or African Americans. An increased incidence of hyperbilirubinemia is seen in newborns from certain geographic areas, particularly areas around Greece. These populations may have glucose-6-phosphate dehydrogenase (G6PD) deficiency, which can cause hemolytic anemia.

On average, newborns produce twice as much bilirubin as do adults because of higher concentrations of circulating erythrocytes and a shorter life span of RBCs (only 70 to 90 days in contrast to 120 days in older children and adults). In addition, the liver's ability to conjugate bilirubin is reduced because of limited production of glucuronyl transferase. Newborns also have a lower plasma-binding capacity for bilirubin because of reduced albumin concentrations compared with older children. Normal changes in hepatic circulation after birth may contribute to excess demands on liver function.

Normally, conjugated bilirubin is reduced to **urobilinogen** by the intestinal flora and excreted in feces. However, the relatively sterile and less motile newborn bowel is initially less effective in excreting urobilinogen. In the newborn intestine, the enzyme β-glucuronidase is able to convert conjugated bilirubin into the unconjugated form, which is subsequently reabsorbed by the intestinal mucosa and transported to the liver. This process, known as **enterohepatic circulation**, or **shunting**, is accentuated in newborns and is thought to be a primary mechanism in physiologic jaundice (Blackburn, 2011). Feeding (1) stimulates peristalsis and produces more rapid passage of meconium, thus diminishing the amount of reabsorption of unconjugated bilirubin, and (2) introduces bacteria to aid in the reduction of bilirubin to urobilinogen. Colostrum, a natural cathartic, facilitates meconium evacuation.

Breastfeeding is associated with an increased incidence of jaundice as a result of two distinct processes. **Breastfeeding-associated jaundice (early-onset jaundice)** begins at 2 to 4 days of age and occurs in approximately 12% to 35% of breastfed newborns (Blackburn, 2011). The jaundice is related to the process of breastfeeding and probably results from decreased caloric and fluid intake by breastfed infants before the milk supply is well established because decreased milk intake is associated with increased enterohepatic circulation of bilirubin (Watchko, 2009). Reduced fluid intake results in dehydration, which also concentrates the bilirubin in the blood.

Breast milk jaundice (late-onset jaundice) begins at age 5 to 7 days and occurs in 2% to 4% of breastfed infants (Blackburn, 2011). Rising levels of bilirubin peak during the second week and gradually diminish. Despite high levels of bilirubin that may persist for 3 to 12 weeks, these infants are well. The jaundice may be caused by factors in the breast milk (pregnanediol, fatty acids, and β-glucuronidase) that either inhibit the conjugation or decrease the excretion of bilirubin. Less

frequent stooling by breastfed infants may allow for an extended time for reabsorption of bilirubin from stools.

Diagnostic Evaluation

The degree of jaundice is determined by serum bilirubin measurements. Normal values of unconjugated bilirubin are 0.2 to 1.4 mg/dl. In newborns, levels must exceed 5 mg/dl before jaundice (icterus) is observable. It is important to note, however, that the evaluation of jaundice is not based solely on serum bilirubin levels but also on the timing of the appearance of clinical jaundice; gestational age at birth; age in days since birth; family history, including maternal Rh factor; evidence of hemolysis; feeding method; infant's physiologic status; and the progression of serial serum bilirubin levels. The following criteria are indicators of pathologic jaundice that, when present, warrant further investigation as to the cause of the jaundice. It is not an all-inclusive list; other factors are also evaluated:

- Persistent jaundice over 2 weeks in a full-term formula-fed infant
- Total serum bilirubin levels over 12.9 mg/dl (term infant) or over 15 mg/dl (preterm infant); the upper limit for breastfed infant is 15 mg/dl
- Increase in serum bilirubin by 5 mg/dl/day
- Direct bilirubin exceeding 1.5 to 2 mg/dl
- Total serum bilirubin level over the 95th percentile for age (in hours) on an hour-specific nomogram (Fig. 9-16)

Risk factors that have been identified and that may place newborns at high risk for hyperbilirubinemia include maternal race (e.g., Asian or Asian American), late preterm birth, jaundice observed in the first 24 hours of life, significant bruising, cephalhematoma, exclusive breastfeeding, blood group incompatibility or hemolytic disease such as G6PD, and history of sibling with hyperbilirubinemia (Watchko, 2009).

Noninvasive monitoring of bilirubin via cutaneous reflectance measurements (**transcutaneous bilirubinometry [TcB]**) allows for repetitive estimations of bilirubin and, when used correctly, may decrease the need for invasive monitoring (Thayyil and Marriott, 2005). The new TcB monitors provide accurate measurements within 2 to 3 mg/dl in most neonatal populations at serum levels below 15 mg/dl (AAP, Subcommittee on Hyperbilirubinemia, 2004). TcB monitors must be used according to published guidelines as a screening tool, not as a predictor of need for therapy; multiple readings over time at a consistent site (e.g., sternum or forehead) are of more value than a single reading. After phototherapy has been initiated, TcB is no longer useful as a screening tool.

The use of hour-specific serum bilirubin levels to predict newborns at risk for rapidly rising levels has now become the standard of care as well as an official recommendation by the AAP, Subcommittee on Hyperbilirubinemia (2004) for the monitoring of healthy neonates of 35 weeks of gestation or older. The use of a nomogram with three levels (high, intermediate, or low risk) of rising total serum bilirubin values assists in the determination of which newborns might need further evaluation after discharge (Bhutani, Johnson, and Keren, 2004; Maisels, Bhutani, Bogen, and others, 2011; Watson, 2009) (see Fig. 9-16, A). The hour-specific bilirubin risk nomogram is used to determine the infant's risk for developing hyperbilirubinemia requiring medical treatment or more frequent screening. Risk factors recognized to place infants in the high-risk category include gestational age of less than 38 weeks, breastfeeding, a sibling who had significant jaundice, and jaundice appearing before discharge (AAP, Subcommittee on Hyperbilirubinemia, 2004; Maisels, Bhutani, Bogen, and others, 2011).

It is also recommended that healthy term infants receive follow-up care and bilirubin risk assessment with TcB or the hour-specific nomogram within 3 days of discharge if discharged at less than

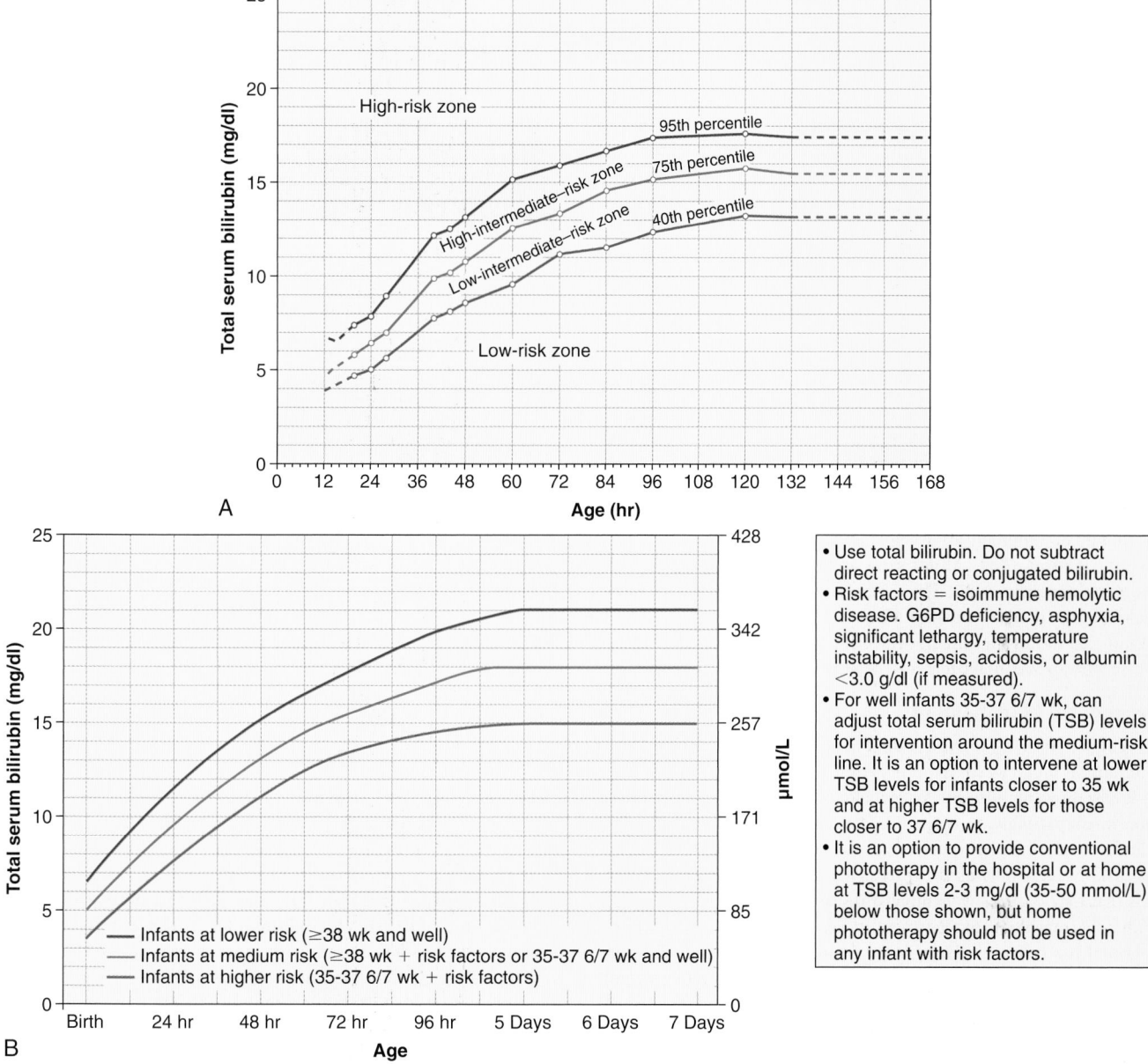

FIG 9-16 A, Nomogram for designation of risk in 2840 well newborns at 36 or more weeks of gestational age with birth weights of 2000 g (4.4 pounds) or more or 35 or more weeks of gestational age and birth weights of 2500 g (5.5 pounds) or more based on the hour-specific serum bilirubin values. (This nomogram should not be used to represent the natural history of neonatal hyperbilirubinemia.) **B,** Guidelines for phototherapy in hospitalized infants of 35 or more weeks of gestation. *G6PD,* Glucose-6-phosphate dehydrogenase. (**A,** From Bhutani VK, Johnson L, Sivieri EM: Predictive ability of a pre-discharge hour-specific serum bilirubin for subsequent significant hyperbilirubinemia in healthy term and near-term newborns, *Pediatrics* 103(1):6–14, 1999. **B,** From American Academy of Pediatrics, Subcommittee on Hyperbilirubinemia: Management of hyperbilirubinemia in the newborn infant 35 or more weeks of gestation, *Pediatrics* 114(1):297–316, 2004.)

24 hours of age. Newborns discharged at 24 to 47.9 hours should receive follow-up evaluation within 4 days (96 hours), and those discharged between 48 and 72 hours should receive follow-up within 5 days (AAP, Subcommittee on Hyperbilirubinemia, 2004). The serum bilirubin may be obtained at the time of the metabolic screening, thus precluding the need for additional blood sampling. The newest guidelines for monitoring and treating neonatal hyperbilirubinemia are published extensively elsewhere, and readers are referred to the AAP,

Subcommittee on Hyperbilirubinemia (2004) reference for an in-depth overview of management guidelines.

Complications

Unconjugated bilirubin is highly toxic to neurons; therefore, an infant with severe jaundice is at risk of developing bilirubin encephalopathy, a syndrome of severe brain damage resulting from the deposition of unconjugated bilirubin in brain cells. Kernicterus describes the yellow staining of the brain cells that may result in bilirubin encephalopathy (Watson, 2009). The damage occurs when the serum concentration reaches toxic levels, regardless of cause. There is evidence that a fraction of unconjugated bilirubin crosses the blood–brain barrier in neonates with physiologic hyperbilirubinemia. When certain pathologic conditions exist in addition to elevated bilirubin levels, there is an increase in the permeability of the blood–brain barrier to unconjugated bilirubin and thus potential irreversible damage. The exact level of serum bilirubin required to cause damage is not yet known.

Multiple factors contribute to bilirubin neurotoxicity; therefore, *serum bilirubin levels alone do not predict the risk of brain injury.* Factors that are known to enhance the development of bilirubin encephalopathy include metabolic acidosis, lowered serum albumin levels, intracranial infections such as meningitis, and abrupt fluctuations in BP. In addition, any condition that increases the metabolic demands for oxygen or glucose (e.g., fetal distress, hypoxia, hypothermia, hypoglycemia) also increases the risk of brain damage at lower serum levels of bilirubin.

The signs of bilirubin encephalopathy are those of CNS depression or excitation. Prodromal symptoms consist of decreased activity, lethargy, irritability, hypotonia, and seizures. Later these subtle findings are followed by development of athetoid cerebral palsy, gaze palsies, and deafness (Watson, 2009). Motor skills are delayed, and dental enamel hypoplasia may also occur. Those who survive may eventually show evidence of neurologic damage, such as cognitive delay, ADHD, delayed or abnormal motor movement (especially ataxia or athetosis), behavior disorders, perceptual problems, or sensorineural hearing loss.

Therapeutic Management

The primary goals in the treatment of hyperbilirubinemia are to identify infants at high risk for hyperbilirubinemia; monitor serum bilirubin levels; prevent bilirubin encephalopathy; and, as in any blood group incompatibility, to reverse the hemolytic process (p. 263). The main form of treatment involves the use of phototherapy. Exchange transfusion is generally used for reducing dangerously high bilirubin levels that may occur with hemolytic disease.

The pharmacologic management of hyperbilirubinemia with phenobarbital has centered primarily on infants with hemolytic disease, and phenobarbital is most effective when given to the mother several days before delivery. Phenobarbital promotes (1) hepatic glucuronyl transferase synthesis, which increases bilirubin conjugation and hepatic clearance of the pigment in bile, and (2) protein synthesis, which may increase albumin for more bilirubin binding sites. However, the use of phenobarbital in either the antenatal or the postnatal period has not proved to be as effective as other treatments in reducing bilirubin. Bilirubin production in newborns can be decreased by inhibiting heme oxygenase—an enzyme needed for heme breakdown (to biliverdin)—with **metalloporphyrins**, especially tin protoporphyrin and tin mesoporphyrin. The use of heme-oxygenase inhibitors provides a preventive approach to hyperbilirubinemia (Watson, 2009).

Intravenous immunoglobulin (IVIG) is effective in reducing bilirubin levels in infants with Rh isoimmunization and ABO incompatibility (Watson, 2009). A systematic review of IVIG demonstrated that it reduced the duration of phototherapy and hospital days in infants with hemolytic disease (Gottstein and Cooke, 2003).

Healthy near-term and full-term infants with jaundice may also benefit from early initiation of feedings and frequent breastfeeding. These preventive measures are aimed at promoting increased intestinal motility, decreasing enterohepatic shunting, and establishing normal bacterial flora in the bowel to effectively enhance the excretion of unconjugated bilirubin.

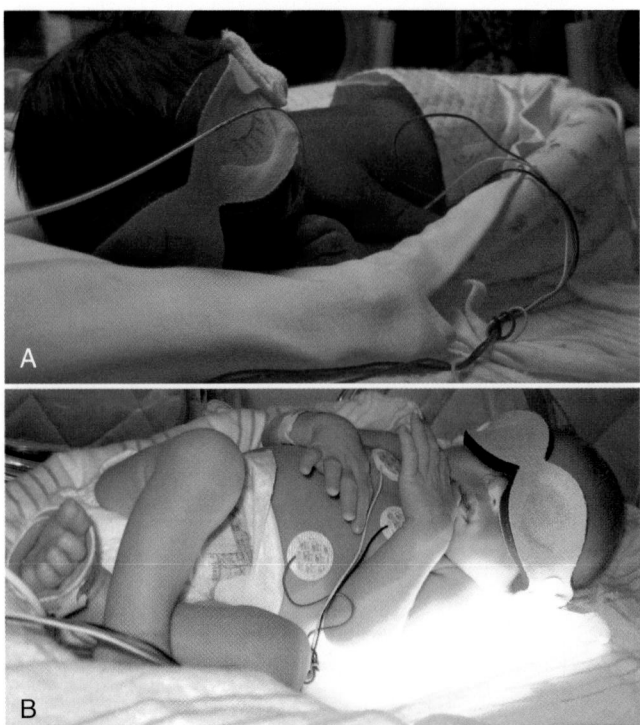

FIG 9-17 A, An infant receiving phototherapy; note the nested boundaries for comfort and eye protection. **B,** A newborn laying on a BiliBlanket, which may be used with overhead lights to provide intensive phototherapy. (Courtesy E. Jacobs, Texas Children's Hospital, Houston.)

Phototherapy consists of the application of a special source of light (irradiance) to the infant's exposed skin (Fig. 9-17). Light promotes bilirubin excretion by **photoisomerization**, which alters the structure of bilirubin to a soluble form (**lumirubin**) for easier excretion.

Studies indicate that blue fluorescent light is more effective than white fluorescent in reducing bilirubin levels. However, because blue light alters the infant's coloration, the normal light of fluorescent bulbs in the spectrum of 420 to 460 nm is often preferred so the infant's skin can be better observed for color (jaundice, pallor, cyanosis) or other conditions. Increasing irradiance to the 430 to 490 nm band provides best results. For phototherapy to be effective, the infant's skin must be fully exposed to an adequate amount of the light source. A diaper and boundary materials for postural support may be left in place; periodically turning the neonate under phototherapy has not been shown to accelerate bilirubin clearance (Stokowski, 2011). When serum bilirubin levels are rapidly increasing or approximating critical levels, intensive phototherapy is recommended. Intensive phototherapy with a higher irradiance is considered to be more effective than standard phototherapy for rapid reduction of serum bilirubin levels (Beachy, 2007). The color of the infant's skin does not influence the efficacy of phototherapy. Best results occur within the first 4 to 6 hours of treatment (Stokowski, 2011). Phototherapy alone is not effective in the management of hyperbilirubinemia when levels are at a critical level or are rising rapidly; it is designed primarily for the treatment of moderate hyperbilirubinemia.

Available commercial phototherapy delivery systems are numerous and include halogen spotlights, light-emitting diodes, fluorescent tubes or bank lights, and fiberoptic mattresses (Stokowski, 2011). A Cochrane review of 24 studies indicated that conventional phototherapy was more effective at lowering serum bilirubin values than fiberoptic lights alone; when two fiberoptic devices were used simultaneously in preterm infants, the therapy was as effective as conventional therapy at reducing serum bilirubin levels. Combination phototherapy (fiberoptic mattress and conventional overhead lights) was found to be more effective than conventional therapy alone. The authors further concluded that fiberoptic phototherapy is a safe and effective alternative to conventional therapy in preterm infants. The authors also pointed out that no trials were available to show that fiberoptic therapy is more effective than conventional phototherapy (Mills and Tudehope, 2005).

The AAP, Subcommittee on Hyperbilirubinemia (2004) practice parameter guidelines provide suggestions for initiating phototherapy (see Fig. 9-16, *B*) and for implementing exchange transfusion in healthy term infants.

Some clinicians believe that preterm infants have a higher risk of developing pathologic jaundice at lower serum bilirubin levels than do healthy term infants because of associated illness factors that may increase the entry of bilirubin into the brain; however, research has failed to confirm this belief (Watchko and Maisels, 2010). Until further research is completed, the recommendations for starting phototherapy in infants weighing less than 1500 g is 5 to 8 mg/dl, 8 to 12 mg/dl for infants weighing 1500 to 1999 g, and 11 to 14 mg/dl for infants weighing 2000 to 2499 g (Watchko and Maisels, 2010). However, each infant should be carefully evaluated with other illness and risk factors in mind rather than depending on absolute values for all infants in a specific group. Prophylactic phototherapy may be used in preterm infants to prevent a significant increase in serum bilirubin levels (Stokowski, 2011).

Phototherapy has not been found to cause long-term adverse effects. The effectiveness of treatment is determined by a decrease in total serum bilirubin levels. Concurrently, the infant's total physical status is assessed continually because the suppression of jaundice by phototherapy may mask signs of sepsis, hemolytic disease, or hepatitis.

Recommendations for prevention and management of early-onset jaundice in breastfed infants include encouraging frequent breastfeeding, preferably every 2 hours; avoiding glucose water, formula, and water supplementation; and monitoring for early stooling. The infant's weight, voiding, and stooling should be evaluated along with the breastfeeding pattern (Lawrence and Lawrence, 2011). Parents are taught to evaluate the number of voids and evidence of adequate breastfeeding after the infant is home and are encouraged to call the primary care practitioner if there are indications the infant is not feeding well, is difficult to arouse for feedings, or is not voiding and stooling adequately (Smith, Donze, and Schuller, 2007).

Phototherapy as a treatment for hyperbilirubinemia is further discussed on p. 262.

Prognosis

Early recognition and treatment of hyperbilirubinemia prevents unnecessary medical therapies, parent–infant separation, breastfeeding disruption and possibly failure, and neurologic damage (bilirubin encephalopathy). Phototherapy is a safe and effective method of decreasing serum bilirubin levels in newborns with mild to moderate hyperbilirubinemia.

Nursing Care Management

The nursing care of infants with jaundice is discussed in the Nursing Process box and in the following section.

Part of the routine physical assessment includes observing for evidence of jaundice at regular intervals. Jaundice is most reliably assessed by observing the infant's skin color from head to toe and the color of

NURSING PROCESS
The Newborn with Jaundice

Assessment
Assess for signs of clinical jaundice. See further assessments on pp. 258 and 261.

Diagnosis (Problem Identification)
After the nursing assessment, a number of nursing diagnoses may be evident. Additional nursing diagnoses that may apply include:
- Risk for Neonatal Jaundice (risk factors include but are not limited to physiologic immaturity of the liver, increased production of unconjugated bilirubin, enterohepatic circulation)
- Risk for Impaired Parent–Infant Attachment (risk factors include separation from parents for treatment of elevated bilirubin levels, eye shields, phototherapy, perception of fragile status of infant)
- Interrupted Breastfeeding related to increasing serum bilirubin levels
- Risk for Deficient Fluid Volume (risk factors include increased ECF volume, immature kidney function, increased body temperature, decreased oral fluid intake, increased fluid losses in stool and urine)
- Risk for Impaired Skin Integrity (risk factors include increased stooling, decreased oral intake, immature skin function, increased body metabolism and fluid losses)
- Interrupted Family Processes related to required treatment and physical separation from infant because of treatment (phototherapy)

Planning
Expected outcomes include:
- Infant will receive appropriate monitoring for jaundice in the newborn period.
- Infant will receive appropriate therapy as needed to reduce serum bilirubin levels.
- Infant will experience no complications from therapy.
- Mother–infant dyad will achieve successful breastfeeding.
- Family will receive emotional support.
- Family will be prepared for home phototherapy (if prescribed).
- Family will receive appropriate education about neonatal jaundice.

Implementation
Numerous nursing interventions are discussed on pp. 261 to 263.

Evaluation
The effectiveness of nursing interventions for the family and infant with jaundice is determined by continual reassessment and evaluation of care based on the following guidelines:
- Observe skin color; review bilirubinometric or laboratory findings.
- Evaluate feedings and elimination pattern.
- Check placement of eye shields; observe skin for signs of dehydration; monitor infant's temperature.
- Interview family members and observe parent–infant interactions.

the sclerae and mucous membranes. Applying direct pressure to the skin, especially over bony prominences such as the tip of the nose or the sternum, causes blanching and allows the yellow stain to be more pronounced. For dark-skinned infants, the color of the sclerae, conjunctiva, and oral mucosa is the most reliable indicator. Also, bilirubin (especially at high levels) is not uniformly distributed in the skin. The nurse should observe the infant in natural daylight for a true assessment of color.

The TcB is a useful screening device and is used to detect neonatal jaundice in full-term infants. Because phototherapy reduces the accuracy of the instrument, its value is limited to assessments made before the initiation of phototherapy. Institutions in which the device is used set up their own criteria based on their experience with their particular instrument. Blood samples are also taken for the measurement of bilirubin in the laboratory.

With short hospital stays, jaundice may appear after discharge. A careful history from the parents may reveal significant familial patterns of hyperbilirubinemia (e.g., older siblings who had jaundice). Other considerations in assessment include the ethnic origin of the family (e.g., higher incidence in Asian infants); type of delivery (e.g., induction of labor); and infant characteristics such as weight loss after birth, gestational age, sex, and the presence of any bruising. The method and frequency of feeding are assessed. Prevention of jaundice may be possible with early introduction of feedings and frequent nursing without supplementation. Every effort is made to provide an optimum thermal environment to reduce metabolic needs.

> **NURSING TIP** While blood is drawn, phototherapy lights are turned off. Blood is transported in a covered tube to avoid a false reading as a result of bilirubin destruction in the test tube.

> **QUALITY PATIENT OUTCOMES: Neonatal Hyperbilirubinemia**
> Total serum bilirubin level will be maintained below high-risk critical value (as determined on the hour-specific total serum bilirubin nomogram).

> ⚠ **NURSING ALERT**
> Evidence of jaundice that appears before the infant is 24 hours of age is an indication for assessing bilirubin levels.

Phototherapy

The infant who receives phototherapy is placed semi-nude (diaper may be left in place) under the light source and periodically evaluated to ensure tolerance to the procedure. After phototherapy has been initiated, frequent serum bilirubin levels (every 6–12 hours) are necessary because visual assessment of jaundice or transcutaneous bilirubin monitoring are no longer considered valid.

Several precautions are instituted to protect the infant during phototherapy. The infant's eyes are shielded by an opaque mask to prevent exposure to the light (see Fig. 9-17). The eye shield should be properly sized and correctly positioned to cover the eyes completely but prevent any occlusion of the nares. The infant's eyelids are closed before the mask is applied because the corneas may become excoriated if they come in contact with the dressing. On each nursing shift, the eyes are checked for evidence of discharge, excessive pressure on the eyelids, and corneal irritation. Eye shields are removed during feedings, which provide the opportunity for visual and sensory stimulation.

Infants who are in an open crib must have a protective Plexiglas shield between them and the overhead fluorescent lights to minimize the amount of undesirable ultraviolet light reaching their skin and to protect them from accidental bulb breakage. Their temperature is closely monitored to prevent hyperthermia or hypothermia. Maintaining the infant in a flexed position with rolled blankets along the sides of the body helps maintain heat and provides comfort.

Accurate documentation is another important nursing responsibility and includes (1) times that phototherapy is started and stopped, (2) proper shielding of the eyes, (3) type of light source (by manufacturer), (3) use of phototherapy in combination with an incubator or open bassinet, (4) photometer measurement of light intensity according to hospital protocol, (5) feeding and elimination pattern, (6) body temperature, and (7) serum bilirubin levels.

Minor side effects for which the nurse should be alert include loose, greenish stools; transient skin rashes; hyperthermia; increased metabolic rate; dehydration; electrolyte disturbances, such as hypocalcemia; and priapism. To prevent or minimize these effects, the temperature is monitored to detect early signs of hypothermia or hyperthermia, and the skin is observed for evidence of dehydration and drying, which can lead to excoriation and breakdown. Oily lubricants or lotions are not used on the skin while the infant is under phototherapy. Infants receiving phototherapy may require additional fluid volume to compensate for insensible and intestinal fluid loss. Breastfeeding or bottle feeding by the parent(s) and parental interaction such as holding is encouraged once phototherapy is initiated provided the infant receives adequate exposure to the treatment. Because phototherapy enhances the excretion of unconjugated bilirubin through the bowel, loose stools may indicate accelerated bilirubin removal. Frequent stooling can cause perianal irritation; therefore, meticulous skin care, especially keeping the skin clean and dry, is essential.

> ⚡ **SAFETY ALERT**
> Parents may be told by some practitioners to place the infant in the sunlight when the infant has jaundice; however, this practice is not recommended. If performed, the infant should only be placed in indirect sunlight (e.g., in a room where sunlight filters through a glass window) because direct sunlight may cause skin burns in a newborn.

After phototherapy is permanently discontinued, there is often a subsequent increase in the serum bilirubin level, often called the rebound effect; this is usually transient and resolves without resuming therapy; however, a follow-up serum bilirubin level should be checked.

Family Support

Parents need reassurance concerning their infant's progress. All the procedures are explained to familiarize them with the benefits and risks. Parents need to be reassured that the naked infant under the bilirubin light is warm and comfortable. Eye shields are removed when the parents are visiting to facilitate the attachment process. The parents can be reassured that the neonate is accustomed to darkness after months of intrauterine existence and benefits a great deal from auditory and tactile stimulation (see Family-Centered Care box).

The initiation of any treatment requires informed consent by the parents for the therapy prescribed; however, in the case of phototherapy, considerable anxiety may rightfully occur when words such as kernicterus and neurologic damage are used to describe possible effects of nontreatment. It is imperative that nurses remain sensitive to parents' feelings and information needs during this process; an important nursing intervention is assessment of the parents' understanding of the treatment involved and clarification of the nature of the therapy.

An important nursing intervention is recognition of breastfeeding jaundice. Lack of familiarity among health professionals has caused many newborns prolonged hospitalization, termination of breastfeeding, and unnecessary phototherapy. Care of the new mother may include supporting successful and frequent breastfeeding. Parents also need reassurance of the benign nature of the jaundice in a healthy infant and encouragement to resume breastfeeding if temporary cessation is prescribed. In some situations, jaundice may increase the

FAMILY-CENTERED CARE

Phototherapy and Parent–Infant Interaction

The traditional use of phototherapy has evoked concerns regarding a number of psychobehavioral issues, including parent–infant separation, potential social isolation, decreased sensorineural stimulation, altered biologic rhythms, altered feeding patterns, and activity changes. Parental anxiety is greatly increased, particularly at the sight of their newborn blindfolded and under special lights. The interruption of breastfeeding for phototherapy is a potential deterrent to successful mother–infant attachment and interaction. Because research has demonstrated that bilirubin catabolism occurs primarily within the first few hours of the initiation of phototherapy, there is increased support for the periodic removal of the infant from treatment for feeding and holding. The benefits of stopping phototherapy for parental feeding and holding outweigh concerns related to the clearance of bilirubin in healthy full-term newborns with mild hyperbilirubinemia. Home phototherapy offers an additional opportunity to foster parent–infant attachment.

risk of the parents' discontinuing breastfeeding and developing the **vulnerable child syndrome**—a belief that their child has experienced a "close call" and is vulnerable to serious injury (see Critical Thinking Case Study box).

Discharge Planning and Home Care

With short hospital stays, mothers and infants may be discharged before evidence of jaundice is present. It is important for the nurse to discuss signs of jaundice with the mother because any clinical symptoms will probably appear at home. Home visits within 2 to 3 days after discharge to evaluate feeding and elimination patterns and jaundice are often routine for some health care organizations. Others may have an outpatient bilirubin clinic or laboratory where the infant can be evaluated by a nurse and weighed and a serum bilirubin can be drawn for evaluation. Assessment of breastfeeding is essential.

If home phototherapy is instituted, the hospital or home health care nurse or medical equipment company representative is usually responsible for teaching the family members and assessing their abilities to implement the treatment safely. General guidelines for home care preparation and education are discussed in Chapter 20. Written instructions and supervision of care—especially the application of eye shields, if needed—are essential. The minor side effects of phototherapy are reviewed, and parents may need instruction in taking axillary temperatures and recording times and amounts of feedings and the number of wet diapers and stools. Regardless of how benign the disorder or the therapy, the parents need support and understanding. Measures should be taken to assist the mother in achieving successful breastfeeding, including consultation with a lactation specialist on an outpatient basis. Phenomenological research showed that mothers of infants who were receiving treatment for jaundice experienced physical and emotional exhaustion, loss of control, distress at the infant's appearance, and a feeling of having been robbed (Brethauer and Carey, 2010). Mothers in the study reported receiving a significant amount of conflicting information about jaundice and feeding from health care professionals. In jaundice associated with breastfeeding, follow-up blood studies are usually required to assess the progress of the jaundice. If temporary cessation of breastfeeding is prescribed, mothers should be taught to pump the breasts every 3 to 4 hours to maintain lactation; the expressed milk is frozen for use after breastfeeding is resumed.

CRITICAL THINKING CASE STUDY

Jaundice

A full-term, 120-hour-old newborn is brought to the urgent care department late in the evening for evaluation of newborn jaundice. A serum bilirubin level was drawn earlier in the day at the birth hospital by heel stick; the results were total bilirubin, 13.6 mg/dl and direct bilirubin, 0.6 mg/dl. The father is concerned because he saw an online medical report saying that newborns could develop brain damage if the bilirubin levels were to increase to high levels. The mother is breastfeeding every 2 to 3 hours, and the newborn has had five wet diapers and three semiliquid stools over the past 18 hours. The newborn's birth weight was 2834 g (6.2 pounds), and her current weight (nude) is 2722 g (6 pounds). On examination, the infant is active and alert, with visibly jaundiced skin and sclerae, intact neurologic reflexes, and a strong suck reflex. The history reveals no prenatal or delivery complications. Apgar scores at 1 and 5 minutes were 8 and 9, respectively, and the initial assessment did not reveal any problems. The mother's blood type is A positive, and the direct Coombs test result is negative. The newborn was discharged from the birth hospital on the second day of life in apparent good health.

Questions

1. Evidence—Is there sufficient evidence to draw any conclusions about the newborn's condition at this time?
2. Assumptions—Describe some underlying assumptions about the following:
   a. Newborn jaundice in a healthy full-term infant
   b. Serum bilirubin levels and the newborn's age in hours; other pertinent laboratory values (may refer to Fig. 9-16, A) to determine the risk zone for the serum bilirubin
   c. Nutritional and excretory function and relation to bilirubin metabolism
   d. The physical status of the infant per assessment data
3. What implications and priorities for nursing care can be drawn at this time?
4. Does the evidence objectively support your argument (conclusion)?

HEMOLYTIC DISEASE OF THE NEWBORN

Hyperbilirubinemia in the first 24 hours of life is most often the result of HDN, an abnormally rapid rate of RBC destruction. Anemia caused by this destruction stimulates the production of RBCs, which in turn provides increasing numbers of cells for hemolysis. Major causes of increased erythrocyte destruction are isoimmunization (primarily Rh) and ABO incompatibility.

Blood Incompatibility

The membranes of human blood cells contain a variety of **antigens**, also known as **agglutinogens**, substances capable of producing an immune response if recognized by the body as foreign. The reciprocal relationship between antigens on RBCs and antibodies in the plasma causes **agglutination** (clumping). In other words, antibodies in the plasma of one blood group (except the AB group, which contains no antibodies) produce agglutination when mixed with antigens of a different blood group. In the **ABO blood group system**, the antibodies occur naturally. In the **Rh system**, the person must be exposed to the Rh antigen before significant antibody formation takes place and causes a sensitivity response known as **isoimmunization**.

Rh Incompatibility (Isoimmunization)

The Rh blood group consists of several antigens (with D being the most prevalent). For simplicity, only the terms **Rh positive** (presence of antigen) and **Rh negative** (absence of antigen) are used in this discussion. The presence or absence of the naturally occurring Rh factor determines the blood type.

Ordinarily, no problems are anticipated when the Rh blood types are the same in both the mother and the fetus or when the mother is Rh positive and the infant is Rh negative. Difficulty may arise when the mother is Rh negative and the infant is Rh positive. Although the maternal and fetal circulations are separate, there is evidence of a bidirectional trafficking of fetal RBCs and cell-free DNA to the maternal circulation (Moise, 2007). More commonly, however, fetal RBCs enter into the maternal circulation at the time of delivery. The mother's natural defense mechanism responds to these alien cells by producing anti-Rh antibodies.

Under normal circumstances, this process of isoimmunization has no effect during the first pregnancy with an Rh-positive fetus because the initial sensitization to Rh antigens rarely occurs before the onset of labor. However, with the increased risk of fetal blood being transferred to the maternal circulation during placental separation, maternal antibody production is stimulated. During a subsequent pregnancy with an Rh-positive fetus, these previously formed maternal antibodies to Rh-positive blood cells may enter the fetal circulation, where they attack and destroy fetal erythrocytes (Fig. 9-18). Multiple gestations, abruptio placentae, placenta previa, manual removal of the placenta, and cesarean delivery increase the incidence of transplacental hemorrhage and subsequent isoimmunization (Diehl-Jones and Fraser Askin, 2010).

Because the condition begins in utero, the fetus attempts to compensate for the progressive hemolysis and anemia by accelerating the rate of erythropoiesis. As a result, immature RBCs (**erythroblasts**) appear in the fetal circulation, hence the term **erythroblastosis fetalis**.

There is wide variability in the development of maternal sensitization to Rh-positive antigens. Sensitization may occur during the first pregnancy if the woman had previously received an Rh-positive blood transfusion. No sensitization may occur in situations in which a strong placental barrier prevents transfer of fetal blood into the maternal circulation. In approximately 10% to 15% of sensitized mothers, there is no hemolytic reaction in the newborn. In addition, some Rh-negative women, even though exposed to Rh-positive fetal blood, are immunologically unable to produce antibodies to the foreign antigen (Neal, 2001).

In the most severe form of erythroblastosis fetalis, **hydrops fetalis**, the progressive hemolysis causes fetal hypoxia; cardiac failure; generalized edema (anasarca); and fluid effusions into the pericardial, pleural, and peritoneal spaces (hydrops). The fetus may be delivered stillborn or in severe respiratory distress. Maternal Rh immunoglobulin (RhIg) administration, early intrauterine detection of fetal anemia by ultrasonography (serial Doppler assessment of the peak velocity in the fetal middle cerebral artery), and subsequent treatment by fetal blood transfusions or high-dose IVIG have dramatically improved the outcome of affected fetuses (Moise, 2008a).

ABO Incompatibility

Hemolytic disease can also occur when the major blood group antigens of the fetus are different from those of the mother. The major blood groups are A, B, AB, and O. In the North American white population, 46% have type O blood, 42% have type A blood, 9% have type B blood, and 3% have type AB blood.

The presence or absence of antibodies and antigens determines whether agglutination will occur. Antibodies in the plasma of one blood group (except the AB group, which contains no antibodies) will produce agglutination (clumping) when mixed with antigens of a different blood group. Naturally occurring antibodies in the recipient's blood cause agglutination of a donor's RBCs. The agglutinated donor cells become trapped in peripheral blood vessels, where they hemolyze, releasing large amounts of bilirubin into the circulation.

The most common blood group incompatibility in the neonate is between a mother with O blood group and an infant with A or B blood group (see Table 9-3 for possible ABO incompatibilities). Naturally occurring anti-A or anti-B antibodies already present in the maternal circulation cross the placenta and attack the fetal RBCs, causing hemolysis. Usually, the hemolytic reaction is less severe than in Rh incompatibility; however, rare cases of hydrops have been reported (Black and Maheshwari, 2009). Unlike the Rh reaction, ABO incompatibility may occur in the first pregnancy. The risk of significant hemolysis in subsequent pregnancies is higher when the first pregnancy is complicated by ABO incompatibility (Sarici, Yurdakok, Serdar, and others, 2002).

Clinical Manifestations

Jaundice may appear shortly after birth (during the first 24 hours) in newborns affected by HDN, and serum levels of unconjugated bilirubin rise rapidly. Anemia results from the hemolysis of large numbers of erythrocytes, and hyperbilirubinemia and jaundice result from the liver's inability to conjugate and excrete the excess bilirubin.

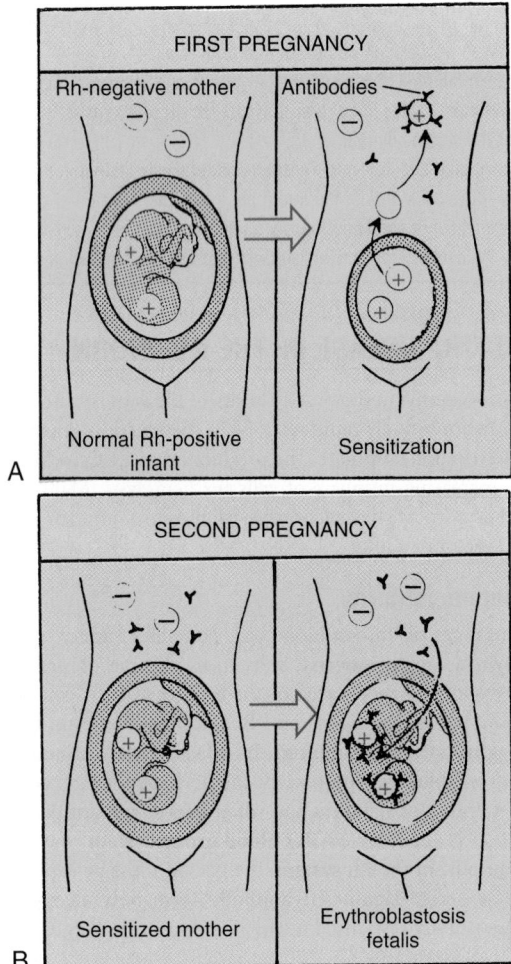

FIG 9-18 Development of maternal sensitization to Rh antigens. **A,** Fetal Rh-positive erythrocytes enter the maternal system. Maternal anti-Rh antibodies are formed. **B,** Anti-Rh antibodies cross the placenta and attack fetal erythrocytes.

FIRST PREGNANCY

Rh-negative mother — Antibodies

Normal Rh-positive infant — Sensitization

A

SECOND PREGNANCY

Sensitized mother — Erythroblastosis fetalis

B

TABLE 9-3	POTENTIAL MATERNAL-FETAL ABO INCOMPATIBILITIES	
MATERNAL BLOOD GROUP	**INCOMPATIBLE FETAL BLOOD GROUP**
O	A or B
B	A or AB
A	B or AB

Most newborns with HDN are not jaundiced at birth. However, hepatosplenomegaly and varying degrees of hydrops may be evident. If the infant is severely affected, signs of anemia (notably, marked pallor) and hypovolemic shock are apparent. Hypoglycemia may occur as a result of pancreatic cell hyperplasia.

Diagnostic Evaluation

Early identification and diagnosis of RhD sensitization are important in the management and prevention of fetal complications. A maternal antibody titer (**indirect Coombs test**) should be drawn at the first prenatal visit. Genetic testing allows early identification of paternal zygosity at the RHD gene locus, thus allowing earlier detection of the potential for isoimmunization and avoiding further maternal or fetal testing (Moise, 2008b). Amniocentesis can be used to test the fetal blood type of a woman whose antibody screen result is positive; the use of polymerase chain reaction may determine the fetal blood type and presence of maternal antibodies. The fetal hemoglobin and hematocrit can also be measured (Moise, 2008b). Chorionic villus sampling has drawbacks that preclude its use, including possible spontaneous abortion of the fetus and fetomaternal hemorrhage, which would essentially make the situation worse. With either method, if the fetus is found to be Rh negative, no further treatment is required. The detection of cell-free fetal DNA in the maternal plasma of RhD-negative women to detect an RhD-positive fetus has been used successfully in the United Kingdom; however, this technology is not yet available in the United States (Finning, Martin, and Daniels, 2009; Moise, 2008b). Such testing would negate the necessity for amniocentesis for fetal blood type.

Ultrasonography is considered an important adjunct in the detection of isoimmunization; alterations in the placenta, umbilical cord, and amniotic fluid volume, as well as the presence of fetal hydrops, can be detected with high-resolution ultrasonography and allow early treatment before the development of erythroblastosis. Doppler ultrasonography of fetal middle cerebral artery peak velocity has been used to detect and measure fetal hemoglobin and, subsequently, fetal anemia (Moise, 2008b). Erythroblastosis fetalis caused by Rh incompatibility can also be monitored by evaluating rising anti-Rh antibody titers in the maternal circulation or by testing the optical density of amniotic fluid ($\Delta OD450$ test) because bilirubin discolors the fluid (Mari, 2000).

The disease in the newborn is suspected on the basis of the timing and appearance of jaundice (see Table 9-2) and can be confirmed postnatally by detecting antibodies attached to the circulating erythrocytes of affected infants (**direct Coombs test or direct antiglobulin test**). The Coombs test may be performed on umbilical cord blood samples from infants born to Rh-negative mothers if there is a history of incompatibility or further investigation is warranted.

Therapeutic Management

The primary aim of therapeutic management of isoimmunization is prevention. Postnatal therapy is usually phototherapy for mild cases of hemolysis and exchange transfusion for more severe forms. Although phototherapy may control bilirubin levels in mild cases, the hemolytic process may continue, causing severe anemia between 7 and 21 days of life. In some institutions, a metalloporphyrin is administered (intramuscular) to decrease the formation of bilirubin in neonates with ABO incompatibility.

Prevention of Rh Isoimmunization

The administration of RhIg, a human gamma globulin concentrate of anti-D, to all unsensitized Rh-negative mothers after delivery or abortion of an Rh-positive infant or fetus prevents the development of maternal sensitization to the Rh factor. The injected anti-Rh antibodies are thought to destroy (by subsequent phagocytosis and agglutination) fetal RBCs passing into the maternal circulation before they can be recognized by the mother's immune system. Because the immune response is blocked, anti-D antibodies and memory cells (which produce the primary and secondary immune responses, respectively) are not formed (Bagwell, 2007; Blackburn, 2011). The inhibition of memory cell formation is especially important because memory cells provide long-term immunity by initiating a rapid immune response after the antigen is reintroduced (McCance and Huether, 2010).

To be effective, RhIg (e.g., RhoGAM) must be administered to unsensitized mothers within 72 hours (but possibly as long as 3-4 weeks) after the first delivery or abortion and repeated after subsequent pregnancies or losses. The administration of RhIg at 26 to 28 weeks of gestation further reduces the risk of Rh isoimmunization. RhIg is not effective against existing Rh-positive antibodies in the maternal circulation.

Studies have demonstrated the effectiveness of IVIG at decreasing the severity of RBC destruction (hemolysis) in HDN and subsequent development of neonatal jaundice (Elalfy, Elbarbary, and Abaza, 2011; Mundy, 2005). IVIG administered to the neonate is believed to attack the maternal cells that destroy neonatal RBCs, slowing the progression of bilirubin production (Mundy, 2005). This therapy, often used in conjunction with phototherapy, may decrease the necessity for exchange transfusion. Maternal administration of high-dose IVIG, alone or in combination with plasmapheresis, decreases the fetal effects of RhD isoimmunization (Moise, 2008b; Urbaniak, 2008).

> ### ⬤ DRUG ALERT!
>
> RhIg is administered intramuscularly, not intravenously, and only to Rh-negative women with a negative Coombs test result—never to the newborn or father.

Intrauterine Transfusion

Infants of mothers already sensitized may be treated by intrauterine transfusion, which consists of infusing blood into the umbilical vein of the fetus. The need for therapy is based on the antenatal diagnosis of isoimmunization by determining the optical density of amniotic fluid (by amniocentesis) as an index of fetal hemolysis or by serial ultrasonography, which may detect the presence of fetal hydrops as early as 16 weeks of gestation. With the advance of ultrasound technology, fetal transfusion may be accomplished directly via the umbilical vein, infusing type O Rh-negative packed RBCs to raise the fetal hematocrit to 40% to 50%; fetal movement and transfusion risks are minimized by administering vecuronium bromide for temporary fetal paralysis. The frequency of intrauterine transfusions may vary according to institution and fetal hydropic status but are most often done every 3 to 4 weeks until the fetus reaches pulmonary maturity at approximately 37 to 38 weeks of gestation (Moise, 2008b). The use of intraperitoneal blood transfusions is used less commonly for isoimmunization because of higher associated fetal risks; however, it may be used when intravascular access is impossible.

Exchange Transfusion

Exchange transfusion, in which the infant's blood is removed in small amounts (usually 5–10 ml at a time) and replaced with compatible blood (e.g., Rh-negative blood), is a standard mode of therapy for treatment of severe hyperbilirubinemia and is the treatment of choice for hyperbilirubinemia and hydrops caused by Rh incompatibility. Exchange transfusion removes the sensitized erythrocytes, lowers the serum bilirubin level to prevent bilirubin encephalopathy, corrects the anemia, and prevents cardiac failure. Indications for exchange transfusion in full-term infants may include a rapidly increasing serum bilirubin level and hemolysis despite intensive phototherapy. The criteria for exchange transfusions in preterm infants vary according to associated illness factors. The AAP, Subcommittee on Hyperbilirubinemia (2004) practice parameter guidelines provide recommendations for initiating phototherapy and for exchange transfusion in infants at 35 weeks of gestation or more. An infant born with hydrops fetalis or signs of cardiac failure is a candidate for immediate exchange transfusion with fresh whole blood.

For exchange transfusion, fresh whole blood is typed and crossmatched to the mother's serum. The amount of donor blood used is usually double the blood volume of the infant, which is approximately 85 ml/kg body weight but is limited to no more than 500 ml. The two-volume exchange transfusion replaces approximately 85% of the neonate's blood.

An exchange transfusion is a sterile surgical procedure. A catheter is inserted into the umbilical vein and threaded into the inferior vena cava. Depending on the infant's weight, 5 to 10 ml of blood is withdrawn within 15 to 20 seconds, and the same volume of donor blood is infused over 60 to 90 seconds. If the blood has been citrated (addition of citrate phosphate dextrose adenine to prevent coagulation), calcium gluconate may be given after the infusion of each 100 ml of donor's blood to prevent hypocalcemia.

Prognosis

The severe anemia of isoimmunization may result in stillbirth, shock, congestive heart failure, or pulmonary or cerebral complications such as cerebral palsy. As a result of early detection and intrauterine treatment, erythroblastotic newborns are seen less often and exchange transfusions for the condition are less common. Despite the availability of effective preventive measures, Rh HDN continues to cause significant fetal morbidity and mortality in the United States.

Nursing Care Management

The initial nursing responsibility is recognizing newborn jaundice. The possibility of hemolytic disease can be anticipated from the prenatal and perinatal history. Prenatal evidence of incompatibility and a positive Coombs test result are cause for increased vigilance for early signs of jaundice in an infant. Data indicate that the use of the hour-specific bilirubin nomogram can be used in infants born at 35 weeks or more with ABO incompatibility and a positive Coombs test result to follow the infant's serum bilirubin to determine the need for additional follow-up after hospital discharge (Schutzman, Sekhon, and Hundalani, 2010).

If an exchange transfusion is required, the nurse prepares the infant and the family and assists the practitioner with the procedure. The infant receives nothing by mouth (NPO) during the procedure; therefore, a peripheral infusion of dextrose and electrolytes is established. The nurse documents the blood volume exchanged, including the amount of blood withdrawn and infused, the time of each procedure, and the cumulative record of the total volume exchanged. Vital signs, monitored electronically, are evaluated frequently and correlated with the removal and infusion of blood. If signs of cardiac or respiratory problems occur, the procedure is stopped temporarily and resumed after the infant's cardiorespiratory function stabilizes. The nurse also observes for signs of blood transfusion reaction and maintains the infant's blood glucose levels and fluid balance.

Throughout the procedure, attention must be given to the infant's thermoregulation. Hypothermia increases oxygen and glucose consumption, causing metabolic acidosis. Not only do these consequences hinder the infant's overall physical ability to withstand the long procedure, but they also inhibit the binding capacity of albumin and bilirubin and the hepatic enzymatic reactions, thus increasing the risk of kernicterus. Conversely, hyperthermia damages the donor erythrocytes, elevating the free potassium content and predisposing the infant to cardiac arrest.

The exchange transfusion is performed with the infant in a radiant warmer. However, the infant is usually covered with sterile drapes that may prevent the radiant heat from sufficiently warming the skin. The blood may also be warmed (using specially designed blood warming devices, never a microwave oven) before infusion.

After the procedure is completed, the nurse inspects the umbilical site for evidence of bleeding. The catheter may remain in place in case repeated exchanges are required.

! NURSING ALERT

Signs of blood exchange transfusion reaction include tachycardia or bradycardia, respiratory distress, dramatic change in BP, temperature instability, and generalized rash.

METABOLIC COMPLICATIONS

High-risk infants are subject to a variety of complications related to physiologic function and the transition to extrauterine life. Prominent among these are fluid and electrolyte derangements, hypoglycemia, and hypocalcemia. These complications often occur concurrently with or as a secondary result of other neonatal disorders and may therefore be difficult to differentiate from other conditions. The major characteristics of hypoglycemia and hypocalcemia are outlined in Table 9-4.

 DRUG ALERT!

Calcium preparations should *never* be administered by bolus rapid infusion in infants.

QUALITY PATIENT OUTCOMES: Neonatal Hypoglycemia
- Maintains serum blood glucose level above 45 mg/dl
- No clinical evidence of hypoglycemia or its effects
- Receives adequate carbohydrate intake

TABLE 9-4   METABOLIC COMPLICATIONS

HYPOGLYCEMIA	HYPOCALCEMIA
Definition	
Blood glucose concentration significantly lower than that in the majority of infants of the same age and weight (usually <45 mg/dl) (see also Adamkin and AAP, Committee on Fetus and Newborn, 2011, for parameters for SGA, late preterm, and IDM or LGA infants)	Abnormally low levels of calcium in circulating blood (see values listed below)
Type	
Increased or impaired glucose utilization—Large or normal-size infants who appear to have hyperinsulinism; infants born to women with diabetes; infants with increased metabolic demands such as those with cold stress, sepsis, or after resuscitation; infants with enzymatic or metabolic endocrine defects **Decreased glucose stores**—Small or growth-restricted infants, preterm infants	**Early onset**—Appears in first 48 hr; appears in preterm infants who experienced perinatal hypoxia or sometimes in infant of diabetic mother **Late onset**—Cow's milk–induced hypocalcemia (neonatal tetany); apparent after first 3–4 days (high phosphorus-to-calcium ratio of cow's milk depresses parathyroid activity, reducing serum calcium levels); infants with intestinal malabsorption, hypoparathyroidism, or hypomagnesemia
Clinical Manifestations	
Vague, often indistinguishable from other newborn conditions **Cerebral signs**—Jitteriness, tremors, twitching, weak or high-pitched cry, lethargy, limpness, apathy, convulsions, and coma **Other**—Cyanosis, apnea, rapid irregular respirations, sweating, eye rolling, poor feeding Signs often transient but recurrent	**Early onset**—Jitteriness, apnea, cyanotic episodes, edema, high-pitched cry, abdominal distention **Late onset**—Twitching, tremors, seizures
Screening	
Bedside monitoring or serum blood glucose for all infants at risk	At-risk infants or those who are symptomatic
Laboratory Diagnosis	
Plasma glucose concentrations <47–50 mg/dl (2.6–2.8 mmol/L) (see also Adamkin and AAP, Committee on Fetus and Newborn, 2011, for parameters for SGA, late preterm, and IDM or LGA infants)	Serum calcium <7.8–8 mg/dl (1.95–2.0 mmol/L) in full-term infant or Ionized calcium <4.4 mg/dl (1.1 mmol/L)
Treatment	
Early feeding (within 1 hour) in normoglycemic and asymptomatic infants (preventive); IV glucose administration if breastfeeding or formula feedings not tolerated or glucose level extremely low (<25 mg/dL)	**Early onset**—Increased appropriate infant formula feedings; administration of calcium supplements (sometimes) **Late onset**—Administration of calcium gluconate orally or intravenously (slowly); vitamin D Correct hypoparathyroidism
Nursing	
Identify infants at risk or with hypoglycemia (e.g., SGA, IUGR, LGA, IDM, late preterm). Reduce environmental factors that predispose to hypoglycemia (e.g., cold stress, respiratory distress). Administer IV dextrose as prescribed. Initiate early breastfeeding or formula feedings in healthy infant. Ensure adequate intake of carbohydrate (breast milk or formula).	Identify infants at risk, or with hypocalcemia. Administer calcium as prescribed.* Observe for signs of acute hypercalcemia (e.g., vomiting, bradycardia). Manipulate environment to reduce stimuli that might precipitate a seizure or tremors (e.g., picking up infant suddenly, sudden jarring of crib).

IDM, Infant of diabetic mother; *IUGR*, intrauterine growth restriction; *IV*, intravenous; *LGA*, large for gestational age; *SGA*, small for gestational age.
*See Drug Alert box, p. 266.

RESPIRATORY DISTRESS SYNDROME

Respiratory distress is a name applied to respiratory dysfunction in neonates and is primarily a disease related to developmental delay in lung maturation. The terms **respiratory distress syndrome (RDS)** and **hyaline membrane disease** are most often applied to this severe lung disorder, which not only is responsible for more infant deaths than any other disease but also carries the highest risk in terms of long-term respiratory and neurologic complications (see Chapter 23 for a discussion of acute RDS). It is seen almost exclusively in preterm infants. The disorder is rare in drug-exposed infants and infants who have been subjected to chronic intrauterine stress (e.g., maternal preeclampsia or hypertension). Respiratory distress of a nonpulmonary origin in neonates may also be caused by sepsis, cardiac defects (structural or functional), exposure to cold, airway obstruction (atresia), intraventricular hemorrhage, hypoglycemia, metabolic acidosis, acute blood loss, and drugs. Pneumonia in the neonatal period may result in respiratory distress caused by bacterial or viral agents and may occur alone or as a complication of RDS.

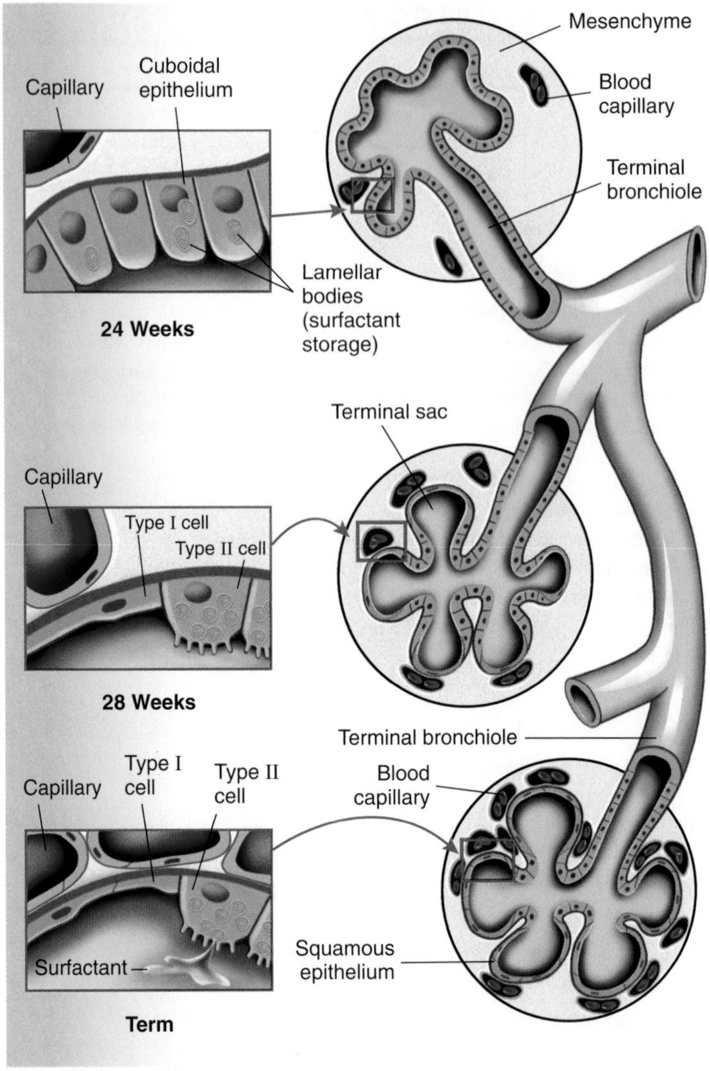

FIG. 9-19 Prenatal development of the alveolar unit. (From McCance K, Huether S: *Pathophysiology: the biological basis for disease in adults and children*, ed 6, St. Louis, 2010, Mosby.)

Pathophysiology

Preterm infants are born before the lungs are fully prepared to serve as efficient organs for gas exchange. This appears to be a critical factor in the development of RDS. The effects of lung immaturity are compounded by the presence of more cartilage in the chest wall, leading to increased compliance of the chest wall, which collapses inward in response to less compliant (stiffer) lung tissue.

There is evidence of fetal respiratory activity before birth. The lungs make feeble respiratory movements, and fluid is excreted through the alveoli. Because the final unfolding of the alveolar septa, which increases the surface area of the lungs, occurs during the last trimester of pregnancy, preterm infants are born with numerous underdeveloped and many uninflatable alveoli. Pulmonary blood flow is limited as a result of the collapsed state of the fetal lungs, particularly poor vascular development in general and an immature capillary network. Because of increased pulmonary vascular resistance (PVR), the major portion of fetal blood is shunted from the lungs by way of the ductus arteriosus and foramen ovale.

At birth, infants must initiate breathing and keep the previously fluid-filled lungs inflated with air. At the same time, the pulmonary capillary blood flow must be increased approximately 10-fold to provide for adequate lung perfusion and to alter the intracardiac pressure that closes the fetal cardiac structures. Most full-term infants successfully accomplish these adjustments, but preterm infants with respiratory distress are unable to do so. Although numerous factors are involved, immaturity of the surfactant system plays a central role.

Surfactant is a surface-active phospholipid secreted by the alveolar epithelium. Acting much like a detergent, this substance reduces the surface tension of fluids that line the alveoli and respiratory passages, resulting in uniform expansion and maintenance of lung expansion at low intraalveolar pressure. Immature development of these functions produces consequences that seriously compromise respiratory efficiency (Fig. 9-19). Deficient surfactant production causes unequal inflation of alveoli on inspiration and the collapse of alveoli on end expiration. Without surfactant, infants are unable to keep their lungs inflated and therefore exert a great deal of effort to reexpand the alveoli with each breath. With increasing exhaustion, infants are able to open fewer and fewer alveoli. This inability to maintain lung expansion produces widespread atelectasis.

In the absence of alveolar stability (normal functional residual capacity) and with progressive atelectasis, PVR increases; with normal lung expansion, it would decrease. Consequently, hypoperfusion to the lung tissue occurs, with a decrease in effective pulmonary blood flow. The increase in PVR causes partial reversion to the fetal circulation, with a right-to-left shunting of blood through the persisting fetal communications—the ductus arteriosus and foramen ovale.

Inadequate pulmonary perfusion and ventilation produce hypoxemia and hypercapnia. Pulmonary arterioles, with their thick muscular layer, are markedly reactive to diminished oxygen concentration. Thus, a decrease in oxygen tension causes vasoconstriction in the pulmonary arterioles that is further enhanced by a decrease in blood pH. This vasoconstriction contributes to a marked increase in PVR. In normal ventilation with increased oxygen concentration, the ductus arteriosus constricts and the pulmonary vessels dilate to decrease PVR.

Prolonged hypoxemia activates anaerobic glycolysis, which produces increased amounts of lactic acid. An increase in lactic acid causes metabolic acidosis; an inability of the atelectatic lungs to blow off excess carbon dioxide produces respiratory acidosis. Acidosis causes further vasoconstriction. With deficient pulmonary circulation and alveolar perfusion, partial pressure of oxygen in arterial blood continues to fall, pH falls, and the materials needed for surfactant production are not circulated to the alveoli.

Diagnostic Evaluation

The diagnosis of RDS is made on the basis of clinical manifestations (Box 9-4) and radiographic studies. Radiographic findings characteristic of RDS include (1) a diffuse granular pattern over both lung fields that closely resembles ground glass and represents alveolar atelectasis and (2) dark streaks, or bronchograms, within the ground glass areas that represent dilated, air-filled bronchioles. It is difficult to distinguish between RDS and pneumonia in infants with respiratory distress. The extent of respiratory function and acid–base balance is determined by blood gas analysis. Criteria for visually evaluating the degree of respiratory distress are illustrated in Figure 9-20. Pulse oximetry and carbon dioxide monitoring, as well as pulmonary function studies, assist in differentiating pulmonary and extrapulmonary illness and are used in the management of RDS.

QUALITY PATIENT OUTCOMES: Neonatal RDS
- Room air or oxygen saturation ≥90%
- Respiratory rate <60 breaths/min
- Blood pH ≥7.35

Therapeutic Management

The treatment of RDS involves immediate establishment of adequate oxygenation and ventilation and supportive care and measures required for any preterm infant, as well as those instituted to prevent further complications associated with preterm birth. The supportive measures most crucial to a favorable outcome are to:

BOX 9-4 CLINICAL MANIFESTATIONS OF RESPIRATORY DISTRESS SYNDROME

Tachypnea (≤80 to 120 breaths/min) initially*
Dyspnea
Pronounced intercostal or substernal retractions (Fig. 9-20)
Fine inspiratory crackles
Audible expiratory grunt
Flaring of the external nares
Cyanosis or pallor

*Not all infants born with respiratory distress syndrome manifest these characteristics; very low–birth-weight and extremely low–birth-weight infants may have respiratory failure and shock at birth because of physiologic immaturity.

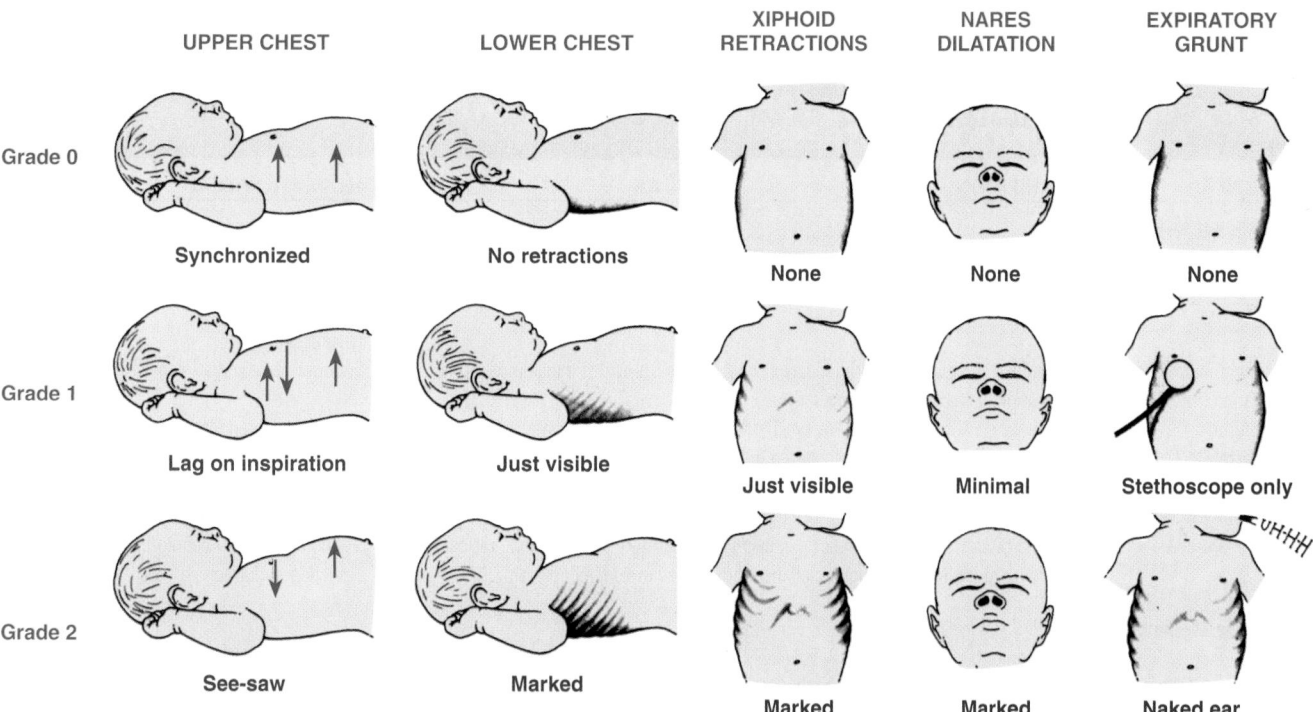

FIG 9-20 Criteria for evaluating respiratory distress. (Modified from Silvermann WA, Anderson DH: A controlled clinical trial of effects of water mist on obstructive respiratory signs, death rate, and necropsy findings among premature infants, *Pediatrics* 17:1, 1956.)

- Maintain adequate ventilation and oxygenation.
- Maintain acid–base balance.
- Maintain a neutral thermal environment.
- Maintain adequate tissue perfusion and oxygenation.
- Prevent hypotension.
- Maintain adequate hydration and electrolyte status.

Nipple and gavage feedings are contraindicated in any situation that creates a marked increase in respiratory rate because of the greater hazards of aspiration. Nutrition is provided by parenteral therapy during the acute stage of the disease, and minimal enteral feeding is provided to enhance maturation of the neonate's gastrointestinal system.

The administration of **exogenous surfactant** to preterm neonates with RDS has become an accepted and common therapy in most neonatal centers worldwide. Numerous clinical trials involving the administration of exogenous surfactant to infants with or at high risk for RDS demonstrate improvements in blood gas values and ventilator settings, decreased incidence of pulmonary air leaks, intraventricular hemorrhage, decreased deaths from RDS, and an overall decreased infant mortality rate (AAP, Committee on Fetus and Newborn, 2008; Stevens and Sinkin, 2007). The overall rates of some associated comorbidities (bronchopulmonary dysplasia, NEC, patent ductus arteriosus) have not decreased with surfactant replacement. Currently, exogenous surfactant is derived from a natural source (e.g., porcine, bovine).

Complications seen with surfactant administration include pulmonary hemorrhage and mucous plugging. Surfactant therapy is also being used in infants with meconium aspiration, infectious pneumonia, sepsis, persistent pulmonary hypertension, and lung hypoplasia concomitant with congenital diaphragmatic hernia (Stevens and Sinkin, 2007). Surfactant may be administered at birth as a preventive or prophylactic treatment of RDS or later on in the course of RDS as a rescue treatment; however, research has demonstrated improved clinical outcomes and fewer adverse effects when surfactant is administered prophylactically to infants at risk for developing RDS (AAP,

Committee on Fetus and Newborn, 2008; Stevens, Harrington, Blennow, and others, 2007). Surfactant is administered via an endotracheal (ET) tube directly into the infant's trachea. Nursing responsibilities with surfactant administration include assistance in the delivery of the product, collection and monitoring of arterial blood gases, scrupulous monitoring of oxygenation with pulse oximetry, and assessment of the infant's tolerance of the procedure. After surfactant is absorbed, there is usually an increase in respiratory compliance that requires adjustment of ventilator settings to decrease mean airway pressure and prevent overinflation or hyperoxemia. Suctioning is usually delayed for an hour or so (depending on the type of surfactant and unit protocol) to allow maximum effects to occur. Studies have shown the benefit of administering surfactant early (prophylactic) in infants at risk for developing RDS, then extubating and placing on nasal continuous positive airway pressure (CPAP); this decreased the overall incidence of bronchopulmonary dysplasia, need for mechanical ventilation, and fewer air leak syndromes (Stevens, Harrington, Blennow, and others, 2007). Research is in progress to investigate the possibility of delivering an aerosolized surfactant (Donn and Sinha, 2008; Mazela, Merritt, and Finer, 2007). This method would decrease the problems associated with current delivery systems (contamination of the airway, interruption of mechanical ventilation, and loss of the drug in the ET tubing from reflux).

The goals of oxygen therapy are to provide adequate oxygen to the tissues, prevent lactic acid accumulation resulting from hypoxia, and at the same time avoid the potentially negative effects of oxygen and barotrauma. Numerous methods have been devised to improve oxygenation (Table 9-5). All require that the gas be warmed and humidified before entering the respiratory tract. If the infant does not require mechanical ventilation, oxygen can be supplied by nasal cannula or via nasal prongs in conjunction with CPAP (see Oxygen Therapy, Chapter 22). If oxygen saturation of the blood cannot be maintained at a satisfactory level and the carbon dioxide level ($PaCO_2$) rises, infants will require ventilatory assistance.

TABLE 9-5	COMMON METHODS FOR ASSISTED VENTILATION IN NEONATAL RESPIRATORY DISTRESS		
METHOD	**DESCRIPTION**		**HOW PROVIDED**
Conventional Methods			
Continuous positive airway pressure (CPAP)	Provides constant distending pressure to airway in spontaneously breathing infant		Nasal prongs Endotracheal tube Face mask Nasal cannula
Intermittent mandatory ventilation (IMV)*	Allows infant to breathe spontaneously at own rate but provides mechanical cycled respirations and pressure at regular preset intervals		Endotracheal intubation and ventilator
Synchronized intermittent mandatory ventilation (SIMV)	Mechanically delivered breaths are synchronized to the onset of spontaneous patient breaths; assist/control mode facilitates full inspiratory synchrony; involves signal detection of onset of spontaneous respiration from abdominal movement, thoracic impedance, and airway pressure or flow changes		Patient-triggered infant ventilator with signal detector and assist/control mode; endotracheal tube
Volume guarantee ventilation	Delivers a predetermined volume of gas using an inspiratory pressure that varies according to the infant's lung compliance (often used in conjunction with SIMV)		Volume guarantee ventilator with flow sensor; endotracheal tube
Alternative Methods			
High-frequency oscillation (HFO)	Application of high-frequency, low-volume, sine-wave flow oscillations to airway at rates between 480 and 1200 breaths/min		Variable-speed piston pump (or loudspeaker, fluidic oscillator); endotracheal tube
High-frequency jet ventilation (HFJV)	Uses a separate, parallel, low-compliant circuit and injector port to deliver small pulses or jets of fresh gas deep into airway at rates between 250 and 900 breaths/min		May be used alone or with low-rate IMV; endotracheal tube

*Also referred to as conventional ventilation (vs. high-frequency ventilation [HFV]).

Prevention

The most successful approach to prevention of RDS is prevention of preterm delivery, especially in elective early delivery and cesarean section. Improved methods for assessing the maturity of the fetal lung by amniocentesis, although not a routine procedure, allow a reasonable prediction of adequate surfactant formation. Because estimation of a delivery date can be miscalculated by as much as 1 month, such tests are particularly valuable when scheduling an elective cesarean section. The combination of maternal steroid administration before delivery and surfactant administration postnatally seems to have a synergistic effect on neonatal lungs, with the net result being a decrease in infant mortality, decreased incidence of intraventricular hemorrhage, fewer pulmonary air leaks, and fewer problems with pulmonary interstitial emphysema and RDS (Warren and Anderson, 2009).

Prognosis

Respiratory distress syndrome is a self-limiting disease. Before the use of surfactant, infants typically experienced a period of deterioration ($\approx$48 hours) and, in the absence of complications, improved by 72 hours. Often heralded by the onset of diuresis, this improvement was attributed primarily to increased production and greater availability of surfactant. With the administration of surfactant, lung compliance begins to improve almost immediately, resulting in lower oxygen requirements and a decreased need for ventilatory support (Stevens and Sinkin, 2007).

Infants with RDS who survive the first 96 hours have a reasonable chance of recovery. However, complications of RDS include associated respiratory conditions and problems associated with prematurity, including patent ductus arteriosus and congestive heart failure, intraventricular hemorrhage, bronchopulmonary dysplasia, retinopathy of prematurity, pneumonia, air leak syndrome, sepsis, NEC, and neurologic sequelae.

Nursing Care Management

Care of infants with RDS involves all of the observations and interventions previously described for high-risk infants. In addition, the nurse is concerned with the complex problems related to respiratory therapy and the constant threat of hypoxemia and acidosis that complicates the care of patients in respiratory difficulty.

The respiratory therapist, an important member of the NICU team, is often responsible for the maintenance of respiratory equipment.

Although it may be the respiratory therapist's responsibility to regulate the apparatus, nurses should understand the equipment and be able to recognize when it is not functioning correctly. The most essential nursing function is to observe and assess the infant's response to therapy. Continuous monitoring and close observation are mandatory because an infant's status can change rapidly and because oxygen concentration and ventilation parameters are prescribed according to the infant's blood gas measurements and pulse oximetry readings.

Changes in oxygen concentration are based on these observations. The amount of oxygen administered, expressed as the fraction of inspired air (FiO_2), is determined on an individual basis according to pulse oximetry or direct or indirect measurement of arterial oxygen concentration. Capillary samples collected from the heel (see Chapter 22 for procedure) are useful for pH and $PaCO_2$ determinations but not for oxygenation status. Continuous transcutaneous or pulse oximetry readings are recorded at least hourly. Blood sampling is performed after ventilator changes for the acutely ill infant and thereafter when clinically indicated.

Mucus may collect in the respiratory tract as a result of the infant's pulmonary condition. Secretions interfere with gas flow and predispose the infant to obstruction of the passages, including the ET tube. Suctioning should be performed only when necessary and should be based on individual infant assessment, which includes auscultation of the chest, evidence of decreased oxygenation, excess moisture in the ET tube, or increased infant irritability. During suctioning, a variety of techniques can be used to minimize complications, including the use of a closed suctioning system (Cifuentes and Carlo, 2007). (See Evidence-Based Practice box.)

❗ NURSING ALERT

Endotracheal suctioning is not an innocuous procedure (it may cause bronchospasm, bradycardia resulting from vagal nerve stimulation, hypoxia, or increased ICP, predisposing the infant to intraventricular hemorrhage) and should never be carried out on a routine basis. Improper suctioning technique can also cause infection, airway damage, or even pneumothoraces.

When nasopharyngeal passages, the trachea, or the ET tube is being suctioned, the catheter should be inserted gently but quickly; intermittent suction is applied as the catheter is withdrawn. Negative airway

Nursing Care Plan—The High-Risk Infant with Respiratory Distress Syndrome

---

EVIDENCE-BASED PRACTICE

Normal Saline Instillation Before Endotracheal or Tracheostomy Suctioning—Helpful or Harmful?

Updated by Olga A. Taylor

Ask the Question
PICOT Question
In intubated children and those with tracheostomy, is normal saline (NS) instillation before suctioning helpful or harmful?

Search for Evidence
Search Strategies
Searched all literature from 1980 to 2011

Databases Used
PubMed, Cochrane Collaboration, MDConsult, BestBETs, PedsCCM, AHRQ

Critically Analyze the Evidence
- Adult studies have found decreased oxygen saturation, increased frequency of nosocomial pneumonia, and increased intracranial pressure (ICP) after instillation of NS before suctioning (Ackerman, 1993; Ackerman and Gugerty, 1990; Bostick and Wendelgass, 1987; Hagler and Traver, 1994; Kinlock, 1999; O'Neal, Grap, Thompson, and others, 2001; Reynolds, Hoffman, Schlichtig, and others, 1990).
- No significant differences in oxygenation, heart rate, or blood pressure were found before or after suctioning in a group of 27 intubated neonates (Shorten, Byrne, and Jones, 1991).
- No adverse effects on lung mechanics were found after NS instillation and suctioning in neonates (Beeram and Dhanireddy, 1992).

Continued

EVIDENCE-BASED PRACTICE

Normal Saline Instillation Before Endotracheal or Tracheostomy Suctioning—Helpful or Harmful?—cont'd

- Children (ages 10 weeks–14 years) experienced significantly greater oxygen desaturation after suctioning if NS was instilled (Ridling, Martin, and Bratton, 2003).
- With tracheostomies, NS should not be instilled before suctioning (American Thoracic Society, 2005).
- Evidence does not support routine instillation of NS in neonates; however, abundant evidence indicates adverse effects of NS instillation (Gardner and Shirland, 2009).
- Evidence indicating the adverse effects of the use of saline for suctioning is lacking in the pediatric population. However, saline should not be routinely used for suctioning infants and children (Morrow and Argent, 2008).
- Endotracheal suctioning performed with saline solution was associated with an increase in episodes of bradycardia, desaturations, and need for increase in the fraction of inspired oxygen (FiO_2) (Trevisanuto, Doglioni, and Zanardo, 2009).
- Potential harms that may be associated with use of NS installation include increased coughing, oxygen desaturation, bronchospasms, tachycardia, pain, anxiety, dyspnea, increased ICP, and loosened bacterial biofilm that may colonize the endotracheal tube (American Association for Respiratory Care, 2010).
- Use of low-sodium solution for airway suctioning in neonates significantly decreased ventilator-associated pneumonia and rates of chronic lung disease (Christensen, Henry, Baer, and others, 2010).

Apply the Evidence: Nursing Implications

There is **moderate quality evidence** with a **strong recommendation** that adverse effects of NS instillation before suctioning in children are similar to those found for adults (Guyatt, Oxman, Vist, and others, 2008). This technique causes a significant reduction in oxygen saturation that can last up to 2 minutes after suctioning. The evidence does not support the use of NS instillation before endotracheal suctioning in children.

QSEN **Quality and Safety Competencies:**
Evidence-Based Practice*

Knowledge

Differentiate clinical opinion from research and evidence-based summaries.

Describe methods for using NS instillation before endotracheal or tracheostomy suctioning.

Skills

Base individualized care plan on patient values, clinical expertise, and evidence.

Integrate evidence into practice on NS instillation before endotracheal or tracheostomy suctioning.

Attitudes

Value the concept of evidence-based practice as integral to determining best clinical practice.

Appreciate strengths and weakness of evidence for NS instillation before endotracheal or tracheostomy suctioning.

References

Ackerman MH: The effect of saline lavage prior to suctioning, *Am J Crit Care* 2(4):326–330, 1993.

Ackerman MH, Gugerty B: The effect of normal saline bolus instillation in artificial airways, *J Soc Otorhinolaryngol Head Neck Nurs* 8:14–17, 1990.

American Association for Respiratory Care: AARC Clinical Practice Guidelines. Endotracheal suctioning of mechanically ventilated patients with artificial airways, *Respir Care* 55(6):758–764, 2010.

American Thoracic Society: Care of the child with a chronic tracheostomy, 2005, retrieved April 17, 2006, from http://www.thoracic.org/sections/publications/statements/pages/respiratory-disease-pediatric/childtrach1–12.html.

Beeram MR, Dhanireddy R: Effects of saline instillation during tracheal suction on lung mechanics in newborn infants, *J Perinatol* 12(2):120–123, 1992.

Bostick J, Wendelgass ST: Normal saline instillation as part of the suctioning procedure: Effects of PaO_2 and amount of secretions, *Heart Lung* 16(5):532–537, 1987.

Christensen RD, Henry E, Baer VL, and others: A low-sodium solution for airway care: results of a multicenter trial, *Respir Care* 5(12):1680–1685, 2010.

Garland DL, Shirland L: Evidence-based guideline for suctioning the intubated neonate and infant, *Neonatal Netw* 28(5):281–302, 2009.

Guyatt GH, Oxman AD, Vist GE, and others: GRADE: An emerging consensus on rating quality of evidence and strength of recommendations, *BMJ* 336(7650):924–926, 2008.

Hagler DA, Traver GA: Endotracheal saline and suction catheters: sources of lower airway contamination, *Am J Crit Care* 3(6):444–447, 1994.

Kinlock D: Instillation of normal saline during endotracheal suctioning: effects on mixed venous oxygen saturation, *Am J Crit Care* 8(4):231–240, 1999.

Morrow BM, Argent AC: A comprehensive review of pediatric endotracheal suctioning: effects, indications, and clinical practice, *Pediatr Crit Care Med* 9(5):465–477, 2008.

O'Neal PV, Grap MJ, Thompson C, and others: Level of dyspnoea experienced in mechanically ventilated adults with and without saline instillation prior to endotracheal suctioning, *Intensive Crit Care Nurs* 17(6):356–363, 2001.

Reynolds P, Hoffman LA, Schlichtig R, and others: Effects of normal saline instillation on secretion volume, dynamic compliance, and oxygen saturation [abstract], *Am Rev Respir Dis* 141:A574, 1990.

Ridling DA, Martin LD, Bratton SL: Endotracheal suctioning with or without instillation of isotonic sodium chloride in critically ill children, *Am J Crit Care* 12(3):212–219, 2003.

Shorten DR, Byrne PJ, Jones RL: Infant responses to saline instillations and endotracheal suctioning, *J Obstet Gynecol Neonatal Nurs* 20(6):464–469, 1991.

Trevisanuto D, Doglioni N, Zanardo V: The management of endotracheal tubes and nasal cannulae: the role of nurses, *Early Hum Dev* 85:S85–S87, 2009.

*Adapted from the QSEN at http://www.qsen.org.

---

pressure should be applied for no more than 10 to 15 seconds because continuous suction removes air from the lungs along with the mucus. It is recommended that the "two-person" suctioning procedure be used on infants who are acutely ill and who do not tolerate any procedure without profound decreases in oxygen saturation, BP, and heart rate. The object of suctioning an artificial airway is to maintain patency of that airway, not the bronchi. Suction applied beyond the ET tube can cause traumatic lesions of the trachea. The use of in-line suction catheters may decrease airway contamination and hypoxia. Evidence-based guidelines for ET suctioning of neonates have been published (Gardner and Shirland, 2009).

The most advantageous positions for facilitating an infant's open airway are on the side with the head supported in alignment by a small folded blanket or, when on the back, positioned to keep the neck slightly extended. With the head in the "sniffing" position, the trachea is opened at its maximum; hyperextension reduces the tracheal diameter in neonates.

Inspection of the skin is part of routine infant assessment. Position changes and the use of water pillows are helpful in guarding against skin breakdown.

Mouth care is especially important when infants are receiving NPO, and the problem is often aggravated by the drying effect of oxygen therapy. Drying and cracking can be prevented by good oral hygiene using sterile water. Irritation to the nares or mouth that occurs from appliances used to administer oxygen (e.g., nasal CPAP) may be reduced by the use of a water-soluble ointment. Routine oral hygiene care in intubated adults and older children has been shown to decerease the incidence of ventilator-associated pneumonia (see Chapter 23).

The nursing care of an infant with RDS is a demanding role; meticulous attention must be given to subtle changes in the infant's oxygenation status. The importance of attention to detail cannot be overemphasized, particularly in regard to medication administration. (See Nursing Care Plan.)

RESPIRATORY COMPLICATIONS

Newborn infants are vulnerable to a variety of pulmonary complications, some requiring oxygen therapy (Table 9-6). For example, the preterm infant is subject to periods of apnea, and in term, late preterm, and postterm infants, intrauterine stress often causes fetuses to pass meconium, which may be aspirated before or during birth. Oxygen therapy, although lifesaving, is not without its hazards. Positive pressure introduced by mechanical apparatus has created an increase in the incidence of ruptured alveoli and subsequent **pneumothorax** and **bronchopulmonary dysplasia (chronic lung disease)**. The use of nasal CPAP decreases the incidence of adverse effects associated with intubation and positive-pressure ventilation in preterm infants with RDS. **Retinopathy of prematurity** is observed almost exclusively in preterm infants and is related primarily to prematurity and oxygen therapy (see Table 9-6). Some evidence supports the resuscitation of asphyxiated newborns with 21% oxygen rather than 100% oxygen; preliminary studies demonstrate no significant neurologic morbidities at 18 to 24 months in newborns resuscitated with 21% oxygen (Saugstad, 2007; Saugstad, Ramji, Irani, and others, 2003). Proponents for room air resuscitation suggest that fewer complications are associated with oxidative stress and hyperoxemia when room air is administered (Vento and Saugstad, 2011). The 2010 American Heart Association Neonatal Resuscitation Guidelines recommend the initiation of neonatal

---

◎ NURSING CARE PLAN

The High-Risk Infant with Respiratory Distress Syndrome

NURSING DIAGNOSIS	PATIENT OUTCOMES	NURSING INTERVENTIONS	RATIONALE
Ineffective Breathing Pattern related to pulmonary, neurologic, vascular, alveolar, and muscular immaturity	High-risk infant will maintain patent airway and ventilatory status adequate for oxygenation.	Position to facilitate airway expansion and prevent collection of secretions (prone position may be preferred in preterm infant to increase chest expansion and oxygenation).	To allow oxygen entry into bronchial tree and alveoli
Child's or Family's Defining Characteristics <u>(Subjective and Objective Data)</u>	**The Following NOC Concepts Apply to These Outcomes**	Closely monitor for deviations from desired breathing pattern—pulse oximetry, arterial blood gases, clinical signs of poor oxygenation, grunting, nasal flaring, apnea, tachypnea, retractions, and cyanosis.	To facilitate proper oxygenation by implementing appropriate therapy such as supplemental oxygen, mechanical ventilation, or change of position
Decreased inspiratory and expiratory pressure	Respiratory Status: Ventilation	Monitor vital signs for change in condition or status such as decreased cardiac output (poor perfusion, mottling, deteriorating ventilation status).	To implement appropriate therapy such as suctioning, supplemental oxygen, or vasopressor drugs
Decreased minute ventilation	Respiratory Status: Gas Exchange		
Use of accessory muscles to breathe	Tissue Perfusion: Pulmonary	Assist with exogenous surfactant administration and monitor patient tolerance or change in status.	To increase alveolar expansion and enhance oxygen–carbon dioxide exchange
Nasal flaring			
Grunting		Suction oropharynx, nasopharynx, trachea, or endotracheal tube only as necessary and based on respiratory assessment.	To remove secretions that may interfere with adequate ventilation and oxygenation
Apnea			
Tachypnea			
Altered chest excursion		Perform gentle chest percussion, vibration, and postural drainage based on assessed need and infant tolerance.	To facilitate drainage and removal of secretions
Respiratory rate: <20 or >60 breaths/min			
		The Following NIC Concepts Apply to These Interventions Vital Signs Monitoring Newborn Monitoring Acid–Base Management Airway Management Chest Physiotherapy Oxygen Therapy Airway Suctioning Energy Management Respiratory Monitoring	

Continued

⊚ NURSING CARE PLAN

The High-Risk Infant with Respiratory Distress Syndrome—cont'd

NURSING DIAGNOSIS	PATIENT OUTCOMES	NURSING INTERVENTIONS	RATIONALE
Ineffective Thermoregulation related to immature neurologic and metabolic temperature control	Infant will maintain stable body temperature (specify range for age).	Place ELBW or VLBW infant in polyethylene wrap or bag immediately after birth (after drying off rapidly). Place newborn in a thermally controlled incubator or radiant warmer.	To control environmental temperature and keep infant's temperature stable
Child's or Family's Defining Characteristics <u>(Subjective and Objective Data)</u>	**The Following NOC Concept Applies to These Outcomes**	Use environmental controls for decreasing body heat loss (plastic heat shield, increased ambient temperature, servo control on warmer or incubator).	To regulate body temperature within acceptable range and minimize heat loss
Reduction in body temperature below normal range	Thermoregulation: Newborn	Place knitted or cloth cap on head.	To prevent heat loss from exposed scalp
Slow capillary refill Cool skin Increased respiratory rate Tachycardia		Monitor axillary temperature as often as necessary or per unit protocol.	To detect necessity for environmental temperature regulation and to determine infant's response to environmental thermoregulation
		Check temperature of newborn in relation to environmental temperature and temperature of heating element.	To detect change in thermoregulatory status, which may indicate a significant disease process such as sepsis
		Monitor vital signs and skin color, perfusion, pulses, and respiratory status.	To detect changes in status that require additional intervention for stabilization
		Monitor for signs of hyperthermia (flushing, tachycardia, altered level of consciousness) and hypothermia (decreased activity; respiratory distress [deterioration]; cool, mottled extremities).	To prevent untoward effects of hyperthermia (fluctuating cerebral perfusion, apnea, increased metabolism with decreased available glucose for vital functions) or hypothermia (increased glucose utilization, lactic acidosis, respiratory compromise)
		Monitor serum glucose levels as necessary or per unit protocol.	To ensure euglycemia is maintained
		The Following NIC Concepts Apply to These Interventions Environmental Management Hypothermia Treatment	
Risk for Impaired Parent–Infant Attachment	Parent(s) will form emotional bond or attachment with newborn.	Encourage parent(s) to hold and make eye contact with newborn as physical status allows.	To minimize effects of physical separation from newborn
Child's or Family's Defining Characteristics <u>(Subjective and Objective Data)</u>		Encourage parent–newborn skin-to-skin contact in delivery room as condition of newborn allows.	To facilitate parent–infant interaction that is meaningful and comforting
Risk Factors	**The Following NOC Concept Applies to These Outcomes**	Explain to parents the newborn's illness in simple terms and expectations for recovery.	To enhance parental knowledge and decrease potential fear of unknown regarding infant's survival and recovery
Separation Preterm infant Physical barriers	Parent–Infant Attachment	Encourage parents to name newborn.	To provide child individual identity
		Encourage parent participation in newborn care activities such as touching infant, expressing and storing maternal breast milk, and talking to infant.	To facilitate parental involvement in attaining the role of parents and decrease feelings of helplessness
		The Following NIC Concepts Apply to These Interventions Infant Care Breastfeeding Assistance Anxiety Reduction Parent Education: Infant	

ELBW, Extremely low–birth-weight; *NIC*, Nursing Interventions Classification; *NOC*, Nursing Outcomes Classification; *VLBW*, very low–birth-weight.

TABLE 9-6	RESPIRATORY COMPLICATIONS		
DESCRIPTION	**CLINICAL MANIFESTATIONS**	**THERAPEUTIC MANAGEMENT**	**NURSING CARE MANAGEMENT**
Meconium Aspiration Syndrome (MAS)			
Aspiration of amniotic fluid containing meconium into fetal or newborn trachea in utero or at first breath	Meconium stained at birth Tachypnea Hypoxia Acidemia Hyperventilation (early) Hypoventilation (later)	Suction hypopharynx after the head is delivered. Infants who are vigorous with strong, stable respiratory effort, good muscle tone, and heart rate >100 beats/min should not undergo tracheal suctioning but should be closely monitored. Infants who demonstrate poor respiratory effort, low heart rate, and poor tone should be rapidly intubated, suctioned appropriately, and resuscitated according to clinical status after suctioning. Monitor for respiratory distress; manage with supplemental oxygen. Prevent acidosis and hypoxemia. May use exogenous surfactant, inhaled nitric oxide, or extracorporeal membrane oxygenation (ECMO).	See Nursing Care Management, Respiratory Distress Syndrome (p. 271).
Apnea of Prematurity			
Lapse of spontaneous breathing for ≥20 seconds, which may or may not be followed by bradycardia, oxygen desaturation, and color change	Persistent apneic spells	Observe for apnea. Check for thermal stability and metabolic problem such as hypoglycemia. Administer caffeine as prescribed. Administer nasal continuous positive airway pressure (CPAP).	Provide continuous electronic monitoring (respiratory and heart rates). Observe for presence of respirations. Observe color. Provide gentle tactile stimulation. Suction nose and oropharynx if still apneic. Apply positive pressure ventilation with bag-valve-mask using the minimum of pressure needed to gently lift rib cage. Assess for and manage any precipitating factors (e.g., temperature instability, abdominal distention, ambient oxygen). Observe for signs of caffeine toxicity: tachycardia (rate ≥180 beats/min) and (later) vomiting, restlessness, irritability. Assess skin (with use of nasal CPAP) for breakdown, irritation at nasal septum.
Pneumothorax			
Presence of extraneous air in pleural space as a result of alveolar rupture	Tachypnea or apnea Systemic hypotension Sudden or persistent oxygen desaturation Grunting, nasal flaring Retractions Absent or diminished breath sounds Shift in point of maximum impulse of heart sounds Bradycardia, cyanosis	Evacuate trapped air in pleural space through needle aspiration or insertion of chest tube. In otherwise healthy term infants who do not require high oxygen concentration or mechanical ventilation, a nitrogen "washout" may be performed with 100% oxygen; this accelerates the resorption of free air in the pleura into the blood; consider benefits and risks of hyperoxygenation.	Maintain close vigilance of infants with respiratory distress and those on assisted ventilation. Provide appropriate care of chest drainage apparatus. Ensure emergency needle aspiration setup is available.

Continued

TABLE 9-6 RESPIRATORY COMPLICATIONS—cont'd

DESCRIPTION	CLINICAL MANIFESTATIONS	THERAPEUTIC MANAGEMENT	NURSING CARE MANAGEMENT
Bronchopulmonary Dysplasia			

Pathologic process related to alveolar damage from lung disease, prolonged exposure to mechanical ventilation, high peak inspiratory pressures and oxygen, and immature alveoli and respiratory tract	Dyspnea
	Barrel chest
	Inability to wean from oxygen or mechanical ventilation after course of respiratory distress syndrome (surfactant deficiency)
	Wheezing
		Prevention:
		  Administer maternal steroids; administer exogenous surfactant postnatally.
		  Provide early detection with pulmonary function tests.
		  Use synchronized or volume guarantee ventilation, decreased inspiratory pressures, or nasal CPAP.
		  Prevent air leaks.
		  Use high-frequency ventilation.
		  Prevent or control respiratory or systemic infections.
		  Minimize use of high oxygen concentrations in neonatal resuscitation and on mechanical ventilation; monitor oxygen saturation and implement resuscitation according to neonate response to low oxygen administration
		Diagnosis established:
		  Support respiratory efforts.
		  Maintain adequate oxygenation and avoid hypoxemia.
		  Administer diuretics, bronchodilators.
		  Provide supplemental oxygen in hospital or home.
			Provide individualized developmental care and enhancement.
			Monitor oxygen saturations closely in preterm infants and avoid hyperoxemia
			Provide opportunities for additional rest during feedings.
			Observe for signs of fluid overload or pulmonary edema.
			Assist with home oxygen therapy as needed.
			Assess susceptibility to upper respiratory tract infections and need for frequent hospitalization for respiratory dysfunction.
			Provide increased caloric density (feedings) with human milk fortifier or protein supplements.

Persistent Pulmonary Hypertension of the Newborn (PPHN)			
Severe pulmonary hypertension and large right-to-left shunt through foramen ovale and ductus arteriosus	Hypoxia Marked cyanosis Tachypnea with grunting and retractions Decreased peripheral pulses and prolonged capillary refill (poor perfusion) Shock	Regulate intravenous (IV) fluids. Provide supplemental oxygen and assisted ventilation. Administer systemic vasodilators such as sildenafil. Maintain acid–base balance. Prevent hypoxemia and hypercarbia. Administer inhaled nitric oxide or ECMO.	See Nursing Care of the High-Risk Newborn and Family (p. 235) and Respiratory Distress Syndrome (p. 267). Provide nursing care to reduce stress to infant, especially noxious stimuli that cause increased oxygen demands. Decrease physical manipulation and disturbance.
Retinopathy of Prematurity			
Severe vascular constriction in the immature retinal vasculature followed by hypoxemia in the retina, which in turn stimulates abnormal vascular proliferation of retinal capillaries into the hypoxic area; as retinal veins dilate and multiply in the direction of the lens, retinal detachment may occur if untreated Multifactorial etiology—preterm birth is major risk factor	Progressive vascular growth of retina Eventual blindness if not treated Diagnosed by ophthalmologic examination	Prevent preterm birth. Provide early screening and detection in infants born at <28 weeks of gestation and weight <1500 g (3.3 pounds). Decrease exposure to bright, direct lighting; although exposure to bright light has not been proven to contribute to retinopathy of prematurity, such exposure is undesirable from a neurobehavioral developmental perspective. Use supplemental oxygen judiciously and monitor oxygen blood levels carefully; prevent wide fluctuations in oxygen blood levels (hyperoxemia and hypoxemia). Arrest vascular proliferation process—cryotherapy or laser photocoagulation; surgical repair of detached retina. Recently, there has been increased interest in the administration of an antivascular endothelial growth factor drug bevacizumab, which arrests the proliferation of vessels and prevents retinal detachment commonly seen in retinopathy of prematurity. If successful, this therapy may preclude the use of laser therapy (Mintz-Hittner and Best, 2009).	See Nursing Care of the High-Risk Newborn and Family (p. 235). Provide preventive care by closely monitoring blood oxygen levels, responding promptly to saturation alarms, and preventing fluctuations in blood oxygen levels. Provide postoperative pain management if surgery is performed. Provide parental education and support. Provide nursing care using principles of individualized developmental care.

ABBREVIATION	TEST	NORMAL VALUES*	DESCRIPTION
pH	Partial pressure of hydrogen	Birth: 7.11–7.36 1 day: 7.29–7.45 Child: 7.35–7.45	Expression of hydrogen ion concentration
PCO_2	Partial pressure of carbon dioxide or carbon dioxide tension	Newborn: 27–40 mm Hg Infant: 27–41 mm Hg Girls: 32–45 mm Hg Boys: 35–48 mm Hg	Measure of carbon dioxide tension; reflects carbonic acid (H_2CO_3) concentrations of plasma
HCO_3^- (serum) arterial	Carbon dioxide content or carbon dioxide combining power	Infant: 21–28 mEq/ml Thereafter: 22–26 mEq/ml	Concentration of base bicarbonate
Base excess	Base excess (whole blood)	Newborn: −2 to −10 Infant: −1 to −7 Child: +2 to −4 Thereafter: +3 to −3	Used to express extent of deviation from normal buffer base concentration; indicates quantity of blood buffers remaining after hydrogen ion is buffered
Anion gap	Anion gap; using chemistry profile and serum bicarbonate	10–12,* (4–11)[†]	Reflects difference between measured cation sodium and anions (also measured) of chloride and bicarbonate

TABLE 9-7   LABORATORY TESTS USED IN ASSESSMENT OF ACID–BASE STATUS

*Huether SE: The cellular environment: fluids and electrolytes, acids and bases. In McCance KL, Huether SE, Brashers VL, and others, editors: *Pathophysiology: the biologic basis for disease in adults and children,* ed 6, St. Louis, 2010, Mosby Elsevier.
[†]Data from Kliegman RM, Stanton BF, St. Geme JW, and others, editors: *Nelson textbook of pediatrics,* ed 19, Philadelphia, 2011, Saunders.

resuscitation using room air (no supplemental oxygen); if the neonate does not improve within 90 seconds, the use of supplemental oxygen is recommended (see Evidence-Based Practice box). Pulse oximetry is recommended to monitor the infant's oxygenation status during resuscitation and to prevent excessive use of oxygen in both term and preterm infants (Kattwinkel, Perlman, Aziz, and others, 2010).

> **QUALITY PATIENT OUTCOMES: Meconium Aspiration Syndrome**
> * Room air oxygen saturation ≥90%
> * Maintains arterial/venous pH ≥7.35

Inhaled nitric oxide (INO) and **extracorporeal membrane oxygenation (ECMO)** are additional therapies used in the treatment of respiratory distress and respiratory failure in neonates. INO is used in term and late preterm infants with conditions such as persistent pulmonary hypertension, meconium aspiration syndrome (see Table 9-6), pneumonia, sepsis, and congenital diaphragmatic hernia to decrease or reverse pulmonary hypertension, pulmonary vasoconstriction, acidosis, and hypoxemia. Nitric oxide is a colorless, highly diffusible gas that can be administered through the ventilator circuit blended with oxygen. INO therapy may be used in conjunction with surfactant replacement therapy, high-frequency ventilation, or ECMO. Although INO is used in preterm infants with respiratory distress and respiratory failure, its use has not proved to be significantly effective in decreasing rates of bronchopulmonary dysplasia or in improving survival rates in preterm infants (Barrington and Finer, 2007; Donohue, Gilmore, Cristofalo, and others, 2011).

Extracorporeal membrane oxygenation may be used in the management of term infants with acute severe respiratory failure for the same conditions as those mentioned for INO. This therapy involves a modified heart–lung machine, although in ECMO the heart is not stopped and blood does not entirely bypass the lungs. Blood is shunted from a catheter in the right atrium or right internal jugular vein by gravity to a servo-regulated roller pump, pumped through a membrane lung where it is oxygenated and through a small heat exchanger and then returned to the systemic circulation via a major artery such

as the carotid artery to the aortic arch. ECMO provides oxygen to the circulation; allows the lungs to "rest"; and decreases pulmonary hypertension and hypoxemia in such conditions as persistent pulmonary hypertension of the newborn, congenital diaphragmatic hernia, sepsis, meconium aspiration, and severe pneumonia.

Acid–Base Imbalance

Many respiratory and metabolic conditions in infants and children may cause an acid–base imbalance. Disease states such as diarrhea (see Chapter 24), RDS, ketoacidosis, bronchopulmonary dysplasia, and respiratory failure may interfere with the body's ability to regulate and maintain acid–base balance. Simply stated, **acidosis** (acidemia) results from either accumulation of acid or loss of base, and **alkalosis** (alkalemia) results from either accumulation of base or loss of acid. Several laboratory tests are used to assess the nature and extent of acid–base disturbances; these are outlined in Table 9-7. To determine the acid–base status, three variables—the respiratory component (PCO_2), the metabolic component (arterial bicarbonate or serum carbon dioxide [HCO_3^-]), and the serum pH—must be determined. In addition, the anion gap may be useful in determining the cause and extent of metabolic acidosis; therefore, serum chemistry is obtained as well. Measurement of any two variables (PCO_2, pH, HCO_3^-) allows computation of the third using the Henderson-Hasselbach equation. A summary of relationships between these and other variables is outlined in Table 9-8.

The pH represents the concentration of hydrogen (H^+) in solution and indicates only whether the imbalance is more acidic or more alkaline. It does not reflect the nature of the imbalance (i.e., whether it is of metabolic or respiratory origin). Body metabolism affects primarily the base bicarbonate (HCO_3^-); therefore, alterations in the concentration of bicarbonate are termed *metabolic disturbances of acid–base balance.* Also, because the amount of carbon dioxide (CO_2) exhaled through the lungs affects the carbonic acid (H_2CO_3), changes in carbonic acid concentration are referred to as *respiratory disturbances.* Consequently, the simple disturbances (those with a single primary cause) are categorized as metabolic acidosis or alkalosis and respiratory acidosis or alkalosis.

EVIDENCE-BASED PRACTICE

Use of Room Air or Low Oxygen for Newborn Stabilization and Resuscitation in the Delivery Room

Olga A. Taylor

Ask the Question
PICOT Question

Is room air or low oxygen better for newborn stabilization and resuscitation in the delivery room?

Search for Evidence
Search Strategies

Search selection included English publications on room air or low oxygen use for newborn stabilization and resuscitation in delivery room in past 3 years.

Database Used

PubMed

Critically Analyze the Evidence

- In infants weighing 1500 g or less, stabilization or resuscitation in the delivery room with fraction of inspired oxygen (FiO_2) below 100% or room air can be initiated without contributing to morbidity (Stola, Schulman, and Perlman, 2009).
- Systematic review of 21% O_2 versus 100% O_2 use for stabilization or resuscitation of newborns found a significant reduction in risk for newborn mortality as well as hypoxic ischemic encephalopathy when 21% O_2 was used (Saugstad, Ramji, Soll, and others, 2008).
- In neonates 24 to 28 weeks' gestational age, resuscitation with 30% O_2 versus 90% O_2 was associated with decreased oxidative stress, inflammation, need for O_2, and risk of bronchopulmonary dysplasia (Vento, Moro, Escrig, and others, 2009).
- In neonates less than or equal to 28 weeks' gestational age, use of a low FiO_2 (≤30%) for resuscitation was found to be safe. The supply of O_2 should be adjusted depending on the response of the newborn (Escrig, Arruza, Izquierdo, and others, 2008).
- In neonates less than or equal to 32 weeks' gestational age, target O_2 saturation was not achieved by 3 minutes of life when room air was used for resuscitation (Wang, Anderson, Leone, and others, 2008).
- Use of heated and humidified air in neonates less than or equal to 32 weeks' gestational age during resuscitation or stabilization in the delivery room minimized postnatal heat loss (te Pas, Lopriore, Dito, and others, 2010).
- Infants receiving 100% O_2 with positive-pressure ventilation and healthy infants transitioned in room air had similar increase in O_2 saturation, but a slower increase in O_2 saturation was observed in infants receiving 100% O_2 free flow (Rabi, Chen, Yee, and others, 2009).
- Newborns with spontaneous circulation (heart rate >60 beats/min) should be stabilized or resuscitated with room air, but asphyxiated newborns with depressed circulation (heart rate <60 beats/min) should be stabilized or resuscitated with 100% O_2 (Ten and Matsiukevich, 2009).
- In very preterm infants (<30 weeks' gestational age) stabilized or resuscitated with 100% O_2, the majority (80%) had SpO_2 95% in the first 10 minutes. Infants stabilized or resuscitated with room air followed a similar course as full-term and preterm newborns when 100% O_2 was administered along with titration against SpO_2. Similar changes in heart rate were observed in both groups (Dawson, Kamlin, Wong, and others, 2009).

- Room air is as effective as 100% O_2 in stabilizing or resuscitating newborns when using short-term outcome measures (Richmond and Goldsmith, 2008).

Apply the Evidence: Nursing Implications

There is **good evidence** with **strong recommendations** for using oxygen of various concentrations for newborn stabilization and delivery room resuscitations (Guyatt, Oxman, Vist, and others, 2008). Factors such as newborn gestational age and heart rate should be taken into consideration when determining oxygen concentration for neonatal resuscitation.

QSEN Quality and Safety Competencies: Evidence-Based Practice*
Knowledge

Differentiate clinical opinion from research and evidence-based summaries.

Describe the various interventions for newborn stabilization and delivery room resuscitations with room air or low oxygen.

Skills

Base individualized care plan on patient values, clinical expertise, and evidence.

Integrate evidence into practice by using interventions for newborn stabilization and delivery room resuscitations with room air or low oxygen.

Attitudes

Value the concept of evidence-based practice as integral to determining best clinical practice.

Appreciate strengths and weakness of evidence for newborn stabilization and delivery room resuscitations with room air or low oxygen.

References

Dawson JA, Kamlin COF, Wong C, and others: Oxygen saturation and heart rate during delivery room resuscitation of infants <30 weeks' gestation with air or 100% oxygen, *Arch Dis Child Fetal Neonatal Ed* 94:F87-F91, 2009.

Escrig R, Arruza L, Izquierdo I, and others: Achievement of targeted saturation values in extremely low gestational age neonates resuscitated with low or high oxygen concentrations: a prospective, randomized trial, *Pediatrics* 121(5):875-881, 2008.

Guyatt GH, Oxman AD, Vist GE, and others: GRADE: An emerging consensus on rating quality of evidence and strength of recommendations, *BMJ*, 336:924-926, 2008.

Rabi Y, Chen SY, Yee WH, and others: Relationship between oxygen saturation and the mode of oxygen delivery used in newborn resuscitation, *J Perinatol* 29:101-105, 2009.

Richmond S, Goldsmith JP: Refining the role of oxygen administration during delivery room resuscitation: what are the future goals? *Semin Fetal Neonatal Med* 13:368-374, 2008.

Saugstad OD, Ramji S, Soll RF, and others: Resuscitation of newborn infants with 21% or 100% oxygen: an updated systematic review and meta-analysis, *Neonatology* 94(3):176-182, 2008.

Stola A, Schulman J, Perlman J: Initiating delivery room stabilization/resuscitation in very low birth weight (VLBW) infants with an FiO2 less than 100% is feasible, *J Perinatol* 29:548-552, 2009.

te Pas AB, Lopriore E, Dito I, and others: Humidified and heated air during stabilization at birth improves temperature in preterm infants, *Pediatrics* 125(6):e1427-e1432, 2010.

Ten VS, Matsiukevich D: Room air or 100% oxygen for resuscitation of infants with prenatal depression, *Curr Opin Pediatr* 21:188-193, 2009.

Vento M, Moro M, Escrig R, and others: Preterm resuscitation with low oxygen causes less oxidative stress, inflammation, and chronic lung disease, *Pediatrics* 124(3):e439-e449, 2009.

Wang CL, Anderson C, Leone TA, and others: Resuscitation of preterm neonates by using room air or 100% oxygen, *Pediatrics* 121(6):1083-1089, 2008.

*Adapted from the QSEN at http://www.qsen.org.

TABLE 9-8	SUMMARY OF SIMPLE ACID–BASE DISTURBANCES (PARTIALLY COMPENSATED)		
DISTURBANCE	**PLASMA PH**	**PLASMA PCO$_2$**	**PLASMA HCO$_3^-$**
Respiratory acidosis	↓	↑	↑
Respiratory alkalosis	↑	↓	↓
Metabolic acidosis	↓	↓	↓
Metabolic alkalosis	↑	↑	↑

When the fundamental acid–base ratio is altered for any reason, the body attempts to correct the deviation. In a simple disturbance, a single primary factor affects one component of the acid–base pair and is usually accompanied by a compensatory or secondary change in the component that is not primarily affected. For example, increased formation of metabolic acid rapidly reduces the bicarbonate in the formation of carbonic acid. The respiratory mechanism immediately attempts to compensate for the imbalance by eliminating the carbonic acid through exhaled carbon dioxide and water. The imbalance is corrected when the kidneys excrete hydrogen and ammonium ions in exchange for reabsorbed sodium bicarbonate.

When the secondary changes (the hyperventilation and renal excretion of hydrogen ions in the preceding example) succeed in preventing a distortion of the acid–base ratio and the pH is restored to normal, the disturbance is described as compensated. The uncompensated state exists when there is no compensatory effect and the pH remains uncorrected. The imbalance is said to be corrected when physiologic mechanisms fully correct the primary abnormality. *Mixed* acid–base imbalances may also occur in diseases states, and the patient will manifest two simultaneous acid–base imbalances rather than a single imbalance. It is not within the scope of this text to discuss the many variations of mixed acid–base imbalances; readers are referred to other published sources for such material (Huether, 2010).

CARDIOVASCULAR COMPLICATIONS

The most serious cardiovascular disorders of newborns are the congenital heart defects. Other conditions that occur in the newborn period are usually related to prematurity (e.g., anemia, patent ductus arteriosus) or other diseases (e.g., respiratory distress). Some of these disorders are outlined in Table 9-9.

NEUROLOGIC COMPLICATIONS

Neurologic injury in newborn infants is common. Newborn infants are particularly vulnerable to ischemic injury caused by variable (both increased and decreased) cerebral blood flow subsequent to asphyxia, and preterm infants, with a fragile cerebrovascular network, are highly prone to periventricular or intraventricular hemorrhage. Fragility and increased permeability of capillaries and prolonged prothrombin time predispose preterm infants to trauma when delicate structures are subjected to the forces of labor. The more common neurologic complications are outlined in Table 9-10.

The highest incidence of abnormal neurologic findings occurs in VLBW infants and those with intracranial hemorrhage. Major neurologic problems, such as cerebral palsy, seizures, and hydrocephalus, are usually diagnosed in the first 2 years of life. Less severe deficits, such as learning disorders, ADHD, and fine and gross motor incoordination,

may not be diagnosed until preschool or even school age. Cerebral palsy is one of the most common neurologic deficits in survivors of prematurity (see Chapter 32).

NEONATAL SEIZURES

Seizures in the neonatal period are usually the clinical manifestation of a serious underlying disease. The most common cause of seizures for term and preterm neonates is hypoxic ischemic encephalopathy secondary to perinatal asphyxia (Volpe, 2008). Although not life threatening as an isolated entity, seizures constitute a medical emergency because they signal a disease process that may produce irreversible cerebral damage. Consequently, it is imperative to recognize a seizure and its significance so that the cause, as well as the seizure, can be treated (Box 9-5).

The features of neonatal seizures are different from those observed in older infants and children. For example, the well-organized, generalized tonic-clonic seizures seen in older children are rare in infants, especially preterm infants. The newborn brain, with its immature anatomic and physiologic status and less cortical organization, is unable to allow ready development and maintenance of a generalized seizure. Instead, signs of seizures in newborns, especially preterm neonates, are subtle and include findings such as lip smacking, tongue thrusting, eye rolling, and arching (Volpe, 2008).

Jitteriness or tremulousness in newborns is a repetitive shaking of an extremity or extremities that may be observed with crying, occur with changes in sleeping state, or is elicited with stimulation. Jitteriness is relatively common in newborns and in a mild degree may be considered normal during the first 4 days of life. Jitteriness can be distinguished from seizures by several characteristics:

- Jitteriness is not accompanied by ocular movement as are seizures.
- Whereas the dominant movement in jitteriness is tremor, seizure movement is clonic jerking that cannot be stopped by flexion of the affected limb.
- Jitteriness is highly sensitive to stimulation, but seizures are not.

Jitteriness may be a sign of hypoglycemia, and infants with jitteriness should have a blood glucose level evaluated.

A tremor is defined as repetitive movements of both hands (with or without movement of legs or jaws) at a frequency of two to five per second and lasting more than 10 minutes. It is common in newborn infants and has a variety of causes, including neurologic damage, hypoglycemia, and hypocalcemia. In most instances, tremors are of no pathologic significance.

Neonatal seizures can be divided into four major types. These classifications are outlined in order of frequency in Table 9-11 and consist of clonic, tonic, subtle, and myoclonic seizures (Volpe, 2008). Clonic, multifocal clonic, and migratory clonic seizures are more common in term infants.

Diagnostic Evaluation

Early evaluation and diagnosis of seizures are urgent. In addition to a careful physical examination, the pregnancy and family histories are investigated for familial and prenatal causes. Blood is drawn for glucose and electrolyte examination, and CSF may be obtained for testing of cell count and differential, protein, glucose, and culture. Electroencephalography (EEG) may help identify subtle seizures but is less helpful in establishing a diagnosis. Other diagnostic procedures, such as CT, MRI, and cerebral ultrasonography, may be indicated. A video EEG may be used to identify seizure activity in some newborns. More extensive metabolic testing may be needed when initial test results do

TABLE 9-9	CARDIOVASCULAR AND HEMATOLOGIC COMPLICATIONS		
DESCRIPTION	**CLINICAL MANIFESTATIONS**	**THERAPEUTIC MANAGEMENT**	**NURSING CARE MANAGEMENT**
Patent Ductus Arteriosus (PDA)			
Failure of ductus arteriosus to close at birth, resulting in shunting of oxygenated blood from aorta through open ductus arteriosus into pulmonary artery, increasing workload on left side of heart and increasing pulmonary vascular congestion (see Chapter 25)	Decreased PaO_2 Increased PCO_2 Recurrent apnea Bounding peripheral pulses Systolic or continuous murmur	Regulate parenteral fluids. Provide respiratory support. Administer course of indomethacin or ibuprofen or perform surgical ductal ligation.	See Nursing Care of the High-Risk Newborn and Family (p. 235).
Anemia			
Hemoglobin (<14 mg/dl) inadequate to carry oxygenated blood to tissues Anemia commonly occurs in ill preterm infants as a result of increased blood sampling and deficient erythropoiesis	Pallor Apnea Tachycardia Diminished activity Poor feeder Poor weight gain Respiratory distress—grunting, nasal flaring, intercostal retractions Respiratory difficulty	Administer volume expanders for hypovolemia at birth (e.g., normal saline). Transfuse with packed red blood cells or administer recombinant human erythropoietin.	Use microsamples for blood tests. Monitor amount of blood drawn for tests. Administer recombinant human erythropoietin as prescribed. Administer iron supplements as prescribed.
Polycythemia or Hyperviscosity Syndrome			

Venous hematocrit ≥65% results in venous stasis in vital organs and risk for microthrombus development	High incidence of:
	  Cardiovascular symptoms (PPHN, cyanosis, apnea)
	  Seizures
	  Hyperbilirubinemia
	  Gastrointestinal abnormalities
		Implement partial exchange transfusion with blood product or appropriate volume expander.
		Provide appropriate therapy for associated problems.
			See Nursing Care of the High-Risk Newborn and Family (p. 235) and Hyperbilirubinemia (p. 256).

Vitamin K Deficiency Bleeding (Formerly Hemorrhagic Disease of the Newborn)			
Bleeding disorder resulting from transient deficiency of vitamin K–dependent blood factors; newborn's sterile gut does not produce adequate amounts of vitamin K	Oozing blood from umbilicus or circumcision Bloody or black stools Hematuria Petechiae	Administer prophylactic vitamin K.	Administer prophylactic vitamin K via intramuscular route. Observe for complications such as bleeding umbilical cord, prolonged circumcision bleeding, and petechiae.

not provide a diagnosis or the history is suggestive of an inherited metabolic disorder.

Therapeutic Management

Treatment is directed toward prevention of neurologic damage and involves correction of metabolic derangements, respiratory and cardiovascular support, and suppression of the seizure activity. The underlying cause is treated (e.g., glucose infusion for hypoglycemia, calcium for hypocalcemia, antibiotics for infection). If needed, respiratory support is provided for hypoxia, and anticonvulsants may be administered, especially when the other measures fail to control the seizures. Phenobarbital, given intravenously or orally, has been the drug of choice and is used if seizures are severe and persistent. Other drugs that may be used are phenytoin (Dilantin) and lorazepam.

Fosphenytoin sodium is a water-soluble prodrug and may also be used for seizures. Fosphenytoin metabolizes to form phenytoin in the body yet can easily be diluted or mixed in dextrose and normal saline and may be given via IV or intramuscular routes. In addition, fosphenytoin does not cause pain during IV administration.

Recent research has shown that therapeutic hypothermia provided by cooling either the infant's head or the whole body reduces the severity of the neurologic damage in hypoxic ischemic encephalopathy when it is applied in the early stages of injury (first 6 hours after delivery) in infants with a gestational age of 35 to 36 weeks or more (Azzopardi, Strohm, Edwards, and others, 2009; Edwards, Brocklehurst, Gunn, and others, 2010; Jacobs, Hunt, Tarnow-Mordi, and others, 2007; Laptook, 2009).

Nursing Care Management

The major nursing responsibilities in the care of infants with seizures are to recognize when the infant is having a seizure so therapy can be instituted, to carry out the therapeutic regimen, and to observe the response to the therapy and any further evidence of seizures or other symptomatology. Assessment and other aspects of care are the same as for all high-risk infants. Parents need to be informed of their infant's status, and the nurse should reinforce and clarify the practitioner's explanations. The infant's behaviors need to be interpreted for the parents, and the infant's responses to the treatment must be anticipated

TABLE 9-10   NEUROLOGIC COMPLICATIONS

DESCRIPTION	CLINICAL MANIFESTATIONS	THERAPEUTIC MANAGEMENT	NURSING CARE MANAGEMENT
Hypoxic-Ischemic Brain Injury			
Nonprogressive neurologic (brain) impairment caused by intrauterine or postnatal asphyxia resulting in hypoxemia or cerebral ischemia	Appears within first 6–12 hr after hypoxic episode	Prevent hypoxia.	See Nursing Care of the High-Risk Newborn and Family (p. 235).
	Seizures	Provide supportive care.	Observe for signs that indicate cerebral hypoxia.
	Abnormal muscle tone (usually hypotonia)	Provide adequate ventilation.	Monitor ventilatory and intravenous therapy.
Hypoxic-ischemic encephalopathy—the resultant cellular damage causes the clinical manifestations	Disturbance of sucking and swallowing	Maintain cerebral perfusion.	Observe for and manage seizures.
	Apneic episodes	Prevent cerebral edema.	Support family.
	Stupor or coma	Treat underlying cause.	Provide guidelines for family management of potential mild to severe neurologic damage.
	Muscular weakness in hips and shoulders (full term), lower limb weakness (preterm)	Administer antiseizure drugs. Initiate therapeutic hypothermia if criteria met (see p. 282).	
Germinal Matrix or Intraventricular Hemorrhage			
Hemorrhage into and around ventricles caused by ruptured vessels as a result of an event that increases cerebral blood flow to area	Sudden deterioration in condition if bleed is large	Supportive care: Provide ventilatory support.	See Nursing Care of the High-Risk Newborn and Family (p. 235).
	Most bleeds initially asymptomatic	Maintain oxygenation.	Prevent increased cerebral blood pressure.
	Tense, bulging anterior fontanel	Regulate fluid and electrolytes, acid–base balance.	Avoid events that may increase or decrease cerebral blood flow (e.g., pain, unnecessary stimulation, endotracheal suctioning, hypoxia, hyperosmolar drugs, rapid volume expansion).
	Neurologic signs: • Twitching • Stupor • Apnea • Seizures	Suppress or prevent seizures.	Elevate head of bed 20–30 degrees; keep head in midline. Support family.
	Evident on cranial ultrasonography or magnetic resonance imaging	Provide ventricular shunting or drainage.	Monitor for posthemorrhagic hydrocephalus after diagnosis. Provide developmental care and enhancement.
Intracranial Hemorrhage			
Subdural	Sudden decrease in hematocrit	See Chapter 28.	Same as for germinal matrix or intraventricular hemorrhage
Subarachnoid	Change in sensorium		
Intracerebellar	Poor feeding		
	See Chapter 28		

BOX 9-5   CAUSES OF NEONATAL SEIZURES

Metabolic
Hypoglycemia, hyperglycemia
Hypocalcemia
Hypernatremia, hyponatremia
Hypomagnesemia
Pyridoxine deficiency
Aminoacidurias (e.g., phenylketonuria, maple syrup urine disease)
Hyperammonemia

Toxic
Uremia
Bilirubin encephalopathy (kernicterus)

Prenatal Infections
Toxoplasmosis
Syphilis
Cytomegalovirus
Herpes simplex
Hepatitis

Postnatal Infections
Bacterial meningitis
Viral meningoencephalitis
Sepsis
Brain abscess

Trauma at Birth
Hypoxic brain injury
Subarachnoid, subdural hemorrhage
Intraventricular hemorrhage

Malformations
Central nervous system agenesis
Hydranencephaly
Tuberous sclerosis

Miscellaneous
Neonatal stroke
Narcotic withdrawal
Degenerative disease
Benign familial neonatal seizures

TABLE 9-11	CLASSIFICATIONS OF NEONATAL SEIZURES
TYPE	**CHARACTERISTICS**
Clonic	Slow, rhythmic jerking movements
	Approximately 1–3/sec
Focal	Involves face, upper or lower extremities on one side of body
	May involve neck or trunk
	Infant is conscious during event
Multifocal	May migrate randomly from one part of the body to another
	Movements may start at different times
Tonic	Extension, stiffening movements
Generalized	Extension of all four limbs (similar to decerebrate rigidity)
	Upper limbs maintained in a stiffly flexed position (resembles decorticate rigidity)
Focal	Sustained posturing of a limb
	Asymmetric posturing of trunk or neck
Subtle	May develop in either full-term or preterm infants but more common in preterm
	Often overlooked by inexperienced observers
	Signs:
	• Horizontal eye deviation
	• Repetitive blinking or fluttering of the eyelids, staring
	• Sucking or other oral–buccal–lingual movements
	• Arm movements that resemble rowing or swimming
	• Leg movements described as pedaling or bicycling
	• Apnea (common)
	Signs may appear alone or in combination
Myoclonic	Rapid jerks that involve flexor muscle groups
Focal	Involves upper extremity flexor muscle group
	No EEG discharges observed
Multifocal	Asynchronous twitching of several parts of the body
	No associated EEG discharges observed
Generalized	Bilateral jerks of upper and lower limbs
	Associated with EEG discharges

Adapted from Volpe J: Neonatal seizures. In Volpe J: *Neurology of the newborn*, ed 4, Philadelphia, 2008, Saunders.
EEG, Electroencephalogram.

and their significance explained. Parents are encouraged to visit their infant and perform the parenting activities consistent with the care plan. Seizures are a frightening phenomenon and generate a great deal of anxiety and fear, which is easily compounded by the justifiable concern of the staff. Providing support and guidance is an important nursing function.

HIGH RISK RELATED TO INFECTIOUS PROCESSES

SEPSIS

Sepsis, or septicemia, refers to a generalized bacterial infection in the bloodstream. Neonates are highly susceptible to infection as a result of diminished nonspecific (inflammatory) and specific (humoral) immunity, such as impaired phagocytosis, delayed chemotactic response, minimal or absent immunoglobulin A and immunoglobulin M (IgA and IgM), and decreased complement levels. Because of infants' poor

response to pathogenic agents, there is usually no local inflammatory reaction at the portal of entry to signal an infection, and the resulting symptoms tend to be vague and nonspecific. Consequently, diagnosis and treatment may be delayed.

Breastfeeding has a protective benefit against infection and should be promoted for all newborns. It is of particular benefit to high-risk neonates. Colostrum contains agglutinins that are effective against gram-negative bacteria.

Sepsis in the neonatal period can be acquired prenatally across the placenta from the maternal bloodstream or during labor from ingestion or aspiration of infected amniotic fluid. Prolonged rupture of the membranes always presents a risk for this type from maternal–fetal transfer of pathogenic organisms. In utero transplacental transfer can occur with organisms and viruses such as cytomegalovirus, toxoplasmosis, and *Treponema pallidum* (syphilis), which cross the placental barrier during the latter half of pregnancy. Intrapartum infection may occur via contact with an infected mother; examples of such infections include herpesvirus and human immunodeficiency virus (HIV).

Early-onset sepsis (less than 3 days after birth) is acquired in the perinatal period; infection can occur from direct contact with organisms from the maternal gastrointestinal and genitourinary tracts. The most common infecting organism in term infants is group B streptococcus (GBS); in preterm infants, it is *Escherichia coli* (Sgro, Shah, Campbell, and others, 2011). Despite the development of maternal screening and prophylaxis, infection rates for early-onset GBS infection remain at approximately 0.3 per 1000 live births (Centers for Disease Control and Prevention, 2007). *E. coli*, which may be present in the vagina, accounts for approximately half of all cases of sepsis caused by gram-negative organisms. GBS is an extremely virulent organism in neonates, with a high (50%) death rate in affected infants. Other bacteria noted to cause early-onset infection include *Haemophilus influenzae*, *Citrobacter* and *Enterobacter* organisms, coagulase-negative staphylococci (ConS), and *Streptococcus viridans* (Stoll, Hansen, Higgins, and others, 2005). Other pathogens that are harbored in the vagina and may infect the infant include gonococci, *C. albicans*, HSV (type II), and *Chlamydia*.

Late-onset sepsis (1–3 weeks after birth) is primarily nosocomial, and the offending organisms are usually staphylococci, *Klebsiella* organisms, enterococci, *E. coli*, and *Pseudomonas* or *Candida* (Stoll, 2011). ConS, considered to be primarily a contaminant in older children and adults, is commonly found to be the cause of septicemia in ELBW and VLBW infants. Bacterial invasion can occur through sites such as the umbilical stump; the skin; mucous membranes of the eye, nose, pharynx, and ear; and internal systems such as the respiratory, nervous, urinary, and gastrointestinal systems. Risk factors for ConS include low birth weight and early gestational age, poor hand hygiene, previous antibiotic exposure, and the presence of central IV lines (Downey, Smith, and Benjamin, 2010).

Postnatal infection is acquired by cross-contamination from other infants, personnel, or objects in the environment. Bacteria that are commonly called "water bugs" (because they are able to grow in water) are found in water supplies, humidifying apparatus, sink drains, suction machines, and most respiratory equipment. Organisms such as ConS, which usually colonize the skin, may infect indwelling venous and arterial catheters used for infusions, blood sampling, and monitoring of vital signs. Neonatal sepsis is most common in infants at risk, particularly preterm infants and infants born after a difficult or traumatic labor and delivery, who are least capable of resisting such bacterial invasion. These organisms are often transmitted by personnel from person to person or object to person by poor hand washing and inadequate housecleaning.

Diagnostic Evaluation

Diagnosis of sepsis is often based on suspicion of presenting clinical signs and symptoms. Because sepsis is so easily confused with other neonatal disorders, the definitive diagnosis is established by laboratory and radiographic examination. Isolation of the specific organism is always attempted through cultures of blood, urine, and CSF. Blood studies may show signs of anemia, leukocytosis, or leukopenia. Leukopenia is usually an ominous sign because of its frequent association with high mortality. An elevated number of immature neutrophils (a left shift), decreased or increased total neutrophils, and changes in neutrophil morphology also suggest an infectious process in the neonate. Other diagnostic data may be helpful in the determination of neonatal sepsis and include C-reactive protein and other acute phase reactants such as serum amyloid A; procalcitonin; and interleukins, specifically interleukin-6 (Ng and Lam, 2010).

Prevention

Several measures are important in the prevention of both early- and late-onset infection. Programs to screen pregnant women for GBS colonization (culture-based) and treatment of those women in labor have dramatically reduced the incidence of GBS infection in neonates (Centers for Disease Control and Prevention, 2007). Screening programs for other maternal infections, including hepatitis B and HIV, have also been recommended. In developed countries, breastfeeding by mothers infected with HIV is not recommended because the virus may be transmitted in breast milk.

Nursery procedures aimed at minimizing the risk of nosocomial infections include the practice of good hand-washing techniques, appropriate isolation precautions where indicated, and the adoption of recommended standards for spacing of infant beds. Strategies such as the early introduction of enteral feeding aimed at reducing the indwelling time of central venous lines have been shown to reduce the risk of nosocomial infection (Borghesi and Stronati, 2008).

Therapeutic Management

In addition to the institution of vigorous therapeutic measures, early recognition (Box 9-6) and diagnosis are essential to increase the infant's chance for survival and reduce the likelihood of permanent neurologic damage. Antibiotic therapy is initiated before laboratory results are available for confirmation and identification of the exact organism. Treatment consists of circulatory support, respiratory support, aggressive administration of antibiotics, and immunotherapy.

Supportive therapy usually involves administration of oxygen (if respiratory distress or hypoxia is evident), careful regulation of fluids, correction of electrolyte or acid–base imbalance, and temporary discontinuation of oral feedings. Blood transfusions may be needed to correct anemia and shock, and electronic monitoring of vital signs and regulation of the thermal environment are mandatory.

Antibiotic therapy is continued for 7 to 10 days if culture results are positive, discontinued in 48 to 72 hours if culture results are negative and the infant is asymptomatic, and most often administered via IV infusion. Antifungal and antiviral therapies are implemented as appropriate, depending on causative agents.

Prognosis

The prognosis for neonatal sepsis is variable. Severe neurologic and respiratory sequelae may occur in ELBW and VLBW infants with early-onset sepsis. Late-onset sepsis and meningitis may also result in poor outcomes for immunocompromised neonates.

BOX 9-6 MANIFESTATIONS OF NEONATAL SEPSIS

General Signs
Infant generally "not doing well"
Poor temperature control—hypothermia, hyperthermia (rare in neonates)

Circulatory System
Pallor, cyanosis, or mottling
Cool, clammy skin
Hypotension
Edema
Irregular heartbeat—bradycardia, tachycardia

Respiratory System
Irregular respirations, apnea, or tachypnea
Cyanosis
Grunting
Dyspnea
Retractions

Central Nervous System
Diminished activity—lethargy, hyporeflexia, coma
Increased activity—irritability, tremors, seizures
Full fontanel
Increased or decreased tone
Abnormal eye movements

Gastrointestinal System
Poor feeding
Vomiting
Diarrhea or decreased stooling
Abdominal distention
Hepatomegaly
Hemoccult-positive stools

Hematopoietic System
Jaundice
Pallor
Petechiae, ecchymosis
Splenomegaly

The introduction of new markers for neonatal sepsis such as acute phase proteins, cytokines, cell surface antigens, and bacterial genomes may prove to be particularly helpful in early differentiation of true sepsis from RDS and in guidance for antibiotic therapy (Arnon and Litmanovitz, 2008). Future experimental methods being explored to combat infection in neonates include monoclonal antibody therapy, fibronectin infusion, and lymphokine enhancement.

Nursing Care Management

Nursing care of infants with sepsis involves observation and assessment as outlined for any high-risk infant. Recognition of the existing problem is of paramount importance; it is usually the nurse who observes and assesses infants and identifies that "something is wrong" with them. Awareness of the potential modes of infection transmission also helps the nurse identify infants at risk for developing sepsis. Much of the care of infants with sepsis involves the medical treatment of the illness. Knowledge of the side effects of the specific antibiotic and proper regulation and administration of the drug are vital.

Prolonged antibiotic therapy poses additional hazards for affected infants. Antibiotics predispose infants to growth of resistant organisms and superinfection from fungal or mycotic agents, such as *C. albicans*. Nurses must be alert for evidence of such complications. Nystatin oral suspension is swabbed on the buccal mucosa for prophylaxis against oral candidiasis.

A number of specimens may be needed to help identify the cause and source of the infection. It is recommended that the fully flexed position be avoided for obtaining spinal fluid and that the side-lying position (modified with neck extension) or sitting position be used instead. Continual cardiorespiratory and pulse oximetry monitoring provides an ongoing assessment of the infant's condition during the procedure.

Part of the total care of infants with sepsis is to decrease any additional physiologic or environmental stress. This includes providing an optimum thermoregulated environment and anticipating potential problems such as dehydration or hypoxia. Precautions are implemented to prevent the spread of infection to other newborns, but to be effective, activities must be carried out by all caregivers. Proper hand washing, the use of disposable equipment (e.g., linens, catheters, feeding supplies, IV equipment), disposal of excretions (e.g., vomitus, stool), and adequate housekeeping of the environment and equipment are essential. Because nurses are the most consistent caregivers involved with sick infants, it is usually their responsibility to see that standard precautions are maintained by everyone.

In recent years ventilator-associated pneumonia has received considerable attention in adult and pediatric intensive care units. Hand hygiene (staff) and oral hygiene (patient) have been shown to decrease the incidence of ventilator-associated pneumonia in children (see Chapter 23).

Another aspect of caring for infants with sepsis involves observation for signs of complications, including meningitis and septic shock, a severe complication caused by toxins in the bloodstream.

NECROTIZING ENTEROCOLITIS

Necrotizing enterocolitis is an acute inflammatory disease of the bowel with increased incidence in preterm infants. The precise cause of NEC is still uncertain, but it appears to occur in infants whose gastrointestinal tracts have experienced vascular compromise. Intestinal ischemia of unknown etiology, immature gastrointestinal host defenses, bacterial proliferation, and feeding substrate are now believed to have a multifactorial role in the etiology of NEC. Prematurity remains the most prominent risk factor in the development of NEC (Schurr and Perkins, 2008).

The damage to mucosal cells lining the bowel wall may be significant. Diminished blood supply to these cells causes their death in large numbers; they stop secreting protective, lubricating mucus; and the thin, unprotected bowel wall is attacked by proteolytic enzymes. Thus, the bowel wall continues to swell and break down; it is unable to synthesize protective IgM, and the mucosa is permeable to macromolecules (e.g., exotoxins), which further hampers intestinal defenses. Gas-forming bacteria invade the damaged areas to produce pneumatosis intestinalis, the presence of gas in the submucosal or subserosal surfaces of the bowel.

A consistent relationship has been observed between the development of NEC and enteric feeding of hypertonic substances (e.g., formula, hyperosmolar medications). It is unclear whether this connection is a result of the formula imposing a stress on an ischemic bowel, serving as a substrate for bacterial growth, or both.

Diagnostic Evaluation

Radiographic studies show a sausage-shaped dilation of the intestine that progresses to marked distention and the characteristic pneumatosis intestinalis—"soapsuds," or the bubbly appearance of thickened bowel wall and ultralumina. There may be air in the portal circulation or free air observed in the abdomen, indicating perforation. Laboratory findings may include anemia, leukopenia, leukocytosis, metabolic acidosis, and electrolyte imbalance. In severe cases, coagulopathy (DIC) or thrombocytopenia may be evident. Organisms are often cultured from blood, although bacteremia or septicemia may not be prominent early in the course of the disease.

Therapeutic Management

Treatment of infants with NEC begins with prevention. Oral feedings may be withheld for at least 24 to 48 hours from infants who are believed to have experienced birth asphyxia. Breast milk is the preferred enteral nutrient because it confers some passive immunity (IgA), macrophages, and lysozymes.

Minimal enteral feedings (trophic feeding, gastrointestinal priming) have gained acceptance with no evidence of increased incidence of NEC. In particular, the use of fresh human milk has been shown to decrease the risk of NEC (Hay, 2008). A systematic review of the role of probiotics such as *Lactobacillus acidophilus* and *Bifidobacterium infantis* administered with enteral feedings for the prevention of NEC has demonstrated a reduced incidence of severe NEC and mortality in preterm infants (Alfaleh, Anabrees, Bassler, and others, 2011). The preferred type and optimal dosing of probiotics remain to be determined.

Medical treatment of infants with confirmed NEC consists of discontinuation of all oral feedings; institution of abdominal decompression via NG suction; administration of IV antibiotics; and correction of extravascular volume depletion, electrolyte abnormalities, acid–base imbalances, and hypoxia. Replacing oral feedings with parenteral fluids decreases the need for oxygen and circulation to the bowel. Serial abdominal radiographs (every 6–8 hours in the acute phase) are taken to monitor for possible progression of the disease to intestinal perforation.

Prognosis

With early recognition and treatment, medical management is increasingly successful. If there is progressive deterioration under medical management or evidence of perforation, surgical resection and anastomosis are performed. Extensive involvement may necessitate surgical intervention and establishment of an ileostomy, jejunostomy, or colostomy. Sequelae in surviving infants include short-bowel syndrome (see Chapter 24), colonic stricture with obstruction, fat malabsorption, and growth failure secondary to intestinal dysfunction. A variety of surgical interventions for NEC are available and depend on the extent of bowel necrosis, associated illness factors, and infant stability. Intestinal transplantation has been successful in some former preterm infants with NEC-associated short-bowel syndrome who had already developed life-threatening total parenteral nutrition–related complications. Transplantation may be a lifesaving option for infants who previously faced high morbidity and mortality. Research is now underway to examine the use of tissue-engineered small intestine (Guner, Chokshi, Petrosyan, and others, 2008).

BOX 9-7 CLINICAL MANIFESTATIONS OF NECROTIZING ENTEROCOLITIS

Nonspecific Clinical Signs
Lethargy
Poor feeding
Hypotension
Vomiting
Apnea
Decreased urinary output
Unstable temperature
Jaundice

Specific Signs
Distended (often shiny) abdomen
Blood in the stools or gastric contents
Gastric retention (undigested formula)
Localized abdominal wall erythema or induration
Bilious vomitus

Nursing Care Management

Nursing responsibilities begin with the prompt recognition of the early warning signs of NEC. Because the signs are similar to those observed in many other disorders of newborns, nurses must constantly be aware of the possibility of this disease in infants who are at high risk for developing NEC (Box 9-7).

When the disease is suspected, the nurse assists with diagnostic procedures and implements the therapeutic regimen. Vital signs, including BP, are monitored for changes that might indicate bowel perforation, septicemia, or cardiovascular shock, and measures are instituted to prevent possible transmission to other infants. It is especially important to avoid rectal temperatures because of the increased danger of perforation. To avoid pressure on the distended abdomen and to facilitate continuous observation, infants are often left undiapered and positioned supine or on the side.

Observe for indications of early development of NEC by checking the appearance of the abdomen for distention (measuring abdominal girth, measuring residual gastric contents before feedings, and listening for bowel sounds) and performing all routine assessments for high-risk neonates.

Conscientious attention to nutritional and hydration needs is essential, and antibiotics are administered as prescribed. The time at which oral feedings are reinstituted varies considerably but is usually at least 7 to 10 days after diagnosis and treatment. Feeding is usually reestablished using human milk, if available.

Because NEC is an infectious disease, one of the most important nursing functions is control of infection. Strict hand washing is the primary barrier to spread, and confirmed multiple cases are isolated. Persons with symptoms of a gastrointestinal disorder should not care for these or any other infants.

Infants who require surgery require the same careful attention and observation as any infant with abdominal surgery, including ostomy care (as applicable). This disorder is one of the most common reasons for performing ostomies on newborns. Throughout the medical and surgical management of infants with NEC, the nurse should be continually alert to signs of complications, such as septicemia, DIC, hypoglycemia, and other metabolic derangements.

HIGH RISK RELATED TO MATERNAL CONDITIONS

The health of fetuses and newborns may be affected by a number of maternal conditions; essentially, any condition affecting the mother also has the potential for negatively affecting the health of the newborn. Pregnancy-induced hypertension or HELLP (hemolysis, elevated liver enzymes, low platelets) syndrome may cause preterm delivery, intrauterine growth restriction (IUGR), asphyxia, and death if it is not detected early and appropriate interventions implemented. It is not within the scope of this text to elaborate on the pathophysiology and treatment of these conditions; however, readers are referred to any one of the excellent maternity texts available for a detailed discussion of these conditions.

INFANTS OF DIABETIC MOTHERS

Before insulin therapy, few women with diabetes were able to conceive; for those who did, the mortality rate for both the mother and the infant was high. The morbidity and mortality of infants of diabetic mothers (IDMs) have been significantly reduced as a result of effective control of maternal diabetes and an increased understanding of fetal disorders. Because infants born to women with gestational diabetes mellitus are at risk for the same complications as IDMs, the following discussion of IDMs includes infants born to women with gestational diabetes mellitus.

The severity of the maternal diabetes affects infant survival. The severity of maternal diabetes is determined by the duration of the disease before pregnancy; age of onset; extent of vascular complications; and abnormalities of the current pregnancy, such as pyelonephritis, diabetic ketoacidosis, pregnancy-induced hypertension, and noncompliance. The single most important factor influencing fetal well-being is the euglycemic status of the mother. It has been found that reasonable metabolic control that begins before conception and continues during the first weeks of pregnancy can prevent malformation in an IDM. Elevated levels of hemoglobin A1c during the periconception period appear to be associated with a higher incidence of congenital malformations. In the case of gestational diabetes, macrosomia is the most common finding; serious complications are rare (Mitanchez, 2010).

Hypoglycemia may appear a short time after birth and in IDMs is associated with increased insulin activity in the blood (see also Table 9-4). The serum glucose level that corresponds to clinical hypoglycemia has not been well defined. Because some infants experience metabolic complications at higher levels than previously thought, some researchers recommend that serum glucose levels be maintained above 45 mg/dl (2.5 mmol/L) in infants with abnormal clinical symptoms and as high as 50 or 60 mg/dl in other infants (Cornblath, Hawdon, Williams, and others, 2000; Deshpande and Ward, 2005). The AAP recommends that symptomatic infants receive treatment if their blood glucose is less than 40 mg/dl (Adamkin and AAP, Committee on Fetus and Newborn, 2011).

Hypoglycemia in IDMs is related to hypertrophy and hyperplasia of the pancreatic islet cells and thus is a transient state of hyperinsulinism. High maternal blood glucose levels during fetal life provide a continual stimulus to the fetal islet cells for insulin production (glucose easily passes the placental barrier from maternal to fetal side; insulin, however, does not cross the placental barrier). This sustained state of hyperglycemia promotes fetal insulin secretion that ultimately leads to excessive growth and deposition of fat, which probably accounts for the infants who are large for gestational age, or macrosomic (Ogata, 2010). IDMs are more likely to have disproportionately large

BOX 9-8   CLINICAL MANIFESTATIONS OF INFANTS OF DIABETIC MOTHERS

- Large for gestational age
- Very plump and full faced
- Abundant vernix caseosa
- Plethora
- Listless and lethargic
- Possibly meconium stained at birth

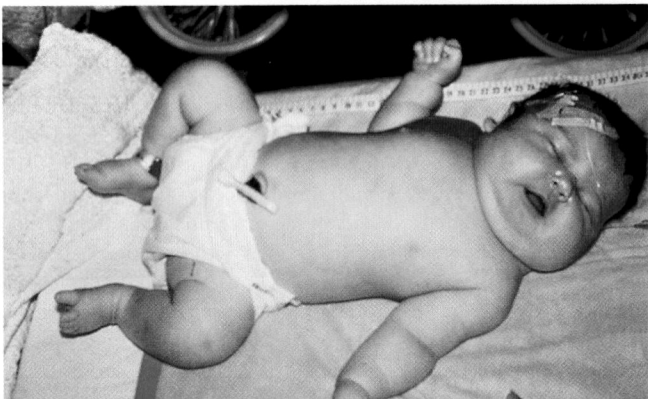

FIG. 9-21 Large-for-gestational age infant. This infant of a diabetic mother weighed 5 kg at birth and exhibits the typical round facies. (From Zitelli BJ, McIntire SC, Nowalk AJ: *Zitelli and Davis' atlas of pediatric physical diagnosis*, ed 6, St. Louis, 2012, Saunders.)

abdominal circumferences and shoulders, leading to an increased risk of shoulder dystocia and birth injury (Dailey and Coustan, 2010). When the neonate's glucose supply is removed abruptly at the time of birth, the continued production of insulin soon depletes the blood of circulating glucose, creating a state of hyperinsulinism and hypoglycemia within 0.5 to 4 hours, especially in infants of mothers with poorly controlled diabetes (formerly class C diabetes or beyond [class D through R]). Precipitous drops in blood glucose levels can cause serious neurologic damage or death.

Infants of diabetic mothers have a characteristic appearance (Box 9-8 and Fig. 9-21). Infants of mothers with advanced diabetes may be small for gestational age, may have IUGR, or may be the appropriate size for gestational age because of the maternal vascular (placental) involvement. There is an increase in congenital anomalies in IDMs in addition to a high susceptibility to hypoglycemia, hypocalcemia, hypomagnesemia, polycythemia, hyperbilirubinemia, cardiomyopathy, and RDS (Dailey and Coustan, 2010). Hyperinsulinemia and hyperglycemia in the diabetic mother may be factors in reducing fetal surfactant synthesis, thus contributing to the development of RDS. Although large, these infants may be delivered before term as a result of maternal complications or increased fetal size.

Congenital hyperinulinism, a condition which causes neonatal macrosomia and profound hypoglycemia, is often present in the neonatal period. However, this condition is usually not associated with maternal diabetes mellitus, but appears to have a genetic etiology; the condition is also associated with syndromes such as Beckwith-Wiedemann syndrome (Sperling, 2011).

Therapeutic Management

The most important management of IDMs is careful monitoring of serum glucose levels and observation for accompanying complications such as RDS. The infants are examined for the presence of any anomalies or birth injuries, and blood studies for determination of glucose, calcium, hematocrit, and bilirubin are obtained on a regular basis.

Because the hypertrophied pancreas is so sensitive to blood glucose concentrations, the administration of oral glucose may trigger a massive insulin release, resulting in rebound hypoglycemia. Therefore, feedings of breast milk or formula begin within the first hour after birth, provided that the infant's cardiorespiratory condition is stable. Approximately half of these infants do well and adjust without complications. Infants born to mothers with poorly controlled diabetes may require IV dextrose infusions. Treatment with 10% dextrose and water (IV) is initiated with the goal of maintaining serum blood glucose levels between 40 and 50 mg/dl (Adamkin and AAP, Committee on Fetus and Newborn, 2011). Oral and IV intake may be titrated to maintain adequate blood glucose levels. Frequent blood glucose determinations are needed for the first 2 to 4 days of life to assess the degree of hypoglycemia present at any given time. Testing blood taken from the heel with calibrated portable reflectance meters (e.g., glucometers) is a simple and effective screening evaluation that can then be confirmed by laboratory examination.

Nursing Care Management

The nursing care of IDMs involves early examination for congenital anomalies, signs of possible respiratory or cardiac problems, maintenance of adequate thermoregulation, early introduction of carbohydrate feedings as appropriate, and monitoring of serum blood glucose levels. The latter is of particular importance because many infants with hypoglycemia may remain asymptomatic. IV glucose infusion requires careful monitoring of the site and the neonate's reaction to therapy; high glucose concentrations (≥12.5%) should be infused via a central line instead of a peripheral site.

Because macrosomic infants are at risk for problems associated with a difficult delivery, they are monitored for birth injuries such as brachial plexus injury and palsy, fractured clavicle, and phrenic nerve palsy. Additional monitoring of the infant for problems associated with this condition (polycythemia, hypocalcemia, poor feeding, and hyperbilirubinemia) is also a vital nursing function.

Some evidence indicates that IDMs have an increased risk of acquiring type 2 diabetes and metabolic syndrome in childhood or early adulthood (Ogata, 2010); therefore, nursing care should also focus on healthy lifestyle and prevention later in life with IDMs.

DRUG-EXPOSED INFANTS*

Maternal habits hazardous to the fetus and neonate include drug addiction, smoking, and alcohol abuse. Occasional withdrawal reactions have been reported in neonates of mothers who use to excess such drugs as barbiturates, alcohol, amphetamines, or antidepressants. Serious reactions are seen in neonates whose mothers abuse psychoactive drugs or are treated with methadone.

---

*Note that the term *addiction* is often associated with behaviors whereby the person seeks the drug(s) to experience a high or euphoria, escape from reality, or satisfy a personal need. Newborns who have been exposed to drugs in utero are not addicted in a behavioral sense, yet they may experience mild to strong physiologic signs as a result of the exposure. Therefore, to say that an infant born to a mother who uses substances is addicted is incorrect; *drug-exposed newborn* is a better term, which implies intrauterine drug exposure.

Narcotics, which have a low molecular weight, readily cross the placental membrane and enter the fetal system. Illicit substances may also be transmitted to the newborn through breast milk. When the mother is a habitual user of opiates, especially OxyContin, heroin, or methadone, the unborn child may also become chemically dependent or passively addicted to the drug, which places such infants at risk during the perinatal and early neonatal periods. **Neonatal abstinence syndrome (NAS)** is the term used to describe the set of behaviors exhibited by infants exposed to narcotics in utero.

Clinical Manifestations

Throughout this section, unless otherwise noted, the information presented refers to drug-exposed neonates in general, regardless of which drug they have been exposed to.

The adverse effects of exposure of a fetus to drugs are varied. They include transient behavioral changes such as alterations in fetal breathing movements and irreversible effects such as fetal death, IUGR, structural malformations, or cognitive impairment. Determining the specific effects of individual drugs on an individual fetus is made difficult by polydrug use, which is common; errors or omissions in reporting drug use; and variations in the strength, purity, and types of additives found in street drugs. Maternal conditions such as poverty, malnutrition, and comorbid conditions such as sexually transmitted infections further compound the difficulty in identifying the presence and consequences of intrauterine drug exposure. Most infants who are exposed to drugs in utero may demonstrate no immediate untoward effects and appear normal at birth. Infants exposed only to heroin may begin to exhibit signs of drug withdrawal within 12 to 24 hours. If mothers have been taking methadone, the signs appear somewhat later—anywhere from 1 or 2 days to 2 to 3 weeks or more after birth. The clinical manifestations may fall into any one or all of the following categories: CNS, gastrointestinal, respiratory, and autonomic nervous system signs (Burgos and Burke, 2009; Kuschel, 2007). The manifestations become most pronounced between 48 and 72 hours of age and may last from 6 days to 8 weeks, depending on the severity of the withdrawal (Box 9-9). Although these infants suck avidly on fists and display an exaggerated rooting reflex, they are poor feeders with uncoordinated and ineffectual sucking and swallowing reflexes.

About 55% to 94% of infants born to narcotic-addicted mothers show signs of withdrawal (Burgos and Burke, 2009). Because of irregular and varying degrees of drug use, quality of drug, and mixed-drug usage by the mother, some infants display mild or variable manifestations. Most manifestations are the vague, nonspecific signs characteristic of all infants in general; therefore, it is important to differentiate between drug withdrawal and other disorders before specific therapy is instituted. Other conditions (e.g., hypocalcemia, hypoglycemia, sepsis) often coexist with the drug withdrawal. Additional signs seen in drug-exposed newborns include loose stools; tachycardia; fever; projectile vomiting; crying; nasal stuffiness; and generalized perspiration, which is unusual in newborns.

Diagnostic Evaluation

Newborn urine, hair, or meconium sampling may be required to identify drug exposure and implement appropriate early interventional therapies aimed at minimizing the consequences of intrauterine drug exposure. Meconium sampling for fetal drug exposure is reported to provide more screening accuracy than urine screening because drug metabolites accumulate in meconium (Kuschel, 2007). Urine toxicology screening may be less accurate because it reflects only recent substance intake by the mother (Albright and Rayburn, 2009). Meconium and hair testing for drug metabolites has the advantages of being

---

BOX 9-9 SIGNS OF WITHDRAWAL IN NEONATES

Neurologic
Irritability
Seizures
Hyperactivity
High-pitched cry
Tremors
Exaggerated Moro reflex
Hypertonicity of muscles

Gastrointestinal
Poor feeding
Diarrhea
Dehydration
Vomiting
Frantic, uncoordinated sucking
Gastric residuals

Autonomic
Diaphoresis
Fever
Mottled skin
Nasal stuffiness

Miscellaneous
Disrupted sleep patterns
Diaphoresis
Tachypnea (>60 breaths/min)
Excoriations (knees, face)
Temperature instability

---

noninvasive, more accurate, and easy to collect. One study examining urine, hair, and meconium samples for drug use found that although all of these tests were reliable to a greater or lesser degree, the single most reliable method for determining prenatal drug use was a careful history collected by an experienced interviewer (Eyler, Behnke, Wobie, and others, 2005).

Therapeutic Management

The treatment of drug-exposed infants initially consists of early identification through maternal history, presenting symptoms of NAS, or toxicology screening when substance abuse is strongly suspected. Early identification and intervention are essential to prevent further adverse effects; early discharge from the birth institution should be postponed until further assessment of the maternal situation and establishment of a treatment plan for the mother and infant. Drug therapies to decrease withdrawal effects include parenteral or oral administration of phenobarbital, buprenorphine, clonidine, methadone, and morphine. A combination of these drugs may be necessary to treat infants exposed to multiple drugs in utero, and careful attention should be given to possible adverse effects of the treatment drugs (Burgos and Burke, 2009).

Prognosis

The prognosis for drug-exposed infants depends on the type and amount of drug(s) taken by the mother and the stage(s) of fetal development in which the drug was taken. The overall mortality rate of infants born to narcotic-addicted mothers is increased, but with early recognition, proper treatment, and long-term follow-up, the morbidity and mortality associated with drug exposure are decreased.

Often, drug-exposed infants exhibit poor brain and body growth at birth; however, at times, infants do not exhibit any signs that indicate exposure to harmful agents, and their condition may therefore be overlooked until symptoms appear later in life. Drug-exposed infants may have chronic feeding problems; irritability; abnormal neurologic responses; abnormal parent–infant interactions; developmental and cognitive delays; learning disabilities in childhood; and behavioral problems, including ADHD.

Nursing Care Management

One of the key factors in the treatment of drug-exposed neonates is early identification of substance abuse in the pregnant woman so treatment can be initiated and side effects minimized. This is especially problematic from a social and legal standpoint because the pregnant woman is often aware of the consequences of admitting to substance abuse and may therefore be less likely to readily admit to the problem for fear of social and legal repercussions. If the mother has had good prenatal care, the practitioner is aware of the problem and may have instituted therapy before delivery. However, a number of mothers deliver their infants without the benefit of adequate care, and the condition is unknown to health care personnel at the time of delivery.

The degree of withdrawal is closely related to the amount of drug the mother has habitually taken, the length of time she has been taking the drug, and her drug level at the time of delivery. The most severe symptoms are observed in the infants of mothers who have taken large amounts of drugs over a long period. In addition, the nearer to the time of delivery that the mother takes the drug, the longer it takes the child to develop withdrawal and the more severe the manifestations. The infant may not exhibit withdrawal symptoms until 7 to 10 days after delivery, by which time most newborns have been discharged from the birth center and caregivers are less likely to recognize signs of irritability and poor feeding as withdrawal, thus predisposing the newborn to abuse or neglect and growth failure (failure to thrive). The infant may be at further risk for subsequent abuse or neglect because of home conditions that preclude adequate newborn care and follow-up.

After the presence of NAS is identified in an infant, nursing care is directed toward treatment of the presenting signs, decreasing stimuli that may precipitate hyperactivity and irritability (e.g., dimming the lights, decreasing noise levels), providing adequate nutrition and hydration, and promoting the mother–infant relationship. Appropriate individualized developmental care is implemented to facilitate self-consoling and self-regulating behaviors. Irritable and hyperactive infants have been found to respond to physical comforting, movement, and close contact. Wrapping infants snugly and rocking and holding them tightly limit their ability to self-stimulate. Arranging nursing activities to reduce the amount of disturbance helps decrease exogenous stimulation.

Breastfeeding is encouraged in mothers who are not using illicit substances, do not have HIV infection, and are compliant with a methadone program; breastfeeding promotes mother–infant bonding, and small quantities of methadone passed through breast milk have not proved to be harmful.

The Neonatal Abstinence Scoring System was developed to monitor infants in an objective manner and evaluate their response to clinical and pharmacologic interventions (Finnegan, 1985). This system is also designed to assist nurses and other health care workers in evaluating the severity of infants' withdrawal symptoms. Another tool that may be used to evaluate withdrawal behavior and treatment in newborns is the Neonatal Withdrawal Inventory developed by Zahorodny, Rom, Whitney, and others (1998); it is important to note that neither of these tools is specific to preterm infants and may not be representative of withdrawal behaviors in such infants (Marcellus, 2002).

The Neonatal Intensive Care Unit Network Neurobehavioral Scale (NNNS) is a comprehensive neurologic and behavioral assessment tool that may be used to identify newborns at risk as a result of intrauterine drug exposure. The tool measures stress or abstinence, state, neurologic status, and muscle tone in the context of the newborn's medical condition at the time of examination. The NNNS may be used for medically stable newborns who are at least 30 weeks of gestation and up to 48 weeks of corrected or conceptional age (Lester, Tronick, and Brazelton, 2004).

Loose stools, poor intake, and regurgitation after feeding predispose these infants to malnutrition, dehydration, skin breakdown, and electrolyte imbalance. In addition, these infants burn up energy with continual activity and increased oxygen consumption at the cellular level. Frequent weighing, careful monitoring of intake and output and electrolytes, and additional caloric supplementation may be necessary. Hyperactive infants must be protected from skin abrasions on the knees, toes, and cheeks that are caused by rubbing on bed linens while in a prone position (awake). Monitoring and recording the activity level and its relationship to other activities, such as feeding and preventing complications, are important nursing functions.

A valuable aid to anticipating problems in the newborn is recognizing substance abuse in the mother. Unless the mother is enrolled in a methadone rehabilitation program, she seldom risks calling attention to her habit by seeking prenatal care. Consequently, infants and mothers are exposed to the additional hazards of obstetric and medical complications. Moreover, the nature of substance use and addiction makes the user susceptible to disorders such as infection (hepatitis B, HIV), foreign body reaction, and the hazards of inadequate nutrition and preterm birth. Methadone treatment does not prevent withdrawal reaction in neonates, but the clinical course may be modified. Also, the intensive psychologic support of mothers is a factor in the treatment and reduction of perinatal mortality. Experience has indicated that these mothers are usually anxious and depressed, lack confidence, have a poor self-image, and have difficulty with interpersonal relationships. They may have a psychologic need for the pregnancy and an infant.

Initial symptoms or the recurrence of withdrawal symptoms may develop after discharge from the hospital; therefore, it is important to establish rapport and maintain contact with the family so they will return for treatment if this occurs. The demands of the drug-exposed infant on the caregiver are enormous and unrewarding in terms of positive feedback. The infants are difficult to comfort, and they cry for long periods, which can be especially trying for the caregiver after the infant's discharge from the hospital. Long-term follow-up to evaluate the status of the infant and family is very important. Sudden infant death syndrome (SIDS) and HIV infection are observed more commonly in infants born to users of methadone and heroin.

Many problems arise in relation to the disposition of infants of drug-dependent mothers. Those who advocate separation of mothers and children argue that the mothers are not capable of assuming responsibility for their infant's care, that child care is frustrating to them, and that their existence is too disorganized and chaotic. Others encourage the mother–infant bond and recommend a protected environment such as a therapeutic community; a halfway house; or continuous ongoing, supportive services in the home after discharge. Careful evaluation and the cooperative efforts of a variety of health professionals are required whether the choice is foster home placement or supportive follow-up care of mothers who keep their infants.

Alcohol Exposure

Alcohol ingestion during pregnancy is associated with both short- and long-term effects on the fetus and newborn. The quantity of alcohol required to produce fetal effects is unclear, but it is known that infants born to heavy drinkers have twice the risk of congenital abnormalities than those born to moderate drinkers (Carlo, 2011). Alcohol withdrawal can occur in neonates, particularly when maternal ingestion occurs near the time of delivery. Signs and symptoms include jitteriness, increased tone and reflex responses, and irritability. Seizures are also common. Fetal effects of alcohol exposure vary from subtle learning disabilities to obvious facial features and growth abnormalities. In 2004, the National Organization on Fetal Alcohol Syndrome (NOFAS) clarified terminology for fetal alcohol exposure by adopting the term *fetal alcohol spectrum disorder (FASD)* as an umbrella term to describe the range of clinical effects. Fetal alcohol syndrome (FAS) falls within this spectrum but is reserved for individuals who display the triad of characteristic facial features, growth restriction, and neurodevelopmental deficits with a confirmed history of maternal alcohol consumption (Banakar, Kudlur, and George, 2009). Craniofacial features include microcephaly, small eyes or short palpebral fissures, a thin upper lip, a flat midface, and an indistinct philtrum. Neurologic problems in FAS children include some degree of IQ deficit, ADHD, diminished fine motor skills, and poor speech. These children have been shown to lack inhibition, have no stranger anxiety, and lack appropriate judgment skills.

Infants who do not display the signs of FAS but are born to mothers who are also heavy alcohol drinkers have significantly more tremors, hypertonia, restlessness, excessive mouthing movements, crying, and inconsolability than infants of substance-abusive mothers who do not consume alcohol during pregnancy. An added concern regarding substance abuse is that many of the mothers often use several drugs, such as tranquilizers, sedatives, amphetamines, phencyclidine, marijuana, and other psychotropic agents.

Cocaine Exposure

Cocaine is a CNS stimulant and peripheral sympathomimetic. Legally, it is classified as a narcotic, but it is not an opioid. The effects on fetuses are secondary to maternal effects, which include increased BP, decreased uterine blood flow, and increased vascular resistance. Consequently, the fetus experiences decreased blood flow and oxygenation because of placental and fetal vasoconstriction. Researchers have concluded that variables such as the mother's lack of prenatal care; poor nutrition; and use of tobacco, alcohol, and other drugs during pregnancy compound the effects of cocaine exposure in the infant (Bandstra, Morrow, Mansoor, and others, 2010).

Infants may appear normal or may show neurologic problems at birth that may continue during the neonatal period. In much of the research literature, these findings were transient, and there has been variable evidence demonstrating permanent sequelae. Either of two types of behavior may emerge as a result of cocaine's effects on fetal development: neurobehavioral depression or excitability. The behaviors of a depressed infant include lethargy, poor suck, hypotonia, a weak cry, and difficulty in arousing. The behaviors of an excitable neonate may include a high-pitched cry, hypertonicity, rigidity, irritability, an inability to be consoled, and an intolerance to changes in routine (Bauer, Langer, Shankaran, and others, 2005; Chiriboga, Kuhn, and Wasserman, 2007).

Sequelae of prenatal cocaine exposure include preterm birth, a smaller head circumference, decreased birth length, and decreased weight. Head growth may be one of the best predictors of long-term development (Bauer, Langer, Shankaran, and others, 2005). Early studies of cocaine exposure identified an increased incidence of gastroschisis, genitourinary anomalies, and periventricular and intraventricular hemorrhage; however, meta-analyses have not confirmed these complications (Bandstra, Morrow, Mansoor, and others, 2010). Heavy cocaine exposure has been shown to result in elevated heart rate and irregular respirations after birth (Schuetze and Eiden, 2006).

Some studies found that long-term sequelae for newborns exposed to cocaine include lower language, motor, and cognitive scores and an increased risk for learning disabilities (Morrow, Culbertson, Accornero, and others, 2006); however, one study revealed no significant differences in the total or verbal IQ scores but did note an increased risk of specific cognitive impairments (Singer, Minnes, Short, and others, 2004). In a study that controlled for other prenatal drug exposures, a dose-related effect of cocaine was found on expressive, receptive, and total language scores at 3, 5, and 12 years of age (Bandstra, Morrow, Accornero, and others, 2011). Other investigators have found that the subtle effects of cocaine on school performance are moderated by the child's environment (Ackerman, Riggins, and Black, 2010). Studies using the Brazelton Neonatal Assessment Scale have again shown inconsistent results with subtle abnormalities in neurobehavioral clusters varying in severity timing and according to levels of exposure (Bandstra, Morrow, Mansoor, and others, 2010).

Therapeutic Management

Treatment of these infants is similar to that for other drug-exposed infants, including reduction of external stimuli; supportive treatment aimed at alleviating symptoms; and, at times, mild sedation.

Nursing Care Management

Nursing care of cocaine-exposed infants is the same as that for other drug-exposed infants. Because they have increased flexor tone, these infants respond to swaddling (Pitts, 2010). Positioning, infant massage, and limited tactile stimulation have been shown to be effective interventions. Significant amounts of cocaine have been found in breast milk (Winecker, Goldberger, Tebbett, and others, 2001); therefore, mothers should be cautioned regarding this hazard to their infants.

Referral to early intervention programs, including child health care, parental drug treatment, individualized developmental care, and parenting education, is essential in promoting optimum outcome for these children. Because these children often live in impoverished environments, they are at high risk for cognitive delays, lack of child health care, and inadequate nutrition and benefit from early intervention programs.

Methamphetamine Exposure

The fetal and neonatal effects of maternal use of methamphetamines in pregnancy are not well known, and findings are often confounded by polydrug use and the effects of the newborn or child's environment. LBW, preterm birth, and anomalies such as cleft lip and palate and cardiac defects have been reported in infants exposed to methamphetamines in utero (Pitts, 2010).

Methamphetamine use has increased significantly in the past 10 years in certain regions of the United States. In a report by Terplan, Smith, Kozloski, and others (2009), 24% of pregnant women admitted to federally funded treatment centers in the United States used methamphetamines in 2006, up from 8% in 1994; 63% of pregnant women using methamphetamines reported using the drug throughout the pregnancy. A higher incidence of preterm delivery and placental abruption was associated with methamphetamine use. In addition, fetal growth restriction (small for gestational age) was slightly higher in methamphetamine-exposed offspring; however, 80% of these neonates' mothers also had significant alcohol and tobacco use.

Study reports vary in the time of clinical manifestations of withdrawal from this drug; one study did not identify any signs of withdrawal in the first 3 days after birth, but long-term data were not collected (Smith, Yonekura, Wallace, and others, 2003). A study of infants exposed to methamphetamine in utero showed that such infants had significantly smaller head circumferences and birth weights than those not exposed; in addition, the exposed infants exhibited withdrawal signs of agitation, vomiting, and tachypnea, which were not observed in the unexposed infants (Chomchai, Na Manorom, Watanarungasan, and others, 2004). After birth, infants may experience abnormal sleep patterns, agitation, poor feeding, and state disorganization (Pitts, 2010).

The long-term effects of methamphetamine exposure on children remains unclear; however, some studies have shown problems with math and language skills. It is postulated that similar to cocaine, methamphetamine exposure may affect areas of the brain responsible for higher order functioning with effects more likely to be manifest when the child reaches school age (Lester and Lagasse, 2010).

Marijuana Exposure

Marijuana has replaced cocaine as the most common illicit drug used by women ages 18 to 44 years (nonpregnant and pregnant) in the United States (Kuczkowski, 2007). Marijuana crosses the placenta; however, specific effects on the fetus have been difficult to determine. Some studies have reported an association between the chronic use of marijuana and a decrease in fetal growth and infant birth weight and length (Kuczkowski, 2007); however, this finding is confounded by cigarette smoking (Bandstra and Accornero, 2011; Schempf, 2007). More subtle effects of major exposure, such as an increase in attention problems, have also been identified (Marroun, Hudziak, Tiemeier, and others, 2011). Compounding the issue of the effects of marijuana, especially among women ages 18 to 30 years (Kuczkowski, 2007), is multidrug use, which combines the harmful effects of marijuana, tobacco, alcohol, opiates, and cocaine. Long-term follow-up studies on exposed infants are needed.

Selective Serotonin Reuptake Inhibitors

Studies estimate that between 15% and 25% of pregnant women experience major depression (Cantor Sackett, Weller, and Weller, 2009; Oberlander, Warburton, Misri, and others, 2006). For many of these women, selective serotonin reuptake inhibitors (SSRIs) provide an important therapeutic benefit; however, these drugs may result in side effects in their newborns. Signs of withdrawal are present in up to one third of infants exposed to SSRIs in utero (Burgos and Burke, 2009). Findings include hypertonia, tremulousness, wakefulness, high-pitched crying, and feeding problems. An increased risk of persistent pulmonary hypertension has been reported in neonates exposed to SSRIs early in pregnancy (Cantor Sackett, Weller, and Weller, 2009); however, this finding has not been consistently reported (Wilson, Zelig, Harvey, and others, 2011). Some SSRIs are transferred into breast milk. Breastfeeding infants whose mothers are taking SSRIs should be monitored for sleep disturbances, irritability, and poor feeding.

MATERNAL INFECTIONS

The range of pathologic conditions produced by infectious agents is large, and the difference between the maternal and fetal effects caused by any one agent is also great. Some maternal infections, especially during early gestation, can result in fetal loss or malformations because the fetus's ability to handle infectious organisms is limited and the fetal immunologic system is unable to prevent the dissemination of infectious organisms to the various tissues.

Not all prenatal infections produce teratogenic effects. Furthermore, the clinical picture of disorders caused by transplacental transfer of infectious agents is not always well defined. Some viral agents can cause remarkably similar manifestations, and it is common to test for all of them when a prenatal infection is suspected. This is the so-called TORCH complex, an acronym for:

T—Toxoplasmosis
O—Other (e.g., hepatitis B, parvovirus, HIV, West Nile)
R—Rubella
C—Cytomegalovirus infection
H—Herpes simplex

To determine the causative agent in a symptomatic infant, tests are performed to rule out each of these infections. The O category may involve testing for several viral infections (e.g., hepatitis B, varicella zoster, measles, mumps, HIV, syphilis, and human parvovirus). Bacterial infections are not included in the TORCH workup because they are usually identified by clinical manifestations and readily available laboratory tests. Gonococcal conjunctivitis (ophthalmia neonatorum) and chlamydial conjunctivitis have been significantly reduced by prophylactic measures at birth (see Chapter 8). The major maternal infections, their possible effects, and specific nursing considerations are outlined in Table 9-12.

Nursing Care Management

One of the major goals in care of infants suspected of having an infectious disease is identification of the causative organism. Standard precautions are implemented according to institutional policy. In suspected cytomegalovirus and rubella infections, pregnant health care personnel are cautioned to avoid contact with these infants. HSV is easily transmitted from one infant to another; therefore, the risk of cross-contamination is reduced or eliminated by wearing gloves for patient contact. The AAP's Red Book: 2009 Report of the Committee on Infectious Diseases (2009) provides guidelines for the type and duration of precautions for most bacterial and viral exposures. Careful hand washing is the most important nursing intervention in reducing the spread of any infection.

Specimens need to be obtained for laboratory examinations, and the infant and parents need to be prepared for diagnostic procedures. When possible, long-term disabilities are prevented by early evaluation and implementation of therapy. The family is taught any special handling techniques needed for the care of their infant and signs of complications or possible sequelae. If sequelae are inevitable, the family will need assistance in determining how they can best cope with the problems, such as assistance with home care, referral to appropriate agencies, or placement in an institution for care. The major goal of nursing care is prevention of these disorders with provision of adequate prenatal care for the expectant mother and precautions regarding exposure to teratogenic infections.

TABLE 9-12   INFECTIONS ACQUIRED FROM THE MOTHER BEFORE, DURING, OR AFTER BIRTH*

FETAL OR NEWBORN EFFECT	TRANSMISSION	NURSING CONSIDERATIONS†
Human Immunodeficiency Virus (HIV) No significant difference between infected and uninfected infants at birth in some instances Embryopathy reported by some observers: • Depressed nasal bridge • Mild upward or downward obliquity of eyes • Long palpebral fissures with blue sclerae • Patulous lips • Ocular hypertelorism • Prominent upper vermilion border See also Chapter 26.	Transplacental; during vaginal delivery; potentially in breast milk	Administer antiviral prophylaxis to the HIV-positive mother beginning at 14 wk of pregnancy. The choice of regimens is determined by examining a number of factors, including the mother's current treatment. Detailed recommendations can be obtained from Perinatal HIV Guidelines Working Group (2011). During labor, *ZDV is recommended for all HIV-infected pregnant women, regardless of the antepartum treatment regimen.* HIV-exposed neonates should receive a 6-wk course of ZDV (consider addition of another antiretroviral drug based on maternal treatment and exposure). Cesarean section in HIV-positive mothers is recommended to reduce transmission. Avoid breastfeeding in HIV-positive mother. For chemoprophylaxis against *Pneumocystis carinii* pneumonia in HIV-exposed infants, drug of choice is trimethoprim–sulfamethoxazole (Bactrim, Septra). Documented routine HIV education and routine testing with consent for all pregnant women in United States are recommended.
Chickenpox (Varicella-Zoster Virus [VZV]) Intrauterine exposure—congenital varicella syndrome: limb dysplasia, microcephaly, cortical atrophy, chorioretinitis, cataracts, cutaneous scars, other anomalies, auditory nerve palsy, motor and cognitive delays Severe symptoms (rash, fever) and higher mortality in infant whose mother develops varicella 5 days before to 2 days after delivery	First trimester (fetal varicella syndrome); perinatal period (infection)	Use varicella zoster immunoglobulin (VariZIG) or IVIG to treat infants born to mothers with onset of disease within 5 days before or 2 days after delivery. Institute isolation precautions in newborn born to mother with varicella up to 21–28 days (latter time if newborn received VariZIG or IVIG after birth) if hospitalized. Prevention—universal immunization of all children with varicella vaccine
Chlamydia Infection (*Chlamydia Trachomatis*) Conjunctivitis, pneumonia	Last trimester or perinatal period	Standard ophthalmic prophylaxis for gonococcal ophthalmia neonatorum (topical antibiotics, silver nitrate, or povidone–iodine) is not effective in treatment or prevention of chlamydial ophthalmia. Treat with oral erythromycin for 14 days.
Coxsackievirus (Group B Enterovirus–Nonpolio) Poor feeding, vomiting, diarrhea, fever; cardiac enlargement, arrhythmias, congestive heart failure; lethargy, seizures, meningeal involvement Mimics bacterial sepsis	Peripartum	Treatment is supportive. Provide IVIG in neonatal infections.
Cytomegalovirus (CMV) Variable manifestation from asymptomatic to severe Microcephaly, cerebral calcifications, chorioretinitis Jaundice, hepatosplenomegaly Petechial or purpuric rash Neurologic sequelae—seizure disorders, sensorimotor deafness, cognitive impairment	Throughout pregnancy	Infection acquired at birth, shortly thereafter, or via human milk is not associated with clinical illness. Affected individuals excrete virus. Virus is detected in urine or tissue by electron microscopy. Pregnant women should avoid close contact with known cases. To treat infection, administer IV antivirals such as ganciclovir to newborn.
Parvovirus B19 (Erythema Infectiosum) Fetal hydrops and death from anemia and heart failure with early exposure Anemia with later exposure No teratogenic effects established Ordinarily, low risk of adverse effect to fetus	Transplacental	First trimester infection has most serious effects. Pregnant health care workers should not care for patients who might be highly contagious (e.g., child with sickle cell anemia, aplastic crisis). Routine exclusion of pregnant women from workplace where disease is occurring is not recommended.

Continued

TABLE 9-12	INFECTIONS ACQUIRED FROM THE MOTHER BEFORE, DURING, OR AFTER BIRTH—cont'd	
FETAL OR NEWBORN EFFECT	**TRANSMISSION**	**NURSING CONSIDERATIONS**[†]
Gonococcal Disease (*Neisseria Gonorrhoeae*) Ophthalmitis Neonatal gonococcal arthritis, septicemia, meningitis	Last trimester or perinatal period	Apply prophylactic medication to eyes at time of birth. Obtain smears for culture. To treat infection, administer penicillin.
Hepatitis B Virus (HBV) May be asymptomatic at birth Acute hepatitis, changes in liver function	Transplacental; contaminated maternal fluids or secretions during delivery	Administer HBIg to all infants of HBsAG-positive mothers within 12 hr of birth; in addition, administer hepatitis B vaccine at separate site. Prevention—universal immunization of all infants with hepatitis B vaccine. (See Immunizations, Chapter 10.)
Listeriosis (*Listeria Monocytogenes*) Maternal infection associated with abortion, preterm delivery, and fetal death Preterm birth, sepsis, and pneumonia seen in early-onset disease; late-onset disease usually manifests as meningitis	Transplacental by ascending infection or exposure at delivery	Hand washing is essential to prevent nosocomial spread. Treat infected newborn with antibiotics—ampicillin and gentamicin.
Rubella, Congenital (Rubella Virus) Eye defects—cataracts (unilateral or bilateral), microphthalmia, retinitis, glaucoma CNS signs—microcephaly, seizures, severe cognitive impairment Congenital heart defects—patent ductus arteriosus Auditory—high incidence of delayed hearing loss IUGR Hyperbilirubinemia, meningitis, thrombocytopenia, hepatomegaly	First trimester; early second trimester	Pregnant women should avoid contact with all affected persons, including infants with rubella syndrome. Emphasize vaccination of all unimmunized prepubertal children, susceptible adolescents, and women of childbearing age (nonpregnant). Caution women against pregnancy for at least 3 mo after vaccination.
Syphilis, Congenital (*Treponema Pallidum*) Stillbirth, prematurity, hydrops fetalis May be asymptomatic at birth and in first few weeks of life or may have multisystem manifestations: hepatosplenomegaly, lymphadenopathy, hemolytic anemia, and thrombocytopenia Copper-colored maculopapular cutaneous lesions (usually after first few weeks of life), mucous membrane patches, hair loss, nail exfoliation, snuffles (syphilitic rhinitis), profound anemia, poor feeding, pseudoparalysis of one or more limbs, dysmorphic teeth (older child)	Transplacental; can be anytime during pregnancy or at birth	This is most severe form of syphilis. Treatment consists of IV penicillin. Diagnostic evaluation depends on maternal serology testing and infant symptoms (American Academy of Pediatrics, 2009).
Toxoplasmosis (*Toxoplasma Gondii*) May be asymptomatic at birth (70%–90% of cases) or have maculopapular rash, lymphadenopathy, hepatosplenomegaly, jaundice, thrombocytopenia Hydrocephaly, cerebral calcifications, chorioretinitis (classic triad) Microcephaly, seizures, cognitive impairment, deafness Encephalitis, myocarditis, hepatosplenomegaly, anemia, jaundice, diarrhea, vomiting, purpura	Throughout pregnancy Predominant host for organism is cats May be transmitted through cat feces or poorly cooked or raw infected meats	Caution pregnant women to avoid contact with cat feces (e.g., emptying cat litter boxes). Administer sulfonamides (trimethoprim–sulfamethoxazole) or pyrimethamine (Daraprim).

CNS, Central nervous system; *HBsAG*, hepatitis B surface antigen; *HBIg*, hepatitis B immunoglobulin; *IUGR*, intrauterine growth restriction; *IV*, intravenous; *IVIG*, intravenous immunoglobulin; *ZDV*, zidovudine.

*This table is not an exhaustive representation of all perinatally transmitted infections. For further information regarding specific diseases or treatment not listed here, refer to American Academy of Pediatrics, Committee on Infectious Diseases, Pickering L, editor: *2009 Red book: report of the Committee on Infectious Diseases*, ed 28, Elk Grove Village, Ill, 2009, Author.

[†]Isolation precautions depend on institutional policy. (See Infection Control, Chapter 22.)

CONGENITAL ANOMALIES*

An appreciation of the basic mechanisms involved in morphogenesis is essential to the understanding of congenital anomalies. Morphogenesis (the study of cell differentiation and development) is a genetically controlled set of events that occurs in precisely timed sequence during embryonic and fetal life. Some of the determinants of normal morphogenesis include the proper migration of cells, a well-timed mitotic rate, and controlled cell death by apoptosis. Disturbances in any of these factors may result in abnormal morphogenesis that can be expressed as various patterns of structural defects (Jones, 2006):

Malformation—Results from deficient formation of tissues. Example: Ventricular septal defects

Deformation—Results from the action of mechanical forces on a normal tissue. These forces may be extrinsic to the developing embryo, such as uterine constraints (especially common during the second trimester of development), or intrinsic, resulting from consequences of a primary malformation. Example: Arthrogryposis, or contraction of the lower limbs

Disruption—Results from the breakdown of previously normal tissue. Example: Amnion disruption sequence (amniotic band sequence)

Dysplasia—Results from abnormal organization of cells within a tissue. Example: Hamartomas

Malformations can be classified according to the defect in morphogenesis, including incomplete morphogenesis, development of accessory tissue, or functional defects. Incomplete morphogenesis may result from lack of development (e.g., vas deferens agenesis, or the absence of a vas deferens), hypoplasia (e.g., micrognathia, or a poorly developed chin), incomplete separation (e.g., syndactyly, or fused digits), incomplete closure (e.g., cleft palate), or persistence of an earlier location (e.g., cryptorchidism, or undescended testes). Development of accessory tissue may result in abnormalities such as polydactyly (supernumerary digits), and functional defects may be the cause of contractures, such as clubfoot.

Congenital anomalies, or birth defects, can be identified prenatally, at birth, or at any point after birth. About 2% to 3% of all births are associated with a major congenital anomaly. Accurate identification of such defects may provide a valuable clue for the presence of or potential for a genetic disorder (Box 9-10).

Overall, genetic disorders can be classified as chromosomal abnormalities (numeric and structural changes in the normal chromosome pattern), gene substitutions or alterations (single-gene and polygenic disorders), and complex (or multifactorial) disorders (those that result from interactions between the individual's genetic predisposition and environmental factors). Chromosomal abnormalities account for approximately 25% of all major birth defects, and single-gene disorders account for approximately 20%. In addition, exposure to known teratogens (agents that cause congenital anomalies) accounts for about 5% of major birth defects. The etiology of the remaining 50% is currently unknown. However, many of these idiopathic birth defects occur in families in patterns similar to complex diseases such as diabetes mellitus and mental illnesses, indicating a possible multifactorial or even polygenic etiology (Nussbaum, McInnes, and Willard, 2007).

The types of malformations that can result from genetic or prenatal environmental causes can be major structural abnormalities with serious medical, surgical, or quality-of-life consequences, or they can be minor anomalies or normal variants with no serious

---

BOX 9-10   ASSESSMENT CLUES TO GENETIC DISORDERS*

Major or minor birth defects (anomalies) and dysmorphic features—Cardiac defect, ear or eye abnormalities, micrognathia, forehead prominence, low-set hairline on forehead or nape of neck, wide-set eyes, epicanthal folds, low-set ears, microcephaly or hydrocephalus

Growth abnormalities—Short stature, overgrowth, asymmetric growth, intrauterine growth restriction, postnatal growth delay

Skeletal abnormalities—Limb abnormalities, asymmetry, scoliosis, pectus excavatum, hyperextensible joints, hypotonic or hypertonic muscle tone, pectus excavatum, finger or joint abnormalities

Vision or hearing problems—Coloboma of the iris, absence of red reflex, cat's eye reflex, hearing deficit, vision deficit, absence of external ear

Metabolic disorders—Unusual odor of breath, urine, or stool; coarse facial features; electrolyte imbalances

Sexual development abnormalities—Ambiguous genitalia (disorders of sex development), small penis, delayed onset of puberty, primary amenorrhea, precocious sexual development, large testicles

Skin disorders—Unusual pigmentation, café-au-lait spots, dry and scaly skin, skin tumors, sparse hair, absent or unusual teeth

Recurrent infection or immunodeficiency—Ear infections, pneumonia

Developmental and speech delays or loss of milestones:
- **Cognitive delays**—Learning disabilities, mild to severe cognitive impairment
- **Behavioral disorders**—Hyperactivity, attention-deficit disorder, autistic-like behavior, aggressive behavior

*Suggests a genetic etiology if two or more findings are present.

---

consequences, such as a sacral dimple, an extra nipple, or a single simian crease of the hand. Malformations can occur in isolation, such as congenital heart defect, or multiple anomalies may be present. A recognized pattern of malformations resulting from a single specific cause is called a syndrome (e.g., Turner syndrome and FAS). A sequence consists of multiple malformations that are caused by a single event with multiple etiologies (Wynshaw-Boris and Biesecker, 2007). An example is the Pierre Robin sequence, which consists of mandibular hypoplasia, a large tongue (glossoptosis), and often subsequent airway compromise.

The identification of a genetic etiology for a birth defect has important implications for knowing:

Diagnosis—What is the disorder?

Etiology—What caused it?

Prognosis—What are the possible consequences?

Therapy—What can be done?

Recurrence risk—Will it happen again?

Prenatal diagnosis—Is testing available for future pregnancies?

Establishing a diagnosis helps the family and health care team develop an awareness of the findings that may be seen with the disorder and to initiate early intervention strategies, including genetic counseling for the parents and extended family. For example, children with DiGeorge, or 22q11 deletion, syndrome may be diagnosed through the identification of the combination of velopharyngeal incompetence and cardiac defects. After the diagnosis of a chromosome microdeletion disorder is made, evaluation for immune function and renal abnormalities can be initiated. Cognitive, speech, and language delays are commonly seen in children with this disorder, and enrollment in early childhood intervention programs should be arranged as soon after diagnosis as possible.

GENETIC ETIOLOGY OF CONGENITAL ANOMALIES

Chromosomal Abnormalities

Chromosomal abnormalities are deviations in either number or structure of chromosomes, and the consequences in either situation can usually be observed in the affected individual. Numeric chromosomal abnormalities can result from the addition of one chromosome to each of the existing pair. Human somatic cells are diploid, with a chromosome complement of 2n = 46. Gametes, both ova and spermatozoa, are haploid cells, with 23 chromosomes each (n = 23). The addition of one haploid complement (23 chromosomes) to a diploid cell will mean that all pairs will now have acquired one chromosome each and are no longer pairs but "trios." The cell is now a triploid cell (3n = 69). This type of configuration, in which one chromosome was equally added to each pair, is termed euploidy and is designated by the suffix -ploidy. Such an enormous increase in chromosome number (46 to 69) represents a large gene imbalance and will likely not be compatible with life. Deviations in chromosome number that are compatible with life, despite resulting in physical or developmental abnormalities, usually involve the gain of one (or few) chromosomes, which are added to an existing pair (only that particular pair becomes a trio). In this case, the chromosome number will increase from the typical 46 to 47 (or 48) through an unequal addition of one (or few) chromosomes to only that specific pair. This unequal addition of one (or few) chromosomes is termed aneuploidy and is designated by the suffix -somy.

The most common type of aneuploidy, from a clinical perspective, is the trisomies. A type of aneuploidy that results from the loss of one member of a chromosome pair is termed a monosomy. The only monosomy that is compatible with life is Turner syndrome, which results from the loss of one of the X chromosomes in women.

Most chromosomal abnormalities in number and structure result from abnormal cell division during germ cell formation or early cell division in the zygote. Structural abnormalities usually involve some degree of chromosome breakage. Fragments broken off a chromosome can be lost (deletion), may rearrange in abnormal configurations, or may attach to another chromosome (translocation). If the rearrangement of fragments between two chromosomes is reciprocal, that is, without loss of genetic material, the resulting configuration is termed a balanced translocation. An individual with a balanced translocation is usually normal in appearance and function but may potentially transmit to the developing offspring the translocation in an unbalanced form, resulting in spontaneous abortion or a child with congenital abnormalities. Therefore, referral for genetic counseling is recommended for individuals found to have a translocation.

Both numeric and structural abnormalities of autosomes and sex chromosomes account for a variety of disorders of infancy and childhood. A few are associated with a group of characteristics that clearly indicate the precise chromosomal anomaly (Table 9-13). The most common is Down syndrome, which is caused by a trisomy of chromosome 21 (see Chapter 19 for a further discussion of Down syndrome). Other known viable autosomal trisomies involve chromosomes 18 (Edwards syndrome) and 13 (Patau syndrome). Although the prognosis for survival after birth is poor, some children with these trisomies have lived for several years. Abnormalities of sex chromosomes are discussed in Chapter 17.

Single-Gene Defects

Single-gene disorders are caused by a mutation or change in a single gene. A single allele of that gene on a chromosome or two alleles of the same (homologous) gene pair on both chromosomes may undergo mutations. For example, one of many genetic variants of cystic fibrosis is caused when two matched pairs of genes on chromosomes 7 carry the cystic fibrosis gene mutation. However, Marfan syndrome occurs when a mutation in the fibrillin gene occurs on one chromosome 15. Single-gene disorders are individually rare but collectively play a significant role in human disease. It is estimated that 6% to 8% of hospitalized children have a single-gene disorder.

Multifactorial Inheritance

Some congenital anomalies are caused by multifactorial inheritance. The concept of multifactorial inheritance has acquired new and expanded importance with the identification of complex disorders. These are disease processes for which the individual has a certain genetic predisposition, but the expression of the gene (disease) depends on its interaction with environmental stimuli. Cleft lip and palate, neural tube defects, and congenital heart defects are some examples of conditions caused by multifactorial inheritance.

DEFECTS CAUSED BY CHEMICAL AGENTS

Prenatal environmental influences from chemicals such as alcohol, medications, or drugs of abuse; infectious disease; or radiation or other environmental influences may be regarded as nongenetic causes of congenital anomalies because these effects can produce congenital structural, functional, or growth defects. An agent that produces congenital malformations or increases their incidence is called a teratogen.

The relationship of the fetal and maternal circulations allows for the interchange of chemical substances across the placental membrane. Many drugs have been suspected of producing congenital malformations, and some have been definitely implicated. Some of the most recognized teratogenic drugs include alcohol, tobacco, antiepileptic medications, isotretinoin (Accutane), lithium, cocaine, and diethylstilbestrol (Table 9-14).

The extent to which chemical agents affect the unborn child depends on the interplay of several factors, including the nature of the agent and its accessibility to the fetus, the gestational age at which exposure occurred, the level and duration of the dosage, and the genetic makeup of the fetus. For example, fetal exposure to valproic acid in the first 3 months of pregnancy may result in congenital anomalies such as neural tube defects, congenital heart defects, and distinctive facial features. The limited metabolic capabilities of the fetal liver and its immature enzyme and transport systems render the unborn child ill equipped for maintaining homeostasis when chemical disturbances are imposed by the mother or the environment. This includes both substances produced by the mother in response to a disease state (e.g., diabetes) and exogenous substances ingested or inhaled by the mother.

The teratogenic effect of drugs is not believed to have an effect on developing tissue until day 15 of gestation, when tissue differentiation begins to take place. Before that time, drugs usually have little effect because they are believed to have an insignificant affinity for undifferentiated tissue. Also, until implantation takes place, at approximately 7 days after conception, the embryo is not exposed to maternal blood that contains the drug. However, some drugs may affect the uterine lining, making it unsuitable for implantation. Drugs administered between days 15 and 90 may produce an effect if the tissue for which the drug has an affinity is in the process of differentiation at that time. After 90 days, when differentiation is complete, most fetal tissues are believed to be relatively resistant to teratogenic effects of drugs. However, the impact on ongoing neurologic development is not known.

TABLE 9-13	COMMON CHROMOSOMAL ABNORMALITIES

ABNORMALITY, CHROMOSOME NOTATION, AND APPROXIMATE INCIDENCE	MAJOR CLINICAL MANIFESTATIONS
Trisomy 21 (Down Syndrome) 47,XY or XX, 21[+] (free trisomy) 46,XY or XX, t(14;21)[+] (translocation) 46,XY or XX/47,XY or XX, 21[+] (mosaic) **Incidence**—1:800 live births*[†]	Brachycephaly with flat occiput; epicanthal folds; small ears, nose, and mouth with protruding tongue; muscular hypotonia; broad, short hands with stubby fingers and transverse palmar crease; broad, stubby feet with wide space between big and second toes; cardiac defects; cognitive impairment; variable life expectancy
Trisomy 18 (Edwards Syndrome) 47,XY or XX, 18[+] **Incidence**—1:7500 live births*	Deformed and low-set ears, micrognathia, rocker-bottom feet, overlapping (index over third) fingers, prominent occiput, hypertelorism, failure to thrive and early death, cognitive impairment
Trisomy 13 (Patau Syndrome) 47,XY or XX, 13[+] **Incidence**—1:22,700 live births*	Multiple anomalies, including cleft lip and palate (frequently bilateral), ear malformations, microphthalmia, polydactyly, eye defects, cognitive impairment, early death
Klinefelter Syndrome 47,XXY (or multiple X, Y) **Incidence**—1:1000 live male births*	Male phenotype, small testes with decreased androgen production, infertility, well-developed genitalia, sparse facial hair, female pubic hair pattern; slightly taller than normal males (longer legs); gynecomastia frequent; voice may not change at puberty **Infrequent abnormalities**—Scoliosis, pectus excavatum, fifth finger clinodactyly, dental anomalies, cardiac anomalies, pulmonary diseases, varicose veins **Intellectual development**—Normal to borderline (IQ, 85), language delay
Turner Syndrome 45,X0 **Incidence**—1:4000 live female births*	Female phenotype, ovarian dysgenesis (streak gonads), short stature, decreased estrogens, infertility, delayed sexual development, webbing of the neck, low posterior neckline, neonatal lymphedema, cubitus valgus, short fourth metacarpals, "shield" chest, divergent nipples, sex chromatin negative, coarctation of the aorta, urinary tract abnormalities, fetal cystic hygroma or hydrops, normal intellectual development

*Data from Nussbaum RL, McInnes RR, Willard HF: *Thompson and Thompson genetics in medicine*, ed 6 (Rev Print), Philadelphia, 2004, Saunders.
[†]Risk related to maternal age: age 30 years = 1:900; age 35 years = 1:385; age 40 years = 1:100; age 45 years and older = 1:25.
From Nussbaum, McInnes, and Willard (2004).

Nursing Care Management

Expectant mothers are cautioned against ingesting any medication without first consulting a practitioner. To help ensure that fewer women will inadvertently take some chemical that might be harmful to their fetuses, labels on medications are now required to include information regarding the possible teratogenic effects of each drug. All women of childbearing age should be educated regarding the effects of chemicals, especially alcohol, on unborn fetuses. FAS is an irreversible condition but is completely preventable. The March of Dimes* and Centers for Disease Control and Prevention[†] have information about prevention tips, and the Genetic Alliance[‡] has information about support groups for families of children with FAS. Genetic counseling is recommended for women who have a concern about a possible teratogen during pregnancy.

---

*1275 Mamaroneck Ave., White Plains, NY 10605; 914-997-4488; http://www.marchofdimes.com.
[†]http://www.cdc.gov/
[‡]4301 Connecticut Ave. NW, Suite 404, Washington, DC 20008; http://www.geneticalliance.org.

NURSING TIP One drug recognized for its carcinogenic effect is diethylstilbestrol. Large doses of this hormone, given to pregnant women in the United States between 1938 and 1971 to prevent abortion, caused adenocarcinoma of the vagina in a significant proportion of the female offspring when they reach adolescence and early adulthood.

▌INBORN ERRORS OF METABOLISM

Inborn errors of metabolism (IEMs) constitute a large number of inherited diseases caused by the absence or deficiency of a substance essential to cellular metabolism, usually an enzyme. When the normal metabolic process is interrupted as a result of a missing enzyme, an accumulation of substances precedes the interruption, the end product of the process is absent, or the process takes an alternate metabolic pathway. The consequence is manifested as an illness. Most IEMs are characterized by abnormal protein, carbohydrate, or fat metabolism.

Newborn screening for IEMs varies from state to state, but all states test for at least seven core disorders, which are phenylketonuria (PKU),

TABLE 9-14	CONGENITAL EFFECTS OF MATERNAL ALCOHOL INGESTION AND TOBACCO SMOKING	
FETAL OR NEWBORN EFFECTS	**COMMENTS AND NURSING CARE MANAGEMENT**	

Alcohol (Fetal Alcohol Spectrum Disorder)

Features vary—infant may not display physical features; involves three main categories:

- Growth failure in utero and after birth, including microcephaly
- Midfacial dysmorphic features
- CNS involvement, including cognitive impairment, irritability, hyperactivity, hypertonia, and behavioral problems

Facial features include hypoplastic maxilla; micrognathia; short palpebral fissures; thinned upper lip; hypoplastic philtrum; short, upturned nose.

One or a combination of these features present in infancy or later (may not appear until later in life).

Children or adults who demonstrate cognitive, behavioral, and psychosocial problems without physical features and growth delay are referred to as having ARND.

Affected infants may display nonspecific signs such as irritability, lethargy, difficulty establishing respirations, seizures, tremors, poor suck reflex, and abdominal distention. Birth defects may occur but are less common.

Diagnosis is made more difficult by a lack of a single biologic marker and may be made based on maternal history of alcohol ingestion.

A number of terms (including ARND and FASD) have been proposed to describe the combination of findings.

Quantity of alcohol consumed is not the determinant; rather, it is the amount consumed in excess of the liver's ability to detoxify the alcohol. Free alcohol has an affinity for brain tissue, hence the CNS symptoms. Ethanol byproducts also contribute to toxicity, as do other substances consumed in addition to alcohol and poor maternal self-care. The effects of alcohol on the fetus occur across a continuum ranging from subtle neurological deficits to full-blown FAS. The term FASD is used to describe the range of clinical presentations ascribed to fetal alcohol exposure.

Early gestation is considered the most vulnerable period; however, exposure at any period may cause subtle damage to the developing fetus.

Effects of alcohol on CNS are not reversible.

FASD is the leading cause of preventable cognitive impairment in the United States.

Early intervention with mothers is aimed at minimizing fetal effects, education, and involvement in prevention and treatment counseling.

Early intervention with newborns focuses on reducing the effects of alcohol exposure on growing child, especially in relation to cognitive deficits and learning disabilities.

Treatment in the neonatal period is similar to that of drug-exposed infants and should involve extensive assessment and individualized developmental care.

Provide resources to help decrease or eliminate alcohol intake. *During Your Pregnancy: Tips for Giving Up Alcohol* is available at the March of Dimes' website.*

Further information is available from the National Organization on Fetal Alcohol Syndrome[†] and Centers for Disease Control and Prevention.[‡]

Maternal Tobacco Smoking

Smoking is associated with significant birth weight deficits; positive dose-response relationship is related to size of fetus.

Two active substances—nicotine and cotinine—are higher in newborns of mothers who smoke than in mothers who do not.

Postnatal growth deficits occur, as do deficits in emotional and behavioral development in the growing child.

Maternal smoking is associated with an increased risk of SIDS, respiratory tract illnesses in childhood, and childhood learning deficits.

There is evidence that even secondhand smoke can be deleterious to unborn fetuses and growing children.

Counseling regarding fetal and postnatal effects should be made available to all pregnant women, and they are encouraged to stop smoking. Smoking cessation during pregnancy decreases the chance of fetal complications.

Encourage pregnant women to enroll in smoking cessation programs.

Evaluate polydrug use in conjunction with smoking.

An increased incidence of perinatal complications leading to preterm birth includes abruptio placentae, placenta previa, and premature rupture of membranes.

Provide resources to help eliminate smoking. *During Your Pregnancy: Tips to Quit (Smoking)* is available from the March of Dimes.*

ARND, Alcohol-related neurodevelopmental disorder; *CNS,* central nervous system; *FAS,* fetal alcohol syndrome; *FASD,* fetal alcohol spectrum disorder; *SIDS,* sudden infant death syndrome.

*http://www.marchofdimes.com.

[†]1200 Eton Court NW, Third Floor, Washington, DC 20007; 202-785-4585; 800 66 NOFAS; http://www.nofas.org.

[‡]Fetal Alcohol Syndrome Branch, Division of Birth Defects, Child Development and Disability and Health, Centers for Disease Control and Prevention, Atlanta, http://www.cdc.gov/ncbddd/fas/index.html.

congenital hypothyroidism (CH), galactosemia, sickle cell disease, thalassemia, congenital adrenal hyperplasia (CAH), and cystic fibrosis (CF).* The purpose of screening is to identify children who may have a condition that benefits from early identification and treatment to prevent cognitive impairment. The screening test is most reliable if the blood sample is taken after the infant has ingested a source of protein for 24 hours. Because of early discharge of newborns,

recommendations for screening include (1) collecting the initial specimen as close as possible to discharge or no later than 7 days, (2) obtaining a subsequent sample by 2 weeks of age if the initial specimen is collected before the newborn is 24 hours old, and (3) designating a primary care provider to all newborns before discharge for adequate newborn screening follow-up (Kaye, Committee on Genetics, Accurso, and others, 2006). A new screening test, tandem mass spectrometry, has the potential for identifying more than 20 IEMs in addition to the standard IEMs. With tandem mass spectrometry, earlier identification of IEMs may prevent further developmental delays and morbidities in affected children (Wilcken, 2010).

*Because newborn screening varies by state and policies change frequently, a good resource is the National Newborn Screening and Genetics Resource Center, http://genes-r-us.uthscsa.edu.

A major concern is that a significantly large number of infants are *not* rescreened for metabolic disorders after early discharge and are at risk for a missed or delayed diagnosis of a treatable disorder. Special consideration must be given to screening infants born at home who have no hospital contact. It is always necessary to confirm the screening results with diagnostic testing.

CONGENITAL HYPOTHYROIDISM

Congenital hypothyroidism may have a number of causes and can be either permanent or transient. Transient CH is frequently associated with maternal Graves disease that was treated with antithyroid drugs. The majority of cases are sporadic (nonhereditary), but approximately 15% of all cases are transmitted as an autosomal dominant trait. The most common pathogenesis is thyroid dysgenesis, mostly with unknown causes. Worldwide, the most common cause of CH resulting in hypothyroidism is iodine deficiency. However, no matter what the cause, the manifestations (Box 9-11) and management are similar. In some conditions, the thyroid deficiency is severe, and manifestations develop early; in others, the symptoms may be delayed for months or years. Early detection and prompt initiation of treatment are essential because their delay will result in various degrees of cognitive impairment, in which the IQ loss has a direct relationship to the time treatment is initiated. If treatment is implemented from 0 to 3 months of age, the mean IQ attained is 89 (range, 64–107); if treatment begins at 3 to 6 months, mean IQ will reach 71 (range, 36–96); treatment initiated after 6 months of age will result in a mean IQ of 54 (range, 25–80).

Results of screening tests in the United States indicate that CH occurs in approximately 1 in 4000 to 1 in 3000 newborns (Kaye, Committee on Genetics, Accurso, and others, 2006). It affects all races and ethnicities, but it is more prevalent among Hispanic and American Indian or Alaskan Native people (1 in 2000 to 1 in 700 newborns) and less prevalent among African Americans (1 in 3200 to 1 in 17,000 newborns). Infants with Down syndrome have a much higher rate of either permanent or transient forms of the disorder (approximately 1 in 140 newborns) (Kaye, Committee on Genetics, Accurso, and others, 2006). Also, a higher incidence of other congenital abnormalities has been observed in infants with CH. Many preterm infants have transient hypothyroidism (hypothyroxinemia) at birth as a result of hypothalamic and pituitary immaturity. Infants born before 28 weeks of gestation may require temporary thyroid hormone replacement. Some screening programs target both primary (thyroid-based) and secondary (pituitary-based) hypothyroidism.

Diagnostic Evaluation

Because CH is one of the most common preventable causes of cognitive impairment, early diagnosis and treatment of this disease are essential interventions. Neonatal screening consists of an initial filter paper blood spot thyroxine (T_4) measurement followed by measurement of thyroid-stimulating hormone (TSH) in specimens with low T_4 values.

Tests are mandatory in all U.S. states and territories. Although a blood sample obtained by heel stick for the spot test is best obtained between 2 and 6 days of age, specimens are usually taken within the first 24 to 48 hours or before discharge as part of a concurrent screen for other metabolic defects. Early screening can result in overdiagnosis (false-positives) but is preferable to missing the diagnosis.

For screening results that show a low level of T_4 (<10%), obtain TSH levels, and if these are elevated (>40 mU/L), further tests to

---

BOX 9-11	CLINICAL MANIFESTATIONS OF CONGENITAL HYPOTHYROIDISM

Birth*
Poor feeding
Lethargy
Prolonged jaundice (>2 weeks)
Respiratory difficulties
Cyanosis
Constipation
Bradycardia
Hoarse cry
Large anterior and posterior fontanels
Postterm
Birth weight over 4000 g (8.8 pounds)

Ages 6 to 9 Weeks†
Depressed nasal bridge
Short forehead
Puffy eyelids
Large tongue
Thick, dry, mottled skin
Coarse, dry, lusterless hair
Abdominal distention
Umbilical hernia
Hyporeflexia
Bradycardia
Hypothermia
Hypotension
Anemia
Widely patent cranial sutures

Older Child
Short stature
Obesity
Varying degrees of intellectual deficits
Abnormal tendon reflexes
Slow, awkward movements

*Clinical manifestations may not be obvious at birth, possibly because of maternal transfer of thyroid hormone to the fetus. Manifestations may be delayed in infants with certain types of familial hypothyroidism and in breastfed infants (may show after weaning).
†If untreated, classical features.

---

determine the cause of the disease should be carried out (AAP and American Thyroid Association, 2006) (see Appendix C for values). Additional tests include serum measurement of T_4, triiodothyronine (T_3), resin uptake, free T_4, and thyroid-bound globulin. Tests of thyroid gland function (thyroid scan and uptake) usually involve oral administration of a radioactive isotope of iodine (^{131}I) and measurement of iodine uptake by the thyroid, usually within 24 hours. In CH, protein-bound iodine, T_4, T_3, and free T_4 levels are low, and thyroid uptake of ^{131}I is decreased. Skeletal radiography is used to assess age.

In newborns, thyroid function studies are elevated in comparison with values in older children; therefore, it is important to document the timing of the tests. In preterm and sick full-term infants, thyroid function tests are usually lower than in healthy full-term infants; a repeat T_4 and TSH may be evaluated after 30 weeks (corrected age) in newborns born before that time and after resolution of the acute illness in sick full-term infants.

Therapeutic Management

Treatment involves lifelong thyroid hormone replacement therapy as soon as possible after diagnosis to abolish all signs of hypothyroidism and reestablish normal physical and mental development. The drug of choice is synthetic levothyroxine sodium (Synthroid, Levothroid). Optimum dosage of L-thyroxine should be able to maintain blood TSH concentration between 0.5 and 2.0 mU/L during the first 3 years of life (AAP and American Thyroid Association, 2006). Regular measurement of thyroxine levels is important in ensuring optimum treatment. Bone age surveys are also performed to ensure optimum growth.

Prognosis

If treatment is started shortly after birth, normal physical growth and intelligence are possible. The most significant factor adversely affecting eventual intellectual development appears to be inadequate treatment, which may be related to noncompliance. On the other hand, prolonged overtreatment can result in future temperament disorders, and close monitoring of adequate hormone replacement is essential, especially in the first 2 to 3 years of life (Selva, Harper, Downs, and others, 2005).

Nursing Care Management

The most important nursing objective is early identification of the disorder. Nurses caring for neonates must be certain that screening is performed, especially in infants who are preterm, discharged early, or born at home. Approximately 10% of cases are detected only by a second screening at 2 to 6 weeks of age. Nurses in community health need to be aware of the earliest signs of the disorder. Parental remarks about an unusually "quiet and good" baby and demonstrated symptoms such as prolonged jaundice, constipation, and umbilical hernia should lead to a suspicion of hypothyroidism, which requires a referral for specific tests.

After the diagnosis is confirmed, parents need an explanation of the disorder and the necessity of lifelong treatment. The child should be referred to a pediatric endocrinologist for care. The importance of compliance with the drug regimen for the child to achieve normal growth and development must be stressed (Kaye, Committee on Genetics, Accurso, and others, 2006). Because the drug is tasteless, it can be crushed and added to formula, water, or food. If a dose is missed, twice the dose should be given the next day. Unless there are maternal contraindicative factors, breastfeeding is acceptable and encouraged in infants with hypothyroidism (Lawrence and Lawrence, 2011). Parents also need to be aware of signs indicating overdose, such as a rapid pulse, dyspnea, irritability, insomnia, fever, sweating, and weight loss. Ideally, they should know how to count the pulse and be instructed to withhold a dose and consult their practitioner if the pulse rate is above a certain value. Signs of inadequate treatment are fatigue, sleepiness, decreased appetite, and constipation.

If the diagnosis was delayed past early infancy, the chance of permanent cognitive impairment is great. Parents need the same guidance in caring for their child as do others who have an offspring with cognitive impairment (see Chapter 19). They need an opportunity to discuss their feelings regarding late recognition of the disorder. Although treatment will not reverse the intellectual deficit, it may prevent further damage. Genetic counseling is important for the rare families in which the etiology of CH is thyroid dyshormonogenesis, which is inherited in an autosomal recessive manner (see Genetic Evaluation and Counseling, p. 301).

PHENYLKETONURIA

Phenylketonuria, an inborn error of metabolism inherited as an autosomal recessive trait (the *PAH* gene is located on chromosome 12q24), is caused by a deficiency or absence of the enzyme needed to metabolize the essential amino acid phenylalanine. Classic PKU is at one end of a spectrum of conditions known as hyperphenylalaninemia. Within the spectrum of hyperphenylalaninemia are conditions with varying degrees of severity depending on the degree of enzyme deficiency. Because rarer forms are a result of a deficiency in other enzymes and are diagnosed and treated differently, the following discussion of PKU is limited to the severe, classic form.

In PKU, the hepatic enzyme phenylalanine hydroxylase, which normally controls the conversion of phenylalanine to tyrosine, is deficient. This results in the accumulation of phenylalanine in the bloodstream and urinary excretion of abnormal amounts of its metabolites, the phenyl acids (Fig. 9-22). One of these phenylketones, phenylacetic acid, gives urine the characteristic musty odor associated with the disease. Another is phenylpyruvic acid, which is responsible for the term phenylketonuria.

Tyrosine, the amino acid produced by the metabolism of phenylalanine, is absent in PKU. Tyrosine is needed to form the pigment melanin and the hormones epinephrine and thyroxine. Decreased melanin production results in similar phenotypes of most individuals with PKU, which is blond hair, blue eyes, and fair skin that is particularly susceptible to eczema and other dermatologic problems. Children with a genetically darker skin color may be red haired or brunette.

The prevalence of PKU varies widely in the United States because different states have different definition criteria for what constitutes hyperphenylalaninemia and PKU. The reported figures for PKU in the United States is one case per 15,000 live births. The disease has a wide variation of incidence by ethnic groups. In Europe, the incidence is 1 in 10,000 births; in Asia and Africa, the prevalence is quite low (Blau, van Spronsen, and Levy, 2010).

Clinical manifestations in untreated PKU include failure to thrive (growth failure); frequent vomiting; irritability; hyperactivity; and unpredictable, erratic behavior. Cognitive impairment is thought to be caused by the accumulation of phenylalanine and presumably by decreased levels of the neurotransmitters dopamine and tryptophan, which affect the normal development of the brain and CNS, resulting in defective myelinization, cystic degeneration of the gray and white matter, and disturbances in cortical lamination. Older children commonly display bizarre or schizoid behavior patterns such as fright reactions, screaming episodes, head banging, arm biting, disorientation, failure to respond to strong stimuli, and catatonia-like positions.

Diagnostic Evaluation*

The objective in diagnosing and treating the disorder is to prevent cognitive impairment. Every newborn should be screened for PKU. The most commonly used test for screening newborns is the Guthrie blood test, a bacterial inhibition assay for phenylalanine in the blood. *Bacillus subtilis*, present in the culture medium, grows if the blood contains an excessive amount of phenylalanine. If performed properly, this test detects serum phenylalanine levels greater than 4 mg/dl (normal value, 1.6 mg/dl), but it will not quantify the results. Other methods for testing include quantitative fluorometric assay and

---

*Always refer patient to a genetic metabolic specialist. For a reference list, visit the American Society of Human Genetics' website, http://www.ashg.org.

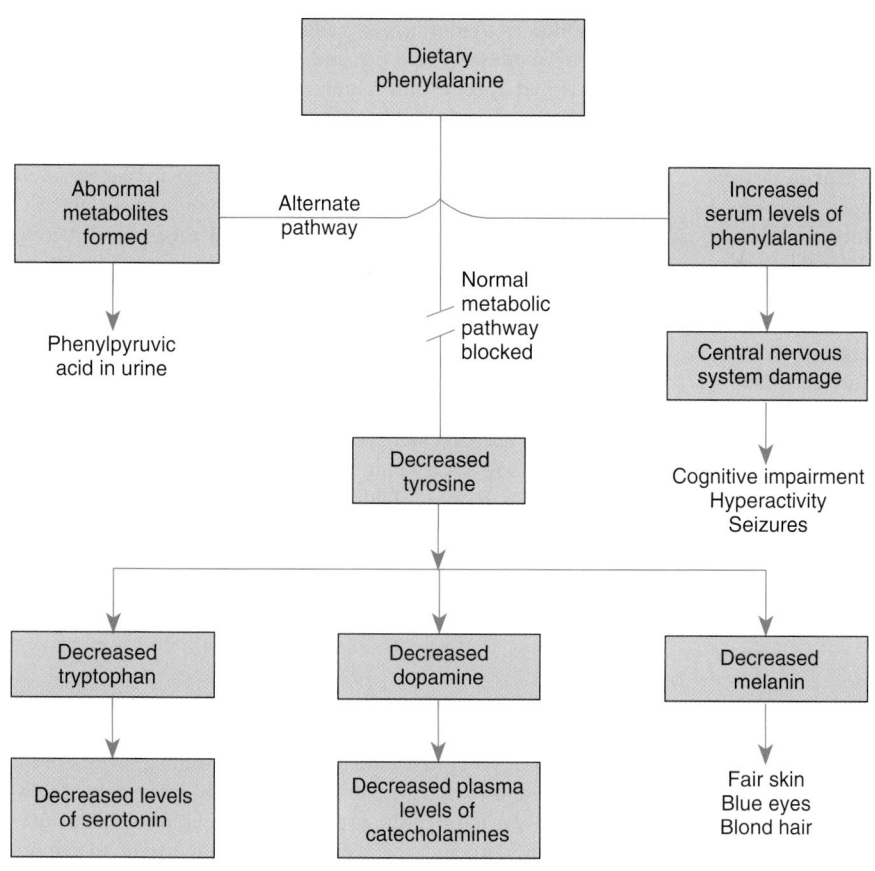

FIG 9-22 Metabolic error and consequences in phenylketonuria.

tandem mass spectrometry, which will give an absolute value. Only fresh heel blood, not cord blood, can be used for the test.

Avoid "layering" the blood specimen on the special Guthrie paper. Layering is placing one drop of blood on top of the other or overlapping the specimen. This practice results in a falsely high reading, or false positive, which will lead the newborn screening department to call the family and physician to arrange for a diagnostic blood phenylalanine test to determine whether the newborn truly has PKU. Best results are obtained by collecting the specimen with a pipette from the heel stick and spreading the blood uniformly over the blot paper.

Because of the possibility of variant forms of hyperphenylalaninemia, PKU cofactor variant screen should be performed in all children diagnosed with PKU. A major concern is that a significant number of infants are not rescreened for PKU after early discharge and are at risk for a missed or delayed diagnosis. Give special consideration to screening infants born at home who have no hospital contact and infants adopted internationally.

Therapeutic Management*

Treatment of PKU involves restricting phenylalanine in the diet. Because the genetic enzyme is intracellular, systemic administration of phenylalanine hydroxylase is of no value. Phenylalanine cannot be eliminated because it is an essential amino acid in tissue growth.

Therefore, dietary management must meet two criteria: (1) meet the child's nutritional need for optimum growth and (2) maintain phenylalanine levels within a safe range (2–6 mg/dl in neonates and children up to 12 years, 2–10 mg/dl through adolescence, and 2–15 mg/dl in adults) (Kaye, Committee on Genetics, Accurso, and others, 2006).

Professionals agree that infants with PKU who have blood phenylalanine levels higher than 10 mg/dl should be started on treatment to establish metabolic control as soon as possible, ideally by 7 to 10 days of age (Kaye, Committee on Genetics, Accurso, and others, 2006). The daily amounts of phenylalanine are individualized for each child and require frequent changes on the basis of appetite, growth and development, and blood phenylalanine and tyrosine levels.

Because all natural food proteins contain phenylalanine and will be limited, the diet must be supplemented with a specially prepared phenylalanine-free formula (e.g., Phenex-1 for infants or Phenex-2 for children and adults).† The phenylalanine-free formula is an amino acid–modified formula essential in the low phenylalanine diet to provide the appropriate protein, vitamins, minerals, and calories for optimal growth and development. Because tyrosine becomes an essential amino acid, the phenylalanine-free formula supplies an adequate amount, but in some cases, additional supplementation may be needed. The phenylalanine-free amino acid–modified formula for infants has all the nutrients necessary for adequate infant growth. Because of the low phenylalanine content of breast milk, total or partial breastfeeding

---

*For more information, contact American Society of Human Genetics, 9650 Rockville Pike, Bethesda, MD 20814; 301-634-7300, 866-HUM-GENE; http://www.ashg.org.

†A resource for dietary management is Acosta PB, Yannicelli S: *The Ross metabolic formula system nutrition support protocols*, ed 4, Columbus, Ohio, 2001, Abbott Nutrition; 800-227-5767; http://abbottnutrition.com.

may be possible with close monitoring of phenylalanine levels (Lawrence and Lawrence, 2011).

When treatment for PKU was first instituted it was believed that phenylalanine withdrawal during only the first 3 years of age would suffice to avoid cognitive impairment and other deleterious manifestations of PKU. However, most clinicians now agree that to achieve optimal metabolic control and outcome, a restricted phenylalanine diet, including medical foods and low-protein products, most likely will be medically required for virtually all individuals with classic PKU for their entire lives (Kaye, Committee on Genetics, Accurso, and others, 2006). Such lifetime reduction of phenylalanine intake is necessary to prevent neuropsychologic and cognitive deficits because even mild hyperphenylalaninemia (20 mg/dl) would produce such effects. To evaluate the effectiveness of dietary treatment, frequent monitoring of blood phenylalanine and tyrosine levels is necessary.

Phenylalanine levels greater than 6 mg/dl in mothers with PKU affect the normal embryologic development of the fetus, including cognitive impairment, cardiac defects, and LBW. It is recommended that phenylalanine levels below 6 mg/dl be achieved at least 3 months before conception in women with PKU (Kaye, Committee on Genetics, Accurso, and others, 2006).

Prognosis

Although many individuals with treated PKU manifest no cognitive and behavioral deficits, many comparisons of individuals with PKU with control participants show lower performance on IQ tests, with larger differences in other cognitive domains; however, their performance is still in the average range. Evidence for differences in behavioral adjustment is inconsistent despite anecdotal reports suggesting greater risk for internalizing psychopathology and attention disorders. In addition, insufficient data are available on the effects of phenylalanine restriction over many decades of life (Kaye, Committee on Genetics, Accurso, and others, 2006). Recent data suggest that treatment with tetrahydrobiopterin in addition to the phenylalanine-restricted diet may be beneficial to PKU patients (Blau, van Spronsen, and Levy, 2010). Total bone mineral density is considerably lower in children who are on a low-phenylalanine diet even though calcium, phosphorus, and magnesium intakes are higher than normal.

Nursing Care Management

The principal nursing considerations involve teaching the family regarding the dietary restrictions. Although the treatment may sound simple, the task of maintaining such a strict dietary regimen is demanding, especially for older children and adolescents. In addition, mothers of children with PKU may have to spend many hours preparing special foods such as low-phenylalanine snacks. Foods with low phenylalanine levels (e.g., vegetables; fruits; juices; some cereals, breads, and starches) must be measured to provide the prescribed amount of phenylalanine. High-protein foods, such as meat and dairy products, are eliminated from the diet. The sweetener aspartame (NutraSweet) should be avoided because it is composed of two amino acids, aspartic acid and phenylalanine, and if used will decrease the amount of natural phenylalanine that is prescribed for the day. However, medications that use aspartame as the sweetener may be used if no other nonaspartame medications are available because the content of the artificial sweetener is minimal or can be counted in the total daily phenylalanine allowance.

Maintaining the diet during infancy presents few problems. Solid foods such as cereal, fruits, and vegetables are introduced as usual to the infant. Difficulties arise as the child gets older. Studies show a gradual decline in diet compliance with consequent increases in blood

phenylalanine levels during early adolescence and young adulthood (Channon, Goodman, Zlotowitz, and others, 2007).

A decreased appetite and refusal to eat may reduce intake of the calculated phenylalanine requirement. The child's increasing independence may also inhibit absolute control of what he or she eats. Either factor can result in decreased or increased phenylalanine levels. During the school years, peer pressure becomes a major force in deterring the child from eating the prescribed foods or abstaining from high-protein foods such as milkshakes and ice cream. Limitations of this diet are best illustrated by an example: a quarter-pound hamburger may provide a 2-day phenylalanine allowance for a school-age child.

The assistance of a registered dietitian is essential. Parents need a basic understanding of the disorder and practical suggestions regarding food selection and preparation.* Meal planning is based on weighing the food on a gram scale; a less accurate method is the exchange list. As soon as children are old enough, usually by early preschool, they should be involved in the daily calculation, menu planning, and formula preparation. Using a computer, voice-activated calculator, cards, or colored beads can help children keep track of the daily allowance of phenylalanine foods. A system of goal setting, self-monitoring, contracts, and rewards can promote compliance in adolescents.

Preparation of the phenylalanine-free formula can present some challenges. The formula tends to be lumpy; mixing the powder with a small amount of water to make a paste and then adding the rest of the required liquid, helps alleviate this problem. A blender or mixer dissolves the powder more easily; a rechargeable hand mixer can be used when traveling. Although the taste is virtually impossible to camouflage, many new products are on the market today. Some of the complete formulas are chocolate, vanilla, strawberry, and orange flavored. Incomplete formulas are also available that do not contain the vitamins and minerals and are plain tasting; these can be added to cold foods instead of mixing them as a formula. Formula bars are convenient for active adolescents. Formula capsules are also available, but the patient would need to take 20 or more capsules per day.

Family Support[†]

In addition to the problem related to a child with a chronic disorder (see Chapter 18), the parents have the burden of knowing that they are carriers of the defect. Genetic counseling is especially important to inform the parents that prenatal testing is now available to detect the presence of the defective gene in heterozygotes. Counseling is also important for adults with PKU to inform them that all of their offspring will be carriers for PKU (see Genetic Evaluation and Counseling, p. 301).

GALACTOSEMIA

Galactosemia is a rare autosomal recessive disorder that results from various gene mutations leading to three distinct enzymatic deficiencies. The most common type of galactosemia (classic galactosemia)

---

*A helpful resource is Schuett V, editor: *Low protein cookery for phenylketonuria*, ed 3, Madison, Wis, 1997, University of Wisconsin Press.
[†]National support groups include the Children's PKU Network, which offers a variety of support services; contact 3790 Via de la Valle, Suite 120, Del Mar, CA 92014; 800-377-6677; e-mail: PKUnetwork@aol.com; http://www.pkunetwork.org, and the National PKU Alliance, contact Christine Brown, Executive Director, PO Box 501, Tomahawk, WI 54487; 715-437-0477; http://www.npkua.org.

results from a deficiency of a hepatic enzyme, galactose 1-phosphate uridyltransferase (GALT), and affects approximately 1 in 50,000 births. The other two varieties of galactosemia involve deficiencies in the enzymes galactokinase (GALK) and galactose 4′-epimerase (GALE); these are extremely rare disorders. All three enzymes (GALT, GALK, and GALE) are involved in the conversion of galactose into glucose.

As galactose accumulates in the blood, several organs are affected. Hepatic dysfunction leads to cirrhosis, resulting in jaundice in the infant by the second week of life. The spleen subsequently becomes enlarged as a result of portal hypertension. Cataracts are usually recognizable by 1 or 2 months of age; cerebral damage, manifested by the symptoms of lethargy and hypotonia, is evident soon afterward. Infants with galactosemia appear normal at birth, but within a few days of ingesting milk (which has a high lactose content), they begin to experience vomiting and diarrhea, leading to weight loss. *E. coli* sepsis is also a common presenting clinical sign. Death during the first month of life is frequent in untreated infants. Occasionally classic galactosemia is seen with milder, chronic manifestations, such as growth failure, feeding difficulty, and developmental delay. This presentation is more frequent among African-American children with galactosemia (Kaye, Committee on Genetics, Accurso, and others, 2006).

Diagnostic Evaluation

Diagnosis is made on the basis of the infant's history, physical examination, galactosuria, increased levels of galactose in the blood, and decreased levels of GALT activity in erythrocytes. The infant may display characteristics of malnutrition; hypoglycemia, jaundice, hepatosplenomegaly, sepsis, cataracts, and decreased muscle tone (Bosch, 2006). Newborn screening for this disease is required in most states. Heterozygotes can also be identified because heterozygotic individuals have significantly lower levels of the essential enzyme.

Therapeutic Management

During infancy, treatment consists of eliminating all milk and lactose-containing formula, including breast milk. Traditionally, lactose-free formulas are used, with soy-protein formula being the feeding of choice; however, some research suggests that elemental formula (galactose-free) may be more beneficial than soy formulas (Zlatunich and Packman, 2005). However, the AAP recommends the use of soy protein–based formula for infants with galactosemia, and it is considerably less expensive than elemental formula (Bhatia, Greer, and Committee on Nutrition, 2008). As the infant progresses to solids, only foods low in galactose should be consumed. Certain fruits are high in galactose, and some dietitians recommend that they be avoided. Food lists should be given to the family to ensure that appropriate foods are chosen.

If galactosemia is suspected, supportive treatment and care are implemented, including monitoring for hypoglycemia, liver failure, bleeding disorders, and *E. coli* sepsis.

Prognosis

Follow-up studies of children treated from birth or within the first 2 months of life after symptoms appear have found long-term complications, such as hypogonadism, cognitive impairment, growth restriction, and verbal and motor delays (Bosch, 2006). These findings have revealed that eliminating sources of galactose does not significantly improve the outcome. New therapeutic strategies, such as enhancing residual transferase activity, replacing depleted metabolites, and using gene replacement therapy, are needed to improve the prognosis for these children.

NURSING CARE GUIDELINES
Common Indications for Referral

Previous child with multiple congenital anomalies; cognitive impairment; or an isolated birth defect, such as neural tube defect, cleft lip, or cleft palate

Family history of a hereditary condition, such as cystic fibrosis, fragile X syndrome, or diabetes

Prenatal diagnosis of advanced maternal age or other indication

Consanguinity

Teratogen exposure, such as to occupational chemicals, medications, or alcohol

Repeated pregnancy loss or infertility

Newly diagnosed abnormality or genetic condition

Before undertaking genetic testing and after receiving results, particularly when testing for susceptibility to late-onset disorders, such as cancer or neurologic disease

As follow-up for a positive newborn test, as with phenylketonuria, or a heterozygote screening test, such as Tay-Sachs disease

From Nussbaum R, McInnes R, Willard H: *Thompson and Thompson genetics in medicine,* ed 6, Philadelphia, 2007, Saunders/Elsevier.

Nursing Care Management*

Nursing interventions are similar to those for PKU except that dietary restrictions are easier to maintain because many more foods are allowed. However, reading food labels carefully for the presence of any form of lactose, especially dairy products, is mandatory. Many drugs, such as some of the penicillin preparations, contain lactose as filler and also must be avoided. Unfortunately, lactose is an unlabeled ingredient in many pharmaceuticals. Therefore, instruct parents to ask their local pharmacist about galactose content of any over-the-counter or prescription medication.

GENETIC EVALUATION AND COUNSELING

Genetic counseling is a communication process concerned with the human problems associated with the occurrence, or risk of occurrence, of a genetic disorder in a family. It involves relaying information about the diagnosis, treatment options, recurrence risk, and availability of prenatal diagnosis. With the completion of the Human Genome Project, the international project to determine the total genetic information in humans, a new era of human genetics is unfolding (International Human Genome Sequencing Consortium, 2004), and it will lead to a better understanding of specifically how genetic variation contributes to health and disease. It is essential that nurses master the basic principles of heredity, understand how heredity contributes to disorders, and be aware of the types of genetic testing available (Table 9-15).

Nurses frequently encounter children with genetic diseases and families in which there is a risk that a disorder may be transmitted to or occur in an offspring. It is a responsibility of nurses to be alert to situations in which persons could benefit from a genetic evaluation and counseling (see Nursing Care Guidelines box), to be aware of the local genetic resources, to aid families in finding services, and to offer

*Information and support for parents can be found at the American Liver Foundation, http://www.liverfoundation.org; and at Parents of Galactosemic Children, Inc., PO Box 2401, Mandeville, LA 74070-2401; 866-900-PGC1; http://www.galactosemia.org.

TABLE 9-15	TYPES OF GENETIC TESTING		
TEST AND METHOD	**SPECIMEN**	**INDICATION**	**COMMENTS**
Chromosome analysis (karyotyping)	Blood, skin, amniocytes, bone marrow	Detection of chromosomal abnormality, sex determination, cancer classification	Almost 100% accuracy for whole or partial chromosomal abnormality; will not detect microdeletions or duplication (submicroscopic chromosome segments), single-gene defects, or multifactorial disorders
Fluorescence in situ hybridization (FISH)	Blood, skin, amniocytes, bone marrow	Detection of microdeletion or duplications of chromosome segments (not visible by chromosome analysis)	A technique that is a cross between chromosome analysis and single-gene DNA tests
Direct DNA mutation detection (polymerase chain reaction, Southern blot, gene sequencing)	Blood, skin, amniocytes	Detection of gene mutation(s) in affected individual for diagnosis, in unaffected carrier, or for presymptomatic diagnosis	Gene location must be mapped, and disease-producing mutations must be characterized; can test single individual
Indirect DNA linkage studies (restriction length fragment polymorphisms, microsatellites, genetic markers)	Blood	Prediction of carrier or presymptomatic status based on inheritance of same chromosome segment as in known affected individual	Must test several family members, including one or two confirmed affected individuals, for testing to be valid
Biochemical	Blood, skin, amniotic fluid, muscle biopsy, urine, stool, cerebrospinal fluid	Detection of metabolic pathway errors, enzyme defects, prenatal neural tube or ventral wall defect	Results may be difficult to interpret if partial pathway error or modified substrate is present. Maternal serum α-fetoprotein levels screen for neural tube and ventral wall defects

DNA, Deoxyribonucleic acid.

support and care for children and families affected by genetic conditions. Local genetic clinics can be located through several sites; for example, GeneTests,* a publicly funded medical genetics information resource developed for physicians and other health care providers, is available at no cost to all interested persons. Another resource is the National Society of Genetic Counselors,† which lists genetic counselors by states in the United States.

Maintaining contact with the family or referring the family to an agency that can provide a sustained relationship, usually the public health agency in their locality, is one of the most important aspects in the care of the patient and family. In a disorder that requires conscientious diet management, such as PKU or galactosemia, it is important to make certain that the family understands and follows the advice. A vital role for nurses is to advocate for the child and family as they make their way through the various specialty clinics. This is especially important for families that are more vulnerable because of cognitive, hearing, language, or financial issues and those who otherwise may have difficulty accessing health services. Nurses can reinforce the genetic information or arrange for additional genetic counseling if a family has additional questions or misunderstandings.

One of the current ethical concerns is the testing of healthy children for carrier status of a genetic condition that either will not have adverse consequences until adulthood or only has reproductive implications. The AAP, Committee on Bioethics (2001, reaffirmed 2008) policy statement does not support the broad use of carrier testing or screening in children or adolescents. When there is no clear medical benefit to testing in childhood, the child should be permitted to wait until adulthood to choose whether or not to be tested. Genetic counseling is recommended to help the family weigh all of the issues.

PSYCHOLOGIC ASPECTS OF GENETIC DISEASE

The diagnosis of a genetic disorder in a child can be a life-altering experience for families. They may have to reassess their perception of "self" and the loss of the dream of the perfect infant. Parents may change educational, employment, and reproductive plans after the diagnosis of a genetic disorder in their child.

Families may need to have the genetic information repeated several times. Families may also encounter ethical or moral dilemmas regarding genetic evaluation and testing options, as well as potential involvement of other family members. Nurses are pivotal caregivers in assessing the family's understanding of the genetic disorder, psychologic responses, and coping mechanisms. Nurses may help families by providing support and attempting to alleviate possible feelings of guilt and by helping the family make the best possible adjustment to the disorder.

It is important to stress that there is nothing shameful about an inherited or congenital defect and to emphasize any appropriate remedy. The thought of a hereditary disorder often creates intrafamily strife, hostility, and marital disharmony, sometimes to the point of family disintegration. Relatives may change their reproductive plans after the diagnosis of a genetic disorder in a member, or the decision to reproduce may be postponed indefinitely on the basis of a disorder in a relative, even a remote one. Although people may understand the information on an intellectual level, they may still harbor fears on an emotional level. Nurses can help the family identify their personal strengths and offer them information about local and national support groups. (The Genetic Alliance‡ is a nonprofit organization that has a database of support groups for genetic conditions.) Finally, it is important to keep in mind that the infant or child has the same basic needs after the diagnosis of a genetic disorder as he or she had before the diagnosis.

*http://www.ncbi.nlm.nih.gov/sites/GeneTests.
†http://www.nsgc.org.

‡http://www.geneticalliance.org.

KEY POINTS

- Birth injuries are usually transient and may involve soft tissue, bone, or nervous tissue.
- High-risk neonates are newborn infants, regardless of gestational age or birth weight, who have a greater than average chance of morbidity or mortality because of conditions or circumstances associated with birth and adjustment to extrauterine life.
- Appropriate developmental care for preterm infants focuses on individualized neurobehavioral assessment, planning, diagnosis, intervention, and reevaluation to foster appropriate growth and maturation in a potentially harmful environment.
- Parents are encouraged to interact with their high-risk infant and gradually assume care of the infant as allowed by the infant's condition.
- Because of their immature physical status, preterm infants need special attention to promote respiratory efforts, maintain body temperature, maintain fluid and electrolyte balance, prevent infection, and provide adequate nutrition for growth.
- Late-preterm infants, by nature of their limited gestation, remain at risk for problems related to thermoregulation, hypoglycemia, hyperbilirubinemia, sepsis, and respiratory function.
- Jaundice is a common transient problem in newborns that results from RBC breakdown that exceeds the ability of the immature liver to metabolize and excrete.
- Preterm infants are subject to a number of complications, including apnea, sepsis, RDS, NEC, and intraventricular hemorrhage.
- Sepsis is a serious condition with generalized nonspecific manifestations that requires immediate intervention involving systemic antibiotics and observation for associated complications.
- Maternal conditions that may pose health risks in the neonatal period include maternal diabetes, perinatal infections, and substance abuse.
- Chromosomal disorders are caused by abnormalities in either chromosomal structure or number.
- Some of the most significant IEMs in the neonatal period include CH, PKU, and galactosemia. Specific population-based newborn screening for IEMs should take place when the incidence of other IEMs is prevalent. Severe cognitive delays can result if these conditions are undiagnosed and untreated.
- Genetic counseling is directed toward providing individuals and families with information needed to make decisions about a course of action appropriate to them.
- Although no cure for genetic disease is presently available, various therapeutic measures are used to modify the basic defect.

REFERENCES

Ackerman JP, Riggins T, Black MM: A review of the effects of prenatal cocaine exposure among school-aged children, *Pediatrics* 125(3):554–565, 2010.

Adamkin DH, American Academy of Pediatrics, Committee on Fetus and Newborn: Postnatal glucose homeostasis in late-preterm and term infants, *Pediatrics* 127(3):575–579, 2011.

Afsar FS: Skin care for preterm and term neonates, *Clin Exp Dermatology* 34(8):855–858, 2009.

Ahmed AH, Sands LP: Effects of pre- and post-discharge interventions on breastfeeding outcomes and weight gain among premature infants, *J Obstet Gynecol Neonatal Nurs* 39(1):53–63, 2010.

Albright BB, Rayburn WF: Substance abuse among reproductive age women, *Obstet Gynecol Clin* 36(4) 891–906, 2009.

Alfaleh K, Anabrees J, Bassler D, Al-Kharfi T: Probiotics for prevention of necrotizing enterocolitis in preterm infants, *Cochrane Database Syst Rev* 2011(3):CD005496, 2011.

Alster TS, Railan D: Laser treatment of vascular birthmarks, *J Craniofac Surg* 17(4):720–723, 2006.

Altimier L: The neonatal intensive care unit (NICU). In Kenner C, Lott J, editors: *Comprehensive neonatal care: an interdisciplinary approach*, ed 4, St. Louis, 2007, Saunders Elsevier.

American Academy of Pediatrics: Breastfeeding and the use of human milk, *Pediatrics* 115(2): 496–506, 2005.

American Academy of Pediatrics, Committee on Bioethics: Ethical issues with genetic testing in pediatrics, *Pediatrics* 107(6):1451–1455, 2001.

American Academy of Pediatrics, Committee on Fetus and Newborn: Surfactant-replacement therapy for respiratory distress in preterm and term neonates, *Pediatrics* 121(2):419–432, 2008.

American Academy of Pediatrics, Committee on Infectious Diseases, Pickering L, editor: *Red book: 2009 Report of the Committee on Infectious Diseases*, ed 27, Elk Grove, Ill, 2009, Author.

American Academy of Pediatrics, Subcommittee on Hyperbilirubinemia: Management of hyperbilirubinemia in the newborn infant 35 or more weeks of gestation (clinical practice guideline), *Pediatrics* 114(1):297–316, 2004.

American Academy of Pediatrics, Task Force on Sudden Infant Death Syndrome: The changing concept of sudden infant death syndrome: diagnostic coding shifts, controversies regarding the sleeping environment, and new variables to consider in reducing risk, *Pediatrics* 116(5):1245–1255, 2005.

American Academy of Pediatrics, American College of Obstetricians and Gynecologists: *Guidelines for perinatal care*, ed 6, Elk Grove Village, Ill, 2007, Author.

American Academy of Pediatrics, American Thyroid Association: Update of newborn screening and therapy for congenital hypothyroidism, *Pediatrics* 117(6):2290–2303, 2006.

Arnon S, Litmanovitz I: Diagnostic tests in neonatal sepsis, *Curr Opin Infect Dis* 21(3):223–227, 2008.

Askin DF, Bakewell-Sachs S, Medoff-Cooper B, and others: *Late preterm infant assessment guide*, Washington, DC, 2007, Association of Women's Health, Obstetric and Neonatal Nurses.

Azzopardi DV, Strohm B, Edwards D, and others: Moderate hypothermia to treat perinatal asphyxial encephalopathy, *N Engl J Med* 361(14):1349–1358, 2009.

Bagwell GA: Hematologic system. In Kenner C, Lott J, editors: *Comprehensive neonatal care: an interdisciplinary approach*, ed 4, St. Louis, 2007, Saunders Elsevier.

Banakar MK, Kudlur NS, George S: Fetal alcohol spectrum disorder (FASD), *Indian J Pediatr* 76(11):1173–1175, 2009.

Bandstra ES, Accornero VH: Infants of substance abusing mothers. In Martin RJ, Fanaroff AA, Walsh MC, editors: *Fanaroff and Martin's neonatal-perinatal medicine: diseases of the fetus and infant*, ed 9, St. Louis, 2011, Elsevier Mosby.

Bandstra ES, Morrow CE, Accornero VH, and others: Estimated effects of in utero cocaine exposure on language development through early adolescence, *Neurotoxicol Teratol* 33(1):25–35, 2011.

Bandstra ES, Morrow CE, Mansoor E, and others: Prenatal drug exposure: infant and toddler outcomes, *J Addict Dis* 29(2):245–258, 2010.

Barrington KJ, Finer NN: Inhaled nitric oxide for preterm infants: a systematic review, *Pediatrics* 120(5):1088–1099, 2007.

Bauer CR, Langer JC, Shankaran S, and others: Acute neonatal effects of cocaine exposure during pregnancy, *Arch Pediatr Adolesc Med* 159(9):824–834, 2005.

Beachy JM: Investigating jaundice in the newborn, *Neonatal Netw* 26(5):327–333, 2007.

Beauman SS, Swanson A: Neonatal infusion therapy: preventing complications and improving outcomes, *Newborn Infant Nurs Rev* 16(4):193–201, 2006.

Beyerlein A, Hadders-Algra M, Kennedy K, and others: Infant formula supplementation with long-chain polyunsaturated fatty acids has no effect on Bayley developmental scores at 18 months of age—IPD meta-analysis of 4 large clinical trials, *J Pediatr Gastroenterol Nutr* 50(1):79–84, 2010.

Bhatia J, Greer F, and Committee on Nutrition: Use of soy protein-based formulas in infant feeding, *Pediatrics* 121(5):1062–1068, 2008.

Bhutani VK, Johnson LH, Keren R: Diagnosis and management of hyperbilirubinemia in the term neonate: for a safer first week, *Pediatr Clin North Am* 51(4):843–861, 2004.

Bissinger RL, Annibale DJ: Thermoregulation in very low–birth-weight infants during the golden hour: results and implications. *Adv Neonatal Care* 10(5):230–238, 2010.

Black LV, Maheshwari A: Disorders of the fetomaternal unit: hematologic manifestations in the fetus and neonate, *Semin Perinatol* 33(1):12–19, 2009.

Blackburn ST: *Maternal, fetal, and neonatal physiology: a clinical perspective*, ed 4, Philadelphia, 2011, Saunders.

Blau N, van Spronsen FJ, Levy HL: Phenylketonuria. *Lancet* 376(9750):1417–1427, 2010.

Borghesi A, Stronati M: Strategies for the prevention of hospital-acquired infections in the neonatal intensive care unit, *J Hosp Infect* 68(4):293–300, 2008.

Bosch AM: Classical galactosaemia revisited, *J Inherit Metab Dis* 29(4):516–525, 2006.

Brethauer M, Carey L: Maternal experience with neonatal jaundice, *MCN Am J Matern Child Nurs* 35(1):8–14, 2010.

Brown VD, Landers S: Heat balance. In Gardner SL, Carter BS, Enzman-Hines M, and others, editors: *Merenstein and Gardner's handbook of neonatal intensive care*, ed 7, St. Louis, 2011, Mosby Elsevier.

Bull MJ, Engle WA, Committee on Injury, Violence and Poison Prevention and the Committee on Fetus and Newborn: Safe transportation of preterm and low birth weight infants at hospital discharge, *Pediatrics* 123(5):1424–1429, 2009.

Burgos AE, Burke BL: Neonatal abstinence syndrome, *NeoReviews* 10(5):e222–e228, 2009.

Byers JF, Waugh WR, Lowman LB: Sound level exposure of high-risk infants in different environmental conditions, *Neonatal Netw* 25(1):25–32, 2006.

Cantor Sackett J, Weller RA, Weller EB: Selective serotonin reuptake inhibitor use during pregnancy and possible neonatal complications, *Curr Psychiatry Rep* 11(3):253–257, 2009.

Carlo WA: Fetal alcohol syndrome: In Kliegman RM, Stanton BF, St. Geme JW, and others, editors: *Nelson textbook of pediatrics*, ed 19, Philadelphia, 2011, Saunders.

Centers for Disease Control and Prevention: Perinatal group B streptococcal disease after universal screening recommendations—United States, 2003–2005, *MMWR Morb Mortal Wkly Rep* 56(28):701–705, 2007.

Channon S, Goodman G, Zlotowitz S, and others: Effects of dietary management of phenylketonuria on long-term cognitive outcome, *Arch Dis Child* 92(3):213–218, 2007.

Chiriboga CA, Kuhn L, Wasserman GA: Prenatal cocaine exposures and dose-related cocaine

effects on infant tone and behavior, *Neurotoxicol Teratol* 29(3):323–330, 2007.

Chomchai C, Na Manorom N, Watanarungasan P, and others: Methamphetamine abuse during pregnancy and its impact on neonates born at Siriraj Hospital, Bangkok, Thailand, *Southeast Asian J Trop Med Public Health* 35(1):228–231, 2004.

Cifuentes J, Carlo W: Respiratory system. In Kenner C, Lott J, editors: *Comprehensive neonatal care: an interdisciplinary approach*, ed 4, St. Louis, 2007, Saunders Elsevier.

Cirgin Ellett ML, Cohen MD, Perkins SM, and others: Predicting the insertion length for gastric tube placement in neonates, *J Obstet Gynecol Neonatal Nurs* 40(4):412–421, 2011.

Conde-Agudelo A, Belizán JM, Diaz-Rossello J: Kangaroo mother care to reduce morbidity and mortality in low birthweight infants. *Cochrane Database of Systematic Reviews* 2011(3): CD002771, 2011.

Cong X, Ludington-Hoe SM, McCain G, and others: Kangaroo care modifies preterm infant heart rate variability in response to heel stick pain: pilot study, *Early Hum Dev* 85(9):561–567, 2009.

Cornblath M, Hawdon JM, Williams A, and others: Controversies regarding definition of neonatal hypoglycemia: suggested operational thresholds, *Pediatrics* 105(5):1141, 2000.

Dailey TL, Coustan DR: Diabetes in pregnancy, *NeoReviews* 11(11):e619–e625, 2010.

de Boer JC, Smit BJ, Mainous RO: Nasogastric tube position and intragastric air collection in a neonatal intensive care population, *Adv Neonatal Care* 9(6):293–298, 2009.

Deshpande S, Ward Platt M: The investigation and management of neonatal hypoglycaemia, *Semin Fetal Neonatal Med* 10(4):351–361, 2005.

Diehl-Jones WL, Fraser Askin D: Hematologic disorders. In Verklan MT, Walden M, editors: *Core curriculum for neonatal intensive care nursing*, ed 4, St. Louis, 2010, Saunders Elsevier.

Dodd VL: Implications of kangaroo care for growth and development in preterm infants, *J Obstet Gynecol Neonatal Nurs* 34(2):218–232, 2005.

Donn SM, Sinha SK: Aerosolized luniactant: a potential alternative to intratracheal surfactant replacement therapy, *Exp Opin Pharmacother* 9(3):475–478, 2008.

Donohue PK, Gilmore MM, Cristofalo E, and others: Inhaled nitric oxide in preterm infants: a systematic review, *Pediatrics* 127(2):e414–e422, 2011.

Dougherty D, Luther M: Birth to breast—a feeding care map for the NICU: Helping the extremely low birth weight infant navigate the course, *Neonat Netw* 27(6):371–377, 2008.

Doumouchtsis SK, Arulkumaran S: Head injuries after instrumental vaginal deliveries, *Curr Opin Obstet Gynecol* 18(2):129–134, 2006.

Downey LC, Smith PB, Benjamin DK Jr: Risk factors and prevention of late-onset sepsis in premature infants, *Early Hum Dev* 86(suppl 1):7–12, 2010.

Durbin DR, AAP, Committee on Injury, Violence, and Poison Prevention: Child passenger safety, *Pediatrics* 127(4):e1050–e1066, 2011.

Edwards AD, Brocklehurst P, Gunn AJ, and others: Neurological outcomes at 18 months of age after moderate hypothermia for perinatal hypoxic ischaemic encephalopathy: synthesis and meta-analysis of trial data, *BMJ* 340:c.363, 2010.

Elalfy MS, Elbarbary NS, Abaza HW: Early intravenous immunoglobulin (two-dose regimen) in the management of severe Rh hemolytic disease of newborn—a prospective randomized controlled trial, *Eur J Pediatr* 170(4):461–467, 2011.

Ellett ML, Croffie JM, Cohen MD, and others: Gastric tube placement in young children, *Clin Nurs Res* 14(3):238–252, 2005.

Engle WA, Tomashek KM, Wallman C, and others: Late-preterm infants: a population at risk, *Pediatrics* 120(6):1390–1401, 2007.

Escobar GJ, Clark RH, Greene JD: Short-term outcomes of infants born at 35 and 36 weeks gestation: we need to ask more questions, *Semin Perinatol* 30(1):28–33, 2006.

Eyler FD, Behnke M, Wobie K, and others: Relative ability of biologic specimens and interviews to detect prenatal cocaine use, *Neurotoxicol Teratol* 27(4):677–687, 2005.

Fanaroff AA: Obstetric management of prematurity. In Martin RJ, Fanaroff AA, Walsh MC, editors: *Fanaroff and Martin's neonatal-perinatal medicine: diseases of the fetus and infant*, ed 9, St. Louis, 2011, Elsevier/Mosby.

Farrington M, Lang S, Cullen L, and others: Nasogastric tube placement verification in pediatric and neonatal patients, *Pediatr Nurs* 35(1):17–24, 2009.

Finnegan LP: Neonatal abstinence. In Nelson N, editor: *Current therapy in neonatal perinatal medicine 1985–1986*, Toronto, 1985, Decker.

Finning K, Martin P, Daniels G: The use of maternal plasma for prenatal RhD blood group genotyping, *Methods Mol Biol* 496:143–157, 2009.

Gardella C, Brown Z: Prevention of neonatal herpes. *BJOG* 118:187–192, 2011.

Gardner DL, Shirland L: Evidence-based guideline for suctioning the intubated neonate and infant, *Neonatal Netw* 28(5):281–302, 2009.

Gardner SL, Carter BS, Enzman-Hines M, Hernandez JA, editors: *Merenstein and Gardner's handbook of neonatal intensive care*, ed 67, St. Louis, 2011, Mosby Elsevier.

Gardner SL, Dickey LA: Grief and perinatal loss. In Gardner SL, Carter BS, Enzman-Hines M, and others, editors: *Merenstein and Gardner's handbook of neonatal intensive care*, ed 67, St. Louis, 2011, Mosby Elsevier.

Gardner SL, Lawrence RA: Breast feeding the neonate with special needs. In Gardner SL, Carter BS, Enzman-Hines M, and others, editors: *Merenstein and Gardner's handbook of neonatal intensive care*, ed 67, St. Louis, 2011, Mosby Elsevier.

Gottstein R, Cooke RW: Systematic review of intravenous immunoglobulin in haemolytic disease of the newborn, *Arch Dis Child Fetal Neonatal Ed* 88(1):F6–10, 2003.

Griffin T: Family-centered care in the NICU, *J Perinat Neonatal Nurs* 20(1):98–102, 2006.

Guner YS, Chokshi N, Petrosyan M, and others: Necrotizing enterocolitis—bench to bedside:

novel and emerging strategies, *SeminPediatr Surg* 17(4):255–265, 2008.

Hale HB, Bae DS, Waters PM: Current concepts in the management of brachial plexus birth injury, *J Hand Surgery* 35(2):322–331, 2009.

Hay WW: Strategies for feeding the preterm infant, *Neonatology* 94(4):245–254, 2008.

Heron M, Hoyert DL, Murphy SL, and others: Deaths: final data for 2006, *National vital statistics reports* 57(14):1–134, 2009.

Hill A: Neurologic problems of the newborn. In Bradley WG, Daroff RB, Fenichel GM, and others, editors. *Neurology in clinical practice*, ed 5, Philadelphia, 2008, Butterworth Heinemann Elsevier.

Holland KE, Drolet BA: Infantile hemangioma. *Ped Clin North Am* 57(5):1069–1083, 2010.

Howard-Salsman KD: Car seat safety for high-risk infants, *Neonatal Netw* 25(2):117–129, 2006.

Hudic I, Fatusic Z, Sinanovic O, and others: Etiological risk factors for brachial plexus palsy, *J Matern Fetal Neonatal Med* 19(10):655–661, 2006.

Huether SE: The cellular environment: fluids and electrolytes, acids and bases. In McCance KL, Huether SE, Brashers VL, and others, editors, *Pathophysiology: the biologic basis for disease in adults and children*, ed 6, St. Louis, 2010, Mosby Elsevier.

Human Milk Banking Association: 2011 guidelines for the establishment and operation of a donor human milk bank, 2011, retrieved June 6, 2011, from http://www.hmbana.org.

International Human Genome Sequencing Consortium: Finishing the euchromatic sequence of the human genome, *Nature* 431:931–945, 2004.

Jacobs S, Hunt R, Tarnow-Mordi W, and others: Cooling for newborns with hypoxic ischaemic encephalopathy, *Cochrane Database Syst Rev* 2007(4):CD003311, 2007.

James SH, Kimberlin DW, Whitley RJ: Antiviral therapy for herpesvirus central nervous system infections: neonatal herpes simplex virus infection, herpes simplex encephalitis, and congenital cytomegalovirus infection, *Antiviral Res* 83(3):207–213, 2009.

Jansen JL: A bereavement model for the intensive care nursery, *Neonatal Netw* 22(3):17–23, 2003.

Johnson CB: Head, eyes, ears, nose, mouth and neck assessment. In Tappero EP, Honeyfield ME, editors: *Physical assessment of the newborn: a comprehensive approach to the art of physical assessment*, ed 4, Santa Rosa, Calif, 2009, NICU Ink.

Jones KL: *Smith's recognizable patterns of human malformation*, ed 4, Philadelphia, 2006, Saunders.

Joyner B, Soto MA, Adam HM: Brachial plexus injury, *Pediatr Rev* 27(6):238–239, 2006.

Kattwinkel JM, Perlman JM, Aziz K, and others: Part 15: neonatal resuscitation: 2010 American Heart Association guidelines for cardiopulmonary resuscitation and emergency cardiovascular care, *Circulation* 122(18 suppl):S909–S919, 2010.

Kaye CI, Committee on Genetics, Accurso F, and others: Newborn screening fact sheets, *Pediatrics* 118(3):e934–e963, 2006.

Kelly M: Kasabach-Merritt syndrome, *Pediatr Clin North Am* 57(5):1085–1089, 2010.

Kemper AR, Mahle WT, Martin GR, and others: Strategies for implementing screening for critical congenital heart disease, *Pediatrics* 128(5):e1259–e1267, 2011.

Kimberlin DW: Herpes simplex virus infections of the newborn, *Semin Perinatol* 31(1):19–25, 2007.

Kuczkowski KM. The effects of drug abuse on pregnancy, *Curr Opin Obstet Gynecol* 19(6):578–585, 2007.

Kuschel C: Managing drug withdrawal in the newborn infant, *Semin Fetal Neonatal Med* 212(2):127–133, 2007.

Laptook AR: Use of therapeutic hypothermia for term infants with hypoxic-ischemic encephalopathy, *Pediatr Clin North Am* 56(3):601–616, 2009.

Lawrence RA, Lawrence RM: *Breastfeeding: a guide for the medical profession*, ed 7, St. Louis, 2011, Mosby.

Lester BM, Lagasse LL. Children of addicted women, *J Addict Dis* 29(2):259–276, 2010.

Lester BM, Tronick EZ, Brazelton TB: The Neonatal Intensive Care Unit Network Neurobehavioral Scale procedures, *Pediatrics* 113(3 suppl):641–667, 2004.

Lewis DA, Sanders LP, Brockopp DY: The effect of three nursing interventions on thermoregulation in low birth weight infants, *Neonatal Netw* 30(3):160–164, 2011.

Liaw JJ, Yang L, Ti Y, and others: Non-nutritive sucking relieves pain for preterm infants during heel stick procedures in Taiwan, *J Clin Nurs* 19(19–20):2741–2751, 2010.

Lund CH, Kuller JM: Integumentary system. In Kenner C, Lott J, editors: *Comprehensive neonatal care: an interdisciplinary approach*, ed 4, St. Louis, 2007, Saunders Elsevier.

Mangurten HH, Puppala BL: Birth injuries. In Martin RJ, Fanaroff AA, Walsh MC, editors: *Fanaroff and Martin's neonatal-perinatal medicine: diseases of the fetus and infant*, ed 9, St. Louis, 2011, Elsevier Mosby.

Marcellus L: Care of substance-exposed infants: the current state of practice in Canadian hospitals, *J Perinat Neonatal Nurs* 16(3):51–68, 2002.

Mari G: Noninvasive diagnosis by Doppler ultrasonography of fetal anemia due to maternal red-cell isoimmunization, *N Engl J Med* 342(1):9–14, 2000.

Marroun HE, Hudziak JJ, Tiemeier H, and others: Intrauterine cannabis exposure leads to more aggressive behavior and attention problems in 18-month-old girls, *Drug Alcohol Depend* 118(2–3):470–474, 2001.

Mazela J, Merritt TA, Finer NN: Aerosolized surfactants, *Curr Opin Pediatr* 19(2):155–162, 2007.

McCain GC, Ludington-Hoe SM, Swinth JY, and others: Heart rate variability responses of a preterm infant to kangaroo care, *J Obstet Gynecol Neonatal Nurs* 34(6):689–694, 2005.

McCall EM, Alderdice FA, Halliday HL, and others: Interventions to prevent hypothermia at birth in preterm and/or low birthweight babies, *Cochrane Database Syst Rev* 2010(3):CD004210, 2010.

McCance K, Huether S: *Pathophysiology: the biological basis for disease in infants and children*, ed 6, St. Louis, 2010, Mosby Elsevier.

McCormick FM, Henderson G, Fahey T, and others: Multinutrient fortification of human breast milk for preterm infants following hospital discharge, *Cochrane Database Syst Rev* 2010(7):CD004866, 2010.

Mills JF, Tudehope D: Fibreoptic phototherapy for neonatal jaundice, *Cochrane Database Syst Rev* 2005(1):CD002060, 2005.

Mintz-Hittner HA, Best LM: Antivascular endothelial growth factor for retinopathy of prematurity, *Curr Opin Pediatr* 21(2):182–187, 2009.

Mitanchez D: Foetal and neonatal complications in gestational diabetes: perinatal mortality, congenital malformations, macrosomia, shoulder dystocia, birth injuries, neonatal complications, *Diabetes Metab* 36(6 Pt 2):617–627, 2010.

Moise KJ: Red cell alloimmunization. In Gabbe SG, Niebyl JR, Simpson KL, editors: *Obstetrics: normal and problem pregnancies*, ed 5, London, 2007, Churchill Livingstone.

Moise KJ: Fetal anemia due to non-Rhesus-D red-cell alloimmunization, *Semin Fetal Neonat Med* 13(4):207–214, 2008a.

Moise KJ Jr: Management of rhesus alloimmunization in pregnancy, *Obstet Gynecol* 112(1):164–176, 2008b.

Morelli JG: Diseases of the neonate. In Kleigman RM, Stanton BF, St. Geme JW, and others, editors: *Nelson textbook of pediatrics*, ed 19, Philadelphia, 2011, Saunders Elsevier.

Morrow CE, Culbertson JL, Accornero VH, and others: Learning disabilities and intellectual functioning in school-aged children with prenatal cocaine exposure, *Dev Neuropsychol* 30(3):905–931, 2006.

Mundy CA: Intravenous immunoglobulin in the management of hemolytic disease of the newborn, *Neonatal Netw* 24(6):17–24, 2005.

Neal JL: RhD isoimmunization and current management modalities, *J Obstet Gynecol Neonatal Nurs* 30(6):589–607, 2001.

Ng PC, Lam HS: Biomarkers for late-onset neonatal sepsis: cytokines and beyond, *Clin Perinatol* 37(3):599–610, 2010.

Nussbaum RL, McInnes RR, Willard HF: *Thompson and Thompson genetics in medicine*, ed 6 (rev reprint), Philadelphia, 2007, Saunders Elsevier.

Nye C: Transitioning premature infants from gavage to breast, *Neonatal Netw* 27(1):7–13, 2008.

Oberlander TF, Warburton W, Misri S, and others: Neonatal outcomes after prenatal exposure to selective serotonin reuptake inhibitor antidepressants and maternal depression using population-based linked health data, *Arch Gen Psychiatry* 63(8):898–906, 2006.

Ogata ES: Problems of the infant of a diabetic mother, *NeoReviews* 11(11):e627–e631, 2010.

Perinatal HIV Guidelines Working Group: Public Health Services Task Force recommendations for use of antiretroviral drugs in pregnant HIV-infected women for maternal health and interventions to reduce perinatal HIV transmission in the United States, September 2011, retrieved March 2, 2012, from http://aidsinfo.nih.gov/Guidelines/HTML/3/perinatal_guidelines/0/.

Pitts K: Perinatal substance abuse. In Verklan MT, Walden M, editors: *Core curriculum for neonatal intensive care nursing*, ed 4, St. Louis, 2010, Saunders Elsevier.

Premji SS, Paes B, Jacobson K, and others: Evidence-based feeding guideline for very low birthweight infants, *Adv Neonatal Care* 2(1):5–18, 2002.

Price AE, Ditaranto P, Yaylali I, and others: Botulinum toxin type A as an adjunct to the surgical treatment of the medial rotation deformity of the shoulder in birth injuries of the brachial plexus, *J Bone Joint Surg Br* 89(3):327–329, 2007.

Quandt D, Schraner T, Ulrich Bucher H, and others: Malposition of feeding tubes in neonates: is it an issue? *J Pediatr Gastroenterol Nutr* 48(5):608–611, 2009.

Reid J: Neonatal subgaleal hemorrhage, *Neonatal Network* 26(4):219–227, 2007.

Renner M: Far from reliable: pH testing in the neonatal intensive care unit, *J Pediatr Nurs* 25(6):580–583, 2010.

Reynolds RM, Thureen PJ: Special circumstances: trophic feeds, necrotizing enterocolitis and bronchopulmonary dysplasia, *Semin Fetal Neonatal Med* 12(1):64–70, 2007.

Sarici SU, Yurdakok M, Serdar MA, and others: An early (sixth-hour) serum bilirubin measurement is useful in predicting the development of significant hyperbilirubinemia and severe ABO hemolytic disease in a selective high-risk population of newborns with ABO incompatibility, *Pediatrics* 109(4):e53, 2002.

Saugstad OD: Optimal oxygenation at birth and in the neonatal period, *Neonatology* 91(4):319–322, 2007.

Saugstad OD, Ramji S, Irani SF, and others: Resuscitation of newborn infants with 21% or 100% oxygen: follow-up at 18 and 24 months, *Pediatrics* 112(2):296–300, 2003.

Schanler RJ, Shulman RJ, Lau C, and others: Feeding strategies for premature infants: randomized trial of gastrointestinal priming and tube-feeding method, *Pediatrics* 103(2):434–439, 1999.

Schempf AH: Illicit drug use and neonatal outcomes: a critical review, *Obstet Gynecol Surv* 62(11):749–757, 2007.

Schierholz E, Walker SR: Responding to traumatic birth: subgaleal hemorrhage, assessment and management during transport, *Adv Neonatal Care* 10(6):311–315, 2010.

Schuetze P, Eiden RD: The association between maternal cocaine use during pregnancy and physiological regulation in 4- to 8-week-old infants: an examination of possible mediators and moderators, *J Pediatr Psychol* 31(1):15–26, 2006.

Schurr P, Perkins EM: The relationship between feeding and necrotizing enterocolitis in very low birth weight infants, *Neonat Netw* 27(6):397–407, 2008.

Schutzman DL, Sekhon R, Hundalani S: Hour-specific bilirubin nomogram in infants with

ABO incompatibility and direct Coombs-positive results, *Arch Pediatr Adolesc Med* 164(12):1158–1164, 2010.

Selva KA, Harper A, Downs A, and others: Neurodevelopmental outcomes in congenital hypothyroidism: comparison of dose and time to reach target T4 and TSH, *J Pediatr* 147(6):775–780, 2005.

Sgro M, Shah PS, Campbell D, and others: Early-onset neonatal sepsis: rate and organism pattern between 2003 and 2008, *J Perinatol* 31(12):794–798, 2011.

Shet A: Congenital and perinatal infections: Throwing new light with an old TORCH. *Indian J Pediatr* 78(1):88–95, 2011.

Sidbury R: Update on vascular tumors of infancy, *Curr Opin Pediatr* 22(4):432–437, 2010.

Singer LT, Minnes S, Short E, and others: Cognitive outcomes of preschool children with prenatal cocaine exposure, *JAMA* 291(20):2448–2456, 2004.

Smith JR, Donze A, Schuller L: An evidence-based review of hyperbilirubinemia in the late preterm infant, with implications for practice: management, follow-up, and breastfeeding support, *Neonatal Netw* 26(6):395–405, 2007.

Smith L, Yonekura ML, Wallace T, and others: Effects of prenatal methamphetamine exposure on fetal growth and drug withdrawal symptoms in infants born at term, *J Dev Behav Pediatr* 24(1):17–23, 2003.

Soll R: Heat loss prevention in neonates, *J Perinatol* 28(suppl 1):S557–S559, 2008.

Sperling MA: Hypoglycemia. In Kliegman RM, Stanton BF, St. Geme JW, and others, editors: *Nelson textbook of pediatrics*, ed 19, Philadelphia, 2011, Saunders.

Stevens TP, Harrington EW, Blennow M, and others: Early surfactant administration with brief ventilation vs. selective surfactant and continued mechanical ventilation for preterm infants with or at risk for respiratory distress syndrome, *Cochrane Database Syst Rev* 2007(4):CD003063, 2007.

Stevens TP, Sinkin RA: Surfactant replacement therapy, *Chest* 131(5):1577–1582, 2007.

Stokowski LA: Fundamentals of phototherapy for neonatal jaundice, *Adv Neonat Care* 11(5S):S10–S21, 2011.

Stoll BJ: Infections of the neonatal infant. In Kliegman RM, Stanton BF, St. Geme JW, and others, editors: *Nelson textbook of pediatrics*, ed 19, Philadelphia, 2011, Saunders.

Stoll BJ, Hansen NI, Higgins RD, and others: Very low birth weight preterm infants with early onset neonatal sepsis: the predominance of gram-negative infections continues in the National Institute of Child Health and Human Development Neonatal Research Network, 2002–2003, *Pediatr Infect Dis J* 24(7):635–639, 2005.

Su CW, Gaskie S, Jamieson B: What is the best treatment for oral thrush in healthy infants? *J Family Pract* 57(7):484–485, 2008.

Symington A, Pinelli J: Developmental care for promoting development and preventing morbidity in preterm infants, *Cochrane Database Syst Rev* 2003(4):CD001814, 2003.

Tappero E: Musculoskeletal system assessment. In Tappero E, Honeyfield MA, editors: *Physical*

assessment of the newborn, ed 4, Santa Rosa, Calif, 2009, NICU Ink.

Terplan M, Smith EJ, Kozloski MJ, and others: Methamphetamine use among pregnant women, *Obstet Gynecol* 113(6):1285–1291, 2009.

Terrin G, Passariello A, Canani RB, and others: Minimal enteral feeding reduces the risk of sepsis in feed-intolerant very low birth weight newborns, *Acta Paediatr* 98(2):31–35, 2009.

Thayyil S, Marriott L: Can transcutaneous bilirubinometry reduce the need for serum bilirubin estimations in term and near term infants? *Arch Dis Child* 90(12):1311–1312, 2005.

Tomashek KM, Shapiro-Mendoza CK, Davidoff MJ, and others: Differences in mortality between late-preterm and term singleton infants in the United States, 1995–2002, *J Pediatr* 151(5):450–456, 2007.

Urbaniak SJ: Noninvasive approaches to the management of RhD hemolytic disease of the fetus and newborn, *Transfusion* 48(1):12–19, 2008.

Vento M, Saugstad OD: Oxygen therapy. In Martin RJ, Fanaroff AA, Walsh MC, editors: *Fanaroff and Martin's neonatal-perinatal medicine: diseases of the fetus and infant*, ed 9, St. Louis, 2011, Elsevier Mosby.

Verklan MT, Lopez SM: Neurologic disorders. In Gardner SL, Carter BS, Enzman-Hines M, and others, editors: *Merenstein and Gardner's handbook of neonatal intensive care*, ed 67, St. Louis, 2011, Mosby Elsevier.

Volpe JJ: *Neurology of the newborn*, ed 5, Philadelphia, 2008, Saunders Elsevier.

Warren JB, Anderson JM: Core concepts: respiratory distress syndrome, *NeoReviews* 10(7):e351–e361, 2009.

Watchko JF: Identification of neonates at risk for hazardous hyperbilirubinemia: emerging clinical insights, *Pediatr Clin North Am* 56(3):671–687, 2009.

Watchko JF, Maisels MJ: Enduring controversies in the management of hyperbilirubinemia in preterm neonates, *Semin Fetal Neonat Med* 15(3):136–140, 2010.

Watson R: Hyperbilirubinemia, *Crit Care Nursing Clinics North Am* 21(1):97–120, 2009.

Westrup B, Sizun J, Lagercrantz H: Family-centered developmental supportive care: a holistic and humane approach to reduce stress and pain in neonates, *J Perinatol* 27(suppl 1):S12–S18, 2007.

Wilcken B: Expanded newborn screening: reducing harm, assessing benefit, *J Inherit Metab Dis* 33(suppl 2):S205–S210, 2010.

Wilson KL, Zelig CM, Harvey JP, and others: Persistent pulmonary hypertension of the newborn is associated with mode of delivery and not with maternal use of selective serotonin reuptake inhibitors, *Am J Perinatol* 28(1):19–24, 2011.

Winecker RE, Goldberger BA, Tebbett IR, and others: Detection of cocaine and its metabolites in breast milk, *J Forensic Sci* 46(5):1221–1223, 2001.

Witt C: Skin assessment. In Tappero EP, Honeyfield ME, editors: *Physical assessment of the newborn*, ed 4, Petaluma, Calif, 2009, NICU Ink.

Woythaler MA, McCormick MC, Smith VC: Late preterm infants have worse 24-month neurodevelopmental outcomes than term infants, *Pediatrics* 127(3):e622–e629, 2011.

Wynshaw-Boris A, Biesecker LG: Dysmorphology. In Kliegman RM, Behrman RE, Jenson HB, and others, editors: *Nelson textbook of pediatrics*, ed 18, Philadelphia, 2007, Saunders.

Zahorodny W, Rom C, Whitney W, and others: The neonatal withdrawal inventory: a simplified score of newborn withdrawal, *Dev Behav Pediatr* 19(2):89–93, 1998.

Zaichkin J: *Newborn intensive care: what every parent needs to know*, ed 3, Elk Grove, Ill, 2010, American Academy of Pediatrics.

Zlatunich CO, Packman S: Galactosaemia: early treatment with an elemental formula, *J Inherit Metab Dis* 28:163–168, 2005.

Health Promotion of the Infant and Family

David Wilson

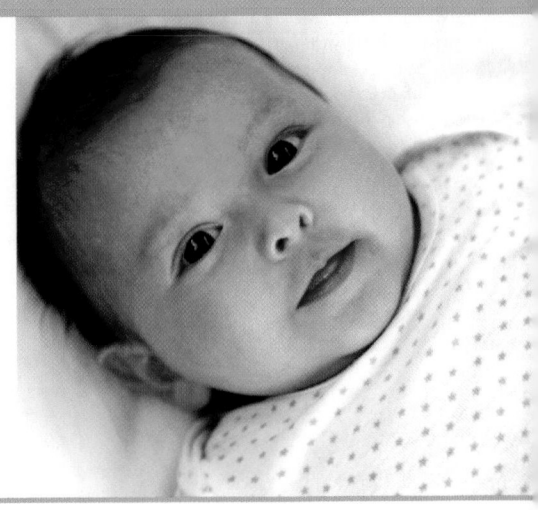

CHAPTER OUTLINE

Promoting Optimal Growth and
   Development, 309
   Biologic Development, 309
      Proportional Changes, 309
      Maturation of Systems, 309
      Fine Motor Development, 315
      Gross Motor Development, 315
   Psychosocial Development: Developing a
      Sense of Trust (Erikson), 318
   Cognitive Development: Sensorimotor
      Phase (Piaget), 319
   Development of Body Image, 320
   Social Development, 320
      Attachment, 320
      Language Development, 321
      Play, 322
   Temperament, 322
      *Childrearing Practices Related to
         Temperament, 323*

Coping with Concerns Related to
   Normal Growth and Development, 323
      Separation and Stranger Fear, 323
      *Alternate Child Care
         Arrangements, 323*
      Limit Setting and Discipline, 324
      *Thumb Sucking and Use of a
         Pacifier, 324*
      Teething, 325
Promoting Optimal Health during
   Infancy, 326
   Nutrition, 326
      The First 6 Months, 326
      The Second 6 Months, 328
      *Selection and Preparation of Solid
         Foods, 328*
      Introduction of Solid Foods, 329
      Weaning, 329
   Sleep and Activity, 330

Dental Health, 330
Immunizations, 330
   Schedule for Immunizations, 330
   *Recommendations for Routine
      Immunizations, 331*
   *Recommendations for Selected
      Immunizations, 339*
   Reactions, 339
   *Contraindications and
      Precautions, 340*
   Administration, 341
Safety Promotion and Injury
   Prevention, 344
      Motor Vehicle Injuries, 344
      Nurse's Role in Injury Prevention, 348
Anticipatory Guidance—Care of
   Families, 350

LEARNING OBJECTIVES

On completion of this chapter the reader will be able to:
- Identify the major biologic, psychosocial, cognitive, and social developments during the first year of life.
- Relate parent–child attachment, separation anxiety, and stranger fear to developmental achievements during infancy.
- Provide anticipatory guidance to parents regarding common parental concerns during infancy.

- Provide parents with feeding recommendations for infants.
- Outline immunization requirements during infancy.
- List general contraindications, precautions, and administration routes for childhood immunizations.
- Provide anticipatory guidance to parents regarding injury prevention based on the infant's developmental achievement.

PROMOTING OPTIMAL GROWTH AND DEVELOPMENT

BIOLOGIC DEVELOPMENT

At no other time in life are physical changes and developmental achievements as dramatic as during infancy. All major body systems undergo progressive maturation, and there is concurrent development of skills that increasingly allow infants to respond to and cope with the environment. Acquisition of these fine and gross motor skills occurs in an orderly head-to-toe and center-to-periphery (cephalocaudal-proximodistal) sequence.

Proportional Changes

During the first year of life, especially the initial 6 months, growth is very rapid. Infants gain 150 to 210 g (≈5–7 oz) weekly until approximately age 5 to 6 months, when the birth weight has at least doubled. An average weight for a 6-month-old child is 7.3 kg (16 pounds). Weight gain slows during the second 6 months. By 1 year of age, the infant's birth weight has tripled, for an average weight of 9.75 kg (21.5 pounds). Infants who are breastfed beyond 4 to 6 months of age typically gain less weight than those who are bottle fed, yet their head circumference is more than adequate. There is evidence that breastfed infants tend to self-regulate energy intake. This self-regulation of intake with breastfeeding (vs. formula [bottle] feeding) is believed to have further significance in the development of childhood obesity and subsequent cardiovascular disease (Grummer-Strawn, Mei, and Centers for Disease Control and Prevention [CDC], 2004; Schack-Nielsen and Michaelsen, 2006). Researchers also found that infants who were bottle fed in early infancy were more likely to empty the bottle or cup of milk in late infancy than infants who were breast fed (Li, Fein, and Grummer-Strawn, 2010).

Height increases by 2.5 cm (1 inch) a month during the first 6 months of life and also slows during the second 6 months. Increases in length occur in sudden spurts, rather than in a slow, gradual pattern. Average height is 65 cm (25.5 inches) at 6 months and 74 cm (29 inches) at 12 months. By 1 year of age, the birth length has increased by almost 50%. This increase occurs mainly in the trunk rather than in the legs and contributes to the characteristic physique of the infant.

Head growth is also rapid. During the first 6 months, head circumference increases approximately 1.5 cm (0.6 inch) per month, but the rate of growth declines to only 0.5 cm (0.2 inch) monthly during the second 6 months. The average size is 43 cm (17 inches) at 6 months and 46 cm (18 inches) at 12 months. By 1 year, head size has increased by almost 33%. Closure of the cranial sutures occurs, with the posterior fontanel fusing by 6 to 8 weeks of age and the anterior fontanel closing by 12 to 18 months of age (average, 14 months).

Expanding head size reflects the growth and differentiation of the nervous system. By the end of the first year, the brain has increased in weight about 2.5 times. Maturation of the brain is exhibited in the dramatic developmental achievements of infancy (Table 10-1). Primitive reflexes are replaced by voluntary, purposeful movement, and new reflexes that influence motor development appear.

The chest assumes a more adult contour, with the lateral diameter becoming larger than the anteroposterior diameter. The chest circumference approximately equals the head circumference by the end of the first year. The heart grows less rapidly than does the rest of the body. Its weight is usually doubled by 1 year of age in comparison with body weight, which triples during the same period. The size of the heart is still large in relation to the chest cavity; its width is approximately 55% of the chest width.

It is important to note that genetic, metabolic, environmental, and nutritional factors strongly influence infant growth; thus, the previous statements are general guidelines only. Use the appropriate infant growth charts reflecting weight for length and head circumference in each case to determine appropriate growth parameters. The World Health Organization growth charts released in 2006 are now recommended as reference growth charts in children 0 to 59 months of age (Grummer-Strawn, Reinold, Krebs, and others, 2010). (See World Health Organization [WHO] growth charts in Appendix A).

Maturation of Systems

Other organ systems also change and grow during infancy. The respiratory rate slows somewhat (see inside back cover) and is relatively stable. Respiratory movements continue to be abdominal. Several factors predispose infants to more severe and acute respiratory problems than older children. The close proximity of the trachea to the bronchi and its branching structures rapidly transmits infectious agents from one anatomic location to another. The short, straight eustachian tube closely communicates with the ear, allowing infection to ascend from the pharynx to the middle ear. In addition, the inability of the immune system to produce immunoglobulin A (IgA) in the mucosal lining provides less protection against infection in infancy than during later childhood.

The heart rate slows (see inside back cover), and the rhythm is often sinus arrhythmia (rate increases with inspiration and decreases with expiration). Blood pressure also changes during infancy (see Appendix E). Systolic pressure rises during the first 2 months as a result of the increasing ability of the left ventricle to pump blood into the systemic circulation. Diastolic pressure decreases during the first 3 months and then gradually rises to values close to those at birth. Fluctuations in blood pressure occur during varying states of activity and emotion.

Significant hematopoietic changes occur during the first year of life (see Appendix B). Fetal hemoglobin (HgbF) is present for the first 5 months, with adult hemoglobin steadily increasing through the first half of infancy. Fetal hemoglobin results in a shortened survival of red blood cells (RBCs) and thus a decreased number of RBCs. A common result at 2 to 3 months of age is physiologic anemia. High levels of fetal hemoglobin are thought to depress the production of erythropoietin, a hormone released by the kidneys that stimulates RBC production.

Maternally derived iron stores are present for the first 5 to 6 months of life and gradually diminish, which also accounts for lowered hemoglobin levels toward the end of the first 6 months. The occurrence of physiologic anemia is not affected by an adequate supply of iron. However, when erythropoiesis is stimulated, iron supplies are necessary for the formation of hemoglobin.

The digestive processes are relatively immature at birth. Although term newborn infants have some limitations in digestive function, human milk has properties that partially compensate for decreased digestive enzymatic activity, thus enabling breastfed infants to receive optimal nutrition during the first several months of life. Saliva is secreted in small amounts, but the majority of the digestive processes do not begin functioning until age 3 months, when drooling is common because of the poorly coordinated swallowing reflex. The enzyme amylase (also called ptyalin) is present in small amounts but usually has little effect on the foodstuffs because of the small amount of time the food stays in the mouth. Gastric digestion in the stomach consists primarily of the action of hydrochloric acid and rennin, an enzyme that acts specifically on the casein in milk to cause the

Text continued on p. 314

TABLE 10-1	GROWTH AND DEVELOPMENT DURING INFANCY				
PHYSICAL	**GROSS MOTOR**	**FINE MOTOR**	**SENSORY**	**VOCALIZATION**	**SOCIALIZATION AND COGNITION**
Age 1 Month Weight gain of 150–210 g (5–7 oz) weekly for first 6 months Height gain of 2.5 cm (1 inch) monthly for first 6 months Head circumference increases by 1.5 cm (0.5 inch) monthly for first 6 months Primitive reflexes present and strong Doll's eye reflex and dance reflex fading Obligatory nose breathing (most infants)	■ Assumes flexed position with pelvis high but knees not under abdomen when prone (at birth, knees flexed under abdomen) ■ Can turn head from side to side when prone; lifts head momentarily from bed (see Fig. 10-3, *A*) Has marked head lag, especially when pulled from lying to sitting position (see Fig. 10-2, *A*) Holds head momentarily parallel and in midline when suspended in prone position Assumes asymmetric tonic neck flex position when supine When held in standing position, body is limp at knees and hips In sitting position, back is uniformly rounded, with absence of head control	Hands predominantly closed Grasp reflex strong Hand clenches on contact with rattle	■ Able to fixate on moving object in range of 45 degrees when held at a distance of 20–25 cm (8–10 inches) Visual acuity approaches 20/100* Follows light to midline Quiets when hears a voice	Cries to express displeasure Makes small, throaty sounds Makes comfort sounds during feeding	Is in sensorimotor phase—stage I, use of reflexes (birth–1 month), and stage II, primary circular reactions (1–4 months) Watches parent's face intently as she or he talks to infant
Age 2 Months Posterior fontanel closed Crawling reflex disappears	■ Assumes less flexed position when prone—hips flat, legs extended, arms flexed, head to side Less head lag when pulled to sitting position (see Fig. 10-2, *B*) Can maintain head in same plane as rest of body when held in ventral suspension When prone, can lift head almost 45 degrees off table When moved to sitting position, head is held up but bends forward (see Fig. 10-5, *B*) Assumes symmetric tonic neck position intermittently	Hands often open Grasp reflex fading	Binocular fixation and convergence to near objects beginning When supine, follows dangling toy from side to point beyond midline Visually searches to locate sounds Turns head to side when sound is made at level of ear	■ Vocalizes, distinct from crying Crying becomes differentiated Coos Vocalizes to familiar voice	■ Demonstrates social smile in response to various stimuli
Age 3 Months Primitive reflexes fading	Able to hold head more erect when sitting but still bobs forward Has only slight head lag when pulled to sitting position Assumes symmetric body positioning Able to raise head and shoulders from prone position to a 45- to 90-degree angle from table; bears weight on forearms When held in standing position, able to bear slight fraction of weight on legs Regards own hand	■ Actively holds rattle but will not reach for it Grasp reflex absent Hands kept loosely open Clutches own hand; pulls at blankets and clothes	■ Follows objects to periphery (180 degrees) ■ Locates sound by turning head to side and looking in same direction Begins to have ability to coordinate stimuli from various sense organs	■ Squeals aloud to show pleasure Coos, babbles, chuckles Vocalizes when smiling "Talks" a great deal when spoken to Less crying during periods of wakefulness	Displays considerable interest in surroundings Ceases crying when parent enters room Can recognize familiar faces and objects, such as feeding bottle Shows awareness of strange situations

TABLE 10-1	GROWTH AND DEVELOPMENT DURING INFANCY—cont'd				
PHYSICAL	**GROSS MOTOR**	**FINE MOTOR**	**SENSORY**	**VOCALIZATION**	**SOCIALIZATION AND COGNITION**
Age 4 Months Drooling begins Moro, tonic neck, and rooting reflexes have disappeared	■ Has almost no head lag when pulled to sitting position (see Fig. 10-2, *C*) ■ Balances head well in sitting position (see Fig. 10-5, *C*) Back less rounded, curved only in lumbar area Able to sit erect if propped up Able to raise head and chest off surface to angle of 90 degrees (see Fig. 10-3, *B*) Assumes predominant symmetric position ■ Rolls from back to side	■ Inspects and plays with hands; pulls clothing or blanket over face in play Tries to reach objects with hand but overshoots Grasps object with both hands Plays with rattle placed in hand and shakes it but cannot pick it up if dropped Can carry objects to mouth	Able to accommodate to near objects Binocular vision fairly well established Can focus on a 1.25-cm (0.5-inch) block Beginning eye–hand coordination	Makes consonant sounds *n, k, g, p, b* ■ Laughs aloud Vocalization changes according to mood	Is in stage III, secondary circular reactions Demands attention by fussing; becomes bored if left alone Enjoys social interaction with people Anticipates feeding when sees bottle or mother if breastfeeding Shows excitement with whole body, squeals, breathes heavily Shows interest in strange stimuli Begins to show memory
Age 5 Months Beginning signs of tooth eruption Birth weight doubles	No head lag when pulled to sitting position When sitting, able to hold head erect and steady Able to sit for longer periods when back is well supported Back straight When prone, assumes symmetric positioning with arms extended ■ Can turn over from abdomen to back When supine, puts feet to mouth	■ Able to grasp objects voluntarily Uses palmar grasp, bidextrous approach Plays with toes Takes objects directly to mouth Holds one cube while regarding a second one	Visually pursues a dropped object Is able to sustain visual inspection of an object Can localize sounds made below ear	Squeals Makes cooing vowel sounds interspersed with consonant sounds (e.g., *ah-goo*)	Smiles at mirror image Pats bottle or breast with both hands More enthusiastically playful but may have rapid mood swings Is able to discriminate strangers from family Vocalizes displeasure when object is taken away Discovers parts of body
Age 6 Months Growth rate may begin to decline Weight gain of 90–150 g (3–5 oz) weekly for next 6 months Height gain of 1.25 cm (0.5 inch) monthly for next 6 months ■ Teething may begin with eruption of two lower central incisors ■ Chewing and biting occur	When prone, can lift chest and upper abdomen off surface, bearing weight on hands (see Fig. 10-3, *C*) When about to be pulled to a sitting position, lifts head Sits in high chair with back straight Rolls from back to abdomen When held in standing position, bears almost all of weight Hand regard absent	Resecures a dropped object Drops one cube when another is given Grasps and manipulates small objects Holds bottle Grasps feet and pulls to mouth	Adjusts posture to see an object Prefers more complex visual stimuli Can localize sounds made above ear Will turn head to the side and then look up or down	■ Begins to imitate sounds ■ Babbling resembles one-syllable utterances—*ma, mu, da, di, hi* Vocalizes to toys, mirror image Takes pleasure in hearing own sounds (self-reinforcement)	Recognizes parents; begins to fear strangers Holds arms out to be picked up Has definite likes and dislikes Begins to imitate (cough, protrusion of tongue) Excites on hearing footsteps ■ Briefly searches for a dropped object (object permanence beginning) Frequent mood swings, from crying to laughing, with little or no provocation

Continued

TABLE 10-1   GROWTH AND DEVELOPMENT DURING INFANCY—cont'd

PHYSICAL	GROSS MOTOR	FINE MOTOR	SENSORY	VOCALIZATION	SOCIALIZATION AND COGNITION
Age 7 Months					
Eruption of upper central incisors	When supine, spontaneously lifts head off surface ■ Sits, leaning forward on both hands (see Fig. 10-5, *D*) When prone, bears weight on one hand Sits erect momentarily Bears full weight on feet (see Fig. 10-6, *A*) When held in standing position, bounces actively	■ Transfers objects from one hand to the other (see Fig. 10-5, *E*) Has unidextrous approach and grasp Holds two cubes more than momentarily Bangs cubes on table Rakes at a small object	■ Can fixate on very small objects Responds to own name Localizes sound by turning head in a curving arch Beginning awareness of depth and space Has taste preferences	■ Produces vowel sounds and chained syllables—*baba, dada, kaka* Vocalizes four distinct vowel sounds "Talks" when others are talking	■ Increasing fear of strangers; shows signs of fretfulness when parent disappears Imitates simple acts and noises Tries to attract attention by coughing or snorting Plays peek-a-boo Demonstrates dislike of food by keeping lips closed Exhibits oral aggressiveness in biting and mouthing Demonstrates expectation in response to repetition of stimuli
Age 8 Months					
Begins to show regular patterns in bladder and bowel elimination Parachute reflex appears (see Fig. 10-4)	■ Sits steadily unsupported (see Fig. 10-5, *E*) Readily bears weight on legs when supported; may stand holding onto furniture Adjusts posture to reach an object	Has beginning pincer grasp using index, fourth, and fifth fingers against lower part of thumb Releases objects at will Rings bell purposely Retains two cubes while regarding third cube Secures an object by pulling on a string Reaches persistently for toys out of reach		Makes consonant sounds *t, d, w* Listens selectively to familiar words Utterances signal emphasis and emotion Combines syllables, such as *dada*, but does not ascribe meaning to them	Increasing anxiety over loss of parent, particularly mother, and fear of strangers Responds to word "no" Dislikes dressing, diaper change
Age 9 Months					
Eruption of upper lateral incisor may begin	Creeps on hands and knees Sits steadily on floor for prolonged time (10 minutes) Recovers balance when leaning forward but cannot do so when leaning sideways ■ Pulls self to standing position and stands holding on to furniture (see Fig. 10-6, *B* and *C*)	■ Uses thumb and index finger in crude pincer grasp (see Fig. 10-1) Preference for use of dominant hand now evident Grasps third cube Compares two cubes by bringing them together	Localizes sounds by turning head diagonally and directly toward sound Depth perception increasing	Responds to simple verbal commands Comprehends "no-no"	Parent (mother) is increasingly important for own sake Shows increasing interest in pleasing parent Begins to show fears of going to bed and being left alone Puts arms in front of face to avoid having it washed

TABLE 10-1	GROWTH AND DEVELOPMENT DURING INFANCY—cont'd				
PHYSICAL	**GROSS MOTOR**	**FINE MOTOR**	**SENSORY**	**VOCALIZATION**	**SOCIALIZATION AND COGNITION**
Age 10 Months					
Labyrinth-righting reflex is strongest when infant is in prone or supine position; is able to raise head	Can change from prone to sitting position Stands while holding on to furniture; sits by falling down Recovers balance easily while sitting While standing, lifts one foot to take a step (see Fig. 10-6, *D*)	Crude release of an object beginning Grasps bell by handle		■ Says "dada," "mama" with meaning Comprehends "bye-bye" May say one word (e.g., "hi," "bye," "no")	Inhibits behavior to verbal command of "no-no" or own name Imitates facial expressions; waves bye-bye Extends toy to another person but will not release it ■ Develops object permanence Repeats actions that attract attention and cause laughter Pulls clothes of another to attract attention Plays interactive games such as pat-a-cake Reacts to adult anger; cries when scolded Demonstrates independence in dressing, feeding, locomotive skills, and testing of parents Looks at and follows picture in a book
Age 11 Months					
Eruption of lower lateral incisor may begin	When sitting, pivots to reach toward back to pick up an object ■ Cruises or walks holding on to furniture or with both hands held	Explores objects more thoroughly (e.g., clapper inside bell) Has neat pincer grasp Drops object deliberately for it to be picked up Puts one object after another into a container (sequential play) Able to manipulate an object to remove it from tight-fitting enclosure		Imitates definite speech sounds	Experiences joy and satisfaction when a task is mastered Reacts to restrictions with frustration Rolls ball to another on request Anticipates body gestures when a familiar nursery rhyme or story is being told (e.g., holds toes and feet in response to "This little piggy went to market") Plays games up-down, "so big," or peek-a-boo Shakes head for "no"

Continued

TABLE 10-1	GROWTH AND DEVELOPMENT DURING INFANCY—cont'd				
PHYSICAL	**GROSS MOTOR**	**FINE MOTOR**	**SENSORY**	**VOCALIZATION**	**SOCIALIZATION AND COGNITION**
Age 12 Months ■ Birth weight tripled ■ Birth length increased by 50% Head and chest circumference equal (head circumference 46 cm [18 inches]) Has six to eight deciduous teeth Anterior fontanel almost closed Landau reflex fading Babinski reflex disappears Lumbar curve develops; lordosis evident during walking	■ Walks with one hand held Cruises well ■ May attempt to stand alone momentarily; may attempt first step alone Can sit down from standing position without help	Releases cube in cup Attempts to build two-block tower but fails Tries to insert a pellet into a narrow-necked bottle but fails Can turn pages in a book, many at a time	Discriminates simple geometric forms (e.g., circle) Amblyopia may develop with lack of binocularity Can follow rapidly moving object Controls and adjusts response to sound; listens for sound to recur	■ Says three to five words besides "dada," "mama" Comprehends meaning of several words (comprehension always precedes verbalization) Recognizes objects by name Imitates animal sounds Understands simple verbal commands (e.g., "Give it to me," "Show me your eyes")	Shows emotions such as jealousy, affection (may hug or kiss on request), anger, fear Enjoys familiar surroundings and explores away from parent Is fearful in strange situation; clings to parent May develop habit of "security blanket" or favorite toy Has increasing determination to practice locomotor skills ■ Searches for an object even if it has not been hidden but searches only where object was last seen

■Milestones that represent essential integrative aspects of development that lay the foundation for the achievement of more advanced skills.
*Degree of visual acuity varies according to vision measurement procedure used.

formation of curds—coagulated semisolid particles of milk. The curds cause the milk to be retained in the stomach long enough for digestion to occur.

Digestion also takes place in the duodenum, where pancreatic enzymes and bile begin to break down protein and fat. Secretion of the pancreatic enzyme amylase, which is needed for digestion of complex carbohydrates, is deficient until about the fourth to sixth month of life. Lipase is also limited, and infants do not achieve adult levels of fat absorption until 4 to 5 months of age. Trypsin is secreted in sufficient quantities to catabolize protein into polypeptides and some amino acids.

The immaturity of the digestive processes is evident in the appearance of stools. During infancy, solid foods (e.g., peas, carrots, corn, raisins) are passed incompletely broken down in the feces. An excess quantity of fiber easily disposes infants to loose, bulky stools.

During infancy, the stomach enlarges to accommodate a greater volume of food. By the end of the first year, infants are able to tolerate three meals a day and an evening bottle and may have one or two bowel movements daily. However, with any type of gastric irritation, infants are vulnerable to diarrhea, vomiting, and dehydration (see Chapter 24).

The liver is the most immature of all the gastrointestinal organs throughout infancy. The ability to conjugate bilirubin and secrete bile is achieved after the first couple of weeks of life. However, the capacities for gluconeogenesis, formation of plasma protein and ketones, storage of vitamins, and deaminization of amino acids remain relatively immature for the first year of life.

Maturation of the suckling, sucking, and swallowing reflexes and the eruption of teeth (see Teething, p. 325) parallel the changes in the gastrointestinal tract and prepare infants for the introduction of solid foods.

The immunologic system undergoes numerous changes during the first year. Full-term newborns receive significant amounts of maternal immunoglobulin G (IgG), which, for approximately 3 months, confers immunity against antigens to which their mothers were exposed. During this time, infants begin to synthesize IgG; approximately 40% of adult levels are reached by 1 year of age. Significant amounts of immunoglobulin M (IgM) are produced at birth, and adult levels are reached by 9 months of age. Secretory IgA is not present at birth but is found in saliva and tears by 2 to 5 weeks. Prebiotic oligosaccharides found in breast milk produce probiotic bacteria such as bifidobacteria and lactobacilli, which in turn stimulate synthesis and secretion of sIgA. Secretory IgA is present in large amounts in colostrum; IgA confers protection to the mucous membranes of the gastrointestinal tract (Blackburn, 2011; Lawrence and Lawrence, 2011) against many bacteria, such as *Escherichia coli*, and viruses such as rubella, poliovirus, and the enteroviruses. The development of the mucosa-associated lymphoid tissue occurs during infancy; in part, this system is believed to prevent colonization and passage of bacteria across the infant's mucosal barrier (Lawrence and Lawrence, 2011). The function and quantity of T lymphocytes, lymphokines, interferon-γ, interleukins, tumor necrosis factor-α, and complement are reduced in early infancy, thus preventing optimal response to certain bacteria and viruses. The production of IgA and immunoglobulins D and E (IgD and IgE) is much more gradual, and maximum levels are not attained until early childhood. Probiotics may have a significant role in helping the gastrointestinal tract establish a "good" bacterial colonization in the gut to prevent many illnesses, including antibiotic-induced diarrhea and possibly *Helicobacter pylori* gastritis (Thomas, Greer, American Academy of Pediatrics [AAP], and others, 2010).

Evidence indicates that vernix caseosa, a white oily substance that coats term infants' bodies and is often found in abundance in creases of the axilla and groin, has innate immunologic properties that serve to protect newborns from infection (Narendran and Hoath, 2006). Vernix also appears to have a role in maintaining the integrity of the stratum corneum and facilitating acid mantle development (Hoath, Pickens, and Visscher, 2006). The epidermis of a full-term infant undergoes maturation during the first month of life; the newborn's skin acts as a barrier to infection, assists in thermal regulation, and prevents transepidermal water loss in term infants.

During infancy, thermoregulation becomes more efficient; the ability of the skin to contract and of muscles to shiver in response to cold increases. The peripheral capillaries respond to changes in ambient temperature to regulate heat loss. The capillaries constrict in response to cold, conserving core body temperature and decreasing potential evaporative heat loss from the skin surface. The capillaries dilate in response to heat, decreasing internal body temperature through evaporation, conduction, and convection. Shivering (thermogenesis) causes the muscles and muscle fibers to contract, generating metabolic heat, which is distributed throughout the body. Increased adipose tissue during the first 6 months insulates the body against heat loss.

A shift in the total body fluid occurs; at birth, 75% of a term infant's body weight is water, and there is an abundance of extracellular fluid (ECF). As the percentage of body water decreases, so does the amount of ECF—from 40% at term to 20% in adulthood. The high proportion of ECF, which is composed of blood plasma, interstitial fluid, and lymph, predisposes the infant to a more rapid loss of total body fluid and, consequently, dehydration. The loss of 5% to 10% of term newborns' initial birth weight in the first 5 days of life is attributed to ECF compartment contraction, enhanced renal tubular function, and rapidly increasing glomerular filtration rate (Blackburn, 2011).

The immaturity of the renal structures also predisposes infants to dehydration and electrolyte imbalance. Complete maturity of the kidneys occurs during the latter half of the second year, when the cuboidal epithelium of the glomeruli becomes flattened. Before this time, the filtration capacity of the glomeruli is reduced. Urine is voided frequently and has a low specific gravity (1.000-1.010). At term, most infants produce and excrete approximately 15 to 60 ml/kg/24 hr, and an output of less than 0.5 ml/kg/hr after 48 hours of age is considered to be oliguria (Blackburn, 2011).

Auditory acuity is at adult levels during infancy. Visual acuity begins to improve, and binocular fixation is established. Binocularity, or the fixation of two ocular images into one cerebral picture (fusion), begins to develop by 6 weeks of age and should be well established by age 4 months. Depth perception (stereopsis) begins to develop by age 7 to 9 months but may not be fully mature until 2 or 3 years of age, thus increasing infants' and younger toddlers' risk of falling.

Fine Motor Development

Fine motor behavior includes the use of the hands and fingers in the prehension (grasp) of objects. Grasping occurs during the first 2 to 3 months as a reflex and gradually becomes voluntary. At 1 month of age, the hands are predominantly closed, and by 3 months, they are mostly open. By this time, infants demonstrate a desire to grasp objects, but they "grasp" objects more with the eyes than with the hands. If a rattle is placed in the hand, infants will actively hold on to it. By 4 months of age, infants regard both a small pellet and the hands and then look from the object to the hands and back again. By 5 months, infants are able to voluntarily grasp objects.

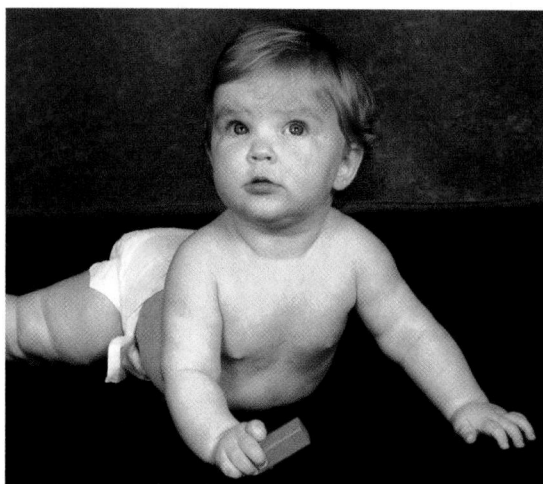

FIG 10-1 Crude pincer grasp at 8 to 10 months. (Photo by Paul Vincent Kuntz, Texas Children's Hospital, Houston.)

By 6 months of age, infants have increased manipulative skill. They hold their bottles, grasp their feet and pull them to their mouths, and feed themselves crackers. By 7 months, they transfer objects from one hand to the other, use one hand for grasping, and hold a cube in each hand simultaneously. They enjoy banging objects and explore the movable parts of toys.

Gradually, the palmar grasp (using the whole hand) is replaced by a pincer grasp (using the thumb and index finger). By 8 to 10 months of age, infants use a crude pincer grasp, and by 11 months, they have progressed to a neat pincer grasp (Fig. 10-1). By 10 months of age, the pincer grasp is sufficiently established to enable infants to pick up raisins and other finger foods. They can deliberately let go of an object and offer it to someone. By 11 months, they put objects into containers and like to remove them. By age 1 year, infants try to build towers of two blocks but fail.

Gross Motor Development
Head Control

Full-term newborns can momentarily hold their heads in midline and parallel when their bodies are suspended ventrally and can lift and turn their heads from side to side when they are prone (see Fig. 8-7). This is not the case when infants are lying prone on a pillow or soft surface; infants do not have the head control to lift their heads out of the depression of the object and therefore risk suffocation in the prone position early in infancy (see Sudden Infant Death Syndrome, Chapter 11). Marked head lag is evident when infants are pulled from a lying to a sitting position. By 3 months of age, infants can hold their heads well beyond the plane of their bodies. By 4 months of age, infants can lift their heads and front portion of their chests approximately 90 degrees above the table, bearing their weight on the forearms. Only slight head lag is evident when infants are pulled from a lying to a sitting position, and by 4 to 6 months, head control is well established (Figs. 10-2 and 10-3).

Rolling Over

Newborns may roll over accidentally because of their rounded backs. The ability to willfully turn from the abdomen to the back occurs around 5 months, and the ability to turn from the back to the abdomen occurs at approximately 6 months. Infants put to sleep on their sides may easily roll over to a prone (face-down) position, thus placing them at higher risk for sudden infant death syndrome (SIDS). It is therefore

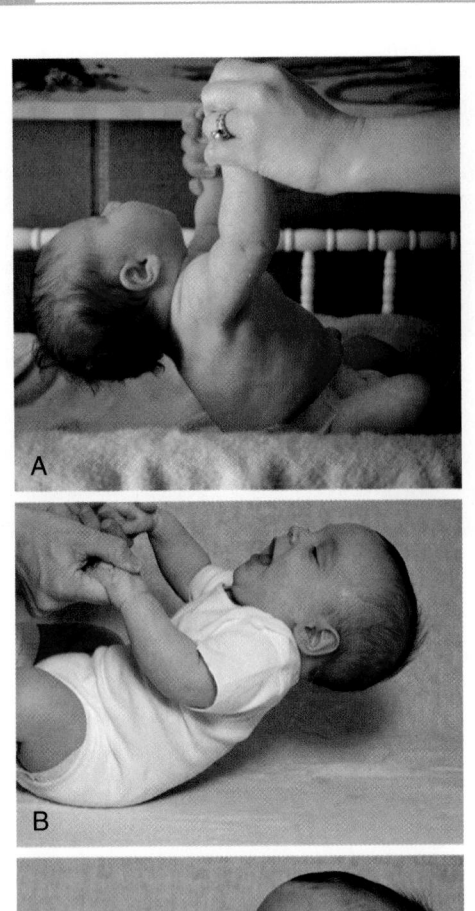

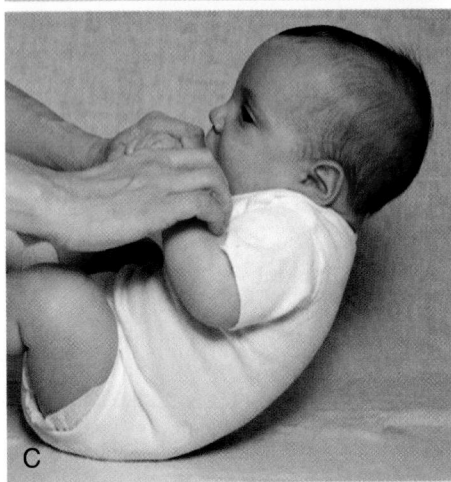

FIG 10-2 Head control while pulled to sitting position. **A,** Complete head lag at 1 month. **B,** Partial head lag at 2 months. **C,** Almost no head lag at 4 months.

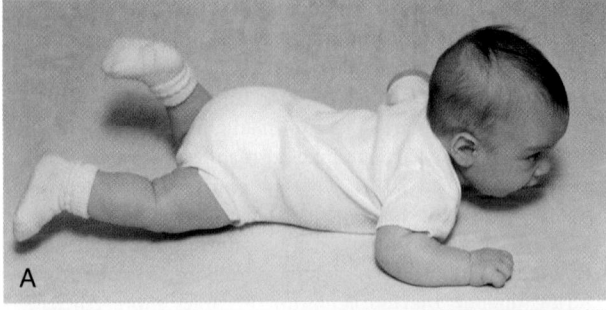

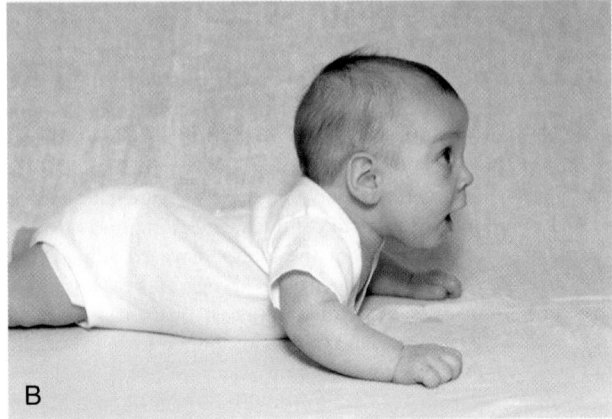

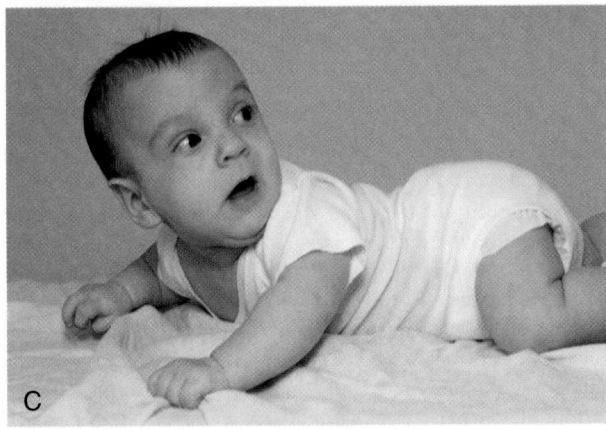

FIG 10-3 Head control while prone. **A,** The infant momentarily lifts the head at 1 month. **B,** The infant lifts the head and chest 90 degrees and bears weight on the forearms at 4 months. **C,** The infant lifts head, chest, and upper abdomen and can bear weight on the hands at 6 months. Note how this position facilitates turning from the abdomen to the back.

important to place infants in a supine position for sleep. While infants are awake, a prone position (tummy time) is acceptable to enhance achievement of milestones such as head control, crawling, creeping, and turning over. It is noteworthy that the parachute reflex (Fig. 10-4), a protective response to falling, appears at approximately 7 months.

<table>
<tr><td>❗</td><td>**NURSING ALERT**</td></tr>
</table>

In the first several months, before the infant can roll over, the head should be positioned on alternating sides to prevent positional plagiocephaly (when asleep or awake in the supine position) (see Chapter 11).

Sitting

The ability to sit follows progressive head control and straightening of the back (Fig. 10-5). For the first 2 to 3 months, the back is uniformly rounded. The convex cervical curve forms at approximately 3 to 4 months of age, when head control is established. The convex lumbar curve appears when the child begins to sit, at about age 4 months. As the spinal column straightens, infants can be propped in a sitting position. By age 7 months, infants can sit alone, leaning forward on their hands for support. By age 8 months, they can sit well while unsupported and begin to explore their surroundings in this position rather than in a lying position. By 10 months, they can maneuver from a prone to a sitting position.

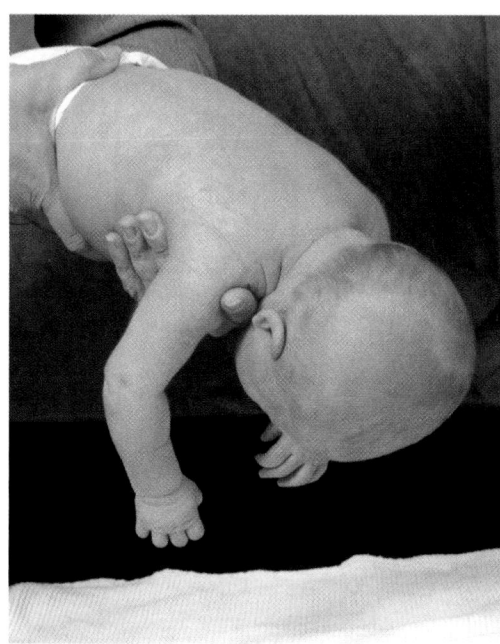

FIG 10-4 Parachute reflex. (Photo by Paul Vincent Kuntz, Texas Children's Hospital, Houston.)

Locomotion

Locomotion involves acquiring the ability to bear weight; propel forward on all four extremities; stand upright with support; cruise by holding on to furniture; and finally, walk alone (Fig. 10-6). Following a cephalocaudal pattern, infants who are 4 to 6 months old have increasing coordination in their arms. Initial locomotion results in infants propelling themselves backward by pushing with their arms. By 6 to 7 months of age, they are able to bear all of their weight on their legs with assistance. Crawling (propelling forward with the belly on the floor) progresses to creeping on hands and knees (with the belly off the floor) by 9 months. At this time, they stand while holding on to furniture and can pull themselves to the standing position, but they are unable to maneuver back down except by falling. By 11 months, they walk while holding on to furniture or with both hands held, and by age 1 year, they may be able to walk with one hand held. A number of infants attempt their first independent steps by their first birthday.

> **! NURSING ALERT**
>
> An infant who does not pull to a standing position by 11 to 12 months of age should be further evaluated for possible developmental dysplasia of the hip (see Chapter 31).

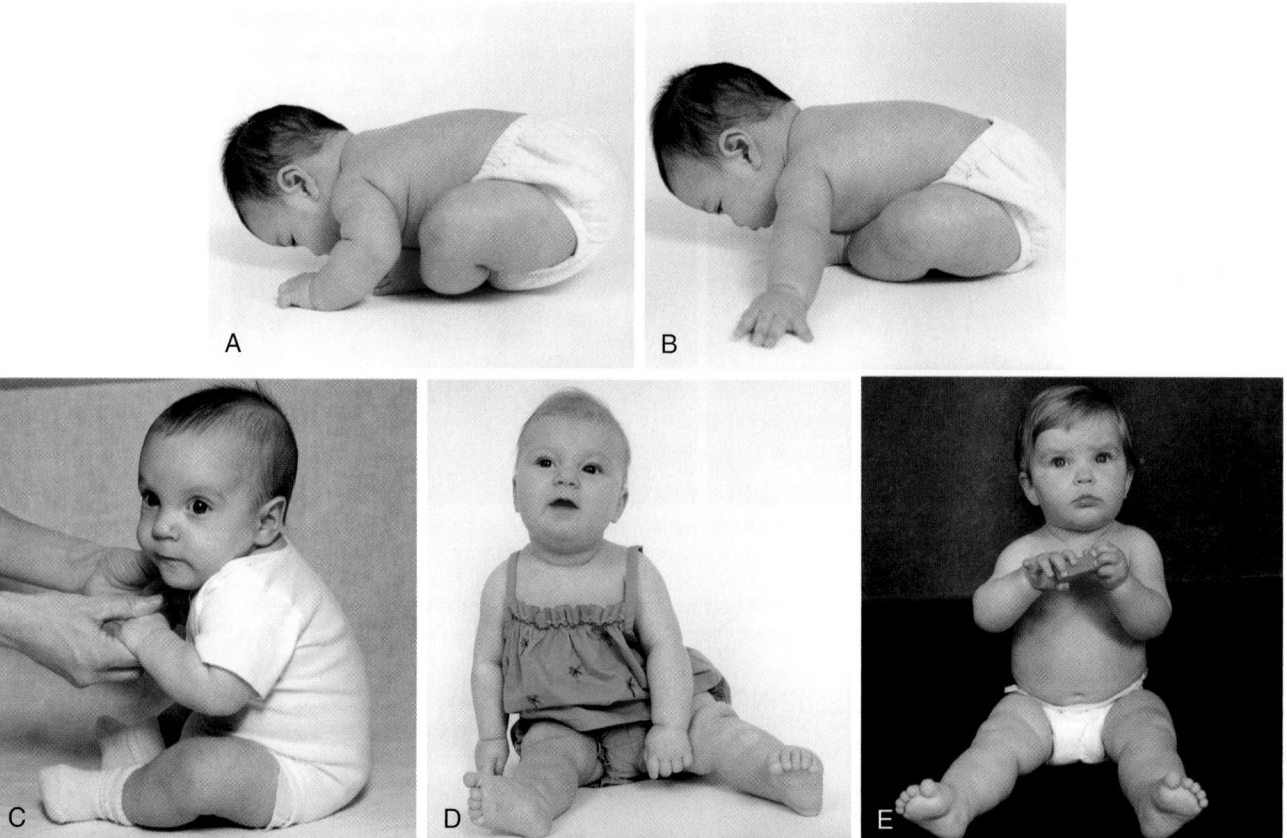

FIG 10-5 Development of sitting. **A,** The back is completely rounded, and the infant has no ability to sit upright at 1 month. **B,** At 2 months, the infant exhibits more control; the back is still rounded, but the infant can try to pull up with some head control. **C,** The back is rounded only in the lumbar area, and the infant is able to sit erect with good head control at 4 months. **D,** The infant can sit alone, leaning on the hands for support, at 7 months. **E,** The infant sits without support at 8 months. Note the transferring of objects that occurs at 7 months. (**B, D,** and **E** photos by Paul Vincent Kuntz, Texas Children's Hospital, Houston.)

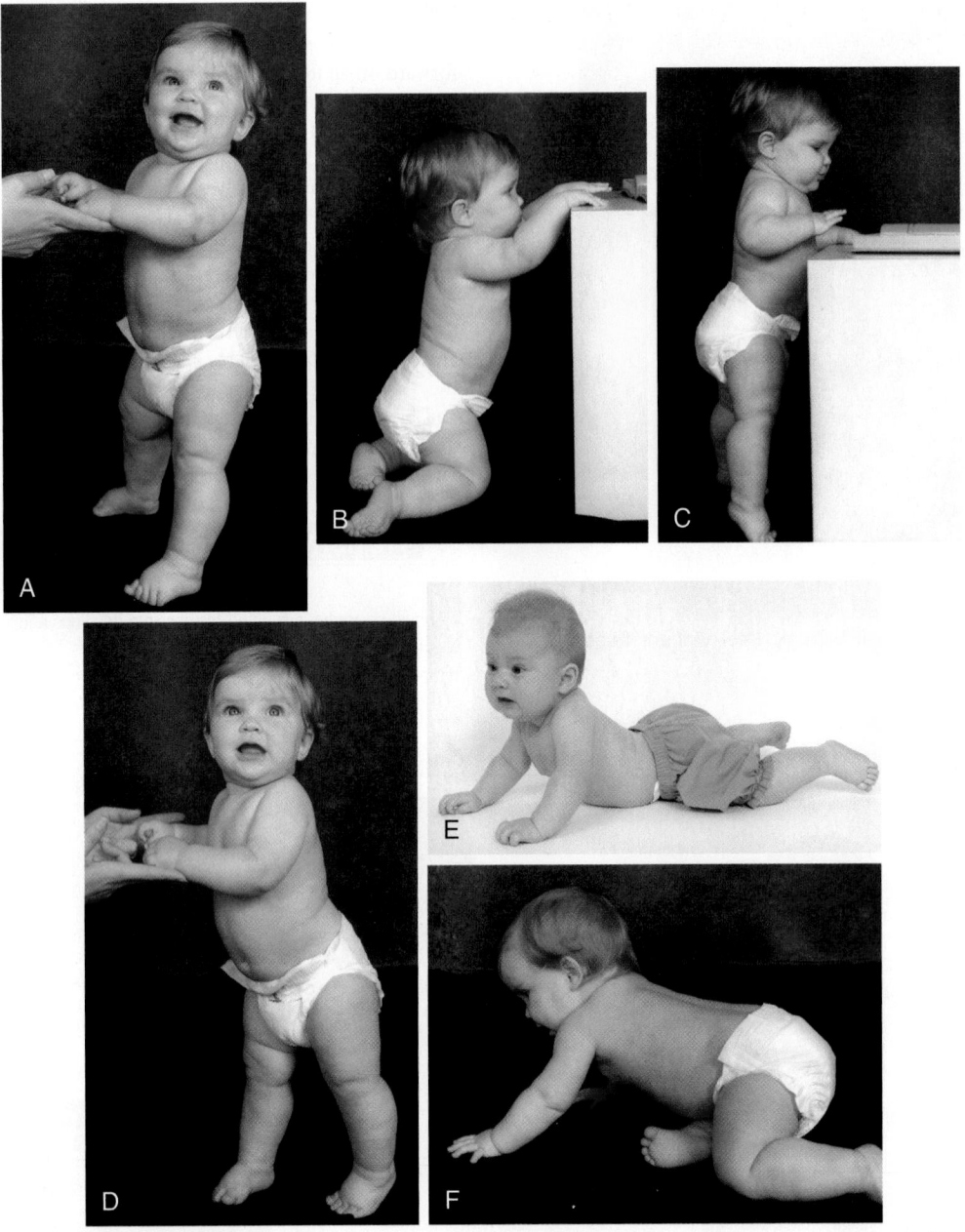

FIG 10-6 Development of locomotion. **A,** The infant bears full weight on the feet by 7 months. **B,** The infant can maneuver from a sitting to a kneeling position. **C,** The infant can stand holding on to furniture at 9 months. **D,** While standing, the infant takes deliberate step at 10 months. **E,** The infant crawls with the abdomen on the floor and pulls self forward at about 7 months and then, **F,** creeps on hands and knees at 9 months. (Photos by Paul Vincent Kuntz, Texas Children's Hospital, Houston.)

PSYCHOSOCIAL DEVELOPMENT: DEVELOPING A SENSE OF TRUST (ERIKSON)

Erikson's phase I (birth to 1 year) is concerned with acquiring a sense of trust while overcoming a sense of mistrust. The trust that develops is a trust of self, of others, and of the world. Infants "trust" that their feeding, comfort, stimulation, and caring needs will be met. The crucial element for the achievement of this task is the quality of both the parent (caregiver)–child relationship and the care the infant receives. The provision of food, warmth, and shelter by itself is inadequate for the development of a strong sense of self. The infant and parent must jointly learn to satisfactorily meet their needs for mutual regulation of

frustration to occur. When this synchrony fails to develop, mistrust is the eventual outcome.

Failure to learn delayed gratification leads to mistrust. Mistrust can result from either too much or too little frustration. If parents always meet their children's needs before the children signal their readiness, infants will never learn to test their ability to control the environment. If the delay is prolonged, infants will experience constant frustration and eventually mistrust others in their efforts to satisfy them. Therefore, consistency of care is essential.

The trust acquired in infancy provides the foundation for all succeeding phases. Trust allows infants a feeling of physical comfort and security, which assists them in experiencing unfamiliar, unknown situations with a minimum of fear. Erikson has divided the first year of life into two oral–social stages. During the first 3 to 4 months, food intake is the most important social activity in which the infant engages. Newborns can tolerate little frustration or delay of gratification. Primary narcissism (total concern for oneself) is at its height.

However, as bodily processes such as vision, motor movements, and vocalization become better controlled, infants use more advanced behaviors to interact with others. For example, rather than cry, infants may put their arms up to signify a desire to be held. The next social modality involves a mode of reaching out to others through grasping. Grasping is initially reflexive, but even as a reflex, it has a powerful social meaning for the parents. The reciprocal response to the infant's grasping is the parents' holding on and touching. There is pleasurable tactile stimulation for both the child and the parents.

Tactile stimulation is extremely important in the total process of acquiring trust. The degree of mothering skill, the quantity of food, or the length of sucking does not determine the quality of the experience. Rather, the total nature of the quality of the interpersonal relationship influences the infant's formulation of trust.

During the second stage, the more active and aggressive modality of biting occurs. Infants learn that they can hold on to what is their own and can more fully control their environment. During this stage, infants may be confronted with one of their first conflicts. If they are breastfeeding, they quickly learn that biting causes the mother to become upset and withdraw the breast. Yet biting also brings internal relief from teething discomfort and a sense of power or control.

This conflict may be solved in a variety of ways. The mother may wean the infant from the breast and begin bottle feeding, or the infant may learn to bite substitute nipples, such as a pacifier, and retain pleasurable breastfeeding. The successful resolution of this conflict strengthens the mother–child relationship because it occurs at a time when infants are recognizing the mother as the most significant person in their life.

COGNITIVE DEVELOPMENT: SENSORIMOTOR PHASE (PIAGET)

The theory most commonly used to explain cognition, or the ability to know, is that of Piaget. The period from birth to 24 months is termed the sensorimotor phase and is composed of six stages; however, because this discussion is concerned with ages birth to 12 months, only the first four stages are discussed. The last two stages occur during the toddler period of 12 to 24 months and are discussed in Chapter 12.

During the sensorimotor phase, infants progress from reflexive behaviors to simple repetitive acts to imitative activity. Three crucial events take place during this phase. The first event involves separation in which infants learn to separate themselves from other objects in the environment. They realize that others besides themselves control the environment and that certain readjustments must take place for mutual satisfaction to occur. This coincides with Erikson's concept of the formation of trust.

The second major accomplishment is achieving the concept of object permanence, or the realization that objects that leave the visual field still exist. A typical example of the development of object permanence is when infants are able to pursue objects they observe being hidden under a pillow or behind a chair (Fig. 10-7). This skill develops at approximately 9 to 10 months of age, which corresponds to the time of increased locomotion skills.

The last major intellectual achievement of this period is the ability to use symbols, or mental representation. The use of symbols allows infants to think of an object or situation without actually experiencing

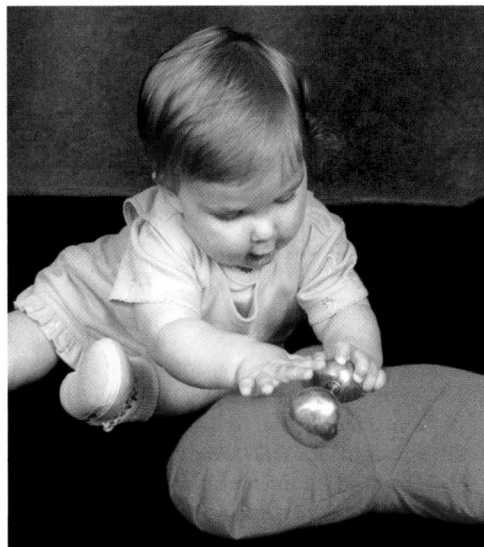

FIG 10-7 A 9-month-old infant is able to find hidden objects under a pillow. (Photo by Paul Vincent Kuntz, Texas Children's Hospital, Houston.)

it. The recognition of symbols is the beginning of the understanding of time and space.

The first stage, from birth to 1 month, is identified by infants' use of reflexes. At birth, infants' individuality and temperament are expressed through the physiologic reflexes of sucking, rooting, grasping, and crying. The repetitious nature of the reflexes is the beginning of associations between an act and a sequential response. When infants cry because they are hungry, a nipple is put in the mouth, and they suck, feel satisfaction, and sleep. They are assimilating this experience while perceiving auditory, tactile, and visual cues. This experience of perceiving certain patterns, or "ordering," provides a foundation for the subsequent stages.

The second stage, primary circular reactions, marks the beginning of the replacement of reflexive behavior with voluntary acts. During the period from 1 to 4 months, activities such as sucking and grasping become deliberate acts that elicit certain responses. The beginning of accommodation is evident. Infants incorporate and adapt their reactions to the environment and recognize the stimulus that produced a response. Previously, they cried until the nipple was brought to the mouth. Now they associate the nipple with the sound of the parent's voice. They accommodate this new piece of information and adapt by ceasing to cry when they hear the voice—before receiving the nipple. What is taking place is realization of causality and recognition of an orderly sequence of events. The environment is taken in with all of the senses and with whatever motor ability is present.

The secondary circular reactions stage is a continuation of primary circular reactions and lasts until 8 months of age. In this stage, the primary circular reactions are repeated and prolonged for the response that results. Grasping and holding now become shaking, banging, and pulling. Shaking is performed to hear a noise, not solely for the pleasure of shaking. The quality and quantity of an act become evident. "More" or "less" shaking produces different responses. Causality, time, deliberate intention, and separateness from the environment begin to develop.

Three new processes of human behavior occur. Imitation requires the differentiation of selected acts from several events. By the second half of the first year, infants can imitate sounds and simple gestures.

Play becomes evident as they take pleasure in performing an act after they have mastered it. Much of infants' waking hours is absorbed in sensorimotor play. Affect (outward manifestation of emotion and feeling) is seen as infants begin to develop a sense of permanence. During the first 6 months, infants believe that an object exists only for as long as they can visually perceive it. In other words, out of sight, out of mind. Affect to external objects is evident when the object continues to be present or remembered even though it is beyond the range of perception. Object permanence is a critical component of parent–child attachment and is seen in the development of stranger anxiety at 6 to 8 months of age (see p. 323).

During the fourth sensorimotor stage, **coordination of secondary schemas and their application to new situations**, infants use previous behavioral achievements primarily as the foundation for adding new intellectual skills to their expanding repertoire. This stage is largely transitional. Increasing motor skills allow for greater exploration of the environment. They begin to discover that hiding an object does not mean that it is gone but that removing an obstacle will reveal the object. This marks the beginning of intellectual reasoning. Furthermore, they can experience an event by observing it, and they begin to associate symbols with events (e.g., "bye-bye" with "Mommy or Daddy goes to work"), but the classification is purely their own. In this stage, they learn from the object itself; this is in contrast to the second stage, in which infants learn from the type of interaction between objects or individuals. Intentionality is further developed in that infants now actively attempt to remove a barrier to the desired (or undesired) action (see Fig. 10-7). If something is in their way, they attempt to climb over it or push it away. Previously, an obstacle would cause them to give up any further attempt to achieve the desired goal.

DEVELOPMENT OF BODY IMAGE

The development of body image parallels sensorimotor development. Infants' kinesthetic and tactile experiences are the first perceptions of their bodies, and the mouth is the principal area of pleasurable sensations. Other parts of their bodies are primarily objects of pleasure—the hands and fingers to suck and the feet to play with. As their physical needs are met, they feel comfort and satisfaction with their bodies. Messages conveyed by their caregivers reinforce these feelings. For example, when infants smile, they receive emotional satisfaction from others who smile back.

Achieving the concept of object permanence is basic to the development of self-image. By the end of the first year, infants recognize that they are distinct from their parents. At the same time, they have increasing interest in their image, especially in the mirror (Fig. 10-8). As motor skills develop, they learn that parts of their bodies are useful; for example, their hands bring objects to their mouths, and their legs help them move to different locations. All of these achievements transmit messages to them about themselves. Therefore, it is important to transmit positive messages to infants about their bodies.

SOCIAL DEVELOPMENT

Infants' social development is initially influenced by their reflexive behavior, such as the grasp, and eventually depends primarily on the interaction between them and their principal caregivers. Attachment to their parents is increasingly evident during the second half of the first year. In addition, tremendous strides are made in communication and personal–social behavior. Whereas crying and reflexive behavior are methods to meet one's needs in early infancy, the social smile is an early step in social communication. This has a profound effect on

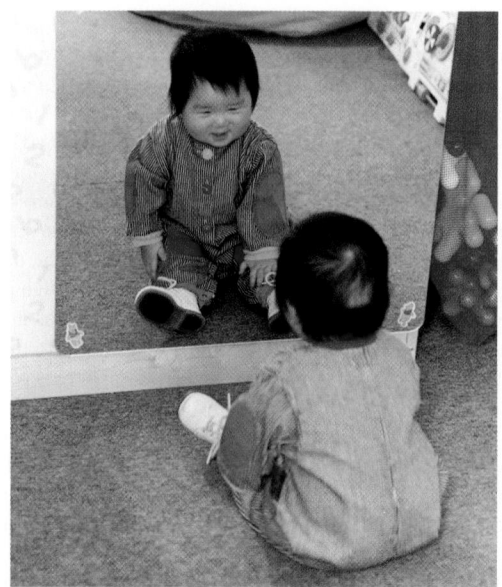

FIG 10-8 A 9-month-old infant enjoying own image in mirror.

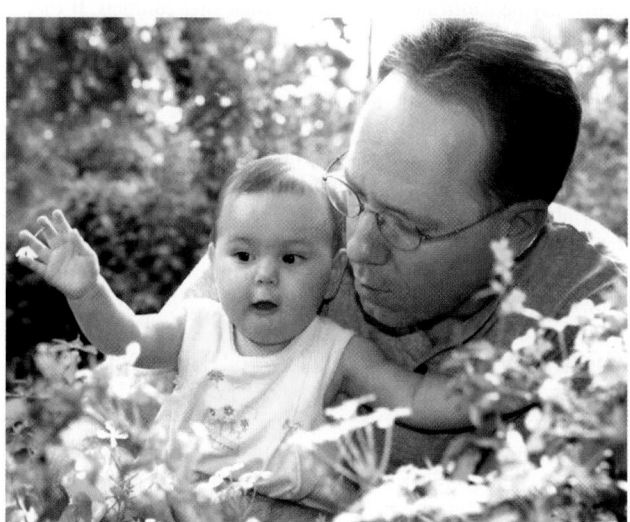

FIG 10-9 Infancy is an important time for attachment to significant others. (Photo by Paul Vincent Kuntz, Texas Children's Hospital, Houston.)

family members and is a tremendous stimulus for evoking continued responses from others. By 4 months, infants laugh aloud.

Play is a major socializing agent and provides stimulation needed to learn from and interact with the environment. By age 6 months, infants are very personable. They play games such as peek-a-boo when their heads are hidden in a towel, they signal their desire to be picked up by extending their arms, and they show displeasure when a toy is removed or their faces are washed.

Attachment

The importance of human physical contact to infants cannot be overemphasized. Parenting is not an instinctual ability but a learned, acquired process. The attachment of parent and child, which often begins before birth and assumes even more importance at birth (see Chapter 8), continues during the first year (Fig. 10-9). In the following discussion of attachment, the term *mother* is used in the broad context of the consistent caregiver with whom the child relates more than anyone else. However, with society's changing social climate and sex-role stereotypes, this person may well be the father or a grandparent. Studies on father–infant attachment demonstrate that stages similar to maternal attachment occur and that fathers are more involved in child care when mothers are employed (although mothers continue to do the majority of infant care). Additional research has shown that inexperienced, first-time fathers are as capable as experienced fathers of developing a close attachment with their infants. Studies of fathers of high-risk infants demonstrate that fathers experience feelings of love and affection toward their offspring during the newborn period; fathers in one study verbalized more positive feelings of love and affection toward their newborns when they were able to have close physical contact such as holding their children (Sullivan, 1999). Fathers have also been reported to have a significant role in supporting mothers in the perinatal period; fathers of high-risk infants reported concern about their mates' well-being in addition to the status of their ill infants (Lundqvist and Jakobsson, 2003). Research demonstrates that fathers develop feelings of attachment with their offspring and that their relationship with the infant is an important factor in the mother's emotional well-being. With many single-parent families in existence, a grandmother (or other significant caretaker) may become the primary caretaker. It is important for nurses to recognize that infant–parent attachments may be present or absent in situations where caretaker roles are less well defined by those involved.

When infants are not provided a safe haven and consistent and loving care, an insecure attachment develops; such infants do not feel they can trust the world in which they live. This insecure attachment may result in psychosocial difficulties as the child grows and may persist even into adulthood. Insecure attachment may also exist in homes where there is domestic violence and maternal postnatal depression.

Attachment progresses during infancy, with the child assuming an increasingly significant role. Two components of cognitive development are required for attachment: (1) the ability to discriminate the mother from other individuals and (2) the achievement of object permanence. Both of these processes prepare infants for an equally important aspect of attachment: separation from the parent. Separation-individuation should occur as a harmonious, parallel process with emotional attachment.

During the formation of attachment to the parent, the infant progresses through four distinct but overlapping stages. For the first few weeks of life, infants respond indiscriminately to anyone. Beginning at approximately 8 to 12 weeks of age, they cry, smile, and vocalize more to the mother than to anyone else but continue to respond to others, whether familiar or not. At approximately 6 months of age, infants show a distinct preference for the mother. They follow her more, cry when she leaves, enjoy playing with her more, and feel most secure in her arms. About 1 month after showing attachment to the mother, many infants begin attaching to other members of the family, most often the father.

Infants acquire other developmental behaviors that influence the attachment process. These include:
- Differential crying, smiling, and vocalization (more to the mother than to anyone else)
- Visual-motor orientation (looking more at the mother, even if she is not close)
- Crying when the mother leaves the room
- Approaching through locomotion (crawling, creeping, or walking)
- Clinging (especially in the presence of a stranger)
- Exploring away from the mother while using her as a secure base

Reactive attachment disorder (RAD) is a psychologic and developmental problem that stems from maladaptive or absent attachment between the infant and parent and may persist into childhood and even adulthood (Zeanah and Fox, 2004). Infants at risk for RAD include those who have been victims of physical or sexual abuse or neglect; infants exposed to parental alcoholism, mental illness, and substance abuse; and infants who have experienced the absence of a consistent primary caregiver as a result of foster care, institutionalization, parental abandonment, or parental incarceration. RAD is a form of extreme insecure attachment. Historically, two different patterns of RAD were described: the emotionally withdrawn–inhibited pattern and an indiscriminate-disinhibited pattern (Zeanah and Fox, 2004). Recently, Zeanah and Gleason (2010) have proposed classifying these two subtypes into separate disorders: disinhibited social engagement disorder of childhood and RAD of infancy or early childhood. These researchers postulate that children who experience grossly inadequate child care will develop severe attachment disorder. Signs of RAD are usually seen before the age of 5 years in infants who had insecure attachments to their mothers or other primary caretakers. Children may manifest behaviors such as not being cuddly with parents, failing to make eye contact with significant others, having poor impulse control, and being destructive to themselves and others. Maltreated and orphaned children may be diagnosed with this complex disorder. Without early intervention, some of these children fail to develop a conscience and develop an antisocial personality disorder that may lead to criminal acts. Children with autism or other pervasive developmental disorders have behaviors that are categorically different from those with RAD (Zeanah and Gleason, 2010).

Separation Anxiety

Between ages 4 and 8 months, infants progress through the first stage of separation-individuation and begin to have some awareness of themselves and their mothers as separate beings. At the same time, object permanence is developing, and infants are aware that their parents can be absent. Therefore, separation anxiety develops and is manifested through a predictable sequence of behaviors.

During the early second half of the first year, infants protest when placed in their cribs, and a short time later, they object when their mothers leave the room. Infants may not notice the mother's absence if they are absorbed in an activity. However, when they realize her absence, they protest. From this point on, they become alert to her activities and whereabouts. By 11 to 12 months, they are able to anticipate her imminent departure by watching her behaviors, and they begin to protest *before* she leaves. At this point, many parents learn to postpone alerting the child to their departure until just before leaving.

Stranger Fear

As infants demonstrate attachment to one person, they correspondingly exhibit less friendliness to others. Between ages 6 and 8 months, fear of strangers and stranger anxiety become prominent and are related to infants' ability to discriminate between familiar and unfamiliar people. Behaviors such as clinging to the parent, crying, and turning away from the stranger are common.

Language Development

Infants' first means of verbal communication is crying. Crying as a biologic sign conveys a message of urgency and signals displeasure, such as hunger. However, crying is also a social event that affects the development of the parent–infant relationship—either by its absence, which usually has a positive effect on parents, or by its presence, which may evoke a negative response or persuade parents to minister to the child's physical or emotional needs.

In the first few weeks of life, crying has a reflexive quality and is mostly related to physiologic needs. Infants cry for 1 to 1.5 hours a day up to 3 weeks of age and then build up to 2, and even 4, hours by 6 weeks. Crying tends to decrease by 12 weeks. It is thought that the increase in crying for no apparent reason during the first few months may be related to the discharge of energy and the maturational changes in the central nervous system. At the end of the first year, infants cry for attention; from fear (especially stranger fear); and from frustration, usually in response to their developing but inadequate motor skills.

Vocalizations heard during crying eventually become syllables and words (e.g., the "mama" heard during vigorous crying). Infants vocalize as early as 5 to 6 weeks of age by making small throaty sounds. By 2 months, they make single vowel sounds such as *ah*, *eh*, and *uh*. By 3 to 4 months, the consonants *n*, *k*, *g*, *p*, and *b* are added, and infants coo, gurgle, and laugh aloud. By 8 months, they imitate sounds; add the consonants *t*, *d*, and *w*; and combine syllables (e.g., "dada"), but they do not ascribe meaning to the word until 10 to 11 months of age. By 9 to 10 months, they comprehend the meaning of the word "no" and obey simple commands. By age 1 year, they can say three to five words with meaning. Because language development is based on expressive skills (ability to make thoughts, ideas, and desires known to others) and receptive skills (ability to understand the words being spoken), it is important that infants are exposed to expressive speech and that infants with delays in achieving milestones are carefully evaluated for potential hearing loss. (See Universal Newborn Hearing Screening, Chapter 8.)

Play

Play during infancy represents the various social modalities observed during cognitive development. The activity of infants is primarily narcissistic and revolves around their own bodies. As discussed under Development of Body Image (p. 320), body parts are primarily objects of play and pleasure.

During the first year, play becomes more sophisticated and interdependent. From birth to 3 months, infants' responses to the environment are global and largely undifferentiated. Play is dependent; pleasure is demonstrated by a quieting attitude (1 month), a smile (2 months), or a squeal (3 months). From 3 to 6 months, infants show more discriminate interest in stimuli and begin to play alone with rattles or soft stuffed toys or with someone else. There is much more interaction during play. By 4 months of age, they laugh aloud, show preference for certain toys, and become excited when food or a favorite object is brought to them. They recognize images in a mirror, smile at them, and vocalize to them.

By 6 months to 1 year, play involves sensorimotor skills. Actual games such as peek-a-boo and pat-a-cake are played. Verbal repetition and imitation of simple gestures occur in response to demonstration. Play is much more selective, not only in terms of specific toys, but also in terms of "playmates." Although play is solitary or one sided, infants choose with whom they will interact. At 6 to 8 months, they usually refuse to play with strangers. Parents are definite favorites, and infants know how to attract their attention. At 6 months, they extend their arms to be picked up; at 7 months, they cough to make their presence known; at 10 months, they pull their parents' clothing; and at 12 months, they call their parents by name. This represents a tremendous advance from the newborn who signaled biologic needs by crying to express displeasure.

Stimulation is as important for psychosocial growth as food is for physical growth. Knowledge of developmental milestones allows nurses to guide parents regarding proper play for infants. It is not sufficient to place a mobile over a crib and toys in a play yard for a child's optimum social, emotional, and intellectual development. Play must provide interpersonal contact and recreational and educational stimulation. Infants need to be *played with*, not merely *allowed to play*. Although the type of play infants engage in is called solitary, this is a figurative, not literal, term to denote one-sided play. The type of toys given to children is much less important than the quality of personal interaction that occurs.

TEMPERAMENT

An infant's temperament or behavioral style influences the type of interaction that occurs between the child and parents, especially the mother, and other family members (see Temperament, Chapter 5). In assessing a child's temperament, the parents' perception of the child and the degree of fit between their expectations and the child's actual temperament are important. The more dissonance, or lack of harmony, between the child's temperament and the parent's ability to accept and deal with the behavior, the more risk for subsequent parent–child conflicts.

Although most behavioral researchers agree that there is a strong biologic component to temperament, researchers also suggest that temperament may be modified by the environment, particularly the family (Wilson, White, Cobb, and others, 2000). Family interaction with the infant is perceived as a circular process wherein each family member affects the others and the family as a unit. With these concepts in mind, the nurse has an important role in helping the family understand the infant's temperament as it relates to family dynamics and the eventual well-being of the child and family unit (Wilson, White, Cobb, and others, 2000).

Some researchers speculate that infant temperament may contribute to maternal depression. Indeed, when there is a lack of reciprocity between the infant and the mother or when the infant's behavior does not meet maternal expectations, there is increased risk for discord. Beck's (2001) meta-analysis found that whereas infant temperament was a mild risk factor for postpartum depression, self-esteem, marital status, socioeconomic status, and unplanned or unwanted pregnancy were much more significant in predicting maternal depression. Fragmented maternal sleep rather than infant temperament was positively correlated to maternal depression in another study (Goyal, Gay, and Lee, 2009). Others (McGrath, Records, and Rice, 2008) found that depressed mothers (vs. nondepressed mothers) rated their infant's temperament at 2 and 6 months of age as more difficult. The researchers stress that depressed mothers need to be identified and assisted in making the transition to motherhood and in developing synchronicity with their newborn infants. Researchers have correlated fussy infant temperament with the introduction of early complementary feedings (at 3 months of age) (Wasser, Bentley, Borja, and others, 2011) and feeding infants foods that may contribute to obesity (Vollrath, Tonstadt, Rothbert, and others, 2011).

The **Revised Infant Temperament Questionnaire (RITQ)** can be used as a screening tool with parents (Carey and McDevitt, 1978). The questionnaire focuses on nine temperament variables, but the 95 questions relate specifically to activities such as sleep, feeding, play, diapering, and dressing. The scores from the RITQ help identify the child's temperamental style. Use of the RITQ is well accepted by parents and should be accompanied by an adequate explanation of the results. In discussing the results, it is best to avoid descriptors such as "difficult"; instead, infants can be described in terms of characteristics such as "intense" or "less predictable." The Early Infancy Temperament

Questionnaire is a 76-item parent questionnaire that was adapted from the RITQ to specifically evaluate temperament characteristics of infants 1 to 4 months old; the RITQ is best suited for infants 4 months old and older (Medoff-Cooper, Carey, and McDevitt, 1993).

Childrearing Practices Related to Temperament

With knowledge of the infant's temperament, nurses are better able to (1) provide parents with background information that will help them see their child in a better perspective, (2) offer a more organized picture of their child's behavior and possibly reveal distortions in their perceptions of the behavior, and (3) guide parents regarding appropriate childrearing techniques.

Knowledge of the developmental sequence allows the nurse to assess normal growth and minor or abnormal deviations. It also helps parents gain realistic expectations of their child's ability and provides guidelines for suitable play and stimulation. Parents who lack knowledge of child growth and development may set inappropriate behavioral expectations for their child. Emphasizing the child's developmental rather than chronologic age strengthens the parent–child relationship by fostering trust and lessening frustration. Therefore, thorough understanding and appreciation of children's growth and development are essential.

Because of the complexity of the developmental process during the first 12 months, Table 10-1 is presented to help organize and clarify the data already discussed. Although all milestones are important, some represent essential integrative aspects of development that lay the foundation for achievement of more advanced skills. These essential milestones are designated by a square (■) in the table. The table represents the average monthly age at which various skills are attained. It must be remembered that although the sequence is the same, the rate will vary among children.

COPING WITH CONCERNS RELATED TO NORMAL GROWTH AND DEVELOPMENT

Separation and Stranger Fear

A number of fears can appear during infancy. However, the fear that causes parents the most concern is fear related to strangers and separation. Although erroneously interpreted by some as a sign of undesirable, antisocial behavior, stranger fear and separation anxiety are important components of a strong, healthy parent–child attachment. Nevertheless, this period can present difficulties for the parent and child. Parents may be more confined to the home because the infant violently protests having babysitters. To accustom the infant to new people, parents are encouraged to have close friends or relatives visit often. This provides other persons with whom the child is comfortable and can give parents time for themselves.

Infants also need opportunities to safely experience strangers. Usually toward the end of the first year, infants begin to venture away from the parent and demonstrate curiosity about strangers. If allowed to explore at their own rate, many infants eventually "warm up." If parents hold the child away from their face, the infant can observe while maintaining close physical contact.

The best approach for the stranger (including nurses) is to talk softly; meet the child at eye level (to appear smaller); maintain a safe distance from the infant; and avoid sudden, intrusive gestures, such as holding out the arms and smiling broadly.

Parents also may wonder whether they should encourage the child's clinging, dependent behavior, especially if there is pressure from others who view this as "spoiling" (see following discussion). Parents need to be reassured that such behavior is healthy, desirable, and necessary for

the child's optimal emotional development. If parents can reassure the infant of their presence, the infant will learn to realize that they are still there even if not physically present. Talking to infants when leaving the room, allowing them to hear one's voice on the telephone, and using transitional objects (e.g., a favorite blanket or toy) reassure them of the parent's continued presence.

Alternate Child Care Arrangements

For many parents, especially working mothers, locating safe and competent child care facilities for infants is an increasingly difficult problem, one that is compounded by the number of mothers working outside the home. Over the past 40 years, there have been variable shifts in child care arrangements; whereas the majority of children are cared for in group centers or other settings, increasingly more children are being cared for in home settings.

The basic types of care are in-home care, either in the parents' or caregivers' home (family daycare), and center-based care, usually in a daycare center. In-home care may consist of a full-time babysitter who lives in the home, a full-time babysitter who comes to the home, cooperative arrangements such as exchange babysitting, or family daycare. A licensed small family child care home typically provides care and protection for up to six children for part of a 24-hour day and does not include informal arrangements such as exchange babysitting or caregivers in the child's own home. The six children may include the family daycare provider's own children younger than 5 years of age living in the home. Large family child care homes may provide care for eight to 12 children. Unfortunately, many family daycare homes operate without a license and may care for large numbers of infants without adequate staff and facilities.

Child center–based care usually refers to a licensed daycare facility that provides care for six or more children for 6 or more hours in a 24-hour day. Work-based group care is another option that is becoming increasingly popular as employers recognize the benefit of providing high-quality and convenient child care to their employees. Sick-child care may also be available for times when children are ill. Such programs are often located in community hospitals or in work settings.

Nurses may fulfill a unique role in guiding parents in locating suitable facilities that have a well-qualified staff. State licensing agencies can help parents identify daycare centers that accept children of specific age groups and are convenient to home and work. Their records are available to the public and provide reports from the health, safety, and fire departments; periodic evaluations from the licensing agency; complaints filed against the center; and qualification of the center's employees. State-licensed programs are supposed to abide by established standards, which represent the minimum requirements and safeguards. However, enforcement of the standards is sometimes inadequate.

Early childhood programs may also belong to a voluntary accreditation system sponsored by National Association for the Education of Young Children (NAEYC), which serves as a model for optimum care.* References from other parents are also helpful, provided that they have

---

*Information about accreditation criteria and procedures of the National Academy for Early Childhood Program Accreditation/NAEYC is available from NAEYC, 1313 L St. NW, Suite 500, Washington, DC 20005; 800-424-2460 or 202-232-8777; http://www.naeyc.org. These criteria are excellent guidelines for evaluating child care facilities. Other resources are (1) *Choosing Quality Child Care: What's Best for Your Family?* and a number of other child care articles and pamphlets from the AAP, 141 Northwest Point Blvd., Elk Grove Village, IL 60007; 847-434-4000; http://aap.org; and (2) Child Care Aware, 800-424-2246; http://www.childcareaware.org.

investigated the center carefully and have remained involved with the agency's activities.

Guidelines for selecting child care facilities are discussed under Preschool and Kindergarten Experience, Chapter 13. The same conscientious attention should be applied to locating competent babysitters. References from other employers are essential, and there is no substitute for observing the interaction between the individual and the child.

Important areas for parents to evaluate are the center's daily program, teacher qualifications, the nurturing qualities of caregivers, student-to-staff ratio, discipline policy, environmental safety precautions, provision of meals, sanitary conditions, adequate indoor and outdoor space per child, and fee schedule. Although fees vary considerably, a program that charges a minimum fee may also be providing minimum services. Parents should arrange to meet the director and some of the employees, especially those who would be caring for the child. Resources to familiarize parents with characteristics of quality child care and checklists to systematically evaluate the center and compare it with other facilities can help parents make successful choices. At all times, the parent should have the right to visit the child, and regular conferences should occur to review the child's progress.

One of the areas that is increasingly important in selecting child care is the center's health practices; however, parents often do not check the center for health and safety features. Evidence shows that children, especially those younger than age 3 years in daycare centers, have more illnesses—especially diarrhea, otitis media, respiratory tract infections (especially if the caregiver smokes), hepatitis A, meningitis, and cytomegalovirus—than children cared for in their homes. The strongest predictor of risk of illness is the number of unrelated children in the room. Proactive infection control measures and education of staff have been effective in reducing the incidence of upper respiratory tract infections, diarrhea, and rotavirus. It has been reported that families that have children in out-of-home child care lose an estimated 13 days of work per year as a result of infections (Brady, 2005). Parents should inquire about the center's policy regarding the attendance and care of sick children.

Limit Setting and Discipline

As infants' motor skills advance and mobility increases, parents are faced with the need to set safe limits to protect the child and establish a positive and supportive parent–child relationship (see Nurse's Role in Injury Prevention, p. 348). Although there are numerous disciplinary techniques, some are more appropriate for this age than others. An effective approach used in disciplining a child is the use of time-out. The basic principles are the same as those discussed in Chapter 3 except that the place for time-out needs to be commensurate with the child's abilities. For example, a play yard is better for most infants than a chair. Although parents may be concerned about instituting discipline during infancy, it is important to stress that the earlier effective disciplinary methods are used, the easier it is to continue these approaches.

Parents must recognize the infant's cognitive and behavioral limitations; adequate protection from hazards must be implemented because infants and toddlers do not understand a cause-and-effect relationship between dangerous objects and physical harm. Additionally, parents may need reassurance that their infant's behavior is exploratory in nature, not oppositional (at this age) and primarily centered on the infant's basic needs of warmth, love, food, security, and comfort. Parents may verbalize that comforting the infant too much or meeting his or her needs will result in a spoiled child; there is no substantial evidence that meeting the infant's basic needs will result in such behaviors later in life. Children innately test limits and explore during the exploratory phase of growth; instead of discouraging exploration,

Pacifier Use and Breastfeeding

O'Connor, Tanabe, Siadaty, and others (2009) reviewed 29 studies and concluded that pacifier use did not adversely affect the duration or exclusivity of breastfeeding. They further concluded that pacifier use and shortened breastfeeding in many studies likely represented a number of other complex factors such as breastfeeding difficulties or intent to wean.

parents should provide safe alternatives, put dangerous household items away, and give children consistent discipline and nurturing.

Effective teaching for injury prevention optimally begins in infancy by helping parents understand the nature of their child's normal development. It must be reiterated continually that infants cry because a need is not being met, not to intentionally irritate an adult. A fussy or irritable infant is a potential victim of shaken baby syndrome (or other bodily harm) because adults and caretakers may not understand the nature of the infant's crying.*

Thumb Sucking and Use of a Pacifier

Sucking is infants' chief pleasure and may not be satisfied by breastfeeding or bottle feeding. It is such a strong need that infants who are deprived of sucking, such as those with a cleft lip repair, suck on their tongues. Some newborns are born with sucking blisters on their hands from in utero sucking activity.

Problems arise when parents are overly concerned about the sucking of the fingers, thumb, or pacifier and attempt to restrain this natural tendency. Before giving advice, nurses should investigate the parents' feelings and base guidance on this information.

Pacifier use, particularly in the early days after birth and in the birth hospital, has gained considerable attention in the scientific literature. Biancuzzo (2003) suggests that it cannot be stated with absolute certainty that pacifier use is bad in every situation but warns of a potential harm in the use of pacifiers based on available evidence. Furthermore, she cautions health care workers to be informed regarding potential harm in pacifier use and to inform parents of the potential. Lawrence and Lawrence (2011) and other experts in breastfeeding recommend that health care workers not introduce pacifiers to breastfed infants unless the parent requests it (see Research Focus box). Pacifier use is not recommended as part of the Baby-Friendly Hospital Initiative (see Box 8-5, p. 215).

Pacifier use has been associated with an increased risk of otitis media in several studies (Niemela, Pihakari, Pokka, and others, 2000; Rovers, Numans, Langenbach, and others, 2008). The AAP and American Academy of Family Physicians recommend use of pacifier during the first 6 months because of the benefit in regard to pain management and prevention of SIDS, but recommend that infants be weaned from the pacifier during the second 6 months of life (Sexton and Natale, 2009). Pacifier use during painful procedures in neonates has been shown to produce an analgesic effect. (See Chapter 7, Pain in Neonates.)

A review of studies by the Joanna Briggs Institute (2005) found an association between pacifier use in infancy and a reduction in breastfeeding and exclusive breastfeeding. However, the authors concluded

---

*One resource for parents and health professionals is the National Center on Shaken Baby Syndrome and the Period of Purple Crying Program®; 1433 North Highway 89, Suite 110, Farmington, UT, 84025; 801-447-9360; http://www.dontshake.org.

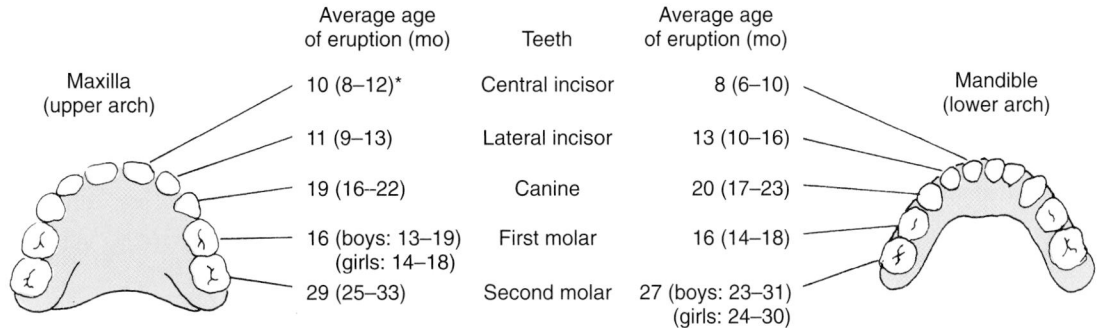

Maxilla (upper arch)	Average age of eruption (mo)	Teeth	Average age of eruption (mo)	Mandible (lower arch)
	10 (8–12)*	Central incisor	8 (6–10)	
	11 (9–13)	Lateral incisor	13 (10–16)	
	19 (16–22)	Canine	20 (17–23)	
	16 (boys: 13–19) (girls: 14–18)	First molar	16 (14–18)	
	29 (25–33)	Second molar	27 (boys: 23–31) (girls: 24–30)	

FIG 10-10 Sequence of eruption of primary teeth. *Range represents ±1 standard deviation, or 67% of subjects studied. (Data from American Dental Association, retrieved August 26, 2011, from http://www.ada.org/2930.aspx?currentTab=1.)

that pacifier use did not cause a reduction in breastfeeding; rather, it was a "marker for socioeconomic, demographic, psychosocial and cultural factors that determine pacifier use and breastfeeding." In addition, the researchers examined studies related to pacifier use and prevention of SIDS; infants put to sleep with a pacifier had a *reduced* risk of SIDS. Because of the limited number of studies correlating pacifier use and increased risk of infections or dental malocclusion, the authors were unable to make any recommendations for or against pacifier use in relation to these practices (Joanna Briggs Institute, 2005).

A recent Cochrane review found that pacifier use in full-term healthy infants started from birth or after lactation was established did not significantly affect the prevalence of duration of exclusive and partial breastfeeding up to 4 months of age (Jaafar, Jahanafar, Angolkar, and others, 2011).

The AAP, Task Force on Sudden Infant Death Syndrome (2005) recommends limited pacifier use in infants, citing the strong evidence for pacifier use at bedtime and nap time and its protective effect in SIDS reduction. The exact mechanism involved in the protection for SIDS is not known. Still, pacifier use should not replace actual feeding or suckling; prohibiting pacifier use will not ensure an increase in the length of breastfeeding, and there should be an emphasis on allowing the infant to control the pace, frequency, and termination of feeding rather than allowing the pacifier (or anything else) to become the focus of the interaction.

To decrease dependence on nonnutritive sucking in young infants, sucking pleasure can be increased by prolonging feeding time. Also, the parent's excessive use of the pacifier to calm the child should be explored. It is not unusual for parents to place a pacifier in the infant's mouth as soon as crying begins, thus reinforcing a pattern of distress–relief.

If the child uses a pacifier, stress safety considerations in purchasing one. During infancy and early childhood, there is no need to restrain nonnutritive sucking of the fingers. Malocclusion may occur if thumb sucking persists past approximately 4 years of age or when the permanent teeth erupt. Some parents may perceive pacifiers as less damaging because they are discarded by 2 to 3 years of age, but thumb sucking may persist well into the school-age years. Both pacifier use and thumb sucking may also have significant cultural variations. Thumb sucking reaches its peak at age 18 to 20 months and is most prevalent when children are hungry, tired, or feeling insecure. Persistent thumb sucking in a listless, apathetic child always warrants investigation. It may be a sign of an emotional problem between the parent and child or of boredom, isolation, and lack of stimulation.

At the time of this writing, there is no evidence that pacifier use and nonnutritive sucking in *preterm infants* has any effect on the initiation and length of breastfeeding. Nonnutritive sucking should not be withheld from preterm infants, especially when used in conjunction with concentrated sucrose for pain management.

Teething

One of the more difficult periods in infants' (and parents') lives is the eruption of the deciduous (primary) teeth, often referred to as teething. The age of tooth eruption shows considerable variation among children, but the order of their appearance is fairly regular and predictable (Fig. 10-10). The first primary teeth to erupt are the lower central incisors, which appear at approximately 6 to 10 months of age (average, 8 months). These are followed closely by the upper central incisors. A quick guide to assessment of deciduous teeth during the first 2 years is: Age of the child in months − 6 = Number of teeth. For example: 8 months of age − 6 = 2 teeth at this time.

Teething is a physiologic process; some discomfort is common as the crown of the tooth breaks through the periodontal membrane. Some children show minimum evidence of teething, such as drooling, gum rubbing, increased finger sucking, or biting on hard objects. Others are very irritable, have difficulty sleeping, and refuse to eat solid foods. Generally, signs of illness such as fever (<38.9° C), vomiting, or diarrhea are not symptoms of teething but of illness and may warrant further investigation. Because teething pain is a result of inflammation, cold is soothing. Giving the child a cold teething ring helps relieve the inflammation (do not freeze liquid-filled teething rings). Several nonprescription topical anesthetic ointments are available, such as Baby Ora-Jel, although parents and health care workers should be aware of the risks of using topical anesthetic products (absorption rates vary in infants) (Markman, 2009). The active ingredient in most of them is benzocaine, which may rarely cause methemoglobinemia. If such products are used, parents are advised to apply them correctly. In the event of persistent irritability that affects sleeping and feeding, systemic analgesics such as acetaminophen or ibuprofen can be given (if age appropriate) for no more than 3 days (Anderson, 2004); however, parents should know that this is a temporary measure and should contact the practitioner if symptoms persist or if the child's condition changes.

The use of teething powders or procedures such as cutting or rubbing the gums with salicylates (aspirin) are discouraged because ingestion of the powder, infection or irritation of the tissue, and ingestion or aspiration of the aspirin can occur. Hard candy may cause accidental choking or aspiration and should be avoided at this age.

PROMOTING OPTIMAL HEALTH DURING INFANCY

NUTRITION

Ideally, discussion of optimal nutrition should begin prenatally with a discussion regarding maternal intake of adequate nutrition in the form of a balanced diet and adequate amounts of protein, vitamins, and minerals, all of which have an impact on the growing fetus. Nurses should encourage and provide information for parents to discuss the options of breastfeeding or bottle feeding the infant well in advance of the delivery date. The choice for either is highly individual and is discussed in Chapter 8. This section is primarily concerned with infant nutrition during the months when growth needs and developmental milestones ready the child for the introduction of solid foods.

Despite adequate availability of optimum nutrient sources, experts are concerned that infants are not fed appropriately. Infants may be given solid foods when their digestive systems are not ready to completely absorb such foods. In addition, drinks that are inappropriate for growing infants may be given in place of enriched infant milk and may only provide "empty" calories and contribute to childhood and adult obesity and place infants at risk for iron deficiency anemia, vitamin D deficiency, and rickets. A survey of infant feeding practices found that about 40% of infants had consumed infant cereal, fruit, or vegetables by 4 months of age despite recommendations that such foods not be introduced until 4 to 6 months (Grummer-Strawn, Scanlon, and Fein, 2008). In the same study, 50% of infants were consuming cake, fried potatoes, candy, and cookies by age 12 months. There is some preliminary evidence that accelerated weight gain in the first 6 months of life may be correlated with obesity later in life (Taveras, Rifas-Shiman, Belfort, and others, 2009). Infant health practices, including nutrition, may have a far-reaching, long-term impact on the child's life. Growth and development could be negatively affected, as could the risk of acquiring certain chronic health conditions. Nurses must be proactive in teaching parents what constitutes appropriate infant nutrition and nutritional habits, which provide the child with an optimum opportunity to grow and develop into a healthy child and adult.

Health care professionals have recently become more aware of the use of complementary and alternative medical therapies in children that may not be as beneficial as touted in various media sources. One concern is children's intake of megavitamins and herbs; parents may assume that the word *natural* in reference to ingredients means the product is safe when this may not be the case. It is important for nurses to be aware of the effects, availability, and practice of complementary therapies and to be able to cogently discuss their use with parents.

The First 6 Months

Human milk is the most desirable complete diet for infants during the first 6 months. A healthy term infant receiving breast milk from a well-nourished mother usually requires no specific vitamin and mineral supplements with a few exceptions. Daily supplements of vitamin D and vitamin B_{12} may be indicated if the mother's intake of these vitamins is inadequate. The AAP (Wagner, Greer, American Academy of Pediatrics Section on Breastfeeding, and others, 2008) recommends that all infants (including those exclusively breastfed) receive a daily supplement of 400 IU of vitamin D beginning in the first few days of life to prevent rickets and vitamin D deficiency. Vitamin D supplementation should occur until the infant is consuming at least 1 L/day (or 1 qt/day) of vitamin D–fortified formula (Wagner, Greer, American Academy of Pediatrics Section on Breastfeeding, and others, 2008).

COMMUNITY FOCUS

Administration of Iron Supplements

- Ideally, iron supplements should be administered between meals for greater absorption.
- Liquid iron supplements may stain the teeth; therefore, administer them with a dropper toward the back of the mouth (side). In older children, administer liquid iron supplements through a straw or rinse the mouth thoroughly after ingestion.
- Avoid administration of liquid iron supplements with whole cow's milk or milk products because they bind free iron and prevent absorption.
- Educate parents that iron supplements will turn stools black or tarry green.
- Iron supplements may cause transient constipation. Caution parents not to switch to a low-iron containing formula or whole milk, which are poor sources of iron and may lead to iron-deficiency anemia (see Iron Deficiency Anemia, Chapter 26).
- In older children, follow liquid iron supplement with a citrus fruit or juice drink (no more than 3–4 oz).
- Avoid administration of iron supplements with foods or drinks that bind iron and prevent absorption (see Iron Deficiency Anemia, Chapter 26).

Non-breastfed infants who are taking less than 1 L/day of vitamin D–fortified formula should also receive a daily vitamin D supplement of 400 IU (see Safety Alert). If the infant is being exclusively breastfed after 4 months (when fetal iron stores are depleted), iron supplementation (1 mg/kg/day) is recommended until appropriate iron-containing complementary foods such as iron-fortified cereal are introduced (Baker, Greer, and AAP Committee on Nutrition, 2010) (see Community Focus box). Infants, whether breastfed or bottle fed, do not require additional fluids, especially water or juice, during the first 4 months of life. Excessive intake of water in infants may result in water intoxication and hyponatremia.

SAFETY ALERT

There are reports of accidental overdoses of liquid vitamin D in infants caused by packaging errors; the syringe for liquid administration may not be labeled clearly for 400 IU. Nurses should educate parents to read syringes and to avoid administering more than 400 IU of vitamin D (FDA Consumer Health Information, 2010).

Fluoride supplementation in exclusively breastfed children is not required for the first 6 months because of the risk of dental fluorosis. However, fluoride supplementation may be necessary if the breastfeeding mother's water supply does not contain the required amount of fluoridation (see p. 330). Even in hot climates, additional water or fluids are not recommended for breastfed infants.

Employed mothers can continue breastfeeding with guidance and encouragement.* Mothers are encouraged to set realistic goals for employment and breastfeeding, with accurate information regarding the costs, risks, and benefits of available feeding options. Barriers encountered by working breastfeeding mothers include lack of employer or coworker support, unavailable or inadequate facilities for

---

*See also *The CDC Guide to Breastfeeding Interventions* (Shealy, Li, Benton-Davis, and others, 2005) at http://www.cdc.gov/breastfeeding/pdf/breastfeeding_interventions.pdf, which includes information for working and breastfeeding.

pumping and storing milk, lack of time to express milk while at work, real or perceived low milk supply, and insufficient time allowed to pump during work (Johnston and Esposito, 2007; Rojjanasrirat, 2004; Shealy, Li, Benton-Davis, and others, 2005). Important themes that emerged in the study by Rojjanasrirat (2004) of working breastfeeding mothers included support (emotional, informational, and instrumental), attitude, and psychologic distress. Johnston and Esposito (2007) found flexible scheduling and increased paid maternity leave time (at least 12 weeks vs. 10 weeks) to be key to encouraging mothers to continue breastfeeding.

Many mothers may find that a program of breast pumping when away from home and bottle feeding the infant the expressed milk with or without formula supplementation is successful. Expressed breast milk may be stored in the refrigerator (4° C [39° F]) without danger of bacterial contamination for up to 5 days (Lawrence and Lawrence, 2011). Although feeding the infant at home may occur on a demand basis, pumping milk away from home may be needed every 3 to 4 hours to maintain adequate supply. Breast milk may be expressed by hand or pump (manual or electric) and stored in an appropriate air-tight glass or plastic container. Expressed breast milk may be frozen (−18° C [0° F] or lower) for up to 6 months (depending on the type of freezer used), but care should be taken to prevent freezer burn (see Lawrence and Lawrence, 2011, for further guidelines on storing and freezing human milk).

In addition to efficient breast pumping, mothers also need child care by a trusted individual or agency and support and assistance from significant others. As with all breastfeeding mothers, these women must have proper nutrition and rest for adequate lactation. Maternal fatigue is considered the biggest threat to successful breastfeeding in employed mothers.

> **! NURSING ALERT**
>
> Warming expressed milk in a microwave decreases the availability of antiinfective properties and vitamin C and causes a separation of milk layers, which affects fat content (Lawrence and Lawrence, 2011). To prevent oral burns from uneven warming of the milk, breast milk should never be thawed or rewarmed in a microwave oven. To thaw the frozen milk, either place the container under a lukewarm water bath (<40.5° C [105° F]) or place it in a refrigerator overnight.

There are reports of an increase in the use of herbs by lactating mothers to increase breast milk supply. The **galactogogues** fenugreek, blessed thistle, fennel, and chaste tree have been purported to increase maternal milk supply, yet few studies support the efficacy or the safety of these herbs in breastfeeding infants; fenugreek has been the most widely studied, yet it may have adverse effects such as colic and diarrhea in breastfeeding infants (Conover and Buehler, 2004; Lawrence and Lawrence, 2011). For a discussion of galactogogues, including those mentioned above, see Appendix P, Protocol 9, in Lawrence and Lawrence (2011).

An acceptable alternative to breastfeeding is commercial iron-fortified formula. Similar to human milk, it supplies all nutrients needed by infants for the first 6 months. Unmodified whole cow's milk, low-fat cow's milk, skim milk, other animal milks, and imitation milk drinks are not acceptable as major sources of nutrition for infants because of their limited digestibility, increased risk of contamination, and lack of components needed for appropriate growth. Whole milk can cause iron-deficiency anemia in infants, possibly as a result of occult gastrointestinal blood loss. Pasteurized whole cow's milk is deficient in iron, zinc, and vitamin C and has a high renal solute load, which makes it undesirable for infants younger than 12 months of age (AAP, Committee on Nutrition, 2009).

> **! NURSING ALERT**
>
> Dietary fat in infants younger than age 6 months should not be restricted unless on specific medical advice. Substituting skim or low-fat milk is unacceptable because the essential fatty acids are inadequate, and the solute concentration of protein and electrolytes, such as sodium, is too high.

The amount of formula per feeding and the number of feedings per day vary among infants. Infants being fed on demand usually determine their own feeding schedule, but some infants may need a more planned schedule based on average feeding patterns to ensure sufficient nutrients. In general, the number of feedings decreases from six at 1 month of age to four or five at 6 months. Regardless of the number of feedings, the total amount of formula ingested will usually level off at about 32 oz (946 ml) per day.

Honey should be avoided in the first 12 months because of the risk of botulism (see Chapter 40); pacifiers should not be coated with honey to encourage the infant to take it. Socializing the infant to food flavors of the family's culture is common in addition to continuing breastfeeding for 2 to 4 years (see Cultural Considerations box).

Bottled water for mixing powdered or concentrated formula is a relatively safe alternative to tap water if available tap water has a high content of contaminants such as lead. Do not assume, however, that bottled water is sterile unless specifically stated on the container. Fluoridated bottled water is not necessary for mixing powdered formula unless the local water source is low in fluoride, in which case fluoride supplementation is recommended after age 6 months (see Dental Health, p. 330).

The addition of solid foods before 4 to 6 months of age is not recommended. During the early months, solid foods are not compatible with the ability of the gastrointestinal tract and infant's nutritional needs. Feeding solids to young infants exposes them to food antigens that may produce food protein allergy. Ample evidence indicates that early introduction of foods other than maternal milk in the first 6 months of life predisposes children to an increased risk for food allergy development; foods known to be allergenic (e.g., peanuts, eggs, fish, seafood) should be introduced later than 12 months according to the child's risk for atopy (AAP, Committee on Nutrition, 2009).

Developmentally, infants are not ready for solid food. The extrusion (protrusion) reflex is strong and often causes them to push food out of the mouth. Infants instinctively suck when given food. Because of their limited motor abilities, infants are unable to deliberately push food away or avoid feeding. Therefore, early introduction of solids is a type of forced feeding that may lead to excessive weight gain and increased predisposition to allergies and iron-deficiency anemia.

> **⊕ CULTURAL CONSIDERATIONS**
>
> **Multicultural Feeding Practices**
>
> Cultural beliefs and values often influence infant-feeding practices. Health care professionals may benefit from understanding the multicultural feeding practices that parents choose for their infants. Traditional feeding practices include offering a variety of liquids or foods, such as sugared wine, water, or honey, during the first few days of life and thereafter.

Parents should be cautioned concerning the use of juices and non-nutritive drinks such as fruit-flavored drinks or carbonated beverages (soda or pop) during this period. Many juices and nonnutritive drinks, although readily available to consumers, do not provide sufficient and appropriate caloric intake for infants younger than 12 months of age; such drinks may replace the nutrients in breast milk or formula and lead to growth or health problems. Fruit juices are not required in the first 6 months; no studies have demonstrated benefits of giving fruit juice to infants.

The Second 6 Months

During the second half of the first year, human milk or formula should optimally continue to be the primary source of nutrition. Fluoride supplementation should begin, depending on the infant's intake of fluoride (in formula mixed with tap water or bottled water [containing fluoride] as appropriate) (see Dental Health, p. 330). If breastfeeding is discontinued, a commercial iron-fortified formula should be substituted. Follow-up or transition formulas marketed for older infants offer no special advantages over other infant formulas and provide excessive protein (AAP, Committee on Nutrition, 2009).

The major change in feeding habits is the addition of solid foods to the infant's diet. Physiologically and developmentally, infants 4 to 6 months of age are in a transition period. By this time, the gastrointestinal tract has matured sufficiently to handle more complex nutrients and is less sensitive to potentially allergenic foods. Tooth eruption is beginning and facilitates biting and chewing. The extrusion reflex has disappeared, and swallowing is more coordinated to allow infants to accept solids easily. Head control is well developed, which permits infants to sit with support and purposely turn their heads away to communicate lack of interest in food. Voluntary grasping and improved eye–hand coordination gradually allow infants to pick up finger foods and feed themselves. Their increasing sense of independence is evident in their desire to hold their bottles and try to "help" during feeding.

Selection and Preparation of Solid Foods

The choice of solid foods to introduce first is variable but should meet the reasons for feeding solids, such as supplying nutrients not found in formula or breast milk. Iron-fortified infant cereal is generally introduced first because of its high iron content (7 mg/3 Tbsp of prepared dry cereal). Commercially prepared ready-to-serve dry cereals for infants include rice, barley, oatmeal, and high-protein cereals; rice is usually suggested as an initial food because of its easy digestibility and low allergenic potential. Cereals such as cream of farina are not used because infant commercial cereals are a better source of iron. Some of the commercial baby cereals are combined with fruit. There is little nutritional benefit from these preparations, and they are more expensive. New foods should be added one at a time; therefore, parents should avoid cereal combinations when beginning a new grain.

Infant cereal (iron fortified) may be mixed with expressed breast milk or water until whole milk is given. After 6 months of age, small amounts of 100% fruit juices can be mixed with the dry cereal; the vitamin C content of the juice enhances the absorption of iron in the cereal. Because of their benefit as a source of iron, infant cereals should be continued until the child is 18 months of age.

Fruit juice can be offered from a cup for its rich source of vitamin C and as a substitute for milk for one feeding a day. Large quantities of certain juices (e.g., apple, pear, prune, sweet cherry, peach, grape) are avoided because they may cause abdominal pain, diarrhea, or bloating in some children. Avoid fruit-flavored drinks,

which may be marketed as juices but contain high concentrations of complex sugars. White grape juice (no more than 5 oz/day) may be better absorbed and safe for infants this age without causing gastrointestinal distress. The AAP, Committee on Nutrition (2009) recommends that fruit juice intake not exceed 4 to 6 oz per day and that juices not be given to infants younger than 4 to 6 months old. Because vitamin C is naturally destroyed by heat, juice is not warmed. Juice containers are always kept covered and refrigerated to prevent further vitamin loss.

The addition of other foods is arbitrary. A common sequence is to introduce strained fruits followed by vegetables and, finally, meats; however, some clinicians prefer to add vegetables before fruit. If foods are introduced early, citrus fruits, meats, and eggs are delayed until after 6 months of age because of their potential to result in allergy. At 6 months, foods such as a cracker or zwieback can be offered as finger and teething foods. By 8 to 9 months, junior foods and nutritious finger foods such as firmly cooked vegetable, raw pieces of fruit, or cheese can be given. By 1 year, well-cooked table foods are served.

The introduction of solid foods into the infant's diet at this age is primarily for taste and chewing experience, not for growth. The majority of infants' caloric needs are derived from the primary milk source (human or formula); therefore, solids should not be perceived as a substitute for milk until the child is older than 12 months. Portion sizes may vary according to the infant's taste. In general, 1 Tbsp per year of age (i.e., $\frac{1}{2}$ to $\frac{3}{4}$ Tbsp for most infants under 12 months) is adequate for most infants. In most cases 2 Tbsp may be served, but because of infants' focus on the texture and feel of the food, smaller amounts will be consumed. Another reason for smaller portions is the concern over feeding habits in early childhood and obesity; early feeding of smaller portions may help prevent the "clean your plate" or "eat all your food or you can't get down from the table" concepts, which are known to contribute to overeating in later life. The addition of solid foods to exclusively breastfed infants' diet does not significantly increase overall caloric intake or weight gain (Dewey, 2001).

Commercially prepared baby foods are the most common type of food served to infants in the United States. They are convenient but sometimes contain added salt or sugar and can be relatively expensive. An alternative is to prepare baby foods at home, which is a simple and inexpensive process. Fruits and vegetables can be steamed in a small amount of water and pureed in a blender or food processor. Many of them, such as ripe banana, can be mashed fine with a fork. Fruits such as apples or pears require little or no water in the cooking process. Vegetables such as carrots, potatoes, or string beans require additional water in the cooking and blending process.

In general, low-calorie milk and foods should be avoided in infants and toddlers unless a strict medically prescribed diet is required. Infants' growth during this phase is crucial to future development, and dietary fat should be curtailed with great caution. At the same time, it is important to recognize that certain types of dietary fat are unacceptable for infants; fried potatoes, candy, ice cream, cake, soda pop and other sweetened drinks, and other such items do not constitute an appropriate amount of fat intake and may contribute to childhood obesity. One suggestion is to limit the *amount* (serving size) of dietary fat in foods provided rather than eliminate them altogether, especially during infancy.

Parents are cautioned to avoid reliance on foods and supplements marketed as iron- or vitamin-fortified as primary sources of minerals. Instead, encourage parents to offer the child a variety of fruits, vegetables, and whole grains, including those known to naturally be rich in iron (Fox, Reidy, Novak, and others, 2006).

Introduction of Solid Foods

When the spoon is first introduced, infants often push it away and appear dissatisfied. Food that is placed on the front of the tongue and pushed out is simply scooped up and refed. As infants become accustomed to the spoon, they will more eagerly accept the food and eventually open the mouth in anticipation (or keep it closed in dislike).

One food item is introduced at intervals of 4 to 7 days to allow for identification of food allergies. New foods are fed in small amounts, from 1 tsp to a few Tbsp. As the amount of solid food increases, the quantity of milk is decreased to less than 1 L/day to prevent overfeeding.

Because feeding is a learning process, as well as a means of nutrition, new foods are given alone to allow the child to learn new tastes and textures. Food should not be mixed in the bottle and fed through a nipple with a large hole. This deprives the child of the pleasure of learning new tastes and developing a discriminating palate. It can also cause problems with poor chewing of food later in life because of lack of experience. Guidelines for the introduction of new foods are given in the Family-Centered Care box.

Weaning

Defined as the process of giving up one method of feeding for another, weaning usually refers to relinquishing the breast or bottle for a cup. In Western societies, this is generally regarded as a major task for infants and is often seen as a potentially traumatic experience. It is psychologically significant because infants are required to give up a major source of oral pleasure and gratification.

Other cultural groups define weaning in relation to significant life events (e.g., teething) or reaching a specific age. No one time for weaning is best for every child, but generally, most infants show signs of readiness during the second half of the first year. It is recommended that weaning occur with the infant's needs as a guide (Lawrence and Lawrence, 2011). Their increasing desire for freedom of movement may lessen their desire to be held close for feedings. They are acquiring more control over their actions and can easily manipulate a cup to their lips (even if it is held upside down!). Imitation becomes a powerful motivator by age 8 or 9 months, and they enjoy using a cup or glass like others do.

Weaning should be gradual by replacing one bottle or breastfeeding session at a time. The nighttime feeding is usually the last feeding to

---

FAMILY-CENTERED CARE
Feeding During the First Year

Birth to 6 Months (Breastfeeding or Bottle Feeding)
Breastfeeding
- Most desirable complete diet for the first half of the first year.*
- A recommended supplement is oral vitamin D (400 IU/day).
- In exclusively breastfed infants 4 months of age and older, recommend an iron supplement of 1 mg/kg/day until iron-rich complementary foods are introduced.

Formula
- Iron-fortified commercial formula is a complete food for the first half of the first year.*
- Requires fluoride supplements (0.25 mg) when the concentration of fluoride in the drinking water is below 0.3 ppm after 6 months of age.
- Evaporated milk formula requires supplements of vitamin C, iron, and fluoride (in accordance with the fluoride content of the local water supply after 6 months of age).

Age 4 to 12 Months (Solid Foods)
- May begin to add solids by 4 to 6 months of age.
- First foods are strained, pureed, or finely mashed.
- Finger foods such as teething crackers, raw fruit, or vegetables can be introduced by 6 to 7 months.
- Chopped table food or commercially prepared junior foods can be started by 9 to 12 months.
- With the exception of cereal, the order of introducing foods is variable; a recommended sequence is fruit, then vegetables, and then meat.
- Introduce one food at a time, usually at intervals of 4 to 7 days, to identify food allergies.
- Introduce solids when the infant is hungry.
- Begin spoon feeding by pushing food to back of tongue because of infants' natural tendency to thrust the tongue forward.
- Use a small spoon with a straight handle; begin with 1 or 2 tsp of food; gradually increase to 2 to 3 Tbsp per feeding.

- As the quantity of solids increases, decrease the quantity of milk to prevent overfeeding. Limit formula or milk to approximately 960 ml (32 oz) daily and fruit juice to less than 180 ml (6 oz) daily.
- Never introduce foods by mixing them with the formula in the bottle.

Cereal—Start at 4 to 6 Months of Age
- Introduce commercially prepared iron-fortified infant cereals and administer daily until 18 months.
- Rice cereal is usually introduced first because of its low allergenic potential.
- Parents can discontinue supplemental iron when iron-fortified cereal is given.

Fruits and Vegetables—Start at 6 to 8 Months of Age
- Applesauce, bananas, and pears are usually well tolerated.
- Avoid fruits and vegetables marketed in cans that are not specifically designed for infants because of variable and sometimes high lead content and addition of salt, sugar, or preservatives.
- Offer fruit juice only from a cup, not a bottle, to reduce the development of early childhood caries. Limit to 4 oz per day or less.

Meat, Fish, and Poultry—Start at 8 to 10 Months of Age
- Avoid fatty meats.
- Prepare by baking, broiling, steaming, or poaching.
- Include organ meats such as liver, which has a high iron, vitamin A, and vitamin B complex content.
- If soup is given, be certain all ingredients are familiar to child's diet.
- Avoid commercial meat and vegetable combinations because their protein content is low.

Eggs and Cheese—Start at 12 Months of Age
- Serve egg yolk hard boiled and mashed, soft cooked, or poached.
- Introduce egg white in small quantities (1 tsp) toward the end of the first year to detect an allergy.
- Use cheese as a substitute for meat and as finger food.

*Breastfeeding or commercial formula feeding for up to 12 months of age is recommended. After 1 year, whole cow's milk can be given.

be discontinued. It is advisable to never allow a child to take a bottle of milk to bed—this is a major cause of caries in deciduous teeth. If breastfeeding is terminated before 5 or 6 months of age, weaning should be to a bottle to provide for the infant's continued sucking needs. If discontinued later, weaning can be directly to a cup, especially by age 12 to 14 months. Any sweet liquid, such as fruit juice, should be given in a cup, and not at bedtime.

SLEEP AND ACTIVITY

Sleep patterns vary among infants, with active infants typically sleeping less than placid children. Generally, by 3 to 4 months of age, most infants have developed a nocturnal pattern of sleep that lasts 9 to 11 hours. The total daily sleep is approximately 15 hours. In a study of Swiss children, Iglowstein, Jenni, Molinari, and others (2003) found that the average number of hours of sleep in 6-month-old infants was 14.2 hours. Consolidation of nocturnal sleep hours occurred during the first 12 months with decreasing daytime sleep and increasing nighttime sleep (11.7 hours) by 1 year of age. The number of naps per day varies, but infants may take one or two naps by the end of the first year. Breastfed infants usually sleep for shorter periods, with more frequent waking, especially during the night, compared with bottle-fed infants (Quillin and Glenn, 2004); the average total sleep for 4-week-old infants in this study was 14 hours. Because of the trend toward breastfeeding, sleep norms such as those previously described, which were based primarily on bottle-fed infants, may not be relevant.

Most infants are naturally active and need no encouragement to be mobile. Problems can arise when devices such as play yards, strollers, commercial swings, and mobile walkers are used excessively. These items restrict movement and prevent infants from exploring and developing gross motor skills. Contrary to popular belief, mobile walkers do not enhance coordination and are dangerous if tipped over or placed near stairs. The AAP, Committee on Injury and Poison Prevention (2001) recommended a ban on the sale of infant walkers because of the large number of injuries. Newer models of infant walkers have been designed to decrease infant injuries. A discussion of sleep problems is found in Chapter 11.

DENTAL HEALTH

Good infant dental hygiene begins with appropriate maternal dental health before and during the pregnancy and counseling during early infancy regarding dietary intake for the promotion of optimum oral hygiene (Douglass, Douglass, and Silk, 2004). Parents are counseled early regarding the risk of feeding practices that increase the risk of poor dental health. Some of these, as previously mentioned, include avoiding propping the milk bottle; giving the milk bottle in the bed; or giving fruit juices in a bottle, especially before 6 months of age. These contribute to enamel erosion and **early childhood caries** (previously called baby bottle tooth decay).

When the primary teeth erupt, cleaning should begin. The teeth and gums are initially cleaned by wiping with a damp cloth; toothbrushing is too harsh for the tender gingiva. The caregiver can stabilize the infant by cradling the child with one arm and using the free hand to cleanse the teeth. Oral hygiene can be made pleasant by singing or talking to the infant. It is recommended that the infant have a brief oral health examination by 6 months of age from a qualified pediatric health practitioner; infants at high risk for caries are identified and oral health counseling is implemented. It is also recommended that the infant have an established dental home by 1 year of age (American Academy of Pediatric Dentistry, 2011). It is generally recommended that a small, soft-bristled toothbrush be used as more teeth erupt and the infant adjusts to the routine of cleaning. Water is preferred to toothpaste, which the infant will swallow (and if the toothpaste is fluoridated, the infant may ingest excessive amounts of fluoride). The American Academy of Pediatric Dentistry (2011) recommends a "smear" of toothpaste for children younger than 2 years and a pea-size amount for those 2 to 5 years old.

Fluoride, an essential mineral for building caries-resistant teeth, is needed beginning at 6 months of age if the infant does not receive water with adequate fluoride content. The AAP, Committee on Nutrition (2009) recommends that children 6 months to 3 years of age take 0.25 mg fluoride daily if water fluoride content is less than 0.3 ppm. The fluoride dosage has been decreased from earlier recommendations because of an increased occurrence of dental fluorosis from excessive fluoride ingestion. If bottled water is used to reconstitute powdered or concentrated formula, it should either be fluoride free or contain low levels of fluoride.

Dietary considerations are also important because habits begun during infancy tend to continue into later years. Avoid foods with concentrated sugar (sucrose) in the infant's diet. Parents need to be counseled regarding the detrimental effects of frequent and prolonged bottle or breastfeeding during sleep, when the milk or other fluid, such as juice, bathes the teeth, producing early childhood caries.

Dietary considerations are also important because habits begun during infancy tend to continue into later years. Foods with concentrated sugar are used sparingly (if at all) in the infant's diet. The practice of coating pacifiers with honey or using commercially available hard-candy pacifiers is discouraged. Besides being cariogenic, honey also may cause infant botulism, and parts of the candy pacifier can be aspirated (see Box 10-1). Parents need to be counseled regarding the detrimental effects of frequent and prolonged bottle feeding or breastfeeding during sleep, when the sweet milk or other fluid, such as juice, bathes the teeth, producing early childhood caries. In addition, carbonated beverages should be avoided in infancy. (See also Chapter 12 for a more extensive discussion of dental care, including early childhood caries.)

IMMUNIZATIONS

One of the most dramatic advances in pediatrics has been the decline of infectious diseases during the twentieth century because of the widespread use of immunization for preventable diseases. Although many of the immunizations can be given to individuals of any age, the recommended primary schedule begins during early infancy and, with the exception of boosters and specific adult and adolescent vaccines, is completed during early childhood. Therefore, health promotion during infancy includes a discussion of childhood immunizations for diphtheria, tetanus, and pertussis; poliovirus; measles, mumps, and rubella; *Haemophilus influenzae* type b; hepatitis B virus; hepatitis A virus; influenza (including H1N1); rotavirus; and chickenpox (varicella). Vaccines that provide protection against meningococcal and pneumococcal infections are also discussed. Selected vaccines generally reserved for children considered at high risk for the disease are discussed here and as appropriate throughout the text. (See also Communicable Diseases, Chapter 14, for a discussion of several of the diseases for which vaccines are available.)

Schedule for Immunizations

In the United States, two organizations—the Advisory Committee on Immunization Practices (ACIP) of the CDC and the Committee on Infectious Diseases of the AAP—govern the recommendations for immunization policies and procedures. In Canada, recommendations are from the National Advisory Committee on Immunization under the authority of the Minister of Health and Public Health Agency of Canada. The policies of each committee are *recommendations*, not rules, and they change as a result of advances in the field of immunology. Nurses need to keep informed of the latest advances and changes in policy (see Community Focus box).

In the United States, the recommended age for beginning primary immunizations of infants is within 2 weeks of birth or, in special circumstances, at birth (Fig. 10-11). Infants born preterm should receive the full dose of each vaccine at the appropriate chronologic age. Recommended schedules for children not immunized during infancy are available at the CDC's website at http://www.cdc.gov/vaccines/schedules/hcp/child-adolescent.html. Table 10-2 describes the recommended vaccine schedule for children in the Canadian provinces and territories.

Children who began primary immunizations at the recommended age but fail to receive all of the doses do not need to begin the series again but instead receive only the missed doses. For situations in which there is doubt that the child will return for immunization according to the optimum schedule, HepA, HepB, DTaP, IPV (poliovirus vaccine), MMR, varicella, and Hib vaccines can be administered simultaneously. Parenteral vaccines are given in separate syringes in different injection sites (AAP, Committee on Infectious Diseases, 2009). The product brand names, routes of administration, and manufacturers for the principal childhood vaccinations are listed at http://www.cdc.gov/vaccines/recs/acip/vac-abbrev.htm#abrv.

Recommendations for Routine Immunizations*
Hepatitis A Virus

Hepatitis A virus (HAV) has been recognized as a significant child health problem, particularly in communities with unusually high infection rates. HAV is spread by the fecal–oral route and from person-to-person contact, by ingestion of contaminated food or water, and rarely by blood transfusion. The illness has an abrupt onset, with fever, malaise, anorexia, nausea, abdominal discomfort, dark urine, and jaundice being the most common clinical signs of infection. In children younger than 6 years of age, who represent approximately one third of all cases of HAV, the disease may be asymptomatic, and jaundice is rarely evident.

Hepatitis A vaccine is now recommended for all children beginning at age 1 year (i.e., 12–23 months). The second dose in the two-dose series may be administered no sooner than 6 months after the first dose. For further information, see Figure 10-11, *A*, footnote 10.

Hepatitis B Virus

Hepatitis B virus (HBV) is a significant pediatric disease because HBV infections that occur during childhood and adolescence can lead to fatal consequences from cirrhosis or liver cancer during adulthood. Up to 90% of infants infected perinatally and 25% to 50% of children infected before age 5 years become HBV carriers. In addition, the incidence of HBV infection increases rapidly during adolescence (AAP, Committee on Infectious Diseases, 2009). It is recommended that newborns receive the HepB vaccine before hospital discharge if the mother

---

*Because of constant changes in the pharmaceutical industry, trade names of single and combination vaccines in this section may differ from those currently available. Readers are encouraged to access the vaccine page of the Center for Biologics Evaluation and Research of the Food and Drug Administration for the latest licensed vaccine trade names at http://www.fda.gov/BiologicsBloodVaccines/Vaccines/default.htm.

Recommended Immunization Schedule for Persons Aged 0 Through 6 Years—United States • 2012
For those who fall behind or start late, see the catch-up schedule*

Vaccine ▼ Age ►	Birth	1 month	2 months	4 months	6 months	9 months	12 months	15 months	18 months	19–23 months	2–3 years	4–6 years	
Hepatitis B[1]	Hep B	HepB			HepB								Range of recommended ages for all children
Rotavirus[2]			RV	RV	RV[2]								
Diphtheria, tetanus, pertussis[3]			DTaP	DTaP	DTaP		see footnote[3]	DTaP				DTaP	
Haemophilus influenzae type b[4]			Hib	Hib	Hib[4]		Hib						Range of recommended ages for certain high-risk groups
Pneumococcal[5]			PCV	PCV	PCV		PCV				PPSV		
Inactivated poliovirus[6]			IPV	IPV		IPV						IPV	
Influenza[7]					Influenza (Yearly)								
Measles, mumps, rubella[8]							MMR			see footnote[8]		MMR	Range of recommended ages for all children and certain high-risk groups
Varicella[9]							Varicella			see footnote[9]		Varicella	
Hepatitis A[10]							Dose 1[10]				HepA Series		
Meningococcal[11]						MCV4 — see footnote[11]							

This schedule includes recommendations in effect as of December 23, 2011. Any dose not administered at the recommended age should be administered at a subsequent visit, when indicated and feasible. The use of a combination vaccine generally is preferred over separate injections of its equivalent component vaccines. Vaccination providers should consult the relevant Advisory Committee on Immunization Practices (ACIP) statement for detailed recommendations, available online at http://www.cdc.gov/vaccines/pubs/acip-list.htm. Clinically significant adverse events that follow vaccination should be reported to the Vaccine Adverse Event Reporting System (VAERS) online (http://www.vaers.hhs.gov) or by telephone (800-822-7967).

1. **Hepatitis B (HepB) vaccine.** (Minimum age: birth)
   At birth:
   - Administer monovalent HepB vaccine to all newborns before hospital discharge.
   - For infants born to hepatitis B surface antigen (HBsAg)–positive mothers, administer HepB vaccine and 0.5 mL of hepatitis B immune globulin (HBIG) within 12 hours of birth. These infants should be tested for HBsAg and antibody to HBsAg (anti-HBs) 1 to 2 months after receiving the last dose of the series.
   - If mother's HBsAg status is unknown, within 12 hours of birth administer HepB vaccine for infants weighing ≥2,000 grams, and HepB vaccine plus HBIG for infants weighing <2,000 grams. Determine mother's HBsAg status as soon as possible and, if she is HBsAg-positive, administer HBIG for infants weighing ≥2,000 grams (no later than age 1 week).
   Doses after the birth dose:
   - The second dose should be administered at age 1 to 2 months. Monovalent HepB vaccine should be used for doses administered before age 6 weeks.
   - Administration of a total of 4 doses of HepB vaccine is permissible when a combination vaccine containing HepB is administered after the birth dose.
   - Infants who did not receive a birth dose should receive 3 doses of a HepB-containing vaccine starting as soon as feasible.
   - The minimum interval between dose 1 and dose 2 is 4 weeks, and between dose 2 and 3 is 8 weeks. The final (third or fourth) dose in the HepB vaccine series should be administered no earlier than age 24 weeks and at least 16 weeks after the first dose.

2. **Rotavirus (RV) vaccines.** (Minimum age: 6 weeks for both RV-1 [Rotarix] and RV-5 [Rota Teq])
   - The maximum age for the first dose in the series is 14 weeks, 6 days; and 8 months, 0 days for the final dose in the series. Vaccination should not be initiated for infants aged 15 weeks, 0 days or older.
   - If RV-1 (Rotarix) is administered at ages 2 and 4 months, a dose at 6 months is not indicated.

3. **Diphtheria and tetanus toxoids and acellular pertussis (DTaP) vaccine.** (Minimum age: 6 weeks)
   - The fourth dose may be administered as early as age 12 months, provided at least 6 months have elapsed since the third dose.

4. **Haemophilus influenzae type b (Hib) conjugate vaccine.** (Minimum age: 6 weeks)
   - If PRP-OMP (PedvaxHIB or Comvax [HepB-Hib]) is administered at ages 2 and 4 months, a dose at age 6 months is not indicated.
   - Hiberix should only be used for the booster (final) dose in children aged 12 months through 4 years.

5. **Pneumococcal vaccines.** (Minimum age: 6 weeks for pneumococcal conjugate vaccine [PCV]; 2 years for pneumococcal polysaccharide vaccine [PPSV])
   - Administer 1 dose of PCV to all healthy children aged 24 through 59 months who are not completely vaccinated for their age.
   - For children who have received an age-appropriate series of 7-valent PCV (PCV7), a single supplemental dose of 13-valent PCV (PCV13) is recommended for:
     — All children 14 through 59 months
     — Children aged 60 through 71 months with underlying medical conditions.
   - Administer PPSV at least 8 weeks after last dose of PCV to children aged 2 years or older with certain underlying medical conditions, including a cochlear implant. See MMWR 2010;59(No. RR-11), available at http://www.cdc.gov/mmwr/pdf/rr/rr5911.pdf.

6. **Inactivated poliovirus vaccine (IPV).** (Minimum age: 6 weeks)
   - If 4 or more doses are administered before age 4 years, an additional dose should be administered at age 4 through 6 years.
   - The final dose in the series should be administered on or after the fourth birthday and at least 6 months after the previous dose.

7. **Influenza vaccines.** (Minimum age: 6 months for trivalent inactivated influenza vaccine [TIV]; 2 years for live, attenuated influenza vaccine [LAIV])
   - For most healthy children aged 2 years and older, either LAIV or TIV may be used. However, LAIV should not be administered to some children, including 1) children with asthma, 2) children 2 through 4 years who had wheezing in the past 12 months, or 3) children who have any other underlying medical conditions that predispose them to influenza complications. For all other contraindications to use of LAIV, see MMWR 2010;59(No. RR-8), available at http://www.cdc.gov/mmwr/pdf/rr/rr5908.pdf.
   - For children aged 6 months through 8 years:
     — For the 2011–12 season, administer 2 doses (separated by at least 4 weeks) to those who did not receive at least 1 dose of the 2010–11 vaccine. Those who received at least 1 dose of the 2010–11 vaccine require 1 dose for the 2011–12 season.
     — For the 2012–13 season, follow dosing guidelines in the 2012 ACIP influenza vaccine recommendations.

8. **Measles, mumps, and rubella (MMR) vaccine.** (Minimum age: 12 months)
   - The second dose may be administered before age 4 years, provided at least 4 weeks have elapsed since the first dose.
   - Administer MMR vaccine to infants aged 6 through 11 months who are traveling internationally. These children should be revaccinated with 2 doses of MMR vaccine, the first at ages 12 through 15 months and at least 4 weeks after the previous dose, and the second at ages 4 through 6 years.

9. **Varicella (VAR) vaccine.** (Minimum age: 12 months)
   - The second dose may be administered before age 4 years, provided at least 3 months have elapsed since the first dose.
   - For children aged 12 months through 12 years, the recommended minimum interval between doses is 3 months. However, if the second dose was administered at least 4 weeks after the first dose, it can be accepted as valid.

10. **Hepatitis A (HepA) vaccine.** (Minimum age: 12 months)
    - Administer the second (final) dose 6 to18 months after the first.
    - Unvaccinated children 24 months and older at high risk should be vaccinated. See MMWR 2006;55(No. RR-7), available at http://www.cdc.gov/mmwr/pdf/rr/rr5507.pdf.
    - A 2-dose HepA vaccine series is recommended for anyone aged 24 months and older, previously unvaccinated, for whom immunity against hepatitis A virus infection is desired.

11. **Meningococcal conjugate vaccines, quadrivalent (MCV4).** (Minimum age: 9 months for Menactra [MCV4-D], 2 years for Menveo [MCV4-CRM])
    - For children aged 9 through 23 months 1) with persistent complement component deficiency; 2) who are residents of or travelers to countries with hyperendemic or epidemic disease; or 3) who are present during outbreaks caused by a vaccine serogroup, administer 2 primary doses of MCV4-D, ideally at ages 9 months and 12 months or at least 8 weeks apart.
    - For children aged 24 months and older with 1) persistent complement component deficiency who have not been previously vaccinated; or 2) anatomic/functional asplenia, administer 2 primary doses of either MCV4 at least 8 weeks apart.
    - For children with anatomic/functional asplenia, if MCV4-D (Menactra) is used, administer at a minimum age of 2 years and at least 4 weeks after completion of all PCV oses.
    - See MMWR 2011;60:72–6, available at http://www.cdc.gov/mmwr/pdf/wk/mm6003. pdf, and Vaccines for Children Program resolution No. 6/11-1, available at http://www. cdc.gov/vaccines/programs/vfc/downloads/resolutions/06-11mening-mcv.pdf, and MMWR 2011;60:1391–2, available at http://www.cdc.gov/mmwr/pdf/wk/mm6040. pdf, for further guidance, including revaccination guidelines.

This schedule is approved by the Advisory Committee on Immunization Practices (http://www.cdc.gov/vaccines/recs/acip), the American Academy of Pediatrics (http://www.aap.org), and the American Academy of Family Physicians (http://www.aafp.org). Department of Health and Human Services • Centers for Disease Control and Prevention

A

FIG 10-11 A, Recommended immunization schedules for persons aged 0 through 6 years—United States, 2012. **B,** Recommended immunization schedules for persons aged 7 through 18 years—United States, 2012. (From Centers for Disease Control and Prevention: Recommended immunization schedules for persons aged 0 through 18 years—United States, 2012, *MMWR Morb Mortal Wkly Rep* 61[05]:1–4, 2012.)

*Catch-up schedule is available at http://www.cdc.gov/vaccines/schedules/hcp/child-adolescent.html.

Recommended Immunization Schedule for Persons Aged 7 Through 18 Years—United States • 2012
For those who fall behind or start late, see the schedule below and the catch-up schedule*

Vaccine ▼ Age ►	7–10 years	11–12 years	13–18 years	
Tetanus, diphtheria, pertussis[1]	1 dose (if indicated)	1 dose	1 dose (if indicated)	Range of recommended ages for all children
Human papillomavirus[2]	see footnote[2]	3 doses	Complete 3-dose series	
Meningococcal[3]	See footnote[3]	Dose 1	Booster at 16 years old	Range of recommended ages for catch-up immunization
Influenza[4]	Influenza (yearly)			
Pneumococcal[5]	See footnote[5]			
Hepatitis A[6]	Complete 2-dose series			Range of recommended ages for certain high-risk groups
Hepatitis B[7]	Complete 3-dose series			
Inactivated poliovirus[8]	Complete 3-dose series			
Measles, mumps, rubella[9]	Complete 2-dose series			
Varicella[10]	Complete 2-dose series			

This schedule includes recommendations in effect as of December 23, 2011. Any dose not administered at the recommended age should be administered at a subsequent visit, when indicated and feasible. The use of a combination vaccine generally is preferred over separate injections of its equivalent component vaccines. Vaccination providers should consult the relevant Advisory Committee on Immunization Practices (ACIP) statement for detailed recommendations, available online at http://www.cdc.gov/vaccines/pubs/acip-list.htm. Clinically significant adverse events that follow vaccination should be reported to the Vaccine Adverse Event Reporting System (VAERS) online (http://www.vaers.hhs.gov) or by telephone (800-822-7967).

1. **Tetanus and diphtheria toxoids and acellular pertussis (Tdap) vaccine.** (Minimum age: 10 years for Boostrix and 11 years for Adacel)
   - Persons aged 11 through 18 years who have not received Tdap vaccine should receive a dose followed by tetanus and diphtheria toxoids (Td) booster doses every 10 years thereafter.
   - Tdap vaccine should be substituted for a single dose of Td in the catch-up series for children aged 7 through 10 years. Refer to the catch-up schedule if additional doses of tetanus and diphtheria toxoid–containing vaccine are needed.
   - Tdap vaccine can be administered regardless of the interval since the last tetanus and diphtheria toxoid–containing vaccine.
2. **Human papillomavirus (HPV) vaccines (HPV4 [Gardasil] and HPV2 [Cervarix]).** (Minimum age: 9 years)
   - Either HPV4 or HPV2 is recommended in a 3-dose series for females aged 11 or 12 years. HPV4 is recommended in a 3-dose series for males aged 11 or 12 years.
   - The vaccine series can be started beginning at age 9 years.
   - Administer the second dose 1 to 2 months after the first dose and the third dose 6 months after the first dose (at least 24 weeks after the first dose).
   - See MMWR 2010;59:626–32, available at http://www.cdc.gov/mmwr/pdf/wk/mm5920.pdf.
3. **Meningococcal conjugate vaccines, quadrivalent (MCV4).**
   - Administer MCV4 at age 11 through 12 years with a booster dose at age 16 years.
   - Administer MCV4 at age 13 through 18 years if patient is not previously vaccinated.
   - If the first dose is administered at age 13 through 15 years, a booster dose should be administered at age 16 through 18 years with a minimum interval of at least 8 weeks after the preceding dose.
   - If the first dose is administered at age 16 years or older, a booster dose is not needed.
   - Administer 2 primary doses at least 8 weeks apart to previously unvaccinated persons with persistent complement component deficiency or anatomic/functional asplenia, and 1 dose every 5 years thereafter.
   - Adolescents aged 11 through 18 years with human immunodeficiency virus (HIV) infection should receive a 2-dose primary series of MCV4, at least 8 weeks apart.
   - See MMWR 2011;60:72–76, available at http://www.cdc.gov/mmwr/pdf/wk/mm6003.pdf, and Vaccines for Children Program resolution No. 6/11-1, available at http://www.cdc.gov/vaccines/programs/vfc/downloads/resolutions/06-11mening-mcv.pdf, for further guidelines.
4. **Influenza vaccines (trivalent inactivated influenza vaccine [TIV] and live, attenuated influenza vaccine [LAIV]).**
   - For most healthy, nonpregnant persons, either LAIV or TIV may be used, except LAIV should not be used for some persons, including those with asthma or any other underlying medical conditions that predispose them to influenza complications. For all other contraindications to use of LAIV, see MMWR 2010;59(No.RR-8), available at http://www.cdc.gov/mmwr/pdf/rr/rr5908.pdf.
   - Administer 1 dose to persons aged 9 years and older.

- For children aged 6 months through 8 years:
  — For the 2011–12 season, administer 2 doses (separated by at least 4 weeks) to those who did not receive at least 1 dose of the 2010–11 vaccine. Those who received at least 1 dose of the 2010–11 vaccine require 1 dose for the 2011–12 season.
  — For the 2012–13 season, follow dosing guidelines in the 2012 ACIP influenza vaccine recommendations.
5. **Pneumococcal vaccines (pneumococcal conjugate vaccine [PCV] and pneumococcal polysaccharide vaccine [PPSV]).**
   - A single dose of PCV may be administered to children aged 6 through 18 years who have anatomic/functional asplenia, HIV infection or other immunocompromising condition, cochlear implant, or cerebral spinal fluid leak. See MMWR 2010:59(No. RR-11), available at http://www.cdc.gov/mmwr/pdf/rr/rr5911.pdf.
   - Administer PPSV at least 8 weeks after the last dose of PCV to children aged 2 years or older with certain underlying medical conditions, including a cochlear implant. A single revaccination should be administered after 5 years to children with anatomic/functional asplenia or an immunocompromising condition.
6. **Hepatitis A (HepA) vaccine.**
   - HepA vaccine is recommended for children older than 23 months who live in areas where vaccination programs target older children, who are at increased risk for infection, or for whom immunity against hepatitis A virus infection is desired. See MMWR 2006;55(No. RR-7), available at http://www.cdc.gov/mmwr/pdf/rr/rr5507.pdf.
   - Administer 2 doses at least 6 months apart to unvaccinated persons.
7. **Hepatitis B (HepB) vaccine.**
   - Administer the 3-dose series to those not previously vaccinated.
   - For those with incomplete vaccination, follow the catch-up recommendations.
   - A 2-dose series (doses separated by at least 4 months) of adult formulation Recombivax HB is licensed for use in children aged 11 through 15 years.
8. **Inactivated poliovirus vaccine (IPV).**
   - The final dose in the series should be administered at least 6 months after the previous dose.
   - If both OPV and IPV were administered as part of a series, a total of 4 doses should be administered, regardless of the child's current age.
   - IPV is not routinely recommended for U.S. residents aged 18 years or older.
9. **Measles, mumps, and rubella (MMR) vaccine.**
   - The minimum interval between the 2 doses of MMR vaccine is 4 weeks.
10. **Varicella (VAR) vaccine.**
   - For persons without evidence of immunity (see MMWR 2007;56[No. RR-4], available at http://www.cdc.gov/mmwr/pdf/rr/rr5604.pdf), administer 2 doses if not previously vaccinated or the second dose if only 1 dose has been administered.
   - For persons aged 7 through 12 years, the recommended minimum interval between doses is 3 months. However, if the second dose was administered at least 4 weeks after the first dose, it can be accepted as valid.
   - For persons aged 13 years and older, the minimum interval between doses is 4 weeks.

This schedule is approved by the Advisory Committee on Immunization Practices (http://www.cdc.gov/vaccines/recs/acip), the American Academy of Pediatrics (http://www.aap.org), and the American Academy of Family Physicians (http://www.aafp.org).
Department of Health and Human Services • Centers for Disease Control and Prevention

B

FIG 10-11, cont'd

TABLE 10-2 CANADIAN IMMUNIZATION SCHEDULES FOR INFANTS AND CHILDREN

A. ROUTINE IMMUNIZATION SCHEDULE FOR INFANTS AND CHILDREN

Age at vaccination	DTaP-IPV[a]	Hib[b]	MMR[c]	Var[d]	HB[e]	Pneu–C-7[f]	Men-C[g]	Tdap[h]	HPV[i]	Inf[j]
Birth	—	—	—	—	—	—	—	—	—	—
2 months	Yes	Yes	—	—	—	Yes	Yes*	—	—	—
4 months	Yes	Yes	—	—	Yes;	Yes	Yes*	—	—	—
6 months	Yes	Yes	—	—	Infancy, 3 doses	Yes	Yes* and	—	—	Yes; 6–23 months, 1–2 doses
12 months	—	—	Yes	Yes	↓	Yes; 12–15 months	Yes	—	—	
18 months	Yes	Yes	Yes or	↓	or		↓	—	—	
4–6 years	Yes	Yes	Yes		↓	—	and	—	—	—
12 years	—	—	—	—	Preteen/teen, 2–3 doses	—	Yes	—	Yes; Females, 9–13 years, 3 doses	—
14–16 years	—	—	—	—	—	—	—	Yes	—	—

B. ROUTINE IMMUNIZATION SCHEDULE FOR CHILDREN <7 YEARS OF AGE NOT IMMUNIZED IN EARLY INFANCY

Timing	DTaP-IPV	Hib	MMR	Var	HB	Pneu–C-7	Men-C	Tdap	HPV
First visit	Yes	Yes	Yes	Yes	Yes	Yes	Yes	—	—
2 months later	Yes	Yes*	Yes	—	Yes	Yes*	—	—	—
2 months later	Yes	—	—	—	—	Yes*	—	—	—
6–12 months later	Yes	Yes*	—	—	Yes	—	—	—	—
4–6 years of age	Yes*	—	—	—	—	—	—	—	—
12 years of age	—	—	—	—	—	—	Yes	—	Yes; Females, 9–13 years, 3 doses
14–16 years of age	—	—	—	—	—	—	—	Yes	—

C. ROUTINE IMMUNIZATION SCHEDULE FOR CHILDREN ≥7 YEARS OF AGE UP TO 17 YEARS OF AGE NOT IMMUNIZED IN EARLY INFANCY

Timing	IPV[k]	MMR	Var	HB	Men-C	Tdap	HPV
First visit	Yes	Yes	Yes	Yes	Yes	Yes	Yes
2 months later	Yes	Yes	Yes*	Yes*	—	Yes	Yes; Females, ≥9 years
6–12 months later	Yes	—	—	Yes	—	Yes	Yes
10 years later	—	—	—	—	—	Yes	—

Modified from Public Health Agency of Canada: Immunization Schedules for Infants and Children, Canada, 2012, The Agency, available at http://www.phac-aspc.gc.ca/im/is-cv/index-eng.php#a. Reproduced with the permission of the Minister of Public Works and Government Services, 2012.

*Asterisks imply that these doses may not be required, depending upon the age of the child or adult.

[a]**Diphtheria, tetanus, acellular pertussis and inactivated polio virus vaccine (DTaP-IPV):** DTaP-IPV(± Hib) vaccine is the preferred vaccine for all doses in the vaccination series, including completion of the series in children who have received one or more doses of DPT (whole cell) vaccine (e.g., recent immigrants). In schedules A and B, the 4–6 year dose can be omitted if the fourth dose was given after the fourth birthday.

[b]***Haemophilus influenzae* type b conjugate vaccine (Hib):** The Hib schedule shown is for the *Haemophilus* b capsular polysaccharide—polyribosylribitol phosphate (PRP) conjugated to tetanus toxoid (PRP-T). For catch up, the number of doses depends on the age at which the schedule is begun. Not usually required past age 5 years.

[c]**Measles, mumps, and rubella vaccine (MMR):** A second dose of MMR is recommended for children at least 1 month after the first dose for the purpose of better measles protection. For convenience, options include giving it with the next scheduled vaccination at 18 months of age or at school entry (4–6 years) (depending on the provincial/territorial policy) or at any intervening age that is practical. In the catch-up schedule (B), the first dose should not be given until the child is ≥12 months old. MMR should be given to all susceptible adolescents and adults.

[d]**Varicella vaccine (Var):** Children aged 12 months to 12 years should receive one dose of varicella vaccine. Susceptible individuals ≥13 years of age should receive two doses at least 28 days apart.

[e]**Hepatitis B vaccine (HB):** Hepatitis B vaccine can be routinely given to infants or pre-adolescents, depending on the provincial/territorial policy. For infants born to chronic carrier mothers, the first dose should be given at birth (with hepatitis B immunoglobulin), otherwise the first dose can be given at 2 months of age to fit more conveniently with other routine infant immunization visits. The second dose should be administered at least 1 month after the first dose, and the third at least 2 months after the second dose, but these may fit more conveniently into the 4 and 6 month immunization visits. A two-dose schedule for adolescents is an option.

TABLE 10-2   CANADIAN IMMUNIZATION SCHEDULES FOR INFANTS AND CHILDREN—cont'd

[f]**Pneumococcal conjugate vaccine–7-valent (Pneu–C-7):** Recommended for all children under 2 years of age. The recommended schedule depends on the age of the child when vaccination is begun.

[g]**Meningococcal C conjugate vaccine (Men-C):** Recommended for children under 5 years of age, adolescents, and young adults. The recommended schedule depends on the age of the individual and the conjugate vaccine used. At least one dose in the primary infant series should be given after 5 months of age. If the provincial/territorial policy is to give Men-C to persons ≥12 months of age, one dose is sufficient.

[h]**Diphtheria, tetanus, acellular pertussis vaccine—adult/adolescent formulation (Tdap):** A combined adsorbed "adult type" preparation for use in people ≥7 years of age, contains less diphtheria toxoid and pertussis antigens than preparations given to younger children and is less likely to cause reactions in older people.

[i]**Human papillomavirus (HPV):** HPV vaccine is recommended for routine use in females between 9 and13 years of age, before the onset of sexual intercourse. The recommended schedule is 3 doses at 0, 2, and 6 months, with a minimum interval of one month between the first two doses. HPV vaccine is also recommended for females between 14 and 26 years who would benefit from the vaccine.

[j]**Influenza vaccine (Inf):** Recommended for all children 6–23 months of age and all persons ≥65 years of age. Previously unvaccinated children <9 years of age require two doses of the current season's vaccine with an interval of at least 4 weeks. The second dose within the same season is not required if the child received one or more doses of influenza vaccine during the previous influenza season.

[k]**IPV Inactivated polio virus**

is hepatitis B surface antigen (HBsAg) negative. Monovalent HepB vaccine should be given as the birth dose; combination vaccine containing HepB may be given for subsequent doses in the series (see also Fig. 10-11, *A*, footnote 1). Both full-term and preterm infants born to mothers whose HBsAg status is positive or unknown should receive HepB and hepatitis B immune globulin (HBIG) vaccines, 0.5 ml, within 12 hours of birth at two different injection sites. Because the immune response to HepB vaccine is not optimum in newborns weighing less than 2000 g (4.4 lb), the first HepB dose should be given to such infants at 1 month as long as the mother's HBsAg status is negative (AAP, Committee on Infectious Diseases, 2009). In the event that a preterm infant is given a dose at birth, the current recommendation is that the infant be given the full series (three additional doses) at 1, 2, and 6 months of age. The AAP, Committee on Infectious Diseases (2009) also encourages immunization of all children by age 11 years.

In the late 1990s, the HepB vaccine contained small amounts of mercury (thimerosal) as a preservative, which generated concern regarding possible mercury poisoning in infants and led to a subsequent decrease in HepB immunization rates in newborns. However, a preservative-free HepB (Recombivax HB, pediatric-adolescent formulation) is available, and the CDC (2005a, 2011a) strongly recommends that HepB immunization occur in newborns before discharge from the birth hospital. To date, studies have not found any association between thimerosal in vaccines and neurologic developmental disorders such as autism spectrum disorder (DeStefano, 2007; Miller and Reynolds, 2009; Price, Thompson, Goodson, and others, 2010) (see Critical Thinking Case Study).

The vaccine is given intramuscularly in the vastus lateralis in newborns or in the deltoid for older infants and children. One study found that needle length affected the immune response of obese adolescents receiving the HepB vaccine; according to this study, obese adolescents immunized with a 1.5-inch (38-mm) needle achieved significantly higher antibody titers to HBV than those immunized with a standard 1-inch needle (Middleman, Anding, and Tung, 2010). Regardless of age, the dorsogluteal site should be avoided because it has been associated with low antibody seroconversion rates, indicating a reduced immune response. No data exist regarding the seroconversion when the ventrogluteal site is used. The vaccine can be safely administered simultaneously at a separate site with DTaP, MMR, and Hib vaccines.

? CRITICAL THINKING CASE STUDY
Childhood Immunizations and Autism

Monica, a 26-year-old mother of two children, aged 8 months and 2 years, brings them to the clinic for a well-child check. When asked if the children are up to date on their immunization schedule, Monica replies that she and her partner have decided not to have the children immunized. She states that a neighbor has a 9-year-old child with autism, and her Internet research and talks with various neighbors have convinced them that autism may possibly be caused by all of the immunizations children are receiving. Monica also points out that her children do not go to daycare and that she plans to home school them; therefore, she believes the risk for communicable disease contraction is low. "Besides, none of our neighborhood kids have ever had any of those diseases like measles or chickenpox because their parents get them immunized," she states. Upon physical examination, the two children appear to be in excellent health, and their previous health history and family health history do not reveal any major health risk factors.

1. Evidence: Is there sufficient evidence to draw any conclusions about Monica's concerns about childhood immunizations?
2. Assumptions: Describe any underlying assumptions about the following:
   a. Childhood immunizations and autism
   b. Monica's reasons for not immunizing her children
   c. The concept of herd immunity
3. What approach would be the best to address Monica's concerns about not immunizing her children?
4. Is there objective evidence to support your conclusions?

Diphtheria

Although cases of diphtheria are rare in the United States, the disease can result in significant morbidity. Respiratory manifestations include respiratory nasopharyngitis or obstructive laryngotracheitis with upper airway obstruction. The cutaneous manifestations of the disease include vaginal, otic, conjunctival, or cutaneous lesions, which are primarily seen in urban homeless persons and in the tropics (AAP, Committee on Infectious Diseases, 2009). Administer a single dose of equine antitoxin intravenously to the child with clinical symptoms because of the often fulminant progression of the disease (AAP, Committee on Infectious Diseases, 2009). Diphtheria vaccine is commonly administered (1) in combination with tetanus and pertussis vaccines

(DTaP) or DTaP and Hib vaccines for children younger than 7 years of age, (2) in combination with a conjugate Hib vaccine (see Fig. 10-11), (3) in a combined vaccine with tetanus (DT) for children younger than 7 years of age who have some contraindication to receiving pertussis vaccine, (4) in combination with tetanus and acellular pertussis (Tdap) for children 11 years and older, or (5) as a single antigen when combined antigen preparations are not indicated. Although the diphtheria vaccine does not produce absolute immunity, protective antitoxin persists for 10 years or more when given according to the recommended schedule, and boosters are given every 10 years for life (see discussion below for adolescent diphtheria and acellular pertussis and tetanus toxoid recommendation). Several vaccines contain diphtheria toxoid (Hib, meningococcal, pneumococcal), but this does not confer immunity to the disease.

Tetanus

Three forms of tetanus vaccine—tetanus toxoid, tetanus immunoglobulin (TIG) (human), and tetanus antitoxin (equine antitoxin)—are available; however, tetanus antitoxin is no longer available in the United States. Tetanus toxoid is used for routine primary immunization, usually in one of the combinations listed for diphtheria, and provides protective antitoxin levels for approximately 10 years.

Tetanus and diphtheria toxoids along with acellular pertussis vaccine (Tdap, adolescent formulation) are now recommended for children ages 11 to 12 years who have completed the recommended DTaP/DTP vaccine series but have not received the tetanus (Td) booster dose. Adolescents 13 to 18 years of age who have not received the Td/Tdap booster should receive a single Tdap booster, provided the routine DTaP/DTP childhood immunization series has been previously received. In response to the increase in cases of pertussis in children, adolescents, and adults, the ACIP now recommends that a Tdap booster be administered regardless of the time interval from the last tetanus- or diptheria-toxoid–containing vaccine (DTaP, DTP, Td, or Tdap). In addition, children ages 7 through 10 years who are not fully vaccinated for pertussis (did not receive 5 doses of DTaP or 4 doses of DTaP with the fourth dose being administered on or after the fourth birthday) should receive a dose of Tdap (CDC, 2011b). Boostrix (Tdap) is currently licensed for children 10 to 18 years of age, and Adacel (Tdap) is licensed for individuals 11 to 64 years of age. For more information see Figure 10-11, *B*, footnote 1.

For wound management, passive immunity is available with TIG. Persons with a history of two previous doses of tetanus toxoid can receive a booster dose of the toxoid. Separate syringes and different sites are used when tetanus toxoid and TIG are given concurrently.

For children older than 7 years who require wound prophylaxis, tetanus immunization may be accomplished by administering Td (adult-type diphtheria and tetanus toxoids). If TIG is not available, the equine antitoxin (not available in the United States) may be administered after appropriate testing for sensitivity. The antitoxin is administered in a separate syringe and at a separate intramuscular site if given concurrently with tetanus toxoid.

Pertussis

Pertussis vaccine is recommended for all children 6 weeks through 6 years of age (up to the seventh birthday) who have no neurologic contraindications to its use. Concerns over outbreaks of the disease in the past decade have prompted discussion about vaccinating infants and adults. Many cases of pertussis have occurred in children younger than 6 months or persons older than 7 years, both groups falling in the category for which pertussis immunization previously was not recommended (CDC, 2005c). The tetanus and diphtheria

toxoids and acellular pertussis vaccine (Tdap) is now recommended at ages 11 to 12 years for children who have completed the DTaP/DTP childhood series. The Tdap is also recommended for adolescents 13 to 18 years old who have not received a tetanus booster (Td) or Tdap dose and have completed the childhood DTaP/DTP series. When the Tdap is used as a booster dose, it may be administered earlier than the previous 5-year interval to provide adequate pertussis immunity (regardless of interval from the last Td dose) (CDC, 2011b). In addition, children ages 7 through 10 years who are not fully vaccinated for pertussis (did not receive five doses of DTaP or four doses of DTaP with the fourth dose being administered on or after the fourth birthday) should receive a dose of Tdap (CDC, 2011b) (see discussion in Tetanus).

Currently, two forms of pertussis vaccine are available in the United States. The whole-cell pertussis vaccine is prepared from inactivated cells of *Bordetella pertussis* and contains multiple antigens. In contrast, the acellular pertussis vaccine contains one or more immunogens derived from the *B. pertussis* organism. The highly purified acellular vaccine is associated with fewer local and systemic reactions than those occurring with the whole-cell vaccine in children of similar age. The acellular pertussis vaccine is recommended for the first three immunizations and is usually given at 2, 4, and 6 months, 15 to 18 months, and 4 to 6 years of age with diphtheria and tetanus (DTaP). Several forms of acellular pertussis vaccine are currently licensed for use in infants, including Daptacel, Pediarix, Kinrix (DTaP and IPV), and Infanrix (diphtheria, tetanus toxoid, and acellular pertussis conjugate). Pentacel is licensed for use in infants 4 weeks old and older; in addition to acellular pertussis, diphtheria, and tetanus, this vaccine also contains inactivated poliovirus (IPV) and Hib conjugate. Either the acellular or whole-cell vaccine may be given for the fourth and fifth doses, but the acellular is preferred. It is also recommended that the first three DTaP vaccinations be from the same manufacturer. The fourth dose may be from a different manufacturer. The child who has received one or more whole-cell vaccines may complete the series of five with the acellular vaccine.

Health care workers who may be susceptible to pertussis as a result of waning immunity and who have potential exposure to children or adults with pertussis should receive a single dose of Tdap (if not previously vaccinated with same) and take the necessary protective precautions against droplet contamination (wear procedural or surgical masks and practice hand washing). The diagnosis of pertussis may be missed or delayed in unvaccinated infants, who often are seen with respiratory distress and apnea without the typical cough. Additional guidelines for prevention and treatment of pertussis among health care workers and close contacts are available from the CDC's website at http://www.cdc.gov/vaccines.

Polio

An all-IPV (IPV vaccine) schedule for routine childhood polio vaccination is now recommended for children in the United States. All children should receive four doses of IPV at 2 months, 4 months, 6 to 18 months, and 4 to 6 years of age (AAP, Committee on Infectious Diseases, 2009).

The change from the exclusive use of oral polio vaccine (OPV) to the exclusive use of IPV is related to the rare risk of vaccine-associated polio paralysis (VAPP) from OPV. The exclusive use of IPV eliminates the risk of VAPP but is associated with an increased number of injections and increased cost. Since IPV usage was instituted in the United States in 2000, no new cases of VAPP have occurred. Pediarix is a combination vaccine containing DTaP, hepatitis B, and IPV; this may be used as the primary immunization beginning at 2 months of age (AAP, Committee on Infectious Diseases, 2009). Kinrix contains DTaP and IPV and it may be used as the fifth dose in the DTaP series and the fourth dose in the IPV series in children ages 4 to 6 years whose previous vaccine doses have been with Infanrix or Pediarix for the first three doses and Infanrix for the fourth dose. As noted earlier, Pentacel is also licensed for use in infants 4 weeks old and older and contains DTaP, Hib, and IPV. Pediarix has been licensed for use in children as young as 6 weeks and contains DTaP, HepB, and IPV.

Measles

The measles (rubeola) vaccine is given at 12 to 15 months of age. During the course of measles outbreaks, the vaccine can be given any time after 6 months of age followed by a second inoculation after age 12 months. The second measles immunization is recommended at 4 to 6 years of age (at school entry) but may be given earlier provided that 4 weeks have elapsed since the administration of the previous dose. Revaccination should occur by 11 to 12 years of age if the measles vaccine was not administered at school entry (4–6 years). Any child who is vaccinated before 12 months of age should receive two additional doses beginning at 12 to 15 months and separated by at least 4 weeks (AAP, Committee on Infectious Diseases, 2009). Revaccination should include all individuals born after 1956 who have not received two doses of measles vaccine after 12 months of age. Individuals born before this date are thought to be immune from exposure to natural measles virus. Because of the continuing occurrence of measles in older children and young adults, identify potentially susceptible adolescents and young adults and immunize them if two doses of measles vaccine have not been administered previously or the person had a confirmed case of the illness. The National Institute of Allergy and Infectious Diseases (NIAID) working with 34 other professional organizations published new evidence-based guidelines for the diagnosis and management of food allergy recommends that children receive the MMR or MMRV (measles, mumps, rubella, and varicella) vaccine despite a history of severe egg allergy reaction (Boyce, Assa'ad, Burks, and others, 2010).

The MMRV vaccine (ProQuad) is an attenuated live virus vaccine and may be given to children 12 months to 12 years of age concurrent with other vaccines. Recent concerns for increased risk of febrile seizures in children 12 months to 23 months of age after administration of MMRV initially prompted the ACIP (CDC, 2008) to remove its recommendation for MMRV being the preferred vaccine (vs. separate injections of MMR and varicella vaccines). However, after further review, the ACIP amended that recommendation and now recommends either administering MMR and varicella vaccines (two separate vaccines) or the MMRV as the first vaccination in children ages 12 to 47 months. The risks and benefits of administering the MMRV vaccine should be fully explained to the parent or caregiver; the risk for a febrile seizure at 5 to 12 days in children 12 to 23 months old remains relatively low and should be weighed with the benefit of one less intramuscular injection (Marin, Broder, Temte, and others, 2010).

Vitamin A supplementation has been effective in decreasing the morbidity and mortality associated with measles in developing countries. A Cochrane review of studies wherein a single dose of vitamin A was administered to children with measles found no decrease in mortality. However, children with measles younger than the age of 2 years who received two doses of vitamin A (200,000 IU) on consecutive days did have decreased mortality rates and a reduced rate of pneumonia-specific mortality (Huiming, Chaomin, and Meng, 2005).

Mumps

Mumps virus vaccine is recommended for children at 12 to 15 months of age and is typically given in combination with measles and rubella.

It should not be administered to infants younger than 12 months because persisting maternal antibodies can interfere with the immune response. Because of continued occurrence of the disease, especially in children 10 to 19 years of age, mumps immunization is recommended for all individuals born after 1957 who may be susceptible to mumps (i.e., those who have no history of having had the disease or vaccine and who have no laboratory evidence of immunity).

Rubella

Rubella is a relatively mild infection in children, but in a pregnant woman, the actual infection presents serious risks to the developing fetus. Therefore, the aim of rubella immunization is actually protection of the unborn child rather than the recipient of the immunization.

Rubella immunization is recommended for all children at 12 to 15 months of age and is administered in a combined form with measles and mumps vaccine. Increased emphasis should also be placed on vaccinating all unimmunized prepubertal children and susceptible adolescents and adult women in the childbearing age group. Because the live attenuated virus may cross the placenta and theoretically present a risk to the developing fetus, rubella vaccine is currently not given to pregnant women. Although this is standard practice, current evidence from women who received the vaccine while pregnant and delivered unaffected offspring indicates that the risk to the fetus is negligible. In addition, there is no reported danger of administering rubella vaccine to a child if the mother is pregnant.

Haemophilus Influenzae Type B

Hib conjugate vaccines protect against a number of serious infections caused by Hib, especially bacterial meningitis, epiglottitis, bacterial pneumonia, septic arthritis, and sepsis (Hib is not associated with the viruses that cause influenza, or "flu"). Hib vaccines that are currently available include PedvaxHIB, Pentacel, and Comvax, which are combination vaccines; Hiberix; and ActHIB. Pentacel is described in the previous section on pertussis. These conjugate vaccines connect Hib to a nontoxic form of another organism, such as meningococcal protein or diphtheria protein. There is no antibody response to these nontoxic proteins, but they significantly improve the antibody response to Hib, especially in infants. The use of combination vaccines provides equivalent immunogenicity and decreases the number of injections an infant receives. However, it is important that they be given to the appropriate-age child. Hiberix is a conjugate vaccine licensed for use as the booster (final) dose of the Hib vaccine series for children ages 15 months to 4 years (CDC, 2009).

When possible, the Hib conjugate vaccine used at the first vaccination should be used for all subsequent vaccinations in the primary series. All Hib vaccines are administered by intramuscular injection using a separate syringe and at a site separate from any concurrent vaccinations. For more information see Figure 10-11, *A*, footnote 4.

> **⚠ NURSING ALERT**
>
> The use of meningococcal and diphtheria proteins in combination vaccines does not mean the child has received adequate immunization for meningococcal or diphtheria illnesses; the child must be given the appropriate vaccine for that specific disease.

Varicella

Administration of the cell-free live-attenuated varicella vaccine is recommended for any susceptible child (one who lacks proof of varicella vaccination or has a reliable history of varicella infection). A single dose of 0.5 ml should be given by subcutaneous injection. The first dose of varicella vaccine is recommended for children ages 12 to 15 months, and to ensure adequate protection, a second varicella vaccine is recommended for children at 4 to 6 years of age. The second varicella vaccine may be administered before 4 years of age as long as a period of 3 months occurs between the first and second doses. Children 13 years of age or older who are susceptible should receive two doses administered at least 4 weeks apart. Children in the same age group (13 to 18 years of age) who have received only one previous varicella vaccine should receive a second varicella vaccine. The AAP, Committee on Infectious Diseases (2009) reports that the two-dose regimen was adopted to protect children who did not have adequate protection with one dose, not because of waning immunity to the vaccine. The combination vaccine MMRV (ProQuad) is licensed for use in children ages 12 months to 12 years of age (see discussion in Measles).

According to the AAP, Committee on Infectious Diseases (2009), children who have received two doses of the varicella vaccine are one third less likely to have breakthrough illness in the first 10 years of immunization in comparison with those who have received one dose. Children who do contract varicella after immunization reportedly have milder cases with fewer vesicles, lower degree of fever, and faster recovery. Antibodies persist for at least 8 years (AAP, Committee on Infectious Diseases, 2009).

The vaccine should be kept frozen in the lyophilic form (stable particles that readily go into solution) and used within 30 minutes of being reconstituted to ensure viral potency.

Varicella vaccine may be administered simultaneously with MMR. However, separate syringes and injection sites should be used. If they are not administered simultaneously, the interval between administration of varicella vaccine and MMR should be at least 1 month. Varicella vaccine may also be given simultaneously with DTaP, IPV, HepB, or Hib (AAP, Committee on Infectious Diseases, 2009). The vaccine is administered subcutaneously. For more information see Figure 10-11, *A*, footnote 9.

Pneumococcal Disease

A seven-valent *Streptococcus pneumoniae* conjugate vaccine (PCV7, or Prevnar) has been used for children under 2 years of age since 2000. Streptococcal pneumococci are responsible for a number of bacterial infections in children younger than 2 years, which may cause serious morbidity and mortality. Among these are generalized infections such as septicemia and meningitis or localized infections such as otitis media, sinusitis, and pneumonia. These illnesses are particularly problematic in children who attend daycare facilities (the incidence in daycare children is two or three times higher than in children not attending out-of-home daycare) and in those who are immunocompromised. Since the introduction of the pneumococcal vaccine, the incidence of vaccine-type invasive pneumococcal disease is reported to have decreased by 99% in the United States (AAP, Committee on Infectious Diseases, 2009). In 2010, a 13-valent pneumococcal vaccine (PCV13 [Prevnar 13]) was licensed for use and is currently recommended as the standard pneumococcal vaccine for children ages 6 weeks to 24 months. Children who have started the PCV series with PCV7 may complete the vaccine series with PCV13 (Nuorti, Whitney, and CDC, 2010).

The PCV13 vaccine is administered at 2, 4, and 6 months, with a fourth dose at 12 to 15 months of age. A single supplemental dose of PCV13 is recommended for children 14 through 59 months who have received an age-appropriate series of PCV7, and a single supplemental dose of PCV13 is also recommended for children ages 60 through 71 months who received a series of PCV7. PCV13 is also recommended for all children under 24 months and in older children (24–71 months) with sickle cell disease; functional or anatomic asplenia; nephrotic syndrome or chronic renal failure; conditions associated with immunosuppression, such as solid organ transplantation, drug therapy, or cytoreduction therapy (including long-term systemic corticosteroid therapy); diabetes mellitus; cochlear implants; congenital immunodeficiency; human immunodeficiency virus (HIV) infection; cerebrospinal fluid leaks; chronic cardiovascular disease (e.g., congestive heart failure or cardiomyopathy); chronic pulmonary disease (e.g., emphysema or cystic fibrosis, but not asthma); chronic liver disease (e.g., cirrhosis); or exposure to living environments or social settings in which the risk of invasive pneumococcal disease or its complications is very high (e.g., Alaskan Native, African-American, and certain American Indian populations) The PCV13 vaccine may be administered in conjunction with all other immunizations in a separate syringe and at a separate intramuscular site. For further information, see Figure 10-11, *A*, footnote 5.

The PPV (pneumococcal polysaccharide [23-valent] vaccine) is not recommended for children younger than 24 months who do not have one of the high-risk conditions described previously. One dose of PPV is recommended in children older than 23 months who have one of the high-risk conditions after primary immunization with PCV7 (see Fig. 10-11.)

Influenza

The influenza vaccine is now recommended annually for children 6 months to 18 years. Influenza vaccine (trivalent inactivated influenza vaccine [TIV]) may be given to any healthy children aged 6 months and older. Children who have a reported anaphylactic hypersensitivity to eggs should not receive the vaccine. The vaccine is administered in early fall before the flu season begins and is repeated yearly for ongoing protection. The intramuscular vaccine is administered as two separate doses 4 weeks apart in first-time recipients younger than the age of 9 years. The dose is 0.25 ml for children ages 6 to 35 months and 0.5 ml for children 3 years and older. Children aged 6 months through 8 years who did not receive any dose of influenza vaccine in the 2010 to 2011 season should receive two doses of vaccine administered at least four weeks apart in the 2011–2012 influenza season (AAP, Committee on Infectious Diseases, 2011b). The vaccine may be given simultaneously with other vaccines but at a separate site. The vaccine is administered yearly because different strains of influenza are used each year in the manufacture of the vaccine. The NIAID 2010 guidelines (Boyce, Assa'ad, Burks, and others, 2010) state that there is insufficient evidence to recommend administering either one of the available influenza vaccines to patients with a history of severe reactions to egg proteins; however, the guidelines also point out that egg protein allergy is relatively common in individuals who would benefit from the influenza vaccine (e.g., children with asthma). Several options for administering the influenza vaccine are described in the literature, and individuals should discuss the risks and benefits with a knowledgeable health care practitioner.

The live attenuated influenza vaccine (LAIV) is an acceptable alternative to the intramuscular trivalent vaccine in specific age groups. The vaccine is given nasally as two doses at least 28 days apart in healthy persons ages 2 to 49 years. Although it is an alternative to the injection, it costs more and may not be covered by insurance companies. Either TIV or LAIV may be given to healthy, nonpregnant persons ages 2 to 49 years (AAP, Committee on Infectious Diseases, 2009). Yearly influenza vaccine should be administered to health care workers and to children ages 6 to 59 months with medical conditions (including asthma, cardiac disease, HIV, diabetes, and sickle cell disease) that place them at risk for influenza-related complications.

The H1N1 virus (swine flu) is a subtype of influenza type A. Previous outbreaks of H1N1 influenza occurred in 1918, and the mortality rates were significant both in the United States and worldwide (AAP, Committee on Infectious Diseases, 2009). The recent pandemic of H1N1 caused significant morbidity and mortality worldwide, particularly in Mexico and the United States. Antigenic shift occurs when influenza A viruses undergo significant changes that result in new infection subtypes; such is the case in the current pandemic. The 2011 to 2012 flu vaccination included the H1N1 virus (AAP, Committee on Infectious Diseases, 2011b). For more information see Figure 10-11, *A*, footnote 7.

Meningococcal Disease

Invasive meningococcal disease continues to be the cause of high morbidity in children in the United States. Infants younger than 1 year of age are particularly susceptible, yet the highest fatalities occur in adolescents (≈20%). There is also evidence that the risk of meningococcal infections is high in college freshmen living in dormitories. Meningococcal infections are also responsible for significant morbidities, including limb or digit amputation, skin scarring, hearing loss, and neurologic disabilities.

Neisseria meningitidis is the leading cause of bacterial meningitis in the United States. It is not recommended that children 2 to 10 years old routinely receive the quadrivalent conjugate vaccine MCV4 (Menactra [MCV4-D] or Menveo [MCV4-CRM]) except those in certain high-risk groups. These include children with terminal complement component deficiency, anatomic or functional asplenia, or HIV and children who travel to or reside in countries where *N. meningitidis* is hyperendemic or epidemic. In such cases, these children should receive two doses of MCV4 at least 8 weeks apart. The minimum age for administration of Menactra is 9 months; for Menveo it is 2 years. Children and adolescents 11 to 12 years of age should receive a single immunization of MCV4 (Menactra or Menveo) and a booster of the same at age 16 to 18 years. For adolescents who received their first dose of MCV4 at age 13 through 15 years, a one-time booster may be given at age 16 through 18 years. Those who receive the first dose of MCV4 at or after age 16 do not need a booster dose of the vaccine (AAP, Committee on Infectious Diseases, 2011a). Others at high risk who should receive MCV4 include college freshmen living in dormitories and military recruits. For further information see Figure 10-11, *A*, footnote 11.

Persons who are at high risk for the disease and received MPSV4 three or more years previously should be vaccinated with MCV4. The vaccine protects against meningococcal disease caused by serogroups A, C, Y, and W-135. MCV4 is administered as an intramuscular injection (0.5 ml) and may be administered in conjunction with other vaccines in a separate syringe and at a separate site. Immunization with MCV4 is contraindicated in persons with hypersensitivity to any components of the vaccine, including diphtheria toxoid, and to rubber latex (part of vial stoppers).

Recommendations for Selected Immunizations

Two additional vaccines are recommended for children and adolescents at high risk for particular diseases. Two rotavirus vaccines, RotaTeq and Rotarix, have been licensed by the U.S. Food and Drug Administration for distribution in the United States. Rotavirus is one of the leading causes of severe diarrhea in infants and young children. RotaTeq is licensed for administration to infants at 6 to 12 weeks of age, with two additional doses administered at 4- to 10-week intervals but not after 32 weeks of age. The dose is 2 ml, and the product must be protected from light until administration (AAP, Committee on Infectious Diseases, 2009). Rotarix (1 ml) may be administered beginning at 6 weeks of age with a second dose at least 4 weeks after the first dose but before 24 weeks of age. Both vaccines are administered orally. (see Figure 10-11, *A*, footnote 2).

Two human papillomavirus (HPV) vaccines have been licensed for use in adolescents; a quadrivalent HPV4 vaccine, Gardasil, has been approved and is recommended for female children and adolescents to prevent HPV-related cervical cancer. The vaccine is administered intramuscularly in three separate doses; the first dose in the series may be given at 11 to 12 years of age (minimum age, 9 years), and the second dose is administered 2 months after the first, with the third dose being given 6 months after the first dose. The HPV4 vaccine may also be administered to boys and men ages 9 to 26 years in a three-dose series to reduce the likelihood of genital warts (CDC, 2010b). The bivalent vaccine (HPV2), Cervarix, is licensed for use in girls and women ages 10 to 25 years for the prevention of HPV-related cervical cancer; this vaccine is given in a three-dose series (CDC, 2010a) (see Fig. 10-11, *B*, footnote 2).

Immunizations that may be used in older children and adolescents in the future and that are being evaluated include vaccines for preventing diseases such as herpes simplex virus, human cytomegalovirus, and Epstein-Barr virus. A vaccine for respiratory syncytial virus is currently being tested in animal models with apparent success. Others, such as the rabies vaccine, are discussed elsewhere in this text.

Reactions

Vaccines for routine immunizations are among the safest and most reliable drugs available. However, minor side effects do occur after many of the immunizations, and, rarely, a serious reaction may result from a vaccine.

With inactivated antigens, such as DTaP, side effects are most likely to occur within a few hours or days of administration and are usually limited to local tenderness, erythema, and swelling at the injection site; low-grade fever; and behavioral changes (drowsiness, fretfulness, eating less, prolonged or unusual cry). Rarely, more severe reactions may occur, especially with pertussis. Reactions to DTaP tend to be more severe if they occurred with a previous immunization; fever, swelling, irritability, and pain are more common after the fourth DTaP vaccination in the series. Acetaminophen may help reduce this discomfort and should be given in an age-appropriate dose and time interval. A recent study of 4- to 6-year-old children receiving the fifth DTaP vaccine in the series were reported to be 78% more likely to have a localized reaction when the vaccine was administered in the deltoid versus the thigh muscle; these findings suggest the thigh should be used to administer this vaccine (Jackson, Yu, Nelson, and others, 2011).

Hib vaccine is one of the safest vaccines available but may be associated with low-grade fever and mild local reactions at the site of injection, which resolve rapidly. Fever (temperature >38.5° C [101.3° F]) may rarely occur.

A number of inactive components are incorporated in vaccines to enhance their effectiveness and safety. Some of these components include preservatives, stabilizers, adjuvants, antibiotics, and purified culture medium proteins to enhance effectiveness. A child may react to the preservative in the vaccine rather than the vaccine component; an example of this is the HepB vaccine, which is prepared from yeast cultures. Yeast hypersensitivity might preclude one from receiving this particular vaccine. Trace amounts of neomycin are used to decrease bacterial growth within certain vaccine preparations, and persons with documented anaphylactic reactions to neomycin should avoid these vaccines. Most vaccine preparations now contain vial stoppers with a

ATRAUMATIC CARE

Immunizations

Needle length is an important factor and must be considered for each individual child; fewer reactions to immunizations are observed when vaccines are given deep into the muscle rather than into subcutaneous tissue. Contrary to previous belief, deep intramuscular tissue has a better blood supply and fewer pain receptors than adipose tissue, thus providing an optimum site for immunizations with fewer side effects (Zuckerman, 2000).

To minimize local reactions from vaccines:

- Recommended needle length for newborn to 2 months is 16 mm (⅝ inch).
- Select a needle of adequate length (25 mm [1 inch] in infants) to deposit the antigen deep in the muscle mass.
- Toddlers and older children require a needle length of 16 to 25 mm (⅝–1 inch) for deltoid, or 25 to 32 mm (1–1¼ inches) for vastus lateralis (Schechter, Zempsky, Cohen, and others, 2007).
- Adolescents require a needle length of 25 to 51 mm (1–2 inches) in the deltoid or vastus lateralis (Schechter, Zempsky, Cohen, and others, 2007) depending on the size of muscle mass.
- Inject into the vastus lateralis or ventrogluteal muscle; the deltoid may be used in children 18 months of age and older.

Use one or more of the following techniques to minimize pain:

- Apply the topical anesthetic EMLA (lidocaine–prilocaine) to the injection site and cover with an occlusive dressing for at least 1 hour.*
- Apply the topical anesthetic LMX4 (4% lidocaine) to the injection site 30 minutes before the injection; there is no evidence that an occlusive dressing is required except to prevent ingestion or accidental application to the eyes in infants (Wong, 2003).
- Apply a vapocoolant spray (e.g., ethyl chloride or FluoriMethane) directly to the skin or to a cotton ball, which is placed on the skin for 15 seconds immediately before the injection (Reis and Holubkov, 1997).

- Evidence indicates that a concentrated oral sucrose solution (24%) and nonnutritive sucking (NNS) (pacifier) decrease the pain related to minor invasive procedures in neonates (Stevens, Johnston, Franck, and others, 1999; Stevens, Yamada, and Ohlsson, 2001). Most studies have focused on heel lance, venipuncture, and circumcision (neonatal period), but one institution has incorporated a neonatal oral sucrose pain protocol for painful procedures, including intramuscular injections (Thompson, 2005). Hatfield (2008) found that 2- and 4-month-old infants who received a 0.6 ml/kg dose of 24% sucrose and NNS 2 minutes before immunization administration had decreased pain behavioral responses compared with a control group of infants who only received sterile water and NNS 2 minutes before the injection. Liaw, Zeng, Yang, and others (2011) found that NNS and oral sucrose provided analgesia to newborns receiving the hepatitis B vaccine. Therefore, it is recommended that a concentrated oral sucrose solution (1–2 ml) be administered orally 2 minutes before the injection, during the injection, and up to 3 minutes after the procedure to decrease neonatal pain with immunizations.
- In preschool children, use distraction, such as telling the child to "take a deep breath and blow and blow and blow until I tell you to stop."
- A combination of pharmacologic and nonpharmacologic interventions, including breastfeeding, oral sucrose, and NNS, have been found to decrease the pain sensation in infants receiving their childhood immunizations (Shah, Taddio, Rieder, and others, 2009) (see Chapter 7).
- NOTE: Changing the needle on the syringe after drawing up the vaccine and before injecting it has not been shown to decrease local reactions. In children 4 to 6 years of age, the administration of sequential injections or simultaneous injections of vaccines did not alter their perceptions of distress, but parents preferred the simultaneous method (Horn and McCarthy, 1999).

*The use of the EMLA patch before administration of diphtheria–tetanus–acellular pertussis–inactivated poliovirus–*Haemophilus influenzae* type b (DTaP-IPV-Hib) and hepatitis B vaccines did not decrease antibody titers in immunized infants and was effective in reducing pain in 6-month-old children (Halperin, Halperin, McGrath, and others, 2002). The EMLA patch is no longer commercially available in the United States.

---

synthetic rubber to prevent latex allergy reactions; however, health care personnel administering vaccines should make sure that the package insert specifies there is no latex in the stopper. In the event that an individual has a severe reaction to a vaccine and subsequent immunizations are required, an allergist may be consulted to determine the best course of action (Schuval, 2003). The influenza vaccine contains small amounts of egg protein; thus, children who have severe allergy to egg should seek the advice of an allergist regarding this vaccine; most children with egg allergy are reported to be likely to develop a tolerance to small amounts over time (Settipane, Siri, and Beltani, 2009). (See discussion in Influenza section.)

Some vaccines contain a preservative, thimerosal, which contains ethylmercury. Concerns regarding possible mercury poisoning in the 1990s prompted many to put off vaccination of infants and small children for fear of childhood developmental problems such as autism. A number of manufacturers have since stopped producing vaccines containing thimerosal. No local hypersensitivity reactions to thimerosal have been recorded, and studies on thimerosal and the potential link to autism or any other pervasive developmental disorder failed to establish a causal relationship between the two (DeStefano, 2007; Hviid, Stellfeld, Wohlfahrt, and others, 2003; Parker, Schwartz, Todd, and others, 2004). The Institute of Medicine (2004), after an in-depth 3-year study, issued a report concluding that there is no link between

autism and the MMR vaccine or vaccines containing the preservative thimerosal.

A commonly observed reaction includes localized erythema and induration, which may occur when the vaccine is not administered deeply enough into the muscle. This reaction can be prevented by ensuring that needle length is appropriate for the child's muscle size. Although many vaccine preparations are commercially available in prepackaged form, the enclosed needle may not be of adequate length to penetrate the muscle in certain children (see Atraumatic Care box and Administration, p. 341).

Unlike the inactivated antigens, live attenuated virus vaccines such as MMR multiply for days or weeks, and unfavorable reactions and vaccine-associated disorders can occur for 30 to 60 days. These reactions are usually mild, although reactions to rubella tend to be more troublesome in older children and adults.

Contraindications and Precautions

Nurses need to be aware of the reasons for withholding immunizations—both for the child's safety in terms of avoiding reactions and for the child's maximum benefit from receiving the vaccine. Unfounded fears and lack of knowledge regarding contraindications can needlessly prevent a child from having protection from life-threatening diseases. Issues that have surfaced regarding vaccines include the misconception that administering combination vaccines may overload the child's immune system; the combined vaccines have undergone rigorous study in relation to side effects and immunogenicity rates after administration. Others may express concern that vaccines are not a part of the individual's natural immunity and that administering too many vaccines may decrease the child's immunity to such diseases. Parents may also voice concerns that vaccines may cause diseases such as asthma, multiple sclerosis, or diabetes mellitus (Kimmel, Burns, Wolfe, and others, 2007). Another concern of parents is the number of vaccines or "shots" given to infants at any given time and the pain and discomfort this may cause.

A contraindication is considered as a condition in an individual that increases the risk for a serious adverse reaction (e.g., not administering a live virus vaccine to a severely compromised child). A precaution is a condition in a recipient that might increase the risk for a serious adverse reaction or that might compromise the ability of the vaccine to produce immunity (National Center for Immunization and Respiratory Diseases, 2011).

The general contraindication for all immunizations is a severe febrile illness. This precaution avoids adding the risk of adverse side effects from the vaccine to an already ill child or mistakenly identifying a symptom of the disease as having been caused by the vaccine. The presence of minor illnesses such as the common cold is not a contraindication. Live virus vaccines are generally not administered to anyone with an altered immune system because multiplication of the virus may be enhanced, causing a severe vaccine-induced illness.

In general, live virus vaccines such as varicella and MMR should not be administered to persons who are severely immunocompromised (National Center for Immunization and Respiratory Diseases, 2011). Another contraindication to live virus vaccines (e.g., MMR and varicella) is the presence of recently acquired passive immunity through blood transfusions, immunoglobulin, or maternal antibodies. Administration of MMR and varicella should be postponed for a minimum of 3 months after passive immunization with immunoglobulins and blood transfusions (except washed RBCs, which do not interfere with the immune response). Suggested intervals between administration of immunoglobulin preparations and MMR and varicella depend on the type of immune product and dosage. If the vaccine and immunoglobulin are given simultaneously because of imminent exposure to disease, the two preparations are injected at sites far from each other. Vaccination should be repeated after the suggested intervals unless there is serologic evidence of antibody production.

A final contraindication is a known allergic response to a previously administered vaccine or a substance in the vaccine. MMR vaccines contain minute amounts of neomycin; measles and mumps vaccines, which are grown on chick embryo tissue cultures, are not believed to contain significant amounts of egg cross-reacting proteins. Therefore, only a history of anaphylactic reaction to neomycin, gelatin, or the vaccine itself is considered a contraindication to their use.

Pregnancy is a contraindication to MMR vaccines, although the risk of fetal damage is primarily theoretic. Breastfeeding is not a contraindication for any vaccine.

Parents must be given appropriate information regarding vaccine safety, benefits, and risks so they can make informed decisions regarding vaccinations for their children (Kimmel, Burns, Wolfe, and others, 2007). The advantage of widespread media coverage on television and the Internet is that information is readily available at any given moment; the disadvantage may rest in the fact that information— rather, misinformation—from questionable sources is also readily available and may influence parents to make decisions that may have

FAMILY-CENTERED CARE

Communicating with Parents About Immunizations

- Provide accurate and user-friendly information on vaccines (the necessity for each one, the disease each prevents, potential adverse effects).
- Realize that the parent is expressing concern for the child's health.
- Acknowledge the parent's concerns in a genuine, empathetic manner.
- Tailor the discussion to the needs of the parent.
- Avoid judgmental or threatening language.
- Be knowledgeable about the benefits of individual vaccines, the common adverse effects, and how to minimize those effects.
- Give the parent the vaccine information statement beforehand and be prepared to answer any questions that may arise.
- Help the parent make an informed decision regarding the administration of each vaccine.
- Be flexible and provide parents with options regarding the administration of multiple vaccines, especially in infants, who must receive multiple injections at 2, 4, and 6 months of age (i.e., allow parents to space the vaccinations at different visits to decrease the total number of injections at each visit; make provisions for office visits for immunization purposes only [does not incur a practitioner fee except for administration of vaccine], provided the child is healthy).
- Involve the parent in minimizing the potential adverse effects of the vaccine (e.g., administering an appropriate dose of acetaminophen 45 minutes before administering the vaccine [as warranted]; applying EMLA [lidocaine–prilocaine] or LMX4 [4% lidocaine] to the injection sites before administration; following up to check on the child if untoward reactions have occurred in the past or parent is especially anxious about the child's well-being).
- Respect the parent's ultimate wishes.

Data from Coyer SM: Understanding parental concerns about immunizations, *J Pediatr Health Care* 16(4):193–196, 2002; Fredrickson DD, Davis TC, Bocchini JA: Explaining the risks and benefits of vaccines to parents, *Pediatr Ann* 30(7):400–406, 2001; and Rosenthal P: Overcoming skepticism toward vaccines: a look at the real benefits and risks, *Consult Pediatr* 4(suppl):S3–S7, 2004.

deleterious consequences for their children's health. In one survey, parents' fear of side effects was the most commonly expressed (52%) reason for vaccination refusal; other common reasons included the belief that the disease was not harmful (26%), religious beliefs (28%), and philosophical reasons (26%) (Fredrickson, Davis, Arnold, and others, 2004). See also Family-Centered Care box. A complete table of childhood vaccines with contraindications is found on the Evolve website.

Administration

The principal precautions in administering immunizations include proper storage of the vaccine to protect its potency and institution of recommended procedures for injection. The nurse must be familiar with the manufacturer's directions for storage and reconstitution of the vaccine. For example, if the vaccine is to be refrigerated, it should be stored on a center shelf, not in the door, where frequent temperature increases from opening the refrigerator can alter the vaccine's potency. For protection against light, the vial can be wrapped in aluminum foil. Periodic checks are established to ensure that no vaccine is used after its expiration date.

The DTaP vaccines contain the adjuvant alum to retain the antigen at the injection site and prolong the stimulatory effect. Because subcutaneous or intracutaneous injection of the adjuvant can cause local irritation, inflammation, or abscess formation, attention to excellent intramuscular injection technique must be used (see Atraumatic Care box, p. 340, and Research Focus box).

One of the most important features of injecting vaccines is adequate penetration of the muscle for deposition of the drug intramuscularly and not subcutaneously. The use of appropriate needle length is an essential component of administering vaccines. In two studies, the use of longer needles significantly decreased the incidence of localized edema and tenderness when vaccines were administered to a group of infants (Diggle and Deeks, 2000; Diggle, Deeks, and Pollard, 2006) (see Evidence-Based Practice box). Similar findings have been recorded for children 4 to 6 years of age receiving the fifth DTaP

vaccine (Jackson, Yu, Nelson, and others, 2011). Cook and Murtagh (2006) found that administration of the pertussis vaccine in the ventrogluteal muscle in children aged 2 months to 18 months was safe and had few localized reactions in comparison to anterolateral thigh administration. Junqueira, Tavares, Martins, and others (2010) found that administration of the hepatitis B vaccine in the ventrogluteal muscle (vs. anterolateral thigh) of 580 infants resulted in a lower incidence of fever and localized reactions. (See Intramuscular Administration, Chapter 22).

The total series requires several injections, and every attempt is made to rotate the sites and administer the injections as painlessly as possible (see Intramuscular Administration, Chapter 22). When two or more injections are given at separate sites, the order of injections is arbitrary. Because allergic reactions can occur after injection of vaccines, appropriate precautions are taken (see Anaphylaxis, Chapter 25).

Nurses often administer vaccines and thus have the responsibility for adequately informing parents of the nature, prevalence, and risks of the disease; the type of immunization product to be used; the expected benefits and the risk of side effects of the vaccine; and the need for accurate immunization records. Referring to immunizations as "baby shots" and limiting the discussion to vague statements about the vaccines are unacceptable practices.

Another important nursing responsibility is accurate documentation. Each child should have an immunization record for parents to keep, especially for families that move frequently. Although immunization rates have increased significantly, health professionals should use every opportunity to encourage complete immunization of all children. Electronic health records and computerized childhood immunization databases may be helpful in maintaining updated records. Blank immunization records may be downloaded from a number of websites,

---

RESEARCH FOCUS

Order of Injections

Ipp, Parkin, Lear, and others (2009) evaluated the administration order of the vaccines diphtheria–tetanus–acellular pertussis–*Haemophilus influenzae* type b (DTaP-Hib) and pneumococcal conjugate vaccine (PCV) and pain perception in 120 infants 2 to 6 months of age. The infants who were given the primary DTaP-Hib vaccine before the PCV vaccine had significantly lower pain scores as measured by the Modified Behavioral Pain Scale than those who received the PCV vaccine first. Both groups of infants were given both vaccines. Additional pain measures included crying as measured by video recording and parent perception of child pain using the Visual Analog Scale. The researchers recommend giving the primary DTaP-Hib vaccine before the PCV to reduce pain in infants receiving routine immunizations.

EVIDENCE-BASED PRACTICE

Appropriate Site, Technique, Needle Size, and Dose for Intramuscular Injections in Infants, Toddlers, and Small Children

Updated by Olga Taylor

Ask the Question
Picot Question
In infants, toddlers, and small children, what are the best site, technique, needle size and gauge, and dosage for intramuscular (IM) injections?

Search the Evidence
Search Strategies
Literature from 1990 to 2009 was reviewed to obtain clinical research studies related to this issue.

Databases Used
CINAHL, PubMed

Critically Analyze the Evidence
Searches reviewed were small studies. There were no randomized trials, double-blinded trials, or large clinical studies addressing the subject of IM injections in children.

Infants and Toddlers
- A 16-mm needle was sufficient to penetrate the anterolateral thigh muscle if the needle is inserted at a 90-degree angle without pinching the muscle in children ages 2, 4, 6, and 18 months (Cook and Murtagh, 2002).
- A 25-mm needle is necessary to penetrate the thigh muscle when a 45-degree injection technique was used. A longer needle length is needed to fully

deposit the medication into the muscle in children ages 2, 4, 6, and 18 months (Cook and Murtagh, 2002).
- In diphtheria–tetanus–pertussis (DTP) immunizations administered to infants 7 months of age or younger, 84.6% of injections were administered at the correct site (anterior thigh); 5.1% dorsogluteal and 2.6% deltoid muscles, which are considered incorrect sites (Daly, Johnston, and Chung, 1992).
- Vaccines containing adjuvant such as aluminum (e.g., DTaP, hepatitis A and B, diphtheria–tetanus [DT or Td]) should be given deep into the muscle to prevent local reactions (AAP, Committee on Infectious Diseases, 2009; CDC, 2002; Petousis-Harris, 2008; Taddio, Ilersich, Ipp, and others, 2009).
- Injecting adjuvant-containing vaccines into subcutaneous tissue increases the incidence of local reactions (Taddio, Ilersich, Ipp, and others, 2009; Zuckerman, 2000).
- Four-month-old infants experienced fewer local side effects (redness, tenderness, and swelling) when immunizations were administered into the anterior aspect of the thigh with a 25-mm (1-inch) needle versus shorter 16-mm (⅝-inch) needle (Diggle and Deeks, 2000).
- Localized vaccine reactions were significantly reduced when long needles (25 mm) were used for infant immunizations (Diggle, Deeks, and Pollard, 2006; Petousis-Harris, 2008).
  - A 16-mm needle may be adequate for injections in small infants, and a 22- to 25-mm (⅞–1 inch) needle can be used in infants 2 months and older (AAP, Committee on Infectious Diseases, 2009).

EVIDENCE-BASED PRACTICE

Appropriate Site, Technique, Needle Size, and Dose for Intramuscular Injections in Infants, Toddlers, and Small Children—cont'd

- A 22- to 32-mm (⅞–1¼-inch) needle is recommended for injections in toddlers if deltoid muscle size is adequate (CDC, 2002).
- A minimum of a 25-mm-long needle is recommended for anterolateral thigh injection in toddlers (CDC, 2002).
- Dorsogluteal muscle should be avoided in infants and toddlers and in smaller preschoolers with smaller muscle mass because of the possibility of damaging the sciatic nerve (AAP, Committee on Infectious Diseases, 2009).
- In children older than 1 year of age, the deltoid muscle is recommended for IM injections. When multiple vaccines are given, two may be given in the thigh (anterior and lateral) because of its larger size (Diggle, 2003).
- Injections in the anterolateral thigh be given at least 2.5 cm (1 inch) apart so local reactions are less likely to overlap (AAP, Committee on Infectious Diseases, 2009).
- No research or supportive data were found regarding the amount of medication to be given at the different sites in infants and toddlers.
- Small and preterm infants may only tolerate up to 0.5 ml in each muscle to prevent local complications, and 1 ml of medication is recommended for infants younger than 12 months; no data can be found to refute or support such a recommendation.

Children and Adolescents

- A 22- to 25-gauge needle for all IM childhood immunizations is recommended (AAP, Committee on Infectious Diseases, 2009; CDC, 2002).
- Deltoid muscle may be used for immunizations in toddlers, older children, and adolescents (AAP, Committee on Infectious Diseases, 2009; CDC, 2002).
- A 16-mm needle for children weighing less than 60 kg and a 25-mm needle for children 60–70 kg is appropriate for IM injections in the deltoid injection site (Koster, Stellato, Kohn, and others, 2009).
- The ventrogluteal site is relatively free of important nerves and vascular structures and is the site of choice for pediatric IM injections in children of all ages; no complications at this site were reported (Beecroft and Kongelbeck, 1994).
- A longer needle (25 mm) was preferred for injection when bunching the skin and injecting; a shorter needle (16 mm) was perceived as causing fewer localized reactions when the injection was administered with the skin being held taut (Groswasser, Kahn, Bouche, and others, 1997).
- Needle length found to be the most significant variable for local reactions in children after injection: a 25-mm needle was associated with fewer localized reactions versus a 16-mm needle (Davenport, 2004).
- In children older than 1 year of age, the deltoid muscle is recommended for IM injections. When multiple vaccines are given, two may be given in the thigh (anterior and lateral) because of its larger size (Diggle, 2003).
- Injections in the anterolateral thigh be given at least 2.5 cm (1 inch) apart so local reactions are less likely to overlap (AAP, Committee on Infectious Diseases, 2009).
- IM injections in the dorsogluteal muscle with longer needles and a 90-degree angle are associated with less reactogenicity (Petousis-Harris, 2008).

Apply the Evidence: Nursing Implications

There is **low-quality evidence** with **strong recommendation** to continue administering IM injections to children in the anterolateral thigh (up to 12 months old), deltoid (12 months and older), and ventrogluteal sites (all ages)

(Guyatt, Oxman, Vist, and others, 2008). Needle length is an important factor in decreasing local reactions; the length should be adequate to deposit the medication into the muscle for IM injections. Recommendations are for a 25-mm (1-inch) needle in infants, a 25- to 32-mm (1–1¼-inch) needle for toddlers, and a 38- to 51-mm (1½–2-inch) needle for older children; preterm and small, emaciated infants may require a shorter needle (16–25 mm [⅝–1 inch]) based on weight and muscle mass size.

QSEN Quality and Safety Competencies:
Evidence-Based Practice*

Knowledge

Differentiate clinical opinion from research and evidence-based summaries.

Describe various methods for identifying appropriate site, technique, needle size, and dose for IM injections in infants, toddlers, and small children.

Skills

Base individualized care plan on patient values, clinical expertise, and evidence.

Integrate evidence into practice by using the techniques for IM injections in clinical care.

Attitudes

Value the concept of evidence-based practice (EBP) as integral to determining best clinical practice.

Appreciate the strengths and weakness of evidence for identifying the appropriate site, technique, needle size, and dose for IM injections in infants, toddlers, and small children.

References

American Academy of Pediatrics, Committee on Infectious Diseases, Pickering L, editor: *2009 Red book: report of the Committee on Infectious Diseases*, ed 28, Elk Grove Village, Ill, 2009, Author.

Beecroft PC, Kongelbeck SR: How safe are intramuscular injections? *AACN Clin Issues* 5(2):207–215, 1994.

Centers for Disease Control and Prevention: General recommendations on immunization, *MMWR Morb Mortal Wkly Rep* 51(RR-2):12–14, 2002.

Cook IF, Murtagh J: Needle length required for intramuscular vaccination of infants and toddlers: an ultrasonographic study, *Aust Fam Phys* 31(3):295–297, 2002.

Daly JM, Johnston W, Chung Y: Injection sites utilized for DPT immunizations in infants, *J Comm Health Nurs* 9(2):87–94, 1992.

Davenport JM: A systematic review to ascertain whether the standard needle is more effective than a longer or wider needle in reducing the incidence of local reaction in children receiving primary immunization, *J Adv Nurs* 46(1):66–77, 2004.

Diggle L: The administration of child vaccines, part 11, childhood vaccinations, *Practice Nurse* 25(12):63–69, 2003.

Diggle L, Deeks J: Effect of needle length on incidence of local reactions to routine immunisation in infants aged 4 months: Randomised controlled trial, *BMJ* 321(7266):931–933, 2000.

Diggle L, Deeks JJ, Pollard AJ: Effect of needle size on immunogenicity and reactogenicity of vaccines in infants: Randomized controlled trial, *BMJ* 333(7568):571, 2006.

Groswasser J, Kahn A, Bouche B, and others: Needle length and injection technique for efficient intramuscular vaccine delivery in infants and children evaluated through an ultrasonographic determination of subcutaneous and muscle layer thickness, *Pediatrics* 100(3 Pt 1):400–403, 1997.

Guyatt GH, Oxman AD, Vist GE, and others: GRADE: An emerging consensus on rating quality of evidence and strength of recommendations, *BMJ* 336(7650):924–926, 2008.

Koster M, Stellato N, Kohn N, and others: Needle length for immunizations of early adolescents as determined by ultrasound, *Pediatrics*, 124:667–672, 2009.

Petousis-Harris H: Vaccine injection technique and reactogenicity—evidence for practice, *Vaccine*, 26:6299–6304, 2008.

Taddio A, Ilersich AL, Ipp M, and others: Physical interventions and injection techniques for reducing injection pain during routine childhood immunizations: systematic review of randomized controlled trials and quasi-randomized controlled trials, *Clin Ther* 31(suppl):S48–S76, 2009.

Zuckerman J: The importance of injecting vaccines into muscle, *BMJ* 321(7271):1237–1238, 2000.

*Adapted from the QSEN at http://www.qsen.org.

including the Immunization Action Coalition,* which has vaccine information and records in a number of languages.

The following information is documented on the medical record: day, month, and year of administration; manufacturer and lot number of vaccine; and the name, address, and title of the person administering the vaccine. Additional data to record are the site and route of administration and evidence that the parent or legal guardian gave informed consent before the immunization was administered. Any adverse reactions after the administration of any vaccine are reported to the Vaccine Adverse Event Reporting System.†

An additional source of vaccine information that must be given to parents (by law; National Childhood Vaccine Injury Act of 1986) before the administration of given vaccines is the vaccine information statement (VIS) for the particular vaccine being administered. Practitioners are required to fully inform families of the risks and benefits of the vaccines. VISs are designed to provide updated information to the adult vaccinee or parents or legal guardians of children being vaccinated regarding the risks and benefits of each vaccine. Questions regarding the information in the VISs should be answered by the practitioner. VISs are available for the following vaccines: anthrax, tetanus, diphtheria, pertussis, MMR, MMRV, IPV, varicella, Hib, influenza, meningococcal, pneumococcal, rabies, shingles, smallpox, yellow fever, Japanese encephalitis, rotavirus, HPV, typhoid, HepA, and HepB. An updated VIS should be provided, and documentation in the patient's chart should state that the VIS was given and include the publication date of the VIS; this represents informed consent when the parent or caregiver gives permission to administer the vaccines. VISs are available from state or local health departments or from the Immunization Action Coalition‡ and CDC.§

In response to the concerns of manufacturers, practitioners, and parents of children with serious vaccine-associated injuries, the National Childhood Vaccine Injury Act of 1986 and the Vaccine Compensation Amendments of 1987 were passed. These laws are designed to provide fair compensation for children who are inadvertently injured and provide greater protection from liability for vaccine manufacturers and providers. For further information, contact the National Vaccine Injury Compensation Program; 800-338-2382; http://www.hrsa.gov/vaccinecompensation.

SAFETY PROMOTION AND INJURY PREVENTION

Injuries are a major cause of death during infancy, especially for children 6 to 12 months old. According to a Canadian survey (Pickett, Streight, Simpson, and others, 2003), the top leading causes of injury to infants were falls, ingestion injuries, and burns. The three leading cause of accidental death injury in infants were suffocation, motor vehicle–related injuries, and drowning (Bernard, Paulozzi, Wallace, and others, 2007). Mack, Gilchrist, and Ballesteros (2007) report that fall-related injuries in the home were the most common reason for emergency department visits in infants ages 0 to 12 months; according to these authors, one infant is injured every 1.5 minutes. In a similar study of infants treated for accidents, beds were commonly listed as being involved, and car seats at 2 months of age and stairs at 12 months were reported to be the cause of the accidental injury (Mack, Gilchrist, and Ballesteros, 2008). According to a recent Cochrane study, one third

of all injuries occur in the home, yet there is insufficient evidence to demonstrate that modification of the home environment has an impact on the rate of injuries (Turner, Arthur, Lyons, and others, 2011). Constant vigilance, awareness, and supervision are essential as children gain increased locomotor and manipulative skills that are coupled with an insatiable curiosity about the environment. Box 10-1 lists the major developmental achievements of each period during infancy and the appropriate injury prevention plan. Table 10-3 lists common types of injuries and associated objects that predispose to such injuries. Suggestions for promoting safety in the home environment are given for specific types of injuries. The acronym SAFE PAD, described in Table 10-3, may be used to identify common types of injuries to infants and older children.

Motor Vehicle Injuries

Automobile injuries are the leading cause of accidental death in children between the ages of 1 and 9 years (Bernard, Paulozzi, Wallace, and others, 2007). A significant number of nonfatal vehicle-related injuries in children between 1 and 4 years of age occur as a result of back-over while children are playing in driveways (CDC, 2005b). In addition, a significant number of infants are injured or die from improper restraint within vehicles, most often from riding on the lap of another occupant. Desapriya, Joshi, Subwarzi, and others (2008) found that falls accounted for a significant proportion of injuries (98%) in infants from birth to 4 months of age as a result of inappropriate use of a car restraint system. Reports indicate that child restraint use decreases with increasing age of children and increasing number of occupants. Lack of proper child restraint continues to be a major factor in fatal accidents involving children. All infants must be secured in federally approved restraints rather than held or placed on the seat of the car. There is no safe alternative.

Infant restraints are designed either as an infant-only model or as a convertible infant–toddler model. Either restraint is a semireclined seat that faces the rear of the car. A rear-facing car seat provides the best protection for the disproportionately heavy head and weak neck of an infant. This position minimizes the stress on the neck by spreading the forces of a frontal crash over the entire back, neck, and head; the spine is supported by the back of the car seat. If the seat were faced forward, the head would whip forward because of the force of the crash, creating enormous stress on the neck (Fig. 10-12). It is now recommended that all infants and toddlers ride in rear-facing car safety seats until they reach the age of 2 years or the height recommended by

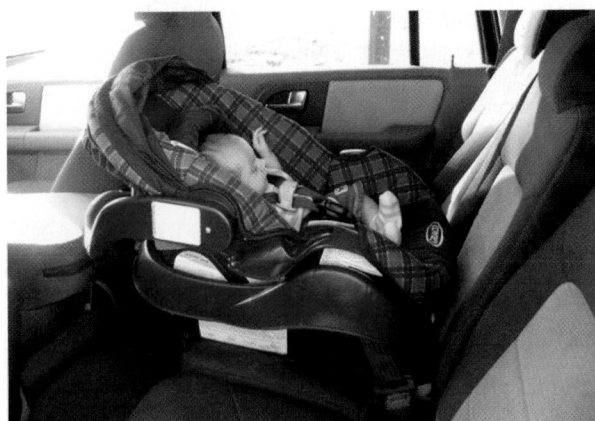

FIG 10-12 Rear-facing infant seat in rear seat of car. The infant is placed in the seat when going home from the hospital. (Courtesy Brian and Mayannyn Sallee, Anchorage, Alaska.)

BOX 10-1 SAFETY PROMOTION AND INJURY PREVENTION DURING INFANCY

Birth to 4 Months
Major Developmental Accomplishments

Exhibits involuntary reflexes (e.g., crawling reflex may propel infant forward or backward; startle reflex may cause the body to jerk)

May roll over

Has increasing eye–hand coordination and voluntary grasp reflex

Injury Prevention
Aspiration

Aspiration is not as great a danger to this age group, but parents should begin practicing safeguarding early (see under Age 4 to 7 Months).

Never shake baby powder directly on infant; place powder in hand and then on infant's skin; store container closed and out of infant's reach.

Hold infant for feeding; do not prop bottle.

Know emergency procedures for choking.

Use pacifier with one-piece construction and loop handle.

Burns

Install smoke detectors in home.

Use caution when warming formula in microwave oven; always check temperature of liquid before feeding.

Check bathwater.

Do not pour hot liquids when infant is close by, such as sitting on lap.

Beware of cigarette ashes that may fall on infant.

Do not leave infant in sun for more than a few minutes; keep skin covered.

Wash flame-retardant clothes according to label directions.

Use cool-mist vaporizers.

Do not leave child in parked car.

Check surface heat of car restraint before placing child in seat.

Suffocation and Drowning

Keep all plastic bags stored out of infant's reach; discard large plastic garment bags after tying in a knot.

Do not cover mattress with plastic.

Use firm mattress and loose blankets with no pillows.

Make certain crib design follows federal regulations and mattress fits snugly—crib slats 2.375 inches (6 cm) apart.*

Position crib away from other furniture and away from radiators.

Do not tie pacifier on a string around infant's neck.

Remove bibs at bedtime.

Never leave infant alone in bath.

Do not leave infant younger than 12 months alone on adult or youth mattress or "beanbag"-type seats.

Motor Vehicles

Transport infant in federally approved, rear-facing car seat, preferably in back seat.†

Do not place infant on seat (of car) or in lap.

Do not place child in a carriage or stroller behind a parked car.

Do not place infant or child in front passenger seat with an air bag.

Do not leave infant unattended in car, especially in environmental temperatures above 70° F.

Falls

Always raise crib rails.

Never leave infant alone on a raised, unguarded surface.

When in doubt as to where to place child, use floor.

Restrain child in infant seat and never leave child unattended while the seat is resting on a raised surface.

Avoid using a high chair until child can sit well with support.

Poisoning

Poisoning is not as great a danger to this age group, but parents should begin practicing safeguards early (see under Age 4 to 7 Months).

Bodily Damage

Keep sharp or jagged objects such as knives and broken glass out of child's reach.

Keep diaper pins closed and away from infant.

Age 4 to 7 Months
Major Developmental Accomplishments

Rolls over

Sits momentarily

Grasps and manipulates small objects

Resecures a dropped object

Has well-developed eye–hand coordination

Can focus on and locate very small objects

Has prominent mouthing (oral fixation)

Can push up on hands and knees

Crawls backward

Injury Prevention
Aspiration

Keep buttons, beads, syringe caps, and other small objects out of infant's reach.

Keep floor free of any small objects.

Do not feed infant hard candy, nuts, food with pits or seeds, or whole or circular pieces of hot dog.

Exercise caution when giving teething biscuits because large chunks may be broken off and aspirated.

Do not feed infant while he or she is lying down.

Inspect toys for removable parts.

Keep baby powder, if used, out of reach.

Avoid storing large quantities of cleaning fluid, paints, pesticides, and other toxic substances.

Discard used containers of poisonous substances.

Do not store toxic substances in food or drink containers.

Discard used button-size batteries; store new batteries in safe area.

Know telephone number of local poison control center (800-222-1222) (usually listed in front of telephone directory).

Suffocation

Keep all latex balloons out of reach.

Remove all crib toys that are strung across crib or play yard when child begins to push up on hands or knees or is 5 months old.

Burns

Keep water faucets out of reach.

Place hot objects (cigarettes, candles, incense) on high surface out of child's reach.

Limit exposure to sun; apply sunscreen.

Falls

Restrain in a high chair.

Keep crib rails raised to full height.

Continued

BOX 10-1   SAFETY PROMOTION AND INJURY PREVENTION DURING INFANCY—cont'd

Motor Vehicles
See under Birth to 4 Months.

Poisoning
Make certain that paint for furniture or toys does not contain lead.
Place toxic substances on a high shelf or in locked cabinet.
Hang plants or place on high surface rather than on floor.
Know telephone number of local poison control center (800-222-1222) (usually listed in front of telephone directory).

Bodily Damage
Give toys that are smooth and rounded, preferably made of wood or plastic.
Avoid long, pointed objects as toys.
Avoid toys that are excessively loud.
Keep sharp objects out of infant's reach.

Age 8 to 12 Months
Major Developmental Accomplishments
Crawls or creeps
Stands, holding on to furniture
Stands alone
Cruises around furniture
Walks
Climbs
Pulls on objects
Throws objects
Is able to pick up small objects; has pincer grasp
Explores by putting objects in mouth
Dislikes being restrained
Explores away from parent
Increasingly understands simple commands and phrases

Injury Prevention
Aspiration
Keep small objects off floor, off furniture, and out of reach of children.
Take care when feeding solid table food to give very small pieces.
Do not use beanbag toys or allow child to play with dried beans.
See also under Age 4 to 7 Months.

Bodily Damage
See under Age 4 to 7 Months.
Avoid placing televisions or other large objects on top of furniture, which may be overturned when infant pulls self to standing position.

Falls
Avoid walkers, especially near stairs.*
Ensure that furniture is sturdy enough for child to pull self to standing position and cruise.
Fence stairways at top and bottom if child has access to either end.*
Dress infant in safe shoes and clothing (soles that do not "catch" on floor, tied shoelaces, pant legs that do not touch floor).

Suffocation and Drowning
Keep doors of ovens, dishwashers, refrigerators, coolers, and front-loading clothes washers and dryers closed at all times.
If storing an unused large appliance, such as a refrigerator, remove the door.
Supervise contact with inflated balloons; immediately discard popped balloons and keep uninflated balloons out of reach.
Fence swimming pools and other bodies of standing water such as decorative fountains; lock gate to swimming pools so only adult can access.
Always supervise when near any source of water, such as cleaning buckets, drainage areas, toilets.
Keep bathroom doors closed.
Eliminate unnecessary pools of water.
Keep one hand on child at all times when in tub.

Poisoning
Administer medications as a drug, not as a candy.
Do not administer medications unless prescribed by a practitioner.
Return medications and poisons to safe storage area immediately after use; replace caps properly if a child-protector cap is used.
Have poison control center number (800-222-1222) on telephone and refrigerator.

Burns
Place guards in front of or around any heating appliance, fireplace, or furnace.
Keep electrical wires hidden or out of reach.
Place plastic guards over electrical outlets; place furniture in front of outlets.
Keep hanging tablecloths out of reach (child may pull down hot liquids or heavy or sharp objects).

*Information on many items such as cribs or walkers is available from U.S. Consumer Product Safety Commission, 800-638-2772; http://www.cpsc.gov/.

---

the car seat manufacturer (AAP, 2011)*. Some infant-only rear-facing infant car safety seats can accommodate children weighing up to a maximum of 35 pounds. Studies indicate that toddlers up to 24 months of age are safer riding in convertible seats in the rear-facing position (Bull and Durbin, 2008; Henary, Sherwood, Crandall, and others, 2007).

The restraint is anchored to the vehicle with the vehicle's seat belt, and the restraint has a harness system for securing the infant. Some harness systems require a clip to keep the shoulder straps correctly positioned. Newer vehicles (manufactured after 1999) have tether straps that attach to anchors in the car seat to better secure the seat and minimize forward movement of the forward-facing convertible seats in the event of an accident. The LATCH (lower anchor and tether for children) system provides car seat anchors between the front cushion and backrest so that the seat belt does not have to be used. Some automobiles have tether straps for rear-facing infant-only seats as well (see Fig 12-12). Although many infant restraints can be recliners, they are used in the car only in the position specified by the manufacturer.

---

*Car seat information is available from the AAP at http://www.aap.org/healthtopics/carseatsafety.cfm; and from the Insurance Institute for Highway Safety, 1005 N. Glebe Road, Suite 800, Arlington, VA 22201; 703-247-1500; fax: 703-247-1588; http://www.iihs.org. The National Highway Traffic Safety Administration, http://www.nhtsa.gov, also provides child passenger safety and air bag safety information for parents.

TABLE 10-3	COMMON INFANT INJURIES, ASSOCIATED RISK FACTORS, AND SAFETY PROMOTION	
SAFE PAD	**RISK FACTORS**	**SUGGESTED SAFETY INTERVENTIONS**
S—Suffocation, Sleep position	Latex balloons	Avoid latex balloons except with close adult supervision.
	Plastic bags	Tie unused plastic bags in a knot and dispose of in a safe container.
	Bed surface (noninfant) such as sofa or adult bed	Avoid placing infants to sleep on sofas, soft bedding, or adult bed.
	Pillows	Avoid use of pillows for sleep.
	Soft cushions and blankets	Clear bedding of soft cushions and blankets.
	Prone sleeping	Place infant to sleep on back at all times.
A—Asphyxia, animal bites	Food items: cylindrical items such as hot dogs, hard candy, peanuts, almonds	Cut hot dogs lengthwise; avoid hard candy in infants and toddlers. Infants should completely chew up each food item in mouth; do not feed more until item is swallowed.
	Toys: small toys such as Legos	As a general rule of thumb, if the toy fits into a toilet paper cardboard roll, it can be swallowed by a small child.
	Small objects: batteries, buttons, beads, dried beans, syringe caps, safety pins	Keep out of reach of infants, who are naturally inquisitive.
	Pacifiers	Pacifiers should be one piece.
	Baby (talc) powder	Avoid shaking powder over infant; if used, place on adult's hand and then place on infant's skin.
	Domestic dogs, cats	Supervise child around domestic animals; teach not to approach dog that is eating, has puppies, or is not feeling well. Animals that are "tame" can be unpredictable. Small children are the right size for most domesticated animals to come face to face. Closely supervise child around visiting pets. (See Pet and Wild Animal Bites, Chapter 30.)
F—Falls	Stairs	Infants like to climb; place childproof gate at top and bottom of stairs.
	Diaper changing table	Infants do not have depth perception and cannot perceive a dangerous height from one that is safe. Never leave infants unattended on a flat surface even if not rolling over.
	Crib, bed-crib sides can fall when infant leans on them	In 2011, a mandate was made to stop selling drop-side infant cribs.*
	Infant carriers	Never leave infant unattended in a carrier on top of a surface such as a shopping cart, clothes dryer, washer, kitchen cabinet; place carrier on floor.
	Car seat restraints	Secure infant in car seat restraint securely and never leave unattended if unrestrained.
	High chair	Restrain infant in high chair; avoid using high chair except for feeding and only if adult supervision is adequate; even restrained infants can squirm out of some restraints and fall.
	Infant walkers	Use only stationary walkers. There is no evidence that walkers help infants "walk" any sooner. Wheeled walkers can easily be propelled off stairs and other platforms such as porches or decks, causing significant injury
	Windows, screens	Avoid placing furniture next to a window. Infants learn to climb and can fall out of open windows, even with screens.
	Television, stereos, sound systems	These must be secured to the stand; infants can pull the stand over, causing the TV or sound system to land on their heads, causing significant injury.
E—Electrical burns or burns	Electrical outlets	Place safety cap over electrical outlets; infants may be burned by placing conductive object into outlet.
	Hot hair combs, curlers	Keep out of reach of infant and keep turned off when not in use.
	Water	Infants may turn on tap or faucet in bathtub and burn self. Lower the water heater to a safe temperature of 49° C (120° F). Before placing infant in tub, check temperature of water and completely turn off faucet so child cannot alter temperature of water. NEVER leave infant unattended in tub or sink of water.
	Fireplace	Place a childproof screen in front of fireplace.
	Stove, hot liquids	Keep top front burners off and keep pot handles turned toward back to avoid infant pulling hot pot onto self and causing burn injuries.
	Cigarettes	Avoid smoking and holding infant on lap while smoking cigar or cigarette.

Continued

TABLE 10-3	COMMON INFANT INJURIES, ASSOCIATED RISK FACTORS, AND SAFETY PROMOTION—cont'd	
SAFE PAD	**RISK FACTORS**	**SUGGESTED SAFETY INTERVENTIONS**
P—Poisoning, ingestions	Medication, ointments, cream, lotions	Medications left in purses or handbags or on a table top can often be ingested by the curious infant.
		Keep Poison Control Center number readily available (800-222-1222).
	Plants: household plants may be a source of accidental poisoning	Keep plants out of child's reach.
	Cleaning solutions	Store in locked cabinet or in top cabinet where there are no drawers or shelves for infant to climb on. Avoid storing cleaning and caustic solutions in containers such as a soda bottle or jar—infants and toddlers cannot differentiate a soda from a caustic drain cleaner.
	Inhalation or oral or nasal ingestion of poisonous or harmful chemicals such as methamphetamine, gasoline, turpentine	Keep gasoline and turpentine stored in a locked cabinet or closet out of child's reach. Avoid storing in containers that are also used to keep drinks or food.
A—Automobile safety	Car or truck and hot weather	An automobile-related hazard for infants is overheating (hyperthermia) and subsequent death when left in a vehicle in hot weather (>26.4° C [80° F]). Infants dissipate heat poorly, and an increase in body temperature may cause death in a few hours. Caution parents against leaving infants in a vehicle alone for *any reason*.
	Air bags	Avoid placing infant in a car restraint behind an air bag. Deactivate the air bag (available in certain models) or place the infant in the back seat in a proper car seat restraint.
	Car seat restraint	See discussion on p. 344.
D—Drowning	Bath tub	NEVER leave infant unattended in tub or sink of water.
	Swimming pools, bird baths, decorative ponds of water, splash pads	Place fence around pools with gate lock that is out of child's reach. Supervise infants in water at ALL times; an infant may drown in as little as 2 inches of water. Swimming lessons are encouraged but are not foolproof for drowning if infant or child hits head on hard object and becomes unconscious as falling into the water.
	5-gal buckets	Keep 5-gal buckets empty of water or elevated out of child's reach.

*A number of parent education pamphlets—such as *Crib Safety Tips* and *Is Your Used Crib Safe?*—are available in English and Spanish from the U.S. Consumer Product Safety Commission, 4330 East West Highway, Bethesda, MD 20814; 800-638-2772; http://www.cpsc.gov.

Severe injuries and deaths in children have occurred from air bags deploying on impact in the front passenger seat. The back seat is the safest area of the car for children. For restraints to be effective, they must be used properly. Dressing the infant in an outfit with sleeves and legs allows the harness to hold the child securely in the seat. A small blanket or towel rolled tightly can be placed on either side of the head to minimize movement and keep the infant's hips against the back of the seat. Padding between the infant's legs and crotch is added to prevent slouching. Thick, soft padding is not placed under the infant or behind the back because during the impact, the padding will compress, leaving the harness straps loose. Preterm infants being discharged home from the hospital should be placed in appropriate car seat restraints as they would be placed in the car and their heart rate and oxygen saturation should be monitored for 90 to 120 minutes to detect any potential problems with airway occlusion. (For further discussion of car seat restraints, see Chapter 12.)

! NURSING ALERT

Rear-facing infant safety seats must not be placed in the front seats of cars equipped with an air bag on the passenger side. If an infant safety seat is placed in the passenger seat with an air bag, the child could be seriously injured if the air bag is released because rear-facing infant seats extend closer to the dashboard.

Nurse's Role in Injury Prevention

The task of injury prevention begins to be appreciated only when the potential environmental dangers to which infants are vulnerable are considered. Injury prevention and parent education should be handled on a growth and developmental basis. It is simply impossible to completely protect infants and small children from all potential dangers without placing them in a sterile, impractical environment. However, a large percentage of childhood deaths continue to occur as a result of preventable injuries (Martin, Kochanek, Strobino, and others, 2005; Schnitzer, 2006). Nurses must be aware of the possible causes of injury in each age group to provide anticipatory, preventive teaching. For example, the nurse should discuss guidelines for injury prevention during infancy (see Box 10-1) before the child reaches the susceptible age group. Preventive teaching ideally begins during pregnancy.

One third of all injuries to children occur in the home, and therefore the importance of safety cannot be overemphasized. The Family-Centered Care box summarizes a home safety checklist that can be presented to parents to increase their awareness of danger areas in the home and assist them in implementing safety devices and practices *before* their absence can inflict injury on infants. Hands-on displays such as cabinet latches or toilet seat locks can familiarize parents with inexpensive, commercial devices that can be used in the home to prevent injuries.

Injury prevention requires protection of the child and education of the caregiver. Nurses in ambulatory care settings, health maintenance centers, and visiting nurse agencies are in a most favorable position for

FAMILY-CENTERED CARE

Child Safety Home Checklist

Safety: Fire, Electrical, Burns
- Guards in front of or around any heating appliance, fireplace, or furnace (including floor furnace)*
- Electrical wires hidden or out of reach*
- No frayed or broken wires; no overloaded sockets
- Plastic guards or caps over electrical outlets; furniture in front of outlets*
- Hanging tablecloths out of reach away from open fires*
- Smoke detectors tested and operating properly
- Kitchen matches stored out of child's reach*
- Large, deep ashtrays throughout house (if used)
- Small stoves, heaters, and other hot objects (cigarettes, candles, coffee pots, slow cookers) placed where they cannot be tipped over or reached by children
- Hot water heater set at 49° C (120° F) or lower
- Pot handles turned toward back of stove and the center of table
- No loose clothing worn near stove
- No cooking or eating hot foods or liquids with child standing nearby or sitting in lap
- All small appliances, such as iron, turned off, disconnected, and placed out of reach when not in use
- Cool, not hot, mist vaporizer used
- Fire extinguisher available on each floor and checked periodically
- Electrical fuse box and gas shutoff accessible
- Family escape plan in case of a fire practiced periodically; fire escape ladder available on upper-level floors
- Telephone number of fire or rescue squad and address of home with nearest cross street posted near phone

Safety: Suffocation and Aspiration
- Small objects stored out of reach*
- Toys inspected for small removable parts or long strings*
- Hanging crib toys and mobiles placed out of reach
- Plastic bags stored away from young child's reach; large plastic garment bags discarded after tying in knots*
- Mattress or pillow not covered with plastic or in manner accessible to child*
- Crib design according to federal regulations (crib slats <2.375 inches [6 cm] apart) with snug-fitting mattress*†
- Crib positioned away from other furniture or windows*
- Portable play yard sides up and locked at all times while in use*
- Accordion-style gates not used*
- Bathroom doors kept closed and toilet seats down*
- Faucets turned off firmly*
- Pool fenced with locked gate
- Proper safety equipment at poolside
- Electronic garage door openers stored safely and garage door adjusted to rise when door strikes object
- Doors of ovens, trunks, dishwashers, refrigerators, and front-loading clothes washers and dryers kept closed*
- Unused appliance, such as a refrigerator, securely closed with lock or doors removed*
- Food served in small, noncylindric pieces*

- Toy chests without lids or with lids that securely lock in open position*
- Buckets and wading pools kept empty when not in use*
- Clothesline above head level
- At least one member of household trained in basic life support (cardiopulmonary resuscitation), including first aid for choking

Safety: Poisoning
- Toxic substances, including batteries, placed on a high shelf, preferably in locked cabinet
- Toxic plants hung or placed out of reach*
- Excess quantities of cleaning fluid, paints, pesticides, drugs, and other toxic substances not stored in home
- Used containers of poisonous substances discarded where child cannot obtain access
- Telephone number of local poison control center (800-222-1222) and home address with nearest cross street posted near phone
- Medicines clearly labeled in childproof containers and stored out of reach
- Household cleaners, disinfectants, and insecticides kept in their original containers separate from food and out of reach
- Smoking in areas away from children

Safety: Falls
- Nonskid mats, strips, or surfaces in tubs and showers
- Exits, halls, and passageways in rooms kept clear of toys, furniture, boxes, and other items that could be obstructive
- Stairs and halls well lighted with switches at both top and bottom
- Sturdy handrails for all steps and stairways
- Nothing stored on stairways
- Treads, risers, and carpeting in good repair
- Glass doors and walls marked with decals
- Safety glass used in doors, windows, and walls
- Gates on top and bottom of staircases and elevated areas, such as porch, fire escape*
- Guardrails on upstairs windows with locks that limit height of window opening and access to areas such as fire escape*
- Crib side rails raised to full height; mattress lowered as child grows*
- Restraints used in high chairs, walkers, or other baby furniture; preferably, walkers not used*
- Scatter rugs secured in place or used with nonskid backing
- Walks, patios, and driveways in good repair

Safety: Bodily Injury
- Knives, power tools, and unloaded firearms stored safely or placed in locked cabinet
- Garden tools returned to storage racks after use
- Pets properly restrained and immunized for rabies
- Swings, slides, and other outdoor play equipment kept in safe condition
- Yard free of broken glass, nail-studded boards, and other litter
- Cement birdbaths placed where young child cannot tip them over*
- Furniture anchored so child cannot pull down on top of self when climbing or pulling to stand

*Safety measures are specific for homes with young children. All safety measures should be implemented in homes where children reside and visit frequently, such as those of grandparents and babysitters.
†Federal regulations are available from the U.S. Consumer Product Safety Commission, 800-638-2772; http://www.cpsc.gov.

injury education. This does not exclude nurses in inpatient facilities, who could use visiting times as an excellent opportunity for discussing this topic. Although early postpartum discharge may be restrictive for parent teaching, this is an excellent opportunity to introduce the family to infant safety and safety for other children as well. Parents should be encouraged to take an infant cardiopulmonary resuscitation (CPR) class to deal effectively with potential problems. This tool further empowers the parents to raise their new infant in the best environment possible.

One approach to teaching injury prevention is to relate why children in various age groups are prone to specific types of injuries. Stressing prevention is just as important as emphasizing the *why* of the injury. However, injury prevention must also be practical. Asking parents for their ideas leads to realistic suggestions that can be followed. For instance, bathroom cleaning agents, cosmetics, and personal care items can be placed on a top shelf in the linen closet, and towels or sheets can be stored on the lower shelves and floor.

If an injury has occurred, the nurse should not be too quick to admonish the parent. Injuries do not always indicate neglect. It is a difficult task to watch children carefully without overprotecting or unnecessarily confining them. Allowing children to explore while maintaining consistent, age-appropriate limits is sound advice.

Parents need to remember that infants and young children cannot anticipate danger or understand when it is or is not present. Additionally, infants have no cognitive concept of cause and effect and therefore cannot relate meaning to experiences or potential dangers. A dead electrical wire may present no actual harm, but if the child is allowed to play with it, a poor behavior is enforced and will be practiced when the child encounters a live wire. Although it is always wise to explain why something is dangerous, it must be remembered that small children need to be physically removed from the situation.

It is not easy to teach safety, supervise closely, and refrain from saying "no" a hundred times a day. Parents become acutely aware of this dilemma as soon as their infants learn to crawl. Preventing injuries

to children is usually the first reason for limit setting and discipline, but limits are also set to prevent damage to valuable household objects. When small children are in the home, dangerous objects must be removed or guarded and valuable articles placed out of reach.

When children are taught the meaning of "no," they should also be taught what "yes" means. Children should be praised for playing with suitable toys, their efforts at behaving or listening should be reinforced, and innovative and creative recreational toys should be provided for them. Infants love to tear paper and avidly pursue books, magazines, or newspapers left on the floor. Instead of always scolding them for destroying a valued book, parents should provide child-safe books (e.g., those constructed of fabric) for them to play with. If they enjoy pots and pans, a cabinet can be arranged with safe utensils for them to explore.

One additional factor must be stressed concerning injury prevention and education. Children are imitators; they copy what they see and hear. *Practicing safety teaches safety*, which applies to parents and their children and to nurses and their clients. Saying one thing but doing another confuses children and can lead to difficulties as the child grows older.

ANTICIPATORY GUIDANCE—CARE OF FAMILIES

Childrearing is no easy task; it presents challenges to both new parents and "seasoned" parents. With society's changing roles and mores combined with a highly mobile population, there is little stability for traditional role models and time-honored methods of raising children. As a result, parents look to professionals for guidance. Nurses are in an advantageous position to render assistance and suggestions. Every phase of a child's life has its particular traumas—toilet training for toddlers, unexplained fears for preschoolers, and identity crises for adolescents. For parents of infants, some challenges center around dependency, discipline, increased mobility, and safety. Major areas for parental guidance during the first year are listed in the Family-Centered Care box.

FAMILY-CENTERED CARE

Guidance During Infant's First Year

First 6 Months

- Teach car safety with use of federally approved restraint, facing rearward, in the middle of the back seat—not in a seat with an air bag.
- Understand each parent's adjustment to newborn, especially mother's postpartum emotional needs.
- Teach care of infant and help parents understand his or her individual needs and temperament and that the infant expresses wants through crying.
- Reassure parents that infant cannot be spoiled by too much attention during the first 4 to 6 months.
- Encourage parents to establish a schedule that meets needs of child and themselves.
- Help parents understand infant's need for stimulation in environment.
- Support parents' pleasure in seeing child's growing friendliness and social response, especially smiling.
- Plan anticipatory guidance for safety.
- Stress need for immunizations.
- Prepare for introduction of solid foods.

Second 6 Months

- Prepare parents for child's "stranger anxiety."
- Encourage parents to allow child to cling to them and avoid long separation from either.
- Guide parents concerning discipline because of infant's increasing mobility.
- Encourage use of negative voice and eye contact rather than physical punishment as a means of discipline.
- Encourage showing most attention when infant is behaving well rather than when infant is crying.
- Teach injury prevention because of child's advancing motor skills and curiosity.
- Encourage parents to leave child with suitable caregiver to allow some free time.
- Discuss readiness for weaning.
- Explore parents' feelings regarding infant's sleep patterns.

KEY POINTS

- Children's biologic development encompasses proportional changes; sensory changes, including binocularity and depth perception; maturation of biologic systems; fine motor development; and gross motor development.
- In Erikson's theory of psychosocial development, the period from birth to 1 year is concerned with acquiring a sense of trust while overcoming a sense of mistrust.
- Piaget's theory of cognitive development, as it applies to infants, focuses on the sensorimotor phase, which includes the use of reflexes, primary circular reactions, secondary circular reactions, and coordination of secondary schemas and their application to new situations.
- Development of body image begins in infancy; by 1 year of age, infants recognize that they are distinct from their parents.
- Infants' social development is guided by attachment, language development, personal–social behavior, and participation in play.
- Temperament influences the type of interaction that occurs between the child and parents and siblings.
- Parents are faced with many concerns, including infant fears, daycare, limit setting and discipline, thumb sucking and pacifier use, and teething.
- Breast milk is the most desirable food for infants during the first 6 months; formula is an acceptable alternative followed by gradual introduction of solid food during the second 6 months. Whole milk is not recommended until after 12 months.
- Solid foods may be introduced between 4 and 6 months, beginning with iron-fortified rice cereal.
- Cleaning the teeth regularly and appropriate dietary intake promote good dental health.
- Recommended routine childhood immunizations include those for HAV and HBV, diphtheria, tetanus, pertussis, polio, measles, mumps, rubella, varicella (chickenpox), pneumococcal infection, meningococcal infection, influenza, and Hib infection.
- Recommended immunizations for selected groups of children include rotavirus and the HPV vaccine.
- Because injuries are a major cause of death during infancy, parents should be alerted to the risks related to aspiration of foreign objects, suffocation, falls, poisoning, burns, and motor vehicle injuries, as well as preventive actions needed to make the environment safe for infants.

REFERENCES

American Academy of Pediatric Dentistry: Guideline on infant oral health care. In *AAPD reference manual, 2010–2011*, 33(6):12, 114, retrieved June 9, 2011, from http://www.aapd.org/media/Policies_Guidelines/G_InfantOralHealthCare.pdf.

American Academy of Pediatrics: Policy statement—child passenger safety, *Pediatrics* 127(4):788–793, 2011.

American Academy of Pediatrics, Committee on Infectious Diseases, Pickering L, editor: *2009 Red book: report of the Committee on Infectious Diseases*, ed 28, Elk Grove Village, Ill, 2009, Author.

American Academy of Pediatrics, Committee on Infectious Diseases: Policy statement—recommendations for the prevention and treatment of influenza in children, 2009–2010, *Pediatrics* 124(4):1216–1226, 2009.

American Academy of Pediatrics, Committee on Infectious Diseases: Recommendations for prevention and control of influenza in children, 2011–2012, *Pediatrics* 128(4): 813–825, 2011a.

American Academy of Pediatrics, Committee on Infectious Diseases: Meningococcal conjugate vaccines policy update: booster dose recommendations, *Pediatrics* 128(6): 1213–1218, 2011b.

American Academy of Pediatrics, Committee on Injury and Poison Prevention: Injuries associated with infant walkers, *Pediatrics* 108(3):790–792, 2001.

American Academy of Pediatrics, Committee on Nutrition: *Pediatric nutrition handbook*, ed 6, Elk Grove Village, Ill, 2009, Author.

American Academy of Pediatrics, Task Force on Sudden Infant Death Syndrome: The changing concept of sudden infant death syndrome: diagnostic coding shifts, controversies regarding the sleeping environment, and new variables to consider in reducing risk, *Pediatrics* 116(5): 1245–1255, 2005.

Anderson JE: "Nothing but the tooth": dispelling myths about teething, *Contemp Pediatr* 21(7): 75–83, 2004.

Baker RD, Greer FR, American Academy of Pediatrics, Committee on Nutrition: Clinical report—diagnosis and prevention of iron deficiency and iron-deficiency anemia in infants and young children (0–3 years of age), *Pediatrics* 126(5):1040–1050, 2010.

Beck CT: Predictors of postpartum depression: an update, *Nurs Res* 50(5):275–285, 2001.

Bernard SJ, Paulozzi LJ, Wallace DL, and others: Fatal injuries among children by race and ethnicity—United States, 1999–2002, *MMWR Surveill Summ* 56(SS-5):1–16, 2007.

Biancuzzo M: *Breastfeeding the newborn: clinical strategies for nurses*, ed 2, St. Louis, 2003, Mosby.

Blackburn ST: *Maternal, fetal, and neonatal physiology: a clinical perspective*, ed 4, Philadelphia, 2011, Saunders.

Boyce JA, Assa'ad A, Burks AW, and others: Guideline for the diagnosis and management of food allergy in the United States: summary of the NIAID-sponsored expert panel report, *J Allergy Clin Immunol* 126(6):1005–1118, 2010.

Brady MT: Infectious disease in pediatric out-of-home child care, *Am J Infect Control* 33(5):276–285, 2005.

Bull MJ, Durbin DR: Rear-facing car safety seats: getting the message right, *Pediatrics* 121(3):619–620, 2008.

Carey WB, McDevitt SC: Revision of the infant temperament questionnaire, *Pediatrics* 61(5): 735–739, 1978.

Centers for Disease Control and Prevention: A comprehensive immunization strategy to eliminate transmission of hepatitis B virus infection in the United States, *MMWR Morb Mortal Wkly Rep* 54(RR-16):1–23, 2005a.

Centers for Disease Control and Prevention: Nonfatal motor-vehicle-related backover injuries among children—United States, 2001–2003, *MMWR Morb Mortal Wkly Rep* 54(06):144–146, 2005b.

Centers for Disease Control and Prevention: Outbreaks of pertussis associated with hospitals—Kentucky, Pennsylvania, and Oregon, 2003, *MMWR Morb Mortal Wkly Rep* 54(03):67–71, 2005c.

Centers for Disease Control and Prevention: Update: Guillain-Barré syndrome among recipients of Menactra meningococcal conjugate vaccine—United States, June 2005–September 2006, *MMWR Morb Mortal Wkly Rep* 55(41):1120–1124, 2006.

Centers for Disease Control and Prevention: Fatal injuries among children by race and ethnicity—United States, 1999–2002, *MMWR Morb Mortal Wkly Rep* 56(SS05):1–16, 2007.

Centers for Disease Control and Prevention: Update: recommendations from the Advisory Committee on Immunization Practices (ACIP) regarding administration of combination MMRV vaccine, *MMWR Morb Mortal Wkly Rep* 57(10):258–260, 2008.

Centers for Disease Control and Prevention: Licensure of a *Haemophilus influenza* type b (Hib) vaccine (Hiberix) and updated recommendations for use of Hib vaccine, *MMWR Morb Mortal Wkly Rep* 58(36): 1008–1009, 2009.

Centers for Disease Control and Prevention: FDA licensure of bivalent humanpapillomavirus vaccine (HPV2, Cervarix) for use in females and updated HPV recommendations from the Advisory Committee on Immunization Practices

(ACIP), *MMWR Morb Mortal Wkly Rep* 59(20):626–629, 2010a.

Centers for Disease Control and Prevention: FDA licensure of quadrivalent human papillomavirus vaccine (HPV4, Gardasil) for use in males and guidance from the Advisory Committee on Immunization Practices (ACIP), *MMWR Morb Mortal Wkly Rep* 59(20):630–632, 2010b.

Centers for Disease Control and Prevention: Recommended immunization schedules for persons aged 0 through 18 years—United States, 2011, *MMWR Morb Mortal Wkly Rep* 60(5):1–4, 2011a.

Centers for Disease Control and Prevention: Updated recommendations for use of tetanus toxoid, reduced diphtheria toxoid and acellular pertussis (Tdap) vaccine from the Advisory Committee on Immunization Practices, 2010, *MMWR Morb Mortal Wkly Rep* 60(01):13–15, 2011b.

Conover E, Buehler BA: Use of herbal agents by breastfeeding women may affect infants, *Pediatr Ann* 33(4):235–240, 2004.

Cook IF, Murtagh J: Ventrogluteal area—a suitable site for intramuscular vaccination in infants and toddlers, *Vaccine* 24(13): 2403–2408, 2006.

DeStefano F: Vaccines and autism: evidence does not support a causal association, *Clin Pharmacol Ther* 82(6):756–759, 2007.

Desapriya EB, Joshi P, Subwarzi S, and others: Infant injuries from child restraint safety seat misuse at British Columbia Children's Hospital, *Pediatr Int* 50(5):674–678, 2008.

Dewey KG: Nutrition, growth, and complementary feeding of the breastfed infant, *Pediatr Clin North Am* 48(1):87–104, 2001.

Diggle L, Deeks J: Effect of needle length on incidence of local reactions to routine immunizations in infants aged 4 months: randomized controlled trial, *BMJ* 321(7266): 931–993, 2000.

Diggle L, Deeks JJ, Pollard AJ: Effect of needle size and immunogenicity and reactogenicity of vaccines in infants: a randomized controlled trial, *BMJ* 333(7568):571, 2006.

Douglass JM, Douglass AB, Silk HJ: A practical guide to infant oral health, *Am Fam Physician* 70(11):2113–2120, 2004.

FDA Consumer Health Information: *Infant overdose risk with liquid vitamin D*, Washington, DC, June 10, 2010, U.S. Food and Drug Administration, retrieved June 9, 2011, from http://www.fda.gov/downloads/ForConsumers/ConsumerUpdates/UCM215586.pdf.

Fox MK, Reidy K, Novak T, and others: Sources of energy and nutrients in the diets of infants and toddlers, *J Am Diet Assoc* 106(1 suppl 1): S28–S42, 2006.

Fredrickson DD, Davis TC, Arnold CL, and others: Childhood immunization refusal: provider and parent perceptions, *Fam Med* 36(6):431–438, 2004.

Goyal D, Gay C, Lee K: Fragmented maternal sleep is more strongly correlated with depressive symptoms than infant temperament at three months postpartum, *Arch Wom Ment Health* 12(4):229–237, 2009.

Grummer-Strawn LM, Mei Z, Centers for Disease Control and Prevention Pediatric Nutrition Surveillance System: Does breastfeeding protect against pediatric overweight? Analysis of longitudinal data from the Centers for Disease Control and Prevention Pediatric Nutrition Surveillance System, *Pediatrics* 113(2):e81–e86, 2004.

Grummer-Strawn LM, Reinold C, Krebs NF, and others: Use of World Health Organization and CDC growth charts for children aged 0–59 months in the United States, *MMWR Recomm Rep* 59(RR-9):1–15, 2010.

Grummer-Strawn LM, Scanlon KS, Fein SB: Infant feeding and feeding transitions during the first year of life, *Pediatrics* 122(suppl 2):S36–S42, 2008.

Halperin BA, Halperin SA, McGrath P, and others: Use of lidocaine-prilocaine patch to decrease intramuscular injection pain does not adversely affect the antibody response to diphtheria–tetanus–acellular pertussis–inactivated poliovirus–*Haemophilus influenzae* type b conjugate and hepatitis B vaccines in infants from birth to 6 months of age, *Pediatr Infect Dis* 21(5):399–405, 2002.

Hatfield LA: Sucrose decreases infant neurobehavioral pain response to immunizations: a randomized controlled trial, *J Nurs Scholarship* 40(3):219–225, 2008.

Henary B, Sherwood CP, Crandall JR, and others: Car safety for children: rear facing for best protection, *Inj Prev* 13(6):398–402, 2007.

Hoath SB, Pickens WL, Visscher MO: The biology of vernix caseosa, *Int J Cosmet Sci* 28(5):319–333, 2006.

Horn MI, McCarthy AM: Children's responses to sequential versus simultaneous immunization injections, *J Pediatr Health Care* 13(1):18–23, 1999.

Huiming Y, Chaomin W, Meng M: Vitamin A for treating measles in children, *Cochrane Database Syst Rev* (4):CD001479, 2005.

Hviid A, Stellfeld M, Wohlfahrt J, and others: Association between thimerosal-containing vaccine and autism, *JAMA* 290(13):1763–1766, 2003.

Iglowstein I, Jenni OG, Molinari L, and others: Sleep duration from infancy to adolescence: reference values and generational trends, *Pediatrics* 111(2):302–307, 2003.

Institute of Medicine: *Immunization safety review: vaccines and autism*, Washington, DC, 2004, National Academies Press.

Ipp M, Parkin PC, Lear N, and others: Order of vaccine injection and infant pain response, *Arch Pediatr Adolesc Med* 163(5):469–472, 2009.

Jaafar SH, Jahanafar S, Angolkar M, and others: Pacifier use versus no pacifier use in breastfeeding term infants for increasing duration of breastfeeding, *Cochrane Database Syst Rev* (3):CD007202, 2011.

Jackson LA, Yu O, Nelson JC, and others: Injection site and risk of medically attended local reactions to acellular pertussis vaccine, *Pediatrics* 127(3):e681–e687, 2011.

Joanna Briggs Institute: Evidence based practice information sheet for health professionals: early childhood pacifier use in relation to breastfeeding, SIDS, infection, and malocclusion, *Best Practice* 9(3):1–6, 2005.

Johnston ML, Esposito N: Barriers and facilitators for breastfeeding among working women in the United States, *J Obstetr Gynecol Neonat Nurs* 36(1):9–20, 2007.

Junqueira ALN, Tavares VR, Martins RMB, and others: Safety and immunogenicity of hepatitis B vaccine administered into ventrogluteal vs. anterolateral thigh sites in infants: a randomised controlled trial, *Int J Nurs Stud* 47(9): 1074–1079, 2010.

Kimmel SR, Burns IT, Wolfe RM, and others: Addressing immunization barriers, benefits, and risks, *J Fam Pract* 56(2):S61–S69, 2007.

Lawrence RA, Lawrence RM: *Breastfeeding: a guide for the medical profession*, ed 7, St. Louis, 2011, Mosby.

Li R, Fein SB, Grummer-Strawn LM: Do infants fed bottles lack self-regulation of milk intake compared with directly breastfed infants? *Pediatrics* 125(6):e1386–e1393, 2010.

Liaw JJ, Zeng WP, Yang L, and others: Nonnutritive sucking and oral sucrose relieve neonatal pain during intramuscular injection of hepatitis vaccine, *J Pain Symptom Manage* 42(6):918–930, Epub 2011.

Lundqvist P, Jakobsson L: Swedish men's experiences of becoming fathers to their preterm infants, *Neonat Netw* 22(6):25–31, 2003.

Mack KA, Gilchrist J, Ballesteros MF: Unintentional injuries among infants age 0–12 months, *J Safety Res* 38(5):609–612, 2007.

Mack KA, Gilchrist J, Ballesteros MF: Injuries among infants treated in the emergency departments in the United States, 2001–2004, *Pediatrics* 121(5):930–937, 2008.

Marin M, Broder KR, Temte JL, and others: Use of combination measles, mumps, rubella, and varicella vaccines: recommendations of the Advisory Committee on Immunization Practices, *MMWR Recomm Rep* 59(RR-3):1–12, 2010.

Markman L: Teething: facts and fiction, *Pediatr Rev* 30(8):e59–e64, 2009.

Martin JA, Kochanek KD, Strobino DM, and others: Annual summary of vital statistics—2003, *Pediatrics* 115(3):619–634, 2005.

McGrath JM, Records K, Rice M: Maternal depression and infant temperament characteristics, *Infant Behav Dev* 31(1):71–80, 2008.

Medoff-Cooper B, Carey WB, McDevitt SC: The early infancy temperament questionnaire, *J Dev Behav Pediatr* 14(4):230–235, 1993.

Middleman AB, Anding R, Tung C: Effect of needle length when immunizing obese adolescents with hepatitis B vaccine, *Pediatrics* 125(3):e508–e512, 2010.

Miller L, Reynolds J: Autism and vaccination—the current evidence, *J Spec Pediatr Nurs* 14(3): 166–172, 2009.

Narendran V, Hoath SB: The skin. In Martin RJ, Fanaroff AA, Walsh MC, editors: *Fanaroff and Martin's neonatal-perinatal medicine*, ed 8, St. Louis, 2006, Mosby.

National Center for Immunization and Respiratory Diseases: General recommendations on immunization: recommendations of the Advisory Committee on Immunization Practices (ACIP), *MMWR Recomm Rep* 60(2):1–64, 2011.

Niemela M, Pihakari O, Pokka T, and others: Pacifier as a risk factor for acute otitis media: a randomized, controlled trial of parental counseling, *Pediatrics* 106(3):483–488, 2000.

Nuorti JP, Whitney CG, Centers for Disease Control and Prevention: Prevention of pneumococcal disease among infants and children—use of 13-valent pneumococcal conjugate vaccine and 23-valent pneumococcal polysaccharide vaccine: recommendations of the Advisory Committee on Immunization Practices (ACIP), *MMWR Recomm Rep* 59(RR-11):1–18, 2010.

O'Connor NR, Tanabe KO, Siadaty MS, and others: Pacifiers and breastfeeding: a systematic review, *Arch Pediatr Adolesc Med* 163(4):378–382, 2009.

Parker SK, Schwartz B, Todd J, and others: Thimerosal-containing vaccines and autistic spectrum disorder: a critical review of published original data, *Pediatrics* 114(3): 793–804, 2004.

Pickett W, Streight S, Simpson K, and others: Injuries experienced by infant children: a population-based epidemiological analysis, *Pediatrics* 111(4 pt 1):e365–e370, 2003.

Price CS, Thompson WW, Goodson B, and others: Prenatal and infant exposure to thimerosal from vaccines and immunoglobulins and risk of autism, *Pediatrics* 126(4):656–664, 2010.

Quillin SI, Glenn LL: Interaction between feeding method and co-sleeping on maternal-newborn sleep, *J Obstet Gynecol Neonatal Nurs* 33(5): 580–588, 2004.

Reis EC, Holubkov R: Vapocoolant spray is equally effective as EMLA cream in reducing immunization pain in school-aged children, *Pediatrics* 100(6):1025, 1997.

Rojjanasrirat W: Working women's breastfeeding experiences, *MCN Am J Matern Child Nurs* 29(4):222–227, 2004.

Rovers MM, Numans ME, Langenbach E, and others: Is pacifier use a risk factor for otitis media? A dynamic cohort study, *Fam Pract* 25(4):233–236, 2008.

Schack-Nielsen L, Michaelsen KF: Breast feeding and future health, *Curr Opin Nutr Metab Care* 9(3):289–296, 2006.

Schechter NL, Zempsky WT, Cohen LL, and others: Pain reduction during pediatric immunizations: evidence-based review and recommendations, *Pediatrics* 119(5):e1184–e1198, 2007.

Schnitzer PG: Prevention of unintentional childhood injuries, *Am Fam Physician* 74(11):1864–1869, 2006.

Schuval S: Avoiding allergic reactions to childhood vaccines (and what to do when they occur), *Contemp Pediatr* 22(4):29–49, 53, 2003.

Settipane RA, Siri D, Bellanti JA: Egg allergy and influenza vaccination, *Allergy Asthma Proc* 30(6):660–665, 2009.

Sexton S, Natale R: Risks and benefits of pacifiers, *Am Fam Physician* 79(8):681–685, 2009.

Shah V, Taddio A, Rieder MJ, and others: Effectiveness and tolerability of pharmacologic and combined interventions for reducing injection pain during routine childhood immunizations: systematic review and meta-analyses, *Clin Ther* 31(Suppl 2):S104–151, 2009.

Shealy KR, Li R, Benton-Davis S, and others: *The CDC guide to breastfeeding interventions*, Atlanta, 2005, U.S. Department of Health and Human Services, Centers for Disease Control and Prevention.

Stevens B, Johnston C, Franck L, and others: The efficacy of developmentally sensitive interventions and sucrose for relieving procedural pain in very low birth weight neonates, *Nurs Res* 48(1):35–43, 1999.

Stevens B, Yamada J, Ohlsson A: Sucrose for analgesia in newborn infants undergoing painful procedures. In *Cochrane Database Syst Rev* (4):CD001069, 2001.

Sullivan JR: Development of father-infant attachment in fathers of preterm infants, *Neonat Netw* 18(7):33–39, 1999.

Taveras EM, Rifas-Shiman SL, Belfort MB, and others: Weight status in the first 6 months of life and obesity at 3 years of age, *Pediatrics* 123(4): 1177–1183, 2009.

Thomas DW, Greer FR, American Academy of Pediatrics, Committee on Nutrition and Section on Gastroenterology, Hepatology, and Nutrition: Probiotics and prebiotics in pediatrics, *Pediatrics* 126(6):1217–1231, 2010.

Thompson DG: Utilizing an oral sucrose solution to minimize neonatal pain, *J Spec Pediatr Nurs* 10(1):3–10, 2005.

Turner S, Arthur G, Lyons RA, and others: Modification of the home environment for the reduction of injuries, *Cochrane Database Syst Rev* (2):CD003600, 2011.

Vollrath ME, Tonstad S, Rothbart MK, and others: Infant temperament is associated with potentially obesogenic diet at 18 months, *Int J Obes* 6(2–2):e408–e414, 2011.

Wagner CL, Greer FR, American Academy of Pediatrics, Section on Breastfeeding, and others: Prevention of rickets and vitamin D deficiency in infants, children, and adolescents, *Pediatrics* 122(5):1142–1148, 2008.

Wasser H, Bentley M, Borja J, and others: Infants perceived as "fussy" are more likely to receive complementary foods before 4 months, *Pediatrics* 127(2):229–237, 2011.

Wilson ME, White MA, Cobb B, and others: Family dynamics, parental-fetal attachment and infant temperament, *J Adv Nurs* 31(1):204–210, 2000.

Wong DL: Topical local anesthetics: two products for pain relief during minor procedures, *Am J Nurs* 103(6):42–45, 2003.

Zeanah CH, Fox NA: Temperament and attachment disorders, *J Clin Child Adolesc Psychol* 33(1):82–87, 2004.

Zeanah CH, Gleason MM: *Reactive attachment disorder: a review for DSM-V*, pp. 1–53, Washington, DC, 2010, American Psychiatric Association, retrieved June 7, 2011, from http://www.dsm5.org/Proposed%20Revision%20Attachments/APA%20DSM-5%20Reactive%20Attachment%20Disorder%20Review.pdf.

Zuckerman J: The importance of injecting vaccines into muscle, *BMJ* 321(7271):1237–1238, 2000.

Health Problems of Infants

David Wilson

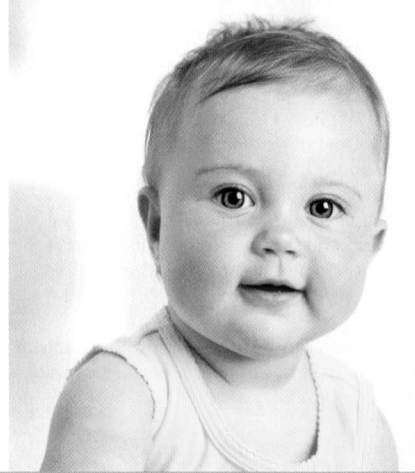

evolve WEBSITE

http://evolve.elsevier.com/wong/essentials
Case Study—Health Problems of Infants
Key Point Summaries
NCLEX-Style Review Questions
Nursing Care Plan—The Child with Growth Failure

CHAPTER OUTLINE

Nutritional Disorders, 354
  Vitamin Imbalances, 355
  Mineral Imbalances, 355
  Nursing Care Management, 356
  Protein-Energy Malnutrition (Severe
    Childhood Undernutrition), 356
    Kwashiorkor, 357
    Marasmus, 357

Food Allergy, 358
  Cow's Milk Allergy, 360
  Growth Failure (Failure to
    Thrive), 362
  Sleep Problems, 364
Positional Plagiocephaly, 366
  Therapeutic Management, 366
  Nursing Care Management, 367

Disorders of Unknown Etiology, 367
  Colic (Paroxysmal Abdominal
    Pain), 367
  Sudden Infant Death Syndrome, 368
    Risk Factors for SIDS, 370
    Protective Factors for SIDS, 370
    Infant Risk Factors, 371
  Apparent Life-Threatening Event, 372

LEARNING OBJECTIVES

On completion of this chapter the reader will be able to:
* Identify children at increased risk of developing nutritional disorders.
* Outline a nutritional counseling plan for vitamin or mineral deficiency or excess.
* Outline a dietary plan for parents when the infant has a cow's milk intolerance.
* List measures that can be used to alleviate colic.
* Plan nursing care that meets the physical and emotional needs of the child and family with growth failure.

* Identify infants at increased risk for sudden infant death syndrome.
* Provide nursing care that meets the immediate and long-term needs of the family that has lost a child from sudden infant death syndrome.
* Identify the stresses and needs of the family whose infant is being monitored for apnea in the home.

NUTRITIONAL DISORDERS

Reports of severe nutritional disorders in childhood in most developed countries are uncommon, yet there often exist small numbers of children who may experience a nutritional deficiency of some kind. The 2008 Feeding Infants and Toddlers Study (FITS) found that usual nutrient intake of infants, toddlers, and preschoolers (ages 0–47 months) met or exceeded energy and protein requirements based on the Dietary Reference Intakes (DRIs) and the 2005 Dietary Guidelines for Americans (Butte, Fox, Briefel, and others, 2010). According to the study, a small but significant number of infants was at risk for inadequate intake of iron and zinc. Dietary fiber intakes in toddlers and preschoolers were low, and saturated fat intakes exceeded recommendations for the majority of preschoolers (Butte, Fox, Briefel, and others,

2010). There are reports of an increased dependence on fortified foods and supplements in toddlers to meet nutritional requirements rather than meeting such needs with a wide variety of fruits, vegetables, and whole grains (Fox, Reidy, Novak, and others, 2006).

The findings of these studies and other similar reports are important for nurses who work with infants and children. Nurses must work to promote healthy nutrition habits early in children's lives through proper education of families and children about healthy lifestyle habits, including diet and exercise for health promotion and prevention of morbidities associated with poor micronutrient intake and sedentary lifestyle.

VITAMIN IMBALANCES

Although true vitamin deficiencies are rare in the United States, subclinical deficiencies are commonly seen in population subgroups in which either maternal or child dietary intake is imbalanced and contains inadequate amounts of vitamins. Vitamin D–deficiency rickets, once rarely seen because of the widespread commercial availability of vitamin D–fortified milk, increased before the turn of the century. Populations at risk include:

- Children who are exclusively breastfed by mothers with an inadequate intake of vitamin D or are exclusively breastfed longer than 6 months without adequate maternal vitamin D intake or supplementation
- Children with dark skin pigmentation who are exposed to minimal sunlight because of socioeconomic, religious, or cultural beliefs or housing in urban areas with high levels of pollution
- Children with diets that are low in sources of vitamin D and calcium
- Individuals who use milk products not supplemented with vitamin D (e.g., yogurt,* raw cow's milk) as the primary source of milk

The American Academy of Pediatrics (AAP) (2008) recommends that infants who are exclusively breastfed receive 400 IU of vitamin D beginning shortly after birth to prevent rickets and vitamin D deficiency. Vitamin D supplementation should continue until the infant is consuming at least 1 L/day (or 1 quart/day) of vitamin D–fortified formula (AAP, 2008). Non-breastfed infants who are taking less than 1 L/day of vitamin D–fortified formula should also receive a daily vitamin D supplement of 400 IU. Inadequate maternal ingestion of cobalamin (vitamin B_{12}) may contribute to infant neurologic impairment when exclusive breastfeeding (past 6 months) is the only source of the infant's nutrition. A correlation between the incidence of childhood upper respiratory infections and vitamin D deficiency has been found, but the implications of the findings have yet to be completely understood (Taylor and Camargo, 2011; Walker and Modlin, 2009).

Children may also be at risk for vitamin deficiencies secondary to disorders or their treatment. For example, vitamin deficiencies of the fat-soluble vitamins A and D may occur in malabsorptive disorders such as cystic fibrosis and short bowel syndrome. Preterm infants may develop rickets in the second month of life as a result of inadequate intake of vitamin D, calcium, and phosphorus. Children receiving high doses of salicylates may have impaired vitamin C storage. Environmental tobacco smoke exposure has been implicated in decreased concentrations of ascorbate in children; therefore, increased intake of sources of vitamin C should be encouraged even in children minimally exposed to environmental tobacco smoke (Preston, Rodriguez, and Rivera,

2006). Children with chronic illnesses resulting in anorexia, decreased food intake, or possible nutrient malabsorption as a result of multiple medications should be carefully evaluated for adequate vitamin and mineral intake in some form (parenteral or enteral).

Children with sickle cell disease are reported to have suboptimal intakes (according to DRI recommendations) of vitamins E and D, folate, calcium, and fiber, which decrease significantly with increasing age. Poor dietary intake was a significant factor in the study's findings (Kawchak, Schall, Zemel, and others, 2007). One study found that children with intestinal failure who were being transitioned from parenteral nutrition to enteral nutrition had at least one vitamin and mineral deficiency; vitamin D was the most common deficiency identified, and zinc and iron were the most common minerals identified as being deficient (Yang, Duro, Zurakowski, and others, 2011).

Vitamin A deficiency has been reported with increased morbidity and mortality in children with measles. However, a Cochrane review of studies wherein a single dose of vitamin A was administered to children with measles found no decrease in mortality. Children with measles younger than the age of 2 years who received two doses of vitamin A (200,000 IU) on consecutive days did have decreased mortality rates and a reduced rate of pneumonia-specific mortality (Huiming, Chaomin, and Meng, 2005). Complications from diarrhea and infections are often increased in infants and children with vitamin A deficiency. Although scurvy (caused by a deficiency of vitamin C) is rare in developed countries, cases have been reported in children who were fed an organic diet deficient in vegetables and fruits (Burk and Molodow, 2007).

An excessive dose of a vitamin is generally defined as 10 or more times the Recommended Dietary Allowance (RDA), although the fat-soluble vitamins, especially vitamins A and D, tend to cause toxic reactions at lower doses. With the addition of vitamins to commercially prepared foods, the potential for hypervitaminosis has increased, especially when combined with the excessive use of vitamin supplements. Hypervitaminosis of A and D presents the greatest problems because these fat-soluble vitamins are stored in the body. High intakes of vitamin A have been linked to physeal growth arrest, which can lead to osteoporosis, fracture, and metaphyseal irregularity (Saltzman and King, 2007). Vitamin D is the most likely of all vitamins to cause toxic reactions in relatively small overdoses. The water-soluble vitamins, primarily niacin, B_6, and C, can also cause toxicity. Poor outcomes in infants (e.g., fatal hypermagnesemia) have been associated with megavitamin therapy with high doses of magnesium oxide, and severe anemia and thrombocytopenia have resulted from megadoses of vitamin A.

One vitamin supplement that is recommended for all women of childbearing age is a daily dose of 0.4 mg of folic acid, the usual RDA. Folic acid taken before conception and during early pregnancy can reduce the risk of neural tube defects such as spina bifida by as much as 70%. Drugs such as oral contraceptives and antidepressants may decrease folic acid absorption; thus, adolescent girls taking such medications should consider supplementation. (See Spina Bifida, Chapter 32.)

MINERAL IMBALANCES

A number of minerals are essential nutrients. The macrominerals refer to those with daily requirements greater than 100 mg and include calcium, phosphorus, magnesium, sodium, potassium, chloride, and sulfur. Microminerals, or trace elements, have daily requirements of less than 100 mg and include several essential minerals and those whose exact role in nutrition is still unclear. The greatest concern

---

*Yogurt does not contain adequate amounts of vitamins A and D yet is an acceptable source of calcium and phosphorus.

with minerals is deficiency, especially iron-deficiency anemia (see Chapter 26). However, other minerals that may be inadequate in children's diets, even with supplementation, include calcium, phosphorus, magnesium, and zinc. Low levels of zinc can cause nutritional growth failure (failure to thrive [FTT]). Some of the macrominerals may be inadvertently overlooked when a child with intestinal failure or recent surgery is making the transition from total parenteral intake to enteral intake.

An imbalance in the intake of calcium and phosphorous may occur in infants who are given whole cow's milk instead of infant formula; neonatal tetany may be observed in such cases. Whole cow's milk is also a poor source of iron, and inadequate intake of iron from other food sources such as iron-fortified cereal may cause iron-deficiency anemia.

The regulation of mineral balance in the body is a complex process. Dietary extremes of mineral intake can cause a number of mineral–mineral interactions that could result in unexpected deficiencies or excesses. For example, excessive amounts of one mineral, such as zinc, can result in a deficiency of another mineral, such as copper, even if sufficient amounts of copper are ingested. Thus, megadose intake of one mineral may cause an inadvertent deficiency of another essential mineral by blocking its absorption in the blood or intestinal wall or by competing with binding sites on protein carriers needed for metabolism.

Deficiencies can also occur when various substances in the diet interact with minerals. For example, iron, zinc, and calcium can form insoluble complexes with phytates or oxalates (substances found in plant proteins), which impair the bioavailability of the mineral. This type of interaction is important in vegetarian diets because plant foods such as soy are high in phytates. Contrary to popular opinion, spinach is not an ideal source of iron or calcium because of its high oxalate content.

Children with certain illnesses are at greater risk for growth failure, especially in relation to bone mineral deficiency as a result of the treatment of the disease, decreased nutrient intake, or decreased absorption of necessary minerals. Those at risk for such deficiencies include children who are receiving or have received radiation and chemotherapy for cancer; children with human immunodeficiency virus (HIV), sickle cell disease, cystic fibrosis, gastrointestinal (GI) malabsorption, or nephrosis; and extremely low–birth-weight (ELBW) and very low–birth-weight (VLBW) preterm infants.

NURSING CARE MANAGEMENT

Identification of adequacy of nutrient intake is the initial nursing goal and requires assessment based on a dietary history and physical examination for signs of deficiency or excess (see Nutrition, Chapter 12, and Nutritional Assessment, Chapter 6). After assessment data are collected, this information is evaluated against standard intakes to identify areas of concern. One source of standard nutrient intakes is the Dietary Reference Intakes (see Chapter 12).

Standardized growth reference charts are used in infants, children, and adolescents to compare and assess growth parameters such as height and head circumference with the percentile distribution of other children at the same ages (Chumlea, 2005). The World Health Organization (WHO) growth chart is a standardized growth reference now recommended for infants and toddlers up to age 24 months. This growth chart includes head circumference, height, and weight references which were derived from healthy children in six different countries around the world. These growth standards are based on the growth of healthy breastfed infants throughout the first year of life. The Centers for Disease Control and Prevention's growth charts are now recommended for children 2 to 19 years of age (Grummer-Strawn, Reinold, Krebs, and others, 2010).

Infants should be breastfed for the first 6 months and preferably for 1 year, be introduced to some solid foods after about 4 to 6 months, and receive iron-fortified cereal for at least 18 months (see Chapter 10). Vitamin B_{12} supplementation is recommended if the breastfeeding mother's intake of the vitamin is inadequate or if she is not taking vitamin supplements (Dunham and Kollar, 2006). If the infant is being exclusively breastfed after 4 months (when fetal iron stores are depleted), iron supplementation (1 mg/kg/day) is recommended until appropriate iron-containing complementary foods such as iron-fortified cereal are introduced (Baker, Greer, and AAP, Committee on Nutrition, 2010). The introduction of solids for vegetarian infants may occur using the same guidelines as for other children (see Nutrition, Chapter 10). A variety of foods should be introduced during the early years to ensure a well-balanced intake. Infants who have particular nutritional deficits should be identified; a multidisciplinary approach should be taken to identify the deficit and the etiology, and to establish a plan with the caregiver to promote adequate growth and development.

PROTEIN-ENERGY MALNUTRITION (SEVERE CHILDHOOD UNDERNUTRITION)

Malnutrition continues to be a major health problem in the world today, particularly in children younger than 5 years of age. However, lack of food is not always the primary cause of malnutrition. In many developing and underdeveloped nations, diarrhea (gastroenteritis) is a major factor. Additional factors are bottle feeding (in poor sanitary conditions), inadequate knowledge of proper child care practices, parental illiteracy, economic and political factors, climate conditions, cultural and religious food preferences, and simply a lack of adequate food. Müller and Krawinkel (2005) point out that poverty is the underlying cause of malnutrition. The most extreme forms of malnutrition, or protein-energy malnutrition (PEM), are kwashiorkor and marasmus. Some authorities suggest that severe malnutrition encompasses more than protein energy deficits and thus prefer the term *severe childhood undernutrition* (SCU). Another term used is *severe acute malnutrition* (SAM). Entities such as the WHO continue to use the term *protein-energy malnutrition*. SCU may also be subdivided into edematous (kwashiorkor) and nonedematous (marasmus) types.

In the United States, milder forms of PEM are seen as a result of primary malnutrition, although the classic cases of marasmus and kwashiorkor may also occur. Unlike in developing countries, where the main reason for PEM is inadequate food, in the United States, PEM occurs despite ample dietary supplies (see Growth Failure [Failure to Thrive], p. 362). PEM may also be seen in persons with chronic health problems such as cystic fibrosis, renal dialysis, cancer, and GI malabsorption; in elderly adults who have chronic malnutrition; and in persons with acute illnesses such as prolonged, untreated anorexia nervosa. Kwashiorkor has been reported in the United States in children fed only a rice beverage diet (Rice Dream) and few solid foods (Katz, Mahlberg, Honig, and others, 2005; Tierney, Sage, and Shwayder, 2010). The rice drink contains 0.13 g of protein per ounce (compared with the 0.5 g found in human milk and infant formulas) and is an inadequate source of nutrition for children. Other reported cases of kwashiorkor in developed countries involved infants who were fed nonstandard infant diets such as flour water, corn porridge, molasses, and nondairy creamer (Katz, Mahlberg, Honig, and others, 2005). Kwashiorkor has also been reported in the United States when infants have been fed inappropriate food as a result of parental (caretaker) nutritional ignorance, a perceived cow's milk–based formula intolerance, family social chaos, or cow's milk intolerance (Liu, Howard, Mancini, and others, 2001). Therefore, it is important that health care workers not assume that PEM cannot occur in developed countries; a comprehensive dietary history should be obtained in any child with clinical features resembling PEM.

Kwashiorkor

Kwashiorkor has been defined as primarily a deficiency of protein with an adequate supply of calories. A diet consisting mainly of starch grains or tubers provides adequate calories in the form of carbohydrates but an inadequate amount of high-quality proteins. Some evidence, however, supports a multifactorial etiology, including cultural, psychologic, and infective factors that may interact to place the child at risk for kwashiorkor. Penny (2003) suggests that kwashiorkor may result from the interplay of nutrient deprivation and infectious or environmental stresses, which produces an imbalanced response to such insults. Kwashiorkor often occurs subsequent to an infectious outbreak of measles and dysentery. There is further evidence that oxidative stress occurs in children with kwashiorkor, resulting in free radical damage, which may precipitate cellular changes, resulting in edema and muscle wasting (Penny, 2003). The role of the essential fatty acid arachidonic acid in lipid metabolism, altered leukotriene production, and oxidative stress in kwashiorkor has yet to be fully understood, but arachidonic acid seems to have an interactive role in its development (Penny, 2003).

Taken from the Ga language (Ghana), the word *kwashiorkor* means "the sickness the older child gets when the next baby is born" and aptly describes the syndrome that develops in the first child, usually between 1 and 4 years of age, when weaned from the breast after the second child is born.

The child with kwashiorkor has thin, wasted extremities and a prominent abdomen from edema (ascites). The edema often masks severe muscular atrophy, making the child appear less debilitated than he or she actually is. The skin is scaly and dry and has areas of depigmentation. Several dermatoses may be evident, partly resulting from the vitamin deficiencies. Permanent blindness often results from the severe lack of vitamin A. Mineral deficiencies are common, especially iron, calcium, and zinc. Acute zinc deficiency is a common complication of severe PEM and results in skin rashes, loss of hair, impaired immune response and susceptibility to infections, digestive problems, night blindness, changes in affective behavior, defective wound healing, and impaired growth. Its depressant effect on appetite further limits food intake. The hair is thin, dry, coarse, and dull. Depigmentation is common, and patchy alopecia may occur.

Diarrhea (persistent diarrhea malnutrition syndrome) commonly occurs from a lowered resistance to infection and further complicates the electrolyte imbalance. Low levels of cytokines (protein cells involved in the primary response to infection) have been reported in children with kwashiorkor, suggesting that such children have a blunted immune response to infection. A large number of deaths in children with kwashiorkor occur in those who develop HIV infection. GI disturbances such as fatty infiltration of the liver and atrophy of the acini cells of the pancreas occur. Anemia is also a common finding in malnourished children. Protein deficiency increases the child's susceptibility to infection, which eventually results in death. Fatal deterioration may be caused by diarrhea and infection or by circulatory failure.

Marasmus

Marasmus results from general malnutrition of both calories and protein. It is common in underdeveloped countries during times of drought, especially in cultures where adults eat first; the remaining food is often insufficient in quality and quantity for the children.

Marasmus is usually a syndrome of physical and emotional deprivation and is not confined to geographic areas where food supplies are inadequate. It may be seen in children with growth failure in whom the cause is not solely nutritional but primarily emotional. Marasmus may be seen in infants as young as 3 months of age if breastfeeding is not successful and there are no suitable alternatives. Marasmic kwashiorkor is a form of PEM in which clinical findings of both kwashiorkor and marasmus are evident; the child has edema, severe wasting, and stunted growth. In marasmic kwashiorkor the child has inadequate nutrient intake and superimposed infection. Fluid and electrolyte disturbances, hypothermia, and hypoglycemia are associated with a poor prognosis.

Marasmus is characterized by gradual wasting and atrophy of body tissues, especially of subcutaneous fat. The child appears to be very old, with loose and wrinkled skin, unlike the child with kwashiorkor, who appears more rounded from the edema. Fat metabolism is less impaired than in kwashiorkor; thus, deficiency of fat-soluble vitamins is usually minimal or absent. In general, the clinical manifestations of marasmus are similar to those seen in kwashiorkor with the following exceptions: with marasmus, there is no edema from hypoalbuminemia or sodium retention, which contributes to a severely emaciated appearance; no dermatoses caused by vitamin deficiencies; little or no depigmentation of hair or skin; moderately normal fat metabolism and lipid absorption; and a smaller head size and slower recovery after treatment.

The child is fretful, apathetic, withdrawn, and so lethargic that prostration frequently occurs. Intercurrent infection with debilitating diseases such as tuberculosis, parasitosis, HIV, and dysentery is common.

Therapeutic Management

The treatment of PEM includes providing a diet with high-quality proteins, carbohydrates, vitamins, and minerals. When PEM occurs as a result of persistent diarrhea, three management goals are identified:

1. Rehydration with an oral rehydration solution that also replaces electrolytes
2. Administration of antibiotics to prevent intercurrent infections
3. Provision of adequate (energy intake) nutrition by either breastfeeding or a proper weaning diet

Local protocols are used in developing countries to deal with PEM. Penny (2003) recommends a three-phase treatment protocol: (1) acute or initial phase in the first 2 to 10 days involving initiation of treatment for oral rehydration, diarrhea, and intestinal parasites; prevention of hypoglycemia and hypothermia; and subsequent dietary management; (2) recovery or rehabilitation (2–6 weeks) focusing on increasing dietary intake and weight gain; and (3) follow-up phase, focusing on care after discharge in an outpatient setting to prevent relapse and promote weight gain, provide developmental stimulation, and evaluate cognitive and motor deficits. In the acute phase, care is taken to prevent fluid overload; the child is observed closely for signs of food or fluid intolerance. The refeeding syndrome may occur if intake progresses too rapidly; cardiac failure may cause sudden death in a child who has been malnourished and refed too rapidly (Grover and Ee, 2009).

Vitamin and mineral supplementation are required in most cases of PEM; vitamin A, zinc, and copper are recommended; iron supplementation is not recommended until the child is able to tolerate a steady food source. In addition, the child is observed for signs of skin breakdown, which should be treated to prevent infection. Breastfeeding is encouraged if the mother and child are able to do so effectively; in some cases, partial supplementation with a modified cow's milk–based formula may be necessary (Penny, 2003).

The WHO (2006) issued a statement recognizing the importance of breastfeeding for the first 6 months in developing countries where HIV is prevalent among childbearing women and children. The WHO recognizes that appropriate sources of food and water for infants may not be available after the 6 months are concluded and that the risk for malnutrition is greater among such children than the theoretical risk of HIV. However, the organization does recommend that breastfeeding continue after 6 months with the introduction of complementary foods, provided they are safe for child consumption. In severely malnourished children, a modest energy food source is given initially followed by a high-protein and energy food source; severely malnourished children will not tolerate a high-energy and high-protein source initially. A number of food sources may be provided to treat PEM. They include oral rehydration solutions (ReSoMal), amino acid–based elemental food, and ready-to-feed foods that do not require the addition of water (to minimize contaminated water consumption); parenteral and oral antibiotics are often part of the standard treatment for PEM (Amadi, Mwiya, Chomba, and others, 2005; Ciliberto, Sandige, Ndehka, and others, 2005).

Nursing Care Management

Because PEM appears early in childhood, primarily in children 6 months to 2 years of age, and is associated with early weaning, low-protein diet, delayed introduction of complementary foods, and frequent infections (Grover and Ee, 2009; Müller and Krawinkel, 2005), it is essential that nursing care focus on *prevention* of PEM through parent education about feeding practices during this crucial period. Prevention should also focus on the nutritional health of pregnant women because this will directly affect the health of their unborn children. Breastfeeding is the optimal method of feeding for the first 6 months. The immune properties naturally found in breast milk not only nourish infants but also help prevent opportunistic infections, which may contribute to PEM. Providing for essential physiologic needs, such as appropriate nutrient intake, protection from infection, adequate hydration, skin care, and restoration of physiologic integrity, is paramount. Additional nursing care focuses on education about and administration of childhood vaccinations to prevent illness, promotion of nutrition and well-being for the lactating mother, encouragement and participation in well-child visits for infants and toddlers, appropriate food sources for children being weaned from breastfeeding, and education regarding sanitation practices to prevent childhood GI diseases.

Poor skin integrity further increases the chance of infections, hypothermia, water loss, and skin breakdown. Tube feedings may be required for infants too weak to breastfeed or bottle feed. Oral rehydration with an approved oral rehydration solution is commonly used in cases of PEM in which diarrhea and infection are not immediately life threatening.

One approach that has gained acceptance for treating childhood malnutrition in developing countries is the home-based use of ready-to-use therapeutic food (RUTF). RUTF is a paste based on peanut butter and dried skim milk with vitamins and minerals; it requires no mixing with water or milk. The packaged RUTF can be stored without refrigeration. Studies have demonstrated improved survival rates in malnourished children (Amthor, Cole, and Manary, 2009; Ciliberto, Sandige, Ndehka, and others, 2005). Some of the reported advantages of home-based (community-based) treatment include that children are not exposed to hospital-acquired infections and may receive the RUTF from village health aides (Kapil, 2009).

It is imperative that nurses be at the forefront in educating and reinforcing healthy nutrition habits in parents of small children to prevent malnutrition. Because children with marasmus may experience emotional starvation as well, care should be consistent with care of children with growth failure (p. 362).

The WHO has published guidelines for the treatment and management of children with severe malnutrition (Ashworth, Khanum, Jackson, and others, 2003; Grover and Ee, 2009). These guidelines include a two-phase program with a 10-step guide to treating the child with malnutrition.

FOOD ALLERGY

In late 2010, the National Institute of Allergy and Infectious Diseases (NIAID), working with 34 other professional organizations, published new evidence-based guidelines for the diagnosis and management of food allergy. A food allergy is defined by the NIAID (Boyce, Assa'ad, Burks, and others, 2010) as "an adverse health effect arising from a specific immune response that occurs reproducibly on exposure to a given food" (2010, p. 1108). Food allergens are defined as specific components of food or ingredients in food such as a protein that are recognized by allergen-specific immune cells eliciting an immune reaction that results in the characteristic symptoms (Boyce, Assa'ad, Burks, and others, 2010). A food intolerance is said to exist when a food or food component elicits a reproducible adverse reaction but does not have an established or likely immunologic mechanism (Boyce, Assa'ad, Burks, and others, 2010). A person may have an immune-mediated allergy to cow's milk protein, but the person who is unable to digest the lactose in cow's milk is considered to be intolerant to cow's milk, not allergic as is the first person described. The NIAID guidelines classify food allergy according to the following: food-induced anaphylaxis, GI food allergies, and specific syndromes; cutaneous reactions to foods; respiratory manifestation; and Heiner syndrome (Boyce, Assa'ad, Burks, and others, 2010). The exact prevalence of food allergies in children is reported to be much lower than what parents report. Approximately 6% of children may experience food allergic reactions in the first 2 to 3 years of life; 1.5% will have an allergy to eggs, 2.5% to cow's milk, and 1.0% to peanuts (Sampson and Leung, 2011). Seafood allergies in children are reported to be low in the United States: 0.2% for fish and 0.5% for crustaceans (Boyce, Assa'ad, Burks, and others, 2010). Diagnosed allergy to milk and eggs was found to be 2.2% in a Danish study and 1.6% in a Norwegian study. The NIAID report further points out that most children will eventually be able to tolerate milk, eggs, soy, and wheat, but far fewer will ever tolerate tree nut and peanuts (Boyce, Assa'ad, Burks, and others, 2010). The NIAID report indicates that 50% to 90% of all presumed food allergies are not actually allergies. The NIAID's (Boyce, Assa'ad, Burks, and others, 2010) guidelines also recommend the following:

- Infants should be exclusively breastfed until 4 to 6 months of age.
- Soy formula is not recommended to prevent the development of food allergy.
- Introduction of complementary foods should not be delayed beyond 6 months of age.
- Hydrolyzed formula (vs. cow's milk) may be used in at-risk infants to prevent or modify food allergy.
- Maternal diet during pregnancy or lactation should not be restricted to prevent food allergy.
- Children should be vaccinated with the MMR (measles, mumps, and rubella) and MMRV (measles, mumps, rubella, and varicella) vaccines (even with egg allergy).
- Patients with severe egg allergy reactions should not receive the influenza vaccine without consulting the primary practitioner for an analysis of the risks vs. benefits.

BOX 11-1   COMMON ALLERGENIC FOODS AND SOURCES

Nuts*—Some chocolates, candy, baked goods, cherry soda (may be flavored with a nut extract), walnut oil

Eggs*—Mayonnaise, creamy salad dressing, baked goods, egg noodles, some cake icing, meringue, custard, pancakes, French toast, root beer

Wheat*—Almost all baked goods, wieners, bologna, pressed or chopped cold cuts, gravy, pasta, some canned soups

Legumes—Peanuts,* peanut butter or oil, beans, peas, lentils

Fish or shellfish*—Cod liver oil, pizza with anchovies, Caesar salad dressing, any food fried in same oil as fish

Soy*—Soy sauce, teriyaki or Worcestershire sauce, tofu, baked goods using soy flour or oil, soy nuts, soy infant formulas or milk, soybean paste, tuna packed in vegetable oil, many margarines

Chocolate—Cola beverages, cocoa, chocolate-flavored drinks

Milk—Ice cream, butter, margarine (if it contains dairy products), yogurt, cheese, pudding, baked goods, wieners, bologna, canned creamed soups, instant breakfast drinks, powdered milk drinks, milk chocolate

Buckwheat—Some cereals, pancakes

Pork, chicken—Bacon, wieners, sausage, pork fat, chicken broth

Strawberries, melon, pineapple—Gelatin, syrups

Corn—Popcorn, cereal, muffins, cornstarch, corn meal, corn bread, corn tortillas, corn syrup

Citrus fruits—Orange, lemon, lime, grapefruit; any of these in drinks, gelatin, juice, or medicines

Tomatoes—Juice, some vegetable soups, spaghetti, pizza sauce, catsup

Spices—Chili, pepper, vinegar, cinnamon

*Most common allergens.

A summary of the NIAID guidelines is provided by McBride (2011).

The clinical manifestations of food allergy may be divided as follows (AAP, 2009):

Systemic—Anaphylactic, growth failure
GI—Abdominal pain, vomiting, cramping, diarrhea
Respiratory—Cough, wheezing, rhinitis, infiltrates
Cutaneous—Urticaria, rash, atopic dermatitis

Food allergies usually occur either as an immunoglobulin E (IgE)–mediated or non–IgE-mediated immune response; some toxic reactions may occur as a result of a toxin found within the food. Food allergy is caused by exposure to allergens, usually proteins (but not the smaller amino acids), that are capable of inducing IgE antibody formation (sensitization) when ingested. Sensitization refers to the initial exposure of an individual to an allergen, resulting in an immune response; subsequent exposure induces a much stronger response that is clinically apparent. Consequently, food allergy typically occurs after the food has been ingested one or more times. The NIAID report (Boyce, Assa'ad, Burks, and others, 2010) indicates that sensitization alone is not sufficient to classify as a food allergy; rather, an immune-mediated response *and* manifestation of specific signs and symptoms are necessary to categorize an individual as having a food allergy. The most common food allergens are listed in Box 11-1.

Oral allergy syndrome occurs when a food allergen (commonly fruits and vegetables) is ingested and there is subsequent edema and pruritus involving the lips, tongue, palate, and throat. Recovery from symptoms is usually rapid. Immediate GI hypersensitivity is an IgE-mediated reaction to a food allergen; reactions include nausea, abdominal pain, cramping, diarrhea, vomiting, anaphylaxis, or all of these. Additional food allergies seen in young children include allergic eosinophilic esophagitis, allergic eosinophilic gastroenteritis, food protein–induced proctocolitis, and food protein–induced enterocolitis.

Food allergy or hypersensitivity may also be classified according to the interval between ingestion and the manifestation of symptoms: immediate (within minutes to hours) or delayed (2–48 hours) (AAP, 2009).

Food allergies can occur at any time but are common during infancy because the immature intestinal tract is more permeable to proteins than the mature intestinal tract, thus increasing the likelihood of an immune response. Allergies in general demonstrate a genetic component: Children who have one parent with allergy have a 50% or greater risk of developing allergy; children who have both parents with allergy have up to a 100% risk of developing allergy. Allergy with a hereditary tendency is referred to as atopy. Some infants with atopy can be identified at birth from elevated levels of IgE in umbilical cord blood.

Deaths have been reported in children who experienced an anaphylactic reaction to food. Onset of the reactions occurred shortly after ingestion (5–30 minutes). In most of the children, the reactions did not begin with skin signs, such as hives, red rash, and flushing, but rather mimicked an acute asthma attack (wheezing, decreased air movement in airways, dyspnea). Watch children with food anaphylaxis closely because a biphasic response has been recorded in a number of cases in which there is an immediate response, apparent recovery, and then acute recurrence of symptoms (Simons, 2009) (see Nursing Alert and Drug Alert). Children with extremely sensitive food allergies should wear a medical identification bracelet and have an injectable epinephrine cartridge (EpiPen) readily available. (See Anaphylaxis, Chapter 25.) Any child with a history of food allergy or previous severe reaction to food should have a written emergency treatment plan, as well as an EpiPen. Note that Benadryl and cetirizine are effective for cutaneous and nasal manifestations but not for airway manifestations (Keet, 2011).

Although the reason is unknown, many children "outgrow" their food allergies, especially to milk and eggs. About 50% of all infants who are intolerant to cow's milk usually develop tolerance by 3 to 5 years of age (Sampson and Leung, 2011). More than half (60%) of infants have an IgE-mediated reaction to cow's milk, and 25% retain sensitivity until the second decade of life. Children who are allergic to more than one food may develop tolerance to each food at a different time. The most common allergens, such as peanuts, are outgrown less readily than other food allergens. Because of the tendency to lose the hypersensitivity, allergenic foods should be reintroduced into the diet after a period of abstinence (usually ≥1 year) to evaluate whether the food can be safely added to the diet. Foods that are associated with severe anaphylactic reactions, however, continue to present a lifelong risk and must be avoided.

! NURSING ALERT

Indications for the administration of **intramuscular** epinephrine in a child with a life-threatening anaphylactic reaction or one who is experiencing severe symptoms include any one of the following (Wang and Sampson, 2007):

- Itching sensation or tightness in throat; hoarseness
- "Barky" cough
- Difficulty swallowing; dyspnea
- Wheezing
- Cyanosis
- Respiratory arrest; mild dysrhythmia or mild hypotension
- Severe bradycardia, hypotension, or cardiac arrest; loss of consciousness

🔴 DRUG ALERT
*Emergency Management of Anaphylaxis**

Drug: Epinephrine 0.001 mg/kg up to maximum of 0.3 mg
Dose: EpiPen Jr (0.15 mg) intramuscularly (IM) for child weighing 8 to 25 kg (17.5–55 lb)
EpiPen (0.3 mg) IM for child weighing 25 kg (55 lb) or more
Observe for adverse reactions: tachycardia, hypertension, irritability, headaches, nausea, and tremors.

*Keet C: Recognition and management of food-induced anaphylaxis, *Pediatr Clin North Am* 58(2):377–388, 2011; Sampson HA, Leung DYM: Adverse reactions to foods. In Kliegman RM, Stanton BF, St. Geme JW, and others, editors: *Nelson textbook of pediatrics,* ed 19, Philadelphia, 2011, Saunders.

Diagnosis and Therapeutic Management

The diagnosis of food allergy is made based on a number of factors, including the occurrence of anaphylaxis or any combination of 37 symptoms listed in the NIAID guidelines within minutes to hours of ingesting food or if such symptoms have occurred after the ingestion of a specific food on one or more occasions. The gold standard is the double-blind, placebo-controlled food challenge; the skin prick test and serum IgE measurements may be used as an adjunct to diagnose food allergy but singly should not be used for the diagnosis. The atopy patch test, intradermal test, and serum IgE test are not recommended for establishing a diagnosis. A single oral food challenge may be used in certain circumstances (Boyce, Assa'ad, Burks, and others, 2010). The management of food allergy consists of avoiding the specific food or ingredient that causes the manifestations. Because children with food allergies (usually two or more) are at risk for inadequate nutrient intake and growth failure, it is recommended that they have an annual nutritional assessment to prevent such problems.

Nursing Care Management

Nursing care of children with potential food allergy consists of assisting in collecting vital health assessment data for the establishment of a diagnosis and assisting with diagnostic tests. It is important for nurses to be informed about food allergy and provide parents and caregivers, as well as older children, with accurate information regarding food allergy.

Educate parents, teachers, and daycare workers regarding signs and symptoms of food allergy and reactions. People with food allergy should avoid unfamiliar foods and restaurants that do not disclose food ingredients. New labeling guidelines require that food additives such as spices and flavoring be clearly labeled on commercially sold, store-bought foods. Hidden ingredients in prepared foods are also potential sources of food allergy.

Children with a history of food allergy may spend a considerable amount of time in daycare; therefore, persons working in daycare centers and other children's settings need to be properly educated regarding recognition and management of severe anaphylactic reactions (see Critical Thinking Case Study box).

Breastfeeding is now considered a primary strategy for avoiding atopy in families with known food allergies; however, there is no evidence that maternal avoidance (during pregnancy or lactation) of cow's milk protein or other dietary products known to cause food allergy will prevent food allergy in children (AAP, 2009; Boyce, Assa'ad, Burks, and others, 2010). Researchers indicate that delaying the introduction of highly allergenic foods past 4 to 6 months of age may not be as protective for food allergy as previously believed (Greer, Sicherer, Burks, and others, 2008). Likewise, studies have shown that

❓ CRITICAL THINKING CASE STUDY
Food Allergy Anaphylaxis

A group of nursing students is holding a health promotion fair at a local elementary school for first, second, and third graders. The nursing students have several booths set up in the school cafeteria. Three second-grade boys are horseplaying in front of one of the booths when one of the boys, Jason, an 8-year-old child, suddenly starts coughing and clutching his throat. The students also observe that he is developing red splotches on his face, neck, and throat and that he is scratching. Jason says, "I'm having trouble breathing!" The school nurse is nearby and comes over to see what the commotion is about. One of the boys with Jason says, "We didn't mean any harm—we were just goofing around when we put peanuts in his trail mix." One of the student nurses says, "He's in obvious distress—what should we do?"

1. Evidence—Is there sufficient evidence to draw any conclusions at this time about Jason's condition?
2. Assumptions—Describe some underlying assumptions about the following:
   a. Clinical manifestations of food allergy.
   b. The emergency treatment of a food allergy "reaction," or anaphylaxis.
   c. Which one of the following interventions would have highest immediate priority?
      1. Call Jason's parents and ask them to come pick him up from school.
      2. Call Jason's family practitioner to obtain orders for medication.
      3. Promptly administer an intramuscular dose of epinephrine.
      4. Call 911 and wait for the emergency response personnel to arrive.
   d. Based on your answer to item 2c, identify the appropriate medication dosage for this child.
3. What implications for nursing care exist in this situation after an intervention in item 2c has been chosen and implemented?
4. Describe the potential results of taking a "Let's observe Jason for a few minutes before we do anything" stance in this scenario.
5. Is there evidence to support your immediate and secondary nursing interventions? Provide objective evidence to support your decisions for action.

soy formula does not prevent allergic disease in infants and children (AAP, 2009).*

Cow's Milk Allergy

Cow's milk allergy (CMA) is a multifaceted disorder representing adverse systemic and local GI reactions to cow's milk protein. Approximately 2.5% of infants develop cow's milk hypersensitivity, with 60% being IgE mediated. It is estimated that 50% of those children may outgrow the hypersensitivity by 3 to 4 years of age (Sampson and Leung, 2011). Some studies suggest that milk allergy may persist and some children may not be able to tolerate milk until they are 16 years of age (AAP, 2009). (This discussion centers on cow's milk protein contained in commercial infant formulas; whole milk is not recommended for infants younger than 12 months of age.) The allergy may be manifested within the first 4 months of life through a variety of signs and symptoms that may appear within 45 minutes of milk ingestion or after several days (Box 11-2). The diagnosis may initially be

*Additional information for parents of infants with food allergies is available from the American Academy of Allergy, Asthma and Immunology, 555 E. Wells St., Suite 1100, Milwaukee, WI 53202; 414-272-6071; http://www.aaaai.org. Additional helpful websites for information on food allergy include MedlinePlus (sponsored by U.S. National Library of Medicine and National Institutes of Health), http://www.nlm.nih.gov/medlineplus; Food Allergy and Anaphylaxis Network, 800-929-4040, http://www.foodallergy.org; NIAID, http://www.niaid.nih.gov/Pages/default.aspx; and http://www.allergicchild.com.

BOX 11-2 COMMON CLINICAL MANIFESTATIONS OF COW'S MILK ALLERGY

Gastrointestinal
Diarrhea
Vomiting
Colic (controversial)
Abdominal pain
Nausea and vomiting
Oral itching
Constipation (controversial)
Gastroesophageal reflux (controversial)
Blood streaked, mucous, loose stools (protein-induced allergic enterocolitis)

Respiratory
Rhinitis
Conjunctivitis
Bronchitis
Asthma
Wheezing
Sneezing
Coughing
Chronic nasal discharge
Asthma exacerbation
Laryngeal edema

Cutaneous
Urticaria
Atopic dermatitis

Systemic
Anaphylaxis

Other Signs and Symptoms
Eczema
Excessive crying
Pallor (from anemia secondary to chronic blood loss in gastrointestinal tract)

testing involves reintroducing small quantities of milk in the diet to detect resurgence of symptoms; at times it involves the use of a placebo so that the parent is unaware of (or "blind" to) the timing of allergen ingestion. A double-blind, placebo-controlled food challenge is the gold standard for diagnosing food allergies such as CMA, yet it may not be used often for diagnosing CMA because of the expense, time involved, and risk for further exposure and anaphylactic reaction (Ewing and Allen, 2005). Careful observation of the child is required during a challenge test because of the possibility of anaphylactic reaction.

Therapeutic Management

Treatment of CMA is elimination of cow's milk–based formula and all other dairy products. For infants fed cow's milk formula, this primarily involves changing the formula to a casein hydrolysate milk formula (Pregestimil, Nutramigen, or Alimentum) in which the protein has been broken down into its amino acids through enzymatic hydrolysis. Although the AAP (2009) recommends the use of extensively hydrolyzed formulas for CMA, many practitioners may start a soy formula instead because of the expense of the hydrolyzed formulas. Approximately 50% of infants who are sensitive to cow's milk protein also demonstrate sensitivity to soy, but soy is less expensive than protein hydrolysate formula. Other choices for children who are intolerant to cow's milk–based formula are the amino acid–based formulas Neocate or EleCare, but their cost is a major consideration. Goat's milk (raw) is not an acceptable substitute because it cross-reacts with cow's milk protein, is deficient in folic acid, has a high sodium and protein content, and is unsuitable as the only source of calories. Some suggest that goat's milk infant formula may be a suitable substitute for cow's milk formula (Basnet, Schneider, Gazit, and others, 2010). Anaphylactic reaction to goat's milk has been noted in an infant who was also allergic to cow's milk (Pessler and Nejat, 2004). Infants usually remain on the milk-free diet for 12 months, after which time small quantities of milk are reintroduced.

Children who have CMA may tolerate extensively heated cow's milk (Nowak-Wegrzyn, Bloom, Sicherer, and others, 2008). One study reports that children with CMA became tolerant to uncooked milk products over time after consuming baked milk products (Kim, Nowak-Wegrzyn, Sicherer, and others, 2011).

Nursing Care Management

The principal nursing objectives are identification of potential CMA and appropriate counseling of parents regarding substitute formulas. Parents often interpret GI symptoms such as spitting up and loose stools or fussiness as indications that the infant is allergic to cow's milk and switch the infant to a variety of formulas in an attempt to resolve the problem.

Parents need much reassurance regarding the needs of nonverbal infants with such an array of symptoms. Endless nights of lost sleep and a crying infant may promote feelings of parenting inadequacy and role conflict, thus aggravating the situation. Nurses can reassure parents that many of these symptoms are common and the reasons are often never found, yet the child does achieve appropriate growth and development. Report acute symptoms to the practitioner for further evaluation. Parents need reassurance that the infant will receive complete nutrition from the new formula and will have no ill effects from the absence of cow's milk.

When solid foods are started, parents need guidance in avoiding milk product. Carefully reading all food labels helps avoid exposure to prepared foods containing milk products. Although labeled as nondairy, milk, cream, and butter substitutes may contain cow's milk protein (Kattan, Cocco, and Järvinen, 2011).

made from the history, although the history alone is not diagnostic. The timing and diversity of clinical manifestations vary greatly. For example, CMA may be manifested as colic (see p. 367), diarrhea, vomiting, GI bleeding, gastroesophageal reflux, chronic constipation, or sleeplessness in an otherwise healthy infant.

Diagnostic Evaluation

A number of diagnostic tests may be performed, including stool analysis for blood, eosinophils, and leukocytes (both frank and occult bleeding can occur from the colitis); serum IgE levels; skin-prick or scratch testing; and radioallergosorbent test (RAST) (measures IgE antibodies to specific allergens in serum by radioimmunoassay). Both skin testing and RAST may help identify the offending food, but the results are not always conclusive. No single diagnostic test is considered definitive for the diagnosis (AAP, 2009). In breastfed infants, cow's milk protein products should be eliminated to improve the diagnostic results (Kattan, Cocco, and Järvinen, 2011).

The most definitive diagnostic strategy is elimination of milk in the diet followed by challenge testing after improvement of symptoms. A clinical diagnosis is made when symptoms improve after removal of milk from the diet and two or more challenge tests produce symptoms (Ewing and Allen, 2005; Kattan, Cocco, and Järvinen, 2011). Challenge

GROWTH FAILURE (FAILURE TO THRIVE)

Growth failure, or failure to thrive (FTT), is a sign of inadequate growth resulting from an inability to obtain or use calories required for growth. FTT has no universal definition, although one of the more common criteria is a weight (and sometimes height) that falls below the fifth percentile for the child's age. Another definition of FTT includes a weight for age (height) z value of less than −2.0 (a z value is a standard deviation value that represents anthropometric data normalizing for sex and age with greater precision than growth percentile curves [Markowitz, Watkins, and Duggan, 2008]). A third way to define FTT is a weight curve that crosses more than 2 percentile lines on a standardized growth chart after previous achievement of a stable growth pattern. Weight for length is reported to be a better indicator of acute undernutrition (Cole and Lanham, 2011). Growth measurements alone are not used to diagnose children with FTT. Rather, the finding of a pattern of persistent deviation from established growth parameters is cause for concern. In addition to lack of consensus on the precise definition of FTT, some advocate for a change in terminology; thus, terms such as *growth failure* and *pediatric undernutrition* are used in the literature for FTT (Locklin, 2005). Another term seen in the literature is *weight or growth faltering*. According to Cole and Lanham (2011), approximately 5% to 10% of children in primary care in the United States have FTT with the majority presenting before the age of 18 months.

Some experts suggest that the previously used classifications of *organic FTT* and *nonorganic FTT* are too simplistic because most cases of growth failure have mixed causes; they suggest that FTT be classified according to pathophysiology in the following categories (Krugman and Dubowitz, 2003):

Inadequate caloric intake—Incorrect formula preparation, neglect, food fads, excessive juice consumption, poverty, breastfeeding problems, behavioral problems affecting eating, or central nervous system problems affecting intake

Inadequate absorption—Cystic fibrosis, celiac disease, vitamin or mineral deficiencies, biliary atresia, or hepatic disease

Increased metabolism—Hyperthyroidism, congenital heart disease, hyperthyroidism, or chronic immunodeficiency

Defective utilization—Genetic anomaly such as trisomy 21 or 18, congenital infection, or metabolic storage diseases

The cause of growth failure is often multifactorial and involves a combination of infant organic disease, dysfunctional parenting behaviors, subtle neurologic or behavioral problems, and disturbed parent–child interactions (Block, Krebs, and Committee on Child Abuse and Neglect and Committee on Nutrition, 2005). However, the primary etiology is inadequate caloric intake, regardless of the cause.

Infants who are born preterm and with VLBW or ELBW, as well as those with intrauterine growth restriction (IUGR), are often referred for growth failure within the first 2 years of life because they typically do not grow physically at the same rate as term cohorts even after discharge from the acute care facility. Catch-up growth has been shown to be much more difficult to achieve in ELBW and VLBW infants. As children, former VLBW and ELBW infants are more likely to have small stature and demonstrate lower cognitive and academic achievement scores than term cohorts (Casey, Whiteside-Mansell, Barrett, and others, 2006).

Other factors that can lead to inadequate caloric intake in infancy include poverty, health or childrearing beliefs such as fad diets, inadequate nutritional knowledge, family stress, feeding resistance, and insufficient breast milk intake. In infants younger than 8 weeks of age, breastfeeding problems as a result of inadequate latch or uncoordinated sucking and swallowing may occur (Cole and Lanham, 2011). One account reports a 6-month-old term infant with FTT as a result of severe ankyloglossia (tongue tie) (Forlenza, Paradise Black, McNamara, and others, 2010).

Diagnostic Evaluation

Diagnosis is initially made from evidence of growth failure. If FTT is recent, the weight, but not the height, is below accepted standards (usually the fifth percentile); if FTT is longstanding, both weight and height are low, indicating chronic malnutrition. Perhaps as important as anthropometric measurements are a complete health and dietary history (including perinatal history), physical examination for evidence of organic causes, developmental assessment, and family assessment. A dietary intake history, either a 24-hour food intake or a history of food consumed over a 3- to 5-day period, is also essential. In addition, explore the child's activity level, parental height, perceived food allergies, and dietary restrictions. An assessment of household organization and mealtime behaviors and rituals is important in the collection of pertinent data. It is often helpful to obtain the growth patterns of the affected child's parents and siblings; these can be compared with norm-referenced standards to evaluate the child's growth (Markowitz, Watkins, and Duggan, 2008). An assessment of the home environment and child–parent interaction may be helpful as well. Other tests (lead toxicity, anemia, stool-reducing substances, occult blood, ova and parasites, alkaline phosphatase, and zinc levels) are selected only as indicated to rule out organic problems. In most cases, laboratory studies are of little diagnostic value (AAP, 2009). To prevent the overuse of diagnostic procedures, consider FTT early in the differential diagnosis. To avoid the social stigma of FTT during the early investigative phase, some health care workers use the term *growth delay* (or *failure*) until the actual cause is established.

Therapeutic Management

The primary management of FTT is aimed at reversing the cause of the growth failure. If malnutrition is severe, the initial treatment is directed at reversing the malnutrition. The goal is to provide sufficient calories to support "catch-up" growth—a rate of growth greater than the expected rate for age.

In addition to adding caloric density to feedings, the child may require multivitamin supplements and dietary supplementation with high-calorie foods and drinks. Any coexisting medical problems are treated.

In most cases of FTT, an interdisciplinary team of physician, nurse, dietitian, child life specialist, occupational therapist, pediatric feeding specialist, and social worker or mental health professional is needed to deal with the multiple problems. Make efforts to relieve any additional stresses on the family by offering referrals to welfare agencies or supplemental food programs. In some cases, family therapy may be required. Temporary placement in a foster home may relieve the family's stress, protect the child, and allow the child some stability if insurmountable obstacles are preventing appropriate family function. Behavior modification aimed at mealtime rituals (or lack thereof) and family social time may be required. Hospitalization admission is indicated for (1) evidence (anthropometric) of severe acute malnutrition, (2) child abuse or neglect, (3) significant dehydration, (4) caretaker substance abuse or psychosis, (5) outpatient management that does not result in weight gain, and (6) serious intercurrent infection (AAP, 2009; Block, Krebs, and Committee on Child Abuse and Neglect and Committee on Nutrition, 2005).

Prognosis

The prognosis for FTT is related to the cause. If the parents have simply not understood the infant's needs, teaching may remedy the child's limited caloric intake and permanently reverse the growth failure. Inadequate or infrequent feeding periods by the infant's primary caretaker, in conjunction with family disorganization, are often observed to be the cause of FTT.

Few long-term studies provide data on the prognosis for children with FTT; however, some studies indicate that children who had FTT as infants had shorter heights, lower weights, and lower scores on measures of psychomotor development than peers (Black, Dubowitz, Krishnakumar, and others, 2007; Rudolf and Logan, 2005). Factors related to poor prognosis are severe feeding resistance, lack of awareness in and cooperation from the parent(s), low family income, low maternal educational level, adolescent mother, preterm birth, IUGR, and early age of onset of FTT. Because later cognitive and motor function is affected by malnourishment in infancy, many of these children are below normal in intellectual development, have poorer language development and less well-developed reading skills, attain lower social maturity, and have a higher incidence of behavioral disturbances (Markowitz, Watkins, and Duggan, 2008). Such findings indicate that a long-term plan and follow-up care are needed for the optimum development of these children.

Nursing Care Management

Caring for the child with FTT presents many nursing challenges, whether treatment takes place in the hospital, clinic, or home. Providing a positive feeding environment, teaching the parents successful feeding strategies, and supporting the child and family are essential components of care.

Nurses play a critical role in the diagnosis of FTT through their assessment of the child, parents, and family interactions. Knowledge of the characteristics of children with FTT and their families is essential in helping identify these children and hastening the confirmation of a diagnosis (Box 11-3). Accurate assessment of initial weight and height and daily weight, as well as recording of all food intake, is mandatory. The nurse documents the child's feeding behavior and the parent–child interaction during feeding, other caregiving activities, and play. One available feeding observation instrument is the Nursing Child Assessment Satellite Training (NCAST) Feeding Scale, which is designed to assess the feeding interaction of infants up to 12 months of age (Barnard, Hammond, Booth, and others, 1993).* (See Nutritional Assessment, Chapter 6.)

The nurse should assess the approximate developmental age on admission by administering an appropriate developmental test. Only after objective measurements are available is a care plan for stimulation outlined. The nursing admission history and ongoing assessment should also focus on the following characteristics that have been identified in many of these children and their parents.

Besides showing signs of malnutrition and delayed social development, children with FTT may exhibit altered behavioral interactions. They may display intense interest in inanimate objects, such as toys, but much less interest in social interactions. They are often watchful of people at a distance but become increasingly distressed as others come closer. They may dislike being touched or held and avoid

---

BOX 11-3   CLINICAL MANIFESTATIONS OF FAILURE TO THRIVE

- Growth failure (see p. 362 for definitions)
- Developmental delays—social, motor, adaptive, language
- Undernutrition
- Apathy
- Withdrawn behavior
- Feeding or eating disorders, such as vomiting, feeding resistance, anorexia, pica, rumination
- No fear of strangers (at age when stranger anxiety is normal)
- Avoidance of eye contact
- Wide-eyed gaze and continual scan of the environment ("radar gaze")
- Stiff and unyielding or flaccid and unresponsive
- Minimal smiling

---

face-to-face contact. However, when held, they protest briefly on being put down and are apathetic when left alone.

Children with growth failure may have a history of difficult feeding, vomiting, sleep disturbance, and excessive irritability. Patterns such as crying during feedings; vomiting; hoarding food in the mouth; ruminating after feeding; refusing to switch from liquids to solids; and displaying aversion behavior, such as turning from food or spitting food, become attention-seeking mechanisms to prolong the attention received at mealtime. In some cases, the child may use feeding as a control mechanism in a poorly organized or chaotic family situation; parents may allow the child to dictate the norms for behavior and feeding because of inexperience with parenting or poor parenting role models. Thus, refusing to eat or only eating high-sugar foods may be the child's norm. In such cases, family therapy is essential to reverse the trend and assist the parents and child in understanding each other's roles.

Some parents are at increased risk for attachment problems because of (1) isolation and social crisis; (2) inadequate support systems, such as teenage and single mothers; and (3) poor parenting role models as a child. Other factors that should be considered are lack of education; physical and mental health problems such as physical and sexual abuse, depression, or drug dependence; immaturity, especially in adolescent parents; and lack of commitment to parenting, such as giving priority to entertainment or employment. Often these parents and their families are under stress and in multiple chronic emotional, social, and financial crises.

Because part of the difficulty between parent and child is dissatisfaction and frustration, the child should have a primary core of nurses (Fig. 11-1). The nurses caring for the child can learn to perceive the child's cues and reverse the cycle of dissatisfaction, especially in the area of feeding.

Because many of these children are responding to stimuli that have led to the negative feeding patterns, the first goal is to structure the feeding environment to encourage eating. Initially, staff members and a feeding specialist may need to feed these children to thoroughly assess the difficulties encountered during the feeding process and to devise strategies that eliminate or minimize such problems. General guidelines for the feeding process are outlined in the Nursing Care Guidelines box.

Four primary goals in the nutritional management of children with FTT are to (1) correct nutritional deficiencies and achieve ideal weight for height, (2) allow for catch-up growth, (3) restore optimum body composition, and (4) educate the parents or primary caregivers regarding the child's nutritional requirements and appropriate feeding

---

*Training is required to use the feeding scale. For information, contact NCAST Programs, University of Washington, PO Box 357920, Seattle, WA 98195; 206-543-8528; e-mail: ncast@u.washington.edu; http://www.ncast.org.

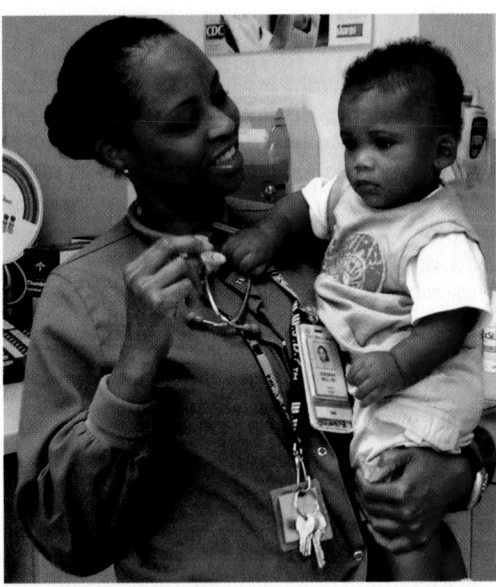

FIG 11-1 A consistent nurse is important in developing trust in infants with failure to thrive.

📋 NURSING CARE GUIDELINES

Feeding Children with Failure to Thrive

Provide a primary core of staff to feed the child. The same nurses are able to learn the child's cues and respond consistently.

Provide a quiet, unstimulating atmosphere. A number of children with colic are very distractible, and their attention is diverted with minimal stimuli. Older children do well at a feeding table; bottle-fed infants children should always be held.

Maintain a calm, even temperament throughout the meal. Negative outbursts may be commonplace in this child's habit formation. Limits on eating behavior definitely need to be provided, but they should be stated in a firm, calm tone. If the nurse is hurried or anxious, the feeding process will not be optimized.

Talk to the child by giving directions about eating. "Take a bite, Lisa" is appropriate and directive. The more distractible the child, the more directive the nurse should be to refocus attention on feeding. Positive comments about feeding are actively given.

Be persistent. This is perhaps one of the most important guidelines. Parents often give up when the child begins negative feeding behavior. Calm perseverance through 10 to 15 minutes of food refusal will eventually diminish negative behavior. Although forced feeding is avoided, "strictly encouraged" feeding is essential.

Maintain a face-to-face posture with the child when possible. Encourage eye contact and remain with the child throughout the meal.

Introduce new foods slowly. Often these children have been exclusively bottle fed. If acceptance of solids is a problem, begin with pureed food and, after it is accepted, advance to junior and regular solid foods.

Follow the child's rhythm of feeding. The child will set a rhythm when the previous conditions are met.

Develop a structured routine. Disruption in other activities of daily living has great impact on feeding responses, so bathing, sleeping, dressing, playing, and feeding are structured. The nurse should feed the child in the same way and place as often as possible. The length of the feeding should also be established (usually 30 minutes).

---

methods (Corrales and Utter, 2005; Maggioni and Lifshitz, 1995). For infants, 24 kcal/oz formulas may be provided to increase caloric intake; older children (1–6 years) may benefit from a 30 kcal/oz formula (AAP, 2009). Other carbohydrate additives include fortified rice cereal and vegetable oil. Because vitamin and mineral deficiencies may occur, multivitamin supplementation, including zinc and iron, is recommended. For toddlers, a high-calorie milk drink such as PediaSure may be used to increase caloric intake. Carefully monitor for signs of intolerance to the formula. Usually only in extreme cases of malnourishment are tube feedings or intravenous therapy required.

Because maladaptive feeding practices often contribute to growth failure, give parents specific step-by-step directions for formula preparation, as well as a written schedule of feeding times. Avoid juices in children with growth failure until adequate weight gain has been achieved with appropriate milk sources; thereafter give no more than 4 oz/day of juice.

Behavior modification techniques may be used with older infants and toddlers to interrupt poor feeding patterns. Feeding times may actually involve "struggles of will" in cases of maladaptive feedings that result in FTT. These behaviors are different from the occasional toddler behavior of food refusal, which is primarily developmental, not pathologic. The association of appropriate food with good or bad behaviors and consequent rewards may be part of the complex problem. In severe cases of malnourishment, tube feedings or intravenous therapy may be required.

In addition to attending to the child's physical needs, the interdisciplinary team must plan care for appropriate developmental stimulation. After an approximate developmental age is established, a planned program of play is begun. Ideally, a child life specialist is involved to implement and supervise the stimulation program. Every effort is made to teach the parent how to play and interact with the child.

Nursing care of these children involves a "family systems" approach. In other words, for the entire family to become healthy, each member must be helped to change. Care of the parents is aimed at helping them improve their self-esteem by acquiring positive, successful parenting skills. Initially, this necessitates providing an environment in which they feel welcomed and accepted. Depending on the cause of FTT, many children are treated on an outpatient basis.

SLEEP PROBLEMS

A number of sleep problems are identified in small children. The two major categories are the **dyssomnias**: the child has trouble either falling or staying asleep at night or has difficulty staying awake during the day. The second category, **parasomnias**, is characterized as confusional arousals, sleepwalking, sleep terrors, nightmares, and rhythmic movement disorders; these typically occur in children 3 to 8 years old (Ward, Rankin, and Lee, 2007) and decline in incidence as the child matures (Davis, Parker, and Montgomery, 2004). This discussion focuses on minor sleep issues in infants such as refusal to go to sleep and frequent waking during the night (Table 11-1). Other sleep disturbances such as obstructive sleep, disordered breathing, and sleep terrors are discussed elsewhere in this text.

Concerns regarding sleep are common during infancy. Sometimes these concerns are as basic as parents' questioning whether the infant needs additional sleep. In this case, it is best to investigate the reason for their concern, stressing the individual needs of each child. Infants who are active during wakeful periods and growing normally are sleeping a sufficient amount of time.

Sleep problems in early infancy have been positively correlated with higher maternal depression scores (Hiscock and Wake, 2001;

TABLE 11-1   SELECTED SLEEP DISTURBANCES DURING INFANCY AND EARLY CHILDHOOD

DISORDER AND DESCRIPTION	MANAGEMENT
Nighttime Feeding Child has a prolonged need for middle-of-night bottle or breastfeeding. Child goes to sleep at breast or with a bottle. Awakenings are frequent (may be hourly). Child returns to sleep after feeding; other comfort measures (e.g., rocking or holding) are usually ineffective.	Increase daytime feeding intervals to 4 hours or more (may need to be done gradually). Offer last feeding as late as possible at night; may need to gradually reduce amount of formula or length of breastfeeding. Offer no bottles in bed. Put to bed awake. When child is crying, check at progressively longer intervals each night; reassure child but do not hold, rock, take to parent's bed, or give bottle or pacifier.
Developmental Nighttime Crying Child age 6–12 months with undisturbed nighttime sleep now wakes abruptly; may be accompanied by nightmares.	Reassure parents that this phase is temporary. Enter room immediately to check on child but keep reassurances brief. Avoid feeding, rocking, taking to parent's bed, or any other routine that may initiate trained nighttime crying.
Refusal to Go to Sleep Child resists bedtime and comes out of room repeatedly. Nighttime sleep may be continuous, but frequent awakenings and refusal to return to sleep may occur and become a problem if parent allows child to deviate from usual sleep pattern.	Evaluate if hour of sleep is too early (child may resist sleep if not tired). Assist parents in establishing consistent before-bedtime routine and enforcing consistent limits regarding child's bedtime behavior. If child persists in leaving bedroom, close door for progressively longer periods. Use reward system with child to provide motivation.
Trained Nighttime Crying (Inappropriate Sleep Associations) Child typically falls asleep in place other than own bed (e.g., rocking chair or parent's bed) and is brought to own bed while asleep; on awakening, cries until usual routine is instituted (e.g., rocking).	Put child in own bed when awake. If possible, arrange sleeping area separate from other family members. When child is crying, check at progressively longer intervals each night; reassure child but do not resume usual routine.
Nighttime Fears Child resists going to bed or wakes during the night because of fears. Child seeks parent's physical presence and falls asleep easily with parent nearby unless fear is overwhelming.	Evaluate if hour of sleep is too early (child may fantasize when nothing to do but think in dark room). Calmly reassure the frightened child; keeping a night light on may be helpful. Use reward system with child to provide motivation to deal with fears. Avoid patterns that can lead to additional problems (e.g., sleeping with child or taking child to parent's room). If child's fear is overwhelming, consider desensitization (e.g., progressively spending longer periods of time alone; consult professional help for protracted fears). Distinguish between nightmares and sleep terrors (confused partial arousals).

Modified from Ferber R: Behavioral "insomnia" in the child, *Psychiatr Clin North Am* 10(4):641–653, 1987.

Hawkins-Walsh, 2003) and poorer general and mental health in both the mother and the father (Goyal, Gay, and Lee, 2009; Martin, Hiscock, Hardy, and others, 2007); therefore, nurses must discuss infant sleep problems with the mother (and family) in addition to other developmental aspects of newborn care. One study found that infants slept less if there was maternal depression during pregnancy, early introduction of solid foods (<4 mo), television viewing of at least 1 hour per day, and attendance at child care outside the home (Nevarez, Rifas-Shiman, Kleinman, and others, 2010).

When a sleeping problem is presented, a careful assessment is essential. Charting sleep habits both before and after interventions is also an important strategy. Questions regarding the frequency and duration of waking, the usual bedtime routine, the number of nighttime feedings, the perceived problem (e.g., how much disruption the behavior generates), and the attempted interventions are important in planning effective approaches designed for the specific sleep problem.

One suggestion given for any type of sleep problem, "Let the child cry until he or she falls asleep," is very difficult to implement and is inappropriate for certain conditions. After the parents relent and console the child, they have only reinforced the crying. This approach is called the "extinction" method and is still used by some; parental consistency is essential for this approach (Moore, Meltzer, and Mindell, 2008).

Another approach to night crying is known as graduated extinction. This involves letting the child cry for progressively longer times between brief parental interventions that consist only of reassurance—not rocking, holding, or using a bottle or pacifier. For example, the parents may check on the child every 5 minutes (of crying) during the first night and progressively extend this interval by 5 minutes on successive nights (Ferber and Kryger, 1995).

Families that cannot tolerate unexpected crying spells while everyone else is asleep can try the two-step approach. Graduated extinction is used during naps and at bedtime until the parents retire for the night. If the child cries during the night, the parents use comforting measures. However, after the child is partially trained, step 2 is initiated—the use of graduated extinction at all times.

Another approach includes the positive routine and faded bedtime. In this approach, the parents schedule some quiet activities close to bedtime to calm the child down for approximately 20 minutes and then place the child to sleep. Gradually, the bedtime is moved 10 to 15 minutes earlier until a suitable bedtime is set. This approach requires parental consistency and cooperation (Moore, Meltzer, and Mindell, 2008). This method is appropriate for toddlers who thrive on rituals and routines. Additional methods for dealing with specific sleep problems may be found in the Moore, Meltzer, and Mindell (2008) reference.

Children who learn to fall asleep on their own at bedtime have longer sustained sleep periods than those who fall asleep with a parent present (Davis, Parker, and Montgomery, 2004). In addition, comforting children outside their own bed at night when they awaken was associated with poor sleep consolidation. Feeding 5-month-old infants after awakening at night has been associated with fewer consecutive sleep hours (Touchette, Petit, Paquet, and others, 2005). The authors of this study recommend parental presence at bedtime until the child is drowsy and then placing the child in his or her own bed for a night's sleep.

The best way to prevent sleep problems is to encourage parents to establish bedtime rituals that do not foster problematic patterns. One of the most constructive is placing infants awake in their own crib. When infants are accustomed to falling asleep somewhere else, such as in their parent's arms, and then being transferred to their crib, they awaken in unfamiliar surroundings and are unable to fall asleep until the routine is repeated. Also, the bed should be used for sleeping only—not as a play yard. It is advisable not to hang playthings over or on the bed; in this way, the child associates the bed with sleep, not with activity. Although the interventions described previously and in Table 11-1 are usually successful, it is much easier to prevent the problem with appropriate counseling during the early months of the infant's life.

POSITIONAL PLAGIOCEPHALY

Since the Back to Sleep campaign began in 1992 advocating nonprone sleeping for infants to prevent sudden infant death syndrome (SIDS), an increase in the incidence of positional plagiocephaly has been observed (AAP, Task Force on Sudden Infant Death Syndrome, 2005; Littlefield, Saba, and Kelly, 2004). The prevalence of positional plagiocephaly at 4 months is reported to range from slightly less than 20% to as much as 48% (Robinson and Proctor, 2009). The term **plagiocephaly** connotes an oblique or asymmetric head; *positional plagiocephaly, deformational plagiocephaly,* or *nonsynostotic plagiocephaly* implies an acquired condition that occurs as a result of cranial molding during infancy (Hummel and Fortado, 2005). Because infants' sutures are not closed, the skull is pliable and, when infants are placed on their backs to sleep, the posterior occiput flattens over time (Fig. 11-2, *A*). A typical bald spot develops, which is usually transient. As a result of prolonged pressure on one side of the skull, that side becomes misshapen; mild facial asymmetry may develop. The sternocleidomastoid muscle may tighten on the preferential side, and torticollis may also develop. Congenital or acquired torticollis may cause plagiocephaly; other causes of deformational plagiocephaly include certain craniofacial syndromes. This discussion centers only on positional plagiocephaly caused by supine sleeping position.

THERAPEUTIC MANAGEMENT

Prevention of positional plagiocephaly may begin shortly after birth by placing the infant to sleep supine and alternating the infant's head position nightly, avoiding prolonged placement in car safety seats and swings, and using prone positioning or "tummy time" for

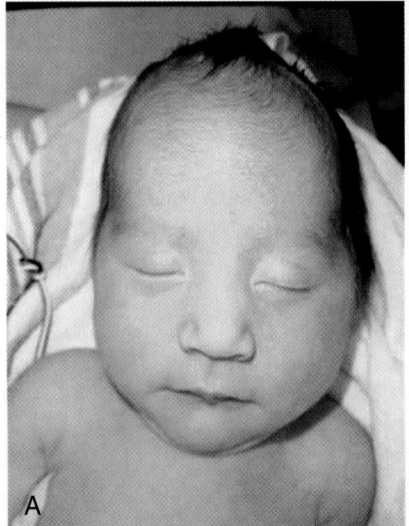
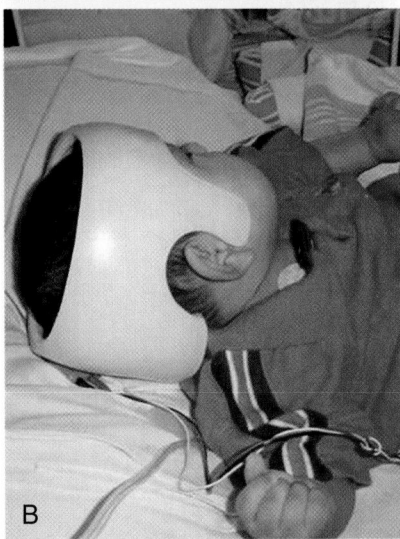

FIG 11-2 A, Plagiocephaly. **B,** Helmet used to correct plagiocephaly. (Courtesy Dr. Gerardo Cabrera-Meza, Department of Neonatology, Baylor College of Medicine, Houston.)

approximately 30 to 60 minutes per day when the infant is awake (Laughlin, Luerssen, Dias, and others, 2011).

Treatment of torticollis and plagiocephaly initially involves exercises to loosen the tight muscle and switching head position sides during feeding, carrying, and sleep. If the plagiocephaly is not resolved within 4 to 8 weeks of physical therapy, a customized helmet may be worn to decrease the pressure on the affected side of the skull (Fig. 11-2, *B*). If no improvement occurs with physical therapy or a molded helmet over a period of 2 to 3 months, the infant may be referred to a pediatric neurosurgeon or craniofacial surgeon; the referral should optimally occur by 4 to 6 months of age (Laughlin, Luerssen, Dias, and others, 2011).

The helmet is worn 23 hours a day for a prescribed period (usually 3 months). Repositioning and physical therapy are said to be more effective when used before the infant can roll over or move his or her head alone (i.e., before approximately 3 to 4 months of age) (Robinson and Proctor, 2009). Reports of developmental delay in infants with positional plagiocephaly (nonsynostotic) vary in regard to outcomes, but current studies do not conclusively prove that such infants are at higher risk for developmental delays (Robinson and Proctor, 2009).

NURSING CARE MANAGEMENT

Minor skull flattening is not considered significant, but parents should learn to prevent plagiocephaly by altering the infant's head position during sleep. Infants should be placed prone on a firm surface during awake time (tummy time), which prevents plagiocephaly and facilitates development of upper shoulder girdle strength; the latter helps in the progressive development of movements such as rolling over and starting to rise up on all fours, which are precursors to crawling and eventually walking. Thirty to sixty minutes of supervised tummy time per day in infants younger than 6 months of age is recommended (Laughlin, Luerssen, Dias, and others, 2011; Robinson and Proctor, 2009).

Despite the perceived increase in the incidence of positional plagiocephaly, the supine sleeping position is still recommended because it has led to a significant decrease in loss of infant lives from SIDS (AAP, Task Force on Sudden Infant Death Syndrome, 2011). Additional measures to prevent positional plagiocephaly include avoiding excessive time spent in car seat restraints, infant seats, and bouncers. Alternating the infant's head position for sleep times can also prevent unilateral molding. When a nurse or parent notices plagiocephaly, a consultation with the primary practitioner is recommended to evaluate the head shape and ascertain the need for early intervention.

Nurses are in a unique position in well-child care settings to encourage parents to follow guidelines for preventing plagiocephaly, demonstrate alternating head placement for sleeping, demonstrate sternocleidomastoid muscle exercises (as appropriate to the condition), and encourage tummy time for infants during awake periods. Most important, nurses should continue to encourage parents to place the infant in a supine sleep position despite the development of plagiocephaly. Nurses can also assist parents in the proper use of a skull-molding helmet and reassure them of the high rate of success with the helmet. Allowing parents to verbalize concerns and feelings related to the health status of the child as well as provision of current best practice is an important nursing function. Parents should not become so alarmed by plagiocephaly that they abandon supine sleeping position for the infant but should consult with the practitioner for further advice.

DISORDERS OF UNKNOWN ETIOLOGY

COLIC (PAROXYSMAL ABDOMINAL PAIN)

Colic is reported to occur in 15% to 40% of all infants (Morin, 2009), yet it has no particular affinity in regard to gender, race, or socioeconomic status (Ellett, 2003). An organic cause may be identified in fewer than 5% of infants seen by physicians because of excessive crying (Roberts, Ostapchuk, and O'Brien, 2004). The condition is generally described as abdominal pain or cramping that is manifested by loud crying and drawing the legs up to the abdomen. Other definitions include variables such as duration of cry greater than 3 hours a day occurring more than 3 days per week and for more than 3 weeks and parental dissatisfaction with the child's behavior. Some studies report an increase in symptoms (fussiness and crying) in the late afternoon or evening (Morin, 2009); however, in some infants, the onset of symptoms occurs at another time. Colic is more common in infants younger than 3 months than in older infants, and infants with difficult temperaments are more likely to be colicky.

Despite the obvious behavioral indications of pain, the infant with colic gains weight and usually thrives. There is no evidence of a residual effect of colic on older children except perhaps a strained parent–child relationship in some cases. In other words, infants who are colicky grow up to be normal children and adults. Colic is self-limiting and in most cases resolves as infants mature, generally around 12 to 16 weeks of age (Lobo, Kotzer, Keefe, and others, 2004; O'Connor, 2009).

Among the theories investigated as potential causes are too rapid feeding, overeating, swallowing excessive air, improper feeding technique (especially in positioning and burping), and emotional stress or tension between the parent and child. Although all of these may occur, there is no evidence that one factor is consistently present. Infants with CMA symptoms have a high rate of colic (44%), and eliminating cow's milk products from the infant's diet can reduce the symptoms. However, there is considerable controversy about the role of allergy and colic because there does not appear to be an increased incidence of atopy in infants with colic (Sicherer, 2003).

Parental smoking, strained parent–infant interaction, lactase deficiency, difficult infant temperament, difficulty regulating emotions, overstimulation, central nervous system immaturity, and neurochemical dysregulation in the brain have also been proposed as potential causes of colic (Ellett, 2003; Neu and Robinson, 2003). A positive association between consumption of fruit juices (carbohydrate malabsorption) and colic has been demonstrated in some cases (Duro, Rising, Cedillo, and others, 2002). Some experts have suggested that gastroesophageal reflux is a cause of colic, but studies have not supported this theory (St. James-Roberts, 2008). The consensus of many experts who study colic is that it is multifactorial and that no single treatment for every colicky infant will be effective in alleviating the symptoms.

Therapeutic Management

Management of colic should begin with an investigation of possible organic causes, such as CMA, intussusception, or other GI problem. If a sensitivity to cow's milk is strongly suspected, a trial substitution of another formula such as an extensively hydrolyzed (Nutramigen, Alimentum, Pregestimil), whey hydrolysate, or amino acid (Neocate, EleCare) formula is warranted. Soy formulas are usually avoided because of the possibility of sensitivity to soy protein as well (AAP, 2009). Oral administration of *Lactobacillus reuteri* to colicky breastfed infants decreased symptoms within 1 week of initiation in one small study (Savino, Pelle, Palumeri, and others, 2007).

When no specific inciting agent can be found, the supportive measures discussed under Nursing Care Management are used.

The use of drugs, including sedatives, antispasmodics, antihistamines, and antiflatulents, is sometimes recommended. The most commonly used sedatives are phenobarbital, hydroxyzine hydrochloride (Atarax), and chloral hydrate. Simethicone (Mylicon) may also help allay the symptoms of colic. However, in most controlled studies, none of these drugs completely reduced the symptoms of colic. Behavioral interventions have not proved effective at reducing the symptoms of colic but have helped parents deal with their crying infants in a more positive manner. The addition of lactase to infant formula has produced mixed results as far as abatement of overall symptoms.

An extensive review of a wide variety of interventions for colic indicates no specific safe remedies are available to alleviate symptoms of colic in every infant. Dietary changes, such as eliminating cow's milk protein from the lactating mother's diet, and behavioral interventions were shown to be effective in helping parents reduce stimulation and respond to the infant's crying, yet these interventions are perceived only as moderately effective (Joanna Briggs Institute, 2008). Administering sucrose was effective at reducing crying in colicky infants for a short period (3–30 minutes) (Joanna Briggs Institute, 2008). A recent position statement by the Canadian Paediatric Society, Nutrition and Gastroenterology Committee (Critch, 2011) concluded that dietary

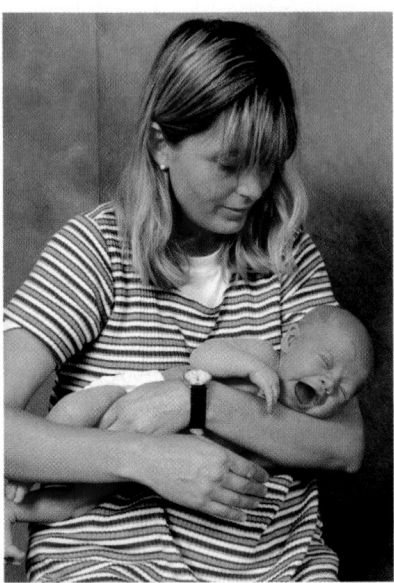

FIG 11-3 The "colic carry" may be comforting to an infant with colic. (Photo by Paul Vincent Kuntz, Texas Children's Hospital, Houston.)

modifications are beneficial in some cases but not all; the use of lactate, probiotics, prebiotics, or soy formula independently to decrease symptoms of colic had insufficient evidence to support their use. The use of complementary medicines for infantile colic, namely fennel extract, herbal tea, and sugar solutions, reportedly lack sufficient evidence to recommend their use (Perry, Hunt, and Ernst, 2011).

Nursing Care Management

The initial step in managing colic is to take a thorough, detailed history of the usual daily events. Areas that should be stressed include (1) the infant's diet; (2) the diet of the breastfeeding mother; (3) the time of day when crying occurs; (4) the relationship of crying to feeding time; (5) the presence of specific family members during crying and habits of family members, such as smoking; (6) activity of the mother or usual caregiver before, during, and after crying; (7) characteristics of the cry (duration, intensity); (8) measures used to relieve crying and their effectiveness; and (9) the infant's stooling, voiding, and sleeping patterns. Of special emphasis is a careful assessment of the feeding process via demonstration by the parent.

If cow's milk sensitivity is suspected, breastfeeding mothers should follow a milk-free diet for a minimum of 3 to 5 days in an attempt to reduce the infant's symptoms. Caution mothers that some nondairy creamers may contain calcium caseinate, a cow's milk protein. If a milk-free diet is helpful, lactating mothers may need calcium supplements to meet the body's requirement. Bottle-fed infants may improve with the same dietary modifications as for infants with CMA (see p. 360). Additional approaches for managing colic are listed in the Family-Centered Care box (see also Fig. 11-3).

One important nursing intervention (before or after an organic cause has been eliminated) is reassuring both parents that they are not doing anything wrong and that the infant is not experiencing any physical or emotional harm. Parents, especially mothers, become easily frustrated with their infant's crying and perceive this as a sign that something is horribly wrong. Additionally, colicky infants may be at increased risk for being shaken by their caregivers and experiencing traumatic brain injury. A survey of fathers of colicky infants revealed that professional assistance was limited. The fathers described the experience of having a colicky infant as similar to falling into an abyss

---

FAMILY-CENTERED CARE
Managing the Colicky Infant

- Place infant prone over a covered hot-water bottle, heated towel, or covered heating pad.
- Massage infant's abdomen.
- Respond immediately to the crying.
- Change infant's position frequently; walk with child's face down and with body across parent's arm, with parent's hand under infant's abdomen, applying gentle pressure.
- Use a front carrier for transporting infant.
- Swaddle infant tightly with a soft, stretchy blanket.
- Place infant in an electric (or wind-up) infant swing.
- Take infant for car rides or outside for a change in environment.
- Use bottles that minimize air swallowing (curved bottle or inner collapsible bag).
- Use a commercial device in the crib that stimulates the vibration and sound of a car ride or plays soothing "noise," in utero sounds, or music.
- Provide smaller, frequent feedings; burp infant during and after feedings using the shoulder position or sitting upright, and place infant in an upright seat after feedings.
- Introduce a pacifier for added sucking.
- In breastfed infants, mother should avoid all milk products for a trial period.
- If household members smoke, avoid smoking near infant; preferably confine smoking activity to outside of home.
- Give appropriate dose of acetaminophen elixir or suppository if suggested by health professional; not recommended for daily use.
- If nothing reduces the crying, place infant in crib and allow to cry; periodically hold and comfort child and put down again.
- Maintain a brief diary of the time of day the crying starts; events going on in household; time, amount, and type of last feeding; length of crying; and characteristics of cry. Although this will not stop the crying, it may help the practitioner identify a possible cause.

---

from which they had to climb with the assistance of family and friends, thus reinforcing the importance of empathetic nurses (Ellett, Appleton, and Sloan, 2009). An empathetic, gentle, and reassuring attitude, in addition to suggestions for treatment, will help allay parents' anxieties, which are usually exacerbated by loss of sleep and preoccupation over the infant's welfare. Colic disappears spontaneously, usually by 3 to 4 months of age, although guarantees should never be given, since it may continue for much longer. Other support persons and extended family members may be enlisted to help the parents during this difficult time.

SUDDEN INFANT DEATH SYNDROME

Sudden infant death syndrome (SIDS) is defined as the sudden death of an infant younger than 1 year of age that remains unexplained after a complete postmortem examination, including an investigation of the death scene and a review of the case history. Since 1992, the incidence of SIDS in the United States has decreased by 53% to an all-time low of 0.57 per 1000 live births in 2002 (AAP, Task Force on Sudden Infant Death Syndrome, 2005). The dramatic decrease is attributed to the Back to Sleep campaign.* SIDS is the third leading cause of infant

---

*Back to Sleep materials may be ordered by contacting the National Institute of Child Health and Human Development Information Resource Center, Back to Sleep, PO Box 3006, Rockville, MD 20847; 800-505-CRIB (2742); fax: 866-760-5947; http://www.nichd.nih.gov/sids.

TABLE 11-2	EPIDEMIOLOGY OF SUDDEN INFANT DEATH SYNDROME
FACTOR	**OCCURRENCE**
Incidence	57 per 100,000 live births (2007)*
Peak age	2–3 mo; 95% occur by 6 mo; preterm infants die from sudden infant death syndrome (SIDS) at mean age of 6 wk later than mean age of death from SIDS for term infants
Sex	Higher percentage of boys affected
Time of death	During sleep
Time of year	Increased incidence in winter
Racial	Greater incidence in African Americans and American Indians (see SIDS, p. 368)
Socioeconomic	Increased occurrence in lower socioeconomic class
Birth	Higher incidence in:
	• Preterm infants, especially infants of extremely and very low birth weight
	• Multiple births†
	• Neonates with low Apgar scores
	• Infants with central nervous system disturbances and respiratory disorders such as bronchopulmonary dysplasia
	• Increasing birth order (subsequent siblings as opposed to firstborn child)
Health status	Infants with a recent history of illness; lower incidence in immunized infants
Sleep habits	Highest risk associated with prone position; use of soft bedding; overheating (thermal stress); cosleeping with adult, especially on sofa or noninfant bed; higher incidence in cosleeping with adult smoker
	Infants cosleeping with adult at higher risk if <11 wk old
Feeding habits	Lower incidence in breastfed infants
Pacifier	Lower incidence in infants put to sleep with pacifier
Siblings	May have greater incidence in siblings of SIDS victims
Maternal	Young age; cigarette smoking, especially during pregnancy; poor prenatal care; substance abuse (heroin, methadone, cocaine). A few studies have shown an increased risk in infants exposed to second-hand environmental tobacco smoke.

Data from American Academy of Pediatrics, Task Force on Infant Sleep Position and Sudden Infant Death Syndrome: Changing concepts of sudden infant death syndrome: implications for infant sleeping environment and sleep position, *Pediatrics* 105(3):650–656, 2000; American Academy of Pediatrics, Task Force on Sudden Infant Death Syndrome: The changing concept of sudden infant Death syndrome: diagnostic coding shifts, controversies regarding the sleeping environment, and new variables to consider in reducing risk, *Pediatrics* 116(5):1245–1255, 2005; and American Academy of Pediatrics, Task Force on Sudden Infant Death Syndrome: SIDS and other sleep-related infant deaths: expansion of recommendations for a safe infant sleeping environment, *Pediatrics* 128(5): 1030–1038, 2011.
*Mathews TJ, MacDorman MF: Infant mortality statistics from the 2007 period linked birth/infant death data set, *Natl Vital Statistics Rep* 59(6): 8–30, 2011.
†Although a rare event, simultaneous death of twins from SIDS can occur.

deaths (birth to 12 months) and the leading cause of postneonatal deaths (between 1 and 12 months). SIDS claimed the lives of 2145 infants in the United States in 2006; preliminary data from 2007 indicate there were 2461 deaths from SIDS (Heron, Hoyert, Xu, and others, 2008; Mathews and MacDorman, 2011). Despite dramatic decreases in SIDS rates, rates for African-American, American Indian, and Alaskan Native infants remains disproportionately higher than for the rest of the population. In 2007 SIDS rates were 2.4 times higher for American Indian mothers and 1.9 times higher for African-American mothers in comparison to non-Hispanic white mothers (Mathews and MacDorman, 2011). It is also important to note that overall infant death rates for 2006 and 2007 were significantly higher for African-American infants (13.59 per 1000 live births) than for Hispanic (5.59 per 1000 live births) or white (5.70 per 1000 live births) infants. Likewise, the percentage of infants born preterm (<37 weeks) was significantly higher (18.5%) in African-American women than in white women (11.7%) (MacDorman and Mathews, 2011). Preterm births rank second as cause of infant death; this trend has been constant since the mid-1990s, when the rates of SIDS deaths significantly decreased in the United States.

The SIDS rate remained fairly static between 1999 and 2001. This has been attributed to improved death scene investigation and determination of non-SIDS causes of postneonatal mortality. In addition, there is speculation that deaths attributed to SIDS during the period of 1992 to 2001 may have been a result of other causes (AAP, Task Force on Sudden Infant Death Syndrome, 2005). Table 11-2 summarizes the major epidemiologic characteristics of SIDS. There has been much debate over the term *SIDS*, yet the definition noted above remains for the time being. Other terms have been developed to explain sudden deaths in infants. Sudden unexpected early neonatal death (SUEND) and sudden unexpected infant death (SUID) share similar features but differ in regards to the timing of death: whereas SUID is considered a death in the postneonatal period, SUEND occurs in the first week of life. The AAP, Task Force on Sudden Infant Death Syndrome (2011) policy statement considers SIDS to be a component of SUID.

Etiology

There are numerous theories regarding the etiology of SIDS; however, the cause remains unknown. One hypothesis is that SIDS is related to a brainstem abnormality in the neurologic regulation of cardiorespiratory control. This maldevelopment affects arousal and physiologic responses to a life-threatening challenge during sleep (AAP, Task Force on Sudden Infant Death Syndrome, 2005). Abnormalities include prolonged sleep apnea, increased frequency of brief inspiratory pauses, excessive periodic breathing, and impaired arousal responsiveness to increased carbon dioxide or decreased oxygen. However, *sleep apnea is not the cause of SIDS*. The vast majority of infants with apnea do not die, and only a minority of SIDS victims have documented apparent life-threatening events (ALTEs) (see Apparent Life-Threatening Event, p. 372). Numerous studies indicate that no association exists between SIDS and any childhood vaccine.

A genetic predisposition to SIDS has been postulated as a cause. In one study, a genetic mutation on chromosome 6q 22.1-22.31 was positively linked to a syndrome of SIDS and dysgenesis of the testis (Puffenberger, Hu-Lince, Parod, and others, 2004).

Risk Factors for SIDS

Maternal smoking during pregnancy has emerged in numerous epidemiologic studies as a major factor in SIDS, and tobacco smoke in the infant's environment after birth has also been shown to have a possible relationship to the incidence of SIDS (AAP, Task Force on Sudden Infant Death Syndrome, 2005, 2011). Data show that exposure to tobacco smoke increased an infant's risk for SIDS 1.9 times over infants not exposed; 59% of SIDS deaths in smoke-exposed infants were attributed to maternal smoking (Anderson, Johnson, and Batal, 2005). It has been postulated that 12% of all SIDS deaths could be prevented with prenatal maternal smoking cessation (Pollack, 2001). Increased nicotine concentrations in lung tissue were found in children who died from SIDS compared with a group of control children (McMartin, Platt, Hackman, and others, 2002).

Cosleeping, or an infant sharing a bed with an adult or older child on a noninfant bed, has been reported to have a positive association with SIDS. One survey found a high association between infant deaths, nonstandard beds (sofa, day bed), and bed sharing; a large percentage of infants were found dead on their backs when bed sharing, suggesting suffocation (Unger, Kemp, Wilkins, and others, 2003). A study from Scotland indicates that the risk for SIDS when bed sharing is significantly increased for infants younger than 11 weeks of age (Tappin, Ecob, and Brooke, 2005). Vennemann, Bajanowski, Brinkmann, and others (2009) identified infant sleeping in the house of a friend or relative and sleeping in the family living room as significant risk factors for SIDS. Other studies correlated higher incidences of SIDS and infant cosleeping with maternal smoking, cosleeping with multiple family members, sleeping on a couch, use of a pillow in the infant's bed, maternal overweight, soft bedding, and unintentional asphyxiation resulting from adult intoxication (overlaying) (AAP, Task Force on Infant Sleep Position and Sudden Infant Death Syndrome, 2000; AAP, Task Force on Sudden Infant Death Syndrome, 2005, 2011; Blair, Sidebotham, Evason-Coombe, and others, 2009; Carroll-Pankhurst and Mortimer, 2001; Hauck, Herman, Donovan, and others, 2003; Li, Zhang, Zielke, and others, 2009; McGarvey, McDonnell, Chong, and others, 2003; Person, Lavezzi, and Wolf, 2002).

Studies from countries other than the United States link sleep habits with an increased risk of SIDS. Prone sleeping may cause oropharyngeal obstruction or affect thermal balance or arousal state. One study found that healthy full-term infants had significantly impaired arousal from active and quiet sleep states when sleeping prone (Horne, Ferens, Watts, and others, 2001). Rebreathing of carbon dioxide by infants in the prone position is also a possible cause of SIDS. Infants sleeping prone and on soft bedding may not be able to move their heads to the side, thus increasing the risk of suffocation and lethal rebreathing. Evidence from other countries and the United States shows an increased incidence of SIDS in infants placed in a side-lying position; thus, the side-lying position is no longer recommended for infants sleeping at home, daycare, or hospitals (unless medically indicated). Most preterm infants being discharged from the hospital should be placed in a supine sleeping position unless special factors predispose them to airway obstruction.

One postulated cause of SIDS has been a prolonged Q-T interval; however, there has been no strong evidence to support this as a cause of SIDS or universal testing of newborns for prolonged Q-T interval (AAP, Task Force on Sudden Infant Death Syndrome, 2005).

Soft bedding such as waterbeds, sheepskins, beanbags, pillows, and quilts should be avoided for infant sleeping surfaces. Bedding items such as stuffed animals and toys should be removed from the crib while the infant is asleep. Head covering by a blanket has also been found to be a risk factor for SIDS, thus supporting the recommendation to avoid extra bed linens and other items (Mitchell, Thompson, Becroft, and others, 2008). Crib bumper pads have not been shown to reduce infant injury and should therefore be avoided (AAP, Task Force on Sudden Infant Death Syndrome, 2011).

In a recent retrospective study of SIDS deaths, Ostfield, Esposito, Perl, and others (2010) found that at least one modifiable risk factor such as those previously listed was present in 96% of the deaths; a total of 78% of the deaths had anywhere from two to seven risk factors.

Protective Factors for SIDS

One study indicated that breastfeeding during the first 16 weeks of life decreased the likelihood of SIDS (Alm, Wennergren, Norvenius, and others, 2002). A subsequent meta-analysis confirmed that exclusive breastfeeding for any period of time decreased the overall risk of SIDS (Hauck, Thompson, Tanabe, and others, 2011). Some studies have found pacifier use in infants to be a protective factor against the occurrence of SIDS; the data for pacifier use in infants in the first year of life are said to be more compelling than data linking pacifier use to the development of dental complications and the inhibition of breastfeeding (AAP, Task Force on Sudden Infant Death Syndrome, 2005, 2011). Therefore, the AAP recommends using a pacifier at naptime and bedtime, using a pacifier only if the infant is breastfeeding successfully, not using a sweetened coating on the pacifier, and avoiding forcing the infant to use the pacifier.

The AAP, Task Force on Sudden Infant Death Syndrome (2005, 2011) recommends that all infants be placed to sleep in the supine (on the back) position. The AAP, Task Force on Sudden Infant Death Syndrome (2011) emphasizes that medically stable preterm infants and infants diagnosed with gastroesophageal reflux (GER) be placed in a supine sleep position unless there is a specific upper airway disorder wherein the risk of death from the condition is greater than the risk of SIDS. The supine sleep position has not demonstrated an increased risk of choking and aspiration in infants, including those with GER (AAP, Task Force on Sudden Infant Death Syndrome, 2011).

Since the Back to Sleep campaign in 1992 advocating nonprone sleeping for infants, an increased incidence of positional plagiocephaly has been observed (see p. 366). It is recommended that an infant's head position be alternated during sleep time to prevent plagiocephaly. Infants may be placed prone during awake periods to prevent positional plagiocephaly and to encourage development of upper shoulder girdle strength (AAP, Task Force on Sudden Infant Death Syndrome, 2005, 2011). Updated childhood immunization status has also been shown to be protective against SIDS.

Although the cause of SIDS is unknown, autopsies reveal consistent pathologic findings, such as pulmonary edema and intrathoracic hemorrhages, that confirm the diagnosis. Consequently, autopsies should be performed on all infants suspected of dying of SIDS, and findings should be shared with the parents as soon as possible after the death. Postmortem findings in SIDS and accidental suffocation or intentional suffocation such as in Munchausen syndrome by proxy (see Child Maltreatment, Chapter 14) are practically the same. Individuals with less experience and training in performing autopsies, such as coroners instead of medical examiners, may not correctly identify some deaths as SIDS. Therefore, mortality statistics can vary in different regions.

Infant Risk Factors

Certain groups of infants are at increased risk for SIDS:

- Low birth weight
- Low Apgar scores
- Recent viral illness
- Siblings of two or more SIDS victims
- Male sex
- Infants of American Indian or African-American ethnicity

No diagnostic tests exist to predict which infants, including those in the above groups, will survive, and home monitoring is no guarantee of survival. Whether subsequent siblings of one SIDS infant are at increased risk for SIDS is unclear. Even if the risk is increased, families have a 99% chance that their subsequent child will *not* die of SIDS. A review of sibling deaths attributed to SIDS in England failed to ascertain a precise risk of recurrence; previous studies suggested a recurrence risk range of 1.7 to 10.1, yet the researchers concluded the studies had too many methodologic flaws to draw any firm conclusions (Bacon, Hall, Stephenson, and others, 2008). Others report that recurrence risks for a SIDS death in a family with a previous infant SIDS death range from 2% to 6% (AAP, Task Force on Sudden Infant Death Syndrome, 2005). *Home monitoring is not recommended* for this group of children, but it is often used by practitioners and may even be requested by parents (AAP, Task Force on Sudden Infant Death Syndrome, 2005, 2011). There is no evidence that home apnea monitoring prevents SIDS (Strehle, Gray, Gopisetti, and others, 2012). Monitoring is best initiated on an individual basis.

Nursing Care Management

Nurses have a vital role in preventing SIDS by educating families about the risk of prone sleeping position in infants from birth to 6 months of age, the use of appropriate bedding surfaces, the association with maternal smoking, and the dangers of cosleeping on noninfant surfaces with adults or other children. Additionally, nurses have an important role in modeling behaviors for parents to foster practices that decrease the risk of SIDS, including placing infants in a supine sleeping position in the hospital. Data indicate that a small percentage of nurses still place healthy infants in a side-lying position in the hospital (Bullock, Mickey, Green, and others, 2004; Thompson, 2005). Statistics for infants being placed in a prone sleeping position in the United States decreased from 70% in 1992 to 13% in 2004 (AAP, Task Force on Sudden Infant Death Syndrome, 2005). One study of neonatal intensive care (NICU) nurses indicated that 52% routinely provided discharge instructions that promote supine sleep positions at home; common nonsupine positions recommended by the nurses included either supine or side or exclusive side-lying sleep position (Aris, Stevens, Lemura, and others, 2006). A survey of level II and III NICU nurses found that nurses still positioned infants in a side-lying position for fear of aspiration (29%), for comfort reasons (28%), and for infant safety (20%) (Grazel, Phalen, and Palomano, 2010). Nurses *must* be proactive in further decreasing the incidence of SIDS; postpartum discharge planning, newborn discharges, follow-up home visits, well-baby clinic visits, and immunization visits provide excellent opportunities to educate parents on these matters.

Many health care workers are concerned that infants placed on the back to sleep will aspirate emesis or mucus, yet studies fail to show an increase in infant deaths, spitting up during sleep, aspiration, asphyxia, or respiratory failure as a result of supine sleep positioning (AAP, Task Force on Sudden Infant Death Syndrome, 2011; Malloy, 2002; Tablizo, Jacinto, Parsley, and others, 2007).

Research findings have important implications for practices that may reduce the risk of SIDS, such as avoiding smoking during pregnancy and near the infant; using the supine sleeping position; avoiding soft, moldable mattresses, blankets, and pillows; avoiding bed sharing; breastfeeding; and avoiding overheating during sleep. Nurses must continue to take every opportunity to advocate for infants by providing information for parents and caretakers about the modifiable risk factors for SIDS which can be implemented to prevent its occurrence across all sectors of the population.

Loss of a child from SIDS presents several crises with which the parents must cope. In addition to grief and mourning the death of their child, the parents must face a tragedy that was sudden, unexpected, and unexplained. The psychologic intervention for the family must deal with these additional variables. This discussion focuses primarily on the objectives of care for families experiencing SIDS rather than on the process of grief and mourning, which is explored in Chapter 18.

Care of the Family of a SIDS Infant

The first persons to arrive at the scene may be the police and emergency medical service personnel. They should handle the situation by asking few questions; giving no indication of wrongdoing, abuse, or neglect; making sensitive judgments concerning any resuscitation efforts for the child; and comforting the family members as much as possible. A compassionate, sensitive approach to the family during the first few minutes can help spare them some of the overwhelming guilt and anguish that commonly follow this type of death.

The medical examiner or coroner may go to the home or place of death and make the death pronouncement; until then, the sleep environment should remain as it was when the infant was initially found (Koehler, 2008). If the infant is not pronounced dead at the scene, he or she may be transported to the emergency department to be pronounced dead by a physician. Usually there is no attempt at resuscitation in the emergency department. While they are in the emergency department, the parents are asked only factual questions, such as when they found the infant, how he or she looked, and whom they called for help. The nurse avoids any remarks that may suggest responsibility, such as "Why didn't you go in earlier?" "Didn't you hear the infant cry out?" "Was the head buried in a blanket?" or "Were the siblings jealous of this child?" It is the coroner's responsibility to document these findings at the scene rather than have parents recount the experience in the emergency department (Koehler, 2008). Parents may also express feelings of guilt about administering cardiopulmonary resuscitation (CPR) correctly or the timing of CPR in relation to finding the infant.

At this time, the physician should initiate the discussion of an autopsy, often with the nurse being present to support the family. The physician or medical examiner, depending on the circumstances, emphasizes that a diagnosis cannot be confirmed until the postmortem examination is completed. Nurses may balk at the idea of requesting an autopsy because of the parents' emotional state; however, an autopsy may clear up possible misconceptions regarding the death. Instructions about the autopsy and funeral arrangements may need to be repeated or put in writing. If the mother was breastfeeding, she needs information about abrupt discontinuation of lactation. The nurse or physician should contact the primary care practitioner for the infant and the mother to avoid any miscommunications or telephone calls at a later date inquiring about the child's health status.

A review of 60 studies shows that parents experiencing perinatal death perceive health care workers' responses as having a significant impact on the parents' grieving process; parents perceived the behavior of many health care workers as thoughtless or insensitive. The findings suggest that nurses and physicians would benefit from more bereavement training (Gold, 2007).

An important aspect of compassionate care for these parents is allowing them to say good-bye to their child. These are the parents' last moments with their child, and they should be as quiet, meaningful, peaceful, and undisturbed as possible. Encourage parents to hold their infant before leaving the emergency department. Because the parents leave the hospital without their infant, it is helpful to accompany them to the car or arrange for someone else to take them home. A debriefing session may help health care workers who dealt with the family and deceased infant to cope with emotions that are often engendered when a SIDS victim is brought into the acute care facility. Comprehensive guidelines have been published for health professionals involved in SIDS investigations to assist the family and at the same time to determine that the infant's death was not the result of other factors such as child maltreatment (AAP, Committee on Child Abuse and Neglect, 2001).

When the parents return home, a competent, qualified professional should visit them as soon after the death as possible. They should receive printed material that contains excellent information about SIDS (available from the national organizations*).

During the initial visit, help the parents gain an intellectual understanding of the condition. The nursing objectives are to assess what the parents have been told about SIDS; what they think happened; and how they explained this to the other siblings, family members, and friends. One question that the nurse will never be able to answer and therefore should not attempt to is, "Why did this happen to our baby?" or "Who is responsible for this tragedy?" These and other questions may linger in the parents' minds for months or even years.

When the unexpected death of a child occurs, it is common for one parent to blame the other for the child's death. Parents may also experience guilt over the child's death; if they had checked earlier, the child might still be alive. It is important that the nurse assist parents in working through these feelings to prevent marital disruption in addition to the loss of the loved child.

Some parents are able to discuss their feelings openly, and the nurse supports this coping skill. However, others may be reluctant to express their grief, and the nurse can encourage the expression of emotions by asking about crying and feeling sad, angry, or guilty. This is an attempt to provoke a display of emotion, not just an admission of a feeling. During this session, help the parents to explore their usual coping mechanisms and, if these are ineffectual, to investigate new approaches. For example, one parent may refrain from discussing the death for fear of upsetting the other parent, but each may need to hear how the other feels.

Ideally, the number of visits and plans for subsequent intervention need to be flexible. Parents facing the question of having a subsequent child will need support. Both the birth of a subsequent child and the survival of that child, especially past the age of death of the previous child, are important transitional stages for parents.

---

*American SIDS Institute, 528 Ravens Way, Naples, FL 34110; 239-431-5425; http://www.sids.org; First Candle, 1314 Bedford Ave., Suite 210, Baltimore, MD 21208; 800-221-7437; http://www.sidsalliance.org; National Sudden and Unexpected Infant/Child Death and Pregnancy Loss Resource Center, Georgetown University, Box 571272, Washington, DC 20057-1272; 866-866-7437, 202-687-7466; http://www.sidscenter.org.

APPARENT LIFE-THREATENING EVENT

An ALTE, formerly referred to as *aborted SIDS death* or *near-miss SIDS*, generally refers to an event that is sudden and frightening to the observer in which the infant exhibits a combination of apnea; change in color (pallor, cyanosis, redness); change in muscle tone (usually hypotonia); and choking, gagging, or coughing and that usually involves a significant intervention and even CPR by the caregiver who witnesses the event (National Institutes of Health Consensus Development Conference, 1987). The definition of ALTE may include apnea, but ALTE may occur without apnea (Silvestri and Weese-Mayer, 2003). It is erroneous to characterize ALTE as a near-miss SIDS incident (Adams, Good, and Defranco, 2009). Infants with ALTE are at increased risk for SIDS; the risk for SIDS may be three to five times greater in infants who experienced an ALTE (Hunt and Hauck, 2011).

Results from the Collaborative Home Infant Monitoring Evaluation (CHIME) study found that apnea and bradycardia occurred at conventional and extreme alarm thresholds in all groups of infants studied—siblings of SIDS infants, infants with ALTEs, symptomatic (of apnea and bradycardia) and asymptomatic preterm infants weighing less than 1750 g (3.8 pounds) at birth, and healthy term infants. Approximately 30% of infants with ALTE were born at less than 37 weeks' gestation. The researchers concluded that many infants experience apnea and bradycardia in each of these groups yet do not die (Jobe, 2001; Ramanathan, Corwin, Hunt, and others, 2001). Furthermore, it was reported that apnea does not appear to be an immediate precursor to SIDS and that cardiorespiratory monitoring is not an effective tool for identifying infants at greater risk for SIDS (AAP, Committee on Fetus and Newborn, 2003). CHIME data indicate that infants with ALTE did not have some of the typical characteristics associated with SIDS infants; these include fewer infants with low birth weight and who are small for gestational age at birth, fewer teenage pregnancies, and a younger infant age at the time of ALTE. The researchers concluded that despite some similar characteristics between ALTE and SIDS, the differences warrant a separate focus on ALTE events (Esani, Hodgman, Ehsani, and others, 2008).

Diagnostic Evaluation

An essential component of the diagnostic process includes a detailed description of the event, including who witnessed the event; where the infant was during the event; and what, if any, activities were involved (e.g., during or after a feeding, riding in a car seat restraint, presence of siblings or any minor children, what clothing the infant was wearing). In addition, a prenatal and postnatal history must be obtained. A short period of observation in the emergency department may be appropriate to observe the infant's respiratory pattern and response to feeding. A careful evaluation of late preterm and preterm infants in the car seat restraints currently in use is essential; upper airway occlusion and subsequent apnea and cyanosis may occur if the infant is not positioned properly (see Chapter 9). Reported diagnoses in infants with ALTE include a neurologic event such as a seizure (30% of cases seen); GI problem, including gastroesophageal reflux (50%); respiratory conditions (20%); and metabolic conditions, cardiac anomaly, or child abuse (each <5%). In some cases, multiple diagnoses may be made (Hall and Zalman, 2005).

In the event that an underlying diagnosis such as those mentioned previously is not established, home monitoring may be recommended. The most commonly used monitoring is continuous recording of cardiorespiratory patterns (cardiopneumogram or pneumocardiogram). Four-channel pneumocardiograms (or multichannel pneumogram) monitor heart rate, respirations (chest impedance), nasal airflow, and

FAMILY-CENTERED CARE

Using Apnea Monitors

Use the monitor as instructed by the practitioner or home monitor equipment company.

Do not adjust the monitor to eliminate false alarms. Adjustments could compromise the monitor's effectiveness.

Place the monitor on a firm surface away from the crib and drapes; plug power cord directly into a wall socket with a three-pronged outlet.

Do not sleep in the same bed as the monitored infant.

Keep pets and children away from the monitor and infant.

Keep the monitor away from possible electrical interferences such as appliances (e.g., electric blankets, televisions, air conditioners, remote telephones).

Be aware that strong signals from nearby radio and television stations, airports, ham radios, cellular phones, or police stations could interfere with the monitor. Check for interference if the monitor is to be operated in these areas.

Check the monitor several times a day to be sure the alarm is working and that it can be heard from room to room. Be certain the caregiver can reach the monitor quickly (in <30 seconds).

Periodically check the monitor's breath detection indicator and battery or charger connections.

Read the monitor's user manual carefully; report problems promptly.

Inform community utility and rescue squads of home monitoring as appropriate.

Keep emergency numbers near phones in the home.

Practice safety precautions:

- Remove leads when infant is not attached to the monitor.
- Unplug the power cord from the electrical outlet when the cord is not plugged into the monitor.
- Use safety covers on electrical outlets to prevent children from inserting objects into a socket.

Data primarily from U.S. Food and Drug Administration: *Safety alert: important tips for apnea monitor users*, Rockville, Md, 1990, U.S. Department of Health and Human Services.

oxygen saturation. A more sophisticated test, polysomnography (sleep study), also records brain waves, eye and body movements, esophageal manometry, and end-tidal carbon dioxide measurements. However, none of these tests can predict risk. Some children with normal results may still have subsequent apneic episodes (see Family-Centered Care box).

Therapeutic Management

The treatment of an infant with an ALTE depends on the underlying condition (see above). Treatment of recurrent apnea (without an underlying organic problem) usually involves continuous home monitoring of cardiorespiratory rhythms and in some cases the use of methylxanthines (respiratory stimulant drugs, such as caffeine). The decision to discontinue the monitoring is based on the infant's clinical condition. A general guideline for discontinuation is when infants with ALTEs have gone 2 or 3 months without significant numbers of episodes requiring intervention.

Newer home apnea monitors allow download of information that assists the practitioner in deciding when to discontinue home monitoring. It is imperative to remember, however, that the home apnea monitor will not predict or prevent SIDS deaths. Furthermore, impedance-based monitors detect chest wall movement and will not detect obstructive apnea unless the episode involves significant bradycardia.

Nursing Care Management

The diagnosis of an ALTE causes great anxiety and concern in parents, and the institution of home monitoring presents additional physical and emotional burdens. Parents of infants on home apnea monitors report experiencing emotional distress, especially depression and hostility, during the first few weeks after hospital discharge (Abendroth, Moser, Dracup, and others, 1999). For parents of a SIDS victim who have a new infant on home apnea monitoring, the anxiety is compounded by the uncertainty of the future of the living child and grief for the lost child. Home apnea monitoring may offer some predictability and control over the current child's survival through the period of uncertainty.

If home monitoring is required, the nurse can be a major source of support to the family in terms of education about the equipment; education regarding observation of the infant's status; and instructions regarding immediate intervention during apneic episodes, including CPR. Several reports indicate that the first week to month after discharge is the most stressful for parents, particularly when the rate of false alarms is high (Bennett, 2002). To help the family cope with the numerous procedures they must learn, adequate preparation before discharge and written instructions are essential. In the first few weeks after discharge, parents may benefit by having a practitioner readily available to answer questions regarding false alarms and for other technical assistance.

Several types of home monitors are available and are set up by either a home monitor equipment company or home health staff. Nurses, especially those involved in the care at home, must become familiar with the equipment, including its advantages and disadvantages. Safety is a major concern because monitors can cause electrical burns and electrocution. The following precautions are recommended:

- Remove leads from infant when not attached to the monitor.
- Unplug the power cord from the electrical outlet when the cord is not plugged into the monitor.
- Use safety covers on electrical outlets to discourage children from inserting objects into sockets.

Siblings should also be supervised when near the infant and taught that the monitor is not a toy. Other safety practices include informing local utility and rescue squads of the home monitoring in case of an emergency. Telephone numbers for these services should be posted in the home.

! NURSING ALERT

If the infant is apneic, gently stimulate the trunk by patting or rubbing it. If the infant is prone, turn to the back and flick the feet. If there is still no response, begin CPR and activate the emergency medical service—"Call 911!" Never vigorously shake the child. No more than 10 to 15 seconds is spent on stimulation before implementing CPR.

Caregivers need detailed information regarding proper attachment of the electrodes to the infant's chest with impedance monitors that detect chest movement. The electrodes are placed in the midaxillary line at a space one or two fingerbreadths below the nipple. For home use, electrodes attached to a belt that is placed around the child's trunk are preferred (Fig. 11-4). The belt is positioned so that the electrodes contact the skin in the same area. Monitors may have memory chips

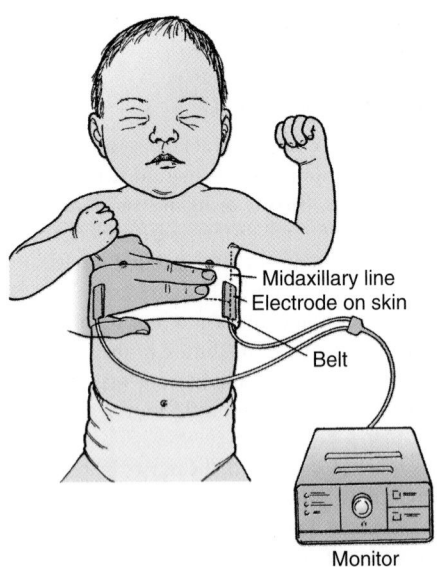

FIG 11-4 Placement of electrodes or belt for apnea monitoring. In small infants, one fingerbreadth may be used.

that allow for event recording, which can be an effective tool in evaluating the use of the monitor, events immediately before and after the ALTE, and reported frequency of alarms.

Monitors are effective only if they are used. They do not prevent death but alert the caregiver to the ALTE in time to intervene. The need

to use the monitor and to respond appropriately to alarms must be stressed. Noncompliance can result in the infant's death.

Family Support

Many of the stresses observed during the home monitoring period are characteristic of families with chronically ill children. The child with an apnea or cardiorespiratory monitor may have additional health care needs such as a gastrostomy, tracheostomy, and myriad medications or treatments that exacerbate the parents' stress. Parents report increased stress, including concern for the child's survival, fear of incompetence in assuming home responsibility, inadequate respite care, lack of time for other children and spouse, social isolation from friends and extended family, constant work, and fatigue. The monitored child is at risk for vulnerable child syndrome, which may lead to lack of parental separation and preferential treatment, causing further family disruption. To deal with these potential effects, nurses need to use the same interventions as those discussed for children with chronic illness and be aware of the need for referral when difficulties are suspected.

To lessen the continuous responsibility of monitoring, other family members, such as grandparents and other immediate family members, should be taught how to manipulate the equipment, read and interpret the signals, and administer CPR. They are encouraged to stay with the infant for regular periods to allow the parents respite. Support groups of other families who have successfully completed monitoring can also be of benefit. Because reliable babysitters are difficult to locate, support group members and nursing students may be potential sources of qualified caregivers.

KEY POINTS

- Common nutritional disorders of infancy and early childhood may result from vitamin and mineral deficiency or excess, PEM, and food allergy.
- Cow's milk allergy may occur in infancy; many children outgrow CMA by the age of 5 years.
- PEM may occur as a complication of underlying disease, lack of parental education about infant nutrition, inappropriate management of food allergy, or incorrect preparation of formula.
- Food allergies in children often have a number of systemic, cutaneous, or local manifestations.
- Anaphylactic reaction to food should be immediately recognized and treated with intramuscular epinephrine.
- Treatment of colic may involve a change in infant feeding practices, correction of a stressful environment, behavior modification, and support of the parent.
- Growth failure or FTT may occur in children who have a chronic illness, or it may occur in a family environment wherein healthy infant feeding practices are poorly managed or understood; FTT is not always associated with a pattern of disturbed mother–infant relationship.

- Common sleep problems that develop during infancy—and that are easily prevented—are associated with night crying and refusal to go to sleep.
- Positional plagiocephaly can be easily prevented by allowing the awake infant to have periods of tummy time and by alternating the infant's head position during sleep.
- SIDS is the third leading cause of infant death in the United States.
- Factors that place infants at high risk for SIDS include prone sleeping position, soft bedding, sleeping in a noninfant bed with an adult or older child, and environmental exposure to smoking.
- Factors that are protective for SIDS include supine sleep position, breastfeeding, pacifier use at bedtime and naptime, and updated immunization status.
- The primary nursing responsibility in care associated with sudden infant death is educating the family of newborns about the risks for SIDS, modeling appropriate behaviors in the hospital such as placing the infant in a supine sleep position, and providing emotional support of the family who has experienced a SIDS loss.
- Infants with ALTEs are carefully evaluated for clues to the underlying cause.
- Home apnea or cardiorespiratory monitors do not prevent SIDS.

REFERENCES

Abendroth D, Moser DK, Dracup K, and others: Do apnea monitors decrease emotional distress in parents of infants at high risk for cardiopulmonary arrest? *J Pediatr Health Care* 13(2):50–57, 1999.

Adams SM, Good MW, Defranco GM: Sudden infant death syndrome, *Am Fam Physician* 79(10):870–874, 2009.

Alm B, Wennergren G, Norvenius SG, and others: Breast-feeding and the sudden infant death

syndrome in Scandinavia, 1992–1995, *Arch Dis Child* 86(6):400–402, 2002.

Amadi B, Mwiya M, Chomba E, and others: Improved nutritional recovery on an elemental diet in Zambian children with persistent diarrhoea and malnutrition, *J Trop Pediatr* 51(1):5–10, 2005.

American Academy of Pediatrics: Prevention of rickets and vitamin D deficiency in infants, children, and adolescents, *Pediatrics* 122(5): 1142–1148, 2008.

American Academy of Pediatrics: *Pediatric nutrition handbook*, ed 6, Elk Grove Village, Ill, 2009, Author.

American Academy of Pediatrics, Committee on Child Abuse and Neglect: Distinguishing sudden infant death syndrome from child abuse fatalities, *Pediatrics* 107(2):437–441, 2001.

American Academy of Pediatrics, Committee on Fetus and Newborn: Apnea, sudden infant death syndrome, and home monitoring, *Pediatrics* 111(4):914–917, 2003.

American Academy of Pediatrics, Task Force on Infant Sleep Position and Sudden Infant Death Syndrome: Changing concepts of sudden infant death syndrome: implications for infant sleeping environment and sleep position, *Pediatrics* 105(3):650–656, 2000.

American Academy of Pediatrics, Task Force on Sudden Infant Death Syndrome: The changing concept of sudden infant death syndrome: diagnostic coding shifts, controversies regarding the sleeping environment, and new variables to consider in reducing risk, *Pediatrics* 116(5): 1245–1255, 2005.

American Academy of Pediatrics, Task Force on Sudden Infant Death Syndrome: SIDS and other sleep-related infant deaths: expansion of recommendations for a safe infant sleeping environment, *Pediatrics* 128(5):1030–1038, 2011.

Amthor RE, Cole SM, Manary MJ: The use of home-based therapy with ready-to-use therapeutic food to treat malnutrition in a rural area during a food crisis, *J Am Diet Assoc* 109(3):464–467, 2009.

Anderson ME, Johnson DC, Batal HA: Sudden infant death syndrome and prenatal maternal smoking: rising attributed risk in the Back to Sleep era, *BMC Med* 3(1):4, 2005.

Aris C, Stevens TP, Lemura C, and others: NICU nurses' knowledge and discharge teaching related to infant sleep position and risk of SIDS, *Adv Neonatal Care* 6(5):281–294, 2006.

Ashworth A, Khanum S, Jackson A, and others: *Guidelines for the inpatient treatment of severely malnourished children*, Geneva, 2003, World Health Organization, retrieved July 2009 from http://www.who.int/nutrition/ publications/severemalnutrition/ 9241546093_eng.pdf.

Bacon CJ, Hall DBM, Stephenson TJ, and others: How common is repeat sudden infant death syndrome? *Arch Dis Child* 93(4):323–326, 2008.

Baker RD, Greer FR, American Academy of Pediatrics Committee on Nutrition: Clinical report—diagnosis and prevention of iron deficiency and iron-deficiency anemia in infants and young children (0–3 years of age), *Pediatrics* 126(5):1040–1050, 2010.

Barnard K, Hammond MA, Booth CL, and others: Measurement and meaning of parent-child interaction. In Morrison F, Lord C, Keating D, editors: *Applied developmental psychology*, vol 3, New York, 1993, Academic Press.

Basnet S, Schneider M, Gazit A, and others: Fresh goat's milk for infants: myths and realities—a review, *Pediatrics* 125(4):e973–e977, 2010.

Bennett AD: Home apnea monitoring for infants: a discussion of primary care issues, *Adv Nurs Pract* 10(3):48–53, 2002.

Black MM, Dubowitz H, Krishnakumar A, and others: Early intervention and recovery among children with failure to thrive: follow-up at age 8, *Pediatrics* 120(1):59–69, 2007.

Blair PS, Sidebotham P, Evason-Coombe C, and others: Hazardous cosleeping environments and risk factors amenable to change: case-control study of SIDS in south west England, *BMJ* 339:b3446, 2009.

Block RW, Krebs NF, American Academy of Pediatrics Committee on Child Abuse and Neglect and Committee on Nutrition: Failure to thrive as a manifestation of child neglect, *Pediatrics* 116(5):1234–1237, 2005.

Boyce JA, Assa'ad A, Burks AW, and others: Guideline for the diagnosis and management of food allergy in the United States: summary of the NIAID-sponsored expert panel report, *J Allergy Clin Immunol* 126(6):1005–1118, 2010.

Bullock LFC, Mickey K, Green J, and others: Are nurses acting as role models for the prevention of SIDS? *MCN Am J Matern Child Nurs* 29(3): 172–177, 2004.

Burk CJ, Molodow R: Infantile scurvy: an old diagnosis revisited with a modern dietary twist, *Am J Clin Dermatol* 8(2):103–106, 2007.

Butte NF, Fox MK, Briefel RR, and others: Nutrient intakes of US infants, toddlers, and preschoolers meet or exceed dietary reference intakes, *J Am Diet Assoc* 110(12 suppl):S27–S37, 2010.

Carroll-Pankhurst C, Mortimer EA: Sudden infant death syndrome, bedsharing, parental weight, and age of death, *Pediatrics* 107(3):530–536, 2001.

Casey PH, Whiteside-Mansell L, Barrett K, and others: Impact of prenatal and/or postnatal growth problems in low birth weight preterm infants on school-age outcomes: an 8-year longitudinal evaluation, *Pediatrics* 118(3): 1078–1086, 2006.

Chumlea WC: Physical growth and maturation. In Samour PQ, King K, editors: *Handbook of pediatric nutrition*, ed 3, Sudbury, Mass, 2005, Jones & Bartlett.

Ciliberto MA, Sandige H, Ndekha MJ, and others: Comparison of a home-based therapy with ready-to-use therapeutic food with standard therapy in the treatment of malnourished Malawin children: a controlled, clinical effectiveness trial, *Am J Clin Nutr* 81(4): 864–870, 2005.

Cole SZ, Lanham JS: Failure to thrive: an update, *Am Fam Physician* 83(7):829–834, 2011.

Corrales KM, Utter SL: Growth failure. In Samour PQ, King K, editors: *Handbook of pediatric nutrition*, ed 3, Sudbury, Mass, 2005, Jones & Bartlett.

Critch JN: Infantile colic: is there a role for dietary interventions? *Paediatr Child Health* 16(1): 47–49, 2011, retrieved June 15, 2011, from http://www.cps.ca/english/statements/N/ InfantileColic.htm.

Davis KF, Parker K, Montgomery GL: Sleep in infants and young children, part 2, common

sleep problems, *J Pediatr Health Care* 18(3): 130–137, 2004.

Dunham L, Kollar L: Vegetarian eating for children and adolescents, *J Pediatr Health Care* 20(1): 27–34, 2006.

Duro D, Rising R, Cedillo M, and others: Association between infantile colic and carbohydrate malabsorption from fruit juices in infancy, *Pediatrics* 109(5):797–805, 2002.

Ellett ML, Appleton MM, Sloan RS: Out of the abyss of colic: a view through the father's eyes, *MCN Am J Matern Child Nurs* 34(3):164–171, 2009.

Ellett MLC: What is known about colic? *Gastroenterol Nurs* 26(2):60–65, 2003.

Esani N, Hodgman JE, Ehsani N, and others: Apparent life-threatening events and sudden infant death syndrome: comparison of risk factors, *J Pediatr* 152(3):A2, 2008.

Ewing WM, Allen PJ: The diagnosis and management of cow milk protein intolerance in the primary care setting, *Pediatr Nurs* 31(6): 486–492, 2005.

Ferber R, Kryger M: *Principles and practice of sleep medicine in the child*, Philadelphia, 1995, Saunders.

Forlenza GP, Paradise Black NM, McNamara EG, and others: Ankyloglossia, exclusive breastfeeding, and failure to thrive, *Pediatrics* 125(6):e1500–e1504, 2010.

Fox M, Reidy K, Novak T, and others: Sources of energy and nutrients in the diets of infants and toddlers, *J Am Diet Assoc* 106(1 suppl 1): S28–S42, 2006.

Gold KJ: Navigating care after a baby dies: a systematic review of parent experiences with health providers, *J Perinatol* 27(4):230–237, 2007.

Goyal D, Gay C, Lee K: Fragmented maternal sleep is more strongly correlated with depressive symptoms than infant temperament at three months postpartum, *Arch Wom Ment Health* 12(4):229–237, 2009.

Grazel R, Phalen AG, Palomano RC: Implementation of the American Academy of Pediatrics recommendations to reduce sudden infant death syndrome risk in neonatal intensive care units: an evaluation of nursing knowledge and practice, *Adv Neonatal Care* 10(6):332–342, 2010.

Greer FR, Sicherer SH, Burks AW, and others: Effects of early nutritional interventions on the development of atopic disease in infants and children: the role of maternal dietary restriction, breastfeeding, timing of introduction of complementary foods, and hydrolyzed formulas, *Pediatrics* 121(1):183–191, 2008.

Grover Z, Ee LC: Protein energy malnutrition, *Pediatr Clin North Am* 56(5):1055–1068, 2009.

Grummer-Strawn LM, Reinold C, Krebs NF, and others: Use of World Health Organization and CDC growth charts for children aged 0–59 months in the United States, *MMWR Recomm Rep* 59(RR-9):1–15, 2010.

Hall KL, Zalman B: Evaluation and management of apparent life threatening events in children, *Am Fam Physician* 71(12):2301–2308, 2005.

Hauck FR, Herman SM, Donovan M, and others: Sleep environment and the risk of sudden infant death syndrome in an urban population: the

Chicago Infant Mortality Study, *Pediatrics* 111(5):1207–1214, 2003.

Hauck FR, Thompson JM, Tanabe KO, and others: Breastfeeding and reduced risk of sudden infant death syndrome: a meta-analysis, *Pediatrics* 128(1):103–110, 2011.

Hawkins-Walsh E: A behavioural infant sleep intervention resolved sleep problems, *Evidence-Based Nurs* 6(1):10–12, 2003.

Heron MP, Hoyert DL, Xu J, and others: Deaths: preliminary data for 2006, National Vital Statistics Report: Centers for Disease Control and Prevention, *Natl Vital Stat Rep* 56(16):1–51, 2008.

Hiscock H, Wake M: Infant sleep problems and postnatal depression: a community-based study, *Pediatrics* 107(6):1317–1322, 2001.

Horne RS, Ferens D, Watts AM, and others: The prone sleeping position impairs arousability in term infants, *J Pediatr* 138(6):793–795, 2001.

Huiming Y, Chaomin W, Meng M: Vitamin A for treating measles in children, *Cochrane Database Syst Rev* (4):CD001479, 2005.

Hummel P, Fortado D: Impacting infant head shapes, *Adv Neon Care* 5(6):329–342, 2005.

Hunt CE, Hauck FR: Sudden infant death syndrome. In Kliegman RM, Stanton BF, St. Geme JW, and others, editors: *Nelson textbook of pediatrics*, ed 19, Philadelphia, 2011, Elsevier/Saunders.

Joanna Briggs Institute: Best practice: the effectiveness of interventions for infant colic, *Best Practice Information Sheet* 12(6):1–4, 2008, retrieved July 20, 2009, from http://www.joannabriggs.edu.au/pdf/BPIScolic.pdf.

Jobe AH: What do home monitors contribute to the SIDS problem [editorial]? *JAMA* 285(17):2244–2245, 2001.

Kapil U: Ready to use therapeutic food (RUTF) in the management of severe acute malnutrition in India, *Indian Pediatr* 46(5):381–382, 2009.

Kattan JD, Cocco RR, Järvinen KM: Milk and soy allergy, *Pediatr Clin North Am* 58(2):407–426, 2011.

Katz KA, Mahlberg MA, Honig PJ, and others: Rice nightmare: kwashiorkor in two Philadelphia-area infants fed Rice Dream beverage, *J Am Acad Dermatol* 52(5 suppl 1):S69–S72, 2005.

Kawchak DA, Schall JI, Zemel BS, and others: Adequacy of dietary intake declines with age in children with sickle cell disease, *J Am Diet Assoc* 107(5):843–848, 2007.

Keet C: Recognition and management of food-induced anaphylaxis, *Pediatr Clin North Am* 58(2):377–388, 2011.

Kim JS, Nowak-Wegrzyn A, Sichere SH, and others: Dietary baked milk accelerates the resolution of cow's milk allergy in children, *J Allergy Clin Immunol* 128(1):125–131.e2, 2011.

Koehler SA: Sudden infant death syndrome deaths: the role of forensic nurses, *J Forensic Nurs* 4(3):141–142, 2008.

Krugman SD, Dubowitz H: Failure to thrive, *Am Fam Physician* 68(5):879–886, 2003.

Laughlin J, Luerssen TG, Dias MS, and others: Prevention and management of positional skull deformities in infants, *Pediatrics* 128(6):1236–1241, 2011.

Li L, Zhang Y, Zielke RH, and others: Observations on increased accidental asphyxia deaths in

infancy while cosleeping in the state of Maryland, *Am J Forensic Med Pathol* 30(4):318–321, 2009.

Littlefield TR, Saba NM, Kelly KM: On the current incidence of deformational plagiocephaly: an estimation based on prospective registration at a single center, *Semin Pediatr Neurol* 11(4):301–304, 2004.

Liu T, Howard RM, Mancini AJ, and others: Kwashiorkor in the United States: fad diets, perceived and true milk allergy, and nutritional ignorance, *Arch Dermatol* 137(5):630–636, 2001.

Lobo ML, Kotzer AM, Keefe MR, and others: Current beliefs and management strategies for treating infant colic, *J Pediatr Health Care* 18(3):115–122, 2004.

Locklin M: The redefinition of failure to thrive from a case study perspective, *Pediatr Nurs* 31(6):474–479, 495, 2005.

MacDorman MF, Mathews TJ: Infant deaths—United States, 2000–2007, *MMWR Surveill Summ* 60(01):49–51, 2011.

Maggioni A, Lifshitz F: Nutritional management of failure to thrive, *Pediatr Clin North Am* 42(4):791–809, 1995.

Malloy MH: Trends in postneonatal aspiration deaths and reclassification of sudden infant death syndrome: impact of the "Back to Sleep" program, *Pediatrics* 109(4):661–665, 2002.

Markowitz R, Watkins JB, Duggan C: Failure to thrive: malnutrition in the pediatric outpatient setting. In Markowitz R, Watkins JB, Duggan C, editors: *Nutrition in pediatrics*, ed 4, Hamilton, Ontario, 2008, BC Decker.

Martin J, Hiscock H, Hardy P, and others: Adverse associations of infant and child sleep problems and parent health: an Australian population study, *Pediatrics* 119(5):947–955, 2007.

Mathews TJ, MacDorman MF: Infant mortality statistics from the 2007 period linked birth/infant death data set, *Natl Vital Statistics Rep* 59(6): 8–30 , 2011.

McBride DL: New food allergy guidelines, *J Pediatr Nurs* 26(3):262–263, 2011.

McGarvey C, McDonnell M, Chong A, and others: Factors relating to the infant's last sleep environment in sudden infant death syndrome in the Republic of Ireland, *Arch Dis Child* 88(12):1058–1064, 2003.

McMartin KI, Platt MS, Hackman R, and others: Lung tissue concentrations of nicotine in sudden infant death syndrome, *J Pediatr* 140(2):205–209, 2002.

Mitchell EA, Thompson JM, Becroft DM, and others: Head covering and the risk for SIDS: findings from the New Zealand and German SIDS case-control studies, *Pediatrics* 121(6):e1478–e1483, 2008.

Moore M, Meltzer LJ, Mindell JA: Bedtime problems and night waking in children, *Prim Care Clin Office Pract* 35(3):569–581, 2008.

Morin K: The challenge of colic in infants, *MCN Am J Matern Child Nurs* 34(3):192, 2009.

Müller O, Krawinkel M: Malnutrition and health in developing countries, *CMAJ* 173(3):279–286, 2005.

National Institutes of Health Consensus Development Conference on Infantile Apnea and Home Monitoring, Sept 29 to Oct 1, 1986, *Pediatrics* 79(2):292–299, 1987.

Neu M, Robinson JA: Infants with colic: their childhood characteristics, *J Pediatr Nurs* 18(1):12–20, 2003.

Nevarez MD, Rifas-Shiman SL, Kleinman KP, and others: Association of early life risk factors with infant sleep duration, *Acad Pediatr* 10(3):187–193, 2010.

Nowak-Wegrzyn A, Bloom KA, Sicherer SH, and others: Tolerance to extensively heated milk in children with cow's milk allergy, *J Allergy Clin Immunol* 122(2):342–347, 2008.

O'Connor NR: Infant formula, *Am Family Physician* 79(7):565–570, 2009.

Ostfield BM, Esposito L, Perl H, and others: Concurrent risks of sudden infant death syndrome, *Pediatrics* 125(3):447–453, 2010.

Penny ME: Protein-energy malnutrition: pathophysiology, clinical consequences, and treatment. In Walker WA, Watkins JB, Duggan C, editors: *Nutrition in pediatrics*, ed 3, Hamilton, Ontario, 2003, Decker.

Perry R, Hunt K, Ernst E: Nutritional supplements and other complementary medicines for infantile colic: a systematic review, *Pediatrics* 127(4):720–733, 2011.

Person TLA, Lavezzi WA, Wolf BC: Cosleeping and sudden unexpected death in infancy, *Arch Pathol Lab Med* 126(3):343–345, 2002.

Pessler F, Nejat M: Anaphylactic reaction to goat's milk in a cow's milk–allergic infant, *Pediatr Allergy Immunol* 15(2):183–185, 2004.

Pollack HA: Sudden infant death syndrome, maternal smoking during pregnancy and effectiveness of smoking cessation intervention, *Am J Public Health* 91(3):432–436, 2001.

Preston AM, Rodriguez C, Rivera C, and others: Influence of environmental tobacco smoke on vitamin C status in children, *Am J Clin Nutr* 77(1):167–172, 2003.

Puffenberger EG, Hu-Lince D, Parod JM, and others: Mapping of sudden infant death with dysgenesis of the testis syndrome (SIDDT) by a SNP genome scan and identification of TSPYL loss of function, *Proc Natl Acad Sci U S A* 101(32):11689–11694, 2004.

Ramanathan R, Corwin MJ, Hunt DE, and others: Cardiorespiratory events recorded on home monitors: comparison of healthy infants with those at increased risk for SIDS, *JAMA* 285(17):2199–2243, 2001.

Roberts DM, Ostapchuk M, O'Brien J: Infantile colic, *Am Fam Physician* 70(4):735–740, 741–742, 2004.

Robinson S, Proctor M: Diagnosis and management of deformational plagiocephaly: a review, *J Neurosurg Pediatr* 3(4):284–295, 2009.

Rudolf MCJ, Logan S: What is the long term outcome for children who fail to thrive? A systematic review, *Arch Dis Child* 90(9):925–931, 2005.

Saltzman MD, King EC: Central physeal arrests as a manifestation of hypervitaminosis A, *J Pediatr Orthop* 27(3):351–353, 2007.

Sampson HA, Leung DYM: Adverse reactions to foods. In Kliegman RM, Stanton BF, St. Geme JW, and others, editors: *Nelson textbook of pediatrics*, ed 19, Philadelphia, 2011, Saunders.

Savino F, Pelle E, Palumeri E, and others: *Lactobacillus reuteri* (American type culture collection strain 55730) versus simethicone in the treatment of infantile colic: a prospective randomized study, *Pediatrics* 119(1):e124–e130, 2007.

Sicherer SH: Clinical aspects of gastrointestinal food allergy in children, *Pediatrics* 111(6 Pt 3): 1609–1616, 2003.

Silvestri JM, Weese-Mayer D: Disorders of respiratory control: apnea and SIDS. In Rudolph CD, Rudolph AM, Hostetter MK, editors: *Rudolph's pediatrics*, ed 21, New York, 2003, McGraw-Hill.

Simons FE: Anaphylaxis: recent advances in assessment and treatment, *J Allergy Clin Immunol* 124(4):625–636, 2009.

St. James-Roberts I: Infant crying and sleeping: helping parents to prevent and manage problems, *Primary Care* 35(3):547–567, 2008.

Strehle EM, Gray WK, Gopisetti S, and others: Can home monitoring reduce mortality in infants at increased risk of sudden infant death syndrome? A systematic review, *Acta Paediatr* 101(1): 8–13, 2012.

Tablizo MA, Jacinto P, Parsley D, and others: Supine sleeping position does not cause clinical aspiration in neonates in hospital newborn nurseries, *Arch Pediatr Adolesc Med* 161(5): 507–510, 2007.

Tappin D, Ecob R, Brooke H: Bedsharing, roomsharing, and sudden infant death syndrome in Scotland: a case-control study, *J Pediatr* 147(1):32–37, 2005.

Taylor CE, Camargo CA: Impact of micronutrients on respiratory infections, *Nutr Rev* 69(5): 259–269, 2011.

Thompson DG: Safe sleep practices for hospitalized infants, *Pediatr Nurs* 31(5):400–403, 409, 2005.

Tierney EP, Sage RJ, Shwayder T: Kwashiorkor from a severe dietary restriction in an 8-month infant in suburban Detroit, Michigan: case report and review of the literature, *Int J Dermatol* 49(5):500–506, 2010.

Touchette E, Petit D, Paquet J, and others: Factors associated with fragmented sleep at night across early childhood, *Arch Pediatr Adolesc Med* 159(3):242–249, 2005.

Unger B, Kemp JS, Wilkins D, and others: Racial disparity and modifiable risk factors among infants dying suddenly and unexpectedly, *Pediatrics* 111(2):e127–e131, 2003.

Vennemann MM, Bajanowski T, Brinkmann B, and others: Sleep environment risk factors for sudden infant death syndrome: the German Sudden Infant Death Syndrome Study, *Pediatrics* 123(4):1162–1170, 2009.

Walker VP, Modlin RL: The vitamin D connection to pediatric infections and immune function, *Pediatr Res* 65(5 Pt 2): 106R–113R, 2009.

Wang J, Sampson HA: Food anaphylaxis, *Clin Exp Allergy* 37(5):651–660, 2007.

Ward TM, Rankin S, Lee KA: Caring for children with sleep problems, *J Pediatr Nurs* 22(4): 283–296, 2007.

World Health Organization: *HIV and infant feeding update*, Geneva, 2006, Author.

Yang CF, Duro D, Zurakowski D, and others: High prevalence of multiple micronutrient deficiencies in children with intestinal failure: a longitudinal study, *J Pediatr* 159(1):39–44.e1, 2011.

Health Promotion of the Toddler and Family

David Wilson

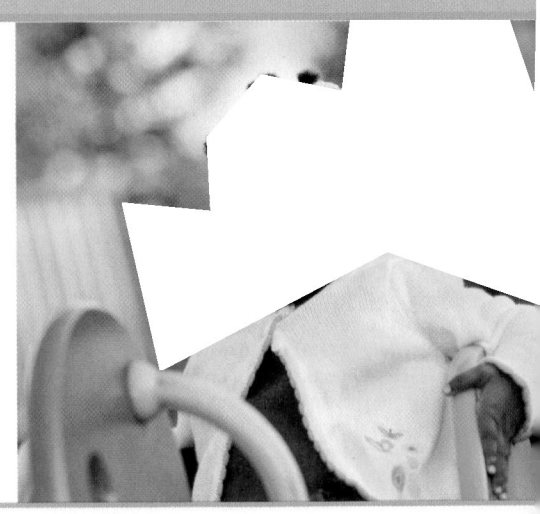

evolve WEBSITE

http://evolve.elsevier.com/wong/essentials
Case Study—Toilet Training/Toddler Development
Key Point Summaries
NCLEX-Style Review Questions

CHAPTER OUTLINE

Promoting Optimal Growth and
Development, 379
  Biologic Development, 379
    Proportional Changes, 379
    Sensory Changes, 379
    Maturation of Systems, 379
    Gross and Fine Motor
      Development, 379
  Psychosocial Development, 380
    Developing a Sense of Autonomy
      (Erikson), 380
  Cognitive Development: Sensorimotor
    and Preoperational Phase
    (Piaget), 380
    Tertiary Circular Reactions, 380
    Invention of New Means Through
      Mental Combinations, 381
    Preoperational Phase, 381
  Spiritual Development, 382

Development of Body Image, 383
Development of Gender Identity, 383
Social Development, 383
    Language, 384
    Personal-Social Behavior, 384
    Play, 384
Coping with Concerns Related to
  Normal Growth and Development, 385
    Toilet Training, 385
    Sibling Rivalry, 389
    Temper Tantrums, 389
    Negativism, 390
    Regression, 390
Promoting Optimal Health During
Toddlerhood, 390
  Nutrition, 390
    Nutritional Counseling, 391
    Dietary Guidelines, 391
    Vegetarian Diets, 392

Complementary and Alternative
  Medicine, 393
Sleep and Activity, 393
Dental Health, 394
    Regular Dental Examinations, 394
    Plaque Removal, 394
    Fluoride, 395
    Dietary Factors, 395
Safety Promotion and Injury
  Prevention, 396
    Motor Vehicle Safety, 396
    Drowning, 401
    Burns, 401
    Accidental Poisoning, 402
    Falls, 402
    Aspiration and Suffocation, 403
    Bodily Injury, 403
Anticipatory Guidance—Care of
  Families, 403

LEARNING OBJECTIVES

On completion of this chapter the reader will be able to:
- Identify the major biologic, psychosocial, cognitive, and social developments during the toddler years.
- Relate separation anxiety and negativism to developmental tasks.
- Recognize readiness for toilet training and offer parents guidelines.
- Help parents foster toddlers' language development.

- Provide parents with guidelines for handling temper tantrums.
- Provide parents with feeding recommendations.
- Outline a preventive dental hygiene plan for toddlers.
- Provide anticipatory guidance to parents regarding injury prevention based on the toddler's developmental achievements.

PROMOTING OPTIMAL GROWTH AND DEVELOPMENT

The term *terrible twos* has often been used to describe the toddler years, the period from 12 to 36 months of age. It is a time of intense exploration of the environment as children attempt to find out how things work; what the word "no" means; and the power of temper tantrums, negativism, and obstinacy. "Getting into things" is their way of learning about their world, especially relationships. Successful mastery of the tasks of this age requires a strong foundation of trust during infancy and frequently necessitates guidance from others when parents and toddlers face the struggles of toilet training, limit setting, and sibling rivalry. Nurses who understand the dynamics of growth and development of toddlers can help families deal effectively with the tasks of this age.

BIOLOGIC DEVELOPMENT

Proportional Changes

Physical growth slows considerably during toddlerhood. The average weight gain is 1.8 to 2.7 kg (4–6 pounds) per year. The average weight at 2 years is 12 kg (26.5 pounds). The birth weight is quadrupled by 2½ years of age. The rate of increase in height also slows. The usual increment is an addition of 7.5 cm (3 inches) per year and occurs mainly in elongation of the legs rather than the trunk. The average height of a 2-year-old child is 86.6 cm (34 inches). In general, adult height is about twice the 2-year-old child's height. Accurate measurement of height and weight during the toddler years should reveal a steady growth curve that is steplike in nature rather than linear (straight), which is characteristic of the growth spurts during the early childhood years.

The rate of increase in head circumference slows somewhat by the end of infancy, and head circumference is usually equal to chest circumference by 1 to 2 years of age. The usual total increase in head circumference during the second year is 2.5 cm (1 inch). Then the rate of increase slows until at age 5 years, the increase is less than 1.25 cm (0.5 inch) per year. The anterior fontanel closes between 1 and 1½ years of age.

Chest circumference continues to increase in size and exceeds head circumference during the toddler years. The chest's shape also changes as the transverse, or lateral, diameter exceeds the anteroposterior diameter. After the second year, the chest circumference exceeds the abdominal measurement, which, in addition to the growth of the lower extremities, makes the child appear taller and leaner. However, toddlers retain a squat, "pot-bellied" appearance because of their less developed abdominal musculature and short legs. The legs retain a slightly bowed or curved appearance during the second year from the weight of the relatively large trunk.

Sensory Changes

Visual acuity of 20/40 is considered acceptable during the toddler years. Full binocular vision is well developed, and any evidence of persistent strabismus requires professional attention as early as possible to prevent amblyopia. Depth perception continues to develop, but because of toddlers' lack of motor coordination, falls from heights continue to be a persistent danger.

The senses of hearing, smell, taste, and touch become increasingly well developed, coordinated with each other, and associated with other experiences. All of the senses are used to explore the environment. Toddlers visually inspect an object by turning it over; they may taste it, smell it, and touch it several times before they are satisfied with their investigation. They shake it to see if it makes noise and vigorously test its durability.

Another example of the integrated function of the senses is toddlers' development of specific taste preferences. Toddlers are much less likely than infants to try new foods because of their appearance, texture, or smell, not just their taste.

Maturation of Systems

Most of the physiologic systems are relatively mature by the end of toddlerhood. The volume of the respiratory tract and growth of associated structures continue to increase during early childhood, lessening some of the factors that predisposed children to frequent and serious infections during infancy. The internal structures of the ear and throat continue to be short and straight, and the lymphoid tissue of the tonsils and adenoids continues to be large. As a result, otitis media, tonsillitis, and upper respiratory tract infections are common. The respiratory and heart rates slow, and the blood pressure increases (see Appendix E and inside back cover). Respirations continue to be abdominal.

Under conditions of moderate variation in temperature, toddlers rarely have the difficulties of young infants in maintaining body temperature. The mature functioning of the renal system serves to conserve fluid under times of stress, decreasing the risk of dehydration.

The digestive processes are fairly complete by the beginning of toddlerhood. The acidity of the gastric contents continues to increase and has a protective function because it is capable of destroying many types of bacteria. Stomach capacity increases to allow for the usual schedule of three meals a day.

One of the more prominent changes of the gastrointestinal system is the voluntary control of elimination. With complete myelination of the spinal cord, control of the anal and urethral sphincters is gradually achieved. The physiologic ability to control the sphincters probably occurs somewhere between ages 18 and 24 months. Bladder capacity also increases considerably. By 14 to 18 months of age, children are able to retain urine for up to 2 hours or longer.

The defense mechanisms of the skin and blood, particularly phagocytosis, are much more efficient in toddlers than in infants. The production of antibodies is well established. However, many young children demonstrate a sudden increase in colds and minor infections when they enter preschool or other group situations, such as daycare, because of their exposure to pathogens.

Rapid growth in neurobehavioral organization contributes to greater regularity of sleep–wake cycles, the diminishing of crying and unexplained fussiness, and the enhanced predictability in mood. Valuable stimulants of early brain development include the various interactions (talking, singing, and playing) between the toddler and caregivers. Adequate nutrition; protection from environmental toxins such as lead, various drugs, and stress; and promotion of good health care all contribute to healthy brain growth.

Gross and Fine Motor Development

The major gross motor skill during the toddler years is the development of locomotion. By 12 to 13 months of age, toddlers walk alone using a wide stance for extra balance, and by 18 months, they try to run but fall easily. Between 2 and 3 years of age, refinement of the upright, biped position is evident in improved coordination and equilibrium. At age 2 years, toddlers can walk up and down stairs, and by age 2½ years, they can jump using both feet, stand on one foot for a second or two, and manage a few steps on tiptoe. By the end of the second year, they can stand on one foot, walk on tiptoe, and climb stairs with alternate footing.

Fine motor development is demonstrated in increasingly skillful manual dexterity. For example, by age 12 months, toddlers are able to grasp a very small object but are unable to release it at will. At 15 months, they can drop a raisin into a narrow-necked bottle. Casting or throwing objects and retrieving them become almost obsessive activities at about 15 months. By 18 months of age, toddlers can throw a ball overhand without losing their balance. By 2 years of age, toddlers use their hands to build towers, and by 3 years of age, they draw circles on paper.

Mastery of gross and fine motor skills is evident in all phases of toddlers' activity, such as play, dressing, language comprehension, response to discipline, social interaction, and propensity for injuries. Activities occur less in isolation and more in conjunction with other physical and mental abilities to produce a purposeful result. For example, the toddler walks to reach a new location, releases a toy to pick it up or to choose a new one, and scribbles to look at the image produced. The possibilities of the exploration, investigation, and manipulation of the environment—and its hazards—are endless.

PSYCHOSOCIAL DEVELOPMENT

Toddlers are faced with the mastery of several important tasks. If the need for basic trust has been satisfied, they are ready to give up dependence for control, independence, and autonomy. Some of the specific tasks to be dealt with include:

- Differentiation of self from others, particularly the mother
- Toleration of separation from parent
- Ability to withstand delayed gratification
- Control over bodily functions
- Acquisition of socially acceptable behavior
- Verbal means of communication
- Ability to interact with others in a less egocentric manner

Mastery of these goals is only begun during late infancy and the toddler years; tasks such as developing interpersonal relationships with others may not be completed until adolescence. However, crucial foundations for successful completion of such developmental tasks are laid during these early formative years.

Developing a Sense of Autonomy (Erikson)

According to Erikson (1963), the developmental task of toddlerhood is acquiring a sense of autonomy while overcoming a sense of doubt and shame. As infants gain trust in the predictability and reliability of their parents, environment, and interactions with others, they begin to discover that their behavior is their own and that it has a predictable, reliable effect on others. Although they realize their will and control over others, they are confronted with the conflict of exerting autonomy and relinquishing the much-enjoyed dependence on others. Whereas exerting their will has definite negative consequences, retaining dependent, submissive behavior is generally rewarded with affection and approval. However, continued dependence creates a sense of doubt regarding their potential capacity to control their actions. This doubt is compounded by a sense of shame for feeling this urge to revolt against others' will and a fear that they will exceed their own capacity for manipulating the environment. Skillful monitoring and balance of controls by parents allows a growing rate of realistic successes and the emergence of autonomy.

Just as infants have the social modalities of grasping and biting, toddlers have the newly gained modality of holding on and letting go. To hold on and let go is evident with the use of the hands; mouth; eyes; and, eventually, the sphincters, when toilet training is begun. These social modalities are expressed constantly in the child's play activities,

such as throwing objects; taking objects out of boxes, drawers, or cabinets; holding on tighter when someone says, "No; don't touch"; and refusing or spitting out food as taste preferences become very strong.

Several characteristics, especially negativism and ritualism, are typical of toddlers in their quest for autonomy. As toddlers attempt to express their will, they often act with negativism, the persistent negative response to requests. The words "no" or "me do" can be their sole vocabulary. Emotions become strongly expressed, usually in rapid mood swings. One minute, toddlers can be engrossed in an activity, and the next minute they might be angry because they are unable to manipulate a toy or open a door. If scolded for doing something wrong, they can have a temper tantrum and almost instantaneously pull at the parent's legs to be picked up and comforted. Understanding and coping with these swift changes is often difficult for parents. Many parents find the negativism exasperating and, instead of dealing constructively with it, give in to it, which further threatens children in their search for learning acceptable methods of interacting with others (see Temper Tantrums, p. 389, and Negativism, p. 390).

In contrast to negativism, which frequently disrupts the environment, ritualism, the need to maintain sameness and reliability, provides a sense of comfort. Toddlers can venture out with security when they know that familiar people, places, and routines still exist. One can easily understand why any change in the daily routine represents such a threat to these children. Without comfortable rituals, they have little opportunity to exert autonomy. Consequently, dependency and regression occur (see Regression, p. 390).

Erikson focuses on the development of the ego, which may be thought of as reason or common sense, during this phase of psychosocial development. Children struggle to deal with the impulses of the id and attempt to tolerate frustration and learn socially acceptable ways of interacting with the environment. The ego is evident as children are able to tolerate delayed gratification. Toddlers also have a rudimentary beginning of the superego, or conscience, which is the incorporation of the morals of society and the process of acculturation.

With the development of the ego, children further differentiate themselves from others and expand their sense of trust within themselves. But as they begin to develop awareness of their own will and capacity to achieve, they also become aware of their ability to fail. This ever-present awareness of potential failure creates doubt and shame. Successful mastery of the task of autonomy necessitates opportunities for self-mastery while withstanding the frustration of necessary limit setting and delayed gratification. Opportunities for self-mastery are present in appropriate play activities, toilet training, the crisis of sibling rivalry, and successful interactions with significant others (Fig. 12-1).

COGNITIVE DEVELOPMENT: SENSORIMOTOR AND PREOPERATIONAL PHASE (PIAGET)

The period from 12 to 24 months of age is a continuation of the final two stages of the sensorimotor phase. During this time, the cognitive processes develop rapidly and at times seem similar to those of mature thinking. However, reasoning skills are still primitive and need to be understood to effectively deal with the typical behaviors of a child of this age.

Tertiary Circular Reactions

In the fifth stage of the sensorimotor phase, tertiary circular reactions (13–18 months of age), the child uses active experimentation to achieve previously unattainable goals (see Cognitive Development, Chapter 10). Newly acquired physical skills are increasingly important

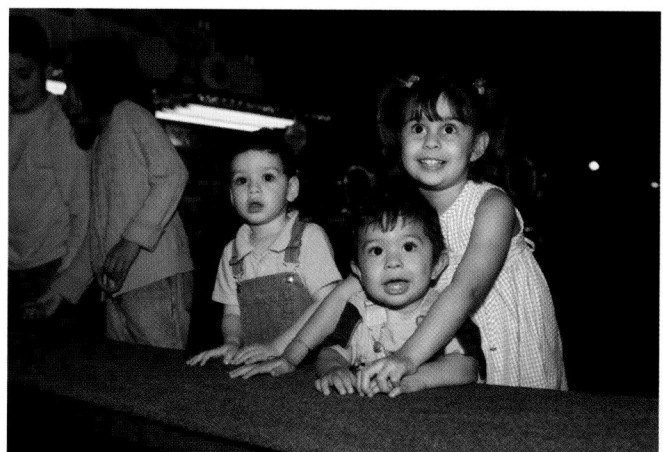

FIG 12-1 Toddlers begin socializing with significant others such as siblings as a part of development. (© 2011 Photos.com, a division of Getty Images. All rights reserved.)

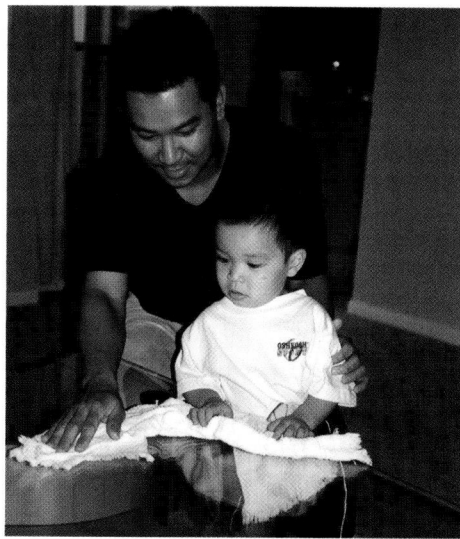

FIG 12-2 Domestic mimicry is common during toddlerhood.

for the function they serve rather than for the acts themselves. Children incorporate the old learning of secondary circular reactions with new skills and apply the combined knowledge to new situations, with emphasis on the results of the experimentation. In this way, there is the beginning of rational judgment and intellectual reasoning. During this stage, there is further differentiation of oneself from objects. This is evident in children's increasing ability to venture away from their parents and to tolerate longer periods of separation.

Awareness of a causal relationship between two events is apparent. After flipping a light switch, toddlers are aware that a reciprocal response occurs. However, they are not able to transfer that knowledge to new situations. Therefore, every time they see what appears to be a light switch, they must reinvestigate its function. Such behavior demonstrates the beginning of *categorizing data into distinct classes and subclasses*. There are innumerable examples of this type of behavior as toddlers continuously explore the same object each time it appears in a new place.

Because classification of objects is still rudimentary, the appearance of an object denotes its function. For example, if the child's toys are stored in a paper bag or large container, that toy receptacle is no different from the garbage pail or laundry basket. If allowed to turn over the toy receptacle, the child will just as quickly do the same to other similar containers because, in the child's mind, there is no difference. Expecting the child to judge which receptacles are permissible to explore and which are not is inappropriate for this age group. Instead, the forbidden object, such as the garbage pail, should be placed out of reach. This has significant implications for prevention of accidents and accidental ingestion of injurious agents.

The discovery of objects as objects leads to the awareness of their spatial relationships. Children are able to recognize different shapes and their relationships to each other. For example, they can fit slightly smaller boxes into each other (nesting) and can place a round object into a hole even if the board is turned around, upside down, or reversed. Children are also aware of space and the relationship of their bodies to dimensions such as height. They will stretch, stand on a low stair or stool, and pull a string to reach an object.

Object permanence has also advanced. Although they still cannot find an object that has been invisibly displaced or moved from under one pillow to another without their seeing the change, toddlers are increasingly aware of the existence of objects behind closed doors, in drawers, and under tables. Parents are usually acutely aware of this

developmental achievement and find high places and locked cabinets the only places that are inaccessible to toddlers.

Invention of New Means Through Mental Combinations

From ages 19 to 24 months, children are in the final sensorimotor stage, invention of new means through mental combinations. During this stage, children complete the more primitive, autistic-like thought processes of infancy and are prepared for the more complex mental operations that occur during the phase of preoperational thought. One of the most dramatic achievements of this stage is in the area of object permanence. Toddlers will now actively search for an object in several potential hiding places. In addition, they can infer a cause when only experiencing the effect. They can infer that an object was hidden in any number of places even if they only saw the original hiding place.

Imitation displays deeper meaning and understanding. There is greater symbolization to imitation. Children are acutely aware of others' actions and attempt to copy them in gestures and in words. Domestic mimicry (imitating household activities) and sex-role behavior become increasingly common during this period and during the second year. Identification with the parent of the same gender becomes apparent by the second year and represents the child's intellectual ability to differentiate different models of behavior and to imitate them appropriately (Fig. 12-2).

The concept of time is still embryonic, but children have some sense of timing in terms of anticipation, memory, and a limited ability to wait. They may listen to the command, "Just a minute," and behave appropriately. However, their sense of timing is exaggerated—1 minute can seem like an hour. Toddlers' limited attention spans also indicate their sense of immediacy and concern for the present.

Preoperational Phase

At approximately 2 years of age, children enter the preconceptual phase of cognitive development, which lasts until about age 4 years. The preconceptual phase is a subdivision of the preoperational phase, which spans ages 2 to 7 years. The preconceptual phase is primarily one of transition that bridges the purely self-satisfying behavior of infancy and the rudimentary socialized behavior of latency. Preoperational thought implies that children cannot think in terms of operations—the ability to manipulate objects in relation to each other in a logical fashion. Rather, toddlers think primarily on the basis of

BOX 12-1 CHARACTERISTICS OF PREOPERATIONAL THOUGHT

Egocentrism—Inability to envision situations from perspectives other than one's own

Example—If a person is positioned between the toddler and another child, the toddler, who is facing the person, will explain that both children can see the middle person's face. The young child is unable to realize that the other person views the middle person from a different perspective, the back.

Implication—Avoid moralizing about "why" something is wrong if it requires an understanding of someone else's feelings or opinion. Telling a child to stop hitting because hitting hurts the other person is often ineffective because, to the aggressor, it feels good to hit someone else. Instead, emphasize that hitting is not allowed.

Transductive reasoning—Reasoning from the particular to the particular

Example—Child refuses to eat a food because something previously eaten did not taste good.

Implication—Accept child's reasoning; offer refused food at different time.

Global organization—Reasoning that changing any one part of the whole changes the entire whole

Example—Child refuses to sleep in his or her room because location of bed has changed.

Implication—Accept child's reasoning; use same bed position or introduce change slowly.

Centration—Focusing on one aspect rather than considering all possible alternatives

Example—Child refuses to eat a food because of its color even though its taste and smell are acceptable.

Implication—Accept child's reasoning.

Animism—Attributing lifelike qualities to inanimate objects

Example—Child scolds stairs for making child fall down.

Implication—Join child in the "scolding." Keep frightening objects out of view.

Irreversibility—Inability to undo or reverse the actions initiated physically

Example—When told to stop doing something, such as talking, child is unable to think of a positive activity.

Implication—State requests or instructions positively (e.g., "Be quiet.").

Magical thinking—Believing that thoughts are all-powerful and can cause events

Examples—Child wishes someone died; then if the person dies, child feels at fault because of the "bad" thought that made the death happen. Calling children "bad" because they did something wrong makes them feel as if they are bad.

Implication—Clarify that thoughts do not make things happen and that child is not responsible.

- Use "I" messages rather than "you" messages to communicate thoughts, feelings, expectations, or beliefs without imposing blame or criticism. Emphasize that the act, not the child, is bad.

Inability to conserve—Inability to understand the idea that a mass can be changed in size, shape, volume, or length without losing or adding to the original mass (instead, children judge what they see by the immediate perceptual clues given to them)

Example—If two lines of equal length are presented in such a way that one appears longer than the other, child will state that one line is longer even if child measures both lines with a ruler or yardstick and finds that each has the same length.

Implication—Change the most obvious perceptual clue to reorient child's view of what is seen.

- Give medicine in a small medicine cup, rather than a large cup, because the child will imagine that the large vessel contains more liquid. If child refuses the medicine in the small cup, pour it into a large cup because the liquid will appear to be less in a tall, wide container.
- Give a large, flat cookie rather than a thick, small one or do the reverse with meat or cheese; child will usually eat larger size of favorite food and smaller size of less favorite food.

their perception of an event. Problem solving is based on what they see or hear directly rather than on what they recall about objects and events. Several characteristics are unique to preoperational thought (Box 12-1).

Within the second year, children increasingly use language symbolically and are concerned with the "why" and "how" of things. For example, a pencil is "something to write with," and food is "something to eat." However, such mental symbolization is closely associated with prelogical reasoning. For instance, a needle is "something that hurts." Such painful experiences take on new significance because memory is associated with the specific event, and fears are likely to develop, such as resistance to people who wear colored uniforms or rooms that look like the practitioner's office. Because of the vulnerability of these early years, it is essential to prepare children for any new experience, whether it is a new babysitter or a visit to the dentist.

SPIRITUAL DEVELOPMENT

Spiritual development in children is often discussed in terms of the child's developmental level because the evolution of spirituality often parallels cognitive development (Elkins and Cavendish, 2004). The child's family and environment strongly influence the child's perception of the world around him or her, and this often includes spirituality. Furthermore, family values, beliefs, customs, and expressions of these influence the child's perception of his or her spiritual self (Elkins

and Cavendish, 2004). Neuman (2011) proposes that Fowler's (1981) stages of faith be used to better understand children and spirituality; she provides an excellent overview of the stages of faith in childhood. The relationship between spirituality, illness in childhood, and nursing has been studied in the context of suffering, terminal illness such as cancer, and end-of-life care. In the past decade, there has been an increased interest in and focus on spiritual care in adults and children as further understanding of the influence of one's spirituality on health, illness, and well-being has progressed.

Toddlers learn about God through the words and the actions of those closest to them. They have only a vague idea of God and religious teachings because of their immature cognitive processes; however, if God is spoken about with reverence, young children associate God with something special. During this period, the assignment of powerful religious symbols and images is strongly influenced by the manner in which it is presented; therein lies the potential for the development of guilt and fear or, conversely, love and companionship with religious symbols (Roehlkepartain, King, Wagener, and others, 2006). Toddlers are said to be in the intuitive-projective phase of Fowler's (1981) faith construct wherein thinking is largely based on fantasy and rather fluid in relation to reality and fantasy. God may be described as being around like air by the toddler because of the fluidity in dividing fantasy and reality (Neuman, 2011).

Toddlers begin to assimilate behaviors associated with the divine (folding hands in prayer). Routines such as saying prayers before meals or at bedtime can be important and comforting. Because toddlers tend to find solace in ritualistic behavior and routines, they incorporate routines associated with religious practices into their behavioral patterns without understanding all of the implications of the rituals until later. Near the end of toddlerhood, when children use preoperational thought, there is some advancement of their understanding of God. Religious teachings, such as reward or fear of punishment (heaven or hell) and moral development (see Chapter 5), may influence their behavior (Fosarelli, 2003).

DEVELOPMENT OF BODY IMAGE

As in infancy, the development of body image closely parallels cognitive development. Developing psychologic understanding provides greater self-awareness, and young children learn to answer the question: "Who am I?" During the second year, children recognize themselves in a mirror and make verbal references to themselves ("Me big"). With increasing motor ability, toddlers recognize the usefulness of body parts and gradually learn their names. They also learn that certain parts of the body have various meanings; for example, during toilet training, the genitalia become significant, and cleanliness is emphasized. By 2 years of age they recognize gender differences and refer to themselves by name and then by pronoun. Gender identity is developed by age 3 years. Also by this time, children begin to remember events with reference to their personal significance, forming an autobiographic memory that helps to establish a continuous identity throughout life's events.

After they begin preoperational thought, toddlers can use symbols to represent objects, but their thinking may lead to inaccuracies. For example, if someone who is pregnant is called "fat," they will describe all "fat" women as having babies. They begin to recognize words used to describe physical appearance, such as *pretty*, *handsome*, or *big boy*. Such expressions eventually influence how children view their own bodies.

Although little research has been done on body image development in young children, it is evident that body integrity is poorly understood and that intrusive experiences are threatening. For example, toddlers forcefully resist procedures such as examining their ears or mouths and having their axillary temperature taken. The procedure itself (e.g., taking vital signs) does not hurt the child, but it represents an intrusion into the child's personal space, which elicits a strong protest. Toddlers also have unclear body boundaries and may associate nonviable parts, such as feces, with essential body parts. This can be seen in a toddler who is upset by flushing the toilet and watching the stool disappear.

Nurses can assist parents in fostering a positive body image in their child by encouraging them to avoid negative labels, such as "skinny arms" or "chubby legs"—self-perceptions that can last a lifetime. Body parts, especially those related to elimination and reproduction, should be called by their correct names. Respect for the body should be practiced.

DEVELOPMENT OF GENDER IDENTITY

Just as toddlers explore their environment, they also explore their bodies and find that touching certain body parts is pleasurable. Genital fondling (masturbation) can occur and involves manual stimulation, as well as posturing movements (especially in young girls) such as tightening of the thighs or mechanical pressure applied to the pubic or suprapubic area. Other demonstrations of pleasurable activities include rocking, swinging, and hugging people and toys. Parental reactions to toddlers' behavior influence the children's own attitudes and

should be accepting rather than critical. If such acts are performed in public, parents should not condone or bring attention to the behavior but should teach the child that it is more acceptable to perform the behavior in private.

Children in this age group are learning vocabulary associated with anatomy, elimination, and reproduction. Certain associations between words and functions become significant and can influence future sexual attitudes. For example, if parents refer to the genitalia as dirty, especially in the context of elimination, this association between "genitalia" and "dirty" may be transferred to sexual functions later in life. Sex-role differences become obvious to children and are evident in much of toddlers' imitative play. Although current research indicates that prenatal exposure to testosterone strongly influences the individual's gender identity, researchers also indicate that there are sensitive periods (e.g., puberty) that may also have an influence on the development of gender identity (Berenbaum and Beltz, 2011; Hines, 2011; Savic, Garcia-Falqueras, and Swaab, 2010). A sense of maleness or femaleness, or gender identity, is formed by age 3 years, and the child's feelings about being male or female begin to form (Fonseca and Greydanus, 2007). Early attitudes are formed about affectionate behaviors between adults from observing parental and other adult intimate or sensual activities. (See also Sex Education, Chapter 13.) The quality of relationships with parents is important to the child's capacity for sexual and emotional relationships later in life.

SOCIAL DEVELOPMENT

A major task of the toddler period is differentiation of the self from significant others, usually the mother. The differentiation process consists of two phases: separation, the children's emergence from a symbiotic fusion with the mother; and individuation, those achievements that mark children's expression of their individual characteristics in the environment. Although the process begins during the latter half of infancy, the major achievements occur during the toddler years.

Toddlers have an increased understanding and awareness of object permanence and some ability to withstand delayed gratification and tolerate moderate frustration. As a result, toddlers react differently to strangers than do infants. The appearance of unfamiliar persons does not represent such a significant threat to their attachment to their mothers. They have learned from experience that parents exist when physically absent. Repetition of events such as going to bed without the parents but waking to find them there again reinforces the reliability of such brief separations. Consequently, toddlers are able to venture away from their parents for brief periods because of the security of knowing that the parents will be there when they return. Verbal and visual reassurance from the parents gradually replaces some of the previous need to be physically close for comfort.

According to Harpaz-Rotem and Bergman (2006), the separation-individuation phase encompasses the phenomenon of rapprochement; as a toddler separates from the mother and begins to make sense of experiences in the environment, he or she is drawn back to the mother for assistance in verbally articulating the meaning of the experiences. Developmentally, the term *rapprochement* means the child moves away and returns for reassurance. If the mother's response to the toddler is inappropriate, the toddler may experience insecurity and confusion.

Transitional objects, such as a favorite blanket or toy, provide security for children, especially when they are separated from their parents, dealing with a new stress, or just fatigued (Fig. 12-3). Security objects often become so important to toddlers that they refuse to let them be taken away. Such behavior is normal; there is no need to

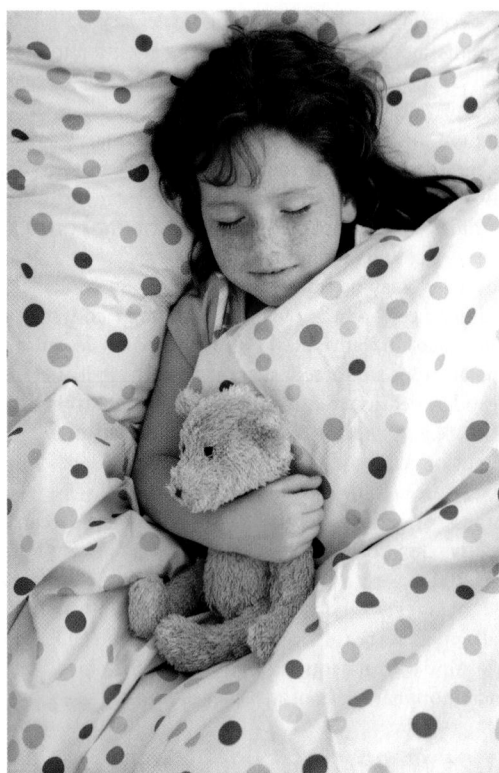

FIG 12-3 Transitional objects, such as a warm and fuzzy stuffed animal, are sources of security to a toddler. (© 2011 Photos.com, a division of Getty Images. All rights reserved.)

discourage this tendency. During separations, such as daycare, hospitalization, or even staying overnight with a relative, transitional objects should be provided to minimize any fear or loneliness.

Learning to tolerate and master brief periods of separation is an important developmental task for children in this age group. In addition, it is a necessary component of parenting because brief periods of separation allow parents to restore their energy and patience and to minimize directing their irritations and frustrations at the children.

Language

The most striking characteristic of language development during early childhood is the increasing level of comprehension. Although the number of words acquired—from about four at 1 year of age to approximately 300 at age 2 years—is notable, the ability to comprehend and understand speech is much greater than the number of words the child can say. Bilingual children can also achieve their early linguistic milestones in each of the languages at the same time and produce a substantial number of semantically corresponding words in each of their two languages from the very first words or signs.

At age 1 year, children use one-word sentences or holophrases. The word "up" can mean "pick me up" or "look up there." For children, the one word conveys the meaning of a sentence, but to others, it may mean many things or nothing. At this age, about 25% of the vocalizations are intelligible. By the age of 2 years, children use multiword sentences by stringing together two or three words, such as the phrases "mama go bye-bye" or "all gone," and approximately 65% of their speech is understandable. By 3 years, children put words together into simple sentences, begin to master grammatical rules, acquire five or six new words daily, know their age and gender, and can count three objects correctly. Looking at books during this period provides an ideal setting

for further language development (Feigelman, 2011). Authorities have evaluated the impact of television viewing on toddler language development and found that those who started watching television at younger than 12 months of age and who watched longer than 2 hours per day had significant language delays (Chonchaiva and Pruksananonda, 2008). Adult–child conversations with infants and toddlers have been shown to positively affect language development; the researchers recommend reading, storytelling, and interactive adult–child communication (Zimmerman, Gilkerson, Richards, and others, 2009). The American Academy of Pediatrics (AAP), Council on Communications and Media (2011) reaffirms that televised or recorded media usage in children less than 2 years of age decreases language skills, as well as the time parents interact with the child. Furthermore, educational programs have not been shown to increase cognitive skills in young children (AAP, Council on Communications and Media, 2011).

Gestures precede or accompany each of the language milestones up to 30 months of age (putting phone to ear, pointing). After sufficient language development, gestures phase out, and the pace of word learning increases (Bates and Dick, 2002).

Personal-Social Behavior

One of the most dramatic aspects of development in the toddler is personal-social interaction. Personal-social behaviors are evident in such areas as dressing, feeding, playing, and establishing self-control. Parents frequently wonder why their manageable, docile, lovable infant has turned into a determined, strong-willed, volatile little tyrant. In addition, the tyrant of the terrible twos can swiftly and unpredictably revert back to the adorable infant. All of this is part of growing up as toddlers acquire a more sophisticated awareness that others' feelings and desires can be different from their own. Through interactions with caregivers, children are able to explore these differences and their consequences.

Toddlers are developing skills of independence, which are evident in all areas of behavior. By 15 months of age, children feed themselves, drink well from a covered cup, and manage a spoon with considerable spilling. By 2 years, they use a spoon well, and by 3 years, they may be using a fork. Between ages 2 and 3 years, they eat with the family and like to help with chores such as setting the table or removing dishes from the dishwasher, but they lack table manners and may find it difficult to sit through the family's entire meal.

In dressing, toddlers also demonstrate strides in independence. Fifteen-month-old children help by putting their arms or feet out for dressing and pull off their shoes and socks. Eighteen-month-old children remove gloves, help with pullover shirts, and may be able to unzip. By age 2 years toddlers remove most articles of clothing and put on socks, shoes, and pants without regard for right or left and back or front. Help is still needed to fasten clothes.

Toddlers also begin to develop concern for the feelings of others and develop an understanding of how adult expectations for behavior apply to specific situations (e.g., causing a sibling to cry while playing rough). As their understanding is fostered, they are able to develop control. Age-appropriate discipline contributes to healthy social and emotional development. Positive reinforcement, redirection, and time-outs are appropriate for most toddlers. Social and emotional problems can develop in the youngest children. Early screening and intervention promote more positive outcomes as young children grow and develop.

Play

Play magnifies toddlers' physical and psychosocial development. Interaction with people becomes increasingly important. The solitary play

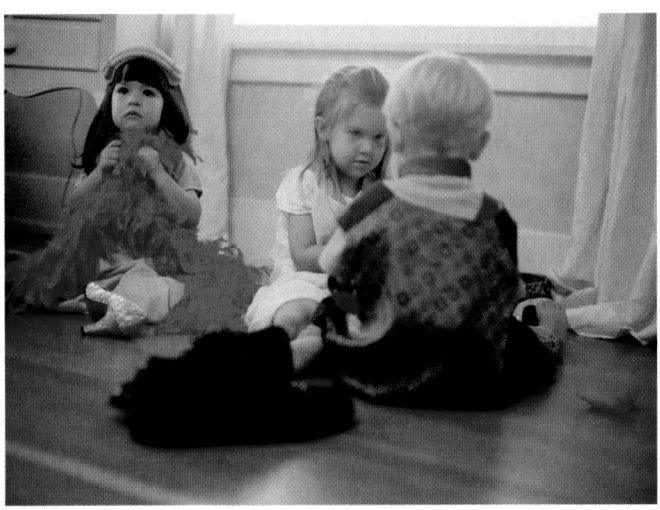

FIG 12-4 Young children enjoy dressing up. (© 2011 Photos.com, a division of Getty Images. All rights reserved.)

of infancy progresses to parallel play—toddlers play alongside, not with, other children. Although sensorimotor play is still prominent, there is much less emphasis on the exclusive use of one sensory modality. Toddlers inspect toys, talk to toys, test toys' strength and durability, and invent several uses for toys. Imitation is one of the most distinguishing characteristics of play and enriches children's opportunity to engage in fantasy. With less emphasis on gender-stereotyped toys, play objects such as dolls, carriages, dollhouses, balls, dishes, cooking utensils, child-size furniture, trucks, and dress-up clothes are suitable for both genders (Fig. 12-4); however, whereas boys may be more interested than girls in activities related to trucks, trailers, action figures, and building blocks, girls may prefer doll-related activities.

Increased locomotive skills make push–pull toys, straddle trucks or cycles, a small gym and slide, balls of various sizes, and riding toys appropriate for energetic toddlers. Finger paints; thick crayons; chalk; blackboard; paper; and puzzles with large, simple pieces use toddlers' developing fine motor skills. Interlocking blocks in various sizes and shapes provide hours of fun and, during later years, are useful objects for creative and imaginative play. The most educational toy is the one that fosters the interaction of an adult with a child in supportive, unconditional play. Toys should not be substitutes for the attention of devoted caregivers, but toys can enhance these interactions (Glassy, Romano, and Committee on Early Childhood, 2003). Parents and other providers are encouraged to allow children to play with a variety of simple toys that foster creative thinking (e.g., blocks, dolls, and clay) rather than passive toys that the child observes (battery-operated or mechanical). Active play time should also be encouraged over the use of computer or video games, which are more passive (Ginsburg and AAP, Committee on Communications, 2007).

Certain aspects of play are related to emerging linguistic abilities. Talking is a form of play for toddlers, who enjoy musical toys such as age-appropriate compact disc (CD) players, "talking" dolls and animals, and toy telephones. Children's television programs are appropriate for some children over age 2 years, who learn to associate words with visual images. However, total media time should be limited to 1 hour or less of quality programming per day. Parents are encouraged to allow the child to engage in unstructured playtime, which is considered much more beneficial than any electronic media exposure (AAP, Council on Communications and Media, 2011). Toddlers also enjoy

"reading" stories from a picture book and imitating the sounds of animals.

Tactile play is also important for exploring toddlers. Water toys, a sandbox with a pail and shovel, finger paints, soap bubbles, and clay provide excellent opportunities for creative and manipulative recreation. Adults sometimes forget the fascination of feeling textures such as slippery cream, mud, or pudding; catching air bubbles; squeezing and reshaping clay; or smearing paints. These types of unstructured activities are as important as educational play to allow children the freedom of expression.

Selection of appropriate toys must involve safety factors, especially in relation to size and sturdiness. The oral activity of toddlers puts them at risk for aspirating small objects and ingesting toxic substances. Parents need to be especially vigilant of toys played with in other children's homes and toys of older siblings. Toys are a potential source of serious bodily damage to toddlers, who may have the physical strength to manipulate them but not the knowledge to appreciate their danger (Stephenson, 2005). Government agencies do not inspect and police all toys on the market. Therefore, adults who purchase play equipment, supervise purchases, or allow children to use play equipment need to evaluate its safety, including toys that are gifts or those that are purchased by the children themselves. Adults should also be alert to notices of toys determined to be defective and recalled by the manufacturers. Parents and health care workers can obtain information on a variety of recalled products and can report potentially dangerous toys and child products to the U.S. Consumer Product Safety Commission* or, in Canada, the Canadian Toy Testing Council.† Printable tips on toy safety are also available from Safe Kids Worldwide (http://www.safekids.org).

Table 12-1 summarizes the major features of growth and development for the age groups of 15, 18, 24, and 30 months.

COPING WITH CONCERNS RELATED TO NORMAL GROWTH AND DEVELOPMENT

Toilet Training

One of the major tasks of toddlerhood is toilet training. Anticipatory guidance and clinical intervention for families surrounding toilet training should begin during routine well-child visits before the child's developmental readiness to toilet train. Preparation and education reveal and allay misconceptions; lead to the development of appropriate expectations; and provide information, guidance, and support to parents for managing this potentially frustrating process.

Voluntary control of the anal and urethral sphincters is achieved sometime after the child is walking, probably between ages 18 and 24 months. However, complex psychophysiologic factors are required for readiness. The child must be able to recognize the urge to let go and hold on and be able to communicate this sensation to the parent. In addition, some motivation is probably involved in the desire to please the parent by holding on rather than pleasing oneself by letting go. Cultural beliefs may also affect the age at which children demonstrate readiness (Feigelman, 2011).

Schmitt (2004) notes that comparative studies over the past 5 decades indicate that children in the 1990s in the United States were toilet trained at a later age (18 months in the 1960s vs. 36 months in the 1990s); one possible contributing factor is the availability and convenience of disposable diapers. Another study found that the child's

---

*800-638-2772; http://www.cpsc.gov (assistance is also available in Spanish).
†1973 Baseline Road, Ottawa, ON K2C 0C7 Canada; 613-228-3155; fax: 613-228-3242; http://www.toy-testing.org.

Case Study—Toilet Training/Toddler Development

TABLE 12-1 **GROWTH AND DEVELOPMENT DURING THE TODDLER YEARS**

PHYSICAL	GROSS MOTOR	FINE MOTOR	SENSORY	LANGUAGE	SOCIALIZATION
Age 15 Months					
Steady growth in height and weight Head circumference, 48 cm (19 inches) Weight, 11 kg (24 pounds) Height, 78.7 cm (31 inches)	Walks without help (usually since age 13 months) Creeps up stairs Kneels without support Cannot walk around corners or stop suddenly without losing balance without support Cannot throw ball without falling Runs clumsily; falls often	Constantly casting objects to floor Builds tower of two cubes Holds two cubes in one hand Releases a pellet into a narrow-necked bottle Scribbles spontaneously Uses cup well but often rotates spoon before it reaches mouth	Able to identify geometric forms; places round object into appropriate hole Binocular vision well developed Displays an intense and prolonged interest in pictures	Uses expressive jargon Says four to six words, including names "Asks" for objects by pointing Understands simple commands May use head-shaking gesture to denote "no" Uses "no" even while agreeing to the request Uses common gestures such as putting cup to mouth when empty	Tolerates some separation from parent Less likely to fear strangers Beginning to imitate parents, such as cleaning house (sweeping, dusting), folding clothes May discard bottle Kisses and hugs parents; may kiss pictures in a book
Age 18 Months					
Picky eater as a result of decreased growth needs and need to assert independence Anterior fontanel closed Physiologically able to control sphincters	Assumes standing position Walks up stairs with one hand held Pulls and pushes toys Jumps in place with both feet Seats self on chair Throws ball overhand without falling	Builds tower of three or four cubes Release, prehension, and reach well developed Turns pages in a book two or three at a time In a drawing, makes stroke imitatively Manages spoon without rotation		Says 10 or more words Points to a common object, such as a shoe or ball, and to two or three body parts Forms word combinations Forms gesture–word combinations (points while naming) Forms gesture–gesture combinations	Expresses emotions; has temper tantrums Great imitator (domestic mimicry) Takes off gloves, socks, and shoes and unzips zippers Temper tantrums may be more evident Beginning awareness of ownership ("My toy") May develop dependence on transitional objects, such as security blanket
Age 24 Months					
Head circumference, 49–50 cm (19.5–20 inches) Chest circumference exceeds head circumference Lateral diameter of chest exceeds anteroposterior diameter Usual weight gain of 1.8–2.7 kg (4–6 pounds) per year Usual gain in height of 10–12.5 cm (4–5 inches) per year Adult height approximately double height at 2 years of age Primary dentition of 16 teeth May demonstrate readiness for beginning daytime control of bowel and bladder	Goes up and down stairs alone with two feet on each step Runs fairly well, with wide stance Picks up object without falling Kicks ball forward without overbalancing	Builds tower of six or seven cubes Aligns two or more cubes like a train Turns pages of book one at a time In drawing, imitates vertical and circular strokes Turns doorknobs; unscrews lids	Accommodation well developed in geometric discrimination; able to insert square block into oblong space	Has a vocabulary of approximately 300 words Uses two- or three-word phrases Uses pronouns "I," "me," "you" Understands directional commands Gives first name; refers to self by name Verbalizes need for toileting, food, or drink Talks incessantly Able to remember and imitate arbitrary sequences of manual actions and gestures	Stage of parallel play Has sustained attention span Temper tantrums decreasing Pulls people to show them something Increased independence from parent Dresses self in simple clothing Develops visual recognition and verbal self-reference ("Me big") Develops awareness that feelings and desires of others may be different and begins to explore implications and consequences

TABLE 12-1	GROWTH AND DEVELOPMENT DURING THE TODDLER YEARS—cont'd					
PHYSICAL	**GROSS MOTOR**	**FINE MOTOR**	**SENSORY**	**LANGUAGE**	**SOCIALIZATION**
Age 30 Months Birth weight quadrupled Primary dentition (20 teeth) completed May have daytime bowel and bladder control	Jumps with both feet Jumps from chair or step Stands on one foot momentarily Takes a few steps on tiptoe	Builds tower of eight cubes Adds chimney blocks to train of block Good hand–finger coordination; holds crayon with fingers rather than fist In drawing, imitates vertical and horizontal strokes; makes two or more strokes for cross; draws circles		Gives first and last name Refers to self by appropriate pronoun Uses plurals Names one color	Separates more easily from parent In play, helps put things away; can carry breakable objects; pushes with good steering Begins to notice gender differences; knows own gender May attend to toilet needs without help except for wiping Emotions expand to include pride, shame, guilt, embarrassment

average age at initiation of toilet training was 20.6 months (Horn, Brenner, Rao, and others, 2006).

Five markers signal a child's readiness to toilet train: bladder readiness, bowel readiness, cognitive readiness, motor readiness, and psychologic readiness (Schmitt, 2004). According to some experts, physiologic and psychologic readiness is not complete until ages 22 to 30 months (Schum, Kolb, McAuliffe, and others, 2002); however, Schmitt (2004) emphasizes that parents should begin preparing their children for toilet training earlier than 30 months. By this time, children have mastered the majority of essential gross motor skills, can communicate intelligibly, are in less conflict with their parents in terms of self-assertion and negativism, and are aware of the ability to control the body and please their parents. There is no universal right age to begin toilet training or an absolute deadline to complete training. An important role for the nurse is to help parents identify the readiness signs in their children (see Nursing Care Guidelines box).* On average, girls are developmentally ready to begin toilet training 2 to 2½ months before boys (Schum, Kolb, McAuliffe, and others, 2002).

Nighttime bladder control normally takes several months to years after daytime training begins. This is because the sleep cycle needs to mature so the child can awake in time to urinate. Feigelman (2011) indicates that bedwetting is normal in girls up to age 4 years and in boys up to age 5 years. Few children have night wetting episodes after daytime dryness is totally achieved; however, children who do not have nighttime dryness by the age of 6 years are likely to require intervention (Mercer, 2003).

Bowel training is usually accomplished before bladder training because of its greater regularity and predictability. The sensation for defecation is stronger than that for urination and easier for children to recognize. A well-balanced diet that includes dietary fiber helps keep stool soft and supports the development and maintenance of regular bowel movements.

A number of techniques are helpful when initiating training, and cultural differences should be considered (see Cultural Considerations

---

*A helpful book is *Guide to Toilet Training*, available from the AAP, 847-434-4000; http://www.aap.org/bookstore. Additional resources are listed in the Schmitt (2004) reference.

 NURSING CARE GUIDELINES

Assessing Toilet Training Readiness

Physical Readiness
Voluntary control of anal and urethral sphincters, usually by 22 to 30 months of age
Ability to stay dry for 2 hours; decreased number of wet diapers; waking dry from nap
Regular bowel movements
Gross motor skills of sitting, walking, and squatting
Fine motor skills to remove clothing

Mental Readiness
Recognizes urge to defecate or urinate
Verbal or nonverbal communicative skills to indicate when wet or has urge to defecate or urinate
Cognitive skills to imitate appropriate behavior and follow directions

Psychologic Readiness
Expresses willingness to please parent
Able to sit on toilet for 5 to 8 minutes without fussing or getting off
Curiosity about adults' or older sibling's toilet habits
Impatience with soiled or wet diapers; desire to be changed immediately

Parental Readiness
Recognizes child's level of readiness
Willing to invest the time required for toilet training
Provides consistency in toileting instructions
Provides positive rewards and encouragement
Avoids the use of punishment for inability to toilet train or for toileting accidents
Absence of family stress or change, such as a divorce, moving, new sibling, or imminent vacation

box). In the United States, some of the options recommended by practitioners include the Brazelton child-oriented approach, the AAP guidelines (which are similar to the Brazelton method), Dr. Spock's training method, and the intensive "toilet-training-in-a-day" (operant conditioning) approach by Azrin and Foxx

Toilet Training

Cultural practices influence the timing, method, and significance of toilet training. For many families in China, the timing is liberal, the method is distinct, and the significance is low. Children are diapered during infancy. Once they are walking, they wear loose pants with a long slit between the legs, and they eliminate on the ground. This practice may continue until the child is 5 years of age. In cold weather, a piece of cloth, like a "curtain," may be inserted. However, the Chinese have a concept that the buttocks are not susceptible to cold, so this is not a common practice.

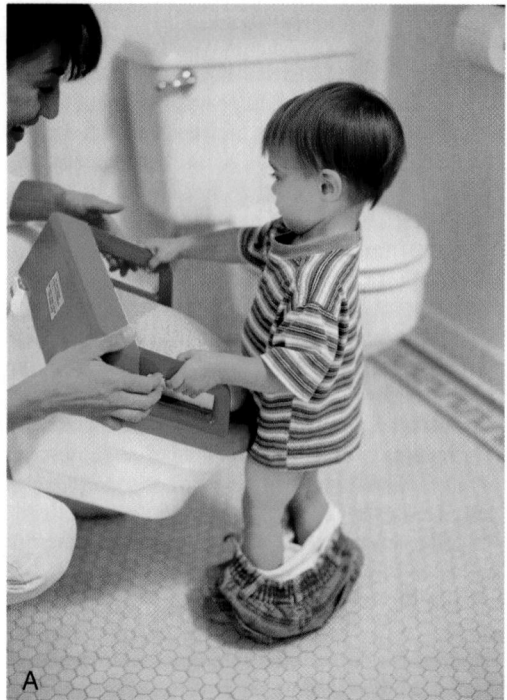

(Choby and George, 2008). An extensive study and review by the Agency for Healthcare Research and Quality in 2006 (Klassen, Kiddoo, Lang, and others, 2006) concluded that the child-oriented method and the Azrin and Foxx methods were effective at toilet training healthy children (Choby and George, 2008). The following discussion of toilet training methods includes suggestions from the child-oriented approach.

Parents should begin the readiness phase of toilet training by teaching the child about how the body functions in relation to voiding and having a stool. Schmitt (2004) suggests that parents talk about how adults and animals perform such functions on a routine basis. Another suggestion is to make toilet training as easy and simple as possible. Important considerations are the selection of the child's clothing and the potty chair or use of the toilet. A freestanding potty chair allows children a feeling of security (Fig. 12-5, *A*). Planting the feet firmly on the floor also facilitates defecation. Another option is a portable seat attached to the regular toilet, which may ease the transition from potty chair to regular toilet. Placing a small bench under the feet helps stabilize the child's position. It is probably best to keep the potty in the bathroom and to let the child observe the excreta being flushed down the toilet to associate these activities with usual practices. If a potty chair is not available, having the child sit facing the toilet tank provides added support (Fig. 12-5, *B*). Practice sessions should be limited to 5 to 8 minutes, and a parent should stay with the child, practicing sanitary habits after every session. Children should be praised for cooperative behavior and successful evacuation. Dressing children in easily removed clothing; using training pants, "pull-on" diapers, or underwear; and encouraging imitation by watching others are other helpful suggestions.

When the child begins to experience regular daytime dryness, parents may experiment with underwear during the day. Daytime accidents are common, particularly during periods of intense activity. Young children become so engrossed in play activity that, if they are not reminded, they will wait until it is too late to reach the bathroom. Therefore, frequent reminders and trips to the toilet are necessary. Parents often forget to plan ahead when their toddlers are being toilet trained; before trips outside the house, it is important to remind children to at least try to urinate to decrease the chance of needing to use the toilet while the car is stuck in traffic.

As the child masters each step of toileting (discussion, undressing, going, wiping, dressing, flushing, and hand washing), he or she gains a sense of accomplishment that parents should reinforce. If the parent–child relationship becomes strained, both may need a break to focus on enjoyable activities together. Regression may coincide with a stressful family situation or the child being pushed too hard and too fast. Regression is a normal part of toilet training and does not mean failure

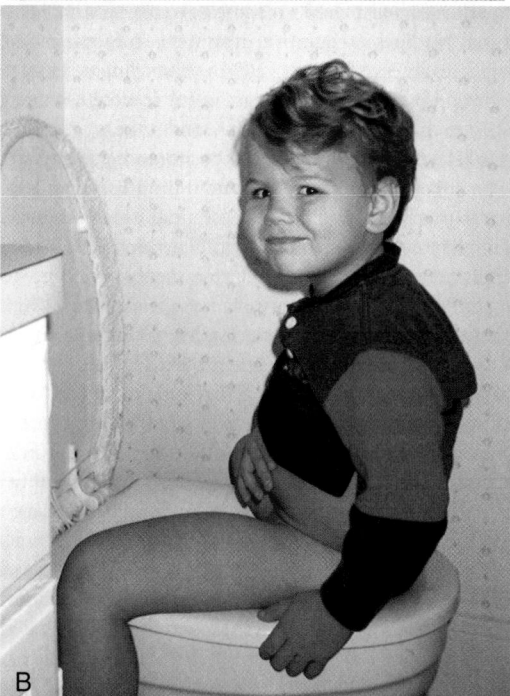

FIG 12-5 A, Children may begin toilet training sitting on a small potty chair. **B,** Sitting in reverse fashion on a regular toilet provides additional security to a young child. (**A,** © 2011 Photos.com, a division of Getty Images. All rights reserved.)

but should be viewed as a temporary setback to a more comfortable place for the child.

Daycare providers also play a role in the support and education of parents regarding toilet training practices. It is important for parents to inform all caregivers of their individual family values and the child's specific needs when planning for training away from home. Ensuring consistency in care of toddlers and ensuring healthy practices in a sanitary environment allow for safe and effective toilet practices in all settings.

Sibling Rivalry

Children have a natural jealousy and resentment toward a new child in the family or toward other children in the family when a parent turns his or her attention from them and interacts with their brother or sister; this is referred to as sibling rivalry.

The arrival of a new infant represents a crisis for even the best-prepared toddlers. They do not hate or resent the infant; rather, they hate the changes that this additional sibling produces, especially the separation from mother during the birth. The parents now share their love and attention with someone else, the usual routine is disrupted, and toddlers may lose their crib or room—all at a time when they thought they were in control of their world. Sibling rivalry tends to be most pronounced in firstborn children, who experience **dethronement** (loss of sole parental attention). It also seems to be most difficult for young children, particularly in terms of mother–child interaction.

Preparation of children for the birth of a sibling is individual but is dictated to some extent by age. For toddlers, *time* is a vague concept. Tomorrow could be yesterday or next week, and a month from now could be never. Preparing children too soon for the birth may lessen their interest by the time the event occurs. A good time to start talking about the baby is when toddlers become aware of the pregnancy and the changes taking place in the home in anticipation of the new member.

Toddlers need to have a realistic idea of what the newborn will be like. Telling them that a new playmate will come home soon sets up unrealistic expectations. Rather, parents should stress the activities that will take place when the baby arrives home, such as diapering, bottle feeding or breastfeeding, bathing, and dressing. At the same time, parents should emphasize which routines will stay the same, such as reading stories or going to the park. If toddlers have had no contact with an infant, it is a good idea to introduce them to one, if feasible. Providing a doll with which toddlers can imitate parental behaviors is another excellent strategy. They can tend to the doll's needs (diapering, feeding) at the same time the parent is performing similar activities for the infant.

A new sibling in the home is stressful, so any additional stresses for the toddler should be avoided or minimized. For example, moving the toddler to a regular bed or to a different room should be done well in advance of the infant's arrival.

Pregnancy is an abstraction for toddlers. They need concrete illustrations of how the baby is growing inside the mother. It is an excellent opportunity for introducing aspects of reproduction in simple terms that the child can comprehend. Seeing simple pictures of the uterus and fetus and feeling the fetus move help the child feel involved in the experience. Children also benefit from classes for siblings that may be part of prenatal sessions.

When the new baby arrives, toddlers keenly feel the changed focus of attention. Visitors may initiate problems when they inadvertently shower the infant with attention and presents while neglecting the older child. Parents can minimize this by alerting visitors to the toddler's needs, having small presents on hand for the toddler, and including the child in the visit as much as possible. The toddler can also help with the care of the newborn by getting diapers and doing other small tasks (Fig. 12-6).

How children exhibit jealousy is complex. Some will hit the infant, push the child off the mother's lap, or pull the bottle or breast from the infant's mouth. For this reason, infants must be protected by parental supervision of the interaction between the siblings. More often,

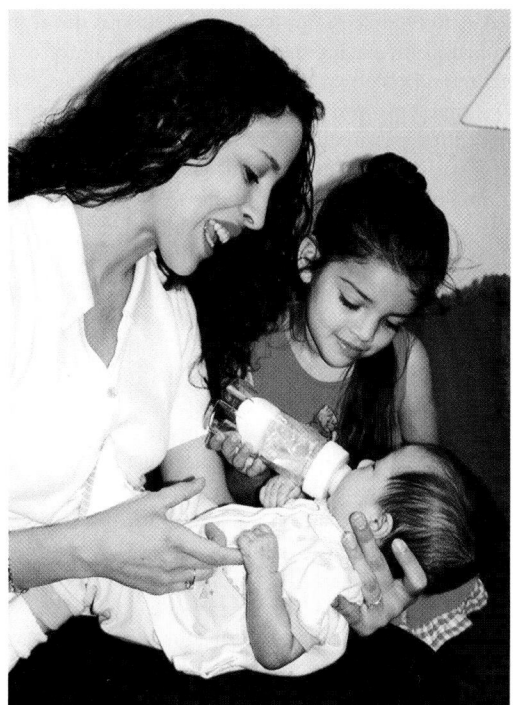

FIG 12-6 To minimize sibling rivalry, parents should include the toddler during caregiving activities.

however, the expressions of hostility and resentment are more subtle and covert. Toddlers may verbally express a wish that the infant "go back inside mommy," or they will revert to more infantile forms of behavior, such as demanding a bottle, soiling their underpants, clinging for attention, using baby talk, or aggressively acting out toward others. The latter is particularly common in preschoolers, who may seem accepting of the new sibling at home but behave poorly in daycare or preschool. This is a form of displacement that says, "I can't let my parents know how I feel, so I will tell you."

Temper Tantrums

Temper tantrums are nearly universal during toddlerhood as independence is established and more complex tasks are attempted that may overwhelm the child emotionally. Toddlers may assert their independence by violently objecting to discipline. They may lie down on the floor, kick their feet, and scream at the top of their lungs. Some have learned the effectiveness of holding their breath until the parent relents. Although holding one's breath may cause fainting from the lack of oxygen, the accumulation of carbon dioxide will stimulate the respiratory control center, resulting in no physical harm. Rarely, breath-holding spells can involve symmetric tonic-clonic movements, which can be frightening to parents; the child recovers quickly when the spell is over, and there is no residual damage (Stein, 2003). Tantrums are an indication of the child's inability to control emotions; toddlers are particularly prone to tantrums because their strong drive for mastery and autonomy is frustrated by adult figures or lack of motor and cognitive skills (Needlman, Howard, and Zuckerman, 1995).

The best approach toward tapering temper tantrums requires parental consistency and developmentally appropriate expectations and rewards. Ensuring consistency among all caregivers in expectations, prioritizing what rules are important, and developing consequences that are reasonable for the child's level of development help manage the behavior. For example, a popular time for a tantrum is before bed. Active toddlers often have trouble slowing down and, when placed in bed, resist staying there. Parents can reinforce consistency and expectations by stating, "After this story, it is bedtime." Starting at 18 months, time-outs work well for managing temper tantrums.

During tantrums, parents should ignore the behavior, provided the behavior is not injurious to the child, such as violently banging the head on the floor. They should continue to be present to provide a feeling of control and security to the child when the tantrum has subsided. At this time, a toy or a favorite activity can be substituted for the request (see also Limit Setting and Discipline, Chapter 3). During periods of no tantrums, parents can practice developmentally appropriate positive reinforcement.

Other suggestions for handling tantrums include the following (Needlman, Howard, and Zuckerman, 1995):
- Offering the child options instead of an "all or none" position
- Picking one's battles carefully and ignoring small skirmishes over unimportant issues
- Giving comfort when the child is able to control his or her emotions but not giving in to the original request
- Praising the child for positive behavior when he or she is not having a tantrum

Temper tantrums are common during the toddler years and essentially represent normal developmental behaviors. However, temper tantrums can be signs of serious problems. Nurses should be alert to situations that require further evaluation.

Negativism

One of the more difficult aspects of rearing children in this age group is their persistent "no" response to every request. The negativism is not an expression of being stubborn or insolent but a necessary assertion of self-control. Children test limits to gain understanding of the world and to learn to modify their behavior to fit the expectations of society. Negativism begins to subside as most children prepare to enter kindergarten.

One method of dealing with the negativism is to reduce the opportunities for a "no" answer. Asking the child, "Do you want to go to sleep now?" is an example of a question that will almost certainly be answered with an emphatic "no." Instead, tell the child that it is time to go to sleep and proceed accordingly. In their attempt to exert control, children like to make choices. When confronted with appropriate choices, such as "You may have a peanut butter and jelly sandwich or chicken noodle soup for lunch," they are more likely to choose one rather than automatically say no. However, if their response is negative, parents should make the choice for the child.

Nurses working with children and parents can assist parents in understanding this concept by role modeling. For example, when the nurse approaches the toddler for taking vital signs, instead of asking, "Can I listen to your heart?" the nurse can say, "I am going to listen to your heart." Because of normal developmental behavior, toddlers first resist having their vital signs taken because it is an intrusion on their bodies. Second, toddlers are most likely going to answer "no," not because they necessarily fear the procedure itself but because of the tendency to answer all questions with a negative response. If the nurse asks the question and the toddler says, "No" but the nurse proceeds anyway, the toddler starts to mistrust the nurse's actions because they contradict his or her words.

Regression

The retreat from one's present pattern of functioning to past levels of behavior is referred to as **regression**. It usually occurs in instances of discomfort or stress when one attempts to conserve psychic energy by reverting to patterns of behavior that were successful in earlier stages of development. Regression is common in toddlers because almost any additional stress hinders their ability to master present developmental tasks. Any threat to their autonomy, such as illness, hospitalization, separation from a parent, disruption of established routines, or adjustment to a new sibling, represents a need to revert to earlier forms of behavior, such as increased dependency; refusal to use the potty chair; temper tantrums; demand for the bottle or pacifier; and loss of newly learned motor, language, social, and cognitive skills.

At first, such regression appears acceptable and comfortable for children, but the loss of newly acquired achievements is frightening and threatening because children are aware of their helplessness. Parents become concerned about regressive behavior and frequently, in their efforts to deal with it, force the child to cope with an additional source of stress: the pressure to live up to expected standards. Brazelton (1999) suggests that these predictable times of regression, or **touchpoints**, are an opportunity to prepare parents for the next step in their child's development.

When regression does occur, the best approach is to ignore it while praising existing patterns of appropriate behavior. Regression is a child's way of saying, "I can't cope with this present stress and perfect this skill as well, but I will if given patience and understanding." For this reason, it is advisable not to attempt new areas of learning when an additional crisis is present or expected, such as beginning toilet training shortly before a sibling is born or during a brief period of hospitalization.

PROMOTING OPTIMAL HEALTH DURING TODDLERHOOD

NUTRITION

During the period from 12 to 18 months of age, the growth rate slows, decreasing the child's need for calories, protein, and fluid. However, the protein (13 g/day) and energy requirements are still relatively high to meet the demands for muscle tissue growth and high activity level. The need for minerals such as iron, calcium, and phosphorus may be difficult to meet, considering the characteristic food habits of children in this age group. Parents may be tempted to rely on vitamin supplementation, rather than a well-balanced diet, to meet these requirements. Toddlers usually require three meals and two snacks per day; however, the portions consumed are generally smaller compared with those of older children.

The 2008 Feeding Infants and Toddlers Study (FITS) (Butte, Fox, Briefel, and others, 2010) found that, in general, toddlers met or exceeded the requirements for daily energy and protein requirements. FITS recommended that toddlers be fed a more balanced diet of vegetables, fruits, and whole grains.

At approximately 18 months of age, most toddlers manifest this decreased nutritional need with a decreased appetite, a phenomenon known as **physiologic anorexia**. They become picky, fussy eaters with strong taste preferences. They may eat large amounts one day and almost nothing the next. Toddlers are increasingly aware of the nonnutritive function of food—the pleasure of eating, the social aspect of mealtime, and the control of refusing food. They are influenced by factors other than taste when choosing food. If a family member refuses to eat something, toddlers are likely to imitate that response. If the plate is overfilled, they are likely to push it away, overwhelmed by its size. If food does not appear or smell appetizing, they will probably not agree to try it. In essence, mealtime is more closely associated with psychologic components than with nutritional ones.

The ritualism of this age also dictates certain principles in feeding practices. Toddlers like to have the same dish, cup, or spoon every time they eat. They may reject a favorite food simply because it is served in a different dish. If one food touches another, they often refuse to eat it. Mixed foods, such as stews or casseroles, are rarely favorites. Because toddlers have unpredictable table manners, it is best to use plastic dishes and cups for both economic and safety reasons. For some children, a regular mealtime schedule also contributes to their desire and need for predictability and ritualism.

Developmentally, by 12 months of age, most children eat many of the same foods prepared for the rest of the family. Some may have mastered using a cup with occasional spilling, although most cannot adeptly use a spoon until 18 months of age or later and generally prefer using their fingers.

Nutritional Counseling

The emphasis on preventing childhood obesity and subsequent cardiovascular disease in the United States has prompted a number of changes in dietary recommendations for children and adults alike. It is now recognized that lifetime eating habits may be established in early childhood, and health care workers are increasingly emphasizing the role of food selection choices, exercise, stress reduction, and other lifestyle choices (tobacco and alcohol use) on the quality of adult life and survival. Conditions such as obesity and cardiovascular disease can be prevented by encouraging healthy eating habits in toddlers and their families.

If food is used as a reward or sign of approval, a child may overeat for nonnutritive reasons. If food is forced and mealtime is consistently unpleasant, the usual pleasure associated with eating may not develop. Mealtimes should be enjoyable rather than times for discipline or family arguments. The social aspect of mealtime may be distracting for young children; therefore, an earlier feeding hour may be appropriate. Young children are unable to sit through a long meal and become restless and disruptive. This is particularly common when children are brought to the table just after active play. Calling them in from play 15 minutes before mealtime allows them ample opportunity to get ready for eating while settling down their active minds and bodies.

The method of serving food also takes on more importance during this period. Toddlers need to have a sense of control and achievement in their abilities. Giving them large, adult-size portions can overwhelm them. In general, what is eaten is much more significant than how much is consumed. Toddlers usually restrict their food preference to four or five main foods and rarely try new foods; in some cases, a toddler may insist on one food such as mashed potatoes for lunch and dinner. Small amounts of meat and vegetables supply greater food value than a large consumption of bread or potato. Serving sizes need to be appropriate for age. Young children tend to like less spicy, bland food, although this is a culturally determined preference. Substitutions can be provided for foods that they do not enjoy, although parents need not cater to all of their desires. Frequent nutritious snacks can replace a meal. Grazing—nibbling and snacking—is a good way to ensure proper nutrition, provided that appropriate foods are offered.

Mastication skills continue to mature, putting children at risk for choking; therefore, large round foods (hot dogs, grapes, peas, carrots, popcorn, fruit gel snacks) should be avoided until the child is able to chew them effectively. Active play while eating should be discouraged to prevent choking. Appetite and food preferences are sporadic. Often the interest in food parallels a growth spurt, so that periods of good eating are interspersed with phases of poor eating. If exposed to the same food every day, a young toddler does not learn how to manage the complex sensory information needed to eat new, more difficult foods (e.g., vegetables with a different texture vs. pureed, slippery fruits). To help prevent "food jags," it is recommended that parents present food in various physical forms. The child may need to progress to eating new foods in a stepwise fashion such as visually tolerating the food, interacting with the food, smelling the food, touching the food, tasting the food, and then eating the food.

Many authorities consider this period of picky eating to be a developmental phase and stress that most toddlers will consume the necessary amount of food required for growth (Cathey and Gaylord, 2004). It has also been suggested that parents plan a nutritionally balanced week instead of day because of the way toddlers restrict food intake in their effort to exert control over their environment (Morin, 2007).

Dietary Guidelines

Dietary guidelines are necessary to promote adequate energy and nutrient intake to support physical, emotional, psychologic, and cognitive development. A number of new dietary guidelines have been developed to address the issue of childhood obesity, sedentary lifestyles, and increase in cardiovascular disease mortality in the United States.

The Institute of Medicine (IOM) (2005) has developed guidelines for nutritional intake that encompass the Recommended Daily Allowances (RDAs) yet extend their scope to include additional parameters related to nutritional intake. The Dietary Reference Intakes (DRIs)* are composed of four categories. These include Estimated Average Requirements (EARs) for age and gender categories, Tolerable Upper-Limit (UL) nutrient intakes that are associated with a low risk of adverse effects, Adequate Intakes (AIs) of nutrients, and new standard RDAs. The guidelines present information about lifestyle factors that may affect nutrient function, such as caffeine intake and exercise, and about how the nutrient may be related to chronic disease. An important factor in the development of the DRIs that affects children, particularly infants 0 to 6 months, is that the AIs are based on the nutrient intake of full-term, healthy, breastfed infants (by well-nourished mothers), which now represents the gold standard for infant nutrition in this age group. In 2010, new DRIs for vitamin D and calcium were released by the IOM.

The 2010 Dietary Guidelines for Americans may also be used to encourage healthy dietary intakes as well as regular exercise designed to decrease obesity and cardiovascular risk factors and subsequent cardiovascular disease, which is now known to occur in young children as well as adults. The 2010 Dietary Guidelines recommend a caloric intake for a moderately active boy, ages 2 to 3 years, of 1000 to 1400 calories per day. The emphasis in the Dietary Guidelines is in decreasing overall fat and sodium intakes and increasing the amount of daily exercise to reduce the incidence of obesity and cardiovascular disease. The 2010 Dietary Guidelines[†] are for children ages 2 years and older. The guidelines encourage a variety of fruits, vegetables, whole grains, and low-fat dairy and nonfat dairy products in addition to fish, beans, and lean meat.

> **NURSING TIP** A general guide to serving sizes for toddlers is 1 tbsp of solid food per year of age, or one fourth to one third of the adult portion size.
> - Use the tablespoon guide for easily measured foods such as vegetables or rice.
> - Use the fraction guide for bread or milk.

---

*http://www.iom.edu/Activities/Nutrition/SummaryDRIs/DRI-Tables.aspx.
†http://www.cnpp.usda.gov/DietaryGuidelines.htm.

Additional resources for dietary counseling include MyPlate*, recently developed by the U.S. Department of Agriculture to replace MyPyramid. This colorful plate shows the five main food groups—fruits, grains, vegetable, protein, and dairy—with the intended purpose to involve children and their families in making appropriate food choices for meals and decrease the incidence of overweight and obesity in the United States. MyPlate provides an online interactive feature that allows the individual to select (click on) an individual food group and see choices for foods in that group. Approximate serving sizes are suggested, and vegetarian substitutions are also provided.

Nutrition during toddlerhood involves a transition as a young toddler is weaned off milk- or formula-based diets. Milk intake, the chief source of calcium and phosphorus, should average two or three servings (24–30 oz) a day. More than a quart of milk consumption daily considerably limits the intake of solid foods, resulting in a deficiency of dietary iron and other nutrients. After 2 years of age, children can be given low-fat milk to reduce daily total fat to less than 30% of calories, saturated fatty acids to less than 10% of calories, and cholesterol to less than 300 mg. Other measures to reduce dietary fat include using lean meats, fat-modified products (e.g., low-fat cheese), and low-fat cooking. Because less fat in children's diets can also mean fewer calories and nutrients, caregivers must know what kinds of food to choose. *Trans* fatty acids and saturated fats, however, should be avoided.

Iron-fortified cereals and iron-rich foods are recommended for all children older than 6 months of age. Parents should be encouraged to provide an iron-rich diet that includes heme and nonheme iron sources (red meats, poultry, fish, green leafy vegetables, dried fruit, beans) and limit whole-milk consumption. Iron supplementation may be necessary in some cases. (See Constipation, Chapter 24, for information on dietary fiber intake for children.)

Calcium and vitamin D are essential for healthy bone development. Adequate Intake of calcium for children 1 to 3 years of age is 500 mg. Whole milk, cheese, yogurt, legumes (beans), and vegetables (broccoli, collard greens, kale) are good sources for calcium. Popular calcium-fortified foods include waffles, cereals and cereal bars, orange juice, and some white breads. Adequate vitamin D intake is essential to prevent rickets; it is now recommended that children and adolescents have an intake of at least 400 IU of vitamin D daily (AAP, 2008). Multivitamin preparations containing 400 IU of vitamin D (by tablet or liquid) are adequate if food intake is poor or exposure to sunlight is minimal; vitamin D–only preparations containing 400 IU are also available commercially (Wagner, Greer, and AAP, Section on Breastfeeding and Committee on Nutrition, 2008). Sources of vitamin D include fish, fish oils, and egg yolks. Fortified cereals, dairy products, and meat are also good sources of zinc and vitamin E.

It is also recommended that toddlers have 1 cup of fruit each day. Vitamin C enhances iron absorption. Toddlers should consume approximately 4 to 6 oz of juice per day. It tastes good to toddlers and is readily available. A 6-oz glass of fruit juice equals one fruit serving; however, juices lack the fiber of whole fruit and should not be a substitution for whole fruit. High intake of juice can contribute to diarrhea, overnutrition or undernutrition, and the development of caries; thus, only 4 to 6 oz of 100% fruit juice per day is recommended for toddlers (AAP, Committee on Nutrition, 2009). Fruit-flavored drinks advertised as juices may not actually contain 100% juice and should be avoided.

Vegetarian Diets

Vegetarian diets have become increasingly popular in the United States because people are concerned about hypertension; cholesterol; obesity; cardiovascular disease; cancer of the stomach, intestine, and colon; and the influence of the animal rights movement. The American Dietetic Association and Dietitians of Canada (2003) issued a statement endorsing vegetarian diets for adults and children; the statement further notes that well-planned vegetarian diets are adequate for all stages of the life cycle and promote normal growth. Children and adolescents on vegetarian diets have the potential for lifelong healthy diets and have been shown to have lower intakes of cholesterol, saturated fat, and total fat and higher intakes of fruits, fiber, and vegetables than nonvegetarians (American Dietetic Association and Dietitians of Canada, 2003).

The major types of vegetarianism are:

Lacto-ovo vegetarians, who exclude meat from their diet but consume dairy products and rarely fish

Lactovegetarians, who exclude meat and eggs but drink milk

Pure vegetarians (vegans), who eliminate all foods of animal origin, including milk and eggs

Macrobiotics, who are even more restrictive than pure vegetarians, allowing only a few types of fruits, vegetables, and legumes

Semi-vegetarians, who consume a lacto-ovo vegetarian diet with some fish and poultry. This is an increasingly popular form of vegetarianism and poses little or no nutritional risk to infants unless dietary fat and cholesterol intake is severely restricted.

Many individuals who are concerned about healthy diets subscribe to vegetarian diets that may not be typified by the above categories. Therefore, during nutritional assessment, it is necessary to clearly list exactly what the diet includes and excludes.*

The major deficiencies that may occur in the stricter vegan diets are inadequate protein for growth; inadequate calories for energy and growth; poor digestibility of many of the bulky natural, unprocessed foods, especially for infants; and deficiencies of vitamin B_6, niacin, riboflavin, vitamin D, iron, calcium, and zinc. Strict vegan diets also require supplements of vitamin B_{12} and vitamin D. Vitamin D is essential if exposure to sunlight is inadequate ($\approx$5 to 15 min/day on the hands, arms, and face of light-skinned persons; slightly more in darker pigmented individuals) or in persons who are dark skinned or who live in northern latitudes or cloudy or smoky areas. Many of these deficiencies can be avoided in children who are not consuming 100% of the RDA of vitamins and minerals with a multivitamin and mineral supplement (Dunham and Kollar, 2006).

Evaluate for iron-deficiency anemia and rickets in children on strict vegetarian and macrobiotic diets; this may occur as a result of consuming plant foods such as unrefined cereals, which impair the absorption of iron, calcium, and zinc. The American Dietetic Association and Dietitians of Canada (2003) and AAP, Committee on Nutrition (2009) recommend iron supplementation of 1 mg/kg/day in infants exclusively breastfed after 4 to 6 months of age by vegetarian mothers and no dietary fat restrictions in vegetarian children younger than age 2 years. Other factors that affect iron absorption are listed in Box 12-2.

Achieving a nutritionally adequate vegetarian diet is not difficult (except with the strictest diets), but it requires careful planning and knowledge of nutrient sources (AAP, Committee on Nutrition, 2009). For children, the lacto-ovo vegetarian diet is nutritionally adequate;

---

*http://www.cnpp.usda.gov/MyPlate.htm.

*Additional information regarding vegetarian diets may be found at the Vegetarian Resource Group; 410-366-8343; http://www.vrg.org. Another helpful resource for adolescents and parents is the KidsHealth website: http://kidshealth.org/parent/nutrition_center/dietary_needs/vegetarianism.html.

BOX 12-2   FACTORS THAT AFFECT IRON ABSORPTION

Increase

Acidity (low pH)—Administer iron between meals (gastric hydrochloric acid).
Ascorbic acid (vitamin C)—Administer iron with juice, fruit, or multivitamin preparation.
Vitamin A
Calcium
Tissue (cellular) need
Meat, fish, poultry
Cooking in cast iron pots

Decrease

Alkalinity (high pH)—Avoid any antacid preparation.
Phosphates—Milk is unfavorable vehicle for iron administration.
Phytates—Found in cereals
Oxalates—Found in many fruits and vegetables (plums, currants, green beans, spinach, sweet potatoes, tomatoes)
Tannins—Found in tea, coffee
Tissue (cellular) saturation
Malabsorptive disorders
Disturbances that cause diarrhea or steatorrhea
Infection

however, the vegan diet requires supplementation with vitamins D and B$_{12}$ for children ages 2 to 12 years.

To ensure sufficient protein in the diet, foods with incomplete proteins (those that do not have all the essential amino acids) must be eaten at the same meal with other foods that supply the missing amino acids. The three basic combinations of foods consumed by vegetarians that generally provide the appropriate amounts of essential amino acids are:

1. Grains (cereal, rice, pasta) and legumes (beans, peas, lentils, peanuts)
2. Grains and milk products (milk, cheese, yogurt)
3. Seeds (sesame, sunflower) and legumes

Additional dietary considerations for young children are found in Chapter 13.

COMPLEMENTARY AND ALTERNATIVE MEDICINE

There are four complementary and alternative medicine (CAM) domains according to the National Center for Complementary and Alternative Medicine (NCCAM); this discussion centers only on one of those—biologically based practices, which include herbs, vitamins, and foods. NCCAM (2010) classifies probiotics as a type of natural product and CAM. Many CAM products are sold over the counter as dietary supplements, but the use of some dietary supplements such as calcium for bone health or a multivitamin supplement are not considered to be CAM (NCCAM, 2010). The NCCAM (2010) reports that natural products are the most commonly used CAM products in children and most often these products are used for chronic conditions such as neck and back pain and for head and chest colds. Other surveys confirm that CAM is often used for children's chronic remedies for which traditional therapy is not effective (Huillet, Erdie-Lalena, Norvell, and others, 2011).

The misuse of vitamins as a part of CAM has the potential for placing some children at risk for health problems. Sawni, Ragothaman, Thomas, and others (2007) noted that of persons reportedly using

CAM, the most common CAM remedies used in children seen in the emergency department were home or folk remedies (59%), herbs (41%), prayer for healing (14%), and massage therapy (10%). A survey in a WIC (Women, Infants, and Children) clinic found that child herbal use was common, especially among Hispanic children attending the clinic. Some of the herbs used by the children in the survey (St. John's wort, dong quai, and kava) have questionable safety (Lohse, Stotts, and Priebe, 2006). A recent study of CAM use in children on a military base found that 23% of parents reported using CAM in their children, with herbal therapy being the most common type of CAM reported; 50% of the parents who used CAM for their children reported the use of vitamins and minerals in amounts that exceeded the RDA (Huillet, Erdie-Lalena, Norvell, and others, 2011).

There is concern that terms often used to market supplements such as megavitamins may mislead parents regarding the actual benefits (or harm) of such therapies. The intention herein is not to discredit the use of CAM such as vitamin supplements; rather, it is to ensure safety and efficacy in children who may experience inadvertent harm. The use of various herbal therapies, or intake of herbs, is also becoming more popular; many of these have been a part of medicine since early days and are beneficial in some cases. Many mind–body CAM therapies (e.g., guided imagery, distraction) have proved beneficial for children undergoing cancer treatment, but the small sample sizes of the groups being studied may preclude generalization to a larger population group until further studies are undertaken (Landier and Tse, 2010).

Herbs known to have adverse effects in children include ephedra, comfrey, and pennyroyal; some herbs may not be harmful taken alone but may counteract or potentiate prescription medications when taken together. Parents should be fully informed of the use of herbs to ensure that there is more benefit than potential harm in the ingredients being used. Health care workers also need to be knowledgeable of the benefits or potential harm in herbs to appropriately counsel parents and address their concerns. Little research has been performed in children on many over-the-counter (OTC) herbal medicines, yet some herbs are known to cause harm in children (Gardiner and Kemper, 2011; Lanski, Greenwald, Perkins, and others, 2003; Loman, 2003). Parents should be cautioned not to exceed the upper limits of vitamin intake according to the new DRIs (see p. 391).*

SLEEP AND ACTIVITY

Total sleep decreases only slightly during the second year and averages about 11 to 12 hours a day. Most children take one nap a day but may relinquish this habit by the end of the second or third year. Children reach an adult pattern of sleep by 3 years of age.

Sleep problems are common, especially going to bed and falling asleep, and are a response to fears and awareness of separation. Toddlers are more prone to having bedtime resistance (refusal to go to bed) and frequent night waking; during later toddlerhood, this group of children may become more resistant about going to bed and express fears about monsters (Meltzer and Mindell, 2006). Fears can be provoked by a child's daily stressors such as pressure to toilet train, moves, sibling birth, experiences of loss, or separation from parents. Establishing a regular bedtime and routine before bedtime is helpful, and providing transitional objects, such as a favorite stuffed animal or blanket,

*Helpful websites for health care and consumer information concerning herbs are NCCAM, http://www.nccam.nih.gov; American Botanical Council, http://abc.herbalgram.org; and Herb Research Foundation, http://www.herbs.org.

can ease the child's insecurity at bedtime (see Fig. 12-3). Children may need a light snack before bedtime; a heavy meal immediately before bedtime may interfere with sleep. Other suggestions to help small children sleep better include keeping the television out of the child's room, making the hour before bedtime a quiet time of reading stories, and avoiding stimulating activities such as computer games and rough-housing (Owens, 2011). Toddlers no longer sleeping in a crib may come out of their rooms after being put to bed. Limit prolonged bedtime rituals by defining a length of time and set of activities (one more story, one more drink). Toddlers who are too immature to respond to the measures identified may need their doorways gated.

A toddler's activity level is high, and there is rarely a problem with too little physical exercise, provided inappropriate restrictions are not instituted. Recently, however, there has been concern that decreased time spent in actual physical play and more time involved with computers and television watching have increased the tendency toward being overweight. This is especially true in large urban centers during the winter months where there may not be adequate "safe" play and physical exercise space. With increasing numbers of young children being cared for outside the home, attention to the kinds of activity provided is important. For example, children with high activity levels may benefit from an environment that encourages vigorous play whether outside or in a large indoor play area.

With increasing numbers of young children being cared for outside the home, attention to the kinds of activity provided is important. For example, children with high activity levels may benefit from an environment in which outdoor play is encouraged. Neurodevelopment is necessary for developing children to participate in activities.

DENTAL HEALTH

Regular Dental Examinations

The American Academy of Pediatric Dentistry (AAPD) (2011a) recommends that every child have an oral health examination by a practitioner by 6 months of age; if the child is in a high-risk category for caries, it is recommended that an initial visit to a dentist or pedodontist (pediatric dentist) occur by age 6 months or within 6 months of the eruption of the first tooth. Every child should have an established dental home by the age of 12 months (AAPD, 2011a). Initial visits to the dentist should be nontraumatizing. Because toddlers react negatively to new and potentially frightening experiences, the initial visit can center around meeting the dentist, seeing the equipment, and sitting in the chair. If the child is cooperative, the dentist may just look at the teeth but reserve a more thorough examination for another visit. Modeling, in which the child observes procedures performed on the parent or a cooperative sibling, can also be effective but may not work on all toddlers.

Plaque Removal

Oral hygiene measures should be implemented according to the suggested schedule noted above to remove plaque, soft bacterial deposits that adhere to the teeth and cause dental caries (decay or cavities) and periodontal (gum) disease. Poor oral hygiene and poor dietary habits are associated with the development of caries in children.

The most effective methods for plaque removal are brushing and flossing. Several brushing techniques exist, although there is no universal agreement regarding the best method. One that is suitable for cleaning the primary teeth is the scrub method. The tips of the bristles are placed firmly at a 45-degree angle against the teeth and gums and moved back and forth in a vibratory motion. The ends of the bristles should be wiggling but not moving forcefully back and forth, which

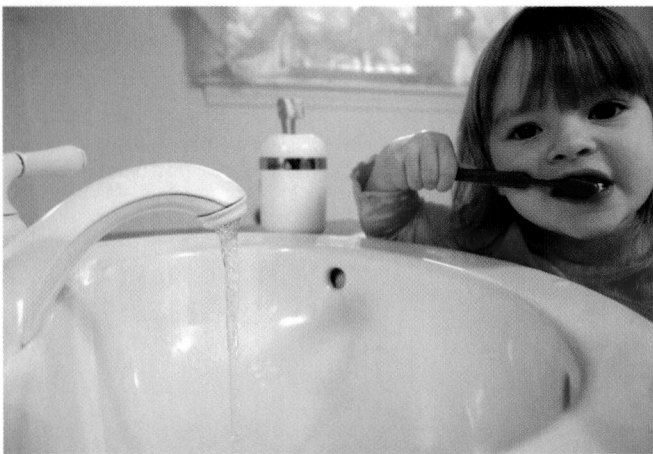

FIG 12-7 Young children can participate in toothbrushing, but parents need to brush all of the child's teeth thoroughly. (© 2011 Photos.com, a division of Getty Images. All rights reserved.)

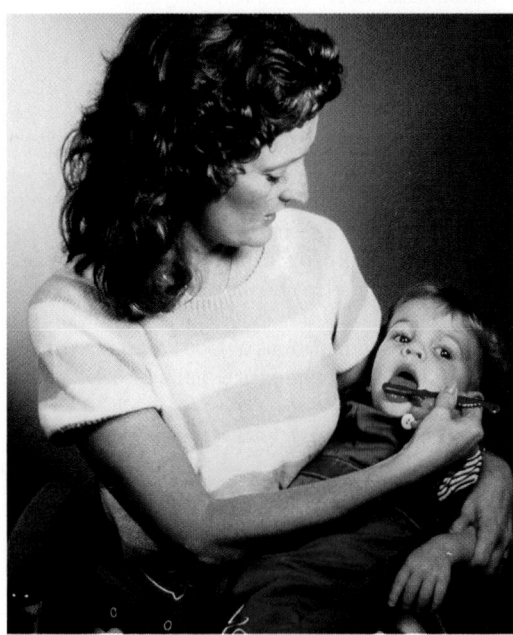

FIG 12-8 The most effective cleaning of teeth is done by parents.

can damage the gums and enamel. All the surfaces of the teeth are cleaned in this manner except the lingual (inner) surfaces of the anterior teeth. To clean these surfaces, the toothbrush is placed vertical to the teeth and moved up and down. Only a few teeth are brushed at one time, using six to eight strokes for each section. A systematic approach is used so that all surfaces are thoroughly cleaned (Fig. 12-7).

For young children, the most effective cleaning is done by parents (Fig. 12-8). Several positions can be used that facilitate access to the mouth and help stabilize the head for comfort:
- Stand with the child's back toward the adult. (When done in front of a bathroom mirror, both the child and the adult can see what is being done in the mirror.)
- Sit on a couch or bed with the child's head resting in the adult's lap.
- Sit on the floor or a stool with the child's head resting between the adult's thighs.

Use one hand to cup the chin and one to brush the teeth. For easier access to back teeth, hold the mouth partially open. After brushing with a fluoridated paste or gel, avoid rinsing the mouth to maximize the beneficial effects of the fluoride (AAPD, 2011b).

> **NURSING TIP**
> - To encourage children to open their mouths, ask them to "tweet like a bird" or to say "cheese" to brush the front teeth, and to "roar like a lion" to brush the back teeth.
> - Sing, tell stories, or talk to children during teeth cleaning to prevent boredom.

For effective cleaning, a small toothbrush with soft, rounded, multitufted nylon bristles that are short and uniform in length is recommended. Nylon bristles dry more rapidly after use and retain their shape better than natural bristles. Toothbrushes are replaced as soon as the bristles are frayed or bent. With young children, brushing may be more easily accomplished using only water because many children dislike the foam from toothpaste, and the foam interferes with visibility. There is also the danger of swallowing fluoridated toothpaste (see following discussion under Fluoride). Introduce toothpaste around 2 years of age and allow children to select the flavor they like to encourage the brushing habit. Use a pea-sized amount of toothpaste for children 2 to 5 years of age (apply across the narrow width of the toothbrush, rather than along its length, to decrease the chance of applying an excessive amount); only a "smear" of toothpaste should be used in children younger than 2 years of age if paste is used.

After the teeth have been cleaned, the teeth are flossed to remove plaque and debris from between the teeth and below the gum margin, where brushing is ineffective. Because young children do not have the dexterity to manipulate dental floss, parents must perform the procedure.

Ideally, the teeth should be cleaned after each meal and especially before bedtime, and the child should be given nothing to eat or drink after the night brushing except water. At times when brushing is impractical, the "swish-and-swallow" method of cleaning the mouth is taught; with a mouthful of water the child rinses the mouth and swallows, repeating the procedure three or four times.*

Fluoride

Fluoride supplementation should be considered for any child older than the age of 6 months whose drinking water is deficient in fluoride. Supplementation based on fluoride concentration of water supply less than 0.3 ppm (parts per million) is 0.25 mg for a child 6 months to 3 years of age and 0.5 mg for a child 3 to 6 years of age (AAPD, 2011b).

Fluoride, a mineral, is found in water, foods, or drinks in which fluoridated water was used as part of the processing system. Because the water fluoridation process and manufacturing of fluoride toothpaste are almost impossible to standardize in the United States, the dosage of fluoride supplements has been lowered to reduce the incidence of fluorosis (Table 12-2). Increased fluoride ingestion leads to enamel protein retention, hypomineralization of the enamel and dentin, and disturbance of crystal formation. The effects caused by this change range from barely discernible white fiberlike lines or spots to gray-brown stains or pitted areas. Parents should be cautioned against regular use of fluoridated water or beverages such as bottled water containing fluoride if the community water supply already has an adequate amount of fluoride.

---

*More detailed information can be obtained from the AAPD, http://www.aapd.org.

TABLE 12-2 FLUORIDE SUPPLEMENTATION*

AGE	WATER FLUORIDE CONTENT (PPM)	
	0.3	0.3–0.6
Birth–6 months	0	0
6 months–3 years	0.25	0
3–6 years	0.50	0.25
6–16 years	1.00	0.50

From American Academy of Pediatric Dentistry: Guideline on fluoride therapy. In *AAPD reference manual 2010–2011*, 2011, retrieved June 19, 2011, from http://www.aapd.org/media/policies.asp.
ppm, Parts per million.
*Fluoride daily doses are given in milligrams.

Topical fluoride treatments (e.g., fluoride varnish) performed in the dental home are also effective in decreasing caries (AAPD, 2011b).

Dietary Factors

Diet is critical to developing good teeth because the carious process depends primarily on fermentable sugars, especially sucrose, and other carbohydrates. Refined table sugar, honey, molasses, corn syrup, and dried fruits such as raisins are highly cariogenic. Complex carbohydrates, such as breads, potatoes, and pasta, also contribute to caries because they lower the plaque pH. Beverages that are commonly consumed by children and adolescents and snacks are also highly cariogenic and may contribute to the incidence of overweight and obesity (AAPD, 2011c).

Ideally, highly cariogenic foods, especially those containing complex sugars, should be eliminated. However, because this is impractical, some suggestions can be helpful. First, *the frequency with which sugar is consumed is more important than the total amount eaten.* Therefore, when sweets are eaten, they are less damaging if consumed immediately after a meal rather than as a snack between meals. When sweets are served as the dessert, the teeth can be cleaned afterward, decreasing the amount of time the sugar is in the mouth.

Second, the form of sugar (sucrose) is important. The more cariogenic foods are those that are sticky or hard because they remain in the mouth longer. Consequently, sucking on lollipops is more cariogenic than eating a chocolate bar. Sometimes the source of the sugar is "hidden," as in numerous prescription and nonprescription drugs and in many popular cereals, including the "all-natural" variety. Reading food labels is essential in eliminating sources of sucrose.

Some snacks do not contribute to tooth decay. Aged cheeses, such as cheddar, may alter the pH and delay bacterial growth. Sugarless gum chewed after eating may actually protect against cavities by stimulating saliva that neutralizes acid.

A special form of tooth decay in children between 18 months and 3 years of age is early childhood caries (ECC) (historically called *nursing caries* or *baby bottle tooth decay*) (Fig. 12-9). This often occurs when a child is routinely given a bottle of milk or juice at naptime or bedtime or uses the bottle as a pacifier while awake. Frequent nocturnal breastfeeding for prolonged periods also leads to extensive destruction of the teeth. The practice of coating pacifiers in honey can also contribute to caries and may be a potential source of botulism. As the sweet liquid pools in the mouth, the teeth are bathed for several hours in this cariogenic environment. Prolonged bottle feeding well into toddler years in some cultures may contribute to significant ECC (Brotanek,

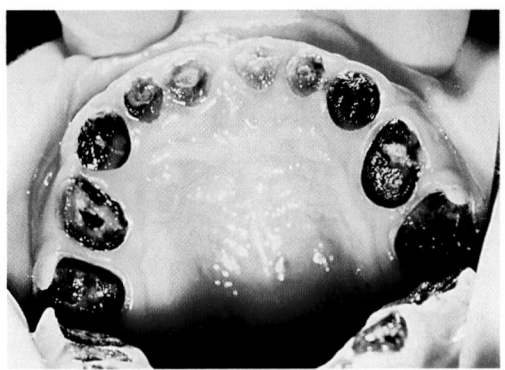

FIG 12-9 Early childhood caries. (Courtesy Bruce Carter, DDS, Texas Children's Hospital, Houston.)

Schroer, Valentyn, and others, 2009). In one group, prolonging bottle feeding into toddlerhood was perceived as "buying time" to decrease the child's crying (Freeman and Stevens, 2008). The maxillary (upper) incisors and molars are affected most because the mandibular (lower) incisors are protected by the lower lip, tongue, and saliva. Severely decayed teeth may require the application of stainless steel bands to preserve the spacing until the permanent teeth erupt.

Early childhood caries is now considered to be an infectious disease of childhood. There is evidence that *Streptococcus mutans* is a highly cariogenic bacteria (AAPD, 2011d). One of the early origins of *S. mutans* is the mother's saliva; infants of mothers with high counts of the bacteria have a greater incidence of ECC. Therefore, it is important to discuss oral hygiene with pregnant women because of its impact on their children's tooth development.

Prevention involves eliminating the bedtime bottle completely, feeding the last bottle before bedtime, substituting a bottle of water for milk or juice, not using the bottle as a pacifier, and never coating pacifiers in sweet substances. Juice in bottles, especially commercially available ready-to-use bottles, is discouraged; these beverages are especially damaging because the sugar is more readily converted to acid. Juice should always be offered in a cup to avoid prolonging the bottle-feeding habit. Toddlers should be encouraged to drink from a cup at the first birthday and weaned from a bottle by 14 months of age. Nurses are in an excellent position to counsel parents regarding the dangers of this habit and other aspects of dental care.*

SAFETY PROMOTION AND INJURY PREVENTION

According to recent data from the Centers for Disease Control and Prevention (CDC) (Borse, Gilchrist, Delinger, and others, 2008), children ages 1 to 4 years had the second highest rate of deaths from accidental injuries in the United States during the period from 2000 to 2006; the group with the highest number of deaths (56%) from accidental injuries were children ages 15 to 19 years. Boys were involved almost twice as often as girls in deaths attributed to unintentional injury. Among children ages 1 to 4 years of age, the leading causes for

---

*Sources of information about nursing caries and other aspects of child dental health include the National Institute of Dental and Craniofacial Research, National Institutes of Health, Bethesda, MD 20892-2190; 301-496-4261; http:// www.nidcr.nih.gov; American Academy of Pediatric Dentistry, 211 E. Chicago Ave., Suite 1700, Chicago, IL 60611; 312-337-2169; http://www.aapd.org; American Dental Association, 211 E. Chicago Ave., Chicago, IL 60611; 312-440-2500; http://www.ada.org/; and Canadian Dental Association, 1815 Alta Vista Drive, Ottawa, ON K1G 3Y6; 613-523–1770; http://www.cda-adc.ca.

death were transportation related (including motor vehicle occupant, pedestrian, and pedal cyclist), drowning, and fires or burns. Deaths from accidental poisoning were higher among infants and adolescents than toddlers. Nonfatal injuries in children ages 1 to 4 years of age occurred as a result of falls (leading cause) followed by being struck by or against something and bites or stings (including dog bites and bee or other insect attacks). Nonfatal drowning injury rates and nonfatal accidental poisoning were higher among children ages 1 to 4 years than any other age group.

A major factor in the critical increase of injuries during early childhood is the unrestricted freedom achieved through locomotion combined with an unawareness of danger within the environment. Toddlers delight in the repetitive use of gross motor skills, and with increasing age, these skills are refined. This age group is also very curious about how things work and exploration of previously unknown or unseen objects and places is common. Toddlers also have not fully developed or understand the cause-and-effect principles older children have and often are unable to gauge danger; poorly developed depth perception may also contribute to falls and tumbles as does the general bodily structure of toddlers.

Nonaccidental trauma is a term used to denote child physical abuse, whether the etiology is suspected or confirmed, without the stigma of the term *child abuse*. Toddlers are at particular risk for nonaccidental trauma because of their tendency to be mobile and curious yet clumsy and uncoordinated; the toddlers' inability to control emotions at times and the tendency toward negativism further place them at high risk for nonaccidental trauma (see Chapter 14).

Specific categories of injuries and appropriate prevention are best understood by associating them with the major growth and developmental achievements of this age (Table 12-3). The discussions of injuries in Chapters 1 and 10 are also relevant to safety concerns at this age.

Motor Vehicle Safety

Motor vehicle injuries cause more accidental deaths in all pediatric age groups after age 1 year than any other type of injury or disease and are responsible for almost half of all accidental deaths among children ages 1 to 4 years. Many of the deaths are caused by injuries within the car when restraints have not been used or have been used improperly. Unrestrained children riding in the vehicle's front seat are at highest risk for injury. Approved restraints properly installed and applied can prevent many fatalities and injuries. Motor vehicle back-over injuries and deaths, along with deaths or serious injury resulting from heat stroke when left in a car, account for a large number of motor vehicle–related injuries in children (CDC, 2005; McLaren, Null, and Quinn, 2005).

Car Restraints

Nurses are responsible for educating parents regarding the importance of car restraints and their proper use. Five types of restraints are available: (1) infant-only devices, (2) convertible models for both infants and toddlers, (3) boosters, (4) safety belts, and (5) devices for children with disabilities (see Chapter 18). Chapter 10 discusses the infant-type restraints; convertible restraints and boosters are included here. Convertible restraints are suitable for infants and toddlers in the rearward-facing position (Fig. 12-10). It is now recommended that all infants and toddlers ride in rear-facing car safety seats until they reach the age of 2 years or the height recommended by the car seat manufacturer (Durbin and Committee on Injury, Violence, Poison Prevention, 2011). Many rear-facing car safety seats can accommodate children weighing up to a maximum of 35 pounds (according to the manufacturer's

TABLE 12-3   INJURY PREVENTION DURING EARLY CHILDHOOD

DEVELOPMENTAL ABILITIES RELATED TO RISK OF INJURY	INJURY PREVENTION
Motor Vehicles	
Walks, runs, and climbs	Use federally approved car restraint per manufacturer's recommendations for weight and height.
Able to open doors and gates	Supervise child while playing outside.
Can ride tricycle	Do not allow child to play on curb or behind a parked car.
Can throw ball and other objects	Do not permit child to play in pile of leaves, snow, or large cardboard container in trafficked area.
	Supervise tricycle riding; have child wear helmet.
	Limit playing in driveways with parked cars or provide physical barriers limiting access.
	Lock fences and doors if not directly supervising children.
	Teach child to obey pedestrian safety rules:
	• Obey traffic regulations; cross only at crosswalks and only when traffic signal indicates it is safe.
	• Stand back a step from the curb until it is time to cross.
	• Look left, right, and left again and check for turning cars before crossing street.
	• Use sidewalks; when there is no sidewalk, walk on the left, facing traffic.
	• Wear light colors at night and attach fluorescent material to clothing.
Drowning	
Able to explore if left unsupervised	Supervise closely when near any source of water, including buckets.
Has great curiosity	Never, under any circumstance, leave unsupervised in bathtub.
Helpless in water; unaware of its danger; depth of water has no significance	Keep bathroom doors closed and lid down on toilet.
	Have fence around swimming pool and lock gate.*
Burns	
Able to reach heights by climbing, stretching, and standing on toes	Turn pot handles toward back of stove.
Pulls objects	Place electric appliances, such as coffee maker and popcorn machine, toward back of counter.
Explores any holes or opening	Place guardrails in front of radiators, fireplaces, and other heating elements.
Can open drawers and closets	Store matches and cigarette lighters in locked or inaccessible area; discard carefully.
Unaware of potential sources of heat or fire	Place burning candles, incense, hot foods, and cigarettes out of reach.
Plays with mechanical objects	Do not let tablecloth hang within child's reach.
	Do not let electric cord from iron or other appliance hang within child's reach.
	Cover electrical outlets with protective plastic caps.
	Keep electrical wires hidden or out of reach.
	Do not allow child to play with electrical appliance, wires, or lighters.
	Stress danger of open flames; teach what "hot" means.
	Always check bathwater temperature; adjust water heater temperature to 49° C (120° F) or lower; do not allow children to play with faucets.
	Apply a sunscreen when child is exposed to sunlight (all year round).
Accidental Poisoning	
Explores by putting objects in mouth	Place all potentially toxic agents, including cosmetics, personal care items, cleaning products, pesticides, and medications, out of reach or in a locked cabinet.
Can open drawers, closets, and most containers	Caution against eating nonedible items, such as plants.
Climbs	Replace medications or poisons immediately in locked cabinet; replace child-guard caps promptly.
Cannot read labels	Administer medications as a drug, not as a candy.
Does not know safe dose or amount	Do not store large surplus of toxic agents.
	Promptly discard empty poison containers; never reuse to store a food item or other poison.
	Teach child not to play in trash containers.
	Never remove labels from containers of toxic substances.
	Know number of nearest poison control center: **800-222-1222.**
Falls	
Able to open doors and some windows	Use window guards; do not rely on screens to stop falls.
Goes up and down stairs	Place gates at top and bottom of stairs.
Depth perception unrefined	Keep doors locked or use childproof doorknob covers at entry to stairs, high porch, or other elevated area, including laundry chute.
	Ensure safe and effective barriers on porches, balconies, decks.
	Remove unsecured or scatter rugs.

*Detailed guidelines for swimming pool safety may be found at http://www.poolsafely.gov.

Continued

TABLE 12-3	**INJURY PREVENTION DURING EARLY CHILDHOOD—cont'd**
DEVELOPMENTAL ABILITIES RELATED TO RISK OF INJURY	**INJURY PREVENTION**
	Apply nonskid decals in bathtub or shower.
	Keep crib rails fully raised and mattress at lowest level.
	Place carpeting under crib and in bathroom.
	Keep large toys and bumper pads out of crib or play yard (child can use these as "stairs" to climb out) and then move to youth bed when child is able to climb out of crib.
	Avoid using mobile walker, especially near stairs.
	Dress in safe clothing (soles that do not "catch" on floor, tied shoelaces, pant legs that do not touch floor).
	Keep child restrained in vehicle; never leave unattended in vehicle or shopping cart.
	Never leave child unattended in high chair.
	Supervise at playgrounds; select play areas with soft ground cover and safe equipment.
Choking and Suffocation	
Puts things in mouth	Avoid large, round chunks of meat, such as whole hot dogs (slice lengthwise into short pieces).
May swallow hard or inedible pieces of food	Avoid fruit with pits, fish with bones, hard candy, chewing gum, nuts, popcorn, grapes, and marshmallows.
	Choose large, sturdy toys without sharp edges or small removable parts.
	Discard old refrigerators, ovens, and so on, and remove the door.
	Install smoke and carbon monoxide alarms; change batteries every 6 months.
	Develop a fire escape plan for the entire family and have drills.
	Keep automatic garage door transmitter in an inaccessible place.
	Select safe toy boxes or chests without heavy, hinged lids.
	Keep venetian blind cords out of child's reach.
	Remove drawstrings from clothing; shorten essential drawstrings to 15.24 cm (6 inches) or less.
	Avoid contact with round, hollow, semirigid plastic items such as half of a plastic ball.
Bodily Injury	
Still clumsy in many skills	Avoid giving sharp or pointed objects (e.g., knives, scissors, or toothpicks) especially when walking or running.
Easily distracted from tasks	Do not allow lollipops or similar objects in mouth when walking or running.
Unaware of potential danger from strangers or other people	Teach safety precautions (e.g., to carry knife or scissors with pointed end away from face).
	Store all dangerous tools, garden equipment, and firearms in locked cabinet.
	Be alert to danger of unsupervised animals and household pets.
	Use safety glass on large glassed areas, such as sliding glass doors.
	Teach child name, address, and phone number and to ask for help from appropriate people (cashier, security guard, policeman) if lost; have identification on child (sewn in clothes, inside shoe).
	Teach stranger safety:
	• Avoid personalized clothing in public places.
	• Never go with a stranger.
	• Tell parents if anyone makes child feel uncomfortable in any way.
	• Always listen to child's concerns regarding others' behavior.
	• Teach child to say "no" when confronted with uncomfortable situations.

specifications).* Studies indicate that toddlers up to 24 months of age are safer riding in convertible seats in the rear-facing position (Bull and Durbin, 2008; Henary, Sherwood, Crandall, and others, 2007). In Sweden, children ride in a rear-facing car safety seat until the age of 4 years, at which time they transition to a booster seat (Durbin and Committee on Injury, Violence, and Poison Prevention, 2011).

Children ages 2 years and older (or those younger than 2 years) who have outgrown the rear-facing height or weight limit for their car safety seat should use a forward-facing car safety seat with a harness up to the maximum height or weight recommended by the manufacturer (Durbin and Committee on Injury, Violence, and Poison Prevention, 2011).

Convertible restraints use different types of harness systems: a **five-point harness** that consists of a strap over each shoulder, one on each

side of the pelvis, and one between the legs (all five come together at a common buckle), as well as a **padded overhead shield** that uses shoulder straps attached to a shield that is held in place by a crotch strap. In some seats, a **T-shield**, a padded triangular shield, attaches to shoulder straps to keep the child safely restrained. With both infant and toddler restraints, it is important not to add extra blankets, head cushions, or padding between the child and the restraint straps that did not come as original equipment because these "add-ons" create spaces of air between the child and the restraint and decrease support for the back, head, and neck. Cars with free-sliding latch plates on the lap or shoulder belt require the use of a metal locking clip to keep the belt in a tight-holding position. The locking clip is threaded onto the belt above the latch plate (Fig. 12-11, *A*). If parents have newer cars with automatic lap and shoulder belts, they need to have additional lap belts installed to properly secure the restraint.

Booster seats are not restraint systems like the convertible devices because they depend on the vehicle belts to hold the child and booster

See footnote on p. 399.

seat in place. Three booster models have been approved by the National Highway Traffic Safety Administration (NHTSA): the high-back belt-positioning seat (Fig. 12-11, *B*), which provides head and neck support for the child riding in a vehicle seat without a head rest; the no-back belt-positioning seat, which should be used only if the vehicle seat has a head rest; and a combination seat, which converts from a forward-facing toddler seat to a booster seat. This last model is equipped with a harness for use by toddlers; the harness may be removed and a shoulder-lap belt used when the child outgrows the harness. The belt-positioning booster seats are used for children who are less than 145 cm (4 feet, 9 inches) tall and who weigh 15.9 kg to 36.3 kg (35–80 pounds, depending on the type of booster seat). In general, school-aged children should ride in a belt-positioning booster seat until approximately 7 to 8 years of age. Note, however, that because children's sizes vary considerably, manufacturer's recommendations should be followed regarding height and weight limitations. A booster seat should be used until the child is able to sit against the back of the seat with feet hanging down and legs bent at the knees. The belt-positioning booster model raises a child higher in the seat, moving the shoulder part of the belt off the neck and the lap portion of the belt off the abdomen onto the pelvis. Children who outgrow the convertible restraint may still be able to ride safely in a booster seat until the midpoint of the head is higher than the vehicle seat back.

Children should use specially designed car restraints until they are 145 cm (4 feet, 9 inches) in height or are 8 to 12 years old (AAP, 2011). Shoulder-lap safety belts should be worn low on the hips, snug, and not on the abdominal area. Children should be taught to sit up straight to allow for proper fit. The shoulder belt is used only if it does not cross the child's neck or face.

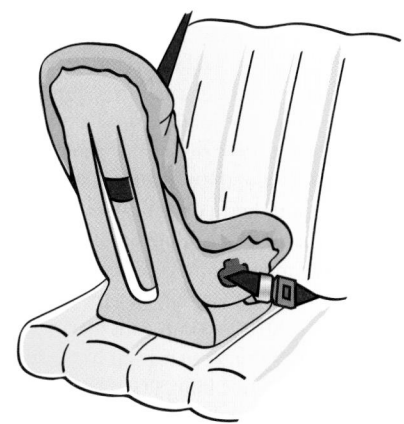

FIG 12-10 Rear-facing convertible car seat.

Shoulder-only automatic belts are designed to protect adults. Children should use the manual shoulder belts in the rear seat. Air bags do not take the place of child safety seats or seat belts and can be lethal to young children. The safest area of the car for children is the back seat. Children who must ride in the passenger side of the front seat with an air bag should be positioned as far back as possible or have the air bag disabled.

For any restraint to be effective, it must be used consistently and properly. Examples of misuse include misrouting the vehicle seat belt through the restraint; failing to use the vehicle seat belt to secure the restraint; failing to use a tether strap; failing to use the restraint's harness system; and incorrectly positioning the child, especially by facing infants forward instead of rearward. To address these issues, nurses must stress correct use of car restraints and rules that ensure compliance (see Family-Centered Care box). Children riding in car safety seats are generally much better behaved than children left unrestrained, which can be a major benefit to parents and should be emphasized as an additional advantage of restraints. Additional information about child safety restraints is available from various sources.*

The LATCH (lower anchors and tethers for children) universal child safety seat system was implemented as a requirement starting in 2002 for all new automobiles and child safety seats. This system provides uniform anchorage consisting of two lower anchorages and one upper anchorage in the rear seat of the vehicle (Fig. 12-12). When used appropriately, the top anchor (tether) strap prevents the child from pitching forward in a crash. If the tether strap is not used, up to 90% of the restraint's protection is lost. Instructions for proper installation of the tether strap and permanent bracket are included with the car restraint. New child safety seats will have a hook, buckle, strap, or other connector that attaches to the anchorage. Seat belts will no longer be used to anchor child safety seats to newer vehicles. The first phase requires all new cars to have an upper anchorage. After fall 2002, all new cars were required to have the entire LATCH system.

Children with disabilities may require a restraint system that secures them appropriately in the event of a crash. Examples of such devices include car bed restraints for infants who cannot tolerate a semireclining position and specially adapted molded-plastic chairs for children who have spica casts. The E-Z-On vest is a special safety harness for larger children with poor trunk control. A HIPPO (Spica

---

*AAP, 141 Northwest Point Blvd., Elk Grove Village, IL 60007; 847-434-4000; http://www.aap.org; and local division of traffic safety or NHTSA, 1200 New Jersey Ave. SE, West Building, Washington, DC 20590; 888-327-4236; http://www.nhtsa.dot.gov.

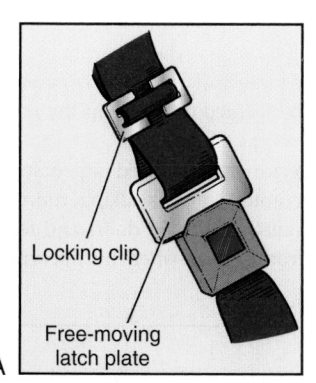

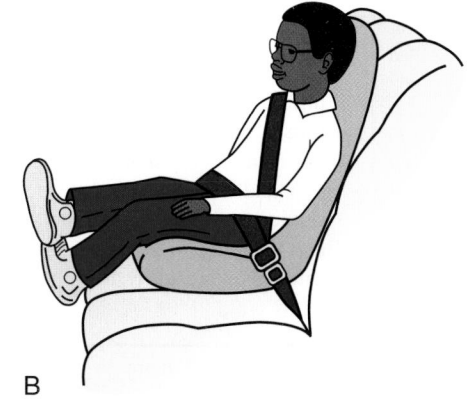

FIG 12-11 A, Locking clip used with free-sliding lap or shoulder belt to keep the belt in a tight-holding position. **B,** Automobile booster seat. Note placement of the shoulder strap (away from the neck and face).

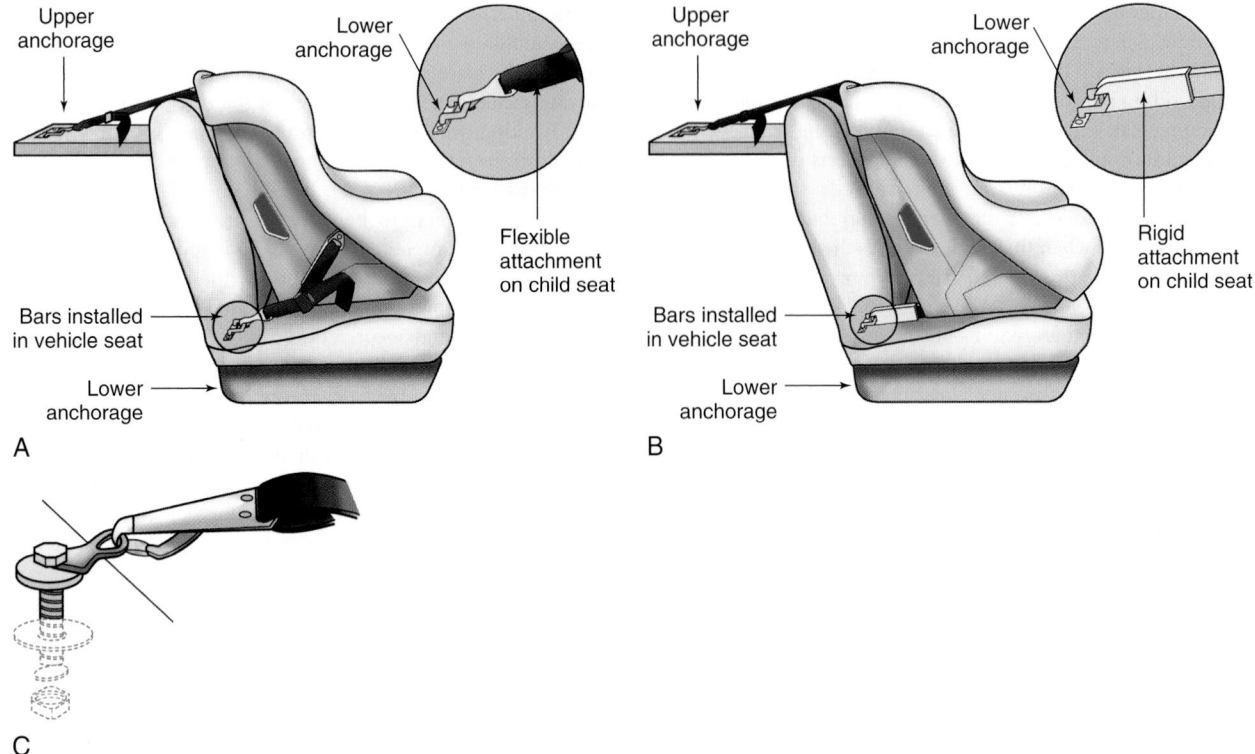

FIG 12-12 LATCH (lower anchors and tethers for children) universal child safety seat system. **A,** Flexible two-point attachment with top tether. **B,** Rigid two-point attachment with top tether. **C,** Top tether. (Courtesy U.S. Department of Transportation, National Highway Traffic Safety Administration.)

FAMILY-CENTERED CARE

Using Car Safety Restraints

- Read manufacturer's directions and follow them exactly.
- Start using car seat when child is infant so he or she will be accustomed to riding restrained.
- Provide favorite toy, stuffed animal, or snack for child while in car seat.
- Anchor car safety seat securely to car's anchoring system and apply harness snugly to child.*
- Do not start the car until everyone is properly restrained.
- Always use the restraint even for short trips.
- If car seat is vinyl and used in a hot car, cover with cloth to prevent skin burns.
- If child begins to climb out or undo the harness, firmly say, "No." It may be necessary to stop the car to reinforce the expected behavior. Use rewards, such as stars or stickers, to encourage cooperation.
- Encourage child to help attach buckles, straps, and shields but always double-check fastenings.
- Decrease boredom on long trips. Keep soft toys in the car for quiet play, talk to child, and point out objects and teach child about them. Stop periodically. If child wishes to sleep, make certain he or she stays in the restraint.
- Insist that others who transport children also follow these safety rules.

*A free car seat restraint inspection may be obtained from a SafeKids inspector. Check for local inspection SafeKids clinics or access website for information: http://www.safekids.org.

Cast) Car Seat is available for transporting children with spica casts; these are sold only in the United States. Additional safety restraints and a listing of distributors are available at the SafetyBeltSafe U.S.A. website.* See also Chapter 9 for a discussion of preterm infants being discharged home and car seat evaluation.

Optimally, children should not ride in the front seat of any car with an activated air bag; if they do, the seat should be pushed as far back as possible to prevent serious harm or critical injury from front seat air bags; in some models the air bag can be disabled. Many of the newer model vehicles have side impact air bags for collision protection; these air bags are reported to be safe as long as the child is in a proper restraint system. NHTSA (2010) recommends that children not lean on chest-only or head-chest combination side air bags. Some of the newer model child car seats include side bumpers at head and neck height to protect children in side-impact collisions. Built-in seats are available in some cars and vans. Built-in seats eliminate installation problems; however, weight and height limits vary. Reinforce that owners must verify with vehicle manufacturers details about built-in seats.

Motor Vehicle—Related Injuries

Injuries may also occur during sudden stops when objects are left unrestrained. On sudden impact, a loose ball becomes a projectile missile. Therefore, all items should be secured or stored in the trunk or behind a barrier such as netting in vans and wagons.

Children older than 3 years of age are often involved in pedestrian traffic injuries. Because of their gross motor skills of walking, running, and climbing and their fine motor skills of opening doors and fence gates, they are likely to be in hazardous areas when unsupervised.

*http://www.carseat.org.

Unaware of danger and unable to approximate the speed of cars, they are hit by moving vehicles. Running after a ball, riding a tricycle, and playing behind a parked car are common activities that may result in a vehicular tragedy.

Toddlers playing in driveways or farmyards are at risk of back-over injury from vehicles in reverse gear. A precaution when children are playing in driveways is attaching to the tricycle a pole with a bright flag that is high enough to be visible through an automobile's back window. Another safeguard is the use of a device that beeps when the vehicle is driven in reverse to alert children to the oncoming car, van, tractor, or truck. Some models now come equipped with rearview motion cameras so the driver can see the driveway clearly while backing out.

Preventing vehicular injuries involves protecting and educating children and adults about the danger of moved or parked vehicles. Children should never ride in the open back of a truck; the danger of falls can be compounded by another vehicle striking the child or by the truck rolling over. In addition, leaving children unsupervised in a parked vehicle, especially in a private driveway, provides an opportunity for the child to release the brake or put the car in gear. Children in bicycle-towed trailers or bicycle-mounted child seats can also be injured by collisions or falls.

One type of injury that has become more commonplace occurs when children crawl into an open trunk and pull it closed. Asphyxia may occur in such cases; therefore, car trunks should not be left open when children are not being supervised. Some cars are equipped with a safety switch that can be activated from inside the trunk to open a closed trunk door.

Another automobile-related hazard for toddlers is overheating (hyperthermia) and subsequent death when left in a vehicle in hot weather (>27° C [80° F]). Small children dissipate heat poorly, and an increase in body temperature can cause death in a few hours. From 1998 to 2011 (June), a total of 506 children died from hyperthermia when left alone in parked cars; in 2010, the total number of child deaths was 49, and it is estimated that an average of 38 children die each year from overheating in cars (Null, 2011). It is estimated that with the ambient temperature at 22° to 35.5° C (72°–96° F), the vehicle interior temperature rises by 10.5° to 11° C (19°–20° F) for each 10 minutes even with a window cracked (Null, 2011). In a study of 171 child fatalities from overheating in a car, 50% of adults who left a child in a car either forgot or were unaware that the child was still in the car. A significant number of those children (32) were left by family members who intended to take the child to daycare but forgot the child in the car at the workplace; 22 children were left in the car by a daycare worker or driver (Guard and Gallagher, 2005). Parents are cautioned against leaving infants alone in a vehicle for *any reason*.

Preventing vehicular injuries involves protecting and educating children about the danger of moving and parked vehicles. Although preschool children are too young to be trusted to always obey, parents should emphasize looking for moving vehicles before crossing the street, recognizing the stop and go colors of traffic lights, and following traffic officers' signals. Physical barriers limiting children from playing near vehicles help prevent these injuries. Most important, what is preached must be practiced. Children learn through imitation, and consistency reinforces learning.

Drowning

The highest rate of drowning in the years 2000 to 2006 was in children ages 0 to 4 years; children ages 12 to 36 months were at highest risk for drowning during the same time period (Weiss and Committee on Injury, Violence, and Poison Prevention, 2010). Drowning deaths in infants occur most commonly in the bathtub and large buckets.

With well-developed skills of locomotion, toddlers are able to reach potentially dangerous areas, such as bathtubs, toilets, buckets, swimming pools, hot tubs, and ponds or lakes. Toddlers' intense drive for exploration and investigation combined with an unawareness of the danger of water and their helplessness in water makes drowning always a viable threat. It is also one category of injury that results in death within minutes, diminishing the chance for rescue and survival. Close adult supervision of children when near any source of water is essential; many drownings in this age group occur when a supervising adult becomes distracted. Teaching swimming and water safety can be helpful but cannot be regarded as sufficient protection. Pool fencing, although critical, does not always deter fast-moving children (see Table 12-3).

Burns

Burns rank second among girls and third among boys in this age group as a cause of accidental death. Toddlers' ability to climb, stretch, and reach objects above their heads makes any hot surface a potential source of danger. Scalds from children pulling pots on top of themselves are a major source of burns. As a precaution, pot handles should be turned toward the back of the stove.

Other sources of heat, such as radiators, fireplaces, accessible furnaces, kerosene heaters, and wood-burning stoves, should have guards placed in front of them. Portable electric heaters must be placed in a high area, well out of reach of climbing young children. Hair curling irons and hot curlers may also be easily reached and can burn the hands of curious toddlers.

Hot objects such as candles, incense, cigarettes, pots of tea or coffee, and irons must be placed away from children. The flame of a candle and the smoke of a cigarette invite investigation. Flame burns represent one of the most fatal types of burns and commonly occur when children play with matches and accidentally set themselves (and the home) on fire. To prevent flame burns, matches and lighters must be stored safely away from children, and parents need to teach children the dangers of playing with such objects. In addition, all homes, apartments, and any other type of dwelling where people sleep should have smoke detectors installed to alert the occupants of a fire. A safety plan for immediate escape is also essential.

Electrical burns represent an immediate danger to children. Young toddlers may explore outlets with conductive articles and wires by mouthing them. Because water is an excellent conductor, the chance for a severe circumoral electrical burn is great. Electrical outlets should have protective guards plugged into them when not in use (Fig. 12-13) or be made inaccessible by having furniture placed in front of them when feasible.

Scald burns are the most common type of thermal injury in children. A scalding burn is often caused by high-temperature tap water, which children come in contact with as a result of turning on the hot-water faucet, falling into a bathtub of hot water, pulling hot pots onto themselves, or suffering deliberate abuse. Limiting household water temperatures to less than 49° C (120° F) is highly recommended. At this temperature, it takes 10 minutes of exposure to the water to cause a full-thickness burn. Conversely, water temperatures of 54° C (130° F), the usual setting of most water heaters, expose household members to the risk of full-thickness burns within 30 seconds. Nurses can help prevent such burns by advising parents of this common household danger and recommending that they readjust their water heaters to a safe temperature.

Sunburns are a year-round concern in certain regions. Children spend a large amount of time outdoors. Their increased mobility makes it difficult to prevent sun exposure. Sunburn can be prevented

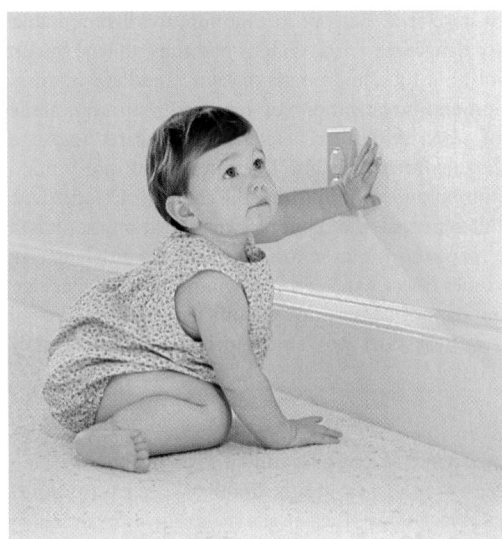

FIG 12-13 Special plastic caps in electrical sockets prevent young fingers from exploring dangerous areas. (© 2011 Photos.com, a division of Getty Images. All rights reserved.)

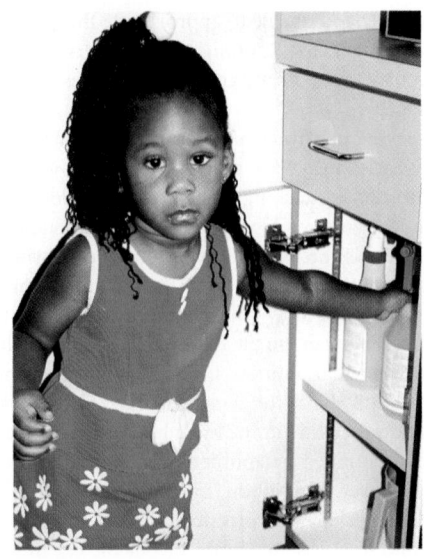

FIG 12-14 Children are most likely to ingest substances that are on their level, such as household cleaning agents stored under sinks; rat poison; or plants.

by applying a sunscreen with a sun protection factor (SPF) of 15 or greater, dressing in protective clothing (wide-brimmed hat, protective cotton clothing with a tight weave), and avoiding sun exposure between 10 AM and 2 PM.

Accidental Poisoning

Toddlers are at the highest risk for accidental poisoning because of the innate curiosity and ability to open "childproof" containers. Mouthing activity continues to be prevalent after 1 year of age, and exploring objects by tasting them is part of children's curious investigation. Toddlers' curiosity and inability to understand logical consequences further place them at risk for ingesting harmful substances. Many household products, medications, and plants can be poisonous if swallowed, if they come in contact with the skin or eyes, or if they are inhaled. Although in many instances poisoning does not result in death, it may cause significant morbidity, such as esophageal stricture from lye ingestion. Toddlers are able to climb most heights, open most drawers or closets, and unscrew most lids. By trial and error, younger children also manage to undo tops of bottles, plastic containers, aerosol cans, and jars, including those with child-resistant lids. Newer forms of drugs, such as transdermal patches and cough-suppressant lozenges, have created additional dangers because they are not packaged with safety caps and the lozenges look like candy.

The major reason for poisoning is improper storage (Fig. 12-14). The guidelines suggested in Chapter 10 apply to children in this age group as well. However, unlike infants, who are confined to certain heights and unable to unlatch child-proof locks, young children manage to find access to many high-level, tight-security places. For this age group, only a locked cabinet is safe.

Recent attention has focused on the use of OTC medications used for cough and colds as a common cause of accidental poisonous ingestion in toddlers. Ingestion of acetaminophen is also a common cause of morbidity because it is found in many combination OTC products; caregivers may unknowingly administer a dose of acetaminophen in addition to an OTC drug containing the product without knowing the danger.

Emergency and preventive measures for accidental poisoning are discussed in Chapter 14. Parents should have ready access to the telephone number for the poison control center (National Poison Center, 800-222-1222) and be prepared to act on the advice of the center.

Falls

Falls are still a hazard to children in this age group, although by the later part of early childhood, gross and fine motor skills are well developed, decreasing the incidence of falls down stairs and from chairs. However, playground injuries are common. Children need to be taught safety at play areas, such as no horseplay on high slides or jungle gyms, sitting on swings, and staying away from moving swings. Passive prevention includes placement of grass, sand, or wood chips under play equipment. Swing seats should be made of plastic, canvas, or rubber and have smooth or rounded edges. Slides should have inclines of no more than 30 degrees, have evenly spaced rungs for climbing, and have protective "tunnels."

The climbing and running of the typical toddler are complicated by the child's total disregard and lack of appreciation for danger. Gates must be placed at both ends of stairs. Accessible windows must have window guards, not screens, to prevent falls to the ground below. Falling from open windows is a major cause of accidental death in urban, lower socioeconomic groups. Doors leading to stairwells or porches must be locked because preschoolers can easily open them. A convenient type of lock is a sliding bar or hook that can be attached to the door and frame at a level higher than the child can reach; such locks also have safety clasps or devices that prevent children from being able to open them. Falls from balconies, porches, decks, and bleachers are all possible for active toddlers. Rails need to be sized appropriately because most children younger than 6 years of age can slip through a 6-inch opening, and none older than 1 year can usually pass through a 4-inch opening.

Cribs and vehicles are other sources of falls. To avoid injury, crib rails should be fully raised, the mattress should be kept at the lowest position, and toys or bumper pads that may be used as steps to climb out should be removed. Ideally, the floor under the crib should be carpeted. Crib, bassinets, and play yards were associated with a large number (66% of all fall injuries to children) of accidental falls (Yeh, Rochette, McKenzie, and others, 2011). The manufacture and sale of drop-side cribs has been banned by the Consumer Product Safety Commission (2010). When children reach a height of 89 cm (35 inches), they should sleep in a bed rather than a crib. If a bunk bed is selected, parents should be aware of possible dangers, including falls from the top bed and from the ladder and head entrapment between the mattress and guardrail or between the supporting mattress slats.

Children can fall from high chairs, shopping carts, carriages, car seats, and strollers if not properly restrained or because of a change in balance created by weighting the object down with heavy objects. Therefore, proper restraint and adequate supervision are essential. Children, especially older infants who are mobile, should not be placed in an infant seat on top of a shopping cart because the infant seat may fall off the cart; the safest place for an infant seat is inside the cart's bed.

Aspiration and Suffocation

Foreign body aspiration is most common during the second year of life. Usually by 1 year of age, children chew well, but they may have difficulty with large pieces of food, such as meat and whole hot dogs, and with hard foods, such as nuts. Young children cannot discard pits from fruit or bones from fish. It takes practice to learn how to chew gum without swallowing it. Gel snacks that are sealed in plastic wrappers can also be difficult to manage, and the plastic wrapper can be aspirated. Therefore, parents must implement the same precautions as discussed for infants regarding food selection (see Chapter 10).

Play objects for toddlers must still be chosen with an awareness of danger from small parts. Large, sturdy toys without sharp edges or removable parts are safest. Small plastic toys such as Legos can cause choking or can be aspirated; such plastic items often do not appear on radiographic films. Balloons, coins, paper clips, pins, bells, button batteries, pull-tabs on cans, thumbtacks, nails, screws, jewelry (especially pierced earrings), and all types of pins are common household objects that can cause significant harm if swallowed or aspirated. Because of the danger of aspiration, parents should be taught emergency procedures for choking (see Airway Obstruction, Chapter 23).

Suffocation from causes seen during infancy is less frequent, but old refrigerators, ovens, and other large appliances are an ever-present threat. Toddlers can climb inside these appliances and, if they close the door behind them, can be trapped inside. Removing all doors before discarding or storing old appliances prevents such tragic deaths. Toddlers may also suffocate when unsafe toy box lids accidentally close on their heads or necks.

Because some of the older heating systems and hot water heaters may emit carbon monoxide, which is undetectable by human smell, each house should have a carbon monoxide detector in addition to a smoke detector.

Bodily Injury

Toddlers are still clumsy in many of their skills and can seriously harm themselves when walking while holding a sharp or pointed object or having food or objects such as spoons in their mouths. Preventing such occurrences is the best approach with toddlers. With preschoolers, teaching safety is most important. The child should be taught that when walking with a pointed object such as a knife or scissors, the pointed end is held away from the face. Dangerous garden or workshop equipment and all firearms should be stored in locked cabinets. Power lawn mowers and weed eaters are especially dangerous because they can throw rocks and other solid items (projectiles), and young children should not be allowed in an area where such tools are in use; nor should they be taken for a ride on a mower or allowed to operate the device. Television tip-overs are a source of head trauma in toddlers and preschool age group (Rutkoski, Sippey, and Gaines, 2011).

Safety education should include respect for firearms and their appropriate use, including nonpowder guns, such as air guns, rifles (BB and pellet), and paintball guns, which can cause serious penetrating injuries. Firearm safety devices such as trigger locks and personalized locks should be used to prevent unintentional firing of guns and subsequent injuries or fatalities. In addition, the child should be warned of and protected against potential danger from animals (see Pet and Wild Animal Bites, Chapter 30).

An additional safeguard for young children is the use of safety glass in doors, windows, and tabletops and the application of decals on glass doors and windows to reduce the likelihood of running through glass. Also, children should not be allowed to run, jump, wrestle, or play ball near glass structures.

A discussion of bodily injury must also include alerting the parent to threats to the child's well-being from adults or other children who might take advantage of the toddler who cannot protect himself- or herself. Because toddlers are often not able to verbalize their emotions and feelings or may not understand inappropriate touching behavior by a family member or friend, it is important for parents to protect children by not leaving them in situations where there is a potential for bodily harm. The "stranger danger" concept is still important to teach, yet statistics show that personal harm more often comes from relatives or family friends who are not considered strangers. Therefore, it is important to discuss appropriate and inappropriate touching (what feels comfortable and what does not) in a manner that will not frighten or overwhelm the child. Child abductions can be prevented with close adult supervision; additional safeguards include screening for risk factors for missing children such as divorce, family discord, and substance abuse. Encourage parents to have a current, high-quality picture of the child. The goal is not to induce fear about such events but to make nurses and parents aware so they can take steps to keep each child safe from bodily harm.

Household safety should be practiced and includes the usual precautions recommended for any age group (see Family-Centered Care box: Child Safety Home Checklist, Chapter 10).

ANTICIPATORY GUIDANCE—CARE OF FAMILIES

Understanding toddlers is fundamental to successful childrearing. Nurses, particularly those in ambulatory or child health centers, are in a favorable position to assist parents in facilitating the tasks and meeting the needs of children in this age group. Prevention yields better results than treatment. Anticipatory guidance is paramount if one wishes to prevent future problems (see Family-Centered Care box).

Advice is sometimes not the sole answer. Actual assistance, such as being available for home visiting or telephone consulting, should be part of the nurse's flexible repertoire of interventions. Whether parents are experiencing the dilemmas of rearing a first or a subsequent child, they benefit from sharing their feelings, frustrations, and satisfactions. They need adult companionship, freedom from childrearing responsibilities, and periodic separations from their children. Part of a nurse's responsibility is to provide opportunities for parents to express their feelings and to meet their physical, mental, and spiritual needs.

FAMILY-CENTERED CARE

Guidance During the Toddler Years

Ages 12 to 18 Months

Prepare parents for expected behavioral changes of toddlers, especially negativism and ritualism.

Assess present feeding habits and encourage gradual weaning from bottle and increased intake of solid foods.

Stress expected feeding changes of physiologic anorexia, food fads and strong taste preferences, need for scheduled routine at mealtimes, inability to sit through an entire meal, and lack of table manners.

Assess sleep patterns at night, particularly habit of a bedtime bottle, which is a major cause of early childhood caries, and procrastination behaviors that delay hour of sleep.

Prepare parents for potential dangers of the home and motor vehicle environment, particularly motor vehicle injuries, drowning, accidental poisoning, and falling injuries; give appropriate suggestions for safeproofing the home.

Discuss need for firm but gentle discipline and ways to deal with negativism and temper tantrums; stress positive benefits of appropriate discipline.

Emphasize importance for both child and parents of brief, periodic separations.

Discuss toys that use developing gross and fine motor, language, cognitive, and social skills.

Emphasize need for dental supervision, types of basic dental hygiene at home, and food habits that predispose to caries; stress importance of supplemental fluoride.

Ages 18 to 24 Months

Stress importance of peer companionship in play.

Explore need for preparation for additional sibling; stress importance of preparing child for new experiences.

Discuss present discipline methods, their effectiveness, and parents' feelings about child's negativism; stress that negativism is important aspect of developing self-assertion and independence and is not a sign of spoiling.

Discuss signs of readiness for toilet training; emphasize importance of waiting for physical and psychologic readiness.

Discuss development of fears, such as darkness or loud noises, and of habits, such as security blanket or thumb sucking; stress normalcy of these transient behaviors.

Prepare parents for signs of regression in time of stress.

Assess child's ability to separate easily from parents for brief periods under familiar circumstances.

Allow parents to express their feelings of weariness, frustration, and exasperation; be aware that it is often difficult to love toddlers at times when they are not asleep!

Point out some of the expected changes of the next year, such as longer attention span, somewhat less negativism, and increased concern for pleasing others.

Ages 24 to 36 Months

Discuss importance of imitation and domestic mimicry and need to include child in activities.

Discuss approaches toward toilet training, particularly realistic expectations and attitude toward accidents.

Stress uniqueness of toddlers' thought processes, especially through their use of language, poor understanding of time, causal relationships in terms of proximity of events, and inability to see events from another's perspective.

Stress that discipline still must be structured and concrete and that relying solely on verbal reasoning and explanation leads to injuries, confusion, and misunderstanding.

Discuss investigation of preschool or daycare center toward completion of second year.

KEY POINTS

- The toddler stage, extending from 12 to 36 months, is a period of intense exploration of the environment.
- Biologic development during the toddler years is characterized by the acquisition of fine and gross motor skills that allow children to master a wide variety of activities.
- Although most of the physiologic systems are mature by the end of toddlerhood, development of certain areas of the brain is still occurring, allowing for greater intellectual capacity.
- Locomotion is the major gross motor skill acquired during toddlerhood followed by increased eye–hand coordination.
- Specific tasks in the psychosocial development of toddlers include differentiating themselves from others, tolerating separation from their parents, coping with delayed gratification, controlling bodily functions, acquiring socially acceptable behavior, communicating verbally, and interacting with others in a less egocentric manner.
- According to Erikson, the major developmental task of toddlerhood is acquiring a sense of autonomy while overcoming a sense of doubt and shame.
- In Piaget's sensorimotor and preoperational phases of development, the toddler experiments by incorporating the old learning

of secondary circular reactions with new skills and applies this knowledge to new situations. There is the beginning of rational judgment, an understanding of causal relationships, and discovery of objects as objects. Preoperational thought is characterized by egocentricism, centration, global organization of thought processes, animism, and irreversibility.
- Language is the major cognitive achievement in toddlerhood.
- The most striking characteristic of language development during early childhood is the increasing level of comprehension.
- Development of body image occurs with increasing motor ability, at which point toddlers recognize the importance and capacity of body parts.
- The two phases of differentiation of self from significant others are separation and individuation.
- Parental concerns during the toddler years include toilet training, coping with sibling rivalry, limit setting and discipline, dealing with temper tantrums, negativism, and regression.
- Effective discipline techniques for toddlers include rewards, ignoring or extinction, and time-outs.
- Nutrition is important at this stage because eating habits established in toddlerhood tend to have long-term effects.

- Food consumption varies among vegetarians; therefore, a detailed dietary intake is essential for planning adequate intakes, particularly in children and pregnant or lactating women.
- Regular dental examinations, fluoride supplementation, removal of plaque, and promotion of a balanced diet with less emphasis on complex carbohydrates and sweetened drinks (soda, artifical juices) and more fruits, grains, and vegetables promote optimum dental health.

- Because of increased locomotion, toddlers are at high risk for sustaining injuries. Fatal injuries are primarily a result of motor vehicle crashes, drownings, and burns. Most of these are accidental and entirely preventable; therefore nurses must take an active part in counseling parents regarding safety and prevention.

REFERENCES

American Academy of Pediatric Dentistry: Guideline on infant oral health care. In *AAPD reference manual 2010–2011* 33(6):12, 114, 2011a, retrieved June 9, 2011, from http://www.aapd.org/media/Policies_Guidelines/G_InfantOralHealthCare.pdf.

American Academy of Pediatric Dentistry: Policy on early childhood caries (ECC): classifications, consequences, and preventive strategies. In *AAPD reference manual 2010–2011* 32(6):41–43, 2011b.

American Academy of Pediatric Dentistry: Policy on use of fluoride. In *AAPD reference manual 2010–2011* 32(6):34–35, 2011c.

American Academy of Pediatric Dentistry: Policy on dietary recommendations for infants, children and adolescents. In *AAPD reference manual 2010–2011* 32(6):48–49, 2011d.

American Academy of Pediatrics: Prevention of rickets and vitamin D deficiency in infants, children, and adolescents, *Pediatrics* 122(5): 1142–1148, 2008.

American Academy of Pediatrics: Car safety seats: a guide for families 2011, 2011, retrieved June 20, 2011, from http://www.healthychildren.org/English/safety-prevention/on-the-go/Pages/Car-Safety-Seats-Information-for-Families.aspx.

American Academy of Pediatrics, Committee on Nutrition: *Pediatric nutrition handbook*, ed 6, Elk Grove Village, Ill, 2009, Author.

American Academy of Pediatrics, Council on Communications and Media: Media use by children younger than 2 years, *Pediatrics* 128(5):1040–1045, 2011.

American Dietetic Association, Dietitians of Canada: Position of the American Dietetic Association and Dietitians of Canada: vegetarian diets, *J Am Diet Assoc* 103(6):748–765, 2003.

Bates E, Dick F: Language, gesture, and the developing brain, *Dev Psychobiol* 40:293–310, 2002.

Berenbaum SA, Beltz AM: Sexual differentiation of human behavior: effects of prenatal and pubertal organizational hormones, *Front Neuroendocrinol* 32(2):183–200, 2011.

Borse NN, Gilchrist J, Delinger AM, and others: *CDC childhood injury report: patterns of unintentional injuries among 0–19 year olds in the United States, 2000–2006*, Atlanta, 2008, Centers for Disease Control and Prevention.

Brazelton TB: How to help parents of young children: the touchpoints model, *J Perinatol* 19(6 pt 2):S6–S7, 1999.

Brotanek JM, Schroer D, Valentyn L, and others: Reasons for prolonged bottle-feeding and iron deficiency among Mexican-American toddlers:

an ethnographic study, *Acad Pediatr* 9(1):17–25, 2009.

Bull MJ, Durbin DR: Rear-facing car safety seats: getting the message right, *Pediatrics* 121(3): 619–620, 2008.

Butte NF, Fox MK, Briefel RR, and others: Nutrient intakes of U.S. infants, toddlers, and preschoolers meet or exceed dietary reference intakes, *J Am Diet Assoc* 110(12, suppl 3):S27–S37, 2010.

Cathey M, Gaylord N: Picky eating: a toddler's continuing approach to mealtime, *Pediatr Nurs* 30(2):101–107, 2004.

Centers for Disease Control and Prevention: Nonfatal motor-vehicle-related backover injuries among children—United States, 2001–2003, *MMWR Morb Mortal Wkly Rep* 54(06):144–146, 2005.

Choby BA, George SA: Toilet training, *Am Family Physician* 78(9):1059–1064, 2008.

Chonchaiva W, Pruksananonda C: Television viewing associates with delayed language development, *Acta Paediatr* 97(7):977–982, 2008.

Consumer Product Safety Commission: Full-size baby cribs and non-full size baby cribs: safety standards, *Fed Reg* 75(248):81766–81788, 2010.

Dunham L, Kollar L: Vegetarian eating for children and adolescents, *J Pediatr Health Care* 20(1): 27–34, 2006.

Durbin DR, Committee on Injury, Violence, and Poison Prevention: Technical report—child passenger safety, *Pediatrics* 127(4):e1050–e1066, 2011.

Elkins M, Cavendish R: Developing a plan for pediatric spiritual care, *Holistic Nurs Pract* 18(4):179–184, 2004.

Erikson EH: *Childhood and society*, ed 2, New York, 1963, Norton.

Feigelman S: The second year. In Kliegman RM, Stanton BF, St. Geme JW, and others, editors: *Nelson textbook of pediatrics*, ed 19, Philadelphia, 2011, Saunders.

Fonseca H, Greydanus DE: Sexuality in the child, teen, and young adult: concepts for the clinician, *Prim Care Clin Office Pract* 34(2):275–292, 2007.

Fosarelli P: Children and the development of faith: implications for pediatric practice, *Contemp Pediatr* 20(1):85–98, 2003.

Fowler JW: *Stages of faith: the psychology of human development and the quest for meaning*, San Francisco, 1981, Harper & Row.

Freeman R, Stevens A: Nursing caries and buying time: an emerging theory of prolonged bottle-feeding, *Community Dent Oral Epidemiol* 36(5):425–433, 2008.

Gardiner P, Kemper KJ: Herbs, complementary therapies, and integrative medicine. In

Kliegman RM, Stanton BF, St. Geme JW, and others, editors: *Nelson textbook of pediatrics*, ed 19, Philadelphia, 2011, Saunders.

Ginsburg KR, American Academy of Pediatrics, Committee on Communications: The importance of play in promoting healthy child development and maintaining strong parent-child bonds, *Pediatrics* 119(1):182–191, 2007.

Glassy D, Romano J, Committee on Early Childhood, Adoption, and Dependent Care: Selecting appropriate toys for young children: the pediatrician's role, *Pediatrics* 111(4): 911–913, 2003.

Guard A, Gallagher SS: Heat related deaths in young children in parked cars: an analysis of 171 fatalities in the United States, 1995–2002, *Inj Prev* 11(1):33–37, 2005.

Harpaz-Rotem I, Bergman A: On an evolving theory of attachment: rapprochement-theory of a developing mind, *Psychoanal Study Child* 61:170–189, 2006.

Henary B, Sherwood CP, Crandall JR, and others: Car safety for children: rear facing for best protection, *Inj Prev* 13(6):398–402, 2007.

Hines M: Gender development and the human brain, *Annu Rev Neurosci* 34:69–88, 2011.

Horn IB, Brenner R, Rao M, and others: Beliefs about the appropriate age for initiating toilet training: are there racial and socioeconomic differences? *J Pediatr* 149(2):165–168, 2006.

Huillet A, Erdie-Lalena C, Norvell D, and others: Complementary and alternative medicine used by children in military pediatric clinics, *J Altern Complement Med* 17(6):531–537, 2011.

Institute of Medicine: *Dietary reference intakes for energy, carbohydrate, fiber, fat, fatty acids, cholesterol, protein, and amino acids*, Washington, DC, 2005, The National Academies Press.

Klassen TP, Kiddoo D, Lang ME, and others: The effectiveness of different methods of toilet training for bowel and bladder control, *Evid Rep Technol Assess (Full Rep)* Dec(147):1–57, 2006.

Landier W, Tse AM: Use of complementary and alternative medical interventions for the management of procedural-related pain, anxiety, and distress in pediatric oncology: an integrative review, *J Pediatr Nurs* 25(6):566–579, 2010.

Lanski SL, Greenwald M, Perkins A, and others: Herbal therapy in a pediatric emergency department population: expect the unexpected, *Pediatrics* 111(5 Pt 1):981–985, 2003.

Lohse B, Stotts JL, Priebe JR: Survey of herbal use by Kansas and Wisconsin WIC participants reveals moderate, appropriate use and identifies herbal education needs, *J Am Diet Assoc* 106(2): 227–237, 2006.

Loman DG: The use of complementary and alternative health care practices among children, *J Pediatr Health Care* 17(2):58–63, 2003.

McLaren C, Null J, Quinn J: Heat stress from enclosed vehicles: moderate ambient temperatures cause significant temperature rise in enclosed vehicles, *Pediatrics* 116(1): e109–e112, 2005.

Meltzer LJ, Mindell JA: Sleep and sleep disorders in children and adolescents, *Psychiatr Clin North Am* 29(4):1059–1076, 2006.

Mercer R: Treating nocturnal enuresis, *Adv Nurs Pract* 11(2):26–31, 2003.

Morin K: Infant nutrition: toddlers: start off on the right foot, *MCN Am J Matern Child Nurs* 32(2):122, 2007.

National Center for Complementary and Alternative Medicine: *What is complementary and alternative medicine?* Bethesda, Md, 2010, National Institutes of Health, National Center for Complementary and Alternative Medicine, retrieved June 19, 2011, from http://nccam.nih. gov/health/whatiscam.

National Highway Transportation Safety Administration: *Air bags: minimize injury: parents and caregivers*, NHTSA ("*Safecar.gov*"), 2010, retrieved June 20, 2011, from http:// www.safercar.gov/Vehicle+Shoppers/Air+Bags/ Side-Impact+Air+Bags#9.

Needlman R, Howard B, Zuckerman B: Helping parents get beyond the terrible 2's, *Patient Care* 29(1):52–61, 1995.

Neuman ME: Addressing children's beliefs through Fowler's stages of faith, *J Pediatr Nurs* 26(1): 44–50, 2011.

Null J: *Hyperthermia deaths of children in vehicles*, 2011, San Francisco State University, Department of Geosciences, retrieved June 20, 2011, from http://www.ggweather.com/ heat.

Owens JA: Sleep medicine. In Kliegman RM, Stanton BF, St. Geme JW, and others, editors. *Nelson textbook of pediatrics*, ed 19, Philadelphia, 2011, Saunders.

Roehlkepartain EC, King PE, Wagener LM, and others, editors: *The handbook of spiritual development in childhood and adolescence*, Thousand Oaks, Calif, 2006, Sage.

Rutkoski JD, Sippey M, Gaines BA: Traumatic television tip-overs in the pediatric population, *J Surg Res* 166(2):199–204, 2011.

Savic I, Garcia-Falqueras A, Swaab DF: Sexual differentiation of the human brain in relation to gender identity and sexual orientation, *Prog Brain Res* 186:41–62, 2010.

Sawni A, Ragothaman R, Thomas RL, and others: The use of complementary/alternative therapies among children attending an urban pediatric emergency department, *Clin Pediatr* 46(1): 36–41, 2007.

Schmitt BD: Toilet training: getting it right the first time, *Contemp Pediatr* 21(3):105–108, 111–112, 115–116, 2004.

Schum TR, Kolb TM, McAuliffe TL, and others: Sequential acquisition of toilet-training skills: a descriptive study of gender and age differences in normal children, *Pediatrics* 109(3):e48, 2002.

Stein MT: Difficult behavior: temper tantrums to conduct disorders. In Rudolph CD, Rudolph AM, Hostetter MK, editors: *Rudolph's pediatrics*, ed 21, New York, 2003, McGraw-Hill.

Stephenson M: Danger in the toy box, *J Pediatr Health Care* 19(3):187–189, 2005.

Wagner CL, Greer FR, American Academy of Pediatrics, Section on Breastfeeding and Committee on Nutrition: Prevention of rickets and vitamin D deficiency in infants, children, and adolescents, *Pediatrics* 122(5):1142–1150, 2008.

Weiss J, Committee on Injury, Violence, and Poison Prevention: Technical report—prevention of drowning, *Pediatrics* 126(1):e253–e262, 2010.

Yeh ES, Rochette LM, McKenzie LB, and others: Injuries associated with cribs, playpens, and bassinets among young children in the U.S.—1990–2008, *Pediatrics* 127(3):479–486, 2011.

Zimmerman FJ, Gilkerson J, Richards JA, and others: Teaching by listening: the importance of adult-child conversations to language development, *Pediatrics* 124(1):342–349, 2009.

Health Promotion of the Preschooler and Family

Rebecca A. Monroe

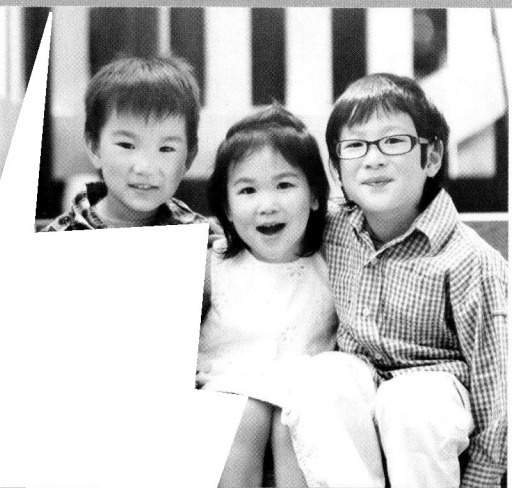

evolve WEBSITE

http://evolve.elsevier.com/wong/essentials
Case Study—Sleep Problems
Key Point Summaries
NCLEX-Style Review Questions

CHAPTER OUTLINE

Promoting Optimal Growth and
  Development, 408
  Biologic Development, 408
    Gross and Fine Motor Skills, 408
  Psychosocial Development, 408
    *Developing a Sense of Initiative
      (Erikson), 408*
  Cognitive Development, 408
    Preoperational Phase (Piaget), 409
  Moral Development, 409
    *Preconventional or Premoral Level
      (Kohlberg), 409*
  Spiritual Development, 409

Development of Body Image, 409
Development of Sexuality, 410
Social Development, 410
  Language, 410
  Personal-Social Behavior, 410
  Play, 411
Coping with Concerns Related to
  Normal Growth and Development, 412
  *Preschool and Kindergarten
    Experience, 412*
  Sex Education, 415
  Fears, 416
  Stress, 416

  Aggression, 416
  Speech Problems, 417
Promoting Optimal Health During the
  Preschool Years, 417
  Nutrition, 417
  Sleep and Activity, 418
    Sleep Problems, 418
  Dental Health, 419
  Injury Prevention, 419
  Anticipatory Guidance—Care of
    Families, 420

LEARNING OBJECTIVES

On completion of this chapter the reader will be able to:
- Identify the major biologic, psychosocial, cognitive, moral, spiritual, and social developments that occur during the preschool years.
- List the benefits of imaginary playmates.
- Prepare preschoolers for preschool or daycare experience.
- Provide parents with guidelines for sex education.

- Provide parents with guidelines for dealing with a child's fears, stresses, aggression, and sleep problems.
- Recognize the causes of stuttering during the preschool years.
- Offer parents suggestions for preventing speech problems.
- Recognize the feeding patterns of preschoolers.
- Provide anticipatory guidance to parents regarding injury prevention based on the preschooler's developmental achievements.

PROMOTING OPTIMAL GROWTH AND DEVELOPMENT

The combined biologic, psychosocial, cognitive, spiritual, and social achievements during the preschool period (3–5 years of age) prepare preschoolers for their most significant change in lifestyle: entrance into school. Their control of bodily functions, experience of brief and prolonged periods of separation, ability to interact cooperatively with other children and adults, use of language for mental symbolization, and increased attention span and memory prepare them for the next major period: the school years. Successful achievement of previous levels of growth and development is essential for preschoolers to refine many of the tasks that were mastered during the toddler years.

BIOLOGIC DEVELOPMENT

The rate of physical growth slows and stabilizes during the preschool years. The average weight is 14.5 kg (32 pounds) at 3 years, 16.7 kg (36.8 pounds) at 4 years, and 18.7 kg (41.5 pounds) at 5 years. The average weight gain per year remains approximately 2 to 3 kg (4.5–6.5 pounds).

Growth in height also remains steady, with a yearly increase of 6.5 to 9 cm (2.5–3.5 inches), and generally occurs by elongation of the legs rather than of the trunk. The average height is 95 cm (37.5 inches) at 3 years, 103 cm (40.5 inches) at 4 years, and 110 cm (43.5 inches) at 5 years.

Physical proportions no longer resemble those of the squat, potbellied toddler. Preschoolers are slender but sturdy, graceful, agile, and posturally erect. There is little difference in physical characteristics according to gender except as dictated by such factors as dress and hairstyle.

Most organ systems can adjust to moderate stress and change. During this period, most children are toilet trained. For the most part, motor development consists of increases in strength and refinement of previously learned skills, such as walking, running, and jumping. However, muscle development and bone growth are still far from mature. Excessive activity and overexertion can injure delicate tissues. Good posture, appropriate exercise, and adequate nutrition and rest are essential for optimal development of the musculoskeletal system.

Gross and Fine Motor Skills

Walking, running, climbing, and jumping are well established by age 36 months. Refinement in eye–hand and muscle coordination is evident in several areas. At age 3 years, preschoolers can ride a tricycle, walk on tiptoe, balance on one foot for a few seconds, and do broad jumps. By age 4 years, children can skip and hop proficiently on one foot (Fig. 13-1) and catch a ball reliably. By age 5 years, children can skip on alternate feet and jump rope and begin to skate and swim.

Fine motor development is evident in the child's increasingly skillful manipulation, such as in drawing and dressing. These skills provide readiness for learning and independence for entry into school.

PSYCHOSOCIAL DEVELOPMENT

Developing a Sense of Initiative (Erikson)

After preschoolers have mastered the tasks of the toddler period, they are ready to face the developmental endeavors of the preschool period. Erikson maintained that the chief psychosocial task of this period is acquiring a sense of initiative. Children are in a stage of energetic learning. They play, work, and live to the fullest and feel a real sense

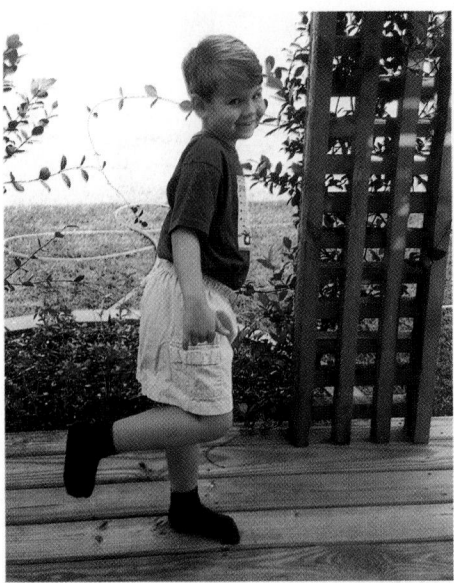

FIG 13-1 A 4-year-old child has sufficient balance to stand or hop on one foot.

🌐 CULTURAL CONSIDERATIONS
Learning Sociocultural Mores

Developing a conscience implies learning the sociocultural mores of the family's heritage. Depending on the type of attitudes conveyed, children will learn not only appropriate behaviors but also tolerant, biased, or prejudicial values concerning their ethnic, religious, and social background and those of other groups. Much of this influence may remain dormant until they associate with children or adults of a different heritage. Then, depending on the particular group, they may be accepted or ostracized for their attitudes.

of accomplishment and satisfaction in their activities. Conflict arises when children overstep the limits of their ability and inquiry and experience a sense of guilt for not having behaved appropriately. Feelings of guilt, anxiety, and fear may also result from thoughts that differ from expected behavior.

A particularly stressful thought is wishing one's parent dead. As a sense of rivalry or competition develops between the child and same-sex parent, the child may think of ways to get rid of the interfering parent. In most situations, this rivalry is resolved when the child strongly identifies with the same-sex parent and peers during the school years. However, if that parent dies before the identification process is completed, the preschooler may be overwhelmed with feelings of guilt for having wished and therefore "caused" the death. Clarifying for children that wishes cannot and do not make events occur is essential in helping them overcome their guilt and anxiety.

Development of the superego, or conscience, begins toward the end of the toddler years and is a major task for preschoolers (see Cultural Considerations box). Learning right from wrong and good from bad is the beginning of morality (see Moral Development).

COGNITIVE DEVELOPMENT

One of the tasks related to the preschool period is readiness for school and scholastic learning. Many of the thought processes of this period are crucial for achieving such readiness, and it is intentional that children begin school between ages 5 and 6 years rather than at an earlier age.

Preoperational Phase (Piaget)

Piaget's cognitive theory does not include a period specifically for children who are 3 to 5 years old. The preoperational phase covers the age span from 2 to 7 years and is divided into two stages: the preconceptual phase, ages 2 to 4 years, and the phase of intuitive thought, ages 4 to 7 years. One of the main transitions during these two phases is the shift from totally egocentric thought to social awareness and the ability to consider other viewpoints. However, egocentricity is still evident. (For a review of the characteristics of preoperational thought, see Chapter 12.)

Language continues to develop during the preschool period. Speech remains primarily a vehicle of egocentric communication. Preschoolers assume that everyone thinks as they do and that a brief explanation of their thinking makes the entire thought understood by others. Because of this self-referenced, egocentric verbal communication, it is often necessary to explore and understand young children's thinking through other, nonverbal approaches. For children in this age group, the most enlightening and effective method is play, which becomes children's way of understanding, adjusting to, and working out life's experiences.

Preschoolers increasingly use language without comprehending the meaning of words, particularly concepts of left and right, causality, and time. Children may use the concepts correctly but only in the circumstances in which they have learned them. For example, they may know how to put on shoes by remembering that the buckle is always on the outside of the foot. However, if different shoes have no buckles, they cannot reason which shoe fits which foot. In other words, they do not understand the concept of *left* and *right*.

Superficially, causality resembles logical thought. Preschoolers explain a concept as they heard it described by others, but their understanding is limited. An example is the concept of time. Because time is still incompletely understood, the child interprets it according to his or her own frame of reference, such as "A long time means until Christmas." Consequently, time is best explained in relationship to an event, such as "Your mother will visit you after you finish your lunch." Avoiding words such as *yesterday*, *tomorrow*, *next week*, or *Tuesday* to express when an event is expected to occur and instead associating time with expected daily events help children learn about temporal relationships while increasing their trust in others' predictions.

Preschoolers' thinking is often described as magical thinking. Because of their egocentrism and transductive reasoning, they believe that thoughts are all-powerful. Such thinking places them in the vulnerable position of feeling guilty and responsible for bad thoughts, which may coincide with the occurrence of a wished event. Their inability to logically reason the cause and effect of illness or an injury makes it especially difficult for them to understand such events.

> ### ❗ NURSING ALERT
>
> Counseling children whose parents are going through a divorce or separation should involve a discussion with the child about his or her role. Because of magical thinking, the child may believe he or she wished the other parent away. The child should be reassured that this is not the case.

Preschoolers believe in the power of words and accept their meaning literally. An example of this type of thinking is calling children "bad" because they did something wrong. In the preschooler's

mind, calling them bad means they are a bad person; thus, it is better to say that their actions were bad by saying, for example, "That was a bad thing to do."

MORAL DEVELOPMENT

Preconventional or Premoral Level (Kohlberg)

Young children's development of moral judgment is at the most basic level. They have little, if any, concern about why something is wrong. They behave because of the freedom or restriction that is placed on actions. In the punishment and obedience orientation, children (ages about 2–4 years) judge whether an action is good or bad depending on whether it results in a reward or a punishment. If children are punished for it, the action is bad. If they are not punished, the action is good regardless of the meaning of the act. For example, if parents allow hitting, the child will perceive that hitting is good because it is not associated with punishment.

From approximately 4 to 7 years of age, children are in the stage of naive instrumental orientation in which actions are directed toward satisfying their needs and, less frequently, the needs of others. They have a concrete sense of justice and fairness during this period of development.

SPIRITUAL DEVELOPMENT

Children generally learn about faith and religion from significant others in their environment, usually from parents and their religious beliefs and practices. However, young children's understanding of spirituality is influenced by their cognitive level. Preschoolers have a concrete concept of a God with physical characteristics, often similar to an imaginary friend. They understand simple Bible stories, memorize short prayers, and imitate the religious practices of their parents without fully understanding the significance of these rituals. Preschoolers benefit from concrete representations of religious practices, such as picture Bible books and small statues, such as those of the Nativity scene.

Development of the conscience is strongly linked to spiritual development. At this age, children are learning right from wrong and behaving correctly to avoid punishment. Wrongdoing provokes feelings of guilt, and preschoolers often misinterpret illness as a punishment for real or imagined transgressions. Observing religious traditions and participating in a religious community can help children cope during stressful periods, such as illness and hospitalization (Speraw, 2006).

DEVELOPMENT OF BODY IMAGE

The preschool years play a significant role in the development of body image. With increasing comprehension of language, preschoolers recognize that individuals have desirable and undesirable appearances. They recognize differences in skin color and racial identity and are vulnerable to learning prejudices and biases. They are aware of the meaning of words such as *pretty* or *ugly*, and they reflect the opinions of others regarding their own appearance. By 5 years of age, children compare their size with that of their peers and can become conscious of being large or short, especially if others refer to them as "so big" or "so little" for their age. Research indicates that girls as young as preschool age already show concern about appearance and weight (Skouteris, McCabe, Swinburn, and others, 2010). Because these are formative years for both boys and girls, parents should make efforts to instill positive principles regarding body image, give their children encouraging feedback regarding their appearance, and emphasize the importance of accepting individuals no matter their differences in appearance.

Despite the advances in body image development, preschoolers have poorly defined body boundaries and little knowledge of their internal anatomy. Intrusive experiences are frightening, especially those that disrupt the integrity of the skin, such as injections and surgery. They fear that if their skin is "broken," all of their blood and "insides" can leak out. Therefore, bandages are critical to "keep everything from coming out."

DEVELOPMENT OF SEXUALITY

Sexual development during these years is an important phase in a person's overall sexual identity and beliefs. Preschoolers are forming strong attachments to the opposite-sex parent while identifying with the same-sex parent. Sex typing, or the process by which an individual develops the behavior, personality, attitudes, and beliefs appropriate for his or her culture and sex, occurs through several mechanisms during this period. Probably the most powerful mechanisms are child-rearing practices and imitations. Gender identification is a result of complex prenatal and postnatal psychologic factors, as well as biologic, social, and genetic factors. Most children are aware of their gender and the expected sets of related behaviors by 1½ to 2½ years of age.

As sexual identity develops beyond gender recognition, modesty may become a concern. Sex-role imitation and "dressing up" like Mommy or Daddy are important activities. Attitudes and the responses of others to role-playing can condition children to views of themselves and others. For example, comments such as "Boys shouldn't play with dolls" can influence a boy's self-concept of masculinity.

Sexual exploration may be more pronounced now than ever before, particularly in terms of exploring and manipulating the genitalia. Questions about sexual reproduction may come to the forefront in preschoolers' search for understanding (see Sex Education, p. 415, and in Chapter 15).

SOCIAL DEVELOPMENT

During the preschool period, the separation-individuation process is completed. Preschoolers have overcome much of the anxiety associated with strangers and the fear of separation of earlier years. They relate to unfamiliar people easily and tolerate brief separations from their parents with little or no protest. However, they still need parental security, reassurance, guidance, and approval, especially when entering preschool or elementary school. Prolonged separation, such as that imposed by illness and hospitalization, is difficult, but preschoolers respond to anticipatory preparation and concrete explanation. They can cope with changes in daily routine much better than toddlers, although they may develop more imaginary fears. Preschoolers gain security and comfort from familiar objects, such as toys, dolls, or photographs of family members. They are able to work through many of their unresolved fears, fantasies, and anxieties through play, especially if guided with appropriate play objects (e.g., dolls, puppets) that represent family members, health care professionals, and other children.

Language

During the preschool years, language becomes more sophisticated and complex and becomes a major mode of communication and social interaction (Fig. 13-2). Through language, preschool children learn to express feelings of frustration or anger without acting them out. Both cognitive ability and environment—particularly, consistent

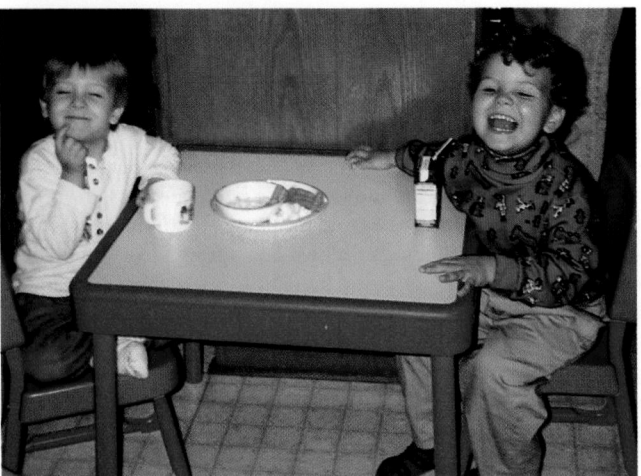

FIG 13-2 Preschool children enjoy friends and often use nonverbal messages to communicate.

role models—influence vocabulary, speech, and comprehension. Vocabulary increases dramatically, from 300 words at age 2 years to more than 2100 words at the end of 5 years. Sentence structure, grammatical usage, and intelligibility also advance to a more adult level. Language development during these early years predicts school readiness (Harrison and McLeod, 2010) and sets the stage for later success in school (Reilly, Wake, Ukoumunne, and others, 2010).

Children between the ages of 3 and 4 years form sentences of about three or four words and include only the most essential words to convey a meaning. Such speech is often termed **telegraphic** for its brevity. Three-year-old children ask many questions and use plurals, correct pronouns, and the past tense of verbs. They name familiar objects, such as animals, parts of the body, relatives, and friends. They can give and follow simple commands. They talk incessantly regardless of whether anyone is listening or answering them. They enjoy musical or talking toys or dolls and imitate new words proficiently.

From ages 4 to 5 years, preschoolers use longer sentences of four or five words and use more words to convey a message, such as prepositions, adjectives, and a variety of verbs. They follow simple directional commands, such as "Put the ball on the chair," but can carry out only one request at a time. They answer questions such as "What do you do when you are hungry?" by describing the appropriate action. The pattern of asking questions is at its peak, and children usually repeat a question until they receive an answer.

By age 6 years, children can use all parts of speech correctly except for deviations from the rule. They can define simple things by describing their use, shape, or general category of classification, rather than simply describing their outward appearance. For example, they define a ball as "round," "something you bounce," or "a toy," rather than only describing its color. They can give some opposites, such as "If Mommy is a woman, Daddy is a man." They can also describe an object according to its composition, such as "A spoon is made of metal."

Personal-Social Behavior

The pervasive ritualism and negativism of toddlerhood gradually diminish during the preschool years. Although self-assertion is still a major theme, preschoolers demonstrate their sense of autonomy differently. They are able to verbalize their request for independence and perform independently because of their much-refined physical and cognitive development. By 4 or 5 years of age, they need little if any assistance with dressing, eating, or toileting (Fig. 13-3). They can also

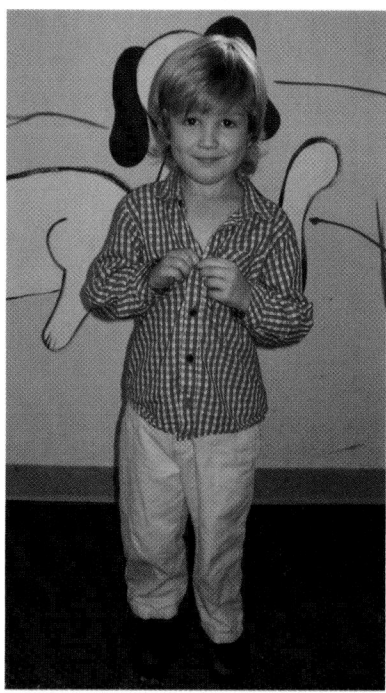

FIG 13-3 Most preschoolers are able to dress themselves but need help with more difficult items of clothing.

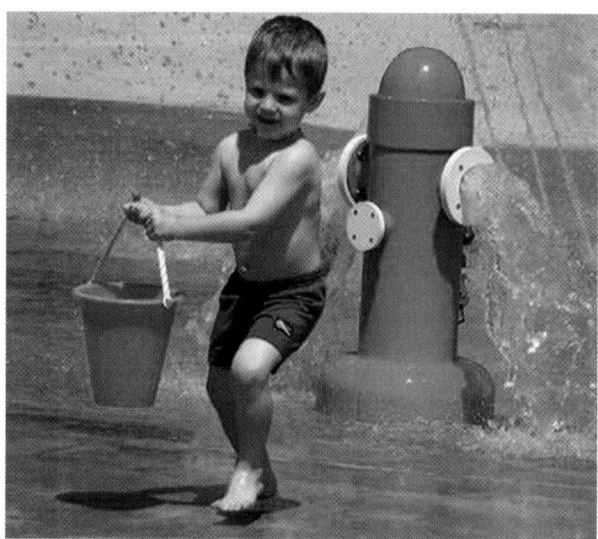

FIG 13-4 Preschoolers enjoy play activities that promote motor skills such as jumping and running. Water play is an exciting activity for preschoolers.

be trusted to obey warnings of danger; however, 3- or 4-year-old children may exceed their boundaries at times.

They are also much more sociable and willing to please. They have internalized many of the standards and values of the family and culture. However, by the end of early childhood, they begin to question parental values and compare them with those of their peer group and other authority figures. As a result, they may be less willing to abide by the family's code of conduct. Preschoolers become increasingly aware of their position and role within the family. Although this is a more secure age for experiencing the addition of another sibling, relinquishing the position of first or youngest is still difficult and requires appropriate preparation. (See Sibling Rivalry, Chapter 12.)

Play

Various types of play are typical of this period, but preschoolers especially enjoy associative play—group play in similar or identical activities but without rigid organization or rules. Play should provide for physical, social, and mental development.

Play activities for physical growth and refinement of motor skills include jumping, running, and climbing. Tricycles, wagons, gym and sports equipment, sandboxes, wading pools, and activities at water parks can help develop muscles and coordination (Fig. 13-4). Activities such as swimming and skating teach safety as well as muscle development and coordination. Children involved in the work of play do not require expensive toys and gadgets to keep them entertained but often enjoy playing with common household items such as a broom handle or even items adults consider junk (boxes, sticks, rocks, and dirt). The imaginative mind of the preschooler enjoys playing for play's sake.

Manipulative, constructive, creative, and educational toys provide for quiet activities, fine motor development, and self-expression. Easy construction sets, large blocks of various sizes and shapes, a counting frame, alphabet or number flash cards, paints, crayons, simple carpentry tools, musical toys, illustrated books, simple sewing or handicraft sets, large puzzles, and clay are suitable toys. Electronic games and

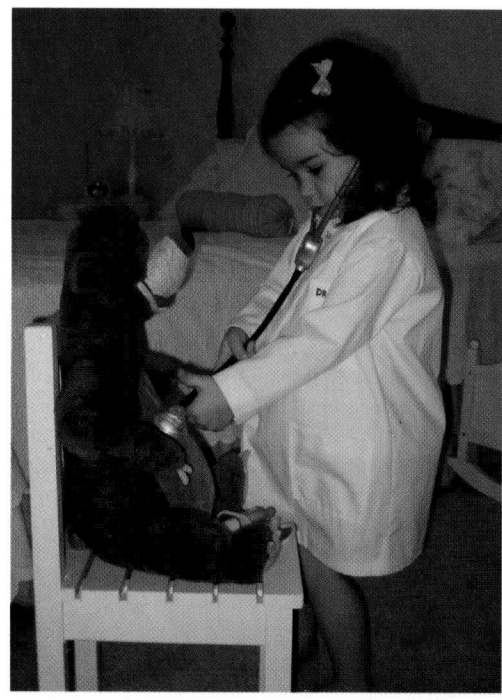

FIG 13-5 Imaginative and imitative play is typical of preschoolers.

computer programs are especially valuable in helping children learn basic skills, such as letters and simple words.

Probably the most characteristic and pervasive preschool activity is *imitative*, *imaginative*, and *dramatic play*. Dress-up clothes, dolls, housekeeping toys, dollhouses, play store toys, telephones, farm animals and equipment, village sets, trains, trucks, cars, planes, hand puppets, and medical kits provide hours of self-expression (Fig. 13-5). Probably at no other time is the reproduction of adult behavior so faithful and absorbing as in 4- and 5-year-old children. Toward the end of the preschool period, children are less satisfied with make-believe or pretend objects and enjoy doing the actual activity, such as cooking and carpentry.

Television and other media also have their place in children's play, although each should be only one part of children's total repertoire of social and recreational activities. Parents and other caregivers should supervise the selection of programs, watch and discuss programs with their children, schedule limited time for television viewing, and set a good example of television viewing (American Academy of Pediatrics [AAP], 2007). Children enjoy and learn from educational programs; however, television viewing may limit time spent in other meaningful activities such as reading, physical activity, and socialization (AAP, 2007).

Although the potential negative effects of television viewing have been well documented in literature, research has also shown that prosocial behavior and later academic achievement can result from viewing educational media during the preschool years; however, positive effects depend on the media content, the age of the viewer, the length of viewing time, and the presence of a coviewing parent (Kirkorian, Wartella, and Anderson, 2008). When parents view media with their children, the activity can become interactive with parents and children discussing program content. Considering the significant increase in media accessibility through various portable electronic devices and cell phones, parents need to be aware of the potential positive and negative effects of media exposure.

Play is so much a part of young children's lives that reality and fantasy become blurred. Make-believe is reality during play and only becomes fantasy when the toys are put away or the dress-up clothes are removed. It is no wonder that imaginary playmates are so much a part of this age period. The appearance of imaginary companions usually occurs between ages 2½ and 3 years, and for the most part, such playmates are relinquished when the child enters school. Differences in birth order and gender have been noted in studies of imaginary companion play. Firstborn children have a higher incidence of imaginary companions, as do young girls; young boys tend to impersonate characters more often (Trionfi and Reese, 2009).

Imaginary companions serve many purposes: They become friends in times of loneliness, they accomplish what the child is still attempting, and they experience what the child wants to forget or remember. It is not unusual for the "friend" to have myriad vices and to be blamed for wrongdoing. Sometimes the child hopes to escape punishment by saying, "My friend George broke the glass." At other times, the child may fantasize that the companion misbehaved and play the role of the parent. This becomes a way of assuming control and authority in a safe situation.

Parents often worry about the imaginary playmates, not realizing how normal and useful they are. Parents need to be reassured that the child's fantasy is a sign of health that helps differentiate make-believe and reality. Parents can acknowledge the presence of the imaginary companion by calling him or her by name and even agreeing to simple requests such as setting an extra place at the table, but they should not allow the child to use the playmate to avoid punishment or responsibility. For example, if the child blames the companion for messing up a room, parents need to state clearly that the child is the only one they see; therefore, the child is responsible for cleaning up.

Children also benefit from play that occurs between them and a parent. Mutual play fosters development from birth through the school years and provides enriched opportunities for learning. Through mutual play, parents can provide tactile and kinesthetic experiences, maximize verbal and language abilities, and offer praise and encouragement for exploration of the world. In addition, mutual play encourages positive interactions between the parent and child, strengthening their relationship.

Table 13-1 summarizes the major developmental achievements for children 3, 4, and 5 years of age.

COPING WITH CONCERNS RELATED TO NORMAL GROWTH AND DEVELOPMENT

Preschool and Kindergarten Experience

Some children are home schooled, but many children attend some type of early childhood program, usually preschool or a daycare center. Group care has become commonplace with the large number of parents currently employed outside the home (see Alternate Child Care Arrangements, Chapter 10). The effects of early education and stimulation on children have increasingly gained recognition. (For a discussion of the effects of daycare on young children, see Working Mothers, Chapter 3.) Because social development widens to include age mates and other significant adults, preschool provides an excellent vehicle for expanding children's experiences with others. It is also excellent preparation for entrance into elementary school.

In preschool or daycare centers, children are exposed to opportunities for learning group cooperation; adjusting to sociocultural differences; and coping with frustration, dissatisfaction, and anger. If activities are tailored to provide mastery and achievement, children increasingly have feelings of success, self-confidence, and personal competence. Whether structured learning is imposed is less important than the social climate, type of guidance, and attitude toward the children that is fostered by the teacher or leader. With a teacher who is aware of preschoolers' developmental abilities and needs, children will learn from the activity that is provided. Most programs incorporate a daily schedule of quiet play, active outdoor activity, group activities such as games and projects, creative or free play, and snack and rest periods. Preschool is particularly beneficial for children who lack a peer-group experience, such as only children, and for children from impoverished homes.

One of the issues that parents face is their children's readiness for preschool or kindergarten. There are no absolute indicators for school readiness, but children's social maturity, especially attention span, is as important as their academic readiness. Using a developmental screening tool that addresses cognitive (especially language), social, and physical milestones can identify children who may benefit from diagnostic testing and early intervention programs before starting school. Parents play an integral role in their children's school readiness. They should promote a positive attitude toward learning, read to their children, encourage their children to participate in a variety of activities to explore their talents and interests, and choose appropriate child care or preschool programs (Hagan, Shaw, and Duncan, 2008).

Nurses and other health care workers can guide parents in selecting enriched social and educational early intervention programs, schools, and child care centers. Careful selection of early childhood education is intrinsic to future learning and development. Licensed and regulated programs are mandated to abide by established standards, which represent minimum requirements and safeguards. Regulation is important to protect children from harm and to promote the conditions essential for a child's healthy development and learning. The National Association for the Education of Young Children (NAEYC) serves as the model for optimal care of small children.*

---

*Information about accreditation criteria and procedures of the NAEYC Academy for Early Childhood Program Accreditation is available from the National Association for the Education of Young Children, 1313 L St. NW, Suite 500, Washington, DC 20005; 800-424-2460 or 202-232-8777; fax: 202-328-1846; http://www.naeyc.org. These criteria are excellent guidelines for evaluating preschools and daycare centers.

TABLE 13-1 GROWTH AND DEVELOPMENT DURING THE PRESCHOOL YEARS

PHYSICAL	GROSS MOTOR	FINE MOTOR	LANGUAGE	SOCIALIZATION	COGNITION	FAMILY RELATIONSHIPS
Age 3 Years						
Usual weight gain of 1.8-2.7 kg (4-6 pounds)	Rides tricycle	Builds tower of nine or 10 cubes	Has vocabulary of about 900 words	Dresses self almost completely if helped with back buttons and told which shoe is right or left	Is in preconceptual phase	Attempts to please parents and conform to their expectations
Average weight of 14.5 kg (32 pounds)	Jumps off bottom step	Builds bridge with three cubes	Uses primarily telegraphic speech	Pulls on shoes	Is egocentric in thought and behavior	Is less jealous of younger sibling; may be opportune time for birth of additional sibling
Usual gain in height of 7.5 cm (3 inches) per year	Stands on one foot for a few seconds	Adeptly places small pellets in narrow-necked bottle	Uses complete sentences of three or four words	Has increased attention span	Has beginning understanding of time; uses many time-oriented expressions, talks about past and future as much as about present, pretends to tell time	Is aware of family relationships and sex-role functions
Average height of 95 cm (37.5 inches)	Goes up stairs using alternate feet; may still come down using both feet on step	In drawing, copies a circle, imitates a cross and names what has been drawn; cannot draw stick figure but may make circle with facial features	Talks incessantly regardless of whether anyone is paying attention	Feeds self completely	Has improved concept of space, as demonstrated by understanding of prepositions and ability to follow directional command	Boys tend to identify more with father or other male figure
May have achieved nighttime control of bowel and bladder	Broad jumps		Repeats sentence of six syllables	Can help to set table; can dry dishes without breaking any	Has beginning ability to view concepts from another perspective	Has increased ability to separate easily and comfortably from parents for short periods
Maximum potential for development of amblyopia	May try to dance, but balance may not be adequate		Asks many questions	May have fears, especially of dark and going to bed		
			Can prepare simple meals, such as cold cereal and milk	Knows own gender and gender of others		
				Play is parallel and associative; begins to learn simple games but often follows own rules; begins to share		
Age 4 Years						
Pulse and respiration rates decrease slightly	Skips and hops on one foot	Uses scissors successfully to cut out picture following outline	Has vocabulary of 1500 words or more	Very independent	Is in phase of intuitive thought	Rebels if parents expect too much, such as impeccable table manners
Growth rate is similar to that of previous year	Catches ball reliably	Can lace shoes but may not be able to tie bow	Uses sentences of four or five words	Tends to be selfish and impatient	Causality is still related to proximity of events	Takes aggression and frustration out on parents or siblings
Average weight of 16.7 kg (36.8 pounds)	Throws ball overhead	In drawing, copies a square, traces a cross and diamond, adds three parts to stick figure	Questioning is at peak	Aggressive physically as well as verbally	Understands time better, especially in terms of sequence of daily events	Do's and don'ts become important
Average height of 103 cm (40.5 inches)	Walks down stairs using alternate footing		Tells exaggerated stories	Takes pride in accomplishments	Unable to conserve matter	May have rivalry with older or younger siblings; may resent older sibling's privileges and younger sibling's invasion of privacy and possessions
Length at birth is doubled			Knows simple songs	Has mood swings	Judges everything according to one dimension, such as height, width, or order	May "run away" from home
			May be mildly profane if associates with older children	Shows off dramatically; enjoys entertaining others	Immediate perceptual clues dominate judgment	Identifies strongly with parent of opposite sex
			Obeys four prepositional phrases, such as *under, on top of, beside, in back of,* or *in front of*	Tells family tales to others with no restraint	Is beginning to develop less egocentrism and more social awareness	Is able to run simple errands outside the home
			Names one or more colors	Still has many fears	May count correctly but has poor mathematic concept of numbers	
			Comprehends analogies, such as "If ice is cold, fire is _____"	Play is associative	Obeys because parents have set limits, not because of understanding of right or wrong	
				Imaginary playmates are common		
				Uses dramatic, imaginative, and imitative devices		
				Sexual exploration and curiosity demonstrated through play, such as being "doctor" or "nurse"		

Continued

TABLE 13-1 GROWTH AND DEVELOPMENT DURING THE PRESCHOOL YEARS—cont'd

PHYSICAL	GROSS MOTOR	FINE MOTOR	LANGUAGE	SOCIALIZATION	COGNITION	FAMILY RELATIONSHIPS
Age 5 Years	Skips and hops on alternate feet	Ties shoelaces	Has vocabulary of about 2100 words	Less rebellious and quarrelsome than at age 4 years	Begins to question what parents think by comparing them with age mates and other adults	Gets along well with parents
Pulse and respiration rates decrease slightly	Throws and catches ball well	Uses scissors, simple tools, or pencil very well	Uses sentences of six to eight words, with all parts of speech	More settled and eager to get down to business	May notice prejudice and bias in outside world	May seek out parent more often than at age 4 years for reassurance and security, especially when entering school
Average weight of 18.7 kg (41.5 pounds)	Jumps rope	In drawing, copies a diamond and triangle; adds seven to nine parts to stick figure; prints a few letters, numbers, or words, such as first name	Names coins (e.g., nickel, dime)	Not as open and accessible in thoughts and behavior as in earlier years	Is more able to view other's perspective but tolerates differences rather than understanding them	Begins to question parents' thinking and principles
Average height of 110 cm (43.5 inches)	Skates with good balance		Names four or more colors	Independent but trustworthy; not foolhardy; more responsible		Strongly identifies with parent of same sex, especially boys with their fathers
Eruption of permanent dentition may begin	Walks backward with heel to toe		Describes drawing or pictures with much comment and enumeration	Has fewer fears; relies on outer authority to control world	May begin to show understanding of conservation of numbers through counting objects regardless of arrangement	Enjoys activities such as sports, cooking, and shopping with parent of same sex
Handedness is established (about 90% are right handed)	Jumps from height of 12 inches and lands on toes		Knows names of days of week, months, and other time-associated words	Eager to do things right and to please; tries to "live by the rules"	Uses time-oriented words with increased understanding	
	Balances on alternate feet with eyes closed		Knows composition of articles, such as "A shoe is made of _____"	Has better manners	Very cautious about factual information regarding world	
			Can follow three commands in succession	Cares for self totally, occasionally needing supervision in dress or hygiene		
				Not ready for concentrated close work or small print because of slight farsightedness and still unrefined eye–hand coordination		
				Play is associative; tries to follow rules but may cheat to avoid losing		

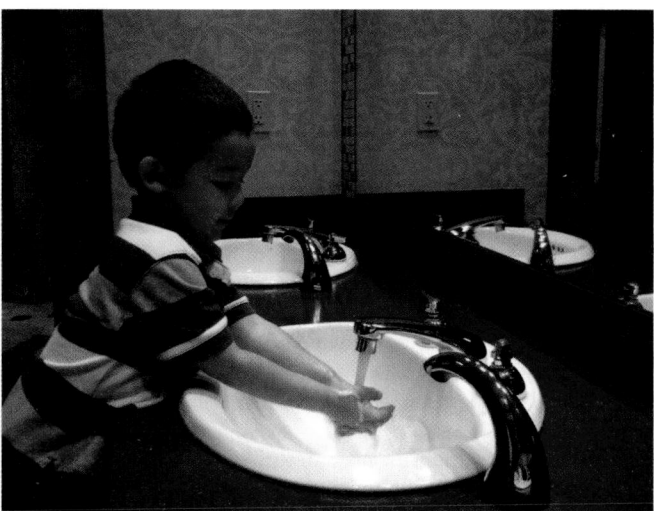

FIG 13-6 Thorough hand washing is the single most effective method of preventing infection.

Areas for parents to evaluate include the facility's daily program, teacher qualifications, staff-to-student ratio, discipline policy, environmental safety precautions, provision of meals, sanitary conditions, adequate indoor and outdoor space per child, and fee schedule. References from other parents help in evaluating a facility, but personal observation of the facility is recommended. Encourage parents to meet the director and some of the employees at a few facilities to make an informed choice.

Evaluation of the facility's health practices is extremely important. Children in daycare centers have more illnesses than children not in daycare centers, especially gastrointestinal tract infections; respiratory tract infections; and hepatitis A, varicella-zoster virus, and cytomegalovirus infections (Nesti and Goldbaum, 2007). Nurses play an important role in infection control. Not only can they advise parents regarding the evaluation of a facility's sanitary practices, but they can also take an active part in educating staff in measures to minimize transmission of infection (Fig. 13-6).

Children need preparation for the preschool or kindergarten experience. For young children, it represents a change from their usual home environment and prolonged separation from their parents. Before children begin school, parents should present the idea as exciting and pleasurable. Talking to children about activities such as painting, building with blocks, or enjoying swings and other outdoor equipment allows children to fantasize about the forthcoming event in a positive manner. When the first day of school arrives, parents should behave confidently. Such behavior requires parents to have resolved their own feelings regarding the experience.

Parents should introduce their child to the teacher and the facility. In some instances, it is helpful for parents to remain with the child for at least part of the first day until the child is comfortable and at ease. Other specific actions that can help reduce separation anxiety include providing the school with detailed information about the child's home environment, such as familiar routines, favorite activities, food preferences, names of siblings or pets, and personal habits. Such information helps the child feel familiar in the strange surroundings. When schools automatically request this information, the parent has a valuable clue to evaluating the quality of the program because the request represents the staff's awareness of each child's needs. Transitional objects, such as a favorite toy, may also help the child bridge the gap from home to school.

Sex Education

Preschoolers have assimilated a tremendous amount of information during their short lifetimes. Although their thinking may not be mature, they search constantly for explanations and reasons that are logical and reasonable to them. The word "why" seems to supplant the word "no," which was common in toddlerhood. It is only natural that as they learn about "me," they will also want to know "Why me?" and "How me?" Questions such as "Where do babies come from?" are as casual as "What makes it rain?" or "Who is that?" It is the way in which questions about procreation are answered that conditions children, even the youngest, to separate these questions from others about their world.

Two rules govern answering sensitive questions about topics such as sex. The first is to *find out what children know and think.* By investigating the theories children have produced as a reasonable explanation, parents can not only give correct information but also help children understand why their explanation is inaccurate. Another reason for ascertaining what the child thinks before offering any information is that the "unasked for" answer may be given. For example, 4-year-old Sally asked her father, "Where did I come from?" Both parents quickly took this inquiry as a clue for offering sex education. After the explanation, Sally exclaimed, "I don't know about all that! All I know is Mary came from New York, and I want to know where I was born."

The second rule for giving information is to *be honest.* It is true that much of the correct information will be forgotten or misunderstood by the preschooler, but the correct information can be restated until the child absorbs and comprehends the facts. Even though the correct anatomic words may be hard to pronounce or even more difficult to remember, they become foundational content for explaining other concepts later on.

Honesty does not imply imparting to children every fact of life or allowing excessive permissiveness in sexual curiosity. When children ask one question, they are looking for one answer. When they are ready, they will ask about the other "unfinished" parts of the story. Sooner or later they will wonder how the "sperm meets the egg" and "how the baby gets out," but during this period, it is best to wait until they ask.

Regardless of whether children are given sex education, they will engage in games of sexual curiosity and exploration. At about 3 years of age, children are aware of the anatomic differences between the sexes and are concerned with how the other "works." This is not really "sexual" curiosity because many children are still unaware of the reproductive function of the genitalia. Their curiosity is for the eliminative function of the anatomy. Little boys wonder how girls can urinate without a penis, so they watch girls go to the bathroom. Because they cannot see anything but the stream of urine coming out, they want to observe further. "Doctor play" is often a game invented for just such investigation. Little girls are no less curious about boys' anatomy. It is intriguing to closely inspect this "thing" that girls do not have.

One question that parents often have is how to handle such sexual curiosity. A positive approach is to neither condone nor condemn the sexual curiosity but to express that if children have questions, they should ask their parents; the parents should then encourage them to engage in some other activity. In this way, children can be helped to understand that there are ways that their sexual curiosity can be satisfied other than through playing investigative games. This in no way condemns the act but stresses alternate methods to seek solutions and answers. Allowing children unrestricted permissiveness only intensifies their anxiety and concern because exploring and searching usually yield little evidence to satisfy their curiosity.

Many excellent books on sex education are available for preschool children at public libraries. The Sexuality Information and Education Council of the United States (SIECUS)* and the AAP† have bibliographies of suggested reading material. Parents should read the book themselves *before* giving or reading them to their children.

Another concern for some parents is masturbation, or self-stimulation of the genitalia. This occurs at any age for a variety of reasons and, if not excessive, is normal and healthy. It is most common at 4 years of age and during adolescence. For preschoolers, it is a part of sexual curiosity and exploration. If parents are concerned about their children masturbating, it is essential for nurses to investigate the circumstances associated with the activity because it may be an expression of anxiety, boredom, or unresolved conflicts. Children who openly and publicly masturbate are inviting a reaction, such as discipline, punishment, or criticism. They may be overwhelmed by their sexual feelings and are asking others to help them channel them into more constructive outlets. Masturbation, similar to other forms of sex play, is a private act, and parents should emphasize this to children when teaching them socially acceptable behavior.

Fears

A great number and variety of real and imagined fears are present during the preschool years, including fear of the dark, being left alone (especially at bedtime), animals (particularly large dogs), ghosts, sexual matters (castration), and objects or persons associated with pain. The exact cause of children's fears is unknown. Parents often become perplexed about handling the fears because no amount of logical persuasion, coercion, or ridicule will send away the ghosts, bogeymen, monsters, and devils. Inappropriate television viewing by preschoolers may increase fears and anxieties because of the inability to separate reality-based experiences from fantasy portrayed on television.

The concept of animism, ascribing lifelike qualities to inanimate objects, helps explain why children fear objects. For example, a child may refuse to use the toilet after watching a television commercial in which the toilet bowl is portrayed as turning into a monster and swallowing a child.

Preschoolers also experience fear of annihilation. Because of poorly defined body boundaries and improved cognitive abilities, young children develop concerns related to loss of body parts. They fear losing body parts with certain medical procedures such as an intravenous insertion or cast application on a limb and may see these procedures as real threats to their existence.

The best way to help children overcome their fears is by actively involving them in finding practical methods to deal with the frightening experience. This may be as simple as keeping a night light on in the child's bedroom for assurance that no monsters lurk in the dark. Exposing children to the feared object in a safe situation also provides a type of conditioning, or desensitization. For instance, children who are afraid of dogs should never be forced to approach or touch one, but they may be gradually introduced to the experience by watching other children play with the animal. This type of modeling, with others demonstrating fearlessness, can be effective if the child is allowed to progress at his or her own rate.

Usually by 5 or 6 years of age, children relinquish many of their fears. Explaining the developmental sequence of fears and their gradual disappearance may help parents feel more secure in handling

preschoolers' fears. Sometimes fears do not subside with simple measures or developmental maturation. When children experience severe fears that disrupt family life, professional help is required.

Stress

Although for parents the preschool years generally are less troublesome than toddlerhood, this period of life presents children with many unique stresses. Some, such as fears, are innate and stem from preschoolers' unique understanding of the world. Others are imposed, such as beginning school. Although minimal amounts of stress are beneficial during the early years to help children develop effective coping skills, excessive stress is harmful. Young children are especially vulnerable because of their limited capacity to cope. Expression of frustration, fear, or anxiety is hampered by inadequate expressive language.

To help parents deal with stress in their children's lives, they must be aware of signs of stress and be helped to identify the source. Any number of stressors may be present, such as the birth of a sibling, marital discord, divorce and separation, relocation, or illness.

The best approach to dealing with stress is prevention—monitoring the amount of stress in children's lives so that levels do not exceed their coping ability. In many instances, structuring children's schedules to allow rest and preparing them for change, such as entering school, is a sufficient measure.

Aggression

The term aggression refers to behavior that attempts to hurt a person or destroy property. Aggression differs from anger, which is a temporary emotional state, but anger may be expressed through aggression. Hyperaggressive behavior in preschoolers is characterized by unprovoked physical attacks on other children and adults, destruction of others' property, frequent intense temper tantrums, extreme impulsivity, disrespect, and noncompliance. Aggression is influenced by a complex set of biologic, sociocultural, and familial variables. Factors that tend to increase aggressive behavior are gender, frustration, modeling, and reinforcement.

Evidence indicates that types of aggression differ between genders. Boys exhibit more physical aggression than girls during preschool years (Benzies, Keown, and Magill-Evans, 2009); however, preschool girls exhibit more relational aggression than preschool boys (Ostrov and Bishop, 2008). Frustration, or the continual thwarting of self-satisfaction by disapproval, humiliation, punishment, or insults, can lead children to act out against others as a means of release. Especially if they fear their parents, these children will displace their anger on others, particularly peers and other authority figures. This type of aggression often applies to children who are well-behaved at home but have a discipline problem at school or are bullies among their playmates.

Modeling, or imitating the behavior of significant others, is a powerful influencing force in preschoolers. Children who see their parents as physically abusive are observing behavior that they come to know as acceptable and therefore may exhibit this behavior with others (Benzies, Keown, and Magill-Evans, 2009). Another aspect of modeling is the "double standard" for acceptable conduct. For example, in some families, aggression is synonymous with masculinity, and boys are encouraged to defend themselves. Television is also a significant source for modeling at this impressionable age. Research indicates there is a direct correlation between media exposure, both violent and educational media, and preschoolers exhibiting physical and relational aggression (Ostrov, Gentile, and Crick, 2006). Therefore, parents should be encouraged to supervise television viewing. The

---

*SIECUS, 1706 R St. NW, Washington, DC 20009; 202-265-2405; fax: 202-462-2340; http://www.siecus.org.
†AAP, 141 Northwest Point Blvd., Elk Grove Village, IL 60007; 847-434-4000; fax: 847-434-8000; http://www.aap.org.

AAP (2007) offers a list of recommendations for healthy television viewing.

Reinforcement can also shape aggressive behavior. Sometimes the reward for aggression is negative (e.g., punishment) yet reinforcing because it brings attention. For example, children who are ignored by a parent until they hit a sibling or the parent learn that this act garners attention.

When children exhibit extreme behaviors, such as aggression, parents may be concerned about the need for professional help. Generally, the difference between "normal" and "problematic" behavior is not the behavior itself but its quantity (number of occurrences), severity (interference with social or cognitive functioning), distribution (different manifestations), onset (when behavior started), and duration (at least 4 weeks).*

Speech Problems

The most critical period for speech development occurs between 2 and 4 years of age. During this period, children are using their rapidly growing vocabulary faster than they can produce the words. Failure to master sensorimotor integrations results in stuttering or stammering as children try to say the word they are already thinking about. This dysfluency in speech pattern is common during language development in children ages 2 to 5 years of age (National Institute on Deafness and Other Communication Disorders, 2010). Stuttering affects boys more frequently than girls, has been shown to have a genetic link, and usually resolves during childhood (Prasse and Kikano, 2008). The National Institute on Deafness and Other Communication Disorders (2010) encourages parents and caregivers of children who stutter to speak slowly and relaxed, refrain from criticizing the child's speech, resist completing the child's sentences, and take time to listen attentively.

The best therapy for speech problems is prevention and early detection. Common causes of speech problems include hearing loss or impairment, oropharyngeal structural anomalies, developmental disorders such as autism, brain injuries and other neuromotor impairments, lack of a verbally stimulating environment, and change in language exposure as in international adoption (Sharp and Hillenbrand, 2008). Referral for further evaluation and treatment may be necessary to prevent a problem from interfering with learning. Anticipatory preparation of parents for expected developmental norms may allay caregiver concerns.

Children pressured into producing sounds ahead of their developmental level may develop dyslalia (articulation problems) or revert to using infantile speech. Prevention involves educating parents regarding the usual achievement of speech production during childhood. The Denver Articulation Screening Exam is an excellent tool for assessing articulation skills of a child and for explaining to parents the expected progression of sounds.

PROMOTING OPTIMAL HEALTH DURING THE PRESCHOOL YEARS†

NUTRITION

Healthy nutrition during childhood should include eating a variety of foods and consuming sufficient energy to promote growth and development while avoiding the development of obesity (Kleinman, 2009). The requirement for calories per unit of body weight continues to decrease slightly to 90 kcal/kg for an average daily intake of 1800 calories. Fluid requirements may also decrease slightly to approximately 100 ml/kg/day but depend on the child's activity level, climatic conditions, and state of health. Protein requirements increase with age, and the recommended intake for preschoolers is 13 to 19 g/day (0.45–0.67 oz/day) (Otten, Hellwig, and Meyers, 2006).

The AAP, Committee on Nutrition recommends the following guidelines for children older than 2 years: saturated fatty acid consumption should be less than 10% of total caloric intake, total fat over several days should be 20% to 30% of total caloric intake, and cholesterol consumption should be less than 300 mg/day (Kleinman, 2009). Research supports the efficacy of following these recommendations, and negative health effects have not been reported (American Heart Association, Gidding, Dennison, and others, 2006). These efforts are important in the prevention of childhood obesity, cardiovascular disease, diabetes, and metabolic syndrome. Evidence is increasing that the incidence of coronary heart disease, obesity, and chronic health problems such as diabetes mellitus can be influenced by early eating patterns (Barlow and Expert Committee, 2007).

While limiting fat consumption, it is also important to ensure diets contain adequate nutrients such as calcium. The recommendation for daily calcium intake for children 1 to 3 years of age is 500 mg, and the recommendation for children 4 to 8 years of age is 800 mg (Otten, Hellwig, and Meyers, 2006). Milk and dairy products are excellent sources of calcium and vitamin D (fortified). Low-fat milk may be substituted, so the quantity of milk may remain the same while limiting fat intake overall.

Excessive consumption of fruit juices and other sweetened beverages has been associated with adverse health effects such as dental caries, gastrointestinal conditions such as chronic diarrhea, and diets poor in nutritive value (Allen and Myers, 2006). The AAP recommends limiting the intake of 100% fruit juice to 4 to 6 oz/day for children ages 1 to 6 years (American Heart Association, Gidding, Dennison, and others, 2006). Parents should be educated regarding nonnutritious fruit drinks, which usually contain less than 10% fruit juice yet are often advertised as healthy and nutritious; sugar content is dramatically increased and often precludes an adequate intake of milk by the child. While counseling parents regarding moderation in fruit juice consumption, providers should offer suggestions for more appropriate sources of nutrients such as ascorbic acid, folate, and potassium. In young children, intake of carbonated beverages that are acidic or that contain high amounts of sugar is also known to contribute to dental caries; large amounts of nonnutritive calories in such beverages may also displace or preclude intake of nutrients necessary for growth.

MyPyramid for Preschoolers is a food guide system created specifically for children ages 2 to 5 years (U.S. Department of Agriculture, Center for Nutrition Policy and Promotion, 2011)‡. This system is comprehensive and provides information for developing a healthy lifestyle at an early age. MyPyramid for Preschoolers includes customizable eating plans and offers information on growth during the preschool years, healthy eating habits, physical activity, and food safety. Parents can use this information to assist their children in making healthy lifestyle choices and to help prevent adverse health conditions secondary to poor nutrition. The importance of role-modeling by parents cannot be overemphasized in regard to food intake and dietary

---

*Information on child development and behavior can be obtained through the AAP, Section on Developmental and Behavioral Pediatrics, http://www.aap.org/sections/dbpeds.

†For a more comprehensive understanding, readers are urged to review Promoting Optimal Health During Toddlerhood, Chapter 12.

‡MyPyramid for Preschoolers information and customizable eating plans are available at http://www.mypyramid.gov/preschoolers.

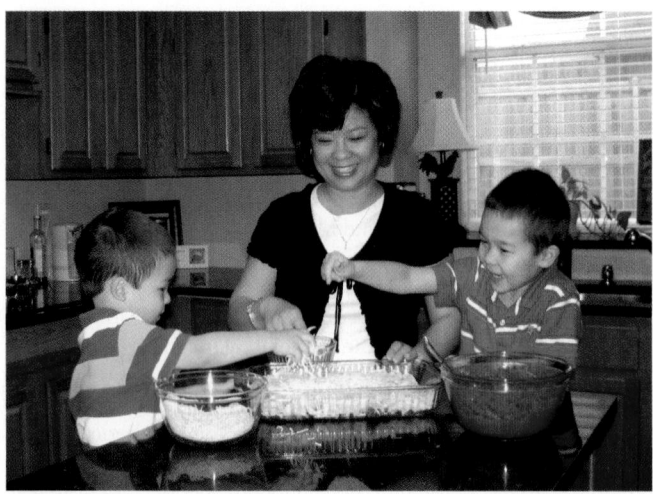

FIG 13-7 Preschool-age children enjoy helping adults and are more likely to try new foods if they can assist in the preparation.

habits; if parents will not eat a particular food or if their dietary habits are poor, children are likely to develop the same habits.

> ### ⚠ NURSING ALERT
>
> Obesity in young children has increased over the past 2 decades. Efforts to provide a healthy diet and to encourage physical activity should begin early to help children achieve optimum health (American Heart Association, Gidding, Dennison, and others, 2006). The 5-2-0-1 framework described by Joy (2008) and inspired by AAP's recommendations, provides a foundation for patient education regarding healthy lifestyle choices. This framework refers to five daily servings of fruits and vegetables, 2 hours or less of screen time, 0 servings of sugar-sweetened beverages, and 1 hour of physical activity per day.

Some preschoolers still have food habits that are typical of toddlers, such as food fads and strong taste preferences. When children reach 4 years of age, they seem to enter another period of finicky eating, which is generally characteristic of the more rebellious behavior of children in this age group. As with toddlers, small portions of each item being served should be offered. The practice of having children remain at the table until the "plate is clean" should be avoided because this may contribute to overeating and the development of poor eating habits that contribute to poor health later in life. By age 5 years, children are more agreeable to trying new foods, especially if they are encouraged by an adult who allows them to help with food preparation or experiment with a new taste or different dish (Fig. 13-7). Mealtimes can become battlegrounds if parents expect perfect table manners.* Usually 5-year-old children are ready for the "social" side of eating, but 3- or 4-year-old children still have difficulty sitting quietly through long family meals.

The amount and variety of foods consumed by young children vary greatly from day to day. Consequently, parents sometimes worry about the quantity and quality of food preschoolers consume. In general, the quality is much more important than the quantity, a fact that should be stressed during nutritional counseling.

*Excellent resources for parents related to mealtimes with toddlers and preschoolers include Jana LA, Shu J: *Food fights: winning the nutritional challenges of parenthood armed with insight, humor, and a bottle of ketchup*, Elk Grove Village, Ill, 2008, AAP; and Satter E: *How to get your kid to eat . . . but not too much*, Boulder, Colo, 1987, Bull Publishing Co.

One way to lessen parental concern is advising parents to keep a weekly record of everything the child eats. In particular, the parents can measure the amount of food, such as setting aside a half cup of vegetables and serving the child from this premeasured amount, to provide a more accurate estimate of food intake at each meal. When parents look at the food chart at the end of the week, they are usually amazed by how much the child has consumed. In general, preschoolers consume only slightly more than toddlers, or about half an adult's portion.

SLEEP AND ACTIVITY

Sleep patterns vary widely, but the average preschooler sleeps about 12 hours a night and infrequently takes daytime naps. Waking during the night is common throughout early childhood and may be related to social and environmental factors rather than developmental or physiologic causes (Moore, Meltzer, and Mindell, 2008). Motor activity levels continue to be high and allow preschoolers to explore their environment, begin learning physical games and sports, and interact with others. Sedentary activities, such as television and video or computer games, are increasingly appealing and can become unhealthy substitutes for active play.

Preschoolers' increased gross motor abilities and coordination allow them to engage in many physical activities, if only at a novice level. Whether young children should begin formalized training in an activity at this early age is controversial. Training programs must consider the child's physical and psychologic immaturity, and readiness to participate in organized sports should be determined individually. The decision to participate should be based on the child's, not the parent's, motivation and enjoyment. The AAP, Committee on Sports Medicine and Fitness and Committee on School Health (2006) encourages free play and a variety of physical activities; however, the AAP also supports organized play when it is developmentally appropriate and occurs in a nonthreatening, fun, and safe environment.

Sleep Problems

The preschool years are a prime time for sleep disturbances. Such disturbances are typically related to increasing autonomy, negative sleep associations, nighttime fears, inconsistent bedtime routines, and lack of limit setting (Moore, Meltzer, and Mindell, 2008). Sleep disturbances may also be caused by nightmares and sleep terrors. Consequences of inadequate sleep include daytime tiredness, irritability and other negative behaviors, hyperactivity, difficulty concentrating, impaired learning ability, poor control of emotions and impulses, and strain on family relationships (Mindell, Kuhn, Lewin, and others, 2006).

Recommendations for handling sleep disturbances are offered only *after* a thorough assessment of the problem. Cultural traditions may dictate sleep practices that are contrary to certain well-accepted professional recommendations; therefore, parents may not perceive a particular sleep practice as a problem.

Interventions differ greatly; for example, **nightmares** (frightening dreams that are followed by full arousal) and **sleep terrors** (partial arousal from deep, nondreaming sleep) require different approaches (Table 13-2).

For children who delay going to bed, a recommended approach involves counseling parents about the importance of a consistent bedtime ritual and emphasizing the normalcy of this type of behavior in young children. Parents should ignore attention-seeking behavior and not take the child into the parents' bed or allow the child to stay up past a reasonable hour. Other measures that may be helpful include keeping a light on in the room, providing transitional objects such as

TABLE 13-2	COMPARISON OF NIGHTMARES WITH SLEEP TERRORS
NIGHTMARES	**SLEEP TERRORS**
Description	
A scary dream; takes place during rapid eye movement (REM) sleep and is followed by full waking	A partial arousal from very deep (stage IV, non-REM) sleep
Time of Distress	
After the dream is over, child wakes and cries or calls, not during the nightmare itself	During the terror itself, child screams and thrashes; afterward is calm
Time of Occurrence	
In the second half of the night, when dreams are most intense	Usually 1–4 hours after falling asleep, when non-REM sleep is deepest
Child's Behavior	
Crying in younger children, fright in all; these behaviors persist even though the child is awake	Initially, child may sit up, thrash, or run in a bizarre manner, with eyes bulging, heart racing, and profuse perspiring; may cry, scream, talk, or moan; there is apparent fright, anger, or obvious confusion, which disappears when child is fully awake
Responsiveness to Others	
Is aware of and reassured by another's presence	Is not very aware of another's presence, is not comforted, and may push person away and scream and thrash more if held or restrained
Return to Sleep	
May be considerably delayed because of persistent fear	Usually rapid; often difficult to keep child awake
Description of Dream	
Yes (if old enough)	No memory of a dream or of yelling or thrashing
Interventions	
Accept dream as real fear. Sit with child; offer comfort, assurance, and sense of protection. Avoid taking child to own bed. Consider professional counseling for recurrent nightmares unresponsive to above approaches.	Observe child for a few minutes *without interfering* until child becomes calm or wakes fully. Intervene only if necessary to protect child from injury. Guide child back to bed if needed. Stress to parents that sleep terrors are a normal, common phenomenon in preschoolers that requires relatively little intervention.

Modified from Ferber R: *Solve your child's sleep problems*, New York, 1985, Simon & Schuster.

a favorite toy, or leaving a drink of water by the bed. Parental consistency is paramount to all treatment approaches.

Helping children slow down *before* bedtime also reduces the resistance to going to bed. One strategy is to establish limited rituals that signal readiness for bed, such as a bath or story. Parents can reinforce the pattern by stating, "After this story, it is bedtime," and consistently carrying out the routine. If anticipated extra stimulation, such as having visitors arrive at bedtime, disrupts this routine, it is advisable to settle children in bed beforehand. Television viewing before bedtime may cause bedtime resistance and delay sleep.

DENTAL HEALTH

By the beginning of the preschool period, the eruption of the deciduous (primary) teeth is complete. Dental care is essential to preserve these temporary teeth and to teach good dental habits (see Chapter 12). Although preschoolers' fine motor control is improved, they still require assistance and supervision with brushing, and flossing should be performed by parents. Professional care and prophylaxis, especially fluoride supplements (if needed), should be continued. The frequency of professional dental care should be based on a child's individual risk assessment, including family history, socioeconomic status, dental development, presence or absence of dental disease,

special health care needs, and dietary habits (Kagihara, Niederhauser, and Stark, 2009). For children cared for away from home, parents should be encouraged to monitor the dental care provided by others, including minimizing cariogenic foods in the diet. Trauma to teeth during this period is common, and prompt evaluation by a dentist is warranted if oral trauma occurs. Preservation of the space previously occupied by an avulsed tooth is necessary for proper eruption of the secondary tooth.

INJURY PREVENTION

Because of improved gross and fine motor skills, coordination, and balance, preschoolers are less prone to falls than are toddlers. They tend to be less reckless; listen more to parental rules; and are aware of potential dangers, such as hot objects, sharp instruments, and dangerous heights. Putting objects in the mouth as part of exploration has all but ceased, although accidental poisoning is still a danger. Pedestrian motor vehicle injuries increase because of activities such as playing in parking lots, driveways, or streets; riding tricycles, bicycles, and other play vehicles; running after balls; or forgetting safety regulations when crossing streets.

In general, the guidelines suggested for injury prevention in Table 12-3 apply to children in this age group as well. However,

FAMILY-CENTERED CARE
Guidance During Preschool Years

Age 3 Years

Prepare parents for child's increasing interest in widening relationships.

Encourage enrollment in preschool.

Emphasize importance of setting limits.

Prepare parents to expect exaggerated tension-reduction behaviors, such as need for a "security blanket."

Encourage parents to offer child choices.

Prepare parents to expect marked changes at 3½ years when child becomes insecure and exhibits emotional extremes.

Prepare parents for normal dysfluency in speech and advise them to avoid focusing on the pattern.

Prepare parents to expect extra demands on their attention as a reflection of child's emotional insecurity and fear of loss of love.

Warn parents that the equilibrium of a 3-year-old child will change to the aggressive, out-of-bounds behavior of a 4-year-old child.

Inform parents to anticipate a more stable appetite with more food selections.

Stress need for protection and education of child to prevent injury (see Safety Promotion and Injury Prevention, Chapter 12).

Age 4 Years

Prepare parents for more aggressive behavior, including motor activity and offensive language.

Prepare parents to expect resistance to parental authority.

Explore parental feelings regarding child's behavior.

Suggest some type of respite for primary caregivers, such as placing child in preschool for part of the day.

Prepare parents for child's increasing sexual curiosity.

Emphasize the importance of realistic limit setting on behavior and appropriate disciplinary techniques.

Prepare parents for the highly imaginative 4-year-old child who indulges in "tall tales" (to be differentiated from lies) and develops imaginary playmates.

Prepare parents to expect nightmares or an increase in them.

Provide reassurance that a period of calmness begins at 5 years of age.

Age 5 Years

Inform parents to expect a tranquil period at 5 years of age.

Help parents prepare the child for entrance into school environment.

Make certain that immunizations are up to date before child enters school.

Suggest that unemployed parental caregivers consider own activities when children begin school.

Suggest swimming lessons for the child.

---

emphasis is now on **education** concerning safety and potential hazards in addition to appropriate protection. This period is an excellent time to start enforcing the use of safety items such as bicycle helmets to prevent head trauma; children are less likely to warm to the idea later in life because of peer pressure. Because preschoolers are great imitators, it is essential that parents set a good example by "practicing what they preach." Children quickly observe discrepancies in what they are told to do and what they see others do. Establishing habits at this time, such as wearing protective equipment, can create long-term safety behaviors.

ANTICIPATORY GUIDANCE—CARE OF FAMILIES

The preschool years present fewer childrearing difficulties than do the earlier years, and this stage of development is facilitated by appropriate anticipatory guidance in the areas already discussed (see Family-Centered Care box). There is a shift in childrearing practices from protection to education. Whereas injury prevention previously focused on safeguarding the immediate environment with less emphasis on reasoning, now the protective guardrails or electrical outlet caps may be replaced by verbal explanations of why danger exists and how to avoid it.

During this period, an emotional transition between parent and child occurs. Although children are still attached to their parents and accept all of their values and beliefs, they are nearing the period of life when they will question previous teachings and prefer the companionship of peers. Entry into school marks a separation from home for parents as well as for children. Parents may need help in adjusting to this change, particularly if one parent has focused his or her daily activities primarily on home responsibilities. All family members must adjust to changes, which is part of the process of growth and development.

KEY POINTS

- The preschool years consist of the period from 3 to 5 years of age, a time that is considered critical for emotional and psychologic development.
- Biologic development in the preschool period is characterized by mature body systems and refinement in gross and fine motor behavior, as evidenced by participation in activities such as running, riding a tricycle, and drawing.
- According to Erikson, acquiring a sense of initiative is the chief psychosocial task of preschoolers. Development of the superego occurs during this period, and conscience begins to emerge.
- According to Piaget, the preschool age is characterized by intuitive or prelogical thinking and a move toward logical thought processes through advanced, complex learning; language; and understanding of causality.

- The seeds of moral development are planted during the preschool period. According to Kohlberg, these children are in the stage of naive instrumental orientation during which they are concerned with satisfying their own needs and, less frequently, the needs of others.
- Social development includes further separation-individuation; more sophisticated language; greater independence; and more complex, imaginative forms of play.
- Areas of special concern to parents during the preschool period are the preschool and kindergarten experience, sex education, fears, stress, and speech problems.
- In selecting an early learning program, parents should inquire about daily activities, teacher qualifications, accreditation, student-to-staff ratio, safety, meals, fees, and health practices.

- Two rules that govern how parents answer questions about sex and other sensitive issues are to find out what the child knows and to be honest.
- Fears constitute a great part of the preschool period; fear of objects or potential annihilation and parent-induced fears are common.
- Preschool aggression may result from frustration, modeling behavior, and reinforcement.

- Hesitancy or dysfluency in speech patterns is a normal characteristic of language development. Speech problems can occur when parents express excessive concern over this pattern.
- Health promotion continues to be directed toward proper nutrition, adequate sleep, proper dental care, and injury prevention.

REFERENCES

Allen RE, Myers AL: Nutrition in toddlers, *Am Fam Physician* 74(9):1527–1532, 2006.

American Academy of Pediatrics: *TV and your family*, 2007, retrieved March 9, 2009, from http://www.aap.org/publiced/BR_TV.htm.

American Academy of Pediatrics, Committee on Sports Medicine and Fitness and Committee on School Health: Active healthy living: prevention of childhood obesity through increased physical activity, *Pediatrics* 117(5):1832–1842, 2006.

American Heart Association, Gidding SS, Dennison BA, and others: Dietary recommendations for children and adolescents: a guide for practitioners, *Pediatrics* 117(2):544–559, 2006.

Barlow SE, Expert Committee: Expert committee recommendations regarding the prevention, assessment, and treatment of child and adolescent overweight and obesity: summary report, *Pediatrics* 120(suppl 4):S164–S192, 2007.

Benzies K, Keown, L, Magill-Evans J: Immediate and sustained effects of parenting on physical aggression in Canadian children aged 6 years and younger, *Can J Psychiatry* 54(1):55–64, 2009.

Hagan JF, Shaw JS, Duncan PM, editors: *Bright futures: guidelines for health supervision of infants, children, and adolescents*, ed 3, Elk Grove Village, Ill, 2008, American Academy of Pediatrics.

Harrison LJ, McLeod S: Risk and protective factors associated with speech and language impairment in a nationally representative sample of 4- to 5-year-old children, *J Speech Lang Hear Res* 53(2):508–529, 2010.

Joy EA: Practical approaches to office-based physical activity promotion for children and adolescents, *Curr Sports Med Rep* 7(6):367–372, 2008.

Kagihara LE, Niederhauser VP, Stark M: Assessment, management, and prevention of early childhood caries, *J Am Acad Nurse Pract* 21(1):1–10, 2009.

Kirkorian HL, Wartella EA, Anderson DR: Media and young children's learning, *Future Child* 18(1):39–61, 2008.

Kleinman RE, editor: *Pediatric nutrition handbook*, ed 6, Elk Grove Village, Ill, 2009, American Academy of Pediatrics.

Mindell JA, Kuhn B, Lewin DS, and others: Behavioral treatment of bedtime problems and night wakings in infants and young children, *Sleep* 29(10):1263–1276, 2006.

Moore M, Meltzer LJ, Mindell JA: Bedtime problems and night wakings in children, *Primary Care Clin Office Pract* 35(3):569–581, 2008.

National Institute on Deafness and Other Communication Disorders, National Institutes of Health: Stuttering, 2010, retrieved January 5, 2011, from http://www.nidcd.nih.gov/health/voice/stutter.htm.

Nesti MMM, Goldbaum M: Infectious diseases and daycare and preschool education, *J Pediatr (Rio J)* 83(4):299–312, 2007.

Ostrov JM, Bishop CM: Preschoolers' aggression and parent-child conflict: a multiinformant and multimethod study, *J Experiment Child Psychol* 99(4):309–322, 2008.

Ostrov JM, Gentile DA, Crick NR: Media exposure, aggression and prosocial behavior during early childhood: a longitudinal study, *Soc Dev* 15(4):612–627, 2006.

Otten JJ, Hellwig JP, Meyers LD, editors: *Dietary reference intakes: the essential guide to nutrient requirements*, Washington, DC, 2006, National Academies Press.

Prasse JE, Kikano GE: Stuttering: an overview, *Am Fam Physician* 77(9):1271–1276, 2008.

Reilly S, Wake M, Ukoumunne OC, and others: Predicting language outcomes at 4 years of age: findings from Early Language in Victoria Study, *Pediatrics* 126(6):1530–1537, 2010.

Sharp HM, Hillenbrand K: Speech and language development and disorders in children, *Pediatr Clin North Am* 55(5):1159–1173, 2008.

Skouteris H, McCabe M, Swinburn B, Hill B: Healthy eating and obesity prevention for preschoolers: a randomized controlled trial, *BMC Public Health* 10:220, 2010.

Speraw S: Spiritual experiences of parents and caregivers who have children with disabilities or special needs, *Issues Mental Health Nurs* 27(2):213–230, 2006.

Trionfi G, Reese E: Good story: children with imaginary companions create richer narratives, *Child Dev* 80(4):1301–1313, 2009.

U.S. Department of Agriculture, Center for Nutrition Policy and Promotion: MyPyramid for preschoolers, 2011, retrieved March 30, 2011, from http://www.mypyramid.gov/preschoolers.

Health Problems of Toddlers and Preschoolers

Kathy McCarthy

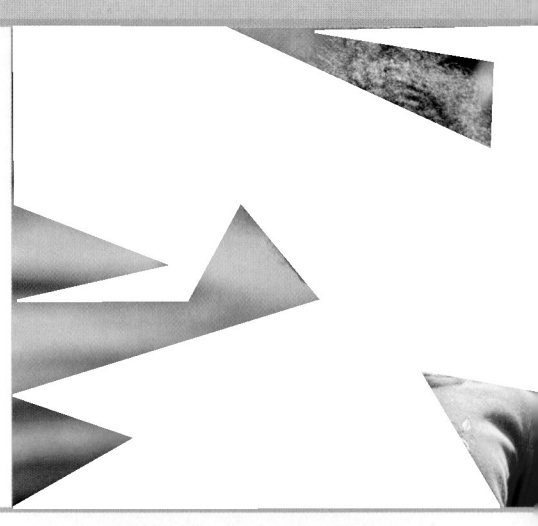

CHAPTER OUTLINE

Infectious Disorders, 423
 Communicable Diseases, 423
 Conjunctivitis, 432
 Stomatitis, 432
Intestinal Parasitic Diseases, 433
 General Nursing Care Management, 433
 Giardiasis, 434
 Enterobiasis (Pinworms), 435
Ingestion of Injurious Agents, 436
 Principles of Emergency Treatment, 437
  Assessment, 437
  Gastric Decontamination, 440
  Prevention of Recurrence, 440

Heavy Metal Poisoning, 441
Lead Poisoning, 441
 Causes of Lead Poisoning, 441
 Screening for Lead Poisoning, 443
Child Maltreatment, 445
Child Neglect, 445
 Types of Neglect, 446
Physical Abuse, 446
 Shaken Baby Syndrome, 446
 Munchausen Syndrome by Proxy, 446
 Factors Predisposing to Physical
  Abuse, 446
Sexual Abuse, 447

Characteristics of Abusers and
 Victims, 447
Initiation and Perpetuation of Sexual
 Abuse, 448
Nursing Care of the Maltreated
 Child, 448
 Caregiver–Child Interaction, 448
 History and Interview, 449
 Physical Assessment, 451

LEARNING OBJECTIVES

On completion of this chapter the reader will be able to:

- Describe the major characteristics of communicable diseases of childhood.
- List three principles of nursing care of children with communicable disease.
- Describe the nursing care of the child with conjunctivitis.
- Distinguish between aphthous stomatitis and herpetic gingivostomatitis.

- Outline a teaching plan designed to prevent transmission of intestinal parasites.
- Identify the principles in the emergency treatment of poisoning.
- Name four sources of lead in the environment.
- Describe the nursing care of the child with lead poisoning.
- State three factors thought to be associated with child abuse.
- State four areas of the history that should arouse suspicion of abuse.
- Describe the nursing care of the abused child.

INFECTIOUS DISORDERS

COMMUNICABLE DISEASES

The incidence of childhood communicable diseases has declined significantly since the advent of immunizations. Serious complications resulting from such infections have been further reduced with the use of antibiotics and antitoxins. However, infectious diseases do occur, and nurses must be familiar with the infectious agent to recognize the disease and to institute appropriate preventive and supportive interventions (Table 14-1). (See also Chapter 30 for a discussion of nursing care for dermatologic conditions.)

Nursing Care Management

Table 14-1 describes the more common communicable diseases of childhood, their therapeutic management, and specific nursing care. The following is a general discussion of nursing care management for communicable diseases. The nursing process for care of the child with a communicable disease is outlined in the Nursing Process box.

Identification of the infectious agent is of primary importance to prevent exposure of susceptible individuals. Nurses in ambulatory care settings, child care centers, and schools are often the first persons to see signs of a communicable disease, such as a rash or sore throat. The nurse must operate under a high index of suspicion for common childhood diseases to identify potentially infectious cases and to recognize diseases that require medical intervention. An example is the common complaint of sore throat. Although most often a symptom of a minor viral infection, it can signal diphtheria or a streptococcal infection, such as scarlet fever. Each of these bacterial conditions requires appropriate medical treatment to prevent serious sequelae.

When a communicable disease is suspected, it is important to assess:

- Recent exposure to a known case
- Prodromal symptoms (symptoms that occur between early manifestations of the disease and its overt clinical syndrome) or evidence of constitutional symptoms, such as a fever or rash (see Table 14-1)
- Immunization history
- History of having the disease

Immunizations are available for many diseases, and infection usually confers lifelong immunity; therefore, the possibility of many infectious agents can be eliminated based on these two criteria.

Prevent Spread

Prevention consists of two components: prevention of the disease and control of its spread to others. Primary prevention rests almost exclusively on immunization. (Chapter 10 discusses the nurse's role in childhood immunization.)

Control measures to prevent spread of disease should include techniques to reduce risk of cross-transmission of infectious organisms between patients and to protect health care workers from organisms harbored by patients. If a child is hospitalized, the facility's policies for infection control should be followed (see Chapter 22). The most important procedure is hand washing. Persons directly caring for children and handling contaminated articles must wash their hands and practice effective Standard Precautions in care of their patients.

Instruct children to practice good hand-washing technique before eating and after toileting. For diseases spread by droplets, instruct the parents in measures to reduce airborne transmission. Children who are old enough should use a tissue to cover their faces during coughing or sneezing; otherwise, the parent should cover children's mouths with tissues and then discard them. Stress the usual hygiene measures of not sharing eating and drinking utensils to the family.

 NURSING PROCESS

Communicable Disease

Assessment

Assess for signs and symptoms of a communicable disease and its consequences. (See Table 14-1 for a discussion of specific communicable diseases.)

Diagnosis (Problem Identification)

After a thorough assessment, several nursing diagnoses are evident:

- Risk for Infection related to susceptible host and infectious agents
- Pain related to skin lesions, malaise
- Impaired Social Interaction related to isolation from peers
- Risk for Impaired Skin Integrity related to scratching from pruritus
- Interrupted Family Processes related to child with an acute illness

Planning

Expected patient outcomes include:

- Child will not spread the infection to others.
- Child will not experience complications.
- Child will have minimum discomfort.
- Child and family will receive adequate emotional support.

Implementation

Numerous intervention strategies are discussed on pp. 423–432.

Evaluation

The effectiveness of nursing interventions for the child with a communicable disease is determined by continual assessment and evaluation of care based on the following guidelines:

- Observe or inquire about family members' use of control measures; observe for signs of disease in household contacts.
- Monitor vital signs, especially temperature; inquire about the identification of high-risk contacts and appropriate isolation of the contacts; observe or inquire about compliance with antibiotic or antiviral therapy.
- Inquire about effectiveness of comfort measures.
- Interview family and child regarding their feelings and concerns, especially when the child returns to school.

! NURSING ALERT

If a child is admitted to the hospital with an undiagnosed exanthema, strict Transmission-Based Precautions (Contact, Airborne, and Droplet) and Standard Precautions are instituted until a diagnosis is confirmed. Childhood communicable diseases requiring these precautions include diphtheria, chickenpox, measles, tuberculosis, adenovirus, *Haemophilus influenza* type b, influenza, mumps, *Mycoplasma pneumonia* infection, pertussis, plague, streptococcal pharyngitis, pneumonia, and scarlet fever (American Academy of Pediatrics, Committee on Infectious Diseases, 2009).

Prevent Complications

Although most children recover without difficulty, certain groups are at risk for serious, even fatal, complications from communicable diseases, especially the viral diseases chickenpox and erythema infectiosum (EI) (fifth disease) caused by human parvovirus (HPV) B19.

Children with immunodeficiency—those receiving steroid or other immunosuppressive therapy, those with a generalized malignancy such as leukemia or lymphoma, and those with an immunologic

Text continues on p. 431

TABLE 14-1 COMMUNICABLE DISEASES OF CHILDHOOD

DISEASE	CLINICAL MANIFESTATIONS	THERAPEUTIC MANAGEMENT AND COMPLICATIONS	NURSING CARE MANAGEMENT
Chickenpox (Varicella) (Fig. 14-1) **Agent**—Varicella-zoster virus (VZV) **Source**—Primary secretions of respiratory tract of infected persons; to a lesser degree, skin lesions (scabs not infectious) **Transmission**—Direct contact, droplet (airborne) spread, and contaminated objects **Incubation period**—2–3 wk, usually 14–16 days **Period of communicability**—Probably 1 day before eruption of lesions (prodromal period) to 6 days after first crop of vesicles when crusts have formed	**Prodromal stage**—Slight fever, malaise, and anorexia for first 24 hr; rash highly pruritic; begins as macule, rapidly progresses to papule and then vesicle (surrounded by erythematous base; becomes umbilicated and cloudy; breaks easily and forms crusts); all three stages (papule, vesicle, crust) present in varying degrees at one time **Distribution**—Centripetal, spreading to face and proximal extremities but sparse on distal limbs and less on areas not exposed to heat (i.e., from clothing or sun) **Constitutional signs and symptoms**—Elevated temperature from lymphadenopathy, irritability from pruritus	**Specific**—Antiviral agent acyclovir (Zovirax); varicella-zoster immune globulin (VariZIG) or immune globulin intravenous (IGIV) after exposure in high-risk children **Supportive**—Diphenhydramine hydrochloride or antihistamines to relieve itching; skin care to prevent secondary bacterial infection Acetaminophen for antipyretic **Complications**—Secondary bacterial infections (abscesses, cellulitis, necrotizing fasciitis, pneumonia, sepsis) Encephalitis Varicella pneumonia (rare in normal children) Hemorrhagic varicella (tiny hemorrhages in vesicles and numerous petechiae in skin) Chronic or transient thrombocytopenia **Preventive**—Childhood immunization	Maintain Standard, Airborne, and Contact Precautions if hospitalized until all lesions are crusted; for immunized child with mild breakthrough varicella, isolate until no new lesions are seen. Keep child in home away from susceptible individuals until vesicles have dried (usually 1 wk after onset of disease), and isolate high-risk children from infected children. Administer skin care: give bath and change clothes and linens daily; administer topical calamine lotion; keep child's fingernails short and clean; apply mittens if child scratches. Keep child cool (may decrease number of lesions). Lessen pruritus; keep child occupied. Remove loose crusts that rub and irritate skin. Teach child to apply pressure to pruritic area rather than scratching it. Avoid use of aspirin (possible association with Reye syndrome).

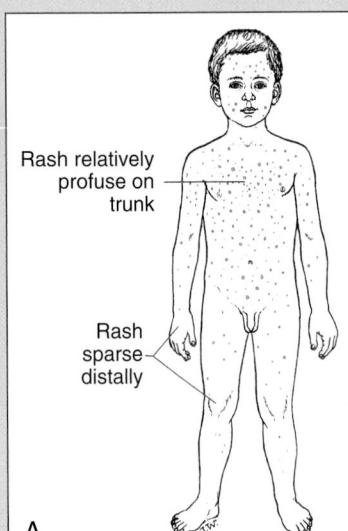

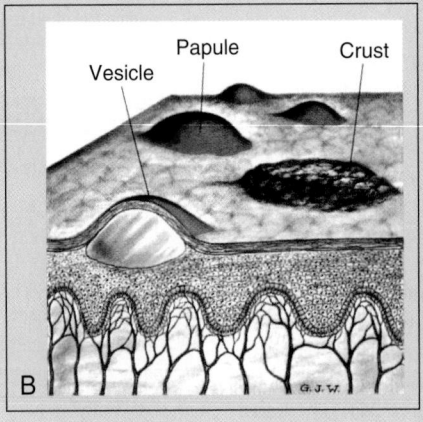

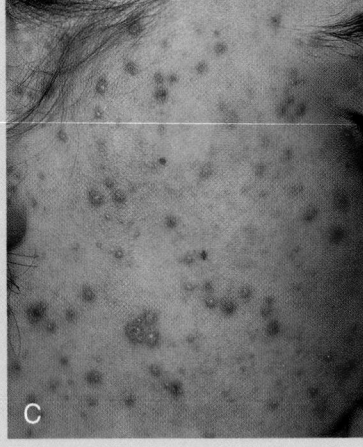

FIG 14-1 Chickenpox (varicella). **A,** Progression of disease. **B,** Simultaneous stages of lesions in chickenpox. **C,** Clinical view. (**C,** From Habif TP: *Clinical dermatology: a color guide to diagnosis and therapy,* ed 5, St. Louis, 2010, Mosby.)

TABLE 14-1 COMMUNICABLE DISEASES OF CHILDHOOD—cont'd

DISEASE	CLINICAL MANIFESTATIONS	THERAPEUTIC MANAGEMENT AND COMPLICATIONS	NURSING CARE MANAGEMENT
Diphtheria **Agent**—*Corynebacterium diphtheriae* **Source**—Discharges from mucous membranes of nose and nasopharynx, skin, and other lesions of infected person **Transmission**—Direct contact with infected person, a carrier, or contaminated articles **Incubation period**—Usually 2–5 days, possibly longer **Period of communicability**—Variable; until virulent bacilli are no longer present (identified by three negative culture results); usually 2 wk but as long as 4 wk	Vary according to anatomic location of pseudomembrane **Nasal**—Resembles common cold, serosanguineous mucopurulent nasal discharge without constitutional symptoms; may have frank epistaxis **Tonsillar–pharyngeal**—Malaise; anorexia; sore throat; low-grade fever; pulse increased above expected for temperature within 24 hr; smooth, adherent, white or gray membrane; lymphadenitis possibly pronounced ("bull's neck"); in severe cases, toxemia, septic shock, and death within 6–10 days **Laryngeal**—Fever, hoarseness, cough, with or without previous signs listed; potential airway obstruction; apprehensive; dyspneic retractions; cyanosis	Equine antitoxin (usually intravenously); preceded by skin or conjunctival test to rule out sensitivity to horse serum Antibiotics (penicillin G procaine or erythromycin) in addition to equine antitoxin Complete bed rest (prevention of myocarditis) Tracheostomy for airway obstruction Treatment of infected contacts and carriers **Complications**—Toxic cardiomyopathy (second to third weeks) Toxic neuropathy **Preventive**—Childhood immunization	Follow Standard and Droplet Precautions until two culture results are negative for *C. diphtheriae*; use Contact Precautions with cutaneous manifestations. Administer antibiotics in a timely manner. Participate in sensitivity testing; have epinephrine available. Administer complete care to maintain bed rest. Use suctioning as needed. Observe respiration for signs of obstruction. Administer humidified oxygen as prescribed.
Erythema Infectiosum (Fifth Disease) (Fig. 14-2) **Agent**—Human parvovirus (HPV) B19 **Source**—Infected persons, mainly school-age children **Transmission**—Respiratory secretions and blood, blood products **Incubation period**—4–14 days; may be as long as 21 days **Period of communicability**—Uncertain but before onset of symptoms in children with aplastic crisis	Rash appears in three stages: **I**—Erythema on face, chiefly on cheeks ("slapped face" appearance); disappears by 1–4 days **II**—About 1 day after rash appears on face, maculopapular red spots appear, symmetrically distributed on upper and lower extremities; rash progresses from proximal to distal surfaces and may last ≥1 wk **III**—Rash subsides but reappears if skin is irritated or traumatized (sun, heat, cold, friction) In children with aplastic crisis, rash usually absent and prodromal illness includes fever, myalgia, lethargy, nausea, vomiting, and abdominal pain Child with sickle cell disease may have concurrent vaso-occlusive crisis	**Symptomatic and supportive**—Antipyretics, analgesics, antiinflammatory drugs Possible blood transfusion for transient aplastic anemia **Complications**—Self-limited arthritis and arthralgia (arthritis may become chronic); more common in women May result in serious complications (anemia, hydrops) or fetal death if mother infected during pregnancy (primarily second trimester) Aplastic crisis in children with hemolytic disease or immunodeficiency Myocarditis (rare)	Isolation of child is not necessary, except hospitalized child (immunosuppressed or with aplastic crises) suspected of HPV infection is placed on Droplet Precautions and Standard Precautions. Pregnant women need not be excluded from workplace where HPV infection is present; they should not care for patients with aplastic crises. Explain low risk of fetal death to those in contact with affected children; assist with routine fetal ultrasonography for detection of fetal hydrops.

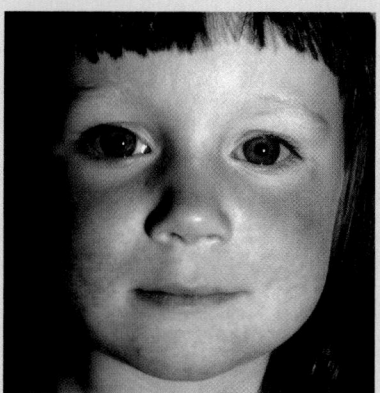

FIG 14-2 Erythema infectiosum. (From Habif TP: *Clinical dermatology: a color guide to diagnosis and therapy*, ed 5, St. Louis, 2010, Mosby.)

Continued

TABLE 14-1	COMMUNICABLE DISEASES OF CHILDHOOD—cont'd		
DISEASE	**CLINICAL MANIFESTATIONS**	**THERAPEUTIC MANAGEMENT AND COMPLICATIONS**	**NURSING CARE MANAGEMENT**
Exanthem Subitum (Roseola Infantum) (Fig. 14-3) **Agent**—Human herpesvirus type 6 (HHV-6; rarely HHV-7) **Source**—Possibly acquired from saliva of healthy adult; entry via nasal, buccal, or conjunctival mucosa **Transmission**—Year round; no reported contact with infected individual in most cases (virtually limited to children <3 yr but peak age is 6–15 mo) **Incubation period**—Usually 5–15 days Period of communicability—Unknown	Persistent high fever for 3–4 days in child who appears well Precipitous drop in fever to normal with appearance of rash **Rash**—Discrete rose-pink macules or maculopapules appearing first on trunk and then spreading to neck, face, and extremities; nonpruritic; fades on pressure; lasts 1–2 days **Associated signs and symptoms**—Cervical and postauricular lymphadenopathy, inflamed pharynx, cough, coryza	Nonspecific Antipyretics to control fever **Complications**—Recurrent febrile seizures (possibly from latent infection of central nervous system that is reactivated by fever) Encephalitis (rare)	Teach parents measures for lowering temperature (antipyretic drugs); ensure adequate parental understanding of specific antipyretic dosage to prevent accidental overdose. If child is prone to seizures, discuss appropriate precautions and possibility of recurrent febrile seizures.

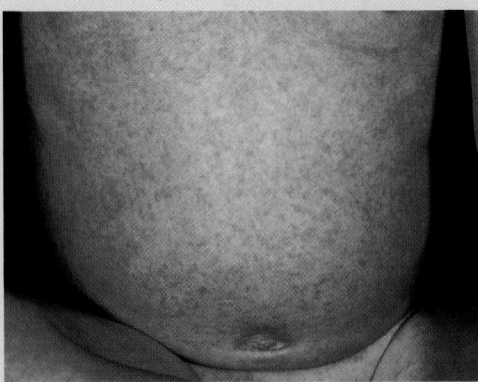

FIG 14-3 Roseola infantum. (From Habif TP: *Clinical dermatology: a color guide to diagnosis and therapy*, ed 5, St. Louis, 2010, Mosby.)

⊖ **Mumps**

Mumps **Agent**—Paramyxovirus **Source**—Saliva of infected persons **Transmission**—Direct contact with or droplet spread from an infected person **Incubation period**—14–21 days **Period of communicability**—Most communicable immediately before and after swelling begins	**Prodromal stage**—Fever, headache, malaise, and anorexia for 24 hr followed by "earache" that is aggravated by chewing **Parotitis**—By third day, parotid gland(s) (either unilateral or bilateral) enlarges and reaches maximum size in 1–3 days; accompanied by pain and tenderness; other exocrine glands (submandibular) may also be swollen	**Preventive**—Childhood immunization **Symptomatic and supportive**—Analgesics for pain and antipyretics for fever Intravenous fluid if needed for child who refuses to drink or vomits because of meningoencephalitis **Complications**—Sensorineural deafness Postinfectious encephalitis Myocarditis Arthritis Hepatitis Epididymoorchitis Oophoritis Pancreatitis Sterility (extremely rare in adult men) Meningitis	Maintain isolation during period of communicability; institute Droplet and Contact Precautions during hospitalization. Encourage rest and decreased activity during prodromal phase until swelling subsides. Give analgesics for pain; if child is unwilling to swallow pills or tablets medication, use elixir form. Encourage fluids and soft, bland foods; avoid foods requiring chewing. Apply hot or cold compresses to neck, whichever is more comforting. To relieve orchitis, provide warmth and local support with tight-fitting underpants.

TABLE 14-1   COMMUNICABLE DISEASES OF CHILDHOOD—cont'd

DISEASE	CLINICAL MANIFESTATIONS	THERAPEUTIC MANAGEMENT AND COMPLICATIONS	NURSING CARE MANAGEMENT
Measles (Rubeola) (Fig. 14-4) **Agent**—Virus **Source**—Respiratory tract secretions, blood, and urine of infected person **Transmission**—Usually by direct contact with droplets of infected person; primarily in the winter **Incubation period**—10–20 days **Period of communicability**—From 4 days before to 5 days after rash appears but mainly during prodromal (catarrhal) stage	**Prodromal (catarrhal) stage**—Fever and malaise, followed in 24 hr by coryza, cough, conjunctivitis, Koplik spots (small, irregular red spots with a minute, bluish white center first seen on buccal mucosa opposite molars 2 days before rash); symptoms gradually increasing in severity until second day after rash appears, when they begin to subside **Rash**—Appears 3–4 days after onset of prodromal stage; begins as erythematous maculopapular eruption on face and gradually spreads downward; more severe in earlier sites (appears confluent) and less intense in later sites (appears discrete); after 3–4 days, assumes brownish appearance, and fine desquamation occurs over area of extensive involvement **Constitutional signs and symptoms**—Anorexia, abdominal pain, malaise, generalized lymphadenopathy	**Preventive**—Childhood immunization. Vitamin A supplementation (see p. 431) **Supportive**—Bed rest during febrile period; antipyretics Antibiotics to prevent secondary bacterial infection in high-risk children **Complications**—Otitis media Pneumonia (bacterial) Obstructive laryngitis and laryngotracheitis Encephalitis (rare but has high mortality)	Maintain isolation until fifth day of rash; if child is hospitalized, institute Airborne Precautions. Encourage rest during prodromal stage; provide quiet activity. **Fever**—Instruct parents to administer antipyretics; avoid chilling; if child is prone to seizures, institute appropriate precautions. **Eye care**—Dim lights if photophobia present; clean eyelids with warm saline solution to remove secretions or crusts; keep child from rubbing eyes. **Coryza, cough**—Use cool-mist vaporizer; protect skin around nares with layer of petrolatum; encourage fluids and soft, bland foods. **Skin care**—Keep skin clean; use tepid baths as necessary.

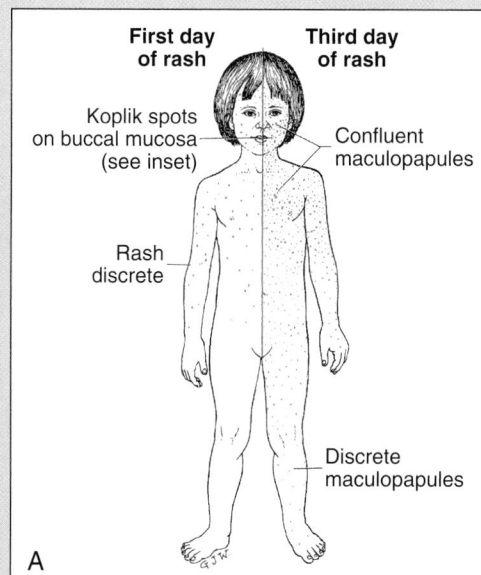

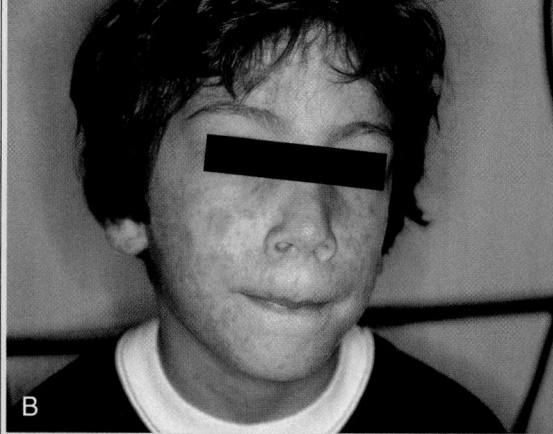

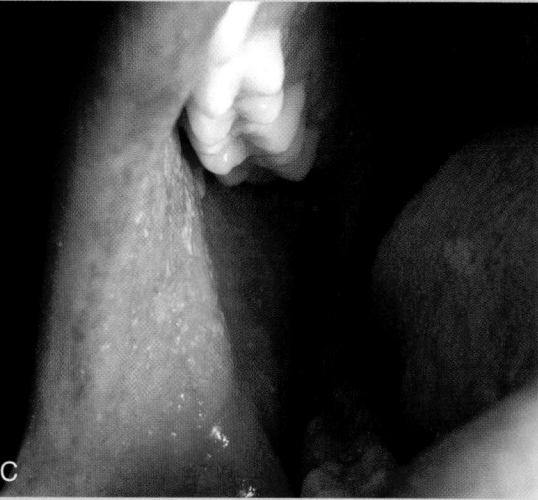

FIG 14-4 Measles (rubeola). **A,** Progression of disease. **B,** Clinical view. **C,** Koplik spots. (**B,** From Paller SA, Mancini AJ: *Hurwitz clinical pediatric dermatology,* ed 4, St. Louis, 2011, Saunders; **C,** From Habif TP: *Clinical dermatology: a color guide to diagnosis and therapy,* ed 5, St. Louis, 2010, Mosby.)

Continued

TABLE 14-1	COMMUNICABLE DISEASES OF CHILDHOOD—cont'd		
DISEASE	**CLINICAL MANIFESTATIONS**	**THERAPEUTIC MANAGEMENT AND COMPLICATIONS**	**NURSING CARE MANAGEMENT**
Pertussis (Whooping Cough) **Agent**—*Bordetella pertussis* **Source**—Discharge from respiratory tract of infected persons **Transmission**—Direct contact or droplet spread from infected person; indirect contact with freshly contaminated articles **Incubation period**—6–20 days; usually 7–10 days **Period of communicability**— Greatest during catarrhal stage before onset of paroxysms	**Catarrhal stage**—Begins with symptoms of upper respiratory tract infection, such as coryza, sneezing, lacrimation, cough, and low-grade fever; symptoms continue for 1–2 wk, when dry, hacking cough becomes more severe **Paroxysmal stage**—Cough most common at night; consists of short, rapid coughs followed by sudden inspiration associated with a high-pitched crowing sound or "whoop"; during paroxysms, cheeks become flushed or cyanotic, eyes bulge, and tongue protrudes; paroxysm may continue until thick mucous plug is dislodged; vomiting frequently follows attack; stage generally lasts 4–6 wk, followed by convalescent stage Infants younger than age 6 mo may not have characteristic whoop cough but have difficulty maintaining adequate oxygenation with amount of secretions, frequent vomiting of mucus and formula or breast milk Pertussis may occur in adolescents and adults with varying manifestations; cough and whoop may be absent; however, as many as 50% of adolescents may have a cough for ≤10 wk (American Academy of Pediatrics, Committee on Infectious Diseases, 2009) Additional symptoms in adolescents include difficulty breathing and posttussive vomiting (See also Immunizations, Chapter 10, for discussion of pertussis immunization schedule.)	**Preventive**—Immunization; current belief is that childhood immunizations for pertussis do not confer lifelong immunity to adolescents and adults, so a pertussis booster is recommended for adolescents (see Chapter 10, Schedule for Immunizations) Antimicrobial therapy (e.g., erythromycin, clarithromycin, azithromycin) **Supportive**—Hospitalization sometimes required for infants, children who are dehydrated, or those who have complications Increased oxygen intake and humidity Adequate fluids Intensive care and mechanical ventilation if needed for infants younger than age 6 mo **Complications**—Pneumonia (usual cause of death in younger children) Apnea (infants <1 yr) Atelectasis Otitis media Seizures Hemorrhage (scleral, conjunctival, epistaxis; pulmonary hemorrhage in neonate) Weight loss and dehydration Hernias (umbilical and inguinal) Prolapsed rectum Complications reported among adolescents include syncope, sleep disturbance, rib fractures, incontinence, and pneumonia (American Academy of Pediatrics, Committee on Infectious Diseases, 2009)	Maintain isolation during catarrhal stage; if child is hospitalized, institute Droplet Precautions. Obtain nasopharyngeal culture for diagnosis. Encourage oral fluids; offer small amount of fluids frequently. Ensure adequate oxygenation during paroxysms; position infant on side to decrease chance of aspiration with vomiting. Provide humidified oxygen; suction as needed to prevent choking on secretions. Observe for signs of airway obstruction (increased restlessness, apprehension, retractions, cyanosis). Encourage compliance with antibiotic therapy for household contacts. Encourage adolescents to obtain pertussis booster (Tdap) (see also Immunizations, Chapter 10). Use Standard Precautions and mask in health care workers exposed to children with persistent cough and high suspicion of pertussis. Cough medicine unlikely to help and not recommended for children younger than age 2 yr (http://www.fda.gov, 2008)
Poliomyelitis **Agent**—Enteroviruses, three types: type 1, most frequent cause of paralysis, both epidemic and endemic; type 2, least frequently associated with paralysis; type 3, second most frequently associated with paralysis	May be manifested in three different forms: **Abortive or inapparent**—Fever, uneasiness, sore throat, headache, anorexia, vomiting, abdominal pain; lasts a few hours to a few days **Nonparalytic**—Same manifestations as abortive but more severe, with pain and stiffness in neck, back, and legs	**Preventive**—Childhood immunization **Supportive**—Complete bed rest during acute phase Mechanical or assisted ventilation in case of respiratory paralysis Physical therapy for muscles after acute stage	Institute Contact Precautions. Administer mild sedatives as necessary to relieve anxiety and promote rest. Participate in physical therapy procedures (use of moist hot packs and range-of-motion exercises).

TABLE 14-1	COMMUNICABLE DISEASES OF CHILDHOOD—cont'd		
DISEASE	**CLINICAL MANIFESTATIONS**	**THERAPEUTIC MANAGEMENT AND COMPLICATIONS**	**NURSING CARE MANAGEMENT**
Source—Feces and oropharyngeal secretions of infected persons, especially young children **Transmission**—Direct contact with persons with apparent or inapparent active infection; spread via fecal–oral and pharyngeal–oropharyngeal routes Vaccine-acquired paralytic polio may occur as a result of the live oral polio vaccination (no longer available in the United States) **Incubation period**—Usually 7–14 days, with range of 5–35 days **Period of communicability**—Not exactly known; virus present in throat and feces shortly after infection and persists for about 1 wk in throat and 4–6 wk in feces	**Paralytic**—Initial course similar to nonparalytic type followed by recovery and then signs of central nervous system paralysis	**Complications**—Permanent paralysis Respiratory arrest Hypertension Kidney stones from demineralization of bone during prolonged immobility	Position child to maintain body alignment and prevent contractures or skin breakdown; use footboard or appropriate orthoses to prevent footdrop; use pressure mattress for prolonged immobility. Encourage child to perform activities of daily living to capability; promote early ambulation with assistive devices; administer analgesics for maximum comfort during physical activity; give high-protein diet and bowel management for prolonged immobility. Observe for respiratory paralysis (difficulty talking, ineffective cough, inability to hold breath, shallow and rapid respirations); report such signs and symptoms to practitioner.
Rubella (German Measles) (Fig. 14-5) **Agent**—Rubella virus **Source**—Primarily nasopharyngeal secretions of person with apparent or inapparent infection; virus also present in blood, stool, and urine **Incubation period**—14–21 days **Period of communicability**—7 days before to about 5 days after appearance of rash **Constitutional signs and symptoms**—Occasionally low-grade fever, headache, malaise, and lymphadenopathy	**Prodromal stage**—Absent in children, present in adults and adolescents; consists of low-grade fever, headache, malaise, anorexia, mild conjunctivitis, coryza, sore throat, cough, and lymphadenopathy; lasts 1–5 days, subsides 1 day after appearance of rash **Rash**—First appears on face and rapidly spreads downward to neck, arms, trunk, and legs; by end of first day, body is covered with discrete, pinkish red maculopapular exanthema; disappears in same order as it began and is usually gone by third day	**Preventive**—Childhood immunization No treatment necessary other than antipyretics for low-grade fever and analgesics for discomfort **Complications**—Rare (arthritis, encephalitis, or purpura); most benign of all childhood communicable diseases; greatest danger is teratogenic effect on fetuses	Institute Droplet Precautions. Reassure parents of benign nature of illness in affected child. Use comfort measures as necessary. Avoid contact with pregnant women. Monitor rubella titer in pregnant adolescents.

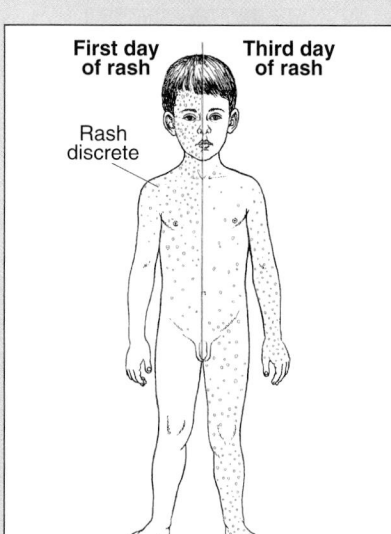

First day of rash Third day of rash

Rash discrete

A

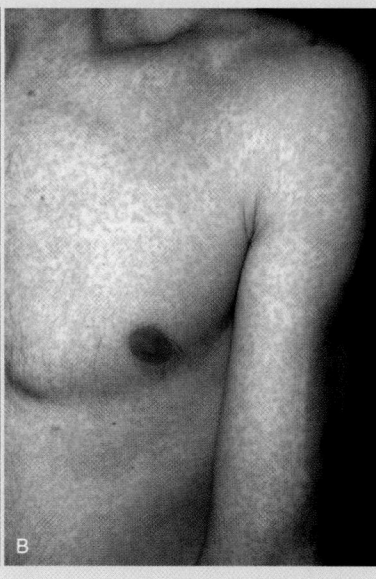

B

FIG 14-5 Rubella (German measles). **A,** Progression of rash. **B,** Clinical view. (**B,** From Habif TP: *Clinical dermatology: a color guide to diagnosis and therapy,* ed 5, St. Louis, 2010, Mosby.)

Continued

TABLE 14-1 COMMUNICABLE DISEASES OF CHILDHOOD—cont'd

DISEASE	CLINICAL MANIFESTATIONS	THERAPEUTIC MANAGEMENT AND COMPLICATIONS	NURSING CARE MANAGEMENT
Scarlet Fever (Fig. 14-6) **Agent**—Group A β-hemolytic streptococci **Source**—Usually from nasopharyngeal secretions of infected persons and carriers **Transmission**—Direct contact with infected person or droplet spread; indirectly by contact with contaminated articles or ingestion of contaminated milk or other food **Incubation period**—2–5 days, with range of 1–7 days **Period of communicability**—During incubation period and clinical illness, ≈10 days; during first 2 wk of carrier phase, although may persist for months	**Prodromal stage**—Abrupt high fever, pulse increased out of proportion to fever, vomiting, headache, chills, malaise, abdominal pain, halitosis **Enanthema**—Tonsils enlarged, edematous, reddened, and covered with patches of exudates; in severe cases appearance resembles membrane seen in diphtheria; pharynx is edematous and beefy red; during first 1–2 days tongue is coated and papillae become red and swollen (white strawberry tongue); by fourth or fifth day, white coat sloughs off, leaving prominent papillae (red strawberry tongue); palate is covered with erythematous punctate lesions **Exanthema**—Rash appears within 12 hr after prodromal signs; red pinhead-sized punctate lesions rapidly become generalized but are absent on face, which becomes flushed with striking circumoral pallor; rash more intense in folds of joints; by end of first wk desquamation begins (fine, sandpaper-like on torso; sheetlike sloughing on palms and soles), which may be complete by ≥3 wk	Full course of penicillin (or erythromycin in penicillin-sensitive children) or oral cephalosporin Antibiotic therapy for newly diagnosed carriers (nose or throat cultures positive for streptococci) **Supportive**—Rest during febrile phase, analgesics for sore throat; antipruritics for rash if bothersome **Complications**—Peritonsillar and retropharyngeal abscess Sinusitis Otitis media Acute glomerulonephritis Acute rheumatic fever Polyarthritis (uncommon)	Institute Standard and Droplet Precautions until 24 hr after initiation of treatment. Ensure compliance with oral antibiotic therapy; intramuscular benzathine penicillin G [Bicillin] may be given. Encourage rest during febrile phase; provide quiet activity during convalescent period. Relieve discomfort of sore throat with analgesics, gargles, lozenges, antiseptic throat sprays, and inhalation of cool mist. Encourage fluids during febrile phase; avoid irritating liquids (certain citrus juices) and rough foods (chips); when child is able to eat, begin with soft diet. Advise parents to consult practitioner if fever persists after beginning therapy. Discuss procedures for preventing spread of infection—discard toothbrush; avoid sharing drinking and eating utensils.

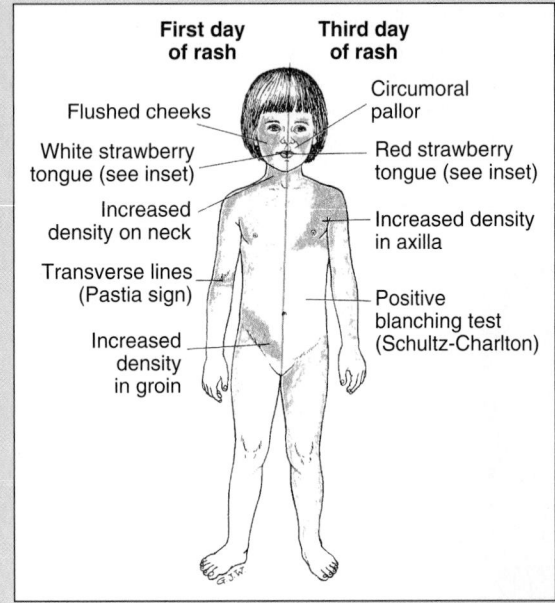
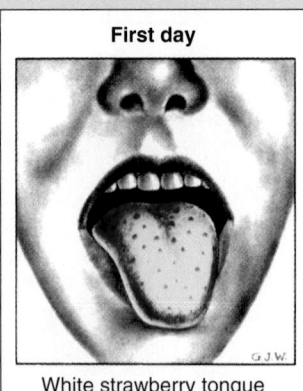
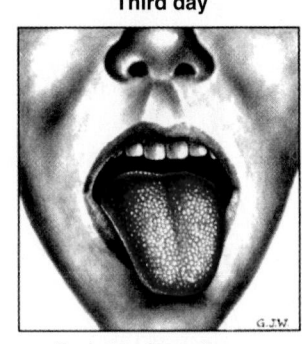

FIG 14-6 Scarlet fever.

disorder—are at risk for viremia from replication of the varicella-zoster virus (VZV)* in the blood. VZV is so named because it causes two distinct diseases: varicella (chickenpox) and zoster (herpes zoster or shingles). Varicella occurs primarily in children younger than 15 years of age. However, it leaves the threat of herpes zoster, an intensely painful varicella that is localized to a single dermatome (body area innervated by a particular segment of the spinal cord). In children, the dermatomes most likely affected by herpes zoster are the cervical and sacral dermatomes (Leung, Robson, and Leong, 2006). Immunocompromised patients and healthy infants younger than 1 year of age (who also have reduced immunity) are at a higher risk for reactivation of VZV causing herpes zoster, probably as a result of a deficiency in cellular immunity (American Academy of Pediatrics [AAP], Committee on Infectious Diseases, 2009; Galea, Sweet, Beninger, and others, 2008). Complications of herpes zoster virus in children include secondary bacterial infection, depigmentation, and scarring. Postherpetic neuralgia in children is uncommon (Leung, Robson, and Leong, 2006).

The use of VCZ immune globulin (VariZIG) or immune globulin intravenous (IGIV) is recommended for children who are immunocompromised, who have no previous history of varicella, and who are likely to contract the disease and have complications as a result (AAP, Committee on Infectious Diseases, 2009). The antiviral agent acyclovir (Zovirax) may be used to treat varicella infections in susceptible immunocompromised persons. It is effective in decreasing the number of lesions; shortening the duration of fever; and decreasing itching, lethargy, and anorexia. Consider oral acyclovir for immunocompromised children without a history of varicella disease, newborns whose mothers had varicella within 5 days before delivery or within 48 hours after delivery, and hospitalized preterm infants with significant varicella exposure (AAP, Committee on Infectious Diseases, 2009).

Children with hemolytic disease, such as sickle cell disease, are at risk for aplastic anemia from EI. HPV B19 infects and lyses red blood cell (RBC) precursors, thus interrupting the production of RBCs. Therefore, the virus may precipitate a severe aplastic crisis in patients who need increased RBC production to maintain normal RBC volumes. Thrombocytopenia and neutropenia may also occur as a result of HPV B19 infection. Fetuses have a relatively high rate of RBC production and immature immune systems; they may develop severe anemia and hydrops as a result of maternal HPV infection. Fetal death rates as a result of HPV B19 have been estimated to be between 2% and 6% (AAP, Committee on Infectious Diseases, 2009).

> **! NURSING ALERT**
>
> Refer children at risk for contracting these communicable diseases to the practitioner immediately in case of known exposure or outbreaks.

In the past decade, the incidence of pertussis has increased, particularly in infants younger than 6 months old and in children 10 to 14 years of age. Early clinical manifestations of pertussis in infants may include gagging, coughing, emesis, and apnea; the typical "whoop" associated with the disease is absent (Teng and Wang, 2011; Wood and McIntyre, 2008). In older children, the disease may manifest as a common cold (see Table 14-1). There is now a recommendation that children ages 11 to 18 years old receive a booster pertussis vaccine (tetanus and acellular pertussis [Tdap]) to prevent the disease. (See Immunizations, Chapter 10.) Because pertussis is contagious, especially among close household members, identify pertussis early and initiate treatment for the child and those who have been exposed. Azithromycin (for infants younger than 1 month old) and clarithromycin or azithromycin is administered to infants and children with pertussis (Teng and Wang, 2011; Wood and McIntyre, 2008).

Prevention of complications from diseases such as diphtheria, pertussis, and scarlet fever requires compliance with antibiotic therapy. With oral preparations, stress the need to complete the entire course of therapy. (See Compliance, Chapter 22.)

Evidence suggests that vitamin A supplementation reduces both morbidity and mortality in measles and that all children with severe measles should receive vitamin A supplements. A single oral dose of 200,000 IU for children at least 1 year old is recommended (use half that dose for children 6 to 12 months of age). The higher dose may be associated with vomiting and headache for a few hours. The dose should be repeated the next day and at 4 weeks for children with ophthalmologic evidence of vitamin A deficiency (AAP, Committee on Infectious Diseases, 2009).

> **! NURSING ALERT**
>
> Although the risk of vitamin A toxicity from these doses (they are 100–200 times the Recommended Dietary Allowance) is relatively low, nurses should instruct parents on safe storage of the drug. Ideally, vitamin A should be dispensed in the age-appropriate unit dose to prevent excessive administration and possible toxicity.

Provide Comfort

Many communicable diseases cause skin manifestations that are bothersome to children. The chief discomfort from most rashes is itching, and measures such as cool baths (usually without soap) and lotions (e.g., calamine) are helpful.

> **! NURSING ALERT**
>
> When lotions with active ingredients such as diphenhydramine in Caladryl are used, they are applied sparingly, especially over open lesions, where excessive absorption can lead to drug toxicity. Use these lotions with caution in children who are simultaneously receiving an oral antihistamine. Cooling the lotion in the refrigerator beforehand often makes it more soothing on the skin than at room temperature.

To avoid overheating, which increases itching, children should wear lightweight, loose, nonirritating clothing and keep out of the sun. If the child persists in scratching, keep the nails short and smooth or use mittens and clothes with long sleeves or legs. For severe itching, antipruritic medication, such as diphenhydramine (Benadryl) or hydroxyzine (Atarax), may be required, especially when the child has trouble sleeping because of itching. Loratadine, cetirizine, and fexofenadine do not cause drowsiness and may be preferred for urticaria during the day.

An elevated temperature is common, and both antipyretic medicine (acetaminophen or ibuprofen) and environmental manipulation are implemented. (See Controlling Elevated Temperatures, Chapter 22.) Acetaminophen is effective in lowering the fever but does not significantly reduce the symptoms of itching, anorexia, abdominal pain, fussiness, or vomiting.

---

*Educational materials may be obtained from the National Shingles Foundation, 603 West 115th St., Suite 371, New York, NY 10025; 212-222-3390; www.vzvfoundation.org.

A sore throat, another frequent symptom, is managed with lozenges, saline rinses (if the child is old enough to cooperate), and analgesics. Because most children are anorectic during an illness, bland foods and increased liquids are usually preferred. During the early stages of the disease, children voluntarily curtail their activity, and although bed rest is beneficial, it should not be imposed unless specifically indicated. During periods of irritability, quiet activity (e.g., reading, music, television, video games, puzzles, coloring) helps distract children from the discomfort.

Support the Child and Family

Most communicable diseases are benign, but they may produce considerable concern and anxiety for parents. Often the occurrence of a disease such as chickenpox is the first time the child is acutely uncomfortable. Parents need assistance to cope with manifestations of the illness, such as intense itching. The family and child need reassurance that recovery is generally rapid. However, visible signs of the dermatosis may be present for some time after the child is well enough to resume usual activities.

CONJUNCTIVITIS

Acute conjunctivitis (inflammation of the conjunctiva) occurs from a variety of causes that are typically age related. In newborns, conjunctivitis can occur from infection during birth, most often from *Chlamydia trachomatis* (inclusion conjunctivitis) or *Neisseria gonorrhoeae*. These organisms, as well as herpes simplex virus (HSV), cause serious ocular damage. In infants, recurrent conjunctivitis may be a sign of nasolacrimal (tear) duct obstruction. A chemical conjunctivitis may occur within 24 hours of instillation of neonatal ophthalmic prophylaxis; the clinical features include mild eyelid edema and a sterile, nonpurulent eye discharge (Fuloria and Kreiter, 2002). In children, the usual causes of conjunctivitis are viral, bacterial, allergic, or related to a foreign body. Bacterial infection accounts for most instances of acute conjunctivitis in children. Diagnosis is made primarily from the clinical manifestations (Box 14-1), although cultures of purulent drainage may be needed to identify the specific cause.

Therapeutic Management

Treatment of conjunctivitis depends on the cause. Viral conjunctivitis is self-limiting, and treatment is limited to removal of the accumulated secretions. Bacterial conjunctivitis has traditionally been treated with topical antibacterial agents such as polymyxin and bacitracin (Polysporin), sodium sulfacetamide (Sulamyd), or trimethoprim and polymyxin (Polytrim). However, in one study of children with acute infective conjunctivitis treated by placebo versus topical chloramphenicol, there was little difference in cure rates; the authors concluded that most children get better without antibiotic treatment (Rose, Harnden, Brueggemann, and others, 2005). Fluoroquinolones, approved for children ages 1 year and older, are viewed by ophthalmologists as the best ophthalmic antimicrobial agents available (Lichtenstein, Rinehart, and Levofloxacin Bacterial Conjunctivitis Study Group, 2003). Drops may be used during the day and an ointment at bedtime because the ointment preparation remains in the eye longer but blurs the vision. Corticosteroids are avoided because they reduce ocular resistance to bacteria.

Nursing Care Management

Nursing care includes keeping the eye clean and properly administering ophthalmic medication. Remove accumulated secretions by wiping from the inner canthus downward and outward away from the opposite eye. Warm, moist compresses, such as a clean washcloth wrung out with hot tap water, are helpful in removing the crusts. Compresses are *not* kept on the eye because an occlusive covering promotes bacterial growth. Medication should be instilled immediately after the eyes have been cleaned and according to correct procedure (see Chapter 22).

Prevention of infection in other family members is an important consideration with bacterial conjunctivitis. Keep the child's washcloth and towel separate from those used by others. Discard tissues used to clean the eye. Instruct the child to refrain from rubbing the eye and to use good hand-washing technique.

> ### BOX 14-1 CLINICAL MANIFESTATIONS OF CONJUNCTIVITIS
>
> **Bacterial Conjunctivitis ("Pink Eye")**
> Purulent drainage
> Crusting of eyelids, especially on awakening
> Inflamed conjunctiva
> Swollen eyelids
>
> **Viral Conjunctivitis**
> Usually occurs with upper respiratory tract infection
> Serous (watery) drainage
> Inflamed conjunctiva
> Swollen eyelids
>
> **Allergic Conjunctivitis**
> Itching
> Watery to thick, stringy discharge
> Inflamed conjunctiva
> Swollen eyelids
>
> **Conjunctivitis Caused by Foreign Body**
> Tearing
> Pain
> Inflamed conjunctiva
> Usually only one eye affected

> ### ! NURSING ALERT
>
> Signs of serious conjunctivitis include reduction or loss of vision, ocular pain, photophobia, exophthalmos (bulging eyeball), decreased ocular mobility, corneal ulceration, and unusual patterns of inflammation (e.g., the perilimbal flush associated with iritis or localized inflammation associated with scleritis). If a patient has any of these signs, refer him or her immediately to an ophthalmologist (Lederman and Lederman, 2003).

STOMATITIS

Stomatitis is inflammation of the oral mucosa, which may include the buccal (cheek) and labial (lip) mucosa, tongue, gingiva, palate, and floor of the mouth. It may be infectious or noninfectious and may be caused by local or systemic factors. In children, aphthous stomatitis and herpetic stomatitis are typically seen. Children with immunosuppression and those receiving chemotherapy or head and neck radiotherapy are at high risk for developing mucosal ulceration and herpetic stomatitis.

Case Study—Bacterial Conjunctivitis

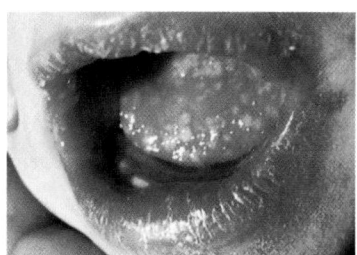

FIG 14-7 Primary gingivostomatitis. (From Thompson JM, McFarland GM, Hirsch JE, and others: *Mosby's clinical nursing,* ed 5, St. Louis, 2002, Mosby.)

Aphthous stomatitis (aphthous ulcer, canker sore) is a benign but painful condition whose cause is unknown. Its onset is usually associated with mild traumatic injury (biting the cheek, hitting the mucosa with a toothbrush, or a mouth appliance rubbing on the mucosa), allergy, or emotional stress. The lesions are painful, small, whitish ulcerations surrounded by a red border. They are distinguished from other types of stomatitis by healthy adjacent tissues, absence of vesicles, and no systemic illness. The ulcers persist for 4 to 12 days and heal uneventfully.

Herpetic gingivostomatitis (HGS) is caused by HSV, most often type 1, and may occur as a primary infection or recur in a less severe form known as **recurrent herpes labialis** (commonly called *cold sores* or *fever blisters*). The primary infection usually begins with a fever; the pharynx becomes edematous and erythematous; and vesicles erupt on the mucosa, causing severe pain (Fig. 14-7). Cervical lymphadenitis often occurs, and the breath has a distinctly foul odor. In the recurrent form, the vesicles appear on the lips, usually singly or in groups. The precipitating factors for the cold sores include emotional stress, trauma (often related to dental procedures), immunosuppression, or exposure to excessive sunlight. The disease can last 5 to 14 days, with varying degrees of severity.

Stomatitis may occur as a manifestation of hand, foot, and mouth disease (HFMD) and herpangina; both manifest with scattered vesicles on the buccal mucosa and are commonly caused by the nonpolio enteroviruses (primarily coxsackieviruses). Children with either HFMD or herpangina often have poor intake as a result of the mouth sores.

Therapeutic Management

Treatment for all types of stomatitis is aimed at relief of symptoms, primarily pain. Acetaminophen and ibuprofen are usually sufficient for mild cases, but with more severe HGS, stronger analgesics such as codeine may be needed. Topical anesthetics are helpful and include over-the-counter preparations such as Orabase, Anbesol, and Kank-A. Lidocaine (Xylocaine Viscous) can be prescribed for children who can keep 1 tsp of the solution in the mouth for 2 to 3 minutes and then expectorate the drug. A mixture of equal parts of diphenhydramine elixir and Maalox (aluminum and magnesium hydroxide) provides mild analgesia, antiinflammatory properties, and a protective coating for the lesions. Sucralfate can also be used as a coating agent for oral mucous membranes. Specific treatment for children within 72 hours of symptom onset and with severe cases of HGS is the use of antiviral agents such as acyclovir (Hudson and Powell, 2009; Phillips, 2008). A recent systematic review found weak evidence that acyclovir is effective in reducing the number of oral lesions, preventing development of new lesions, and decreasing difficulty with eating and drinking (Nasser, Fedorowicz, Khoshnevisan, and others, 2008).

Nursing Care Management

The chief nursing goals for children with stomatitis are relief of pain and prevention of spread of the herpes virus. Analgesics and topical anesthetics are used as needed to provide relief, especially before meals to encourage food and fluid intake. For younger infants and toddlers who cannot swish and swallow, apply the diphenhydramine and Maalox solution with a cotton-tipped applicator before feedings to minimize pain. Educating parents regarding the use of these medications is important to maintain adequate hydration in children whose mouths are too sore to take liquids. Drinking bland fluids through a straw is helpful in avoiding the painful lesions. Encourage mouth care; the use of a very soft bristle toothbrush or disposable foam-tipped toothbrush provides gentle cleaning near ulcerated areas.

Careful hand washing is essential when caring for children with HGS. Because the infection is autoinoculable, children should keep their fingers out of their mouths; contaminated hands can infect other body parts. Very young children may require elbow restraints to ensure compliance. Articles placed in the mouth should be cleaned thoroughly. Newborns and individuals with immunosuppression should not be exposed to infected children.

> ⚠ **NURSING ALERT**
>
> When examining herpetic lesions, wear gloves. The virus easily enters breaks in the skin and can cause herpetic whitlow of the fingers.

Because herpes infection is often associated with sexual transmission, explain to parents and older children that HGS is usually caused by type 1 HSV, the type not associated with sexual activity.

INTESTINAL PARASITIC DISEASES

Intestinal parasitic diseases, including helminths (worms) and protozoa, constitute the most frequent infections in the world. In the United States, the incidence of intestinal parasitic disease, especially giardiasis, has increased among young children who attend daycare centers. Young children are especially at risk because of typical hand–mouth activity and uncontrolled fecal activity.

Various infecting organisms cause intestinal parasitic diseases in humans. This discussion is limited to the two most common parasitic infections among children in the United States: giardiasis and pinworms. Table 14-2 describes the outstanding features of selected helminths that belong to the family of nematodes.

GENERAL NURSING CARE MANAGEMENT

Nursing responsibilities related to intestinal parasitic infections involve assistance with identification of the parasite, treatment of the infection, and prevention of initial infection or reinfection. Laboratory examination of substances containing the worm, its larvae, or ova can identify the organism. Most are identified by examining fecal smears from the stools of persons suspected of harboring the parasite. Fresh specimens are best for revealing parasites or larvae; therefore, take collected specimens directly to the laboratory for examination. If this is not possible, place the specimen in a container with a preservative. Parents need clear instructions on obtaining an adequate sample and the number of samples required (see Stool Specimens, Chapter 22). In most parasitic infections, other family members, especially children, may be examined to identify those who are similarly affected.

TABLE 14-2 SELECTED INTESTINAL PARASITES

CLINICAL MANIFESTATIONS	COMMENTS
Ascariasis—*Ascaris lumbricoides* (Common Roundworm) Light infections—Asymptomatic Heavy infections—Anorexia, irritability, nervousness, enlarged abdomen, weight loss, fever, intestinal colic Severe infections—Intestinal obstruction, appendicitis, perforation of intestine with peritonitis, obstructive jaundice, lung involvement (pneumonitis)	Transferred to mouth by way of contaminated food, fingers, or toys Largest of the intestinal helminths Affects principally young children 1–4 yr of age Prevalent in warm climates
Hookworm Disease—*Necator americanus* Light infections in well-nourished individuals—No problems Heavier infections—Mild to severe anemia, malnutrition May be itching and burning followed by erythema and a papular eruption in areas to which the organism migrates	Transmitted by discharging eggs on the soil, which are picked up, causing infection from direct skin contact with contaminated soil Recommend wearing shoes, although children playing in contaminated soil expose many skin surfaces
Strongyloidiasis—*Strongyloides stercoralis* (Threadworm) Light infection—Asymptomatic Heavy infection—Respiratory signs and symptoms; abdominal pain, distention; nausea and vomiting; diarrhea (large, pale stools, often with mucus) Life threatening in children with weakened immunologic defenses	Transmission is same as for hookworm except autoinfection common Older children and adults affected more often than young children Severe infections may lead to severe nutritional deficiency
Visceral Larva Migrans—*Toxocara canis* (Dogs) **Intestinal Toxocariasis—*Toxocara cati* (Cats)** Depends on reactivity of infected individual May be asymptomatic except for eosinophilia Specific diagnosis difficult	Transmitted by direct contamination of hands from contact with dog, cat, or objects or by ingestion of soil Keep dogs and cats away from areas where children play; sandboxes especially important transmission areas Periodic deworming of diagnosed dogs and cats Control of dog and cat population
Trichuriasis—*Trichuris trichiura* (Whipworm) Light infections—Asymptomatic Heavy infections—Abdominal pain and distention, diarrhea	Transmitted from contaminated soil, vegetables, toys, and other objects Most frequent in warm, moist climates Occurs most often in undernourished children living in unsanitary conditions

After the diagnosis is confirmed and appropriate treatment is planned, parents need further explanation and reinforcement. Compliance in terms of drug therapy and other measures, such as thorough hand washing, is essential for eradication of the parasite. The family needs to understand the nature of transmission and that in some cases the medication must be repeated in 2 weeks to 1 month to kill organisms hatched since initial treatment.

The nurse's most important function is preventive education of children and families regarding hygiene and health habits. Thorough hand washing before eating or handling food and after using the toilet is the most important precautionary method. The Family-Centered Care box lists other preventive practices.

GIARDIASIS

Giardiasis is caused by the protozoan *Giardia lamblia* (also called *Giardia intestinalis, Giardia duodenalis,* and *Lamblia intestinalis*). It is the most common intestinal parasitic pathogen in the United States. Child care centers and institutions providing care for persons with developmental disabilities are common sites for urban giardiasis, and the children may pass cysts for months. Also consider giardiasis in those with a history of recent travel to an endemic area (Shields, Gleim, and Beach, 2008; Yoder and Beach, 2010).

FAMILY-CENTERED CARE
Preventing Intestinal Parasitic Disease

- Always wash hands and fingernails with soap and water before eating and handling food and after toileting.
- Avoid placing fingers in mouth and biting nails.
- Discourage children from scratching bare anal area.
- Use superabsorbent disposable diapers to prevent leakage.
- Change diapers as soon as soiled and dispose of diapers in closed receptacle out of children's reach.
- Do not rinse cloth or disposable diapers in toilet.
- Disinfect toilet seats and diaper-changing areas; use dilute household bleach (10% solution) or ammonia (Lysol) and wipe clean with paper towels.
- Drink only treated water or bottled water, especially if camping.
- Wash all raw fruits and vegetables and food that has fallen on the floor.
- Avoid growing foods in soil fertilized with human or untreated animal excreta.
- Teach children to defecate only in a toilet, not on the ground.
- Keep dogs and cats away from playgrounds and sandboxes.
- Avoid swimming in pools frequented by diapered children.
- Wear shoes outside.

BOX 14-2 CLINICAL MANIFESTATIONS OF GIARDIASIS

Infants and young children:
- Diarrhea
- Vomiting
- Anorexia
- Growth failure (failure to thrive) if chronic exposure

Children older than 5 years of age:
- Abdominal cramps
- Intermittent loose stools
- Constipation

Stools that are malodorous, watery, pale, and greasy

Spontaneous resolution of most infections in 4 to 6 weeks

Rare, chronic form:
- Intermittent loose, foul-smelling stools
- Possibility of abdominal bloating, flatulence, sulfur-tasting belches, epigastric pain, vomiting, headache, and weight loss

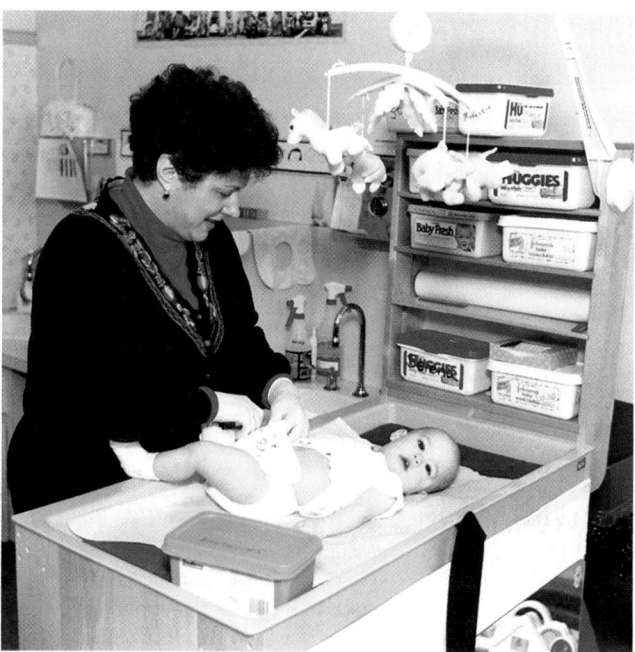

FIG 14-8 Prevention of giardiasis, especially in daycare centers, requires sanitary practices during diaper changes, such as discarding paper diapers in a covered receptacle, changing paper covers on the diaper-changing surface, and having facilities for hand washing nearby. Note: Soiled cloth diapers and clothing should be stored in a plastic bag for transport home.

The potential for transmission is great because the cysts—the non-motile stage of the protozoa—can survive in the environment for months. Chief modes of transmission are person to person; food; and animals, especially puppies. Contaminated water, especially in mountain lakes and streams and swimming or wading pools frequented by diapered infants, are common sources of transmission. In children, person-to-person transmission is the most likely cause. Recent studies indicate swimming pool filters and interactive water fountains to be sites of contamination (Eisenstein, Bodager, and Ginzl, 2008; Shields, Gleim, and Beach, 2008). Although individuals infected with giardiasis may be asymptomatic, common symptoms include abdominal cramps and diarrhea (Box 14-2).

Diagnosis of giardiasis may be made by microscopic examination of stool specimens or duodenal fluid or by identification of *G. lamblia* antigens in these specimens by techniques such as enzyme immunoassay (EIA). Because the *Giardia* organisms live in the upper intestine and are excreted in a highly variable pattern, repeated microscopic examination of stool specimens may be required to identify trophozoites (active parasites) or cysts. Duodenal specimens are obtained by direct aspiration, biopsy, or the string test. In the string test, the child swallows a gelatin capsule with a nylon string attached. Several hours later, the string is withdrawn, and the contents are sent for laboratory analysis. With the availability of EIA techniques to identify *Giardia* antigens in stool specimens, other tests are being used less often.

Therapeutic Management

The drugs of choice for treatment of giardiasis are metronidazole (Flagyl), tinidazole (Tindamax), and nitazoxanide (Alinia). Tinidazole is said to have an 80% to 100% cure rate after a single dose (AAP, Committee on Infectious Diseases, 2009). Metronidazole and tinidazole have a metallic taste and gastrointestinal side effects, including nausea and vomiting; nitazoxanide does not have a bitter taste and should be taken with food to avoid gastrointestinal symptoms. Albendazole is also used to treat the disease and reportedly has fewer side effects than metronidazole (AAP, Committee on Infectious Diseases, 2009).

The most important nursing consideration is prevention of giardiasis and education of parents, child care center staff, and others who assume the daily care of small children. Attention to meticulous sanitary practices, especially during diaper changes, is essential (see

Family-Centered Care box and Fig. 14-8). Nurses can play an important role in educating parents of small children and daycare staff regarding appropriate sanitation practices (see Preschool and Kindergarten Experience, Chapter 13). In addition, discourage young children who are infected or who have diarrhea from swimming in community or private pools until they are infection free. Lakes and streams may contain high numbers of *Giardia* spore cysts, which can be swallowed in the water. Discourage children from swimming in stagnant bodies of water and in water where there are known infected children swimming when there is a high chance of swallowing water. *Giardia* organisms are said to be resistant to chlorine (Eisenstein, Bodager, and Ginzl, 2008). Encourage parents to take small children to the restroom frequently when swimming, avoid letting children in diapers in swimming areas, and change diapers away from the water source. (See also Centers for Disease Control and Prevention [CDC] information on recreational water illnesses, http://www.cdc.gov/healthywater/swimming.) After children are infected, family education regarding drug administration is essential.

ENTEROBIASIS (PINWORMS)

Enterobiasis, or pinworms, caused by the nematode *Enterobius vermicularis*, is the most common helminthic infection in the United States. It is universally present in temperate climatic zones and may infect more than 30% of all children at any one time. Crowded conditions, such as in classrooms and daycare centers, favor transmission.

Infection begins when the eggs are ingested or inhaled (the eggs float in the air). The eggs hatch in the upper intestine and then mature and migrate through the intestine. After mating, adult females migrate out the anus and lay eggs (AAP, Committee on Infectious Diseases,

BOX 14-3 CLINICAL MANIFESTATIONS OF PINWORMS

Intense perianal itching (principal symptom); evidence of itching in young children includes:
- General irritability
- Restlessness
- Poor sleep
- Bedwetting
- Distractibility
- Short attention span

Perianal dermatitis and excoriation secondary to itching
If worms migrate, possible vaginal (vulvovaginitis) and urethral infection

2009). The movement of the worms on skin and mucous membrane surfaces causes intense itching. As the child scratches, eggs are deposited on the hands and underneath the fingernails. The typical hand-to-mouth activity of youngsters makes them especially prone to reinfection. Pinworm eggs persist in the indoor environment for 2 to 3 weeks, contaminating anything they contact, such as toilet seats, doorknobs, bed linen, underwear, and food. Except for the intense rectal itching associated with pinworms, the clinical manifestations are nonspecific (Box 14-3).

Diagnostic Evaluation

Diagnosis is most commonly made from the tape test (see Nursing Care Management). Repeated tests to collect eggs may be necessary, and if there is a possibility that other family members may be infected, a tape test should be performed on them.

Therapeutic Management

The drugs available for treatment of pinworms include mebendazole (Vermox), pyrantel pamoate (Pin-Rid, Antiminth), and albendazole. The drug of choice is mebendazole, which is safe, effective, and convenient, with few side effects. However, it is not recommended for children younger than 2 years of age. If pyrvinium pamoate is prescribed, advise parents that the drug stains stool and vomitus bright red, as well as clothing or skin that comes in contact with the drug; it is available without prescription and should not be used in children younger than 2 years without consulting a primary practitioner. Because pinworms are easily transmitted, all household members are treated. The dose of antiparasitic medication should be repeated in 2 weeks to completely eradicate the parasite and prevent reinfection.

Nursing Care Management

Direct nursing care at identifying the parasite, eradicating the organism, and preventing reinfection. Parents need clear, detailed instructions for the tape test. A loop of transparent (not "frosted" or "magic") tape, sticky side out, is placed around the end of a tongue depressor, which is then firmly pressed against the child's perianal area. A convenient, commercially prepared tape is also available for this purpose. Pinworm specimens are collected in the morning as soon as the child awakens and *before* the child has a bowel movement or bathes. The procedure may need to be performed on 3 or more consecutive days before eggs are collected. Parents are instructed to place the tongue blade in a glass jar or loosely in a plastic bag so it can be brought in for microscopic examination. For specimens collected in the hospital, practitioner's office, or clinic, place the tape smoothly on a glass slide, sticky side down, for examination.

Adherence to the drug regimen is usually excellent because only one or two doses are needed. The family should be reminded of the need to take a second dose in 2 weeks to ensure eradication of the eggs.

To prevent reinfection, washing all clothes and bed linens in hot water and vacuuming the house may be recommended. However, there is little documentation on the effectiveness of these measures because pinworms survive on many surfaces. Helpful suggestions include hand washing after toileting and before eating, keeping the child's fingernails short to minimize the chance of ova collecting under the nails, dressing children in one-piece sleeping outfits, and daily showering rather than tub bathing. Inform families that recurrence is common. Treat repeated infections in the same manner as the first one.

INGESTION OF INJURIOUS AGENTS

Since the passage of the Poison Prevention Packaging Act of 1970, which requires that certain potentially hazardous drugs and household products be sold in child-resistant containers, the incidence of poisonings in children has decreased dramatically. However, despite these advances, poisoning remains a significant health concern, with most cases (51.9% in 2009) occurring in children younger than 6 years of age (Bronstein, Spyker, Cantilena, and others, 2010). The home environment lends itself to injury in this vulnerable age group of children (Dessypris, Dikalioti, Skalkidis, and others, 2009). Although pharmaceuticals such as analgesics, cough and cold preparations, topical preparations, antibiotics, vitamins, gastrointestinal preparations, hormones, and antihistamines are frequently the agents of poisonings, a variety of other substances can also poison children. The most frequently ingested poisons include (Bronstein, Spyker, Cantilena, and others, 2010; Franklin and Rodgers, 2008):[*]

- Cosmetics and personal care products (perfume, cologne, aftershave)
- Cleaning products (hypochlorite [household] bleach, pine oil disinfectants)
- Plants (nontoxic gastrointestinal irritants, oxalates) (Box 14-4)
- Foreign bodies, toys, and miscellaneous substances (desiccants, thermometers, bubble-blowing solutions)

Children are exposed to toxic substances more frequently than any other age group (Eldridge, Van Eyk, and Kornegay, 2007). Many poisonings reflect the ready accessibility of the products in the home, where more than 90% of poisonings occur. A significant number of poisonings take place elsewhere, such as in a grandparent's or friend's home, in a school, or in a health care facility.

The developmental characteristics of young children predispose them to poisoning by ingestion. Infants and toddlers explore their environment through oral experimentation. Because their sense of taste is not discriminating at this age, they ingest many unpalatable substances. In addition, toddlers and preschoolers are developing autonomy and initiative, which increase their curiosity and noncompliant behavior. Imitation is also a powerful motivator, especially when combined with a lack of awareness of danger.

This section is primarily concerned with the immediate emergency treatment of ingestion of injurious agents. Box 14-5 summarizes specific management of corrosive, hydrocarbon, acetaminophen, salicylate, iron, and plant poisoning. Because of the importance of lead poisoning among young children, ingestion of lead is discussed separately. Appropriate suggestions for poison prevention are discussed on p. 440 and in Chapter 12.

---

[*]The most common substances in each category are in parentheses. Substances ingested are not necessarily the most toxic but often are readily available.

BOX 14-4 POISONOUS AND NONPOISONOUS PLANTS

Poisonous Plants (Toxic Parts)

Apple (leaves, seeds)
Apricot (leaves, stem, seed pits)
Azalea (all parts)
Buttercup (all parts)
Castor (bean or seeds—extremely toxic)
Cherry (wild or cultivated) (twigs, seeds, foliage)
Daffodil (bulbs)
Dumbcane (dieffenbachia) (all parts)
Elephant ear (all parts)
English ivy (all parts)
Foxglove (leaves, seeds, flowers)
Holly (berries and leaves)
Hyacinth (bulbs)
Ivy (leaves)
Mistletoe* (berries, leaves)
Oak tree (acorn, foliage)
Philodendron (all parts)
Plum (pit)
Poinsettia† (leaves)
Poison ivy, poison oak (leaves, stems, sap, fruit, smoke from burning plants)
Pokeweed, pokeberry (roots, berries, leaves [when eaten raw])

Pothos (all parts)
Rhubarb (leaves)
Tulip (bulbs)
Water hemlock (all parts)
Wisteria (seeds, pods)
Yew (all parts)

Nonpoisonous Plants

African violet
Aluminum plant
Asparagus fern
Begonia
Boston fern
Christmas cactus
Coleus
Gardenia
Grape ivy
Jade plant
Piggyback begonia
Piggyback plant
Prayer plant
Rubber tree
Snake plant
Spider plant
Swedish ivy
Wax plant
Weeping fig
Zebra plant

*Eating one or two berries or leaves is probably nontoxic.
†Mildly toxic if ingested in massive quantities.

PRINCIPLES OF EMERGENCY TREATMENT

A poisoning may or may not require emergency intervention, but in every instance medical evaluation is necessary to initiate appropriate action. Advise parents to call the poison control center (PCC) *before* initiating any intervention. Parents should post the local PCC telephone number (usually listed in the front of the telephone directory) near each phone in the house* (see Emergency Treatment box).

Based on the initial telephone assessment, the PCC counsels the parents to begin treatment at home or to take the child to an emergency facility. When a call is taken, the name and telephone number of the caller are recorded to reestablish contact if the connection is interrupted. Because most poisonings are managed in the home, expert advice is essential in minimizing adverse effects. When the exact quantity or type of ingested toxin is not known, admission to a health care facility with pediatric emergency treatment services for laboratory evaluation and surveillance during the time after ingestion is critical.

Assessment

The first and most important principle in dealing with a poisoning is to treat the child first, not the poison. This requires an immediate concern for life support. Vital signs are taken, and respiratory or circulatory support is instituted as needed. The child's condition is routinely reevaluated. Because shock is a complication of several types of household poisons, particularly corrosives, measures to reduce the effects of shock are important, beginning with the CABs (circulation, airway, and breathing support measures) of resuscitation. Establishing and maintaining vascular access for rapid intravascular volume expansion is vital in the treatment of pediatric shock.

*Also available by calling 800-222-1222 or online at American Association of Poison Control Centers, http://www.aapcc.org.

✚ EMERGENCY TREATMENT

Poisoning

1. Assess the victim:
   - Initiate cardiorespiratory support if needed (circulation, airway, breathing).
   - Take vital signs; reevaluate routinely.
   - Treat associated complications.
2. Terminate exposure:
   - Empty mouth of pills, plant parts, or other material.
   - Flush eyes continuously with normal saline (or room-temperature tap water at home) for 15 to 20 minutes.
   - Flush skin and wash with soap and a soft cloth; remove contaminated clothes, especially if a pesticide, acid, alkali, or hydrocarbon is involved.
   - Bring victim of an inhalation poisoning into fresh air.
3. Identify the poison:
   - Question the victim and witnesses.
   - Look for environmental clues (empty container, nearby spill, odor on breath) and save all evidence of poison (container, vomitus, urine).

- In absence of other evidence, be alert to signs and symptoms of potential poisoning in the absence of other evidence, including symptoms of ocular or dermal exposure.
- Call the poison control center or other competent emergency facility for immediate advice regarding treatment.

4. Prevent poison absorption:
   - Place the child in a side-lying, sitting, or kneeling position with the head below the chest to prevent aspiration.
   - Administer activated charcoal if ordered (unless used repeatedly, usual dose is 1 g/kg unless the amount of toxin is known), administer drug antidote, or perform gastric lavage.

BOX 14-5   SELECTED POISONINGS IN CHILDREN

Corrosives (Strong Acids or Alkalis)
Drain, toilet, and oven cleaners
Electric dishwasher detergent (liquid because of higher pH, is more hazardous than granular)
Mildew remover
Batteries
Clinitest tablets
Denture cleaners
Bleach

Clinical Manifestations
Severe burning pain in the mouth, throat, and stomach
White, swollen mucous membranes; edema of the lips, tongue, and pharynx (respiratory obstruction)
Violent vomiting (hemoptysis)
Drooling and inability to clear secretions
Signs of shock
Anxiety and agitation

Comments
Household bleach is a frequently ingested corrosive but rarely causes serious damage.
Liquid corrosives cause more damage than granular preparations.

Treatment
Inducing emesis is contraindicated (vomiting redamages the mucosa).
Contact the poison control center (PCC) immediately. If the PCC or medical advice and treatment not immediately available, it may be appropriate to dilute corrosive with water or milk (usually ≤120 ml [4 oz]).
Do not neutralize. Neutralization can cause an exothermic reaction (which produces heat and causes increased symptoms or produces a thermal burn in addition to a chemical burn).
Maintain patent airway as needed.
Administer analgesics.
Do not allow oral intake.
Esophageal stricture may require repeated dilations or surgery.

Hydrocarbons
Gasoline
Kerosene
Lamp oil
Mineral seal oil (found in furniture polish)
Lighter fluid
Turpentine
Paint thinner and remover (some types)

Clinical Manifestations
Gagging, choking, and coughing
Nausea
Vomiting
Alterations in sensorium, such as lethargy
Weakness
Respiratory symptoms of pulmonary involvement
- Tachypnea
- Cyanosis
- Retractions
- Grunting

Comments
Immediate danger is aspiration (even small amounts can cause bronchitis and chemical pneumonia).
Gasoline, kerosene, lighter fluid, mineral seal oil, and turpentine cause severe pneumonia.

Treatment
Inducing emesis is generally contraindicated.
Gastric decontamination and emptying are questionable even when the hydrocarbon contains a heavy metal or pesticide; if gastric lavage must be performed, a cuffed endotracheal tube should be in place before lavage because of a high risk of aspiration.
Symptomatic treatment of chemical pneumonia includes high humidity, oxygen, hydration, and antibiotics for secondary infection.

Acetaminophen
Clinical Manifestations
Occurs in four stages:
1. Initial period (2–4 hours after ingestion)
   - Nausea
   - Vomiting
   - Sweating
   - Pallor
2. Latent period (24–36 hours)
   - Patient improves
3. Hepatic involvement (may last ≤7 days and be permanent)
   - Pain in right upper quadrant
   - Jaundice
   - Confusion
   - Stupor
   - Coagulation abnormalities
4. Patients who do not die in hepatic stage gradually recover.

Comments
This is the most common accidental drug poisoning in children.
It occurs from acute ingestion.
Toxic dose is 150 mg/kg or greater in children.
Because of multiple formulations and concentrations, chronic acetaminophen toxicity is a significant problem.
Parents should be counseled to read product packaging carefully and to consult a health care professional to avoid inappropriate dosing.

Treatment
Antidote *N*-acetylcysteine can usually be given orally but is first diluted in fruit juice or soda because of the antidote's offensive odor.
Given as 1 loading dose and usually 17 maintenance doses in different dosages.
May be given intravenously, but use is investigational.

Aspirin (Acetylsalicylic Acid [ASA])
Clinical Manifestations
Acute poisoning
- Nausea
- Disorientation
- Vomiting
- Dehydration
- Diaphoresis
- Hyperpnea
- Hyperpyrexia

BOX 14-5 SELECTED POISONINGS IN CHILDREN—cont'd

- Oliguria
- Tinnitus
- Coma
- Convulsions

Chronic poisoning

- Same as above but subtle onset (often mistaken for viral illness)
- Dehydration, coma, and seizures may be more severe
- Bleeding tendencies

Comments

May be caused by acute ingestion (severe toxicity occurs with 300–500 mg/kg).

May be caused by chronic ingestion (i.e., >100 mg/kg/day for ≥2 days); can be more serious than acute ingestion.

Time to peak serum salicylate level can vary with enteric aspirin or the presence of concretions (bezoars).

Treatment

Hospitalization is necessary for severe toxicity.

Emesis, lavage, activated charcoal, or cathartic may be used.

Lavage will not remove concretions of ASA.

Activated charcoal is important early in ASA toxicity.

Sodium bicarbonate transfusions are used to correct metabolic acidosis, and urinary alkalinization may be effective in enhancing elimination; urinary alkalinization is difficult to achieve.

Be aware of the risk for fluid overload and pulmonary edema.

Use external cooling for hyperpyrexia.

Administer anticonvulsants.

Provide oxygen and ventilation for respiratory depression.

Administer vitamin K for bleeding.

In severe cases, hemodialysis (not peritoneal dialysis) is used.

Iron

Mineral supplement or vitamin containing iron

Clinical Manifestations

Occurs in five stages:

1. Initial period ($\frac{1}{2}$–6 hours after ingestion; if child does not develop gastrointestinal symptoms in 6 hours, toxicity is unlikely)
   - Vomiting
   - Hematemesis
   - Diarrhea
   - Hematochezia (bloody stools)
   - Gastric pain
2. Latency (2–12 hours): patient improves
3. Systemic toxicity (4–24 hours)
   - Metabolic acidosis
   - Fever
   - Hyperglycemia
   - Bleeding
   - Shock
   - Death (may occur)

4. Hepatic injury (48–96 hours)
   - Seizures
   - Coma
5. Rarely, pyloric stenosis develops at 2 to 5 weeks.

Comments

Factors related to frequency of iron poisoning include:

- Widespread availability
- Packaging of large quantities in individual containers
- Lack of parental awareness of iron toxicity
- Resemblance of iron tablets to candy (e.g., M&Ms)

Toxic dose is based on the amount of elemental iron in various salts (sulfate, gluconate, fumarate), which ranges from 20% to 33%; ingestions of 60 mg/kg are considered dangerous.

Treatment

Use emesis or lavage.

For toxic doses, lavage may be necessary for all chewable tablets or liquids if spontaneous vomiting has not occurred.

Chelation therapy with deferoxamine should be used in severe intoxication (may turn urine red to orange).

If intravenous deferoxamine is given too rapidly, hypotension, facial flushing, rash, urticaria, tachycardia, and shock may occur; stop the infusion, maintain the intravenous line with normal saline, and notify the practitioner immediately.

Plants

Plants listed in Box 14-4

Clinical Manifestations

Depends on type of plant ingested

May cause local irritation of oropharynx and entire gastrointestinal tract

May cause respiratory, renal, and central nervous system symptoms

Topical contact with plants can cause dermatitis

Comments

Plants are some of the most frequently ingested substances.

They rarely cause serious problems, although some plant ingestions can be fatal.

Plants can also cause choking and allergic reactions.

Treatment

Induce emesis.

Wash from skin or eyes.

Provide supportive care as needed.

The emergency department nurse's responsibility is to be prepared for immediate intervention with all of the necessary equipment. Because time and speed are critical factors in recovery from serious poisonings, anticipation of potential problems and complications may mean the difference between life and death.

Gastric Decontamination

Although pediatric poison ingestions are common, they rarely result in significant morbidity or mortality (Bronstein, Spyker, Cantilena, and others, 2010; Greene, Harris, and Singer, 2008). Consider using gastrointestinal decontamination (GID) only after careful evaluation of the potential toxicity of the poison and the risks versus benefits. When GID is needed, the immediate treatment is to remove the ingested poison by adsorbing the toxin with activated charcoal (AC), performing gastric lavage, or increasing bowel motility (catharsis). Because of continuing controversy regarding the use of these methods, treat each toxic ingestion individually (Eldridge, Van Eyk, and Kornegay, 2007; Madden, 2008). Specific antidotes may be administered for certain poisonings.

Syrup of ipecac, an emetic that exerts its action through irritation of the gastric mucosa and by stimulation of the vomiting center, is no longer recommended for routine treatment of poison ingestion (AAP, Committee on Infectious Diseases, 2009; Criddle, 2007; Greene, Harris, and Singer, 2008; Sheffield and Serwint, 2008).

> ### ! NURSING ALERT
>
> Ipecac is not recommended for routine poison treatment intervention in the home (AAP, 2009; Criddle, 2007; Greene, Harris, and Singer, 2008; Sheffield and Serwint, 2008).

Medications such as calcium channel blockers and benzodiazepines either produce a rapid onset of adverse symptoms (e.g., sedation, seizures, coma) or exaggerate the vagal response induced by gagging, which can lead to significant bradycardia. Under either circumstance, uncontrolled vomiting becomes an undesirable and unsafe event.

A more commonly used method of GID is the use of activated charcoal (AC), an odorless, tasteless, fine black powder that adsorbs many compounds, creating a stable complex (Frithsen and Simpson, 2010; Sheffield and Serwint, 2008). AC is mixed with water or a saline cathartic to form a slurry. Slurries are neither gritty nor distasteful but resemble black mud. To increase the child's acceptance of AC, the nurse should mix it with diet soda and serve it through a straw in an opaque container with a cover (e.g., a disposable coffee cup and lid) or an ordinary cup covered with aluminum foil or placed inside a small paper bag. In one small study, healthy adolescents preferred the taste of AC mixed with cola or chocolate milk mixture instead of water (Cheng and Ratnapalan, 2007). For small children, a nasogastric tube may be required to administer AC (Greene, Harris, and Singer, 2008).

There is discussion of the use of AC in the home for pediatric poison ingestion. The evidence is not clear regarding the risk versus benefit of home AC administration (Eldridge, Van Eyk, and Kornegay, 2007). Potential complications from the use of AC include aspiration (usually in patients with impaired gag reflexes), constipation, and intestinal obstruction (in multiple doses) (Sheffield and Serwint, 2008). Superactivated charcoal products for gastric decontamination are often more palatable and just as effective (Criddle, 2007).

If the child is admitted to an emergency facility, gastric lavage may be performed to empty the stomach of the toxic agent; however, this procedure can be associated with serious complications (gastrointestinal perforation, hypoxia, aspiration), and it is no longer recommended in all cases of ingestion. There is no conclusive evidence that gastric lavage decreases morbidity (Criddle, 2007; Greene, Harris, and Singer, 2008; Sheffield and Serwint, 2008). In addition, gastric lavage may be of little benefit if used later than 1 hour after ingestion (Frithsen and Simpson, 2010; Greene, Harris, and Singer, 2008). Conditions that may be appropriate for the use of gastric lavage include presentation within 1 hour of ingestion of a toxin, ingestion in patient who has decreased gastrointestinal motility, the ingestion of a toxic amount of sustained-release medication, and a massive or life-threatening amount of poison (Criddle, 2007; Madden, 2008). When gastric lavage is used, the patient requires a protected airway, possible sedation, and the largest diameter tube that can be inserted to facilitate passage of gastric contents.

In a minority of poisonings, specific antidotes are available to counteract the poison. They are highly effective and should be available in all emergency facilities. The supply of antidotes should be checked routinely and replaced as used or according to expiration dates. Antidotes available to treat toxin ingestion include *N*-acetylcysteine for acetaminophen poisoning, oxygen for carbon monoxide inhalation, naloxone for opioid overdose, flumazenil (Romazicon) for benzodiazepines (diazepam [Valium], midazolam [Versed]) overdose, digoxin immune Fab (Digibind) for digoxin toxicity, amyl nitrate for cyanide, and antivenin for certain poisonous bites.

Prevention of Recurrence

The ultimate objective is to prevent poisonings from occurring or recurring. Home safety education improves poison prevention practices (Kendrick, Smith, Sutton, and others, 2008). Research supports the effectiveness of parent education on preventing unintentional injuries (Kendrick, Barlow, Hampshire, and others, 2007; Kendrick, Coupland, Mulvaney, and others, 2007). One effective counseling method is first to discuss the difficulties of constantly watching and safeguarding young children (see Family-Centered Care box). In this way, the challenging task of raising children can lead to a discussion of injury prevention as part of the parental role. This approach also incorporates contributory causes for the incident, such as inadequate support systems; marital discord; discipline techniques (especially use of physical punishment); and any disruption in the family or family activities, such as vacations, moves, visitors, illnesses, or births. A visit to the home, especially after repeat poisonings, is recommended as part of the follow-up care to assess hazards, including family factors, and to evaluate appropriate injury-proofing measures. One method of

> ### FAMILY-CENTERED CARE
> #### *Poisoning*
>
> A poisoning is more than a physical emergency for the child—it also usually represents an emotional crisis for the parents, particularly in terms of guilt, self-reproach, and insecurity in the parenting role. The emergency department is no place to admonish the family for negligence, lack of appropriate supervision, or failure to injury proof the home. Rather, it is a time to calm and support the child and parents while unaccusingly exploring the circumstances of the injury. If the nurse prematurely attempts to discuss ways of preventing such an incident from recurring, the parents' anxiety will block out any suggestions or offered guidance. Therefore, it is preferable for the nurse to delay the discussion until the child's condition is stabilized or, if the child is discharged immediately after emergency treatment, to make a public health referral or send a packet of information.

NURSING CARE GUIDELINES

Poison Prevention

- Assess possible contributing factors in occurrence of injury, such as discipline, parent–child relationship, developmental ability, environmental factors, and behavior problems.
- Institute anticipatory guidance for possible future injuries based on child's age and developmental level.
- Initiate referral to appropriate agency to evaluate home environment and need for injury-proofing measures.
- Provide assistance with environmental manipulation, such as lead removal, when necessary.
- Educate parents regarding safe storage of toxic substances.
- Advise parents to take drugs out of sight of children.
- Teach children the hazards of ingesting nonfood items.
- Advise parents against using plants for teas or medicine.
- Discuss problems of discipline and children's noncompliance and offer strategies for effective discipline.
- Instruct parents regarding correct administration of drugs for therapeutic purposes and to discontinue drug if there is evidence of mild toxicity.
- Advise parents to contact the Poison Control Center (800-222-1222) or practitioner immediately when a poisoning occurs.
- Tell them to post the number of the regional poison control center with an emergency phone list by the telephone.
- They should include by the telephone the home address with nearest cross street in case an ambulance is needed. (In an emergency, family members may not remember the house address, and babysitters may not be aware of the information.)

BOX 14-6 SOURCES OF LEAD*

- Lead-based paint in deteriorating condition
- Lead solder
- Lead crystal
- Battery casings
- Lead fishing sinkers
- Lead curtain weights
- Lead bullets
- Some of these may contain lead:
  - Ceramic ware
  - Water
  - Pottery
  - Pewter
  - Dyes
  - Industrial factories
  - Vinyl mini-blinds
  - Playground equipment
  - Collectible toys
- Some imported toys or children's metal jewelry
- Artists' paints
- Pool cue chalk
- Occupations and hobbies involving lead:
  - Battery and aircraft manufacturing
  - Lead smelting
  - Brass foundry work
  - Radiator repair
  - Construction work
  - Bridge repair work
  - Painting contracting
  - Mining
  - Ceramics work
  - Stained-glass making
  - Jewelry making

*The U.S. Consumer Product Safety Commission issues alerts and recalls for products that contain lead and may unexpectedly pose a hazard to young children. Additional information may be obtained from Alliance for Healthy Homes, http://www.afhh.org.

insomnia, gingivitis, diarrhea, anorexia, weight loss). The classic form of mercury poisoning is called **acrodynia** (or "painful extremities").

! NURSING ALERT

Mercury thermometers are no longer recommended because if they are broken, the inhaled vapors can cause toxicity. To prevent inhalation, clean up spilled mercury quickly, using disposable towels and rubber gloves and washing the hands well afterward.

Heavy metals have an affinity for certain essential tissue chemicals, which must remain free for adequate cell functioning. When metals are bound to these substances, cellular enzyme systems are inactivated. Treatment involves **chelation**, use of a chemical compound that combines with the metal for rapid and safe excretion.

LEAD POISONING

Poisoning from lead has been a problem throughout history and throughout the world. In the United States, the problem became apparent in the early 1900s when white lead was added to paints and when tetraethyl lead was added to gasoline as an antiknock compound. Lead content in paint was decreased in 1950, and in 1978, the use of lead in household paint was banned. The use of lead in paint and leaded gasoline has been banned in the United States. After this change in policy, the average blood lead level (BLL) in the United States for people ages 1 to 74 years dropped from 12.8 mcg/dl in 1980 to 1.9 mcg/dl in 1999 (AAP, Committee on Environmental Health, 2005). However, children continue to be exposed to lead; an estimated 1.6% of U.S. children had BLLs of more than 10 mcg/dl in 2002, and almost 14% had BLLs of 5 to 9 mcg/dl (Levin, Brown, Kashtock, and others, 2008).

Causes of Lead Poisoning

Although there are numerous sources of lead (Box 14-6), in most instances of acute childhood lead poisoning, the source is nonintact

identifying risk areas is to ask specific questions or to have the parent complete a questionnaire designed to isolate factors that predispose children to poisoning. Another approach is to encourage parents to bend down to the child's eye level and survey the home environment for potential hazards. Have the parents try to open cabinets and reach shelves to access poisons.

Passive measures (those that do not require active participation) have been the most successful in preventing poisoning and include using child-resistant closures and limiting the number of tablets in one container. However, these measures alone are not sufficient to prevent poisoning because most toxic agents in the home do not have safety closures. Therefore, active measures (those that require participation) are essential. The Nursing Care Guidelines box lists the guidelines for preventing the occurrence or recurrence of a poisoning.

HEAVY METAL POISONING

Heavy metal poisoning can occur from the ingestion of a variety of substances, the most common being lead. Other sources that are important in terms of children are iron and mercury. Mercury toxicity, a rare form of heavy metal poisoning, has occurred in children from a variety of sources, such as broken thermometers or thermostats, broken fluorescent light bulbs, disk batteries, topical medications, gas regulators, cathartics, and interior latex house paint (Bose-O'Reilly, McCarthy, Steckling, and others. 2010; Clifton, 2007). Elemental mercury (also called metallic mercury or quicksilver) is nontoxic if ingested and if the gastrointestinal tract is healthy (e.g., has no fistulas). However, mercury is volatile at room temperature and enters the bloodstream after it is inhaled, causing toxicity (tremors, memory loss,

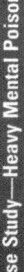

lead-based paint in an older home or lead-contaminated bare soil in the yard. Microparticles of lead gain entrance into a child's body through ingestion or inhalation and, in the case of an exposed pregnant woman, by placental transfer. When measured, a mother's lead level is nearly the same as that of her unborn child. However, although the level of lead may not be harmful to adult women, it can be harmful to fetuses.

Whereas inhalation exposure usually occurs during renovation and remodeling activities in the home, ingestion happens during normal day-to-day play and mouthing activities. Sometimes a child will actually swallow loose chips of lead-based paint because it has a sweet taste. Water and food may also be contaminated with lead. A child does not need to eat loose paint chips to be exposed to the toxin; normal hand-to-mouth behavior, coupled with the presence of lead dust in the environment that has settled over decades, is the usual method of poisoning (AAP, Committee on Environmental Health, 2005; Bose-O'Reilly, McCarthy, Steckling, and others, 2010; Erickson and Thompson, 2005; Frazer, 2008).

Because of family, cultural, or ethnic traditions, a source of lead may be a routine part of life for a child. Nurses must educate themselves about the practices of their patients and identify when such products may be a source of lead. The use of pottery or dishes containing lead may be an issue, as may the use of folk remedies for stomachaches or the use of some cosmetics (see Cultural Considerations box). Children of immigrants and internationally adopted children may have been exposed to sources of lead before arrival in the United States and should also be carefully evaluated for lead exposure (Woolf, Goldman, and Bellinger, 2007). Other risk factors for having an elevated BLL include living in poverty, being younger than 6 years of age, dwelling in urban areas, and living in older rental homes where lead decontamination may not be a priority. Nurses are often in a position to observe or elicit information about these practices and educate families about their potential harm.

Pathophysiology and Clinical Manifestation

Lead can affect any part of the body, including the renal, hematologic, and neurologic systems (Fig. 14-9). Of most concern for young children is the developing brain and nervous system, which are more vulnerable than those of older children and adults. Lead in the body moves via an equilibration process between the blood, the soft tissues and organs, and the bones and teeth. Lead ultimately settles in the bones and teeth, where it remains inert and in storage. This makes up the largest portion of the body burden, approximately 75% to 90%. At the cellular level, it competes with molecules of calcium, interfering with the regulating action of calcium. In the brain, lead disrupts the biochemical processes and may have a direct effect on the release of neurotransmitters, may cause alterations in the blood–brain barrier, and may interfere with the regulation of synaptic activity (Lidsky and Schneider, 2006).

There is a relationship between anemia and lead poisoning. Children who are iron deficient absorb lead more readily than those with sufficient iron stores. Lead can interfere with the binding of iron onto the heme molecule. This sometimes creates a picture of anemia even though the child is not iron deficient. Lead toxicity to the erythrocytes leads to the release of the enzyme erythrocyte protoporphyrin (EP). Because EP is not sensitive to BLLs of less than about 16 to 25 mcg/dl, it is no longer used as a screening test. Therefore, the BLL test is currently used for screening and diagnosis. However, elevation of the EP level (>35 mcg/dl of whole blood) is a good indicator of toxicity from lead and reflects the length of exposure and body burden of lead in an individual child.

Although adults have been shown to experience adverse renal effects from occupational lead exposure, few studies document renal effects in children except at extremely high lead levels. One can hypothesize that lead can affect the renal integrity of children as well as adults. Therefore, the renal system of a child is still considered a potential target for the harmful effects of lead.

The lead levels identified in children have declined since the initiation of screening for children at risk for lead poisoning. With earlier intervention, the most prevalent effects have changed. Since the late 1960s, children have rarely died of lead poisoning, and seizures or cognitive impairment have become less likely. However, even mild and moderate lead poisoning can cause a number of cognitive and behavioral problems in young children, including aggression, hyperactivity, impulsivity, delinquency, disinterest, and withdrawal. Long-term neurocognitive signs of lead poisoning include developmental delays, lowered intelligence quotient (IQ), reading skill deficits, visual-spatial problems, visual-motor problems, learning disabilities, and lower academic success. Chronic lead toxicity may also affect physical growth and reproductive efficiency (Woolf, Goldman, and Bellinger, 2007).

⊕ CULTURAL CONSIDERATIONS

Sources of Lead

In some cultures, the use of traditional ethnic remedies that contain lead may increase children's risk of lead poisoning. These remedies include:

Azarcon (Mexico)—For digestive problems; a bright orange powder; usual dose is 0.25 to 1 tsp, often mixed with oil, milk, or sugar or sometimes given as a tea; sometimes a pinch is added to a baby bottle or tortilla dough for preventive purposes

Greta (Mexico)—A yellow-orange powder used in the same way as azarcon

Paylooah (Southeast Asia)—Used for rash or fever; an orange-red powder given as 0.5 tsp straight or in a tea

Surma (India)—Black powder applied to the inner lower eyelid that is used as a cosmetic to improve eyesight

Unknown ayurvedic (Tibet)—Small, gray-brown balls used to improve slow development; two balls are given orally three times a day

Tamarindo jellied, fruit candy (Mexico)—Fruit candy packaged in paper wrappers that contain high lead levels

Lozeena (Iraq)—A bright orange powder used to color meat and rice

Modified from Centers for Disease Control and Prevention: Lead poisoning associated with use of traditional ethnic remedies—California, 1991–1992, *MMWR Morb Mortal Wkly Rep* 42(27): 521–524, 1993; Centers for Disease Control and Prevention: Lead poisoning associated with imported candy and powdered food coloring—California and Michigan, *MMWR Morb Mortal Wkly Rep* 47(48):1041–1043, 1998; Centers for Disease Control and Prevention: Childhood lead poisoning associated with tamarind candy and folk remedies—California, 1992–2000, *MMWR Morb Mortal Wkly Rep* 51(31):684–686, 2002.

⚠ NURSING ALERT

Acute signs of lead poisoning include nausea, vomiting, constipation, anorexia, and abdominal pain. Additional clinical manifestations are hypophosphatemia, glycosuria, and aminoaciduria (Erickson and Thompson, 2005).

Diagnostic Evaluation

Children with lead poisoning rarely have symptoms even at levels requiring chelation therapy. A diagnosis of lead poisoning is based only on the lead testing of a venous blood specimen from a venipuncture. The collection process is important. Blood must be collected carefully

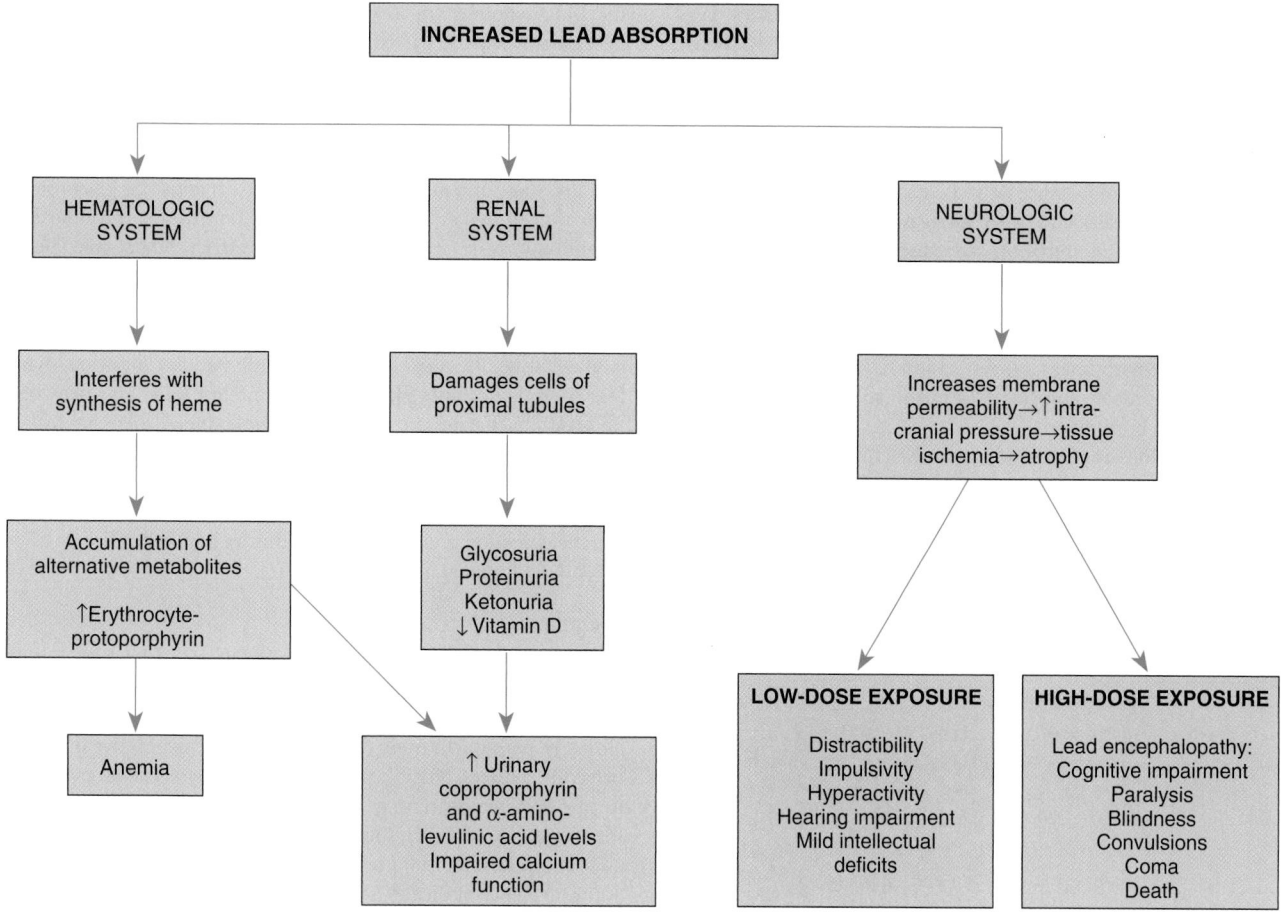

FIG 14-9 Main effects of lead on body systems.

to avoid contamination by lead on the skin. The level of concern for an elevated BLL has dropped from 80 mcg/dl in 1950 to 5 mcg/dl today (CDC Advisory Committee on Childhood Lead Poisoning Prevention, 2012; Heavey, 2008).

Anticipatory Guidance

Anticipatory guidance lends support to primary prevention efforts. The CDC (2005) recommends that the following information be made available to families beginning during prenatal care, at 3 to 6 months, and at 1 year of age:

- Hazards of lead-based paint in older housing
- Ways to control lead hazards safely
- How to choose safe toys
- Hazards accompanying repainting and renovation of homes built before 1978
- Other exposure sources, such as traditional remedies, that might be relevant for a family

There has been recent concern regarding toys and other imported items children play with that were found to contain lead. Parents should carefully evaluate the source of the toy (manufacturer) or item the child may play with and not assume it is safe because it is sold in a U.S. market. The U.S. Consumer Product Safety Commission (http://www.cpsc.gov) is an excellent resource for parents and caregivers concerned about the safety of a given toy or product that may be harmful.

Screening for Lead Poisoning

When primary prevention fails, secondary prevention screening efforts for elevated BLLs can identify children much earlier than in the past.

Guidelines recommend universal or targeted screening (Levin, Brown, Kashtock, and others, 2008). This need is established using blood lead surveillance and other risk factor data collected over time to establish the status and risk of children throughout the state. In areas without available data, universal screening is recommended.

Universal screening should be done at ages 1 and 2 years. Any child between the ages of 3 and 6 years who has not been previously screened should also be tested. All children with risk factors should be screened more often.

Targeted screening is acceptable when an area has been determined by existing data to have less risk. Children should be screened when they live in a high-risk geographic area or are members of a group determined to be at risk (e.g., Medicaid recipients) or if their family cannot answer "no" to the following personal risk questions:

- Does your child live in or regularly visit a house that was built before 1950?
- Does your child live in or regularly visit a house built before 1978 with recent or ongoing renovations or remodeling within the past 6 months?
- Does your child have a sibling or playmate who has or had lead poisoning?

Therapeutic Management

The degree of concern, urgency, and need for medical intervention change as the lead level increases. Education is one of the most important elements of the treatment process. Areas that the nurse needs to discuss with the family of every child who has an elevated BLL

(≥5 mcg/dl) include (CDC Advisory Committee on Childhood Lead Poisoning Prevention, 2012; Heavey, 2008; Levin, Brown, Kashtock, and others, 2008):

- The child's BLL and what it means
- Potential adverse health effects of an elevated BLL
- Sources of lead exposure and suggestions on how to reduce exposure, such as the importance of wet cleaning to remove lead dust on floors, windowsills, and other surfaces
- Importance of good nutrition in reducing the absorption and effects of lead; for persons with poor nutritional patterns, adequate intake of calcium and iron and importance of regular meals
- Need for follow-up testing to monitor the child's BLL
- Results of an environmental investigation if applicable
- Hazards of improper removal of lead paint (dry sanding, scraping, or open-flame burning)

Treatment actions vary depending on the child's BLL. Based on a diagnosis from a venous BLL test, the CDC (2002) recommends the following actions:

BLOOD LEAD LEVEL (BLL) (mcg/dl)	ACTION
<5	Reassess or rescreen in 1 year. If exposure status changes, do this sooner.
5–14	Provide family with lead poisoning education, follow-up testing, and social service referral if necessary.
15–19	Provide family with lead poisoning education (dietary and environmental), follow-up testing, and social service referral as needed; if BLL persists, initiate actions for BLL of 20–44 mcg/dl.
20–44	Provide coordination of care, clinical management, environmental investigation, and lead hazard control.
45–69	Within 48 hours, provide coordination of care and clinical management, including treatment, environmental investigation, and lead hazard control. The child must not remain in a lead-hazardous environment if resolution is to occur.
≥70	*Immediately* provide medical treatment and begin coordination of care, clinical management, environmental investigation, and lead hazard control.

Chelation Therapy

Chelation is the term used for removing lead from circulating blood and, theoretically, some lead from organs and tissues. It is unclear whether chelation affects lead stores in bones. Although not an antidote in the truest sense, it does serve a similar purpose in that the toxic substance or poison is removed from the body. However, chelation does not counteract any effects of the lead.

Historically, two chelating agents have been used consistently: calcium disodium edetate (CaNa₂EDTA, or calcium EDTA) and succimer (Chemet, *meso*-2,3-dimercaptosuccinic acid [DMSA]). British antilewisite (BAL, dimercaprol, dimercaptopropanol) is used in conjunction with EDTA. All of the agents have potential toxic side effects and contraindications. Renal, hepatic, and hematologic parameters should be monitored.

Because of the equilibration process between blood, soft tissues, and other sites in the body, there is often a rebound of the BLL after chelation. After the body burden of lead is reduced enough to stabilize the BLL, rebound will cease. Multiple chelation treatments may be necessary. Adequate hydration is essential during therapy because the chelates are excreted via the kidneys.

British antilewisite must not be used in the presence of a glucose 6-phosphate dehydrogenase deficiency or peanut allergy, nor should it be given in conjunction with iron. It is never used as a single-agent therapy, only in conjunction with EDTA. It must be given only at a deep intramuscular site. EDTA should be given intravenously over several hours or, when necessary to restrict fluids, may be given intramuscularly.

Succimer is given orally over a 19-day course of treatment. The capsule is opened and sprinkled on a small amount of food or may be swallowed whole. Adverse effects include nausea, vomiting, diarrhea, loss of appetite, rash, elevated liver function tests, and neutropenia. Because the chelates are excreted via the kidneys, adequate hydration is essential.

An oral chelating agent, d-penicillamine, is sometimes used to treat lead poisoning, but low doses should be used in children. Monitoring of renal function and blood counts during administration is essential (Woolf, Goldman, and Bellinger, 2007).

Prognosis

Although most of the pathophysiologic effects of lead are reversible, the most serious consequences of both high and low lead exposure are the effects on the central nervous system. In children with lead encephalopathy, permanent brain damage can result in cognitive impairment, behavior changes, possible paralysis, and seizures. However, moderate-to low-dose exposure may also cause permanent neurologic deficits. Increased distractibility, short attention span, impulsivity, reading disabilities, and school failure have been associated with lead exposure. Some evidence indicates that treatment of moderate levels of lead poisoning can result in cognitive improvement (AAP, Committee on Environmental Health, 2005; CDC Advisory Committee on Childhood Lead Poisoning Prevention, 2007).

Nursing Care Management

The primary nursing goal in lead poisoning is to prevent the child's initial or further exposure to lead. For children with low-level exposure, this requires identifying the sources of lead in the environment. Careful history taking is the most useful and most valuable tool and should concentrate on the personal risk questions (see p. 443). Suggestions for reducing lead in the child's environment are listed in the Community Focus box.

For children who undergo chelation therapy, the nurse prepares them for the injections and makes all efforts to reduce injection pain. Chelating agents are administered deeply into a large muscle mass (see Atraumatic Care box). To lessen the pain from EDTA, the local anesthetic procaine is injected with the drug. Rotation of sites is essential to prevent the formation of painful areas of fibrotic tissue. Because EDTA and lead are toxic to the kidneys, keep records of intake and output and assess the results of urinalysis to monitor renal functioning.

> **! NURSING ALERT**
>
> Use extreme caution with chelating agents. Incidences of child death from hypocalcemia have been recorded when Na₂EDTA was substituted for CaNa₂EDTA and used as a chelating agent (Centers for Diseases Control and Prevention, 2006).

COMMUNITY FOCUS

Reducing Blood Lead Levels

- Make certain children do not have access to peeling paint or chewable surfaces painted with lead-based paint, especially windowsills and wells.
- If a house was built before 1960 (possibly before 1980) and has hard-surface floors, wet mop them at least once per week. Wipe other hard surfaces (e.g., windowsills, baseboards). If there are loose paint chips in an area, such as a window well, use a wet disposable cloth to pick up and discard them. Do not vacuum hard-surfaced floors or windowsills or wells because this spreads dust. Use vacuum cleaners with agitators to remove dust from rugs rather than vacuum cleaners with suction only. If a rug is known to contain lead dust and cannot be washed, it should be discarded.
- Wash and dry children's hands and faces frequently, especially before eating.
- Wash toys and pacifiers frequently.
- If soil around home is or is likely to be contaminated with lead (e.g., if the home was built before 1960 or is near a major highway), plant grass or other ground cover; plant bushes around outside of the house so children cannot play there.
- During remodeling of older homes, follow correct procedures. Be certain that children and pregnant women are not in the home, day or night, until the process is completed. After deleading, thoroughly clean the house using cleaning solution to a damp mop and dust before inhabitants return.
- In areas where lead content of water exceeds the drinking water standard and a particular faucet has not been used for 6 hours or more, "flush" the cold-water pipes by running the water until it becomes as cold as it will get (30 seconds to 2 minutes). The more time water has been sitting in pipes, the more lead it may contain.
- *Use only cold water* for consumption (drinking, cooking, and especially for reconstituting powder infant formula). Hot water dissolves lead more quickly than cold water and thus contains higher levels of lead. It is acceptable to use first-flush water for nonconsumption uses.
- Have water tested by a competent laboratory. This action is especially important for apartment dwellers; flushing may not be effective in high-rise buildings and in other buildings with lead-soldered central piping.
- Do not store food in open cans, particularly if cans are imported.
- Do not use pottery or ceramic ware that was inadequately fired or is meant for decorative use for food storage or service. Do not store drinks or food in lead crystal.
- Avoid folk remedies and cosmetics that contain lead.
- Make certain that home exposure is not occurring from parental occupations or hobbies. Household members employed in occupations such as lead smelting should shower and change into clean clothing before leaving work. Construction and lead abatement workers may also bring home lead contaminants.
- Ensure that children eat regular meals because more lead is absorbed on an empty stomach.
- Ensure that children's diets contain sufficient iron and calcium and not excessive fat.

Modified from Centers for Disease Control and Prevention: *Preventing lead poisoning in young children*, Atlanta, 2005, Author.

! NURSING ALERT

Calcium EDTA is always administered when there is adequate urinary output. Children receiving the drug intramuscularly must be able to maintain adequate oral intake of fluids.

ATRAUMATIC CARE

Lead Chelation Therapy

To lessen the pain from intramuscular injection of calcium disodium edetate (CaNa$_2$EDTA or calcium EDTA), the local anesthetic procaine is injected with the drug. Apply topical anesthetic cream such as eutectic mixture of local anesthetic (e.g., lidocaine-prilocaine [EMLA]) or LMX4 (4% lidocaine) over the puncture site before the injection of EDTA and British antilewisite (BAL) (time per manufacturer's guidelines). Administer intravenous EDTA whenever possible.

Discharge planning for children with lead poisoning must include thorough education of families regarding safety from lead hazards, clear instructions regarding medication administration and follow-up, and confirmation that the child will be discharged to a home without lead hazards. Although the nurse must use caution to avoid alarming parents unnecessarily, it is important that they know the risk implications for their child's behavior and cognitive functions. Nurses should observe the development and behavior of children who are hospitalized. Thoroughly evaluate any concerns that are identified. Referral to a child development or speech and language specialist may be necessary.

As in any situational crisis, parents need support and understanding if their child is treated for lead poisoning. Many families at the highest risk for lead poisoning have the fewest resources to comply with measures such as relocation or removal of lead from the environment where the child experiences exposure.

CHILD MALTREATMENT

The broad term *child maltreatment* includes intentional physical abuse or neglect, emotional abuse or neglect, and sexual abuse of children, usually by adults. It is one of the most significant social problems affecting children. In 2007, child protective service (CPS) agencies in the United States confirmed that an estimated 794,000 children were victims of child maltreatment. Of the confirmed cases, about 11% suffered physical abuse, 8% sexual abuse, 60% neglect, and 4% psychologic maltreatment or emotional abuse. In 2007, there were an estimated 1760 child fatalities as a result of child abuse and neglect (U.S. Department of Health and Human Services, 2009). Reported statistics only partially represent the actual incidence of child maltreatment because many cases are believed to go unreported.*

CHILD NEGLECT

Child neglect is the most common form of maltreatment. More than half of all reported cases are associated with deprivation of necessities, and 34% of deaths from maltreatment are in this group (U.S. Department of Health and Human Services, 2009). Neglect is generally defined as the failure of a parent or other person legally responsible for the child's welfare to provide for the child's basic needs and an adequate level of care.

Important contributing factors for child neglect are lack of knowledge of child's needs, lack of resources, and caregiver substance abuse.

---

*Additional information is available from the Children's Bureau, Administration for Children and Families, 370 L'Enfant Promenade SW, Washington, DC 20447; 800-422-4453; http://www.acf.hhs.gov.

For example, neglectful parents often demonstrate poor parenting skills. They may be unaware that an infant needs to be fed every 3 to 4 hours, may not know what to feed the child, and may have insufficient funds to buy food. The most serious lack of knowledge is failure to recognize emotional nurturing as an essential need of children. (See also Growth Failure [Failure to Thrive], Chapter 11.)

Types of Neglect

Neglect takes many forms and can be classified broadly as physical or emotional maltreatment. Physical neglect involves the deprivation of necessities, such as food, clothing, shelter, supervision, medical care, and education. Emotional neglect generally refers to failure to meet the child's needs for affection, attention, and emotional nurturance.

Neglect may also include lack of intervention for or fostering of maladaptive behavior, such as delinquency or substance abuse. Emotional abuse or psychologic maltreatment, an even more difficult aspect of maltreatment to define, refers to the deliberate attempt to destroy or significantly impair a child's self-esteem or competence. Emotional abuse may take the form of rejecting, isolating, terrorizing, ignoring, corrupting, verbally assaulting, or overpressuring the child (Nelms, 2001).

PHYSICAL ABUSE

The deliberate infliction of physical injury on a child, usually by the child's caregiver, is termed *physical abuse*. Legal definitions of physical abuse are found in state and federal statutes. The Child Abuse Prevention and Treatment Act of 1996 defines abuse as "any recent act or failure to act that results in imminent risk of serious harm, death, serious physical or emotional harm of a child (<18 years) by a parent or caregiver who is responsible for the child's welfare." Each state defines abuse according to its reporting laws. Minor physical injury is responsible for more reported cases of maltreatment than major physical injury, but major physical abuse causes more deaths. Despite the importance of the problem, a universally accepted definition of what constitutes minor and major physical abuse does not exist. Rather, each state in the United States defines abuse according to its individual reporting laws.

Shaken Baby Syndrome

Shaken baby syndrome (SBS) is a serious form of child abuse caused by violent shaking of infants and young children and is one form of abusive head trauma. Physicians commonly use more general terms, including *abusive head trauma, inflicted head injury,* or *neuroinflicted brain injury;* these terms do not assume the mechanism of injury but rather describe the injury itself (AAP, Committee on Child Abuse and Neglect, 2009; Chiesa and Duhaime, 2009). This violent shaking would be easily recognized by others as dangerous (AAP, Committee on Child Abuse and Neglect, 2009) and is most often a result of the caregiver's frustration with crying (Castiglia, 2001). Every year in the United States, an estimated 1200 to 1400 children are shaken, and of these victims, 25% to 30% die as a result of their injuries. The rest have lifelong complications (National Center on Shaken Baby Syndrome, n.d.).

It is important to understand what happens in SBS. Infants have a large head-to-body ratio, weak neck muscles, and a large amount of water in the brain. Violent shaking causes the brain to rotate within the skull, resulting in shearing forces that tear blood vessels and neurons. The characteristic injuries that occur are intracranial bleeding (subdural and subarachnoid hematomas) and, in approximately 85%

of cases, retinal hemorrhages, which are classic results of repetitive acceleration–deceleration head trauma (Levin, 2009). Injuries may also include fractures of the ribs and long bones. Most often there are no signs of external injury. SBS is often not an isolated event, and in one study, 45% of the children with inflicted traumatic brain injury caused by shaking showed some evidence of prior injury (Ewing-Cobb, Kramer, Prasad, and others, 1998). Victims of SBS can be seen with a variety of symptoms, from generalized flulike symptoms to unresponsiveness with impending death (Miehl, 2005). Many of the presenting symptoms, such as vomiting, irritability, poor feeding, and listlessness, are often mistaken for common infant and childhood ailments. In more severe forms, presenting symptoms may include seizures, posturing, alterations in level of consciousness, apnea, bradycardia, or death. The long-term outcomes of SBS include seizure disorders; visual impairments, including blindness; developmental delays; hearing loss; cerebral palsy; and mild to profound mental, cognitive, or motor impairments (Walls, 2006). Nurses can take an active role in prevention of SBS by teaching all caregivers about crying and techniques to cope with inconsolable crying (Carbaugh, 2004).

> **! NURSING ALERT**
>
> Stress to parents the danger of shaking infants (shaking can cause SBS). Education must include coping mechanisms on caring for children with inconsolable crying.

Munchausen Syndrome by Proxy

Munchausen syndrome by proxy (MSBP), also known as medical child abuse or factitious disorder by proxy, is a rare but serious form of child abuse in which caregivers deliberately exaggerate or fabricate histories and symptoms or induce symptoms. It is a form of child maltreatment that may include physical, emotional, and psychologic abuse for the gratification of the caregiver. In most cases, the perpetrator is the biologic mother, with some degree of health care knowledge and training. Health care providers can become easily misled and unknowingly enable the perpetrator (Leider, Irving, Mauricio, and others, 2005). Because of the history of symptoms provided by the caregiver, the child endures painful and unnecessary medical testing and procedures. Common symptoms presented are seizures, nausea and vomiting, diarrhea, and altered mental status; they are usually witnessed only by the perpetrator.

Considerations when determining whether a child is a victim of MSBP include:

- Is the child's condition consistent with the reported history?
- Does diagnostic evidence support the reported history?
- Has anyone other than the caregiver witnessed the symptoms?
- Is treatment being provided primarily because of the caregiver's demands?

The resolution of symptoms after separation from the perpetrator confirms the diagnosis.

Factors Predisposing to Physical Abuse

The causes of child abuse are multifaceted. Child maltreatment occurs across all socioeconomic, religious, cultural, racial, and ethnic groups (Goldman, Salus, Wolcott, and others, 2003). Three risk factors are commonly identified in child abuse: parental characteristics, characteristics of the child, and environmental characteristics. However, no single factor or group of factors is predictive of abuse. Rather, the interaction of these factors is thought to increase the risk of abuse occurring in a particular family.

Parental Characteristics

Some identified characteristics occur more frequently in parents who abuse their children and are therefore considered risk factors. Younger parents more often are abusers of their children. Single-parent families are at higher risk for abuse, and in single-parent families that include an unrelated partner, the partner is sometimes the abuser, although a biologic parent is most commonly the perpetrator (U.S. Department of Health and Human Services, 2009).

Abusive families are often socially isolated and have few supportive relationships. They often have additional stressors such as low-income circumstances with little education. Parents with substance abuse problems pose a greater risk for abuse and neglect because of a variety of factors. The additional stressors of substance abuse with the demands of normal care of children create situations in which abuse and neglect can occur because these parents have impaired judgment and may react with violence while under the influence of drugs or alcohol (Wells, 2009). With little or no available support system and concurrent stressors imposed by the child or environment, these parents are vulnerable to additional crises of any nature and may strike out at the child as a method of releasing their frustration and anxiety.

Other factors identified in abusive parents include low self-esteem and little knowledge of appropriate parenting skills. Parenting skills are learned behaviors, and parents who grew up with poor parental role models may have difficulty parenting their own children. Approximately one third of parents who were maltreated as children will subject their children to similar maltreatment (Gara, Allen, Herzog, and others, 2000).

Characteristics of the Child

The onus for child abuse is always on the abuser. However, children who are abused do have some common characteristics. Children from birth to 1 year of age are at highest risk for being abused (U.S. Department of Health and Human Services, 2009). Infants and small children require constant attention and must have all their needs met by others. This can result in parental or caregiver fatigue that results in striking out at the child with physical force, shaking the child, or ignoring the child's needs.

The physical and emotional demands placed on the parents or caregiver of an unwanted, brain-damaged, hyperactive, or physically disabled child may overwhelm them, resulting in abuse. Children with disabilities may not understand that abusive behaviors are not appropriate, so they may not tell others or defend themselves. Premature infants may be at risk for maltreatment because of failure of parent–child bonding during early infancy, increased physical needs, or irritability. One child may be singled out in an abusive family. Removing that child from the home often places the other siblings at risk for abuse. Therefore, no child is safe if left in the abusive environment unless the parents can be helped to learn new parenting skills, to meet the children's needs, and to release their frustration through alternatives other than attacking their children.

Environmental Characteristics

The environment is a significant part of the potentially abusive situation. A typical environment is one of chronic stress, including problems of divorce, poverty, unemployment, poor housing, frequent relocation, alcoholism, and drug addiction. Increased exposure between children and parents, such as that which occurs in crowded living conditions, also increases the likelihood of abuse.

Although most reporting of abuse has been from lower socioeconomic populations, as stated before, child abuse is not a problem of any one societal group. Stresses imposed by poverty predispose lower

socioeconomic families to abusive situations, and abuse in these groups is more likely to be reported. However, concealed crises may also be present in upper-class families. Families who have substitute caregivers such as daycare providers and babysitters may also be at risk for child abuse, especially if the family has not fully evaluated the caregiver. Nurses need to be aware of all these factors to identify the less obvious examples of child abuse and neglect.

SEXUAL ABUSE

Sexual abuse is one of the most devastating types of child maltreatment, and estimates indicate that it has increased significantly during the past decade (U.S. Department of Health and Human Services, 2009). Some of the apparent increase is because of increased awareness (Putnam, 2003).

As with all forms of child maltreatment, no universal definition for sexual abuse exists. Definitions of sexual abuse cover a range of acts including involvement of children in sexual acts they do not understand, to which they cannot give consent, or that violate social taboos (Finkel and DeJong, 2001). The Child Abuse and Prevention Act defines sexual abuse as "the use, persuasion, or coercion of any child to engage in sexually explicit conduct (or any simulation of such conduct) or producing any visual depiction of such conduct, or rape, molestation, prostitution, or incest with children."

Sexual abuse includes the following types of sexual maltreatment (see also Sexual Assault [Rape], Chapter 17):

Incest—Any physical sexual activity between family members; blood relationship is not required (abusers can include stepparents, unrelated siblings, grandparents, uncles, and aunts); does not include sexual relations between legally sanctioned partners, such as spouses

Molestation—A vague term that includes "indecent liberties," such as touching, fondling, kissing, single or mutual masturbation, or oral–genital contact

Exhibitionism—Indecent exposure, usually exposure of the genitalia by an adult man to children or women

Child pornography—Arranging and photographing, in any media, sexual acts involving children, alone or with adults or animals, regardless of consent by the child's legal guardian; also may denote distribution of such material in any form with or without profit

Child prostitution—Involving children in sex acts for profit and usually with changing partners

Pedophilia—Literally means "love of child" and does not denote a type of sexual activity but rather the preference of an adult for prepubertal children as the means of achieving sexual excitement

Characteristics of Abusers and Victims

Anyone, including siblings and mothers, can be sexual abusers, but a typical abuser is a man whom the victim knows. Offenders come from all levels of society. Adults comprise 80% of sexual abuse offenders, with the remaining 20% being made of adolescents and preadolescents (Johnson, 2004). Many offenders hold full-time jobs, are active in community affairs, and may not have prior criminal records (Finkel and DeJong, 2001). Offenders often are employed (or volunteers) in positions such as teaching or coaching that bring them into contact with young girls and boys. Child sexual abuse may be generational unless discovered and stopped (Johnson, 2004). Offenders may commit many assaults before being caught.

Incestuous relationships between father or stepfather and daughter are generally prolonged, and the victims are usually reluctant to report the situation because of fear of retaliation and fear that they will not

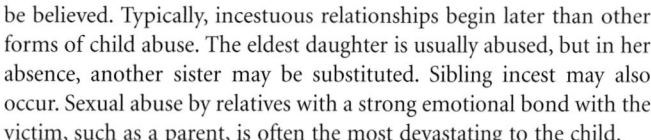

BOX 14-7 **METHODS USED TO PRESSURE CHILDREN INTO SEXUAL ACTIVITY**

- The child is offered gifts or privileges or has privileges withheld.
- The adult misrepresents moral standards by telling the child that it is "okay to do."
- Isolated and emotionally and socially impoverished children are enticed by adults who meet their needs for warmth and human contact.
- The successful sex offender pressures the victim into secrecy by describing it as a "secret between us" that other people would take away if they found out.
- The offender plays on the child's fears, including fear of punishment by the offender, fear of repercussions if the child tells, and fear of abandonment or rejection by the family.

 NURSING CARE GUIDELINES

Talking with Children Who Reveal Abuse

- Provide a private time and place to talk.
- Do not promise not to tell; tell them that you are required by law to report the abuse.
- Do not express shock or criticize their family.
- Use their vocabulary to discuss body parts.
- Avoid using any leading statements that can distort their report.
- Reassure them that they have done the right thing by telling.
- Tell them that the abuse is not their fault and that they are not bad or to blame.
- Determine their immediate need for safety.
- Let the child know what will happen when you report.

be believed. Typically, incestuous relationships begin later than other forms of child abuse. The eldest daughter is usually abused, but in her absence, another sister may be substituted. Sibling incest may also occur. Sexual abuse by relatives with a strong emotional bond with the victim, such as a parent, is often the most devastating to the child.

Boys are also victims of both intrafamilial and extrafamilial abuse. Compared with female victims, male victims are much less likely to report abuse, and they may suffer much greater emotional harm from incestuous relationships. Boys are likely to be subjected to anal penetration and oral–genital contact. They often have subtle physical findings and are abused by a father, stepfather, or mother's boyfriend.

Significant risk factors for child sexual abuse include parental unavailability, lack of emotional closeness and flexibility, social isolation, emotional deprivation, and communication difficulties. Most sexual abuse is committed by men and by persons known to the child, with family members constituting up to two thirds of the perpetrators (Christian, Lavelle, DeJong, and others, 2000). Around 20% to 25% of child sexual abuse cases involve penetration or oral–genital contact. In 2007, more than 35% of sexual abuse victim were between 12 and 15 years of age (U.S. Department of Health and Human Services, 2009).

Initiation and Perpetuation of Sexual Abuse

The cycle of sexual abuse often starts insidiously unless it involves an isolated attack, such as rape. Often offenders spend time with the victims to gain their trust before initiating any sexual contact. Most victims are then pressured into being an accessory to the sexual activity through various means (Box 14-7) and may be unaware that sexual activity is part of the offer. Children may not reveal the truth for fear that their parents would not believe them if they told, especially if the offender is a trusted member of the family. Some fear that they will be blamed for the situation, and many young children with limited vocabulary have difficulty describing the activity when they do have the courage or opportunity to reveal the abuse.

Incest most frequently occurs between fathers and daughters, but it may also be between grandfather and granddaughter or brother and sister. Brother–sister incest has been found to be just as damaging as father–daughter abuse (Cyr, Wright, McDuff, and others, 2002). Victims may take years to disclose this abuse. However, not all incestuous relationships follow this pattern of silence. Reports of father–daughter incest during child custody conflicts have become more common and have raised serious concerns regarding the possibility of false accusation. Rather than tolerating or denying the child's sexual abuse, the other parent (usually the mother) is typically the chief accuser.

NURSING CARE OF THE MALTREATED CHILD

A critical responsibility of health professionals is identifying abusive situations as early as possible. Nurses who increase their knowledge of the different types of abuse and neglect and underlying causes will enhance their ability to identify, intervene, and prevent children from maltreatment and neglect (Giardino and Giardino, 2003). The characteristics that may predispose members of some families to commit abuse can serve as a framework for assessing vulnerability but are never predictive of actual abuse. A careful, detailed history and interview combined with a thorough physical examination are the diagnostic tools needed to identify abuse. Nurses have a special role because they may be the first person to see the child and parent and are the consistent caregivers if the child is hospitalized (see Nursing Care Guidelines box).

In interviewing the child and family, the nurse must be careful to avoid biasing the child's retelling of the events. Some experts suggest that health professionals limit the interview to the child's physical and mental health concerns and leave topics of the family's social, legal, or other problems to the police or the CPS (Kellogg, 2005; McClain, Giardet, Lahoti, and others, 2000). If this is not possible, make an effort to coordinate the interview process so that all pertinent health care professionals can be present for the interview.

Recognition of abuse or neglect necessitates a familiarity with both physical and behavioral signs that suggest maltreatment (Box 14-8). No one indicator can be used to diagnose maltreatment. It is a pattern or combination of indicators that should arouse suspicion and lead to further investigation. It is important to note that some situations, such as bleeding disorders, osteogenesis imperfecta, or sudden infant death syndrome, may be misinterpreted as abuse. Also, some cultural practices, such as cupping or coin rubbing (see Health Practices, Chapter 4), may mimic physical abuse. Unintentional injuries, such as burns from metal buckles on car seats, bruising from seat belts, or spiral fractures from a twist and fall injury, may also be wrongly diagnosed as abuse. Normal variants, such as mongolian spots and congenital anomalies of genitalia, can be mistaken for abuse.

Caregiver–Child Interaction

The nurse can use the initial contact with the family to assess the interaction between the caregiver and the child. Observations of the caregivers should include emotional support for the child, attentiveness to the child's needs, and concern for the child's injury. Although caregivers and children may vary in responses to a stressful event, note

BOX 14-8 WARNING SIGNS OF ABUSE

- Child has physical evidence of abuse or neglect, including previous injuries.
- History is incompatible with the pattern or degree of injury, such as bilateral skull fractures after being dropped.
- Explanation of how injury occurred is vague or the parent or guardian is reluctant to provide information.
- The patient is brought in with a minor, unrelated complaint, and significant trauma is found.
- Histories are contradictory among caregivers.
- The mechanism of injury provided is not possible given age or developmental level of the patient, such as 6-month-old turning on hot water.
- Bruising or other injury is present in a nonmobile patient.
- The patient's affect is inappropriate in relation to the extent of injury.
- Evidence of abusive or neglectful parent–child interaction is present.
- The parent, guardian, or custodian disappears after bringing in the patient for trauma or a patient with suspicious injury is brought in by an unrelated adult.
- The patient has multiple fractures of differing ages.
- There was a delay in seeking care.
- The parent or caregiver discloses that abuse has or may have occurred.
- The patient makes an outcry of abuse or neglect.

an unusual caregiver–child relationship and factor this into the overall evaluation of the child.

Certain behavioral responses of the parents to their child and to the interviewer should alert the nurse to the possibility of maltreatment. Abusive parents may have difficulty showing concern toward their child. They may be unable or unwilling to comfort the child. Abusers may blame the child for the injuries or belittle him or her for being clumsy or stupid. When interacting with health care workers, the parent may become hostile or uncooperative. During the child's hospitalization, they may not participate in the child's care and may show little concern for his or her progress, eventual discharge, or need for follow-up care.

Abused children's responses to their parents or the injury may also support the suspicion of abuse. Although no one pattern is typical, extremes of behavior may be observed. Children may be unresponsive to the parent or excessively clinging and intolerant of separation. They may be overly attached to the abusive parent, possibly in the hope of preventing any upset that may precipitate anger and another attack. During care of the injury, children may be passive and accepting of the discomfort or uncooperative and fearful of any physical contact. They may avoid eye contact. Some children maintain a wary watchfulness of all strangers; some shy away from strangers as if frightened; others are unusually affectionate and outgoing.

History and Interview
Child Physical Abuse

It is often difficult to distinguish child maltreatment from accidental injuries. Caregivers whose history of events may be deceptive or incomplete and children who are nonverbal may make the assessment more complex. A purposeful, skilled history and appropriate interview questions help the nurse ensure the right course of action. Knowledge of mechanism of injury and child development is essential. Cases of abuse are often detected when the child or caregiver history of events does not match with physical findings. Children who are verbal can often give a history of the injury. Separating the child from the caregiver may provide a more reliable history. It is important to ask

nonleading, open-ended questions. The history should include a narrative of the injury from both caregiver and child (if verbal). Date, time, and location where the injury took place along with who was present at the time of the injury are essential questions. Family history for bleeding and bone disorders is important. Box 14-8 outlines areas of history that are concerning for abuse.

Neglect and Emotional Abuse

Each child may manifest different responses to neglect, depending on the situation and developmental age of the child. The goal of the interview is to determine whether the child is in a safe environment and whether the caregiver has the skills and resources to care for the child. It is often difficult to determine whether the circumstances constitute poor parenting skills or true neglect. Box 14-9 lists flags for behaviors to look for in neglected and abused children.

Sexual Abuse

An essential component to identifying sexual abuse is the interview. Several dynamics may impede the child's revelation of sexual abuse. Child sexual abuse is often perpetrated by someone known to the child, including family members. In some cases, the child may have been sworn to secrecy. The child may have been told that no one will believe the story or that his or her family would be harmed if he or she told someone about the abuse. Small children may imitate behaviors they have had perpetrated on themselves or have seen others do. The nurse must be able to recognize normal, age-related sexual curiosity and self-stimulating behaviors. Typically, children do not act out specific details of the sexual act or perform intrusive acts on others unless they have sexual knowledge beyond their normal age-related development. (Johnson, 2004).

Children's reports of sexual abuse may vary from contradictory stories to unwavering versions of the experience. Stories that sound contradictory may reflect the child's experiences in several instances of abuse. Also, children who repeatedly tell identical facts may have been prompted to do so.

Increasing evidence suggests that the types of interrogation children are exposed to after reports of sexual abuse shape their thinking. To avoid biasing the interaction, nurses must be skillful interviewers when questioning children who may be victims of abuse. Medical records should include verbatim statements made by the child and interviewer that reflect appropriate nonleading questions and statements (Hornor, 2001; Kellogg, 2005; McClain, Girardet, Lahoti, and others, 2000). The child may not be emotionally ready to discuss the abuse. Establishing rapport with the child is essential to gaining his or her trust. Interviews should not be rushed. Engaging the child in play activities while encouraging conversation may help the child discuss the abuse. It may take several interviews or psychologic counseling for the child to be forthcoming about the abuse. Information regarding the last sexual contact is important because it determines the need for a forensic evaluation. Children who have been sexually abused within the past 72 to 96 hours should be considered for forensic testing.

Unfortunately, there is no typical profile of the victim, and the nurse must have a high index of suspicion to identify these children. Physical signs vary and may include any of those listed for sexual abuse. The victim may exhibit various behavioral manifestations, but none of these behaviors is diagnostic. When abused children exhibit these behaviors, the signs may be incorrectly attributed to the normal stresses of childhood, especially in older school-age children or adolescents. Even signs considered most predictive of sexual abuse, such as certain genital findings, sexually inappropriate behavior for age, enactment of adult sexual activity, and intense focus on sexual activity (e.g.,

BOX 14-9 CLINICAL MANIFESTATIONS OF POTENTIAL CHILD MALTREATMENT

Physical Neglect
Suggestive Physical Findings
Growth failure
Signs of malnutrition, such as thin extremities, abdominal distention, lack of subcutaneous fat
Poor personal hygiene
Unclean or inappropriate dress
Evidence of poor health care, such as delayed immunization, untreated infections, frequent colds
Frequent injuries from lack of supervision

Suggestive Behaviors
Dull and inactive affect; excessively passive or sleepy
Self-stimulatory behaviors, such as finger sucking or rocking
Begging or stealing food
Absenteeism from school
Substance abuse
Vandalism or shoplifting

Emotional Abuse and Neglect
Suggestive Physical Findings
Growth failure
Eating or feeding disorder
Enuresis
Sleep disorder

Suggestive Behaviors
Self-stimulatory behaviors, such as biting, rocking, or sucking
During infancy, lack of social smile and stranger anxiety
Withdrawal from environment and people
Unusual fearfulness
Antisocial behavior, such as destructiveness, stealing, cruelty to animals or people
Extremes of behavior, such as overcompliant and passive or aggressive and demanding
Lags in emotional and intellectual development, especially language
Suicide attempts

Physical Abuse
Suggestive Physical Findings
Bruises and welts (may be in various stages of healing)
• On face, lips, mouth, back, buttocks, thighs, or areas of torso
• Regular patterns descriptive of object used, such as belt buckle, hand, wire hanger, chain, wooden spoon, squeeze or pinch marks
• May be present in various stages of healing
Burns
• On soles, palms, back, or buttocks
• Patterns descriptive of object used, such as round cigar or cigarette burns; sharply demarcated areas from immersion in scalding water; rope burns on wrists or ankles from being bound; burns in the shape of an iron, radiator, or electric stove burner
• Absence of "splash" marks and presence of symmetric burns
• Stun gun injury: lesions circular, fairly uniform (≤0.5 cm), and paired about 5 cm apart
Fractures and dislocations
• Skull, nose, or facial structures
• Injury denoting type of abuse, such as spiral fracture or dislocation from twisting of an extremity or whiplash from shaking the child
• Multiple new or old fractures in various stages of healing

Lacerations and abrasions
• On backs of arms, legs, torso, face, or external genitalia
• Unusual symptoms, such as abdominal swelling, pain, and vomiting from punching
• Descriptive marks such as from human bites or pulling out of hair
Chemical
• Unexplained repeated poisoning, especially drug overdose
• Unexplained sudden illness, such as hypoglycemia from insulin administration

Suggestive Behaviors
Wary of physical contact with adults
Apparent fear of parents or going home
Lying very still while surveying environment
Inappropriate reaction to injury, such as failure to cry from pain
Lack of reaction to frightening events
Apprehensive when hearing other children cry
Indiscriminate friendliness and displays of affection
Superficial relationships
Acting-out behavior, such as aggression, to seek attention
Withdrawal behavior

Sexual Abuse
Suggestive Physical Findings
Bruises, bleeding, lacerations, or irritation of external genitalia, anus, mouth, or throat
Torn, stained, or bloody underclothing
Pain on urination or pain, swelling, and itching of genital area
Penile discharge
Sexually transmitted disease, nonspecific vaginitis
Difficulty in walking or sitting
Unusual odor in the genital area
Recurrent urinary tract infections
Presence of sperm
Pregnancy in young adolescent

Suggestive Behaviors
Sudden emergence of sexually related problems, including excessive or public masturbation, age-inappropriate sexual play, promiscuity, or overtly seductive behavior
Withdrawn behavior, excessive daydreaming
Preoccupation with fantasies, especially in play
Poor relationships with peers
Sudden changes, such as anxiety, loss or gain of weight, clinging behavior
In incestuous relationships, excessive anger at mother for not protecting daughter
Regressive behavior, such as bedwetting or thumb sucking
Sudden onset of phobias or fears, particularly fears of the dark, men, strangers, or particular settings or situations (e.g., undue fear of leaving the house or staying at the daycare center or the babysitter's house)
Running away from home
Substance abuse, particularly of alcohol or mood-elevating drugs
Profound and rapid personality changes, especially extreme depression, hostility, and aggression (often accompanied by social withdrawal)
Rapidly declining school performance
Suicidal attempts or ideation

masturbation), do not always indicate that sexual abuse has occurred. Conversely, abused children may not demonstrate more knowledge of sexual activity than nonabused children. However, one difference in the abused children's explanation of sexual activity may be unusual affective responses. For example, abused children may have an increased incidence of sleep disorders, temper tantrums, and depression.

> **! NURSING ALERT**
>
> When children report potentially sexually abusive experiences, take their reports seriously but also cautiously to avoid alarming the child or falsely accusing someone.

Physical Assessment
Child Physical Abuse

The goal of the physical assessment for child physical abuse is identification of all injuries. A system approach ensures that the whole body is evaluated. In instances of severe abuse and injuries, the assessment should begin with a rapid assessment of airway, breathing, circulation, and neurologic systems. A systematic head-to-toe examination follows. Attention to areas often overlooked, such as the scalp, behind the ears, and the frenulum, is essential. The child's exterior genital area and posterior surface should be completely examined.

Record the location and a detailed description of all injuries. Note the color, size, and location of all bruising. Burn documentation should include the location, pattern, demarcation lines, and presence of eschar or blisters. Diagrams of the injuries using a body diagram form are helpful. If possible, obtain photographs of the injuries using a measurement tool.

Not all forms of physical abuse have obvious signs. Intraabdominal organ injury from blunt trauma to the abdomen can occur without signs of external abdominal bruising. Nurses should consider intraabdominal injury in infants and children who have any other signs of abuse.

> **! NURSING ALERT**
>
> Incompatibility between the history and the injury is probably the most important criterion on which to base the decision to report suspected abuse.

All evidence collected must adhere to strict guidelines for legal purposes; the chain of custody must be appropriately maintained with local law enforcement personnel. Documentation on the chain of custody form should include the names of persons collecting and receiving evidence (e.g., photographs and DNA samples), types of evidence collected and received, and date of receipt (Kaczor, Pierce, Makoroff, and others, 2006; Kellogg, 2005).

Neglect and Emotional Abuse

Neglect from deprivation of necessities is easier to identify than emotional neglect or psychologic maltreatment because physical signs are usually evident. Assessment of the child's height, weight, nutritional status, hygiene, and age-appropriate interactions is important for the overall picture of potential neglect. Emotional maltreatment may be readily suspected, but it is difficult to substantiate. Physical signs are often nonspecific, and nurses must rely on behavioral indicators, which range from depression to acting-out behavior, to help identify a possibly abusive situation. Any persistent and unexplained change in the child's behavior is an important clue to possible emotional abuse.

Sexual Abuse

Identifying instances of sexual abuse is particularly difficult because, often, few if any obvious physical indications of the activity exist. Physical signs vary and may include any of those listed in Box 14-9 for sexual abuse. The goal of the physical examination is to document genital findings. In most cases, the genital examination findings are normal, which does not mean that sexual abuse did not occur. Fondling or genital-to-genital contact without penetration may leave no physical findings. Forensic evidence obtained directly from a prepubertal victim's body diminishes greatly after 24 hours, with the best chance for evidence collection coming from bed linens or the child's underwear (Christian, Lavelle, DeJong, and others, 2000). The female genital examination should include a description of the vulva, hymen, and surrounding tissue. Abnormal findings of concern are injuries to the posterior vulva or the lower half of the hymeneal ring or abrasions, bruising, or bleeding of the genital or anal tissue. It is often helpful to use a magnifying instrument (colposcope) to detect subtle injuries. There are many variants of normal findings for female genital anatomy, so it is recommended that the examination be done by a practitioner experienced with these types of cases. Contrary to popular myth, the size of the hymeneal opening is not predictive of the likelihood of sexual abuse (Christian and Rubin, 2002). For male victims, swelling, abrasions, or bruising of the genital tissue raises concerns for abuse. Examine the anal area for symmetry, tone, fissures, or scars. Genital tissue heals very quickly and most often without scars. Therefore, unless the child is seen within a few days of injury, the genital tissue may appear normal. In addition, the vaginal and anal mucosa is elastic; therefore, penetration without disruption of tissue is possible. This defies another myth that there is always evidence of female virginity. Consider the collection of specimens for determining the presence of sexually transmitted infections, which may have been contracted during the sexual contact.

A number of nursing diagnoses are prominent in the nursing care of the maltreated child and family, and others specific to individual cases become evident. The Nursing Care Plan on p. 452 describes the expected outcomes.

Nursing Care Management
Protect the Child from Further Abuse

Initially, identification of instances of suspected abuse or neglect is essential. The nurse may come in contact with abused children in an emergency department, practitioner's office, home, daycare center, or school.

> **! NURSING ALERT**
>
> The priority is to remove the child from the abusive situation to prevent further injury.

All states and provinces in North America have laws for mandatory reporting of child maltreatment. Suspected child abuse is reported to the local authorities.* Referrals usually come to the state child welfare department and are assigned to a caseworker in an agency such as CPS. After a referral has been made, a caseworker is assigned to investigate the report. Based on the findings, the child is left in the home or temporarily removed.

---

*Telephone numbers are usually listed under "Child Abuse" in the business white pages of the local directory or you can call the emergency child abuse hotline: 800-422-4453 (800-4-A-CHILD).

NURSING CARE PLAN

The Child Who Is Maltreated

NURSING DIAGNOSIS	PATIENT OUTCOMES	NURSING INTERVENTIONS	RATIONALE
Risk for Trauma related to child, caregiver(s), environment	Child will not experience any maltreatment.	Observe child for physical and behavioral evidence of abuse.	To detect abuse and protect the child
	Child will be protected from further abuse.	Report suspicions to appropriate authorities.	To comply with laws requiring health care providers to report suspicions of maltreatment to child protective services
Child's or Family's Defining Characteristics (Subjective and Objective Data)	Child will be able to express feelings about returning to home or foster home.	Assist in removing child from unsafe environment.	
Physical Neglect	Child and family, including foster parents if appropriate, will be prepared for discharge.	Refer family to social agencies.	To prevent further injury or neglect
Failure to thrive		Collaborate with multidisciplinary team.	To provide assistance for physical needs to help prevent physical neglect
Malnutrition		Keep factual, objective records of child's and parents' behaviors.	
Poor hygiene		Be aware of signs for continued abuse or neglect.	To provide counseling and education so parents learn appropriate parenting skills
Poor health care	**The Following NOC Concepts Apply to These Outcomes**	Help parents identify circumstances that precipitate an abused act.	
Frequent injuries	Abuse Protection Support	Assist families with realizing abuse or neglect has occurred.	To involve several disciplines providing expertise in prevention of future neglect or abuse
Emotional Neglect	Abuse Recovery: Physical, Sexual		To facilitate documentation and action planning by authorities
Failure to thrive	Anxiety Control	**The Following NIC Concepts Apply to These Interventions**	To prevent further injury or neglect
Enuresis	Fear Control	Abuse Protection Support: Child	To promote more effective parenting skills
Sleep disorders	Coping	Coping Enhancement	
	Safety Behavior: Personal	Environment Management: Violence Prevention	To promote awareness of what has happened
Physical Abuse	Home Physical Environment		
Bruises			
Burns			
Fractures or dislocation			
Lacerations			
Intracranial hemorrhage			
Sexual Abuse			
Torn or bloody underclothing			
Bruises, bleeding, lacerations of external genitalia, anus, mouth, or throat			
Genital discharge or odor			
Recurrent urinary tract infection			
Fear or Anxiety related to negative interpersonal interaction, repeated maltreatment, powerlessness, potential loss of parents	Child will exhibit minimal fear and anxiety.	Provide consistent caregiver during hospitalization.	To promote trust
	Child will engage in positive relationships with caregivers.	Demonstrate acceptance of child.	To minimize feelings of shame and guilt
		Praise child's abilities.	To promote self-esteem
	Child will grieve loss of parent.	Treat child as one with a specific physical problem, not as an "abused" victim.	To promote self-esteem and minimize feelings of guilt
Child's or Family's Defining Characteristics (Subjective and Objective Data)		Avoid asking too many questions.	To avoid upsetting child by probing investigation; to avoid interfering with interrogation
Withdrawn and depressed	**The Following NOC Concepts Apply to These Outcomes**	Use play to communicate.	
Change in behavior		Encourage child to talk about feelings.	To allow child to communicate thoughts and feelings
Inappropriate responses	Anxiety Control	Provide a private time and place to talk.	
Fear of strangers	Fear Control	Help child grieve for loss of parents if parental rights are terminated.	To facilitate coping
Lack of engagement with others	Coping	Encourage introduction of foster parents before placement if possible.	To foster trust
No response to painful interventions			To support child who will likely be attached to parents despite the abuse
May not cry or ask for food when hungry		Offer and encourage food intake at usual times.	To give child time to adjust
			To promote adequate nutrition
		The Following NIC Concepts Apply to These Interventions	
		Active Listening	
		Calming Technique	
		Counseling	
		Presence	
		Therapeutic Play	
		Distraction	

NIC, Nursing Interventions Classification; *NOC,* Nursing Outcomes Classification.

NURSING CARE GUIDELINES
Recording Assessment Data in Suspected Abuse

History of Injury

Date, time, and place of occurrence

Sequence of events with recorded times

Presence of witnesses, especially person caring for child at time of incident

Time lapse between occurrence of injury and initiation of treatment

Interview with child when appropriate, including verbal quotations and information from drawing or other play activities

Interview with parent, witnesses, and other significant persons, including verbal quotations

Description of parent–child interactions (verbal interactions, eye contact, touching, parental concern)

Name, age, and condition of other children in home (if possible)

Physical Examination

Location, size, shape, and color of bruises; approximate location, size, and shape on drawing of body outline

Distinguishing characteristics, such as a bruise in the shape of a hand or a round burn (possibly caused by cigarette)

Symmetry or asymmetry of injury; presence of other injuries

Degree of pain; any bone tenderness

Evidence of past injuries; general state of health and hygiene

Developmental level of child; screening test (see Developmental Assessment, Chapter 5)

A court proceeding may be necessary before the child can be placed outside the home or when parental rights are to be terminated. When the courts are involved, they usually require firsthand testimony by the referring parties. Nurses may be subpoenaed to appear in court, or their notes may be introduced as evidence in court hearings. Accurate and factual documentation is essential. Behaviors are described, not interpreted, and are recorded daily to establish a progress record (see Nursing Care Guidelines box). Conversations among the nurse, child, and parent are recorded verbatim as much as possible.

Support the Child

Children suspected of being abused are often hospitalized for medical management of their injuries and to allow further assessment of their safety needs. The needs of these children are the same as those of any hospitalized child. The child should be treated as a child with the usual physical needs, developmental tasks, and play interests—not as a victim of abuse. The goal of the nurse–child relationship is to provide a role model for the parents in helping them to relate positively and constructively to their child and to foster a therapeutic environment for the child in his or her reprieve from the abusing situation.

Support the Family

The nurse also encourages the child's relationship with nonoffending parents. The nurse does not become a substitute parent but rather acts as a role model for parents in helping them to relate positively and constructively to their child. When parental ignorance of childrearing practices has played a part in the abuse, the nurse can educate the parent regarding children's physical and emotional needs. Because of the parents' own childrearing, they may not be aware of nonviolent methods of discipline, such as time-outs. They may also need help in dealing with their frustration so they do not vent anger on the child. Because these parents may be sensitive to criticism or resistant to authority figures, teaching is implemented through demonstration and

example rather than through lecturing. Praise any competent parenting abilities they demonstrate to promote their sense of parental adequacy.

Advise family members to encourage the child to resume normal activities and observe the child for signs of distress. (See Posttraumatic Stress Disorder, Chapter 17.) Children express their feelings primarily through behavior. Parents should be alert for changes in behavior that indicate distress resulting from the incident, such as remaining in the house, refusal to go to school, changes in sleeping patterns, and frequency of dreams and nightmares.

Referral to appropriate social service agencies is also essential. Many abusive parents live in poverty, and the daily stresses imposed by their circumstances are overwhelming. Seek resources for financial aid, improved housing, and child care. Self-help groups also provide important services. Groups such as Parents Anonymous* (a group for parents who have abused or fear that they may abuse their child but only in terms of physical abuse, not sexual abuse) are accepting and nonjudgmental.

Plan for Discharge

Discharge planning should begin as soon as the legal disposition for placement has been decided, which may be temporary foster home placement, return to the parents, or permanent termination of parental rights. The latter is the most drastic solution, but it is necessary in situations of life-threatening abuse. Whenever children are sent to a foster home or juvenile institution, they must be allowed an opportunity to express their feelings. No matter how severe the abuse, they usually mourn the loss of their parents. They need help to understand why they must not return home and that this new home is in no way a punishment. Whenever possible, foster parents are encouraged to visit in the hospital, and the nurse should take an active role in helping the new parents understand the child, as well as the child's health care needs because studies have shown that the health care needs of children in foster care often go unmet (Mekonnen, Noonan, and Rubin, 2009).

Prevent Abuse

Prevention of child maltreatment has been an extremely difficult goal. However, nurses have played an important role in such programs. For example, home visits to primiparas who were teenagers, unmarried, or of low socioeconomic status were noted to be an effective preventive measure (Eckenrode, Ganzel, Henderson, and others, 2000; McMillian, 2000). The nurses provided information on normal child growth and development and routine health care needs, served as informal support persons, and referred families to appropriate services when a need for assistance was identified. The Nurse-Family Partnership is one such program that has demonstrated evidence-based interventions resulting in the prevention of child maltreatment (Donelan-McCall, Eckenrode, and Olds, 2009).

Nurses in a variety of settings can implement similar activities. For example, nurses in prenatal clinics can prepare expectant families for adjustment to parenthood. Nursery and postpartum nurses can foster the attachment process by encouraging parents to hold and look at their infant, as well as teaching coping mechanisms for prolonged crying. Nurses in neonatal intensive care units can minimize the effects of separation by encouraging parents to visit and can help parents become comfortable caring for their child. Nurses in ambulatory settings can teach parents appropriate methods of bathing, feeding, toileting, disciplining, and preventing injuries while stressing the normal

---

*675 W. Foothill Blvd., Suite 220, Claremont, CA 91711; 909-621-6184; http://www.parentsanonymous.org.

FAMILY-CENTERED CARE

Preventing and Dealing with Sexual Abuse of Children

Sexual assault of children is much more common than most people realize. It may be preventable if children have good preparation. *To provide protection and preparation:*

- Pay careful attention to who is around children. (Unwanted touch may come from someone liked and trusted.)
- Back up a child's right to say no.
- Encourage communication by taking seriously what children say.
- Take a second look at signals of potential danger.
- Refuse to leave children in the company of those who are not trusted.
- Include information about sexual assault when teaching about safety.
- Provide specific definitions and examples of sexual assault.
- Remind children that even "nice" people sometimes do mean things.
- Urge children to tell about *anybody* who causes them to be uncomfortable.
- Prepare children to deal with bribes, threats, and possible physical force.
- Virtually eliminate secrets between children and parents.
- Teach children how to say no, ask for help, and control who touches them and how.
- Model self-protective and limit-setting behavior for children.

If it ever becomes necessary to help a child recover from a sexual assault:

- Listen carefully to understand the child.
- Support the child for telling through praise, belief, sympathy, and lack of blame.
- Know local resources and choose help carefully.
- Provide opportunities to talk about the assault.
- Provide opportunities for the entire family to go through a recovery process.

Sexual assault affects everyone. To help deal with this social problem:

- Provide care and support to those who have been victimized.
- Recognize that offenders may not change behavior even with intervention.
- Organize neighborhood programs to support each other's efforts to protect children.
- Encourage schools to provide information about sexual assault as a problem of health and safety.
- Organize community groups to support educational treatment and law enforcement programs.

Modified from Adams C, Fay J: *No more secrets: protecting your child from sexual assault,* San Luis Obispo, Calif, 1981, Impact.

needs and developmental characteristics of children. Nurses must be sensitive to parental needs for attention, reassurance, and reinforcement and should refer parents to community services and self-help groups.

Unlike preventive efforts for neglect and physical abuse, which have been aimed at the potential offender, prevention of child sexual abuse has centered on education of children to protect themselves. Materials are available for parents that describe sexual abuse and its prevention.* Helpful games such as "What if the babysitter wants to wrestle and hug but tells you to keep it a secret?" can be used to explore dangerous situations in advance and help children learn the importance of saying "no." They need reassurance that no matter what the other person says or does, the parents want to know about it and will not punish them. Even if children participate in the activity before telling their parents,

they must be reassured that it was not their fault. It is equally important to teach children safety in terms of potential risk situations. Several suggestions for parents regarding protecting and educating children against possible molestation are presented in the Family-Centered Care box. The nurse is frequently in a position to discuss the topic of abuse with parents and to provide guidelines. In addition, parents need to be made aware that "nice" people, including friends and relatives, can be offenders; parents should carefully observe how others act toward the child. A sudden change in the child's behavior and a response such as "I don't like Uncle anymore" are clues to investigate the relationship. In the event of any doubt, prevent further solitary encounters with this person and the child. It is sometimes to the child's great misfortune that parents do not take certain comments seriously, such as "He hugs me too tight" or "I don't want to go with him." Casual parental statements such as "He just loves you" or "You do whatever adults tell you to do" can place children in jeopardy. Health professionals must alert parents to such dangers and guide them toward an appreciation of the problem, providing concrete guidelines toward child education and protection (see Nursing Care Plan).

*Sources of information are Prevent Child Abuse America, 228 S. Wabash Ave., 10th Floor, Chicago, IL 60604; 312-663-3520 or 800-Children; http://www.preventchildabuse.org; and American Humane, 63 Inverness Drive East, Englewood, CO 80112; 800-227-4645 (outside Colorado) or 303-792-9900; http://www.americanhumane.org.

KEY POINTS

- Common infectious disorders during early childhood include communicable diseases, intestinal parasitic infections, conjunctivitis, and stomatitis.
- Nursing goals in the treatment of a communicable disease are identification, prevention of transmission, provision of comfort, and prevention of complications.
- Intestinal parasitic diseases constitute the most common infections in the world; giardiasis and enterobiasis are the most widespread parasitic infections among children in the United States.

- Although the incidence of poisoning has decreased in the past 30 years as a result of more stringent packaging regulations, childhood poisoning remains a serious health concern.
- The major principles of treatment for poisoning include assessment and the CABs (circulation, airway, and breathing support), minimization of poison absorption, prevention of complications, family support, and prevention of recurrence.
- Communication with the area PCC is essential in the treatment of any poisoning.

- Acetaminophen poisoning is the most common accidental drug poisoning among children and occurs primarily from acute overdose.
- The most important factor contributing to lead poisoning is its availability in the child's environment. Lead-based paint is the most toxic source of lead.
- Because of increasing awareness of the detrimental effects of low levels of lead on the developing nervous system, acceptable BLLs have been decreasing and now are at less than 5 mcg/dl.
- Child maltreatment may take the form of physical abuse or neglect, emotional abuse or neglect, or sexual abuse.
- Parental, child, and environmental characteristics are criteria that may predispose children to maltreatment.
- Identification of abuse entails securing evidence of maltreatment, taking a history pertaining to the incident, and assessing parental and child behaviors.
- The reported incidence of sexual abuse has increased in the past decade; common forms are incest, molestation, rape, exhibitionism, child pornography, child prostitution, and pedophilia.

REFERENCES

American Academy of Pediatrics, Committee on Child Abuse and Neglect: Abusive head trauma in infants and children, *Pediatrics* 123(5):1409–1411, 2009.

American Academy of Pediatrics, Committee on Infectious Diseases, Pickering L, editor: *Red book: 2009 report of the Committee on Infectious Diseases*, ed 28, Elk Grove Village, Ill, 2009, Author.

Bose-O'Reilly S, McCarthy KM, Steckline N, and others: Mercury exposure and children's health, *Curr Probl Pediatr Adolesc Health Care* 40(8):186–215, 2010.

Bronstein AC, Spyker DA, Cantilena LR Jr, and others: 2009 Annual report of the American Association of Poison Control Centers' National Poison Data System (NPDS): 27th annual report, *Clin Toxicol (Phila)* 48(10):979–1178, 2010.

Carbaugh SF: The long road home: understanding shaken baby syndrome, *Adv Neonatal Care* 4:105–117, 2004.

Castiglia R: Shaken baby syndrome, *J Pediatr Health Care* 15(2):78–80, 2001.

CDC Advisory Committee on Childhood Lead Poisoning Prevention: *CDC response to Advisory Committee on Childhood Lead Poisoning Prevention recommendations in "Low level lead exposure harms children: a renewed call of primary prevention,"* 2012, retrieved May 17, 2012, from http://www.cdc.gov/nceh/lead/ACCLPP/CDC_Response_Lead_Exposure_Recs.pdf.

Centers for Disease Control and Prevention: *Managing elevated blood lead levels among young children: recommendations from the Advisory Committee on Childhood Lead Poisoning Prevention*, Atlanta, 2002, Author.

Centers for Disease Control and Prevention: *Statewide plan for childhood blood lead screening*, Atlanta, 2005, Author.

Centers for Disease Control and Prevention: Deaths associated with hypocalcemia from chelation therapy—Texas, Pennsylvania, and Oregon, 2003–2005, *MMWR Morb Mortal Wkly Rep* 55(08):204–207, 2006.

Centers for Disease Control and Prevention Advisory Committee on Childhood Lead Poisoning Prevention: Interpreting and managing blood lead levels <10 ug/dL in children and reducing childhood exposures to lead, *MMWR Morb Mortal Wkly Rep* 56(47):1241, 2007.

Cheng A, Ratnapalan S: Improving the palatability of activated charcoal in pediatric patients, *Pediatr Emerg Care* 23(6):384–386, 2007.

Chiesa A, Duhaime A: Abusive head trauma, *Pediatr Clin North Am* 56(2):317–331, 2009.

Christian CW, Lavelle JM, DeJong AR, and others: Forensic evidence findings in prepubertal victims of sexual assault, *Pediatrics* 106:100–104, 2000.

Christian CW, Rubin DM: Sexual abuse. In Giardino AP, Giardino ER, editors: *Recognition of child abuse for the mandated reporter*, St. Louis, 2002, GW Medical Publishing.

Clifton JC: Mercury exposure and public health, *Pediatr Clin North Am* 54(2):237–269, 2007.

Criddle LM: An overview of pediatric poisonings, *AACN Adv Crit Care* 18(2):109–118, 2007.

Cyr M, Wright J, McDuff P, and others: Intrafamilial sexual abuse: brother-sister incest does not differ from father-daughter and stepfather-stepdaughter incest, *Child Abuse Negl* 26(9):957–973, 2002.

Dessypris N, Dikalioti SK, Skalkidis I, and others: Combating unintentional injury in the United States: lessons learned from the ICD-10 classification period, *J Trauma* 66(2):519–525, 2009.

Donelan-McCall N, Eckenrode J, Olds D: Home visiting for the prevention of child maltreatment: lessons learned during the past 20 years, *Pediatr Clin North Am* 56(2):389–403, 2009.

Eckenrode J, Ganzel B, Henderson C, and others: Preventing child abuse and neglect with a program of nurse home visitation: the limiting effects of domestic violence, *JAMA* 284(11):1385–1391, 2000.

Eisenstein L, Bodager D, Ginzl D: Outbreak of giardiasis and cryptosporidiosis associated with a neighborhood interactive water fountain—Florida, 2006, *J Environ Health* 71(3):18–22, 2008.

Eldridge DL, Van Eyk J, Kornegay C: Pediatric toxicology, *Emerg Med Clin North Am* 25(2):283–308, 2007.

Erickson L, Thompson T: A review of a preventable poison: pediatric lead poisoning, *J Soc Pediatr Nurs* 10(4):171–182, 2005.

Ewing-Cobb L, Kramer L, Prasad M, and others: Neuroimaging, physical, and developmental findings after inflicted and noninflicted traumatic brain injury in young children, *Pediatrics* 102:300–307, 1998.

Finkel MA, DeJong AR: Medical findings in child sexual abuse. In Reece RM, Ludwig S, editors: *Child abuse medical diagnosis and management*, Philadelphia, 2001, Lippincott Williams & Wilkins.

Franklin RL, Rodgers GB: Unintentional child poisonings treated in United States hospital emergency departments: national estimates of incident cases, population-based poisoning rates, and product involvement, *Pediatrics* 122(6):1244–1251, 2008.

Frazer L: Soil in the city: a prime source of lead. *Environ Health Perspect* 116(12):A522, 2008.

Frithsen I, Simpson W: Recognition and management of acute medication poisoning, *Am Fam Physician* 81(3):316–323, 2010.

Fuloria M, Kreiter S: The newborn examination, part I, emergencies and common abnormalities involving the skin, head, neck, chest, and respiratory and cardiovascular systems, *Am Fam Physician* 65(1):61–68, 2002.

Galea SA, Sweet A, Beninger P, and others: The safety profile of varicella vaccine: a 10-year review, *J Infect Dis* 197(suppl 2):S165–S169, 2008.

Gara MA, Allen LA, Herzog EP, and others: The abused child as parent: the structure and content of physically abused mothers' perceptions of their babies, *Child Abuse Negl* 24(5):627–639, 2000.

Giardino ER, Giardino AP, editors: *Nursing approach to the evaluation of child maltreatment*, St. Louis, 2003, GW Medical Publishing.

Goldman J, Salus MK, Wolcott D, and others: What factors contribute to child abuse and neglect? In *A coordinated response to child abuse and neglect: the foundation for practice*, Child Welfare Information Gateway, 2003, retrieved June 26, 2011, from http://www.childwelfare.gov/pubs/usermanuals/foundation/foundatione.cfm.

Greene S, Harris C, Singer J: Gastrointestinal decontamination of the poisoned patient, *Pediatr Emerg Care* 24(3):176–189, 2008.

Heavey E: Lead poisoning in children: still a threat, *Nursing* 38(12):17–18, 2008.

Hornor G: Repeated sexual abuse allegations: a problem for primary care providers, *J Pediatr Health Care* 15(2):71–76, 2001.

Hudson B, Powell C: Towards evidence based medicine for paediatricians: does oral acyclovir improve clinical outcome in immunocompetent children with primary herpes simplex gingivostomatitis? *Arch Dis Child* 94(2): 165–167, 2009.

Johnson CF: Child sexual abuse, *Lancet* 364(9432): 462–470, 2004.

Kaczor K, Pierce MC, Makoroff K, and others: Bruising and physical child abuse, *Clin Pediatr Emerg Med* 7(3):153–160, 2006.

Kellogg N: The evaluation of sexual abuse in children, *Pediatrics* 116(2):506–512, 2005.

Kendrick D, Barlow J, Hampshire A, and others: Parenting interventions for the prevention of unintentional injuries in childhood, *Cochrane Database Syst Rev* 17(4):CD006020, 2007.

Kendrick D, Coupland C, Mulvaney C, and others: Home safety education and provision of safety equipment for injury prevention, *Cochrane Database Syst Rev* 24(1):CD005014, 2007.

Kendrick D, Smith S, Sutton A, and others: Effect of education and safety equipment on poisoning-prevention practices and poisoning: systematic review, meta-analysis and meta-regression, *Arch Dis Child* 93(7):599–608, 2008.

Lederman C, Lederman M: Ophthalmologic emergencies. In Crain EF, Gershel JC, editors: *Clinical manual of emergency pediatrics,* ed 4, New York, 2003, McGraw-Hill.

Leider HS, Irving SY, Mauricio R, and others: Munchausen syndrome by proxy: a case report, *AACN Clin Issues* 16(2):178–184, 2005.

Leung AK, Robson WL, Leong AG: Herpes zoster in childhood, *J Pediatr Health Care* 20(5):1783–1785, 2006.

Levin A: Retinal hemorrhages: advances in understanding, *Pediatr Clin North Am* 56(2):333–344, 2009.

Levin R, Brown MJ, Kashtock ME, and others: Lead exposures in U.S. children, 2008: implications for prevention, *Environ Health Perspect* 116(10):1285–1293, 2008, retrieved March 25, 2011, from http://www.ncbi.nlm.nih.gov/pmc/articles/PMC2569084/?tool=pubmed.

Lichtenstein SJ, Rinehart M: Levofloxacin Bacterial Conjunctivitis Study Group: efficacy and safety of 0.5% levofloxacin ophthalmic solution for the treatment of bacterial conjunctivitis in pediatric patients, *J AAPOS* 7(5):317–324, 2003.

Lidsky TI, Schneider JS: Adverse effects of childhood lead poisoning: the clinical neuropsychological perspective, *Environ Res* 100(1):284–293, 2006.

Madden MA: Responding to pediatric poisoning, *Nursing* 38(8):52–55, 2008.

McClain N, Giardet R, Lahoti S, and others: Evaluation of sexual abuse in the pediatric patient, *J Pediatr Health Care* 14(3):93–102, 2000.

McMillian H: Child maltreatment: what we know in the year 2000, *Can J Psychiatry* 45(8):702–709, 2000.

Mekonnen R, Noonan K, Rubin D: Achieving better healthcare outcomes for children in foster care, *Pediatr Clin North Am* 56(2):405–415, 2009.

Miehl NJ: Shaken baby syndrome, *J Forensic Nurs* 1(3):111–117, 2005.

Nasser M, Fedorowicz Z, Khoshnevisan MH, and others: Acyclovir for treating primary herpetic gingivostomatitis, *Cochrane Database Syst Rev* Oct 8(4):CD006700, 2008.

National Center on Shaken Baby Syndrome: *All about SBS/AHT,* n.d., retrieved July 10, 2011, from http://www.dontshake.org/sbs.php?topNavID= 2&subNavID=10.

Nelms BC: Emotional abuse: helping prevent the problem, *J Pediatr Health Care* 15(3):103–104, 2001.

Phillips B: Towards evidence-based medicine for paediatricians, *Arch Dis Child Educ Pract Ed* 93(4):129, 2008.

Putnam FW: Ten year update review: child sexual abuse, *J Am Acad Child Adolesc Psychiatry* 42(3):269–278, 2003.

Rose PW, Harnden A, Brueggemann AB, and others: Chloramphenicol treatment for acute infective conjunctivitis in children in primary care: a randomized double-blind placebo-controlled trial, *Lancet* 366(9479):37–43, 2005.

Sheffield P, Serwint JR: Emetics, cathartics, and gastric lavage, *Pediatr Rev* 29(6):214–215, 2008.

Shields JM, Gleim ER, Beach MJ: Prevalence of *Cryptosporidium* spp. and *Giardia intestinalis* in swimming pools, Atlanta, *Emerg Infect Dis* 14(6):948–950, 2008.

Teng MS, Wang NW: Whooping cough: management and diagnosis of pertussis. *Pediatric Emergency Medicine Reports,* Health Reference Center Academic, March 1, 2011, retrieved May 15, 2011, from http://www.find.galegroup.com.ezproxyhost.library.tmc.edu/gtx/start.do?prodId=HRCA&userGroupName=txshracd2509.

U.S. Department of Health and Human Services, Administration on Children, Youth and Families: *Child maltreatment 2007,* Washington, DC, 2009, U.S. Government Printing Office.

Walls C: Shaken baby syndrome education: a role for nurse practitioners working with families of small children, *J Pediatr Health Care* 20(5):304–310, 2006.

Wells K: Substance abuse and child maltreatment, *Pediatr Clin North Am* 56(2):354–362, 2009.

Wood N, McIntyre P: Pertussis: review of epidemiology, diagnosis, management and prevention, *Paediatr Respir Rev* 9(3):201–212, 2008.

Woolf AD, Goldman R, Bellinger DC: Update on clinical management of childhood lead poisoning, *Pediatr Clin North Am* 54(2): 271–294, 2007.

Yoder JS, Beach MJ: Centers for Disease Control and Prevention (CDC): giardiasis surveillance—United States, 2006–2008, *MMWR Surveill Summ* 59(SS06):15–25, 2010.

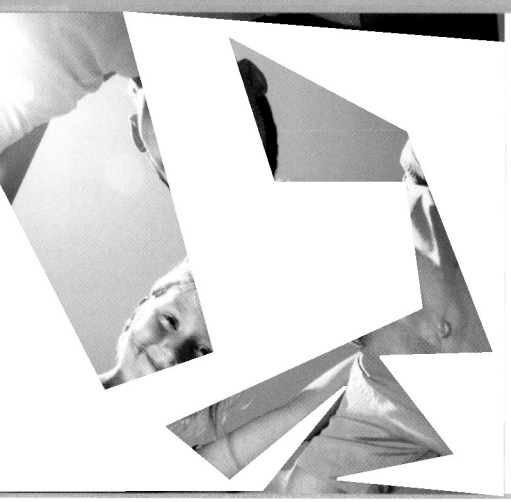

Health Promotion of the School-Age Child and Family

Cheryl C. Rodgers

⊖volve WEBSITE

http://evolve.elsevier.com/wong/essentials
Case Study—Injury Prevention
Key Points Summaries
NCLEX-Style Review Questions
Pediatric Assessment Video Clips

CHAPTER OUTLINE

Promoting Optimal Growth and
Development, 458
  Biologic Development, 458
    Proportional Changes, 458
    Maturation of Systems, 458
    Prepubescence, 459
  Psychosocial Development:
    Developing a Sense of Industry
    (Erikson), 459
  Cognitive Development (Piaget), 460
  Moral Development (Kohlberg), 460
  Spiritual Development, 460
  Social Development, 460
    *Social Relationships and
    Cooperation, 462*

Relationships with Families, 463
  Play, 463
Developing a Self-Concept, 464
  Developing a Body Image, 464
Coping with Concerns Related to
  Normal Growth and Development, 464
    School Experience, 464
    Latchkey Children, 466
    Limit Setting and Discipline, 466
    Dishonest Behavior, 466
    Stress and Fear, 467
Promoting Optimal Health During the
School Years, 468
  Nutrition, 468
  Sleep and Rest, 468

Exercise and Activity, 468
  Sports, 469
  Acquisition of Skills, 469
Dental Health, 469
  Dental Problems, 470
Sex Education, 470
  Nurse's Role in Sex Education, 471
School Health, 471
Injury Prevention, 472
Anticipatory Guidance—Care of
  Families, 472

LEARNING OBJECTIVES

On completion of this chapter the reader will be able to:
- Describe the physical, cognitive, and moral changes that take place during the middle childhood years.
- Describe ways to help a child develop a sense of accomplishment.
- Demonstrate an understanding of the changing interpersonal relationships of school-age children.
- Discuss the role of the peer group in the socialization of the school-age child.

- Discuss the role of schools in the development and socialization of the school-age child.
- Outline an appropriate health teaching plan for the school-age child.
- Plan a sex education session for a group of school-age children.
- Identify the causes and discuss the preventive aspects of injury in middle childhood.

PROMOTING OPTIMAL GROWTH AND DEVELOPMENT

The segment of the life span that extends from age 6 to approximately age 12 has a variety of labels, each of which describes an important characteristic of the period. These middle years are most often referred to as **school-age** or the **school years**. This period begins with entrance into the school environment, which has a significant impact on development and relationships.

Physiologically the middle years begin with the shedding of the first deciduous tooth and end at puberty with the acquisition of the final permanent teeth (with the exception of the wisdom teeth). Before 5 or 6 years of age, children have progressed from helpless infants to sturdy, complicated individuals with an ability to communicate, conceptualize in a limited way, and become involved in complex social and motor behaviors. Physical growth is also rapid during the preschool-age years. In contrast, the period of middle childhood, between the rapid growth of early childhood and the prepubescent growth spurt, is a time of gradual growth and development with more even progress in both physical and emotional aspects.

BIOLOGIC DEVELOPMENT

During middle childhood, growth in height and weight assumes a slower but steady pace as compared with the earlier years. Between ages 6 and 12 years, children grow an average of 5 cm (2 inches) per year to gain 30 to 60 cm (1–2 feet) in height and almost double their weight, increasing 2 to 3 kg (4.5–6.5 pounds) per year. The average 6-year-old child is about 116 cm (45.7 inches) tall and weighs about 21 kg (46 pounds); the average 12-year-old child is about 150 cm (59 inches) tall and weighs approximately 40 kg (88 pounds). During this period, girls and boys differ little in size, although boys tend to be slightly taller and somewhat heavier than girls. Toward the end of the school-age years, both boys and girls begin to increase in size, although most girls begin to surpass boys in both height and weight, to the acute discomfort of both girls and boys.

Proportional Changes

School-age children are more graceful than they were as preschoolers, and they are steadier on their feet. Their body proportions take on a slimmer look, with longer legs, varying body proportion, and a lower center of gravity. Posture improves over that of the preschool period to facilitate locomotion and efficiency in using the arms and trunk. These proportions make climbing, bicycle riding, and other activities easier. Fat gradually diminishes, and its distribution patterns change, contributing to the thinner appearance of children during the middle years.

Accompanying the skeletal lengthening and fat diminution is an increase in the percentage of body weight represented by muscle tissue. By the end of this age period, both boys and girls double their strength and physical capabilities, and their steady and relatively consistent development of coordination increases their poise and skill. However, this increased strength can be misleading. Although strength increases, muscles are still functionally immature when compared with those of adolescents, and they are more readily damaged by muscular injury caused by overuse.

The most pronounced changes that indicate increasing maturity in children are a decrease in head circumference in relation to standing height, a decrease in waist circumference in relation to height, and an increase in leg length in relation to height. These observations often provide a clue to a child's degree of physical maturity and have proved

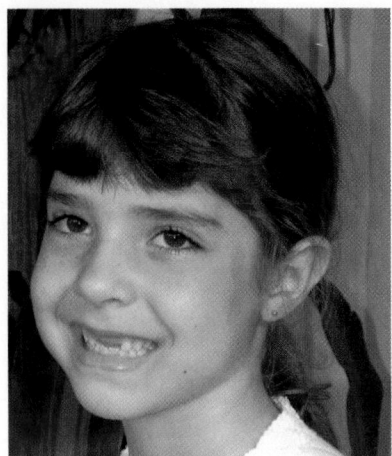

FIG 15-1 Middle childhood is the stage of development when deciduous teeth are shed.

useful in predicting readiness for meeting the demands of school. There appears to be a correlation between physical indications of maturity and success in school.

Specific physiologic and anatomic characteristics are typical of children in middle childhood. Facial proportions change as the face grows faster in relation to the remainder of the cranium. The skull and brain grow very slowly during this period and increase little in size. Because all of the primary (deciduous) teeth are lost during this age span, middle childhood is sometimes known as the **age of the loose tooth** (Fig. 15-1). The early years of middle childhood, when the new secondary (permanent) teeth appear too large for the face, are known as the **ugly duckling stage**.

Maturation of Systems

Maturity of the gastrointestinal system is reflected in fewer stomach upsets; better maintenance of blood glucose levels; and an increased stomach capacity, which permits retention of food for longer periods. School-age children do not need to be fed as promptly or as frequently as preschool-age children. Caloric needs are less than they were in the preschool years.

Physical maturation is evident in other body tissues and organs. **Bladder capacity**, although differing widely among individual children, is generally greater in girls than in boys. The **heart** grows more slowly during the middle years and is smaller in relation to the rest of the body than at any other period of life. Heart and respiratory rates steadily decrease, and blood pressure increases from ages 6 to 12 years (see Appendix E and inside back cover).

The **immune system** becomes more competent in its ability to localize infections and to produce an antibody–antigen response. However, children have several infections in the first 1 to 2 years of school because of increased exposure to other children.

Bones continue to ossify throughout childhood but yield to pressure and muscle pulls more readily than with mature bones. Children need ample opportunity to move around, but they should observe caution in carrying heavy loads. For example, they should shift books or tote bags from one arm to the other. Backpacks distribute weight more evenly than tote bags.

Wider differences between children are observed at the end of middle childhood than at the beginning. These differences become increasingly apparent and, if they are extreme or unique, may create emotional problems. The associated characteristics of height and weight relationships, rapid or slow growth, and other important

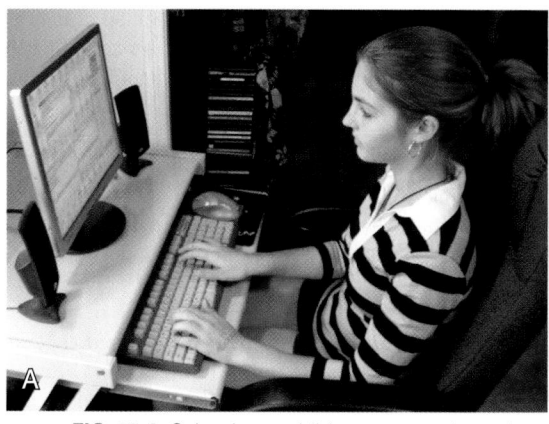 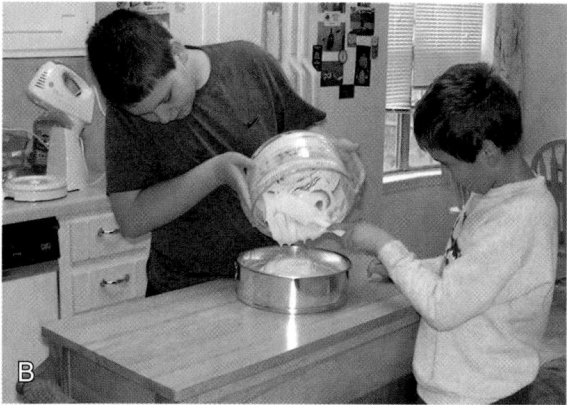

FIG 15-2 School-age children are motivated to complete tasks. **A,** Working alone. **B,** Working with others.

features of development should be explained to children and their families. Physical maturity is not necessarily correlated with emotional and social maturity. Seven-year-old children who look like 10-year-old children will, in fact, think and act like 7-year-old children. To expect behaviors appropriate for the older age is unrealistic and can be detrimental to their development of competence and self-esteem. Conversely, to treat 10-year-old children who look young physically as though they were younger is an equal disservice to them.

Prepubescence

Preadolescence is the period of approximately 2 years that begins at the end of middle childhood and ends with the thirteenth birthday. Because puberty signals the beginning of the development of secondary sex characteristics, prepubescence typically occurs during preadolescence.

Toward the end of middle childhood, the discrepancies in growth and maturation between boys and girls become apparent. On the average, there is a difference of approximately 2 years between girls and boys in the age of onset of pubescence. This is a period of rapid growth in height and weight, especially for girls.

There is no universal age at which children assume the characteristics of prepubescence. The first physiologic signs appear at about 9 years of age (particularly in girls) and are usually clearly evident in 11- to 12-year-old children. Although preadolescent children do not want to be different, variability in physical growth and physiologic changes among children of the same sex and between the two sexes is often striking at this time. This variability, especially in relation to the onset of secondary sexual characteristics, is of great concern to preadolescents. Either early or late appearance of these characteristics is a source of embarrassment and uneasiness to both sexes.

Preadolescence is a period of considerable overlapping of developmental characteristics of both middle childhood and early adolescence. However, several unique characteristics set this period apart from others. Generally, puberty begins at 10 years in girls and 12 years in boys, but it can be normal for either sex after the age of 8 years. Boys experience little visible sexual maturation during preadolescence.

PSYCHOSOCIAL DEVELOPMENT: DEVELOPING A SENSE OF INDUSTRY (ERIKSON)

Freud described middle childhood as the latency period, a time of tranquility between the Oedipal phase of early childhood and the eroticism of adolescence. During this time, children experience relationships with same-sex peers following the indifference of earlier years

and preceding the heterosexual fascination that occurs for most boys and girls in puberty.

Successful mastery of Erikson's first three stages of psychosocial development is important in terms of development of a healthy personality. Successful completion of these stages requires a loving environment within a stable family unit. These experiences prepare the child to engage in experiences and relationships beyond the intimate family group.

A sense of industry or a stage of accomplishment is achieved somewhere between age 6 years and adolescence. School-age children are eager to develop skills and participate in meaningful and socially useful work. They acquire a sense of personal and interpersonal competence; receive the systematic instruction prescribed by their individual cultures; and develop the skills needed to become useful, contributing members of their social communities.

Interests expand in the middle years, and with a growing sense of independence, children want to engage in tasks that can be carried through to completion (Fig. 15-2). They gain satisfaction from independent behavior in exploring and manipulating their environment and from interaction with peers. Often the acquisition of skills provides a way to achieve success in social activities. Reinforcement in the form of grades, material rewards, additional privileges, and recognition provides encouragement and stimulation.

A sense of accomplishment also involves the ability to cooperate, to compete with others, and to cope effectively with people. Middle childhood is the time when children learn the value of doing things with others and the benefits derived from division of labor in the accomplishment of goals. Peer approval is a strong motivating power.

The danger inherent in this period of development is the occurrence of situations that might result in a sense of inferiority. Children with physical and mental limitations may be at a disadvantage in the acquisition of certain skills. When the reward structure is based on evidence of mastery, children who are incapable of developing these skills risk feeling inadequate and inferior. Even children without chronic disabilities may experience feelings of inadequacy in some areas. No child is able to do everything well, and children must learn that they will not be able to master every skill they attempt. All children, even children who usually have positive attitudes toward work and their own abilities, will feel some degree of inferiority when they encounter specific skills that they cannot master.

Children need and want real achievement. Children achieve a sense of industry when they have access to tasks that need to be done and they are able to complete the tasks well despite individual differences in their innate capacities and emotional development.

COGNITIVE DEVELOPMENT (PIAGET)

When children enter the school years, they begin to acquire the ability to relate a series of events to mental representations that can be expressed both verbally and symbolically. This is the stage Piaget describes as concrete operations, when children are able to use thought processes to experience events and actions. The rigid, egocentric view of the preschool years is replaced by mental processes that allow children to see things from another's point of view.

During this stage, children develop an understanding of relationships between things and ideas. They progress from making judgments based on what they see (perceptual thinking) to making judgments based on what they reason (conceptual thinking). They are able to master symbols and to use their memories of past experiences to evaluate and interpret the present.

One cognitive task of school-age children is mastering the concept of conservation (Fig. 15-3). At an early age (5–7 years), children grasp the concept of reversibility of numbers as a basis for simple mathematics problems (e.g., 2 + 4 = 6 and 6 − 4 = 2). They learn that simply altering their arrangement in space does not change certain properties of the environment, and they are able to resist perceptual cues that suggest alterations in the physical state of an object. For example, they recognize that changing the shape of a substance such as a lump of clay does not alter its total mass. They no longer perceive a tall, thin glass of water as containing a greater volume than a short, wide glass; they can distinguish between the weight of items regardless of their size. They recognize that size is not necessarily related to weight or volume. There is a developmental sequence in children's capacity to conserve matter. Conservation of mass usually is accomplished first, weight some time later, and volume last.

School-age children also develop classification skills. They can group and sort objects according to the attributes they share, place things in a sensible and logical order, and hold a concept in mind while making decisions based on that concept. Another characteristic of middle childhood is that children derive enjoyment from classifying and ordering their environment. They become occupied with collections of objects, such as stickers, shells, dolls, cars, cards, and stuffed animals. They may even begin to order friends and relationships (e.g., best friend, second best friend).

They develop the ability to understand relational terms and concepts, such as bigger and smaller; darker and paler; heavier and lighter; to the right of and to the left of; and more than and less than. They view family relationships in terms of reciprocal roles (e.g., to be a brother, one must have a sibling).

School-age children learn the alphabet and the world of symbols called *words*, which can be arranged in terms of structure and their relationship to the alphabet. They learn to tell time, to see the relationship of events in time (history) and places in space (geography), and to combine time and space relationships (geology and astronomy).

The ability to read is acquired during the school years and becomes the most significant and valuable tool for independent inquiry. Children's capacity to explore, imagine, and expand their knowledge is enhanced by reading.

MORAL DEVELOPMENT (KOHLBERG)

As children move from egocentrism to more logical patterns of thought, they also move through stages in the development of conscience and moral standards. Young children do not believe that standards of behavior come from within themselves but that rules are established and set down by others. During the preschool years, children adopt and internalize the moral values of their parents. They learn standards for acceptable behavior, act according to these standards, and feel guilty when they violate them. Although children 6 or 7 years of age know the rules and behaviors expected of them, they do not understand the reasons behind them. Rewards and punishments guide their judgment; a "bad act" is one that breaks a rule or causes harm. Young children believe that what other people tell them to do is right and that what they themselves think is wrong. Consequently, children 6 or 7 years old may interpret accidents or misfortunes as punishment for "bad" acts.

Older school-age children are able to judge an act by the intentions that prompted it rather than just its consequences. Rules and judgments become less absolute and authoritarian and begin to be founded on the needs and desires of others. For older children, a rule violation is likely to be viewed in relation to the total context in which it appears. The situation, as well as the morality of the rule itself, influences reactions. Although younger children judge an act only according to whether it is right or wrong, older children take into account different points of view. They are able to understand and accept the concept of treating others as they would like to be treated.

SPIRITUAL DEVELOPMENT

Children at this age think in concrete terms but are avid learners and have a great desire to learn about their God. They picture God as human and use adjectives such as "loving" and "helping" to describe their deity. They are fascinated by the concepts of hell and heaven, with a developing conscience and concern about rules. They may fear going to hell for misbehavior. School-age children want and expect to be punished for misbehavior and, when given the option, tend to choose a punishment that "fits the crime." However, they may view illness or injury as a punishment for a real or imagined misdeed. The beliefs and ideals of family and religious persons are more influential than those of their peers in matters of faith.

School-age children begin to learn the difference between the natural and the supernatural but have difficulty understanding symbols. Consequently, religious concepts must be presented to them in concrete terms. Prayer or other religious rituals comfort them, and if these activities are a part of their daily lives, they can help them cope with threatening situations. Their petitions to their God in prayers tend to be for tangible rewards. Although younger children expect their prayers to be answered, as they get older, they begin to recognize that this does not always occur, and they become less concerned when their prayers are not answered. They are able to discuss their feelings about their faith and how it relates to their lives (see Cultural Considerations box).

SOCIAL DEVELOPMENT

One of the most important socializing agents in the school-age years is the peer group. In addition to parents and schools, the peer group

⊕ CULTURAL CONSIDERATIONS
Religious Orientation

Many schools and communities have a Judeo-Christian orientation toward prayer, holidays, and values. This may result in conflict and discomfort for children of other religious or ethnic groups. Sensitivity must be exercised so as not to offend and confuse children from other religious backgrounds, such as the Buddhist, Hindu, and Muslim faiths, and those with no religious backgrounds.

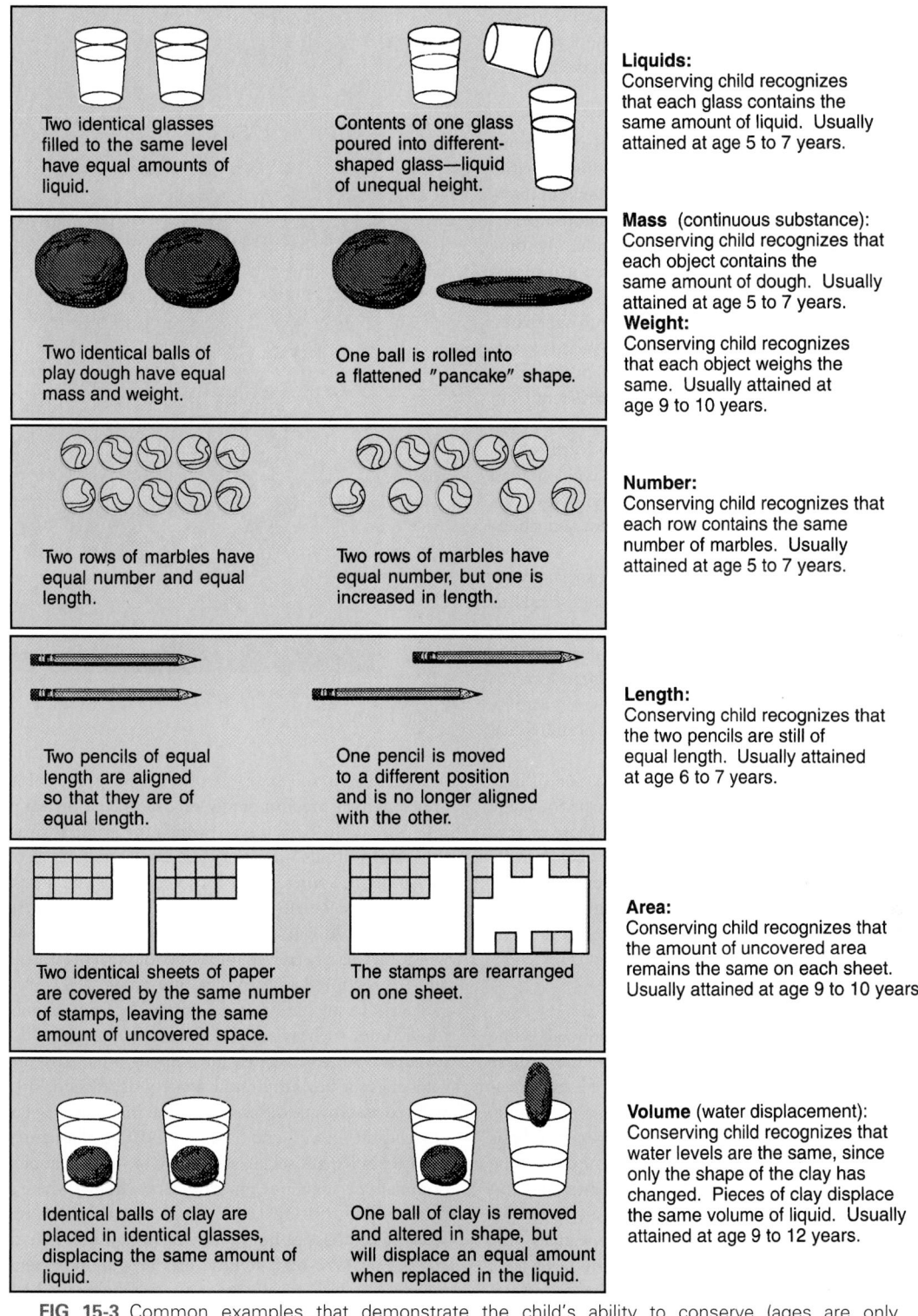

Liquids:
Conserving child recognizes that each glass contains the same amount of liquid. Usually attained at age 5 to 7 years.

Two identical glasses filled to the same level have equal amounts of liquid.

Contents of one glass poured into different-shaped glass—liquid of unequal height.

Mass (continuous substance): Conserving child recognizes that each object contains the same amount of dough. Usually attained at age 5 to 7 years.
Weight:
Conserving child recognizes that each object weighs the same. Usually attained at age 9 to 10 years.

Two identical balls of play dough have equal mass and weight.

One ball is rolled into a flattened "pancake" shape.

Number:
Conserving child recognizes that each row contains the same number of marbles. Usually attained at age 5 to 7 years.

Two rows of marbles have equal number and equal length.

Two rows of marbles have equal number, but one is increased in length.

Length:
Conserving child recognizes that the two pencils are still of equal length. Usually attained at age 6 to 7 years.

Two pencils of equal length are aligned so that they are of equal length.

One pencil is moved to a different position and is no longer aligned with the other.

Area:
Conserving child recognizes that the amount of uncovered area remains the same on each sheet. Usually attained at age 9 to 10 years.

Two identical sheets of paper are covered by the same number of stamps, leaving the same amount of uncovered space.

The stamps are rearranged on one sheet.

Volume (water displacement): Conserving child recognizes that water levels are the same, since only the shape of the clay has changed. Pieces of clay displace the same volume of liquid. Usually attained at age 9 to 12 years.

Identical balls of clay are placed in identical glasses, displacing the same amount of liquid.

One ball of clay is removed and altered in shape, but will displace an equal amount when replaced in the liquid.

FIG 15-3 Common examples that demonstrate the child's ability to conserve (ages are only approximate).

conveys a substantial amount of information to its members. Peer groups have a culture of their own with secrets, traditions, and codes of ethics that promote feelings of solidarity and detachment from adults. Through peer relationships, children learn how to deal with dominance and hostility, how to relate to persons in positions of leadership and authority, and how to explore ideas and the physical environment.

Peer group identification is an important factor in gaining independence from parents. The aid and support of the group provide children with enough security to risk the moderate parental rejection brought about by small victories in the development of independence.

A child's concept of the appropriate sex role is also influenced by relationships with peers. During the early school years, few gender differences exist in the play experiences of children. Both girls and boys share games and other activities. However, in the later school years, the differences in the play of boys and girls become more marked.

Social Relationships and Cooperation

Daily relationships with peers provide important social interactions for school-age children. For the first time, children join group activities with unrestrained enthusiasm and steady participation. Previous interactions were limited to short periods under considerable adult supervision. With increased skills and wider opportunities, children become involved with one or more peer groups in which they can gain status as respected members.

Valuable lessons are learned from daily interaction with age mates. First, children learn to appreciate the numerous and varied points of view that are represented in the peer group. As children interact with peers who see the world in ways that are somewhat different from their own, they become aware of the limits of their own point of view. Because age mates are peers and are not forced to accept each other's ideas as they are expected to accept those of adults, other children have a significant influence on decreasing the egocentric outlook of the child. Consequently, children learn to argue, persuade, bargain, cooperate, and compromise to maintain friendships.

Second, children become increasingly sensitive to the social norms and pressures of the peer group. The peer group establishes standards for acceptance and rejection, and children are often willing to modify their behavior to be accepted by the group. The need for peer approval becomes a powerful influence toward conformity. Children learn to dress, talk, and behave in a manner acceptable to the group. A variety of roles, such as class joker or class hero, may be assumed by individual children to gain approval from the group.

Third, the interaction among peers leads to the formation of intimate friendships between same-sex peers. The school-age period is the time when children have "best friends" with whom they share secrets, private jokes, and adventures; they come to one another's aid in times of trouble. In the course of these friendships, children also fight, threaten each other, break up, and reunite. These relationships, in which the child experiences love and closeness with a peer, may be important as a foundation for relationships in adulthood (Fig. 15-4).

Clubs and Peer Groups

One of the outstanding characteristics of middle childhood is the formation of formalized groups, or clubs. A prominent feature of these groups is the rigid rules imposed on the members. There is exclusiveness in the selection of persons who have the privilege of joining. Acceptance in the group is often determined on a pass–fail basis according to social or behavioral criteria. Conformity is the core of the group structure. There are often secret codes, shared interests, and special modes of dress, and each child must abide by a standard of behavior established by the members. Conforming to the rules provides children with feelings of security and relieves them of the responsibility of making decisions. By merging their identities with those of their peers, children are able to move from the family group to an outside group as a step toward seeking further independence. Peer groups and clubs allow children to substitute conformity to a peer group for conformity to a family at a time when children are still too insecure to function independently.

During the early school years, groups are usually small and loosely organized, with changing membership and no formal structure. The clubs and groups usually do not display elements of cooperation and order that are seen in groups of older children. In general, girls' groups are less formalized than boys' are, and although there may be a mixture

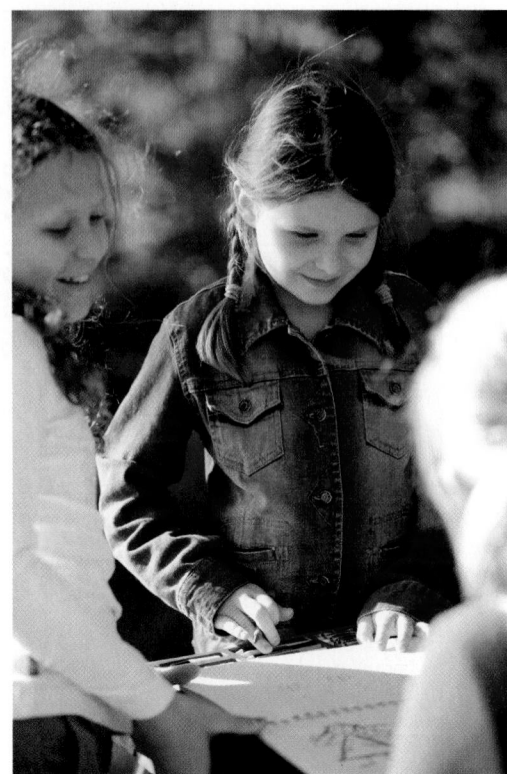

FIG 15-4 School-age children enjoy engaging in activities with a "best friend."

of both sexes in the early school years, the groups of later school years are composed predominantly of children of the same sex. Common interests are the basis around which the group is structured.

Peer-group identification and association are essential to a child's socialization. Poor relationships with peers and a lack of group identification can contribute to bullying. **Bullying** is any recurring activity that intends to cause harm, distress, or control towards another in which there is a perceived imbalance of power between the aggressor(s) and the victim (Lamb, Pepler, and Craig, 2009). Although bullying can occur in any setting, it most often occurs at school during unstructured times such as recess (Arseneault, Bowes, and Shakoor, 2010). Children who are targeted for bullying often have internalizing characteristics such as withdrawal, anxiety, depression, low self-esteem, and reduced assertiveness that may make them an easy target for bullying (Arseneault, Bowes, and Shakoor, 2010). Bullies are generally defiant toward adults, antisocial, and likely to break school rules. They have dominant personalities, may come from homes where parental involvement and nurturing are lacking, and may experience or witness violence or abuse at home (Bowes, Arseneault, Maughan, and others, 2009). Boys who bully tend to use physical force, referred to as *direct bullying*, but girls usually use indirect bullying methods, such as exclusion, gossip, or rumors (Arseneault, Bowes, and Shakoor, 2010). Cyberbullying is a new form of bullying and involves the use of cellular telephones, digital cameras, or social networking Internet sites to cause distress on an individual (American Academy of Pediatrics [AAP], Committee on Injury, Violence, and Poison Prevention, 2009).

The long-term consequences of bullying are significant. Chronic bullies seem to continue their behaviors into adulthood, negatively influencing their ability to develop and maintain relationships. Victims of bullying often experience psychological distress such as worry, sadness, anxiety, depression, and nightmares and can have increased self-harm behaviors, social isolation, suicidal ideation, and violent behaviors (Arseneault, Bowes, and Shakoor, 2010). School personnel play an important role in implementing antibullying interventions in schools; however, research has recognized that involving the whole family in antibullying programs greatly increases success (Arseneault, Bowes, and Shakoor, 2010).

There are also dangers in peer group attachments that are too strong. Peer pressures force some children to take risks or engage in behaviors that are against their better judgment. A child's membership in a gang is associated with marked increases in serious delinquent behavior (Fisher, Montgomery, and Gardner, 2008). Peer group activities that result in unlawful or criminal gang violence are increasing in the United States. An integration of family-centered and school-based programs is needed to reduce the influences for children to become affiliated with gangs.

Relationships with Families

Although the peer group is influential and necessary for normal child development, parents are the primary influence in shaping their children's personalities, setting standards for behavior, and establishing value systems. Family values usually take precedence over peer value systems. Although children may appear to reject parental values while testing the new values of the peer group, ultimately they retain and incorporate into their own value systems the parental values they have found to be of worth.

In the middle school years, children want to spend more time in the company of peers, and they often prefer peer group activities to family activities. This can be disturbing to parents. Children become intolerant and critical of their parents, especially when their parents' ways deviate from those of the group. They discover that parents can be wrong, and they begin to question the knowledge and authority of their parents, who were previously considered to be all-knowing and all-powerful.

Although increased independence is the goal of middle childhood, children are not prepared to abandon all parental control. They need and want restrictions placed on their behavior, and they are not prepared to cope with all of the problems of their expanding environment. They feel more secure knowing there is an authority figure to implement controls and restrictions. Children may complain loudly about restrictions and try to break down parental barriers, but they are uneasy if they succeed in doing so. They respect adults who prevent them from acting on every urge. Children view this behavior as an expression of love and concern for their welfare.

Children also need their parents to be adults, not friends. Sometimes parents, hurt by their children's rejection, attempt to maintain their love and gratitude by assuming the role of "pals." Children need the stable, secure strength provided by mature adults to whom they can turn during troubled relationships with peers or stressful changes in their world. With a secure base in a loving family, children are able to develop the self-confidence and maturity needed to break loose from the group and stand independently.

Play

Play takes on new dimensions that reflect a new stage of development in the school years. Play involves increased physical skill, intellectual ability, and fantasy. In addition, children develop a sense of belonging to a team or club by forming groups and cliques.

Rules and Rituals

The need for conformity in middle childhood is strongly manifested in the activities and games of school-age children. In the preschool years, children's games were either invented for them or played in the company of a friend or an adult. Now children begin to see the need for rules, and their games have fixed and unvarying rules that may be bizarre and extraordinarily rigid. Part of the enjoyment of the game is knowing the rules because knowing means belonging. Conformity and ritual permeate their play and are also evident in their behavior and language. Childhood is full of chants and taunts, such as "Eeeny, meeny, miney, mo," "Last one is a rotten egg," and "Step on a crack, break your mother's back." Children derive a sense of pleasure and power from such sayings, which have been handed down with few changes through generations.

Team Play

A more complex form of play that evolves from the need for peer interaction is team games and sports. A referee, umpire, or person of authority may be required so that the rules can be followed more accurately. Team play teaches children to modify or exchange personal goals for goals of the group; it also teaches them that division of labor is an effective strategy for attaining a goal. Children learn about competition and the importance of winning—an attribute highly valued in the United States.

Team play can also contribute to children's social, intellectual, and skill growth. Children work hard to develop the skills needed to become team members, to improve their contribution to the group, and to anticipate the consequences of their behavior for the group. Team play helps stimulate cognitive growth because children are called on to learn many complex rules, make judgments about those rules, plan strategies, and assess the strengths and weaknesses of members of their own team and members of the opposing team.

Quiet Games and Activities

Although play at this age is highly active, school-age children also enjoy quiet and solitary activities. The middle years are the time for collections, which constitute another ritual. Young school-age children's collections are an odd assortment of unrelated objects in messy, disorganized piles. Collections of later school years are more orderly; selective; and organized in scrapbooks, on shelves, or in boxes.

School-age children become fascinated with complex board, card, or computer games that they can play alone, with a best friend, or with a group. As in all games, adherence to the rules is fanatic. Disagreements over rules can cause much discussion and argument but are easily resolved by reading the rules of the game.

The newly acquired skill of reading becomes increasingly satisfying as school-age children expand their knowledge of the world through books (Fig. 15-5). School-age children never tire of stories and, as with preschool children, love to have stories read aloud. They also enjoy sewing, cooking, carpentry, gardening, and creative activities such as painting. Many creative skills such as music and art, as well as athletic skills such as swimming, karate, dancing, and skating, are learned during these years and continue to be enjoyed into adolescence and adulthood (Fig. 15-6).

Ego Mastery

Play affords children the means to acquire mastery over themselves, their environment, and others. Through play, children can feel as big, as powerful, and as skillful as their imaginations will allow. They can also feel in control and attain vicarious mastery and power over whomever and whatever they choose. School-age children still need the opportunity to use large muscles in exuberant outdoor play and the freedom to exert their newfound autonomy and initiative. They need space in which to exercise large muscles and to deal with tensions,

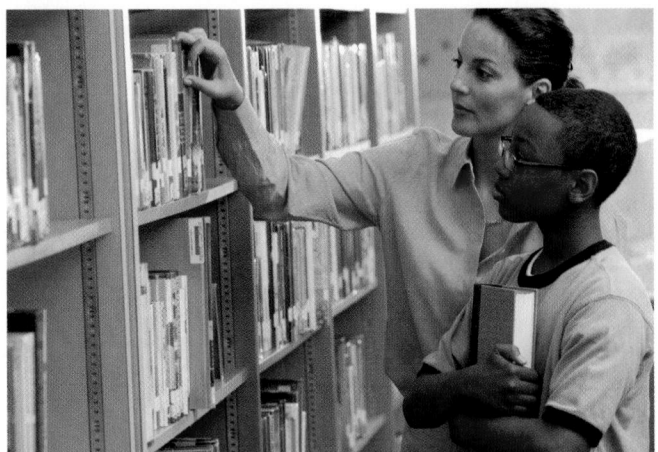

FIG 15-5 Selecting a book with the assistance of an adult.

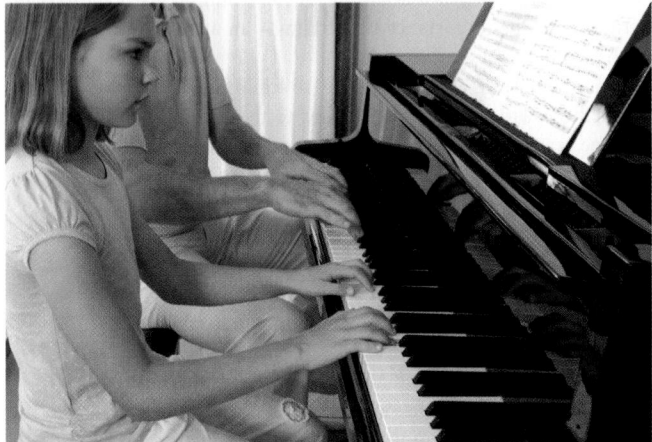

FIG 15-6 School-age children take pride in learning new skills.

frustrations, and hostility. Physical skills practiced and mastered in play help them develop a feeling of personal competence, which contributes to a sense of accomplishment and provides status in their peer group.

DEVELOPING A SELF-CONCEPT

The term **self-concept** refers to a conscious awareness of self-perceptions, such as one's physical characteristics, abilities, values, self-ideals and expectancy, and idea of self in relation to others. It also includes one's body image, sexuality, and self-esteem. Although primary caregivers continue to exert influence on children's self-evaluation, the opinions of peers and teachers provide valuable input during middle childhood. With the emphasis on skill building and broadened social relationships, children are continually engaged in the process of self-evaluation.

Significant adults can often manage to unobtrusively manipulate the environment so that children experience success. Each small success increases a child's self-image. The more positive children feel about themselves, the more confident they will be in trying for success in the future. All children profit from feeling that they are in some way special to a significant adult. A positive self-concept makes children feel likeable, worthwhile, and capable of significant contributions. These feelings lead to self-respect, self-confidence, and happiness. Negative feelings lead to self-doubt.

Developing a Body Image

School-age children have a relatively accurate and positive perception of their physical selves, but in general, they like their physical selves less as they grow older. The head appears to be the most important part of the school-age child's perceived image of self, with hair and eye color the characteristics used most frequently to describe the physical self.

Body image is influenced, but not solely determined, by significant others. The number of significant others that influences children's perception of themselves increases with age. Children are acutely aware of their own bodies, the bodies of their peers, and those of adults. They are also aware of deviations from the norm. Physical impairments, such as hearing or visual defects, ears that "stick out," or birthmarks, assume great importance. Increasing awareness of these differences, especially when accompanied by unkind comments and taunts from others, may cause a child to feel inferior and less desirable. This is especially true if the defect interferes with the child's ability to participate in games and activities.

Table 15-1 summarizes the major developmental achievements of the school-age years.

COPING WITH CONCERNS RELATED TO NORMAL GROWTH AND DEVELOPMENT

School Experience

School serves as the agent for transmitting the values of society to each succeeding generation of children. School is also the setting for relationships with peers. After the family, schools are the second most important socializing agent in the lives of children.

Entrance into school causes a sharp break in the structure of the child's world. For many children, it is their first experience in conforming to a group pattern imposed by an adult who is not a parent and who has responsibility for too many children to be constantly aware of each child as an individual. Children want to go to school and usually adapt to the new conditions with little difficulty. Successful adjustment is related to the child's physical and emotional maturity and the parent's readiness to accept the separation associated with school entrance. Unfortunately, some parents express their unconscious attempts to delay the child's maturity by clinging behavior, particularly with their youngest child.

By the time they enter school, most children have a fairly realistic concept of what school involves. They receive information regarding the role of a student from parents, siblings, playmates, and the media. In addition, most children have had some experience with daycare, preschool, or kindergarten. Middle-class children have fewer adjustments to make and less to learn about expected behavior because schools tend to reflect dominant middle-class customs and values. If the child has attended a preschool program, the focus of the preschool program also affects the child's adjustment. Some preschool programs provide custodial care only, but others emphasize emotional, social, and intellectual development.

Classmates have a significant impact on the socialization of children. School is the first time that most children become members of a large group of individuals their own age. Peer relationships become increasingly important and influential as children proceed through school. The specific influence exerted by the peer group depends on the background, interests, and abilities of the individual child.

Teachers

Children respond best to teachers who possess the characteristics of a warm, loving parent. Teachers in the early grades perform many of the activities formerly assumed by the parent, such as recognizing the

TABLE 15-1 GROWTH AND DEVELOPMENT DURING THE SCHOOL-AGE YEARS

PHYSICAL AND MOTOR	MENTAL	ADAPTIVE	PERSONAL-SOCIAL
Age 6 Years			
Height and weight gain continues slowly	Develops concept of numbers	At table, uses knife to spread butter or jam on bread	Can share and cooperate better
Weight, 16–26.3 kg (35.5–58 pounds)	Can count 13 pennies	At play, cuts, folds, pastes paper; sews crudely if needle is threaded	Has great need for children of own age
Height, 106.7–122 cm (42–48 inches)	Knows whether it is morning or afternoon		Will cheat to win
Central mandibular incisors erupt	Defines common objects such as fork and chair in terms of their use	Takes bath without supervision; performs bedtime activities alone	Often engages in rough play
Loses first tooth	Obeys three commands in succession	Reads from memory; enjoys oral spelling game	Often jealous of younger brother or sister
Gradual increase in dexterity	Knows right and left hands		Does what adults are seen doing
Active age; constant activity	Says which is pretty and which is ugly of a series of drawings of faces	Likes table games, checkers, simple card games	May have occasional temper tantrums
Often returns to finger feeding	Describes the objects in a picture rather than simply enumerating them	Giggles a lot	Is a boaster
More aware of hand as a tool	Attends first grade	Sometimes steals money or attractive items	Is more independent, probably an influence of school
Likes to draw, print, color		Has difficulty owning up to misdeeds	Has own way of doing things
Vision reaches maturity		Tries out own abilities	Increases socialization
Age 7 Years			
Begins to grow at least 5 cm (2 inches) in height per year	Notices that certain items are missing from pictures	Uses table knife for cutting meat; may need help with tough or difficult pieces	Is becoming a real member of the family group
Weight, 17.7–30 kg (39–66.5 pounds)	Can copy a diamond		Takes part in group play
Height, 112–130 cm (44–51 inches)	Repeats three numbers backward	Brushes and combs hair acceptably without help	Boys prefer playing with boys; girls prefer playing with girls
Maxillary central incisors and lateral mandibular incisors erupt	Develops concept of time; reads ordinary clock or watch correctly to nearest quarter hour; uses clock for practical purposes	Likes to help and have a choice	Spends a lot of time alone; does not require a lot of companionship
More cautious in approaches to new performances		Is less resistant and stubborn	
Repeats performances to master them	Attends second grade		
Jaw begins to expand to accommodate permanent teeth	More mechanical in reading; often does not stop at the end of a sentence; skips words such as "it," "the," and "he"		
Ages 8 to 9 Years			
Continues to gain 5 cm (2 inches) in height per year	Gives similarities and differences between two things from memory	Makes use of common tools such as hammer, saw, screwdriver	Is easy to get along with at home
Weight, 19.5–39.5 kg (43–87 pounds)	Counts backward from 20 to 1; understands concept of reversibility	Uses household and sewing utensils	Likes the reward system
Height, 117–142 cm (46–56 inches)	Repeats days of the week and months in order; knows the date	Helps with routine household tasks such as dusting, sweeping	Dramatizes
Lateral incisors (maxillary) and mandibular cuspids erupt	Describes common objects in detail, not merely their use	Assumes responsibility for share of household chores	Is more sociable
Movement fluid; often graceful and poised	Makes change out of a quarter	Looks after all of own needs at table	Is better behaved
Always on the go; jumps, chases, skips	Attends third and fourth grades	Buys useful articles; exercises some choice in making purchases	Is interested in boy–girl relationships but will not admit it
Increased smoothness and speed in fine motor control; uses cursive writing	Reads more; may plan to wake up early just to read	Runs useful errands	Goes about home and community freely, alone or with friends
Dresses self completely	Reads classic books but also enjoys comics	Likes pictorial magazines	Likes to compete and play games
Likely to overdo; hard to quiet down after recess	More aware of time; can be relied on to get to school on time	Likes school; wants to answer all the questions	Shows preference in friends and groups
More limber; bones grow faster than ligaments	Can grasp concepts of parts and whole (fractions)	Is afraid of failing a grade; is ashamed of bad grades	Plays mostly with groups of own sex but is beginning to mix
	Understands concepts of space, cause and effect, nesting (puzzles), conservation (permanence of mass and volume)	Is more critical of self	Develops modesty
	Classifies objects by more than one quality; has collections	Takes music and sport lessons	Compares self with others
	Produces simple paintings or drawings		Enjoys organizations, clubs, and group sports

Continued

TABLE 15-1	GROWTH AND DEVELOPMENT DURING THE SCHOOL-AGE YEARS—cont'd		
PHYSICAL AND MOTOR	**MENTAL**	**ADAPTIVE**	**PERSONAL-SOCIAL**
Ages 10 to 12 Years Weight, 24.5–58 kg (54–128 pounds) Height, 127–162.5 cm (50–64 inches) Posture is more similar to an adult's; will overcome lordosis Remainder of teeth will erupt and tend toward full development (except wisdom teeth) **Girls**—Pubescent changes may begin to appear; body lines soften and round out **Boys**—Slow growth in height and rapid weight gain; may become obese in this period	Writes brief stories Attends fifth to seventh grades Writes occasional short letters to friends or relatives on own initiative Uses telephone for practical purposes Responds to magazine, radio, or other advertising Reads for practical information or own enjoyment—stories or library books of adventure or romance, animal stories	Makes useful tools or does easy repair work Cooks or sews in small way Raises pets Washes and dries own hair; is responsible for a thorough job of cleaning hair but may need reminding to do so Is sometimes left alone at home for an hour or so Is successful in looking after own needs or those of other children left in his or her care	Loves friends; talks about them constantly Chooses friends more selectively; may have a "best friend" Enjoys conversation Develops beginning interest in opposite sex Is more diplomatic Likes family; family really has meaning Likes mother and wants to please her in many ways Demonstrates affection Likes father, who is admired and may be idolized Respects parents

child's personal needs (e.g., the need to go to the bathroom, need for help with clothing) and helping to develop their social behavior (e.g., manners).

Teachers, like parents, are concerned about the child's psychologic and emotional welfare. Although the functions of teachers and parents differ, both place constraints on behavior and both are in a position to enforce standards of conduct. However, the teacher's primary responsibility involves stimulating and guiding children's intellectual development, as opposed to providing for their physical welfare beyond the school setting.

Teachers serve as models that children try to emulate. Children seek their teachers' approval and avoid their disapproval. The teacher is a significant person in the life of the early school-age child, and hero worship of a teacher may extend into late childhood and preadolescence. Teachers who make supportive statements that reassure or commend children, use accepting and clarifying statements that help children refine ideas and feelings, and provide assistance that aids children with their own problem solving contribute to the development of a positive self-concept in the school-age child.

Parents

Parents share responsibility for helping children achieve their maximum potential. Parents can supplement the school program in numerous ways (see Family-Centered Care box). Cultivating responsibility is the goal of parental assistance. Being responsible for schoolwork helps children learn to keep promises, meet deadlines, and succeed at their jobs as adults. Responsible children may occasionally ask for help (e.g., with a spelling list), but usually they prefer to think through their work by themselves. Excessive pressure or lack of encouragement from parents may inhibit the development of these desirable traits.

Latchkey Children

The term **latchkey children** is used to describe children who are left to care for themselves before or after school without the supervision of an adult. The large numbers of single-parent families and working mothers, together with the lack of available child care, have created a stress-provoking situation for many school-age children. Some of these children may have a chronic illness as well.

Inadequate adult supervision after school leaves children at greater risk for injury and delinquent behavior. In some instances, outside activities are curtailed, and relationships with peers may be significantly diminished. Latchkey children may feel more lonely, isolated, and fearful than children who have someone to care for them. To cope with their fears and anxieties while alone, these children may devise strategies such as hiding, playing the television at a loud volume, or using pets for comfort.

Many communities and persons concerned about the welfare of latchkey children are trying to help these children and their parents deal with this potentially serious problem. Some communities and employers have implemented after-school programs or telephone "hotlines" that provide check-in and reassurance for children. Nurses should be aware of these community services and encourage parents to teach self-help skills to these children.

Limit Setting and Discipline

Many factors influence the amount and manner of discipline and limit setting imposed on school-age children. Some of these factors are the parents' psychosocial maturity, the parents' childhood and childrearing experiences, the children's temperament, the context of the children's misconduct, and the children's response to rewards and punishments. When children develop an ability to see a situation from another's point of view, they are also able to understand the effects of their reactions on others and themselves.

Discipline should take place in a positive, supportive environment with the use of strategies to instruct and guide desired behaviors and eliminate undesired behaviors (Knox, 2010). Reasoning is an effective technique for middle school–age children. With advancing cognitive skills, they are able to benefit from more complex disciplinary strategies. For example, withholding privileges, requiring compensation, imposing penalties, and contracting can be used with great success. Problem solving is the best approach to limit setting, and children themselves can be included in the process of determining appropriate disciplinary measures.

Dishonest Behavior

During middle childhood, children may engage in what is considered to be antisocial behavior. Previously well-behaved children may engage

♦ FAMILY-CENTERED CARE
Helping Children in School

General Guidelines

Be supportive—provide companionship; share ideas and thoughts.

Be positive—every child should experience some success each day.

Share an interest in reading—use the library; discuss books they are reading.

Support and encourage activity rather than passivity.

Encourage originality—help children make their own projects from discarded articles or other available materials.

Foster the development of hobbies and collections.

Encourage children to wonder and reflect during free time.

Encourage family experiences and trips to places of interest.

Encourage questions—help children discover sources for information or places to explore and investigate.

Stimulate creative thinking and problem solving—help children try out new solutions to problems without fear of making mistakes.

Use rewards rather than punishment.

Specific Guidelines

Meet the teacher at the beginning of school and plan to visit the school to see what is taught and expected.

Send the child to school every day. Teachers are concerned when parents make other plans for their children; it conveys the impression that school is unimportant.

Demonstrate an interest in what the child is learning.

Demonstrate an interest in content and growth more than in grades.

Make it clear to the child that schoolwork is between the child and the teacher; the teacher and child should set goals for better school performance to allow the child to feel responsible for school successes and failures.

Take advantage of situations that support and reinforce school learning.

Share information with teachers that will help them understand the child better.

Communicate with the teacher if there appears to be a problem; avoid waiting for a scheduled conference.

Provide a quiet, well-lit area for study that is safe from interruption; do not allow television or radio.

Avoid dictating a study time but do enforce rules, such as no television until homework is done; accept the child's word that work is complete.

Help with homework should focus on explaining the question, not giving the answer.

Teach the child to break large tasks (e.g., a report) into smaller, manageable tasks spread over the allotted time rather than attempting the entire project the night before it is to be completed.

Limit home tutoring to special circumstances, such as when the teacher requests parental assistance after a child's prolonged absence.

Request special help for children with learning problems.

Support the school staff by showing respect for both the school system and the teacher, at least in the child's presence.

in lying, stealing, and cheating. Such behaviors are disturbing and challenging to parents.

Lying can occur for a number of reasons. By the time children enter school, they still "tell stories," often exaggerating a story or situation as a means of impressing their family or friends. However, during middle childhood, children become able to distinguish between fact and fantasy. If children do not develop this characteristic, parents need to teach them what is real and what is make-believe.

Young children may lie to escape punishment or to get out of some difficulty even when their misbehavior is evident. Older children may lie to meet expectations set by others to which they have been unable to measure up. However, most children know that lying and cheating are wrong, and they are concerned when it is observed in their friends. They are quick to tell on others when they detect cheating.

Parents need to be reassured that all children lie occasionally and that sometimes children may have difficulty separating fantasy from reality. Parents should be helped to understand the importance of being truthful in their relationships with children.

Cheating is most common in young children 5 to 6 years of age. They find it difficult to lose at a game or contest, so they may cheat to win. They have not yet realized that this behavior is wrong, and they do it almost automatically. This behavior usually disappears as they mature. However, because children model observed behaviors, parents need to be aware of their own behavior. When parents set examples of honesty, children are more likely to conform to these standards.

As with other ethically related behavior, stealing is not unexpected in younger children. Between 5 and 8 years of age, children's sense of property rights is limited, and they tend to take things simply because they are attracted to them or to take money for what it will buy. They are equally likely to give away something valuable that belongs to them. When young children are caught and punished, they are penitent— they "didn't mean to" and "promise to never do it again"—but they are likely to repeat the performance the following day. Often they not only steal but also lie about their behavior or attempt to justify it with excuses. It is seldom helpful to trap children into admission by asking directly if they committed the offense. Children do not take responsibility for these behaviors until the end of middle childhood. Stealing can be an indication that something is seriously wrong or lacking in the child's life. For example, children may steal to make up for love or another satisfaction that they feel is lacking. In most situations, it is wise not to attempt to attach a hidden or deep meaning to the stealing. An admonition, together with an appropriate and reasonable punishment, such as having the older child pay back the money or return the stolen items, takes care of most cases. Most children can be taught to respect the property rights of others with little difficulty despite numerous temptations and opportunities. If children's personal rights are respected, they are likely to respect the rights of others. Some children simply need more time to learn the rules regarding private property.

Stress and Fear

Children today experience significant amounts of stress, which can cause long-term adjustment and health problems. Stress in childhood comes from a variety of sources such as conflict within the family, interpersonal relationships, and poverty. The school environment and participation in multiple organized activities can be additional sources of stress. The demands from coaches and parents, in addition to school requirements and pressure from teachers to do well on proficiency testing, can cause unrealistic expectations on school-age children (Schredl, Biernelt, Roos, and others, 2008). In addition, with the increased exposure to sexuality and provocative clothing and behaviors, children of this age group may feel pressured to have a girlfriend or boyfriend, which their maturity level cannot handle and which causes additional stress (McLeod and Knight, 2010).

The increasing violence in society has infiltrated into the school setting. In the present information age in which tragedy is broadcast daily in the media, children come to school knowing more about the latest world events than any previous generation of children. Many children know other children who have been killed or children who have brought weapons to school. School-age children can be victims of bullying, verbal insults, unwanted sexual remarks, damaged or stolen property, and physical abuse in the school environment (Fredland, 2008).

To help children cope with stress, parents, teachers, and health care providers need to frequently reassure children that they are safe, have honest and open communication, encourage children to express their feelings, and provide time for unstructured play (Washington, 2009). Adults must recognize signs that indicate a child is undergoing stress, identify the source of the stress promptly, and refer those children who need specialized treatment.

> **! NURSING ALERT**
>
> The nurse who observes the following signs of stress in a child should explore the situation further:
> - Stomach pains or headache
> - Changes in sleep patterns or nightmares
> - Bedwetting
> - Changes in eating habits
> - Aggressive or stubborn behavior
> - Withdrawal or reluctance to participate
> - Regression to earlier behaviors (e.g., thumb sucking)
> - Trouble concentrating or changes in academic performance

Children 7 to 12 years of age are capable of identifying their own physiologic responses to stress. Common physiologic signs of stress include tight muscles, hot or red in the face, jittery, fast heartbeat, breathing difficulties, headache, neck pain, and abdominal pain (Washington, 2009). Children should be taught to recognize these signs as indicators of stress and to use techniques to manage their stress. Children can learn relaxation techniques such as deep-breathing exercises, progressive relaxation of muscle groups, and positive imagery to immediately reduce stress (Kostenius and Ohrling, 2009). Encouraging them to "blow off steam" through physical activity reduces tension and anxiety. Children can be encouraged to observe effective coping strategies in others and adopt them for their own use (Kostenius and Ohrling, 2009). When an effective strategy has been developed for one situation, parents can show the child how to transfer the coping strategy or technique to other situations.

In addition to stress, school-age children experience a wide variety of fears, including fear of the dark, excessive worry about past behavior, self-consciousness, social withdrawal, and an excessive need for reassurance. These fears are considered normal for children this age. During the middle-school years, children become less fearful of body safety than they were as preschoolers, but they still fear being hurt, being kidnapped, or having to undergo surgery. They also fear death and are fascinated by all the aspects of death and dying. The fears of noises, darkness, storms, and dogs lessen, but new fears related predominantly to school and family bother children during this time.

PROMOTING OPTIMAL HEALTH DURING THE SCHOOL YEARS

NUTRITION

Although caloric needs are diminished in relation to body size during middle childhood, resources are being laid down at this time for the increased growth needs of adolescence. Parents and children need to be aware of the value of a balanced diet to promote growth because children usually eat what their family members eat. The quality of the child's diet depends on the family's pattern of eating.

Likes and dislikes established at an early age continue in middle childhood, although preferences for single foods subside, and children develop a taste for a variety of foods. However, the easy availability of fast-food restaurants, the influence of the mass media, and the temptation of "junk food" make it easy for children to fill up on empty calories. Foods that do not promote growth, such as sugars, starches, and excess fats, are common in school-age children's diets. The easy availability of high-calorie foods, combined with the tendency toward more sedentary activities, has also contributed to an epidemic of childhood obesity. This problem is discussed further in Chapter 17.

Parents are unable to monitor what their children eat when they are away from home. A parent may pack a lunch for school but is unaware of how much is eaten, traded, sold, or thrown away. Nutrition education can and should be integrated in the curriculum throughout the school years. Important aspects of nutrition education include the U.S. Food and Drug Administration's MyPlate; elements of a wholesome diet; and how food products are grown, processed, and prepared. However, school cafeterias may not always provide healthy, nutritious meals. School nurses can take an active role in nutrition education by working with teachers to plan and implement units on nutrition instruction and by working with parents and children to give nutritional guidance.

SLEEP AND REST

The amount of sleep and rest required during middle childhood is highly individualized. The amount of sleep depends on the child's age, activity level, and state of health. The growth rate slows in the school-age years, and less energy is expended in growth than during preceding years.

School-age children usually do not require naps, but they do need to sleep approximately 11 hours at age 5 years and 9 hours at age 12 years each night (Smaldone, Honig, and Byrne, 2007). Although fewer bedtime problems occur during these years, occasional difficulties are still associated with the bedtime ritual. Usually children 6 or 7 years old exhibit few bedtime problems, and encouraging quiet activity before bedtime, such as coloring or reading, facilitates the task of going to bed. However, most children in middle childhood must be reminded frequently to go to bed; 8- to 9-year-old children and 11-year-old children are particularly resistant. Often these children are unaware that they are tired; if they are allowed to remain up later than usual, they are fatigued the following day. Sometimes bedtime resistance can be resolved by allowing a later bedtime as the child gets older. Twelve-year-old children usually offer no resistance at bedtime; some even retire early to read a book or listen to music.

EXERCISE AND ACTIVITY

The improved capabilities and adaptability of school-age children permit greater speed and effort in motor activities. Larger, stronger muscles permit longer and increasingly strenuous play without exhaustion. School-age children acquire the coordination, timing, and concentration that are required to participate in adult-type activities, but they may lack the strength, stamina, and control of adolescents and adults. They can engage in a greater amount of physical activity during the school years. However, parents, teachers, and coaches must remember that although children this age are large and appear strong, they may not be ready for strenuous competitive athletics.

All growing children need regular exercise and opportunities for satisfying experiences consistent with individual likes and dislikes. Appropriate activities during the school-age years include running, jumping rope, swimming, roller skating, ice skating, dancing, and bicycle riding. Positive reinforcement achieved by experiencing increasingly smooth, rhythmic, and efficient use of the body conditions the child toward regular physical activity. Exercise is essential for muscle development and tone, refinement of balance and coordination, increased strength and endurance, and stimulation of body functions and metabolic processes. Children need ample space to run, jump, skip, and climb in addition to safe indoor and outdoor facilities and equipment. Most children have abundant energy and need little encouragement to engage in physical activity. Children with disabling conditions or those who hesitate to become involved in active play (e.g., obese children) require special assessment and help so that activities appeal to them and are compatible with their limitations while also meeting their developmental needs.

Sports

Considerable controversy surrounds the trend toward early participation in competitive athletics and the amount and type of competitive sports that are appropriate for children in the elementary grades. The current view is that virtually every child is suited for some sport, and authorities do not discourage participation if children are matched to the type of sport appropriate to their abilities and to their physical and emotional constitution. School-age children enjoy competition (Fig. 15-7). However, teachers and coaches must understand the physical limitations of children this age and teach them the proper techniques and safety measures needed to avoid injuries. A safe and appropriate sport can be identified for even the most unskilled and uncompetitive child, including children with chronic illnesses and

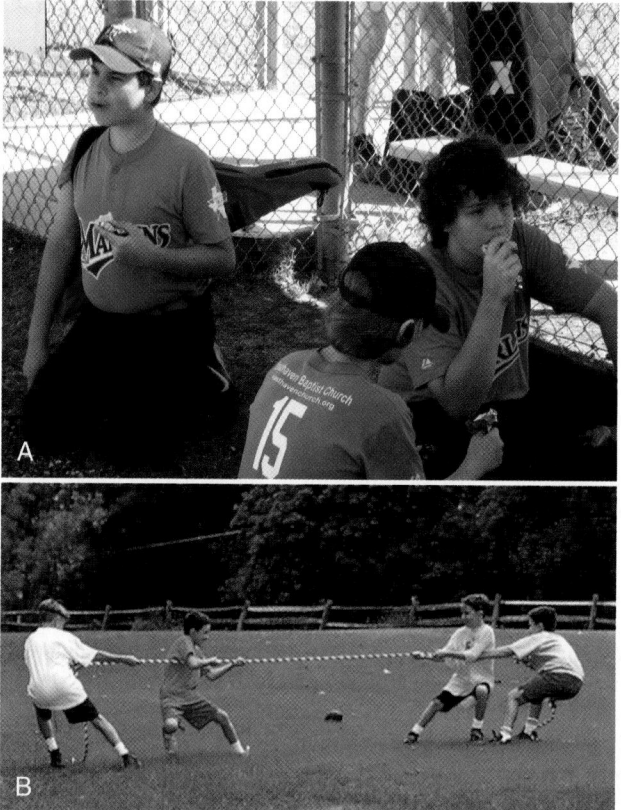

FIG 15-7 The activities engaged in by school-age children vary according to interest and opportunity. **A,** Little League competitors. **B,** Playing tug-of-war.

mental retardation. Common activities for school-age children include baseball, soccer, gymnastics, and swimming. Equipment must be maintained in safe condition, and protective apparatus should be worn to prevent serious injury (see Traumatic Injury, Chapter 31).

During the school-age years, girls have the same basic body structure as boys and have a similar response to systematic exercise training. However, at puberty, boys become larger and have more muscle mass, and at this stage, it is usually recommended that girls compete only against other girls. Before puberty, there is no essential difference in strength and size between girls and boys, making these precautions unnecessary.

Preadolescence is a time to teach fundamental motor skills; develop fitness in a practical, safe, and gradual manner; and promote healthy attitudes and values. Activities should include both practice sessions and unstructured play; the actual game or event should be managed in a manner that stresses mastery of the sport and enhancement of self-image rather than winning or pleasing others. All children should have an opportunity to participate, and special ceremonies should recognize all participants, not just individuals who excel in sports or athletics.

Acquisition of Skills

School-age children demonstrate increasing fine motor abilities and complex artistic skills. Handedness is well established by the beginning of the school years, and children make great strides in writing and drawing during this period. It is a time of energetic and vibrant creative productivity. With the tools of language and reading, children create poems, stories, and plays. With more advanced fine motor skills, they are able to master an unlimited variety of handicrafts, such as ceramics, needlework, woodworking, and beadwork. They avidly pursue these skills in solitude; with a friend; or through organized groups such as boys' or girls' clubs or special interest groups that use crafts or other activities as a means to occupy, entertain, and educate children.

School-age children are capable of assuming responsibility for their own needs, although their distaste for soap and water and "dress" clothes is legendary. School-age children can and want to assume their share of household tasks, which usually are related to the male and female roles that have been defined by their culture. Many children also assume responsibility for tasks outside the home, such as babysitting, mowing lawns, or paper routes.

DENTAL HEALTH

The first permanent (secondary) teeth erupt at about 6 years of age, beginning with the 6-year molar, which erupts posterior to the deciduous molars. Other permanent teeth appear in approximately the same order as eruption of the primary teeth (see Teething, Chapter 10) and follow shedding of the deciduous teeth (Fig. 15-8). With the appearance of the second permanent (12-year) molar, most permanent teeth are present. Permanent dentition is more advanced in girls than in boys.

Because the permanent teeth erupt during the school-age years, dental hygiene and regular attention to dental caries are important parts of health supervision during this period (see Dental Health, Chapter 12). Correct brushing techniques should be taught or reinforced, and the role that fermentable carbohydrates play in production of dental caries should be emphasized. It is important to be alert to possible malocclusion problems that may result from irregular eruption of permanent teeth and that may impair function. Regular dental supervision and continued fluoride supplementation are integral parts of the health maintenance program.

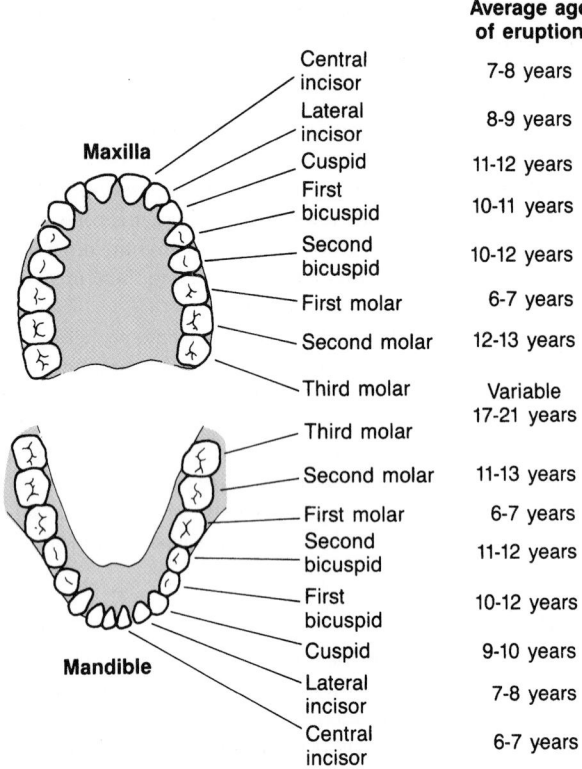

	Average age of eruption
Maxilla	
Central incisor	7-8 years
Lateral incisor	8-9 years
Cuspid	11-12 years
First bicuspid	10-11 years
Second bicuspid	10-12 years
First molar	6-7 years
Second molar	12-13 years
Third molar	Variable 17-21 years
Third molar	Variable 17-21 years
Second molar	11-13 years
First molar	6-7 years
Second bicuspid	11-12 years
First bicuspid	10-12 years
Cuspid	9-10 years
Mandible Lateral incisor	7-8 years
Central incisor	6-7 years

FIG 15-8 Sequence of eruption of the secondary teeth. (Data from Dean JA, McDonald RE, Avery DR: *McDonald and Avery dentistry for the child and adolescent*, ed 9, St. Louis, 2011, Mosby.)

The most effective means of preventing dental caries is proper oral hygiene. Children should be taught to perform their own dental care with the supervision and guidance of the parents. Parents should learn the correct brushing technique with their children, and they should monitor their child's efforts until the child can assume full responsibility.

Teeth should be brushed after meals, after snacks, and at bedtime. Children who brush their teeth frequently and become accustomed to the feel of a clean mouth at an early age usually maintain the habit throughout life. For school-age children with mixed and permanent dentition, the best toothbrush is one with soft nylon bristles and an overall length of about 21 cm (6 inches). Several methods of brushing have been described and recommended for children, but there is no conclusive evidence that one method is superior to another. Thorough cleaning is more important than the specific technique used. The dentist should assess factors such as the manipulative skills and special needs of the child and suggest the most appropriate brushing technique and regimen. Flossing follows brushing. Parents should perform the flossing until children acquire the manual dexterity required (usually at about 8 or 9 years of age).

Dental Problems

Limited or inadequate dental care results in the most common dental problems: dental caries, malocclusion, and periodontal disease. Trauma, especially tooth avulsion, is another important dental problem. All of these conditions benefit from early intervention to prevent tooth loss.

Dental caries (cavities) is the principal oral problem in children and adolescents. Reducing the incidence and consequences of dental caries is extremely important in childhood. If untreated, dental caries can result in total destruction of the involved teeth. The prevalence rate of caries increases steadily across the life span; whereas 28% of children ages 2 to 5 years have caries, 59% of children 7 years of age have caries (Wagner and Oskouian, 2008).

Dental caries is a multifactorial disease involving susceptible teeth, cariogenic microflora, and an appropriate oral environment. The incidence of lesions and the likelihood of progressive invasion vary considerably and depend on a number of factors being present in the right combination. Because many children are exposed to health care but not dental care, oral inspection is an integral part of the physical assessment of every child. If there is any evidence of dental caries or other unhealthy dental state, the child should be referred for dental services. An alarming number of children do not receive regular dental supervision, and a significant number reach adulthood without dental examinations or treatment by a dentist.

Periodontal disease, an inflammatory and degenerative condition involving the gums and tissues supporting the teeth, often begins in childhood and accounts for a significant amount of tooth loss in adulthood. The more common periodontal problems are gingivitis (simple inflammation of the gums) and periodontitis (inflammation of the gums and loss of connective tissue and bone in the supporting structures of the teeth). Gingivitis, the most prevalent periodontal disease, is a reversible inflammatory disease that can begin in early childhood and is most often associated with the buildup of plaque on the teeth. Management is directed toward prevention by conscientious brushing and flossing, including the use of fluoride. Children should see a dentist at any signs of inflammation or irritation.

Malocclusion occurs when teeth of the upper and lower dental arches do not approximate in the proper relationships. As a result, the physiologic function of chewing is less effective, and the cosmetic effect is displeasing. Teeth that are uneven, crowded, or overlapping are unable to meet their counterparts in the opposite jaw in the appropriate relationships and may be predisposed to disease in later years.

Orthodontic treatment is most successful when it is started in the late school-age or early teenage years after the last primary teeth have been shed and before growth ceases. However, referral should be made as soon as malocclusion is evident because some deformities can be corrected at an earlier age.

Dental injury may occur in childhood and includes fractures of varying degrees of severity, chipping, dislocation, or avulsion. All tooth injuries require prompt treatment by a competent dentist to prevent permanent displacement or loss. Delayed examination and diagnosis of tooth damage can result in infection or pulp involvement. Because it can affect the remaining teeth, replacement of the lost tooth is needed to maintain normal alignment and position of the other teeth.

A tooth that is avulsed (exarticulated, or "knocked out") should be replanted by the child, parent, or nurse and stabilized as soon as possible so the blood supply to the tooth can be reestablished and the tooth kept alive (see Emergency Treatment box). A tooth that is replanted promptly has a good survival rate. Avulsed primary teeth are usually not reimplanted.

As with all injuries to the mouth, an avulsed tooth causes a large amount of bleeding, which is frightening to children and their families; therefore, the nurse or anyone faced with dental trauma should be prepared to provide support and reassurance during the dental trauma.

SEX EDUCATION

Many children experience some form of sex play during or before preadolescence as a response to normal curiosity, not as a result of love or sexual urges. Children are experimentalists by nature, and sex play

✚ EMERGENCY TREATMENT

Avulsed Permanent Tooth

Recover tooth.

Hold tooth by crown; avoid touching root area.

If tooth is dirty, rinse it gently under running water or saline; be certain to insert stopper in sink or basin (to avoid tooth loss).

To Reimplant the Tooth

Insert tooth into socket; be certain that the lip side (or convex surface) is facing front.

Have child maintain tooth in place by slowly biting down on a piece of gauze.

Transport child to dentist immediately.

Avoid sudden stops or sharp turns to prevent dislodging tooth.

If Reluctant to Reimplant the Tooth

Place avulsed tooth in suitable medium for transport:

- Cold milk
- Saliva—under child's or parent's tongue

If child is holding tooth in the mouth, avoid sudden stops to prevent swallowing tooth.

DO NOT FORGET TO TAKE THE TOOTH.

---

is incidental and transitory. Any adverse emotional consequences or guilt feelings depend on how the behavior is managed by the parents, if it is discovered, or whether children view their actions as wrong in the eyes of significant persons, particularly the parents.

The child's attitude toward sex is acquired indirectly at an early age. Initial curiosity about differences in body structure between boys and girls and between children and adults arises in the preschool years. Middle childhood is an ideal time for formal sex education, and many authorities believe that the topic is best presented from a life span approach. Information about sexual maturation and the process of reproduction minimizes children's uncertainty, embarrassment, and feelings of isolation that often accompany puberty.

An important component of ongoing sex education is effective communication with parents. If parents either repress the child's sexual curiosity or avoid dealing with it, the sexual information that the child receives may be acquired almost entirely from peers. When peers are the primary source of sexual information, it is transmitted and exchanged in secret conversation and contains a large amount of misinformation.

Nurse's Role in Sex Education

No matter where nurses practice, they can provide information on human sexuality to both parents and children. To discuss the topic adequately, nurses must have an understanding of the physiologic aspects of sexuality; knowledge of the cultural and societal values; and an awareness of their own attitudes, feelings, and biases about sexuality.

When presenting sexual information to school-age children, nurses should treat sex as a normal part of growth and development. Questions should be answered honestly, matter of factly, and to the same extent as questions about other topics. Answers should be at the child's level of understanding. There may be times when boys and girls should be taught content separately.

Children need help to differentiate sex and sexuality. Exercises on clarifying values, identifying role models, engaging in problem-solving skills, and practicing responsibility are important to prepare children for early adolescence and puberty. In addition, children need

explanations of sexual information that is provided via the media or jokes. Information concerning pregnancy; contraceptives; and sexually transmitted diseases, including human immunodeficiency virus and human papillomavirus, should be presented in simple, accurate terms.

Preadolescents need precise and concrete information that will allow them to answer questions such as, "What if I start my period in the middle of class?" or "How can I keep people from telling I have an erection?" It is important to tell children what they want to know and what they can expect to happen as they become mature sexually.

During encounters with parents, nurses can be open and available for questions and discussion. They can set an example by the language they use in discussing body parts and their function and by the way in which they deal with problems that have emotional overtones, such as exploratory sex play and masturbation. Parents need help to understand normal behaviors and to view sexual curiosity in their children as a part of the developmental process. Assessing the parents' level of knowledge and understanding of sexuality provides cues to their need for supplemental information that will prepare them for the increasingly complex explanations they will need to provide as their children grow older.

SCHOOL HEALTH

Child health maintenance is ultimately the responsibility of the parents; however, the public schools and health departments in the United States have contributed to the improvement of child health by providing a healthful school environment, health services, and health education that emphasize sound health practices. Most of these functions constitute major components of community health services and involve large amounts of public funds and large numbers of health professionals, including nurses.

A school health program is involved in ongoing health maintenance through assessment, screening, and referral activities. Routine health services provided by most schools include health appraisal, emergency care, safety education, communicable disease control, counseling, and follow-up care. Health education of school-age children is directed toward providing knowledge of health and influencing habits, attitudes, and conduct in relation to health and injury prevention.

Traditionally, school nurses were viewed as the individuals who detected diseases in the school, applied bandages, and cared for students who were ill or injured. Although these functions remain important parts of the school nurse's job, the role has expanded considerably. Today, school nurses manage and coordinate all the care required by regular students and students with special health care needs. In many settings, school health services have enlarged into family health centers that meet the needs of not only school-age children but also their families and the community. In these settings, school nurse practitioners provide health care that includes assessment of physical, psychomedical, psychoeducational, behavioral, and learning problems, as well as comprehensive well-child care (AAP, 2008).

The passage of the Education for All Handicapped Children Act and its amendments (Public Laws 94-142 and 99-457) mandated the integration of children with chronic illnesses and disabilities into the least restrictive environments, including regular classrooms whenever possible. School nurses are responsible for the medical and nursing needs of these children while they are in the school setting. School nurses develop, implement, and evaluate individualized health care plans for these children. Not all schools have a school nurse, and the use of unlicensed assistive personnel (UAP) is needed in some cases. After appropriate training and supervision, UAPs can provide standardized routine health care to students. Delegation and supervision of UAP requires skillful nursing assessment, effective communication, and professional judgment (AAP, Council on School Health, 2009).

INJURY PREVENTION

Because school-age children have developed more refined muscular coordination and control and can apply their cognitive capacities to their behavior, the number of injuries in middle childhood is diminished compared with the number in early childhood. The most common cause of severe injury and death in school-age children is motor vehicle crashes—either as a pedestrian or passenger (Centers for Disease Control and Prevention [CDC], 2010). It is important that nurses continue to emphasize three automobile safety measures that have been found to reduce the severity of injuries: effective car restraint systems, door-lock mechanisms, and appropriate passenger seating locations in the motor vehicle. The rear vehicle seat is the safest place for children younger than the age of 13 years and booster seats should be used until 8 years of age (CDC, 2010).

School-age children's desire for riding bicycles increases the risk of injury on streets. Other serious injuries include accidents on skateboards, roller skates, in-line skates, scooters, and other sports equipment. All-terrain vehicles (ATVs) are popular with children but are unstable, difficult to handle, and responsible for a large number of childhood injuries. Several national organizations have developed policy and position statements to discourage the use of ATVs in any child younger than the age of 16 years (American Pediatric Surgical Association, 2009).

Most injuries occur in or near the home or school. The most effective means of prevention is education of the child and family regarding the hazards of risk taking and the improper use of equipment. Safety helmets, protective eye and mouth shields, and protective padding are strongly recommended for children engaging in active sports even though they may not be required equipment. Falls from bicycles are the cause of a significant number of head injuries in school-age children, and the most important aspect of bicycle safety is to encourage children to wear protective helmets (Fig. 15-9) (Okun and Adam, 2008).

Physically active school-age children are also highly susceptible to cuts and abrasions, and the incidence of childhood fractures, strains, and sprains is high. Trampoline injuries are highest in children 5 through 14 years and account for numerous fractures, sprains, and head injuries. Trampolines in the home environment, routine physical education classes, or outdoor playgrounds are not recommended for children of any age (Eberl, Schalamon, Singer, and others, 2009). Serious injuries are discussed elsewhere in the book: burns (Chapter 30), eye trauma (Chapter 19), near drowning (Chapter 28),

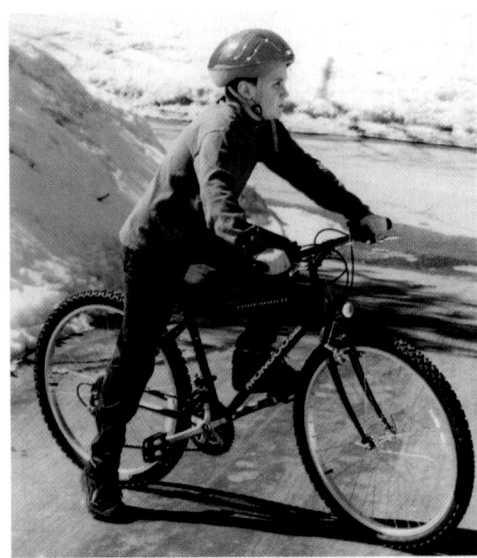

FIG 15-9 The right size bike is important. The child should be able to sit on the bike and place the balls of both feet on the ground. The foot should comfortably reach and manipulate the pedal in the down position. Wearing a protective helmet is mandatory. The helmet should be positioned so it sits low on the forehead and parallel to the ground when the head is held upright. It should not rock back and forth or shift from side to side. The strap should fasten securely under the chin.

and head injuries (Chapter 28). The prevalence of injuries depends on the dangers present in the environment, the protection offered by adults, and children's behavior patterns. Table 15-2 lists characteristics of school-age children that make them prone to injury and suggestions for injury prevention. Family-Centered Care boxes provide guidelines for bicycle, skateboard, and in-line skate safety and guidance during the school years.

ANTICIPATORY GUIDANCE—CARE OF FAMILIES

Parents of the school-age child must share their child's time with the increasingly important peer group. Experiences with the peer group prepare school-age children for the broader world of relationships and increased independence from their parents. Parents must learn to provide support as unobtrusively as possible without feeling rejected, hurt, or angry. The nurse can help parents of the school-age child by providing anticipatory guidance and reassurance throughout this period (see Family-Centered Care box).

TABLE 15-2	INJURY PREVENTION DURING THE SCHOOL-AGE YEARS
DEVELOPMENTAL ABILITIES RELATED TO RISK OF INJURY	**INJURY PREVENTION**
Motor Vehicle Crashes	
Is increasingly involved in activities away from home	Educate child regarding proper use of seat belts while a passenger in a vehicle.
Is excited by speed and motion	Maintain discipline while a passenger in a vehicle (e.g., keep arms inside, do not lean against doors, do not interfere with driver).
Is easily distracted by environment	Remind parents and children that no one should ride in the bed of a pickup truck.
Can be reasoned with	Emphasize safe pedestrian behavior.
	Insist on child wearing safety apparel (e.g., helmet) when applicable, such as riding bicycle, motorcycle, moped, or all-terrain vehicle (see Family-Centered Care box, p. 474).

TABLE 15-2	INJURY PREVENTION DURING THE SCHOOL-AGE YEARS—cont'd

DEVELOPMENTAL ABILITIES RELATED TO RISK OF INJURY	INJURY PREVENTION
Drowning	
Is apt to overdo	Teach child to swim.
May work hard to perfect a skill	Teach basic rules of water safety.
Has cautious, but not fearful, gross motor actions	Select safe and supervised places to swim.
	Check sufficient water depth for diving.
Likes swimming	Swim with a companion.
	Use an approved flotation device.
	Advocate for legislation requiring fencing around pools.
	Learn cardiopulmonary resuscitation.
Burns	
Has increasing independence	Make certain home has smoke detectors.
Is adventurous	Set water heaters to 48.9° C (120° F) to avoid scald burns.
Enjoys trying new things	Instruct child in behavior in areas involving contact with potential burn hazards (e.g., gasoline, matches, bonfires or barbecues, lighter fluid, firecrackers, cigarette lighters, cooking utensils, chemistry sets).
	Instruct child to avoid climbing or flying kite around high-tension wires.
	Instruct child in proper behavior in the event of fire (e.g., fire drills at home and school).
	Teach child safe cooking (use low heat; avoid any frying; be careful of steam burns, scalds, or exploding foods, especially from microwaving).
Poisoning	
Adheres to group rules	Educate child regarding hazards of taking nonprescription drugs and chemicals, including aspirin and alcohol.
May be easily influenced by peers	Teach child to say "no" if offered illegal or dangerous drugs or alcohol.
Has strong allegiance to friends	Keep potentially dangerous products in properly labeled receptacles, preferably out of reach.
Bodily Damage	
Has increased physical skills	Help provide facilities for supervised activities.
Needs strenuous physical activity	Encourage playing in safe places.
Is interested in acquiring new skills and perfecting attained skills	Keep firearms safely locked up except under adult supervision.
	Teach proper care of, use of, and respect for devices with potential danger (e.g., power tools, firecrackers).
Is daring and adventurous, especially with peers	Teach children not to tease or surprise dogs, invade their territory, take dogs' toys, or interfere with dogs' feeding.
Frequently plays in hazardous places	Stress eye, ear, or mouth protection when using potentially hazardous objects or devices or when engaging in potentially hazardous sports.
Confidence often exceeds physical capacity	Do not permit use of trampolines except as part of supervised training.
Desires group loyalty and has strong need for friends' approval	Teach safety regarding use of corrective devices (glasses); if child wears contact lenses, monitor duration of wear to prevent corneal damage.
Delights in physical activity	Stress careful selection, use, and maintenance of sports and recreation equipment, such as skateboards and in-line skates (see Family-Centered Care box, p. 474).
Takes risks	Emphasize proper conditioning, safe practices, and use of safety equipment for sports or recreational activities.
Is likely to overdo	Caution against engaging in hazardous sports, such as those involving trampolines.
Growth in height exceeds muscular growth and coordination	Use safety glass and decals on large glassed areas, such as sliding glass doors.
	Use window guards to prevent falls.
	Teach name, address, and phone number and emphasize that child should ask for help from appropriate people (e.g., cashier, security guard, police) if lost; have identification on child (e.g., sewn in clothes, inside shoe).
	Teach stranger safety:
	• Avoid personalized clothing in public places.
	• Caution child to never go with a stranger.
	Have child tell parents if anyone makes child feel uncomfortable in any way.
	Always listen to child's concerns regarding others' behavior.
	Teach child to say "no" when confronted by uncomfortable situations.

FAMILY-CENTERED CARE

Bicycle Safety

- Always wear a properly fitted bicycle helmet that is approved by the U.S. CPSC; encourage parents to look for the CPSC approval sticker on the inside liner of the helmet.
- Replace a helmet every 5 years or sooner if manufacturer recommends it. Never use a damaged or outgrown helmet.
- Ride bicycles with traffic and away from parked cars.
- Ride single file.
- Walk bicycles through busy intersections only at crosswalks.
- Give hand signals well in advance of turning or stopping.
- Keep as close to the curb as practical.
- Watch for drain grates, potholes, soft shoulders, loose dirt, and gravel.
- Keep both hands on handlebars except with signaling.
- Never ride double on a bicycle.
- Do not carry packages that interfere with vision or control; do not drag objects behind a bike.
- Watch for and yield to pedestrians.
- Watch for cars backing up or pulling out of driveways; be especially careful at intersections.
- Look left, right, and then left before turning into traffic or roadway.
- Never hitch a ride on a truck or other vehicle.
- Learn rules of the road and respect for traffic officers.
- Obey all local ordinances.
- Wear shoes that fit securely while riding.
- Wear light colors at night and attach fluorescent material to clothing and bicycle.
- Equip the bicycle with proper lights and reflectors.
- Be certain the bicycle is the correct size for rider (see Fig. 15-9).
- Have the bicycle inspected to ensure good mechanical condition.
- Children riding as passengers must wear appropriate-size helmets and sit in specially designed protective seats.

Modified from American Academy of Pediatrics, Committee on Injury and Poison Prevention: Bicycle helmets, *Pediatrics* 122(2):450, 2008. *CPSC,* Consumer Product Safety Commission.

FAMILY-CENTERED CARE

Skateboard, In-Line Skate, and Scooter Safety

- Children younger than 5 years of age should not use skateboards or in-line skates because they are not developmentally prepared to protect themselves from injury. Children ages 6 to 10 years should use these only with close adult supervision.
- Children younger than 8 years should ride scooters only with close adult supervision.
- Children who ride skateboards, in-line skates, or scooters should wear helmets and other protective equipment, especially on their knees, wrists, and elbows, to prevent injury.
- Skateboards, in-line skates, and scooters should never be used near traffic or in streets. Their use should be prohibited at night. Activities that bring skateboards together (e.g., "catching a ride") are especially dangerous.
- Some types of use, such as riding homemade ramps on hard surfaces, may be particularly hazardous.

Data from Brudvik C: Injuries caused by small wheel devices, *Prev Sci* 7:313–320, 2006; and American Academy of Pediatrics, Committee on Injury and Poison Prevention: In-line skating injuries in children and adolescents, *Pediatrics* 123:1421–2422, 2009.

FAMILY-CENTERED CARE

Guidance During School Years

Age 6 Years

Prepare parents to expect strong food preferences and frequent refusal of specific food items.

Prepare parents to expect an increasingly ravenous appetite.

Prepare parents for emotionality as child experiences erratic mood changes.

Help parents anticipate continued susceptibility to illness.

Teach injury prevention and safety, especially bicycle safety.

Encourage parents to respect child's need for privacy and to provide a separate bedroom for child, if possible.

Prepare parents for child's increasing interests outside the home.

Help parents understand the need to encourage child's interactions with peers.

Ages 7 to 10 Years

Prepare parents to expect improvement in health with fewer illnesses but warn them that allergies may increase or become apparent.

Prepare parents to expect an increase in minor injuries.

Emphasize caution in selecting and maintaining sports equipment and reemphasize safety.

Prepare parents to expect increased involvement with peers and interest in activities outside the home.

Emphasize the need to encourage independence while maintaining limit setting and discipline.

Prepare mothers to expect more demands at 8 years.

Prepare fathers to expect increasing admiration at 10 years; encourage father–child activities.

Prepare parents for prepubescent changes in girls.

Ages 11 to 12 Years

Help parents prepare child for body changes of pubescence.

Prepare parents to expect a growth spurt in girls.

Make certain child's sex education is adequate with accurate information.

Prepare parents to expect energetic but stormy behavior at 11 years, becoming more even-tempered at 12 years.

Encourage parents to support child's desire to "grow up" but to allow regressive behavior when needed.

Prepare parents to expect an increase in child's masturbation.

Instruct parents that the amount of rest the child needs may increase.

Help parents educate child regarding experimentation with potentially harmful activities.

Health Guidance

Help parents understand the importance of regular health and dental care for the child.

Encourage parents to teach and model sound health practices, including diet, rest, activity, and exercise.

Stress the need to encourage children to engage in appropriate physical activities.

Emphasize providing a safe physical and emotional environment.

Encourage parents to teach and model safety practices.

KEY POINTS

- Middle childhood, also known as the school years, is the period of life that extends from 6 to 12 years of age.
- Although growth is slower than in previous years, there is a steady gain in height and weight, with maturation of body systems; primary teeth are lost and replaced by permanent teeth.
- A major task during the middle school years is developing a sense of industry or accomplishment (Erikson).
- Piaget's period of concrete operations refers to the school-age period when children are able to use their thought processes to experience events and actions and make judgments based on reasoning.
- The child develops a conscience and is able to understand and adhere to rules and standards set by others.
- Entertaining different points of view, becoming sensitive to social norms, and forming peer friendships are important features of social development during the school years.
- Cooperative play, team activities, and the acquisition of skills are prime elements of play during the school years; rules and rituals assume greater importance.
- Parental concerns during middle childhood include lying, cheating, stealing, and school achievement.
- The availability of junk foods, irregular family meals, and schedules of working parents often interfere with optimal nutrition.
- Dental care is important during this time; potential dental problems include caries, periodontal disease, malocclusion, and dental injury.
- Increased socialization and media exposure make the school years an ideal time for sex education.
- School health programs ideally include health appraisal, emergency care, safety education, communicable disease control, counseling, guidance, and health education with adjustment to individual student needs.
- Injury prevention is directed toward safety education, provision of safe play areas and equipment, and well-supervised sports activities.

REFERENCES

American Academy of Pediatrics, Committee on Injury, Violence, and Poison Prevention: Policy statement: role of the pediatrician in youth violence prevention, *Pediatrics* 124(1):393–402, 2009.

American Academy of Pediatrics, Council on School Health: Role of the school nurse in providing school health services, *Pediatrics* 121(5):1052–1056, 2008.

American Academy of Pediatrics, Council on School Health: Policy statement guidance for the administration of medication in school, *Pediatrics* 124(4):1244–1251, 2009.

American Pediatric Surgical Association, Trauma Committee: Position statement on the use of all-terrain vehicles by children and youth, *J Pediatr Surg* 44:1638–1639, 2009.

Arseneault L, Bowes L, Shakoor S: Bullying victimization in youths and mental health problems: 'much ado about nothing?' *Psychol Med* 40:717–729, 2010.

Bowes L, Arseneault L, Maughan B, and others: School, neighborhood, and family factors are associated with children's bullying involvement: a nationally representative longitudinal study,

J Am Acad Child Adolesc Psychiatry 48(5):545–553, 2009.

Centers for Disease Control and Prevention, National Center for Injury Prevention and Control: Child passenger safety, 2010, Centers for Disease Control and Prevention, retrieved January 14, 2011, from http://www.cdc.gov/ncipc/factsheets/childpas.htm.

Eberl R, Schalamon J, Singer G, and others: Trampoline-related injuries in childhood, *Eur J Pediatr* 168:1171–1174, 2009.

Fisher H, Montgomery P, Gardner F: Opportunities provision for preventing youth gang involvement for children and young people (7–16), *Cochrane Database Syst Rev* (2):CD007002, 2008.

Fredland N: Nurturing hostile environments, the problem of school violence, *Fam Community Health* 31(suppl 18):S32–S41, 2008.

Knox M: On hitting children: A review of corporal punishment in the United States, *J Pediatr Health Care* 24(2):103–107, 2010.

Kostenius C, Ohrling K: Being relaxed and powerful: children's lived experiences of coping with stress, *Child Soc* 23:203–213, 2009.

Lamb J, Pepler D, Craig W: Approach to bullying and victimization, *Can Fam Physician* 55:356–390, 2009.

McLeod J, Knight S: The association of socioemotional problems with early sexual initiation, *Perspect Sex Reprod Health* 42(2):93–101, 2010.

Okun A, Adam H: Safety on bicycles, skateboards, scooters, and skates, *Pediatr Rev* 29(10):366–367, 2008.

Schredl M, Biernelt J, Roos K, and others: Nightmares and stress in children, *Sleep Hypnosis* 10(1):19–25, 2008.

Smaldone A, Honig J, Byrne M: Sleepless in America: inadequate sleep and relationships to health and well-being of our nation's children, *Pediatrics* 119(suppl 1):S29–S37, 2007.

Wagner R, Oskouian R: The ECC epidemic, *Contemp Pediatr* 25(9):60–79, 2008.

Washington T: Psychological stress and anxiety in middle to late childhood and early adolescence: manifestations and management, *J Pediatr Nurs* 24(4):302–313, 2009.

Health Promotion of the Adolescent and Family

Linda M. Kollar

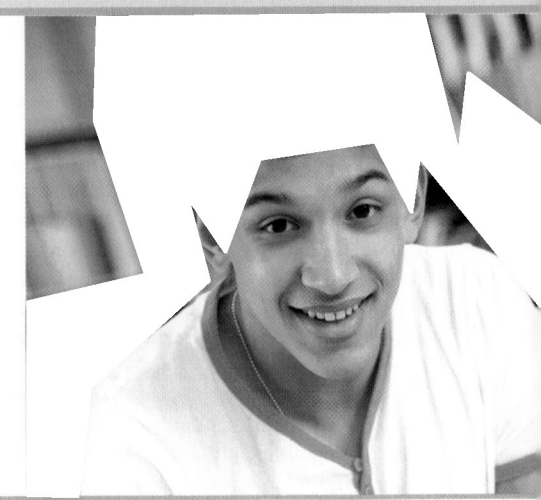

CHAPTER OUTLINE

Promoting Optimal Growth and
  Development, 477
  Biologic Development, 477
    Hormonal Changes of Puberty, 477
    Sexual Maturation, 477
    Physical Growth, 478
    Physiologic Changes, 481
  Psychosocial Development, 481
    *Developing a Sense of Identity
      (Erikson), 481*
  Cognitive Development (Piaget), 482
  Moral Development (Kohlberg), 482
  Spiritual Development, 482
  Social Development, 483
    Relationships with Parents, 483
    Relationships with Peers, 483
    Interests and Activities, 484

Adolescent Sexuality, 485
Development of Self-Concept and Body
  Image, 486
    Responses to Puberty, 487
Promoting Optimal Health During
  Adolescence, 487
  Immunizations, 488
  Nutrition, 489
    *Eating Habits and
      Behavior, 489*
  Sleep and Rest, 490
    Exercise and Activity, 490
  Dental Health, 491
  Personal Care, 491
    Vision, 491
    Hearing, 491
    Posture, 491

Body Art, 492
Tanning, 492
Stress Reduction, 492
Sexuality Education and Guidance, 493
Safety Promotion and Injury
  Prevention, 493
    Motor Vehicle–Related Injuries, 493
    Firearms, 494
    Sports Injuries, 495
Anticipatory Guidance—Care of
  Families, 495

LEARNING OBJECTIVES

On completion of this chapter the reader will be able to:
- Describe the physical changes that occur at puberty.
- Discuss the reactions of the adolescent to physical changes that take place at puberty.
- Demonstrate an understanding of the processes by which adolescents develop a sense of identity.
- Develop an education session on sexuality for a group of adolescents.
- Discuss the significance of the changing interpersonal relationships and the role of the peer group during adolescence.

- Outline a health teaching plan for adolescents.
- Describe the process by which adolescents develop their sexual identities.
- Identify the causes and discuss the preventive aspects of injuries during adolescence.
- Discuss the impact of social media on the social development of adolescents.

PROMOTING OPTIMAL GROWTH AND DEVELOPMENT

Adolescence is a period of transition between childhood and adulthood—a time of rapid physical, cognitive, social, and emotional maturation as boys prepare for manhood and girls prepare for womanhood (see Cultural Considerations box). The precise boundaries of adolescence are difficult to define, but this period is customarily viewed as beginning with the gradual appearance of secondary sex characteristics at about 11 or 12 years of age and ending with cessation of body growth at 18 to 20 years.

Several terms are used to refer to this stage of growth and development. Puberty refers to the maturational, hormonal, and growth process that occurs when the reproductive organs begin to function and the secondary sex characteristics develop. This process is sometimes divided into three stages: prepubescence, the period of about 2 years immediately before puberty when the child is developing preliminary physical changes that herald sexual maturity; puberty, the point at which sexual maturity is achieved, marked by the first menstrual flow in girls but by less obvious indications in boys; and postpubescence, a 1- to 2-year period after puberty during which skeletal growth is completed and reproductive functions become fairly well established. Adolescence, which literally means "to grow into maturity," is generally regarded as the psychologic, social, and maturational process initiated by the pubertal changes. It involves three distinct subphases: early adolescence (ages 11–14), middle adolescence (ages 15–17), and late adolescence (ages 18–20). The term teenage years is used synonymously with *adolescence* to describe ages 13 through 19 years.

BIOLOGIC DEVELOPMENT

The physical changes of puberty are primarily the result of hormonal activity under the influence of the central nervous system, although all aspects of physiologic functioning are mutually interacting. The obvious physical changes are noted in increased physical growth and in the appearance and development of secondary sex characteristics; less obvious are physiologic alterations and neurogonadal maturity, accompanied by the ability to procreate. Physical distinction between the sexes is made on the basis of distinguishing characteristics. Primary sex characteristics are the external and internal organs that carry out the reproductive functions (e.g., ovaries, uterus, breasts, penis).

🌐 CULTURAL CONSIDERATIONS
The Adolescent Years

Other societies in which adolescence is seen as part of the life cycle may have ideas very different from those of American culture about how the adolescent years are to be spent. For example, some societies discourage contact between adolescent boys and girls. Sexual experimentation is outlawed, and all grown children, men and women, remain in their parents' homes until they wed. In the United States, we tend to believe that the way our culture is organized is the way all cultures are or should be organized, but of course, this is not so. Each society is unique. The way we describe adolescence, the way we experience it, and the predisposition of our adolescents toward violence are peculiar to our American culture.

Modified from Prothrow-Stith D: *Deadly consequences: how violence is destroying our teenage population and a plan to begin solving the problem,* New York, 1993, HarperCollins.

Secondary sex characteristics are the changes that occur throughout the body as a result of hormonal changes (e.g., voice alterations, development of facial and pubertal hair, fat deposits) but that play no direct part in reproduction.

Hormonal Changes of Puberty

The events of puberty are caused by hormonal influences and controlled by the anterior pituitary (adenohypophysis) in response to a stimulus from the hypothalamus. Stimulation of the gonads has a dual function:

1. Production and release of gametes—production of sperm in the male and maturation and release of ova in the female
2. Secretion of sex-appropriate hormones—estrogen and progesterone from the ovaries (female) and testosterone from the testes (male)

The ovaries, testes, and adrenals secrete sex hormones. These hormones are produced in varying amounts by both sexes throughout the life span. The adrenal cortex is responsible for the small amounts secreted before the pubescent years, but the sex hormone production that accompanies maturation of the gonads is responsible for the biologic changes observed during puberty.

Estrogen, the feminizing hormone, is found in low quantities during childhood. This hormone is secreted in slowly increasing amounts until about age 11 years. In males, this gradual increase continues through maturation. In females, the onset of estrogen production in the ovary causes a pronounced increase that continues until about 3 years after the onset of menstruation, at which time it reaches a maximum level that continues throughout the reproductive life of the female.

Androgens, the masculinizing hormones, are also secreted in small and gradually increasing amounts up to about 7 or 9 years of age, at which time there is a more rapid increase in both sexes, especially boys, until about age 15 years. These hormones appear to be responsible for most of the rapid growth changes of early adolescence. With the onset of testicular function, the level of androgens (principally testosterone) in males increases over that in females and continues to increase until a maximum is attained at maturity.

Sexual Maturation

The visible evidence of sexual maturation is achieved in an orderly sequence, and the state of maturity can be estimated on the basis of the appearance of these external manifestations. The age at which these changes are observed and the time required to progress from one stage to another may vary among children. The time from the appearance of breast buds to full maturity may be $1\frac{1}{2}$ to 6 years for adolescent girls. It may take 2 to 5 years for male genitalia to reach adult size. The stages of development of secondary sex characteristics and genital development have been defined as a guide for estimating sexual maturity and are referred to as the Tanner stages (Box 16-1). The usual sequence of appearance of maturational changes is presented in Box 16-2.

Sexual Maturation in Girls

In most girls, the initial indication of puberty is the appearance of breast buds, an event known as thelarche, which occurs between 8 and 13 years of age (Fig. 16-1). This is followed in approximately 2 to 6 months by growth of pubic hair on the mons pubis, known as adrenarche (Fig. 16-2). In a minority of normally developing girls, however, pubic hair may precede breast development. The average age of thelarche for white girls is 10 years, with a range of 8 to 12.75 years; for African-American girls, the average age of thelarche is earlier, around 9 years, with a range of 7 to 11 years (Herman-Giddens, 2006).

Animation—Ovarian Growth

BOX 16-2 USUAL SEQUENCE OF MATURATIONAL CHANGES

Girls

Breast changes
Rapid increase in height and weight
Growth of pubic hair
Appearance of axillary hair
Menstruation (usually begins 2 years after first signs)
Abrupt deceleration of linear growth

Boys

Enlargement of testicles
Growth of pubic hair, axillary hair, hair on upper lip, hair on face and elsewhere on body (facial hair usually appears about 2 years after appearance of pubic hair)
Rapid increase in height
Changes in the larynx and consequently the voice (usually take place along with growth of penis)
Nocturnal emissions
Abrupt deceleration of linear growth

The average age of thelarche for Hispanic girls falls somewhere between the other two groups.

The initial appearance of menstruation, or **menarche**, occurs about 2 years after the appearance of the first pubescent changes, approximately 9 months after attainment of peak height velocity, and 3 months after attainment of peak weight velocity. There is evidence that girls are developing secondary sex characteristics at a younger age with differences between white and African-American girls. The explanation for this is not yet clear but appears to be influenced by being overweight as well as environmental influences. The normal age range of menarche is usually 10½ to 15 years, with the average age being 12 years, 4 months for North American girls (Wu, Mendola, and Buck, 2002). Ovulation and regular menstrual periods usually occur 6 to 14 months after menarche. Girls may be considered to have **pubertal delay** if breast development has not occurred by age 13 years or if menarche has not occurred within 4 years of the onset of breast development.

Sexual Maturation in Boys

The first pubescent changes in boys are testicular enlargement accompanied by thinning, reddening, and increased looseness of the scrotum (Fig. 16-3). These events usually occur between 9½ and 14 years of age. Early puberty is also characterized by the initial appearance of pubic hair. Penile enlargement begins, and testicular enlargement and pubic hair growth continue throughout midpuberty. During this period, there is also increasing muscularity, early voice changes, and

development of early facial hair. Temporary breast enlargement and tenderness, **gynecomastia**, are common during midpuberty, occurring in up to one third of boys. The spurts in height and weight occur concurrently toward the end of midpuberty. For most boys, breast enlargement disappears within 2 years. By late puberty, there is a definite increase in the length and width of the penis, testicular enlargement continues, and first ejaculation occurs. Axillary hair develops, and facial hair extends to cover the anterior neck. Final voice changes occur secondary to the growth of the larynx. Concerns about **pubertal delay** should be considered for boys who exhibit no enlargement of the testes or scrotal changes by 13½ to 14 years of age or if genital growth is not complete 4 years after the testicles begin to enlarge.

Physical Growth

A constant phenomenon associated with sexual maturation is a dramatic increase in growth. The final 20% to 25% of height is achieved during puberty, and most of this growth occurs during a 24- to 36-month period—the adolescent **growth spurt**. This accelerated growth occurs in all children but, as in other areas of development, is highly variable in age of onset, duration, and extent. The growth spurt begins earlier in girls, usually between ages 9½ and 14½ years; on average it begins between ages 10½ and 16 years in boys. During this period, the average boy gains 10 to 30 cm (4–12 inches) in height and 7 to 30 kg (15.5–66 pounds) in weight. The average girl, in whom the growth spurt is slower and less extensive, gains 5 to 20 cm (2–8 inches) in height and 7 to 25 kg (15.5–55 pounds) in weight. Growth in height typically ceases 2 to 2½ years after menarche in girls and at age 18 to 20 years in boys.

This increase in size is acquired in a characteristic sequence. Growth in length of the extremities and neck precedes growth in other areas, and because these parts are the first to reach adult length, the hands and feet appear larger than normal during adolescence. Increases in hip and chest breadth take place in a few months followed several months later by an increase in shoulder width. These changes are followed by increases in length of the trunk and depth of the chest. This sequence of changes is responsible for the characteristic long-legged, gawky appearance of early adolescent children.

Sex Differences in General Growth Patterns

Sex differences in general growth and distribution patterns are apparent in skeletal growth, muscle mass, adipose tissue, and skin. **Skeletal growth** differences between boys and girls are apparently a function of hormonal effects at puberty and are evident primarily in limb length. The earlier cessation of growth in girls is caused by epiphyseal unity under the potent effect of estrogen secretion, and the hormonal effect on female bone growth is much stronger than the similar effect of testosterone in boys. In boys, the prolonged growth period before puberty and the less rapid epiphyseal closure are reflected in their greater overall height and longer arms and legs. Other skeletal differences are increased shoulder width in boys and broader hip development in girls.

Hypertrophy of the laryngeal mucosa and enlargement of the larynx and vocal cords occur in both boys and girls to produce **voice changes**. Girls' voices become slightly deeper and considerably fuller, but the effect in boys is striking. The change in the voice of adolescent boys occurs between Tanner stages 3 and 4, with the voice often shifting uncontrollably from deep to high tones in the middle of a sentence. The average lengthening of the vocal cords is 10.9 mm (0.4 inch) for boys and 4.2 mm (0.17 inch) for girls.

Growth of **lean body mass**, principally muscle, which tends to occur after the bone growth spurt, takes place steadily during

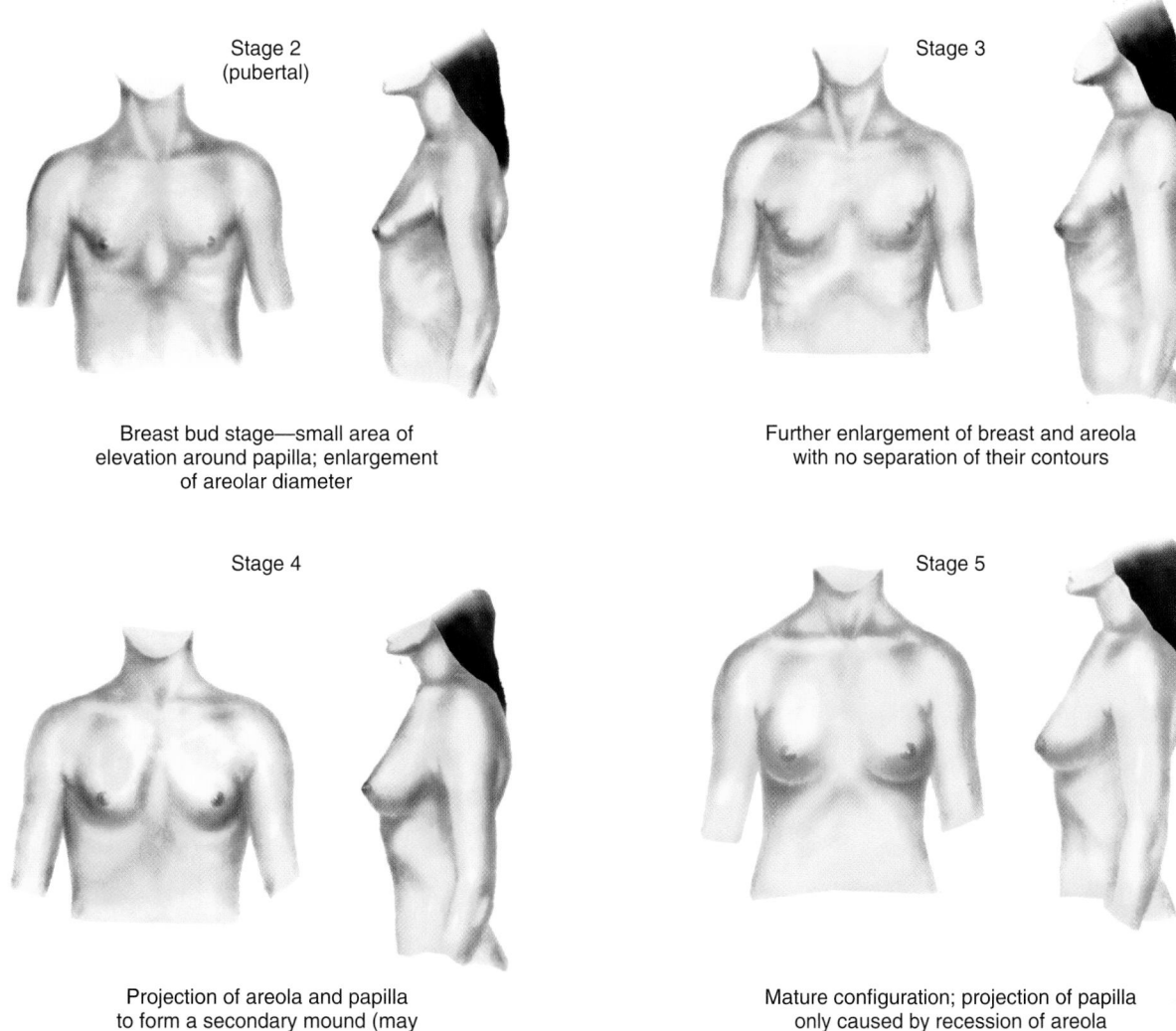

Stage 2
(pubertal)

Breast bud stage—small area of
elevation around papilla; enlargement
of areolar diameter

Stage 3

Further enlargement of breast and areola
with no separation of their contours

Stage 4

Projection of areola and papilla
to form a secondary mound (may
not occur in all girls)

Stage 5

Mature configuration; projection of papilla
only caused by recession of areola
into general contour

FIG 16-1 Development of breasts in girls. The average age span is 8 to 13 years. Stage 1 (prepubertal—elevation of papilla only) is not shown. (Modified from Marshall WA, Tanner JM: Variations in pattern of pubertal changes in girls, *Arch Dis Child* 44[235]:291–303, 1969; and Daniel WA, Paulshock BZ: A physician's guide to sexual maturity, *Patient Care* 13:122–124, 1979.)

adolescence. Lean body mass is both quantitatively and qualitatively greater in boys than in girls at comparable stages of pubertal development. Muscle development, under the influence of androgenic hormones, increases steadily. Muscles become remarkably well developed in boys, but in girls, muscle mass increase is proportionate to general tissue growth.

Nonlean body mass, primarily fat, is also increased but follows a less orderly pattern. There may be a transient increase in subcutaneous fat just before the skeletal growth spurt, especially in boys. This is followed 1 to 2 years later by a modest to marked decrease, which is again more marked in boys. Later, variable amounts of fat are deposited to fill out and contour the mature physique in patterns characteristic of the adolescent's sex, particularly in the regions over the thighs, hips, and buttocks and around the breast tissue. It should be noted, however, that pediatric obesity is steadily on the increase in the United States, and obesity can change the timing and sequence of puberty. Girls with thelarche as the first sign of puberty have earlier menarche and greater body fat and body mass index (BMI) at menarche than girls with

adrenarche as the first pubertal sign. This may have long-term effects for increased risk of adult adiposity and obesity (Biro, Lucky, Simbarti, and others, 2003). Kaplowitz (2008) states that evidence indicates a causal relationship between obesity and onset of early puberty in girls rather than earlier puberty causing an increase in body fat; no correlations between body fat and earlier puberty in boys have been reported.

Hormonal influences during puberty cause acceleration in growth and maturation of the skin and its structural appendages. Sebaceous glands become extremely active at this time, especially those on the genitalia and in the "flush areas" of the body (i.e., face, neck, shoulders, upper back, and chest). This increased activity and the structural nature of the glands are extremely important in the pathogenesis of a common problem of puberty: acne (see Chapter 30). The eccrine sweat glands, present almost everywhere on the human skin, become fully functional and respond to emotional as well as thermal stimulation. Heavy sweating appears to be more pronounced in boys than in girls. The apocrine sweat glands, nonfunctional in childhood, reach secretory capacity during puberty. Unlike the eccrine sweat glands, the

Stage 1
(prepubertal)

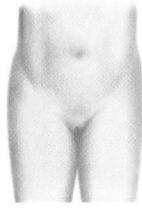

No pubic hair; essentially the same as
during childhood; no distinction between
hair on pubis and over the abdomen

Stage 2

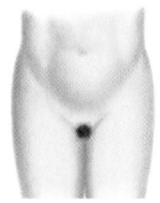

Sparse growth of long, straight, downy, and
slightly pigmented hair extending along labia;
between stages 2 and 3 begins to appear on pubis

Stage 3

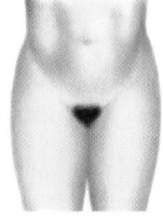

Hair darker, coarser, and curly and
spread sparsely over entire pubis in
the typical female triangle

Stage 4

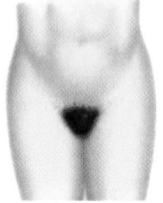

Pubic hair denser, curled, and adult in distribution
but less abundant and restricted to the pubic area

Stage 5

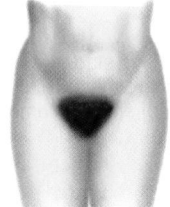

Hair adult in quantity, type, and pattern
with spread to inner aspect of thighs

FIG 16-2 Growth in pubic hair in girls. The average age span for stages 2 through 5 is 11 to 14 years. (Modified from Marshall WA, Tanner JM: Variations in pattern of pubertal changes in girls, *Arch Dis Child* 44[235]:291–303, 1969; and Daniel WA, Paulshock BZ: A physician's guide to sexual maturity, *Patient Care* 13:122–124, 1979.)

Stage 1
(prepubertal)

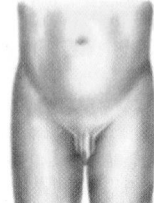

No pubic hair; essentially the same as
during childhood; no distinction between
hair on pubis and over the abdomen

Stage 2 (pubertal)

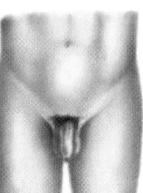

Initial enlargement of scrotum and testes;
reddening and textural changes of scrotal skin;
sparse growth of long, straight, downy, and
slightly pigmented hair at base of penis

Stage 3

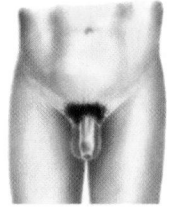

Initial enlargement of penis, mainly in
length; testes and scrotum further enlarged;
hair darker, coarser, and curly and spread
sparsely over entire pubis

Stage 4

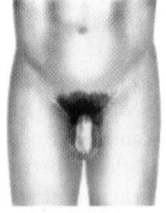

Increased size of penis with growth in diameter and
development of glans; glans larger and broader; scrotum
darker; pubic hair more abundant with curling but
restricted to pubic area

Stage 5

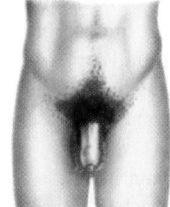

Testes, scrotum, and penis adult in size and shape;
hair adult in quantity and type with spread to inner
surface of thighs

FIG 16-3 Developmental stages of secondary sex characteristics and genital development in boys. The average age span is 12½ to 16 years. (Modified from Marshall WA, Tanner JM: Variations in pattern of pubertal changes in boys, *Arch Dis Child* 45[239]:13–23, 1970; and Daniel WA, Paulshock BZ: A physician's guide to sexual maturity, *Patient Care* 13:122–124, 1979.)

apocrine glands are limited in distribution and grow in conjunction with hair follicles in the axillae, around the areola of the breast, around the umbilicus, on the external auditory canal, and in the genital and anal regions. Apocrine glands secrete a thick substance as a result of emotional stimulation that, when acted on by surface bacteria, becomes highly odoriferous.

Body hair assumes characteristic distribution patterns and changes texture during puberty. Under the influence of gonadal and adrenal androgens, hair coarsens, darkens, and lengthens at sites related to secondary sex characteristics. Pubic and axillary hair appears in both sexes, although pubic hair is more extensive in males than in females. Beard, mustache, and body hair on the chest, upward along the linea alba, and sometimes on other areas (e.g., back and shoulders) appears in males and is androgen dependent. Extremity hair appears in varying amounts in both males and females but is also more prolific in males.

Physiologic Changes

A number of physiologic functions are altered in response to some of the pubertal changes. The size and strength of the heart, blood volume, and systolic blood pressure increase, and the pulse rate and basal heat production decrease (see Appendix E and inside back cover). Blood volume, which has increased steadily during childhood, reaches a higher value in boys than in girls, a fact that may be related to the increased muscle mass in pubertal boys. Adult values are reached for all formed elements of the blood. Respiratory rate and basal metabolic rate, decreasing steadily throughout childhood, reach the adult rate in adolescence. Respiratory volume and vital capacity are increased and to a far greater extent in males than in females. During this period, physiologic responses to exercise change drastically: performance improves, especially in boys, and the body is able to make the physiologic adjustments needed for normal functioning after exercise is completed. These capabilities are a result of the increased size and strength of muscles and the increased level of cardiac, respiratory, and metabolic functioning.

PSYCHOSOCIAL DEVELOPMENT

Developing a Sense of Identity (Erikson)

Traditional psychosocial theory holds that the developmental crisis of adolescence leads to the formation of a sense of identity. Throughout childhood, individuals have been going through the process of identification as they concentrate on various parts of the body at specific times. During infancy, children identify themselves as being separate from the mother; during early childhood they establish gender role identification with the appropriate-sex parent; and in later childhood, they establish who they are in relation to others. In adolescence, they come to see themselves as distinct individuals, somehow unique and separate from every other individual.

Adolescence begins with the onset of puberty and extends to relative physical and emotional stability at or near graduation from high school. During this time, adolescents are faced with the crisis of group identity versus alienation. In the period that follows, individuals strive to attain autonomy from the family and develop a sense of personal identity as opposed to role diffusion. A sense of group identity appears to be essential to the development of a personal identity. Young adolescents must resolve questions concerning relationships with a peer group before they are able to resolve questions about who they are in relation to family and society.

Group Identity

During the early stage of adolescence, pressure to belong to a group is intensified. Teenagers find it essential to belong to a group from which

they can derive status. Belonging to a crowd helps adolescents establish the differences between themselves and their parents. They dress as the group dresses and wear makeup and hairstyles according to group criteria, all of which are different from those of the parental generation. Language, music, and dancing reflect a culture that is exclusive to adolescents. When adults begin to emulate these fashions and interests, the style changes immediately. The evidence of adolescent conformity to the peer group and nonconformity to the adult group provides teenagers with a frame of reference for self-assertion and rejection of the identity of their parents' generation. To be different is to be unaccepted and alienated from the group.

Individual Identity

The quest for personal identity is part of the ongoing identification process. As adolescents establish identity within a group, they also attempt to incorporate multiple body changes into a concept of the self. Body awareness is part of self-awareness. In their search for identity, adolescents consider the relationships that have developed between themselves and others in the past, as well as the directions they hope to take in the future.

Significant others hold expectations for the behavior of adolescents. Often these expectations or demands are persistent enough that individuals make certain decisions that they would not make if they were solely responsible for identity formation. Adolescents may find it too easy to slip into the roles expected by others without incorporating their own personal goals or questioning decisions. Thus, individuals may become what parents or others wish them to be based on these premature decisions. Young persons might form a negative identity when society or their culture provides them with a self-image that is contrary to the values of the community. Labels such as "juvenile delinquent," "hoodlum," or "failure" are applied to certain adolescents, who then accept and live up to these labels with behaviors that validate and strengthen them.

The process of evolving a personal identity is time consuming and fraught with periods of confusion, depression, and discouragement. Determining an identity and a place in the world is a critical and perilous feature of adolescence (see Critical Thinking Case Study). However,

---

? CRITICAL THINKING CASE STUDY
Discussing the Future

Jeremy, age 17 years, will be graduating from high school in the spring. His mother, a single parent, tells you that she is concerned because graduation is quickly approaching and Jeremy has made no plans for what he will do with his life after graduation. Whenever Jeremy mentions the topic, his mother tells him, "This is what you must do" and begins to outline the steps he must take. Jeremy just walks away. She asks, "What should I do?" What advice should you give Jeremy's mother?

Questions
1. Evidence—Is there sufficient evidence to draw any conclusions about what advice to give Jeremy's mother?
2. Assumptions—Describe an underlying assumption about each of the following issues:
   a. Adolescents and the search for personal identity
   b. The influence of others on the adolescent's search for personal identity
   c. Ways to communicate with adolescents
3. What implications and priorities for nursing care can be drawn at this time?
4. Does the evidence objectively support your argument (conclusion)?

as the pieces gradually shift and settle into place, a positive identity emerges. Role diffusion results when the individual is unable to formulate a satisfactory identity from the multiplicity of aspirations, roles, and identifications.

Sex-Role Identity

Adolescence is the time for consolidation of a sex-role identity. During early adolescence, the peer group begins to communicate expectations regarding heterosexual relationships, and as development progresses, adolescents encounter expectations for mature sex-role behavior from both peers and adults. Expectations vary from culture to culture, among geographic areas, and among socioeconomic groups.

Emotionality

Adolescents vacillate in their emotional states between considerable maturity and childlike behavior. One minute they are exuberant and enthusiastic; the next minute they are depressed and withdrawn. Unpredictable but essentially normal, mood swings are common during this time. As the tension is relieved, emotion is brought under control, and individuals retreat to review what has happened, to attempt to master their anger, and to grow in their ability to control their emotions and gain from the new experience. Because of these mood swings, adolescents are frequently labeled as unstable, inconsistent, and unpredictable. Little things can cause an emotional upheaval and, depending on the teenager's interpretation, can mean a great deal.

Teenagers are better able to control their emotions in later adolescence. They can approach problems more calmly and rationally, and although they are still subject to periods of sadness, their feelings are less vulnerable, and they begin to demonstrate the more mature emotions of later adolescence. Whereas early adolescents react immediately and emotionally, older adolescents can control their emotions until socially acceptable times and places for expression present themselves. They are still subject to heightened emotion, and when it is expressed, their behavior reflects feelings of insecurity, tension, and indecision.

COGNITIVE DEVELOPMENT (PIAGET)

Cognitive thinking culminates with the capacity for abstract thinking. This stage, the period of formal operations, is Piaget's fourth and last stage. Adolescents are no longer restricted to the real and actual, which was typical of the period of concrete thought; now they are also concerned with the possible. They think beyond the present. Without having to center attention on the immediate situation, they can imagine a sequence of events that might occur, such as college and occupational possibilities; how things might change in the future, such as relationships with parents; and the consequences of their actions, such as dropping out of school. At this time, their thoughts can be influenced by logical principles rather than just their own perceptions and experiences. They become increasingly capable of scientific reasoning and formal logic.

Adolescents are capable of mentally manipulating more than two categories of variables at the same time. For example, they can consider the relationship between speed, distance, and time in planning a trip. They can detect logical consistency or inconsistency in a set of statements and evaluate a system or set of values in a more analytic manner. For instance, they question the parent who insists on honesty in the youngster but at the same time cheats on an income tax report or expense account.

In adolescence, young people begin to consider both their own thinking and the thinking of others. They wonder what opinion others have of them, and they are able to imagine the thoughts of others. With this capacity comes the ability to differentiate between others' thoughts and their own and to interpret the thoughts of others more accurately. They are able to understand that few concepts are absolute or independent of other influencing factors. As they become aware that other cultures and communities have different norms and standards from their own, it becomes easier for them to accept members of these other cultures, and the decision to behave in their own culture in an accepted manner becomes a more conscious commitment.

MORAL DEVELOPMENT (KOHLBERG)

Although younger children merely accept the decisions or point of view of adults, adolescents, to gain autonomy from adults, must substitute their own set of morals and values. When old principles are challenged but new independent values have not yet emerged to take their place, young people search for a moral code that preserves their personal integrity and guides their behavior, especially in the face of strong pressure to violate the old beliefs. Their decisions involving moral dilemmas must be based on an internalized set of moral principles that provides them with the resources to evaluate the demands of the situation and to plan actions that are consistent with their ideals.

Late adolescence is characterized by serious questioning of existing moral values and their relevance to society and the individual. Adolescents can easily take the role of another. They understand duty and obligation based on reciprocal rights of others and the concept of justice that is founded on making amends for misdeeds and repairing or replacing what has been spoiled by wrongdoing. However, they seriously question established moral codes, often as a result of observing that adults verbally ascribe to a code but do not adhere to it.

SPIRITUAL DEVELOPMENT

As adolescents move toward independence from parents and other authorities, some begin to question the values and ideals of their families. Others cling to these values as a stable element in their lives as they struggle with the conflicts of this turbulent period. Adolescents need to work out these conflicts for themselves, but they also need support from authority figures or peers for their resolution.

Adolescents are capable of understanding abstract concepts and of interpreting analogies and symbols. They are able to empathize, philosophize, and think logically. Most teens search for ideals and speculate about illogical statements and conflicting ideologies. Their tendency toward introspection and emotional intensity often makes it difficult for others to know what they are thinking. They tend to keep their thoughts private, fearing that no one will understand these feelings that they perceive to be unique and special. However, they may reveal deep spiritual concerns. They need support and encouragement in their struggle for understanding and the freedom to question without censure.

Generally, the stated importance of participation in organized religion declines somewhat during the adolescent years. More high school students than postsecondary school young people attend religious services regularly, and, not surprisingly, the younger the adolescents, the more likely they are to view religion as being important to them. Among older adolescents, the importance of organized religion declines more among college students than among those not in college. Late adolescence appears to be a time when individuals reexamine and reevaluate many of the beliefs and values of their childhood. Consistent with developmental changes in value autonomy, the religious beliefs of young people are likely to become more personalized and less bound to the traditional religious practices they may have been exposed to when they were younger.

Greater levels of religiosity and spirituality are associated with fewer high-risk behaviors and more health-promoting behaviors, especially for youth living in environments lacking positive influences (Regnerus and Glen, 2003). Nurses play an important role for teens by providing an opportunity to discuss issues regarding spirituality.

SOCIAL DEVELOPMENT

To achieve full maturity, adolescents must free themselves from family domination and define an identity independent of parental authority. However, this process is fraught with ambivalence on the part of both teenagers and their parents. Adolescents want to grow up and to be free of parental restraints, but they are fearful as they try to comprehend the responsibilities that are linked with independence. Feelings of immortality and exemption from the consequences of risk-taking behavior, although viewed as negative, can serve an important developmental function at this time. These feelings give adolescents the courage to separate from their parents and become independent. Part of this emancipation involves developing social relationships outside the family that help teenagers identify their role in society. Adolescence is a time of intense sociability and often a time of equally intense loneliness. Acceptance by peers, a few close friends, and the secure love of a supportive family are requisites for interpersonal maturation.

Relationships with Parents

During adolescence, the parent–child relationship changes from one of protection–dependency to one of mutual affection and equality. The process of achieving independence often involves turmoil and ambiguity as both parent and adolescent learn to play new roles and work toward this end while at the same time resolving the often painful series of rifts essential to establishing the ultimate relationship.

Most behavior observed in the adolescent is related to the struggle for independence and the external restrictions and checks that are placed on this spontaneous maturation process. On the one hand, adolescents are accepted as maturing preadults. They are allowed privileges heretofore denied, and they are provided with increasing responsibilities. On the other hand, because of their unpredictability and insecurity in evaluating situations and making sound judgments, they must conform to regulations and restrictions set by adults. This state of affairs is particularly exemplified by the struggle between parents and adolescents concerning the nightly curfew.

As teenagers assert their rights for grown-up privileges, they frequently create tensions within the home. They resist parental control, and conflicts can arise from almost any situation or any subject. Favorite topics of dispute include use of the home telephone, Internet use, the need for a personal cellular telephone, manners, dress, chores and duties, homework, disrespectful behavior, friendships, dating and relationships, money, automobiles, alcohol and other substance abuse, and time schedules. Present in these areas of conflict are the overriding arguments that "Everyone else has one" or is allowed the desired item or privilege and the ever-present assertions that "You don't understand me or trust me" and "You always treat me like a baby." Spoken or unspoken, parents' reactions consist of "Is this all the thanks I get for what I have done for you?"

Teenagers' earliest attempts to achieve emancipation from parental controls are manifested in a period of rejection of the parents. They absent themselves from home and family activities and spend an

---

👪 FAMILY-CENTERED CARE

Communication with Adolescents: The Art of Listening

Conflicts between parents and their adolescents are often a result of a natural characteristic of parenthood: the desire to protect one's offspring from harm or from simply doing something stupid or embarrassing or something they may later regret. Teenagers sometimes bounce their thoughts and ideas off adults. At times, they really want some feedback; at other times, they simply want to elicit a reaction.

I found it easy to listen openly, thoughtfully, and without interrupting when my teenagers' friends discussed troublesome topics. However, one day, when one of my own teenagers had a similar conversation with me, the parent part kicked in. I felt responsible and spoke my piece on the spot.

This brought communication to a halt and resulted in defensiveness. It was a long time before my child tried to talk to me about anything controversial again.

The next time one of my teenagers started a similar conversation, I decided to try to trick myself. Throughout the entire conversation, I told myself over and over again to act as if this were not my teenager but rather someone else's child. I found this actually worked quite well, and I was able to listen without interrupting. I continue to use the system, sometimes with more success than at other times.

—Mother of four

---

increasing amount of time with the peer group. They confide less in their parents, but parents continue to play an important role in the personal and health-related decision making of adolescents.

With advancing adolescence, teenagers become more competent, and with this competence comes a need for more autonomy. Although they may be psychologically prepared for independence, they are often thwarted in their efforts by lack of money or other parental barriers. Conflict arises in relation to the teenagers' outside activities and the elements of privacy and trust. Parental monitoring remains important throughout adolescence and may have a direct influence on adolescent sexual and substance use behavior. Parents should be guided toward an authoritative style of parenting in which authority is used to guide the adolescent while allowing developmentally appropriate levels of freedom and providing clear, consistent messages regarding expectations. Authoritative style of parenting has been shown to have both immediate and long-term protective effects toward adolescent risk reduction (DeVore and Ginsburg, 2005). However, to gain the trust of adolescents, parents must respect their adolescent's privacy and show an honest and sincere interest in what the adolescent believes and feels (see Family-Centered Care box).

Relationships with Peers

Although parents remain the primary influence in their lives, for the majority of teenagers, peers assume a more significant role in adolescence than they did during childhood. The peer group serves as a strong support to teenagers, individually and collectively, providing them with a sense of belonging and a feeling of strength and power. The peer group forms the transitional world between dependence and autonomy.

Peer Group

Adolescents are usually social, gregarious, and group minded. Thus, the peer group has an intense influence on adolescents' self-evaluation and behavior. To gain acceptance by a group, younger teenagers tend

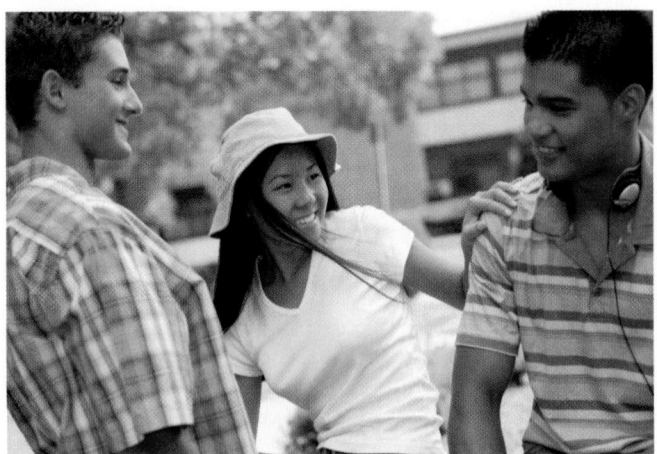

FIG 16-4 Teenagers like to gather in small groups. (© 2011 Photos.com, a division of Getty Images. All rights reserved.)

to conform completely in such things as mode of dress, hairstyle, taste in music, and vocabulary. Teenagers use the peer group as a yardstick of what is normal.

The school is psychologically important to adolescents as a focus of social life. Teenagers usually distribute themselves into a relatively predictable social hierarchy. They know to which groups they and others belong. A sense of school connectedness and optimal social connectedness is associated with positive outcomes for school completion, positive mood, and decreased high-risk behavior in adolescents (Bond, Butler, Thomas, and others, 2007). School connectedness is correlated with caring teachers and the absence of prejudice or discrimination from peers. A sense of school connectedness is less dependent on class size, attendance, academic preparation, and parental involvement (Maes and Lievens, 2003).

Within the larger groups are smaller, distinct, and exclusive crowds or cliques of selected close friends who are emotionally attached to one another. The selection is based on common tastes, interests, and background. Although cliques may become formalized, most remain informal and small. However, each has an identifying feature that proclaims its difference from others and its solidarity within itself in much the same manner as the adolescent generation as a whole sets itself apart from the adult generation. Cliques are usually made up of one sex, and girls tend to be more cliquish than boys and to have a greater need for close friendships (Fig. 16-4). Within the intimacy of the group, adolescents gain support in learning about themselves, consideration for the feelings of others, and increased ego development and self-reliance.

To belong is of utmost importance; thus, adolescents behave in a way that will ensure their establishment in a group. Adolescents are highly susceptible to social approval, acceptance, and demands. To be ignored or criticized by peers creates feelings of inferiority, inadequacy, and incompetence.

Best Friends

Personal friendships of the one-on-one variety usually develop between same-sex adolescents. This relationship is closer and more stable than it is in middle childhood, and it is important in the quest for identity. A best friend is the best audience on whom to try out possible roles and identities that an adolescent wants to test. Best friends may try a role together, each providing support for the other. Each cares about what the other thinks and feels. Because a sense of intimacy grows within a permanent relationship, the stability of this same-sex

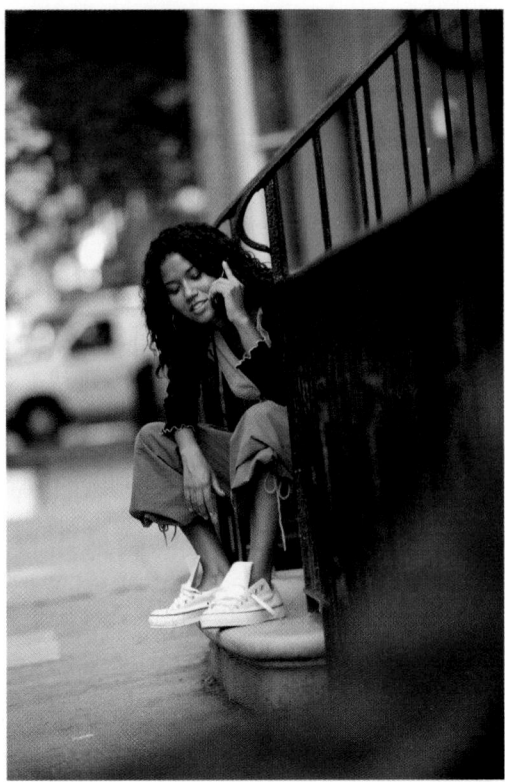

FIG 16-5 Cell phones allow adolescents to talk for hours with their peers. (© 2011 Photos.com, a division of Getty Images. All rights reserved.)

friendship is an important link in the progress toward an intimate relationship in young adulthood.

Interests and Activities

Adolescents spend a large amount of time engaging in leisure-time activities. As teenagers progress through the developmental stages of adolescence, these leisure-time activities move from being family centered to being peer centered. In addition to providing teenagers with fun and enjoyment, leisure-time activities assist in the development of social, physical, and cognitive skills. Leisure-time activities also allow teenagers the opportunity to learn to set priorities and structure their time (Fig. 16-5).

The role of social media and advanced technology are nowhere more prominent than in the lives of today's adolescents. The widespread availability of the Internet and access to social networking websites such as Facebook, chatrooms, free e-mail, blogs, and Twitter have created "virtual" communities and ways for young people to interact with others; web cameras even allow those interactions to include real-time video communication. Cellular telephones offer more mobile opportunities to talk on the phone, send text messages or instant messaging, send photos, or use video phone capabilities.

Internet chatrooms and social networking sites have created a more public arena for trying out identities and developing interpersonal skills with a wider network of people, occasionally with anonymity. This can create opportunities for young people who have a limited access to friends (because of rural location, shyness, or rare chronic conditions) to interact with people like themselves. However, most adolescents appear to be using the online social environment to interact with the same peers they spend their day with at school.

Text messaging via cell phones has become a common activity and can sometimes be disruptive during school. In addition, both the online and the text environment can create opportunities for cyberbullying, where teens engage in insults, harassment, and publicly humiliating statements online or on cell phones. In addition, there is increased danger of adolescents coming in contact and sharing personal information with sexual predators who pose as adolescents in an attempt to make personal contact with underage victims or engage them in sexting (sending sexually explicit or suggestive pictures or messages online) (Dowdell, Burgess, and Flores, 2011).

Today, many adolescents must learn to juggle their time between school, activities, and the responsibilities of a job. Adolescent work experiences provide many benefits, including time management, teamwork skills, and increased income. However, many jobs available to teenagers do not provide opportunities to apply the skills they learn in school, and jobs often have high demands for quick work with low rewards. Few apprentice opportunities are available for teenagers. It is generally recommended that adolescents limit their work to no more than 20 hours per week during the school year.

ADOLESCENT SEXUALITY

Sexual activity is common by the late teen years, but only 13% of teens have ever had vaginal sex by age 15 years. The average age of sexual initiation is about age 17 years. The top three reasons teenagers report for waiting to have sex include religious or moral beliefs, desire to postpone motherhood, and "haven't found the right person yet" (Abma, Martinez, and Copen, 2010).

Adolescence represents a critical time in the development of sexuality. Hormonal, physical, cognitive, and social changes that occur during adolescence all have an impact on sexual development. Of all the developmental changes that affect adolescent sexuality, none is more obvious than the impact of puberty. Adolescents must come to terms with hormonal influences, physiologic manifestations such as menstruation and ejaculation, and physical changes such as breast and genital development. All of these changes have a profound impact on the way teenagers perceive their bodies (i.e., body image). In addition to transitions in body image, increasing levels of pubertal hormones contribute to increased levels of sexual motivation among both boys and girls.

Changes in sexual motivations and feelings, happening at the same time as shifts in cognitive skills, contribute to painful conjectures ("Is what I'm feeling normal?"), self-conscious concern ("Am I good-looking enough?"), and hypothetical thinking ("What if she wants to have sex?"). The emergence of formal operational thinking also increases adolescents' decision-making capabilities concerning sexual issues. As they mature, teenagers become better able to think through potential risks and benefits of sexual behaviors before they engage in any behavior. Older adolescents may also be able to conceptualize more long-term consequences of present behaviors. One of the important tasks of adolescence is to incorporate sexuality successfully into close, intimate relationships. This task is made possible by the advanced cognitive abilities that emerge over the course of adolescence.

Part of adolescent identity formation involves the development of **sexual identity**. As they begin to integrate changes involved with puberty, young adolescents also develop emotional and social identities separate from their families'. For young adolescents, the process of sexual identity development usually involves forming close friendships with same-sex peers, with whom they may experiment sexually, often to satisfy curiosity. Sexual activity among young teenagers varies by gender. Masturbation provides an opportunity for sexual

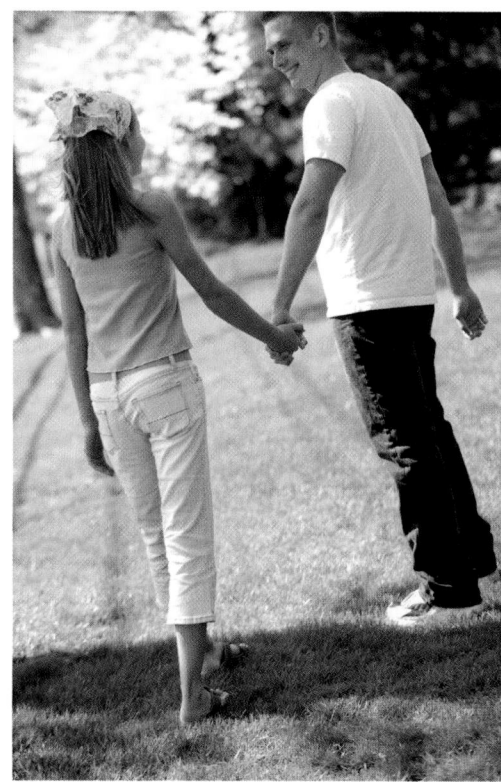

FIG 16-6 Heterosexual relationships are important for most adolescents. (© 2011 Photos.com, a division of Getty Images. All rights reserved.)

self-exploration; participation in this behavior is influenced by learned cultural attitudes and sex-role expectations.

Many teenagers begin to make a shift from relationships with same-sex peers to intimate relationships with members of the opposite sex during middle adolescence (Fig. 16-6). Opposite-sex relationships typically begin with peer activities involving both boys and girls. Pairing off as couples becomes more common as middle adolescence progresses. The type and degree of seriousness of partner relationships vary. Initial relationships are usually noncommittal, extremely mobile, and seldom characterized by any deep romantic attachments. Sexual activity becomes more common during middle adolescence. The relationship between love and sexual expression is brought into focus during middle adolescence. Most young people oppose exploitation, pressure, or force in sex as well as sex solely for the sake of physical enjoyment without a personal relationship. Adolescents find it hard to believe that sex can exist without love; therefore, they view each relationship as real love.

An integrated sexual identity often emerges during late adolescence as individuals incorporate sexual experiences, feelings, and knowledge. For most, this identity is consistent with their own physical and mental capacities and with societal limits and expectations. Most older adolescents identify themselves as being predominantly heterosexual; about 3% of males and 8% of females identify themselves as bisexual or homosexual (Mosher, Chandra, and Jones, 2005). Whatever their sexual orientation, most older teenagers possess the capacity to have intimate relationships that satisfy the emotional and sexual needs of both partners.

Sexual orientation is an important aspect of sexual identity. Sexual orientation is defined as a pattern of sexual arousal or romantic attraction toward persons of the opposite gender (heterosexual), of the same gender (homosexual, often called gay or lesbian), or of both genders (bisexual). Sexual orientation encompasses several dimensions, including attraction, fantasy, actual sexual behavior, and self-labeling or group affiliation. In individuals, the direction and intensity of each dimension are not necessarily consistent with any of the others. For example, individuals may be attracted most strongly to their same gender, fantasize about both genders, have sexual activity only with the opposite gender, and identify as gay or lesbian. Other individuals may engage in same-gender sexual behavior and fantasize about both genders but identify as heterosexual. As with all aspects of sexual identity, the dimensions of sexual orientation are influenced by cultural meaning and expectation, by gender, by peer groups, and by other environmental contexts.

Adolescence is the period during which individuals commonly begin to identify their sexual orientation as part of their developing sexual identity. However, this identification process can be profoundly influenced by cultural beliefs and values, by societal and family pressures, or by a lack of similar peers. The majority of adolescents eventually report an orientation toward exclusively heterosexual relationships. For adolescents whose orientation encompasses any same-gender dimensions, the identity process during adolescence can be complicated, especially when community norms disapprove of orientations other than heterosexual. Adolescents who have witnessed harassment or violence directed at gay, lesbian, and bisexual people, for example, may be reluctant to self-identify even when their attractions and behaviors are exclusively same-gender or bisexual.

The development of sexual orientation as part of sexual identity includes several developmental milestones during late childhood and throughout adolescence. These milestones do not necessarily occur in the same order for everyone, nor are they completed in the same amount of time. They include (1) the realization of romantic or erotic attraction to people of one (or both) genders; (2) erotic daydreaming about one or both genders; (3) romantic partners or dates without sexual activity; (4) sexual activity with people of the preferred gender or genders (also, for some teens, sexual activity with a nonpreferred gender, out of curiosity or through social pressure); (5) self-identification of the orientation that best fits one's current circumstances and understanding; (6) publicly self-identifying that orientation, usually to intimate friends and family first and then the wider social group; and (7) an intimate, committed sexual relationship with a person of the gender appropriate to one's orientation.

There is no evidence that gay, lesbian, or bisexual adults are more or less likely to create long-term, stable relationships than are heterosexual couples. It should be noted that bisexual adolescents and adults do not generally engage in sexual relationships with both genders concurrently; self-identification as bisexual usually refers to the ability to be attracted to either gender but does not imply that such a person requires partners of both genders or that one must be equally attracted to and have sexual experience with both genders in order to be bisexual.

Although the order of these milestones varies greatly among adolescents, adolescents who identify as gay, lesbian, or bisexual tend to publicly self-identify later than heterosexual peers. Without positive gay, lesbian, or bisexual role models or a supportive peer group, sexual-minority teens can feel isolated, and they may not share their orientation with anyone for fear of rejection or violence (see Critical Thinking Case Study box). A comparison of bisexual youth and heterosexual youth found that bisexual adolescents, especially girls, reported lower levels of connection to family and school than did heterosexual adolescents. Nurses should be alert to these lower levels of protective relationships for bisexual youth because it may lead to poor health outcomes (Saewyc, Homma, Skay, and others, 2009).

☒ CRITICAL THINKING CASE STUDY
Discussing Sexual Orientation with Adolescents

John, a 17-year-old adolescent, comes into the school-based clinic and tells the nurse practitioner that he thinks he is gay. Based on this information, answer the following questions:

Questions
1. Evidence—Is there sufficient evidence to draw any conclusions about John's statement regarding his sexual orientation at this time?
2. Assumptions—Describe an underlying assumption about each of the following issues:
   a. Development of sexual orientation in adolescents
   b. Society's reaction to homosexuality
   c. Health care professionals and adolescent sexuality
3. What is the most appropriate response by the nurse practitioner to John's statement?
4. Does the published evidence support your argument (conclusion)?

DEVELOPMENT OF SELF-CONCEPT AND BODY IMAGE

The sudden growth that takes place in early adolescence creates feelings of confusion for adolescents. They have lost the security of a familiar body and feel uncomfortable with their altered body. Consequently, they may try to either hide their body or advertise it, or they may alternate between the two extremes. Teenagers are acutely aware of their appearance as they begin to acquire images of themselves as adults, but they see discrepancies between their ideal and actual skills and abilities.

Adolescents are continually comparing themselves with their peers and making judgments about their own normality based on these observations. Pubertal children feel most comfortable when they are just like their friends and age mates. Perceived defects or deviations from the group average are threatening to their idealized image. Any blemish is likely to be magnified out of proportion, and any delay of the visible evidence of maturity is cause for worry. Unfortunately, this is also the time when the hormonal effect of the sebaceous glands produces acne, which creates problems for many adolescents. To adolescents, even the most insignificant pimple may be viewed as a gross disfigurement. The advent of chronic disease or a permanent physical disability has special significance during adolescence and creates additional stresses for both adolescents with the condition and health care providers.

Experts have determined that the body image established during adolescence is the one that individuals retain throughout life. Much of adolescents' search for identity takes place before a mirror as they try to read from the reflected features just who they are and what they look like to other people. Adolescents practice facial expressions and postures, try out hair arrangements, worry about pimples, and in other ways attempt to assess the best means to achieve a maximum effect—to reveal the "true self."

The **self-concept** becomes more differentiated as adolescents acquire a more complex picture of themselves, one that takes situational factors into account. The self-concept gradually becomes more individualized and more distinct from the concepts of others. Although younger teenagers describe themselves in terms of similarities with peers, as adolescence advances, young people describe themselves in terms of their special characteristics.

Responses to Puberty

The response to the physical changes of pubertal growth and development differs depending on the stage of development. Young adolescents become preoccupied with the rapid changes in their bodies and are interested in the anatomy, physiology, and function of their sexual organs. Boys must also confront the sexual feelings and tensions that accompany puberty, and the appearance of nocturnal emissions may be puzzling, troublesome, or embarrassing. Unless the boy has been prepared in advance, he may find it difficult to discuss his feelings with his parents and may turn to his friends for information and guidance. Many girls also are concerned over the rapid changes in their body. Some girls perceive the increase in weight and associated fat deposition as evidence of obesity and may indulge in fad diets. Although many girls look forward to menstruation and take this event in stride, others may find the first menstrual period a distressing and frightening event. All teenagers, regardless of gender, are concerned with the question, "Am I normal?" To answer this question, they compare their body with the bodies of their peers and with images in the media. This leads to a great deal of uncertainty about their appearance and attractiveness.

If an adolescent does not enter puberty at the same time as his or her peers, considerable inner conflict may occur. Early-maturing girls and boys have higher rates of sexual risk-taking behaviors, delinquency, and substance abuse than their on-time peers (Costello, Sung, Worthman, and others, 2007; Lynne, Graber, Nichols, and others, 2007). Nurses who work with adolescents must provide teaching and health care interventions that are appropriate for the chronologic and cognitive development of the adolescent rather than the stage of physical maturation.

As growth and development proceed through middle adolescence, the rapid body changes diminish, and adolescents have time to try to make their bodies more attractive. Adolescents strive to achieve the perfect body within their own cultural norms. The "right" clothes and hairstyle become very important. By late adolescence, the heightened concern with body image has ended and is replaced with a general comfort with the body.

The changes that occur during the early, middle, and late phases of adolescence are summarized in Table 16-1.

PROMOTING OPTIMAL HEALTH DURING ADOLESCENCE

The major causes of morbidity and mortality in adolescence are not diseases but health-damaging behaviors. New sources of morbidity in adolescence include injury (primarily motor vehicle related), depression, violence, sexually transmitted infections, and pregnancy; obesity may begin in childhood or adolescence, with secondary health consequences becoming evident in adolescence. Health promotion for this age group consists mainly of teaching and guidance to avoid risk-taking activities and health-damaging behaviors. Adolescence provides an opportunity for teenagers to incorporate healthy lifestyle behaviors that will benefit them not only during the teenage years but also throughout the life span.

Effective health education for adolescents should incorporate a developmentally appropriate, multifaceted approach. Motivational interviewing has been shown to improve adherence to health care advice by using a collaborative approach (Gance-Cleveland, 2007). Education alone is not enough to change behavior. Effective programs must include opportunities to improve communication skills and enhance their social network to make more positive connections (Tuttle, Campbell-Heider, and David, 2006).

 NURSING CARE GUIDELINES

Interviewing Adolescents

- Ensure confidentiality and privacy; interview adolescent without his or her parents.
- Show concern for adolescent's perspective, saying: "First, I'd like to talk about your main concerns" and "I'd like to know what you think is happening."
- Offer a nonthreatening explanation for the questions you ask, such as: "I'm going to ask a number of questions to help me better understand your health."
- Maintain objectivity; avoid assumptions, judgments, and lectures.
- Ask open-ended questions when possible; move to more directive questions if necessary.
- Begin with less sensitive issues and proceed to more sensitive ones.
- Use language that both the adolescent and you understand. Clarify terms, such as "having sex."
- Restate: reflect back to adolescents what they have said along with feelings that may be associated with their descriptions.

CRITICAL THINKING CASE STUDY

Respecting Privacy

Jamie, a 17-year-old girl, arrives at the adolescent clinic with her mother, Mrs. S., for a routine history and physical examination with the nurse practitioner. As the nurse practitioner walks with Jamie to an examination room, Mrs. S. whispers to the nurse practitioner, "I need to speak with you in private." How should the nurse practitioner respond to Mrs. S.'s request?

Questions

1. Evidence—Is there sufficient evidence to formulate a response to Jamie's mother?
2. Assumptions—Describe an underlying assumption about each of the following topics:
   a. The role of the adolescent in health care
   b. The role of the parents in the health of their adolescent
   c. Adolescents and confidentiality
3. What priorities or implications for nursing care should be established at this time?
4. Does the evidence support your conclusion?

As adolescents develop, they are able to assume additional responsibility for their own health, including maintaining health practices, taking prescribed medications, keeping appointments, and performing procedures when necessary. Health professionals who work with adolescents should consider their increasing independence and responsibility while maintaining privacy and ensuring confidentiality (see Nursing Care Guidelines box and Critical Thinking Case Study box). Parents should also respect their teenager's independence and move toward the role of consultant about health issues while maintaining some level of involvement throughout adolescence.

Several professional organizations have published guidelines aimed at improving and maintaining health care for adolescents and young adults. The American Academy of Pediatrics (AAP), American Academy of Family Physicians, American Medical Association, and U.S. Preventive Services Task Force have similar guidelines for health supervision of adolescents. These guidelines emphasize the need to provide health services to adolescents that meet their physical and

TABLE 16-1 GROWTH AND DEVELOPMENT DURING ADOLESCENCE		
EARLY ADOLESCENCE (11–14 YEARS)	**MIDDLE ADOLESCENCE (15–17 YEARS)**	**LATE ADOLESCENCE (18–20 YEARS)**
Growth		
Rapidly accelerating growth	Growth decelerating in girls	Physically mature
Reaches peak velocity	Stature reaches 95% of adult height	Structure and reproductive growth almost complete
Secondary sex characteristics appear	Secondary sex characteristics well advanced	
Cognition		
Explores newfound ability for limited abstract thought	Developing capacity for abstract thinking	Established abstract thought
Clumsy groping for new values and energies	Enjoys intellectual powers, often in idealistic terms	Can perceive and act on long-range options
Comparison of "normality" with peers of same sex	Concern with philosophic, political, and social problems	Able to view problems comprehensively
		Intellectual and functional identity established
Identity		
Preoccupied with rapid body changes	Modifies body image	Body image and gender role definition nearly secured
Trying out various roles	Very self-centered; increased narcissism	Mature sexual identity
Measurement of attractiveness by acceptance or rejection of peers	Tendency toward inner experience and self-discovery	Phase of consolidation of identity
Conformity to group norms	Has a rich fantasy life	Stability of self-esteem
	Idealistic	Comfortable with physical growth
	Able to perceive future implications of current behavior and decisions; variable application	Social roles defined and articulated
Relationships with Parents		
Defining independence–dependence boundaries	Major conflicts over independence and control	Emotional and physical separation from parents completed
Strong desire to remain dependent on parents while trying to detach	Low point in parent–child relationship	Independence from family with less conflict
No major conflicts over parental control	Greatest push for emancipation; disengagement	Emancipation nearly secured
	Final and irreversible emotional detachment from parents; mourning	
Relationships with Peers		
Seeks peer affiliations to counter instability generated by rapid change	Strong need for identity to affirm self-image	Peer group recedes in importance in favor of individual friendship
Upsurge of close, idealized friendships with members of the same sex	Behavioral standards set by peer group	Testing of romantic relationships against possibility of permanent alliance
Struggle for mastery takes place within peer group	Acceptance by peers extremely important—fear of rejection	Relationships characterized by giving and sharing
	Exploration of ability to attract opposite sex	
Sexuality		
Self-exploration and evaluation	Multiple plural relationships	Forms stable relationships and attachment to another
Limited dating, usually group	Internal identification of heterosexual, homosexual, or bisexual attractions	Growing capacity for mutuality and reciprocity
Limited intimacy	Exploration of "self appeal"	Dating as a romantic pair
	Feeling of "being in love"	May publicly identify as gay, lesbian, or bisexual
	Tentative establishment of relationships	Intimacy involves commitment rather than exploration and romanticism
Psychologic Health		
Wide mood swings	Tendency toward inner experiences; more introspective	More constancy of emotion
Intense daydreaming	Tendency to withdraw when upset or feelings are hurt	Anger more likely to be concealed
Anger outwardly expressed with moodiness, temper outbursts, and verbal insults and name calling	Vacillation of emotions in time and range	
	Feelings of inadequacy common; difficulty in asking for help	

emotional needs. They place great import on provision of health care by health care providers who are trained in meeting the adolescents' needs. The American Medical Association issued a comprehensive set of recommendations, the *Guidelines for Adolescent Preventive Services* (GAPS), intended to provide a framework for providers who have one-on-one contact with adolescents in clinical settings (American Medical Association, 1997). The following discussion is an overview of the

GAPS topics and provides specific recommendations related to screening, guidance, and immunizations.

IMMUNIZATIONS

An immunization update is an important part of adolescent preventive care. Obtaining a record of the teenager's prior immunizations is important. The Tdap (tetanus, diphtheria, acellular pertussis) vaccine is recommended for adolescents 11 to 18 years old who have not received a tetanus booster (Td) or Tdap dose and have completed the childhood DTaP/DTP series. When the Tdap is used as a booster dose, it may be administered at any time earlier than the previous 5-year interval to provide adequate pertussis immunity (regardless of interval from the last Td dose) (Centers for Disease Control and Prevention [CDC], 2011). Meningococcal vaccine (MCV4) should be given to adolescents 11 to 12 years of age with a booster dose at age 16 years. If not previously vaccinated, they should receive 1 dose at age 13 through 18 years (CDC, 2012).

The quadrivalent human papillomavirus (HPV) vaccine or the bivalent HPV vaccine is recommended for the prevention of cervical precancers and cancers for girls beginning at ages 11 to 12 years and at the physician's discretion as early as age 11 years (AAP, Committee on Infectious Diseases, 2012). The quadrivalent HPV vaccine is recommended for males aged 11 through 12 years to reduce their likelihood of genital warts; the vaccine may be given as early as age 9 years at the physician's discretion. Each one of the HPV vaccines is administered in a three-dose series; it is important to follow the recommended dose intervals for optimal effectiveness.

All adolescents who have not previously received three doses of hepatitis B vaccine should be vaccinated against hepatitis B virus. The hepatitis A vaccine should be given to adolescents who live in areas where vaccination programs target older children or who are at increased risk for infection or for whom immunity against hepatitis A is desired. Annual influenza vaccination with either the live attenuated influenza vaccine or the trivalent influenza vaccine is recommended for all children and adolescents. All adolescents should also be assessed for previous history of varicella infection or vaccination. Vaccination with the varicella vaccine is recommended for those with no previous history; for those with no previous infection or history, the varicella vaccine may be given in two doses 4 or more weeks apart to adolescents 13 years or older. (See also Immunizations, Chapter 10.) Adolescents should receive a tuberculin skin test if they have been exposed to active tuberculosis (TB), have lived in a homeless shelter, have been incarcerated, have lived in or come from an area with a high prevalence of TB, or currently work in a health care setting.

NUTRITION

The rapid and extensive increase in height, weight, muscle mass, and sexual maturity of adolescence is accompanied by increased nutritional requirements. Because nutritional needs are closely related to the increase in body mass, the peak requirements occur in the years of maximum growth, during which the body mass almost doubles. The caloric and protein requirements during this time are higher than at almost any other time of life. As a result of this increased anabolic need, the adolescent is highly sensitive to caloric restrictions.

Current guidelines for caloric intake are provided by a number of sources. The Dietary Reference Intakes (DRIs) provide age-specific guidelines for nutrients (see Chapters 6 and 12). The 2010 Dietary Guidelines for Americans* recommend specific caloric intakes for adolescents based on their levels of activity (sedentary, moderately active, and active) as well as a recommendation to decrease the amount of fat to approximately 25% to 36% of total daily intake. A recent change in guidelines is reflected in the new MyPlate,† which takes the place of

MyPyramid as a scheme for eating a balanced diet of the five main food groups—fruits, grains, protein, vegetables, and dairy products. Recent guidelines by the National Heart Lung and Blood Institute (NHLBI) include dietary recommendations to reduce the risk of cardiovascular disease. Included in these guidelines for adolescents is a total daily fat intake of 25% to 30% of estimated energy requirements, with emphasis on a reduction of saturated fat and avoidance of *trans* (unsaturated) fat. The guidelines also address the need for an increased intake of dietary fiber, consumption of 3 meals per day, avoidance of tobacco, and routine screening for hyperlipidemia and hypertension in children and adolescents. Estimated energy requirements for adolescents of both genders are provided based on 3 levels of activity: sedentary, moderately active, and active (NHLBI, 2011). Caloric intake can be tailored to meet adolescents' increased growth needs as well as activity level such as involvement in sports. Additional guidelines recommend the reduction in added sugars; adolescents consume most of their added sugars in sweetened beverages such as soda and energy and sports drinks (Van Horn, Johnson, Flickinger, and others, 2010).

Adolescents usually have sufficient intake of protein to meet their needs except for those who limit their food intake because of economic problems or in an attempt to lose weight. There is a substantial increase in the need for the minerals calcium, iron, and zinc during periods of rapid growth: calcium for skeletal growth, iron for expansion of muscle mass and blood volume, and zinc for the generation of both skeletal and bone tissue. The Estimated Average Requirement for calcium in adolescents 14 to 18 years of age is 1100 mg (Institute of Medicine, 2010). Girls with heavy or frequent menses may be especially susceptible to iron deficiency resulting from blood loss. Calcium intake from food sources is essential during adolescence to assist in the prevention of osteoporosis. Eventual bone mass is a balance between the amount of bone laid down during adolescence and the amount later lost with aging. Overall, osteoporosis is a result of polygenic and multiple environmental factors such as nutrition, economics, and exercise (Ongphiphadhanakul, 2007). Dietary intervention should promote the regular consumption of breakfast and a balanced intake of a variety of foods.

Eating Habits and Behavior

Eating and attitudes toward food are primarily family centered during early and middle childhood, and food habits are largely related to cultural and individual family preferences and patterns. With adolescence and the move toward independence, family influences on the child diminish. Children's interests, attitudes, and routines are altered as an increasing number of meals are eaten away from home. These changes are largely a result of the high value that teenagers place on peer acceptability and sociability. Their peers easily influence their eating habits.

Pressure for time and commitments to activities adversely affect teenagers' eating habits. Omitting breakfast or eating a breakfast that is nutritionally poor in quality is frequently a problem. Snacks, usually selected on the basis of accessibility rather than nutritional merit, become increasingly a part of the habitual eating pattern during adolescence (Fig. 16-7). Excess intake of calories, sugar, fat, cholesterol, and sodium is common among adolescents and is found in all income and racial or ethnic groups and both genders. Inadequate intake of certain vitamins (folic acid, vitamin B_6, vitamin A) and minerals (iron, calcium, zinc) is also evident, particularly among girls and teenagers of low socioeconomic status. In combination with other factors, these dietary patterns could result in increased risk for obesity and chronic diseases such as heart disease, osteoporosis, and some types of cancer later in life. Maximum bone mass is also acquired during adolescence;

---

*Dietary Guidelines for Americans, Institute of Medicine, available at http://www.health.gov/dietaryguidelines.
†MyPlate, http://www.choosemyplate.gov.

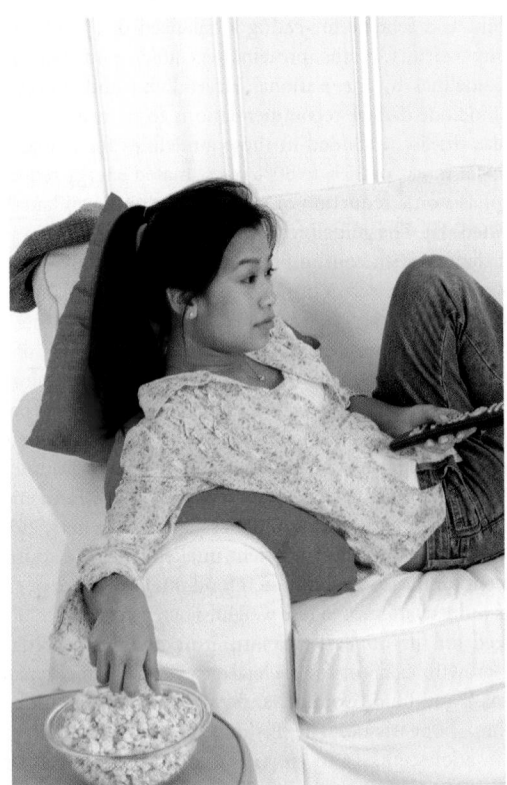

FIG 16-7 Snacking on empty calories is common among adolescents, especially during inactivity. (© 2011 Photos.com, a division of Getty Images. All rights reserved.)

therefore, the calcium deposited during these years determines the risk of osteoporosis. Milk is usually passed over in favor of soft drinks.

Overeating or undereating during adolescence presents special problems. When they experience the normal increase in weight and fat deposition of the growth spurt, teenage girls often resort to dieting. The desire for a slim figure and a fear of becoming "fat" prompt teenage girls to embark on nutritionally inadequate reducing regimens that drain their energy and deprive their growing bodies of essential nutrients. They resort to diets on their own or with peers in an effort to conform. Many adopt current fad diets and are victims of food misinformation. Boys are less inclined to undereat. They are more concerned about gaining size and strength. However, they tend to eat foods high in calories but low in other essential nutrients.

Obesity is increasing among both children and adolescents in the United States. Poor dietary habits and increasingly sedentary lifestyles have caused this obesity epidemic. Currently 16.9% of children ages 2 to 19 years are obese. The vast majority (90%) of obese adolescents remain obese into their 30s: 94% of women overall and 88% of men (Gordon-Larsen, The, and Adair, 2010).

Health problems traditionally thought of as adult comorbities of obesity, including type 2 diabetes mellitus, obstructive sleep apnea, and nonalcoholic steatohepatitis, are occurring in adolescents. Lifestyle changes necessary for adolescents to lose weight require the involvement of family members who provide support and encourage active participation.

Hypertension and Hyperlipidemia

As adolescents experience sexual maturation, along with increases in height and weight, blood pressure increases from the onset of adolescence and continues to rise until the end of pubertal growth. This trend is especially apparent among males. Approximately 1% of adolescents have sustained hypertension, defined as a blood pressure greater than the 95th percentile of standards. The detection of hypertension during adolescence is important because hypertension is one of the major preventable risk factors for adult cardiovascular disease. With increasing levels of obesity, there have been reports of increasing incidence of hypertension among adolescents (Hansen, Gunn, and Kaelber, 2007; LaRosa and Meyers, 2010). Screening for hypertension and associated risk factors should take place annually beginning at age 3 years. Specific guidelines for monitoring and treatment of hypertension in adolescents are found in the 2011 NHLBI summary report (see also Chapter 25).

Along with hypertension, smoking, and obesity, elevated serum cholesterol and triglyceride levels are major risk factors for the development of adult cardiovascular disease.

The NHLBI (2011) recently issued a recommendation for universal lipid (nonfasting or fasting) screening of all children and adolescents between the ages of 9 and 11 years, and again between the ages of 17 and 21 years. Low-density lipoprotein (LDL) cholesterol–lowering drug therapy is recommended for children and adolescents 10 years of age and older whose LDL remains elevated after 6 months to 1 year on a restricted fat diet, lifestyle modification (exercise), and weight management (NHLBI, 2011). Additional information and practice guidelines for monitoring cholesterol levels and initiation of LDL cholesterol–lowering medication as well as specific dietary modifications are found in the 2011 NHLBI summary report at http://www.nhlbi.nih.gov/guidelines/cvd_ped/summary.htm#chap5.

Nursing Care Management

Adolescents should receive at a minimum an annual assessment of weight, height, and BMI for age plotted on a standard growth reference chart. Healthy dietary habits should be discussed with all adolescents. The frequency of eating at fast-food and other restaurants, consumption of sweetened beverages, and consumption of excessive portion sizes should be identified. In addition to food intake, the nurse should assess the level of physical activity, sedentary behaviors, and sleep patterns. Readiness to change; environmental supports and barriers; and family history of diabetes, heart disease, and early stroke must be considered when planning nutritional education and guidance. Nurses in the school setting can assist in advocating for comprehensive nutritional services for preschool through grade 12 students.

SLEEP AND REST

Teenagers vary in their need for sleep and rest. Rapid physical growth, the tendency toward overexertion, and the overall increased activity of this age contribute to fatigue in adolescents. During growth spurts, the need for sleep is increased. Their propensity for staying up late makes it difficult to arise in the morning, and they may sleep late at every opportunity. Adequate sleep and rest at this time are important to a total health regimen.

Exercise and Activity

Although today's youth are less fit than children 20 years ago, adolescents probably spend more time and energy practicing and participating in sports activities than members of any other age group. Many adolescents participate in sports within school settings (Fig. 16-8). School-based, health-oriented physical education may provide both immediate effects of the activity and sustained effects through encouragement of lifelong activity patterns. High schools continue to cut physical education classes, with only half of high school students

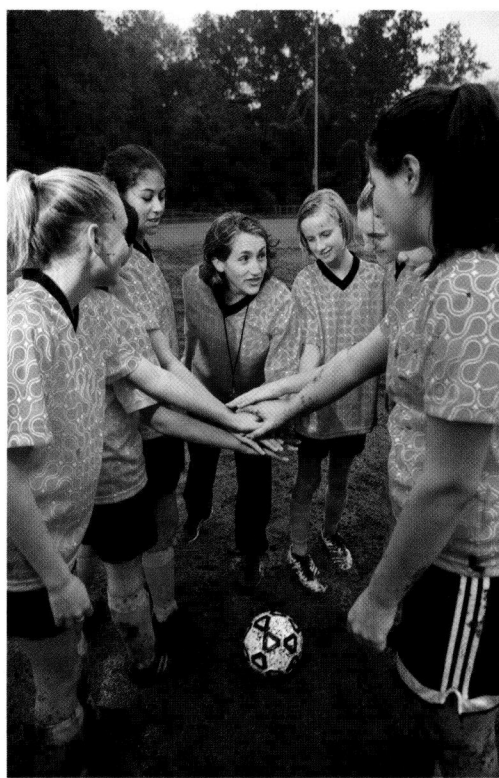

FIG 16-8 Adolescents should be encouraged to participate in activities that contribute to lifelong physical fitness. (© 2011 Photos.com, a division of Getty Images. All rights reserved.)

attending physical education classes in 2005. Fewer than half of students attended these classes daily, and the majority of classes included only 20 minutes of exercise (CDC, 2006). To improve health outcomes, school-age children and adolescents should engage in 60 minutes or more of moderate to vigorous physical activity daily (U.S. Department of Health and Human Services, 2008).

The practice of sports, games, and even dancing contributes significantly to growth and development, the education process, and better health. These activities provide exercise for growing muscles, interactions with peers, and a socially acceptable means of enjoying stimulation and conflict. In addition, competitive activities help teenagers in the process of self-appraisal and the development of self-respect and concern for others. Because physical fitness appears to be a major influence on one's lifelong health status, children should be encouraged to participate in activities that contribute to lifelong physical fitness. Nurses can encourage participation as a way to promote health and build self-esteem. However, adolescents should not be encouraged to engage in physical activities that are beyond their physical or emotional capacity (see Sports Participation and Injury, Chapter 31).

DENTAL HEALTH

Dental health should not be neglected during adolescence, although the rate of caries formation is not as great as in childhood. Dental care is an aspect of preventive care that is not received by substantial proportions of children in the United States. It is recommended that an evaluation for caries take place at a minimum of every year and optimally at 6-month intervals. Pit and fissure sealants are a safe and effective technique for dental caries prevention. Early adolescence is usually when corrective orthodontic appliances are worn, and these are frequently a source of embarrassment and concern to youngsters. Reassurance regarding the temporary nature of the annoyance and anticipation of an improved appearance help adolescents tolerate the inconvenience. It is also important to reinforce the orthodontist's directions regarding use and care of the appliances and to emphasize careful attention to toothbrushing during this time (see also Chapters 12 and 15). During late adolescence, an evaluation of the third molars (wisdom teeth) should take place to determine appropriate management (American Academy of Pediatric Dentistry, 2011).

PERSONAL CARE

Body-conscious teenagers are highly amenable to discussion and counseling about personal care and hygiene. Body changes associated with puberty bring special needs for cleanliness. The hyperactive sebaceous glands and newly functioning apocrine glands make frequent bathing or showering a necessity, and underarm deodorants assume an important place in personal care. Adolescents discover that hair requires more frequent shampooing, and girls often have questions about hair removal, use of cosmetics, and menstrual hygiene. Peer group discussions center on the advantages of particular products or methods. Adolescents are continually bombarded with messages from the media regarding the best way to enhance their popularity and attractiveness. Nurses are in a position to help them evaluate the relative merits of commercial products.

Vision

Regular vision testing is an important part of health care and supervision during adolescence. During adolescence, visual refractive difficulties reach a peak that is not exceeded until the fifth decade of life. The increased demands of schoolwork make adequate vision essential for academic success. Consequently, teenagers are more likely to be referred for visual evaluation. The need for corrective lenses can create psychologic problems for teenagers if they believe that glasses spoil their appearance or do not fit their body image. Contact lenses may be a preferred solution; a variety of lenses are now available at fairly reasonable prices. For some, the impact of a visual defect, no matter how slight, may be stressful.

Hearing

Considerable concern has focused on current teenage practices that cause hearing damage. Cochlear damage from relatively continuous exposure to the loud sound levels of rock music has been documented. The popularity of personal music players with lightweight earphones that are inserted into the ear canal is of particular concern to health care professionals. When these units are used for extended periods, permanent hearing loss can occur. Although appeals for more judicious use are not always successful, teenagers should be informed of the risk. Efforts directed toward legislating legal limits to the noise exposure that can be achieved through the sets may be another possible solution. (See Chapter 19 for a discussion of noise-related hearing loss.)

Posture

Many adolescents demonstrate altered posture. Rapid skeletal growth is often associated with slower muscular growth, and as a result, some teenagers may appear awkward or slump and fail to stand or sit upright. However, some postural defects of adolescence require early medical intervention. Scoliosis is a defect of the spine that occurs frequently in adolescence and is more common in girls than in boys (see Idiopathic Scoliosis, Chapter 31). The majority of cases are idiopathic, and the defect manifests as a painless curvature of the spine. Fortunately, most of these spinal curvatures will not require treatment. However, because there is no way to predict which curvatures will progress, all curvatures of the spine should be referred for further evaluation.

Body Art

Body art (piercing and tattooing) is an aspect of adolescent identity formation. The skin has become the latest source of parent–adolescent conflict. Adolescents often seek body art as an expression of their personal identity and style. Tattoos may mark significant life events such as new relationships, births, and deaths. Piercing the ear, nose, nipple, eyebrow, navel, penis, or tongue may sometimes create a health problem. It is a nursing responsibility to caution girls and boys against having piercing performed by friends, parents, or themselves. Although in most cases piercings have few, if any, serious side effects, there is always a risk of complications such as infection, cyst or keloid formation, bleeding, dermatitis, or metal allergy. Using the same unsterilized needle to pierce body parts of multiple teenagers presents the same risk of human immunodeficiency virus (HIV), hepatitis C, and hepatitis B virus transmission as occurs with other needle-sharing activities.

A qualified operator using proper sterile technique should perform the procedure. This is especially important if an adolescent has a history of diabetes, allergies, or skin disorders. Adolescents should be informed about the approximate time for healing after body piercing and the care of the pierced area during and after healing. Some body sites need extra precautions. For example, cartilage (ear, nose) has a poor blood supply and heals slowly and scars easily; nipple piercing puts adolescents at risk for breast abscesses. Finally, migration of the piercing is common with naval and other flat skin surface piercing. Piercing guns should not be used for piercing anything other than the earlobe because guns place the piercing too deeply.

The presence of body art in the form of tattoos and branding is common among adolescents and young adults. Professionals as well as amateur artists administer tattoos. The risk to adolescents receiving tattoos is low. The greatest risk is for the tattoo artist, who comes in contact with the client's blood. Adolescents who are amateur tattoo artists benefit from discussions about standard precautions and the hepatitis B vaccination. Many states either have no regulations or do not enforce existing regulations of piercing and tattooing facilities. The local health department is a source of information about local regulatory requirements. The CDC has an excellent website that outlines safety concerns for persons performing and receiving body art (http://www.cdc.gov/features/bodyart/).

Tanning

The quest for an attractive appearance leads many teenagers to excessive sunbathing and artificial means for tanning. However, this practice has serious long-term risks, and adolescents should be educated regarding the detrimental effects of sunlight on the skin (see Sunburn, Chapter 30). Long-term effects include premature aging of the skin; increased risk of skin cancer; and, in susceptible individuals, phototoxic reactions.

The increasing popularity of artificial tanning has prompted concern from health professionals regarding the use of sunlamps and tanning machines. The long-term effects of tanning machines are similar to those of the sun; dermatologists do not recommend suntanning by this means. Those who insist on using tanning equipment should be warned that goggles must be worn in tanning booths to prevent serious corneal burning. Education on the use of sunscreens, including hypoallergenic products, with a sun protective factor (SPF) of at least 15 and a nonalcohol base without lanolin, parabens, or fragrance, is important. Broad-spectrum sunscreens that protect against both ultraviolet A and B (UV-A and UV-B) are the most effective. Self-tanning creams safely stimulate the appearance of a tan; however, teens using these products should be cautioned that with sun exposure, protection is still required. Targeting health education messages to adolescents and incorporating educational components relating to sun protection behaviors in school health curricula and in health care visits will increase adolescents' knowledge and awareness.

STRESS REDUCTION

The multiple changes occurring in adolescence can result in great stress (Fig. 16-9 and Box 16-3). Adolescents are faced with pressures from peers that often involve taking serious health risks, including pressures for sexual experimentation; use of drugs, alcohol, and cigarettes; and potentially dangerous physical activities.

Early-maturing girls and late-maturing children are especially sensitive to the stresses of being different from their peers. Many feel intense anxiety over their identity. Both early- and late-maturing children feel out of place among their classmates, but slow-maturing children appear to experience the most pronounced inner turmoil and may be hesitant to voice their concerns. Slow-maturing adolescents need support and reassurance that they are not abnormal and need only be patient until the time comes when they, too, will mature physically.

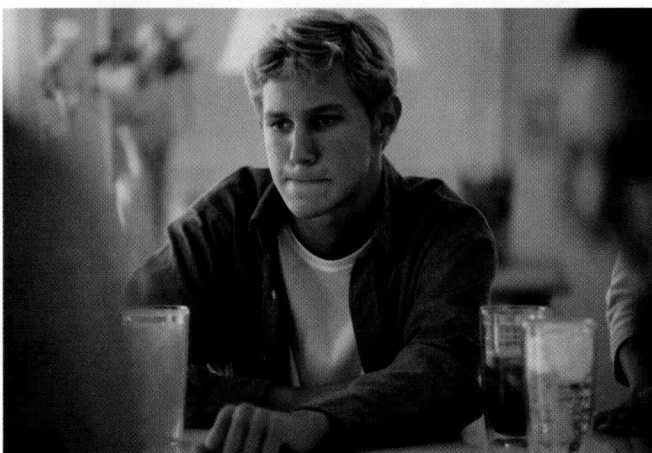

FIG 16-9 Adolescents use being alone as a method of coping with stress. Health care professionals need to assess whether this indicates clinical depression. (© 2011 Photos.com, a division of Getty Images. All rights reserved.)

BOX 16-3 AREAS OF STRESS IN ADOLESCENCE

- Body image
- Sexuality conflicts
- Scholastic pressures
- Competitive pressures
- Relationships with parents
- Relationships with siblings
- Relationships with peers
- Finances
- Decisions about present and future roles
- Career planning
- Ideologic conflicts

SEXUALITY EDUCATION AND GUIDANCE

The average American teenager spends more than 7 hours every day in front of some type of media. This potentially exposes them to unrealistic sexual messages and images, usually without adult supervision or interaction. Research has demonstrated that adolescents whose parents limit their television viewing are less likely to engage in earlier sex (AAP, Council on Communications and Media, 2010). In addition, social media use is a routine part of contemporary adolescents daily lives, and there are many positive benefits including enhancing communication, social connection, and computer skills. However, some evidence indicates that there are often online expressions of sexual experimentation, including sending and receiving sexually explicit messages, photographs, or images via cell phones and computers (O'Keeffe and Clarke-Pearson, 2011). All media sources provide adolescents potential exposure to information that may be inaccurate, riddled with cultural and moral judgments, and not very helpful.

The responsibility for providing sexuality education has been assumed by parents; schools; churches; community agencies such as Planned Parenthood Federation of America, Inc.;* and health professionals, especially nurses. Many adolescents perceive nurses, especially school nurses, as individuals who possess important information and who are willing to discuss sex with them. To be able to discuss the topic adequately, nurses must have not only an understanding of the physiologic aspects of sexuality and a knowledge of cultural and societal values but also an awareness of their own attitudes, feelings, and biases about sexuality.

Comprehensive information about sexuality education is offered by the Sexuality Information and Education Council of the United States (SIECUS)† and the Sex Information and Education Council of Canada.‡ The SIECUS maintains that every sexuality education program should present the topic from six aspects, including biologic, social, health, personal adjustments and attitudes, interpersonal associations, and the establishment of values.

Whether nurses counsel young people on an individual basis, in mixed groups, or in groups segregated by gender makes little difference. Ideally, boys and girls should be able to discuss sexuality objectively with one another and in groups, but this is not always possible. The differences in the rate of maturation between boys and girls and among different members of the same sex often make it desirable to discuss certain aspects of sexuality in segregated groups for early adolescents. As a rule, the need for separate discussion groups diminishes as young people mature.

Sexuality education should consist of instruction concerning normal body functions and should be presented in a straightforward manner using correct terminology. When discussing sex and sexual activities, nurses should use simple but correct language, not street language, highly scientific terminology, or evasive jargon. After they understand the meaning of biologic terms such as uterus, testicles, and vagina, most teenagers prefer to use them in their discussions.

Many girls arrive at menarche with ambivalent attitudes, myths, and illogical beliefs. Even girls adequately prepared for menstruation do not always understand its relationship to the total process of reproduction. Many are under the incorrect impression that the "safe" time for sexual intercourse is midway between menstrual periods.

Teenagers' curiosity and desire for information extend beyond the need for anatomic and physiologic knowledge. They need to know more than the mechanics of conception, pregnancy, and birth. Adolescents, girls in particular, want answers to questions such as "What is it like?" "Does it hurt?" "What happens when . . . ?" and "Is it all right if you . . . ?" Boys are often concerned about the fallacy that a relationship exists between penis size and sexual function. They need reassurance that masturbation is a normal and common practice, that some degree of homosexuality in early adolescence is not unusual, and that oral–genital relations can be normal substitutes for intercourse.

Teenagers need to discuss intercourse, alternative methods of sexual satisfaction, and how to resist peer pressure. With the increased incidence of sexually transmitted infections, especially HIV infection, the topic of "safe sex," especially abstinence or the use of condoms, is essential. Role-playing can help teenagers learn effective approaches to dealing with difficult situations. Sex and sexuality cannot be taught without discussions of mature decision making, sexual responsibility, and values clarification. Adolescents may receive inaccurate and ambiguous messages regarding sexual behavior; for example, an adolescent may be told that abstinence from vaginal intercourse will prevent transmission of a sexually transmitted infection. Accurate and unbiased information regarding sexual practices should be provided in a setting wherein the adolescent feels comfortable asking questions without being degraded or made to feel uncomfortable for seeking information.

Adolescents need role models and life experiences with delayed gratification. Most important, they need problem-solving experience and decision-making skills so they can anticipate the positive and negative outcomes of their decisions. With this type of assistance, teenagers can become sexually responsible young adults.

SAFETY PROMOTION AND INJURY PREVENTION

Physical injuries are the greatest single cause of death in the adolescent age group and claim more lives than all other causes combined. The most vulnerable ages are 15 to 24 years, when accidental injuries account for about 60% of deaths in boys and 40% of deaths in girls. These figures remain fairly constant from year to year and are significant because almost all fatal injuries are preventable.

During adolescence, peak physical, sensory, and psychomotor function gives teenagers a feeling of strength and confidence that they have never experienced before, and the physiologic changes of puberty give impetus to many basic instinctual forces. One manifestation of this is an increase in energy that simply must be discharged through action, often at the expense of logical thinking and other control mechanisms. Their propensity for risk-taking behavior plus feelings of indestructibility make adolescents especially prone to injuries. Some of the developmental characteristics of teenagers and injury prevention suggestions are outlined in Box 16-4.

Motor Vehicle–Related Injuries

Adolescents' newly acquired ability to drive and the normal developmental need for independence and freedom make automobiles an attractive part of their lives. Motor vehicle crashes are the single greatest source of unintentional injury and death in young people in the United States. Many factors contribute to the higher rate of crashes among teen drivers, including lacking driving experience and maturity, following too closely, driving too fast, having other teen passengers in the car, and using alcohol. Young drivers' elevated crash risk is highest between ages 16 and 17 years but persists through age 19 or 20 years. These data lend support to efforts in the United States to delay full

---

*434 West 33rd St., New York, NY 10001; 800-230-PLAN (7526); http://www.plannedparenthood.org.
†90 John St., Suite 402, New York, NY 10038; 212-819-9770; http://www.siecus.org.
‡850 Coxwell Ave., Toronto, ON M4C 5R1; 416-466-5304; http://www.sieccan.org.

BOX 16-4   INJURY PREVENTION DURING ADOLESCENCE

Developmental Abilities Related to Risk of Injury

Need for independence and freedom

Testing independence

Age permitted to drive a motor vehicle (varies from state to state)

Inclination for risk taking

Feeling of indestructibility

Need for discharging energy, often at expense of logical thinking and other control mechanisms

Strong need for peer approval

Attempting hazardous maneuvers

Peak incidence for practice and participation in sports

Access to more complex tools, objects, and locations

Can assume responsibility for own actions

Injury Prevention
Motor or Nonmotor Vehicles
Pedestrian

Emphasize and encourage safe pedestrian behavior.

- At night, walk with a friend.
- If someone is following you, go to nearest place with people.
- Do not walk in secluded areas; take well-traveled walkways.

Passenger

Promote appropriate behavior while riding in a motor vehicle. Refuse to ride with an impaired person or one who is driving recklessly.

Driver

Provide competent driver education; encourage judicious use of vehicle; discourage drag racing or playing chicken; maintain vehicle in proper condition (e.g., brakes, tires).

Teach and promote safety and maintenance of two- and three-wheeled vehicles.

Promote and encourage wearing of safety apparel such as a helmet and long trousers.

Reinforce the dangers of drugs, including alcohol, when operating a motor vehicle.

Discourage distractions while driving—cell phone talking or texting, eating, smoking, or reading.

Drowning

Teach nonswimmers to swim.

Teach basic rules of water safety.

- Judicious selection of places to swim
- Sufficient water depth for diving
- Swimming with a companion
- No alcohol with water sports

Burns

Reinforce proper behavior in areas with burn hazards (gasoline, electric wires, fires).

Advise regarding excessive exposure to natural or artificial sunlight (ultraviolet burn).

Discourage smoking.

Encourage use of sunscreen.

Poisoning

Educate in hazards of drug use, including alcohol.

Falls

Teach and encourage general safety measures in all activities.

Bodily Damage

Promote acquisition of proper instruction in sports and use of sports equipment.

Instruct in safe use of and respect for firearms and other devices with potential danger (e.g., power tools, firecrackers).

Provide and encourage use of protective equipment when using potentially hazardous devices.

Promote access to or provision of safe sports and recreational facilities.

Be alert for signs of depression (potential suicide).

Discourage use of hazardous sports equipment (e.g., trampoline, surfboards).

Instruct regarding proper use of corrective devices (e.g., glasses, contact lenses, hearing aids).

Encourage and foster judicious application of safety principles and prevention.

---

licensure beyond age 16 years. There is also evidence that graduated licensing systems that phase in unsupervised driving in higher-risk situations such as nighttime driving and having passengers in the car are effective in decreasing the motor vehicle crash risk for adolescents (McCartt, Mayhew, Braitman, and others, 2009).

There has been recent attention on distracted teenage driving and cell phone talking or texting while driving. Studies have shown that drivers using handheld devices are considerably more distracted and spend less time looking at the road or paying attention to driving conditions (Hosking, Young, and Regan, 2009).

Nurses should educate teenagers and their parents about the risk of driving while drinking alcohol or of riding in an automobile with a drunk driver. Many families arrange a no-questions-asked ride home to prevent an adolescent from riding with a drunk driver. Families should also require adolescents to log several hours of supervised practice driving before taking the car out alone. Educational efforts should also discuss that the major risk for death in a motor vehicle crash is failure to use a safety restraint.

Other Vehicle Injuries

The increasing use of motorcycles, all-terrain vehicles, jet skis, and snowmobiles has caused an increase in injuries among young people who are below the legal age for driving automobiles. Many adolescents ride bicycles without helmets and without lights at night, and the overwhelming majority of deaths from bicycle injuries (primarily head injuries) involve teenagers. In-line skating and skateboarding without protective gear also contribute to a significant number of traumatic brain injuries in U.S. adolescents and young people.

Firearms

Firearms are the major cause of intentional fatal injuries in the United States. Adolescence is the peak age for being either a victim or an offender in an injury involving a firearm. Gun carrying among adolescents is on the rise and is not limited to the stereotypic inner-city youth. Family members and acquaintances are a common source of guns for young people. Gun availability in the home is strongly linked to unintentional death and injury to children (Glatt, 2005). In addition, the presence of a gun in the home increases the risk of adolescent suicide and homicide. All families should be assessed for the presence of a gun in the home and informed of this risk. They must take preventive action to ensure that the guns are never loaded, that guns are locked up in a safe place, and that ammunition is stored and locked up separately in a location accessible only to appropriate adults.

Sports Injuries

Because the degree of physical maturation, size, coordination, and endurance varies greatly among adolescents of the same age, sports competition among young people who differ greatly in strength and agility is unfair and hazardous. Matching candidates for sports should be done relative to physical maturity, height, weight, and physical fitness and skills, particularly in sports involving rigorous body contact. Age is a less important consideration.

Every sport has some potential for injury, whether one participates in serious competition or engages in the activity for pure enjoyment. Overuse injuries are common in adolescents and result in more time missed from the activity than fractures. The increase in strength and vigor in adolescence may tempt adolescents to overextend themselves. Injuries sustained in sports or recreational activities can involve any part of the body and range from relatively minor cuts, bruises, and abrasions to totally incapacitating central nervous system injuries or death (see Chapter 31).

Nursing Care Management

Injury prevention is an ongoing part of nursing responsibility throughout the childhood years. Anticipatory guidance to parents and children regarding the expected problems and hazards related to growth and development does not end as children approach maturity. They need education in basic safety precautions, instruction in skills required in the performance of activities such as sports, instruction in handling motor vehicles, and information about using proper protective equipment and properly maintaining equipment. During adolescence, however, health and safety education and guidance are more effective when the young people are involved directly. Parents and health professionals can emphasize the importance of safety during performance of activities and the proper conditioning and preparation for sports.

Prevention can occur on a variety of levels. Safety advocacy, public policy changes, and legislation can curtail injuries. Examples of such approaches are laws that mandate wearing seat belts, prohibiting hand-held cell phone usage while the car is in motion, using helmets while driving moving vehicles other than automobiles, keeping the legal drinking age at 21 years, and instituting curfews for teen drivers. In addition to improvements in the environment, health education for teenagers and significant adults is essential. Helping adolescents understand their need for engaging in risky behavior, exploring possible negative outcomes, and weighing possible alternatives are critical components of injury prevention.

ANTICIPATORY GUIDANCE—CARE OF FAMILIES

Both adolescents and their parents are often confused and perplexed about the changes and behavior of this stage of development. Parents need support and guidance to help them through this trying time. They need to understand the changes taking place and to accept the expected behaviors that accompany the process of detachment. Parents may need help to "let go" and to promote the changed relationship from one of dependence to one of mutuality (see Family-Centered Care boxes).

FAMILY-CENTERED CARE

Guidance During Adolescence

Encourage Parents To:
Accept adolescent as a unique individual.
Respect adolescent's ideas, likes and dislikes, and wishes.
Be involved with school functions and attend adolescent's performances, whether they are sporting events or school plays.
Listen and try to be open to teenager's views even when they disagree with parental views.
Avoid criticism about no-win topics.
Provide opportunity for choosing options and accept natural consequences of these choices.
Allow young persons to learn by doing even when choices and methods differ from those of adults.
Provide adolescent with clear, reasonable limits.
Clarify house rules and consequences for breaking them. Adhere to the rules (even though it hurts!).
Let society's rules and consequences teach responsibility outside the home.
Allow increasing independence within limitations of safety and well-being.
Respect adolescent's privacy.
Try to share adolescent's feelings of joy or sorrow.
Respond to feelings as well as words.
Be available to answer questions, give information, and provide companionship.
Try to make communication clear.
Avoid comparisons with siblings.
Assist adolescent in selecting appropriate career goals and preparing for adult roles.
Welcome adolescent's friends into the home and treat them with respect.
Provide unconditional love and acceptance.
Be willing to apologize when mistaken.

Be Aware That Adolescents:
Are subject to turbulent, unpredictable behavior.
Are struggling for independence.
Are extremely sensitive to feelings and behavior that affect them.
May receive a different message from what was sent.
Consider friends extremely important.
Have a strong need to belong.

FAMILY-CENTERED CARE

Family Rules for Adolescents

U.S. society does little to help adolescents mature and separate. Americans have remarkably few rites of passage that mark the stages of life. Few ceremonies and tests are practiced to determine eligibility for specific adult privileges. Obtaining a driver's license, graduating from high school, and reaching legal age for drinking are among the few milestones that exist. U.S. society also does not have many generally agreed-on social dictums. When is the right age to begin dating? What is a reasonable curfew? Should an 18-year-old adolescent be allowed to stay out all night? There are few areas of general agreement. Every family makes up its own rules, influenced, but uninstructed, by the society at large. Many families have great difficulty with this process.

Modified from Prothrow-Stith D: *Deadly consequences: how violence is destroying our teenage population and a plan to begin solving the problem*, New York, 1993, HarperCollins.

KEY POINTS

- Adolescence is considered as beginning with the gradual appearance of secondary sex characteristics at about 11 or 12 years of age and ending with cessation of body growth at 18 to 20 years.
- Biologic development during puberty is characterized by increased activity of the pituitary gland, which results in sexual maturity and the appearance of secondary sex characteristics.
- According to Erikson, the major developmental crisis of adolescence is establishing a sense of identity.
- Cognitive development in adolescence includes abstract thought, thinking beyond the present, logical reasoning, and a sense of idealism.
- Development of body image is closely tied to body changes and social interactions.
- According to Kohlberg's theory of moral development, adolescents begin to question existing moral values and learn to make choices.

- Spiritual development is characterized by the questioning of family values and ideals, a move to more philosophic thinking, and an emphasis on personal religion.
- Adolescents' relationships with their parents may be strained; the influence of the peer group increases, and intimate relationships assume importance.
- Teenagers demonstrate a wide variety of interests, and their increased physical and cognitive skills allow them to engage in increasingly difficult and complex activities.
- Adolescents' emotions fluctuate.
- Nutritional needs, especially for calcium, zinc, and iron, may not be met by teenagers' eating habits as they begin to make independent food choices.
- Motor vehicle injuries are the primary cause of death from injury in the adolescent years.

REFERENCES

Abma JC, Martinez GM, Copen CE: Teenagers in the United States: Sexual activity, contraceptive use, and childbearing, National Survey of Family Growth 2006–2008, National Center for Health Statistics, *Vital Health Stat* 23(30), 2010.

American Academy of Pediatric Dentistry: Guideline on periodicity of examination, preventive dental services, anticipatory guidance/counseling and oral treatment for infants, children, and adolescents, *AAPD Reference Manual 2010–2011* 32(6):93–100, 2011.

American Academy of Pediatrics, Committee on Infectious Diseases: HPV vaccine recommendations, *Pediatrics* 129(3):602–605, 2012.

American Academy of Pediatrics, Council on Communications and Media: Policy statement: sexuality, contraception and the media, *Pediatrics* 126(3):576–582, 2010.

American Medical Association: *Guidelines for adolescent preventive services (GAPS)*, Chicago, 1997, Author.

Biro FM, Lucky AW, Simbarti LA, and others: Pubertal maturation in girls and the relationship to anthropometric changes: pathways through puberty, *J Pediatr* 142(6): 643–646, 2003.

Bond L, Butler H, Thomas L, and others: Social and school connectedness in early secondary school as predictors of late teenage substance use, mental health, and academic outcomes, *J Adolesc Health* 40(4):357.e9–357.e18, 2007.

Centers for Disease Control and Prevention: Youth risk behavior surveillance—United States, 2005, *MMWR Morb Mortal Wkly Rep* 55(SS-5):1–108, 2006.

Centers for Disease Control and Prevention: Updated recommendations for use of tetanus toxoid, reduced diphtheria toxoid and acellular pertussis (Tdap) vaccine from the Advisory Committee on Immunization Practices, 2010, *MMWR Morb Mortal Wkly Rep* 60(01):13–15, 2011.

Centers for Disease Control and Prevention: Recommended immunization schedules for persons aged 0 through 18 years—United States, 2012, *MMWR Morb Mortal Wkly Rep* 61(5):1–4, 2012.

Costello EJ, Sung M, Worthman C, and others: Pubertal maturation and the development of alcohol use and abuse, *Drug Alcohol Depend* 88(Suppl 1):S50–S59, 2007.

DeVore ER, Ginsburg KR: The protective effects of good parenting on adolescents, *Curr Opin Pediatr* 17(4):460–465, 2005.

Dowdell EB, Burgess AW, Flores JR: Online social networking patterns among adolescents, young adults, and sexual offenders, *American J Nurs* 111(7):28–36, 2011.

Gance-Cleveland B: Motivational interviewing: improving patient education, *J Pediatr Health* 21(2):81–88, 2007.

Glatt K: Child-to-child unintentional injury and death from firearms in the United States: what can be done? *J Pediatr Nurs* 10(6):448–452, 2005.

Gordon-Larsen P, The NS, Adair LS: Longitudinal trends in obesity in the United States from adolescence to the third decade of life, *Obesity* 18:1801–1804, 2010.

Hansen ML, Gunn PW, Kaelber DC: Underdiagnosis of hypertension in children and adolescents, *JAMA* 298(8):874–879, 2007.

Herman-Giddens ME: Recent data on pubertal milestones in United States children: the secular trend toward earlier development, *Int J Androl* 29(1):241–246, 2006.

Hosking SG, Young KL, Regan MA: The effects of text messaging on young drivers, *Hum Factors* 51(4):582–592, 2009.

Institute of Medicine: *Report at a glance: dietary reference intakes for calcium and vitamin D*, 2010, Institute of Medicine, retrieved June 20, 2011, from http://www.iom.edu/Reports/2010/Dietary-Reference-Intakes-for-Calcium-and-Vitamin-D/Report-Brief.aspx.

Kaplowitz PB: Link between body fat and the timing of puberty, *Pediatrics* 121(Suppl 3):S208–S217, 2008.

LaRosa C, Meyers K: Epidemiology of hypertension in children and adolescents, *J Med Liban* 58(3):132–136, 2010.

Lynne SD, Graber JA, Nichols TR, and others: Links between pubertal timing, peer influences and externalizing behaviors among urban students followed through middle school, *J Adolesc Health* 40(2): 181.e7–13, 2007.

Maes L, Lievens J: Can the school make a difference? A multilevel analysis of adolescent risk and health behaviour, *Soc Sci Med* 56(3):517–529, 2003.

McCartt AT, Mayhew DR, Braitman KA, and others: Effects of age and experience on young driver crashes: review of recent literature, *Traffic Inj Prev* 10:209–219, 2009.

Mosher WD, Chandra A, Jones J: Sexual behavior and selected health measures: men and women 15–44 years of age, United States, 2002, *Adv Data* 15(362):1–55, 2005.

National Heart Lung Blood Institute: Expert panel on integrated guidelines for cardiovascular health and risk reduction in children and adolescents: Summary report. U.S. Department of Health and Human Services, 2011, NHLBI, Bethesda, Md., retrieved January 3, 2012, from http://www.nhlbi.nih.gov/guidelines/cvd_ped/summary.htm#chap5.

O'Keeffe SG, Clarke-Pearson KC: Clinical report—the impact of social media on children, adolescents and families, *Pediatrics* 127(4): 800–804, 2011.

Ongphiphadhanakul B: Osteoporosis: the role of genetics and the environment, *Forum Nutr* 60:158–167, 2007.

Regnerus MD, Glen HE: Religion and vulnerability among low risk adolescents, *Soc Sci Res* 32(4): 633–658, 2003.

Saewyc EM, Homma Y, Skay CL, and others: Protective factors in the lives of bisexual adolescents in North America, *Am J Pub Health* 99(1):110–117, 2009.

Tuttle J, Campbell-Heider N, David TM: Positive adolescent life skills training for high-risk teens:

results of a group intervention study, *J Pediatr Health* 20(3):184–191, 2006.

U.S. Department of Health and Human Services: *2008 physical activity guidelines for Americans,* retrieved April 5, 2011, from http://www.health. gov/PAGuidelines/guidelines.

Van Horn L, Johnson RK, Flickinger BD, and others: Translation and implementation of added sugars consumption recommendations: a conference report from the American Heart Association Added Sugars Conference 2010, *Circulation* 122(23):2470–2490, 2010.

Wu T, Mendola P, Buck GM: Ethnic differences in the presence of secondary sex characteristics and menarche among U.S. girls: the Third National Health and Nutrition Examination Survey, 1988–1994, *Pediatrics* 10(4):752–757, 2002.

Health Problems of School-Age Children and Adolescents

Linda M. Kollar, Kristine Jordan, and David Wilson

evolve WEBSITE

http://evolve.elsevier.com/wong/essentials
Animation—Pelvic Inflammatory Disease
**Case Studies—Attention-Deficit/Hyperactivity Disorder; Obesity;
   Teen Smoking**

Key Points Summaries
NCLEX-Style Review Questions
Nursing Care Plan—The Adolescent with an Eating Disorder

CHAPTER OUTLINE

Health Problems of School-Age
   Children, 499
   Problems Related to Elimination, 499
      Enuresis, 499
      Encopresis, 500
   School-Age Disorders with Behavioral
      Components, 501
      Attention-Deficit/Hyperactivity
         Disorder and Learning
         Disability, 501
      Posttraumatic Stress Disorder, 504
      School Phobia, 505
      Bullying, 505
      Conversion Reaction, 506
      Childhood Depression, 506
      Childhood Schizophrenia, 507

Health Problems of Adolescents, 507
   Altered Growth and Maturation, 507
      Sex Chromosome Abnormalities, 508
   Disorders Related to the Reproductive
      System, 508
      Amenorrhea, 508
      Dysmenorrhea, 509
      Vaginitis, 509
      Disorders of the Male Reproductive
         System, 510
      Gynecomastia, 510
   Health Problems Related to
      Sexuality, 510
      Adolescent Pregnancy, 511
      Contraception, 511
      Sexually Transmitted Infections, 514

Pelvic Inflammatory Disease, 514
   Sexual Assault (Rape), 516
Nutrition and Eating Disorders, 517
   Obesity, 517
   Anorexia Nervosa and Bulimia
      Nervosa, 523
   Lactose Intolerance, 526
Adolescent Disorders with a Behavioral
   Component, 527
   Substance Abuse, 527
   Suicide, 531

LEARNING OBJECTIVES

On completion of this chapter the reader will be able to:
- Outline a plan of care for the child with an elimination problem.
- Describe the most common causes of physical growth or maturation failure in later childhood.
- Demonstrate an understanding of common disorders of the male and female reproductive systems.
- Demonstrate an understanding of health problems related to adolescent sexuality.

- Outline a plan for discussing sexuality issues with adolescents.
- Outline a plan of care for the adolescent with an eating disorder.
- Discuss the manifestations and nursing management of selected emotional or behavioral problems in school children and adolescents.

HEALTH PROBLEMS OF SCHOOL-AGE CHILDREN

PROBLEMS RELATED TO ELIMINATION

Enuresis

Enuresis (bedwetting), or nocturnal enuresis, is a common and troublesome disorder that is defined as intentional or involuntary passage of urine into bed (usually at night) in children who are beyond the age when voluntary bladder control should normally have been acquired. The inappropriate voiding of urine must occur at least twice a week for at least 3 months, and the chronologic or developmental age of the child must be at least 5 years. The predominant symptom is urgency that is immediate and accompanied by acute discomfort, restlessness, and urinary frequency. In addition, the urinary incontinence must not be related to the direct physiologic effects of a substance (e.g., diuretics) or a general medical condition (e.g., diabetes mellitus or diabetes insipidus, spina bifida, seizure disorder, or sickle cell disease).

Enuresis is more common in boys; nocturnal bedwetting usually ceases between 6 and 8 years of age. Enuresis can also be defined as primary (bedwetting in children who have never been dry for extended periods) or secondary (the onset of wetting after a period of established urinary continence). The passage of urine may occur only during nighttime sleep with the child remaining dry during the day (monosymptomatic), or it may be polysymptomatic, wherein the child has daytime urinary urgency and an occasional daytime accident in conjunction with other conditions such as sleep apnea, urinary tract infection, neurologic impairment, constipation, or emotional stressors (Berry, 2006; Katz and DeMaso, 2011). The nocturnal, monosymptomatic type is most common. The condition may be particularly distressing to adolescents, who may refuse therapy. Although enuresis may occur during the daytime, the following discussion primarily focuses on nocturnal enuresis.

Before psychogenic factors are considered, organic causes that may be related to enuresis should be ruled out. These include structural disorders of the urinary tract; urinary tract infection; neurologic deficits; disorders that increase the normal output of urine, such as diabetes; and disorders that impair the concentrating ability of the kidneys, such as chronic renal failure or sickle cell disease. A bladder volume of 300 to 350 ml (10–12 oz) is sufficient to hold a night's urine. Normal bladder capacity (in ounces) is the child's age plus 2 (up to age 14 years). In other cases, enuresis is influenced by emotional factors, although it is doubtful that they are causative factors. Parents report that these children sleep more soundly than other children; however, the depth of sleep has not been identified as the cause of nocturnal enuresis (Berry, 2006; Elder, 2011). Nocturnal enuresis has a strong familial tendency.

Therapeutic techniques used to manage nocturnal enuresis include medications, complementary and alternative medicine techniques such as hypnotherapy, restriction or elimination of fluids after the evening meal, avoidance of caffeinated and sugar-containing beverages after 4 PM, purposeful interruption of sleep to void, motivational therapy, and various devices designed to establish a conditioned reflex response to waken the child at the initiation of voiding (alarms).

Drug therapy is increasingly being prescribed to treat enuresis. Three types of drugs are used: tricyclic antidepressants (TCAs), antidiuretics, and antispasmodics. The selection depends on the interpretation of the cause. The drug used most frequently is the TCA imipramine (Tofranil), which exerts an anticholinergic action in the bladder to inhibit urination. The dosage and time of administration are individualized, and the drug is given in amounts sufficient to lighten sleep but not to cause wakefulness. Some practitioners prescribe low doses, which reduces bedwetting in two thirds of children. However, it is important to note that almost all children relapse when the medication is stopped. The suggested length of treatment is 6 to 8 weeks followed by gradual withdrawal over 4 weeks. Because overdosage of this drug is especially dangerous, caution parents about safe use and the need to keep supplies of the drug from the reach of younger siblings.

Anticholinergic drugs, especially oxybutynin, reduce uninhibited bladder contractions and may be helpful for children with daytime urinary frequency. Success has also been achieved with desmopressin acetate (DDAVP) nasal spray, an analog of vasopressin, which reduces nighttime urinary output to a volume less than functional bladder capacity. Typically, the child receives two sprays before bedtime. The medication is generally well tolerated but may cause nasal irritation or, rarely, headache or nausea. A preparation of desmopressin acetate is also available in tablet form. This preparation is as effective and safe as the nasal spray but avoids the problem of nasal irritation.

These drugs are considered second-line management, and parents should be cautioned not to think that these agents will cure the condition; parents are also advised of the drug's side effects (Katz and DeMaso, 2011; Sethi, Bhargava, and Shipra, 2005).

Nursing Care Management

No matter what techniques are used, the nurse can help both children and parents understand the problem of enuresis, the treatment plan, and the difficulties they may encounter in the process. Essential to the success of any method is the supportive management of parents and their children. Both need encouragement and patience. The problem is discussed with both the parent and the child because all treatments involve and require the child's active participation. In some treatment interventions, the child is in charge of the intervention; therefore, parents must learn to support the child rather than intervene themselves. For example, children can strip their wet linens, limit fluids, and use the toilet before bedtime. Parents should encourage the child to maintain a regular bowel evacuation regimen; constipation can contribute to nocturnal enuresis (Katz and DeMaso, 2011). A calendar with wet and dry nights may be helpful to motivate the child to stay dry and maintain a positive perspective on the problem; positive rewards are also helpful (Box 17-1).

Parents need to understand that punishment such as scolding, shaming, and threatening is contraindicated because of its negative emotional impact and limited success in reducing the behavior. Positive reinforcement of the desired behavior may be beneficial. Children need to believe that they are helping themselves, and they need to sustain feelings of confidence and hope. Many parents believe that enuresis is caused by an emotional disturbance and fear that they have somehow produced the situation by improper childrearing practices. They need reassurance that bedwetting is not a manifestation of emotional disturbance and does not represent willful misbehavior. Encourage parents to be patient, to be understanding, and to communicate love and support to the child.

Communication with children is directed toward eliminating the emotional impact of the problem, relieving feelings of shame and guilt and the burden of parental disapproval, building self-confidence, and motivating children toward independent control. More important, the nurse can provide consistent support and encouragement to help children through the inconsistent and unpredictable treatment process. Children need to believe that they are helping themselves and to maintain feelings of confidence and hope.

Parents should also be taught to observe for side effects of any medications used. All children with primary enuresis should be encouraged to void before bedtime and diapering should be avoided.

BOX 17-1 SUGGESTIONS FOR MANAGING NOCTURNAL ENURESIS*

Have child empty bladder immediately before going to bed.

Restrict fluids at nighttime meal to 7 to 8 oz (depending on age of child and previous activities).

Avoid fruit and juice drinks after 4 PM.

Avoid caffeinated or carbonated beverages after 4 PM.

Offer only sips of water before bedtime if child wants a drink before going to bed.

Allow child to wear regular sleepwear and avoid use of diapers or pull-ups.

Consider using environmental modifications such as a nightlight in the bathroom or bedroom (move furniture so child's path to bathroom is not obstructed; avoid the top bunk of bunk beds).

Avoid scolding, threatening, embarrassing, or teasing child if a nighttime accident occurs.

Keep a calendar of wet and dry nights (e.g., use smiley or frowny faces and allow child to choose the appropriate "face" for the night).

Encourage parents to use positive reinforcements for dry nights.

Encourage the child to avoid holding urine during daytime.

If bedwetting occurs, have child participate in changing his or her bedclothing and personal clothing but explain that it is not a punishment for the accident.

Wake up child at a predetermined time every night and have him or her go to the bathroom; remain with child during the process and accompany child back to bed. (If bedwetting incidents occur, keep a diary of the times they occur based on the alarm and wake the child around that time.)

Encourage parents to maintain a positive attitude and to be patient with child.

Increase dietary fiber in child's diet.

Encourage child to have a bowel movement on a regular basis (constipation may contribute to enuresis).

Encourage liberal intake of water throughout the daytime.

Data from Drutz JE, Tu ND: Patient information: bedwetting in children, *UptoDate*, 2011, retrieved July 20, 2011, from http://www.uptodate.com/contents/patient-information-bedwetting-in-children?view=print; Elder JS: Voiding dysfunction. In Kliegman RM, Stanton BF, St. Geme JW, and others, editors: *Nelson textbook of pediatrics*, ed 19, Philadelphia, 2011, Saunders; Fera P, Santos Lelis MA, Quadros Glashan R, and others: Behavioral interventions in primary enuresis: experience report in Brazil, *Urol Nurs* 22(4):257–262, 2002; Katz ER, DeMaso D: Enuresis (bed-wetting). In Kliegman RM, Stanton BF, St. Geme JW, and others, editors: *Nelson textbook of pediatrics*, ed 19, Philadelphia, 2011, Saunders.

*These guidelines should be reserved for children ages 7 years and older.

Encopresis

Encopresis is the repeated voluntary or involuntary passage of feces of normal or near-normal consistency in places not appropriate for that purpose according to the individual's own sociocultural setting. The event must occur at least once per month for at least 3 months, and the chronologic or developmental age of the child must be at least 4 years. The fecal incontinence must not be caused by any physiologic effect, such as a laxative, or a general medical condition.

Primary encopresis is identified by age 4 years when a child has not achieved fecal continence. Secondary encopresis is fecal incontinence occurring in a child older than 4 years of age after a period of established fecal continence. The disorder is more common in boys than in girls.

One of the most common causes of encopresis is constipation, which may be precipitated by environmental change, such as having a new sibling, moving to a new house, changing schools, or even having to use new or unfamiliar toilet facilities. Chronic, severe constipation has a tendency to impair the usual movement and contractions of the colon, which can lead to fecal obstruction. Abnormalities in the digestive tract (e.g., Hirschsprung disease, anorectal lesions, malformations, rectal prolapse) and medical conditions such as hypothyroidism, hypokalemia, hypercalcemia, lead intoxication, myelomeningocele, cerebral palsy, muscular dystrophy, and irritable bowel syndrome are also associated with constipation, which can lead to encopresis. Voluntary retention of stool may also follow an incident of painful defecation (e.g., in a child with anal fissures). Involuntary retention may be produced by emotional problems caused by the encopresis, which sets up a fear–pain cycle and results in learned abnormal defecation patterns. Psychogenic encopresis, in which the soiling is caused by emotional problems, is often related to a disturbed mother–child relationship.

Normally, children and adolescents have one or two soft-formed stools per day. Children with soiling problems tend to form large-bore stools, which are painful to excrete. Therefore, they tend to avoid defecation and withhold stooling. Stool held in the rectum and sigmoid colon loses water and progressively hardens, which causes successively more painful bowel movements and a stretched rectal vault. Over time, the child will lose the urge to defecate on his or her own (Montgomery, 2008). A pain–retention–pain cycle is established. Many children have diarrhea or loose leakage in their clothing and pass small amounts of hard stool, which suggests leakage around an impaction.

Children may experience exacerbations with transitions in the school setting. Some reasons for developing retentive tendencies at this time are fear of using school bathrooms, a busy schedule, and the interruption of an established time schedule for bowel evacuation. Children may also react to stress with bowel dysfunction.

Therapeutic management consists of determining the cause of the soiling and using appropriate interventions to correct the problem. To determine the cause, perform a complete physical examination, including a rectal examination. Abdominal radiography may be done to determine the severity of impaction. Dietary modifications, stool softeners, and a toilet ritual that encourages the child to establish normal defecation are used. Fecal impaction is relieved by lubricants such as mineral oil; osmotic laxatives such as lactulose, sorbitol, or polyethylene glycol (PEG or MiraLax); and magnesium hydroxide. Customary dosages are usually insufficient. Mineral oil should be avoided in children who have dysphagia or vomiting to prevent aspiration. Dietary changes may be helpful, including elimination of milk and dairy products and consumption of increased amounts of high-fiber foods, such as fruits, vegetables, and cereals, as well as increased fluids (see Chapter 24). Behavior therapy may be indicated to eliminate any fear that has developed as a result of painful defecation. Psychotherapeutic intervention with the child and the family may become necessary.

Nursing Care Management

A thorough history of the soiling is essential, including when soiling began, how often it occurs and under what circumstances, and whether the child uses the toilet successfully at all. Because the parents and child are reluctant to volunteer information, direct questioning about the soiling is more successful.

Education regarding the physiology of normal defecation, toilet training as a developmental process, and the treatment outlined for the particular family is a prerequisite to a successful outcome. The regimen prescribed for stimulating elimination is explained to parents. Bowel retraining with mineral oil, a high-fiber diet, and a regular toileting routine is essential in treating encopresis or chronic constipation.

Encourage the child to sit on the toilet 10 to 15 minutes after meals for intervals of 10 to 15 minutes. Provide a quiet activity for the child and make sure the toilet is comfortable and in a nonthreatening environment. Placing a footstool below the feet may relax the abdomen and make the child more comfortable. Enemas may be needed for impactions in children with neurologic impairments and those with severe impactions, but long-term use prevents children from assuming responsibility for defecation. Initially, stool lubricants such as mineral oil may be given, but stimulant cathartics often cause abdominal cramps that can frighten children. Osmotic laxatives such as lactulose, sorbitol, or polyethylene glycol and magnesium hydroxide may be prescribed. Positive reinforcement such as giving stickers, praising the child, and awarding special activities may encourage the child to participate in the bowel regimen. Adequate fluid intake for the child is essential; many children play hard and forget to drink water or appropriate amounts of fluids, leading to a decrease in the formation of soft stool. Increase dietary fiber in meals and with fiber snacks that do not contain sugar (or <5 g). Many of the fast foods consumed by children, namely burgers, fries, and pizza, may also tend to be more constipating and should be minimized.

Family counseling is directed toward reassurance that most problems resolve successfully, although the child may have relapses during periods of stress, such as vacations or illness. If encopresis persists beyond occasional relapses, the condition needs to be reevaluated. Explain behavior modification techniques and assist the family with a plan suited to the particular situation (see Family-Centered Care box).

SCHOOL-AGE DISORDERS WITH BEHAVIORAL COMPONENTS

Attention-Deficit/Hyperactivity Disorder and Learning Disability

Attention-deficit/hyperactivity disorder (ADHD) refers to developmentally inappropriate degrees of inattention, impulsiveness, and hyperactivity. To be diagnosed as ADHD, the symptoms must have been present in children 4 to 18 years of age and must be present in more than one major setting (American Academy of Pediatrics [AAP], Clinical Practice Guideline, 2011). In addition, the persistence of developmentally inappropriate and marked inattention must not be a symptom of another disorder (American Psychiatric Association [APA],

2000). A learning disability (LD) refers to a heterogeneous group of disorders manifested by significant difficulties in the acquisition and use of listening, speaking, reading, writing, reasoning, or mathematic skills.

Learning disabilities and ADHD affect every aspect of the child's life but are most obvious in the classroom. Early identification of affected children is important because the characteristics of these disorders significantly interfere with the normal course of emotional and psychologic development. Many children develop maladaptive behavior patterns that impede psychosocial adjustment while they try to cope with cognitive dysfunction. Their behavior evokes negative responses from others, and repeated exposure to negative feedback adversely affects their self-concept. The characteristics of ADHD affect the child's written and adaptive skills, social status, and self-esteem (Cunningham and Jensen, 2011; Myers, Eisenhauer, and Ryan, 2003).

Diagnostic Evaluation

The behaviors exhibited by children with ADHD are not unusual. The difference lies in the quality of motor activity and developmentally inappropriate inattention, impulsivity, and hyperactivity that children display. The manifestations may be numerous or few, mild or severe, and vary with the child's developmental level. Any given child will not have every manifestation that is characteristic of the syndrome, and the degree of severity is highly variable. Mild manifestations of the symptoms may not be apparent in some educational and family environments, but severe symptomatology will be recognizable in most environments. Every child with ADHD is different from all other children with ADHD. The clinical manifestations of ADHD are outlined in Box 17-2.

Most behavioral manifestations are apparent at an early age, but the LDs may not become evident until the child enters school. The disorder is unpredictable; it may remit spontaneously at any age, and the number of years that a child will require treatment is unknown.

A major clinical manifestation is distractibility. The stimuli may come from external sources or internal sources. Children frequently demonstrate immaturity relative to chronologic age. Selective attention is often seen in which the child has difficulty attending to "nonpreferred" tasks, such as completing chores or finishing homework. The child may not consider the consequences of behavior, may take excessive physical risks (often beginning early in life), and may demonstrate inappropriate social skills.

Children with ADHD demonstrate one of three subtypes (APA, 2000).

1. **Combined type**—Six (or more) symptoms of inattention and six (or more) symptoms of hyperactivity-impulsivity have persisted for at least 6 months. Most children and adolescents with the disorder have the combined type.

2. **Predominantly inattentive type**—Six (or more) symptoms of inattention (but fewer than six symptoms of hyperactivity-impulsivity) have persisted for at least 6 months.

3. **Predominantly hyperactive-impulsive type**—Six (or more) symptoms of hyperactivity-impulsivity (but fewer than six symptoms of inattention) have persisted for at least 6 months. Inattention may often still be a significant clinical feature in such cases.

The diagnosis is established based on the APA's (2000) *Diagnostic and Statistical Manual of Mental Disorders (DSM-IV-TR)* characteristics and a thorough evaluation. It is important to emphasize the need for a complete and thorough multidisciplinary evaluation of the child, incorporating the efforts of the pediatrician (often a developmental pediatrician or pediatric neurologist), psychologist, pediatric nurse, classroom teacher, reading and math specialist, special education

---

BOX 17-2 DIAGNOSTIC CRITERIA FOR ATTENTION-DEFICIT/ HYPERACTIVITY DISORDER

A. Either (1) or (2):

(1) six (or more) of the following symptoms of **inattention** have persisted for at least 6 months to a degree that is maladaptive and inconsistent with developmental level:

(a) often fails to give close attention to details or makes careless mistakes in schoolwork, work, or other activities

(b) often has difficulty sustaining attention in tasks or play activities

(c) often does not seem to listen when spoken to directly

(d) often does not follow through on instructions and fails to finish school work, chores, or duties in the workplace (not due to oppositional behavior or failure to understand instructions)

(e) often has difficulty organizing tasks and activities

(f) often avoids, dislikes, or is reluctant to engage in tasks that require sustained mental effort (such as schoolwork or homework)

(g) often loses things necessary for tasks or activities (e.g., toys, school assignments, pencils, books, or tools)

(h) is often easily distracted by extraneous stimuli

(i) is often forgetful in daily activities

(2) six (or more) of the following symptoms of **hyperactivity-impulsivity** have persisted for at least 6 months to a degree that is maladaptive and inconsistent with developmental level:

Hyperactivity

(a) often fidgets with hands or feet or squirms in seat

(b) often leaves seat in classroom or in other situations in which remaining seated is expected

(c) often runs about or climbs excessively in situations in which it is inappropriate (in adolescents or adults, may be limited to subjective feelings of restlessness)

(d) often has difficulty playing or engaging in leisure activities quietly

(e) is often "on the go" or often acts as if "driven by a motor"

(f) often talks excessively

Impulsivity

(g) often blurts out answers before questions have been completed

(h) often has difficulty awaiting turn

(i) often interrupts or intrudes on others (e.g., butts into conversations or games)

B. Some hyperactive-impulsive or inattentive symptoms that caused impairment were present before age 7 years.

C. Some impairment from the symptoms is present in two or more settings (e.g., at school [or work] and at home).

D. There must be clear evidence of clinically significant impairment in social, academic, or occupational functioning.

E. The symptoms do not occur exclusively during the course of a Pervasive Developmental Disorder, Schizophrenia, or other Psychotic Disorder and are not better accounted for by another mental disorder (e.g., Mood Disorder, Anxiety Disorder, Dissociative Disorders, or a Personality Disorder).

From American Psychiatric Association: *Diagnostic and statistical manual of mental disorders*, ed 4, text rev (DSM-IV TR), Washington, DC, 2000, Author.

---

teacher, possibly a speech therapist, and the child's parents. The clinicians and professionals must first determine whether the child's behavior is age appropriate or truly problematic.

A history, both medical and developmental, and a description of the child's behavior should be obtained from as many observers of the child as possible, especially the parents and teachers, along with the health professionals involved. Descriptions of the child's behavior in home and school situations should be included. In obtaining descriptive material, the interviewer must question the observers carefully because some persons, especially parents, may be so concerned with gross behaviors that they overlook less distressing but equally important symptoms. For example, parents may report a "colicky" infant, a child who began to run soon after walking, a toddler who was compelled to touch everything in sight, and a child who resisted sleep until exhausted. A pregnancy and birth history may provide clues to a situation that might have produced an episode of hypoxia.

A physical examination, including vision and hearing screening and a detailed neurologic evaluation, will help rule out any severe neurologic disorders. Psychologic testing, especially projective tests, is valuable in identifying visual-perceptual difficulties, problems with spatial organization, and other phenomena that suggest cortical or diencephalic involvement, and it helps to identify the child's intelligence and achievement levels.

Behavioral checklists and adaptive scales are also helpful in measuring social adaptive functioning in children with ADHD. Psychiatric disorders, medical problems, and traumatic experiences are ruled out, including lead poisoning, seizures, partial hearing loss, psychosis, and witnessing of sexual activity or violence.

Therapeutic Management

Management of the child with ADHD usually involves multiple approaches that include family education and counseling, medication, proper classroom placement, environmental manipulation, and behavioral therapy or psychotherapy for the child. Interventions for children with LD are primarily educational.

Pharmacologic Therapy. The most frequently used medications are the psychostimulants: methylphenidate hydrochloride (Ritalin) and dextroamphetamine sulfate (Dexedrine). The majority of patients with ADHD are treated with the psychostimulant methylphenidate (AAP, Clinical Practice Guideline, 2011). Psychostimulants cause an increase in dopamine and norepinephrine levels that leads to stimulation of the inhibitory system of the central nervous system (CNS). Children are given a small dosage initially, and the dosage is gradually increased until the desired response is achieved. Children who receive stimulants should be monitored carefully for the development of tics during initial treatment, and stimulants should be avoided in children who have a history of ticlike behaviors, a family history of Tourette syndrome (TS), or ADHD combined with TS.

The stimulant dextroamphetamine may be used in children younger than 6 years of age to treat ADHD, but evidence of its safety and efficacy in young children and adolescents has been questioned. Lisdexamfetamine (Vyvanse) reportedly has less substance abuse potential than dextroamphetamine; the former is only metabolized to dextroamphetamine after ingestion, thus it may be more suitable for children and adolescents who may abuse dextroamphetamine (AAP, Clinical Practrice Guideline, 2011). Other medications include the mixed amphetamine salts (Adderall) which are available in extended release form. In some cases a nonstimulant may be added to the medication regimen with a stimulant to achieve optimal therapeutic effects. Many of the stimulant drugs are available in short-acting and long-acting form to better meet the child's need for therapeutic management. An additional consideration in the administration of medications is the child's ability to swallow pills; since some come in capsule form they can be sprinkled on applesauce (Ryan-Krause, 2011).

Other nonstimulant medications which are recommended by the AAP, Clinical Practice Guideline (2011) include the selective norepinephrine reuptake inhibitor atomoxitine (Strattera) and the selective

🔍 CRITICAL THINKING CASE STUDY

Attention-Deficit/Hyperactivity Disorder

Johnnie, age 8 years, is a third grader who was recently diagnosed with ADHD. He has been taking the drug methylphenidate (Ritalin) for about 1 month. In the short time that Johnnie has been taking this medication, his math teacher has noticed an improvement in his performance in math class. He is receiving a grade of B instead of his previous grades of D on most math quizzes. The math teacher has also noted that Johnnie is socializing more with his classmates and that he now has a "best friend" in math class. Johnnie usually receives his methylphenidate from the school nurse before lunch. Yesterday Johnnie's mother told the school nurse that he has not eaten his lunch for the past week and that he is not hungry.

What important issues regarding Johnnie's medication should the nurse consider in her discussions with Johnnie's mother?

Questions

1. Evidence—Is there sufficient evidence to draw conclusions about Johnnie's medication from his behavior?
2. Assumptions—Describe some underlying assumptions about the following:
   a. Pharmacologic action of methylphenidate in ADHD
   b. Side effects of methylphenidate
   c. Management of side effects
3. What implications for nursing care can be drawn at this time?
4. Does the evidence objectively support your conclusion?

ADHD, Attention-deficit/hyperactivity disorder.

---

alpha adrenergic agonists—guanfacine (Tenex, Intuniv) and clonidine. Both of these are available in extended release form but are reported to have limited evidence of their efficacy and safety in preschool children with ADHD (AAP, Clinical Practice Guideline, 2011).

It is important to remember that these medications are not prescribed based on the child's weight (except atomoxitine), but on resolution of the symptoms; therefore, it is important to follow the child closely and evaluate for therapeutic effects as well as potential side effects. Regularly scheduled reevaluation of the child is essential with all of these medications to determine medication effectiveness, detect and evaluate any side effects, monitor development and health status (especially growth and blood pressure), and assess family interaction (see Critical Thinking Case Study box). Children on stimulant drugs for ADHD should undergo an extensive physical examination and history, including a family history of cardiac disease or cardiac problems. Currently, electrocardiography screening is only recommended for children with ADHD taking stimulant drugs who have a close member with a history of cardiac arrhythmia or structural heart defect (Perrin, Friedman, Knilans, and others, 2008). Medication therapy alone is not adequate to manage the child's symptoms, and other treatment modalities such as behavioral therapy should also be utilized for successful treatment.

Behavioral Therapy. Behavioral therapy focuses on the prevention of undesired behavior. The nurse should help families identify new appropriate contingencies and reward systems to meet the child's developing needs. They may also receive instruction in effective parenting skills, such as delivering positive reinforcement, rewarding small increments of desired behaviors, and providing age-appropriate consequences (e.g., time-out, response cost). Use of organizational charts for completing self-care activities and use of a word processor instead of manually writing assignments are emphasized. Through collaborative teamwork, parents learn techniques to help the child become more successful at home and in school.

Counseling or therapy can be helpful for children who demonstrate signs of anxiety or depression. Therapy can help children develop healthier self-esteem and practice problem-solving strategies. Adolescents may benefit from group work focusing on social skill development. Parents of children with ADHD can face a lot of stress, and therapy may be indicated for parents and other family members.

Multimodal Treatment. The results of several studies suggest that multimodal treatment involving the use of pharmacotherapy and behavioral intervention as well as close follow-up and feedback from school personnel is more effective than intensive behavioral treatment alone (Selekman, 2010).

Environmental Manipulation. Encourage families to learn how to modify the environment to allow the child to be more successful. Consistency is especially important for children with ADHD. Consistency between families and teachers in terms of reinforcing the same goals is essential. Fostering improved organizational skills requires a more highly structured environment than most children need. Children should be encouraged to make more appropriate choices and to take responsibility for their actions.

Other helpful interventions include teaching parents how to make organizational charts (e.g., listing all activities that must be performed before leaving for school) and decrease distractions in the environment while the child is completing homework (e.g., turning off the television, having a consistent study area equipped with needed supplies) and helping parents to understand ways to model positive behaviors and problem solving. The focus is on strategies to help the child succeed and cope with deficits while emphasizing strengths.

Appropriate Classroom Placement. Children with ADHD need an orderly, predictable, and consistent classroom environment with clear and consistent rules. Homework and classroom assignments may need to be reduced, and more time may need to be allotted for tests to allow the child to complete the task. Verbal instructions should be accompanied by visual references such as written instructions on the blackboard. Schedules may need to be arranged so that academic subjects are taught in the morning when the child is experiencing the effects of the morning dose of medication. Low-interest and high-interest classroom activities should be intermingled to maintain the child's attention and interest. Regular and frequent breaks in activity are helpful because sitting in one place for an extended time may be difficult. Computers are helpful for children who have difficulty with writing (dysgraphia) and fine motor skills; in such children, handwriting will *not* improve. They need to find alternatives to physical competition that requires coordination of movement.

If the child has an LD, special training activities may be accomplished in self-contained classes limited to six to eight children, in special resource rooms with equipment and teaching teams, by mobile consultants who move from room to room to provide assistance to teachers and children, and in special first-grade programs in which high-risk children receive special attention to prevent or reduce the need for services as they progress. The purpose of programs for children with LDs is to assist them toward more successful achievement, personal adjustment, and retention in the regular classroom. Additional behavioral, educational, and environmental strategies for children and adolescents with ADHD are listed in the Selekman (2010) reference.

Growth and Development. Children with ADHD who are taking stimulant medications need to be assessed for the achievement of appropriate growth and development milestones at least every 6 months (Pliszka and AACAP Work Group, 2007; Selekman, 2010).

FAMILY-CENTERED CARE
A Child's Perception of Taking Ritalin at School

I feel embarrassed by having to leave class early to go take my medication. The other kids always ask where I'm going and why. It would be better if we could leave class at the same time as everyone else, go take the medication, and then just be a little late to the next class. Students don't ask why people are late for class, only why they leave early. It also bothers me when kids tell other kids, "Go take a pill" and other mean things just because someone is acting up.

What could nurses and teachers do to help? Most kids do not understand why other kids have to take medication. I think it would help if a nurse or teacher talked with the other kids and explained why some children take the medication and how ADHD affects people. That way there would be more understanding among all the kids.

—Marissa White, age 16 years

The side effects of these drugs often include appetite suppression, nausea, and vomiting; suppression of growth acceleration and sleep disturbances have also been recorded in children taking stimulant drugs (Selekman, 2010).

Prognosis. With appropriate intervention, ADHD is relatively stable through early adolescence for most children. Some children experience decreased symptoms during late adolescence and adulthood, but a significant number of these children carry their symptoms into adulthood. The goal for children with LDs is to help them identify their areas of weakness and learn to compensate for them.

Nursing Care Management

Nurses, especially school nurses, are active participants in all aspects of management of children with ADHD and LDs. Nurses in the community work with families and school personnel on a long-term basis to help plan and implement therapeutic regimens and to evaluate the effectiveness of therapy. They coordinate services and serve as a liaison between health and education professionals directly involved in the child's therapy program. School nurses understand the child's special needs and work with teachers (see Family-Centered Care box). Nurses in any setting (community, school, hospital, practitioner's office) provide support and guidance to children and families during the difficult period of the child's growing up with a disabling condition.

Management begins with an explanation to the parents and the child about the diagnosis, including the nature of the problem and the practitioner's concept of the underlying CNS basis for the disorder. Most parents are confused and feel some measure of guilt. To some parents, a diagnosis of ADHD is confirmation of the fear that their child has some irreversible, serious disease; to others, it is a relief. All need the opportunity to vent their feelings and suspicions. A common complaint of parents is that health professionals do not listen to what they have to say about their children. The health professional should focus on building self-esteem by encouraging the family to focus on developing their child's strengths (e.g., sport, hobbies, and talents) rather than just weaknesses (Jellinek, 2008).

Parents need to be informed of the possible side effects of medications. The psychostimulants have similar side effects that include weight loss, abdominal pain, headaches, decreased appetite, sleeplessness, increased crying and irritability, nervous stimulation, and cardiovascular stimulation. The use of caffeine decreases the efficacy of these drugs, and insulin requirements may also be altered. If decreased appetite is a concern, giving the psychostimulants with or after meals rather than before, encouraging consumption of nutritious snacks in the evening when the effects of the medication are decreasing, and serving frequent small meals with healthy "on the go" snacks are helpful interventions. Sleeplessness is reduced by administering medication early in the day.

Children and adolescents with ADHD are at increased risk for accidents and unintentional injuries because of their impulsivity and decreased judgment of dangerous activities. Therefore, measures should be taken to protect such children from personal injury (Selekman, 2010).

Children taking tricyclic antidepressants display a dramatic increase in the incidence of dental caries. The marked anticholinergic action of the drugs increases saliva viscosity and produces a dry mouth. Emphasis on rigorous dental hygiene, conscientious home fluoride treatments, regular visits to the dentist, limited intake of refined carbohydrates, and use of artificial saliva is an important nursing function. The child should drink plenty of fluids and be well hydrated.

Parents often express concern that their children will become addicted to the psychostimulants or the antidepressant drugs. Both types of drugs have the potential for abuse, and all children taking these drugs should be monitored closely for psychologic dependence, tolerance, depression, and other adverse behavior changes or idiosyncratic effects. Most children with ADHD are not interested in abusing their drugs because the effect of the drugs in these children is opposite that produced in normal individuals. However, caution parents to keep these drugs safely stored away from young children who may inadvertently ingest them and adolescents who may abuse these drugs.

Parents need information about the prognosis and an understanding of the treatment plan. The greater their understanding of the disorder and its effects, the more likely they will be to carry out the recommended program of therapy. It is important that they understand that the therapy is not necessarily a panacea and that it will extend over a long period. This has particular significance for changes they need to make in environmental management. Reading material to help the child and family can be obtained from a variety of sources.

Posttraumatic Stress Disorder

Posttraumatic stress disorder (PTSD) refers to the development of characteristic symptoms after exposure to an extremely traumatic experience or catastrophic event. The traumatic experience is typically life threatening to oneself or a significant other and may involve grotesque mutilation or death, serious injury, or physical coercion (e.g., an assault, a natural disaster, sexual abuse, witnessing violence). It is important to note that PTSD is not limited to children who have lived in "war-torn" countries. Events such as automobile, school, or recreational accidents and bullying have also been identified as causes of PTSD. The characteristic symptoms are persistent reexperiencing of the traumatic event, avoidance of stimuli associated with the event or trauma, numbing of general responsiveness, and increased arousal.

Acute PTSD is diagnosed if the symptoms are present after the first month but before the third month after the initial traumatic event. Acute stress disorder may also occur with acute PTSD. Chronic PTSD is diagnosed if the symptoms persist beyond 3 months (Cohen and AACAP Work Group on Quality Issues, 2010).

The response to the event takes place in three stages. The **initial response** involves intense arousal, which usually lasts for a few minutes to 1 or 2 hours. The stress hormones are at the maximum as the individual prepares for "fight or flight." A prolonged arousal phase may indicate psychosis.

The second phase, which lasts approximately 2 weeks, is one in which defense mechanisms are mobilized. It is a period of calm in which the event appears to have produced no impression. The child feels numb, and stress hormone secretion is absent. Defense mechanisms are less adaptive to specific situations and may not be what the situation demands. Denial that anything is wrong is a frequently observed defense mechanism.

The third phase is one of coping and consciously directed inquiry, which normally extends over 2 to 3 months. The victims want to know what happened and appear to be getting worse when actually they are getting better. Numerous psychologic symptoms, such as depression, repetitive phenomena, phobic symptoms, anxiety, and conversion reactions, may be present. Children frequently display repetitive actions. They play out the situation over and over again in an attempt to come to terms with their fear. Flashbacks are common. This phase can be self-perpetuating, and a prolonged reaction can develop into an obsession with the traumatic event. Some traumatic effects remain indefinitely.

Trauma-focused psychotherapy is considered first-line therapy, and selective serotonin reuptake inhibitor (SSRI) drugs may be considered on an individual basis. Rebirthing therapies or restrictive treatments that bind or withhold water or food are not recommended (Cohen and AACAP Work Group on Quality Issues, 2010). A practice parameter for the assessment and management of PTSD in children and adolescents is published elsewhere (Cohen and AACAP Work Group on Quality Issues, 2010).

Nursing Care Management

Children need to deal with all traumatic events. Their reactions depend heavily on their social environment and the way in which their caretaking adults react to the event. In the second phase of PTSD, the appropriateness of the defense mechanism must be assessed, and children must be assisted in application of their defense. If children do not engage in some catharsis or if their defense phase is prolonged, they need referral for special psychologic help.

Coping is a learned response, and children in the third phase can be helped to deal with their fear. Children usually are willing to accept reasoning. Those who are assisted in their catharsis and allowed expression will survive without serious lasting effects. They should be encouraged to play out the stress and to discuss their feelings about the event. If they are unable to do this, they may become obsessed with the traumatic event and require professional help. Conversion reactions are common obsessive behaviors in children with PTSD.

Children need professional help if any of the phases of PTSD are prolonged. Boys tend to have a prolonged defense phase more often than girls. Occasionally, the event will be unrecognized, and the affected child will engage in what is considered to be unusual behavior. Children exhibiting any sudden change in behavior need to be assessed for a traumatic event. When the change in behavior is traced to a traumatic event, treatment can be implemented.

Nurses in settings such as the emergency department, pediatric intensive care unit, and neonatal intensive care unit should also recognize that parents of children who experience a traumatic acute trauma, life-threatening illness, or chronic illness may experience symptoms of PTSD; PTSD may occur more often in mothers than in fathers; however, some evidence indicates that fathers may have delayed symptoms (Mowery, 2011). Appropriate nursing interventions include allowing parents to discuss their feelings about the incident or threat (to themselves or their children), encourage support from other parents in similar situations, avoid interjecting one's own experience or feelings, and evaluate the child's reaction to the parents' symptoms (Mowery, 2011).

School Phobia

Children, other than beginning students, who resist going to school or who demonstrate extreme reluctance to attend school for a sustained period as a result of severe anxiety or fear of school-related experiences are said to have school phobia. The terms *school refusal* and *school avoidance* are also used to describe this behavior. School phobia occurs in children of all ages, but it is more common in children 10 years of age and older. School avoidance behaviors occur in both boys and girls and in children from all socioeconomic levels.

Anxiety that frequently verges on panic is a constant manifestation, and children can develop symptoms as a protective mechanism to keep them from facing the situation that distresses them. Physical symptoms are prominent and may affect any part of the body; they include anorexia, nausea, vomiting, diarrhea, dizziness, headache, leg pains, and abdominal pains. Children may even develop a low-grade fever. A striking feature of school phobia is the prompt subsiding of symptoms when it is evident that the child can remain at home. Another significant observation is absence of symptoms on weekends and holidays unless they are related to other places such as Sunday school or parties. Occasional mild reluctance to attend school is common among schoolchildren, but if the fear continues for longer than a few days, it must be considered a serious problem.

The onset is usually sudden and precipitated by a school-related incident. By taking a careful history, nurses find out whether a poor attendance record is caused by trivial reasons.

Nursing Care Management

Treatment for school phobia depends on the cause. The primary goal is to return the child to school. The longer a child is permitted to stay out of school, the more difficult it is for the child to reenter. Parents must be convinced gently but firmly that immediate return is essential and that it is their responsibility to insist on school attendance.

A school reentry protocol may be necessary for the child with severe symptoms. In reentry programs, the child role-plays routines involved in getting ready for school and that occur at school. Relaxation techniques are also used. The child usually goes to school initially for a half day and then progresses to a full day. Often the school nurse is asked to provide support to the parents and the teacher during the reentry process. If the problem persists, professional help is recommended.

Bullying

Bullying is a form of aggression wherein a person asserts power over another who is considered weaker through social, emotional, and physical means. The consequences of bullying include depression, long-term psychopathology, suicidality, psychosomatic symptoms, and psychoses. Bullying involves aggression in which the behavior is intended to harm or embarrass the victim, it occurs repeatedly over time, and there is an imbalance of power with the bully exerting dominance over the victim (Liu and Graves, 2011). The behavior may be carried out by one person or several who isolate the victim for purposes of harming and embarrassing through an imbalance of power. Bullying may be perceived by some as a normal social developmental step in childhood and in some cases the bully may perceive the behavior as being fun rather than harmful. Some may view bullying with a "boys will be boys" attitude and ignore the behavior. Research has shown that bullying occurs more often in boys although girls may also be involved in what is called *relational bullying*, which is a more subtle and indirect form of bullying. Bullying is more common in middle school than in high school children (Powell and Ladd, 2010; CDC, 2011a).

Most bullying occurs in and around the school; therefore, there has been more emphasis on recognizing and dealing with the behaviors in schools.* Interventions should include recognition of the behavior in both the bully and the victim and protection of the victim as well as stopping the behavior altogether. In order to be effective, behavioral changes from the bully and social changes in the school environment with the assistance of parents and adults in the school should occur. The school nurse and community nurse are likely to come in contact with victims and bullies alike; the practitioner may also be involved in caring for the physical and emotional health of the victim. School and community-lead programs to heighten awareness of the consequences of bullying are reported to have been ineffective in stopping bullying; however, further studies are needed (Liu and Graves, 2011).

Conversion Reaction

Conversion reaction, also known as hysteria, hysterical conversion reaction, and childhood hysteria, is a psychophysiologic disorder with a sudden onset that can usually be traced to a precipitating environmental event. The disorder is observed with equal frequency in both sexes in childhood, but affected girls outnumber affected boys during adolescence. The manifestations involve primarily the voluntary musculature and special senses and include abdominal pain, fainting, pseudoseizures, paralysis, headaches, and visual field restriction. Once considered rare in childhood, the disorder occurs more frequently than has generally been acknowledged. The most commonly observed symptom is seizure activity, which can be differentiated from symptoms of neurogenic origin by formal tests, the most useful of which is normal electroencephalogram findings.

Many children with conversion reaction have experienced a major family crisis before the onset of symptoms, such as loss of a parent or other significant person through death, divorce, or moving. The families of children with conversion reaction characteristically display problems in communication and depression or hypochondriasis in a parent.

Educating the child and family regarding the cause of emotional stresses or feelings and alternative approaches to coping with stress may alleviate the child's symptoms. If deep personality problems are evident, psychiatric consultation is indicated. Nursing care is similar to that for the child with recurrent abdominal pain (see also Chapter 24).

Childhood Depression

Depression in childhood is often difficult to detect because children may be unable to express their feelings and tend to act out their problems and concerns. Some states of depression are temporary, such as acute depression precipitated by a traumatic event. The event might include a period of hospitalization; loss of a parent through death or separation; or loss of a significant relationship with something (a pet), a person (a friend, significant other, or family member), or a place (move from a familiar home, neighborhood, or city). Children with depression may demonstrate a variety of behaviors; symptoms must be present for one year to establish the diagnosis of major depressive disorder in children and adolescents (Calles, 2007) (Box 17-3). Most

---

*Resources on bullying include the following: www.eyesonbullying.org and http://webcast.hrsa.gov/archives/mchb/director/112009/200911Bully.pdf.

BOX 17-3   CHARACTERISTICS OF CHILDREN WITH DEPRESSION

Behavior

Predominantly sad facial expression with absence or diminished range of affective response

Solitary play or work; tendency to be alone; disinterest in play

Withdrawal from previously enjoyed activities and relationships

Lowered grades in school; lack of interest in doing homework or achieving in school

Diminished motor activity; tiredness, fatigue

Tearfulness or crying; irritability

Dependent and clinging or aggressive and disruptive

Internal States

Utterance of statements reflecting lowered self-esteem, sense of hopelessness, or guilt

Suicidal ideations

Physiology

Constipation

Nonspecific complaints of not feeling well

Change in appetite resulting in weight loss or gain

Alterations in sleeping pattern, sleeplessness, or hypersomnia

---

responses in children are not sustained and can be modified with social and family support.

More serious and less common are the depressive responses to more chronic stress and loss. These are frequently observed in children with chronic illness or disability. There is no apparent precipitating event, but there is often a history of frequent disruptions in important relationships. A history of depressive illness in one or both parents during the child's lifetime is also common. Manifestations in the child are similar to those observed in acute reactions, but they occur more frequently and extend over a longer period.

Nursing Care Management

Depressed children are managed by a health team that is especially prepared in the care of children with mental health disorders. Treatment is highly individualized and undertaken in the least restrictive environment. Suicidal children are admitted to the hospital for protection if the family is unable to provide constant monitoring. Pharmacotherapy may involve TCAs or SSRIs such as fluoxetine, trazodone (Desyrel), sertraline, and paroxetine (Paxil), as well as bupropion (Wellbutrin) and venlafaxine (Effexor). There have been reports that antidepressant medications may cause increased suicidal thinking and behaviors in pediatric patients. This prompted the U.S. Food and Drug Administration (FDA) to require black box drug labeling detailing potential suicide-related risks for pediatric patients; this warning was updated, and it was noted that the risk of suicide was highest among adolescents and young adults ages 18 to 24 years. Some data suggest that the suicide rate among adolescents on therapeutic doses of SSRIs was lower than among those who were not being treated with antidepressant medication (Gibbons, Hur, Bhaumik, and others, 2006). However, the issue remains controversial because study results are mixed, and further studies are needed (Walter and DeMaso, 2011). Patients taking SSRIs should be followed closely (once a week) for the first 4 weeks of therapy before a dose increase is made; thereafter it is recommended that follow-up occur biweekly and children and

Critical Thinking Exercise—Depression

adolescents with a risk for suicidality be referred for specialized treatment (Walter and DeMaso, 2011).

Nurses should be aware that depression is a problem that can be easily overlooked in children and one that can interrupt normal growth and development. Recognizing depression and suicidal tendencies in depressed adolescents and making appropriate referrals are important nursing functions. Identification of a depressed child requires a careful history (health, growth and development, social and family health); interviews with the child; and observations by the nurse, parents, and teachers. If antidepressants are prescribed, the child and family need to know that antidepressants must be at a therapeutic level for 2 to 4 weeks to achieve a beneficial effect. The child and family also need to monitor the child for side effects of the specific drug prescribed and any interactions with other drugs (see also Suicide, p. 530).

Childhood Schizophrenia

Childhood schizophrenia is a term that refers to severe deviations in ego functioning and is generally reserved for psychotic disorders that appear in children younger than 15 years of age. Childhood schizophrenia is a rare illness among children in the general population; among children with mental illness, only about 2 in every 1000 have childhood schizophrenia.

Childhood schizophrenia is characterized by symptoms that last for at least 6 months and that seriously interfere with the child's functioning in school, at home, or in other social situations. The basic disturbance is a lack of contact with reality and the subsequent development of a world of the child's own. Other areas of development that may be impaired include cognition, perception, emotion, language, and physical motor control. The most common manifestations involve language disturbances, impaired interpersonal relationships, and inappropriate affect (outward expression of emotion). Treatment involves management of the symptoms, prevention of relapse, and social and occupational rehabilitation of the young person. Antipsychotic drugs that may be used include haloperidol, clozapine, chlorpromazine, olanzapine, quetiapine fumarate, and risperidone. Family interventions and family therapy often result in improvements in psychotic symptoms, thought disorders, and social functioning among children with schizophrenia.

Nursing Care Management

Nursing of psychotic children is a highly specialized area. However, nurses should be alert to the possibility that schizophrenia can occur in children and refer children who consistently demonstrate abnormal behavior to a psychiatrist for evaluation. In addition, nurses need to teach family members of children taking antipsychotic drugs to observe for possible side effects. Common side effects of these drugs include dizziness; drowsiness; tachycardia; hypotension; and extrapyramidal effects, such as abnormal movements and seizures.

HEALTH PROBLEMS OF ADOLESCENTS
ALTERED GROWTH AND MATURATION

The absence of physical or sexual maturation at a time when other children are experiencing positive evidence of sexual development and its associated spurt in growth and physical strength is an important concern to both the parents and their affected child. In most instances, the delay in development is a simple physiologic or constitutional delay of growth and puberty (Nwosu and Lee, 2008) that represents one end of the normal genetically influenced variation of pubertal growth. These adolescents go through a delayed but normal puberty and finally catch up in their late teens with their more rapidly

developing age mates. Growth delay may be proportionate or disproportionate; both require careful evaluation by a multidisciplinary team. Less benign causes of delayed development may be endocrine disorders such as growth hormone deficiency, a disease process such as human immunodeficiency virus (HIV) or chronic malabsorption, or a chromosomal abnormality such as Turner syndrome. Additional causes of delayed development include asthma, cystic fibrosis, malabsorption syndromes, cardiac anomalies, and chronic renal conditions. Skeletal disorders that affect growth in stature are those described as dwarfism. Most disorders are caused by congenital defects, such as achondroplasia, and by inborn errors of metabolism such as Hurler syndrome or Hunter syndrome.

The rate of maturation is important during the school years, but at puberty, it assumes significant proportions to both teens and their parents. Girls and boys who lag behind their peers in physical maturation are painfully aware of their difference in growth. Adolescent girls with delayed maturation may feel out of place among companions whose hips and breasts are developing, feel cheated if they have not yet menstruated, and be frightened about being abnormal. Adolescent boys with delayed maturation may feel inferior and small compared with their more muscular companions with whom they can no longer compete physically. Serial measurements of height and weight, as well as other anthropometric data, are obtained and plotted on standard growth charts to determine the pattern of growth and to compare the individual child with the norms for his or her age group (see Appendix A). When children are in the extremes of height ranges, it is important to compare their height with those of their parents.

Psychosocial, or deprivation dwarfism (also known as psychosocial failure to thrive or psychosocial short stature) is a stress-induced growth failure. It is defined as growth restriction, usually below the third percentile, in children older than 2 years of age that is caused by environmental (emotional) stress and is associated with a marked delay in physical growth, delayed developmental skills, and immature behavior. When these children are removed from the deprived environment, their growth proceeds at a normal or increased rate.

Management of growth delay in childhood and adolescence includes continued medical observation, attention to general health and nutrition, and psychologic support. Growth hormone is often recommended to treat growth hormone deficiency (see Hypopituitarism, Chapter 29).

Nursing Care Management

Deviation from the normal course of puberty is a significant concern for affected adolescents. For some adolescents, this concern assumes monumental proportions. Many cases of delayed development are caused by simple constitutional delay of growth and puberty, and the child can be assured that normal development will eventually take place.

One difficulty related to a size that is incongruent with chronologic and mental age is the manner in which others relate to the child. People often respond to children with short stature as though they were younger than their age. Consequently, these children may react with babyish or juvenile behavior, thus establishing a circular pattern of behavior and response. Conversely, children who are tall or physically advanced for their age are frequently treated as though they were more advanced than their years. They are often considered clumsy, cognitively delayed, or immature when they perform according to the normal behavioral expectations for their age.

Listening to distressed adolescents and conveying interest and concern are important interventions. Slowly maturing adolescents

TABLE 17-1 COMMON SEX CHROMOSOME DISORDERS

SYNDROME	CHROMOSOMAL NOTATION	PHENOTYPE	FREQUENCY (LIVE BIRTHS)	CLINICAL MANIFESTATIONS
Turner	45,X or 45,XO	Female	1 : 10,000 female births	Short stature; webbed neck; low posterior hairline; shield-shaped chest with widely spaced nipples; sterile; no development of secondary sex characteristics; urinary tract abnormalities; normal intellectual development
Triple X, or superfemale	47,XXX (can also be 48,XXXX or 49,XXXXX)	Female	1 : 1000 female births	Normal female characteristics; usually tall; variable mental capacity and behavior; at risk for impaired language, learning difficulties; fertile
Jacob, XYY male	47,XYY (can also be 48,XYYY or mosaic)	Male	1 : 1000 male births	Usually normal sexual development; tendency to be tall with long head; poor coordination; offspring chromosomally normal; previously thought to have aggressive tendencies, but well-controlled studies refuted this hypothesis
Klinefelter	47,XXY (or 48,XXYY, 48,XXXY, 49,XXXXY, and so on, mosaics)	Male	1 : 1000 male births	Tall with long legs; hypogenitalism; sterile; male secondary sex characteristics may be deficient; may demonstrate aberrant behavior; may have learning disabilities; 80% have gynecomastia

need support and reassurance that they are unique individuals who have an important contribution to society that is equally as important as that of their peers. Counseling and therapy are individualized for each youth. Encouraging these children to focus on the positive aspects of their bodies and personalities and to adopt sound health practices and practice good grooming fosters a more positive self-image.

Sex Chromosome Abnormalities

Most sex chromosome abnormalities are caused by an alteration in sex chromosome number (Table 17-1). The majority of these conditions are caused by nondisjunction. An alteration in the number of sex chromosomes usually does not produce the profound defects that are associated with the autosomal disorders (trisomies). Intelligence may be normal or low normal, or the child may have some LDs. Moderate or severe cognitive impairment is less common.

Turner Syndrome

Turner syndrome is caused by absence of one of the X chromosomes. Most girls who have this disorder have one X chromosome missing from all cells (45,XO). This disorder may be recognized at birth if the newborn has a webbed neck, low posterior hairline, widely spaced nipples, and edema of the hands and feet. Individuals with mosaic Turner syndrome do not have the classic physical features (Nwosu and Lee, 2008). This condition is often diagnosed in preschool children because growth is restricted or delayed around 3 to 4 years of age. In some cases, it may be diagnosed at puberty because of three features: short stature, delayed sexual development, and amenorrhea; individuals with Turner syndrome are generally infertile. They may also have difficulty with peer relationships and understanding social cues. They frequently exhibit behavioral problems, especially immature, socially isolated behavior. Diagnosis is confirmed on the basis of a negative sex chromatin test result.

Therapy is individualized for these girls and consists primarily of female hormone treatment and psychologic counseling for both the child and the parents. Linear growth can be increased by the administration of growth hormone if therapy is begun early. Estrogen therapy is initiated during the usual time for puberty to promote the development of secondary sex characteristics. Responses to estrogen therapy vary from girl to girl, but gradual feminization is accomplished to some degree in most individuals.

Klinefelter Syndrome

Klinefelter syndrome, the most common of all sex chromosome disorders, is caused by the presence of one or more additional X chromosomes and only one Y chromosome. Most males with this syndrome have a chromosome complement of 47,XXY. The disorder is infrequently diagnosed before puberty, at which time varying degrees of failure of adolescent virilization occur. Some males are not diagnosed until they appear for evaluation for infertility. All have absence of sperm in the semen (azoospermia), small firm testes, and defective development of secondary sex characteristics (gynecomastia, hypogonadism). In 80% of these boys, there is a chromatin-positive buccal smear, and the extra chromosome is apparent on chromosome analysis.

Cognitive impairment is a frequent clinical finding and appears to be related to the number of X chromosomes. Boys may also have gross motor skill difficulties, developmental language delays, poor verbal skills, reduced auditory memory, shyness, passivity, behavioral problems, and school difficulties. Therapy is directed toward enhancing the masculine characteristics through administration of testosterone.

Nursing Care Management

The nursing care of children with Turner or Klinefelter syndrome is primarily supportive. Nurses assist in the diagnosis, explain tests and therapies, and provide support and encouragement to the child and family. Because both disorders render the individual unable to reproduce, psychologic counseling is an important aspect of care. In young adults, marriage and sexual relationships are possible, but alternative reproductive options, such as artificial insemination and adoption, should be discussed.

DISORDERS RELATED TO THE REPRODUCTIVE SYSTEM

Amenorrhea

Menarche, or the first menstrual period, occurs relatively late in female pubertal development. Although girls vary in the onset and rate of progression of pubertal development, the sequence and tempo should be the same. When an adolescent is seen with a complaint of absence of menses, a careful history of the timing of her pubertal development will help to determine if there is a need for further evaluation or if reassurance is all that is necessary.

Primary amenorrhea is an absence of secondary sex characteristics and no uterine bleeding by 14 to 15 years of age or absence of uterine bleeding with secondary sex characteristics by 16 years of age (Master-Hunter and Heiman, 2006). No uterine bleeding after attaining a sexual maturity rating of 5 on the Tanner scale for 1 year (see Chapter 16) or after breast development for 4 years is also considered primary amenorrhea (AAP and American College of Obstetricians and Gynecologists [ACOG], 2006). The cause of primary amenorrhea may be anatomic, hormonal, genetic, or idiopathic. A thorough patient and family history and physical examination provide clues to the etiology.

Secondary amenorrhea is defined as the absence of menses for 6 months or at least three cycles after menstruation was previously established. Irregular menstrual cycles are common within the first year or two after menarche. These early cycles may be anovulatory, resulting in regular, irregular, or absent bleeding; however, cycle lengths outside the range of 21 to 45 days should be investigated (AAP and ACOG, 2006). Girls with a later onset of menarche take longer to establish regular ovulatory cycles.

Pregnancy is the most common cause of secondary amenorrhea and should be ruled out in both types of amenorrhea even if the adolescent denies sexual activity. Other factors that disturb the hypothalamic–pituitary–gonadal axis and cause secondary amenorrhea include physical or emotional stress; sudden environmental change; hyperthyroidism or hypothyroidism; polycystic ovary syndrome; chronic illness; extreme weight loss or gain; intensive exercise; anorexia nervosa or bulimia; ovarian disturbance; and use of extrinsic pharmacologic agents, especially phenothiazines, contraceptive steroids, and heroin.

Dysmenorrhea

A certain amount of discomfort during the first day or two of the menstrual flow is extremely common. Most girls experience cramping, abdominal pain, backache, and leg ache, but in a few cases, the pain is intolerable and incapacitating. Primary dysmenorrhea is painful menses not related to any pelvic disease or condition. Secondary dysmenorrhea is defined as painful menses with a pathologic condition such as endometriosis, salpingitis, or congenital anomalies of the müllerian system.

Primary dysmenorrhea usually begins at the time of menarche or within 6 to 12 months. The pain begins with menstrual flow or hours before the onset of bleeding each month, usually continuing for 48 to 72 hours. The exact etiology is unknown, but the pain is clearly related to ovulatory cycles. An overproduction of uterine prostaglandins has been implicated; women with dysmenorrhea have higher levels of prostaglandins. Overproduction of vasopressin (a hormone that stimulates the contraction of muscular tissue) may also contribute to dysmenorrhea.

A careful history should include the onset of symptoms; the duration, type of pain, and relationship to menstrual flow; the age at menarche; family history of dysmenorrhea; and sexual history. The nurse should also ask about previous treatments, including dosages of medications. Associated symptoms such as nausea, vomiting, diarrhea, and leg and back pain are helpful for diagnosis and treatment. Depending on the results of the history, the physical examination may include a gynecologic examination.

Therapeutic Management

First-line treatment for adolescents with dysmenorrhea is the administration of nonsteroidal antiinflammatory drugs (NSAIDs), which block the formation of prostaglandins for 2 to 3 days of the menstrual cycle. Girls should be instructed to begin the medication at the first sign of cramping or bleeding. Girls with regular menstrual cycles benefit from beginning the medication 1 or 2 days before the onset of their menses. The medications should be taken with food. If an NSAID such as ibuprofen is not effective, another NSAID should be tried because some women receive relief from different NSAIDs (Stoelting-Gettelfinger, 2010).

Cyclic estrogen therapy and oral contraceptives are also effective. Simple exercises such as pelvic rocking, assuming the knee–chest position, and breathing exercises may be beneficial. Adequate personal hygiene, participation in regular activities, and methods to decrease stress should be discussed with the adolescent. Dietary changes, supplements, and herbal medications are often used to treat dysmenorrhea. Exercise is widely believed to alleviate dysmenorrhea by improving pelvic blood flow and stimulating the release of β-endorphins, which have an analgesic effect.

Randomized controlled clinical trials (RCTs) have demonstrated that vitamins B_1 and E are effective in the treatment of dysmenorrhea (Dennehy, 2006).

Nursing Care Management

All adolescent girls need reassurance that menstruation is a normal function. When nurses are asked for advice regarding menstrual problems, they have a valuable opportunity to engage in health teaching concerning menstrual physiology; hygiene; and the importance of a well-balanced diet, exercise, and general health maintenance. Health teaching can dispel myths about menstruation and femininity. When assessment indicates a potential problem and the need for evaluation, referral to an appropriate practitioner, health service, or clinic may be necessary.

If a gynecologic examination is necessary, the nurse can play a supportive role for the adolescent girl. Whether it is her first experience or not, she is often filled with apprehension. Almost all adolescents are extremely self-conscious about their bodies and the changes taking place. They need continuing support in the form of anticipatory guidance regarding what to expect and suggestions of what to do to relax during the procedure. Most girls favor a semisitting position, which has the additional advantage of allowing eye contact during the procedure. Sometimes a pillow helps the patient feel more comfortable and less vulnerable. The provision of a mirror for the girl to see what is taking place if she so desires helps the examiner explain various aspects of anatomy. When possible, it is important to respect the adolescent's request for a female provider and to have her mother or other supportive person present if she desires.

Vaginitis

Vaginitis can be caused by physical, chemical, or infectious agents. Leukorrhea is the term used to describe a glutinous, gray-white discharge, which can be caused by physical, chemical, or infectious agents.

Physical causes may include a forgotten tampon; chemical irritants include bubble baths, douching, deodorant pads, and tampons. Removing the offending material or discontinuing use of the irritating substance is usually all that is necessary to treat physical or chemical vaginitis. Infectious vaginitis can be caused by *Candida* fungi (yeast), *Trichomonas* protozoa parasites, or bacteria. Diagnosis is confirmed with microscopic evaluation of vaginal secretions, vaginal culture, or rapid testing methods. Treatment varies depending on the infectious agent.

Health teaching is important in the prevention and management of vaginitis. Adolescent girls need reassurance that increased vaginal mucus can occur at the time of ovulation, before menstruation, or with sexual excitement. Many teenage girls mistake these variations as signs of infection. Girls should be taught to wipe from front to back after toileting and to realize that vaginitis can result from irritation, foreign objects, and sexual activity. Nurses should stress the importance of an evaluation to determine the exact cause.

Disorders of the Male Reproductive System

Many obvious anomalies, such as hypospadias, hydrocele, phimosis, and cryptorchidism, are identified with corrective measures instituted during early childhood. The most frequent problems related to the reproductive organs in later childhood are:

- Infections, such as urethritis (see Urinary Tract Infection, Chapter 27)
- Hematuria
- Penile problems, such as nonretractable foreskin in uncircumcised males, drug-induced priapism, carcinoma, and trauma
- Scrotal conditions, such as varicocele (elongation, dilation, and tortuosity of the veins superior to the testicle)
- Testicular torsion (a condition in which the testicle hangs free from its vascular structures, which can result in partial or complete venous occlusion with rotation)

Tumors of the testes are not common (≈8000 cases per year in the United States [Feldman, Bosl, Sheinfeld, and others, 2008]), but when manifested in adolescence, they are generally malignant and demand immediate evaluation. Testicular cancer is the most common solid tumor in adolescent boys and men 15 to 34 years of age. The usual presenting symptom for testicular cancer is a heavy, hard, painless mass (either smooth or nodular) that is palpated on the testis. If a firm swelling is noted, the adolescent should be evaluated by ultrasonography and immediately referred for direct biopsy if the mass is found to be solid.

Treatment involves surgical removal of the affected testicle (orchiectomy) and adjacent lymph nodes (if affected) and possibly chemotherapy and radiation. Fertility may be regained after chemotherapy and surgery; however, sperm banking before the initiation of chemotherapy is recommended. Assisted reproduction is also an option, and successful paternity is reported to be between 50% and 85% (Feldman, Bosl, Sheinfeld, and others, 2008).

Nursing Care Management

Adolescent boys are also self-conscious about their changing bodies and need preparation for a genital examination. The most successful approach is to assume a matter-of-fact attitude toward the examination, explain precisely what will take place, and maintain a continuous commentary about what is being done and the findings at each phase of the examination.

The routine health assessment of every adolescent boy should include teaching about testicular cancer and how to perform a testicular self-examination (TSE) every month. This rare malignancy is curable if detected early. Nurses are in an ideal position to teach TSE in a manner that is respectful of the adolescent boy's anxieties and that promotes early treatment (see Critical Thinking Case Study box).

In the TSE, each testicle is examined individually, preferably after a warm bath or shower, when scrotal skin is more relaxed, using the thumbs and fingers of both hands and applying a small amount of firm, gentle pressure. The normal testicle is a firm organ with a smooth, egg-shaped contour; the epididymis is palpated as a raised swelling on the superior aspect of the testicle and should not be taken for an abnormality.

❓ CRITICAL THINKING CASE STUDY
Testicular Self-Examination

At a recent faculty meeting, Paul, the pediatric nurse practitioner who runs the school-based health clinic, presented his plan for a class on TSE to be delivered to the sophomore boys. Several teachers questioned the value of providing such a class when there is limited time to deliver content relating to "routine academic subjects." What important issues regarding testicular cancer and TSE should Paul use to justify providing this class to the sophomore boys?

Questions

1. Evidence—Is there sufficient evidence to justify teaching sophomore boys about TSE?
2. Assumptions—Describe the underlying assumption about each of the following:
   a. Detection of testicular cancers in adolescence
   b. Usual presenting symptom of testicular cancer
   c. Knowledge of genital anatomy among adolescent boys
   d. Ways to teach adolescent boys about their anatomy
3. What priorities and implications for nursing care can be drawn at this time?
4. Does the evidence support your conclusion?

TSE, Testicular self-examination.

Gynecomastia

Male breasts, although not strictly part of the male reproductive system, respond to hormonal changes. Some degree of bilateral or unilateral breast enlargement occurs frequently in boys during puberty. It is estimated that approximately half of adolescent boys have transient gynecomastia, usually lasting less than 1 year, which subsides spontaneously with achievement of male development. A careful assessment of the pubertal stage at the onset of gynecomastia; medication history, including anabolic steroids; and the exclusion of renal, liver, thyroid, and endocrine disorders or dysfunction allow the examiner to reassure the adolescent that the changes are pubertal gynecomastia and that no further assessment is indicated. Gynecomastia may also be drug induced; calcium channel blockers, cancer chemotherapeutic agents, histamine$_2$-receptor blockers, and oral ketoconazoles have all been shown to cause the condition.

If the condition persists or is extensive enough to cause embarrassment or excessive stress in the young boy, plastic surgery may be indicated for cosmetic and psychologic considerations. Administration of testosterone has no effect on breast development or regression and may aggravate the condition.

Nursing Care Management

Treatment usually consists of assurance to the adolescent and his parents that this is a benign and temporary situation. A physical examination with palpation is necessary to differentiate gynecomastia from increased adiposity caused by being overweight. Adolescents who are distressed about physical integrity and masculinity may benefit from the knowledge that this condition occurs in more than 50% of all adolescent boys.

HEALTH PROBLEMS RELATED TO SEXUALITY

Sexual activity is common among late adolescents; by age 19 years, 7 of 10 adolescents have had sexual intercourse. Many serious health consequences are associated with adolescent sexual activity, including unplanned pregnancy and sexually transmitted infections (STIs); additional health problems may arise from an increased number of sexual partners over time and incomplete education regarding sexual practices in adolescents. Health professionals must understand the issues related to adolescent sexual activity and the psychosocial dynamics that influence them.

Adolescent Pregnancy

The teenage pregnancy rate has been on an overall downward trend for all races since the peak of 117 per 1000 that occurred in 1990 (Kost, Henshaw, and Carlin, 2010). In 2009, preliminary data showed an adolescent pregnancy rate of 39.1 births per 1000 women 15 to 19 years of age (Centers for Disease Control and Prevention [CDC], 2011b). The decline is attributed to increased condom and contraception use as well as a delay in the initiation of sexual activity for adolescents. However, adolescent birth rates still remain high in the United States compared with those in other developed countries (AAP, Committee on Adolescence, 2005; CDC, 2011b). Teens who postpone the initiation of sexual intercourse decrease their risk for STIs, including HIV.

The reduction in teen pregnancy is an important national goal because of the risk for negative outcomes for both mothers and their children. A wide range of factors put adolescents at risk for pregnancy, including having sex with an older partner; the type of contraception used; living in poverty; having a mother who was a teen parent; school failure; lack of access to confidential health care; and living in a poor community where access to education, health care, and work may not be optimal.

With better facilities available for care, the mortality associated with teenage pregnancies is decreasing, but morbidity remains high. Teenage girls and their unborn infants are at greater risk for complications of both pregnancy and delivery. The most frequent complications are premature labor and low-birth-weight infants, high neonatal mortality, iron-deficiency anemia, fetopelvic disproportion, and prolonged labor. The pregnancies of adolescents younger than 15 years old are more frequently complicated by obstetric problems and neonatal morbidity and mortality than those of adolescents ages 15 to 19 years. The increased risk has traditionally been thought to be related to incomplete growth and physiologic immaturity. However, pregnancy can take place only after the girl has achieved an advanced state of growth and sexual maturity. Therefore, concerns are dietary habits, substance use (especially cigarettes), STIs, the effects of poverty, and a late onset of prenatal care.

Nursing Care Management

A pregnant teenager needs careful assessment by the nurse to determine the level of social support available to her and her partner. The adolescent needs to make many important decisions and may not have the life experience to know how to cope with this stress. Whenever possible, guidance from the adults in her life will be invaluable. Information about options to continue the pregnancy and parent the child, continue the pregnancy with adoption, or terminate the pregnancy with abortion should be given in a nonjudgmental manner. If the adolescent chooses to continue the pregnancy, prenatal care should be initiated as soon as possible. No matter what the teenager decides, nutrition information will be necessary. Information should also be provided regarding the pregnant adolescent's nutritional status and health care needs related to the unborn fetus' condition. Because adolescent nutrition habits may vary, it is important to stress that the mother's overall health status will ultimately influence that of her newborn. Myths such as "you can now eat for two" must be addressed. The diet must provide sufficient nutrients to meet growth needs of

both the prospective mother and the unborn child without the threat of excessive weight gain or fetal malnutrition.

> ## ! NURSING ALERT
>
> All pregnant women should take a vitamin and mineral supplement to ensure the Recommended Dietary Allowance for folic acid (0.4 mg [400 mcg] daily) to help prevent neural tube defects. (See Neural Tube Defects [Meningomyelocele], Prevention, Chapter 32.) Initiation before pregnancy has been shown to have the most benefit. Consider a multivitamin for all sexually active women.

Contraception

Family planning services have developed and expanded during recent years, but the need for contraceptive services as part of the health care of adolescents remains great. The birth control pill and condom remain the most popular methods for adolescents; 3-month injectable contraception is more popular among lower-income adolescents. Adolescents commonly delay seeking contraceptive information. The typical interval from onset of sexual intercourse until the first visit for contraception is 1 year. A pregnancy scare is usually the precipitating event for the contraception appointment. Counseling about contraceptive options should be conducted in a manner that is consistent with the cognitive level of the adolescent. The adolescent should be given accurate information about the risks and benefits of each method before making a choice.

Many teenagers feel ambivalent regarding their sexual activity and avoid many contraceptives because their use seems too premeditated and implies that sex is planned rather than a spontaneous activity. Most of these girls believe that sex is all right if it is not planned. This may often play a role in adolescents delaying contraception, waiting for a relationship that is "close enough." A close relationship would allow adolescents to accept and acknowledge their sexual activity.

The choice of a safe and effective contraceptive method must be suited to the individual (Table 17-2). The choice is based on preference after the adolescent is informed of the benefits and disadvantages. Motivation is necessary for most methods. For example, the pill is effective if used correctly, but the adolescent must remember to take the pill at approximately the same time every day. For many young women, a medroxyprogesterone injection (Depo-Provera) is an ideal choice because it is extremely effective and is administered every 12 weeks, but side effects such as weight gain and decreased bone mineralization may make it undesirable. Sexually active adolescents need to know that contraceptive devices other than condoms do not prevent STIs. Condom use is still important and must be discussed with all sexually and non–sexually active adolescents.

Confidentiality is a critical issue when discussing contraception with adolescents. Privacy is important to adolescents as they struggle to forge a personal identity and establish social relationships. Adolescents are particularly concerned about the judgments of others. The predominant belief among many health professionals is that parental notification is important but that the "parents' rights" view is not necessarily sensitive to the health needs and basic rights of youth. No evidence substantiates the belief that providing contraceptive guidance contributes to sexual irresponsibility and promiscuity.

Nursing Care Management

Nurses are often involved in providing education about contraception. Such education is ideally combined with ongoing sex education. Although sexual abstinence is a highly desirable form of contraception for teenagers, nurses working with adolescents must recognize that teens feel multiple pressures to engage in sexual intercourse.

TABLE 17-2	ADVANTAGES AND DISADVANTAGES OF CONTRACEPTIVE METHODS IN ADOLESCENTS	
METHOD	**ADVANTAGES**	**DISADVANTAGES**
Behavioral Methods		
Abstinence	100% effective in preventing STIs and pregnancy	Peer pressure to conform
		Relatively high failure rate from noncompliance
Withdrawal (coitus interruptus)	No medical visit necessary	High failure rate
Withdrawal of penis before ejaculation		Some seminal fluid often released before ejaculation
		Ejaculate at vaginal orifice may enter vagina
		No STI protection
Calendar method	Teaches adolescent girls about their menstrual cycle	High failure rate
Refrain from intercourse during fertile period (time of ovulation)	Encourages couple participation	Requires a regular, predictable menstrual cycle (irregular menses are common for first 2 years after menarche)
		No STI protection
Barrier Methods		
Condom	Minimal side effects	Requires consistent use
	Easy to use	Requires premeditated intent for sexual union
	Available without prescription	May decrease sensation
	Portable	Misuse results in failure
	Provides protection against STIs	Decreased spontaneity
Male—Penile covering to trap sperm	Spermicidal condoms increase effectiveness for pregnancy and STI prevention	Latex sensitivity or allergies in a small percentage of people
	Inexpensive compared with female condom	Improper use may lead to pregnancy or development of STI
Female—Inserted into vagina with base covering part of perineum; may be inserted 8 hours before intercourse	Female participation	May be difficult to insert
	Made of polyurethane; no latex sensitivities and can be used with oil-based lubricants	Coital dependent
	Provides protection from STIs	Noisy
Diaphragm	Can be fitted in virgins	High failure rate in adolescents because of inconvenience of use
Cervical covering to prevent sperm from reaching egg	Low failure rate when used correctly	Requires consistent use
Must be used in conjunction with spermicidal jelly	Few contraindications	Requires fitting and instruction by medical personnel
	May be reused	Requires premeditated intent for sexual union
May be inserted 4–6 hours before intercourse		Requires body awareness and comfort with touching oneself for insertion
If inserted early, should be checked for placement before coitus		Minimal STI protection
		May increase incidence of urinary tract infection
Lea's shield	Non latex (silicone)	Less effective in women who have delivered a baby
Reusable vaginal contraceptive made of silicone; elliptical bowl placed in vagina up to 48 hours before sexual intercourse; removed 8 hours after intercourse	Reusable	Requires prescription
	Very effective in nulliparous women	No STI protection
	Simple fitting	More effective if spermicidal cream is used
		May increase incidence of urinary tract infection
Cervical cap	May be inserted hours before intercourse	Available in only four sizes
Soft rubber dome with a firm but pliable rim; fits over base of the cervix close to the junction of the cervix and vaginal fornices	Insertion and removal similar to diaphragm	Must remain in place at least 6 hours after intercourse but no longer than 48 hours
		Not recommended for women with abnormal Papanicolaou test result, history of toxic shock syndrome, or difficulty with proper fitting
		No STI protection

TABLE 17-2	ADVANTAGES AND DISADVANTAGES OF CONTRACEPTIVE METHODS IN ADOLESCENTS—cont'd	
METHOD	**ADVANTAGES**	**DISADVANTAGES**
Chemicals		
Spermicidal foam, jelly, cream, and suppositories Substance inserted into vagina to kill sperm	Available without prescription Inexpensive Easy to use No major health concerns	High failure rate unless combined with condom Possible for sperm to be ejaculated directly into uterine os, bypassing spermicide in vagina Must be used shortly before coitus; therefore requires interruption of sexual experience Repeated sexual union requires repeated application Requires premeditated intent for sexual union Messy Nonoxynol-9 associated with increased transmission of HIV to women; should not be used with anal sex in male partner sex for same reason No STI protection
Hormonal Methods		
Oral contraceptives Estrogen and progesterone-like compounds Inhibit ovulation by blocking release of gonadotropins from anterior pituitary gland	99% effective if used correctly Safe for adolescents Method of choice for most adolescents Administered by mouth Becomes a ritual not associated with sexual activity Regulates menses, decreases dysmenorrhea and acne, decreases menstrual flow Prevents ovarian and endometrial cancers Prevents functional ovarian cysts	Higher failure rate in adolescents than in older women Need to follow precise instructions; requires continued motivation, consistent use Requires prescription Price substantial for teenager No STI protection Possible side effects include headaches, missed or scanty periods, breakthrough bleeding, blood clot Increased rates of *Chlamydia*
Medroxyprogesterone acetate (Depo-Provera) Progestin that suppresses hormonal cycle and prevents ovulation Injection given every 3 months	No interruption of intercourse Invisible method	No STI protection Possible side effects include significant weight gain, decreased bone density, decreased HDLs, irregular menses or amenorrhea, decreased libido, depression Fertility perhaps delayed after discontinuation Must return to care provider every 3 months for injection Food and Drug Administration recommends discontinuation after 2 years because of decreased bone density
Ortho Evra transdermal system 4.5-cm square patch with norelgestromin and ethinyl estradiol Hormonal patch applied to skin weekly for 3 weeks per month Suppresses ovulation, thickens cervical mucus, and thins endometrium	88.2% effective in perfect users Simple to use Regular menstrual cycles Not associated with sexual activity Avoids first-pass metabolism, resulting in more constant levels	Not recommended for women >90 kg (198 pounds) Possible side effects include skin reaction at site, nausea, headache, dysmenorrhea, and breast tenderness Slight increase in risk of blood clot formation over combination oral contraceptive pill Patch may be visible No STI protection
NuvaRing Etonogestrel plus ethinyl estradiol Soft flexible transparent ring placed in vagina for 3 weeks Suppresses ovulation	99.3% effective Immediate return to ovulation at discontinuation May leave in place during sexual intercourse Avoids first-pass metabolism, resulting in more constant levels No spermicide needed No vaginal erosion No weight gain	Device may be felt by female or partner during sexual intercourse Device may fall out Possible side effects include headache, vaginitis, leukorrhea, nausea, and breakthrough bleeding May have late withdrawal bleeding requiring placement of ring during menses No STI protection
Levonorgestrel intrauterine system (Mirena) T-shape intrauterine device that releases 20 mcg/d of levonorgestrel Inserted within 7 days of menses and remains in place for 5 years Thickens cervical mucus and inhibits sperm mobility and function	>99% effective Effectively prevents fertilization, resulting in low rates of ectopic pregnancy Reduced length and quantity of menstrual bleeding Reduced dysmenorrhea No weight gain	Risk of perforation at time of insertion 2%–12% expulsion rate Not recommended in nulliparous women or women not in monogamous relationships Possible side effects include abdominal pain, headache, vaginal discharge, and breast pain No STI protection

Continued

TABLE 17-2	ADVANTAGES AND DISADVANTAGES OF CONTRACEPTIVE METHODS IN ADOLESCENTS—cont'd	
METHOD	**ADVANTAGES**	**DISADVANTAGES**
Letonogestrel implant (Implanon) 40×2 mm implanted rod Progestin-only method Suppresses ovulation	>99% effective Efficacy not user dependent Provides 3 years of protection Single rod insertion and removal Palpable but not visible after insertion	Irregular menstrual bleeding Other less common side effects include headache, vaginitis, weight gain (1.7 kg [3.7 pounds] at 2 years) No STI protection
Emergency or Postcoital Contraception Emergency contraception works in one of three ways: by suppressing or delaying ovulation, by preventing the meeting of sperm and egg, or by preventing implantation **Progestin-only pill given within 72 hours of intercourse** *or* **Insertion of a copper-releasing intrauterine device** up to 7 days after unprotected intercourse	Useful in unplanned sexual intercourse or contraceptive failure May be given in advance for emergency use Available without prescription for adults	No STI protection May cause nausea if combination method used May change timing of next menstrual cycle

HDL, High-density lipoprotein; *HIV,* human immunodeficiency virus; *STI,* sexually transmitted infection.

Postponing sexual involvement requires effective communication and decision-making skills. Adolescents benefit from role-playing refusal skills and opportunities to practice making decisions in a safe environment. Information about safe sex must be provided, and role-playing how to discuss condom use with a partner is helpful to teenagers.

Education concerning contraception should be provided in both oral and written form. All available methods, including their benefits, disadvantages, and side effects, should be discussed. Concrete, concise language must be used, demonstrations of how to use the contraceptive should be provided, and adolescents should repeat all instructions in their own words. If teenagers are using oral contraceptive pills, they should be encouraged to use a daily activity as a reminder or cue to take the pill. A knowledgeable phone triage person should be available for questions and concerns. Parents or other important adults may be included in all discussions, with the adolescent's permission.

Sexually Transmitted Infections

Sexually active adolescents are at increased risk (compared with adults) for the acquisition of STIs. Physiologically, the adolescent girl's cervix has a large ectropion, which is composed of columnar epithelial cells that are much more susceptible to STIs, especially human papillomavirus (HPV) and *Chlamydia* infection. Adolescents' immune systems also contribute to the increased risk because adolescents have not had an opportunity to develop resistance to these organisms. Behavioral factors contributing to increased risk include initiating sexual intercourse at an early age, having multiple sexual partners concurrently, having serial short-term monogamous relationships, failing to use barrier protection consistently and correctly, and experiencing difficulty accessing health care (Workowski, Berman, and CDC, 2010). A listing of common STIs is included in Table 17-3.

The rates of *Chlamydia* and gonorrhea are reported to be highest among adolescent girls ages 15 to 19 years, and high rates of HPV exist in the adolescent population (Workowski, Berman, and CDC, 2010). Whereas much emphasis has been placed on prevention of HIV in the past decade, other STIs have received little attention in regards to prevention. Lack of awareness regarding one's susceptibility to STIs

when engaged in unprotected sexual activity, be it oral, anal, or vaginal intercourse, is perhaps one of the greatest dangers adolescents face.

Therapeutic Management

Effective treatment of both male and female adolescents with STIs involves administration of the appropriate therapeutic agent. Treatment of sexual partners is also an essential part of therapy. Adolescents need help to develop strategies to inform their partners and to abstain from sex until all partners have completed treatment.

A totally effective prophylaxis against infection is not yet available; therefore, preventive efforts must be directed toward finding and treating affected persons, locating and examining contacts of affected persons, educating young people regarding the facts of the disease and its spread, and encouraging the use of condoms in sexually active young people.

Nursing Care Management

Nursing responsibilities encompass all aspects of STI education, confidentiality, prevention, and treatment. Part of the sex education of young people should include providing information about STIs, including their symptoms and treatment, and dispelling the myths associated with their mode of transmission. Many vulnerable adolescents are uninformed or misinformed about STIs.

Primary prevention efforts for STIs include encouraging abstinence and postponing sexual involvement, encouraging condom use, and ensuring vaccination for hepatitis A and B and HPV. Nurses play a role in secondary prevention by helping to identify early cases and referring adolescents for treatment. Nurses can also be involved in tertiary prevention by decreasing the medical and psychologic effects of STIs; conducting support groups for adolescents with HIV, herpes simplex virus, and HPV infections; and assisting pregnant adolescents in obtaining adequate prenatal screening and treatment of STIs.

Pelvic Inflammatory Disease

Pelvic inflammatory disease (PID) is an infection of the upper genital tract (endometrium, fallopian tubes, and ovaries), most

Animation—Pelvic Inflammatory Disease

TABLE 17-3	SELECTED SEXUALLY TRANSMITTED INFECTIONS*	
MANIFESTATIONS	**THERAPY**	**NURSING CARE MANAGEMENT**

Gonorrhea (*Neisseria gonorrhoeae*)
Male—Urethritis (dysuria with profuse yellow discharge, frequency, urgency, nocturia) or pharyngitis
Female—Cervicitis (postpubertal); may be associated with discharge, dysuria, dyspareunia, vulvovaginitis (prepubertal), or pharyngitis
	For uncomplicated urogenital and anorectal gonorrhea:
	  Single intramuscular dose of ceftriaxone†
	  or
	  Single oral dose of cefixime
		Instruct patient to abstain from sexual intercourse for 7 days after single-dose treatment.
		Test and treat for other STIs
		Find and treat sexual contacts.
		Educate young people regarding facts of the disease and its spread.
		Encourage use of condoms in sexually active young people.

Chlamydia (*Chlamydia trachomatis*) **Male**—Meatal erythema, tenderness, itching, dysuria, urethral discharge; or no symptoms **Female**—Mucopurulent cervical exudate with erythema, edema, congestion; or no symptoms	Azithromycin or doxycycline If pregnant—azithromycin	Same as above Rescreen women 3–4 months after treatment; repeat infection elevates risk for PID.
Syphilis (*Treponema pallidum*) **Primary stage**—Chancre, a hard, painless, red, sharply defined lesion with indurated base, raised border, eroded surface, and scanty yellow discharge; usually located on the penis, vulva, or cervix **Secondary stage**—Systemic influenza-like symptoms and lymphadenopathy, rash; usually appears 1–3 weeks after healing of chancre	Penicillin G (parenteral—benzathine, aqueous procaine, or aqueous crystalline)	Instruct patients to use condoms to avoid spread or infection with other organisms. Identify sexual contacts of infected person(s). Test women in pregnancy and prior to delivery (VDRL and RPR). Evaluate newborn for presence of disease if mother is untreated.
Herpes Progenitalis (Genital Herpes Simplex Virus) Small (usually painful) vesicles on genital area, buttocks, and thighs; itching is usually the initial symptom; when vesicles break, shallow, circular, extremely painful lesions remain	No known cure Acyclovir, famciclovir, or valacyclovir May need suppressive therapy for recurrences	Instruct patients to use condoms to avoid spread or infection with other organisms. Infection can be transmitted to infant during birth. Evaluate maternal history and observe infant for signs or symptoms. Cultures may be obtained in newborn.
Trichomoniasis (*Trichomonas vaginalis*) Pruritus and edema of external genitalia; foul-smelling, greenish vaginal discharge; sometimes postcoital bleeding May be asymptomatic, especially in men	Oral metronidazole or oral tinidazole	Patient should not consume alcohol while taking medication and for at least 48 hours after the last dose. Sexual partners should be treated.

Human Papillomavirus
Warts found on any part of male or female genitalia
	Patient applied:
	  Podofilox solution (0.5%) or gel or imiquimod (5%) cream
	Provider applied:
	  Podophyllin resin 10%–25% in compound tincture of benzoin
	  Freezing with liquid nitrogen or cryoprobe (cryotherapy)
	  Trichloroacetic acid or bichloroacetic acid 80%–90%
	  Laser therapy or intralesional interferon or surgical removal
		An acceptable alternative is to forgo treatment and await spontaneous resolution.
		Treatments are usually painful; analgesics may be needed, and steroid cream may provide relief.
		Vaccine available for prevention (see Chapter 10).

Acquired Immunodeficiency Syndrome (Human Immunodeficiency Virus) See Chapter 26.	Numerous antiviral medications to delay viral replication and progression of disease in the pregnant woman and to prevent transmission of virus to newborn.	See Chapter 26.

PID, Pelvic inflammatory disease; *RPR,* rapid plasma reagin; *STI,* sexually transmitted infection; *VDRL,* Venereal Disease Research Laboratory.
*Updated information on specific treatment of STIs may be accessed at http://www.cdc.gov/STI/treatment.
†Centers for Disease Control and Prevention: Update to CDC's *Sexually transmitted disease treatment guidelines, 2006*: fluoroquinolones no longer recommended for treatment of gonococcal infections, *MMWR Morb Mortal Wkly Rep* 56(14):332–336, 2007.

commonly caused by sexually transmitted bacteria, such as *Neisseria gonorrhoeae*, *Chlamydia trachomatis*, and a variety of other anaerobic bacteria.

The long-term effects of PID include infertility because of tubal scarring, ectopic pregnancy, and chronic abdominal pain. It is estimated that each year 1 million women of reproductive age experience an episode of PID, with approximately 20% of cases occurring in teenagers. Women younger than age 25 years have a 1 in 8 chance of experiencing PID compared with those older than age 25 years, whose risk is 1 in 80.

Presenting symptoms in adolescents may be generalized, including fever; abdominal pain; urinary tract symptoms; and vague influenza-like manifestations, such as malaise, nausea, diarrhea, or constipation. A pelvic examination is indicated for every sexually active woman who complains of lower abdominal pain to evaluate for the possibility of PID.

Pelvic inflammatory disease is of major concern to nurses because of its devastating effects on the reproductive tract. Approximately 25% of women experiencing PID may have short-term complications, such as acute abscess formation in the fallopian tubes (tubo-ovarian abscess), or long-term complications, such as chronic pelvic pain, dyspareunia (painful coitus), or adhesion formation. Most significant, however, is the increased risk for ectopic pregnancy or infertility, which results from tubal scarring.

Prevention is the primary concern of health care professionals. Barrier contraceptive methods, such as condoms, seem to offer the best protection for preventing STIs and PID. Sexually active female teenagers should be screened every 6 months to detect asymptomatic STIs, and treatment should be initiated to prevent PID and all associated complications. Reinfection with *Chlamydia* organisms is associated with a higher incidence of PID. Women who have had a *Chlamydia* infection should be rescreened for *Chlamydia* 3 months after treatment.

Sexual Assault (Rape)

Typically, stranger rape is what comes to mind when one thinks of sexual assault; however, more than half of assaults are committed by someone known to the survivor. Although both males and females can be sexually assaulted, females are at greatest risk. Adolescents are at high risk for sexual assault; other high-risk groups include survivors of childhood sexual or physical abuse; persons who are disabled; persons with substance abuse problems; sex workers; persons who are poor or homeless; and persons living in prisons, institutions, or areas of military conflict. Sexual assault remains underreported for multifactorial reasons (Luce, Schrager, and Gilchrist, 2010).

An understanding of the legal definitions of sexual assault, rape, acquaintance rape, and statutory rape is essential for the nurse to identify, treat, and manage adolescent victims (Box 17-4).

Statutory rape laws have been revised in many states across the country. The motivation for tougher laws and greater enforcement is to decrease teen pregnancy, increase male responsibility, and decrease welfare dependency. Traditionally, statutory rape laws have been concerned with the protection of girls. In the past 20 years, many laws have been rewritten to be gender neutral. Statutory rape laws require reporting to child protective services or local law enforcement. One risk of strict statutory rape enforcement is that girls may not seek health care for reproductive care, prenatal care, or domestic violence. Young people may fear not only for themselves but also for their partners. However, sexual coercion of teens by adults remains a problem and results in STIs and adolescent pregnancy.

BOX 17-4 DEFINITIONS OF SEXUAL ASSAULTS

Sexual assault—Comprehensive term that includes various types of forced or inappropriate sexual activity. Sexual assault includes both physical and psychologic coercion as well as touch, penetration, and other sexual contact.

Rape—Forced sexual intercourse that occurs by physical force or psychologic coercion. Rape includes vaginal, anal, or oral penetration by body parts or inanimate objects.

Acquaintance rape (date rape)—Applied to situations in which the assailant and victim know each other.

Statutory rape—Consensual sexual contact by a person 18 years of age or older with a person under the age of consent or unable to consent because of developmental disability. Age of consent varies by state.

In the United States, it is illegal for anyone to have sexual intercourse with a child younger than the age of 12 years. These laws protect the health and safety of children incapable of protecting themselves. When consensuality is considered in statutory rape laws and cases, it implies that adolescents are morally and socially responsible for sexual contact that occurs with adults. This does not afford adolescents the same protections provided to children younger than the age of 12 years (Kandakai and Smith, 2007).

Nurses can obtain information about their state statutory rape reporting responsibilities from state or local child protective services agencies, legal counsel, rape crisis organizations, state or local law enforcement agencies, or the state nurses' association. The limits of confidentiality should be clearly reviewed with each adolescent patient before beginning the interview about sexual activity.

Diagnostic Evaluation

Rape victims may exhibit a variety of reactions (Box 17-5), and the circumstances of the initial medical evaluation may be frightening and stressful. The initial contact with the rape victim must be supportive because the interrogation and associated activities have the potential to add to the trauma of the sexual assault. First of all, the victim needs to know that she (or he) is (1) all right and (2) not being blamed for the situation.

It is important to obtain a clear account of the circumstances of an alleged rape without forcing the victim to relive a painful experience. Information includes the date, time, location, and an accurate description of any type of sexual contact. The physical examination is carried out as soon as possible because physical evidence deteriorates rapidly. The victim should not bathe or shower before the examination.

! NURSING ALERT

It is common for rape victims to delay seeking help, especially in cases of acquaintance or date rape. Nurses can be most supportive by acknowledging the painful and sometimes confusing feelings that surround such experiences and by focusing on the fact that the victim is seeking assistance now.

The young person is always told in advance in understandable terms exactly what to expect in the way of tests and procedures, and the explanation is accompanied by strong emotional support. The victim is examined thoroughly, including nongenital areas, for evidence of injury that might substantiate the use of force.

BOX 17-5 CLINICAL MANIFESTATIONS OF RAPE VICTIMS

May Display a Variety of Emotions and Behaviors:
Hysterical crying
Giggling
Agitation
Feelings of degradation
Anger and rage
Helplessness
Nervousness
Rapid mood swings
Appearing calm and controlled (masking inner turmoil)
Confused
Self-blame
Fear—of the rape and of injury

Evidence of Physical Force From:
Roughness
Nonbrutal beating (slapping)
Brutal beating (slugging, kicking, beating repeatedly with fists)
Choking or gagging

Medical Examination Provides Evidence Of:
Penetration
Ejaculation
Use of force

FAMILY-CENTERED CARE
Supporting the Rape Victim's Parents

In addition to the needs of the adolescent rape victim, the nurse should also be sensitive to the needs and reactions of the adolescent's parents. Some parents will be angry and blame the adolescent; others will feel guilty and embarrassed. Many reactions can be expected at the time of the incident, ranging from despair to extreme agitation. Frequently, the parents require as much support and reassurance as the victim. Agitated, angry, or incapacitated parents are unable to provide support for their adolescent. Meeting their needs can foster their ability to support the teenager during the crisis.

The forensic examination of a sexual assault victim must follow strict legal requirements. The medical record may provide key evidence for the legal case. Practitioners specially trained for rape examination should be used when possible. Nurses are often members of this group and are known as sexual assault nurse examiners (SANEs). Evaluation for STIs is an important part of the evaluation. The following procedures are recommended for the initial examination: nucleic acid amplified testing (NAATs) for *Chlamydia* and gonorrhea; wet mount and culture or point-of-care testing of a vaginal swab specimen for trichomoniasis; and a serum sample for HIV infection, hepatitis B, and syphilis. Decisions to perform these tests should be made on an individual basis. Repeat testing for *Chlamydia* and gonorrhea can be done at 2 weeks if prophylactic treatment was not administered. Serologic tests for syphilis and HIV infection can be repeated 6 weeks, 3 months, and 6 months after the assault if infection in the assailant could not be ruled out (Workowski, Berman, and CDC, 2010).

Prophylactic treatment for *Chlamydia*, gonorrhea, and trichomoniasis is recommended. Vaccination for hepatitis B should be administered if the patient has not been previously vaccinated. Follow-up doses of vaccine should be administered 1 to 2 and 4 to 6 months after the first dose. Female victims should be provided with emergency contraception. The recommendation for HIV prophylaxis varies depending on the geographic area, the circumstances of the assault, and the known HIV status of the perpetrator. The CDC (Workowski, Berman, and CDC, 2010) maintains updates and recommendations for treatment of STIs incurred as a result of sexual assault.*

Therapeutic Management

Adolescents who have been raped arrive at the emergency department or practitioner's office under a variety of circumstances. They are usually brought by parents, friends, or police officers, but some may seek medical help on their own. It is advisable to obtain parental consent for examination, but the examination may be performed without parental consent if the adolescent is mature and the parents are unavailable. A female observer or chaperone should be present during the history and examination of female victims who are examined by a male practitioner. Whether a parent should be present during the examination is determined on an individual basis. The parent's presence is usually encouraged if the parent is supportive and the young person agrees.

Nursing Care Management

Many of the approaches that have been described for sexually abused children (see Chapter 14) also apply to adolescents. Sexual assault is a devastating experience with long-lasting effects. The primary goal of nursing care is to avoid inflicting further stress on the adolescent, who is often angry, confused, frightened, embarrassed, and filled with self-blame. The nurse must do everything possible to reduce the stress of the interrogation and examination. Although most health professionals and law enforcement officers are sensitive to the needs of adolescents and attempt to make the process as nonstressful as possible, the nurse should be alert to cues that indicate the victim is being overstressed.

Follow-up care of the rape victim is essential and extends over a long period. The health-compromising responses to sexual assault include PTSD, anxiety, and depression. PTSD is the most common mental health sequelae of sexual violence with rates of 33% to 45% among women (Campbell, Dworkin, and Cabral, 2009). Aside from the universal need for emotional support, the needs of rape victims vary widely and depend on the nature of the incident, the victim's age when the rape occurred, the physical and emotional injuries sustained by the victim, the legal actions being considered as a result, the resources available for informal support, and the anticipated reactions of persons in the informal support network (see Family-Centered Care box).†

NUTRITION AND EATING DISORDERS

Obesity

Few problems in childhood and adolescence are so obvious to others, are so difficult to treat, and have such long-term effects on health as obesity. Several different definitions have been proposed for obesity and overweight. Obesity has been defined as an increase in body weight resulting from an excessive accumulation of body fat relative to lean

---

*http://www.cdc.gov/std/treatment/2010/default.htm.

†For information about local organizations, contact National Organization for Victim Assistance, Courthouse Square, 510 King St., Suite 424, Alexandria, VA 22314; 800-879-6682 or 703-535-6682; http://www.trynova.org.

body mass. Overweight refers to the state of weighing more than average for height and body build. Currently, the body mass index (BMI) measurement is recommended as the most accurate method for screening children and adolescents for obesity. The BMI measurement is strongly associated with subcutaneous and total body fat and with skinfold thickness measurements. It is also highly specific for children with the greatest amount of body fat. Pediatric growth charts that include BMI for age and gender are available from the CDC.* Children with BMIs between the 85th and 95th percentiles are considered overweight, and obesity is defined by a BMI greater than or equal to the 95th percentile (Gahagan, 2011).

Regardless of the definition used, the number of overweight children in the United States is increasing and has reportedly reached epidemic status (Spruijt-Metz, 2011). Approximately 12.5 million children are overweight or obese (Ogden, Carroll, and Flegal, 2008). Numerous studies dating back to the early 1960s have documented childhood overweight through comprehensive evaluations of dietary intake, physical activity, and anthropometric measures (CDC using the various National Health Examination Surveys [NHANES], I, II, III, and IV) (Ogden, Carroll, and Flegal, 2008; Ogden, Kuczmarski, Flegal, and others, 2002; Ogden, Troiano, Briefel, and others, 1997). In children ages 6 to 11 years, the prevalence of childhood overweight remained fairly constant between 1963 and 1974 at approximately 4% and 5.5%, respectively. However, recent NHANES surveys have seen these numbers steadily climb to reach 17% in both 6- to 11-year-old children and 12- to 19-year-old children (Ogden, Carroll, and Flegal, 2008). African-American and Hispanic children and youth are disproportionately represented by a higher prevalence of overweight and obesity (23.1% and 21.0%, respectively) compared with non-Hispanic white children (15.9%) (Ogden, Carroll, and Flegal, 2008). A study of 9464 American Indian schoolchildren ages 5 to 18 years found that 39% were overweight, and a further review of tribes across the United States found that 30% to 46% of American Indians were at risk for overweight (Hardy, Harrell, and Bell, 2004).

Because adult obesity is associated with increased mortality and morbidity from a variety of complications, both physical and psychologic, adolescent obesity is a serious condition. Research indicates that overweight children and adolescents are at risk for continuing to be obese as adults, thereby experiencing the health and social consequences of obesity much earlier than children and adolescents of normal weight. Parental obesity increases the risk of overweight by two- to threefold (Baker, Barlow, Cochran, and others, 2005). The probability that overweight school-age children will become obese adults is estimated at 50%, and the likelihood that overweight adolescents will become obese adults is estimated at 70% to 80% (National Institute for Health Care Management Foundation, 2003).

Obesity in childhood and adolescence has been related to elevated blood cholesterol, high blood pressure, respiratory disorders, orthopedic conditions, cholelithiasis, some types of adult-onset cancer, nonalcoholic fatty liver disease (NAFLD), and type 2 diabetes mellitus. The incidence of metabolic syndrome was 50% in a study group of overweight and obese adolescents (Weiss, Dziura, Burgert, and others, 2004). Common emotional consequences of obesity include poor body image, low self-esteem, social isolation, and feelings of depression and rejection (Sjöberg, Nilsson, and Leppert, 2005).

Etiology and Pathophysiology

Obesity results from a caloric intake that consistently exceeds caloric requirements and expenditure and may involve a variety of

*http://www.cdc.gov/growthcharts.

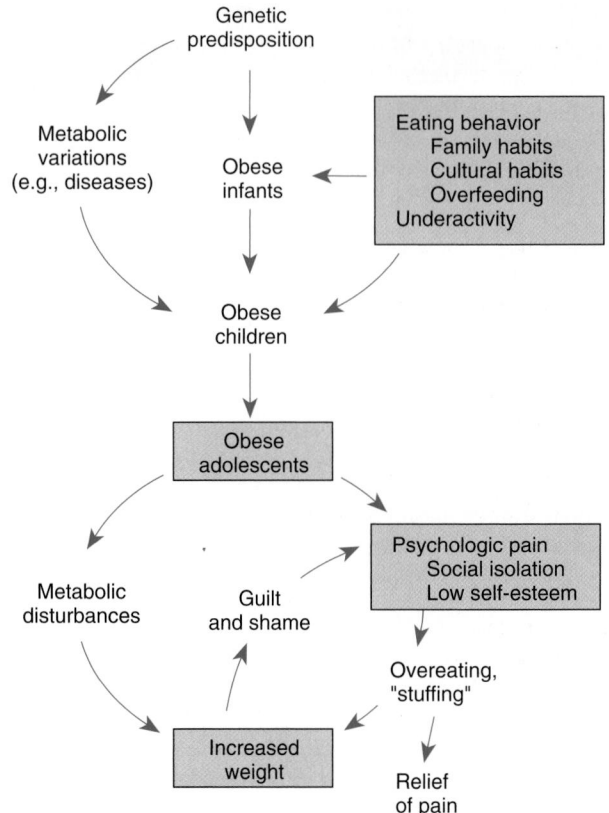

FIG 17-1 Complex relationships in obesity.

interrelated influences, including metabolic, hypothalamic, hereditary, social, cultural, and psychologic factors (Fig. 17-1). Because the etiology of obesity is multifactorial, the treatment requires multilevel interventions.

A balance between energy intake and energy expenditure is a critical factor in regulating body weight. Factors that raise energy intake or decrease energy expenditure by even small amounts can have a long-term impact on the development of overweight and obesity. For example, a positive balance of one serving of a sweetened juice or soft drink (≈120 kcal) per day would produce a 50-kg (110-pound) increase in body mass over a 10-year period (Hill, Wyatt, Reed, and others, 2003).

Familial influence is an epidemiologic consideration in regard to children's weight. Twin studies suggest that approximately 35% to 50% of the tendency toward obesity is inherited (Beaty, 2007). Twin studies have also suggested that this tendency is a combination of genetic and environmental factors. Mothers seem to play a greater role in the gestational weight of their children (Jaquet, Swaminathan, Alexander, and others, 2005). When both parents are obese, there is a 60% to 80% increase in the likelihood of the child becoming obese (Koeppen-Schomerus, Wardle, and Plomin, 2001; Wardle, Carnell, Haworth, and others, 2008). The specific influences of genes and environment within developing children are not well defined. The increasing rates of obesity within genetically stable populations suggest that environmental and some perinatal factors (e.g., bottle feeding) are contributors to the current increases in childhood obesity (National Institute for Health Care Management Foundation, 2003).

Birth weight does not seem to be a long-term contributing factor in detection and prediction of childhood obesity (Kain, Corvalán, Lera, and others, 2009; McCarthy, Hughes, Tilling, and others, 2007); obese children do not have higher birth weights than nonobese children. There is, however, a high correlation between childhood adiposity and parental adiposity (Boney, Verma, Tucker, and others, 2005; Bouchard, 2009; Li, Kaur, Choi, and others, 2005). One study found that the best determinant of adult obesity was the child's weight at 5 years of age or an increased weight gain from 1 to 5 years of age (McCarthy, Hughes, Tilling, and others, 2007).

Fewer than 5% of the cases of childhood obesity can be attributed to an underlying disease. Such diseases include hypothyroidism; adrenal hypercorticoidism; hyperinsulinism; and dysfunction or damage to the CNS as a result of tumor, injury, infection, or vascular accident. Obesity is a frequent complication of muscular dystrophy, paraplegia, Down syndrome, spina bifida, and other chronic illnesses that limit mobility.

A major focus of obesity research has been on appetite regulation. The expression of appetite is chemically coded in the hypothalamus by distinctive circuitry. Orexigenic substances produce signals that promote eating behaviors, and anorexigenic substances promote the cessation of eating behaviors. Feedback loops between signals have been identified where one signal peptide is able to alter the secretion of another signal peptide. No one signal has been identified as the gatekeeper of appetite. It is apparent that an entire network of signals, including their frequency and amplitude, is responsible for triggering eating behaviors.

There is little evidence to support a relationship between obesity and "low metabolism." Small differences may exist in regulation of dietary intake or metabolic rate between obese and nonobese children that could lead to an energy imbalance and inappropriate weight gain, but these small differences are difficult to accurately quantify. No differences in basal metabolic rate, sleeping metabolic rate, respiratory quotient, heart rate, or total energy expenditure have been found in normal weight children with or without a familial predisposition to overweight (Baker, Barlow, Cochran, and others, 2005). Whereas in childhood, overeating is the dominant feature in obesity, in adult life, reduced physical activity with normal intake is more likely.

The tendency toward obesity is manifested whenever environmental conditions are favorable to excessive caloric intake, such as an abundance of food, limited access to low-fat foods, reduced or minimum physical activity, and snacking combined with excessive television viewing. Family and cultural eating patterns, as well as psychologic factors, play important roles; many families and cultures consider fat to be an indication of good health. It is common for obese children to have families that emphasize large meals or admonish children for leaving food on their plates. Parents may have an exaggerated concept of the amount of food children require and expect them to eat more than they need. The prevalence of obesity shows a marked difference between upper and lower class children, with differences often becoming apparent before 6 years of age. Lower socioeconomic groups have a greater prevalence of obesity, especially in girls. Physical activity may also be influenced by sociocultural factors.

Some community factors that influence activity patterns include unsafe neighborhoods that keep children from playing outside. Many communities lack affordable and accessible areas for low-income youth to be active, thus limiting opportunities for young people to participate in physical activities. Social policies also contribute to obesity. The increased availability of high-fat foods, pricing strategies that promote unhealthy food choices, and overzealous food advertising that targets children and adolescents with high-fat and high-sugar foods are some examples.

Institutional factors also influence patterns of obesity and decreased physical activity. Many school policies allow students to leave

school for lunch. Vending machines in school often are filled with high-fat and high-calorie foods and soft drinks. Although well-balanced, nutritious school lunches may be available to students, they often opt for less nutritious choices such as high-fat snacks.

Physical inactivity has also been identified as an important contributing factor in the development and maintenance of childhood overweight. There is little doubt that physical activity has decreased in elementary and secondary schools in the United States in past years; however, there have been positive attempts to incorporate more physical activity into schools within the past several years. Consequently, most of children's physical activity must occur within the family or outside of school. Decreased physical activity within the family is a powerful influence on children because children imitate their parents and other adults. Parental obesity and low levels of physical activity are correlated with decreased physical activity in children.

The growing attraction and availability of many sedentary activities, including television, handheld video games, computers, and the Internet, have also greatly influenced the amount of time that children spend participating in sedentary behaviors. When combining television viewing with video games, it is estimated that children may spend as much as 6 hours per day on various media, which takes time away from meaningful activities such as exercise and reading (Roberts and Foehr, 2008). The AAP (2011) recently issued a policy statement encouraging parents to limit media viewing in children to 2 hours or less per day. The AAP asserts that media time, especially advertisements of food products, has a direct correlation with the increased incidence of childhood obesity in the United States.

Psychologic factors also affect eating patterns. In infancy, children experience relief from discomfort through feeding and learn to associate eating with a sense of well-being, security, and the comforting presence of a nurturing person. Eating is soon associated with the feeling of being loved. In addition, the pleasurable oral sensation of sucking provides a connection between emotions and early eating behavior. Many parents use food as a positive reward for desired behaviors. This practice may become a habit, and the child may continue to use food as a reward, a comfort, and a means of dealing with depression or hostility. Many individuals eat when they are not hungry or in response to boredom, loneliness, sadness, depression, or tiredness. Difficulty in determining feelings of satiety can lead to weight problems and may compound the factor of eating in response to emotional rather than physical hunger cues.

Eating behaviors are closely related to memory. Memory and appetite are chemically encoded, with each individual having his or her own circuitry relating to eating behaviors. Similar to memory, the circuitry can be modified over time (Feldman, Friedman, and Sleisenger, 2002).

Diagnostic Evaluation

A careful history is obtained regarding the development of obesity, and a physical examination is performed to differentiate simple obesity from increased fat that results from organic causes. A family history of obesity, diabetes, coronary heart disease, and dyslipidemia should be obtained for all children who are overweight or at risk for overweight. Specific information from the patient and family about the effects of obesity on daily functioning—for example, problems with nighttime breathing and sleep, daytime sleepiness, joint pain, ability to keep up with family activities and peers at school—is helpful. The physical examination should focus on identifying comorbid conditions and identifiable causes of obesity. For some, psychologic assessment, by interviews and standardized personality tests, may provide insight into the personality and emotional problems that contribute to obesity and that might interfere with therapy.

It is useful to estimate the degree of obesity to determine the component of body weight that can be modified. All of the following methods have been used to assess obesity: BMI, body weight, weight–height ratios, weight–age ratios, hydrostatic (underwater) weight, skinfold measurements, bioelectrical analysis, computed tomography, magnetic resonance imaging, and neutron activation. Each of these methods has advantages and disadvantages. Hydrostatic, or underwater, weighing provides the most accurate measurement of lean body weight.

Body mass index is currently considered the best method to assess weight in children and adolescents. The calculation is based on the individual's height and weight. In adults, BMI definitions are fixed measures without regard for sex and age. The BMI in children and adolescents varies to accommodate age- and gender-specific changes in growth. The formula for BMI calculation is:

$$\frac{\text{Weight in pounds} \div \text{Height in inches} \times 703}{\text{Height in inches}}$$

Body mass index measures in children and adolescents are plotted on growth charts that enable health care professionals to determine BMI for age for the patient (see Appendix A).

The initial assessment of obese children and adolescents should include screening to evaluate for comorbidities. The history is an important guide to determine the workup. A complete physical examination is important. Some areas to focus on include (1) skin for stretch markings and discolorations (e.g., acanthosis nigricans), (2) joints for swelling and evidence of pain, and (3) airway for evidence of obstruction and enlarged tonsils. Basic laboratory studies include a fasting lipid panel; fasting insulin level; fasting glucose hepatic enzymes, including γ-glutamyltransferase (GGT); and in some institutions, hemoglobin A1c. Other studies, such as a sleep study, metabolic studies, and radiographic evaluations, may be added based on the history and physical examination. These assessments may determine whether the patient needs a referral to specialty services for more focused evaluation and treatment, such as endocrinology (insulin resistance, diabetes), hepatology (elevated liver enzymes, NAFLD), orthopedics (Blount disease), or pulmonary medicine (sleep-disordered breathing, noninvasive continuous positive airway pressure).

Therapeutic Management

The best approach to the management of obesity is a preventive one. Early recognition and control measures are essential before the child or adolescent reaches an obese state. Health care providers must educate families about the medical complications of obesity, and families are encouraged to be involved in the treatment plan.

The treatment of obesity is difficult. Many approaches do not achieve long-term success. The average individual only loses about 5% to 10% of his or her weight with available therapies. Losing weight can have a significant positive effect on many comorbidities, but unfortunately, the lost weight is frequently regained in a year or two.

Diet modification is an essential part of weight reduction programs. Dietary counseling is directed toward improving the nutritional quality of the diet rather than toward dietary restriction. Children and adolescents should avoid fad diets. Most dietitians and nutrition experts recommend a diet with no *trans* fats, low-saturated fat, moderate total fat (≤30%), and a half plate of fruits and vegetables daily, consistent with the My Plate* food guide for children. Also, promoting high-fiber foods and avoiding highly refined starches and sugars decrease caloric intake. The Dietary Guidelines for Americans[†] may

---

*http://www.choosemyplate.gov/index.html.
[†]http://www.health.gov/dietaryguidelines.

BOX 17-6 RECOMMENDED BEHAVIORS FOR PREVENTING OBESITY

In counseling adolescents whose body mass index is between the 5th and 84th percentiles, physicians and health care providers should recommend the following steps to prevent obesity:

- Limit consumption of sugar-sweetened beverages.
- Consume recommended quantities of fruits and vegetables.
- Limit television and other screen time to no more than 2 hours per day.
- Remove television and computer screens from primary sleeping areas.
- Eat breakfast daily.
- Limit eating at restaurants.
- Have frequent family meals in which parents and youth eat together.
- Limit portion sizes.

Adapted from Davis DM, Gance-Cleveland B, Hassink S, and others: Recommendations for prevention of childhood obesity, *Pediatrics* 120 (suppl):S229–S253, 2007.

---

be used as a guide for caloric intake for adolescents concerned about weight control; these guidelines also emphasize daily exercise in weight management for children and adolescents. Many programs recommend using a food diary as a helpful tool to increase awareness of food choices and eating behaviors. The goal is to encourage the individual to make healthy choices in food selection and discourage eating food by habit or to appease boredom. Box 17-6 contains helpful suggestions.

In patients with severe obesity, strict diets have been used, such as the protein-sparing modified fast, a hypocaloric, ketogenic diet that is designed to provide enough protein to minimize loss of lean body mass during weight loss. Such diets need to be closely monitored and should be used only with multidisciplinary teams that include a physician, nutritionist, and behavioral therapist. Generally, the diet consists of 1.5 to 2.5 g of protein per kilogram. The intake of carbohydrates is low enough to induce ketosis. The benefits of the diet are relatively rapid weight loss and anorexia induced by ketosis. Potential complications include protein losses, hypokalemia, hypoglycemia, inadequate calcium intake, and orthostatic hypotension. Potassium and calcium supplements and adequate calorie-free beverages can minimize these complications (Baker, Barlow, Cochran, and others, 2005). It is difficult to sustain such diets over the long term, and the long-term outcomes of using these diets have not been established.

Researchers continue searching for medications that will successfully treat obesity. The FDA has approved sibutramine, an appetite suppressant for use in adolescents 16 years and older for the treatment of obesity (U.S. Preventive Services Task Force, 2010). Orlistat, a lipase inhibitor, has been approved for adolescents 12 to 18 years of age who have BMIs more than 2 units above the 95th percentile for age and gender; however, side effects of the drug include fatty or oily stools and possible malabsorption of fat-soluble vitamins (Kanekar and Sharma, 2010). There are currently no drugs approved for use in overweight or obese children younger than the age of 12 years. Other drugs have been used to promote weight loss in children with certain conditions such as metformin in obese adolescents with insulin resistance and hyperinsulinism, octreotide for hypothalamic obesity caused by intracranial tumors, growth hormone in children with Prader-Willi syndrome, and leptin for congenital leptin deficiency.

Combining behavioral modifications with pharmacologic therapy in children 12 years and older have produced mixed results referent to total weight loss maintained over a significant period of time

(U.S. Preventive Services Task Force, 2010). Reports suggest modest benefits with moderate-to-high behavioral interventions (measured in number of contact hours) in decreasing mean BMI of children and adolescents involved in such programs over a period of 6 to 12 months (Whitlock, O'Connor, Williams, and others, 2010). Programs including family-based behavioral modification, dietary modification, and exercise have been shown to be successful in reducing obesity in some children (AAP, 2006).

Bariatric surgery may be the only practical alternative for increasing numbers of severely overweight adolescents who have failed organized attempts to lose or maintain weight loss through conventional nonoperative approaches and who have serious life-threatening conditions. Until recently, there were few studies in adolescents that suggested surgical weight loss improved the early mortality of patients with severe obesity. In the past 5 years, there has been an increase in bariatric surgery among teens, especially involving the laparoscopic adjustable gastric band procedure (although the FDA has not approved its use in adolescents). The laparoscopic Roux-en-Y gastric bypass is commonly performed for weight loss in adolescents. Data suggest that bariatric surgery in adolescents results in sustained weight loss, a decrease in BMI, and a decrease in the incidence of comorbidities such as type 2 diabetes (Barnett, 2011). Best practice recommendations for childhood and adolescent weight loss surgery are published elsewhere (Pratt, Lenders, Dionne, and others, 2009). Physicians must define clear, realistic, and restrictive guidelines to apply with younger patients when surgery is considered. Candidates for surgery should be referred to centers that offer a multidisciplinary team experienced in the management of childhood and adolescent obesity. The surgery should be performed by surgeons who have participated in subspecialty training in bariatric medical and surgical care as detailed by the American College of Surgeons and the American Society for Metabolic and Bariatric Surgery.

Nursing Care Management

Nurses play a key role in the adherence and maintenance phases of many weight reduction programs. Nurses assess, manage, and evaluate the progress of many overweight adolescents. They also play an important role in recognizing potential weight problems and assisting parents and adolescents in preventing obesity. The nursing process in the care of adolescents with obesity or overweight is outlined in the Nursing Process box.

The presence of obesity may not be obvious from appearance alone. Regular assessment of height and weight and computation of the BMI facilitate early recognition. Published guidelines are available for childhood obesity prevention and treatment (Barlow and Expert Committee, 2007). Children with BMIs greater than or equal to the 95th percentile for age and sex should receive in-depth medical assessment. Children with BMIs in the 85th to 95th percentile range should be evaluated for secondary complications, such as diabetes, hypertension and hyperlipidemia, and family history. Evaluation includes a height and weight history of the adolescent and family members, eating habits, appetite and hunger patterns, and physical activities. A psychosocial history is also helpful in understanding the impact of obesity on the child's life.

Before initiating a treatment plan, it is important to be certain that the family is ready for change. Lack of readiness may result in failure, frustration, and reluctance to address the problem in the future. The nurse should explore with adolescents the reasons behind the desire to lose weight because motivation to lose weight is the key to success. Adolescents need to take personal responsibility for their dietary habits and physical activity. Young persons who are forced by their parents to

NURSING PROCESS
The Child or Adolescent Who Is Overweight or Obese

Assessment

The nurse assists in determining the child or adolescent's body mass index, gathers appropriate anthropometric data, uses standardized growth charts to plot growth, and obtains a comprehensive health history. Further information that is appropriate to obtain in the assessment includes a 24-hour food intake history, family health history, and lifestyle practices that affect the child or adolescent's well-being. The health interview and nutritional assessment often provide clues and guidelines for further investigation.

Diagnosis (Problem Identification)

Several nursing diagnoses are identified after a thorough assessment:
- Situational Low Self-Esteem
- Imbalanced Nutrition: More Than Body Requirements
- Risk for Injury
- Risk-Prone Health Behavior
- Disturbed Personal Identity

Planning

Expected patient outcomes for the adolescent with an eating disorder include:
- Child or adolescent will develop a positive self-image.
- Adolescent will willingly engage in behaviors to reverse effects of cardiovascular disease.
- Healthy personal identity will be achieved.
- Healthy eating patterns will be adopted.
- Adolescent will assume control for changes in lifestyle designed to lose weight.
- Child or adolescent will remain injury free.

Implementation

Numerous intervention strategies are discussed on pp. 520–522.

Evaluation

The effectiveness of nursing interventions is determined by continual reassessment and evaluation of nursing care based on the following observational guidelines:
- Perform a nutritional assessment, measure weight, review diet and nutritional intake (e.g., log), interview adolescent regarding food and eating behaviors, observe eating behaviors.
- Interview adolescent regarding self-perceptions, observe behavior, confer with psychologist and other members of the interdisciplinary team regarding evidence of progress.
- Observe adolescent's behavior and interview him or her regarding attitudes, concerns, and behaviors.

seek help are seldom motivated, become rebellious, and are unwilling to control their dietary intake.

Nutritional Counseling. Preventing an increase in body fat during growth is a realistic approach. This is often accomplished by adjusting four aspects of eating: (1) reducing the quantity eaten by purchasing, preparing, and serving smaller portions; (2) altering the quality consumed by substituting low-calorie, low-fat foods for high-calorie foods (especially for snacks); (3) eating regular meals and snacks, particularly breakfast; and (4) altering situations by severing associations between eating and other stimuli, such as eating while watching television.

The most successful diets are those that use ordinary foods in controlled portions rather than diets that require the avoidance of specific foods.

Teach adolescents and parents how to incorporate favorite foods into their diet and to select satisfying substitutes. Dieting teens should eat what the rest of the family eats but less of it. When parents buy and prepare smaller amounts, they eliminate tempting second helpings and leftovers. To maintain a healthy diet, it is necessary to encourage the consumption of high-nutrient foods such as fruits, vegetables, whole grains, and low-fat dairy protein products. Keep calories and fat to a healthy level without being significantly restricted. To be successful, a dietary program should be nutritionally sound with sufficient satiety value, produce the desired weight loss, and be accompanied by nutrition education and continued support. Children and adolescents should not initiate a reduction diet without health assessment and counseling. Davis, Gance-Cleveland, Hassink, and colleagues (2007) describe steps to approaching behavior change with youth (Box 17-7).

Behavioral Therapy. Altering eating behavior and eliminating inappropriate eating habits are essential to weight reduction, especially in maintaining long-term weight control. Most behavioral modification programs include the following concepts:

- A description of the behavior to be controlled, such as eating habits
- Attempts to modify and control the stimuli that govern eating
- Development of eating techniques designed to control speed of eating
- Positive reinforcement for these modifications through a suitable reward system that does not include food

Box 17-6 includes specific strategies to modify eating habits.

Group Involvement. Commercial groups (e.g., Weight Watchers) and diet workshops composed primarily of adults may be helpful to some teenagers; however, a peer group is often more effective. Teenage groups include summer camps designed for obese young people and conducted by health professionals, school groups organized and led by a school nurse, and groups associated with special clinics.

These groups are concerned not only with weight loss but also with the development of a positive self-image and the encouragement of physical activity. Nutrition education, diet planning, and the improvement of social skills are essential components of these groups. Improvement is determined by positive changes in all aspects of behavior.

Family Involvement. There is a definite connection among family environment, interaction, and obesity. The nurse needs to educate parents in the purposes of the therapeutic measures and their role in management. The family needs nutrition education and counseling regarding the reinforcement plan, alterations in the food environment, and ways to maintain proper attitudes. They can support their child in efforts to change eating behaviors, food intake, and physical activity.

Research indicates that family meals may also play a role in decreasing obesity and high-risk behaviors among adolescents by promoting healthy eating habits; however, more quality research is needed to clarify the protective role of such interactions in regards to adolescent obesity (Fulkerson, Story, Mellin, and others, 2006; Fulkerson, Neumark-Sztainer, Hannan, and others, 2008; Larson, Neumark-Sztainer, Hannan, and others, 2007).

Parents can also affect the child's eating habits by decreasing media time viewed by the entire family and by discussing food advertisements that promote unhealthy food and eating habits.

Physical Activity. The current recommendation for physical activity for children and adolescents is to participate in a combined total of 60 minutes of physical activity daily; this can be moderate- to vigorous-intensive exercise or activity (U.S. Department of Health and Human Services, 2008). Regular physical activity is incorporated into all weight reduction programs. Any form of increased physical activity is beneficial, provided that the activities are age appropriate and enjoyable. Recommendations for physical activity need to consider the current health status and developmental level of the child or adolescent. The best choice for exercise is any form that is enjoyable and likely to be sustainable. Aerobic and endurance exercises help oxidize body fats. Light exercises such as walking may provide an opportunity for the family to increase time together and increase caloric expenditure. Walking for 30 minutes each day and decreasing caloric intake by 500 calories per day may significantly reduce the risk of chronic disease. Weight training can increase the basal metabolic rate and replace fat mass with muscle mass. However, weight training is not generally recommended for prepubertal children until they have reached physical and skeletal maturity. In prepubertal children, increasing outdoor playtime is likely to be beneficial. Many children find exercise videos and treadmills boring and may not continue these activities. There are a great variety of physical activities to choose from that are likely to appeal to different people. Team sports and individual sports such as dance, bike riding, swimming, and karate are some examples. Limiting

---

BOX 17-7 PEDIATRIC OBESITY PREVENTION PROTOCOL FOR PRIMARY CARE

Step 1: Assess

Explain and conduct assessments of:

- Weight, height, and body mass index percentile
- Dietary intake (fruit, vegetables, sweetened beverages, and fast food)
- Activity (screen time, moderate to vigorous activity)
- Eating behaviors (breakfast, portion sizes, family meals)

Provide and elicit feedback on body mass index and behaviors found to be inside and outside the optimal range.

Step 2: Set Agenda

Explore interest in changing behaviors not in the optimal range.

Agree on target behaviors with the patient and caregiver.

Step 3: Assess Motivation and Confidence

With regard to interest in changing weight status or behaviors, assess:

- Willingness
- Perceived importance
- Confidence in having success

Probe the patient regarding ratings of willingness, perceived importance, and confidence to explore the advantages and disadvantages of changing.

Step 4: Summarize and Probe Possible Changes

Summarize the advantages and disadvantages of change.

Query possible next steps.

Offer ideas for getting started in making a change as needed.

Summarize the change plan.

Provide positive feedback.

Step 5: Schedule Follow-Up Visit

If a change plan is made, agree on a follow-up appointment within a specified number of weeks or months.

If no change plan is made, agree to revisit the topic within a specific number of weeks or months.

Adapted from Davis DM, Gance-Cleveland B, Hassink S, and others: Recommendations for prevention of childhood obesity, *Pediatrics* 120(suppl):S229–S253, 2007.

sedentary activities such as television viewing (while eating snacks!) is the most effective way to encourage physical activity.

Prevention. Weight loss programs do not enjoy the success of therapeutic interventions for other disorders. Gradual accumulation of adipose tissue during childhood establishes a pattern of eating that is difficult to reverse in adolescence. Prevention of obesity should begin in early childhood with the development of healthy eating habits, including breastfeeding, regular exercise patterns, and a positive relationship between parents and children. Prevention of adolescent obesity is best accomplished by early identification of obesity in the preschool, school-age, and preadolescent periods. Health care professionals should encourage frequent health care visits for children who are overweight or obese and incorporate a dietary history and counseling into each well-infant, well-child, and well-adolescent visit.*

Anorexia Nervosa and Bulimia Nervosa

Anorexia nervosa (AN) is an eating disorder characterized by a refusal to maintain a minimally normal body weight and by severe weight loss in the absence of obvious physical causes. Approximately 5% of adolescent girls in the United States have AN, and 5% to 10% of all cases occur in boys and men (AAP, Committee on Adolescence, 2010). The average age of onset is 13 years, but the disorder can occur as early as 10 years of age and as late as 25 years of age. Individuals with AN are described as perfectionists, academically high achievers, conforming, and conscientious. Typically, they have high energy levels even with marked emaciation. Patients with AN may eventually develop bulimia.

Bulimia (from the Greek meaning "ox hunger") refers to an eating disorder similar to AN. Bulimia nervosa (BN) is observed more commonly in older adolescent girls and young women; boys and men with bulimia are less common. BN patients may be of average or slightly above average weight. BN is characterized by repeated episodes of binge eating followed by inappropriate compensatory behaviors, such as self-induced vomiting; misuse of laxatives, diuretics, or other medications; fasting; or excessive exercise (AAP, Committee on Adolescence, 2010). The binge behavior consists of secretive, frenzied consumption of large amounts of high-calorie (or "forbidden") foods during a brief time (usually <2 hours). The binge is counteracted by a variety of weight control methods (purging). These binge–purge cycles are followed by self-deprecating thoughts, a depressed mood, and an awareness that the eating pattern is abnormal. Nonpurging bulimic individuals may use other inappropriate compensatory behaviors such as fasting or excessive exercising but do not regularly engage in self-induced vomiting or the abuse of laxatives, enemas, or diuretics (APA, 2000).

Although persons with BN have many issues in common with those who have other eating disorders, impulse control and satiety regulation are important problems in BN. Many individuals with BN begin with only occasional binges and purges "just for fun," enjoying the control over their weight while eating amounts of food that would normally produce obesity. As the condition progresses, the frequency of binges increases, the amount of food consumed increases, and they gradually lose control over the binge–purge cycle. The frequency of binging can be anywhere from once per week to seven or eight times per day. Because persons with BN usually binge on high-calorie foods, especially sweets, ice cream, and pastries, insulin production is stimulated to cope with the added carbohydrates. When the food is vomited, the unused insulin stimulates hunger and the desire to eat.

A third eating disorder, identified as eating disorder not otherwise specified (EDNOS), has components of both AN and BN with varying degrees of symptomatology that are not always characteristic of the established diagnostic criteria for AN and BN (American Dietetic Association, 2006). Binge eating disorder (BED) is a type of EDNOS. Persons with BED may diet in an attempt to control their weight but without the extreme weight control compensatory practices of vomiting, laxative use, diuretics, and excessive exercise (American Dietetic Association, 2006; Forman, 2011).

Another type of eating disorder, avoidant/restrictive food intake disorder (ARFID), has been proposed and is scheduled to appear in the APA's *DSM-V* classification of eating disorders of children. In this disorder, there is an apparent lack of interest in eating or food with significant weight loss, nutritional deficiency, and dependence on enteral feeding; there is also significant interference with psychosocial functioning in this disorder, and it is not associated with AN or BN (APA, 2010).

Etiology and Pathophysiology

The etiology of these disorders remains unclear. There is a distinct psychologic component, and the diagnosis is based primarily on psychologic and behavioral criteria. Dieting appears to be common to the initiation of both AN and BN. The disorders appear to be caused by a combination of genetic, neurochemical, psychodevelopmental, and sociocultural factors. The dominant aspects of AN are a relentless pursuit of thinness and a fear of fatness, usually preceded by a period of mood disturbances and behavior changes.

Weight loss may be triggered by a typical adolescent crisis such as the onset of menstruation or a traumatic interpersonal incident that precipitates serious, out-of-control dieting. Situations of severe family stress (e.g., parental separation or divorce) or circumstances in which the adolescent perceives a lack of personal control (e.g., teasing at school, changing schools, or going to college) may precipitate a desire for control and the decision not to eat. Frequently, there is an exaggerated misinterpretation of the normal fat deposition characteristic of early adolescence or anxiety because of comments that the adolescent is putting on weight.

Many experts have associated the development of an eating disorder with family characteristics such as an adolescent perception of high parental expectations for achievement and appearance, difficulty managing conflict and poor communication styles, enmeshment and occasionally estrangement among family members, devaluation of the mother or the maternal role, and marital tension. Families struggling with an eating disorder have been characterized as often having difficulties responding positively to the changing physical and emotional needs of the adolescent. Family stress of any kind may become a significant factor in the development of an eating disorder (Forman, 2011).

Society's emphasis and the media's focus on tall, thin individuals may also play a role. Studies evaluating the possible association of eating disorders and sexual abuse have been conflicting. Childhood sexual abuse may be a factor in some cases of AN.

Patients with eating disorders commonly have psychiatric problems, including affective disorder, anxiety disorder, obsessive-compulsive disorder (OCD), and personality disorder. Adult women with eating disorders were found to have higher rates of obsessive-compulsive behavior traits in their childhoods. Patients with eating disorders have also been found to have higher reported rates of substance abuse, with alcohol problems being more common in those with BN than AN (Forman, 2011). It is important to note that many of the clinical findings are directly related to the state of starvation and improve with weight gain.

---

*For additional information on prevention of obesity in childhood, visit the IOM website, www.iom.edu/obesityyoungchildren.

Nursing Care Plan—The Adolescent with an Eating Disorder

BOX 17-8 CLINICAL MANIFESTATIONS OF ANOREXIA NERVOSA

- Severe and profound weight loss
- Secondary amenorrhea (if menarche attained)
- Primary amenorrhea (if menarche not attained)
- Sinus bradycardia
- Low body temperature
- Hypotension
- Intolerance to cold
- Dry skin and brittle nails
- Appearance of lanugo hair
- Thinning hair
- Abdominal pain
- Bloating
- Constipation
- Fatigue
- Lightheadedness
- Evidence of muscle wasting (cachectic appearance)
- Bone pain with exercise

TABLE 17-4 CHARACTERISTICS OF INDIVIDUALS WITH EATING DISORDERS

FACTORS	ANOREXIA NERVOSA	BULIMIA
Food	Turns away from food to cope	Turns to food to cope
Personality	Introverted	Extroverted
	Avoids intimacy	Seeks intimacy
	Negates feminine role	Aspires to feminine role
Behavior	"Model" child	Often acts out
	Obsessive-compulsive	Impulsive
School	High achiever	Variable school performance
Control	Maintains rigid control	Loses control
Body image	Body image distortion	Less frequent body image distortion
Health	Denies illness	Recognizes illness
		Health fluctuates
Weight	Body weight <85% of expected norm	Within 2.3–7 kg (5–15 lb) of normal body weight or may be overweight
Sexuality	Usually not sexually active	Often sexually active

Many sports and artistic endeavors that emphasize leanness (e.g., ballet and running) and sports in which the scoring is partly subjective (e.g., gymnastics) have been associated with a higher incidence of eating disorders such as AN. The term female athlete triad, characterized by disordered eating behavior, amenorrhea, and osteoporosis, has been applied to young women with restrictive eating disorders and amenorrhea (Landry, 2011).

A genetic role has been postulated for eating disorders; a significant number of young women with a first-degree relative having an eating disorder were at a significantly higher rate of having an eating disorder (Forman, 2011). However, some consider these eating disorders to not be a direct result of family inheritance but rather a secondary effect of the manifestations of conditions such as anxiety, depression, and OCD "that may be modulated through the internal milieu of puberty" (Landry, 2011).

Diagnostic Evaluation

Diagnosis of AN is made on the basis of clinical manifestations (Box 17-8) and conformity to the criteria established by the APA (2000). Diagnosis of BN is confirmed, according to the APA's *DSM* (2000), by at least two binge eating episodes per week for the preceding 3 months. Characteristics of BN and AN are listed in Table 17-4.

A complete history and physical examination are important to rule out other causes of weight loss. The medical assessment of an eating disorder focuses on the complications of altered nutritional status and purging. A careful history assesses weight changes, dietary patterns, and the frequency and severity of purging and excessive exercise. The patient's weight and height should be measured and evaluated for appropriateness according to standard weight for height, age, and sex determined according to the percentile of his or her expected body weight or BMI.

The diagnosis of eating disorder is made clinically, but additional laboratory diagnostic tests may be obtained to identify malnutrition or other associated complications. Additional diagnostic measures may include a complete blood count to evaluate for anemia and other hematologic abnormalities; erythrocyte sedimentation rate or C-reactive protein to detect evidence of inflammation; electrolytes as well as calcium, magnesium, phosphorus, blood urea nitrogen, and

creatinine; urinalysis, including specific gravity; and bone density studies for osteopenia, which is commonly observed in patients with AN. In patients with prolonged amenorrhea, human chorionic gonadotropin is assessed to determine the presence of pregnancy. Other tests for patients with amenorrhea include thyroid function tests and measurement of serum prolactin and follicle-stimulating hormone to help rule out prolactinoma (hormone-secreting pituitary tumor), hyperthyroidism, hypothyroidism, or ovarian failure. In addition, a comprehensive cardiac evaluation is often recommended in those with AN. Further diagnostic tests may be required based on the history and findings from these diagnostic tests.

Screening Tools. All patients in high-risk categories for eating disorders should be screened during routine office visits. The medical history is most important for diagnosing eating disorders because the physical examination findings may be normal, especially early in the illness. A number of screening questionnaires are available to assist with the interview. For example, with the Scoff Questionnaire, 1 point is scored for every "yes." A score of 2 or more indicates a likely case of AN or BN. The questions related to the mnemonic SCOFF are (1) Do you make yourself *sick* because you feel uncomfortably full? (2) Do you worry that you have lost *control* over how much you eat? (3) Have you recently lost more than 6.4 kg (14 pounds or *one* stone) in a 3-month period? (4) Do you believe yourself to be *fat* when others say that you are too thin? and (5) Would you say that *food* dominates your life? (Morgan, Reid, and Lacey, 1999).

Therapeutic Management

The treatment and management of AN involve three major goals: (1) reinstitution of normal nutrition or reversal of the severe state of malnutrition, (2) resolution of disturbed patterns of family interaction, and (3) individual psychotherapy to correct deficits and distortions in psychologic functioning. The treatment of eating disorders requires the cooperative efforts of an interdisciplinary team composed of a primary practitioner, nurse, dietitian, and mental health provider with pediatric and adolescent health care experience. Because of the psychogenic nature of the disorder, the treatment may be long. Recent studies suggest that family-based therapy is more effective than individual cognitive behavioral therapy in reducing the maladaptive eating behaviors in adolescents with AN (Lock, 2010).

Most adolescents are treated on an outpatient basis, but those with problems requiring immediate medical attention, such as severe malnutrition or electrolyte or psychiatric disturbances (severe depression or suicidal ideation), require hospitalization. Persons with BN may benefit from cognitive behavioral therapy, other psychotherapy, antidepressant medications, or a combination of antidepressant medication and psychotherapy (Kreipe, 2011).

Nutrition Therapy. The most important goal is to treat any life-threatening malnutrition and to restore dietary stability and weight gain. This may require the administration of tube feedings or intravenous fluids if the malnutrition is severe. In most cases, it is best to reintroduce food and snacks slowly in a stepwise manner. A reasonable goal is to reach an eventual intake of 2000 to 3000 kcal per day and a weight gain of 0.22 to 0.45 kg (0.5–1 pound) per week (American Dietetic Association, 2006). When restoring nutrition, health professionals must avoid the refeeding syndrome, which consists of cardiovascular, neurologic, and hematologic complications that occur when nutritional replacement is given too rapidly. This syndrome can be avoided with slow refeeding and the addition of phosphorus when total body phosphorus is depleted. Treatment goal weights are individualized and based on age, height, stage of puberty, premorbid weight, and previous growth charts. In young women who have reached menarche, resumption of menses is an objective measure of return to biologic health.

Dietary interventions are combined with behavioral therapy to improve the underlying psychologic misconceptions about weight loss. Another aspect of treatment is to relieve the anxiety related to eating and the depression that accompanies the disorder. The administration of antianxiety or antidepressant medications is beneficial. However, when these drugs are used, patients should be carefully monitored for cardiovascular side effects.

Cognitive Behavioral Therapy. Behavioral interventions are often necessary to encourage patients to accomplish the desired caloric intake and weight gain. Weight restoration as an outpatient is accomplished with behavioral contracts negotiated between the therapists and patient. The goal is to increase the patient's feelings of control and responsibility toward achieving recovery. The contract can stipulate at what weight tube feedings will be implemented. Individual psychotherapy is aimed at helping the young person resolve the adolescent identity crisis, particularly as it relates to a distorted body image. If the disorder is related to a dysfunctional family situation, therapy is most successful when it is started soon after the onset of illness and directed toward disengagement and redirection of malfunctioning processes in the family.

Pharmacotherapy. Pharmacotherapy in the treatment of AN has been disappointing so far. None of the RCTs have shown improvement in weight gain in adults treated with pharmacotherapy, and no studies have been conducted in children and adolescents (Golden and Attia, 2011). The few studies that have been done have primarily evaluated medications' efficacy in the treatment of comorbid disorders such as OCD and depression. Anxiolytic medications may be helpful before meals to relieve some patients' anxiety.

Tricyclic antidepressants and fluoxetine belong to a group of medications known as SSRIs, which have been more successful when used with BN. There is also some evidence that TCAs such as desipramine, imipramine, and amitriptyline; monoamine oxidase inhibitors; and buspirone are more effective compared with a placebo in decreasing binging and vomiting in patients with BN. Some of the latter

CRITICAL THINKING CASE STUDY
Anorexia Nervosa

Jane is a 13-year-old girl whose grades have been excellent and whom the teachers describe as a "model student." Recently, Jane's teacher told the nurse practitioner that Jane's parents were in the middle of a "messy divorce." In addition, several of Jane's friends told the nurse practitioner that they are concerned about Jane because she runs every day at lunchtime and seldom eats lunch with them. Jane told her friends that she gained weight over the winter months and that she is running because she wants to qualify for the track team this spring. At the time of her routine health interview and sports physical examination, the nurse practitioner notes that Jane's oral temperature is 36° C (96.8° F) and that she weighs 34 kg (75 pounds). Jane has lost 9 kg (20 pounds) since her last sports physical. Jane tells the nurse practitioner that she has not had her menstrual period for 3 months.

Questions
1. Evidence—Is there sufficient evidence to draw any conclusions about Jane's behavior?
2. Assumptions—Describe some underlying assumptions about the following:
   a. Personality characteristics of individuals with AN
   b. Factors influencing the development of AN
   c. Clinical manifestations of AN
   d. Treatment of AN
3. What priorities for nursing care should be established for Jane at this time?
4. Does the evidence support your conclusion?

AN, Anorexia nervosa.

medications, however, may have side effects which may preclude their utility in such patients (Golden and Attia, 2011). Topiramate, an antiepileptic agent, and the selective serotonin antagonist ondansetron have demonstrated some benefit in treating patients with BN. As with AN, pharmacotherapy should be an adjunct to behavioral therapy.

Nursing Care Management

Nurses need to adopt and maintain a kind and supportive yet firm manner in managing the care of the adolescent with eating disorders without creating a passive-dependent attitude. The individual requires sustained support and reassurance to cope with ambivalent feelings related to body concept and the desire to be seen as cooperative, reliable, and worthy of receiving kindness. Encouraging the adolescent with education and activities that strengthen self-esteem facilitates the resocialization process and promotes social acceptance among peers.

It is important for nurses to be aware of the physical side effects of AN. Patients frequently limit their fluid intake. Urinary tract problems are common, and ketones and protein may be detected in the urine as a result of breakdown of fat and protein. Vital sign instability can be severe and can include orthostatic hypotension; the pulse becomes irregular, and the rate decreases markedly. Electrolyte imbalances can be life threatening and bradycardia and hypothermia can result in cardiac arrest (see Critical Thinking Case Study box).

The team responsible for the management of young people with AN arranges a carefully structured environment. First, there must be consistency. The team decides on an approach and adheres to it. The plan is structured with reality testing regarding caloric intake and body image perception as an essential component. The team members provide a unified front to avoid any possibility of manipulation or inconsistency. Second, all team members are involved; responsibility for the program cannot be left to one person. The role and boundaries of each member are clearly spelled out. Third, continuity of team members is important; it is helpful to have the same team members all the time.

Fourth, communication among team members is essential. Communication with the patient regarding what is expected is also important. Sometimes the limit setting may seem unreasonable; if the adolescent does not understand the rationale for the limits, he or she may sabotage the entire program. It is also important to communicate with the family. Fifth, the plan must provide for support of the adolescent, the family, and team members. The adolescent's efforts should be supported, and positive feedback should be provided for accomplishments made in normalizing eating habits. Meetings are held to discuss the feelings and concerns of the patient, immediate caregivers, and team members.

A **behavioral contract**, an agreement that the adolescent makes with others to change a maladaptive behavior, has proved to be effective in some cases. The written contract is constructed by the therapeutic team and approved and signed by the adolescent. Unless the adolescent agrees to its terms, the contract can become the source of a power struggle. However, it can be an effective tool that places the responsibility for weight gain or other behavioral change on the adolescent.

Family-based therapy is often used in the treatment of adolescent eating disorders, specifically in the treatment of AN. In particular, the Maudsley approach aims to help parents rediscover their own resources and take an active role in their children's recovery. Encourage families to explore how it has become problematic to follow the normal developmental course of their family life cycle by looking at how the eating disorder and the interactional patterns in the family have become entangled.

Nursing care of the adolescent with BN is similar to care of the patient with AN. Acute care involves careful monitoring of fluid and electrolyte alterations and observation for signs of cardiac complications. Nutritional consultation and follow-up care are essential. The nurse should encourage the adolescent and family members to structure the environment to reduce the binging behavior. Getting rid of binge foods; restricting eating to one room of the house; not engaging in other activities while eating; and substituting exercise, crafts, visualization, and relaxation techniques for binging are helpful interventions.

Nurses, patients, and families can find assistance and information from several organizations. The American Anorexia/Bulimia Association, Inc.,* provides information, referrals, counseling, and activities aimed at combating eating disorders. The National Association of Anorexia Nervosa and Associated Eating Disorders[†] provides counseling, referral, and self-help programs for young people with AN. The National Eating Disorders Association[‡] provides information and support services for both patients and families.

Lactose Intolerance

Lactose intolerance refers to at least four different entities that involve a deficiency of the enzyme **lactase**, which is needed for the hydrolysis or digestion of lactose in the small intestine; lactose is hydrolyzed into glucose and galactose. **Congenital lactase deficiency** occurs soon after birth after the newborn has consumed lactose-containing milk (human

milk or commercial formula). This inborn error of metabolism involves the complete absence or severely reduced presence of lactase, is extremely rare, and requires a lifelong lactose-free or extremely reduced lactose diet.

Primary lactase deficiency, sometimes referred to as late-onset lactase deficiency, is the most common type of lactose intolerance and is manifested usually after 4 or 5 years of age, although the time of onset is variable. Ethnic groups with a high incidence of lactase deficiency include Asians, southern Europeans, Arabs, Israelis, and African Americans; Scandinavians tend to have the lowest incidence. Lactose malabsorption manifests as lactose intolerance and is characterized by an imbalance between the ability for lactase to hydrolyze the ingested lactose and the amount of lactose ingested (Heyman and AAP, Committee on Nutrition, 2006).

Secondary lactase deficiency may occur secondary to damage of the intestinal lumen, which decreases or destroys the enzyme lactase. Cystic fibrosis; sprue; celiac disease; kwashiorkor; and infections such as giardiasis, HIV, or rotavirus may cause a temporary or permanent lactose intolerance.

Developmental lactase deficiency refers to the relative lactase deficiency observed in preterm infants of less than 34 weeks of gestation (Heyman and AAP, Committee on Nutrition, 2006).

The primary symptoms of lactose intolerance include abdominal pain, bloating, flatulence, and diarrhea after the ingestion of lactose. The onset of symptoms occurs within 30 minutes to several hours of lactose consumption. Lactose intolerance is often perceived as an allergy, and in several studies with reports of acute gastrointestinal symptoms ascribed to lactose intolerance, measurement of lactase activity is normal.

Lactose intolerance may be diagnosed on the basis of the history and improvement with a lactose-reduced diet. The breath hydrogen test is used to positively diagnose the condition. Breath samples in lactose-deficient individuals will yield a higher percentage of hydrogen ($\geq$20 ppm [parts per million] above baseline). In infants, lactose malabsorption may be diagnosed by evaluating fecal pH and reducing substances; fecal pH in infants is usually lower than in older children, but an acidic pH may indicate malabsorption (Heyman and AAP, Committee on Nutrition, 2006).

Treatment of lactose intolerance is elimination of offending dairy products; however, some advocate decreasing amounts of dairy products rather than total elimination, especially in small children (Heyman and AAP, Committee on Nutrition, 2006). In infants, lactose-free or low-lactose formula offers no special advantages over lactose-containing formula except in those who are severely malnourished (Heyman and AAP, Committee on Nutrition, 2006).

One concern is that dairy avoidance in children and adolescents with lactose intolerance will contribute to reduced bone mineral density and osteoporosis (AAP, 2009; Suchy, Brannon, Carpenter, and others, 2010). Evidence indicates that dietary lactose enhances calcium absorption and that lactose-free diets may negatively affect bone mineralization (Heyman and AAP, Committee on Nutrition, 2006). It is recommended that individuals with lactose maldigestion who do not experience lactose intolerance symptoms continue to consume small amounts of dairy products with meals to prevent reduced bone mass density and subsequent osteoporosis. Some evidence indicates that **probiotics** (food preparations containing microorganisms such as *Lactobacillus*, which alter the gastrointestinal microflora and thus are beneficial to the host) improve lactose intolerance when live cultures are fermented in dairy products (de Vrese and Schrezenmeir, 2008). The positive attributes of probiotics for those with lactose maldigestion include delayed gastrointestinal transit (slower than milk), positive

---

*800-522-2230; http://orgs.tigweb.org/american-anorexia-bulimia-association.
[†]Helpline 630-577-1330, available 9 AM to 5 PM Central Time, Monday to Friday; e-mail: anadhelp@anad.org; http://www.anad.org.
[‡]603 Stewart St., Suite 803, Seattle, WA 98101; 800-931-2237; http://www.edap.org.

👪 FAMILY-CENTERED CARE
Controlling Symptoms of Lactose Intolerance

- In infants, substitute lactose-free or soy-based formula for cow's milk–based formula or human milk (only after a diagnosis of congenital lactose deficiency or secondary lactase intolerance is made).
- Limit milk consumption to one to two glasses per day.
- Drink milk with other foods rather than alone.
- Eat hard cheese, cottage cheese, or yogurt instead of drinking milk.
- Use enzyme tablets (Lactaid, Lactrase, Dairy Ease) to metabolize the lactose in milk or supplement the body's own lactase (add tablets to milk or sprinkle on dairy products such as ice cream).
- Eat small amounts of dairy foods daily to help colonic bacteria adapt to ingested lactose.
- Include a probiotic (yogurt or cultured [fermented] milk) in meal or as a snack that has *Lactobacillus* or *Bifidobacterium* organisms.
- Take a calcium supplement if unable to consume any dairy products such as cheese.

effects on intestinal and colonic microflora, and a reduction of maldigestion symptoms.

Most people are able to tolerate small amounts of lactose (≈1 cup of milk per day) even in the presence of deficient lactase activity (Heyman and AAP, Committee on Nutrition, 2006; Suchy, Brannon, Carpenter, and others, 2010) and should be encouraged to continue their intake of dairy products in small amounts to obtain much-needed nutrients. Milk taken at meals may be better tolerated than when taken alone (see Family-Centered Care box). Pretreated milk (with microbial-derived lactase) is reported to be effective in improving lactose absorption. Because dairy products are a major source of calcium and vitamin D, supplementation of these nutrients is needed to prevent deficiency. Yogurt contains inactive lactase enzyme, which is activated by the temperature and pH of the duodenum; this lactase activity substitutes for the lack of endogenous lactase. Fresh, plain yogurt may be tolerated better than frozen or flavored yogurt; hard cheeses, lactase-treated dairy products, and lactase tablets taken with dairy products are also viable options. An important distinction between lactose intolerance and food allergy is that lactose intolerance will not manifest as an anaphylactic-type reaction.

Nursing Care Management

Nursing care is similar to the interventions discussed for cow's milk allergy in Chapter 11 and includes explaining the dietary restrictions to the family; identifying alternate sources of calcium such as yogurt and calcium supplementation; explaining the importance of supplementation; and discussing sources of lactose, especially hidden sources such as its use as a bulk agent in certain medications, and ways of controlling the symptoms (see Family-Centered Care box). Parents are advised to check with the pharmacist regarding this possibility when obtaining medication.

ADOLESCENT DISORDERS WITH A BEHAVIORAL COMPONENT

Substance Abuse

Although experimentation with drugs during childhood and adolescence is widespread, most children and teens do not become high-risk users. *Monitoring the Future* has been providing long-term research about the rates of substance use among adolescents, young adults, and adults since 1975. The 2010 survey found that marijuana use and acceptance of marijuana use has been on the rise since 2007. Alcohol use has been on the decline since the early 1980s and reached historically low levels in 2010. Cigarette use was on a steady decline since the mid-1990s but showed some increase in 2010, which followed a leveling off of the perceived risk of cigarette use. The use of illicit drugs other than marijuana has shown minimal change. However, 15% of 12th graders in 2010 reported the use of prescription drugs without medical supervision (Johnston, O'Malley, Bachman, and others, 2011).

Drug abuse, misuse, and addiction are culturally defined and are voluntary behaviors. Drug tolerance and physical dependence are involuntary physiologic responses to the pharmacologic characteristics of drugs, such as opioids and alcohol. Consequently, an individual can be addicted to a narcotic with or without being physically dependent. A person can also be physically dependent on a narcotic without being addicted (e.g., patients who use opioids to control pain).

Motivation

Most drug use begins with experimentation. The drug may be used only once, may be used occasionally, or may become part of a drug-centered lifestyle. Children and adolescents initiate drug use out of curiosity. Adolescents who use drugs may fall into one of two broad categories—experimenters and compulsive users—or they may fall into a third category somewhere on the continuum between these extremes, referred to as recreational users, principally of drugs such as marijuana, cocaine, alcohol, and prescription drugs. For many, the goal is peer acceptance; these users fit more closely with the experimenting, intermittent users. For others, the goal is intoxication or the sustained intense effects from using a particular drug; these users resemble the compulsive users. These users may engage in periodic heavy use, or binges. The groups of greatest concern to health care workers are those whose patterns of use involve high doses or mixed drugs with the danger of overdose and compulsive users with the threat of dependence, withdrawal syndromes, and altered lifestyle.

Types of Drugs Abused

Any drug can be abused, and most are potentially harmful to adolescents still going through formative life experiences. Although rarely considered drugs by society, the chemically active substances frequently abused are the xanthines and theobromines contained in chocolate, tea, coffee, and colas. Ethyl alcohol and nicotine are other drugs that are legal and socially sanctioned. Any of these substances can produce mild to moderate euphoric or stimulant effects and can lead to physical and psychologic dependence.

Drugs with mind-altering abilities that are available on the "street" and are of medical and legal concern are the hallucinogenic, narcotic, hypnotic, and stimulant drugs. In addition, health professionals are concerned about the use of alcohol and volatile substances that are inhaled to achieve altered sensation (e.g., gasoline, antifreeze, plastic model airplane cement, typewriter correction fluid, organic solvents). Recently, abuse of prescription and synthetic drugs such as oxycodone, alprazolam (Xanax), and amphetamine-dextroamphetamine (Adderall) has become a concern for professionals who work with children and adolescents.

Many of the prescription drugs are available at a decreased cost compared with the more exotic drugs of abuse and are often found in the medicine or kitchen cabinet at home. Websites also promote the "safe use" of some psychoactive drugs and supply information on new "designer" drugs that are not detectable on a standard urine drug screening test.

Tobacco. Cigarette smoking has been on a slow decline since the peak in 1999 despite multiple efforts, including increased costs,

COMMUNITY FOCUS

Early Sexual Maturation, Alcohol, and Cigarettes

Smoking cigarettes and drinking alcohol among adolescents are complex behaviors that are not explained by any one cause or factor. Some theorists and investigators believe there is a relationship between biologic maturation and these risk-taking behaviors. For example, young girls who are sexually mature at an earlier age than their peers are often attracted to older girls and boys who may engage in risk-taking behaviors. If older teens smoke, drink, and drive while under the influence of alcohol with no adverse consequences (e.g., no motor vehicle crashes), young girls may believe that they, too, will be safe while smoking, drinking, or riding in an automobile with friends who are drinking.

Although parents and nurses cannot influence the time of biologic maturation, they can identify young girls who are at risk for the initiation of risk-taking behaviors because of early puberty. Parents need to understand that an early-maturing daughter might be uncomfortable with her body, and they should take advantage of opportunities to build her self-esteem. Parental sensitivity to the importance of peer group acceptance and parental support of a teenage daughter who feels left out or different are crucial. School nurses can provide anticipatory guidance to these girls and help them to role-play coping strategies for situations that involve offers to smoke and drink. In addition, school nurses can provide information about physical development during puberty and emphasize the fact that not all teenagers mature at the same time or rate.

Teachers, coaches, and church leaders can provide opportunities for these girls to "fit in" with their same-age peers through activities that stress mutual goals. For example, an early-maturing girl is typically taller than her age mates and can be an asset in sports such as basketball and track-and-field events.

---

changes in community attitudes about smoking among adults, media campaigns with counter-advertising, and tobacco-free environments (CDC, 2010a). Use of all tobacco products among youth did not change between 2006 and 2009 (CDC, 2010b).

Although the number of adult and adolescent smokers has declined in recent years, cigarette smoking is still considered the chief avoidable cause of death. The hazards of smoking at any age are undisputed; however, a preventive approach to teenage smoking is especially important. Because of its addictive nature, smoking begun in childhood and adolescence can result in a lifetime habit, with increased morbidity and early mortality.

The effects of secondhand smoke exposure are also well known and include increased incidence of low birth weight and subsequent illness, increased incidence of sudden infant death syndrome (maternal smoking during and after pregnancy), increased incidence of acute lower respiratory tract infections, and exacerbation of asthma symptoms (wheezing, cough, phlegm, breathlessness) in children with asthma (U.S. Department of Health and Human Services, 2006).

Etiology. Teenagers begin smoking for a variety of reasons, including imitation of adult behavior; peer pressure; a desire to imitate behaviors and lifestyles portrayed in movies and advertisements; and a desire to control weight, especially among young women. Teenagers who do not smoke usually have family members and friends who do not smoke or who oppose smoking. Most teens who refrain from smoking have a desire to succeed in academics or athletics (particularly high-performance sports, such as basketball, swimming, and track) and plans to go to college (see Community Focus box). Although smoking among college students has increased in recent years, rates of smoking are highest among adolescents who do not complete high school.

Smokeless Tobacco. The term *smokeless tobacco* refers to tobacco products that are placed in the mouth but not ignited (e.g., snuff and chewing tobacco). This substitute for cigarettes continues to pose a hazard to adolescents, although use had steadily declined by about 50% since the peak prevalence in 1995; the 2010 data showed a slight increase. Children and adolescents continue to recognize the risk of smokeless tobacco and have expressed high rates of disapproval (Johnston, O'Malley, Bachman, and others, 2011). These products have also been proved to be carcinogenic, and regular use can cause dental problems, foul-smelling breath, and tooth erosion or loss.

Nursing Care Management. Prevention of regular smoking in teenagers is the most effective way to reduce the overall incidence of smoking. A variety of methods have been used. Posters, charts, displays, statistics, and the use of examples of actual damaged lungs to communicate the hazards of smoking all have their supporters and doubters. Some schools also use films and demonstrations in science classes.

For the most part, smoking prevention programs that focus on the negative, long-term effects of smoking on health have been ineffective. Youth-to-youth programs and those emphasizing the immediate effects are more effective but primarily in improving teenagers' attitudes toward not smoking. Because smoking and smoking-related behaviors are social symbols, antismoking campaigns must address the norms of potential smokers. Anything that ridicules or threatens the social norms of the peer group can be unproductive or counterproductive. Investigators have found that teaching resistance to peer pressure to smoke is effective in early adolescence. Although the effects of these programs may decrease with time, the effects can be enhanced in older adolescents by presenting information in class instead of simply handing out written material to the students.

Two areas of focus for antismoking programs are peer-led programs and use of media in smoking prevention (e.g., CDs, videotapes, and films). Peer-led programs emphasizing the social consequences of smoking have proved most successful. If a significant number of influential peers can "sell" their classmates on the idea that the habit is not popular, the followers will imitate their behavior. Such programs emphasize short-term rather than long-term consequences (e.g., the effects of smoking on personal appearance, such as unattractive stains on teeth and hands and unpleasant odor of breath and clothing).

The impact of school-based antismoking programs can be strengthened by expanding these programs to include parents, mass media, youth groups, and community organizations. For example, mass media efforts that involve antismoking radio campaigns have been identified as the most cost-effective mass media intervention.

Smoking bans in schools also accomplish several goals: (1) they discourage students from starting to smoke, (2) they reinforce knowledge of the health hazards of cigarette smoking and exposure to environmental tobacco smoke, and (3) they promote a smoke-free environment as the norm (see Community Focus box).

Alcohol. Acute or chronic abuse of alcohol (ethanol) is responsible for many acts of violence, suicide, accidental injury, and death. Alcohol drinking is likely to begin in the middle school years and increases with age. By 18 years of age, 80% to 90% of adolescents have tried alcohol. Ethanol is a depressant that reduces inhibitions against aggressive and sexual acting out. Severe physical and psychologic symptoms accompany abrupt withdrawal, and long-term use leads to slow tissue destruction, especially of the brain and liver cells. The most noticeable effects of alcohol occur within the CNS and include changes in cognitive and autonomic functions such as judgment, memory, learning ability, and other intellectual capacities. Young people with alcoholism often drink alone and cannot control their use of alcohol. They often

🏠 COMMUNITY FOCUS

Nonsmoking Strategies

Nurses who work in schools, hospitals, and community agencies can take advantage of all opportunities to provide education about the dangers of smoking, to discourage smoking initiation by children and adolescents, to encourage smoking cessation, and to promote smoke-free environments. In particular, school nurses must be alert to the vulnerability of young preteens when they enter middle school. These nurses are in an ideal position to assess stress, personal conflict, weight concerns, peer pressures, and other factors that place preteens at risk for smoking initiation. Nurses should serve as counselors to student, teacher, and parent groups and as advocates for anti-smoking legislative efforts. Several additional strategies are recommended*:

- Provide only brief information about long-term health consequences (e.g., cardiovascular, cancer risks).
- Discuss immediate physiologic consequences (e.g., changes in heart rate, blood pressure, respiratory symptoms, blood carbon monoxide concentrations).
- Mention alternatives to smoking that also establish a self-image that appears independent, mature, or sophisticated (e.g., weightlifting; running; dancing; joining a boys or girls club; volunteering for a hospital or political, religious, or community group).
- Mention the negative effects in detail (e.g., earlier wrinkling of skin; yellow stains on teeth and fingers; tobacco odor on breath, hair, and clothing).
- Mention the increasing ostracism of smokers by nonsmokers, both legal and informal, in the workplace and in public places.
- Mention the increasing evidence that secondhand smoke is injurious to the health of nonsmokers who are regularly exposed, especially small children.
- Acknowledge that many adults who were enticed to start smoking as teenagers because of its social benefits now wish they could stop smoking.
- Give cooperative adolescents effective arguments to deal with peer pressure (e.g., by not smoking, a teenager demonstrates independence and nonconformity, traits normally prized by youth).
- Request posters or pamphlets from local agencies (e.g., American Cancer Society, American Heart Association, American Lung Association) to display in prominent places at school.

*The Centers for Disease Control and Prevention has information on the effects of tobacco, smoking cessation, and tobacco control programs: 1600 Clifton Rd., Atlanta, GA 30333; 800-232-4636; e-mail: tobaccoinfo@cdc.gov; http://www.cdc.gov/tobacco.

rely on the substance as a defense against depression, anxiety, fear, or anger. Not all of these characteristics are observed in adolescents who are abusing alcohol, but if several signs are evident, the child or adolescent should be considered at risk. Referral to a health care professional and detoxification therapy may be necessary. Information about alcohol and answers to questions are available through the Alcohol Hotline.* Other groups that provide support and counseling for families are Al-Anon, Ala-Teen, Ala-Tot, and Alcoholics Anonymous (an organization that has listings in all local telephone directories).

Cocaine. Although cocaine is not pharmacologically considered a narcotic, it is legally categorized as such. Cocaine is available in two forms: water-soluble cocaine hydrochloride, which is administered by "snorting" or intravenous injection, and nonsoluble alkaloid (freebase) cocaine, which is used primarily for smoking. Crack, or "rock," is a

purer, more menacing form of the drug. It can be produced cheaply and smoked in either water pipes or mentholated cigarettes.

Cocaine creates a sense of euphoria, or an indefinable high. Withdrawal does not produce the dramatic symptoms observed in withdrawal from other substances. The effects are those commonly seen in depression, including lack of energy and motivation, irritability, appetite changes, psychomotor delay, and irregular sleep patterns. More serious symptoms include cardiovascular manifestations and seizures. Physical withdrawal should not be confused with the so-called crash after a cocaine high, which consists of a long period of sleep. Answers to questions about the risks of using cocaine are available at the National Cocaine Hotline,* which also provides referrals to support groups and treatment centers.

Narcotics. Narcotic drugs include opiates, such as heroin and morphine, and opioids (opiate-like drugs), such as hydromorphone (Dilaudid), hydrocodone, fentanyl, meperidine (Demerol), and codeine. These drugs produce a state of euphoria by removing painful feelings and creating a pleasurable experience and a sense of success accompanied by clouding of the consciousness and a dreamlike state. Physical signs of narcotic abuse include constricted pupils; respiratory depression; and, often, cyanosis. Needle marks may be visible on the arms or legs in chronic users. Physical withdrawal from opiates is extremely unpleasant unless controlled with supervised tapering doses of the opioid or substitution of methadone.

As important as the physical effects are the indirect consequences related to the illegal status of narcotic use and the problems associated with securing the drug (e.g., the time-consuming searches to obtain the drug and the often illegal methods used to meet the high cost of purchasing it). Health problems also result from self-neglect of physical needs (nutrition, cleanliness, dental care); overdose; contamination; and infection, including HIV and hepatitis B and C infection.

Central Nervous System Depressants. Central nervous system depressants include a variety of hypnotic drugs that produce physical dependence and withdrawal symptoms on abrupt discontinuation. They create a feeling of relaxation and sleepiness but impair general functioning. Drugs in this category include barbiturates, nonbarbiturates, and alcohol. Barbiturates combined with alcohol produce a profound depressant effect. Flunitrazepam (Rohypnol), known as the "date rape drug," is a recent hypnotic drug abused by adolescents. Many women and men report being raped after unknowingly being given Rohypnol in a drink. Rohypnol is 10 times more powerful than diazepam (Valium). It produces prolonged sedation, a feeling of well-being, and short-term memory loss.

Central Nervous System Stimulants. Amphetamines and cocaine do not produce strong physical dependence and can be withdrawn without much danger. However, psychologic dependence is strong, and acute intoxication can lead to violent aggressive behavior or psychotic episodes characterized by paranoia, uncontrollable agitation, and restlessness. When combined with barbiturates, the euphoric effects are particularly addictive.

Methamphetamine can be snorted, injected, swallowed, or smoked and produces a burst of energy in its users, along with intense, alternating attacks of boldness and paranoia. It provokes excitement far more intense than that caused by cocaine. The drug, with the street names *crank*, *meth*, and *crystal*, is inexpensive and has a longer period of action than cocaine. Instead of a short (few minutes) high, as achieved with cocaine, a user can remain "up" for hours on a similar dose of crank.

*Toll free 866-925-4030.

*800-COCAINE (800-262-2463).

Health care professionals are concerned about the use of various volatile substances, or inhalants such as gasoline, model airplane cement, and organic solvents; these substances are inhaled by the user to achieve an altered sensation, and the most recent surveillance has indicated a modest increase in use after nearly a decade of decline. Adolescents breathe or place these substances into paper or plastic bags or soda cans from which they rebreathe the fumes to produce a feeling of euphoria and altered consciousness. These substances contain chemical solvents and are extremely hazardous. Dusters contain Freon, a substance that can cause fatal cardiac arrhythmias. Inhalants are the only substance that has a higher incidence of use among young adolescents. This is probably related to the fact that the products are readily available and may be the only substances available for young teens. Many young children are unaware of the dangers of "sniffing" or "huffing." In addition to rapid loss of consciousness and respiratory arrest, these substances may cause visual scanning problems, language deficiencies, motor instability, memory deficits, and attention and concentration problems.

Mind-Altering Drugs. Hallucinogens (psychedelics, psychotomimetics, psychotropics, or illusionogenics) are drugs that produce vivid hallucinations and euphoria. These drugs do not produce physical dependence, and they can be abruptly withdrawn without ill effect. However, the acute and long-term effects are variable, and in some individuals, the dissociative behavior may be prolonged. Cannabis (marijuana, hashish) and lysergic acid diethylamide (LSD) are also included in this category of drugs.

Nursing Care Management and Therapeutic Management

Nurses who have contact with children and adolescents are in an excellent position to provide information about substance abuse and to serve as patient advocates. Nurses most often encounter young drug abusers when they are (1) experiencing overdose or withdrawal symptoms, (2) manifesting bizarre behavior or confusion secondary to drug ingestion, (3) worried that they are or will become addicted, or (4) worried about a friend or family member who is addicted.

In particular, nurses who care for hospitalized adolescents need to know if these youths use drugs compulsively. Drug withdrawal can seriously complicate other illnesses. Nurses should be alert for any physical or behavioral clues that indicate the onset of withdrawal or the effects of drugs. School nurses and nurses who work in the community play an essential role in identifying children, adolescents, and families with substance abuse problems. The school nurse may be the first to identify a child or adolescent who has ingested a particular drug by the child's erratic behavior in class or on the school grounds (see Critical Thinking Case Study box). Early identification of those at risk for substance abuse problems is an essential aspect of prevention. Pediatric health care professionals also prevent substance abuse by creating trusting relationships so that children and adolescents feel comfortable asking questions about drugs and health professionals can alert them to websites and other aspects of society that encourage experimentation with drugs.

Acute Care. Adolescents experiencing toxic drug effects or withdrawal symptoms are usually seen initially in the emergency department. Experienced emergency department personnel are familiar with the management of acute drug toxicity and the signs, symptoms, and behavioral characteristics associated with a variety of substances. When the drug is questionable or unknown, knowledge of these factors facilitates management and treatment. Often, observation or description of the child's or adolescent's behavior is more valuable than reports by patients or their friends.

❓ CRITICAL THINKING CASE STUDY
Prescription Medication Abuse in Adolescence

An eighth-grade teacher calls the school nurse, Sally, to her classroom and reports that a girl is behaving "strangely"; the girl slept most of the period before lunch and has not participated in class discussions. Sally, RN, takes the girl to her office and performs an initial assessment. Upon assessment, the girl demonstrates short-term memory lapse and has slightly slurred speech, and her pupillary reaction to light is delayed; her blood pressure is 112/68 mm Hg, respirations are 14 breaths/min and regular, and heart rate is 102 beats/min. She denies taking any pills or liquid initially but then states she had a migraine on arrival to school and a friend gave her two blue pills to help with the headache. She refuses to say who gave her the pills and does not know what they were but thought they were Tylenol. She states that she does not know where her mother and father are but thinks they are at work.

Questions
1. Evidence—Is there sufficient evidence for Sally to implement a plan of care for this adolescent?
2. What should Sally's next course of action involve? What is her professional responsibility in this case?
3. Assumptions—Describe the underlying assumptions about the following:
   a. The school nurse's physical assessment findings
   b. The misuse of prescription medications by adolescents
4. What nursing priorities and implications for care can be made at this time? What type of care should the eighth grader receive?

The treatment for drug toxicity or withdrawal varies according to the drug and the method used. Every effort is made to determine the type, time of ingestion, amount of drug taken, mode of administration, and factors related to the onset of presenting symptoms. It is helpful to know the individual's pattern of use. For example, if two types of drugs are involved, they may require different treatments. Historically, gastric lavage has been used when the drug has been ingested recently and the cough reflex is intact, but it is of little value when the drug has been administered by the intravenous ("mainlined") or intranasal ("sniffed") route. More commonly, the administration of a drug antidote such as naloxone and the early (within 1–2 hours of ingestion) administration of activated charcoal may be used for opioid overdose. Because the actual content of most street drugs is highly questionable, other pharmaceutical agents are administered with caution except perhaps the narcotic antagonists in cases of suspected opiate overdoses. It is also necessary to assess for possible trauma sustained while the patient was under the influence of the drug.

Long-Term Management. A major factor in the treatment and rehabilitation of young drug users is careful assessment in the nonacute stage to determine the function that the drug plays in the adolescent's life. The motivation phase is directed toward exploring the factors that influence drug use. It also involves establishing a feeling of self-worth and a commitment to self-help in the teen.

Rehabilitation begins when adolescents decide that they can and are willing to change. Rehabilitation involves fostering healthy interdependent relationships with caring and supportive adults and exploring alternate mechanisms for problem solving while simultaneously reducing or eliminating drug use. Persons working with troubled youth must be prepared for recidivism, or the tendency to relapse, and maintain a plan for reentry into the treatment process.

Family Support. Most treatment programs for substance abusers are based on adult 12-step models such as Alcoholics Anonymous.

Research is needed to determine whether these adult models are effective for adolescents. Tough Love* is one program that is based on the conviction that parents have the right and responsibility to be the policymakers in the family, to set limits on the behavior of their children, and to take control of the household from out-of-control adolescents. The premise is that allowing teenagers to experience the negative consequences of their behavior will bring them closer to accepting help or changing their behavior. Another group that provides support and counseling for families experiencing substance abuse and seeking strategies to cope with their children is Parents Anonymous.[†] Another source of information is the Substance Abuse and Mental Health Services Administration's National Clearinghouse for Alcohol and Drug Information.[‡]

Prevention. Nurses play an important role in education efforts, as well as in individual observation, assessment, and therapy related to substance abuse. In recent years, a variety of educational programs have been applied with promising results. The most effective prevention strategies are those that are part of a broader, more general effort to promote overall health and success. Health-compromising behaviors are often interconnected and have common antecedents. Prevention efforts that focus on changing only one behavior (e.g., alcohol, other drug use) are less likely to be successful. Successful programs are those that have promoted parenting skills, social skills among distractible children, academic achievement, and skills to resist peer pressure.

Peer pressure is a powerful tool and can be used effectively in substance abuse prevention. A group that has had some success in reducing injury from drunk driving is Students Against Destructive Decisions (SADD).[§] Techniques used by this group include peer counseling, parental guidelines for teenage parties, and community awareness. Nurses should encourage the formation of SADD chapters in the high schools in their communities.

Suicide

Suicide is defined as the deliberate act of self-injury with the intent that the injury results in death. Most experts distinguish among suicidal ideation, suicide attempt (or parasuicide), and suicide.

Suicidal ideation involves a preoccupation with thoughts about committing suicide and may be a precursor to suicide. Although it is common for adolescents to experience occasional suicidal thoughts, expressions of preoccupation with suicide should be taken seriously, and an assessment should be conducted for appropriate referral. A suicide attempt is intended to cause injury or death. The term parasuicide is used to refer to behaviors ranging from gestures to serious attempts to kill oneself. *Parasuicide* is a preferred term because it makes no reference to intent and because a person's motive may be too difficult or complex to determine. However, all parasuicidal activity should be taken seriously.

! NURSING ALERT

A history of a previous suicide attempt is a serious indicator for possible suicide completion in the future. Studies of adolescent suicides have found that as many as half of the adolescents had made previous attempts.

Results from the Youth Risk Behavior Surveillance, 2009, indicated that 6.3% of students nationwide had attempted suicide at least once during the 12 months preceding the survey; the range of suicide attempts by adolescents across the states varied from 4.32% to 12.8% (Eaton, Kann, Kinchen, and others, 2010). The overall incidence of youth suicide has decreased since 1992, yet the CDC and other experts note that the incidence is still too high. Approximately 11% of the students in this survey reported that they had made a specific plan to attempt suicide in the 12 months preceding the survey. Suicide is currently the third leading cause of death during the teenage years, surpassed only by death from motor vehicle crashes and homicides (see Chapter 1).

Etiology

Individual, family, and social or environmental factors have all been implicated in suicide. The single most important individual factor is the presence of an active psychiatric disorder (depression, bipolar disorder, psychosis, substance abuse, or conduct disorder). Alcohol use in particular has been associated with more than 50% of suicides (Shain and Committee on Adolescence, 2007). For some teens, suicide becomes the final pathway for release from their psychiatric and social problems. Child and adolescent suicide victims are reported to have higher rates not only of depression but also of conduct disorders; bipolar disorders; substance abuse; interpersonal problems with parents; and a family history of depression, substance abuse, and suicidal behavior.

Gay, lesbian, and bisexual adolescents are at particularly high risk for suicide attempts, especially if raised in an environment where they are denied support systems (Saewyc, Skay, Hynds, and others, 2007) (see Community Focus box). Family factors influencing suicide include

🏠 COMMUNITY FOCUS

Suicide, Sexual Identity, and Sexual Orientation

A significant number of teenage suicides occur among homosexual youths. Gay or lesbian adolescents who live in families or communities that do not accept homosexuality are likely to experience low self-esteem, self-loathing, depression, and hopelessness. Such internalization, without treatment and support, can lead to substance abuse and, eventually, suicide. Youths most at risk are those who struggle with gender identity issues such as gay identity formation at a young age, intrapersonal conflict regarding sexuality, and nondisclosure of orientation to others.

Supportive parents, friends, or relationships serve as protective factors against suicide. However, many gay, lesbian, and bisexual adolescents do not feel supported, understood, or accepted by their friends, parents, and families. Nurses who interact with adolescents must be aware of the association between suicide and adolescent homosexuality and gender nonconformity. School nurses may be the first individuals to discuss issues of sexual identity and orientation with adolescents or their families. In their professional capacity, nurses can also serve as support persons for these adolescents. Nurses can provide guidance and resources to families so that they know and understand how best to nurture and support their child.

Nurses must also capitalize on opportunities or experiences that promote the healthy development of self-esteem in youths who choose nontraditional sexual orientation. Educational programs to raise the level of consciousness about the risk factors for and warning signs of suicide are one example. Another possibility could be programs conducted in or outside of school that are designed to foster peer relationships and competency in social skills among high-risk adolescents and young adults, such as support groups and social organizations for these young people.

---

*http://www.toughlove.com.
[†]675 W. Foothill Blvd., Suite 220, Claremont, CA 91711; 909-621-6184; http://www.parentsanonymous.org.
[‡]1 Choke Cherry Road, Rockville, MD 20857; 877-SAMHSA-7; http://ncadi.samhsa.gov.
[§]255 Main St., Marlborough, MA 01752; 877-SADD-INC; http://www.sadd.org.

parental loss; family disruption; a family history of suicide, depression, substance abuse, or emotional disturbance; child abuse or neglect; unavailable parents; poor communication and isolation within the family; family conflict; and unrealistically high parental expectations or parental indifference with low expectations. Families who respect individuality, are cohesive and caring, balance discipline with a supportive and understanding relationship, have good systems of communication, and have at least one attentive and caring parent available to the child protect adolescents from suicidal outcomes. Social or environmental risk factors include incarceration, isolation, acute loss of a boyfriend or girlfriend, lack of future options, and availability of firearms in the home.

Methods

Firearms are by far the most commonly used instruments in completed suicides among males and females (Shain and Committee on Adolescence, 2007). For adolescent males, the second and third most common means of suicide are hanging and overdose, respectively; for females, the second and third most common means are overdose and strangulation, respectively.

The most common method of suicide *attempt* is overdose or ingestion of a potentially toxic substance, such as drugs. The second most common method of suicide attempt is self-inflicted laceration.

! NURSING ALERT

Given what is known about youth suicide, nurses should ask parents, especially those with at-risk teenagers, if firearms are available in the house and, if so, recommend their removal. Parents must ensure that their children—especially those who are depressed, have poor problem-solving skills, or use drugs or alcohol—do not have access to firearms. Parents must also be educated on the warning signs of suicide (Box 17-9).

Motivation

Suicidal ideation is common in adolescents. It represents numerous fantasies, such as relief from suffering, a means of gaining comfort and sympathy, or a means of revenge against those who have hurt them. Adolescents have the erroneous perception that the act of suicide will evoke remorse and pity and that they will be able to return and witness the grief. Angry children who are unable to directly punish those who have injured or insulted them may take revenge on those who love them through self-destruction ("They'll be sorry when they find me dead"; "They'll be sorry they were mean to me").

For adolescents who are severely depressed, suicide seems to be the only release from their despair. These adolescents rarely provide evidence of their intent and frequently conceal their suicidal thoughts. Many adolescents, however, tell their peers of their suicidal thoughts or plans but avoid telling adults. Social isolation is a significant factor in distinguishing adolescents who will kill themselves from those who will not. It is also more characteristic of those who complete suicide than of those who make attempts or threats.

The frequency of contagion, or copycat suicides (i.e., an increase in youth suicide that occurs after the suicide of one teenager is publicized) is disturbing and may indicate that teenagers perceive suicide as glamorous. In addition, young people may not realize the finality of suicide because they have become desensitized from constantly viewing violence and death on television.

Diagnostic Evaluation

Depression is common among adolescents who attempt suicide. Depression is characterized by both subjective symptoms and objective

BOX 17-9 WARNING SIGNS OF SUICIDE

- Preoccupation with themes of death—focuses on morbid thoughts
- Wants to give away cherished possessions
- Talks of own death or desire to die
- Loss of energy—loss of interest, listlessness
- Exhaustion without obvious cause
- Changes in sleep patterns—too much or too little
- Increased irritability, argumentativeness, or stubbornness
- Physical complaints—recurrent stomachaches, headaches
- Repeated visits to physician, nurse practitioner, or emergency department for treatment of injuries
- Reckless behavior
- Antisocial behavior—engages in drinking, uses drugs, fights, commits acts of vandalism, runs away from home, becomes sexually promiscuous
- Sudden change in school performance—lowered grades, cutting classes, dropping out of activities
- Resists or refuses to go to school
- Remains distant, sad, remote—flat affect, frozen facial expression
- Describes self as worthless
- Sudden cheerfulness following deep depression
- Social withdrawal from friends, activities, interests that were previously enjoyed
- Impaired concentration
- Dramatic change in appetite

signs that reflect the adolescent's sadness and despair. Adolescents describe feelings of sadness, despair, helplessness, hopelessness, boredom, loss of interest, and isolation. They may also feel self-reproach, self-deprecation, and guilt. Subjective symptoms of depression or specific changes in behavior place an adolescent at risk for suicide.

Therapeutic Management

Threats of suicide should always be taken seriously. There has been a tendency to dismiss suicide attempts as impulsive acts resulting from temporary crises or depression. If a suicide attempt fails to draw attention to his or her problems or makes them worse, the child or adolescent may conclude that suicide is the only answer. Children and adolescents need to know that someone cares and must be provided with swift and efficient crisis intervention. Although ordinary practitioners can manage an acute depressive reaction without difficulty, the adolescent who has made a serious attempt or has a specific plan for suicide should receive immediate attention and competent psychiatric care.

Youths who are actively suicidal need inpatient care, monitoring, and treatment. Medications for depression and bipolar disorder often take several weeks to reach therapeutic dosages. The time until medications and therapy begin to take effect can be trying for the adolescent and the family. It is important to encourage families to support their teen in adherence to the regimen prescribed. The SSRIs are often prescribed for depression, but teens who are taking such medications need careful, frequent monitoring.

! NURSING ALERT

Adolescents who express suicidal feelings and have a specific plan should be monitored at all times. They should not have access to firearms, prescription or over-the-counter drugs, belts, scarves, shoestrings, sharp objects, matches, or lighters. If they are intoxicated, they must be restrained or placed in a protective environment until a psychiatrist or psychologist can assess them.

Nursing Care Management

Nurses play a pivotal role in reducing adolescent suicide. Nurses have the opportunity to provide anticipatory guidance to parents and adolescents. They can teach parents to be supportive and to develop positive communication patterns that help teens feel connected with and loved by their families. To foster healthy development, parents can be encouraged to provide teens with creative outlets and to assist young people in accepting strong emotions—pain, anger, and frustration—as a normal part of the human experience.

Care of suicidal adolescents includes early recognition, management, and prevention. The most important aspect of management is the recognition of warning signs that indicate that an adolescent is troubled and might attempt suicide. The nurse must take any suicidal remarks seriously and not leave the young person alone until the degree of suicidality is assessed. A mnemonic for the assessment process is SLAP: specificity, lethality, accessibility, and proximity. The first step (specificity) is to ask adolescents whether they feel suicidal or as though they would like to take their own lives. If so, have they chosen a means of suicide, and do they have a specific plan? The second stage of assessment (lethality) involves determining the lethality of the methods available to them. Do they plan to use a gun or knife? Have they chosen highly lethal medications, hanging, or carbon monoxide poisoning? The third stage (accessibility) involves determining the availability of the means of suicide, and the fourth stage (proximity) involves assessing whether they have determined a time to commit suicide and when.

Health professionals must be alert to the signs of depression, and anyone who exhibits such behavior should be referred for thorough psychologic assessment. Depression is manifested differently in children and adolescents than in adults. In teens, it may be masked by impulsive aggressive behaviors. Defiance, disobedience, behavior problems, and psychosomatic disturbances can indicate underlying depression, suicidal ideation, and impending suicide attempts.

> **! NURSING ALERT**
>
> No threat of suicide should be ignored or challenged. Threats are a symptom that must be taken seriously. Too often, suicidal threats or minor attempts are confused with bids for attention. It is also a mistake to be lulled into a false sense of security when an adolescent's depression is suddenly or apparently relieved. The improvement in attitude may mean that the adolescent has made the decision and found the means to carry out the threat.

Peers and other confidants are valuable observers and excellent sources of information about potential suicide attempts. They may not be able to diagnose depression, but they are able to sense when a friend has undergone a marked personality change. It is important to emphasize that the peer who detects any changes in a friend is a potential rescuer and should not remain silent about the observations. Friendship does not imply collusion. A peer who believes that a friend may be suicidal should alert someone who can help (e.g., a parent, teacher, guidance counselor, school nurse).

Routine health assessments of adolescents should include questions that assess the presence of suicidal ideation or intent. The following questions can be asked (Greydanus and Pratt, 1995):

1. Do you consider yourself more a happy person, an unhappy person, or somewhere in the middle?
2. Have you ever been so unhappy or upset that you felt like being dead?
3. Have you ever thought about hurting yourself?
4. Have you ever developed a plan to hurt yourself or kill yourself?
5. Have you ever attempted to kill yourself?

If adolescents answer "yes" to questions 2, 3, or 4, they should be asked if they feel that way now to assess for current suicidality. If teens say they have attempted suicide in the past, assess the number of times and ask them to describe what they were feeling, which method they used, what happened, if they would make a similar attempt, and how they would handle their despair now. Any previous suicide attempt indicates an increased risk for a future attempt. The risk of a suicide attempt in the near future increases as the frequency of suicidal ideation increases.

> **! NURSING ALERT**
>
> The National Suicide Prevention Lifeline (800-273-TALK [8255]; in Spanish, 888-628-9454) offers someone to talk to 24/7.

If children or adolescents express suicidal intent, nurses make a contract, asking them to sign an agreement that they will not attempt suicide during an agreed-on period and that they will call the 24-hour crisis line immediately if they feel that they cannot keep to their contract. The amount of time an adolescent feels comfortable contracting is usually an indication of his or her risk and stability.

Because a suicide attempt is frequently an outgrowth of family distress, it is essential to intervene with the family. It is important to assess family interactions and to recognize disturbed relationships. The most effective approach is recognition of susceptible adolescents during the early stages of family distress so that family counseling can be started. Prevention must be directed toward improving childrearing practices through support and education of parents and changing societal conditions that generate defeat, despair, and maladaptive behavior.

Although confidentiality is an essential part of adolescent counseling, in the case of self-destructive behaviors, confidentiality cannot be honored. Suicidal behavior is reported to the family and other professionals, and adolescents are informed that this will be done. Such action conveys an important message to the youth: that the professionals understand and care.

Many schools have instituted suicide prevention programs. These programs include services such as drop-in counseling and a peer counseling telephone line. Information can also be obtained from the American Association of Suicidology.*

---

*5221 Wisconsin Ave. NW, Washington, DC 20015; 202-237-2280; http://www.suicidology.org.

▌ KEY POINTS

- Alterations in growth and maturation may be manifested as short or tall stature, precocious puberty, or delayed sexual development.
- The most frequent health problems related to the female reproductive system involve menstrual dysfunction.
- Health problems related to sexuality include pregnancy, sexual assault, and STIs; prevention includes sex education and contraceptive counseling.
- Eating disorders observed in middle and late childhood include obesity, AN, and BN.

KEY POINTS—cont'd

- Lactose intolerance is a developmental disorder in which there is reduced lactase activity in the intestine, which causes bloating, abdominal distention, and flatulence shortly after the ingestion of lactose. Most persons with lactose malabsorption are able to consume approximately 1 cup of milk per day without having these signs and symptoms.
- Behavior problems in middle childhood can result from ADHD, enuresis, encopresis, school phobia, childhood depression, conversion reaction, and childhood schizophrenia.
- Signs of depression in children and adolescents are often subtle and require astute observation by parents and health professionals.

- The substances abused by children and adolescents include alcohol, marijuana, narcotics, opiates, CNS depressants or stimulants, inhalants, and mind-altering drugs.
- Tobacco smoking is a significant problem among teenagers; reasons for smoking include social pressures, mass media influence, and a need to develop a self-concept.
- Suicide, the deliberate act of self-injury with the intent to kill, is often associated with depression, substance abuse, difficulties in coping with stress, an affective disorder, or a disturbed family environment.

REFERENCES

American Academy of Pediatrics: Active healthy living: prevention of childhood obesity through increased physical activity, *Pediatrics* 117(5): 1834–1842, 2006.

American Academy of Pediatrics: *Pediatric nutrition handbook*, ed 6, Elk Grove Village, Ill, 2009, Author.

American Academy of Pediatrics: Policy statement—children, adolescents, obesity, and the media, *Pediatrics* 128(1):201–208, 2011.

American Academy of Pediatrics, Clinical Practice Guideline: ADHD: clinical practice guideline for the diagnosis, evaluation, and treatment of attention-deficit/hyperactivity disorder in children and adolescents, *Pediatrics* 128(5): 1007–1022, 2011.

American Academy of Pediatrics, Committee on Adolescence: Adolescent pregnancy: current trends and issues, *Pediatrics* 116(1):281–286, 2005.

American Academy of Pediatrics, Committee on Adolescence: Identification and management of eating disorders in children and adolescents, *Pediatrics* 126(6):1240–1253, 2010.

American Academy of Pediatrics, American College of Obstetricians and Gynecologists: Menstruation in girls and adolescents: using the menstrual cycle as a vital sign, *Pediatrics* 118(5):2245–2250, 2006.

American Dietetic Association: Position of the American Dietetic Association: Nutrition intervention in the treatment of anorexia nervosa, bulimia nervosa, and other eating disorders, *J Am Diet Assoc* 106(12):2073–2082, 2006.

American Psychiatric Association: *Diagnostic and statistical manual of mental disorders*, ed 4 (text rev) (DSM-IV TR), Washington, DC, 2000, Author.

American Psychiatric Association: *DSM-V development: proposed revisions*, Arlington, Va, 2010, Author, retrieved on July 20, 2011, from http://www.dsm5.org/ProposedRevisions/Pages/proposedrevision.aspx?rid=110.

Baker S, Barlow S, Cochran W, and others: Overweight children and adolescents: a clinical report of the North American Society for Pediatric Gastroenterology, Hepatology and Nutrition, *J Pediatr Gastroenterol Nutr* 40:533–543, 2005.

Barlow SE, Expert Committee: Expert Committee recommendations regarding the prevention, assessment, and treatment of child and adolescent overweight and obesity: summary report, *Pediatrics* 120(suppl 4):S164–S192, 2007.

Barnett SJ: Contemporary surgical management of the obese adolescent, *Curr Opin Pediatr* 23(3): 351–355, 2011.

Beaty TH: Invited commentary: two studies of genetic control of birth weight where large data sets were available, *Am J Epidemiol* 165:753–755, 2007.

Berry AK: Helping children with nocturnal enuresis: the wait-and-see approach may not be in everyone's interest, *Am J Nurs* 106(8):56–63, 2006.

Boney C, Verma A, Tucker R, and others: Metabolic syndrome in childhood: association with birth weight, maternal obesity, and gestational diabetes mellitus, *Pediatrics* 115:290–296, 2005.

Bouchard C: Childhood obesity: are genetic differences involved? *Am J Clin Nutr* 89(5): 1494S–1501S, 2009.

Calles JL: Depression in children and adolescents, *Prim Care Clin Office Pract* 34(2):243–258, 2007.

Campbell R, Dworkin E, Cabral G: An ecological model of the impact of sexual assault on women's mental health, *Trauma Violence Abuse* 10(3):225–246, 2009.

Centers for Disease Control and Prevention: Bullying among middle school and high school students—Massachusetts, 2009, *MMWR Weekly* 60(15):465–471, 2011a.

Centers for Disease Control and Prevention: Cigarette use among high school students—United States, 1991–2009, *MMWR Morb Mortal Wkly Rep* 59(26):797–801, 2010a.

Centers for Disease Control and Prevention: Tobacco use among middle and high school students—United States, 2000–2009, *MMWR Morb Mortal Wkly Rep* 59(33):1063–1068, 2010b.

Centers for Disease Control and Prevention: Vital signs: teen pregnancy—United States, 1991–2009, *MMWR Morb Mortal Wkly Rep* 60(13):414–420, 2011b.

Cohen JA, AACAP Work Group on Quality Issues: Practice parameter for the assessment and treatment of children and adolescents with posttraumatic stress disorder, *J Am Acad Child Adolesc Psychiatry* 49(4):414–430, 2010.

Cunningham NR, Jensen P: Attention-deficit/hyperactivity disorder. In Kliegman RM, Stanton BF, St. Geme JW, and others, editors: *Nelson textbook of pediatrics*, ed 19, Philadelphia, 2011, Saunders.

Davis DM, Gance-Cleveland B, Hassink S, and others: Recommendations for prevention of childhood obesity, *Pediatrics* 120(Suppl): S229–S253, 2007.

Dennehy CE: The use of herbs and dietary supplements in gynecology: an evidence-based review, *J Midwifery Womens Health* 51(6):402–409, 2006.

de Vrese M, Schrezenmeir J: Probiotics, prebiotics, and synbiotics, *Adv Biochem Eng Biotechnol* 111:1–66, 2008.

Eaton DK, Kann L, Kinchen S, and others: Youth risk behavior surveillance—United States, 2009, *MMWR Surveill Summ* 59(SS05):1–142, 2010.

Elder JS: Voiding dysfunction. In Kliegman RM, Stanton BF, St. Geme JW, and others, editors: *Nelson textbook of pediatrics*, ed 19, Philadelphia, 2011, Saunders.

Feldman DR, Bosl GJ, Sheinfeld J, and others: Medical treatment of advanced testicular cancer, *JAMA* 299(6):672–684, 2008.

Feldman M, Friedman LS, Sleisenger MH, editors: Obesity: a historical perspective and disease prevalence estimates. In *Sleisenger and Fordtran's gastrointestinal and liver disease*, ed 7, Philadelphia, 2002, Saunders.

Forman SF: Eating disorders: epidemiology, pathogenesis, and clinical features, *UpToDate*, 2011, retrieved July 22, 2011, from http://www.uptodate.com/contents/eating-disorders-epidemiology-pathogenesis-and-overview-of-clinical-features.

Fulkerson JA, Neumark-Sztainer D, Hannan P, and others: Family meal frequency and weight status among adolescents: cross-sectional and 5-year longitudinal associations, *Obesity* 16(11): 2529–2534, 2008.

Fulkerson JA, Story M, Mellin A, and others: Family dinner meal frequency and adolescent development: relationships with developmental assets and high-risk behaviors, *J Adolesc Health* 39(3):337–345, 2006.

Gahagan S: Overweight and obesity. In Kliegman RM, Stanton BF, St. Geme JW, and others, editors: *Nelson textbook of pediatrics*, ed 19, Philadelphia, 2011, Saunders.

Gibbons RD, Hur K, Bhaumik DK, and others: The relationship between antidepressant prescription rates and rate of early adolescent suicide, *Am J Psychiatry* 163(11):1898–1904, 2006.

Golden NH, Attia E: Psychopharmacology of eating disorders in children and adolescents, *Pediatr Clin North Am* 58(1):121–138, 2011.

Greydanus DE, Pratt HD: Emotional and behavioral disorders of adolescence, part 2, *Adolesc Health Update* 8(1):1–8, 1995.

Hardy LR, Harrell JS, Bell RA: Overweight in children: definitions, measurements, confounding factors, and health consequences, *J Pediatr Nurs* 19(6):376–383, 2004.

Heyman MB, American Academy of Pediatrics Committee on Nutrition: Lactose intolerance in infants, children, and adolescents, *Pediatrics* 118(3):1279–1286, 2006.

Hill JO, Wyatt HR, Reed GW, and others: Obesity and the environment: where do we go from here? *Science* 299(5608):853–855, 2003.

Jaquet D, Swaminathan S, Alexander GR, and others: Significant paternal contribution to the risk of small for gestational age, *BJOG* 112:1539, 2005.

Jellinek M: ADHD treatments: going beyond the meds, *Contemp Pediatr* 25(5):39–48, 2008.

Johnston LD, O'Malley, PM, Bachman JG, and others: *Monitoring the Future national results on adolescent drug use: overview of key findings, 2010.* Ann Arbor, 2011, Institute for Social Research, The University of Michigan.

Kain J, Corvalán C, Lera L, and others: Accelerated growth in early life and obesity in preschool Chilean children, *Obesity* 17(8):1603–1608, 2009.

Kandakai TL, Smith LC: Denormalizing a historical problem: teen pregnancy, policy and public health action, *Am J Health Behav* 31(2):170–180, 2007.

Kanekar A, Sharma M: Pharmacological approaches for management of child and adolescent obesity, *J Clin Med Res* 2(3):105–111, 2010.

Katz ER, DeMaso D: Enuresis (bed-wetting). In Kliegman RM, Stanton BF, St. Geme JW, and others, editors: *Nelson textbook of pediatrics*, ed 19, Philadelphia, 2011, Saunders.

Koeppen-Schomerus G, Wardle J, Plomin R: A genetic analysis of weight and overweight in 4-year-old twin pairs, *Int J Obes Relat Metab Dis* 25(6):838–844, 2001.

Kost K, Henshaw S, Carlin L: U.S. teenage pregnancies. *Birth and abortions: national and state trends and trends by race and ethnicity*, 2010, retrieved February 10, 2011, from http://www.guttmacher.org/pubs/USTPtrends.pdf.

Kreipe RE: Eating disorders. In Kliegman RM, Stanton BF, St. Geme JW, and others, editors: *Nelson textbook of pediatrics*, ed 19, Philadelphia, 2011, Saunders.

Landry GL: Female athletes: menstrual problems and the risk of osteopenia. In Kliegman RM, Stanton BF, St. Geme JW, and others, editors: *Nelson textbook of pediatrics*, ed 19, Philadelphia, 2011, Saunders.

Larson NI, Neumark-Sztainer D, Hannan PJ, and others: Family meals during adolescence are associated with higher diet quality and healthful meal patterns during young adulthood, *J Am Diet Assoc* 107(9):1502–1510, 2007.

Li C, Kaur H, Choi WS, and others: Additive interactions of maternal prepregnancy BMI and breast-feeding on childhood overweight, *Obesity Res* 13:362–371, 2005.

Liu J, Graves N: Childhood bullying: A review of constructs, concepts, and nursing implications, *Public Health Nurs* 28(6):556–568, 2011.

Lock J: Treatment of adolescent eating disorders: progress and challenges, *Minerva Psichiatr* 51(3):207–216, 2010.

Luce H, Schrager S, Gilchrist V: Sexual assault of women, *Family Physician* 81(4):489–495, 2010.

Master-Hunter T, Heiman DL: Amenorrhea: evaluation and treatment, *Am Fam Physician* 73(8):1374–1382, 2006.

McCarthy A, Hughes R, Tilling K, and others: Birth weight; postnatal, infant, and childhood growth; and obesity in young adulthood: evidence from the Barry Caerphilly Growth Study, *Am J Clin Nutr* 86(4):907–913, 2007.

Montgomery DF: Management of constipation and encopresis in children, *J Pediatr Health Care* 22(3):199–204, 2008.

Morgan JF, Reid F, Lacey JH: The SCOFF questionnaire: assessment of a new screening tool for eating disorders, *BMJ* 319(7223):1467–1468, 1999.

Mowery BD: Post-traumatic stress disorder (PTSD) in parents: is this a significant problem? *Pediatr Nurs* 37(2):89–92, 2011.

Myers SM, Eisenhauer NJ, Ryan ME: ADHD: it is real, and it can be treated. *Clin Advisor* 6(3):15–25, 2003.

National Institute for Health Care Management Foundation: *Childhood obesity: advancing effective prevention and treatment: an overview for health professionals*, prepared for National Institute for Health Care Management Foundation Forum, Washington, DC, April 9, 2003.

Nwosu BU, Lee MM: Evaluation of short and tall stature in children, *Am Fam Physician* 78(5):597–604, 2008.

Ogden CL, Carroll MD, Flegal KM: High body mass index for age among U.S. children and adolescents, 2003–2006, *JAMA* 299(20):2401–2405, 2008.

Ogden CL, Kuczmarski RJ, Flegal KM, and others: Centers for Disease Control and Prevention 2000 growth charts for the United States: improvements to the 1977 National Center for Health Statistics version, *Pediatrics* 109(1):141–142, 2002.

Ogden CL, Troiano RP, Briefel RR, and others: Prevalence of overweight among preschool children in the United States, 1971 through 1994, *Pediatrics* 99(4):e1, 1997.

Perrin JM, Friedman RA, Knilans TK, and others: Cardiovascular monitoring and stimulant drugs for attention-deficit/hyperactivity disorder, *Pediatrics* 122(2):451–453, 2008.

Pliszka S, AACAP Work Group on Quality Issues: Practice parameter for the assessment and treatment of children, adolescents, and adults with attention-deficit/hyperactivity disorder, *J Am Acad Child Adolesc Psychiatry* 46(7):894–921, 2007.

Powell MD, Ladd LD: Bullying: a review of the literature and implications for family therapists, *Am J Fam Ther* 38(3):189–206, 2010.

Pratt JSA, Lenders CM, Dionne EA, and others: Best practice updates for pediatric/adolescent weight loss surgery, *Obesity* 17(5):901–910, 2009.

Roberts DF, Foehr UG: Children and electronic media, *Future Child* 8(1):235–253, 2008.

Ryan-Krause P: Attention deficit hyperactivity disorder: part III, *J Pediatr Health Care* 25(1):50–56, 2011.

Saewyc EM, Skay CL, Hynds P, and others: Suicidal ideation and attempts among adolescents in North American school-based surveys: are bisexual youth at increasing risk? *J LGBT Health Res* 3:25–36, 2007.

Selekman J: Attention-deficit/hyperactivity disorder. In Jackson P, Vessey JA, Schapiro NA, editors: *Primary care of children with chronic conditions*, ed 5, St. Louis, 2010, Mosby.

Sethi S, Bhargava S, Shipra PM: Nocturnal enuresis: a review, *J Pediatr Neurol* 3(1):11–18, 2005.

Shain BN, Committee on Adolescence: Suicide and suicide attempts in adolescents, *Pediatrics* 120(3):669–676, 2007.

Sjöberg RL, Nilsson KW, Leppert J: Obesity, shame, and depression in school-aged children: a population-based study, *Pediatrics* 116(3):e389–e393, 2005.

Spruijt-Metz D: Etiology, treatment and prevention of obesity in childhood and adolescence: a decade in review, *J Res Adolesc* 21(1):129–152, 2011.

Stoelting-Gettelfinger W: A case study and comprehensive differential diagnosis and care plan for the three Ds of women's health: primary dysmenorrheal, secondary dysmenorrheal, and dyspareunia, *J Am Acad Nurse Pract* 22(10):513–522, 2010.

Suchy FJ, Brannon PM, Carpenter TO, and others: National Institutes of Health consensus development conference: lactose intolerance and health, *Ann Intern Med* 152(12):792–796, 2010, retrieved June 22, 2011, from http://consensus.nih.gov/2010/lactose.htm.

U.S. Department of Health and Human Services: *The health consequences of involuntary exposure to tobacco smoke: a report of the surgeon general*, Washington, DC, 2006, Author.

U.S. Department of Health and Human Services: Active children and adolescents. In *2008 physical activity guidelines for Americans*, Washington, DC, Author, retrieved July 20, 2011, from http://www.health.gov/paguidelines/guidelines/chapter3.aspx.

U.S. Preventive Services Task Force: Screening for obesity in children and adolescents: U.S. Preventive Services Task Force recommendation statement, *Pediatrics* 125(2):361–367, 2010.

Walter HJ, DeMaso DR: Major depression. In Kliegman RM, Stanton BF, St. Geme JW, and others, editors: *Nelson textbook of pediatrics*, ed 19, Philadelphia, 2011, Saunders.

Wardle J, Carnell S, Haworth CMA, and others: Evidence for a strong genetic influence on childhood adiposity despite the force of the obesogenic environment, *Am J Clin Nutr* 87(2):398–404, 2008.

Weiss R, Dziura J, Burgert TS, and others: Obesity and the metabolic syndrome in children and adolescents, *N Engl J Med* 350(23):2362–2374, 2004.

Whitlock EP, O'Connor EA, Williams SB, and others: Effectiveness of weight management interventions in children: a targeted systematic review for the USPSTF, *Pediatrics* 125(2):e396–e418, 2010.

Workowski KA, Berman S, Centers for Disease Control and Prevention: Sexually transmitted diseases treatment guidelines, 2010, *MMWR Recomm Rep* 59(RR-12):1–112, 2010.

Quality of Life for Children Living with Chronic or Complex Diseases

Sharron L. Docherty, Raymond Barfield, Cheryl Thaxton, and Debra Brandon

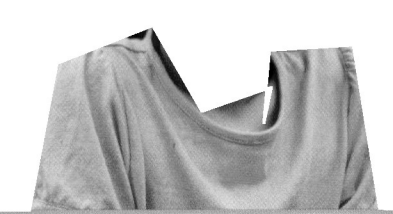

evolve WEBSITE

http://evolve.elsevier.com/wong/essentials

Case Study—The Dying Child

Key Point Summaries

NCLEX-Style Review Questions

Nursing Care Plan—The Child Who Is Terminally Ill or Dying

CHAPTER OUTLINE

Perspectives on the Care of Children and Families Living with or Dying from Chronic or Complex Diseases, 537

Scope of the Problem, 537

Trends in Care, 538

Developmental Focus, 538

Family-Centered Care, 538

Family–Health Care Provider Communication, 538

Establishing Therapeutic Relationships, 538

The Role of Culture in Family-Centered Care, 538

Shared Decision Making, 539

Normalization, 539

Managed Care, 540

The Family of the Child with a Chronic or Complex Condition, 540

Impact of the Child's Chronic Illness, 540

Parents, 540

Siblings, 541

Coping with Ongoing Stress and Periodic Crises, 542

Concurrent Stresses Within the Family, 542

Coping Mechanisms, 542

Parental Empowerment, 542

Assisting Family Members in Managing Their Feelings, 543

Shock and Denial, 543

Adjustment, 543

Reintegration and Acknowledgment, 544

Establishing a Support System, 544

The Child with a Chronic or Complex Condition, 545

Developmental Aspects, 545

Coping Mechanisms, 545

Hopefulness, 547

Health Education and Self-Care, 547

Responses to Parental Behavior, 547

Type of Illness or Condition, 547

Nursing Care of the Family and Child with a Chronic or Complex Condition, 548

Assessment, 548

Provide Support at the Time of Diagnosis, 548

Support the Family's Coping Methods, 549

Parents, 549

Parent-to-Parent Support, 551

Advocate for Empowerment, 551

The Child, 551

Siblings, 551

Educate About the Disorder and General Health Care, 552

Activities of Daily Living, 552

Safe Transportation, 552

Primary Health Care, 552

Promote Normal Development, 552

Early Childhood, 553

School Age, 553

Adolescence, 554

Establish Realistic Future Goals, 554

Perspectives on the Care of Children at the End of Life, 555

Principles of Palliative Care, 555

Decision Making at the End of Life, 555

Ethical Considerations in End-of-Life Decision Making, 555

Physician–Health Care Team Decision Making, 557

Parental Decision Making, 557

The Dying Child, 557

Treatment Options for Terminally Ill Children, 558

Nursing Care of the Child and Family at the End of Life, 560

Nursing Care Plan: The Child Who Is Terminally Ill or Dying, 560

Fear of Pain and Suffering, 560

Pain and Symptom Management, 562

Parents' and Siblings' Need for Education and Support, 563

Fear of Dying Alone or of Not Being Present When the Child Dies, 563

Fear of Actual Death, 564

Home Deaths, 564

Hospital Deaths, 564

Organ or Tissue Donation and Autopsy, 565

Grief and Mourning, 565

Parental Grief, 565

Sibling Grief, 565

Nurses' Reactions to Caring for Dying Children, 566

LEARNING OBJECTIVES

On completion of this chapter the reader will be able to:

- Identify the scope of and changing trends in care of children with special needs.
- Identify the major reactions of and effects on the family of a child with a special need.
- Define the stages of adjustment to the diagnosis of a chronic condition.

- Recognize the impact of the illness or condition on the developmental stages of childhood.
- Outline nursing interventions that promote the family's optimal adjustment to the child's chronic disorder.
- Outline nursing interventions that support the family at the time of death.
- Define the usual symptoms of normal grief.

PERSPECTIVES ON THE CARE OF CHILDREN AND FAMILIES LIVING WITH OR DYING FROM CHRONIC OR COMPLEX DISEASES

SCOPE OF THE PROBLEM

Advances in medical and nursing care, such as the increasing viability of extremely preterm infants, the portability of life-sustaining technology (e.g., total parental nutrition, ventilatory support), and life-extending treatments for children with conditions that previously would have led to an early death (e.g., malignancies, genetic conditions) (Burke and Alverson, 2010), have led to an exponential rise in the prevalence of children with complex and chronic diseases. These children have complex conditions involving several organ systems and require multiple specialists, technologic supports, and community services to assist them to function to their healthiest potential. The complex, high level of skill required to meet their daily health care needs and the continuous nature and potential volatility of the condition sets this group apart from the broader population of children with special health care needs (Harrigan, Ratliffe, Patrinos, and others, 2002; Rehm and Bradley, 2005). A range of terms, such as *medically complex*, *technology dependent*, and *multiply handicapped*, have been used to describe this vulnerable population of children (Carnevale, Rehm, Kirk, and others, 2008; Cohen, Friedman, Nicholas, and others, 2008; Harrigan, Ratliffe, Patrinos, and others, 2002; Miles, Holditch-Davis, Burchinal, and others, 1999; O'Brien and Wegner, 2002; Watson, Townsley, and Abbot, 2002). Frequent and prolonged hospitalizations; complex and multisystem health and developmental needs; and reliance on technology and care that cross hospital, clinic, and home settings are the key characteristics that all of these terms seek to signify about the children they are used to represent (Harrigan, Ratliffe, Patrinos, and others, 2002).

The nature and severity of childhood chronic and complex conditions is widely heterogeneous. Table 18-1 is a nonexhaustive sampling of conditions organized by specialty. However, it is the health and developmental consequences of these diagnoses, such as ongoing functional impairment; neurodevelopmental disability; dependence on medical technology; and the need for ongoing skilled, supportive care from health care providers and family members, that render these children and families as particularly vulnerable. The impact of chronic and complex illness in children is wide ranging. Although many authors have described the rise in prevalence that has come about because of advances in medical care (Cohen, Friedman, Nicholas, and others, 2008; Council on Children with Disabilities, 2005; Haffner and Schurman, 2001; Mentro, 2003), accurate estimates of the numbers of affected families are not known (Carnevale, Rehm, Kirk, and others,

2008). These conditions present most families with additional tasks, responsibilities, and concerns (Ray, 2002). A child's activity level and developmental opportunities can be affected. Days can be lost from school. Children with complex chronic conditions may be at increased risk for behavior or emotional problems. Parents may lose days from work, experience financial strain, and be challenged both emotionally and physically as they cope with care of the child.

Siblings are also affected by having a "different" brother or sister and may simultaneously feel guilt and anger or jealousy toward their ill sibling. Clinicians need to know that siblings of children with chronic illnesses are at risk for negative psychological effects (Sharpe and Rossiter, 2002). Parents need encouragement and assistance with understanding the reactions of siblings to having a chronically ill family member (e.g. behavioral regression, anxiety, withdrawal, apathy). Additionally, secondary losses such as the ability to participate in extracurricular activities or social events occur because of routines imposed by the affected child's chronic condition.

TABLE 18-1	CHRONIC CONDITIONS OF CHILDHOOD
SPECIALTY	**EXAMPLES OF CHRONIC CONDITIONS**
Cardiology	Complex congenital heart disease, congestive heart failure, cardiac dysrhythmias, Kawasaki disease, rheumatic fever, hyperlipidemia
Endocrinology	Diabetes, congenital adrenal hyperplasia, Cushing syndrome
Gastroenterology	Short bowel syndrome, biliary atresia, inflammatory bowel disease, hepatitis, cirrhosis, peptic ulcer disease, celiac disease
Hematology	Sickle cell anemia, thalassemia, aplastic anemia, hereditary anemias, hemophilia
Immunology	Immune deficiency, human immunodeficiency virus, Wiskott-Aldrich syndrome, severe combined immunodeficiency disease
Nephrology	Prune belly syndrome, renal disease
Neurology	Cerebral palsy, ataxia telangiectasia, muscular dystrophy, seizure disorder, spina bifida, traumatic brain injury
Oncology	Brain tumor, leukemia, lymphoma, solid tumors, bone tumors, rare tumors
Pulmonology	Asthma, chronic lung disease, cystic fibrosis, tuberculosis
Rheumatology	Systemic lupus erythematosus, juvenile rheumatoid arthritis, dermatomyositis

TRENDS IN CARE

Developmental Focus

Focusing on the child's developmental level rather than chronologic age or diagnosis emphasizes the child's abilities and strengths rather than disabilities. Attention is directed to normalizing experiences, adapting the environment, and promoting coping skills. Nurses often are in vital positions to redirect attention from the pathologic model with its focus on weaknesses and problems to the developmental model to meet the unique needs of the child and family.

A developmental focus also considers family development. The life cycle of the family unit reflects changing ages and needs of family members, as well as changing external demands. A family member's serious illness can cause significant stress or crisis at any stage of the family life cycle. Just as with individual development, family development may be interrupted or even regress to an earlier level of functioning. Nurses can use the concept of family development to plan meaningful interventions and evaluate care (see Developmental Theory, Chapter 3).

Family-Centered Care

Children's physical and emotional health, as well as their cognitive and social functioning, is strongly influenced by how well their families function (Schor, 2003). The importance of family-centered care—a philosophy that considers the family as the constant in the child's life—is especially evident in the care of children with special needs (see also Family-Centered Care, Chapter 1). As parents learn about the child's health care needs, they often become experts in delivering care. Health care providers, including nurses, are adjuncts to the child's care and need to form partnerships with parents. Effective communication and negotiation between parents and nurses are essential to forming trusting and effective partnerships and finding the best ways to meet the needs of the child and family (Corlett and Twycross, 2006). Collaborative relationships are characterized by communication, dialogue, active listening, awareness, and acceptance of others' differences (Schor, 2003).

Family–Health Care Provider Communication

The disclosure of a serious chronic or complex condition of a child is one of the most stressful aspects of communication between families and health care professionals. Often, parents have suspected for some time that something is wrong with their child and believe that their concerns were minimized or ignored by health care professionals (Smaldone and Ritholz, 2011; Thomlinson, 2002; Whitehead and Gosling, 2003). After a diagnosis is made, numerous studies have shown that parents are not always satisfied with the way in which information is given. Factors that influence parent dissatisfaction with communication include disrespectful attitudes, breaking bad news in an insensitive manner, withholding information, and changing a treatment course without preparing the child and family (Hsiao, Evan, and Zeltzer, 2007). Conversely, parents report satisfaction when they perceived health care providers to be available, demonstrate competence, and engage the child and parent in care decision making (Hsiao, Evan, and Zeltzer, 2007). Similar factors are important in communication of changes in the child's condition throughout the course of the illness.

Providing information to families with a chronically ill child should be a process of repeated discussions to allow the family to process the information and their reactions to that information and allow them to ask for clarification and further information. Nurses play an important role in ensuring that families' needs are met during discussions related to the child's diagnosis, condition, and treatment. This requires assessment regarding how much information the family is comfortable with, what they understand of the information already given to them, and how they are coping with the information both cognitively and emotionally. Nurses should ensure that the appropriate health care professionals address any concerns or further questions that families may have.

Establishing Therapeutic Relationships

Another important aspect of family-centered care of children with chronic and complex conditions is establishing a therapeutic relationship with the child and family, which has been shown to predict improved health-related outcomes (Denboba, McPherson, Kenney, and others, 2006). Families, most often the mother, take on enormous responsibility in providing technical care and symptom management of their child's condition outside the health care institution (O'Brien and Wegner, 2002; Raina, O'Donnell, Rosenbaum, and others, 2005; Swallow and Jacoby, 2001). To build successful therapeutic relationships with families, it is necessary for nurses to recognize parents' expertise with regard to their child's condition and needs. Care conferences, especially multidisciplinary meetings that include the family and key health professionals, provide an opportunity for sharing ideas and expressing feelings or concerns. Health care environments for children with serious illnesses are fraught with obstacles that serve as barriers to successful therapeutic relationships with families. For example, the complex, multidisciplinary care required is often characterized by fragmented, noncohesive approaches to care. Continuity of care can be a challenge in acute care hospitals today, and this makes it difficult to establish relationships and understand communication styles.

Individual discussions, especially with the case manager, primary nurse, clinical nurse specialist, or nurse practitioner, help establish a consistent and flexible care plan that can prevent conflicts or deal with these conflicts before they disrupt care. In family-centered care, the goal is to maintain the integrity of the leadership role and support the family during times of crisis or stress.

The Role of Culture in Family-Centered Care

Issues of culture, ethnicity, and race affect access to services, utilization, and follow-through with referrals and recommendations (Coker, Rodriguez, and Flores, 2010; van Dyck, Kogan, McPherson, and others, 2004; Wise, Wampler, Chavkin, and others, 2002; Wood, Smith, Romero, and others, 2002; Zuvekas and Taliaferro, 2003). For some ethnic and minority populations, cultural understandings of illness, the structure of family life, social roles for individuals with disabilities, and other factors related to the perception of children may differ from those of mainstream American culture. These factors may affect family needs and family choices regarding the care of their child with special needs.

Although culture cannot completely explain how an individual will think and act, understanding cultural perspectives can help the nurse anticipate and understand why families may make certain decisions. Cultural attributes such as values and beliefs regarding illness or chronic condition and its causation, social roles for people who are ill or disabled, family structure, the role of children, childrearing practices, self versus group orientation, spirituality, and time orientation also affect a family's response to illness or chronic condition in a child (Carnevale, Alexander, Davis, and others, 2006; Carter, 2002; Marshall, Olsen, Mandleco, and others, 2003; Rehm, 1999; Sterling and Peterson, 2003).

When parents are informed of their child's chronic illness, interpreters familiar with both culture and language should be used. Children, family members, and friends of the family should not be used as translators because their presence may prevent parents from openly discussing the issues. When working with people of cultural backgrounds different from their own, nurses must listen carefully with an initial goal of understanding and articulating the family's perspective. The ability to interpret the mainstream medical culture to the family is also important. Furthermore, every effort is made to incorporate traditional cultural beliefs of a family into treatment plans. It is important to keep in mind that "cultural norms" may not always apply to every family from a shared background. Nurses who assess the unique needs of each family, listen, and keep themselves open to novel ways of meeting the individual needs of the child and family will likely be successful in establishing a therapeutic relationship. Developing a care plan in conjunction with the family, considering their preferences and priorities, is an important first step in formulating a plan that best meets the family's needs, no matter what their cultural background (Ahmann, 1994; Coker, Rodriguez, and Flores, 2010; Ochieng, 2003).

Shared Decision Making

Shared decision making among the child, family, and health care team can result from open, honest, culturally sensitive communication and the establishment of a therapeutic relationship among the family and health care providers. In a shared decision-making model, the health care professionals provide honest, clear information regarding diagnosis, prognosis, treatment options, and risk–benefit assessment. The patient and family then share information with the health care team regarding important family values, acceptable levels of discomfort or inconvenience, and the ability to comply with treatments being recommended (Charles, Gafni, and Whelan, 1997; Kon, 2010). This process allows them to discuss all options in terms of the risks and benefits to the child and family, the prognosis or expected course of the illness, and the impact on the family's resources (Box 18-1). Together the parents and health care team can make decisions that are best for the family and child at the time the decision is made (Kon, 2010).

Normalization

Normalization refers to the efforts family members make to create a normal family life, their perceptions of the consequences of these efforts, and the meanings they attribute to their management efforts (Knafl, Darney, Gallo, and others, 2010). For chronically ill children, such efforts may include attending school, pursuing hobbies and recreational interests, and achieving employment and a level of independence. For their families, it may entail adapting the family routine to accommodate the ill or disabled child's health and physical needs (McDougal, 2002).

Children with chronic and complex conditions and their families face numerous challenges in achieving normalization. Families move between the "normal" of living with the experience of chronic

---

BOX 18-1 FACILITATING SHARED DECISION MAKING

- Continually assess the impact of the child's illness and treatment on the family.
- Provide honest, accurate information regarding the trajectory of the disease, anticipated complications, and prognostic information.
- Discuss what the family desires for the child's quality of life.
- Avoid personal opinion or judgment of the family's questions and decisions.
- Be aware of nurses' personal and cultural assumptions and the ways these assumptions impact communication, decision making, and judgment.

---

childhood illness and the "normal" of the healthy outside world; they often redefine "normal" based on their particular experiences, needs, and circumstances (Deatrick, Knafl, Murphy-Moore, 1999; Gantt, 2002; Nelson, 2002). Normalization may be an important mediator of illness-related stressors (e.g., treatment demands, uncertainty) on family outcomes

Nurses can assist families in normalizing their lives by assessing the family's everyday life, social support systems, coping strategies, family cohesiveness, and family and community resources. Interventions could include encouraging families to reduce stress through delegation of care and family tasks, identifying ways to incorporate care into current routines, structuring the home environment to encourage the child's engagement in age-appropriate activities, and ensuring families have access to appropriate community support services (Jokinen, 2004; Shepard and Mahon, 2000). Being supportive of the child's illness and treatment and actively including the family in all aspects of care will improve their self-esteem and promote further development (Shepard and Mahon, 2000).

Home care represents the return to a system and set of priorities in which family values are as important in the care of a child with a chronic health problem as they are in the care of other children. Home care seeks to achieve goals that are consistent with the developmental model (Stein, 1985):

- Normalize the life of the child, including those with technologically complex care, in a family and community context and setting.
- Minimize the disruptive impact of the child's condition on the family.
- Foster the child's maximum growth and development.

With appropriate training and support, families provide complex procedures and treatments in the home. Parents are challenged to retain a homelike setting among monitors, ventilators, and other sophisticated equipment. Throughout the text, home care is discussed as appropriate for specific conditions. The process of transition from hospital to home is elaborated on in Chapters 20 and 21.

Paralleling normalization and home care is the process of mainstreaming, or integrating children with disabilities into regular classrooms. Just as the home is the natural environment for children, so school must also be included as an essential component of children's overall physical, intellectual, and social development. Children who attend school have the advantages of learning and socializing with a wide group of peers. There is an increased focus on individualization as plans are made to meet the academic needs of these children along with those of the rest of the students.

A variety of supplemental programs have been designed in the school system to accommodate special needs, both at school age and younger, through early intervention, which consists of any sustained and systematic effort to assist children from birth to age 3 years with disabilities and who are developmentally vulnerable. This change and increasing opportunities for normalization for children with disabilities in large part have resulted from the passage of (1) the Education for All Handicapped Children Act of 1975 (Public Law 94-142) and its 1990 amendments (Public Law 101-476), which changed the name of the act to the Individuals with Disabilities Education Act (IDEA); (2) the Education of the Handicapped Act Amendments of 1986 (Public Law 99-457), which directs states to develop and implement statewide comprehensive, coordinated, multidisciplinary interagency programs of early intervention services for infants and toddlers with disabilities, as well as support services for their families; and (3) the Americans with Disabilities Act of 1990. Nurses can provide parents with information about these laws and in some cases may participate in the development of individualized educational programs (IEPs) or individualized family service plans (IFSPs) for children with disabilities.

Managed Care

Managed care programs have become the major form of health care provision in the United States (Jackson, 2000). This model of care has brought both opportunities and challenges with respect to the care of children with chronic and complex conditions. Although managed care may promote continuity and coordination of care for children and families with private insurance, it has had an unfavorable impact on relatively resource-limited families caring for children with complex chronic illnesses (Huffman, Brat, Chamberlain, and other, 2010). Children rely on adults for access to health care and follow-up with treatment regimens, making it necessary to manage the child's care in the context of the family (McPherson, Weissman, Strickland, and others, 2004; van Dyck, Kogan, McPherson, and others, 2004).

THE FAMILY OF THE CHILD WITH A CHRONIC OR COMPLEX CONDITION

A major goal in working with the family of a child with chronic or complex illness is to support the family's coping and promote their optimal functioning throughout the child's life. Long-term, comprehensive, family-centered approaches extend beyond supporting the child and family during the critical periods of diagnosis and hospitalization. Rather, comprehensive care involves forming parent–professional partnerships that can support a family's adaptation across the trajectory of the illness to the many changes that may be necessary in day-to-day life, determine expectations of and for the child, and provide a long-term perspective (Box 18-2).

The impact of a child's medical or developmental condition is often experienced over time, initially as a crisis at the time of diagnosis, which may occur at birth, after a long period of diagnostic testing, or immediately after a tragic injury. The impact may also be felt before the diagnosis is made, when parents are aware that something is wrong with their child but before medical confirmation (Thomlinson, 2002; Whitehead and Gosling, 2003).

The diagnosis and initial discharge home are critical times for parents (Coffey, 2006). Several factors can make it particularly difficult, including a long duration of uncertainty in the diagnostic process, negative perceptions of chronic illness, insufficient information, and lack of mutual trust between parents and their child's health care team (Garwick, Patterson, Bennett, and others, 1995; Monterosso, Kristjanson, Aoun, and others, 2007; Nuutila and Salanterä, 2006). Parental feelings of shock, helplessness, isolation, fear, and depression

are common (Coffey, 2006; Nuutila and Salanterä, 2006). Throughout the first year, parents struggle to accept the child's diagnosis, care, and uncertainty of the future (Coffey, 2006). Providing explicit and uncomplicated information to parents in an empathic way (Nuutila and Salanterä, 2006); assessing the family's daily routine, living conditions, background knowledge, skills and abilities, and coping behaviors; and evaluating the family's understanding of the information can encourage optimal support at the time of diagnosis and initial discharge home. It is also necessary to reassess parents' needs for information and support on a routine basis (Nuutila and Salanterä, 2006).

Other critical times include the exacerbation of the child's physical symptoms, which increases parental care. These crises often involve medical intervention and rehospitalization. Frequently, the child does not return to his or her precrisis level of functioning, and parents and family must adapt to new care needs and schedules. Instability may also follow transition points on the illness trajectory. For example, changes in caregivers and significant chronologic age milestones can increase parental stress, and advocating for the child during these times is essential. Supporting parents, respecting their stress and emotions, and acknowledging their role as team members in the care of their child are important aspects of nursing care (Coffey, 2006; Nuutila and Salanterä, 2006).

IMPACT OF THE CHILD'S CHRONIC ILLNESS

Each member of a family who has a child with a chronic or complex illness is affected by the experience (Sullivan-Bolyai, Sadler, Knafl, and others, 2003). The effects on the parents and their responses may be so intense that they directly influence the other members' reactions and the child's own coping.

Parents

In addition to the stress of grieving for the loss of a perfect child, parents are affected by whether or not they receive positive feedback from interactions with their child. Many parents feel satisfaction and fulfillment from the parenting role. For others, parenting may be a series of unrewarding experiences that contribute to feelings of inadequacy and failure (Box 18-3). These responses may be most evident in parents who are responsible for the child's care. For example, parents may become preoccupied with their ability to carry out certain procedures, overlooking the child's personal comfort and satisfaction or

---

BOX 18-2 **ADAPTIVE TASKS OF PARENTS HAVING CHILDREN WITH CHRONIC CONDITIONS**

1. Accept the child's condition.
2. Manage the child's condition on a day-to-day basis.
3. Meet the child's normal developmental needs.
4. Meet the developmental needs of other family members.
5. Cope with ongoing stress and periodic crises.
6. Assist family members to manage their feelings.
7. Educate others about the child's condition.
8. Establish a support system.

From Canam C: Common adaptive tasks facing parents of children with chronic conditions, *J Adv Nurs* 18:46–53, 1993.

BOX 18-3 **ANTICIPATED PARENTAL STRESS POINTS**

Diagnosis of the condition—Parents require considerable education while dealing with an emotional response.

Developmental milestones—Times that children normally achieve walking, talking, and self-care are delayed or impossible for the child.

Start of schooling—Particularly stressful are situations in which appropriate schooling will not be in a regular class placement.

Reaching the ultimate attainment—Parents must handle situations such as realizing that ambulation will be impossible or that the child will not learn to read.

Adolescence—Issues such as sexuality and independence become prominent.

Future placement—Decisions about placement must be made when the child becomes an adult or when the parents can no longer care for the child.

Death of the child

failing to offer praise for anything less than perfect cooperation or performance. They may pursue a frustrating activity until they achieve "success"—long after the child has become irritable and uncooperative. As a result, parents can become caught in a pattern of interaction that is mutually unrewarding and minimally productive. This situation may become exacerbated by disagreements or lack of support from other family members and judgment from caregivers and others in the community. For these parents, several strategies may be helpful, including education regarding what can reasonably be expected of their child, assistance in identifying the child's strengths, praise for a parental job well done, and respite care so that parents can renew their energies.

Parental Roles

Parenting a child with a complex chronic condition requires much more than raising a typical child. In addition to attending to the routine aspects of parenting, parents of chronically ill children take on the added responsibility of performing complex technical care and symptom management, advocating for their child, and seeking and coordinating health and social services for their ill or disabled child (Kirk, Glendinning, and Callery, 2005). These added responsibilities must then be balanced with the needs of other family members, extended family and friends, and personal health and obligations to minimize consequences to the overall functioning of the family (Coffey, 2006; Ray, 2002). Enormous demands may be placed on parental time, energy, and financial resources.

Often one parent or partner remains at home to manage existing family responsibilities while the other remains with the ill child. The partner who is not included in the caregiving activities may feel neglected because all of the attention is directed toward the child and be resentful that he or she is not sufficiently informed to be competent in the care. Without active participation in the child's care, the parent has little appreciation of the time and energy involved in performing these activities. When this partner does attempt to participate, the other parent may criticize the less skillful efforts. As a result, communication and support for each other may be adversely affected.

The nurse can assist parents in avoiding role conflicts by providing anticipatory guidance early on. Teaching should address stressors often identified as having an impact on the marriage, including (1) the burden of care at home assumed by primarily one parent, (2) the financial burden, (3) the fear of the child dying, (4) pressure from relatives, (5) the hereditary nature of the disease (if applicable), and (6) fear of pregnancy. Other causes of tension may center on the inconveniences associated with care, such as long waits for an appointment, lack of parking near care facilities, or lack of overnight accommodations. Certainly, these last stressors are within health professionals' domain to minimize, if not eliminate.

Mother–Father Differences

Mothers and fathers in the same family often adjust and cope differently as parents of a child with a complex condition. Whereas some mothers experience a peaks-and-valleys periodic crisis pattern, most fathers tend to experience a steady, gradual recovery. Some research suggests that mothers of children with certain conditions may be more susceptible to psychologic distress and fatigue than fathers (Tong, Kandala, Haig, and others, 2002). Mothers are most often the primary caregiver and are more likely than fathers to give up their jobs to care for their children, often resulting in social isolation (Coffey, 2006). Whereas mothers often have greater needs for social support and positive appraisal of the situation, fathers are more likely to use self-controlling behaviors to cope (Goldbeck, 2001; Mastroyannopoulou, Stallard, Lewis, and others, 1997).

Fathers of children with disabilities struggle with issues that may be distinct from those of the mothers (Swallow, Macfadyen, Santacroce, and others, 2011). Fathers may think that their role of protector is challenged because they do not know how to help and cannot protect their family from the seemingly overwhelming recurring problems. With today's increased emphasis on fathers' involvement in the lives of their children, this loss is felt more profoundly than in the past. The extensive stresses in the family can leave fathers feeling depressed, weak, guilty, powerless, isolated, embarrassed, and angry. Fearful that they will lose control or be viewed as weak or ineffectual, however, fathers often hide their feelings and display an outward confidence that may lead others to believe that everything is fine. Fathers worry about what the future holds for their children, their ability to manage the increasing financial burden, and the daily disruptions of the entire family (Davies, Gudmundsdottir, Worden, and others, 2004; Swallow, Macfadyen, Santacroce, and others, 2011). Some fathers escape in their work as a means of dulling the pain. Common coping strategies are problem oriented and include praying, getting information, looking at options, and weighing choices in addition to withdrawal (Mastroyannopoulou, Stallard, Lewis, and others, 1997).

Single-Parent Families

Single-parent families are of special concern. The absence of a parent may result from divorce or death, or the parents may never have married. As the only parent of a child who may require extensive, sophisticated, and lifelong care, the single parent may feel an enormous burden. Available financial and emotional resources may already be stretched to the limit. A special effort should be made to assist the single parent in finding financial and support services that can ease the burden of care. Nurses can also assist the single parent in identifying helping roles that may be acceptable to relatives and friends.

Siblings

Results of studies on how siblings are affected by having a brother or sister with a complex condition are unclear (Anderson and Davis, 2011; Barlow and Ellard, 2006). Generally, evidence shows a negative effect on siblings of children with chronic illnesses compared with siblings of healthy children (Gold, Treadwell, Weissman, and others, 2011). Siblings of children with chronic illnesses report psychosocial problems more often than their peers (Gold, Treadwell, Weissman, and others, 2011; Rossiter and Sharpe, 2001). A number of factors increase the risk of negative effects for siblings of ill children. Responsibility for caregiving, differential treatment by parents, and limitations in family resources and recreational time are often the experiences of siblings of ill or disabled children (Lobato and Kao, 2002) (Box 18-4).

An important factor in sibling adjustment and coping is information and knowledge regarding their brother's or sister's illness or complex condition. What siblings piece together or overhear is often much worse than the truth. Often they imagine gruesome things regarding the experiences related to the illness, treatment, and hospitalization (Shepard and Mahon, 2000). Latino siblings have reported less accurate information about their siblings' condition than non-Latino siblings (Lobato, Kao, and Plante, 2005). Parents are usually in the best position to impart information, although they are often overwhelmed with the medical crisis at hand (Fleitas, 2000). Nurses can encourage parents to talk with the siblings about how they perceive their sick brother or sister and to be accepting of the siblings' feelings. Nurses can be ideal educators and counselors of siblings during the course of their brother's or sister's illness (Shepard and Mahon, 2000) (see Family-Centered Care box).

BOX 18-4 SUPPORTING SIBLINGS OF CHILDREN WITH SPECIAL NEEDS

Promote Healthy Sibling Relationships

Value each child individually and avoid comparisons. Remind each child of his or her positive qualities and contribution to other family members.

Help siblings see the differences and similarities between themselves and the child with special needs. Create a climate in which children can achieve successes without feeling guilty.

Teach siblings ways to interact with the child.

Seek to be fair in terms of discipline, attention, and resources; require the affected child to do as much for himself or herself as possible.

Let siblings settle their own differences; intervene only to prevent siblings from hurting one another.

Legitimize reasonable anger. Even children with special needs behave badly sometimes.

Respect a sibling's reluctance to be with or to include the child with special needs in activities.

Help Siblings Cope

Listen to siblings to let them know that their thoughts and suggestions are valued.

Praise siblings when they have been patient, have sacrificed, or have been particularly helpful. Do not expect siblings to always act in this manner.

Acknowledge the personal strengths siblings have and their ability to cope with stress successfully.

Provide age-appropriate information about the child's condition and update it when appropriate.

Let teachers know what is happening so they can be understanding and helpful.

Recognize special stress times for siblings and plan to minimize negative effects.

Schedule special time with siblings; have a friend or family member substitute when parent is unavailable.

Encourage siblings to join or help establish a sibling support group.

Use the services of professionals when needed. If parent feels that such a service is necessary, it should be provided in as vigorous a manner as a service for the child with special needs.

Involve Siblings

Seek out ways to realistically include siblings in the care and treatment of the child with special needs.

Limit caregiving responsibilities and give recognition when siblings perform them.

Develop a library of children's books on special needs.

Invite siblings to attend meetings to develop plans for the child with special needs (e.g., individualized educational program, individualized family service plan).

Discuss future plans with them.

Solicit their ideas on treatment and service needs.

Have them visit professionals who work with the child.

Help them develop competencies to teach the child new skills.

Provide opportunities for siblings to advocate for the child.

Allow siblings to set their own pace for learning and involvement.

Data from Powell T, Ogle P: Brothers and sisters—a special part of exceptional families, Baltimore, 1985, Paul H Brooks; Spokane Washington Deaconess Medical Center, Pediatric Oncology Unit: Tips for dealing with siblings, Candlelighters Childhood Cancer Found Q Newslett 11(3,4):7, 1987; and Carlson J, Leviton A, Mueller M: Services to siblings: an important component of family-centered practice, ACCH Advocate 1(1):53–56, 1993.

FAMILY-CENTERED CARE
Reflection of an Older Brother

My youngest sister, Kerry, was on an apnea monitor 3 years ago, when I was 15. I was never embarrassed about Kerry being on the monitor, except for the time it went off in church and everyone turned around to look at us.

Joey Bellino
Oldest sibling of an infant on an apnea monitor
Washington, DC

COPING WITH ONGOING STRESS AND PERIODIC CRISES

Professionals can help families cope with stress by providing anticipatory guidance, providing emotional support, assisting the family in assessing and identifying specific stressors, aiding the family in developing coping mechanisms and problem-solving strategies, and working collaboratively with parents so that they become empowered in the process (Anderson and Davis, 2011).

Concurrent Stresses Within the Family

The ability to deal with the overwhelming stress of a chronic illness is challenged further when additional stresses are present. Stressors may be situational or developmental. They may be related to marital difficulties, sibling needs, homelessness, or social isolation. Some families may simultaneously be struggling with a family member's alcohol or other drug problem. Even relatively minor stressors, such as arranging care for siblings, managing the home, and traveling to distant treatment centers, can challenge a family's ability to cope successfully.

Most families, regardless of their income or insurance coverage, have financial concerns. The costs of caring for a child with a complex illness can be overwhelming. Nurses and social workers can help a family review various options for financial assistance, including insurance, managed care, or health maintenance organization policies; Medicaid; Supplemental Security Income; Women, Infants, and Children program (WIC); the state Program for Children with Special Health Needs; disease-related associations; and local philanthropic organizations.

Coping Mechanisms

Coping mechanisms are behaviors aimed at reducing the tension caused by a crisis. **Approach behaviors** are coping mechanisms that result in movement toward adjustment and resolution of the crisis. **Avoidance behaviors** result in movement away from adjustment and represent maladaptation to the crisis. Several approach and avoidance behaviors used in coping with a chronic illness are listed in the Nursing Care Guidelines box. None of the indexes can be used singly to assess the possible success or failure in resolving the crisis. Each behavior must be viewed in the context of all of the variables affecting the family. For example, the observation of several avoidance behaviors in an emotionally healthy family may denote significantly less risk to the successful resolution of the crisis than an equal number of avoidance behaviors in an individual who has few available supports.

Parental Empowerment

Empowerment can be seen as a process of recognizing, promoting, and enhancing competence. For parents of children with chronic conditions, empowerment may occur gradually as strength and capabilities are drawn on to master the child's care, manage family life, and plan for the future. Advocating for the child and developing parent–professional partnerships are part of taking charge (Ray, 2002).

ASSISTING FAMILY MEMBERS IN MANAGING THEIR FEELINGS

Although some previous research has postulated stages of adaptation to a chronic illness, there is a great deal of individual variation in responses to the diagnosis, adjustments made, and time frames for coming to terms with a diagnosis. It is important that professionals recognize and respect a wide range of reactions and coping mechanisms. In fact, members of the family of a child with a complex chronic condition may experience a number of difficult emotions, including fear, guilt, anger, resentment, and anxiety. Learning to manage these emotions promotes adaptive coping (see Nursing Care Guidelines box). Support from professionals, other family members, and friends can assist family members in managing their feelings. The following discussion examines some common phases of adjustment and emotional reactions.

 NURSING CARE GUIDELINES

Assessing Coping Behaviors

Approach Behaviors

Asks for information regarding diagnosis and child's present condition

Seeks help and support from others

Anticipates future problems; actively seeks guidance and answers

Endows the chronic illness or complex condition with meaning

Shares burden of disorder with others

Plans realistically for the future

Acknowledges and accepts child's awareness of diagnosis and prognosis

Expresses feelings such as sorrow, depression, and anger and realizes reason for the emotional reaction

Realistically perceives child's condition; adjusts to changes

Recognizes own growth through passage of time, such as earlier denial and nonacceptance of diagnosis

Verbalizes possible loss of child

Avoidance Behaviors

Fails to recognize seriousness of child's condition despite physical evidence

Refuses to agree to treatment

Intellectualizes about the illness but in areas unrelated to child's condition

Is angry and hostile to members of the staff regardless of their attitude or behavior

Avoids staff, family members, or child

Entertains unrealistic future plans for child with little emphasis on the present

Is unable to adjust to or accept a change in progression of disease

Continually looks for new cures with no perspective toward possible benefit

Refuses to acknowledge child's understanding of disease and prognosis

Uses magical thinking and fantasy; may seek "occult" help

Places complete faith in religion to point of relinquishing own responsibility

Withdraws from outside world; refuses help

Punishes self because of guilt and blame

Makes no change in lifestyle to meet needs of other family members

Resorts to excessive use of alcohol or drugs to avoid problems

Verbalizes suicidal intents

Is unable to discuss possible loss of child or previous experiences with death

---

Shock and Denial

The initial diagnosis of a chronic illness or complex condition is often met with intense emotion and is characterized by shock, disbelief, and sometimes denial, especially if the disorder is not obvious, as in chronic illness. Denial as a defense mechanism is a necessary cushion to prevent disintegration and is a normal response to grieving for any type of loss. Probably all family members experience various degrees of adaptive denial as they learn of the impact that the diagnosis has on their lives.

Shock and denial can last from days to months, sometimes even longer. Examples of denial that may be exhibited at the time of diagnosis include:

- Physician shopping
- Attributing the symptoms of the actual illness to a minor condition
- Refusing to believe the diagnostic tests
- Delaying consent for treatment
- Acting happy and optimistic despite the revealed diagnosis
- Refusing to tell or talk to anyone about the condition
- Insisting that no one is telling the truth, regardless of others' attempts to do so
- Denying the reason for admission
- Asking no questions about the diagnosis, treatment, or prognosis

Generally, these mechanisms should be respected as short-term responses that allow individuals to distance themselves from the tremendous emotional impact and to collect and mobilize their energies toward goal-directed, problem-solving behaviors.

In children, the importance of denial has repeatedly been demonstrated as a factor in their positive coping with the diagnosis. Denial allows the child to maintain hope in the face of overwhelming odds and to function adaptively and productively. Similar to hope, denial may be an adaptive mechanism for dealing with loss that persists until a family or patient is ready or needs other responses.

Denial is probably the least understood and most poorly dealt-with reaction. Health professionals typically label denial as maladaptive and act inappropriately by attempting to strip it away by repeated and sometimes blunt explanations of the prognosis. However, denial becomes maladaptive only when it prevents recognition of treatment or rehabilitative goals necessary for the child's optimal survival or development.

Adjustment

For most families, adjustment gradually follows shock and is usually characterized by an open admission that the condition exists. This stage may be accompanied by several responses, which are normal parts of the adaptation process. Probably the most universal of these feelings are **guilt** and **self-accusation**. Guilt is often greatest when the cause of the disorder is directly traceable to the parent, as in genetic diseases or accidental injury. However, it can occur even without any scientific or realistic basis for parental responsibility. Frequently, the guilt stems from a false assumption that the child's condition is a result of personal failure or wrongdoing, such as not doing something correctly during pregnancy or the birth. Guilt may also be associated with cultural or religious beliefs. Some parents are convinced that they are being punished for some previous misdeed. Others may see the illness as a trial sent by God to test their religious strength and faith. With correct information, support, and time, most parents master guilt and self-accusation. The ability to master resentful and self-accusatory feelings of having "caused" the child's disorder is a crucial factor in determining the parents' acceptance of their child.

Children, too, may interpret their serious illness as retribution for past misbehavior. The nurse should be particularly sensitive to the child who passively accepts all painful procedures. This child may believe that such acts are inflicted as deserved punishment. It is vital that parents and health care professionals reassure children that their illnesses are not their fault.

Other common and normal reactions to a diagnosis are **bitterness** and **anger**. Anger directed inward may be evident as self-reproaching or punitive behavior, such as neglecting one's health and verbally degrading oneself. Anger directed outward may be manifested in either open arguments or withdrawal from communication and may be evident in the person's relationship with any number of individuals, such as the spouse, the child, and siblings. Passive anger toward the ill child may be evident in decreased visiting, refusal to believe how sick the child is, or an inability to provide comfort. Among the most common targets for parental anger are members of the staff. Parents may complain about the nursing care, the insufficient time physicians spend with them, or the lack of skill of those who draw blood or start intravenous infusions.

Children are apt to respond with anger as well, and this includes the affected child and the well siblings. Children are aware of the loss engendered by their illness or complex condition and may react angrily to the restrictions imposed or the feelings of being different. Siblings may also feel anger and resentment toward the ill child and parents for the loss of routine and parental attention. It is difficult for older children and almost impossible for younger children to comprehend the plight of the affected child. Their perception is of a brother or sister who has the undivided attention of their parents, is showered with cards and gifts, and is the focus of everyone's concern.

During the period of adjustment, four types of parental reactions to the child influence the child's eventual response to the disorder:

Overprotection in which the parents fear letting the child achieve any new skill, avoid all discipline, and cater to every desire to prevent frustration

Rejection in which the parents detach themselves emotionally from the child but usually provide adequate physical care or constantly nag and scold the child

Denial in which the parents act as if the disorder does not exist or attempt to have the child overcompensate for it

Gradual acceptance in which the parents place necessary and realistic restrictions on the child, encourage self-care activities, and promote reasonable physical and social abilities

Reintegration and Acknowledgment

For many families, the adjustment process culminates in the development of realistic expectations for the child and reintegration of family life with the illness or complex condition in a manageable perspective. Because a large portion of this phase is one of grief for a loss, total resolution is not possible until the child dies or leaves home as an independent adult. Therefore, one can regard adjustment as "increased comfort" with everyday living rather than a complete resolution.

This adjustment phase also involves social reintegration in which the family broadens its activities to include relationships outside of the home with the child as an acceptable and participating member of the group. This last criterion often differentiates the reaction of gradual acceptance during the adjustment period from total acceptance or perhaps is more descriptive of the acknowledgment process.

Many parents of children with chronic illnesses experience **chronic sorrow**, feelings of sorrow and loss that recur in waves over time. As the child's condition progresses, parents experience repeated losses that represent further declines and new caregiving demands. Consequently, families must be assessed on an ongoing basis and offered appropriate support and resources as their needs change over time (Bettle and

Latimer, 2009; Gordon, 2009). This represents a critical period of time as the nursing and medical team approach and support provided during this period of time can directly impact the experience of complicated grief after the death of the child. Complicated grief (Meert, Shear, Newth, and others, 2011), characterized as persistent distress and chronic stress response, may last 6 months or longer after the death of a child and has a significant impact on quality of life of the family left behind. Complicated grief has been proposed as a new diagnostic entity to be included in the fifth edition of the *Diagnostic and Statistical Manual of Mental Disorders* (Meert, Shear, Newth, and others, 2011).

ESTABLISHING A SUPPORT SYSTEM

The diagnosis of a child with a complex chronic condition is a major situational crisis that affects the entire family system. However, families can experience positive outcomes as they successfully deal with the many challenges that accompany a child with chronic illness (Hungerbuehler, Vollrath, and Landolt, 2011).

One nursing goal is to assess which families are at greater or lesser risk for succumbing to the effects of the crisis. Several variables— available support system, perception of the event, coping mechanisms, reactions to the child, available resources, and concurrent stresses within the family—influence the resolution of a crisis. Although most families cope well, the needs of families at risk are great. If they receive emotional support and guidance early, there is an increased likelihood that they will also cope successfully.

Although it is easy to assume that families of children with the most severe illnesses or disabilities would have the poorest adjustment, the severity of the condition reflects only one part of the overall picture. The level of adjustment is significantly influenced by the **functional burden** on the individual family (Stein, 1985). This concept considers the issues related to caring for and living with the child in relation to the family's resources and ability to cope (Box 18-5). The family of a child with a high level of technology dependence demanding complex care yet having many resources and coping skills may adjust more successfully to the child's situation than the family of a child with a less serious condition and few resources to counterbalance.

Intrafamilial resources, social support from friends and relatives, parent-to-parent support, parent–professional partnerships, and community resources interweave to provide a flexible web of support for families of children with chronic conditions.

BOX 18-5 **CONCEPT OF FUNCTIONAL BURDEN**

Impact of the Child with Special Needs

The child's need for medical and nursing care

The child's fixed deficits

The child's age-appropriate dependency in activities of daily living

The disruptions in the family routine caused by the care

The psychologic burden of the prognosis on the family

Family Resources and Ability to Cope

The family's physical resources

The family's emotional resources

The family's educational resources

The family's social supports and available help

The competing demands for family members' time and energy

Data from Stein REK: Home care: a challenging opportunity, *Child Health Care* 14(2):90–95, 1985.

THE CHILD WITH A CHRONIC OR COMPLEX CONDITION

The child's reaction to chronic illness depends to a great extent on his or her developmental level, temperament, and available coping mechanisms; on the reactions of family members or significant others; and, to a lesser extent, on the condition itself. A child's conceptual understanding of his or her own illness is based not only on age and developmental level but also on the duration and type of experience accumulated with the disease. Knowledge of these variables is essential in providing the kind of information and support needed by these children to cope with an often overwhelming situation.

DEVELOPMENTAL ASPECTS

The impact of a complex chronic illness is influenced by the age at onset. Chronic illness affects children of all ages, but the developmental aspects of each age group dictate particular stresses and risks for the child. The nurse must also recognize that children need to redefine their condition and its implications as they develop and grow. For example, appearance, skills, and abilities are highly valued by peers (Fig. 18-1); a teenager who is limited in any of these qualities is subject to rejection. This is especially marked when an illness interferes with sexual attractiveness.

Children's developmental concepts of illness are discussed in Chapter 21. An understanding of these developmental factors facilitates planning care to support the child and minimize the risks. Developmental aspects of chronic illness on children are described in Table 18-2.

COPING MECHANISMS

Children with chronic conditions tend to use five distinct patterns of coping (Box 18-6). Children with more positive and accepting attitudes about their chronic illness use a more adaptive coping style characterized by optimism, competence, and compliance. They show fewer behavior problems at home and at school. The two maladaptive coping patterns—"Feels different and withdraws" and "Is irritable, is moody, and acts out"—are associated with poorer adaptation; children using these strategies have poorer self-concepts, more negative attitudes

about their conditions, and more behavior problems at home and at school.

Well-adapted children gradually learn to accept their physical limitations and find achievement in a variety of compensatory motor and intellectual pursuits. They function well at home, at school, and with peers. They have an understanding of their disorder that allows them to accept their limitations, assume responsibility for their care, and assist in treatment and rehabilitation regimens. They express appropriate emotions, such as sadness, anxiety, and anger, at times of exacerbations but confidence and guarded optimism during periods of clinical stability (Fig. 18-2). They are able to identify with other similarly affected individuals, promoting positive self-images and displaying pride and self-confidence in their ability to master a productive, successful life despite their illnesses.

BOX 18-6   COPING PATTERNS USED BY CHILDREN WITH SPECIAL NEEDS

Develops competence and optimism—Accentuates the positive aspects of the situation and concentrates more on what he or she has or can do than on what is missing or on what he or she cannot do; is as independent as possible

Feels different and withdraws—Sees self as being different from other children because of the chronic health condition; views being different as negative; sees self as less worthy than others; focuses on things he or she cannot do and sometimes overrestricts activities needlessly

Is irritable, is moody, and acts out—Uses proactive and self-initiated coping behaviors, although usually counterproductive in that the behaviors are not ego enhancing or socially responsible and do not result in desired outcomes; acts out irritability, which may or may not be associated with condition's symptoms

Complies with treatment—Takes necessary medications, treatments; adheres to activity restrictions; also uses behaviors that indicate developing independence (e.g., assumes responsibility for taking medication)

Seeks support—Talks with adults, children, physicians, and nurses; develops plans to handle problems as they occur; uses downward comparison (i.e., realizes that others have it worse)

Modified from Austin J, Patterson J, Huberty T: Development of the Coping Health Inventory for children, *J Pediatr Nurs* 6(3):166–174, 1991.

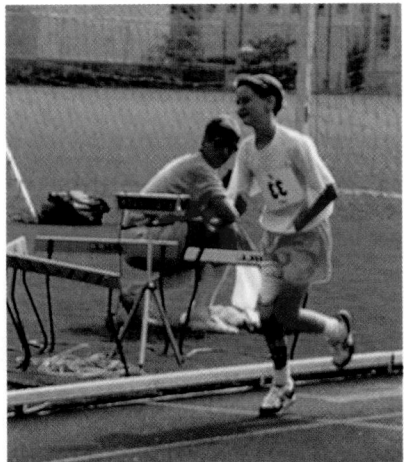

FIG. 18-1 Children with any type of impairment should have the opportunity to develop their skills. (Courtesy Poyo/Hinton Photography.)

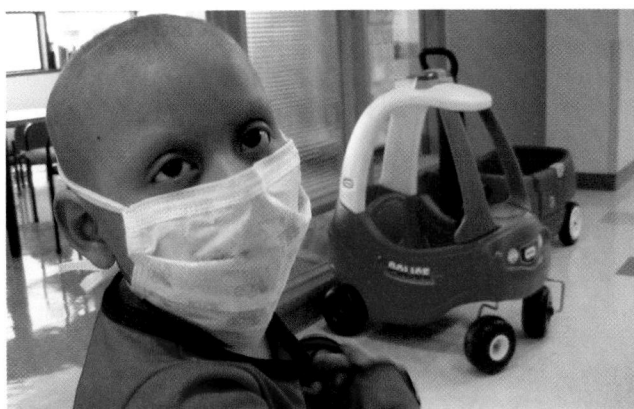

FIG. 18-2 Periods of sadness and anger are appropriate in the child's adjustment to a chronic illness or disability, especially during exacerbations of the disorder.

TABLE 18-2	DEVELOPMENTAL EFFECTS OF CHRONIC ILLNESS OR DISABILITY ON CHILDREN	
DEVELOPMENTAL TASKS	**POTENTIAL EFFECTS OF CHRONIC ILLNESS OR DISABILITY**	**SUPPORTIVE INTERVENTIONS**
Infancy		
Develop a sense of trust	Multiple caregivers and frequent separations, especially if hospitalized	Encourage consistent caregivers in hospital or other care settings.
	Deprived of consistent nurturing	Encourage parental presence, "rooming in" during hospitalization, and participation in care.
Bond, or attach, to parent	Delayed because of separation; parental grief for loss of "dream" child; parental inability to accept the condition, especially a visible defect	Emphasize healthy, perfect qualities of infant. Help parents learn special care needs of infant for them to feel competent.
Learn through sensorimotor experiences	More exposure to painful experiences than pleasurable ones	Expose infant to pleasurable experiences through all senses (touch, hearing, sight, taste, movement).
	Limited contact with environment from restricted movement or confinement	Encourage age-appropriate developmental skills (e.g., holding bottle, finger feeding, crawling).
Begin to develop a sense of separateness from parent	Increased dependency on parent for care	Encourage all family members to participate in care to prevent overinvolvement of one member.
	Overinvolvement of parent in care	Encourage periodic respite from demands of care responsibilities.
Toddlerhood		
Develop autonomy	Increased dependency on parent	Encourage independence in as many areas as possible (e.g., toileting, dressing, feeding).
Master locomotor and language skills	Limited opportunity to test own abilities and limits	Provide gross motor skill activity and modification of toys or equipment, such as modified swing or rocking horse.
Learn through sensorimotor experience; beginning preoperational thought	Increased exposure to painful experiences	Give choices to allow simple feeling of control (e.g., choice of what book to look at, what kind of sandwich to eat). Institute age-appropriate discipline and limit setting. Recognize that negative and ritualistic behaviors are normal. Provide sensory experiences (e.g., water play, sandbox play, finger painting).
Preschool Age		
Develop initiative and purpose Master self-care skills	Limited opportunities for success in accomplishing simple tasks or mastering self-care skills	Encourage mastery of self-help skills. Provide devices that make tasks easier (e.g., self-dressing).
Begin to develop peer relationships	Limited opportunities for socialization with peers; may appear "like a baby" to age mates	Encourage socialization (e.g., inviting friends to play, daycare experience, trips to park).
	Protection within tolerant and secure family, causing child to fear criticism and withdraw	Provide age-appropriate play, especially associative play opportunities. Emphasize child's abilities; dress appropriately to enhance desirable appearance.
Develop sense of body image and sexual identification	Awareness of body centering on pain, anxiety, and failure Sex-role identification focused primarily on mothering skills	Encourage relationships with same-sex and opposite-sex peers and adults.
Learn through preoperational thought (magical thinking)	Guilt (thinking he or she caused the illness or disability or is being punished for wrongdoing)	Help child deal with criticisms; realize that too much protection prevents child from realities of world. Clarify that cause of child's illness or disability is not his or her fault or a punishment.
School Age		
Develop a sense of accomplishment	Limited opportunities to achieve and compete (e.g., many school absences, inability to join regular athletic activities)	Encourage school attendance; schedule medical visits at times other than school; encourage child to make up missed work.
Form peer relationships	Limited opportunities for socialization	Educate teachers and classmates about child's condition, abilities, and special needs. Encourage sports activities (e.g., Special Olympics). Encourage socialization (e.g., Girl Scouts, Campfire, Boy Scouts, 4-H Club; having a best friend or club membership).
Learn through concrete operations	Incomplete comprehension of the imposed physical limitations or treatment of the disorder	Provide child with information about his or her condition. Encourage creative activities (e.g., VSA Arts).

TABLE 18-2	DEVELOPMENTAL EFFECTS OF CHRONIC ILLNESS OR DISABILITY ON CHILDREN—cont'd	
DEVELOPMENTAL TASKS	**POTENTIAL EFFECTS OF CHRONIC ILLNESS OR DISABILITY**	**SUPPORTIVE INTERVENTIONS**
Adolescence		
Develop personal and sexual identity	Increased sense of feeling different from peers and reduced ability to compete with peers in appearance, abilities, special skills	Help child realize that many of the difficulties the teenager is experiencing are part of normal adolescence (rebelliousness, risk taking, lack of cooperation, hostility toward authority).
Achieve independence from family	Increased dependency on family; limited job or career opportunities	Provide instruction on interpersonal and coping skills. Encourage increased responsibility for care and management of the disease or condition (e.g., assuming responsibility for making and keeping appointment [ideally alone], sharing assessment and planning stages of health care delivery, contacting resources). Discuss planning for future and how condition can affect choices.
Form heterosexual relationships	Limited opportunities for heterosexual friendships; less opportunity to discuss sexual concerns with peers Increased concern with issues such as why did he or she get the disorder and whether he or she will marry and have a family	Encourage socialization with peers, including peers with special needs and those without special needs. Encourage activities appropriate for age (e.g., attending mixed-sex parties, sports activities, driving a car). Be alert to cues that signal readiness for information regarding implications of condition on sexuality and reproduction. Emphasize good appearance and wearing stylish clothes, use of makeup. Understand that adolescent has same sexual needs and concerns as any other teenager.
Learn through abstract thinking	Decreased opportunity for earlier stages of cognition impeding achievement of level of abstract thinking	Provide instruction on decision making, assertiveness, and other skills necessary to manage personal plans.

Hopefulness

Children, particularly adolescents, are sensitive to the presence or absence of hope. Hopefulness is an internal quality that mobilizes humans into goal-directed action that may be satisfying and life sustaining. A sense of hopefulness can produce increased participation in health-seeking behaviors and an improved sense of well-being (Ritchie, 2001).

Health Education and Self-Care

Health education is an intervention that promotes coping. Children need information about their condition, the therapeutic plan, and how the disease or the therapy might affect their particular situation. Children nearing puberty also need to understand the maturation process and how their chronic illness may alter this event. For example, a youngster with Crohn disease should understand that this disorder is associated with growth failure and delayed puberty, a child with diabetes needs to know that hormonal changes and increased growth needs will alter food and insulin requirements at this time, and a sexually active girl with sickle cell anemia or systemic lupus erythematosus needs to be aware of the risks of pregnancy. The information should not be given all at once but should be timed appropriately to meet the changing needs of the youngsters, and it should be described and repeated as often as the situation demands.

RESPONSES TO PARENTAL BEHAVIOR

Parental behavior toward the child is one of the most important factors influencing the child's adjustment. Children's perceptions of their mothers' support and maternal perceptions of the psychosocial impact of the child's chronic illness on the family were shown to be two of the greatest predictors of children's psychologic adjustment (Immelt, 2006). In addition, family organization and illness-related support and involvement of the parents influence children's adjustment to chronic illness (Schor, 2003). They often display pride and confidence in their ability to cope successfully with the challenges imposed by their disorder. Anticipatory guidance by the nurse and encouragement of normalizing practices may assist parents in facilitating positive adjustment in their children.

TYPE OF ILLNESS OR CONDITION

The type of illness or condition also influences the child's emotional response. Interestingly, children with *more* severe disorders often cope better than those with milder conditions. However, the presence of multiple conditions may place a child at risk for more behavioral problems (Newacheck and Halfon, 1998). Considering children's cognitive ability and their delay in achieving abstract thinking until adolescence, it is likely that an obvious condition is easier to accept because its limitations are concrete. For example, children who are blind or have physical disabilities are constantly reminded of their inability to run. However, children with cardiac defects not only live by rules they do not understand but also only vaguely and occasionally sense their illness, such as when they try to run and experience dyspnea and fatigue. Therefore, some chronic illnesses pose special threats to children.

The onset of a disabling condition may generate a state of confusion for children, who may have trouble differentiating between actual bodily functions and their image of their bodies. They may also experience problems in identifying themselves and those extensions of self (e.g., wheelchairs, braces, crutches, other mechanical or prosthetic devices) and may have difficulty in accepting functional aids.

NURSING CARE OF THE FAMILY AND CHILD WITH A CHRONIC OR COMPLEX CONDITION

ASSESSMENT

Because the nurse may meet a family during any phase of the adjustment process, several assessment areas are important. The family's ability to cope with previous stresses influences the current situation, and answers to questions about their usual coping skills are enlightening. Knowledge of concurrent stresses, such as financial, marital or nonmarital, and career or unemployment, helps identify families who may have fewer resources to cope with the child's needs.

Finally, awareness of the family members' reactions to the child and the illness or condition is important. Sample questions that the nurse and family can use to evaluate the support system, perception of the illness, coping mechanisms, resources, and concurrent stresses are listed in Table 18-3. Because factors affecting the family's response may change at any point during the illness, assessment must be a continuous process.

Special challenges exist in assessing the child's feelings about having a chronic condition. Chapter 6 presents several approaches to encourage children to discuss their feelings about their conditions. The nurse should use a variety of communication techniques, such as drawing and play, as assessment tools rather than relying solely on parental reports. Often, children are neglected partners in their care, and their unique needs are not identified (Dixon-Woods, Young, and Henry, 1999; Young, Dixon-Woods, Windridge, and others, 2003).

The needs of working parents and siblings also should be assessed, a goal that requires flexibility in scheduling appointments to include these important family members. When working parents know that their input is valuable, they will often change their work schedule to meet with a health professional. Because siblings can be of any age, the use of appropriate communication strategies for assessment must be considered. Nonverbal techniques such as those discussed in Chapter 6 should be considered for these children.

PROVIDE SUPPORT AT THE TIME OF DIAGNOSIS

The diagnosis is a critical time for parents and can influence how they perceive their health care providers throughout care. Although they may not hear or remember all that is said to them, they frequently sense a certain attitude of acceptance, rejection, hope, or despair that may influence their ability to absorb the shock and begin adapting to the family's altered future.

Parents may be encouraged to be together when they are informed of their child's condition, thus avoiding the problem of one parent having to interpret complex findings and deal with the initial emotional reaction of the other. The informing session should take place in a private, comfortable setting free of distractions and interruptions in an atmosphere in which the parents feel free to express their emotions (Fig. 18-3). Their emotional needs are acknowledged by showing acceptance of such expressions as crying, sadness, anger, and disappointment. Emotional support is offered by having tissues available if a family member cries and demonstrating through facial and body

TABLE 18-3	ASSESSMENT OF FACTORS AFFECTING FAMILY ADJUSTMENT
FACTORS AFFECTING ADJUSTMENT	**ASSESSMENT QUESTIONS**
Available Support System	
Status of marital relationship	To whom do you talk when you have something on your mind? (If answer is not the spouse, ask for the reason.)
Alternate support systems	When something is worrying you, what do you do?
	What helps you most when you are upset?
Ability to communicate	Does talking seem to help when you feel upset?
Perception of the Illness or Disability	
Previous knowledge of disorder	Have you ever heard the word (name of diagnosis) before? Tell me about it (if answer is yes).
Imagined cause of disorder	What are your thoughts about the causes of the disorder?
Effects of illness or disability on family	How has your child's illness or disability affected you and your family?
	How has your lifestyle changed?
Coping Mechanisms	
Reactions to previous crises	Tell me one time you've had another crisis (problem, bad time) in your family. How did you solve that problem?
Reactions to the child	Do you find yourself being a little more cautious with this child than with your other children?
Childrearing practices	Do you feel as comfortable disciplining this child as your other children?
Influence of religion	Has your religion or faith been of help to you? Tell me how (if answer is yes).
Attitudes	How is this child different from the siblings or other children of similar age?
	Describe your child's personality. Is it easy, difficult, or in between?
	When you think of your child's future, what thoughts come to mind?
Available Resources	
	What parts of your child's care are causing the most difficulty for you or your family?
	What services are available to help?
	What services do you need that currently are not available?
Concurrent Stresses	
	What other problems are you facing now? (Be specific; ask about financial, marital, sibling, and extended family or friends concerns.)

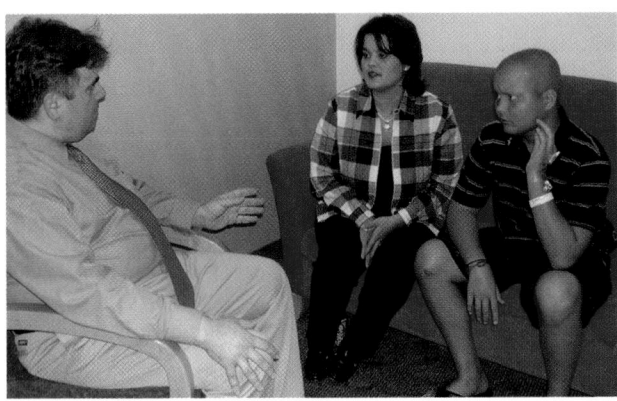

FIG. 18-3 Information sessions should take place in a private, comfortable setting free of distractions and interruptions.

language that indeed this is a difficult and painful period. Although touching is a powerful expression of empathy, it must be used wisely. For example, it can prematurely terminate free expression of feelings, especially when combined with statements such as "Everything will be all right." Nurses should also be aware of cultural issues regarding touching (see Chapter 4).

Parents should receive the kind of information they desire. This can be assessed by asking questions such as "Do you prefer to hear detailed information?" Parents or other family members may have different preferences regarding the amount of information they wish to hear. Most parents want a clear, simple explanation of the diagnosis; a prediction of possible futures for the child; advice on what to do next; an opportunity to ask questions; a warm, sympathetic listener; and, most important, time. Understanding of explanations is elicited with such questions as "Do you see what I mean?" or "Is this clear to you?" Technical terms are used with simple definitions. If the parents are unaware of the term, they are given written literature or at least a written summary of the diagnosis.

> **NURSING TIP** Develop a glossary of commonly used terms, acronyms, and abbreviations to distribute to parents. The list can stand alone or become a part of patient or parent handbooks.

Finally, the informing conference does not end with the presentation of devastating news. Instead, the child's strengths, appealing behaviors, and potential for development are stressed, as are available rehabilitation efforts or treatments. Parents can be encouraged to view their experiences as a series of challenges that they are capable of handling, particularly with available professional feedback. The parents are assured that the nurse will be available to answer questions and to provide further assistance as needed.

The preceding discussion relates primarily to the initial informing interview. However, because of the need for long-term follow-up, it is only one in a series of continuing discussions. In all interactions, the family's input is solicited and incorporated into the care plan. Some situations require consideration of special problems (see Nursing Care Guidelines box).

SUPPORT THE FAMILY'S COPING METHODS

For the family to meet the stresses of optimally adjusting to the child's condition, each member must be individually supported so that the family system is strong. Although the family can indefinitely support

a member who is in need of assistance, its greatest strength lies in every member supporting each other. The nurse should bear in mind that the family member in greatest need is not necessarily the affected child but may be a parent or sibling who is dealing with stresses that require intervention.

Parents

The nurse can provide support by being attentive to families' responses to their children. Mothers and fathers need to experience success, joy, and pride in their children to give the support they need. Children, too, require support for their interactions, adjustments, and efforts. They must be reinforced for attempts to get to know their care providers and to communicate their needs to them.

It is important for nurses to examine their attitudes to determine their ability to engage in parent–professional partnerships. An essential characteristic is the belief that parents are equal to professionals and are experts regarding their child (see Nursing Care Guidelines box).

Communication among all family members is encouraged. Parent group sessions can help parents verbalize thoughts and feelings to each other but often do not take into account siblings' or the child's viewpoint. Therefore, the nurse may need to set up a family session, such as during a home or clinic visit. Although the ideal situation is to have all the members present at one time, often this is not possible. Inviting members to participate at various visits is an appropriate alternative.

Parents can be encouraged to discuss their feelings toward the child, the impact of this event on their marriage, and associated stresses such as financial burdens. For most families, regardless of their income or insurance coverage, financial concerns exist. The costs of caring for a child with special needs can be overwhelming. In addition, the family wage earner may have to sacrifice job opportunities to remain close to a medical facility or to avoid losing insurance benefits.*

The nurse regards fathers as able, effective parents who are competent and capable of coping with the challenges they face. Every effort is made to include the father in visits, such as to the nursery, clinic, special school, and stimulation programs. The father is included in the assessment process, with specific emphasis on having him describe the child's strengths and difficulties. It is not unusual to find two parents who have differing views of the child's abilities, especially in the area of developmental disabilities.

Numerous volunteer and community resources are available that provide assistance, rehabilitation, equipment, and funding for a variety of health problems.† National and local disease-oriented organizations may provide needed assistance and support to families that qualify. Many of these are discussed elsewhere in the text under the specific diagnosis. State and federal departments of health, mental health, social service, and labor may be able to help locate appropriate regional resources. For example, state programs for Children with Special Health Needs (formerly Crippled Children's Services) provide financial assistance for children with many disabling conditions. Local and

---

*Information regarding financial issues is available from the Federation for Children with Special Needs, 1135 Tremont St., Suite 420, Boston, MA 02120; 617-236-7210; http://www.fcsn.org.

†General sources of information are the Clearinghouse on Disability Information, 550 12th St. SW, Room 5133, Washington, DC 20202-2550; 202-245-7307; http://www.ed.gov; and National Dissemination Center for Children with Disabilities, PO Box 1492, Washington, DC 20013; 202-884-8411 or 800-695-0285; http://www.nichcy.org. A comprehensive list of books and pamphlets for parents and teachers is available from the Easter Seals, 230 W. Monroe St., Suite 1800, Chicago, IL 60606; 312-726-6200; http://www.easterseals.com. In Canada: Council of Canadians with Disabilities, 926–294 Portage Ave., Winnipeg, MB R3C 0B9; 204-947-0303; http://www.ccdonline.ca.

NURSING CARE GUIDELINES

Situations Requiring Special Consideration

Congenital Anomaly

Tension in the delivery room conveys the sense that something is seriously wrong. Communication is often delayed while the physician is involved with the mother's care. The manner in which the infant is presented may well set the tone for the early parent–child relationship.

Clarify role with physician in regard to revealing information to enable immediate parental support.

Explain to parents briefly in simple language what the defect is and something concerning the immediate prognosis before showing them the infant, when they are more ready to "hear" what is said.

Be aware of nonverbal communication. Parents watch facial expressions of others for signs of revulsion or rejection.

Present infant as something precious.

Emphasize well-formed aspects of infant's body.

Allow time and opportunity for parents to express their initial response.

Encourage parents to ask questions and provide honest, straightforward answers without undue optimism or pessimism.

Cognitive Impairment

Unless cognitive impairment (or mental retardation) is associated with other physical problems, it is often easy for parents to miss clues to its presence or to make defensive excuses regarding the diagnosis.

Plan situations that help parents become aware of the problem.

Encourage parents to discuss their observations of child but withhold diagnostic opinions.

Focus on what the child can do and appropriate interventions to promote progress (e.g., infant stimulation programs) to involve parents in their child's care while helping them gain an awareness of the child's condition.

Physical Disability

If loss of motor or sensory ability occurs during childhood, the diagnosis is readily apparent. The challenge lies in helping the child and parents over the period of shock and grief and toward the phase of acceptance and reintegration.

Institute early rehabilitation (e.g., using a prosthetic limb, learning to read braille, learning to read lips).

Be aware that physical rehabilitation usually precedes psychologic adjustment.

When the cause of the disability is accidental, avoid implying that parents or child was responsible for the injury but allow them the opportunity to discuss feelings of blame.

Encourage expression of feelings (see Communication Techniques, Chapter 6).

Chronic Illness

Realization of the true impact may take months or years. Conflict over parents' versus child's concerns may result in serious problems. When condition is inherited, parents may blame themselves or child may blame the parents.

Help each family member gain an appreciation of the others' concerns.

Discuss hereditary aspect of condition with parents at time of diagnosis to lessen guilt and accusatory feelings.

Encourage child to express feelings by using third-person technique (e.g., "Sometimes when a person has an illness that was passed on by the parents, that person feels angry or bitter toward them").

Multiple Disabilities

The child or parent may require additional time for the shock phase and may be able to attend to only one diagnosis before hearing significant information regarding other disorders.

Acknowledge parents' understanding and acceptance of all diagnoses, especially when an obvious and more hidden disability coexists.

Appreciate the devastating consequences of more than one disability for a child, especially if they interfere with expressive-receptive abilities.

Terminal Illness

Parents require much support to deal with their own feelings and guidance in how to tell the child the diagnosis. They may want to conceal the diagnosis from the child. They may believe that the child is too young to know, will not be able to cope with the information, or will lose hope and the will to live.

Approach the subject of disclosure in a positive way by asking, "How will you tell your child about the diagnosis?"

Help parents understand the disadvantages of not telling the child (e.g., deprives child of the opportunity to discuss feelings openly and ask questions, incurs the risk of child learning the truth from outside and sometimes less tactful sources, may lessen child's trust and confidence in the parents after learning the truth).

Guide parents to see the potential problems involved in fostering a conspiracy.

Offer parents guidelines for how and what to tell the child about the disease or the possibility of death. Explanations should be tailored to child's cognitive ability, be based on knowledge child already has, and be honest. Honesty must be tempered with concern for child's feelings.

Assure parents that telling a child the name of the illness and the reason for treatment instills hope, provides support from others, and serves as a foundation for explaining and understanding subsequent events.

Acknowledge that being honest is not always easy because the truth may prompt the child to ask other distressing questions, such as "Am I going to die?" However, even this difficult question must be answered.

 NURSING CARE GUIDELINES

Developing Successful Parent–Professional Partnerships

Promote primary nursing; in nonhospital settings, designate a case manager.

Acknowledge parents' overall competence and their unique expertise with their child.

Respect parents' time as having value equal to that of other members of child's health care team.

Explain or define any medical, technical, or discipline-specific terms.

Tell families, "I am not sure" or "I don't know" when appropriate.

Facilitate family's effectiveness in team meetings (e.g., provide parents with same information as other participants).

national sources of respite care and medical daycare may be useful to families. Nurses should become acquainted with those in their communities and with vocational programs for special groups.

Parent-to-Parent Support

Just being with another parent who has shared similar experiences is helpful. It may not need to be a parent of a child with the same diagnosis because parents in the process of adjusting to a child with special needs—or finding respite services, educational or rehabilitative services, special equipment vendors, and financial counseling—tread a common path. If the agency does not have a parent staff position, the nurse can contact parent groups that will often send a representative. Another strategy is to ask another parent to talk to the parents. The nurse should seek out a parent who is a good listener, has a nonjudgmental approach to differences in families, and possesses good advocacy and problem-solving skills.

The parent self-help group is another way to promote parent-to-parent support.* Group members feel less alone and have the opportunity to observe both coping and mastery role modeling from other members. Parents' groups are rich resources for information. Even if parents are unable to attend meetings, they can still benefit from group newsletters and other literature that often accompany membership. The nurse can foster parent participation in self-help groups by serving as a referral agent, a group advisory board member, a resource person, a group member, or an assistant in founding a group. Sometimes all that is required in starting a group is identifying one or two parents as leaders; sharing with them the names, telephone numbers, and addresses of other families who have expressed both an interest and a willingness to release their phone number and address; and guiding them in how to initiate a first meeting.

Advocate for Empowerment

Nurses can advocate for methods that foster opportunities for parent empowerment. For example, nurses can suggest reimbursement for travel and child care plus stipends to enable parents' voices to be heard at meetings and conferences. They can encourage parent membership on committees and advisory boards. They can keep parents informed of pending legislation on child health issues or take action when parents inform them.

The Child

Through ongoing contacts with the child, the nurse (1) observes the child's responses to the disorder, ability to function, and adaptive behaviors within the environment and with significant others; (2) explores the child's own understanding of his or her illness or condition; and (3) provides support while the child learns to cope with his or her feelings. Children are encouraged to express their concerns rather than allowing others to express them for them because open discussions may reduce anxiety (see Nursing Care Guidelines box).

One of the most important interventions is alleviating the child's feeling of being different and normalizing his or her life as much as possible (see Nursing Care Guidelines box). Whenever possible, the nurse assists the family in assessing the child's daily routine for indications of a need for normalizing practices. For example, the child who remains in a bedroom all day requires a restructured daily routine to provide activities in different parts of the house, such as eating in the kitchen or dining room with the family. Such children may also be

---

*Information about self-help groups and books and pamphlets are available from the National Self-Help Clearinghouse, 365 Fifth Ave., Suite 3300, New York, NY 10016; 217-817-1822; http://www.selfhelpweb.org.

 NURSING CARE GUIDELINES
Encouraging Expression of Emotion

Describe the behavior—"You seem angry at everyone."
Give evidence of understanding—"Being angry is only natural."
Give evidence of caring—"It must be difficult to endure so many painful procedures."
Help focus on feelings—"Maybe you wonder why this happened to your child."

 NURSING CARE GUIDELINES
Promoting Normalization

Preparation—Prepare child in advance for changes that may occur from the chronic or complex condition.
 Example—Tell the child in advance the possible side effects of drug therapy.
Participation—Include child in as many decisions as possible, especially those relating to his or her care regimen.
 Example—The child is responsible for taking medications or scheduling home treatments.
Sharing—Allow both family members and child's peers to be a part of the care regimen whenever possible.
 Examples—Give the child his or her medication when the other siblings receive their vitamins.
 The parent cooks the same menu for the whole family.
 If the child is invited to another's home, the parent advises the family of the child's dietary restrictions.
Control—Identify areas where child can be in control so that feelings of uncertainty, passivity, and helplessness are decreased.
 Example—The child identifies activities that are appropriate to his or her energy level and chooses to rest when fatigued.
Expectation—Apply the same family rules to the child with a complex chronic illness as to the well siblings or peers.
 Example—The child is disciplined, is expected to fulfill household responsibilities, and attends school in accordance with abilities.

---

deprived of social, recreational, and academic activities that can be better accommodated by applying normalization practices. For example, home and out-of-home health-related treatments should be planned at times that least interfere with normal daily activities.

Children who are concerned that their condition detracts from their physical attractiveness need attention focused on the normal aspects of appearance and capabilities. Health professionals help strengthen and consolidate the self-image by emphasizing the normal while allowing children to express anger, isolation, fear of rejection, feelings of sadness, and loneliness. The children need positive reinforcement for compliance and any evidence of improvement. Anything that might improve attractiveness and contribute to a positive self-image is used, such as makeup for a teenager with a scar, clothing that disguises a prosthesis, or a hairstyle or wig to cover a deformity or lost hair.

Siblings

The presence of a child with special needs in a family may result in parents paying less attention to the other children. Siblings may respond by developing negative attitudes toward the child or by expressing anger in different forms. The nurse can help by using anticipatory guidance, questioning the parents about what they believe is the best way to have siblings respond to the child, and guiding them through ways to meet their other children's needs for attention. This questioning should take place before serious negative effects occur.

Siblings may also experience embarrassment associated with having a brother or sister with a chronic or complex condition. Parents are then faced with the difficulty of responding to this embarrassment in an understanding and appropriate manner without punishing the siblings for how they feel. Parents are encouraged to talk with the siblings about how they view their affected sibling. For example, siblings of a child with developmental disabilities may express fears about their ability to bear normal children. Adolescents in particular may not be able to discuss these vital issues with their parents and may prefer to consult with the nurse. Many siblings benefit from sharing their concerns with other young people who are experiencing a similar situation. Support groups for siblings can help decrease isolation, promote expression of feelings, and provide examples of effective coping skills.

Many parents express concern about when and how to inform the other children in the family about a sibling's illness or disability. The answer depends on each child's level of sophistication and understanding. However, it is usually best to inform the siblings before a neighbor or other nonfamily member does so. Uninformed siblings may fantasize or develop apprehensions that are out of proportion to the child's actual condition. Furthermore, if parents choose to be silent or deceptive about the issue, they are setting a negative precedent for the siblings to follow rather than encouraging the siblings to cope with the experience in a healthy and nurturing way.

The nurse is sensitive to the reactions of siblings and whenever possible intervenes to promote more positive adjustment. For example, siblings often mention that they are expected to take on additional responsibilities to help the parents care for the child. It is not unusual for them to express a positive reaction to assuming the extra duties but a negative response to feeling unappreciated for doing so. Such feelings can often be minimized by encouraging siblings to discuss this with the parents and by suggesting to parents ways of showing gratitude, such as an increase in allowance; special privileges; and, most significantly, verbal praise.

EDUCATE ABOUT THE DISORDER AND GENERAL HEALTH CARE

Educating the family about the disorder is actually an extension of revealing the diagnosis. Education involves not only supplying technical information but also discussing how the condition will affect the child. Parents may be able to digest only so much information at a time. It may be helpful to provide essential information and then follow by asking, "What else would you like to know about your child's condition?" Responding to parents' questions and concerns ensures that their information needs are met.

Activities of Daily Living

Parents also need guidance in how the condition may interfere with or alter activities of daily living, such as eating, dressing, sleeping, and toileting. One area frequently affected is nutrition. Common problems are undernutrition resulting from food being inappropriately restricted or loss of appetite, vomiting, or motor deficits that interfere with feeding; overnutrition may also occur, usually because of a caloric intake in excess of energy expenditure or boredom and lack of stimulation in other areas. Although the child requires the same basic nutrients as other children, the daily requirements may differ. Special nutritional considerations are discussed as appropriate throughout the text.

Safe Transportation

Modifications may also be needed regarding car safety. Children with conditions such as low birth weight (see Discharge Planning and Home Care, Chapter 9) or orthopedic, neuromuscular, or respiratory impairments often cannot safely use conventional car restraints. For example, children with hip spica casts cannot sit properly in child safety seats (see Developmental Dysplasia of the Hip, Chapter 31). Modifications can be made to some commercial models, and for older children, a special vest is available that secures the child to the back seat in a lying-down position.*

If a child requires a wheelchair, the family should consult the wheelchair manufacturer for specific instructions regarding safe car transportation. Considerations for wheelchairs used with vehicle transportation must address securing both the wheelchair and the occupant in the wheelchair. Wheelchairs should be secured facing forward with tie downs at four points. The tie-down system should be dynamically crash tested, as should the occupant securement system that secures the child in the wheelchair. For example, use of trays is not recommended for transportation. With children who must travel with additional medical equipment, this equipment (e.g., oxygen, monitors, or ventilators) should be anchored to the floor or underneath the vehicle seat or wheelchair. Soft padding should be added around the equipment to reduce movement. A second adult should be present to monitor the condition of a medically fragile child while traveling.

Primary Health Care

Children with special needs require all the usual health care recommended for any child. Attention to injury prevention, immunizations, dental health, and regular physical examinations is essential. Nurses can play an important role in reminding parents of these aspects of care that are so often neglected when the concern is focused on the child's chronic condition. Specific discussions of nutrition, sleep and activity, dental health, and injury prevention are presented in the chapters on health promotion for specific age groups. Immunizations are discussed in Chapter 10.

Parents also need to be aware of the importance of communicating the child's condition in the event of a medical emergency. Young children are unable to give information about their disorders, and although older children may be reliable sources, after an accident, they may be physically unable to speak. Therefore, all children with any type of chronic condition that may affect medical care should wear some type of identification, such as a Medic Alert bracelet,† or carry a card in their wallet that lists the medical condition and a phone number for emergency medical records and other personal information.

PROMOTE NORMAL DEVELOPMENT

Aside from knowledge of the condition and its effect on the child's abilities, the family must be guided toward fostering appropriate development in their child. Although each stage may take longer to achieve, parents are guided toward helping the child fully realize his or her potential in preparation for the next developmental stage. Table 18-2 outlines developmental aspects of complex conditions and supportive interventions. With appropriate planning and knowledge of strategies

---

*Information on car safety restraints for children with special needs is available from the Automotive Safety Program, 575 West Drive, Room 004, Indianapolis, IN 46202; 800-543-6227 or 317-274-2997; http://www.preventinjury.org.
†MedicAlert Foundation International, 2323 Colorado Ave., Turlock, CA 95382; 888-633-4298; http://www.medicalert.org.

BOX 18-7 CHARACTERISTICS OF PARENTAL OVERPROTECTION

Sacrifices self and rest of family for the child

Continually helps the child even when the child is capable

Is inconsistent with regard to discipline or uses no discipline; frequently applies different rules to the siblings

Is dictatorial and arbitrary, making decisions without considering the child's wishes, such as keeping the child from attending school

Hovers and offers suggestions; calls attention to every activity; overdoes praise

Protects the child from every possible discomfort

Restricts play, often because of fear that the child will be injured

Denies the child opportunities for growing up and assuming responsibility, such as learning to give own medications or perform treatments

Does not understand the child's capabilities and sets goals too high or too low

Monopolizes the child's time, such as sleeping with the child, permitting few friends, or refusing participation in social or educational activities

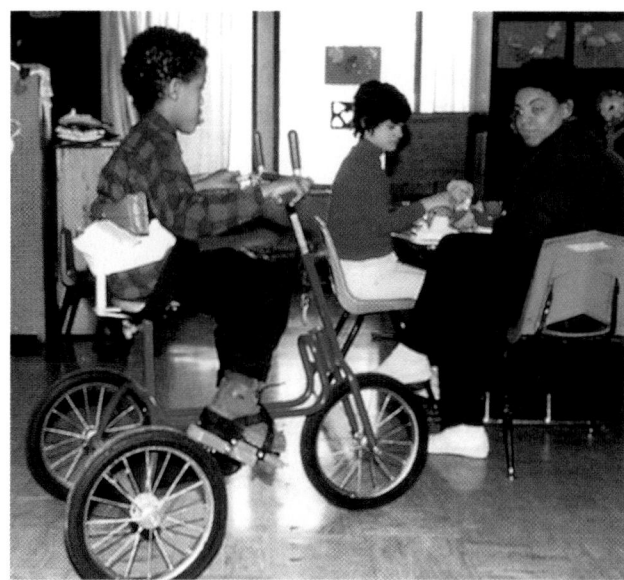

FIG. 18-4 A modified tricycle with block pedals, self-adhesive straps for support, and a modified seat and handle bars can help a child with disabilities gain mobility.

to improve the child's functional abilities, most children can live fulfilling and productive lives.

One important aspect of promoting normal development is to encourage the child's self-care abilities in both activities of daily living and the medical regimen. An assessment of the child's age and physical, emotional, and mental capacities, as well as the support and structure provided by the family, should be considered in determining the appropriate level of self-care in the medical regimen. Even toddlers can be involved in their own care by holding supplies for the parent during a procedure. Over time, children should be encouraged toward greater autonomy in the self-care arena.

Early Childhood

During infancy, the child is achieving basic **trust** through a satisfying, intimate, consistent relationship with his or her parents. However, affected children's early existence may be stressful, chaotic, and unsatisfying. Consequently, they may need more parental support and expressions of affection to achieve trust. Likewise, the parents require assistance in finding ways to meet the infant's needs, such as how to hold a rigid or flaccid infant, how to feed a child with tongue thrust or episodes of dyspnea, and how to stimulate a child who seems incapable of achieving any skills. If hospitalizations are frequent or prolonged, every effort is made to preserve the parent–child relationship (see also Chapter 21). Hospital policies should promote visitation by and involvement of families.

During early childhood, the goal is to achieve **separation** from parents, **autonomy**, and **initiative**. However, the natural parental response to having a sick child is overprotection (Box 18-7). Parents need help in realizing the importance of brief separations of the child from them and from others involved in the child's care and of providing social experiences outside the home whenever possible. Respite care, which provides temporary relief for family members, can be essential in allowing caregivers time away from the daily burdens.

Young children also need the opportunity to develop **independence**. Frequently, the child is able to learn self-help skills, such as holding a bottle, finger feeding, and removing simple articles of clothing, but the parent continues to perform the act. The nurse can guide parents to the usual milestones expected from the child. When a child is unable to perform a skill independently, functional aids should be

used. With innovation, many adaptations can be implemented in children's environments to increase their mobility and independence and allow them to play like other children their age. For example, with slight modifications, a child with physical limitations may be able to ride a tricycle (Fig. 18-4).

Another critical component for normal child development is **discipline**. Discipline and guidance serve several purposes, such as providing children with boundaries on which to test out their behavior and teaching them socially acceptable behavior. Resentment and hostility can arise among siblings if different standards are applied to each child. The nurse's responsibility is to help parents learn successful methods of managing a child's behaviors before they become problems (see Limit Setting and Discipline, Chapter 3).

School Age

For school-age children, the major tasks are entry into school and achieving a sense of **industry**. Although the importance of school in the life of all children is well known, school absences are significantly higher among children with chronic illnesses than among their healthy peers. The more school absences the child experiences, the more difficult it is to resume attendance, and school phobia may result. The child should return to school as soon as possible after diagnosis or treatments.

Preparation for entry into or resumption of school is best accomplished through a team approach with the parents, child, teacher, school nurse, and primary nurse in the hospital. Ideally, this planning should begin before hospital discharge, provided that the child is well enough to resume usual activities. A structured plan should be developed, with attention to aspects of care that must be continued during school hours, such as administration of medication or other treatments.

Children also need preparation before entering or resuming school. Having a tutor in the hospital or home as soon as children are physically able helps them realize that school will continue and gives them time to consider this prospect (Fig. 18-5). They need to investigate possible answers to the many questions others will ask. One method of anticipatory preparation is to role-play, with the child as the

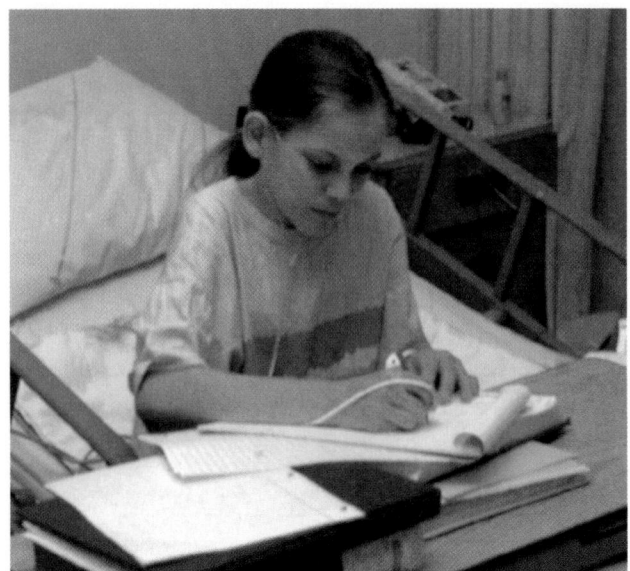

FIG. 18-5 Children with disabilities should continue their schooling as soon as their condition permits.

"returned pupil" and the nurse or parent as "other schoolmates." If the child returns to school with some obvious physical change, such as hair loss, amputation, or a visible scar, the nurse might also ask questions about these alterations to prompt preparatory responses from the child.

Classroom peers also need preparation, and a joint plan of the teacher, nurse, and child is best. At a minimum, classmates should be given a description of the child's condition, prepared for any visible changes in the child, and allowed an opportunity to ask questions. The child should have the option of attending this session. As the child's condition changes, particularly if the illness is potentially fatal, school personnel, including the students, need periodic appraisal of the child's status and preparation for what to expect.

Children with special needs are encouraged to maintain or reestablish relationships with peers and to participate according to their capabilities in any age-appropriate activities. Alternative activities may be substituted for those that are impossible or that place a strain on the child's condition. Programs such as the Special Olympics* offer children an opportunity to compete with their peers and to achieve athletic skill. Summer camps† allow children to associate with peers and develop a wide variety of skills. Children with special needs can derive enormous benefits from expressive activities, such as art, music, poetry, dance, and drama. With adaptive equipment and imagination, children can participate in a variety of activities. Organizations such as VSA Arts allow children to celebrate and share their accomplishments.‡ Children

---

*1133 19th St. NW, Washington, DC 20036; 202-628-3630; http://www. specialolympics.org. Several pamphlets on sports and recreation for children with disabilities are available from Easter Seals (see footnote, p. 549) and American Alliance for Health, Physical Education, Recreation and Dance, 1900 Association Drive, Reston, VA 20191; 703-476-3400 or 800-213-7193; http:// www.aahperd.org.

†A directory of private and paying camps for children with a variety of chronic illnesses and general physical disabilities is available from the American Camp Association, 5000 State Road 67 North, Martinsville, IN 46151-7902; 765-342-8456; http://www.acacamps.org.

‡VSA Arts has affiliate chapters in all 50 states and in selected sites internationally; yearly festivals are held throughout the world. Information is available from VSA Arts, 818 Connecticut Avenue NW, Suite 600, Washington, DC 20006; 202-628-2800 or 800-933-8721; http://www.vsarts.org.

---

need the opportunity to interact with healthy peers and to engage in activities with groups or clubs composed of similarly affected agemates. Such organizations as ostomy clubs, diabetes clubs, and cerebral palsy groups share information and provide support related to the special problems the members face.

Adolescence

Adolescence can be a particularly difficult period for the teenager and family. All of the needs discussed previously apply to this age group as well. Developing **independence** or **autonomy**, however, is a major task for the adolescent as planning for the future becomes a prominent concern. Although the emphasis in the past has been on achieving independence from physical assistance, recent developments in the fields of special education, adolescent development, and family systems suggest redefining autonomy in terms of individuals' capacities to take responsibility for their own behavior, to make decisions regarding their own lives, and to maintain supportive social relationships. Given this understanding, even individuals with severe impairments can be viewed as autonomous if they perceive their own needs and take responsibility for meeting them, either directly or by engaging the assistance of others. As adolescents become more autonomous, the nurse can help them articulate their needs, participate in developing their own care plans, and discover and express how others can be of greatest assistance.

Physical symptoms are high on teenagers' list of health-related concerns. Because adolescence is a time of enormous physical and emotional changes, it is important for the nurse to distinguish between body changes that are related to the child's complex condition and those that are a result of normal body development. It can be a great comfort for teenagers with disabling conditions to know that many of the changes they experience are normal developmental outcomes.

A sense of feeling different from peers can lead to loneliness, isolation, and depression. Participation in groups of teenagers with chronic conditions or disabilities can alleviate feelings of isolation and smooth the transition to a meaningful relationship with one person in adulthood.

ESTABLISH REALISTIC FUTURE GOALS

One of the most difficult adjustments is setting realistic future goals for the child that are based on the child's own goals and values. Sometimes the impact of this decision does not surface until the child finishes school or the parents approach retirement, when a crisis can arise because of disruption of all of the family roles and relationships that maintained stability.

Planning for the future should be a gradual process. All along, the parents should cultivate realistic vocations for the child. For example, if children have physical disabilities, they are directed to intellectual, artistic, or musical pursuits. Children with developmental disabilities are taught manual skills. In this way, the child's development proceeds in the direction of self-support through gainful employment.

With prolonged survival, young people with chronic illnesses must deal with new decisions and problems, such as marriage, employment, and insurance coverage. With appropriate guidance, individuals with disabilities can attain gainful employment, marriage, and a family. For those whose conditions are genetic, counseling is needed regarding future offspring. Prospective spouses often benefit from an opportunity to discuss their feelings regarding marriage to an individual with continued health needs and possibly a limited life span. Health insurance coverage is a critical issue for chronically ill children because of their enormous health care costs over time. The Affordable Care Act allows young adults to remain on their parents insurance until 26 years of age and prevents private insurance carriers from denying them coverage. Life insurance is another dilemma, especially when children have serious conditions, such as congenital heart anomalies.

PERSPECTIVES ON THE CARE OF CHILDREN AT THE END OF LIFE

Although most childhood illnesses and many injuries and other trauma respond favorably to treatment, some do not. When a child and family face a prolonged and life-limiting illness, health professionals must confront the challenge of providing the best possible care to meet the physical, psychologic, spiritual, and emotional needs of the child and family during the uncertain course of the illness and at the time of death. When death is sudden and unexpected, nurses are challenged to respond to grief and shock in families and provide comfort and support in the absence of a prior relationship.

Many factors affect the causes of death that nurses are likely to encounter in children, including developmental factors, medical advances and technology, and changing social patterns. In infants, the leading causes of death are congenital anomalies, respiratory distress syndrome, disorders related to short gestation and low birth weight, and sudden infant death syndrome (Arias, MacDorman, Strobino, and others, 2003) (see Chapter 1). The leading causes of death in children 5 to 9 years of age include injuries (accidents), malignant neoplasms, congenital anomalies, assault (homicide), and heart disease. In children 10 to 14 years of age, suicide is the third leading cause of death after injuries (accidents) and malignant neoplasms. In youths 15 to 19 years of age, assault (homicide), suicide, malignant neoplasms, and heart disease follow accidents as the most prevalent causes of death (Anderson and Smith, 2005).

A child who is diagnosed with a life-threatening illness or who is suffering serious, life-threatening trauma needs medical diagnosis and intervention, as well as nursing assessment and care—sometimes for a short time and sometimes over a lengthy period. When cure is no longer possible and life-prolonging measures result in pain and distress to the child, parents need information about care options that are available to assist them in deciding how they want the remaining time with their child to be managed by the health care team. It is important that families are reassured that although their child cannot be cured, active care will continue to be provided to maintain the child's comfort. Support is provided to assist the child and family during the dying process. As a result, nurses may care for children and families who are making the difficult transition from curative or restorative treatments to palliative care.

PRINCIPLES OF PALLIATIVE CARE

Palliative care involves a multidisciplinary approach to the care of children living with or dying from chronic, complex, or potentially life-limiting conditions with a primary focus on symptom control, supportive care, and quality of life rather than on cure or life prolongation in the absence of the possibility of a cure (Field and Behrman, 2004). The World Health Organization (WHO) (1996) defines **palliative care** as the "active total care of patients whose disease is not responsive to curative treatment. Control of pain, of other symptoms, and of psychological, social and spiritual problems is paramount. The goal of palliative care is the achievement of the best possible quality of life for patients and their families." This goal is certainly compatible with care for patients who are pursuing curative or life-prolonging therapy. Therefore, there should be a distinction between palliative care

and end-of-life care: end of life care is a part of palliative care, but the goals of palliative care extend to all aspects of a patient's quality of life and can be established early in the trajectory of a patient's disease. The WHO (1998) amended the definition of palliative care for children to include:

- Palliative care for children is the active total care of the child's body, mind, and spirit and involves giving support to the family.
- It begins when illness is diagnosed and continues regardless of whether or not a child receives treatment directed at the disease.
- Health providers must evaluate and alleviate the child's physical, psychological, and social distress.
- Effective palliative care requires a broad multidisciplinary approach that includes the family and makes use of available community resources; it can be successfully implemented even if resources are limited.
- It can be provided in tertiary care facilities, in community health centers, and even in children's homes.

Palliative care interventions do not serve to hasten death; rather, they provide pain and symptom management, attention to issues faced by the child and family with regard to death and dying, and promotion of optimal functioning and quality of life during the time the child has remaining. The implementation of neonatal and pediatric palliative care consulting services within hospitals has led to enhanced quality of life and end-of-life care for children and their families and support for their care providers (Jennings, 2005; Pierucci, Kirby, and Leuthner, 2001). Several principles are hallmarks of palliative care.

The child and family are considered the unit of care. The death of a child is an extremely stressful event for a family because it is out of the natural order of things. Children represent health and hope, and their death calls into question the understanding of life. A multidisciplinary team of health care professionals consisting of social workers, chaplains, nurses, personal care aides, and physicians skilled in caring for dying patients assist the family by focusing care on the complex interactions among physical, emotional, social, and spiritual issues.

Palliative care seeks to create a therapeutic environment as home-like as possible, if not in the child's own home. Through education and support of family members, an atmosphere of open communication is provided regarding the child's dying process and its impact on all members of the family (see Evidence-Based Practice box).

DECISION MAKING AT THE END OF LIFE

Discussions concerning the possibility that a child's illness or condition is not curable and that death is an inevitable outcome cause everyone involved a great deal of stress. Physicians, other members of the health care team, and families must consider all information regarding the child's situation and make decisions that all parties agree to and that will have a profound impact on the child and family.

Ethical Considerations in End-of-Life Decision Making

A number of ethical concerns arise when parents and health care professionals are deciding on the best course of care for the dying child. Many parents and health care providers are concerned that not offering treatment that would cause potential pain and suffering but might extend life would be considered euthanasia or assisted suicide. To eliminate such concerns, it is necessary to understand the various terms. **Euthanasia** involves an action carried out by a person other than the patient to end the life of the patient suffering from a terminal condition. The intent of this action is based on the belief that the act is "putting the person out of his or her misery"; this action has also been called **mercy killing**. **Assisted suicide** occurs when someone

EVIDENCE-BASED PRACTICE
Pediatric Pain and Symptom Management at the End of Life

Ask the Question
Picot Question
In children, what is the pain and symptom experience at the end of life?

Search for the Evidence
Search Strategies
Published studies from 2000 to 2005 using the subject terms *child, palliative care, pain,* and *symptoms* were identified and examined. Retrospective descriptive studies dominated the findings describing infants' and children's end-of-life experiences through the use of medical record reviews and provider and parental surveys.

Databases Used
PubMed, CINAHL

Critically Analyze the Evidence
Children experienced an average of 11 symptoms during their last week of life (Drake, Frost, and Collins, 2003). Pain, dyspnea, and fatigue were the most frequently documented symptoms experienced by most children at the end of life (Bradshaw, Hinds, Lensing, and others, 2005; Carter, Howenstein, Gilmer, and others, 2004; Drake, Frost, and Collins, 2003; Hongo, Chieko, Okada, and others, 2003). Children and their parents report high distress with pain and symptoms at the end of life. Parents reported pain and suffering as one of the most important factors in deciding to withhold or withdraw life support from their child in the pediatric intensive care unit (Meert, Thurston, and Sarnaik, 2000).

Documentation was scarce related to symptom management. Morphine was the most commonly prescribed pain medication (Drake, Frost, and Collins, 2003; Hongo, Chieko, Okada, and others, 2003). Parents reported their children as experiencing high levels of pain near the end of life (Contro, Larson, Scofield, and others, 2002). Physicians were more likely than nurses or parents to report that a child's pain and symptoms were well managed at the end of life, but the majority of both provider groups believed the child's physical management was difficult (Andresen, Seecharan, and Toce, 2004; Wolfe, Grier, Klar, and others, 2000).

Barriers to the adequate provision of pediatric palliative care include developmental issues specific to infants and children; symptoms, their causes, how they are related, and effective treatment strategies; lack of education; and reimbursement issues (Harris, 2004). Physicians report reliance on trial and error as they learn to care for children at the end of life and the need for specialty consults with palliative care service providers (Hilden, Emanuel, Fairclough, and others, 2001).

Apply the Evidence: Nursing Implications
There is **moderate-quality evidence** with a **strong recommendation** (Guyatt, Oxman, Vist, and others, 2008) for better pain management at the end of life. Although the philosophy of palliative care encompasses pain and symptom management for infants and children who may not outlive their disease, the provision of that care to ease suffering and provide comfort to those who will die continues to lag. Studies show that children experience significant pain and other distressing symptoms at the end of life that are not well managed. Discrepancies in perceptions of infants' and children's pain and suffering continue to exist between providers and parents. Barriers to the provision of pediatric palliative care exist. Improvements are needed in the management of pain and symptoms at the end of life for infants and children.

QSEN Quality and Safety Competencies:
Evidence-Based Practice*
Knowledge
Differentiate clinical opinion from research and evidence-based summaries.
Describe common symptoms experienced at the end of life.

Skills
Base individualized care plan on patient values, clinical expertise, and evidence.
Integrate evidence into practice by carefully assessing pain and other symptoms in children at the end of life.

Attitudes
Value the concept of evidence-based practice as integral to determining best clinical practice.
Appreciate strengths and weakness of evidence for symptom assessment and management at the end of life.

References
Andresen EM, Seecharan GA, Toce SS: Provider perceptions of child deaths, *Arch Pediatr Adolesc Med* 158:430–435, 2004.
Bradshaw G, Hinds PS, Lensing S, and others: Cancer-related deaths in children and adolescents, *J Palliat Med* 8(1):86–95, 2005.
Carter BS, Howenstein BS, Gilmer MJ, and others: Circumstances surrounding the deaths of hospitalized children: opportunities for pediatric palliative care, *Pediatrics* 114(3):361–366, 2004.
Contro N, Larson J, Scofield S, and others: Family perspectives on the quality of pediatric palliative care, *Arch Pediatr Adolesc Med* 156:1–29, 2002.
Drake R, Frost J, Collins JJ: The symptoms of dying children, *J Pain Symptom Manage* 26(1):594–603, 2003.
Guyatt GH, Oxman AD, Vist GE, and others: GRADE: an emerging consensus on rating quality of evidence and strength of recommendations, *BMJ* 336:924–926, 2008.
Harris B: Palliative care in children with cancer: which child and when? *J Natl Cancer Institute Mono* 32:144–149, 2004.
Hilden JM, Emanuel EJ, Fairclough DL, and others: Attitudes and practices among pediatric oncologists regarding end-of-life care: results of the 1998 American Society of Clinical Oncology Survey, *J Clin Oncol* 19(1):205–212, 2001.
Hongo T, Chieko W, Okada S, and others: Analysis of the circumstances at the end of life in children with cancer: symptoms, suffering and acceptance, *Pediatr Int* 45:60–64, 2003.
Meert KL, Thurston CS, Sarnaik AP: End-of-life decision-making and satisfaction with care: parental perspectives, *Pediatr Crit Care Med* 1(2):179–185, 2000.
Wolfe J, Grier HE, Klar N, and others: Symptoms and suffering at the end of life in children with cancer, *N Engl J Med* 342(5):326–333, 2000.

*Adapted from the QSEN at http://www.qsen.org/.

provides the patient with the means to end his or her life and the patient uses that means to do so. The important distinction between these two actions involves who is actually acting to end the person's life.

The American Nurses Association *Code of Ethics for Nurses* (2001) does not support the active intent on the part of a nurse to end a person's life. However, it does permit the nurse to provide interventions to relieve symptoms in the dying patient even when the interventions involve substantial risks of hastening death. When the prognosis for a patient is poor and death is the expected outcome, it is ethically acceptable to withhold or withdraw treatments that may cause pain and suffering and provide interventions that promote comfort and quality of life. Therefore, providing palliative care for patients is the ethically correct choice in such a circumstance.

Physician–Health Care Team Decision Making

Decisions by physicians regarding care are often made on the basis of the progression of the disease or amount of trauma, the availability of treatment options that would provide cure from disease or restoration of health, the impact of such treatments on the child, and the child's overall prognosis (Davis and Eng, 1998). Often the main determinants prompting physicians to discuss end-of-life issues and options for children with critical illnesses include the child's age, premorbid cognitive condition and functional status, pain or discomfort, probability of survival, and quality of life (Masri, Farrell, Lacroix, and others, 2000). When the physician discusses this information openly with families, a shared decision-making process can occur regarding **do not resuscitate (DNR) orders** and care that is focused on the comfort of the child and family during the dying process.

Unfortunately, many families are not given the option of terminating treatment and pursuing care that is focused on comfort and quality of life when cure is unlikely, and staff may be reluctant to raise the question of DNR orders. This occurs for a number of reasons, including the belief that not being able to "save" a child is a "failure." Also, the physician and other members of the health care team may lack knowledge of and experience with the principles of palliative care (Field and Behrman, 2004; Sahler, Frager, Levetown, and others, 2000; Sumner, 2003).

Parental Decision Making

Rarely are families prepared to cope with the numerous decisions that must be made when a child is dying. When the death is unexpected, as in the case of an accident or trauma, the confusion of emergency services and possibly an intensive care setting presents challenges to parents as they are asked to make difficult choices. If the child has either experienced a life-threatening illness such as cancer or lived with a chronic illness that has now reached its terminal phase, parents are often unprepared for the reality of their child's impending death (see Family-Centered Care box). Numerous studies have found that families facing the impending death of a child depend on information provided to them by the health care team, particularly an honest appraisal of the child's prognosis, to make difficult decisions regarding care options for their children (Hinds, Oakes, Furman, and others, 2001; James and Johnson, 1997; Wolfe, Friebert, and Hilden, 2002).

As the group of health professionals that is most involved with families, nurses are in an excellent position to ensure that families are presented with the options available to them. The nurse's first responsibility is to explore the family's wishes. This is best done in concert with the physician but at times may need to be initiated by the nurse. Statements such as "Tell me about your thoughts for the type of care you want your child to receive when he is dying" or "Have you considered the types of interventions you would like us to use when your child is near death?" can begin discussion of this sensitive but critical aspect of terminal care.

The Dying Child

Children need honest and accurate information about their illness, treatments, and prognosis; this information needs to be given in clear, simple language. In most situations, this best occurs as a gradual process over time characterized by increasingly open dialogue among parents, professionals, and the child (Young, Dixon-Woods, Windridge, and others, 2003). Providing an atmosphere of open communication early in the course of an illness facilitates answering difficult questions as the child's condition worsens. Providing appropriate literature about the disease, as well as the experience of illness and possible death, is also helpful. Exactly how and when to involve

FAMILY-CENTERED CARE
Family of the Dying Child

No matter whether you have a PhD or many children, when your child dies, it is a new experience, and nothing can prepare you for it. Like so many things in life, experience is the best teacher.

Three of our children have died, and by the time the third was dying, we handled many things differently. We learned a lot about dignity and the rights of the child and family. For example, at first, we didn't know that we had a right to have our child die at home. We also didn't understand pain medications and that if children are taking these medicines and are still in agony, they have not overdosed on the medication.

We learned a lot about case management. With our first two children, lots of different people were making decisions and disagreeing about what was best and what should be done. No one had primary authority. With our third child, one doctor took a primary role. Any questions and problems were handled by one person. I could call him 24 hours a day. It made a lot of difference, and I felt our concerns and needs were better heard and respected.

The nurses caring for our third child at home enabled me to step back and just be his mommy. When I could do this, I realized that we were fighting so hard for his life that we weren't really letting him die. His nurses had worked with him for a long time and really loved him. It was hard for them when we decided to let him die. In his last several days, we wanted a lot of family time with our son, and I think the nurses felt left out. Something about their reaction to our increased time with him in the last few days made us feel guilty. If we had all been able to communicate a little more openly, I would have understood that they needed more time with him at the end, too. Everyone's needs could have been met.

Jeni Stepanek
Mother
Upper Marlboro, Md.

children in decisions regarding care during their dying process and death is an individual matter. The child's age or developmental level is an important consideration in the process (Table 18-4). In general, parents should be asked how they would like their child to be told of his or her prognosis, and they should be included in his or her care. Some parents may request that their child not be told that he or she is dying even if the child asks. This often places health care providers in a difficult situation. Children, even at a young age, are perceptive. Even if they are not told outright that they are dying, they realize that something is seriously wrong and that it involves them. Often, helping parents understand that honesty and shared decision making between them and their child are important to the child's and family's emotional health will encourage parents to allow discussion of dying with their child. Parents may require professional support and guidance in this process from a nurse, social worker, or child life specialist who has a good relationship with the child and family.

If given the opportunity, children will tell others how much they want to know. Asking questions such as "If the disease came back, would you want to know?" "Do you want others to tell you everything even if the news isn't good?" or "If someone were not getting better [or more directly, "were dying"], do you think he would want to know?" helps children set the limits of how much truth they can accept and cope with. Children need time to process many feelings and much information so that they can assimilate and ideally accept the inevitable fact of mortality.

Care of dying adolescents requires the nurse to become knowledgeable about any possible delays or alterations in normal growth and development. Legal and ethical issues also come to the forefront with respect to the age at which an adolescent should have autonomy in decision making with regard to care and treatment. Effective communication among the patient, family, and health care team is an important part of optimal care for dying adolescents (Freyer, 2004).

Treatment Options for Terminally Ill Children

Based on the child and family's decision regarding their wishes for terminal care, they have several options from which to choose.

Hospital

Families may choose to remain in the hospital to receive care if the child's illness or condition is unstable and home care is not an option or the family is uncomfortable with providing care at home. If a family chooses to remain at the hospital for terminal care, the setting should be made as homelike as possible. Families are encouraged to bring familiar items from the child's room at home. In addition, there should be a consistent and coordinated care plan for the child's and family's comfort.

Home Care

Some families prefer to take their child home and receive services from a home care agency. Generally, these services entail periodic nursing visits to administer a treatment or provide medications, equipment, or supplies. The child's care continues to be directed by the primary physician. Home care is often the option chosen by physicians and families because of the traditional view that a child must be considered to have a life expectancy of less than 6 months to be referred to hospice care. Fortunately, a number of hospice organizations are expanding their services to children based on the presence of a life-limiting disease process for which cure is not possible rather than on the sole criteria of a limited time-projected prognosis.

TABLE 18-4	CHILDREN'S UNDERSTANDING OF AND REACTIONS TO DEATH	
CONCEPTS OF DEATH	**REACTIONS TO DEATH**	**NURSING CARE MANAGEMENT**
Infants and Toddlers		
Death has least significance to children younger than 6 months of age. After parent–child attachment and trust are established, the loss, even if temporary, of the significant person is profound. Prolonged separation during the first several years is thought to be more significant in terms of future physical, social, and emotional growth than at any subsequent age. Toddlers are egocentric and can only think about events in terms of their own frame of reference—living. Their egocentricity and vague separation of fact and fantasy make it impossible for them to comprehend absence of life. Instead of understanding death, this age group is affected more by any change in lifestyle.	With the death of someone else, they may continue to act as though the person is alive. As children grow older, they will be increasingly able and willing to let go of the dead person. Ritualism is important; a change in lifestyle could be anxiety producing. This age group reacts more to the pain and discomfort of a serious illness than to the probable fatal prognosis. This age group also reacts to parental anxiety and sadness.	Help parents deal with their feelings, allowing them greater emotional reserves to meet the needs of their children. Encourage parents to remain as near to child as possible yet be sensitive to parents' needs. Maintain as normal an environment as possible to retain ritualism. If a parent has died, encourage having consistent caregiver for child. Promote primary nursing.
Preschool Children		
Preschoolers believe their thoughts are sufficient to cause death; the consequence is the burden of guilt, shame, and punishment. Their egocentricity implies a tremendous sense of self-power and omnipotence. They usually have some understanding of the meaning of death. Death is seen as a departure, a kind of sleep. They may recognize the fact of physical death but do not separate it from living abilities. Death is seen as temporary and gradual; life and death can change places with one another. They have no understanding of the universality and inevitability of death.	If they become seriously ill, they conceive of the illness as a punishment for their thoughts or actions. They may feel guilty and responsible for the death of a sibling. Greatest fear concerning death is separation from parents. They may engage in activities that seem strange or abnormal to adults. Because they have fewer defense mechanisms to deal with loss, young children may react to a less significant loss with more outward grief than to the loss of a very significant person. The loss is so deep, painful, and threatening that the child must deny it for a time to survive its overwhelming impact. Behavior reactions such as giggling, joking, attracting attention, or regressing to earlier developmental skills indicate children's need to distance themselves from tremendous loss.	Help parents deal with their feelings, allowing them greater emotional reserves to meet the needs of their children. Help parents understand behavioral reactions of their children. Encourage parents to remain near the child as much as possible to minimize the child's great fear of separation from parents. If a parent has died, encourage having a consistent caregiver for child. Promote primary nursing.

TABLE 18-4	CHILDREN'S UNDERSTANDING OF AND REACTIONS TO DEATH—cont'd	
CONCEPTS OF DEATH	**REACTIONS TO DEATH**	**NURSING CARE MANAGEMENT**
School-Age Children Children still associate misdeeds or bad thoughts with causing death and feel intense guilt and responsibility for the event. Because of their higher cognitive abilities, they respond well to logical explanations and comprehend the figurative meaning of words. They have a deeper understanding of death in a concrete sense. They particularly fear the mutilation and punishment they associate with death. They personify death as the devil, a monster, or the bogeyman. They may have naturalistic or physiologic explanations of death. By age 9 or 10 years, children have an adult concept of death, realizing that it is inevitable, universal, and irreversible.	Because of their increased ability to comprehend, they may have more fears, for example: • The reason for the illness • Communicability of the disease to themselves or others • Consequences of the disease • The process of dying and death itself Their fear of the unknown is greater than their fear of the known. The realization of impending death is a tremendous threat to their sense of security and ego strength. They are likely to exhibit fear through verbal uncooperativeness rather than actual physical aggression. They are interested in postdeath services. They may be inquisitive about what happens to the body.	Help parents deal with their feelings, allowing them greater emotional reserves to meet the needs of their children. Encourage parents to remain near child as much as possible yet be sensitive to parents' needs. Because of children's fear of the unknown, anticipatory preparation is important. Because the developmental task of this age is industry, interventions of helping children maintain control over their bodies and increasing their understanding allow them to achieve independence, self-worth, and self-esteem and avoid a sense of inferiority. Encourage children to talk about their feelings and provide aggressive outlets. Encourage parents to honestly answer questions about dying rather than avoiding the subject or fabricating euphemisms. Encourage parents to share their moments of sorrow with their children. Provide preparation for postdeath services.
Adolescents Adolescents have a mature understanding of death. They are still influenced by remnants of magical thinking and are subject to guilt and shame. They are likely to see deviations from accepted behavior as reasons for their illness.	Adolescents straddle transition from childhood to adulthood. They have the most difficulty in coping with death. They are least likely to accept cessation of life, particularly if it is their own. Concern is for the present much more than for the past or the future. They may consider themselves alienated from their peers and unable to communicate with their parents for emotional support, feeling alone in their struggle. Adolescents' orientation to the present compels them to worry about physical changes even more than the prognosis. Because of their idealistic view of the world, they may criticize funeral rites as barbaric, money making, and unnecessary.	Help parents deal with their feelings, allowing them greater emotional reserves to meet the needs of their children. Avoid alliances with either parent or child. Structure hospital admission to allow for maximum self-control and independence. Answer adolescents' questions honestly, treating them as mature individuals and respecting their needs for privacy, solitude, and personal expressions of emotions. Help parents understand their child's reactions to death and dying, especially that concern for present crises, such as loss of hair, may be much greater than for future ones, including possible death.

Hospice Care

Parents should be offered the option of caring for their child at home during the final phases of an illness with the assistance of a hospice organization. Hospice is a community health care organization that specializes in the care of dying patients by combining the hospice philosophy with the principles of palliative care. Hospice philosophy regards dying as a natural process and care of dying patients as including management of the physical, psychosocial, and spiritual needs of the patient and family. Care is provided by a multidisciplinary group of professionals in the patient's home or an inpatient facility that uses the hospice philosophy. Hospice care for children was introduced in the 1970s, and a number of community hospice organizations now accept children into their care (Davies, Davis, and Sibert, 2003; Faulkner and Armstrong-Dailey, 1997; Forrester, 2003; Winkler and Mardegian, 2001). Collaboration between the child's primary treatment team and the hospice care team is essential to the success of hospice care. Families may continue to see their primary care physicians as they choose.*

Hospice care is based on a number of important concepts that significantly set it apart from hospital care:
- Family members are usually the principal caregivers and are supported by a team of professional and volunteer staff.
- The priority of care is comfort. The child's physical, psychosocial, and spiritual needs are considered. Pain and symptom control are

*For more information, contact National Hospice and Palliative Care Organization, 1700 Diagonal Road, Suite 625, Alexandria, VA 22314; 703-837-1500; fax: 703-837-1233; http://www.nho.org; and Children's Hospice International, 1101 King St., Suite 360, Alexandria, VA 22314; 703-684-0330 or 800-24-CHILD; http://www.chionline.org.

primary concerns, and no extraordinary efforts are used to attempt a cure or prolong life.

- The family's needs are considered to be as important as those of the patient.
- Hospice is concerned with the family's postdeath adjustment, and care may continue for a year or more.

The goal of hospice care is for children to live life to the fullest without pain, with choices and dignity, in the familiar environment of their home, and with the support of their family. Hospice care is covered under state Medicaid programs and by most insurance plans. The service provides home visits from nurses; social workers; chaplains; and, in some cases, physicians. Medications, medical equipment, and any necessary medical supplies are all provided by the hospice organization providing care.

With children, the home has been the more common environment for implementing the hospice concept; it benefits the family in a variety of ways. Children who are dying are allowed to remain with those they love and with whom they feel secure. Many children who were thought to be in imminent danger of death have gone home and lived longer than expected. Siblings can feel more involved in the care and often have more positive perceptions of the death. Parental adaptation is often more favorable, demonstrated by their perceptions of how the experience at home affected their marriage, social reorientation, religious beliefs, and views on the meaning of life and death.

If the home is chosen for hospice care, the child may or may not die in the home. Reasons for final admission to a hospital vary but may be related to the parents' or siblings' wish to have the child die outside the home; exhaustion on the part of the caregivers; and physical problems such as sudden, acute pain or respiratory distress.

NURSING CARE OF THE CHILD AND FAMILY AT THE END OF LIFE

Regardless of where the child is cared for during the terminal stage of illness, both the child and the family usually experience fear of (1) pain and suffering, (2) dying alone (child) or not being present when the child dies (parent), and (3) actual death. Nurses can help families by lessening their fears through attention to the care needs of the child and family (see Nursing Care Plan).

FEAR OF PAIN AND SUFFERING

The presence of unrelieved pain in a terminally ill child can have detrimental effects on the quality of life experienced by the child and family. Parents feel that having their child in pain is unendurable and results in feelings of helplessness and a sense that they must be present and vigilant to get the necessary pain medications. Persistent pain also has an impact on the family as a whole. Nurses can alleviate the fear

NURSING CARE PLAN
The Child Who Is Terminally Ill or Dying

NURSING DIAGNOSIS	PATIENT OUTCOMES	NURSING INTERVENTIONS	RATIONALE
Anxiety related to fear or worry about dying	Child and family will receive appropriate emotional support during the terminal phase of the child's illness.	Encourage family to remain near child as much as possible.	To provide support through the presence of a loved one
Child's or Family's Defining Characteristics (Subjective and Objective Data) Unstable emotions Aggressive behavior Withdrawn behavior Depression	Child will express fears and anxiety related to dying. Family will support the child's ability to express fears and anxiety. Child and family will be informed of symptoms to expect as child nears the end of life. Child and family will be informed of procedures and therapies necessary to promote comfort. Child and family will be able to cope with the dying process.	Encourage child to talk about feelings; help the family as they encourage child to express feelings. Provide safe, acceptable outlets for aggression and for grieving. Answer questions as honestly as possible while maintaining a positive, hopeful approach. Explain progression of physical symptoms as child nears the end of life. Explain all procedures and therapies, especially physical effects child will experience. Help child distinguish between consequences of treatment and manifestations of the disease. Structure hospital or home environment to allow for maximum self-control and independence within the limitations imposed by child's developmental level and physical condition.	To provide a sense of closeness and understanding among family members To establish that anger and sadness are normal reactions To promote trust as a major strength for therapeutic relationships To promote trust and decrease anxiety To decrease fear of the unknown, which may be more of a concern than the actual procedure or therapy To focus on interventions that can minimize discomfort To minimize fear and loss of control
	The Following NOC Concepts Apply to These Outcomes Anxiety Self-Control Coping Fear Self-Control	**The Following NIC Concepts Apply to These Interventions** Active Listening Coping Enhancement Simple Relaxation Touch	

NIC, Nursing Interventions Classification; *NOC,* Nursing Outcomes Classification.

NURSING CARE PLAN

The Child Who Is Terminally Ill or Dying—cont'd

NURSING DIAGNOSIS	PATIENT OUTCOMES	NURSING INTERVENTIONS	RATIONALE
Chronic Pain related to disease process **Child's or Family's Defining Characteristics** **(Subjective and Objective Data)** Crying Withdrawal Aggression Fear of touch Fear of movement	Child will exhibit minimal or no evidence of physical discomfort. Family will be able to participate in the child's care without causing discomfort. Family will be able to provide comfort measures for child. **The Following NOC Concepts Apply to These Outcomes** Comfort Level Pain Control	Assess child's level of comfort. Provide pain management around the clock. Assess child for symptoms associated with pain or its treatment. Provide stool softener, laxative, or diphenhydramine as needed. Provide nonpharmacologic interventions child prefers. Administer anticholinergic drugs as needed. Encourage family to provide comfort measures the child prefers. Provide soothing surroundings for child. Avoid excessive noise and light. Ensure pleasant smell, touch, temperature. Place all commodities within easy reach of the child. Use gentle touch when required to perform physical procedures. Avoid pressure on painful areas. Avoid pressure on bony prominences and painful sites. Use pillows and other supports to prop child in a comfortable position. Place absorbent pads under hips if the child is incontinent. Limit care to essential needs. **The Following NIC Concepts Apply to These Outcomes** Analgesic Administration Patient-Controlled Analgesia Positioning Simple Massage Sleep Enhancement Simple Relaxation Therapy	To ensure child is treated for changes in pain To prevent the recurrence or escalation of pain To ensure child is treated for symptoms accompanying pain or its management To prevent or treat symptoms related to pain or its management To aid pharmacologic management of pain, helping to prevent recurrence or escalation of pain and accompanying symptoms To reduce secretions and lessen "death rattle," which can be distressing to family To provide comfort To minimize irritation and maximize comfort To minimize discomfort from movement To minimize pain when possible To make it easier for the child to breathe To prevent skin breakdown To minimize fatigue
Anticipatory Grieving related to impending loss of child **Child's or Family's Defining Characteristics** **(Subjective and Objective Data)** Parents' feelings and physical responses of loss and depression Parents' feelings of loss of control and uncertainty Child's or sibling's feelings and physical responses of loss and depression Child's or sibling's feelings of loss of control and uncertainty	Family will express fears, concerns, and any special desires for terminal care. Family will demonstrate an understanding of their children's needs. Family members will be actively involved in their child's care. Family members will seek resources needed to assist them during the grieving process. **The Following NOC Concept Applies to These Outcomes** Family Coping	Discuss with the family and child the grieving process and differences in grieving among men, women, and children. Provide opportunities for family members to express emotions independently or together as desired. Facilitate child's or sibling's expression of emotions through art or play activities. Help parents and siblings deal with their feelings about the child's death. Encourage parents to remain as near the child as possible. Provide family with information regarding the child's status. Provide family with information on common behavioral reactions. Encourage family's assistance with child's care.	To facilitate understanding of what family members are feeling and experiencing To provide an outlet for their emotions To facilitate expression of their emotions To provide support To allow parents to feel they are doing something for their child To promote understanding and communication To promote understanding of their children's behaviors To assist with coping and minimize loss of control

Continued

NURSING CARE PLAN

The Child Who Is Terminally Ill or Dying—cont'd

NURSING DIAGNOSIS	PATIENT OUTCOMES	NURSING INTERVENTIONS	RATIONALE
		Provide information to family on how to maintain own health care needs.	To give families the approval to take care of themselves
		Provide as much privacy as possible without isolating family from nurse's care.	To provide dignity for the grieving process
		Assist family in assessing their needs for referral services.	To facilitate support for families
		Encourage parents to honestly answer children's questions about dying.	To decrease children's fear and anxiety
		Provide resources for family to facilitate discussions with children about dying.	To provide support and facilitate parents' discussion
		Encourage parents to share their moments of sorrow with their children.	To promote grief expression of children
		Assist family and child with memory-making opportunities.	To facilitate emotions and sharing between family and child
		Assist child as needed to complete any unfinished business.	To facilitate support of child
		Discuss with parents appropriate involvement of siblings.	To prevent siblings from feeling excluded
		Identify family's religious and cultural beliefs related to death.	To provide support and spiritual care
		Provide preparation for postdeath services.	To provide support and guidance
		Discuss with parents the frequent need of children to be given permission to die.	To provide support and guidance
		Discuss with family their preferences for care if death is imminent.	To allow families to be in control
		Facilitate appropriate spiritual care in accordance with family's beliefs or affiliations.	To provide support
		Provide support for families who choose home care for their child.	To allow families to choose where the child is to die and provide guidance for this to occur

The Following NIC Concepts Apply to These Outcomes
Anticipatory Guidance
Anxiety Reduction
Caregiver Support
Counseling
Family Support
Family Therapy

of pain and suffering by providing interventions aimed at treating the pain and symptoms associated with the terminal process in children.

Pain and Symptom Management

Pain control for children in the terminal stages of illness or injury must be given the highest priority. Despite ongoing efforts to educate physicians and nurses on pain management strategies in children, studies have reported that children continue to be undermedicated for their pain (Wolfe, Grier, Klar, and others, 2000). Nearly all children experience some amount of pain in the terminal phase of their illness. The current standard for treating children's pain follows the WHO's analgesic stepladder (1996), which promotes tailoring the pain interventions to the child's level of reported pain. Children's pain

should be assessed frequently and medications adjusted as necessary. Pain medications should be given on a regular schedule, and extra doses for breakthrough pain should be available to maintain comfort. Opioid drugs such as morphine should be given for severe pain, and the dose should be increased as necessary to maintain optimal pain relief. Techniques such as distraction, relaxation techniques, and guided imagery (Lambert, 1999) should be combined with drug therapy to provide the child and family strategies to control pain (see Chapter 7 for further discussion of pain management strategies).

In addition to pain, children experience a variety of symptoms during their terminal course as a result of their disease process or as a side effect of medicines used to manage pain or other symptoms. These symptoms include fatigue, nausea and vomiting, constipation, anorexia, dyspnea, congestion, seizures, anxiety, depression, restlessness, agitation, and confusion (Hellsten, Hockenberry, Lamb, and others, 2000; Wolfe, Friebert, and Hilden, 2002). Each of these symptoms should be aggressively managed with appropriate medications or treatments and with interventions such as repositioning, relaxation, massage, and other measures to maintain the child's comfort and quality of life.

Occasionally, children require very high doses of opioids to control pain. This may occur for several reasons. Children on long-term opioid pain management can become **tolerant** of the drug, meaning that it is necessary to give more drugs to maintain the same level of pain relief. This should not be confused with **addiction**, which is a psychologic dependence on the side effects of opioids. Addiction is not a factor in managing terminal pain in children. Other obvious reasons for requiring increased doses of opioids include progression of disease and other physiologic experiences of pain. It is important to understand that there is no maximum dose that can be given to control pain. However, nurses often express concern that administering doses of opioids that exceed what they are familiar with will hasten the child's death. The **principle of** double effect (Box 18-8) addresses such concerns. It provides an ethical standard that supports the use of interventions intended to relieve pain and suffering even though there is a foreseeable possibility that death may be hastened (Rousseau, 2001). In cases in which the child is terminally ill and in severe pain, using large doses of opioids and sedatives to manage pain is justified when no other treatment options are available that would relieve the pain but make the risk of death less likely (Hawryluck and Harvey, 2000). See Chapter 7 for an extensive discussion of pain assessment and management.

Parents' and Siblings' Need for Education and Support

Parents are the primary caregivers when the child is at home, and nurses providing care to the child and family need to teach the family about the medications being given to the child, how to administer medications, and the use of nonpharmacologic techniques. Parents are kept informed of all medications and treatments given to a child in the hospital, and they are encouraged to participate in the child's care to the extent that they desire. This empowers parents and provides a sense of control over the child's comfort and well-being, reducing their fear that their child will be in pain or suffering as he or she is dying. Additionally, better bereavement outcomes (e.g., adaptive coping; family cohesion; less anxiety, stress, and depression) have been reported by parents who were actively involved in the care of their child (Goodenough, Drew, Higgins, and others, 2004; Lauer, Mulhern, Schell, and others, 1989). The grief work of fathers in particular seems to be facilitated when their child dies in the home setting. This finding may be related to the increased opportunity of working fathers to provide care to and spend time with their child at home versus the hospital setting.

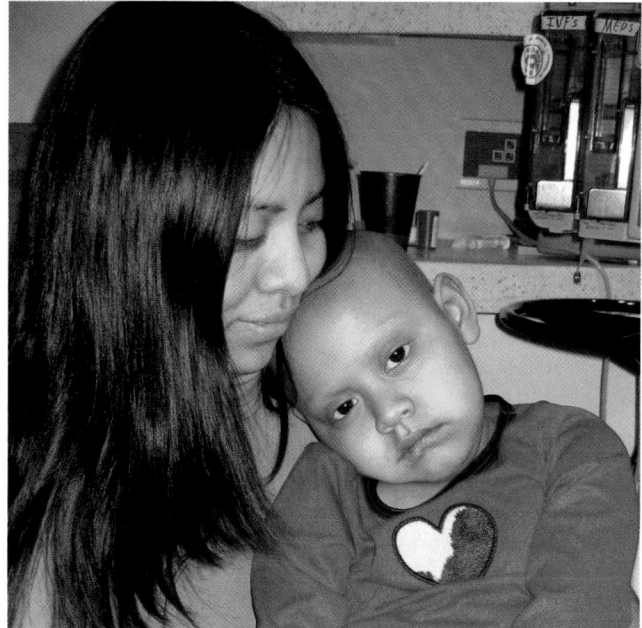

FIG. 18-6 For a dying child, there is no greater comfort than the security and closeness of a parent.

Siblings may feel isolated and displaced during the time that their brother or sister is dying. Parents devote the majority of their time to the care and comfort of the dying child, causing siblings to feel left out of the parent–sick child relationship. Siblings may become resentful of their sick sibling and begin to feel guilty or ashamed about such feelings (Murray, 1999). Nurses can assist the family by helping the parents identify ways to involve siblings in the caring process, perhaps by bringing some supplies or favorite toy, game, or food item. Parents should also be encouraged to schedule time to spend with the other children during which their focus is on them. Helping parents identify a trusted friend or family member who can sit with the ill child for a short period will allow them to attend to their own needs or those of their other children.

FEAR OF DYING ALONE OR OF NOT BEING PRESENT WHEN THE CHILD DIES

When a child is being cared for at home, the burden of care on parents and family members can be great. Often, as the child's condition declines, family members begin the "death vigil." Rarely is a child left alone for any length of time. This can be exhausting for family members, and nurses can assist the family by helping them arrange shifts so that friends or family members can be present with the child and allow others to rest. If the family has limited resources, community organizations such as hospice or churches often have volunteers who are willing to visit and sit with children. It is important that whoever is sitting with the child be aware of when the parent(s) would like to be notified to return to the child's bedside (Fig. 18-6).

When a child is dying in the hospital, the parents should be given full access to the child at all times. If the parents need to leave, they should be provided with a pager or other means of immediate communication and alerted if staff members note any change in the child that may indicate imminent death. Nurses should advocate for parents' presence in intensive care and emergency departments and attend to the parents' needs for food, drinks, comfortable chairs, blankets, and pillows.

BOX 18-9 PHYSICAL SIGNS OF APPROACHING DEATH

Loss of sensation and movement in the lower extremities, progressing toward the upper body

Sensation of heat, although the body feels cool

Loss of senses:
- Tactile sensation decreasing
- Sensitivity to light
- Hearing the last sense to fail

Confusion, loss of consciousness, slurred speech

Muscle weakness

Loss of bowel and bladder control

Decreased appetite and thirst

Difficulty swallowing

Change in respiratory pattern:
- Cheyne-Stokes respirations (waxing and waning of depth of breathing with regular periods of apnea)
- "Death rattle" (noisy chest sounds from accumulation of pulmonary and pharyngeal secretions)

Weak, slow pulse; decreased blood pressure

FEAR OF ACTUAL DEATH

Home Deaths

The majority of children receiving hospice care die at home, often in their own room with family, pets, and loved possessions around them. The physical process of dying can be distressing to parents because often the child slowly becomes less alert in the days before the actual death. The nurse can assist the family by providing them with information about what changes will occur as the child progresses through the dying process (Box 18-9). During this time, nursing visits often become more frequent and longer in duration to provide the family with additional support as the death nears. The most distressing change for parents to observe is the change in the respiratory pattern. In the final hours of life, the dying patient's respirations may become labored, with deep breaths and long periods of apnea, referred to as Cheyne-Stokes respirations. Families are reassured that this is not distressing to the child and that it is a normal part of the dying process. However, the use of opioids can slow the respirations to make the child breathe more easily, and scopolamine, usually applied as a topical patch, can help reduce noisy respirations known as the "death rattle." Noisy respirations are more likely to occur if the child is overhydrated.

All families have the option of admitting their child to the hospital if they feel unable to deal with the death. The child who dies at home must be pronounced dead; hospice programs typically have provisions so that this proceeds smoothly. In some circumstances, the police may be notified, with an explanation of the circumstances to prevent unnecessary concern regarding abuse. Providing the police with the number of the responsible practitioner is usually all that is necessary to confirm the cause of death.

Hospital Deaths

Children dying in the hospital of terminal illnesses who are receiving supportive care interventions experience a similar process. Again, increased nursing presence and attendance to the child's and family's needs provide comfort and support for many families.

Death resulting from accident or trauma or acute illness in settings such as the emergency department or intensive care unit often requires the active withdrawal of some form of life-supporting intervention, such as a ventilator or bypass machine. These situations often raise difficult ethical issues (Sine, Sumner, Gracy, and others, 2001), and parents are often less prepared for the actual moment of death. Nurses can assist these parents by providing detailed information about what will happen as supportive equipment is withdrawn, ensuring that appropriate pain medications are administered to prevent pain during the dying process and allowing the parents time before the start of the withdrawal to be with and speak to their child. It is important that the nurse attempt to control the environment around the family at this time by providing privacy, asking if they would like to play music, softening lights and monitor noises, and arranging for any religious or cultural rituals that the family may want performed.

After the child's death, the family should be allowed to remain with the body and hold or rock the child if they desire. After the nurse has removed all tubes and equipment from the body, the parents should be given the option of assisting with the preparation of the body, such as bathing and dressing. It is important for the nurse to determine whether the family has any specific needs because many cultures have adopted specific methods for coping with and mourning death, and impeding these practices may interfere with the grieving process (Clements, Vigil, Manno, and others, 2003).

At some point, the nurse discusses whether the family has made preparations for the burial service and whether the staff can help in any way. Parents often have concerns about the funeral, such as siblings' involvement in the death rituals. Although no absolute answers exist regarding the question of siblings attending the funeral or burial services, the consensus is that the surviving children benefit from being involved in these events. However, children need preparation for postdeath services. They should be told what to expect, particularly how the deceased person will look if the coffin is open; allowed their private time to say good-bye; and permitted to stay as long as they wish. Ideally, the parents should prepare the siblings. If the parents' grief prevents this communication, a significant family member or friend should substitute (see Family-Centered Care box).

FAMILY-CENTERED CARE
Children Need to Say Good-Bye

As a nurse and grief counselor, I conduct grief workshops with children who have experienced the death of someone special. Children often communicate their feelings of being excluded through drawings. They may draw a picture of the dying person in a hospital bed that is raised too high for them to see the person's face clearly. Sometimes children reveal that they did not get to say good-bye because a family member told them, for example, "You don't want to see your grandma this way. She is too sick for you to visit." If the special person died at home, the children had to stay in their room when the funeral home staff took away the body.

I have learned never to underestimate the importance of allowing children to be involved with the dying person and the significance of a child's loss. Once, when I asked a 6-year-old girl to draw a picture with the theme "This is what I was doing when my _____ died," she drew a picture and completed the sentence with "when my home died." Her grandmother had been like her mother; to the child, her home was gone. We need to give children the choice of being included in the family's activities of saying good-bye.

Barbara Bilderback, MS, MA, RN
Bereavement Supervisor, Saint Francis Hospice
Tulsa, Okla.

ORGAN OR TISSUE DONATION AND AUTOPSY

For some families, organ or tissue donation may be a meaningful act—one that benefits another human being despite the loss of their child. Unfortunately, initiating a discussion about tissue donation is often stressful for staff, and there may be confusion regarding whose responsibility this is. In centers in which transplants are performed, a full-time transplant coordinator is usually available to inform the family about organ donation and to take care of details. If such services are not available, the staff needs to determine which members should discuss this topic with the family. Ideally, the person who knows the family best, knows when the death is expected, or has the opportunity to spend time with the family when the death is unexpected takes the role. Often nurses are in an optimal position to suggest tissue donation after consultation with the attending physician. When possible, the topic should be raised before death occurs. The request should be made in a private and quiet area of the hospital and should be simple and direct, with questions such as "Are you a donor family?" or "Have you ever considered organ donation?"

Many states have legislated a mandatory request for organ or tissue donation when a child dies, especially if the patient is brain dead. Written consent from the family is required before donation can proceed. When requests for organ donation are made, health care practitioners must address common misunderstandings families have about brain death and organ donation (Franz, DeJong, Wolfe, and others, 1997). Training health care professionals on sensitive approaches to requests for organ donation has been shown to increase families' willingness to consent to organ donation (American Academy of Pediatrics, 2002; Evanisko, Beasley, Brigham, and others, 1998). The option to donate organs should always be separate from the communication of impending or actual death.

Nurses need to be aware of common questions about organ donation to help families make an informed decision. Healthy children who die unexpectedly are excellent candidates for organ donation. Children with cancer, chronic disease, or infection and those who have suffered prolonged cardiac arrest may not be suitable candidates, although this is individually determined. The nurse should ask whether organ donation was discussed with the child or whether the child ever expressed such a wish. Any number of body tissues or organs can be donated (skin, corneas, bone, kidney, heart, liver, pancreas), and their removal does not mutilate or desecrate the body or cause any suffering. The family may have an open casket, and there is no delay in the funeral. There is no cost to the donor family, but organ donation does not eliminate funeral or cremation responsibilities. Most religions permit organ donation as long as the recipient benefits from the transplant, although Orthodox Judaism forbids it.

In cases of unexplained death, violent death, or suspected suicide, autopsy is required by law. In other instances, it may be optional, and parents should be informed of this choice. The procedure, as well as forms that require signing, should be explained. The family should know that the child can be in an open casket after an autopsy.

GRIEF AND MOURNING

Grief is a process, not an event, of experiencing physiologic, psychologic, behavioral, social, and spiritual reactions to the loss of a child. Grief is highly individualized, encompassing a broad range of manifestations from person to person. It is a natural and expected reaction to loss. It is neither orderly nor predictable. Grieving in any form is necessary for healing to occur. When death is the expected or a possible outcome of a disorder, the child and family members may experience anticipatory grief. Anticipatory grief may be manifested in varying behaviors and intensities and may include denial, anger, depression, and other psychologic and physical symptoms.

Anticipatory guidance may assist grieving family members. Health care professionals should emphasize that grief reactions such as hearing the dead person's voice, feeling distant from others, or seeking reassurance that they did everything possible for the lost person are normal, necessary, and expected. They in no way signify poor coping, insanity, or an approaching mental breakdown. On the contrary, such behaviors signify that the survivor is working through the acute grief. They are a necessary part of grief work. Anticipatory guidance regarding the mourning process may help families recognize the normalcy of their experiences.

It is important to recognize that some family members may experience complicated grief. Complicated grief reactions (>1 year after the loss) include such symptoms as intense intrusive thoughts, pangs of severe emotion, distressing yearnings, feelings of excessive loneliness and emptiness, unusual sleep disturbance, and maladaptive levels of loss of interest in personal activities (Meert, Shear, Newth, and others, 2011). Bereaved persons experiencing such prolonged and complicated grief should be referred to an expert in grief and bereavement counseling.

Another important aspect of grief is the individual nature of the grief experience. Each member of the family will experience the grief of the child's death in his or her own way based on the particular relationship with that child. This can create potential conflict for families because each family member has expectations that the other family members should feel and grieve as they do. Nurses caring for families experiencing grief should be aware of the different grieving styles and help the family learn to recognize and support the uniqueness of each other's grief.

Parental Grief

Parental grief after the death of a child has been found to be the most intense, complex, long-lasting, and fluctuating grief experience compared with that of other bereaved individuals. Although parents experience the primary loss of their child, many secondary losses are felt such as the loss of part of one's self, hopes and dreams for the child's future, the family unit, prior social and emotional community supports, and often spousal support. It is common for parents of the same child to experience different grief reactions.

Studies with bereaved parents have shown that grieving does not end with the severing of the bond with the deceased child but rather involves a continuing bond between the parent and the deceased child (Klass, 2001). Parental resolution of grief is a process of integrating the dead child into daily life in which the pain of losing a child is never completely gone but lessens. There are occasions of brief relapse but not to the degree experienced when the loss initially occurred. Thus, parental grief work is never completed and is a timeless process of accommodating the new reality of being without a child as it changes over time (Davies, 2004). A child's death can also challenge the marital relationship in several ways. Maternal and paternal reactions often differ (Birenbaum, Stewart, and Phillips, 1996; Moriarty, Carroll, and Cotroneo, 1996; Vance, Najman, Thearle, and others, 1995). Different grieving styles between the couple may hinder communication and support for each other. Differing needs and expectations can place a strain on the marriage.

Sibling Grief

Each child grieves in his or her own way and on his or her own timeline. Children, even adolescents, grieve differently than adults. Adults

---

📋 NURSING CARE GUIDELINES

*Supporting Grieving Families**

General

Stay with the family; sit quietly if they prefer not to talk; cry with them if desired.

Accept the family's grief reactions; avoid judgmental statements (e.g., "You should be feeling better by now").

Avoid offering rationalizations for the child's death (e.g., "Your child isn't suffering anymore").

Avoid artificial consolation (e.g., "I know how you feel," or "You are still young enough to have another baby").

Deal openly with feelings such as guilt, anger, and loss of self-esteem.

Focus on feelings by using a feeling word in the statement (e.g., "You're still feeling all the pain of losing a child").

Refer the family to an appropriate self-help group or for professional help if needed.

At the Time of Death

Reassure the family that everything possible is being done for the child if they want lifesaving interventions.

Do everything possible to ensure the child's comfort, especially relieving pain.

Provide the child and family with the opportunity to review special experiences or memories in their lives.

Express personal feelings of loss or frustrations (e.g., "We will miss him so much," "We tried everything; we feel so sorry that we couldn't save her").

Provide information that the family requests and be honest.

Respect the emotional needs of family members, such as siblings, who may need brief respites from the dying child.

Make every effort to arrange for family members, especially the parents, to be with the child at the moment of death if they want to be present.

Allow the family to stay with the dead child for as long as they wish and to rock, hold, or bathe the child.

Provide practical help when possible, such as collecting the child's belongings.

Arrange for spiritual support based on the family's religious beliefs; pray with the family if no one else can stay with them.

Postdeath

Attend the funeral or visitation if there was a special closeness with the family.

Initiate and maintain contact (e.g., sending cards, telephoning, inviting them back to the unit, making a home visit).

Refer to the dead child by name; discuss shared memories with the family.

Discourage the use of drugs and alcohol as a method of escaping grief.

Encourage all family members to communicate their feelings rather than remaining silent to avoid upsetting another member.

Emphasize that grieving is a painful process that often takes years to resolve.

*"Family" refers to all significant persons involved in the child's life, such as the parents, siblings, grandparents, and other close relatives or friends.

---

and children differ more widely in their reactions to death than in their reactions to any other phenomenon. Children of all ages grieve the loss of a loved one, and their understanding and reactions to death depend on their age and developmental level. Children grieve for a longer duration, revisiting their grief as they grow and develop new understandings of death. However, they do not grieve 100% of the time. They grieve in spurts and can be emotional and sad in one instance and then, just as quickly, off and playing. Children express their grief through play and behavior. Children can be exquisitely attuned to their parents' grief and will try to protect them by not asking questions or by trying not to upset them. This can set the stage for the sibling to try to become the "perfect child." Children exhibit many of the grief reactions of adults, including physical sensations and illnesses, anger, guilt, sadness, loneliness, withdrawal, acting out, sleep disturbances, isolation, and search for meaning. Again, nurses should be attentive for signs that siblings are struggling with their grief and provide guidance to parents when possible.

At times, family members may need assistance in their grieving (see Nursing Care Guidelines box). Communication with the bereaved family is essential, but often nurses do not know what to say and feel helpless in offering words of comfort. The most supportive approach is to avoid judging the family's reactions or offering advice or rationalizations and to focus on feelings. Perhaps the most valuable supportive measure the nurse can perform for families is to listen. Families understand that no words will relieve their pain; all they want is acceptance, understanding, and respect for their grief.

It is important for families to understand that mourning takes a long time. Whereas acute grief may last only weeks or months, resolving the loss is measured in years. Holidays and anniversaries can be particularly difficult, and people who previously had been supportive may now expect the family to have "adjusted." Consequently, prolonged mourning is often silent and lonely.

Many families never receive the support and guidance that could help them resolve the loss. A plan for regular follow-up with bereaved families can be beneficial. At minimum, one follow-up phone call or meeting with the family should be arranged. Families can also be referred to self-help groups. When such groups are not available, nurses can be instrumental in bringing families together or facilitating parent and sibling groups. Formal bereavement programs or bereavement counseling can be helpful as well.

NURSES' REACTIONS TO CARING FOR DYING CHILDREN

The death of a patient is one of the most stressful aspects of critical care and oncology nursing (see Family-Centered Care box).* Nurses experience reactions to a fatal illness that are very similar to the responses of family members, including denial, anger, depression, guilt, and ambivalent feelings.

---

*Other sources of publications on life-threatening illness and death are the Compassionate Friends, PO Box 3696, Oak Brook, IL 60522-3696; 630-990-0010 or 877-969-0010; http://www.compassionatefriends.org; Centering Corporation, 7230 Maple St., Omaha, NE 68134; 866-218-0101; http://www.centering.org; Children's Hospice International, 1104 King St., Suite 360, Alexandria, VA 22314; 800-24-CHILD or 703-684-0330; e-mail: info@chionline.org; http://www.chionline.org; and National Cancer Institute, Cancer Information Service, Building 21, Room 10A29, Bethesda, MD 20892-2580; 800-422-6237; http://www.cancer.gov.

FAMILY-CENTERED CARE

A Dying Child: A Nurse's Perspective

Claire was unresponsive with slow, gasping breathing. Her mother asked me what I thought was happening. I replied honestly, "Your baby is dying because of her brain tumor." The mother put her arms around me and cried. We arranged for Claire to be baptized.

Honesty. As painful as the loss of a child is, my job is to assist the family through this experience. Although I usually wait until a private moment, such as driving home, I found tears streaming down my face as family and friends gathered for Claire's baptism. I went into the kitchen to compose myself, only to find several of my colleagues crying as well. Saying good-bye to a dying child will always be a difficult but shared experience.

Jeanne O'Connor Egan, RN, MSN
Pediatric Clinical Specialist, Children's Hospital
Washington, DC

Strategies that can assist nurses in maintaining the ability to work effectively in these settings include maintaining good general health, developing well-rounded interests, using distancing techniques such as taking time off when needed, developing and using professional and personal support systems, cultivating the capacity for empathy, focusing on the positive aspects of the caregiver role, and basing nursing interventions on sound theory and empiric observations. Attending shared-remembrance rituals assists some nurses in resolving grief (Davis and Eng, 1998). Similarly, attending the funeral services can be a supportive act for both the family and the nurse and in no way detracts from the professionalism of care.

KEY POINTS

- Trends in the treatment of children with chronic illnesses and disabilities have focused on developmental age, the child's strengths and uniqueness, family-centered care, normalization, early discharge, home care, mainstreaming, and early intervention.
- In response to the child with chronic conditions, parents may be affected by feelings of inadequacy and failure; excessive demands on time, energy, and financial resources; and strain on the marital relationship.
- Families' reactions to chronic conditions are manifested in the following stages: shock and denial, adjustment, reintegration, and acknowledgment.
- The child's reaction to chronic conditions depends on the child's developmental level, coping mechanisms, others' reactions, and the illness itself.
- Assessment of the family's adjustment to a child's chronic illness, disability, or death includes the availability of a support system, their perception of the event, their coping mechanisms, concurrent stressors, and their response to the child.
- To help parents cope with their child's chronic and complex conditions, nurses must offer attentiveness, humanistic support, solicitation of suggestions for care, facilitation of communication, verbalization of feelings, and referral to volunteer and community agencies.
- Supporting the child involves encouraging self-expression, alleviating feelings of being different, and strengthening the child's self-image.
- Children's concept of death is determined by their cognitive ability and their experience with life-threatening illness.

- Young children see death as temporary and reversible and mainly fear separation.
- School-age children view death as irreversible but not necessarily inevitable and may fear mutilation.
- Children beyond 9 to 10 years of age realize that death is irreversible, universal, and inevitable but may resist the thought of their own death.
- Siblings have special needs, including the need for information, reassurance about their own health status, assurance that they are not responsible for the illness or death, and support for their own grieving process.
- Special needs of the family facing the unexpected death of a child include support while awaiting news of the child's status; a sensitive pronouncement of death; acknowledgment of feelings of denial, guilt, and anger; an opportunity to view the body; and referrals for support.
- Special decisions at the time of dying and death may involve hospital or hospice care, visualization of the body, tissue donation and autopsy, and siblings' attendance at the funeral.
- Acute grief is a syndrome with intense and distressing psychologic and somatic symptoms that appear at the time of death.
- In dealing with stress related to the dying patient, the nurse can cope successfully through self-awareness, consciousness raising, knowledge and practice, an available support system, and maintenance of general good health and by focusing on the positive rewards of involvement with dying children and their families.

REFERENCES

Ahmann E: "Chunky stew:" appreciating cultural diversity while providing health care for children, *Pediatr Nurs* 20(3):320–324, 1994.

American Academy of Pediatrics, Committee on Hospital Care and Section on Surgery: Pediatric organ donation and transplantation, *Pediatrics* 109(5):982–984, 2002.

American Nurses Association: *Code of ethics for nurses with interpretive statements*, Washington, DC, 2001, ANA Publishing.

Anderson RN, Smith BL: Deaths: leading causes, *Natl Vital Stat Rep* 53(17):1–89, 2005.

Anderson T, Davis C: Evidence-based practice with families of chronically ill children: a critical literature review, *J Evid Based Soc Work* 8(4):416–425, 2011.

Arias E, MacDorman MF, Strobino DM, and others: Annual summary of vital statistics—2002, *Pediatrics* 112(6):1215–1230, 2003.

Barlow JH, Ellard DR: The psychosocial well-being of children with chronic disease, their parents and siblings: an overview of the research evidence base, *Child Care Health Dev* 32(1): 19–31, 2006.

Bettle AM, Latimer MA: Maternal coping and adaptation: a case study examination of chronic sorrow in caring for an adolescent with a progressive neurodegenerative disease, *Can J Neurosci Nurs* 31(4):15–21, 2009.

Birenbaum LK, Stewart BJ, Phillips DS: Health status of bereaved parents, *Nurs Res* 45(2): 105–109, 1996.

Burke RT, Alverson B: Impact of children with medically complex conditions, *Pediatrics* 126(4):789–790, 2010.

Carnevale FA, Alexander E, Davis M, and others: Daily living with distress and enrichment: the moral experience of families with ventilator-assisted children at home, *Pediatrics* 117(1): e48–e60, 2006.

Carnevale FA, Rehm RS, Kirk S, and others: What we know (and don't know) about raising children with complex continuing care needs, *J Child Health Care* 12:4–6, 2008.

Carter B: Chronic pain in childhood and the medical encounter: professional ventriloquism and hidden voices, *Qual Health Res* 12:28–41, 2002.

Charles C, Gafni A, Whelan T: Shared decision making in the medical encounter: what does it mean? *Soc Sci Med* 44:681–692, 1997.

Clements PT, Vigil GJ, Manno MS, and others: Cultural perspectives of death, grief, and bereavement, *J Psychosoc Nurs Ment Health Serv* 41(7):18–26, 2003.

Coffey JS: Parenting a child with chronic illness: a metasynthesis, *Pediatr Nurs* 32(1):51–59, 2006.

Cohen E, Friedman J, Nicholas DB, and others: A home for medically complex children: the role of hospital programs, *J Health Care Quality* 30(3):7–15, 2008.

Coker TR, Rodriguez MA, Flores G: Family-centered care for U.S. children with special health care needs: who gets it and why? *Pediatrics* 125(6):1159–1167, 2010.

Corlett J, Twycross A: Negotiation of parental roles within family-centered care: a review of the research, *J Clin Nurs* 15(10):1308–1316, 2006.

Council on Children with Disabilities: Care coordination in the medical home: integrating health and related systems of care for children with special health care needs, *Pediatrics* 116(5):1238–1244, 2005.

Davies B, Gudmundsdottir M, Worden B, and others: "Living in the dragon's shadow": fathers' experiences of a child's life-limiting illness, *Death Studies* 28(2):111–135, 2004.

Davies R: New understandings of parental grief: literature review, *J Adv Nurs* 46(5):506–513, 2004.

Davies R, Davis B, Sibert J: Parents' stories of sensitive and insensitive care by paediatricians in the time leading up to and including diagnostic disclosure of a life-limiting condition in their child, *Child Care Health Dev* 29(1): 77–82, 2003.

Davis B, Eng B: Special issues in bereavement and staff support. In Doyle D, Hanks GWC, MacDonald N, editors: *Oxford textbook of palliative medicine*, ed 2, Oxford, 1998, Oxford University Press.

Deatrick JA, Knafl KA, Murphy-Moore C: Clarifying the concept of normalization, *Image J Nurs Sch* 31:209–214, 1999.

Denboba D, McPherson MG, Kenney MK, and others: Achieving family and provider partnerships for children with special health care needs, *Pediatrics* 118(4):1607–1615, 2006.

Dixon-Woods M, Young B, Henry D: Partnerships with children, *BMJ* 319:778–780, 1999.

Evanisko MJ, Beasley CL, Brigham LE, and others: Readiness of critical care physicians and nurses to handle requests for organ donation, *Am J Crit Care* 7(1):4–12, 1998.

Faulkner KW, Armstrong-Dailey A: Care of the dying child. In Pizzo PA, Poplack DG, editors: *Principles and practice of pediatric oncology*, Philadelphia, 1997, Lippincott-Raven.

Field MJ, Behrman RE, editors: *When children die: improving palliative and end-of-life care for children and their families*, Washington, DC, 2004, National Academies Press.

Fleitas J: When Jack fell down … Jill came tumbling after: siblings in the web of illness and disability, *MCN Am J Matern Child Nurs* 25:267–273, 2000.

Forrester L: One to one care in children's hospice, *Nurs Times* 99(16):44–45, 2003.

Franz HG, DeJong W, Wolfe SM, and others: Explaining brain death: a critical feature of the donation process, *J Transplant Coord* 7(1):14–21, 1997.

Freyer DR: Care of the dying adolescent: special considerations, *Pediatrics* 113(2):381–388, 2004.

Gantt L: As normal a life as possible: mothers and their daughters with congenital heart disease, *Health Care Women Int* 23(5):481–491, 2002.

Garwick AW, Patterson J, Bennett FC, and others: Breaking the news: how families first learn about their child's chronic condition, *Arch Pediatr Adolesc Med* 149(9):991–997, 1995.

Gold JI, Treadwell M, Weissman L, and others: The mediating effects of family functioning on psychosocial outcomes in healthy siblings of children with sickle cell disease, *Pediatr Blood Cancer* 57(6):1055–1061, 2011.

Goldbeck L: Parental coping with the diagnosis of childhood cancer: gender effects, dissimilarity within couples, and quality of life, *Psychooncology* 10:325–335, 2001.

Goodenough B, Drew D, Higgins S, and others: Bereavement outcomes for parents who lose a child to cancer: are place of death and sex of parent associated with differences in psychological functioning? *Psychooncology* 13(11):779–791, 2004.

Gordon J: An evidence-based approach for supporting parents experiencing chronic sorrow, *Pediatr Nurs* 35(2):115–119, 2009.

Haffner JC, Schurman SJ: The technology dependent child, *Pediatr Clin North Am* 48:751–764, 2001.

Harrigan RC, Ratliffe C, Patrinos ME, and others: Medically fragile pediatric patients: an integrative review of the literature and recommendations for future research, *Issues Compr Pediatr Nurs* 25:1–20, 2002.

Hawryluck LA, Harvey WR: Analgesia, virtue, and the principle of double effect, *J Palliat Care* 16(suppl):S24–S30, 2000.

Hellsten MB, Hockenberry M, Lamb D, and others: *End-of-life care for children*, Austin, Tex, 2000, Texas Cancer Council.

Hinds PS, Oakes L, Furman W, and others: End-of-life decision making by adolescents, parents, and healthcare providers in pediatric oncology: research to evidence-based practice guidelines, *Cancer Nurs* 24:122–134, 2001.

Hsiao JL, Evan EE, Zeltzer LK: Parent and child perspectives on physician communication in pediatric palliative care, *Palliat Support Care* 5(4):355–365, 2007.

Huffman LC, Brat GA, Chamberlain LJ, and others: Impact of managed care on publicly insured children with special health care needs, *Acad Pediatr* 10(1):48–55, 2010.

Hungerbuehler I, Vollrath ME, Landolt MA: Posttraumatic growth in mothers and fathers of children with severe illnesses, *J Health Psychol* 16(8):1259–1267, 2011.

Immelt S: Psychological adjustment in young children with chronic medical conditions, *J Pediatr Nurs* 21(5):362–377, 2006.

Jackson PL: The primary care provider and children with chronic conditions. In Jackson PL, Vessey PA, editors: *Primary care of the child with a chronic condition*, ed 3, St. Louis, 2000, Mosby.

James L, Johnson B: The needs of parents of pediatric oncology patients during the palliative care phase, *J Pediatr Oncol Nurs* 14(2):83–95, 1997.

Jennings PD: Providing pediatric palliative care through a pediatric supportive care team, *Pediatr Nurs* 31(3):195–200, 2005.

Jokinen P: The family life-path theory: a tool for nurses working in partnership with families, *J Child Health Care* 8(2):124–133, 2004.

Kirk S, Glendinning C, Callery PJ: Parent or nurse? The experience of being the parent of a technology-dependent child, *Adv Nurs* 51(5):456–464, 2005.

Klass D: The inner representation of the dead child in the psychic and social narratives of bereaved parents. In Neimeyer RA, editor: *Meaning reconstruction and the experience of loss*, Washington, DC, 2001, American Psychological Association.

Knafl KA, Darney BG, Gallo AM, and others: Parental perceptions of the outcome and meaning of normalization, *Res Nurs Health* 33(2):87–98, 2010.

Kon AA: The shared decision-making continuum, *JAMA* 304(8):903–904, 2010.

Lambert S: Distraction, imagery, and hypnosis techniques for management of children's pain, *J Child Fam Nurs* 2(1):5–15, 1999.

Lauer ME, Mulhern RK, Schell MJ, and others: Long-term follow-up of parental adjustment following a child's death at home or hospital, *Cancer* 63(5):988–994, 1989.

Lobato DJ, Kao BT: Integrated sibling–parent group intervention to improve sibling knowledge and adjustment to chronic illness and disability, *J Pediatr Psychol* 27:711–716, 2002.

Lobato DJ, Kao BT, Plante W: Latino sibling knowledge and adjustment to chronic illness, *J Fam Psychol* 19(4):625–632, 2005.

Marshall ES, Olsen SF, Mandleco BL, and others: "This is a spiritual experience": perspectives of Latter-Day Saint families living with a child with disabilities, *Qual Health Res* 13:57–76, 2003.

Masri C, Farrell CA, Lacroix J, and others: Decision making and end-of-life care in critically ill children, *J Palliative Care* 16(suppl):S45–S52, 2000.

Mastroyannopoulou K, Stallard P, Lewis M, and others: The impact of childhood non-malignant life threatening illness on parents: gender differences and predictors of parental adjustment, *J Child Psychol Psychiatry* 38(7):823–829, 1997.

McDougal J: Promoting normalization in families with preschool children with type 1 diabetes, *J Spec Pediatr Nurs* 7(3):113–120, 2002.

McPherson M, Weissman G, Strickland BB, and others: Implementing community-based systems of services for child and youths with special health care needs: how well are we doing? *Pediatrics* 113(5):1538–1544, 2004.

Meert KL, Shear K, Newth CJ, and others: Follow-up study of complicated grief among parents eighteen months after a child's death in the pediatric intensive care unit, *J Palliat Med* 14(2):207–214, 2011.

Mentro A: Health care policy for medically fragile pediatric patients, *J Pediatr Nurs* 18(4):22, 2003.

Miles M, Holditch-Davis D, Burchinal M, and others: Distress and growth outcomes in mothers of medically fragile infants, *Nurs Res* 48:129–140, 1999.

Monterosso L, Kristjanson LJ, Aoun S, and others: Supportive and palliative care needs of families of children with life-threatening illnesses in Western Australia: evidence to guide the development of a palliative care service, *Palliat Med* 1(8):689–696, 2007.

Moriarty H, Carroll R, Cotroneo M: Differences in bereavement reactions within couples following the death of a child, *Res Nurs Health* 19:461–469, 1996.

Murray JS: Siblings of children with cancer: a review of the literature, *J Pediatr Oncol Nurs* 16(1):25–34, 1999.

Nelson AM: A metasynthesis: mothering other-than-normal children, *Qual Health Res* 12:515–530, 2002.

Newacheck PW, Halfon N: Prevalence and impact of disabling chronic conditions in childhood, *Am J Public Health* 88(4):610–617, 1998.

Nuutila L, Salanterä S: Children with a long-term illness: parents' experiences of care, *J Pediatr Nurs* 21(2):153–160, 2006.

O'Brien ME, Wegner CB: Rearing the child who is technology dependent: perceptions of parents and home care nurses, *J Spec Pediatr Nurs* 7:7–15, 2002.

Ochieng BM: Minority ethnic families and family-centered care, *J Child Health Care* 7(2):123–132, 2003.

Pierucci RL, Kirby RS, Leuthner SR: End-of-life for neonates and infants: the experience and effects of a palliative care consultation service, *Pediatrics* 108(3):653–660, 2001.

Raina P, O'Donnell M, Rosenbaum P, and others: The health and well-being of caregivers of children with cerebral palsy, *Pediatrics* 115(6): e626–e636, 2005.

Ray LD: Parenting and childhood chronicity: making visible the invisible work, *J Pediatr Nurs* 17(6):424–438, 2002.

Rehm RS: Religious faith in Mexican-American families dealing with chronic childhood illness, *Image J Nurs Sch* 31:33–38, 1999.

Rehm RS, Bradley JF: The search for social safety and satisfaction in families raising children with complex chronic conditions, *J Fam Nurs* 11(1): 59–78, 2005.

Ritchie MA: Self-esteem and hopefulness in adolescents with cancer, *J Pediatr Nurs* 16:35–42, 2001.

Rossiter L, Sharpe D: The siblings of individuals with mental retardation: a quantitative integration of the literature, *J Child Fam Studies* 10(1):65–84, 2001.

Rousseau P: Ethical and legal issues in palliative care, *Prim Care* 28:391–400, 2001.

Sahler O, Frager G, Levetown M, and others: Medical education about end-of-life care in the pediatric setting: principles, challenges, and opportunities, *Pediatrics* 105:575–584, 2000.

Schor EL: Family pediatrics: report of the Task Force on the Family, *Pediatrics* 111:1541–1571, 2003.

Sharpe D, Rossiter L: Siblings of children with a chronic illness: a meta-analysis, *J Pediatr Psychol* 27:699–710, 2002.

Shepard MP, Mahon MM: Chronic conditions and the family. In Jackson PL, Vessey JA, editors: *Primary care of the child with a chronic condition*, ed 3, St. Louis, 2000, Mosby.

Sine D, Sumner L, Gracy D, and others: Pediatric extubation: "pulling the tube," *J Palliat Med* 4:519–524, 2001.

Smaldone A, Ritholz MD: Perceptions of parenting children with type 1 diabetes diagnosed in early childhood, *J Pediatr Health Care* 25(2):87–95, 2011.

Stein REK: Home care: a challenging opportunity, *Child Health Care* 14(2):90–95, 1985.

Sterling YM, Peterson JW: Characteristics of African American women caregivers of children with asthma, *MCN Am J Matern Child* 28:32–38, 2003.

Sullivan-Bolyai S, Sadler L, Knafl KA, and others: Great expectations: a position description for parents as caregivers, part I, *Pediatr Nurs* 29(6):52–56, 2003.

Sumner LH: Lighting the way: improving the way children die in America, *Caring* 22:14–18, 2003.

Swallow V, Macfadyen A, Santacroce SJ, and others: Fathers' contributions to the management of their child's long-term medical condition: a narrative review of the literature, *Health Expect* 2011, in press.

Swallow VM, Jacoby A: Mothers' evolving relationships with doctors and nurses during the chronic childhood illness trajectory, *J Adv Nurs* 36:755–764, 2001.

Thomlinson EH: The lived experience of families of children who are failing to thrive, *J Adv Nurs* 39:537–545, 2002.

Tong H, Kandala G, Haig AJ, and others: Physical functioning in female caregivers of children with physical disabilities compared with female caregivers of children with a chronic medical condition, *Arch Pediatr Adolesc Med* 156:1138–1142, 2002.

Vance JC, Najman JM, Thearle MJ, and others: Psychological changes in parents eight months after the loss of an infant from stillbirth, neonatal death, or sudden infant death syndrome—a longitudinal study, *Pediatrics* 96(5):933–938, 1995.

Van Dyck PC, Kogan MD, McPherson MG, and others: Prevalence and characteristics of children with special health care needs, *Arch Pediatr Adolesc Med* 158(9):884–890, 2004.

Watson D, Townsley R, Abbott D: Exploring multi-agency working in services to disabled children with complex health care needs and their families, *J Clin Nurs* 11:367–375, 2002.

Whitehead LC, Gosling V: Parent's perceptions of interactions with health professionals in the pathway to gaining a diagnosis of tuberous sclerosis (TS) and beyond, *Res Dev Disabil* 24:109–119, 2003.

Winkler WD, Mardegian CA: Completing the continuum of care: the growth of a pediatric hospice program, *Caring* 20:22–25, 2001.

Wise PH, Wampler NS, Chavkin W, and others: Chronic illness among poor children enrolled in the temporary assistance for needy families program, *Am J Public Health* 92:1458–1461, 2002.

Wolfe J, Friebert S, Hilden J: Caring for children with advanced cancer integrating palliative care, *Pediatr Clin North Am* 49(5):1043–1062, 2002.

Wolfe J, Grier HE, Klar N, and others: Symptoms and suffering at the end of life in children with cancer, *N Engl J Med* 342(5):326–333, 2000.

Wood PR, Smith LA, Romero D, and others: Relationships between welfare status, health insurance status, and health and medical care among children with asthma, *Am J Public Health* 92:1446–1452, 2002.

World Health Organization: *Cancer pain relief and palliative care*, Geneva, 1996, Author.

World Health Organization: *Definition of palliative care for children*, 1998, retrieved June 20, 2011, from http://www.who.int/cancer/palliative/definition/en.

Young B, Dixon-Woods M, Windridge KC, and others: Managing communication with young people who have a potentially life threatening chronic illness: qualitative study of patients and parents, *BMJ* 326(7384):305, 2003.

Zuvekas SH, Taliaferro GS: Pathways to access: health, insurance, the health care delivery system and racial/ethnic disparities, 1996–1999, *Health Affairs* 22(2):139–153, 2003.

Impact of Cognitive or Sensory Impairment on the Child and Family

Rosalind Bryant

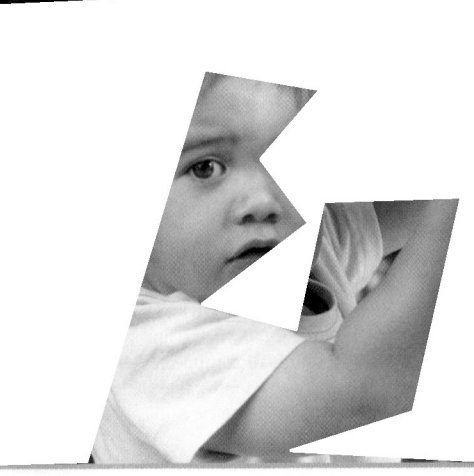

evolve WEBSITE

http://evolve.elsevier.com/wong/essentials
Case Study—Down Syndrome
Key Point Summaries
NCLEX-Style Review Questions
Nursing Care Plan—The Child with Impaired Cognitive Function

CHAPTER OUTLINE

Cognitive Impairment, 571
  General Concepts, 571
  Nursing Care of Children with Impaired
    Cognitive Function, 572
    Educate Child and Family, 572
    Teach Child Self-Care Skills, 573
    Promote Child's Optimal
      Development, 573
    Encourage Play and Exercise, 573
    Provide Means of Communication, 574

Establish Discipline, 574
Encourage Socialization, 575
Provide Information on
  Sexuality, 575
Help Family Adjust to Future
  Care, 575
Care for Child During
  Hospitalization, 575
Assist in Measures to Prevent Cognitive
  Impairment, 576

Down Syndrome, 576
Fragile X Syndrome, 578
Sensory Impairment, 579
  Hearing Impairment, 579
  Visual Impairment, 584
  Hearing–Visual Impairment, 589
  Retinoblastoma, 589
  Autism Spectrum Disorders, 590

LEARNING OBJECTIVES

On completion of this chapter the reader will be able to:
- Define the classifications of intellectual disability.
- Define *developmental delay.*
- Outline nursing interventions for the child with cognitive impairment that promote optimal development, including during hospitalization.
- Identify the major biologic and cognitive characteristics of children with Down syndrome.
- Outline nursing interventions for children with Down syndrome.
- Identify the major characteristics associated with fragile X syndrome.

- List the general classifications of hearing impairment and the effect on speech.
- Outline nursing interventions for children with hearing impairment, including during hospitalization.
- List the common types of visual impairments in children.
- Outline nursing interventions for children with visual impairment, including during hospitalization.
- Outline nursing interventions for children with retinoblastoma.
- Outline nursing interventions for children with an autism spectrum disorder.

COGNITIVE IMPAIRMENT

GENERAL CONCEPTS

Cognitive impairment (CI) is a general term that encompasses any type of mental difficulty or deficiency. In this chapter, the term is used synonymously with *intellectual disability* and replaces the term mental retardation (MR), defined by the American Association on Intellectual and Developmental Disabilities (AAIDD, 2010). Although the needs and concerns of the family are a primary focus throughout the chapter, readers are encouraged to review Chapter 18, which details the family's adjustment to disabilities in general.

The definition of intellectual disability in children consists of three components: intellectual functioning, functional strengths and weaknesses, and age younger than 18 years at time of diagnosis. Intellectual functioning is measured by the intelligence quotient (IQ) of 70 to 75 or below. The child with an intellectual disability must demonstrate functional impairment in at least 2 of 10 different adaptive skill areas: communication, self-care, home living, social skills, leisure, health and safety, self-direction, functional academics, community use, and work (American Psychiatric Association, 2000) or have deficits in one or more adaptive domains (AAIDD, 2010). The classification system by the AAIDD allows for identification of the individual's specific needs in four established dimensions of care (Box 19-1). Careful evaluation to identify the needs of individuals with CI is focused on promoting habilitation for each person. It is anticipated that the functional capabilities of children with CI will improve over time when support is provided.

Diagnosis and Classification

The diagnosis of CI is usually made after a period of suspicion, by professionals or the family, that the child's developmental progress is delayed. In some cases, it is confirmed at birth because of recognition of distinct syndromes, such as Down syndrome and fetal alcohol syndrome. At the other extreme, the diagnosis is made when problems such as speech delays arouse concern. In all cases, a high index of suspicion for developmental delay and behavioral signs (Box 19-2) is necessary for early diagnosis; routine developmental screening can assist in early identification (see Chapter 5). Delays are typically seen in gross and fine motor and speech development, although the latter is most predictive. Developmental delay can be described as any significant lag in a child's physical, cognitive, behavioral, emotional, or social development when compared against developmental norms. CI is a permanent impairment encompassing cognitive ability and adaptive behavior that are functioning significantly below average (see Box 19-2). In the absence of clear-cut evidence of CI, it is more appropriate to use a diagnosis of developmental delay.

Results of standardized tests are used in making the diagnosis of intellectual disability (or MR) based on cognitive deficits. Tests for assessing adaptive behaviors include the Vineland Social Maturity Scale and the AAMR Adaptive Behavior Scale. Informal appraisal of adaptive behavior may be made by those fully acquainted with the child (e.g., teachers, parents, other care providers). Frequently these observations lead parents to seek evaluation of the child's development.

A more useful approach for clinical application is classification based on educational potential or symptom severity. For educational purposes, the mildly impaired group (educable MR) constitutes about 85% of all people with CI, and the group with moderate levels of CI (trainable MR) accounts for about 10% of the intellectually disabled population (American Psychiatric Association, 2000; Katz and Lazcano-Ponce, 2008; Walker and Johnson, 2006) (Table 19-1). Although nurses may be familiar with the approximate range of IQ for classifying severity, they should refrain from using numbers as the criterion for assessing or evaluating the child's abilities because numbers are of little value in counseling parents or training these children.

Etiology

The causes of severe CI are primarily genetic, biochemical, and infectious. Although the etiology is unknown in the majority of cases, familial, social, environmental, and organic causes may predominate. Among individuals with CI, a sizable proportion of the cases are linked to Down syndrome, fragile X syndrome, or fetal alcohol syndrome. General categories of events that may lead to CI include (Katz and Lazcano-Ponce, 2008; Walker and Johnson, 2006):

- Infection and intoxication, such as congenital rubella, syphilis, maternal drug consumption (e.g., fetal alcohol syndrome), chronic lead ingestion, or kernicterus
- Trauma or physical agent (i.e., injury to the brain experienced during the prenatal, perinatal, or postnatal period)
- Inadequate nutrition and metabolic disorders, such as phenylketonuria or congenital hypothyroidism
- Gross postnatal brain disease, such as neurofibromatosis and tuberous sclerosis
- Unknown prenatal influence, including cerebral and cranial malformations, such as microcephaly and hydrocephalus
- Chromosomal abnormalities resulting from radiation; viruses; chemicals; parental age; and genetic mutations, such as Down syndrome and fragile X syndrome
- Gestational disorders, including prematurity, low birth weight, and postmaturity
- Psychiatric disorders that have their onset during the child's developmental period up to age 18 years, such as autism spectrum disorders (ASDs)

BOX 19-1   **DIMENSIONS OF CARE FOR INTELLECTUALLY DISABLED PATIENTS**

Dimension I—Intellectual functioning and adaptive skills
Dimension II—Psychologic and emotional considerations
Dimension III—Physical, health, and etiology considerations
Dimension IV—Environmental considerations

BOX 19-2   **EARLY BEHAVIORAL SIGNS SUGGESTIVE OF COGNITIVE IMPAIRMENT**

Dysmorphic features (e.g., Down syndrome, fragile X syndrome)
Irritability or unresponsiveness to contact
Abnormal eye contact
Gross motor delay
Decreased alertness to voice or movement
Language difficulties or delay
Feeding difficulties

Modified from Shapiro B, Batshaw M: Mental retardation (intellectual disability). In Kliegman RM, Behrman RE, Jenson HB, editors: *Nelson textbook of pediatrics,* ed 18, Philadelphia, 2007, Saunders; Wilks T, Gerber J, Erdie-Lalena C: Developmental milestones: cognitive development, *Pediatr Rev* 31(9):364–367, 2010.

TABLE 19-1 CLASSIFICATION OF COGNITIVE IMPAIRMENT		
LEVEL (IQ)*	**PRESCHOOL (BIRTH–5 YEARS)—MATURATION AND DEVELOPMENT**	**SCHOOL AGE (6–21 YEARS)—TRAINING AND EDUCATION**	**ADULT (≥21 YEARS)—SOCIAL AND VOCATIONAL ADEQUACY**

LEVEL (IQ)*	**PRESCHOOL (BIRTH–5 YEARS)—MATURATION AND DEVELOPMENT**	**SCHOOL AGE (6–21 YEARS)—TRAINING AND EDUCATION**	**ADULT (≥21 YEARS)—SOCIAL AND VOCATIONAL ADEQUACY**
Mild—50–55 to ≈70–75	Often not noticed as delayed by casual observer but is slower to walk, feed self, and talk than most children; follows same sequence in development as normal children	Can acquire practical skills and useful reading and arithmetic to a third- to sixth-grade level with special education; can be guided toward social conformity; achieves mental age of 8–12 years	Can usually achieve social and vocational skills adequate to self-maintenance; may need occasional guidance and support when under unusual social or economic stress; can adjust to marriage but not childrearing
Moderate—35–40 to 50–55	Noticeable delays in motor development, especially in speech; responds to training in various self-help activities	Can learn simple communication, elementary health and safety habits, and simple manual skills; does not progress in functional reading or arithmetic; achieves mental age of 3–7 years	Can perform simple tasks under sheltered conditions; participates in simple recreation; travels alone in familiar places; usually incapable of self-maintenance
Severe—20–25 to 35–40	Marked delay in motor development; little or no communication skills; may respond to training in elementary self-care (e.g., self-feeding)	Usually walks, barring specific disability; has some understanding of speech and some response; can profit from systematic habit training; achieves mental age of toddler	Can conform to daily routines and repetitive activities; needs continuing direction and supervision in protective environment
Profound—below 20–25	Gross delay; minimum capacity for functioning in sensorimotor areas; needs total care	Obvious delays in all areas of development; shows basic emotional responses; may respond to skillful training in use of legs, hands, and jaws; needs close supervision; achieves mental age of young infant	May walk; needs complete custodial care; has primitive speech; usually benefits from regular physical activity

IQ, intelligence quotient.

*Data from American Psychiatric Association: *Diagnostic and statistical manual of mental disorders*, ed 4 (text rev) (DSM-IV TR), Washington, DC, 2000, Author; and Rittey CD: Learning difficulties: what the neurologist needs to know, *J Neurol Neurosurg Psychiatry* 74(suppl 1):30–36, 2005.

- Environmental influences, including evidence of a deprived environment associated with a history of intellectual disability among parents and siblings

NURSING CARE OF CHILDREN WITH IMPAIRED COGNITIVE FUNCTION

Nurses play a major role in identifying children with CI. In the newborn and early infancy periods, few signs are present, with the exception of Down syndrome (p. 576). After this age, however, delayed developmental milestones are the major clues to CI. In addition, nurses must have a high index of suspicion for early behavior patterns that may suggest CI (see Box 19-2). Parental concerns, such as delayed development compared with siblings, need to be taken seriously. All children should receive regular developmental assessment, and the nurse is often the person responsible for performing such assessments (see Chapter 5). When delays are found, the nurse must use sensitivity and discretion in revealing this finding to parents.

Educate Child and Family

To teach children with CI, it is necessary to investigate their learning abilities and deficits. This is important for the nurse who may be involved in a home care program or who may be caring for the child in a health care setting. The nurse who understands how these children learn can effectively teach them basic skills or prepare them for various health-related procedures.

Children with CI have a marked deficit in their ability to discriminate between two or more stimuli because of difficulty in recognizing the relevance of specific cues. However, these children can learn to discriminate if the cues are presented in an exaggerated, concrete form

and if all extraneous stimuli are eliminated. For example, the use of colors to emphasize visual cues or the use of singing or rhymes to stress auditory cues can help them learn. Their deficit in discrimination also implies that concrete ideas are learned much more effectively than abstract ideas. Therefore, demonstration is preferable to verbal explanation, and learning should be directed toward mastering a skill rather than understanding the scientific principles underlying a procedure.

Another cognitive deficit is in short-term memory. Whereas children of average intelligence can remember several words, numbers, or directions at one time, children with CI are less able to do so. Therefore, they need simple, one-step directions. Learning through a step-by-step process requires a task analysis in which each task is separated into its necessary components and each step is taught completely before proceeding to the next activity.

One critical area of learning that has had a tremendous impact on education for cognitively impaired individuals is motivation. Programs based on the motivational principles of behavior modification, using positive reinforcement for specific tasks or behaviors, have demonstrated marked improvement in children's ability to learn. Advances in technology have greatly aided in providing reinforcement, especially in children with severe disabilities and who may have physical disabilities that limit their range of capabilities. For example, with the use of specially designed switches, children are given control of some event in the environment, such as turning on the television (Fig. 19-1). The television picture becomes the reinforcement for activating the switch. Repetitive use of these switches provides an early, simplistic association with a technical device that may progress to increasingly complex aids.

Early intervention program is a systematic program of therapy, exercises, and activities designed to address developmental delays in disabled children to help achieve their full potentials (American

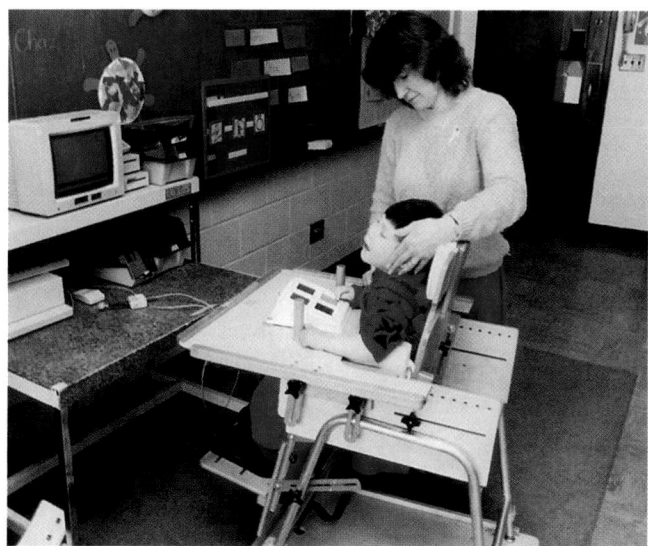

FIG. 19-1 A push panel allows a child with cognitive impairment to turn a computer on and off.

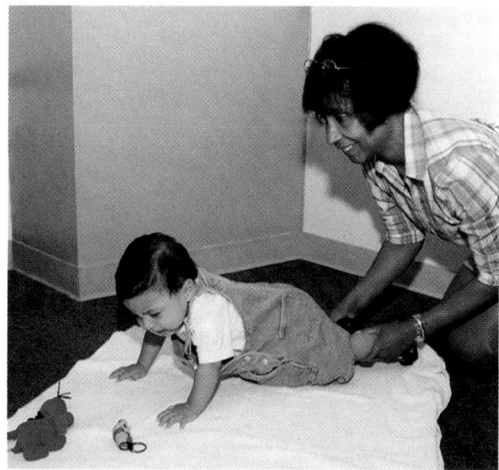

FIG. 19-2 Placing an attractive object outside the child's reach encourages crawling movements. (Courtesy James DeLeon, Texas Children's Hospital, Houston.)

Academy of Pediatrics [AAP], Committee on Genetics, 2001; National Down Syndrome Society, 2011a; Weijerman and de Winter, 2010). Considerable evidence indicates that these programs are valuable for cognitively impaired children. Nurses working with these families need to be aware of the types of programs in their community. Under the Individuals with Disabilities Education Act (IDEA) of 1990 (Public Law 101-476), states are encouraged to provide full early intervention services and are required to provide educational opportunities for all children with disabilities from birth to 21 years of age. Services may be provided under state Programs for Children with Special Health Needs or Head Start, or by private organizations such as National Down Syndrome Society,* Easter Seals,† or the Arc of the United States.‡ Parents should inquire about these programs by contacting the appropriate agencies. The child's education should begin as soon as possible. As children grow older, their education should be directed toward vocational training that prepares them for as independent a lifestyle as possible within their scope of abilities.

Teach Child Self-Care Skills

When a child with CI is born, parents need assistance in promoting normal developmental skills that are almost automatically learned by other children. These include self-care skills such as feeding, toileting, dressing, and grooming. Teaching these skills requires a basic knowledge of the developmental sequence in learning the skills demonstrated by children of average intelligence. For example, children with subaverage intelligence would not be expected to dress themselves as early as unaffected youngsters.

Teaching self-care skills also necessitates a working knowledge of the individual steps needed to master a skill. For example, before beginning a self-feeding program, the nurse performs a task analysis. After a task analysis, the child is observed in a particular situation, such as eating, to determine what skills are possessed and the child's developmental readiness to learn the task. Family members are included in this process because their "readiness" is as important as the child's. Numerous self-help aids are available to facilitate independence and can help eliminate some of the difficulties of learning, such as using a plate with suction cups to prevent accidental spills.*

Promote Child's Optimal Development

Optimal development involves more than achieving independence. It requires appropriate guidance for establishing acceptable social behavior and personal feelings of self-esteem, worth, and security. These attributes are not simply learned through a stimulation program. Rather, they must arise from the genuine love and caring that exist among family members. However, families need guidance in providing an environment that fosters optimal development. Often the nurse can provide assistance in these areas of childrearing.

Another important area for promoting optimal development and self-esteem is ensuring the child's physical well-being. Any congenital defects, such as cardiac, gastrointestinal, or orthopedic anomalies, should be repaired. Plastic surgery may be considered when the child's appearance can be substantially improved. Dental health is significant, and orthodontic and restorative procedures can improve facial appearance immensely.

Encourage Play and Exercise

Children who are cognitively impaired have the same needs for recreation and exercise as other children. However, because of the children's slower development, parents may be less aware of the need to provide such activities. Therefore, the nurse guides parents toward selection of suitable play and exercise activities. Because play has been discussed for children in each age group in earlier chapters, only the exceptions are presented here (Fig. 19-2).

The type of play is based on the child's developmental age, although the need for sensorimotor play may be prolonged for several years. Parents should use every opportunity to expose the child to as many

---

*Information on early intervention programs in each state is available from the National Down Syndrome Society, 666 Broadway, 8th Floor, New York, NY 10012-2317; 800-221-4602; fax: 212-979-2873; email: info@ndss.org; http://www.ndss.org.
†233 South Wacker Drive., Suite 2400, Chicago, IL 60606-4802; 800-221-6827; TTY: 312-726-4258; fax: 312-726-1494; http://www.easterseals.com.
‡1010 Wayne Ave., Suite 650, Silver Spring, MD 20910; 301-565-3842 or 800-433-5255; fax: 301-565-5342; http://www.thearc.org.

---

*A resource for a variety of self-help equipment is Sammons Preston, PO Box 5071, Bolingbrook, IL 60440-5071; 800-323-5547; fax: 800-547-4333; http://www.sammonspreston.com. In Canada: 800-665-9200.

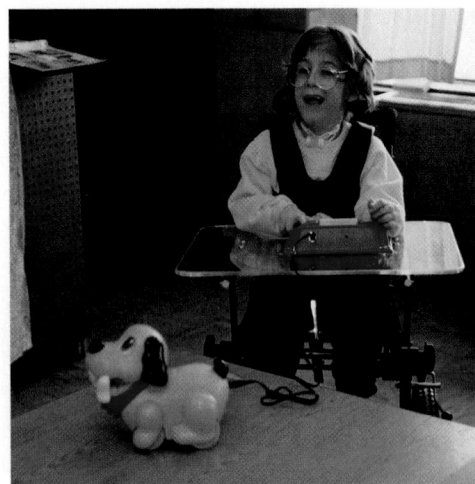

FIG. 19-3 A manual switch allows a child with cognitive impairment to play with a battery-operated toy.

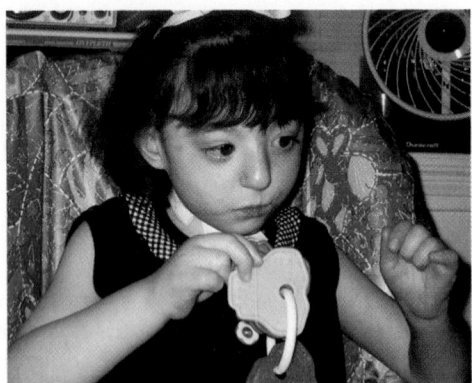

FIG. 19-4 A favorite toy provides stimulation for a young child.

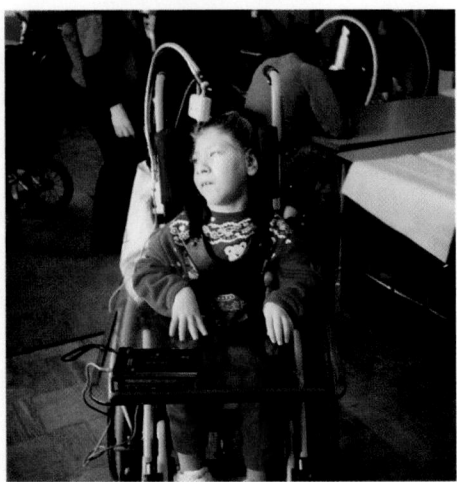

FIG. 19-5 A child with cognitive and physical impairments can activate electronic and communication equipment by moving a device near her head.

different sounds, sights, and sensations as possible. Appropriate play includes musical mobiles, stuffed toys, water play, floating toys, a rocking chair or horse, a swing, bells, and rattles. The child should be taken on outings, such as trips to the grocery store or shopping center; other people should be encouraged to visit in the home; and the child should be related to directly, such as by cuddling, holding, rocking, talking to the child in the en face (face-to-face) position, and giving "rides" on the parents' shoulders.

Toys are selected for their recreational and educational value. For example, a large inflatable beach ball is a good water toy; it encourages interactive play and can be used to learn motor skills, such as balance, rocking, kicking, and throwing. A doll with removable clothes and different types of closures can help the child learn dressing skills. Musical toys that mimic animal sounds or respond with social phrases are excellent ways of encouraging speech. Toys should be simple in design so the child can learn to manipulate them without help. For children with severe cognitive and physical impairment, electronic switches can be used to allow them to operate toys (Fig. 19-3).

Suitable activities for physical activity are based on the child's size, coordination, physical fitness and maturity, motivation, and health (Fig. 19-4). Some children may have physical problems that prevent participation in certain sports, such as atlantoaxial instability in children with Down syndrome (p. 576). These children often have greater success in individual and dual sports than in team sports and enjoy themselves most with children of the same developmental level. The

Special Olympics* provides these children with a unique competitive opportunity.

Safety is a major consideration in selecting recreational and exercise activities. For example, toys that may be appropriate developmentally may present dangers to a child who is strong enough to break them or use them incorrectly.

Provide Means of Communication

Verbal skills are typically delayed more than other physical skills. Speech requires hearing and interpretation (**receptive skills**) and facial muscle coordination (**expressive skills**). Because both types of skills may be impaired, these children need frequent audiometric testing and should be fitted with hearing aids if indicated. In addition, they may need help in learning to control their facial muscles. For example, some children may need tongue exercises to correct the tongue thrust or gentle reminders to keep the lips closed.

Nonverbal communication may be appropriate for some of these children, and various devices are available. For the child without associated physical disabilities, a talking picture board is helpful. For children with physical limitations, several adaptations or types of communication devices are available to facilitate selection of the appropriate picture or word (Fig. 19-5). Some children may be taught sign language or **Blissymbols**—a highly stylized system of graphic symbols representing words, ideas, and concepts. Although the symbols require education to learn their meaning, no reading skill is needed. The symbols are usually arranged on a board, and the person points or uses some type of selector to convey a message.

Establish Discipline

Discipline must begin early. Limit-setting measures need to be simple, consistently applied, and appropriate for the child's mental age. Control measures are based primarily on teaching a specific behavior rather than on understanding the reasons behind it. Stressing moral lessons is of little value to a child who lacks the cognitive skills to learn from

---

*1133 19th St. NW, Washington, DC 20036; 800-700-8585 or 202-628-3630; fax: 202-824-0200; http://www.specialolympics.org. (Website includes listing of state offices.) In Canada: Special Olympics Canada, 60 St. Clair Ave. E, Suite 700, Toronto, ON M4T 1N5; 416-927-9050; fax: 416-927-8475; http://www.specialolympics.ca.

self-criticism or from a lesson based on previous wrong-doing. Behavior modification, especially reinforcement of desired actions, and time-out are appropriate forms of behavior control.

Encourage Socialization

Acquiring social skills is a complex task, as is learning self-care procedures. Active rehearsals with role-playing and practice sessions and positive reinforcement for desired behavior have been the most successful approaches. Parents should be encouraged early to teach their child socially acceptable behavior: waving goodbye, saying "hello" and "thank you," responding to his or her name, greeting visitors, and sitting modestly. The teaching of socially acceptable sexual behavior is especially important to minimize sexual exploitation. Parents also need to expose the child to strangers so that he or she can practice manners because there is no automatic transfer of learning from one situation to another.

Dressing and grooming are also important aspects of socialization. A child who is dressed in age-appropriate clothing and is well groomed is much more likely to be accepted and to develop good self-esteem. Clothes should be clean, up-to-date, and well fitted. Many attractive outfits can be adapted with self-adhering fasteners and elastic openings to facilitate self-dressing.

As soon as possible, parents should enroll the child in appropriate preschool programs. Not only do these programs provide education and training, but they also offer an opportunity for social experiences among the children. As children grow older, they should have peer experiences similar to those of other children, including group outings, sports, and organized activities such as scouts and Special Olympics. Nurses can assess the child's abilities and encourage others (e.g., parents, teachers) to promote developmentally appropriate peer interaction (Johnson and Walker, 2006; National Down Syndrome Society, 2011a; Shapiro and Batshaw, 2007).

Provide Information on Sexuality

Adolescence may be a particularly difficult time for the family, especially in terms of the child's sexual behavior, possibility of pregnancy, future plans to marry, and ability to be independent. Frequently, little anticipatory guidance has been offered parents to prepare the child for physical and sexual maturation. The nurse can help in this area by providing parents with information about sexuality education that is geared to the child's developmental level. For example, adolescent girls need a *simple* explanation of menstruation and instructions on personal hygiene during the menstrual cycle.

These adolescents also need practical sexual information regarding anatomy, physical development, and conception.* Because of their easy persuasion and lack of judgment, they need a well-defined, concrete code of conduct. The subtleties of social sexual behavior are less beneficial than specific instructions for handling certain situations. For example, an adolescent should be firmly told never to go alone anywhere with any person that he or she does not know well. To protect him or her from abusive sexual activities, parents must closely observe their teenager's activities and associates. The question of contraceptive protection for these adolescents is often a parental concern.

Parents of these adolescents are often concerned about the advisability of marriage between two individuals with intellectual disabilities. There is no conclusive answer; each situation must be judged individually. In some instances, marriage is possible, but parenthood may not be desirable because of the complexity of childrearing and the potential problem of perpetuating mental deficiency. The nurse should discuss this topic with parents and with the prospective couple, stressing suitable living accommodations and contraceptive methods to prevent pregnancy. If children are conceived, these parents require specialized assistance in learning to meet the needs of their offspring (Johnson and Walker, 2006).

Help Family Adjust to Future Care

Not all families are able to cope with home care of their affected child, especially one who is severely or profoundly impaired or has multiple disabilities. Older parents may not be able to assume care responsibilities after they reach retirement or older age. For these parents, the decision regarding residential placement is a difficult one, and the availability of such facilities varies widely. The nurse working with a family should help them investigate and evaluate various programs in addition to assisting them in adjusting to the decision for placement.

Care for Child During Hospitalization

Caring for the child during hospitalization can be a special challenge. Frequently, nurses are unfamiliar with children who are cognitively impaired, and they may cope with their feelings of insecurity and fear by ignoring or isolating the child. Not only is this approach non-supportive, but it may also be destructive for the child's sense of self-esteem and optimal development, and it may hamper the parents' ability to cope with the stress of the experience. One method that successfully avoids this nontherapeutic approach is the use of the mutual participation model in planning the child's care. Parents are encouraged to stay with their child but should not be made to feel as if the responsibility is totally theirs.

When the child is admitted, a detailed history is taken (see Chapter 21), especially in terms of all self-care activity. During the interview, the child's developmental age is assessed. It is best to avoid asking directly about IQ levels because this may make the parents uncomfortable and often tells little about the child's actual abilities. Questions are approached positively. For example, rather than asking, "Is your child toilet trained yet?" the nurse may state, "Tell me about your child's toileting habits." The assessment should also focus on any special devices the child uses, effective measures of limit setting, unusual or favorite routines, and any behaviors that may require intervention. If the parent states that the child engages in self-injurious activities (e.g., head banging, self-biting), the nurse should inquire about events that precipitate them and techniques (e.g., distraction, medication) that the parents use to manage them (Johnson and Walker, 2006; Oliver and Richards, 2010).

The nurse also assesses the child's functional level of eating and playing; ability to express needs verbally; progress in toilet training; and relationship with objects, toys, and other children. The child is encouraged to be as independent as possible in the hospital.

Realizing that the child may be lonely in the hospital, the nurse makes certain that toys and other activities are provided. The child is placed in a room with other children of approximately the same developmental age, preferably a room with only two beds to avoid overstimulation. The nurse discusses with the other parents the child's abilities and introduces the parents and children to each other. By the nurse's example of treating the child with dignity and respect, others who may be fearful of what they do not understand are encouraged to accept the child.

Procedures are explained to the child through methods of communication that are at the appropriate cognitive level. Generally,

---

*Sources of information on sexuality and conception are the Arc of the United States (see footnote, p. 573) and Planned Parenthood Federation of America, 434 W. 33rd St., New York, NY 10001; 212-541-7800 or 800-230-7526; fax: 212-245-1845; http://www.plannedparenthood.org.

explanations should be simple, short, and concrete, emphasizing what the child will experience *physically*. Demonstration either through actual practice or with visual aids is always preferable to verbal explanation. The nurse repeats instructions often and evaluates the child's understanding by asking questions such as "What will it feel like?" "Show me how you must lie," or "Where will the dressing be?" Parents are included in preprocedural teaching for their own learning and to help the nurse learn effective methods of communicating with the child.

During hospitalization, the nurse should also focus on growth-promoting experiences for the child. For example, hospitalization may be an excellent opportunity to emphasize to parents abilities that the child does have but has not had the opportunity to practice, such as self-dressing. It may also be an opportunity for social experiences with peers, group play, or new educational and recreational activities. For example, one child who had the habit of screaming and kicking demonstrated a definite decrease in those behaviors after he learned to pound pegs and use a punching bag. Through social services, the parents may become aware of specialized programs for the child. Hospitalization may also offer parents a respite from everyday care responsibilities and an opportunity to discuss their feelings with a concerned professional.

Assist in Measures to Prevent Cognitive Impairment

Besides having a responsibility to families with a child with CI, nurses also need to be involved in programs aimed at preventing CI. Many of the familial, social, and environmental factors known to cause mild impairment are preventable. Counseling and education can reduce or eliminate such factors (e.g., poor nutrition, cigarette smoking, chemical abuse), which increase the risk of prematurity and intrauterine growth restriction. Interventions are directed toward improving maternal health by educating women regarding the dangers of chemicals, including prenatal alcohol exposure, which affects organogenesis, craniofacial development, and cognitive ability (Defendi, 2010; Wilton and Plane, 2006). Other preventive strategies that play an important role include adequate prenatal care; optimal medical care of high-risk newborns; rubella immunization; genetic counseling and prenatal screening, especially in terms of Down or fragile X syndrome; use of folic acid supplements to prevent neural tube defects during pregnancy and during the childbearing years; newborn screening for treatable inborn errors of metabolism, such as congenital hypothyroidism, phenylketonuria, and galactosemia; and early appropriate therapies and rehabilitation services for children with developmental disabilities.

DOWN SYNDROME

Down syndrome is the most common chromosomal abnormality of a generalized syndrome, occurring in 1 in 691 to 1000 live births (National Down Syndrome Society, 2011b; Weijerman and de Winter, 2010). It occurs in people of all races and economic levels.

Etiology

The cause of Down syndrome is not known, but evidence from cytogenetic and epidemiologic studies supports the concept of multiple causality. Approximately 95% of all cases of Down syndrome are attributable to an extra chromosome 21 (group G), thus the name nonfamilial trisomy 21 (National Down Syndrome Society, 2011b; Walker and Johnson, 2006). Although children with trisomy 21 are born to parents of all ages, there is a statistically greater risk in older women, particularly those older than 35 years of age. For example, in women 35 years of age, the chance of conceiving a child with Down

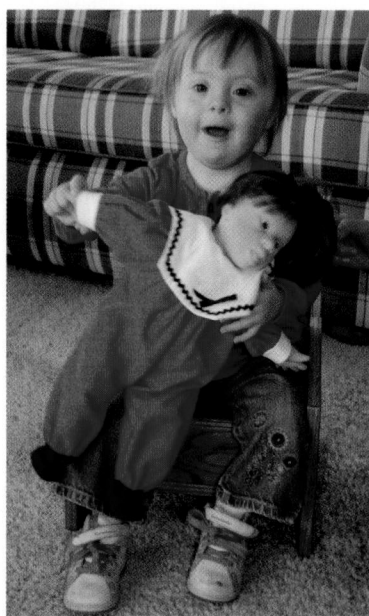

FIG. 19-6 Down syndrome in an infant. Note the infant's small, square head with upward slant to the eyes; flat nasal bridge; protruding tongue; mottled skin; and hypotonia.

syndrome is about 1 in 350 live births, but in women age 40 years, it is about 1 in 100. However, the majority (≈80%) of infants with Down syndrome are born to women younger than age 35 years because younger women have higher fertility rates (National Down Syndrome Society, 2011b). About 3% to 4% of the cases may be caused by translocation of chromosomes 15 and 21 or 22. This type of genetic aberration is usually hereditary and is not associated with advanced parental age. From 1% to 2% of affected persons demonstrate mosaicism, which refers to a mixture of normal and abnormal cell types. The degree of cognitive and physical impairment is related to the percentage of cells with the abnormal chromosome makeup.

Diagnostic Evaluation

Down syndrome can usually be diagnosed by the clinical manifestations alone (Box 19-3 and Fig. 19-6), but a chromosome analysis should be done to confirm the genetic abnormality.

Several physical problems are associated with Down syndrome. Many of these children have congenital heart malformations, the most common being septal defects. Respiratory tract infections are prevalent and, when combined with cardiac anomalies, are the chief causes of death, particularly during the first year of life. Hypotonicity of chest and abdominal muscles and dysfunction of the immune system probably predispose the child to the development of respiratory tract infection. Other physical problems include thyroid dysfunction, especially congenital hypothyroidism, and an increased incidence of leukemia.

Therapeutic Management

Although no cure exists for Down syndrome, a number of therapies are advocated, such as surgery to correct serious congenital anomalies (e.g., heart defects, strabismus). These children also benefit from evaluative echocardiography soon after birth and regular medical care. Evaluation of sight and hearing is essential, and treatment of otitis media is required to prevent auditory loss, which can influence cognitive function. Periodic testing of thyroid function is recommended, especially if growth is severely delayed. Children participating in sports

BOX 19-3   CLINICAL MANIFESTATIONS OF DOWN SYNDROME

Head and Eyes
Separated sagittal suture*
Brachycephaly
Rounded and small skull
Flat occiput
Enlarged anterior fontanel
Oblique palpebral fissures (upward, outward slant)*
Inner epicanthal folds
Speckling of iris (Brushfield spots)

Nose and Ears
Small nose*
Depressed nasal bridge (saddle nose)*
Small ears and narrow canals
Short pinna (vertical ear length)
Overlapping upper helices
Conductive hearing loss

Mouth and Neck
High, arched, narrow palate*
Protruding tongue
Hypoplastic mandible
Delayed teeth eruption and microdontia
Alignment teeth abnormalities common
Periodontal disease
Neck skin excess and laxity*
Short and broad neck

Chest and Heart
Shortened rib cage
Twelfth rib anomalies
Pectus excavatum or carinatum
Congenital heart defects common (e.g., atrial septal defect, ventricular septal defect)

Abdomen and Genitalia
Protruding, lax, and flabby abdominal muscles
Diastasis recti abdominis
Umbilical hernia
Small penis
Cryptorchidism
Bulbous vulva

Hands and Feet
Broad, short hands and stubby fingers
Incurved little finger (clinodactyly)
Transverse palmar crease
Wide space between big and second toes*
Plantar crease between big and second toes*
Broad, short feet and stubby toes

Musculoskeleton and Skin
Short stature
Hyperflexibility and muscle weakness*
Hypotonia
Atlantoaxial instability
Dry, cracked, and frequent fissuring
Cutis marmorata (mottling)

Other
Reduced birth weight
Learning difficulty (average intelligence quotient of 50)
Hypothyroidism common
Impaired immune function
Increased risk of leukemia
Early-onset dementia (in one third)

*Most common findings in modified chart (Pueschel, 1999).

that may involve stress on the head and neck, such as gymnastics, diving, butterfly stroke in swimming, high jump, and soccer, should be evaluated radiologically for atlantoaxial instability. Symptoms of the disorder include neck pain, weakness, and torticollis. Affected children are at risk for spinal cord compression.

! NURSING ALERT

Report immediately any child with the following signs of spinal cord compression:
• Persistent neck pain
• Loss of established motor skills and bladder or bowel control
• Changes in sensation

Prognosis

Life expectancy for those with Down syndrome has improved in recent years but remains lower than for the general population. More than 80% survive to age 60 years and beyond (National Down Syndrome Society, 2011b; Weijerman and de Winter, 2010). As the prognosis continues to improve for these individuals, it will be important to provide for their long-term health care and social and leisure needs.

Nursing Care Management
Support Family at Time of Diagnosis

Because of the unique physical characteristics, infants with Down syndrome are usually diagnosed at birth, and parents should be informed of the diagnosis at this time. Parents usually prefer that both of them be present during the informing interview so they can support one another emotionally. They appreciate receiving reading material about the syndrome* and being referred to others for help or advice, such as parent groups or professional counseling.

After parents are aware of the diagnosis, they are confronted with the crisis of losing their perfect or dream child and grieving for and accepting their reality child. Consequently, the parents' responses to the child may greatly influence decisions regarding future care. Whereas some families willingly take the child home, others consider immediate residential placement. The nurse must carefully answer questions

*Sources of information include the Arc of the United States (see footnote, p. 573); the AAIDD, 444 N. Capitol Street NW, Suite 846, Washington, DC 20001-1512; 800-424-3688; fax: 202-387-2193; http://www.aamr.org; the National Down Syndrome Society (see footnote, p. 573); and the National Down Syndrome Congress, 1370 Center Drive, Suite 102, Atlanta, GA 30338; 800-232-6372 or 770-604-9500; http://www.ndsccenter.org.

CRITICAL THINKING CASE STUDY

Diagnosis of Down Syndrome

The parents of Melissa, a newborn diagnosed as having Down syndrome, ask the nurse, "What are we supposed to do with her?" They further state that they already have three other children at home.

Questions

1. Evidence—Is there sufficient evidence to draw conclusions about the parents' concerns regarding their newborn daughter?
2. Assumptions—Describe an underlying assumption about each of the following:
   a. Newborn diagnosed with Down syndrome
   b. Parental care of a newborn with Down syndrome
   c. Newborn with Down syndrome and older siblings
3. What priorities for the nursing response should be established?
4. Does the evidence support your nursing intervention?

regarding developmental potential. Institutionalization is no longer an option. For families unable or unready to choose taking the newborn home, specialized foster care and adoption are other options (see Critical Thinking Case Study box).

Assist Family in Preventing Physical Problems

Many of the physical characteristics of infants with Down syndrome present nursing problems. The hypotonicity of muscles and hyperextensibility of joints complicate positioning. The limp, flaccid extremities resemble the posture of a rag doll; as a result, holding the infant is difficult and cumbersome. Sometimes parents perceive this lack of molding to their bodies as evidence of inadequate parenting. The extended body position promotes heat loss because more surface area is exposed to the environment. Parents are encouraged to swaddle or wrap the infant tightly in a blanket before picking up the child to provide security and warmth. The nurse also discusses with parents their feelings concerning attachment to the child, emphasizing that the child's lack of clinging or molding is a physical characteristic, not a sign of detachment or rejection.

Decreased muscle tone compromises respiratory expansion. In addition, the underdeveloped nasal bone causes a chronic problem of inadequate drainage of mucus. The constant stuffy nose forces the child to breathe by mouth, which dries the oropharyngeal membranes, increasing the susceptibility to upper respiratory tract infections. Measures to lessen these problems include clearing the nose with a bulb-type syringe, rinsing the mouth with water after feedings, increasing fluid intake, and using a cool-mist vaporizer to keep the mucous membranes moist and the secretions liquefied. Other helpful measures include changing the child's position frequently, performing postural drainage with percussion if necessary, practicing good hand washing, and properly disposing of soiled articles such as tissues. If antibiotics are ordered, the nurse stresses the importance of completing the full course of therapy for successful eradication of the infection and prevention of growth of resistant organisms.

Inadequate drainage resulting in pooling of mucus in the nose also interferes with feeding. Because the child breathes by mouth, sucking for any length of time is difficult. When eating solids, the child may gag on the food because of mucus in the oropharynx. Parents are advised to clear the nose before each feeding; give small, frequent feedings; and allow opportunities for rest during mealtime.

The protruding tongue also interferes with feeding, especially of solid foods. Parents need to know that the tongue thrust is not an indication of refusal to feed but a physiologic response. Parents are advised to use a small but long, straight-handled spoon to push the food toward the back and side of the mouth. If food is thrust out, it should be refed.

Dietary intake needs supervision. Decreased muscle tone affects gastric motility, predisposing the child to constipation. Dietary measures such as increased fiber and fluid promote evacuation. The child's eating habits may need careful scrutiny to prevent obesity. Height and weight measurements should be obtained on a serial basis, especially during infancy. Because these children grow more slowly than the general pediatric population's trends, special growth charts developed for these children should be used (AAP, Committee on Genetics, 2001; National Down Syndrome Society, 2011c).

During infancy, the child's skin is pliable and soft. However, it gradually becomes rough and dry and is prone to cracking and infection. Skin care involves the use of minimum soap and application of lubricants. Lip balm is applied to the lips, especially when the child is outdoors, to prevent excessive chapping.

Assist in Prenatal Diagnosis and Genetic Counseling

Prenatal diagnosis of Down syndrome is possible through chorionic villus sampling and amniocentesis because chromosome analysis of fetal cells can detect the presence of trisomy or translocation. However, analysis will not identify sporadic cases in young women when there is no indication for prenatal testing. Testing for low maternal serum α-fetoprotein, high chorionic gonadotropin, low unconjugated estriol levels, maternal serum fetal cell markers, and measurement of the first trimester nuchal transparency ultrasound marker may identify an affected fetus in women, who can then undergo amniocentesis (Bahado-Singh and Argoti, 2010; Benn and Chapman, 2009; National Down Syndrome Society, 2011b).

Prenatal testing and genetic counseling should be offered to women of advanced maternal age and those who have a family history of the disorder. If prenatal testing indicates that the fetus is affected, the nurse must allow the parents to express their feelings concerning elective abortion and support their decision to terminate or proceed with the pregnancy.

FRAGILE X SYNDROME

Fragile X syndrome is the most common inherited cause of CI and the second most common genetic cause of CI after Down syndrome. It has been described in all ethnic groups and races; the incidence of affected boys is 1 in 3600, the incidence of affected girls is 1 in 4000 to 6000, the incidence of carrier girls is 1 in 100 to 260, and the incidence of carrier boys is 1 in 250 to 800 worldwide (Hagerman, 2008; National Fragile X Foundation, 2010).

The syndrome is caused by an abnormal gene on the lower end of the long arm of the X chromosome. Chromosome analysis may demonstrate a fragile site (a region that fails to condense during mitosis and is characterized by a nonstaining gap or narrowing) in the cells of affected males and females and in carrier females. This fragile site has been determined to be caused by a gene mutation that results in excessive repeats of nucleotide in a specific deoxyribonucleic acid (DNA) segment of the X chromosome. The number of repeats in a normal individual is between 6 and 50. An individual with 50 to 200 base-pair repeats is said to have a permutation and is therefore a carrier. When passed from a parent to a child, these base-pair repeats can expand from 200 or more, which is termed a full mutation. This expansion occurs only when a carrier mother passes the mutation to her

BOX 19-4   CLINICAL MANIFESTATIONS OF FRAGILE X SYNDROME

Physical Features

Increased head circumference
Long, wide, or protruding ears
Long, narrow face with prominent jaw
Strabismus
Mitral valve prolapse, aortic root dilation
Hypotonia
Enlarged testicles (postpubertally)

Behavioral Features

Mild to severe cognitive impairment
Speech delay; may be rapid speech with stuttering and word repetition
Short attention span, hyperactivity
Hypersensitivity to taste, sounds, touch
Intolerance to change in routine
Autistic-like behaviors such as social anxiety and gaze aversion

offspring; it does not occur when a carrier father passes the mutation to his daughters.

The inheritance pattern has been termed X-linked dominant with reduced penetrance. This is in distinct contrast to the classic X-linked recessive pattern in which all carrier females are normal, all affected males have symptoms of the disorder, and no males are carriers. Consequently, genetic counseling of affected families is more complex than that for families with a classic X-linked disorder, such as hemophilia. Prenatal diagnosis of the fragile X gene mutation is now possible with direct DNA testing in a family with an established history using amniocentesis or chorionic villus sampling (National Fragile X Foundation, 2010). Both affected sexes are capable of transmitting the fragile X disorder.

Clinical Manifestations

The classic trend of physical findings in adult men with fragile X syndrome consists of a long face with a prominent jaw (prognathism); large, protruding ears; and large testes (macroorchidism). In prepubertal children, however, these features may be less obvious, and behavioral manifestations may initially suggest the diagnosis (Box 19-4). In carrier females, the clinical manifestations are extremely varied.

Therapeutic Management

Fragile X syndrome has no cure. Medical treatment may include the use of serotonin agents such as carbamazepine (Tegretol) or fluoxetine (Prozac) to control violent temper outbursts and the use of central nervous system stimulants or clonidine (Catapres) to improve attention span and decrease hyperactivity. Protein replacement and gene therapy are treatment options that are being investigated (Kuehn, 2011).

All affected children require referral to early intervention program (speech and language therapy, occupational therapy, and special education assistance) and multidisciplinary assessment, including cardiology, neurology, and orthopedic anomalies.

Prognosis

Individuals with fragile X syndrome are expected to live a normal life span. Their CI may be improved by behavioral and educational interventions that usually begin in preschool-age children.

Nursing Care Management

Because CI is a fairly consistent finding in individuals with fragile X syndrome, the care given to these families is the same as for any child with CI. Because the disorder is hereditary, genetic counseling is necessary to inform parents and siblings of the risks of transmission. In addition, any male or female with unexplained or nonspecific mental impairment should be referred for genetic testing and, if needed, counseling. Families with a member affected by the disorder should be referred to the National Fragile X Foundation.*

SENSORY IMPAIRMENT

HEARING IMPAIRMENT

Hearing impairment is one of the most common disabilities in the United States. An estimated one to six per 1000 well infants have hearing loss of varying degrees (AAP, Task Force on Newborn and Infant Hearing, 1999; Gifford, Holmes, and Bernstein, 2009). For infants admitted to neonatal intensive care units, the incidence rises sharply to approximately two to four per 100 neonates (AAP, Task Force on Newborn and Infant Hearing, 1999). In the United States, there are about 1 million children with hearing impairment ranging in age from birth to 21 years, and almost one third of these children have other disabilities, such as visual or cognitive deficits.

Definition and Classification

Hearing impairment is a general term indicating disability that may range in severity from slight to profound hearing loss. *Slight to moderately severe hearing loss* describes a person who has residual hearing sufficient to enable successful processing of linguistic information through audition, generally with the use of a hearing aid. *Severe to profound hearing loss* describes a person whose hearing disability precludes successful processing of linguistic information through audition with or without a hearing aid. Hearing-impaired persons who are speech impaired tend not to have a physical speech defect other than that caused by the inability to hear.

Hearing defects may be classified according to etiology, pathology, or symptom severity. Each is important in terms of treatment, possible prevention, and rehabilitation.

Etiology

Hearing loss may be caused by a number of prenatal and postnatal conditions. These include a family history of childhood hearing impairment, anatomic malformations of the head or neck, low birth weight, severe perinatal asphyxia, perinatal infection (cytomegalovirus, rubella, herpes, syphilis, toxoplasmosis, bacterial meningitis), chronic ear infection, cerebral palsy, Down syndrome, prolonged neonatal oxygen supplementation or administration of ototoxic drugs (Botelho, Bouzada, de Resende, and others, 2010; Haddad, 2007; Robertson, Howarth, Bork, and others, 2009; Weijerman and de Winter, 2010).

In addition, high-risk neonates who survive formerly fatal prenatal or perinatal conditions may be susceptible to hearing loss from the disorder or its treatment. For example, sensorineural hearing loss may be a result of continuous humming noises or high noise levels associated with incubators, oxygen hoods, or intensive care units, especially when combined with the use of potentially ototoxic antibiotics.

*PO Box 37, Walnut Creek, CA 94597; 800-688-8765 or 925-938-9300; fax: 925-938-9315; http://www.fragilex.org.

Environmental noise is a special concern. Sounds loud enough to damage sensitive hair cells of the inner ear can produce irreversible hearing loss. Very loud, brief noise, such as gunfire, can cause immediate, severe, and permanent loss of hearing. Longer exposure to less intense but still hazardous sounds, such as loud persistent music via headphones, sound systems, concerts, or industrial noises, may also produce hearing loss (Daniel, 2007; Henderson, Testa, and Hartnick, 2011). Loud noises combined with the toxic substances such as smoking or secondhand smoke produce a synergistic effect on hearing that causes hearing loss (Fabry, Davila, Arheart, and others, 2011; Mohammadi, Mazhari, Mehrparvar, and others, 2009).

Pathology

Disorders of hearing are divided according to the location of the defect. Conductive or middle-ear hearing loss results from interference of transmission of sound to the middle ear. It is the most common of all types of hearing loss and most frequently a result of recurrent serous otitis media. Conductive hearing impairment involves mainly interference with loudness of sound.

Sensorineural hearing loss involves damage to the inner ear structures or the auditory nerve. The most common causes are congenital defects of inner ear structures or consequences of acquired conditions, such as kernicterus, infection, administration of ototoxic drugs, or exposure to excessive noise. Sensorineural hearing loss results in distortion of sound and problems in discrimination. Although the child hears some of everything going on around him or her, the sounds are distorted, severely affecting discrimination and comprehension.

Mixed conductive-sensorineural hearing loss results from interference with transmission of sound in the middle ear and along neural pathways. It frequently results from recurrent otitis media and its complications.

Central auditory imperception includes all hearing losses that are not linked to defects in the conductive or sensorineural structures. They are usually divided into organic or functional losses. In the organic type of central auditory imperception, the defect involves the reception of auditory stimuli along the central pathways and the expression of the message into meaningful communication. Examples are aphasia, the inability to express ideas in any form, either written or verbal; agnosia, the inability to interpret sound correctly; and dysacusis, difficulty in processing details or discriminating among sounds. In the functional type of hearing loss, no organic lesion exists to explain a central auditory loss. Examples of functional hearing loss are conversion hysteria (an unconscious withdrawal from hearing to block remembrance of a traumatic event), infantile autism, and childhood schizophrenia.

Symptom Severity

Hearing impairment is expressed in terms of a decibel (dB), a unit of loudness (Table 19-2); hearing is measured at various frequencies, such as 500, 1000, and 2000 cycles/sec, the critical listening speech range. Hearing impairment can be classified according to hearing threshold level (the measurement of an individual's hearing threshold by means of an audiometer) and the degree of symptom severity as it affects speech (Table 19-3). These classifications offer only general guidelines regarding the effect of the impairment on any individual child because children differ greatly in their ability to use residual hearing.

Therapeutic Management
Conductive Hearing Loss

Treatment of hearing loss depends on the cause and type of hearing impairment. Many conductive hearing defects respond to medical or

TABLE 19-2	INTENSITY OF SOUNDS EXPRESSED IN DECIBELS
DECIBELS	**REPRESENTATIVE SOUND**
0	Softest sound normal ear can hear
10	Heartbeat, rustling of leaves
20	Whisper at 1.5 m (5 feet)
30–45	Normal conversation
60	Noise in average restaurant
70–80	Street noises
80	Loud radio in home
90–100	Train
120	Thunder, loud music (e.g., rock concerts)
140	Jet plane during departure
>140	Pain threshold

TABLE 19-3	CLASSIFICATION OF HEARING IMPAIRMENT BASED ON SYMPTOM SEVERITY
HEARING LEVEL (dB)	**EFFECT**
Slight—16–25	Has difficulty hearing faint or distant speech
	Usually is unaware of hearing difficulty
	Likely to achieve in school but may have problems
	No speech defects
Mild to moderate—26–55	May have speech difficulties
	Understands face-to-face conversational speech at 0.9–1.5 m (3–5 ft)
Moderately severe—56–70	Unable to understand conversational speech unless loud
	Considerable difficulty with group or classroom discussion
	Requires special speech training
Severe—71–90	May hear a loud voice if nearby
	May be able to identify loud environmental noises
	Can distinguish vowels but not most consonants
	Requires speech training
Profound—91	May hear only loud sounds
	Requires extensive speech training

dB, Decibels.

surgical treatment, such as antibiotic therapy for acute otitis media or insertion of tympanostomy tubes for chronic otitis media. When the conductive loss is permanent, hearing can be improved with the use of a hearing aid to amplify sound.

The nurse should be familiar with the types, basic care, and handling of hearing aids, especially when the child is hospitalized.* Types of aids include those worn in or behind the ear, models incorporated into an eyeglass frame, and types worn on the body with a wire connection to the ear (Fig. 19-7). One of the most common problems with a hearing aid is acoustic feedback, an annoying whistling sound usually caused by improper fit of the ear mold. Sometimes the whistling may be at a frequency that the child cannot hear but that is

---

*Information about hearing aids is available from the International Hearing Society, 16880 Middlebelt Road, Suite 4, Livonia, MI 48154; 800-521-5247 or 734-522-7200; fax: 734-522-0200; http://ihsinfo.org.

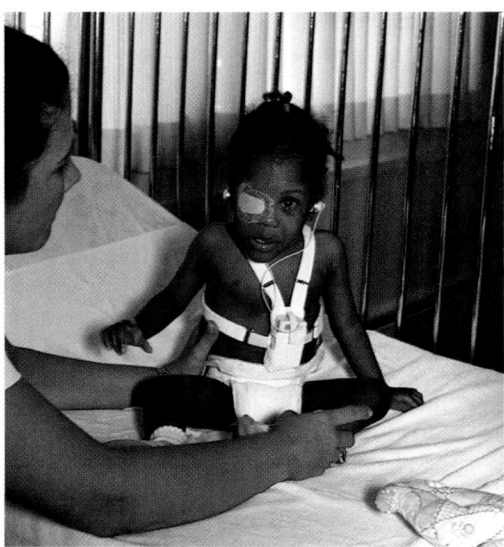

FIG. 19-7 On-the-body hearing aids are convenient for young children, such as this child with severe bilateral hearing loss. Note eye patching for strabismus.

annoying to others. In this case, if children are old enough, they are told of the noise and asked to readjust the aid.

> **NURSING TIP** To reduce or eliminate whistling from a hearing aid, try removing and reinserting the aid, making certain that no hair is caught between the ear mold and the canal, cleaning the ear mold or ear, or lowering the volume of the aid.

As children grow older, they may be self-conscious about the device. Effort may be made to make the aid inconspicuous, such as styling the hair to cover behind-the-ear or in-the-ear models and encourage the use of attractive frames for glasses with connected hearing aids. Give children responsibility for the care of the device as soon as they are able because fostering independence is a primary goal of rehabilitation.

> **⚠ NURSING ALERT**
>
> Stress to parents the importance of storing batteries for hearing aids in a safe location out of reach of children and teaching children not to remove the battery from the hearing aid (or supervising young children when they do so). Battery ingestion requires immediate emergency management.

Sensorineural Hearing Loss

Treatment for sensorineural hearing loss is much less satisfactory. Because the defect is not one of intensity of sound, hearing aids are of less value in this type of defect. The use of **cochlear implants*** (a surgically implanted prosthetic device) provides a sensation of hearing for individuals who have severe or profound hearing loss (Gifford, Holmes, and Bernstein, 2009; Zeng and Liu, 2006). Children with sensorineural hearing loss have lost or damaged some or all of their hair cells or auditory nerve fibers. Often these children cannot benefit from

*Hearing Enrichment Language Program of the Hough Ear Institute, 3434 N.W. 56th St., Oklahoma City, OK 73112; 405-945-7186; fax: 405-947-6266; http://www.integris-health.com/INTEGRIS/en-US/Specialties/EarInstitute/HELP.

conventional hearing aids because they only amplify sound that cannot be processed by a damaged inner ear. A cochlear implant bypasses the hair cells to directly stimulate surviving auditory nerve fibers so that they can send signals to the brain. These signals can be interpreted by the brain to produce sound and sensations (Baldassari, Schmidt, Schubert, and others, 2009; Gifford, Holmes, and Bernstein, 2009).

Multichanneled implants are now available. This more sophisticated device stimulates the auditory nerve at a number of locations with differently processed signals. This type of stimulation allows a person to use the pitch information present in speech signals, leading to better understanding of speech. The trend is toward early use of cochlear implants, usually by 18 months of age, to give the child maximum opportunity to develop listening, language, and speaking skills.

Nursing Care Management

Assessment of children for hearing impairment is a critical nursing responsibility. Identification of hearing loss within the first 3 to 6 months of life is essential to improve the language and educational outcomes for children with hearing impairments (Gifford, Holmes, and Bernstein, 2009; Tierney and Brown, 2008). The Joint Committee on Infant Hearing (2000) issued guidelines on auditory screening of newborns and infants to detect early hearing loss and implement intervention programs. Auditory testing is presented in Chapter 6.

At birth, the nurse can observe the neonate's response to auditory stimuli, as evidenced by the startle reflex, head turning, eye blinking, and cessation of body movement. The infant may vary in the intensity of the response, depending on the state of alertness. However, a consistent absence of a reaction should lead to suspicion of hearing loss. Box 19-5 summarizes other clinical manifestations of hearing impairment in infants.

Children who are profoundly hearing impaired are much more likely to be diagnosed during infancy than less severely affected ones. If the defect is not detected during early childhood, it likely will become evident during entry into school, when the child has difficulty learning. Unfortunately, some of these children are mistakenly placed in special classes for students with learning disabilities or CI. Therefore, it is essential that the nurse suspect a hearing impairment in any child who demonstrates the behaviors listed in Box 19-5.

> **⚠ NURSING ALERT**
>
> When parents express concern about their child's hearing and speech development, refer the child for a hearing evaluation. Absence of well-formed syllables (*da, na, yaya*) by 11 months of age should result in immediate referral.

During early childhood, the primary importance of hearing impairment is the effect on speech development. A child with a mild conductive hearing loss may speak fairly clearly but in a loud, monotone voice. A child with a sensorineural defect usually has difficulty in articulation. The toddler will need guidance on how to play with others, and safety issues must be considered. Communication may be difficult, leading to frustration when words are not understood. For example, an inability to hear higher frequencies may result in the word *spoon* being pronounced "poon." Children with articulation problems need to have their hearing tested.

Lipreading

Even though the child may become an expert at lipreading, only about 40% of the spoken word is understood, less if the speaker has an accent,

BOX 19-5 CLINICAL MANIFESTATIONS OF HEARING IMPAIRMENT

Infants

Lack of startle or blink reflex to a loud sound
Failure to be awakened by loud environmental noises
Failure to localize a source of sound by 6 months of age
Absence of babble or voice inflections by age 7 months
Lack of response to the spoken word; failure to follow verbal directions
Response to loud noises as opposed to the voice

Children

Use of gestures rather than verbalization to express desires, especially after age 15 months
Failure to develop intelligible speech by age 24 months
Monotone and unintelligible speech; lessened laughter
Vocal play, head banging, or foot stamping for vibratory sensation
Yelling or screeching to express pleasure, needs, or annoyance
Asking to have statements repeated or answering them incorrectly
Greater response to facial expression and gestures than to verbal explanation
Avoidance of social interaction; prefer to play alone
Inquiring, sometimes confused facial expression
Suspicious alertness alternating with cooperation
Frequently stubbornness because of lack of comprehension
Irritability at not making themselves understood
Shy, timid, and withdrawn behavior
Frequently appear "dreamy" or "in a world of their own" or exhibit inattentiveness

mustache, or beard. Exaggerating pronunciation or speaking in an altered rhythm further reduces comprehension. Parents can help the child understand the spoken word by using the suggestions in the Nursing Care Guidelines box. The child learns to supplement the spoken word with sensitivity to visual cues, primarily body language and facial expression (e.g., tightening the lips, muscle tension, eye contact). Health care providers should consider not putting on the surgical mask if a child with hearing impairment is able to lipread. Someone who is able to translate using sign language should always be with the child.

Cued Speech

This method of communication is an adjunct to straight lipreading. It uses hand signals to help the child with a hearing impairment distinguish between words that look alike when formed by the lips (e.g., mat, bat). It is most often used by children with hearing impairments who are using speech rather than those who are nonverbal.

Sign Language

Sign language, such as **American Sign Language (ASL)** or **British Sign Language (BSL)**, is a visual gestural language that uses hand signals that roughly correspond to specific words and concepts in the English language. Family members are encouraged to learn signing because using or watching hands requires much less concentration than lipreading or talking. Also, a symbol method enables some children to learn more and to learn faster.

Speech Language Therapy

The most formidable task in the education of a child who is profoundly hearing impaired is learning to speak. Speech is learned through a multisensory approach using visual, tactile, kinesthetic, and auditory stimulation. Parents are encouraged to participate fully in the learning process.

Additional Aids

Everyday activities present problems for older children with hearing impairment. For example, they may not be able to hear the telephone, doorbell, or alarm clock. Several commercial devices are available to help them adjust to these dilemmas. Flashing lights can be attached to a telephone or doorbell to signal its ringing. Trained hearing ear dogs can provide great assistance because they alert the person to sounds, such as someone approaching, a moving car, a signal to wake up, or a child's cry. Special **teletypewriters** or **telecommunications devices for the deaf (TDD or TTY)** help people with impaired hearing communicate with each other over the telephone; the typed message is conveyed via the telephone lines and displayed on a small screen.*

Any audiovisual medium presents dilemmas for these children, who can see the picture but cannot hear the message. However, with **closed captioning** a special decoding device is attached to the television, and the audio portion of a program is translated into subtitles that appear on the screen.†

Socialization

As children learn to compensate for their lack of hearing, they become extremely perceptive to visual and vibratory changes. Children often know when another person wants to talk to them because the person will walk close by but not pass. They learn to be alert to other people approaching them by seeing their shadows or feeling the vibrations of their footsteps. They are acutely aware of facial expressions and may comprehend unspoken messages more quickly than the spoken word.

Socialization is extremely important to children's development. If children attend a special school for the hearing impaired, they are able to socialize with peers in that setting. Classmates become a potential source of close friendships because they communicate more easily among themselves. Encourage parents to promote these relationships whenever possible.

Children with a hearing impairment may need special help with school or social activities. For children wearing hearing aids, background noise should be kept to a minimum. Because many of these children are able to attend regular classes, the teacher may need assistance in adapting methods of teaching for the child's benefit. The school nurse is often in an optimal position to emphasize methods of facilitated communication, such as lipreading (see Nursing Care Guidelines box). Because group projects and audiovisual teaching aids may hinder the child's learning, these educational methods should be carefully evaluated.

In a group setting, it is helpful for the other members to sit in a semicircle in front of the child. Because one of the difficulties in following a group discussion is that the child is unaware of who will speak next, someone should point out each speaker. Speakers can also be given numbers, or their names can be written down as each person

---

*Other sources of information on several aspects of hearing loss and on the International Parents' Organization are the Alexander Graham Bell Association for the Deaf and Hard of Hearing, 3417 Volta Place NW, Washington, DC 20007; voice: 202-337-5220; TTY: 202-337-5221; fax: 202-337-8314; http://www.agbell.org; and Canadian Hearing Society, 271 Spadina Road, Toronto, ON M5R 2V3; voice: 416-928-2500; TTY: 416-964-0023; fax: 416-928-2506; http://www.chs.ca.

†Additional information is available from the National Captioning Institute, 3725 Concord Pkwy., Suite 100, Chantilly, VA 20151; voice/TTY: 703-917-7600; fax: 703-917-9853; http://www.ncicap.org.

NURSING CARE GUIDELINES

Facilitating Lipreading

Attract child's attention before speaking; use light touch to signal speaker's presence.

Stand close to child.

Face child directly or move to a 45-degree angle.

Stand still; do not walk back and forth or turn away to point or look elsewhere.

Establish eye contact and show interest.

Speak at eye level and with good lighting on speaker's face.

Be certain nothing interferes with speech patterns, such as chewing food or gum.

Speak clearly and at a slow and even rate.

Use facial expression to assist in conveying messages.

Keep sentences short.

Rephrase message if child does not understand the words.

CRITICAL THINKING CASE STUDY

Hearing Impairment

Four-year-old Jason has a severe congenital hearing impairment. Jason has been admitted to the outpatient surgery PACU after a herniorrhaphy and regional block. As he emerges from anesthesia, he becomes more and more agitated.

Questions

1. Evidence—Is there sufficient evidence to draw conclusions about Jason's increasing agitation after surgery?
2. Assumptions—Describe an underlying assumption about each of the following:
   a. Severe congenital hearing impairment in a preschool child
   b. Preschooler with severe congenital hearing impairment awakening in the PACU after surgery
   c. Preschooler with severe congenital hearing impairment awakening from herniorrhaphy and after regional block
3. What priorities for nursing care should be established for Jason?
4. Does the evidence support your nursing intervention?

PACU, Postanesthesia care unit.

talks. If one person writes down the main topic of the discussion, the child is able to follow lipreading more closely. Such suggestions can increase the child's ability to participate in sports, organizations such as Scouts, and group projects.

Support Child and Family

After the diagnosis of hearing impairment is made, parents need extensive support to adjust to the shock of learning about their child's disability and an opportunity to realize the extent of the hearing loss. If the hearing loss occurs during childhood, the child also requires sensitive, supportive care during the long and often difficult adjustment to this sensory loss. Early rehabilitation is one of the best strategies for fostering adjustment. However, progress in learning communication may not always coincide with emotional adjustment. Depression or anger is common, and such feelings are a normal part of the grieving process. (See also Chapter 18 for an extensive discussion of the emotional support of the child and family.)

Care for the Child During Hospitalization

The needs of the hospitalized child with impaired hearing are the same as those of any other child, but the disability presents special challenges to the nurse (see Critical Thinking Case Study box). For example, verbal explanations must be supplemented by tactile and visual aids, such as books or actual demonstration and practice. Children's understanding of the explanation needs to be constantly reassessed. If their verbal skills are poorly developed, they can answer questions through drawing, writing, or gesturing. For example, if the nurse is attempting to clarify where a spinal tap is done, the child is asked to point to where the procedure will be done on the body. Because these children often need more time to grasp the full meaning of an explanation, the nurse needs to be patient, allowing ample time for understanding.

When communicating with the child, the nurse should use the same principles as those outlined for facilitating lipreading. Ideally, nurses without foreign accents should be assigned to the child. The child's hearing aid is checked to ensure that it is working properly. If it is necessary to awaken the child at night, the nurse should gently shake the child or turn on the hearing aid before arousing the child. The nurse should always make certain that the child can see him or her before any procedures, even routine ones such as changing a diaper or regulating an infusion. It is important to remember that the child may not be aware of one's presence until alerted through visual or tactile cues.

Ideally, parents are encouraged to room with the child. However, it must be conveyed to them that this is not to serve as a convenience to the nurse but as a benefit to the child. Although the parents' aid can be enlisted in familiarizing the child with the hospital and explaining procedures, the nurse also talks directly to the youngster, encouraging expression of feelings about the experience. If the child's speech is difficult to understand, the nurse makes an effort to become familiar with his or her pronunciation of words. Parents often can be helpful by explaining the child's usual speech habits. Nonverbal communication devices that use pictures or words that the child can point to are also available. Such boards can also be made by drawing pictures or writing the words of common needs on cardboard, such as *parent, food, water,* or *toilet.*

The nurse has a special role as child advocate and is in a strategic position to alert other health team members and other patients to the child's special needs regarding communication. For example, the nurse should accompany other practitioners on visits to the child's room to ensure that they speak to the child and that the child understands what is said. Caregivers sometimes forget that the child has the abilities to perceive and learn despite a hearing loss, and consequently they communicate only with the parents. As a result, the child's needs and feelings remain unrecognized and unmet.

Because children with impaired hearing may have difficulty forming social relationships with other children, the child is introduced to roommates and encouraged to engage in play activities. The hospital setting can provide growth-promoting opportunities for social relationships. With the assistance of a child life specialist, the child can learn new recreational activities, experiment with group games, and engage in therapeutic play. The use of puppets, dollhouses, role-playing with dress-up clothes, building with a hammer and nails, finger painting, and water play can help the child express feelings that previously were suppressed.

Assist in Measures to Prevent Hearing Impairment

A primary nursing role is prevention of hearing loss. Because the most common cause of impaired hearing is chronic otitis media, it is essential that appropriate measures be instituted to treat existing infections and prevent recurrences (see Chapter 23). Children with a history of ear or respiratory infections or any other condition known to increase the risk of hearing impairment should receive periodic auditory testing.

To prevent the causes of hearing loss that begin prenatally and perinatally, pregnant women need counseling regarding the necessity of early prenatal care, including genetic counseling for known familial disorders; avoidance of all ototoxic drugs, especially during the first trimester; tests to rule out syphilis, rubella, or blood incompatibility; medical management of maternal diabetes; strict control of alcohol intake; adequate dietary intake; and avoidance of smoke exposure. The necessity of routine immunization during childhood to eliminate the possibility of acquired sensorineural hearing loss from rubella, mumps, or measles (encephalitis) is stressed.

Excessive noise pollution is a well-established cause of sensorineural hearing loss. The nurse should routinely assess the possibility of environmental noise pollution and advise children and parents of the potential danger. When individuals engage in activities associated with high-intensity noise, such as flying model airplanes, target shooting, or snowmobiling, they should wear ear protection such as earmuffs or earplugs. Even common household equipment, such as lawn mowers, vacuum cleaners, and cordless telephones, can be harmful.

> **! NURSING ALERT**
>
> Suspect hazardous noise if the listener experiences (1) difficulty in communication while hearing the sound, (2) ringing in the ears (tinnitus) after exposure to the sound, or (3) muffled hearing after leaving the sound.

VISUAL IMPAIRMENT

Visual impairment is a common problem during childhood. In the United States, the prevalence of serious visual impairment in the pediatric population is estimated at 30 to 64 children per 100,000 population. Vision impairment such as refractive error, strabismus, and amblyopia occur in 5% to 10% of all preschoolers, who are usually identified through vision screening programs (Rahi, Cumberland,

Perkham, and others, 2010; Tingley, 2007; U.S. Preventive Services Task Force, 2011). The nurse's role is one of assessment, detection, prevention, referral, and (in some instances) rehabilitation.

Definition and Classification

Visual impairment is a general term that encompasses both partial sight and legal blindness. Partial sight or partial visual impairment is defined as a visual acuity between 20/70 and 20/200. The child can generally use normal-sized print because near vision is almost always better than distance vision. Legal blindness or severe permanent visual impairment is defined as a visual acuity of 20/200 or lower or a visual field of 20 degrees or less in the better eye. It is important to keep in mind that legal blindness is not a medical diagnosis but a legal definition. Educational and governmental agencies in the United States use the legal definition of blindness to determine tax status, eligibility for entrance into special schools, eligibility for financial aid, and other benefits.

Etiology

Visual impairment can be caused by a number of genetic and prenatal or postnatal conditions. These include perinatal infections (herpes, *Chlamydia*, gonococci, rubella, syphilis, toxoplasmosis); retinopathy of prematurity; trauma; postnatal infections (meningitis); and disorders such as sickle cell disease, juvenile rheumatoid arthritis, Tay-Sachs disease, albinism, and retinoblastoma. In many instances, such as with refractive errors, the cause of the defect is unknown.

Refractive errors are the most common types of visual disorders in children. The term refraction means bending and refers to the bending of light rays as they pass through the lens of the eye. Normally, light rays enter the lens and fall directly on the retina. However, in refractive disorders, the light rays either fall in front of the retina (myopia) or beyond it (hyperopia). Other eye problems, such as strabismus, may or may not include refractive errors, but they are important because, if untreated, they result in severe permanent visual impairment from amblyopia. These, along with other less frequent visual disorders, are summarized in Box 19-6. In addition to these disorders, other visual problems can be a result of infection or trauma.

BOX 19-6 TYPES OF VISUAL IMPAIRMENT

Refractive Errors

Myopia
Nearsightedness—Ability to see objects clearly at close range but not at a distance

Pathophysiology
Results from eyeball that is too long, causing images to fall in front of the retina

Clinical Manifestations
Headaches
Dizziness
Excessive eye rubbing
Head tilt or forward head thrusts
Difficulty in reading or doing other close work
Clumsiness; walking into objects
Blinking more than usual or irritability when doing close work
Inability to see objects clearly
Poor school performance, especially in subjects that require demonstration, such as arithmetic

Treatment
Corrected with biconcave lenses that focus rays on retina
May be corrected with laser surgery

Hyperopia
Farsightedness—Ability to see objects at a distance

Pathophysiology
Results from eyeball that is too short, causing image to focus beyond retina

Clinical Manifestations
Because of accommodative ability, child can usually see objects at all ranges
Most children normally hyperopic until about 7 years of age

Treatment
When required, corrected with convex lenses that focus rays on retina
May be corrected with laser surgery

Astigmatism
Unequal curvatures in refractive apparatus

BOX 19-6 TYPES OF VISUAL IMPAIRMENT—cont'd

Pathophysiology
Results from unequal curvatures in cornea or lens that cause light rays to bend in different directions

Clinical Manifestations
Depend on severity of refractive error in each eye
Possible clinical manifestations of myopia

Treatment
Corrected with special lenses that compensate for refractive errors
May be corrected with laser surgery

Anisometropia
Different refractive strength in each eye

Pathophysiology
May develop amblyopia as weaker eye is used less

Clinical Manifestations
Depend on severity of refractive error in each eye
Possible clinical manifestations of myopia

Treatment
Treated with corrective lenses, preferably contact lenses, to improve vision in each eye so they work as a unit
May be corrected with laser surgery

Amblyopia
Lazy eye—Reduced visual acuity in one eye

Pathophysiology
Results when one eye does not receive sufficient stimulation
Each retina receives different images, resulting in diplopia (double vision)
Brain accommodates by suppressing less intense image
Visual cortex eventually does not respond to visual stimulation, with resultant loss of vision in that eye

Clinical Manifestations
Poor vision in affected eye

Treatment
Preventable if treatment of primary visual defect, such as anisometropia or strabismus, begins before 6 years of age

Strabismus
"Squint" or malalignment of eyes
Esotropia—Inward deviation of eye
Exotropia—Outward deviation of eye

Pathophysiology
May result from muscle imbalance or paralysis, poor vision, or congenital defect
Because visual axes are not parallel, brain receives two images, and amblyopia can result

Clinical Manifestations
Squints eyelids together or frowns
Difficulty in focusing from one distance to another
Inaccurate judgment in picking up objects
Unable to see print or moving objects clearly
Closing one eye to see

Tilting head to one side
If combined with refractive errors, may see any of the manifestations listed for refractive errors
Diplopia
Photophobia
Dizziness
Headaches

Treatment
Depends on cause of strabismus
May involve occlusion therapy (patching stronger eye) or surgery to increase visual stimulation to weaker eye
Early diagnosis essential to prevent vision loss

Cataracts
Opacity of crystalline lens

Pathophysiology
Prevents light rays from entering eye and refracting on retina

Clinical Manifestations
Gradual decrease in ability to see objects clearly
Possible loss of peripheral vision
Nystagmus (with severe permanent visual impairment)
Gray opacities of lens
Strabismus
Absence of red reflex

Treatment
Requires surgery to remove cloudy lens and replace lens (with intraocular lens implant, removable contact lens, prescription glasses)
Must be treated early to prevent severe permanent visual impairment from amblyopia

Glaucoma
Increased intraocular pressure

Pathophysiology
Congenital type results from defective development of some component related to flow of aqueous humor
Increased pressure on optic nerve causes eventual atrophy and severe permanent visual impairment

Clinical Manifestations
Loss of peripheral vision—mostly seen in acquired types
Possible bumping into objects
Perception of halos around objects
Possible complaint of pain or discomfort (pain, nausea, or vomiting if sudden rise in pressure)
Eye redness
Excessive tearing (epiphora)
Photophobia
Spasmodic winking (blepharospasm)
Corneal haziness
Enlargement of eyeball (buphthalmos)

Treatment
Requires surgical treatment (goniotomy) to open outflow tracts
May require more than one procedure

Trauma

Trauma is a common cause of visual impairment in children. Injuries to the eyeball and adnexa (supporting or accessory structures, such as eyelids, conjunctiva, or lacrimal glands) can be classified as penetrating or nonpenetrating. Penetrating wounds are most often a result of sharp instruments, such as sticks, knives, or scissors, or propulsive objects, such as firecrackers, guns, arrows, or slingshots. Nonpenetrating injuries may be a result of foreign objects in the eyes, lacerations, a blow from a blunt object such as a ball (baseball, softball, basketball, racquet sports) or fist, or thermal or chemical burns.

Treatment is aimed at preventing further ocular damage and is primarily the responsibility of the ophthalmologist. It involves adequate examination of the injured eye (with the child sedated or anesthetized in severe injuries); appropriate immediate intervention, such as removal of the foreign body or suturing of the laceration; and prevention of complications, such as administration of antibiotics or steroids and complete bed rest to allow the eye to heal and blood to reabsorb (see Emergency Treatment box). The prognosis varies according to the type of injury. It is usually guarded in all cases of penetrating wounds because of the high risk of serious complications.

Infections

Infections of the adnexa and structures of the eyeball or globe may occur in children. The most common eye infection is conjunctivitis (see Chapter 14). Treatment is usually with ophthalmic antibiotics. Severe infections may require systemic antibiotic therapy. Steroids are used cautiously because they exacerbate viral infections such as herpes simplex, increasing the risk of damage to the involved structures.

Nursing Care Management

Assessment of children for visual impairment is a critical nursing responsibility. Discovery of a visual impairment as early as possible is essential to prevent social, physical, and psychologic damage to the child. Assessment involves (1) identifying those children who by virtue of their history are at risk, (2) observing for behaviors that indicate a vision loss, and (3) screening all children for visual acuity and signs of other ocular disorders such as strabismus. This discussion focuses on clinical manifestations of various types of visual problems (see Box 19-6). Vision testing is discussed in Chapter 6.

Infancy

At birth, the nurse should observe the neonate's response to visual stimuli, such as following a light or object and cessation of body movement. The infant may vary in the intensity of the response, depending on the state of alertness.

Of special importance in detecting visual impairment during infancy are the parents' concerns regarding visual responsiveness in their child. Their concerns, such as lack of eye contact from the infant, must be taken seriously. During infancy, the child should be tested for strabismus. Lack of binocularity after 4 months of age is considered abnormal and must be treated to prevent amblyopia.

> **! NURSING ALERT**
>
> Suspect visual impairment in an infant who does not react to light and in a child of any age if the parents express concern.

Childhood

Because the most common visual impairment during childhood is refractive errors, testing for visual acuity is essential. The school nurse

---

> **✚ EMERGENCY TREATMENT**
>
> ### Eye Injuries
>
> **Foreign Object**
> Examine eye for presence of a foreign body (evert upper eyelid to examine upper eye).
> Remove a freely movable object with pointed corner of gauze pad lightly moistened with water.
> Do not irrigate eye or attempt to remove a penetrating object (see Penetrating Injuries).
> Caution child against rubbing eye.
>
> **Chemical Burns**
> Irrigate eye copiously with tap water for 20 minutes.
> Evert upper eyelid to flush thoroughly.
> Hold child's head with eye under a tap of running lukewarm water.
> Take child to emergency department.
> Have child rest with eyes closed.
> Keep room darkened.
>
> **Ultraviolet Burns**
> If skin is burned, patch both eyes (make certain eyelids are completely closed); secure dressing with Kling bandages wrapped around head rather than with tape.
> Have child rest with eyes closed.
> Refer to an ophthalmologist.
>
> **Hematoma ("Black Eye")**
> Use a flashlight to check for gross hyphema (hemorrhage into anterior chamber; visible fluid meniscus across iris; more easily seen in light-colored than in brown eyes).
> Apply ice for first 24 hours to reduce swelling if no hyphema is present.
> Refer to an ophthalmologist immediately if hyphema is present.
> Have child rest with eyes closed.
>
> **Penetrating Injuries**
> Take child to emergency department.
> Never remove an object that has penetrated eye.
> Follow strict aseptic technique in examining eye.
> Observe for:
> - Aqueous or vitreous leaks (fluid leaking from point of penetration)
> - Hyphema
> - Shape and equality of pupils, reaction to light, prolapsed iris (not perfectly circular)
>
> Apply a Fox shield if available (not a regular eye patch) and apply patch over unaffected eye to prevent bilateral movement.
> Maintain bed rest with child in a 30-degree Fowler position.
> Caution child against rubbing eye.
> Refer to an ophthalmologist.

usually assumes major responsibility for vision testing in schoolchildren. Besides refractive errors, the nurse should be aware of signs and symptoms that indicate other ocular problems. If a referral is made to the family requesting further eye testing, the nurse is responsible for follow-up concerning the recommendation.

The shock of learning that their child has severe permanent visual impairment precipitates an immense crisis for families. The family is encouraged to investigate appropriate stimulation and educational programs for their child as soon as possible. Sources of information include state commissions for the visually impaired, local schools for children with visual impairments, the American Foundation for the Blind,* the National Federation of the Blind,† the National Association for Parents of Children with Visual Impairments,‡ the National Association for Visually Handicapped,§ the American Council of the Blind,‖ and CNIB.¶

Promote Parent–Child Attachment

A crucial time in the life of visual impaired infants is when they and their parents are getting acquainted with each other. Pleasurable patterns of interaction between the infant and parents may be lacking if there is not enough reciprocity. For example, if the parent gazes fondly at the infant's face and seeks eye contact but the infant fails to respond because he or she cannot see the parent, a troubled cycle of responses may occur. The nurse can help parents learn to look for other cues that indicate the infant is responding to them, such as whether the eyelids blink; whether the activity level accelerates or slows; whether respiratory patterns change, such as faster or slower breathing, when the parents come near; and whether the infant makes throaty sounds when the parents speak to the infant. In time, parents learn that the infant has unique ways of relating to them. They are encouraged to show affection using nonvisual methods, such as talking or reading, cuddling, and walking the child.

Promote Child's Optimal Development

Promoting the child's optimum development requires rehabilitation in a number of important areas. These include learning self-help skills and appropriate communication techniques to become independent. Although nurses may not be directly involved in such programs, they can provide direction and guidance to families regarding the availability of programs and the need to promote these activities in their child.

Development and Independence

Motor development depends on sight almost as much as verbal communication depends on hearing. From earliest infancy, parents are encouraged to expose the infant to as many visual-motor experiences as possible, such as sitting supported in an infant seat or swing and being given opportunities for holding up the head, sitting unsupported, reaching for objects, and crawling.

Despite visual impairment, the child can become independent in all aspects of self-care. The same principles used for promoting independence in sighted children apply, with additional emphasis on nonvisual cues. For example, the child may need help in dressing, such as special arrangement of clothing for style coordination and braille tags to distinguish colors and prints.

The severe permanent visual impaired child also must learn to become independent in navigational skills. The two main techniques are the **tapping method** (use of a cane to survey the environment for direction and to avoid obstacles) and **guides**, such as a sighted human guide or a dog guide, such as a Seeing Eye dog. Children who are partially sighted may benefit from ocular aids, such as a monocular telescope.

Play and Socialization

Children with severe permanent visual impairments do not learn to play automatically. Because they cannot imitate others or actively explore the environment as sighted children do, they depend much more on others to stimulate and teach them how to play. Parents need help in selecting appropriate play materials, especially those that encourage fine and gross motor development and stimulate the senses of hearing, touch, and smell. Toys with educational value are especially useful, such as dolls with various clothing closures.

Children with severe permanent visual impairments have the same needs for socialization as sighted children. Because they have little difficulty in learning verbal skills, they are able to communicate with age mates and participate in suitable activities. The nurse should discuss with parents opportunities for socialization outside the home, especially regular preschools. The trend is to include these children with sighted children to help them adjust to the outside world for eventual independence.

To compensate for inadequate stimulation, these children may develop self-stimulatory activities, such as body rocking, finger flicking, or arm twirling. Discourage such habits because they delay the child's social acceptance. Behavior modification is often successful in reducing or eliminating self-stimulatory activities.

Education

The main obstacle to learning is the child's total dependence on nonvisual cues. Although the child can learn via verbal lecturing, he or she is unable to read the written word or to write without special education. Therefore, the child must rely on **braille**, a system that uses raised dots to represent letters and numbers. The child can then read braille with the fingers and can write messages using a braille writer. However, unless others read braille, this system is not useful for communicating with others. A more portable system for written communication is the use of a braille slate and stylus or a microcassette tape recorder. A recorder is especially helpful for leaving messages for others and taking notes during classroom lectures. For mathematic calculations, portable calculators with voice synthesizers are available.*

Records and tapes are significant sources of reading material other than braille books, which are large and cumbersome. The Library of Congress† has talking books, braille books, and a special records program, which are available at many local and state libraries and directly from the Library of Congress. The talking book machine and tape player are provided at no cost to families, and there is no postage fee for returning the materials. Recording for the Blind and Dyslexic‡ also provides texts and tapes of books, which are helpful for secondary

---

*Two Penn Plaza, Suite 1102, New York, NY 10021; 800-232-5463 or 212-502-7600; fax: 212-502-7777; http://www.afb.org.
†200 E. Wells St., Baltimore, MD 21230; 410-659-9314; fax: 410-685-5653; http://www.nfb.org.
‡PO Box 317, Watertown, MA 02471; 800-562-6265; fax: 617-972-7444; http://www.napvi.org.
§22 W. 21st St., 6th Floor, New York, NY 10010; 212-889-3141; fax: 212-727-2931; http://www.navh.org.
‖2200 Wilson Blvd., Suite 650, Arlington, VA 22201; 800-424-8666; 202-467-5081; fax: (202) 465-5085; http://www.acb.org.
¶1929 Bayview Ave., Toronto, ON M4G 3E8; Canada: 800-563-2642; fax: 416-480-7700; http://www.cnib.ca.

*A catalog of numerous products for people with vision problems is available from American Foundation for the Blind (see previous footnote) and from Lighthouse International, 111 E. 59th St., New York, NY 10022-1202; 212-821-9200 or 800-829-0500; TTY: 212-821-9713; fax: 212-821-9707; http://www.lighthouse.org.
†National Library Service for the Blind and Physically Handicapped, Library of Congress, 1291 Taylor St. NW, Washington, DC 20011; 202-707-5100; 888-657-7323; TTD: 202-707-0744; fax: 202-707-0712; http://www.loc.gov/nls. (A state listing of libraries for readers with severe permanent visual impairments and physical disabilities, as well as other reference circulars, is available from this office.)
‡20 Roszel Road, Princeton, NJ 08540; 800-221-4792 or 866-RFBD-585; http://www.rfbd.org.

and college students who are blind. A means of writing is learning to use a home computer with a voice synthesizer that can be adapted to speak each letter or word typed.

Children with partial sight benefit from specialized visual aids that produce a magnified retinal image. The basic devices are accommodation (e.g., bringing the object closer), special plus lenses, handheld and stand magnifiers, telescopes, video projection systems, and large print. Special equipment is available to enlarge print. Information about services for the partially sighted is available from the National Association for Visually Handicapped and American Foundation for the Blind. Children with diminished vision often prefer to do close work without their glasses and compensate by bringing the object very near to their eyes. This should be allowed. The exception is children with vision in only one eye, who should always wear glasses for protection.

Care for the Child During Hospitalization

Because nurses are more likely to care for children who are hospitalized for procedures that involve temporary loss of vision than for children who have severe permanent visual impairments, the following discussion concentrates primarily on the needs of such children. The nursing care objectives in either situation are to (1) reassure the child and family throughout every phase of treatment, (2) orient the child to the surroundings, (3) provide a safe environment, and (4) encourage independence. Whenever possible, the same nurse should care for the child to ensure consistency in the approach.

When sighted children temporarily lose their vision, almost every aspect of the environment becomes bewildering and frightening. They are forced to rely on nonvisual senses for help in adjusting to the visual impairment without the benefit of any special training. Nurses have a major role in minimizing the effects of temporary loss of vision. They need to talk to the child about everything that is occurring, emphasizing aspects of procedures that are felt or heard. They should approach the child by always identifying themselves as soon as they enter the room. Because unfamiliar sounds are especially frightening, these are explained. Parents are encouraged to room with their child and participate in the care. Familiar objects, such as a teddy bear or doll, should be brought from home to help lessen the strangeness of the hospital. As soon as the child is able to be out of bed, he or she is oriented to the immediate surroundings. If the child is able to see on admission, this opportunity is taken to point out significant aspects of the room. The child is encouraged to practice ambulating with the eyes closed to become accustomed to this experience.

The room is arranged with safety in mind. For example, a stool or chair is placed next to the bed to help the child climb in and out of bed. The furniture is always placed in the same position to prevent collisions. Cleaning personnel are reminded of the need to keep the room in order. If the child has difficulty navigating by feeling the walls, a rope can be attached from the bed to the point of destination, such as the bathroom. Attention to details such as well-fitting slippers and robes that do not drag on the floor is important in preventing tripping. Unlike children who have permanent visual impairments, children with temporary visual impairments are not familiar with navigating with a cane.

The child is encouraged to be independent in self-care activities, especially if the visual loss may be prolonged or potentially permanent. For example, during bathing, the nurse sets up all of the equipment and encourages the child to participate. At mealtimes, the nurse explains where each food item is on the tray, opens any special containers, prepares cereal or toast, and encourages the child in self-feeding. Favorite finger foods, such as sandwiches, hamburgers, hot dogs, or pizza, may be good selections. The child is praised for efforts at being

cooperative and independent. Any improvements made in self-care, no matter how small, are stressed.

Appropriate recreational activities are provided, and if a child life specialist is available, such planning is done jointly. Because children with temporary visual impairment have a wide variety of play experiences to draw on, they are encouraged to select activities. For example, if they like to read, they may enjoy being read to. If they prefer manual activity, they may appreciate playing with clay or building blocks or feeling different textures and naming them. If they need an outlet for aggression, activities such as pounding or banging on a drum can be helpful. Simple board and card games can be played with a "seeing partner" or an opponent who helps with the game. They should have familiar toys from home to play with because familiar items are more easily manipulated than new ones. If parents want to bring presents, they should be objects that stimulate hearing and touch, such as a radio, music box, or stuffed animal.

Occasionally, children who are visually impaired come to the hospital for procedures to restore their vision. Although this is an extremely happy time, it also requires intervention to help them adjust to sight. They need an opportunity to take in all that they see. They should not be bombarded with visual stimuli. They may need to concentrate on people's faces or their own to become accustomed to this experience. They often need to talk about what they see and to compare the visual images with their mental ones. The children may also go through a period of depression, which must be respected and supported. The nurse or parents should encourage the child to discuss how it feels to see, especially in terms of seeing themselves.

Newly sighted children also need time to adjust and engage in activities that were impossible before. For example, they may prefer to use braille to read rather than learning a new "visual approach" because of familiarity with the touch system. Eventually, as they learn to recognize letters and numbers, they will integrate these new skills into reading and writing. However, parents and teachers must be careful not to push them before they are ready. This applies to social relationships and physical activities as well as learning situations.

Assist in Measures to Prevent Visual Impairment

An essential nursing goal is to prevent visual impairment. This involves many of the same interventions discussed for hearing impairments:

- Prenatal screening for pregnant women at risk, such as those with rubella or syphilis infection and family histories of genetic disorders associated with visual loss
- Adequate prenatal and perinatal care to prevent prematurity
- Periodic screening of all children, especially newborns through preschoolers, for congenital and acquired visual impairments caused by refractive errors, strabismus, and other disorders
- Rubella immunization of all children
- Safety counseling regarding the common causes of ocular trauma, including safe practices when working with, playing with, and carrying objects such as scissors, knives, and balls

> **! NURSING ALERT**
>
> A helmet with a face mask should be required for children playing football, hockey, and baseball.

After detection of eye problems, the nurse has a responsibility to prevent further ocular damage by ensuring that corrective treatment is used. For children with strabismus, this often necessitates occlusion patching of the stronger eye. Compliance with the procedure is greatest during the early preschool years. It is more difficult to encourage school-age children to wear the occlusive patch because the poor visual acuity of the uncovered weaker eye interferes with school work and the patch sets them apart from their peers. In school, they benefit from being positioned favorably (closer to the white board or other visual media) and allowed extra time to read or complete an assignment. If treatment of the eye disorder requires instillation of ophthalmic medication, the family is taught the correct procedure (see Chapter 22).

For children with refractive errors, the nurse helps them adjust to wearing glasses. Young children who often pull off glasses benefit from temporal pieces that wrap around the ears or an elastic strap attached to the frames and around the back of the head to hold the glasses on securely. After children appreciate the value of clear vision, they are more likely to wear the corrective lenses.

Glasses should not interfere with any activity. Special protective guards are available during contact sports to prevent accidental injury, and all corrective lenses should be made from safety glass, which is shatterproof. Often, corrective lenses improve visual acuity so dramatically that children are able to compete more effectively in sports. This in itself is a tremendous inducement to continue wearing glasses.

Contact lenses are a popular alternative, especially for adolescents. Several types are available, such as hard lenses, including gas-permeable ones, and soft lenses, which may be designed for daily or extended wear. Contact lenses offer several advantages over glasses, such as greater visual acuity, total corrected field of vision, convenience (especially with the extended-wear type), and optimal cosmetic benefit. Unfortunately, they are usually more expensive and require much more care than glasses, including considerable practice to learn techniques for insertion and removal. If they are prescribed, the nurse can be helpful in teaching parents or older children how to care for the lenses.

Because trauma is the leading cause of visual impairment, the nurse has the major responsibility of preventing further eye injury until specific treatment is instituted. The major principles to follow when caring for an eye injury are outlined in the Emergency Treatment box on p. 586. Because patients with a serious eye injury fear visual impairment, the nurse should stay with the child and family to provide support and reassurance.

HEARING–VISUAL IMPAIRMENT

The most traumatic sensory impairment is loss of both vision and hearing, which may have profound effects on the child's development. These losses interfere with the normal sequence of physical, intellectual, and psychosocial growth. Although such children often achieve the usual motor milestones, their rate of development is slower. These children learn communication only with specialized training. Finger spelling is one desirable method often taught to these children. Words are spelled letter by letter into the child's hand, and the child spells into the other person's hand. Some children with hearing–visual impairment, especially those with residual hearing or sight, can learn to speak. Whenever possible, speech is encouraged because it allows communication with other individuals.

The future prospects for children with hearing–visual impairment are, at best, unpredictable. Congenital hearing–visual impairment may be accompanied by other physical or neurologic problems, which further diminish the child's learning potential. The most favorable prognosis is for children who have acquired hearing–visual impairment with few, if any, associated disabilities. Their learning capacity is greatly potentiated by their developmental progress before the sensory impairments. Although total independence, including gainful vocational training, is the goal, some children with hearing–visual impairment are unable to develop to this level. They may require lifelong

---

BOX 19-7   CLINICAL MANIFESTATIONS OF RETINOBLASTOMA

White eye reflex (most common sign)
Strabismus (second most common sign)
Red, painful eye, often with glaucoma
Severe permanent visual impairment (late sign)

---

parental or residential care. The nurse working with such families helps them deal with future goals for the child, including possible alternatives to home care during the parents' advancing years.

RETINOBLASTOMA

Retinoblastoma, which arises from the retina, is the most common congenital malignant intraocular tumor of childhood. Approximately 11 cases per million occur annually, primarily in children younger than 5 years of age. Retinoblastoma is caused by a mutation in a gene and may occur sporadically or be inherited (Hurwitz, Shields, Shields, and others, 2011; Parulekar, 2010). Retinoblastoma develops when the mutated gene is unable to produce the natural signals to stop the growth of retinal cells. Of all cases, the majority are nonhereditary and unilateral, with the remainder divided between hereditary and unilateral, and hereditary and bilateral. Hereditary retinoblastomas are transmitted with few exceptions as an autosomal dominant trait with high but incomplete penetrance (Hurwitz, Shields, Shields, and others, 2011; Parulekar, 2010).

Diagnostic Evaluation

Retinoblastoma has few grossly obvious signs (Box 19-7). Typically the most common sign is observed by the parent as a whitish "glow" in the pupil, known as the white reflex or leukokoria. Leukokoria represents visualization of the tumor as the light momentarily falls on the mass (Fig. 19-8). The second most common sign of retinoblastoma is acquired strabismus (Hurwitz, Shields, Shields, and others, 2011; Phan and Stout, 2010).

The first step in diagnosis is carefully listening to and recognizing the significance of reports from family members regarding suspected abnormalities within the eye. Eye abnormalities, including white reflex, strabismus, decreased vision, and persistent painful erythematous eyes, are referred to an ophthalmologist. Definitive diagnosis is usually based on ophthalmoscopic examination with the patient under general anesthesia. Imaging studies, including ultrasonography and computed tomography of the orbit, are done to determine the extent of the disease.

Therapeutic Management

Treatment of retinoblastoma is complex. Enucleation may be used to treat advanced disease with optic nerve invasion in which there is no hope for salvage of vision. Irradiation can be used when there is vitreous seeding and chemotherapy has been used more recently to decrease the size of the tumor that would then allow treatment with local therapies such as plaque brachytherapy (surgical implantation of an iodine-125 applicator on the sclera until the maximum radiation dose has been delivered to the tumor), photocoagulation (use of a laser beam to destroy retinal blood vessels that supply nutrition to the tumor), and cryotherapy (freezing of the tumor, which destroys the microcirculation to the tumor and the cells themselves through microcrystal formation). Vincristine, carboplatin, and etoposide are the agents most commonly used.

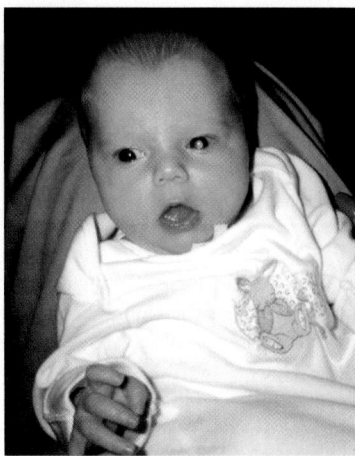

FIG. 19-8 White reflex. Whitish appearance of lens is produced as light falls on the tumor mass in the left eye.

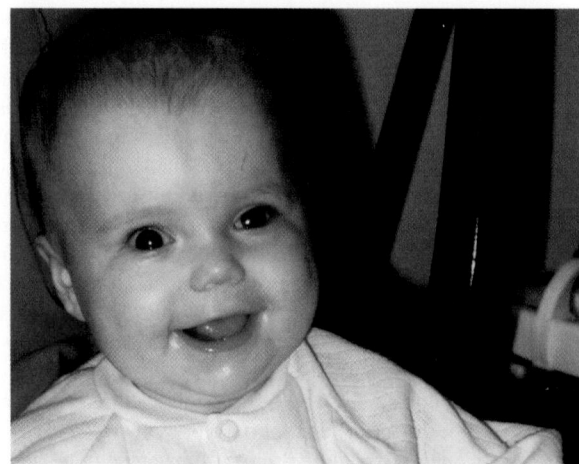

FIG. 19-9 The same infant with a left prosthetic eye.

The use of chemotherapy in advanced disease is controversial and has not shown improved survival. Drugs that may be used in the treatment of metastatic disease include vincristine, cyclophosphamide, doxorubicin, cisplatin, carboplatin, and etoposide. In the case of central nervous system (CNS) disease, intrathecal chemotherapy may be administered (Hurwitz, Shields, Shields, and others, 2011; Lanzkowsky, 2005).

Prognosis

The overall prognosis for retinoblastoma is favorable; with early appropriate treatment, the survival rate is nearly 95% for both unilateral and bilateral tumors. Retinoblastoma is one of the tumors that may spontaneously regress. Of major concern in long-term survivors is the development of decreased visual acuity; facial disfiguration; and secondary tumors, especially osteogenic sarcoma, other sarcomas, and melanoma. Children with bilateral disease (hereditary form) are more likely to develop secondary cancers than are children with unilateral disease. It is thought that these individuals are predisposed to developing cancer and that radiation increases their risk.

Nursing Care Management

One of the most important nursing goals is to have a high index of suspicion for this rare malignancy. If parents report noticing a strange light in the eye or expression, these concerns must be taken seriously. Families with a history of retinoblastoma require follow-up, and the nurse can be instrumental in reminding parents of appointments and the importance of genetic counseling

Because the tumor is usually diagnosed in infants or very young children, most of the preparation for diagnostic tests and treatment involves parents. After indirect ophthalmoscopy, the child may not see clearly, or the eyes may be sensitive to light because of pupillary dilation. The parents are made aware of these normal reactions before the procedure.

The treatment plan may include focal intraocular therapy with or without chemotherapy; external-beam radiation; and, if necessary, enucleation. Enucleation is the treatment of choice if there is extensive disease threatening metastasis or no chance for useful vision. The enucleation procedure and the positive benefits of a prosthesis are explained to the parents. Showing them pictures of another child with an artificial eye may help them adjust to the thought of disfigurement (Fig. 19-9).

After surgery the parents are prepared for the child's facial appearance. An eye patch is in place, and the child's face may be edematous or ecchymotic. Parents often fear seeing the surgical site because they imagine a cavity in the skull. A surgically implanted sphere maintains the shape of the eyeball, and the implant is covered with conjunctiva. When the eyelids are open, the exposed area resembles the mucosal lining of the mouth. After the child is fitted for a prosthesis, usually within 3 weeks, the facial appearance returns to normal. Initial instructions for care of the prosthesis are given by the ocularist who fits and manufactures the device.

Care of the socket is minimal and easily accomplished. The wound itself is clean and has little or no drainage. If an antibiotic ointment is prescribed, it is applied in a thin line on the surface of the tissues of the socket. To cleanse the site, an irrigating solution may be ordered and is instilled daily or more frequently *before* application of the antibiotic ointment. The dressing, consisting of an eye pad taped over the surgical site, is changed daily. After the socket has healed completely, a dressing is no longer necessary, although it is a preventive measure against infection.

AUTISM SPECTRUM DISORDERS

Autism spectrum disorders (ASDs) are complex neurodevelopmental disorders of unknown etiology composed of qualitative alterations in social interaction and verbal impairment with repetitive, restricted, and stereotype behavioral patterns (American Psychological Association, 2000; Amin, Smith, and Wang, 2011; Grynszpan, Nadel, Constant, and others, 2011).

Autism spectrum disorder impairments range from mild to severe (Johnson, 2008). ASD is manifested during early childhood, primarily from 18 to 36 months of age. It occurs in 1 in 100 to 150 children in the United States; is about four times more common in boys than in girls (although girls are more severely affected); and is not related to socioeconomic level, race, or parenting style (Centers for Disease Control and Prevention, 2009; Johnson, 2008; Shah, Dalton, and Boris, 2007).

Etiology

The cause of ASD is unknown. Researchers are investigating a number of theories, including a link between hereditary, genetic, and medical problems. Immune and environmental factors (e.g., viral infections)

may interact with the genetic susceptibility to increase the incidence of ASD (Bloom-DiCicco, Lord, Zwaigenbaum, and others, 2006). Individuals with ASD may have abnormal electroencephalograms, epileptic seizures, delayed development of hand dominance, persistence of primitive reflexes, metabolic abnormalities (elevated blood serotonin), cerebellar vermal hypoplasia (part of the brain involved in regulating motion and some aspects of memory), and infantile abnormal head enlargement (Dawson, 2007; Rutter, 2011).

The strong evidence for a genetic basis in twins is consistent with an autosomal recessive pattern of inheritance. Twin studies demonstrate a high concordance (60%–96%) for monozygotic (identical) twins and less than 5% concordance for dizygotic (nonidentical) twins. In addition, between 5% and 16% of boys with ASD are positive for the fragile X chromosome (Clifford, Dissanayake, Bui, and others, 2007).

There is a relatively high risk of recurrence of ASD in families with one affected child (Rutter, 2011; Schaefer and Lutz, 2006; Yoder, Stone, and Walden, 2009). Several genes have been suggested as possible causative factors in ASD (Dawson, 2007; Kolevzon, Gross, and Reichenberg, 2007).

The scientific evidence to date supports that there is no link between measles, mumps, and rubella (MMR) and thimerosal-containing vaccines and ASDs (Price, Thompson, Goodson, and others, 2010; Schultz, 2010) (see Evidence-Based Practice box). ASD has been reported in association with a number of conditions such as fragile X syndrome, tuberous sclerosis, metabolic disorders, fetal rubella syndrome, *Haemophilus influenzae* meningitis, and structural brain anomalies (Dawson, 2007). Recent reports have retrospectively tied ASD to prenatal and perinatal events such as maternal and paternal ages over 40 years (for fathers, 1 in 116 births; for mothers, 1 in 123 births), uterine bleeding during pregnancy, low Apgar score, fetal distress, and neonatal hyperbilirubinemia (Amin, Smith, and Wang, 2011; Croen, Najjar, Fireman, and others, 2007; Kolevzon, Gross, and Reichenberg, 2007; Rutter, 2011). These same researchers, however, urge caution in interpreting these findings.

Clinical Manifestations and Diagnostic Evaluation

Children with ASD demonstrate several peculiar and often seemingly bizarre characteristics, primarily in social interactions, communication, and behavior. One hallmark characteristic is the inability to maintain eye contact with another person. Parents of autistic children have noted that their infants had difficulties with eye contact, avoidance of body contact, and language delay at a very early age (Belschner, 2007; Golnik and Maccabee-Ryaboy, 2010; Kirchner, Hatri, Heekeren, and others, 2011). Children with ASD also display limited functional play and may interact with toys in an unusual or odd manner (Belschner, 2007). Children with ASD may have significant gastrointestinal symptoms. Constipation is a common symptom and can be associated with acquired megarectum in children with ASD (Buie, Campbell, Fuchs, and others, 2010). Other clinical manifestations typically seen in children with autism are described in Box 19-8.

Children with autism do not always have the same manifestations, from mild forms requiring minimal supervision to severe forms in which self-abusive behavior is common. The majority (50%–70%) of children with autism have some degree of CI, with scores typically in the moderate to severe range. More girls than boys tend to have very low intelligence scores. Despite their relatively moderate to severe disability, some children with autism (known as **savants**) excel in particular areas, such as art, music, memory, mathematics, or perceptual skills such as puzzle building.

BOX 19-8   DIAGNOSTIC CRITERIA FOR AUTISM SPECTRUM DISORDERS

A. A total of six (or more) items from (1), (2), and (3), with at least two from (1) and one each from (2) and (3):

(1) Qualitative impairment in social interaction, as manifested by at least two of the following:

(a) Marked impairment in the use of multiple nonverbal behaviors such as eye-to-eye gaze, facial expression, body postures, and gestures to regulate social interaction

(b) Failure to develop peer relationships appropriate to developmental level

(c) A lack of spontaneous seeking to share enjoyment, interests, or achievements with other people (e.g., by a lack of showing, bringing, pointing out objects of interest)

(d) Lack of social or emotional reciprocity

(2) Qualitative impairments in communication as manifested by at least one of the following:

(a) Delay in or total lack of the development of spoken language (not accompanied by an attempt to compensate through alternative modes of communication such as gestures or mime)

(b) In individuals with adequate speech, marked impairment in the ability to initiate or sustain a conversation with others

(c) Stereotyped and repetitive use of language or idiosyncratic language

(d) Lack of varied, spontaneous make-believe play or social imitative play appropriate to developmental level

(3) Restricted repetitive and stereotyped patterns of behavior, interests, and activities as manifested by at least one of the following:

(a) Encompassing preoccupation with one or more stereotyped and restricted patterns of interest that is abnormal either in intensity or focus

(b) Apparently inflexible adherence to specific, nonfunctional routines or rituals

(c) Stereotyped and repetitive motor mannerisms (e.g., hand or finger flapping or twisting, complex whole-body movements)

(d) Persistent preoccupation with parts of objects

B. Delays or abnormal functioning in at least one of the following areas, with onset before age 3 years: (1) social interaction, (2) language as used in social communication, or (3) symbolic or imaginative play.

C. The disturbance is not better accounted for by Rett disorder or childhood disintegrative disorder.

From American Psychiatric Association: *Diagnostic and statistical manual of mental disorders*, ed 4, rev trans (DSM-IV TR), Washington, DC, 2000, Author.

NURSING TIP Claims of beneficial results from the use of secretin, a peptide hormone that stimulates pancreatic secretion, have not been substantiated by scientific study (Shah, Dalton, and Boris, 2007; Welch, Ludwig, Opler, and others, 2006).*

Speech and language delays are also common in children with ASD. Any child who does not display such language skills as babbling or gesturing by 12 months, single words by 16 months, and two-word phrases by 24 months is recommended for immediate hearing and

---

*Additional information on secretin may be found by contacting the Autism Society, 4340 East-West Hwy., Suite 350, Bethesda, MD 20814-3067; 800-3AUTISM or 301-657-0881; http://www.autism-society.org.

EVIDENCE-BASED PRACTICE

Thimerosal-Containing Vaccines and Autism Spectrum Disorders

Rosalind Bryant

Ask the Question
Picot Question

Is the incidence of ASDs increased in children receiving vaccines containing thimerosal?

Search for the Evidence
Search Strategies

Published studies from 2001 to early 2011 focused on the pediatric population and restricted to the English language

Databases Used

PubMed, Cochrane Collaboration, MD Consult, Vaccine Adverse Events Reporting System (VAERS) database, American Academy of Pediatrics, Autism Research Institute

Critically Analyze the Evidence

Evidence does not support an association between autism and mercury exposure from the pharmaceutical preservative thimerosal used in vaccinations until 2001.

- A Cochrane systematic review of 31 studies evaluating trivalent MMR in healthy individuals up to 15 years of age found no evidence that MMR is associated with autism (Demicheli, Jefferson, Rivetti, and others, 2005). Two other reviews made similar conclusions. Two other reviews found no evidence to support an association between ASDs and thimerosal-containing vaccines (Parker, Schwartz, Todd, and others, 2004; Schultz, 2010).
- Two large studies in Europe found no evidence that childhood vaccination with thimerosal-containing vaccines was associated with the development of ASDs. One longitudinal study evaluated more than 14,000 children in the United Kingdom. The mercury exposure from thimerosal-containing vaccines was recorded and calculated at ages 3, 4, and 6 months and compared with cognitive and behavioral-developmental assessments performed from 6 to 91 months of age (Heron, Golding, and the ALSPAC study team, 2004). The second study, a cohort of 467,450 children in Denmark, compared the incidence of ASDs in children vaccinated with thimerosal-containing vaccines with the incidence of ASDs in children vaccinated with a thimerosal-free formulation of the same vaccine.
- Smaller case-control studies have also found no relationships between childhood vaccination with thimerosal-containing vaccines and the development of ASDs (Baird, Pickles, Simonoff, and others, 2007; Hviid, Stellfeld, Wohlfahrt, and others, 2003; Price, Thompson, Goodson, and others, 2010).
- In 2004, the Institute of Medicine (2004) completed an update to the review of the evidence and concluded that the epidemiologic evidence supports the rejection of a causal relationship between thimerosal exposure from childhood vaccines and the onset of autism. Based on guidelines established by the U.S. Food and Drug Administration (2010) and other government monitoring agencies, no children will be exposed to excessive mercury from childhood vaccines.

Apply the Evidence: Nursing Implications

There is **moderate-quality evidence** with a **strong recommendation** (Guyatt, Oxman, Vist, and others, 2008) of vaccines and no link between vaccines containing thimerosal and autism or other neurodevelopmental disorders.

QSEN Quality and Safety Competencies:
Evidence-Based Practice*
Knowledge

Differentiate clinical opinion from research and evidence-based summaries.

Compare research summaries that provide evidence of the lack of association between vaccines containing thimerosal and autism or other neurodevelopmental disorders.

Skills

Base individualized care plan on patient values, clinical expertise, and evidence.

Integrate evidence into practice by sharing results with parents regarding the benefits of vaccinating their children and the evidence regarding lack of association between immunizations and autism disorders.

Attitudes

Value the concept of evidence-based practice as integral to determining best clinical practice.

Appreciate strengths and weakness of the evidence that confirms the lack of a link between vaccines containing thimerosal and autism or other neurodevelopmental disorders.

References

Baird A, Pickles A, Simonoff E, and others: Measles vaccination and antibody response in autism spectrum disorders, *Arch Dis Child* 93:832–837, 2007.

Demicheli V, Jefferson T, Rivetti A, and others: Vaccines for measles, mumps and rubella in children, *Cochrane Database Syst Rev* (4):CD004407, 2005

Guyatt GH, Oxman AD, Vist GE, and others: GRADE: an emerging consensus on rating quality of evidence and strength of recommendations, *BMJ* 336:924–926, 2008.

Heron J, Golding J, ALSPAC study team: Thimerosal exposure in infants and developmental disorders: a prospective cohort study in the United Kingdom does not support a causal association, *Pediatrics* 114(3):577–583, 2004.

Hviid A, Stellfeld M, Wohlfahrt J, and others: Association between thimerosal-containing vaccine and autism, *JAMA* 290(13):1763–1766, 2003.

Institute of Medicine: *Immunization safety review: vaccines and autism*, Washington, DC, 2004, National Academies Press.

Parker SK, Schwartz B, Todd J, and others: Thimerosal-containing vaccines and autistic spectrum disorder: a critical review of published original data, *Pediatrics* 114(3):793–804, 2004.

Price CS, Thompson WW, Goodson B, and others: Prenatal and infant exposure to thimerosal from vaccines and immunoglobulins and risk of autism, *Pediatrics* 126:656–664, 2010.

Schultz ST: Does thimerosal or other mercury exposure increase the risk for autism? *Acta Neurobiol Exp* 70:187–195, 2010.

U.S. Food and Drug Administration: *Vaccines, blood and biologics: thimerosal in vaccines*, 2010, retrieved April 3, 2011, from http://www.fda.gov/BiologicsBloodVaccines/SafetyAvaukbility/vaccineSafety/UCM096228.

ASD, Autism spectrum disorder; *MMR*, measles, mumps, and rubella.
*Based on QSEN at http://www.qsen.org.

---

language evaluation. A sudden deterioration in extant expressive speech is also a red-flag event for further evaluation.

Early recognition, referral, diagnosis, and intensive early intervention tend to improve outcomes for children with ASD (Dawson, Rogers, Munson, and others, 2009; Golnik and Maccabee-Ryaboy, 2010; Zwaigenbaum, 2010). Unfortunately, diagnosis is often not made until 2 to 3 years after symptoms are first recognized, which is based on the diagnostic criteria of *Diagnostic and Statistical Manual of Mental Disorders* (*DSM-IV-TR*) (see Box 19-8).

Prognosis

Autism spectrum disorder is usually a severely disabling condition. However, some children improve with acquisition of language skills and communication with others (Golnik and Maccabee-Ryaboy, 2010;

Zwaigenbaum, 2010). Some ultimately achieve independence, but most require lifelong adult supervision. Aggravation of psychiatric symptoms occurs in about half of the children during adolescence, with girls having a tendency for continued deterioration.

Early recognition of behaviors associated with ASD is critical to implement appropriate interventions and family involvement. The prognosis is most favorable for children with higher intelligence, functional speech, and less behavioral impairment (Shah, Dalton, and Boris, 2007; Solomon, Buaminger, and Rogers, 2011).

Nursing Care Management

Therapeutic intervention for children with ASD is a specialized area involving professionals with advanced training. Although there is no cure for ASD, numerous therapies have been used. The most promising results have been through highly structured and intensive behavior modification programs. In general, the objective in treatment is to promote positive reinforcement, increase social awareness of others, teach verbal communication skills, and decrease unacceptable behavior. Providing a structured routine for the child to follow is a key in the management of ASD.

When these children are hospitalized, the parents are essential to planning care and ideally should stay with the child as much as possible. Nurses should recognize that not all children with ASD are the same and that they require individual assessment and treatment. Decreasing stimulation by using a private room, avoiding extraneous auditory and visual distractions, and encouraging the parents to bring in possessions the child is attached to may lessen the disruptiveness of hospitalization. Because physical contact often upsets these children, minimal holding and eye contact may be necessary to avoid behavioral outbursts. Care must be taken when performing procedures on, administering medicine to, and feeding these children because they may be either fussy eaters who willfully starve themselves or gag to prevent eating, or indiscriminate hoarders who swallow any available edible or inedible items, such as a thermometer. Eating habits of ASD children may be particularly problematic for families and may involve food refusal accompanied by mineral deficiencies, mouthing objects, eating nonedibles, and smelling and throwing food (Belschner, 2007; Caronna, Augustyn, and Zuckerman, 2007; Herndon, DiGuiseppi, Johnson, and others, 2009).

Children with ASD need to be introduced slowly to new situations, with visits with staff caregivers kept short whenever possible. Because these children have difficulty organizing their behavior and redirecting their energy, they need to be told directly what to do. Communication should be at the child's developmental level, brief, and concrete.

Family Support

Autism spectrum disorder, as with so may other chronic conditions, involves the entire family and often becomes "a family disease." Nurses can help alleviate the guilt and shame often associated with this disorder by stressing what is known from a biologic standpoint and by providing family support. It is imperative to help parents understand that they are not the cause of the child's condition.

Parents need expert counseling early in the course of the disorder and should be referred to the Autism Society website.* The society provides information about education, treatment programs and techniques, and facilities such as camps and group homes. Other helpful resources for parents of children with ASD are the local and state departments of mental health and developmental disabilities; these organizations provide important programs and in-school programs throughout the United States for children with ASD.

As much as possible, the family is encouraged to care for the child in the home. With the help of family support programs in many states, families are often able to provide home care and assist with the educational services the child needs. As the child approaches adulthood and the parents become older, the family may require assistance in locating a long-term placement facility.

---

*See footnote on p. 591.

KEY POINTS

- The AAIDD defines *intellectual disability* as significantly subaverage general intellectual functioning existing concurrently with deficits in adaptive behavior and manifested during the developmental period.
- Causes of severe CI are primarily genetic, biochemical, and infectious. Whereas mild CI is associated primarily with familial, social, and environmental causes, severe CI is more likely to be associated with specific syndromes.
- Education of children with CI emphasizes sensory and verbal discrimination, improvement of short-term memory, motivation, and technologic support.
- Optimal development may be promoted through family guidance regarding play, communication, discipline, socialization, and sexuality.
- Prevention of CI focuses on support for preterm neonates and other high-risk newborns, rubella immunization, genetic counseling, and maternal education regarding the risks of chemical use (e.g., alcohol ingestion) and the importance of adequate nutrition.
- Down syndrome, a chromosomal abnormality, is characterized by mild to moderate range of CI (most often), physical characteristics, slowed language development, congenital anomalies, sensory problems, and diminished growth and sexual development.

- Fragile X syndrome is characterized by CI and phenotypic findings in affected boys. It is considered the most common hereditary cause and the second leading chromosomal cause of CI after Down syndrome.
- Hearing disorders may be classified according to the location of the defect: conductive, sensorineural, mixed conductive-sensorineural, and central auditory imperception.
- Rehabilitation for hearing loss involves parent education and support, hearing aids, lipreading, sign language, speech therapy, and promotion of socialization.
- Prevention of hearing loss includes treatment of infection, universal newborn screening and child auditory testing, immunization, pregnancy and genetic counseling, and reduction of noise pollution.
- Common visual impairments in childhood include refractive errors, amblyopia, strabismus, cataracts, glaucoma, trauma, and infections.
- Prevention of visual impairment focuses on prenatal screening, prenatal and perinatal care, periodic vision screening, immunization, and safety counseling.
- Nursing goals in visual rehabilitation include helping the family and child adjust to the child's visual impairment, promoting parent–child attachment, fostering optimal development and

KEY POINTS—cont'd

- independence, providing for play and socialization, and being aware of educational facilities.
- For a child undergoing ocular surgery, nursing care is aimed at reassuring the child and family throughout treatment, orienting the child to the surroundings, providing a safe environment, and encouraging independence.
- Retinoblastoma is a rare congenital malignant tumor; its most common clinical manifestations are white pupil reflex and strabismus.
- ASDs are a complex neurodevelopmental disorder of brain function accompanied by a broad range and severity of intellectual and behavioral deficits.

REFERENCES

American Academy of Pediatrics, Committee on Genetics: Health supervision for children with Down syndrome, *Pediatrics* 107(2):442–449, 2001.

American Academy of Pediatrics, Task Force on Newborn and Infant Hearing: Newborn and infant hearing loss: detection and intervention, *Pediatrics* 103(2):527–530, 1999.

American Association on Intellectual and Developmental Disabilities: *Intellectual disability: definition, classification, and systems of supports*, ed 11, Washington, DC, 2010, Author.

American Psychiatric Association: *Diagnostic and statistical manual of mental disorders*, ed 4 (text rev) (DSM-IV TR), Washington, DC, 2000, Author.

Amin SB, Smith T, Wang H: Is neonatal jaundice associated with autism spectrum disorders: a systematic review, *J Autism Dev Disord* 29:1169–1176, 2011.

Bahado-Singh RO, Argoti P: An overview of first-trimester screening for chromosomal abnormalities, *Clin Lab Med* 30:545–555, 2010.

Baldassari CM, Schmidt C, Schubert CM, and others: Receptive language outcomes in children after cochlear implantation, *Otolaryngol Head Neck Surg* 140:114–119, 2009.

Belschner RA: Stop, assess and motivate: the SAM approach to autism spectrum disorder, *Am J Nurse Pract* 11(4):43–50, 2007.

Benn PA, Chapman AR: Practical and ethical considerations of noninvasive prenatal diagnosis, *JAMA* 301(2), 2009.

Bloom-DiCicco E, Lord C, Zwaigenbaum L, and others: The development neurobiology of autism spectrum disorder, *J Neurosci* 26(26):6897–6906, 2006.

Botelho FA, Bouzada MCF, de Resende LM, and others: Prevalence of hearing impairment in children at risk, *Braz J Otorhinolaryngol* 76(6):739–744, 2010.

Buie T, Campbell DB, Fuchs GJ, and others: Evaluation, diagnosis, and treatment of gastrointestinal disorders in individuals with ASDs: a consensus report, *Pediatrics* 125(suppl 1):S1–S18, 2010.

Caronna EB, Augustyn M, Zuckerman B: Revisiting parental concerns in the age of autism spectrum disorders, *Arch Pediatr Adolesc Med* 161:406–407, 2007.

Centers for Disease Control and Prevention: Prevalence of autism spectrum disorders: autism and developmental disorders monitoring network—United States, 2006, *MMWR Surveill Summ* 58(SS10):1–20, 2009.

Clifford S, Dissanayake C, Bui QM, and others: Autism spectrum phenotype in males and females with fragile X full mutation and permutation, *J Autism Dev Disord* 37:738–747, 2007.

Croen LA, Najjar DV, Fireman B, and others: Maternal and paternal age and the risk of autism spectrum disorders, *Arch Pediatr Adolesc Med* 161:334–340, 2007.

Daniel E: Noise and hearing loss: a review, *J School Health* 77(5):225–231, 2007.

Dawson G: Despite major challenges, autism research continues to offer hope, *Arch Pediatr Adolesc Med* 161:411–412, 2007.

Dawson G, Rogers S, Munson J, and others: Randomized, controlled trial of an intervention for toddlers with autism: the early start Denver model, *Pediatrics* 125:e17–e23, 2009.

Defendi GL: Fetal alcohol spectrum disorder: how to recognize the various manifestations, *Consult Ped* 9(10):343–351, 2010.

Fabry DA, Davila EP, Arheart KL, and others: Secondhand smoke exposure and the risk of hearing loss, *Tobacco Control* 20:82–85, 2011.

Gifford KA, Holmes MG, Bernstein HH: Hearing loss in children, *Pediatr Rev* 30(6):207–216, 2009.

Golnik A, Maccabee-Ryaboy N: Autism: clinical pearls for primary care, *Contemp Pediatr* 42–60, Nov 2010.

Grynszpan O, Nadel J, Constant J, and others: A new virtual environment paradigm for high-functioning autism intended to help attentional disengagement in a social context, *J Phys Ther Educ* 25(1):42–47, 2011.

Haddad J: Hearing loss. In Kliegman RM, Behrman RE, Jenson HB, and others, editors: *Nelson textbook of pediatrics*, ed 18, Philadelphia, 2007, Saunders.

Hagerman RJ: The fragile X prevalence paradox, *J Med Genet* 45:498–499, 2008.

Henderson E, Testa MA, Hartnick C: Prevalence of noise-induced hearing-threshold shifts and hearing loss among U.S. youths, *Pediatrics* 127(1):e39–e46, 2011.

Herndon AC, DiGuiseppi C, Johnson SL, and others: Does nutritional intake differ between children and autism spectrum disorders and children with typical development? *J Autism Dev Disord* 39:212–222, 2009.

Hurwitz RL, Shields CL, Shields JA, and others: Retinoblastoma. In Pizzo PA, Poplack DG, editors: *Principles and practice of pediatric oncology*, ed 6, Philadelphia, 2011, Lippincott.

Johnson CP: Recognition of autism before age 2 years, *Pediatr Rev* 29(3):86–96, 2008.

Johnson CP, Walker WO: Mental retardation: management and prognosis, *Pediatr Rev* 27(7):249–256, 2006.

Joint Committee on Infant Hearing: Year 2000 position statement: principles and guidelines for early hearing detection and intervention programs, *Pediatrics* 106(4):798–817, 2000.

Katz G, Lazcano-Ponce E: Intellectual disability: definition, etiological factors, classification, diagnosis, treatment and prognosis, *Salud Publica de Mexico* 50(suppl 2):S132–S141, 2008.

Kirchner JC, Hatri A, Heekeren HR, and others: Autistic symptomatology, face processing abilities, and eye fixation patterns, *J Autism Dev Disord* 41:158–167, 2011.

Kolevzon A, Gross R, Reichenberg A: Prenatal and perinatal risk factors for autism: a review and integration of findings, *Arch Pediatr Adolesc Med* 161:326–333, 2007.

Kuehn BM: Scientists find promising therapies for fragile X and Down syndromes, *JAMA* 305(4):344–346, 2011.

Lanzkowsky P: *Manual of pediatric hematology and oncology*, ed 4, San Diego, 2005, Academic Press.

Mohammadi S, Mazhari MM, Mehrparvar AH, and others: Cigarette smoking and occupational noise-induced hearing loss, *Eur J Public Health* 20(4):452–455, 2009.

National Down Syndrome Society: *Education, development, and community life*, 2011a, retrieved January 18, 2011, from http://www.ndss.org.

National Down Syndrome Society: *About Down syndrome*, 2011b, retrieved January 18, 2011, from http://www.ndss.org.

National Down Syndrome Society: *Heathcare*, 2011c, retrieved January 18, 2011, from http://www.ndss.org.

National Fragile X Foundation: *Prevalence of fragile X syndrome*, 2010, retrieved January 18, 2011, from http://www.fragilex.org/html/prevalence.htm.

Oliver C, Richards C: Self-injurious behavior in people with intellectual disability, *Curr Opin Psychiatr* 23:412–416, 2010.

Parulekar MV: Retinoblastoma—current treatment and future direction, *Early Hum Dev* 86:619–625, 2010.

Phan IT, Stout T: Retinoblastoma presenting as strabismus and leukocoria, *J Pediatr* 157:858, 2010.

Price CS, Thompson WW, Goodson B, and others: Prenatal and infant exposure to thimerosal from vaccines and immunoglobulins and risk of autism, *Pediatrics* 126:656–664, 2010.

Pueschel SM: The child with Down syndrome. In Levine MD, Carey WB, Crocker AC, editors: *Developmental-behavioral pediatrics*, ed 3, Philadelphia, 1999, Saunders.

Rahi JS, Cumberland PM, Peckham CS, and others: Improving detection of blindness in childhood: the British childhood vision impairment study, *Pediatrics* 126:e895–e903, 2010.

Robertson CMT, Howarth TM, Bork DLR, and others: Permanent bilateral sensory and neural hearing loss of children after neonatal intensive care because of extreme prematurity: a thirty-year study, *Pediatrics* 123(5):e797–e807, 2009.

Rutter ML: Progress in understanding autism: 2007–2010, *J Autism Dev Disord* 41:395–404, 2011.

Schaefer GB, Lutz RE: Diagnostic yield in the clinical genetic evaluation of autism spectrum disorders, *Genet Med* 8(9):549–556, 2006.

Schultz ST: Does thimerosal or other mercury exposure increase the risk for autism? *Acta Neurobiol Exp* 70:187–195, 2010.

Shah PE, Dalton R, Boris NW: Pervasive developmental disorders and childhood psychosis. In Kliegman RM, Behrman RE, Jenson HB, and others, editors: *Nelson textbook of pediatrics*, ed 18, Philadelphia, 2007, Saunders.

Shapiro BK, Batshaw ML: Mental retardation (intellectual disability). In Kliegman RM, Behrman RE, Jenson HB, and others, editors: *Nelson textbook of pediatrics*, ed 18, Philadelphia, 2007, Saunders.

Solomon M, Buaminger N, Rogers SJ: Abstract reasoning and friendship in high functioning preadolescents with autism spectrum disorders, *J Autism Dev Disord* 41:32–43, 2011.

Tierney CD, Brown PJ: Development of children who have hearing impairment, *Pediatr Rev* 29(12):e72–e73, 2008.

Tingley DH: Vision screening essentials: screening today for eye disorders in the pediatric patient, *Pediatr Rev* 28(2):54–61, 2007.

U.S. Preventive Services Task Force: Vision screening for children 1 to 5 years of age, *Pediatrics* 127:340–346, 2011.

Walker WO, Johnson CP: Mental retardation: overview and diagnosis, *Pediatr Rev* 27(6):204–212, 2006.

Weijerman ME, de Winter JP: Clinical practice: the care of children with Down syndrome, *Eur J Pediatr* 169:1445–1452, 2010.

Welch MG, Ludwig RJ, Opler M, and others: Secretin's role in the cerebellum: A larger biological context and implications for developmental disorders, *Cerebellum* 5:2–6, 2006.

Wilton G, Plane MB: The family empowerment network: a service model to address the needs of children and families affected by fetal alcohol spectrum disorders, *Pediatr Nurs* 32(4):299–305, 2006.

Yoder P, Stone WL, Walden T: Predicting social impairment and ASD diagnostic in younger siblings of children with autism spectrum disorder, *J Autism Dev Disord* 39:1381–1391, 2009.

Zeng FG, Liu S: Speech perception in individuals with auditory neuropathy, *J Speech Lang Hearing Res* 49:367–380, 2006.

Zwaigenbaum L: Advances in the early detection of autism, *Curr Opin Neurol* 23:97–102, 2010.

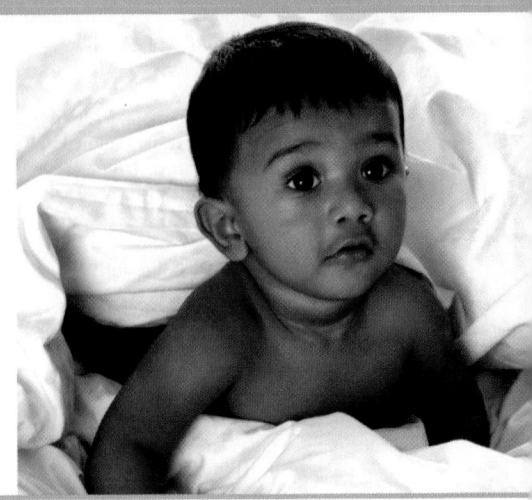

evolve WEBSITE

http://evolve.elsevier.com/wong/essentials
Case Study—Home Care
Key Point Summaries
NCLEX-Style Review Questions

CHAPTER OUTLINE

General Concepts of Home Care, 596
   Home Care Trends, 597
   Effective Home Care, 598
   Discharge Planning and Selection of a
     Home Care Agency, 599
   Care Coordination (Case
     Management), 600

Role of the Nurse, Training, and
   Standards of Care, 601
Family-Centered Home Care, 603
   Diversity in Home Care, 603
   Parent–Professional Collaboration, 604
   The Nursing Process, 605

Promotion of Optimum Development,
   Self-Care, and Education, 606
Safety Issues in the Home, 608
Family-to-Family Support, 609

LEARNING OBJECTIVES

On completion of this chapter the reader will be able to:
- Differentiate home care from hospice care.
- List at least three factors contributing to the increasing emphasis on home care services.
- Describe case management/care coordination and its importance in home care.
- List general principles of a family-centered assessment and planning process.

- Identify five key characteristics of collaborative relationships.
- Describe approaches to promoting optimal development, self-care, and education in home care.
- Outline six areas in need of attention for promoting safety in home care.

GENERAL CONCEPTS OF HOME CARE

The heart of any home is the family. For home care nurses working with pediatric patients this is especially true, as it is the family who nurtures and raises the child. Hence, home care is a family-centered practice. The approach is multidisciplinary and holistic in nature. Body-mind-spirit interventions support quality of life for the child and integrity of the family unit (Arango, 2011). Family-centered home care also reflects ongoing socioeconomic and technologic influences that move the care of the child from the hospital to the home setting (Smith, Piamjariyakul, Yadrich, and others, 2010).

Many children with special health care needs may be cared for in the home setting after their medical condition has stabilized. Although there is limited evidence on the ability of home care to reduce hospital admissions and emergency department visits, home care programs lead to greater parent satisfaction, improved quality of life, and a reduction in length of hospital stay (Cooper, Wheeler, Woolfenden, and others, 2006).

Nursing education has also shifted to incorporate a broader focus on community and home health nursing. Nurses wishing to work in the home care setting must develop pertinent skills for this challenging subspecialty. Duties may include well-baby visits and discussing

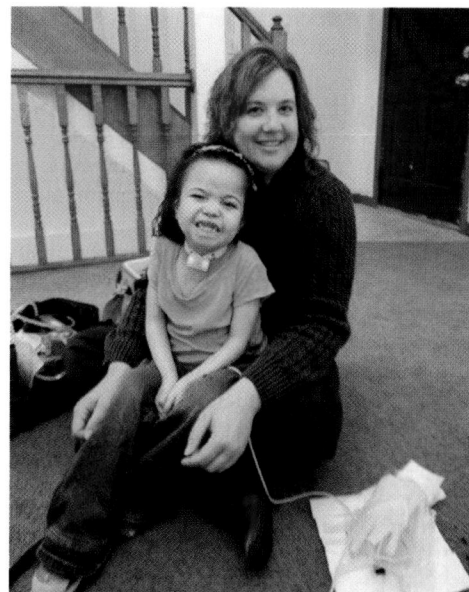

FIG 20-1 A BJC Hospice Wings Pediatric Palliative Care and Hospice program nurse meets with one of the children benefiting from services in their own home. (Photo courtesy BJC Hospice, St. Louis.)

immunizations, caring for an acutely or chronically ill child with possible dependence on medical technology, caring for a child with physical and/or mental disabilities, or preparing the family and child for his or her eventual death (Rice, 2006). In addition, the home milieu and general environment must be an aspect of every home care nursing assessment (Takaro, Krieger, Song, and others, 2011).

Home care is not a new concept in pediatrics. As discussed in this chapter, home care refers to care provided for children with simple or complex health care needs and their families in their places of residence for the purpose of promoting, maintaining, or restoring health or for maximizing the level of independence while minimizing the effects of disability and illness, including terminal illness.

Home care differs from hospice care, which is a program of palliative and supportive care services that provides physical, psychologic, social, and spiritual care for dying persons, their families, and other loved ones (Fig. 20-1). Hospice services are available both in the home and in inpatient settings and are discussed more fully in Chapter 18. End-of-life care and planning should be considered for any child with a terminal diagnosis. Some patients may be admitted for end-of-life home care services before being ready for admission to hospice services. Many hospice programs have admission criteria that do not permit therapies such as intravenous antibiotics, total parenteral nutrition, or enteral feedings that the family may wish to continue. It is therefore important to discuss the type of care the family wishes for the child early in discharge planning to clarify expectations and goals for home care (Wilson, 2004).

HOME CARE TRENDS

Numerous factors have influenced the shift toward home-based health care. Providing high-quality home health care for children generally requires parental desire and ability, professional assistance, and community preparedness (Rice, 2011). A natural family environment optimizes growth and development when stress is minimized and support is maximized.

Advances in medical technology have resulted in increased survival for children with congenital and acquired illnesses. Preterm infants or children who are ventilator dependent were once cared for indefinitely in an intensive care unit or long-term care facility. These children are now able to live with their families in their own homes (Feudtner, Villareale, Morray, and others, 2005). Safe and effective noninvasive ventilation modes and airway clearance devices and methods have also increased the home care of children with neuromuscular diseases. The survival of such children into adulthood has been enhanced by improvements in antibiotic therapy, evidence-based practices, more effective airway clearance techniques, and greater portability of technologic devices that were once impossible to transport into the home environment.

Children with cancer, kidney disorders, cystic fibrosis, spina bifida, cardiac and respiratory disorders, gastrointestinal disorders, neurodegenerative diseases, and human immunodeficiency virus (HIV) infection may have ongoing health care needs as a result of the disease, its treatment, or side effects of treatment (Balaguer and Gonzalez de Dios, 2008; Davis, 2006; Stevens, McKeever, Law, and others, 2006). Parents frequently face ongoing stressors after a child's hospitalization for diagnosis and treatment. Subsequent needs may include reinforcing teachings about the disease process, addressing the child's physical care needs, providing emotional support during this change in parental role, and teaching in a low-stress environment. Home-based nutrition programs are useful, safe, and well tolerated in children. Sufficient evidence indicates that these programs provide a better quality of life, decrease cost of therapy, and improve survival (DiBaise and Scolapio, 2007; Howard, 2006).

Improving the quality of life for both the child and the family is one of the driving forces in the efforts to move technology-dependent children from the hospital to the home setting. The concept of normalization describes the process whereby families of children with chronic illness over time begin to perceive the child and their family life as normal (Knafl and Deatrick, 2002). This has important implications for pediatric home care nurses in relation to the assessment of family function and understanding of family dynamics. The normalized family tends to be more flexible with treatments and incorporates the child with a disability or illness into the routines of daily living (Knafl and Deatrick, 2002). However, as part of this process, home care nurses should be aware that parents may experience chronic sorrow as a parental stressor. Gordon (2009) describes chronic sorrow as a normal grief response associated with a living loss (the loss of a healthy child) that is cyclical in nature. When encountering family expressions of chronic sorrow such as guilt and depression, home care nurses should develop evidence-based strategies to facilitate positive coping. Such strategies may include journaling, exercise, support groups, and professional counseling (Gordon, 2009).

The cost of care is an important factor in the health care delivery system today. Shorter inpatient stays are a reaction in part to the overwhelming cost of lengthy hospitalizations. Children either are not admitted to the hospital at all or are returned home as soon as possible after their illness. Home-based nursing care has decreased the length of hospital stays (Cooper, Wheeler, Woolfenden, and others, 2006). Shifting the financial burden from acute care to home care agencies is an attractive alternative to third-party reimbursers. Likewise, a portion of the financial burden is shifted to the family as caregivers. The family may be forced to absorb the costs of certain medications, supplies, transportation, shelter, utilities, food, laundry, housekeeping, and a portion of the nursing care. Over time, the care of chronically ill children can cause a financial burden to the family. Families may use up lifetime insurance benefits quickly, the primary caregiver may be unable to work, and many costs of health care are simply not covered by other means (Smith, Piamjariyakul, Yadrich, and others, 2010).

Home health care of children, however, is not restricted to children with chronic health care needs. Short-term intermittent therapies such as phototherapy, apnea monitoring, chemotherapy, and intravenous antibiotic administration may be successfully provided in a home setting rather than in an acute care setting. One study found that children who moved into an asthma-friendly home experienced large decreases in asthma morbidity and trigger exposure which often resulted in hospitalization (Takaro, Krieger, Song, and others, 2011). (See Asthma, Chapter 23.)

With the increased demand for nurses in home care and pervasive short supply, increasing attention has focused on the role of the family caregiver in providing home care. A recent survey by the National Alliance for Caregiving (2009) revealed that 30% of U.S. households have a person being cared for by another family member; this represents care above and beyond the daily routine care of the family household.

Primary caregiver responsibilities for the child in the home include:

- **Managing the illness** (providing daily hands-on care; monitoring the child's medical condition; and educating others, including extended family, to care for the child)
- **Identifying, accessing, and coordinating resources** (locating appropriate resources in the community to meet the child's needs and the needs of the family as the child's caregiver)
- **Maintaining the integrity of the family unit** (continuing to nurture the family unit, including siblings' needs, husband–wife relationships, and household maintenance)
- **Maintaining self** (managing chronic sorrow; balancing caregiver responsibilities with own physical, emotional, mental, and personal needs; recognizing stressors and potential caregiver burnout)

Home care nurses should recognize family responsibilities as areas for potential stress and, again, assist family in finding resources for respite and positive coping.

The American Academy of Pediatrics (AAP) supports the philosophy of permanency planning, wherein children with special health care needs obtain permanent family placement and ongoing relationship with caring adults (Johnson, Kastner, and AAP, 2005). Within this framework, the child's home environment with the child's family is perceived as the best place for the child to be reared. If the family is unable to support the child because of poor resources or family structure, options include extended family members, birth family plus an unrelated family sharing parental responsibilities, or two unrelated families sharing parental responsibilities. In addition, adoptive families may participate in care of the child with special health care needs. The AAP further stresses the importance of providing the child's family with adequate resources and support to promote family well-being (Johnson, Kastner, and AAP, 2005).

Respite care for caregivers of children with special care needs has been slow in its development and availability, although respite care centers are now common for adults. Respite care provides temporary relief to parents and allows a break from the responsibilities of caring for the child on a daily basis. Such care for ventilator-dependent children and those with skilled technologic care requirements is lacking throughout the United States. Respite care of children is still primarily done in the home. For example, a trusted and trained grandparent or extended family member along with private duty services may be called in to give the family a break from caring for the child.

Nurses can play an important role in advocating for the provision of high-quality respite care so families and caregivers can maintain appropriate family function, care for themselves, and continue to care for the child as necessary.

EFFECTIVE HOME CARE

Providing home-based care for children gives the nurse an opportunity to assess and interact with the family in its environment. This assessment can provide the health care team with valuable information about safety, support systems, nutrition, parental ability, and actual health care practices. This valuable information will inform future decisions for individualized care and realistic outcomes.

Pediatric home care nurses have two distinct areas of implementation of care. Nurses who perform intermittent skilled nursing visits may see many different types and numbers of patients each day. These nurses typically have a caseload assigned to them and accept responsibility for implementing the care plan. This mode of nursing care is the most commonly used today as a result of personnel shortages and decreased reimbursement. Most home visits now focus on helping the patient and caregiver achieve independence with care in the home, including home care by therapists, home infusion teaching by nurses, and care management, rather than direct provision of physical care.

Nurses who perform private-duty nursing or block nursing are usually assigned individual patients, and they remain in the home for a predetermined time (e.g., 8- or 12-hour blocks). The care plan is implemented over the course of the time in the home.

Required nursing skills depend on patient need, parental ability, complexity of family, and the home environment. In both types of home care, the pediatric nurse is responsible for assessing the patient and family and evaluating the appropriateness of the care plan (Box 20-1).

Consideration of the caregiver's willingness, ability, and limitations are of utmost importance when assessing the appropriateness of the care plan. It is vital to ensure that patients and families have adequate back-up support and access to resources such as social services. An increasing concern in pediatric home health care is obtaining a managing practitioner. Declining reimbursement and short hospital stays have increased patients' rapid movement through the continuum of care. For example, a patient may be seen in the emergency department or neonatal intensive care unit and then discharged to home care without ever seeing a primary care physician. It is therefore imperative that the provision of care for home patients involves multidisciplinary cooperation and communication among health care workers.

From technology dependence to pain management to wound care, pediatric nurses are appropriate professionals to meet children's health care needs at home. High-quality multidisciplinary care (e.g., a respiratory therapist and social worker) can have a significant, positive impact on family coping and child outcomes (Box 20-2) (Rice, 2006).

DISCHARGE PLANNING AND SELECTION OF A HOME CARE AGENCY

Identifying appropriate local community resources is critical to a successful transfer to home care (Box 20-3). The ultimate goal of discharge planning is for the family to become familiar with the child's needs and to be competent in providing that care. A discharge plan should include emergency management and provision of social and emotional support. General guidelines for discharge that allow for family individuality provide for ideal outcomes.

The AAP (Johnson, Kastner, and AAP, 2005) emphasizes that the goal for a home health care program for infants, children, or

BOX 20-1 INTERMITTENT SKILLED NURSING

Health Care Need

Child at risk—Parental substance abuse, growth failure, social or family situation potentially detrimental to child's well-being

Chronically ill but medically stable child with multiple care needs

Skilled procedures—Regularly scheduled injections or infusions, ostomy care, burn, care, dressing changes, phototherapy

Reinforcement of home care teaching; evaluation of caregiver's skills

Technology-dependent child (e.g., ventilator or tracheostomy, home total parenteral nutrition, or enteral feedings by pump)

Chronically ill child with multiple skilled nursing needs

Well-baby visit (e.g., postpartum home care)

Hospice child

Intervention

Regularly scheduled visits to assess patient status, evaluate home environment, teach care provider skills, determine status of growth and development, set goals with family for positive health outcomes

As-needed home visits during illness exacerbation to assess physical status and determine appropriate intervention

Assistance with transportation of child to ambulatory center or practitioner's office for evaluation and diagnostic services

Regular visits of limited duration to perform skilled nursing intervention, assess parental ability and desire to perform procedure, teach procedure technique, supervise parental performance of procedure

Assessment of patient status (body–mind–spirit); evaluation of safety of home environment; teaching, evaluation, and reinforcement of caregiver skills; determination of status of growth and development; goal setting with family for positive health outcomes

BOX 20-2 SERVICES THAT SUPPORT EFFECTIVE HOME CARE

- Adequate family training and preparation
- Primary care physician willing to oversee medical aspects of home care
- Professional caregivers trained in relevant nursing and communication skills
- Developmental intervention (e.g., physical, occupational, and speech therapy; early intervention)
- Appropriately designed and well-maintained equipment
- Supportive therapies (e.g., respiratory therapy, parenteral therapy, nutritional support)
- Adequate social and psychological support services
- High-quality respite care
- Appropriate home renovation
- Telephone service in the home
- Appropriate transportation
- Appropriate locally available emergency facilities
- Competent case management services
- Safe home environment (electricity, refrigeration, cleanliness)

BOX 20-3 CHARACTERISTICS OF A HIGH-QUALITY PEDIATRIC HOME CARE AGENCY

- Fully trained pediatric staff to provide for all aspects of care (nursing, rehabilitation therapies, pharmacy, dietitian, social work, home medical equipment)
- Prompt, responsive staff with 24-hour availability
- Family-centered care
- Comprehensive continuing education programs
- Certification of local, state, and federal regulatory agencies
- Accreditation by The Joint Commission or Community Health Accreditation Program

Data from Dittbrenner H: Pediatric home care as a viable new service, *Caring* 18(2):12–15, 1998; and Lovejoy D: *Making the transition to home health nursing: a practice guide*, New York, 1997, Springer.

NURSING TIP If home care equipment is different from hospital equipment, have the portable equipment delivered to the hospital to allow family use before discharge.

Much of the success of home care, particularly for children who are dependent on medical technology or who have complex medical problems, depends on careful planning and preparation. General principles of discharge planning and the transition to home care are presented in Chapter 26. Discharge planning must begin early; should be based on criteria of child and family readiness; must be a multidisciplinary process, including representatives from acute care facilities, home care, and community settings; and must involve the family.

Predischarge assessment (Box 20-4) and planning should include:
- The child's medical, nursing, educational, and other therapeutic needs (respiratory, pharmaceutical)
- Family members' (including siblings') education and training, coping skills, and adjustment needs (including transportation of equipment and child)
- Community readiness in areas such as availability of equipment, appropriate nursing and other personnel, educational and developmental services, respite care, and emergency plans
- Emergency care and transport plan
- Financial arrangements
- Infection control practices (clean technique is most often emphasized for procedural care)
- Plan for follow-up medical care (designated medical home equipment company and pharmacy)

Creative financial planning, including negotiating arrangements with the insurance company, health maintenance or managed care organization, and public programs, may be required.

Early involvement of the home care agency in the discharge planning process promotes continuity of care and a smooth transition from hospital to home (Box 20-5). Before discharge, a general plan, sometimes called an individualized home care plan, should be developed with multidisciplinary input. This care plan should address the range of needs identified as part of the comprehensive predischarge assessment.

One method of providing home care instructions is with video recordings. After the family masters the procedures, consider recording their performance on video. Visual learning is most helpful for people

adolescents with chronic conditions or disabilities is the provision of community-based, culturally effective, comprehensive, and cost-effective health care within a nurturing home environment that maximizes the capabilities of the individual and minimizes the effects of the disabilities.

BOX 20-4 EXAMPLE OF PREDISCHARGE ASSESSMENT FOR A TECHNOLOGY-DEPENDENT INFANT

The Child's Family

Identification and training of primary caretakers

Identification and training of caretakers for respite and emergency care

Parent employment status while caring for child at home

Family financial picture, especially if one parent must stop working

Sibling preparation

Availability of psychosocial support services

Technical Equipment and Supplies for the Home

Home care company's availability and experience

Home care company's coordination of services with local health care provider and others

Twenty-four-hour availability and coverage for unexpected situations

Community Nursing and Support Services

Availability, training, and experience

Adequacy of number of personnel to meet needs

Additional training of staff, if needed

Twenty-four-hour availability of ambulance services

Physical Environment of the Home

Adequacy of space for equipment and supplies

Heavy equipment (e.g., ventilator, oxygen tanks, compressor) accessibility

Layout of home (e.g., number of floors, stairways, room accessibility, room sizes)

Location and layout of bedrooms

Adequacy of apartment building elevator and fire escape

Telephone access

Type of transportation family uses

Possibility of modifying living space to minimize invasiveness of technology without isolating child

Adequacy of heating and cooling systems

Adequacy of electrical system to accommodate equipment

Infection control measures

Emergency Plan

Identification and training of those involved

Written implementation plan: who, what, where, when, how (include telephone numbers)

Notification of utility companies for priority repairs and maintenance

Notification of emergency medical unit (911)

Emergency drill

Primary Care Provider

Identification of local primary provider or pediatrician who is able to assume direct care responsibility and coordinate other care providers

Inclusion of local provider in discharge planning

Needs of local provider before child's discharge

Alternate provider if primary is unavailable

Adapted from Bakewell-Sachs S, Porth S: Discharge planning and home care of the technology-dependent infant, *J Obstet Gynecol Neonatal Nurs* 24(1):77–83, 1995.

BOX 20-5 CRITICAL HOME CARE REFERRAL INFORMATION

- Scheduled medications
- Durable medical equipment
- Medical supplies
- Transportation needs
- Adaptive equipment
- Rehabilitation therapies (occupational, physical, and speech therapy)
- Psychologic counseling
- Social work referral
- Nursing care
- Respite plans
- Key family members
- Demographic information
- Reimbursement information

Modified from Townsend JL: Assessment of the child and family. In Votroubek WL, Townsend JL, editors: *Pediatric home care*, ed 2, Gaithersburg, MD, 1997, Aspen.

who cannot read or who are not fluent in English. Additionally, Internet resources are encouraged.

The plans for transition from hospital to home should include family members (ideally two persons) both learning and demonstrating all aspects of the child's care in the hospital. An in-hospital trial period, during which parents provide total care for the child, is generally beneficial. The home care nurse plays an important role in assessing this experience with the family. A predischarge home visit offers the home care nurse the opportunity to meet the family and help them assess their own preparedness and that of the home environment. It also helps them to discuss plans for arranging the child's equipment at home (see Fig. 20-1), reinforce prior discharge teaching, and implement any additional teaching that is necessary (AAP, 2008).

A comprehensive discharge plan includes the care plan, specific written instructions to facilitate continuity, and detailed information about home care outcomes.

CARE COORDINATION (CASE MANAGEMENT)

Traditional definitions of case management generally focus on cost control, attainment of desired clinical outcomes, and monitoring and evaluation of care provided. However, for optimum home care of children who are technology dependent, case management (or care coordination) should be viewed more broadly.

Changes in health care over the past 3 decades have not only improved survival and decreased morbidity among children with special health care needs but also heralded higher costs for health care and services provided. As a result, insurance companies have focused on reducing services to contain costs. The advent of managed care and fee-for-service reimbursement has changed the outlook for families desiring to have the child in the home. Often services are provided by multiple organizations and multiple vendors with different missions and lack of consistent single systems linking home health care. In addition, eligibility criteria for receiving funding and services are complex and vary from one state to another. As a result, coordination of home care can be challenging, frustrating, and complicated for the family (AAP, Council on Children with Disabilities, 2005).

The concept of care coordination is to link children with special home health care needs (and their families) to services and resources in a coordinated effort to provide the child with optimum care

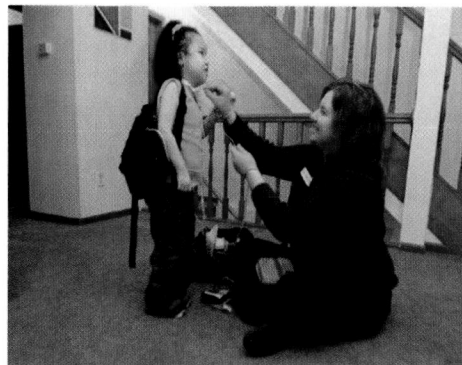

FIG 20-2 Tracheostomy care in the home setting requires technical skill and knowledge of childhood development. (Photo courtesy BJC Hospice, St. Louis.)

(AAP, Council on Children with Disabilities, 2005). Care coordination has several purposes. Its primary goal is ensuring continuity for the child and family across hospital, home, educational, therapeutic, and other settings. Other goals involve facilitating timely access to services and enhancing child and family well-being. Care should be coordinated among multiple providers to reduce the complexity of care for the child, reduce fragmentation of care, prevent duplication of services, and decrease the burden of care for the family. Case managers from a number of agencies may be involved in the patient's care, which may add to the parents' confusion. The home care nurse may assume the role of care coordinator and should make efforts to coordinate all case managers for meetings with the family to minimize confusion and prevent duplication. Care coordination should ensure that the child's medical, nursing, and health maintenance needs, as well as financial issues, psychosocial concerns, and educational needs of the child and family, are addressed (AAP, Council on Children with Disabilities, 2005).

Care coordination is most effective if a single person works with the family to accomplish the many tasks and responsibilities involved (Box 20-6). The nurse case manager should be knowledgeable about community resources, including:

- Primary, secondary, and tertiary health care services
- Speech, language, hearing, and vision resources
- Respite care services
- Financial assistance programs
- Parent groups
- Advocacy groups
- Local, state, and federal public officials
- Transportation services
- Private-sector individuals with an interest in children with disabilities

With a greater focus on outcomes of home health care, the nurse case manager has to be resourceful and skilled in communication at a number of levels. A valuable tool for nurse case managers is the care path, which is a multidisciplinary care plan aimed at measuring the quality of patient care outcomes derived from standardized patient outcomes. The care path evaluates the quality of patient care with respect to cost-effectiveness and timeliness. (For samples of home care clinical care paths, see Rice, 2006.) Care paths may also be used to help nurses and other health care workers learn home care. Nurses should share care paths with the family members involved in patient care to provide direction and help the family see the eventual goals of care.

Although professionals must always see part of their role as ensuring that integrated, coordinated care is provided, care coordination should promote the family's role as primary decision maker and enhance the family's capability to meet the special needs of the child and the family unit. Families may choose to be involved to varying degrees in coordinating their child's care. Many parents take on increasing responsibility for care coordination over time. Encourage and support families in this role. Home care nurses and case managers should be aware that the termination of private-duty or home care nursing can be a difficult transition for which families may need preparation. A gradual reduction in services provided allows patients and families to adjust favorably to the changes. Care coordination by office-based nurses for children and youth with special health care needs decreased emergency department visits and periodic office visits, thus significantly decreasing the cost of health care; increased health care costs were associated with more physician-dependent care coordination activities among such children (Antonelli, Stille, and Antonelli, 2008).

ROLE OF THE NURSE, TRAINING, AND STANDARDS OF CARE

The home care nurse must share a level of technical expertise with the critical care nurse while being able to adapt equipment, procedures, and the nursing process to the home setting (Fig. 20-2) (Cervasio, 2010; Rice, 2011). (See Chapters 22 and 23 for specific technical skills that may be required in home care practice.) The need for technical expertise must be matched by knowledge of child development and the ability to work creatively with the child who is challenged by chronic illness and technology dependence. When practicing in the home, the home care nurse must be comfortable making independent nursing judgments and problem solving with no immediate assistance. At the same time, the nurse must have excellent interpersonal skills; an ability to work with other professionals and the family; and, most important, respect for family autonomy. Patient outcomes are more readily achieved with a balance of nursing skills that demonstrates clinical excellence; adaptability; accountability; and the ability to develop positive relationships with patients, families, and practitioners (Box 20-7).

When working with a home care agency, nurses should expect to receive patient placements appropriate to their expertise. They should also expect to receive orientation to the skills and knowledge base of the home care nursing specialty and subsequent continuing education to develop as expert practitioners. The minimum initial orientation should include the individual patient's care plan and equipment needs; the agency's policies and procedures, including procedures for addressing any problems that may occur when care is provided in the home; legal liability issues; and documentation procedures. The orientation should place strong emphasis on issues specific to home care. For

---

BOX 20-7   QUALITIES OF A PEDIATRIC HOME CARE NURSE

- Demonstrates flexibility in skills and case management (care coordination)
- Recognizes that the nurse is a guest in the home
- Respects family culture and adapts appropriately
- Works as an interdisciplinary team member
- Demonstrates expertise in pediatric care (assessment and technical skills)
- Possesses and uses effective communication skills

---

example, the nursing care plan should be based on information obtained about the environment, family dynamics, and health-related behaviors. The multidisciplinary care path may assist nurses, technicians, other health care providers involved in the child's care, and the family, serving as a focal point for achievement of patient and family outcomes.

Reimbursement-driven documentation in home care differs from documentation practices in the hospital setting. Increasingly, documentation must be written in specific ways to qualify for reimbursement.

Supervision of practice, including occasional site visits by a nursing supervisor, should be provided. Mentoring or precepting is ideal. Because of the unique practice environment of home care nurses, it is important for an agency to facilitate sharing among peers to decrease work-related stress, increase job satisfaction, and support high-quality patient care.

Public or private home care agencies that participate in the Medicare or Medicaid programs must be certified by a federally designated state certification body and abide by federal and state regulations. Additionally, the American Nurses Association has developed standards of nursing practice for public health and home care nurses (American Nurses Association, 2007a, 2007b). Generalist and clinical specialist certification in both home health and community health is offered by the American Nurses Credentialing Center,* a subsidiary of the American Nurses Association. The Hospice and Palliative Nurses Association offers certification in hospice nursing. Despite important differences between pediatric and adult care in the home, as of this writing, no national standards specific to pediatric home care practice have been developed. Nursing practice in pediatric home care should be guided by published guidelines, textbooks, peer-reviewed articles, and written standards of care for pediatric patients. Professional nursing organizations such as Infusion Nurses Society, National Association of Neonatal Nurses, Society of Pediatric Nurses, Association of Pediatric Hematology/Oncology Nurses, National Association of Pediatric Nurse Practitioners, and others have published standards of care that apply to pediatric home health nursing practice (Box 20-8).

A quality improvement program is an important component of an effective home care agency. Evidence-based practice is rapidly becoming an important aspect of home health care, as is benchmarking, in which the product or practice (in this case, patient outcome) is compared with other agencies' outcomes and practices to determine best practice; this allows agencies to see how they measure compared with other similar agencies (Yoder-Wise, 2011). The OASIS (Outcome and Assessment Information Set), as part of Medicare, has been established for adults in home health care; however, as of this writing, no

---

BOX 20-8   SELECTED RESOURCES FOR HOME CARE

American Academy of Pediatrics
141 Northwest Point Blvd.
Elk Grove Village, IL 60007
847-434-4000
Fax: 847-434-8000
http://www.aap.org

Association of Maternal and Child Health Programs
2030 M St. NW, Suite 350
Washington, DC 20036
202-775-0436
Fax: 202-775-0061
http://www.amchp.org

Children's Hospice International
1101 King St., Suite 360
Alexandria, VA 22314
800-2-4-CHILD, 703-684-0330
http://www.chionline.org

Father's Network
Kindering Center, 16120 NE Eighth St.
Bellevue, WA 98008-3937
425-653-4286
http://www.fathersnetwork.org

National Association for Home Care and Hospice
228 Seventh St. SE
Washington, DC 20003
202-547-7424
Fax: 202-547-3540
http://www.nahc.org

National Dissemination Center for Children with Disabilities
1825 Connecticut Ave. NW, Suite 700
Washington, DC 20009
Voice/TTY: 800-695-0285, 202-884-8200
Fax: 202-884-8441
http://www.nichcy.org

National Hospice and Palliative Care Organization
1731 King St., Suite 100
Alexandria, VA 22314
703-837-1500
http://www.nhpco.org/templates/1/homepage.cfm

Pediatric Home Care Association of America
Division of National Association for Home Care and Hospice (see contact information above); special feature on website is peds@home, an electronic newsletter

PediatricNursing.com
Health resources for parents
http://www.pediatricnursing.com/parents

Sibling Support Project
http://www.siblingsupport.org

---

*8515 Georgia Ave., Suite 400, Silver Spring, MD 20910-3492; 800-284-2378; http://www.nursecredentialing.org.

such data exist for children younger than age 18 years. As a part of OASIS, home health care quality measures have been established to measure patient care outcomes for Medicare reimbursement purposes. Other certification and licensing organizations that may oversee and regulate practice in home health care include The Joint Commission, Centers for Medicare and Medicaid Services, Occupational Safety and Health Administration, and Community Health Accreditation Program. The Health Insurance Portability and Accountability Act of 1996 guidelines affect the manner in which patient records are handled in home health care to ensure patient confidentiality. Ongoing changes in home care legislation and reimbursement are expected (Rice, 2011).

FAMILY-CENTERED HOME CARE

Technology dependence, chronic illness, and complex care requirements cross social, cultural, spiritual, and economic boundaries. Regardless of a family's background, the nurse must respect family values in the provision of home care services. The home is the family's domain, and the child is at home because the family's central role is to nurture and raise the child. The ultimate responsibility for managing the child's health, developmental, and emotional needs lies with the family.

The home care nurse must respect and encourage the family's central role in care of the child and must collaborate with the family in efforts to care for the child. Family-centered nursing practice is essential in the home setting. Family-centered care has become the acknowledged standard of care for children with special health care needs.

The philosophic basis for family-centered practice is the recognition that the family is the constant in the child's life, but the service systems and personnel within those systems fluctuate. Professionals working with families of children with complex chronic problems must respect the family's central, caring role; their knowledge; and their particular and unique expertise. Families have the most intimate knowledge of the child's strengths and abilities, the challenges of providing care, and the abilities and needs of other family members (Arango, 2011). Believing that no one knows the child better than the family is critical to the success of any health care plan.

DIVERSITY IN HOME CARE

Respect for varied family structures and for racial, ethnic, cultural, and socioeconomic diversity among families is essential in home care. Home care nurses work in close relationships with family members throughout the course of an illness (see Family-Centered Care box). The nurse must assess and respect the family's background and lifestyle choices. Pay particular attention to communication. The meaning of the words used and the way in which they are said may affect people of various cultural groups in different ways. Take volume of speech and language style into consideration as part of a family cultural assessment.

> **NURSING TIP** One should not assume that everyone who speaks English can read the language. Color-coded medication bottles, written schedules, and pillboxes or oral syringes may aid compliance with prescription administration. Pictures or special symbols may be helpful when providing instructions for procedures and medication administration.

The home care nurse must also pay particular attention to nonverbal communication. Body language, eye contact, and degree of physical contact have different meanings within a particular culture.

 FAMILY-CENTERED CARE

Developing Relationships with Culturally Diverse Families

I work in the inner city, and my home care patients come from a variety of racial and ethnic backgrounds. I am Caucasian, from Australia. Often, when I first visit a family, there is an initial coolness or apprehension toward me. This is understandable because I am a stranger, and perhaps families think I'll judge them in one way or another. By the end of the first visit, however, there is usually a smile as I leave. By the second visit, they often greet me with a smile at the door, and by the third visit we usually have a friendship, trust, and an ease of communication.

If I'm working on a case for an extended time, I use a holistic nursing approach. This involves being aware of how the child's illness affects the entire family. As I listen over many weeks to their fears and questions, and often as I share faith perspectives, a bond begins to form. I find it a privilege to share in their joys and their pain, and I feel rewarded by the trust that they invest in me.

Julie Edgerton, RN
Home Care Nurse
Children's National Medical Center
Washington, DC

 COMMUNITY FOCUS

Spiritual Assessment

Children are spiritual beings, but their expression of spirituality may be limited by adults' ability to understand how they feel (Mueller, 2010). Spiritual distress in children may be evidenced by (Mueller, 2010):

- Expressing a lack of hope or verbalizations of sorrow
- Refusing interactions with family, spiritual leaders, or friends
- Verbalizing a desire to be separated from their support system or expressing feelings of alienation
- Demonstrating an inability to pray or participate in religious activity
- Expressing feelings of anger toward God or feelings of hopelessness and suffering

Families may also differ in their cultural view of children, health care, childrearing practices, and illness and its causes and meaning. The family's health care practices and beliefs may influence the level of investment a family makes in the child's care. The family's religion or spirituality also can have a major influence on a family's response to the child's special health care needs. Some families look for spiritual meaning and purpose for the illness. Other families may choose to reject past religious ties. In some cultures, religion and beliefs about health care and illness are closely intertwined (McEvoy, 2003); thus, it is important that home care nurses assess the relationships among culture, religion, and the family's beliefs about the child's illness (see Community Focus box).

The home care nurse, aware that personal values drive behavior, must learn about the family's culture, ask questions without implying judgment, interpret the mainstream medical culture for the family, and help families design interventions that meet their preferences. When possible, use culture-specific teaching materials. Most important, verify that the family understands what their physician has told them (see Complementary and Alternative Therapy box).

Respect for family diversity and an awareness of the family's stages of development and of adjustment to a child's illness assist the home

Use of Complementary and Alternative Medicine in Children

A wide variety of CAM strategies are used in home setting by adults. In such settings, use of CAM by the children is also common. Prayer, herbal remedies, acupuncture, massage, meditation, breathing, music, therapeutic storytelling, and art therapy are but a sample of the variety of therapies used in North American households (Rice, 2006).

CAM, Complementary and alternative medicine.

care nurse in recognizing and promoting family strengths and in respecting various coping mechanisms. Labels such as *dysfunctional, difficult,* and *noncompliant* can reinforce negative expectations and shape the behaviors of both parents and professionals. On the other hand, identifying, emphasizing, and building on family strengths and coping mechanisms are strategies that promote a central goal in the nursing care of the child and family: family empowerment. The home care nurse working with families should remain flexible and open minded because new family strengths may emerge over time, and coping mechanisms may wax and wane with the stresses of caring for a child with serious or multiple problems.

PARENT–PROFESSIONAL COLLABORATION

Family-centered nursing practice is built on a foundation of parent–professional collaboration, which represents a dynamic shift from the traditional unidirectional relationships between health care providers and families. The Collaborative Family Healthcare Coalition has developed core competencies for professionals collaborating with families (McDaniel and Campbell, 1996). Collaborative caring allows the nurse and family to work together and share outcomes in a deep and meaningful way. This approach, essential in the home care setting, is characterized by the following (Kellett and Mannion, 1999):

- Encouraging activities to develop self-confidence and self-esteem
- Displaying increased awareness of and respect for family caregivers
- Recognizing that families vary in defining their role
- Demonstrating an ability to understand the family's approach to caregiving
- Sharing perspectives, not just tasks and functions
- Supporting family in their primary, irreplaceable role as caregiver
- Exchanging expertise in providing care to the child
- Assisting family in recognizing their contributions as worthwhile
- Identifying strengths and resources of child and family
- Negotiating options, priorities, and preferences
- Assisting with coping by allowing family to find meaning in caring for child at home

Communication with the family should not be intrusive. There is no need to collect information from the family that can be obtained from the child's records. The nurse should explain to the family the reason for questions, particularly those that the family may perceive as intrusive, and should tell families who will have access to the information. The nurse must also assure families that they have a right to expect confidentiality in regard to the data collected. When working in the home, the nurse must respect the privacy of family communications that may be overheard.

Communication with family members should include sharing with the family, in a supportive manner, complete and unbiased information about all aspects of the child's condition and care. Parents often

Knowledgeable Parents

It is not unusual for parents, particularly those whose children have chronic illnesses or complex care regimens, to be more knowledgeable about their child's condition than a nurse who is assigned to the child's care. This can be disconcerting for both the parents and the nurse. It is important to remember and reinforce that regardless of the condition, the parents will always know more about their child than the professional caring for the child. The nurse and parents can set goals for care in an atmosphere of mutual respect. If the parents' goal is respite from prolonged caregiving, they are less likely to want to give long explanations about the child's care, and it may be more appropriate for the nurse to seek assistance from an experienced peer. If the parents wish to maintain maximum participation in care delivery, the nurse and the parents can negotiate the collaboration.

When teaching parents to perform complex chronic care regimens at home, advise them to expect to know more about their child's care than professionals who may come to assist them, whether it is home health, hospital, or outpatient personnel. At the same time, assure them that various professionals, experienced in working with a multitude of families, will have a scientific knowledge base and a wealth of options for addressing and solving care problems.

Teresa L. Hall, MS, RN
Hathaway Children's Services
Sylmar, Calif.

feel overwhelming frustration when trying to obtain accurate information about their child's illness and its management. Parents want information given slowly and repeated as necessary over time; they want explanations in terms they can understand; and they want the opportunity to ask questions, which should be answered in a straightforward manner. Stating "I don't know" or "I'll find out" is better than pretending to know or giving excuses.

Nurses can make plans with the parents to gather relevant information when necessary. Nurses should share information with families in a way that has meaning in their cultural context. Many parents report a preference for interactions with professionals who communicate empathy and concern. Families vary in the amount of information they prefer regarding their child's status. Home care nurses should restrict their communications with other professionals to clinically relevant information about the family.

On occasion, parents and nurses may disagree about proper procedures for the child's care. Nurses should respect parental preferences in any situation that does not pose danger or risk for the child (see Family-Centered Care box). If parents wish to alter a treatment plan that is part of medical orders, the nurse should ask that they negotiate the change with the practitioner because the nurse must follow the written medical orders. If they cannot resolve disagreements, contact a home care supervisor or case manager (care coordinator) to assist with problem solving. Increasingly, home care agencies are developing ethics committees and policies for managing difficult situations such as treatment refusal (see Critical Thinking Case Study box).

A tool that might be helpful to the pediatric home care nurse is the Caregiver Strain Index, a 13-item assessment designed to ascertain caregiver stress and subsequently develop appropriate strategies for individual and family coping (Sullivan, 2003). For further information on conflict resolution, see Askew, Williams, Rachel, and others (2008).

In addition to maintaining a sense of control over their child's care, families need to control their home and personal lives. For this reason,

CRITICAL THINKING CASE STUDY

Family-Centered Home Care and Conflicts

A family wants to begin oral feeding of their 3-year-old daughter, Sarah, who is ventilator dependent, has a tracheostomy, and is being tube fed through a skin-level gastrostomy feeding tube. The mother, who is Sarah's primary caretaker, is adamant about starting oral feedings so Sarah can be more like other children her age. One day the mother asks you, the nurse case manager overseeing the child's home care, to feed Sarah baby food by mouth to see how she tolerates the feeding. The child is alert and sociable yet cannot communicate her wishes except through crying and whining. She has a seizure disorder and has had several episodes of aspiration pneumonia since birth. Sarah appears to have a considerable amount of tongue thrusting and lots of oral mucus that must be suctioned frequently to prevent aspiration; her cough reflex is compromised and usually only elicited with tracheal suctioning.

1. Evidence—Is there sufficient evidence to draw any conclusions about the issue of feeding Sarah at this time?
2. Assumptions—Describe some underlying assumptions about the following:
   a. Sarah's readiness for oral feedings
   b. Sarah's ability to tolerate oral feedings
   c. The mother's request for Sarah to start oral feedings
3. What implications and priorities for nursing care may be drawn at this time?
4. Does the evidence objectively support your conclusion?

nurses should discuss "house rules" with the family and address issues such as the physical environment, private areas in the home, responsibility for maintaining the child's environment, and interactions with siblings (see Nursing Care Guidelines box).

Home care nursing encourages a close and rewarding relationship with the family. One of the most important aspects of this relationship is maintaining professional boundaries and a therapeutic role that is supportive of the client and family but does not cross the line of nursing professionalism (Wright, 2006) (see Critical Thinking Case Study box, p. 606).

THE NURSING PROCESS

The most recent American Nurses Association (2007a) standards for home health care nursing practice include six standards of practice, which are the components of the nursing process: assessment, diagnosis, outcomes identification, planning, implementation, and evaluation (Gorski, 2008). In the home, the family is a partner in each step of the nursing process. Assessment should address family strengths and resources, as well as the child's health status (Box 20-9).* The principles of communication discussed previously guide data collection. The nurse shares observations neutrally without value judgment and in a way that preserves the family's own role in decision making.

All information gathered as part of the assessment process is shared with the family. The nurse should recognize that the family's perception of their most important need will generally guide their behavior and consume their attention and energy. Family priorities should guide the planning process.

*Self-report instruments to help families identify concerns, priorities, resources, and sources of support include Family Needs Survey, which is available from FPG Child Development Institute, CB 8180, Chapel Hill, NC 27599; 919-966-0857 or can be downloaded from http://www.fpg.unc.edu.

NURSING CARE GUIDELINES

Negotiating "House Rules" for Home Care

House Rules

Parking—Specify where the nurse should park and any community regulations.

Access—Specify where the nurse enters the home. Is knocking or ringing the bell preferred?

Personal belongings—Where does the nurse store own coat, boots, and so on? Does the family prefer slippers to shoes in the home?

Meals—Where can the nurse store own food? Note: This is important given the cultural diversity of families.

Radio and television—Identify preferences regarding usage. Remember, this may help nurses remain awake at night.

Patient room—The nurse is responsible for the child's immediate environment. Maintaining a clean working area and cleaning up the room at the end of the shift are the nurse's responsibility.

Telephone—Agency policy may dictate that all personal calls be limited to brief periods. Clarify expectations regarding mobile phone use in the home setting by the nurse. Note: Many nurses do need to check in with home at some interval during the evening, but this practice should not interfere with the nurse's responsibility to the child and family in her or his care.

Visitors—Identify who may enter the home when the parents are away (e.g., child's friends or grandparents). A list of names should be available.

Privacy—Describe what parts of the home are off limits to the nurse and at what times.

Child

Routine—Specify times for playtime, bathtime, and bedtime. To what extent does the parent want to participate in these routines?

Mealtime—Specify where the family wants the child fed; if tube fed, specify a preference as to how and where it is done.

Clothing—Identify who picks out the child's clothes. Identify where the laundry is and who is responsible for washing the sick child's clothing.

Discipline—Discuss specific guidelines for discipline.

Homework—Discuss when it should be done and who is responsible for ensuring it is completed.

Siblings

Discipline—Establish guidelines regarding how parents should be informed of siblings' conflicts and how discipline should be handled. Note: Parents or another caregiver must be in the home when siblings are home.

Patient care—Be specific regarding how children can help with the child's care. Discuss any concerns regarding behavior that may compromise the child's or siblings' safety.

Nursing

Parental notification—Specify what information the family wishes to be aware of immediately and what can wait until they are home.

Limits of responsibility—Specify duties the nurse may not perform, such as transporting the child to care facilities or babysitting the child or siblings not under the nurse's care.

Environment—Discuss the need to have adequate lighting, a comfortable working area, and safe environment for the nurse.

NURSING TIP At each visit, physically handle and look at all medications. Check them against the medical orders and read the labels. As needed, do pill counts from visit to visit. There may be discrepancies, duplications, or changes between hospitalizations or follow-up visits. Clarify medications' purposes, effects, and dosages for the family.

? CRITICAL THINKING CASE STUDY
Maintaining Therapeutic Boundaries

As the home care nurse who has been working with a 4-year-old ventilator-dependent child, Derek, weekly for about 5 months, you are aware that the parents have become increasingly argumentative with each other. Most of the arguments are about whether Mr. Jones helps enough with the child's care and the house cleaning. Mr. Jones works full time at one job and then supplements the family income by working at a part-time job every weekend. Mrs. Jones complains to you about her husband's lack of involvement with the child and his care. Derek requires constant care, and the family has many expenses related to his physical care; the child is severely developmentally impaired and is not expected to improve significantly despite numerous medical interventions. He is the only child, although Mrs. Jones stated at one time that they wanted to have many children.

1. Evidence—Is there sufficient evidence to draw any conclusions about the family situation at this time?
2. Assumptions—Describe some underlying assumptions about:
   a. Home care of the child with a chronic, terminal condition (see p. 596)
   b. Impact of the chronic condition, child's prognosis, and required care on the parents
   c. Status of the marriage relationship between Mr. and Mrs. Jones
3. What implications and priorities for nursing care may be drawn at this time?
4. Does the evidence objectively support your conclusion?

BOX 20-9   SAMPLE FAMILY ASSESSMENT QUESTIONS

- What are the child's and family's experiences and expectations of disease or illness?
- How does that affect the current situation?
- Is the current coping status a reflection of a new condition, the same chronic condition, or a new phase in a chronic condition?
- How can the nurse address family needs and promote health among all family members?
- What specific nursing interventions will facilitate a healthy response to child and family limitations caused by the illness?
- What are the goals of care?

Modified from Gedaly-Duff, Helms ML: Family child health nursing. In Hanson SMH, Boyd ST, editors: *Family health care nursing*, Philadelphia, 1996, Davis.

The nurse should outline both short- and long-term goals, and the child, family, and professionals involved should agree on them. The care plan should integrate various disciplines that may be involved with the child to eliminate duplication and coordinate and consolidate care requirements. Cross-training of professionals and a multidisciplinary mode of treatment are also useful when a child has multiple and complex care requirements. For example, certain physical or occupational therapy routines may be incorporated into the child's morning nursing procedures, or speech therapy interventions may be conducted by the parent or nurse around eating times so the entire day is not occupied by procedures. A written schedule of daily routines should be developed and followed by all caregivers. Ratcliff (2007) stresses the importance of the written care plan for the ventilator-dependent child in the home to ensure that the care being given is consistent; written instructions regarding the frequency of equipment

FAMILY-CENTERED CARE
What I Learned About Home Care

I learned many things as a result of having home care for four children over a period of 8 years. Two of the major areas I learned about were communication and families' rights. It took a long time to learn some of these things.

Initially, I tried hard to be sensitive to the professionals and often put my own feelings and needs aside. It took a while to learn that I could stand up for myself and my family and that my child could continue to receive good care. One area important to me was to have nurses withhold judgment on our parenting style, even if they might have parented differently.

Communication needs to be open and two way. Families and nurses ought to tell each other what is going well. For example, "Thanks for keeping the room so neat while you're here" can help a nurse see a family's appreciation. There was so little I could do as just "Mommy" that it really meant a lot to me when nurses would say, "That's such a cute outfit you picked out for him today." Communicating about little things, even inconsequential topics such as favorite television shows, makes it easier to communicate about more important things and about problems. Communication has to be open about problems, too.

Jeni Stepanek
Mother
Upper Marlboro, Md.

cleaning, chest physiotherapy, and reused versus discarded supplies assist in providing consistent care.

Goals of care and achievement of established outcomes are supported by intervention strategies that reflect normalization (see Chapter 18) and the interests and abilities of the child and family. Nurses can help the family explore a range of alternative strategies, services, and resources so the family can choose the best match for their situation.

Family participation in evaluating a home care plan can occur on several levels. Families and care providers should regularly review the goals of care and update the care plan as required. The nurse can ask the family open-ended questions at regular intervals to assess their opinions on the effectiveness of care. As part of the evaluation process, acknowledge families for their successes and accomplishments. Finally, give families an opportunity to evaluate individual home care nurses, the home care agency, and other service providers periodically. The evaluation should address the nurse's knowledge, skills, and respect for the family's choices. The agency should use these evaluations to improve quality of care (see Family-Centered Care box).

Technologic trends that influence the nursing process in home care include the use of laptop computers (notebooks) to document the home visit and mobile telephones and other small handheld computers that store large amounts of data (tablet computers), including addresses, appointments, patient tracking systems, textbooks, and pharmacologic databases. Internet and e-mail services, which increase patient–practitioner accessibility and communication, and telemedicine or telehealth, which has various features, including electronic systems that can transmit physiologic data directly to the practitioner via the telephone, also influence the nursing process (Cady, Kelly, and Finkelstein, 2008; Vasquez, 2008). Telephone triage has become standard in many health care institutions, and standards for pediatric triage have been published elsewhere. Concerns with the increasing use of technology in health care are cost, governmental regulations and patient care standards, liability and malpractice issues, ethics, and confidentiality matters (Rice, 2006). In addition, the use of any technology

BOX 20-10   INCORPORATING DEVELOPMENTAL SUPPORT INTO THE HOME CARE PLAN

Example: 6-month-old infant with a history of 24-week prematurity; currently using cardiorespiratory monitor, oxygen via nasal cannula, and nasogastric feeding tube

Outcome Criteria

Age-appropriate growth—developmental activities promoted with normal parameters achieved

Absence of growth and development deficits for age within limits imposed by illness

Intervention

Assess growth and development with the Denver II Developmental Assessment.

Reassess growth and development every 4 weeks.

Provide consistent caregiver.

Instruct parents in normal growth and development for child's age, reasons for delay, and anticipated outcomes.

Inform parents of age-related play and other activities that enhance growth and development and provide stimulation.

Consult with physical, occupational, and speech therapists to incorporate recommendations in daily routines.

Provide visual, auditory, and tactile stimulation, including mobiles with or without color, music, toys, books, and television.

Hold, rock, pat, and talk to child.

Data from Klijanowicz AS: Care of high-risk infant. In Votroubek WL, Townsend JL, editors: *Pediatric home care*, ed 2, Gaithersburg, Md, 1997, Aspen; Jaffe M: *Pediatric nursing care plans*, ed 2, Englewood, Col, 1998, Skidmore-Roth; and Luxner K, Jaffe M: *Delmar's pediatric nursing care plans*, ed 3, Clifton Park, NY, 2004, Thomson Delmar Learning.

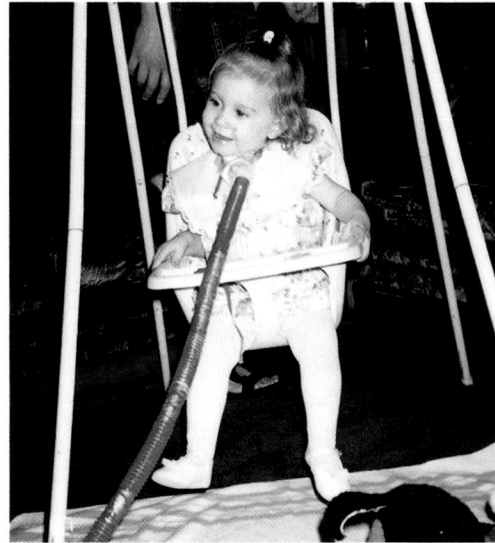

FIG 20-3 The use of lengthy tubing facilitates a child's freedom of movement.

raises concerns regarding the nurse–patient relationship (high tech–low touch) and the nurse's role.

PROMOTION OF OPTIMUM DEVELOPMENT, SELF-CARE, AND EDUCATION

There is little question that living at home offers most children with complex medical problems great social and emotional advantages over living in hospitals and other institutional settings. However, in infancy and throughout the developmental stages, a child's medical condition and dependence on medical technology can place constraints on and pose challenges to normal development. For example, the child may have lengthy and repeated hospitalizations; developmental regression can occur in response to stress; fatigue may result from an underlying pathologic condition, the exacerbation of an illness, or medication side effects; and equipment requirements may impede mobility, exploration, and independence. The challenge of providing support for normal development in a child who is chronically ill and technology dependent is to maximize the opportunities for developmentally appropriate experiences while respecting the limits of the medical condition and the equipment requirements.

Home care plans are designed to promote optimum child development through assessment, planning, and referrals, and through interventions that address normalization issues and self-care (Box 20-10). General principles for a family-centered assessment and planning

process are addressed earlier in this chapter and are also applied in developmental assessment and planning.

Some parents may not pursue early developmental intervention because they do not believe their child needs the services. In these cases, professionals need to explain the child's developmental needs in ways that are meaningful from the parents' own cultural and socio-economic perspectives. Only then can parents make truly informed decisions. After the parents have been fully informed of the child's condition, likely developmental sequelae, and the expected benefits of intervention, developmental goals outlined by the child and family should guide planning and intervention.

Several principles underlie the appropriate developmental intervention plans for children with complex medical problems. First, understanding a child's medical condition ensures that the nurse and family can plan to maximize developmental opportunities at times when the child has the most energy and endurance while noting stress signals that determine the child's tolerance for type, intensity, and duration of activity. Second, plans for developmental support must be flexible and tailored to the individual child's abilities, interests, and needs. Third, familiarity with the child's medical equipment facilitates the planning of creative ways to meet the child's developmental needs. For example, the use of lengthy oxygen tubing allows the active toddler freedom of movement during the day (Fig. 20-3), portable equipment of any type facilitates family outings, and mounting a ventilator to a wheelchair allows the school-age child and adolescent greater independence.

Chapter 18 discusses the impact of chronic illness on development. Behaviors that the nurse may observe in children receiving home care that need to be addressed include:

Infants—Crying, withdrawal, detachment, inability to achieve developmental milestones

Toddlers—Inactivity; sadness; screaming; regressive behavior; delays in motor, speech, or social skills

Preschoolers—Temper tantrums, refusal to comply with routines, refusal to eat or participate in self-care

School-age children—Expression of loneliness, boredom, isolation, depression, or worry about school absences; altered physical growth

Adolescents—Dependency, uncooperativeness, withdrawal, fear of loss of peer status or acceptance at school, altered image

Promoting coping and capability can reduce stress and contribute to mental health and self-esteem in a child with a chronic illness. The extent to which a child is involved in his or her own care depends on many factors, including parental comfort and support and the child's developmental age, level of interest, and physical ability. Self-care, both in activities of daily living and in regard to the medical condition, is important. The goal for self-care in activities of daily living should be attaining age-appropriate competence. Some modifications in the environment, the medical equipment, or the techniques for daily activities may be required to promote and support self-care. Effective teaching for self-care focuses on the child's own level of conceptual understanding. The nurse can enhance teaching through the use of dolls, models and diagrams, simple explanations, and repetition.

Educational planning is important for the child who has a chronic medical condition. Federal laws ensure that all children receive a public education. Before age 3 years, children with developmental delays are eligible for an **early intervention program**. The child can receive rehabilitation therapies as appropriate (physical, occupational, or speech therapy). After age 3 years, the local school system is responsible for providing this education. Some children may be eligible for special education preschools. The home care nurse should refer the family to local educational programs.

Each family is entitled to an individualized family service plan (IFSP), or individualized care plan, to help ensure early intervention. All states in the United States provide agencies that develop IFSPs; each state's plan can easily be accessed on the Internet by entering the term *individualized (or individual) family service plan* in an Internet search engine such as Yahoo! or Google. The IFSP provides the child with a disability, from birth to age 3 years, with a plan for integrating early intervention and rehabilitation, based on the child's and family's needs.

When a child requiring special medical care is to be placed in an educational setting, the parents, child, school health coordinator, educational evaluation team, and education and administrative staff should meet to determine safe and appropriate placement and the necessary services and personnel to enable the child to attend school in the least restrictive environment. Training of education staff and caregivers is essential to ensuring the child's safety in the educational setting.* Special assistance can also be beneficial in reintegrating previously schooled children, such as those with cancer, into the school setting. The home care nurse may need to assist parents in developing the skills necessary to advocate effectively for their child in the educational system.

SAFETY ISSUES IN THE HOME

Safety is an important consideration in pediatric home care, and the nurse should include this in the home care plan.

> **NURSING TIP** Arrangements should be made to ensure that, in case of emergencies, the family has adequate methods of communicating (e.g., telephone) with properly trained emergency medical personnel. A mobile (cellular) phone may be used in place of a local telephone, but it is advisable to check with the local emergency facilities regarding policies for cell phone use and emergency 911 calls.

---

*A thorough discussion of training issues, content, and guidelines for care in the school is provided in Porter S, Bierle T, Haynie M, and others, editors: *Children and youth assisted by medical technology in educational settings: guidelines for care*, ed 2, Baltimore, 1997, Paul H. Brookes.

The telephone and electric companies (if the use of medical equipment requires electricity) must be notified to place the family on a priority service list. In this way, the family will learn of any anticipated interruptions in service and will receive priority in reinstatement of interrupted services. Prior contact with rescue squad and local emergency facility personnel can help ensure prompt and appropriate interventions if required. This is especially important if the family lives in a rural location that may not be familiar to local emergency responders. It is recommended that a map be given to local authorities with key landmarks and intersections for rapid access to the home.

Before hospital discharge, develop and review emergency protocols with the parents and professional caregivers. After an emergency plan is developed with the family, it is helpful to print it and have it in a central location for easy access and referral. The emergency plan should include assigned responsibilities (family members). In the case of a technology-dependent child, it may be helpful to occasionally have a fire drill evacuation to work out any problems in the system. Performing the skill rather than just discussing the actions may help participants in time of emergency recall the steps involved. Post cardiopulmonary resuscitation guidelines, if appropriate, near the child's bedside or in another accessible location. As applicable, instruct the family to tape a one size smaller extra tracheostomy tube on the wall over the headboard of the child's bed. Place a list of emergency telephone numbers near each home phone and include the numbers of the rescue squad, emergency department, managing physician(s), nursing agency, and equipment vendor(s) or providers. Specifically, instruct the family to tape the plan on the front of their refrigerator for quick and easy access. Additional issues to consider are advance directives and out-of-hospital do not resuscitate orders (may vary by state), as indicated. If the patient and family desire an advance directive to be enforced, specific guidelines must be followed and could potentially prevent undesired lifesaving measures for children with terminal illnesses.

Infection control in the home setting should not be overlooked. Although the child may be exposed to fewer organisms than in the acute care setting, it is still important to maintain "clean" and "dirty" areas to protect the child, family members, and caregivers. Needle and sharps disposal should be a priority in home care (see Community Focus box). The home health care agency should have in place policies and procedures for infection control in relation to disposal of contaminated dressings and sharps for the protection of its employees. Impenetrable needle disposal containers should be available for the protection of those in the household and the community. Hand hygiene is the cornerstone of infection control, and the nurse and family should identify appropriate areas and items in the home setting for hand hygiene to be carried out with ease. Personal protective equipment may be required in some cases; these items should be available to the caretakers as well as the nurse. Some medical equipment may be washed with an appropriate disinfectant and reused to decrease cost of care; however, appropriate infection control practices should not be compromised to save money.

Another aspect of safety relates to the provision of care by appropriately trained individuals. Family members should receive thorough training in the child's care requirements and have the opportunity to demonstrate knowledge and confidence before hospital discharge. Children with complex medical care needs are often admitted to an acute care center for nonmedical reasons, including parents' lack of training and inability to care for a child with complex medical needs (Schanwald, 2005). One study found that although technology-dependent children cared for in the home received adequate care, the time demands of such care had negative effects on the caregiver's

🏠 COMMUNITY FOCUS

Safe Disposal of Needles and Lancets

The growing number of persons being cared for in home settings has increased the amount of medical waste that communities must properly dispose of to prevent accidental needlesticks and the spread of diseases such as hepatitis and human immunodeficiency virus. Many states have programs to assist with the disposal of sharps such as needles and lancets to prevent environmental contamination and accidental mishaps involving needle exposures. Contact one of the resources listed below to obtain further information about needle disposal in your state or discuss the proper disposal of sharp medical equipment with your health professional.

If your state or community does not have programs for safe needle disposal, an option is to place sharps such as needles or lancets in a rigid container such as a bleach bottle or aluminum coffee can. Place the lid on the container to prevent accidental needle exposure. Store the container on a top bedroom shelf or closet out of reach of children. When the container is about three-quarters full and ready to be discarded, you may add to it a liquid mixture such as cement or plaster to harden the contents and prevent needle exposure. Special devices that break off the needle into a rigid container are also available in some communities.

Additional information is available at Coalition for Safe Community Needle Disposal, 800-643-1643, http://www.safeneedledisposal.org and Environmental Protection Agency, http://www.epa.gov/wastes/nonhaz/industrial/medical/med-govt.pdf.

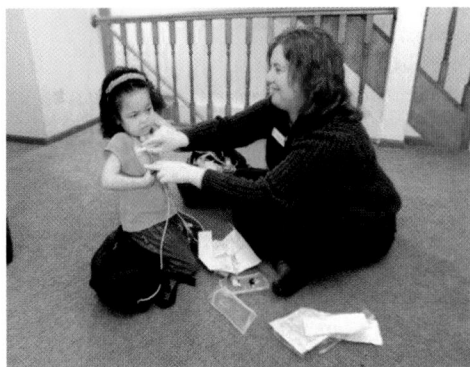

FIG 20-4 An implanted port is accessed in the home care setting. (Photo courtesy BJC Hospice, St. Louis.)

school, employment, and social life; a shortage of skilled caregivers often leads to disrupted sleep patterns and increased stress (Heaton, Noyes, Sloper, and others, 2005). Professional staff caring for the child should have the appropriate background and training for the child's particular care needs (Boroughs and Dougherty, 2009). Because of the child's body size, special skill and caution are required in the performance of procedures (e.g., gastrostomy feedings, tracheostomy suctioning) and in monitoring the use of equipment (e.g., ventilator settings, intravenous flow rates, and total fluid volumes) (see Chapters 22, 23, and 25) (Fig. 20-4).

The activity level and curiosity of young children raise additional safety considerations in the provision of home care. All medications, needles, syringes, and contaminated materials must be securely stored well out of the reach of curious hands. Make arrangements for the disposal of sharp items or contaminated materials with the home health agency. Pay special attention to childproofing the control panels on ventilators, pumps, monitors, and other equipment. The use of

clear plastic tape, covers, or panels to cover control knobs or buttons reduces the risk of accidental changes in settings. Much of the medical equipment now in use has special lock-out capabilities to prevent someone from accidentally altering settings. Keep electrical cords short and out of reach and use safety covers on any open outlets. Unplug equipment when not in use and store any wires (e.g., lead wires for an apnea monitor) out of reach. (See Chapter 11 for use of apnea monitors in the home.)

Care at night poses other safety concerns. Parents and other caregivers need to be able to clearly hear monitor, ventilator, or pump alarms at night. They can use an inexpensive intercom system or baby monitor. Take steps to prevent accidental strangulation by apnea, oximeter, or cardiac monitor wires or lengthy intravenous tubing during sleep.

> **NURSING TIP** Coiling extra tubing and taping it at the exit site, as well as running wires or tubes out the bottoms of pajamas or the back of one-piece pajamas, are precautions against strangulation.

Safe transportation is a vital concern. Wheelchairs and other medical equipment must be properly secured to the vehicle, including vans and buses. Appropriate child restraints must be used. If necessary, an extra adult should be present to monitor the child while in transit. Information on car seat safety and transportation for children with disabilities is available from Riley Hospital for Children at 800-KID-N-CAR. The local public health department is a resource for current guidelines for child car seats as well as equipment transportation. Additionally, the AAP (Bull, Engle, and AAP, 2009) has recently issued new guidelines for the safe transportation of preterm and low-birth-weight infants.

FAMILY-TO-FAMILY SUPPORT

Family-to-family support networks can be an important source of emotional and instrumental support and empowerment for families of children with chronic health problems. Family-to-family support does not replace professional sources of support but rather is a unique resource that promotes family strengths through shared experience.

Families will most likely experience increased emotional stress as the result of living with and caring for a child with disabilities. Parents and families of technology-dependent children reported that they felt isolated from the community when caring for the child in the home; the parents believed the community as a whole was not supportive of the child's needs, suggesting that the child's life was not worth maintaining. The families reported an overall theme in their lives of living daily with distress and enrichment (Carnevale, Alexander, Davis, and others, 2006).

Identifying meaningful sources of support can make a difference in coping abilities. Montagnino and Mauricio (2004) surveyed a group of mothers who were providing home care for children with a tracheostomy and gastrostomy. The researchers found that the mothers experienced significant anxiety, and social interaction within and outside the family was disrupted as a result of the child's condition. The authors recommended that families of children with special health care needs network with other parents in similar conditions through online and local support groups to prevent social disruption and maintain a sense of family normalcy despite the child's condition.

Baum (2004) surveyed caregivers of children with special health care needs about the value of an Internet parent support group. The researcher used stress and coping theory as a guide for measuring perceived satisfaction and a number of other characteristics. The survey indicated that parents were satisfied with the information obtained through the Internet support group, and improved caregiver–child relationship was the strongest outcome factor. The author suggests that undesirable results may also be obtained via such an Internet group and that the quality of such support groups should be carefully evaluated by those involved.

The nurse can assist the family in increasing their involvement in community social networks. For example, a referral to a parent support group may meet an individual family's needs. The nurse should inform the parents of the group's goals so the family can determine whether they might benefit from this connection. In addition, informal support networks can be extremely beneficial. A link to a family in the same or a similar situation allows the sharing of common experiences. This in itself may decrease the sense of isolation and provide a connection with someone who can really identify with family struggles. Positive outcomes can include understanding, empathizing, problem solving, or just talking to someone who will listen.

The nurse should remember that the needs of each family member differ. The care plan should acknowledge each family member's needs (mother, father, siblings, grandparents). Peer support for school-age children and adolescents with complex care needs may be beneficial. These connections can include letter writing, e-mails, social networking such as text messaging, Twitter and Facebook participation, telephone calls, and specialty camping programs. Most school-age children and adolescents just want to be accepted by their peers and fit in as a part of the group. Same-age peers may at first be distant to children with disabilities, but this is likely out of fear and lack of understanding. Helping others see that they have the same dreams, desires, goals, and interests promotes group cohesiveness and understanding.

KEY POINTS

- Effective home care depends on many factors, including the child's medical stability; the family's willingness, training, and ability to accommodate the child's care requirements; and professional, financial, and community support.
- Comprehensive, multidisciplinary discharge planning should begin early and should include the family and a home care coordinator in addition to hospital personnel.
- Thorough education and training of the family or primary caregiver can ease the transition to home.
- Care coordination ensures continuity of care, prevents duplication of services, and reduces fragmentation of services. The family may assume responsibility for varying degrees of care coordination over time.
- The home care nurse must possess a high level of technical expertise while being able to adapt equipment, procedures, and the nursing process to the sometimes unpredictable home milieu.
- Federal standards apply to agencies that participate in Medicare or Medicaid; standards of practice by the American Nurses Association and other professional nursing organizations can guide nurses in the home setting.

- Family-centered nursing practice is applied in the home setting; nurses should respect diversity in family structures, cultural backgrounds, strengths, and coping mechanisms.
- Collaborative relationships between parents and home care providers are characterized by communication, dialogue, active listening, awareness and acceptance of differences, and negotiation.
- The nursing process is adapted to involve the family in each step and to preserve the family's central role in decision making.
- House rules agreed on by the nurse, child, and family allow the family to maintain a feeling of control over their own environment when professionals are present.
- Individualized home care plans are designed to promote optimum development of the child and to focus on normalization, the impact of the child's medical condition and technologic requirements on development, self-care, and educational needs.
- Safety in the provision of home care services involves emergency preparations and protocols, appropriate training of family and home care personnel, and the safe use and childproofing of medical equipment.
- Family-to-family support networks can provide emotional and instrumental support and encourage family empowerment.

REFERENCES

American Academy of Pediatrics: Hospital discharge of the high-risk neonate, *Pediatrics* 122(5):1119–1126, 2008.

American Academy of Pediatrics, Council on Children with Disabilities: Care coordination in the medical home: integrating health and related systems of care for children with special health care needs, *Pediatrics* 116(5):1238–1244, 2005.

American Nurses Association: *Home health nursing scope and standards of practice*, Washington, DC, 2007a, Author.

American Nurses Association: *Public health nursing scope and standards of practice*, Washington, DC, 2007b, Author.

Antonelli RC, Stille CJ, Antonelli DM: Care coordination for children and youth with special health care needs: a descriptive, multisite study of activities, personnel, costs,

and outcomes, *Pediatrics* 122(1):e209–e216, 2008.

Arango P: Family-centered care, *Acad Pediatr* 10(2):14–18, 2011.

Askew R, Williams PR, Rachel M, and others: Resolving conflict in the home care setting, *Home Healthcare Nurse* 26(10):589–593, 2008.

Balaguer A, Gonzalez de Dios J: Home intravenous antibiotics for cystic fibrosis, *Cochrane Database Syst Rev* 16(3):CD001917, 2008.

Baum LS: Internet parent support groups for primary caregivers of a child with special health care needs, *Pediatr Nurs* 30(5):381–388, 401, 2004.

Boroughs D, Dougherty JA: Care of technology-dependent children in the home, *Home Healthcare Nurse* 27(1):37–42, 2009.

Bull MJ, Engle WA, American Academy of Pediatrics, Committee on Injury, Violence, and

Poison Prevention and Committee on Fetus and Newborn: Safe transportation of preterm and low birth weight infants at hospital discharge, *Pediatrics* 123(5):1424–1429, 2009.

Cady R, Kelly A, Finkelstein S: Home telehealth for children with special healthcare needs, *J Telemed Telecare* 14(4):173–177, 2008.

Carnevale FA, Alexander E, Davis M, and others: Daily living with distress and enrichment: the moral experience of families with ventilator-assisted children at home, *Pediatrics* 117(1):e48–e60, 2006.

Cervasio K: The role of the pediatric home healthcare nurse: one case study approach in New York City, *Home Healthcare Nurse* 28(7):424–431, 2010.

Cooper C, Wheeler DM, Woolfenden SR, and others: Specialist home-based nursing services for children with acute and chronic illnesses,

Cochrane Database Syst Rev 18(4):CD004383, 2006.

Davis C: Safe on the home watch, *Nurs Stand* 20(34):20–22, 2006.

DiBaise JK, Scolapio JS: Home parenteral and enteral nutrition, *Gastroenterol Clin North Am* 36(1):123–144, 2007.

Feudtner C, Villareale V, Morray NL, and others: Technology-dependence among patients discharged from a children's hospital: a retrospective cohort study, *BMC Pediatrics* 5(8):1–8, 2005.

Gordon J: An evidenced-based approach for supporting parents experiencing chronic sorrow, *Pediatr Nurs* 35(2):115–119, 2009.

Gorski L: Implementing home health standards in clinical practice: an overview of the updated standards, *Home Healthcare Nurse* 26(5): 308–316, 2008.

Heaton J, Noyes J, Sloper P, and others: Families' experiences of caring for technology-dependent children: a temporal perspective, *Health Soc Care Community* 13(5):441–450, 2005.

Howard L: Home parenteral nutrition: survival, cost, and quality of life, *Gastroenterology* 130(2 suppl 1):S52-S59, 2006.

Johnson CP, Kastner TA, American Academy of Pediatrics, Committee on Children with Disabilities: Helping families raise children with special health care needs at home, *Pediatrics* 115(2):507–511, 2005.

Kellett UM, Mannion J: Meaning in caring: reconceptualizing the nurse–family carer relationship in community practice, *J Adv Nurs* 29(3):697–703, 1999.

Knafl KA, Deatrick JA: The challenges of normalization for families of children with chronic conditions, *Pediatr Nurs* 28(1):49–53, 56, 2002.

McDaniel SH, Campbell TL: Training for collaborative family healthcare, *Fam Syst Health* 14(2):147–150, 1996.

McEvoy M: Culture and spirituality as an integrated concept in pediatric care, *MCN Am J Matern Child Nurs* 28(1):39–43, 2003.

Montagnino BA, Mauricio RV: The child with a tracheostomy and gastrostomy: parental stress and coping in the home—a pilot study, *Pediatr Nurs* 30(5):373–380, 401, 2004.

Mueller C: Spirituality in children: understanding and developing interventions, *Pediatr Nurs* 36(4):197–208, 2010.

National Alliance for Caregiving: *The Evercare Survey of the economic downturn and its impact on family caregiving*, Bethesda, Md, 2009, Author, retrieved February 20, 2010, from http://www.caregiving.org/data/EVC_Caregivers_Economy_Report%20 FINAL_4–28–09.

Ratcliff JD: Home health admission and care of a pediatric ventilator-dependent client, *Home Healthcare Nurse* 25(1):34–40, 2007.

Rice R: Case management and leadership strategies in home care. In Rice R, editor: *Home care nursing practice: concepts and application*, ed 4, St. Louis, 2006, Mosby.

Rice R: *Home care trends and challenges,* Presentation for Missouri League for Nurses, Spring 2011.

Schanwald PR: Gaps in pediatric care, *Caring* 25(9):20–25, 2005.

Smith C, Piamjariyakul U, Yadrich D, and others: Complex home care part III: economic impact on family caregiver quality of life and patients' clinical outcomes, *Nurs Econ* 28(6):393–414, 2010.

Stevens B, McKeever P, Law MP, and others: Children receiving chemotherapy at home: perceptions of children and parents, *J Pediatr Oncol Nurs* 23(5):276–285, 2006.

Sullivan T: Caregiver Strain Index, *Home Healthcare Nurse* 21(3):197–198, 2003.

Takaro T, Krieger J, Song L, and others: The breathe-easy home: the impact of asthma-friendly home construction on clinical outcomes and trigger exposure, *Am J Pub Health* 101(1):55–62, 2011.

Vasquez MS: Down to the fundamentals of telehealth and home healthcare nursing, *Home Healthcare Nurse* 26(5):280–287, 2008.

Wilson H: HIPAA: the big picture for home care and hospice, *Home Health Care Manage Pract* 16(2):127–137, 2004.

Wright LD: Professional boundaries in home care, *Home Healthcare Nurse* 24(10):672–675, 2006.

Yoder-Wise P: *Leading and managing in nursing,* ed 5, St. Louis, 2011, Mosby.

Family-Centered Care of the Child During Illness and Hospitalization

Tara Merck and Patricia McElfresh

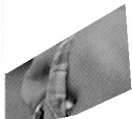

evolve WEBSITE

http://evolve.elsevier.com/wong/essentials
Key Point Summaries
NCLEX-Style Review Questions
Nursing Care Plan—The Child Undergoing Surgery

CHAPTER OUTLINE

Stressors of Hospitalization and Children's Reactions, 613
  Separation Anxiety, 613
    Early Childhood, 614
    Later Childhood and Adolescence, 614
  Loss of Control, 615
    Infants, 615
    Toddlers, 615
    Preschoolers, 615
    School-Age Children, 615
    Adolescents, 616
  Effects of Hospitalization on the Child, 616
    Individual Risk Factors, 616
    Beneficial Effects of Hospitalization, 617
Stressors and Reactions of the Family of the Child Who Is Hospitalized, 617
  Parental Reactions, 617
  Sibling Reactions, 617

Nursing Care of the Child Who Is Hospitalized, 617
  Preparation for Hospitalization, 617
    Admission Assessment, 618
    Preparing the Child for Admission, 618
  Nursing Interventions, 621
    Preventing or Minimizing Separation, 621
    Parental Absence During Infant Hospitalization, 621
    Minimizing Loss of Control, 622
    Preventing or Minimizing Fear of Bodily Injury, 623
    Providing Developmentally Appropriate Activities, 624
    Providing Opportunities for Play and Expressive Activities, 624
    Maximizing Potential Benefits of Hospitalization, 626

Nursing Care of the Family, 627
  Supporting Family Members, 627
  Providing Information, 628
  Encouraging Parent Participation, 628
  Preparing for Discharge and Home Care, 629
Care of the Child and Family in Special Hospital Situations, 629
  Ambulatory or Outpatient Setting, 629
  Isolation, 630
  Emergency Admission, 631
  Intensive Care Unit, 631

LEARNING OBJECTIVES

On completion of this chapter the reader will be able to:
- Identify the stressors of illness and hospitalization for children during each developmental stage.
- List essential priorities of nursing care upon a child's admission to the hospital.
- Review nursing interventions that prevent or minimize the stress of separation during hospitalization.
- Discuss nursing interventions that minimize the stress of loss of control during hospitalization.

- Describe nursing interventions that minimize the fear of bodily injury during hospitalization.
- Outline nursing interventions that support parents, siblings, and family during a child's illness and hospitalization.
- Describe nursing interventions needed when children are admitted to special units such as the emergency department.

STRESSORS OF HOSPITALIZATION AND CHILDREN'S REACTIONS

Often, illness and hospitalization are the first crises children must face. Especially during the early years, children are particularly vulnerable to these stressors because (1) stress represents a change from the usual state of health and environmental routine and (2) children have a limited number of coping mechanisms to resolve stressors. Major stressors of hospitalization include separation, loss of control, bodily injury, and pain. Children's reactions to these crises are influenced by their developmental age; their previous experience with illness, separation, or hospitalization; their innate and acquired coping skills; the seriousness of the diagnosis; and the support system available. Children also expressed fears caused by the unfamiliar environment or lack of information; child–staff relations; and the physical, social, and symbolic environment (Samela, Salanterä, and Aronen, 2009).

SEPARATION ANXIETY

The major stress from middle infancy throughout the preschool years, especially for children ages 6 to 30 months, is separation anxiety, also called anaclitic depression. The principal behavioral responses to this stressor during early childhood are summarized in Box 21-1. During the stage of protest, children react aggressively to the separation from the parent. They cry and scream for their parents, refuse the attention of anyone else, and are inconsolable in their grief (Fig. 21-1). In contrast, through the stage of despair, the crying stops, and depression is evident. The child is much less active, is uninterested in play or food, and withdraws from others (Fig. 21-2).

The third stage is detachment, also called denial. Superficially, it appears that the child has finally adjusted to the loss. The child becomes more interested in the surroundings, plays with others, and seems to form new relationships. However, this behavior is the result of resignation and is not a sign of contentment. The child detaches from the parent in an effort to escape the emotional pain of desiring the parent's presence and copes by forming shallow relationships with others, becoming increasingly self-centered, and attaching primary importance to material objects. This is the most serious stage in that reversal of the potential adverse effects is less likely to occur after detachment is established. However, in most situations, the temporary separations imposed by hospitalization do not cause such prolonged parental absences that the child enters into detachment. In addition, considerable evidence suggests that even with stressors such as separation, children are remarkably adaptable, and permanent ill effects are rare.

Although progression to the stage of detachment is uncommon, the initial stages are frequently observed even with brief separations from either parent. Unless health team members understand the meaning of each stage of behavior, they may erroneously label the behaviors as positive or negative. For example, they may see the loud crying of the protest phase as "bad" behavior. Because the protests increase when a stranger approaches the child, they may interpret that reaction as meaning they should stay away. During the quiet, withdrawn phase of despair, health team members may think that the child is finally "settling in" to the new surroundings, and they may see the detachment

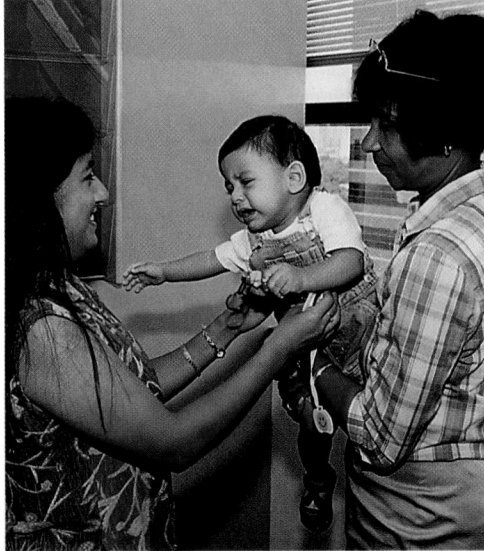

FIG 21-1 In the protest phase of separation anxiety, children cry loudly and are inconsolable in their grief for the parent. (Courtesy James DeLeon, Texas Children's Hospital, Houston.)

BOX 21-1   MANIFESTATIONS OF SEPARATION ANXIETY IN YOUNG CHILDREN

Stage of Protest
Behaviors observed during later infancy include:
- Cries
- Screams
- Searches for parent with eyes
- Clings to parent
- Avoids and rejects contact with strangers

Additional behaviors observed during toddlerhood include:
- Verbally attacks strangers (e.g., "Go away")
- Physically attacks strangers (e.g., kicks, bites, hits, pinches)
- Attempts to escape to find parent
- Attempts to physically force parent to stay

Behaviors may last from hours to days.

Protest, such as crying, may be continuous, ceasing only with physical exhaustion.

Approach of stranger may precipitate increased protest.

Stage of Despair
Observed behaviors include:
- Is inactive
- Withdraws from others
- Is depressed, sad
- Lacks interest in environment
- Is uncommunicative
- Regresses to earlier behavior (e.g., thumb sucking, bedwetting, use of pacifier, use of bottle)

Behaviors may last for variable length of time.

Child's physical condition may deteriorate from refusal to eat, drink, or move.

Stage of Detachment
Observed behaviors include:
- Shows increased interest in surroundings
- Interacts with strangers or familiar caregivers
- Forms new but superficial relationships
- Appears happy

Detachment usually occurs after prolonged separation from parent; it is rarely seen in hospitalized children.

Behaviors represent a superficial adjustment to loss.

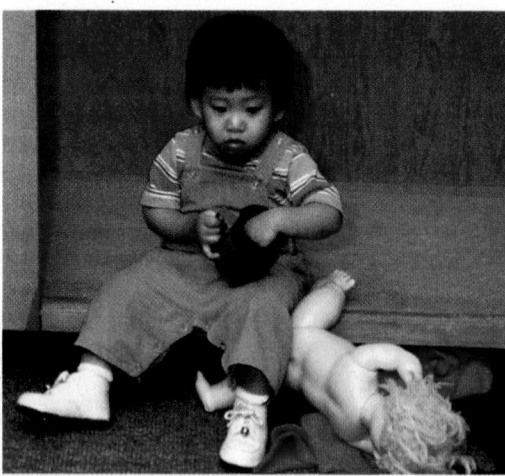

FIG 21-2 During the despair phase of separation anxiety, children are sad, lonely, and uninterested in food and play.

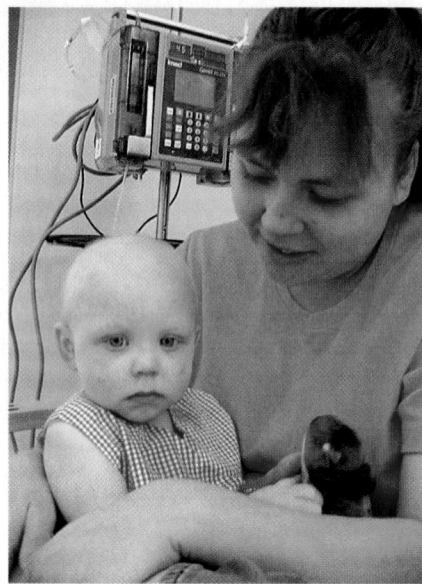

FIG 21-3 Young children may appear withdrawn and sad even in the presence of a parent. (Courtesy E. Jacob, Texas Children's Hospital, Houston.)

behaviors as proof of a "good adjustment." The faster this stage is reached, the more likely it is that the child will be regarded as the "ideal patient."

Because children seem to react "negatively" to visits by their parents, uninformed observers feel justified in restricting parental visiting privileges. For example, during the protest stage, children outwardly do not appear happy to see their parents (Fig. 21-3). In fact, they may even cry louder. If they are depressed, they may reject their parents or begin to protest again. Often they cling to their parents in an effort to ensure their continued presence. Consequently, such reactions may be regarded as "disturbing" the child's adjustment to the new surroundings. If the separation has progressed to the phase of detachment, children will respond no differently to their parents than they would to any other person.

Such reactions are distressing to parents, who are unaware of their meaning. If parents are regarded as intruders, they will see their absence as "beneficial" to the child's adjustment and recovery. They may respond to the child's behavior by staying for only short periods, visiting less frequently, or deceiving the child when it is time to leave. The result is a destructive cycle of misunderstanding and unmet needs.

Early Childhood

Separation anxiety is the greatest stress imposed by hospitalization during early childhood. If separation is avoided, young children have a tremendous capacity to withstand any other stress. During this age period, the typical reactions just described are seen. However, children in the toddler stage demonstrate more goal-directed behaviors. For example, they may plead with the parents to stay and physically try to keep the parents with them or try to find parents who have left. They may demonstrate displeasure on the parents' return or departure by having temper tantrums; refusing to comply with the usual routines of mealtime, bedtime, or toileting; or regressing to more primitive levels of development. However, temper tantrums, bedwetting, or other behaviors may also be expressions of anger, a physiologic response to stress, or symptoms of illness.

Because preschoolers are more secure interpersonally than toddlers, they can tolerate brief periods of separation from their parents and are more inclined to develop substitute trust in other significant adults. However, the stress of illness usually renders preschoolers less able to cope with separation; as a result, they manifest many of the stage behaviors of separation anxiety, although in general, the protest behaviors are more subtle and passive than those seen in younger children. Preschoolers may demonstrate separation anxiety by refusing to eat, experiencing difficulty in sleeping, crying quietly for their parents, continually asking when the parents will visit, or withdrawing from others. They may express anger indirectly by breaking their toys, hitting other children, or refusing to cooperate during usual self-care activities. Nurses need to be sensitive to these less obvious signs of separation anxiety in order to intervene appropriately.

Later Childhood and Adolescence

Previous research, usually based on adult recollections, indicated that the family does not play as important a role for school-age children as it does during the toddler and preschool years. However, in a recent study that asked children about their fears when hospitalized, children listed their greatest fears regarding hospitalization as being separated from family and friends, being in an unfamiliar environment, receiving investigations or treatments, and losing self-determination or choices (Coyne, 2006). In a qualitative study of children ages 5 to 9 years, children described hospitalization in stories that focused on being alone and feeling scared, angry, or sad. These children also described the need for protection and companionship while hospitalized (Wilson, Megel, Enenbach, and others, 2010).

Although school-age children are better able to cope with separation in general, the stress and often accompanying regression imposed by illness or hospitalization may increase their need for parental security and guidance. This is particularly true for young school-age children who have only recently left the safety of the home and are struggling with the crisis of school adjustment. Middle and late school-age children may react more to the separation from their usual activities and peers than to the absence of their parents. These children have a high level of physical and mental activity that frequently finds no suitable outlets in the hospital environment, and even when they dislike school, they admit to missing its routine and worry that they will not be able to compete or "fit in" with their classmates when they return. Feelings of loneliness, boredom, isolation, and depression are common. Such reactions may occur more as a result of separation than of concern over the illness, treatment, or hospital setting.

School-age children may need and desire parental guidance or support from other adult figures but may be unable or unwilling to ask for it. Because the goal of attaining independence is so important to them, they are reluctant to seek help directly, fearing that they will appear weak, childish, or dependent. Cultural expectations to "act like a man" or to "be brave and strong" weigh heavily on these children, especially boys, who tend to react to stress with stoicism, withdrawal, or passive acceptance. Often the need to express hostile, angry, or other negative feelings finds outlets in alternate ways, such as irritability and aggression toward parents, withdrawal from hospital personnel, inability to relate to peers, rejection of siblings, or subsequent behavioral problems in school.

For adolescents, separation from home and parents may produce varied emotions, ranging from difficulty coping to welcoming the event. However, loss of peer-group contact may pose a severe emotional threat because of loss of group status, inability to exert group control or leadership, and loss of group acceptance. Deviations within peer groups are poorly tolerated, and although group members may express concern for the adolescent's illness or need for hospitalization, they continue their group activities, quickly filling the gap of the absent member. During the temporary separation from their usual group, ill adolescents may benefit from group associations with other hospitalized teens.

LOSS OF CONTROL

One of the factors influencing the amount of stress imposed by hospitalization is the amount of control that persons perceive themselves as having. Lack of control increases the perception of threat and can affect children's coping skills. Many hospital situations decrease the amount of control a child feels. Although the usual sensory stimulations are lacking, the additional hospital stimuli of sight, sound, and smell may be overwhelming. Without an insight into the type of environment conducive to children's optimal growth, the hospital experience can at best temporarily slow development and at worst permanently restrict it. Because children's needs vary greatly depending on their age, the major areas of loss of control in terms of physical restriction, altered routine or rituals, and dependency are discussed for each age group.

Infants

Infants are developing the most important attribute of a healthy personality—trust. Trust is established through consistent, loving care by a nurturing person. Infants attempt to control their environment through emotional expressions, such as crying or smiling. In the hospital setting, cues may be missed or misinterpreted, and routines may be established to meet the hospital staff's needs instead of the infant's needs. Inconsistent care and deviations from the infant's daily routine may lead to mistrust and a decreased sense of control.

Toddlers

Toddlers are striving for autonomy, and this goal is evident in most of their behaviors: motor skills, play, interpersonal relationships, activities of daily living, and communication. When their egocentric pleasures meet with obstacles, toddlers react with negativism, especially temper tantrums. Any restriction or limitation of movement, such as the simple act of making toddlers lie down, can cause forceful resistance and noncompliance.

Loss of control also results from altered routines and rituals. Toddlers rely on the consistency and familiarity of daily rituals to provide a measure of stability and control in their complex world of growing and developing. The experience of hospitalization or illness severely limits their sense of expectation and predictability because practically every detail of the hospital environment differs from that of the home.

Toddlers' main areas for rituals include eating, sleeping, bathing, toileting, and play. When the routines are disrupted, difficulties can occur in any or all of these areas. The principal reaction to such change is regression. For example, when mealtime and food choices differ from those at home, toddlers often refuse to eat, demand a bottle, or ask others to feed them. Although regression to earlier forms of behavior may seem to increase toddlers' security and comfort, in reality, it is threatening for them to relinquish their most recently acquired achievements.

Enforced dependency is a chief characteristic of the sick role and accounts for the numerous instances of toddler negativism. For example, rigid schedules, different clothes, altered caregiving activities, unfamiliar surroundings, separation from parents, and medical procedures take away toddlers' control over their world. Although most toddlers initially react negatively and aggressively to such dependency, prolonged loss of autonomy may result in passive withdrawal from interpersonal relationships and regression in all areas of development. Therefore, the effects of the sick role are most severe in instances of chronic, long-term illnesses or in those families who foster the sick role despite the child's improved state of health.

Preschoolers

Preschoolers also experience loss of control caused by physical restriction, altered routines, and enforced dependency. However, their specific cognitive abilities, which make them feel all-powerful, also make them feel out of control. This loss of control in the context of their sense of self-power is a critical influencing factor in their perception of and reaction to separation, pain, illness, and hospitalization.

Preschoolers' egocentric and magical thinking limits their ability to understand events because they view all experiences from their own self-referenced (egocentric) perspective. Without adequate preparation for unfamiliar settings or experiences, preschoolers' fantasy explanations for such events are usually more exaggerated, bizarre, and frightening than the facts. One typical fantasy to explain the illness or hospitalization is that it represents punishment for real or imagined misdeeds. In response to such thinking, the child usually feels shame, guilt, and fear.

Preschoolers' preoperational thinking means that they understand explanations only in terms of real events. Purely verbal instructions are often inadequate for them because they are unable to abstract and synthesize beyond what their senses tell them. When combined with their egocentric and magical thinking, this characteristic may lead them to interpret messages according to their particular past experiences. Even with the best preparation for a procedure, they may misconstrue the details.

Preschoolers use transductive reasoning as they lack understanding of *cause-and-effect relationships*. For example, if preschoolers perceive that nurses inflict pain, preschoolers will think that every nurse or everyone wearing a similar uniform will also inflict pain.

School-Age Children

Because of their striving for independence and productivity, school-age children are particularly vulnerable to events that may lessen their feeling of control and power. In particular, altered family roles; physical disability; fears of death, abandonment, or permanent injury; loss of peer acceptance; lack of productivity; and inability to cope with stress according to perceived cultural expectation may result in loss of control.

Because of the nature of the patient role, many routine hospital activities seize individual power and identity. For school-age children, dependent activities such as enforced bed rest, use of a bedpan, inability to choose a menu, lack of privacy, help with a bed bath, or transport by a wheelchair or stretcher can be direct threats to their security. Although all of these procedures seem routine and inconsequential, they allow no freedom of choice to children who want to "act grown up." However, when children are allowed to exert a measure of control, regardless of how limited it may be, they generally respond well to any procedure. For example, some of the most cooperative, satisfied, and contented patients are school-age children who help make their beds, choose their schedule of activities, and assist in their own care. An increased sense of control usually results from a feeling of usefulness and productivity.

In addition to the hospital environment, illness may also cause a feeling of loss of control. One of the most significant problems of children in this age group is boredom. When physical or enforced limitations curtail their usual ability to care for themselves or to engage in favorite activities, school-age children generally respond with depression, hostility, or frustration. Keeping a normally active child on bed rest is difficult. However, emphasizing areas of control and capitalizing on quiet activities, particularly hobbies such as building models or playing age-appropriate video or board games, promote their adjustment to physical restriction.

Adolescents

Adolescents' struggle for independence, self-assertion, and liberation centers on the quest for personal identity. Anything that interferes with this poses a threat to their sense of identity and results in a loss of control. Illness, which limits their physical abilities, and hospitalization, which separates them from their usual support systems, constitute major situational crises.

The patient role fosters dependency and depersonalization. Adolescents may react to dependency with rejection, uncooperativeness, or withdrawal. They may respond to depersonalization with self-assertion, anger, or frustration. Regardless of the response elicited, hospital personnel often regard them as difficult, unmanageable patients. Parents may not be a source of help because these behaviors serve to isolate them further from understanding the adolescent. Although peers may visit, they may not be able to offer the kind of support and guidance needed. Sick adolescents often voluntarily isolate themselves from age mates until they feel they can compete on an equal basis and meet group expectations. As a result, ill adolescents may be left with virtually no support system.

Loss of control also occurs for many of the reasons discussed for school-age children. However, adolescents are more sensitive to potential instances of loss of control and dependency than are younger children. For example, both groups seek information about their physical status and rely heavily on anticipatory preparation to decrease fear and anxiety. However, adolescents react not only to the kinds of information supplied them but also to the means by which it is conveyed. They may feel threatened by others who convey facts in a condescending manner. Adolescents want to know that others can relate to them on their own level. This necessitates a careful assessment of their intellectual abilities, previous knowledge, and present needs. It may also require the nurse's willingness to learn the adolescent's language.

EFFECTS OF HOSPITALIZATION ON THE CHILD

Children may react to the stresses of hospitalization before admission, during hospitalization, and after discharge. A child's concept of illness is even more important than age and intellectual maturity in predicting the level of anxiety before hospitalization (Clatworthy, Simon, and Tiedeman, 1999). This may or may not be affected by the duration of the condition or prior hospitalizations; therefore, nurses should avoid overestimating the illness concepts of children with prior medical experience (Box 21-2).

Individual Risk Factors

A number of risk factors make certain children more vulnerable than others to the stresses of hospitalization (Box 21-3). Rural children may exhibit significantly greater degrees of psychological upset than urban children, possibly because urban children have opportunities to become familiar with a local hospital. Because separation is such an important issue surrounding hospitalization for young children, children who are active and strong willed tend to fare better when hospitalized than youngsters who are passive. Consequently, nurses should be alert to children who passively accept all changes and requests; these children may need more support than "oppositional" children.

BOX 21-2   POSTHOSPITAL BEHAVIORS IN CHILDREN

Young Children

They show initial aloofness toward parents; this may last from a few minutes (most common) to a few days.

This is frequently followed by dependency behaviors:
- Tendency to cling to parents
- Demands for parents' attention
- Vigorous opposition to any separation (e.g., staying at preschool or with a babysitter)

Other negative behaviors include:
- New fears (e.g., nightmares)
- Resistance to going to bed, night waking
- Withdrawal and shyness
- Hyperactivity
- Temper tantrums
- Food peculiarities
- Attachment to blanket or toy
- Regression in newly learned skills (e.g., self-toileting)

Older Children

Negative behaviors include:
- Emotional coldness followed by intense, demanding dependence on parents
- Anger toward parents
- Jealousy toward others (e.g., siblings)

BOX 21-3   RISK FACTORS THAT INCREASE CHILDREN'S VULNERABILITY TO THE STRESSES OF HOSPITALIZATION

"Difficult" temperament
Lack of fit between child and parent
Age (especially between 6 months and 5 years)
Male gender
Below-average intelligence
Multiple and continuing stresses (e.g., frequent hospitalizations)

The stressors of hospitalization may cause young children to experience short- and long-term negative outcomes. Adverse outcomes may be related to the length and number of admissions, multiple invasive procedures, and the parents' anxiety. Common responses include regression, separation anxiety, apathy, fears, and sleeping disturbances, especially for children younger than 7 years of age (Melnyk, 2000). Supportive practices, such as family-centered care and frequent family visiting, may lessen the detrimental effects of such admissions. Nurses should attempt to identify children at risk for poor coping strategies (Small, 2002).

Changes in the Pediatric Population

The pediatric population in hospitals has changed dramatically over the past 2 decades. With a growing trend toward shortened hospital stays and outpatient surgery, a greater percentage of the children hospitalized today have more serious and complex problems than those hospitalized in the past. Many of these children are fragile newborns and children with severe injuries or disabilities who have survived because of major technologic advances yet have been left with chronic or disabling conditions that require frequent and lengthy hospital stays. The nature of their conditions increases the likelihood that they will experience more invasive and traumatic procedures while they are hospitalized. These factors make them more vulnerable to the emotional consequences of hospitalization and result in their needs being significantly different from those of the short-term patients of the past (see Chapter 18 for further discussion on children with special needs). The majority of these children are infants and toddlers, the age group most vulnerable to the effects of hospitalization.

Concern in recent years has focused on the increasing length of hospitalization because of complex medical and nursing care, elusive diagnoses, and complicated psychosocial issues. Without special attention devoted to meeting children's psychosocial and developmental needs in the hospital environment, the detrimental consequences of prolonged hospitalization may be severe.

Beneficial Effects of Hospitalization

Although hospitalization can be and usually is stressful for children, it can also be beneficial. The most obvious benefit is the recovery from illness, but hospitalization also can present an opportunity for children to master stress and feel competent in their coping abilities. The hospital environment can provide children with new socialization experiences that can broaden their interpersonal relationships. The psychological benefits need to be considered and maximized during hospitalization. Appropriate nursing strategies to achieve this goal are presented on p. 621.

STRESSORS AND REACTIONS OF THE FAMILY OF THE CHILD WHO IS HOSPITALIZED

PARENTAL REACTIONS

The crisis of childhood illness and hospitalization affects every member of the family. Parents' reactions to illness in their child depend on a variety of factors. Although one cannot predict which factors are most likely to influence their response, a number of variables have been identified (Box 21-4). (See also Chapter 18.)

Recent research has identified common themes among parents whose children were hospitalized, including feeling an overall sense of helplessness, questioning the skills of staff, accepting the reality of hospitalization, needing to have information explained in simple

---

BOX 21-4   FACTORS AFFECTING PARENTS' REACTIONS TO THEIR CHILD'S ILLNESS

Seriousness of the threat to the child
Previous experience with illness or hospitalization
Medical procedures involved in diagnosis and treatment
Available support systems
Personal ego strengths
Previous coping abilities
Additional stresses on the family system
Cultural and religious beliefs
Communication patterns among family members

---

language, dealing with fear, coping with uncertainty, and seeking reassurance from caregivers. This reassurance involves staff being compassionate, expressing concern for the child, and attending to detail in the child's care (Stranton, 2004).

SIBLING REACTIONS

Siblings' reactions to a sister's or brother's illness or hospitalization are discussed in Chapter 18 and differ little when a child becomes temporarily ill. Siblings experience loneliness, fear, and worry, as well as anger, resentment, jealousy, and guilt. Illness may also result in children's loss of status within either their family or their social group. Various factors have been identified that influence the effects of the child's hospitalization on siblings. Although these factors are similar to those seen when a child has a chronic illness, Craft (1993) reported that the following factors regarding siblings are related specifically to the hospital experience and increase the effects on the sibling:

- Being younger and experiencing many changes
- Being cared for outside the home by care providers who are not relatives
- Receiving little information about their ill brother or sister
- Perceiving that their parents treat them differently compared with before their sibling's hospitalization

Parents are often unaware of the number of effects that siblings experience during the sick child's hospitalization and the benefit of simple interventions to minimize such effects, such as explicit explanations about the illness and provisions for the siblings to remain at home. Sibling visitation is usually beneficial to the patient, sibling, and parent but should be evaluated on an individual basis. Siblings should be prepared for the visit with developmentally appropriate information and be given the opportunity to ask questions.

NURSING CARE OF THE CHILD WHO IS HOSPITALIZED

PREPARATION FOR HOSPITALIZATION

Children and families require individualized care to minimize the potential negative effects of hospitalization. One method that can decrease negative feelings and fear in children is preparation for hospitalization. The rationale for preparing children for the hospital experience and related procedures is based on the principle that a fear of the unknown (fantasy) exceeds fear of the known. When children do not have paralyzing fear to cope with, they are able to direct their energies toward dealing with the other, unavoidable stresses of hospitalization.

Although preparation for hospitalization is a common practice, there is no universal standard or program for all settings. The preparation process may be elaborate with tours, puppet shows, and playtime with miniature hospital equipment; it may involve the use of books, videos, or films; or it may be limited to a brief description of the major aspects of any hospital stay. No consensus exists on the timing of preparation. Some authorities recommend preparing children 4 to 7 years of age about 1 week in advance so they can assimilate the information and ask questions. For older children, the time may be longer. However, for young children, who may begin to fantasize about what they observed, 1 or 2 days before admission is sufficient time for anticipatory preparation. The length of the session should be tailored to the children's attention span—the younger the child, the shorter the program. The optimal approach is one that is individualized for each child and family.

Regardless of the specific type of program, all children, even those who have been hospitalized before, benefit from an introduction to the environment and routine of the unit. Sometimes it is not possible to prepare children and families for hospitalization, such as in the event of sudden, acute illness. However, care should be taken to orient the child and family to hospital routines, establish expectations, and allow for questions.

> **NURSING TIP** In many hospitals, child life specialists—health care professionals with extensive knowledge of child growth and development and of the special psychosocial needs of children who are hospitalized and their families—help prepare children for hospitalization, surgery, and procedures. Although the structure of a program may vary depending on the size of the pediatric facility, the patient population, and the availability of ancillary services, the two primary program objectives for child life are consistent: (1) to reduce the stress and anxiety related to the hospitalization or health care–related experiences and (2) to promote normal growth and development in the health care setting and at home (Thompson, 2009).

A collaborative effort between the nurse, child life specialist, and other members of the child's health care team helps ensure the best possible hospital experience for the child and family.

Admission Assessment

The nursing admission history refers to a systematic collection of data about the child and family that allows the nurse to plan individualized care. The nursing admission history presented in Box 21-5 is organized according to the Functional Health Patterns outlined by Gordon (2002) (see Nursing Diagnosis, Chapter 1). This assessment framework is a guideline for formulating nursing diagnoses. One of the main purposes of the history is to assess the child's usual health habits at home to promote a more normal environment in the hospital. Therefore, questions related to activities of daily living in the nutritional–metabolic, elimination, sleep–rest, and activity–exercise patterns are a major part of the assessment. The questions found under the health perception–health management pattern are directed toward evaluation of the child's preparation for hospitalization and are key factors in determining whether additional preparation is needed. The questions included in the self-perception–self-concept and role–relationship patterns offer insight into the child's potential reaction to hospitalization, especially in terms of separation.

The nurse should also inquire about the use of any medications at home, including complementary medicine practices (Box 21-6). In a

> ### ❓ CRITICAL THINKING CASE STUDY
> **Complementary and Alternative Medicine**
>
> Maria, a 13-year-old Hispanic girl, has had severe nosebleeds. She is admitted to the hospital for a complete workup in an attempt to determine the cause. Her parents and grandparents have gathered around her bed. When you enter her room to begin admitting procedures, you notice an unusual scent. Maria's mother is rubbing the contents from an unfamiliar bottle of liquid on Maria. Meanwhile, the grandmother is rubbing Maria's head. She is startled at your entry and drops something on the floor near your feet. You bend over to pick it up and discover that it is a penny.
>
> **Questions**
> 1. Evidence—Is there sufficient evidence to draw any conclusions?
> 2. Assumptions—What are some underlying assumptions that may be drawn from the data about the following:
>   a. Complementary or alternative medical remedies
>   b. The role of ethnic or folk remedies in modern health care practice
>   c. The nurse's role in cases where alternative medicine is practiced (vs. traditional medicine)
> 3. What implications and priorities for nursing care can be drawn at this time?
> 4. Does the evidence objectively support your argument (conclusion)?

study of children with cancer, 42% had used alternative or complementary therapies simultaneously with or after conventional treatments (Fernandez, Pyesmany, and Stutzer, 1999). It is important that the use of any herbal or complementary therapy be noted in a preoperative assessment because of possible anesthesia or surgical complications related to herbal products (Flanagan, 2001) (see Critical Thinking Case Study box).

In addition to completing the nursing admission history, nurses should also perform a physical assessment (see Chapter 6) before planning care. At the very least, the nurse's physical assessment of the child should include observation of the body for any bruises, rashes, signs of neglect, deformities, or physical limitations. The nurse should also listen to the heart and lungs to assess overall physical status. For example, it is impossible to evaluate improvement in respiratory function in a child admitted with pulmonary disease unless there are baseline data with which to compare subsequent findings.

Preparing the Child for Admission

The preparation that children require on the day of admission depends on the kind of prehospital counseling they have received. If they have been prepared in a formalized program, they usually know what to expect in terms of initial medical procedures, inpatient facilities, and nursing staff. However, prehospital counseling does not preclude the need for support during procedures such as obtaining blood specimens, x-ray tests, or physical examination. For example, undressing young children before they feel comfortable in their new surroundings can be upsetting. Causing needless anxiety and fear during admission may adversely affect the nurse's establishment of trust with these children. Therefore, nursing assistance during the admission procedure is vital regardless of how well prepared any child is for the experience of hospitalization. In addition, spending this time with the child gives the nurse an opportunity to evaluate the child's understanding of subsequent procedures (Fig. 21-4). Ideally, a primary nurse is assigned whenever possible to allow for individualized care and to provide a substitute support person for the child.

When a child is admitted, nurses follow several fairly universal admission procedures (Box 21-7). The minimum considerations for

BOX 21-5 NURSING ADMISSION HISTORY ACCORDING TO FUNCTIONAL HEALTH PATTERNS*

Health Perception–Health Management Pattern

Why has your child been admitted?

How has your child's general health been?

What does your child know about this hospitalization?

- Ask the child why he or she came to the hospital.
- If the answer is "For an operation or for tests," ask the child to tell you about what will happen before, during, and after the operation or tests.

Has your child ever been in the hospital before?

- How was that hospital experience?
- What things were important to you and your child during that hospitalization? How can we be most helpful now?

What medications does your child take at home?

- Why are they given?
- When are they given?
- How are they given (if a liquid, with a spoon; if a tablet, swallowed with water; or other)?
- Does your child have any trouble taking medication? If so, what helps?
- Is your child allergic to any medications?

What, if any, forms of complementary medicine practices are being used?

Nutrition–Metabolic Pattern

What is the family's usual mealtime?

Do family members eat together or at separate times?

What are your child's favorite foods, beverages, and snacks?

- Average amounts consumed or usual size of portions
- Special cultural practices, such as family eats only ethnic food

What foods and beverages does your child dislike?

What are your child's feeding habits (bottle, cup, spoon, eats by self, needs assistance, any special devices)?

How does your child like the food served (warmed, cold, one item at a time)?

How would you describe your child's usual appetite (hearty eater, picky eater)?

- Has being sick affected your child's appetite? In what ways?

Are there any known or suspected food allergies?

Is your child on a special diet?

Are there any feeding problems (excessive fussiness, spitting up, colic); any dental or gum problems that affect feeding?

- What do you do for these problems?

Elimination Pattern

What are your child's toileting habits (diaper, toilet trained—day only or day and night, use of word to communicate urination or defecation, potty chair, regular toilet, other routines)?

What is your child's usual pattern of elimination (bowel movements)?

Do you have any concerns about elimination (bedwetting, constipation, diarrhea)?

- What do you do for these problems?

Have you ever noticed that your child sweats a lot?

Sleep–Rest Pattern

What is your child's usual hour of sleep and awakening?

What is your child's schedule for naps; length of naps?

Is there a special routine before sleeping (bottle, drink of water, bedtime story, night light, favorite blanket or toy, prayers)?

Is there a special routine during sleep time, such as waking to go to the bathroom?

What type of bed does your child sleep in?

Does your child have a separate room or share a room; if shares, with whom?

Does your child sleep with someone or alone (e.g., sibling, parent, other person)?

What is your child's favorite sleeping position?

Are there any sleeping problems (falling asleep, waking during night, nightmares, sleep walking)?

Are there any problems in awakening and getting ready in the morning?

- What do you do for these problems?

Activity–Exercise Pattern

What is your child's schedule during the day (preschool, daycare center, regular school, extracurricular activities)?

What are your child's favorite activities or toys (both active and quiet interests)?

What is your child's usual television-viewing schedule at home?

What are your child's favorite programs?

Are there any television restrictions?

Does your child have any illness or disabilities that limit activity? If so, how?

What are your child's usual habits and schedule for bathing (bath in tub or shower, sponge bath, shampoo)?

What are your child's dental habits (brushing, flossing, fluoride supplements or rinses, favorite toothpaste); schedule of daily dental care?

Does your child need help with dressing or grooming, such as hair combing?

Are there any problems with these patterns (dislike of or refusal to bathe, shampoo hair, or brush teeth)?

- What do you do for these problems?

Are there special devices that your child requires help in managing (eyeglasses, contact lenses, hearing aid, orthodontic appliances, artificial elimination appliances, orthopedic devices)?

NOTE: Use the following code to assess functional self-care level for feeding, bathing and hygiene, dressing and grooming, toileting:

0—Full self-care

I—Requires use of equipment or device

II—Requires assistance or supervision from another person

III—Requires assistance or supervision from another person and equipment or device

IV—Is totally dependent and does not participate

Cognitive–Perceptual Pattern

Does your child have any hearing difficulty?

- Does the child use a hearing aid?
- Have "tubes" been placed in your child's ears?

Does your child have any vision problems?

- Does the child wear glasses or contact lenses?

Does your child have any learning difficulties?

What is the child's grade in school?

For information on pain, see Chapter 7.

Self-Perception–Self-Concept Pattern

How would you describe your child (e.g., takes time to adjust, settles in easily, shy, friendly, quiet, talkative, serious, playful, stubborn, easygoing)?

What makes your child angry, annoyed, anxious, or sad? What helps?

How does your child act when annoyed or upset?

What have your child's experiences been with and reactions to temporary separation from you (parent)?

*The focus of the admission history is the child's psychosocial environment. Most of the questions are worded in terms of parental responses. Depending on the child's age, they should be addressed directly to the child when appropriate.

Continued

Does your child have any fears (places, objects, animals, people, situations)?
- How do you handle them?

Do you think your child's illness has changed the way he or she thinks about him- or herself (e.g., more shy, embarrassed about appearance, less competitive with friends, stays at home more)?

Role–Relationship Pattern

Does your child have a favorite nickname?

What are the names of other family members or others who live in the home (relatives, friends, pets)?

Who usually takes care of your child during the day and night (especially if other than parent, such as babysitter, relative)?

What are the parents' occupations and work schedules?

Are there any special family considerations (adoption, foster child, stepparent, divorce, single parent)?

Have any major changes in the family occurred lately (death, divorce, separation, birth of a sibling, loss of a job, financial strain, mother beginning a career, other)? Describe child's reaction.

Who are your child's play companions or social groups (peers, younger or older children, adults, or prefers to be alone)?

Do things generally go well for your child in school or with friends?

Does your child have "security" objects at home (pacifier, bottle, blanket, stuffed animal or doll)? Did you bring any of these to the hospital?

How do you handle discipline problems at home? Are these methods always effective?

Does your child have any condition that interferes with communication? If so, what are your suggestions for communicating with your child?

Will your child's hospitalization affect the family's financial support or care of other family members (e.g., other children)?

What concerns do you have about your child's illness and hospitalization?

Who will be staying with your child while hospitalized?

How can we contact you or another close family member outside of the hospital?

Sexuality–Reproductive Pattern

(Answer questions that apply to your child's age group.)

Has your child begun puberty (developing physical sexual characteristics, menstruation)? Have you or your child had any concerns?

Does your daughter know how to do breast self-examination?

Does your son know how to do testicular self-examination?

How have you approached topics of sexuality with your child?

Do you think you might need some help with some topics?

Has your child's illness affected the way he or she feels about being a boy or a girl? If so, how?

Do you have any concerns with behaviors in your child, such as masturbation, asking many questions or talking about sex, not respecting others' privacy, or wanting too much privacy?

Initiate a conversation about an adolescent's sexual concerns with open-ended to more direct questions and using the terms "friends" or "partners" rather than "girlfriend" or "boyfriend":
- Tell me about your social life.
- Who are your closest friends? (If one friend is identified, could ask more about that relationship, such as how much time they spend together, how serious they are about each other, if the relationship is going the way the teenager hoped.)
- Might ask about dating and sexual issues, such as the teenager's views on sexuality education, "going steady," "living together," or premarital sex.
- Which friends would you like to have visit in the hospital?

Coping–Stress Tolerance Pattern

(Answer questions that apply to your child's age group.)

What does your child do when tired or upset?
- If upset, does your child want a special person or object?
- If so, explain.

If your child has temper tantrums, what causes them, and how do you handle them?

Whom does your child talk to when worried about something?

How does your child usually handle problems or disappointments?

Have there been any big changes or problems in your family recently? If so, how have you handled them?

Has your child ever had a problem with drugs or alcohol or tried to commit suicide?

Do you think your child is "accident prone?" If so, explain.

Value–Belief Pattern

What is your religion?

How is religion or faith important in your child's life?

What religious practices would you like continued in the hospital (e.g., prayers before meals or bedtime; visit by minister, priest, or rabbi; prayer group)?

BOX 21-6 **COMPLEMENTARY MEDICINE PRACTICES AND EXAMPLES**

Nutrition, diet, and lifestyle or behavioral health changes—Macrobiotics, megavitamins, diets, lifestyle modification, health risk reduction and health education, wellness

Mind–body control therapies—Biofeedback, relaxation, prayer therapy, guided imagery, hypnotherapy, music or sound therapy, massage, aromatherapy, education therapy

Traditional and ethnomedicine therapies—Acupuncture, ayurvedic medicine, herbal medicine, homeopathic medicine, American Indian medicine, natural products, traditional Asian medicine

Structural manipulation and energetic therapies—Acupressure, chiropractic medicine, massage, reflexology, rolfing, therapeutic touch, Qi Gong

Pharmacologic and biologic therapies—Antioxidants, cell treatment, chelation therapy, metabolic therapy, oxidizing agents

Bioelectromagnetic therapies—Diagnostic and therapeutic application of electromagnetic fields (e.g., transcranial electrostimulation, neuromagnetic stimulation, electroacupuncture)

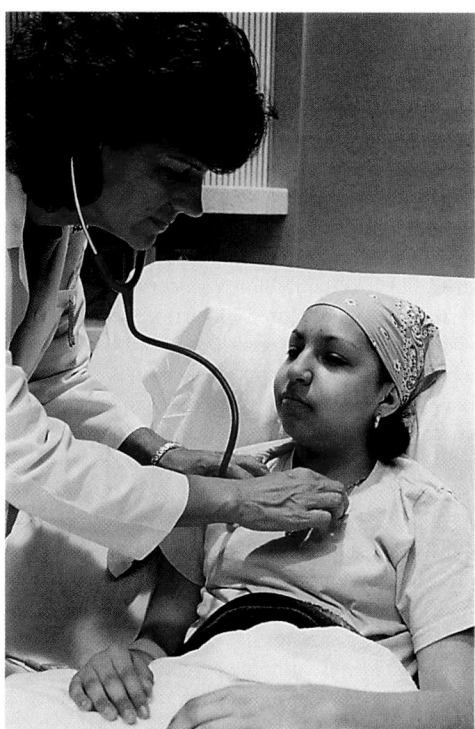

FIG 21-4 The initial admission procedures give the nurse an opportunity to get to know the child and to assess the child's understanding of the hospital experience.

BOX 21-7   GUIDELINES FOR ADMISSION

Preadmission

Assign a room based on developmental age, seriousness of diagnosis, communicability of illness, and projected length of stay.

Prepare roommate(s) for the arrival of a new patient; when children are too young to benefit from this consideration, prepare parents.

Prepare room for child and family, with admission forms and equipment nearby to eliminate need to leave child.

Admission

Introduce primary nurse to child and family.

Orient child and family to inpatient facilities, especially to assigned room and unit; emphasize positive areas of pediatric unit.

Room—Explain call light, bed controls, television, bathroom, telephone, and so on.

Unit—Direct to playroom, desk, dining area, or other areas.

Introduce family to roommate and his or her parents.

Apply identification band to child's wrist, ankle, or both (if not already done).

Explain hospital regulations and schedules (e.g., visiting hours, mealtimes, bedtime, limitations [give written information if available]).

Perform nursing admission history (see Box 21-5).

Take vital signs, blood pressure, height, and weight.

Obtain specimens as needed and order needed laboratory work.

Support child and assist practitioner with physical examination (for purposes of nursing assessment).

---

room assignment are age, sex, and nature of the illness. No absolute rules govern room selection, but in general, placing children of the same age group and with similar types of illness in the same room is both psychologically and medically advantageous. However, there are many exceptions. For example, a child in traction may be therapeutic for another child confined to bed because of a serious illness. A child who is independent despite physical disabilities may help another child with similar or different limitations, and the parents of the child with disabilities may achieve deeper insight and acceptance of their child's disorder.

Age grouping is especially important for adolescents. Many hospitals make an effort to place teenagers on their own unit or in a separate designated section of the pediatric or general unit whenever possible.

NURSING INTERVENTIONS

Preventing or Minimizing Separation

A primary nursing goal is to prevent separation, particularly in children younger than 5 years of age. Many hospitals have developed a system of family-centered care. This philosophy of care recognizes the integral role of the family in a child's life and acknowledges the family as an essential part of the child's care and illness experience. The family is considered to be partners in the care of the child (Smith and Conant Rees, 2000) (see Chapter 1). Family-centered care also supports the family by establishing priorities based on the needs and values of the family unit (Lewandowski and Tesler, 2003).

At the very least, most hospitals welcome parents at any time. Many provide facilities such as a chair or bed for at least one person per child, unit kitchen privileges, and other amenities that create a welcoming atmosphere for parents. However, not all hospitals provide such amenities, and parents' own schedules may prevent rooming-in. In such instances, strategies to minimize the effects of separation must be implemented.

Nurses must have an appreciation of the child's separation behaviors. As discussed earlier, the phases of protest and despair are normal. The child is allowed to cry. Even if the child rejects strangers, the nurse provides support through physical presence. Presence is defined as spending time being physically close to the child while using a quiet tone of voice, appropriate choice of words, eye contact, and touch in ways that establish rapport and communicate empathy. If behaviors of detachment are evident, the nurse maintains the child's contact with the parents by frequently talking about them; encouraging the child to remember them; and stressing the significance of their visits, telephone calls, or letters. The use of cellular phones can increase the contact between the hospitalized child and parents or other significant family members and friends. However, wireless technology devices may not be compatible with medical equipment, and use may be restricted in certain areas within the hospital.

Parental Absence During Infant Hospitalization

Familiar surroundings also increase the child's adjustment to separation. If the parents cannot stay with the child, they should leave favorite articles from home with the child, such as a blanket, toy, bottle, feeding utensil, or article of clothing. Because young children associate such inanimate objects with significant people, they gain comfort and reassurance from these possessions. They make the association that if the parents left this, the parents will surely return. Placing an identification band on the toy lessens the chances of its being misplaced and provides a symbol that the toy is experiencing the same needs as the child. Other reminders of home include photographs and recordings of family members reading a story, singing a song, saying prayers before bedtime, relating events at home, or taking a "talking walk" through the home. These reminders can be played at lonely times, such as on awakening or before sleeping. Some units allow pets to visit, which can have therapeutic benefits for a child. Older children also appreciate familiar articles from home, particularly photographs, a radio, a favorite toy or game, and their own pajamas. Often the importance of treasured objects to school-age children is overlooked or criticized. However, many school-age children have a special object to which they formed an attachment in early childhood. Therefore, such treasured or transitional objects can help even older children feel more comfortable in a strange environment.

The strange sights, smells, and sounds in the hospital that are commonplace for the nurse can be frightening and confusing for children. It is important for the nurse to try to evaluate stimuli in the environment from the child's point of view (considering also what the child may see or hear happening to other patients) and to make every effort to protect the child from frightening and unfamiliar sights, sounds, and equipment. The nurse should offer explanations or prepare the child for experiences that are unavoidable. Combining familiar or comforting sights with the unfamiliar can relieve much of the harshness of medical equipment.

Helping children maintain their usual contacts also minimizes the effects of separation imposed by hospitalization. This includes continuing school lessons during the illness and confinement, visiting with friends either directly or through letter writing or telephone calls, and participating in stimulating projects whenever possible (Fig. 21-5). For extended hospitalizations, youngsters enjoy personalizing the hospital room to make it "home" by decorating the walls with posters and cards, rearranging the furniture, and displaying a collection or hobby.

Minimizing Loss of Control

Feelings of loss of control result from separation, physical restriction, changed routines, enforced dependency, and magical thinking. Although some of these cannot be prevented, most can be minimized through individualized planning of nursing care.

Promoting Freedom of Movement

Younger children react most strenuously to any type of physical restriction or immobilization. Although temporary immobilization may be necessary for some interventions such as maintaining an intravenous line, most physical restriction can be prevented if the nurse gains the child's cooperation.

For young children, particularly infants and toddlers, preserving parent–child contact is the best means of decreasing the need for or stress of restraint. For example, almost the entire physical examination can be done in a parent's lap with the parent hugging the child for procedures such as an otoscopic examination. For painful procedures, the nurse should assess the parents' preferences for assisting, observing, or waiting outside the room.

Environmental factors may also restrict movement. Keeping children in cribs or play yards may not represent immobilization in a concrete sense, but it certainly limits sensory stimulation. Increasing mobility by transporting children in carriages, wheelchairs, carts, or wagons provides them with a sense of freedom.

In some cases, physical restraint or isolation is necessary because of the child's medical diagnosis. In these cases, the environment can be altered to increase sensory freedom (e.g., moving the bed toward the window; opening window shades; providing musical, visual, or tactile activities).

Maintaining the Child's Routine

Altered daily schedules and loss of rituals are particularly stressful for toddlers and early preschoolers and may increase the stress of separation. The nursing admission history provides a baseline for planning care around the child's usual home activities. A frequently neglected aspect of altered routines is the change in the child's daily activities. A typical child's day, especially during the school years, is structured with specific times for eating, dressing, going to school, playing, and sleeping. However, this time structure vanishes when the child is hospitalized. Although nurses have a set schedule, the child is frequently unaware of it, and the new schedules that are imposed may be rigid. For example, some units have uniform nap times and bedtimes for all children, but others allow children to stay up late at night. Many children obtain significantly less sleep in the hospital than at home; the primary causes are a delay in sleep onset and early termination of sleep because of hospital routines. Not only are hours of sleep disrupted, but waking hours are spent in passive activities. For example, few institutions impose any limits on the amount of time the child spends watching television. This may lead to children's being less "tired" at bedtime and delay the onset of sleep.

One technique that can minimize the disruption in the child's routine is establishing a daily schedule. This approach is most suitable for non–critically ill school-age and adolescent children who have mastered the concept of time. It involves scheduling the child's day to include all those activities that are important to the child and nurse, such as treatment procedures, schoolwork, exercise, television, playroom, and hobbies. Together, the nurse, parent, and child then plan a daily schedule with times and activities written down (Fig. 21-6). This is left in the child's room, and a clock or watch is available for the child's

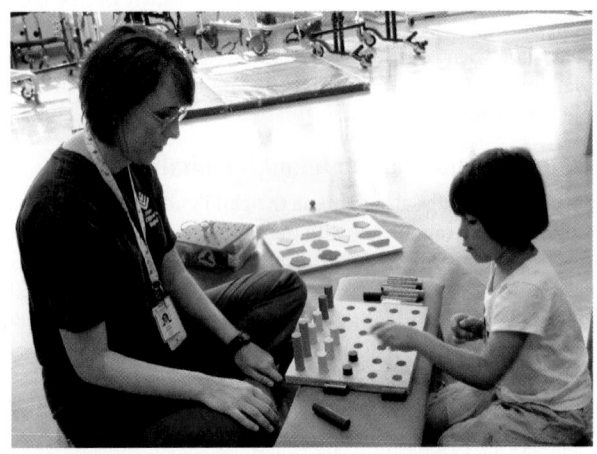

FIG 21-5 For extended hospitalizations, children enjoy doing projects to occupy time.

Eric's Daily Schedule		
7:30 AM – Breakfast, morning bath	3:00 PM – Tutor (M, W, F)	
	– Study time (T, Th)	
9:00 – Medications, dressing change	4:00 – Physical therapy	
	5:30 – Dinner	
11:00 – Physical therapy	9:00 – Medications, dressing change	
12:00 PM – Lunch		
	9:15 – Bedtime	

FIG 21-6 Time structuring is an effective strategy for normalizing the hospital environment and increasing the child's sense of control.

use. Whenever possible, a calendar is also constructed with special events marked, such as favorite television programs, visits by friends or relatives, events in the playroom, and holidays or birthdays. If specific changes in treatment are expected (e.g., "beginning physical therapy in 2 days"), these are added.

> **NURSING TIP** Ask the young child to select or draw pictures or symbols to represent daily or weekly fun activities (e.g., favorite television programs, family visits, and playroom times). Draw a clock face with the hands of the clock depicting the time each event will occur next to the child's representation. Have the child compare the clock on the schedule with a clock or watch in the room. When the two match, the child knows it is time for a favorite activity.

Encouraging Independence

The dependent role of the hospitalized patient imposes tremendous feelings of loss on older children. Principal interventions should focus on respect for individuality and the opportunity for decision making. Although these sound simple, their efficacy lies with nurses who are flexible and tolerant. It is also important for the nurse to empower the patient while not feeling threatened by a sense of lessened control.

Enabling children's control involves helping them maintain independence and promoting the concept of self-care. **Self-care** refers to the practice of activities that individuals personally initiate and perform on their own behalf in maintaining life, health, and well-being (Orem, 2001). Although self-care is limited by the child's age and physical condition, most children beyond infancy can perform some activities with little or no help. Whenever possible, these activities are encouraged in the hospital. Other approaches include jointly planning care, time structuring, wearing street clothes, making choices in food selections and bedtime, continuing school activities, and rooming with an appropriate age mate.

Promoting Understanding

Loss of control can occur from feelings of having too little influence on one's destiny or from sensing overwhelming control or power over fate. Although preschoolers' cognitive abilities predispose them most to magical thinking and delusions of power, all children are vulnerable to misinterpreting causes for stresses such as illness and hospitalization.

Most children feel more in control when they know what to expect because the element of fear is reduced. Anticipatory preparation and provision of information help to lessen stress and increase understanding (see Preparation for Diagnostic and Therapeutic Procedures, Chapter 22).

Informing children of their rights while hospitalized fosters greater understanding and may relieve some of the feelings of powerlessness they typically experience. An increasing number of hospitals and organizations have developed a patient "bill of rights" that is prominently displayed throughout the hospital or is presented to children and their families on admission (Box 21-8).

Preventing or Minimizing Fear of Bodily Injury

Beyond early infancy, all children fear bodily injury from mutilation, bodily intrusion, body image change, disability, or death. In general, preparation of children for painful procedures decreases their fears and increases cooperation. Modifying procedural techniques for children in each age group also minimizes fear of bodily injury. For example, because toddlers and young preschoolers are traumatized by insertion of a rectal thermometer, axillary temperatures or temperatures taken

---

> ### BOX 21-8   BILL OF RIGHTS FOR CHILDREN AND TEENS
>
> In this hospital, you and your family have the right to:
> - Respect and personal dignity
> - Care that supports you and your family
> - Information you can understand
> - Quality health care
> - Emotional support
> - Care that respects your need to grow, play, and learn
> - Make choices and decisions

From Association for the Care of Children's Health: *A pediatric bill of rights*, Bethesda, MD, 1991, Author.

---

with electronic or tympanic membrane devices can effectively be substituted. Whenever procedures are performed on young children, the most supportive intervention is to do the procedure as quickly as possible while maintaining parent–child contact.

Because of toddlers' and preschool children's poorly defined body boundaries, the use of bandages may be particularly helpful. For example, telling children that the bleeding will stop after the needle is removed does little to relieve their fears, but applying a small Band-Aid usually reassures them. The size of bandages is also significant to children in this age group; the larger the bandage, the more importance is attached to the wound. Watching their surgical dressings become successively smaller is one way young children can measure healing and improvement. Prematurely removing a dressing may cause these children considerable concern for their well-being. Specific pain management strategies are discussed in Chapter 7.

For children who fear mutilation of body parts, it is essential that the nurse repeatedly stress the reason for a procedure and evaluate the child's understanding. For example, explaining cast removal to preschoolers may seem simple enough, but children's comprehension of the details may vary considerably from the explanation. Asking the child to draw a picture of what they foresee happening presents substantial evidence of how they perceive events.

Children may fear bodily injury from a great variety of sources. Imaging machines, strange equipment used for examination, unfamiliar rooms, and awkward positions can be perceived as potentially hazardous. In addition, thoughts and actions can be imagined sources of bodily damage. Therefore, it is important to investigate imagined reasons, particularly of a sexual nature, for illness. Because children may fear revealing such thoughts, using techniques such as drawing or doll play may elicit previously undisclosed misconceptions.

Older children fear bodily injury of both internal and external origins. For example, school-age children are aware of the significance of the heart and may fear the actual operation as much as the pain, the stitches, and the possible scar. Adolescents may express concern about the actual procedure but be much more anxious over the resulting scar.

Children can grasp information only if it is presented on or close to their level of cognitive development. This necessitates an awareness of the words used to describe events or processes. For example, young children told that they are going to have a CAT (i.e., CT, computed tomography) scan may wonder, "Will there be cats? Or something that scratches?" It is clearer to describe the procedure in simple terms and explain what the letters of the common name stand for. Therefore, to prevent or alleviate fears, nurses must be keenly aware of the medical terminology and vocabulary that they use every day.

When children are upset about their illness, their perception can be changed by (1) providing a somewhat different and less negative account of the disease or (2) offering an explanation that is characteristic of the next stage of cognitive development. An example of the first strategy is reassuring a preschooler who fears that after a tonsillectomy, another sore throat means a second operation. Explaining that after tonsils are "fixed" they do not need fixing again can help relieve the fear. An example of the latter strategy is to explain that germs made the tonsils sick and even though germs can cause another sore throat, they cannot cause the tonsils to ever be sick again. This higher-level explanation is based on the school-age child's concept of germs as a cause of disease.

Providing Developmentally Appropriate Activities

A primary goal of nursing care for the child who is hospitalized is to minimize threats to the child's development. Many strategies (e.g., minimizing separation) have been discussed and may be all that the short-term patient requires. However, children who experience prolonged or repeated hospitalization are at greater risk for developmental delays or regression. The nurse who provides opportunities for the child to participate in developmentally appropriate activities further normalizes the child's environment and helps reduce interference with the child's ongoing development (see Normalization, Chapter 18).

Interference with normal development may have long-term implications for developing infants and toddlers. The nurse plays a primary role in identifying children at risk and helping to plan, implement, and evaluate developmental intervention (see Chapters 10 and 12).

School is an integral part of the school-age child's and adolescent's development. Accreditation standards for hospitals serving children consider access to appropriate educational services a key factor in the accreditation decision process when a child's treatment requires a significant absence from school (The Joint Commission, 2011). The nurse can encourage children to resume schoolwork as quickly as their condition permits, help them schedule and protect a selected time for studies, and help the family coordinate hospital educational services with their children's schools. Children should have the opportunity to continue art and music classes, as well as their academic subjects.

To meet the unique developmental needs of adolescents, special units may be developed that provide privacy, increased socialization, and appropriate activities for these young people. Typically, these units can be set apart from the general pediatric facility so that the teenagers do not share space with younger children, who are often perceived as a threat to their maturity.

In caring for adolescent patients, it is essential to provide flexible routines and activities, such as more group activity, wearing of street clothes, and access to the items so critical to adolescents—wireless technology devices, MP3 players, DVD players, computers, e-mail, electronic video game systems, and high-definition televisions. Because adolescents' food habits are rarely limited to the three traditional meals a day, a ready supply of snacks should be available. However, the most important benefit of these units is increased socialization with peers. In addition, staff members usually enjoy working with this age group and are able to establish the trust that is so essential for communication.

> **NURSING TIP** When adolescents must share a common activity room with younger patients, referring to the area as the "activity" room rather than the "playroom" may entice them to visit the room and participate in activities.

Although regression is expected and normal for all age groups, nurses have the responsibility for fostering the child's growth and

---

> ### BOX 21-9 FUNCTIONS OF PLAY IN THE HOSPITAL
>
> Provides diversion and brings about relaxation
> Helps the child feel more secure in a strange environment
> Lessens the stress of separation and the feeling of homesickness
> Provides a means for release of tension and expression of feelings
> Encourages interaction and development of positive attitudes toward others
> Provides an expressive outlet for creative ideas and interests
> Provides a means for accomplishing therapeutic goals (see Use of Play in Procedures, Chapter 22)
> Places child in active role and provides opportunity to make choices and be in control

development. Hospitalization can become a significant opportunity for learning and advancing. Extended hospitalizations for long-term chronic illness or situations of failure to thrive, abuse, or neglect represent instances in which regression must be seen as an adjustment period to be followed by plans for promoting appropriate developmental skills.

Providing Opportunities for Play and Expressive Activities

Play is one of the most important aspects of a child's life and one of the most effective tools for managing stress. Because illness and hospitalization constitute crises in a child's life and often involve overwhelming stresses, children need to act out their fears and anxieties as a means of coping with these stresses. Play is essential to children's mental, emotional, and social well-being; however, play does not stop when children are ill or in the hospital. On the contrary, play in the hospital serves many functions (Box 21-9). Of all hospital facilities, no room probably alleviates the stressors of hospitalization more than the playroom (or activity room). In the playroom, children temporarily distance themselves from their illness, hospitalization, and the associated stressors. This room should be a safe haven for children, free from medical or nursing procedures (including medication administration), strange faces, and probing questions. The playroom then becomes a sanctuary in an otherwise frightening environment.

Engaging in play activities gives children a sense of control. In the hospital environment, most decisions are made for the child; play and other expressive activities offer the child much-needed opportunities to make choices for themselves. Even if a child chooses not to participate in a particular activity, the nurse has offered the child a choice, perhaps one of only a few real choices the child has had that day.

Hospitalized children typically have lower energy levels than healthy children of the same age. Therefore, children may not appear engaged and enthusiastic about an activity even though they are enjoying the experience. Activities may need to be adjusted or limited based on the child's age, endurance, and any special needs.

Diversional Activities

Almost any form of play can be used for diversion and recreation, but the activity should be selected on the basis of the child's age, interests, and limitations (Fig. 21-7). Children do not necessarily need special direction for using play materials. All they require is the raw materials with which to work and adult approval and supervision to help keep their natural enthusiasm or expression of feelings from getting out of control. Small children enjoy a variety of small, colorful toys that they

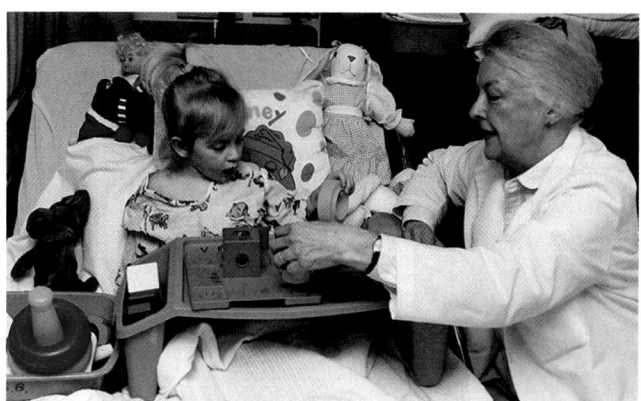

FIG 21-7 Play materials for children in the hospital need to be appropriate for their age, interests, and limitations.

can play with in bed or in their room or more elaborate play equipment, such as playhouses, sandboxes, rhythm instruments, or large boxes and blocks that may be a part of the hospital playroom.

Games that can be played alone or with another child or an adult are popular with older children, as are puzzles; reading material; quiet, individual activities, such as sewing, stringing beads, and weaving; and Lego blocks and other building materials. Assembling models is an excellent pastime, but one should make certain that all pieces and necessary materials are included in the package so the child is not disappointed and frustrated.

Well-selected books are of infinite value to children. Children never tire of stories; having someone read aloud gives them endless hours of pleasure and is of special value to children who have limited energy to expend in play. A radio, DVD player, electronic games, and television, included among most hospital room equipment, are useful tools for entertaining children. Computers with access to the Internet can provide diversion, educational opportunities, and online support groups.

When supervising play for ill or convalescent children, it is best to select activities that are simpler than would normally be chosen for the child's specific developmental level. These children usually do not have the energy to cope with more challenging activities. Other limitations also influence the type of activities. Special consideration must be given to children who are confined in terms of movement, have a restricted extremity, or are isolated. Toys for isolated children must be disposable or need to be disinfected after every use.

Toys

Parents of hospitalized children often ask nurses about the types of toys that would be best to bring for their child. Although parents often want to buy new toys for the hospitalized child to offer cheer and comfort, it is often better to wait to bring new things, especially in the case of younger children. Small children need the comfort and reassurance of familiar things, such as the stuffed animal the child hugs for comfort and takes to bed at night. These familiar items are a link with home and the world outside the hospital. All toys brought into the hospital should be assessed for safety.

Large numbers of toys often confuse and frustrate small children. A few small, well-chosen toys are usually preferred to one large, expensive one. Children who are hospitalized for an extended time benefit from changes. Rather than a confusing accumulation of toys, older toys should be replaced periodically as interest wanes.

A highly successful diversion for a child who is hospitalized for a length of time and whose parents are unable to visit frequently is

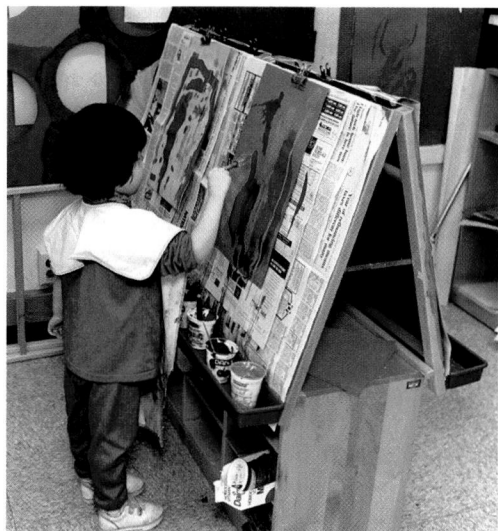

FIG 21-8 Drawing and painting are excellent media for expression.

having the parents bring a box with several small, inexpensive, brightly wrapped items with a different day of the week printed on the outside of each package. The child will eagerly anticipate the time for opening each one. If the parents know when their next visit will be, they can provide the number of packages that corresponds to the time between visits. In this way, the child knows that the diminishing packages also represent the anticipated visit from the parent.

Expressive Activities

Play and other expressive activities provide one of the best opportunities for encouraging emotional expression, including the safe release of anger and hostility. Nondirective play that allows children freedom for expression can be tremendously therapeutic. Therapeutic play, however, should not be confused with play therapy, a psychological technique reserved for use by trained and qualified therapists as an interpretative method with emotionally disturbed children. Therapeutic play, on the other hand, is an effective, nondirective modality for helping children deal with their concerns and fears, and at the same time, it often helps the nurse gain insights into children's needs and feelings.

Tension release can be facilitated through almost any activity; with younger ambulatory children, large-muscle activity such as use of tricycles and wagons is especially beneficial. Much aggression can be safely directed into pounding and throwing games or activities. Beanbags are often thrown at a target or open receptacle with surprising vigor and hostility. A pounding board is used with enthusiasm by young children; clay and play dough are beneficial for use at any age.

Creative Expression

Although all children derive physical, social, emotional, and cognitive benefits from engaging in art and other creative activities, children's need for such activities is intensified when they are hospitalized. Drawing and painting are excellent media for expression. Children are more at ease expressing their thoughts and feelings through art because humans think first in images and later learn to translate these images into words. Children need only to be supplied with the raw materials, such as crayons and paper, large brushes and an ample supply of newsprint supported on easels, or materials for finger painting (Fig. 21-8).

Children can work individually or work together on a group project, such as a mural painted on a long piece of paper.

Although interpretation of children's drawings requires special training, observing changes in a series of the child's drawings over time can be helpful in assessing psychosocial adjustment and coping. The nurse can use children's drawings, stories, poetry, and other products of creative expression as a springboard for discussion of thoughts, fears, and understanding of concepts or events (see Communication Techniques, Chapter 6). A child's drawing before surgery, for example, may reveal unvoiced concerns about mutilation, body changes, and loss of self-control.

Nurses can incorporate opportunities for musical expression into routine nursing care. For example, simple musical instruments, such as bracelets with bells, can be placed on infants' legs for them to shake to accompany mealtime music or dressing changes. Dance and movement suggestions may encourage a child to ambulate.

Holidays provide stimulus and direction for unlimited creative projects. Children can participate in decorating the pediatric unit; making pictures and decorations for their rooms gives the children a sense of pride and accomplishment. This is especially beneficial for children who are immobilized and isolated. Making gifts for someone at home helps to maintain interpersonal ties.

Dramatic Play

Dramatic play is a well-recognized technique for emotional release, allowing children to reenact frightening or puzzling hospital experiences. Through use of puppets, replicas of hospital equipment, or some actual hospital equipment, children can act out the situations that are a part of their hospital experience. Dramatic play enables children to learn about procedures and events that concern them and to assume the roles of the adults in the hospital environment.

Puppets are universally effective for communicating with children. Most children see them as peers and readily communicate with them. Children will tell the puppet feelings that they hesitate to express to adults. Puppets can share children's own experiences and help them to find solutions to their problems. Puppets dressed to represent figures in the child's environment—for example, a physician, nurse, child patient, therapist, and members of the child's own family—are especially useful. Small, appropriately attired dolls are equally effective in encouraging the child to play out situations, although puppets are usually best for direct conversation.

Play must consider medical needs, but at times, a procedure can be postponed briefly to allow the child to complete a special activity (see Critical Thinking Case Study box). Play must consider any limitations imposed by the child's condition. For example, small children may eat paste and other creative media; therefore, a child who is allergic to wheat should not be given finger paint made from wallpaper paste or modeling dough made with flour. A child on a restricted salt intake should not play with modeling dough because salt is one of its major constituents. At home, the play program can be planned around the therapy regimen. However, play can be satisfactorily incorporated into the child's care if the nurse and others involved allow some flexibility and use creativity in planning for play.

Maximizing Potential Benefits of Hospitalization

Although hospitalization generally represents a stressful time for children and families, it also represents an opportunity for facilitating positive change within the child and among family members. For some families, the stress of a child's illness, hospitalization, or both can lead to strengthening of family coping behaviors and the emergence of new coping strategies.

❓ CRITICAL THINKING CASE STUDY
Playroom and Hospital Procedures

Joel, an 8-year-old with cystic fibrosis, has been hospitalized numerous times with complications from the condition. He is playing a board game with his brother, sister, and several other children in the playroom on the pediatric unit. A pediatric phlebotomist enters the playroom and says, "Joel, I need to take some blood. I can see that you are playing a game, so I'll just do it while you play. It will just take a minute." The playroom is usually off limits for invasive procedures. As Joel's nurse, you are aware that Dr. Lung wants the results of the laboratory studies as soon as possible to make a decision about the course of therapy.

Questions

1. Evidence—Is there sufficient evidence to draw any conclusions about this situation at this time?
2. Assumptions—What are some underlying assumptions about the following:
   a. Children and painful procedures such as venipunctures
   b. The function of play in a hospitalized child
   c. The priority in performing the procedure
   d. Implications of performing the procedure in the playroom
3. What implications and priorities for nursing care can be drawn at this time (i.e., what will you do)?
4. Does the evidence objectively support your argument (conclusion)?

Fostering Parent–Child Relationships

The crisis of illness or hospitalization can mobilize parents into more acute awareness of their child's needs. For example, hospitalization provides opportunities for parents to learn more about their children's growth and development. When parents are helped to understand children's usual reactions to stress, such as regression or aggression, they are not only better able to support the child through the hospital experience but also may extend their insights into childrearing practices after discharge.

Difficulties in parent–child relationships that existed before hospitalization that are characterized by feeding problems, negative behavior, and sleep disturbances may decrease during hospitalization. The temporary cessation of such problems sometimes alerts parents to the role they may be playing in propagating the negative behavior. With assistance from health professionals, parents can restructure ways of relating to their children to foster more positive behavior.

Hospitalization may also represent a temporary reprieve or refuge from a disturbed home. Typically, abused or neglected children's dramatic physical and social improvement during hospitalization is proof of the benefits and potential growth that can occur during hospitalization. These children temporarily are able to seek support, reassurance, and security from new relationships, particularly with nurses and hospitalized peers.

Providing Educational Opportunities

Illness and hospitalization represent excellent opportunities for children and other family members to learn more about their bodies, each other, and the health professions. For example, during a hospital admission for a diabetic crisis, the child may learn about the disease; the parents may learn about the child's needs for independence, normalcy, and appropriate limits; and each of them may find a new support system in the hospital staff.

Illness or hospitalization can also help older children in choosing a career. Frequently, children have impressions of physicians or nurses that are disproportionately positive or negative. Actual experience with different health professionals can influence their attitude about health professionals and even a decision regarding a career in health care.

Promoting Self-Mastery

The experience of facing a crisis such as illness or hospitalization, coping successfully with it, and maturing as a result of it constitutes an opportunity for self-mastery. Younger children have the chance to test fantasy versus reality fears. They realize that they were not abandoned, mutilated, or punished. In fact, they were loved, cared for, and treated with respect for their individual concerns. It is not unusual for children who have undergone hospitalization or surgery to tell others that "it was nothing" or to display proudly their scars or bandages. For older children, hospitalization may represent an opportunity for decision making, independence, and self-reliance. They are proud of having survived the experience and may feel a genuine self-respect for their achievements. Nurses can facilitate such feelings of self-mastery by emphasizing aspects of personal competence in the child and not focusing on uncooperative or negative behavior.

Providing Socialization

Hospitalization may offer children a special opportunity for social acceptance. Lonely, asocial, and even delinquent children find a sympathetic environment in the hospital. Children who have a physical disability or are in some other way "different" from their age mates may find an accepting social peer group (Fig. 21-9). Although this does not always spontaneously occur, nurses can structure the environment to foster a supportive child group. For example, selection of a compatible roommate can help children gain a new friend and learn more about themselves. Forming relationships with significant members of the health care team, such as the physician, nurse, child life specialist, or social worker, can greatly enhance children's adjustment in many areas of life.

Parents may also encounter a new social group in other parents who have similar problems. The waiting room or hallway "self-help" groups are inherent to every institution. Parents meet while in the hospital or clinic and discuss their children's illnesses and treatments. Nurses can capitalize on this informal gathering by encouraging parents to discuss collectively their concerns and feelings. Nurses can also refer parents to organized parent groups or can use the help and support of parents of recovered hospitalized patients. It is important that nurses emphasize to families that each child responds differently to disease, treatments, and care. Any questions raised during group discussions should be clarified with a nurse or physician.

NURSING CARE OF THE FAMILY

Although it is not possible to predict exactly which factors are most likely to have an effect on a family's reactions, important variables are (1) the seriousness of the child's illness, (2) the family's previous experience with hospitalization, and (3) the medical procedures involved in the diagnosis and treatment. Important information is also obtained in the nursing admission history (see Box 21-5).

SUPPORTING FAMILY MEMBERS

Support involves the willingness to stay and listen to parents' verbal and nonverbal messages. Sometimes the nurse does not give this support directly. For example, the nurse may offer to stay with the child to allow the parents time alone or may discuss with other family members the parents' need for extra relief. Often relatives and friends want to help but do not know how. Suggesting ways, such as babysitting, preparing meals, doing laundry, or transporting the siblings to school, can prompt others to help reduce the responsibilities that burden parents.

Support may also be provided through the clergy. Parents with deep religious beliefs may appreciate the counsel of a clergy member, but because of their stress, they may not have sufficient energy to initiate the contact. Nurses can be supportive by arranging for clergy to visit, upholding parents' religious beliefs, and respecting the individual meaning and significance of those beliefs (Feudtner, Haney, and Dimmers, 2003).

Support involves accepting cultural, socioeconomic, and ethnic values. For example, health and illness are defined differently by various ethnic groups. For some, a disorder that has few outward manifestations of illness, such as diabetes, hypertension, or cardiac problems, is not a sickness. Consequently, following a prescribed treatment may be seen as unnecessary. Nurses who appreciate the influences of culture are more likely to intervene therapeutically. (See also Cultural Influences, Chapter 4.)

Parents need help in accepting their own feelings toward the ill child. If given the opportunity, parents often disclose their feelings of loss of control, anger, and guilt. They often resist admitting to such feelings because they expect others to disapprove of behavior that is less than perfect. Unfortunately, health personnel, including nurses, sometimes do exercise little tolerance for deviation from the norm. This only increases the psychological impact of a child's illness on family members. Helping parents identify the specific reason for such feelings and emphasizing that each is a normal, expected, and healthy response to stress may reduce the parents' emotional burden.

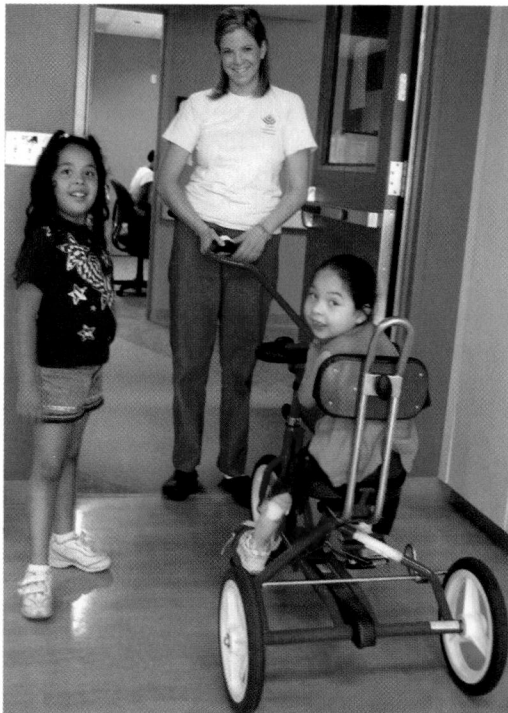

FIG 21-9 Placing children of the same age group with similar illnesses near each other on the unit is both psychologically and medically supportive. (Courtesy E. Jacob, Texas Children's Hospital, Houston.)

Supporting Siblings During Hospitalization

Trade off staying at the hospital with spouse or have a surrogate who knows the siblings well stay in the home.

Offer information about the child's condition to young siblings as well as older siblings; respect the sibling who avoids information as a means of coping with the situation.

Arrange for children to visit their brother or sister in the hospital if possible.

Encourage phone visits and mail between brothers and sisters; provide children with phone numbers, writing supplies, and stamps.

Help each sibling identify an extended family member or friend to be their support person and provide extra attention during parental absence.

Make or buy inexpensive toys or trinkets for siblings, one gift for each day the child will be hospitalized.

- Wrap each gift separately and place them in a basket, box, or other container at the child's bedside.
- Instruct siblings to open one gift at bedtime and to remember that he or she is in their parent's thoughts.

If the child's condition is stable and distance is not prohibitive, plan a special time at home with the siblings or have spouse or another relative or friend bring the children to meet parent(s) at a restaurant or other location near the hospital.

- Have extended family members or friends schedule a visit to the child in the hospital during parental absence.
- Arrange a pass for the child to leave the hospital to join the family if the child's condition permits.

Modified from Craft M, Craft J: Perceived changes in siblings of hospitalized children: a comparison of sibling and parent reports, *Child Health Care* 18(1):42–48, 1989; Rollins J: *Brothers and sisters: a discussion guide for families*, Landover, MD, 1992, Epilepsy Foundation of America.

Family-centered care also addresses the needs of siblings. Support may involve preparing siblings for hospital visits, assessing their adjustment, and providing appropriate interventions or referrals when needed. The Family-Centered Care box suggests ways that parents can support siblings during hospitalization.

PROVIDING INFORMATION

One of the most important nursing interventions is providing information about (1) the disease, its treatment, prognosis, and home care; (2) the child's emotional and physical reactions to illness and hospitalization; and (3) the probable emotional reactions of family members to the crisis.

For many families, the child's illness is the first contact they have with the hospital experience. Often parents are not prepared for the child's behavioral reactions to hospitalization, such as separation behaviors, regression, aggression, and hostility. Providing the parents with information about these normal and expected behavioral responses can lessen the parents' anxiety during the hospital admission. The family is equally unfamiliar with hospital rules, which often compounds their confusion and anxiety. Therefore, the family needs clear explanations about what to expect and what is expected of them.

Parents also need to be aware of the effects of illness on the family and strategies that prevent negative changes. Specifically, parents should keep the family well informed and communicate with everyone as much as possible. They should treat all the children equally and as

normally as before the illness occurred. Discipline, which initially may be lessened for the ill child, should be continued to provide a measure of security and predictability. When ill children know that their parents expect certain standards of conduct from them, they feel certain that they will recover. Conversely, when all limits are removed, they fear that something catastrophic will happen.

Helping parents understand the meaning of posthospitalization behaviors in the sick child is necessary for them to tolerate and support such behaviors. In addition, parents should be forewarned of the common reactions after discharge (see Box 21-2). Parents who do not expect such reactions may misinterpret them as evidence of the child's "being spoiled" and demand perfect behavior at a time when the child is still reacting to the stress of illness and hospitalization. If the behaviors, especially the demand for attention, are dealt with in a supportive manner, most children are able to relinquish them and assume prior levels of functioning.

Nurses should also prepare parents for the reactions of siblings—particularly anger, jealousy, and resentment. Older siblings may deny such reactions because they provoke feelings of guilt. However, everyone needs outlets for emotions, and the repressed feelings may surface as problems in school or with age mates, as psychosomatic illnesses, or in delinquent behavior.

Probably one of the most neglected areas of communication involves giving information to siblings. Frequently, age becomes the only factor that leads to an awareness of this problem because older children may begin to ask questions or request explanations. Even in this situation, however, the information may be seriously inadequate. Children in every age group deserve some explanation of the sibling's illness or hospitalization. In addition, nurses can minimize a sibling's fear of also getting sick or having caused the illness.

ENCOURAGING PARENT PARTICIPATION

Preventing or minimizing separation is a key nursing goal with the child who is hospitalized, but maintaining parent–child contact is also beneficial for the family. One of the best approaches is encouraging parents to stay with their child and to participate in the care whenever possible. Although some health facilities provide special accommodations for parents, the concept of rooming in can be instituted anywhere. The first requirement is the staff's positive attitude toward parents. A negative attitude toward parent participation can create barriers to collaborative working relationships.

When hospital staff genuinely appreciates the importance of continued parent–child attachment, they foster an environment that encourages parents to stay. When parents are included in the care planning and understand that they are a contributing factor to the child's recovery, they are more inclined to remain with their child and have more emotional reserves to support themselves and the child through the crisis. An empowerment model of helping allows the nurse to focus on parents' strengths and seek ways to promote growth and family functioning so that the parents become empowered in caring for their child. Strategies such as bedside reporting that allow parents to be involved in the discussion of the child's current status are moving health care settings closer to family-centered care (Anderson and Mangino, 2006). Liaison nursing roles in tertiary care settings are also focused on improving communication between parents and health care providers (Caffin, Linton, and Pellegrini, 2007).

Because the mother tends to be the usual family caregiver, she usually spends more time in the hospital than the father. However, not all parents feel equally comfortable assuming responsibility for their child's care. Some may be under such great emotional stress that they need a temporary reprieve from total participation in caregiving activities. Others may feel insecure in participating in specialized areas of care, such as bathing the child after surgery. On the other hand, some mothers may feel a great need to control their child's care. This seems particularly true of young mothers, who have recently established their role as a parent; mothers of children too young to verbalize their needs; and ethnic minority mothers when the hospital setting is predominantly staffed by nonminority personnel. Individual assessment of each parent's preferred involvement is necessary to prevent the effects of separation while supporting parents in their needs as well.

With lifestyles and gender roles changing, fathers may assume all or some of the usual "mothering" roles in the household. In these cases, it may be the father–child relationship that requires preservation. Fathers need to be included in the care plan and respected for their parental role. For some fathers, the child's hospitalization may represent an opportunity to alter their usual caregiving role and increase their involvement. In single-parent families, the caregiver may not be a parent but an extended family member, such as a grandparent or aunt.

One of the potential problems with continuous parent involvement is neglect of the parent's need for sleep, nutrition, and relaxation. Often the sleeping accommodations are limited to a chair, and sleep is disrupted by nursing procedures. Encouraging the parents to leave for brief periods, arranging for sleeping quarters on the unit but outside the child's room, and planning a schedule of alternating visits with another family member can minimize the stresses for the parent.

All too often, nurses respond to parent participation by abandoning their patient responsibilities. Nurses need to restructure their roles to complement and augment the caregiving functions of parents (Hopia, Tomlinson, Paavilainen, and others, 2005). Even in units structured to provide care by parents, parents frequently feel anxiety in their caregiving responsibilities; those more involved in direct care may feel more anxiety than those less involved in direct care. Therefore, 24-hour responsibility may be too much for some parents. Assistance and relief by nursing personnel should always be available to these families, and nurses may need to work diligently to establish the strong bond of trust some parents need to take advantage of these opportunities.

PREPARING FOR DISCHARGE AND HOME CARE

Most hospitalizations necessitate some type of discharge preparation. Often this involves education of the family for continued care and follow-up in the home. Depending on the diagnosis, this may be relatively simple or highly complex. Preparing the family for home care demands a high degree of competence in planning and implementing discharge instructions.

Nurses are often key individuals in initiating and carrying out the discharge process. They collaborate with others in the planning and implementation phases to ensure appropriate care after hospitalization. Throughout the hospitalization, the nurse should be aware of the need for discharge planning and those assessment factors that affect the family's ability to provide home care. A thorough assessment of the family and home environment should be performed to ensure that the family's emotional and physical resources are sufficient to manage the tasks of home care. (For a discussion of family and home assessment strategies, see Chapter 6.) In addition to adequate family resources, an investigation of community services, including respite care, is needed to ensure that appropriate support agencies are available, such as emergency facilities, home health agencies, and equipment vendors. Financial resources are also a consideration. To

coordinate the immense task of assessment and to plan implementation, a care coordinator or manager should be appointed early in the discharge process.

The preparation for hospital discharge and home care begins during the admission assessment. Short- and long-term goals are established to meet the child's physical and psychosocial needs. For children with complex care needs, discharge planning focuses on obtaining appropriate equipment and health care personnel for the home. Discharge planning is also concerned with treatments that parents or children are expected to continue at home. In planning appropriate teaching, nurses need to assess (1) the actual and perceived complexity of the skill, (2) the parents' or child's ability to learn the skill, and (3) the parents' or child's previous or present experience with such procedures.

The teaching plan incorporates levels of learning, such as observing, participating with assistance, and finally acting without help or guidance. The skill is divided into discrete steps, and each step is taught to the family member until it is learned. Return demonstration of the skill is requested before new skills are introduced. A record of teaching and performance provides an efficient checklist for evaluation. All families need to receive detailed *written* instructions about home care, with telephone numbers for assistance, before they leave the hospital. Communication between the nurse performing discharge planning and home health care is essential for ensuring a smooth transition for the child and family.

After the family is competent in performing the skill, they are given responsibility for the care. When possible, the family should have a transition or trial period to assume care with minimal health care supervision. This may be arranged on the unit; during a home pass; or in a facility, such as a motel, near the hospital. Such transitions provide a safe practice period for the family, with assistance readily available when needed, and are especially valuable when the family lives far from the hospital.

In many instances, parents need only simple instructions and understanding of follow-up care. However, the often overwhelming care assumed by some families, coupled with other stressors they may be experiencing, necessitates continued professional support after discharge. A follow-up home visit or telephone call gives the nurse an opportunity to individualize care and provide information in perhaps a less stressful learning environment than the hospital. Appropriate referrals and resources may include visiting nurse or home health agencies, private nurse services, the school system, a physical therapist, a mental health counselor, a social worker, and any number of community agencies. Sharing the important issues surrounding the child's and family's needs is essential. Referral summaries should be concise, specific, and factual. When numerous support services are required, periodic collaboration among the professionals involved and the family is an excellent strategy to ensure efficient usage and comprehensive delivery of services.

CARE OF THE CHILD AND FAMILY IN SPECIAL HOSPITAL SITUATIONS

In addition to a general pediatric unit, children may be admitted to special facilities such as an ambulatory or outpatient setting, an isolation room, or intensive care.

AMBULATORY OR OUTPATIENT SETTING

The ambulatory or outpatient setting provides needed medical services for the child while eliminating the necessity of overnight

---

FAMILY-CENTERED CARE

Discharge from Ambulatory Settings

1. Before beginning, explain that all instructions will also be presented in writing for the family to refer to later.
2. Provide an overview of the typical trajectory (expected pattern) of recovery.
3. Discuss expected progression of the child's activity level during the post-discharge period (e.g., "Mary will probably sleep for the rest of the day and feel kind of tired most of tomorrow but will be back to her usual activities the next day").
4. Explain which activities the child is allowed and what is not permitted (e.g., bed rest, bathing).
5. Discuss dietary restrictions, being very specific and giving examples of "clear fluids" or what is meant by a "full liquid diet."
6. Discuss nausea and vomiting, if applicable, explaining how much is "normal" and what to do if more occurs (e.g., "Juan may be sick to his stomach and vomit. This is normal. However, if he vomits more than three times, please call us at this number right away.").
7. Discuss fever and appropriate comfort measures, explaining how much fever is considered "normal," and specifically what to do if the child goes beyond the range.
8. Explain the amount, location, and kind of pain or discomfort the child may experience.
   - Give any prescribed medication before leaving the facility.
   - Send a pain scale home with the family.
   - Explain how much pain and discomfort is "normal" and what to do if the child surpasses that level or if pain management interventions are unsuccessful.
   - Discuss pain management, including dosage for pain medications and details on how to administer them.
   - Describe appropriate nonpharmacologic comfort measures, such as holding, rocking, or swaddling.
9. Provide information about each medication that the child will be taking at home.
   - Review the details, including dose and route.
   - Demonstrate how to administer medications, if necessary (e.g., how to take outer packaging off suppositories, how to insert).
   - Discuss guidelines for requesting other medications.
   - Request that all prescriptions be filled and given to the family before discharge.
10. Make certain the family has all of the equipment and supplies (e.g., gauze and tape for dressing changes) they will need at home.
11. Discuss complications that may occur and the steps to take if they do.
12. Ensure that appropriate measures are in place for safe transport home.
    - Remind family to use a seat belt or car seat for the child.
    - Determine if there will be one person whose sole responsibility is helping ensure the child's safety and comfort during transport.
    - Discuss measures the driver may need to take if this is impossible (e.g., be certain a basin is within the child's reach in case vomiting occurs; take a route that permits slower traffic and has places along the roadside to stop if necessary).
    - Determine the availability of a blanket, pillow, and cup with a lid and straw for the child's use in the car.
13. Provide emergency phone numbers for the family to call with any concerns.
14. Explain that the family will be contacted (give an approximate time) to follow up on the child but that they should not hesitate to call if concerns arise before then.
15. Ask the family and child, if appropriate, if they have any questions and problem solve with family members to meet their unique needs.

---

admission. The benefits of ambulatory care are (1) minimized stressors of hospitalization, especially separation from the family; (2) reduced chances of infection; and (3) increased cost savings. Admission to the ambulatory or outpatient hospital setting usually is for surgical or diagnostic procedures, such as insertion of tympanostomy tubes, hernia repair, adenoidectomy, tonsillectomy, cystoscopy, or bronchoscopy.

In the ambulatory or outpatient setting, adequate preparation is particularly challenging. Ideally, the child and parents should receive preadmission preparation, including a tour of the facility and a review of the day's events. Parents need information in advance to help prepare the child and themselves for surgery and enable them to care for the child at home after the procedure. Parents also appreciate suggestions for items to bring to the hospital, such as blankets or stuffed animals. When preadmission preparation is not possible, time should be allowed on the day of the procedure for children to become acquainted with their surroundings and for nurses to assess, plan, and implement appropriate teaching.

Explicit discharge instructions are important after outpatient surgery (see Family-Centered Care box and Preparing for Discharge and Home Care, p. 629). Parents need guidelines on when to call their practitioner regarding a change in the child's condition. A follow-up telephone call system allows for nurses to check on the child's progress within 48 to 72 hours after discharge. It also provides an opportunity for the nurse to review discharge information and answer questions.

NURSING TIP Help the family prepare for the transportation home by offering these suggestions:
- Have a blanket and pillow in the car. (Always use the car safety restraint system.)
- Take a basin or plastic bag in case of vomiting.
- Use a cup with a cap and straw for the child to drink fluids (except in cases of oral facial surgery in which a straw may be contraindicated).
- Give any prescribed pain medication before leaving facility.
- Provide parents verbal and written information regarding potential side effects of pain medication for which they should be vigilant after discharge.

ISOLATION

Admission to an isolation room increases all of the stressors typically associated with hospitalization. There is further separation from familiar persons; additional loss of control; and added environmental changes, such as sensory deprivation and the strange appearance of visitors. Orientation to time and place is affected. These stressors are compounded by children's limited understanding of isolation. Preschool children have difficulty understanding the rationale for isolation because they cannot comprehend the cause-and-effect relationship between germs and illness. They are likely to view isolation as punishment. Older children understand the causality better but still require information to decrease fantasizing or misinterpretation.

When a child is placed in isolation, preparation is essential for the child to feel in control. With young children, the best approach is a simple explanation, such as "You need to be in this room to help you get better. This is a special place to make all the germs go away. The germs made you sick, and you could not help that."

All children, but especially younger ones, need preparation in terms of what they will see, hear, and feel in isolation. Therefore, they are shown the mask, gloves, and gown and are encouraged to "dress up" in them. Playing with the strange apparel lessens the fear of seeing "ghostlike" people walk into the room. Before entering the room, nurses and other health personnel should introduce themselves and let the child see their faces before donning masks. In this way, the child associates them with significant experiences and gains a sense of familiarity in an otherwise strange and lonely environment.

When the child's condition improves, appropriate play activities are provided to minimize boredom, stimulate the senses, provide a real or perceived sense of movement, orient the child to time and place, provide social interaction, and reduce depersonalization. For example, the environment can be manipulated to increase sensory freedom by moving the bed toward the door or window. Opening window shades; providing musical, visual, or tactile toys; and increasing interpersonal contact can substitute mental mobility for the limitations of physical movement. Rather than dwelling on the negative aspects of isolation, the child can be encouraged to view this experience as challenging and positive. For example, the nurse can help the child look at isolation as a method of keeping others out and letting only special people in. Children often think of intriguing signs for their doors, such as "Enter at your own risk." These signs also encourage people "on the outside" to talk with the child about the ominous greeting.

> **NURSING TIP** Have the child select a place he or she would like to visit. Help the child decorate the bed and equipment to suit the theme (e.g., truck, circus tent, spaceship, sky). At a set time each day, pretend to go with the child to the special place. Consider including props such as a suitcase or picnic basket.

EMERGENCY ADMISSION

One of the most traumatic hospital experiences for the child and parents is an emergency admission. The sudden onset of an illness or the occurrence of an injury leaves little time for preparation and explanation. Sometimes the emergency admission is compounded by admission to an intensive care unit (ICU) or the need for immediate surgery. However, even in instances requiring only outpatient treatment, the child is exposed to a strange, frightening environment and to experiences that may elicit fear or cause pain.

There is a wide discrepancy between what constitutes a medically defined emergency and a client-defined emergency. A growing concern is the use of major emergency departments for routine primary care health visits. To offset overcrowding in emergency departments, many facilities have minor emergency units or pediatric minor emergency units for after-hours health care. Telephone triage for minor illnesses for patients is also emerging as a health care delivery mode to differentiate illnesses such as a common cold from true life-threatening conditions that require immediate practitioner attention and intervention. Other factors contributing to the overuse of emergency departments (as opposed to the primary practitioner's office) include the increasing number of uninsured persons and households where both parents work full time and cannot afford to take time off during the day to take the sick child to a practitioner.

In pediatric populations, most visits to an emergency department are for respiratory infections, skin conditions, gastrointestinal disorders, and trauma such as poisoning accounting for the remainder of cases. The most common reason parents give for bringing the child to the emergency department is concern about the illness worsening. However, practitioners may not think that the progressive symptoms necessitate immediate or emergency care. One of the nurse's primary goals is to assess the parents' perception of the event and their reasons for considering it serious or life threatening.

Lengthy preparatory admission procedures are often inappropriate for emergency situations. In such instances, nurses must focus their nursing interventions on the essential components of admission counseling (Box 21-10) and complete the process as soon as the child's condition has stabilized.

Unless an emergency is life threatening, children need to participate in their care to maintain a sense of control. Because emergency departments are frequently hectic, there is a tendency to rush through procedures to save time. However, the extra few minutes needed to allow children to participate may save many more minutes of useless resistance and uncooperativeness during subsequent procedures. Other supportive measures include ensuring privacy, accepting various emotional responses to fear or pain, preserving parent–child contact, explaining all events before or as they occur, and personally remaining calm. Pain management strategies are discussed in Chapter 7.

At times, because of the child's physical condition, little or no preparatory counseling for emergency hospitalization can be done. In such situations, counseling subsequent to the event has therapeutic value. The counseling should focus on evaluating children's thoughts regarding admission and related procedures. It is similar to precounseling techniques; however, instead of supplying information, the nurse listens to the explanations offered by the child. Projective techniques such as drawing, doll play, or storytelling are especially effective. The nurse then bases additional information on what has already been understood.

INTENSIVE CARE UNIT

Admission to an ICU can be traumatic for both the child and parents (Fig. 21-10). The nature and severity of the illness and the

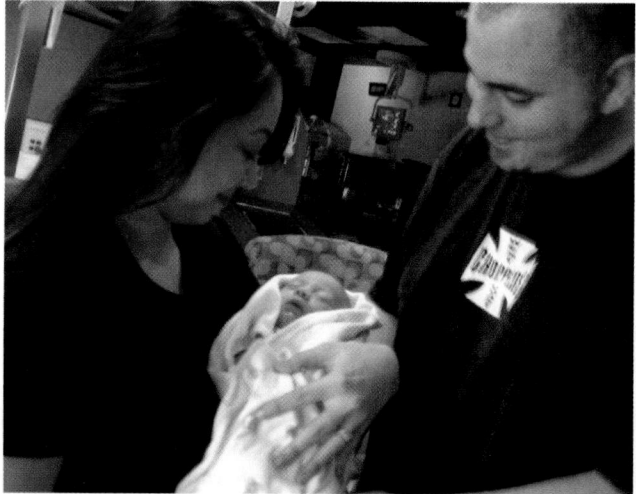

FIG 21-10 Parental presence during hospitalization provides emotional support for the child and increases the parent's sense of empowerment in the caregiver role. (Courtesy E. Jacob, Texas Children's Hospital, Houston.)

BOX 21-10 GUIDELINES FOR SPECIAL HOSPITAL ADMISSION*

Emergency Admission

Lengthy preparatory admission procedures are often impossible and inappropriate for emergency situations.

Focus assessment on airway, breathing, and circulation; weigh child whenever possible for calculation of drug dosages.

Unless an emergency is life threatening, children need to participate in their care to maintain a sense of control.

Focus on essential components of admission counseling, including:
- Appropriate introduction to the family
- Use of child's name, not terms such as "honey" or "dear"
- Determination of child's age and some judgment about developmental age (If the child is of school age, asking about the grade level will offer some evidence of intellectual ability.)
- Information about child's general state of health, any problems that may interfere with medical treatment (e.g., allergies), and previous experience with hospital facilities
- Information about the chief complaint from both the parents and the child

Admission to Intensive Care Unit (ICU)

Prepare child and parents for elective ICU admission, such as for postoperative care after cardiac surgery.

Prepare child and parents for unanticipated ICU admission by focusing primarily on the sensory aspects of the experience and on usual family concerns (e.g., persons in charge of child's care, schedule for visiting, area where family can stay).

Prepare parents regarding child's appearance and behavior when they first visit child in ICU.

Accompany family to bedside to provide emotional support and answer questions.

Prepare siblings for their visit; plan length of time for sibling visitation; monitor siblings' reactions during visit to prevent them from becoming overwhelmed.

Encourage parents to stay with their child:
- If visiting hours are limited, allow flexibility in schedule to accommodate parental needs.
- Give family members a written schedule of visiting times.
- If visiting hours are liberal, be aware of family members' needs and suggest periodic respites.
- Assure family they can call the unit at any time.

Prepare parents for expected role changes and identify ways for parents to participate in child's care without overwhelming them with responsibilities:
- Help with bath or feeding.
- Touch and talk to child.
- Help with procedures.

Provide information about child's condition in understandable language:
- Repeat information often.
- Seek clarification of understanding.
- During bedside conferences, interpret information for family members and child or, if appropriate, conduct report outside room.

Prepare child for procedures even if it involves explanation while procedure is performed.

Assess and manage pain; recognize that a child who cannot talk, such as an infant or child in a coma or on mechanical ventilation, can be in pain.

Establish a routine that maintains some similarity to daily events in child's life whenever possible:
- Organize care during normal waking hours.
- Keep regular bedtime schedules, including quiet times when television or radio is lowered or turned off.
- Provide uninterrupted sleep cycles (60 minutes for infants; 90 minutes for older children).
- Close and open drapes and dim lights to allow for day and night.
- Place curtain around bed for privacy.
- Orient child to day and time; have clocks or calendars in easy view for older children.

Schedule a time when child is left undisturbed (e.g., during naps, visit with family, playtime, or favorite program).

Provide opportunities for play.

Reduce stimulation in environment:
- Refrain from loud talking or laughing.
- Keep equipment noise to a minimum:
  - Turn alarms as low as safely possible.
  - Perform treatments requiring equipment at one time.
  - Turn off bedside equipment that is not in use, such as suction and oxygen.
  - Avoid loud, abrupt noises.

*See also Box 21-7.

---

circumstances surrounding the admission are major factors, especially for parents. Parents experience significantly more stress when the admission is unexpected rather than expected. Stressors for the child and parent are described in Box 21-11. Although several studies have described what parents perceive as most stressful, the most effective strategy may be to simply ask parents what is stressful and implement interventions that will enhance their ability to cope (Board and Ryan-Wenger, 2003). Assessment should be repeated periodically to account for changes in perceptions over time. The use of daily patient goal sheets has been successful in improving communication among health care providers caring for children in the ICU (Agarwal, Frankel, Tourner, and others, 2008; Phipps and Thomas, 2007). By clearly defining daily patient care goals, health care providers believed that care was improved.

The family's emotional needs are paramount when a child is admitted to an ICU. A major stressor for parents of a child in the ICU is the child's appearance (Latour, van Goudoever, and Hazelzet, 2008).

Although the same interventions discussed earlier for the stressors of separation and loss of control apply here, additional interventions may also benefit the family and child (see Box 21-11). In a qualitative study of 19 parents of 10 children in an ICU, parents reported that they simply wanted nurses to nurture the child in the same way the family would (Harbaugh, Tomlinson, and Kirschbaum, 2004). Nurse behaviors that exemplified caring and affection were perceived as helpful in decreasing stress. Behaviors perceived as not helpful included separating the child from the parents and communicating poorly with parents. Therefore, even critical care must be centered on the family. It is important that visiting hours be liberal and flexible enough to accommodate parental needs and involvement.

Critically ill children become the focus of the parents' lives, and parents' most pressing need is for information. They want to know if their child will live and, if so, whether the child will be the same as before. They need to know why various interventions are being done for the child, that the child is being treated for pain or is comfortable,

---

BOX 21-11   NEONATAL OR PEDIATRIC INTENSIVE CARE UNIT STRESSORS FOR THE CHILD AND FAMILY

Physical Stressors

Pain and discomfort (e.g., injections, intubation, suctioning, dressing changes, other invasive procedures)

Immobility (e.g., use of restraints, bed rest)

Sleep deprivation

Inability to eat or drink

Changes in elimination habits

Environmental Stressors

Unfamiliar surroundings (e.g., crowding)

Unfamiliar sounds

- Equipment noise (e.g., monitors, telephone, suctioning, computer printout)
- Human sounds (e.g., talking, laughing, crying, coughing, moaning, retching, walking)

Unfamiliar people (e.g., health care professionals, patients, visitors)

Unfamiliar and unpleasant smells (e.g., alcohol, adhesive remover, body odors)

Constant lights (disturb day–night rhythms)

Activity related to other patients

Sense of urgency among staff

Unkind or thoughtless comments from staff

Psychologic Stressors

Lack of privacy

Inability to communicate (if intubated)

Inadequate knowledge and understanding of situation

Severity of illness

Parental behavior (expression of concern)

Social Stressors

Disrupted relationships (especially with family and friends)

Concern with missing school or work

Play deprivation

Data primarily from Tichy AM, Braam CM, Meyer TA, and others: Stressors in pediatric intensive care units, *Pediatr Nurs* 14(1):40–42, 1988.

---

and that the child may be able to hear them even though not awake. When parents first visit the child in the ICU, they need preparation regarding the child's appearance. Ideally, the nurse should accompany the parents to the bedside to provide emotional support and answer any questions.

Despite the stresses normally associated with ICU admission, a special security develops from being carefully monitored and receiving individualized care. Therefore, planning for transition to the regular unit is essential and should include:

- Assignment of a primary nurse on the regular unit
- Continued visits by the ICU staff to assess the child's and parents' adjustment and to act as a temporary liaison with the nursing staff
- Explanation of the differences between the two units and the rationale for the change to less intense monitoring of the child's physical condition
- Selection of an appropriate room, such as one that is close to the nursing station, and a compatible roommate

KEY POINTS

- Children are particularly vulnerable to the stressors of illness and hospitalization because stress represents a change from the usual state of health and routine and because they possess limited coping mechanisms.
- The three stages of separation anxiety are protest, despair, and detachment.
- Feelings of loss of control are caused by unfamiliar environmental stimuli, physical restriction, altered routine, and dependency.
- Fear of bodily pain may be manifested in the following ways: infants—facial expressions and body movements; toddlers—intense emotional upset and physical resistance; preschoolers—aggression, verbal expression, and dependency; school-age children—precise verbalization of pain, passive requests for support or help, and procrastination technique; and adolescents—self-control and limited movement.
- Because of their separation from significant people, children who are hospitalized may lack the opportunity to form new attachments in the strange environment of the hospital and exhibit negative behaviors after discharge.
- Nursing care of children in the hospital is aimed at preventing or minimizing separation, decreasing loss of control, minimizing fear of bodily injury, using play or expressive activities to lessen stress, and maximizing the potential benefits of hospitalization.

- The nurse can maximize potential benefits of hospitalization by fostering parent–child relations, providing educational opportunities, promoting self-mastery, and encouraging socialization.
- Family reactions are influenced by the seriousness of the illness, experience with illness or hospitalization and diagnostic or therapeutic procedures, available support systems, personal ego strengths, coping abilities, presence of additional stressors, cultural and religious beliefs, and family communication patterns.
- Fear of contracting illness, their younger age, a close relationship with the ill sibling, substitute child care, minimal explanation of the illness, and perceived changes in parenting all increase the deleterious effects of a brother's or sister's illness and hospitalization on siblings.
- Nursing care of the family involves listening to parents' verbal and nonverbal messages; providing clergy support; accepting cultural, socioeconomic, and ethnic values; giving information to families and siblings; and preparing for discharge and home care.
- Admission to an outpatient setting, emergency department, isolation room, or ICU requires additional intervention strategies to meet the child's and family's needs.

REFERENCES

Agarwal S, Frankel L, Tourner S, and others: Improving communication in a pediatric intensive care unit using daily patient goal sheets, *J Crit Care* 23(2):227–235, 2008.

Anderson CD, Mangino RR: Nurse shift report: who says you can't talk in front of the patient? *Nurs Adm Q* 30(2):112–122, 2006.

Board R, Ryan-Wenger N: Stressors and symptoms of mothers with children in the PICU, *J Pediatr Nurs* 18(3):195–201, 2003.

Caffin CL, Linton S, Pellegrini J: Introduction of a liaison nurse role in a tertiary paediatric ICU, *Intensive Crit Care Nurs* 23(4):226–233, 2007.

Clatworthy S, Simon K, Tiedeman ME: Child drawing: hospital—an instrument designed to measure the emotional status of hospitalized school-aged children, *J Pediatr Nurs* 14(1):2–9, 1999.

Coyne I: Children's experiences of hospitalization, *J Child Health Care* 10(4):326–336, 2006.

Craft MJ: Siblings of hospitalized children: assessment and intervention, *J Pediatr Nurs* 8(5):289–297, 1993.

Fernandez C, Pyesmany A, Stutzer C: Alternative therapies in childhood cancer, *N Engl J Med* 340(7):569–570, 1999.

Feudtner HJ, Haney J, Dimmers MA: Spiritual care needs of hospitalized children and their families: a national survey of pastoral care providers' perceptions, *Pediatrics* 111(1):e67–e72, 2003.

Flanagan K: Preoperative assessment: safety considerations for patients taking herbal products, *J Perianesth Nurs* 16(1):19–26, 2001.

Gordon M: *Manual of nursing diagnosis*, ed 10, St. Louis, 2002, Mosby.

Harbaugh BL, Tomlinson PS, Kirschbaum M: Parents' perceptions of nurses' caregiving behaviors in the pediatric intensive care unit, *Issues Compr Pediatr Nurs* 27(3):163–178, 2004.

Hopia H, Tomlinson PS, Paavilainen E, and others: Child in hospital: family experiences and expectations of how nurses can promote family health, *J Clin Nurs* 14(2):212–222, 2005.

The Joint Commission: *Comprehensive accreditation manual for hospitals (CAMH)*, Oakbrook Terrace, Ill, 2011, Author.

Latour JM, van Goudoever JB, Hazelzet JA: Parent satisfaction in the pediatric ICU, *Pediatr Clin North Am* 55(3):779–790, 2008.

Lewandowski LA, Tesler MD: *Family centered care: putting it into action*, Washington, DC, 2003, American Nurses Association.

Melnyk BM: Intervention studies involving parents of hospitalized young children: an analysis of the past and future recommendations, *J Pediatr Nurs* 15(1):4–13, 2000.

Orem D: *Nursing: concepts of practice*, ed 5, New York, 2001, Mosby.

Phipps LM, Thomas NJ: Hepatitis C: the use of a daily goals sheet to improve communication in the paediatric intensive care unit, *Intensive Crit Care Nurs* 23(5):264–271, 2007.

Samela M, Salanterä S, Aronen E: Child-reported hospital fears in 4 to 6 year-old-children, *Pediatr Nurs* 35(5):269–276, 303, 2009.

Small L: Early predictors of poor coping outcomes in children following intensive care hospitalization and stressful medical encounters, *Pediatr Nurs* 28(4):393–401, 2002.

Smith T, Conant Rees HL: Making family-centered care a reality, *Semin Nurs Manage* 8(3):136–142, 2000.

Stranton KM: Parents' experiences of their child's care during hospitalization, *J Cult Divers* 11(1):4–11, 2004.

Thompson R: *The handbook of child life: a guide for pediatric psychosocial care*, Springfield, Ill, 2009, Charles C Thomas.

Wilson ME, Megel ME, Enenbach L, and others: The voices of children: stories about hospitalization, *J Pediatr Health Care* 24(2): 95–102, 2010.

Pediatric Variations of Nursing Interventions

Terri L. Brown

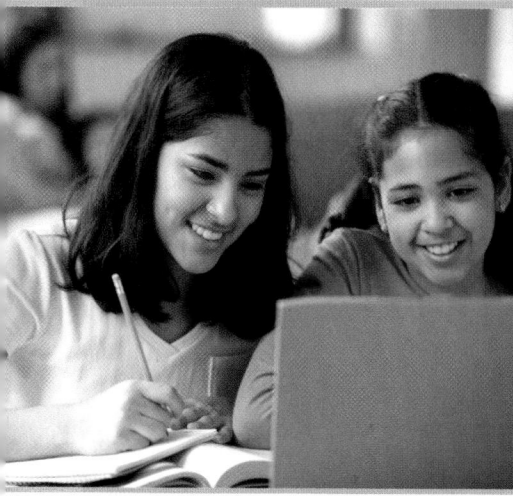

evolve WEBSITE

http://evolve.elsevier.com/wong/essentials

Animations—Central Venous Access via Femoral Vein; Central Venous Access via Jugular Vein; Foley Catheter Insertion; IV Line Placement; Lumbar Puncture, Infant; PICC Line Placement; Tracheostomy

Case Study—Pediatric Procedures

Key Points Audio Summaries

NCLEX-Style Review Questions

Nursing Care Plan—The Child with Elevated Body Temperature

CHAPTER OUTLINE

General Concepts Related to Pediatric Procedures, 636

Informed Consent, 636
 Requirements for Obtaining Informed Consent, 636
 Eligibility for Giving Informed Consent, 637
Preparation for Diagnostic and Therapeutic Procedures, 637
 Psychologic Preparation, 637
 Physical Preparation, 641
 Performance of the Procedure, 641
 Postprocedural Support, 642
 Use of Play in Procedures, 642
 Preparing the Family, 642
Surgical Procedures, 642
 Preoperative Care, 642
 Postoperative Care, 645
Compliance, 646
 Compliance Strategies, 647
Skin Care and General Hygiene, 647
Maintaining Healthy Skin, 647
Bathing, 648
Oral Hygiene, 649
Hair Care, 649
Feeding the Sick Child, 649
Controlling Elevated Temperatures, 650
Family Teaching and Home Care, 651
Safety, 652
Environmental Factors, 652
 Toys, 652
 Preventing Falls, 653

Infection Control, 653
Transporting Infants and Children, 654
Restraining Methods and Therapeutic Holding, 655
 Mummy Restraint or Swaddle, 656
 Jacket Restraint, 656
 Arm and Leg Restraints, 656
 Elbow Restraint, 656
Positioning for Procedures, 657
Femoral Venipuncture, 657
Extremity Venipuncture or Injection, 657
Lumbar Puncture, 657
Bone Marrow Aspiration or Biopsy, 658
Collection of Specimens, 658
Fundamental Procedure Steps Common to All Procedures, 658
Urine Specimens, 658
 Clean-Catch Specimens, 659
 Twenty-Four-Hour Collection, 659
 Bladder Catheterization and Other Techniques, 660
Stool Specimens, 662
Blood Specimens, 662
Respiratory Secretion Specimens, 664
Administration of Medication, 665
Determination of Drug Dosage, 665
 Checking Dosage, 665
 Identification, 665
 Preparing the Parents, 665
 Preparing the Child, 665

Oral Administration, 665
 Preparation, 666
 Administration, 666
Intramuscular Administration, 667
 Selecting the Syringe and Needle, 667
 Determining the Site, 667
 Administration, 671
Subcutaneous and Intradermal Administration, 671
Intravenous Administration, 671
 Peripheral Intermittent Infusion Device, 672
 Central Venous Access Device, 673
Nasogastric, Orogastric, and Gastrostomy Administration, 676
Rectal Administration, 678
Optic, Otic, and Nasal Administration, 679
Aerosol Therapy, 680
Family Teaching and Home Care, 680
Maintaining Fluid Balance, 681
Measurement of Intake and Output, 681
 Special Needs When the Child Is NPO, 681
Parenteral Fluid Therapy, 681
 Site and Equipment, 681
 Safety Catheters and Needleless Systems, 682
 Infusion Pumps, 683
 Securement of a Peripheral Intravenous Line, 684

CHAPTER OUTLINE—cont'd

Removal of a Peripheral Intravenous Line, 684
Complications, 687
Procedures for Maintaining Respiratory Function, 687
Inhalation Therapy, 687
Oxygen Therapy, 687
Monitoring Oxygen Therapy, 688
End-Tidal Carbon Dioxide Monitoring, 689

Bronchial (Postural) Drainage, 689
Chest Physical Therapy, 689
Intubation, 690
Mechanical Ventilation, 690
Tracheostomy, 690
Chest Tube Procedures, 693
Alternative Feeding Techniques, 694
Gavage Feeding, 695
Preparations, 695
Procedure, 695

Gastrostomy Feeding, 698
Nasoduodenal and Nasojejunal Tubes, 700
Total Parenteral Nutrition, 701
Family Teaching and Home Care, 701
Procedures Related to Elimination, 701
Enema, 701
Ostomies, 702
Family Teaching and Home Care, 702

LEARNING OBJECTIVES

On completion of this chapter the reader will be able to:

- Identify instances in which informed consent is required and in which minors may be considered emancipated.
- Formulate general guidelines for preparing children for procedures, including surgery.
- Implement play in therapeutic procedures.
- List general strategies for enhancing compliance in children and families.
- Outline general hygiene and care procedures for hospitalized children.
- Implement feeding techniques that encourage food and fluid intake.

- Describe methods of reducing the temperature in a child with fever or hyperthermia.
- Describe systems that can be used for infection control.
- Describe safe methods of administering oral, parenteral, rectal, optic, otic, and nasal medications to children.
- Identify nursing responsibilities in maintaining fluid balance.
- Demonstrate correct procedures for postural drainage and tracheostomy care.
- Describe the procedures involved in providing nutrition via gavage, gastrostomy, and parenteral routes.
- Describe the procedures involved in administering an enema and ostomy care to children.

GENERAL CONCEPTS RELATED TO PEDIATRIC PROCEDURES

INFORMED CONSENT

Before undergoing any invasive procedure, the patient or the patient's legal surrogate must receive sufficient information on which to make an informed health care decision. Informed consent should include the expected care or treatment; potential risks, benefits, and alternatives; and what might happen if the patient chooses not to consent. To obtain valid informed consent, health care providers must meet the following three conditions:

1. The person must be capable of giving consent; he or she must be over the age of majority (usually age 18 years) and must be considered competent (i.e., possessing the mental capacity to make choices and understand their consequences).
2. The person must receive the information needed to make an intelligent decision.
3. The person must act voluntarily when exercising freedom of choice without force, fraud, deceit, duress, or other forms of constraint or coercion.

The patient has the right to accept or refuse any health care. If a patient is treated without consent, the hospital or health care provider may be charged with assault and held liable for damages.

Requirements for Obtaining Informed Consent

Written informed consent of the parent or legal guardian is usually required for medical or surgical treatment of a minor, including many diagnostic procedures. One universal consent is not sufficient. Separate informed permissions must be obtained for each surgical or diagnostic procedure, including:

- Major surgery
- Minor surgery (e.g., cutdown, biopsy, dental extraction, suturing a laceration [especially one that may have a cosmetic effect], removal of a cyst, closed reduction of a fracture)
- Diagnostic tests with an element of risk (e.g., bronchoscopy, angiography, lumbar puncture, cardiac catheterization, bone marrow aspiration)
- Medical treatments with an element of risk (e.g., blood transfusion, thoracentesis or paracentesis, radiotherapy)

Other situations that require patient or parental consent include:

- Photographs for medical, educational, or public use
- Removal of the child from the health care institution against medical advice
- Postmortem examination, except in unexplained deaths, such as sudden infant death, violent death, or suspected suicide
- Release of medical information

Decision making involving the care of older children and adolescents should include the patient's **assent** (if feasible), as well as the parent's consent. Assent means the child or adolescent has been informed about the proposed treatment, procedure, or research and is willing to permit a health care provider to perform it. Assent should include:

- Helping the patient achieve a developmentally appropriate awareness of the nature of his or her condition
- Telling the patient what he or she can expect
- Making a clinical assessment of the patient's understanding
- Soliciting an expression of the patient's willingness to accept the proposed procedure

Health care providers should use multiple methods to provide information, including age-appropriate methods (e.g., videos, peer discussion, diagrams, and written materials). The nurse should provide an assent form for the child to sign, and the child should keep a copy.

By including the child in the decision-making process and gaining his or her acceptance, staff members demonstrate respect for the child. Assent is not a legal requirement but an ethical one to protect the rights of children.

Eligibility for Giving Informed Consent
Informed Consent of Parents or Legal Guardians

Parents have full responsibility for the care and rearing of their minor children, including legal control over them. As long as children are minors, their parents or legal guardians are required to give informed consent before medical treatment is rendered or any procedure is performed. If the parents are married to each other, consent from only one parent is required for non-urgent pediatric care. If the parents are divorced, consent usually rests with the parent who has legal custody (Berger and American Academy of Pediatrics [AAP], Committee on Medical Liability, 2003). Parents also have a right to withdraw consent later.

Evidence of Consent

Regulations on obtaining informed consent vary from state to state, and policies differ at each health care facility. It is the physician's legal responsibility to explain the procedure, risks, benefits, and alternatives. The nurse witnesses the patient's, parent's, or legal guardian's signature on the consent form and may reinforce what the patient has been told. A signed consent form is the legal document that signifies that the process of informed consent has occurred. If parents are unavailable to sign consent forms, verbal consent may be obtained via the telephone in the presence of two witnesses. Both witnesses record that informed consent was given and by whom. Their signatures indicate that they witnessed the verbal consent.

Informed Consent of Mature and Emancipated Minors

State laws differ with regard to the age of majority, the age at which a person is considered to have all the legal rights and responsibilities of an adult. In most states, 18 years is the age of majority. Competent adults can give informed consent on their own behalf. An **emancipated minor** is one who is legally under the age of majority but is recognized as having the legal capacity of an adult under circumstances prescribed by state law, such as pregnancy, marriage, high school graduation, independent living, or military service.

Treatment Without Parental Consent

Exceptions to requiring parental consent before treating minor children occur in situations in which children need urgent medical or surgical treatment and a parent is not readily available to give consent or refuses to give consent. For example, a child may be brought to an emergency department accompanied by a grandparent, child care provider, teacher, or others. In the absence of parents or legal guardians, persons in charge of the child may be given permission by the parents to give informed consent by proxy. In emergencies, including danger to life or the possibility of permanent injury, appropriate care should not be withheld or delayed because of problems obtaining consent (AAP, 2003; Berger and AAP, Committee on Medical Liability, 2003). The nurse should document any efforts made to obtain consent.

Refusal to give consent can occur when the treatment, such as blood transfusions, conflicts with the parents' religious beliefs. All states recognize such exceptions and have statutory procedures to permit treatment if the life or health of such a minor is in jeopardy or if delayed treatment would create a risk to the minor's health. Evaluation for child abuse or neglect can occur without parental consent and without notification to the state before evaluation in most states.

Adolescents, Consent, and Confidentiality

The Health Insurance Portability and Accountability Act of 1996 (HIPAA) was passed to help protect and safeguard the security and confidentiality of health information. Because adolescents are not yet adults, parents have the right to make most decisions on their behalf and receive information. Adolescents, however, are more likely to seek care in a setting in which they believe their privacy will be maintained. All 50 states have enacted legislation that entitles adolescents to consent to treatment without the parents' knowledge to one or more "medically emancipated" conditions such as sexually transmitted infections, mental health services, alcohol and drug dependency, pregnancy, and contraceptive advice (AAP, 2003; Anderson, Schaechter, and Brosco, 2005; Tillett, 2005). Consent to abortion is controversial, and statutes vary widely by state. State law preempts HIPAA regardless of whether that law prohibits, mandates, or allows discretion about a disclosure.

Informed Consent and Parental Right to the Child's Medical Chart

Some state statutes give parents the unrestricted right to a copy of children's medical records. In states without statutes, the best practice is to allow parents to review or have a copy of minors' charts under reasonable circumstances. Practitioners should avoid restrictive requirements such as review permitted only in the presence of a clinician. Rather, an appropriate practitioner should be available to answer any questions that parents may have during their reviews.

PREPARATION FOR DIAGNOSTIC AND THERAPEUTIC PROCEDURES

Technologic advances and changes in health care have resulted in more pediatric procedures being performed in a variety of settings. Many procedures are both stressful and painful experiences. For most procedures, the focus of care is psychologic preparation of the child and family. However, some procedures require the administration of sedatives and analgesics.

Psychologic Preparation

Preparing children for procedures decreases their anxiety, promotes their cooperation, supports their coping skills and may teach them new ones, and facilitates a feeling of mastery in experiencing a potentially stressful event. Many institutions have developed preadmission teaching programs designed to educate the pediatric patient and family by offering hands-on experience with hospital equipment, the procedure performed, and departments they will visit. Preparatory methods may be formal, such as group preparation for hospitalization. Most preparation strategies are informal, focus on providing information about the experience, and are directed at stressful or painful procedures. The most effective preparation includes the provision of sensory-procedural information and helping the child develop coping skills, such as imagery, distraction, or relaxation.

The Nursing Care Guidelines boxes describe general guidelines for preparing children for procedures along with age-specific guidelines that consider children's developmental needs and cognitive abilities. In addition to these suggestions, nurses should consider the child's temperament, existing coping strategies, and previous experiences in individualizing the preparatory process. Children who are distractible and highly active or those who are "slow to warm up" may need individualized sessions—shorter for active children and more slowly paced for shy children. Whereas youngsters who tend to cope well may need more emphasis on using their present skills, those who appear to cope less adequately can benefit from more time devoted to simple coping

NURSING CARE GUIDELINES
Preparing Children for Procedures

- Determine details of exact procedure to be performed.
- Review parents' and child's present understanding.
- Base teaching on developmental age and existing knowledge.
- Incorporate parents in the teaching if they desire, especially if they plan to participate in care.
- Inform parents of their supportive role during procedure, such as standing near child's head or in child's line of vision and talking softly to child, as well as typical responses of children undergoing the procedure.
- Allow for ample discussion to prevent information overload and ensure adequate feedback.
- Use concrete, not abstract, terms and visual aids to describe procedure. For example, use a simple line drawing of a boy or girl and mark the body part that will be involved in the procedure. Use nonthreatening but realistic models.*
- Emphasize that no other body part will be involved.
- If the body part is associated with a specific function, stress the change or noninvolvement of that ability (e.g., after tonsillectomy, child can still speak).
- Use words and sentence length appropriate to child's level of understanding (a rule of thumb for the number of words in a child's sentence is equal to his or her age in years plus 1).
- Avoid words and phrases with dual meanings (see Table 22-1, p. 641) unless child understands such words.
- Clarify all unfamiliar words (e.g., "Anesthesia is a *special* sleep").
- Emphasize sensory aspects of procedure—what child will feel, see, hear, smell, and touch and what child can do during procedure (e.g., lie still, count out loud, squeeze a hand, hug a doll).
- Allow child to practice procedures that will require cooperation (e.g., turning, deep breathing, using an incentive spirometry).
- Introduce anxiety-inducing information last (e.g., starting an intravenous line).
- Be honest with child about unpleasant aspects of a procedure but avoid creating undue concern. When discussing that a procedure may be uncomfortable, state that it feels differently to different people.
- Emphasize end of procedure and any pleasurable events afterward (e.g., going home, seeing parents).
- Stress positive benefits of procedure (e.g., "After your tonsils are fixed, you won't have as many sore throats").
- Provide a positive ending, praising efforts at cooperation and coping.

*Soft-sculptured dolls and customized adapters and overlays for preparing children and families about procedures and as teaching models for technical care are available from Legacy Products, Inc., 508 S. Green St., PO Box 267, Cambridge City, IN 47327; 800-238-7951; e-mail: info@legacyproductsinc.com; http://www.legacyproductsinc.com.

NURSING TIP Prepare a basket, toy chest, or cart to keep near the treatment area. Items ideal for the basket include a Slinky; a sparkling "magic" wand (sealed, acrylic tube partially filled with liquid and suspended metallic confetti); a soft foam ball; bubble solution; party blowers; pop-up books with foldout, three-dimensional scenes; real medical equipment, such as a syringe, adhesive bandages, and alcohol packets; toy medical supplies or a toy medical kit; marking pens; a note pad; and stickers. Have the child choose an item to help distract and relax during the procedure. After the procedure, allow the child to choose a small gift, such as a sticker, or to play with items, such as medical equipment.

Children differ in their "information-seeking dimension." Some actively ask for information about the intended procedure, but others characteristically avoid information. Parents can often guide nurses in deciding how much information is enough for the child because parents know whether the child is typically inquisitive or satisfied with short answers. Asking older children their preferences about the amount of explanation is also important.

The exact timing of the preparation for a procedure varies with the child's age and the type of procedure. No exact guidelines govern timing, but in general, the younger the child, the closer the explanation should be to the actual procedure to prevent undue fantasizing and worrying. With complex procedures, more time may be needed for assimilation of information, especially with older children. For example, the explanation for an injection can immediately precede the procedure for all ages, but preparation for surgery may begin the day before for young children and a few days before for older children, although the nurse should elicit older children's preferences.

Establish Trust and Provide Support

The nurse who has spent time with and established a positive relationship with a child usually finds it easier to gain cooperation. If the relationship is based on trust, the child will associate the nurse with caregiving activities that give comfort and pleasure most of the time rather than discomfort and stress. If the nurse does not know the child, it is best for the nurse to be introduced by another staff person whom the child trusts. The first visit with the child should not include any painful procedure and ideally should focus on the child first and then on an explanation of the procedure.

Parental Presence and Support

Children need support during procedures, and for young children, the greatest source of support is the parents. They represent security, protection, safety, and comfort. Several studies have reported a positive impact on parental distress and satisfaction and no difference in technical complications when parents remain with children (Piira, Sugiura, Champion, and others, 2005). Controversy exists regarding the role parents should assume during the procedure, especially if discomfort is involved. Several professional associations support the option of family presence during invasive procedures (AAP, American College of Emergency Physicians, O'Malley, and others, 2006; American Association of Critical Care Nurses, 2006; Emergency Nurses Association, 2005). The nurse should assess the parents' preferences for assisting, observing, or waiting outside the room, as well as the child's preference for parental presence. Respect the child's and parents' choices. Give parents who wish to stay appropriate explanation about the procedure and coach them about where to sit or stand and what to say or do to help the child through the procedure. Support parents who do not

strategies, such as relaxing, breathing, counting, squeezing a hand, or singing. Children with previous health-related experiences still need preparation for repeat or new procedures; however, the nurse must assess what they know, correct their misconceptions, supply new information, and introduce new coping skills as indicated by their previous reactions. Especially for painful procedures, the most effective preparation includes providing sensory-procedural information and helping the child develop coping skills, such as imagery or relaxation (see Nursing Care Guidelines box, p. 639).

NURSING CARE GUIDELINES

Age-Specific Preparation of Children for Procedures Based on Developmental Characteristics

Infant—Developing Trust and Sensorimotor Thought

Attachment to Parent

Involve parent in procedure if desired.*

Keep parent in infant's line of vision.

If parent is unable to be with infant, place familiar object with infant (e.g., stuffed toy).

Stranger Anxiety

Have usual caregivers perform or assist with procedure.*

Make advances slowly and in a nonthreatening manner.

Limit number of strangers entering room during procedure.*

Sensorimotor Phase of Learning

During procedure, use sensory soothing measures (e.g., stroking skin, talking softly, giving pacifier).

Use analgesics (e.g., topical anesthetic, intravenous opioid) to control discomfort.*

Cuddle and hug infant after stressful procedure; encourage parent to comfort infant.

Increased Muscle Control

Expect older infants to resist.

Restrain adequately.

Keep harmful objects out of reach.

Memory for Past Experiences

Realize that older infants may associate objects, places, or persons with prior painful experiences and will cry and resist at the sight of them.

Keep frightening objects out of view.*

Perform painful procedures in a separate room, not in crib (or bed).*

Use nonintrusive procedures whenever possible (e.g., axillary or tympanic temperatures, oral medications).*

Imitation of Gestures

Model desired behavior (e.g., opening mouth).

Toddler—Developing Autonomy and Sensorimotor to Preoperational Thought

Use same approaches as for infant plus the following.

Egocentric Thought

Explain procedure in relation to what child will see, hear, taste, smell, and feel.

Emphasize those aspects of procedure that require cooperation (e.g., lying still).

Tell child it is okay to cry, yell, or use other means to express discomfort verbally.

Designate one health care provider to speak during procedure. Hearing more than one can be confusing to a child*

Negative Behavior

Expect treatments to be resisted; child may try to run away.

Use firm, direct approach.

Ignore temper tantrums.

Use distraction techniques (e.g., singing a song *with* child).

Restrain adequately.

Animism

Keep frightening objects out of view (young children believe objects have lifelike qualities and can harm them).

Limited Language Skills

Communicate using gestures or demonstrations.

Use a few simple terms familiar to child.

Give child one direction at a time (e.g., "Lie down" and then "Hold my hand").

Use small replicas of equipment; allow child to handle equipment.

Use play; demonstrate on doll but avoid child's favorite doll because child may think doll is really "feeling" procedure.

Prepare parents separately to avoid child's misinterpreting words.

Limited Concept of Time

Prepare child shortly or immediately before procedure.

Keep teaching sessions short (≈5–10 minutes).

Have preparations completed before involving child in procedure.

Have extra equipment nearby (e.g., alcohol swabs, new needle, adhesive bandages) to avoid delays.

Tell child when procedure is completed.

Striving for Independence

Allow choices whenever possible but realize that child may still be resistant and negative.

Allow child to participate in care and to help whenever possible (e.g., drink medicine from a cup, hold a dressing).

Preschooler—Developing Initiative and Preoperational Thought

Egocentric

Explain procedure in simple terms and in relation to how it affects child (as with toddler, stress sensory aspects).

Demonstrate use of equipment.

Allow child to play with miniature or actual equipment.

Encourage "playing out" experience on a doll both before and after procedure to clarify misconceptions.

Use neutral words to describe the procedure (see Table 22-1, p. 641).

Increased Language Skills

Use verbal explanation but avoid overestimating child's comprehension of words.

Encourage child to verbalize ideas and feelings.

Limited Concept of Time and Frustration Tolerance

Implement same approaches as for toddler but may plan longer teaching session (10–15 minutes); may divide information into more than one session.

Illness and Hospitalization Viewed as Punishment

Clarify why each procedure is performed; child will find it difficult to understand how medicine can make him or her feel better and can taste bad at the same time.

Ask child thoughts regarding why a procedure is performed.

State directly that procedures are never a form of punishment.

Animism

Keep equipment out of sight except when shown to or used on child.

Fears of Bodily Harm, Intrusion, and Castration

Point out on drawing, doll, or child where procedure is performed.

Emphasize that no other body part will be involved.

Use nonintrusive procedures whenever possible (e.g., axillary temperatures, oral medication).

*Applies to any age.

Continued

🔲 NURSING CARE GUIDELINES

Age-Specific Preparation of Children for Procedures Based on Developmental Characteristics—cont'd

Apply an adhesive bandage over puncture site.
Encourage parental presence.
Realize that procedures involving genitalia provoke anxiety.
Allow child to wear underpants with gown.
Explain unfamiliar situations, especially noises or lights.

Striving for Initiative

Involve child in care whenever possible (e.g., hold equipment, remove dressing).
Give choices whenever possible but avoid excessive delays.
Praise child for helping and attempting to cooperate; never shame child for lack of cooperation.

School-Age Child—Developing Industry and Concrete Thought
Increased Language Skills; Interest in Acquiring Knowledge
Explain procedure using correct scientific and medical terminology.
Explain procedure using simple diagrams and photographs.
Discuss why procedure is necessary; concepts of illness and bodily functions are often vague
Explain function and operation of equipment in concrete terms.
Allow child to manipulate equipment; use doll or another person as model to practice using equipment whenever possible (doll play may be considered childish by older school-age child).
Allow time before and after procedure for questions and discussion.

Improved Concept of Time
Plan for longer teaching sessions (≈20 minutes).
Prepare up to 1 day in advance of procedure to allow for processing of information.

Increased Self-Control
Gain child's cooperation.
Tell child what is expected.
Suggest several ways of maintaining control the child may select from (e.g., deep breathing, relaxation, counting).

Striving for Industry
Allow responsibility for simple tasks (e.g., collecting specimens).
Include child in decision making (e.g., time of day to perform procedure, preferred site).

Encourage active participation (e.g., removing dressings, handling equipment, opening packages).

Developing Relationships with Peers
Prepare two or more children for same procedure or encourage one to help prepare another.
Provide privacy from peers during procedure to maintain self-esteem.

Adolescent—Developing Identity and Abstract Thought
Increasing Abstract Thought and Reasoning
Discuss why procedure is necessary or beneficial.
Explain long-term consequences of procedures; include information about body systems working together.
Realize adolescent may fear death, disability, or other potential risks.
Encourage questioning regarding fears, options, and alternatives.

Consciousness of Appearance
Provide privacy; describe how the body will be covered and what will be exposed.
Discuss how procedure may affect appearance (e.g., scar) and what can be done to minimize it.
Emphasize any physical benefits of procedure.

Concern More with Present Than with Future
Realize that immediate effects of procedure are more significant than future benefits.

Striving for Independence
Involve adolescent in decision making and planning (e.g., time, place, individuals present during procedure, clothing, whether they will watch procedure).
Impose as few restrictions as possible.
Explore what coping strategies have worked in the past; they may need suggestions of various techniques.
Accept regression to more childish methods of coping.
Realize that adolescent may have difficulty accepting new authority figures and may resist complying with procedures.

Developing Peer Relationships and Group Identity
Same as for school-age child but assumes even greater significance.
Allow adolescents to talk with other adolescents who have had the same procedure.

---

want to be present in their decision and encourage them to remain close by so they can be available to support the child immediately after the procedure. Parents should also know that someone will be with their child to provide support. Ideally, this person should inform the parents after the procedure about how the child did.

Provide an Explanation

Age-appropriate explanations are one of the most widely used interventions for reducing anxiety in children undergoing procedures. Before performing a procedure, explain what is to be done and what is expected of the child. The explanation should be short, simple, and appropriate to the child's level of comprehension. Long explanations may increase anxiety in a young child. When explaining the procedure to parents with the child present, the nurse uses language

appropriate to the child because unfamiliar words can be misunderstood (Table 22-1). If the parents need additional preparation, it is done in an area away from the child. Teaching sessions are planned at times most conducive to the child's learning (e.g., after a rest period) and for the usual span of attention.

Special equipment is not necessary for preparing a child, but for young children who cannot yet think conceptually, using objects to supplement verbal explanation is important. Allowing children to handle actual items that will be used in their care, such as a stethoscope, sphygmomanometer, or oxygen mask, helps them develop familiarity with these items and reduces the fear often associated with their use. Miniature versions of hospital items such as gurneys and x-ray and intravenous (IV) equipment can be used to explain what the children can expect and permit them to safely experience situations that are

TABLE 22-1	SELECTING NONTHREATENING WORDS OR PHRASES
WORDS AND PHRASES TO AVOID	**SUGGESTED SUBSTITUTIONS**
Shot, bee sting, stick	Medicine under the skin
Organ	Special place in body
Test	To see how (specify body part) is working
Incision, cut	Special opening
Edema	Puffiness
Stretcher, gurney	Rolling bed, bed on wheels
Stool	Child's usual term
Dye	Special medicine
Pain	Hurt, discomfort, "owie," "boo-boo," sore, achy, scratchy
Deaden	Numb, make sleepy
Fix	Make better
Take (as in "take your temperature")	See how warm you are
Take (as in "take your blood pressure")	Check your pressure; hug your arm
Put to sleep, anesthesia	Special sleep so you won't feel anything
Catheter	Tube
Monitor	Television screen
Electrodes	Stickers, ticklers
Specimen	Sample

> **NURSING TIP** Use photographs of children in different areas of the hospital (e.g., radiology department, operating room) to give children a more realistic idea of equipment they may encounter.

unfamiliar and potentially frightening. Written and illustrated materials are also valuable aids to preparation.*

Physical Preparation

One area of special concern is the administration of appropriate sedation and analgesia before stressful procedures. Chapter 7 describes sedative medications used for procedures.

Performance of the Procedure

Supportive care continues during the procedure and can be a major factor in a child's ability to cooperate. Ideally, the same nurse who explains the procedure should perform or assist with the procedure. Before beginning, all equipment is assembled, and the room is readied to prevent unnecessary delays and interruptions that increase the child's anxiety. Minimizing the number of people present during the procedure also can decrease the child's anxiety.

> **NURSING TIP** To avoid a delay during a procedure, have extra supplies handy. For example, have tape, bandages, alcohol swabs, and an extra needle when performing an injection or venipuncture.

---

*Preparatory materials include Going to the Hospital and Going to the Doctor, available from Family Communications, 4802 Fifth Ave., Pittsburgh, PA 15213; 412-687-2990; http://www.fci.org; Hospital Friends, available from Centering Corporation, 7230 Maple St., Omaha, NE 68134; 866-218-0101; http://www.centering.org. Other resources include *Berenstein Bears Go to the Doctor* and *Berenstein Bears Visit the Dentist* (New York, Random House).

To promote long-term coping and adjustment, give special consideration to the patient's age, coping skills, and procedure to be performed in determining where a procedure will occur. Treatment rooms should be used for procedures requiring sedation, such as bone marrow aspirates and lumbar punctures (LPs) in younger children. Traumatic procedures should never be performed in "safe" areas, such as the playroom. If the procedure is lengthy, avoid conversation that could be misinterpreted by the child. As the procedure is nearing completion, the nurse should inform the child that it is almost over in language the child understands.

Expect Success

Nurses who approach children with confidence and who convey the impression that they expect to be successful are less likely to encounter difficulty. It is best to approach a child as though cooperation is expected. Children sense anxiety and uncertainty in an adult and respond by striking out or actively resisting. Although it is not possible to eliminate such behavior in every child, a firm approach with a positive attitude tends to convey a feeling of security to most children.

Involve the Child

Involving children helps to gain their cooperation. Permitting choices gives them some measure of control. However, a choice is given only in situations in which one is available. Asking children, "Do you want to take your medicine now?" leads them to believe they have an option and provides them the opportunity to legitimately refuse or delay the medication. This places the nurse in an awkward, if not impossible, position. It is much better to state firmly, "It's time to drink your medicine now." Children usually like to make choices, but the choice must be one that they do indeed have (e.g., "It's time for your medicine. Do you want to drink it plain or with a little water?").

Many children respond to tactics that appeal to their maturity or courage. This also gives them a sense of participation and achievement. For example, preschool children will be proud that they can hold the dressing during the procedure or remove the tape. The same is true for school-age children, who often cooperate with minimal resistance.

Provide Distraction

Distraction is a powerful coping strategy during painful procedures (Uman, Chambers, McGrath, and others, 2006). It is accomplished by focusing the child's attention on something other than the procedure. Singing favorite songs, listening to music with a headset, counting aloud, or blowing bubbles to "blow the hurt away" are effective techniques. (For other nonpharmacologic interventions, see Chapter 7.)

> **NURSING TIP** Help the child select and practice a coping technique before the procedure. Consider having the parent or some other supportive person, such as a child life specialist, "coach" the child in learning and using the coping skill.

Allow Expression of Feelings

The child should be allowed to express feelings of anger, anxiety, fear, frustration, or any other emotion. It is natural for children to strike out in frustration or to try to avoid stress-provoking situations. The child needs to know that it is all right to cry. Behavior is children's primary means of communication and coping and should be permitted unless it inflicts harm on them or those caring for them.

Postprocedural Support

After the procedure, the child continues to need reassurance that he or she performed well and is accepted and loved. If the parents did not participate, the child is united with them as soon as possible so they can provide comfort.

Encourage Expression of Feelings

Planned activity after the procedure is helpful in encouraging constructive expression of feelings. For verbal children, reviewing the details of the procedure can clarify misconceptions and garner feedback for improving the nurse's preparatory strategies. Play is an excellent activity for all children. Infants and young children should have the opportunity for gross motor movement. Older children are able to vent their anger and frustration in acceptable pounding or throwing activities. Play-Doh is a remarkably versatile medium for pounding and shaping. Dramatic play provides an outlet for anger and places the child in a position of control, in contrast to the position of helplessness in the real situation. Puppets also allow the child to communicate feelings in a nonthreatening way. One of the most effective interventions is therapeutic play, which includes well-supervised activities such as permitting the child to give an injection to a doll or stuffed toy to reduce the stress of injections (Fig. 22-1).

Positive Reinforcement

Children need to hear from adults that they did the best they could in the situation—no matter how they behaved. It is important for children to know that their worth is not being judged on the basis of their behavior in a stressful situation. Reward systems, such as earning stars, stickers, or a badge of courage, are appealing to children.

Returning to the child a short while after the procedure helps the nurse strengthen a supportive relationship. Relating with the child in a relaxed and nonstressful period allows him or her to see the nurse not only as someone associated with stressful situations but also as someone with whom to share pleasurable experiences.

Use of Play in Procedures

The use of play is an integral part of relationships with children. As such, its value in specific situations is discussed throughout this book,

such as in Chapter 21 in relation to hospitalization. Many institutions have elaborate and well-organized play areas and programs under the direction of child life specialists. Other institutions have limited facilities. No matter what the institution provides for children, nurses can include play activities as part of nursing care. Play can be used to teach, express feelings, or achieve a therapeutic goal. Consequently, it should be included in preparing children for and encouraging their cooperation during procedures. Play sessions after procedures can be structured, such as directed toward needle play, or general, with a wide variety of equipment available for children to play with.

Routine procedures such as measuring blood pressure and oral administration of medication may be of concern to children. Box 22-1 describes suggestions for incorporating play into nursing procedures and activities for the hospitalized child that facilitate learning and adjustment to a new situation.

Preparing the Family

The process of patient education involves giving the family information about the child's condition, the regimen that must be followed and why, and other health teaching as indicated. The goal of this education is to enable the family to modify behaviors and adhere to the regimen that has been mutually established (see Nursing Care Guidelines box below).

If equipment will be needed at home (e.g., suction machines, syringes), begin making the necessary arrangements in advance so that discharge can proceed smoothly. Whenever possible, make arrangements for the family to use the same equipment in the home that they are using in the hospital. This allows them to become familiar with the items. In addition, the staff can help troubleshoot the equipment in a controlled environment. Plan the teaching sessions well in advance of the time the family will be responsible for performing the care. The more complex the procedure, the more time is needed for training.

Review the instructions with family members (see Nursing Care Guidelines box, p. 643). Encourage note taking if they desire. Allow ample practice time under supervision. At least one family member, but preferably two members, should demonstrate the procedure before they are expected to care for the child at home. Provide the family with the telephone numbers of resource individuals who are available to assist them in the event of a problem.

SURGICAL PROCEDURES

Preoperative Care

Children experiencing surgical procedures require both psychologic and physical preparation. An important concern is restriction of food

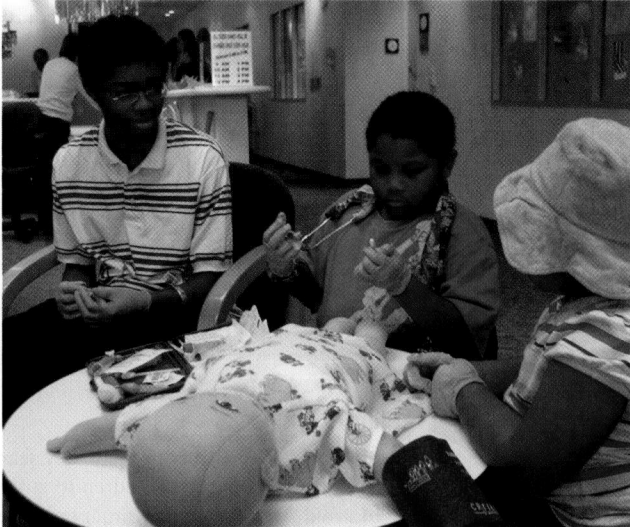

FIG 22-1 Playing with medical objects provides children with the opportunity to play out fears and concerns with supervision by a nurse or child life specialist.

📋 **NURSING CARE GUIDELINES**

General Principles of Family Education

- Establish a rapport with the family.
- Avoid using *any* specialized terms or jargon. Clarify all terms with the family.
- When possible, allow family members to decide how they want to be taught (e.g., all at once or over a day or two). This gives the family a chance to incorporate the information at a rate that is comfortable.
- Provide accurate information to the family about the illness.
- Assist family members in identifying obstacles to their ability to comply with the regimen and in identifying the means to overcome those obstacles. Then help family members find ways to incorporate the plan into their daily lives.

BOX 22-1 PLAY ACTIVITIES FOR SPECIFIC PROCEDURES

Fluid Intake
Make ice pops using child's favorite juice.

Cut gelatin into fun shapes.

Make a game out of taking a sip when turning page of a book or in games such as Simon Says.

Use small medicine cups; decorate the cups.

Color water with food coloring or powdered drink mix.

Have a tea party; pour at a small table.

Let child fill a syringe and squirt it into mouth or use it to fill small decorated cups.

Cut straws in half and place in a small container (much easier for child to suck liquid).

Use a "crazy" straw.

Make a "progress poster"; give rewards for drinking a predetermined quantity.

Deep Breathing
Blow bubbles with a bubble blower.

Blow bubbles with a straw (no soap).

Blow on a pinwheel, feather, whistle, harmonica, balloon, or party blower.

Practice band instruments.

Have a blowing contest using balloons,* boats, cotton balls, feathers, marbles, ping-pong balls, pieces of paper; blow such objects on a table top over a goal line, over water, through an obstacle course, up in the air, against an opponent, or up and down a string.

Suck paper or cloth from one container to another using a straw.

Dramatize stories such as "I'll huff and puff and blow your house down" from the "Three Little Pigs."

Do straw-blowing painting.

Take a deep breath and "blow out the candles" on a birthday cake.

Use a little paint brush to "paint" nails with water and blow nails dry.

Range of Motion and Use of Extremities
Throw beanbags at a fixed or movable target or throw wadded-up paper into a wastebasket.

Touch or kick Mylar balloons held or hung in different positions (if child is in traction, hang balloon from a trapeze).

Play "tickle toes"; have the child wiggle them on request.

Play Twister game or Simon Says.

Play pretend and guessing games (e.g., imitate a bird, butterfly, or horse).

Have tricycle or wheelchair races in safe area.

Play kickball or throw ball with a soft foam ball in a safe area.

Position bed so that child must turn to view television or doorway.

Climb wall with fingers like a "spider."

Pretend to teach aerobic dancing or exercises; encourage parents to participate.

Encourage swimming if feasible.

Play video games or pinball (fine motor movement).

Play hide and seek: hide toy somewhere in bed (or room if ambulatory) and have child find it using specified hand or foot.

Provide clay to mold with fingers.

Paint or draw on large sheets of paper placed on floor or wall.

Encourage combing own hair; play "beauty shop" with "customer" in different positions.

Soaks
Play with small toys or objects (cups, syringes, soap dishes) in water.

Wash dolls or toys.

Pick up marbles or pennies* from bottom of bath container.

Make designs with coins on bottom of container.

Pretend a boat is a submarine by keeping it immersed.

Read to child during soaks; sing with child; or play game, such as cards, checkers, or other board game (if both hands are immersed, move board pieces for child).

Sitz bath: give child something to listen to (music, stories) or look at (View-Master, book).

Punch holes in bottom of plastic cup, fill with water, and let it "rain" on child.

Injections
Let child handle syringe, vial, and alcohol swab and give an injection to doll or stuffed animal.

Use syringes to decorate cookies with frosting, squirt paint, or target shoot into a container.

Draw a "magic circle" on area before injection; draw smiling face in circle after injection but avoid drawing on puncture site.

Allow child to have a "collection" of syringes (without needles); make "wild" creative objects with syringes.

If multiple injections or venipunctures are planned, make a "progress poster"; give rewards for predetermined number of injections.

Have child count to 10 or 15 during injection.

Ambulation
Give child something to push:
- Toddler: push-pull toy
- School-age child: wagon or a doll in a stroller or wheelchair
- Adolescent: decorated intravenous stand

Have a parade; make hats, drums, and so on.

Extending Environment (e.g., for Patients in Traction)
Make bed into a pirate ship or airplane with decorations.

Put up mirrors so patient can see around room.

Move bed frequently to playroom, hallway, or outside.

*Small objects such as marbles and coins, as well as gloves and balloons, are unsafe for young children because of possible aspiration. Latex products also carry the risk of an allergic reaction.

NURSING CARE GUIDELINES
Family Preparation for Procedures

Family education for specific procedures is included throughout this unit. General concepts applicable to most family education sessions include the following:
- Name of the procedure
- Purpose of the procedure
- Length of time anticipated to complete the procedure
- Anticipated effects
- Signs of adverse effects
- Assess the family's level of understanding
- Demonstrate and have family return demonstration (if appropriate)

TABLE 22-2	FASTING RECOMMENDATIONS TO REDUCE THE RISK OF PULMONARY ASPIRATION*	
INGESTED MATERIAL	**MINIMUM FASTING PERIOD (HR)**[†]	
Clear liquids[‡]	>2	
Breast milk	4	
Infant formula	6	
Nonhuman milk[§]	6	
Light meal[¶]	6	

From American Society of Anesthesiologists: Practice guidelines for preoperative fasting and the use of pharmacologic agents to reduce the risk of pulmonary aspiration: application to healthy patients undergoing elective procedures, *Anesthesiology* 90(3):896–905, 1999.
*These recommendations apply to healthy patients who are undergoing elective procedures. They are not intended for women in labor. Following the guidelines does not guarantee that complete gastric emptying has occurred.
[†]Fasting periods noted in chart apply to all ages.
[‡]Examples of clear liquids include water, fruit juices without pulp, carbonated beverages, clear tea, and black coffee.
[§]Because nonhuman milk is similar to solids in gastric emptying time, the amount ingested must be considered when determining appropriate fasting period.
[¶]A light meal typically consists of toast and clear liquids. Meals that include fried or fatty foods or meat may prolong gastric emptying time. Both the amount and type of foods ingested must be considered when determining an appropriate fasting period.

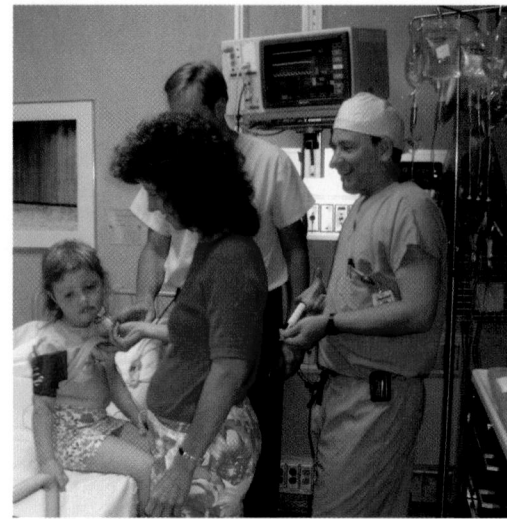

FIG 22-2 Parental presence during induction of anesthesia can minimize the child's and parents' anxiety during the preoperative period.

and fluids before surgery to avoid aspiration during anesthesia. Infants require special attention to fluid needs. They should not be without oral fluids for an extended period preoperatively to avoid glycogen depletion and dehydration. Table 22-2 contains current preoperative fasting guidelines.

In general, psychologic preparation is similar to that discussed earlier for any procedure and uses many of the same techniques used in preparing a child for hospitalization, such as films, books, brochures, play, and tours (see Chapter 21). Stress points before and after surgery include the admission process, blood tests, injection of preoperative medication (if prescribed), transport to the operating room, the mask on the face during induction, and the stay in the postanesthesia care unit (PACU). Wearing a hospital gown without the security of underpants or pajama bottoms can also be traumatic. Therefore, these articles of clothing should be allowed to be worn into the operating room and removed after induction of anesthesia. Children are at higher risk of ineffective response to anesthesia because of higher anxiety associated with stranger anxiety (infants), separation anxiety (toddlers and preschoolers), and fear of injury or death (adolescents) (Romino, Keatley, Secrest, and others, 2005).

Psychologic intervention consisting of systematic preparation, rehearsal of the forthcoming events, and supportive care at each of these points has shown to be more effective than a single-session preparation or consistent supportive care without systematic preparation and rehearsal (Kain, Caldwell-Andrews, Mayes, and others, 2007). A family-centered preoperative preparation program may consist of a tour of the perioperative areas with short explanations of the events 5 to 7 days before surgery, a video to take home and review a couple of times with additional explanations and demonstrations of perioperative processes, a mask to take home and practice with, pamphlets to guide parents on supporting children during induction, phone calls

to coach parents on preparing children 1 or 2 days before surgery, and toys and supplies in the holding area. Therapeutic play is an effective strategy in preparing children, and increased familiarity with medical procedures decreases anxiety (Li, Lopez, and Lee, 2007).

Parental Presence

Some institutions support parental presence during induction of anesthesia (Fig. 22-2). Appropriate education is essential to help parents understand the stages of anesthesia, what to expect, and how to support their child. When parents choose not to or are not allowed to attend the induction, leaving a favorite possession with the child and uniting the child and parents as soon as possible after surgery (preferably in the PACU) are important interventions. During surgery, the family should have a designated place to wait and should be kept informed of the child's progress. They also should know where and when they can visit the child after surgery.

According to research conducted by Kain, Caldwell-Andrews, Mayes, and colleagues (2007), benefits of well-prepared children and parents along with parental presence during induction of anesthesia include reduced anxiety for children and parents, lower doses of postoperative analgesia, lower incidence of severe emergence delirium symptoms, and shorter discharge time for short procedures. Other studies have not universally supported these benefits. Concern exists regarding the appropriateness of this practice for all parents. Some parents may become upset by the rapid succession of induction events, by observing their child becoming limp, and by leaving the child in the care of strangers. Even though some parents may become anxious, most control their anxiety, do not disrupt the induction, and support the child (Munro and D'Errico, 2000). Whereas parents who are anxious before surgery tend to become even more anxious after the induction, the reverse is true of parents with little anxiety.

Preoperative Sedation

Historically, the most upsetting event for children has been the preoperative injection. An increasing number of anesthesiologists use preoperative sedative premedication, usually midazolam (Versed), and parental presence for children undergoing surgery (Kain, Caldwell-Andrews, Krivutza, and others, 2004).

The goals for using preoperative medications include (1) anxiety reduction, (2) amnesia, (3) sedation, (4) antiemetic effect, and (5) reduction of secretions (Manworren and Fledderman, 2000). (Chapter 7 includes a discussion of pain management strategies for children undergoing surgery.) When drugs are administered, they should be delivered atraumatically via oral or IV routes. Numerous preanesthetic drug regimens are used with children, and no consensus exists on the optimal method. If children have no preoperative pain, are well prepared psychologically for surgery, and have their parents nearby, however, preoperative medication may be unnecessary.

Postoperative Care

Various psychologic and physical interventions and observations help prevent or minimize possible unpleasant effects from anesthesia and the surgical procedure. Although the incidence of serious postoperative complications in healthy children undergoing surgery is less than 1% (Maxwell and Yaster, 2000), continuous monitoring of the child's cardiopulmonary status is essential during the immediate postoperative period. Postanesthesia complications such as airway obstruction, postextubation croup, laryngospasm, and bronchospasm make maintaining a patent airway and maximum ventilation critical.

Monitoring the patient's oxygen saturation and providing supplemental oxygen as needed, maintaining body temperature, and promoting fluid and electrolyte balance are important aspects of immediate postoperative care. Vital signs are continuously monitored, and each vital sign is evaluated in terms of side effects from anesthesia, shock, or respiratory compromise (Table 22-3).

A change in vital signs that demands immediate attention in the perioperative period is caused by malignant hyperthermia (MH), a potentially fatal pharmacogenetic disorder involving a defective

TABLE 22-3	POTENTIAL CAUSES OF POSTOPERATIVE VITAL SIGN ALTERATIONS IN CHILDREN		
ALTERATION	**POTENTIAL CAUSE**		**COMMENTS**
Heart Rate			
Increase	Decreased perfusion (shock) Elevated temperature Pain Respiratory distress (early) Medications (atropine, morphine, epinephrine)		Heart rate may increase to maintain cardiac output.
Decrease	Hypoxia Vagal stimulation Increased intracranial pressure Respiratory distress (late) Medications (neostigmine [Prostigmin])		Bradycardia is of more concern in young child than tachycardia.
Respiratory Rate			
Increase	Respiratory distress Fluid volume excess Hypothermia Elevated temperature Pain		Body responds to respiratory distress primarily by increasing rate.
Decrease	Anesthetics, opioids Pain		Decreased respiratory rate from opioids may be compensated for by increased depth of respiration.
Blood Pressure			
Increase	Excess intravascular volume Increased intracranial pressure Carbon dioxide retention Pain Medication (ketamine, epinephrine)		This is serious in premature infants because it increases risk of intraventricular hemorrhage.
Decrease	Vasodilating anesthetic agents (halothane, isoflurane, enflurane) Opioids (e.g., morphine)		Decreased blood pressure is late sign of shock because of elasticity and constriction of vessels to maintain cardiac output.
Temperature			
Increase	Shock (late sign) Infection Environmental causes (warm room, excess coverings) Malignant hyperthermia		Fever associated with infection usually occurs later than fever of noninfectious origin. Absence of fever does not rule out infection, especially in infants. Malignant hyperthermia requires immediate treatment.
Decrease	Vasodilating anesthetic agents (halothane, isoflurane, enflurane) Muscle relaxants Environmental causes (cool room) Infusion of cool fluids or blood		Neonates are especially susceptible to hypothermia, with serious or fatal consequences.

From Smith DP: *Comprehensive child and family nursing skills*, St. Louis, 1991, Mosby.

calcium channel in the sarcoplasmic reticulum membrane. In susceptible children, inhaled anesthetics and the muscle relaxant succinylcholine trigger the disorder, producing hypermetabolism. Symptoms of MH include hypercarbia (increasing end-tidal carbon dioxide), elevated temperature, tachycardia, tachypnea, acidosis, muscle rigidity, and rhabdomyolysis (Rosenberg, Davis, and James, 2007). A family or previous history of sudden high fever associated with a surgical procedure and myotonia increase the risk for MH. Children who have successfully undergone prior surgery without adverse effects may still be considered susceptible.

Treatment of MH includes immediate discontinuation of the triggering agent, hyperventilation with 100% oxygen, and IV dantrolene sodium. If the child is hyperthermic, initiate cooling measures such as ice packs to the groin, axillae, and neck and iced nasogastric (NG) lavage. The surgery may be discontinued or if it is emergent, it may be continued with a different anesthetic agent. The patient should be transferred to an intensive care unit for at least 36 hours and is closely monitored for stabilization of vital signs, metabolic state, and possible recurrence of symptoms.

Managing pain is a major nursing responsibility after surgery. The nurse should assess pain frequently and administers analgesics to provide comfort and facilitate cooperation with postoperative care such as ambulation and deep breathing. Opioids are the most commonly used analgesics. Routinely scheduled IV analgesics, patient-controlled analgesia, and epidural infusions, rather than as-needed orders, provide excellent analgesia in postoperative pediatric patients.

Because respiratory tract infections are a potential complication of anesthesia, make every effort to aerate the lungs and remove secretions. The lungs are auscultated regularly to identify abnormal sounds or any areas of diminished or absent breath sounds. To prevent pneumonia, encourage respiratory movement with incentive spirometers or other motivating activities (see Box 22-1). If these measures are presented as games, the child is more likely to comply. The child's position is changed every 2 hours, and deep breathing is encouraged.

> **NURSING TIP** Because deep breathing is usually painful after surgery, be certain that the child has received analgesics. Have the child splint the operative site (depending on its location) by hugging a small pillow or a favorite stuffed animal.

During the recovery period, spend some time with the child to assess his or her perceptions of surgery. Play, drawing, and storytelling are excellent methods of discovering the child's thoughts. With such information, the nurse can support or correct the child's perceptions and boost his or her self-esteem for having endured a stressful procedure.

Many pediatric patients are discharged shortly after surgery. Preparation for discharge begins with the preadmission preparation visit. The nurse should discuss instructions for postoperative care and review them throughout the perioperative visit. After discharge, the nursing staff often makes phone calls to check the patient's status. Patient education and compliance with discharge instructions can also be assessed during these phone calls (Barnes, 2000) (see Nursing Care Guidelines box).

COMPLIANCE

Compliance, also termed **adherence**, refers to the extent to which the patient's behavior coincides with the prescribed regimen in terms of taking medication, following diets, or executing other lifestyle changes.

📋 NURSING CARE GUIDELINES
Postoperative Care

- Ensure that preparations are made to receive child:
  - Bed or crib is ready.
  - Intravenous pumps and poles, suction apparatus, and oxygen flow meter are at bedside.
- Obtain baseline information:
  - Take vital signs, including blood pressure; keep blood pressure cuff in place and deflated to lessen disturbance to child.
  - Take and record vital signs more frequently if any value fluctuates.
  - Inspect operative area.
  - Check dressing if present.
    - Outline any bleeding area on dressing or cast with pen.
    - Reinforce, but do not remove, loose dressing.
    - Observe areas below surgical site for blood that may have drained toward bed.
    - Assess for bleeding and other symptoms in areas not covered with a dressing, such as throat after tonsillectomy.
  - Assess skin color and characteristics.
  - Assess level of consciousness and activity.
- Notify physician of any irregularities in child's condition.
- Assess for evidence of pain. (See Pain Assessment, Chapter 7.)
- Review surgeon's orders after completing initial assessment and check that any preoperative orders, such as seizure or cardiac medications, have been reordered and can be given by available routes (oral preparations may be contraindicated).
- Monitor vital signs as ordered and more often if indicated.
- Check dressings for bleeding or other abnormalities.
- Check bowel sounds.
- Observe for signs of shock, abdominal distention, and bleeding.
- Assess for bladder distention.
- Observe for signs of dehydration.
- Detect presence of infection:
  - Take vital signs every 2 to 4 hours as ordered.
  - Collect or request needed specimens.
  - Inspect wound for signs of infection—redness, swelling, heat, pain, and purulent drainage.

In developing strategies to improve compliance, the nurse must first assess level of compliance. Because many children are too young to assume partial or total responsibility for their care, parents are usually primarily responsible for home management.

Factors relating to the care setting are important in ensuring compliance and should be considered in planning strategies to improve compliance. Basically, any aspect of the health care setting that increases the family's satisfaction with the physical setting and the relationship with the practitioner positively influences adherence to the treatment regimen. However, the more complex, expensive, inconvenient, and disruptive the treatment protocol, the less likely the family is to comply. During long-term conditions that involve multiple treatments and considerable rearrangement of lifestyle, compliance is severely affected.

Although it is helpful to know those factors that influence compliance, assessment must include more direct measurement techniques. A number of methods exist, each with advantages and disadvantages. The most successful approach includes a combination of at least two of the following methods:

Clinical judgment—This is subject to bias and inaccuracy unless the nurse carefully evaluates the criteria used in assessment.

Self-reporting—Most people overestimate their compliance by about 20% even when they admit to lapses.

Direct observation—This is difficult to use outside the health care setting, and awareness of being observed frequently affects performance.

Monitoring appointments—Keeping appointments indirectly indicates compliance with the prescribed care.

Monitoring therapeutic response—Few treatments yield directly measurable results (e.g., decreased blood pressure, weight loss); record on a graph or chart.

Pill counts—The nurse counts the number of pills remaining in the original container and compares the number missing with the number of times the medication should have been taken. Although this is a simple method, families may forget to bring the container or deliberately alter the number of pills to avoid detection. This method is also poorly suited to liquid medication. Another technique is the use of pill container caps that record every opening as a presumptive dose.

Chemical assay—For certain drugs, such as digoxin, measurement of plasma drug levels provides information on the amount of drug recently ingested. However, this method is expensive, indicates only short-term compliance, and requires precise timing of the assay for accurate results.

Compliance Strategies

Strategies to improve compliance involve interventions that encourage families to follow the prescribed treatment regimen. Some evidence suggests that higher levels of self-esteem and increased autonomy favorably affect adolescent compliance (Kyngas, Kroll, and Duffy, 2000). However, family factors are important, and characteristics associated with good compliance include family support, family reminders, good communication, and expectations for successful completion of the therapeutic regimen. No one approach is always successful, and the best results occur when at least two strategies are used.

Organizational strategies involve the care setting and the therapeutic plan. This may involve increasing the frequency of appointments, designating a primary practitioner, reducing the cost of medication by prescribing generic brands, reducing the treatment's disruption of the family's lifestyle, and using "cues" to minimize forgetting. Numerous devices are available commercially or can be improvised for cueing, such as pill dispensers; watches with alarms; charts to record completed therapy; messages on the refrigerator or morning coffee pot; and treatment schedules that incorporate the treatment plan into the daily routine, such as physical therapy after the evening bath.

The nurse instructs the family about the treatment plan. Although education is an important factor in enhancing compliance and patients who are more knowledgeable about their condition are more likely to comply, education alone does not ensure compliant behavior. The nurse should incorporate teaching principles known to enhance understanding and retention of material. Written materials are essential, especially in any regimen requiring multiple or complex treatments, and they need to be understandable to the average individual, who reads at about the fourth-grade level. Involvement of the immediate and extended family (e.g., grandparents) in education sessions may enhance compliance.

Treatment strategies relate to the child's refusal or inability to take the prescribed medication. The family may also have difficulty following a prescribed treatment regimen. They may remember and understand the instructions but may not be able to give the medicine as prescribed. Assess the reason for refusal. For example, the child may not be able to swallow pills. In this case, perhaps pills could be crushed or a liquid medication substituted (always review medication to ensure that crushing is acceptable before giving this instruction).

Assess the treatment and medication schedule to determine whether it is reasonable for a home situation. Although an every-6-hour or every-8-hour schedule is reasonable for hospitals, a parent would have difficulty getting up once or twice nightly. Instead the patient could take a medication during the day at times that would be easy to remember.

Behavioral strategies are designed to modify behavior directly. Nurses can use several effective strategies with children to encourage the desired behavior. Positive reinforcement is one strategy that strengthens the behavior. One example of this is the child earning stars or tokens, which can be exchanged for a special privilege or gift. At times, however, disciplinary techniques, such as time-out for young children or withholding privileges for older children, may be needed to improve compliance.

SKIN CARE AND GENERAL HYGIENE

MAINTAINING HEALTHY SKIN

Maintaining an IV line, removing a dressing, positioning a child in bed, changing a diaper, using electrodes, or using restraints have the potential to contribute to skin injury. General guidelines for skin care are listed in the Nursing Care Guidelines box. (Specific guidelines for skin care of neonates are provided in Chapter 9 under Skin Care.)

Assessment of the skin is easiest to accomplish during the bath. Examine for early signs of injury. Risk factors include impaired mobility, protein malnutrition, edema, incontinence, sensory loss, anemia, infection, failure to turn the patient, and intubation. Critically ill children are at a higher risk of pressure ulcers and skin breakdown because they often have several risk factors combined. The incidence in these children has been reported as high as 27% (Curley, Quigley, and Lin, 2003). Identification of risk factors helps to determine children who need a more thorough skin assessment. Several risk assessment scales are available for use in pediatrics, such as the Braden Q Scale (Curley, Razmus, Roberts, and others, 2003) and the Glamorgan Scale (Willock, Baharestani, and Anthony, 2009). Assessment should occur within 24 hours of admission to identify pressure ulcers and wounds that occurred before admission. Pressure ulcers in children typically occur on the occiput, ears, sacrum, and scapula (Amlung, Miller, and Bosley, 2001); the heels and sacrum are common sites in adults.

When capillary blood flow is interrupted by pressure, the blood flows back into the tissue when the pressure is relieved. As the body attempts to reoxygenate the area, a bright red flush appears. This *reactive hyperemia*, or flush, is the earliest sign of tissue compromise and pressure-related ischemia. If pressure is prolonged, reactive hyperemia will not be sufficient to revitalize ischemic tissue. Pressure ulcers in hospitalized children are uncommon, with reported rates of 1% to 13% (Noonan, Quigley, and Curley, 2006). Risk factors associated with pressure ulcers in pediatric intensive care unit patients include edema, length of stay, increasing positive end-expiratory pressure, lack of turning, use of a specialty bed in the turning mode, and weight loss (McCord, McElvain, Sachdeva, and others, 2004). Medical devices such as pulse oximeter probes, bilevel and continuous positive airway pressure masks, oxygen cannulas, orthotics, and casts can also cause pressure ulcers.

NURSING CARE GUIDELINES

Skin Care

- Keep skin free of excess moisture (e.g., urine or fecal incontinence, wound drainage, excessive perspiration).
- Cleanse skin with mild nonalkaline soap or soap-free cleaning agents for routine bathing.
- Provide daily cleansing of eyes, oral and diaper or perineal areas, and any areas of skin breakdown.
- Apply non–alcohol-based moisturizing agents after cleansing to retain moisture and rehydrate skin.
- Use minimum amount of tape and adhesives. On very sensitive skin, use a protective, pectin-based or hydrocolloid skin barrier between skin and tape or adhesives.
- Place pectin-based or hydrocolloid skin barriers directly over excoriated skin. Leave barrier undisturbed until it begins to peel off or for 5 to 7 days. With wet, oozing excoriations, place a small amount of stoma powder on site, remove excess powder, and apply skin barrier. Hold barrier in place for several minutes to allow barrier to soften and mold to skin surface.
- Alternate electrode and probe placement sites and thoroughly assess underlying skin typically every 8 to 24 hours.
- Eliminate pressure secondary to medical devices such as tracheostomy tubes, wheelchairs, braces, and gastrostomy tubes.
- Be certain fingers or toes are visible whenever extremity is used for intravenous (IV) or arterial line.
- Use a draw sheet to move child in bed or onto a stretcher; do not drag child from under the arms.
- Position in neutral alignment; pillows, cushions, or wedges may be needed to prevent hip abduction and pressure to bony prominences, such as heels, elbows, and sacral and occipital areas. When child is positioned laterally, pillows or cushions between the knees, under the head, and under the upper arm will help promote neutral body alignment. Avoid donut cushions because they can cause tissue ischemia. Elevate the head of bed 30 degrees or less to reduce pressure unless contraindicated.
- Do not massage reddened bony prominences because this can cause deep tissue damage; provide pressure relief to those areas instead.
- Routinely assess the child's nutritional status. A child who is NPO (nothing by mouth) for several days and is receiving only IV fluid is nutritionally at risk, which can also affect the skin's ability to maintain its integrity. Consider parenteral nutrition.

Pressure ulcers are staged to classify the amount of tissue damage that has occurred.* Necrotic tissue must be removed so the tissue depth can accurately be assessed. Accurate documentation of redness or obvious skin breakdown is essential. Color, size (diameter and depth), location, presence of sinus tracts, odor, exudate, and response to treatment are observed and recorded at least daily. (For treatment of wounds, see Chapter 30.)

Pressure ulcers can develop when the pressure on the skin and underlying tissues is greater than the capillary closing pressure, causing capillary occlusion. If the pressure remains unrelieved, vessels can collapse, resulting in tissue anoxia and cellular death. Pressure ulcers most often occur over bony prominences. These lesions are usually very deep (stage IV), extending into subcutaneous tissue or even more deeply into muscle, tendon, or bone.

A pressure reduction device reduces pressure but does not prevent pressure from causing capillary closure; therefore, turning and repositioning are always included when using these devices. Most of these items are overlays that are placed on top of the regular mattress. A **pressure-relief device** maintains pressure below that which would cause capillary closure. These devices are usually high-technology beds that are used for patients who have multiple problems and cannot be turned effectively.

Friction and shear contribute to pressure ulcers. **Friction** occurs when the surface of the skin rubs against another surface, such as bed sheets. The skin may have the appearance of an abrasion. The skin damage is usually limited to the epidermal and upper layers. It most often occurs over the elbows, heels, or occiput. Prevention of friction injury includes the use of customized splinting over infants' heels; gel pillows under the heads of infants and toddlers; moisturizing agents; transparent dressings over susceptible areas; and soft, smooth bed linens and clothing (Baharestani and Ratliff, 2007). By itself, friction does not cause tissue necrosis, but when it acts with gravity, it results in shear injury.

Shear is the result of the force of gravity pushing down on the body and friction of the body against a surface, such as the bed or chair. For example, when a patient is in the semi-Fowler position and begins to slide to the foot of the bed, the skin over the sacral area remains in the same place because of the resistance of the bed surface. The blood vessels in the area are stretched and may cause small-vessel thrombosis and tissue death (Bryant and Doughty, 2000). Prevention of shear injury includes using lift sheets when repositioning a patient, elevating the bed no more than 30 degrees for short periods, and using the knee gatch to interrupt the pull of gravity on the body toward the foot of the bed.

Epidermal stripping results when the epidermis is unintentionally removed when tape is removed. These lesions are usually shallow and irregularly shaped. Babies are at increased risk for epidermal injury. Prevention includes using no tape when possible, securing dressings with laced binders (Montgomery straps) or stretchy netting (Spandage or stockinette). Using porous or low-tack tapes (e.g., Medipore, paper, hydrogel), using alcohol-free skin sealants (No Sting Barrier Film), or picture framing wounds with hydrocolloid or wafer barriers (e.g., DuoDERM, Coloplast, Stomahesive) and then taping on top of the barrier also will reduce epidermal stripping.

Tape is placed so that there is no tension, traction, or wrinkles on the skin. To remove tape, slowly peel the tape away while stabilizing the underlying skin. Adhesive remover may be used to break the adhesive bond but may be drying to the skin. Avoid adhesive removers in preterm neonates because absorption rates vary and toxicity may occur. Remove the adhesive with water to prevent absorption and irritation. Wetting the tape with water or alcohol-based foam hand cleansers may facilitate removal.

Chemical factors can also lead to skin damage. Fecal incontinence, especially when mixed with urine; wound drainage; or gastric drainage around gastrostomy tubes can erode the epidermis. The skin can quickly progress from redness to denudement if exposure continues. Moisture barriers, gentle cleansing as soon after exposure as possible, and skin barriers can be used to prevent damage caused by chemical factors. In addition, foam dressings that wick moisture away from the skin are helpful around gastrostomy tubes and tracheostomy sites.

BATHING

Most infants and children can be bathed in a basin at the bedside or on the bed in a standard bathtub or shower. For infants and young

---

*Staging of pressure ulcers and guidelines for prevention and management of pressure ulcers are available from the National Pressure Ulcer Advisory Panel, http://npuap.org.

children confined to bed, use the towel method. Immerse two towels in a dilute soap solution and wring them damp. With the child lying supine on a dry towel, place one damp towel on top of the child and use it to gently clean the body. Discard the towel and dry the child and turn him or her prone. Repeat the procedure using the second damp towel. Commercially available bath cloths may also be used.

Infants and small children are never left unattended in a bathtub, and infants who are unable to sit alone are securely held with one hand during the bath. The nurse securely supports the infant's head with one hand or grasps the infant's farther arm while the head rests comfortably on the nurse's arm. Children who are able to sit without assistance need only close supervision and a pad placed in the bottom of the tub to prevent slipping and loss of balance.

School-age children and adolescents may shower or bathe. Nurses need to use judgment regarding the amount of supervision the child requires. Some can assume this responsibility unaided, but others need someone in constant attendance. Children with cognitive impairments, physical limitations such as severe anemia or leg deformities, or suicidal or psychotic problems (who may commit bodily harm) require close supervision.

Areas that require special attention are the ears, between skinfolds, the neck, the back, and the genital area. The genital area should be carefully cleansed and dried, with particular care given to skinfolds. In uncircumcised boys, usually those older than 3 years of age, the foreskin should be gently retracted, the exposed surfaces cleansed, and the foreskin then replaced. If the condition of the glans indicates inadequate cleaning, such as accumulated smegma, inflammation, phimosis, or foreskin adhesions, teaching proper hygiene is indicated. In the Vietnamese and Cambodian cultures, the foreskin is traditionally not retracted until adulthood. Older children have a tendency to avoid cleaning the genitalia; therefore, they may need a gentle reminder.

ORAL HYGIENE

Mouth care is an integral part of daily hygiene and should be continued in the hospital. For some young children, this is their first introduction to the use of a toothbrush. Infants and debilitated children require the nurse or a family member to perform mouth care. Although young children can manage a toothbrush and are encouraged to use it, most need assistance to perform satisfactorily. Older children, although capable of brushing and flossing without assistance, sometimes need to be reminded.

HAIR CARE

Children should have their hair brushed and combed at least once daily. The hair is styled for comfort and in a manner pleasing to the child and parents. The hair should not be cut without parental permission, although clipping hair to provide access to a scalp vein for IV insertion may be necessary.

If children are hospitalized for more than a few days, the hair may need shampooing. With infants, the hair may be washed during the daily bath or less frequently. For most children, washing the hair and scalp once or twice weekly is sufficient unless there is an indication for more frequent washing, such as after a high fever and profuse sweating. Adolescents normally have increased oily sebaceous secretions that require frequent hair care and more frequent shampoos.

Almost any child can be transported to an accessible sink for shampooing. Those who are unable to be transported can receive a shampoo in their beds with adequate protection, specially adapted equipment or positioning, or dry shampoo caps. When necessary, a shampoo basin may be used or the child may be positioned near the edge of the bed, towels placed under the shoulders, a large plastic garbage bag draped at the edge of the bed with one open end under the shoulders, and the hair placed inside the opening. The other end is opened and placed in a collection container. Water can be transported in a basin.

For African-American children with curly hair, most standard combs are inadequate and may cause hair breakage and discomfort. Use a special comb with widely spaced teeth. It is also much easier to comb the hair after shampooing when it is wet. Use a special hair dressing or pomade, which usually has a coconut oil base. Rub the preparation on the hands and then transfer it to the hair to make it more pliable and manageable. Consult the child's parents regarding the preparation to use on the child's hair and ask if they can provide some for use during the child's hospitalization. Petroleum jelly should not be used. If braiding or plaiting the hair, weave it loosely while the hair is damp. The hair tightens as it dries, which could result in tension folliculitis.

FEEDING THE SICK CHILD

Loss of appetite is a symptom common to most childhood illnesses. Because an acute illness is usually short, the nutritional state is seldom compromised. Urging food on the sick child may precipitate nausea and vomiting. In most cases, children can usually determine their own need for food.

Refusing to eat may also be one way children can exert power and control in an otherwise helpless situation. For young children, loss of appetite may be related to depression caused by separation from their parents. Parents' concern with eating can intensify the problem. Forcing a child to eat meets with rebellion and reinforces the behavior as a control mechanism. Encourage parents to relax any pressure during an acute illness. Although it is best to provide high-quality nutritious foods, the child may desire foods and liquids that contain mostly empty or nonnutritional calories. Some well-tolerated foods include gelatin, diluted clear soups, carbonated drinks, flavored ice pops, dry toast, and crackers. Even though these substances are not nutritious, they can provide necessary fluid and calories.

Dehydration is always a hazard when children have a fever or anorexia, especially when accompanied by vomiting or diarrhea. Fluids should not be forced, and the child is not awakened to take fluids. Forcing fluids may create the same difficulties as urging the child to eat unwanted food. Gentle persuasion with preferred beverages will usually meet with success. Using play techniques can also be effective (see Nursing Care Guidelines box).

An understanding of children's feeding habits can also increase food consumption. For example, if children are given all their food at one time, they generally eat the dessert first. Likewise, if they are presented with large portions, they often push the food away because the amount overwhelms them. If young children are not supervised during mealtime, they tend to play with the food rather than eat it. Therefore, nurses should present food in the usual order, such as soup first followed by small portions of meat, potatoes, and vegetables and ending with dessert.

When the child is feeling better, appetite usually begins to improve. It is best to take advantage of any hungry period by serving high-quality foods and snacks. If the child still refuses to eat, offer nutritious fluids, such as prepared breakfast drinks. Parents can help by bringing in food items from home, especially if the family's cultural eating habits differ from the hospital food. A clinical dietitian may be consulted for alternative food choices.

NURSING CARE GUIDELINES

Feeding a Sick Child

Take a dietary history (see Chapter 6) and use information to make eating time as similar to eating at home as possible.

Encourage parents or other family members to feed child or to be present at mealtimes.

Make mealtimes pleasant; avoid any procedures immediately before or after eating; make certain child is rested and pain free.

Serve small, frequent meals rather than three large meals or serve three meals and nutritious between-meal snacks.

Provide finger foods for young children.

Involve children in food selection and preparation whenever possible.

Serve small portions and serve each course separately, such as soup first followed by meat, potatoes, and vegetables and ending with dessert. With young children, camouflage size of food by cutting meat thicker so less appears on plate or by folding a cheese slice in half. Offer second helpings.

Ensure a variety of foods, textures, and colors.

Provide food selections that are favorites of most children, such as peanut butter and jelly sandwiches, hot dogs, hamburgers, macaroni and cheese, pizza, spaghetti, tacos, fried chicken, corn, and fruit yogurt.

Avoid foods that are highly seasoned, have strong odors, or are all mixed together unless typical of cultural practices.

Provide fluid selections that are favorites of most children, such as fruit punch, cola, ginger ale, sweetened tea, flavored ice pops, sherbet, ice cream, milk, milkshakes, pudding, gelatin, clear broth, or creamed soups.

Offer nutritious snacks, such as frozen yogurt or pudding, ice cream, oatmeal or peanut butter cookies, hot cocoa, cheese slices, pieces of raw vegetable or fruit, and dried fruit or cereal.

Make food attractive and different; for example:
- Serve a "picnic lunch" in a paper bag.
- Pack food in a Chinese take-out container; decorate container.
- Put a "face" or a "flower" on a hamburger or sandwich with pieces of vegetable.
- Use a cookie cutter to shape a sandwich.
- Serve pudding, yogurt, or juice frozen as an ice pop.
- Make Slurpies or snow cones by pouring flavored syrup on crushed ice.
- Add food coloring to water or milk.
- Serve fluids through brightly colored or unusually shaped straws.
- Make "bowtie" sandwiches by cutting them in triangles and placing two points together.
- Slice sandwiches into "fingers."
- Grate mounds of cheese.
- Cut apples horizontally to make circles.
- Put a banana on a hot dog bun and spread with peanut butter.
- Break uncooked spaghetti into toothpick lengths and skewer cheese, cold meat, vegetables, or fruit chunks.

Praise children for what they do eat.

Do not punish children for not eating by removing their dessert or putting them to bed.

When children are placed on special diets, such as clear liquids after surgery or during episodes of diarrhea, assessment of their intake and readiness to advance to more complex foods is essential.

Regardless of the type of diet, charting the amount consumed is an important nursing responsibility. Descriptions need to be detailed and accurate, such as "4 oz of orange juice, one pancake, and 8 oz of milk."

Comments such as "ate well" or "ate poorly" are inadequate. Charting the percentage of the meal eaten is also inadequate unless food is measured before serving.

If the parents are involved in the child's care, encourage them to keep a list of everything the child eats. Using a premeasured cup for fluids ensures a more accurate estimate of intake. A comparison of the intake at each meal can isolate food deficiencies, such as insufficient intake of meat or vegetables. Behaviors associated with mealtime also identify possible factors influencing appetite. For example, the observation, "Child eats well when with other children but plays with food if left alone in room" helps the nurse plan mealtime activities that stimulate the child's appetite.

Although sick children's appetites may be poor and not characteristic of their home eating habits, the hospital stay provides numerous opportunities for nurses to assess the family's knowledge of good nutrition and to implement teaching as needed to improve nutritional intake.

CONTROLLING ELEVATED TEMPERATURES

An elevated temperature, most frequently from fever but occasionally caused by hyperthermia, is one of the most common symptoms of illness in children. This manifestation is a great concern to parents. To facilitate an understanding of fever, the following terms are defined:

Set point—The temperature around which body temperature is regulated by a thermostat-like mechanism in the hypothalamus

Fever (hyperpyrexia)—An elevation in set point such that body temperature is regulated at a higher level; may be arbitrarily defined as temperature above 38° C (100.4° F)

Hyperthermia—Body temperature exceeding the set point, which usually results from the body or external conditions creating more heat than the body can eliminate, such as in heat stroke, aspirin toxicity, seizures, or hyperthyroidism

Body temperature is regulated by a thermostat-like mechanism in the hypothalamus. This mechanism receives input from centrally and peripherally located receptors. When temperature changes occur, these receptors relay the information to the thermostat, which either increases or decreases heat production to maintain a constant set point temperature. However, during an infection, pyrogenic substances cause an increase in the body's normal set point, a process that is mediated by prostaglandins. Consequently, the hypothalamus increases heat production until the core temperature reaches the new set point.

During the fever (febrile) state, shivering and vasoconstriction generate and conserve heat during the chill phase of fever, raising central temperatures to the level of the new set point. The temperature reaches a plateau when it stabilizes in the higher range. When the temperature is greater than the set point or when the pyrogen is no longer present, a crisis, or defervescence, of the temperature occurs.

Most fevers in children are of brief duration with limited consequences and are viral in origin. When fever is caused by bacteria, endotoxins are produced that activate the inflammatory process and produce fever (Rote, Huether, and McCance, 2000). Fever has physiologic benefits, including increased white blood cell activity, interferon production and effectiveness, and antibody production and enhancement of some antibiotic effects (Considine and Brennan, 2007). Contrary to popular belief, neither the rise in temperature nor its response to antipyretics indicates the severity or etiology of the infection, which casts doubt on the value of using fever as a diagnostic or prognostic indicator.

Therapeutic Management

Treatment of elevated temperature depends on whether it is attributable to a fever or hyperthermia. Because the set point is normal in hyperthermia but increased in fever, different approaches must be used to lower body temperature successfully.

Fever

The principal reason for treating fever is the relief of discomfort. Relief measures include pharmacologic and environmental intervention. The most effective intervention is the use of antipyretics to lower the set point.

Antipyretics include acetaminophen, aspirin, and nonsteroidal antiinflammatory drugs (NSAIDs). Acetaminophen is the preferred drug. Aspirin should not be given to children because of its association in children with influenza virus or chickenpox and Reye syndrome. One nonprescription NSAID, ibuprofen, is approved for fever reduction in children as young as 6 months of age. The dosage is based on the initial temperature level: 5 mg/kg of body weight for temperatures less than 39.2° C (102.6° F) or 10 mg/kg for temperatures greater than 39.2° C. The recommended dosage for pain is 10 mg/kg every 6 to 8 hours, and the recommended maximum daily dose for pain and fever is 40 mg/kg. The duration of fever reduction is generally 6 to 8 hours and is longer with the higher dose.

The recommended doses of acetaminophen should never be exceeded. Acetaminophen should be given every 4 hours but no more than five times in 24 hours. Because body temperature normally decreases at night, three or four doses in 24 hours will control most fevers. The temperature is usually retaken 30 minutes after the antipyretic is given to assess its effect but should not be repeatedly measured. The child's level of discomfort is the best indication for continued treatment.

The nurse can use environmental measures to reduce fever if they are tolerated by the child and if they do not induce shivering. Shivering is the body's way of maintaining the elevated set point by producing heat. Compensatory shivering greatly increases metabolic requirements above those already caused by the fever.

Traditional cooling measures, such as wearing minimum clothing; exposing the skin to air; reducing room temperature; increasing air circulation; and applying cool, moist compresses to the skin (e.g., the forehead), are effective if used approximately 1 hour after an antipyretic is given so the set point is lowered. Cooling procedures such as sponging or tepid baths are ineffective in treating febrile children (these measures are effective for hyperthermia) either when used alone or in combination with antipyretics, and they cause considerable discomfort (Axelrod, 2000).

Seizures associated with a fever occur in 3% to 4% of all children, usually in those between 6 months and 6 years of age. About 30% of children have subsequent febrile seizures; a younger age at onset and a family history of febrile seizures are associated with increased incidence of recurring episodes. There is little evidence to support the use of antipyretic drugs or anticonvulsants to prevent a second febrile seizure; nursing intervention should focus on ways to provide care and comfort during a febrile illness. Simple febrile seizures lasting less than 10 minutes do not cause brain damage or other debilitating effects (Jones and Jacobsen, 2007; Sadleir and Scheffer, 2007). (See Febrile Seizures, Chapter 28.)

Hyperthermia

Unlike in fever, antipyretics are of no value in hyperthermia because the set point is already normal. Consequently, cooling measures are used. Cool applications to the skin help reduce the core temperature. Cooled blood from the skin surface is conducted to inner organs and tissues, and warm blood is circulated to the surface, where it is cooled and recirculated. The surface blood vessels dilate as the body attempts to dissipate heat to the environment and facilitate this cooling process.

Commercial cooling devices, such as cooling blankets or mattresses, are available to reduce body temperature. Place the patient on the bed and cover with a sheet or lightweight blanket. Frequent temperature monitoring is essential to prevent excessive cooling of the body.

Traditionally, cool compresses decrease high temperature. For tepid tub baths, it is usually best to start with warm water and gradually add cool water until the desired water temperature of 37° C (98.6° F) is reached to acclimate the child to the lower water temperature. Generally, the temperature of the water only has to be 1° C (or 2° F) less than the child's temperature to be effective. The child is placed directly in the tub of tepid water for 15 to 20 minutes while water is gently squeezed from a washcloth over the back and chest or gently sprayed over the body from a sprayer. In the bed or crib, cool washcloths or towels are used, exposing only one area of the body at a time. Continue sponging for approximately 20 minutes.

After the tub or sponge bath, the child is dried and dressed in lightweight pajamas, a nightgown, or a diaper and placed in a dry bed. The child is dried by gently rubbing the skin surface with a towel to stimulate circulation. The temperature is retaken 30 minutes after the tub or sponge bath. The tub or sponge bath should not be continued or restarted until the skin surface is warm or if the child feels chilled. Chilling causes vasoconstriction, which defeats the purpose of the cool applications. In this condition, little blood is carried to the skin surface; the blood remains primarily in the viscera to become heated.

Whether a temperature elevation in the critically ill child is caused by fever or hyperthermia, it should be treated aggressively. The metabolic rate increases 10% for every 1° C increase in temperature and three to five times during shivering, thus increasing oxygen, fluid, and caloric requirements. If the child's cardiovascular or neurologic system is already compromised, these increased needs are especially hazardous. In all children with an elevated temperature, attention to adequate hydration is essential. Most children's needs can be met through additional oral fluids.

FAMILY TEACHING AND HOME CARE

Fever is one of the most common problems for which parents seek health care. High levels of parental anxiety (fever phobia) surrounding potential complications of fever such as seizures and dehydration are prevalent and can result in overusing antipyretics (Purssell, 2008). Parents need to know that sponging is indicated for elevated temperatures from hyperthermia rather than fever and that ice water and alcohol are inappropriate, potentially dangerous solutions (Axelrod, 2000). Parents should know how to take the child's temperature, how to read the thermometer accurately, and when to seek professional care (see Family-Centered Care box). Some of the newer temperature-measuring devices, such as plastic strip or digital thermometers, may be better suited for home use. (See Temperature, Chapter 6.) If the use of acetaminophen or ibuprofen is indicated, the parents need instructions in administering the drug. Emphasize accuracy in both the amount of drug given and the time intervals at which the drug is administered. Along with reduced activity, encourage small, frequent sips of clear liquids. Dress the child in light clothing; use a light blanket for children who are cold or shivering (Walsh and Edwards, 2006).

Nursing Care Plan—The Child with Elevated Body Temperature

The Child with Fever

Call Office Immediately If:
Your child is younger than 2 months old.
The fever is over 40.6° C (105° F).
Your child looks or acts very sick, including a stiff neck, persistent vomiting, purplish spots on the skin, confusion, trouble breathing after you have cleaned his or her nose, or inability to be comforted.

Call Within 24 Hours If:
The fever is between 40° and 40.6° C (104° and 105° F), especially if your child is younger than 2 years old.
Your child has had a fever for more than 24 hours without an obvious cause or location of infection.
Your child has had a fever for more than 3 days.
Your child has burning or pain with urination.
Your child has a history of febrile seizures.
The fever went away for more than 24 hours and then returned.
You have other concerns or questions.

Modified from Schmitt BD: *Instructions for pediatric patients,* ed 2, Philadelphia, 1999, Saunders.

SAFETY

Safety is an essential component of any patient's care, but children have special characteristics that require an even greater concern for safety. Because small children in the hospital are separated from their usual environment and do not possess the capacity for abstract thinking and reasoning, it is the responsibility of everyone who comes in contact with them to maintain protective measures throughout their hospital stay. Nurses need to understand the age level at which each child is operating and plan for safety accordingly.

Identification bands are particularly important for children. Infants and unconscious patients are unable to tell or respond to their names. Toddlers may answer to any name or to a nickname only. Older children may exchange places, give an erroneous name, or choose not to respond to their own names as a joke, unaware of the hazards of such practices.

ENVIRONMENTAL FACTORS

All of the environmental safety measures for the protection of adults apply to children, including good illumination, floors that are clear of fluid and objects that might contribute to falls, and nonskid surfaces in showers and tubs. All staff members should be familiar with the area-specific fire plan. Elevators and stairways should be made safe.

All windows should be secured. Window blind and curtain cords should be out of reach with split cords to prevent strangulation. Pacifiers should not be tied around the neck or attached to an infant by string.

Electrical equipment should be in good working order and used only by personnel familiar with its use. It should not be in contact with moisture or situated near tubs. Electrical outlets should have covers to prevent burns in small children, whose exploratory activities may extend to inserting objects into the small openings.

Staff members should practice proper care and disposal of small objects such as syringe caps, needle covers, and temperature probes. Staff also must carefully check bathwater before placing the child in it

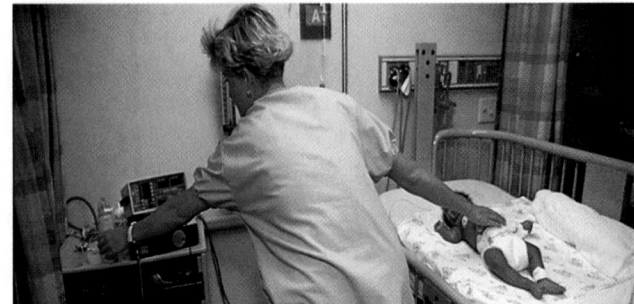

FIG 22-3 The nurse maintains hand contact when her back is turned.

and never leave children alone in a bathtub. Infants are helpless in water, and small children (and some older ones) may turn on the hot water faucet and be severely burned.

Furniture is safest when it is scaled to the child's proportions, is sturdy, and is well balanced to prevent its being easily tipped over. A special hazard for children is the danger of entrapment under an electronically controlled bed when it is activated to descend. Infants and small children must be securely strapped into infant seats, feeding chairs, and strollers. Baby walkers should not be used because they provide access to hazards, resulting in burns, falls, and poisonings. Infants; young children; and children who are weak, paralyzed, agitated, confused, sedated, or cognitively impaired are never left unattended on treatment tables, on scales, or in treatment areas. Even premature infants are capable of surprising mobility; therefore, portholes in incubators must be securely fastened when not in use.

Crib sides up should always be raised and fastened securely. Use cribs that meet federal safety standards (http://www.cpsc.gov/info/cribs/index.html). Anyone attending an infant or small child on a stretcher or table should never turn away without maintaining hand contact with the child, that is, keeping one hand on the child's back or abdomen to prevent rolling, crawling, or jumping from the open crib (Fig. 22-3). A child who is likely to climb over the sides of the crib is safest when placed in a specially constructed crib with a cover over the top. Never tie nets to the movable crib sides or use knots that do not permit quick release.

The safest sleeping position to prevent sudden infant death syndrome is wholly supine (AAP, Task Force on Sudden Infant Death Syndrome, 2005). No pillows should be placed in a young infant's crib while the infant is sleeping.

Toys

Toys play a vital role in the everyday lives of children, and they are no less important in the hospital setting. Nurses are responsible for assessing the safety of toys brought to the hospital by well-meaning parents and friends. Toys should be appropriate to the child's age, condition, and treatment. For example, if the child is receiving oxygen, electrical or friction toys or equipment are not safe because sparks can cause oxygen to ignite. Inspect toys to ensure they are nonallergenic, washable, and unbreakable and that they have no small, removable parts that can be aspirated or swallowed or can otherwise inflict injury on a child. All objects within reach of children younger than 3 years of age should pass the choke tube test. A toilet paper roll is a handy guide. If a toy or object fits into the cylinder (items <1¼ inches across or balls <1¾ inches in diameter), it is a potential choking danger to the child. Latex balloons pose a serious threat to children of all ages. If the balloon breaks, a child may put a piece of the latex in his or her mouth. If it is aspirated or swallowed, the latex piece is difficult to remove, resulting in choking. Latex balloons should never be permitted in the hospital setting.

Preventing Falls

Falls prevention begins with identification of children most at risk for falls. Pediatric hospitals use various methods to identify a child's risk of falls (Child Health Corporation of America, 2009). After a risk assessment is performed, multiple interventions are needed to minimize pediatric patients' risk of falling, including education of patient, family, and staff.

To identify children at risk of falling, perform a fall risk assessment on patients on admission and throughout hospitalization. Risk factors for hospitalized children include:

- Medication effects—Postanesthesia or sedation; analgesics or narcotics, especially in those who have never had narcotics in the past and in whom effects are unknown
- Altered mental status—Secondary to seizures, brain tumors, or medications
- Altered or limited mobility—Reduced skill at ambulation secondary to developmental age, disease process, tubes, drains, casts, splints, or other appliances; new to ambulation with assistive devices such as walkers or crutches
- Postoperative children—Risk of hypotension or syncope secondary to large blood loss, a heart condition, or extended bed rest
- History of falls
- Infants or toddlers in cribs with side rails down or on the daybed with family members

Once children at risk of falls have been identified, alert other staff members by posting signs on the door and at the bedside, applying a special colored armband labeled "Fall Precautions," labeling the chart with a sticker, or documenting information on the chart.

Prevention of falls requires alterations in the environment, including:

- Keep the bed in the lowest position with the brakes locked and the side rails up.
- Place the call bell within reach.
- Ensure that all necessary and desired items are within reach (e.g., water, glasses, tissues, snacks).
- Offer toileting on a regular basis, especially if the patient is taking diuretics or laxatives.
- Keep lights on at all times, including dim lights while sleeping.
- Lock wheelchairs before transferring patients.
- Ensure that the patient has an appropriate size gown and nonskid footwear. Do not allow gowns or ties to drag on the floor during ambulation.
- Keep the floor clean and free of clutter. Post a "wet floor" sign if the floor is wet.
- Ensure that the patient has glasses on if he or she normally wears them.

Preventing falls also relies on age-appropriate education of patients. Assist the child with ambulation even though he or she may have ambulated well before hospitalization. Patients who have been lying in bed need to get up slowly, sitting on the side of the bed before standing.

The nurse also needs to educate family members:

- Call the nursing staff for assistance and do not allow patients to get up independently.
- Keep the side rails of the crib or bed up whenever patient is in the crib or bed.
- Do not leave infants on the daybed; put them in the crib with the side rails up.

- When all family members need to leave the bedside, notify the staff and ensure that the patient is in the bed or crib with the side rails up and call bell within reach (if appropriate).

INFECTION CONTROL

According to the Centers for Disease Control and Prevention (CDC), approximately 2 million patients each year develop nosocomial (hospital-acquired) infections. These infections occur when there is interaction among patients, health care personnel, equipment, and bacteria (Quality, equipment hold keys to infection control, 2006). Nosocomial infections are preventable if caregivers practice meticulous cleaning and disposal techniques.

Standard precautions synthesize the major features of universal (blood and body fluid) precautions (designed to reduce the risk of transmission of bloodborne pathogens) and body substance isolation (designed to reduce the risk of transmission of pathogens from moist body substances). Standard precautions involve the use of barrier protection, such as gloves, goggles, gown, or mask, to prevent contamination from (1) blood; (2) all body fluids, secretions, and excretions except sweat, regardless of whether they contain visible blood; (3) nonintact skin; and (4) mucous membranes. Standard precautions are designed for the care of all patients to reduce the risk of transmission of microorganisms from both recognized and unrecognized sources of infection.

Transmission-based precautions are designed for patients with documented or suspected infection or colonization (presence of microorganisms in or on patient but without clinical signs and symptoms of infection) with highly transmissible or epidemiologically important pathogens for which additional precautions beyond standard precautions are needed to interrupt transmission in hospitals. There are three types of transmission-based precautions: airborne precautions, droplet precautions, and contact precautions. They may be combined for diseases that have multiple routes of transmission (Box 22-2). They are to be used in addition to standard precautions.

Airborne precautions reduce the risk of airborne transmission of infectious agents. Airborne transmission occurs by dissemination of either airborne droplet nuclei (small-particle residue [<5 mm] of evaporated droplets that may remain suspended in the air for long periods) or dust particles containing the infectious agent. Microorganisms carried in this manner can be dispersed widely by air currents and may become inhaled by or deposited on a susceptible host within the same room or over a longer distance from the source patient, depending on environmental factors. Special air handling and ventilation are required to prevent airborne transmission. Airborne precautions apply to patients with known or suspected infection with pathogens transmitted by the airborne route such as measles, varicella, and tuberculosis.

Droplet precautions reduce the risk of droplet transmission of infectious agents. Droplet transmission involves contact of the conjunctivae or the mucous membranes of the nose or mouth of a susceptible person with large-particle droplets (>5 mm) containing microorganisms generated from a person who has a clinical disease or who is a carrier of the microorganism. Droplets are generated from the source person primarily during coughing, sneezing, or talking and during procedures such as suctioning and bronchoscopy. Transmission requires close contact between source and recipient persons because droplets do not remain suspended in the air and generally travel only short distances, usually 3 feet or less, through the air. Because droplets do not remain suspended in the air, special air handling and ventilation are not required to prevent droplet transmission. Droplet precautions apply to any patient with known or suspected infection with pathogens that can be transmitted by infectious droplets (see Box 22-2).

Contact precautions reduce the risk of transmission of microorganisms by direct or indirect contact. Direct-contact transmission involves skin-to-skin contact and physical transfer of microorganisms to a susceptible host from an infected or colonized person, such as occurs when turning or bathing patients. Direct-contact transmission also can occur between two patients (e.g., by hand contact). Indirect contact transmission involves contact of a susceptible host with a contaminated intermediate object, usually inanimate, in the patient's environment. Contact precautions apply to specified patients known or suspected to be infected or colonized with microorganisms that can be transmitted by direct or indirect contact.

> ## ! NURSING ALERT
>
> The most common piece of medical equipment, the stethoscope, can be a potent source of harmful microorganisms and nosocomial infections.

Nurses caring for young children are frequently in contact with body substances, especially urine, feces, and vomitus. Nurses need to exercise judgment concerning situations when gloves, gowns, or masks are necessary. For example, nurses should wear gloves and possibly gowns for changing diapers when there are loose or explosive stools. Otherwise, the plastic lining of disposable diapers provides a sufficient barrier between the hands and body substances.

Antimicrobial-resistant organisms are causing increasing numbers of nosocomial infections. In hospitals, patients are the most significant sources of methicillin-resistant *Staphylococcus aureus*, and the main mode of transmission is patient to patient via the hands of a health care provider (Eaton, 2005; Quality, equipment hold keys to infection control, 2006). Hand washing is the most critical infection control practice.

During feedings, wear gowns if the child is likely to vomit or spit up, which often occurs during burping. When wearing gloves, wash the hands thoroughly after removing the gloves because gloves fail to provide complete protection. The absence of visible leaks does not indicate that the gloves are intact.

Another essential practice of infection control is that all needles (uncapped and unbroken) are disposed of in a rigid, puncture-resistant container located near the site of use. Consequently, these containers are installed in patients' rooms. Because children are naturally curious, extra attention is needed in selecting a suitable type of container and a location that prevents access to the discarded needles (Fig. 22-4). The use of needleless systems allows secure syringe or IV tubing attachment to vascular access devices without the risk of needlestick injury to the child or nurse.

TRANSPORTING INFANTS AND CHILDREN

Infants and children need to be transported within the unit and to areas outside the pediatric unit. Infants and small children can be carried for short distances within the unit, but for more extended trips, the child should be securely transported in a suitable conveyance.

Small infants can be held or carried in the horizontal position with the back supported and the thigh grasped firmly by the carrying arm (Fig. 22-5, *A*). In the football hold, the infant is carried on the nurse's arm with the head supported by the hand and the body held securely between the nurse's body and elbow (Fig. 22-5, *B*). Both of these holds leave the nurse's other arm free for activity. The infant also can be held in the upright position with the buttocks on the nurse's forearm and the front of the body resting against the nurse's chest. The infant's head

---

BOX 22-2 TYPES OF PRECAUTIONS AND PATIENTS REQUIRING THEM

Standard Precautions for Prevention of Transmission of Pathogens

Use standard precautions for the care of all patients.

Airborne Precautions

In addition to standard precautions, use airborne precautions for patients known or suspected to have serious illnesses transmitted by airborne droplet nuclei. Examples of such illnesses include measles, varicella (including disseminated zoster), and tuberculosis.

Droplet Precautions

In addition to standard precautions, use droplet precautions for patients known or suspected to have serious illnesses transmitted by large-particle droplets. Examples of such illnesses include:

- Invasive *Haemophilus influenzae* type b disease, including meningitis, pneumonia, epiglottitis, and sepsis
- Invasive *Neisseria meningitidis* disease, including meningitis, pneumonia, and sepsis
- Other serious bacterial respiratory tract infections spread by droplet transmission, including diphtheria (pharyngeal), mycoplasmal pneumonia, pertussis, pneumonic plague, streptococcal pharyngitis, pneumonia, and scarlet fever in infants and young children
- Serious viral infections spread by droplet transmission, including adenovirus, influenza, mumps, parvovirus B19, and rubella

Contact Precautions

In addition to standard precautions, use contact precautions for patients known or suspected to have serious illnesses easily transmitted by direct patient contact or by contact with items in the patient's environment. Examples of such illnesses include:

- Gastrointestinal, respiratory, skin, or wound infections or colonization with multidrug-resistant bacteria judged by the infection control program based on current state, regional, or national recommendations, to be of special clinical and epidemiologic significance
- Enteric infections with a low infectious dose or prolonged environmental survival, including *Clostridium difficile*; for diapered or incontinent patients: enterohemorrhagic *Escherichia coli* O157:H7, *Shigella* organisms, hepatitis A, or rotavirus
- Respiratory syncytial virus, parainfluenza virus, or enteroviral infections in infants and young children.
- Skin infections that are highly contagious or that may occur on dry skin, including diphtheria (cutaneous), herpes simplex virus (neonatal or mucocutaneous), impetigo, major (noncontained) abscesses, cellulitis or decubitus, pediculosis, scabies, staphylococcal furunculosis in infants and young children, zoster (disseminated or in the immunocompromised host)
- Viral or hemorrhagic conjunctivitis
- Viral hemorrhagic infections (Ebola, Lassa, or Marburg)

Modified from Siegel JD, Rhinehart E, Jackson M, and others, 2007 Guideline for isolation precautions: preventing transmission of infectious agents in healthcare settings, available at http://www.cdc.gov/hicpac/pdf/isolation/Isolation2007.pdf.

and shoulders are supported by the nurse's other arm in case the infant moves suddenly (Fig. 22-5, *C*). Older infants are able to hold their heads erect but are still subject to sudden movements.

The method of transporting children depends on their age, condition, and destination. Older children are safe in wheelchairs or on stretchers. Younger children can be transported in a crib, on a stretcher, in a wagon with raised sides, or in a wheelchair with a safety belt. Stretchers should be equipped with high sides and a safety belt, both of which are secured during transport.

Special care is needed in transporting critically ill patients in the hospital. Critically ill children should always be transported on a stretcher or bed (rather than carried) by at least two staff members with monitoring continued during transport. A blood pressure monitor (or standard blood pressure cuff), pulse oximeter, and cardiac monitor/defibrillator should accompany every patient (Warren, Fromm, Orr, and others, 2004). Airway equipment and emergency medications should accompany the patient.

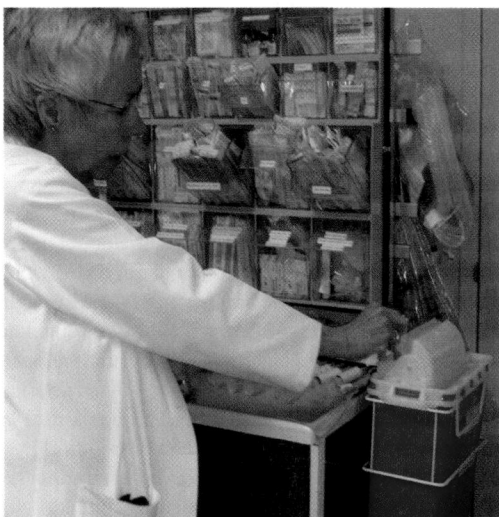

FIG 22-4 To prevent needlestick injuries, used needles (and other sharp instruments) are not capped or broken and are disposed of in a rigid, puncture-resistant container located near site of use. Note placement of container to prevent children's access to contents.

RESTRAINING METHODS AND THERAPEUTIC HOLDING

The Joint Commission (Joint Commission on Accreditation of Healthcare Organizations, 2001) defines restraint as "any method, physical or mechanical, which restricts a person's movement, physical activity, or normal access to his or her body." Before initiating restraints, the nurse completes a comprehensive assessment of the patient to determine whether the need for a restraint outweighs the risk of not using one. Restraints can result in loss of dignity, violation of patient rights, psychologic harm, physical harm, and even death.

Consider alternative methods first and document them in the patient's record. Some examples of alternative measures include bringing a child to the nurses' station for continuous observation, providing diversional activities such as music, encouraging the participation of the parents, or therapeutic holding. Therapeutic holding is the use of a secure, comfortable, temporary holding position that provides close physical contact with the parent or caregiver for 30 minutes or less. The use of restraints can often be avoided with adequate preparation of the child; parental or staff supervision of the child; or adequate protection of a vulnerable site, such as an infusion device.

The nurse needs to assess the child's development, mental status, potential to hurt others or self, and safety. The nurse is responsible for selecting the least restrictive type of restraint. Using less restrictive restraints is often possible by gaining the cooperation of the child and parents. Examples of less restrictive restraints are provided in Table 22-4.

The two types of restraints used with children are classified as medical-surgical and behavioral restraints. When a standard or protocol states that immobilization is required 100% of the time as a part of the procedure or postprocedural care process, the restraint device is considered a part of routine care. For example, the postoperative use of elbow restraints after a cleft lip repair, if written in the protocol or standard of care and used for 100% of patients, would not fall under The Joint Commission or Centers for Medicare and Medicaid Services mandates concerning restraints.

Medical-surgical restraints are used for children with an artificial airway or airway adjunct for delivery of oxygen, indwelling catheters, tubes, drains, lines, pacemaker wires, or suture sites. The medical-surgical restraint is used to ensure that safe care is given to the patient.

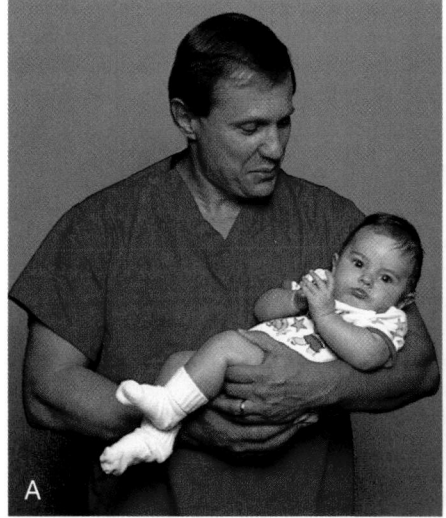 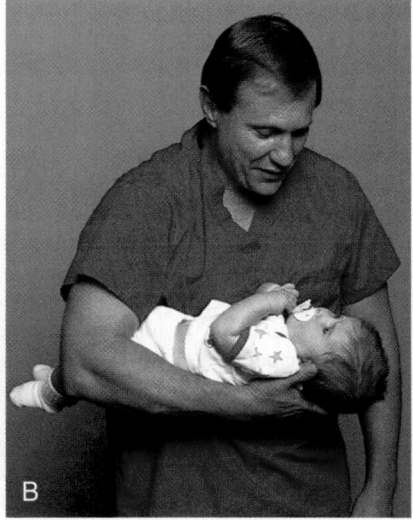 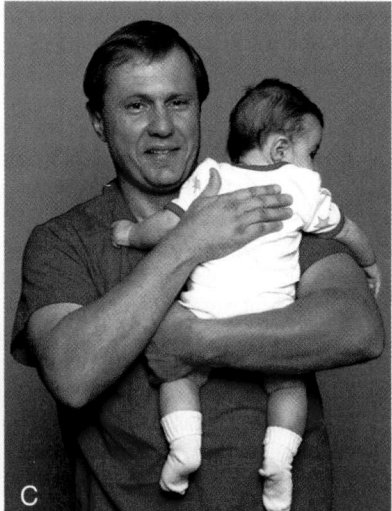

FIG 22-5 Transporting infants. **A,** The infant's thigh firmly grasped in the nurse's hand. **B,** Football hold. **C,** Back supported.

TABLE 22-4	RESTRAINING CHILDREN: LESS RESTRICTIVE TO MORE RESTRICTIVE TECHNIQUES

TECHNIQUE OR DEVICE	LESS RESTRICTIVE TO MORE RESTRICTIVE					
Extremities						
Sleeves	X					
Hand mitts, mittens	X					
Stockinette		X				
Elbows (no-no's)			X			
Arm board				X		
One or two limbs					X	
Three or four limbs						X
Chest and Body						
Belts, safety belts	X					
Posey vest, safety jacket			X			
Mummy restraint						X
Papoose board						X
Environment						
Side rails		X				
Crib tops		X				
Seclusion						X
Other						
Chemical						X

Adapted from Selekman J, Snyder B: Uses of and alternatives to restraints in pediatric settings, *AACN Clin Issues* 7(4):603–610, 1996.

The potential risks of the restraint are offset by the potential benefit of providing safer care. Medical-surgical restraints may be instituted for any of the following reasons:
- Risk for interruption of therapy used to maintain oxygenation or airway patency
- Risk of harm if indwelling catheter, tube, drain, line, pacemaker wire, or sutures are removed, dislodged, or ruptured
- Patient confusion, agitation, unconsciousness, or developmental inability to understand direct requests or instructions

Medical-surgical restraints can be initiated by an individual order or by protocol; the use of the protocol must be authorized by an individual order. The order for continued use of restraints must be renewed each day. Patients are monitored at least every 2 hours.

Behavioral restraints are limited to situations with a significant risk of patients physically harming themselves or others because of behavioral reasons and when nonphysical interventions are not effective. Before initiating a behavioral restraint, the nurse should assess the patient's mental, behavioral, and physical status to determine the cause for the child's potentially harmful behavior. If behavioral restraints are indicated, a collaborative approach involving the patient (if appropriate), the family, and the health care team should be used. An order must be obtained as soon as possible but no longer than 1 hour after the initiation of behavioral restraints. Behavioral restraints for children must be reordered every 1 to 2 hours based on age. A licensed independent practitioner must conduct an in-person evaluation within 1 hour and again every 4 hours until restraints are discontinued. Children in behavioral restraints must be continuously observed and assessed every 15 minutes. Assessment components include signs of injury associated with applying restraint, nutrition and hydration, circulation and range-of-motion of extremities, vital signs, hygiene and elimination, physical and psychologic status and comfort, and readiness for discontinuation of restraint. The nurse must use clinical judgment in setting a schedule for when each of these parameters needs to be evaluated because every parameter must be assessed during each 15-minute physical assessment.

Restraints with ties must be secured to the bed or crib frame, not the side rails. Suggestions for increasing safety and comfort while the child is in a restraint include leaving one finger breadth between skin and the device and tying knots that allow for quick release. The nurse can also increase safety by ensuring the restraint does not tighten as the child moves and decreasing wrinkles or bulges in the restraint. Placing jacket restraints over an article of clothing; placing limb restraints below waist level, below knee level, or distal to the IV; and tucking in dangling straps also increase safety and comfort.

Mummy Restraint or Swaddle

When an infant or small child requires short-term restraint for examination or treatment that involves the head and neck (e.g., venipuncture, throat examination, gavage feeding), a papoose board with straps or a mummy wrap effectively controls the child's movements. A blanket or sheet is opened on the bed or crib with one corner folded to the center. The infant is placed on the blanket with the shoulders at the fold and feet toward the opposite corner. With the infant's right arm straight down against the body, the right side of the blanket is pulled firmly across the infant's right shoulder and chest and secured beneath the left side of the body. The left arm is placed straight against the infant's side, and the left side of the blanket is brought across the shoulder and chest and locked beneath the body on the right side. The lower corner is folded and brought over the body and tucked or fastened securely with safety pins. Safety pins can be used to fasten the blanket in place at any step in the process. To modify the mummy restraint for chest examination, bring the folded edge of the blanket over each arm and under the back and then fold the loose edge over and secure it at a point below the chest to allow visualization and access to the chest (Fig. 22-6, *A*).

Jacket Restraint

A jacket restraint is sometimes used to keep the child safe in various chairs. The jacket is put on the child with the ties in back so the child is unable to manipulate them. The jacket restraint is also useful as a means for maintaining the child in a desired horizontal position. The long tapes, secured to the understructure of the crib, keep the child inside the crib.

Arm and Leg Restraints

Occasionally, the nurse needs to restrain one or more extremities or limit their motion. Several commercial restraining devices are available, including disposable wrist and ankle restraints (Fig. 22-6, *B*). Restraints must be appropriate to the child's size and padded to prevent undue pressure, constriction, or tissue injury; and the extremity must be observed frequently for signs of irritation or impaired circulation. The ends of the restraints are never tied to the side rails because lowering the rail will disturb the extremity, frequently with a jerk that may hurt or injure the child.

Elbow Restraint

Sometimes it is important to prevent the child from reaching the head or face (e.g., after lip surgery or when a scalp vein infusion is in place

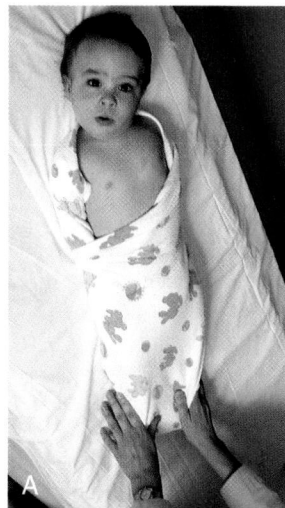

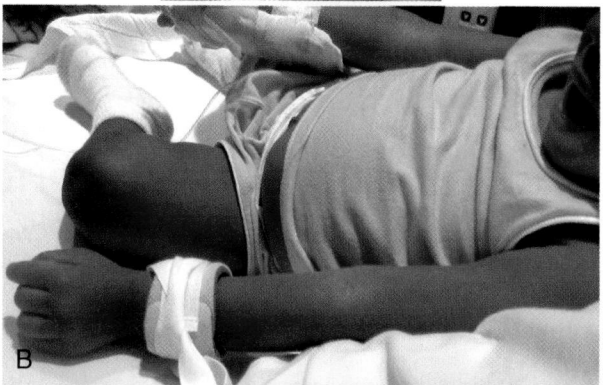

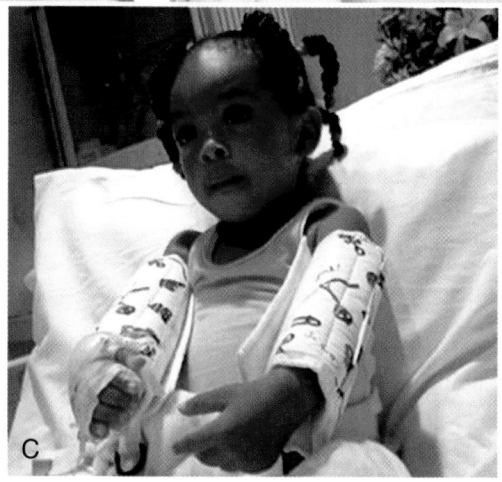

FIG 22-6 Restraint examples from most restrictive to least restrictive. **A,** Mummy restraint. **B,** Wrist restraints. **C,** Elbow restraints.

or to prevent scratching in skin disorders). Elbow restraints fashioned from a variety of materials function well (Fig. 22-6, *C*). Commercial elbow restraints are available. An improvised form of elbow restraint consists of a piece of muslin long enough to reach comfortably from just below the axilla to the wrist with a number of vertical pockets into which tongue depressors are inserted. The restraint is wrapped around the arm and secured with tapes or pins. It may be necessary to pin the top of the restraint to the undershirt sleeve to prevent the restraint from slipping.

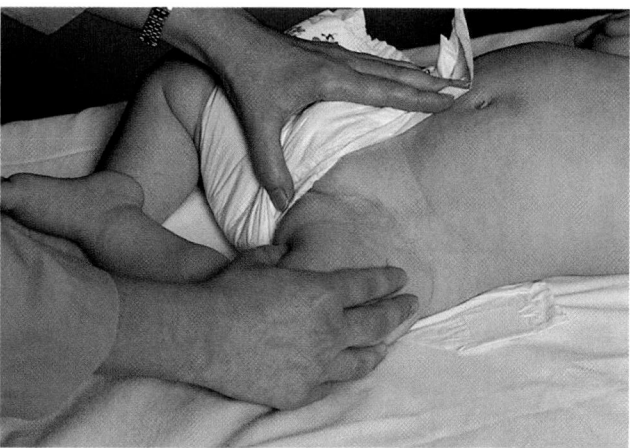

FIG 22-7 Positioning infant for femoral venipuncture.

POSITIONING FOR PROCEDURES

Infants and small children are unable to cooperate for many procedures. Therefore, the nurse is responsible for minimizing their movement and discomfort with proper positioning. Older children usually need only minimal, if any, restraint. Careful explanation and preparation beforehand and support and simple guidance during the procedure are usually sufficient. For painful procedures, the child should receive adequate analgesia and sedation to minimize pain and the need for excessive restraint. For local anesthesia, use buffered lidocaine to reduce the stinging sensation or a topical anesthetic. (See Pain Management, Chapter 7.)

FEMORAL VENIPUNCTURE

The nurse places the child supine with the legs in a frog position to provide extensive exposure of the groin area. The infant's legs can be effectively controlled by the nurse's forearms and hands (Fig. 22-7). Only the side used for the venipuncture is uncovered so that the practitioner is protected if the child urinates during the procedure. Apply pressure to the site to prevent oozing from the site.

EXTREMITY VENIPUNCTURE OR INJECTION

The most common sites of venipuncture are the veins of the extremities, especially the arm and hand. A convenient position is to place the child in the parent's (or assistant's) lap with the child facing the parent and in the straddle position. Next, place the child's arm for venipuncture on a firm surface, such as a treatment table. The nurse can partially stabilize the child's outstretched arm and have the parent hug the child's upper body, preventing movement; the nurse can then use the parent's arm to immobilize the venipuncture site. This type of restraint also comforts the child because of the close body contact and allows each person to maintain eye contact (Fig. 22-8).

LUMBAR PUNCTURE

Pediatric LP sets contain smaller spinal needles, but sometimes the practitioner will specify a different size or type of needle. The technique for LP in infants and children is similar to that in adults, although modifications are suggested in neonates, who have less distress in a side-lying position with modified neck extension than in flexion or a sitting position.

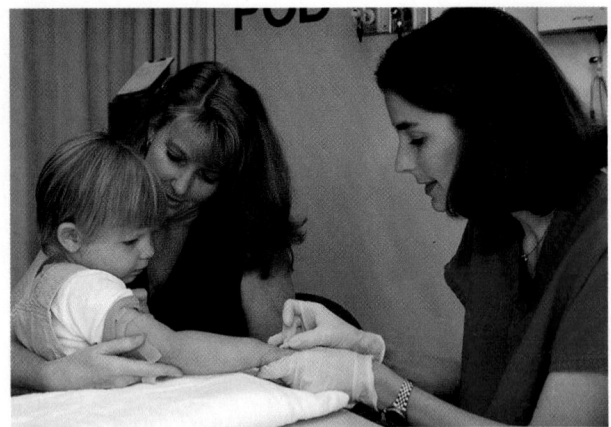

FIG 22-8 Therapeutic holding of child for extremity venipuncture with parental assistance.

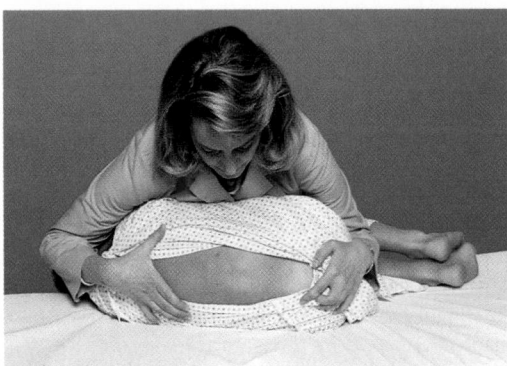

FIG 22-9 Side-lying position for lumbar puncture.

Children are usually easiest to control in the side-lying position, with the head flexed and the knees drawn up toward the chest. Even cooperative children need to be held gently to prevent possible trauma from unexpected, involuntary movement. They can be reassured that, although they are trusted, holding will serve as a reminder to maintain the desired position. It also provides a measure of support and reassurance to them.

A flexed sitting or side-lying position may be used, depending on the child's ability to cooperate and whether sedation will be used. In the sitting position with the hips flexed, the interspinous space is maximized (Abo, Chen, Johnston, and others, 2010). The child is placed with the buttocks at the edge of the table. The nurse's hands immobilize the infant's arms and legs. Neck flexion is not necessary (Fig. 22-9).

> **! NURSING ALERT**
>
> The sitting position may interfere with chest expansion and diaphragm excursion, and in infants the soft, pliable trachea may collapse. Therefore, observe the child for difficulty with breathing.

Specimens and spinal fluid pressure are obtained, measured, and sent for analysis in the same manner as for adult patients. Take vital signs as ordered and observe the child for any changes in level of consciousness, motor activity, and other neurologic signs. Post-LP headache may occur and is related to postural changes; this is less severe when the child lies flat. Headache is seen much less frequently in young children than in adolescents.

BONE MARROW ASPIRATION OR BIOPSY

The position for a bone marrow aspiration or biopsy depends on the chosen site. In children, the posterior or anterior iliac crest is most frequently used, but in infants, the tibia may be selected because it is easy to access the site and hold the child.

If the posterior iliac crest is used, the child is positioned prone. Sometimes a small pillow or folded blanket is placed under the hips to facilitate obtaining the bone marrow specimen. Children should receive adequate analgesia or anesthesia to relieve pain. If the child might awaken, he or she may need to be held, preferably by two people—one person to immobilize the upper body and a second person to immobilize the lower extremities.

▋ COLLECTION OF SPECIMENS

Many of the specimens needed for diagnostic examination of children are collected in much the same way as they are for adults. Older children are able to cooperate if given proper instruction regarding what is expected of them. Infants and small children, however, are unable to follow directions or control body functions sufficiently to help in collecting some specimens.

FUNDAMENTAL PROCEDURE STEPS COMMON TO ALL PROCEDURES

The following steps are very important for every procedure and should be considered fundamental aspects of care. These steps, although important, are not listed in each of the specimen collection procedures.

1. Assemble the necessary equipment.
2. Identify the child using two patient identifiers (e.g., patient name and medical record or birth date; neither can be a room number). Compare the same two identifiers with the specimen container and order.
3. Perform hand hygiene, maintain aseptic technique, and follow standard precautions.
4. Explain the procedure to parents and child according to the developmental level of the child; reassure the child that the procedure is not a punishment.
5. Provide atraumatic care and position the child securely.
6. Prepare area with antiseptic agent.
7. Place specimens in appropriate containers and apply a patient identification label to the specimen container in the presence of the child and family.
8. Discard puncture device in puncture-resistant container near the site of use.
9. Wash the procedural preparation agent off if povidone–iodine is used, if skin is sensitive, and for infants.
10. Remove gloves and perform hand hygiene after the procedure. Have children wash their hands if they have helped.
11. Praise the child for helping.
12. Document pertinent aspects of the procedure, such as number of attempts, site and amount of blood or urine withdrawn, as well as type of test performed.

URINE SPECIMENS

Older children and adolescents can use a bedpan or urinal or can be trusted to follow directions for collection in the bathroom. However, they may have special needs. School-age children are cooperative but curious. They are concerned about the reasons behind things and are likely to ask questions regarding the disposition of their specimen and what one expects to discover from it. Self-conscious adolescents may be reluctant to carry a specimen through a hallway or waiting room and appreciate a paper bag for disguising the container. The presence of menses may be an embarrassment or a concern to teenage girls; therefore, it is a good idea to ask them about this and make adjustments as necessary. The specimen can be delayed or a notation made on the laboratory slip to explain the presence of red blood cells.

Preschoolers and toddlers are usually unable to void on request. It is often best to offer them water or other liquids that they enjoy and wait about 30 minutes until they are ready to void voluntarily.

> **NURSING TIP** In infants, wipe the abdomen with an alcohol pad and fan it dry; the cooling effect often causes voiding within 2 minutes. Apply pressure over the suprapubic area or stroke the paraspinal muscles (along the spine) to elicit the Perez reflex; in infants 4 to 6 months of age, this reflex causes crying, extension of the back, flexion of the extremities, and urination.

Children will better understand what is expected if the nurse uses familiar terms, such as "pee-pee," "wee-wee," or "tinkle." Some have difficulty voiding in an unfamiliar receptacle. Potty chairs or a potty hat placed on the toilet is usually satisfactory. Toddlers who have recently acquired bladder control may be especially reluctant because they undoubtedly have been admonished for "going" in places other than those approved by parents. Enlisting the parents' help usually leads to success. For infants and toddlers who are not toilet trained, special urine collection bags with self-adhering material around the opening at the point of attachment are used. To prepare the infant, the genitalia, perineum, and surrounding skin are washed and dried thoroughly because the adhesive will not stick to a moist, powdered, or oily skin surface. The collection bag is easiest to apply if attached first to the perineum, progressing to the symphysis pubis (Fig. 22-10). With girls, the perineum is stretched taut during application to ensure a leakproof fit. With boys, the penis and sometimes the scrotum are placed inside the bag. The adhesive portion of the bag must be firmly applied to the skin all around the genital area to avoid leakage. The bag is checked frequently and removed as soon as the specimen is available because the moist bag may become loosened on an active child. For some types of urine testing, such as specific gravity, ketones, glucose, and protein, the nurse can aspirate urine directly from the diaper. If the urine is not tested within 30 minutes, the specimen is refrigerated or placed in a sterile container with a preservative. Superabsorbent disposable diapers may absorb all urine and may also produce a false crystalluria. Specific gravity measurements are accurate for up to

4 hours provided that the disposable diapers are kept folded. Urine samples collected by the cotton ball method were accurate for pH and specific gravity and were atraumatic to the skin of newborns (Burke, 1995).

> **NURSING TIP** When using a urine collection bag, cut a small slit in the diaper and pull the bag through to allow room for urine to collect and to facilitate checking on the contents. To obtain small amounts of urine, use a syringe without a needle to aspirate urine directly from the diaper. If diapers with absorbent gelling material that trap urine are used, place a small gauze dressing, some cotton balls, or a urine collection device inside the diaper to collect urine and aspirate the urine with a syringe.

At times, parents may be asked to bring a urine sample to a health care facility for examination, especially when infants are unable to void during an outpatient visit. In these instances, parents need instructions on applying the collection device and storing the specimen. Ideally, the specimen should be brought to the designated place as soon as possible. If there is a delay, the sample should be refrigerated and the lapsed time reported to the examiner.

Clean-Catch Specimens

Clean-catch specimen traditionally refers to a urine sample obtained for culture after the urethral meatus is cleaned and the first few milliliters of urine are voided (midstream specimen). In girls, the perineum is wiped with an antiseptic pad from front to back. In boys, the tip of the penis is cleansed.

Twenty-Four-Hour Collection

For a 24-hour collection, collection bags are required in infants and small children. Older children require special instruction about notifying someone when they need to void or have a bowel movement so that urine can be collected separately and is not discarded. Some older school-age children and adolescents can take responsibility for collection of their own 24-hour specimens and can keep output records and transfer each voiding to the 24-hour collection container.

The collection period always starts and ends with an empty bladder. At the time the collection begins, instruct the child to void and discard the specimen. All urine voided in the subsequent 24 hours is saved in a container with a preservative or is placed on ice. Twenty-four hours from the time the precollection specimen was discarded, the child is again instructed to void, the specimen is added to the container, and the entire collection is taken to the laboratory.

Infants and small children who are bagged for 24-hour urine collection require a special collection bag. Frequent removal and

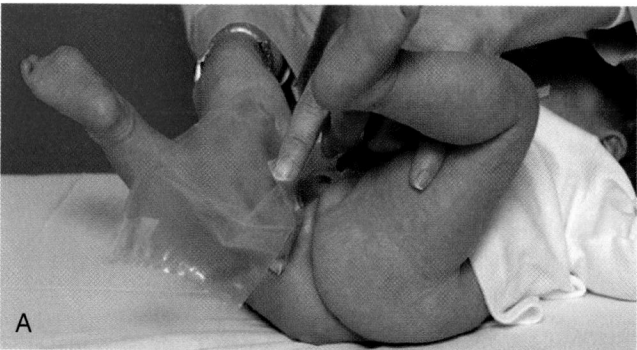
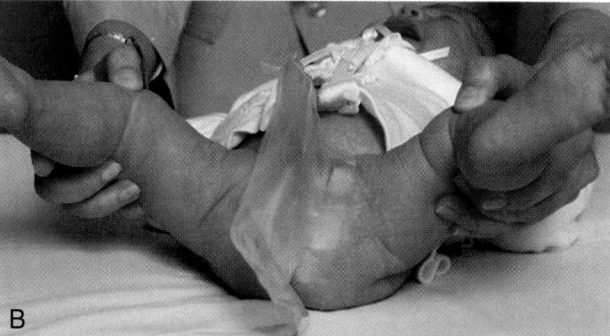

FIG 22-10 Application of urine collection bag. **A,** On female infants, the adhesive portion is applied to the exposed and dried perineum first. **B,** The nag adheres firmly around the perineal area to prevent urine leakage.

replacement of adhesive collection devices can produce skin irritation. A thin coating of sealant, such as Skin-Prep, applied to the skin helps to protect it and aids adhesion (unless its use is contraindicated, such as in premature infants or children with irritated skin). Plastic collection bags with collection tubes attached are ideal when the container must be left in place for a time. These can be connected to a collecting device or emptied periodically by aspiration with a syringe. When such devices are not available, a regular bag with a feeding tube inserted through a puncture hole at the top of the bag serves as a satisfactory substitute. However, take care to empty the bag as soon as the infant urinates to prevent leakage and loss of contents. An indwelling catheter may also be placed for the collection period.

Bladder Catheterization and Other Techniques

Bladder catheterization or suprapubic aspiration is used when a specimen is urgently needed or a child is unable to void or otherwise provide an adequate specimen. In infants younger than 3 months of age who are febrile, urine specimens should be collected by bladder catheterization (McGillivray, Mok, Mulrooney, and others, 2008). The AAP recommends that urine collected by the bag can be used to determine whether it is necessary to obtain a catheterized urine specimen for culture (Wald, 2005).

Preparation for catheterization includes instruction on pelvic muscle relaxation whenever possible. The toddler, preschooler, or younger child should blow on a pinwheel and press the hips against the bed or procedure table during catheterization to relax the pelvic and periurethral muscles. The nurse describes the location and function of the pelvic muscles briefly to the older child or adolescent. The patient then contracts and relaxes the pelvic muscles, and the relaxation procedure is repeated during catheter insertion. If the patient vigorously contracts the pelvic muscles when the catheter reaches the striated sphincter (proximal urethra in boys and midurethra in girls), catheter insertion is temporarily stopped. The catheter is neither removed nor advanced; instead, the child is helped to press the hips against the bed or examining table and relax the pelvic muscles. The catheter is then gently advanced into the bladder (Gray, 1996).

Catheterization is a sterile procedure, and standard precautions for body substance protection should be followed. If the catheter is to remain in place, a Foley catheter is used. Table 22-5 gives guidelines for choosing the appropriate-size catheter and length of insertion. The supplies needed for this procedure include sterile gloves, sterile lubricant anesthetic, the appropriate-size catheter, povidone–iodine (Betadine) swabs or an alternative cleansing agent and 4 × 4-inch gauze squares, a sterile drape, and a syringe with sterile water if a Foley catheter is used. Test the balloon of the Foley catheter by injecting sterile water before catheter insertion.

Adolescent boys and children with a history of urethral surgery may be catheterized with a coudé-tipped catheter. Children with myelodysplasia and those who have been identified as being sensitive or allergic to latex are catheterized with catheters manufactured from an alternative material. When an indwelling catheter is indicated for urinary drainage, a lubricious-coated or silicone catheter is selected because these materials produce less irritation of the urethral mucosa compared with Silastic or latex catheters when left in place for more than 72 hours.

A 2% lidocaine lubricant with applicator is assembled according to the manufacturer's instructions, and several drops of the lubricant are placed at the meatus. The child is advised that the lubricant is used to reduce any discomfort associated with inserting the catheter and that introduction of the catheter into the urethra will produce a sensation of pressure and a desire to urinate (Gray, 1996) (see Evidence-Based Practice box).

In male patients, grasp the penis with the nondominant hand and retract the foreskin. In uncircumcised newborns and infants, the foreskin may be adhered to the shaft; use care when retracting. If the penis is pendulous, place a sterile drape under the penis. Using the sterile hand, swab the glans and meatus three times with povidone–iodine. Gently introduce the tip of the lidocaine jelly applicator into the urethra 1 to 2 cm (0.4–0.8 inch) so that the lubricant flows only into the urethra; insert 5 to 10 ml 2% lidocaine lubricant into the urethra and hold it in place for 2 to 3 minutes by gently squeezing the distal penis. Lubricate the catheter and insert it into the urethra while gently stretching the penis and lifting it to a 90-degree angle to the body. Resistance may occur when the catheter meets the urethral sphincter. Ask the patient to inhale deeply and advance the catheter. Do not force a catheter that does not easily enter the meatus, particularly if the child has had corrective surgery. For indwelling catheters, after urine is obtained, advance the catheter to the hub, inflate the balloon with sterile water, pull it back gently to test inflation, and connect it to the closed drainage system. Cleanse the glans and meatus and replace retracted foreskin. If blood is seen at any time during the procedure, discontinue the procedure and notify the practitioner.

In female patients, place a sterile drape under the buttocks. Use the nondominant hand to gently separate and pull up the labia minora to visualize the meatus. Swab the meatus from front to back three times using a different povidone–iodine swab each time. Place 1 to 2 ml 2% lidocaine lubricant on the periurethral mucosa and insert the lubricant 1 to 2 ml into the urethral meatus. Delay catheterization for 2 to 3 minutes to maximize absorption of the anesthetic into the periurethral and intraurethral mucosa. Add lubricant to the catheter and gently insert it into the urethra until urine returns; then advance the catheter an additional 2.5 to 5 cm (1–2 inches). When using an indwelling Foley catheter, inflate the balloon with sterile water and gently pull back; then connect to a closed drainage system. Cleanse the meatus and labia (see Cultural Considerations box). Because the use of lidocaine jelly can increase the volume of intraurethral lubricant, urine return may not be as rapid as when minimal lubrication is used.

TABLE 22-5	STRAIGHT CATHETER OR FOLEY CATHETER*	
	SIZE (LENGTH OF INSERTION [CM]) FOR GIRLS	**SIZE (LENGTH OF INSERTION [CM]) FOR BOYS**
Term neonate	5–6 (5)	5–6 (6)
Infant–3 yr	5–8 (5)	5–8 (6)
4–8 yr	8 (5–6)	8 (6–9)
8 yr–prepubertal	10–12 (6–8)	8–10 (10–15)
Pubertal	12–14 (6–8)	12–14 (13–18)

*Foley catheters are approximately 1 Fr size larger because of the circumference of the balloon. Example: 10-Fr Foley catheter = ≈12-Fr calibration.

⚡ SAFETY ALERT

Do not advance the catheter too far into the bladder. Knotting of catheters and tubes within the bladder has been reported in several case studies. Feeding tubes should not be used for urinary catheterization because they are more flexible, longer, and prone to knotting compared with commercially designed urinary catheters (Foster, Ritchey, and Bloom, 1992; Gonzalez and Palmer, 1997; Kilbane, 2009; Levison and Wojtulewicz, 2004; Lodha, Ly, Brindle, and others, 2005; Turner, 2004).

EVIDENCE-BASED PRACTICE

The Use of Lidocaine Lubricant for Urethral Catheterization

Ask the Question

Picot Question

In children, does a lidocaine lubricant decrease the pain associated with urethral catheterization?

Search for the Evidence

Search Strategies

Search selection criteria included English-language publications, research-based studies, and review articles on use of the lidocaine lubricant before urethral catheterization.

Databases Used

Cochrane Collaboration, PubMed, MD Consult, BestBETs, American Academy of Pediatrics

Critically Analyze the Evidence

- Smith and Adams (1998) surveyed 46 children's hospitals to determine the existence of standardized practice guidelines for urethral catheter insertion in children. Only 54% of the institutions had a written policy providing guidelines for the procedure, and practices had wide variations.
- Gray (1996) published a review of strategies to minimize distress associated with urethral catheterization in children and supported intraurethral instillation of a local anesthetic that contains 2% lidocaine before catheter insertion.
- One prospective, double-blind, placebo-controlled trial evaluated the use of lidocaine lubricant for discomfort in 20 children before urethral catheterization. Lidocaine lubricant instilled into the urethra significantly reduced pain and distress during urethral catheterization (Gerard, Cooper, Duethman, and others, 2003).
- A placebo-controlled, double-blind, randomized controlled trial of 115 children younger than 2 years of age found no significant difference when 2% lidocaine gel was compared with a nonanesthetic lubricant. The lubricant was applied to the genital mucosa for 2 to 3 minutes and liberally applied to the catheter but not instilled into the urethra (Vaughn, Paton, Bush, and others, 2005).

Apply the Evidence: Nursing Implications

There is **moderate-quality evidence** with a **weak recommendation** (Guyatt, Oxman, Vist, and others, 2008) for using a lidocaine lubricant to decrease pain associated with urethral catheterization

Although only one published research study was found to support the use of anesthetic before urethral catheterization, the study found significant reductions in procedural pain. Several publications support its effectiveness in clinical practice. Transurethral instillation of 2% lidocaine gel before urethral catheterization may be considered.

QSEN **Quality and Safety Competencies: Evidence-Based Practice***

Knowledge

Differentiate clinical opinion from research and evidence-based summaries.

Describe use of buffered lidocaine for pain reduction during urethral catheterization.

Skills

Base individualized care plan on patient values, clinical expertise, and evidence.

Integrate evidence into practice by using buffered lidocaine for pain reduction during urethral catheterization in children.

Attitudes

Value the concept of evidence-based practice as integral to determining best clinical practice.

Appreciate the strengths and weakness of evidence for using buffered lidocaine for pain reduction during urethral catheterization in children.

References

Gerard LL, Cooper CS, Duethman KS, and others: Effectiveness of lidocaine lubricant for discomfort during pediatric urethral catheterization, *J Urol* 170:564–567, 2003.

Gray M: Atraumatic urethral catheterization of children, *Pediatr Nurs* 22(4):306–310, 1996.

Guyatt GH, Oxman AD, Vist GE, and others: GRADE: an emerging consensus on rating quality of evidence and strength of recommendations, *BMJ* 336:924–926, 2008.

Smith AB, Adams LL: Insertion of indwelling urethral catheters in infants and children: a survey of current nursing practice, *Pediatr Nurs* 24(3):229–234, 1998.

Vaughn H, Paton EA, Bush A, and others: Does lidocaine gel alleviate the pain of bladder catheterization in young children? A randomized, controlled trial, *Pediatrics* 116(4):917–920, 2005.

*Adapted from the QSEN at http://www.qsen.org.

⊕ CULTURAL CONSIDERATIONS

Bladder Catheterization

Parents may be upset when their child is catheterized. Aside from the trauma the child experiences, some parents may fear that the procedure affects the daughter's virginity. To correct this misconception, the family may benefit from a detailed explanation of the genitourinary anatomy, preferably with a model that shows the separate vaginal and urethral openings. The nurse can also indicate that catheterization has no effect on virginity.

Suprapubic aspiration is mainly used when the bladder cannot be accessed through the urethra (e.g., with some congenital urologic birth defects) or to reduce the risk of contamination that may be present when passing a catheter. With the advent of small catheters (5- and 6-French straight catheters), the need for suprapubic aspiration has decreased. Access to the bladder via the urethra has a much higher success rate than suprapubic aspiration, in which success depends on the practitioner's skill at assessing the location of the bladder and the amount of urine in the bladder.

Suprapubic aspiration involves aspirating bladder contents by inserting a 20- or 21-gauge needle in the midline approximately 1 cm (0.4 inch) above the symphysis pubis and directed vertically downward. The nurse prepares the skin as for any needle insertion, and the bladder should contain an adequate volume of urine. This can be

ATRAUMATIC CARE

Bladder Catheterization or Suprapubic Aspiration

- Use distraction to help the child relax (e.g., blowing bubbles, deep breathing, singing a song).
- Use lidocaine jelly to anesthetize the area before insertion of the catheter. EMLA cream (a eutectic mix of lidocaine and prilocaine) or LMX cream (lidocaine) may lessen an infant's discomfort as the needle passes through the skin for suprapubic aspiration, but care should be taken that the site is thoroughly cleaned and prepped before the procedure.
- Children often become agitated at being restrained for either procedure. Use comfort measures through touch and voice, both during and after the procedure, to help reduce the child's distress.

assumed if the infant has not voided for at least 1 hour or the bladder can be palpated above the symphysis pubis. This technique is useful for obtaining sterile specimens from young infants because the bladder is an abdominal organ and is easily accessed. Suprapubic aspiration is painful; therefore, pain management during the procedure is important (see Atraumatic Care box).

STOOL SPECIMENS

Stool specimens are frequently collected from children to identify parasites and other organisms that cause diarrhea, assess gastrointestinal function, and check for occult (hidden) blood. Ideally, stool should be collected without contamination with urine, but in children wearing diapers, this is difficult unless a urine bag is applied. Children who are toilet trained should urinate first, flush the toilet, and then defecate into the toilet or a bedpan (preferably one that is placed on the toilet to avoid embarrassment) or a commercial potty hat.

> **NURSING TIP** To obtain a stool specimen, place plastic wrap over the toilet bowl before defecation. Use a tongue depressor or disposable spoon or knife to collect the stool.

Stool specimens should be large enough to obtain an ample sampling, not merely a fecal fragment. Specimens are placed in an appropriate container, which is covered and labeled. If several specimens are needed, mark the containers with the date and time and keep them in a specimen refrigerator. Exercise care in handling the specimen because of the risk of contamination.

BLOOD SPECIMENS

Whether the specimen is collected by the nurse or by others, the nurse is responsible for making certain that specimens, such as serial examinations and fasting specimens, are collected on time and that the proper equipment is available. Collecting, transporting, and storing specimens can have a major impact on laboratory results.

Venous blood samples can be obtained by venipuncture or by aspiration from a peripheral or central access device. Withdrawing blood specimens through peripheral lock devices in small peripheral veins has varying degrees of success. Although it avoids an additional venipuncture for the child, attempting to aspirate blood from the peripheral lock may shorten the life of the device. However, the nurse can use central lines to withdraw blood samples (see Evidence-Based Practice box and Atraumatic Care box, p. 664). When using an IV

infusion site for specimen collection, consider the type of fluid being infused. For example, a specimen collected for glucose determination would be inaccurate if removed from a catheter through which glucose-containing solution was being administered.

The needed specimens are quickly collected, and pressure is applied to the puncture site with dry gauze until bleeding stops. The arm should be extended, not flexed, while pressure is applied for a few minutes after venipuncture in the antecubital fossa to reduce bruising. The nurse then covers the site with an adhesive bandage. In young children, adhesive bandages pose an aspiration hazard, so avoid using them or remove the adhesive bandage as soon as the bleeding stops. Applying warm compresses to ecchymotic areas increases circulation, helps remove extravasated blood, and decreases pain.

Arterial blood samples are sometimes needed for blood gas measurement, although noninvasive techniques, such as transcutaneous oxygen monitoring and pulse oximetry, are used frequently. Arterial samples may be obtained by arterial puncture using the radial, brachial, or femoral arteries or from indwelling arterial catheters. Assess adequate circulation before arterial puncture by observing capillary refill or performing the **Allen test**, a procedure that assesses the circulation of the radial, ulnar, or brachial arteries. Because unclotted blood is required, use only heparinized collection tubes or syringes. In addition, no air bubbles should enter the tube because they can alter blood gas concentration. Crying, fear, and agitation affect blood gas values; therefore, make every effort to comfort the child. Pack the blood samples in ice to reduce blood cell metabolism and take it to the laboratory immediately.

> **NURSING TIP** To obtain a blood specimen from a central venous line or peripheral lock when the infusion solution may interfere with the test results, first aspirate a quantity of blood equal to the volume of fluid in the catheter and discard and then aspirate the blood sample. For a blood culture, use the first sample of blood because organisms are most likely to collect within the catheter itself.

Take capillary blood samples from children by finger stick. A common method for taking peripheral blood samples from infants younger than 6 months of age is by a heel stick. Before the blood sample is taken, warm the heel for 3 minutes and cleanse the area with alcohol. Holding the infant's foot firmly with the free hand, the nurse then punctures the heel with an automatic lancet device. An automatic device delivers a more precise puncture depth and is less painful than using a lance (Vertanen, Fellman, Brommels, and others, 2001). A surgical blade of any kind is contraindicated. An example of a safe device is the BD Quickheel Safety Lancet. The Tenderfoot Preemie device* was compared with the Monolet lancet and was found to be safer than the lancet and required fewer heel punctures, less collection time, and lower recollection rates (Kellam, Sacks, Wailer, and others, 2001). Shepherd, Glenesk, Niven, and others (2005) reported that the Tenderfoot device was more effective and safer than a lancet for newborn screening tests. Although obtaining capillary blood gases is a common practice, these measures may not accurately reflect arterial values.

The most serious complications of infant heel puncture are necrotizing osteochondritis from lancet penetration of the underlying

---

*The Tenderfoot Preemie device is manufactured by ITC, Edison, NJ; http://www.itcmed.com/tenderfoot.shtml.

EVIDENCE-BASED PRACTICE

Obtaining Blood Specimens from Central Venous Catheters in Children

Joy Hesselgrave; updated by Olga A. Taylor

Ask the Question
Picot Question
In children, do blood specimens obtained from central venous catheters using the discard, reinfusion, or push–pull method yield more accurate samples?

Search for the Evidence
Search Strategies
Search selection criteria included English-language research-based publications within the past 15 years on pediatric blood specimen collection from central venous access.

Databases Used
National Guideline Clearinghouse (AHRQ), Cochrane Collaboration, Joanna Briggs Institute, PubMed, TRIP database Plus, MD Consult, PedsCCM, BestBETs

Critically Analyze the Evidence
- Benefits of sampling blood from central venous access devices (CVADs) include a decrease in anxiety, discomfort, and dissatisfaction for patients that is associated with venipuncture (Infusion Nurses Society, 2011).
- Risks of sampling blood from CVAD include catheter-related bloodstream infection and occlusion (Infusion Nurses Society, 2011).
- Questionable drug levels in samples obtained from CVADs have been reported. Retesting using venipuncture should be considered (Infusion Nurses Society, 2011; Mogayzel, Pierce, Mills, and others, 2008, Wright, Al-Sallami, Jackson, and others, 2010).
- The push–pull method eliminates loss of blood and decreases the amount of times the central line is accessed (Barton, Chase, Latham, and others, 2004).
- In nonneutropenic pediatric patients (2–20 years old), discard specimen, routinely reinfused, was collected using the usual clean procedure and an exaggerated unclean alternative procedure. Neither the sterile specimens nor the unclean specimens grew organisms, suggesting that the reinfusion of the blood specimen would be safe. Clots in the discard specimen were not evaluated (Hinds, Wentz, Hughes, and others, 1991).
- Thirty bone marrow transplant units were surveyed to evaluate how blood samples were drawn from CVADs. The patient age range was 5 to 16 years. A total of 75% units used the discard method (volume of discard, 0.5–10 ml; average, 4–6 ml), 14% used the reinfusion method, and 11% used the push–pull or mixing method (Keller, 1994).
- The discard method should be used when drawing blood samples from CVADs. The discard volume should be 1.5 to 2 times the fill volume of the CVAD (Infusion Nurses Society, 2011).
- The discard method is most widely reported, with disadvantages including blood loss, blood exposure risk for clinicians, and the potential to confuse the discard specimen for the blood sample (Frey, 2003).
- When obtaining blood from CVADs, discarding blood is not necessary for obtaining accurate laboratory results (Adlard, 2008).
- The reinfusion method does not deplete blood volume but risks blood exposure for clinicians and the potential to reinfuse a contaminated specimen or clots in the discard volume (Frey, 2003).
- The incidence of hemolysis, hemodilution, and bloodstream infections did not increase with the push–pull method (Adlard, 2008).
- Push–pull or mixing method demonstrates accuracy for other than coagulation and drug levels and reduces blood loss and clinician exposure risk (Frey, 2003).

Apply the Evidence: Nursing Implications
There is **moderate-quality evidence** with a **strong recommendation** (Guyatt, Oxman, Vist, and others, 2008) for obtaining blood specimens from central venous catheters in children. There is limited pediatric research that clearly supports any particular central line blood sampling method as being superior. All three methods yield accurate results and appear safe. The discard method is the most frequently reported in the literature and benchmarking. However, if there is a concern about blood volume, the push–pull or reinfusion method should be considered. If the catheter has multiple lumens, use the distal lumen for laboratory specimen collection. Infusions should be stopped and lumens clamped before blood sampling. Cleanse the injection cap with antiseptic agent and allow it to dry before drawing laboratory specimens. Attach a syringe or stopcock (depending on specimen method selected) to the injection cap, not directly to the catheter hub. The injection cap at the catheter hub should be removed only if blood cultures are drawn.

QSEN Quality and Safety Competencies: Evidence-Based Practice*
Knowledge
Differentiate clinical opinion from research and evidence-based summaries.

Describe methods for obtaining blood specimens from central venous catheters in children.

Skills
Base individualized care plan on patient values, clinical expertise, and evidence.

Integrate evidence into practice by using appropriate technique when obtaining blood specimens from central venous catheters in children.

Attitudes
Value the concept of evidence-based practice as integral to determining best clinical practice.

Appreciate the strengths and weakness of evidence for obtaining blood specimens from central venous catheters in children.

References
Adlard K: Examining the push–pull method of blood sampling from central venous access devices, *J Pediatr Oncol Nurs* 25(4):200–207, 2008.

Barton S, Chase T, Latham B, and others: Comparing two methods to obtain blood specimens from pediatric central venous catheters, *J Pediatr Oncol Nurs* 21(6):320–326, 2004.

Frey M: Drawing blood samples from vascular access devices, *J Infus Nurs* 26(5):285–293, 2003.

Guyatt GH, Oxman AD, Vist GE, and others: GRADE: An emerging consensus on rating quality of evidence and strength of recommendations, *BMJ* 336(7650):924–926, 2008.

Hinds PS, Wentz T, Hughes W, and others: An investigation of the safety of the blood reinfusion step used with tunneled venous access devices in children with cancer, *J Pediatr Oncol Nurs* 8(4):59–64, 1991.

Infusion Nurses Society: Infusion nursing standards of practice, *J Infus Nurs* 34(1S):S63–S64, 2011.

Keller CA: Methods of drawing blood samples through central venous catheters in pediatric patients undergoing bone marrow transplant: results of a national survey, *Oncol Nurs Forum* 21(5):879–884, 1994.

Mogayzel PJ, Pierce E, Mills J, and others: Accuracy of tobramycin levels obtained from central venous access devices in patients with cystic fibrosis is technique dependent, *Pediatr Nurs* 34(6):464–467, 2008.

Wright DFB, Al-Sallami HS, Jackson PM, and others: Falsely elevated vancomycin plasma concentrations sampled from central venous implantable catheters (portacaths), *Br J Clin Pharmacol* 70(5):769–772, 2010.

*Adapted from the QSEN at http://www.qsen.org.

Guidelines for Skin and Vessel Punctures

To reduce the pain associated with heel, finger, venous, or arterial punctures:

- Apply EMLA (a eutectic mix of lidocaine and prilocaine) topically over the site if time permits (>60 minutes). LMX cream (lidocaine) also may be used and requires a shorter application time (30 minutes). To remove the transparent dressing atraumatically, grasp opposite sides of the film and pull the sides away from each other to stretch and loosen the film. After the film begins to loosen, grasp the other two sides of the film and pull. Use iontophoresis (Numby Stuff) over the site if time permits (8–20 minutes, depending on the amount of current), a vapocoolant spray, or buffered lidocaine (injected intradermally near the vein with a 30-gauge needle) to numb the skin.
- Use nonpharmacologic methods of pain and anxiety control (e.g., ask the child to take a deep breath when the needle is inserted and again when the needle is withdrawn, to exhale a large breath or blow bubbles to "blow hurt away," or to count slowly and then faster and louder if pain is felt).
- Keep all equipment out of sight until used.
- Enlist parents' presence or assistance if they wish.
- Restrain child *only as needed* to perform the procedure safely; use therapeutic holding (p. 655).
- Allow the skin preparation to dry completely before penetrating the skin.
- Use the smallest gauge needle (e.g., 25 gauge) that permits free flow of blood; a 27-gauge needle can be used for obtaining 1 to 1.5 ml of blood and for prominent veins (needle length is only 1.25 cm [0.5 inch]).
- If possible, avoid putting an IV line in the dominant hand or the hand the child uses to suck the thumb.
- Use an automatic lancet device for precise puncture depth of the finger or heel; press the device lightly against the skin; avoid steadying the finger against a hard surface.
- Have a "two-try" only policy to reduce excessive insertion attempts—two operators each have two insertion attempts. If insertion is not successful after four punctures, consider alternative venous access, such as a PICC; have

a policy for identifying children with difficult access and appropriate interventions (e.g., most experienced operator for the first attempt, use transilluminator or ultrasonography for insertion guidance).

For Multiple Blood Samples

- Use an intermittent infusion device (saline lock) to collect additional samples from an existing IV line; consider PICC lines early, not as a last resort.
- Coordinate care to allow several tests to be performed on one blood sample using micromethods of testing.
- Anticipate tests (e.g., drug levels, chemistry, immunoglobulin levels) and ask the laboratory to save blood for additional testing.

For Heel Lancing in Newborns

- Heel lancing has shown to be more painful than venipuncture (Shah and Ohlsson, 2007); consider venipuncture when the amount of blood from the heel would require much squeezing (e.g., genetic screening tests).
- The effectiveness of EMLA is controversial, although application of 0.5 g for 30 minutes four times a day in preterm infants was found to be safe (Essink-Tebbes, Wuis, Liem, and others, 1999).
- Place diapered newborn against mother's bare chest in skin-to-skin contact 10 to 15 minutes before and during heel lance (Gray, Watt, and Blass, 2000).
- During the procedure, administer sucrose and encourage the newborn to suck a pacifier. When commercially manufactured 24% sucrose solution is unavailable, add 1 tsp of table sugar to 20 ml of sterile water. Use this solution to coat the pacifier or administer 2 ml to the tongue 2 minutes before the procedure. (See Evidence-Based Practice Box, Reduction of Minor Procedural Pain in Infants, Chapter 7.)
- One study found that breastfeeding during a neonatal heel lance was more effective than sucrose in reducing pain (Codipietro, Ceccarelli, and Ponzone, 2008).

IV, Intravenous; *PICC,* peripherally inserted central catheter.

calcaneus bone, infection, and abscess of the heel. To avoid osteochondritis, the puncture should be no deeper than 2 mm and should be made at the outer aspect of the heel. The boundaries of the calcaneus can be marked by an imaginary line extending posteriorly from a point between the fourth and fifth toes and running parallel with the lateral aspect of the heel and another line extending posteriorly from the middle of the great toe and running parallel with the medial aspect of the heel (Fig. 22-11). Repeated trauma to the walking surface of the heel can cause fibrosis and scarring that may interfere with locomotion.

No matter how or by whom the specimen is collected, children, even some older ones, fear the loss of their blood. This is particularly true for children whose condition requires frequent blood specimens. They mistakenly believe that blood removed from their body is a threat to their lives. Explaining to them that their body continuously produces blood provides them a measure of reassurance. When the blood is drawn, a comment such as, "Just look how red it is. You're really making a lot of nice red blood," confirms this information and affords them an opportunity to express their concern. An adhesive bandage gives them added assurance that the vital fluids will not leak out through the puncture site.

Children also dislike the discomfort associated with venous, arterial, and capillary punctures. Children have identified these procedures as the ones most frequently causing pain during hospitalization and an arterial puncture as being one of the most painful of all procedures

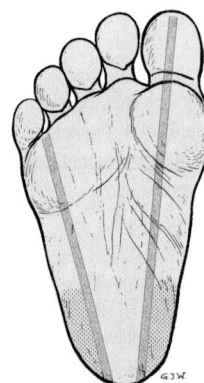

FIG 22-11 Puncture site (colored stippled area) on the sole of an infant's foot.

experienced. Toddlers are most distressed by venipuncture followed by school-age children and then adolescents. Consequently, nurses need to institute pain reduction techniques to lessen the discomfort of these procedures. (See Pain Management, Chapter 7.)

RESPIRATORY SECRETION SPECIMENS

Collection of sputum or nasal discharge is sometimes required for the diagnosis of respiratory infections, especially tuberculosis and respiratory syncytial virus (RSV). Older children and adolescents are able to cough as directed and supply sputum specimens when given proper directions. The nurse must make it clear to them that a coughed specimen, not mucus cleared from the throat, is needed. It is helpful to demonstrate a deep cough. Infants and small children are unable to follow directions to cough and will swallow any sputum produced; therefore, gastric washings (lavage) may be used to collect a sputum specimen. Sometimes a satisfactory specimen can be obtained using a suction device such as a mucus trap if the catheter is inserted into the trachea and the cough reflex elicited. A catheter inserted into the back of the throat is not sufficient. For children with a tracheostomy, a specimen is easily aspirated from the trachea or major bronchi by attaching a collecting device to the suction apparatus.

Nasal washings are usually obtained to diagnose an infection of RSV. The child is placed supine, and 1 to 3 ml of sterile normal saline is instilled with a sterile syringe (without needle) into one nostril. The contents are aspirated using a small, sterile bulb syringe and are placed in a sterile container. Another method uses a syringe with 5 cm (2 inches) of 18- to 20-gauge tubing. The saline is quickly instilled and then aspirated to recover the nasal specimen. To prevent any additional discomfort, all of the equipment should be ready before beginning the procedure.

Other respiratory secretion collection methods include naso-pharyngeal swabs to diagnose *Bordetella* pertussis and throat cultures. The nurse swabs both the tonsils and the posterior pharynx when obtaining a throat culture. The swab stick is inserted into the culture tube. Some culture kits require squeezing an ampule to release the culture medium.

ADMINISTRATION OF MEDICATION

DETERMINATION OF DRUG DOSAGE

Nurses must have an understanding of the safe dosages of medications they administer to children, as well as the expected actions, possible side effects, and signs of toxicity. Unlike with adult medications, there are few standardized pediatric dosage ranges, and with a few exceptions, drugs are prepared and packaged in average adult-dosage strengths.

Factors related to growth and maturation significantly alter an individual's capacity to metabolize and excrete drugs. Immaturity or defects in any of the important processes of absorption, distribution, biotransformation, or excretion can significantly alter the effects of a drug. Newborn and premature infants with immature enzyme systems in the liver (where most drugs are broken down and detoxified), lower plasma concentrations of protein for binding with drugs, and immaturely functioning kidneys (where most drugs are excreted) are particularly vulnerable to the harmful effects of drugs. Beyond the newborn period, many drugs are metabolized more rapidly by the liver, necessitating larger doses or more frequent administration. This is particularly important in pain control, when the dosage of analgesics may need to be increased or the interval between doses decreased.

Various formulas involving age, weight, and body surface area (BSA) as the basis for calculations have been devised to determine children's drug dosages. Because the administration of medication is a nursing responsibility, nurses need to have not only knowledge of drug action and patient responses but also resources for estimating safe dosages for children. Children's dosages are most often expressed in units of measure per body weight (mg/kg). Some medications, such as chemotherapy, are more precisely dosed using BSA. The ratio of BSA to weight varies inversely with length; therefore, an infant who is shorter and weighs less than an older child or adult has relatively more BSA than would be expected from the weight. BSA is based on the West nomogram and is easily determined using conversion programs widely available on the Internet.

Checking Dosage

Administering the correct dosage of a drug is a shared responsibility between the practitioner who orders the drug and the nurse who carries out that order. Children react with unexpected severity to some drugs, and ill children may be especially sensitive to drugs. When a dose is ordered that is outside the usual range or when there is some question regarding the preparation or the route of administration, the nurse should check with the prescribing practitioner before proceeding with the administration because the nurse is legally liable for any drug administered.

Even when it has been determined that the dosage is correct for a particular child, many drugs are potentially hazardous or lethal. Most facilities have regulations requiring specified drugs to be double checked by another nurse before giving them to the child. Among drugs that require such safeguards are antiarrhythmics, anticoagulants, chemotherapeutic agents, and insulin. Others frequently included are epinephrine, opioids, and sedatives. Even if this precaution is not mandatory, nurses are wise to take such precautions. Errors in decimal point placement may occur and may result in a 10-fold or greater dosage error.

Identification

Before the administration of any medication, the child must be correctly identified using two identifiers (e.g., name and medical record number or birth date). With an infant, young child, or nonverbal child, the parent or guardian (if present) can verify the child's identity. After verbal verification of the child's identity (by the parent, guardian, or child), the identification (ID) band should be verified using two identifiers. Bedside computers to scan the ID bracelet for electronic record updating may also be used.

Preparing the Parents

Nearly all parents have given some type of medication to their child and can describe the approaches they have found successful. In some cases, it is less traumatic for the child if a parent gives the medication, provided that the nurse prepares the medication and supervises its administration. Children being given daily medications at home are accustomed to the parent's functioning in this capacity and are less likely to fuss than if a stranger administers the medication. Individual decisions need to be made regarding parental presence and participation, such as holding the child during injections.

Preparing the Child

Every child requires psychologic preparation for parenteral administration of medication and supportive care during the procedure (see p. 637). Even if children have received several injections, they rarely become accustomed to the discomfort and have as much right as any other child to understanding and patience from those giving the injection.

ORAL ADMINISTRATION

The oral route is preferred for administering medications to children because of the ease of administration. Most medications are dissolved or suspended in liquid preparations. Although some children are able to swallow or chew solid medications at an early age, solid preparations

ATRAUMATIC CARE

Encouraging a Child's Acceptance of Oral Medication

- Give the child a flavored ice pop or small ice cube to suck to numb the tongue before giving the drug.
- Mix the drug with a small amount (≈1 tsp) of sweet-tasting substance, such as honey (except in infants because of the risk of botulism), flavored syrups, jam, fruit purees, sherbet, or ice cream; avoid essential food items because the child may later refuse to eat them.
- Give a "chaser" of water, juice, soft drink, or ice pop or frozen juice bar after the drug.
- If nausea is a problem, give a carbonated beverage poured over finely crushed ice before or immediately after the medication.
- When medication has an unpleasant taste, have the child pinch the nose and drink the medicine through a straw. Much of what we taste is associated with smell.
- Flavorings such as apple, banana, and bubble gum (e.g., FLAVORx) can be added at many pharmacies at nominal additional cost. An alternative is to have the pharmacist prepare the drug in a flavored, chewable troche or lozenge.*
- Infants will suck medicine from a needleless syringe or dropper in small increments (0.25–0.5 ml) at a time. Use a nipple or special pacifier with a reservoir for the drug.

*For information about compounding drugs, contact Technical Staff, Professional Compounding Centers of America, 9901 S. Wilcrest Drive, Houston, TX 77099; 800-331-2498; http://www.pccarx.com.

are not recommended for young children because of the danger of aspiration.

Most pediatric medications come in palatable and colorful preparations for added ease of administration. Some have a slightly unpleasant aftertaste, but most children swallow these liquids with little, if any, resistance. Complaints of dislike from the child can be accepted and the taste camouflaged whenever possible. Most pediatric units have preparations available for this purpose (see Atraumatic Care box).

Preparation

The devices available to measure medicines are not always sufficiently accurate for measuring the small amounts needed in pediatric nursing practice. Molded plastic cups offer reasonable accuracy in measuring moderate doses of liquids; paper cups, on the other hand, are likely to have irregularly shaped or crumpled bottoms and retain considerable amounts of thick medication. Measures less than 1 tsp are impossible to determine accurately with a medicine cup.

The teaspoon is an inaccurate measuring device and is subject to error. Teaspoons vary greatly in capacity, and different persons using the same spoon will pour different amounts. Therefore, measure a drug ordered in teaspoons in milliliters; the established standard is 5ml/tsp. A convenient hollow-handled medicine spoon is available to accurately measure and administer the drug. Household measuring spoons can also be used when other devices are not available. A device called the Medibottle has shown to be more effective in delivering oral medication to infants than an oral syringe (Kraus, Stohlmeyer, Hannon, and others, 2001).

Another unreliable device for measuring liquids is the dropper, which varies to a greater extent than the teaspoon or measuring cup. The volume of a drop varies according to the viscosity (thickness) of the liquid measured. Viscous fluids produce much larger drops than thin liquids. Many medications are supplied with caps or droppers designed for measuring each specific preparation. These are accurate when used to measure that specific medication but are not reliable for measuring other liquids. Emptying dropper contents into a medicine cup invites additional error. Because some of the liquid clings to the sides of the cup, a significant amount of the drug can be lost.

The most accurate means for measuring small amounts of medication is the plastic disposable syringe, especially the tuberculin syringe for volumes less than 1 ml. Not only does the syringe provide a reliable measure, but it also serves as a convenient means for transporting and administering the medication. The medication can be placed directly into the child's mouth from the syringe.

Young children and some older children have difficulty swallowing tablets or pills. Because a number of drugs are not available in pediatric preparations, tablets need to be crushed before being given to these children. Commercial devices* are available, or simple methods can be used for crushing tablets. Not all drugs can be crushed (e.g., medication with an enteric or protective coating or formulated for slow release).

The nurse can teach children who must take solid oral medication for an extended period to swallow tablets or capsules. Training sessions include using verbal instruction, demonstration, reinforcement for swallowing progressively larger candy or capsules, no attention for inappropriate behavior, and gradual withdrawal of guidance after children can swallow their medication.

Because pediatric doses often require dividing adult preparations of medication, the nurse may be faced with the dilemma of accurate dosage. With tablets, only those that are scored can be halved or quartered accurately. If the medication is soluble, the tablet or contents of a capsule can be mixed in a small premeasured amount of liquid and the appropriate portion given. For example, if half a dose is required, the tablet is dissolved in 5 ml of water, and 2.5 ml is given.

Administration

Although administering liquids to infants is relatively easy, the nurse must take care to prevent aspiration. While holding the infant in a semireclining position, place the medication in the mouth from a spoon, plastic cup, dropper, or syringe (without a needle). It is best to place the dropper or syringe along the side of the infant's tongue and administer the liquid slowly in small amounts, waiting for the child to swallow between deposits.

> **NURSING TIP** In infants up to 11 months of age and children with neurologic impairments, blowing a small puff of air in the face frequently elicits a swallow reflex.

Medicine cups can be used effectively for older infants who are able to drink from a cup. Because of the natural outward tongue thrust in infancy, medications may need to be retrieved from the lips or chin and refed. Allowing the infant to suck the medication that has been placed in an empty nipple or inserting the syringe or dropper into the side of the mouth, parallel to the nipple, while the infant nurses is another convenient method for giving liquid medications to infants. Medication is not added to the infant's formula feeding because the child may subsequently refuse the formula. Dispose of any plastic covers that may be on the ends of syringes because these covers are choking hazards.

*Several styles of pill crushers are available from Trademark Medical, 449 Sovereign Court, St. Louis, MO 63011; 800-325-9044; http://www.trademarkmedical.com.

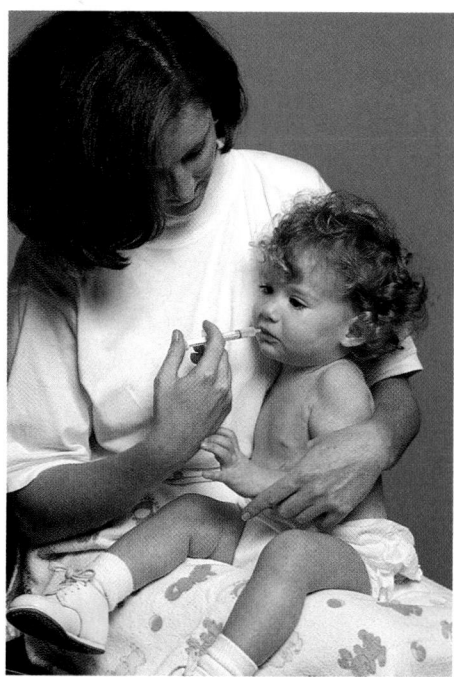

FIG 22-12 A nurse partially restrains a child for easy and comfortable administration of oral medication.

Young children who refuse to cooperate or resist consistently despite explanation and encouragement may require mild physical coercion. If so, it is carried out quickly and carefully. Make every effort to determine why the child resists and explain the reasons for the coercion in such a way that the child knows it is being carried out for his or her well-being and is not a form of punishment. There is always a risk in using even mild forceful techniques. A crying child can aspirate a medication, particularly when lying on the back. If the nurse holds the child in the lap with the child's right arm behind the nurse, the left hand firmly grasped by the nurse's left hand, and the head securely cradled between the nurse's arm and body, the medication can be slowly poured into the mouth (Fig. 22-12).

INTRAMUSCULAR ADMINISTRATION

Selecting the Syringe and Needle

The volume of medication prescribed for small children and the small amount of tissue available for injection necessitate selection of a syringe that can measure small amounts of solution. For volumes less than 1 ml, the tuberculin syringe, calibrated in 0.01-ml increments, is appropriate. Minute doses may require the use of a 0.5-ml, low-dose syringe. These syringes, along with specially constructed needles, minimize the possibility of inadvertently administering incorrect amounts of a drug because of dead space, which allows fluid to remain in the syringe and needle after the plunger is pushed completely forward. A minimum of 0.2 ml of solution remains in a standard needle hub; therefore, when very small amounts of two drugs are combined in the syringe, such as mixtures of insulin, the ratio of the two drugs can be altered significantly. Measures that minimize the effect of dead space are (1) when two drugs are combined in the syringe, always draw them up in the same order to maintain a consistent ratio between the drugs, (2) use the same brand of syringe (dead space may vary between brands), and (3) use one-piece syringe units (needle permanently attached to the syringe).

Dead space is also an important factor to consider when injecting medication because flushing the syringe with an air bubble adds an additional amount of medication to the prescribed dose. This can be hazardous when very small amounts of a drug are given. Consequently, flushing is not recommended, especially when less than 1 ml of medication is given. Syringes are calibrated to deliver a prescribed drug dose, and the amount of medication left in the hub and needle is not part of the syringe barrel calibrations. Certain drugs such as iron dextran and diphtheria and tetanus toxoid may cause irritation when tracked into the subcutaneous tissue. The Z-track method is recommended for use in infants and children rather than an air bubble. Changing the needle after withdrawing the fluid from the vial is another technique to minimize tracking.

The needle length must be sufficient to penetrate the subcutaneous tissue and deposit the medication into the body of the muscle. The needle gauge should be as small as possible to deliver the fluid safely. Smaller-diameter (25- to 30-gauge) needles cause the least discomfort, but larger gauges are needed for viscous medication and prevention of accidental bending of longer needles (see Evidence-Based Practice box).

Determining the Site

Factors to consider when selecting a site for an intramuscular (IM) injection on an infant or child include:

- The amount and character of the medication to be injected
- The amount and general condition of the muscle mass
- The frequency or number of injections to be given during the course of treatment
- The type of medication being given
- Factors that may impede access to or cause contamination of the site
- The child's ability to assume the required position safely

Older children and adolescents usually pose few problems in selecting a suitable site for IM injections, but infants, with their small and underdeveloped muscles, have fewer available sites. It is sometimes difficult to assess the amount of fluid that can be safely injected into a single site. Usually 1 ml is the maximum volume that should be administered in a single site to small children and older infants. The muscles of small infants may not tolerate more than 0.5 ml. As the child approaches adult size, the nurse can use volumes approaching those given to adults. However, the larger the amount of solution, the larger the muscle at the injection site must be.

Injections must be placed in muscles large enough to accommodate the medication, while avoiding major nerves and blood vessels. The IM immunization site recommended by the CDC, World Health Organization, and AAP for infants is the anterolateral thigh or vastus lateralis (Table 22-6). However, in two studies, immunizations at the ventrogluteal site have been found to have fewer local reactions and fever (Cook and Murtagh, 2003; Junqueira, Tavares, Martins, and others, 2010). Cook and Murtagh (2003) also found fewer systemic reactions (irritability and persistent crying or screaming) and greater parental acceptance for the ventrogluteal site. The ventrogluteal site is relatively free of major nerves and blood vessels, is a relatively large muscle with less subcutaneous tissue than the dorsal site, has well-defined landmarks for safe site location, and is easily accessible in several positions. Distraction and prevention of unexpected movement may be more easily achieved by placing the child supine on a parent's lap for ventrogluteal site use (Cook and Murtagh, 2006).

The deltoid muscle, a small muscle near the axillary and radial nerves, can be used for small volumes of fluid in children as young as 18 months of age. Its advantages are less pain and fewer side effects

EVIDENCE-BASED PRACTICE

Appropriate Site, Technique, Needle Size, and Dose for Intramuscular Injections in Infants, Toddlers, and Small Children

Updated by Olga A. Taylor

Ask the Question

Picot Question

In infants, toddlers, and small children, what are the best site, technique, needle size and gauge, and dosage for intramuscular (IM) injections?

Search for the Evidence

Search Strategies

Literature from 1990 to 2011 was reviewed to obtain clinical research studies related to this issue.

Databases Used

CINAHL, PubMed

Critically Analyze the Evidence

Searches reviewed were small studies. There were no randomized trials, double-blind trials, or large clinical studies addressing the subject of IM injections in children.

Infants and Toddlers

- A 16-mm needle was sufficient to penetrate the anterolateral thigh muscle if the needle was inserted at a 90-degree angle without pinching the muscle in children ages 2, 4, 6, and 18 months (Cook and Murtagh, 2002).
- A 25-mm needle was necessary to penetrate the thigh muscle when a 45-degree injection technique was used. Longer needle length was needed to fully deposit the medication into the muscle in children ages 2, 4, 6, and 18 months (Cook and Murtagh, 2002).
- For diphtheria–tetanus–pertussis (DTP) immunizations administered to infants 7 months of age and younger, 84.6% of injections were administered at the correct site (anterior thigh); 5.1% dorsogluteal and 2.6% deltoid muscles were administered at the incorrect sites (Daly, Johnston, and Chung, 1992).
- Vaccines containing adjuvant such as aluminum (e.g., DTaP, hepatitis A and B, diphtheria–tetanus [DT or Td]) should be given deep into the muscle to prevent local reactions (American Academy of Pediatrics [AAP], Committee on Infectious Diseases and Pickering, 2009; Centers for Disease Control and Prevention [CDC], 2002; Petousis-Harris, 2008; Taddio, Ilersich, Ipp, and others, 2009).
- Injecting adjuvant-containing vaccines into subcutaneous tissue increases the incidence of local reactions (Taddio, Ilersich, Ipp, and others, 2009; Zuckerman, 2000).
- Four-month-old infants experienced fewer local side effects (redness, tenderness, and swelling) when immunizations were administered into the anterior aspect of the thigh with a 25-mm (1-inch) needle versus shorter 16-mm ⅝-inch) needle (Diggle and Deeks, 2000).
- Localized vaccine reactions were significantly reduced when long needles (25 mm) were used for infant immunizations (Diggle, Deeks, and Pollard, 2006; Petousis-Harris, 2008).
- A 16-mm needle may be adequate for injections in small infants, and a 22- to 25-mm (⅞- to 1-inch) needle can be used in infants 2 months and older (AAP, Committee on Infectious Diseases and Pickering, 2009).
- A 22- to 32-mm (⅞- to 1¼-inch) needle is recommended for injections in toddlers if deltoid muscle size is adequate (CDC, 2002).
- A minimum of a 25-mm-long needle is recommended for anterolateral thigh injection in toddlers (CDC, 2002).

- Dorsogluteal muscle should be avoided in infants and toddlers and in smaller preschoolers with smaller muscle mass because of the possibility of damaging the sciatic nerve (AAP, Committee on Infectious Diseases and Pickering, 2009).
- In children older than age 1 year, deltoid muscle is recommended for IM injections. When multiple vaccines are given, two may be given in the thigh (anterior and lateral) because of its larger size (Diggle, 2003).
- Injections in the anterolateral thigh should be given at least 2.5 cm (1 inch) apart so local reactions are less likely to overlap (AAP, Committee on Infectious Diseases and Pickering, 2009).
- No research or supportive data were found regarding the amount of medication to be given at the different sites in infants and toddlers.
- Small and preterm infants may only tolerate up to 0.5 ml in each muscle to prevent local complications, and 1 ml of medication is recommended for infants less than 12 months; no data can be found to refute or support such a recommendation.

Children and Adolescents

- A 22- to 25-gauge needle for all IM childhood immunizations is recommended (AAP, Committee on Infectious Diseases and Pickering, 2009; CDC, 2002).
- Deltoid muscle may be used for immunizations in toddlers, older children, and adolescents (AAP, Committee on Infectious Diseases and Pickering, 2009; CDC, 2002).
- 16-mm for children <60 kg and 25-mm needle for children 60–70 kg is appropriate for IM injections in the deltoid injection site (Koster, Stellato, Kohn, and others, 2009).
- Ventrogluteal site is relatively free of important nerves and vascular structures and is the site of choice for pediatric IM injections in children of all ages; no complications at this site were reported (Beecroft and Kongelbeck, 1994).
- Longer needles (25 mm) were preferred for injection when bunching the skin and injecting; shorter needles (16 mm) were perceived as causing fewer localized reactions when the injection was administered with the skin being held taut (Groswasser, Kahn, Bouche, and others, 1997).
- Needle length found to be the most significant variable for local reactions in children after injection: 25-mm needle was associated with fewer localized reactions versus 16-mm needle (Davenport, 2004).
- In children older than age 1 year, deltoid muscle is recommended for IM injections. When multiple vaccines are given, two may be given in the thigh (anterior and lateral) because of its larger size (Diggle, 2003).
- Injections in the anterolateral thigh should be given at least 2.5 cm (1 inch) apart so local reactions are less likely to overlap (AAP, Committee on Infectious Diseases and Pickering, 2009).
- IM injections in the buttocks with longer needles using a 90-degree angle are associated with less reactogenicity (Petousis-Harris, 2008).

Apply the Evidence: Nursing Implications

There is **low-quality evidence** with a **strong recommendation** (Guyatt, Oxman, Vist, and others, 2008) to continue administering IM injections to children in the anterolateral thigh (up to 12 months old), deltoid (12 months and older), and ventrogluteal site. Needle length is an important factor in decreasing local reactions; the length should be adequate to deposit the medication into

EVIDENCE-BASED PRACTICE

Appropriate Site, Technique, Needle Size, and Dose for Intramuscular Injections in Infants, Toddlers, and Small Children—cont'd

the muscle for IM injections. Recommendations are for a 25-mm (1-inch) needle for infants, a 25- to 32-mm (1- to 1¼-inch) needle for toddlers, and a 38- to 51-mm (1½- to 2-inch) needle for older children; preterm and small emaciated infants may require a shorter needle (16 to 25 mm [⅝ to 1 inch]) based on weight and muscle mass size.

QSEN Quality and Safety Competencies:
Evidence-Based Practice*
Knowledge

Differentiate clinical opinion from research and evidence-based summaries.

Describe various methods for identifying the appropriate site, technique, needle size, and dose for IM injections in infants, toddlers, and small children.

Skills

Base individualized care plan on patient values, clinical expertise, and evidence.

Integrate evidence into practice by using the techniques for IM injections in clinical care.

Attitudes

Value the concept of evidence-based practice as integral to determining best clinical practice.

Appreciate the strengths and weakness of evidence for identifying appropriate site, technique, needle size, and dose for IM injections in infants, toddlers, and small children.

*Adapted from the QSEN at http://www.qsen.org.

References

American Academy of Pediatrics, Committee on Infectious Diseases, Pickering L, editor: *Red book: report of the Committee on Infectious Diseases*, ed 28, Elk Grove Village, Ill, 2009, Author.

Beecroft PC, Kongelbeck SR: How safe are intramuscular injections? *AACN Clin Issues* 5(2):207–215, 1994.

Centers for Disease Control and Prevention: General recommendations on immunization, *MMWR Morb Mortal Wkly Rep* 51(RR-2):12–14, 2002.

Cook IF, Murtagh J: Needle length required for intramuscular vaccination of infants and toddlers: an ultrasonographic study, *Austral Fam Phys* 31(3):295–297, 2002.

Daly JM, Johnston W, Chung Y: Injection sites utilized for DPT immunizations in infants, *J Comm Health Nurs* 9(2):87–94, 1992.

Davenport JM: A systematic review to ascertain whether the standard needle is more effective than a longer or wider needle in reducing the incidence of local reaction in children receiving primary immunization, *J Adv Nurs* 46(1):66–77, 2004.

Diggle L: The administration of child vaccines, part 11, childhood vaccinations, *Practice Nurse* 25(12):63–69, 2003.

Diggle L, Deeks J: Effect of needle length on incidence of local reactions to routine immunisation in infants aged 4 months: randomised controlled trial, *BMJ* 321(7266):931–933, 2000.

Diggle L, Deeks JJ, Pollard AJ: Effect of needle size on immunogenicity and reactogenecity of vaccines in infants: randomized controlled trial, *BMJ* 333(7568):571, 2006.

Groswasser J, Kahn A, Bouche B, and others: Needle length and injection technique for efficient intramuscular vaccine delivery in infants and children evaluated through an ultrasonographic determination of subcutaneous and muscle layer thickness, *Pediatrics* 100(3 Pt 1):400–403, 1997.

Guyatt GH, Oxman AD, Vist GE, and others: GRADE: an emerging consensus on rating quality of evidence and strength of recommendations, *BMJ* 336(7650):924–926, 2008.

Koster M, Stellato N, Kohn N, and others: Needle length for immunizations of early adolescents as determined by ultrasound, *Pediatrics*, 124:667–672, 2009.

Petousis-Harris H: Vaccine injection technique and reactogenicity—evidence for practice, *Vaccine*, 26:6299–6304, 2008.

Taddio A, Ilersich AL, Ipp M, and others: Physical interventions and injection techniques for reducing injection pain during routine childhood immunizations: systematic review of randomized controlled trials and quasi-randomized controlled trials, *Clin Ther* 31(suppl):S48–S76, 2009.

Zuckerman J: The importance of injecting vaccines into muscle, *BMJ* 321(7271):1237–1238, 2000.

TABLE 22-6 INTRAMUSCULAR INJECTION SITES IN CHILDREN

SITE	DISCUSSION
Vastus Lateralis 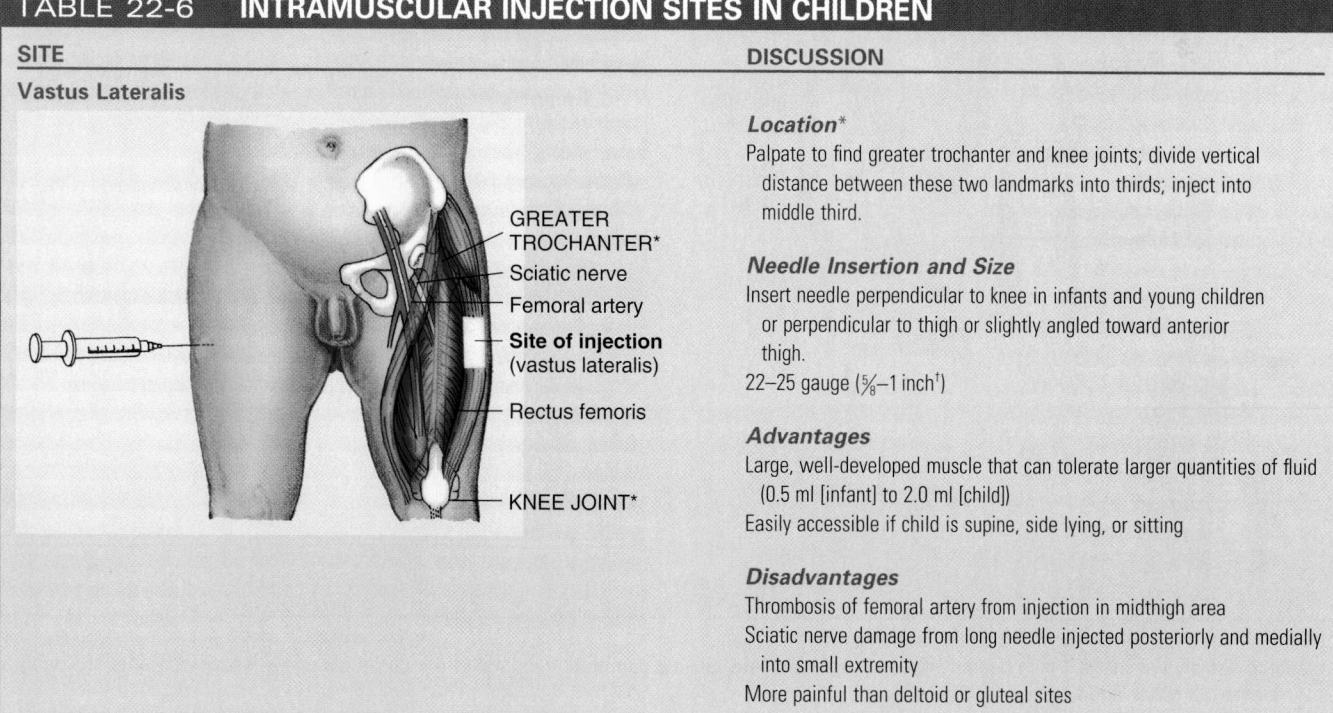 GREATER TROCHANTER* Sciatic nerve Femoral artery **Site of injection** (vastus lateralis) Rectus femoris KNEE JOINT*	**Location*** Palpate to find greater trochanter and knee joints; divide vertical distance between these two landmarks into thirds; inject into middle third. **Needle Insertion and Size** Insert needle perpendicular to knee in infants and young children or perpendicular to thigh or slightly angled toward anterior thigh. 22–25 gauge (⅝–1 inch†) **Advantages** Large, well-developed muscle that can tolerate larger quantities of fluid (0.5 ml [infant] to 2.0 ml [child]) Easily accessible if child is supine, side lying, or sitting **Disadvantages** Thrombosis of femoral artery from injection in midthigh area Sciatic nerve damage from long needle injected posteriorly and medially into small extremity More painful than deltoid or gluteal sites

Continued

TABLE 22-6 INTRAMUSCULAR INJECTION SITES IN CHILDREN—cont'd

SITE	DISCUSSION

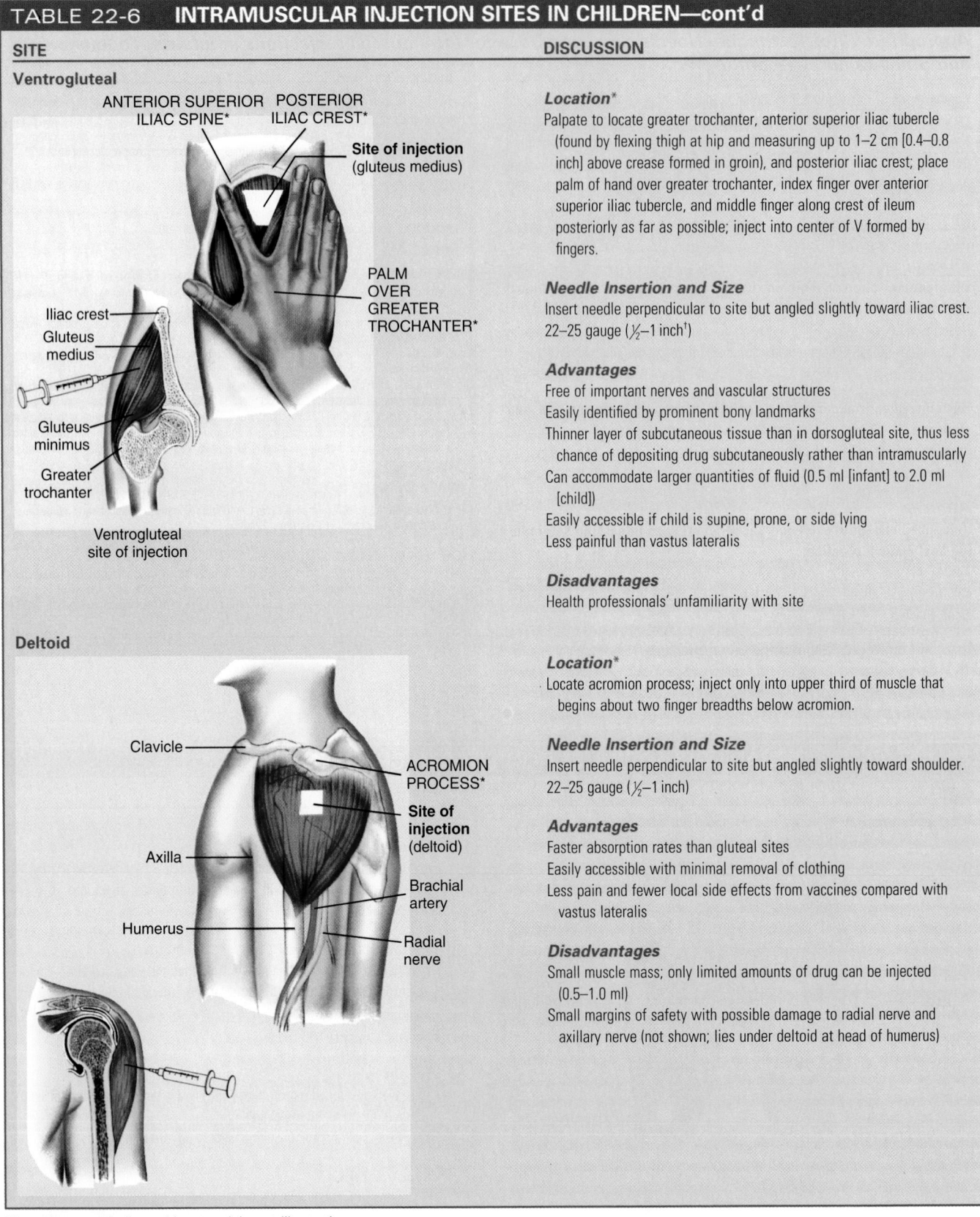

Ventrogluteal

ANTERIOR SUPERIOR ILIAC SPINE* POSTERIOR ILIAC CREST*

Site of injection (gluteus medius)

Iliac crest
Gluteus medius

PALM OVER GREATER TROCHANTER*

Gluteus minimus

Greater trochanter

Ventrogluteal site of injection

Deltoid

Clavicle

ACROMION PROCESS*

Site of injection (deltoid)

Axilla

Brachial artery

Humerus

Radial nerve

Ventrogluteal

Location*

Palpate to locate greater trochanter, anterior superior iliac tubercle (found by flexing thigh at hip and measuring up to 1–2 cm [0.4–0.8 inch] above crease formed in groin), and posterior iliac crest; place palm of hand over greater trochanter, index finger over anterior superior iliac tubercle, and middle finger along crest of ileum posteriorly as far as possible; inject into center of V formed by fingers.

Needle Insertion and Size

Insert needle perpendicular to site but angled slightly toward iliac crest. 22–25 gauge (½–1 inch†)

Advantages

Free of important nerves and vascular structures
Easily identified by prominent bony landmarks
Thinner layer of subcutaneous tissue than in dorsogluteal site, thus less chance of depositing drug subcutaneously rather than intramuscularly
Can accommodate larger quantities of fluid (0.5 ml [infant] to 2.0 ml [child])
Easily accessible if child is supine, prone, or side lying
Less painful than vastus lateralis

Disadvantages

Health professionals' unfamiliarity with site

Deltoid

Location*

Locate acromion process; inject only into upper third of muscle that begins about two finger breadths below acromion.

Needle Insertion and Size

Insert needle perpendicular to site but angled slightly toward shoulder. 22–25 gauge (½–1 inch)

Advantages

Faster absorption rates than gluteal sites
Easily accessible with minimal removal of clothing
Less pain and fewer local side effects from vaccines compared with vastus lateralis

Disadvantages

Small muscle mass; only limited amounts of drug can be injected (0.5–1.0 ml)
Small margins of safety with possible damage to radial nerve and axillary nerve (not shown; lies under deltoid at head of humerus)

*Locations are indicated by asterisks on illustrations.
†Research has shown that a 1-inch needle is needed for adequate muscle penetration in infants 4 months old and possibly in infants as young as 2 months old (Cook and Murtagh, 2002).

from the injectate (as observed with immunizations), compared with the vastus lateralis. Table 22-6 summarizes the three major injection sites and illustrates the location of the preferred IM injection sites for children.

Administration

Although injections that are executed with care seldom cause trauma to children, there have been reports of serious disability related to IM injections in children. Repeated use of a single site has been associated with fibrosis of the muscle with subsequent muscle contracture. Injections close to large nerves, such as the sciatic nerve, have been responsible for permanent disability, especially when potentially neurotoxic drugs are administered. One of the difficulties in administering the opaque preparations, such as penicillin G (Bicillin), is that aspirated blood cannot be detected at the bottom of the syringe, thus increasing the risk of injecting into a blood vessel. When such drugs are injected, use great care in locating the correct site. When aspirating, the nurse should look for blood at the top of the syringe near the plunger because blood may be drawn up through the column of penicillin. One study of IM injection techniques revealed that the straighter the path of needle insertion (e.g., 90-degree angle), the less displacement and shear to tissue, causing less discomfort (Katsma and Smith, 1997).

A reported potential hazard with medication in glass ampules is the presence of glass particles in the ampule after the container is broken. When the medication is withdrawn into the syringe, the glass particles are also withdrawn and subsequently injected into the patient. As a precaution, medication from glass ampules is only drawn through a needle with a filter.

Most children are unpredictable, and few are totally cooperative when receiving an injection. Even children who appear to be relaxed and constrained can lose control under the stress of the procedure. It is advisable to have someone available to help hold the child if needed. Because children often jerk or pull away unexpectedly, the nurse should carry an extra needle to exchange for the contaminated one so the delay is minimal. The child, even a small one, is told that he or she is receiving an injection (preferably using a phrase such as "putting the medicine under the skin"), and then the procedure is carried out as quickly and skillfully as possible to avoid prolonging the stressful experience. Invasive procedures such as injections are especially anxiety provoking in young children, who may associate any assault to the "behind" with punishment. Because injections are painful, the nurse should use excellent injection techniques and effective pain reduction measures to reduce discomfort (see Nursing Care Guidelines box).

Small infants offer little resistance to injections. Although they squirm and may be difficult to hold in position, they can usually be restrained without assistance. A larger infant's body can be securely restrained between the nurse's arm and body. To inject into the body of a muscle, the nurse firmly grasps the muscle mass between the thumb and fingers to isolate and stabilize the site (Fig. 22-13). However, in obese children, it is preferable to first spread the skin with the thumb and index finger to displace subcutaneous tissue and then grasp the muscle deeply on each side.

If medication is given around the clock, the nurse must wake the child. Although it may seem easier to surprise the sleeping child and do it quickly, this can cause the child to fear going back to sleep. When awakened first, children will know that nothing will be done to them unless they are forewarned. The Nursing Care Guidelines box summarizes administration techniques that maximize safety and minimize the discomfort often associated with injections.

A needleless injection system (e.g., Biojector) delivers IM or subcutaneous injections without the use of a needle and eliminates the

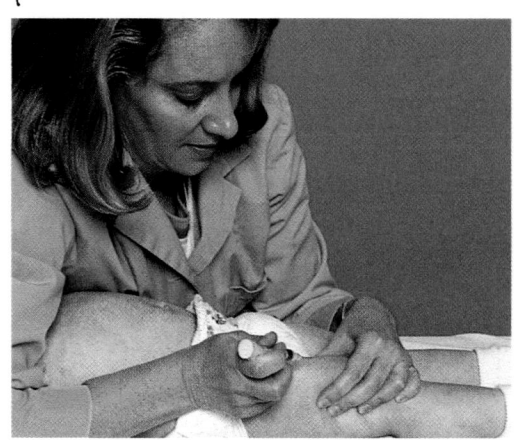

FIG 22-13 Holding a small child for intramuscular injection. Note how the nurse isolates and stabilizes the muscle.

risk of accidental needle puncture. This needle-free injection system uses a carbon dioxide cartridge to power the delivery of medication through the skin. Although it is not painless, it may reduce pain and the anxiety of seeing the needle.

SUBCUTANEOUS AND INTRADERMAL ADMINISTRATION

Subcutaneous and intradermal injections are frequently administered to children, but the technique differs little from the method used with adults. Examples of subcutaneous injections include insulin, hormone replacement, allergy desensitization, and some vaccines. Tuberculin testing, local anesthesia, and allergy testing are examples of frequently administered intradermal injections.

Techniques to minimize the pain associated with these injections include changing the needle if it pierced a rubber stopper on a vial, using 26- to 30-gauge needles (only to inject the solution), and injecting small volumes (≤0.5 ml). The angle of the needle for the subcutaneous injection is typically 90 degrees. In children with little subcutaneous tissue, some practitioners insert the needle at a 45-degree angle. However, the benefit of using the 45-degree angle rather than the 90-degree angle remains controversial.

Although subcutaneous injections can be given anywhere there is subcutaneous tissue, common sites include the center third of the lateral aspect of the upper arm, the abdomen, and the center third of the anterior thigh. Some practitioners believe it is not necessary to aspirate before injecting subcutaneously; for example, this is an accepted practice in the administration of insulin. Automatic injector devices do not aspirate before injecting.

When giving an intradermal injection into the volar surface of the forearm, the nurse should avoid the medial side of the arm, where the skin is more sensitive.

> **NURSING TIP** Families often need to learn injection techniques to administer medications, such as insulin, at home. Begin teaching as early as possible to allow the family the maximum amount of practice time.

INTRAVENOUS ADMINISTRATION

The IV route for administering medications is frequently used in pediatric therapy. For some drugs, it is the only effective route. This method is used for giving drugs to children who:

IV Line Placement

NURSING CARE GUIDELINES

Intramuscular Administration of Medication

Apply EMLA (a eutectic mix of lidocaine and prilocaine) or LMX cream (lidocaine) topically over site if time permits. (See Pain Management, Chapter 7.)

Prepare medication.

- Select appropriately sized needle and syringe.
- If withdrawing medication from an ampule, use a needle equipped with a filter that removes glass particles; then use a new, nonfilter needle for injection.
- Maximum volume to be administered in a single site is 1 ml for older infants and small children.
- Have medication at room temperature before injection.

Determine site of injection (see Table 22-6); make certain that muscle is large enough to accommodate volume and type of medication.

- For infants and small or debilitated children, use the vastus lateralis or ventrogluteal muscles; the dorsogluteal muscle is insufficiently developed to be a safe site for infants and small children.

Obtain sufficient help in restraining child.

Explain briefly what is to be done and, if appropriate, what child can do to help.

Expose injection area for unobstructed view of landmarks.

Select a site where skin is free of irritation and danger of infection; palpate for and avoid sensitive or hardened areas.

With multiple injections, rotate sites.

Place child in a lying or sitting position; child is not allowed to stand because landmarks are more difficult to assess, restraint is more difficult, and the child may faint and fall.

- **Ventrogluteal**—on side with upper leg flexed and placed in front of lower leg
- **Vastus lateralis**—supine, lying on side, or sitting

Use a new, sharp needle (not one that has pierced rubber stopper on vial) with smallest diameter that permits free flow of the medication.

Grasp muscle firmly between thumb and fingers to isolate and stabilize muscle for deposition of drug in its deepest part; in obese children, spread skin with thumb and index finger to displace subcutaneous tissue and grasp muscle deeply on each side.

Allow skin preparation to dry completely before penetrating skin.

Decrease perception of pain.

- Distract child with conversation.
- Give child something on which to concentrate (e.g., squeezing a hand or side rail, pinching own nose, humming, counting, yelling "Ouch!").
- Spray vapocoolant (e.g., ethyl chloride or fluoromethane) on site before injection, place a cold compress or wrapped ice cube on site about 1 minute before injection, or apply cold to contralateral site.
- Have child hold a small adhesive bandage and place it on puncture site after intramuscular injection is given.

Insert needle quickly using a dartlike motion at a 90-degree angle unless contraindicated.

Avoid tracking any medication through superficial tissues:

- Replace needle after withdrawing medication.
- Use the Z-track or air-bubble technique as indicated.
- Avoid any depression of the plunger during insertion of the needle.

Aspirate for blood.

- If blood is found, remove syringe from site, change needle, and reinsert into new location.
- If no blood is found, inject medication slowly into a relaxed muscle.

Remove needle quickly; hold gauze firmly against skin near needle when removing it to avoid pulling on tissue.

Apply firm pressure to site after injection; massage site to hasten absorption unless contraindicated, as with irritating drugs.

Place a small adhesive bandage on puncture site; with young children, decorate it by drawing a smiling face or other symbol of acceptance.

Hold and cuddle young child and encourage parents to comfort child; praise older child.

Allow expression of feelings.

Discard syringe and uncapped, uncut needle in puncture-resistant container located near site of use.

Record time of injection, drug, dose, and injection site.

- Have poor absorption as a result of diarrhea, vomiting, or dehydration
- Need a high serum concentration of a drug
- Have resistant infections that require parenteral medication over an extended time
- Need continuous pain relief
- Require emergency treatment

The nurse needs to consider several factors in relation to IV medication. When a drug is administered intravenously, the effect is almost instantaneous and further control is limited. Most drugs for IV administration require a specified minimum dilution, rate of flow, or both, and many drugs are highly irritating or toxic to tissues outside the vascular system. In addition to the precautions and nursing observations commonly related to IV therapy, factors to consider when preparing and administering drugs to infants and children by the IV route include:

- Amount of drug to be administered
- Minimum dilution of drug and whether child is fluid restricted
- Type of solution in which drug can be diluted
- Length of time over which drug can be safely administered
- Rate limitations of child, vascular system, and infusion equipment

- Time that this or another drug is to be administered
- Compatibility of all drugs that child is receiving intravenously
- Compatibility with infusion fluids

Before any IV infusion, check the site of insertion for patency. Never administer medications with blood products. Only one antibiotic should be administered at a time. Extra fluids needed to administer IV medications can be problematic for infants and fluid-restricted children. Syringe pumps are often used to deliver IV medication because they minimize fluid requirements and more precisely deliver small volumes of medication compared with large-volume infusion pumps. Regardless of the technique, the nurse must know the minimum dilutions for safe administration of IV medications to infants and children.

Peripheral Intermittent Infusion Device

The **peripheral lock**, also known as an **intermittent infusion device** or **saline** or **heparin lock**, is an alternative to a keep-open infusion when extended access to a vein is required without the need for continuous fluid. It is most frequently used for intermittent infusion of medication into a peripheral venous route. A short, flexible catheter is used as the lock device, and a site is selected where there will be minimal movement, such as the forearm. The catheter is inserted and secured in the same manner as for any IV infusion device, but the hub is occluded with a stopper or injection cap.

The type of device used may vary, and the care and use of the peripheral lock are carried out according to the protocol of the institution or unit. However, the general concept is the same. The catheter remains in place and is flushed with saline after infusion of the medication. See the Evidence-Based Practice box and Table 22-7 on flushing with normal saline or heparin.

Children may be discharged with a peripheral lock in place to continue receiving medications without hospitalization; this is usually reserved for children who require medications on a short-term basis and are referred to a home-based infusion company. Those with chronic illnesses who require repeated blood sampling or medications, long-term chemotherapy, or frequent hyperalimentation or antibiotic therapy are best managed with a central venous catheter.

Central Venous Access Device

Central venous access devices (CVADs) have several different characteristics. Factors that can influence the type of CVAD include the reason for placement of the catheter (diagnosis), length of therapy, risk to the patient in placement of the catheter, and availability of resources to assist the family in maintaining the catheter.

Short-term or nontunneled catheters are used in acute care, emergency, and intensive care units. These catheters are made of polyurethane and are placed in large veins such as the subclavian, femoral, or jugular. Insertion is by surgical incision or large percutaneous threading. A chest x-ray film should be taken to verify placement of the catheter tip before administration of fluids or medications.

TABLE 22-7	INTRAVENOUS CATHETER FLUSHES FOR LINES WITHOUT CONTINUOUS FLUID INFUSIONS
Peripheral lines (Hep-Lock or saline locks)	NS* after medications or every 8 hr for dormant lines; instill 2½ times tubing volume 24-g catheters: NS* or heparin 2 units/ml 2 ml
Midline	Heparin 10 units/ml; 3 ml in a 10-ml syringe[†] after medications or every 8 hr if dormant Newborns: heparin 1–2 units/ml to run continuously at ordered rate
External central line (nonimplanted, nontunneled, tunneled, or PICC)	Heparin 10 units/ml; 3 ml in a 10-ml syringe[†] after medications or once daily if dormant Newborns: heparin 2 units/ml; 2–3 ml after medications or to check line patency OR heparin 1–2 units/ml to run continuously at ordered rate
Totally implanted central line (TIVAS, implanted port)	Heparin 10 units/ml; 5 ml after medications or once daily if dormant and accessed; if not accessed, heparin 100 units/ml; 5 ml every month
Arterial and central venous pressure continuous monitored lines	Heparin 2 units/ml in 55-ml syringe to run continuously at 1 ml/hr

NS, Normal saline; *PICC*, peripherally inserted central catheter; *TIVAS*, totally implantable venous access device.
*Use 5% dextrose in water when medication is incompatible with saline.
[†]Smaller syringes may be used when flush is delivered by a pump.

EVIDENCE-BASED PRACTICE

Normal Saline or Heparinized Saline Flush Solution in Pediatric Intravenous Lines

Updated by Olga A. Taylor

Ask the Question
Picot Question
Is there a significant difference in the longevity of IV intermittent infusion locks in children when NS is used as a flush instead a HS solution?

Search for the Evidence
Search Strategies
Selection criteria included evidence during the years 1992 to 2011 with the following terms: saline versus heparin intermittent flush, children's heparin lock flush, heparin lock patency, peripheral venous catheter in children.

Databases Used
CINAHL, PubMed

Critically Analyze the Evidence
- In trials of HS administration versus NS, placebo, or no treatment in neonates, no strong evidence regarding the effectiveness and safety of heparin in prolonging catheter life was found (Shah, Ng, and Sinha, 2005).
- No significant statistical difference was found between HS and NS flushes for maintaining catheter patency in children (Hanrahan, Kleiber, and Berends, 2000; Hanrahan, Kleiber, and Fagan, 1994; Heilskov, Kleiber, Johnson, and others, 1998; Kotter, 1996; Mok, Kwong, and Chan, 2007; Schultz, Drew, and Hewitt, 2002).

- Increased incidence of pain or erythema was associated with HS flushing of infusion devices (Hanrahan, Kleiber, and Fagan, 1994; McMullen, Fioravanti, Pollack, and others, 1993; Nelson and Graves, 1998; Robertson, 1994).
- Increased patency or longer dwell times were found with HS solutions versus NS in 24-gauge catheters (Beecroft, Bossert, Chung, and others, 1997; Danek and Noris, 1992; Gyr, Burroughs, Smith, and others, 1995; Hanrahan, Kleiber, and Berends, 2000; Mudge, Forcier, and Slattery, 1998; Tripathi, Kaushik, and Singh, 2008).
- Younger children and preterm neonates with lower gestational ages were associated with shorter patency of IV catheters (McMullen, Fioravanti, Pollack, and others, 1993; Paisley, Stamper, Brown, and others, 1997; Robertson, 1994; Tripathi, Kaushik, and Singh, 2008).
- Infusion devices flushed with NS lasted longer than those flushed with HS (Goldberg, Sankaran, Givelichian, and others, 1999; Le Duc, 1997; Nelson and Graves, 1998).
- When measured and reported, the length of time between flushing peripheral devices affected the dwell time (Crews, Gnann, Rice, and others, 1997; Gyr, Burroughs, Smith, and others, 1995).
- Preterm neonates are at higher risk for development of clotting problems as a result of heparin; none of the studies cited anticoagulation-associated complications with HS (Klenner, Fusch, Rakow, and others, 2003).
- 0.9% sodium chloride injection is safe for maintaining patency of peripheral locks in adults and children older than age 12 years (American Society of Hospital Pharmacists, 2006).

Continued

EVIDENCE-BASED PRACTICE

Normal Saline or Heparinized Saline Flush Solution in Pediatric Intravenous Lines—cont'd

- Either preservative-free heparin or preservative-free 0.9% sodium chloride may be used to flush a peripheral IV; however, catheter patency may be maintained by flushing with saline when converting from continuous to intermittent use (Infusion Nurses Society, 2006).
- After each catheter use, peripheral catheters should be locked with preservative-free 0.9% sodium chloride (Infusion Nurses Society, 2011).
- No recommendation is made for use of preservative-free 0.9% sodium chloride versus heparin for locking peripheral catheters (Infusion Nurses Society, 2011).

Apply the Evidence: Nursing Implications

There is **low-quality evidence** with a **weak recommendation** (Guyatt, Oxman, Vist, and others, 2008) for using NS versus HS flush solution in pediatric IV lines. Further research is still needed with larger samples of children, especially preterm neonates, using small-gauge catheters (24 gauge) and other gauge catheters flushed with NS and HS as intermittent infusion devices only (no continuous infusions). Variables to be considered include catheter dwell time; medications administered; period between regular flushing and flushing associated with medication administration; pain, erythema, and other localized complications; concentration and amount of HS used; flush method (positive-pressure technique vs. no specific technique); reason for IV device removal; and complications associated with either solution. NS is a safe alternative to HS flush in infants and children with intermittent IV locks larger than 24 gauge; smaller neonates may benefit from HS flush (longer dwell time), but the evidence is inconclusive for all weight ranges and gestational ages.

[QSEN] Quality and Safety Competencies:
Evidence-Based Practice*

Knowledge

Differentiate clinical opinion from research and evidence-based summaries.

Describe methods for using NS or HS flush solution in pediatric IV lines.

Skills

Base individualized care plan on patient values, clinical expertise, and evidence.

Integrate evidence into practice on NS or HS flush solution in pediatric IV lines.

Attitudes

Value the concept of evidence-based practice as integral to determining best clinical practice.

Appreciate the strengths and weakness of evidence for NS or HS flush solution in pediatric IV lines.

References

American Society of Hospital Pharmacists Commission on Therapeutics: ASHP therapeutic position statement on the institutional use of 0.9% sodium chloride injection to maintain patency of peripheral indwelling intermittent infusion devices, *Am J Health Syst Pharm* 63(13):1273–1275, 2006.

Beecroft PC, Bossert E, Chung K, and others: Intravenous lock patency in children: dilute heparin versus saline, *J Pediatr Pharm Practice* 2(4):211–223, 1997.

Crews BE, Gnann KK, Rice MH, and others: Effects of varying intervals between heparin flushes on pediatric catheter longevity, *Pediatr Nurs* 23(1):87–91, 1997.

Danek GD, Noris EM: Pediatric IV catheters: efficacy of saline flush, *Pediatr Nurs* 18(2):111–113, 1992.

Goldberg M, Sankaran R, Givelichian L, and others: Maintaining patency of peripheral intermittent infusion devices with heparinized saline and saline: a randomized double blind controlled trial in neonatal intensive care and a review of literature, *Neonat Intensive Care* 12(1):18–22, 1999.

Guyatt GH, Oxman AD, Vist GE, and others: GRADE: An emerging consensus on rating quality of evidence and strength of recommendations, *BMJ* 336(7650):924–926, 2008.

Gyr P, Burroughs T, Smith K, and others: Double blind comparison of heparin and saline flush solutions in maintenance of peripheral infusion devices, *Pediatr Nurs* 21(4):383–389, 1995.

Hanrahan KS, Kleiber C, Berends S: Saline for peripheral intravenous locks in neonates: Evaluating a change in practice, *Neonat Netw* 19(2):19–24, 2000.

Hanrahan KS, Kleiber C, Fagan C: Evaluation of saline for IV locks in children, *Pediatr Nurs* 20(6):549–552, 1994.

Heilskov J, Kleiber C, Johnson K, and others: A randomized trial of heparin and saline for maintaining intravenous locks in neonates, *J Soc Pediatr Nurs* 3(3):111–116, 1998.

Infusion Nurses Society: *Policies and procedures for infusion nursing*, ed 3, Norwood, Mass, 2006, Author.

Infusion Nurses Society: Infusion nursing standards of practice, *J Infus Nurs* 34(1S):S63–S64, 2011.

Klenner AF, Fusch C, Rakow A, and others: Benefit and risk of heparin for maintaining peripheral venous catheters in neonates: a placebo-controlled trial, *J Pediatr* 143(6):741–745, 2003.

Kotter RW: Heparin vs. saline for intermittent intravenous device maintenance in neonates, *Neonat Netw* 15(6):43–47, 1996.

Le Duc K: Efficacy of normal saline solution versus heparin solution for maintaining patency of peripheral intravenous catheters in children, *J Emerg Nurs* 23(4):306–309, 1997.

McMullen A, Fioravanti ID, Pollack D, and others: Heparinized saline or normal saline as a flush solution in intermittent intravenous lines in infants and children, *MCN Am J Matern Child Nurs* 18(2):78–85, 1993.

Mok E, Kwong TK, Chan ME: A randomized controlled trial for maintaining peripheral intravenous lock in children, *Int J Nurs Pract* 13(1):33–45, 2007.

Mudge B, Forcier D, Slattery MJ: Patency of 24-gauge peripheral intermittent infusion devices: a comparison of heparin and saline flush solutions, *Pediatr Nurs* 24(2):142–149, 1998.

Nelson TJ, Graves SM: 0.9% Sodium chloride injection with and without heparin for maintaining peripheral indwelling intermittent infusion devices in infants, *Am J Heath Syst Pharm* 55:570–573, 1998.

Paisley MK, Stamper M, Brown T, and others: The use of heparin and normal saline flushes in neonatal intravenous catheters, *J Pediatr Nurs* 23(5):521–527, 1997.

Robertson J: Intermittent intravenous therapy: a comparison of two flushing solutions, *Contemp Nurs* 3(4):174–179, 1994.

Schultz AA, Drew D, Hewitt H: Comparison of normal saline and heparinized saline for patency of IV locks in neonates, *Appl Nurs Res* 15(1):28–34, 2002.

Shah PS, Ng E, Sinha AK: Heparin for prolonging peripheral intravenous catheter use in neonates, *Cochrane Database Syst Rev* (4):CD002774, 2005.

Tripathi S, Kaushik V, Singh V: Peripheral IVs: factors affecting complications and patency—a randomized controlled trial, *J Infus Nurs* 31(3):182–188, 2008.

HS, Heparinized saline; *IV,* intravenous; *NS,* normal saline.

*Adapted from the QSEN at http://www.qsen.org.

Animation—PICC Line Placement

⊖ **Peripherally inserted central catheters (PICCs)** can be used for short-term to moderate-length therapy. These catheters consist of silicone or polymer material and are placed by specially trained nurses, physicians, or interventional radiologists (Gamulka, Mendoza, and Connolly, 2005). The most common insertion site is above the antecubital area using the median, cephalic, or basilic vein. The catheter is threaded either with or without a guidewire into the superior vena cava. PICCs can be trimmed before insertion, and the decision can be made to insert the catheter midline, which is considered between the insertion site and the axilla. If the catheter is threaded midline, total parenteral nutrition (TPN) or any other drug known to irritate a peripheral vein (e.g., chemotherapy drugs) should not be administered. The high concentration of glucose in TPN makes it irritating to the vessel; it should be infused through a central catheter.

The decision to insert a PICC needs to be made before several attempts at IV insertion are done. When the antecubital veins have been punctured repeatedly, they are not considered candidates for this type of catheter. Because this catheter is the least costly and has less chance of complications than other CVADs, it is an excellent choice for many pediatric patients.

TABLE 22-8	COMPARISON OF LONG-TERM CENTRAL VENOUS ACCESS DEVICES	
DESCRIPTION	**BENEFITS**	**CARE CONSIDERATIONS**
Tunneled Catheter (e.g., Hickman or Broviac Catheter)		
Silicone, radiopaque, flexible catheter with open ends or VitaCuffs (biosynthetic material impregnated with silver ions) on catheter(s) enhances tissue ingrowth May have more than one lumen	Reduced risk of bacterial migration after tissue adheres to cuff One or two Dacron cuff Easy to use for self-administered infusions Removal requires pulling catheter from site (nonsurgical procedure)	Requires daily heparin flushes Must be clamped or have clamp nearby at all times Must keep exit site dry Heavy activity restricted until tissue adheres to cuff Water sports may be restricted (risk of infection) Risk of infection still present Protrudes outside body; susceptible to damage from sharp instruments and may be pulled out; may affect body image More difficult to repair Patient or family must learn catheter care
Groshong Catheter		
Clear, flexible, silicone, radiopaque catheter with closed tip and two-way valve at proximal end Dacron cuff or VitaCuff on catheter enhances tissue ingrowth May have more than one lumen	Reduced time and cost for maintenance care; no heparin flushes needed Reduced catheter damage; no clamping needed because of two-way valve Increased patient safety because of minimal potential for blood backflow or air embolism Reduced risk of bacterial migration after tissue adheres to cuff Easily repaired Easy to use for self-administered intravenous infusions	Requires weekly irrigation with normal saline Must keep exit site dry Heavy activity restricted until tissue adheres to cuff Water sports may be restricted (risk of infection) Risk of infection still present Protrudes outside body; susceptible to damage from sharp instruments and may be pulled out; can affect body image Patient or family must learn catheter care
Implanted Ports (e.g., Port-A-Cath, Infus-A-Port, Mediport, Norport, Groshong Port)		
Totally implantable metal or plastic device that consists of self-sealing injection port with top or side access with preconnected or attachable silicone catheter that is placed in large blood vessel	Reduced risk of infection Placed completely under the skin and therefore much less likely to be pulled out or damaged No maintenance care and reduced cost for family Heparinized monthly and after each infusion to maintain patency (only Groshong port requires saline) No limitations on regular physical activity, including swimming Dressing needed only when port accessed with Huber needle that is not removed No or only slight change in body appearance (slight bulge on chest)	Must pierce skin for access; pain with insertion of needle; can use local anesthetic (EMLA, LMX) or intradermal buffered lidocaine before accessing port Special noncoring needle (Huber) with straight or angled design must be used to inject into port Skin preparation needed before injection Difficult to manipulate for self-administered infusions Catheter may dislodge from port, especially if child "plays" with port site (twiddler syndrome) Vigorous contact sports generally not allowed Removal requires surgical procedure

EMLA, Eutectic mix of lidocaine and prilocaine; *LMX,* lidocaine.

> ❗ **NURSING ALERT**
>
> Most PICC lines are not sutured into place, so care is needed when changing the dressing.

> ❗ **NURSING ALERT**
>
> When working with tunneled catheters, PICCs, and peripheral IVs, avoid the use of any scissors around the tubing or dressing. Removal is best accomplished using fingers and much patience. In the event that a tunneled catheter is cut, use a padded clamp to clamp the catheter proximal to the exit site to avoid blood loss. Repair kits are available, which may save the catheter and avoid surgery to replace a cut catheter.

Long-term CVADs include tunneled catheters and implanted infusion ports (Table 22-8 and Fig. 22-14). They may have single, double, or triple lumens. Several lumens (multilumen) catheters allow more than one therapy to be administered at the same time. Reasons to use multilumen catheters include repeated blood sampling, TPN, administration of blood products or infusion of large quantities or concentrations of fluids, administration of incompatible drugs or fluids at the same time (through different lumens), and central venous pressure monitoring.

With any of the central venous catheters, medication is easily instilled through the injection cap. Maintenance of the catheter includes dressing changes, flushing to maintain patency, and prevention of occlusion or dislodgment.

With the implanted device, the port must be palpated for placement and stabilized, the overlying skin cleansed, and only special noncoring Huber needles used to pierce the port's diaphragm on the top or side, depending on the style. To avoid repeated skin punctures, a special infusion set with a Huber needle and extension tubing with a Luer connection can be used (see Fig. 22-14). With this attached, the injection procedure is the same as for an intermittent infusion device or a central venous catheter. To prevent infection, meticulous aseptic technique must be used any time the devices are entered, including

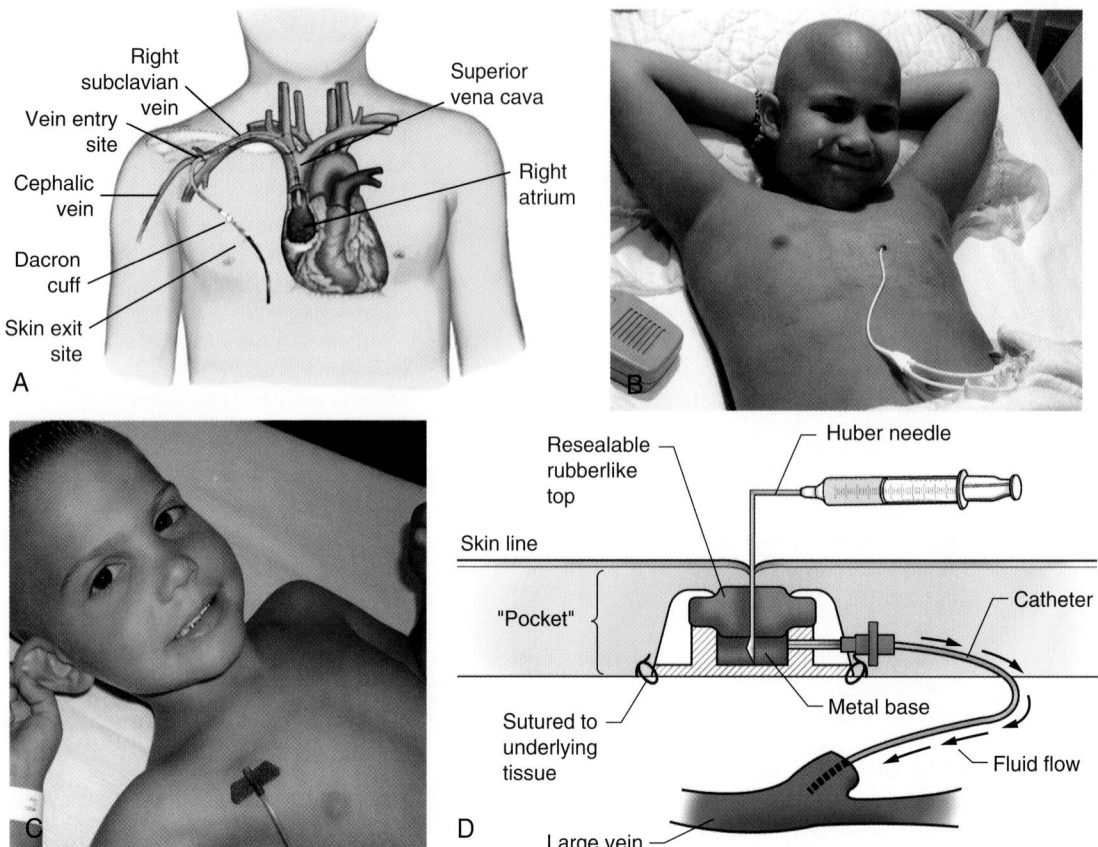

FIG 22-14 Venous access devices. **A,** External central venous catheter insertion and exit site. **B,** Child with a external central venous catheter (dressing removed for photo). **C,** Child with an implanted port with a Huber needle in place (dressing removed for photo). **D,** Side view of an implanted port.

instillation of heparin or saline to prevent clotting. There should be a protocol stating that the Huber needle needs to be changed at established intervals, usually 5 to 7 days.

The children and parents are taught the procedure for care of the CVAD before discharge from the hospital, including preparation and injection of the prescribed medication, the flush, and dressing changes. A protective device may be recommended for some active children to prevent their accidentally dislodging the needle. Many children take responsibility for preparing and administering medications. Both verbal and written step-by-step instructions are provided for the learners. See the Evidence-Based Practice box for CVAD site care.

> **NURSING TIP** A pocket sewn on the inside of a T-shirt provides a place in which to coil the catheter line while the child is at play if a dressing is not used.

Infection and catheter occlusion are two of the most common complications of central venous catheters. They require treatment with antibiotics for infection and a fibrinolytic agent, such as alteplase, for thrombus formation (Blaney, Shen, Kerner, and others, 2006; Fisher, Deffenbaugh, Poole, and others, 2004; Kerner, Garcia-Careaga, Fisher, and others, 2006; Shen, Li, Murdock, and others, 2003). Uncapping can be prevented by taping the cap securely to the catheter and the clamped line to the dressing. Leaks can be prevented by using a

smooth-edged clamp only. The parents are cautioned to keep scissors away from the child to prevent accidental cutting of the catheter. If the catheter leaks, the parents are instructed to tape it above the leak and then clamp the catheter at the taped site. The child should be taken to the practitioner as soon as possible to prevent infection or clotting after a catheter leak.

> ⚠ **NURSING ALERT**
>
> If a central venous catheter is accidentally removed, apply pressure to the entry site to the vein, not the exit site on the skin.

NASOGASTRIC, OROGASTRIC, AND GASTROSTOMY ADMINISTRATION

When a child has an indwelling feeding tube or a gastrostomy, oral medications are usually given via that route. An advantage of this method is the ability to administer oral medications around the clock without disturbing the child. A disadvantage is the risk of occluding, or clogging, the tube, especially when giving viscous solutions through small-bore feeding tubes. The most important preventive measure is adequate flushing after the medication is instilled (see Nursing Care Guidelines box).

EVIDENCE-BASED PRACTICE

Central Venous Catheter Site Care

Brandi Horvath; updated by Olga A. Taylor

Ask the Question
Picot Question

In children with CVCs, is chlorhexidine gluconate a more effective antiseptic solution than povidone–iodine in preventing CVC-related site infections and bacteremia?

Search the Evidence
Search Strategies

Search selection criteria included English-language publications within the past 10 years and research-based articles on catheter site care and chlorhexidine.

Databases Used

The National Guideline Clearinghouse (AHRQ), Centers for Disease Control and Prevention (CDC), Cochrane Collaboration, Joanna Briggs Institute, PubMed, Infusion Nurses Society, Oncology Nurses Society, MD Consult, BestBETs, TRIP Database Plus

Critically Analyze the Evidence
Chlorhexidine Gluconate versus Povidone–Iodine

- Use of 2% chlorhexidine for disinfecting catheter site before insertion (allowing it to dry) is preferred, but tincture of iodine, an iodophor, or 70% alcohol can be used. Iodine needs to remain on the skin for at least 2 minutes or until dry (Infusion Nurses Society, 2011a, 2011b; O'Grady, Alexander, Dellinger, and others, 2002).
- No recommendations can be made for the use of chlorhexidine in infants younger than 2 months of age, use of topical antibiotic ointments or creams because of the potential to promote fungal infections and antimicrobial resistance, or use of impregnated catheters and chlorhexidine sponge dressings to reduce the incidence of infection (Infusion Nurses Society, 2011a, 2011b; O'Grady, Alexander, Dellinger, and others, 2002).
- Avoid use of sponges in infants younger than 7 days and younger than 26 weeks' gestation. Replace the catheter-site dressing when it becomes damp, loosened, or soiled or when inspection of the site is necessary (O'Grady, Alexander, Dellinger, and others, 2002).
- Replace dressings used on short-term CVC sites every 2 days for gauze dressings and at least every 7 days for transparent dressings except in pediatric patients in whom the risk for dislodging the catheter outweighs the benefit of changing the dressing (Infusion Nurses Society, 2011a; O'Grady, Alexander, Dellinger, and others, 2002).
- Use of alcohol, chlorhexidine gluconate, povidone–iodine, and tincture of iodine (allow to dry) is recommended. If using povidone–iodine, do not apply alcohol as a second antiseptic (Infusion Nurses Society, 2006, 2011a, 2011b; Marlowe, Mistry, Coffin, and others, 2010).
- Dress the vascular access site with sterile gauze and cover it with sterile transparent dressings. Gauze dressings should be changed every 48 hours (Camp-Sorrell, 2004; Infusion Nurses Society, 2006, 2011a, 2011b).
- Semipermeable transparent dressings should be changed at least every 5 to 7 days; the interval depends on the dressing material, age and condition of the patient, infection rate reported by the organization, environmental conditions, and manufacturer's labeled uses and directions (Infusion Nurses Society, 2006, 2011a, 2011b).

- Chlorhexidine for preinsertion and postinsertion site catheter care was found superior to alcohol and povidone–iodine (Camp-Sorrell, 2004; Carson, 2004; Chaiyakunapruk, Veenstra, Lipsky, and others, 2002).
- Routine application of antibiotic ointment is not recommended because of the risk of fungal infections and antimicrobial resistance.
- For bone marrow transplant recipients, chlorhexidine is the recommended antisepsis for prevention of catheter-related infection (Zitella, 2003).
- In pediatric hemopoietic stem cell transplant patients, use of 2% chlorhexidine in 70% isopropanol resulted in a sustained decrease in catheter-related infections (Soothill, Bravery, Ho, and others, 2009).
- Neonates weighing 1500 g or more and 7 days of age or older tolerated use of chlorhexidine gluconate; however, some chlorhexidine gluconate was absorbed cutaneously (Garland, Alex, Uhing, and others, 2009).
- Neonates and infants with Biopatch (chlorhexidine sponge dressings) had a substantial decrease in colonized catheter tips compared with the group that used standard dressings. Biopatch was associated with localized contact dermatitis in infants of very low birth weight (Garland, Alex, Mueller, and others, 2001).
- Skin disinfection before CVC insertion and daily dressing changes with propanol–chlorhexidine followed by povidone–iodine was associated with the lowest rate of microbial catheter colonization (Langgartner, Linde, Lehn, and others, 2004).
- Patients with chlorhexidine-impregnated CVC dressing (Biopatch) had a significantly reduced risk of CVC colonization compared with patients with transparent dressing alone (Levy, Katz, Solter, and others, 2005; Onder, Chandar, Coakley, and others, 2009).
- In children older than 2 years of age, use of chlorhexidine-impregnated dressing should be considered as an extra prevention measure for catheter-related bloodstream infection (Infusion Nurses Society, 2011a).

Other Antiseptics

- Use of ethanol locks in children on parental nutrition (median age, 18.3 months) significantly decreased the rate of CVC infections (9.9 per 1000 to 2.1 per 1000 catheter days) (Jones, Hull, Richardson, and others, 2010).
- In pediatric patients with hemophilia (3, 11, and 13 years of age), ethanol lock therapy cleared catheter-related infection (Rajpurkar, Boldt-Macdonald, Mclenon, and others, 2009).
- In pediatric cancer patients, taurolidin/citrate (TauroLock) reduced catheter-related blood infections (Simon, Ammann, Wiszniewsky, and others, 2008).

Apply the Evidence: Nursing Implications

There is **moderate-quality evidence** with a **strong recommendation** (Guyatt, Oxman, Vist, and others, 2008) for CVC care. Two percent chlorhexidine should be used for catheter site antisepsis. Two percent chlorhexidine should be used with caution in premature and low–birth-weight infants. Chlorhexidine-impregnated sponges (Biopatch) should be used around the catheter site except in low–birth-weight infants in the first 2 weeks of life.

QSEN Quality and Safety Competencies:
Evidence-Based Practice*
Knowledge

Differentiate clinical opinion from research and evidence-based summaries.
Describe methods for CVC care.

CVC, Central venous catheter.
*Adapted from the QSEN at http://www.qsen.org.

Continued

EVIDENCE-BASED PRACTICE

Central Venous Catheter Site Care—cont'd

Skills

Base individualized care plan on patient values, clinical expertise, and evidence.

Integrate evidence into practice by using appropriate CVC care.

Attitudes

Value the concept of evidence-based practice as integral to determining best clinical practice.

Appreciate the strengths and weakness of evidence for CVC care.

References

Camp-Sorrell D, editor: *Access device guidelines: recommendations for nursing practice and education*, ed 2, Pittsburgh, 2004, Oncology Nursing Society.

Carson S: Chlorhexidine versus povidone-iodine for central venous catheter site care in children, *J Pediatr Nurs* 19(1):74–80, 2004.

Chaiyakunapruk N, Veenstra D, Lipsky B, and others: Chlorhexidine compared with povidone-iodine solution for vascular catheter-site care: A meta-analysis, *Ann Intern Med* 136(11):792–801, 2002.

Garland J, Alex C, Mueller C, and others: A randomized trial comparing povidone-iodine to a chlorhexidine-impregnated dressing for prevention of central venous catheter infections in neonates, *Pediatrics* 107(6):1431–1436, 2001.

Garland JS, Alex CP, Uhing MR, and others: Pilot trial to compare tolerance of chlorhexidine gluconate to povidone-iodine antisepsis for central venous catheter placement in neonates, *J Perinatol* 29:808–813, 2009.

Guyatt GH, Oxman AD, Vist GE, and others: GRADE: An emerging consensus on rating quality of evidence and strength of recommendations, *BMJ* 336(7650):924–926, 2008.

Infusion Nurses Society: Infusion nursing standards of practice, *J Infus Nurs* 34(1S):S63–S64, 2011a.

Infusion Nurses Society: *Policies and procedures for infusion nursing*, ed 4, South Norwood, Mass, 2011b, Author.

Jones BA, Hull MA, Richardson DS, and others: Efficacy of ethanol locks in reducing central venous catheter infections in pediatric patients with intestinal failure, *J Pediatr Surg* 45:1287–1293, 2010.

Langgartner J, Linde H, Lehn N, and others: Combined skin disinfection with chlorhexidine/propanol and aqueous povidone-iodine reduces bacterial colonisation of central venous catheters, *Intensive Care Med* 30(6):1081–1088, 2004.

Levy I, Katz J, Solter E, and others: Chlorhexidine-impregnated dressing for prevention of colonization of central venous catheters in infants and children: a randomized controlled study, *Pediatr Infect Dis* 24(8):676–679, 2005.

Marlowe L, Mistry RD, Coffin S, and others: Blood culture contamination rates after skin antisepsis with chlorhexidine gluconate versus povidone-iodine in a pediatric emergency department, *Infect Control Hosp Epidemiol* 31(2):171–176, 2010.

O'Grady N, Alexander M, Dellinger EP, and others: Guidelines for the prevention of intravascular catheter-related infections, *MMWR Morb Mortal Wkly Rep* 51(RR-10):1–29, 2002.

Onder AM, Chandar J, Coakley S, and others: Controlling exit site infections: does it decrease the incidence of catheter-related bacteremia in children on chronic hemodialysis? *Hemodial Int* 13:11–18, 2009.

Rajpurkar M, Boldt-Macdonald K, Mclenon R, and others: Ethanol lock therapy for the treatment of catheter-related infections in haemophilia patients, *Haemophilia* 15:1267–1271, 2009.

Simon A, Ammann RA, Wiszniewsky G, and others: Taurolidine-citrate lock solution (TauroLock) significantly reduces CVAD-associated gram-positive infections in pediatric cancer patients, *BMC Infect Dis* 8:102–109, 2008.

Soothill JS, Bravery K, Ho A: A fall in bloodstream infections followed a change to 2% chlorhexidine in 70% isopropanol for catheter connection antisepsis: a pediatric single center before/after study on a hemopoietic stem cell transplant ward, *Am J Infect Control* 37:626–630, 2009.

Zitella L: Central venous catheter site care for blood and marrow transplant recipients, *Clin J Oncol Nurs* 7(3):289–298, 2003.

NURSING CARE GUIDELINES

Nasogastric, Orogastric, or Gastrostomy Medication Administration in Children

Use elixir or suspension (rather than tablet) preparations of medication whenever possible.

Dilute viscous medication or syrup with a small amount of water if possible.

If administering tablets, crush tablet to a fine powder and dissolve drug in a small amount of warm water.

Never crush enteric-coated or sustained-release tablets or capsules.

Avoid oily medications because they tend to cling to side of tube.

Do not mix medication with enteral formula unless fluid is restricted. If adding a drug:

* Check with pharmacist for compatibility.
* Shake formula well and observe for any physical reaction (e.g., separation, precipitation).
* Label formula container with name of medication, dosage, date, and time infusion started.

Check for correct placement of nasogastric or orogastric tube (see Nursing Care Guidelines box, p. 697).

Attach syringe (with adaptable tip but without plunger) to tube.

Pour medication into syringe.

Unclamp tube and allow medication to flow by gravity.

Adjust height of container to achieve desired flow rate (e.g., increase height for faster flow).

As soon as syringe is empty, pour in water to flush tubing.

* Amount of water depends on length and gauge of tubing.
* Determine amount before administering any medication by using a syringe to fill completely an unused nasogastric or orogastric tube with water. Amount of flush solution is usually 1.5 times this volume.
* With certain drug preparations (e.g., suspensions), more fluid may be needed.

If administering more than one drug at the same time, flush tube between each medication with clear water.

Clamp tube after flushing unless tube is left open.

RECTAL ADMINISTRATION

The rectal route for administration is less reliable but is sometimes used when the oral route is difficult or contraindicated. It is also used when oral preparations are unsuitable to control vomiting. Some of the drugs available in suppository form are acetaminophen, aspirin, sedatives, analgesics (morphine), and antiemetics. The difficulty in using the rectal route is that unless the rectum is empty at the time of insertion, the absorption of the drug may be delayed, diminished, or prevented by the presence of feces. Sometimes the drug is later evacuated, securely surrounded by stool.

Remove the wrapping on the suppository and lubricate the suppository with warm water (water-soluble jelly may affect medication absorption). Rectal suppositories are traditionally inserted with the apex (pointed end) foremost. Reverse contractions or the pressure

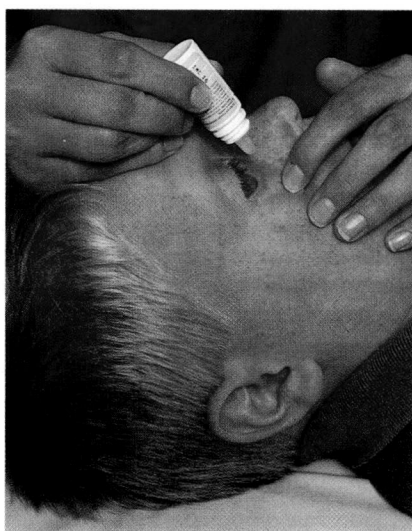

FIG 22-15 Administering eye drops.

Instilling eye drops in infants can be difficult because they often clench the eyelids tightly closed. One approach is to place the drops in the nasal corner where the eyelids meet. The medication pools in this area, and when the child opens the eyelids, the medication flows onto the conjunctiva. For young children, playing a game can be helpful, such as instructing the child to keep the eyes closed to the count of three and then open them, at which time the drops are quickly instilled. Ointment can be applied by gently pulling down the lower eyelid and placing the ointment in the lower conjunctival sac.

DRUG ALERT

If both eye ointment and drops are ordered, give drops first, wait 3 minutes, and then apply the ointment to allow each drug to work. When possible, administer eye ointments before bedtime or naptime because the child's vision will be blurred temporarily.

Ear drops are instilled with the child in the prone or supine position and the head turned to the appropriate side. For children younger than 3 years of age, the external auditory canal is straightened by gently pulling the pinna downward and straight back. The pinna is pulled upward and back in children older than 3 years of age. To place the drops deep into the ear canal without contaminating the tip of the dropper, place a disposable ear speculum in the canal and administer the drops through the speculum. Position the bottle so that the drops fall against the side of the ear canal. After instillation, the child should remain lying on the unaffected side for a few minutes. Gentle massage of the area immediately anterior to the ear facilitates the entry of drops into the ear canal. The use of cotton pledgets prevents medication from flowing out of the external canal. However, they should be loose enough to allow any discharge to exit from the ear. Premoistening the cotton with a few drops of medication prevents the wicking action from absorbing the medication instilled in the ear.

Nose drops are instilled in the same manner as in the adult patient. Remove mucus from the nose with a clean tissue or a washcloth. Unpleasant sensations associated with medicated nose drops are minimized when care is taken to position the child with the head extended well over the edge of the bed or pillow (Fig. 22-16). Depending on size, infants can be positioned in the football hold (see Fig. 22-5, *B*), in the nurse's arm with the head extended and stabilized between the nurse's body and elbow and the arms and hands immobilized with the nurse's hands, or with the head extended over the edge of the bed or a pillow. After instillation of the drops, the child should remain in position for 1 minute to allow the drops to come in contact with the nasal surfaces. Insert nasal spray dispensers into the naris vertically and then angle them to avoid trauma to the septum and to direct medication toward the inferior turbinate.

gradient of the anal canal may help the suppository slip higher into the canal. Using a glove or finger cot, quickly but gently insert the suppository into the rectum beyond both of the rectal sphincters. Then hold the buttocks together firmly to relieve pressure on the anal sphincter until the urge to expel the suppository has passed, which occurs within 5 to 10 minutes. Sometimes the amount of drug ordered is less than the dose available. The irregular shape of most suppositories makes the process of dividing them into a desired dose difficult if not dangerous. If it must be halved, it should be cut lengthwise. However, there is no guarantee that the drug is evenly dispersed throughout the petrolatum base.

If medication is administered via a retention enema, the same procedure is used. Drugs given by enema are diluted in the smallest amount of solution possible to minimize the likelihood of being evacuated.

OPTIC, OTIC, AND NASAL ADMINISTRATION

There are few differences in administering eye, ear, and nose medication to children and to adults. The major difficulty is in gaining children's cooperation. Older children need only an explanation and direction. Although the administration of optic, otic, and nasal medication is not painful, these drugs can cause unpleasant sensations, which can be eliminated with various techniques.

To instill eye medication, place the child supine or sitting with the head extended and ask the child to look up. Use one hand to pull the lower eyelid downward; the hand that holds the dropper rests on the head so that it may move synchronously with the child's head, thus reducing the possibility of trauma to a struggling child or dropping medication on the face (Fig. 22-15). When the lower eyelid is pulled down, a small conjunctival sac is formed; apply the solution or ointment to this area rather than directly on the eyeball. Another effective technique is to pull the lower eyelid down and out to form a cup effect, into which the medication is dropped. Gently close the eyelids to prevent expression of the medication. Wipe excess medication from the inner canthus outward to prevent contamination to the contralateral eye.

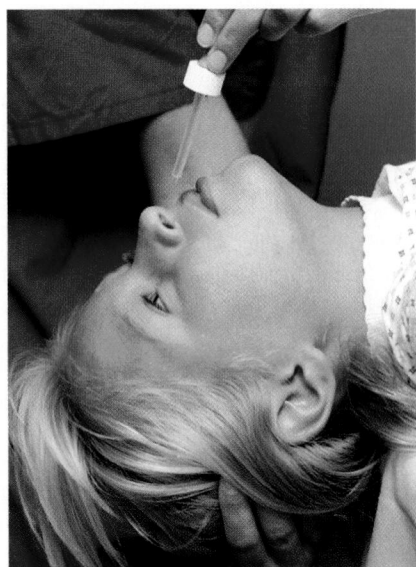

FIG 22-16 Proper position for instilling nose drops.

AEROSOL THERAPY

Aerosol therapy can be effective in depositing medication directly into the airway. The value of aerosolized water, or "mist therapy," is controversial. This route of administration can be useful in avoiding the systemic side effects of certain drugs and in reducing the amount of drug necessary to achieve the desired effect. Bronchodilators, steroids, mucolytics, and antibiotics, suspended in particulate form, can be inhaled so that the medication reaches the small airways. Aerosol therapy is particularly challenging in children who are too young to cooperate with controlling the rate and depth of breathing. Administration of this therapy requires skill, patience, and creativity.

⚠ DRUG ALERT

Medications can be aerosolized or nebulized with air or with oxygen-enriched gas. The **metered-dose inhaler (MDI)** is a self-contained, handheld device that allows for intermittent delivery of a specified amount of medication. Many bronchodilators are available in this form and are successfully used by children with asthma. For children younger than 5 or 6 years, a **spacer device** attached to the MDI can help with coordination of breathing and aerosol delivery. It also allows the aerosolized particles to remain in suspension longer. Handheld nebulizers discharge a medicated mist into a small plastic mask, which the child holds over the nose and mouth. To avoid particle deposition in the nose and pharynx, the child is instructed to take slow, deep breaths through an open mouth during the treatment. For home use, an air compressor is necessary to force air through the liquid medication to form the aerosol. Compact, portable units can be obtained from health equipment companies.

Assessment of breath sounds and work of breathing should be done before and after treatments. Young children who become upset by having a mask held close to the face may become fatigued with fighting the procedure and may actually appear worse during and immediately after the therapy. It may be necessary to spend a few minutes calming the child after the procedure and allowing the vital signs to return to baseline to accurately assess changes in breath sounds and work of breathing.

FAMILY TEACHING AND HOME CARE

The nurse usually assumes responsibility for preparing families to administer medications at home. The family should understand why the child is receiving the medication and the effects that might be expected, as well as the amount, frequency, and length of time the drug is to be administered. Instruction should be carried out in an unhurried, relaxed manner, preferably in an area away from a busy ward or office.

Instruct the caregiver carefully regarding the correct dosage. Some persons have difficulty understanding medical terminology, and just because they nod or otherwise indicate they understand, the nurse should not assume that the message is clear. It is important to ascertain their interpretation of a teaspoon, for example, and to be certain they have acceptable devices for measuring the drug. If the drug is packaged with a dropper, syringe, or plastic cup, the nurse should show or mark the point on the device that indicates the prescribed dose and demonstrate how the dose is drawn up into a dropper or syringe, measured, and the bubbles eliminated. If the nurse has any doubts about the parent's ability to administer the correct dose, the parent should give a return demonstration. This is essential when the drug has potentially serious consequences from incorrect dosage, such as insulin or digoxin, or when more complex administration is required, such as parenteral injections. When teaching a parent to give an injection, the nurse must allot adequate time for instruction and practice.

Home modifications are often necessary because the availability of equipment or assistance can differ from the hospital setting. For example, the parent may need guidance in devising methods that allow one person to hold the child and safely give the drug.

NURSING TIP To administer oral, nasal, or optic medication when only one person is available to hold the child, use the following procedure:
- Place child supine on a flat surface (bed, couch, floor).
- Sit facing child so child's head is between operator's thighs and child's arms are under operator's legs.
- Place lower legs over child's legs to restrain lower body, if necessary.
- To administer oral medication, place a small pillow under child's head to reduce risk of aspiration.
- To administer nasal medication, place a small pillow under child's shoulders to aid flow of liquid through nasal passages.

The nurse should clarify with parents the time that the drug is to be administered. For instance, when a drug is prescribed in association with meals, the number of meals that the family is accustomed to eating influences the amount of drug the child receives. Does the family have meals twice a day or five times a day? When a drug is to be given several times during the day, together the nurse and parents can work out a schedule that accommodates the family's routine. This is particularly significant if a drug must be given at equal intervals throughout a 24-hour period. For example, telling parents that the child needs 1 tsp of medicine four times a day is subject to misinterpretation because the parents may routinely schedule the doses at incorrect times. Instead, a preplanned schedule based on 6-hour intervals should be set up with the number of days required for the therapeutic dosage listed. Modification should also be made to accommodate sleep schedules. Written instructions should accompany all drug prescriptions.

MAINTAINING FLUID BALANCE

MEASUREMENT OF INTAKE AND OUTPUT

Accurate measurements of fluid intake and output (I&O) are essential to the assessment of fluid balance. Measurements from all sources—including gastrointestinal and parenteral I&O from urine, stools, vomitus, fistulas, NG suction, sweat, and drainage from wounds—must be taken and considered. Although the practitioner usually indicates when I&O measurements are to be recorded, it is a nursing responsibility to keep an accurate I&O record on certain children, including those:

- Receiving IV therapy
- Who underwent major surgery
- Receiving diuretic or corticosteroid therapy
- With severe thermal burns or injuries
- With renal disease or damage
- With congestive heart failure
- With dehydration
- With diabetes mellitus
- With oliguria
- In respiratory distress
- With chronic lung disease

Infants and small children who are unable to use a bedpan and those who have bowel movements with every voiding require the application of a collecting device. If collecting bags are not used, wet diapers or pads are carefully weighed to ascertain the amount of fluid lost. This includes liquid stool, vomitus, and other losses. The volume of fluid in milliliters is equivalent to the weight of the fluid measured in grams. The specific gravity as a measure of osmolality assists in assessing the degree of hydration.

In infants with diapers, weigh all dry diapers to be used and note in an indelible marker the dry weight of the diaper; when there is fluid (urine or liquid stool) in the diaper, the amount of output can be approximated by subtracting the weight of the dry diaper from the weighed amount of the wet diaper.

Disadvantages of the weighed-diaper method of fluid measurement include (1) an inability to differentiate one type of loss from another because of admixture, (2) loss of urine or liquid stool from leakage or evaporation (especially if the infant is under a radiant warmer), and (3) additional fluid in the diaper (superabsorbent disposable type) from absorption of atmospheric moisture (in high-humidity incubators).

Special Needs When the Child Is NPO

Infants or children who are unable or not permitted to take fluids by mouth (NPO) have special needs. To ensure that they do not receive fluids, a sign can be placed in some obvious place, such as over their beds or on their shirts, to alert others to the NPO status. To prevent the temptation to drink, fluids should not be left at the bedside.

Oral hygiene, a part of routine hygienic care, is especially important when fluids are restricted or withheld. For young children who cannot brush their teeth or rinse their mouth without swallowing fluid, the mouth and teeth can be cleaned and kept moist by swabbing with saline-moistened gauze.

The child who is fluid restricted presents an equal challenge. Limiting fluids is often more difficult for the child than being NPO, especially when IV fluids are also eliminated. To make certain the child does not drink the entire amount allowed early in the day, the daily allotment is calculated to provide fluids at periodic intervals throughout the child's waking hours. Serving the fluids in small containers gives the illusion of larger servings. No extra liquid is left at the bedside.

PARENTERAL FLUID THERAPY

Site and Equipment

The site selected for peripheral intravenous (PIV) infusion depends on accessibility and convenience. Although it is possible to use any accessible in older children, the child's developmental, cognitive, and mobility needs must be considered when selecting a site. Ideally, in older children, the superficial veins of the forearm should be used, leaving the hands free. An older child can help select the site and thereby maintain some measure of control. For veins in the extremities, it is best to start with the most distal site and avoid the child's favored hand to reduce the disability related to the procedure. Restrict the child's movements as little as possible—avoid a site over a joint in an extremity, such as the antecubital space. In small infants, a superficial vein of the hand, wrist, forearm, foot, or ankle is usually most convenient and most easily stabilized (Fig. 22-17). Foot veins should be avoided in children learning to walk and in children already walking. Superficial veins of the scalp have no valves, insertion is easy, and they can be used in infants up to about 9 months of age, but they should be used only when other site attempts have failed. A transilluminator (Fig. 22-18) can aid in finding and evaluating veins for access (see Evidence-Based Practice box).

Selection of a scalp vein may require clipping the area around the site to better visualize the vein and provide a smoother surface on which to tape the catheter hub and tubing. Clipping a portion of the infant's hair is upsetting to parents; therefore, they should be told what to expect and reassured that the hair will grow in again rapidly (save the hair because parents often wish to keep it). Remove as little as possible directly over the insertion site and taping surface. A rubber band slipped onto the head from brow to occiput will usually suffice as a tourniquet, although if the vessel is visible, a tourniquet may not be necessary.

Situations may occur in which rapid establishment of systemic access is vital, and venous access may be hampered by peripheral

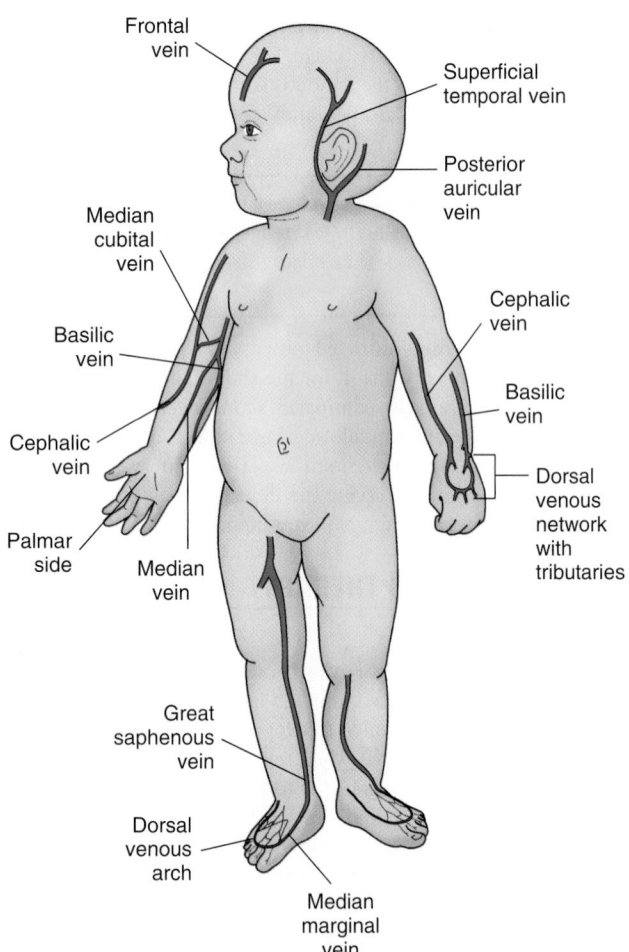

FIG 22-17 Preferred sites for venous access in infants.

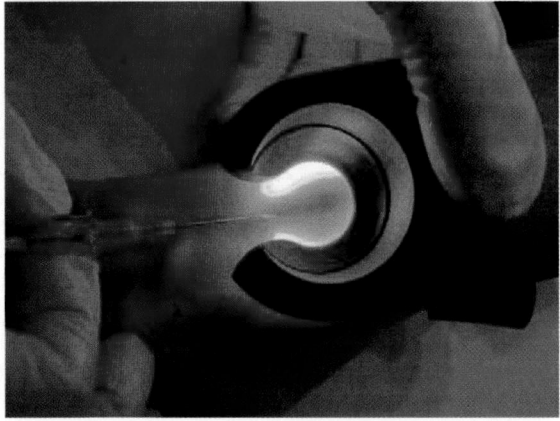

FIG 22-18 Transilluminator: low-heat light-emitting diode (LED) light placed on the skin to illuminate veins; an opening allows cannulation of vein. (Courtesy of Professor Mark Waltzman, Children's Hospital, Boston.)

circulatory collapse, hypovolemic shock (secondary to vomiting or diarrhea, burns, or trauma), cardiopulmonary arrest, or other conditions (de Caen, Reis, and Bhutta, 2008; Hazinski, Zaritsky, Nadkarni, and others, 2002). **Intraosseous infusion** provides a rapid, safe, and lifesaving alternate route for administration of fluids and medications until intravascular access can be attained, especially in children who are 6 years of age and younger.

A large-bore needle, such as a bone marrow aspiration needle (e.g., Jamshidi) or an intraosseous needle (e.g., Cook), is inserted into the medullary cavity of a long bone, most often the proximal tibia. This procedure is usually reserved for children who are unconscious or for those who are receiving analgesia because the procedure is painful. Local anesthesia should be used for semiconscious patients. Observe the dependent tissue closely for swelling because extravasation may be hidden under the leg, and compartment syndrome may result.

For most IV infusions in children, a 22- to 24-gauge catheter may be used if therapy is expected to last less than 5 days. The smallest gauge and shortest length catheter that will accommodate the prescribed therapy should be chosen. The length of the catheter may be directly related to infection or embolus formation—the shorter the catheter, the fewer the complications. The gauge of the catheter should maintain adequate flow of the infusate into the cannulated vein while allowing adequate blood flow around the catheter walls to promote proper hemodilution of the infusate.

Determining the best catheter for the patient early in the therapy provides the best chance of avoiding catheter-related complications. As the length of therapy increases, decisions regarding the type of infusion device (short peripheral, midline, PICC, or central venous catheter) should be explored. Guidelines such as flow charts and algorithms are available to help in these decisions.

Safety Catheters and Needleless Systems

Over-the-needle IV catheters with hollow-bore needles carry a high risk for transmission of bloodborne pathogens from needlestick injuries. Safety catheters prevent accidental needlesticks with the use of over-the-needle IV catheters (Whitby, McLaws, and Slater, 2008).

Needleless IV systems are designed to prevent needlestick injuries during administration of IV push medications and IV piggyback medications. Some needleless devices can be used with any tubing, but others require use of the entire IV delivery system for compatibility. Needleless IV systems rely on prepierced septa that are accessed by blunted plastic cannulas or systems that use valves that open and close a fluid path when activated by insertion of a syringe.

Blunt plastic cannulas and preslit injection port sites (Fig. 22-19) eliminate the need for steel needles and conventional injection port sites but remain accessible via hypodermic needles, a drawback except in emergent situations. Systems that do not permit needled access enhance safety by preventing health care workers from attempting to use needles. A syringe with a blue spike is available to access a single-dose vial (see Fig. 22-19, *A*). The preslit injection port sites are identified by a white ring surrounding the port; this ring alerts users that the system is needleless (see Fig. 22-19, *B*). Syringes are available with the blunt plastic cannula for accessing these sites (see Fig. 22-19, *C*). A lever lock (see Fig. 22-19, *D*) or threaded lock cannula (see Fig. 22-19, *E*) attaches to an IV line, IV Y site, or peripheral intermittent infusion device. A preslit universal vial adapter (not pictured) provides access to standard multiple-dose vials, and syringe cannulas are then used to access the adapter. Valve technology allows syringes and IV tubing to connect directly in-line without the use of an adapter.

> **! NURSING ALERT**
>
> Misconnections of tubing have occurred, resulting in patient deaths. Many needleless IV systems allow other types of tubing such as blood pressure and oxygen tubing to connect and instill air directly into the IV line. Before tubing is connected or reconnected to a patient, trace it completely from the patient to the point of origin for verification.

EVIDENCE-BASED PRACTICE
Use of Transillumination Devices in Obtaining Vascular Access

Jennifer L. Sanders; updated by Olga A. Taylor

Ask the Question
Picot Question
Do transillumination devices decrease the number of attempts needed to obtain vascular access in children?

Search the Evidence
Search Strategies
Search selection criteria included English-language publications within the past 30 years and research-based articles on children undergoing venipuncture.

Databases Used
PubMed, Cochrane Collaboration, MD Consult, BestBETs

Critically Analyze the Evidence
- Transillumination aids in decreasing the number of access attempts (Curran, 1980; Dinner, 1992; Goren, Laufer, Yativ, and others, 2001; Katsogridakis, Seshadri, Sullivan, and others, 2005; Kuhns, Martin, Gildersleeve, and others, 1975).
- Ultrasound screening and guidance improves safety and efficacy of vascular access in neonate and pediatric patients (Arul, Livingstone, Bromley, and others, 2009, 2010; Detaille, Pirotte, Veyckemans, 2010; Samoya, 2010).
- Transillumination was used to decrease the number of peripheral intravenous (PIV) attempts; PIV access of infants and obese children was easier for staff (Kuhns, Martin, Gildersleeve, and others, 1975).
- Small superficial veins that were not previously visualized or palpated were visualized using the transillumination device (Kuhns, Martin, Gildersleeve, and others, 1975).
- No incidents of burns were reported when the transillumination device was used for up to 20 minutes in neonates (Curran, 1980).
- Using two fiberoptic lights as a venous transilluminator resulted in successful PIV access on the first attempt because of the increased visualization of the superficial venous anatomy (Dinner, 1992).
- In infants ages 2 to 36 months, PIV access using a simple otoscope for transillumination was successful on the first attempt for 39 of 40 patients (Goren, Laufer, Yativ, and others, 2001).
- Patients that received PIV access with transillumination using Veinlite were more likely to have a successful IV insertion on the first or second attempt (Katsogridakis, Seshadri, Sullivan, and others, 2005).

Apply the Evidence: Nursing Implications
There is **low-quality evidence** with a **strong recommendation** (Guyatt, Oxman, Vist, and others, 2008) for using transillumination before venous access to decrease the number of attempts needed for successful venous access. Education and practice in this technique are needed for success. Because the veins stand out so clearly with transillumination, they appear more superficial than they are. An assistant may be needed to hold the device when using the transilluminator to obtain PIV access. The heat and temperature of the transilluminator should be monitored to prevent injury to the patient's skin. Appropriate equipment should be used to increase the likelihood of visualization of the vasculature.

QSEN Quality and Safety Competencies:
Evidence-Based Practice*
Knowledge
Differentiate clinical opinion from research and evidence-based summaries.
Describe method of using transillumination before venous access to decrease the number of attempts needed for successful venous access.

Skills
Base individualized care plan on patient values, clinical expertise, and evidence.
Integrate evidence into practice by using transillumination before venous access to decrease the number of attempts needed for successful access.

Attitudes
Value the concept of evidence-based practice as integral to determining best clinical practice.
Appreciate the strengths and weakness of evidence for using transillumination before attempting venous access.

References
Arul GS, Lewis N, Bromley P, and others: Ultrasound-guided percutaneous insertion of Hickman lines in children. Prospective study of 500 consecutive procedures, *J Pediatr Surg*, 44:1371–1376, 2009.
Arul GS, Livingstone H, Bromley P, and others: Ultrasound-guided percutaneous insertion of 2.7 Fr tunneled Broviac lines in neonates and small infants, *Pediatr Surg Int*, 26:815–818, 2010.
Curran JS: A restraint and transillumination device for neonatal-arterial/venipuncture: efficacy and thermal safety, *Pediatrics* 66(1):128–130, 1980.
Detaille T, Pirotte T, Veyckemans F: Vascular access in the neonate, *Best Pract Res Clin Anaesthesiol* 24:203–418, 2010.
Dinner M: Transillumination to facilitate venipuncture in children [letter to editor], *Anesthesiol Analg* 74(3):467–477, 1992.
Goren A, Laufer J, Yativ N, and others: Transillumination of the palm for venipuncture in infants, *Pediatr Emerg Care* 17(2):130–131, 2001.
Guyatt GH, Oxman AD, Vist GE, and others: GRADE: An emerging consensus on rating quality of evidence and strength of recommendations, *BMJ* 336(7650):924–926, 2008.
Katsogridakis Y, Seshadri R, Sullivan C, and others: *Veinlite transillumination in the pediatric emergency department: a therapeutic interventional trial*, retrieved August 2005 from http://www.veinlite.com/public.html.
Kuhns LR, Martin AJ, Gildersleeve S, and others: Intense transillumination for infant venipuncture, *Radiology* 116(3):734–735, 1975.
Samoya SW: Real-time ultrasound-guided peripheral vascular access in pediatric patients, *Anesth Analg* 111:823–824, 2010.

*Adapted from the QSEN at http://www.qsen.org.

Infusion Pumps

A variety of infusion pumps are available and used in nearly all pediatric infusions to accurately administer medication and minimize the possibility of overloading the circulation. It is important to calculate the amount to be infused in a given length of time, set the infusion rate, and monitor the apparatus frequently (at least every 1 to 2 hours) to make certain that the desired rate is maintained, the integrity of the system remains intact, the site remains intact (free of redness, edema, infiltration, or irritation), and the infusion does not stop. Continuous infusion pumps, although convenient and efficient, are not without risks. Overreliance on the accuracy of the machine can cause either too much or too little fluid to be infused; therefore, its use does not eliminate careful periodic assessment by the nurse. Excess pressure can build up if the machine is set at a rate faster than the vein is able to accommodate (or continues to pump when the needle is out of the lumen).

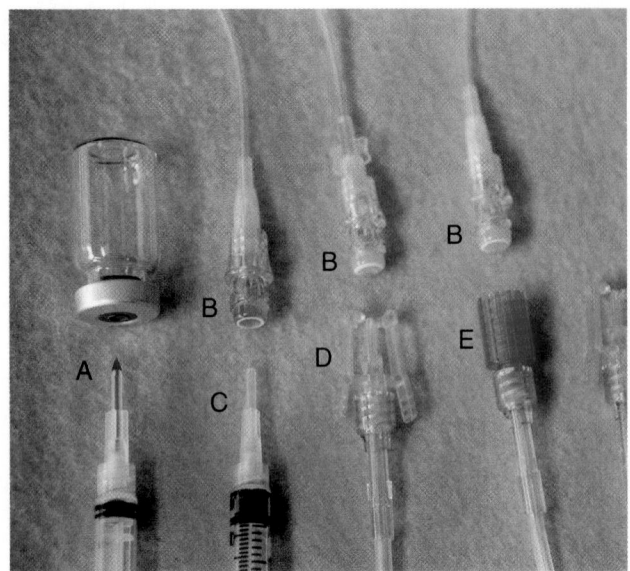

FIG 22-19 Interlink intravenous access systems. **A,** Blue spike syringe. **B,** Preslit injection port (needleless). **C,** Blunt plastic cannula syringe. **D,** Lever lock cannula. **E,** Threaded lock cannula.

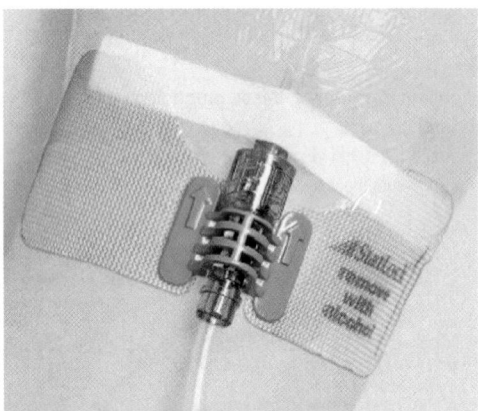

FIG 22-20 StatLock securement devices enhance peripheral intravenous line dwell time and decrease phlebitis.

Securement of a Peripheral Intravenous Line

To maintain the integrity of the IV line, adequate protection of the site is required. The catheter hub is firmly secured at the puncture site with a transparent dressing and commercial securement device (e.g., StatLock) (Fig. 22-20) or clear nonallergenic tape. Transparent dressings are ideal because the insertion site is easily observed. Minimal tape should be used at the puncture site and on about 1 to 2 inches of skin beyond the site to avoid obscuring the insertion site for early detection of infiltration.

A protective cover is applied directly over the catheter insertion site to protect the infusion site. Easy access to the IV site for frequent (hourly) assessments must be considered (Infusion Nurses Society, 2006). Improvised plastic cups that are cut in half with the ridged edges covered with tape should not be used because they have injured patients. A commercial site protector, I.V. House, is available in different sizes (Fig. 22-21). Its ventilation holes prevent moisture from accumulating under the dome. This device is designed to protect the IV site and allows for visibility of the site. The device also minimizes use of padded boards, splints, or other restraints and tape and maintains skin

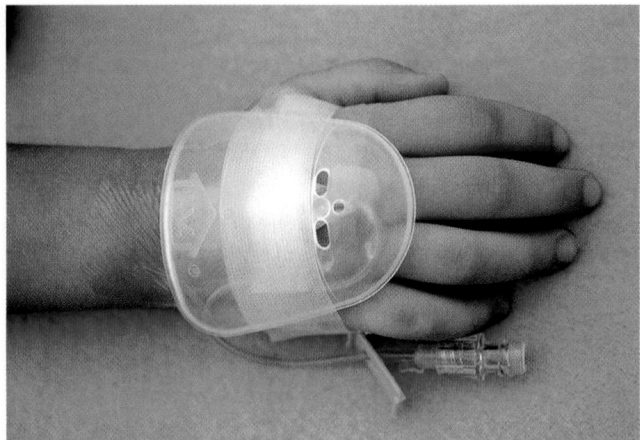

FIG 22-21 I.V. House used to protect the intravenous site.

integrity. The connector tubing or extension tubing can be looped to make it small enough to fit under the protective cover to prevent accidental snagging of the catheter. It is important to safely secure the IV tubing to prevent infants and children from becoming entangled in the tubing and from accidentally pulling the catheter or needle out. Securing the tubing in this manner also eliminates movement of the catheter hub at the insertion site (mechanical manipulation). A colorful and interesting sticker can be applied to the protecting device to add a positive note to the procedure.

Finger and toe areas are left unoccluded by dressings or tape to allow for assessment of circulation. The thumb is never immobilized because of the danger of contractures with limited movement later on. An extremity should never be encircled with tape. The use of roll gauze, self-adhering stretch bandages (Coban), and Ace bandages can cause the same constriction and hide signs of infiltration.

> **! NURSING ALERT**
>
> Opaque covering should be avoided; however, if any type of opaque covering is used to secure the IV line, the insertion site and extremity distal to the site should be visible to detect an infiltration. If these sites are not visible, they must be checked frequently to detect problems early.

Traditionally, padded boards and splints have been used to partially immobilize the IV site. Padded boards and splints and restraints were appropriate when metal needles were inserted into the vein to prevent the sharp end from puncturing the vessel, especially at a joint. With the more recent use of soft, pliable catheters, arm or leg boards may not be necessary and have several disadvantages. They obscure the IV site, can constrict the extremity, may excoriate the underlying tissue and promote infection, can cause a contracture of a joint, restrict useful movement of the extremity, and are uncomfortable. Unfortunately, no research has been conducted to demonstrate their proposed benefit of increasing dwell time (patency of the IV line). Adequate securement should eliminate the need for padded boards in most circumstances. Older children who are alert and cooperative can usually be trusted to protect the IV site (see Evidence-Based Practice boxes).

Removal of a Peripheral Intravenous Line

When it comes time to discontinue an IV infusion, many children are distressed by the thought of catheter removal. Therefore, they need a careful explanation of the process and suggestions for helping.

Peripheral Intravenous Care

Joy Hesselgrave; updated by Olga A. Taylor

Ask the Question
Picot Question

What site preparation and stabilization measures for PIV catheters are optimum for preventing complications and extending dwell time in children?

Search for the Evidence
Search Strategies

Search selection criteria included English-language and research-based publications within the past 20 years on PIV catheter site care.

Databases Used

National Guidelines Clearinghouse (AHQR), Cochrane Collaboration, Joanna Briggs Institute, PubMed, TRIP Database Plus, MD Consult, PedsCCM, BestBETs.

Critically Analyze the Evidence
Site Preparation

- The skin should be disinfected with an appropriate antiseptic before PIV catheter insertion; allow it to dry before catheter insertion (Infusion Nurses Society, 2011a, 2011b; O'Grady, Alexander, Dellinger, and others, 2002; Registered Nurses' Association of Ontario, 2008).
- A 2% chlorhexidine-based preparation is preferred, but tincture of iodine, an iodophor, or 70% alcohol can be used. There is no recommendation for the use of chlorhexidine in infants younger than 2 months old (Infusion Nurses Society, 2011a; O'Grady, Alexander, Dellinger, and others, 2002).
- Cleansing the skin with a preparation that combines alcohol with either chlorhexidine gluconate or povidone–iodine before PIV catheter insertion is recommended (Infusion Nurses Society, 2006, 2011a, 2011b).
- All disinfectants have risks for neonates. Chlorhexidine gluconate with alcohol should not be used in neonates; aqueous chlorhexidine or povidone–iodine should be used in premature infants. Remove cleansers from infants using sterile water or normal saline to prevent absorption of the disinfectant (Association of Women's Health, Obstetric and Neonatal Nurses, 2007).

Stabilization or Securement Devices

- PIV catheters must be stabilized for easy monitoring and evaluation of the access site; to promote delivery of therapy; and to prevent damage, dislodgement, or migration of the catheter (Infusion Nurses Society, 2011a; Registered Nurses' Association of Ontario, 2008).
- To avoid catheter movement and damage, the catheter and hub should be secured firmly with Steri-Strips and clear occlusive dressing; tape should not be placed directly to the catheter (Infusion Nurses Society, 2011a; Paulson and Miller, 2008).
- The catheter site should be assessed every 7 to 8 hours to ensure that the catheter has not migrated (Infusion Nurses Society, 2011a; Paulson and Miller, 2008).
- The traditional transparent dressing (Tegaderm) and tape group had a 65% complication rate (dislodgments, infiltration, and phlebitis) versus a 20% complication rate in the transparent dressings and a catheter securement device (StatLock) group, indicating a 45% reduction in overall PIV therapy complications in the StatLock group (Wood, 1997).

- When comparing tape, StatLock, and Hub-Guard for a 96-hour PIV protocol change, it was found that PIV catheters with StatLock produced a statistically significant improved survival rate (52%) compared with tape (8%) or Hub-Guard (9%) (Smith, 2006).

Dwell Time

- In pediatric patients, PIV catheters may remain in place until a complication occurs or the therapy is complete (O'Grady, Alexander, Dellinger, and others, 2002).
- In pediatric patients with PIV catheters, the overall risk of PIV catheter complications was extremely low and would not be reduced substantially by routine catheter replacement (Shimandle, Johnson, Baker, and others, 1999).
- Evidence is insufficient regarding the effect of heparin use for extending PIV catheter use in neonates (Shah, Ng, and Sinha, 2005).
- An increase in complications and obstructions of PIV catheters was related to younger patient age, insertion into the wrist and scalp, and use of a 24-gauge catheter (Tripathi, Kaushik, and Singh, 2008).

Apply the Evidence: Nursing Implications

There is **low-quality evidence** with a **strong recommendation** (Guyatt, Oxman, Vist, and others, 2008) for site preparation and stabilization measures for PIV catheters in children. For children older than 2 months of age, chlorhexidine is the preferred skin cleanser. For younger infants, non–alcohol-based cleansers are preferred and should be removed with sterile water or sterile normal saline to prevent absorption. The most distal vein on the extremity that allows the child optimum movement (avoid over the joint) should be selected. Veins on the scalp may be used in infants. Subsequent PIV catheters should be proximal to the previous IV site. If the child is mobile, consider using a securement or protection device (e.g., StatLock, HubGuard, Ray-Marshall Shield, IV House, IV Shield, IV Pro). Discontinue the PIV catheter if complications occur or when it is no longer needed.

QSEN Quality and Safety Competencies:
Evidence-Based Practice*
Knowledge

Differentiate clinical opinion from research and evidence-based summaries.

Describe methods for site preparation and stabilization measures of PIV catheters for preventing complications and extending dwell time in children.

Skills

Base individualized care plan on patient values, clinical expertise, and evidence.

Integrate evidence into practice by using techniques for site preparation and stabilization measures for PIV catheters in children.

Attitudes

Value the concept of evidence-based practice as integral to determining best clinical practice.

Appreciate the strengths and weakness of evidence for site preparation and stabilization measures for PIV catheters in children.

PIV, Peripheral intravenous.
*Adapted from the QSEN at http://www.qsen.org.

Continued

EVIDENCE-BASED PRACTICE

Peripheral Intravenous Care—cont'd

References

Association of Women's Health, Obstetric and Neonatal Nurses: *Neonatal skin care 2nd edition evidence-based clinical practice guideline*, Washington, DC, 2007, Author.

Guyatt GH, Oxman AD, Vist GE, and others: GRADE: An emerging consensus on rating quality of evidence and strength of recommendations, *BMJ* 336(7650):924–926, 2008.

Infusion Nurses Society: Infusion nursing standards of practice, *J Infus Nurse* 34(1S), 2011a.

Infusion Nurses Society: *Policies and procedures for infusion nursing*, ed 4, South Norwood, Mass, 2011b, Author.

O'Grady N, Alexander M, Dellinger E, and others: Guidelines for the prevention of intravascular catheter–related infections, *MMWR Morb Mortal Wkly Rep* 51(32), 2002.

Paulson PR, Miller KM: Neonatal peripherally inserted central catheters: recommendations for prevention of insertion and postinsertion complications, *Neonatal Netw* 27:245–257, 2008.

Registered Nurses' Association of Ontario: *Care and maintenance to reduce vascular access complications, guideline supplement*, Toronto, 2008, Author.

Shah PS, Ng E, Sinha AK: Heparin for prolonging peripheral intravenous catheter use in neonates, *Cochrane Database Syst Rev* (4):CD002774, 2005.

Shimandle R, Johnson D, Baker M, and others: Safety of peripheral intravenous catheters in children, *Infect Control Hosp Epidemiol* 20:736–740, 1999.

Smith B: Peripheral intravenous catheter dwell times: a comparison of three securement methods for implementation of a 96-hour scheduled change protocol, *J Infus Nurs* 29(1):14–17, 2006.

Tripathi S, Kaushik V, Singh V: Peripheral IVs: factors affecting complications and patency—a randomized controlled trial, *J Infus Nurs* 31:182–188, 2008.

Wood D: A comparative study of two securement techniques for short peripheral intravenous catheters, *J Intraven Nurs* 20(6):280–285, 1997.

EVIDENCE-BASED PRACTICE

Frequency of Changing Intravenous Administration Sets

Brandi Horvath; updated by Olga A. Taylor

Ask the Question

Picot Question

In children, should IV administration sets be changed at 24, 48, 72, or 96 hours to safely prevent patient infection while containing costs?

Search the Evidence

Search Strategies

Search selection criteria included English-language publications within the past 10 years and research-based articles on frequency of changing IV administration sets.

Databases Used

National Guideline Clearinghouse (AHRQ), Cochrane Collaboration, Joanna Briggs Institute, PubMed, Infusion Nurses Society, Oncology Nurses Society, MD Consult, BestBETs, TRIP Database Plus, PedsCCM

Critically Analyze the Evidence

- Replacing IV administration sets every 96 hours or with catheter change, except for fluids that enhance microbial growth, is recommended (Camp-Sorreli, 2004; Gillies, O'Riordan, Wallen, and others, 2005; Infusion Nurses Society, 2011a, 2011b).
- For IV administration sets including blood or blood products and lipids, changing the sets every 24 hours is recommended (Camp-Sorreli, 2004; Gillies, O'Riordan, Wallen, and others, 2005; Infusion Nurses Society, 2011a).
- IV administration sets for crystalloids should be changed at no more than 72-hour intervals (O'Grady, Alexander, Dellinger, and others, 2002).
- Replace tubing used to administer blood and blood products or lipid emulsions within 24 hours of starting the infusion (O'Grady, Alexander, Dellinger, and others, 2002).
- Continuously infusing IV administration sets should be replaced no more frequently than every 72 hours (Alexander, 2006; Infusion Nurses Society, 2011a).
- Administration sets used intermittently should be changed every 24 hours (Alexander, 2006; Infusion Nurses Society, 2006, 2011a, 2011b).
- Secondary piggyback sets may be changed no more frequently than every 72 hours when attached to a continuously infusing line; after being detached from the primary set, they should be changed at 24 hours; exceptions: sets used with lipids (change at 24 hours if continuous or after each unit if intermittently infused) and blood or blood components (change at the end of

4 hours if continuous or after each intermittent component) (Alexander, 2006; Infusion Nurses Society, 2011a, 2011b).

Apply the Evidence: Nursing Implications

There is **moderate-quality evidence** with a **strong recommendation** (Guyatt, Oxman, Vist, and others, 2008) for replacing IV administration sets every 96 hours; replacing tubing used for lipid emulsions, blood, and blood products every 24 hours; and replacing blood tubing with in-line filters after 2 units or 4 hours, whichever comes first.

QSEN **Quality and Safety Competencies:**

Evidence-Based Practice*

Knowledge

Differentiate clinical opinion from research and evidence-based summaries.

Describe methods for frequency of changing IV administration sets in children.

Skills

Base individualized care plan on patient values, clinical expertise, and evidence.

Integrate evidence into practice by using techniques for frequency of changing IV administration sets in children.

Attitudes

Value the concept of evidence-based practice as integral to determining best clinical practice.

Appreciate the strengths and weakness of evidence for frequency of changing IV administration sets in children.

References

Alexander M, editor: Infusion nursing standards of practice, *J Infus Nurs* 29(1S):S48–S50, 2006.

Camp-Sorreli D, editor: *Access device guidelines: recommendations for nursing practice and education*, ed 2, Pittsburgh, 2004, Oncology Nursing Society.

Gillies D, O'Riordan L, Wallen M, and others: Optimal timing for intravenous administration set replacement, *Cochrane Database Syst Rev* (4):CD003588, 2005.

Guyatt GH, Oxman AD, Vist GE, and others: GRADE: an emerging consensus on rating quality of evidence and strength of recommendations, *BMJ* 336(7650):924–926, 2008.

Infusion Nurses Society: Infusion nursing standards of practice, *J Infus Nurse* 34(1S), 2011a.

Infusion Nurses Society: *Policies and procedures for infusion nursing*, ed 4, South Norwood, Mass, 2011b, Author.

O'Grady N, Alexander M, Dellinger E, and others: Guidelines for the prevention of intravascular catheter-related infections, *MMWR Morb Mortal Wkly Rep* 51(RR-10):1–29, 2002.

IV, Intravenous.

*Adapted from the QSEN at http://www.qsen.org.

Encouraging children to remove or help remove the tape from the site provides them with a measure of control and often fosters their cooperation. The procedure consists of turning off any pump apparatus, occluding the IV tubing, removing the tape, pulling the catheter out of the vessel in the opposite direction of insertion, and exerting firm pressure at the site. A dry dressing (adhesive bandage strip) is placed over the puncture site. The use of adhesive-removal pads can decrease the pain of tape removal, but the skin should be washed after use to avoid irritation. To remove transparent dressings (e.g., OpSite, Tegaderm), pull the opposing edges parallel to the skin to loosen the bond. Inspect the catheter tip to ensure the catheter is intact and that no portion remains in the vein.

> **! NURSING ALERT**
>
> Consider the child's age, development, and neurologic status, as well as the predictability of the child (how the child responds to painful treatments), when determining the need for assistance to maintain safety. Manual removal of tape is the preferred method. Only if absolutely necessary should a small cut be made in the tape, using bandage scissors, to facilitate its removal. Before cutting the tape:
> * Ensure that all digits are visible.
> * Remove any barrier that hinders visibility, such as a protective covering.
> * Protect the child's skin and digits by sliding own finger(s) between the tape and the child's skin so that the scissors do not touch the patient.
> * Cut on the tape on the medial aspect (thumb side) of the extremity.

Complications

The same precautions regarding maintenance of asepsis, prevention of infection, and observation for infiltration are carried out with patients of any age. However, infiltration is more difficult to detect in infants and small children than in adults. The increased amount of subcutaneous fat and the amount of tape used to secure the catheter often obscure the early signs of infiltration. When the fluid appears to be infusing too slowly or ceases, the usual assessment for obstruction within the apparatus—kinks, screw clamps, shutoff valve, and positioning interference (e.g., a bent elbow)—often locates the difficulty. When these actions fail to detect the problem, it may be necessary to carefully remove some of the dressing to obtain a clear view of the venipuncture site. Dependent areas, such as the palm and undersides of the extremity or the occiput and behind the ears, are examined.

Whenever possible, the IV infusion should be placed in an extremity to which the identification band (or bracelet) is not attached. Serious circulatory impairment can result from infiltrated solution distal to the band, which acts as a tourniquet, preventing adequate venous return. To check for return blood flow through the catheter, the tubing is removed from the infusion pump, and the bag is lowered below the level of the infusion site. Resistance during flushing or aspiration for blood return also indicates that the IV infusion may have infiltrated surrounding tissue. A good blood return, or lack thereof, is not always an indicator of infiltration in small infants. Flushing the catheter and observing for edema, redness, or streaking along the vein are appropriate for assessment of the IV.

Intravenous therapy in pediatrics tends to be difficult to maintain because of mechanical factors such as vascular trauma resulting from the catheter, the insertion site, vessel size, vessel fragility, pump pressure, the patient's activity level, operator skill and insertion technique, forceful administration of boluses of fluid, and infusion of irritants or vesicants through a small vessel. These factors cause infiltration and extravasation injuries. Infiltration is defined as inadvertent administration of a nonvesicant solution or medication into surrounding tissue. Extravasation is defined as inadvertent administration of vesicant solution or medication into surrounding tissue (Infusion Nurses Society, 2006). A vesicant or sclerosing agent causes varying degrees of cellular damage when even minute amounts escape into surrounding tissue. Guidelines are available for determining the severity of tissue injury by staging characteristics, such as the amount of redness, blanching, the amount of swelling, pain, the quality of pulses below infiltration, capillary refill, and warmth or coolness of the area (Infusion Nurses Society, 2006).*

Treatment of infiltration or extravasation varies according to the type of vesicant. Guidelines are available outlining the sequence of interventions and specific treatment of infiltration or extravasation with antidotes.

> **! NURSING ALERT**
>
> When infiltration or extravasation is observed (signs include erythema, pain, edema, blanching, streaking on the skin along the vein, and darkened area at the insertion site), immediately stop the infusion, elevate the extremity, notify the practitioner, and initiate the ordered treatment as soon as possible. Remove the IV line when it is no longer needed (e.g., after infusing an antidote).

Phlebitis, or inflammation of the vessel wall, may also develop in children who require IV therapy. Lamagna and MacPhee (2004) describe three types of phlebitis: mechanical (caused by rapid infusion rate, manipulation of the IV), chemical (caused by medications), and bacterial (caused by staphylococcal organisms). The initial sign of phlebitis is erythema (redness) at the insertion site. Pain may or may not be present.

Peripheral intravenous catheters are the most commonly used intravascular device. Heavy cutaneous colonization of the insertion site is the single most important predictor of catheter-related infection with all types of short-term, percutaneously inserted catheters. Phlebitis, largely a mechanical rather than infectious process, remains the most important complication associated with the use of peripheral venous catheters.†

> **! NURSING ALERT**
>
> The most effective ways to prevent infection of an IV site are to cleanse hands between each patient, wear gloves when inserting a catheter, and closely inspect the insertion site and physical condition of the dressing. Proper education of the patient and family regarding signs and symptoms of an infected site can help prevent infections from going unnoticed.

PROCEDURES FOR MAINTAINING RESPIRATORY FUNCTION

INHALATION THERAPY

Oxygen Therapy

Oxygen is administered for hypoxemia and may be delivered by mask, nasal cannula, face tent, hood, face mask, or ventilator. The mode of

---

*Guidelines for determining tissue injury severity are available from the Infusion Nurses Society, 315 Norwood Park South, Norwood, MA 02062; 781-440-9408; http://www.ins1.org.
†Guidelines for prevention of intravascular device–related infections are available from the CDC, 1600 Clifton Road, Atlanta, GA 30333; 404-639-1515; http://www.cdc.gov/ncidod/dhqp/gl_intravascular.html.

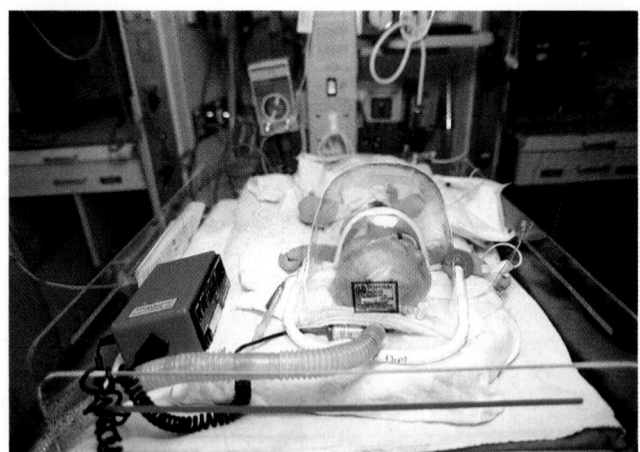

FIG 22-22 Oxygen administered to an infant by means of a plastic hood. Note the oxygen analyzer (blue machine).

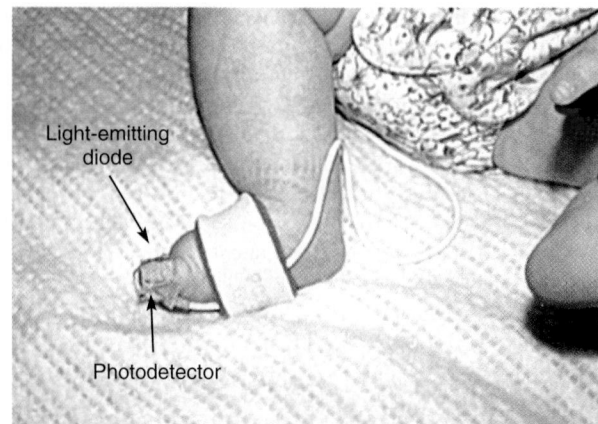

FIG 22-23 Oximeter sensor on the great toe. Note that the sensor is positioned with a light-emitting diode (LED) opposite the photodetector. The cord is secured to the foot to minimize movement of the sensor.

delivery is selected on the basis of the concentration needed and the child's ability to cooperate in its use. Oxygen therapy is frequently administered in the hospital, although increasing numbers of children are receiving oxygen in the home. Oxygen is dry and therefore must be humidified.

Oxygen delivered to infants is well tolerated by using a **plastic hood** (Fig. 22-22). At least 4 to 5 L/min of flow is necessary to maintain oxygen concentrations and remove the exhaled carbon dioxide. The humidified oxygen should not be blown directly into the infant's face. Older, cooperative infants and children can use a **nasal cannula** or **prongs**, which can supply a concentration of oxygen of about 50%.

Oxygen masks are available in pediatric sizes but may not be well tolerated in children because a snug fit is required to ensure adequate oxygen delivery. A face tent or bucket is often better tolerated because this soft piece of plastic sits beneath the child's chin and allows oxygen to be directed to the mouth and nose without enclosure (Curley and Moloney-Harmon, 2001). **Oxygen tents** (croup tents) are rarely used today in developed countries. Oxygen concentration is difficult to control, and the child's clothing can become saturated with water from the humidification and cause hypothermia.

💊 DRUG ALERT

Oxygen Toxicity

Prolonged exposure to high oxygen tensions can damage some body tissues and functions. The organs most vulnerable to the adverse effects of excessive oxygenation are the retinas of extremely preterm infants and the lungs of persons at any age.

❗ NURSING ALERT

Inspect all toys for safety and suitability (e.g., vinyl or plastic, not stuffed items that absorb moisture and are difficult to keep dry). The high-level oxygen environment makes any source of sparks (e.g., mechanical or electrical toys) a potential fire hazard.

Oxygen-induced carbon dioxide narcosis is a physiologic hazard of oxygen therapy that may occur in persons with chronic pulmonary disease, such as cystic fibrosis. In these patients, the respiratory center has adapted to the continuously higher arterial carbon dioxide tension

($PaCO_2$) levels, and therefore hypoxia becomes the more powerful stimulus for respiration. When the arterial oxygen tension (PaO_2) level is elevated during oxygen administration, the hypoxic drive is removed, causing progressive hypoventilation and increased $PaCO_2$ levels, and the child rapidly becomes unconscious. Carbon dioxide narcosis can also be induced by the administration of sedation in these patients.

Monitoring Oxygen Therapy

Pulse oximetry is a continuous, noninvasive method of determining oxygen saturation (SaO_2) to guide oxygen therapy. A sensor composed of a light-emitting diode (LED) and a photodetector is placed in opposition around a foot, hand, finger, toe, or earlobe, with the LED placed on top of the nail when digits are used (Fig. 22-23). The diode emits red and infrared lights that pass through the skin to the photodetector. The photodetector measures the amount of each type of light absorbed by functional hemoglobins. Hemoglobin saturated with oxygen (oxyhemoglobin) absorbs more infrared light than does hemoglobin not saturated with oxygen (deoxyhemoglobin). Pulsatile blood flow is the primary physiologic factor that influences accuracy of the pulse oximeter. In infants, reposition the probe at least every 3 to 4 hours to prevent pressure necrosis; poor perfusion and very sensitive skin may necessitate more frequent repositioning.

Another noninvasive method is **transcutaneous monitoring (TCM)**, which provides continuous monitoring of transcutaneous partial pressure of oxygen in arterial blood ($tcPaO_2$) and, with some devices, of carbon dioxide in arterial blood ($tcPaCO_2$). An electrode is attached to the warmed skin to facilitate arterialization of cutaneous capillaries. The site of the electrode must be changed every 3 to 4 hours to avoid burning the skin, and the machine must be calibrated with every site change. TCM is used frequently in neonatal intensive care units, but it may not reflect PaO_2 in infants with impaired local circulation or in older infants whose skin is thicker.

Oximetry is insensitive to hyperoxia because hemoglobin approaches 100% saturation for all PaO_2 readings greater than approximately 100 mm Hg, which is a dangerous situation for preterm infants at risk for developing retinopathy of prematurity (see Chapter 9). Therefore, preterm infants being monitored with oximetry should have their upper limits identified, such as 90% to 95%, and a protocol should be established for decreasing oxygen when saturations are high.

Oximetry offers several advantages over TCM. Oximetry (1) does not require heating the skin, thus reducing the risk of burns;

(2) eliminates a delay period for transducer equilibration; and (3) maintains an accurate measurement regardless of the patient's age or skin characteristics or the presence of lung disease.

> **! NURSING ALERT**
>
> It is important to make certain that sensor connectors and oximeters are compatible. Wiring that is incompatible can generate considerable heat at the tip of the sensor, causing second- and third-degree burns under the sensors. Pressure necrosis can also occur from sensors attached too tightly. Therefore, inspect the skin under the sensor frequently.

Applying the sensor correctly is essential for accurate SaO_2 measurements. Because the sensor must identify every pulse beat to calculate the SaO_2, movement can interfere with sensing. Some devices synchronize the SaO_2 reading with the heartbeat, thereby reducing the interference caused by motion. Sensors are not placed on extremities used for blood pressure monitoring or with indwelling arterial catheters because pulsatile blood flow may be affected.

> **NURSING TIP** **Infant**—Secure the sensor to the great toe and tape the wire to the sole of the foot (or use a commercial holder that fastens with a self-adhering closure). Place a snugly fitting sock over the foot but check the site frequently for color, temperature, and pulse.
> **Child**—Secure the sensor securely to the index finger and tape the wire to the back of the hand.

Ambient light from ceiling lights and phototherapy, as well as high-intensity heat and light from radiant warmers, can interfere with readings. Therefore, the sensor should be covered to block these light sources. IV dyes; green, purple, or black nail polish; nonopaque synthetic nails; and possibly ink used for footprinting can also cause inaccurate SaO_2 measurements. The dyes should be removed or, in the case of porcelain nails, a different area used for the sensor. Skin color, thickness, and edema do not affect the readings.

Blood gas measurements are sensitive indicators of change in respiratory status in acutely ill patients. They provide valuable information regarding lung function, lung adequacy, and tissue perfusion. The pH, $PaCO_2$, HCO_3, and PaO_2 levels can provide information about whether the child is compensating and guide critical treatment decisions.

END-TIDAL CARBON DIOXIDE MONITORING

End-tidal CO_2 ($ETCO_2$) monitoring measures exhaled carbon dioxide noninvasively. Capnometry provides a numeric display, and capnography provides a graph over time. Continuous capnometry is available in many bedside physiologic monitors as well as stand-alone monitors. $ETCO_2$ differs from pulse oximetry in that it is more sensitive to the mechanics of ventilation rather than oxygenation. Hypoxic episodes can be prevented through the early detection of hypoventilation, apnea, or airway obstruction.

Children who are experiencing an asthma exacerbation, receiving procedural sedation, or who are mechanically ventilated may have $ETCO_2$ monitoring. Special sampling cannulas are used for nonintubated patients, and a small device is placed between the endotracheal (ET) tube and the ventilator tubing in intubated patients. Although $ETCO_2$ monitoring is not a substitute for arterial blood gases, it does have the information of providing ventilation information continuously and noninvasively. Normal $ETCO_2$ values are 30 to 43 mm Hg, which is slightly lower than normal arterial PCO_2 of 35 to 45 mm Hg.

During cardiopulmonary resuscitation (CPR), $ETCO_2$ values consistently below 15 mm Hg indicate ineffective compressions or excessive ventilation. Changes in waveform and numeric display follow changes in ventilation by a very few seconds and precede changes in respiratory rate, skin color, and pulse oximetry values.

For years, disposable colormetric $ETCO_2$ detectors have been used to assess ET tube placement. A color change with each exhaled breath when there is adequate systemic perfusion indicates that the tube is in the lungs. These devices do not provide numbers or graphic representation and do not provide the same early detection of hypoventilation as the continuous quantitative monitors.

Additional uses of $ETCO_2$ monitoring have limited supporting research. Although waveform analysis does not yet have standardized nomenclature, some clinicians use the angles of the waveform coupled with the quantitative value of $ETCO_2$ to classify the severity of asthma exacerbations. The severity of diabetic ketoacidosis (Fearon and Steele, 2002) and acidosis from gastroenteritis (Nagler, Wright, and Krauss, 2006) has also been researched in children and is used in some facilities.

When there is a change in the $ETCO_2$ value or waveform, assess the patient quickly for adequate airway, breathing, and circulation. Sedated patients may be hypoventilating and need stimulation. Intubated patients may need suctioning, have self-extubated or dislodged the tube, or have equipment failure or disconnection. Patients with asthma may have a worsening condition. Problems with the $ETCO_2$ monitoring system can include a kink in the sample line or disconnection. In general, check the patient first and then the equipment.

BRONCHIAL (POSTURAL) DRAINAGE

Bronchial drainage is indicated whenever excessive fluid or mucus in the bronchi is not being removed by normal ciliary activity and cough. Positioning the child to take maximum advantage of gravity facilitates removal of secretions. Postural drainage can be effective in children with chronic lung disease characterized by thick mucus, such as cystic fibrosis.

Postural drainage is carried out three or four times daily and is more effective when it follows other respiratory therapy, such as bronchodilator or nebulization medication. Bronchial drainage is generally performed before meals (or 1 to 1½ hours after meals) to minimize the chance of vomiting and is repeated at bedtime. The duration of treatment depends on the child's condition and tolerance; it usually lasts 20 to 30 minutes. Several positions facilitate drainage from all major lung segments).

CHEST PHYSICAL THERAPY

Chest physical therapy (CPT) usually refers to the use of postural drainage in combination with adjunctive techniques that are thought to enhance the clearance of mucus from the airway. These techniques include manual percussion, vibration, and squeezing of the chest; cough; forceful expiration; and breathing exercises. Special mechanical devices are also currently used to perform CPT (e.g., vest-type percussors). Postural drainage in combination with forced expiration has been shown to be beneficial.

Common techniques used in association with postural drainage include manual percussion of the chest wall and percussion with mechanical devices such as a high-frequency handheld chest compression device. A "popping," hollow sound, not a slapping sound, should be the result. The procedure should be done over the rib cage only and should be painless. Percussion can be performed with a soft circular mask (adapted to maintain air trapping) or a percussion cup marketed especially for the purpose of aiding in loosening secretions. CPT is contraindicated when patients have pulmonary hemorrhage, pulmonary embolism, end-stage renal disease, increased intracranial pressure, osteogenesis imperfecta, or minimal cardiac reserves.

INTUBATION

Rapid-sequence intubation (RSI) is commonly performed in pediatric (and some neonatal) patients to induce an unconscious, neuromuscular blocked condition to avoid the use of positive-pressure ventilation and the risk of possible aspiration (Bottor, 2009). Atropine, fentanyl, and vecuronium or rocuronium are drugs commonly used during RSI. In neonates, ET tube intubation is often a stressful event, and hypoxia and pain are commonly associated with routine intubation; RSI in neonates may serve to prevent such adverse events (Bottor, 2009).

Indications for intubation include:

- Respiratory failure or arrest, agonal or gasping respirations, apnea
- Upper airway obstruction
- Significant increase in work of breathing, use of accessory muscles
- Potential for developing partial or complete airway obstruction—respiratory effort with no breath sounds, facial trauma, and inhalation injuries
- Potential for or actual loss of airway protection, increased risk for aspiration
- Anticipated need for mechanical ventilation related to chest trauma, shock, increased intracranial pressure
- Hypoxemia despite supplemental oxygen
- Inadequate ventilation

In preparation for intubation, the child should be preoxygenated with 100% oxygen using an appropriately sized bag and mask. Only uncuffed ET tubes should be used in children younger than 8 years of age (Curley and Moloney-Harmon, 2001). Air or gas delivered directly to the trachea must be humidified. During intubation, the cardiac rhythm, heart rate, and oxygen saturation should be monitored continuously with audible tones. ET tube placement should be verified by at least one clinical sign and at least one confirmatory technology:

- Visualization of bilateral chest expansion
- Auscultation over the epigastrium (breath sounds should not be heard) and the lung fields bilaterally in the axillary region (breath sounds should be equal and adequate)
- Water vapor in the tube (helpful; not definitive)
- Color change on end-tidal carbon dioxide detector during exhalation after at least 3 to 6 breaths or waveform/value verification with continuous capnography
- Chest radiography

Apply a protective skin barrier and secure the ET tube with tape or a securement device. An NG tube is typically inserted after intubation.

MECHANICAL VENTILATION

Endotracheal intubation can be accomplished by the nasal (nasotracheal), oral (orotracheal), or direct tracheal (tracheostomy) routes. Although it is more difficult to place, nasotracheal intubation is preferred to orotracheal intubation because it facilitates oral hygiene and provides more stable fixation, which reduces the complication of tracheal erosion and the danger of accidental extubation.

Basic ongoing assessment of the mechanically ventilated patient includes observing the chest rise and fall for symmetry, bilateral breath sounds equal or unchanged from last assessment, level of consciousness, capillary refill and skin color, and vital signs. A heart rate that is too fast or too slow is a possible indication of hypoxemia, air leak, or low cardiac output. Pulse oximetry and end-tidal carbon dioxide monitoring is also routine along with periodic arterial blood gas analysis. If sudden deterioration of an intubated patient occurs, consider the following etiologies.

DOPE*

Displacement—the tube is not in the trachea or has moved into a bronchus (right mainstream most common)

Obstruction—secretions or kinking of the tube

Pneumothorax—chest trauma, barotraumas, or noncompliant lung disease

Equipment failure—check the oxygen source, Ambu bag, and ventilator

Verify placement again during each transport and when patients are moved to different beds

To maintain skin integrity in the mechanically ventilated patient, reposition the patient at least every 2 hours as the patient's condition tolerates. Apply a hydrocolloid barrier to protect the facial cheeks. Place gel pillows under pressure points such as occiput, heels, elbows, and shoulders. Allow no tubes, lines, wires, or wrinkles in bedding under the patient. Provide meticulous skin care.

Provide analgesia and sedation as needed. Use a system for communication that includes sign boards, pointing, and opening and closing eyes. To maintain safety, use soft restraints if necessary to maintain a critical airway.

Ventilator-associated pneumonia is a complication that can be prevented through the use of aggressive hand hygiene, oral care, and elevation of the head of the bed between 30 and 45 degrees (unless contraindicated). Enteral nutrition is often provided to decrease the risk of bacterial translocation. Routinely assess the patient's intestinal motility (e.g., by auscultating for bowel sounds and measuring residual gastric volume or abdominal girth) and adjust the rate and volume of enteral feeding to avoid regurgitation. In high-risk patients (decreased gag reflex, delayed gastric emptying, gastroesophageal reflux, severe bronchospasm), postpyloric (duodenal or jejunal) feeding tubes are often used. To prevent the aspiration of pooled secretions, suction hypopharynx before suctioning the ET tube, before repositioning the ET tube, and before repositioning the patient. Prevent ventilator circuits' condensate from entering ET tube or in-line medication nebulizers.

Assess readiness to extubate daily. Indications that a child is ready to be extubated include an improvement in underlying condition, hemodynamic stability, and mechanical support no longer being necessary. Assess level of consciousness and ability to maintain a patent airway by mobilizing pulmonary secretions through effective coughing. Maintain NPO status 4 hours before extubation. After extubation, monitor for respiratory distress, which may develop within minutes or hours. Signs of postintubation respiratory distress include stridor, hoarseness, increased work of breathing, unstable vital signs, and desaturations.

Tracheostomy

A tracheostomy is a surgical opening in the trachea; the procedure may be done on an emergency basis or may be an elective one, and it may be combined with mechanical ventilation. Pediatric tracheostomy tubes are usually made of plastic or Silastic (Fig. 22-24). The most common types are the Hollinger, Jackson, Aberdeen, and Shiley tubes.

---

*American Heart Association, 2010.

Animation—Tracheostomy

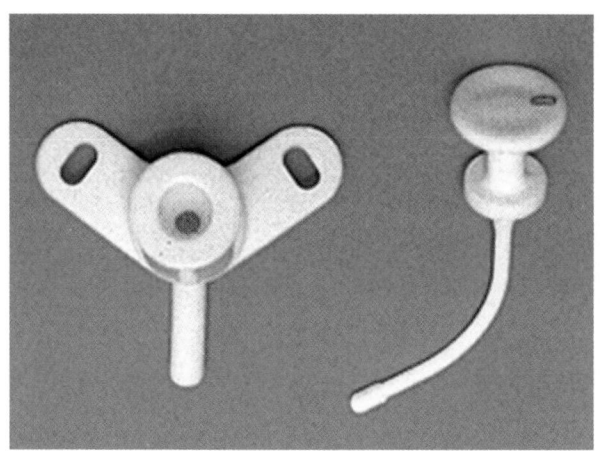

FIG 22-24 Silastic pediatric tracheostomy tube and obturator.

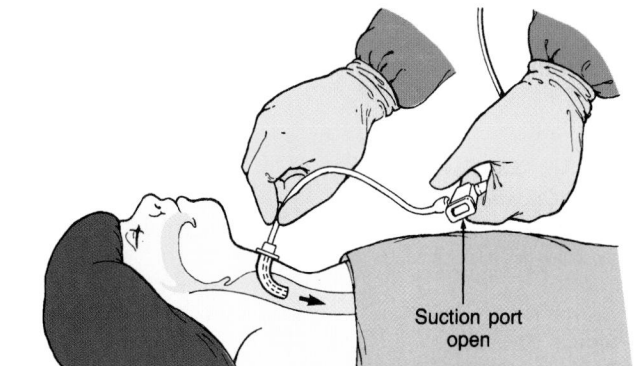

Suction port
open

FIG 22-25 Tracheostomy suction catheter insertion. Note that the catheter is inserted just to the end of the tracheostomy tube.

These tubes are constructed with a more acute angle than adult tubes, and they soften at body temperature, conforming to the contours of the trachea. Because these materials resist the formation of crusted respiratory secretions, they are made without an inner cannula.

Children who have undergone a tracheostomy must be closely monitored for complications such as hemorrhage, edema, aspiration, accidental decannulation, tube obstruction, and the entrance of free air into the pleural cavity. The focuses of nursing care are maintaining a patent airway, facilitating the removal of pulmonary secretions, providing humidified air or oxygen, cleansing the stoma, monitoring the child's ability to swallow, and teaching while simultaneously preventing complications.

Because the child may be unable to signal for help, direct observation and use of respiratory and cardiac monitors are essential. Respiratory assessments include breath sounds and work of breathing, vital signs, tightness of the tracheostomy ties, and the type and amount of secretions. Large amounts of bloody secretions are uncommon and should be considered a sign of hemorrhage. The practitioner should be notified immediately if this occurs.

The child is positioned with the head of the bed raised or in the position most comfortable to the child with the call light easily available. Suction catheters, suction source, gloves, sterile saline, sterile gauze for wiping away secretions, scissors, an extra tracheostomy tube of the same size with ties already attached, another tracheostomy tube one size smaller, and the obturator are kept at the bedside. A source of humidification is provided because the normal humidification and filtering functions of the airway have been bypassed. IV fluids ensure adequate hydration until the child is able to swallow sufficient amounts of fluids.

Suctioning

The airway must remain patent and may require frequent suctioning during the first few hours after a tracheostomy to remove mucous plugs and excessive secretions. Proper vacuum pressure and suction catheter size are important to prevent atelectasis and decrease hypoxia from the suctioning procedure. Vacuum pressure should range from 60 to 100 mm Hg for infants and children and from 40 to 60 mm Hg for preterm infants. Unless secretions are thick and tenacious, the lower range of negative pressure is recommended. Tracheal suction catheters are available in a variety of sizes. The catheter selected should have a diameter that is half the diameter of the tracheostomy tube. If the catheter is too large, it can block the airway. The catheter is constructed with a side port so that the catheter is introduced without suction and

removed while simultaneous intermittent suction is applied by covering the port with the thumb (Fig. 22-25). The catheter is inserted just to the end of the tracheostomy tube. The practice of instilling sterile saline in the tracheostomy tube before suctioning is not supported by research and is no longer recommended (see Evidence-Based Practice box).

> **NURSING TIP** In a closed suction system, a suction catheter is directly attached to the ventilator tubing. This system has several advantages. First, there is no need to disconnect the patient from the ventilator, which allows for better oxygenation. Second, the suction catheter is enclosed in a plastic sheath, which reduces the risk that the nurse will be exposed to the patient's secretions.

> **! NURSING ALERT**
>
> Suctioning should require no more than 5 seconds. Counting one one-thousand, two one-thousand, three one-thousand, and so on while suctioning is a simple means for monitoring the time. Without a safeguard, the airway may be obstructed for too long. Hyperventilating the child with 100% oxygen before and after suctioning (using a bag–valve–mask or increasing the fraction of inspired oxygen concentration [FiO_2] ventilator setting) may be performed to prevent hypoxia. Closed tracheal suctioning systems that allow for uninterrupted oxygen delivery may also be used.

The child is allowed to rest for 30 to 60 seconds after each aspiration to allow oxygen saturation to return to normal; then the process is repeated until the trachea is clear. Suctioning should be limited to about three aspirations in one period. Oximetry is used to monitor suctioning and prevent hypoxia.

> **! NURSING ALERT**
>
> Suctioning is carried out only as often as needed to keep the tube patent. Signs of mucus partially occluding the airway include an increased heart rate, a rise in respiratory effort, a drop in SaO_2, cyanosis, and an increase in the positive inspiratory pressure on the ventilator.

In the acute care setting, aseptic technique is used during care of the tracheostomy. Secondary infection is a major concern because the air entering the lower airway bypasses the natural defenses of the upper airway. Gloves are worn during the aspiration procedure, although a

EVIDENCE-BASED PRACTICE

Normal Saline Instillation Before Endotracheal or Tracheostomy Suctioning—Helpful or Harmful?

Updated by Olga A. Taylor

Ask the Question
Picot Question
In intubated children and those with tracheostomy, is NS instillation before suctioning helpful or harmful?

Search for the Evidence
Search Strategies
Searched all literature from 1980 to 2011

Databases Used
PubMed, Cochrane Collaboration, MDConsult, BestBETs, PedsCCM, AHRQ

Critically Analyze the Evidence
- Adult studies have found decreased oxygen saturation, increased frequency of nosocomial pneumonia, and increased intracranial pressure after instillation of NS before suctioning (Ackerman, 1993; Ackerman and Gugerty, 1990; Bostick and Wendelgass, 1987; Hagler and Traver, 1994; Kinlock, 1999; O'Neal, Grap, Thompson, and others, 2001; Reynolds, Hoffman, Schlichtig, and others, 1990).
- No significant differences in oxygenation, heart rate, or blood pressure were found before or after suctioning in a group of 27 intubated neonates (Shorten, Byrne, and Jones, 1991).
- No adverse effects on lung mechanics were found after NS instillation and suctioning in neonates (Beeram and Dhanireddy, 1992).
- Children (ages 10 weeks to 14 years) experienced significantly greater oxygen desaturation after suctioning if NS was instilled (Ridling, Martin, and Bratton, 2003).
- With tracheostomies, NS should not be instilled before suctioning (American Thoracic Society, 2005).
- Evidence does not support routine instillation of NS in neonates; however, abundant evidence indicates the adverse effects of NS instillation (Gardner and Shirland, 2009).
- Evidence indicating the detriment of the use of saline for suctioning is lacking in the pediatric population. However, saline should not be routinely used for suctioning infants and children (Morrow and Argent, 2008).
- Endotracheal (ET) suctioning performed with saline solution was associated with an increase in episodes of bradycardia, desaturations, and need for increase in the fraction of inspired oxygen (Trevisanuto, Doglioni, and Zanardo, 2009).
- Potential harms that may be associated with use of NS installation include increased coughing, oxygen desaturation, bronchospasms, tachycardia, pain, anxiety, dyspnea, increased intracranial pressure, and loosened bacterial biofilm that may colonize the ET tube (American Association for Respiratory Care, 2010).
- Use of low-sodium solution for airway suctioning in neonates significantly decreased VAP and rates of chronic lung disease (Christensen, Henry, Baer, and others, 2010).

Apply the Evidence: Nursing Implications
There is **moderate-quality evidence** with a **strong recommendation** (Guyatt, Oxman, Vist, and others, 2008) that adverse effects of NS instillation before suctioning in children are similar to those found in adults. This technique

causes a significant reduction in oxygen saturation that can last up to 2 minutes after suctioning. The evidence does not support the use of NS instillation before ET suctioning in children.

QSEN Quality and Safety Competencies:
Evidence-Based Practice*
Knowledge
Differentiate clinical opinion from research and evidence-based summaries.
Describe methods for using NS instillation before ET or tracheostomy suctioning.

Skills
Base individualized care plan on patient values, clinical expertise, and evidence.
Integrate evidence into practice on NS instillation before ET or tracheostomy suctioning.

Attitudes
Value the concept of evidence-based practice as integral to determining best clinical practice.
Appreciate the strengths and weakness of evidence for normal saline instillation before ET or tracheostomy suctioning.

References
Ackerman MH: The effect of saline lavage prior to suctioning, *Am J Crit Care* 2(4):326–330, 1993.

Ackerman MH, Gugerty B: The effect of normal saline bolus instillation in artificial airways, *J Soc Otorhinolaryngol Head Neck Nurs* 8:14–17, 1990.

American Association for Respiratory Care: AARC Clinical Practice Guidelines. Endotracheal suctioning of mechanically ventilated patients with artificial airways, *Respir Care* 55(6):758–764, 2010.

American Thoracic Society: *Care of the child with a chronic tracheostomy*, 2005, retrieved April 17, 2006, from http://www.thoracic.org/sections/publications/statements/pages/respiratory-disease-pediatric/childtrach1–12.html.

Beeram MR, Dhanireddy R: Effects of saline instillation during tracheal suction on lung mechanics in newborn infants, *J Perinatol* 12(2):120–123, 1992.

Bostick J, Wendelgass ST: Normal saline instillation as part of the suctioning procedure: effects of PaO$_2$ and amount of secretions, *Heart Lung* 16(5):532–537, 1987.

Christensen RD, Henry E, Baer VL, and others: A low-sodium solution for airway care: results of a multicenter trial, *Respir Care* 5(12):1680–1685, 2010.

Gardner DL, Shirland L: Evidence-based guideline for suctioning the intubated neonate and infant, *Neonat Netw* 28(5):281–302, 2009.

Guyatt GH, Oxman AD, Vist GE, and others: GRADE: an emerging consensus on rating quality of evidence and strength of recommendations, *BMJ* 336(7650):924–926, 2008.

Hagler DA, Traver GA: Endotracheal saline and suction catheters: sources of lower airway contamination, *Am J Crit Care* 3(6):444–447, 1994.

Kinlock D: Instillation of normal saline during endotracheal suctioning: effects on mixed venous oxygen saturation, *Am J Crit Care* 8(4):231–240, 1999.

Morrow BM, Argent AC: A comprehensive review of pediatric endotracheal suctioning: effects, indications, and clinical practice, *Pediatr Crit Care Med* 9(5):465–477, 2008.

O'Neal PV, Grap MJ, Thompson C, and others: Level of dyspnoea experienced in mechanically ventilated adults with and without saline instillation prior to endotracheal suctioning, *Intensive Crit Care Nurs* 17(6):356–363, 2001.

Reynolds P, Hoffman LA, Schlichtig R, and others: Effects of normal saline instillation on secretion volume, dynamic compliance, and oxygen saturation [abstract], *Am Rev Respir Dis* 141:A574, 1990.

Ridling DA, Martin LD, Bratton SL: Endotracheal suctioning with or without instillation of isotonic sodium chloride in critically ill children, *Am J Crit Care* 12(3):212–219, 2003.

Shorten DR, Byrne PJ, Jones RL: Infant responses to saline instillations and endotracheal suctioning, *J Obstet Gynecol Neonatal Nurs* 20(6):464–469, 1991.

Trevisanuto D, Doglioni N, Zanardo V: The management of endotracheal tubes and nasal cannulae: the role of nurses, *Early Hum Dev* 85:S85–S87, 2009.

NS, Normal saline; *VAP*, ventilator-associated pneumonia.
*Adapted from the QSEN at http://www.qsen.org.

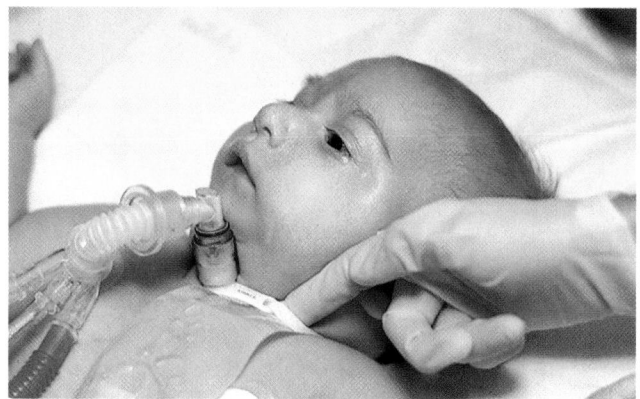

FIG 22-26 Tracheostomy ties are snug but allow one finger to be inserted.

sterile glove is needed only on the hand touching the catheter. A new tube, gloves, and sterile saline solution are used each time.

Routine Care

The tracheostomy stoma requires daily care. Assessments of the stoma area include observations for signs of infection and breakdown of the skin. The skin is kept clean and dry, and crusted secretions around the stoma may be gently removed with half-strength hydrogen peroxide. Hydrogen peroxide should not be used with sterling silver tracheostomy tubes because it tends to pit and stain the silver surface. The nurse should be aware of wet tracheostomy dressings, which can predispose the peristomal area to skin breakdown. Several products are available to prevent or treat excoriation. The Allevyn tracheostomy dressing is a hydrophilic sponge with a polyurethane back that is highly absorptive. Other possible barriers to help maintain skin integrity include the use of hydrocolloid wafers (e.g., DuoDERM CGF, Hollister Restore) under the tracheostomy flanges, as well as extra-thin hydrocolloid wafers under the chin.

The tracheostomy tube is held in place with tracheostomy ties made of a durable, nonfraying material. The ties are changed daily and when soiled. Ties fastened with self-adhering Velcro closures are commonly used. If Velcro ties are not available, cotton ties are looped through the flanges and tied snugly in a triple knot at the side of the neck before the soiled ties are cut and removed. The ties should be tight enough to allow just a fingertip to be inserted between the ties and the neck (Fig. 22-26). It is easier to ensure a snug fit if the child's head is flexed rather than extended while the ties are being secured.

Routine tracheostomy tube changes are usually carried out weekly after a tract has been formed to minimize the formation of granulation tissue. The first change is usually performed by the surgeon; subsequent changes are performed by the nurse and, if the child is discharged home with the tracheostomy, by either a parent or a visiting nurse. Ideally, two caregivers participate in the procedure to assist with positioning the child.

Changing the tracheostomy tube is accomplished using sterile technique. Tube changes should occur before meals or 2 hours after the last meal. Continuous feedings should be turned off at least an hour before a tube change. The new sterile tube is prepared by inserting the obturator and attaching new ties. The child may be suctioned if necessary before the procedure and then restrained and positioned with the neck slightly extended. One caregiver removes the old ties and removes the tube from the stoma. The new tube is inserted gently into the stoma (using a downward and forward motion that follows the curve of

the trachea), the obturator is removed, and the ties are secured. The adequacy of ventilation must be assessed after a tube change because the tube can be inserted into the soft tissue surrounding the trachea; therefore, breath sounds and respiratory effort are carefully monitored.

Supplemental oxygen is always delivered with a humidification system to prevent drying of the respiratory mucosa. Humidification of room air for an established tracheostomy can be intermittent if secretions remain thin enough to be coughed or suctioned from the tracheostomy. Direct humidification via a tracheostomy mask can be provided during naps and at night so the child is able to be up and around unencumbered during much of the day. Room humidifiers are also used successfully.

The inner cannula, if used, should be removed with each suctioning, cleaned with sterile saline and pipe cleaners to remove crusted material, dried thoroughly, and reinserted.

Emergency Care: Tube Occlusion and Accidental Decannulation

Occlusion of the tracheostomy tube is life threatening, and infants and children are at greater risk than adults because of the smaller diameter of the tube. Maintaining patency of the tube is accomplished with suctioning and routine tube changes to prevent the formation of crusts that can occlude the tube.

> ### ! NURSING ALERT
>
> Life-threatening occlusion is apparent when the child displays signs of respiratory distress and a suction catheter cannot be passed to the end of the tube despite several attempts and instillation of saline. This situation requires an immediate tube change.

Accidental decannulation also requires immediate tube replacement. Some children have a fairly rigid trachea, so the airway remains partially open when the tube is removed. However, others have malformed or flexible tracheal cartilage, which causes the airway to collapse when the tube is removed or dislodged. Because many infants and children with upper airway problems have little airway reserve, if replacement of the dislodged tube is impossible, a smaller-sized tube should be inserted. If the stoma cannot be cannulated with another tracheostomy tube, oral intubation should be performed.

CHEST TUBE PROCEDURES

A chest tube is placed to remove fluid or air from the pleural or pericardial space. Chest tube drainage systems collect air and fluid while inhibiting backflow into the pleural or pericardial space. Indications for chest tube placement include pneumothorax, hemothorax, chylothorax, empyema, pleural or pericardial effusion, and prevention of accumulation of fluid in the pleural and pericardial space after cardiothoracic surgery. Nursing responsibilities include assisting with chest tube placement, managing chest tubes, and assisting with chest tube removal.

Before chest tube insertion, assess hematologic and coagulation studies for any risk of bleeding during the procedure. Notify the physician of abnormal findings. Prepare the drainage system with sterile water as described in the package insert (some systems may not require this step). Administer pain and sedation medications as ordered. Monitor airway, breathing, circulation, and pulse oximetry throughout the procedure.

After the tube has been inserted and connected to the chest drainage system, secure the tubing so it does not become disconnected. If suction is required, use connection tubing to join the drainage system to a wall suction adapter and adjust suction on the drainage system as ordered (usually −10 to −20 cm H_2O). There should be gentle, continuous bubbling in the suction control chamber. Place occlusive dressing over the chest tube insertion site per hospital policy. Note the date, time, and your initials on the dressing. If gauze is used, use presplit gauze; "homemade" split gauze may leave loose threads in the wound. Ensure that the drainage system is positioned below the patient's chest and secured to the floor or bed. Keep the drainage tubing free of dependent loops. Obtain a chest radiograph to confirm placement of the chest tube. Ensure that daily chest radiographs are scheduled to monitor placement of the chest tube as well as resolution of the pneumothorax or effusion.

Disposable chest drainage systems typically consist of three chambers next to one another in one drainage unit (Fig. 22-27). The fluid collection chamber collects drainage from the patient's pleural or pericardial space. The water seal chamber is directly connected to the fluid collection chamber and acts as a one-way valve, protecting patients from air returning to the pleural or pericardial space. The suction chamber may be a dry suction or calibrated water chamber. It is connected to external vacuum suction set to the amount of suction ordered and controls the amount of suction patients experience.

Assess for blood clots and fibrin strands in tubes with sanguinous or serosanguineous drainage and ensure that there are no obstructions to drainage in the tube. Maintain chest tube clearance per hospital policy. Milking or stripping of chest tubes is not recommended for chest tube clearance because of the high negative intrathoracic pressure that is created. However, some special circumstances warrant chest tube clearance with these methods, such as maintaining chest tube patency while a patient is bleeding. Notify the physician immediately if chest tube obstruction is suspected. Generally, chest tubes should not be clamped. However, it may be necessary to clamp a chest tube when exchanging the collection chamber or to determine the site of an air leak (see Nursing Care Guidelines box).

ALTERNATIVE FEEDING TECHNIQUES

Some children are unable to take nourishment by mouth because of anomalies of the throat, esophagus, or bowel; impaired swallowing capacity; severe debilitation; respiratory distress; or unconsciousness. These children are frequently fed by way of a tube inserted orally or nasally into the stomach (**orogastric [OG]** or **NG gavage**) or duodenum–jejunum (**enteral gavage**) or by a tube inserted directly into the stomach (**gastrostomy**) or jejunum (**jejunostomy**). Such feedings may be intermittent or by continuous drip. Feeding resistance, a problem that may result from any long-term feeding method that bypasses the mouth, is discussed in Chapter 9. During gavage or gastrostomy feedings, infants are given a pacifier. Nonnutritive sucking has several advantages, such as increased weight gain and decreased crying. However, only pacifiers with a safe design can be used to prevent the possibility of aspiration. Using improvised pacifiers made from bottle nipples is not a safe practice.

When a child is concurrently receiving continuous-drip gastric or enteral feedings and parenteral (IV) therapy, the potential exists for inadvertent administration of the enteral formula through the circulatory system. The possibility for error increases when the parenteral solution is a fat emulsion, a milky-appearing substance. Safeguards to prevent this potentially serious error include:

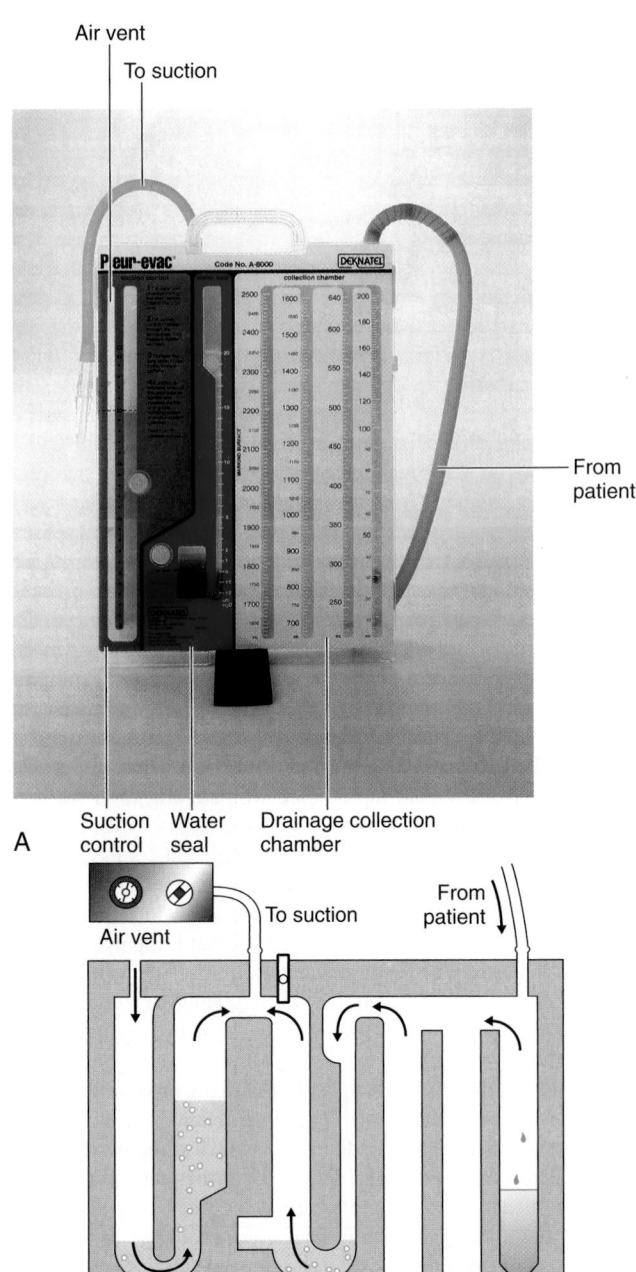

FIG 22-27 A, The Pleur-Evac drainage system, a commercial three-bottle chest drainage device. **B,** Schematic of the drainage device. (From Ignatavicius DD, Workman LM: *Medical-surgical nursing: patient-centered collaborative care,* ed 7, Philadelphia, 2013, Saunders Elsevier.)

- Use a separate, specifically designed enteral feeding pump mounted on a separate pole for continuous-feeding solutions.
- Label all tubing of continuous enteral feeding with brightly colored tape or labels.
- Use specifically designed continuous-feeding bags to contain the solutions instead of parenteral equipment, such as a burette.
- Whenever access or connections are made, trace the tubing all the way from the patient to the bag to ensure that the correct tubing source is selected.

NURSING CARE GUIDELINES

Ongoing Patient and Chest Drainage System Assessment

Drainage type (sanguinous, serosanguineous, serous, chylous, empyemic), color, amount, consistency. If there is a marked decrease in the amount of drainage, assess for drainage around the chest tube insertion site.

Dressing clean, dry, and intact.

Chest tube sutures are intact.

Prescribed amount of suction is applied.

Water level is at 2 cm. If the water column is too high, the flow of air from the chest may be impeded.

Bubbling in the water seal chamber is normal if the chest tube was placed to evacuate a pneumothorax. The bubbling will stop when the pneumothorax has resolved.

Fluctuations may be seen in the water column because of changes in intra-thoracic pressure. Substantial fluctuations may reflect changes in a patient's respiratory status.

Signs and symptoms of infection or skin breakdown.

Palpate for the presence of subcutaneous air.

Interventions

Notify the physician of any changes in the quantity or quality of drainage.

If 3 ml/kg/hr or greater of sanguinous drainage occurs for 2 to 3 consecutive hours after cardiothoracic surgery, it may indicate active hemorrhaging and warrants immediate attention of the physician.

Change dressing and perform site care per hospital policy. Typically, a minimal, occlusive dressing is applied.

When the collection chamber is almost full, exchange existing drainage system with a new one per manufacturer's instructions using sterile technique.

To lower the water column, depress the manual vent on the back of the unit until the water level reaches 2 cm. *Do not depress the filtered manual vent when the suction is not functioning or connected.*

If evacuation of a pneumothorax was not the indication for placement of the chest tube, bubbling in the water seal chamber may be the result of a break in the chest drainage system. Identify the break in the system by briefly clamping the system between the drainage unit and the patient. When the clamp is placed between the unit and the break in the system, the bubbling will stop. Tighten any loose connections. If the air leak is suspected to be at the patient's chest wall, notify the physician.

Encourage patient ambulation. Secure chest tube drainage system to prevent chest tube dislodgment from patient or disconnection from drainage system.

GAVAGE FEEDING

Infants and children can be fed simply and safely by a tube passed into the stomach through either the nares or the mouth. The tube can be left in place or inserted and removed with each feeding. In older children, it is usually less traumatic to tape the tube securely in place between feedings. When this alternative is used, the tube should be removed and replaced with a new tube according to hospital policy, specific orders, and the type of tube used. Meticulous hand washing is practiced during the procedure to prevent bacterial contamination of the feeding, especially during continuous-drip feedings.

Preparations

The equipment needed for gavage feeding includes:

- A suitable tube selected according to the child's size, the viscosity of the solution being fed, and anticipated duration of treatment
- A receptacle for the fluid; for small amounts, a 10- to 30-ml syringe barrel or Asepto syringe is satisfactory; for larger amounts a 60-ml syringe with a catheter tip is more convenient
- A 10-ml barrel syringe to aspirate stomach contents after the tube has been placed
- Water or water-soluble lubricant to lubricate the tube; sterile water is used for infants
- Paper or nonallergenic tape to mark the tube and to attach the tube to the infant's or child's cheek (and nose if placed through the nares)
- pH paper to determine the correct placement in the stomach
- The solution for feeding

Not all feeding tubes are the same. Polyethylene and polyvinyl-chloride types lose their flexibility and need to be replaced frequently, usually every 3 or 4 days. Polyurethane and silicone tubes remain flexible, so they can remain in place up to 30 days. Advantages of small-bore tubes include a reduced incidence of pharyngitis, otitis media, aspiration, and discomfort. Disadvantages include difficulty during insertion (may require a stylet or metal guide wire), collapse of the tube during aspiration of gastric contents to test for correct placement, dislodgment during forceful coughing, migration out of position, knotting, occlusion, and unsuitability for thick feedings.

Procedure

Infants are easier to control if they are first wrapped in a mummy restraint (see Fig. 22-6, *A*). Even tiny infants with random movements can grasp and dislodge the tube. Preterm infants do not ordinarily require restraint, but if they do, a small blanket folded across the chest and secured beneath the shoulders is usually sufficient. Be careful so that breathing is not compromised.

Whenever possible, the infant should be held and provided with a means for nonnutritive sucking during the procedure to associate the comfort of physical contact with the feeding. When this is not possible, gavage feeding is carried out with the infant or child on the back or toward the right side and the head and chest elevated. Feeding the child in a sitting position helps maintain placement of the tube in the lowest position, thus increasing the likelihood of correct placement in the stomach.

Although the most accurate method for testing tube placement is radiography, this practice is not always possible before each feeding. Research indicates that bedside assessment of gastrointestinal aspirate color and pH is useful in predicting feeding tube placement (see Evidence-Based Practice box). If doubt exists regarding correct placement, consult the practitioner. The Nursing Care Guidelines box describes the procedure for gavage feeding.

Studies evaluating NG and OG tube length in infants and children found that age-specific methods for predicting the distance based on height is a more accurate estimate of internal distance to the stomach (Beckstrand, Ellett, and McDaniel, 2007; Klasner, Luke, and Scalzo, 2002). The morphologic measure most commonly used by clinicians, nose–ear–xiphoid distance, is often too short to locate the entire tube pore span in the stomach. However, the nose–ear–midxiphoid umbilicus span approached the accuracy of the age-specific prediction equations and is easier to use in a clinical setting. The best option is to adapt the nose–ear–midxiphoid umbilicus

EVIDENCE-BASED PRACTICE

Confirming Nasogastric Tube Placement in Pediatric Patients

Marilyn Hockenberry; updated by Olga Taylor

Ask the Question
Picot Question
In children, how should correct placement of NG tubes be assessed during hospitalization?

Search for the Evidence
Search Strategies
Search selection criteria included English-language, research-based articles, and children and adolescents requiring NG tube placement. Search areas included aspirate, auscultation and radiology methods, NG tube length prediction methods, age-related height-based methods, and accurate NG tube placement. Searches excluded newborns and preterm infants.

Databases Used
PubMed, Cochrane Collaboration, MDConsult, Joanna Briggs Institute, AHRQ-National Guideline Clearinghouse, TRIP database Plus, PedsCCM, BestBETS

Critically Analyze the Evidence
Studies compared various methods used to evaluate correct placement of the NG tube.

Accurate NG Tube Length Measurement
• Children 8 years, 4 months of age or younger: use age-related height-based equation for NG length predictions.
• Children older than 8 years, 4 months of age, short stature or when you cannot obtain accurate height: use nose–ear–midxiphoid–umbilicus (NEMU) (Beckstrand, 1990; Beckstrand, Cirgin-Ellett, and McDaniel, 2007; Ellett, Beckstrand, Welch, and others, 1992; Strobel, Byrne, Ament, and others, 1979).

Nonradiologic Verification Methods
• A pH of 6 or less supports that the tip of the tube is in the gastric location (Ellett and Beckstrand, 1999; Ellett, Croffie, Cohen, and others, 2005; Huffman, Pieper, Jarczyk, and others, 2004; Metheny and Stewart, 2002; Metheny, Reed, Wiersema, and others, 1993; Metheny, Stewart, Smith, and others, 1997, 1999; Neumann, Meyer, Dutton, and others, 1995; Nyqvist, Sorell, and Ewald, 2005; Phang, Marsh, Barlows, and others, 2004; Westhus, 2004).
• A pH greater than 5 does not reliably predict correct distal tip location. This may indicate respiratory or esophageal placement or the presence of medications to suppress acid secretion. Gastric aspirate pH means are statistically significantly lower compared with means from intestinal and respiratory pH aspirates (Ellett, Croffie, Cohen, and others, 2005; Metheny and Stewart, 2002; Metheny, Stewart, Smith, and others, 1997, 1999; Phang, Marsh, Barlows, and others, 2004; Westhus, 2004).

Visual Inspection of Aspirate
• Visual inspection is less accurate than pH to confirm placement. Aspirate colors are specific to the intended placement location. Gastric contents are clear, off-white, or tan or may be brown-tinged if blood is present. Respiratory secretions may look the same. Intestinal contents are often bile stained, light to dark yellow, or greenish-brown (Metheny, Reed, Berglund, and others, 1994; Metheny and Stewart, 2002; Metheny, Stewart, Smith, and others, 1999; Phang, Marsh, Barlows, and others, 2004; Westhus, 2004).

Enzyme Testing
• Aspirate testing of enzyme levels for bilirubin, pepsin, and trypsin is highly accurate but limited to laboratory assessment (Ellett, Croffie, Cohen, and others, 2005; Metheny and Stewart, 2002; Metheny, Stewart, Smith, and others, 1999; Westhus, 2004).

CO_2 Monitoring
• CO_2 monitoring is a reliable method to determine incorrect tube placement in the respiratory tract; it requires a capnograph monitor (Ellett, Croffie, Cohen, and others, 2005; Metheny and Stewart, 2002; Metheny, Stewart, Smith, and others, 1999).

Gastric Auscultation
• Auscultation as a verification tool is reliable only 60% to 80% of the time and should not be used without additional methods (Ellett and Beckstrand, 1999; Metheny, McSweeney, Wehrle, and others, 1990; Neumann, Meyer, Dutton, and others, 1995).
• Using aspirate and non-aspirate NG tube placement verification methods in combination increases the likelihood for accurate NG tube placement to 97% to 99%, similar to the radiologic chest radiography gold standard of 99% (Ellett and Beckstrand, 1999; Ellett, Croffie, Cohen, and Perkins, 2005; Metheny and Stewart, 2002; Metheny, Reed, Berglund, and others, 1994; Metheny, Reed, Wiersema, and others, 1993; Metheny, Stewart, Smith, and others, 1999; Neumann, Meyer, Dutton, and others, 1995; Phang, Marsh, Barlows, and others, 2004; Westhus, 2004).

Apply the Evidence: Nursing Implications
There is **moderate-quality evidence** with a **strong recommendation** (Guyatt, Oxman, Vist, and others, 2008) that a combination of verification methods to confirm NG tube placement will reduce the required number of x-rays in children (Cincinnati Children's Hospital Medical Center, 2009). These methods include pH testing and visual inspection of the pH aspirate. There is also good evidence that improving the accuracy of predicting NG tube length before insertion will enhance the precision of successful NG tube placement. Auscultation is used in combination with other NG tube verification methods.

QSEN Quality and Safety Competencies: Evidence-Based Practice*
Knowledge
Differentiate clinical opinion from research and evidence-based summaries.
Describe the various verification methods to confirm NG tube placement.

Skills
Base individualized care plan on patient values, clinical expertise, and evidence.
Integrate evidence into practice by using the techniques for NG tube placement verification in clinical care.

Attitudes
Value the concept of evidence-based practice as integral to determining best clinical practice.
Appreciate the strengths and weakness of evidence for confirming NG tube placement.

NG, Nasogastric.
*Adapted from the QSEN at http://www.qsen.org.

EVIDENCE-BASED PRACTICE

Confirming Nasogastric Tube Placement in Pediatric Patients—cont'd

References

Beckstrand J: The distance to the stomach for feeding tube placement in children predicted from regression on height, *Res Nurs Health* 13:411–420, 1990.

Beckstrand J, Cirgin-Ellett M, McDaniel A: Predicting internal distance to the stomach for positioning nasogastric and orogastric feeding tubes in children, *J Adv Nurs* 59:274–289, 2007.

Ellett M, Beckstrand J, Welch J, and others: Predicting the distance for gavage tube placement in children, *Pediatr Nurs* 18:119–121, 1992.

Ellett ML, Croffie JM, Cohen MD, and others: Gastric tube placement in young children, *Clin Nurs Res* 14:238–252, 2005.

Guyatt GH, Oxman AD, Vist GE, and others: GRADE: an emerging consensus on rating quality of evidence and strength of recommendations, *BMJ*, 336:924–926, 2008.

Huffman S, Pieper P, Jarczyk KS, and others: Methods to confirm feeding tube placement: application of research in practice, *Pediatr Nurs* 30:10–13, 2004.

Metheny N, McSweeney M, Wehrle MA, and others: Effectiveness of the auscultatory method in predicting feeding tube location, *Nurs Res* 39:262–267, 1990.

Metheny N, Reed L, Berglund B, and others: Visual characteristics of aspirates from feeding tubes as a method for predicting tube location, *Nurs Res* 43:282–287, 1994.

Metheny N, Reed L, Wiersema L, and others: Effectiveness of pH measurements in predicting feeding tube placement: an update, *Nurs Res* 42:324–331, 1993.

Metheny NA, Stewart BJ: Testing feeding tube placement during continuous tube feedings, *Appl Nurs Res* 15:254–258, 2002.

Metheny NA, Stewart BJ, Smith L, and others: pH and concentrations of pepsin and trypsin in feeding tube aspirates as predictors of tube placement, *JPEN J Parenter Enteral Nutr* 21:279–285, 1997.

Metheny NA, Stewart BJ, Smith L, and others: pH and concentration of bilirubin in feeding tube aspirates as predictors of tube placement, *Nurs Res* 48:189–197, 1999.

Neumann MJ, Meyer CT, Dutton JL, and others: Hold that x-ray: aspirate pH and auscultation prove tube placement, *J Clin Gastroenterol* 20:293–295, 1995.

Nyqvist KH, Sorell A, Ewald U: Litmus tests for verification of feeding tube location in infants: evaluation of their clinical use, *J Clin Nurs* 14:486–495, 2005.

Phang JS, Marsh WA, Barlows TG, and others: Determining feeding tube location by gastric and intestinal pH values, *Nutr Clin Pract* 19:640–644, 2004.

Strobel CT, Byrne WJ, Ament ME, and others: Correlation of esophageal lengths in children with height: application to the Tuttle test without prior esophageal manometry, *J Pediatr* 94:81–84, 1979.

Westhus N: Methods to test feeding tube placement in children, *MCN Am J Matern Child Nurs* 29:282–291, 2004.

NURSING CARE GUIDELINES

Nasogastric Tube Feedings in Children

Place child supine with head slightly hyperflexed or in a sniffing position (nose pointed toward ceiling).

Measure the tube for approximate length of insertion and mark the point with a small piece of tape.

Insert a tube that has been lubricated with sterile water or water-soluble lubricant through either the mouth or one of the nares to the predetermined mark. Because most young infants are obligatory nose breathers, insertion through the mouth causes less distress and helps stimulate sucking. In older infants and children, the tube is passed through the nose and alternated between nostrils. An indwelling tube is almost always placed through the nose.

- When using the nose, slip the tube along the base of the nose and direct it straight back toward the occiput.
- When entering through the mouth, direct the tube toward the back of the throat (see Fig. 22-28, *B*).
- If the child is able to swallow on command, synchronize passing the tube with swallowing.

Confirm placement (see Evidence-Based Practice box).

Stabilize the tube by holding or taping it to the cheek, not to the forehead, because of possible damage to the nostril. To maintain correct placement, measure and record the amount of tubing extending from the nose or mouth to the distal port when the tube is first positioned. Recheck this measurement before each feeding.

Warm the formula to room temperature. Do not microwave! Pour formula into the barrel of the syringe attached to the feeding tube. To start the flow, give a gentle push with the plunger but then remove the plunger and allow the fluid to flow into the stomach by gravity. The rate of flow should not exceed 5 ml every 5 to 10 minutes in premature and very small infants and 10 ml/min in older infants and children to prevent nausea and regurgitation. The rate is determined by the diameter of the tubing and the height of the reservoir containing the feeding and is regulated by adjusting the height of the syringe. A usual feeding may take 15 to 30 minutes to complete.

Flush the tube with sterile water (1 or 2 ml for small tubes to 5 to 15 ml or more for large ones), or see discussion of flushing for administering medication through nasogastric tubes in the Nursing Care Guidelines box (p. 678) to clear it of formula.

Cap or clamp indwelling tubes to prevent loss of feeding.

- If the tube is to be removed, first pinch it firmly to prevent escape of fluid as the tube is withdrawn. Withdraw the tube quickly.

Position the child with the head elevated 30 to 45 degrees or on the right side for 30 to 60 minutes in the same manner as after any infant feeding to minimize the possibility of regurgitation and aspiration. If the child's condition permits, bubble the youngster after the feeding.

Record the feeding, including the type and amount of residual, the type and amount of formula, and how it was tolerated.

- For most infant feedings, any amount of residual fluid aspirated from the stomach is refed to prevent electrolyte imbalance, and the amount is subtracted from the prescribed amount of feeding. For example, if the infant is to receive 30 ml and 10 ml is aspirated from the stomach before the feeding, the 10 ml of aspirated stomach contents is refed along with 20 ml of feeding. Another method can be used in children. If residual fluid is more than one fourth of the last feeding, return the aspirate and recheck in 30 to 60 minutes. When residual fluid is less than one fourth of the last feeding, give the scheduled feeding. If large amounts of aspirated fluid persist and the child is due for another feeding, notify the practitioner.

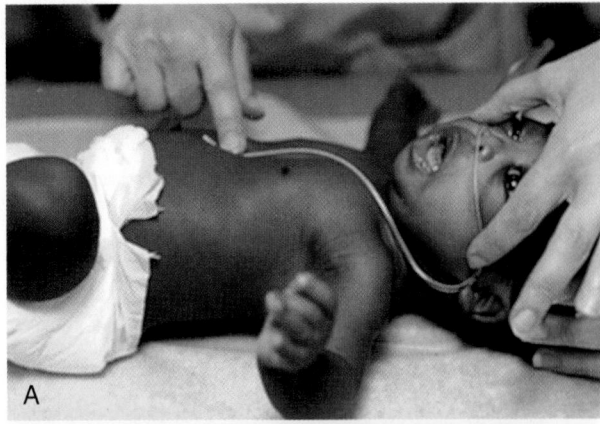

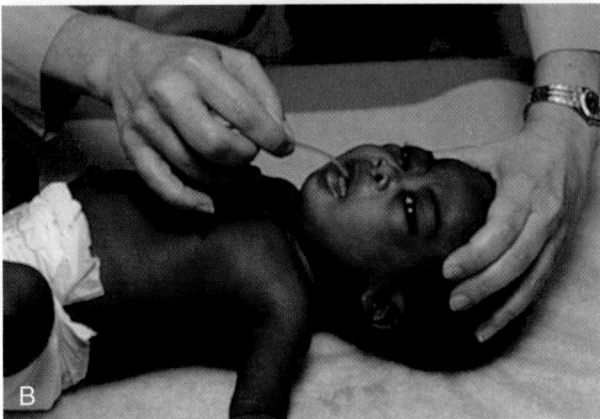

FIG 22-28 Gavage feeding. **A,** Measuring the tube for orogastric feeding from the tip of the nose to the earlobe and to the midpoint between the end of the xiphoid process and the umbilicus. **B,** Inserting the tube.

measurement for NG or OG tube length (Fig. 22-28, *A*) (see Nursing Care Guidelines box).

Ellett and Beckstrand (1999) found significant tube placement errors (43.5%) in a study of 39 hospitalized children. Children who were comatose or semicomatose, were inactive, had swallowing difficulty, or had Argyle tubes experienced increased tube placement errors. Findings supported the effectiveness of radiographs in documenting tube placement.

In a survey of 113 level II and III nurseries, 98% of the nurseries measured from the nose or mouth to the earlobe and then to the xiphoid process to calculate the length of the feeding tube for placement in preterm infants. For very low–birth-weight infants, daily weight can be used to predict insertion length. Until more definitive data are available, no method that results in a shorter distance than these methods should be used.

GASTROSTOMY FEEDING

Feeding by way of gastrostomy, or G tube, is often used for children in whom passage of a tube through the mouth, pharynx, esophagus, and cardiac sphincter of the stomach is contraindicated or impossible. It is also used to avoid the constant irritation of an NG tube in children who require tube feeding over an extended period. A gastrostomy tube may be placed with the child under general anesthesia or

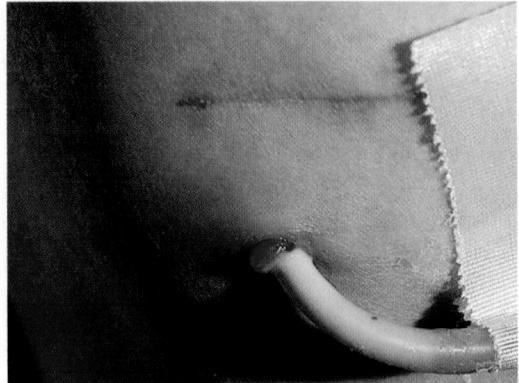

FIG 22-29 Appearance of healthy granulation tissue around a stoma.

percutaneously using an endoscope with the patient sedated and under local anesthesia (percutaneous endoscopic gastrostomy [PEG]). The tube is inserted through the abdominal wall into the stomach about midway along the greater curvature and secured by a purse-string suture. The stomach is anchored to the peritoneum at the operative site. The tube used can be a Foley, wing-tip, or mushroom catheter. Immediately after surgery, the catheter may be left open and attached to gravity drainage for 24 hours or more.

Direct postoperative care of the wound site toward prevention of infection and irritation. Cleanse the area at least daily or as often as needed to keep the area free of drainage. After healing, meticulous care is needed to keep the area surrounding the tube clean and dry to prevent excoriation and infection. Daily applications of antibiotic ointment or other preparations may be prescribed to aid in healing and prevent irritation. Exercise care to prevent excessive pull on the catheter that might cause widening of the opening and subsequent leakage of highly irritating gastric juices. Secure the tube to the abdomen, leaving a small loop of tubing at the exit site to prevent tension on the site (see Evidence-Based Practice box).

Granulation tissue may grow around a gastrostomy site (Fig. 22-29). This moist, beefy red tissue is not a sign of infection. However, if it continues to grow, the excess moisture can irritate the surrounding skin.

For children receiving long-term gastrostomy feeding, a **skin-level device** (e.g., MIC-KEY, Bard Button) offers several advantages. The small, flexible silicone device protrudes slightly from the abdomen, is cosmetically pleasing, affords increased comfort and mobility to the child, is easy to care for, and is fully immersible in water. The one-way valve at the proximal end minimizes reflux and eliminates the need for clamping. However, the skin-level device requires a well-established gastrostomy site and is more expensive than the conventional tube. In addition, the valve may become clogged. When functioning, the valve prevents air from escaping; therefore, the child may require frequent bubbling. With some devices, during feedings, the child must remain fairly still because the tubing easily disconnects from the opening if the child moves. With other devices, extension tubing can be securely attached to the opening (Fig. 22-30). The feeding is instilled at the other end of the tubing in a manner similar to that for a regular gastrostomy. The extension tubing may also have a separate medication port. Both the feeding and the medication ports have plugs attached. Some skin-level devices require a special tube to be able to decompress the stomach (to check residual or decompress air).

EVIDENCE-BASED PRACTICE

Skin Care: Prevention and Management of Gastrostomy Button and Gastrostomy Tube Breakdown

Caterina Nicole Landry, Andrea J. Harrison, Mary Hershey Pascual, and Barbara Montagnino

Ask the Question
Picot Question

In children with skin breakdown around the gastrostomy device (tube or skin-level button), what are the recommended interventions for management of skin issues?

Search for the Evidence
Search Strategies

Search selection criteria included English-language publications on children and adults published on gastrostomy, care practice guidelines, and manufacturer product information.

Databases Used

Cochrane Collaboration Database, Joanna Briggs Institute, Proquest, PubMed, Scopus, National Guideline Clearinghouse (AHRQ), SUMSearch, CINAHL, Wound Ostomy and Continence Nurses Society, American Pediatric Surgical Nurses Association, patient and family listservs

Critically Analyze the Evidence
Skin Care of the Gastrostomy Tube

- The American Pediatric Surgical Nurses Association (2006) recommends cleaning the skin around the gastrostomy twice daily and as needed with warm soap and water and keeping the area dry. It is important to remove crusted areas around the G tube. Diluted half-strength hydrogen peroxide may be used to clean for the first 2 weeks.
- The Wound Ostomy and Continence Nurses Society (2008) clinical guidelines identify the use of hydrogen peroxide as one of the possible causes of hypergranulation tissue. The guidelines recommend routine assessment of the site and keeping the skin around the G tube dry to prevent complications.
- McClave and Neff (2006) suggest cleaning the skin around the G tube with mild antibacterial soap and water. The use of hydrogen peroxide is discouraged because it is corrosive to the skin and leads to excessive drying of the tissue. Prompt treatment of skin irritation is vital in preventing further skin breakdown.
- Borkowski (2004, 2005) discourages the use of hydrogen peroxide because it can cause skin irritation and may be cytotoxic, disrupting wound healing. The author recommends gently cleaning the skin with water and patting dry because aggressive cleaning around the G tube may also interfere with the healing process.
- Product information by the manufacturer of MIC-KEY (Kimberly-Clark, 2006) advises cleaning the skin around the G button with soap and water using a soft cotton tip applicator or washcloth. The document recommends inspecting the skin daily and reporting any complications to a health care provider.

Skin Barriers

- The Wound Ostomy and Continence Nurses Society (2008) clinical guidelines recommend the use of barrier ointments such as zinc oxide and non-alcohol skin barrier film to control leakage. If skin irritation is present, the guidelines recommend adding absorptive powders and skin barrier wafers to help manage leakage and promote healing.
- Borkowski (2004, 2005) uses protective barriers such as zinc oxide and petrolatum to provide skin protection. For maceration around the stoma, the use of a solid skin barrier (pectin-based wafer Stomahesive) to provide an environment for protection and healing of the skin is recommended.

Stabilization

- The Wound Ostomy and Continence Nurses Society (2008) recommends that the stabilizer be placed on the skin without excessive tension and pulling. If a long tube is not stabilized, it can increase the risk for infection, cause hyperplasia, and lead to skin breakdown.
- In three patients with peristomal irritation caused by G tube mobility, Borkowski (2004) successfully managed two patients by applying a stabilization method to the G tube. In the third patient, despite the author's recommendation, the family refused to stabilize the G tube and preferred to treat the irritation with protective barrier ointments only. This finding illustrates the need to individualize care. There was no follow-up reported in the article regarding the success of the family's methods.
- McClave and Neff (2006) reported on their experience with percutaneous endoscopic gastrostomy (PEG) tubes. PEG tubes have increased risk for mobility and migration, which leads to ulceration and enlargement of the stoma. This can be prevented by stabilizing the tube.
- Crawley-Coha (2004) strongly recommends the use of stabilizing techniques to promote healing postoperatively and prevent dislodgment. In active children, the use of additional products such as elastic wraps and flexible dressings to immobilize the gastrostomy device is recommended.

Hypergranulation

- In a longitudinal study of 40 children with G tubes, granulation tissue occurred two times more often in children with long tube devices than those who had skin-level devices (Thorne, Radford, Onyskiw, and others, 1998).
- In a prospective study of eight patients, granulation tissue was the complication that prompted the most hospital and physician visits. Granulation tissue affected five patients (63%). Although families and caregivers were educated about the potential complications, this did not eliminate unscheduled health care contacts (Crosby and Duerksen, 2007).
- Borkowski (2004, 2005) recommends the use of triamcinolone (0.5%–0.1%) cream as a less painful alternative to the traditional silver nitrate sticks. Polyurethane foam may be used to absorb moisture and keep the skin dry to prevent further breakdown. One 2 × 2 gauze may be placed to create a snug fit for an ill-fitting low-profile device and assist with keeping the skin dry. Stabilization of the tube is a priority to prevent the development of hypergranulation.
- In the experience of Crawley-Coha (2004), hypergranulation tissue can occur regardless of type of G tube placed and method of stabilization used. Treatment options include the application of silver nitrate, sharp débridement, and topical steroids. This author used triamcinolone cream (0.5%) three times a day with great success for the previous 6 years. In some patients, polyurethane foam dressing is also used to manage hypergranulation tissue.
- The Wound Ostomy and Continence Nurses Society's (2008) clinical guidelines recommend managing hypergranulation by stabilizing the tube, keeping the peristomal area dry by applying polyurethane foam, and using triamcinolone (0.5%) three times a day. Silver nitrate may also be used for hypergranulation.

Individualizing Care

- Borkowski (2004) acknowledges that when children with G tubes develop complications despite family education on alternative management options,

Continued

Skin Care: Prevention and Management of Gastrostomy Button and Gastrostomy Tube Breakdown—cont'd

families may have chosen to continue to use familiar techniques. The care plan for managing complications should consider the child's developmental age, activity level, and parental preferences.

- Crawley-Coha (2004) recommends providing parents with individualized written instructions before discharge. Ongoing support should be provided by the child's medical team. To assist with transition to the home, information on support groups for patients with G tubes may be offered (e.g., Oley Foundation, http://www.oley.org).

Apply the Evidence: Nursing Implications

There is **very low-quality evidence** with a **strong recommendation** for the following (Guyatt, Oxman, Vist, and others, 2008):

1. Use mild soap and water to clean the peristomal area.
2. If skin irritation or breakdown is noted, use appropriate skin barriers:
   - Zinc oxide–based ointment, petrolatum-based ointment, or non-alcohol skin barrier for prevention or treatment of breakdown
   - Solid pectin-based wafer for maceration
3. Stabilize long G tube using one of the three methods: commercial stabilization device, polyurethane foam, or the H tape method.
4. Request an order for triamcinolone cream for short-term treatment of hypergranulation.
5. Individualize skin care management.

QSEN Quality and Safety Competencies:
Evidence-Based Practice*
Knowledge

Differentiate clinical opinion from research and evidence-based summaries.

Recommend interventions for management of skin breakdown around the gastrostomy device (tube or skin-level button).

Skills

Base individualized care plan on patient values, clinical expertise, and evidence.

Integrate evidence into practice by using recommend interventions for management of skin breakdown around the gastrostomy device (tube or skin-level button).

Attitudes

Value the concept of evidence-based practice as integral to determining best clinical practice.

Appreciate the strengths and weakness of evidence for using interventions for management of skin breakdown around the gastrostomy device (tube or skin-level button).

References

American Pediatric Surgical Nurses Association: *Gastrostomy*, 2006, retrieved December 17, 2008, from http://data.memberclicks.com/site/aps/GASTROSTOMY.doc.

Borkowski S: Similar gastrostomy peristomal skin irritations in three pediatric patients, *J Wound Ostomy Contin Nurs* 31(4):201–206, 2004.

Borkowski S: G tube care: managing hypergranulation tissue, *Nursing* 35(8):24, 2005.

Crawley-Coha T: A practical guide for the management of pediatric gastrostomy tubes based on 14 years of experience, *J Wound Ostomy Contin Nurs* 31(4):193–200, 2004.

Crosby J, Duerksen D: A prospective study of tube- and feeding-related complications in patients receiving long-term home enteral nutrition, *J Parenter Enter Nutr* 31(4):274–277, 2007.

Guyatt GH, Oxman AD, Vist GE, and others: GRADE: an emerging consensus on rating quality of evidence and strength of recommendations, *BMJ* 336:924–926, 2008.

Kimberly-Clark: *MIC-KEY: low profile gastrostomy feeding tube—your guide to proper care*, 2006, retrieved December 10, 2008, from http://kchealthcare.com/docs/R8201B%20MIC-KEY%20Care%20guide%20English.pdf.

McClave S, Neff R: Care and long-term maintenance of percutaneous endoscopic gastrostomy tubes [electronic version], *J Parenter Enter Nutr* 30(1):S27–S38, 2006.

Thorne S, Radford J, Onyskiw J, and others: A comparative longitudinal study of gastrostomy devices in children [electronic version], *West J Nurs Res* 20(2):145–165, 1998.

Wound Ostomy and Continence Nurses Society: *Management of gastrostomy tube complications for the pediatric and adult patient*, 2008, retrieved December 2, 2008, from http://wwwwocn.org/WOCN_Library.

*Adapted from the QSEN at http://www.qsen.org.

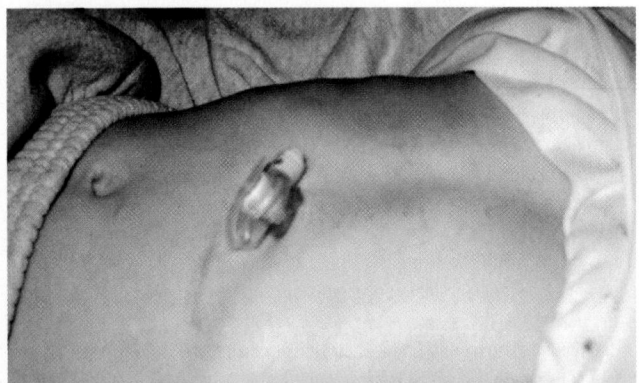

FIG 22-30 Child with a skin-level gastrostomy device (MIC-KEY), which provides for secure attachment of extension tubing to the gastrostomy opening.

Feeding of water, formula, or pureed foods is carried out in the same manner and rate as for gavage feeding. A mechanical pump may be used to regulate the volume and rate of feeding. After feedings, the infant or child is positioned on the right side or in the Fowler position, and the tube may be clamped or left open and suspended between feedings, depending on the child's condition. A clamped tube allows more mobility but is only appropriate if the child can tolerate intermittent feedings without vomiting or prolonged backup of feeding into the tube. Sometimes a Y tube is used to allow for simultaneous decompression during feeding. If a Foley catheter is used as the gastrostomy tube, apply very slight tension. The tube is securely taped to maintain the balloon at the gastrostomy opening and prevent leakage of gastric contents and the tube's progression toward the pyloric sphincter, where it may occlude the stomach outlet. As a precaution, the length of the tube is measured postoperatively and then remeasured each shift to be certain it has not slipped. The nurse can make a mark above the skin level to further ensure its placement. When the gastrostomy tube is no longer needed, it is removed; the skin opening usually closes spontaneously by contracture.

NASODUODENAL AND NASOJEJUNAL TUBES

Children at high risk for regurgitation or aspiration such as those with gastroparesis, mechanical ventilation, or brain injuries may require placement of a postpyloric feeding tube. A trained practitioner inserts the nasoduodenal or nasojejunal tube because of the risk of misplacement and potential for perforation in tubes requiring a stylet. Accurate placement is verified by radiography. Small-bore tubes may easily clog.

Flush the tube when feeding is interrupted, before and after medication administration, and routinely every 4 hours or as directed by institutional policy. Tube replacement should be considered monthly to ensure optimal tube patency. Continuous feedings are delivered by a mechanical pump to regulate their volume and rate. Bolus feeds are contraindicated. Tube displacement is suspected in children showing signs of feeding intolerance such as vomiting. In these cases, stop the feedings and notify the practitioner.

TOTAL PARENTERAL NUTRITION

Total parenteral nutrition provides for the total nutritional needs of infants and children whose lives are threatened because feeding by way of the gastrointestinal tract is impossible, inadequate, or hazardous.

Total parenteral nutrition therapy involves IV infusion of highly concentrated solutions of protein, glucose, and other nutrients. The solution is infused through conventional tubing with a special filter attached to remove particulate matter or microorganisms that may have contaminated the solution. The highly concentrated solutions require infusion into a vessel with sufficient volume and turbulence to allow for rapid dilution. The wide-diameter vessels selected are the superior vena cava and innominate or intrathoracic subclavian veins approached by way of the external or internal jugular veins. The highly irritating nature of concentrated glucose precludes the use of the small peripheral veins in most instances. However, dilute glucose–protein hydrolysates that are appropriate for infusing into peripheral veins are being used with increasing frequency. When peripheral veins are used, intralipid becomes the major calorie source. For long-term alimentation, central venous catheters are usually used.

The major nursing responsibilities are the same as for any IV therapy and include control of sepsis, monitoring of the infusion rate, and assessment of the patient. The TPN solution must be prepared under rigid aseptic conditions, which is best accomplished by specially trained technicians. Specially trained nurses should change the solution and tubing and redress the infusion using meticulous aseptic precautions. In some institutions, this may be a nursing responsibility. If so, the procedure is carried out according to hospital protocol.

The infusion is maintained at a constant rate by means of an infusion pump to ensure the proper concentrations of glucose and amino acids. Accurate calculation of the rate is required to deliver a measured amount in a given length of time. Because alterations in flow rate are relatively common, the drip should be checked frequently to ensure an even, continuous infusion. The TPN infusion rate should not be increased or decreased without the practitioner being informed because alterations can cause hyperglycemia or hypoglycemia.

General assessments, such as vital signs, input and output measurements, and checking results of laboratory tests, facilitate early detection of infection or fluid and electrolyte imbalance. Additional amounts of potassium and sodium chloride are often required in hyperalimentation; therefore, observation for signs of potassium or sodium deficit or excess is part of nursing care. This is rarely a problem except in children with reduced renal function or metabolic defects. Hyperglycemia may occur during the first day or two as the child adapts to the high-glucose load of the hyperalimentation solution. Although hyperglycemia occurs infrequently, insulin may be required to help the body adjust. When this occurs, nursing responsibilities include blood glucose testing. To prevent hypoglycemia when the hyperalimentation is disconnected, the rate of the infusion and the amount of insulin are decreased gradually.

TABLE 22-9	ADMINISTRATION OF ENEMAS TO CHILDREN	
AGE	**AMOUNT (ML)**	**INSERTION DISTANCE**
Infant	120–240	2.5 cm (1 inch)
2–4 yr	240–360	5 cm (2 inches)
4–10 yr	360–480	7.5 cm (3 inches)
11 yr	480–720	10 cm (4 inches)

FAMILY TEACHING AND HOME CARE

When alternative feedings are needed for an extended period, the family needs to learn how to feed the child with an NG, gastrostomy, or TPN feeding regimen. The same principles apply as discussed earlier in this chapter for compliance, especially in terms of education, and in Chapter 21 for discharge planning and home care. Plan ample time for the family to learn and perform the procedures under supervision before they assume full responsibility for the child's care. Refer the family to community agencies that provide support and practical assistance. The Oley Foundation* is a nonprofit research and education organization that assists persons receiving enteral nutrition and home TPN.

PROCEDURES RELATED TO ELIMINATION

ENEMA

The procedure for giving an enema to an infant or child does not differ essentially from that for an adult except for the type and amount of fluid administered and the distance for inserting the tube into the rectum (Table 22-9). Depending on the volume, use a syringe with rubber tubing, an enema bottle, or an enema bag.

An isotonic solution is used in children. Plain water is not used because, being hypotonic, it can cause rapid fluid shift and fluid overload. The Fleet enema (pediatric or adult sized) is not advised for children because of the harsh action of its ingredients (sodium biphosphate and sodium phosphate). Commercial enemas can be dangerous to patients with megacolon and to dehydrated or azotemic children. The osmotic effect of the Fleet enema may produce diarrhea, which can lead to metabolic acidosis. Other potential complications are extreme hyperphosphatemia, hypernatremia, and hypocalcemia, which may lead to neuromuscular irritability and coma (Walton, Thomas, Aly, and others, 2000).

> **NURSING TIP** If prepared saline is not available, the nurse can make some by adding 1 tsp of table salt to 500 ml (1 pint) of tap water.

Because infants and young children are unable to retain the solution after it is administered, the buttocks must be held together for a short time to retain the fluid. The enema is administered and expelled while the child is lying with the buttocks over the bedpan and with the head and back supported by pillows. Older children are ordinarily able to hold the solution if they understand what to do and if they are not expected to hold it for too long. The nurse should have the bedpan handy or, for ambulatory children, ensure that the bathroom

---

*214 Hun Memorial, MC-28, Albany Medical Center, Albany, NY 12208; 800-776-OLEY; http://www.oley.org.

is available before beginning the procedure. An enema is an intrusive procedure and thus threatening to preschool children; therefore, a careful explanation is especially important to ease possible fear.

A preoperative bowel preparation solution given orally or through an NG tube is increasingly being used instead of an enema. The polyethylene glycol–electrolyte lavage solution (GoLYTELY) mechanically flushes the bowel without significant absorption, thereby avoiding potential fluid and electrolyte imbalances. NuLYTELY, a modification of GoLYTELY, has the same therapeutic advantages as GoLYTELY and was developed to improve on the taste. Another effective oral cathartic is magnesium citrate solution.

OSTOMIES

Children may require stomas for various health problems. The most frequent causes in infants are necrotizing enterocolitis and imperforate anus and, less often, Hirschsprung disease. In older children the most frequent causes are inflammatory bowel disease, especially Crohn disease (regional enteritis), and ureterostomies for distal ureter or bladder defects.

Care and management of ostomies in older children differ little from the care of ostomies in adult patients. The major emphasis in pediatric care is preparing the child for the procedure and teaching care of the ostomy to the child and family. The basic principles of preparation are the same as for any procedure (see p. 637). Simple, straightforward language is most effective together with the use of illustrations and a replica model (e.g., drawing a picture of a child with a stoma on the abdomen and explaining it as "another opening where bowel movements [or any other term the child uses] will come out"). At another time, the nurse can draw a pouch over the opening to demonstrate how the contents are collected. Using a doll to demonstrate the process is an excellent teaching strategy, and special books are available.

Children with ileostomies are fitted immediately after surgery with an appliance to protect the skin from the proteolytic enzymes in the liquid stool. Infants may not be fitted with a pouch in the immediate postoperative period. When stomal drainage is minimal, as is often the case in small or preterm infants, a gauze dressing will suffice. Give your parents a choice of caring for the colostomy with or without an appliance. Pediatric appliances are available in a variety of sizes to ensure an adequate fit.*

Ostomy equipment consists of a one- or two-piece system with a hypoallergenic skin barrier to maintain peristomal skin integrity. The pouch should be large enough to contain a moderate amount of stool and flatus but not so large as to overwhelm the infant or child. A backing helps minimize the risk of skin breakdown from moisture trapped between the skin and pouch. Avoid small clips and rubber bands to prevent choking in young children.

Protection of the peristomal skin is a major aspect of stoma care. Well-fitting appliances are important to prevent leakage of contents. Before applying the appliance, prepare the skin with a skin sealant that is allowed to dry. Then apply stoma paste around the base of the stoma or to the back of the wafer. The sealant and paste work together to prevent peristomal skin breakdown.

In infants with a colostomy left unpouched, skin care is similar to that of any diapered child. However, protect the peristomal skin with a barrier substance (e.g., zinc oxide ointment [Sensi-Care] or a mixture of zinc oxide ointment and stoma powder [Stomahesive]). A diaper larger than the one usually worn may be needed to extend upward over the stoma and absorb drainage. If the skin becomes inflamed, denuded, or infected, the care is similar to the interventions used for diaper dermatitis (see Chapter 30). A zinc-based product helps protect healthy skin, heal excoriated skin, and minimize pain associated with skin breakdown. The skin protectant adheres to denuded, weeping skin. The nurse can apply zinc-based products over topical antifungal and antibacterial agents if infection is present. No-sting barrier film is a skin sealant that has no alcohol base and can be used on open skin without stinging.

With young children, preventing them from pulling off the pouch is also an important consideration. One-piece outfits keep exploring hands from reaching the pouch, and the loose waist avoids any pressure on the appliance. Keeping the child occupied with toys during the pouch change is also helpful. As children mature, encourage their participation in ostomy care. Even preschoolers can assist by holding supplies, pulling paper backings from the appliance, and helping clean the stoma area. Toilet training for bladder control needs to begin at the appropriate time as for any other child.

Older children and adolescents should eventually have total responsibility for ostomy care just as they would for usual bowel function. During adolescence, concerns for body image and the ostomy's impact on intimacy and sexuality emerge. The nurse should stress to teenagers that the presence of a stoma need not interfere with their activities. These youngsters can choose which ostomy equipment is best suited to their needs. Attractively designed and decorated pouch covers are well liked by teenagers.

Children with familial adenomatous polyposis may require a colectomy with ileoanal reservoir to prevent or treat carcinoma of the colon. Peristomal skin care for these children is particularly challenging because of increased liquid stools, increased digestive enzymes that may cause skin breakdown, and the stoma being at skin level rather than raised. Additional care with this condition includes close monitoring of fluid and electrolyte status and increased incidence of bowel obstruction.

An enterostomal therapy nurse specialist is an important member of the health care team and will have additional suggestions and assistance with skin care information and ostomy pouching options. The nurse can obtain further information by contacting the Wound, Ostomy and Continence Nurses Society.†

FAMILY TEACHING AND HOME CARE

Because these children are almost always discharged with a functioning colostomy, preparation of the family should begin as early as possible in the hospital. The nurse instructs the family in the application of the device (if used), care of the skin, and appropriate action in case skin problems develop. Early evidence of skin breakdown or stomal complications, such as ribbonlike stools, excessive diarrhea, bleeding, prolapse, or failure to pass flatus or stool, is brought to the attention of the physician, nurse, or stoma specialist. The same principles are applied as discussed earlier in this chapter for compliance, especially in terms of education, and in Chapter 21 for discharge planning and home care.

---

*Parents may find the following pamphlets helpful: *A Parent's Guide to Necrotizing Enterocolitis* and *Parent's Guide to Ostomy Care for Children*, available from ConvaTec (http://www.convatec.com).

†888-224-9626; http://www.wocn.org.

KEY POINTS

- Informed consent is valid when the person is capable of giving consent (is over the age of majority and is competent), is supplied with information needed to make an intelligent decision, and acts voluntarily when exercising freedom of choice.
- Informed consent is needed for major surgery, minor surgery, and diagnostic tests and medical treatments with an element of risk.
- The major principles in psychologic preparation of the child for surgery are to establish trust, provide support, and give an explanation in easy-to-understand terms.
- Preparation for procedures should be based on developmental characteristics of the child and family, emphasizing the importance of the parents' role.
- Most parents and children want to be together during stressful procedures and should be offered this opportunity, with guidance on how the parent can comfort the child.
- The use of play activities to provide teaching about necessary nursing and medical interventions is an effective tool for use with children.
- In the performance of a procedure, the nurse should expect success, involve the child when possible in the procedure, provide distraction, and allow for expression of feelings.
- Proper positioning of infants and small children for procedures is essential to minimize movement and discomfort.
- In giving postprocedural support, the nurse should encourage children to express their feelings and praise them for completion of the procedure.
- Stressful times before and after surgery that produce anxiety in children are admission, blood tests, injection of preoperative medication (if used), transportation to the operating room, and return from the PACU.
- Assessment of compliance entails measuring factors that affect compliance through clinical judgment, self-reporting, direct observation, monitoring of appointments and therapeutic response, pill counts, and chemical assay.
- Compliance strategies may be classified as organizational, educational, and behavioral.
- Knowledge of the ill child's eating habits and favorite foods can help in maintaining adequate nutrition.
- Skin care is essential to prevent skin breakdown.

- Control of fever may be accomplished by administration of antipyretics; hyperthermia is controlled by environmental means (minimum clothing, increased air circulation, hypothermia mattress, or cool compresses).
- Infection control is based on two systems. Standard precautions provide protection when the infected person is undiagnosed. Transmission-based precautions add extra interventions for patients diagnosed with or suspected of having an infection.
- Ensuring safety in the hospital setting is a major concern and can be achieved through environmental measures, infection control measures, limit setting, and safe transportation.
- Restraints are used cautiously and require a medical order. Therapeutic hugging can avoid the use of restraints.
- Factors that affect drug dosage determination are growth and maturation, difficulty in evaluating drug response, and BSA.
- Family teaching regarding medication administration includes telling parents why the child is receiving the drug; its possible effects; and the amount, frequency, and length of time the drug is to be administered.
- The preferred sites for IM injection in children are the vastus lateralis and ventrogluteal areas.
- Intermittent venous access is accomplished by a peripheral intermittent infusion device, a PICC, a central venous catheter, or an implanted port.
- Several safety catheters and needleless device systems are available to reduce the risk of needlestick injuries in patients and caregivers.
- Nursing assessment of fluid and electrolyte disturbances entails observation of general appearance, vital signs, and measurement of I&O.
- Oxygen can be administered by hood, mask, nasal cannula, prongs, or face tent.
- Tracheostomy suctioning involves premeasured insertion of the catheter, application of suction for 5 seconds when withdrawing the catheter, and supplemental oxygen before and after suctioning.
- Alternative forms of feeding include gavage feeding, gastrostomy feeding, and TPN.
- In the care of children with ostomies, nurses play an important role in family support and instruction in care of the stoma site.

REFERENCES

Abo A, Chen L, Johnston P, and others: Positioning for lumbar puncture in children evaluated by bedside ultrasound, *Pediatrics* 125:e1149–e1153, 2010.

American Academy of Pediatrics: Consent for emergency medical services for children and adolescents, *Pediatrics* 111(3):703–706, 2003.

American Academy of Pediatrics, Committee on Pediatric Emergency Medicine, American College of Emergency Physicians, Pediatric Emergency Medicine Committee, O'Malley P, and others: Patient- and family-centered care and the role of the emergency physician providing care to a child in the emergency department, *Pediatrics* 118(5):2242–2244, 2006.

American Academy of Pediatrics, Task Force on Sudden Infant Death Syndrome: The changing concept of sudden infant death syndrome:

diagnostic coding shifts, controversies regarding the sleeping environment, and new variables to consider in reducing risk, *Pediatrics* 116(5): 1245–1255, 2005.

American Association of Critical Care Nurses: Practice alert: family presence during CPR and invasive procedures, 2006, retrieved July 7, 2009, from http://www.aacn.org.

American Heart Association: 2010 American Heart Association guidelines for CPR and ECC, *Circulation* 122(suppl 2), 2010.

Amlung SR, Miller WL, Bosley LM: The 1999 national pressure ulcer prevalence survey: a benchmarking approach, *Adv Skin Wound Care* 14:297–301, 2001.

Anderson SL, Schaechter J, Brosco JP: Adolescent patients and their confidentiality: staying within legal bounds, *Contemp Pediatr* 22(7):54, 2005.

Axelrod P: External cooling in the management of fever, *Clin Infect Dis* 31(suppl 5):S224–S229, 2000.

Baharestani MM, Ratliff CR: Pressure ulcers in neonates and children: an NPUAP white paper, *Adv Skin Wound Care* 20(4):208–220, 2007.

Barnes S: Not a social event: the follow-up phone call, *J Perianesth Nurs* 14(4):223–255, 2000.

Beckstrand J, Ellett MLC, McDaniel A: Predicting internal distance to the stomach for positioning NG and OG feeding tubes in children, *J Adv Nurs* 59(3):274–289, 2007.

Berger JE, American Academy of Pediatrics, Committee on Medical Liability: Consent by proxy for nonurgent pediatric care, *Pediatrics* 112(5):1186–1195, 2003.

Blaney M, Shen V, Kerner JA, and others: Alteplase for the treatment of central venous catheter occlusion in children: results of a prospective, open-label, single-arm study (the Cathflo Activase Pediatric Study), *J Vasc Interv Radiol* 17(11 Pt 1):1745–1751, 2006.

Bottor LT: Rapid sequence intubation in the neonate, *Adv Neonat Care* 9(3):111–117, 2009.

Bryant RA, Doughty D, editors: *Acute and chronic wounds: nursing management*, ed 2, St. Louis, 2000, Mosby.

Burke N: Alternative methods for newborn urine sample collection, *Pediatr Nurs* 21(6):546–549, 1995.

Child Health Corporation of America: Pediatric falls: state of the science, *Pediatr Nurs* 35(4): 227–231, 2009.

Codipietro L, Ceccarelli M, Ponzone A: Breastfeeding or oral sucrose solution in term neonates receiving heel lance: a randomized, controlled trial, *Pediatrics* 122(3):e716–e721, 2008.

Considine J, Brennan D: Effect of an evidence-based education programme on ED discharge advice for febrile children, *J Clin Nurs* 16:1687–1694, 2007.

Cook IF, Murtagh J: Comparative reactogenicity and parental acceptability of pertussis vaccines administered into the ventrogluteal area and anterolateral thigh in children aged 2, 4, 6, and 18 months, *Vaccine* 4(21):3330–3334, 2003.

Cook IF, Murtagh J: Ventrogluteal area—a suitable site for intramuscular vaccination of infants and toddlers, *Vaccine* 24(13):2403–2408, 2006.

Curley MAQ, Moloney-Harmon PA: *Critical care nursing of infants and children*, ed 2, Philadelphia, 2001, Saunders.

Curley MAQ, Quigley SM, Lin M: Pressure ulcers in pediatric intensive care: incidence and associated factors, *Pediatr Crit Care Med* 4:284–290, 2003.

Curley MAQ, Razmus IS, Roberts KE, and others: Predicting pressure ulcer risk in pediatric patients: the Braden Q scale, *Nurs Res* 52:22–33, 2003.

de Caen AR, Reis A, Bhutta A: Vascular access and drug therapy in pediatric resuscitation, *Pediatr Clin North Am* 55(4):909–927, 2008.

Eaton L: Hand washing is more important than cleaner wards in controlling MRSA, *BMJ* 330(7497):922, 2005.

Ellett ML, Beckstrand J: Examination of gavage tube placement in children, *J Soc Pediatr Nurs* 4(2):51–60, 1999.

Emergency Nurses Association: *Family presence at the bedside during invasive procedures and resuscitation*, 2005, retrieved July 7, 2009, from http://www.ena.org.

Essink-Tebbes CM, Wuis EW, Liem KD, and others: Safety of lidocaine-prilocaine cream application four times a day in premature neonates: a pilot study, *Eur J Pediatr* 158(5):421–423, 1999.

Fearon DM, Steele DW: End-tidal carbon dioxide predicts the presence and severity of acidosis in children with diabetes, *Acad Emerg Med* 9(12): 1373–1379, 2002.

Fisher AA, Deffenbaugh C, Poole RL, and others: The use of alteplase for restoring patency to occluded central venous access devices in infants and children, *J Infus Nurs* 27(3):171–174, 2004.

Foster H, Ritchey M, Bloom D: Adventitious knots in urethral catheters: report of 5 cases, *J Urol* 148(5):1496–1498, 1992.

Gamulka B, Mendoza C, Connolly B: Evaluation of a unique, nurse-inserted, peripherally inserted central catheter program, *Pediatrics* 6(115): 1602–1606, 2005.

Gonzalez CM, Palmer LS: Double-knotted feeding tube in a child's bladder, *Urology* 49(5):772. 1997.

Gray L, Watt L, Blass EM: Skin-to-skin contact is analgesic in healthy newborns, *Pediatrics* 105(1):110–111, 2000, retrieved June 10, 2009, from http://www.pediatrics.org/cgi/content/full/105/1/E14.

Gray M: Atraumatic urethral catheterization of children, *Pediatr Nurs* 22(4):306–310, 1996.

Hazinski MF, Zaritsky AL, Nadkarni VM, and others: *PALS provider manual*, Dallas, 2002, American Heart Association.

Infusion Nurses Society: *Policies and procedures for infusion nursing*, ed 3, Norwood, Mass, 2006, Author.

Joint Commission on Accreditation of Healthcare Organizations: *Comprehensive accreditation manual for hospitals: restraint and seclusion standards, TX7.1-TX7.5.5*, Oakbrook Terrace, Ill, 2001, Author.

Jones T, Jacobsen SJ: Childhood febrile seizures: overview and implications, *Int J Med Sci* 4(2): 110–114, 2007.

Junqueira AL, Tavares VR, Martins RM, and others: Safety and immunogenicity of hepatitis B vaccine administered into ventrogluteal vs. anterolateral thigh sites in infants: a randomized controlled trial, *Int J Nurs Stud* 47(9): 1074–1079, 2010.

Kain ZN, Caldwell-Andrews AA, Krivutza DM, and others: Trends in the practice of parental presence during induction of anesthesia and the use of preoperative sedative premedication in the United States, 1995–2002: results of a follow-up national survey, *Anesth Analg* 98(5):1252–1259, 2004.

Kain ZN, Caldwell-Andrews AA, Mayes LC, and others: Family-centered preparation for surgery improves perioperative outcomes in children, *Anesthesiology* 106(1):65–74, 2007.

Katsma D, Smith G: Analysis of needle path during intramuscular injection, *Nurs Res* 46(5): 288–292, 1997.

Kellam B, Sacks LM, Wailer JL, and others: Tenderfoot Preemie vs a manual lancet: a clinical evaluation, *Neonatal Netw* 20(7): 31–36, 2001.

Kerner JA, Garcia-Careaga MG, Fisher AA, and others: Treatment of catheter occlusion in pediatric patients, *J Parenter Enteral Nutr* 30(suppl 1):S73–S81, 2006.

Kilbane BJ: Images in emergency medicine. Knotting of a urinary catheter, *Ann Emerg Med* 53(5):e3–4, 2009.

Klasner AE, Luke DA, Scalzo AJ: Pediatric orogastric and nasogastric tubes: a new formula evaluated, *Ann Emerg Med* 39(3): 268–272, 2002.

Kraus D, Stohlmeyer LA, Hannon DR, and others: Effectiveness and infant acceptance of the Rx Medibottle versus the oral syringe, *Pharmacotherapy* 21(4):416–423, 2001.

Kyngas H, Kroll T, Duffy M: Compliance in adolescents with chronic diseases: a review, *J Adolesc Health* 26:379–388, 2000.

Lamagna P, MacPhee M: Phlebitis and infiltration: troubleshooting pediatric peripheral IVs, *Nurse Week (Heartland ed)* 5(4):20, 26, 28, 2004.

Levison J, Wojtulewicz J: Adventitious knot formation complicating catheterization of the infant bladder, *J Paediatr Child Health* 40(8): 493–494, 2004.

Li HCW, Lopez V, Lee TLI: Psychoeducational preparation of children for surgery: the importance of parental involvement, *Patient Educ Counsel* 65:34–41, 2007.

Lodha A, Ly L, Brindle M, and others: Intraurethral knot in a very-low-birth-weight infant: Radiological recognition, surgical management and prevention, *Pediatr Radiol* 35(7):713–716, 2005.

Manworren R, Fledderman M: Preparation of the child and family for surgery. In Wise BV, McKenna C, Garvin G, and others, editors: *Nursing care of the general pediatric surgical patient*, Gaithersburg, Md, 2000, Aspen.

Maxwell LG, Yaster M: Perioperative management issues in pediatric patients, *Anesthesiol Clin North Am* 18(3):601–632, 2000.

McCord S, McElvain V, Sachdeva R, and others: Risk factors associated with pressure ulcers in the pediatric intensive care unit, *J Wound Ostomy Continence Nurs* 31(4):179–183, 2004.

McGillivray D, Mok E, Mulrooney E, and others: A head-to-head comparison: "clean-void" bag versus catheter urinalysis in the diagnosis of urinary tract infection in young children, *J Pediatr* 147(4):451–456, 2008.

Munro H, D'Errico FC: Parental involvement in perioperative anesthetic management, *J Perianesth Nurs* 15(6):397–400, 2000.

Nagler J, Wright R, Krauss B: End-tidal carbon dioxide as a measure of acidosis among children with gastroenteritis, *Pediatrics* 118(1):260–267, 2006.

Noonan C, Quigley S, Curley MAQ: Skin integrity in hospitalized infants and children: a prevalence survey, *J Pediatr Nurs* 21(6):445–453, 2006.

Piira T, Sugiura T, Champion GD, and others: The role of parental presence in the context of children's medical procedures: a systematic review, *Child Care Health Dev* 31(2):233–243, 2005.

Purssell E: Parental fever phobia and its evolutionary correlates, *J Clin Nurs* 18:210–218, 2008.

Quality, equipment hold keys to infection control, *ED Manage* 18(2):19–21, 2006.

Romino SL, Keatley VM, Secrest J, and others: Parental presence during anesthesia induction in children, *AORN J* 81(4):780–792, 2005.

Rosenberg H, Davis M, James D: Malignant hyperthermia, *Orphanet J Rare Dis* 2:21, 2007.

Rote N, Huether S, McCance K: Infections and alterations in immunity and inflammation. In Huether S, McCance K, editors: *Understanding pathophysiology*, ed 2, St. Louis, 2000, Mosby.

Sadleir LG, Scheffer IE: Febrile seizures, *BMJ* 334:307–311, 2007.

Shah V, Ohlsson A: Venepuncture versus heel lance for blood sampling in term neonates, *Cochrane Database Syst Rev* (4):CD001452, 2007.

Shen V, Li X, Murdock M, and others: Recombinant tissue plasminogen activator (alteplase) for restoration of function to occluded central venous catheters in pediatric patients, *J Pediatr Hematol Oncol* 25(1):38–45, 2003.

Shepherd AJ, Glenesk A, Niven CA, and others: A Scottish study of heel-prick blood sampling in newborn babies, *Midwifery* 22(2):158–168, 2005.

Tillett J: Adolescents and informed consent: ethical and legal issues, *J Perinat Neonat Nurs* 19(2):112–121, 2005.

Turner TW: Intravesical catheter knotting: an uncommon complication of urinary catheterization, *Pediatr Emerg Care* 20(2):115–117, 2004.

Uman LS, Chambers CT, McGrath PJ, and others: Psychological interventions for needle-related procedural pain and distress in children and adolescents, *Cochrane Database Syst Rev* (4):CD005179, 2006.

Vertanen H, Fellman V, Brommels M, and others: An automatic incision device for obtaining blood samples from the heels of the preterm infants causes less damage than a conventional manual lancet, *Arch Dis Child Fetal Neonatal Educ* 84:F53–F55, 2001.

Wald ER: To bag or not to bag, *J Pediatr* 174(4):418–419, 2005.

Walsh A, Edwards H: Management of childhood fever by parents: literature review, *J Adv Nurs* 54(2):217–222, 2006.

Walton DM, Thomas DC, Aly HZ, and others: Morbid hypocalcemia associated with phosphate enema in a 6-week-old infant, *Pediatrics* 106:e37, 2000.

Warren J, Fromm RE Jr, Orr RA, and others: Guidelines for the inter- and intrahospital transport of critically ill patients, *Crit Care Med* 32(1):256–262, 2004.

Whitby M, McLaws ML, Slater K: Needlestick injuries in a major teaching hospital: the worthwhile effect of hospital-wide replacement of conventional hollow-bore needles, *Am J Infect Control* 36(3):180–186, 2008.

Willock J, Baharestani M, Anthony D: The development of the Glamorgan paediatric pressure ulcer risk assessment scale, *J Wound Care* 18(1):17–21, 2009.

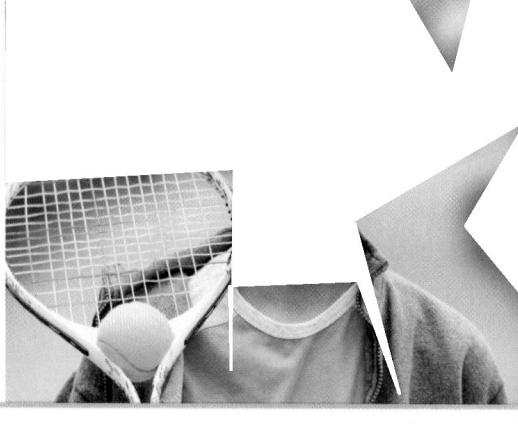

evolve WEBSITE

http://evolve.elsevier.com/wong/essentials

Animations—Asthma; Bag Ventilation; Bronchi and Bronchioles; Intubation; Intubation in Infant; Intubation, Incorrect Placement; Lung Sounds; Pediatric CPR; Pneumonia; Respiratory Failure, Infant

Case Studies—Acute Epiglottitis; Asthma; Bronchiolitis; Cystic Fibrosis; Mononucleosis; Tonsillitis

Key Point Summaries

NCLEX-Style Review Questions

Nursing Care Plans—The Child with Acute Respiratory Infection; The Child with Asthma; The Child with Bronchiolitis and Respiratory Syncytial Virus (RSV) Infection; The Child with Cystic Fibrosis; The Child with Respiratory Failure; The Child with Tonsillectomy

CHAPTER OUTLINE

Respiratory Infection, 707
  Nursing Care Plan: The Child with Acute
    Respiratory Tract Infection, 711
Upper Respiratory Tract Infections, 710
  Acute Viral Nasopharyngitis, 710
  Acute Streptococcal Pharyngitis, 714
  Tonsillitis, 715
  Influenza, 716
  Otitis Media, 717
  Infectious Mononucleosis, 719
Croup Syndromes, 720
  Acute Epiglottitis, 721
  Acute Laryngotracheobronchitis, 722
  Acute Spasmodic Laryngitis, 723
  Bacterial Tracheitis, 723
Infections of the Lower Airways, 723
  Bronchitis, 723
  Respiratory Syncytial Virus and
    Bronchiolitis, 723

Pneumonias, 725
  Viral Pneumonia, 726
  Primary Atypical Pneumonia, 726
  Bacterial Pneumonia, 726
Other Infections of the Respiratory
  Tract, 728
  Pertussis (Whooping Cough), 728
  Tuberculosis, 729
Pulmonary Dysfunction Caused by
  Noninfectious Irritants, 731
  Foreign Body Aspiration, 731
  Aspiration Pneumonia, 732
  Pulmonary Edema, 733
  Acute Respiratory Distress Syndrome
    and Acute Lung Injury, 733
  Smoke Inhalation Injury, 734
  Environmental Tobacco Smoke
    Exposure, 735

Long-Term Respiratory Dysfunction, 736
  Asthma, 736
    *Nursing Care Plan: The Child with
      Acute Asthma Exacerbation, 742*
    *Nursing Care Plan: The Child with
      Asthma, 745*
  Cystic Fibrosis, 747
  Obstructive Sleep-Disordered
    Breathing, 754
Respiratory Emergency, 754
  Respiratory Failure, 754
  Cardiopulmonary Resuscitation, 755
    Resuscitation Procedure, 755
  Airway Obstruction, 758
    Infants, 758
    Children, 759

LEARNING OBJECTIVES

On completion of this chapter the reader will be able to:
- Identify the factors leading to respiratory tract infection in infants and young children.
- Contrast the effects of various respiratory infections observed in infants and children.
- Describe the postoperative nursing care of a child with a tonsillectomy.

- Outline a nursing care plan for a child with croup.
- Describe priorities of nursing care for a child with acute otitis media.
- Identify priorities of nursing care for an infant with respiratory syncytial virus bronchiolitis.
- Describe the various therapeutic measures to relieve the symptoms of asthma.

- Outline a plan for teaching home care management of a child with asthma.
- Describe the physiologic effects of cystic fibrosis on the gastrointestinal and pulmonary systems.

- Outline a care plan for a child with cystic fibrosis.
- List the major signs of respiratory distress in infants and children.
- Describe emergent procedures for the relief of foreign body obstruction in an infant or child.

RESPIRATORY INFECTION

Infections of the respiratory tract are described according to the anatomic area of involvement. The upper respiratory tract, or upper airway, consists of the oronasopharynx, pharynx, larynx, and upper part of the trachea. The lower respiratory tract consists of the lower trachea, mainstem bronchi, segmental bronchi, subsegmental bronchioles, terminal bronchioles, and alveoli. In this discussion, the trachea is considered with lower tract disorders, and infections of the epiglottis and larynx are categorized as croup syndromes. However, respiratory infections seldom fall into discrete anatomic areas. Infections often spread from one structure to another because of the contiguous nature of the mucous membrane lining the entire tract. Consequently, respiratory tract infections involve several areas rather than a single structure, although the effect on one area may predominate in any given illness.

Etiology and Characteristics

Respiratory tract infections account for the majority of acute illnesses in children. The etiology and course of these infections are influenced by the age of the child, the season, living conditions, and preexisting medical problems.

Infectious Agents

The respiratory tract is subject to a wide variety of infective organisms. Most infections are caused by viruses, particularly respiratory syncytial virus (RSV), nonpolio enteroviruses (coxsackieviruses A and B), adenoviruses, parainfluenza viruses, and human metapneumoviruses. Other agents involved in primary or secondary invasion include group A β-hemolytic streptococci (GABHS), staphylococci, *Haemophilus influenzae*, *Chlamydia trachomatis*, *Mycoplasma* organisms, and pneumococci.

Age

Healthy full-term infants younger than age 3 months are presumed to have a lower infection rate than older infants because of the protective function of maternal antibodies; however, infants may be susceptible to specific respiratory tract infections, namely pertussis, during this period. The infection rate increases from 3 to 6 months of age, the time between the disappearance of maternal antibodies and the infant's own antibody production. The viral infection rate remains high during the toddler and preschool years. By 5 years of age, viral respiratory tract infections are less frequent, but the incidence of *Mycoplasma pneumoniae* and GABHS infections increases. The amount of lymphoid tissue increases throughout middle childhood, and repeated exposure to organisms confers increasing immunity as children grow older.

Some viral or bacterial agents produce a mild illness in older children but severe lower respiratory tract illness or croup in infants. For example, pertussis causes a relatively harmless tracheobronchitis in childhood but is a serious disease in infancy.

Size

Anatomic differences influence the response to respiratory tract infections. The diameter of the airways is smaller in young children and subject to considerable narrowing from edematous mucous membranes and increased production of secretions. Organisms may move rapidly down the shorter respiratory tract of younger children, causing more extensive involvement. The relatively short and open eustachian tube in infants and young children allows pathogens easy access to the middle ear.

Resistance

The ability to resist pathogens depends on several factors. Deficiencies of the immune system place the child at risk for infection. Other conditions that decrease resistance are malnutrition, anemia, fatigue, and chilling of the body. Conditions that weaken defenses of the respiratory tract and predispose children to infection also include allergies (e.g., allergic rhinitis), preterm birth, bronchopulmonary dysplasia (BPD), asthma, history of RSV infection, cardiac anomalies that cause pulmonary congestion, and cystic fibrosis (CF). Daycare attendance and exposure to secondhand smoke increase the likelihood of infection.

Seasonal Variations

The most common respiratory pathogens appear in epidemics during the winter and spring months. Mycoplasmal infections occur more often in autumn and early winter. Whereas infection-related asthma occurs more frequently during cold weather, winter and early spring are typically "RSV season."

Clinical Manifestations

Infants and young children, especially those between 6 months and 3 years of age, react more severely to acute respiratory tract infections than older children. Young children display a number of generalized signs and symptoms as well as local manifestations (Box 23-1).

Nursing Care Management

Assessment of the respiratory system follows the guidelines described in Chapter 6 (for assessment of the ears, nose, mouth and throat, chest, and lungs). The assessment should include respiratory rate, depth and rhythm, heart rate, oxygenation, hydration status, body temperature, activity level, and level of comfort. Special attention should also be given to the components and observations listed in Box 23-2. A noninvasive pulse oximeter (oxygen saturation) measurement should be performed on *all* children as part of the routine physical assessment. The nursing process in the care of the child with acute respiratory tract infection is outlined in the Nursing Process box.

Ease Respiratory Efforts

Many acute respiratory tract infections are mild and cause few symptoms. Although children may feel uncomfortable and have a "stuffy"

Nursing Care Plan—The Child with Acute Respiratory Infection

Animations—Bronchi and Bronchioles; Lung Sounds

BOX 23-1 **SIGNS AND SYMPTOMS ASSOCIATED WITH RESPIRATORY TRACT INFECTIONS IN INFANTS AND SMALL CHILDREN**

Fever
May be absent in newborn infants
Greatest at ages 6 months to 3 years
May reach 39.5° to 40.5° C (103°–105° F) even with mild infections
Often appears as first sign of infection
May lead to listlessness and irritability, with altered activity pattern (usually decreased)
Tendency to develop high temperatures with infection in certain families
May precipitate febrile seizure (see Chapter 28)

Poor Feeding and Anorexia
Common in infants during breastfeeding or bottle feeding
Common with most childhood illnesses
Frequently the initial evidence of illness
Persists to a greater or lesser degree throughout febrile stage of illness; often extends into convalescence

Vomiting
Common in small children with illness
Clue to onset of infection
May precede other signs by several hours
Usually short lived but may persist during the illness

Diarrhea
Usually mild, transient diarrhea but may become severe
Often accompanies viral respiratory infections
Frequent cause of dehydration

Abdominal Pain
Common complaint
Sometimes indistinguishable from pain of appendicitis
May be caused by mesenteric lymphadenitis
May be linked to muscle spasms from vomiting, especially in nervous, tense child

Nasal Blockage
Small nasal passages of infants easily blocked by mucosal swelling and exudation
Can interfere with respiration and feeding in infants
May contribute to the development of otitis media and sinusitis

Nasal Discharge
Frequent occurrence
May be thin and watery (rhinorrhea) or thick and purulent
Depends on the type or stage of infection
Associated with itching
May irritate upper lip and skin surrounding the nose

Cough
Common feature
May be evident only during acute phase
May persist several months after a disease

Respiratory Sounds
Sounds associated with respiratory disease:
- Cough
- Hoarseness
- Grunting
- Stridor
- Wheezing
Auscultation:
- Wheezing
- Crackles
- Absence of breath sounds (movement of air)

Sore Throat
Frequent complaint of older children
Young children (unable to describe symptoms) may not complain even when highly inflamed
Often accompanied by refusal to take oral fluids or solids

Meningismus
Meningeal signs without infection of the meninges
Occurs with abrupt onset of fever
Accompanied by:
- Headache
- Pain and stiffness in the back and neck
Subsides as body temperature decreases

---

nose and some mucosal swelling, respiratory distress occurs infrequently. Interventions delivered at home are usually sufficient to relieve minor discomfort and ease respiratory efforts. However, in some cases, the infant or child may require close observation by health professionals for adequate oxygenation and fluid and electrolyte status.

Warm or cool mist is a common therapeutic measure for symptomatic relief of respiratory discomfort. The moisture soothes inflamed membranes and is beneficial when there is hoarseness or laryngeal involvement. The use of steam vaporizers in the home is often discouraged because of the hazards related to their use and limited evidence to support their efficacy.

A time-honored method (albeit not evidence based!) of producing steam is the shower. Running a shower of hot water into the empty bathtub or open shower stall with the bathroom door closed produces a quick source of steam. Keeping a child in this environment for approximately 10 to 15 minutes humidifies inspired air and can help

relieve symptoms. A small child can be held on the lap of a parent or other adult. Older children can sit in the bathroom under the supervision of an adult.

Promote Rest

Children who have an acute febrile illness usually have limited activity. One of the cardinal signs that the child is feeling better is the increase in activity; this may, however, be temporary if a high fever returns after a few hours of increased activity. Children should be encouraged to rest or play quietly to avoid exacerbating symptoms.

Promote Comfort

Older children are usually able to manage nasal secretions with little difficulty. For very young infants, who normally breathe through their noses, an infant nasal aspirator or a bulb syringe is helpful in removing nasal secretions, especially before being put to bed to sleep and before

BOX 23-2   COMPONENTS FOR ASSESSING RESPIRATORY FUNCTION

Respirations

The pattern of respirations is observed for rate, depth, ease, and rhythm of breathing:

Rate—Rapid (**tachypnea**), normal, or slow for the particular child

Depth—Normal depth, too shallow (**hypopnea**), too deep (**hyperpnea**); usually estimated from the amplitude of thoracic and abdominal excursion

Ease—Effortless, labored (**dyspnea**), orthopnea (difficult breathing except in upright position), associated with intercostal or substernal retractions (inspiratory "sinking in" of soft tissues in relation to the cartilaginous and bony thorax), **pulsus paradoxus** (blood pressure falling with inspiration and rising with expiration), nasal flaring, head bobbing (head of sleeping child with suboccipital area supported on caregiver's forearm bobbing forward in synchrony with each inspiration), grunting, wheezing, or stridor

Labored breathing—Continuous, intermittent, becoming steadily worse, sudden onset, at rest or on exertion, associated with wheezing or grunting, associated with pain

Rhythm—Variation in rate and depth of respirations

Other Observations

In addition to respirations, particular attention is addressed to:

Evidence of infection—Check for elevated temperature; enlarged cervical lymph nodes; inflamed mucous membranes; and purulent discharges from the nose, ears, or lungs (sputum).

Cough—Observe the characteristics of the cough (if present), under what circumstances the cough is heard (e.g., night only, on arising), nature of the cough (paroxysmal with or without wheeze, "croupy" or "brassy"), frequency of cough, association with swallowing or other activity, character of the cough (moist and dry), productivity.

Wheeze—Observe character of wheezing: expiratory or inspiratory, high pitched or musical, prolonged, slowly progressive or sudden, association with labored breathing.

Cyanosis—Note distribution (peripheral, perioral, facial, trunk, and face), degree, duration, association with activity.

Chest pain—This may be a complaint of older children. Note location and circumstances: localized or generalized; referral to base of neck or abdomen; dull or sharp; deep or superficial; association with rapid, shallow respirations or grunting.

Nasal mucus—Whereas older children may provide sample by blowing nose or provide sputum sample by coughing, young children may need use of bulb suction, wall suction, DeLee mucus trap, or baby nasal aspirator (attaches to wall suction tubing and fits on small nose) to provide a sample. Note volume, color, viscosity, and odor.

Bad breath (**halitosis**)—May be associated with some upper airway infections but is more common in mouth breathers.

◎ NURSING PROCESS

The Child with Acute Respiratory Tract Infection

Assessment

Assessment of the respiratory system follows the guidelines described in Chapter 6 (for nose, ears, mouth and throat, chest, and lungs). In addition, special attention is given to the observations outlined in Box 23-1 and the components in Box 23-2.

Diagnoses (Problem Identification)

After a thorough assessment, several nursing diagnoses are evident. Other nursing diagnoses may be apparent in individual cases.

- Ineffective Breathing Pattern related to inflammatory process
- Impaired Gas Exchange related to hypoxemia or hypercapnia
- Ineffective Airway Clearance related to mechanical obstruction, inflammation, increased secretions
- Risk for Infection related to presence of infectious organisms, presence of optimum medium (mucus, sputum) for growth of infectious agents
- Activity Intolerance related to inflammatory process, imbalance between oxygen supply and demand
- Altered Family Processes related to child's illness

Planning

Expected patient outcomes include:

- Child will have adequate oxygenation.
- Child will demonstrate effective clearance of secretions.
- Optimum patient comfort will be achieved.
- Child will have effective respirations.
- Child will have adequate fluid and nutrient intake.

Implementation

Numerous intervention strategies are discussed on pp. 707-710.

Evaluation

The effectiveness of nursing interventions is determined by continual reassessment and evaluation of care based on the following observational guidelines:

- Observe child's respiratory effort and chest movements.
- Observe child's behavior and activity.
- Observe other family members and contacts for evidence of infection.
- Take temperature, respiratory rate, pulse oximetry reading, blood pressure, and heart rate.
- Observe for signs of adequate hydration.
- Assess complications, such as dehydration, weight loss, or spread of infection to other areas of the body.
- Observe family's behavior and interview members regarding their feelings and concerns.

---

feeding. This practice, preceded by instillation of saline nose drops as needed, may clear nasal passages and promote feeding. Saline nose drops can be prepared at home by dissolving 1 tsp of salt in 1 pint of warm water.

For older infants and children who can tolerate decongestants, vasoconstrictive nose drops may be administered 15 to 20 minutes before feeding and at bedtime. Two drops are instilled, and because this shrinks only the anterior mucous membranes, two more drops are instilled 5 to 10 minutes later. Phenylephrine 0.25% (for infants and children older than 6 months of age), ephedrine 1% (for children older than 6 years of age), or oxymetazoline 0.05% (for children older than 6 years of age) are sometimes prescribed. Older cooperative children

often prefer nasal sprays. They are taught to compress the plastic container at the moment of inspiration while occluding the other nostril. Bottles of nose drops should be used for only one child and one illness because they are easily contaminated with bacteria and viruses. To avoid rebound congestion, nose drops or sprays should not be administered for more than 3 days. To prevent cross-contamination with nose drops, draw the nose spray solution into a clean tuberculin syringe. Inject the nose spray solution into the child's nostrils using the blunt syringe.

Hot or cold applications sometimes provide relief for children with painful cervical adenitis. An ice bag or heating pad applied to the neck may decrease the discomfort, but safety precautions must be observed to prevent burns. The ice bag or heating device must be covered, and the heating pad should not be set at high settings.

Prevent Spread of Infection

Careful hand washing is important when caring for children with respiratory tract infections. Older children should use a tissue or their arm to cover their noses and mouths when they cough or sneeze, dispose of the tissues properly, and wash their hands. Remembering to cover the nose or mouth is often difficult for small children. Used tissues should be immediately thrown into the wastebasket and not allowed to accumulate in a pile. Children with respiratory tract infections should not share drinking cups, eating utensils, washcloths, or towels. Well individuals generally should not touch their eyes or noses with unwashed hands. Parents should try to remove affected children from contact with other children. Parents should also keep affected children out of school or daycare settings to prevent the spread of infection. This may be a problem when living arrangements are crowded and the family has several children. An effort should be made to teach well children to stay away from ill children, to wash their hands frequently, and to avoid eating and drinking from the same utensils or cups.

Reduce Body Temperature

If the child has a significantly elevated body temperature, controlling the fever is important. Parents should know how to take a child's temperature and read a thermometer accurately. Nurses should not assume that all parents can read a thermometer and should provide education when needed.

If the practitioner prescribes acetaminophen or ibuprofen (for infants and children 6 months and older), parents will need instruction on how to administer it. Most parents can read the label and calculate the desired dosage, but parents of infants and toddlers require detailed instruction and dosing parameters. It is important to emphasize accuracy in determining both the amount of drug to be given and the time intervals for administration.

Cool liquids are encouraged to reduce the temperature and minimize the chances of dehydration (see Controlling Elevated Temperatures, Chapter 22).

> ### ! NURSING ALERT
>
> Parents are cautioned regarding over-the-counter combination "cold" remedies because these often include acetaminophen. Careful calculation of both the acetaminophen given separately and the acetaminophen in combination medications is necessary to avoid an overdose.

Promote Hydration

Dehydration is a potential complication when children have respiratory tract infections and are febrile or anorectic, especially when vomiting or diarrhea is present. Infants are especially prone to fluid and electrolyte deficits when they have a respiratory illness because a rapid respiratory rate that accompanies such illnesses precludes adequate oral fluid intake. In addition, the presence of fever increases the total body fluid turnover in infants. If the infant has nasal secretions, this further prevents adequate respiratory effort by blocking the narrow nasal passages when the infant reclines to bottle feed or breastfeed and ceases the compensatory mouth breathing effort, thus causing the child to limit intake of fluids. Adequate fluid intake is encouraged by offering small amounts of favorite fluids (clear liquids if vomiting) at frequent intervals. Oral rehydration solutions, such as Infalyte or Pedialyte, should be considered for infants, and water or a low-carbohydrate (≤5 g per 8 oz) flavored drink should be considered for older children. Fluids with caffeine (tea, coffee) are avoided because these may act as diuretics and promote fluid loss. Sports drinks and energy drinks are not recommended for oral rehydration (American Academy of Pediatrics [AAP], 2011). Breastfeeding infants should continue to be breastfed because human milk confers some degree of protection from infection (see Chapter 8). Fluids should not be forced, and children should not be awakened to take fluids. Forcing fluids creates the same problem as urging unwanted food. Gentle persuasion with preferred beverages or sugar-free popsicles is usually more successful. Younger children may like to drink smaller amounts from a plastic medicine cup.

To assess their child's level of hydration (see Chapters 9 and 24), parents are advised to observe the frequency of voiding and to notify the nurse or practitioner if there is insufficient voiding. Counting the number of wet diapers in a 24-hour period is a satisfactory method to assess output in infants and toddlers. In the hospital, diapers are weighed to assess output, which should be at least 1 ml/kg/hr up to 30 kg in weight. Then it should be at least 30 ml per hour in patients weighing more than 30 kg. The practitioner should be notified if the urine output is low.

Provide Nutrition

Loss of appetite is characteristic of children with acute infections. In most cases, children can be permitted to determine their own need for food. Many children show no decrease in appetite, and others respond well to foods such as gelatin, popsicles, and soup (see Feeding the Sick Child, Chapter 22). Urging solid foods for children who are sick may precipitate nausea and vomiting and cause an aversion to feeding that may extend into the convalescent period and beyond.

Provide Family Support and Home Care

Young children with respiratory tract infections are irritable and difficult to comfort; therefore, the family needs support, encouragement, and practical suggestions concerning comfort measures and administration of medication. In addition to antipyretics and nose drops, the child may require antibiotic therapy. Parents of children receiving oral antibiotics must understand the importance of regular administration and of continuing the drug for the prescribed length of time regardless of whether the child appears ill. Parents are cautioned against giving their children any medications that are not approved by the health practitioner and are cautioned to avoid giving antibiotics left over from a previous illness or prescribed for another child. Administering unprescribed antibiotics can produce serious side effects and adverse reactions (see Chapter 22 for administration of medications and teaching parents). See Nursing Care Plan.

UPPER RESPIRATORY TRACT INFECTIONS

ACUTE VIRAL NASOPHARYNGITIS

Acute nasopharyngitis, or the equivalent of the "common cold," is caused by the rhinovirus, RSV, adenoviruses, enteroviruses, influenza virus, and parainfluenza virus. Symptoms are more severe in infants and children than in adults. Fever is common in young children, and older children have low-grade fevers, which appear early in the course of the illness. Other clinical manifestations are listed in Box 23-3. Symptoms may last up to 10 days.

⊚ NURSING CARE PLAN

The Child with Acute Respiratory Tract Infection

NURSING DIAGNOSIS	PATIENT OUTCOMES	NURSING INTERVENTIONS	RATIONALE
Ineffective Breathing Pattern related to inflammatory process	Child's respirations will be nonlabored.	Position child for maximal ventilatory efficiency and airway patency.	To allow increased chest expansion
		Position child to facilitate drainage of secretions.	To maintain patent airway and prevent airway obstruction
Child's Defining Characteristics (Subjective and Objective Data)	**The Following NOC Concept Applies to These Outcomes**	Provide humidified oxygen as prescribed.	To improve oxygenation
Use of accessory muscles to breathe	Respiratory Status: Airway Patency, Ventilation	Monitor oxygenation status, including vital signs, for changes in condition.	To determine need for additional interventions
Dyspnea		Suction airway (nose, trachea) as necessary.	To remove secretions and maintain airway patency
Shortness of breath			
Nasal flaring			
Altered chest excursion		Administer prescribed antibiotics (if bacterial).	To treat infection source
Assumption of three-point position (tripod)		Administer bronchodilator medications as prescribed.	To promote bronchodilation and improve ventilation
Respiratory rate outside normal parameter for child's age (increased or decreased rate)		Administer antiinflammatory medications as prescribed.	To decrease airway inflammation and inflammatory response
		Assist with coughing.	To remove secretions and clear airway
		The Following NIC Concepts Apply to These Interventions	
		Aspiration Precautions	
		Positioning	
		Respiratory Monitoring Surveillance	
		Oxygen Therapy	
		Airway Suctioning	
		Vital Signs Monitoring	
		Cough Enhancement	
Ineffective Airway Clearance related to inflammation, mechanical obstruction, increased secretions	Child's airways will remain patent.	Position child to facilitate drainage of secretions.	To prevent airway obstruction
		Perform chest percussion and postural drainage only as prescribed.	To loosen and remove secretions
Child's Defining Characteristics (Subjective and Objective Data)	**The Following NOC Concepts Apply to These Outcomes**	Suction airway as necessary.	To remove secretions
Dyspnea	Aspiration Control	Provide humidified oxygen as prescribed.	To moisten secretions and prevent airway drying
Difficulty vocalizing	Airway Patency		
Orthopnea		Assist with coughing (as developmentally or age appropriate).	To remove secretions
Adventitious breath sounds (crackles, wheezing, rhonchi)		Avoid throat examination if epiglottitis is suspected.	To prevent airway compromise
Cough ineffective or absent		Assure child (as appropriate) all measures will be taken to ensure adequate airway is maintained.	To allay anxiety
Restlessness			
Changes in respiratory rate and rhythm		Implement comfort measures such as allowing parental presence, parental holding, favorite blanket or stuffed animal at side; explain all procedures beforehand.	To reduce anxiety and decrease effects of medical therapy, including hospitalization if required
		The Following NIC Concepts Apply to These Interventions	
		Cough Enhancement	
		Positioning	
		Chest Physiotherapy	
		Vital Signs Monitoring	
		Anxiety Reduction	

NIC, Nursing Interventions Classification; *NOC,* Nursing Outcomes Classification.

Continued

◎ NURSING CARE PLAN

The Child with Acute Respiratory Tract Infection—cont'd

NURSING DIAGNOSIS	PATIENT OUTCOMES	NURSING INTERVENTIONS	RATIONALE
Risk for Injury related to presence (only as indicated) of infective organisms **Child's/Family's Defining Characteristics (Subjective and Objective Data)** Tissue hypoxia Abnormal blood profile People or provider (nosocomial agents) Mode of transport Developmental age	Child will remain free from complications of infection. **The Following NOC Concept Applies to These Outcomes** Risk Control	Maintain aseptic environment using sterile suction equipment and technique. Implement and practice standard precautions. Implement contact and airborne precautions as indicated. Obtain (secretion, tissue, or blood) specimen as indicated and prescribed. Encourage child and family contacts to practice frequent hand washing and avoid hand-to-eye and hand-to-mouth contact. Teach child (as age appropriate) and family how to decrease spread of organisms through coughing and other secretions (e.g., by covering mouth when coughing; disposing of secretions to avoid cross-contamination). Administer antibiotic or antiviral medications as prescribed. Administer fever reduction medication(s) as indicated or prescribed. Monitor and assess for signs and symptoms of secondary complications: hypoxia, skin breakdown, poor nutrient and fluid intake, increased work of breathing, deteriorating cardiorespiratory status. Encourage small amounts of oral clear liquids as condition allows. **The Following NIC Concepts Apply to These Interventions** Risk Identification Environmental Management Infection Control Parent Education	To prevent spread of infectious organisms in child and family To identify infective organism To prevent spread of infection To prevent spread of infection To treat infection source To promote comfort if fever is present To implement therapy for prevention of secondary complications To promote hydration
Interrupted Family Processes related to child's illness, hospitalization, and medical or therapeutic regimen **Child's/Family's Defining Characteristics (Subjective and Objective Data)** Communication patterns Participation in decision making Availability for emotional support Expressions of conflict within family Patterns and rituals	Family will demonstrate ability to cope with child's illness. **The Following NOC Concepts Apply to These Outcomes** Family Functioning Family Normalization Parenting	Encourage family to remain with child. Promote family-centered care. Explain procedures and therapeutic regimen to family. Keep family informed of child's status. Encourage family involvement in child's care. Provide support and referral for continued support as necessary. **The Following NIC Concepts Apply to These Interventions** Caregiver Support Family Support Coping Enhancement Emotional Support Financial Resource Assistance	To decrease effects of separation To promote family integrity To provide accurate information regarding therapy and child's condition To promote family sense of control and involvement in care

NIC, Nursing Interventions Classification; *NOC,* Nursing Outcomes Classification.

BOX 23-3   CLINICAL MANIFESTATIONS OF ACUTE NASOPHARYNGITIS AND PHARYNGITIS

Nasopharyngitis
Younger Children
Fever
Irritability, restlessness
Poor feeding and decreased fluid intake
Sneezing
Nasal mucus (abundant) causing mouth breathing
Vomiting or diarrhea

Older Children
Dryness and irritation of nose and throat initially
Nasal discharge causing mouth breathing
Sneezing, chilling
Muscle aches
Cough (sometimes)

Physical Assessment Signs
Edema and vasodilation of mucosa

Pharyngitis
Younger Children
Fever
General malaise
Anorexia
Moderate sore throat
Headache

Older Children
Fever (may reach 40° C [104° F])
Headache
Anorexia
Dysphagia
Abdominal pain
Vomiting

Physical Assessment Signs
Younger Children
Mild to moderate hyperemia

Older Children
Mild to bright red, edematous pharynx
Hyperemia of tonsils and pharynx; may extend to soft palate and uvula
Often abundant follicular exudate that spreads and coalesces to form pseudomembrane on tonsils
Cervical glands enlarged and tender

Therapeutic Management

Children with nasopharyngitis are managed at home. There is no specific treatment, and effective vaccines are not available. Antipyretics may be indicated for mild fever and discomfort (see Chapter 22 for management of fever). Rest is recommended. The provision of a humidified environment and increasing oral fluids may be beneficial to some children with a cold. Decongestants may be prescribed for children and infants older than 12 months of age to shrink swollen nasal passages (they should be used with caution in infants younger than 1 year of age).

Cough suppressants containing dextromethorphan should be used with caution (cough is a protective way of clearing secretions) but may be prescribed for a dry, hacking cough, especially at night. However, some preparations contain 22% alcohol and can cause adverse effects such as confusion, hyperexcitability, dizziness, nausea, and sedation. Parents should monitor the child carefully for potential adverse effects. Recent concerns regarding serious side effects of cough and cold preparations in young children, particularly infants, and lack of convincing evidence that such medications are effective in reducing symptoms have prompted recommendations by health experts to carefully evaluate the benefits and risks of recommending such preparations for children younger than 6 years of age (Ryan, Brewer, and Small, 2008). Over-the-counter cold preparation such as pseudoephedrine and some antihistamines are not appropriate for the treatment of the common cold in infants and toddlers; these may cause serious side effects in such children and have been associated with death in infants (Rimsza and Newberry, 2008; Ryan, Brewer, and Small, 2008).

Antihistamines are largely ineffective in treatment of nasopharyngitis. These drugs have a weak atropine-like effect that dries secretions, but they can cause drowsiness or, paradoxically, have a stimulatory effect on children. There is no support for the usefulness of expectorants, and antibiotics are usually not indicated because most infections are viral.

Prevention

Nasopharyngitis is so widespread in the general population that it is impossible to prevent. Children are more susceptible because they have not yet developed resistance to many viruses. Young infants and those with decreased resistance and pulmonary illness are subject to serious complications, so attempts should be made to protect them from exposure.

Nursing Care Management

A cold is often the parents' first introduction to an illness in their infant. Most discomfort of nasopharyngitis is related to the nasal obstruction, especially in small infants. Elevating the head of the bed or crib mattress assists with drainage of secretions. Suctioning and vaporization may also provide relief. Saline nose drops and gentle suction with a bulb syringe before feeding and sleep time may be useful.

Maintaining adequate fluid intake is essential. Although a child's appetite for solid foods is usually diminished for several days, it is important to offer appropriate fluids to prevent dehydration.

Because nasopharyngitis is spread from secretions, the best means for prevention is avoiding contact with affected persons. This goal is difficult to accomplish in family settings, classrooms, and daycare centers. Family members with a cold should try to "keep it to themselves" by carefully disposing of tissues; not sharing towels, glasses, or eating utensils; covering the mouth and nose with tissues when coughing or sneezing; and washing the hands thoroughly after nose blowing or sneezing. The most frequent carriers of infection are the human hands, which deposit viruses on doorknobs, faucets, and everyday objects. Children should be taught to wash their hands thoroughly and avoid touching their eyes, noses, and mouths.

Family Support

Support and reassurance are important elements of care for families of young children with recurrent upper respiratory infections (URIs). Because URIs are frequent in children younger than 3 years of age, families may feel they are on an endless roller coaster of illness. They need reassurance that frequent colds are a normal part of childhood and that by 5 years of age, their children will have developed immunity to many viruses. When children spend time in daycare centers, their infection rate is higher than if they are cared for in the home because of increased exposure. Parents should know the signs of respiratory complications and should notify a health professional if complications occur or the child does not improve within 2 or 3 days (Box 23-4).

ACUTE STREPTOCOCCAL PHARYNGITIS

Children who experience GABHS infection of the upper airway (**strep throat**) are at risk for **rheumatic fever (RF)**, an inflammatory disease of the heart, joints, and central nervous system (CNS) (see Chapter 25), and **acute glomerulonephritis (AGN)**, an acute kidney infection (see Chapter 27). Permanent damage can result from these sequelae, especially RF. GABHS may also cause skin manifestations, including impetigo and pyoderma.

Clinical Manifestations

Group A β-hemolytic streptococci infection is generally a relatively brief illness that varies in severity from subclinical (no symptoms) to severe toxicity. The onset is often abrupt and characterized by pharyngitis, headache, fever, and abdominal pain. The tonsils and pharynx may be inflamed and covered with exudate (Fig. 23-1), which usually appear by the second day of illness. However, streptococcal infections should be suspected in children older than 2 years of age who have pharyngitis without exudate or nasal symptoms. The tongue may appear edematous and red (strawberry tongue), and the child may have a fine sandpaper rash on the trunk, axillae, elbows, and groin seen in **scarlet fever** (caused by a strain of group A streptococcus). The uvula is edematous and red. Anterior cervical lymphadenopathy (in ≈30%-50% of cases) usually occurs early, and the nodes are often tender. Pain can be relatively mild to severe enough to make swallowing difficult. Clinical manifestations usually subside in 3 to 5 days unless complicated by sinusitis or parapharyngeal, peritonsillar, or retropharyngeal abscess. Nonsuppurative complications may appear after the onset of GABHS—AGN in about 10 days and RF in an average of 18 days.

Children who are GABHS carriers may have a positive throat culture but often experience a coincidental viral illness. Although antibiotic administration is not indicated for most GABHS carriers, some conditions require antibiotic therapy; these are published in the AAP's *Red Book* (AAP, Committee on Infectious Diseases and Pickering, 2009).

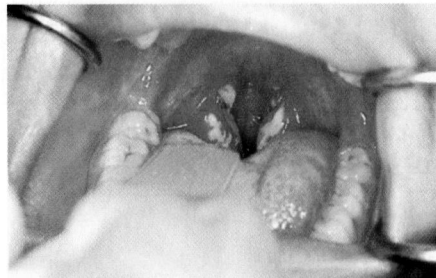

FIG 23-1 Tonsillitis and pharyngitis. (Courtesy Dr. Edward L. Applebaum, Head, Department of Otolaryngology, University of Illinois Medical Center, Chicago.)

Diagnostic Evaluation

Although 80% to 90% of all cases of acute pharyngitis are viral, a throat culture or rapid streptococcal identification test should be performed to rule out GABHS. Most streptococcal infections are short-term illnesses, and antibody responses (e.g., antistreptolysin-O titer) appear later than symptoms and are useful only for retrospective diagnosis.

Rapid identification of GABHS with diagnostic test kits (rapid antigen detection test) is possible in the office or clinic setting. Because of the high specificity of these rapid tests, a positive test result generally does not require throat culture confirmation. However, the sensitivities of these kits vary considerably, and a confirmatory throat culture is recommended in patients who have a negative test result (AAP, Committee on Infectious Diseases and Pickering, 2009).

Therapeutic Management

If streptococcal sore throat infection is present, oral penicillin is prescribed in a dose sufficient to control the acute local manifestations and to maintain an adequate level for at least 10 days to eliminate any organisms that might remain to initiate RF symptoms. Penicillin does not prevent the development of AGN in susceptible children; however, it may prevent the spread of a nephrogenic strain of GABHS to others in the family. Penicillin usually produces a prompt response within 24 hours. Patients who have a history of RF or who remain symptomatic after a full course of antibiotics may require a follow-up throat swab.

Intramuscular (IM) benzathine penicillin G is an appropriate therapy, but it is painful and is not the first choice for children. Oral erythromycin is indicated for children who are allergic to penicillin. Other antibiotics used to treat GABHS are azithromycin, clarithromycin, oral cephalosporins, amoxicillin, and amoxicillin with clavulanic acid (AAP, Committee on Infectious Diseases and Pickering, 2009).

Nursing Care Management

The nurse often obtains a throat swab for culture or rapid antigen testing and instructs the parents about administering oral antibiotics and analgesics as prescribed. Cold or warm compresses to the neck may provide relief. In children who can cooperate, warm saline gargles may offer relief of throat discomfort. Acetaminophen and ibuprofen may be effective in decreasing the throat pain; liquid preparations or chewable forms may be preferable because of the pain associated with swallowing. Pain may interfere with oral intake, and children should not be forced to eat, but fluid intake is essential. Cool liquids or ice chips may be more acceptable than solids.

Special emphasis is placed on correct administration of oral medication and completion of the course of antibiotic therapy (see Administration of Medication, and Compliance, Chapter 22). If an injection is required, it must be administered deep into a large muscle mass (e.g., vastus lateralis or ventrogluteal muscle). To prevent pain, application of a topical anesthetic cream such as EMLA (an eutectic mixture of lidocaine and prilocaine) over the injection site 2½ hours before the injection or LMX4 (4% lidocaine) over the site 30 minutes before the injection is helpful (see Administration of Medication: Intramuscular Administration, Chapter 22). The injection site may be tender for 1 to 2 days.

Children are considered infectious to others at the onset of symptoms and up to 24 hours after initiation of antibiotic therapy, but they should not return to school or daycare until they have been taking antibiotics for a full 24-hour period. Nurses should remind the children to discard their toothbrushes and replace them with new ones after they have been taking antibiotics for 24 hours. Orthodontic appliances should be washed thoroughly because they may harbor the organisms. Parents are cautioned to prevent other household members, especially if immunocompromised, from having close contact with the sick child and avoid sharing drinking or eating items.

If the child continues to have a high fever that does not respond to antipyretics, has an extremely sore throat, refuses liquids, and appears toxic 24 to 48 hours after starting antibiotics, further evaluation by the practitioner is recommended.

> ### 💊 **DRUG ALERT!**
>
> Never administer penicillin G procaine or penicillin G benzathine suspensions intravenously (they may cause embolism or toxic reaction with ensuing death in minutes). Instead, administer these medications deep into the muscle tissue to decrease localized reactions and pain.

TONSILLITIS

 The tonsils are masses of lymphoid tissue located in the pharyngeal cavity. They filter and protect the respiratory and alimentary tracts from invasion by pathogenic organisms and play a role in antibody formation. Although their size varies, children generally have much larger tonsils than adolescents or adults. This difference is thought to be a protective mechanism because young children are especially susceptible to URIs.

Pathophysiology

Several pairs of tonsils are part of a mass of lymphoid tissue encircling the nasal and oral pharynx, known as the Waldeyer tonsillar ring (Fig. 23-2). The palatine, or faucial, tonsils are located on either side of the oropharynx behind and below the pillars of the fauces (opening from the mouth). A surface of the palatine tonsils is usually visible during oral examination. The palatine tonsils are those removed during tonsillectomy. The pharyngeal tonsils, also known as the adenoids, are located above the palatine tonsils on the posterior wall of the nasopharynx. Their proximity to the nares and eustachian tubes causes difficulties in instances of inflammation. The lingual tonsils are located at the base of the tongue. The tubal tonsils, found near the posterior nasopharyngeal opening of the eustachian tubes, are not part of the Waldeyer tonsillar ring.

Etiology

Tonsillitis often occurs with pharyngitis. Because of the abundant lymphoid tissue and the frequency of URIs, tonsillitis is a common cause of illness in young children. The causative agent may be viral or bacterial.

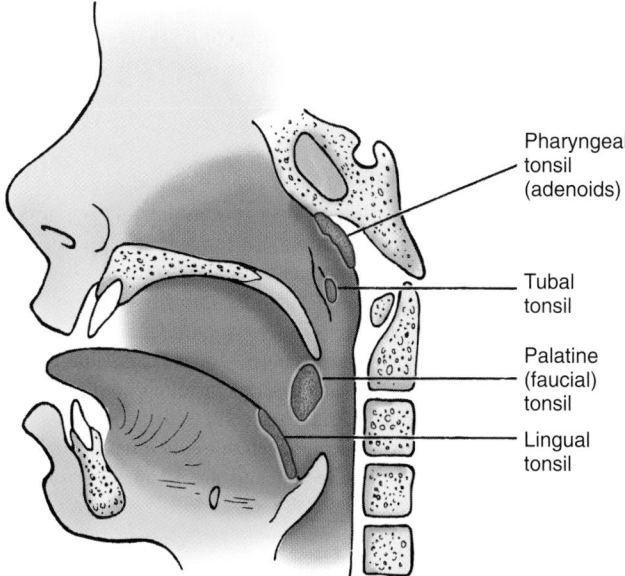

FIG 23-2 Location of various tonsillar masses.

Clinical Manifestations

The manifestations of tonsillitis are caused by inflammation. As the palatine tonsils enlarge from edema, they may meet in the midline (kissing tonsils), obstructing the passage of air or food. The child has difficulty swallowing and breathing. When enlargement of the adenoids occurs, the space behind the posterior nares becomes blocked, making it difficult or impossible for air to pass from the nose to the throat. As a result, the child breathes through the mouth.

Therapeutic Management

Because tonsillitis is self-limiting, treatment of viral pharyngitis is symptomatic. Throat cultures positive for GABHS infection warrant antibiotic treatment. It is important to differentiate between viral and streptococcal infection in febrile exudative tonsillitis. Because most infections are of viral origin, early rapid tests can eliminate unnecessary antibiotic administration.

Tonsillectomy is the surgical removal of the palatine tonsils. Absolute indications for a tonsillectomy are recurrent peritonsillar abscess, airway obstruction, tonsillitis resulting in febrile convulsions, and tonsils requiring tissue pathology (American Academy of Otolaryngology—Head and Neck Surgery, 2011). Relative indications include three or more tonsil infections per year, persistent foul taste or breath caused by chronic tonsillitis, unilateral tonsil hypertrophy presumed to be malignant, and chronic tonsillitis in a streptococcus carrier who fails to respond to antibiotics (American Academy of Otolaryngology—Head and Neck Surgery, 2011).

Adenoidectomy (the surgical removal of the adenoids) is recommended for children who have hypertrophied adenoids that obstruct nasal breathing; additional indications for adenoidectomy include recurrent adenoiditis and sinusitis, chronic otitis media (OM) with effusion (especially if associated with hearing loss), airway obstruction and subsequent sleep-disordered breathing, persistent mouth-breathing, nasal speech, and recurrent nasopharyngitis (Benninger and Walner, 2007a). For some children, the effectiveness of tonsillectomy or adenoidectomy is modest and may not justify the risk of surgery. In practice, many physicians rely on individualized decision making and do not subscribe to an absolute set of eligibility criteria for these surgical procedures. Contraindications to either tonsillectomy or adenoidectomy are (1) cleft palate because the tonsils help minimize escape of air during speech, (2) acute infections at the time of surgery because locally inflamed tissues increase the risk of bleeding, (3) uncontrolled systemic diseases or blood dyscrasias, and (4) poor anesthetic risk.

Nursing Care Management

Nursing care involves providing comfort and minimizing activities or interventions that precipitate bleeding. Patients with sleep-disordered breathing require close monitoring of airway and breathing postoperatively. A soft to liquid diet is preferred. A cool-mist vaporizer keeps the mucous membranes moist during periods of mouth breathing. Warm salt-water gargles, throat lozenges, and analgesic–antipyretic drugs such as acetaminophen are used to promote comfort. Often opioids are needed to reduce pain for the child to drink. Combination nonopioid and opioid elixirs such as acetaminophen with codeine or with hydrocodone (Lortab) relieve pain and should be given routinely every 4 hours.

If surgery is required, the child requires the same psychologic preparation and physical care as for any other surgical procedure (see Chapters 21 and 22). Most tonsillectomy and adenoidectomy (T&A) surgeries now take place in outpatient settings; however, the priorities of preoperative and postoperative care remain the same. The following discussion focuses on postoperative nursing care for T&A, although both procedures may not be performed.

Until they are fully awake, the child is placed on his or her abdomen or side to facilitate drainage of secretions. Routine suctioning is avoided, but when performed, it is done carefully to avoid trauma to the oropharynx. When alert, the child may prefer sitting up. The child is discouraged from coughing frequently, clearing the throat, blowing the nose, and any other activity that may aggravate the operative site.

Some secretions are common, particularly dried blood from surgery. All secretions and vomitus are inspected for evidence of fresh bleeding (some blood-tinged mucus is expected). Dark brown (old) blood is usually present in the emesis, in the nose, and between the teeth. If parents do not expect this, they often become frightened at a time when they need to be calm and reassuring.

The throat is sore after surgery. An ice collar may provide relief, but many children find it bothersome and refuse to use it. Most children experience moderate pain after a T&A and need pain medication regularly for at least the first few days. Analgesics may be given rectally or intravenously to avoid the oral route. Because the pain is continuous, analgesics should be administered at regular intervals even at night (see Pain Management, Chapter 7). An antiemetic such as ondansetron (Zofran) may be administered postoperatively if nausea or vomiting is present.

Food and fluids are restricted until the child is fully alert and there are no signs of hemorrhage. Cool water, crushed ice, flavored ice pops, or diluted fruit juice may be given, but fluids with a red or brown color are avoided to distinguish fresh or old blood in emesis from the ingested liquid. Citrus juice may cause discomfort and is usually poorly tolerated. Soft foods, particularly gelatin, cooked fruits, sherbet, soup, and mashed potatoes, are started on the first or second postoperative day or as the child tolerates feeding. The pain from surgery often inhibits fluid intake, reinforcing the need for adequate pain control. Milk, ice cream, and pudding are usually not offered because milk products coat the mouth and throat and may cause the child to clear the throat, which can initiate bleeding.

Postoperative hemorrhage is uncommon but can occur in up to 5% of patients up to 14 days after surgery. The nurse observes the throat directly for evidence of bleeding; using a good source of light; and, if necessary, carefully inserting a tongue depressor. Other signs of hemorrhage are tachycardia, pallor, frequent clearing of the throat or swallowing by a younger child, and vomiting of bright red blood. Restlessness, an indication of hemorrhage, may be difficult to differentiate from general discomfort after surgery. Decreasing blood pressure is a late sign of shock.

Surgery may be required to ligate a bleeding vessel. Airway obstruction may also occur as a result of edema or accumulated secretions and is indicated by signs of respiratory distress, such as stridor, drooling, restlessness, agitation, increasing respiratory rate, and progressive cyanosis. Suction equipment and oxygen should be available after tonsillectomy.

> ### ! NURSING ALERT
>
> The most obvious early sign of bleeding is the child's continuous swallowing of the trickling blood. While the child is sleeping, note the frequency of swallowing. If continuous bleeding is suspected, notify the surgeon immediately.

Family Support and Home Care

Discharge instructions include (1) avoiding irritating and highly seasoned foods, (2) avoiding gargles or vigorous toothbrushing, (3) avoiding coughing or clearing of the throat or putting objects in the mouth (e.g., a straw), (4) using analgesics or an ice collar for pain, and (5) limiting activity to decrease the potential for bleeding. Chewing gum may prevent throat and ear pain in older children. Objectionable mouth odor and slight ear pain with a low-grade fever are common for 5 to 10 days postoperatively. However, persistent severe earache, fever, or cough requires medical evaluation. Most children are ready to resume normal activity within 1 to 2 weeks after the operation. The child's voice may sound different postoperative, especially if the tonsils were large.

Hemorrhage may occur after surgery as a result of tissue sloughing from the healing process. Any sign of bleeding warrants immediate medical attention.

INFLUENZA

Influenza, or the "flu," is caused by three orthomyxoviruses, which are antigenically distinct: types A and B, which cause epidemic disease, and type C, which is unimportant from an epidemiologic standpoint. Influenza is spread from one individual to another by direct contact (large-droplet infection) or by articles recently contaminated by nasopharyngeal secretions. There is no predilection for a specific age group, but attack rates are highest in young children who have had no previous contact with a strain. Influenza is frequently most severe in infants. During epidemics, infection among school-age children is believed to be a major source of transmission in a community. The disease is more common during the winter months and has a 1- to 3-day incubation period. Affected persons are most infectious for 24 hours before and after the onset of symptoms. The virus has a peculiar affinity for epithelial cells of the respiratory tract mucosa, where it destroys ciliated epithelium with metaplastic hyperplasia of the tracheal and bronchial epithelium with associated edema. The alveoli may also become distended with a hyaline-like material. The viruses can be isolated from nasopharyngeal secretions early after the onset of infection, and serologic tests identify the type by complement fixation or the subgroups by hemagglutination inhibition.

H1N1 (swine flu) is a subtype of influenza type A. In 2009, a pandemic of H1N1 caused significant morbidity and mortality, particularly in Mexico and the United States; it was declared at an end in

August 2010. A *pandemic* is defined by the World Health Organization (2011) as the spread of a new disease to which the population has little or no immunity and that spreads rapidly from human to human. The signs and symptoms of H1N1 flu are the same as those mentioned below for influenza. H1N1 vaccine was combined with the seasonal influenza vaccine in the 2011 to 2012 season.

Clinical Manifestations

The manifestations of influenza may be subclinical, mild, moderate, or severe. Most patients have a dry throat and nasal mucosa, a dry cough, and a tendency toward hoarseness. A flushed face, photophobia, myalgia, hyperesthesia, and sometimes exhaustion and lack of energy accompany a sudden onset of fever and chills. Subglottal croup is common, especially in infants. The symptoms of influenza last for 4 or 5 days. Complications include severe viral pneumonia (often hemorrhagic); encephalitis; and secondary bacterial infections such as OM, sinusitis, or pneumonia.

Therapeutic Management

Uncomplicated influenza in children usually requires only symptomatic treatment, including acetaminophen or ibuprofen for fever and sufficient fluids to maintain hydration. Amantadine hydrochloride (Symmetrel) has been effective in reducing symptoms associated with type A disease if administered within 24 to 48 hours after their onset; the symptoms associated with influenza are reportedly shortened by 24 hours, but the drug does not "cure" the disease. It is ineffective against type B or C influenza or other viral diseases. It should not be given to children younger than 1 year of age but is recommended for unvaccinated high-risk children.

Rimantadine has been approved for the treatment of flu symptoms in children and adults, but it is effective only for type A virus; this drug is taken orally in tablet or syrup twice daily for 7 days. It cannot be used for children younger than 1 year of age.

Zanamivir can be used for treatment of influenza in patients 7 years of age and older and for prophylaxis of influenza in patients 5 years of age and older. Both medications must also be started within 48 hours of symptom onset. Zanamivir is an inhaled medication effective for type A and B influenza. The drug is taken twice daily for 5 days and is administered by a specially designed oral inhaler (Diskhaler).

A fourth drug, oseltamivir (Tamiflu), is a neuraminidase inhibitor that may be administered orally for 5 days to children older than 1 year of age (and adults) to decrease the flu symptoms; as with other antiviral drugs, this drug must be taken within 2 days of the onset of symptoms. It is reported to be effective for types A and B influenza (AAP, Committee on Infectious Diseases and Pickering, 2009). Bronchospasm and a decline in lung function can occur when zanamivir is used in patients with underlying airway disease such as asthma or chronic obstructive pulmonary disease (COPD). At the time of this writing, oseltamivir and zanamivir are the only antiviral medications recommended for treatment during the 2011-2012 flu season because of widespread resistance to amantidine and rimantidine (AAP, Committee on Infectious Diseases, 2011).

Prevention

The influenza vaccine is now recommended annually for children 6 months to 18 years of age (completed). Influenza vaccine (trivalent inactivated influenza vaccine [TIV]) may be given to healthy children 6 months old and older. The TIV vaccines are safe and effective provided the antigens in the vaccine correlate with the circulating influenza viruses (see Immunizations, Chapter 10) but are contraindicated in patients who developed Guillain-Barré syndrome within 6 weeks of receiving the vaccine in the past. The live-attenuated influenza vaccine (LAIV) is a nasal spray flu vaccine approved by the U.S. Food and Drug Administration (FDA) that is licensed for administration in persons ages 2 to 49 years. However, this preparation contains a live virus and should not be used in individuals who are immunocompromised, have reactive airway disease, are receiving immunosuppressive therapy, have a febrile illness, are receiving aspirin therapy, have a chronic respiratory condition, have received a live vaccine in the previous 28 days, are or could be pregnant, or have a history of Guillain-Barré syndrome. Patients who have had anaphylactic reactions to egg protein should not receive either influenza vaccine.

Nursing Care Management

Nursing care is the same as for any child with a URI, including implementing measures to relieve symptoms. The greatest danger to affected children is development of a secondary infection. Prolonged fever or the appearance of fever during early convalescence is a sign of secondary bacterial infection and should be reported to the practitioner for antibiotic therapy. Children with influenza (or other similar viruses) should not receive aspirin because of its possible link with Reye syndrome.

OTITIS MEDIA

Otitis media is one of the most prevalent diseases of early childhood. Its incidence is highest in the winter months. Many cases of bacterial OM are preceded by a viral respiratory infection. The two viruses most likely to precipitate OM are RSV and influenza. Most episodes of acute otitis media (AOM) occur in the first 24 months of life, but the incidence decreases with age except for a small increase at age 5 or 6 years when children enter school. OM occurs infrequently in children older than 7 years of age. Preschool-age boys are affected more frequently than preschool-age girls. Children who have siblings or parents with a history of chronic OM have a higher incidence of OM. Children living in households with many members (especially smokers) are more likely to have OM than those living with fewer persons. Passive smoking increases the risk of persistent middle ear effusion by enhancing attachment of the pathogens that cause otitis to the respiratory epithelium in the middle ear space, by prolonging the inflammatory response, and by impeding drainage through the eustachian tube (AAP, 2004a). Family socioeconomic status and extent of exposure to other children are the two most important identifiable risk factors for the occurrence of OM (AAP, 2004a).

OM has been defined in a variety of ways. The standard terminology used to define OM is outlined in Box 23-5, and AOM treatment guidelines have been published (AAP, 2004a, 2004b).

Etiology

Streptococcus pneumoniae, H. influenzae, and *Moraxella catarrhalis* are the three most common bacteria causing AOM. The etiology of noninfectious OM is unknown, but OM may occur because of blocked eustachian tubes, which results in negative ear pressure. Fluid is pulled from the mucosal lining, which accumulates and becomes colonized by infectious organisms. Predisposing factors include URIs, allergies, Down syndrome, cleft palate, daycare attendance, exposure to secondhand smoke, and bottle propping during feeding. Infants fed breast milk have a lower incidence of OM than formula-fed infants. Breastfeeding may protect infants against respiratory viruses and allergy because it contains secretory immunoglobulin A, which limits the exposure of the eustachian tube and middle ear mucosa to microbial pathogens and foreign proteins. Reflux of milk up the eustachian tubes is less likely in breastfed infants because of the semivertical positioning during breastfeeding compared with bottle feeding.

Pathophysiology

Otitis media is primarily a result of malfunctioning eustachian tubes. Eustachian tubes have three functions relative to the middle ear: (1) protection of the middle ear from nasopharyngeal secretions, (2) drainage of secretions produced in the middle ear into the nasopharynx, and (3) ventilation of the middle ear to equalize air pressure within the middle ear and atmospheric pressure in the external ear canal and to replenish oxygen that has been absorbed.

Mechanical or functional obstruction of the eustachian tube causes accumulation of secretions in the middle ear. Intrinsic obstruction can be caused by infection or allergy; extrinsic obstruction is usually a result of enlarged adenoids or nasopharyngeal tumors. When the passage is not totally obstructed, contamination of the middle ear can take place by reflux, aspiration, or insufflation during crying, sneezing, nose blowing, and swallowing when the nose is obstructed.

Diagnostic Evaluation

Careful assessment of tympanic membrane mobility with a pneumatic otoscope is essential to differentiate AOM from OM with effusion (OME) (AAP, 2004b). A diagnosis of AOM is made if visual inspection of the tympanic membrane reveals a purulent discolored effusion and a bulging or full, opacified, or reddened immobile membrane. Some practitioners also consider the presence of acute onset of less than 48 hours of ear pain with the above criteria to be a diagnostic factor in AOM. An immobile tympanic membrane or an orange, discolored membrane indicates OME. Clinical symptoms of otitis are also helpful in making the diagnosis (Box 23-6). In AOM, symptoms such as acute onset of ear pain, fever, and a bulging yellow or red tympanic membrane are usually present. In OME, these symptoms may be absent, and other nonspecific symptoms such as rhinitis, cough, or diarrhea are often present (AAP, 2004a, 2004b).

Therapeutic Management

Treatment for AOM is one of the most common reasons for antibiotic use in the ambulatory setting. Recently, however, concerns about drug-resistant *S. pneumoniae* and other drug resistances have led infectious disease authorities to recommend careful and judicious use of antibiotics for the treatment of this illness. Current literature indicates that waiting up to 72 hours for spontaneous resolution is safe and appropriate management of AOM in healthy infants older than 6 months and children (AAP, 2004a; Bhetwal and McConaghy, 2007). Furthermore, some reviews of the treatment of AOM reveal no clear evidence that antibiotics improve outcomes in children younger than 2 years of age with uncomplicated AOM. However, the watchful waiting approach is not recommended for children younger than 2 years of age who have persistent acute symptoms of fever and severe ear pain (Kerschner, 2011). In addition, all cases of AOM in infants younger than 6 months

of age should be treated with antibiotics because of their immature immune systems and the potential for infection with bacteria.

When antibiotics are warranted, oral amoxicillin in high doses (80-90 mg/kg/day divided twice daily) is the treatment of choice for initial episodes of AOM in children who have not received antibiotics within the past month (AAP, 2004a; Bhetwal and McConaghy, 2007). The recommendation for the duration of antibiotic therapy in severe AOM is 10 to 14 days; in children 6 years and older with uncomplicated AOM or with a moderate or mild infection, a 5- to 7-day course may be sufficient (AAP, Committee on Infectious Diseases and Pickering, 2009).

Second-line antibiotics used to treat OM include amoxicillin–clavulanate; azithromycin; and cephalosporins such as cefdinir, cefuroxime, and cefpodoxime. IM ceftriaxone is used if the causative organism is a highly resistant pneumococcus or if the parents are noncompliant with the therapy. An important consideration with the use of single-dose IM injections is the pain involved in this therapy. One strategy to minimize pain at the injection site is to reconstitute the cephalosporin with 1% lidocaine. A topical analgesic cream such as EMLA or LMX4 can also be applied to the site beforehand to reduce pain. The use of steroids, decongestants, and antihistamines to treat AOM is not recommended.

Supportive care or symptomatic treatment of AOM includes treating the fever and pain. For fever or discomfort associated with OM, analgesic–antipyretic drugs such as acetaminophen or ibuprofen may be given. The practitioner may prescribe topical pain relief drops such as benzocaine drops. Antibiotic ear drops have no value in treating AOM.

Myringotomy, a surgical incision of the eardrum, may be necessary to alleviate the severe pain of AOM. A myringotomy is also performed to provide drainage of infected middle ear fluid in the presence of complications (mastoiditis, labyrinthitis, or facial paralysis) or to allow purulent middle ear fluid to drain into the ear canal for culture. A minimally invasive laser-assisted myringotomy procedure may be performed in outpatient settings. These procedures should only be performed by ear, nose, and throat (ENT) specialists.

Tympanostomy tube placement and adenoidectomy are surgical procedures that may be done to treat recurrent chronic OM (defined as three bouts in 6 months, six in 12 months, or six by 6 years of age). Tympanostomy tubes are pressure-equalizer (PE) tubes or grommets that facilitate continued drainage of fluid and allow ventilation of the middle ear. They are inserted to treat severe eustachian tube dysfunction, OM with effusion, or complications of OM (mastoiditis, facial nerve paralysis, brain abscess, labyrinthitis). Adenoidectomy is not recommended for treatment of AOM and is performed only in children with recurrent AOM or chronic OME with postnasal obstruction, adenoiditis, or chronic sinusitis.

In some children, residual middle ear effusions remain after episodes of AOM. Some children have fluid that persists in the middle ear for weeks or months. Antibiotics are not required for initial treatment of OME but may be indicated for children with persistent effusion for more than 3 months (AAP, 2004a). Placement of tympanostomy tubes is recommended after a total of 4 to 6 months of bilateral effusion with a bilateral hearing deficit (AAP, 2004b). This therapy allows for mechanical drainage of the fluid, which promotes healing of the membrane and prevents scar formation and loss of elasticity. Myringotomy with or without insertion of PE tubes should not be performed for initial management of OME but may be recommended for children who have recurrent episodes of OME with a long cumulative duration (AAP, 2004b).

Otitis media with effusion is frequently associated with mild to moderate impairment of hearing; therefore, a hearing test should also be performed if OME persists for 3 months or more or if there is evidence of language or learning delays. Follow-up examinations of children with chronic OME should be maintained on a 3- to 6-month basis until the OME is resolved, a significant hearing loss is identified, or structural defect of the tympanic membrane or middle ear is identified (AAP, 2004a). Children with hearing loss should be referred to an otolaryngologist and should receive a speech and language evaluation as necessary.

Prevention

Routine immunization with the pneumococcal conjugate vaccine PCV7 (Prevnar 7) has reduced the incidence of AOM in some infants and children (AAP, Committee on Infectious Diseases and Pickering, 2009). In 2010, the FDA approved a new conjugate vaccine, Prevnar 13, which replaces Prevnar 7. The vaccine is administered as a four-dose series beginning at 2 months of age; infants and children who have started the series with Prevnar 7 may complete the series with Prevnar 13 (Centers for Disease Control and Prevention [CDC], 2010).

Parents are encouraged to reduce risk factors for AOM by breast-feeding infants for at least the first 6 months of life, avoid propping the bottle, decrease or discontinue pacifier use after 6 months, and prevent exposure to tobacco smoke (AAP, 2004a).

Nursing Care Management

Nursing objectives for children with AOM include (1) relieving pain, (2) facilitating drainage when possible, (3) preventing complications or recurrence, (4) educating the family in care of the child, and (5) providing emotional support to the child and family.

Analgesic drugs such as acetaminophen (all ages) and ibuprofen (6 months of age and older) are used to treat mild pain. For more severe pain, the AAP (2004a) guidelines recommend a stronger analgesic such as codeine.

If the ear is draining, the external canal may be cleaned with sterile cotton swabs or pledgets coupled with topical antibiotic treatment. If ear wicks or lightly rolled sterile gauze packs are placed in the ear after surgical treatment, they should be loose enough to allow accumulated drainage to flow out of the ear; otherwise, infection may be transferred to the mastoid process. The wicks need to stay dry during shampoos or baths. Occasionally, drainage is so profuse that the auricle and the skin surrounding the ear become excoriated from the exudate. This is usually prevented by frequent cleansing and application of various moisture barriers (e.g., Proshield Plus), zinc oxide–based products, or petrolatum jelly (e.g., Vaseline).

Tympanostomy tubes may allow water to enter the middle ear, but recommendations for earplugs are inconsistent. Research indicates that swimming without earplugs poses a slight increased risk of infection (Goldstein, Mandel, Kurs-Lasky, and others, 2005). However, lake and river water is potentially contaminated, and wearing earplugs while swimming in a lake prevents total flooding of the external canal. Bathwater and shampoo water should be kept out of the ear, if possible, because soap reduces the surface tension of water and facilitates entry through the tube. Parents should be aware of the appearance of a grommet (usually a tiny, white, plastic spool-shaped tube) so that they can recognize it if it falls out. They are reassured that this is normal and requires no immediate intervention, although they should notify the practitioner.

Prevention of recurrence requires adequate education regarding antibiotic therapy. The symptoms of pain and fever usually subside within 24 to 48 hours, but nurses must emphasize that all of the prescribed medication should be taken. Parents should be aware that potential complications of OM, such as hearing loss, can be prevented with adequate treatment and follow-up care.

Parents also need anticipatory guidance regarding methods to reduce the risks of OM, especially in children younger than 2 years of age. Reducing the chances of OM is possible with simple measures, such as sitting or holding an infant upright for feedings, maintaining routine childhood immunizations, and exclusively breastfeeding until at least 6 months of age. Propping bottles is discouraged to avoid pooling of milk while the child is in the supine position and to encourage human contact during feeding. Additional recommendations include avoiding washing the child's hair with bathtub water (use fresh water from the tap, with the child sitting) and avoiding exposure to bacteria that are found in stagnant water such as that in inflatable and small swimming pools (these often do not contain chemicals that are bacteriostatic). Eliminating tobacco smoke and known allergens is also recommended. Early detection of middle ear effusion is essential to prevent complications. Infants and preschool children should be screened for effusion, and all schoolchildren, especially those with learning disabilities, should be tested for hearing deficits related to a middle ear effusion.

INFECTIOUS MONONUCLEOSIS

Infectious mononucleosis is an acute, self-limiting infectious disease that is common among adolescents. Symptoms include fever, exudative pharyngitis, lymphadenopathy, hepatosplenomegaly, and an increase in atypical lymphocytes. The course is usually mild but occasionally can be severe or, rarely, accompanied by serious complications.

Etiology and Pathophysiology

The herpes-like Epstein-Barr virus (EBV) is the principal cause of infectious mononucleosis. It appears in both sporadic and epidemic forms, but the sporadic cases are more common. The mechanism of spread has not been proven, but it is believed to be transmitted in saliva by direct intimate contact, although it survives in saliva for many hours

BOX 23-7	CLINICAL MANIFESTATIONS OF INFECTIOUS MONONUCLEOSIS

Early Signs
Headache
Epistaxis
Malaise
Fatigue
Chills
Low-grade fever
Loss of appetite
Puffy eyes

Acute Disease
Cardinal Features
Fever
Sore throat
Cervical adenopathy

Common Features
Splenomegaly (may persist for several months)
Palatine petechiae
Macular eruption (especially on trunk)
Exudative pharyngitis or tonsillitis
Hepatic involvement to some degree, often associated with jaundice

outside of the body. The incubation period after exposure is approximately 30 to 50 days (AAP, Committee on Infectious Diseases and Pickering, 2009).

Diagnostic Tests

The onset of symptoms may be acute or insidious and may appear anywhere from 10 days to 6 weeks after exposure. The presenting symptoms vary greatly in type, severity, and duration (Box 23-7). The clinical manifestations of infectious mononucleosis are usually less severe (often subclinical or unapparent), and the convalescent phase is shorter in younger children than in older children and young adults. Heterophil antibody tests (Paul-Brunell or Monospot) determine the extent to which the patient's serum will agglutinate sheep red blood cells; the response in these tests is primarily to immunoglobulin M, which is present in the first 2 weeks of the illness in adolescents. The spot test (Monospot) is a slide test of venous blood that has high specificity. It is rapid, sensitive, inexpensive, and easy to perform, and has the advantage over the Paul-Brunell test that it can detect significant agglutinins at lower levels, thus allowing earlier diagnosis. Blood is usually obtained for the test by finger puncture or venous sampling and is placed on special paper. If the blood agglutinates, forming fragments or clumps, the test result is positive for the infection.

Therapeutic Management

No specific treatment exists for infectious mononucleosis. A mild analgesic is often sufficient to relieve the headache, fever, and malaise. Rest is encouraged for fatigue but is not imposed for any specific period. Affected persons are instructed to regulate activities according to their own tolerance unless complicating factors are present. Contact sports are discouraged in the presence of splenomegaly.

Antibiotics are contraindicated unless β-hemolytic streptococci are present (amoxicillin or ampicillin can cause a rash in patients with

EBV infection). If sore throat is severe, effective therapies include gargles; hot drinks; anesthetic troches; or analgesics, including opioids. Corticosteroids have been used to treat respiratory distress from significant tonsillar inflammation, myocarditis, hemolytic anemia, thrombocytopenia, and neurologic complications; however, routine use of steroids is not recommended (AAP, Committee on Infectious Diseases and Pickering, 2009).

Prognosis

The course of this disease is usually self-limiting and uncomplicated. Acute symptoms often disappear within 7 to 10 days, and persistent fatigue subsides within 2 to 4 weeks. Some adolescents may need to restrict their activities for 2 to 3 months, but the disease rarely extends for longer periods. The child is encouraged to maintain limited exercise to prevent deconditioning.

Nursing Care Management

Nursing responsibilities are directed toward providing comfort measures to relieve symptoms and helping affected adolescents and their families to determine appropriate activities for the stage of the disease. The child is advised to limit exposure to persons outside the family, especially during the acute phase of illness. It may be more comfortable to limit intake to liquids during the acute phase; milkshakes are a good alternative to solid foods on a temporary basis. Throat pain may be severe enough to require an analgesic such as acetaminophen, ibuprofen, or even codeine. Careful nursing assessment of swallowing ability is essential to detect serious airway edema and airway compromise.

> **! NURSING ALERT**
>
> Advise the family to seek medical evaluation of the child or adolescent if:
> - Breathing becomes difficult.
> - Severe abdominal pain develops.
> - Sore throat pain is so severe that the child is unable drink liquids.
> - Respiratory stridor is observed.

CROUP SYNDROMES

Croup is a general term applied to a symptom complex characterized by hoarseness, a resonant cough described as "barking" or "brassy" (croupy), varying degrees of inspiratory stridor, and varying degrees of respiratory distress resulting from swelling or obstruction in the region of the larynx. Acute infections of the larynx are important in infants and small children because of their increased incidence in these age groups and because the small diameter of the airway in infants and children places them at risk for significant narrowing with inflammation.

Croup syndromes can affect the larynx, trachea, and bronchi. However, laryngeal involvement often dominates the clinical picture because of the severe effects on the voice and breathing. Croup syndromes are described according to the primary anatomic area affected (i.e., epiglottitis [or supraglottitis], laryngitis, laryngotracheobronchitis [LTB], and tracheitis). In general, LTB occurs in very young children, and epiglottitis is more common in older children. A comparison of croup syndromes is provided in Table 23-1.

With widespread immunization programs aimed at preventing *H. influenzae* type b, the cause of most cases of croup in the United States is attributed to viruses, namely parainfluenza virus, human metapneumovirus, influenza types A and B, adenovirus, and measles.

TABLE 23-1   COMPARISON OF CROUP SYNDROMES

	ACUTE EPIGLOTTITIS	ACUTE LARYNGOTRACHEOBRONCHITIS (LTB)	ACUTE SPASMODIC LARYNGITIS	ACUTE TRACHEITIS
Age group affected	2–5 years but varies	Infant or child younger than 5 years	1–3 years	1 month–6 years
Etiologic agent	Bacterial	Viral	Viral with allergic component	Viral or bacterial with allergic component
Onset	Rapidly progressive	Slowly progressive	Sudden; at night	Moderately progressive
Major symptoms	Dysphagia	URI	URI	URI
	Stridor aggravated when supine	Stridor	Croupy cough	Croupy cough
	Drooling	Brassy cough	Stridor	Purulent secretions
	High fever	Hoarseness	Hoarseness	High fever
	Toxic appearance	Dyspnea	Dyspnea	No response to LTB therapy
	Rapid pulse and respirations	Restlessness	Restlessness	
		Irritability	Symptoms awakening child but disappearing during day	
		Low-grade fever	Tendency to recur	
		Nontoxic appearance		
Treatment	Airway protection	Racemic epinephrine	Cool mist	Antibiotics
	Racemic epinephrine	Corticosteroids	Reassurance	Fluids
	Corticosteroids	Fluids		
	Fluids	Reassurance		
	Antibiotics			
	Reassurance			

URI, Upper respiratory infection.

ACUTE EPIGLOTTITIS

A presumptive diagnosis of acute epiglottitis, or acute supraglottitis, is a medical emergency. It is a serious obstructive inflammatory process that occurs predominantly in children 2 to 5 years but can occur from infancy to adulthood. The obstruction is supraglottic as opposed to the subglottic obstruction of laryngitis. The responsible organism is usually *H. influenzae*. LTB and epiglottitis do not occur together.

Clinical Manifestations

The onset of epiglottitis is abrupt, and it can rapidly progress to severe respiratory distress. The child usually goes to bed asymptomatic to awaken later, complaining of sore throat and pain on swallowing. The child has a fever; appears sicker than clinical findings suggest; and insists on sitting upright and leaning forward with the chin thrust out, mouth open, and tongue protruding (tripod position). Drooling of saliva is common because of the difficulty or pain on swallowing and excessive secretions.

> **! NURSING ALERT**
>
> Three clinical observations that are predictive of epiglottitis are absence of spontaneous cough, presence of drooling, and agitation.

The child is irritable; extremely restless; and has an anxious, apprehensive, and frightened expression. The voice is thick and muffled, with a froglike croaking sound on inspiration, but the child is not hoarse. Suprasternal and substernal retractions may be evident. The child seldom struggles to breathe, and slow, quiet breathing provides better air exchange. The sallow color of mild hypoxia may progress to frank cyanosis. The throat is red and inflamed, and a distinctive large, cherry red, edematous epiglottis is visible on careful throat inspection.

> **! NURSING ALERT**
>
> Throat inspection should be attempted only when immediate endotracheal intubation can be performed if needed.

Therapeutic Management

The course of epiglottitis may be fulminant, with respiratory obstruction appearing suddenly. Progressive obstruction leads to hypoxia, hypercapnia, and acidosis followed by decreased muscle tone; reduced level of consciousness; and, when obstruction becomes more or less complete, a rather sudden death.

The child who is suspected of having epiglottitis should be examined in a setting where emergency airway equipment is readily available. Examination of the throat with a tongue depressor is contraindicated until experienced personnel and equipment are available to proceed with immediate intubation or tracheostomy in the event that the examination precipitates further or complete obstruction (see Critical Thinking Case Study box).

Nasotracheal intubation or tracheostomy is usually considered for the child with epiglottitis with severe respiratory distress. It is recommended that the intubation or tracheostomy and any invasive procedure, such as starting an intravenous (IV) infusion, be performed in an area where emergency airway maintenance can be easily and quickly accomplished. Humidified oxygen is administered as necessary either via mask in older children or flow-by in younger children to avoid further agitation (see Evidence-Based Practice Box, p. 727). Whether or not there is an artificial airway, the child requires intensive observation by experienced personnel. The epiglottal swelling usually decreases after 24 hours of antibiotic therapy (ceftriaxone sodium or alternate cephalosporin), and the epiglottis is near normal by the third day. Intubated children are generally extubated at this time. The use of corticosteroids for reducing edema may be beneficial during the early treatment phase.

CRITICAL THINKING CASE STUDY

Croup Syndrome

Kim, a 5-year-old girl, is admitted to the emergency department in the early evening hours with a sore throat, pain on swallowing, drooling, and a fever of 39° C (102.2° F). She looks ill; her skin is flushed; she is agitated; and she prefers to sit up, leaning on her arms. According to the child's mother, she has not had anything to eat or drink in 2 or 3 days. What nursing interventions should the nurse implement in this situation?

Questions

1. Evidence—Is there sufficient evidence to draw any conclusions about Kim's condition at this time?
2. Assumptions—Describe some underlying assumptions about each of the following:
   a. Epiglottitis in children
   b. Symptoms of epiglottitis
   c. Precautions to be taken when a child has suspected epiglottitis
   d. Immediate nursing interventions when caring for a child with epiglottitis
3. What priorities for nursing care can be drawn at this time?
4. Does the evidence objectively support your argument (conclusion)?

Children with suspected bacterial epiglottitis are given antibiotics intravenously followed by oral administration to complete a 7- to 10-day course. Family contacts with children younger than 4 years of age and any contacts younger than 4 years of age are treated with rifampin for 4 days (AAP, Committee on Infectious Diseases and Pickering, 2009).

Nursing Care Management

Epiglottitis is a serious and frightening disease for the child and family. It is important to act quickly but calmly and to provide support without increasing anxiety. The child is allowed to remain in the position that provides the most comfort and security, and the parents are reassured that everything possible is being done to obtain relief for their child.

! NURSING ALERT

When epiglottitis is suspected, the nurse should not attempt to visualize the epiglottis directly with a tongue depressor or take a throat culture but should refer the child for medical evaluation immediately.

Acute care of the child is the same as that described later for the child with LTB. Continuous monitoring of respiratory status, including pulse oximetry (and blood gases if the patient is intubated), is an important part of nursing observations, and the IV infusion is maintained as described in Chapter 22.

ACUTE LARYNGOTRACHEOBRONCHITIS

Laryngotracheobronchitis is the most common croup syndrome. It primarily affects children younger than 5 years of age, and the causative organisms are viral agents, particularly the parainfluenza virus types 2 and 3, human metapneumovirus, RSV, and influenza A and B. Other causative agents include *M. pneumoniae*, pneumococcus, and staphylococcus. The disease is usually preceded by a URI, which gradually descends to adjacent structures. It is characterized by a gradual onset of low-grade fever, and the parents often report that the child went to bed and later awoke with a barky, brassy cough. Inflammation of the mucosa lining the larynx and trachea causes a narrowing of the airway. When the airway is significantly narrowed, the child inspires air past the obstruction and into the lungs, producing the characteristic inspiratory stridor and suprasternal retractions. Other classic manifestations include cough and hoarseness. Respiratory distress in infants and toddlers may be manifested by nasal flaring, intercostal retractions, tachypnea, and continuous stridor. The typical child with LTB develops the classic barking or seal-like cough and acute stridor after several days of rhinitis. When the child is unable to inhale a sufficient volume of air, symptoms of hypoxia become evident. Obstruction that is severe enough to prevent adequate ventilation and exhalation of carbon dioxide can cause respiratory acidosis and eventually respiratory failure.

Therapeutic Management

The major objective in medical management is maintaining the airway and providing adequate respiratory exchange. Children with mild croup (no stridor at rest) can be managed at home. Parents are taught the signs of respiratory distress and instructed to summon professional help early if needed. Children with labored respirations and stridor or other respiratory symptoms should receive medical attention.

The application of humidity with cool mist provides relief for most children. A cool-air vaporizer can be used at home. In the hospital, a nebulized mist for older infants and toddlers may be used to provide increased humidity and supplemental oxygen. However, controversy surrounds the use of mist therapy to treat croup. Studies have failed to demonstrate any improvement in subglottic edema with mist therapy (Moore and Little, 2006). A ride in the car with the windows down may help relieve symptoms.

Nebulized epinephrine (racemic epinephrine) is often used in children with severe disease, stridor at rest, retractions, or difficulty breathing. The α-adrenergic effects cause mucosal vasoconstriction and subsequently decrease subglottic edema. The onset of action is rapid, and the peak effect is observed in 2 hours. Children may be discharged home following racemic epinephrine after a 2- to 3-hour period of observation for return of acute symptoms.

Oral steroids have proven effective in the treatment of croup (often as a single dose); IM dexamethasone may be given to children who are unable to tolerate oral dosing. Nebulized budesonide may be administered in conjunction with IM dexamethasone.

In severe cases of LTB, the administration of heliox may be used to reduce the work of breathing and relieve airway obstruction. It reduces airway turbulence but is not recommended as a standard treatment of croup.

Nursing Care Management

The most important nursing function in the care of children with LTB is continuous, vigilant observation and accurate assessment of respiratory status. Pulse oximetry is commonly used for monitoring oxygenation status. Changes in therapy are frequently based on the nurses' observations and assessments, the child's response to therapy, and tolerance of procedures. The trend away from early intubation of children with LTB emphasizes the importance of nursing observations and the ability to recognize impending respiratory failure so that intubation can be implemented without delay.

! NURSING ALERT

Early signs of impending airway obstruction include increased pulse and respiratory rate; substernal, suprasternal, and intercostal retractions; flaring nares; and increased restlessness.

Infants or small children find that being treated with cool mist, coughing, having laryngeal spasms, and needing IV therapy are additional sources of distress. In many acute care facilities, the infant is allowed to be held by the parent; if cool mist is used in the treatment, it can be administered through a tube held in front of the patient while the child is held on the parent's lap.

Children with mild croup are allowed to drink the beverages they like as long as their respiratory status is stable, and parents are encouraged to try whatever comforting measures work best (e.g., holding their child, rocking, singing). If the child is unable to take oral fluids, IV fluids may be required, and steroids may need to be given intravenously.

The rapid progression of croup, the alarming sound of the cough and stridor, and the child's apprehensive behavior and ill appearance combine to create a frightening experience for the parents and family. The family should be allowed to remain with their child as much as possible.

Parents need frequent reassurance provided in a calm, quiet manner and education regarding what they can do to make their child more comfortable. Home care includes monitoring for worsening symptoms, continued humidity, adequate hydration, and nourishment.

ACUTE SPASMODIC LARYNGITIS

Acute spasmodic laryngitis (spasmodic croup) is distinct from laryngitis and LTB and is characterized by recurrent paroxysmal attacks of laryngeal obstruction that occur chiefly at night. Signs of inflammation are absent or mild, and it is followed by an uneventful recovery. The child feels well the next day. Some children appear to be predisposed to the condition; allergies or hypersensitivities may be implicated in some cases. Management is the same as for infectious croup.

BACTERIAL TRACHEITIS

Bacterial tracheitis, an infection of the mucosa of the upper trachea, is a distinct entity with features of both croup and epiglottitis. The disease occurs in children younger than 3 years of age and may cause airway obstruction that is severe enough to cause respiratory arrest. It is believed to be a complication of LTB, and although *Staphylococcus aureus* is the most frequent organism responsible, *M. catarrhalis*, *S. pneumoniae*, and *H. influenzae* have also been implicated.

Many of the manifestations of bacterial tracheitis are similar to those of LTB but are unresponsive to LTB therapy. The child has a history of previous URI with croupy cough, stridor unaffected by position, toxicity, absence of drooling, and high fever. Thick, purulent tracheal secretions are common, and respiratory difficulties are secondary to these copious secretions. The child's white cell count will be elevated. Children with this condition may develop a life-threatening upper airway obstruction, respiratory failure, acute respiratory distress syndrome (ARDS), and multiple organ dysfunction (Hopkins, Lahiri, Salerno, and others, 2006).

Therapeutic Management and Nursing Care Management

Bacterial tracheitis requires vigorous management with oxygen therapy, antipyretics, and antibiotics. Many children require endotracheal intubation and mechanical ventilation; patients are closely monitored for impending respiratory failure if not intubated. Early recognition to prevent life-threatening airway obstruction is essential.

INFECTIONS OF THE LOWER AIRWAYS

The reactive portion of the lower respiratory tract includes the bronchi and bronchioles in children. Cartilaginous support of the large airways is not fully developed until adolescence. Consequently, the smooth muscle in these structures represents a major factor in the constriction of the airway, particularly in the bronchioles, the portion that extends from the bronchi to the alveoli. Table 23-2 compares some of the major features of bronchial and bronchiolar infections.

BRONCHITIS

Bronchitis (sometimes referred to as tracheobronchitis) is inflammation of the large airways (trachea and bronchi), which is frequently associated with URIs. Viral agents are the primary cause of the disease, although *M. pneumoniae* is a common cause in children older than 6 years of age. A dry, hacking, nonproductive cough that worsens at night and becomes productive in 2 or 3 days characterizes this condition.

Bronchitis is a mild, self-limiting disease that requires only symptomatic treatment, including analgesics, antipyretics, and humidity. Cough suppressants may be useful to allow rest but can interfere with clearance of secretions. Most patients recover uneventfully in 5 to 10 days. It can be associated with other underlying conditions such as CF and bronchiectasis and can become chronic in nature (cough >3 months). Adolescents with bronchitis should be screened for tobacco or marijuana use.

RESPIRATORY SYNCYTIAL VIRUS AND BRONCHIOLITIS

Bronchiolitis is a common, acute viral infection with maximum effect at the bronchiolar level. The infection occurs primarily in winter and early spring. By age 3 years, most children have been infected at least once. RSV infection is the most frequent cause of hospitalization in children younger than 1 year old. In addition, severe RSV infections in the first year of life represent a significant risk factor for the development of asthma up to age 13 years (Chávez-Bueno, Mejías, Jafri, and others, 2005). RSV infection may also occur in children older than 1 year of age who have a chronic or serious disabling illness. Although most cases of bronchiolitis are caused by RSV, adenoviruses and parainfluenza viruses are also implicated; recently, human metapneumovirus has also been associated with bronchiolitis in children. It can also rarely be caused by *M. pneumoniae*.

Respiratory syncytial virus is transmitted from exposure to contaminated secretions. RSV can live on fomites for several hours and on hands for 30 minutes (AAP, Committee on Infectious Diseases and Pickering, 2009). The incubation period is 2 to 8 days.

Pathophysiology

Respiratory syncytial virus affects the epithelial cells of the respiratory tract. The ciliated cells swell, protrude into the lumen, and lose their cilia. RSV produces a fusion of cell membranes, forming a giant cell. The bronchiolar mucosa swells, and lumina are subsequently filled with mucus and exudate. The walls of the bronchi and bronchioles are infiltrated with inflammatory cells, and peribronchiolar interstitial pneumonitis is usually present. The varying degrees of intraluminal obstruction lead to hyperinflation, obstructive emphysema resulting from partial obstruction, and patchy areas of atelectasis. Dilation of bronchial passages on inspiration allows sufficient space for intake of air, but narrowing of the passages on expiration prevents air from

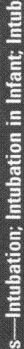

Case Study—Bronchiolitis

Animations—Intubation; Intubation in Infant; Intubation, Incorrect Placement

TABLE 23-2	COMPARISON OF CONDITIONS AFFECTING THE BRONCHI		
	ASTHMA*	**BRONCHITIS**	**BRONCHIOLITIS**
Description	Exaggerated response of bronchi to a trigger such as URI, animal dander, cold air, exercise Bronchospasm, exudation, and edema of bronchi, airway obstruction Inflammatory response	Usually occurs in association with URI Seldom an isolated entity	Most common infectious disease of lower airways Maximum obstructive impact at bronchiolar level
Age group affected	Infancy to adolescence	First 4 years of life	Usually children 2 to 12 mo of age; rare after age 2 yr Peak incidence, ≈age 6 mo
Etiologic agents	Most often viruses such as RSV in infants but may be any of a variety of URI pathogens	Usually viral Other agents (e.g., bacteria, fungi, allergic disorders, airborne irritants) can trigger symptoms	Viruses, predominantly RSV; also adenoviruses, parainfluenza viruses, human metapneumovirus, and *Mycoplasma pneumoniae*
Predominant characteristics	Wheezing, cough	Persistent dry, hacking cough (worse at night) becoming productive in 2–3 days	Labored respirations, poor feeding, cough, tachypnea, retractions and flaring nares, emphysema, increased nasal mucus, wheezing, may have fever
Treatment	Inhaled corticosteroids, bronchodilators, leukotriene modifiers, allergen and "triggers" control, long-term anti-inflammatory medications	Cough suppressants if needed	Supplemental oxygen if saturations ≤90%; bronchodilators (optional) Suctioning nasopharynx Ensure adequate fluid intake Maintain adequate oxygenation

RSV, Respiratory syncytial virus; *URI,* upper respiratory infection.
*See Asthma, p. 736.

BOX 23-8	SIGNS AND SYMPTOMS OF RESPIRATORY SYNCYTIAL VIRUS

Initial
Rhinorrhea
Pharyngitis
Coughing, sneezing
Wheezing
Possible ear or eye drainage
Intermittent fever

With Progression of Illness
Increased coughing and wheezing
Tachypnea and retractions
Cyanosis

Severe Illness
Tachypnea, >70 breaths/min
Listlessness
Apneic spells
Poor air exchange; poor breath sounds

leaving the lungs. Thus, air is trapped distal to the obstruction and causes progressive overinflation (emphysema).

Clinical Manifestations

The illness usually begins with a URI after an incubation of about 5 to 8 days. Symptoms such as rhinorrhea and low-grade fever often appear first. OM and conjunctivitis may also be present. In time, a cough may develop. If the disease progresses, it becomes a lower respiratory tract infection and manifests typical symptoms (Box 23-8). Infants may have several days of URI symptoms or no symptoms except slight lethargy, poor feeding, or irritability.

When the lower airway is involved, classic manifestations include signs of altered air exchange, such as wheezing, retractions, crackles, dyspnea, tachypnea, and diminished breath sounds. Apnea may be the first recognized indicator of RSV infection in very young infants (younger than 1 month old).

Diagnostic Evaluation

Identification has been simplified by the development of tests done on nasopharyngeal secretions, using either a rapid immunofluorescent antibody–direct fluorescent antibody (DFA) staining or an enzyme-linked immunosorbent assay (ELISA) for RSV antigen detection (see Respiratory Secretion Specimens, Chapter 22). Hyperinflation of the lungs is generally seen on the chest radiograph.

Therapeutic Management

Children with bronchiolitis are treated symptomatically with humidified oxygen, adequate fluid intake, airway maintenance, and medications. Most children with bronchiolitis can be managed at home. Hospitalization is usually recommended for children with respiratory distress and those who cannot maintain adequate hydration. Other reasons for hospitalization include complicating conditions, such as underlying lung or heart disease or associated debilitated states, or a home environment where adequate management is questionable. An infant who is tachypneic or apneic, has marked retractions, seems listless, has a history of poor fluid intake, or is dehydrated should be closely observed for respiratory failure.

Humidified oxygen is administered in concentrations sufficient to maintain adequate oxygenation (SpO_2) at or above 90% as measured by pulse oximetry. The administration of humidified mist may be used. Routine chest percussion and postural drainage (formerly CPT) is not recommended; infants with abundant nasal secretions benefit from periodic suctioning. Fluids by mouth may be contraindicated because of tachypnea, weakness, and fatigue; therefore, IV fluids may be used until the acute stage of the disease has passed. Nasogastric fluids may be required if the infant is unable to tolerate oral fluids and a peripheral IV is difficult to establish.

Clinical assessments, noninvasive oxygen monitoring, and blood gas values may guide therapy. Medical therapy for bronchiolitis is primarily supportive and aimed at decreasing airway hyperresonance and inflammation and promoting adequate fluid intake. Bronchodilators may provide short-term benefits, yet overall significant improvement in the child's condition is not always appreciable. A single dose of bronchodilator therapy is often prescribed to assess for a clinical response. If it improves symptoms, it may be prescribed on an ongoing basis. If no response is evident, no further doses are given. Racemic epinephrine has been shown to produce modest improvement in ventilation status. Corticosteroids and antihistamines have not been shown to be effective in controlled studies and are not recommended for routine use. Antibiotics are not part of the treatment of RSV unless there is a coexisting bacterial infection such as OM (AAP, 2006). Additional recommendations in the AAP (2006) practice guideline are to encourage breastfeeding; avoid passive tobacco smoke exposure; and promote preventive measures, including hand washing.

Ribavirin, an antiviral agent (synthetic nucleoside analog), is the only specific therapy approved for hospitalized children; however, use of this drug is controversial because of concerns about the high cost, aerosol route of administration, potential toxic effects among exposed health care personnel (teratogenicity), and conflicting results of efficacy trials (AAP, 2006; Chávez-Bueno, Mejías, Jafri, and others, 2005; Ventre and Randolph, 2007).

Prevention of Respiratory Syncytial Virus Infection

The only product available in the United States for prevention of RSV is palivizumab (Synagis), a monoclonal antibody, which is given monthly in an IM injection to prevent hospitalization associated with RSV. According to the AAP (Meissner and Bocchini, 2009), candidates for palivizumab include infants born before 32 weeks' gestation, infants with chronic lung disease, infants born at 32 to less than 35 weeks' gestation who attend daycare or have a sibling under 5 years, children younger than 2 years of age with hemodynamically significant congenital heart disease, and children with severe immunodeficiencies (e.g., severe combined immunodeficiency or acquired immunodeficiency syndrome [AIDS]). Prophylaxis for RSV should be initiated at the onset of the RSV season and terminated at the end of the season (November to March). Additional age and condition recommendations are outlined in the AAP practice guideline (2006).

 DRUG ALERT!

The lyophilized powder form of palivizumab should be administered within 6 hours of being reconstituted with sterile water because it is preservative free. A new liquid form of the drug may be available for future use.

QUALITY PATIENT OUTCOMES: Bronchiolitis
- Room air or O_2 saturation ≥90%
- Respiratory rate ≤60 breaths/min
- Adequate oral fluid intake

Nursing Care Management

Children admitted to the hospital with suspected RSV infection are usually assigned separate rooms or grouped with other RSV-infected children. Contact and standard precautions are used, including hand washing, not touching the nasal mucosa or conjunctiva, and using gloves and gowns when entering the patient's room; droplet precautions are also recommended. Other isolation procedures of potential benefit are those aimed at diminishing the number of hospital personnel, visitors, and uninfected children in contact with the child. Another measure is to make patient assignments so that nurses assigned to children with RSV are not caring for other patients who are considered high risk.

Infants with RSV often have copious nasal secretions, making breathing and breastfeeding or bottle feeding difficult. This engenders concerns that the child will lose weight or stop breastfeeding altogether. Encourage breastfeeding mothers to continue feeding the infant or, if feedings are contraindicated because of the acuity of the illness, mothers should pump their milk and store it appropriately for later use (see Chapter 8). Parents are taught how to instill normal saline drops into the nares and suction the mucus with a bulb syringe or portable suction machine, before feedings and before bedtime so the child may eat and rest better; unfortunately, no medications appropriate for infants can help with these symptoms. To address the issue of decreased fluid intake, parents may offer small amounts of fluids frequently to maintain adequate hydration. Infants may cough or vomit as the secretions settle in the stomach and make them prone to emesis of such secretions.

Additional nursing care is aimed at monitoring oxygenation with pulse oximetry, ensuring any bronchodilator therapy is optimized by using a small mask for delivery, and providing information for the parent and family regarding the infant's status. For the most part, infants recover quickly from the disease and resume normal daily activities, including fluid intake. Such infants are at risk for further episodes of wheezing that may or may not involve another RSV infection; parents, however, may be concerned that the infant has another serious case of RSV.

PNEUMONIAS

Pneumonia, inflammation of the pulmonary parenchyma, is common in childhood but occurs more frequently in early childhood. Clinically, pneumonia may occur either as a primary disease or as a complication of another illness. The causative agent is either inhaled into the lungs directly or comes from the bloodstream.

The most useful classification of pneumonia is based on the etiologic agent (e.g., viral, bacterial, mycoplasmal, or aspiration of foreign substances) (see Aspiration Pneumonia, p. 732). Many organisms can cause pneumonia and these vary according to the child's age (Ranganathan and Sonnappa, 2009):

Neonates—Group B streptococci, gram-negative enteric bacteria, cytomegalovirus, *Ureaplasma urealyticum*, *Listeria monocytogenes*, *C. trachomatis*

Infants—RSV, parainfluenza virus, influenza virus, adenovirus, metapneumovirus, *S. pneumoniae*, *H. influenzae*, *M. pneumoniae*, *Mycobacterium tuberculosis*

Preschool children——RSV, parainfluenza virus, influenza virus, adenovirus, metapneumovirus, *S. pneumoniae*, *H. influenzae*, *M. pneumoniae*, *M. tuberculosis*

School-age children—*M. pneumoniae*, *Chlamydia pneumoniae*, *M. tuberculosis*, and respiratory viruses

Histomycosis, coccidioidomycosis, and other fungi also cause pneumonia. Pneumonitis is a localized acute inflammation of the lung without the toxemia associated with lobar pneumonia.

The clinical manifestations of pneumonia vary depending on the etiologic agent, the child's age, the child's systemic reaction to the infection, the extent of the lesions, and the degree of bronchial and bronchiolar obstruction. The causative agent is identified from the clinical history, the child's age, the general health history, the physical examination, radiography, and the laboratory examination.

BOX 23-9   GENERAL SIGNS OF PNEUMONIA

Fever—Usually high
Respiratory
- Cough—Unproductive to productive with white sputum
- Tachypnea
- Breath sounds—Crackles, decreased breath sounds, rales
- Dullness with percussion
- Chest pain
- Retractions
- Nasal flaring
- Pallor to cyanosis (depends on severity)

Chest radiography—Diffuse or patchy infiltration with peribronchial distribution
Behavior—Irritability, restlessness, malaise, lethargy
Gastrointestinal—Anorexia, vomiting, diarrhea, abdominal pain

Viral Pneumonia

Viral pneumonias, which occur more frequently than bacterial pneumonias, are seen in children of all ages and are often associated with viral URIs. Viruses that cause pneumonia include RSV in infants and parainfluenza, influenza, human metapneumovirus, enterovirus, and adenovirus in older children. Differentiation among viruses is usually made by clinical features such as child's age, medical history, season of the year, and radiographic and laboratory examination (Box 23-9).

Viral infections of the respiratory tract render the affected child more susceptible to secondary bacterial invasion, especially when there is denuded bronchial mucosa. Treatment is symptomatic and includes measures to promote oxygenation and comfort, such as oxygen administration with cool mist, antipyretics for fever management, monitoring fluid intake, and family support. Antimicrobial therapy is usually reserved for children in whom a bacterial infection is demonstrated by appropriate cultures.

Primary Atypical Pneumonia

Atypical pneumonia refers to pneumonia that is caused by pathogens other than the traditionally most common and readily cultured bacteria (e.g., *S. pneumoniae*). In the category of atypical pneumonias, *M. pneumoniae* is the most common cause of community-acquired pneumonia in children 5 years of age or older (Rafei and Lichenstein, 2006). It occurs in the fall and winter months and is more prevalent in crowded living conditions. Most affected persons recover from acute illness at home in 7 to 10 days with symptomatic treatment followed by 1 week of convalescence. The incubation period is 2 to 3 weeks, but the cough may last several weeks.

Chlamydial pneumonia, caused by *C. trachomatis*, can occur in infants and generally appears between 3 and 19 weeks of age. The infant contracts this from the infected genital tract of the mother at birth.

Erythromycin (for those younger than 9 years of age), azithromycin, and clarithromycin are the primary agents used for treating atypical pneumonia.

Bacterial Pneumonia

S. pneumoniae is the most common bacterial pathogen responsible for community-acquired pneumonia in both children and adults (Rafei and Lichenstein, 2006). Other bacteria that cause pneumonia in children are pneumococcus, group A streptococcus, *S. aureus*, *M. catarrhalis*, and *C. pneumoniae*.

Beyond the neonatal period, bacterial pneumonias display distinct clinical patterns that facilitate their differentiation from other forms of pneumonia. The onset of illness is abrupt and generally follows a viral infection that disturbs the natural defense mechanisms of the upper respiratory tract.

The child with bacterial pneumonia usually appears ill. Symptoms include fever, malaise, rapid and shallow respirations, cough, and chest pain. The pain of pneumonia may be referred to the abdomen in young children and confused with appendicitis. Chills and meningeal symptoms (meningism) without meningitis are common.

Most older children with pneumonia can be treated at home if the condition is recognized and treatment is initiated early. Antibiotic therapy, rest, liberal oral intake of fluid, and administration of an antipyretic for fever are the principal therapeutic measures. Chest percussion and postural drainage may be indicated; however, this is controversial. Follow-up examination is recommended for small infants and toddlers. Hospitalization is indicated when pleural effusion or empyema accompanies the disease, when respiratory distress occurs, in situations in which compliance with therapy is estimated to be poor, in infants younger than 1 month old, and when there are chronic illnesses such as congenital heart disease or BPD (Rafei and Lichenstein, 2006). IV fluids may be necessary to ensure adequate hydration, and oxygen is required if the child is in respiratory distress; some children may require initial therapy with parenteral antibiotics because of the severity of illness.

Prevention

In February 2010, a 13-valent pneumococcal conjugate vaccine (PCV13) was approved for use in children ages 6 weeks to 71 months to protect against 13 pneumococcal serotypes. The Advisory Committee on Immunization Practices (ACIP) recommends routine vaccination with PCV13 of all children ages 2 to 59 months, children ages 60 to 71 months with underlying medical conditions that increase their risk for pneumococcal disease or complications, and children who previously received one or more doses of PCV7 (CDC, 2010). (See Immunizations, Chapter 10.)

Complications

At present, the classic features and clinical course of pneumonia are seen infrequently because of early and vigorous antibiotic and supportive therapy. However, some children, especially infants, with staphylococcal or GABHS pneumonia develop empyema, pyopneumothorax, or tension pneumothorax. AOM and pleural effusion are common in children with pneumococcal pneumonia (Box 23-10) (see Evidence-Based Practice box).

Continuous closed chest drainage may be instituted when purulent fluid is aspirated. If a large amount of purulent drainage is obtained, an appropriate antibiotic may be instilled into the chest cavity, and chest drainage is discontinued for approximately 1 hour after the instillation. Closed drainage via a chest tube is continued until drainage fluid is minimal, which rarely requires more than 5 to 7 days. Sometimes repeated pleural taps are sufficient to remove fluid; however, if the purulent drainage accumulates rapidly and is highly viscous, continuous drainage is preferred. Thoracotomy with open debridement of the infected lung tissue may be required; if empyema and pneumothorax tend to recur, a partial thoracoscopic lobectomy may be performed. Alternatively, video-assisted thoracoscopy (VATS) and intrapleural fibrinolytic therapy may preclude the use of open debridement and thoracotomy (Sandora and Sectish, 2011).

EVIDENCE-BASED PRACTICE

Nursing Interventions for Prevention of Ventilator-Associated Pneumonia in Children

Olga A. Taylor

Ask the Question
Picot Question
What nursing interventions prevent VAP in children?

Search for the Evidence
Search Strategies
Search selection included English-language publications on nursing interventions for prevention of VAP in children and adolescents.

Databases Used
PubMed, AHRQ

Critically Analyze the Evidence
- Implementation of VAP bundle resulted in a decreased VAP rate from 5.6 infections per 1000 ventilator days at baseline to 0.3 per 1000 ventilator days (Bigham, Amato, Bondurrant, and others, 2009).
- Common VAP prevention interventions include (Bigham, Amato, Bondurrant, and others, 2009; Garland, 2010; Morrow, Argent, Jeena, and others, 2009; Norris, Barnes, and Roberts, 2009):
  - Change ventilator circuits and in-line suction catheters only when soiled.
  - Every 2 to 4 hours, drain condensate from ventilator circuit (use heated wire circuits to reduce rainout).
  - Rinse oral suction devices after use and store in a nonsealed plastic bag at the bedside.
  - Hand hygiene should be used before and after contact with ventilator circuit.
  - Wear PPE before providing care to patients when soiling from respiratory secretions is anticipated.
  - Every 2 to 4 hours, follow unit mouth care policy.
  - Unless contraindicated, elevate head of bed to 30 to 45 degrees.
  - Before repositioning patient, always drain ventilator circuit.
  - For patients older than 12 years old, when possible, use ET tube with dorsal lumen above ET cuff to help suction secretions above the cuff.
  - Evaluate daily for possible extubation.
  - Avoid reintubation.
  - Provide deep vein thrombosis and peptic ulcer disease prophylaxis.
- Infants in supine position (infant lying on back with ET tube held upright in the vertical position) had increased colony counts or new organisms in tracheal aspirate than infants in lateral position (infant lying on side with ET tube at same level as the trachea) (Aly, Badawy, El-Kholy, and others, 2008).
- Staff education on VAP and improvements to practice changes can have a substantial impact on reducing VAP (Garland, 2010; Richardson, Hines, Dixon, and others, 2010; Turton, 2008).
- A 7-day versus 3-day ventilator circuit change was not associated with increased VAP rates (Samransamruajkit, Jirapaiboonsuk, Siritantiwat, and others, 2010).
- Use of low-sodium solution for airway care was associated with a decrease in VAP as well as chronic lung disease (Christensen, Henry, Baer, and others, 2010).
- In bronchoalveolar lavage fluid, PAI-1 levels can aid in early diagnosis of VAP (Srinivasan, Song, Wiener-Kronish, and others, 2011).

- Reduced mortality rates were observed in patients with VAP when silver-coated ET tube was used versus uncoated ET tube (Afessa, Shorr, Anzueto, and others, 2010).

Apply the Evidence: Nursing Implications
There is **good evidence** with a **strong recommendation** (Guyatt, Oxman, Vist, and others, 2008) for use of interventions to prevent VAP in children. Some prevention methods included in VAP bundles are hand hygiene, oral hygiene, use of PPE, elevation of head of bed 30 to 45 degrees, and more. Staff education and engagement in VAP prevention initiatives is important.

QSEN Quality and Safety Competencies:
Evidence-Based Practice*
Knowledge
Differentiate clinical opinion from research and evidence-based summaries.
Describe the various interventions for prevention of VAP in children.

Skills
Base individualized care plan on patient values, clinical expertise, and evidence.
Integrate evidence into practice by using interventions for prevention of VAP.in children.

Attitudes
Value the concept of evidence-based practice as integral to determining best clinical practice.
Appreciate strengths and weakness of evidence for preventions of VAP in children.

References
Afessa B, Shorr AF, Anzueto AR, and others: Association between a silver-coated endotracheal tube and reduced mortality in patients with ventilator-associated pneumonia, *Chest* 137(5): 1015–1021, 2010.
Aly H, Badawy M, El-Kholy A, and others: Randomized, controlled trial on tracheal colonization of ventilated infants: can gravity prevent ventilator-associated pneumonia? *Pediatrics* 122:770–774, 2008.
Bigham MT, Amato R, Bondurrant P, and others: Ventilator-associated pneumonia in the pediatric intensive care unit: characterizing the problem and implementing a sustainable solution, *J Pediatr* 154:582–587, 2009.
Christensen RD, Henry E, Baer VL, and others: A low-sodium solution for airway care: results of a multicenter trial, *Respir Care* 55(12):1680–1685, 2010.
Garland JS: Strategies to prevent ventilator-associated pneumonia in neonates, *Clin Perinatol* 37:629–643, 2010.
Guyatt GH, Oxman AD, Vist GE, and others: GRADE: an emerging consensus on rating quality of evidence and strength of recommendations, *BMJ*, 336:924–926, 2008.
Morrow BM, Argent AC, Jeena PM, and others: Guideline for the diagnosis, prevention and treatment of paediatric ventilator-associated pneumonia, *S Afr Med J* 99(4):255–267, 2009.
Norris SC, Barnes AK, Roberts TD: When ventilator-associated pneumonias haunt your NICU—one unit's story, *Neonatal Netw* 28(1):59–66, 2009.
Richardson M, Hines S, Dixon G, and others: Establishing nurse-led ventilator-associated pneumonia surveillance in paediatric intensive care, *J Hosp Infect* 75(3):220–224, 2010.
Samransamruajkit R, Jirapaiboonsuk S, Siritantiwat S, and others: Effective of frequency of ventilator circuit changes (3 vs 7 days) on the rate of ventilator-associated pneumonia in PICU, *J Crit Care* 25:56–61, 2010.
Srinivasan R, Song Y, Wiener-Kronish J, and others: Plasminogen activation inhibitor concentrations in bronchoalveolar lavage fluid distinguishes ventilator-associated pneumonia from colonization in mechanically ventilated pediatric patients, *Pediatr Crit Care Med* 12(1):21–27, 2011.
Turton P: Ventilator-associated pneumonia in paediatric intensive care: a literature review, *Nurs Crit Care* 13(5):241–248, 2008.

ET, Endotracheal; *PAI,* plasminogen activation inhibitor; *PPE,* personal protection equipment; *VAP,* ventilator-associated pneumonia.
*Adapted from the QSEN at http://www.qsen.org.

BOX 23-10 PNEUMOTHORAX

Pneumothorax occurs when there is an accumulation of air in the pleural space; this air increases intrapleural pressure, making it more difficult to expand the affected lung and thus the clinical manifestations of dyspnea, chest pain and often back pain, labored respirations, tachycardia, and decreased oxygen saturation. In neonates and infants on mechanical ventilation, the first clinical signs of a pneumothorax are oxygen desaturation and hypotension. The three major types of pneumothorax are tension, spontaneous, and traumatic. The definitive diagnosis of pneumothorax is a chest radiograph. The emergent treatment involves needle aspiration of the air within the pleural space; subsequently a chest tube to closed drainage is usually inserted to prevent the reaccumulation of air. *Pleural effusion* occurs when there is an excessive accumulation of fluid in the pleural space. The diagnosis is made by chest radiography, and the treatment involves evacuation of the fluid by needle aspiration followed by insertion of a chest tube to closed drainage.

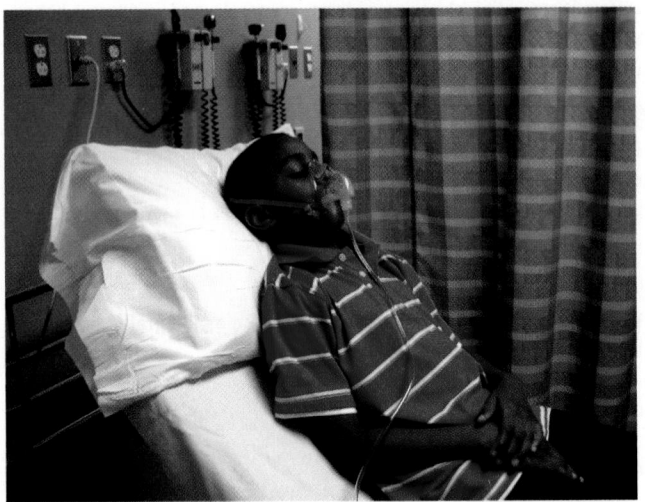

FIG 23-3 Child placed in semierect position is often more comfortable, and this position enhances diaphragmatic expansion.

Nursing Care Management

Nursing care of the child with pneumonia is primarily supportive and symptomatic but necessitates thorough respiratory assessment and administration of supplemental oxygen (as required), fluids, and antibiotics. The child's respiratory rate, rhythm and depth, oxygenation, general disposition, and level of activity are frequently assessed. To prevent dehydration, fluids are frequently administered intravenously during the acute phase.

Nursing care of the child with a chest tube requires close attention to respiratory status, as noted previously; the chest tube and drainage device used are monitored for proper function (i.e., drainage is not impeded, vacuum setting is correct, tubing is free of kinks, dressing covering chest tube insertion site is intact, water seal is maintained [if used], and chest tube remains in place). Movement in bed and ambulation with a chest tube are encouraged according to the child's respiratory status, but children require frequent doses of analgesia. Supplemental oxygen may be required in the acute phase of the illness and may be administered by nasal cannula, face mask, flow-by, or face tent. Children are usually more comfortable in a semierect position (Fig. 23-3) but should be allowed to determine the position of comfort. Lying on the affected side if the pneumonia is unilateral ("good lung up") splints the chest on that side and reduces the pleural rubbing that often causes discomfort. Fever is controlled by the cool environment and administration of antipyretic drugs. Children, especially infants, with ineffectual cough or difficulty handling secretions may require suctioning to maintain a patent airway. A simple bulb suction syringe is usually sufficient for clearing the nares and nasopharynx of infants, but mechanical suction should be readily available if needed. A noninvasive suction device (BBG nasal aspirator) may be used to suction the infant's nares without the danger of causing nasal trauma; the device may be connected to mechanical suction for best results. Older children can usually handle secretions without assistance. Chest percussion, postural drainage, and nebulized bronchodilator treatments may be prescribed depending on the child's condition. Chest percussion and postural drainage currently lacks empirical support for improving the child's condition or decreasing the length of stay in children with community-acquired pneumonia. For the child being cared for at home, the nurse educates the parent regarding observation for worsening symptoms, antibiotic and antipyretic administration, and encouragement of oral fluid intake. If the child is ill, solid foods may be rejected; fluid intake is encouraged until the child feels well enough to eat solids. Return to school or daycare is usually permitted according to the type of pneumonia, severity of illness, and practitioner recommendation. It should be emphasized that the infection may be transmitted to other children with close contact.

The hospitalized child may be apprehensive, and the treatments and tests are frightening and stress producing. It is important to involve the entire family in the care as appropriate and to encourage questions and facilitate effective communication. Reducing anxiety and apprehension reduces psychologic distress in the child, and when the child is more relaxed, the respiratory efforts are lessened. Easing respiratory efforts makes the child less apprehensive, and encouraging the presence of the caregiver provides the child with a source of comfort and support.

OTHER INFECTIONS OF THE RESPIRATORY TRACT

PERTUSSIS (WHOOPING COUGH)

Pertussis, or whooping cough, is an acute respiratory tract infection caused by *Bordetella pertussis*, which in the past primarily occurred in children younger than 4 years of age who were not immunized. It is highly contagious and is particularly threatening in young infants, who have a higher morbidity and mortality rate. It can result in encephalopathy, seizures, and pneumonia. Infants younger than 6 months of age may not come in to the practitioner with the typical cough; in this age group, apnea is a common presenting manifestation (AAP, Committee on Infectious Diseases and Pickering, 2009). Likewise, older children are known to manifest the disease with a persistent cough and the absence of the characteristic whoop (see Table 14-1 for signs, symptoms, and management of pertussis). The incidence is highest in the spring and summer months, and a single attack confers lifetime immunity. The resurgence of pertussis in the United States, particularly among children age 10 years and older, has prompted concerns of the long-term effects of the pertussis vaccine. Consequently, two acellular pertussis booster vaccines have been approved for children: Boostrix (for persons ages 10 to 64 years) and Adacel (for persons ages 11 to 64 years). (See also Immunizations, Chapter 10.) Most children with pertussis can be managed at home; care is supportive in nature, including encouraging adequate hydration and administering antipyretics. When coughing spasms occur in small children, they can be frightening for the parent and family in an unvaccinated child. Admission to the hospital occurs if respiratory symptoms are severe or if apnea occurs. Treatment with antibiotics (erythromycin, clarithromycin, or azithromycin) in the catarrhal stage may result in a milder form of the infection, but treatment also prevents spread to others (AAP, Committee on Infectious Diseases and Pickering, 2009). Family contacts may also be treated. Pertussis symptoms usually last for 6 to 10 weeks but may persist for longer.

TUBERCULOSIS

Tuberculosis (TB) is the second leading cause of death from an infectious disease. Ten million to 15 million persons in the United States are infected with TB. Case rates of TB for all ages are higher in urban, low-income areas and among non-white racial and ethnic groups. In recent years, foreign-born children have accounted for more than one fourth of newly diagnosed cases of TB in children 14 years of age or younger in the United States (AAP, Committee on Infectious Diseases and Pickering, 2009). The following groups have the greatest rates of latent TB infection: immigrants, international adoptees, refugees from or travelers to high-prevalence regions (Asia, Africa, Latin America, and countries of the former Soviet Union), homeless individuals, and inmates of correctional facilities (AAP, Committee on Infectious Diseases and Pickering, 2009).

Tuberculosis is caused by *M. tuberculosis*, an acid-fast bacillus. Children are susceptible to the human (*M. tuberculosis*) and the bovine (*Mycobacterium bovis*) organisms. In parts of the world where TB in cattle is not controlled or milk is not pasteurized, the bovine type is a common source of infection.

Certain factors influence the degree to which the organism produces an altered state in the host. These factors include heredity (resistance to the infection may be genetically transmitted), gender (higher rates in adolescent girls), age (lower resistance in infants; higher incidence during adolescence), stress (emotional or physical), nutritional status, and intercurrent infection (especially human immunodeficiency virus [HIV], measles, and pertussis). Children with HIV infection have an increased incidence of TB disease, and all children with TB should be tested for HIV.

The source of TB infection in children is usually an infected member of the household or a frequent visitor to the home such as a babysitter or domestic worker. The airway is the usual portal of entry for the organism. In the lungs, a proliferation of epithelial cells surrounds and encapsulates the multiplying bacilli in an attempt to wall it off, thus forming the typical tubercle. Extension of the primary lesion at the original site causes progressive tissue destruction as it spreads within the lung, discharges material from foci to other areas of the lungs (e.g., bronchi, pleura), or produces pneumonia. Erosion of blood vessels by the primary lesion can cause widespread dissemination of the tubercle bacillus to near and distant sites (miliary TB). Extrapulmonary (miliary) TB may be manifested as malaise, fever, weight loss, superior lymphadenitis, meningitis, hepatomegaly, splenomegaly, and osteoarthritis (AAP, Committee on Infectious Diseases and Pickering, 2009). With the exception of meningitis, the treatment for extrapulmonary TB may be the same drug regimen as for pulmonary TB. Infants and children younger than 3 years of age are more likely to develop miliary TB.

Diagnostic Evaluation

Diagnosis is based on information derived from physical examination, history, tuberculin skin testing, radiographic examinations, and cultures of the organism. The clinical manifestations of the disease are extremely variable (Box 23-11).

BOX 23-11   CLINICAL MANIFESTATIONS OF TUBERCULOSIS

May be asymptomatic or produce a broad range of symptoms:
- Fever
- Malaise
- Anorexia
- Weight loss
- Cough (may or may not be present; progresses slowly over weeks to months)
- Aching pain and tightness in the chest
- Hemoptysis (rare)

With progression:
- Increasing respiratory rate
- Poor expansion of lung on the affected side
- Diminished breath sounds and crackles
- Dullness to percussion
- Persistent fever
- Generalized symptoms
- Pallor, anemia, weakness, and weight loss

The tuberculin skin test (TST) is the most important indicator of whether a child has been infected with the tubercle bacillus. The standard dose of purified protein derivative (PPD) is 5 tuberculin units, which is administered using a 27-gauge needle and a 1-ml syringe intradermally into the volar aspect of the forearm. Creation of a visible wheal is crucial to accurate testing. The AAP (AAP, Committee on Infectious Diseases and Pickering, 2009) recommends that administration of the TST and interpretation of the results be performed and read only by specially educated health care professionals. Universal testing of all children for TB is no longer recommended. A targeted testing method is employed wherein only children and adolescents at high risk for contracting the disease, in addition to patients at risk for progression to TB disease, are screened. A risk factor questionnaire has been developed to facilitate screening pediatric populations at high risk; factors on the questionnaire include a close association with persons having latent or active disease, foreign birth, or foreign travel (Pediatric Tuberculosis Collaborative Group, 2004). The entire questionnaire is available in the Pediatric Tuberculosis Collaborative Group (2004) reference or online at http://www.sfdph.org/dph/files/TBdocs/PediatricTBRiskAssessQuest_2006.pdf. Recommendations for TST of children are listed in Box 23-12.

A positive reaction indicates that the individual has been infected and has developed sensitivity to the tubercle bacillus. The test is usually positive 2 to 10 weeks after initial infection with the organism. It does not, however, confirm the presence of active disease. Once an individual reacts positively, he or she will always react positively. A previously negative reaction that becomes positive indicates that the person has been infected since the previous test. Guidelines for interpreting the TST are listed in Box 23-13. Prompt radiographic evaluation of all children with a positive TST reaction is recommended.

The term latent tuberculosis infection (LTBI) is used to indicate infection in a person who has a positive TST, no physical findings of disease, and normal chest radiograph findings. The majority of children are asymptomatic when a positive skin test result is found, and most of them do not go on to develop the disease. The term tuberculosis disease or clinically active TB is used when a child has clinical symptoms or radiographic manifestations caused by the *M. tuberculosis* organism. A diagnosis of TB disease represents recent transmission of the *M. tuberculosis* organism and is an urgent event for public health.

BOX 23-12 TUBERCULIN SKIN TEST (TST) RECOMMENDATIONS FOR INFANTS, CHILDREN, AND ADOLESCENTS*

Children for Whom Immediate TST Is Indicated

Contacts of persons with confirmed or suspected contagious tuberculosis (contact investigation).

Children with radiographic or clinical findings suggesting tuberculosis disease.

Children immigrating from endemic countries (e.g., Asia, Middle East, Africa, Latin America).

Children with travel histories to endemic countries or significant contact with indigenous persons from such countries.[†]

Children Who Should Have Annual TST[‡]

Children infected with human immunodeficiency virus (HIV).

Incarcerated adolescents.

Children Who Some Experts Recommend Should Be Tested Every 2 to 3 Years

Children with ongoing exposure to the following people: HIV-infected people, homeless people, residents of nursing homes, institutionalized adolescents or adults, users of illicit drugs, incarcerated adolescents or adults, migrant farm workers; foster children with exposure to adults in the preceding high-risk groups are included.

Children Who Some Experts Recommend Should Be Considered for TST at 4 to 6 and 11 to 16 Years

Children whose parents immigrated (with unknown TST status) from regions of the world with high prevalence of tuberculosis; continued potential exposure by travel to the endemic areas or household contact with persons from the endemic areas (with unknown TST status) should be an indication for repeat TST.

Children at Increased Risk for Progression of Infection to Disease

Children with other medical risk factors, including diabetes mellitus, chronic renal failure, malnutrition, and congenital or acquired immunodeficiencies, deserve special consideration. Without recent exposure, these people are not at increased risk of acquiring tuberculosis infection. Underlying immune deficiencies associated with these conditions theoretically would enhance the possibility for progression to severe disease. Initial histories of potential exposure to tuberculosis should be included for all of these patients. If these histories or local epidemiologic factors suggest a possibility of exposure, immediate and periodic TST should be considered. **An initial TST should be performed before initiation of immunosuppressive therapy, including prolonged steroid administration, for any child with an underlying condition that necessitates immunosuppressive therapy.**

From American Academy of Pediatrics, Committee on Infectious Diseases, Pickering L, editor: *Red book: 2009 report of the Committee on Infectious Diseases,* ed 28, Elk Grove Village, Ill, 2009, Author.

*Bacille Calmette-Guérin (BCG) immunization is not a contraindication to TST.

[†]If child is well, TST should be delayed for up to 10 weeks after return.

[‡]Initial tuberculin skin testing is done at the time of diagnosis or circumstance, beginning as early as 3 months of age.

BOX 23-13 DEFINITION OF POSITIVE TUBERCULIN SKIN TEST (TST) RESULTS IN INFANTS, CHILDREN, AND ADOLESCENTS*

Induration ≥5 mm

Children in close contact with known or suspected contagious cases of tuberculosis disease

Children suspected to have tuberculosis disease:
- Findings on chest radiography consistent with active or previously active tuberculosis
- Clinical evidence of tuberculosis disease[†]

Children receiving immunosuppressive therapy, including immunosuppressive doses of corticosteroids or who have immunosuppressive conditions, including HIV infection

Induration ≥10 mm

Children at increased risk of disseminated disease:
- Children younger than 4 years of age
- Children with other medical risk conditions, including Hodgkin disease, lymphoma, diabetes mellitus, chronic renal failure, or malnutrition

Children at increased risk of exposure to TB:
- Children born or whose parents were born in high-prevalence (TB) regions of the world
- Children frequently exposed to adults who are HIV infected, homeless, users of illicit drugs, residents of nursing homes, incarcerated or institutionalized, or migrant farm workers
- Children who travel to high-prevalence (TB) regions of the world

Induration ≥15 mm

Children 4 years of age or older without any risk factors

From American Academy of Pediatrics, Committee on Infectious Diseases, Pickering L, editor: *Red book: 2009 report of the Committee on Infectious Diseases,* ed 28, Elk Grove Village, Ill, 2009, Author.

HIV, Human immunodeficiency virus; *TB,* tuberculosis.

*These definitions apply regardless of previous Bacille Calmette-Guérin (BCG) immunization; erythema at the TST site does not indicate a positive test result. TSTs should be read at 48 to 72 hours after placement.

[†]Evidence by physical examination or laboratory assessment that would include tuberculosis in the working differential diagnosis (e.g., meningitis).

Prompt evaluation, treatment, and identification and treatment of contacts are key components to managing TB.

Therapeutic Management

Medical management of TB disease in children consists of adequate nutrition, pharmacotherapy, prevention of unnecessary exposure to other infections that further compromise the body's defenses, and sometimes surgical procedures. Family members and other contacts should also be assessed for symptoms by public health and treated accordingly.

The recommended drug regimen for LTBI in children and adolescents includes a daily dose of isoniazid (INH) for 9 months or alternatively two or three times per week with **direct observation of therapy (DOT)** if daily treatment is not possible. DOT means that a health care worker or other responsible, mutually agreed-on individual is present when medications are administered to the patient. Rifampin (daily for 6 months; alternatively DOT twice weekly for 6 months) may be used to treat the child or adolescent who is INH resistant (AAP, Committee on Infectious Diseases and Pickering, 2009).

For the child with clinically active TB, the goal is to achieve sterilization of the tuberculous lesion. Recommended drug therapy for treating TB disease includes combinations of INH, rifampin, and pyrazinamide (PZA). The AAP (AAP, Committee on Infectious Diseases and Pickering, 2009) recommends a 6-month regimen consisting of INH, rifampin, and PZA given daily for the first 2 months followed by INH and rifampin given two or three times a week by DOT for the remaining 4 months. DOT decreases the rates of relapse, treatment failures, and drug resistance and is recommended for treatment of children and adolescents with TB in the United States.

If the child is suspected of having multidrug-resistant TB, a fourth medication such as streptomycin (IM injection only) or ethambutol is added. Optimal therapy for TB in children with HIV infection has not been established, and consultation with a specialist is advised. Therapy should always include at least three drugs initially and be continued for at least 9 months. INH, rifampin, and PZA usually with ethambutol or an aminoglycoside should be given for at least the first 2 months. The three-drug regimen can be used after drug-resistant disease is excluded.

Surgical procedures may be required to remove the source of infection in tissues that are inaccessible to pharmacotherapy or that are destroyed by the disease. Orthopedic procedures may be performed for correction of bone deformities, and bronchoscopy may be done for removal of a tuberculous granulomatous polyp.

Prognosis

Most children recover from primary TB infection and are often unaware of its presence. However, very young children have a higher incidence of disseminated disease. TB is a serious disease during the first 2 years of life, during adolescence, and in children who are HIV positive. Except in cases of tuberculous meningitis, death seldom occurs in treated children. Antibiotic therapy has decreased the death rate and the hematogenous spread from primary lesions.

Prevention

The only definite means to prevent TB is to avoid contact with the tubercle bacillus. Maintaining an optimal state of health with adequate nutrition and avoiding fatigue and debilitating infections promote natural resistance but do not prevent infection. Pasteurization and routine testing of milk and elimination of diseased cattle have reduced the incidence of bovine TB.

Limited immunity can be produced by administration of bacille Calmette-Guérin (BCG), a live vaccine containing bovine bacilli with reduced virulence (attenuated). In most instances, positive tuberculin reactions develop after inoculation with BCG. The distribution of BCG is controlled by local or state health departments, and the vaccine is not used extensively, even in areas with a high prevalence of disease. BCG vaccination is not generally recommended for use in the United States. However, it may be recommended for long-term protection of infants and children with negative TST results who are not infected with HIV and who (1) are at high risk for continuing exposure to persons with infectious pulmonary TB or (2) are continuously exposed to persons with TB who have bacilli resistance to both INH and rifampin when the child cannot be removed from the environment or given antituberculosis drug therapy (AAP, Committee on Infectious Diseases and Pickering, 2009).

Nursing Care Management

Children with TB receive their nursing care in ambulatory settings, outpatient departments, schools, and public health settings. Most children are not contagious and require only standard precautions. Children with no cough and negative sputum smears can be hospitalized in a regular patient room. However, airborne precautions and a negative-pressure room are required for children who are contagious and hospitalized with active TB disease. Infection control for hospital personnel in contagious cases should include the use of a personally fitted air-purifying N95 or N100 respirator (PAPR) for all patient contacts.

Asymptomatic children with TB can attend school or daycare facilities if they are receiving pharmacotherapy. They can return to regular activities as soon as effective therapy has been instituted, adherence to therapy has been documented, and clinical symptoms have diminished. Children receiving pharmacotherapy for TB can receive measles and other age-appropriate live virus vaccines unless they are receiving high-dose corticosteroids, are severely ill, or have specific contraindications to immunization.

Skin tests must be carried out correctly to obtain accurate results. The tuberculin is injected intradermally with the bevel of the needle pointing upward. A wheal 6 to 10 mm in diameter should form between the layers of the skin when the solution is injected properly. If the wheal is not formed, the procedure is repeated. The volar or dorsal surface of the forearm is the usual injection site. The reaction to the skin test is determined in 48 to 72 hours; reactions occurring after 72 hours should be measured and considered the result. The size of the transverse diameter of induration, not the erythema, is measured. The diameter transverse to the long axis of the forearm is the only one standardized for measurement purposes (AAP, Committee on Infectious Diseases and Pickering, 2009).

Sputum specimens are difficult or impossible to obtain from infants and young children because they swallow any mucus coughed from the lower respiratory tract. The best means for obtaining material for smears or culture is by gastric washing (i.e., aspiration of lavaged contents from the fasting stomach with a nasogastric tube). The procedure is carried out and the specimen obtained early in the morning before the customary breakfast time. In some cases, an induced sputum specimen may be obtained by administering aerosolized normal saline for 10 to 15 minutes followed by chest percussion and postural drainage and suctioning of the nasopharynx for sputum collection.

Because the success of therapy depends on compliance with the drug regimen, parents are instructed about the importance and rationale for DOT. Case finding in the community and follow-up of known contacts—individuals from whom the affected child may have acquired the disease and persons who may have been exposed to the child with the disease—are essential control measures.

PULMONARY DYSFUNCTION CAUSED BY NONINFECTIOUS IRRITANTS

FOREIGN BODY ASPIRATION

Small children characteristically explore matter with their mouths and are prone to aspirate foreign bodies (FBs). Small children also place objects such as beads, paper clips, small magnets, or food items in the nose, which can easily be aspirated into the trachea. FB aspiration can occur at any age but is most common in children 1 to 3 years of age. Severity is determined by the location, type of object aspirated, and extent of obstruction. For example, dry vegetable matter, such as a seed, nut, or piece of carrot or popcorn, that does not dissolve and that may swell when wet creates a particularly difficult problem. The high fat content of potato chips and peanuts may cause the added risk of lipoid pneumonia. "Fun foods" are the worst offenders in terms of potential for choking. Offending foods in the order of frequency of choking are hot dogs, round candies, peanuts or other nuts, grapes, cookies or biscuits, other meats, caramels, carrots, peas, apples, celery, popcorn, sunflower seeds, orange seeds, cherry pits, watermelon seeds, gum, and peanut butter. Other items include burst latex balloons, plastic or glass beads, marbles, pen or marker caps, button or disc batteries, and coins. Objects such as small lithium or cadmium batteries may cause esophageal or tracheal corrosion.

Diagnostic Evaluation

The diagnosis of FB aspiration is suspected on the basis of the history and physical signs. Initially, a FB in the air passages produces choking, gagging, wheezing, or coughing. Laryngotracheal obstruction most commonly causes dyspnea, cough, stridor, and hoarseness because of decreased air entry. Up to half of all children with FB ingestion may be asymptomatic. Cyanosis may occur if the obstruction becomes worse. Bronchial obstruction usually produces cough (frequently paroxysmal), wheezing, asymmetric breath sounds, decreased airway entry, and dyspnea. When an object is lodged in the larynx, the child is unable to speak or breathe. If the obstruction progresses, the child's face may become livid, and if the obstruction is total, the child can become unconscious and die of asphyxiation. If obstruction is partial, hours, days, or even weeks may pass without symptoms after the initial period. Secondary symptoms are related to the anatomic area in which the object is lodged and are usually caused by a persistent respiratory tract infection distal to the obstruction. FB aspiration should also be suspected in the presence of acute or chronic pulmonary lesions. Often, by the time secondary symptoms appear, the parents have forgotten the initial episode of coughing and gagging. Nasal FBs often manifest by unilateral purulent drainage that does not improve with time.

Radiographic examination reveals opaque FBs but is of limited use in localizing nonradiographic matter. Bronchoscopy is required for a definitive diagnosis of objects in the larynx and trachea. Fluoroscopic examination is valuable in detecting FBs in the bronchi. The mainstay of diagnosis and management of FBs is endoscopy. If there is doubt about the presence of an FB, endoscopy can be diagnostic and therapeutic.

Therapeutic Management

Foreign body aspiration may result in life-threatening airway obstruction, especially in infants because of the small diameters of their airways. Current recommendations for the emergency treatment of the choking child include the use of abdominal thrusts for children older than 1 year of age and back blows and chest thrusts for children younger than 1 year of age (see Airway Obstruction, p. 758).

A FB is rarely coughed up spontaneously. Most frequently, it must be removed instrumentally by endoscopy. Endoscopy and bronchoscopy require sedation with an agent such as IV propofol or midazolam. The procedure is carried out as quickly as possible because the progressive local inflammatory process triggered by the foreign material hampers removal. A chemical pneumonia soon develops, and vegetable matter begins to macerate within a few days, making it even more difficult to remove. After removal of the FB, the child is usually observed for any complications such as laryngeal edema and then discharged home within a matter of hours if vital signs are stable and recovery is satisfactory.

Nursing Care Management

A major role of nurses caring for a child who has aspirated an FB is to recognize the signs of FB aspiration, observe for worsening of respiratory symptoms, and implement immediate measures to relieve an emergency obstruction. Choking on food or other material should not be fatal. Back blows and chest thrusts in infants and abdominal thrusts in children are simple procedures that can be used by both health professionals and laypersons to save lives. To aid a child who is choking, nurses must recognize the signs of distress. A blind sweep of the child's mouth should never be performed because it may lodge the agent farther into the airway. Not every child who gags or coughs while eating is truly choking.

> **! NURSING ALERT**
>
> The child in severe distress (1) cannot speak, (2) becomes cyanotic, and (3) collapses. These three signs indicate that the child is truly choking and requires immediate action. The child can die within 4 minutes.

Prevention

Nurses are in a position to teach prevention in a variety of settings. They can educate parents singly or in groups about hazards of aspiration in relation to the developmental level of their children and encourage them to teach their children safety. Parents should be cautioned about behaviors that their children might imitate (e.g., holding foreign objects, such as pins, nails, and toothpicks, in their lips or mouth). (Prevention based on the child's age is discussed in Chapters 10 and 12.)

ASPIRATION PNEUMONIA

Aspiration pneumonia occurs when food, secretions, inert materials, volatile compounds, or liquids enter the lung and cause inflammation and a chemical pneumonitis. Aspiration of fluid or foods is a particular hazard in the child who has difficulty with swallowing or is unable to swallow because of paralysis, weakness, debility, congenital anomalies, or absent cough reflex or in the child who is force-fed, especially while crying or breathing rapidly. Clinical signs of the aspiration of oral secretions may not be distinguishable from those of other forms of acute bacterial pneumonia. For example, if vegetable matter has been aspirated, manifestations may not appear for several weeks after the event. Classic symptoms include an increasing cough or fever with foul-smelling sputum, deteriorating oxygenation, evidence of infiltrates on chest radiographs, and other signs of lower airway involvement. These deviations may persist for weeks, however, while the child starts to feel better. Rarely, aspiration causes immediate death from asphyxia; more often, the irritated mucous membrane becomes a site for secondary bacterial infection. In addition to fluids, food, vomitus, and nasopharyngeal secretions, other substances that may cause pneumonia are hydrocarbons, lipids, powder, and contrast dye or barium. The severity of the lung injury depends on the pH of the aspirated material.

Nursing Care Management

Care of the child with aspiration pneumonia is the same as that described for the child with pneumonia from other causes. However, the major focus of nursing care is on prevention of aspiration. Proper feeding techniques should be carried out, and preventive measures should be used to prevent aspiration of any material that might enter the nasopharynx. The presence of a nasogastric feeding tube or a history of gastroesophageal reflux disease places the child at risk of aspiration. Nasogastric tubes used for feedings should be checked before the initiation of bolus feedings; continuous nasogastric tube feedings should also be evaluated periodically for proper tube placement. Children who are at risk for swallowing difficulties as a result of illness, physical debilitation, anesthesia, or sedation are kept NPO (nothing by mouth) until they can properly swallow fluids effectively. The child may receive nutrition by alternate means such as an enteral feeding tube. The child who is at risk for vomiting and incapable of protecting the airway should be positioned in a side-lying recovery position (see Fig. 23-18). Educating parents on its prevention is important.

PULMONARY EDEMA

Pulmonary edema (PE) is the movement of fluid into the alveoli and interstitium of the lungs caused by extravasation of fluid from the pulmonary vasculature (Mazor and Green, 2011). There are two main types of PE, cardiogenic and noncardiogenic.

Cardiogenic (hydrostatic, hemodynamic) PE is caused by an increase in pulmonary capillary pressure because of an increase in pulmonary venous pressure. It can be caused by excessive IV fluid administration, left ventricular failure, heart valve disorder (aortic regurgitation, aortic stenosis, mitral regurgitation), myocardial ischemia, myocarditis, sepsis, acute tachydysrhythmia, or coronary arteriosclerosis (Sovari and Ooi, 2008).

Noncardiogenic PE is caused by various conditions that result in increased pulmonary capillary permeability. Some subtypes of noncardiogenic PE include permeability PE (caused by ARDS or acute lung injury [ALI]), high altitude PE (caused by rapid ascension to heights above 12,000 feet), or neurogenic PE (after CNS insult such as seizures, head injury, or cerebral hemorrhage). Some less common forms of PE are reperfusion PE (after removal of thromboemboli from the lung or a lung transplant), reexpansion PE (caused by rapid reexpansion of a collapsed lung), or PE that results from opiate overdose (methadone or heroin), salicylate toxicity (chronic), aspiration (FB inhalation), inhalation injuries, near drowning, pulmonary embolism, viral infections, or pulmonary veno-occlusive disease. Other causes include aspiration, traumatic injury, organ dysfunction caused by sepsis, multiorgan failure, alcoholism or substance abuse, pregnancy (eclampsia), chronic renal impairment, malnutrition, hypertension, or a blood transfusion (transfusion-related ALI).

Pathophysiology

Fluid flows from the pulmonary vasculature into the alveolar interstitial space and then returns to the systemic circulation in a normal lung. Movement of this fluid is controlled by the net difference between hydrostatic and osmotic pressures and the permeability of the capillary membrane (Sovari and Ooi, 2008). Increased pulmonary hydrostatic pressure or increased permeability of the vascular membrane results in movement of fluid into the alveoli and interstitium of the lung. The pulmonary lymph system normally drains away any fluid from the alveoli, but when the amount of fluid present in the alveoli exceeds lymph drainage, PE occurs.

Symptoms include extreme shortness of breath, cyanosis, tachypnea, diminished breath sounds, anxiety, agitation, confusion, diaphoresis, orthopnea, respiratory crackles, expiratory wheezing (in young infants), heart murmur, S3 gallop, cool peripheries, jugular venous distension, nocturnal dyspnea, cough, pink frothy sputum (if severe), tachycardia, hypertension, and hypotension (if caused by left ventricle dysfunction).

Therapeutic Management

Management of PE depends on the cause but can include oxygen therapy, peak end-expiratory pressure (PEEP) via continuous positive airway pressure (CPAP), and intubation with ventilatory support if respiratory failure occurs. If ventricular failure is the cause, medications such as diuretics, digoxin, positive inotropes, and vasodilators (nitroglycerin) may be started, and the child may be placed on a fluid and sodium restriction. Morphine may be prescribed to relieve dyspnea. The primary goal of management is to determine why it occurred and treat the underlying condition.

Nursing Care Management

Nursing care of the child with PE is similar to that for any other respiratory condition. Pulse oximetry is monitored, and vital signs are observed closely for any deterioration. The nurse should note changes in SaO_2, end-tidal CO_2, and arterial blood gas (ABG) values. An ongoing assessment of the child's cardiopulmonary status is needed by checking lung sounds and observing respiratory rate, rhythm, depth, and effort. Oxygen, medications, and other respiratory treatments are administered as prescribed. Close monitoring of intake and output, electrolytes, and comfort are important. The child should be monitored for restlessness, anxiety, and air hunger. Placing the child in a high Fowler position may help with lung expansion. Because this position places pressure on bony prominences in the sacrum and hips, pressure areas must be relieved at intervals. Most of the care of PE occurs in the intensive care unit, which is anxiety provoking for the child and family. They should be given the opportunity to express their fears and anxieties and to ask questions. (For other nursing care activities, see the section on ARDS and ALI.)

ACUTE RESPIRATORY DISTRESS SYNDROME AND ACUTE LUNG INJURY

Ⓔ Acute lung injury and ARDS are potentially life-threatening inflammatory lung conditions that may occur in both children and adults. The syndromes may be caused by direct injury to the lungs or by systemic insults that lead indirectly to lung injury, categorized by acute onset of bilateral infiltrates consistent with PE, but there is no indication of elevated left atrial pressure. They result in hypoxemia and respiratory failure. Sepsis, trauma, viral pneumonia, aspiration, fat emboli, drug overdose, reperfusion injury after lung transplantation, smoke inhalation, and near-drowning, among others, have been associated with ALI and ARDS. Both conditions are characterized by respiratory distress and hypoxemia that occur within 72 hours of a serious injury or surgery in a person with previously normal lungs. Acute pulmonary inflammation with alveolar capillary membrane destruction results in significant hypoxemia. Mechanical ventilation is often required.

Diagnostic criteria were established by the American European Consensus Conference (Bernard, Artigas, Brigham, and others, 1994) and include radiographic evidence of bilateral alveolar infiltrates, the absence of left-sided heart failure and hypoxemia. Hypoxemia is expressed in terms of the ratio of partial pressure of oxygen (PaO_2) to the fraction of inspired oxygen (FiO_2) (P/F ratio). ALI is differentiated from the more severe syndrome of ARDS by the severity of hypoxemia. In ALI, the P/F ratio is less than or equal to 300; in ARDS, the P/F ratio is less than or equal to 200. ARDS is the most severe in the spectrum of illnesses in relation to the degree of hypoxemia.

Pathologically, the hallmark of ARDS is increased permeability of the alveolar-capillary membrane that results in PE. During the acute phase of ARDS, inflammatory mediators cause damage to the alveolo-capillary membrane, with an increasing pulmonary capillary permeability with resulting interstitial edema. Later stages are characterized by pneumocyte and fibrin infiltration of the alveoli, with the start of either the healing process or fibrosis. When fibrosis occurs, the child may demonstrate respiratory distress and the need for mechanical ventilation. In ARDS, the lungs become stiff as a result of surfactant inactivation; gas diffusion is impaired; and eventually, bronchiolar mucosal swelling and congestive atelectasis occur. The net effect is decreased functional residual capacity, pulmonary hypertension (see Chapter 25), and increased intrapulmonary right-to-left shunting of pulmonary blood flow. Surfactant secretion is reduced, and the atelectasis and fluid-filled alveoli provide an excellent medium for bacterial growth. Hypoxemia or increased work of breathing may require ventilatory support.

The child with ARDS may first demonstrate only symptoms caused by an injury or infection, but as the condition deteriorates, hyperventilation, tachypnea, increasing respiratory effort, cyanosis, and decreasing oxygen saturation occur. At times, the developing hypoxemia is not responsive to oxygen administration.

Treatment involves supportive measures to maintain adequate oxygenation and pulmonary perfusion, treatment of infection (or the precipitating cause), and maintenance of adequate cardiac output. After the underlying cause has been identified, specific treatment (e.g., antibiotics for infection) is initiated. Many patients require mechanical ventilatory support. This is usually achieved invasively (i.e., with endotracheal intubation), but occasionally non-invasive ventilation is used in milder cases. Patients requiring invasive mechanical ventilation usually require sedation, at least initially, to allow for ventilatory synchrony. Fluid administration to maintain adequate intravascular volume and end-organ perfusion must be balanced against the desire to decrease lung fluid to improve oxygenation. The provision of adequate nutrition, maintenance of patient comfort, and prevention of complications such as gastrointestinal ulceration are essential. Psychological support of the patient and family is also important.

It has been demonstrated that inappropriate use of mechanical ventilatory support may worsen the lung injury by causing volutrauma, barotrauma, atelectrauma, and biotrauma to the injured lungs. Protective ventilatory strategies using low tidal volumes (6 ml/kg ideal body weight) have been demonstrated to improve outcomes in adults and theoretically are also appropriate in children. PEEP is applied to decrease atelectasis and maintain an "open" lung. Permissive hypercapnia may also be used. Other strategies used in the support of patients with ARDS include use of the prone position, inhaled nitric oxide, inhaled prostaglandins, high-frequency oscillatory ventilation, and extracorporeal membrane support (ECMO), although evidence to support these therapies is scant.

Prognosis

The prognosis for patients with ARDS is improving. Nonetheless, the mortality rate remains high, and in children, it ranges from 18% to 49% (Albuali, Singh, Fraser, and others, 2007; Randolph, 2009). The precipitating disorder influences the outcome; the worst prognosis is associated with uncontrolled sepsis, bone marrow transplantation, cancer, and multisystem involvement with hepatic failure. Children who recover may have persistent cough and exertional dyspnea.

Nursing Care Management

The child with ARDS is cared for in the intensive care unit during the acute stages of illness. Nursing care involves close monitoring of oxygenation and respiratory status as well as assessment of cardiac output,

perfusion, fluid and electrolyte balance, and renal function (urinary output). Acid-base status and pulse oximetry are important evaluation tools. Diuretics may be administered to reduce pulmonary fluid, and vasodilators may be administered to decrease pulmonary vascular pressure. Nutritional support is often required because of the prolonged acute phase of the illness. Nursing management also includes monitoring the effects of the numerous parenteral fluids and drugs used to stabilize the child and monitoring for changes in the child's hemodynamic status. Most children with ARDS require invasive monitoring via a central venous catheter. The nursing care of the child with ARDS also involves close observance of skin condition, prevention of skin breakdown by pressure area relief, and passive range of motion for prevention of muscle atrophy and contractures. Respiratory distress is a frightening situation for both the child and the parents, and attention to their psychologic needs is a major element in the care of these children. The child is often sedated during the acute phase of the illness, and weaning from sedation requires close monitoring for anxiety reduction and comfort.

SMOKE INHALATION INJURY

A number of noxious substances that may be inhaled are toxic to humans. They are primarily products of incomplete combustion and cause more deaths from fires than flame injuries. The severity of the injury depends on the nature of the substances generated by the material burned, whether the victim is confined in a closed space, and the duration of contact with the smoke. Three distinct syndromes of pulmonary complications may occur in children with inhalation injury: (1) early carbon monoxide (CO) poisoning, airway obstruction, and PE; (2) ARDS occurring at 24 to 48 hours or later in some cases; and (3) late complications of bronchopneumonia and pulmonary emboli (Antoon and Donovan, 2011). Smoke inhalation results in three types of injury: heat, chemical, and systemic.

Heat injury involves thermal injury to the upper airway. Air has low specific heat; therefore, the injury goes no farther than the upper airway. Reflex closure of the glottis prevents injury to the lower airway.

Chemical injury involves gases that may be generated during the combustion of materials such as clothing, furniture, and floor coverings. Acids, alkalis, and their precursors in smoke can produce chemical burns. These substances can be carried deep into the respiratory tract, including the lower respiratory tract, in the form of insoluble gases. Soluble gases tend to dissolve in the upper respiratory tract.

Synthetic materials are especially toxic, producing gases such as oxides of sulfur and nitrogen, acetaldehyde, formaldehyde, hydrocyanic acid, and chlorine. Heated plastics are the source of extremely toxic vapors, including chlorine and hydrochloric acid from polyvinyl-chloride, and hydrocarbons, aldehydes, ketones, and acids from polyethylene. Irritant gases such as nitrous oxide and carbon dioxide combine with water in the lungs to form corrosive acids; aldehydes cause denaturation of proteins, cellular damage, and edema of pulmonary tissues. Chemical burns to the airways are similar to burns on the skin, except they are painless because the tracheobronchial tree is relatively insensitive to pain.

Inhalation of small amounts of noxious irritants produces alveolar and bronchiolar damage that can lead to obstructive bronchiolitis. Severe exposure causes further injury, including alveolocapillary damage with hemorrhage, necrotizing bronchiolitis, inhibited secretion of surfactant, and formation of hyaline membranes—manifestations of ARDS.

Systemic injury occurs from gases that are nontoxic to the airways (e.g., CO, hydrogen cyanide). However, these gases cause injury and death by interfering with or inhibiting cellular respiration. CO is responsible for more than half of all fatal inhalation poisonings in the United States. CO is a colorless, odorless gas with an affinity for hemoglobin 230 times greater than that of oxygen. When it enters the bloodstream, CO combines readily with hemoglobin to form carboxyhemoglobin (COHb). Because it is released less readily, tissue hypoxia reaches dangerous levels before oxygen is available to meet tissue needs.

> ### ! NURSING ALERT
>
> The oxygen saturation (SaO_2) obtained by pulse oximetry will be normal because the device measures only oxygenated and deoxygenated hemoglobin; it does not measure dysfunctional hemoglobin, such as COHb.

Accidental CO poisoning is most often a result of exposure to fumes of heaters or smoke from structural fires, although poorly ventilated recreational vehicles with improperly operated or maintained gas lamps or stoves and cooking in underventilated areas with charcoal grills are also frequent causes. CO is produced by incomplete combustion of carbon or carbonaceous material such as wood or charcoal.

The signs and symptoms of CO poisoning are secondary to tissue hypoxia and vary with the level of COHb. Mild manifestations include headache, visual disturbances, irritability, and nausea; more severe intoxication causes confusion, hallucinations, ataxia, and coma. The bright, cherry red lips and skin often described are less often observed; pallor and cyanosis are seen more frequently.

Therapeutic Management

Treatment of children with smoke inhalation injury is largely symptomatic. The most widely accepted treatment is placing the child on humidified 100% oxygen as quickly as possible and monitoring for signs of respiratory distress and impending failure. Baseline ABGs and COHb levels are obtained. PaO_2 may be within normal limits unless there is marked respiratory depression. If CO poisoning is confirmed, 100% oxygen is continued until COHb levels fall to the nontoxic range of about 10%. If CO poisoning is severe, the patient may benefit from hyperbaric oxygen therapy. Hyperbaric oxygen therapy may be useful in the treatment of neurologic complications related to CO poisoning. Pulmonary care may be facilitated by bronchodilators, inhaled corticosteroids, humidification, and chest percussion and postural drainage to enhance the removal of necrotic material, minimize bronchoconstriction, and avoid atelectasis. Bronchoscopy may be needed to clear heavy secretions.

Respiratory distress may occur early in the course of smoke inhalation as a result of hypoxia, or patients who are breathing well on admission may suddenly develop respiratory distress. Therefore, intubation equipment should be readily available. Transient edema of the airways can occur at any level in the tracheobronchial tree. Assessment and localization of the obstruction should be accomplished before severe swelling of the head, neck, or oropharynx occurs. Intubation is often necessary when (1) severe burns in the area of the nose, mouth, and face increase the likelihood of developing oropharyngeal edema and obstruction; (2) vocal cord edema causes obstruction; (3) the patient has difficulty handling secretions; and (4) progressive respiratory distress requires artificial ventilation. Controversy surrounds tracheostomy, but many prefer this procedure when the obstruction is proximal to the larynx and reserve nasotracheal intubation for lower tract involvement.

Nursing Care Management

Nursing care of the child with inhalation injury is the same as that for any child with respiratory distress. Vital signs and other respiratory assessments (oxygenation, work of breathing, acid-base status) are performed frequently, and the pulmonary status is carefully observed and maintained. Chest percussion and postural drainage is often part of the therapy, as well as mechanical ventilation if needed. Fluid requirements for children experiencing inhalation injury are greater than for those with surface burns alone; however, one concern is the development of PE. Therefore, accurate monitoring of fluid intake and output is essential.

In addition to observation and management of the physical aspects of inhalation injury, the nurse also deals with the psychologic needs of a frightened child and distraught parents. As with any accidental injury, the parents may feel overwhelming guilt even when the injury occurred through no fault of their own. Parents need support, reassurance, and information regarding the child's condition, treatment, and progress.

The nurse can provide anticipatory guidance and education families on prevention of inhalation injuries and the importance of CO detectors in the home.

ENVIRONMENTAL TOBACCO SMOKE EXPOSURE

Numerous investigations indicate that parental or family smoking is an important cause of morbidity in children. Children exposed to (second-hand) passive or environmental tobacco smoke have an increased number of respiratory illnesses, increased respiratory symptoms (i.e., cough, sputum, and wheezing), and reduced performance on pulmonary function tests (PFTs). AOM and OME are also increased in children who have smoking parents. Indoor exposure to tobacco smoke has been linked to asthma in children. Among children with asthma, there is an association between parental cigarette smoking and asthma exacerbations, trips to the emergency department (ED), medication use, and impaired recovery after hospitalization for acute asthma. Maternal cigarette smoking is associated with increased respiratory symptoms and illnesses in children; decreased fetal growth; increased deliveries of low–birth-weight, preterm, and stillborn infants; and a greater incidence of sudden infant death syndrome (SIDS). Antenatal maternal smoking has emerged as a significant risk factor for SIDS (AAP, Task Force on Sudden Infant Death Syndrome, 2005). The risk for diagnosis of early-onset asthma in the first 3 years of life is associated with in utero exposure to maternal smoking; grandmaternal smoking was also associated with an increased risk of early-onset asthma in the grandchild even if the mother did not smoke during pregnancy (Li, Langholz, Salam, and others, 2005). Exposure to tobacco smoke during childhood may also contribute to the development of chronic lung disease in the adult.

Nursing Care Management

Nurses must provide information about the hazards of environmental smoke exposure in all of their interactions with children and their family members. This information is especially important for children with respiratory and allergic illnesses. In families in which smokers refuse to quit, appropriate guidance is provided for reducing smoke in the child's environment (see Family-Centered Care box). Nurses should set an example for children and families and become advocates for "no smoking" ordinances in public places, prohibition of advertising tobacco products in the media, and inclusion of health warnings of sidestream smoke on tobacco products.* Nurses have an important role in providing parents with affordable smoking cessation education

---

*For further information on the effects of second-hand smoke on child health, go to http://www.cdc.gov/Features/WorldCancerDay.

FAMILY-CENTERED CARE

Decreasing Childhood Exposure to Environmental Tobacco Smoke

- Maintain a smoke-free home.
- Avoid exposing an infant to environmental smoke.
- Use an air-purifying filter in the home where smoking is unavoidable.
- Encourage exclusive breastfeeding for the first 6 months.
- If smoking cessation is in progress by breastfeeding mother, suggest she change upper clothing after smoking and before breastfeeding infant.
- Do not smoke around children.
- Change clothing after smoking and before holding an infant in close proximity. Suggest wearing a removable outer garment for smoking that is removed on return to the house or when in contact with the child.
- Restrict smoking to an isolated area of the house or outside the house where the children do not play or sleep.
- Do not smoke in motor vehicles with children.
- Do not smoke in rooms children use.
- Do not allow visitors to smoke in the home.

resources, including the appropriate use of smoking cessation pharmacologic aids (Sheahan and Free, 2005). Nurses also have a role in educating adolescents about avoiding using tobacco products or smoking marijuana.

LONG-TERM RESPIRATORY DYSFUNCTION

ASTHMA

Asthma is a chronic inflammatory disorder of the airways characterized by recurring symptoms, airway obstruction, and bronchial hyperresponsiveness (National Asthma Education and Prevention Program [NAEPP], 2007). In susceptible children, inflammation causes recurrent episodes of wheezing, breathlessness, chest tightness, and cough, especially at night or in the early morning. The airflow limitation or obstruction is reversible either spontaneously or with treatment. Inflammation causes an increase in bronchial hyperresponsiveness to a variety of stimuli (NAEPP, 2007). Recognition of the key role of inflammation has made the use of antiinflammatory agents, especially inhaled steroids, a major component in the treatment of asthma.

Asthma is classified into four categories based on the symptom indicators of disease severity. These categories are intermittent, mild persistent, moderate persistent, and severe persistent. Symptoms increase in frequency or intensity until the last category of severe persistent asthma (Box 23-14). These categories provide a stepwise approach to the pharmacologic management, environmental control, and educational interventions needed for each category (NAEPP, 2007). These categories emphasize the multifaceted aspect of the disease for consideration of effects on present quality of life and functional capacity and the future risk of adverse events (NAEPP, 2007).

Asthma prevalence, morbidity, and mortality are increasing in the United States, especially among African Americans (Akinbami, Moorman, Garbe, and others, 2009). These increases may result from worsening air pollution, poor access to medical care, or underdiagnosis and undertreatment. Asthma is the most common chronic disease of childhood, the primary cause of school absences, and the third leading cause of hospitalizations in children younger than the age of 15 years. Although the onset of asthma may occur at any age, 80% to 90% of

BOX 23-14 ASTHMA SEVERITY CLASSIFICATION IN CHILDREN*

Step 5 OR 6: Severe Persistent Asthma
Continual symptoms throughout the day
Frequent nighttime symptoms (>1 time/wk ages 0–4 and 7 nights/wk, ages 5 and older)
PEF: <60%
FEV$_1$: <75% of predicted value
Interference with normal activity: extremely limited
Use of short-acting β-agonist for symptom control: several times a day

Step 3 OR 4: Moderate Persistent Asthma
Daily symptoms
Nighttime symptoms: 3 to 4 times a month (ages 0–4 years), >1/wk but not nightly (ages 5–11 years)
PEF: 60% to 80% of predicted value (ages 5 and over)
FEV$_1$: 75% to 80% (ages 5 and over)
PEF variability: >30%
Interference with normal activity: some limitation
Use of short-acting β-agonist for symptom control: daily

Step 2: Mild Persistent Asthma
Symptoms >2 times/wk but <1 time/day
Nighttime symptoms: 1 to 2 times a month (ages 0–4 years), 3 to 4 times a month (ages 5–11 years)
PEF or FEV$_1$: ≥80% of predicted value
PEF variability: 20% to 30%
Interference with normal activity: minor limitation
Use of short-acting β-agonist for symptom control: >2 days/wk but not daily

Step 1: Intermittent Asthma
Symptoms ≤2 days/wk
Nighttime symptoms (awakenings): ≤2 nights per month
PEF or FEV$_1$: ≤80% of predicted value
PEF variability: <20%
Interference with normal activity: none
Use of short-acting β-agonist for symptom control: <2 days/wk

From National Asthma Education and Prevention Program: *Guidelines for the diagnosis and management of asthma: summary report 2007,* retrieved June 24, 2011, from http://www.nhlbi.nih.gov/guidelines/asthma/index.htm.
FEV$_1$, Forced expiratory volume in 1 second; *PEF,* peak expiratory flow.
*The presence of one clinical feature of severity is sufficient to place a patient in that category. An individual should be assigned to the most severe grade in which any feature occurs. The characteristics in this table are general and may overlap because asthma is highly variable. An individual's classification may change over time. Risk factors for each category are not presented in this table. See the original table referenced below for additional classification data. Asthma treatment should not be based on this table.

children have their first symptoms before 4 or 5 years of age. Boys are affected more frequently than girls until adolescence, when the trend reverses.

Etiology

Studies of children with asthma indicate that allergies influence both the persistence and the severity of the disease. In fact, atopy, or the genetic predisposition for the development of an immunoglobulin E (IgE)–mediated response to common aeroallergens, is the strongest identifiable predisposing factor for developing asthma (NAEPP, 2007). However, 20% to 40% of children with asthma have no evidence of allergic disease. In addition to allergens, other substances and conditions can serve as triggers that may exacerbate asthma (Box 23-15). Evidence shows that viral respiratory infections, including RSV infection, may also have a significant role in the development and expression of asthma (NAEPP, 2007).

Pathophysiology

There is general agreement that inflammation contributes to heightened airway reactivity in asthma. The mechanisms contributing to airway inflammation are multiple and involve a number of different pathways. It is unlikely that asthma is caused by either a single cell or a single inflammatory mediator; rather, it appears that asthma results from complex interactions among inflammatory cells, mediators, and the cells and tissues present in the airways (NAEPP, 2007). However, recognition of the importance of inflammation has made the use of anti-inflammatory agents a key component of asthma therapy.

Another important component of asthma is bronchospasm and obstruction. The mechanisms responsible for the obstructive symptoms in asthma include (1) inflammatory response to stimuli; (2) airway edema and accumulation and secretion of mucus; (3) spasm of the smooth muscle of the bronchi and bronchioles, which decreases the caliber of the bronchioles; and (4) airway remodeling, which causes permanent cellular changes (NAEPP, 2007) (Fig. 23-4).

Airflow is determined by the size of the airway lumen, degree of bronchial wall edema, mucus production, smooth muscle contraction, and muscle hypertrophy. Bronchial constriction is a normal reaction to foreign stimuli, but with asthma, it is abnormally severe, producing impaired respiratory function. Because the bronchi normally dilate and elongate during inspiration and contract and shorten on expiration, the respiratory difficulty is more pronounced during the expiratory phase of respiration.

Increased resistance in the airway causes forced expiration through the narrowed lumen. The volume of air trapped in the lungs increases as airways are functionally closed at a point between the alveoli and the lobar bronchi. This trapping of gas forces the individual to breathe at higher and higher lung volumes. Consequently, the person with asthma fights to inspire sufficient air. This expenditure of effort for breathing causes fatigue, decreased respiratory effectiveness, and increased oxygen consumption. The inspiration occurring at higher lung volumes hyperinflates the alveoli and reduces the effectiveness of the cough. As the severity of obstruction increases, there is a reduced alveolar ventilation with carbon dioxide retention; hypoxemia; respiratory acidosis; and, eventually, respiratory failure.

Chronic inflammation may also cause permanent damage (airway remodeling) to airway structures, which cannot be prevented by and is not responsive to current treatments (NAEPP, 2007).

BOX 23-15   TRIGGERS TENDING TO PRECIPITATE OR AGGRAVATE ASTHMA EXACERBATIONS

- Allergens
  - Outdoor—Trees, shrubs, weeds, grasses, molds, pollens, air pollution, spores
  - Indoor—Dust or dust mites, mold, cockroach antigen
- Irritants—Tobacco smoke, wood smoke, odors, sprays
- Exposure to occupational chemicals
- Exercise
- Cold air
- Changes in weather or temperature
- Environmental change—Moving to new home, starting new school, and so on
- Colds and infections
- Animals—Cats, dogs, rodents, horses
- Medications—Aspirin, NSAIDs, antibiotics, beta-blockers
- Strong emotions—Fear, anger, laughing, crying
- Conditions—Gastroesophageal reflux, tracheoesophageal fistula
- Food additives—Sulfite preservatives
- Foods—Nuts, milk or other dairy products
- Endocrine factors—Menses, pregnancy, thyroid disease

NSAID, Nonsteroidal anti-inflammatory drug.

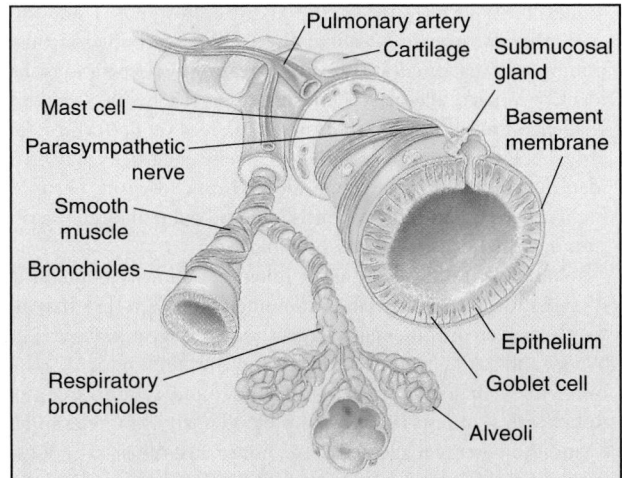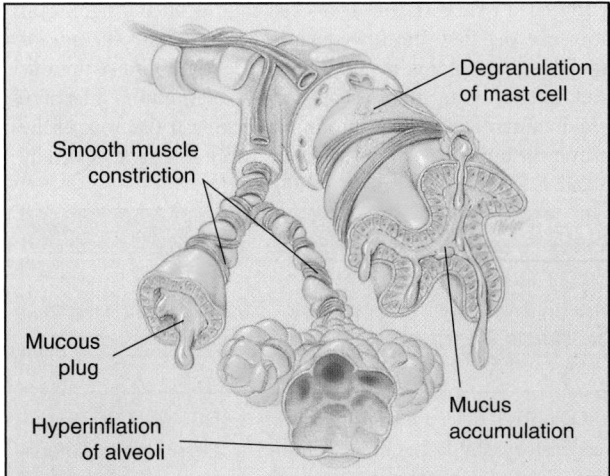

A

B

FIG 23-4 Airway obstruction caused by asthma. **A,** A normal lung. **B,** Bronchial asthma: thick mucus, mucosal edema, and smooth muscle spasm causing obstruction of small airways; breathing becomes labored, and expiration is difficult. (Modified from Des Jardins T, Burton GG: *Clinical manifestations and assessment of respiratory disease,* ed 3, St. Louis, 1995, Mosby.)

BOX 23-16 CLINICAL MANIFESTATIONS OF ASTHMA

Cough
Hacking, paroxysmal, irritative, and nonproductive
Becomes rattling and productive of frothy, clear, gelatinous sputum

Respiratory-Related Signs
Shortness of breath
Prolonged expiratory phase
Audible wheeze
May have a malar flush and red ears
Lips deep, dark red color
May progress to cyanosis of nail beds or circumoral cyanosis
Restlessness
Apprehension
Prominent sweating as the attack progresses
Older children sitting upright with shoulders in a hunched-over position, hands on the bed or chair, and arms braced (tripod)
Speaking with short, panting, broken phrases

Chest
Hyperresonance on percussion
Coarse, loud breath sounds
Wheezes throughout the lung fields
Prolonged expiration
Crackles
Generalized inspiratory and expiratory wheezing; increasingly high pitched

With Repeated Episodes
Barrel chest
Elevated shoulders
Use of accessory muscles of respiration
Facial appearance—flattened malar bones, dark circles beneath the eyes, narrow nose, prominent upper teeth

Diagnostic Evaluation

The classic manifestations of asthma are dyspnea, wheezing, and coughing. An attack may develop gradually or appear abruptly and may be preceded by a URI. The age of the child is often a significant factor because the first attack frequently occurs before the age of 5 years, with some children manifesting clinical signs and symptoms in infancy. In infancy, an attack usually follows a respiratory infection. Some children may experience a prodromal itching at the front of the neck or over the upper part of the back just before an attack, especially if the attack is related to allergies (Box 23-16).

! NURSING ALERT

Shortness of breath with air movement in the chest restricted to the point of absent breath sounds (silent chest) accompanied by a sudden rise in respiratory rate is an ominous sign indicating ventilatory failure and imminent respiratory arrest.

The diagnosis is determined primarily on the basis of clinical manifestations, history, physical examination, and, to a lesser extent, laboratory tests. Generally, chronic cough in the absence of infection or diffuse wheezing during the expiratory phase of respiration is sufficient to establish a diagnosis.

Pulmonary function tests provide an objective method of evaluating the presence and degree of lung disease, as well as the response to

📋 NURSING CARE GUIDELINES
*Interpreting Peak Expiratory Flow Rates**

- **Green (80%–100% of personal best)** signals all clear. Asthma is under reasonably good control. No symptoms are present, and the routine treatment plan for maintaining control can be followed.
- **Yellow (50%–79% of personal best)** signals caution. Asthma is not well controlled. An acute exacerbation may be present. Maintenance therapy may need to be increased. Call the practitioner if the child stays in this zone.
- **Red (<50% of personal best)** signals a medical alert. Severe airway narrowing may be occurring. A short-acting bronchodilator should be administered. Notify the practitioner if the peak expiratory flow rate does not return immediately and stay in yellow or green zones.

*These zones are guidelines only. Specific zones and management should be individualized for each child.

therapy. Spirometry can generally be performed reliably on children by the age of 5 or 6 years. The NAEPP (2007) recommends that spirometry testing be done at the time of initial assessment of asthma, after treatment is initiated and symptoms have stabilized, and at least every 1 to 2 years to assess the maintenance of airway function.

Another measurement to consider is the peak expiratory flow rate (PEFR), which measures the maximum flow of air that can be forcefully exhaled in 1 second. PEFR is measured in liters per minute using a peak expiratory flow meter (PEFM). Three zones of measurement are typically used to interpret PEFR. The zone system is patterned after a traffic light to make the categories easy to understand and remember (see Nursing Care Guidelines box). Each child needs to establish his or her personal best value. A personal best value should be established during a 2- to 3-week period when the child's asthma is stable. During this period, the child records the PEFR at least twice a day. After the personal best value has been established, the child's current PEFR on any occasion can be compared with the personal best value. Although it can be a helpful tool in assessing a child's asthma control, it is important to note that its results depend on the child's ability to use the PEFM and willingness to participate. In some cases, a low PEFR may not truly mean that the child's asthma is poorly controlled. Each individual child's PEFR varies according to age, height, sex, and race.

Bronchoprovocation testing, direct exposure of the mucous membranes to a suspected antigen in increasing concentrations, helps to identify inhaled allergens. Exposure to methacholine (methacholine challenge), histamine, or cold or dry air may be performed to assess airway responsiveness or reactivity. Exercise challenges may be used to identify children with exercise-induced bronchospasm. These tests are highly specific and sensitive but should be done under close observation in a qualified laboratory or clinic.

Skin prick testing (SPT) and serological testing (with quantification of sIgE) for allergen-specific immunoglobulin E (sIgE) may be used to identify environmental allergens which trigger asthma (Sicherer, Wood, and AAP Section on Allergy and Immunology, 2012). It is recommended that all patients with year-round asthma symptoms be tested with skin tests or laboratory blood analysis to determine sensitization to perennial allergens (e.g., house dust mites, cats, dogs, cockroaches, molds, and fungus) (NAEPP, 2007).

In addition to these tests, other tests may be performed, including laboratory tests (complete blood count [CBC] with differential) and chest radiographs. The CBC may show a slight elevation in the white blood cell count during acute asthma, but elevations to more than

12,000/mm^3 or an increased percentage of band cells may indicate a respiratory tract infection. The presence of eosinophilia of greater than 500/mm^3, on the other hand, tends to suggest an allergic or inflammatory disorder.

Frontal and lateral radiographs may show infiltrates and hyperexpansion of the airways, with the anteroposterior diameter on physical examination indicating an increased diameter (suggestive of barrel chest). Additional diagnostic tests for conditions such as gastroesophageal reflux may be carried out to determine whether they may contribute to asthma symptoms. Radiography may assist in ruling out a respiratory tract infection.

Therapeutic Management

The overall goals of asthma management are to maintain normal activity levels, maintain normal pulmonary function, prevent chronic symptoms and recurrent exacerbations, provide optimum drug therapy with minimum or no adverse effects, and assist the child in living as normal and happy a life as possible. This includes facilitating the child's social adjustments in the family, school, and community and normal participation in recreational activities and sports. To accomplish these goals, several treatment principles need to be followed (NAEPP, 2007):

- A continuous care approach with regular visits to the health care provider is necessary to control symptoms and prevent exacerbations.
- Prevention of exacerbations includes avoiding triggers, avoiding allergens, and using medications as needed.
- Therapy includes efforts to reduce underlying inflammation and to relieve or prevent symptomatic airway narrowing.
- Therapy includes patient education, environmental control, pharmacologic management, and the use of objective measures to monitor the severity of disease and guide the course of therapy.

Allergen Control

Nonpharmacologic therapy is aimed at the prevention and reduction of exposure to airborne allergens and irritants. House dust mites and other components of house dust are frequent agents identified in children who are allergic to inhalants. The cockroach, another common household inhabitant, is an important allergen in many locations. Exterminating live cockroaches, carefully cleaning kitchen floors and cabinets, putting food away after eating, and taking trash out in the evening are essential measures to control cockroaches. The mouse allergen is the most recent allergen to be identified in the homes of inner-city children with asthma. The role of cat and dog dander in allergen-induced asthma has also been studied. Although some studies suggest sensitized persons should carefully evaluate having such pets in the household, the overall data are inconsistent on the effect of cat or dog exposure and subsequent asthma development (Chen, Tischer, Schnappinger, and others, 2010). Additional sources of pollutants include ozone, particulate matter produced by tobacco smoke, woodburning stoves, pesticides, lead, mold spores, nitrogen dioxide, and sulfur dioxide; these are believed to contribute to asthma morbidity in children and should be avoided or minimized. Living in homes close to busy roads, damp homes with mold, and exposure to tobacco smoke are significant contributing factors in the development of asthma in infants and small children (Heinrich, 2011).

Skin testing identifies specific allergens so steps can be taken to eliminate or avoid them. Often, simply removing the offending environmental allergens or irritants (e.g., removing carpeting from the home of a child sensitive to mold and dust particles) will decrease the frequency of asthma episodes. Dehumidifiers or air conditioners may control nonspecific factors that trigger an episode, such as extremes of temperature.

Drug Therapy

Pharmacologic therapy is used to prevent and control asthma symptoms, reduce the frequency and severity of asthma exacerbations, and reverse airflow obstruction. A stepwise approach is recommended based on the severity of the child's asthma. Because inflammation is considered an early and persistent feature of asthma, therapy is directed toward long-term suppression of inflammation.

Asthma medications are categorized into two general classes: long-term control medications (preventive medications) to achieve and maintain control of inflammation, and quick-relief medications (rescue medications) to treat symptoms and exacerbations (NAEPP, 2007).

Quick-relief and long-term medications are often used in combination. Inhaled corticosteroids, cromolyn sodium and nedocromil, long-acting β_2-agonists, methylxanthines, and leukotriene modifiers are used as long-term control medications. Short-acting β_2-agonists, anticholinergics, and systemic corticosteroids are used as quick-relief or rescue medications.

Many asthma medications are given by inhalation with a nebulizer or a metered-dose inhaler (MDI). The MDI should always be attached to a spacer, especially when an inhaled corticosteroid is administered to prevent yeast infections in the mouth. The spacer and holder can be equipped with a mask or a mouthpiece. Pharmaceutical companies are currently mandated to produce inhalers that do not contain chlorofluorocarbons (CFCs) as the propellant because CFCs have been linked to damage and depletion of the earth's ozone level. Several currently available CFC-free MDI devices use dry powder (and are called dry powder inhalers); these include the Diskus inhaler and the Turbuhaler. These devices are breath activated, and the child needs to inhale as quickly and deeply as possible to use them effectively. The Diskhaler and Aerosolizer are similar, but with the Aerosolizer, the medication must be loaded into the inhaler before use. Children who have difficulty using MDIs or other inhalers can receive their asthma medications via a nebulizer, which administers the medication via compressed air or oxygen. Children are instructed to breathe normally with the mouth open to provide a direct route to the trachea.

Corticosteroids are anti-inflammatory drugs used to treat reversible airflow obstruction, control symptoms, and reduce bronchial hyperresponsiveness in chronic asthma. Inhaled corticosteroids are used as first-line therapy in children older than 5 years of age. Clinical studies of corticosteroids have indicated significant improvement of all asthma parameters, including decreases in symptoms, emergency visits, and medication requirements (NAEPP, 2007).

Corticosteroids may be administered parenterally, orally, or by inhalation. Oral medications are metabolized slowly, with an onset of action up to 3 hours after administration and peak effectiveness occurring within 6 to 12 hours. Oral systemic steroids may be given for short periods of time (e.g., 3- or 10-day "bursts") to gain prompt control of inadequately controlled persistent asthma or to manage severe persistent asthma. These drugs should be given in the lowest effective dose. These medications have few side effects (cough, dysphonia, and oral thrush), and strong evidence indicates that they improve the long-term outcomes for children of all ages with mild or moderate persistent asthma. Some studies have monitored children for 6 years after starting inhaled corticosteroids, and they indicate that when used at recommended doses, they do not have long-term significant effects on growth, bone mineral density, ocular toxicity, or suppression of the adrenal–pituitary axis (NAEPP, 2007). However, primary care providers should frequently monitor the growth of children and adolescents taking corticosteroids to assess the systemic effects of these drugs and make appropriate reductions in dosages or changes to other types of asthma therapy when necessary. Inhaled corticosteroids include budesonide and fluticasone.

β-Adrenergic agonists (short acting) (primarily albuterol, levalbuterol [Xopenex]**,** and terbutaline) are used for treatment of acute exacerbations and for the prevention of exercise-induced bronchospasm. These drugs bind with the β-receptors on the smooth muscle of airways, where they activate adenylate cyclase and convert adenosine monophosphate (AMP) to cyclic AMP (cAMP). It is believed that the increased cAMP enhances binding of intracellular calcium to the cell membrane, reducing the availability of calcium and thus allowing smooth muscle to relax. Other effects of the drug help stabilize mast cells to prevent release of mediators. Most β-adrenergics used in asthma therapy affect predominantly the β₂-receptors, which help eliminate bronchospasm. β₁-receptor effects, such as increased heart rate and gastrointestinal disturbances, have been minimized. Albuterol is given orally (liquid or pill) or via a nebulizer or inhaler. Levalbuterol is given via nebulizer only. Terbutaline is given orally, via nebulizer, subcutaneously, or intravenously. The inhaled drugs have a more rapid onset of action than oral forms. Inhalation also reduces troublesome systemic side effects, including irritability, tremor, nervousness, and insomnia.

Salmeterol (Serevent) is a long-acting β₂-agonist (bronchodilator) that is used twice a day (no more frequently than every 12 hours). This drug is added to antiinflammatory therapy and used for long-term prevention of symptoms, especially nighttime symptoms, and exercise-induced bronchospasm. Salmeterol is not used in children younger than 12 years of age, and it is not used to treat acute symptoms or exacerbations. The 2007 NAEPP guidelines recommend the addition of a long-acting β₂-agonist (e.g., Salmeterol) to a low- or medium-dosage inhaled corticosteroid to improve lung function and asthma symptoms and decrease the need for a short-acting β₂-agonist. Currently, the FDA is requiring studies be conducted by drug manufacturers to evaluate the safety of long-acting β₂-agonists (LABAs) when combined with inhaled corticosteroids versus inhaled corticosteroids alone. LABAs can increase the risk of severely worsening asthma symptoms, potentially leading to hospitalizations and death (FDA, 2011).

Theophylline is a methylxanthine drug used for decades to relieve symptoms and prevent asthma attacks; however, it is now used primarily in the ED when the child is not responding to maximal therapy. Therapeutic levels should be obtained with this drug because it has a narrow therapeutic window.

Cromolyn sodium is a medication used in maintenance therapy for asthma. It stabilizes mast cell membranes; inhibits activation and release of mediators from eosinophil and epithelial cells; and inhibits the acute airway narrowing after exposure to exercise, cold dry air, and sulfur dioxide. It does not result in immediate relief of symptoms and has minimal side effects (occasional coughing on inhalation of the powder formulation). It may be given via nebulizer or MDI. **Nedocromil sodium** inhibits the bronchoconstrictor response to inhaled antigens and inhibits the activity of and release of inflammatory cell types such as histamine, leukotrienes, and prostaglandins. The drug has few side effects and is used for maintenance therapy in asthma; it is not effective for reversal of acute exacerbations and is not used in children younger than 5 years of age.

Leukotrienes are mediators of inflammation that cause increases in airway hyperresponsiveness. Leukotriene modifiers (e.g., zafirlukast [Accolate] and montelukast sodium [Singulair]) block inflammatory and bronchospasm effects. These drugs are not used to treat acute episodes but are given orally in combination with β-agonists and steroids to provide long-term control and prevent symptoms in mild persistent asthma. Montelukast is approved for children 12 months old and older, and zafirkulast is approved for children 7 years and older.

Anticholinergics (atropine and ipratropium [Atrovent]) may also be used for relief of acute bronchospasm. However, these drugs have adverse side effects that include drying of respiratory secretions, blurred vision, and cardiac and CNS stimulation. The primary anticholinergic drug used is ipratropium, which does not cross the blood–brain barrier and therefore elicits no CNS effects. Ipratropium, when used in combination with albuterol, has been shown to be effective during acute severe asthma in significantly improving lung function and reducing hospitalizations in children coming to the ED.

A fairly new asthma drug, omalizumab (Xolair), is a **monoclonal antibody** that blocks the binding of IgE to mast cells. Blocking this interaction eventually inhibits the inflammation that is associated with asthma. It is used in patients with moderate to persistent asthma who have confirmed perennial aeroallergen sensitivity and have had poor control of symptoms on inhaled steroids. Many patients with asthma are atopic and possess specific IgE antibodies to allergens responsible for airway inflammation. Xolair has been approved for use in children 12 years and older. The drug is administered once or twice a month by subcutaneous injection. Efficacy of omalizumab is not immediate. Clinical trials report that response to the drug was not evident before 12 weeks (Strunk and Bloomberg, 2006). The drug is expensive (Courtney, McCarter, and Pollart, 2005), however, and there have been reported cases of severe anaphylactic reactions. In early 2007, the FDA added a "black box warning" to the drug, which highlights the risk of anaphylaxis. In 2009, the FDA reported an increase in cardiovascular and cerebrovascular adverse events related to its use (FDA, 2009).

Some children with severe asthma and a history of severe life-threatening episodes may need a primary care practitioner prescription for an EpiPen (subcutaneous injectable epinephrine).

Exercise

Exercise-induced bronchospasm (EIB) is an acute, reversible, usually self-terminating airway obstruction that develops during or after vigorous activity, reaches its peak 5 to 10 minutes after stopping the activity, and usually stops in another 20 to 30 minutes. Patients with EIB have cough, shortness of breath, chest pain or tightness, wheezing, and endurance problems during exercise, but an exercise challenge test in a laboratory is necessary to make the diagnosis.

The problem is rare in activities that require short bursts of energy (e.g., baseball, sprints, gymnastics, skiing) and more common in those that involve endurance exercise (e.g., soccer, basketball, distance running). Swimming is well tolerated by children with EIB because they are breathing air fully saturated with moisture and because of the type of breathing required in swimming.

Children with asthma are often excluded from exercise by parents, teachers, and practitioners, as well as by the children themselves because they are reluctant to provoke an attack. However, this practice can seriously hamper peer interaction and physical health. Exercise is advantageous for children with asthma, and most children can participate in activities at school and in sports with minimal difficulty, provided their asthma is under control. Appropriate prophylactic treatment with β-adrenergic agents or cromolyn sodium before exercise usually permits full participation in strenuous exertion.

Breathing Exercises

Breathing exercises and physical training help produce physical and mental relaxation, improve posture, strengthen respiratory musculature, and develop more efficient patterns of breathing. For motivated children, breathing exercises and controlled breathing are of value in preventing overinflation and improving efficiency of the cough. However, these exercises are not recommended during acute, uncomplicated exacerbation of asthma.

Hyposensitization

The role of hyposensitization in childhood asthma has become controversial. In the past, immunotherapy was used for seasonal allergies and when single substances were identified as the offending allergen. It is not recommended for allergens that can be eliminated, such as foods, drugs, and animal dander.

The NAEPP guidelines (2007) recommend immunotherapy for asthma patients in the following situations:
- When there is evidence of a relationship between asthma symptoms and unavoidable exposure to an allergen to which the patient is sensitive
- When symptoms occur all year or at least during a major portion of the year
- When symptom control is difficult with drug therapy because multiple medications are required, the patient is not responsive to available drugs, or the patient refuses to take the medications

Injection therapy is usually limited to clinically significant allergens. The initial dose of the offending allergen(s), based on the size of the skin reaction, is injected subcutaneously. The amount is increased at weekly intervals until a maximum tolerance is reached, after which a maintenance dose is given at 4-week intervals. This may be extended to 5- or 6-week intervals during the off-season for seasonal allergens. Successful treatment is continued for a minimum of 3 years and then stopped. If no symptoms appear, acquired immunity is assumed; if symptoms recur, treatment is reinstituted. Hyposensitization injections should be administered only with emergency equipment and medications readily available in the event of an anaphylactic reaction.

Status Asthmaticus

Status asthmaticus is a medical emergency that can result in respiratory failure and death if untreated. Children who continue to display respiratory distress despite vigorous therapeutic measures, especially the use of sympathomimetics (e.g., albuterol, epinephrine), are considered to be in status asthmaticus. The condition may develop gradually or rapidly, often coincident with complicating conditions, such as pneumonia or a respiratory virus, that can influence the duration and treatment of the exacerbation.

> **! NURSING ALERT**
>
> A child with asthma who sweats profusely, remains sitting upright, and refuses to lie down is in severe respiratory distress. Also, a child who suddenly becomes agitated or an agitated child who suddenly becomes quiet may have serious hypoxia and requires immediate intervention.

Therapy for status asthmaticus is aimed at improving ventilation, decreasing airway resistance and relieving bronchospasm, correcting dehydration and acidosis, allaying child and parent anxiety related to the severity of the event, and treating any concurrent infection. Humidified oxygen is recommended and should be given to maintain an oxygen saturation greater than 90%. Inhaled aerosolized short-acting β_2-agonists are recommended for all patients. Three treatments of β_2-agonists spaced 20 to 30 minutes apart are usually given as initial therapy, and continuous administration of β_2-agonists may be initiated. A systemic corticosteroid (oral, IV, or IM) may also be given to decrease the effects of inflammation. An anticholinergic agent such as ipratropium bromide may be added to the aerosolized solution of the β_2-agonist. Anticholinergics have been shown to result in additional bronchodilation in patients with severe airflow obstruction. An IV infusion is often initiated to provide a means for hydration and to administer medications. Correction of dehydration, acidosis, hypoxia, and electrolyte disturbance is guided by frequent determination of arterial pH, blood gases, and serum electrolytes.

Additional therapies in acute asthma attacks include the use of IV magnesium sulfate, a potent muscle relaxant that acts to decrease inflammation and improves pulmonary function and peak flow rate among pediatric patients treated in the ED with moderate to severe asthma. Heliox may be administered to decrease airway resistance and thereby decrease the work of breathing; heliox can be delivered via a nonrebreathing face mask from premixed tanks, which may be blended in a stand-alone unit or within a ventilator. Heliox may be used in acute exacerbations as an adjunct to β_2-agonist and IV corticosteroid therapy to improve pulmonary function until the two latter medications have time to take full effect in decreasing bronchospasm; whereas the effects of heliox are usually seen within 20 minutes of administration, other drugs may take longer to exert the desired effect. Ketamine, a dissociative anesthetic, is believed to cause smooth muscle relaxation and decrease airway resistance caused by severe bronchospasm in acute asthma; it may be administered as an adjunct to other therapies mentioned previously.

Antibiotics should not be used to treat acute asthma attacks except when a bacterial infection resulting from another condition such as pneumonia or sinusitis is present (NAEPP, 2007). A child suspected of having status asthmaticus is usually seen in the ED and is often admitted to a pediatric intensive care unit for close observation and continuous cardiorespiratory monitoring. A key component in the prevention of morbidity is helping the child, parents, teachers, coaches, and other adults recognize features of deteriorating respiratory status, use the correct rescue drugs effectively, and immediately place the child with deteriorating respiratory status into the care of health care professionals instead of waiting to see if the asthma gets better on its own. For the child going into early status asthmaticus, immediate medical care is required to irreversible respiratory failure and possible death (see Nursing Care Plan).

Prognosis

Although deaths from asthma have been relatively uncommon since the 1980s, the rate of death from asthma increased steadily in the United States until it peaked in the mid-1990s. Asthma-related deaths decreased between 1996 and 2005 by approximately 3.9% per year (Akinbami, Moorman, Garbe, and others, 2009). Data for the year 2008 indicate a significant increase in asthma symptoms, ED visits, and hospitalization among boys from birth to 4 years of age. African-American children have hospitalization and death rates three times higher than those of white and Hispanic children (Liu, Covar, Spahn, and others, 2011). Most asthma deaths in children occur in the home, school, or community before lifesaving medical care can be administered.

Some children's asthma symptoms may improve at puberty, but up to two thirds of children with asthma continue to have symptoms through puberty and into adulthood. The prognosis for control or disappearance of symptoms varies in children from those who have rare and infrequent attacks to those who are constantly wheezing or are subject to status asthmaticus. In general, when symptoms are severe and numerous, when symptoms have been present for a long time, and

◎ NURSING CARE PLAN

The Child with Acute Asthma Exacerbation

NURSING DIAGNOSIS	PATIENT OUTCOMES	NURSING INTERVENTIONS	RATIONALE
Ineffective Airway Clearance related to inflammation and constriction (spasm) of the bronchial tree	Child will exhibit effective ventilatory capacity (specify). Child will breathe easily without dyspnea.	Allow child to assume position of comfort (tripod or other).	To promote maximum ventilatory function
		Administer oxygen by face mask to maintain oxygen saturation >90%.	To enhance oxygenation of tissues
Child's Defining Characteristics (Subjective and Objective Data)	**The Following NOC Concepts Apply to These Outcomes**	Provide reassurance that symptoms will be managed and air hunger will subside.	To decrease anxiety related to hypoxia
Dyspnea	Airway Patency	Administer rescue medications (as prescribed) (NAEPP, 2007):	To open constricted airways and allow air exchange
Diminished breath sounds (air movement)	Asthma Control	• Inhaled β_2-agonist by metered-dose inhaler or aerosolized nebulization (up to three treatments in first 60 minutes) OR	To maintain adequate tissue oxygenation
Adventitious breath sounds (wheezing)	Anxiety Control	• Inhaled high-dose β_2-agonist (albuterol) and anticholinergic (ipratropium bromide [as age appropriate]) in nebulized form with oxygen (as necessary to keep saturation >90%)	
Difficulty vocalizing			
Changes in respiratory rate and rhythm		• Oral corticosteroid	
(Related Factors)		Assess child's response to rescue medications.	To determine need for more aggressive interventions
Allergen exposure			
Allergic airway		Administer rescue medications ordered as appropriate until optimum response is obtained.	To control asthma symptoms
Respiratory tract infection			
		Observe for exacerbation of asthma symptoms.	To prevent recurrence of acute episode
		Encourage small amounts of clear oral fluids as condition allows.	To maintain hydration
		For severe, unresponsive exacerbation, initiate peripheral intravenous line.	To maintain hydration and administer medications
		Titrate or wean oxygen concentration according to patient's response to rescue medications (based on work of breathing and oxygen saturation).	To prevent hyperoxemia
		Collaboratively evaluate cause of asthma exacerbation and treat if infection.	To prevent recurrence
		Provide discharge instructions for continued control of asthma symptoms.	To educate for management of symptoms and prevention of exacerbations
		• Review home medication use.	
		• Review written action plan for asthma symptom control.	To provide sense of control
		• Review signs and symptoms requiring immediate medical attention.	To enhance self-esteem
		• Control or eradicate allergens, irritants, and other precipitating factors.	
		• Follow up with practitioner.	
		The Following NIC Concepts Apply to These Interventions	
		Positioning	
		Anxiety Reduction	
		Vital Signs Monitoring	
		Surveillance	
		Medication Administration: Inhalation, Oral Administration	
		Infection Control	
		Fluid Management	
		Fever Treatment	

NIC, Nursing Interventions Classification; *NOC,* Nursing Outcomes Classification.

when there is a family history of allergy, there is a greater likelihood of a poor prognosis. Risk factors that may predict the persistence of symptoms into childhood (from infancy) include atopy, male gender, exposure to environmental tobacco, and maternal history of asthma. Many children who outgrow their exacerbations continue to have airway hyperresponsiveness and cough as adults. Furthermore, airway hyperresponsiveness in adults appears to be associated with decreased lung function.

The adolescent age group appears to be the most vulnerable, with the greatest increase occurring in children 10 to 14 years of age. No reliable data exist to explain this increase. Factors that have been postulated include exposure of atopic persons to more allergens (particularly in large urban centers), change in severity of the disease, abuse of drug therapy (toxicity), failure of families and practitioners to recognize the severity of asthma, and psychologic factors such as denial and refusal to accept the disease. On the other hand, studies have shown that children living in rural areas and farming communities have a decreased incidence of asthma and allergy (Liu, Covar, Spahn, and others, 2011).

Risk factors for asthma deaths include early onset, frequent attacks, difficult-to-manage disease, adolescence, history of respiratory failure, psychologic problems (refusal to take medications), dependency on or misuse of asthma drugs (high use), presence of physical stigmata (barrel chest, intercostal retractions), and abnormal PFT results.

Nursing Care Management
Provide Acute Asthma Care

Children who are admitted to the hospital with acute asthma are ill, anxious, and uncomfortable. The importance of continual observation and assessment cannot be overemphasized.

When β$_2$-agonists, supplemental oxygen, and corticosteroids are given, the child is monitored closely and continuously for relief of respiratory distress and signs of side effects or toxicity. Pulse oximetry is monitored along with rate and depth of breathing, auscultation of air movement, adventitious sounds, and any signs of respiratory distress (e.g., nasal flaring, tachypnea, retractions). The child on

supplemental oxygen requires intermittent or continuous oxygenation monitoring depending on severity of respiratory compromise and initial oxygenation status. The child in status asthmaticus should be placed on continuous cardiorespiratory (including blood pressure) and pulse oximetry monitoring. Oral fluid intake may be limited during the acute phase; IV fluid replacement may be required to provide adequate tissue hydration.

Older children may be more comfortable standing (Fig. 23-5), sitting upright, or leaning slightly forward (Fig. 23-6). Shortness of breath makes talking difficult.

The calm, efficient presence of a nurse helps reassure children that they are safe and will be cared for during this stressful period. It is important to assure children that they will not be left alone and that their parents are allowed to remain with them. Parents need reassurance and want to be informed of their child's condition and therapies. They may believe that they have in some way contributed to the child's

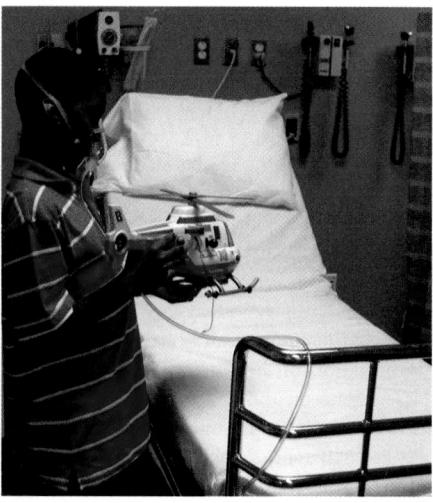

FIG 23-5 A child with asthma is allowed play activity as tolerated.

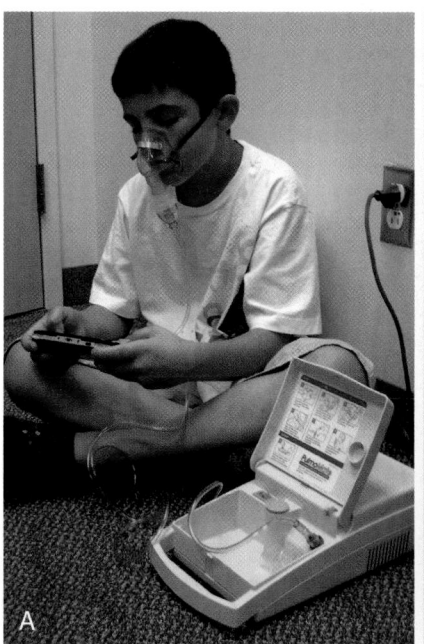
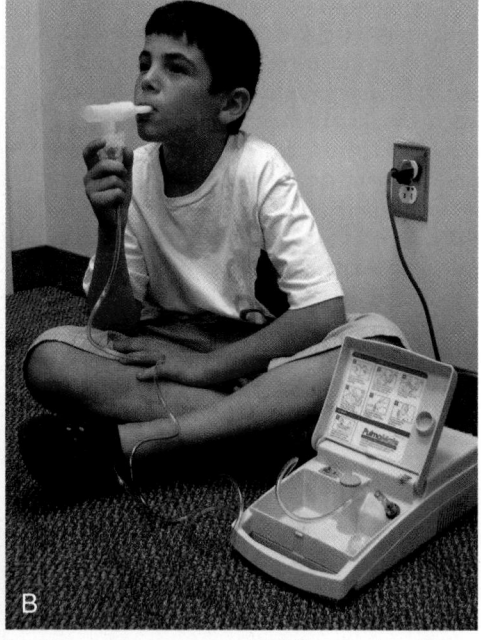

FIG 23-6 Children with asthma may take a nebulized aerosol treatment with **(A)** a mask or **(B)** mouthpiece. (Courtesy Texas Children's Hospital, Houston.)

condition or could have prevented the episode. Reassurance regarding their efforts expended on the child's behalf and their parenting capabilities can help alleviate their stress. Efforts to reduce parental apprehension will also reduce the child's distress. Anxiety is easily communicated to the child from parents and members of the staff.

Provide Long-Term Asthma Care

The nursing care of the child with asthma begins with a review of the child's health history; the home, school, and play environment; parent and child attitudes about the child's condition; and a comprehensive physical assessment with focus on the respiratory system. Nursing care of children with asthma involves both acute and long-term care. Nurses who are involved with children in the home, hospital, school, outpatient clinic, or practitioner's office play an important role in helping children and their families learn to live with the condition. The disease can be managed so that it does not require hospitalization or interfere with family life, physical activity, or school attendance. The nursing process in the care of the child with asthma is outlined in the Nursing Care Plan.

Physical assessment of asthma involves the same observations and techniques described in Chapter 6. In addition, the nurse notes and evaluates physical characteristics of a chronic respiratory condition, including chest configuration (e.g., barrel chest), posturing, and type of breathing. A history of the current and previous episodes and precipitating factors or events is important.

Nurses may perform a variety of functions in asthma care. These may include asthma education in the primary care setting and in schools and other community settings, care of the child with asthma in the acute care setting, ambulatory care, and intensive care. Nurses also obtain information on how asthma affects the child's everyday activities and self-concept, the child's and family's adherence to the prescribed therapy, and their personal treatment goals. Every effort is made to build a partnership between the child and family and the health care team, and effective communication is an essential part of this partnership. In particular, the child and family's satisfaction with asthma control and with the quality of care should be assessed. The nurse should also assess the child and family's perception of the severity of the disease and their level of social support.

One of the major emphases of nursing care is outpatient management by the family. Parents are taught how to prevent exacerbations, to recognize and respond to symptoms of bronchospasm, to maintain health and prevent complications, and to promote normal activities. The nurse should determine any cultural or ethnic beliefs or practices that influence self-management and that may necessitate modifications in educational approaches to meet the family's needs. Inconsistent home care, on the part of either the child or the parents, often leads to unnecessary ED visits for management (Volpe, Smith, and Sultan, 2011). Parents and older children often need education reinforced about the maintenance aspect of asthma management; children benefit from drug therapy even when asthma manifestations are not evident.

Avoid Allergens

One goal of asthma management is avoidance of an exacerbation. Parents need to know how to avoid allergens that precipitate asthma episodes. The nurse assists the parent in modifying the environment to reduce contact with the offending allergen(s). Parents are cautioned to avoid exposing a sensitive child to excessive cold, wind, and other extremes of weather; smoke (open fire or tobacco); sprays; scents; and other irritants. Foods known to provoke symptoms should be eliminated from the diet.

Approximately 2% to 6% of children with asthma are sensitive to aspirin; therefore, nurses should caution parents to use other analgesic–antipyretic drugs for discomfort or fever and to read package labeling. Although aspirin is rarely given to children in the United States, salicylate compounds are in other common medicines such as Pepto-Bismol. Children with aspirin-induced asthma may also be sensitive to nonsteroidal anti-inflammatory drugs and tartrazine (yellow dye number 5, a common food coloring).

> ### ! NURSING ALERT
>
> Parents are encouraged to avoid administering aspirin to any child unless specifically recommended by and under the supervision of a health practitioner. Acetaminophen is safe for children and is the analgesic of choice.

Relieve Bronchospasm

Teach parents and older children to recognize early signs and symptoms of an impending attack so it can be controlled before symptoms become distressing. Most children can recognize prodromal symptoms well before an attack (≈6 hours) and implement preventive therapy. Objective signs that parents may observe include rhinorrhea, cough, low-grade fever, irritability, itching (especially in front of the neck and chest), apathy, anxiety, sleep disturbance, abdominal discomfort, and loss of appetite. A variety of easy-to-use, inexpensive PEFMs are available for use in the home and at school to assess changes in pulmonary function (see Family-Centered Care box). In general, children 5 years of age and older are able to use a PEFM successfully. However, young children need to be supervised while they are learning to use their PEFM, and their technique should be checked frequently to ensure it is correct. Children should use the same peak flow meter over time because different brands can give significantly different values. The use of a PEFM provides objective monitoring regarding the severity of asthma and can decrease asthma episodes, health care visits, and missed school days (Burkhart, Rayens, Revelette, and others, 2007).

Children who use a nebulizer, MDI, Diskus, or Turbuhaler to deliver drugs need to learn how to use the device correctly. The MDI device (Fig. 23-7) delivers medication directly to the airways; therefore, the child needs to learn to breathe slowly and deeply for better distribution to narrowed airways (see Family-Centered Care box on p. 746).

> ### 👪 FAMILY-CENTERED CARE
> #### *Instructions for Use of a Peak Expiratory Flow Meter*
>
> 1. Before each use, make certain the sliding marker or arrow on the PEFM points to zero or is at the bottom of the numbered scale.
> 2. Stand up straight.
> 3. Remove gum or any food from the mouth.
> 4. Close your lips tightly around the mouthpiece. Be sure to keep your tongue away from the mouthpiece.
> 5. Blow out as hard and as quickly as you can, a "fast, hard puff."
> 6. Note the number by the marker on the numbered scale.
> 7. Repeat entire routine three times; wait 30 seconds between each routine.
> 8. Record the highest of the three readings, not the average.
> 9. Measure the PEFR close to the same time and same way each day (e.g., morning and evening; before or 15 minutes after taking medication).
> 10. Keep a chart of your PEFRs.

PEFM, Peak expiratory flow meter; *PEFR,* peak expiratory flow rate.

⊚ NURSING CARE PLAN

The Child with Asthma

NURSING DIAGNOSIS	PATIENT OUTCOMES	NURSING INTERVENTIONS	RATIONALE
Risk for Suffocation related to interaction between individual and triggering factors (allergens, respiratory tract infection, exercise, irritants, emotions, temperature changes)	Child will have adequate airway exchange. Family and child will assume responsibility for asthma symptom management.	Assist child and family in recognizing factors such as allergens, irritants, temperature changes, and upper respiratory infections that trigger asthma symptoms.	To avoid asthma exacerbations
		Assist child (according to developmental age) and family in recognizing early signs of an asthmatic episode (use PEFM).	To control symptoms with medication
Child's Defining Characteristics (Subjective and Objective Data)	**The Following NOC Concepts Apply to These Outcomes**	Educate child and family in the use of inhaled corticosteroids and bronchodilator.	To control symptoms and minimize shortness of breath
Wheezing	Asthma Control	Educate child and family regarding proper use of rescue medications in case of asthma exacerbation.	To prevent illness exacerbations and hospitalization; to prevent side effects from improper use of certain asthma drugs
Dry cough	Anxiety Control		
Labored respirations	Child Development		
Dyspnea			
Intercostal retractions		Educate child and family regarding the proper use of MDI with spacer, aerosolized nebulizer, and PEFM (know child's personal best).	To help child and family effectively manage asthma symptoms independently
Complaints of tightness in chest, shortness of breath			
Bronchial inflammation and airway constriction		**The Following NIC Concepts Apply to These Interventions**	
		Respiratory Monitoring	
		Administering Inhaled Medications	
		Risk Identification	
		Family Integrity Promotion	
		Energy Management	
		Coping Enhancement	
		Environmental Management	
Interrupted Family Processes related to child with a chronic illness	Family will cope with effects of the disease. Family will provide child an appropriate protective environment.	Provide family and child (as age appropriate) with explanations about the disease and management.	To provide adequate information To provide realistic expectations
		Cooperate with family to develop a written action plan for asthma management.	To provide family and child sense of control
Child's/Family's Defining Characteristics (Subjective and Objective Data)		Discuss facilitators and barriers to effective asthma management.	To assist family members in understanding their role as being vital in the management of asthma
Anxiety	**The Following NOC Concepts Apply to These Outcomes**		
Disruptive family interactions with child and members	Family Support	Encourage family and child (as age appropriate) to discuss the impact of the illness on the family's lifestyle.	To provide opportunity to verbalize frustrations and challenges of having a child with a chronic illness
Family conflicts	Family Normalization		
Inadequate child support		Evaluate family resources for asthma management in relation to the following:	To enhance family's ability to cope with child's chronic illness
Child's health status ignored		• Access to health care	
Family ignoring other members' needs for those of the child with asthma		• Medication availability in home and school (or daycare as appropriate)	
		• Allergen exposure control and eradication	
		The Following NIC Concepts Apply to These Interventions	
		Emotional Support	
		Anticipatory Guidance	
		Family Involvement Promotion	
		Financial Resource Assistance	
		Decision-Making Support	
		Mutual Goal Setting	

MDI, Metered-dose inhaler; *NIC,* Nursing Interventions Classification; *NOC,* Nursing Outcomes Classification; *PEFM,* peak expiratory flow meter.

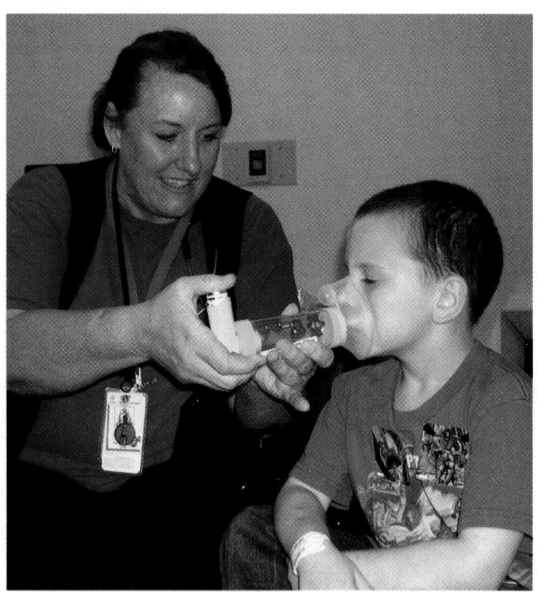

FIG 23-7 Child using metered-dose inhaler with spacer and face mask.

A spacer or AeroChamber device should be used with MDI inhalers. These devices allow the parent or child to deliver the medication from the MDI and slowly inhale it. Spacers also help prevent yeast infections in the mouth when corticosteroids are inhaled via an MDI.

The child and parents also need to be cautioned about the adverse effects of prescribed drugs and the dangers of overuse of β_2-agonists. They should know that it is important to use these drugs when needed but not indiscriminately or as a substitute for avoiding the symptom-provoking allergen.

> **! NURSING ALERT**
>
> Long-acting β-adrenergic inhalers (salmeterol) should be used only as directed (usually every 12 hours) and not more frequently. They are not intended to relieve acute asthmatic symptoms.

The family should obtain a PEFM and learn to use this device to monitor the child's asthma if the child is 5 years of age and older. A written asthma action plan that includes the three peak flow meter zones and the child's asthma medications may be obtained from the child's primary care provider. A home asthma action plan may reduce the risk of asthma death by 70% (Liu, Covar, Spahn, and others, 2011). Medications used for asthma exacerbations are also included in the asthma plan. This action plan should be used to make decisions about asthma management at home and at school. The nurse may assist the child and family in understanding the written action plan, emphasizing

 FAMILY-CENTERED CARE

Use of a Metered-Dose Inhaler*

Steps for Checking How Much Medicine Is in the Canister
1. If the canister is new, it is full.
2. If the canister has been used repeatedly, it might be empty. (Check product label to see how many inhalations should be in each canister.)
3. The most accurate way to determine how many doses remain in an MDI is to count and record each actuation as it is used.
4. Many dry powder inhalers have a dose-counting device or dose indicator on the canister to let you know when the canister is empty.
5. Do not place inhalers with hydrofluoroalkanes in water to check fill because it will destroy them.

Steps for Using the Inhaler with Mouthpiece
1. Remove the cap and hold inhaler upright.
2. Shake the inhaler.
3. Attach spacer, as appropriate.
4. Tilt the head back slightly and breathe out slowly.
5. With the inhaler in an upright position, insert the mouthpiece:
   a. About 3 to 4 cm (1–1½ inches) from the mouth or
   b. Into the mouth, forming an airtight seal between the lips and the mouthpiece
6. At the end of a normal expiration, depress the top of the inhaler canister firmly to release the medication (into the mouth) and breathe in slowly (about 3 to 5 seconds). Relax the pressure on the top of the canister.
7. Hold the breath for at least 5 to 10 seconds to allow the aerosol medication to reach deeply into the lungs.
8. Remove the inhaler and breathe out slowly through the nose.

9. Wait 1 minute between puffs (if an additional puff is needed) when using a bronchodilator.

Steps for Using the Inhaler with an AeroChamber (see Figure 23-7)
1. Remove the cap and hold inhaler upright.
2. Shake the inhaler.
3. Attach the AeroChamber.
4. With the inhaler in an upright position, insert the mouthpiece into the back of the AeroChamber.
5. Apply the AeroChamber mask to child's face and make sure there is a good seal.
6. Have child breathe slow regular breaths. Depress the top of the inhaler canister firmly to release the medication (into the AeroChamber) as the child breathes slowly in and out. Relax the pressure on the top of the canister.
7. Hold the AeroChamber in place over the child's face until six breaths have been taken. Give one puff at a time.
8. Remove the inhaler and AeroChamber.
9. Wait 1 minute between puffs (if an additional puff is needed) when using a bronchodilator.

Common Problems for Children Using Inhalers
- Child refuses or resists treatment.
- Inhalation is too rapid.
- Child is unable to coordinate the spray with inhalation.
- Breath is not held long enough after inhalation.

MDI, Metered-dose inhaler.
*Inhaled dry powder such as budesonide (Pulmicort) requires a different inhalation technique. To use a dry powder inhaler, the base of the device is turned until a click is heard. It is important to close the mouth tightly around the mouthpiece of the inhaler and inhale rapidly.

that the child and family determine the success of the plan, not the health professionals. Teach parents how to read labels on prepared foods and snacks to determine the presence of allergens.

The child should be protected from a respiratory tract infection that can trigger an attack or aggravate the asthmatic state, especially in young children whose airways are mechanically smaller and more reactive. Annual influenza vaccinations are recommended for all children. Pneumococcal vaccines should also be maintained. Equipment used for the child, such as nebulizers, must be kept absolutely clean to decrease the chances of contamination with bacteria and fungi.

Breathing exercises and controlled breathing are taught and encouraged for motivated children, and the nurse should provide information concerning activities that promote diaphragmatic breathing, side expansion, and improved mobility of the chest wall. Play techniques that can be used for younger children to extend their expiratory time and increase expiratory pressure include blowing cotton balls or a ping-pong ball on a table, blowing a pinwheel, blowing bubbles, or preventing a tissue from falling by blowing it against the wall.

Self-care and asthma self-management programs are important in helping the child and family cope with asthma. They are based on the following principles:

- Asthma is a common disease that can be controlled with appropriate drug therapy, environmental control, education, and management skills.
- It is much easier to prevent than to treat an asthma episode, and adherence to a therapeutic program is necessary to prevent exacerbations
- Children with asthma can live full and active lives.

Self-contained programs and brochures for patient education are available from the Asthma and Allergy Foundation of America* and the American Lung Association.† The National Heart, Lung, and Blood Institute‡ provides educational materials for asthma education in the school setting and also copies of the *Guidelines for the Diagnosis and Management of Asthma* for the practitioner (NAEPP, 2007). Another publication designed for health care practitioners, *Pediatric Asthma: Promoting Best Practice*, can be obtained from the American Academy of Allergy Asthma and Immunology.§

Support Child or Adolescent and Family

The nurse working with children with asthma can provide support in a number of ways. Many children voice frustration because their exacerbations interfere with their daily activities and social lives. Children need education on their condition and reassurance from the health team that they can learn to control and cope with their asthma and live a normal life.

Children in disruptive family situations (divorce, separation, violence, custodial battles) may disregard their daily asthma medication regimen or may be at higher risk as a result of neglect by adults who are in charge of their care. Adolescents struggling with a sense of identity and body image often regard asthma as a condition that will "go away," especially if there is a time lapse between symptoms, and may abandon the therapeutic regimen. Referral for counseling and

guidance is appropriate where the child's or adolescent's life is potentially in harm's way and the therapeutic regimen for asthma is abandoned due to personal or family crises.

The task of living day to day with affected children involves the entire family. There are periodic crises and the ever-present threat of a crisis, requiring parental vigilance; sleepless nights; frequent trips to the provider, ED, or hospital; and often overwhelming medical expenses. Throughout these stresses, parents are encouraged to promote as normal a life as possible for their children.

CYSTIC FIBROSIS

Cystic fibrosis is inherited as an autosomal recessive trait; the affected child inherits the defective gene from both parents, with an overall risk of one in four if both parents carry the gene. The mutated gene responsible for CF is located on the long arm of chromosome 7. This gene codes a protein of 1480 amino acids called the **cystic fibrosis transmembrane regulator (CFTR)**. The CFTR protein is related to a family of membrane-bound glycoproteins. The glycoproteins constitute a cAMP-activated chloride channel and regulate other chloride and sodium channels at the surfaces of the epithelial cells.

Pathophysiology

Cystic fibrosis is characterized by several clinical features, which are increased viscosity of mucous gland secretions, a striking elevation of sweat electrolytes, an increase in several organic and enzymatic constituents of saliva, and abnormalities in autonomic nervous system function. Although both sodium and chloride are affected, the defect appears to be primarily a result of abnormal chloride movement; the CFTR appears to function as a chloride channel. Children with CF demonstrate an increase in sodium and chloride in both saliva and sweat. This characteristic is the basis for the sweat chloride diagnostic test. The sweat electrolyte abnormality is present from birth, continues throughout life, and may be unrelated to the severity of the disease or the extent to which other organs are involved.

The primary factor, and the one that is responsible for many of the clinical manifestations of the disease, is mechanical obstruction caused by the increased viscosity of mucous gland secretions (Fig. 23-8). Instead of forming a thin, freely flowing secretion, the mucous glands produce a thick mucoprotein that accumulates and dilates them. Small passages in organs such as the pancreas and bronchioles become obstructed as secretions precipitate or coagulate to form concretions in glands and ducts. The earliest postnatal manifestation of CF is often **meconium ileus** in the newborn, in which the small intestine is blocked with thick, puttylike, tenacious, mucilaginous meconium.

In the pancreas, the thick secretions block the ducts, eventually causing **pancreatic fibrosis**. This blockage prevents essential pancreatic enzymes from reaching the duodenum, which causes marked impairment in the digestion and absorption of nutrients. The disturbed function is reflected in bulky stools that are frothy from undigested fat (**steatorrhea**) and foul smelling from putrefied protein (**azotorrhea**).

The incidence of diabetes mellitus (cystic fibrosis–related diabetes [CFRD]) is greater in CF children than in the general population, which may be caused by changes in pancreatic architecture and diminished blood supply over time. CFRD is reported to be the most common complication associated with CF; by age 30 years, approximately 50% of people with CF will develop diabetes, which is associated with increased morbidity (sixfold) and mortality and poor lung function (O'Riordan, Dattani, and Hindmarsh, 2010). The primary characteristic of CFRD is severe insulin deficiency as a result of β-cell

*8201 Corporate Drive, Suite 1000, Landover, MD 20785; 800-7-Asthma; http://www.aafa.org.
†1301 Pennsylvania Ave NW, Suite 800, Washington, DC 20004; 800-548-8252; national headquarters: 202-785-3385; http://www.lungusa.org.
‡NHLBI Health Information Center, PO Box 30105, Bethesda, MD 20824-0105; 301-592-8573; fax: 240-629-3246; http://www.nhlbi.nih.gov.
§555 E. Wells St., Suite 1100, Milwaukee, WI 53202; 414-272-6071; http://aaaai.org.

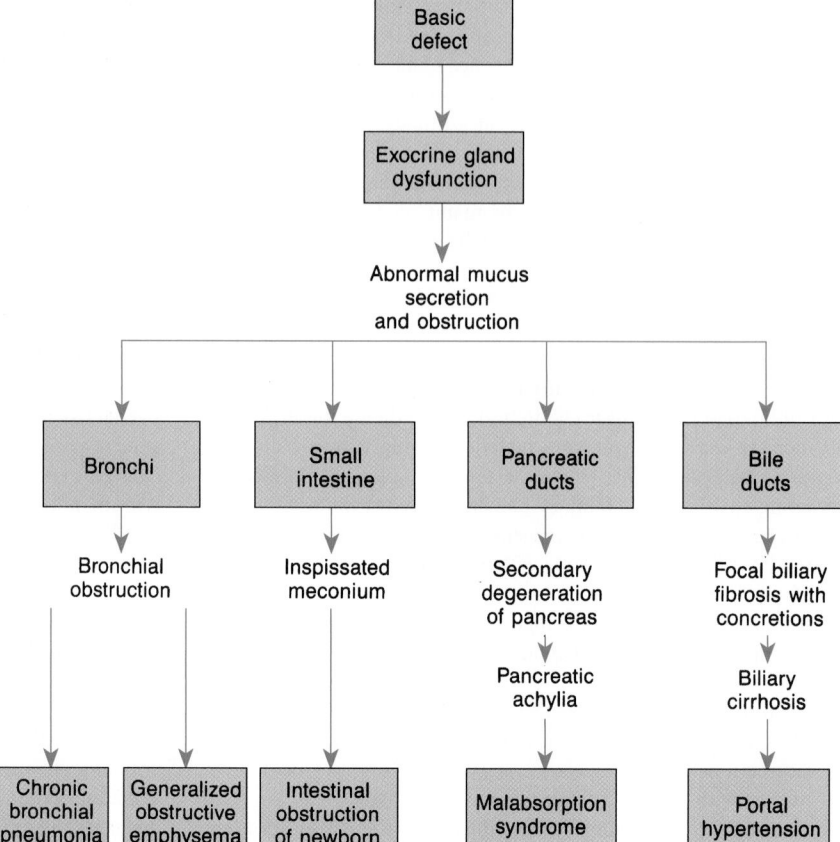

FIG 23-8 Various effects of exocrine gland dysfunction in cystic fibrosis.

dysfunction; however, CFRD also may demonstrate fluctuating insulin resistance, especially during acute illness. Thus, CFRD has characteristics of both type 1 diabetes mellitus and type 2 diabetes mellitus but is considered to be its own entity (Moran, Brunzell, Cohen, and others, 2010; O'Riordan, Dattani, and Hindmarsh, 2010). The positive correlation between nutritional status and optimal pulmonary function in patients with CF has been described; the presence of adequate insulin appears to be a key factor in maintaining an adequate nutritional status. Experts continue to recommend a high-fat, high-calorie diet in CF patients, and at this time there is no evidence to support a change in this diet for patients with CFRD (O'Riordan, Dattani, and Hindmarsh, 2010). Dietary guidelines are described further in the Borowitz, Baker, and Stallings (2002) reference.

A common gastrointestinal complication associated with CF is **prolapse of the rectum**, which occurs in infancy and childhood and is related to large, bulky stools; malnutrition; and increased intraabdominal pressure secondary to paroxysmal cough. Affected children of all ages are subject to intestinal obstruction from inspissated or impacted feces. Gumlike masses can obstruct the bowel and produce a partial or complete obstruction, a condition that is referred to as **distal intestinal obstruction syndrome**.

Pulmonary complications are present in almost all children with CF, but the onset and extent of involvement are variable. Symptoms are produced by stagnation of mucus in the airways, with eventual bacterial colonization leading to destruction of lung tissue. The abnormally viscous and tenacious secretions are difficult to expectorate and gradually obstruct the bronchi and bronchioles, causing scattered areas of bronchiectasis, atelectasis, and hyperinflation. The stagnant mucus also offers a favorable environment for bacterial growth. The most common pathogens are *Pseudomonas aeruginosa*, *Burkholderia cepacia*, *S. aureus*, *H. influenzae*, *Escherichia coli*, and *Klebsiella pneumoniae*.

The reproductive systems of both males and females with CF are affected. Females with CF have normal fallopian tubes and ovaries. Fertility can be inhibited by highly viscous cervical secretions, which act as a plug, blocking sperm entry. Women with CF who become pregnant have an increased incidence of premature labor and delivery and infant low birth weight. Favorable nutritional status and pulmonary function are positively correlated with favorable pregnancy outcomes. Most men (95%) with CF are sterile, which may be caused by blockage of the vas deferens with abnormal secretions or by failure of normal development of the wolffian duct structures (vas deferens, epididymis, and seminal vesicles), resulting in decreased or absent sperm production.

Growth and development are often affected in children with moderate to severe forms of CF. Physical growth may be restricted as a result of decreased absorption of nutrients, including vitamins and fat; increased oxygen demands for pulmonary function; and delayed bone growth. The usual pattern is one of growth failure (failure to thrive) with increased weight loss despite an increased appetite and gradual deterioration of the respiratory system. Clinical manifestations of CF are listed in Box 23-17.

Diagnostic Evaluation

Traditionally, the diagnosis of CF was based on a positive sweat chloride test result, absence of pancreatic enzymes, radiography, COPD, and family history. Newer diagnostic methods make it possible to diagnose CF early in infancy so therapies can be implemented to increase the child's overall survival and quality of life. In addition to

BOX 23-17 CLINICAL MANIFESTATIONS OF CYSTIC FIBROSIS

Meconium Ileus*
Abdominal distention
Vomiting
Failure to pass stools
Rapid development of dehydration

Gastrointestinal Manifestations
Large, bulky, loose, frothy, extremely foul-smelling stools
Voracious appetite (early in disease)
Loss of appetite (later in disease)
Weight loss
Marked tissue wasting
Failure to grow
Distended abdomen
Thin extremities
Sallow skin
Evidence of deficiency of fat-soluble vitamins A, D, E, and K
Anemia

Pulmonary Manifestations
Initial signs:
    Wheezy respirations
    Dry, nonproductive cough
Eventually:
    Increased dyspnea
    Paroxysmal cough
    Evidence of obstructive emphysema and patchy areas of atelectasis
Progressive involvement:
    Overinflated, barrel-shaped chest
    Cyanosis
    Clubbing of fingers and toes
    Repeated episodes of bronchitis and bronchopneumonia

*In about 10% of cases.

the sweat chloride test and factors listed above, diagnosis may be confirmed by any one of the following: newborn screening, DNA identification of mutant genes, and abnormal nasal potential difference measurement.

Universal newborn screening for CF has been proposed yet remains controversial because many states lack the resources for such screening programs. All 50 states have passed legislation requiring that all newborns be screened for CF. The newborn screening test consists of an immunoreactive trypsinogen (IRT) analysis performed on a dried spot of blood, which may be followed by direct analysis of DNA for the presence of the ΔF508 mutation or other mutations on the same dried blood spot. Benefits of early screening and detection include earlier nutritional intervention for identified infants; disadvantages include the parental anxiety false-positive results may generate. Children who were identified and treated early in infancy with aggressive nutritional support had improved height and weight well into adolescence. Although the technology is available to conduct carrier screening for the general population, this issue remains controversial, and widespread implementation of carrier screening programs is not recommended. An in utero diagnosis of CF is also possible based on detection of two CF mutations in the fetus.

The consistent finding of abnormally high sodium and chloride concentrations in the sweat is a unique characteristic of CF. Parents may report that their infant tastes "salty" when they kiss him or her. The quantitative sweat chloride test (pilocarpine iontophoresis) involves stimulating the production of sweat with a special device (involves stimulation with 3-mA electric current), collecting the sweat on filter paper, and measuring the sweat electrolytes. The quantitative analysis requires a sufficient volume of sweat (>75 mg). Two separate samples are collected to ensure the reliability of the test for any individual. Normally, sweat chloride content is less than 40 mEq/L, with a mean of 18 mEq/L. A chloride concentration greater than 60 mEq/L is diagnostic of CF; in infants younger than 3 months, a sweat chloride concentration greater than 40 mEq/L is highly suggestive of CF. In some situations, DNA testing may be substituted for the sweat test. The presence of a mutation known to cause CF on each CFTR gene predicts with a high degree of certainty that the individual has CF; however, multiple CFTR mutations may also be present and detected with DNA assay.

Chest radiography reveals characteristic patchy atelectasis and obstructive emphysema. PFTs are sensitive indexes of lung function, providing evidence of abnormal small airway function in CF. Other diagnostic tools that may aid in diagnosis include stool fat or enzyme analysis. Stool analysis requires a 72-hour sample with accurate recording of food intake during that time. Radiographs, including a contrast (dye) enema, are used for diagnosis of meconium ileus.

Therapeutic Management

Improved survival among patients with CF during the past 2 decades is attributable largely to antibiotic therapy and improved nutritional and respiratory management. Goals of CF therapeutic management are to (1) prevent or minimize pulmonary complications, (2) ensure adequate nutrition for growth, (3) encourage appropriate physical activity, and (4) promote a reasonable quality of life for the child and the family. A multidisciplinary approach to treatment is needed to accomplish these goals.

Management of Pulmonary Problems

Management of pulmonary problems is directed toward prevention and treatment of pulmonary infection by improving ventilation, removing mucopurulent secretions, and administering antimicrobial agents. Many children develop respiratory symptoms by 3 years of age. The large amounts and viscosity of respiratory secretions in children with CF contribute to the likelihood of respiratory tract infections. Recurrent pulmonary infections in children with CF result in greater damage to the airways; small airways are destroyed, causing bronchiectasis.

The most common pathogens responsible for pulmonary infections are *P. aeruginosa*, *B. cepacia*, *S. aureus*, *H. influenzae*, *E. coli*, and *K. pneumoniae*. *P. aeruginosa* and *B. cepacia* are particularly pathogenic for children with CF, and infections with these organisms are difficult to clear from the system. In addition, children with CF who are chronically colonized with these organisms have poorer survival rates than children who are not colonized. Colonization and infection with methicillin-resistant *S. aureus* (MRSA) has recently emerged as a critical factor in lung infection and pulmonary function in patients with CF. Patients with MRSA require longer hospitalization and multiple antibiotic regimens (Ren, Morgan, Konstan, and others, 2007). Fungal colonization with *Candida* or *Aspergillus* organisms in the respiratory tract is also common in CF patients.

Until recently, CPT has been the cornerstone of airway clearance; however, other airway clearance therapies (ACTs) have replaced this modality; these treatments often require more active involvement by the patient (Newton, 2009). The ACTs include the following:

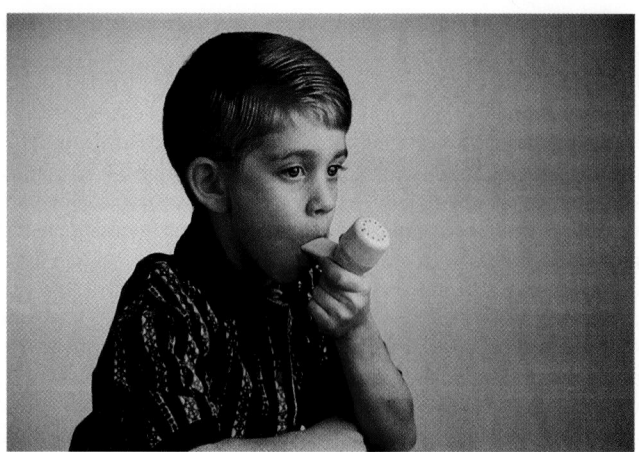

FIG 23-9 Child using a Flutter mucus clearance device. (Courtesy Scandipharm, Inc.)

percussion and postural drainage, positive expiratory pressure (PEP), active-cycle-of-breathing technique, autogenic drainage, oscillatory PEP, high-frequency chest compressions (HFCC), and exercise. Studies have demonstrated that no particular ACT has any advantage over the other in relation to outcomes of sputum production; however, it is recommended that individualized assessment occur to determine the best ACT for each patient (Flume, Robinson, O'Sullivan, and others, 2009). It is not within the scope of this chapter to discuss the many different ACTs.

Airway clearance therapies such as percussion and postural drainage are usually performed on average twice daily (on rising and in the evening) and more frequently if needed, especially during pulmonary infection. The Flutter mucus clearance device is a small handheld plastic pipe with a stainless-steel ball on the inside that facilitates removal of mucus (Fig. 23-9). It has the advantage of increasing sputum expectoration and being used without an assistant. Handheld percussors may be used to loosen secretions. Another method to clear mucus is high-frequency chest compression in which the child temporarily wears a mechanical vest device that provides high-frequency chest wall oscillation. Some children and adolescents with an implantable port may experience localized pain with the vest.

Patients with CF have been found to regress when conventional percussion and postural drainage is discontinued. Forced expiration, or "huffing," with the glottis partially closed helps move secretions from the small airways so that subsequent coughing can move secretions forcefully from the large airways. Several studies indicate that this maneuver enhances the pulmonary function of patients with CF. Autogenic drainage involves a variety of breathing techniques, which older children can use to force mucus in lower lobes up into the airways so it can be successfully expelled. Another mucus-clearing technique involves use of a positive expiratory pressure mask; this technique involves breathing into a mask attached to a one-way valve, which creates resistance—as the patient exhales, the airway is kept open by the pressure, and mucus is forced into the upper airway for expulsion.

Bronchodilator medication delivered in an aerosol opens bronchi for easier expectoration and is administered before percussion and postural drainage when the patient exhibits evidence of reactive airway disease or wheezing. Another aerosolized medication is recombinant human deoxyribonuclease (DNase, known generically as dornase alfa [Pulmozyme]), which decreases the viscosity of mucus. It is well tolerated and has no major adverse effects; minor reactions are voice alterations and laryngitis. This medication, given daily via nebulization generally before or with percussion and postural drainage, has resulted in improvements in spirometry, PFTs, dyspnea scores, and perceptions of well-being and has reduced the viscosity of sputum.

Nebulized hypertonic saline (6%–7%) has been shown to be effective in improving airway hydration and increases mucus clearance in patients with CF; this treatment, however, causes bronchospasm and may not be recommended for patients with severe disease (Redding, 2009).

Physical exercise is an important adjunct to daily ACT. Exercise stimulates mucus excretion and provides a sense of well-being and increased self-esteem. Any aerobic exercise that the patient enjoys should be encouraged. The ultimate aim of exercise is to increase lung vital capacity, remove secretions, increase pulmonary blood flow, and maintain healthy lung tissue for effective ventilation.

Pulmonary infections are treated as soon as they are recognized. In CF patients, characteristic signs of pulmonary infection—fever, tachypnea, and chest pain—may be absent; therefore, a careful history and physical examination are essential. The presence of anorexia, weight loss, and decreased activity alerts the practitioner to pulmonary infection and the need for an antibiotic regimen. Aerosolized antibiotics such as tobramycin, ticarcillin, and gentamicin are beneficial for patients with frequent pulmonary exacerbations (Redding, 2009). It is common for a hospitalized child with CF to be prescribed as many as two or three antibiotics and one antifungal medication to treat coexisting pulmonary infections.

Intravenous antibiotics may be administered at home as an alternative to hospitalization. The use of peripherally inserted central catheters (PICCs) for the administration of antibiotics in children with CF is a viable option with limited complications and fewer needle punctures to obtain blood specimens and to maintain often lengthy treatment with parenteral antibiotics. Alternatively, an implanted port offers the advantage of access for blood draws and antibiotic infusion. When pulmonary function does not improve with outpatient management, hospitalization may be recommended for continued antibiotic therapy and vigorous postural drainage. Some institutions hospitalize patients for IV antibiotic therapy and percussion and postural drainage periodically (a "tune up") to keep them well. Oxygen administration is used for children with acute episodes but must be used cautiously because many children with CF have chronic carbon dioxide retention, and the unsupervised use of oxygen can be harmful (see Oxygen Therapy, Chapter 22). With repeated infection and inflammation, bronchial cysts and emphysema may develop. These cysts may rupture, resulting in a pneumothorax.

> **! NURSING ALERT**
>
> Signs of a pneumothorax are usually nonspecific and include tachypnea, tachycardia, dyspnea, pallor, and cyanosis. A subtle drop in oxygen saturation (measured by pulse oximetry) may be an early sign of pneumothorax.

Blood streaking of the sputum is usually associated with increased pulmonary infection and often requires no specific treatment. Hemoptysis greater than 250 ml/24 hr for an older child (less for a younger child) indicates a potentially life-threatening event and needs to be treated immediately. Sometimes bleeding can be controlled with bed rest, IV antibiotics, replacement of acute blood loss, IV conjugated estrogens (Premarin) or vasopressin (Pitressin), and correction of any coagulation defects with vitamin K or fresh-frozen plasma. If hemoptysis persists, the site of bleeding should be localized via bronchoscopy and cauterized or embolized.

Treatment of nasal polyps includes intranasal corticosteroids, oral antihistamines, and decongestants. If these measures are ineffective, surgical interventions may be necessary.

Because pulmonary damage in patients with CF is believed to be caused by the inflammatory process that occurs with frequent infections, the use of corticosteroids has been studied; however, treatment with corticosteroids for prolonged periods has been associated with linear growth restriction, glucose tolerance abnormalities, and cataract formation. Anti-inflammatory medications such as ibuprofen are becoming more important in the treatment of CF, but careful monitoring for adverse effects (gastrointestinal bleeding) is essential.

Management of Gastrointestinal Problems

The principal treatment for pancreatic insufficiency is replacement of pancreatic enzymes, which are administered with meals and snacks to ensure that digestive enzymes are mixed with food in the duodenum. Enteric-coated products prevent the neutralization of enzymes by gastric acids, thus allowing activation to occur in the alkaline environment of the small bowel. The amount of enzymes depends on the severity of the insufficiency, the child's response to enzyme replacement, and the practitioner's philosophy. Usually one to five capsules are administered with a meal, and a smaller amount is taken with snacks. Capsules can be swallowed whole or taken apart and the contents sprinkled on a small amount of food to be taken at the beginning of the meal. The amount of enzyme is adjusted to achieve normal growth and a decrease in the number of stools to one or two per day. Pancreatic enzymes should be taken within 30 minutes of eating. The enteric-coated beads should not be chewed or crushed because destroying the enteric coating can lead to inactivation of the enzymes and excoriation of oral mucosa. The powder form should be used cautiously because inhalation of the powder may precipitate acute bronchospasm and, if mixed with food, predigests the food, making it unpalatable.

Children with CF require a well-balanced, high-protein, high-caloric diet (because of their impaired intestinal absorption). In fact, they often require up to 150% of the recommended daily allowances to meet their needs for growth. Breastfeeding with enzyme supplementation should be continued whenever possible for parents who prefer this method and, when necessary, supplemented with a higher-calorie-per-ounce formula. For formula-fed infants, commercial cow's milk–based formulas are usually adequate, although frequently a partially hydrolysated formula with medium-chain triglycerides (e.g., Pregestimil, Alimentum) may be recommended. Enzymes are mixed into cereal or fruit, such as applesauce. Because the uptake of fat-soluble vitamins is decreased, water-miscible forms of these vitamins (A, D, E, and K) are given along with multivitamins and the enzymes. When high-fat foods are eaten, the child is encouraged to add extra enzymes. Growth failure despite adequate nutritional support may indicate deterioration of pulmonary status. Patients with CF may experience frequent anorexia as a result of the copious amounts of mucus produced and expectorated, persistent cough, effect of medications, fatigue, and sleep disruption. They may be placed on nighttime supplemental gastrostomy or nasogastric tube feedings or rarely parenteral alimentation in an effort to build up nutritional reserves if there has been a history of inability to maintain weight.

Meconium ileus and meconium ileus equivalent, or total or partial intestinal obstruction, can occur at any age. Constipation is often the result of a combination of malabsorption (either from inadequate pancreatic enzyme dosage or a failure to take the enzymes), decreased intestinal motility, and abnormally viscous intestinal secretions. These problems usually do not require surgical interventions and may be

treated with GoLYTELY or Colyte (osmotic solutions given orally or by nasogastric tubes), other laxatives, stool softeners, or rectal administration of meglumine diatrizoate (Gastrografin).

Rectal prolapse occurs only in a small number of individuals; fewer are affected as result of early diagnosis and administration of pancreatic enzymes (Egan, 2011). The first episode of rectal prolapse is frightening to both the parents and child. Its reduction usually requires immediate guidance and intervention, which is managed by simply guiding the rectum back into place with a gloved, lubricated finger. Further management usually involves attempting to decrease the bulk of daily stools through enzyme replacement.

Children with CF often experience transient or chronic gastroesophageal reflux, which should be treated with the appropriate histamine-receptor antagonist and gastrointestinal motility drug, dietary modifications, and an upright position after feedings and meals (Hazle, 2010).

Management of Endocrine Problems

The management of CFRD is critical in the therapeutic treatment of the child with CF. CFRD presents a combination of insulin resistance and insulin deficiency, with unstable glucose homeostasis in the presence of acute lung infection and treatment. Children with CFRD require close monitoring of blood glucose and administration of insulin, as well as diet and exercise management; quarterly glycosylated hemoglobin (A1c) measurements are recommended. Children with CF may be at increased risk for glucose management problems as a result of decreased nutrient absorption, anorexia, and severity of pulmonary illness. The prevalence of CFRD increases with age, and there is increased morbidity and mortality among children with CFRD compared with those without. Microvascular complications such as retinopathy and nephropathy may occur in children and adolescents with CFRD (O'Riordan, Dattani, and Hindmarsh, 2010). However, ketoacidosis is reported to be rare in individuals with CFRD (Egan, 2011). Children with CFRD should perform self blood glucose monitoring (SBGM) three times daily and should be on an insulin regimen. Target glucose levels should be the same as for any other patient with diabetes. There is no evidence that oral glycemic agents are effective. During acute CF exacerbations, the nondiabetic child should be monitored closely for hyperglycemia; glycosylated hemoglobin is reportedly a poor predictor of CFRD, so an oral glucose tolerance test is the preferred screening tool (Moran, Brunzell, Cohen, and others, 2010).

Bone health is of concern in children and adults with CF. The pancreatic insufficiency of CF and chronic steroid use present potential risks for less than optimum bone growth in such children. Assessment of bone health by history and bone mass density evaluation should be considered in assessing the child's (age 8 years and older) health status to detect and prevent osteoporosis and osteopenia.

Prognosis

The median predicted survival age for the CF patient in 2008 was 37.4 years, and approximately 45% of patients are 18 and older (Cystic Fibrosis Foundation, 2009). Lung, heart, pancreas, and liver transplantation have increased survival rates among some CF patients. Heart–lung and double-lung procedures have been successfully performed in children with advanced pulmonary vascular disease and hypoxia. The obstacles surrounding this technique are availability of donated organs; complications from surgery; pulmonary infections; and recurrence of obstructive bronchiolitis, which decreases transplanted lung function.

There is increasing evidence that two pharmacologic agents act as correctors and potentiators to override the CFTR defect and maintain adequate airway surface liquid layer as well as to correct abnormal chloride and sodium channels to reduce mucus production. These pharmaco-therapeutic approaches have been shown to offer clinical benefits for persons with delta F508 mutation (Cuthbert, 2011; Kim Chiaw, Eckford, and Bear, 2011). With advances in technology, parents and adolescents are challenged to set future goals that may include college, careers, social relationships, and marriage. Concurrently, they are faced with increasing morbidity and higher rates of CF complications as they grow older.

Nursing Care Management

Assessment of the child with CF involves both pulmonary and gastrointestinal observations. Pulmonary assessment is the same as that described for asthma, with special attention to lung sounds, observation of cough, and evidence of decreased activity or fatigue. Gastrointestinal assessment primarily involves observing the frequency and nature of the stools and abdominal distention. The nurse should also be alert to evidence of growth failure (e.g., weight loss, muscle wasting, pallor, anorexia, decreased activity [from baseline norm]). Family members are interviewed to determine the child's eating and eliminating habits and to confirm a history of frequent respiratory tract infections or bowel obstruction in infancy.

The nurse assesses the newborn for feeding and stooling patterns, which may indicate a potential problem such as meconium ileus. The nurse also participates in diagnostic testing such as the initial newborn screening, IRT, DNA analysis, or sweat chloride test.

Parents need careful explanations of the disease, how it might affect their family, and what they can do to provide the best possible care for their child. It is crucial to involve the parents in the follow-up for early diagnostic testing; the neonate may require several follow-up visits in the first few weeks of life if initial test results are not conclusive.

The uncertainty, fear, and initial shock associated with the diagnosis are overwhelming to parents. They must face the impact of the chronic, life-threatening nature of the disease and the prospect of intensive treatment, for which they must assume a major part of the responsibility and for which they are ill prepared. They often fear that they will be unable to provide the care the child needs. One of the most difficult aspects of the diagnosis is the implications inherent in its etiology (i.e., the recognition that each parent contributed the gene responsible for the defect).

Hospital Care

Most patients with CF require hospitalization only for treatment of pulmonary infection, uncontrolled diabetes, or a coexisting medical problem that cannot be treated on an outpatient basis. Therefore, when patients with CF are hospitalized, standard precautions with meticulous hand washing should be implemented to decrease the nosocomial spread of organisms to the CF patient and between hospitalized CF patients (especially when MRSA is prevalent). Contact precautions may be required for specific infections.

When the child with CF is hospitalized for diagnosis or treatment of pulmonary complications, aerosol therapy, percussion and postural drainage are instituted or continued. Respiratory therapists often initiate, supervise, and provide these treatments; however, it is the nurse's responsibility to monitor the patient's tolerance to the procedure and evaluate the effectiveness of the procedure in relation to treatment goals. The nurse may at times administer aerosol therapy, perform chest percussion and postural drainage, assist with ACTs such as the mechanical vest, and teach breathing exercises. Chest percussion and postural drainage should not be performed before or immediately after meals. Planning percussion and postural drainage so it does not coincide with meals is difficult in the hospital situation but is essential to the effectiveness of this treatment.

Nursing assessments, including observation of respiratory pattern, work of breathing, and lung auscultation, are vital assessments. Noninvasive pulse oximetry provides valuable data about the patient's oxygenation status. Supplemental oxygen therapy is administered to the child with mild or moderate respiratory distress, and the child requires frequent assessment of the tolerance to the procedure.

One of the nursing challenges in the care of the child with CF is encouraging compliance with the therapeutic medication regimen, which often involves a significant number of medications; pancreatic enzymes; vitamins A, D, E, and K; oral antifungals for *Candida* infection; antihistamines; anti-inflammatory agents; and oral antibiotics. This may be overwhelming to the child. Factor in multiple inhaled bronchodilators, chest percussion and postural drainage and aerosol treatments, blood glucose monitoring and insulin administration, various other medications, and increased mucus production during the acute phase, and it is common for the child with CF to rebel and be noncompliant with this regimen. Gentle coaxing, positive reinforcement, and frank negotiation may be required to enlist cooperation for effective medication compliance.

The diet for the child with CF represents another challenge; careful planning with a registered pediatric dietitian and the child's input may help decrease the loss of appetite and weight loss that are often part of the condition. Children in the early stages of CF often have a good appetite. With infection and increased lung involvement, their appetite diminishes, and eventually it becomes a challenge to tempt failing appetites. When dietary intake fails to meet the child's needs for growth, enteral feedings or supplements may be considered. These feedings may be administered via a gastrostomy tube during the night to minimize the disruption of daily activities, including school. A skin-level feeding gastrostomy affords the child few activity restrictions and minimum disruption of body image compared with a nasogastric tube or conventional gastrostomy tube. The child and parents are encouraged to not perceive this therapy as a last-ditch effort but as an adjunct therapy to maintain optimum growth and prevent excessive weight loss. Some children have a nasogastric tube placed before bedtime and receive enteral feeds overnight; the tube is removed in the morning so that it does not interfere with regular activities.

The child or adolescent needs support during the many treatments and tests that are a part of the hospitalization. IV fluids, IV antibiotics and antifungals, PICC line placement or port accessing, and blood tests are almost always a part of the acute care treatment, and the child soon associates hospitalization with these stress-provoking procedures.

Depression, anxiety, and disturbed self-image may occur in children and adolescents with CF; older adolescents and young adults with severe symptoms may be especially prone to depression as a result of the realization of the poor prognosis and the reality of unmet life expectations and goals.

Providing support to both the child and the family is essential. Skilled nursing care and sympathetic attention to the emotional needs of the child and family help them cope with the stresses associated with repeated respiratory tract infections and hospitalizations.

Home Care

Most children and adolescents with CF can be managed at home. The goals of care include normalization and daily activities, including school and peer involvement. The care plan should be flexible so that family activities are disrupted as little as possible. Parents may initially require assistance finding and contacting durable medical equipment companies that will provide home care equipment. They also need opportunities to learn how to use the equipment and to solve problems they may encounter while delivering therapy at home (see Chapter 20).

Patients and family members need education about the preferred diet of nutritious meals with tolerated fat, increased protein and carbohydrate, and the administration of pancreatic enzymes. For infants and young children, the enzymes can be mixed with pureed fruit, such as applesauce, and fed with a spoon. Capsules are usually suitable for older children. It is important to stress to parents that the enzymes, in the amount regulated to the child's needs, should be administered at the beginning of all meals and snacks. For enteral feeds administered overnight, enzymes are generally administered at the start and finish of the feeds.

One of the most important aspects of educating parents for home care is teaching techniques for the removal of mucus (ACT, vest, forced expiration) and breathing exercises. The success of a therapy program depends on conscientious performance of these treatments regularly as prescribed. The number of times these therapies are performed each day is determined on an individual basis, and often parents readily learn to adjust the number and intensity of the treatments to the child's needs. For pulmonary infection, home IV antibiotics may be prescribed pending verification of insurance coverage and availability of an agency with adequate staff to perform multiple daily home antibiotic infusions. With use of the venous access devices, such as PICC lines, and implanted ports, the parents and child can be taught the technique of direct administration into the IV line.

Families also need information about medications and possible side effects. Children receiving multiple antibiotics may require serum drug levels to ensure therapeutic dosing.

If the child has CFRD, education on self blood glucose monitoring, insulin therapy, diet control, and possible complications related to these is needed. Follow up with a pediatric endocrinologist is recommended.

Children and adolescents with CF should receive routine primary care with special attention to diet, growth and development, and immunizations. Primary care providers should be alert to any weight loss or flattening in the growth curve associated with loss of appetite, which could indicate a pulmonary exacerbation in children with CF. Anticipatory guidance concerning issues of discipline, how to incorporate aspects of the treatment regimen into the school environment, and delayed pubertal development are also important considerations for the primary care provider.

Home palliative care for the child or adolescent with CF who is in the terminal stages may be carried out with the assistance of palliative care or hospice as appropriate (see Chapter 18).

The nurse can assist the family in contacting resources that provide help to families with affected children. Various special child health services, many local clinics, private agencies, service clubs, and other community groups often offer equipment and medications either free or at reduced rates. The Cystic Fibrosis Foundation* has chapters throughout the United States that provide education and services to families and professionals.

Family Support

One of the most challenging aspects of providing care for the family of a child or adolescent with CF is meeting the emotional needs of the child and family. The diagnosis, treatment, and prognosis for CF are often associated with many problems and frustrations. The diagnosis can evoke feelings of guilt and self-recrimination in parents.

The long-range problems for an infant, child, or adolescent with CF are those encountered in any chronic illness (see Chapter 18). Both the child and the family must make many adjustments, the success of which depends on their ability to cope and on the quality and quantity of support they receive from outside sources. It is often the nurse who assesses the home situation, organizes and coordinates these services, and collects the data needed to evaluate the effectiveness of the services.

The persistent need for treatment several times a day places tremendous strain on the family. When the child is young, a family member must perform postural drainage and other ACTs. Children often balk at these treatments, and the parents are placed in the position of insisting on adherence. The stress and anxiety related to this routine may produce feelings of resentment in both the child and the family members. When possible, occasional trusted respite care should be available to allow parents to leave the situation for short periods without undue anxiety about the child's welfare.

The affected child or adolescent may become resentful about the disease, its relentless routine of therapy, and the necessary curtailment it places on activities and relationships. The child's activities are interrupted or built around treatments, medications, and diet. This imposes hardships and influences the child's quality of life. The child should be encouraged to attend school, seek employment when old enough, and join age-appropriate peer groups to foster a life that is as normal and productive as possible. Sports are often an important part of the child and adolescent's life; interaction with peers includes valuable life experiences, especially to adolescents. The child or adolescent with CF should be encouraged to participate in sports activities in as much as physical and pulmonary health allows. Exercise is encouraged to increase pulmonary vital capacity, promote muscle development, and enhance cardiovascular function.

As the disease progresses, however, family stress should be expected, and the patient may become angry and may resist medical therapy. It is important for the nurse to recognize the family's changing needs and the grief they may experience as the CF worsens. Families should be made aware of resources for counseling. Patients need to be guided into activities that enable them to express anger, sorrow, and fear without guilt.

Transition to Adulthood

As life expectancy continues to rise for children and adolescents with CF, issues related to marriage, sexuality, childbearing, and career choice become more pressing. Male patients must be informed at some point that they will often be unable to produce offspring. It is important that the distinction be made between sterility and impotence. Normal sexual relationships can be expected. Female patients may be able to bear children but should be informed of the possible deleterious effects on the respiratory system created by the burden of pregnancy. They also need to know that their children will be carriers of the CF gene. Adolescent females may need counseling concerning the use of oral contraceptives and other contraceptive options (Hazle, 2010).

---

*6931 Arlington Road, Bethesda, MD 20814-3205; 301-951-4422 or 800-FIGHT CF; http://www.cff.org. In Canada: Canadian Cystic Fibrosis Foundation, 2221 Yonge St., Suite 601, Toronto, ON M4S 2B4; 800-378-2233 (toll free in Canada only), http://www.cysticfibrosis.ca. For information about specialized medications, especially dornase alfa, and equipment for CF and other pulmonary diseases, contact the Cystic Fibrosis Services Pharmacy, 6931 Arlington Road, 2nd floor, Bethesda, MD; 800-541-4959; http://www.cfservicespharmacy.com.

Adolescents with CF are encouraged to take personal ownership and management of the illness to maximize their life's potential. Many adolescents and young persons with the illness enroll in college or vocational and technical training school and complete degrees either by distance learning or by attending a local school. Young people are encouraged to set life goals and live normal lives to the extent their illness allows.

Anticipatory grieving and other aspects related to care of a child with a terminal illness are also part of nursing care. For example, it is important to prepare the child and family members for end-of-life decisions and care when appropriate.

OBSTRUCTIVE SLEEP-DISORDERED BREATHING

Pediatric obstructive sleep-disordered breathing reportedly affects between 10% and 12% of children ages 2 to 8 years; obstructive sleep apnea may occur in as many as 2% of all children (Benninger and Walner, 2007b). Obstructive sleep-disordered breathing is said to form a continuum of sleep-disordered breathing ranging from partial obstruction of the upper airway to continuous episodes of complete upper airway obstruction, with the most severe form being obstructive sleep apnea syndrome (OSAS) (Benninger and Walner, 2007b). OSAS is defined by the American Thoracic Society (1996) as a disorder of breathing during sleep with prolonged partial upper airway obstruction or complete obstruction that disrupts normal respiration during sleep and normal sleep patterns. Common symptoms include nightly snoring, interrupted or disturbed sleep patterns, enuresis, and daytime neurobehavioral problems (AAP, 2002). OSAS is to be distinguished from primary snoring, which is snoring without obstructive apnea, frequent sleep arousals, or abnormalities in gas exchange (AAP, 2002). Children with OSAS usually do not exhibit daytime sleepiness as do adults, with the possible exception of obese children. If left untreated, obstructive sleep-disordered breathing may result in complications such as growth failure, cor pulmonale, pulmonary hypertension, poor learning, behavioral problems, attention-deficit/hyperactivity disorder, and death.

The diagnosis of obstructive sleep-disordered breathing is made by a sleep study (polysomnography), which provides evidence of sleep disturbance, respiratory pauses, and changes in oxygenation. The six-channel polysomnography can be performed in children of all ages with videotaping or audiotaping, and abbreviated (vs. full night sleep study) polysomnography may be useful; however, this latter method does not predict the severity of OSAS (AAP, 2002). Polysomnography can distinguish between OSAS and primary snoring (Owens, 2011).

A common treatment for sleep-disordered breathing in children is adenotonsillectomy, provided there is evidence of adenotonsillar hypertrophy (Benninger and Walner, 2007b). However, evidence indicates that this procedure may not be as successful in children with obesity as previously reported (Witmans and Young, 2011). Complications of these surgical interventions are discussed previously in this chapter. CPAP and bilevel positive airway pressure (BiPAP) may be helpful in older children with sleep-disordered breathing whose condition persists after surgical intervention. CPAP or BiPAP is a long-term therapy with frequent assessments to evaluate the required amount of pressure and the overall effectiveness of the intervention.

Surgical interventions such as tracheotomy may be required for children with craniofacial syndromes, such as Goldenhar, Pierre Robin, Apert, and Crouzon syndromes, in which there is partial or complete upper airway obstruction.

Nursing care of the child with sleep-disordered breathing involves early detection by observation of the infant's or child's sleep patterns and active participation in the diagnostic polysomnography. Important nursing roles are inserting the pH probe into the esophagus, ensuring accurate placement by radiography, and monitoring the sleep study and the patient's response to diagnostic therapy. Counseling families of children with sleep-disordered breathing may involve dietary counseling for exercise programs and weight management, use of the CPAP or BiPAP equipment, and direct postoperative care after the surgical intervention of tonsillectomy or adenoidectomy. Some children may resist wearing the CPAP or BiPAP devices and will need encouragement to do this. The nurse can be instrumental in helping the child and family cope with the chronic illness diagnosis if intervention such as CPAP or BiPAP is required.

RESPIRATORY EMERGENCY

RESPIRATORY FAILURE

Effective pulmonary gas exchange requires clear airways, normal lungs and chest wall, and adequate pulmonary circulation. Anything that affects these functions or their relationships can compromise respiration. In general, the term respiratory insufficiency is applied to two situations: (1) when there is increased work of breathing but gas exchange function is near normal and (2) when normal blood gas tensions cannot be maintained and hypoxemia and acidosis develop secondary to carbon dioxide retention.

Respiratory failure is defined as the inability of the respiratory apparatus to maintain adequate oxygenation of the blood with or without carbon dioxide retention. This process involves pulmonary dysfunction that generally results in impaired alveolar gas exchange, which can lead to hypoxemia or hypercapnia. Respiratory failure is the most common cause of cardiopulmonary arrest in children. Respiratory arrest is the complete cessation of respiration. Apnea is the cessation of breathing for more than 20 seconds or for a shorter period when associated with hypoxemia or bradycardia. Apnea can be (1) central, in which respiratory efforts are absent; (2) obstructive, in which respiratory efforts are present; and (3) mixed, in which both central and obstructive components are present (see Apparent Life-Threatening Event, Chapter 11). Respiratory dysfunction may have an abrupt or an insidious onset. Respiratory failure can occur as an emergency situation or may be preceded by gradual and progressive deterioration of respiratory function. Most clinical manifestations are nonspecific and are affected by variations among individual patients and differences in the severity and duration of inadequate gas exchange.

Diagnostic Evaluation

The diagnosis of respiratory failure is determined by the combined application of three sources of information:
1. Presence or history of a condition that might predispose the patient to respiratory failure
2. Observation of respiratory failure
3. Measurement of ABGs, including pH

Nursing observation and judgment are vital to the recognition and early management of respiratory failure. Nurses must be able to assess a situation and initiate appropriate action within moments. Signs of respiratory failure are listed in Box 23-18.

Therapeutic Management

The interventions used in the management of respiratory failure are often dramatic, requiring special skills and emergency procedures. If respiratory arrest occurs, the primary objectives are to recognize the situation and immediately initiate resuscitative measures, such as

BOX 23-18 CLINICAL MANIFESTATIONS OF RESPIRATORY FAILURE

Cardinal Signs
Restlessness
Tachypnea
Tachycardia
Diaphoresis

Early but Less Obvious Signs
Mood changes, such as euphoria or depression
Headache
Altered depth and pattern of respirations
Hypertension
Exertional dyspnea
Anorexia
Increased cardiac output and renal output
CNS symptoms (decreased efficiency, impaired judgment, anxiety, confusion, restlessness, irritability, depressed level of consciousness)
Flaring nares
Chest wall retractions
Expiratory grunt
Wheezing or prolonged expiration

Signs of More Severe Hypoxia
Hypotension or hypertension
Altered vision
Somnolence
Stupor
Coma
Dyspnea
Depressed respirations
Bradycardia
Cyanosis, peripheral or central

CNS, Central nervous system.

airway positioning, administration of oxygen, cardiopulmonary resuscitation (CPR), suctioning, CPAP or BiPAP, or intubation. When the situation is not an arrest, the suspicion of respiratory failure is confirmed by assessment; the severity may be defined by ABG analysis. Interventions such as administering supplemental oxygen, positioning, stimulation, suctioning, and early intubation may avert an arrest. When the severity is established, an attempt is made to determine the underlying cause by thorough evaluation.

The principles of management are to (1) maintain ventilation and maximize oxygen delivery, (2) correct hypoxemia and hypercapnia, (3) treat the underlying cause, (4) minimize extrapulmonary organ failure, (5) apply specific and nonspecific therapy to control oxygen demands, and (6) anticipate complications. Monitoring the patient's condition closely is critical.

Nursing Care Management

For families whose child has a respiratory arrest, support is aimed at keeping the family informed of the child's status and helping them cope with a near-death experience or an actual death (see Chapter 18). Knowing that their child requires CPR is a frightening and often overwhelming experience for parents. Uncertainty regarding the outcome—both mortality and morbidity—is a primary concern. Traditionally, family members are not allowed to be present during resuscitation efforts in the ED. However, studies indicate that family presence

during emergencies alleviates the family's anger about being separated from the patient during a crisis, reduces their anxiety, eliminates doubts about what was done to help the patient, and facilitates the grieving process if the patient dies (Mangurten, Scott, Guzzetta, and others, 2006).

Regardless of whether an institution permits parental presence during CPR, nurses must consider the needs, fears, and concerns of family members during this situation. If family presence is not permitted during CPR, nurses should arrange for someone to remain with the family. After the child's recovery or death, the family will continue to need support and thorough medical information regarding lifesaving measures, the prognosis if the child survives, and the cause of death if the child dies.

CARDIOPULMONARY RESUSCITATION

Cardiac arrest in children is less often of cardiac origin than from prolonged hypoxemia secondary to inadequate oxygenation, ventilation, and circulation (shock). Some causes of cardiac arrest include injuries, suffocation (e.g., FB aspiration), smoke inhalation, or infection. Respiratory arrest is associated with a better survival rate than cardiac arrest. After cardiac arrest occurs, the outcome of resuscitative efforts is poor.

Apnea signals the need for rapid, vigorous action to prevent cardiac arrest. In such situations, nurses must initiate action immediately and notify emergency personnel. In the hospital, emergency equipment must be available and easily accessible in all patient care areas. The status of emergency equipment must be checked at least once daily. Regardless of the cause of the arrest, basic procedures are carried out and modified somewhat according to the child's size.

Rescuers who have infections that may be transmitted by blood or saliva or who believe they have been exposed to such an infection should not perform mouth-to-mouth resuscitation if a barrier device or mask with a one-way valve is not available. If CPR efforts are anticipated in the workplace or other out-of-hospital settings, rescuers should have access to these devices.

Outside the hospital situation, the first action in an emergency is to quickly assess the extent of any injury and determine whether the child is unconscious. A child who is struggling to breathe but conscious should be transported immediately to an advanced life support (ALS) facility, with the child maintaining whatever position affords the most comfort. Attempting to transport a child by automobile wastes valuable time in obtaining help. Transportation by an emergency medical service (EMS) is recommended. Services in most large communities can institute ALS immediately or en route to a medical facility.

An unconscious child is managed with care to prevent additional trauma if a head or spinal cord injury has been sustained (see Spinal Cord Injury, Chapter 32).

Resuscitation Procedure

In 2010, the American Heart Association (AHA) implemented some changes in CPR guidelines. It stipulates that compressions only (no breaths) should be used when the rescuer is "untrained or trained and not proficient" (Travers, Rea, Bobrow, and others, 2010). However, if there is a respiratory arrest and the cause is asphyxia, then ventilations should be provided. Historically, the sequence for CPR was A-B-C (airway, breathing or ventilation, and chest compressions [or circulation]), but the latest guidelines have changed this recommended sequence to C-A-B to reduce the amount of time to the initiation of chest compressions (Fig. 23-10). Some modifications were also made to the depth of compressions, which now should be at least one third

Animation—Pediatric CPR

Component	RECOMMENDATIONS		
	Adults	**Children**	**Infants**
Recognition	Unresponsive (for all ages)		
	No breathing or no normal breathing (ie, only gasping)	No breathing or only gasping	
	No pulse palpated within 10 seconds for all ages (HCP only)		
CPR sequence*	C-A-B		
Compression rate	At least 100/min		
Compression depth	At least 2 inches (5 cm)	At least ⅓ AP diameter About 2 inches (5 cm)	At least ⅓ AP diameter About 1½ inches (4 cm)
Chest wall recoil	Allow complete recoil between compressions HCPs rotate compressors every 2 minutes		
Compression interruptions	Minimize interruptions in chest compressions Attempt to limit interrruptions to <10 seconds		
Airway	Head tilt–chin lift (HCP suspected trauma: jaw thrust)		
Compression-to-ventilation ratio (until advanced airway placed)	30:2 1 or 2 rescuers	30:2 Single rescuer 15:2 2 HCP rescuers	
Ventilations: when rescuer untrained or trained and not proficient	Compressions only		
Ventilations with advanced airway (HCP)	1 breath every 6-8 seconds (8-10 breaths/min) Asynchronous with chest compressions About 1 second per breath Visible chest rise		
Defibrillation	Attach and use AED as soon as available. Minimize interruptions in chest compressions before and after shock; resume CPR beginning with compressions immediately after each shock.		

Abbreviations: AED, automated external defibrillator; AP, anterior-posterior; CPR, cardiopulmonary resuscitation; HCP, healthcare provider.
*Excluding the newly born, in whom the etiology of an arrest is nearly always asphyxial.
NOTE: Newborn/neonatal information not included.

FIG 23-10 Summary of basic life support maneuvers for infants, children, and adults. (From Hazinski MF, Chameides L, Hemphill RR, and others: *Highlights of the 2010 American Heart Association guidelines for CPR and ECC*, retrieved March 4, 2012, from http://www.heart.org/idc/groups/heart-public/@wcm/@ecc/documents/downloadable/ucm_317350.pdf.)

of the anteroposterior diameter of the chest (4 cm in infants and 5 cm in older children). The AHA stipulates that having rescuers stop to detect a pulse is not reliable and wastes time. Instead, rescuers should start CPR in an adult if unresponsive and not breathing or not breathing normally or if they failed to detect a pulse within 10 seconds. The "look, listen, and feel for breathing" practice is no longer recommended. Chest compressions should be at a rate of *at least* 100 per minute. Each breath should be delivered at a rate of 1 breath every 6 to 8 seconds. The automatic external defibrillator (AED) is used as a part of the treatment of cardiorespiratory arrest in children older than 1 year of age.

An update was made to the recommendation of AED or defibrillation use. The AHA stipulates that a manual defibrillator is preferred to an AED for defibrillation of infants. If a manual defibrillator is not available, an AED equipped with a pediatric dose attenuator is preferred. If neither is available, an AED without a pediatric dose attenuator may be used (Travers, Rea, Bobrow, and others, 2010). There is

still limited evidence to support the safety of AED use in infants, but it may be safe and effective in this group. Appropriate-sized pediatric pads must be used for small children. Health care providers are advised to give children 1 year and older a defibrillatory shock after providing approximately five cycles of CPR (≈2 minutes of cycles of 30 compressions and two ventilations by the lone rescuer), provided the AED is sensitive to pediatric rhythms, the device is capable of delivering a pediatric dose of 2 to 4 joules/kg, and a shockable rhythm (usually ventricular fibrillation) is present. In a hospital situation in which weight-based defibrillation dosing is possible, manual defibrillation is the mode of choice instead of AED. When using an AED, health care providers are advised to give adults and children older than 8 years of age a defibrillatory shock within 5 minutes of collapse outside the hospital and within 3 minutes in the hospital.

If two rescuers are present, one rescuer should begin CPR while the second rescuer activates the EMS system by calling 9-1-1 and obtaining an AED. Pediatric rescuers provide five cycles of basic life support

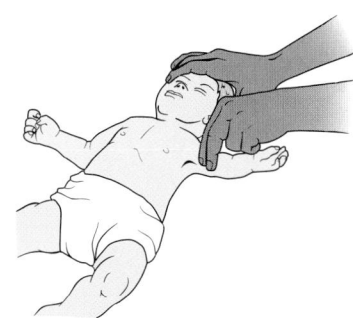

FIG 23-11 Locating the brachial pulse in an infant.

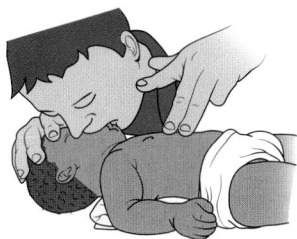

FIG 23-12 Combining chest compressions with breathing in infant.

(≈2 minutes) before activating EMS; each cycle consists of 30 chest compressions and two ventilations. Because pediatric arrests are most commonly caused by respiratory arrest, maintaining ventilation is key.

Pulse Check

During an emergent situation, palpating the pulse can be a challenge. The patient should be reassessed for a pulse every 2 minutes of CPR. The pulse should not be assessed for longer than 10 seconds. The carotid is the most central and accessible artery in children older than 1 year of age, but the femoral pulse may also be used. An infant's short and often fat neck makes the carotid pulse difficult to palpate. Therefore, in an infant, it is preferable to use the brachial pulse, located on the inner side of the upper arm midway between the elbow and the shoulder (Fig. 23-11). Absence of a carotid or brachial pulse is considered sufficient indication to begin external cardiac massage. *Lay rescuers are not taught to check the pulse but are taught to look for signs of circulation (e.g., normal breathing, coughing, or air movement) in response to rescue breaths.*

Chest Compression

External chest compression consists of serial, rhythmic compressions of the chest to maintain circulation to vital organs until the child achieves spontaneous vital signs or ALS can be provided. *Chest compressions are always interspersed with ventilation of the lungs.** For optimal compressions, it is essential that the child's spine is supported on a firm surface during compressions of the sternum and that sternal pressure is forceful but not traumatic. The child's head is positioned for optimal airway opening using the head tilt–chin lift maneuver if the cervical spine is stable and no neck injuries are present. It is essential to prevent overextension of the head of small infants because this tends to close the flexible trachea.

The placement of the fingers for compression in infants is at a point on the lower sternum just below the intersection of the sternum and an imaginary line drawn between the nipples (Fig. 23-12). Compressions on the child 1 to 8 years of age are applied to the lower half of the sternum (Fig. 23-13). Sternal compression to infants is applied with two fingers on the sternum, exerting a firm downward thrust; for children, pressure is applied with the heel of one hand or two hands, depending on the child's size. Current AHA (Travers, Rea, Bobrow, and others, 2010) guidelines include the addition of the two-thumb encircling hands technique for chest compressions for infants when two health care providers are present. In the two-thumb technique, one of the two rescuers places both thumbs side by side over the lower half of the infant's sternum; the remaining fingers encircle the infant's chest

---

*The AHA recommends that laypersons who witness an adult cardiac arrest perform continuous chest compressions (push hard, push fast) without ventilations (Berg, Hemphill, Abella, and others, 2010).

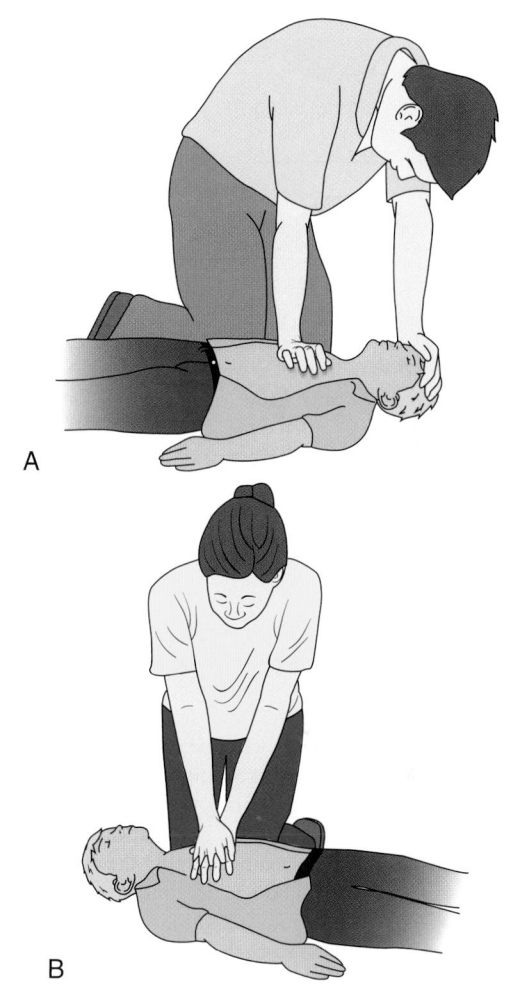

FIG 23-13 Chest compressions in child: one hand for a smaller child **(A)** and two hands for a larger child **(B)**.

and support the back. The two-thumb technique is not taught to lay rescuers and is not practical for a health care provider working alone.

Lone-rescuer CPR is continued at the ratio of two breaths to 30 compressions for all ages until signs of recovery appear. These signs include palpable peripheral pulses, return of pupils to normal size, the disappearance of mottling and cyanosis, and possibly return of spontaneous respiration. When two rescuers are present, they should deliver two breaths to each 15 compressions.

Open the Airway

For effective CPR the victim is placed on the back on a firm, flat surface using appropriate precautions. With loss of consciousness, the tongue, which is attached to the lower jaw, may relax and fall back, obstructing the airway. To open the airway, the head is positioned with a

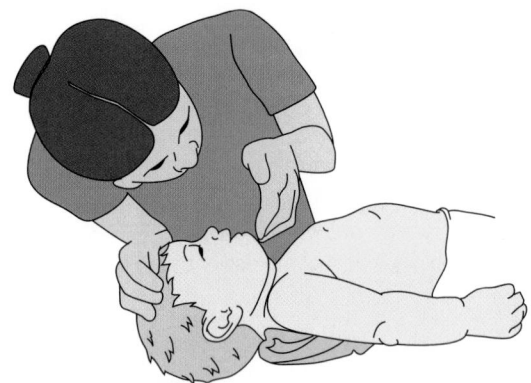

FIG 23-14 Open the airway using the head tilt–chin lift maneuver and check breathing.

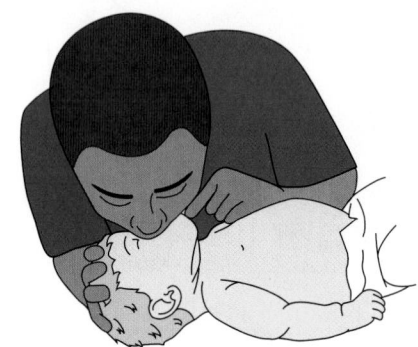

FIG 23-15 Mouth-to-mouth and nose breathing for an infant.

head tilt–chin lift maneuver (if stable cervical spine) by the lay rescuer. Health professionals should open the airway using either a head tilt–chin lift or jaw thrust (if an unstable cervical spine) maneuver. A head tilt is accomplished by placing one hand on the victim's forehead and applying firm, backward pressure with the palm to tilt back the head. The fingers of the free hand are placed under the bony portion of the lower jaw near the chin to lift and bring the chin forward (chin lift). This supports the jaw and helps tilt the head back (Fig. 23-14).

The jaw thrust is accomplished by grasping the angles of the victim's lower jaw and lifting with both hands, one on each side, displacing the mandible upward and outward. *The jaw thrust is recommended only for health care workers.* In suspected neck injuries, the jaw thrust method should be used while the cervical spine is completely immobilized. After a patent airway has been restored by removal of foreign material and secretions (if indicated) and if the child is not breathing, maintenance of the airway is continued, and rescue breathing is initiated.

Give Breaths

To ventilate the lungs in the infant (from birth to 1 year of age), the bag valve mask (BVM) or operator's mouth is placed in such a way that both the mouth and the nostrils are covered (Fig. 23-15) using the E-C technique. The thumb and index finger of the nondominant hand secure the mask on the patient's face (forming a C) while the first three fingers of the same hand are used to lift the jaw (forming an E). Children (older than 1 year of age) are ventilated through the mouth while the nostrils are firmly pinched for airtight contact; alternatively, bag and mask ventilation is optimal.

The volume of air in an infant's lungs is small, and the air passages are considerably smaller, with resistance to flow potentially higher than in adults. The rescuer should deliver small puffs of air and assess the rise of the chest to ensure that overinflation does not occur. A gentle rise of the chest is a sufficient indicator of adequate inflation and indicates that the airway is clear. Breaths should be given over 1 second with sufficient volume to make the chest rise. If the chest does not rise, reposition the head or jaw and try again.

Medications

Medications are an important adjunct to CPR, especially cardiac arrest, and are used during and after resuscitation in children. Medications are used to (1) correct hypoxemia, (2) increase perfusion pressure during chest compression, (3) stimulate spontaneous or more forceful myocardial contraction, (4) accelerate cardiac rate, (5) correct metabolic acidosis, and (6) suppress ventricular ectopy.

Appropriate fluid therapy is initiated immediately in the hospital or by EMS personnel during transport (see Parenteral Fluid Therapy, Chapter 22, and Shock, Chapter 25). A complete supply of emergency medications is kept and maintained in all EMS vehicles and on all hospital units. The supply is checked on a regular basis (usually once a day at minimum). When administering drugs during CPR (or a "code"), use a saline flush or other compatible flush solution between medications to prevent drug interactions. Document all drugs, dosages, and the time and route of administration.

AIRWAY OBSTRUCTION

Attempts at clearing the airway should be considered for (1) children in whom aspiration of an FB is witnessed or strongly suspected and (2) unconscious, nonbreathing children whose airways remain obstructed despite the usual maneuvers to open them. When aspiration is strongly suspected, the child is encouraged to continue coughing as long as the cough remains forceful. In a conscious choking child, attempt to relieve the obstruction only if:

- The child is unable to make any sounds.
- The cough becomes ineffective.
- There is increasing respiratory difficulty with stridor.

! NURSING ALERT

Blind finger sweeps are avoided in infants and children younger than 8 years old.

Infants

A combination of back blows (over the spine between the shoulder blades) and chest thrusts (on the sternum, the same location as for chest compressions) is recommended to relieve the FB obstruction in infants (Fig. 23-16). A choking infant is placed face down over the rescuer's arm with the head lower than the trunk and the head supported. For additional support, the rescuer should support the arm firmly against the thigh. Up to five quick, sharp back blows are delivered between the infant's shoulder blades with the heel of the rescuer's hand. Less force is required than would be applied to an adult. After delivery of the back blows, the rescuer's free hand is placed flat on the infant's back so that the infant is "sandwiched" between the two hands, making certain the neck and chin are well supported. While the rescuer maintains support with the infant's head lower than the trunk, the infant is turned and placed supine on the rescuer's thigh, where up to five quick downward chest thrusts are applied in rapid succession in the same location as external chest compressions described for CPR. Back blows and chest thrusts are continued until the object is removed

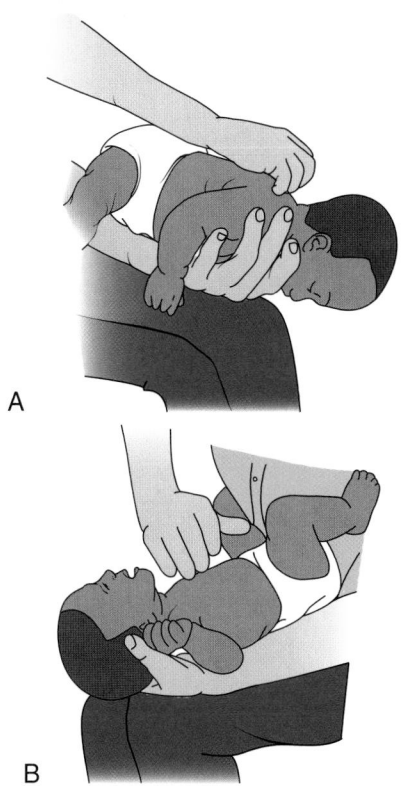

FIG 23-16 Relief of foreign body obstruction in infant. **A,** Back blows. **B,** Chest thrusts.

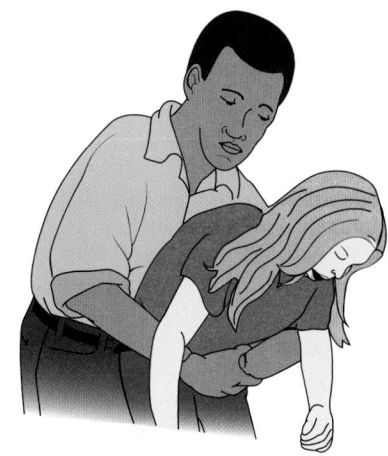

FIG 23-17 Abdominal thrusts in standing child for relief of foreign body obstruction.

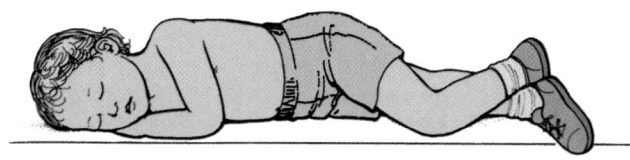

FIG 23-18 Recovery position for a child after a respiratory emergency.

or the infant becomes unconscious. At that time, CPR should be initiated.

Children

A series of subdiaphragmatic abdominal thrusts (Heimlich maneuver) is recommended for children older than 1 year of age. The maneuver creates an artificial cough that forces air—and with it, the FB—out of the airway. The procedure is carried out with the child in a standing, sitting, or lying position (Fig. 23-17). In a conscious choking child, upward thrusts are delivered to the upper abdomen with the fisted hand at a point just below the rib cage. To prevent damage to the internal organs, the rescuer's hands should not touch the xiphoid process of the sternum or the lower margins of the ribs. Up to five thrusts are repeated in rapid succession until the FB is expelled.

It is neither necessary nor desirable to squeeze or compress the arms during the procedure. It is not a punch or a bear hug. The child

may vomit after relief of the obstruction and should be positioned to prevent aspiration. After breathing is restored, the child should receive medical attention and be assessed for complications. If the child is coughing, allow him or her to relieve the obstruction this way.

The success of the technique is primarily a result of the obstruction occurring at the end of a maximum respiration. The victim is most likely to choke on food during inspiration; therefore, the tidal volume plus expiratory reserve volume is present in the lungs. When pressure is exerted on the diaphragm by the maneuver, the food bolus is ejected with considerable force by this trapped air.

If the victim is breathing or resumes effective breathing after emergency interventions, place him or her in the recovery position—move the head, shoulders, and torso simultaneously and turn onto the side. The leg not in contact with the ground may be bent and the knee moved forward to stabilize the victim (Fig. 23-18). The victim should not be moved in any way if trauma is suspected and should not be placed in the recovery position if rescue breathing or CPR is required.

KEY POINTS

- Acute infection of the respiratory tract is the most common cause of illness in infancy and childhood.
- The incidence and severity of respiratory tract infections are influenced by the infectious agents involved, the child's age, any underlying medical conditions, and the child's natural defenses.
- Common respiratory tract infections of childhood include nasopharyngitis, pharyngitis (including tonsillitis), influenza, infectious mononucleosis, and OM.
- Croup syndromes involve acute inflammation and variable degrees of obstruction of the epiglottis, larynx, or trachea.

- The primary goals in the care of children with croup are observation for signs of respiratory distress and relief of laryngeal obstruction.
- Common infections of the lower airways are bacterial tracheitis, bronchitis, and RSV bronchiolitis.
- Pneumonias are classified according to site (lobar, bronchial, or interstitial) or by etiologic agent (viral, bacterial, mycoplasmal) or are associated with aspiration of foreign material.
- In TB, susceptibility to the bacillus can be influenced by heredity, age, stress, poor nutrition, and intercurrent infection.

■ KEY POINTS—cont'd

- Second-hand smoke exposure is a major environmental pollutant contributing to respiratory illness in children.
- Asthma is the leading cause of chronic illness in children.
- General therapeutic management of asthma includes assessment of asthma severity, allergen control, drug therapy, symptom management, and sometimes hyposensitization.
- Support for the family of the child with asthma includes education about the disease and its therapy and facilitation of self-management.
- CF is the most common inherited disease in children.
- The diagnosis of CF is based on newborn screening finding of elevated IRT, DNA analysis showing a CFTR mutation, and a positive sweat chloride test result (increased sweat electrolyte content).

- Choking and respiratory failure are respiratory emergencies that require immediate intervention.
- The sequence for CPR in infants, children, and adults is C-A-B (compressions, airway, breathing).
- Abdominal thrusts are used in children in whom FB obstruction is witnessed or strongly suspected. A combination of back blows and chest thrusts is used for infants with FB obstruction.
- In a conscious choking child, attempts to relieve the obstruction are used only if the child is unable to make any sounds, the cough becomes ineffective, or the child has increasing respiratory difficulty with stridor.

REFERENCES

Akinbami LJ, Moorman JE, Garbe PL, and others: Status of childhood asthma in the United States, 1980–2007, *Pediatrics* 123(suppl 3):S131–S145, 2009.

Albuali WH, Singh RN, Fraser DD, and others: Have changes in ventilation practice improved outcome in children with acute lung injury? *Pediatr Crit Care Med* 8(4):324–330, 2007.

American Academy of Otolaryngology—Head and Neck Surgery: Clinical practice guideline: tonsillectomy in children, *Bulletin* 19:6, 2011.

American Academy of Pediatrics: Clinical practice guideline: diagnosis and management of childhood obstructive sleep apnea syndrome, *Pediatrics* 109(4):704–712, 2002.

American Academy of Pediatrics: Clinical practice guidelines: diagnosis and management of acute otitis media, *Pediatrics* 113(5):1451–1465, 2004a.

American Academy of Pediatrics: Clinical practice guidelines: otitis media with effusion, *Pediatrics* 113(5):1412–1429, 2004b.

American Academy of Pediatrics: Clinical practice guideline: diagnosis and management of bronchiolitis, *Pediatrics* 118(4):1774–1793, 2006.

American Academy of Pediatrics: Clinical report—sports drinks and energy drinks for children and adolescents: are they appropriate? *Pediatrics* 127(6):1182–1189, 2011.

American Academy of Pediatrics, Committee on Infectious Diseases, Pickering L, editor: *Red book: 2009 report of the Committee on Infectious Diseases*, ed 28, Elk Grove Village, Ill, 2009, Author.

American Academy of Pediatrics, Committee on Infectious Diseases: Recommendations for prevention and control of influenza in children, 2011–2012, *Pediatrics* 128(4): 813–824, 2011.

American Academy of Pediatrics, Task Force on Sudden Infant Death Syndrome: The changing concept of sudden infant death syndrome: diagnostic coding shifts, controversies regarding the sleeping environment, and new variables to consider in reducing risk, *Pediatrics* 116(5): 1245–1255, 2005.

American Thoracic Society: Standards and indications for cardiopulmonary sleep studies in children, *Am J Resp Crit Care Med* 153(2):866–878, 1996.

Antoon AY, Donovan MK: Burn injuries. In Kliegman RM, Stanton BF, St. Geme JW, and others, editors: *Nelson textbook of pediatrics*, ed 19, Philadelphia, 2011, Saunders.

Benninger M, Walner D: Coblation: improving outcomes for children following adenotonsillectomy, *Clin Cornerstone* 9(suppl 1):S13–S23, 2007a.

Benninger M, Walner D: Obstructive sleep-disordered breathing in children, *Clin Cornerstone* 9(suppl 1):S6–S12, 2007b.

Berg RA, Hemphill R, Abella BS, and others: Part 5: adult basic life support: 2010 American Heart Association guidelines for cardiopulmonary resuscitation and emergency cardiovascular care, *Circulation* 122(suppl 3):S685–S705, 2010.

Bernard GR, Artigas A, Brigham KL, and others: Report of the American-European consensus conference on ARDS: definitions, mechanisms, relevant outcomes and clinical trial coordination. The Consensus Committee, *Intensive Care Med* 20:225–232, 1994.

Bhetwal N, McConaghy JR: The evaluation and treatment of children with acute otitis media, *Primary Care* 34(1):59–70, 2007.

Borowitz D, Baker RD, Stallings V: Consensus report on nutrition for pediatric patients with cystic fibrosis, *J Pediatr Gastroenterol Nutr* 35(3):246–259, 2002.

Burkhart PV, Rayens MK, Revelette WR, and others: Improved health outcomes with peak flow monitoring for children with asthma, *J Asthma* 44(2):137–142, 2007.

Centers for Disease Control and Prevention: Licensure of a 13-valent pneumococcal conjugate vaccine (PCV13) and recommendations for use among children—Advisory Committee on Immunization Practices (ACIP), 2010, *MMWR Wkly* 59(9):258–261, 2010.

Chávez-Bueno S, Mejías A, Jafri H, and others: Respiratory syncytial virus: old challenges and new approaches, *Pediatr Ann* 34(1):62–68, 2005.

Chen CM, Tischer C, Schnappinger M, and others: The role of cats and dogs in asthma and allergy—a systematic review, *Int J Hyg Environm Health* 213(1):1–31, 2010.

Courtney AU, McCarter DF, Pollart SM: Childhood asthma: treatment update, *Am Fam Physician* 71(10):1959–1968, 2005.

Cuthbert AW: New horizons in the treatment of cystic fibrosis, *Br J Pharmacol* 163(1):173–183, 2011.

Cystic Fibrosis Foundation: *Frequently asked questions*, Bethesda, Md, 2009, Author, retrieved July 23, 2009, from http://www.cff.org/AboutCF/Faqs.

Egan M: Cystic fibrosis. In Kliegman RM, Stanton BF, St. Geme JW, and others, editors: *Nelson textbook of pediatrics*, ed 19, Philadelphia, 2011, Saunders.

Flume PA, Robinson KA, O'Sullivan BP, and others: Cystic fibrosis pulmonary guidelines: airway clearance therapies, *Respir Care* 54(4): 522–537, 2009.

Food and Drug Administration: Early communication about an ongoing safety review of omalizumab (marketed as Xolair), 2009, retrieved April 20, 2011, from http://www.fda.gov/Drugs/DrugSafety/PostmarketDrugSafetyInformationforPatientsandProviders/DrugSafetyInformationforHealthcareProfessionals/ucm172218.htm.

Food and Drug Administration: Long-acting beta-agonists (LABAs): new safe use requirements, 2011, retrieved April 20, 2011, from http://www.fda.gov/Safety/MedWatch/SafetyInformation/SafetyAlertsforHumanMedicalProducts/ucm201003.htm.

Goldstein NA, Mandel EM, Kurs-Lasky M, and others: Water precautions and tympanostomy tubes: a randomized, controlled trial, *Laryngoscope* 115(2):324–330, 2005.

Hazle LA: Cystic fibrosis. In Allen PJ, Vessey JA, Schapiro NA, editors, *Primary care of the child with a chronic condition*, ed 5, St. Louis, 2010, Mosby.

Heinrich J: Influence of indoor factors in dwellings on the development of childhood asthma, *Int J Hyg Environm Health* 214(1):1–25, 2011.

Hopkins A, Lahiri T, Salerno R, and others: Changing epidemiology of life-threatening upper airway infections: the reemergence of bacterial tracheitis, *Pediatrics* 118(4):1418–1421, 2006.

Kerschner JE: Otitis media. In Kliegman RM, Stanton BF, St. Geme JW, and others, editors: *Nelson textbook of pediatrics*, ed 19, Philadelphia, 2011, Saunders.

Kim Chiaw P, Eckford PD, Bear CE: Insights into the mechanisms underlying CFTR channel activity, the molecular basis for cystic fibrosis and strategies for therapy, *Essays Biochem* 50(1):233–248, 2011.

Li YF, Langholz B, Salam MT, and others: Maternal and grandmaternal smoking patterns are associated with early childhood asthma, *Chest* 127(4):1232–1241, 2005.

Liu AH, Covar RA, Spahn JD, and others: Childhood asthma. In Kliegman RM, Stanton BF, St. Geme JW, and others, editors: *Nelson textbook of pediatrics*, ed 19, Philadelphia, 2011, Saunders.

Mangurten J, Scott SH, Guzzetta CE, and others: Effects of family presence during resuscitation and invasive procedures in a pediatric emergency department, *J Emerg Nurs* 32(3): 225–233, 2006.

Mazor R, Green TP: Pulmonary edema. In Kliegman RM, Stanton BF, St. Geme JW, and others, editors: *Nelson textbook of pediatrics*, ed 19, Philadelphia, 2011, Saunders.

Meissner HC, Bocchini JA: Reducing RSV hospitalizations: AAP modifies recommendation for use of palivizumab in high-risk infants, young children, *AAP News* 30(7):1–2, 2009.

Moore M, Little P: Humidified air inhalation for treating croup, *Cochrane Database Syst Rev* 19(3):CD002870, 2006.

Moran A, Brunzell C, Cohen RC, and others: Clinical care guidelines for cystic fibrosis-related diabetes: a position statement of the American Diabetes Association and a clinical practice guideline of the Cystic Fibrosis Foundation endorsed by the Pediatric Endocrine Society, *Diabetes Care* 33(12):2697–2708, 2010.

National Asthma Education and Prevention Program: Guidelines for the diagnosis and management of asthma, August 2007, retrieved March 7, 2008, from http://www.nhlbi.nih.gov/guidelines/asthma/index.htm.

Newton TJ: Respiratory care of the hospitalized patient with cystic fibrosis, *Respir Care* 54(6): 769–775, 2009.

O'Riordan SMP, Dattani MT, Hindmarsh PC: Cystic fibrosis-related diabetes in childhood, *Horm Res Paediatr* 73(1):15–24, 2010.

Owens JA: Sleep medicine. In Kliegman RM, Stanton BF, St. Geme JW, and others, editors: *Nelson textbook of pediatrics*, ed 19, Philadelphia, 2011, Saunders.

Pediatric Tuberculosis Collaborative Group: Targeted tuberculin skin testing and treatment of latent tuberculosis infection in children and adolescents, *Pediatrics* 114(4 suppl):1175–1201, 2004.

Rafei K, Lichenstein R: Airway infectious disease emergencies, *Pediatr Clin North Am* 53(2): 215–242, 2006.

Randolph AG: Management of acute lung injury and acute respiratory distress syndrome in children, *Crit Care Med* 37(8):2448–2454, 2009.

Ranganathan SC, Sonnappa S: Pneumonia and others respiratory infections, *Pediatr Clin North Am* 56(1):135–156, 2009.

Redding GJ: Bronchiectasis in children, *Pediatr Clin North Am* 56(1):157–171, 2009.

Ren CL, Morgan WJ, Konstan KW, and others: Presence of methicillin resistant *Staphylococcus aureus* in respiratory cultures from cystic fibrosis patients is associated with lower lung function, *Pediatr Pulmonol* 42(6):513–518, 2007.

Rimsza ME, Newberry S: Unexpected infant deaths associated with use of cough and cold medications, *Pediatrics* 122(2):e318–e322, 2008.

Ryan T, Brewer M, Small L: Over-the-counter cough and cold medication use in young children, *Pediatr Nurs* 34(2):174–180, 184, 2008.

Sandora TJ, Sectish TC: Community-acquired pneumonia. In Kliegman RM, Stanton BF, St. Geme JW, and others, editors: *Nelson textbook of pediatrics*, ed 19, Philadelphia, 2011, Saunders.

Sheahan SL, Free TA: Counseling parents to quit smoking, *Pediatr Nurs* 31(2):98–108, 2005.

Sicerer SH, Wood RA, AAP Section on Allergy and Immunology: Allergy testing in childhood: Using allergen-specific IgE tests, *Pediatrics* 129(1):193–197, 2012.

Sovari AA, Ooi HH: Cardiogenic pulmonary edema, 2008, retrieved April 8, 2011, from http://emedicine.medscape.com/article/157452-overview#a0104.

Strunk RC, Bloomberg GR: Omalizumab for asthma, *N Engl J Med* 354(25):2689–2695, 2006.

Travers AH, Rea TD, Bobrow BJ, and others: Part 4: CPR overview: 2010 American Heart Association guidelines for cardiopulmonary resuscitation and emergency cardiovascular care, *Circulation* 122(suppl 3):S676–S684, 2010.

Ventre K, Randolph AG: Ribavirin for respiratory syncytial virus infection of the lower respiratory tract in infants and young children, *Cochrane Database Syst Rev* 24(1):CD000181, 2007.

Volpe DI, Smith MF, Sultan K: Managing pediatric asthma exacerbations in the ED, *Am J Nurs* 111(2):48–53, 2011.

Witmans M, Young R: Update on pediatric sleep-disordered breathing, *Pediatr Clin North Am* 58(3):571–589, 2011.

World Health Organization: Global alert and response (GAR): pandemic preparedness, 2011, retrieved April 26, 2011, from http://www.who.int/csr/disease/influenza/pandemic/en/.

CHAPTER

24

The Child with Gastrointestinal Dysfunction

Debi S. Lammert, Kristina D. Wilson, and David Wilson

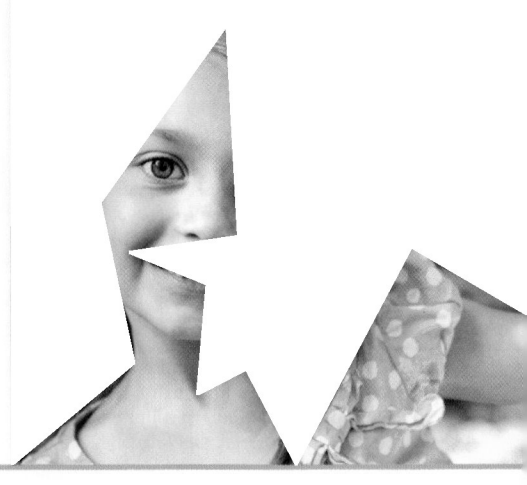

evolve WEBSITE

http://evolve.elsevier.com/wong/essentials

Animations—Appendicitis; Digestive Tract, Passage of Food; Intestines; Intussusception; Volvulus, Pediatric

Case Studies—Acute Diarrhea; Appendicitis; Cleft Lip and Palate; Dehydration; Dehydration and Diarrhea; Gastroenteritis; Gastrointestinal Problems; Hepatitis

Key Point Summaries

NCLEX-Style Review Questions

Nursing Care Plans—The Child with Acute Diarrhea (Gastroenteritis); The Child with Appendicitis; The Child with Cleft Lip and/or Cleft Palate; The Child with Fluid and Electrolyte Disturbances

CHAPTER OUTLINE

Distribution of Body Fluids, 763
  Changes in Fluid Volume Related to Growth, 763
    Water Balance in Infants, 763
  Disturbances of Fluid and Electrolyte Balance, 764
    Water Intoxication, 764
    Dehydration, 764
Gastrointestinal Dysfunction, 771
  Disorders of Motility, 771
    Diarrhea, 771
    Constipation, 778
    Hirschsprung Disease, 779
    Vomiting, 781
    Gastroesophageal Reflux, 782
  Recurrent and Functional Abdominal Pain, 784

Inflammatory Disorders, 785
  Acute Appendicitis, 785
    Nursing Care Plan: The Child with Appendicitis, 787
  Meckel Diverticulum, 786
  Inflammatory Bowel Disease, 789
  Peptic Ulcer Disease, 792
Hepatic Disorders, 794
  Acute Hepatitis, 794
  Cirrhosis, 797
  Biliary Atresia, 798
Structural Defects, 800
  Cleft Lip and Cleft Palate, 800
  Esophageal Atresia and Tracheoesophageal Fistula, 803
  Hernias, 805

Obstructive Disorders, 805
  Hypertrophic Pyloric Stenosis, 805
  Intussusception, 809
  Malrotation and Volvulus, 810
  Anorectal Malformations, 810
Malabsorption Syndromes, 812
  Celiac Disease (Gluten-Sensitive Enteropathy), 813
  Short-Bowel Syndrome, 815

LEARNING OBJECTIVES

On completion of this chapter the reader will be able to:
- Describe the characteristics of infants that affect their ability to adapt to fluid loss or gain.
- Formulate a care plan for the infant with acute diarrhea.
- Compare and contrast the inflammatory diseases of the gastrointestinal tract.
- Describe the nursing care of the child with hepatitis.
- Formulate a plan for teaching parents preoperative and postoperative care of the child with a cleft lip or palate.
- Formulate a care plan for the child with an obstructive disorder.
- Identify nutritional therapies for the child with a malabsorption syndrome.

DISTRIBUTION OF BODY FLUIDS

The distribution of body fluids, or total body water (TBW), involves the presence of intracellular fluid (ICF) and extracellular fluid (ECF). Water is the major constituent of body tissues, and the TBW in an individual ranges from 45% (in late adolescence) to as much as 75% in term newborns or 90% in extremely preterm infants of total body weight.

Whereas the ICF refers to the fluid contained within the cells, the ECF is the fluid outside the cells. The ECF is further broken down into several components: intravascular (contained within the blood vessels), interstitial (surrounding the cell; the location of most ECF), and transcellular (contained within specialized body cavities such as cerebrospinal, synovial, and pleural fluid). Whereas in a newborn about 50% of the body fluid is contained within the ECF, 30% of a toddler's body fluid is contained within the ECF.

Maintenance water requirement is the volume of water needed to replace obligatory fluid loss such as that from insensible water loss (through the skin and respiratory tract), evaporative water loss, and losses through urine and stool formation. The amount and type of these losses may be altered by disease states such as fever (with increased sweating), diarrhea, gastric suction, and pooling of body fluids in a body space.

Nurses should be alert for altered fluid requirements in various conditions:

Increased requirements:
- Fever (add 12% per rise of 1° C)
- Vomiting, diarrhea
- High-output kidney failure
- Diabetes insipidus
- Diabetic ketoacidosis
- Burns
- Shock
- Tachypnea
- Radiant warmer (preterm infant)
- Phototherapy (infants)
- Postoperative bowel surgery (gastroschisis, omphalocele)

Decreased requirements:
- Congestive heart failure
- Syndrome of inappropriate antidiuretic hormone
- Mechanical ventilation
- After surgery
- Oliguric renal failure
- Increased intracranial pressure

Basal maintenance calculations for required body water are based on the body's requirements for water in a normometabolic state at rest; estimated fluid requirements are then increased or decreased from these parameters based on increased or decreased water losses, such as with elevated body temperature (increased) or heart failure (decreased). Daily maintenance fluid requirements for infants, toddlers, and older children are listed in Table 24-1. These requirements are not appropriate for neonates.

Maintenance fluids contain both water and electrolytes and can be estimated from the child's age, body weight, degree of activity, and body temperature. Basal metabolic rate (BMR) is derived from standard tables and adjusted for the child's activity, temperature, and disease state. For example, for afebrile patients at rest, the maintenance water requirement is approximately 100 ml for each 100 kcal expended. Children with fluid losses or other alterations require adjustment of these basic needs to accommodate abnormal losses of both water and electrolytes as a result of a disease state. For example, insensible losses increase when basal expenditure increases by fever or hypermetabolic states. Hypometabolic states, such as hypothyroidism and hypothermia, decrease the BMR.

The percentage of TBW varies among individuals and in adults and older children is related primarily to the amount of body fat. Consequently, females, who have more body fat than males, and obese persons tend to have less water content in relation to weight.

CHANGES IN FLUID VOLUME RELATED TO GROWTH

The fetus is composed primarily of water with little tissue substance. As the organism grows and develops, a progressive decrease occurs in TBW with the fastest rate of decline taking place during fetal life. The changes in water content and distribution that occur with age reflect the changes that take place in the relative amounts of bone, muscle, and fat making up the body. At maturity, the percentage of TBW is somewhat higher in the male than in the female and is probably a result of the differences in body composition, particularly fat and muscle content.

Another important aspect of growth change as it corresponds to water distribution is related to the ICF and ECF compartments. In the fetus and prematurely born infants, the largest proportion of body water is contained in the ECF compartment. As growth and development proceed, the proportion within this fluid compartment decreases as the ICF and cell solids increase. The ECF diminishes rapidly from approximately 40% of body weight at birth to less than 30% at 1 year of age. The different effects on boys and girls become apparent at puberty.

Water Balance in Infants

Compared with older children and adults, infants and young children have a greater need for water and are more vulnerable to alterations in fluid and electrolyte balance. Infants have a greater fluid intake and output relative to size. Water and electrolyte disturbances occur more frequently and more rapidly, and infants and children adjust less promptly to these alterations.

The fluid compartments in infants vary significantly from those in adults, primarily because of an expanded extracellular compartment. The extracellular fluid (ECF) compartment constitutes more than half the TBW at birth and has a greater relative content of extracellular sodium and chloride. Infants lose a large amount of fluid at birth and maintain a larger amount of ECF than adults until about 2 years of age. This contributes to greater and more rapid water loss during this age period.

Fluid losses create compartment deficits that are reflected throughout the duration of dehydration. In general, approximately 60% of fluid is lost from the ECF, and the remaining 40% comes from the intracellular fluid (ICF). The amount of fluid lost from the ECF increases with acute illness and decreases with chronic loss.

Fluid losses vary with age and are divided into insensible, urinary, and fecal losses. Approximately two thirds of insensible losses occur through the skin; the remaining third is lost through the respiratory tract. Heat and humidity, body temperature, and respiratory rate influence insensible fluid loss. Infants and children have a greater tendency to become highly febrile than do adults. Fever increases insensible water loss approximately 7 ml/kg/24 hr for each degree rise in temperature above 37.2° C (99° F). Fever and increased surface area relative to volume are factors that contribute to greater insensible fluid losses in young patients.

TABLE 24-1	DAILY MAINTENANCE FLUID REQUIREMENTS*
BODY WEIGHT (KG)	**AMOUNT OF FLUID PER DAY**
1–10	100 ml/kg
11–20	1000 ml plus 50 ml/kg for each kg >10 kg
>20	1500 ml plus 20 ml/kg for each kg >20 kg

*Not appropriate for neonatal use.

Body Surface Area

The infant's relatively greater body surface area (BSA) allows larger quantities of fluid to be lost in insensible perspiration through the skin. It is estimated that the BSA of preterm neonates is five times greater, and that of newborns is two to three times greater, than that of older children or adults. The proportionately longer gastrointestinal (GI) tract in infancy is another source of fluid loss, especially from diarrhea.

Basal Metabolic Rate

The rate of metabolism in infancy is significantly higher than in adulthood because of the larger BSA in relation to the mass of active tissue. Consequently, there is a greater production of metabolic wastes that must be excreted by the kidneys. Any condition that increases metabolism causes greater heat production, insensible fluid loss, and an increased need for water for excretion. The BMR in infants and children is higher to support growth.

Kidney Function

The kidneys of infants are functionally immature at birth and are inefficient in excreting waste products of metabolism. Of particular importance for fluid balance is the inability of the infant's kidneys to concentrate or dilute urine, to conserve or excrete sodium, and to acidify urine. Infants are less able to handle large quantities of solute-free water than are older children, and infants are more likely to become dehydrated when given concentrated formulas or overhydrated when given excessive water or dilute formula.

Fluid Requirements

Infants ingest and excrete a greater amount of fluid per kilogram of body weight than do older children. Because electrolytes are excreted with water and infants have a limited ability for conservation, maintenance requirements include both water and electrolytes. The daily exchange of ECF in infants is greatly increased over that of older children, leaving infants with little fluid volume reserve in dehydrated states. Fluid requirements depend on hydration status, size, environmental factors, and underlying disease. Daily maintenance fluid requirements are shown in Table 24-1.

DISTURBANCES OF FLUID AND ELECTROLYTE BALANCE

Disturbances of fluids and their solute concentration are closely interrelated. Alterations in fluid volume affect the electrolyte component, and changes in electrolyte concentration influence fluid movement. Because intracellular water and electrolytes move to and from the ECF compartment, any imbalance in the ICF is reflected by an imbalance in the ECF. Disturbances in the ECF involve either an excess or a deficit of fluid or electrolytes. Of these, fluid loss occurs more frequently.

Depletion of ECF, usually caused by gastroenteritis, is one of the most common problems encountered in infants and children. Until modern techniques for fluid replacement were perfected, gastroenteritis was one of the chief causes of infant mortality. Fluid and electrolyte problems related to specific diseases and their management are discussed throughout the book where appropriate. The major fluid disturbances, their usual causes, and clinical manifestations are listed in Table 24-2. Problems of fluid and electrolyte disturbance always involve both water and electrolytes; therefore, replacement includes administration of both calculated on the basis of ongoing processes and laboratory serum electrolyte values.

Water Intoxication

Water intoxication, or fluid volume excess, is observed less often than dehydration. However, it is important that nurses and others who care for children be alert to this possibility in certain situations. Children who ingest excessive amounts of electrolyte-free water develop a concurrent decrease in serum sodium accompanied by central nervous system (CNS) symptoms. There is a large urinary output, and because water moves into the brain more rapidly than sodium moves out, the child may also exhibit irritability, somnolence, headache, vomiting, diarrhea, or generalized seizures. The affected child usually appears well hydrated but may be edematous or even dehydrated.

Fluid intoxication can occur during acute intravenous (IV) fluid replacement, too rapid dialysis, tap water enemas, feeding of incorrectly mixed formula, or excess water ingestion or with too rapid reduction of glucose levels in diabetic ketoacidosis. Patients with CNS infections occasionally retain excessive amounts of water. Administration of inappropriate hypotonic solutions (e.g., 0.45% sodium chloride) may cause a rapid reduction in sodium and result in symptoms of water excess or overload.

Infants are especially vulnerable to fluid volume excess. Their thirst mechanism is not well developed; therefore, they are unable to "turn off" fluid intake appropriately. A decreased glomerular filtration rate does not allow for repeated excretion of a water excess, and antidiuretic hormone (ADH) levels may not be maximally reduced. Consequently, infants are unable to excrete a water excess effectively.

Administration of inappropriately prepared formula is one of the more common causes of water intoxication in infants. Families who cannot afford to buy enough formula may dilute the formula to increase the volume or even substitute water for the formula. A family may run out of formula and dilute the remaining amount to make it last until they are able to purchase more. In addition, water is sometimes used for pacification when the infant is crying or fussy. Water intoxication can also occur in infants who receive overly vigorous hydration during a febrile illness.

A number of clinicians have reported water intoxication in children after swimming lessons. Although they hold their breath, some children apparently swallow a large amount of water during repeated submersion. Anticipatory guidance to parents should include a discussion of swimming instruction and advice to stop a lesson if the child swallows unusual amounts of water or exhibits any symptoms of hyponatremia (see Table 24-2).

Dehydration

Dehydration is a common body fluid disturbance in infants and children and occurs whenever the total output of fluid exceeds the total intake, regardless of the cause. Dehydration may result from a number of diseases that cause insensible fluid losses through the skin and respiratory tract, through increased renal excretion, and through the GI tract. Although dehydration can result from impaired oral intake, it is often a result of abnormal losses, such as those that occur in vomiting or diarrhea, when oral intake only partially compensates for the

TABLE 24-2   DISTURBANCES OF SELECT FLUID AND ELECTROLYTE BALANCE

MECHANISMS AND SITUATIONS	MANIFESTATIONS	MANAGEMENT AND NURSING CARE
Water Depletion Failure to absorb or reabsorb water Complete or sudden cessation of intake or prolonged diminished intake: • Neglect of intake by self or caregiver—confused, psychotic, unconscious, or helpless • Loss from gastrointestinal tract—vomiting, diarrhea, nasogastric suction, fistula Disturbed body fluid chemistry: inappropriate ADH secretion Excessive renal excretion: glycosuria (diabetes) Loss through skin or lungs: • Excessive perspiration or evaporation—febrile states, hyperventilation, increased ambient temperature, increased metabolic activity (BMR) • Impaired skin integrity—transudate from injuries • Hemorrhage Iatrogenic: • Overzealous use of diuretics • Improper perioperative IV fluid replacement • Use of radiant warmer or phototherapy	General symptoms depend to some extent on proportion of electrolytes lost with water Thirst Variable temperature—increased (infection) Dry skin and mucous membranes Poor skin turgor Poor perfusion (decreased pulse, prolonged capillary refill time) Weight loss Fatigue Diminished urinary output Irritability and lethargy Tachycardia Tachypnea Altered level of consciousness, disorientation Laboratory findings: • Increased hematocrit • Variable serum electrolytes • Low serum bicarbonate (CO_2) • Variable urine volume • Increased BUN • Increased serum osmolality	Provide replacement of fluid losses commensurate with volume depletion. Provide maintenance fluids and electrolytes. Determine and correct cause of water depletion. Measure fluid intake and output. Monitor vital signs. Monitor urine specific gravity. Monitor body weight. Monitor serum electrolytes.
Water Excess Water intake in excess of output: • Excessive oral intake of solute-free water • Hypotonic fluid overload • Plain water enemas Failure to excrete water in presence of normal intake: • Kidney disease • Syndrome of Inappropriate Secretion of Antidiuretic Hormone • Heart failure • Malnutrition	Edema: • Generalized • Pulmonary (moist rales or crackles) • Intracutaneous (noted especially in loose areolar tissue) Elevated venous pressure Hepatomegaly Slow, bounding pulse Weight gain Lethargy Increased spinal fluid pressure CNS manifestations (seizures, coma) Laboratory findings: • Low urine specific gravity • Decreased serum electrolytes • Decreased hematocrit • Variable urine volume	Limit fluid intake. Administer diuretics. Monitor vital signs. Monitor neurologic signs as necessary. Determine and treat cause of water excess. Analyze laboratory electrolyte measurements. Implement seizure precautions.
Sodium Depletion (Hyponatremia) Prolonged low-sodium diet Decreased sodium intake Fever Excess sweating Increased water intake without electrolytes Tachypnea; prolonged (infants) Cystic fibrosis Burns and wounds Vomiting, diarrhea, nasogastric suction, fistulas Adrenal insufficiency Renal disease DKA Malnutrition	Associated with water loss: • Same as with water loss—dehydration, weakness, dizziness, nausea, abdominal cramps, apprehension • Mild—apathy, weakness, nausea, weak pulse • Moderate—decreased blood pressure, lethargy Laboratory findings: • Sodium concentration <130 mEq/L (may be normal if volume loss) • Urine specific gravity depends on water deficit or excess	Determine and treat cause of sodium deficit. Administer IV fluids with appropriate saline concentration. Monitor fluid intake and output.

Continued

TABLE 24-2 DISTURBANCES OF SELECT FLUID AND ELECTROLYTE BALANCE—cont'd

MECHANISMS AND SITUATIONS	MANIFESTATIONS	MANAGEMENT AND NURSING CARE
Sodium Excess (Hypernatremia)		
High salt intake—enteral or IV	Intense thirst	Determine and treat cause of sodium excess.
Renal disease	Dry, sticky mucous membranes	Administer IV fluids as prescribed.
Fever	Flushed skin	Measure fluid intake and output.
Insufficient breast milk intake in neonate	Temperature possibly increased	Monitor laboratory data.
(dehydration hypernatremia)	Hoarseness	Monitor neurologic status.
High insensible water loss:	Oliguria	Ensure adequate intake of breast milk and provide
• Increased temperature	Nausea and vomiting	lactation assistance with new mother–baby pair
• Increased humidity	Possible progression to disorientation, seizures,	before hospital discharge.
• Hyperventilation	muscle twitching, nuchal rigidity, lethargy at rest,	
• Diabetes insipidus	hyperirritability when aroused	
• Hyperglycemia	Laboratory findings:	
	• Serum sodium concentration ≥150 mEq/L	
	• High plasma volume	
	• Alkalosis	
Potassium Depletion (Hypokalemia)		
Starvation	Muscle weakness, cramping, stiffness, paralysis,	Determine and treat cause of potassium deficit.
Clinical conditions associated with poor food intake	hyporeflexia	Monitor vital signs, and ECG.
Malabsorption	Hypotension	Administer supplemental potassium. Assess for
IV fluid without added potassium	Cardiac arrhythmias, gallop rhythm	adequate renal output before administration.
Gastrointestinal losses—diarrhea, vomiting, fistulas,	Tachycardia or bradycardia	For IV replacement, administer potassium slowly.
nasogastric suction	Ileus	Always monitor ECG for IV bolus potassium
Diuresis	Apathy, drowsiness	replacement.
Administration of diuretics	Irritability	For oral intake, offer high-potassium fluids and
Administration of corticosteroids	Fatigue	foods.
Diuretic phase of nephrotic syndrome	Laboratory findings:	Evaluate acid–base status.
Healing stage of burns	• Decreased serum potassium concentration	
Potassium-losing nephritis	≤3.5 mEq/L	
Hyperglycemic diuresis (e.g., diabetic ketoacidosis)	• Abnormal ECG—notched or flattened T waves,	
Familial periodic paralysis	decreased ST segment, premature ventricular	
IV administration of insulin in DKA	contractions	
Alkalosis		
Potassium Excess (Hyperkalemia)		
Renal disease	Muscle weakness, flaccid paralysis	Determine and treat cause of potassium excess.
Renal failure	Twitching	Monitor vital signs, including ECG.
Adrenal insufficiency (Addison disease)	Hyperreflexia	Administer exchange resin, if prescribed.
Associated with metabolic acidosis	Bradycardia	Administer IV fluids as prescribed.
Too rapid administration of IV potassium chloride	Ventricular fibrillation and cardiac arrest	Administer IV insulin (if ordered) to facilitate
Transfusion with old donor blood	Oliguria	movement of potassium into cells.
Severe dehydration	Apnea—respiratory arrest	Monitor potassium levels.
Crushing injuries	Laboratory findings:	Evaluate acid–base status.
Burns	• High serum potassium concentration	
Hemolysis	≥5.5 mEq/L	
Dehydration	• Variable urine volume	
Potassium-sparing diuretics	• Flat P wave on ECG, peaked T waves, widened	
Increased intake of potassium (e.g., salt substitutes)	QRS complex, increased PR interval	

ADH, Antidiuretic hormone; *BMR,* basal metabolic rate; *BUN,* blood urea nitrogen; *CNS,* central nervous system; *DKA,* diabetic ketoacidosis; *ECG,* electrocardiogram; *IV,* intravenous.

abnormal losses. Other significant causes of dehydration include diabetic ketoacidosis and burns.

Types of Dehydration

The pathophysiology of dehydration is understood by recognizing that the distribution of water between the ECF and ICF spaces depends on active transport of potassium into and sodium out of cells by energy-requiring processes. Sodium is the chief solute in ECF and is the primary determinant of ECF volume. Sodium is considered a unique electrolyte in that water balance determines sodium concentration; when water is lost and sodium concentration becomes elevated compensatory mechanisms in the kidney stop ADH secretion so water is retained. The thirst mechanism (not fully functional in infants) is also stimulated so water is replaced, thus increasing the total body water content and returning sodium to a normal level (Greenbaum, 2011). Potassium is primarily found inside the cell (intracellular) but small amounts are also found in extracellular fluid. Sodium depletion in diarrhea occurs in two ways: out of the body in stool and into the ICF compartment to replace potassium to maintain electrical equilibrium.

Dehydration is classified into three categories on the basis of osmolality and depends primarily on the serum sodium concentration: (1) isotonic, (2) hypotonic, and (3) hypertonic.

Isotonic (isosmotic or isonatremic) dehydration, the primary form of dehydration in children, occurs in conditions in which electrolyte and water deficits are present in approximately balanced proportions. Water and sodium are lost in approximately equal amounts. The observable fluid losses are not necessarily isotonic because losses from other avenues make adjustments so that the sum of all losses, or the net loss, is isotonic. There is no osmotic force between the ICF and the ECF, so the major loss is sustained from the ECF compartment. This significantly reduces the plasma volume and the circulating blood volume, which affects the skin, muscles, and kidneys. Shock is the greatest threat to life, and children with isotonic dehydration display symptoms characteristic of hypovolemic shock. Plasma sodium remains within normal limits, between 130 and 150 mEq/L.

Hypotonic (hyposmotic or hyponatremic) dehydration occurs when the electrolyte deficit exceeds the water deficit, leaving the serum hypotonic. Because ICF is more concentrated than ECF in hypotonic dehydration, water moves from the ECF to the ICF to establish osmotic equilibrium. This movement further increases the ECF volume loss, and shock is a frequent finding. Because there is a greater proportional loss of ECF in hypotonic dehydration, the physical signs tend to be more severe with smaller fluid losses than with isotonic or hypertonic dehydration. Serum sodium concentration is less than 130 mEq/L.

Hypertonic (hyperosmotic or hypernatremic) dehydration results from water loss in excess of electrolyte loss and is usually caused by a proportionately larger loss of water or a larger intake of electrolytes. This type of dehydration is the most dangerous and requires more specific fluid therapy. Hypertonic diarrhea may occur in infants who are given fluids by mouth that contain large amounts of solute, or in children who receive high-protein nasogastric (NG) tube feedings that place an excessive solute load on the kidneys. In hypertonic dehydration, fluid shifts from the lesser concentration of the ICF to the ECF. Plasma sodium concentration is greater than 150 mEq/L.

Because the ECF volume is proportionately larger, hypertonic dehydration consists of a greater degree of water loss for the same intensity of physical signs. Shock is less apparent. However, CNS disturbances, including alterations in consciousness, poor ability to focus attention, lethargy, increased muscle tone with hyperreflexia, and hyperirritability to stimuli, are more likely to occur. CNS changes are serious and may result in permanent damage.

Degree of Dehydration

Diagnosis of the type and degree of dehydration is necessary to develop an effective plan of therapy. The degree of dehydration has been described as a percentage of body weight dehydrated: mild—less than 3% in older children or less than 5% in infants; moderate—5% to 10% in infants and 3% to 6% in older children; and severe—more than 10% in infants and more than 6% in older children (Greenbaum, 2011). Water constitutes only 60% to 70% of an infant's weight. However, adipose tissue contains little water and is highly variable in individual infants and children. A more accurate means of describing dehydration is to reflect acute loss (time frame of ≤48 hours) in milliliters per kilogram of body weight. For example, a loss of 50 ml/kg is considered to be a mild fluid loss, but a loss of 100 ml/kg produces severe dehydration. Weight is the most important determinant of the percent of total body fluid loss in infants and younger children. However, often the pre-illness weight is unknown. Other predictors of fluid loss include a changing level of consciousness (irritability to lethargy), altered response to stimuli, decreased skin elasticity and turgor, prolonged capillary refill (>2 sec), increased heart rate, and sunken eyes and fontanels.

Clinical signs provide clues to the extent of dehydration (Table 24-3). The earliest detectable sign is usually tachycardia followed by dry skin and mucous membranes, sunken fontanels, signs of circulatory failure (coolness and mottling of extremities), loss of skin elasticity, and prolonged capillary filling time (Table 24-4).

TABLE 24-3	**EVALUATING EXTENT OF DEHYDRATION**		
	LEVEL OF DEHYDRATION		
CLINICAL SIGNS	**MILD**	**MODERATE**	**SEVERE**
Weight loss—infants	3%–5%	6%–9%	≥10%
Weight loss—children	3%–4%	6%–8%	10%
Pulse	Normal	Slightly increased	Very increased
Respiratory rate	Normal	Slight tachypnea (rapid)	Hyperpnea (deep and rapid)
Blood pressure	Normal	Normal to orthostatic (>10 mm Hg change)	Orthostatic to shock
Behavior	Normal	Irritable, more thirsty	Hyperirritable to lethargic
Thirst	Slight	Moderate	Intense
Mucous membranes*	Normal	Dry	Parched
Tears	Present	Decreased	Absent, sunken eyes
Anterior fontanel	Normal	Normal to sunken	Sunken
External jugular vein	Visible when supine	Not visible except with supraclavicular pressure	Not visible even with supraclavicular pressure
Skin*	Capillary refill >2 sec	Slowed capillary refill (2–4 sec [decreased turgor])	Very delayed capillary refill (>4 sec) and tenting; skin cool, acrocyanotic or mottled
Urine	Decreased	Oliguria	Oliguria or anuria

Data from Jospe N, Forbes G: Fluids and electrolytes—clinical aspects, *Pediatr Rev* 17(11):395–403, 1996 and Steiner MJ, DeWalt DA, Byerly JS: Is this child dehydrated? *JAMA* 291(22):2746–2754, 2004.
*These signs are less prominent in patients who have hypernatremia.

TABLE 24-4 CLINICAL MANIFESTATIONS OF DEHYDRATION

MANIFESTATION	ISOTONIC (LOSS OF WATER AND SODIUM)	HYPOTONIC (LOSS OF SODIUM IN EXCESS OF WATER)	HYPERTONIC (LOSS OF WATER IN EXCESS OF SODIUM)
Skin			
Color	Gray	Gray	Gray
Temperature	Cold	Cold	Cold or hot
Turgor	Poor	Very poor	Fair
Feel	Dry	Clammy	Thickened, doughy
Mucous membranes	Dry	Slightly moist	Parched
Tearing and salivation	Absent	Absent	Absent
Eyeball	Sunken	Sunken	Sunken
Fontanel	Sunken	Sunken	Sunken
Body temperature	Subnormal or elevated	Subnormal or elevated	Subnormal or elevated
Pulse	Rapid	Very rapid	Moderately rapid
Respirations	Rapid	Rapid	Rapid
Behavior	Irritable to lethargic	Lethargic or comatose; seizures	Marked lethargy with extreme hyperirritability on stimulation

Compensatory mechanisms attempt to maintain fluid volume by adjusting to these losses. Interstitial fluid moves into the vascular compartment to maintain the blood volume in response to hemoconcentration and hypovolemia, and vasoconstriction of peripheral arterioles helps maintain pumping pressure. When fluid losses exceed the body's ability to sustain blood volume and blood pressure, circulation is seriously compromised, and the blood pressure falls. This results in tissue hypoxia with accumulation of lactic acid, pyruvate, and other acid metabolites, which contribute to the development of metabolic acidosis.

Renal compensation is impaired by reduced blood flow through the kidneys, and little urine is formed. Increased serum osmolality stimulates the secretion of ADH to conserve fluid and initiates the renin–angiotensin mechanisms in the kidney, causing further vasoconstriction. Aldosterone is released to promote sodium retention and conserve water in the kidneys. If dehydration increases in severity, urine formation is greatly diminished, and metabolites and hydrogen ions that are normally excreted by this route are retained.

Shock, a common manifestation of severe depletion of ECF volume, is preceded by tachycardia and signs of poor perfusion and tissue oxygenation (by pulse oximeter readings). Peripheral circulation is poor as a result of reduced blood volume; therefore, the skin is cool and mottled, with decreased capillary filling after blanching. Impaired kidney circulation often leads to oliguria and azotemia. Although low blood pressure may accompany other symptoms of shock, in infants and young children, it is usually a late sign and may herald the onset of cardiovascular collapse.

Diagnostic Evaluation

To initiate a therapeutic plan, several factors must be determined:
- The degree of dehydration based on physical assessment
- The type of dehydration based on the pathophysiology of the specific illness responsible for the dehydrated state
- Specific physical signs other than general signs
- Initial plasma sodium concentrations
- Serum bicarbonate concentration (CO_2)
- Any associated electrolyte (especially serum potassium) and acid–base imbalances (as indicated)

Initial and regular ongoing evaluations assess the patient's progress toward equilibrium and the effectiveness of therapy.

In the examination of an infant or younger child, one of the most important determinants of the extent of dehydration is body weight because this can assist in determining the percentage of total body fluid lost; however, because the pre-illness weight is often unknown, clinical manifestations must be evaluated. Important clinical manifestations include changing sensorium (irritability to lethargy); decreased response to stimuli; integumentary changes (decreased elasticity and turgor); prolonged capillary refill; increased heart rate; sunken eyes; and, in infants, sunken fontanels. Using multiple predictors increases the sensitivity of assessing the fluid deficit, and early studies have shown a reasonably high degree of agreement between experienced observers in assessment of the level of dehydration. Objective signs of dehydration are present at a fluid deficit of less than 5%.

Laboratory data are said to be useful only when results are significantly abnormal (Emond, 2009). Urine specific gravity, urine ketones, and urinary output during rehydration are reportedly unreliable assessments for determining dehydration in children (Steiner, Nager, and Wang, 2007). Shock, tachycardia, and very low blood pressure are common features of severe depletion of ECF volume (see Shock, Chapter 25).

Therapeutic Management

Medical management is directed at correcting the fluid loss or deficit and treating the underlying cause. When the child is alert, awake, and not in danger, correction of dehydration may be attempted with oral fluid administration. Mild cases of dehydration can be managed at home by this method. Several commercial rehydration fluids are available for use (Table 24-5). Oral rehydration management consists of replacement of fluid loss over 4 to 6 hours, replacement of continuing losses, and provision for maintenance fluid requirements. In general, a mildly dehydrated child may be given 50 ml/kg of oral rehydration solution (ORS), and a child with moderate dehydration may be given 100 ml/kg of ORS. A child with fluid losses from diarrhea may be given 10 ml/kg for each stool. Amounts and rates are determined from body weight and the severity of dehydration and are increased if rehydration is incomplete or if excess losses continue until the child is well hydrated and the basic problem is under control.

The child may not be thirsty even though dehydrated and may refuse oral fluids initially for fear of continued emesis (if occurring) or because of decreased strength, oral stomatitis, or thrush. In such

TABLE 24-5   COMPOSITION OF SOME ORAL REHYDRATION SOLUTIONS

FORMULA	NA (MEQ/L)	K (MEQ/L)	CL (MEQ/L)	BASE (MEQ/L)	GLUCOSE (G/L)
Pedialyte (Abbott)*	45	20	35	30 (citrate)	25
Rehydralyte (Abbott)	75	20	65	30 (citrate)	25
Infalyte (Mead Johnson)	50	25	45	34 (citrate)	30
World Health Organization†	90	20	80	30 (bicarbonate)	20

Cl, Chloride; *K*, potassium; *Na*, sodium.

*Note that many generic products are available with compositions identical to Pedialyte.

†Must be reconstituted with 1 L water.

children, rehydration may proceed by administering 2 to 5 ml of ORS by a syringe or small medication cup every 2 to 3 minutes until the child is able to tolerate larger amounts; if the child has emesis, administering small amounts (5–10 ml) of ORS every 5 minutes or so may help overcome fluid deficit, and the emesis will often lessen over time. Oral administration of ondansetron (Zofran) to children with acute gastroenteritis and vomiting may reduce emesis and increase time to oral rehydration, thus preventing IV therapy. Oral rehydration therapy (ORT) is effective for treating mild or moderate dehydration in children, is less expensive, and involves fewer complications than parenteral therapy (American Academy of Pediatrics [AAP], Committee on Infectious Diseases and Pickering, 2009).

> **NURSING TIP** Enhance the flavor of an ORS such as Pedialyte (unflavored) by adding 1 tsp of unsweetened powder Kool-Aid to each 60 to 90 ml of ORS. Older children may take a small Popsicle orally instead of fluids that require drinking. Many commercially available Popsicles are relatively inexpensive, contain small amounts of sucrose, and contain approximately 40 to 50 ml of fluid. Frozen oral hydration may be accepted by some children when conventional ORS is rejected.

Parenteral Fluid Therapy. Parenteral fluid therapy is initiated whenever the child is unable to ingest sufficient amounts of fluid and electrolytes to (1) meet ongoing daily physiologic losses, (2) replace previous deficits, and (3) replace ongoing abnormal losses. Patients who usually require IV fluids are those with severe dehydration, those with uncontrollable vomiting, those who are unable to drink for any reason (e.g., extreme fatigue, coma), and those with severe gastric distention.

Because dehydration constitutes a great threat to life, the first priority is the restoration of circulation by rapid expansion of the ECF volume to treat or prevent shock. IV administration of fluid begins immediately, although the exact nature of the dehydration and the serum electrolyte values may not initially be known. The solution selected is based on what is known regarding the probable type and cause of the dehydration. This usually involves an isotonic solution such as 0.9% sodium chloride or lactated Ringer solution, both of which are close to the body's serum osmolality of 285 to 300 mOsm/kg and do not contain dextrose (which is contraindicated in the early treatment stages of diabetic ketoacidosis).

Parenteral rehydration therapy has three phases. The initial therapy is used to expand ECF volume quickly and to improve circulatory and renal function. During initial therapy, an isotonic solution is used at a rate of 20 ml/kg, given as an IV bolus over 20 minutes, and repeated as necessary after assessment of the child's response to therapy (Ford, 2009; Friedman, 2010). Subsequent therapy is used to replace deficits, meet maintenance water and electrolyte requirements, and catch up with ongoing losses. Water and sodium requirements for the deficit, maintenance, and ongoing losses are calculated at 8-hour intervals, taking into consideration the amount of fluids given with the initial boluses and the amount administered during the first 24-hour period. With improved circulation during this phase, water and electrolyte deficits can be evaluated, and acid–base status can be corrected either directly through the administration of fluids or indirectly through improved renal function. Potassium is withheld until kidney function is restored and assessed and circulation has improved (see Evidence-Based Practice box).

The final phase of therapy allows the patient to return to normal and begin oral feedings, with a gradual correction of total body deficits. The potassium loss in ICF is replaced slowly by way of the ECF. The body fat and protein stores are replaced through diet. If the child is unable to eat or if feeding aggravates a chronic condition, IV maintenance fluids are provided.

Although the initial phase of fluid replacement is rapid in both isotonic and hypotonic dehydration, it is contraindicated in hypertonic dehydration because of the risk of water intoxication, especially in the brain cells, specifically the central pontine cells. Central pontine myelinolysis may occur with an overcorrection of fluid deficit and an overly rapid correction of serum sodium concentration. Whereas there is an apparent lag time for sodium to reach a steady state when diffusing in and out of brain cells, water diffuses almost instantaneously. Consequently, rapid administration of fluid causes equally rapid diffusion of water into the dehydrated brain cells, causing marked cerebral edema. Because ECF volume is maintained relatively well in hypertonic as opposed to the other types of dehydration, shock is not a usual manifestation.

Nursing Care Management

Nursing observation and intervention are essential for detection and therapeutic management of dehydration. A variety of circumstances cause fluid losses in infants and small children, and changes can take place quickly. An important nursing responsibility is observation for signs of dehydration. Nursing assessment should begin with observation of general appearance and proceed to more specific observations. Conditions in which dehydration may develop quickly include diarrhea; vomiting; sweating; fever; disorders such as diabetic ketoacidosis, renal disease, and cardiac anomalies; administration of certain drugs (e.g., diuretics and steroids); and trauma (major surgery, burns, and other extensive injury).

Whether the child is at home, in the practitioner's office or clinic, or in the hospital, nursing assessment is an essential part of the nursing care plan. The assessment of suspected or potential fluid and electrolyte disturbance begins with the observation of general appearance. Ill children usually have drawn expressions, have dry mucous membranes and lips, and "look sick." Loss of appetite is one of the first behaviors

EVIDENCE-BASED PRACTICE

Normal Saline or Heparinized Saline Flush Solution in Pediatric Intravenous Lines

Updated by Olga A. Taylor

Ask the Question
Picot Question
Is there a significant difference in the longevity of IV intermittent infusion locks in children when NS is used as a flush instead of a HS solution?

Search for the Evidence
Search Strategies
Selection criteria included evidence during the years 1992 to 2008 with the following terms: saline versus heparin intermittent flush, children's heparin lock flush, heparin lock patency, and peripheral venous catheter in children.

Databases Used
CINAHL, PubMed

Critically Analyze the Evidence
- In trials of HS administration versus NS, placebo, or no treatment in neonates, no strong evidence regarding the effectiveness and safety of heparin in prolonging catheter life was found (Shah, Ng, and Sinha, 2005).
- No significant statistical difference was found between HS and NS flushes for maintaining catheter patency in children (Hanrahan, Kleiber, and Berends, 2000; Hanrahan, Kleiber, and Fagan, 1994; Heilskov, Kleiber, Johnson, and others, 1998; Kotter, 1996; Mok, Kwong, and Chan, 2007; Schultz, Drew, and Hewitt, 2002).
- Increased incidence of pain or erythema was associated with HS flushing of infusion devices (Hanrahan, Kleiber, and Fagan, 1994; McMullen, Fioravanti, Pollack, and others, 1993; Nelson and Graves, 1998; Robertson, 1994).
- Increased patency or longer dwell times were found with HS solutions versus NS in 24-gauge catheters (Beecroft, Bossert, Chung, and others, 1997; Danek and Noris, 1992; Gyr, Burroughs, Smith, and others, 1995; Hanrahan, Kleiber, and Berends, 2000; Mudge, Forcier, and Slattery, 1998; Tripathi, Kaushik, and Singh, 2008).
- Younger children and preterm neonates with lower gestational ages were associated with shorter patency of IV catheters (McMullen, Fioravanti, Pollack, and others, 1993; Paisley, Stamper, Brown, and others, 1997; Robertson, 1994; Tripathi, Kaushik, and Singh, 2008).
- Infusion devices flushed with NS lasted longer than those flushed with HS (Goldberg, Sankaran, Givelichian, and others, 1999; Le Duc, 1997; Nelson and Graves, 1998).
- When measured and reported, the length of time between flushing peripheral devices affected dwell time (Crews, Gnann, Rice, and others, 1997; Gyr, Burroughs, Smith, and others, 1995).
- Preterm neonates are at higher risk for development of clotting problems as a result of heparin; none of the studies cited anticoagulation-associated complications with HS (Klenner, Fusch, Rakow, and others, 2003).
- 0.9% sodium chloride injection is safe for maintaining patency of peripheral locks in adults and children older than age 12 years (American Society of Hospital Pharmacists, 2006).
- Either preservative-free heparin or preservative-free 0.9% sodium chloride may be used to flush a peripheral IV; however, catheter patency may be maintained by flushing with saline when converting from continuous to intermittent use (Infusion Nurses Society, 2006).
- After each catheter use, peripheral catheters should be locked with preservative-free 0.9% sodium chloride (Infusion Nurses Society, 2011).
- No recommendation is made for use of preservative-free 0.9% sodium chloride versus heparin for locking peripheral catheters (Infusion Nurses Society, 2011).

Apply the Evidence: Nursing Implications
There is **low quality evidence** with a **weak recommendation** (Guyatt, Oxman, Vist, and others, 2008) for using NS versus HS flush solution in pediatric IV lines. Further research is still needed with larger samples of children, especially preterm neonates using small-gauge catheters (24 gauge) and other gauge catheters flushed with NS and HS as intermittent infusion devices only (no continuous infusions); variables to be considered include catheter dwell time; medications administered; the period between regular flushing and flushing associated with medication administration; pain, erythema, or other localized complications; the concentration and amount of HS used; flush method (positive pressure technique versus no specific technique); the reason for IV device removal; and complications associated with either solution. NS is a safe alternative to HS flush in infants and children with intermittent IV locks larger than 24 gauge; smaller neonates may benefit from HS flush (longer dwell time), but the evidence is inconclusive for all weight ranges and gestational ages.

QSEN Quality and Safety Competencies:
Evidence-Based Practice*
Knowledge
Differentiate clinical opinion from research and evidence-based summaries.
Describe methods for using NS or HS flush solution in pediatric IV lines.

Skills
Base individualized care plan on patient values, clinical expertise, and evidence.
Integrate evidence into practice on NS or HS flush solution in pediatric IV lines.

Attitudes
Value the concept of evidence-based practice as integral to determining best clinical practice.
Appreciate strengths and weakness of evidence for NS or HS flush solution in pediatric IV lines.

References
American Society of Hospital Pharmacists Commission on Therapeutics: ASHP therapeutic position statement on the institutional use of 0.9% sodium chloride injection to maintain patency of peripheral indwelling intermittent infusion devices, *Am J Health Syst Pharm* 63(13):1273–1275, 2006.
Beecroft PC, Bossert E, Chung K, and others: Intravenous lock patency in children: dilute heparin versus saline, *J Pediatr Pharm Practice* 2(4):211–223, 1997.
Crews BE, Gnann KK, Rice MH, and others: Effects of varying intervals between heparin flushes on pediatric catheter longevity, *Pediatr Nurs* 23(1):87–91, 1997.
Danek GD, Noris EM: Pediatric IV catheters: efficacy of saline flush, *Pediatr Nurs* 18(2):111–113, 1992.
Goldberg M, Sankaran R, Givelichian L, and others: Maintaining patency of peripheral intermittent infusion devices with heparinized saline and saline: A randomized double blind controlled trial in neonatal intensive care and a review of literature, *Neonatal Intensive Care* 12(1):18–22, 1999.
Guyatt GH, Oxman AD, Vist GE, and others: GRADE: an emerging consensus on rating quality of evidence and strength of recommendations, *BMJ* 336(7650):924–926, 2008.
Gyr P, Burroughs T, Smith K, and others: Double blind comparison of heparin and saline flush solutions in maintenance of peripheral infusion devices, *Pediatr Nurs* 21(4):383–389, 1995.
Hanrahan KS, Kleiber C, Berends S: Saline for peripheral intravenous locks in neonates: evaluating a change in practice, *Neonat Netw* 19(2):19–24, 2000.

HS, Heparinized saline; *IV,* intravenous; *NS,* normal saline.
*Adapted from the QSEN at http://www.qsen.org.

EVIDENCE-BASED PRACTICE

Normal Saline or Heparinized Saline Flush Solution in Pediatric Intravenous Lines—cont'd

Hanrahan KS, Kleiber C, Fagan C: Evaluation of saline for IV locks in children, *Pediatr Nurs* 20(6):549–552, 1994.

Heilskov J, Kleiber C, Johnson K, and others: A randomized trial of heparin and saline for maintaining intravenous locks in neonates, *J Soc Pediatr Nurs* 3(3):111–116, 1998.

Infusion Nurses Society: *Policies and procedures for infusion nursing*, ed 3, Norwood, Mass, 2006, Author.

Infusion Nurses Society: Infusion nursing standards of practice, *J Infus Nurs* 34(1S):S63–S64, 2011.

Klenner AF, Fusch C, Rakow A, and others: Benefit and risk of heparin for maintaining peripheral venous catheters in neonates: a placebo-controlled trial, *J Pediatr* 143(6):741–745, 2003.

Kotter RW: Heparin vs. saline for intermittent intravenous device maintenance in neonates, *Neonat Netw* 15(6):43–47, 1996.

Le Duc K: Efficacy of normal saline solution versus heparin solution for maintaining patency of peripheral intravenous catheters in children, *J Emerg Nurs* 23(4):306–309, 1997.

McMullen A, Fioravanti ID, Pollack D, and others: Heparinized saline or normal saline as a flush solution in intermittent intravenous lines in infants and children, *MCN Am J Matern Child Nurs* 18(2):78–85, 1993.

Mok E, Kwong TK, Chan ME: A randomized controlled trial for maintaining peripheral intravenous lock in children, *Int J Nurs Pract* 13(1):33–45, 2007.

Mudge B, Forcier D, Slattery MJ: Patency of 24-gauge peripheral intermittent infusion devices: A comparison of heparin and saline flush solutions, *Pediatr Nurs* 24(2):142–149, 1998.

Nelson TJ, Graves SM: 0.9% Sodium chloride injection with and without heparin for maintaining peripheral indwelling intermittent infusion devices in infants, *Am J Heath Syst Pharm* 55:570–573, 1998.

Paisley MK, Stamper M, Brown T, and others: The use of heparin and normal saline flushes in neonatal intravenous catheters, *J Pediatr Nurs* 23(5):521–527, 1997.

Robertson J: Intermittent intravenous therapy: a comparison of two flushing solutions, *Contemp Nurs* 3(4):174–179, 1994.

Schultz AA, Drew D, Hewitt H: Comparison of normal saline and heparinized saline for patency of IV locks in neonates, *Appl Nurs Res* 15(1):28–34, 2002.

Shah PS, Ng E, Sinha AK: Heparin for prolonging peripheral intravenous catheter use in neonates, *Cochrane Database Syst Rev* (4):CD002774, 2005.

Tripathi S, Kaushik V, Singh V: Peripheral IVs: factors affecting complications and patency—A randomized controlled trial, *J Infus Nurs* 31(3):182–188, 2008.

observed in most childhood illnesses, and the infant's or child's activity level is diminished from baseline or usual activities. The cry of an ill infant is less vigorous, often whining, and higher pitched than usual. The child is irritable, seeks the parent's comfort and attention, and displays purposeless movements and inappropriate responses to people and familiar objects. In some cases, the child may not protest advances by the health care worker and procedures such as taking vital signs or starting an IV infusion. These are signs that the child truly feels bad and that the condition is serious and immediate intervention is necessary. As the child's illness and level of dehydration become more severe, irritability progresses to lethargy and even unconsciousness.

Assess capillary filling time by pinching the abdominal skin, chest, arm or leg and estimating the time it takes for the blood to return. Capillary filling time in mild dehydration is less than 2 seconds, increasing to more than 4 seconds in severe dehydration. The technique is effective in children of all ages. However, it can be altered in the presence of heart failure, which affects circulation time, and hypertonic dehydration, in which fluid loss is primarily intracellular. Additional clinical signs observed in children with dehydration include cool mottled extremities, sunken eyes, tachypnea, and changes in sensorium.

When caring for the ill child, assess the vital signs as often as every 15 to 30 minutes and record weight frequently during the initial phase of therapy. It is important to use the same scale each time the child is weighed and to predetermine the weight of any equipment or devices that must remain attached during the weighing process, including elbow restraints, and any clothing the child might be wearing. Take routine weights at the same time each day.

Accurate measurements of fluid intake and output are vital to the assessment of dehydration. This includes oral and parenteral intake and losses from urine, stools, vomiting, fistulas, NG suction, sweat, and wound drainage:

Urine—Frequency, color, consistency, and volume (when weighing diapers, ≈1 g of wet diaper weight equals 1 ml of urine)

Stools—Frequency, volume, and consistency

Vomitus—Volume, frequency, and type

Sweating—Can be only estimated from frequency of clothing and linen changes

In addition to fluid intake and output, the following observations assist in assessment of dehydration:

Vital signs—Temperature (normal, elevated, or lowered depending on degree of dehydration), pulse (tachycardia), respirations (hyperpnea), and blood pressure (hypotension)

Skin—Color, temperature, turgor, presence or absence of edema, and capillary refill

Mucous membranes—Moisture, color, and presence and consistency of secretions

Body weight—Decreased in relation to degree of dehydration

Fontanel (infants)—Sunken, soft, or normal

Sensory alterations—Presence of thirst (only in older child)

At home, advise parents to observe the number of times and how much the child voids. A newborn may be expected to void at least once in the first 24 hours, two or three times in the second 24 hours of life, three or four times in the third and fourth days of life, and a minimum of five or six times by the fifth and sixth days; if intake is adequate, an infant 5 to 6 days old and older may be expected to have a minimum of six to eight voidings per day (AAP, Committee on Infectious Diseases and Pickering, 2009). Infants younger than 1 year of age may void every 1 to 2 hours; toddlers urinate approximately every 3 hours. As children get older, they void less frequently. Instruct the parents to notify the nurse or clinician if the child appears to be voiding an insufficient amount or persistently losing fluid through vomiting or diarrhea.

For nursing interventions, see discussion under specific disorders in this chapter.

GASTROINTESTINAL DYSFUNCTION

The extensive surface area of the GI tract and its digestive function represent the major means of exchange between the human organism and the environment. Disorders that impair the functional integrity of the GI system have the potential for causing serious alterations in fluid and electrolyte balance. Disorders that involve GI losses of large amounts of fluid, absorption disorders, inflammatory disorders, and decreased or excessive water intake have the potential for causing fluid and electrolyte imbalance in infants and children.

DISORDERS OF MOTILITY

Diarrhea

Diarrhea is a symptom that results from disorders involving digestive, absorptive, and secretory functions. Diarrhea is caused by abnormal intestinal water and electrolyte transport. Worldwide, there are an estimated 1.3 billion episodes of diarrhea each year. Approximately 24% of all deaths in children living in developing countries are related to diarrhea and dehydration. Most children living in developed

Case Study—Animations: Digestive Tract, Passage of Food; Intestines

Case Study—Gastrointestinal Problems

countries who have gastroenteritis have mild forms. However, in the United States, approximately 200,000 children younger than age 5 years are hospitalized and approximately 200 children younger than 5 years die of diarrhea and dehydration each year (Malek, Curns, Holman, and others, 2006; Staat, 2006).

Diarrheal disturbances involve the stomach and intestines (gastroenteritis), the small intestine (enteritis), the colon (colitis), or the colon and intestines (enterocolitis). Diarrhea is classified as acute or chronic.

Acute diarrhea, a leading cause of illness in children younger than 5 years of age, is defined as a sudden increase in frequency and a change in consistency of stools, often caused by an infectious agent in the GI tract. It may be associated with upper respiratory or urinary tract infections, antibiotic therapy, or laxative use. Acute diarrhea is usually self-limited (<14 days' duration) and subsides without specific treatment if dehydration does not occur. Acute infectious diarrhea (infectious gastroenteritis) is caused by a variety of viral, bacterial, and parasitic pathogens (Table 24-6).

Chronic diarrhea is defined as an increase in stool frequency and increased water content with a duration of more than 14 days. It is often caused by chronic conditions such as malabsorption syndromes, inflammatory bowel disease (IBD), immunodeficiency, food allergy, lactose intolerance, or chronic nonspecific diarrhea or as a result of inadequate management of acute diarrhea.

Intractable diarrhea of infancy is a syndrome that occurs in the first few months of life, persists for longer than 2 weeks with no recognized pathogens, and is refractory to treatment. The most common cause is acute infectious diarrhea that was not managed adequately.

Chronic nonspecific diarrhea (CNSD), also known as irritable colon of childhood and toddlers' diarrhea, is a common cause of chronic diarrhea in children 6 to 54 months of age. These children have loose stools, often with undigested food particles, and diarrhea lasting longer than 2 weeks' duration. Children with CNSD grow normally and have no evidence of malnutrition, no blood in their stool, and no enteric infection. Dietary indiscretions and food sensitivities have been linked to chronic diarrhea. The excessive intake of juices and artificial sweeteners such as sorbitol, a substance found in many commercially prepared beverages and foods, may be a factor.

Etiology

Most pathogens that cause diarrhea are spread by the fecal–oral route through contaminated food or water or are spread from person to person where there is close contact (e.g., daycare centers). Lack of clean water, crowding, poor hygiene, nutritional deficiency, and poor sanitation are major risk factors, especially for bacterial or parasitic pathogens. The increased frequency and severity of diarrheal disease in infants is also related to age-specific alterations in susceptibility to pathogens. For example, the immune systems of infants have not been exposed to many pathogens and have not acquired protective antibodies. Worldwide, the most common causes of acute gastroenteritis are infectious agents, viruses, bacteria, and parasites. In developed nations, viruses, primarily rotavirus, cause 70% to 80% of infectious diarrhea.

Rotavirus is the most important cause of serious gastroenteritis among children and a significant nosocomial (hospital-acquired) pathogen, accounting for 55,000 to 70,000 hospitalizations annually (Centers for Disease Control and Prevention [CDC], 2008; Staat, 2006). Rotavirus disease is most severe in children 3 to 24 months of age. Children younger than 3 months of age have some protection from the disease because of maternally acquired antibodies. Approximately 25% of severe cases of rotavirus occur in older children.

Salmonella, Shigella, and Campylobacter organisms are the most frequently isolated bacterial pathogens. Salmonella has the highest occurrence in infants; Giardia and Shigella have the highest incidence among toddlers. Shigella infection is uncommon in the United States, accounting for fewer than 5% of diarrheal illnesses in infants and toddlers. Campylobacter infection has a bimodal presentation (highest in children younger than 12 months of age with a second rise in incidence

TABLE 24-6	**INFECTIOUS CAUSES OF ACUTE DIARRHEA**		
AGENTS	**PATHOLOGY**	**CHARACTERISTICS**	**COMMENTS**
Viral			
Rotavirus Incubation—48 hr Diagnosis—EIA	Fecal–oral transmission Seven groups (A–G)—Most group A virus replicates in mature villus epithelial cells of small intestine, leading to (1) imbalance in ratio of intestinal fluid absorption to secretion and (2) malabsorption of complex carbohydrates	Mild to moderate fever Vomiting followed by onset of foul-smelling watery stools Fever and vomiting generally abate in ≈2 days, but diarrhea persists 5–7 days	Most common cause of diarrhea in children younger than 5 yr of age; infants 6–12 mo most vulnerable; affects all ages; usually milder in children older than 3 yr of age Immunocompromised children at greater risk for complications Peak occurrences in winter months Important cause of nosocomial infections Two preventive vaccines available (see Chapter 10)
Norwalk-like organisms Also called caliciviruses Incubation—12–48 hr Diagnosis—EIA	Fecal–oral; contaminated water Pathology similar to that of rotavirus; affects villus epithelial cells of small intestine, leading to (1) imbalance in ratio of intestinal fluid absorption to secretion and (2) malabsorption of complex carbohydrates	Abdominal cramps, nausea, vomiting, malaise, low-grade fever, watery diarrhea without blood; duration 2–3 days; tends to resemble so-called food poisoning symptoms with nausea predominating	Affects all ages Multiple strains often named for the location of outbreak (e.g., Norwalk, Sapporo, Snow Mountain, Montgomery)

TABLE 24-6	INFECTIOUS CAUSES OF ACUTE DIARRHEA—cont'd		
AGENTS	**PATHOLOGY**	**CHARACTERISTICS**	**COMMENTS**
Bacterial			
Escherichia coli Incubation—3–4 days; variable depending on strain Diagnosis—SMAC agar positive for blood, but fecal leukocytes absent or rare	*E. coli* strains produce diarrhea as a result of enterotoxin production, adherence, or invasion (enterotoxigenic-producing *E. coli*, enterohemorrhagic *E. coli*, enteroaggregative *E. coli*)	Watery diarrhea 1–2 days, then severe abdominal cramping and bloody diarrhea Can progress to hemolytic uremic syndrome; shock	Foodborne pathogen Traveler's diarrhea Highest incidence in summer Cause of nursery epidemics Symptomatic treatment Antibiotics may worsen course Avoid antimotility agents and opioids
***Salmonella* groups** (nontyphoidal) Gram-negative rods, nonencapsulated nonsporulating Incubation—6–72 hr Diagnosis—gram stain, stool culture	Invasion of mucosa in the small and large intestine, edema of the lamina propria, focal acute inflammation with disruption of the mucosa and microabscesses	Nausea, vomiting, colicky abdominal pain, bloody diarrhea, fever; symptoms variable (mild to severe) May have headache and cerebral manifestations (e.g., drowsiness confusion, meningismus, seizures) Infants may be afebrile and nontoxic May result in life-threatening septicemia and meningitis Nausea and vomiting typically of short duration; diarrhea may persist as long as 2–3 wk Typically shed virus for average of 5 wk; cases reported up to 1 yr	Incidence highest in warm months (July–November); foodborne outbreaks common Usually transmitted person to person but may transmit via undercooked meats or poultry; about half of cases caused by poultry and poultry products In children, related to pets (e.g., dogs, cats, hamsters, turtles) Communicable as long as organisms are excreted Antibiotics not recommended in uncomplicated cases Antimotility agents also not recommended—prolong transit time and carrier state Incidence decreasing over past 10 yr
Salmonella typhi Produces enteric fever—systemic syndrome Incubation—usually 7–14 days but could be 3–30 days depending on size of inoculum Diagnosis—positive blood cultures; also sometimes positive stool and urine cultures Late stage—positive bone marrow culture	Bloodstream invasion; after ingestion, organism attaches to microvilli of ileal brush borders, and bacteria invade the intestinal epithelium via Peyer patches Next, organism is transported to intestinal lymph nodes and enters bloodstream via thoracic ducts, and circulating organism reaches reticuloendothelial cells, causing bacteremia	Manifestations dependent on age Abdominal pain, diarrhea, nausea, vomiting, high fever, lethargy Must be treated with antibiotics	Incidence much lower in developed countries; about 400 cases/yr in United States; 65% of U.S. cases acquired via international cases Ingestion of foods and water contaminated with human feces is most common mode of transmission Congenital and intrapartum transmission possible Two vaccines available
***Shigella* groups** Gram-negative nonmotile anaerobic bacilli Incubation—1–7 days Diagnosis—stool culture loaded with polymorphonuclear leukocytes	Enterotoxins—invades the epithelium with superficial mucosal ulcerations	Children appear sick Symptoms begin with fever, fatigue, anorexia Crampy abdominal pain preceding watery or bloody diarrhea Symptoms usually subside in 5–10 days	Most cases in children younger than 9 yr, with about one third of cases in children ages 1–4 wk Antibiotics shorten illness and lower mortality All patients at risk for dehydration Acute symptoms may persist for 1 wk Antidiarrheal medications not recommended because they may predispose patient to toxic megacolon
***Yersinia* enterocolitis** Incubation—dose dependent, 1–3 wk Diagnosis—stool culture, ELISA Patients have leukocytosis, elevated ESR	Pathology poorly understood; possibly caused by production of enterotoxin	Mucoid diarrhea, sometimes bloody; abdominal pain suggestive of appendicitis; fever, vomiting	Seen more frequently in the winter months Transmitted by pets and food Antibiotics usually do not alter the clinical course in uncomplicated cases; antibiotics used in complicated infections and compromised hosts

Continued

TABLE 24-6   INFECTIOUS CAUSES OF ACUTE DIARRHEA—cont'd

AGENTS	PATHOLOGY	CHARACTERISTICS	COMMENTS
Campylobacter jejuni Microaerophilic, motile, gram-negative bacilli Incubation—1–7 days Ability to cause illness appears dose related Diagnosis—stool culture, sometimes blood culture Commonly found in GI tract of wild or domestic animals	Not fully understood, possibly (1) adherence to intestinal mucosa by toxin, (2) invasion of the mucosa in the terminal ileum and colon, (3) translocation in which the organisms penetrate the mucosa and replicate in the lamina propria	Fever, abdominal pain, diarrhea that can be bloody, vomiting Watery, profuse, foul-smelling diarrhea Clinically similar to infection by *Salmonella* or *Shigella* organisms Fecal–oral transmission	Most infections in humans relate to consumption of contaminated foods or water, such as undercooked meats, particularly chicken Also acquired from contaminated household pets (e.g., dogs, cats, hamsters) Bimodal peaks in infants younger than 1 yr of age and again at ages 15–29 yr Antibiotics do not prolong the carriage of bacteria and may eliminate organism more quickly Erythromycin is the drug of choice Antimotility agents not recommended because they tend to prolong symptoms
Vibrio cholerae Gram-negative, motile, curved bacillus living in bodies of salt water Incubation—1–3 days Diagnosis—stool culture	Enters via oral route in contaminated food or water; if survives acid stomach environment, travels to the small intestine, adheres to the mucosa, and produces toxin	Onset abrupt; vomiting, watery diarrhea without cramping or tenesmus Dehydration can occur quickly	More prevalent in developing countries Rehydration most important treatment Antibiotics can shorten diarrhea Despite continued efforts, still no vaccine
Clostridium difficile Gram-positive anaerobic bacillus with the ability to produce spores Diagnosis—by detecting *C. difficile* toxin in stool culture	Produces two important toxins (A and B) Toxin binds to the enterocyte surface receptor, resulting in altered permeability, protein synthesis, and direct cytotoxicity	Mostly mild watery diarrhea lasting a few days Some prolonged diarrhea and illness May cause pseudomembranous colitis Some individuals extremely ill with high fever, leukocytosis, hypoalbuminemia	Associated with alteration of normal intestinal flora by antibiotics Adults tend to have more severe symptoms than children Treatment with antibiotics (metronidazole) in mildly to moderately symptomatic patients; for nonresponders, give vancomycin Resistant strains have developed Relapse common
Clostridium perfringens Anaerobic, gram-positive, spore-producing bacilli Incubation—8–24 hr	Toxins produced in the intestine after ingestion of organism	Acute onset—watery diarrhea, crampy abdominal pain Fever, nausea, and vomiting are rare Duration of illness usually 24 hr	Transmitted by contaminated food products, most often meats and poultry Usually self-limiting and medical intervention not needed Oral rehydration usually sufficient Antibiotics serve no purpose and should not be used
Clostridium botulinum Gram-positive anaerobic spore-producing bacilli Incubation—12–26 hr (range, 6 hr–8 days) Diagnosis—to detect toxin, submit blood and stool culture to special laboratory (usually state health department)	Botulism caused by binding of toxin to the neuromuscular junction	Clinical presentation related to age and the strain of the botulism GI—abdominal pain, cramping, and diarrhea Other strains—respiratory compromise, CNS symptoms	Transmitted in contaminated food products Can be acquired via wound infection Treatment is supportive care and neutralization of the toxin Infant botulism—primarily in infants <12 mo; source previously found in honey; signs of constipation, poor feeding, weakness, absent deep tendon reflexes and other CNS manifestations; administer botulinum immune globulin (see Chapter 32)
Staphylococcus organisms Gram-positive nonmotile, aerobic or facultative anaerobic bacteria Incubation—generally short, 1–8 hr Diagnosis—identify organism in food, blood, pus, aspirate	Direct tissue invasion and production of toxin	Clinical presentation dependent on site of entry In food poisoning, profuse diarrhea, nausea, and vomiting	Transmitted in inadequately cooked or refrigerated foods Self-limiting Symptomatic treatment

CNS, Central nervous system; *EIA,* enzyme immunoassay; *ELISA,* enzyme-linked immunosorbent assay; *ESR,* erythrocyte sedimentation rate; *GI,* gastrointestinal; *SMAC,* Sorbitol MacConkey.

at age 15 to 19 years). *Giardia* and *Cryptosporidium* organisms are parasites. *Giardia* infection represents 15% of nondysenteric illness in the United States; *Cryptosporidium* infection is often associated with outbreaks in young children in daycare centers. *Plesiomonas* and *Yersinia* are also parasites that are frequently responsible for causing diarrhea that lasts more than 10 days in previously healthy adolescents. (See also Intestinal Parasitic Diseases, Chapter 14.)

Antibiotic administration is frequently associated with diarrhea because antibiotics alter the normal intestinal flora, resulting in an overgrowth of other bacteria such as *Clostridium difficile*. National rates of *C. difficile* almost doubled between 1997 and 2006; highest rates were in children 1 to 4 years of age (Zilberberg, Tillotson, and McDonald, 2010), and it has become more virulent with a high rate of recurrence and treatment failure (Bakken, 2009; DuPont, 2011). Antibiotic-associated diarrhea can also be caused by *Salmonella* organisms, *Clostridium porringers* type A, and *Staphylococcus aureus* pathogens.

Pathophysiology

Invasion of the GI tract by pathogens results in increased intestinal secretion as a result of enterotoxins, cytotoxic mediators, or decreased intestinal absorption secondary to intestinal damage or inflammation. Enteric pathogens attach to the mucosal cells and form a cuplike pedestal on which the bacteria rest. The pathogenesis of the diarrhea depends on whether the organism remains attached to the cell surface, resulting in a secretory toxin (noninvasive, toxin-producing, noninflammatory type diarrhea), or penetrates the mucosa (systemic diarrhea). Noninflammatory diarrhea is the most common diarrheal illness, resulting from the action of enterotoxin that is released after attachment to the mucosa. The most serious and immediate physiologic disturbances associated with severe diarrheal disease are (1) dehydration, (2) acid–base imbalance with acidosis, and (3) shock that occurs when dehydration progresses to the point that circulatory status is seriously impaired.

Diagnostic Evaluation

Evaluation of a child with acute gastroenteritis begins with a careful history that seeks to discover the possible cause of diarrhea, to assess the severity of symptoms and the risk of complications, and to elicit information about current symptoms indicating other treatable illnesses that could be causing the diarrhea. The history should include questions about recent travel, exposure to untreated drinking or washing water sources, contact with animals or birds, daycare center attendance, recent treatment with antibiotics, or recent diet changes. History questions should also explore the presence or absence of other symptoms such as fever and vomiting, frequency and character of stools (e.g., watery, bloody), urinary output, dietary habits, and recent food intake.

Extensive laboratory evaluation is not indicated in children who have uncomplicated diarrhea and no evidence of dehydration because most diarrheal illnesses are self-limiting. Laboratory tests are indicated for children who are severely dehydrated and receiving IV therapy. Watery, explosive stools suggest glucose intolerance; foul-smelling, greasy, bulky stools suggest fat malabsorption. Diarrhea that develops after the introduction of cow's milk, fruits, or cereal may be related to enzyme deficiency or protein intolerance. Neutrophils or red blood cells in the stool indicate bacterial gastroenteritis or IBD. The presence of eosinophils suggests protein intolerance or parasitic infection. Stool cultures should be performed only when blood, mucus, or polymorphonuclear leukocytes are present in the stool, when symptoms are severe, when there is a history of travel to a developing country, and

when a specific pathogen is suspected. Gross blood or occult blood may indicate pathogens such as *Shigella*, *Campylobacter*, or hemorrhagic *Escherichia coli* strains. An enzyme-linked immunosorbent assay (ELISA) may be used to confirm the presence of rotavirus or *Giardia* organisms. If there is a history of recent antibiotic use, the stool should be tested for *C. difficile* toxin. When bacterial and viral culture results are negative and when diarrhea persists for more than a few days, stools should be examined for ova and parasites. A stool specimen with a pH of less than 6 and the presence of reducing substances may indicate carbohydrate malabsorption or secondary lactase deficiency. Stool electrolyte measurements may help identify children with secretory diarrhea.

The serum bicarbonate (CO_2) may be useful when combined with other clinical signs. In the presence of metabolic acidosis an anion gap may be helpful to distinguish between types of metabolic imbalance. Obtain a complete blood count (CBC), serum electrolytes, creatinine, and blood urea nitrogen (BUN) in the child who has moderate to severe dehydration or who requires hospitalization. The hemoglobin, hematocrit, creatinine, and BUN levels are usually elevated in acute diarrhea and should normalize with rehydration.

Therapeutic Management

The major goals in the management of acute diarrhea include (1) assessment of fluid and electrolyte imbalance, (2) rehydration, (3) maintenance fluid therapy, and (4) reintroduction of an adequate diet. Infants and children with acute diarrhea and dehydration should be treated first with oral rehydration therapy (ORT). ORT is one of the major worldwide health care advances. It is more effective, safer, less painful, and less costly than IV rehydration. The AAP, World Health Organization, and CDC all recommend ORT as the treatment of choice for most cases of dehydration caused by diarrhea (CDC, 2003) (Box 24-1). Oral rehydration solutions (ORSs) enhance and promote the reabsorption of sodium and water, and studies indicate that these solutions greatly reduce vomiting, volume loss from diarrhea, and the duration of the illness. ORSs, including reduced osmolarity ORS, are available in the United States as commercially prepared solutions and are successful in treating the majority of infants with dehydration. Guidelines for rehydration recommended by the AAP are included in Table 24-7.

After rehydration, ORS may be used during maintenance fluid therapy by alternating the solution with a low-sodium fluid such as breast milk or commercial infant formula. In older children, ORS can be given and a regular diet continued. Ongoing stool losses should be

---

BOX 24-1   MODEL FOR REHYDRATION

- Rehydration solution should consist of 75 to 90 mEq/L of sodium (Na^+).
- Give 40 to 50 ml/kg of rehydration solution over 4 hours.
- Replacement and maintenance solution should consist of 40 to 60 mEq/L of Na^+.
- Reevaluate the need for further rehydration; initiate maintenance therapy using maintenance formulations, with daily volumes not to exceed 150 ml/kg/day.
- In children with diarrhea without significant dehydration, the maintenance phase may be initiated without the need for rehydration solution.
- If additional fluids are needed, use low-salt fluids such as breast milk or water.

Modified from Centers for Disease Control and Prevention: Managing acute gastroenteritis among children: oral rehydration, maintenance, and nutritional therapy, *MMWR Recommend Rep* 52(RR-16):1–16, 2003.

Case Studies—Acute Diarrhea; Gastroenteritis

TABLE 24-7	**TREATMENT OF ACUTE DIARRHEA**			
DEGREE OF DEHYDRATION	**SIGNS AND SYMPTOMS**	**REHYDRATION THERAPY***	**REPLACEMENT OF STOOL LOSSES**	**MAINTENANCE THERAPY**
Minimal	Increased thirst Slightly dry buccal mucous membranes	ORS, 50 ml/kg over 4 hr ORS, give 5–10 ml every 2–3 minutes	<10 kg: 60–120 ml per vomiting or diarrheal episode; >10 kg: 120–140 ml ORS per episode of vomiting or diarrhea	Breastfeeding, if established, should continue; give regular infant formula if tolerated. If lactose intolerance suspected, give undiluted lactose-free formula (or half-strength lactose-containing formula for brief period only); infants and children who receive solid food should continue their usual diet.
Mild to moderate	Loss of skin turgor, dry buccal mucous membranes, sunken eyes, sunken fontanel	ORS, 100 ml/kg within 4 hr	Same as above	
Severe	Signs of moderate dehydration plus one of following: rapid, thready pulse; cyanosis; rapid breathing; lethargy; or coma	IV fluids (Ringer lactate; 0.9 NS), 20 ml/kg bolus over 30 minutes and repeat until pulse and state of consciousness return to normal; then maintenance fluids with dextrose and 0.45 NS; add K+ after renal function adequate; give 50–100 ml/kg or ORS	Same as above	

Modified from Centers for Disease Control and Prevention: Managing acute gastroenteritis among children: oral rehydration, maintenance, and nutritional therapy, *MMWR Recommend Rep* 52(RR-16):1–16, 2003.
IV, Intravenous; *K+*, potassium; *NS*, normal saline; *ORS,* oral rehydration solution.
*If no signs of dehydration are present, rehydration therapy is not necessary. Proceed with maintenance therapy and replacement of stool losses.

replaced on a 1:1 basis with ORS. If the stool volume is not known, approximately 10 ml/kg (4–8 oz) of ORS should be given for each diarrheal stool. Liquids such as sports drinks, tea, juices, or carbonated beverages are not appropriate for ORT in small children.

Solutions for oral hydration are useful in most cases of dehydration, and vomiting is not a contraindication. A child who is vomiting should be given an ORS at frequent intervals and in small amounts. For young children, the caregiver may give the fluid with a spoon or small syringe in 5- to 10-ml increments every 1 to 5 minutes. An ORS may also be given via NG or gastrostomy tube infusion. Infants without clinical signs of dehydration do not need ORT. They should, however, receive the same fluids recommended for infants with signs of dehydration in the maintenance phase and for ongoing stool losses. The use of probiotics in tandem with rehydration therapy reduces the duration and stool frequency in acute infectious diarrhea (Allen, Martinez, Gregorio, and others, 2010).

Prevention

Two rotavirus vaccines are now available for children. Human-bovine reassortant rotavirus vaccine (RotaTeq) became available in 2006, and live-attenuated human rotavirus vaccine (Rotarix) may be used to prevent this infectious diarrheal disease. Infants should receive three doses of RotaTeq oral vaccine at 2, 4, and 6 months of age. Two doses of Rotarix will induce protective immunity and may be administered at 2 and 4 months of age (AAP, Committee on Infectious Diseases and Pickering, 2009) (see Immunizations, Chapter 10). Population-based studies show a reduction of diarrhea-associated hospitalizations by as much as 40% to 80% in the years after rotavirus vaccination (Chang, Smith, Tserenpuntsag, and others, 2010; Yen, Tate, Wenk, and others, 2011). Breastfeeding during the first 6 months of life has been found to have a protective effect against rotavirus infection (Plenge-Bönig, Soto-Ramirez, Karmaus, and others, 2010).

Early reintroduction of nutrients is desirable and is gaining more widespread acceptance. Continued feeding or early reintroduction of a normal diet has no adverse effects and actually lessens the severity

> **! NURSING ALERT**
>
> Diarrhea is not managed by encouraging intake of clear fluids by mouth, such as fruit juices, carbonated soft drinks, and gelatin. These fluids usually have a high carbohydrate content, a very low electrolyte content, and a high osmolality. Caffeinated soda is avoided because caffeine is a mild diuretic and may lead to increased loss of water and sodium. Chicken or beef broth is not given because it contains excessive sodium and inadequate carbohydrate. A BRAT diet (bananas, rice, applesauce, and toast or tea) is contraindicated for children and especially for infants with acute diarrhea because this diet has little nutritional value (low in energy and protein), is high in carbohydrates, and is low in electrolytes (AAP, Committee on Infectious Diseases and Pickering, 2009).

and duration of the illness and improves weight gain compared with the gradual reintroduction of foods (AAP, Committee on Infectious Diseases and Pickering, 2009; Bhutta, 2011). Infants who are breastfeeding should continue to do so, and ORS should be used to replace ongoing losses in these infants. Formula-fed infants should resume their formula; if it is not tolerated, a lactose-free formula may be used for a few days. In older children, a regular diet, including milk, can generally be offered after rehydration has been achieved. In toddlers, there is no contraindication to continuing soft or pureed foods. A diet of easily digestible foods such as cereals, cooked vegetables, and meats is adequate for older children.

In cases of severe dehydration and shock, IV fluids are initiated whenever the child is unable to ingest sufficient amounts of fluid and electrolytes to (1) meet ongoing daily physiologic losses, (2) replace previous deficits, and (3) replace ongoing abnormal losses. Patients who usually require IV fluids are those with severe dehydration, those with uncontrollable vomiting, those who are unable to drink for any reason (e.g., extreme fatigue, coma), and those with severe gastric distention.

The IV solution for fluid replacement is selected on the basis of what is known regarding the probable type and cause of the dehydration—usually a saline solution (0.9 normal saline [NS] or lactated Ringer solution for rapid volume replacement (see Parenteral Fluid Therapy, p. 769).

After the severe effects of dehydration are under control, specific diagnostic and therapeutic measures are begun to detect and treat the cause of the diarrhea. The use of antibiotic therapy in children with acute gastroenteritis is controversial. Antibiotics may shorten the course of some diarrheal illnesses (e.g., those caused by *Shigella* organisms). However, most bacterial diarrheas are self-limiting, and the diarrhea often resolves before the causative organism can be determined. Antibiotics may prolong the carrier period for bacteria such as *Salmonella* spp. Antibiotics may be considered, however, in patients with immunosuppression, severe symptoms, or persistent disease and in patients who have had transplantation (Jabbar and Wright, 2003) (see Intestinal Parasitic Diseases, Chapter 14). Antimotility drugs such as loperamide are not recommended in children, and antiemetic drugs such as the phenothiazines are not recommended because of their side effects. Because of the self-limiting nature of vomiting and its tendency to improve when dehydration is corrected, the use of antiemetic agents have historically not been recommended; however, ondansetron has few side effects and may be administered if vomiting persists and interferes with ORT (Bhutta, 2011).

Nursing Care Management

The management of most cases of acute diarrhea takes place in the home with education of the caregiver. Caregivers are taught to monitor for signs of dehydration (especially the number of wet diapers or voidings) and the amount of fluids taken by mouth and to assess the frequency and amount of stool losses. Education relating to ORT, including the administration of maintenance fluids and replacement of ongoing losses, is important (see Critical Thinking Case Study). ORS should be administered in small quantities at frequent intervals. Vomiting is not a contraindication to ORT unless it is severe. Information concerning the introduction of a normal diet is essential. Parents need to know that a slightly higher stool output initially occurs with continuation of a normal diet and with ongoing replacement of stool losses. The benefits of a better nutritional outcome with fewer complications and a shorter duration of illness outweigh the potential increase in stool frequency. Parents' concerns should be addressed to ensure adherence to the treatment plan.

If the child with acute diarrhea and dehydration is hospitalized, an accurate weight must be obtained, as well as careful monitoring of fluid intake and output. The child may be placed on parenteral fluid therapy with nothing by mouth (NPO) for 12 to 48 hours, but the trend is to start small amounts of oral fluids to tolerance unless there are other illness factors which preclude ORT. Monitoring the IV infusion is an important nursing function. The nurse must ensure that the correct fluid and electrolyte concentration is infused, that the flow rate is adjusted to deliver the desired volume in a given time, and that the IV site is maintained.

Accurate measurement of output is essential to determine whether renal blood flow is sufficient to permit the addition of potassium to the IV fluids. The nurse is responsible for examination of stools and collection of specimens for laboratory examination (see Collection of Specimens, Chapter 22). Care should be taken when obtaining and transporting stools to prevent possible spread of infection. Stool specimens should be transported to the laboratory in appropriate containers and media.

Diarrheal stools are highly irritating to the perianal skin, and extra care is needed to protect the skin of the diaper region from excoriation (see Diaper Dermatitis, Chapter 30). Taking the temperature rectally

---

⚲ **CRITICAL THINKING CASE STUDY**
Diarrhea

A mother brings her 8-month-old infant, Mary, to the primary care clinic. The mother reports that Mary has had a "cold" for about 2 days, and this morning she began to vomit and has had diarrhea for the past 8 hours. The mother states that Mary is still breastfeeding, but that she is not taking as much milk as usual, and she is having three times as many stools as usual (the stools are watery in consistency). When the nurse practitioner examines Mary, she notes that her temperature is 38° C (100.4° F), her pulse and blood pressure are in the normal range, her mucous membranes are moist, and she has tears when she cries. The nurse practitioner also notes that Mary's weight has not changed from what it was when she was seen in the clinic 2 weeks ago for her well-child visit. What interventions should the nurse practitioner include in her initial management of Mary?

Questions
1. Evidence—Is there sufficient evidence for the nurse practitioner to draw any conclusions for her initial plan of management?
2. Assumptions—Describe some underlying assumptions about:
   a. Clinical manifestations of various levels of dehydration
   b. Management of acute diarrhea
   c. Breastfeeding and the management of acute diarrhea
   d. Use of antidiarrheal medications for acute diarrhea
3. What nursing interventions should the nurse practitioner implement at this time?
4. Does the evidence support the nurse practitioner's conclusion?

---

is usually avoided because it stimulates the bowel, increasing passage of stool.

Support for the child and family involves the same care and consideration given to all hospitalized children (see Chapter 21). Parents are kept informed of the child's progress and instructed in the use of frequent and proper hand washing and the disposal of soiled diapers, clothes, and bed linens. Everyone caring for the child must be aware of "clean" areas and "dirty" areas, especially in the hospital, where the sink in the child's room is used for many purposes. Soiled diapers and linens should be discarded in receptacles close to the bedside.

Prevention

The best intervention for diarrhea is prevention. The fecal–oral route spreads most infections, and parents need information about preventive measures such as personal hygiene, protection of the water supply from contamination, and careful food preparation.

⚠ **NURSING ALERT**

To reduce the risk of bacteria transmitted via food, encourage parents to:
- Quickly freeze or refrigerate all ground meat and other perishable foods.
- Never thaw food on the counter or let it sit out of the refrigerator for more than 2 hours.
- Wash hands, utensils, and work areas with hot, soapy water after contact with raw meat to keep bacteria from spreading.
- Check ground meat with a fork to make certain no pink is showing before taking a bite.
- Cook all dishes made with ground meat until brown or gray inside or to an internal temperature of 71° C (160° F).
- Use soap or a weak chlorine bleach solution to wash all fruits and vegetables that are unable to be peeled.

Nursing Care Plan—The Child with Acute Diarrhea (Gastroenteritis)

Meticulous attention to perianal hygiene, disposal of soiled diapers, proper hand washing, and isolation of infected persons also minimize the transmission of infection (see Infection Control, Chapter 22).

Parents need information about preventing diarrhea while traveling. They are cautioned against giving their children adult medications that are used to prevent traveler's diarrhea. Until vaccines or other prophylactic measures are proved to be safe for children, the best measure during travel to areas where water may be contaminated is to allow children to drink only bottled water and carbonated beverages (from the container through a straw supplied from home). Tap water, ice, unpasteurized dairy products, raw vegetables, unpeeled fruits, meats, and seafood should also be avoided.

The expected outcomes are described in the Nursing Process box.

Constipation

Constipation is an alteration in the frequency, consistency, or ease of passing stool. It is defined as a decrease in bowel movement frequency or trouble defecating for more than 2 weeks (Philichi, 2008). Constipation is an alteration in the frequency, consistency, or ease of passing stool. Parents often define constipation as passing less than three stools per week. It may also be defined as painful bowel movements, which are often blood streaked or include the retention of stool, with or without soiling, even with a stool frequency of more than three stools per week (Loening-Baucke and Pashankar, 2006). The frequency of bowel movements, however, is not considered a diagnostic criterion because it varies widely among children. Having extremely long intervals between defecation is obstipation. Constipation with fecal soiling is encopresis.

Constipation may arise secondary to a variety of organic disorders or in association with a wide range of systemic disorders. Structural disorders of the intestine, such as strictures, ectopic anus, and Hirschsprung disease (HD), may be associated with constipation. Systemic disorders associated with constipation include hypothyroidism, hypercalcemia resulting from hyperparathyroidism or vitamin D excess, and chronic lead poisoning. Constipation may be associated with use of drugs such as antacids, diuretics, antiepileptics, antihistamines, opioids, and iron supplementation. Spinal cord lesions may be associated with loss of rectal tone and sensation. Affected children are prone to chronic fecal retention and overflow incontinence.

The majority of children have idiopathic or functional constipation because no underlying cause can be identified. Chronic constipation may occur as a result of environmental or psychosocial factors or a combination of both. Transient illness, stool withholding and avoidance secondary to painful or negative experiences with stooling, and dietary intake with decreased fluid and fiber all play a role in the etiology of constipation.

Newborn Period

Normally, newborn infants pass a first meconium stool within 24 to 36 hours of birth. Any infant who does not do so should be assessed for evidence of intestinal atresia or stenosis, HD, hypothyroidism, meconium plug, or meconium ileus. Meconium plug is caused by meconium that has reduced water content and is usually evacuated after digital examination but may require irrigations with a hypertonic solution or contrast medium.

Meconium ileus, the initial manifestation of cystic fibrosis, is the luminal obstruction of the distal small intestine by abnormal meconium. Treatment is the same as for a meconium plug; early surgical intervention may be needed to evacuate the small intestine.

NURSING PROCESS
The Child with Diarrhea

Assessment
Observe the infant's or child's general appearance and behavior. Assess for dehydration, such as decreased urinary output; weight loss; dry mucous membranes; poor skin turgor; sunken fontanel; and pale, cool, dry skin. With severe dehydration, increased pulse and respiration, decreased blood pressure, and a prolonged capillary refill time (>2 seconds) may indicate impending shock (see Table 24-4).

A history provides information about probable etiologic agents, such as introduction of a new food, exposure to infectious agents, travel to an area of high susceptibility, contact with foods that might have been contaminated, and contact with pets known to be sources of enteric infections. An allergic, drug, and dietary history may indicate food allergies, use of laxatives or antibiotics, or sources of excess sorbitol and fructose (e.g., apple juice).

Diagnosis (Problem Identification)
After a thorough assessment, several nursing diagnoses are evident:
- Deficient Fluid Volume related to diarrhea (GI) losses, inadequate intake
- Risk for Infection related to microorganisms invading GI tract
- Impaired Skin Integrity related to irritation caused by frequent, loose stools

Planning
Expected patient outcomes include:
- Infant or child will maintain adequate hydration.
- Infant or child will maintain appropriate nutrition for age.
- Infant or child will not spread infection (if etiologic agent) to others.
- Family will receive appropriate support and education, especially regarding home care.
- Caregivers will verbalize understanding of home care regimen, available support, and resources.

Implementation
Numerous intervention strategies are discussed on pp. 775–778.

Evaluation
The effectiveness of nursing interventions for the family and the child with diarrhea is determined by continual assessment and evaluation of care based on the following guidelines:
- Monitor fluid losses with careful intake and output measurements and daily weights.
- Monitor food intake, especially calories.
- Observe for evidence of complications from underlying disease (specify) or therapy.
- Observe and interview family to determine extent and effectiveness of care.

GI, Gastrointestinal.

Infancy

The onset of constipation frequently occurs during infancy and may result from organic causes such as HD, hypothyroidism, and strictures. It is important to differentiate these conditions from functional constipation. Constipation in infancy is often related to dietary practices. It is less common in breastfed infants, who have softer stools than bottle-fed infants. Breastfed infants may also have decreased stools because of more complete digestion of breast milk with little residue. When constipation occurs with a change from human milk or modified cow's milk to whole cow's milk (12 months old and older), simple measures such as adding or increasing the amount of cereal, vegetables,

CRITICAL THINKING CASE STUDY

Constipation

Harry, an 8-month-old infant, is seen by the pediatric nurse practitioner for his well-child visit. Harry's mother states that he usually has one hard stool every 4 or 5 days, which causes discomfort when the stool is passed. He has also had one episode of diarrhea and two episodes of ribbonlike stools. Abdominal distention and vomiting have not accompanied the constipation, and Harry's growth has been appropriate for his age. Currently, his diet consists of formula only. Harry's mother reports that the infrequent passage of hard stools began approximately 6 weeks ago when she stopped breastfeeding. Which interventions should the nurse practitioner include in the initial management of Harry's problem?

Questions

1. Evidence—Is there sufficient evidence for the nurse practitioner to draw any conclusions about the management of Harry's problem?
2. Assumptions—Describe some underlying assumptions about:
   a. Causes of constipation in infants
   b. Factors associated with functional constipation in infants
   c. Management of functional constipation in infants
3. What interventions should the nurse practitioner implement at this time?
4. Does the evidence support these interventions?

and fruit in the infant's diet usually corrects the problem. When a bottle-fed infant passes a hard stool that results in an anal fissure, stool-withholding behaviors may develop in response to pain on defecation (see Critical Thinking Case Study).

Childhood

Most constipation in early childhood is attributable to environmental changes or normal development when a child begins to attain control over bodily functions. A child who has experienced discomfort during bowel movements may deliberately try to withhold stool. Over time, the rectum accommodates to the accumulation of stool, and the urge to defecate passes. When the bowel contents are ultimately evacuated, the accumulated feces are passed with pain, thus reinforcing the desire to withhold stool.

Constipation in school-age children may represent an ongoing problem or a first-time event. The onset of constipation at this age is often the result of environmental changes, stresses, and changes in toileting patterns. A common cause of new-onset constipation at school entry is fear of using the school bathrooms, which are noted for their lack of privacy. Early and hurried departure for school immediately after breakfast may also impede bathroom use.

The management of simple constipation consists of a plan to promote regular bowel movements. Often this is as simple as changing the diet to provide more fiber and fluids, eliminating foods known to be constipating, and establishing a bowel routine that allows for regular passage of stool. An increase in dietary fiber is recommended as a treatment for constipation in the healthy child. The amount of fiber for different aged children varies by various authorities but the formula of "age + 5 g" daily intake of fiber is recommended for children age 3 years and older (Kranz, Brauchla, Slavin, and others, 2012). The Dietary Reference Intake (DRI) Average Intake (AI) for children ages 4 to 8 years is 25 g of fiber daily. AI dietary fiber intake recommendations for boys ages 9 to 13 years are 31 g/day and are 26 g/day for girls of the same age and up to age 18 years. For boys ages 14 to 18 years, the AI for fiber intake is 38 g/day.

Stool-softening agents such as docusate or lactulose may also be helpful. Polyethylene glycol (PEG) 3350 without electrolytes (Miralax) is a chemically inert polymer that has been introduced as a new laxative in recent years. It is tolerated well by children because it can be mixed in a beverage of choice (Loening-Baucke and Pashankar, 2006). If other symptoms such as vomiting, abdominal distention, or pain and evidence of growth failure are associated with the constipation, the condition should be investigated further.

Nursing Care Management

Constipation tends to be self-perpetuating. A child who has difficulty or discomfort when attempting to evacuate the bowels has a tendency to retain the bowel contents, and this may initiate a vicious cycle. Nursing assessment begins with an accurate history of bowel habits; diet; events associated with the onset of constipation; drugs or other substances that the child may be taking; and the consistency, color, frequency, and other characteristics of the stool. If there is no evidence of a pathologic condition, the major task is to educate the parents regarding normal stool patterns and to participate in the education and treatment of the child.

Dietary modifications are essential in preventing constipation. During infancy, simply increasing the carbohydrate (sucrose or corn syrup) in the infant's formula may relieve the problem. During childhood, the diet should contain increased amounts of fiber and fluid. Parents benefit from guidance in selecting foods that facilitate bowel movements (Box 24-2). They need reassurance concerning the benign nature of the condition. It is also important to discuss their attitudes and expectations regarding toilet habits.

When constipation persists despite dietary intervention, more aggressive management may be necessary. It is important to differentiate an acute episode of constipation from chronic functional constipation, which can result from chronic stool-withholding behavior. As the rectal vault becomes distended over time, further complications such as fecal impaction and encopresis may develop (see Chapter 17).

Hirschsprung Disease

Hirschsprung disease is a congenital anomaly that results in mechanical obstruction from inadequate motility of part of the intestine. It accounts for about one fourth of all cases of neonatal intestinal obstruction. The incidence is 1 in 5000 live births. It is four times more common in males than in females and follows a familial pattern in a small number of cases. Mutations in the *RET* protooncogene have been found in 17% to 38% of children with short-segment HD and in 70% to 80% of those with long-segment involvement (Dasgupta and Langer, 2004). In more than 80% of cases, the aganglionosis is restricted to the internal sphincter, rectum, and a few centimeters of the sigmoid colon and is termed *short-segment disease* (Theocharatos and Kenny, 2008).

Pathophysiology

The pathology of HD relates to the absence of ganglion cells in the affected areas of the intestine, resulting in a loss of the rectosphincteric reflex and an abnormal microenvironment of the cells of the affected intestine (Theocharatos and Kenny, 2008). The term *congenital aganglionic megacolon* describes the primary defect, which is the absence of ganglion cells in the myenteric plexus of Auerbach and the submucosal plexus of Meissner (Fig. 24-1).

The absence of ganglion cells in the affected bowel results in a lack of enteric nervous system stimulation, which decreases the internal sphincter's ability to relax. Unopposed sympathetic stimulation of the intestine results in increased intestinal tone. In addition to the

BOX 24-2 FIBER CONTENT OF SELECT FOODS

FOOD	SERVING SIZE	GRAMS OF FIBER
Apple, raw, with skin	1 apple	3.3
Apricot, dried, uncooked	10 halves	2.6
Bananas, ripe, raw	1 banana	3.1
Beans, baked, canned	1 cup	10.4
Beans, pinto, mature seeds*	1 cup	15.4
Beets*	1 cup	3.4
Blackberries, raw	1 cup	7.6
Blueberries, raw	1 cup	3.5
Bread, mixed grain (includes whole grain)	1 slice	1.6
Broccoli*	1 cup	5.1
Brussels sprouts*	1 cup	4.1
Cabbage*	1 cup	2.8
Carrots*	1 cup	4.7
Cereals, ready-to-eat, General Mills, Cheerios	1 cup	3.6
Cereals, ready-to-eat, General Mills, Raisin Nut Bran	1 cup	5.1
Cereals, ready-to-eat, Kellogg's All Bran, original	½ cup	8.8
Cereals, ready-to-eat, Kellogg's Raisin Bran	1 cup	7.3
Collards*	1 cup	5.3
Dates, daglet noor	1 cup	14.2
Lentils, mature seeds*	1 cup	15.6
Lima beans, large, mature*	1 cup	13.2
Oat bran, cooked	1 cup	5.7
Pears, raw	1 pear	5.1
Peas, green, frozen*	1 cup	8.8
Raisins, seedless	1 cup	5.4
Spinach*	1 cup	4.3
Vegetables, mixed, frozen*	1 cup	8.0
Wheat flour, whole grain	1 cup	14.6
Wheat flour, white, all-purpose, enriched	1 cup	3.5

Modified from USDA National Nutrient Database for Standard Reference, Release 17, Fiber, total dietary content of selected foods per common measure, sorted alphabetically, retrieved January 25, 2012, from http://www.nal.usda.gov/fnic/foodcomp/Data/SR17/wtrank/sr17a291.pdf.
*Cooked, boiled, drained, no salt.

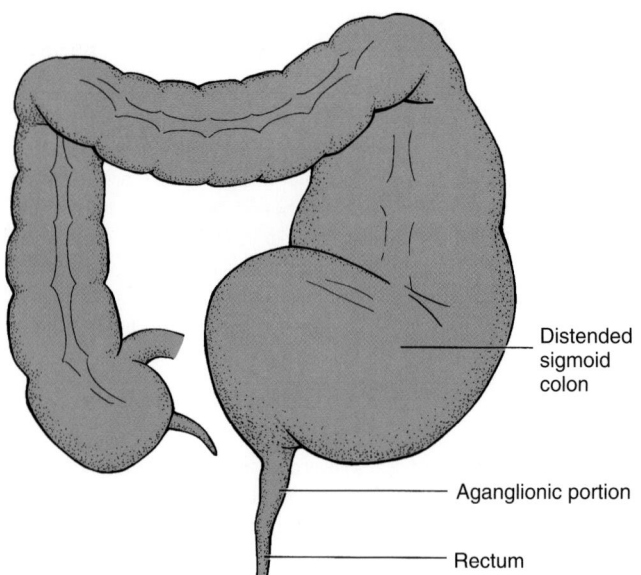

FIG 24-1 Hirschsprung disease.

Distended sigmoid colon

Aganglionic portion

Rectum

BOX 24-3 CLINICAL MANIFESTATIONS OF HIRSCHSPRUNG DISEASE

Newborn Period
Failure to pass meconium within 24 to 48 hours after birth
Refusal to feed
Bilious vomiting
Abdominal distention

Infancy
Growth failure
Constipation
Abdominal distention
Episodes of diarrhea and vomiting
Signs of enterocolitis
  Explosive, watery diarrhea
  Fever
  Appears significantly ill

Childhood
Constipation
Ribbonlike, foul-smelling stools
Abdominal distention
Visible peristalsis
Easily palpable fecal mass
Undernourished, anemic appearance

contraction of the abnormal bowel and the resulting lack of peristalsis, there is a loss of the rectosphincteric reflex. Normally, when a stool bolus enters the rectum, the internal sphincter relaxes and the stool is evacuated. In HD, the internal sphincter does not relax. In most cases, the aganglionic segment includes the rectum and some portion of the distal colon. However, the entire colon or part of the small intestine may be involved. Occasionally, skip segments or total intestinal aganglionosis may occur.

Diagnostic Evaluation

Most children with HD are diagnosed in the first few months of life. Clinical manifestations vary according to the age when symptoms are recognized and the presence of complications, such as enterocolitis (Box 24-3). A neonate usually is seen with distended abdomen, feeding intolerance with bilious vomiting, and delay in the passage of meconium. Typically, 95% of normal term infants pass meconium in the first 24 hours of life, but fewer than 10% of infants with HD do so. In older children, a careful history is helpful. Radiographs, an unprepped barium enema, and anorectal manometric examinations assist in the differential diagnosis, which is confirmed by a full-thickness rectal biopsy demonstrating the absence of ganglion cells in the myenteric and submucosal plexuses.

Therapeutic Management

The majority of children with HD require surgery rather than medical therapy with frequent enemas (Levitt, Martin, Olesevich, and others, 2009). After the child is stabilized with fluid and electrolyte replacement, if needed, surgery is performed, with a high rate of success. Surgical management consists primarily of the removal of the aganglionic portion of the bowel to relieve obstruction, restore normal motility, and preserve the function of the external anal sphincter. The transanal Soave endorectal pull-through procedure is often performed and consists of pulling the end of the normal bowel through the muscular sleeve of the rectum, from which the aganglionic mucosa has been removed (Huang, Zheng, and Xiao, 2008). With earlier diagnosis, the proximal bowel may not be extremely distended, thus allowing for a primary pull-through or one-stage procedure and eliminating the need for a temporary colostomy. Simpler operations, such as an anorectal myomectomy, may be indicated in very short–segment disease.

Prognosis. After the pull-through procedure, anal stricture and incontinence may occur and require further therapy, including dilations or bowel retraining therapy. Constipation and fecal incontinence are chronic problems in a significant proportion of patients after surgical correction for HD (Levitt, Martin, Olesevich, and others, 2009). As these children grow older, this can significantly affect their quality of life (Mills, Konkin, Milner, and others, 2008).

Nursing Care Management

The nursing concerns depend on the child's age and the type of treatment. If the disorder is diagnosed during the neonatal period, the main objectives are to (1) help the parents adjust to a congenital defect in their child, (2) foster infant–parent bonding, (3) prepare them for the medical-surgical intervention, and (4) assist them in colostomy care after discharge.

Preoperative Care. The child's preoperative care depends on the age and clinical condition. A child who is malnourished may not be able to withstand surgery until his or her physical status improves. Often this involves symptomatic treatment with enemas; a low-fiber, high-calorie, and high-protein diet; and in severe situations, the use of total parenteral nutrition (TPN).

Physical preoperative preparation includes the same measures that are common to any surgery (see Surgical Procedures, Chapter 22). In newborns, whose bowels are sterile, no additional preparation is necessary. However, in other children, preparation for the pull-through procedure involves emptying the bowels with saline enemas and decreasing bacterial flora with oral or systemic antibiotics and colonic irrigations using antibiotic solution. Enterocolitis is the most serious complication of HD. Emergency preoperative care includes frequent monitoring of vital signs and blood pressure for signs of shock; monitoring fluid and electrolyte replacements, as well as plasma or other blood derivatives; and observing for symptoms of bowel perforation, such as fever, increasing abdominal distention, vomiting, increased tenderness, irritability, dyspnea, and cyanosis.

Because progressive distention of the abdomen is a serious sign, the nurse measures abdominal circumference with a paper tape measure, usually at the level of the umbilicus or at the widest part of the abdomen. The point of measurement is marked with a pen to ensure reliability of subsequent measurements. Abdominal measurement can be obtained with the vital sign measurements and is recorded in serial order so that any change is obvious. To reduce stress to the acutely ill child when frequent measurements of abdominal circumference are needed, the tape measure can be left in place beneath the child rather than removed each time.

The child's age dictates the type and extent of psychologic preparation. When a colostomy is performed, the child who is of preschool age is told about the procedure in concrete terms with the use of visual aids (see Chapter 22). It is important to time explanations appropriately to prevent the anxiety and confusion that could result from too much information. It is also important to stress to parents and older children that the colostomy for HD is temporary unless so much bowel is involved that a permanent ileostomy must be performed. In most instances, the extent of bowel resection is known before surgery, although the nurse should be aware of cases when doubt exists concerning repair. The nurse should remember that although a temporary colostomy is favorable in terms of future health and adjustment, it requires additional surgery, which may be stressful to parents and children.

Postoperative Care. Postoperative care is the same as that for any child or infant with abdominal surgery (see Surgical Procedures, Chapter 22). When a colostomy is part of the corrective procedure, stomal care is a major nursing task (see Ostomies, Chapter 22). To prevent contamination of an infant's abdominal wound with urine, the diaper should be placed below the dressing. A Foley catheter may be used in the immediate postoperative period to divert the flow of urine away from the abdomen.

Discharge Care. After surgery, parents need instruction concerning colostomy care. Even a preschooler can be included in the care by handing articles to the parent, rolling up the colostomy pouch after it is emptied, or applying barrier preparations to the surrounding skin. Although the diagnosis of HD is less frequent in school-age children and adolescents, children this age can often be involved in colostomy care to the point of total responsibility.

An enterostomal therapy nurse can provide expert assistance in planning home care. If families require financial assistance and psychologic support, referral to a social worker, home health care agency, or community health nurse provides continuity of care.

Vomiting

Vomiting is the forceful ejection of gastric contents through the mouth. It is a well-defined, complex, coordinated process that is under CNS control and is often accompanied by nausea and retching. Vomiting may be divided into two categories: nonbilious and bilious. Some small intestinal reflux is common in all vomiting. In nonbilious vomiting, the majority of bile drains into the more distal portions of the intestine. If an obstruction is present, nonbilious vomiting suggests a more proximal obstruction. Bilious vomiting implies a disorder of motility or distal physical blockage. Causes of nonbilious vomiting include infectious, inflammatory, metabolic or endocrinologic, neurologic, and psychologic causes and obstructive lesions such as pyloric stenosis. Causes of bilious vomiting include intestinal atresia and stenosis, malrotation with or without volvulus, ileus, intussusception, intestinal duplication, mass lesions, incarcerated inguinal hernia, and appendicitis. Vomiting may also be associated with other processes, including acute infectious diseases, increased intracranial pressure, toxic ingestion, food intolerance and allergies, mechanical obstruction of the GI tract, metabolic disorders, and psychogenic problems. Vomiting is common in childhood, is usually self-limiting, and requires no specific treatment. However, complications may occur, including acute fluid volume loss (dehydration) and electrolyte disturbances, malnutrition, aspiration, and Mallory-Weiss syndrome (small tears in the distal esophageal mucosa).

Vomiting is a well-recognized response to psychologic stress. During stress, adrenaline levels rise and may stimulate the chemoreceptor trigger zone. Nausea and vomiting are likely a protective mechanism to remove toxins from the system. Vomiting may follow GI infection or toxic ingestion, or it can be a learned behavioral response.

Cyclic vomiting syndrome is a rare disorder characterized by bouts of vomiting that can last from hours to several days (McRonald and Fleisher, 2005). The cause of this syndrome is unknown (Bullard and Page, 2005).

Therapeutic Management

Management is directed toward detection and treatment of the cause of the vomiting and prevention of complications from the loss of fluid. Fluids are administered in the same manner and in a similar electrolyte composition to those administered for diarrhea. Although most children respond to these measures, antiemetic drugs may be needed. Antiemetics such as ondansetron (Zofran) and trimethobenzamide (Tigan) block receptors in the chemoreceptor trigger zone; others such as metoclopramide (Reglan) enhance gastroduodenal peristalsis; still others such as promethazine (Phenergan) compete for H_1-receptor sites. For children who are prone to motion sickness, it is helpful to administer an appropriate dose of dimenhydrinate (Dramamine) before a trip.

Nursing Care Management

The major focus of nursing care is observation and reporting of vomiting behavior and associated symptoms and the implementation of measures to reduce the vomiting. Accurate assessment of the type of vomiting, the appearance of the vomitus, and the child's behavior in association with the vomiting helps to establish a diagnosis.

Nursing interventions are determined by the cause of the vomiting. When the vomiting is a manifestation of improper feeding methods, establishing proper techniques through teaching and example will usually correct the situation. If vomiting is believed to be an indication of obstruction, food is usually withheld or special feeding techniques are implemented. In situations in which vomiting is related to concurrent infection, dietary indiscretion, or emotional factors, efforts are directed toward maintaining hydration or preventing dehydration.

The thirst mechanism is the most sensitive guide to fluid needs, and *ad libitum* administration of a glucose-electrolyte solution to an alert child will restore water and electrolytes satisfactorily. It is important to include carbohydrate to spare body protein and avoid ketosis resulting from exhaustion of glycogen stores. Small, frequent feedings of fluids or foods are preferred. After vomiting has stopped, more liberal amounts of fluids are offered followed by gradual resumption of the regular diet.

The vomiting infant or child is positioned on the side or semireclining to prevent aspiration and observed for evidence of dehydration. It is important to emphasize the need for the child to brush the teeth or rinse the mouth after vomiting to dilute hydrochloric acid that comes in contact with the teeth. A flavored mouthwash or tooth brushing will freshen the mouth. Careful monitoring of fluid and electrolyte status is necessary to prevent an electrolyte disturbance.

Gastroesophageal Reflux

Gastroesophageal reflux (GER) is defined as the transfer of gastric contents into the esophagus. This phenomenon is physiologic, occurring throughout the day, most frequently after meals and at night; therefore, it is important to differentiate GER from **gastroesophageal reflux disease (GERD)**. GERD represents symptoms or tissue damage that result from GER. Approximately 50% of infants younger than 2 months old are reported to have GER (Suwandhi, Ton, and Schwarz, 2006). This "physiologic" GER usually resolves spontaneously by 1 year of age.

Certain conditions predispose children to a high prevalence of GERD, including neurologic impairment, hiatal hernia, repaired esophageal atresia (EA), and morbid obesity (Suwandhi, Ton, and Schwarz, 2006). Sandifer syndrome is an uncommon condition, usually occurring in young children, characterized by repetitive stretching and arching of the head and neck that can be mistaken for a seizure. This maneuver likely represents a physiologic neuromuscular response attempting to prevent acid refluxate from reaching the upper portion of the esophagus (Cavataio and Guandalini, 2005).

Infants who are prone to develop GER include premature infants and infants with bronchopulmonary dysplasia. Children who have had tracheoesophageal or EA repairs, extracorporeal membrane oxygenation (ECMO), neurologic disorders, scoliosis, asthma, cystic fibrosis, or cerebral palsy are also prone to developing GER. The clinical manifestations of GER are listed in Box 24-4.

Pathophysiology

Although the pathogenesis of GER is multifactorial, its primary causative mechanism likely involves inappropriate transient relaxation of the lower esophageal sphincter (LES) (Suwandhi, Ton, and Schwarz, 2006). Factors that increase abdominal pressure such as coughing and sneezing, scoliosis, and overeating may contribute to GERD. Whereas esophageal symptoms are caused by inflammation from the acid in the

---

BOX 24-4 CLINICAL MANIFESTATIONS AND COMPLICATIONS OF GASTROESOPHAGEAL REFLUX

Symptoms in Infants
Spitting up, regurgitation, vomiting (may be forceful)
Excessive crying, irritability, arching of the back with neck extension, stiffening
May be "silent" (no clinical signs observed)
Weight loss, growth failure (failure to thrive)
Respiratory problems (cough, wheeze, stridor, gagging, choking with feedings)
Hematemesis
Apnea or ALTE

Symptoms in Children
Heartburn
Abdominal pain
Noncardiac chest pain
Chronic cough
Dysphagia
Nocturnal asthma
Recurrent pneumonia

Complications
Esophagitis
Esophageal stricture
Laryngitis
Recurrent pneumonia
Anemia
Barrett esophagus

Adapted from Rudolph CD, Mazur LJ, Liptak GS, and others: Guidelines for evaluation and treatment of gastroesophageal reflux in infants and children: recommendations of the North American Society for Pediatric Gastroenterology and Nutrition, *J Pediatr Gastroenterol Nutr* 32(suppl 2):S1–S31, 2001.
ALTE, Apparent life-threatening event.

gastric refluxate, reactive airway disease (RAD) may result from stimulation of airway reflexes by the acid refluxate.

Diagnostic Evaluation

The history and physical examination are usually sufficiently reliable to establish the diagnosis of GER. However, the upper GI series is helpful in evaluating the presence of anatomic abnormalities (e.g., pyloric stenosis, malrotation, annular pancreas, hiatal hernia, esophageal stricture). The 24-hour intraesophageal pH monitoring study is the gold standard in the diagnosis of GER (Suwandhi, Ton, and Schwarz, 2006). Endoscopy with biopsy may be helpful to assess the presence and severity of esophagitis, strictures, and Barrett esophagus and to exclude other disorders such as Crohn disease. Scintigraphy (gastroesophageal) detects radioactive substances in the esophagus after a feeding of the compound and assesses gastric emptying. It can differentiate between aspiration of gastric contents from reflux vs. aspiration from poor oropharyngeal muscle coordination. A modified barium swallow study with video fluoroscopy may also be used as a diagnostic tool for this condition.

Therapeutic Management

Therapeutic management of GER depends on its severity. No therapy is needed for the infant who is thriving and has no respiratory complications. Avoidance of certain foods that exacerbate acid reflux (e.g., caffeine, citrus, tomatoes, alcohol, peppermint, spicy or fried foods), lifestyle modifications in children (e.g., weight control if indicated; small, more frequent meals; smoking cessation), and feeding maneuvers in infants (e.g., thickened feedings, upright positioning) can improve mild GER symptoms. Thickened feedings do not improve pH scores on 24-hour intraesophageal monitoring but may decrease the number of vomiting episodes. Feedings thickened with 1 tsp to 1 Tbsp of rice cereal per ounce of formula may be recommended. This may benefit infants who are underweight as a result of GERD. Continuous NG feedings may be necessary for infants with severe reflux and growth failure until surgery can be performed. Elevating the head of the bed 30 degrees or placing the infant in an infant seat elevated 30 degrees for 1 hour after feedings may decrease GER. Prone positioning of infants also decreases episodes of GER but is recommended only with extreme caution when the risk of GERD complications exceeds the risk of sudden infant death syndrome (Cavataio and Guandalini, 2005). The AAP, Task Force on Sudden Infant Death Syndrome (2005) recommends supine positioning for sleep (see Chapter 11). If the prone position is used, parents need to be cautioned to avoid soft bedding. If cow milk protein sensitivity is suspected, a brief trial of extensively hydrolyzed formula may alleviate reflux symptoms; changes in formula however should occur under medical supervision. A weight loss program may be necessary for children with GERD symptoms that occur as a result of obesity.

Pharmacologic therapy may be used to treat infants and children with GERD. Both H_2-receptor antagonists (cimetidine [Tagamet], ranitidine [Zantac], or famotidine [Pepcid]) and proton pump inhibitors (PPIs; esomeprazole [Nexium], lansoprazole [Prevacid], omeprazole [Prilosec], pantoprazole [Protonix], and rabeprazole [Aciphex]) reduce gastric hydrochloric acid secretion and may stimulate some increase in LES tone. Use of available prokinetic drugs (e.g., bethanechol [Urecholine] and metoclopramide) remains controversial. Careful analyses of published data have failed to demonstrate clinical efficacy in modifying the natural history or therapeutic outcomes of GER in childhood (Suwandhi, Ton, and Schwarz, 2006).

Surgical management of GER is reserved for children with severe complications, such as recurrent aspiration pneumonia, apnea, severe

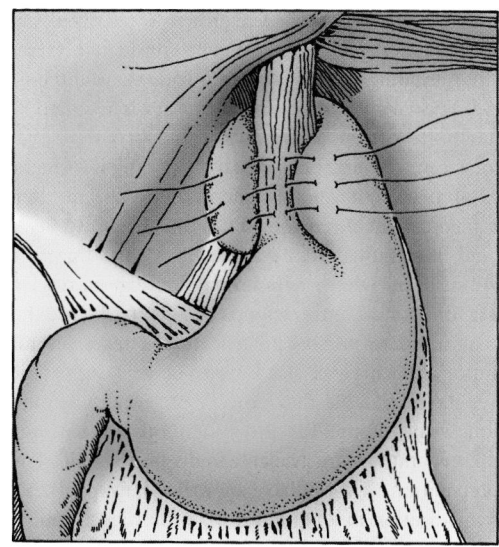

FIG 24-2 Nissen fundoplication sutures passing through esophageal musculature.

esophagitis, or growth failure, and for children who have failed to respond to medical therapy. The Nissen fundoplication (Fig. 24-2) is the most common surgical procedure, which is commonly performed laparoscopically with outcomes of decreased time to feedings, better cosmetic results, less pain, and fewer complications (Kane, 2009). This surgery involves passage of the gastric fundus behind the esophagus to encircle the distal esophagus. Long-term complications from fundoplication include breakdown of the wrap, small bowel obstruction, gas-bloat syndrome, infection, retching, and dumping syndrome.

Nursing Care Management

Nursing care is directed at (1) identifying children with symptoms suggestive of GER; (2) educating parents regarding home care, including feeding, positioning, and medications when indicated; and (3) caring for the child undergoing surgical intervention. For the majority of infants, parental reassurance of the benign nature of the condition and its relationship to physiologic maturity is the most important intervention. To help parents cope with the inconvenience of dealing with a child who spits up or regurgitates frequently, simple tips such as using bibs and protective clothes during feeding and prone positioning when holding the infant after feeding are beneficial.

It is important to educate and reassure parents about positioning. In the past, recommendations encouraged upright positioning during sleeping for both infants and older children. The supine position for sleeping continues to be recommended by the AAP, Task Force on Sudden Infant Death Syndrome (2005). Parents should not place infants on their sides as an alternative to fully supine sleeping, and avoidance of soft bedding and soft objects in the bed is important. Rescheduling of the family's routine may be required to accommodate more frequent feeding times. If parents thicken formula with cereal, they should also enlarge the nipple opening for easier sucking. Usually, breastfeeding may continue, and the mother may provide more frequent feeding times or express the milk for thickening with rice cereal. Parents should avoid feeding the child spicy foods or any foods that they find aggravate symptoms in general and avoid caffeine, chocolate, tobacco smoke, and alcohol when breastfeeding. Other practical advice includes advising the parents to avoid vigorous play after feedings and to avoid feeding just before bedtime.

When regurgitation is severe and growth is restricted, continuous NG tube or gastrostomy feedings may be considered; these feedings decrease the amount of emesis and provide constant buffering of gastric acid. Special preparation of caregivers is required when this type of nutritional therapy is indicated.

The nurse can support the family by providing information about all aspects of treatment. Parents often require specific information about the medications given for GER. PPIs are most effective when administered 30 minutes before breakfast so that the peak plasma concentrations occur with mealtime. If they are given twice a day, the second best time for administration is 30 minutes before the evening meal. Parents need to be reassured because it takes several days of administration to achieve a steady state of acid suppression. They may not see the results that they expect right away. A number of new formulations available in PPIs allow for more efficient administration. Some preparations are available in dissolvable pills. Powder and granule preparations are available as well. Many pharmacies compound the medication in a liquid form for administration.

Postoperative nursing care after the Nissen fundoplication is similar to that for other types of laparoscopic or open abdominal surgery.

RECURRENT AND FUNCTIONAL ABDOMINAL PAIN

Recurrent abdominal pain (RAP) or chronic abdominal pain is a complaint of childhood that is often attributed to psychogenic causes, although it can be a symptom of either psychosomatic or organic disease. The Rome III diagnostic criteria recognize four distinct entities of RAP in childhood: (1) functional dyspepsia, (2) irritable bowel syndrome, (3) abdominal migraine, and (4) childhood functional abdominal pain (Bufler, Gross, and Uhlig, 2011). Functional abdominal pain (FAP) is characterized by intermittent or continuous abdominal pain occurring at least once a week for at least 2 months before the diagnosis that interferes with daily activities and is accompanied by other functional symptoms that do not involve the GI system (Bufler, Gross, and Uhlig, 2011; Rasquin, Di Lorenzo, Forbes, and others, 2006). The disorder affects school-age children 4 to 18 years of age but is more common in children after the age of 8 years, and it occurs more often in girls than in boys (Scholl and Allen, 2007).

Abdominal migraine is characterized by discrete, paroxysmal episodes of severe dull, periumbilical abdominal pain with one of the accompanying manifestations: anorexia, nausea, vomiting, or pallor. The pain may last anywhere from 1 to 72 hours, and in between episodes the child is completely pain free (Hershey, 2011). In the following discussion, the term RAP is used to indicate the general concept of chronic or RAP in childhood before the diagnosis of functional abdominal pain.

Etiology and Pathophysiology

Only a minority of children and adolescents with RAP have an organic basis for their pain. Organic causes include IBD, peptic ulcer disease (PUD), lactose intolerance, pelvic inflammatory disease, urinary tract infection, and pancreatitis. Psychogenic causes of abdominal pain, such as school phobia, depression, acute reactive anxiety, and conversion reaction, account for a small number of cases. Most children with RAP have FAP.

In cases in which no organic disorder is identifiable, the abdominal pain of RAP has been attributed to dysfunction. Dysfunctional conditions causing RAP include constipation, chronic stool retention, overeating, irritable colon, and intestinal gas with heightened awareness of intestinal motility or dysmotility. Normally, intestinal contents arrive at the distal portion of the intestine with a relatively high fluid content, and fluid is extracted in the distal colon and rectum. If the normally relaxed distal intestine fails to relax and prevents the flow of its contents toward the rectum, the resulting excessive distention and spasms of the distal intestinal musculature produce pressure on nerve endings, causing pain.

The symptoms of RAP may result from multiple causes, and it is important to assess a number of factors that could place a child at risk for this condition. These include (1) somatic predisposition, dysfunction, or disorder; (2) lifestyle and habit, including routines, diet, and life tempo; (3) temperament and learned response patterns, such as the child's behavior style, personality, and learned coping skills; and (4) milieu and critical events (i.e., the child's intimate surroundings [familial, social, and cultural norms] and unexpected sources of stress or gratification).

Diagnostic Evaluation

After an organic cause has been excluded, diagnostic evaluation may proceed using the Rome III criteria established in 2006 (Rasquin, Di Lorenzo, Forbes, and others, 2006). Diagnosis is based on a complete family history, the child's health history, physical examination, and laboratory tests. The family history may provide evidence of a hereditary disorder or mimicry of adult symptoms. The child is evaluated for evidence of an organic basis for symptoms, such as pain that radiates to the back, pain that awakens the child from sleep, persistent right upper or right lower quadrant pain, unexplained or recurrent fever, weight loss, GI blood loss, significant vomiting, chronic severe diarrhea, or family history of IBD (AAP, Subcommittee on Chronic Abdominal Pain 2005). Pain is assessed for location, quality, frequency, duration, any associated symptoms, alleviating factors, and exacerbating factors.

Therapeutic Management

Treatment involves providing reassurance and reducing or eliminating symptoms. Hospitalization may be necessary, and the child frequently shows improvement in the hospital environment. Initial efforts are directed toward ruling out organic causes of the pain, relieving discomfort, and attempting to determine the situations that precipitate attacks.

Emphasize a high-fiber diet, psyllium bulk agents, lubricants such as mineral oil, and bowel training for pain associated with bowel patterns. Treatment may also include acid-reduction therapy for pain associated with dyspepsia; antispasmodic agents, smooth muscle relaxants, or low doses of psychotropic agents for pain. Dietary modifications may include removal of dairy products, fructose, and gluten for 2 to 3 weeks to rule out lactose intolerance, sensitivity to high sugar content, and celiac disease. Other treatments include cognitive-behavior therapy and biofeedback.

For functional abdominal pain, however, evidence indicates that treatments such as probiotics, medications, a high-fiber diet, and a low-lactose diet have failed to demonstrate therapeutic benefits in randomized clinical trials; cognitive-behavior therapy is reported to achieve the best results with FAP (Bufler, Gross, and Uhlig, 2011).

Nursing Care Management

The nurse can be instrumental in assessment and management of RAP in children. Many techniques used in a routine assessment elicit information that might help identify factors that contribute to the child's symptoms. Evaluate the child's social and psychologic adjustment and obtain the details of the pain directly from the child. Questions that provide clues to parent–child relationships and the way the family deals with angry feelings provide information for diagnosis and management. Relationships with peers, school problems, and other concerns of the child need to be explored. Note any evidence of depression.

After the diagnosis has been established, the parents and the child need an explanation of the pain, which can be compared to a skeletal muscle cramp, "charley horse," or headache for easier comprehension. Reassurance that the symptoms are not unique to their child and that the pain is rarely associated with a severe disease can help relieve parental fears and anxieties.

Discuss a high-fiber diet with the child and family (see Constipation) and emphasize bowel training. The child is encouraged to establish a pattern of sitting on the toilet for 10 to 15 minutes immediately after breakfast to take advantage of the increased colonic activity after meals. If necessary, have the child use stimulatory suppositories to induce early morning defecation.

After the parents have been reassured that there is no organic cause for the pain, they need guidance on what to do during a pain episode. Often they feel helpless and anxious, which tends to compound the child's distress. The simple measure of having the child rest in a peaceful, quiet environment and providing comfort will often relieve the symptoms in a short time. Application of a heating pad may also ease the discomfort (see Nonpharmacologic [Pain] Management, Chapter 7). If pain is not relieved by these simple measures, teach parents how to administer antispasmodics, if prescribed. For example, if pain is precipitated by meals, having the child take the medication 20 to 30 minutes before mealtime may prevent an episode.

The most valuable assistance that the nurse can provide is support and reassurance to the family. When open communication is established and families are able to see a relationship between stress-provoking situations and the child's symptoms, the chance for remedial action is enhanced. Follow-up care and continued support are essential because the symptoms tend to remit and exacerbate; therefore, the availability of a supportive health professional can be a source of comfort to the child and family.

INFLAMMATORY DISORDERS

ACUTE APPENDICITIS

Appendicitis, inflammation of the vermiform appendix (blind sac at the end of the cecum), is the most common cause of emergency abdominal surgery in childhood. In the United States, 60,000 to 80,000 cases are diagnosed each year. The average age of children with appendicitis is 10 years, with boys and girls equally affected before puberty. Classically, the first symptom of appendicitis is periumbilical pain followed by nausea, right lower quadrant pain, and later vomiting with fever (Kwok, Kim, and Gorelick, 2004). Perforation of the appendix can occur within approximately 48 hours of the initial complaint of pain. At the time of initial presentation, about one third of all cases involve an already perforated appendix. Complications from appendiceal perforation include major abscess, phlegmon, enterocutaneous fistula, peritonitis, and partial bowel obstruction (Kwok, Kim, and Gorelick, 2004). A phlegmon is an acute suppurative inflammation of subcutaneous connective tissue that spreads.

Etiology

The cause of appendicitis is obstruction of the lumen of the appendix, usually by hardened fecal material (fecalith). Swollen lymphoid tissue, frequently occurring after a viral infection, can also obstruct the appendix. Another rare cause of obstruction is a parasite such as *Enterobius vermicularis*, or pinworms, which can obstruct the appendiceal lumen.

Pathophysiology

With acute obstruction, the outflow of mucus secretions is blocked, and pressure builds within the lumen, resulting in compression of blood vessels. The resulting ischemia is followed by ulceration of the epithelial lining and bacterial invasion. Subsequent necrosis causes perforation or rupture with fecal and bacterial contamination of the peritoneal cavity. The resulting inflammation spreads rapidly throughout the abdomen (peritonitis), especially in young children, who are unable to localize infection. Progressive peritoneal inflammation results in functional intestinal obstruction of the small bowel (ileus) because intense GI reflexes severely inhibit bowel motility. Because the peritoneum represents a major portion of total body surface, the loss of ECF to the peritoneal cavity may lead to electrolyte imbalance and hypovolemic shock.

Diagnostic Evaluation

Diagnosis is not always straightforward. Fever, vomiting, abdominal pain, and an elevated white blood cell (WBC) count are associated with appendicitis but are also seen in IBD, pelvic inflammatory disease, gastroenteritis, urinary tract infection, right lower lobe pneumonia, mesenteric adenitis, Meckel diverticulum, and intussusception. Prolonged symptoms and delayed diagnosis often occur in younger children, in whom the risk of perforation is greatest because of their inability to verbalize their complaints.

The diagnosis is based primarily on the history and physical examination. Pain, the cardinal feature, is initially generalized (usually periumbilical); however, it usually descends to the lower right quadrant. The most intense site of pain may be at McBurney point, located at a point midway between the anterior superior iliac crest and the umbilicus. Rebound tenderness is not a reliable sign and is extremely painful to the child. Referred pain, elicited by light percussion around the perimeter of the abdomen, indicates peritoneal irritation. Movement, such as riding over bumps in an automobile or wheelchair, aggravates the pain. In addition to pain, significant clinical manifestations include fever, a change in behavior, anorexia, and vomiting (Box 24-5).

Laboratory studies usually include a CBC; urinalysis (to rule out a urinary tract infection); and, in adolescent females, serum human chorionic gonadotropin (to rule out an ectopic pregnancy). A WBC count greater than 10,000/mm³ and a C-reactive protein (CRP) are common but are not necessarily specific for appendicitis. An elevated

---

BOX 24-5   CLINICAL MANIFESTATIONS OF APPENDICITIS

- Right lower quadrant abdominal pain
- Fever
- Rigid abdomen
- Decreased or absent bowel sounds
- Vomiting (typically follows onset of pain)
- Constipation or diarrhea
- Anorexia
- Tachycardia
- Rapid, shallow breathing
- Pallor
- Lethargy
- Irritability
- Stooped posture (guarding)

Case Study—Appendicitis

Animation—Appendicitis

percentage of bands (often referred to as "a shift to the left") may indicate an inflammatory process. CRP is an acute-phase reactant that rises within 12 hours of the onset of infection.

Computed tomography (CT) has become the imaging technique of choice, although ultrasonography may also be helpful in diagnosing appendicitis. A CT scan result is considered positive in the presence of enlarged appendiceal diameter; appendiceal wall thickening; and peri-appendiceal inflammatory changes, including fat streaks, phlegmon, and fluid collection (Vissers and Lennarz, 2010).

> **! NURSING ALERT**
>
> Signs of peritonitis, in addition to fever, include sudden relief from pain after perforation; a subsequent increase in pain (usually diffuse and accompanied by rigid guarding of the abdomen); progressive abdominal distention; tachycardia; rapid, shallow breathing; pallor; chills; and irritability.

Therapeutic Management

Treatment of appendicitis before perforation includes rehydration, antibiotics, and surgical removal of the appendix (appendectomy). Laparoscopic surgery is now commonly used to treat nonperforated acute appendicitis (Aiken and Oldham, 2011); however, this approach may also be used for perforated cases by some surgeons. Recovery is rapid and, if no complications occur, the hospital stay is short. A one-time dose of antibiotics may be administered intravenously before surgery.

Ruptured Appendix

Management of the child diagnosed with peritonitis caused by a ruptured appendix often begins preoperatively with IV administration of fluid and electrolytes, systemic antibiotics, and NG suction. Postoperative management includes IV fluids, continued administration of antibiotics, and NG suction for abdominal decompression until intestinal activity returns. Sometimes surgeons close the wound after irrigation of the peritoneal cavity. At other times, the wound is left open (delayed closure) to prevent wound infection. A Penrose drain may be used to permit transperitoneal drainage.

Prognosis

Complications are uncommon after a simple appendectomy. The mortality rate for perforating appendicitis has improved from nearly certain death a century ago to 0.3% or less at present (Aiken and Oldham, 2011). Early recognition of the illness is essential to prevent complications.

Nursing Care Management

Because abdominal pain is the most common childhood complaint with appendicitis, it is important to assess the severity of pain (see Pain Assessment, Chapter 7). One of the most reliable estimates is the degree of change in behavior. Younger, nonverbal children will assume a rigid, motionless, side-lying posture with the knees flexed on the abdomen, and there is decreased range of motion of the right hip. Older children may exhibit all of these behaviors while complaining of abdominal pain. They can always indicate a point at which the pain is worse than at any other location.

> **! NURSING ALERT**
>
> Whenever appendicitis is suspected, be aware of the danger of administering laxatives or enemas or applying heat to the area. Such measures stimulate bowel motility and increase the risk of perforation.

Postoperative Care

Postoperative care for the nonperforated appendix is the same as for most abdominal procedures. Care of the child with a ruptured appendix and peritonitis involves more complex care, and the course of recovery is considerably longer. The child is maintained on IV fluids, NPO, and the NG tube is kept on low continuous gastric decompression until there is evidence of intestinal activity. Listening for bowel sounds and observing for other signs of bowel activity (e.g., passage of flatus or stool) are part of the routine assessment. Management of IV therapy is the same as for any child receiving fluids and parenteral antibiotics. A drain is often placed in the wound during surgery, and frequent dressing changes with meticulous skin care are essential to prevent excoriation of the area surrounding the surgical site. Wound care includes irrigation with antibacterial solution or saline. Montgomery straps or a wound binder may be used when the wound is left open postoperatively to facilitate dressing changes and prevent frequent placement and removal of tape on sensitive skin.

Management of pain from the incision and repeated dressing changes and irrigations are an essential part of the child's care. Psychologic care of the child and parents is similar to that used in other emergency situations (see Emergency Admission, Chapter 21). Parents and older children need to express their feelings and concerns regarding the events surrounding the illness and hospitalization. The nurse can provide education and psychosocial support to promote adequate coping and alleviate anxiety for both the child and the family (see Nursing Care Plan).

MECKEL DIVERTICULUM

Meckel diverticulum is a remnant of the fetal omphalomesenteric duct, which connects the yolk sac with the primitive midgut during fetal life (Olson, Kim, and Donnelly, 2009). Normally, the structure is obliterated by the seventh to eighth week of gestation, when the placenta replaces the yolk sac as the source of nutrition for the fetus. Failure of obliteration may result in an omphalomesenteric fistula (a fibrous band connecting the small intestine to the umbilicus), known as Meckel diverticulum.

Meckel diverticulum is a true diverticulum because it arises from the antimesenteric border of the small intestine and includes all layers of the intestinal wall. The position of the diverticulum varies, but it is usually found within 40 to 50 cm (16–20 inches) of the ileocecal valve.

Meckel diverticulum is the most common congenital malformation of the GI tract and is present in 2% to 4% of the population, with more frequent occurrence in boys than girls (Menezes, Tareen, Saeed, and others, 2008). Often it exists without ever causing symptoms.

Pathophysiology

Bleeding, obstruction, or inflammation causes the symptomatic complications of Meckel diverticulum. Gastric mucosa is the most common ectopic tissue found in a Meckel diverticulum. Bleeding, which is the most common problem in children, is caused by peptic ulceration or perforation because of the unbuffered acidic secretion. Several mechanisms may cause obstruction (Olson, Kim, and Donnelly, 2009). Intussusception may be led by Meckel diverticulum. Obstruction may also be caused by entanglement of the small intestine around a fibrous cord, by trapping of a loop of intestine under the band, by incarceration within a hernia sac, or by volvulus of the intestinal segment containing the diverticulum. Diverticulitis occurs when peptic ulceration or obstruction leads to inflammation.

◉ NURSING CARE PLAN

The Child with Appendicitis

NURSING DIAGNOSIS	PATIENT OUTCOMES	NURSING INTERVENTIONS	RATIONALE
Acute Pain related to inflamed appendix **Child's Defining Characteristics (Subjective and Objective Data)** Crying Guarding abdomen Limited movement Withdrawal Refusal to eat or drink Fever Increased pulse	The child will have no pain or pain will be reduced to a level acceptable to child. **The Following NOC Concepts Apply to This Outcome** Comfort Level Pain Control Pain: Disruptive Effects	Allow child to choose position most comfortable (usually legs flexed). Provide small pillow or stuffed animal for abdomen. Administer analgesia on ATC basis in the first 24 hours postoperatively. Teach child (as age appropriate) use of PCA pump. **The Following NIC Concepts Apply to These Interventions** Analgesic Administration Positioning Presence Coping Enhancement Pain Management	To promote the most comfortable position To splint the abdomen To provide pain relief To minimize breakthrough pain
Risk for Infection related to possibility of rupture before surgery and open wound after surgery (if open procedure is performed) **Child's Defining Characteristics (Subjective and Objective Data)** Abdominal pain Fever Rebound tenderness Nausea and vomiting Anorexia Increased WBC count Fluid around the appendix visualized on ultrasound imaging	Child will be free of signs and symptoms of peritonitis. Signs of peritonitis will be recognized early. **The Following NOC Concepts Apply to These Outcomes** Infection Status Wound Healing	Monitor wound status and integrity and type of dressing (e.g., dressing dry, intact; saline or antiseptic solution irrigation or soaks [wet-to-dry] required for open wound]). Specify interval for dressing change. Monitor vital signs, including temperature, pulse oximeter, and blood pressure at least every 4 hours in stable child and more often in child with rupture. Monitor bowel function, including bowel sounds and passage of flatus. Monitor wound drain(s) in relation to proper function, amount, and character of drainage (specify time interval). Encourage early ambulation postoperatively with assistance after administration of analgesia. Set in bedside chair at least twice a day. For child on lengthy bedrest, place antiembolism devices. For child with NG tube, monitor status of NG and suction apparatus to ensure proper function and skin care where anchored. Administer antibiotics as prescribed. Ensure adequacy and function of IV fluid infusion. Provide dietary instructions for foods that provide sufficient calories and protein for growth (once able to eat). **The Following NIC Concepts Apply to These Interventions** Medication Management Laboratory Data Interpretation Vital Signs Monitoring Wound Care Infection Protection	To detect infection and plan interventions To prevent infection at surgical site To promote tissue healing To detect fever or hemodynamic instability and plan necessary intervention To evaluate bowel status and function postoperatively To evaluate wound status and healing To decrease accumulation of flatus and abdominal distention and promote early return of proper bowel function To improve circulation, decrease flatus, and promote bowel function To prevent DVT To prevent nausea and vomiting; to promote drainage of GI secretions and acid To prevent wound infection To promote appropriate fluid intake To support an appropriate diet that can increase wound healing

ATC, Around-the-clock; *DVT,* deep vein thrombosis; *PCA,* patient-controlled analgesia.

Continued

⊙ NURSING CARE PLAN

The Child with Appendicitis—cont'd

NURSING DIAGNOSIS	PATIENT OUTCOMES	NURSING INTERVENTIONS	RATIONALE
Risk for Deficient Fluid Volume related to decreased intake fluid and losses secondary to loss of appetite, vomiting	Child will receive sufficient fluids to replace losses. Child will exhibit signs of adequate hydration (specify).	Maintain NPO status as prescribed. For child with uncomplicated appendectomy (nonperforation), encourage intake of small amounts of ice chips and then progress to clear fluids as prescribed.	To minimize losses through vomiting and minimize abdominal distention To promote fluid intake and bowel function
Child's Defining Characteristics (Subjective and Objective Data) Dry mucous membranes Loss of skin turgor Sunken eyes, sunken fontanel Rapid thready pulse, rapid breathing Lethargy	**The Following NOC Concepts Apply to These Outcomes** Electrolyte and Acid–Base Balance Fluid Balance	Maintain integrity of infusion site for IV fluids. Administer IV fluids and electrolytes as prescribed. Monitor fluid intake and output. **The Following NIC Concepts Apply to These Interventions** Acid–Base Monitoring Electrolyte Monitoring Fluid Monitoring Fluid Management IV Therapy Laboratory Data Interpretation Vital Signs Monitoring	To infuse fluids and electrolytes To replace fluid losses To assess hydration status and renal function
Surgical Recovery, Delayed because of absence of bowel motility	Child will not experience abdominal distention or vomiting caused by delayed bowel mobility.	Maintain NPO status in early postoperative period. Maintain NG tube decompression as necessary (if used). Assess abdomen for distention, tenderness, flatus, and presence of bowel sounds. Monitor passage of flatus and stool.	To prevent abdominal distention and vomiting To remove gastric acid and secretions To assess presence of peristalsis (bowel function) To assess for resumption of bowel motility
Child's Defining Characteristics (Subjective and Objective Data) Abdominal distention Nausea and vomiting Absence of bowel sounds Abdominal tenderness No passage of stools	**The Following NOC Concept Applies to This Outcome** Immobility Consequences: Physiological	Ambulate in room and sit in chair a minimum of three times daily. **The Following NIC Concepts Apply to These Interventions** Bowel Management Flatulence Reduction Positioning	To increase movement, systemic circulation, and peristalsis

GI, Gastrointestinal; *IV,* intravenous; *NG,* nasogastric; *NIC,* Nursing Interventions Classification; *NOC,* Nursing Outcomes Classification; *NPO,* nothing by mouth; *WBC,* white blood cell.

Diagnostic Evaluation

Diagnosis is usually based on the history, physical examination, and radiographic studies. Meckel diverticulum is often a diagnostic challenge. Radionucleotide scintigraphy (Meckel scan) is most often used but is less reliable in the presence of bleeding (Menezes, Tareen, Saeed, and others, 2008). CT scan, wireless capsule endoscopy, and mesenteric angiography may be used to investigate complications of Meckel diverticulum (Thurley, Halliday, Somers, and others, 2009). Laboratory studies are usually part of the general workup to rule out any bleeding disorder and to evaluate the severity of the anemia.

The most common clinical presentation in children includes painless rectal bleeding, abdominal pain, or signs of intestinal obstruction (Box 24-6). Bleeding, which may be mild or profuse, often appears as dark red or "currant jelly" stools; bleeding may be significant enough to cause hypotension.

BOX 24-6 CLINICAL MANIFESTATIONS OF MECKEL DIVERTICULUM

Abdominal Pain
Similar to appendicitis
May be vague and recurrent

Bloody Stools*
Painless
Bright or dark red with mucus ("currant jelly" stool)
In infants, rectal bleeding sometimes accompanied by pain

Sometimes
Severe anemia
Shock

*Often a presenting sign.

Therapeutic Management

The standard treatment is surgical removal of the diverticulum. When severe hemorrhage increases the surgical risk, interventions to correct hypovolemic shock, such as blood replacement, IV fluids, and oxygen, may be necessary. Antibiotics may be used preoperatively to control infection. If intestinal obstruction has occurred, appropriate preoperative measures are used to reverse electrolyte imbalances and prevent abdominal distention.

Prognosis

If this condition is diagnosed and treated early, full recovery is likely. The mortality rate of untreated Meckel diverticulum ranges from 2.5% to 15%. Complications of untreated Meckel diverticulum include GI hemorrhage and bowel obstruction.

Nursing Care Management

Nursing objectives are the same as for any child undergoing surgery (see Chapter 22). When intestinal bleeding is present, specific preoperative considerations include (1) frequent monitoring of vital signs including blood pressure, (2) keeping the child on bed rest, and (3) recording the approximate amount of blood lost in stools.

Postoperatively, the child requires IV fluids and an NG tube for decompression and evacuation of gastric secretions. Because the onset of illness is usually rapid, psychologic support is important, as in other acute conditions, such as appendicitis. It is important to remember that massive rectal bleeding is usually traumatic to both the child and the parents and may significantly affect their emotional reaction to hospitalization and surgery.

INFLAMMATORY BOWEL DISEASE

Inflammatory bowel disease (IBD) is a term used to refer to two major forms of chronic intestinal inflammation: Crohn disease (CD) and ulcerative colitis (UC). CD and UC have similar epidemiologic, immunologic, and clinical features, but they are distinct disorders (Table 24-8).

In addition to GI symptoms, both CD and UC are characterized by extraintestinal and systemic inflammatory responses. Exacerbations and remissions without complete resolution are also characteristics of IBD. Growth failure, which is particularly common in CD, is an important problem unique to the pediatric population. CD is also more disabling, has more serious complications, and is often less amenable to medical and surgical treatment than is UC. Because UC is confined to the colon, theoretically it may be cured by a colectomy.

TABLE 24-8	CLINICAL MANIFESTATIONS OF INFLAMMATORY BOWEL DISEASES	
CHARACTERISTICS	**ULCERATIVE COLITIS**	**CROHN DISEASE**
Rectal bleeding	Common	Uncommon
Diarrhea	Often severe	Moderate to severe
Pain	Less frequent	Common
Anorexia	Mild or moderate	May be severe
Weight loss	Moderate	May be severe
Growth restriction	Usually mild	May be severe
Anal and perianal lesions	Rare	Common
Fistulas and strictures	Rare	Common
Rashes	Mild	Mild
Joint pain	Mild to moderate	Mild to moderate

The prevalence of IBD is between 12 and 40 per 100,000 persons, with 25% of these individuals being diagnosed before 20 years of age (Wong, Clark, Garnett, and others, 2009). Over the past 30 years, the incidence of CD has risen, but the incidence of UC in children has remained stable. Children 6 to 17 years of age with CD appear to have a more complicated disease course compared with that of 0- to 5-year-old children (Gupta, Bostrom, Kirschner, and others, 2008).

Etiology

Despite decades of research, the etiology of IBD is not completely understood, and there is no known cure. There is evidence to indicate a multifactorial etiology. Research is focused on theories of defective immunoregulation of the inflammatory response to bacteria or viruses in the GI tract in individuals with a genetic predisposition (Silbermintz and Markowitz, 2006). Whereas in CD the chronic immune process is characterized by a T-helper 1 cytokine profile, in UC the response is more humoral and mediated by T-helper 2 cells (Silbermintz and Markowitz, 2006).

Development of IBD has a genetic influence. Several IBD susceptibility genes have now been identified through family and twin studies. Family-based genetic studies have linked chromosome 6 in UC and the *NOD2* gene in CD (Sauer and Kugathasan, 2010).

Pathophysiology of Ulcerative Colitis

The inflammation found with UC is limited to the colon and rectum, with the distal colon and rectum the most severely affected. Inflammation affects the mucosa and submucosa and involves continuous segments along the length of the bowel with varying degrees of ulceration, bleeding, and edema. Thickening of the bowel wall and fibrosis are unusual, but longstanding disease can result in shortening of the colon and strictures. Extraintestinal manifestations are less common in UC than in CD. Toxic megacolon is the most dangerous form of severe colitis.

Pathophysiology of Crohn Disease

The chronic inflammatory process of CD involves any part of the GI tract from the mouth to the anus but most often affects the terminal ileum. The disease involves all layers of the bowel wall (transmural) in a discontinuous fashion, meaning that between areas of intact mucosa, there are areas of affected mucosa (skip lesions). The inflammation may result in ulcerations; fibrosis; adhesions; stiffening of the bowel wall; stricture formation; and fistulas to other loops of bowel, bladder, vagina, or skin.

Diagnostic Evaluation

The diagnosis of UC and CD comes from the history, physical examination, laboratory evaluation, and other diagnostic procedures. Laboratory tests include a CBC to evaluate anemia and an erythrocyte sedimentation rate (ESR) or CRP to assess the systemic reaction to the inflammatory process. Levels of total protein, albumin, iron, zinc, magnesium, vitamin B_{12}, and fat-soluble vitamins may be low in children with CD. Stools are examined for blood, leukocytes, and infectious organisms. A serologic panel is often used in combination with clinical findings to diagnose IBD and to differentiate between CD and UC. Observational studies on the utility of blood tests to detect perinuclear antineutrophilic cytoplasmic antibodies (pANCA) and anti–*Saccharomyces cerevisiae* antibodies (ASCA) showed that the combination is specific but not sensitive for diagnosing UC (Reese, Constantinides, Simillis, and others, 2006).

In patients with CD, an upper GI series with small bowel follow-through assists in assessing the existence, location, and extent of disease. Upper endoscopy and colonoscopy with biopsies are an integral part of diagnosing IBD (Langan, Gotsch, Krafczyk, and others, 2007). Endoscopy allows direct visualization of the surface of the GI tract so that the extent of inflammation and narrowing can be evaluated. CT and ultrasonography also may be used to identify bowel wall inflammation, intraabdominal abscesses, and fistulas. CD lesions may pierce the walls of the small intestine and colon, creating tracts called fistulas between the intestine and adjacent structures such as the bladder, anus, vagina, or skin.

Therapeutic Management

The natural history of the disease continues to be unpredictable and characterized by recurrent flare-ups that can severely impair patients' physical and social functioning (Vernier-Massouille, Balde, Salleron, and others, 2008). The goals of therapy are to (1) control the inflammatory process to reduce or eliminate the symptoms, (2) obtain long-term remission, (3) promote normal growth and development, and (4) allow as normal a lifestyle as possible. Treatment is individualized and managed according to the type and the severity of the disease, its location, and the response to therapy.

Medical Treatment

The goal of any treatment regimen is first to induce remission of acute symptoms and then to maintain remission over time. 5-Aminosalicylates (5-ASAs) are effective in the induction and maintenance of remission in mild to moderate UC. Mesalamine, olsalazine, and balsalazide are now preferred over sulfasalazine because of reduced side effects (headache, nausea, vomiting, neutropenia, and oligospermia). Suppository and enema preparations of mesalamine are used to treat left-sided colitis. These drugs decrease inflammation by inhibiting prostaglandin synthesis. 5-ASAs can be used to induce remission in mild CD. Corticosteroids, such as prednisone and prednisolone, are indicated in induction therapy in children with moderate to severe UC and CD. These drugs inhibit the production of adhesion molecules, cytokines, and leukotrienes. Although these drugs reduce the acute symptoms of IBD, they have side effects related to long-term use, including growth suppression (adrenal suppression), weight gain, and decreased bone density. High doses of IV corticosteroids may be administered in acute episodes and tapered according to clinical response. Budesonide, a synthetic corticosteroid, is designed for controlled release in the ileum and is indicated for ileal and right-sided colitis; budesonide has fewer side effects than prednisone and prednisolone (Silbermintz and Markowitz, 2006). Rectal steroid therapy (enemas and foam-based preparations) are available for both induction and maintenance therapy in left-sided colitis.

Immunomodulators, such as azathioprine and its metabolite 6-mercaptopurine (6-MP), are used to induce and maintain remission in children with IBD who are steroid resistant or steroid dependent and in treating chronic draining fistulas. They block the synthesis of purine, thus inhibiting the ability of DNA and RNA to hinder lymphocyte function, especially that of T cells. Side effects include infection, pancreatitis, hepatitis, bone marrow toxicity, arthralgia, and malignancy. Methotrexate is also useful in inducing and maintaining remission in CD patients unresponsive to standard therapies. Cyclosporine and tacrolimus have both been effective in inducing remission in severe steroid-dependent UC. 6-MP or azathioprine is then used to maintain remission. Patients taking immunomodulating medications require regular monitoring of their CBC and differential to assess for changes that reflect suppression of the immune system because many of the side effects can be prevented or managed by dose reduction or discontinuation of medication.

Antibiotics, such as metronidazole and ciprofloxacin, may be used as an adjunctive therapy to treat complications such as perianal disease or small bowel bacterial overgrowth in CD. Side effects of these drugs are peripheral neuropathy, nausea, and a metallic taste.

Biologic therapies act to regulate inflammatory and antiinflammatory cytokines. With the emergence of the biologic agents, specifically the use of antitumor necrosis factor–α (TNF-α) agents such as adalimumab, progress has been made in targeting specific pathogenetic mechanisms and achieving a more prolonged clinical response (Hyams and Markowitz, 2005; Ricart, García-Bosch, Ordás, and others, 2008). TNF-α is believed to influence active inflammation.

Nutritional Support

Nutritional support is important in the treatment of patients with IBD. Growth failure is a common serious complication, especially in CD. Growth failure is characterized by weight loss, alteration in body composition, restricted height, and delayed sexual maturation. Malnutrition causes the growth failure, and its etiology is multifactorial. Malnutrition occurs as a result of inadequate dietary intake, excessive GI losses, malabsorption, drug–nutrient interaction, and increased nutritional requirements. Inadequate dietary intake occurs with anorexia and episodes of increased disease activity. Excessive loss of nutrients (protein, blood, electrolytes, and minerals) occurs secondary to intestinal inflammation and diarrhea. Carbohydrate, lactose, fat, vitamin, and mineral malabsorption, as well as vitamin B_{12} and folic acid deficiencies, occur with disease episodes and with drug administration and when the terminal ileum is resected. Finally, nutritional requirements are increased with inflammation, fever, fistulas, and periods of rapid growth (e.g., adolescence).

The goals of nutritional support include (1) correction of nutrient deficits and replacement of ongoing losses, (2) provision of adequate energy and protein for healing, and (3) provision of adequate nutrients to promote normal growth. Nutritional support includes both enteral and parenteral nutrition (PN). A well-balanced, high-protein, high-calorie diet is recommended for children whose symptoms do not prohibit an adequate oral intake. There is little evidence that avoiding specific foods influences the severity of the disease. Supplementation with multivitamins, iron, and folic acid is recommended.

Special enteral formulas, given either by mouth or continuous NG infusion (often at night), may be required. Elemental formulas are completely absorbed in the small intestine with almost no residue. A diet consisting only of elemental formula not only improves nutritional status but also induces disease remission, either without steroids or with a diminished dosage of steroids required. An elemental diet is a safe and potentially effective primary therapy for patients with CD. Unfortunately, remission is not sustained when NG feedings are discontinued unless maintenance medications are added to the treatment regimen.

Total parenteral nutrition has also improved nutritional status in patients with IBD. Short-term remissions have been achieved after TPN, although complete bowel rest has not reduced inflammation or added to the benefits of improved nutrition by TPN. Nutritional support is less likely to induce a remission in UC than in CD. Improvement of nutritional status is important, however, in preventing deterioration of the patient's health status and in preparing the patient for surgery.

Surgical Treatment

Surgery is indicated for UC when medical and nutritional therapies fail to prevent complications. Surgical options include a subtotal colectomy and ileostomy that leaves a rectal stump as a blind pouch. A reservoir pouch is created in the configuration of a J or S to help improve continence postoperatively. An ileoanal pull-through preserves the normal pathway for defecation. Pouchitis, an inflammation of the surgically created pouch, is the most common late complication of this procedure and had been reported to occur in up to 50% of cases. In many cases, UC can be cured with a total colectomy.

Surgery may be required in children with CD when complications cannot be controlled by medical and nutritional therapy. Segmental intestinal resections are performed for small bowel obstructions, strictures, or fistulas. Partial colonic resection is not curative, and the disease often recurs.

Prognosis

Inflammatory bowel disease is a chronic disease. Relatively long periods of quiescent disease may follow exacerbations. The outcome is influenced by the regions and severity of involvement, as well as by appropriate therapeutic management. Malnutrition, growth failure, and bleeding are serious complications. The overall prognosis for UC is good.

The development of colorectal cancer (CRC) is a long-term complication of IBD. In UC, the cumulative incidence of CRC is 2.5% after 20 years, increasing to 10.8% after 30 years (Rutter, Saunders, Wilkinson, and others, 2006). Surveillance colonoscopy with multiple biopsies should begin approximately 10 years after diagnosis of UC or Crohn colitis and continue every 1 to 2 years (Rubin and Kavitt, 2006). Removal of the diseased colon prevents development of CRC. In CD, however, surgical removal of the affected colon does not prevent cancer from developing elsewhere in the GI tract.

Nursing Care Management

The nursing considerations in the management of patients with IBD extend beyond the immediate period of hospitalization. These interventions involve continued guidance of families in terms of (1) managing diet; (2) coping with factors that increase stress and emotional lability; (3) adjusting to a disease of remissions and exacerbations; and (4) when indicated, preparing the child and parents for the possibility of diversionary bowel surgery.

Because nutritional support is an essential part of therapy, encouraging the anorexic child to consume sufficient quantities of food is often a challenge. Successful interventions include involving the child in meal planning; encouraging small, frequent meals or snacks rather than three large meals a day; serving meals around medication schedules when diarrhea, mouth pain, and intestinal spasm are controlled; and preparing high-protein, high-calorie foods such as eggnog, milkshakes, cream soups, puddings, or custard (if lactose is tolerated). (See Feeding the Sick Child, Chapter 22.) Using bran or a high-fiber diet for active IBD is questionable. Bran, even in small amounts, has been shown to worsen the condition. Occasionally, the occurrence of aphthous stomatitis further complicates adherence to dietary management. Mouth care before eating and the selection of bland foods help relieve the discomfort of mouth sores.

When NG feedings or TPN is indicated, nurses play an important role in explaining the purpose and the expected outcomes of this therapy. The nurse should acknowledge the anxieties of the child and family members and give them adequate time to demonstrate the skills necessary to continue the therapy at home if needed (see Critical Thinking Case Study).

The importance of continued drug therapy despite remission of symptoms must be stressed to the child and family members. Failure to adhere to the pharmacologic regimen can result in exacerbation of the disease (see Compliance, Chapter 22). Unfortunately, exacerbation

of IBD can occur even if the child and family are compliant with the treatment regimen; this is difficult for the child and family to cope with.

Family Support

The nurse should attend to the emotional components of the disease and assess any sources of stress. Frequently, the nurse can help children adjust to problems of growth restriction, delayed sexual maturation, dietary restrictions, feelings of being "different" or "sickly," inability to compete with peers, and necessary absence from school during exacerbations of the illness (see Impact of the Child's Chronic Illness, Chapter 18).

If a permanent colectomy-ileostomy is required, the nurse can teach the child and family how to care for the ileostomy. The nurse can also emphasize the positive aspects of the surgery, particularly accelerated growth and sexual development, permanent recovery, and the eliminated risk of colonic cancer in UC, as well as the normality of life despite bowel diversion. Introducing the child and parents to other ostomy patients, especially those who are the same age, can be effective in fostering eventual acceptance. Whenever possible, continent ostomies should be offered as options to the child, although they are not performed in all centers in the United States.

Because of the chronic and often lifelong nature of the disease, families benefit from the educational services provided by organizations such as the Crohn's and Colitis Foundation of America (CCFA).* If diversionary bowel surgery is indicated, the United Ostomy

---

? CRITICAL THINKING CASE STUDY
Inflammatory Bowel Disease

Susan, a 13-year-old girl, was admitted to the hospital because of bloody diarrhea, abdominal pain, and weight loss. After a thorough evaluation, including laboratory tests, radiographic studies, and gastrointestinal endoscopy procedures, the diagnosis of CD was made. Medical treatment, including corticosteroid drugs and nutritional support, was implemented during this hospitalization.

Susan has improved considerably and is to be discharged home this week. Enteral formula administered by continuous nighttime NG tube infusion will be continued at home, and both Susan and her family are eager to learn how to perform these feedings. You are the nurse responsible for Susan's discharge planning. Which interventions relating to these feedings should you include in Susan's preparations for discharge?

Questions
1. Evidence—Are there sufficient data to formulate any specific interventions for discharge?
2. Assumptions—Describe some underlying assumptions about:
   a. The goals of nutritional support for children with CD
   b. Teaching required by an adolescent or family member who is administering NG tube feedings at home
   c. Psychosocial issues related to CD
3. What are the priorities for discharge planning at this time?
4. Does the evidence support your conclusion?

CD, Crohn disease; *NG,* nasogastric.

Associations of America (UOAA)* and the Wound, Ostomy and Continence Nurses Society† are available to assist with ileostomy care and provide important psychologic support through their self-help groups. Adolescents often benefit by participating in peer-support groups, which are sponsored by the CCFA.

PEPTIC ULCER DISEASE

Peptic ulcers may be classified as acute or chronic, and PUD is a chronic condition that affects the stomach or duodenum. Ulcers are described as gastric or duodenal and as primary or secondary. A gastric ulcer involves the mucosa of the stomach; a duodenal ulcer involves the pylorus or duodenum. Most primary ulcers occur in the absence of a predisposing factor and tend to be chronic, occurring more frequently in the duodenum. Secondary or stress ulcers result from the stress of a severe underlying disease or injury (e.g., severe burns, sepsis, increased intracranial pressure, severe trauma, multisystem organ failure) and are more frequently acute and gastric.

About 1.7% of children in general pediatric practices have PUD, and the disease represents about 3.4% per 10,000 of pediatric hospital admissions. Primary ulcers are more common in children older than 6 years, and stress ulcers are more common in infants younger than 6 months. Except for very young children, the incidence is two to three times greater in boys than in girls.

Etiology

The exact cause of PUD is unknown, although infectious, genetic, and environmental factors are important. There is an increased familial incidence, and the disease is increased in persons with blood group O.

There is a significant relationship between the bacterium *Helicobacter pylori* and ulcers. *H. pylori* is a microaerophilic, gram-negative, slow-growing, spiral-shaped, and flagellated bacterium known to colonize the gastric mucosa in about half of the population of the world (Sung, Kuipers, and El-Serag, 2009). *H. pylori* synthesizes the enzyme urease, which hydrolyses urea to form ammonia and carbon dioxide. Ammonia then absorbs acid to form ammonium, thus raising the gastric pH. *H. pylori* may cause ulcers by weakening the gastric mucosal barrier and allowing acid to damage the mucosa. It is believed that it is acquired via the fecal–oral route, and this hypothesis is supported by finding viable *H. pylori* in feces.

In addition to ulcerogenic drugs, both alcohol and smoking contribute to ulcer formation. There is no conclusive evidence to implicate particular foods, such as caffeine-containing beverages or spicy foods, but polyunsaturated fats and fiber may play a role in ulcer formation. Psychologic factors may play a role in the development of PUD, and stressful life events, dependency, passiveness, and hostility have all been implicated as contributing factors.

Pathophysiology

Most likely, the pathology is caused by an imbalance between the destructive (cytotoxic) factors and defensive (cytoprotective) factors in the GI tract. The toxic mechanisms include acid, pepsin, medications such as aspirin and nonsteroidal anti-inflammatory drugs (NSAIDs),

bile acids, and infection with *H. pylori*. The defensive factors include the mucus layer, local bicarbonate secretion, epithelial cell renewal, and mucosal blood flow. Prostaglandins play a role in mucosal defense because they stimulate both mucus and alkali secretion. The primary mechanism that prevents the development of peptic ulcer is the secretion of mucus by the epithelial and mucous glands throughout the stomach. The thick mucus layer acts to diffuse acid from the lumen to the gastric mucosal surface, thus protecting the gastric epithelium. The stomach and the duodenum produce bicarbonate, decreasing acidity on the epithelial cells and thereby minimizing the effects of the low pH. When abnormalities in the protective barrier exist, the mucosa is vulnerable to damage by acid and pepsin. Exogenous factors, such as aspirin and NSAIDs, cause gastric ulcers by inhibition of prostaglandin synthesis.

Zollinger-Ellison syndrome may occur in children who have multiple, large, or recurrent ulcers. This syndrome is characterized by hypersecretion of gastric acid, intractable ulcer disease, and intestinal malabsorption caused by a gastrin-secreting tumor of the pancreas.

Diagnostic Evaluation

Diagnosis is based on the history of symptoms, physical examination, and diagnostic testing. The focus is on symptoms such as epigastric abdominal pain, nocturnal pain, oral regurgitation, heartburn, weight loss, hematemesis, and melena (Box 24-7). History should include questions relating to the use of potentially causative substances such as NSAIDS, corticosteroids, alcohol, and tobacco. Laboratory studies may include a CBC to detect anemia, stool analysis for occult blood,

---

BOX 24-7   CHARACTERISTICS OF PEPTIC ULCERS

Neonates
Usually gastric and secondary ulcers
Commonly a history of preterm or postterm birth, severe respiratory distress, sepsis, hypoglycemia, or an intraventricular hemorrhage
Perforation may lead to massive bleeding

Infants to 3-Year-Old Children
Most likely to have a secondary ulcer located equally in the stomach or duodenum
Primary ulcers less common and usually located in stomach
Likely to be noticed in relation to illness, surgery, or trauma
Hematemesis, melena, or perforation

2- to 6-Year-Old Children
Primary or secondary ulcers
Located equally in stomach and duodenum
Perforation more likely in secondary ulcers
Periumbilical pain, poor eating, vomiting, irritability, nighttime wakening, hematemesis, melena

Children 6 Years and Older
Usually primary and most often duodenal ulcers
More typical of adult type
Chance of recurrence greater
Often associated with *Helicobacter pylori*
Epigastric pain or vague abdominal pain
Nighttime wakening, hematemesis, melena, and anemia possible

---

*UOAA, PO Box 512, Northfield, MN 55057-0512; 800-826-0826; http://www.ostomy.org. In Canada: United Ostomy Association of Canada, 344 Bloor Street West, Suite 501, Toronto, ON M5S 3A7; 416-595-5452; fax: 888-969-9698, 416-595-9924; http://www.ostomycanada.ca.
†15000 Commerce Pkwy., Suite C, Mt. Laurel, NJ; 888-224-9626; http://www.wocn.org.

liver function tests (LFTs), ESR, or CRP to evaluate IBD; amylase and lipase to evaluate pancreatitis; and gastric acid measurements to identify hypersecretion. A lactose breath test may be performed to detect lactose intolerance.

Radiographic studies such as an upper GI series may be performed to evaluate obstruction or malrotation. An upper endoscopy is the most reliable procedure to diagnose PUD. A biopsy can determine the presence of *H. pylori*. A blood test can also identify the presence of the antigen to this organism. The ^{13}C-urea breath test measures bacterial colonization in the gastric mucosa. This test is used to screen for *H. pylori* in adults and children. Polyclonal and monoclonal stool antigen tests are an accurate, noninvasive method both for the initial diagnosis of *H. pylori* and for the confirmation of its eradication after treatment (Gisbert, de la Morena, and Abraira, 2006).

Diagnosis is based on the history (pattern of pain) and physical examination. Frequently, a history of epigastric and periumbilical pain accompanies PUD. However, children often find it difficult to describe the location of their pain and frequently indicate the location by moving their hand in a circular movement all around the stomach area. Asking the child to take one finger and point to the area where it hurts the most often helps to identify the location of the pain. Pain may also be elicited during the examination with palpation. Routine laboratory studies to diagnose PUD include a CBC with differential, ESR, blood chemistry studies, urinalysis, and stool analysis to identify anemia or inflammation and to rule out infection. A ^{13}C-urea breath test is often performed to determine the presence of antibodies to *H. pylori*. An upper GI series is rarely helpful in identifying ulcers in children; fiberoptic endoscopy is the most reliable way to detect PUD in children. Direct visualization of the gastric and duodenal mucosa with biopsy to determine the presence of *H. pylori* is the most commonly used and effective way to arrive at the diagnosis.

Therapeutic Management

The major goals of therapy for children with PUD are to relieve discomfort, promote healing, prevent complications, and prevent recurrence. Management is primarily medical and consists of administration of medications to treat the infection and to reduce or neutralize gastric acid secretion.

Antacids are beneficial medications to neutralize gastric acid.

Histamine (H$_2$) receptor antagonists (antisecretory drugs) act to suppress gastric acid production. Cimetidine (Tagamet), ranitidine (Zantac), and famotidine (Pepcid) are examples of these medications. These medications have few side effects, although cimetidine has multiple drug interactions and should therefore be used with caution.

Proton pump inhibitors, such as omeprazole and lansoprazole, act to inhibit the hydrogen ion pump in the parietal cells, thus blocking the production of acid. These agents have been shown to be effective in children and adolescents but not in infants (van der Pol, Smits, van Wijk, and others, 2011). Long-term side effects are not fully known but may include decreased bone density with long-term use because of reduced gastric absorption of calcium and hypergastrinemia of unknown significance (Hassall, Owen, Kerr, and others, 2011). With short-term use, these agents appear to be well tolerated and have infrequent side effects (e.g., headache, diarrhea, nausea, and vomiting).

Mucosal protective agents, such as sucralfate and bismuth-containing preparations, may be prescribed for PUD. Sucralfate is an aluminum-containing agent that forms a protective barrier over ulcerated mucosa to protect against acid and pepsin. Sucralfate is available in both pill and liquid forms. Because sucralfate blocks the absorption of other medications, it should be given separately from other medications.

Bismuth compounds are sometimes prescribed for the relief of ulcers, but they are used less frequently than PPIs. Although these compounds inhibit the growth of microorganisms, the mechanism of their activity is poorly understood. In combination with antibiotics, bismuth is effective against *H. pylori*. Although concern has been expressed about the use of bismuth salts in children because of potential side effects, none of these side effects has been reported when these compounds have been used in the treatment of *H. pylori* infection.

Triple-drug therapy is the standard first-line treatment regimen for *H. pylori* (O'Connor, Gisbert, and O'Morain, 2009). Combination therapy has demonstrated 90% effectiveness in eradication of *H. pylori* compared with antibiotic monotherapy. Examples of drug combinations used in triple therapy are (1) bismuth, clarithromycin, and metronidazole; (2) lansoprazole, amoxicillin, and clarithromycin; and (3) metronidazole, clarithromycin, and omeprazole. The benefits of the use of probiotics as an adjunct to treatment remain unclear, with conflicting literature on their effect on eradication and minimizing side effects (O'Connor, Gisbert, and O'Morain, 2009).

Common side effects of medications include diarrhea, nausea, and vomiting. In addition to medications, children with PUD should have a nutritious diet and avoid caffeine. Warn adolescents about gastric irritation associated with alcohol use and smoking.

Children with an acute ulcer who have developed complications, such as massive hemorrhage, require emergency care. The administration of IV fluids, blood, or plasma depends on the amount of blood loss. Replacement with whole blood or packed cells may be necessary for significant loss.

Surgical intervention may be required for complications such as hemorrhage, perforation, or gastric outlet obstruction. Ligation of the source of bleeding or closure of a perforation is performed. A vagotomy and pyloroplasty may be indicated in children with recurring ulcers despite aggressive medical treatment.

Prognosis

The long-term prognosis for PUD is variable. Many ulcers are successfully treated with medical therapy; however, primary duodenal peptic ulcers often recur. Complications such as GI bleeding can occur and extend into adult life. The effect of maintenance drug therapy on long-term morbidity remains to be established with further studies.

Nursing Care Management

The primary nursing goal is to promote healing of the ulcer through compliance with the medication regimen. If an analgesic–antipyretic is needed, acetaminophen, not aspirin or NSAIDs, is used. Critically ill neonates, infants, and children in intensive care units (ICUs) should receive H$_2$ blockers to prevent stress ulcers.

💊 DRUG ALERT

H$_2$ Blockers

Critically ill children receiving IV H$_2$ blockers should have their gastric pH values checked at frequent intervals.

For nonhospitalized children with chronic illnesses, consider the role stress plays. In children, many ulcers occur secondary to other conditions, and the nurse should be aware of family and environmental conditions that may aggravate or precipitate ulcers. Children may benefit from psychologic counseling and from learning how to cope constructively with stress.

HEPATIC DISORDERS

ACUTE HEPATITIS

Etiology

Hepatitis is an acute or chronic inflammation of the liver that can result from several different causes. One cause is infection. Many types of hepatitis are caused by viruses such as the hepatitis viruses, Epstein-Barr virus (EBV), cytomegalovirus (CMV), and human immunodeficiency virus (HIV). Other causes of hepatitis are nonviral (abscess, amebiasis), autoimmune, metabolic, chemical, neoplastic, anatomic (choledochal duct cyst and biliary atresia [BA]), hemodynamic (shock, congestive heart failure), and idiopathic (sclerosing cholangitis and Reye syndrome). The following six viruses cause 90% of cases of viral hepatitis (Table 24-9):

1. Hepatitis A virus (HAV)
2. Hepatitis B virus (HBV)
3. Hepatitis C virus (HCV)

TABLE 24-9	COMPARISON OF TYPES A, B, AND C HEPATITIS		
CHARACTERISTICS	**TYPE A**	**TYPE B**	**TYPE C**
Incubation period	15–50 days; average, 25–30 days	30–180 days; average, 50 days	2 weeks–6 months; average, 6–7 weeks
Period of communicability	Believed to be later half of incubation period to the first week after the onset of clinical illness	Variable Virus in blood or other body fluids during late incubation period and acute stage of disease; may persist in carrier state for years to lifetime	Begins before onset of symptoms May persist in carrier state for years
Mode of transmission	Principal route—fecal-oral Rarely—parenteral	Principal route—parenteral Less frequent route—oral, sexual, any body fluid Perinatal transfer—transplacental blood (last trimester); at delivery; or during breastfeeding, especially if mother has cracked nipples	Principal route—parenteral Nonparenteral spread possible
Clinical features			
Onset	Usually rapid, acute	More insidious	Usually insidious
Fever	Common and early	Less frequent	Less frequent
Anorexia	Common	Mild to moderate	Mild to moderate
Nausea and vomiting	Common	Sometimes present	Mild to moderate
Rash	Rare	Common	Sometimes present
Arthralgia	Rare	Common	Rare
Pruritus	Rare	Sometimes present	Sometimes present
Jaundice	Present (many cases anicteric)	Present	Present
Immunity	Present after one attack; no crossover to type B or C	Present after one attack; no crossover to type A or C	Present after one attack; no crossover to type A or B
Carrier state	No	Yes	Yes
Chronic infection	No	Yes	Yes
Prophylaxis			
Immune globulin (IG)	Passive immunity Successful, especially in early incubation period and preexposure prophylaxis	Passive immunity Inconsistent benefits; probably of no use	Not currently recommended by CDC
HAV vaccine	Two inactivated vaccines approved for children ages 2–18 years: Havrix and Vaqta; given in a two-dose schedule (6–12 months between doses); TWINRIX contains both HAV and HBV (for patients 18 years old and older)		
HBV immune globulin (HBIG)	No benefit	Passive immunity	No benefit
HBV vaccine	No benefit	Postexposure protection possible if given immediately after definite exposure Provides active immunity Universal vaccination recommended for all newborns	No benefit
Mortality rate	0.1%–0.2%	0.5%–2.0% in uncomplicated cases; may be higher in complicated cases	1%–2% in uncomplicated cases; may be higher in complicated cases

CDC, Centers for Disease Control and Prevention; *HAV,* hepatitis A virus; *HBV,* hepatitis B virus.

4. Hepatitis D virus (HDV)
5. Hepatitis E virus (HEV)
6. Hepatitis G virus (HGV)

Hepatitis A

Hepatitis A incidence in the United States has declined 92%, from 12 cases per 100,000 population in 1995 to less than 1 case per 100,000 population in 2009, the lowest rate ever recorded. Declines were greatest among children and in states where routine vaccination of children was recommended beginning in 1999 (Daniels, Grytdal, Wasley, and others, 2009). The virus is spread directly or indirectly by the fecal–oral route by ingestion of contaminated foods, direct exposure to infected fecal material, or close contact with an infected person. The virus is particularly prevalent in developing countries with poor living conditions, inadequate sanitation, crowding, and poor personal hygiene practices. The spread of HAV has been associated with improper food handling and high-risk areas such as households with infected persons, residential centers for people with disabilities, and daycare centers. The average incubation period is about 4 weeks, with a range of 15 to 50 days. Fecal shedding of the virus can occur for 2 to 3 weeks before and for 1 week after the onset of jaundice. During this time, although the individual is asymptomatic, the virus is most likely to be transmitted. Infants with HAV infection are likely to be asymptomatic (anicteric hepatitis). Children often have diarrhea, and their symptoms are frequently attributed to gastroenteritis. Only 1 in 12 young children develops jaundice. Most adults develop clinical signs with icteric hepatitis. The prognosis of HAV infection is usually good, and complications are rare.

Hepatitis B

Hepatitis B can be an acute or chronic infection, ranging from an asymptomatic, limited infection to fatal, fulminant (rapid and severe) hepatitis. There are no environmental or animal reservoirs for HBV. Humans are the main source of infections. HBV may be transmitted parenterally, percutaneously, or transmucosally. Hepatitis B surface antigen (HBsAg) has been found in all body fluids, including feces, bile, breast milk, sweat, tears, vaginal secretions, and urine, but only blood, semen, and saliva have been found to contain infectious HBV particles. HBV infection from human bites has been documented, but transmission from feces has not. HBV has been acquired after blood transfusion, but the likelihood of this has been reduced through blood product screening procedures. Adults whose occupations are associated with considerable exposure to blood or blood products, such as health care workers, are at an increased risk of contracting HBV.

Most HBV infection in children is acquired perinatally. Transmission from mother to infant during the perinatal period (e.g., blood exposure during delivery) results in chronic infection in 70% to 90% of infants if the mother is positive for HBsAg and HBeAg (AAP, Committee on Infectious Diseases and Pickering, 2009; Tran, 2009). Perinatal infection occurs during the birthing process when the infant comes in contact with maternal body fluids, most likely blood. It is still not known if the virus enters infants via mucosal membranes, the intestinal tract, or skin abrasions. HBsAg has been detected in breast milk, but it is not clear whether HBV infection is transmitted through ingested breast milk or from swallowed maternal blood from injured nipples (Tran, 2009). Infants and children who are not infected during the perinatal period remain at high risk for acquiring person-to-person transmission from their mothers during the first 5 years of life.

Hepatitis B virus infection occurs in children and adolescents in specific high-risk groups, which are (1) individuals with hemophilia or other disorders who have received multiple transfusions, (2) children and adolescents involved in IV drug abuse, (3) institutionalized children, (4) preschool children in endemic areas, and (5) individuals engaged in heterosexual activity or sexual activity with homosexual men. The incubation period for HBV infection ranges from 45 to 160 days with an average of 120 days (AAP, Committee on Infectious Diseases and Pickering, 2009). HBV infection can cause a carrier state and lead to chronic hepatitis with eventual cirrhosis or hepatocellular carcinoma in adulthood.

Hepatitis C

Hepatitis C virus is transmitted parenterally through exposure to blood and blood products from HCV-infected persons (AAP, Committee on Infectious Diseases and Pickering, 2009). The most common risk factors associated with HCV acquisition are injections, drug use, having received a blood product before 1992 (e.g., hemophilia), and having multiple sex partners. Recent improvements in donor screening and inactivation procedures for blood products such as the factor concentrates used for patients with hemophilia have significantly reduced the risk of transmission through blood products. The mechanism of nonparenteral or nonpercutaneous transmission of HCV is uncertain. Sexual transmission among monogamous couples and among family contacts is uncommon. Maternal coinfection with HIV has been associated with increased risk of perinatal transmission of HCV and may depend on the HCV genotype and the serum titer of maternal HCV-RNA. All persons with HCV antibody or HCV-RNA in their blood are considered to be infectious (AAP, Committee on Infectious Diseases and Pickering, 2009).

The clinical course is variable. The incubation period for HCV ranges from 14 to 180 days with an average of 45 days. The natural history of the disease in children is not well defined. Some children may be asymptomatic, but hepatitis C can become a chronic condition and can cause cirrhosis and hepatocellular carcinoma. About 60% to 70% of individuals infected with HCV develop chronic disease. Infection with HCV is the leading reason for liver transplantation in the United States (AAP, Committee on Infectious Diseases and Pickering, 2009).

Hepatitis D

Hepatitis D occurs in children already infected with HBV. HDV is a defective RNA virus that requires the helper function of HBV. The incubation period is from 2 to 8 weeks. Both acute and chronic forms of hepatitis D tend to be more severe than hepatitis B and can lead to cirrhosis. HDV infection occurs mostly in drug abusers, individuals with hemophilia, and persons immigrating from endemic areas.

Hepatitis E

Hepatitis E is enterically transmitted non-A, non-B hepatitis. Transmission may occur through the fecal–oral route or from contaminated water. The incubation period is 2 to 9 weeks. This illness is uncommon in children, does not cause chronic liver disease, is not a chronic condition, and has no carrier state. However, it can be a devastating disease among pregnant women, with an unusually high case-fatality rate (10%) (AAP, Committee on Infectious Diseases and Pickering, 2009).

Hepatitis G

Hepatitis G virus is a bloodborne virus that may also be transmitted by organ transplantation. High-risk groups include transfusion recipients, IV drug users, and individuals infected with HCV. Individuals with the virus are often asymptomatic, and most infections are chronic. The incubation period is unknown.

Pathophysiology

Pathologic changes occur primarily in the parenchymal cells of the liver and result in variable degrees of swelling; infiltration of liver cells by mononuclear cells; and subsequent degeneration, necrosis, and fibrosis. Structural changes within the hepatocyte account for altered liver functions, such as impaired bile excretion, elevated transaminase levels, and decreased albumin synthesis. The disorder may be self-limiting with regeneration of liver cells without scarring, leading to a complete recovery. However, some forms of hepatitis do not result in complete return of liver function. These include fulminant hepatitis, which is characterized by a severe, acute course with massive destruction of the liver tissue causing liver failure and high mortality within 1 to 2 weeks, and subacute or chronic active hepatitis, which is characterized by progressive liver destruction, uncertain regeneration, scarring, and potential cirrhosis.

The progression of liver disease is characterized pathologically by four stages: (1) stage one is characterized by mononuclear inflammatory cells surrounding small bile ducts; (2) in stage two, there is proliferation of small bile ductules; (3) stage three is characterized by fibrosis or scarring; and (4) stage four is cirrhosis.

Clinical Manifestations

The clinical manifestations and course of uncomplicated acute viral hepatitis are similar for most of the hepatitis viruses. Usually the prodromal, or *anicteric*, phase (absence of jaundice) lasts 5 to 7 days. Anorexia, malaise, lethargy, and easy fatigability are the most common symptoms. Fever may be present, especially in adolescents. Nausea, vomiting, and epigastric or right upper quadrant abdominal pain or tenderness may occur. Arthralgia and skin rashes may occur and are more likely in children with hepatitis B than those with hepatitis A. The transaminases, rather than bilirubin, are often elevated in acute hepatitis, and hepatomegaly may be present. Some mild cases of acute viral hepatitis do not cause symptoms or can be mistaken for influenza.

In young children, most of the prodromal symptoms disappear with the onset of jaundice, or the icteric phase. Many children with acute viral hepatitis, however, never develop jaundice. If jaundice occurs, it is often accompanied by dark urine and pale stools. Pruritus may accompany jaundice and can be bothersome for children.

Children with chronic active hepatitis may be asymptomatic but more commonly have nonspecific symptoms of malaise, fatigue, lethargy, weight loss, or vague abdominal pain. Hepatomegaly may be present, and the transaminases are often very high, with mild to severe hyperbilirubinemia.

Fulminant hepatitis is primarily caused by HBV or HCV. Many children with fulminant hepatitis develop characteristic clinical symptoms and rapidly develop manifestations of liver failure, including encephalopathy, coagulation defects, ascites, deepening jaundice, and an increasing WBC count. Changes in mental status or personality indicate impending liver failure. Although children with acute hepatitis may have hepatomegaly, a rapid decrease in the size of the liver (indicating loss of tissue due to necrosis) is a serious sign of fulminant hepatitis. Complications of fulminant hepatitis include GI bleeding, sepsis, renal failure, and disseminated coagulopathy.

Diagnostic Evaluation

⊜ Diagnosis is based on the history; physical examination; and serologic markers for hepatitis A, B, and C. No LFT is specific for hepatitis, but serum aspartate (AST) and serum aminotransferase (ALT) levels are markedly elevated. Serum bilirubin levels peak 5 to 10 days after clinical jaundice appears. Histologic evidence from liver biopsy may be required to establish the diagnosis and to assess the severity of the liver disease. Serologic markers indicate the antibodies or antigens formed in response to the specific virus and confirm the diagnosis. Serum immunologic tests are not available to detect HAV antigen, but there are two HAV antibody tests: anti-HAV immunoglobulin G (IgG) and immunoglobulin M (IgM). Anti-HAV antibodies are present at the onset of the disease and persist for life. A positive anti-HAV antibody test result indicates acute infection, immunity from past infection, passive antibody acquisition (e.g., from transfusion, serum immunoglobulin infusion), or immunization. To diagnose an acute or recent HAV infection, a positive anti-HAV IgM test result that is present with the onset of the disease and that persists for only 2 or 3 days is required.

Diagnosis of hepatitis B is confirmed by the detection of various hepatitis virus antigens and the antibodies that are produced in response to the infection. These antibodies and antigens and their significance include:

HBsAg—HBsAg (found on the surface of the virus), indicating ongoing infection or carrier state

Anti-HBs—Antibody to surface antigen HbsAg, indicating resolving or past infection

HBcAg—Hepatitis B core antigen (found on the inner core of the virus), detected only in the liver

Anti-HBc—Antibody to core antigen HbcAg, indicating ongoing or past infection

HBeAg—Hepatitis Be antigen (another component of the HBV core), indicating active infection

Anti-HBe—Antibody to HbeAg, indicating resolving or past infection

IgM anti-HBc—IgM antibody to core antigen

Tests are available for detection of all the HBV antigens and antibodies except HBcAg. HBsAg is detectable during acute infection. The presence of HBsAg indicates that the individual has been infected with the hepatitis virus. If the infection is self-limiting, HBsAg disappears in most patients before serum anti-HBs can be detected (termed the *window phase of infection*). IgM anti-HBc is highly specific in establishing the diagnosis of acute infection, as well as during the window phase in older children and adults. However, IgM anti-HBc usually is not present in perinatal HBV infection (AAP, Committee on Infectious Diseases and Pickering, 2009). Neonatal infection is most likely to occur in infants born to mothers who are HbeAg positive. In contrast, hepatitis B is much less likely to occur in infants whose mothers are HbsAg positive but HbeAg negative and who have antibodies to HBeAg.

Clinical improvement is usually associated with a decrease in or disappearance of these antigens followed by the appearance of their antibodies. For example, anti-HBc of the IgM class often occurs early in the disease followed by a rise in anti-HBc of the IgG class. Because the antibodies persist indefinitely, they are used to identify the carrier state (individuals with HBV who have no clinical disease but are able to transmit the organism). Persons with chronic HBV infection have circulating HBsAg and anti-HBc, and on rare occasions, anti-HBsAg is present. Both anti-HBs and anti-HBc are detected in persons with resolved infection, but anti-HBs alone is present in individuals who have been immunized with the HBV vaccine.

Hepatitis C virus RNA is the earliest serologic marker for HCV. HCV-RNA can be detected during the incubation period before symptoms of HCV disease are expressed. A positive HCV-RNA result indicates active infection, and persistence of HCV-RNA indicates chronic infection. A negative test result correlates with resolution of the disease.

HCV-RNA is also used to determine patient response to antiviral therapy for HCV.

The history of all patients should include questions to seek evidence of (1) contact with a person known to have hepatitis, especially a family member; (2) unsafe sanitation practices, such as contaminated drinking water; (3) ingestion of certain foods, such as clams or oysters (especially from polluted water); (4) multiple blood transfusions; (5) ingestion of hepatotoxic drugs, such as salicylates, sulfonamides, antineoplastic agents, acetaminophen, and anticonvulsants; and (6) parenteral administration of illicit drugs or sexual contact with a person who uses these drugs.

Therapeutic Management

Treatment options for viral hepatitis are limited. The goals of management include early detection, support and monitoring of the disease, recognition of chronic liver disease, and prevention of spread of the disease. No specific effective therapy for either acute or chronic hepatitis B or hepatitis C exists. Special high-protein, high-carbohydrate, low-fat diets are generally not of value. The use of corticosteroids alone or with immunosuppressive drugs is not advocated in the treatment of chronic viral hepatitis. However, steroids have been used to treat chronic autoimmune hepatitis. Hospitalization is required in the event of coagulopathy or fulminant hepatitis. Human interferon-α has been used in the treatment of chronic hepatitis B and C in adults and is being used to treat these infections in children. Therapy for hepatitis depends on the severity of inflammation and the cause of the disorder.

A number of antiviral medications are being used currently to treat HBV and HCV (Degertekin and Lok, 2009). Telbivudine is more potent than lamivudine but is associated with a high rate of antiviral resistance compared with entecavir or tenofovir. Combined therapy with lamivudine and adefovir reduces the rate of antiviral resistance compared with lamivudine monotherapy. Individualizing dose and duration of pegylated interferon and ribavirin according to on-treatment virologic response may improve sustained virologic response rates. Several specifically targeted antiviral therapies, notably protease and polymerase inhibitors, are promising but must be used in combination with pegylated interferon and ribavirin. These agents have multiple side effects, and patients require regular monitoring and support. Many products are under current investigation in clinical trials, largely with adult patients.

Prevention

Proper hand washing and standard precautions prevent the spread of viral hepatitis. Prophylactic use of standard immune globulin is effective in preventing hepatitis A in situations of preexposure (e.g., anticipated travel to areas where HAV is prevalent) or within 2 weeks of exposure.

Hepatitis B immune globulin (HBIG) is effective in preventing HBV infection after one-time exposures such as accidental needle punctures or other contact of contaminated material with mucous membranes and should be given to newborns whose mothers are HbsAg positive. HBIG is prepared from plasma that contains high titers of antibodies against HBV. HBIG should be given within 72 hours of exposure.

Vaccines have been developed to prevent HAV and HBV infection (see Table 24-9). HBV vaccination is recommended for all newborns and for high-risk groups. HAV is recommended for infants starting at 12 months of age. (See Immunizations, Chapter 10.) In addition, the AAP (AAP, Committee on Infectious Diseases and Pickering, 2009) recommends universal immunization of all adolescents with the HBV

vaccine. Because HDV cannot be transmitted in the absence of HBV infection, it is possible to prevent HDV infection by preventing HBV infection. Routine serologic testing for anti-HCV of children born to women previously identified as being infected with HCV is also recommended (AAP, Committee on Infectious Diseases and Pickering, 2009).

Prognosis

The prognosis for children with hepatitis is variable and depends on the type of virus and the child's age and immunocompetence. Hepatitis A and E are usually mild, brief illnesses with no carrier state. Hepatitis B can cause a wide spectrum of acute and chronic illness. Infants are more likely than older children to develop chronic hepatitis. Hepatocellular carcinoma during adulthood is a potentially fatal complication of chronic HBV infection. Hepatitis C frequently becomes chronic, and cirrhosis may develop in these children. Limited data concerning hepatitis G suggest that the rate of progression to cirrhosis with this virus may be very low. The highest mortality occurs in hepatitis D. Viral hepatitis causes approximately 50% of the cases of fulminant hepatic failure. The mechanism by which fulminant hepatic failure occurs is not well understood, and survival varies.

Nursing Care Management

Nursing objectives depend largely on the severity of the hepatitis, the medical treatment, and factors influencing the control and transmission of the disease. Because children with mild viral hepatitis are frequently cared for at home, it is often the nurse's responsibility to explain any medical therapies and infection control measures. When further assistance is needed for parents to comply with instructions, a community health nursing referral is necessary.

Encourage a well-balanced diet and a schedule of rest and activity adjusted to the child's condition. Because the child with HAV is not infectious within 1 week after the onset of jaundice, the child may feel well enough to resume school shortly thereafter. Caution parents about administering any medication to the child because normal doses of many drugs may become dangerous because of the liver's inability to detoxify and excrete them.

Standard precautions are followed when children are hospitalized. However, these children are not usually isolated in a separate room unless they are fecally incontinent or their toys and other personal items are likely to become contaminated with feces. Discourage children from sharing their toys.

Hand washing is the single most effective measure in prevention and control of hepatitis in any setting. Parents and children need an explanation of the usual ways in which HAV (fecal–oral route) and HBV (parenteral route) are spread. Parents should also be aware of the recommendation for universal vaccination against HBV for newborns and adolescents (see Chapter 10).

In young people with HBV infection who have a known or suspected history of illicit drug use, the nurse has the responsibility of helping them realize the associated dangers of drug abuse, stressing the parenteral mode of transmission of hepatitis, and encouraging them to seek counseling through a drug program.

CIRRHOSIS

Cirrhosis occurs at the end stage of many chronic liver diseases, including biliary atresia (BA) and chronic hepatitis. Cirrhosis can also result from infectious, autoimmune, or toxic factors and from chronic diseases such as hemophilia and cystic fibrosis. A cirrhotic liver is irreversibly damaged.

Clinical manifestations of cirrhosis include jaundice, poor growth, anorexia, muscle weakness, and lethargy. Ascites, edema, GI bleeding, anemia, and abdominal pain may be present in children with impaired intrahepatic blood flow. Pulmonary function may be impaired because of pressure against the diaphragm caused by hepatosplenomegaly and ascites. Dyspnea and cyanosis may occur, especially on exertion. Intrapulmonary arteriovenous shunts may develop, which can also cause hypoxemia. Spider angiomas and prominent blood vessels on the upper torso are often present.

Therapeutic Management

There is no successful treatment to arrest the progression of cirrhosis. The goals of management include monitoring liver function and managing specific complications such as esophageal varices and malnutrition. Assessment of the child's degree of liver dysfunction is important so the child can be evaluated for transplantation at the appropriate time.

Liver transplantation has improved the prognosis substantially for many children with cirrhosis. The combination of new immunosuppressive medications and new surgical techniques has resulted in 83% to 91% 1-year survival rates in many large hospital centers and 5-year survival rates of 82% to 83% (Kamath and Olthoff, 2010). The policy governing the allocation of livers for transplantation by the United Network for Organ Sharing allows patients with acute fulminant liver failure, plus those with failed liver grafts and the sickest pediatric patients, to be placed at the top of the network's transplantation lists. Although this change has benefited many pediatric patients, the shortage of available donors for children continues to dictate transplantation decisions, and many children continue to die while waiting for a suitable donor.

Nutritional support is an important therapy for children with cirrhosis and malnutrition. Supplements of fat-soluble vitamins are often required, and mineral supplements may be indicated. In some instances, aggressive nutritional support in the form of continuous tube feedings or PN may be necessary.

Esophageal and gastric varices are life-threatening complications of portal hypertension. Acute hemorrhage is managed with IV fluids, blood products, vasopressin, and gastric lavage. Balloon tamponade with a Sengstaken-Blakemore tube may be indicated. Endoscopic sclerotherapy and endoscopic banding ligation are also effective therapies for esophageal and gastric varices.

Ascites can be managed by sodium restriction and diuretics. Severe ascites with respiratory compromise can be managed with administration of albumin or by paracentesis.

Although the full mechanism of hepatic encephalopathy is unknown, failure of the damaged liver to remove endogenous toxins, such as ammonia, plays a role. Treatment is directed at limiting the ammonia formation and absorption that occur in the bowel, especially with the drugs neomycin and lactulose. Because ammonia is formed in the bowel by the action of bacteria on ingested protein, neomycin reduces the number of intestinal bacteria so less ammonia is produced. The fermentation of lactulose by colonic bacteria produces short-chain fatty acids which lower the colonic pH, thereby inhibiting bacterial metabolism. This decreases the formation of ammonia from bacterial metabolism of protein.

Prognosis

The success of liver transplantation has revolutionized the approach to liver cirrhosis. Liver failure and cirrhosis are indications for transplantation. Retransplantation occurs in 10% to 30% of recipients because of primary nonfunction or hepatic artery thrombosis;

 FAMILY-CENTERED CARE
End-Stage Liver Disease

In many cases, the child and family must cope with an uncertain progression of the disease. The only hope for long-term survival may be liver transplantation. Transplantation can be successful, but the waiting period may be long, and there are many more children in need of organs than there are donors. The procedure is expensive and is performed only at designated medical centers, which are often far from the family's home. The nurse should recognize the unique stresses of coping with end-stage liver disease and waiting for transplantation and assist the family in coping with these stressors. The assistance of social workers and support from other parents can be beneficial.

rejection of the transplanted graft is seen in approximately 60% of children who have a liver transplant (Kamath and Olthoff, 2010). About 20% of infants who undergo portoenterostomy survive into adulthood with their native liver; more than half of patients undergoing portoenterostomy normalize their bilirubin within 6 months, and 5-year survival rates after portoenterostomy (with native liver) are reported to be about 60% (Pakarinen and Rintala, 2011). Careful monitoring of the child's condition and quality of life are necessary to evaluate the need for and timing of transplantation (see Family-Centered Care box).

Nursing Care Management

Several factors influence nursing care of the child with cirrhosis, including the cause of the cirrhosis, the severity of complications, and the prognosis. The prognosis is often poor unless successful liver transplantation occurs. Therefore, nursing care of the child is similar to that for any child with a life-threatening illness (see Chapter 18). Hospitalization is required when complications such as hemorrhage, severe malnutrition, or hepatic failure occur. Nursing assessments are directed at monitoring the child's condition, and interventions are aimed at treatment of specific complications. If liver transplantation is an option, the family needs support and assistance to cope.

BILIARY ATRESIA

Biliary atresia, or extrahepatic biliary atresia (EHBA), is a progressive inflammatory process that causes both intrahepatic and extrahepatic bile duct fibrosis, resulting in eventual ductal obstruction. The incidence of BA is approximately 1 in 10,000 to 15,000 live births (A-Kader and Balistreri, 2011; Kelly and Davenport, 2007). Associated malformations include polysplenia, intestinal atresia, and malrotation of the intestine. BA, if untreated, usually leads to cirrhosis, liver failure, and death in the first 2 years of life.

Etiology and Pathophysiology

The exact cause of BA is unknown, although immune mechanisms or viral injury may be responsible for the progressive process that results in complete obliteration of the bile ducts. BA is not seen in fetuses or stillborn or newborn infants. This suggests that BA is acquired late in gestation or in the perinatal period and is manifested a few weeks after birth. The majority of cases of BA (85%) have a complete obliteration of the extrahepatic biliary tree at or above the porta hepatis (A-Kader and Balistreri, 2011).

Jaundice, manifesting with yellow discoloration of the skin or sclerae, is the most common early symptom of BA. Jaundice, indicating cholestasis (the accumulation of compounds that cannot be excreted because of occlusion or obstruction of the biliary tree), can be visible at a total serum bilirubin concentration as low as 5.0 mg/dl. An abnormal direct bilirubin has been designated as greater than 1.0 mg/dl if the total bilirubin is less than 5 mg/dl or a value of direct bilirubin that represents more than 20% of the total bilirubin if it is greater than 5 mg/dl (Emerick and Whitington, 2006). Direct hyperbilirubinemia first appears after the resolution of physiologic jaundice (see Chapter 9). Jaundice is often associated with pale stool and dark urine. Histologic study demonstrates bile duct remnants and a progressive inflammatory process. In the fetal embryonic form of BA, which represents 10% to 35% of cases, there is a congenital absence of biliary ductal patency and an absence of bile duct remnants. Many infants have associated congenital anomalies. Varying degrees of cholestasis occur, resulting in retention of irritants and toxins. Injury to the liver occurs as the result of the inflammation caused by the cholestasis.

Diagnostic Evaluation

Early diagnosis is the key to the survival of children with BA. Infants who undergo surgery in the first 60 days of life have an 80% chance of establishing bile flow. Between 60 to 90 days of life, the chance of reestablishing flow drops to 50%, and after 90 days to 10% (Chen, Chang, Du, and others, 2006). The typical infant is thriving, appears well, and has only very mild jaundice during the first 6 to 8 weeks (Emerick and Whitington, 2006) but soon begins failing to grow. Several clinical signs may indicate the presence of BA (Box 24-8). Blood tests should include a CBC, electrolytes, bilirubin, and liver enzymes. Additional laboratory analyses, including α_1-antitrypsin level, TORCH titers (see Maternal Infections, Chapter 9), hepatitis serology, α-fetoprotein, urine CMV, and a sweat test, are indicated to rule out other conditions that cause persistent cholestasis and jaundice. Abdominal ultrasonography allows inspection of the liver and biliary system. Hepatobiliary scintigraphy demonstrates biliary patency but does not provide diagnostic certainty. Endoscopic retrograde cholangiopancreatography is performed in very young infants. This procedure, which is done using general anesthesia, has an 80% reported diagnostic accuracy. Percutaneous liver biopsy is highly reliable when the biopsy contains specimens from a number of portal areas. Definitive diagnosis of BA is obtained during surgical laparotomy and an intraoperative cholangiogram.

BOX 24-8 CLINICAL MANIFESTATIONS OF EXTRAHEPATIC BILIARY ATRESIA

Jaundice
- Earliest manifestation and most striking feature of disorder
- First observed in sclera
- Usually not apparent until age 2 to 3 weeks after resolution of neonatal jaundice

Dark yellow urine
Stools lighter than expected or white or tan
Hepatomegaly and abdominal distention common
Splenomegaly occurs later
Poor fat metabolism results in:
- Poor weight gain
- Growth failure (failure to thrive)

Pruritus
Irritability; difficulty comforting infant

Therapeutic Management

The primary treatment of BA is **hepatic portoenterostomy (Kasai procedure)** in which a segment of intestine is anastomosed to the resected porta hepatis to attempt bile drainage. A Roux-en-Y jejunal limb is then anastomosed to the porta hepatis (a Y-shaped anastomosis performed to provide bile drainage without reflux). This procedure has several variations. Bile drainage is achieved in approximately 80% to 90% of infants who undergo surgery when younger than 8 weeks of age (A-Kader and Balistreri, 2011). However, progressive cirrhosis still occurs in many children, necessitating liver transplantation. Prophylactic antibiotics are given after the Kasai procedure to minimize the risk of ascending cholangitis.

Medical management of BA is primarily supportive. It includes nutritional support with infant formulas that contain medium-chain triglycerides and essential fatty acids. Supplementation with fat-soluble vitamins (A, D, E, K); a multivitamin; and minerals, including iron, zinc, and selenium, is usually required. Aggressive nutritional support in the form of continuous gastrostomy feedings or TPN may be indicated for moderate to severe growth failure; the enteral solution should be low in sodium. Phenobarbital may be prescribed after hepatic portoenterostomy to stimulate bile flow, and ursodeoxycholic acid may be used to decrease cholestasis and the intense pruritus from jaundice. In cases of advanced liver dysfunction, management is the same as in infants with cirrhosis.

Prognosis

Untreated BA results in progressive cirrhosis and death in most children by 2 years of age. The Kasai procedure improves the prognosis but is not a cure. Biliary drainage can often be achieved if the surgery is done before the intrahepatic bile ducts are destroyed. Long-term survival has been reported in children who receive the Kasai procedure; however, even with successful bile drainage, many children ultimately develop liver failure.

Advances in surgical techniques and the use of immunosuppressive and antifungal drugs have improved the success of transplantation. The major obstacle continues to be a shortage of donor livers. Reduced-size, split-liver transplantation, retransplantation, and increased public awareness may improve donor organ availability in the future.

Nursing Care Management

Nursing interventions for the child with BA include support of the family before, during, and after surgical procedures and education regarding the treatment plan. In the postoperative period of a portoenterostomy, nursing care is similar to that after major abdominal surgery. Teaching includes the proper administration of medications. Administration of nutritional therapy, including special formulas, vitamin and mineral supplements, gastrostomy feedings, or PN, is an essential nursing responsibility. Growth failure in such infants is common, and increased metabolic needs combined with ascites, pruritus, and nutritional anorexia constitute a challenge for care. The nurse teaches caregivers how to monitor and administer nutritional therapy in the home. Pruritus may be a significant problem that is addressed by drug therapy or comfort measures such as baths in colloidal oatmeal compounds and trimming of fingernails. The risk of complications of BA, such as cholangitis, portal hypertension, GI bleeding, and ascites, should be explained to the caregivers.

Children and their families also need psychosocial support. The uncertain prognosis, discomfort, and waiting for transplantation produce stress, and hospitalizations, pharmacologic therapy, and nutritional therapy impose financial burdens on the family. Families can receive help from the Children's Liver Association for Support

Services,* an organization that provides educational materials, programs, and support systems, and the American Liver Foundation.†

STRUCTURAL DEFECTS

CLEFT LIP AND CLEFT PALATE

Clefts of the lip (CL) and palate (CP) are facial malformations that occur during embryonic development and are the most common congenital deformities in the United States. They may appear separately or, more often, together. CL results from failure of the maxillary and median nasal processes to fuse; CP is a midline fissure of the palate that results from failure of the two palatal processes to fuse.

The palate can be divided into the primary and secondary palates. The primary palate consists of the medial portion of the upper lip and the portion of the alveolar ridge that contains the central and lateral incisors. The secondary palate consists of the remaining portion of the hard palate and all of the soft palate. CL may vary from a small notch in the upper lip to a complete cleft extending into the base of the nose, including the lip and the alveolar ridge (Fig. 24-3). CL can be unilateral or bilateral. Deformed dental structures are associated with CL. Isolated CP occurs in the midline of the secondary palate and may also vary from a bifid uvula (the mildest form of CP) to a complete cleft extending from the soft palate to the hard palate.

Cleft lip and palate (CL/P) is more common than CP alone and varies by ethnicity. The occurrence is 1 in 1000 births in whites, 1.7 in 1000 births in Asians, 3.6 in 1000 births in American Indians, and 1 in 2000 births in African Americans (Moller and Glaze, 2009). CP occurs alone in only 1 in 2500 cases and does not display variation by ethnicity (Wilkins-Haug, 2010). CL/P tends to be more common in boys, and isolated CP occurs more frequently in girls.

Etiology

Cleft deformities may be an isolated anomaly, or they may occur with a recognized syndrome. CL/P and CP are distinct from isolated CP. Clefts of the secondary palate alone are more likely to be associated with syndromes than are isolated CL or CL/P.

Most cases of CL and CP have multifactorial inheritance, which is generally caused by a combination of genetic and environmental factors. Researchers do not yet know which gene(s) are responsible for clefting or to what extent environmental factors impact the developing structures. Exposure to teratogens such as alcohol, cigarette smoking, anticonvulsants, steroids, and retinoids are associated with higher rates of oral clefting. Folate deficiency is also a risk factor for clefting.

Pathophysiology

Cleft deformities represent a defect in cell migration that results in a failure of the maxillary and premaxillary processes to come together between the fourth and tenth weeks of embryonic development. Although often appearing together, CL and CP are distinct malformations embryologically, occurring at different times during the developmental process. Merging of the primary palate (upper lip and alveolus bilaterally) is completed by the seventh week of gestation. Fusion of the secondary palate (hard and soft palate) takes place later, between the seventh and tenth weeks of gestation. In the process of migrating to a horizontal position, the palates are separated by the tongue for a

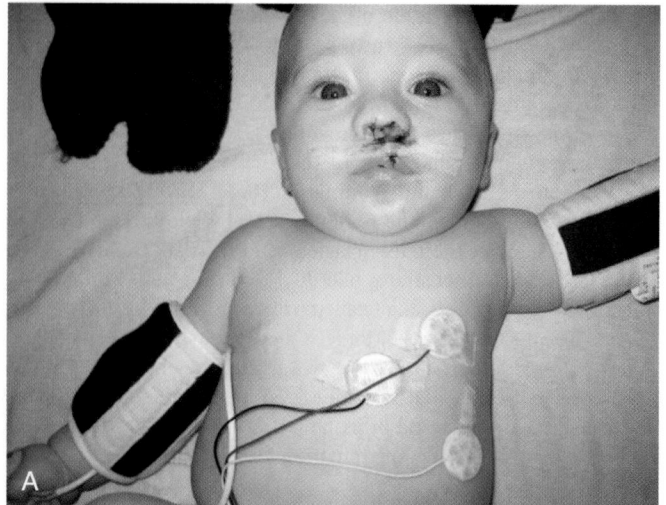

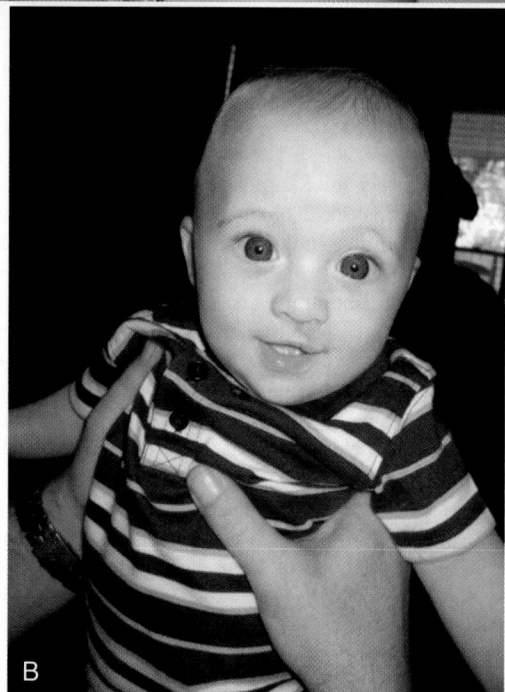

FIG 24-3 **A,** Cleft lip repair at age 16 weeks. Note the elbow restraints. **B,** Cleft lip 3 weeks after surgical repair. (Photos courtesy E. Danks.)

short time. If there is delay in this movement or if the tongue fails to descend soon enough, the remainder of development proceeds, but the palate never fuses.

Diagnostic Evaluation

Cleft lip and CL/P are apparent at birth. The defect may elicit severe emotional reactions in parents. CP is less obvious than CL and may not be detected immediately without a thorough assessment of the mouth. CP is identified through visual examination of the oral cavity or when the examiner places a gloved finger directly on the palate. Clefts of the hard and soft palate form a continuous opening between the mouth and the nasal cavity. The severity of the CP has an impact on feeding; the infant is unable to create suction in the oral cavity that is necessary for feeding. However, in most cases, the infant's ability to swallow is normal.

*25379 Wayne Mills Place, Suite 143, Valencia, CA 91355; 877-679-8256; http://www.classkids.org.
†75 Maiden Lane, Suite 603, New York, NY 10038; 212-668-1000; http://www.liverfoundation.org/education/info/biliaryatresia.

Prenatal diagnosis with fetal ultrasonography is not reliable until the soft tissues of the fetal face can be visualized at 13 to 14 weeks. About 20% to 30% of infants with CL and CL/P are prenatally diagnosed through ultrasonography (Robbins, Damiano, Druschel, and others, 2010), although infants with CP only are rarely diagnosed prenatally.

Therapeutic Management

Treatment of the child with CL and CP involves the cooperative efforts of a multidisciplinary health care team, including pediatrics, plastic surgery, orthodontics, otolaryngology, speech/language pathology, audiology, nursing, and social work. Management is directed toward closure of the cleft(s), prevention of complications, and facilitation of normal growth and development in the child.

Surgical Correction of Cleft Lip

Cleft lip repair typically occurs at most centers between 2 and 3 months of age. Most physicians adhere to the "rule of tens": the infant must be 10 weeks old, weigh 10 pounds, and have a hemoglobin of 10. The two most common procedures for repair of CL are the Tennison-Randall triangular flap (Z-plasty) and the Millard rotational advancement technique. The difference between these two is that the Tennison-Randall procedure crosses the philtral line and the Millard procedure advances a triangle of tissue in the upper third of the lip and does not cross the midline. Surgeons often use a combination of these two techniques to address individual differences. Improved surgical techniques have minimized scar retraction, and in the absence of infection or trauma, healing occurs with little scar formation (see Fig. 24-3). Nasoalveolar molding may also be used to bring the cleft segments closer together before definitive CL repair, reducing the need for CL revision. Optimal cosmetic results, however, may be difficult to obtain in severe defects. Additional revisions may be necessary at a later age.

Surgical Correction of Cleft Palate

Cleft palate repair typically occurs between 6 and 12 months. There is concern that early CP repair interferes with skeletal growth of the midface, but postponing palate closure beyond the child's first words may result in increased speech disorders (Chapman, Hardin-Jones, and Goldstein, 2008). The most common techniques to repair CP include the Veau-Wardill-Kilner V-Y pushback procedure and the Furlow double-opposing Z-plasty. Approximately 20% to 30% of children with repaired CP will need a secondary surgery to improve velopharyngeal closure for speech. Secondary procedures may include palatal lengthening, pharyngeal flap, sphincter pharyngoplasty, or posterior pharyngeal wall augmentation. If the child is not a candidate for surgical revision to improve velopharyngeal function, prosthetic management should be considered.

Prognosis

Children with CL may require multiple surgeries to achieve optimal aesthetic outcomes but are not at risk for increased speech problems. Although some children with CP and CL/P do not require speech therapy, many have some degree of speech impairment that requires speech therapy at some point throughout childhood. Articulation errors result from a history of velopharyngeal dysfunction, incorrect articulatory placement, improper tooth alignment, and varying degrees of hearing loss. Improper drainage of the middle ear as a result of inefficient function of the Eustachian tube relating to the history of CP contributes to recurrent otitis media, which leads to conductive hearing loss in many children with CP; many children with clefts will have pressure-equalization tubes placed. Extensive orthodontics and prosthodontics may be needed to correct malposition of the teeth and maxillary arches. Academic achievement, social adjustment, and behavior should be monitored, particularly in children with syndromic cleft conditions.

Nursing Care Management

The immediate nursing problems for an infant with CL/P deformities are related to feeding. Parents of newborns with clefts place high priority on learning how to feed their infants and identify when they are sick, but they also express interest in learning about the infant's "normal" features (Young, O'Riordan, Goldstein, and others, 2001). Whenever possible, they should be referred to a comprehensive CP team.

Feeding

Feeding the infant with a cleft presents a challenge to nurses and parents. Growth failure in infants with CL/P or CP has been attributed to preoperative feeding difficulties. After surgical repair, most infants who have isolated CL, CP, or CL/P with no associated syndromes gain weight or achieve adequate weight and height for age.

Cleft lip may interfere with an infant's ability to achieve an adequate anterior lip seal. An infant with an isolated CL typically has no difficulty breastfeeding because the breast tissue is able to conform to the cleft. If bottle fed, an infant with an isolated CL may have greater success using bottles with a wide base of the nipple, such as a Playtex nurser or a NUK (orthodontic) nipple. Cheek support (squeezing the cheeks together to decrease the width of the cleft) may be useful in improving lip seal during feeding.

Infants with CP and CL/P are often unable to feed using conventional methods before surgical management. La Leche League International reports that "over time, lactation consultants have found that feeding exclusively at the breast is a difficult goal for all but a few infants with uncorrected cleft palates" (Cleft Palate Foundation, 2009). CP reduces the infant's ability to suck, which interferes with breastfeeding and traditional bottle feeding. Modifications to positioning, bottle selection, and feeder supportive techniques can help infants with CP feed efficiently. Begin by positioning an infant with CP in an upright position with the head supported by the caregiver's hand or cradled in the arm; this position allows gravity to assist with the flow of the liquid so it is swallowed instead of resulting in a loss of liquid through the nose.

Suction is almost certainly impaired in infants with CP because the velum is unable to elevate and separate the oral nasal cavities while generating adequate negative intraoral pressure. Several types of bottles work well with infants unable to generate adequate suction, including the Special Needs Feeder (formerly Haberman), the Pigeon bottle, and the Mead-Johnson Cleft Palate Nurser. The Special Needs Feeder and the Pigeon bottles use a one-way flow valve that allows the infant to feed successfully by compressing the nipple with either the intact segments of the palate and the mandible or tongue. With the one-way flow valve in place, the liquid flows into the oral cavity rather than back into the bottle chamber when the nipple is compressed. The Special Needs Feeder also has a large nipple chamber that allows the feeder to provide extra assistance by squeezing the chamber if needed. The tip of the Special Needs Feeder has a slit cut, which allows the feeder to control the flow of liquid by positioning the slit vertically or horizontally within the mouth, which can reduce choking and gagging. The Pigeon bottle has a bulbous tip that fits naturally into the oral cavity with a Y-cut nipple that increases the flow of liquid. The third bottle, the Mead Johnson Cleft Palate Nurser, is a squeezable bottle with a long, thin X-cut nipple; this bottle requires the feeder to

Nursing Care Plan—The Child with Cleft Lip and/or Cleft Palate rhythmically squeeze the bottle throughout the feeding and does not require the infant to actively compress the nipple during the feeding.

Infants with clefts tend to swallow excessive air during feedings, so it is important to pause during feedings and burp the infant. Some CP specialists advocate for the use of feeding obturators to assist with feeding; these devices may increase compression surfaces within the oral cavity but do not improve feeding efficiency or growth within the first year of life (Masarei, Wade, Mars, and others, 2007).

Regardless of the feeding method used, the mother should begin feeding the infant as soon as possible, preferably after the initial nursery feeding. When maternal feeding is initiated early, the mother can help to determine the method best suited to her and the infant and can become adept in the technique before discharge from the hospital.

Preoperative Care

In preparation for surgical repair, parents may be taught to use alternative feeding systems (e.g., syringes) several days before surgery.

Postoperative Care

The major efforts in the postoperative period are directed toward protecting the operative site. For CL, parents may be advised to apply petroleum jelly to the operative site for several days after surgery. For CL, CP, or CL/P, elbow immobilizers may be used to prevent the infant from rubbing or disturbing the suture line; they are applied immediately after surgery and may be used for 7 to 10 days. Some centers advocate using a syringe for feeding for 7 to 10 days after CL or CP repair. Adequate analgesia is required to relieve postoperative pain and to prevent restlessness. Feeding is resumed when tolerated. An upright or infant seat position is helpful in the immediate postoperative period (especially for infants who have difficulty handling secretions). Avoid the use of suction or other objects in the mouth, such as tongue depressors, thermometers, pacifiers, spoons, and straws.

The older infant or child may be discharged on a blenderized or soft diet, and parents are instructed to continue the diet until the surgeon directs them otherwise. Parents are cautioned against allowing the child to eat hard items (e.g., toast, hard cookies, and potato chips) that can damage the repaired palate. The expected outcomes are described in the Nursing Process box.

Long-Term Care

Children with CL/P often require a variety of services during recovery. Family members need support and encouragement by health professionals and guidance in activities that facilitate a normal outcome for their child. Parents frequently cite financial stress as a difficult issue. With the combined efforts of the family and the health team, most children achieve a satisfactory outcome. Many children with CL/P have

---

◎ NURSING PROCESS

The Child with a Cleft Lip or Cleft Palate

Assessment

The lip defect is visible at birth, and assessment involves describing the location and extent of the defect; the CP is evaluated by visualization during crying. CP without CL is detected by palpating the palate with the gloved finger during the newborn assessment. The emotional impact of the birth of a child with a cosmetic and functional disability is especially traumatic to the family. Consequently, nursing assessment is also concerned with the family's emotional reaction.

Diagnosis (Problem Identification)

After a thorough assessment, several nursing diagnoses are evident:

- Altered Nutrition: Less Than Body Requirements related to deficient oral intake and inability to suck effectively (preoperative CL/CP)
- Risk for Altered Parenting related to infant with a highly visible physical defect
- Risk for Trauma of the surgical site related to infant's hand-to-mouth activity
- Altered Nutrition: Less Than Body Requirements related to difficulty eating after surgical procedure
- Pain related to tissue trauma
- Altered Family Processes related to child's hospitalization and surgical correction of physical defect

Planning

The goals of care are related to preoperative care, short-term postoperative care, and long-term management. Goals for the infant and family include:

Preoperative Care

- Family will cope with the impact of an infant with a defect.
- Infant will receive optimum nutrition.
- Infant will be prepared for surgery.

Postoperative Care

- Infant will experience no trauma and minimal or no pain.
- Infant will receive optimum nutrition.
- Infant will experience no complications.
- Infant and family will receive adequate support.
- Family will be prepared for care at home and long-term needs of a child with CP.

Implementation

Numerous intervention strategies are discussed on pp. 801-803.

Evaluation

The effectiveness of nursing interventions for the family and the child who has CL/CP is determined by continual assessment and evaluation of care based on the following guidelines:

Preoperative Care

- Observe and interview family members about their understanding, feelings, and concerns regarding the defect, any anticipated surgery, and their interactions with the infant.
- Observe infant during feeding.
- Complete preoperative checklist.

Postoperative Care

- Inspect operative site for evidence of infection, bleeding, sloughing, or irritation.
- Observe for behavioral and physiologic indicators of pain and response to analgesics.
- Observe infant during feeding, measure intake and output, and weigh infant daily.
- Observe and interview family regarding their understanding and concerns about the infant, including long-term needs.

CL, Cleft lip; *CP,* cleft palate.

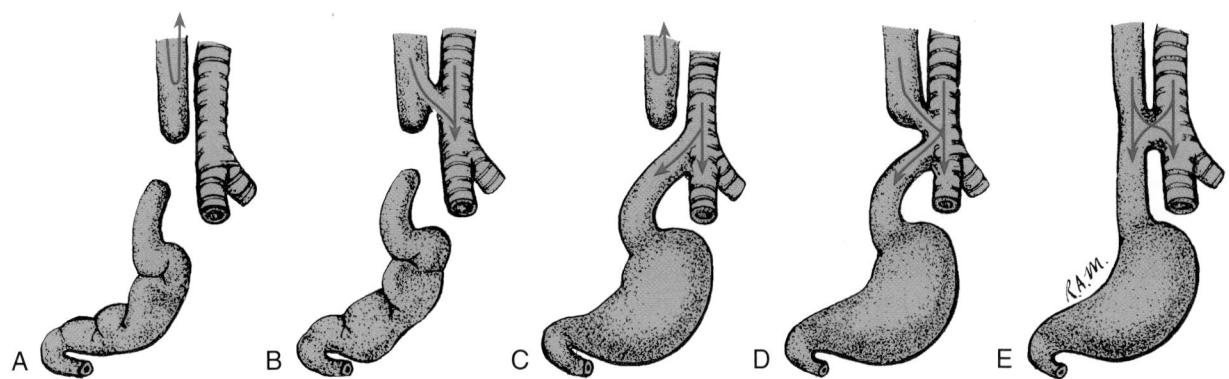

FIG 24-4 **A** to **E,** Five most common types of esophageal atresia and tracheoesophageal fistula.

surgical correction that creates a near normal–appearing lip and permits good function of the palate for speech and feeding. Parents need to understand the function of speech therapy and the purpose and care of all orthodontic appliances, as well as the importance of establishing good mouth care and proper brushing habits.

Throughout the child's development, an important goal is the development of a healthy personality and self-esteem. Many communities have CP parents' groups that offer help and support to families. Agencies that provide services and information for children with CL/P and their families include the American Cleft Palate–Craniofacial Association (http://www.acpa-cpf.org), the Cleft Palate Foundation (http://www.cleftline.org), Cleft Advocate (http://www.cleftadvocate.org), the March of Dimes (http://www.marchforbabies.org), and various state children's medical services.

ESOPHAGEAL ATRESIA AND TRACHEOESOPHAGEAL FISTULA

Congenital EA and tracheoesophageal fistula (TEF) are rare malformations that represent a failure of the esophagus to develop as a continuous passage and a failure of the trachea and esophagus to separate into distinct structures. These defects may occur as separate entities or in combination (Fig. 24-4), and without early diagnosis and treatment, they pose a serious threat to the infant's well-being.

Etiology

Esophageal atresia with or without an associated TEF is the most common esophageal malformation, occurring in approximately 90% of the 1 in 4000 affected neonates (Khan and Orenstein, 2011). There appears to be an equal sex incidence, but the birth weight of most affected infants is significantly lower than average, and the incidence of preterm birth is high. A history of maternal polyhydramnios is present in approximately 50% of infants with the defect.

Approximately 50% of the cases of EA/TEF are a component of VATER or VACTERL association, acronyms used to describe associated anomalies (VATER for *v*ertebral defects, imperforate *a*nus, *t*racheo-*e*sophageal fistula, and *r*adial and *r*enal dysplasia; and VACTERL for *v*ertebral, *a*nal, *c*ardiac, *t*racheal, *e*sophageal, *r*enal, and *l*imb) (Khan and Orenstein, 2011).

Pathophysiology

The cause of EA/TEF is unknown. In the most frequently encountered form of EA and TEF (80%–95% of cases), the proximal esophageal segment terminates in a blind pouch, and the distal segment is connected to the trachea or primary bronchus by a short fistula at or near

the bifurcation (see Fig. 24-4, *C*). The second most common variety (5%–8%) consists of a blind pouch at each end, widely separated and with no communication to the trachea (see Fig. 24-4, *A*). An H-type EA refers to an otherwise normal trachea and esophagus connected by a fistula (4%–5%) (see Fig. 24-4, *E*). Extremely rare anomalies involve a fistula from the trachea to the upper esophageal segment (0.8%) (see Fig. 24-4, *B*) or to both the upper and lower segments (0.7%–6%) (see Fig. 24-4, *D*).

Diagnostic Evaluation

The disorder is suspected on the basis of clinical manifestations (Box 24-9). EA should also be suspected in cases of maternal polyhydramnios. Although the diagnosis is established on the basis of clinical signs and symptoms, the exact type of anomaly is determined by radiographic studies. A radiopaque catheter is inserted into the hypopharynx and advanced until it encounters an obstruction. Chest radiographs are taken to ascertain esophageal patency or the presence and level of a blind pouch. Sometimes fistulas are not patent, which makes them more difficult to diagnose. The presence of gas in the stomach or small bowel is indicative of a coexisting TEF.

Therapeutic Management

The treatment of patients with EA and TEF includes maintenance of a patent airway, prevention of pneumonia, gastric or blind pouch decompression, supportive therapy, and surgical repair of the anomaly.

When EA with a TEF is suspected, the infant is immediately deprived of oral intake, IV fluids are initiated, and the infant is positioned to facilitate drainage of secretions and decrease the likelihood of aspiration. Accumulated secretions are suctioned frequently from the mouth and pharynx. A double-lumen catheter should be placed into the upper esophageal pouch and attached to intermittent or continuous low suction. The infant's head is kept upright to facilitate removal of fluid collected in the pouch and to prevent aspiration of gastric contents. Broad-spectrum antibiotic therapy is often instituted if there is a concern about aspiration of gastric contents.

Most malformations can be corrected surgically in one operation or in two or more staged procedures. The success depends on early diagnosis before complications occur and on the presence and severity of associated anomalies and illness factors, including preterm birth. With measures instituted to prevent aspiration pneumonia and to ensure adequate hydration and nutrition, surgery may be postponed to allow for more effective treatment of pneumonia and physiologic stabilization so the infant can better withstand the complex surgery. The delay also offers an opportunity for further evaluation and assessment to rule out any associated anomalies and to optimize respiratory support.

The surgery consists of a thoracotomy with division and ligation of the TEF and an end-to-end or end-to-side anastomosis of the esophagus. A chest tube may be inserted to drain intrapleural air and fluid. For infants who are not stable enough to undergo definitive repair or those with a lengthy gap between the proximal and distal esophagus, a staged operation is preferred that involves gastrostomy, ligation of the TEF, and constant drainage of the esophageal pouch. A delayed esophageal anastomosis is usually attempted after several weeks to months. Thoracoscopic repair of EA/TEF is being used successfully, thus negating the need for a thoracotomy and minimizing associated postoperative complications and morbidities (MacKinlay, 2009; Rothenberg, 2009).

If an esophageal anastomosis cannot be accomplished, a cervical esophagostomy (to allow drainage of saliva through a stoma in the neck) and gastrostomy are performed.

A primary anastomosis may be impossible because of insufficient length of the two segments of esophagus. This occurs if the distance between the two segments is 3 to 4 cm (1.2–1.6 inches) or greater; this is often referred to as *long-gap EA* (Khan and Orenstein, 2011). In these cases, an esophageal replacement procedure using a part of the colon or gastric tube interposition may be necessary to bridge the missing esophageal segment.

Tracheomalacia may occur as a result of weakness in the tracheal wall that exists when a dilated proximal pouch compresses the trachea early in fetal life. It may also occur as a result of inadequate intratracheal pressure causing abnormal tracheal development. Clinical signs of tracheomalacia include a barking cough, stridor, wheezing, recurrent respiratory tract infections, cyanosis, and sometimes apnea. Tracheomalacia may occur in up to 75% of children with EA/TEF but may be clinically significant in only 10% to 20% of infants with EA/TEF; surgical intervention with aortopexy or stent placement is required in severe cases (Achildi and Grewal, 2007; Fayoux and Sfeir, 2011).

Prognosis

The survival rate is nearly 100% in otherwise healthy children. Most deaths are the result of extreme prematurity or other lethal associated anomalies. Potential complications after the surgical repair of EA and TEF depend on the type of defect and surgical correction. Complications of repair include an anastomotic leak, strictures caused by tension or ischemia, esophageal motility disorders causing dysphagia, respiratory compromise, and GER. Anastomotic esophageal strictures may cause dysphagia, choking, and respiratory distress. The strictures are often treated with routine esophageal dilation. Feeding difficulties are often present for months or years postoperatively, and the infant must be monitored closely to ensure adequate weight gain, growth, and

development. In some cases, laparoscopic fundoplication may be required. At times, the infant must be fed via gastrostomy or jejunostomy to provide adequate caloric intake.

Nursing Care Management

Nursing responsibility for detection of this serious malformation begins immediately after birth. For an infant with the classic signs and symptoms of EA, the major concern is the establishment of a patent airway and prevention of further respiratory compromise. Cyanosis is usually a result of laryngeal spasm caused by overflow of saliva into the larynx from the proximal esophageal pouch or aspiration; it normally resolves after removal of the secretions from the oropharynx by suctioning. The passage of a small-gauge orogastric feeding tube via the mouth into the stomach during the initial nursing physical assessment is helpful to rule out EA or other obstructive defects.

> **! NURSING ALERT**
>
> Any infant who has an excessive amount of frothy saliva in the mouth or difficulty with secretions and unexplained episodes of apnea, cyanosis, or oxygen desaturation should be suspected of having an EA or TEF and referred immediately for medical evaluation.

Preoperative Care

The nurse carefully suctions the mouth and nasopharynx and places the infant in an optimum position to facilitate drainage and avoid aspiration. The most desirable position for a newborn who is suspected of having the typical EA with a TEF (e.g., type C) is supine (or sometimes prone) with the head elevated on an inclined plane of at least 30 degrees. This positioning minimizes the reflux of gastric secretions at the distal esophagus into the trachea and bronchi, especially when intraabdominal pressure is elevated.

It is imperative to immediately remove any secretions that can be aspirated. Until surgery, the blind pouch is kept empty by intermittent or continuous suction through an indwelling double-lumen or Replogle catheter passed orally or nasally to the end of the pouch. In some cases, a percutaneous gastrostomy tube is inserted and left open so that any air entering the stomach through the fistula can escape, thus minimizing the danger of gastric contents being regurgitated into the trachea. The gastrostomy tube is emptied by gravity drainage. Feedings through the gastrostomy tube and irrigations with fluid are contraindicated before surgery in an infant with a distal TEF.

Nursing interventions include respiratory assessment, airway management, thermoregulation, fluid and electrolyte management, and PN support.

Often the infant must be transferred to a hospital with a specialized care unit and pediatric surgical team. The nurse advises the parents of the infant's condition and provides them with necessary support and information.

Postoperative Care

Postoperative care for these infants is the same as for any high-risk newborn. The infant is returned to a radiant warmer or isolette, the double-lumen NG catheter is attached to low-suction or gravity drainage, PN is provided, and the gastrostomy tube (if applicable) is returned to gravity drainage until feedings are tolerated. If a thoracotomy is performed and a chest tube is inserted, attention to the appropriate function of the closed drainage system is imperative. Pain management in the postoperative period is important even if only a thoracoscopic approach is used. In the first 24 to 36 hours, the nurse should provide pain management for the neonate just as for an adult undergoing a similar procedure. (See Pain in Neonates, Chapter 7.) Tracheal suction should only be done using a premeasured catheter and with extreme caution to avoid injury to the suture line.

If tolerated, gastrostomy feedings may be initiated and continued until the esophageal anastomosis is healed. Before oral feedings are initiated and the chest tube is removed, a contrast study or esophagram will verify the integrity of the esophageal anastomosis.

The nurse must carefully observe the initial attempt at oral feeding to make certain the infant is able to swallow without choking. Until the infant is able to take a sufficient amount by mouth, oral intake may need to be supplemented by bolus or continuous gastrostomy feedings. Ordinarily, infants are not discharged until they can take oral fluids well. The gastrostomy tube may be removed before discharge or maintained for supplemental feedings at home.

Special Problems

Upper respiratory tract complications are a threat to life in both the preoperative and the postoperative periods. In addition to pneumonia, there is a constant danger of respiratory distress resulting from atelectasis, pneumothorax, and laryngeal edema. Any persistent respiratory difficulty after removal of secretions is reported to the surgeon immediately. The infant is monitored for anastomotic leaks, as evidenced by purulent chest tube drainage, increased WBC count, and temperature instability.

In the infant awaiting esophageal replacement surgery, the catheter is removed, and the upper esophageal segment is drained through a cervical esophagostomy. An esophagostomy is difficult to care for because the skin becomes irritated by moisture from the continuous discharge of saliva. Frequent removal of drainage and application of a layer of protective ointment may remedy the problem. A dressing or ostomy appliance may be applied to collect the drainage, and an enterostomal therapist can provide additional guidance to prevent or treat skin breakdown.

For an infant who requires esophageal replacement, nonnutritive sucking is provided by a pacifier. Sometimes small amounts of water or formula are given orally, and although the liquid drains from the esophagostomy, this process allows the infant to develop mature sucking patterns. Other appropriate oral stimulation prevents feeding aversion. Infants who remain NPO for an extended period or who have not received oral stimulation have difficulty eating by mouth after corrective surgery and may develop oral hypersensitivity and food aversion. They require patient, firm guidance to learn how to take food into the mouth and swallow after repair. A referral to a multidisciplinary feeding behavior program is often necessary.

Some infants with EA/TEF may require periodic esophageal dilations on an outpatient basis. Discharge education should include instructions about feeding techniques in the child with a repaired esophagus, including a semi-upright feeding position, small feedings, and observation for adequacy of swallowing (regurgitation, cyanosis, choking). Tracheomalacia is often a complication, and parents are educated regarding the signs and symptoms of this condition, which include a barking cough, stridor, wheezing, recurrent respiratory tract infections, cyanosis, and sometimes apnea and ALTE (acute life-threatening event) (see Chapter 11). GER may also occur when feedings resume and may contribute to reactive airway disease with wheezing and labored respirations as the prominent clinical manifestations. Problems with thriving and gaining weight may occur in the first 5 years of life in the child with EA/TEF, especially if the infant is born preterm, and the nurse should be alert to the achievement of developmental milestones that indicate a need for early intervention and multidisciplinary referral.

As with any congenital anomaly, parents need support in adjusting to the child's condition (see Chapter 18). One difficulty is the immediate transfer of the sick newborn to the ICU and the length of hospitalization. Encouraging parents to visit the infant, participate in care when appropriate, and express their feelings regarding the infant's condition facilitates the attachment process. The nurse in the ICU should assume responsibility for ensuring that the parents are kept fully informed of the infant's progress.

Preparing parents for discharge involves teaching them skills they will need at home. Parents are taught to observe for behaviors that indicate the need for suctioning and for signs of respiratory distress and constriction of the esophagus (e.g., poor feeding, dysphagia, drooling, regurgitation of undigested food). Discharge planning also includes obtaining the necessary equipment and home nursing services to provide home care.

HERNIAS

A **hernia** is a protrusion of a portion of an organ or organs through an abnormal opening. The danger from herniation arises when the organ protruding through the opening is constricted to the extent that circulation is impaired or when the protruding organs encroach on and impair the function of other structures. An inguinal hernia that cannot be reduced easily is called an **incarcerated hernia**. A **strangulated inguinal hernia** is one in which the blood supply to the herniated organ is impaired. The herniations of concern are those that protrude through the diaphragm, the abdominal wall, or the inguinal canal (see also Genitourinary Tract Disorders and Defects, Chapter 27). The hernias of significance to the pediatric age groups are outlined in Table 24-10. The abdominal wall defects gastroschisis and omphalocele are considered separately in Table 24-11.

OBSTRUCTIVE DISORDERS

Obstruction in the GI tract occurs when the passage of nutrients and secretions is impeded by a constricted or occluded lumen or when there is impaired motility (**paralytic ileus**). Obstructions may be congenital or acquired. Many congenital obstructions such as atresia, imperforate anus, meconium plug, and meconium ileus usually appear in the neonatal period. Other obstructions of congenital etiology such as malrotation, HD, pyloric stenosis, volvulus, incarcerated hernia, and Meckel diverticulum appear after the first few weeks of life. Intestinal obstruction from acquired causes such as intussusception and tumors may occur in infancy or childhood. Intestinal obstructions from any cause are characterized by similar signs and symptoms (Box 24-10).

HYPERTROPHIC PYLORIC STENOSIS

Hypertrophic pyloric stenosis (HPS) occurs when the circumferential muscle of the pyloric sphincter becomes thickened, resulting in elongation and narrowing of the pyloric channel. This produces an outlet obstruction and compensatory dilation, hypertrophy, and hyperperistalsis of the stomach. This condition usually develops in the first 2 to 5 weeks of life, causing projectile nonbilious vomiting, dehydration, metabolic alkalosis, and growth failure. The precise etiology is unknown. The reported incidence is 1 to 3 per 1000 live births with a male-to-female ratio of 4 to 6:1. There is a genetic predisposition, and siblings and offspring of affected persons are at increased risk of developing HPS. It is more common in full-term than in preterm infants and is seen less frequently in African-American and Asian infants than in white infants.

TABLE 24-10	SUMMARY OUTLINE OF HERNIAS	
MANIFESTATIONS AND TYPE	**DIAGNOSTIC EVALUATION**	**NURSING CARE MANAGEMENT**
Congenital Diaphragmatic Protrusion of abdominal organs through opening in diaphragm, commonly on left side, causing severe respiratory compromise and inability to adequately expand affected lung, which may be hypoplastic	**Symptoms**—Commonly severe respiratory distress at birth or within a few hours; tachypnea, cyanosis, dyspnea, a scaphoid abdomen; absent breath sounds on affected side; impaired cardiac output; possible symptoms of shock, severe acidosis Milder cases may be seen after birth without severe respiratory distress **Diagnosis**—Suspected on basis of symptoms, confirmed by radiographic study; often diagnosed prenatally as early as 25th week of gestation	**Therapeutic:** Provide prompt recognition, resuscitation, and stabilization. Avoid bag and mask ventilation in diagnosed or suspected CDH because this fills stomach with air and further compromises respiratory function. Provide supportive treatment of respiratory distress and correction of pulmonary hypertension and persistence of fetal circulation; correct acidosis*; endotracheal intubation; GI decompression. Additional treatments to reverse pulmonary hypertension may involve administration of inhaled nitric oxide, use of high-frequency oscillation, sildenafil, or ECMO. Perform surgical reduction of hernia and repair of defect after respiratory status is stable (corrected acidosis*; pulmonary hypertension). **Nursing:** *Preoperative:* Monitor respiratory status; provide supplemental oxygen; assist with and monitor mechanical ventilation. Monitor cardiovascular status; support with inotropes may be necessary. Reduce stimulation—environmental and nursing care activities (cluster care to prevent constant interruptions). Maintain NG suction, oxygen, and IV fluids. Administer medications: sedation, muscular paralysis, inotropes, sildenafil (to reverse pulmonary hypertension). *Postoperative:* Carry out routine postoperative care and observation for acutely ill infant. Relieve pain and provide comfort. Support family because this is a critical illness.
Hiatal **Sliding**—Protrusion of an abdominal structure (usually stomach) through esophageal hiatus	**Symptoms**—Dysphagia, growth failure, vomiting, neck contortions, frequent unexplained respiratory problems, bleeding; usually associated with GER; may cause gastric volvulus and obstruction **Diagnosis**—Made by fluoroscopy	**Therapeutic:** Manage GER symptoms; provide patient positioning, pharmacologic treatment, and dietary management. Surgical treatment is necessary when complications are related to GER despite medical management. **Nursing:** Be alert to significant signs and carry out routine postoperative care.
Abdominal **Umbilical**—Weakness in abdominal wall around umbilicus; incomplete closure of abdominal wall, allowing intestinal contents to protrude through opening	**Symptoms**—Noted by inspection and palpation of the abdomen High incidence in preterm and African-American infants Usually closes spontaneously by 1–2 years of age	**Therapeutic:** No treatment is necessary for small defects. Operative repair if persists to age 4–6 years or if defect is >1.5–2.0 cm by age 2 years; cosmetic repair in some cases. Strangulation requires immediate attention. **Nursing:** Discourage use of home remedies (e.g., belly bands, coins). Reassure parents.

CDH, Congenital diaphragmatic hernia; *ECMO*, extracorporeal membrane oxygenation; *GER*, gastroesophageal reflux; *GI*, gastrointestinal; *IV*, intravenous; *NG*, nasogastric.
*Some experts advocate for permissive hypercapnia and mild acidosis during acute phase of illness.

Pathophysiology

The circular muscle of the pylorus thickens as a result of hypertrophy (increased size) and hyperplasia (increased mass). This produces severe narrowing of the pyloric canal between the stomach and the duodenum, causing partial obstruction of the lumen (Fig. 24-5, *A*). Over time, inflammation and edema further reduce the size of the opening, resulting in complete obstruction. The hypertrophied pylorus may be palpable as an olivelike mass in the upper abdomen. Pyloric stenosis is not a congenital disorder. Substantial evidence supports decreased expression of neuronal nitric oxide synthase in the nerve fibers of the

TABLE 24-11   ABDOMINAL WALL DEFECTS

DEFECT	SYMPTOMS	NURSING MANAGEMENT
Omphalocele Protrusion of intraabdominal viscera into base of umbilical cord; sac covered with peritoneum without skin	Usually obvious on inspection; however, small omphalocele may appear to be a hematoma in umbilical cord Observe for associated congenital malformations	**Therapeutic:** Surgical repair of defect **Nursing:** *Preoperative:* Protect defect from trauma or drying. Keep sac or viscera moist with saline-soaked dressings. Maintain thermoregulation. Carry out routine care of IV fluid infusion. Administer prophylactic antibiotics as prescribed. Provide nasogastric suction for gastric decompression. Keep patient NPO. Assess for associated birth defects such as CL or CP. *Postoperative:* Monitor vital signs and BP. Pain management Bowel decompression—NG tube IV fluid intake Monitor return of bowel function.
Gastroschisis Protrusion of intraabdominal contents through defect in abdominal wall lateral to umbilical ring; there is no peritoneal sac covering the exposed bowel	Defect obvious at delivery if not detected prenatally by ultrasonography	**Therapeutic:** Surgical repair of defect. For large lesions, provide gradual reduction of abdominal contents via Siloh pouch before surgical closure. **Nursing:** *Preoperative:* Keep sac covered with a bowel bag to prevent trauma, drying of viscera. NG decompression Maintain thermoregulation. Monitor electrolyte status. Administer IV fluids. Administer antibiotics. Observe exposed bowel for signs of necrosis or constriction at exit site. *Postoperative:* Monitor vital signs and BP. Bowel decompression with NG tube IV fluids Pain management Monitor surgical closure site (if bowel reduced) for infection. Monitor lower extremities for pulses and circulation (in case of vena cava compression by large bowel in small abdominal cavity). Monitor for return of bowel function and peristalsis. In event of Siloh pouch, nursing care should also include monitoring vital signs, keeping pouch clean, and aseptic technique with dressing changes (if not done by surgeon). Monitor lower extremities for circulation (as above). Provide emotional support for parents. Long-term problems associated with feeding and weight gain for gastroschisis and large omphalocele.

BP, Blood pressure; *CL,* cleft lip; *CP,* cleft palate; *IV,* intravenous; *NG,* nasogastric; *NPO,* nothing by mouth.

pyloric circular muscle in infants with HPS (Hunter and Liacouras, 2011). In most cases, HPS is an isolated lesion; however, it may be associated with intestinal malrotation, esophageal and duodenal atresia, and anorectal anomalies. HPS has also been linked to the administration of erythromycin in the first few weeks of life as well as eosinophilic gastroenteritis, Apert syndrome, Cornelia de Lange syndrome, Zellweger syndrome, trisomy 18, and Smith-Lemli-Opitz syndrome (Hunter and Liacouras, 2011).

Diagnostic Evaluation

The diagnosis of HPS is often made after the history and physical examination. The olivelike mass is easily palpated when the stomach is empty, the infant is quiet, and the abdominal muscles are relaxed. Vomiting usually occurs 30 to 60 minutes after feeding and becomes projectile as the obstruction progresses. Emesis is nonbilious, usually consisting of stale milk. These infants may become dehydrated and appear malnourished if an early diagnosis is not established.

BOX 24-10   CLINICAL MANIFESTATIONS OF INTESTINAL OBSTRUCTION

Colicky abdominal pain—From peristalsis attempting to overcome the obstruction

Abdominal distention—As a result of accumulation of gas and fluid above the level of the obstruction

Vomiting—Often the earliest sign of a high obstruction; a later sign of lower obstruction (may be bilious or feculent)

Constipation and obstipation—Early signs of low obstructions; later signs of higher obstructions

Dehydration—From losses of large quantities of fluid and electrolytes into the intestine

Rigid and boardlike abdomen—From increased distention

Bowel sounds—Gradually diminish and cease

Respiratory distress—Occurs as the diaphragm is pushed up into the pleural cavity

Shock—Caused by plasma volume diminishing as fluids and electrolytes are lost from the bloodstream into the intestinal lumen

Sepsis—Caused by bacterial proliferation with invasion into the circulation

BOX 24-11   CLINICAL MANIFESTATIONS OF HYPERTROPHIC PYLORIC STENOSIS

Projectile vomiting
- May be ejected 3 to 4 feet from the child when in a side-lying position or 1 foot or more when in a supine position
- Usually occurs shortly after a feeding but may not occur for several hours
- May occur after each feeding or appear intermittently
- Nonbilious vomitus that may be blood tinged

Infant hungry, avid feeder; eagerly accepts a second feeding after vomiting episode

No evidence of pain or discomfort except that of chronic hunger

Weight loss or failure to gain weight

Signs of dehydration

Distended upper abdomen

Readily palpable olive-shaped tumor in the epigastrium just to the right of the umbilicus

Visible gastric peristaltic waves that move from left to right across the epigastrium

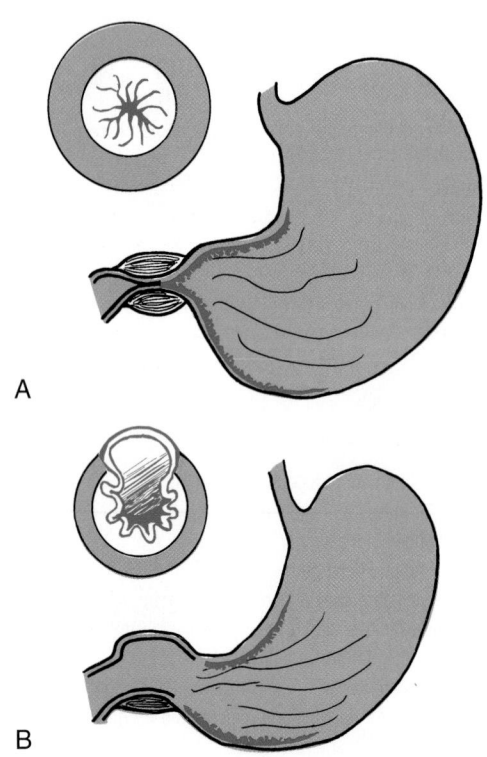

FIG 24-5 Hypertrophic pyloric stenosis. **A,** Enlarged muscular area nearly obliterates the pyloric channel. **B,** Longitudinal surgical division of the muscle down to the submucosa establishes an adequate passageway.

If the diagnosis is inconclusive from the history and physical signs (Box 24-11), ultrasonography will demonstrate an elongated, sausage-shaped mass with an elongated pyloric channel. If ultrasonography fails to demonstrate a hypertrophied pylorus, an upper GI radiography should be done to rule out other causes of vomiting. Laboratory findings reflect the metabolic alterations (hypochloremic metabolic alkalosis) created by severe depletion of both fluid and electrolytes and hydrogen ions from extensive and prolonged vomiting. Hyperbilirubinemia (unconjugated) may also be present and often resolves after surgical correction of the obstruction occurs (Hunter and Liacouras, 2011).

Therapeutic Management

Surgical relief of the pyloric obstruction by pyloromyotomy is the standard therapy for this disorder. Preoperatively, the infant must be rehydrated and metabolic alkalosis corrected with parenteral fluid and electrolyte administration. Replacement fluid therapy usually delays surgery for 24 to 48 hours. The stomach is decompressed with an NG tube. In infants with no evidence of fluid and electrolyte imbalance, surgery is performed without delay.

The surgical procedure is often performed by laparoscope and consists of a longitudinal incision through the circular muscle fibers of the pylorus down to, but not including, the submucosa (pyloromyotomy, sometimes called Fredet-Ramstedt procedure) (Fig. 24-5, *B*). The procedure has a high success rate. Laparoscopic surgery through a single small incision often results in a shorter surgical time, more rapid postoperative feeding, and shorter hospital stay (Sola and Neville, 2009).

Feedings are usually begun 4 to 6 hours postoperatively, beginning with small, frequent feedings of an electrolyte solution such as Pedialyte or sterile water. If clear fluids are retained, about 24 hours after surgery formula is started in the same small increments. The amount and the interval between feedings are gradually increased until a full feeding schedule is reinstated, which usually takes about 48 hours.

Prognosis

Most infants recover completely and rapidly after pyloromyotomy. Postoperative complications include persistent pyloric obstruction and, rarely, wound dehiscence.

Nursing Care Management

The diagnosis of HPS is considered in very young infants who appear alert but fail to gain weight and have a history of vomiting after feedings. Assessment is based on observation of eating behaviors and evidence of other characteristic clinical manifestations.

Preoperative Care

Preoperatively, the emphasis is placed on restoring hydration and electrolyte balance. Infants are usually given no oral feedings and receive IV fluids with glucose and electrolyte replacement based on laboratory serum electrolyte values and clinical appearance.

Observations also include assessment of vital signs, particularly those that might indicate fluid or electrolyte imbalances. These infants are prone to metabolic alkalosis from loss of hydrogen ions and to potassium, sodium, and chloride depletion. The skin, mucous membranes, and daily weight are assessed for alterations in hydration status and water gain or loss.

If stomach decompression is used preoperatively, the nurse is responsible for ensuring that the tube is patent and functioning properly and for measuring and recording the type and amount of drainage. Parental involvement is encouraged and promoted.

Postoperative Care

Postoperative vomiting is common, and most infants, even with successful surgery, exhibit some vomiting during the first 24 to 48 hours. IV fluids are administered until the infant is taking and retaining adequate amounts by mouth. Much of the same care that was instituted before surgery is continued postoperatively, including observation of vital signs, monitoring of IV fluids, and careful monitoring of fluid intake and output. In addition, the infant is observed for responses to the stress of surgery and for evidence of pain. Appropriate analgesics should be given around the clock because pain is continuous. The surgical incision(s) is inspected for drainage or erythema, and any signs of infection are reported to the surgeon. A surgical adhesive may be used for incision closure, and parents are instructed regarding the care of the incision and any dressings before discharge.

Feedings are usually instituted soon after surgery, beginning with clear liquids advancing to formula or breast milk as tolerated. Observation and recording of feedings and the infant's responses to feedings are a vital part of postoperative care. Care of the operative site consists of observation for any drainage or signs of inflammation and care of the incision.

Parents are encouraged to remain with their child and become involved in the child's care. Vomiting of a projectile nature is frightening to parents, and they often believe that they may have done something wrong or that surgery was not successful. Most parents need support and reassurance that the condition is caused by a structural problem and is in no way a reflection on their parenting skills and capacities.

INTUSSUSCEPTION

Intussusception is the most common cause of intestinal obstruction in children between the ages of 3 months and 3 years (Waseem and Rosenberg, 2008). Intussusception is more common in boys than in girls and is more common in children with cystic fibrosis. Although specific intestinal lesions occur in a small percentage of the children, generally the cause is not known. More than 90% of intussusceptions do not have a pathologic lead point, such as a polyp, lymphoma, or Meckel diverticulum. The idiopathic cases may be caused by hypertrophy of intestinal lymphoid tissue secondary to viral infection

Pathophysiology

Intussusception occurs when one segment of the bowel telescopes into another segment, pulling the mesentery with it. The mesentery is compressed and angled, resulting in lymphatic and venous obstruction. As the edema from the obstruction increases, pressure within the area of intussusception increases. When the pressure equals the arterial

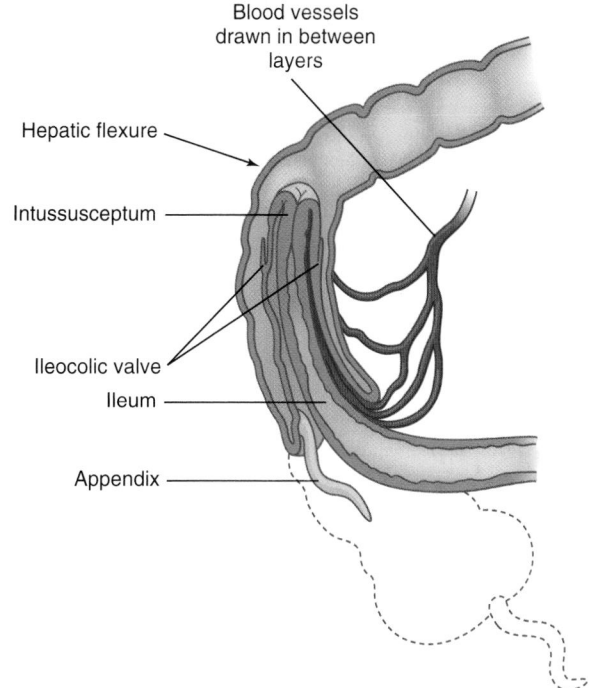

FIG 24-6 Ileocecal intussusception.

pressure, arterial blood flow stops, resulting in ischemia and the pouring of mucus into the intestine. Venous engorgement also leads to leaking of blood and mucus into the intestinal lumen, forming the classic currant jelly–like stools. The most common site is the ileocecal valve (ileocolic), where the ileum invaginates into the cecum and then further into the colon (Fig. 24-6). Other forms include ileoileal (one part of the ileum invaginates into another section of the ileum) and colocolic (one part of the colon invaginates into another area of the colon) intussusceptions, usually in the area of the hepatic or splenic flexure or at some point along the transverse colon.

> **! NURSING ALERT**
>
> The classic triad of intussusception symptoms (abdominal pain, abdominal mass, bloody stools) is present in fewer than 15% of children (Chu and Liacouras, 2011). Children might also be initially seen with screaming, irritability, lethargy, vomiting, diarrhea or constipation, fever, dehydration, and shock. Because intussusception is potentially life threatening, the nurse should be aware of alternate presentations, observe these children closely, and refer them for further evaluation.

Diagnostic Evaluation

Frequently, subjective findings lead to the diagnosis (Box 24-12), which can be confirmed by ultrasonography. Spontaneous reduction occurs in up to 10% of patients.

Therapeutic Management

Conservative treatment consists of radiologist-guided pneumoenema (air enema) with or without water-soluble contrast or ultrasound-guided hydrostatic (saline) enema, the advantage of the latter being that no ionizing radiation is needed (Huppertz, Soriano-Gabarro, Grimprel, and others, 2006). Recurrence of intussusception after conservative treatment is uncommon. Herwig, Brenkert, and Losek (2009) found that hospitalized children needed minimal interventions after undergoing enema-reduced intussusception.

BOX 24-12   **CLINICAL MANIFESTATIONS OF INTUSSUSCEPTION**

Sudden acute abdominal pain
Child screaming and drawing the knees onto the chest
Child appearing normal and comfortable between episodes of pain
Vomiting
Lethargy
Passage of red, currant jelly–like stools (stool mixed with blood and mucus)
Tender, distended abdomen
Palpable sausage-shaped mass in upper right quadrant
Empty lower right quadrant (Dance sign)
Eventual fever, prostration, and other signs of peritonitis

Intravenous fluids, NG decompression, and antibiotic therapy may be used before hydrostatic reduction is attempted. If these procedures are not successful, the child may require surgical intervention. Surgery involves manually reducing the invagination and, when indicated, resecting any nonviable intestine. Laparoscopic surgical repair is commonly performed.

Prognosis

Nonoperative reduction is successful in approximately 80% of cases (Huppertz, Soriano-Gabarro, Grimprel, and others, 2006). Surgery is required for patients in whom the nonoperative reduction is unsuccessful. With early diagnosis and treatment, serious complications and death are uncommon.

Nursing Care Management

The nurse can help establish a diagnosis by listening to the parent's description of the child's physical and behavioral symptoms. It is not unusual for parents to state that they thought something was seriously wrong before others shared their concerns. The description of the child's severe colicky abdominal pain combined with vomiting is a significant sign of intussusception.

As soon as a possible diagnosis of intussusception is made, the nurse prepares the parents for the immediate need for hospitalization, the nonsurgical technique of hydrostatic reduction, and the possibility of surgery. It is important to explain the basic defect of intussusception. A model of the defect is easily demonstrated by pushing the end of a finger on a rubber glove back into itself or using the example of a telescoping rod. The principle of reduction by hydrostatic pressure can be simulated by filling the glove with water, which pushes the "finger" into a fully extended position.

Physical care of the child does not differ from that for any child undergoing abdominal surgery. Even though nonsurgical intervention may be successful, the usual preoperative procedures, such as maintenance of NPO status, routine laboratory testing (CBC and urinalysis), signed parental consent, and preanesthetic sedation, are performed. For the child with signs of electrolyte imbalance, hemorrhage, or peritonitis, additional preparation, such as replacement fluids, whole blood or plasma, and NG suctioning, may be needed. Before surgery, the nurse monitors all stools.

! **NURSING ALERT**

Passage of a normal brown stool usually indicates that the intussusception has reduced itself. This is immediately reported to the practitioner, who may choose to alter the diagnostic and therapeutic care plan.

Postprocedural care includes observations of vital signs, blood pressure, intact sutures and dressing, and the return of bowel sounds. After spontaneous or hydrostatic reduction, the nurse observes for passage of water-soluble contrast material (if used) and the stool patterns because the intussusception may recur. Children may be admitted to the hospital or monitored on an outpatient basis. A recurrence of intussusception is treated with the conservative reduction techniques described above, but a laparotomy is considered for multiple recurrences.

Because hospitalization may be the child's first separation from the parents, it is important to preserve the parent–child relationship by encouraging rooming-in or extended visiting. It may be the parents' first experience with hospitalization, necessitating their preparation for procedures such as IV therapy, frequent vital sign and blood pressure monitoring, dressings, and NPO status. More commonly, the child may be seen in the emergency department and treatment initiated there with eventual discharge home in uncomplicated cases (Gilmore, Reed, and Tenenbein, 2011). Because of the rapidity of the onset, diagnosis, and treatment, parents may feel stunned or numb. They may ask few questions, or they may constantly make inquiries, sometimes the same ones several times. Because of the circumstances surrounding this condition, be accepting and understanding of the parents' reactions.

MALROTATION AND VOLVULUS

Malrotation of the intestine is caused by the abnormal rotation of the intestine around the superior mesenteric artery during embryologic development. Malrotation may manifest in utero or may be asymptomatic throughout life. Infants may have intermittent bilious vomiting, RAP, distention, or lower GI bleeding. Malrotation is the most serious type of intestinal obstruction because, if the intestine undergoes complete volvulus (the intestine twisting around itself), compromise of the blood supply will result in intestinal necrosis, peritonitis, perforation, and death.

Diagnostic Evaluation

It is imperative that malrotation and volvulus be diagnosed promptly and surgical treatment instituted quickly. An upper GI series is the definitive procedure to diagnose this condition.

Therapeutic Management

Surgery is indicated to remove the affected area. Because of the extensive nature of some lesions, short-gut syndrome is a postoperative complication.

Nursing Care Management

Preoperatively, the nursing care is the same as that provided to an infant or child with intestinal obstruction. Postoperatively, the nursing care is similar to that provided to the infant or child who has undergone abdominal surgery.

ANORECTAL MALFORMATIONS

Anorectal malformations are among the more common congenital malformations caused by abnormal development, with an incidence of approximately 1 in 5000 births (Levitt and Peña, 2007). These malformations may range from simple anal stenosis to include other associated complex anomalies of genitourinary (GU) and pelvic organs, which may require extensive treatment for fecal, urinary, and sexual function. Anorectal malformations may occur in isolation or as a part of the VACTERL association (see p. 803). These anomalies are classified according to the newborn's gender and abnormal anatomic features, including GU defects.

The anus and rectum originate from an embryologic structure called the cloaca. Lateral growth of the cloaca forms the urorectal septum that separates the rectum dorsally from the urinary tract ventrally. The rectum and urinary tract separate completely by the seventh week of gestation. Anomalies that occur reflect the stage of development of these processes.

Rectal atresia and stenosis occur when the anal opening appears normal, there is a midline intergluteal groove, and usually no fistula exists between the rectum and urinary tract. Rectal atresia is a complete obstruction (inability to pass stool) and requires immediate surgical intervention. Rectal stenosis may not become apparent until later in infancy when the infant has a history of difficult stooling, abdominal distention, and ribbonlike stools.

A persistent cloaca is a complex anorectal malformation in which the rectum, vagina, and urethra drain into a common channel opening into the perineum (Fig. 24-7, A).

Imperforate anus includes several forms of malformation without an obvious opening (Fig. 24-7, B). Frequently, a fistula (an abnormal communication) leads from the distal rectum to the perineum or GU system (Fig. 24-8, A, B, and C). The fistula may be evidenced when meconium is evacuated through the vaginal opening, the perineum below the vagina, the male urethra, or the perineum under the scrotum. The presence of meconium on the perineum does not indicate anal patency. A fistula may not be apparent at birth, but as peristalsis increases, meconium is forced through the fistula into the urethra or onto the newborn's perineum.

Anorectal anomalies are classified according to gender and abnormal anatomic features, including GU and associated pelvic anomalies (Box 24-13). The classification of high, intermediate, and low may also be used; the level of rectal descent is determined by the relationship of the termination of the bowel to the puborectalis sling of the levator ani musculature. About 50% of children with anorectal anomalies have a urologic problem.

Diagnostic Evaluation

The diagnosis of an anorectal malformation is based on the physical finding of an absent anal opening. Other symptoms may include abdominal distention, vomiting, absence of meconium passage, or presence of meconium in the urine. Additional physical findings with an anorectal malformation are a flat perineum and the absence of a midline intergluteal groove. The appearance of the perineum alone does not accurately predict the extent of the defect and associated

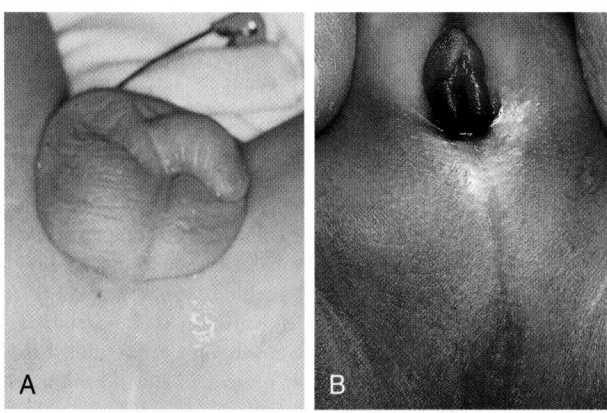

FIG 24-7 **A,** No visible external opening forms in high imperforate anus defect. Absence of the intergluteal cleft is also common, frequently associated with sacral agenesis. **B,** Imperforate anus in a girl, commonly associated with cloaca anomaly, which manifests as a single perineal opening on the perineum. (From Zitelli BJ, McIntire SC, Nowalk AJ: *Zitelli and Davis' atlas of pediatric physical diagnosis*, ed 6, St. Louis 2012, Saunders.)

BOX 24-13   CLASSIFICATION OF ANORECTAL MALFORMATIONS

Male Defects
Perineal fistula
Rectourethral bulbar fistula
Rectourethral prostatic fistula
Rectovesicular (bladder neck) fistula
Imperforate anus without fistula
Rectal atresia and stenosis

Female Defects
Perineal fistula
Vestibular fistula
Imperforate anus without fistula
Rectal atresia and stenosis
Cloaca

From Peña A, Hong A: Advances in the management of anorectal malformations, *Am J Surg* 180(5):370–376, 2000.

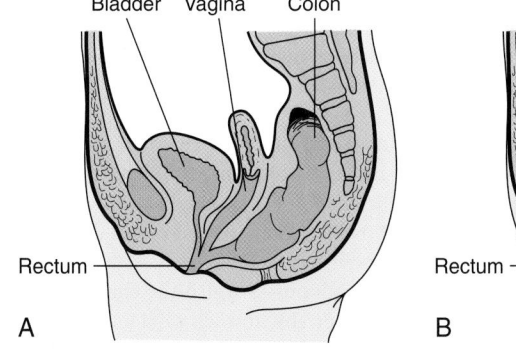
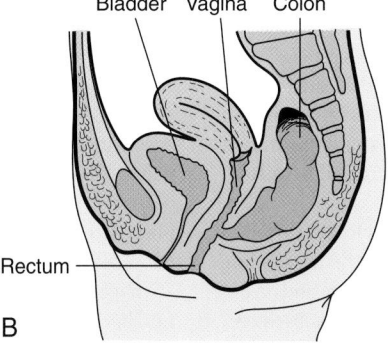
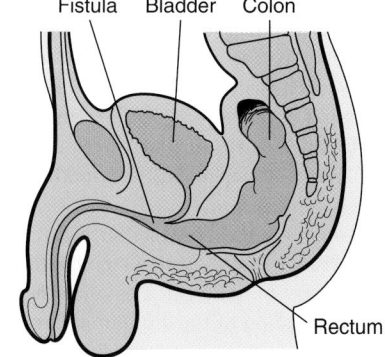

FIG 24-8 Anorectal malformations. **A,** Typical cloaca (female). **B,** Low rectovaginal fistula (female). **C,** Rectourethral bulbar fistula (male)

anomalies. GU and spinal-vertebral anomalies associated with anorectal malformations should be considered when an anomaly is noted. EA with or without TEF, cardiac defects, and neural tube defects or vertebral anomalies may occur in association with anorectal malformations, and the infant should be carefully evaluated for the presence of these and other anomalies.

A perineal fistula may be diagnosed by clinical observation. The presence of a prominent anal dimple and a band of skin tissue commonly known as a bucket handle is indicative of a perineal fistula (Levitt and Peña, 2007). Abdominal and pelvic ultrasonography is performed to further evaluate the infant's anatomic malformation. An IV pyelogram and a voiding cystourethrogram are performed to evaluate associated anomalies involving the urinary tract. Other diagnostic examinations that may be performed include pelvic magnetic resonance imaging, radiography, ultrasonography, and fluoroscopic examination of pelvic anatomic contents and lower spinal anatomy.

Therapeutic Management

The primary management of anorectal malformations is surgical. After the defect has been identified, take steps to rule out associated life-threatening defects, which need immediate surgical intervention. Provided no immediate life-threatening problems exist, the newborn is stabilized and kept NPO for further evaluation. IV fluids are provided to maintain glucose and fluid and electrolyte balance. The current recommendation is that surgery be delayed at least 24 hours to properly evaluate for the presence of a fistula and possibly other anomalies (Levitt and Peña, 2007).

The surgical treatment of anorectal malformations varies according to the defect but usually involves one or possibly a combination of several of the following procedures: anoplasty, colostomy, posterior sagittal anorectoplasty (PSARP) or other pull-through with colostomy, and colostomy (take-down) closure. The Nursing Care Management discussion below outlines some aspects of preoperative and postoperative care.

A primary laparoscopic repair (without colostomy) of anorectal malformations is being performed successfully in some centers. This minimizes surgical risks, associated morbidity, and postoperative pain management.

Nursing Care Management

The first nursing responsibility is assisting in identification of anorectal malformations. A newborn who does not pass stool within 24 hours after birth or has meconium that appears at a location other than the anal opening requires further assessment. Preoperative care includes diagnostic evaluation, GI decompression, bowel preparation, and IV fluids.

For the newborn with a perineal fistula, an anoplasty is performed, which involves moving the fistula opening to the center of the sphincter and enlarging the rectal opening. Postoperative nursing care after anoplasty is primarily directed toward healing the surgical site without other complications. A program of anal dilations is usually initiated when the child returns for the 2-week check-up. Feedings are started soon after surgical repair, and breastfeeding is encouraged because it causes less constipation.

In neonates with anomalies such as cloaca (girls), rectourethral prostatic fistula (boys), and vestibular fistula (girls), a descending colostomy may be performed to allow fecal elimination and avoid fecal contamination of the distal imperforate section and subsequent urinary tract infection in infants with urorectal fistulas. With a colostomy, postoperative nursing care is directed toward maintaining appropriate skin care at the stoma sites (both distal and proximal),

managing postoperative pain, and administering IV fluids and antibiotics. In some centers, this condition is treated surgically when the child is stable and an adequate weight gain is observed; a descending colostomy may not be performed in such cases. Postoperative NG decompression may be required with laparotomy, and nursing care focuses on maintenance of appropriate drainage. (See Chapter 22 for colostomy care.)

The PSARP is a common surgical procedure for the repair of anorectal malformations in infants approximately 1 to 2 months after the initial colostomy. Preoperative PSARP care often involves irrigation of the distal stoma to prevent fecal contamination of the operative site. During this time, parents must be given accurate yet simple information regarding the infant's appearance postoperatively and expectations as to their level of involvement in the child's care.

In the PSARP procedure, the repair is made via a posterior midline sacral approach to dissect the different muscle groups involved without damaging strategic innervation of pelvic structures so that optimum postoperative bowel continence is achieved. A laparotomy may be required if the rectum is unidentifiable by the posterior approach. Additional management after successful repair involves a program of anal dilations, colostomy closure, and a bowel management program.

Parents are instructed in perineal and wound care or care of the colostomy as needed. Anal dilations may be necessary for some infants. Parents should observe stooling patterns and observe for signs of anal stricture or complications. Information on dietary modifications and administration of medications is included in counseling. Nurses have a vital role in helping families of a child with an anorectal malformation provide optimum care so that bowel management is successful and quality of life enhanced for the child and family.

Family Support, Discharge Planning, and Home Care

Long-term follow-up is important for children with complex malformations. After the definitive pull-through procedure, toilet training is delayed, and complete continence is seldom achieved at the usual age of 2 to 3 years. Prevention of constipation is important, and breastfeeding is encouraged postoperatively. If a cow's milk–based formula is used, a mild laxative may be prescribed. Bowel habit training, diet modification, and administration of stool softeners or fiber are important aspects of bowel management. Optimum bowel function may not be achieved until late childhood or adolescence. Support and reassurance are important during the slow progression to normal function.

Parents are instructed in perineal and wound care or care of the colostomy. Parents are advised to observe stooling patterns and notify the physician if there are any signs of anal stricture or complications.

MALABSORPTION SYNDROMES

Chronic diarrhea and malabsorption of nutrients characterize malabsorption syndromes. An important complication of malabsorption syndromes in children is growth failure. Most cases are classified according to the location of the supposed anatomic or biochemical defect. The term celiac disease is often used to describe a symptom complex with four characteristics: (1) steatorrhea (fatty, foul, frothy, bulky stools), (2) general malnutrition, (3) abdominal distention, and (4) secondary vitamin deficiencies.

Digestive defects are conditions in which the enzymes necessary for digestion are diminished or absent, such as (1) cystic fibrosis, in which pancreatic enzymes are absent; (2) biliary or liver disease, in which bile flow is affected; or (3) lactase deficiency, in which there is congenital or secondary lactose intolerance.

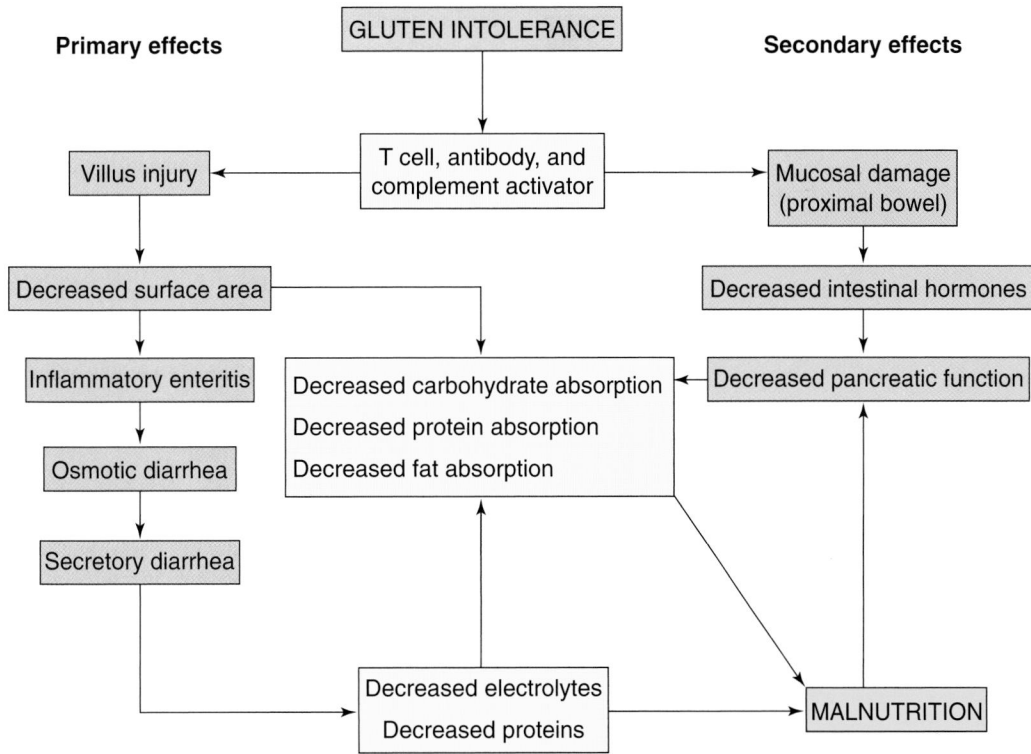

FIG 24-9 Pathophysiology of gluten-sensitive enteropathy.

Absorptive defects are conditions in which the intestinal mucosal transport system is impaired. This may occur because of a primary defect (e.g., celiac disease) or secondary to inflammatory disease of the bowel that results in impaired absorption because bowel motility is accelerated (e.g., UC). Obstructive disorders (e.g., HD) also cause secondary malabsorption from enterocolitis.

Anatomic defects, such as extensive resection of the bowel or **short-bowel syndrome (SBS)**, affect digestion by decreasing the transit time of substances and affect absorption by severely compromising the absorptive surface.

CELIAC DISEASE (GLUTEN-SENSITIVE ENTEROPATHY)

Celiac disease, also known as gluten-induced enteropathy, gluten-sensitive enteropathy, and celiac sprue, is a permanent intestinal intolerance to dietary wheat gliadin and related proteins that produces mucosal lesions in genetically susceptible individuals. It is second only to cystic fibrosis as a cause of malabsorption in children.

The incidence is variable and has been reported in 1 in 3000 to 1 in 4000 people. The disease is seen more frequently in Europe than in the United States. It is more prevalent in women than men and is rarely reported in Asians or African Americans. Although the exact cause is unknown, it is now generally accepted that celiac disease is an immunologically mediated small intestine enteropathy. The mucosal lesions contain features that suggest both humoral and cell-mediated immunologic overstimulation.

Pathophysiology

Celiac disease is characterized by villous atrophy in the small bowel in response to the protein gluten (Maki and Lohi, 2004). Gluten is found in wheat, barley, rye, and oat grains. When individuals are unable to digest the gliadin component of gluten, an accumulation of a toxic substance that is damaging to the mucosal cells occurs. Damage to the mucosa of the small intestine leads to villous atrophy, hyperplasia of the crypts, and infiltration of the epithelial cells with lymphocytes. Villous atrophy leads to malabsorption caused by the reduced absorptive surface area.

Genetic predisposition is an essential factor in the development of celiac disease. Membrane receptors involved in preferential antigen presentation to CD4+ T cells play a crucial role in the immune response characteristic of celiac disease. Genes located on the HLA region of chromosome 6, namely *HLA-DQ2* or *HLA-DQ8*, are found in almost 100% of those affected with celiac disease (Murdock and Johnston, 2005). When the inflammatory reaction is activated by gluten, CD4+ T cells produce cytokines, which are likely to contribute to the intestinal damage. The damage consists of infiltration of the lamina propria, crypt hyperplasia, and villous atrophy and flattening. With sufficient villous atrophy, malabsorption occurs (Fig. 24-9).

Classic symptoms of celiac disease are GI manifestations usually noted several months after the introduction of gluten-containing grains into the diet, typically between the ages of 6 months and 2 years (Box 24-14). Typically, children are seen with impaired growth, chronic diarrhea, abdominal distention, muscle wasting with hypotonia, poor appetite, and lack of energy. The clinical manifestations are usually insidious and chronic. The first evidence may be growth failure and diarrhea. Less typical presentation has been observed in children ages 5 to 7 years who have abdominal pain; nausea; vomiting; bloating; constipation; or extraintestinal manifestations, including iron deficiency anemia, short stature, pubertal delay, dental enamel defects, alopecia, and abnormal LFT results. Older children have been found to have osteoporosis. Untreated celiac disease can evolve into

BOX 24-14 CLINICAL MANIFESTATIONS OF CELIAC DISEASE

Impaired Fat Absorption
Steatorrhea (excessively large, pale, oily, frothy stools)
Exceedingly foul-smelling stools

Impaired Nutrient Absorption
Malnutrition
Muscle wasting (especially prominent in legs and buttocks)
Anemia
Anorexia
Abdominal distention

Behavioral Changes
Irritability
Uncooperativeness
Apathy

Celiac Crisis*
Acute, severe episodes of profuse watery diarrhea and vomiting
May be precipitated by:
• Infections (especially gastrointestinal)
• Prolonged fluid and electrolyte depletion
• Emotional disturbance

*In very young children.

celiac crisis, characterized by abdominal distention, explosive watery diarrhea, and dehydration with electrolyte imbalance, leading to hypotensive shock and lethargy.

Diagnostic Evaluation

The diagnosis of celiac disease is based on a biopsy of the small intestine demonstrating the characteristic changes of villous atrophy with hyperplasia of the crypts and abnormal surface epithelium while the patient is eating adequate amounts of gluten and a full clinical remission after gluten is withdrawn (Branski and Troncone, 2011; Dieterich, Esslinger, and Schuppan, 2003). Within 1 or 2 days of instituting the diet, most children with celiac disease demonstrate a favorable response, including weight gain and improved appetite. Within a few weeks, there is resolution of the diarrhea and steatorrhea.

Commercially available serologic tests for celiac disease include antigliadin antibodies of both the immunoglobulin A and G classes (IgA and IgG); antiendomysium IgA; and antitissue transglutaminase IgA (anti-TG2) and IgG antibodies for screening first-degree relatives of known celiac disease patients and those with known celiac disease–associated disorders such as type 1 diabetes, thyroiditis, arthritis, primary biliary cirrhosis, Down syndrome, Turner syndrome, Williams syndrome, and osteopenia or osteoporosis. False-positive results are likely when only one serologic test is used because patients with these disorders can also test positive for these antibodies. Use of more than one test increases diagnostic accuracy (Gelfond and Fasano, 2006). Ruling out total IgA deficiency is necessary to minimize false-negative results.

Therapeutic Management

Treatment of patients with chronic celiac disease is primarily dietary. Although the diet is called "gluten free," it is actually *low* in gluten because it is impossible to remove every source of this protein. Because gluten is found primarily in the grains of wheat and rye but also in smaller quantities in barley and oats, these four foods are eliminated. Corn and rice become substitute grain foods.

Children with untreated celiac disease may have lactose intolerance, especially if their mucosal lesions are extensive. Lactose intolerance usually improves as the mucosa heals with gluten withdrawal. Specific nutritional deficiencies, such as iron, folic acid, and fat-soluble vitamin deficiencies, are treated with appropriate supplements.

Prognosis

Celiac disease is regarded as a chronic disease. The most severe symptoms usually occur in early childhood and again in adult life. Strict dietary avoidance of gluten prevents symptoms and may minimize the risk of developing lymphoma, especially of the small intestine, the most serious complication of the disease.

Nursing Care Management

The main nursing consideration is helping the child adhere to the dietary regimen. This requires a wheat-, barley-, and rye-free diet; oats may be safe for most patients but contamination with other gluten products may occur in harvesting; therefore, caution should be exercised with oats. Children who have silent celiac disease, without clinical manifestations, should also adhere to a strict gluten-free diet (Branski and Troncone, 2011). Considerable time is involved in explaining the disease process to the child and parents, the specific role of gluten in aggravating the disorder, and the foods that must be restricted. It is difficult to maintain a diet indefinitely when the child has no symptoms and temporary transgressions result in no difficulties. However, the majority of individuals who relax their diet will experience a relapse of their disease and possibly exhibit growth restriction, anemia, or osteomalacia. There is also the risk of developing malignant lymphoma of the small intestine or other GI malignancies.

Although the chief source of gluten is cereal and baked goods, grains are frequently added to processed foods as thickeners or fillers. To compound the difficulty, gluten is added to many foods as hydrolyzed vegetable protein, which is derived from cereal grains. The nurse must advise parents of the necessity of reading all label ingredients carefully to avoid hidden sources of gluten.

Many of children's favorite foods contain gluten, including bread, cake, cookies, crackers, donuts, pies, spaghetti, pizza, prepared soups, some processed ice cream, many types of chocolate candy, milk preparations such as malts, hot dogs, luncheon meats, meat gravy, and some prepared hamburgers. Many of these products can be eliminated from an infant's or young child's diet fairly easily, but monitoring the diet of a school-age child or adolescent is more difficult. Luncheon preparation away from home is particularly difficult because bread, luncheon meats, and instant soups are not allowed. For families on restricted food budgets, the diet adds an additional financial burden because many inexpensive and convenient foods cannot be used.

In addition to restricting gluten, other dietary alterations may be necessary. For example, in some children who have more severe mucosal damage, the digestion of disaccharides is impaired, especially in relation to lactose. Therefore, these children often need a temporarily lactose-free diet, which necessitates eliminating all milk products. In general, dietary management includes a diet high in calories and proteins with simple carbohydrates such as fruits and vegetables but low in fats. Because the bowel is inflamed as a result of the pathologic processes in absorption, the child must avoid high-fiber foods, such as nuts, raisins, raw vegetables, and raw fruits with skin, until inflammation has subsided.

It is important to stress long-range complications and to remind parents of the child's physical status before dietary treatment and the dramatic improvement after treatment. The nurse can be instrumental in allowing the child to express concerns and frustration while focusing on ways in which the child can still feel normal. Encourage the child and parents to find new recipes using suitable ingredients, such as Mexican or Chinese dishes that use corn or rice. Consult a registered dietitian to provide children and their families with detailed dietary instructions and education.*

Several resources are available to assist children and parents in all aspects of coping with celiac disease. The Celiac Sprue Association/United States of America† provides support and guidance to families and supplies educational materials concerning a gluten-free diet, food sources, recipes, and travel information.

SHORT-BOWEL SYNDROME

Short-bowel syndrome is a malabsorptive disorder that occurs as a result of decreased mucosal surface area, usually because of extensive resection of the small intestine. Malabsorption may be exacerbated by other factors, such as bacterial overgrowth and dysmotility. The most common causes of SBS in children are necrotizing enterocolitis, volvulus, jejunal atresias, and gastroschisis. Other causes include midgut volvulus and diffuse small bowel CD in older children. Less frequent causes include trauma to the GI tract and total colonic aganglionosis (HD) with extension into the small bowel.

The definition of SBS includes two important findings: (1) decreased intestinal surface area for absorption of fluid, electrolytes, and nutrients; and (2) a need for PN (Goday, 2009). The prognosis for infants with SBS has improved dramatically in the past 20 to 30 years as a result of advances in PN and enteral feeding.

Therapeutic Management

The goals of therapy for infants and children with SBS include (1) preserve as much length of bowel as possible during surgery; (2) maintain optimum nutritional status, growth, and development while intestinal adaptation occurs; (3) stimulate intestinal adaptation with enteral feeding; and (4) minimize complications related to the disease process and therapy (Goday, 2009).

Nutritional support is the long-term focus of care for children with SBS (Sadlier, 2008). The initial phase of therapy includes PN as the primary source of nutrition. The second phase is the introduction of enteral feeding, which usually begins as soon as possible after surgery. Elemental formulas containing glucose, sucrose and glucose polymers, hydrolyzed proteins, and medium-chain triglycerides facilitate absorption. Usually these formulas are given by continuous infusion through an NG or gastrostomy tube. As the enteral feedings are advanced, the PN solution is decreased in terms of calories, amount of fluid, and total hours of infusion per day.

The final phase of nutritional support occurs when growth and development are sustained exclusively by enteral feedings. When PN is discontinued, there is a risk of nutritional deficiency secondary to malabsorption of fat-soluble vitamins (A, D, E, and K) and trace minerals (iron, selenium, and zinc). Obtain serum vitamin and mineral

levels and require enteral supplementation of vitamins and minerals. Pharmacologic agents have been used to reduce secretory losses. H_2 blockers, PPIs, and octreotide inhibit gastric or pancreatic secretion. Cholestyramine is often prescribed to improve diarrhea that is associated with bile salt malabsorption. Growth factors have also been used to hasten adaptation and to enhance mucosal growth, but these uses are still experimental.

Numerous complications are associated with SBS and long-term PN. Infectious, metabolic, and technical complications can occur. Catheter sepsis can occur after improper care of the catheter. The GI tract can also be a source of microbial seeding of the catheter. Bowel atrophy may foster increased intestinal permeability of bacteria. A lack of adequate sites for central lines may become a significant problem for the child in need of long-term PN. Hepatic dysfunction, hepatomegaly with abnormal LFTs, and cholestasis may also occur (Diamond, Sterescu, Pencharz, and others, 2009).

Bacterial overgrowth is likely to occur when the ileocecal valve is absent or when stasis exists as a result of a partial obstruction or a dilated segment of bowel with poor motility. Alternating cycles of broad-spectrum antibiotics are used to reduce bacterial overgrowth. This treatment may also decrease the risk of bacterial translocation and subsequent central venous catheter infections. Other complications of bacterial overgrowth and malabsorption include metabolic acidosis and gastric hypersecretion.

Many surgical interventions, including intestinal valves, tapering enteroplasty or stricturoplasty, intestinal lengthening, and interposed segments, have been used to slow intestinal transit, reduce bacterial overgrowth, or increase mucosal surface area. Intestinal transplantation has been performed successfully in children. Only children with a permanent dependence on PN or severe complications of long-term PN are candidates for transplantation.

Prognosis

The prognosis for infants with SBS has improved with advances in PN and with the understanding of the importance of intraluminal nutrition. Improved surgical techniques for the management of therapy-related problems and the development of more specific immunosuppressive medications for transplantation have all contributed to improved management. The prognosis depends in part on the length of the residual small intestine. An intact ileocecal valve also improves the prognosis. Infants and children with SBS die from PN-related problems, such as fulminant sepsis or severe PN cholestasis.

Nursing Care Management

The most important components of nursing care are administration and monitoring of nutritional therapy. During PN therapy, care must be taken to minimize the risk of complications related to the central venous access device (i.e., catheter infections, occlusions, dislodgment, or accidental removal). Care of the enteral feeding tubes and monitoring of enteral feeding tolerance are also important nursing responsibilities.

When long-term PN is required, preparing the family for home care is a major nursing responsibility that should be initiated early to prevent a lengthy hospitalization with subsequent problems such as family dysfunction and developmental delays. Many infants and children can be successfully cared for at home with enteral nutrition and PN when the family is prepared and provided with adequate support services. Follow-up by a multidisciplinary nutritional support service is essential. The nurse plays an active and important role in the success of a home nutrition program. Home infusion companies provide

---

*A booklet, *Pointers for Parents: Coping with Celiac Sprue*, provides information on shopping, cooking, and living with an affected child and is available from the Clinical Dietetics Department, Children's Memorial Hospital, 2300 Children's Plaza, Chicago, IL 60614; 773-880-4793.
†PO Box 31700, Omaha, NE 68131-0700; 877-CSA-4CSA or 402-558-0600; http://www.csaceliacs.org. In Canada: Canadian Celiac Association, 5025 Orbitor Dr., Suite 400, Mississauga, ON L4W 4Y5; 800-363-7296; 905-507-6208; http://www.celiac.ca.

portable equipment, which enables the child and family to maintain a more normal lifestyle.

Many infants with SBS have an intestinal ostomy performed at the time of the initial bowel resection. Routine ostomy care is another important nursing responsibility. Because infants and children with SBS have chronic diarrhea, perineal skin irritation is often a problem after ostomy closure. Frequent diaper changes, gentle perineal cleansing, and protective skin ointments help prevent skin breakdown.

When hospitalization is prolonged, the child's developmental and emotional needs must be met. This often requires special planning to promote normal family adjustment and adaptation of the hospital routines. Care of hospitalized children is discussed in Chapter 21.

█ KEY POINTS

- Infants are subject to fluid depletion because of their greater surface area relative to body mass, high rate of metabolism, and immature kidney function.
- Dehydration can be classified as isotonic, hypotonic, and hypertonic.
- Vomiting and diarrhea account for significant fluid depletion, especially in infants and small children.
- The amount, frequency, and characteristics of stool and vomitus are important nursing observations.
- Diarrhea can be caused by an inflammatory process of infectious origin, a toxic reaction to ingestion of poisonous substances, dietary indiscretions, or infections outside the alimentary tract. The primary treatment of diarrhea is the use of ORS.
- HD requires surgical removal of aganglionic segments of bowel.
- Postoperative care of the child with abdominal surgery involves assessing for the return of bowel function and providing hydration and nutrition, IV fluids, pain management, wound care, and psychologic support.
- Nursing care of GER is aimed at identifying children with suggestive symptoms, helping parents with home care feeding and positioning, administering medications to minimize the symptoms, and caring for the child undergoing surgical intervention.
- Although the cause of appendicitis is poorly understood, it is typically a result of obstruction of the lumen, usually by a fecalith. Common signs and symptoms are right lower quadrant abdominal pain, tenderness, and fever.
- Meckel diverticulum is a congenital malformation of the GI tract characterized by bloody stools.
- IBD refers to UC and CD. Chronic diarrhea is the most common feature. It is treated by dietary management and medication, although surgery is needed in some cases.
- Peptic ulcers are poorly understood, but contributing factors include interference with the normal protective mechanisms of the mucosal lining and the presence of *H. pylori*.
- Viral hepatitis is caused by six types of virus: HAV, HBV, HCV, HDV, HEV, and HGV.

- Whereas HAV is spread by the fecal–oral route, HBV and HCV are transmitted primarily by the parenteral route. The most effective measure in prevention and control of hepatitis in any setting is hand washing.
- Structural disorders of the GI tract include CL, CP, EA with TEF, anorectal malformations, and BA.
- BA is a serious disorder, often causing progressive liver failure, which requires eventual liver transplantation.
- CL deformities are repaired at the earliest opportunity; CP repair may be delayed to take advantage of growth changes.
- Management of CP involves a multidisciplinary approach involving professionals from surgery, medicine, nursing, social work, dentistry, speech-language pathology, and audiology.
- Hernias related to the GI tract can be minor (umbilical) or life threatening (congenital diaphragmatic).
- The two major abdominal wall defects are gastroschisis and omphalocele.
- General signs of bowel obstruction include colicky abdominal pain, nausea and vomiting, abdominal distention, and decreased stool output.
- HPS is recognized by characteristic projectile vomiting, malnutrition, dehydration, and a palpable mass in the epigastrium and is relieved by pyloromyotomy.
- Intussusception is one of the most common causes of intestinal obstruction during infancy and is characterized by abdominal pain and blood in stools. Treatment is either nonsurgical hydrostatic reduction or surgical reduction.
- Malabsorption syndromes are disorders associated with some degree of impaired digestion or absorption. They include digestive defects, absorptive defects, and anatomic defects.
- Celiac disease is characterized by an intolerance to gluten. It is thought to be either an inborn error of metabolism or an immunologic response.
- SBS is characterized by a loss of intestine resulting in a diminished ability to absorb a regular diet normally. Specialized enteral nutrition and PN is a major element of care for these children.

REFERENCES

A-Kader HH, Balistreri WF: Neonatal cholestasis. In Kliegman RM, Stanton BF, St. Geme JW, and others, editors: *Nelson textbook of pediatrics*, ed 19, Philadelphia, 2011, Saunders.

Achildi A, Grewal H: Congenital anomalies of the esophagus, *Otolaryngol Clin North Am* 40(1): 219–244, 2007.

Aiken JJ, Oldham KT: Acute appendicitis. In Kliegman RM, Stanton BF, St. Geme JW, and others, editors: *Nelson textbook of pediatrics*, ed 19, Philadelphia, 2011, Saunders.

Allen SJ, Martinez EG, Gregorio GV, and others: Probiotics for treating acute infectious diarrhea, *Cochrane Database Syst Rev* 10(11):CD003048, 2010.

American Academy of Pediatrics, Committee on Infectious Diseases, Pickering L, editor: *Red book: report of the Committee on Infectious Diseases*, ed 28, Elk Grove Village, Ill, 2009, Author.

American Academy of Pediatrics, Subcommittee on Chronic Abdominal Pain: Chronic abdominal pain in children, *Pediatrics* 153(3):812–815, 2005.

American Academy of Pediatrics, Task Force on Sudden Infant Death Syndrome: The changing concept of sudden infant death syndrome: diagnostic coding shifts, controversies regarding the sleep environment and new variables to consider in reducing risk, *Pediatrics* 116(5): 1245–1255, 2005.

Bakken JS: Fecal bacteriotherapy for *Clostridium difficile* infection, *Anaerobe* 15(6):285–289, 2009.

Bhutta ZA: Acute gastroenteritis in children. In Kliegman RM, Stanton BF, St. Geme JW, and others, editors: *Nelson textbook of pediatrics,* ed 19, Philadelphia, 2011, Saunders.

Branski D, Troncone R: Gluten-sensitive enteropathy (celiac disease). In Kliegman RM, Stanton BF, St. Geme JW, and others, editors: *Nelson textbook of pediatrics,* ed 19, Philadelphia, 2011, Saunders.

Bufler P, Gross M, Uhlig HH: Recurrent abdominal pain in childhood, *Deutsches Arztebl Int* 108(17): 295–304, 2011.

Bullard J, Page NE: Cyclic vomiting syndrome: a disease in disguise, *Pediatr Nurs* 31(1):27–29, 2005.

Cavataio F, Guandalini S: Gastroesophageal reflux. In Guandalini S, editor: *Essential pediatric gastroenterology and nutrition,* New York, 2005, McGraw-Hill.

Centers for Disease Control and Prevention: Managing acute gastroenteritis among children: oral rehydration, maintenance, and nutritional therapy. *MMWR Recommend Rep* 52(RR-16): 1–16, 2003.

Centers for Disease Control and Prevention: Delayed onset and diminished magnitude of rotavirus activity—United States, November 2007–May 2008. *MMWR Morb Mortal Wkly Rep* 57(25):697–700, 2008.

Chang HG, Smith PF, Tserenpuntsag B, and others: Reduction in hospitalizations for diarrhea and rotavirus infections in New York state following introduction of rotavirus vaccine, *Vaccine* 28(3):754–758, 2010.

Chapman, KL, Hardin-Jones, MA, Goldstein JA, and others: Timing of palatal surgery and speech outcome. *Cleft Palate Craniofac J* 45(3):297–308, 2008.

Chen S-M, Chang M-H, Du J-C, and others: Screening for biliary atresia by infant stool color card in Taiwan, *Pediatrics* 117(4):1147–1154, 2006.

Chu A, Liacouras CA: Ileus, adhesions, intussusceptions, and closed-loop obstructions. In Kliegman RM, Stanton BF, St. Geme JW, and others, editors: *Nelson textbook of pediatrics,* ed 19, Philadelphia, 2011, Saunders.

Cleft Palate Foundation: Factsheet: what about breastfeeding, Chapel Hill, NC, 2009, Author, retrieved April 24, 2011, from http://www.cleftline.org.

Daniels D, Grytdal S, Wasley A, and others: Surveillance for acute viral hepatitis—United States, 2007, *MMWR Surveill Summ* 58(3):1–27, 2009.

Dasgupta R, Langer JC: Hirschsprung disease, *Curr Probl Surg* 41(12):949–988, 2004.

Degertekin B, Lok AS: Update on viral hepatitis: 2008, *Curr Opin Gastroenterol* 25(3):180–185, 2009.

Diamond IR, Sterescu A, Pencharz PB, and others: Changing the paradigm: omegaven for the treatment of liver failure in pediatric short bowel syndrome, *J Pediatr Gastroenterol Nutr* 48(2):209–215, 2009.

Dieterich W, Esslinger B, Schuppan D: Pathomechanisms in celiac disease, *Int Arch Allergy Immunol* 132(2):98–108, 2003.

DuPont HL: The search for effective treatment of *Clostridium difficile* infection, *N Engl J Med* 364(5):473–475, 2011.

Emerick KM, Whitington PF: Neonatal liver disease, *Pediatr Ann* 35(4):281–286, 2006.

Emond S: Dehydration in infants and young children, *Ann Emerg Med* 53(3):395–397, 2009.

Fayoux P, Sfeir R: Management of severe tracheomalacia, *J Pediatr Gastroenterol Nutr* 52(Suppl 1):S33–S34, 2011.

Ford DM: Fluid, electrolyte, and acid-base disorders. In Hay WW, Levin MJ, Sondheimer JM, and others, editors: *Current diagnosis and treatment,* ed 19, Philadelphia, 2009, McGraw Hill.

Friedman A: Fluid and electrolyte therapy: a primer, *Pediatr Nephrol* 25(5):843–846, 2010.

Gelfond D, Fasano A: Celiac disease in the pediatric population, *Pediatr Ann* 35(4):275–279, 2006.

Gilmore AW, Reed M, Tenenbein M: Management of childhood intussusceptions after reduction by enema, *Am J Emerg Med* 29(9):1136–1140, 2011.

Gisbert JP, de la Morena F, Abraira V: Accuracy of monoclonal stool antigen test for the diagnosis of *H. pylori* infection: a systematic review and meta-analysis, *Am J Gastroenterol* 101(8): 1921–1930, 2006.

Goday PS: Short bowel syndrome: how short is too short? *Clin Perinatol* 36(1):101–110, 2009.

Greenbaum LA: Electrolyte and acid-base disorders. In Kliegman RM, Stanton BF, St. Geme JW, and others, editors: *Nelson textbook of pediatrics,* ed 19, Philadelphia, 2011, Saunders.

Gupta N, Bostrom AG, Kirschner BS, and others: Presentation and disease course in early-compared to later-onset pediatric Crohn's disease, *Am J Gastroenterol* 103(8):2092–2098, 2008.

Hassall E, Owen D, Kerr W, and others: Gastric histology in children treated with proton pump inhibitors long term, with emphasis on enterochromaffin cell-like hyperplasia, *Aliment Pharmacol Ther* 4(33):829–836, 2011.

Hershey AD: Migraine. In Kliegman RM, Stanton BF, St. Geme JW, and others, editors: *Nelson textbook of pediatrics,* ed 19, Philadelphia, 2011, Saunders.

Herwig K, Brenkert T, Losek JD: Enema-reduced intussusception management: is hospitalization necessary? *Pediatr Emerg Care* 25(2):74–77, 2009.

Huang Y, Zheng S, Xiao X: A follow-up study on postoperative function after a transanal Soave 1-stage endorectal pull-through procedure for Hirschsprung's disease, *J Pediatr Surg* 43(9): 1691–1695, 2008.

Hunter AK, Liacouras CA: Pyloric stenosis and other congenital anomalies of the stomach. In Kliegman RM, Stanton BF, St. Geme JW, and others, editors: *Nelson textbook of pediatrics,* ed 19, Philadelphia, 2011, Saunders.

Huppertz H-I, Soriano-Gabarro M, Grimprel E, and others: Intussusception among young children in Europe, *Pediatr Infect Dis J* 25(1): S22–S29, 2006.

Hyams JS, Markowitz JR: Can we alter the natural history of Crohn disease in children? *J Pediatr Gastroenterol Nutr* 40(3):262–272, 2005.

Jabbar A, Wright RA: Gastroenteritis and antibiotic-associated diarrhea, *Primary Care* 30(1):63–80, 2003.

Kamath BM, Olthoff KM: Liver transplantation in children: update 2010, *Pediatr Clin North Am* 57(2):401–414, 2010.

Kane TD: Laparoscopic Nissen fundoplication, *Minerva Chir* 64(2):147–157, 2009.

Kelly DA, Davenport M: Current management of biliary atresia, *Arch Dis Child* 92(12):1132–1135, 2007.

Khan S, Orenstein SR: Esophageal atresia and tracheoesophageal fistula. In Kliegman RM, Stanton BF, St. Geme JW, and others, editors: *Nelson textbook of pediatrics,* ed 19, Philadelphia, 2011, Saunders.

Kranz S, Brauchla M, Slavin JL, and others: What do we know about dietary fiber intake in children and health? The effects of fiber intake on constipation, obesity, and diabetes in children, *Adv Nutr* 3(1): 47–53, 2012.

Kwok MY, Kim MK, Gorelick MH: Evidence-based approach to the diagnosis of appendicitis in children, *Pediatr Emerg Care* 20(10):690–698, 2004.

Langan RC, Gotsch PB, Krafczyk MA, and others: Ulcerative colitis: diagnosis and treatment, *Am Fam Physician* 76:1323–1330, 2007.

Levitt MA, Martin CA, Olesevich M, and others: Hirschsprung disease and fecal incontinence: Diagnostic and management strategies, *J Pediatr Surg* 44(1):271–277, 2009.

Levitt MA, Peña A: Anorectal malformations, *Orphanet J Rare Dis* 2:33, 2007.

Loening-Baucke V, Pashankar DS: A randomized, prospective, comparison study of polyethylene glycole 3350 without electrolytes and milk of magnesia for children with constipation and fecal incontinence, *Pediatrics* 118(2):528–535, 2006.

MacKinlay GA: Esophageal atresia surgery in the 21st century, *Semin Pediatr Surg* 18(1):20–22, 2009.

Maki M, Lohi O: Celiac disease. In Walker WA, Goulet O, Kleinman RE, and others, editors: *Pediatric gastrointestinal disease: pathophysiology, diagnosis, management,* ed 4, Hamilton, Ont, 2004, Decker.

Malek MA, Curns AT, Holman RC, and others: Diarrhea- and rotavirus-associated hospitalizations among children less than 5 years of age: United States, 1997 and 2000, *Pediatrics* 117(6):1887–1892, 2006.

Masarei AG, Wade A, Mars M, and others: A randomized control trial investigating the effect of presurgical orthopedics on feeding in infants with cleft lip and/or cleft palate, *Cleft Palate Craniofac J* 44(2):182–193, 2007.

McRonald FE, Fleisher DR: Anticipatory nausea in cyclical vomiting, *BMC Pediatr* 5(1):3, 2005.

Menezes M, Tareen F, Saeed A, and others: Symptomatic Meckel's diverticulum in children: a 16-year review, *Pediatr Surg Int* 24(5):575–577, 2008.

Mills JLA, Konkin DE, Milner R, and others: Long-term bowel function and quality of life in children with Hirschsprung's disease, *J Pediatr Surg* 43(5):899–905, 2008.

Moller KT, Glaze LE, editors: *Cleft lip and palate: interdisciplinary issues and treatment,* Austin, Tex, 2009, Pro-Ed.

Murdock AM, Johnston SD: Diagnostic criteria for coeliac disease: time for change?

Eur J Gastroenterol Hepatol 17(1):41–43, 2005.

O'Connor A, Gisbert J, O'Morain C: Treatment of *Helicobacter pylori* infection, *Helicobacter* 14(suppl 1):46–51, 2009.

Olson DE, Kim YW, Donnelly LF: CT findings in children with Meckel diverticulum, *Pediatr Radiol* 39(7):659–663, 2009.

Pakarinen MP, Rintala RJ: Surgery of biliary atresia, *Scand J Surg* 100(1):49–53, 2011.

Philichi L: When the going gets tough: pediatric constipation and encopresis, *Gastroenterol Nurs* 31(2):121–130, 2008.

Plenge-Bönig A, Soto-Ramirez N, Karmaus W, and others: Breastfeeding protects against gastroenteritis due to rotavirus in infants, *Eur J Pediatr* 169(12):1471–1476, 2010.

Rasquin A, Di Lorenzo C, Forbes D, and others: Childhood functional gastrointestinal disorders: child/adolescent, *Gastroenterology* 130(5): 1527–1537, 2006.

Reese GE, Constantinides VA, Simillis C, and others: Diagnostic precision of anti–*Saccharomyces cerevisiae* antibodies and perinuclear antineutrophil cytoplasmic antibodies in inflammatory bowel disease, *Am J Gastroenterol* 101:2410–2422, 2006.

Ricart E, García-Bosch O, Ordás I, and others: Are we giving biologics too late? The case for early versus late use, *World J Gastroenterol* 14(36): 5523–5527, 2008.

Robbins JM, Damiano P, Druschel CM, and others: Prenatal diagnosis of orofacial clefts: association with maternal satisfaction, team care, and treatment outcomes, *Cleft Palate Craniofac J* 47(5):476–481, 2010.

Rothenberg SS: Experience with thoracoscopic tracheal surgery in infants and children, *J Laparoendosc Adv Surg Tech A* 19(5):671–674, 2009.

Rubin DT, Kavitt RT: Surveillance for cancer and dysplasia in inflammatory bowel disease, *Gastroenterol Clin North Am* 35(3):581–604, 2006.

Rutter MD, Saunders BP, Wilkinson KH, and others: Thirty-year analysis of colonoscopic surveillance program for neoplasia in ulcerative colitis, *Gastroenterology* 130(4):1030–1038, 2006.

Sadlier C: Intestinal failure and long-term parenteral nutrition in children, *Paediatr Nurs* 20(10):37–43, 2008.

Sauer CG, Kugathasan S: Pediatric inflammatory bowel disease: highlighting pediatric differences in IBD, *Med Clin North Am* 94(1):35–52, 2010.

Scholl J, Allen PJ: A primary care approach to functional abdominal pain, *Pediatr Nurs* 33(3):247–259, 2007.

Silbermintz A, Markowitz J: Inflammatory bowel diseases, *Pediatr Ann* 35(4):268–274, 2006.

Sola JE, Neville HL: Laparoscopic vs open pyloromyotomy: a systematic review and meta-analysis, *J Pediatr Surg* 44(8):1631–1637, 2009.

Staat MA: What is the disease burden associated with rotavirus? In *The management and prevention of rotavirus*, Thorofare, NJ, 2006, Vindico Medical Education.

Steiner MJ, Nager AL, Wang VJ: Urine specific gravity and other urinary indices: inaccurate tests for dehydration, *Pediatr Emerg Care* 23(5):298–303, 2007.

Sung JJ, Kuipers EJ, El-Serag HB: Systematic review: the global incidence and prevalence of peptic ulcer disease, *Aliment Pharmacol Ther* 29(9):938–946, 2009.

Suwandhi E, Ton MN, Schwarz SM: Gastroesophageal reflux in infancy and childhood, *Pediatr Ann* 35(4):259–266, 2006.

Theocharatos S, Kenny SE: Hirschsprung's disease: current management and prospects for transplantation of enteric nervous system progenitor cells, *Early Hum Dev* 84(12): 801–804, 2008.

Thurley PD, Halliday KE, Somers JM, and others: Radiological features of Meckel's diverticulum and its complications, *Clin Radiol* 64(2): 109–118, 2009.

Tran TT: Management of hepatitis B in pregnancy: weighing the options, *Cleve Clin J Med* 76(suppl 3):S25–S29, 2009.

Van der Pol RJ, Smits MJ, van Wijk MP, and others: Efficacy of proton pump inhibitors in children with gastroesophageal reflux disease: a systematic review, *Pediatrics* 127(5):925–935, 2011.

Vernier-Massouille G, Balde M, Salleron J, and others: Natural history of pediatric Crohn's disease: a population-based cohort study, *Gastroenterology* 135(4):1106–1113, 2008.

Vissers RJ, Lennarz WB: Pitfalls in appendicitis, *Emerg Med Clin North Am* 28(1):103–118, 2010.

Waseem M, Rosenberg HK: Intussusception, *Pediatr Emerg Care* 24(11):793–800, 2008.

Wilkins-Haug L: Prenatal diagnosis of orofacial clefts, *UptoDate*, September 29, 2010, retrieved April 23, 2011, from http://www.uptodate.com.

Wong AP, Clark AL, Garnett EA, and others: Use of complementary medicine in pediatric patients with inflammatory bowel disease: results from a multicenter survey, *J Pediatr Gastroenterol Nutr* 48(1):55–60, 2009.

Yen C, Tate JE, Wenk JD, and others: Diarrhea-associated hospitalizations among U.S. children over 2 rotavirus seasons after vaccine introduction, *Pediatrics* 127(1):e9–e15, 2011.

Young JL, O'Riordan M, Goldstein JA, and others: What information do parents of newborns with cleft lip, palate, or both want to know? *Cleft Palate Craniofac J* 38:55–58, 2001.

Zilberberg MD, Tillotson GS, McDonald C: *Clostridium difficile* infections among hospitalized children, United States, 1997–2006, *Emerg Infect Dis* 16(4):604–609, 2010.

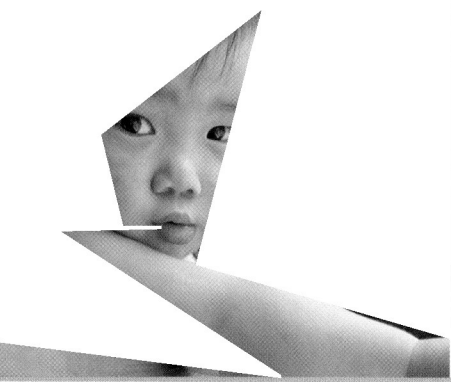

The Child with Cardiovascular Dysfunction

Margaret L. Schroeder, Amy Delaney, and Annette L. Baker

evolve WEBSITE

CHAPTER OUTLINE

Cardiovascular Dysfunction, 820
  History and Physical
    Examination, 820
Congenital Heart Disease, 823
  Circulatory Changes at Birth, 823
  Altered Hemodynamics, 824
  Classification of Defects, 824
    *Defects with Increased Pulmonary
      Blood Flow, 825*
    Obstructive Defects, 825
    *Defects with Decreased Pulmonary
      Blood Flow, 827*
    Mixed Defects, 830
Clinical Consequences of Congenital Heart
  Disease, 830
  Heart Failure, 830
    *Nursing Care Plan: The Child with
      Heart Failure, 837*
  Hypoxemia, 840

Nursing Care of the Family and Child with
  Congenital Heart Disease, 843
  Help the Family Adjust to the
    Disorder, 843
  Educate the Family About the
    Disorder, 843
  Help the Family Manage the Illness at
    Home, 844
  Prepare the Child and Family for
    Invasive Procedures, 845
  Provide Postoperative Care, 845
    Observe Vital Signs, 845
    Maintain Respiratory Status, 846
    Monitor Fluids, 846
    *Provide Rest and Progressive
      Activity, 847*
    *Provide Comfort and Emotional
      Support, 847*
  Plan for Discharge and Home Care, 847

Acquired Cardiovascular Disorders, 848
  Bacterial (Infective) Endocarditis, 848
  Rheumatic Fever, 849
  Hyperlipidemia
    (Hypercholesterolemia), 850
  Cardiac Dysrhythmias, 853
  Pulmonary Artery Hypertension, 854
  Cardiomyopathy, 855
Heart Transplantation, 856
Vascular Dysfunction, 857
  Systemic Hypertension, 857
  Kawasaki Disease (Mucocutaneous
    Lymph Node Syndrome), 858
  Shock, 860
  Anaphylaxis, 862
  Septic Shock, 863
  Toxic Shock Syndrome, 864

LEARNING OBJECTIVES

On completion of this chapter the reader will be able to:

- Design a plan for assisting children during cardiac diagnostic procedures.
- Demonstrate an understanding of the hemodynamics, distinctive manifestations, and therapeutic management of congenital heart disease.
- Outline a care plan for an infant or child with heart failure.
- Describe the care for a child who has hypoxia.
- Describe the care for an infant or a child with a congenital heart defect and its surgical repair.

- Discuss the nurse's role in helping the child and family cope with congenital heart disease.
- Differentiate between rheumatic fever and rheumatic heart disease.
- List the criteria for selected cholesterol screening of children.
- Discuss the assessment and management of hypertension in children and adolescents.
- Outline a care plan for a child with Kawasaki disease.
- Describe the emergency treatment for shock, including anaphylaxis.

CARDIOVASCULAR DYSFUNCTION

Cardiovascular disorders in children are divided into two major groups, congenital heart disease and acquired heart disorders. Congenital heart disease (CHD) includes primarily anatomic abnormalities present at birth that result in abnormal cardiac function. The clinical consequences of congenital heart defects fall into two broad categories, heart failure (HF) and hypoxemia. Acquired cardiac disorders are disease processes or abnormalities that occur after birth and can be seen in the normal heart or in the presence of congenital heart defects. They result from various factors, including infection, autoimmune responses, environmental factors, and familial tendencies. The pathophysiology review found in Figure 25-1 describes the flow of blood through the heart.

HISTORY AND PHYSICAL EXAMINATION

Taking an accurate health history is an important first step in assessing an infant or child for possible heart disease. Parents may have specific concerns, such as an infant with poor feeding or fast breathing, or a 7-year-old who can no longer keep up with friends on the soccer field. Others may not realize that their child has a medical problem because their baby has always been pale and fussy.

Asking details about the mother's health history, pregnancy, and birth history is important in assessing infants. Mothers with chronic health conditions, such as diabetes or lupus, are more likely to have infants with heart disease. Some medications, such as phenytoin (Dilantin), are teratogenic to fetuses. Maternal alcohol use or illicit drug use increases the risk of congenital heart defects. Exposures to infections, such as rubella, early in pregnancy may result in congenital anomalies. Infants with low birth weight resulting from intrauterine growth restriction are more likely to have congenital anomalies. High-birth-weight infants have an increased incidence of heart disease.

A detailed family history is also important. There is an increased incidence of congenital cardiac defects if either parent or a sibling has a heart defect. Some diseases, such as Marfan syndrome, and some cardiomyopathies are hereditary. A family history of frequent fetal loss, sudden infant death, and sudden death in adults may indicate heart disease. Congenital heart defects are seen in many syndromes such as Down and Turner syndromes.

The physical assessment of suspected cardiac disease begins with observation of general appearance and then proceeds with more specific observations. The following are supplementary to the general assessment techniques described for physical examination of the chest and heart in Chapter 6:

Inspection

Nutritional state—Failure to thrive or poor weight gain is associated with heart disease.

Color—Cyanosis is a common feature of CHD, and pallor is associated with poor perfusion.

Chest deformities—An enlarged heart sometimes distorts the chest configuration.

Unusual pulsations—Visible pulsations of the neck veins are seen in some patients.

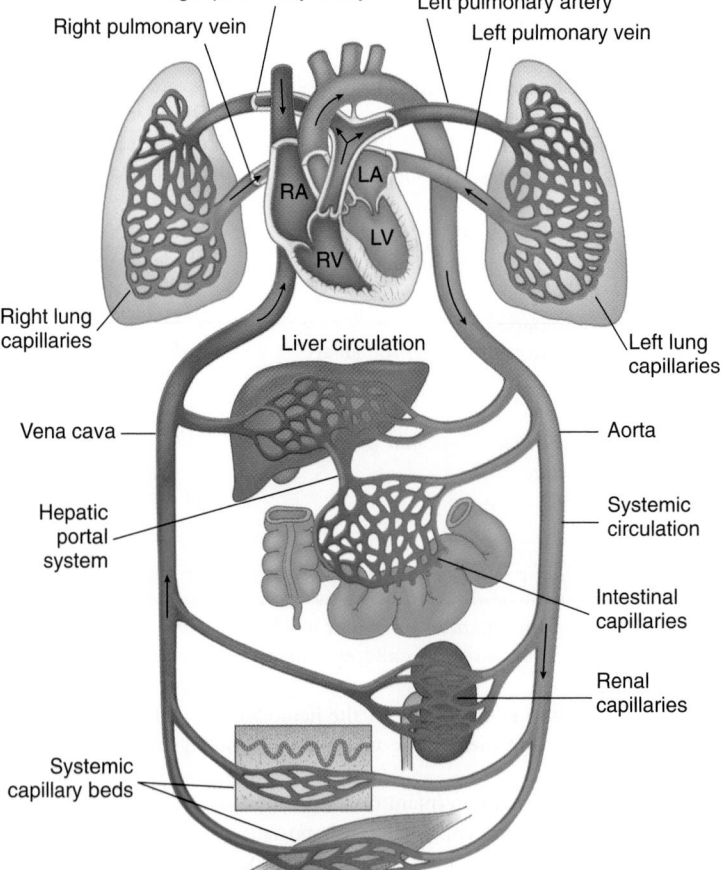

FIG 25-1 Diagram showing serially connected pulmonary and systemic circulatory systems and how to trace the flow of blood. Right heart chambers propel unoxygenated blood through the systemic circulation. *LA,* Left atrium; *LV,* left ventricle; *RA,* right atrium; *RV,* right ventricle. (From McCance KL, Heuther SE: *Pathophysiology: the biological basis for disease in adults and children,* ed 6, St. Louis, 2010, Mosby.)

TABLE 25-1   PROCEDURES FOR CARDIAC DIAGNOSIS

PROCEDURE	DESCRIPTION
Chest radiography (x-ray)	Provides information on heart size and pulmonary blood flow patterns
ECG	Graphic measure of electrical activity of heart
Holter monitor	24-hour continuous ECG recording used to assess dysrhythmias
Echocardiography	Use of high-frequency sound waves obtained by a transducer to produce an image of cardiac structures
Transthoracic	Done with transducer on chest
M-mode	One-dimensional graphic view used to estimate ventricular size and function
Two-dimensional	Real-time, cross-sectional views of heart used to identify cardiac structures and cardiac anatomy
Doppler	Identifies blood flow patterns and pressure gradients across structures
Fetal	Imaging fetal heart in utero
TEE	Transducer placed in esophagus behind heart to obtain images of posterior heart structures or in patients with poor images from chest approach
Cardiac catheterization	Imaging study using radiopaque catheters placed in a peripheral blood vessel and advanced into heart to measure pressures and oxygen levels in heart chambers and visualize heart structures and blood flow patterns
Hemodynamics	Measures pressures and oxygen saturations in heart chambers
Angiography	Use of contrast material to illuminate heart structures and blood flow patterns
Biopsy	Use of special catheter to remove tiny samples of heart muscle for microscopic evaluation; used in assessing infection, inflammation, or muscle dysfunction disorders; also to evaluate for rejection after heart transplant
EPS	Special catheters with electrodes employed to record electrical activity from within heart; used to diagnose rhythm disturbances
Exercise stress test	Monitoring of heart rate, blood pressure, ECG, and oxygen consumption at rest and during progressive exercise on a treadmill or bicycle
Cardiac MRI	Noninvasive imaging technique; used in evaluation of vascular anatomy outside of heart (e.g., COA, vascular rings), estimates of ventricular mass and volume; uses for MRI are expanding

COA, Coarctation of the aorta; *ECG,* electrocardiography; *EPS,* electrophysiology; *MRI,* magnetic resonance imaging; *TEE,* transesophageal echocardiography.

Respiratory excursion—This refers to the ease or difficulty of respiration (e.g., tachypnea, dyspnea, expiratory grunt).

Clubbing of fingers—This is associated with cyanosis.

Palpation and Percussion

Chest—These maneuvers help discern heart size and other characteristics (e.g., thrills) associated with heart disease.

Abdomen—Hepatomegaly or splenomegaly may be evident.

Peripheral pulses—Rate, regularity, and amplitude (strength) may reveal discrepancies.

Auscultation

Heart rate and rhythm—Listen for fast heart rates (tachycardia), slow heart rates (bradycardia), and irregular rhythms.

🅔 **Character of heart sounds**—Listen for distinct or muffled sounds, murmurs, and additional heart sounds.

Diagnostic Evaluation

A variety of invasive and noninvasive tests may be used in the diagnosis of heart disease (Table 25-1). Some of the more common diagnostic tools that require nursing assessment and intervention are described here.

Electrocardiogram

Bedside cardiac monitoring with the electrocardiogram (ECG) is commonly used in pediatrics, especially in the care of children with heart disease. The bedside monitor provides valuable information about heart rate and rhythm through a graphic display of the ECG tracing and a digital display. An alarm can be set with parameters for individual patient requirements and will sound if the heart rate is above or below the set parameters. Gelfoam electrodes are commonly used and placed on the right side of the chest (above the level of the heart) and on the left side of the chest, and a ground electrode is placed on the abdomen. Electrodes should be changed every 1 or 2 days because they irritate the skin. Bedside monitors are an adjunct to patient care and should never be substituted for direct assessment and auscultation of heart sounds. The nurse should assess the patient, not the monitor.

> **NURSING TIP** Electrodes for cardiac monitoring are often color coded: white for right, green (or red) for ground, and black for left. Always check to ensure that these colors are placed correctly.

Echocardiography

Echocardiography is one of the most frequently used tests for detecting cardiac dysfunction in children. Recent improvements in echocardiographic techniques have made it increasingly possible to confirm the diagnosis without resorting to cardiac catheterization. In more and more cases, a prenatal diagnosis of CHD can be made by fetal echocardiography.

Echocardiography involves the use of ultra-high-frequency sound waves to produce an image of the heart's structure. A transducer placed directly on the chest wall delivers repetitive pulses of ultrasound and processes the returned signals (echoes).

Although the test is noninvasive, painless, and associated with no known side effects, it can be stressful for children. The child must lie quietly in the standard echocardiographic positions; crying, nursing, or sitting up often leads to diagnostic errors or omissions. Therefore, infants and young children may need a mild sedative; older children benefit from psychologic preparation for the test. The distraction of a video or movie is often helpful.

Animation—Heart Sounds

Cardiac Catheterization

Cardiac catheterization is an invasive diagnostic procedure in which a radiopaque catheter is inserted through a peripheral blood vessel into the heart. The catheter is usually introduced through percutaneous technique, in which the catheter is threaded through a large-bore needle that is inserted into the vein. The catheter is guided through the heart with the aid of fluoroscopy. After the tip of the catheter is within a heart chamber, contrast material is injected, and films are taken of the dilution and circulation of the material (angiography). Types of cardiac catheterizations include:

Diagnostic catheterizations—These studies are used to diagnose congenital cardiac defects, particularly in symptomatic infants and before surgical repair. They are divided into right-sided catheterizations, in which the catheter is introduced through a vein (usually the femoral vein) and threaded to the right atrium (most common), and left-sided catheterizations, in which the catheter is threaded through an artery into the aorta and into the heart.

Interventional catheterizations (therapeutic catheterizations)—A balloon catheter or other device is used to alter the cardiac anatomy. Examples include dilating stenotic valves or vessels or closing abnormal connections (Table 25-2).

Electrophysiology studies—Catheters with tiny electrodes that record the impulses of the heart directly from the conduction system are used to evaluate dysrhythmias and sometimes destroy accessory pathways that cause some tachydysrhythmias.

Nursing Care Management

Cardiac catheterization has become a routine diagnostic procedure and may be done on an outpatient basis. However, it is not without risks, especially in neonates and seriously ill infants and children. Possible complications include acute hemorrhage from the entry site (more likely with interventional procedures because larger catheters are used), low-grade fever, nausea, vomiting, loss of pulse in the catheterized extremity (usually transient, resulting from a clot, hematoma, or intimal tear), and transient dysrhythmias (generally catheter induced) (Uzark, 2001). Rare risks include stroke, seizures, tamponade, and death.

Preprocedural Care

A complete nursing assessment is necessary to ensure a safe procedure with minimum complications. This assessment should include accurate height (essential for correct catheter selection) and weight. Obtaining a history of allergic reactions is important because some of the contrast agents are iodine based. Specific attention to signs and symptoms of infection is crucial. Severe diaper rash may be a reason to cancel the procedure if femoral access is required. Because assessment of pedal pulses is important after catheterization, the nurse should assess and mark the pulses (dorsalis pedis, posterior tibial) before the child goes to the catheterization room. The presence and quality of pulses in both feet are clearly documented. Baseline oxygen saturation using pulse oximetry in children with cyanosis is also recorded.

Preparing the child and family for the procedure is the joint responsibility of the patient care team. School-age children and adolescents benefit from a description of the catheterization laboratory and a chronologic explanation of the procedure, emphasizing what they will see, feel, and hear. Older children and adolescents may bring earphones and favorite music so they can listen during the catheterization procedure. Preparation materials such as picture books, videotapes, or tours of the catheterization laboratory may be helpful. Preparation should be geared to the child's developmental level. The child's caregivers often benefit from the same explanations. Additional information, such as

TABLE 25-2	CURRENT INTERVENTIONAL CARDIAC CATHETERIZATION PROCEDURES IN CHILDREN
INTERVENTION	**DIAGNOSIS**
Balloon atrioseptostomy—Use well established in newborns; may also be done under echocardiographic guidance	Transposition of great arteries Some complex single-ventricle defects
Balloon dilation—Treatment of choice	Valvular pulmonic stenosis Branch pulmonary artery stenosis Congenital valvular aortic stenosis Rheumatic mitral stenosis Recurrent coarctation of aorta Further follow-up required in: Native coarctation of aorta in patients older than 7 months Congenital mitral stenosis
Coil occlusion—Accepted alternative to surgery	PDA (<4 mm)
Transcatheter device closure—Several devices used in clinical trials	ASD
Amplatzer septal occluder—Approved for ASD closure	ASD
VSD devices—Used in clinical trials	VSDs
Stent placement	Pulmonary artery stenosis Coarctation of the aorta in adolescents Use to treat other lesions investigational
RF ablation	Some tachydysrhythmias

Data from Allen HD, Beekman RH 3rd, Garson A Jr, and others: Pediatric therapeutic cardiac catheterization: AHA scientific statement, *Circulation* 97:609–625, 1998; updated from Rome J, Kreutzer J: Pediatric interventional catheterization: reasonable expectations and outcomes, *Pediatr Clin North Am* 51:1589–1610, 2004.

ASD, Atrial septal defect; *PDA,* patent ductus arteriosus; *RF,* radiofrequency; *VSD,* ventricular septal defects.

the expected length of the catheterization, description of the child's appearance after catheterization, and usual postprocedure care, should be outlined. (See also Prepare the Child and Family for Invasive Procedures, p. 845.)

Methods of sedation vary among institutions and may include oral or intravenous (IV) medications (see Chapter 22). The child's age, heart defect, clinical status, and type of catheterization procedure planned are considered when sedation is determined. General anesthesia may be needed for some interventional procedures. Children are allowed nothing by mouth (NPO) for 4 to 6 hours or more before the procedure according to institutional guidelines. Infants and patients with polycythemia may need IV fluids to prevent dehydration and hypoglycemia.

Postprocedural Care

Patients may recover from the procedure in a recovery unit; their hospital room; or, occasionally, an intensive care unit (ICU). Patients are placed on a cardiac monitor and a pulse oximeter for the first few hours

FAMILY-CENTERED CARE
After Cardiac Catheterization

Remove pressure dressing the day after catheterization. Cover site with an adhesive bandage strip for several days.

Keep site clean and dry. Avoid tub baths for several days; patient may shower.

Observe site for redness, swelling, drainage, and bleeding. Monitor for fever. Notify practitioner if these occur.

Avoid strenuous exercise for several days; patient may attend school.

Resume regular diet without restrictions.

Use acetaminophen or ibuprofen for pain.

Keep follow-up appointments per practitioner's instruction.

Modified from Children's Hospital (Boston) Cardiovascular Program, 1996.

of recovery. The most important nursing responsibility is observation of the following for signs of complications:

- **Pulses**, especially below the catheterization site, for equality and symmetry (Pulse distal to the site may be weaker for the first few hours after catheterization but should gradually increase in strength.)
- **Temperature and color of the affected extremity** because coolness or blanching may indicate arterial obstruction
- **Vital signs**, which are taken as frequently as every 15 minutes, with special emphasis on heart rate, which is counted for 1 full minute for evidence of dysrhythmias or bradycardia
- **Blood pressure (BP)**, especially for hypotension, which may indicate hemorrhage from cardiac perforation or bleeding at the site of initial catheterization
- **Dressing**, for evidence of bleeding or hematoma formation in the femoral or antecubital area
- **Fluid intake**, both IV and oral, to ensure adequate hydration (Blood loss in the catheterization laboratory, the child's NPO status, and diuretic actions of dyes used during the procedure put children at risk for hypovolemia and dehydration.)
- **Blood glucose levels** for hypoglycemia, especially in infants, who should receive dextrose-containing IV fluids

! NURSING ALERT

If bleeding occurs, direct continuous pressure is applied 2.5 cm (1 inch) above the percutaneous skin site to localize pressure over the vessel puncture.

Depending on hospital policy, the child may be kept in bed with the affected extremity maintained straight for 4 to 6 hours after venous catheterization and 6 to 8 hours after arterial catheterization to facilitate healing of the cannulated vessel. If younger children have difficulty complying, they can be held in the parent's lap with the leg maintained in the correct position. The child's usual diet can be resumed as soon as tolerated, beginning with sips of clear liquids and advancing as the condition allows. The child is encouraged to void to clear the contrast material from the blood. Generally, there is only slight discomfort at the percutaneous site. To prevent infection, the catheterization area is protected from possible contamination. If the child wears diapers, the dressing can be kept dry by covering it with a piece of plastic film and sealing the edges of the film to the skin with tape. However, the nurse must be careful to continue observing the site for any evidence of bleeding (see Family-Centered Care box and Critical Thinking Case Study).

? CRITICAL THINKING CASE STUDY
Cardiac Catheterization

Tommy, a 3-year-old boy with tetralogy of Fallot, has just returned to his hospital room from the cardiac catheterization recovery room. His mother calls you to the bedside to tell you that he is vomiting and bleeding. You arrive to find Tommy anxious, pale, crying, and sitting in a puddle of blood.

Questions
1. Evidence—Is there sufficient evidence to draw conclusions about Tommy's situation?
2. Assumptions—Describe an underlying assumption about each of the following:
   a. Risks of cardiac catheterization
   b. Association between vomiting and bleeding after cardiac catheterization
   c. Concerns related to acute blood loss
3. What priorities for nursing care should be established for Tommy?
4. Does the evidence support your nursing interventions?

CONGENITAL HEART DISEASE

The incidence of CHD in children is approximately 5 to 8 per 1000 live births (Park, 2008). About 2 or 3 in 1000 infants will be symptomatic during the first year of life with significant heart disease that requires treatment (Hoffman and Kaplan, 2002). CHD is the major cause of death (other than prematurity) in the first year of life. Although there are more than 35 well-recognized cardiac defects, the most common heart anomaly is ventricular septal defect (VSD).

The exact cause of most congenital cardiac defects is unknown. Most are thought to be a result of multiple factors, including a complex interaction of genetic and environmental influences. Some risk factors are known to be associated with increased incidence of congenital heart defects. Maternal risk factors include chronic illnesses such as diabetes or poorly controlled phenylketonuria, alcohol consumption, and exposure to environmental toxins and infections. Family history of a cardiac defect in a parent or sibling increases the likelihood of a cardiac anomaly. The risk of CHD increases if a first-degree relative (parent or sibling) is affected. The familial risk is higher with left-sided obstructive lesions.

Congenital heart anomalies are often associated with chromosomal abnormalities, specific syndromes, or congenital defects in other body systems. Down syndrome (trisomy 21) and trisomies 13 and 18 are highly correlated with congenital heart defects. Syndromes associated with heart defects include DiGeorge syndrome, a syndrome characterized by deletion of part of chromosome 22q11 (interrupted aortic arch, truncus arteriosus, tetralogy of Fallot, and posterior malaligned VSDs); Noonan syndrome (pulmonic valve anomalies and cardiomyopathy); Williams syndrome (aortic and pulmonic stenosis); and Holt-Oram syndrome (upper limb anomalies and atrial septal defect [ASD]). Extracardiac defects such as tracheoesophageal fistula, renal abnormalities, and diaphragmatic hernia are seen in association with heart anomalies.

CIRCULATORY CHANGES AT BIRTH

Blood carrying oxygen and nutritive materials from the placenta enters the fetal system through the umbilicus via the large umbilical vein. The blood then travels to the liver, where it divides. Part of the blood enters the portal and hepatic circulation of the liver, and the

Animation—Fetal Circulation

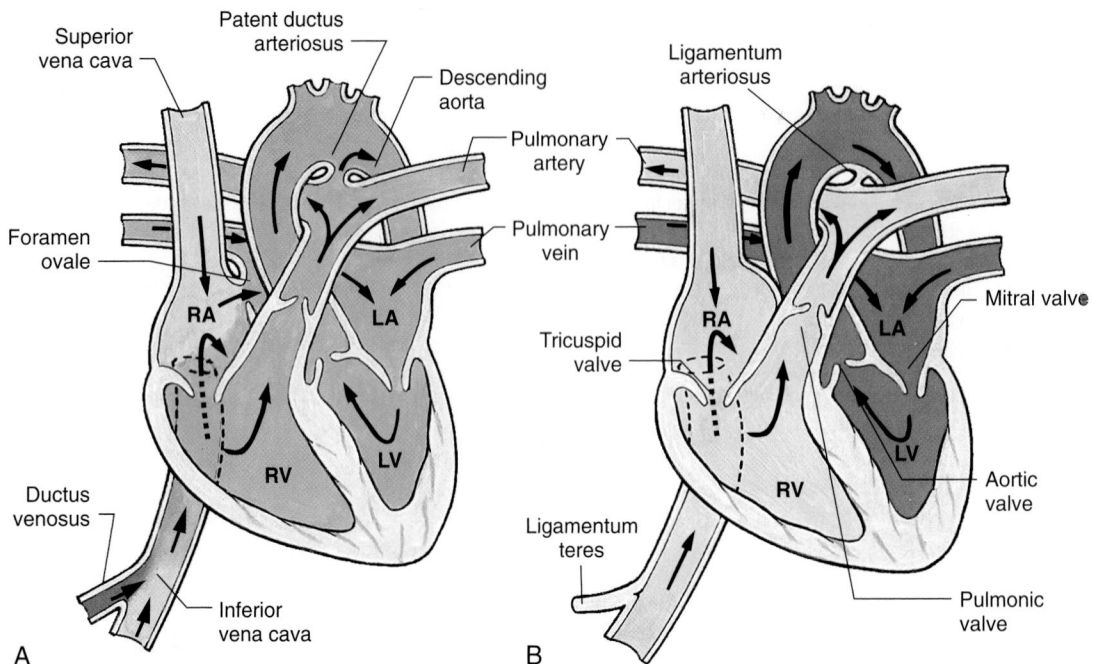

FIG 25-2 Changes in circulation at birth. **A,** Prenatal circulation. **B,** Postnatal circulation. *Arrows* indicate direction of blood flow. Although four pulmonary veins enter the left atrium (LA), for simplicity, this diagram shows only two. *LV,* Left ventricle; *RA,* right atrium; *RV,* right ventricle.

remainder travels directly to the inferior vena cava (IVC) by way of the ductus venosus. Oxygenated blood enters the heart by way of the IVC. Because of the higher pressure of blood entering the right atrium, it is directed posteriorly in a straight pathway across the right atrium and through the foramen ovale to the left atrium. In this way, the better-oxygenated blood enters the left atrium and ventricle to be pumped through the aorta to the head and upper extremities. Blood from the head and upper extremities entering the right atrium from the superior vena cava is directed downward through the tricuspid valve into the right ventricle. From there it is pumped through the pulmonary artery, where the major portion is shunted to the descending aorta via the ductus arteriosus. Only a small amount flows to and from the non-functioning fetal lungs (Fig. 25-2, *A*).

Before birth, the high pulmonary vascular resistance created by the collapsed fetal lung causes greater pressures in the right side of the heart and the pulmonary arteries. At the same time, the free-flowing placental circulation and the ductus arteriosus produce a low vascular resistance in the remainder of the fetal vascular system. With the cessation of placental blood flow from clamping of the umbilical cord and the expansion of the lungs at birth, the hemodynamics of the fetal vascular system undergo pronounced and abrupt changes (Fig. 25-2, *B*).

With the first breath, the lungs are expanded, and increased oxygen causes pulmonary vasodilation. Pulmonary pressures start to fall as systemic pressures, given the removal of the placenta, start to rise. Normally, the foramen ovale closes as the pressure in the left atrium exceeds the pressure in the right atrium. The ductus arteriosus starts to close in the presence of increased oxygen concentration in the blood and other factors.

ALTERED HEMODYNAMICS

To appreciate the physiology of heart defects, it is necessary to understand the role of pressure gradients, flow, and resistance within the circulation. As blood is pumped through the heart, it (1) flows from an area of high pressure to one of low pressure and (2) takes the path of least resistance. In general, the higher the pressure gradient, the faster the rate of flow; the higher the resistance, the slower the rate of flow.

Normally, the pressure on the right side of the heart is lower than that on the left side, and the resistance in the pulmonary circulation is less than that in the systemic circulation. Vessels entering or exiting these chambers have corresponding pressures. Therefore, if an abnormal connection exists between the heart chambers (e.g., a septal defect), blood will necessarily flow from an area of higher pressure (left side) to one of lower pressure (right side). Such a flow of blood is termed a left-to-right shunt. Anomalies resulting in cyanosis may result from a change in pressure so that the blood is shunted from the right to the left side of the heart (right-to-left shunt) because of either increased pulmonary vascular resistance or obstruction to blood flow through the pulmonic valve and artery. Cyanosis may also result from a defect that allows mixing of oxygenated and deoxygenated blood within the heart chambers or great arteries, such as occurs in truncus arteriosus.

CLASSIFICATION OF DEFECTS

There are typically two classification systems used to categorize congenital heart defects. Traditionally, cyanosis, a physical characteristic, has been used as the distinguishing feature, dividing anomalies into acyanotic defects and cyanotic defects. In clinical practice, this system is problematic because children with acyanotic defects may develop cyanosis. Also, more often, those with cyanotic defects may appear pink and have more clinical signs of HF.

A more useful classification system is based on hemodynamic characteristics (blood flow patterns within the heart). These blood flow patterns are (1) increased pulmonary blood flow; (2) decreased pulmonary blood flow; (3) obstruction to blood flow out of the heart;

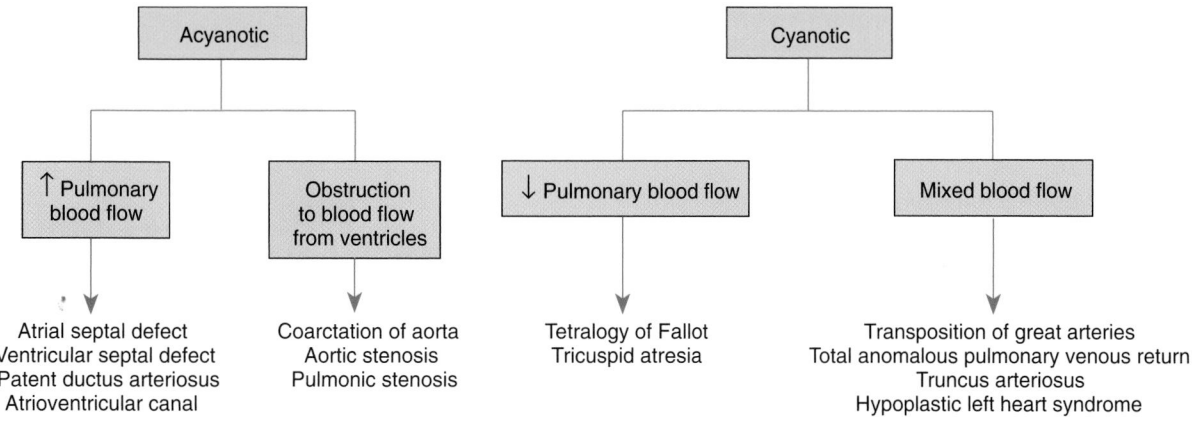

FIG 25-3 Comparison of acyanotic-cyanotic and hemodynamic classification systems of congenital heart disease.

and (4) mixed blood flow, in which saturated and desaturated blood mix within the heart or great arteries. As a comparison, Figure 25-3 outlines both classification systems. With the hemodynamic classification system, the clinical manifestations of each group are more uniform and predictable. Defects that allow blood flow from the higher pressure left side of the heart to the lower pressure right side (left-to-right shunt) result in increased pulmonary blood flow and cause heart failure (HF). Obstructive defects impede blood flow out of the ventricles; whereas obstruction on the left side of the heart results in HF, severe obstruction on the right side causes cyanosis. Defects that cause decreased pulmonary blood flow result in cyanosis. Mixed lesions present a variable clinical picture based on the degree of mixing and amount of pulmonary blood flow; hypoxemia (with or without cyanosis) and HF usually occur together. Using this classification system, the clinical presentation and management of the most common defects are outlined in the following sections and Box 25-1.

The outcomes of surgical treatment for patients with moderate to severe disease are variable. Patient risk factors for increased morbidity and mortality include prematurity or low birth weight, a genetic syndrome, multiple cardiac defects, a noncardiac congenital anomaly, and age at time of surgery (neonates are a higher risk group). For example, aortic stenosis or coarctation manifesting in the first week of life is more severe and carries a higher mortality than if it becomes apparent at 1 year of age. Outcomes for surgical repair of similar congenital heart defects also vary among treatment centers. In general, the outcomes of surgical procedures have steadily improved in the past decade, with mortality rates for many severe defects below 10% and a decrease in the incidence of complications and length of hospital stay.

Defects with Increased Pulmonary Blood Flow

In this group of cardiac defects, intracardiac communications along the septum or an abnormal connection between the great arteries allows blood to flow from the higher pressure left side of the heart to the lower pressure right side of the heart (Fig. 25-4). Increased blood volume on the right side of the heart increases pulmonary blood flow at the expense of systemic blood flow. Clinically, patients demonstrate signs and symptoms of HF. ASD, VSD, and patent ductus arteriosus are typical anomalies in this group (see Box 25-1).

Obstructive Defects

Obstructive defects are those in which blood exiting the heart meets an area of anatomic narrowing (stenosis), causing obstruction to blood flow. The pressure in the ventricle and in the great artery before

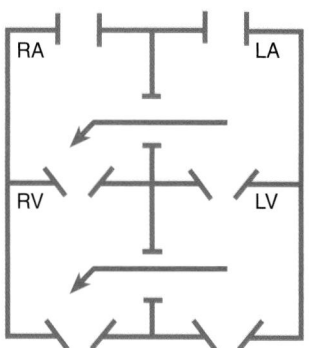

FIG 25-4 Hemodynamics in defects with increased pulmonary blood flow. *LA,* Left atrium; *LV,* left ventricle; *RA,* right atrium; *RV,* right ventricle.

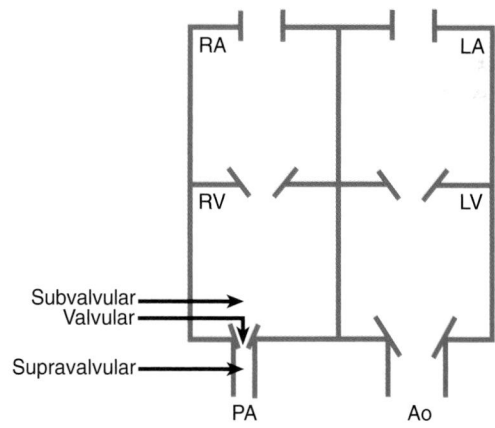

FIG 25-5 Obstruction to ventricular ejection can occur at the valvular level (shown), below the valve (subvalvular), or above the valve (supravalvular). Pulmonary stenosis is shown here. *Ao,* Aorta; *LA,* left atrium; *LV,* left ventricle; *PA,* pulmonary artery; *RA,* right atrium; *RV,* right ventricle.

the obstruction is increased, and the pressure in the area beyond the obstruction is decreased. The location of the narrowing is usually near the valve (Fig. 25-5), as follows:

Valvular—At the site of the valve itself

Subvalvular—Narrowing in the ventricle below the valve (also referred to as the ventricular outflow tract)

Supravalvular—Narrowing in the great artery above the valve

BOX 25-1 DEFECTS WITH INCREASED PULMONARY BLOOD FLOW

Atrial Septal Defect

Description—Abnormal opening between the atria, allowing blood from the higher pressure left atrium to flow into the lower pressure right atrium. There are three types of ASD:

Ostium primum (ASD 1)—Opening at lower end of septum; may be associated with mitral valve abnormalities

Ostium secundum (ASD 2)—Opening near center of septum

Sinus venosus defect—Opening near junction of superior vena cava and right atrium; may be associated with partial anomalous pulmonary venous connection

Pathophysiology—Because left atrial pressure slightly exceeds right atrial pressure, blood flows from the left to the right atrium, causing an increased flow of oxygenated blood into the right side of the heart. Despite the low pressure difference, a high rate of flow can still occur because of low pulmonary vascular resistance and the greater distensibility of the right atrium, which further reduces flow resistance. This volume is well tolerated by the right ventricle because it is delivered under much lower pressure than with a VSD. Although there is right atrial and ventricular enlargement, cardiac failure is unusual in an uncomplicated ASD. Pulmonary vascular changes usually occur only after several decades if the defect is left unrepaired.

Clinical manifestations—Patients may be asymptomatic. They may develop HF. There is a characteristic systolic murmur with a fixed split second heart sound. There may also be a diastolic murmur. Patients are at risk for atrial dysrhythmias (probably caused by atrial enlargement and stretching of conduction fibers) and pulmonary vascular obstructive disease and emboli formation later in life from chronically increased pulmonary blood flow.

Surgical treatment—Surgical patch closure (pericardial patch or Dacron patch) is done for moderate to large defects. Open repair with cardiopulmonary bypass is usually performed before school age. In addition, the sinus

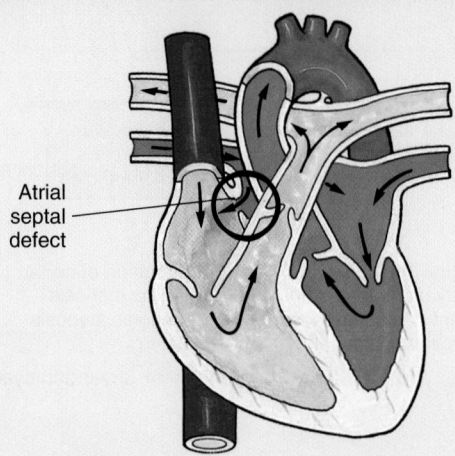

Atrial septal defect

venosus defect requires patch placement, so the anomalous right pulmonary venous return is directed to the left atrium with a baffle. ASD 1 type may require mitral valve repair or, rarely, replacement of the mitral valve.

Nonsurgical treatment—ASD 2 closure with a device during cardiac catheterization is becoming commonplace and can be done as an outpatient procedure. The Amplatzer Septal Occluder is most commonly used. Smaller defects that have a rim around them for attachment of the device can be closed with a device; large, irregular defects without a rim require surgical closure. Successful closure in appropriately selected patients yields results similar to those from surgery but involves shorter hospital stays and fewer complications. Patients receive low-dose aspirin for 6 months (Rome and Kreutzer, 2004).

Prognosis—Operative mortality is very low (<1%).

Ventricular Septal Defect

Description—Abnormal opening between the right and left ventricles. May be classified according to location: membranous (accounting for 80%) or muscular. May vary in size from a small pinhole to absence of the septum, which results in a common ventricle. VSDs are frequently associated with other defects, such as pulmonary stenosis, transposition of the great vessels, PDA, atrial defects, and COA. Many VSDs (20%–60%) close spontaneously. Spontaneous closure is most likely to occur during the first year of life in children having small or moderate defects. A left-to-right shunt is caused by the flow of blood from the higher pressure left ventricle to the lower pressure right ventricle.

Pathophysiology—Because of the higher pressure within the left ventricle and because the systemic arterial circulation offers more resistance than the pulmonary circulation, blood flows through the defect into the pulmonary artery. The increased blood volume is pumped into the lungs, which may eventually result in increased pulmonary vascular resistance. Increased pressure in the right ventricle as a result of left-to-right shunting and pulmonary resistance causes the muscle to hypertrophy. If the right ventricle is unable to accommodate the increased workload, the right atrium may also enlarge as it attempts to overcome the resistance offered by incomplete right ventricular emptying.

Clinical manifestations—HF is common. There is a characteristic loud holosystolic murmur heard best at the left sternal border. Patients are at risk for BE and pulmonary vascular obstructive disease.

Surgical treatment

Palliative—Pulmonary artery banding (placement of a band around the main pulmonary artery to decrease pulmonary blood flow) may be done in infants with multiple muscular VSDs or complex anatomy. Improvements in surgical techniques and postoperative care make complete repair in infancy the preferred approach.

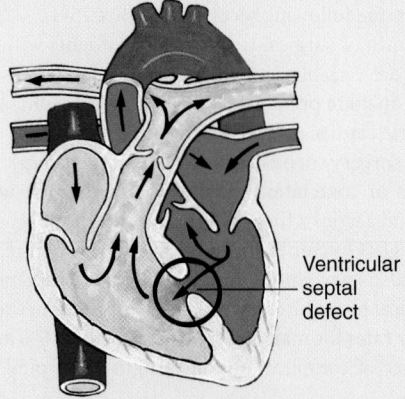

Ventricular septal defect

Complete repair (procedure of choice)—Small defects are repaired with sutures. Large defects usually require that a knitted Dacron patch be sewn over the opening. CPB is used for both procedures. The approach for the repair is generally through the right atrium and the tricuspid valve. Postoperative complications include residual VSD and conduction disturbances.

Nonsurgical treatment—Device closure during cardiac catheterization is being performed in some centers under investigational protocols. One device has been approved for closure of muscular defects, and another is in clinical trials. Early results are encouraging, with successful defect closure and few complications (Rome and Kreutzer, 2004).

Prognosis—Risks depend on the location of the defect, the number of defects, and the presence of other associated cardiac defects. Single-membranous defects are associated with low mortality (<2%); multiple muscular defects can carry a higher risk (Jacobs, Mavroudis, Jacobs, and others, 2004).

BOX 25-1   DEFECTS WITH INCREASED PULMONARY BLOOD FLOW—cont'd

Atrioventricular Canal Defect

Description—Incomplete fusion of the endocardial cushions. Consists of a low ASD that is continuous with a high VSD and clefts of the mitral and tricuspid valves, which create a large central AV valve that allows blood to flow between all four chambers of the heart. The directions and pathways of flow are determined by pulmonary and systemic resistance, left and right ventricular pressures, and the compliance of each chamber, although flow is generally from left to right. It is the most common cardiac defect in children with Down syndrome.

Pathophysiology—The alterations in hemodynamics depend on the severity of the defect and the child's pulmonary vascular resistance. Immediately after birth, while the newborn's pulmonary vascular resistance is high, there is minimum shunting of blood through the defect. When this resistance falls, left-to-right shunting occurs, and pulmonary blood flow increases. The resultant pulmonary vascular engorgement predisposes the child to development of HF.

Clinical manifestations—Patients usually have moderate to severe HF. There is a loud systolic murmur. There may be mild cyanosis that increases with crying. Patients are at high risk for developing pulmonary vascular obstructive disease.

Surgical treatment

Palliative—Pulmonary artery banding is occasionally done in small infants with severe symptoms. Complete repair in infancy is most common.

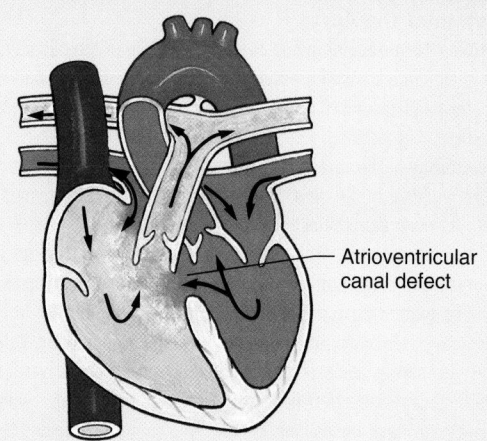

Atrioventricular canal defect

Complete repair—Surgical repair consists of patch closure of the septal defects and reconstruction of the AV valve tissue (either repair of the mitral valve cleft or fashioning of two AV valves). Postoperative complications include heart block, HF, mitral regurgitation, dysrhythmias, and pulmonary hypertension.

Prognosis—Operative mortality is less than 5% (Jacobs, Mavroudis, Jacobs, and others, 2004). A potential later problem is mitral regurgitation, which may require valve replacement.

Patent Ductus Arteriosus

Description—Failure of the fetal ductus arteriosus (artery connecting the aorta and pulmonary artery) to close within the first weeks of life. The continued patency of this vessel allows blood to flow from the higher pressure aorta to the lower pressure pulmonary artery, which causes a left-to-right shunt.

Pathophysiology—The hemodynamic consequences of PDA depend on the size of the ductus and the pulmonary vascular resistance. At birth, the resistance in the pulmonary and systemic circulations is almost identical, so that the resistance in the aorta and pulmonary artery is equalized. As the systemic pressure comes to exceed the pulmonary pressure, blood begins to shunt from the aorta across the duct to the pulmonary artery (left-to-right shunt). The additional blood is recirculated through the lungs and returned to the left atrium and left ventricle. The effects of this altered circulation are increased workload on the left side of the heart, increased pulmonary vascular congestion and possibly resistance, and potentially increased right ventricular pressure and hypertrophy.

Clinical manifestations—Patients may be asymptomatic or show signs of HF. There is a characteristic machinery-like murmur. A widened pulse pressure and bounding pulses result from runoff of blood from the aorta to the pulmonary artery. Patients are at risk for BE and pulmonary vascular obstructive disease in later life from chronic excessive pulmonary blood flow.

Medical management—Administration of indomethacin (a prostaglandin inhibitor) has proved successful in closing a PDA in preterm infants and some newborns.

Surgical treatment—Surgical division or ligation of the patent vessel is performed via a left thoracotomy. In a newer technique, video-assisted

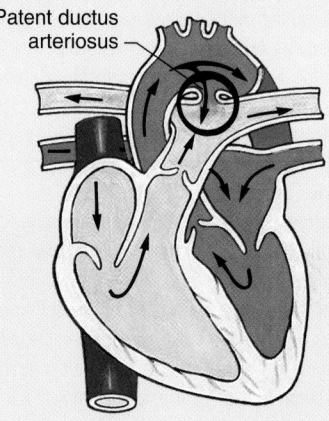

Patent ductus arteriosus

thoracoscopic surgery, a thoracoscope and instruments are inserted through three small incisions on the left side of the chest to place a clip on the ductus. The technique is used in some centers and eliminates the need for a thoracotomy, thereby speeding postoperative recovery.

Nonsurgical treatment—Coils to occlude the PDA are placed in the catheterization laboratory in many centers. Preterm or small infants (with small-diameter femoral arteries) and patients with large or unusual PDAs may require surgery.

Prognosis—Both surgical and nonsurgical procedures can be done at low risk with less than 1% mortality. PDA closure in very preterm infants has a higher mortality rate because of the additional significant medical problems.

ASD, Atrial septal defect; *AV*, atrioventricular; *BE*, bacterial endocarditis; *COA*, coarctation of the aorta; *CPB*, cardiopulmonary bypass; *HF*, heart failure; *PDA*, patent ductus arteriosus; *VSD*, ventricular septal defect.

Coarctation of the aorta (narrowing of the aortic arch), aortic stenosis, and pulmonic stenosis are typical defects in this group (Box 25-2). Hemodynamically, there is a pressure load on the ventricle and decreased cardiac output. Clinically, infants and children exhibit signs of HF. Children with mild obstruction may be asymptomatic. Rarely, as in severe pulmonic stenosis, hypoxemia may be seen.

Defects with Decreased Pulmonary Blood Flow

In this group of defects, there is obstruction of pulmonary blood flow and an anatomic defect (ASD or VSD) between the right and left sides of the heart (Fig. 25-6). Because blood has difficulty exiting the right side of the heart via the pulmonary artery, pressure on the right side

BOX 25-2 OBSTRUCTIVE DEFECTS

Coarctation of the Aorta

Description—Localized narrowing near the insertion of the ductus arteriosus, which results in increased pressure proximal to the defect (head and upper extremities) and decreased pressure distal to the obstruction (body and lower extremities).

Pathophysiology—The effect of a narrowing within the aorta is increased pressure proximal to the defect (upper extremities) and decreased pressure distal to it (lower extremities).

Clinical manifestations—The patient may have high blood pressure and bounding pulses in the arms, weak or absent femoral pulses, and cool lower extremities with lower blood pressure. There are signs of HF in infants. In infants with critical coarctation, the hemodynamic condition may deteriorate rapidly with severe acidosis and hypotension. Mechanical ventilation and inotropic support are often necessary before surgery. Older children may experience dizziness, headaches, fainting, and epistaxis resulting from hypertension. Patients are at risk for hypertension, ruptured aorta, aortic aneurysm, and stroke.

Surgical treatment—Surgical repair is the treatment of choice for infants younger than 6 months of age and for patients with long-segment stenosis or complex anatomy; it may be performed for all patients with coarctation. Repair is by resection of the coarcted portion with an end-to-end anastomosis of the aorta or enlargement of the constricted section using a graft of prosthetic material or a portion of the left subclavian artery. Because this defect is outside the heart and pericardium, cardiopulmonary bypass is not required, and a thoracotomy incision is used. Postoperative hypertension is treated with intravenous sodium nitroprusside, esmolol, or milrinone followed by oral medications, such as ACE inhibitors or beta blockers. Residual permanent hypertension after repair of COA seems to be related to age and time of repair. To prevent both hypertension at rest and exercise-provoked systemic hypertension after repair, elective surgery for COA is advised within the first

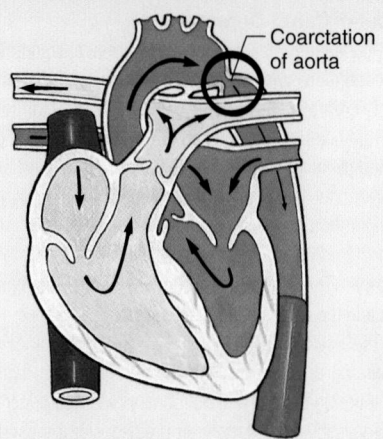
Coarctation of aorta

2 years of life. There is a 15% to 30% risk of recurrence in patients who underwent surgical repair as infants (Beekman, 2001). Percutaneous balloon angioplasty techniques have proved to be effective in relieving residual postoperative coarctation gradients.

Nonsurgical treatment—Balloon angioplasty is being performed as a primary intervention for COA in older infants and children. In adolescents, stents may be placed in the aorta to maintain patency. Recent studies have demonstrated that balloon angioplasty is effective in children and that aneurysm formation is rare. The high restenosis rate in young infants limits its application in this group (Rome and Kreutzer, 2004).

Prognosis—Mortality is less than 5% in patients with isolated coarctation; the risk is increased in infants with other complex cardiac defects (Jacobs, Mavroudis, Jacobs, and others, 2004).

Aortic Stenosis

Description—Narrowing or stricture of the aortic valve, causing resistance to blood flow in the left ventricle, decreased cardiac output, left ventricular hypertrophy, and pulmonary vascular congestion. The prominent anatomic consequence of AS is the hypertrophy of the left ventricular wall, which eventually leads to increased end-diastolic pressure, resulting in pulmonary venous and pulmonary arterial hypertension. Left ventricular hypertrophy also interferes with coronary artery perfusion and may result in myocardial infarction or scarring of the papillary muscles of the left ventricle, which causes mitral insufficiency. Valvular stenosis, the most common type, is usually caused by malformed cusps that result in a bicuspid rather than tricuspid valve or fusion of the cusps. Subvalvular stenosis is a stricture caused by a fibrous ring below a normal valve; supravalvular stenosis occurs infrequently. Valvular AS is a serious defect for the following reasons: (1) the obstruction tends to be progressive; (2) sudden episodes of myocardial ischemia, or low cardiac output, can result in sudden death; and (3) surgical repair rarely results in a normal valve. This is one of the rare instances in which strenuous physical activity may be curtailed because of the cardiac condition.

Pathophysiology—A stricture in the aortic outflow tract causes resistance to ejection of blood from the left ventricle. The extra workload on the left ventricle causes hypertrophy. If left ventricular failure develops, left atrial pressure will increase; this causes increased pressure in the pulmonary veins, which results in pulmonary vascular congestion (pulmonary edema).

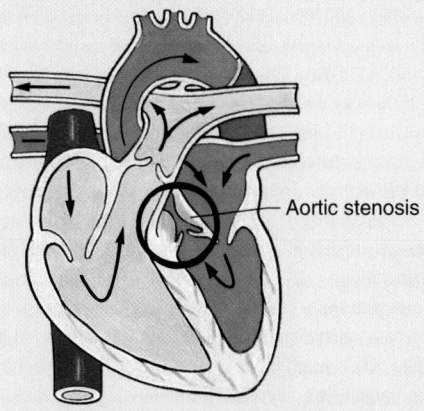
Aortic stenosis

Clinical manifestations—Newborns with critical AS demonstrate signs of decreased cardiac output with faint pulses, hypotension, tachycardia, and poor feeding. Children show signs of exercise intolerance, chest pain, and dizziness when standing for a long period. A systolic ejection murmur may or may not be present. Patients are at risk for BE, coronary insufficiency, and ventricular dysfunction.

BOX 25-2   OBSTRUCTIVE DEFECTS—cont'd

Valvular Aortic Stenosis

Surgical treatment—Aortic valvotomy is performed under inflow occlusion. Used rarely because balloon dilation in the catheterization laboratory is the first-line procedure. Newborns with critical AS and small left-sided structures may undergo a stage 1 Norwood procedure (see Hypoplastic Left Heart Syndrome, Box 25-4).

Prognosis—Aortic valve replacement offers a good treatment option and may lead to normalization of left ventricular size and function (Arnold, Ley-Zaporozhan, Ley, and others, 2008). Results of aortic valvotomy in older children are very good, with mortality and morbidity close to 0% (Shanmugam, MacArthur, and Pollock, 2005). However, aortic valvotomy remains a palliative procedure, and approximately 25% of patients require additional surgery within 10 years for recurrent stenosis. A valve replacement may be required at the second procedure. An aortic homograft with a valve may also be used (extended aortic root replacement), or the pulmonary valve may be moved to the aortic position and replaced with a homograft valve (Ross procedure).

Nonsurgical treatment—The narrowed valve is dilated using balloon angioplasty in the catheterization laboratory. This procedure is usually the first intervention.

Prognosis—Complications include aortic insufficiency or valvular regurgitation, tearing of the valve leaflets, and loss of pulse in the catheterized limb.

⊖ Subvalvular Aortic Stenosis

Surgical treatment—Procedure may involve incising a membrane if one exists or cutting the fibromuscular ring. If the obstruction results from narrowing of the left ventricular outflow tract and a small aortic valve annulus, a patch may be required to enlarge the entire left ventricular outflow tract and annulus and replace the aortic valve; this is known as the Konno procedure.

Prognosis—Mortality from surgical repairs of subvalvular AS is less than 5% in major centers; however, about 20% of these patients develop recurrent subaortic stenosis and require additional surgery (Freed, 2001).

Pulmonic Stenosis

Description—Narrowing at the entrance to the pulmonary artery. Resistance to blood flow causes right ventricular hypertrophy and decreased pulmonary blood flow. Pulmonary atresia is the extreme form of PS in that there is total fusion of the commissures and no blood flows to the lungs. The right ventricle may be hypoplastic.

Pathophysiology—When PS is present, resistance to blood flow causes right ventricular hypertrophy. If right ventricular failure develops, right atrial pressure will increase, and this may result in reopening of the foramen ovale, shunting of unoxygenated blood into the left atrium, and systemic cyanosis. If PS is severe, HF occurs, and systemic venous engorgement will be noted. An associated defect such as a PDA partially compensates for the obstruction by shunting blood from the aorta to the pulmonary artery and into the lungs.

Clinical manifestations—Patients may be asymptomatic; some have mild cyanosis or HF. Progressive narrowing causes increased symptoms. Newborns with severe narrowing are cyanotic. A loud systolic ejection murmur at the upper left sternal border may be present. However, in severely ill patients, the murmur may be much softer because of decreased cardiac output and shunting of blood. Cardiomegaly is evident on chest radiography. Patients are at risk for BE.

Surgical treatment—In infants, transventricular (closed) valvotomy (Brock procedure). In children, pulmonary valvotomy with CPB. Need for surgical treatment is rare with widespread use of balloon angioplasty techniques.

Nonsurgical treatment—Balloon angioplasty in the cardiac catheterization laboratory to dilate the valve. A catheter is inserted across the stenotic pulmonic valve into the pulmonary artery, and a balloon at the end of the catheter is inflated and rapidly passed through the narrowed opening (see figure at right). The procedure is associated with few complications and has proved to be highly effective. It is the treatment of choice for discrete PS in most centers and can be done safely in neonates.

Prognosis—The risk is low for both surgical and nonsurgical procedures; mortality is lower than 1% and slightly higher in neonates (Latson, 2001). Both balloon dilation and surgical valvotomy leave the pulmonic valve incompetent because they involve opening the fused valve leaflets; however, these patients are clinically asymptomatic. Long-term problems with restenosis or valve incompetence may occur.

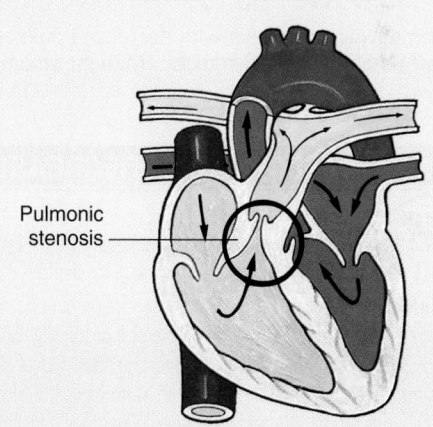

Pulmonic stenosis

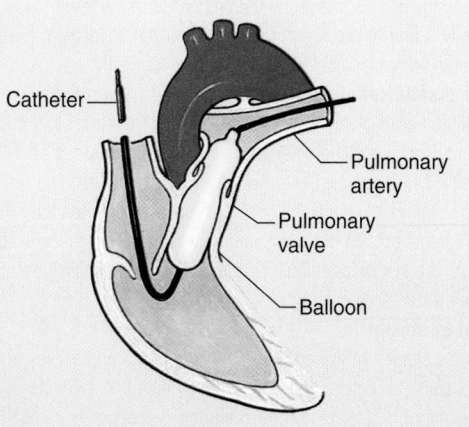

Catheter — Pulmonary artery — Pulmonary valve — Balloon

ACE, Angiotensin-converting enzyme; *AS,* aortic stenosis; *BE,* bacterial endocarditis; *COA,* coarctation of the aorta; *CPB,* cardiopulmonary bypass; *HF,* heart failure; *PDA,* patent ductus arteriosus; *PS,* pulmonic stenosis.

increases, exceeding left-sided pressure. This allows desaturated blood to shunt right to left, causing desaturation in the left side of the heart and in the systemic circulation. Clinically, these patients have hypoxemia and usually appear cyanotic. Tetralogy of Fallot and tricuspid atresia are the most common defects in this group (Box 25-3).

Mixed Defects

Many complex cardiac anomalies are classified together in the mixed category (Box 25-4) because survival in the postnatal period depends on mixing of blood from the pulmonary and systemic circulations within the heart chambers. Hemodynamically, fully saturated systemic

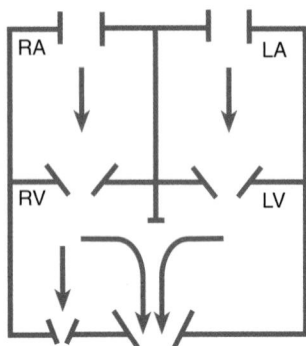

FIG 25-6 Hemodynamic defects with decreased pulmonary blood flow. *LA,* Left atrium; *LV,* left ventricle; *RA,* right atrium; *RV,* right ventricle.

blood flow mixes with the desaturated pulmonary blood flow, causing a relative desaturation of the systemic blood flow. Pulmonary congestion occurs because the differences in pulmonary artery pressure and aortic pressure favor pulmonary blood flow. Cardiac output decreases because of a volume load on the ventricle. Clinically, these patients have a variable picture that combines some degree of desaturation (although cyanosis is not always visible) and signs of HF. Some defects, such as transposition of the great arteries, cause severe cyanosis in the first days of life and later cause HF. Others, such as truncus arteriosus, cause severe HF in the first weeks of life and mild desaturation.

CLINICAL CONSEQUENCES OF CONGENITAL HEART DISEASE

HEART FAILURE

HF is the inability of the heart to pump an adequate amount of blood to the systemic circulation at normal filling pressures to meet the body's metabolic demands. In children, HF most frequently occurs secondary to structural abnormalities (e.g., septal defects) that result in increased blood volume and pressure within the heart. It can also result from myocardial failure in which the contractility of the ventricle is impaired. This can occur with cardiomyopathy, dysrhythmias, or severe electrolyte disturbances. HF can also occur because of excessive demands on a normal heart muscle, such as sepsis or severe anemia.

BOX 25-3   DEFECTS WITH DECREASED PULMONARY BLOOD FLOW

Tetralogy of Fallot

Description—The classic form includes four defects: (1) VSD, (2) PS, (3) overriding aorta, and (4) right ventricular hypertrophy.

Pathophysiology—The alteration in hemodynamics varies widely, depending primarily on the degree of PS but also on the size of the VSD and the pulmonary and systemic resistance to flow. Because the VSD is usually large, pressures may be equal in the right and left ventricles. Therefore, the shunt direction depends on the difference between pulmonary and systemic vascular resistance. If pulmonary vascular resistance is higher than systemic resistance, the shunt is from right to left. If systemic resistance is higher than pulmonary resistance, the shunt is from left to right. PS decreases blood flow to the lungs and consequently the amount of oxygenated blood that returns to the left side of the heart. Depending on the position of the aorta, blood from both ventricles may be distributed systemically.

Clinical manifestations—Some infants may be acutely cyanotic at birth; others have mild cyanosis that progresses over the first year of life as the PS worsens. There is a characteristic systolic murmur that is often moderate in intensity. There may be acute episodes of cyanosis and hypoxia, called *blue spells* or *tet spells* (see p. 841). Anoxic spells occur when the infant's oxygen requirements exceed the blood supply, usually during crying or after feeding. Patients are at risk for emboli, seizures, and loss of consciousness or sudden death after an anoxic spell.

Surgical treatment

Palliative shunt—In infants who cannot undergo primary repair, a palliative procedure to increase pulmonary blood flow and increase oxygen saturation may be performed. The preferred procedure is a modified Blalock-Taussig shunt operation, which provides blood flow to the pulmonary arteries from the left or right subclavian artery via a tube graft (see Table 25-4, p. 842). In general, however, shunts are avoided because they may result in pulmonary artery distortion.

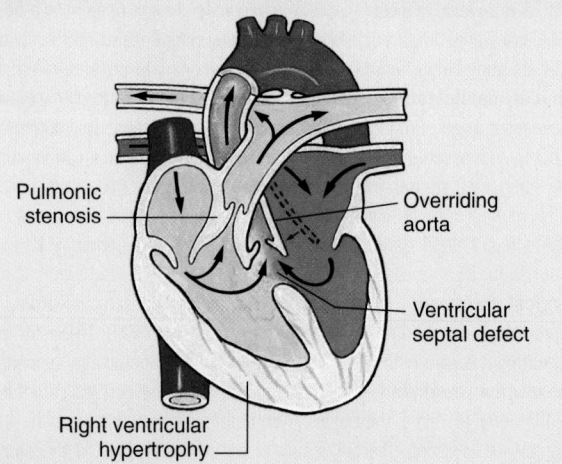

Pulmonic stenosis

Overriding aorta

Ventricular septal defect

Right ventricular hypertrophy

Complete repair—Elective repair is usually performed in the first year of life. Indications for repair include increasing cyanosis and the development of hypercyanotic spells. Complete repair involves closure of the VSD and resection of the infundibular stenosis, with placement of a pericardial patch to enlarge the RVOT. In some repairs, the patch may extend across the pulmonary valve annulus (transannular patch), making the pulmonary valve incompetent. The procedure requires a median sternotomy and the use of cardiopulmonary bypass.

Prognosis—The operative mortality for total correction of tetralogy of Fallot is less than 3% (Jacobs, Mavroudis, Jacobs, and others, 2004). With improved surgical techniques, there is a lower incidence of dysrhythmias and sudden death; surgical heart block is rare. Heart failure may occur postoperatively.

BOX 25-3 DEFECTS WITH DECREASED PULMONARY BLOOD FLOW—cont'd

Tricuspid Atresia

Description—The tricuspid valve fails to develop; consequently there is no communication from the right atrium to the right ventricle. Blood flows through an ASD or a patent foramen ovale to the left side of the heart and through a VSD to the right ventricle and out to the lungs. The condition is often associated with PS and TGA. There is complete mixing of unoxygenated and oxygenated blood in the left side of the heart, which results in systemic desaturation, and varying amounts of pulmonary obstruction, which causes decreased pulmonary blood flow.

Pathophysiology—At birth, the presence of a patent foramen ovale (or other atrial septal opening) is required to permit blood flow across the septum into the left atrium; the PDA allows blood flow to the pulmonary artery into the lungs for oxygenation. A VSD allows a modest amount of blood to enter the right ventricle and pulmonary artery for oxygenation. Pulmonary blood flow usually is diminished.

Clinical manifestations—Cyanosis is usually seen in the newborn period. There may be tachycardia and dyspnea. Older children have signs of chronic hypoxemia with clubbing.

Therapeutic management—For neonates whose pulmonary blood flow depends on the patency of the ductus arteriosus, a continuous infusion of prostaglandin E$_1$ is started at 0.1 mcg/kg/min until surgical intervention can be arranged.

Surgical treatment—Palliative treatment is the placement of a shunt (pulmonary–to–systemic artery anastomosis) to increase blood flow to the lungs. If the ASD is small, an atrial septostomy is performed during cardiac catheterization. Some children have increased pulmonary blood flow and require pulmonary artery banding to lessen the volume of blood to the lungs. A bidirectional Glenn shunt (cavopulmonary anastomosis) may be performed at 4 to 9 months as a second stage.

Modified Fontan procedure—Systemic venous return is directed to the lungs without a ventricular pump through surgical connections between the right atrium and the pulmonary artery. A fenestration (opening) is sometimes made in the right atrial baffle to relieve pressure. The patient must have normal ventricular function and a low pulmonary vascular resistance for the procedure to be successful. The modified Fontan procedure separates oxygenated and unoxygenated blood inside the heart and eliminates the excess volume load on the ventricle but does not restore normal anatomy or hemodynamics. This operation is also the final stage in the correction of many complex defects with a functional single ventricle, including hypoplastic left heart syndrome.

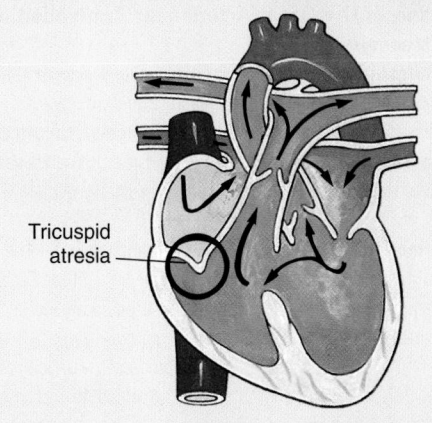

Tricuspid atresia

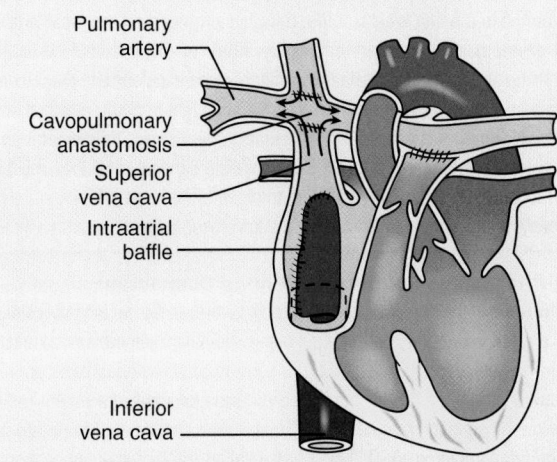

Pulmonary artery
Cavopulmonary anastomosis
Superior vena cava
Intraatrial baffle
Inferior vena cava

Prognosis—Surgical mortality is less than 5% (Jacobs, Mavroudis, Jacobs, and others, 2004); the rate increases when the anatomy is more complex and other risk factors are present. Postoperative complications include dysrhythmias, systemic venous hypertension, pleural and pericardial effusions, and ventricular dysfunction. Long-term concerns are the development of protein-losing enteropathy, atrial dysrhythmias, late ventricular dysfunction, and developmental delays.

ASD, Atrial septal defect; *PDA,* patent ductus arteriosus; *PS,* pulmonic stenosis; *RVOT,* right ventricular outflow tract; *TGA,* transposition of the great arteries; *VSD,* ventricular septal defect.

BOX 25-4 MIXED DEFECTS

Transposition of the Great Arteries, or Transposition of the Great Vessels

Description—The pulmonary artery leaves the left ventricle, and the aorta exits from the right ventricle with no communication between the systemic and pulmonary circulations.

Pathophysiology—Associated defects such as septal defects or PDA must be present to permit blood to enter the systemic circulation or the pulmonary circulation for mixing of saturated and desaturated blood. The most common defect associated with TGA is a patent foramen ovale. At birth, there is also a PDA, although in most instances, this closes after the neonatal period. Another associated defect may be a VSD. The presence of a VSD increases the risk of HF because it permits blood to flow from the right to the left ventricle, into the pulmonary artery, and finally to the lungs. However, it also produces high pulmonary blood flow under high pressure, which can result in high pulmonary vascular resistance.

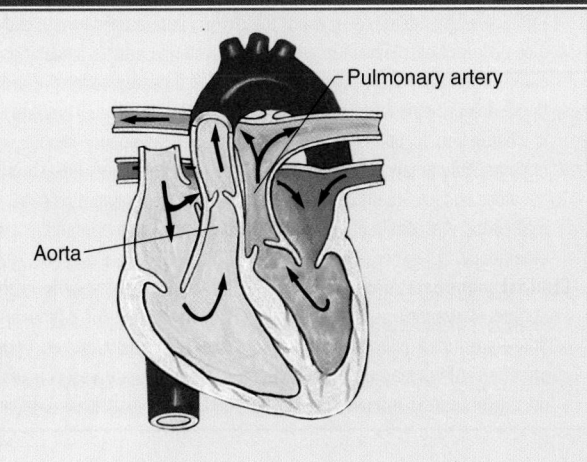

Pulmonary artery
Aorta

Continued

BOX 25-4 MIXED DEFECTS—cont'd

Transposition of the Great Arteries, or Transposition of the Great Vessels

Clinical manifestations—Depend on the type and size of the associated defects. Newborns with minimum communication are severely cyanotic and have depressed function at birth. Those with large septal defects or a PDA may be less cyanotic but have symptoms of HF. Heart sounds vary according to the type of defect present. Cardiomegaly is usually evident a few weeks after birth.

Therapeutic management (to provide intracardiac mixing)—The administration of intravenous prostaglandin E₁ may be initiated to keep the ductus arteriosus open to temporarily increase blood mixing and provide an oxygen saturation of 75% or to maintain cardiac output. During cardiac catheterization or under echocardiographic guidance, a balloon atrial septostomy (Rashkind procedure) may also be performed to increase mixing by opening the atrial septum.

Surgical treatment—An arterial switch procedure is the procedure of choice performed in the first weeks of life. It involves transecting the great arteries and anastomosing the main pulmonary artery to the proximal aorta (just above the aortic valve) and anastomosing the ascending aorta to the proximal pulmonary artery. The coronary arteries are switched from the proximal aorta to the proximal pulmonary artery to create a new aorta. Reimplantation of the coronary arteries is critical to the infant's survival, and they must be reattached without torsion or kinking to provide the heart with its supply of oxygen. The advantage of the arterial switch procedure is the reestablishment of normal circulation, with the left ventricle acting as the systemic pump. Potential complications of the arterial switch include narrowing at the great artery anastomoses and coronary artery insufficiency.

Intraatrial baffle repairs—Intraatrial baffle repairs are rarely performed, although many adolescents and adults survive today with repairs that were done more than 15 years ago. An intraatrial baffle is created to divert venous blood to the mitral valve and pulmonary venous blood to the tricuspid valve using the patient's atrial septum (Senning procedure) or a prosthetic material (Mustard procedure). A disadvantage is the continuing role of the right ventricle as the systemic pump and the late development of right ventricular failure and rhythm disturbances. Other potential postoperative complications include loss of normal sinus rhythm, baffle leaks, and ventricular dysfunction.

Rastelli procedure—This procedure is the operative choice in infants with TGA, VSD, and severe PS. It involves closure of the VSD with a baffle, so that left ventricular blood is directed through the VSD into the aorta. The pulmonic valve is then closed, and a conduit is placed from the right ventricle to the pulmonary artery to create a physiologically normal circulation. Unfortunately, this procedure requires multiple conduit replacements as the child grows.

Prognosis—Operative mortality is less than 2% (Jacobs, Mavroudis, Jacobs, and others, 2004). Potential long-term problems include suprapulmonic stenosis and neoaortal dilation and regurgitation.

Total Anomalous Pulmonary Venous Connection

Description—Rare defect characterized by failure of the pulmonary veins to join the left atrium. Instead, the pulmonary veins are abnormally connected to the systemic venous circuit via the right atrium or various veins draining toward the right atrium, such as the SVC. The abnormal attachment results in mixed blood being returned to the right atrium and shunted from the right to the left through an ASD. TAPVC (also called total anomalous pulmonary venous return or total anomalous pulmonary venous drainage) is classified according to the pulmonary venous point of attachment as follows:

Supracardiac—Attachment above the diaphragm, such as to the SVC (most common form) (see Fig. 25-10, p. 842)

Cardiac—Direct attachment to the heart, such as to the right atrium or coronary sinus

Infradiaphragmatic—Attachment below the diaphragm, such as to the IVC (most severe form)

Pathophysiology—The right atrium receives all the blood that normally would flow into the left atrium. As a result, whereas the right side of the heart hypertrophies, the left side, especially the left atrium, may remain small. An associated ASD or patent foramen ovale allows systemic venous blood to shunt from the higher pressure right atrium to the left atrium and into the left side of the heart. As a result, the oxygen saturation of the blood in both sides of the heart (and ultimately in the systemic arterial circulation) is the same. If the pulmonary blood flow is large, pulmonary venous return is also large, and the amount of saturated blood is relatively high. However, if there is obstruction to pulmonary venous drainage, pulmonary venous return is impeded, pulmonary venous pressure rises, and pulmonary interstitial edema develops and eventually contributes to HF. Infradiaphragmatic TAPVC is often associated with obstruction to pulmonary venous drainage and is a surgical emergency.

Clinical manifestations—Most infants develop cyanosis early in life. The degree of cyanosis is inversely related to the amount of pulmonary blood flow—the more pulmonary blood, the less cyanosis. Children with unobstructed TAPVC may be asymptomatic until pulmonary vascular resistance decreases during infancy, increasing pulmonary blood flow with resulting signs of HF. Cyanosis becomes worse with pulmonary vein obstruction; when obstruction occurs, the infant's condition usually deteriorates rapidly. Without intervention, cardiac failure will progress to death.

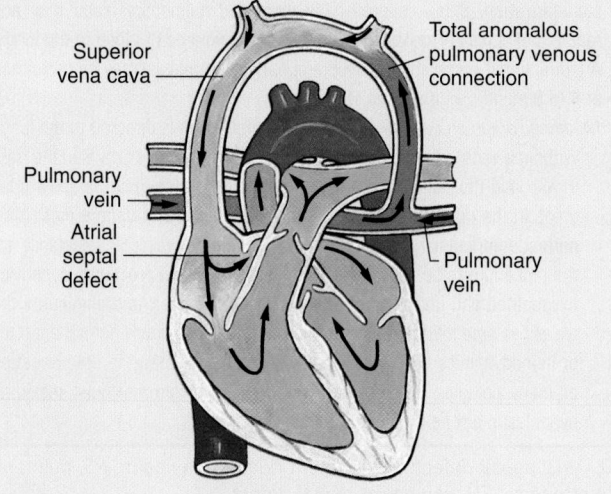

Surgical treatment—Corrective repair is performed in early infancy. The surgical approach varies with the anatomic defect. In general, however, the common pulmonary vein is anastomosed to the back of the left atrium, the ASD is closed, and the anomalous pulmonary venous connection is ligated. The cardiac type is most easily repaired; the infradiaphragmatic type carries the highest morbidity and mortality because of the higher incidence of pulmonary vein obstruction. Potential postoperative complications include reobstruction; bleeding; dysrhythmias, particularly heart block; pulmonary artery hypertension; and persistent heart failure.

Prognosis—Mortality for all types is less than 10% (Jacobs, Mavroudis, Jacobs, and others, 2004) and is lowest for the cardiac type; morbidity increases with the presence of pulmonary vein obstruction.

BOX 25-4   MIXED DEFECTS—cont'd

Truncus Arteriosus

Description—Failure of normal septation and division of the embryonic bulbar trunk into the pulmonary artery and the aorta, which results in development of a single vessel that overrides both ventricles. Blood from both ventricles mixes in the common great artery, which leads to desaturation and hypoxemia. Blood ejected from the heart flows preferentially to the lower-pressure pulmonary arteries, so that pulmonary blood flow is increased and systemic blood flow is reduced. There are three types:

Type I—A single pulmonary trunk arises near the base of the truncus and divides into the left and right pulmonary arteries.

Type II—The left and right pulmonary arteries arise separately but in close proximity and at the same level from the back of the truncus.

Type III—The pulmonary arteries arise independently from the sides of the truncus.

Pathophysiology—Blood ejected from the left and right ventricles enters the common trunk so that pulmonary and systemic circulations are mixed. Blood flow is distributed to the pulmonary and systemic circulations according to the relative resistances of each system. The amount of pulmonary blood flow depends on the size of the pulmonary arteries and the pulmonary vascular resistance. Generally, resistance to pulmonary blood flow is less than systemic vascular resistance, which results in preferential blood flow to the lungs. Pulmonary vascular disease develops at an early age in patients with truncus arteriosus.

Clinical manifestations—Most infants are symptomatic with moderate to severe HF and variable cyanosis, poor growth, and activity intolerance. There is a holosystolic murmur at the left sternal murmur with a diastolic murmur present if truncal regurgitation is present. Thirty-five percent of patients have 22q11 deletions (Goldmuntz, Clark, Mitchell, and others, 1998).

Surgical treatment—Early repair is performed in the first month of life. It involves closing the VSD so that the truncus arteriosus receives the outflow

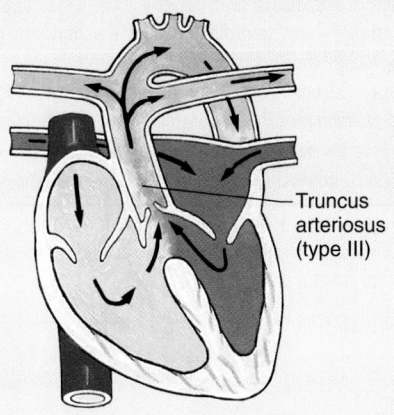

Truncus arteriosus (type III)

from the left ventricle and excising the pulmonary arteries from the aorta and attaching them to the right ventricle by means of a homograft. Currently, homografts (segments of cadaver aorta and pulmonary artery that are treated with antibiotics and cryopreserved) are preferred over synthetic conduits to establish continuity between the right ventricle and pulmonary artery. Homografts are more flexible and easier to use during the procedure and appear less prone to obstruction. Postoperative complications include persistent heart failure, bleeding, pulmonary artery hypertension, dysrhythmias, and residual VSD. Because conduits are not living tissue, they will not grow along with the child and may also become narrowed with calcifications. One or more conduit replacements will be needed in childhood.

Prognosis—Mortality is greater than 10%; future operations are required to replace the conduits.

Hypoplastic Left Heart Syndrome

Description—Underdevelopment of the left side of the heart, resulting in a hypoplastic left ventricle and aortic atresia. Most blood from the left atrium flows across the patent foramen ovale to the right atrium, to the right ventricle, and out the pulmonary artery. The descending aorta receives blood from the PDA supplying systemic blood flow.

Pathophysiology—An ASD or patent foramen ovale allows saturated blood from the left atrium to mix with desaturated blood from the right atrium and to flow through the right ventricle and out into the pulmonary artery. From the pulmonary artery, the blood flows both to the lungs and through the ductus arteriosus into the aorta and out to the body. The amount of blood flow to the pulmonary and systemic circulations depends on the relationship between the pulmonary and systemic vascular resistances. The coronary and cerebral vessels receive blood by retrograde flow through the hypoplastic ascending aorta.

Clinical manifestations—The patient has mild cyanosis and signs of HF until the PDA closes and then progressive deterioration with cyanosis and decreased cardiac output, leading to cardiovascular collapse. The condition is usually fatal in the first months of life without intervention.

Therapeutic management—Neonates require stabilization with mechanical ventilation and inotropic support preoperatively. A prostaglandin E₁ infusion is needed to maintain ductal patency and ensure adequate systemic blood flow.

Surgical treatment—A multiple-stage approach is used. The first stage is a Norwood procedure, which involves an anastomosis of the main pulmonary artery to the aorta to create a new aorta, shunting to provide pulmonary blood flow (usually with a modified Blalock-Taussig shunt), and creation of a large

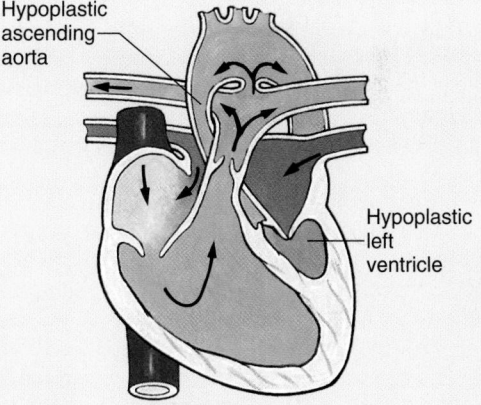

Hypoplastic ascending aorta

Hypoplastic left ventricle

ASD. Postoperative complications include imbalance of systemic and pulmonary blood flow, bleeding, low cardiac output, and persistent heart failure. A new modification of the first stage repair is the use of a right ventricle–to–pulmonary artery homograft conduit instead of a shunt to supply pulmonary blood flow (Sano procedure). The second stage is often a bidirectional Glenn shunt procedure (see Fig. 25-10, p. 842) or a hemi-Fontan operation. Both involve anastomosing the SVC to the right pulmonary artery so SVC flow bypasses the right atrium and flows directly to the lungs. The procedure is usually done at 3 to 6 months of age to relieve cyanosis and reduce the volume load on the right ventricle. The final repair is a modified Fontan procedure (see Tricuspid Atresia, Box 25-3).

Continued

BOX 25-4   MIXED DEFECTS—cont'd

Hypoplastic Left Heart Syndrome

Transplantation—Heart transplantation in the newborn period is another option for these infants. Problems include the shortage of newborn organ donors, risk of rejection, long-term problems with chronic immunosuppression, and infection (see Heart Transplantation, p. 856).

Prognosis—For the first-stage repair, survival rates vary widely in different centers. Much progress has been made, and some experienced centers are

reporting mortality rates of about 10% (Tweddell, Hoffman, Mussatto, and others, 2002), but a large multicenter series reports a mortality rate of about 30% (Jacobs, Mavroudis, Jacobs, and others, 2004). Long-term problems with repair include worsening ventricular function, tricuspid regurgitation, recurrent aortic arch narrowing, dysrhythmias, and developmental delays. There is a risk of mortality between surgical procedures. The mortality for the later two operations is less than 5%.

ASD, Atrial septal defect; *HF,* heart failure; *IVC,* inferior vena cava; *PDA,* patent ductus arteriosus; *PS,* pulmonic stenosis; *SVC,* superior vena cava; *TAPVC,* total anomalous pulmonary venous connection; *TGA,* transposition of the great arteries; *VSD,* ventricular septal defect.

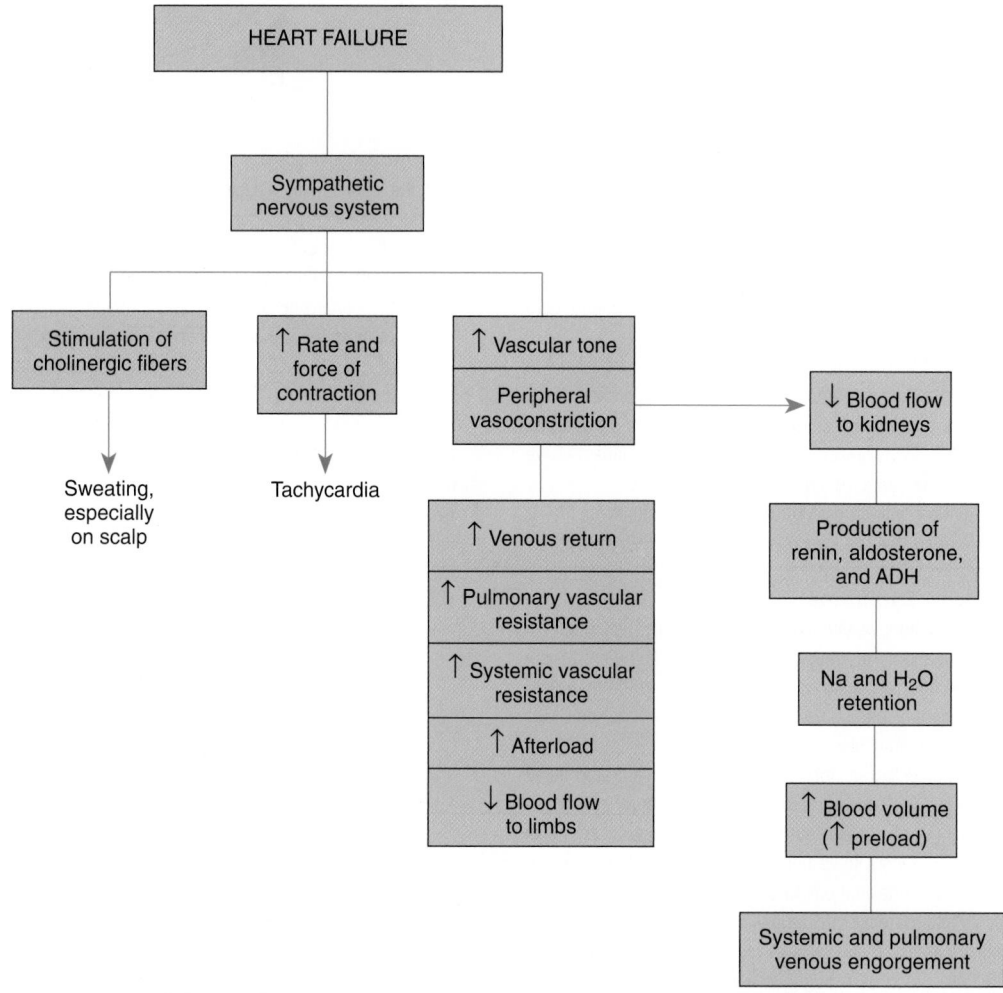

FIG 25-7 Pathophysiology of heart failure. *ADH,* Antidiuretic hormone.

Pathophysiology

Heart failure is often separated into two categories, right-sided and left-sided failure. In **right-sided failure**, the right ventricle is unable to pump blood effectively into the pulmonary artery, resulting in increased pressure in the right atrium and systemic venous circulation. Systemic venous hypertension causes hepatosplenomegaly and occasionally edema. In **left-sided failure**, the left ventricle is unable to pump blood into the systemic circulation, resulting in increased pressure in the left atrium and pulmonary veins. The lungs become congested with blood, causing elevated pulmonary pressures and pulmonary edema.

Although each type of HF produces different signs and symptoms, clinically, it is unusual to observe solely right- or left-sided failure in children. Because each side of the heart depends on adequate function of the other side, failure of one chamber causes a reciprocal change in the opposite chamber.

If the abnormalities precipitating HF are not corrected, the heart muscle becomes damaged. Despite compensatory mechanisms, the heart is unable to maintain an adequate cardiac output. Decreased blood flow to the kidneys continues to stimulate sodium and water reabsorption, leading to fluid overload, increased workload on the heart, and congestion in the pulmonary and systemic circulations (Fig. 25-7).

BOX 25-5 CLINICAL MANIFESTATIONS OF HEART FAILURE

Impaired Myocardial Function
Tachycardia
Sweating (inappropriate)
Decreased urinary output
Fatigue
Weakness
Restlessness
Anorexia
Pale, cool extremities
Weak peripheral pulses
Decreased blood pressure
Gallop rhythm
Cardiomegaly

Pulmonary Congestion
Tachypnea
Dyspnea
Retractions (infants)
Flaring nares
Exercise intolerance
Orthopnea
Cough, hoarseness
Cyanosis
Wheezing
Grunting

Systemic Venous Congestion
Weight gain
Hepatomegaly
Peripheral edema, especially periorbital
Ascites
Neck vein distention (children)

Clinical Manifestations

The signs and symptoms of HF can be divided into three groups: (1) impaired myocardial function, (2) pulmonary congestion, and (3) systemic venous congestion (Box 25-5). Because these hemodynamic changes occur from different causes and at differing times, the clinical presentation may vary among children.

Diagnostic Evaluation

Diagnosis is made on the basis of clinical symptoms such as tachypnea and tachycardia at rest, dyspnea, retractions, activity intolerance (especially during feeding in infants), weight gain caused by fluid retention, and hepatomegaly. Chest radiography demonstrates cardiomegaly and increased pulmonary blood flow. Ventricular hypertrophy appears on the ECG. An echocardiogram is done to determine the cause of HF such as a congenital heart defect or poor ventricular function.

Therapeutic Management

The goals of treatment are to (1) improve cardiac function (increase contractility and decrease afterload), (2) remove accumulated fluid and sodium (decrease preload), (3) decrease cardiac demands, and (4) improve tissue oxygenation and decrease oxygen consumption. For most infants diagnosed with HF, the cause is CHD. Infants are stabilized on medical therapy and then referred for surgical repair. Today many children are being surgically repaired in the neonatal and early

infancy stages before the onset of HF symptoms (Margossian, 2008). For children newly diagnosed with HF, the cause may be worsening ventricular function following a previous cardiac repair, cardiomyopathy, arrhythmia, or other conditions. In addition to management of HF, the underlying cause is treated if possible.

Improve Cardiac Function

Two groups of drugs are used to enhance myocardial function in HF: (1) digitalis glycosides (digoxin), which improve contractility, and (2) angiotensin-converting enzyme (ACE) inhibitors, which reduce the afterload on the heart and thus make it easier for the heart to pump. Myocardial efficiency is improved through administration of digitalis glycosides. The beneficial effects are increased cardiac output, decreased heart size, decreased venous pressure, and relief of edema. In children, digoxin (Lanoxin) is used almost exclusively because of its more rapid onset. It is available as an elixir (0.05 mg/ml) for oral administration. For infants, the dose is calculated in micrograms (1000 mcg = 1 mg).

Treatment consists of a digitalizing dosage, given orally or intravenously in divided doses over 24 hours to produce optimal cardiac effects, and a maintenance dosage, given orally twice a day to maintain blood levels. During digitalization, the child is monitored by means of an ECG to observe for the desired effects (prolonged PR interval and reduced ventricular rate) and detect side effects, especially dysrhythmias.

Another group of drugs used in the treatment of HF, the ACE inhibitors, inhibit the normal function of the renin–angiotensin system in the kidney. The ACE inhibitors block the conversion of angiotensin I to angiotensin II so that, instead of vasoconstriction, vasodilation occurs. Vasodilation results in decreased pulmonary and systemic vascular resistance, decreased BP, and a reduction in afterload. It also reduces the secretion of aldosterone, which reduces preload by preventing volume expansion from fluid retention and decreases the risk of hypokalemia. Common medications used in children are captopril (Capoten), enalapril (Vasotec), and lisinopril. The principal side effects of ACE inhibitors are hypotension, cough, and renal dysfunction.

β-Blockers, specifically metoprolol and carvedilol (Coreg), are the newest medications to be added to the treatment of some children with chronic HF. The α- and β-adrenergic receptors are blocked, causing decreased heart rate, decreased BP, and vasodilation. It has been shown to decrease morbidity and mortality in some adults with HF and is being used selectively in children. Side effects included dizziness, headache, and hypotension.

Cardiac resynchronization therapy (CRT) using biventricular pacing is an effective treatment in adult patients with HF and is beginning to be applied in the pediatric population. With pharmacologic therapies described above, CRT has the potential to improve cardiac function in this group of patients, including those with a single ventricle (Cecchin, Frangini, Brown, and others, 2009; Dubin, Janousek, Rhee, and others, 2005).

! NURSING ALERT

Because ACE inhibitors also block the action of aldosterone, the addition of potassium supplements or spironolactone (Aldactone) to the drug regimen of patients taking diuretics is usually not needed and may cause hyperkalemia.

Remove Accumulated Fluid and Sodium

Treatment consists of diuretics, possible fluid restriction, and possible sodium restriction. Diuretics are the mainstay of therapy to eliminate excess water and salt to prevent reaccumulation. The most frequently used agents are listed in Table 25-3. Because furosemide and the

TABLE 25-3 DIURETICS USED IN HEART FAILURE

ACTIONS	COMMENTS	NURSING CARE MANAGEMENT
Furosemide (Lasix)—Blocks reabsorption of sodium and water in proximal renal tubule and interferes with reabsorption of sodium	Drug of choice in severe HF Causes excretion of chloride and potassium (hypokalemia may precipitate digitalis toxicity)	Begin to record output as soon as drug is given. Observe for dehydration caused by profound diuresis. Observe for side effects (nausea and vomiting, diarrhea, ototoxicity, hypokalemia, dermatitis, postural hypotension). Encourage foods high in potassium or give potassium supplements. Monitor chloride and acid–base balance with long-term therapy. Observe for signs of digoxin toxicity.
Chlorothiazide (Diuril)—Acts directly on distal tubules to decrease sodium, water, potassium, chloride, and bicarbonate absorption	Less frequently used drug Causes hypokalemia, acidosis from large doses	Observe for side effects (nausea, weakness, dizziness, paresthesia, muscle cramps, skin eruptions, hypokalemia, acidosis). Encourage foods high in potassium or give potassium supplements.
Spironolactone (Aldactone)—Blocks action of aldosterone, which promotes retention of sodium and excretion of potassium	Weak diuretic Has potassium-sparing effect; frequently used with thiazides, furosemide Poorly absorbed from GI tract Takes several days to achieve maximum actions	Observe for side effects (skin rash, drowsiness, ataxia, hyperkalemia). Do not administer potassium supplements.

GI, Gastrointestinal; *HF,* heart failure.

thiazides are potassium-losing diuretics, potassium supplements may be prescribed, and rich dietary sources of the electrolyte are encouraged.

> **! NURSING ALERT**
>
> A fall in the serum potassium level enhances the effects of digitalis, increasing the risk of digoxin toxicity. Increased serum potassium levels diminish digoxin's effect. Therefore, serum potassium levels must be carefully monitored.

Fluid restriction may be required in the acute stages of HF and must be carefully calculated to avoid dehydrating the child, especially if cyanotic CHD and significant polycythemia are present. Infants rarely need fluid restrictions because HF makes feeding so difficult that they struggle to take maintenance fluids.

Sodium-restricted diets are used less often in children than in adults to control HF because of their potential negative effects on the child's appetite and ultimate growth. If salt intake is restricted, additional table salt and highly salted foods are avoided.

Decrease Cardiac Demands

To lessen the workload on the heart, metabolic needs are minimized by (1) providing a neutral thermal environment to prevent cold stress in infants, (2) treating any existing infections, (3) reducing the effort of breathing (by placement in semi-Fowler position), (4) using medication to sedate an irritable child, and (5) providing for rest and decreasing environmental stimuli.

Improve Tissue Oxygenation

The preceding measures serve to increase tissue oxygenation, either by improving myocardial function or by lessening tissue oxygen demands. In addition, supplemental cool humidified oxygen may be administered to increase the amount of available oxygen during inspiration. Oxygen administration is especially helpful in patients with pulmonary edema, intercurrent respiratory tract infections, and increased pulmonary vascular resistance (oxygen is a vasodilator that decreases pulmonary vascular resistance).

> **! NURSING ALERT**
>
> Oxygen is a drug and is administered only with an appropriate order. There are some uncommon circumstances in patients with complex hemodynamics in which oxygen can be detrimental.

An oxygen hood, nasal cannula, or face tent is used to deliver oxygen. Nasal cannulas are ideal for long-term oxygen administration because the child can be ambulatory and can easily eat and drink. Cool humidification is necessary to counteract the drying effect of oxygen. The amount of cool humidity is carefully regulated to prevent chilling.

> **QUALITY PATIENT OUTCOMES: Heart Failure**
> - Adequate cardiac output
> - Decreased cardiac demands
> - Improved respiratory function
> - No evidence of fluid excess
> - Adequate support and education

Nursing Care Management

The infant or child with HF may be acutely ill, and some may require intensive care until the symptoms improve. Expert nursing care is essential to reduce the cardiac demands that strain the failing heart muscle. During this time, the child and family require emotional support. Although the objectives of nursing care are the same, interventions differ depending on the child's age (see Nursing Care Plan).

Assist in Measures to Improve Cardiac Function

The nurse's responsibility in administering digoxin includes calculating and administering the correct dosage, observing for signs of toxicity, and instituting parental teaching regarding drug administration at home. The child's apical pulse is always checked before administering digoxin. As a general rule, the drug is not given if the pulse is below 90 to 110 beats/min in infants and young children or below 70 beats/min in older children (the cutoff point for adults is 60 beats/min). However, because the pulse rate varies in children in different age

NURSING CARE PLAN

The Child with Heart Failure

NURSING DIAGNOSIS	PATIENT OUTCOMES	NURSING INTERVENTIONS	RATIONALE
Decreased Cardiac Output related to structural defect, myocardial dysfunction, altered hemodynamics **Child's Defining Characteristics (Subjective and Objective Data)** Tachycardia Tachypnea Ineffective peripheral circulation, cool extremities Hypotension Rapid, weak peripheral pulses Prolonged capillary refill, longer than 2 or 3 seconds Narrow pulse pressure Distended neck veins in older children Cardiomegaly revealed on chest radiograph Gallop rhythm Edema Rapid weight gain Feeding difficulty Irritability	Child will have adequate cardiac output as evidenced by: • Heart rate within acceptable range (state specific range) • Respiratory rate within acceptable range (state specific range) • Skin warm to touch • Strong and equal peripheral pulses • Blood pressure normal for age • Brisk capillary refill within 2 or 3 seconds • Lack of distended neck veins • Normal sinus rhythm • Lack of edema • Adequate urinary output (state specific; 1–2 ml/kg/hr) • Age-appropriate weight gain on standardized growth curve • Successful feeding Child or family will be able to state at least four characteristics of heart failure such as: • Rapid heart rate • Fast breathing • Cool extremities • Puffiness (edema) • Fussiness • Decreased appetite Child or family will be able to state knowledge of care regarding: • Medication administration • Head elevated positioning • Sufficient rest periods • Monitoring of intake and output • When to contact health care provider **The Following NOC Concepts Apply to These Outcomes** Cardiac Pump Effectiveness Knowledge: Illness Care Tissue Perfusion: Cardiac	Assess and record heart rate, respiratory rate, blood pressure, and any signs or symptoms of decreased cardiac output (listed under defining characteristics) every 2 to 4 hours and as necessary. Administer cardiac drugs on schedule. Assess and record any side effects or any signs and symptoms of toxicity. Follow hospital protocol for administration. Keep accurate record of intake and output. Weigh child or infant on same scale at same time of day as previously. Document results and compare to previous weight. Administer diuretics on schedule. Assess and record effectiveness and any side effects noted. Elevate head of bed at a 30- to 45-degree angle. Offer small, frequent feedings to infant's or child's tolerance. Organize nursing care to allow child or infant uninterrupted rest. Educate child and family about characteristics of HF. Assess and record teaching session. Educate child and family about care such as medication administration. Assess and record results and family's participation in care. **The Following NIC Concepts Apply to These Interventions** Cardiac Care Fluid Management Medication Administration Positioning Parent/Child Education Vital Signs Monitoring	To detect change in vital signs and child's physical status that reflect altered cardiac output To avoid dangers inherent in failure to administer cardiac drugs as prescribed and to perform careful assessment before administration To detect HF, which causes decreased urinary output To monitor for weight increases, which may indicate excess fluid accumulation To eliminate excess water and salt because fluid retention commonly occurs with HF To promote maximum chest expansion To increase caloric intake and compensate for fatigue during feeding and increased metabolic rate because of poor cardiac function To allow adequate rest because poor cardiac output decreases energy level and lowers tolerance to activity To promote measures to improve cardiac function and decrease demands To promote safety and minimize medication side effects

Continued

⊚ NURSING CARE PLAN

The Child with Heart Failure—cont'd

NURSING DIAGNOSIS	PATIENT OUTCOMES	NURSING INTERVENTIONS	RATIONALE
Ineffective Breathing Pattern related to pulmonary congestion, decreased cardiac output	Child will have effective breathing pattern as evidenced by: • Respiratory rate within acceptable range (state specific range) • Clear and equal breath sounds bilaterally anteriorly and posteriorly • Pink or tan color • Absence of nasal flaring, retractions, cough, and head bobbing • Unlabored breath sounds • Tolerance of activities appropriate for age	Assess and record respiratory rate, breath sounds, and any signs or symptoms of ineffective pattern (listed under characteristics) every 2 to 4 hr and as needed.	To detect indicators of worsening HF
Child's Defining Characteristics (Subjective and Objective Data) Tachypnea Dyspnea Retractions Crackles Shortness of breath		Administer humidified oxygen in correct amount and route of delivery. Record percent of oxygen and route of delivery. Assess and record child's response to therapy.	To reduce respiratory distress by easing respiratory effort
Cyanosis Pallor	Child or family will be able to state four characteristics of ineffective breathing pattern such as:	Keep head of bed elevated at a 30- to 45-degree angle.	To promote maximum chest expansion
Mottling Nasal flaring Grunting Head bobbing Cough	• Color change from pink or tan to pale, dusky, or blue	Suction if child has ineffective cough or is unable to manage secretions. Assess and record amount and characteristics of secretions.	To maintain patent airway to promote respiratory expansion
Use of accessory muscles Activity intolerance	• Fast breathing • Change in amount or characteristics of secretions	Assess and record oxygen saturation every 2 to 4 hours and as needed.	To evaluate pulmonary effectiveness
	• Retractions, head bobbing • Ineffective cough • Decreased or altered activity level	Educate child and family about characteristics of ineffective breathing pattern. Assess and record results.	To promote measures to improve breathing effort
	Child or family will be able to state knowledge of care regarding: • Positioning to facilitate respiratory effort • Oxygen administration • When to contact health care provider	Educate child and family about care. Assess and record results and family participation in care.	To promote safety and minimize medication side effects
	The Following NOC Concepts Apply to These Outcomes Activity Tolerance Knowledge: Illness Care Respiratory Status: Gas Exchange Tissue Perfusion: Pulmonary	**The Following NIC Concepts Apply to These Interventions** Airway Management Airway Suctioning Chest Physiotherapy Family Involvement Promotion Health Education	

HF, Heart failure; *NIC,* Nursing Interventions Classification; *NOC,* Nursing Outcomes Classification.

groups, the written drug order should specify at what heart rate the drug is withheld. The nurse should also use judgment in evaluating the pulse rate. If it is significantly lower than the previous recording, the dose should be withheld until the practitioner is notified.

The apical rate is taken because a pulse deficit (radial pulse rate lower than apical) may be present with decreased cardiac output. It is auscultated for 1 full minute to evaluate alterations in rhythm. If the child is monitored by means of an ECG, a rhythm strip is obtained and attached to the chart for rate and rhythm analysis, such as abnormal lengthening of the PR interval (>50% increase over predigitalization interval) and dysrhythmias.

Digoxin is a potentially dangerous drug because of its narrow margin of safety of therapeutic, toxic, and lethal doses. Many toxic responses are extensions of its therapeutic effects. Therefore, the nurse must maintain a high index of suspicion for signs of toxicity when administering digoxin (Box 25-6).

Because digoxin toxicity can occur from accidental overdose, great care must be taken in properly calculating and measuring the dosage. When converting milligrams to micrograms to milliliters, the nurse carefully checks the placement of the decimal point because an error causes a significant change in dosage. For example, 0.1 mg is 10 times the dosage of 0.01 mg.

BOX 25-6 COMMON SIGNS OF DIGOXIN TOXICITY IN CHILDREN

Gastrointestinal
Nausea
Vomiting
Anorexia

Cardiac
Bradycardia
Dysrhythmias

👪 FAMILY-CENTERED CARE

Administering Digoxin

Give digoxin at regular intervals, usually every 12 hours, such as at 8 AM and 8 PM.

Administer the drug carefully by slowly directing it to the side and back of the mouth.

Do not mix the drug with foods or other fluids because refusal to consume these results in inaccurate intake of the drug.

If the child has teeth, give water after administering the drug; whenever possible, brush the teeth to prevent tooth decay from the sweetened liquid.

If a dose is missed, do not give an extra dose or increase the dose. Stay on the same medication schedule.

If the child vomits, do not give a second dose.

If more than two consecutive doses have been missed, notify the physician or other designated practitioner.

Frequent vomiting, poor feeding, or slow heart rate can be signs of toxicity; if they occur, contact the physician.

If the child becomes ill, notify the physician or other designated practitioner immediately.

Keep digoxin in a safe place, preferably in a locked cabinet.

In case of accidental overdose of digoxin, call the nearest poison control center immediately.

❗ NURSING ALERT

Infants rarely receive more than 1 ml (50 mcg or 0.05 mg) of digoxin in one dose; a higher dose is an immediate warning of a dosage error. To ensure safety, compare the calculation with another staff member's calculation before giving the drug.

These same principles are taught to parents in preparation for discharge, although the correct dose in milliliters is usually specified on the container, thus reducing potential errors in calculation. The nurse watches the parent measure the elixir in the dropper and stresses the level mark as the meniscus of the fluid that is observed at eye level. Other instructions for administering digoxin are listed in the Family-Centered Care box.

Parents are also advised of the signs of toxicity. According to the practitioner's preference, they may be taught to take the pulse before giving the drug. A return demonstration of the procedure from the parents or another principal caregiver is included as part of the teaching plan. Their level of anxiety in counting the pulse is assessed because overconcern about the heart rate may result in excessive withholding of the drug.

Monitor Afterload Reduction

For patients receiving ACE inhibitors for afterload reduction, the nurse should carefully monitor BP before and after dose administration, observe for symptoms of hypotension, and notify the practitioner if BP is low. Numerous medications affecting the kidney can potentiate renal dysfunction, so children taking multiple diuretics and an ACE inhibitor require careful assessment of serum electrolytes and renal function.

Decrease Cardiac Demands

The infant requires rest and conservation of energy for feeding. Every effort is made to organize nursing activities to allow for uninterrupted periods of sleep. Whenever possible, parents are encouraged to stay with their infant to provide the holding, rocking, and cuddling that help children sleep more soundly. To minimize disturbing the infant, changing bed linens and complete bathing are done only when necessary. Feeding is planned to accommodate the infant's sleep and wake patterns. The child is fed at the first sign of hunger, such as when sucking on fists, rather than waiting until he or she cries for a bottle because the stress of crying exhausts the limited energy supply. Because infants with HF tire easily and may sleep through feedings, smaller feedings every 3 hours may be helpful. Gavage feedings may be instituted to provide adequate nutrition and allow the infant to rest.

Every effort is made to minimize unnecessary stress. Older children need an explanation of what is happening to them to decrease anxiety about their illness and necessary treatments such as cardiac monitoring, oxygen administration, and medications. Outlining a plan for the day, preparing the child for tests and procedures, providing quiet activities, and providing adequate rest periods are all helpful interventions with older children. Some infants and children require sedation during the acute phase of illness to allow them to rest.

Temperature is carefully monitored because hyperthermia or hypothermia increases the need for oxygen. Febrile states are reported to the physician because infection must be promptly treated. Maintaining body temperature is of special importance in children who are receiving cool, humidified oxygen and in infants, who tend to be diaphoretic and lose heat by way of evaporation.

Skin breakdown from edema is prevented with a change of position every 2 hours (from side to side while in semi-Fowler position) and use of a pressure-relieving mattress or bed. The skin, especially over the sacrum, is checked for evidence of redness from pressure.

Reduce Respiratory Distress

Careful assessment, positioning, and oxygen administration can reduce respiratory distress. Respirations are counted for 1 full minute during a resting state. Any evidence of increased respiratory distress is reported because this may indicate worsening HF.

Infants are positioned to encourage maximum chest expansion, with the head of the bed elevated; they should sit up in an infant seat or be held at a 45-degree angle. Children prefer to sleep on several pillows and remain in a semi-Fowler or high-Fowler position during waking hours. Safety restraints, such as those used with infant seats, are applied low on the abdomen and loosely enough to provide both safety and maximum expansion.

The infant or child is often given humidified supplemental oxygen via oxygen hood or tent, nasal cannula, or mask. The child's response to oxygen therapy is carefully evaluated by noting respiratory rate, ease of respiration, color, and especially oxygen saturation as measured by oximetry.

Respiratory tract infections can exacerbate HF and should be appropriately treated and prevented if possible. The child should be protected from persons with respiratory tract infections and have a noninfectious roommate. Good hand washing is practiced before and after caring for any hospitalized child. Antibiotics may be given to combat respiratory tract infection. The nurse ensures that the drug is given at equally divided times over a 24-hour schedule to maintain high blood levels of the antibiotic.

Maintain Nutritional Status

Meeting the nutritional needs of infants with HF or serious cardiac defects is a nursing challenge. The metabolic rate of these infants is greater because of poor cardiac function and increased heart and respiratory rates. Their caloric needs are greater than those of the average infant because of their increased metabolic rate, yet their ability to take in adequate calories is hampered by their fatigue. Feeding for a fragile infant with serious CHD is similar to exercising for an adult, and these infants often do not have the energy or cardiac reserve to do extra work. The nurse seeks measures to enable the infant to feed easily without excess fatigue and to increase the caloric density of the formula.

The infant should be well rested before feeding and fed soon after awakening so as not to expend energy on crying. A 3-hour feeding schedule works well for many infants. (Feeding every 2 hours does not provide enough rest between feedings, and a 4-hour schedule requires an increased volume of feeding, which many infants are unable to take.) The feeding schedule should be individualized to the infant's needs. A feeding goal of 150 ml/kg/day and at least 120 kcal/kg/day is common for newborns with significant heart disease (Steltzer, Rudd, and Pick, 2005). A soft preemie nipple or a slit in a regular nipple to enlarge the opening decreases the infant's energy expenditure while sucking. Infants should be well supported and fed in a semiupright position. Infants may need to rest frequently and may need to have the jaw and cheeks stroked to encourage sucking. Generally, giving an infant about a half hour to complete a feeding is reasonable. Prolonging the feeding time can exhaust the infant and decrease the rest period between feedings.

Infants with feeding difficulties are often gavage fed using a nasogastric tube to supplement their oral intake and ensure adequate calories. If they are very stressed and fatigued, in respiratory distress, or tachypneic to 80 to 100 breaths/min, oral feedings may be withheld and all nutrition given by gavage feedings. Gavage feedings are usually a temporary measure until the infant's medical status improves and nutritional needs can be met through oral feedings. Some infants with severe HF, neurologic deficits, or significant gastroesophageal reflux may need placement of a gastrostomy tube to allow adequate nutrition.

The caloric density of formulas is frequently increased by concentration and then adding Polycose, medium-chain triglyceride oil, or corn oil. Infant formulas provide 20 kcal/oz, and the use of additives can increase the calories to 30 kcal/oz or more. This allows the infant to obtain more calories despite a smaller volume intake of formula. The caloric density of the formula needs to be increased slowly (by 2 kcal/oz/day) to prevent diarrhea or formula intolerance. Breastfeeding mothers are encouraged to provide the infant with alternating feedings of breast milk and high-calorie formulas. Some lactating mothers prefer to feed the child expressed breast milk that has been fortified with Similac or Enfamil powder, Polycose, or corn oil to increase caloric intake. A diet plan specific to the individual infant's needs is calculated and prescribed by the nutritionist in collaboration with the other health personnel. The nurse needs to reinforce this information with the parents as necessary.

Assist in Measures to Promote Fluid Loss

When diuretics are given, the nurse records fluid intake and output and monitors body weight at the same time each day to evaluate benefit from the drug. Because profound diuresis may cause dehydration and electrolyte imbalance (loss of sodium, potassium, chloride, bicarbonate), the nurse observes for signs indicating either complication, as well as signs and symptoms suggesting reactions to the drugs. Diuretics should be given early in the day to children who are toilet trained to avoid the need to urinate at night. If potassium-losing diuretics are given, the nurse encourages foods high in potassium, such as bananas, oranges, whole grains, legumes, and leafy vegetables and administers prescribed supplements. Serum potassium levels are checked frequently.

> **NURSING TIP** Mix the elixir with fruit juice (red punch or grape juice works well) to disguise the bitter taste and to prevent intestinal irritation from a concentrated solution.

Fluid restriction is rarely necessary in infants because of their difficulty in feeding. However, if fluids are restricted, the nurse plans fluid intake schedules for a 24-hour period, allowing for most fluids during waking hours. Toddlers and preschoolers should be given small amounts of liquid in small cups so the containers appear full. Older children's cooperation is gained by placing them in charge of recording their fluid intake.

If salt is limited, the nurse discusses food sources of sodium with the family and discourages their bringing salt-containing treats to the child. At mealtimes, the child's tray is checked to make sure the appropriate diet is given.

Support Child and Family

HF is a serious complication of heart disease. Parents and older children are usually acutely aware of the critical nature of the condition. Because stress places additional demands on cardiac function, the nurse should focus on reducing anxiety through anticipatory preparation, frequent communication with the parent regarding the child's progress, and constant reassurance that everything possible is being done.

Home care involves many of the same interventions discussed under Plan for Discharge and Home Care (p. 847). The nurse teaches the family about the medications that need to be administered and alerts them to the signs of worsening HF that require medical attention, such as increased sweating, decreased urinary output (noted in fewer wet diapers or infrequent use of the toilet), or poor feeding. Every effort is made to improve the family's adherence to the medication schedule by adapting the schedule to their usual home routines, avoiding medications during the night, making it as simple as possible, and using charts or visual aids to remember when to give medications (see Chapter 22). Written instructions regarding correct administration of digoxin are essential (see Family-Centered Care box, p. 839), including an explanation regarding signs of toxicity.

If HF is the end stage of a severe heart defect, the nurse cares for this child as for any child who is terminally ill, using the principles discussed in Chapter 18.

HYPOXEMIA

Hypoxemia refers to an arterial oxygen tension (or pressure, PaO_2) that is less than normal and can be identified by a decreased arterial saturation or a decreased PaO_2. Hypoxia is a reduction in tissue oxygenation that results from low oxygen saturations and PaO₂ and results in impaired cellular processes. Cyanosis is a blue discoloration in the mucous membranes, skin, and nail beds of the child with reduced oxygen saturation. It results from the presence of deoxygenated hemoglobin (hemoglobin not bound to oxygen) in a concentration of 5 g/dl of blood. Cyanosis is usually apparent when arterial oxygen saturations are 80% to 85%. Determination of cyanosis is subjective. It can vary depending on skin pigment, quality of light, color of the room, or clothing worn by the child. The presence of cyanosis may not accurately reflect arterial hypoxemia because both oxygen saturation and the amount of circulating hemoglobin are involved. Children with severe anemia may not be cyanotic despite severe hypoxemia because the hemoglobin level may be too low to produce the characteristic blue color. Conversely, patients with polycythemia may appear cyanotic despite a near-normal PaO₂. Heart defects that cause hypoxemia and cyanosis result from desaturated venous blood (blue blood) entering the systemic circulation without passing through the lungs.

Clinical Manifestations

Over time, two physiologic changes occur in the body in response to chronic hypoxemia: polycythemia and clubbing. Polycythemia, an increased number of red blood cells, increases the oxygen-carrying capacity of the blood. However, anemia may result if iron is not readily available for the formation of hemoglobin. Polycythemia increases the viscosity of the blood and crowds out clotting factors. Clubbing, a thickening and flattening of the tips of the fingers and toes, is thought to occur because of chronic tissue hypoxemia and polycythemia (Fig. 25-8). Infants with mild hypoxemia may be asymptomatic except for cyanosis and exhibit near-normal growth and development. Those with more severe hypoxemia may exhibit fatigue with feeding, poor weight gain, tachypnea, and dyspnea. Severe hypoxemia resulting in tissue hypoxia is manifested by clinical deterioration and signs of poor perfusion.

Hypercyanotic spells, also referred to as blue spells or tet spells because they are often seen in infants with tetralogy of Fallot, may occur in any child whose heart defect includes obstruction to pulmonary blood flow and communication between the ventricles. The infant becomes acutely cyanotic and hyperpneic because sudden infundibular spasm decreases pulmonary blood flow and increases right-to-left shunting (the proposed mechanism in tetralogy of Fallot). Spells, rarely seen before 2 months of age, occur most frequently in the first year of life. They occur more often in the morning and may be preceded by feeding, crying, defecation, or stressful procedures. Because profound hypoxemia causes cerebral hypoxia, hypercyanotic spells require prompt assessment and treatment to prevent brain damage or possibly death.

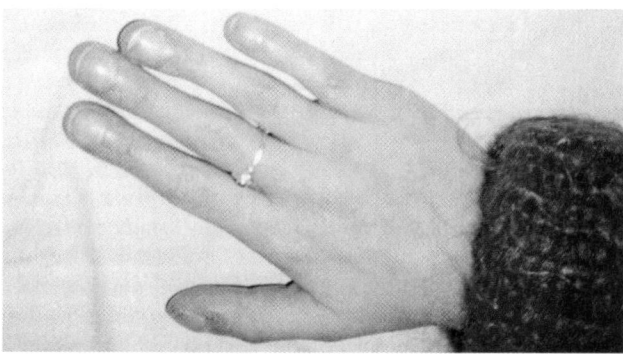

FIG 25-8 Clubbing of the fingers.

Persistent cyanosis as a result of cyanotic heart defects places the child at risk for significant neurologic complications. Cerebrovascular accident (CVA, stroke), brain abscess, and developmental delays (especially in motor and cognitive development) may result from chronic hypoxia.

Diagnostic Evaluation

Cyanosis in a newborn can be the result of cardiac, pulmonary, metabolic, or hematologic disease, although cardiac and pulmonary causes occur most often. To distinguish between the two, a hyperoxia test is helpful. The infant is placed in a 100% oxygen environment, and blood parameters are monitored. A PaO₂ of 100 mm Hg or higher suggests lung disease, and a PaO₂ lower than 100 mm Hg suggests cardiac disease (Park, 2008). An accurate history, a chest radiograph, and especially an echocardiogram contribute to the diagnosis of cyanotic heart disease.

Therapeutic Management

Newborns generally exhibit cyanosis within the first few days of life as the ductus arteriosus, which provided pulmonary blood flow, begins to close. Prostaglandin E₁, which causes vasodilation and smooth muscle relaxation, thus increasing dilation and patency of the ductus arteriosus, is administered intravenously to reestablish pulmonary blood flow. The use of prostaglandins has been lifesaving for infants with ductus-dependent cardiac defects. The increase in oxygenation allows the infant to be stabilized and have a complete diagnostic evaluation performed before further treatment is needed.

Hypercyanotic spells occur suddenly, and prompt recognition and treatment are essential. In the hospital setting, spells are often seen during blood drawing or IV insertion, when the child is highly agitated, or after cardiac catheterization. Treatment of a hypercyanotic spell is outlined in the Nursing Care Guidelines box. Morphine, administered subcutaneously or through an existing IV line, helps reduce infundibular spasm. A spell indicates the need for prompt surgical treatment if possible. In infants with defects not amenable to surgical repair, a shunt may be created surgically to increase blood flow to the lungs. Several commonly used shunt procedures are described in Table 25-4 and Figure 25-9.

The cyanotic infant and child are well hydrated to keep the hematocrit and blood viscosity within acceptable limits to reduce the risk of CVAs. The infant is monitored closely for anemia because of the risk of CVAs and the reduced arterial oxygen-carrying capacity that occurs. Iron supplementation and possibly blood transfusion are used as needed.

Respiratory tract infections or reduced pulmonary function from any cause can worsen hypoxemia in the cyanotic child. Aggressive pulmonary hygiene, chest physical therapy, administration of antibiotics, and use of oxygen to improve arterial saturations are important interventions.

Nursing Care Management

The general appearance of infants and children with significant cyanosis poses unique concerns. Blue lips and fingernails are obvious signs of their hidden cardiac defect. Clubbing and small, thin stature in older children further indicate severe heart disease. Adolescents are especially concerned about their body image; children with cyanosis are often teased about their appearance and singled out as different. Many children, when asked what surgery will do, reply, "Make me pink." Their joy and excitement after surgery are evident when they see their pink fingers. Parents are often fearful of their child's bluish color because cyanosis is usually associated with lack of oxygen and severe

TABLE 25-4	SELECTED SHUNT PROCEDURES FOR CHILDREN WITH CARDIAC DEFECTS
SHUNT TYPE	**COMMENTS**
Modified Blalock-Taussig shunt—Subclavian artery to pulmonary artery using Gore-Tex or Impra tube graft	Shunt flow sometimes excessive, requiring use of diuretics Possibility of thrombosis; aspirin usually prescribed postoperatively Easy to ligate at time of definitive correction Shunt size fixed and may become too small as child grows
Sano Modification—Right ventricular to pulmonary artery using Gore-Tex	Prevents diastolic runoff of systemic blood into the pulmonary arteries Provides a higher diastolic blood pressure and seemingly better coronary perfusion Used in place of the Modified Blalock-Taussig shunt in the Norwood procedure
Central shunt—Ascending aorta to main pulmonary artery using Gore-Tex graft	Length of shunt acts to restrict blood flow; possibility of symptoms of HF; diuretic therapy sometimes required Uncommon; used when modified Blalock-Taussig shunt cannot be used Easy to insert and remove at time of repair Possibility of thrombosis; aspirin usually prescribed postoperatively
Bidirectional Glenn shunt (cavopulmonary anastomosis)—SVC to side of right pulmonary artery; blood flow to both lungs	Done as a second shunt; often used as a staging step to a Fontan procedure Can be incorporated into eventual modified Fontan procedure Relieves severe cyanosis and decreases volume overload on ventricle Carries risk of embolic events (mixing defect); aspirin often prescribed Pulmonary arteriovenous fistulas may occur months or years later, causing desaturation (uncommon finding)

HF, Heart failure; *SVC,* superior vena cava.

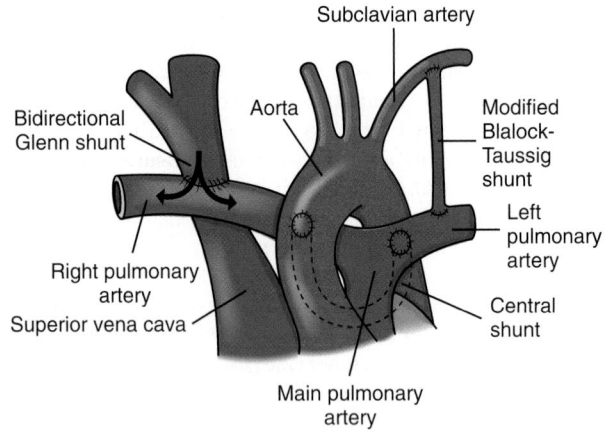

FIG 25-9 Schematic diagram of cardiac shunts.

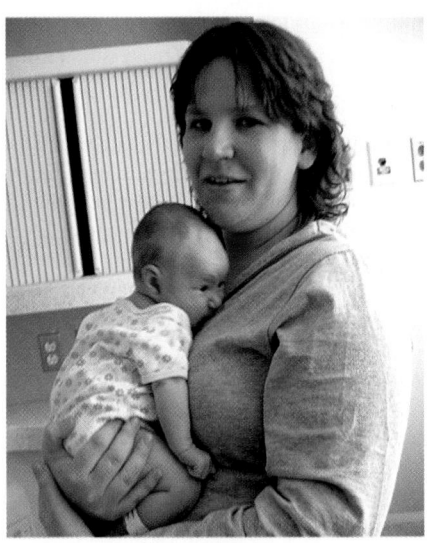

FIG 25-10 Infant held in a knee–chest position.

illness. They also must deal with comments from relatives, friends, and strangers about their child's abnormal color. They need a simple explanation of hypoxemia and cyanosis and reassurance that cyanosis does not imply a lack of oxygen to the brain. Their questions and fears need to be addressed in a calm, supportive manner, and positive aspects of their child's growth and development are emphasized. They are taught the treatment for hypercyanotic spells (see Nursing Care Guidelines box).

Dehydration must be prevented in children with hypoxemia because it potentiates the risk of CVAs. Fluid status is carefully monitored, with accurate intake and output and daily weight measurements. Maintenance fluid therapy is the minimum requirement, supplemental fluids should be readily available, and gavage feeding or IV hydration is given to children unable to take adequate oral fluids. Fever, vomiting, and diarrhea can cause dehydration and require prompt treatment. Parents are instructed in the importance of adequate fluid intake and measures to prevent dehydration. An oral electrolyte solution should be available at home in the event that the infant is unable to tolerate the usual formula. The practitioner should be notified of fever, vomiting, diarrhea, or other problems.

 NURSING CARE GUIDELINES

Treating Hypercyanotic Spells

Place infant in knee–chest position (Fig. 25-10).
Use a calm, comforting approach.
Administer 100% oxygen by blow-by.
Give morphine subcutaneously or through an existing IV line.
Begin IV fluid replacement and volume expansion if needed.
Repeat morphine administration.

IV, Intravenous.

Preventive measures and accurate assessment of respiratory infection are important nursing considerations. Any compromise in pulmonary function will increase the infant's hypoxemia. Good hand washing and protection from individuals with an obvious respiratory tract infection are important. Aggressive pulmonary hygiene, treatment with antibiotics or antiviral agents as indicated, and supplemental oxygen to decrease hypoxemia are necessary measures. Infants may

early postoperative neurologic status, microcephaly, type of cardiac lesions, length of deep hypothermic circulatory arrest, age at surgery, and length of ICU stay were predictors of developmental delay.

Recent efforts to limit the time of deep hypothermic circulatory arrest and provide better neuroprotection during infant surgery may improve outcomes in the future. Although most children with serious heart disease are within the normal range for IQ, there is a higher incidence of neurodevelopmental deficits in children after heart surgery than in the normal population, specifically in speech and language, fine motor skills, and cognitive processes (Majnemer and Limperopoulos, 1999). Severe neurologic problems such as cerebral palsy, epilepsy, and mental retardation are uncommon.

PREPARE THE CHILD AND FAMILY FOR INVASIVE PROCEDURES

Chapter 22 provides an extensive discussion of the principles for preparing children for invasive procedures. The American Heart Association published a scientific statement "Recommendations for Preparing Children and Adolescents for Invasive Cardiac Procedures" (LeRoy, Elixson, O'Brien, and others, 2003), which addresses issues specific to the child with heart disease. The following discussion highlights some important aspects of preparation for cardiac catheterization and cardiac surgery.

The expected outcomes for preprocedure preparation include reducing anxiety, improving patient cooperation with procedures, enhancing recovery, developing trust with caregivers, and improving long-term emotional and behavioral adjustments after procedures (LeRoy, Elixson, O'Brien, and others, 2003). Important factors to consider in planning preparation strategies are the child's cognitive development, previous hospital experiences, the child's temperament and coping style, the timing of preparation, and the involvement of the parents. The most beneficial preparation strategies usually combine information giving and coping skills training such as conscious breathing exercises, distraction techniques, guided imagery, or other behavioral interventions.

Outpatient preoperative and precatheterization workups are common for most elective procedures. Children are then admitted on the morning of the procedure. Preprocedure teaching is often done in the clinic setting or at home and may include a tour of the ICU and inpatient facilities. Children of different ages and developmental levels require different amounts of information and different approaches. Whereas young children should be prepared close in time to the event, older children and adolescents may benefit from teaching several weeks in advance. Parents should be included in the preparation session to support their child and learn about upcoming events.

Topics to include in preoperative or precatheterization preparation include information on the environment, equipment, and procedures that the child will encounter during and after the procedure. Many information-giving techniques can be used such as verbal and written information, hospital tours, preoperative classes, picture books, or videos. Information about what the child will see, hear, and feel should be included, especially for older children and adolescents. Some of the sensory experiences of being in an ICU or catheterization laboratory include sights (monitors, many people, a lot of equipment), sounds (beeping noises, alarms, voices), and sensations (lines and dressings, tape, discomfort, thirst). Familiar aspects of the environment, such as BP cuffs, stethoscopes, or oximeter probes, are reviewed, and new equipment, such as monitors, IV lines, and oxygen masks, are described. Comforting aspects of the environment, such as play areas, chairs for parents, and televisions, are emphasized. Many patients who will

be sedated during catheterization or receive narcotic pain relievers after surgery will have minimal recall of that period and will not need detailed information about the equipment or procedures used. Information should be specific to the planned procedure for each patient.

A discussion of ways the child can cope with the experience should be included. For a young child, bringing a familiar stuffed animal or comfort object will help relieve anxiety, and advising an older child to bring headphones and favorite music to the catheterization laboratory will help distract him or her during the procedure. Recovery topics after catheterization include lying still to prevent bleeding at the catheter site, advancing diet, controlling pain, and monitoring. After surgery, the nurse reviews the importance of ambulation, coughing, deep breathing, drinking, and eating and describes pain management and monitoring routines. Simple coping strategies for use during painful procedures should be reviewed; these include distraction techniques such as counting, blowing, singing, and telling stories.

Children and their families should have a choice about an ICU tour. Exposure to the ICU environment can actually increase anxiety in some children, particularly young children, those with previous hospital experiences, and those who are highly anxious (LeRoy, Elixson, O'Brien, and others, 2003). Usually the day before the procedure is ample time to allow the child to ask questions and to prevent undue fantasizing about the experience. The child should be protected from the frightening sights in the unit; equipment not in view postoperatively, such as equipment located behind or below the bed, needs less attention. The child and parents are encouraged to ask questions or to explore further any equipment in the room, but they should not be pushed to assimilate more information than they are able.

Preoperative physical care differs little, if any, from that for any other surgery and is discussed in Chapter 22. The child should be assured that the parents will be there when the child wakes up; they should be allowed to accompany their child as far as possible to the operating suite (see Surgical Procedures, Chapter 22). After all of the equipment and procedures have been explained, it is important to talk about "getting well" and going home.

PROVIDE POSTOPERATIVE CARE

Immediate postoperative care is usually provided by specially trained nurses in ICUs. Many of the procedures, such as arterial pressure and central venous pressure (CVP) monitoring, and the observations related to vital functions require advanced educational training (readers should refer to critical care texts for further information). However, nurses caring for the child before surgery and during the convalescent period need to be familiar with the major principles of care. Selected complications that may occur postoperatively are described in Box 25-7.

Observe Vital Signs

Vital signs and BP are recorded frequently until stable. Heart rate and respirations are counted for 1 full minute, compared with the ECG monitor, and recorded with activity. The heart rate is normally increased after surgery. The nurse observes cardiac rhythm and notifies the practitioner of any changes in regularity. Dysrhythmias may occur postoperatively secondary to anesthetics, acid–base and electrolyte imbalance, hypoxia, surgical intervention, or trauma to conduction pathways (pp. 845–846).

At least hourly, the lungs are auscultated for breath sounds. Diminished or absent sounds may indicate an area of atelectasis or a pleural effusion or pneumothorax, which necessitates further medical

---

BOX 25-7 **SELECTED COMPLICATIONS AFTER CARDIAC SURGERY AND TREATMENT APPROACHES**

Cardiac

Heart failure—Digoxin, diuretics (see p. 839)

Low cardiac output—Intravenous inotropes (see Shock, p. 860)

Dysrhythmias—Identification, drug treatment, possible pacing, cardioversion (see p. 853)

Tamponade (blood or fluid in the pericardial space constricting the heart)—Prompt removal of fluid by pericardiocentesis

Respiratory

Atelectasis—Chest physical therapy, coughing, deep breathing, ambulation

Pulmonary edema—Diuretics

Pleural effusions—Diuretics, possible chest tube drainage

Pneumothorax—Possible chest tube drainage

Neurologic

Seizures—Assessment, antiepileptic drugs

Cerebrovascular accident (stroke), cerebral edema, neurologic deficits—Assessment and treatment

Infectious Disease

Infections (especially wound, pneumonia, otitis media, and sepsis)—Antibiotics

Hematologic

Anemia—Iron supplementation, possible transfusion

Postoperative bleeding—Initially, clotting factors, blood products; may need repeat surgery to locate and ligate source of bleeding

Other

Postpericardiotomy syndrome (syndrome of fever, leukocytosis, friction rub, pericardial and pleural effusions, and lethargy seen about 7 to 21 days after cardiac surgery; possible viral or autoimmune etiologies)—Antipyretics, diuretics, antiinflammatory medications

---

assessment. Temperature changes are typical during the early postoperative period. Hypothermia is expected immediately after surgery from hypothermia procedures, effects of anesthesia, and loss of body heat to the cool environment. During this period, the child is kept warm to prevent additional heat loss. Infants may be placed under radiant heat warmers. During the next 24 to 48 hours the body temperature may rise to 37.7° C (100° F) or slightly higher as part of the inflammatory response to tissue trauma. After this period, an elevated temperature is most likely a sign of infection and warrants immediate investigation for probable cause.

Intraarterial monitoring of BP is commonly done after open-heart surgery. A catheter is passed into the radial artery or other artery, and the other end is attached to an electronic monitoring system, which provides a continuous recording of the BP. The intraarterial line is maintained with a low-rate, constant infusion of heparinized saline to prevent clotting.

Several IV lines are inserted preoperatively, including a peripheral IV to give fluids and medications and a central venous line, usually in a large vessel in the next, to measure CVP. Additional, intracardiac monitoring lines are sometimes placed intraoperatively in the right atrium, left atrium, or pulmonary artery. Intracardiac lines allow assessment of pressures inside the cardiac chambers, providing vital information about volume status, cardiac output, and ventricular

function. All lines must be cared for using strict aseptic technique, and patients must be carefully assessed for bleeding at the time of line removal.

Maintain Respiratory Status

Infants usually require mechanical ventilation in the immediate postoperative period. Early extubation in the operating room or early postoperative period is becoming more common. Children, especially those not requiring cardiopulmonary bypass, may be extubated in the operating room or in the first few postoperative hours. Suctioning is performed only as needed and performed carefully to avoid vagal stimulation (which can trigger cardiac dysrhythmias) and laryngospasm, especially in infants. Suctioning is intermittent and maintained for no more than 5 seconds at a time to avoid depleting the oxygen supply. Supplemental oxygen is administered with a manual resuscitation bag before and after the procedure to prevent hypoxia. The heart rate is monitored after suctioning to detect changes in rhythm or rate, especially bradycardia. The child should always be positioned facing the nurse to permit assessment of the child's color and tolerance of the procedure.

When weaning and extubation are completed, humidified oxygen is delivered by mask, hood, or nasal cannula to prevent drying of mucosa. The child is encouraged to turn and deep breathe at least hourly. Measures are used to enhance ventilation and decrease pain, such as splinting of the operative site and use of analgesics. Chest tubes are inserted into the pleural or mediastinal space during surgery or in the immediate postoperative period to remove secretions and air to allow reexpansion of the lung. Drainage is checked hourly for color and quantity. Immediately after surgery the drainage may be bright red, but afterward, it should be serous. The largest volume of drainage occurs in the first 12 to 24 hours and is greater in extensive heart surgery.

! **NURSING ALERT**

Chest tube drainage greater than 3 ml/kg/hr for more than 3 consecutive hours or 5 to 10 ml/kg in any 1 hour is excessive and may indicate postoperative hemorrhage. The surgeon should be notified immediately because cardiac tamponade can develop rapidly and is life threatening.

Chest tubes are usually removed on the first to third postoperative day. Removal of chest tubes is a painful, frightening experience. Analgesics such as morphine sulfate, often combined with midazolam (Versed), should be given before the procedure. Older children are forewarned that they will feel a sharp, momentary pain. After the suture is cut, the tubes are quickly pulled out at the end of full inspiration in the extubated patient to prevent intake of air into the pleural cavity. (In the intubated patient, the tubes are pulled out on inspiration because the lungs are stented open with the positive pressure ventilation.) A purse-string suture (placed when the tubes were inserted) is pulled tight to close the opening. A petrolatum-covered gauze dressing is immediately applied over the wound and securely taped on all four sides to the skin so that an airtight seal is formed. It is left on for 1 or 2 days. Breath sounds are checked to assess for a pneumothorax, a possible complication of chest tube removal. A chest radiograph is usually obtained after removal to evaluate for possible pneumothorax or pleural effusion.

Monitor Fluids

Intake and output of all fluids must be accurately calculated. Intake is primarily IV fluids; however, a record of fluid used to flush the arterial and CVP lines or to dilute medications is also kept. Output includes hourly recordings of urine (usually a Foley catheter is inserted and attached to a closed collecting device), drainage from chest and nasogastric tubes, and blood drawn for analysis. Renal failure is a potential risk from a transient period of low cardiac output.

> **! NURSING ALERT**
>
> The signs of renal failure are decreased urinary output (<1 ml/kg/hr) and elevated levels of blood urea nitrogen and serum creatinine.

Fluids are restricted during the immediate postoperative period to prevent hypervolemia, which places additional demands on the myocardium, predisposing the patient to cardiac failure. If the child is to be extubated within the first 24 to 48 hours, fluids are provided primarily intravenously. If the child is to be intubated longer, fluids may be given via a nasogastric or nasojejunal tube to optimize nutrition and gut motility. Approximately 4 hours after extubation, enteral fluids may be reinitiated in the setting of a stable hemodynamic and respiratory status. To monitor fluid retention, the child is weighed daily, and the same scale is used at approximately the same time each day to avoid errors in measurement. Fluid restriction may be imposed even when oral fluids are given. The nurse calculates the distribution over a 24-hour period based on the child's preoperative weight and drinking habits. The distribution should allow for most fluid to be given during the child's most wakeful and active periods.

Provide Rest and Progressive Activity

After heart surgery, rest should be provided to decrease the workload of the heart and promote healing. The simplest way to ensure individualized, efficient, high-quality care is to plan at the beginning of the shift the nursing procedures to be done, with periods of rest identified. The schedule should be shared with parents to allow them to visit at the most advantageous times, such as after a rest period when no special treatments are anticipated.

A progressive schedule of ambulation and activity is planned, based on the child's preoperative activity patterns and postoperative cardiovascular and pulmonary function. Ambulation is initiated early, usually by the second postoperative day, when chest tubes, arterial lines, and assisted ventilatory equipment have been removed. Activity progresses from sitting on the edge of the bed and dangling the legs to standing up and sitting in a chair. Heart rate and respirations are carefully monitored to assess the degree of cardiac demand imposed by each activity. Tachycardia, dyspnea, cyanosis, desaturation, progressive fatigue, and dysrhythmias indicate the need to limit further energy expenditure.

Provide Comfort and Emotional Support

Heart surgery is both painful and frightening for children, and comfort is a primary nursing concern. Several types of incisions are used by the cardiac surgeon. A median sternotomy is most common, following the sternum down the center of the chest. A ministernotomy opens the lower sternum. A thoracotomy incision is most uncomfortable because it goes through muscle tissue. It allows access to the side of the chest through an incision from under the arm around the back to the scapula.

Most patients need IV analgesics for pain control during the immediate postoperative period. Patient-controlled analgesia may be used with children old enough to understand the concept. Nonsteroidal antiinflammatory drugs (NSAIDs) such as ketorolac (Toradol) may be used intravenously. Paralyzing agents may also be used with the analgesics for children who are hemodynamically unstable.

After extubation and removal of lines and tubes, pain can be satisfactorily controlled with oral medications such as ibuprofen, codeine with acetaminophen (Tylenol No. 3), or oxycodone and acetaminophen. Acetaminophen alone provides adequate pain relief for most children at discharge. Sternotomy incisions are usually well tolerated, with some discomfort when walking and coughing. Thoracotomy incisions are usually more painful because the incision is through muscle; a more aggressive pain management plan with around-the-clock medications for several days is often necessary to allow for adequate rest, ambulation, and pulmonary hygiene.

In addition to pharmacologic pain control, every effort is made to minimize the discomfort of procedures, such as using a firm pillow or favorite stuffed animal placed against the chest incision during movement and performing treatments *after* pain medication is given, preferably at a time that coincides with the drug's peak effect. Nonpharmacologic measures are used to lessen the perception of pain, and parents are encouraged to comfort their child as much as possible. (See also Pain Assessment; Pain Management, Chapter 7.)

Children may become depressed after surgery. This is thought to be caused by preoperative anxiety, postoperative psychologic and physiologic stress, and sensory overstimulation. Typically, the child's disposition improves on leaving the ICU.

Children may also be angry and uncooperative after surgery as a response to the physical pain and to the loss of control imposed by the surgery and treatments. They need an opportunity to express feelings, either verbally or through activity. Children often regress in their behavior during the stress of surgery and hospitalization. They also may express feelings of anger or rejection toward their parents. The nurse can support the parents by being available for information and explaining all of the procedures to them. The first few postoperative days are particularly difficult because parents see their child in pain and realize the potential risks from surgery. They often are overwhelmed by the physical environment of the ICU and feel useless because they can do so little for their child. The nurse can minimize such feelings by including parents in caregiving activities and comfort and play activities, providing information about the child's condition, and being sensitive to their emotional and physical needs. The importance of their presence in making the child feel more secure is stressed even if they do not provide physical care.

> **QUALITY PATIENT OUTCOMES: Congenital Heart Disease**
> - Improved cardiac function
> - Prevention of fluid and sodium overload
> - Decreased cardiac demands
> - Improved oxygenation
> - Reduced respiratory distress

PLAN FOR DISCHARGE AND HOME CARE

Ideally, discharge planning begins on admission for cardiac surgery and includes an assessment of the parents' adjustment to the child's altered state of health. Neonates need additional screening tests (e.g., newborn metabolic screen and hearing tests) and may need immunizations before discharge (Dodds and Merle, 2005). The family will need both verbal and written instructions on medication, nutrition, activity restrictions, subacute bacterial endocarditis (SBE), return to school, wound care, and signs and symptoms of infection or complications (see Family-Centered Care box). Referrals to community agencies may be warranted to assist parents in the transition from the hospital to home and to reinforce the teaching.

Topics to Include in Discharge Teaching After Cardiac Surgery

- Medication teaching (for digoxin, see Family-Centered Care box, p. 839)
- Activity restrictions
- Diet and nutrition
- Wound care (including dressings, if any; suture removal; bathing)
- Bacterial (infective) endocarditis prophylaxis (see Box 25-9)
- Follow-up appointments (cardiologist, primary care provider)
- Community agencies as needed (visiting nurse service, early developmental intervention)
- When to call practitioner; signs and symptoms of postoperative problems
- Review of cardiac defect and surgical repair

The parents will also need clear instructions on when to seek medical care for complications and how to contact the health care provider. Follow-up with the cardiologist and primary care provider is also arranged before discharge. Parents should have a summary, including their child's medical condition, medications, and health care providers available for emergencies. Appropriate identification, such as a Medic-Alert device, is indicated for children with a pacemaker or a heart transplant and for those receiving anticoagulation therapy or antidysrhythmic medication.

Although surgical correction of heart defects has improved dramatically, it is still not possible to completely repair many of the complex anomalies. For many children, repeat procedures are required to replace conduits or grafts or to manage complications such as restenosis. Consequently, the long-term prognosis is uncertain, and full recovery is not always possible. For these families, medical follow-up and continued emotional support are essential. The nurse can often serve as an important primary health professional and as a resource for referrals when needed.

ACQUIRED CARDIOVASCULAR DISORDERS

BACTERIAL (INFECTIVE) ENDOCARDITIS

Bacterial endocarditis (BE), or subacute bacterial endocarditis (SBE), is now commonly referred to as infective endocarditis (IE). IE is an infection of the inner lining of the heart (endocardium), generally involving the valves. Although it can occur without underlying heart disease, it is most often a sequela of bacteremia in children with acquired or congenital anomalies of the heart or great vessels. It especially affects children with valvular abnormalities, prosthetic valves, shunts, recent cardiac surgery with invasive lines, and rheumatic heart disease with valve involvement. The most common causative agents are *Staphylococcus aureus* and *Streptococcus viridans*; other causative agents include gram-negative bacteria and fungi such as *Candida albicans*.

Pathophysiology

Organisms may enter the bloodstream from any site of localized infection. In the past, endocarditis was believed to be highly associated with invasive procedures; however, endocarditis is most likely to occur from routine exposure to bacteremia associated with usual daily activities, although it can also occur after procedures such as dental work (*S. viridans*; after invasive procedures involving the gastrointestinal and genitourinary tracts); after cardiac surgery, especially if synthetic

BOX 25-8 CLINICAL MANIFESTATIONS OF INFECTIVE ENDOCARDITIS

Onset usually insidious
Unexplained fever (low grade and intermittent)
Anorexia
Malaise
Weight loss
Characteristic findings caused by extracardiac emboli formation:
- Splinter hemorrhages (thin black lines) under the nails
- Osler nodes (red, painful intradermal nodes found on pads of phalanges)
- Janeway lesions (painless hemorrhagic areas on palms and soles)
- Petechiae on oral mucous membranes
May be present:
- Heart failure
- Cardiac dysrhythmias
- New murmur or change in previously existing one

material is used (valves, patches, conduits); or from long-term indwelling catheters. The microorganisms grow on the endocardium, forming vegetations (verrucae), deposits of fibrin, and platelet thrombi. The lesion may invade adjacent tissues, such as the aortic and mitral valves, and may break off and embolize elsewhere, especially in the spleen, kidney, and central nervous system (CNS).

Diagnostic Evaluation

The diagnosis of IE is suspected on the basis of clinical manifestations (Box 25-8). The most commonly used guidelines for diagnosis use the revised Duke criteria, which outline major and minor criteria consistent with IE (Li, Sexton, Mick, and others, 2000). Several laboratory findings may suggest IE (e.g., ECG changes [prolonged PR interval], radiographic evidence of cardiomegaly, anemia, elevated erythrocyte sedimentation rate [ESR], leukocytosis, microscopic hematuria). Vegetations on the valve and abnormal valve function can often be visualized by echocardiography. Definitive diagnosis rests on growth and identification of the causative agent in the blood. A diagnosis of culture-negative IE is made when the patient has echocardiographic or clinical evidence of IE but no organism can be cultured (Ferrieri, 2002).

Therapeutic Management

Treatment should be instituted immediately and consists of administration of high doses of appropriate antibiotics intravenously for 2 to 8 weeks. Blood cultures are taken periodically to evaluate the response to antibiotic therapy.

Prevention involves administration of prophylactic antibiotic therapy 1 hour before certain procedures that are associated with the risk of entry of organisms in very high–risk patients. Recent guidelines recommend prophylaxis only in patients with the highest risk of poor outcome if they develop endocarditis (Box 25-9). Drugs of choice for prophylaxis include amoxicillin, ampicillin, clindamycin, cephalexin, cefadroxil, azithromycin, and clarithromycin.

QUALITY PATIENT OUTCOMES: Bacterial (Infective) Endocarditis
- Prevention in high-risk patients with antibiotic prophylaxis
- Early recognition and treatment

Nursing Care Management

Ideally, the objective of nursing care is to counsel parents of high-risk children concerning the signs and symptoms of endocarditis and, in certain cases, the need for prophylactic antibiotic therapy before procedures such as dental work. The family's dentist should be advised of the child's cardiac diagnosis as an added precaution to ensure preventive treatment. SBE prophylaxis is now reserved for very high–risk patients. Many patients who met criteria established in the past may not require prophylaxis under the new guidelines (Wilson, Taubert, Gewitz, and others, 2007) (see Box 25-9). Parents should be counseled regarding the rationale for discontinuing prophylaxis and should be educated as to the fact that their child is still at higher risk for IE than the general population. It is important that all children with congenital or acquired heart disease maintain the highest level of oral health to reduce the chance of bacteremia from oral infections.

Parents should also have a high index of suspicion regarding potential infections. Without unduly alarming them, the nurse stresses that any unexplained fever, weight loss, or change in behavior (lethargy, malaise, anorexia) must be brought to the practitioner's attention. Such symptoms should not be self-diagnosed as a cold or flu. Early diagnosis and treatment are important in preventing further cardiac damage, embolic complications, and growth of resistant organisms.

Treatment of endocarditis requires long-term parenteral drug therapy. In many cases, IV antibiotics may be administered at home with nursing supervision. Nursing goals during this period are (1) preparation of the child for IV infusion, usually with an intermittent-infusion device and several venipunctures for blood cultures; (2) observation for side effects of antibiotics, especially inflammation along venipuncture sites; (3) observation for complications, including embolism and HF; and (4) education regarding the importance of follow-up visits for cardiac evaluation, echocardiographic monitoring, and blood cultures.

RHEUMATIC FEVER

Rheumatic fever (RF) is a poorly understood inflammatory disease that occurs after infection with group A β-hemolytic streptococcal (GABHS) pharyngitis. It occurs most often in late school-age children and adolescents and is rare in adults. It is a self-limited illness that involves the joints, skin, brain, serous surfaces, and heart. Cardiac valve damage (referred to as rheumatic heart disease) is the most significant complication of RF. The mitral valve is most often affected. In developed countries, RF and rheumatic heart disease have become uncommon. However, RF remains a devastating problem in developing countries.

Etiology

Strong evidence supports a relationship between upper respiratory tract infection with GABHS and subsequent development of RF (usually within 2–6 weeks). In almost all cases of RF, a previous infection with GABHS can be documented by laboratory evidence of rising antibody titers. Prevention or treatment of GABHS infection prevents RF.

Diagnostic Evaluation

Diagnosis continues to be based on a set of guidelines known as the modified Jones criteria (Guidelines for the diagnosis of rheumatic fever, 1992). These guidelines were reviewed and again endorsed by the American Heart Association in 2002 and continue to be used to this date (Ferrieri, 2002). The updated Jones criteria suggest that the presence of two major manifestations or one major and two minor manifestations, with supportive evidence of recent streptococcal infection, indicates a high probability of RF (see Nursing Care Guidelines box).

Children suspected of having RF are tested for streptococcal antibodies. The most reliable and best standardized test is an elevated or rising antistreptolysin O (ASO or ASLO) titer, which occurs in 80% of children with RF. Additional antistreptococcal antibody titers may be sent if ASO titers are negative. Acute-phase reactants, ESR, and C-reactive protein (CRP) are usually elevated as well.

Therapeutic Management

The goals of medical management are (1) eradication of hemolytic streptococci, (2) prevention of permanent cardiac damage, (3) palliation of the other symptoms, and (4) prevention of recurrences of RF. Penicillin is the drug of choice or an alternative in penicillin-sensitive children (Gerber, Baltimore, Eaton, and others, 2009). Salicylates are used to control the inflammatory process, especially in the joints, and reduce the fever and discomfort. Bed rest is recommended during the acute febrile phase but need not be strict.

Children who have had acute RF are susceptible to recurrent RF for the rest of their lives and should be followed medically because repeated infections are likely to result in rheumatic heart disease.

Prophylactic treatment against recurrence of RF (secondary prevention) is started after the acute therapy and involves monthly intramuscular injections of benzathine penicillin G (1.2 million units), two daily oral doses of penicillin (200,000 units), or one daily dose of sulfadiazine (1 g). The current American Heart Association guidelines recommend secondary prophylaxis for all patients diagnosed with RF. The exact length of secondary prophylaxis is based on whether or not a patient has residual heart disease. In RF with carditis, prophylaxis is recommended for 5 years or until age 21 years. In the setting of carditis, prophylaxis is recommended for 10 years or until 21 years old. In the setting of RF with carditis and residual heart disease, prophylaxis can continue until the age of 40 years and may be indicated indefinitely

NURSING CARE GUIDELINES

Diagnosis of Initial Attack of Rheumatic Fever (Jones Criteria, 1992 Update)*

Major Manifestations
Carditis
Tachycardia out of proportion to degree of fever
Cardiomegaly
New murmurs or change in preexisting murmurs
Muffled heart sounds
Pericardial friction rub
Chest pain
Changes in ECG (especially prolonged PR interval)

Polyarthritis
Swollen, hot, red, painful joint(s)
After 1 to 2 days, different joint(s) affected
Favors large joints—knees, elbows, hips, shoulders, wrists

Erythema Marginatum
Erythematous macules with clear center and wavy, well-demarcated border
Transitory
Nonpruritic
Primarily affects trunk and extremities (inner surfaces)

Chorea (St. Vitus Dance, Sydenham Chorea)
Sudden aimless, irregular movements of extremities
Involuntary facial grimaces
Speech disturbances

Emotional lability
Muscle weakness (can be profound)
Muscle movements exaggerated by anxiety and attempts at fine motor activity; relieved by rest

Subcutaneous Nodes
Nontender swelling
Located over bony prominences
May persist for some time and then gradually resolve

Minor Manifestations
Clinical Findings
Arthralgia
Fever

Laboratory Findings
Elevated acute-phase reactants
- ESR
- CRP
- Prolonged PR interval

Supporting Evidence of Antecedent Group A Streptococcal Infection
Positive throat culture or rapid streptococcal antigen test result
Elevated or rising streptococcal antibody titer

From Guidelines for the diagnosis of rheumatic fever, Jones criteria, 1992 update, Special Writing Group of the Committee on Rheumatic Fever, Endocarditis, and Kawasaki Disease of the Council on Cardiovascular Disease in the Young of the American Heart Association, *JAMA* 268:2069–2073, 1992.
CRP, C-reactive protein; *ECG*, electrocardiogram; *ESR*, erythrocyte sedimentation rate.
*If supported by evidence of preceding group A streptococcal infection, the presence of two major manifestations or of one major and two minor manifestations indicates a high probability of acute rheumatic fever.

depending on the individual's risk (Gerber, Baltimore, Eaton, and others, 2009).

QUALITY PATIENT OUTCOMES: Rheumatic Fever
- GABHS tonsillopharyngitis identified and treated
- Early recognition and treatment to prevent cardiac valve damage
- Recurrence prevented with prophylaxis compliance

Nursing Care Management

The objectives of nursing care for the child with RF are to (1) encourage compliance with drug regimens, (2) facilitate recovery from the illness, (3) provide emotional support, and (4) prevent the disease. Because compliance is a major concern in long-term drug therapy, every effort is made to encourage adherence to the therapeutic plan (see Compliance, Chapter 22). When compliance is poor, monthly injections may be substituted for daily oral administration of antibiotics, and children need preparation for this often-dreaded procedure.

Interventions during home care are primarily concerned with providing rest and adequate nutrition. Usually, after the febrile stage is over, children can resume moderate activity, and their appetite improves. If carditis is present, the family must be aware of any activity restrictions and may need help in choosing less strenuous activities for the child.

One of the most disturbing and frustrating manifestations of the disease is chorea. The onset is gradual and may occur weeks to months after the illness; it sometimes even occurs in children who have not been diagnosed with RF. It may be mistaken for nervousness, clumsiness, behavioral changes, inattentiveness, and learning disability. It is usually a source of great frustration to the child because the movements, incoordination, and weakness severely limit physical ability. Of utmost importance is stressing to parents and schoolteachers the involuntary, sudden nature of the movements; that the chorea is transitory; and that all manifestations eventually disappear.

Nurses also have a role in prevention, primarily in screening school-age children for sore throats caused by GABHS. This may involve actively participating in throat culture screening programs or in referring children with a possible streptococcal infection for testing.

HYPERLIPIDEMIA (HYPERCHOLESTEROLEMIA)

Hyperlipidemia is a general term for excessive lipids (fat and fatlike substances); hypercholesterolemia refers to excessive cholesterol in the blood. Dyslipidemia is a term used to describe all abnormalities in lipid metabolism, including low levels of high-density lipoprotein (HDL) or "good" cholesterol. High lipid or cholesterol levels play an important role in producing atherosclerosis (fatty plaque on the arteries), which eventually can lead to coronary artery disease, a primary cause of morbidity and mortality in the adult population. A presymptomatic phase of atherosclerosis can begin in childhood. Preventive cardiology focuses on the screening and management of lipid levels in childhood. The goal is to identify children at high risk and intervene early.

Cholesterol is part of the lipoprotein complex in plasma that is essential for cellular metabolism. Triglycerides, natural fats synthesized from carbohydrates, are used for energy. Both are major lipids transported on lipoproteins, a combination of lipids and proteins, which include:

Low-density lipoproteins (LDLs)—These contain low concentrations of triglycerides, high levels of cholesterol, and moderate levels of protein. LDL is the major carrier of cholesterol to the cells. Cells use cholesterol for synthesis of membranes and steroid production. Elevated circulating LDL is a strong risk factor in cardiovascular disease.

High-density lipoproteins (HDLs)—These contain very low concentrations of triglycerides, relatively little cholesterol, and high levels of protein. They transport free cholesterol to the liver for excretion in the bile. High levels of HDL are thought to protect against cardiovascular disease.

Diagnostic Evaluation

Hyperlipidemia is diagnosed on the basis of analysis of blood for a full lipid profile, drawn after a 12-hour fast. Hyperlipidemia can have a familial, genetic basis, or a lifestyle component, or can be caused by secondary problems, such as hypothyroidism. In children with elevated cholesterol levels, a screening thyroid-stimulating hormone is also measured once to rule out hypothyroidism as a cause of secondary hypercholesterolemia. Additional blood work is individualized based on other risk factors. In overweight children, a fasting glucose level may be obtained to assess for risk factors associated with metabolic syndrome, which is a combination of multiple symptoms that are associated with increased cardiovascular risk in adults. Blood samples should be collected after having the child sit for 5 minutes, and the tourniquet should be applied immediately before the needle puncture because posture and vascular stasis may affect results. Diagnostic values for acceptable, borderline, and high total cholesterol and LDL cholesterol levels are listed in Table 25-5.

Recent guidelines from the AAP (Daniels, Greer, and Committee on Nutrition, 2008) continue to recommend a strategy that combines two complementary approaches: (1) a population approach that aims to lower the average levels of blood cholesterol among all American children through population-wide changes in nutrient intake and eating patterns and (2) an individualized approach based on selective screening (see Evidence-Based Practice box).

Therapeutic Management

The first step in the treatment of high cholesterol is oriented to lifestyle modification. The AAP (Daniels, Greer, and Committee on Nutrition, 2008) guidelines continue to advocate the benefits of a heart-healthy diet for all children. Children with known elevated cholesterol should have individual nutritional counseling by a nutritionist with expertise in pediatric lipids.

Research continues to support the benefit of diets low in saturated fats. Current thinking favors a "Mediterranean"-type diet. Whole grains, fruits, and vegetables form the foundation of this diet. In addition, this diet allows the use of monounsaturated fats, such as olive oil and canola oil, which have beneficial effects on HDL cholesterol values. The use of these fats also makes the diet more realistic. Patients who have elevated triglycerides, especially in the setting of an elevated body mass index (BMI), should receive targeted counseling related to decreasing their intake of simple carbohydrates. Daily aerobic exercise of at least 60 minutes a day 5 days a week is also recommended for children with high cholesterol. In addition, patients and parents should be counseled regarding the negative effects of smoking (both first- and secondhand).

For children with severe hypercholesterolemia who fail to respond to dietary modifications, drug therapy may be necessary. Pharmacologic therapy is recommended for children older than the age of 8 years who have LDL cholesterol greater than 190 mg/dl without other risk factors or over 160 mg/dl in patients with two or more other risk factors. In young people with other risk factors, such as diabetes, medication can be considered when LDL values are greater than 130 mg/dl. The use of medication in young people needs to be a cooperative decision with the parents. Parents should understand what data are available about statin use in young people because long-term evidence-based practice is not practical or available for this population. In the past, bile acid–binding resins were the only class of drugs recommended for treatment of younger children. This class of drug acts by binding bile acids in the intestinal lumen. Because they are not absorbed by the intestine, resin binders do not produce systemic toxicity and are safe for children. Cholestyramine (Questran) and colestipol (Colestid) are both powders that are mixed with water or juice just before ingestion. Unfortunately, the vast majority of patients do not get adequate reduction in LDL cholesterol from bile acid–binding resins. Many cannot tolerate the medication because of the taste; gritty texture; and side effects, the most significant being constipation, abdominal pain, gastrointestinal bloating, flatulence, and nausea. The most recent guidelines on lipid abnormalities in children give the option for treatment with statins if pharmacologic therapy is indicated using the previously outlined guidelines for treatment (Daniels, Greer, and Committee on Nutrition, 2008; McCrindle, Urbina, Dennison, and others, 2007). Statins are much more effective than other drugs at lowering LDL cholesterol. To a lesser degree, they also help lower triglycerides levels and can raise HDL cholesterol. Statins work by inhibiting the enzyme necessary for cholesterol synthesis. Statins are most effective when taken in the evening and are started at the lowest possible dose in young people. Blood work should be followed closely in children and adolescents and usually includes a fasting lipid profile, liver function tests, and creatinine kinase repeated at 4- and 8-week intervals initially and with dosage changes.

Patients beginning therapy with a statin should be counseled regarding rare but potentially serious side effects such as rhabdomyolysis, elevated transaminases, and elevated creatinine kinase. Patients

TABLE 25-5	CLASSIFICATION OF CHOLESTEROL LEVELS IN CHILDREN FROM FAMILIES WITH A HISTORY OF HEART DISEASE	
CATEGORY	TOTAL CHOLESTEROL (mg/dl)	LDL CHOLESTEROL (mg/dl)
Acceptable	<170	<110
Borderline	170–199	110–129
High	≥200	≥130

Adapted from Daniels SR, Greer FR, and the Committee on Nutrition: Lipid screening and cardiovascular health in childhood, *Pediatrics* 122:198–208, 2008.
LDL, Low-density lipoprotein.

EVIDENCE-BASED PRACTICE
Cholesterol Screening for Children

Updated by Olga A. Taylor

Ask the Question
PICOT Question
Should cholesterol screening be performed in children?

Search for the Evidence
Search Strategies
The literature was searched to locate clinical research studies related to this issue. Selection criteria included English-language publications within the past 10 years, research-based articles (level 3 or lower), and infant and child populations.

Databases Used
PubMed, Cochrane Collaboration, MD Consult, Joanna Briggs Institute, National Guidelines Clearinghouse (AHRQ), TRIP Database Plus, PedsCCM, BestBETs

Critically Analyze the Evidence
- In late 2011, an expert panel of the National Heart, Lung, and Blood Institute (NHLBI) made a recommendation that lipid screening be performed on all children ages 9 to 11 years; this recommendation was based on evidence that as many as 30% to 60% of children with dyslipidemia might be missed when screening is performed by family history alone (National Heart, Lung, and Blood Institute, 2011). The expert panel's guidelines also include comprehensive screening and treatment guidelines for children with cardiovascular disease risk factors.
- Diagnosis of obesity is paramount in enhancing care of obese pediatric patients. Current laboratory (cholesterol or glucose) screening rates (10%) are inadequate in the outpatient setting (Patel, Madsen, Maselli, and others, 2010).
- Testing for cardiovascular risk factors: HDL cholesterol, LDL cholesterol, fasting glucose, blood pressure, OGTT, thyrotropin, and ALT should be considered in pediatric patients with increased waist circumference and even normal BMI (l'Allemand-Jander, 2010).
- In obese children, LDL cholesterol, HDL cholesterol, total cholesterol, and triglycerides are significantly different from subjects who are not obese (Simsek, Balta, Balta, and others, 2010).
- Serum triglyceride levels are a predictive risk factor of carotid intima-media thickness (Simsek, Balta, Balta, and others, 2010).
- In children and adolescents (12–19 years old) fasting non-HDL cholesterol levels were strongly associated with metabolic syndrome. A non-HDL cholesterol threshold of 120 mg/dl indicated borderline risk for metabolic syndrome, and a threshold of 145 mg/dl indicated high metabolic syndrome risk (Li, Ford, McBride, and others, 2011).
- Cholesterol levels in childhood are a major population predictor for adult cholesterol levels (Daniels, Greer, and Committee on Nutrition, 2008).
- Precursors of atherosclerosis are present in young people. The atherosclerotic process begins early in life with early phases characterized by the development of fatty streaks in the vessels (PDAY study) (Enos, Holmes, and Beyer, 1953; Strong, Malcom, McMahan, and others, 1999).
- Atherosclerosis is related to the presence and degree of cardiovascular risk factors in adults (Berenson, Srinivasan, Bao, and others, 1998).
- Most severely affected children come from families with a high incidence of early heart disease. Children whose genetic family history is unknown should also be screened (AAP, Committee on Nutrition, 1998).

- Universal cholesterol screening in children would identify all individuals with dyslipidemia. Using solely the family history to identify subjects for cholesterol screening missed individuals with moderate dyslipidemia and those with potentially genetic dyslipidemia (Ritchie, Murphy, Ice, and others, 2010).

Apply the Evidence: Nursing Implications
There are strong recommendations (Guyatt, Oxman, Vist, and others, 2008) that lipid screening should be performed on all children 9–11 years of age. The NHLBI guidelines have been endorsed by the American Academy of Pediatrics (AAP, 2011).

QSEN Quality and Safety Competencies:
Evidence-Based Practice*
Knowledge
Differentiate clinical opinion from research and evidence-based summaries.
Describe use of cholesterol screening in children.

Skills
Base individualized care plan on patient values, clinical expertise, and evidence.
Integrate evidence into practice by using cholesterol screening in children.

Attitudes
Value the concept of evidence-based practice as integral to determining best clinical practice.
Appreciate strengths and weakness of evidence for using cholesterol screening in children.

References
American Academy of Pediatrics: Expert panel on integrated guidelines for cardiovascular health and risk reduction in children and adolescents: summary report, *Pediatrics* 128(suppl 5):S213–S256, 2011.
Berenson GS, Srinivasan SR, Bao W, and others: Association between multiple cardiovascular risk factors and atherosclerosis in children and young adults, *N Engl J Med* 338(23):1650–1656, 1998.
Daniels SR, Greer FR, Committee on Nutrition: Lipid screening and cardiovascular health in childhood, *Pediatrics* 122:198–208, 2008.
Enos WF, Holmes RH, Beyer J: Coronary disease among United States soldiers killed in action in Korea, *JAMA* 152(12):1090–1093, 1953.
Guyatt GH, Oxman AD, Vist GE, and others: GRADE: an emerging consensus on rating quality of evidence and strength of recommendations, *BMJ* 336:924–926, 2008.
l'Allemand-Jander D: Clinical diagnosis of metabolic and cardiovascular risk in overweight children: early development of chronic diseases in the obese child, *Int J Obes* 34(suppl 2):S32–S36, 2010.
Li C, Ford ES, McBride PE, and others: Non-high-density lipoprotein cholesterol concentration is associated with the metabolic syndrome among US youth aged 12–19 years, *J Pediatr* 158(2):201–207, 2011.
National Heart, Lung, and Blood Institute: *Expert panel on integrated guidelines for cardiovascular health and risk reduction in children and adolescents*, November 2011, retrieved May 31, 2012, from http://www.nhlbi.nih.gov/guidelines/cvd_ped/.
Patel AI, Madsen KA, Maselli JH, and others: Underdiagnosis of pediatric obesity during outpatient preventive care visits, *Acad Pediatr* 10(6):406–409, 2010.
Ritchie SK, Murphy EC, Ice C, and others: Universal versus targeted blood cholesterol screening among youth: the CARDIAC project, *Pediatrics* 126(2):260–265, 2010.
Simsek E, Balta H, Balta Z, and others: Childhood obesity-related cardiovascular risk factors and carotid intima-media thickness, *Turk J Pediatr*, 52(6):602–611, 2010.
Strong JP, Malcom GT, McMahan CA, and others: Prevalence and extent of atherosclerosis in adolescents and young adults: implications for prevention from the Pathobiological Determinants of Atherosclerosis in Youth Study, *JAMA* 281(8):727–735, 1999.

ALT, Alanine aminotransferase; *BMI,* body mass index; *HDL,* high-density lipoprotein; *KD,* Kawasaki disease; *LDL,* low-density lipoprotein; *MI,* myocardial infarction; *OGTT,* oral glucose tolerance test.; *PDAY,* Pathobiological Determinants of Atherosclerosis in Youth.
*Adapted from the QSEN at http://www.qsen.org.

should discontinue their medication and contact their practitioner if they develop dark urine or new muscle aches. Statin medications are not safe during pregnancy; therefore, sexually active adolescents need to take adequate birth control measures. Very long–term studies are unlikely to be available over decades; however, in the shorter-term studies that have been completed, statins seem to have a similar safety profile for children as they do for adults (McCrindle, Urbina, Dennison, and others, 2007).

Nursing Care Management

Nurses play an important role in the screening, education, and support of children with lipid abnormalities and their families. When a child is referred to a preventive cardiology clinic, it is essential that the family be adequately prepared for the first visit. Generally, the parents will be asked to keep a dietary history of the child before this visit. Sometimes they will need to complete a questionnaire regarding the child's normal dietary habits during the preceding year. Families should be instructed to keep their child fasting for at least 12 hours before screening. Last, parents should be aware that lipids should not be drawn within 3 weeks of a febrile illness because doing so can affect cholesterol values. It is important to schedule the blood test early in the morning and to arrange for nourishment immediately thereafter. At the visit, a full family history should be taken, including the health of both parents and all first-degree relatives. Specific questions should be asked regarding early heart disease, hypertension, strokes (CVAs), sudden death, hyperlipidemia, diabetes, and endocrine abnormalities.

Parents and extended families should be educated about cholesterol and lipid abnormalities. This education should include a brief introduction of the different lipoprotein categories, including cholesterol, HDL, LDL, and triglycerides. Also, behavioral risk factors for heart disease, such as smoking and exercise, should be reviewed. For management to be effective, parents and patients need to understand that the rationale for dietary or pharmacologic intervention is prevention of future cardiovascular disease.

Stringent dietary guidelines may become an issue of control and a source of great stress for many families. A child with a lipid disorder should not be viewed as having a disease. Rather, the positive aspects of healthy eating, regularly exercising, and avoiding smoking should be emphasized. Basic dietary changes should be encouraged for the whole family so the affected child is not singled out. Cultural differences must be considered and recommendations individualized. Substitution rather than elimination needs to be emphasized. Visual aids (e.g., test tubes depicting the amount of fat in a hot dog or the number or packs of sugar in a glass of juice) are often helpful, especially for children. Diets should be flexible and individually tailored by a nutritionist who is experienced in lipid disorders. Dietary recommendations need to meet the nutritional demands of growing children while providing benefit to the overall profile. Parents are encouraged to participate in dietary and educational sessions, ask questions, and share ideas and experiences.

Parents often feel guilty about the hereditary component of hyperlipidemia. Many also believe they have failed if the diet alone is not making a significant difference in their child's lipid profile. They need to be reassured that a dietary approach alone is often not sufficient, especially for children with significantly elevated values.

Parents of children who require pharmacologic therapy need to understand the purpose, dosage, and possible side effects of the various drugs. Medication schedules should remain flexible and should not interfere with the child's daily activities. Follow-up phone calls by the nurse between visits allow parents to discuss their concerns and ask any questions that have arisen.

CARDIAC DYSRHYTHMIAS

Dysrhythmias, or abnormal heart rhythms, can occur in children with structurally normal hearts, as features of some congenital heart defects, and in patients after surgical repair of congenital heart defects. They are also seen in patients with cardiomyopathy and with cardiac tumors. They can occur secondary to metabolic and electrolyte imbalances. They can be classified in several ways, including by heart rate characteristics (bradycardia and tachycardia) and by the origin of the dysrhythmia in the atria or ventricles. Some dysrhythmias are well tolerated and self-limiting. Others may cause decreased cardiac output with associated symptoms. Some dysrhythmias can cause sudden death. Treatment depends on the cause of the dysrhythmia and its severity.

Many advances have been made in the diagnosis and treatment of pediatric dysrhythmias in the past decade. Improvements in technology have allowed better diagnosis, the development of ablation techniques, and the expansion of pacemaker capabilities. New antidysrhythmic medications have proven safe and effective in children. Radiofrequency ablation has offered a cure for some dysrhythmias. Pediatric electrophysiology has become a highly specialized field, and students should consult more detailed sources for an in-depth discussion. The following sections address diagnostic studies and provide a general discussion of the most common tachycardia (supraventricular tachycardia [SVT]) and the most common bradycardia (complete heart block) that require treatment in the pediatric population.

Diagnostic Evaluation

Nurses must be familiar with the standards of normal heart rate for the particular age group (see inside back cover). An initial nursing responsibility is recognition of an abnormal heartbeat, either in rate or rhythm. When a dysrhythmia is suspected, the apical rate is counted for 1 full minute and compared with the radial rate, which may be lower because not all of the apical beats are felt. Consistently, high or low heart rates should be regarded as suspicious. The patient should be placed on a cardiac monitor with recording capabilities. A 12-lead ECG yields more information than the monitor recording and should be done as soon as possible.

The basic diagnostic procedure is the ECG, including 24-hour Holter monitoring. Electrophysiologic cardiac catheterization allows for identification of the conduction disturbance and immediate investigation of drugs that may control the dysrhythmia. Another procedure that may be used is transesophageal recording. An electrode catheter is passed to the lower esophagus and, when in position at a point proximal to the heart, is used to stimulate and record dysrhythmias.

Dysrhythmias can be classified according to various criteria, such as effect on heart rate and rhythm, as follows:

Bradydysrhythmias—Abnormally slow rate
Tachydysrhythmias—Abnormally rapid rate
Conduction disturbances—Irregular heart rate

Bradydysrhythmias

Sinus bradycardia (slower than normal rate) in children can be attributed to the influence of the autonomic nervous system, as with hypervagal tone, or in response to hypoxia and hypotension. Sinus bradycardias are also known to develop after some complex cardiac surgical repairs involving extensive atrial suture lines such as atrial baffle repairs (Mustard and Senning repairs) and the Fontan procedure.

Complete atrioventricular (AV) block is also referred to as complete heart block. This can be either congenital (occurring in children with structurally normal hearts) or acquired after surgery to repair cardiac defects. AV blocks are most often related to edema around the conduction system and resolve without treatment. Temporary epicardial wires are placed in most patients at surgery; if a rhythm disturbance occurs, temporary pacing can be used. Several days after surgery, the health practitioner removes the wires by pulling slowly and deliberately down on them from the site of insertion.

Some children may need a permanent pacemaker. The pacemaker takes over or assists in the heart's conduction function. The implantation of a pacemaker, in the operating room or possibly the catheterization laboratory, is usually a low-risk procedure. The pacemaker is made up of two basic parts, the pulse generator and the lead. The pulse generator is composed of the battery and the electronic circuitry. The lead is an insulated, flexible wire that conducts the electrical impulse from the pulse generator to the heart. Two types of leads are available, transvenous and epicardial. After the lead has been attached to the heart, a small incision is made, and a pocket is formed under the muscle to house and protect the generator. Continuous ECG monitoring is necessary during the recovery phase to assess pacemaker function. The nurse should be aware of the programmed rate and expected individual generator variations. The pacemaker insertion site is monitored for signs of infection. Analgesics are given for pain.

Pacemaker functions have become more sophisticated, and some models can adjust the heart rate to activity demands or be programmed for overdrive pacing or cardioversion.

Discharge teaching includes information about the signs and symptoms of infection, general wound care, and activity restrictions. Parents, and patients if they are old enough, should be taught to take a pulse and know the settings of the pacemaker. If the patient's low rate is set at 80 beats/min and the heart rate is only 68 beats/min, there is a possible problem with the pacemaker that needs to be investigated. Instructions for telephone transmission of ECG readings are also given. Telephone transmission can be used to transmit ECG strips and to monitor battery life and pacemaker function. The pacemaker generator will have to be replaced periodically because of battery depletion. Children with pacemakers should wear a Medic-Alert device, and their parents should have a paper identification card with specific pacer data in case of an emergency. Cardiopulmonary resuscitation (CPR) instruction is suggested for parents.

Tachydysrhythmias

Sinus tachycardia (an abnormally fast heart rate) secondary to fever, anxiety, pain, anemia, dehydration, or any other etiologic factor requiring increased cardiac output should be ruled out before diagnosing an increased heart rate as pathologic. SVT is the most common tachydysrhythmia found in children and refers to a rapid regular heart rate of 200 to 300 beats/min. As many as 1 in 250 children experience SVT (Schlente, Boramanand, and Funk, 2008). The onset of SVT is often sudden, the duration is variable, and the rhythm may end abruptly and convert back to a normal sinus rhythm. Clinical signs in infants and young children are poor feeding, extreme irritability, and pallor. Children may experience palpitations, dizziness, chest pain, and diaphoresis. If SVT is sustained, signs of HF may be seen.

The treatment of SVT depends on the degree of compromise imposed by the dysrhythmia (see Critical Thinking Case Study). In some cases, vagal maneuvers, such as applying ice to the face, massaging the carotid artery (on one side of the neck only), or having an older child perform a Valsalva maneuver (e.g., exhaling against a closed glottis, blowing on a thumb as if it were a trumpet for 30 to 60 seconds), have terminated SVT. If vagal maneuvers fail or the child is hemodynamically unstable, adenosine (a drug that impairs AV conduction) may be used. Adenosine is given by rapid IV push with a saline bolus immediately after the drug because of its very short

> ## ⓘ CRITICAL THINKING CASE STUDY
> ### *Supraventricular Tachycardia*
>
> You are working in the emergency department when a father comes through the doors, crying, carrying his 1-month-old infant. The infant is awake and very irritable. The father reports that the infant has not been feeding well for the past 6 hours, and the father has noticed sweating (diaphoresis) with attempted feeds. No history of fever is noted. Further assessment reveals a diaphoretic, crying infant with a respiratory rate of 60 breaths/min, BP of 60/40 mm Hg, and heart rate that is too fast to count by auscultation. When the infant is attached to the cardiorespiratory monitor, the heart rate is 220 beats/min, nonvariable, with an oxygen saturation of 97%. Capillary refill time is slightly prolonged at 3 seconds, and femoral pulses are palpable but weak.
>
> **Questions**
> 1. Evidence—Is there sufficient evidence to draw conclusions about this infant?
> 2. Assumptions—Describe an underlying assumption about each of the following:
>   a. Symptoms associated with heart failure
>   b. An infant younger than 3 months with poor feeding
>   c. Tachyarryhthmias in infants
> 3. What priorities for nursing care should be established?
> 4. Does the evidence support your nursing interventions?

BP, Blood pressure.

half-life. If this is unsuccessful or cardiac output is compromised, esophageal overdrive pacing or synchronized cardioversion (delivering an electrical shock to the heart) can be used in the intensive care setting. Sedation is needed for both procedures. Cardioversion should never be done in a conscious patient. More long-term pharmacologic treatment includes digoxin or possibly propranolol (Inderal) or amiodarone for severe or recurrent SVT.

A primary focus of nursing care is education of the family regarding the symptoms of SVT and its treatment. SVT may occur again despite therapy. Parents should be taught to take a radial pulse for a full minute. If medication is prescribed, instructions regarding accurate dosage and the importance of administering the correct dose at specified intervals are stressed.

Radiofrequency ablation has become first-line therapy for some types of SVT. The procedure is done in the cardiac catheterization laboratory and begins with mapping of the conduction system to identify the dysrhythmia focus. A catheter delivering radiofrequency current is directed at the site, and the area is heated to destroy the tissue in the area. These are lengthy procedures, often lasting 6 to 8 hours, and sedation or general anesthesia is required. Preparation is similar to that for cardiac catheterization. Another procedure, cryoablation, is also used in treatment of SVT. Liquid nitrous oxide is used to cool a catheter to subfreezing temperatures, which then destroys the tissue of target by freezing.

PULMONARY ARTERY HYPERTENSION

Pulmonary artery hypertension (PAH) describes a group of rare disorders that result in an elevation of pulmonary artery pressure above 25 mm Hg at rest after the neonatal period (Barst, 1999). These disorders are poorly understood, and until recently, there was no treatment beyond supportive care. PAH is a progressive, eventually fatal disease for which there is no known cure. It can be difficult to diagnose in the early stages. Often when patients become symptomatic and a diagnosis is made, their disease is rapidly progressing, treatment is unsuccessful, and death occurs within several years. There is now evidence of a genetic basis for some PAH; some mutations localized to chromosome 2 have been identified in about half of patients with familial PAH (Lane, Machado, Pauciulo, and others, 2000).

Pulmonary artery hypertension affects the small pulmonary arteries and is characterized by vascular narrowing leading to an increase in pulmonary vascular resistance. Generally, these abnormalities result in remodeling of the pulmonary circulation, characterized by occlusion of the lumen in medium and small pulmonary arteries because of cellular proliferation (Michelakis, Wilkins, and Rabinovitch, 2008). Why some children develop the disease and others do not is unclear. There are many possible causes of PAH. Cardiac causes occur primarily in patients with a large left-to-right shunt producing increased pulmonary blood flow. If these defects are not repaired early, the high pulmonary flow will cause changes in the pulmonary artery vessels, and the vessels will lose their elasticity. Other causes of PAH include hypoxic lung diseases, thromboembolic diseases causing pulmonary vascular obstruction, collagen vascular diseases, and exposure to toxic substances. Many of the patients have no identifiable cause for PAH and have primary or idiopathic PAH.

Clinical Manifestations

The clinical manifestations include dyspnea with exercise, chest pain, and syncope. Dyspnea is the most common symptom and is caused by impaired oxygen delivery. Chest pain is the result of coronary ischemia in the right ventricle from severe hypertrophy. Syncope reflects a limited cardiac output leading to decreased cerebral blood flow. Right-sided heart dysfunction is steadily progressive, and when symptoms of venous congestion and edema are present, the prognosis is poor.

Therapeutic Management

Although no cure is known, several therapies have shown promise in slowing the progression of the disease and improving quality of life. In general, situations that may exacerbate the disease and cause hypoxia, such as exercise and high altitudes, are avoided. Supplemental oxygen, especially at night while sleeping, is commonly used to relieve hypoxia. Patients are at risk for thromboembolic events leading to pulmonary emboli, so anticoagulation with warfarin (Coumadin) is often prescribed.

Vasodilator therapy (which relaxes vascular smooth muscle and reduces pulmonary artery pressure) can prolong survival of patients with PAH. Oral calcium channel blockers have been successful in some children. For patients who are nonresponders in vasodilator testing, a new oral drug, bosentan, an endothelin-receptor antagonist, is now available that reduces pulmonary artery pressure and resistance and is safe and well tolerated in children (Barst, Ivy, Dingemanse, and others, 2003). It has been used in combination with IV prostacyclin.

Continuous IV prostacyclin has been used with some success in children who did not respond to oral therapy. Both of these therapies, although promising, have been used in only small numbers of patients and are expensive. Lung transplantation may be another treatment option.

QUALITY PATIENT OUTCOMES: Hypertension
- Underlying cause of hypertension identified
- Blood pressure control maintained
- Dietary practices and lifestyle changes effectively used to control hypertension
- Compliance with medication regimen, if prescribed

CARDIOMYOPATHY

Cardiomyopathy refers to abnormalities of the myocardium in which the cardiac muscles' ability to contract is impaired. Cardiomyopathies are relatively rare in children. Possible etiologic factors include familial or genetic causes, infection, deficiency states, metabolic abnormalities, and collagen vascular diseases. Most cardiomyopathies in children are considered primary or idiopathic, in which the cause is unknown and the cardiac dysfunction is not associated with systemic disease. Some of the known causes of secondary cardiomyopathy are anthracycline toxicity (the antineoplastic agents doxorubicin [Adriamycin] and daunomycin), hemochromatosis (from excessive iron storage), Duchenne muscular dystrophy, Kawasaki disease (KD), collagen diseases, and thyroid dysfunction.

Cardiomyopathies can be divided into three broad clinical categories according to the type of abnormal structure and dysfunction present: dilated cardiomyopathy, hypertrophic cardiomyopathy, and restrictive cardiomyopathy.

Dilated cardiomyopathy is characterized by ventricular dilation and greatly decreased contractility, resulting in symptoms of HF. This is the most common type of cardiomyopathy in children. Its cause is often unknown. The clinical findings are of HF with tachycardia, dyspnea, hepatosplenomegaly, fatigue, and poor growth. Dysrhythmias may be present and may be more difficult to control with worsening HF.

Hypertrophic cardiomyopathy is characterized by an increase in heart muscle mass without an increase in cavity size, usually occurring in the left ventricle and associated with abnormal diastolic filling. It is a familial autosomal dominant genetic abnormality in most cases and is probably the most common genetically transmitted cardiovascular disease (Maron, 2001). The expression of clinical disease varies greatly among patients. Clinical symptoms usually appear in school-age period or adolescence and may include anginal chest pain, dysrhythmias, and syncope. One recent study confirmed that unexplained syncope in the childhood age group (younger than 18 years of age) with known hypertrophic cardiomyopathy had a 60% cumulative risk of sudden death within 5 years of the syncopal event (Spirito, Autore, Rapezzi, and others, 2009). Presentation in infancy includes signs of HF and has a poor prognosis. The ECG demonstrates left ventricular hypertrophy, often with ST-T changes. The echocardiogram is most helpful and demonstrates asymmetric septal hypertrophy and an increase in left ventricular wall thickness, with a small left ventricle cavity.

Restrictive cardiomyopathy, which is rare in children, describes a restriction to ventricular filling caused by endocardial or myocardial disease or both. It is characterized by diastolic dysfunction and absence of ventricular dilation or hypertrophy. Symptoms are similar to those of HF (see p. 835).

Therapeutic Management

Treatment is directed toward correcting the underlying cause whenever feasible. However, in most affected children, this is not possible, and treatment is aimed at managing HF (p. 835) and dysrhythmias. Digoxin, diuretics, and aggressive use of afterload reduction agents have been found to be helpful in managing symptoms in those with dilated cardiomyopathy. Practice guidelines for the management of HF in children have recently been outlined and provide an in-depth review of available therapies (Rosenthal, Chrisant, Edens, and others, 2004). Digoxin and inotropic agents are usually not helpful in the other forms of cardiomyopathy because increasing the force of contraction may exacerbate the muscular obstruction and actually impair ventricular ejection. β-Blockers such as propranolol and calcium channel blockers such as verapamil (Calan) have been used to reduce left ventricular outflow obstruction and improve diastolic filling in those with hypertrophic cardiomyopathy.

Careful monitoring and treatment of dysrhythmias are essential. The placement of an automatic implantable cardioverter defibrillator (AICD) should be considered for patients at high risk of sudden death because of ventricular dysrhythmias. Anticoagulants may be given to reduce the risk of thromboemboli, a complication of the sluggish circulation through the heart. For worsening HF and signs of poor perfusion, IV inotropic or vasodilating drugs may be needed. Severely ill children may require mechanical ventilation, oxygen administration, and IV medications. Heart transplantation may be a treatment option for patients who have worsening symptoms despite maximum medical therapy.

Nursing Care Management

Because of the poor prognosis in many children with cardiomyopathy, nursing care is consistent with that for any child with a life-threatening disorder (see Chapter 18). One of the most difficult adjustments for the child (especially normally active youngsters with hypertrophic cardiomyopathy) may be the realization of failing health and the need for restricted activity. The child should be included in decisions regarding activity and allowed to discuss feelings, particularly if the disease follows a progressively fatal course. After symptoms of HF or dysrhythmias develop, the same nursing interventions are implemented as discussed on pp. 836–840. If heart transplantation is considered, the needs of the child and family are great in terms of psychologic preparation and postoperative care. The nurse plays an important role in assessing the family's understanding of the procedure and long-term consequences. Children of school age and older should be fully informed to give their assent to the procedure (see Informed Consent, Chapter 22).

HEART TRANSPLANTATION

Heart transplantation has become a treatment option for infants and children with worsening HF and a limited life expectancy despite maximum medical and surgical management. Indications for heart transplantation in children are cardiomyopathy and end-stage CHD. It is also an option for patients with some forms of complex congenital cardiac defects, such as hypoplastic left heart syndrome, for whom conventional surgical approaches have a high mortality rate.

The heart transplant procedure may be orthotopic or heterotopic. Orthotopic heart transplantation refers to removing the recipient's own heart and implanting a new heart from a donor who has had brain death but a healthy heart. The donor and recipient are matched by weight and blood type. Heterotopic heart transplantation refers to leaving the recipient's own heart in place and implanting a new heart to act as an additional pump, or "piggyback" heart; this type of transplant is rarely done in children.

Before transplantation, potential recipients undergo a careful cardiac evaluation to determine if there are any other medical or surgical options to improve the patient's cardiac status. Other organ systems are assessed to identify problems that might increase the risk of or preclude transplantation. A psychosocial evaluation of the patient and family is done to assess family function, support systems, and ability to comply with the complex medical regimen after the transplant. Support services to help the family successfully care for their child are provided when possible. Parents and older adolescents need extensive education about the risks and benefits of transplantation so they can make an informed decision. Patients are listed on a national computer network organized by the United Network for Organ Sharing to match donors and recipients. (See also Organ or Tissue Donation and Autopsy, Chapter 18.)

Although the total number of pediatric candidates on the waiting list has steadily increased from 1739 in 1997, in 2009 the number of pediatric candidates was 134 active on the waiting list, according to the Scientific Registry of Transplant Recipients (SRTR, 2011). The 1-year graft survival rate for pediatric heart transplants performed in 2008 was 87.5% (SRTR, 2011).

Waiting list mortality remains high, particularly in the smallest children. Recent progress in suitable ventricular assist devices for use in children as a bridge to transplantation has made outcomes to survival for cardiac transplantation more successful (Blume, Naftel, Bastardi, and others, 2006). A multicenter study using the U.S. Scientific Registry of Transplant Recipients was recently conducted (Almond, Thiagarajian, Piercy, and others, 2009). Among 3098 children listed for a heart transplant between 1999 and 2006, the median age was 2 years. Sixty percent of patients were listed as a top status (30% ventilated and 18% on supportive measures), and of those children, 17% died, 63% received transplants, 8% recovered, and 12% remained listed. These numbers concluded that U.S. waiting time remains high in the current era, and high-risk groups in these categories could benefit from emerging cardiac assist devices, such as extracorporeal membrane oxygenation and ventricular assist devices.

The posttransplant course is complex. Although heart function is greatly improved or normal after transplantation, the risk of rejection is serious. The leading cause of death in the first 3 years after heart transplantation is rejection, with the greatest risk in the first 6 months (Blume, 2003). Rejection of the heart is diagnosed primarily by endomyocardial biopsy in older children. Serial echocardiograms are often used in infants and young children to reduce the need for invasive biopsies. Immunosuppressants must be taken for life and have many systemic side effects. Triple-drug therapy for immunosuppression with a calcineurin inhibitor (cyclosporine or tacrolimus), steroids, and azathioprine is most commonly used in pediatric patients, although mycophenolate mofetil is being used more frequently and replacing azathioprine. Steroids are weaned in the first year and may be discontinued in some patients.

Infection is always a risk. Potential long-term problems that may limit survival include chronic rejection, causing coronary artery disease; renal dysfunction and hypertension resulting from cyclosporine administration; lymphoma; and infection. Coronary artery disease is the leading cause of death among late survivors of heart transplantation (Boucek, Aurora, Edwards, and others, 2007). In the short term, after successful transplantation, children are able to return to full participation in age-appropriate activities and appear to adapt well to their new lifestyle. Transplantation is not a cure because patients must live with the lifetime consequences of chronic immunosuppression.

NURSING CARE MANAGEMENT

Successfully caring for a child after a heart transplant requires the expertise and dedication of many members of the health care team. Nurses play vital roles in assessment, coordination of care, psychosocial support, and patient and family education. The heart transplant recipient must be carefully monitored for signs of rejection, infection, and the side effects of the immunosuppressant medications. The patient's and family's psychosocial well-being also needs to be assessed to identify issues such as increased family stress, depression, substance abuse, and school problems. Noncompliance with an intense medication regimen, especially during adolescence, can lead to serious medical problems and can be fatal. Immunosuppressants and nursing implications are discussed in Chapter 27 in relation to renal transplantation. Care of the immunosuppressed child is reviewed in Chapter 26. Psychosocial concerns and appropriate interventions for the child with a life-threatening disorder are presented in Chapter 18.

The first 6 months to 1 year after the transplant are most intense because the risk of complications is greatest and the patient and family are adjusting to a new lifestyle. Patients are monitored closely by the health care team, with frequent visits and laboratory tests. Care is usually shared between local health care providers and the transplant center. Many patients are able to return to school and other age-appropriate activities within 2 to 3 months after the transplant.

VASCULAR DYSFUNCTION

SYSTEMIC HYPERTENSION

Hypertension is defined as the consistent elevation of BP beyond values considered to be the upper limits of normal. The two major categories are essential hypertension (no identifiable cause) and secondary hypertension (subsequent to an identifiable cause). In recent years, there has been increasing interest in this disorder in adolescents and children. Hypertension in children and adolescents is defined as having a systolic or diastolic BP that consistently falls at or over the 95th percentile. This group is further delineated as follows:

Stage 1 hypertension includes patients who have BP readings between the 95th and 99th percentiles.

Stage 2 hypertension includes patients with BP readings over the 99th percentile plus 5 mm Hg.

An additional group includes children and adolescents who have prehypertension (or high-normal BP). This prehypertensive group includes those with BP readings that fall consistently between the 90th and 95th percentiles. *The Fourth Report on the Diagnosis, Evaluation, and Treatment of High Blood Pressure in Children and Adolescents* outlines in detail the identification, testing, and treatment recommendations for young people with high BP (National High Blood Pressure Education Program Working Group on High Blood Pressure in Children and Adolescents, 2004).

Etiology

Most instances of hypertension observed in young children occur secondary to a structural abnormality or an underlying pathologic process, although this is being challenged by screening programs of relatively healthy children. The most common cause of secondary hypertension is renal disease followed by cardiovascular, endocrine, and some neurologic disorders. As a rule, the younger the child and the more severe the hypertension, the more likely it is to be secondary.

The causes of essential hypertension are undetermined, but evidence indicates that both genetic and environmental factors play a role. The incidence of hypertension has been shown to be higher in children whose parents are hypertensive. African Americans have a higher incidence of hypertension than whites, and in African Americans it develops earlier, is frequently more severe, and results in death at an earlier age. Environmental factors that contribute to the risk of developing hypertension include obesity, salt ingestion, smoking, and stress.

Diagnostic Evaluation

From the increasing numbers of hypertensive or potentially hypertensive children and adolescents being identified, a BP determination

---

BOX 25-10   CLINICAL MANIFESTATIONS OF HYPERTENSION

Adolescents and Older Children
Frequent headaches
Dizziness
Changes in vision

Infants or Young Children
Irritability
Head banging or head rubbing
Waking up screaming in the night

---

should be a routine part of annual assessment in healthy children older than age 3 years. BP readings should be done in children younger than 3 years old who have high-risk family histories or those with individual risk factors, including CHD, kidney disease, malignancy, transplant, certain neurologic problems, or systemic illnesses known to cause hypertension. Although clinical manifestations associated with hypertension depend largely on the underlying cause, some observations can provide clues to the examiner that an elevated BP may be a factor (Box 25-10). In infants and very young children who cannot communicate symptoms, observation of behavior provides clues, although gross behavioral changes may not be apparent until complications are present.

No definitive cutoff values are used in the diagnosis of hypertension in the pediatric patient. The *Fourth Report on the Diagnosis, Evaluation, and Treatment of High Blood Pressure in Children and Adolescents* (National High Blood Pressure Education Program Working Group on High Blood Pressure in Children and Adolescents, 2004) provides normative data for children (see Appendix E). BP tables now include the 50th, 90th, 95th, and 99th percentiles for BP readings based on age, gender, and height percentiles. These guidelines are based on auscultatory readings, and therefore this is currently the preferred method of assessment. These charts take into account differences in body height. It is therefore important to note that a child who is large for his or her age may normally have a higher BP than a child of average size. Before a diagnosis is made, BP should be measured on at least three separate occasions. An ambulatory BP monitor may be ordered if "white-coat hypertension" is suspected. These are useful in that they provide BP readings over a 24-hour period. There are different normative values for ambulatory BP readings (Urbina, Alpert, Flynn, and others, 2008).

A careful medical history and family history should be obtained to screen for other relatives with hypertension or other cardiovascular risk factors. In children with suspected hypertension, initial laboratory data include a urinalysis, renal function studies such as creatinine and blood urea nitrogen, a lipid profile, complete blood count, and electrolytes. Depending on the severity of hypertension, additional testing may be indicated. Testing may include a retinal examination, renal ultrasonography to measure kidney size and Doppler flow to detect the possibility of a renal causes, and an ECG and an echocardiogram to evaluate the presence of end-organ involvement such as left ventricular hypertrophy. Further testing for a secondary cause may be indicated based on individual circumstances, especially in children with significant hypertension and normal initial screening test findings.

Oral contraceptives can be a cause of hypertension because of their pressor effects. A trial off of oral contraceptives may be indicated; however, other options of contraceptives should be discussed before this decision is made (see Chapter 17).

Therapeutic Management

Therapy for secondary hypertension involves diagnosis and treatment of the underlying cause. Children and adolescents with consistently elevated BP readings from no known cause or those with secondary hypertension not amenable to surgical correction may be treated with a combination of nonpharmacologic and pharmacologic interventions. Dietary practices and lifestyle changes are important in the control of hypertension both for children and for adults. Nonpharmacologic measures, such as weight control in overweight patients, increased exercise, limited salt intake, and avoidance of stress and smoking, carry no risk and should be instituted as first-line therapy except in severe cases in which pharmacologic therapy may be indicated as well.

Drug therapy is instituted with caution in children with significant elevations of BP resistant to nonpharmacologic intervention. The treatment should begin with one drug and should add other drugs if control is not obtained. The oral antihypertensive drugs used in children include the β-blockers, ACE inhibitors, calcium channel blockers, angiotensin-receptor blockers, and diuretics. The goal is to achieve a normotensive state throughout the day without accompanying drug side effects.

Nursing Care Management

Blood pressure measurement should always be a part of the routine assessment of children older than age 3 years and patients younger than 3 years who are considered to be at high risk for hypertension. To obtain an accurate reading, care is taken to quiet the child or relax the adolescent while the measurement is recorded to avoid false readings caused by excitement. BP should be measured in the sitting position with the arm at the level of the heart. Initial evaluation should also include four extremity pressures (in the supine position) to rule out coarctation of the aorta. The chief cause of falsely elevated BP readings is the use of improperly fitting, narrow cuffs. Therefore, attention to correct measurement technique is essential (see Blood Pressure, Chapter 6).

Nursing counseling and guidance of affected children are challenges. Education aimed at understanding hypertension and its implication over the life span is essential in promoting patient and family compliance with both nonpharmacologic and pharmacologic therapies (see Compliance, Chapter 22).

Home BP measurements can facilitate surveillance in youngsters with chronic hypertension and can document the effectiveness of therapy. A family member can be instructed in how to take and record accurate BP measurements, thus decreasing the number of trips to a health care facility. This individual needs to understand when to contact the practitioner regarding elevated values. The school nurse can often be a valuable resource in monitoring BP. The nurse plays an important role in assessing individual families and providing targeted information regarding nonpharmacologic modes of intervention, such as diet, weight loss, smoking cessation, and exercise programs. If extensive dietary counseling is required, the child should be referred to a nutritionist with expertise in working with children and adolescents. Exercise regimens should be individualized but should emphasize the benefits of regular aerobic exercise. Schoolchildren and young adolescents generally prefer team sports rather than individual training, which they may view as a burden rather than an enjoyable activity. If peers and family members can be encouraged to participate in any of the management strategies, the child's compliance is likely to be greater.

If drug therapy is prescribed, the nurse needs to provide information to the family regarding the reasons for it, how the drug works, and possible side effects. General instructions for antihypertensive drugs include:

- Rise slowly from a horizontal position and avoid sudden position changes.
- Take drugs as prescribed.
- Maintain adequate hydration.
- Notify the practitioner if unpleasant side effects occur but do not discontinue the drug.
- Avoid alcohol and stay on the prescribed diet.

The need for follow-up is stressed, especially because antihypertensive therapy can sometimes be safely discontinued if BP remains under control over time.

KAWASAKI DISEASE (MUCOCUTANEOUS LYMPH NODE SYNDROME)

Kawasaki disease is an acute systemic vasculitis of unknown cause. It is seen in every racial group, and about 75% of the cases occur in children younger than the age of 5 years, with peak incidence in the toddler age group. The acute disease is self-limited; however, without treatment, approximately 20% of children develop coronary artery dilation or aneurysm formation. Infants younger than 1 year of age are most seriously affected by KD and are at the greatest risk for heart involvement, although an increased incidence has also been reported in older children, perhaps because of later diagnosis in many.

The etiology of KD is unknown. It is not spread by person-to-person contact; however, several factors support infectious etiologic factors. It is often seen in geographic and seasonal outbreaks, with most cases reported in the late winter and early spring (Newburger, Takahashi, Gerber, and others, 2004).

Pathophysiology

The principal area of concern in KD is the cardiovascular system. During the initial stage of the illness, extensive inflammation of the arterioles, venules, and capillaries occurs, causing many of the clinical symptoms. In addition, segmental damage to the medium-sized muscular arteries, mainly the coronary arteries, can occur, resulting in the formation of coronary artery aneurysms in some children. When death occurs, which is very rare (in <0.17% of cases), it is usually the result of myocardial ischemia from coronary thrombosis or years later from severe scar formation and stenosis in coronary aneurysms (Wilder, Palinkas, Kao, and others, 2007).

Clinical Manifestations

Because no specific diagnostic test exists for KD, the diagnosis is established on the basis of clinical findings and associated laboratory results (Box 25-11). These criteria should be used as guidelines. It is important to note that many children with KD do not fulfill standard diagnostic criteria, and infants often have an incomplete presentation. It is therefore important to consider KD as a possible diagnosis in any infant or child with prolonged elevated temperature that is unresponsive to antibiotics and is not attributable to another cause.

Kawasaki disease manifests in three phases: acute, subacute, and convalescent. The acute phase begins with the abrupt onset of a high fever that is unresponsive to antibiotics and antipyretics. The child then develops the remaining diagnostic symptoms. Symptoms may come and go and are not always present simultaneously, although the fever is persistent throughout. During this stage, the child is typically *very* irritable. The subacute phase begins with resolution of the fever and lasts until all clinical signs of KD have disappeared. During this phase, the child is at greatest risk for the development of coronary

---

| BOX 25-11 | **DIAGNOSTIC CRITERIA FOR KAWASAKI DISEASE** |

Child must have fever for more than 5 days along with four of five clinical criteria* (diagnosis may be made on day 4 by an experienced clinician if child has all the clinical criteria):

1. Changes in the extremities: in the acute phase edema, erythema of the palms and soles; in the subacute phase, periungual desquamation (peeling) of the hands and feet
2. Bilateral conjunctival injection (inflammation) without exudation
3. Changes in the oral mucous membranes, such as erythema of the lips, oropharyngeal reddening; or "strawberry tongue" (large papillae are exposed)
4. Polymorphous rash
5. Cervical lymphadenopathy (one lymph node >1.5 cm)

*Kawasaki disease can be diagnosed with fewer clinical criteria when coronary artery changes are noted.

---

artery aneurysms. Echocardiograms are used to monitor myocardial and coronary artery status. A baseline echocardiogram should be obtained at the time of diagnosis for comparison with future studies. Irritability persists during this phase. In the convalescent phase, all of the clinical signs of KD have resolved, but the laboratory values have not returned to normal. This phase is complete when all blood values are normal (6–8 weeks after onset). At the end of this stage, the child has regained his or her usual temperament, energy, and appetite.

Cardiac Involvement

Long-term complications of KD include the development of coronary artery aneurysms, disrupting blood flow. Children with larger aneurysms have the potential for myocardial infarction, which can result from thrombotic occlusion of a coronary aneurysm. Affected coronary arteries dilate progressively, reaching their maximal diameter approximately 1 month from the onset of fever. Over time, as the damaged vessel tries to heal, stenosis of the aneurysm may develop and may lead to myocardial ischemia. Most of the morbidity and mortality occur in children affected with the largest aneurysms (giant aneurysms >8 mm or z-score >10). Symptoms of acute myocardial infarction in children are often confusing and may include abdominal pain, vomiting, restlessness, inconsolable crying, pallor, and shock as well as chest pain or pressure (noted less in younger children). In the initial phase of the illness, children with KD may have signs or symptoms related to inflammation of the myocardium, including myocarditis, valvulitis, or arrhythmias.

Therapeutic Management

The current treatment of children with KD includes high-dose IV gamma globulin (IVGG) along with salicylate therapy. IVGG has been demonstrated to be effective at reducing the incidence of coronary artery abnormalities when given within the first 10 days of the illness and ideally in the first 7 days of illness. A single, large infusion of 2 g/kg over 10 to 12 hours is recommended. Retreatment with IVGG is indicated in patients who continue with fever after treatment.

Aspirin is given initially in an antiinflammatory dose (80–100 mg/kg/day in divided doses every 6 hours) to control fever and symptoms of inflammation. After fever has subsided, aspirin is continued at an antiplatelet dose (3–5 mg/kg/day). Low-dose aspirin is continued in patients without echocardiographic evidence of coronary abnormalities until the platelet count has returned to normal (6–8 weeks). If the child develops coronary abnormalities, salicylate therapy is continued

indefinitely. Additional anticoagulation (e.g., clopidogrel [Plavix], enoxaparin [Lovenox], or warfarin) may be indicated in children who have medium-sized or giant coronary artery aneurysms.

Prognosis

Most children with KD recover fully after treatment. However, when cardiovascular complications occur, serious morbidity may result. The prognosis for patients is strongly related to the extent of coronary damage, with patients who have giant aneurysms being at the highest risk for complications.

QUALITY PATIENT OUTCOMES: Kawasaki Disease
- Early diagnosis and treatment
- Prevention of cardiovascular complications

Nursing Care Management

In the initial phase, the nurse must monitor the child's cardiac status carefully. Intake and output and daily weight measurements are recorded. Although the child may be reluctant to eat and therefore may be partially dehydrated, fluids need to be administered with care because of the usual finding of myocarditis. The child should be assessed frequently for signs of HF, including decreased urinary output, gallop rhythm (an additional heart sound), tachycardia, and respiratory distress.

Administration of IVGG should follow the same guidelines as for any blood product, with frequent monitoring of vital signs. Patients must be watched for allergic reactions. Cardiac status must be monitored because of the large volume being administered to patients who may have diminished left ventricular function.

The majority of nursing care focuses on symptomatic relief. To minimize skin discomfort, cool cloths; unscented lotions; and soft, loose clothing are helpful. During the acute phase, mouth care, including lubricating ointment to the lips, is important for mucosal inflammation. Clear liquids and soft foods can be offered.

Patient irritability is perhaps the most challenging problem. These children need a quiet environment that promotes adequate rest. Their parents need to be supported in their efforts to comfort an often inconsolable child. They may need time away from their child, and nurses can often provide respite care for the family. Parents need to understand that irritability is a hallmark of KD and that they need not feel guilty or embarrassed about their child's behavior.

Discharge Teaching

Parents need accurate information about the progression of KD, including the importance of follow-up monitoring and when they should contact their practitioner. Irritability is likely to persist for up to 2 months after the onset of symptoms. Periungual desquamation (peeling of the hands and feet) begins in the second and third weeks. Usually the fingers peel first followed by the feet. The peeling is painless, but the new skin may be tender. Arthritis, especially of the larger weight-bearing joints, may occur and persist for several weeks, although it is temporary. Children are typically most stiff in the mornings, during cold weather, and after naps. Passive range-of-motion exercises in the bathtub are often helpful in increasing flexibility. Any live immunizations (e.g., measles, mumps, and rubella; varicella) should be deferred for 11 months after the administration of gamma globulin because the body might not produce the appropriate amount of antibodies to provide lifelong immunity. The decision to give the varicella (chickenpox) vaccine while the child is receiving aspirin therapy is made individually by the practitioner. Temperature should be recorded after discharge, and the occurrence of fever should be communicated to the health care provider.

Parents of children with large aneurysms should be educated as to the unlikely but real possibility of myocardial infarction, as well as the signs and symptoms of cardiac ischemia in a child. At discharge, the ultimate cardiac sequelae is generally not fully known because vessels do not reach their maximum diameter until 4 to 6 weeks after the onset of KD. CPR should be taught to parents of children with known severe coronary artery sequelae.

Long-Term Follow-up

The frequency and type of followup is based on the presence or absence of coronary damage. The long-term outlook for children without aneurysms is promising. Increased incidence of early heart disease in this population is not observed with over 30 years of follow-up. However, the literature regarding subtle effects of inflammation on the vessels is conflicting, and it is recommended that these children be screened and treated for the presence of coronary risk factors as they grow older. They should have a cholesterol screen performed; BP monitored; and education recommending a heart-healthy lifestyle, including exercise, a heart-healthy diet, and avoidance of smoking. This group of patients is seen at infrequent intervals, approximately every 5 years depending on the institution. In patients with aneurysms, follow-up focuses on the prevention and early detection of coronary ischemia in patients. Noninvasive modalities of coronary imaging, such as cardiac computed tomography angiography, magnetic resonance imaging, echocardiography, and stress testing, are used as much as possible. Patients with coronary aneurysms may require long-term antiplatelet or anticoagulation and possibly β-blocker therapy or other therapies, depending on the severity of coronary involvement.

SHOCK

Shock, or circulatory failure, is a complex clinical syndrome characterized by inadequate tissue perfusion to meet the metabolic demands of the body, resulting in cellular dysfunction and eventual organ failure. Although the causes are different, the physiologic consequences are the same and include hypotension, tissue hypoxia, and metabolic acidosis. Circulatory failure in children is a result of hypovolemia, altered peripheral vascular resistance, or pump failure. Types of shock are listed in Box 25-12.

Pathophysiology

A healthy child's circulatory system is able to transport oxygen and metabolic substrates to body tissues, which require a constant source for these essential needs. The cardiac output and distribution to the various body tissues can change rapidly in response to intrinsic (myocardial and intravascular) or extrinsic (neuronal) control mechanisms. In shock states, these mechanisms are altered or challenged.

Reduced blood flow, as in hypovolemic shock, causes diminished venous return to the heart, low CVP, low cardiac output, and hypotension. Vasomotor centers in the medulla are signaled, causing a compensatory increase in the force and rate of cardiac contraction and constriction of arterioles and veins, thereby increasing peripheral vascular resistance. Simultaneously, the lowered blood volume leads to the release of large amounts of catecholamines, antidiuretic hormone, adrenocorticosteroids, and aldosterone in an effort to conserve body fluids. This causes reduced blood flow to the skin, kidneys, muscles, and viscera to shunt the available blood to the brain and heart. Consequently, the skin feels cold and clammy, there is poor capillary filling,

---

BOX 25-12   TYPES OF SHOCK

Hypovolemic
Characteristics
Reduction in size of vascular compartment
Falling blood pressure
Poor capillary filling
Low CVP

Most Frequent Causes
Blood loss (hemorrhagic shock)—Trauma, gastrointestinal bleeding, intracranial hemorrhage
Plasma loss—Increased capillary permeability associated with sepsis and acidosis, hypoproteinemia, burns, peritonitis
Extracellular fluid loss—Vomiting, diarrhea, glycosuric diuresis, sunstroke

Distributive
Characteristics
Reduction in peripheral vascular resistance
Profound inadequacies in tissue perfusion
Increased venous capacity and pooling
Acute reduction in return blood flow to the heart
Diminished cardiac output

Most Frequent Causes
Anaphylaxis (anaphylactic shock)—Extreme allergy or hypersensitivity to a foreign substance
Sepsis (septic shock, bacteremic shock, endotoxic shock)—Overwhelming sepsis and circulating bacterial toxins
Loss of neuronal control (neurogenic shock)—Interruption of neuronal transmission (spinal cord injury)
Myocardial depression and peripheral dilation—Exposure to anesthesia or ingestion of barbiturates, tranquilizers, opioids, antihypertensive agents, or ganglionic blocking agents

Cardiogenic
Characteristic
Decreased cardiac output

Most Frequent Causes
After surgery for congenital heart disease
Primary pump failure—Myocarditis, myocardial trauma, biochemical derangements, heart failure
Dysrhythmias—Supraventricular tachycardia, atrioventricular block, and ventricular dysrhythmias; secondary to myocarditis or biochemical abnormalities (occasionally)

CVP, Central venous pressure.

---

and glomerular filtration rate and urinary output are significantly reduced.

As a result of impaired perfusion, oxygen is depleted in the tissue cells, causing them to revert to anaerobic metabolism, producing lactic acidosis. The acidosis places an extra burden on the lungs as they attempt to compensate for the metabolic acidosis by increasing the respiratory rate to remove excess carbon dioxide. Prolonged vasoconstriction results in fatigue and atony of the peripheral arterioles, which leads to vessel dilation. Venules, which are less sensitive to vasodilator substances, remain constricted for a time, causing massive pooling in the capillary and venular beds, which further depletes blood volume.

Complications of shock create further hazards. CNS hypoperfusion may eventually lead to cerebral edema, cortical infarction, or intraventricular hemorrhage. Renal hypoperfusion causes renal ischemia with possible tubular or glomerular necrosis and renal vein thrombosis. Reduced blood flow to the lungs can interfere with surfactant secretion and result in acute respiratory distress syndrome, which is characterized by sudden pulmonary congestion and atelectasis with formation of a hyaline membrane. Gastrointestinal tract bleeding and perforation are always possibilities after splanchnic ischemia and necrosis of intestinal mucosa. Metabolic complications of shock may include hypoglycemia, hypocalcemia, and other electrolyte disturbances.

Diagnostic Evaluation

The etiology of shock can be discerned from the history and the physical examination. The severity of the shock is determined by measurements of vital signs, including CVP and capillary filling (Box 25-13). Shock can be regarded as a form of compensation for circulatory failure. Because of the progressive nature of shock, it can be divided into the following three stages or phases:

1. **Compensated shock**—Vital organ function is maintained by intrinsic compensatory mechanisms; blood flow is usually normal or increased but generally uneven or maldistributed in the microcirculation.
2. **Decompensated shock**—Efficiency of the cardiovascular system gradually diminishes until perfusion in the microcirculation becomes marginal despite compensatory adjustments. The outcomes of circulatory failure that progress beyond the limits of compensation are tissue hypoxia, metabolic acidosis, and eventual dysfunction of all organ systems.

BOX 25-13   CLINICAL MANIFESTATIONS OF SHOCK

Compensated
Apprehensiveness
Irritability
Unexplained tachycardia
Normal blood pressure
Narrowing pulse pressure
Thirst
Pallor
Diminished urinary output
Reduced perfusion of extremities

Decompensated
Confusion and somnolence
Tachypnea
Moderate metabolic acidosis
Oliguria
Cool, pale extremities
Decreased skin turgor
Poor capillary filling

Irreversible
Thready, weak pulse
Hypotension
Periodic breathing or apnea
Anuria
Stupor or coma

---

3. **Irreversible, or terminal, shock**—Damage to vital organs, such as the heart or brain, is of such magnitude that the entire organism will be disrupted regardless of therapeutic intervention. Death occurs even if cardiovascular measurements return to normal levels with therapy.

At all stages, the principal differentiating signs are observed in the (1) degree of tachycardia and perfusion to the extremities, (2) level of consciousness, and (3) BP. Additional signs or modifications of these more universal signs may be present depending on the type and cause of the shock. Initially, the child's ability to compensate is effective; therefore, early signs are subtle. As the shock state advances, signs are more obvious and indicate early decompensation.

Additional signs may be present, depending on the type and cause of the shock. In early septic shock, there are chills, fever, and vasodilation, with increased cardiac output that results in warm, flushed skin (hyperdynamic, or "hot," shock). A later and ominous development is disseminated intravascular coagulation (DIC) (see Chapter 26), the major hematologic complication of septic shock. Anaphylactic shock is frequently accompanied by urticaria and angioneurotic edema, which is life threatening when it involves the respiratory passages (see Anaphylaxis, below).

Laboratory tests that assist in assessment are blood gas measurements, pH, and sometimes liver function tests. Coagulation tests are evaluated when there is evidence of bleeding, such as oozing from a venipuncture site, bleeding from any orifice, or petechiae. Cultures of blood and other sites are indicated when there is a high suspicion of sepsis. Renal function tests are performed when impaired renal function is evident.

Therapeutic Management

Treatment of shock consists of three major interventions: (1) ventilation, (2) fluid administration, and (3) improvement of the pumping action of the heart (vasopressor support). The first priority is to establish an airway and administer oxygen. After the airway is ensured, circulatory stabilization is the major concern. Establishment of adequate IV access, ideally with multilumen central lines, is essential to deliver fluids and medications.

Ventilatory Support

The lung is the organ that is most sensitive to shock. Decreased distribution or redistribution of blood flow to respiratory muscles plus the increased work of breathing can rapidly lead to respiratory failure. Critically ill patients are unable to maintain an adequate airway. To place the lung at rest and improve ventilation, tracheal intubation is initiated early with positive-pressure ventilation. Supplemental oxygen is always given as soon as possible. Blood gases and pH are monitored frequently.

Increased extravascular lung water caused by edema contributes to the development of respiratory complications. Therapy is directed toward maintaining normal arterial blood gas measurements, normal acid–base balance, and circulation. Efforts are made to remove fluid and prevent its accumulation with the use of diuretics.

Cardiovascular Support

In most cases, rapid restoration of blood volume is all that is needed for resuscitation of the child in shock. An isotonic crystalloid solution (normal saline or Ringer lactate) is the fluid of choice; colloids such as albumin are also used. Successful resuscitation is reflected by an increase in BP and a reduction in heart rate; increased cardiac output results in improved capillary circulation and skin color. CVP measurements of right atrial pressure help guide fluid therapy, and urinary output measurement is an important indicator of adequacy of circulation. Correction of acidosis, hypoxemia, hypoglycemia, hypothermia, and any metabolic derangements is mandatory.

Temporary pharmacologic support may be required to enhance myocardial contractility, reverse metabolic or respiratory acidosis, and maintain arterial pressure. The principal agents used to improve cardiac output and circulation are catecholamines, such as dopamine (Intropin) and epinephrine (Adrenalin). Vasodilators that are sometimes used include nitroprusside (Nipride) and milrinone.

QUALITY PATIENT OUTCOMES: Shock
- Oxygen content of blood optimized
- Cardiac output improved
- Oxygen demand reduced
- Metabolic abnormalities corrected
- Type of shock identified and treated

Nursing Care Management

The child who is in shock requires intensive observation and care. *The initial action is to ensure adequate tissue oxygenation.* The nurse should be prepared to administer oxygen by the appropriate route and to assist with any intubation and ventilatory procedures indicated. Other procedures and activities that require immediate attention are establishing an IV line, weighing the child, obtaining baseline vital signs, placing an indwelling catheter, obtaining blood gases and other measurements, and administering medications as indicated. The child is best positioned flat with the legs elevated.

! NURSING ALERT

Early clinical signs of shock include apprehension, irritability, normal BP, narrowing pulse pressure (difference between diastolic and systolic BP), thirst, pallor, diminished urinary output, unexplained mild tachycardia, and decreased perfusion of the hands and feet.

The nurse's responsibilities are to monitor the IV infusion, intake and output, vital signs (including CVP), and general systems assessments on a routine basis. IV medications are titrated according to patient responses, and vital signs are taken every 15 minutes during the critical periods and thereafter as needed. Urinary output is measured hourly; blood gases, hematocrit, pH, and electrolytes are monitored frequently to assess the child's status and the efficacy of therapy. An apnea and cardiac monitor is attached and monitored continuously. In the initial stages of acute shock, more than one nurse is often needed to manage all of the necessary activities that must be carried out simultaneously (see Emergency Treatment box).

Throughout the intense activity, support for the family must not be overlooked. Someone should contact family members at frequent intervals to inform them about what is being done and whether there is any progress. Ideally, someone should remain with the parents to serve as a liaison between them and the intensive care team. However, this is not always feasible in such a critical situation. As soon as possible, the family should be allowed to see the child. A member of the clergy or a social worker may be called to help provide comfort and support.

ANAPHYLAXIS

Anaphylaxis is the acute clinical syndrome resulting from the interaction of an allergen and a patient who is hypersensitive to that allergen.

When the antigen enters the circulatory system, a generalized reaction rapidly takes place. Vasoactive amines (principally histamine or a histamine-like substance) are released and cause vasodilation, bronchoconstriction, and increased capillary permeability.

Severe reactions are immediate in onset; are often life threatening; and frequently involve multiple systems, primarily the cardiovascular, respiratory, gastrointestinal, and integumentary systems. Exposure to the antigen can be by ingestion, inhalation, skin contact, or injection. Examples of common allergens associated with anaphylaxis include drugs (e.g., antibiotics, chemotherapeutic agents, radiologic contrast media), latex, foods, venom from bees or snakes, and biologic agents (antisera, enzymes, hormones, blood products).

! NURSING ALERT

Penicillin allergy is associated with immediate onset (within 1 hour of administration) or accelerated onset (1–72 hours after administration) of skin eruption, especially a urticarial rash, or more serious symptoms such as laryngeal edema or anaphylactic shock.

Clinical Manifestations

The onset of clinical symptoms usually occurs within seconds or minutes of exposure to the antigen, and the rapidity of the reaction is directly related to its intensity: the sooner the onset, the more severe the reaction. The reaction may be preceded by symptoms of uneasiness, restlessness, irritability, severe anxiety, headache, dizziness, paresthesia, and disorientation. The patient may lose consciousness. Cutaneous signs of flushing and urticaria are common early signs followed by angioedema, most notable in the eyelids, lips, tongue, hands, feet, and genitalia.

Bronchiolar constriction may follow, causing narrowing of the airway; pulmonary edema and hemorrhage also may occur. Laryngeal edema with severe acute upper airway obstruction may be life threatening and requires rapid intervention. Shock occurs as a result of mediator-induced vasodilation, which causes capillary permeability and loss of intravascular fluid into the interstitial space. Sudden hypotension and impaired cardiac output with poor perfusion are seen.

Therapeutic Management

Successful outcome of anaphylactic reactions depends on rapid recognition and institution of treatment. The goals of treatment are to provide ventilation, restore adequate circulation, and prevent further exposure by identifying and removing the cause when possible.

A mild reaction with no evidence of respiratory distress or cardiovascular compromise can be managed with subcutaneous administration of antihistamines, such as diphenhydramine (Benadryl) and epinephrine.

Moderate or severe distress presents a potentially life-threatening emergency. Establishing an airway is the first concern, as with all shock states. Epinephrine is given subcutaneously or intravenously as an antihistamine and to support the cardiovascular system and increase BP. Other routes for giving epinephrine are intramuscular and via the airway, either nebulized or injected through an endotracheal tube. In severe anaphylaxis, epinephrine by any route is better than none. Fluids are given to restore blood volume. Additional vasopressors may be given to improve cardiac output.

Prevention of a reaction is preferable. Preventing exposure is more easily accomplished in children known to be at risk, including those with (1) a history of previous allergic reaction to a specific antigen; (2) a history of atopy; (3) a history of severe reactions in immediate

✚ EMERGENCY TREATMENT

Shock

Ventilation
Establish airway; be prepared for intubation.
Administer oxygen, usually 100% by mask.

Fluid Administration
Restore fluid volume as ordered.

Cardiovascular Support
Administer vasopressors (epinephrine 1:1000, 0.01 mg/kg subcutaneously; maximum dose of 0.5 mg; may repeat if needed).

General Support
Keep child flat with legs raised above level of heart.
Keep child warm and calm.

---

family members; and (4) a reaction to a skin test, although skin tests are not available for all allergens. Desensitization may be recommended in certain cases.

QUALITY PATIENT OUTCOMES: Anaphylaxis
- Early recognition of symptoms
- Airway patency maintained
- Adequate circulation restored and maintained
- Further exposure to allergic agent prevented

Nursing Care Management

When an anaphylactic reaction is suspected, both immediate intervention and preparation for medical therapy are nursing responsibilities. Ventilation is ensured by placing the child in a head-elevated position, unless contraindicated by hypotension, to facilitate breathing and administer oxygen. If the child is not breathing, CPR is initiated and emergency medical services are summoned.

If the cause can be determined, measures are implemented to slow the spread of the offending substance. An IV infusion is established immediately. Emergency medications are given intravenously whenever possible; however, epinephrine may be given subcutaneously (see Emergency Treatment box). Vital signs and urinary output are monitored frequently. Medications are administered as prescribed, with regular assessment to monitor effectiveness and to detect signs of side effects of medication and fluid overload.

To prevent an anaphylactic reaction, parents are always asked about possible allergic responses to foods, latex, medications, and environmental conditions. These are displayed prominently on the patient's chart. The specific allergen is noted, as are the type and severity of the reaction. Parents are excellent historians, especially when the child has displayed a pronounced reaction to a substance. Drugs, including related drugs (e.g., penicillin, nafcillin), and other items, such as latex, that have produced a reaction previously are *never* used. If the child is allergic to insect venom, the family is instructed to purchase an emergency kit to be kept with the child at all times. Both the family and the child, if the child is old enough, are taught how to use the equipment. The patient should carry medical identification at all times.

SEPTIC SHOCK

Sepsis and septic shock are caused by an infectious organism (Maar, 2004). Normally, an infection triggers an inflammatory response in a

---

BOX 25-14   DEFINITIONS OF SYSTEMIC INFLAMMATORY RESPONSE SYNDROME, INFECTION, SEPSIS, AND SEVERE SEPSIS

SIRS—The presence of at least two of the following four criteria, one of which must be abnormal temperature or leukocyte count:
1. Core temperature of more than 38.5° C (101.3° F) or less than 36° C (96.8° F).
2. Tachycardia, defined as a mean heart rate more than 2 SD above normal for age in the absence of external stimulus, chronic drugs, or painful stimuli; or otherwise unexplained persistent elevation over a 0.5- to 4-hour period; or, for children younger than 1 year old: bradycardia, defined as a mean heart rate less than the 10th percentile for age in the absence of external vagal stimulus, β-blocker drugs, or congenital heart disease; or otherwise unexplained persistent depression over a 0.5-hour period.
3. Mean respiratory rate more than 2 SD above normal for age or mechanical ventilation for an acute process not related to underlying neuromuscular disease or the receipt of general anesthesia.
4. Leukocyte count elevated or depressed for age (not secondary to chemotherapy-induced leukopenia) or more than 10% immature neutrophils.

Infection—A suspected or proven (by positive culture, tissue stain, or PCR test) infection caused by any pathogen; or a clinical syndrome associated with a high probability of infection. Evidence of infection includes positive findings on clinical examination, imaging, or laboratory tests (e.g., white blood cells in a normally sterile body fluid, perforated viscus, chest radiograph consistent with pneumonia, petechial or purpuric rash, or purpura fulminans).

Sepsis—SIRS in the presence of or as a result of suspected or proven infection.

Severe sepsis—Sepsis plus cardiovascular organ dysfunction or ARDS or two or more other organ dysfunctions.

From Goldstein B, Giroir B, Randolph A, and others: International Pediatric Sepsis Consensus Conference: definitions for sepsis and organ dysfunction in pediatrics, *Pediatr Crit Care Med* 6(1):2–8, 2005; used with permission.
ARDS, Acute respiratory distress syndrome; *PCR,* polymerase chain reaction; *SD,* standard deviations; *SIRS,* systemic inflammatory response syndrome.

---

local area, which results in vasodilation, increased capillary permeability, and eventually elimination of the infectious agent. The widespread activation and systemic release of inflammatory mediators is called the systemic inflammatory response syndrome (SIRS). Box 25-14 provides the exact definitions for SIRS, infection, sepsis, and severe sepsis. SIRS can occur in response to both infectious and noninfectious (e.g., trauma, burns) causes. When caused by infection, it is called sepsis. Septic shock is defined as sepsis with organ dysfunction and hypotension.

Most of the physiologic effects of shock occur because the exaggerated immune response triggers more than 30 different mediators that result in diffuse vasodilation, increased capillary permeability, and maldistribution of blood flow. This impairs oxygen and nutrient delivery to the cells, resulting in cellular dysfunction. If the process continues, multiple-organ dysfunction occurs and may result in death. Table 25-6 includes the age-specific vital signs and laboratory values reflective of septic shock in children.

The incidence of septic shock is increasing in adults and children (Arnal and Stein, 2003), possibly as a result of greater numbers of

TABLE 25-6	AGE-SPECIFIC VITAL SIGNS AND LABORATORY VARIABLES IN SEPTIC SHOCK*				
	HEART RATE (BEATS/MIN)		**RESPIRATORY RATE (BREATHS/MIN)**	**LEUKOCYTE COUNT (LEUKOCYTES × 103/MM³)**	**SYSTOLIC BLOOD PRESSURE (MM HG)**
AGE GROUP	**TACHYCARDIA**	**BRADYCARDIA**			
0 days–1 week	>180	<100	>50	>34	<65
1 week–1 month	>180	<100	>40	>19.5 or <5	<75
1 month–1 year	>180	<90	>34	>17.5 or <5	<100
2–5 years	>140	N/A	>22	>15.5 or <6	<94
6–12 years	>130	N/A	>8	>13.50 or <4.5	<105
13–<18 years	>110	N/A	>4	>11 or <4.5	<117

From Goldstein B, Giroir B, Randolph A, and others: International Pediatric Sepsis Consensus Conference: definitions for sepsis and organ dysfunction in pediatrics, *Pediatr Crit Care Med* 6(1):2–8, 2005; used with permission.
N/A, Not applicable.
*Lower values for heart rate, leukocyte count, and systolic blood pressure are for 5th percentile, and upper values for heart rate, respiratory rate, or leukocyte count are for 95th percentile.

immunosuppressed patients, more widespread use of invasive devices in seriously ill patients, increased awareness of the diagnosis, and a growing number of resistant microorganisms.

Three stages have been identified in septic shock. In early septic shock, the patient has chills, fever, and vasodilation with increased cardiac output, which results in warm, flushed skin that reflects vascular tone abnormalities and hyperdynamic, warm, or hyperdynamic-compensated responses. BP and urinary output are normal. The patient has the best chance for survival in this stage. The second stage—the normodynamic, cool, or hyperdynamic-decompensated stage—lasts only a few hours. The skin is cool, but pulses and BP are still normal. Urinary output diminishes, and the mental state becomes depressed. With advancing disease, certain signs of circulatory decompensation that deteriorate to signs of circulatory collapse are indistinguishable from late shock of any cause. In the hypodynamic, or cold, stage of shock, cardiovascular function progressively deteriorates even with aggressive therapy. The patient has hypothermia, cold extremities, weak pulses, hypotension, and oliguria or anuria. Patients are severely lethargic or comatose. Multiorgan failure is common. This is the most dangerous stage of shock.

Management of septic shock involves measures to provide hemodynamic stability and adequate oxygenation to the tissues and the use of antimicrobials to treat the infectious organism. As with other forms of shock, hemodynamic stability is achieved with fluid volume resuscitation and inotropic agents as needed. Providing adequate oxygenation often requires intubation and mechanical ventilation, supplemental oxygen, sedation, and paralysis to decrease the work of breathing. Septic shock involves activation of complement proteins that promote clumping of the granulocytes in the lung. The granulocytes can release chemicals that can cause direct lung injury to the pulmonary capillary endothelium. This causes a fluid leak into the alveoli, which causes stiff, noncompliant lungs. DIC and multiorgan dysfunction may also occur and require prompt assessment and management.

Newer therapies are being developed to modify the host immune response by attempting to block various mediators, thereby interrupting the inflammatory cascade.

Early identification of the symptoms of septic shock is critical to patient survival. A high index of suspicion is required in all critically ill patients who are at greater risk for sepsis because of multiple invasive lines and devices, poor nutrition, and impaired immune function. Subtle alterations in tissue perfusion and unexplained tachypnea and tachycardia often are early warning signs. Identification of the infectious agent and prompt treatment are also critical to patient survival. Broad-spectrum antibiotics should be given, and the site of infection should be removed if possible (e.g., drain abscesses, remove indwelling lines). Patients should be managed in an ICU in which continuous monitoring and sophisticated cardiac and respiratory support are available. Multidisciplinary collaboration is essential in managing these critically ill patients.

TOXIC SHOCK SYNDROME

Toxic shock syndrome (TSS) is a relatively rare condition caused by the toxins produced by the *Staphylococcus* bacteria. First described in 1978, TSS can cause acute multisystem organ failure and a clinical picture that resembles septic shock. TSS became well known in 1980 because of the striking relationship between the disease and tampon use (Nakase, 2000). An aggressive health education campaign about the dangers of prolonged tampon use and a change in the chemical composition of tampons have markedly reduced the incidence of TSS in menstruating women. Cases of TSS have also been reported in men, older women, and children.

Diagnostic Evaluation

Diagnosis is established on the basis of the criteria established by the Centers for Disease Control and Prevention's toxic case definition (Box 25-15). A history of tampon use contributes to the diagnosis. Additional laboratory tests include cultures from blood, the vagina, the cervix, and any discharge. Other laboratory tests are those that facilitate the management of shock.

Therapeutic Management

The management of patients with TSS is the same as management of shock of any cause and may range from supportive care in mild cases to hospitalization and intensive care in severe cases. Appropriate parenteral antibiotics are usually administered after cultures are obtained.

Nursing Care Management

Because the disease is relatively rare, the major efforts of nursing are directed toward prevention. The association between the disease and the use of tampons provides some direction for education. Avoiding the use of tampons offers the most certain preventive measure,

BOX 25-15   CRITERIA FOR DEFINITION OF TOXIC SHOCK SYNDROME

1. Fever of 38.9° C (102° F) or higher
2. Presence of diffuse macular erythroderma
3. Desquamation, particularly of palms and soles, 1 to 2 weeks after onset of illness
4. Hypotension, defined as a systolic blood pressure of 90 mm Hg or less for adults and below the 5th percentile for children younger than 16 years of age; or an orthostatic drop in diastolic blood pressure of 15 mm Hg or more with a change from lying to sitting; or orthostatic syncope; or orthostatic dizziness

5. Involvement of three or more of the following organ systems: GI, muscular, mucous membrane, renal, hepatic, hematologic, or CNS

Toxic shock syndrome is probable when four of the five major criteria are fulfilled. In addition, if blood and cerebrospinal fluid cultures are obtained, they must be negative for any organisms other than *Staphylococcus aureus*. Serologic tests for Rocky Mountain spotted fever, leptospirosis, and measles also must be negative.

Modified from American Academy of Pediatrics, Committee on Infectious Diseases, Pickering L, editor: *Red book: 2006 report of the Committee on Infectious Diseases*, ed 27, Elk Grove Village, Ill, 2006, Author.
CNS, Central nervous system; *GI*, gastrointestinal.

although this approach is probably unacceptable to most adolescent girls, who prefer the freedom, comfort, and inconspicuousness that tampons afford.

Adolescent girls who use tampons can be taught general hygiene measures, such as good hand washing and careful insertion to avoid vaginal abrasion. It is wise to modify their use, alternating with sanitary napkins—perhaps using the napkins during the night, when at home during the day, and when flow is slight. Young girls are advised not to use super-absorbent tampons and not to leave any tampon in the body for more than 4 to 6 hours.

▌ KEY POINTS

- CHD is the most common form of cardiac disease in children.
- Major categories to investigate in the cardiac history are poor weight gain, poor feeding habits, and fatigue during feeding; frequent respiratory tract infections and difficulties; and evidence of exercise intolerance.
- The most common tests used in assessing cardiac function are radiography, ECG, echocardiography, and cardiac catheterization.
- Cardiac catheterization procedures can be divided into three groups: (1) diagnostic procedures, including angiography, that measure pressures and saturations to establish cardiac diagnosis; (2) interventional procedures, in which catheters or balloon devices are used to correct cardiac defects; and (3) electrophysiology studies, in which catheters with electrodes are used to evaluate dysrhythmias.
- Diagnostic cardiac catheterization provides important information about oxygen saturation of blood within the chambers and great vessels, pressure changes, changes in cardiac output or stroke volume, and anatomic abnormalities.
- Several prenatal factors may predispose children to CHD; these include maternal rubella during pregnancy, maternal alcoholism, maternal age older than 40 years, and maternal type 1 diabetes.
- Congenital heart defects can be divided into four main groups, as determined by hemodynamic patterns: (1) defects that result in increased pulmonary blood flow, (2) obstructive defects, (3) defects that result in decreased pulmonary blood flow, and (4) mixed defects.
- Clinical consequences of congenital heart defects include HF and hypoxemia. A child can have both hypoxemia and HF, although usually they occur independently.
- Clinical manifestations of HF are impaired myocardial function (tachycardia, cardiomegaly), pulmonary congestion (dyspnea, tachypnea, orthopnea, cyanosis), and systemic congestion (hepatosplenomegaly, edema, distended veins).
- Nursing measures in the care of a child with HF are to assist in improving cardiac function, decrease cardiac demands, reduce respiratory distress, maintain nutritional status, promote fluid loss, and provide family support.

- Clinical manifestations of hypoxemia are cyanosis, polycythemia, clubbing, and delayed growth and development. The child is at increased risk for hypercyanotic spells, CVAs, brain abscess, and BE.
- Caring for the child with CHD and the family requires helping them to adjust to the disorder and to cope with the effects of the defect and fostering growth-promoting family relationships.
- Preoperative care of the child with a congenital heart defect involves introducing the child and family to the hospital and preparing them for preoperative and postoperative procedures.
- Providing postoperative care includes observing vital signs and arterial and venous pressures, maintaining respiratory status, allowing maximum rest, providing comfort, monitoring fluids, planning for progressive activities, giving emotional support, observing for complications of surgery, and planning for discharge and home care.
- Acquired cardiovascular disorders include BE, RF, hyperlipidemia (hypercholesterolemia), KD, and cardiac dysrhythmias.
- Prevention of BE in certain children with CHD involves administration of prophylactic antibiotics when specific procedures are performed.
- Acute RF is a systemic inflammatory disease that can damage the cardiac valves and is associated with previous GABHS infection. Its incidence has increased in some areas of the United States.
- Cholesterol screening in children is controversial; currently, children with known risk factors for hyperlipidemia are screened and treated as needed. The influence of childhood cholesterol levels on later development of coronary artery disease is under investigation.
- Common dysrhythmias in children include slow rhythms (bradycardias, heart block) and fast rhythms (sinus tachycardia, SVT).
- Heart transplantation has been extended to infants and children with cardiomyopathy and complex congenital heart defects involving ventricular dysfunction, such as hypoplastic left heart syndrome.
- Education of the child with hypertension and the family focuses on drug therapy, diet control, and appropriate exercise.

KEY POINTS—cont'd

- KD is an extensive inflammation of small vessels and capillaries that may progress to involve the coronary arteries, causing aneurysm formation. The administration of gamma globulin is an important aspect of treatment.
- Emergency treatment for shock includes ensuring ventilation; administering vasopressors, fluids, blood, and antibiotics as needed; and providing supportive measures such as correct positioning, warmth, and psychologic reassurance to the child and family.
- Persons at risk for anaphylaxis may be identified by a history of previous allergic reaction, history of atopy, history of severe reactions in family, and positive skin test to the allergen.
- Nursing management of the patient with TSS focuses on prevention primarily through education concerning safe tampon use.

REFERENCES

Almond C, Thiagarajian RR, Piercy GE, and others: Waiting list mortality among children listed for heart transplantation in the United States, *Circulation* 119:717–727, 2009.

American Academy of Pediatrics, Committee on Infectious Diseases, Pickering L, editor: *2009 Red book: report of the Committee on Infectious Diseases*, ed 28, Elk Grove Village, Ill, 2009, Author.

Arnal LE, Stein F: Pediatric septic shock: why has mortality decreased? The utility of goal-directed therapy, *Semin Pediatr Infect Dis* 14(2):165–172, 2003.

Arnold R, Ley-Zaporozhan J, Ley S, and others: Outcome after mechanical aortic valve replacement in children and young adults, *Ann Thorac Surg* 85(2):604–610, 2008.

Barst RJ: Recent advances in the treatment of pediatric pulmonary artery hypertension, *Pediatr Clin North Am* 46(2):333–345, 1999.

Barst RJ, Ivy D, Dingemanse J, and others: Pharmacokinetics, safety, and efficacy of bosentan in pediatric patients with pulmonary artery hypertension, *Clin Pharmacol Ther* 73:372–382, 2003.

Beekman RH: Coarctation of the aorta. In Allen HD, Driscoll DJ, Shaddy RE, and others, editors: *Moss and Adams' heart disease in infants, children and adolescents*, ed 6, Philadelphia, 2001, Lippincott Williams & Wilkins.

Bellinger DC, Wypij D, duPlessis AJ, and others: Neurodevelopmental status at eight years in children with dextro-transposition of the great arteries: the Boston Circulatory Arrest Trial, *J Thorac Cardiovasc Surg* 126:1385–1396, 2003.

Blume ED: Current status of heart transplantation in children: update 2003, *Pediatr Clin North Am* 50:1375–1391, 2003.

Blume ED, Naftel DC, Bastardi HJ, and others: Outcomes of children bridged to heart transplantation with ventricular assist devices: a multi-institutional study, *Circulation* 113:2313–2319, 2006.

Boucek MM, Aurora P, Edwards LB, and others: The Registry of the International Society for Heart and Lung Transplantation: tenth official pediatric heart transplantation report—2007, *J Heart Lung Transplant* 26(8):796–807, 2007.

Cecchin F, Frangini PA, Brown DW, and others: Cardiac resynchronization therapy (and multisite pacing) in pediatrics and congenital heart disease: five years experience in a single institution, *J Cardiovasc Electrophysiol* 20 (1):58–65, 2009.

Daniels SR, Greer FR, Committee on Nutrition: Lipid screening and cardiovascular health in childhood, *Pediatrics* 122:198–208, 2008.

Dodds KM, Merle C: Discharging neonates with congenital heart disease after cardiac surgery: a practical approach, *Clin Perinatol* 32:1031–1042, 2005.

Dubin AM, Janousek J, Rhee E, and others: Resynchronization therapy in pediatric and congenital heart disease patients, *J Am Coll Cardiol* 46(12):2277–2283, 2005.

Ferrieri P: Jones Criteria Working Group: proceedings of the Jones Criteria Workshop, *Circulation* 106:2521–2523, 2002.

Freed MD: Aortic stenosis. In Allen HD, Driscoll DJ, Shaddy RE, and others, editors: *Moss and Adams' heart disease in infants, children, and adolescents*, ed 6, Philadelphia, 2001, Lippincott Williams & Wilkins.

Gerber MA, Baltimore RS, Eaton CB, and others: Prevention of rheumatic fever and diagnosis and treatment of acute streptococcal pharyngitis: a scientific statement from the American Heart Association, *Circulation* 119:1541–1551, 2009.

Goldmuntz E, Clark BJ, Mitchell LE, and others: Frequency of 22q11 deletion in patients with conotruncal defects, *J Am Coll Cardiol* 32:492–498, 1998.

Guidelines for the diagnosis of rheumatic fever, Jones criteria, 1992 update, Special Writing Group of the Committee on Rheumatic Fever, Endocarditis, and Kawasaki Disease of the Council on Cardiovascular Disease in the Young of the American Heart Association, *JAMA* 268:2069–2073, 1992.

Hoffman JIE, Kaplan S: The incidence of congenital heart disease, *J Am Coll Cardiol* 39:1890–1900, 2002.

Jacobs JP, Mavroudis C, Jacobs ML, and others: Lessons learned from the data analysis of the second harvest (1998–2001) of the Society of Thoracic Surgeons (STS) Congenital Heart Surgery Database, *Eur J Cardiothorac Surg* 26(1):18–37, 2004.

Lane KB, Machado RD, Pauciulo MW, and others: Heterozygous germline mutations in BMPR2 encoding a TGF-beta receptor, causing familial primary pulmonary hypertension: the International PPH Consortium, *Nat Genet* 26:81–84, 2000.

Latson LA: Critical pulmonic stenosis, *J Intervent Cardiol* 14(3):345–350, 2001.

LeRoy S, Elixson EM, O'Brien P, and others: Recommendations for preparing children and adolescents for invasive cardiac procedures: AHA Scientific Statement, *Circulation* 108:2550–2564, 2003.

Li JS, Sexton DJ, Mick N, and others: Proposed modifications to the Duke criteria for the diagnosis of infective endocarditis, *Clin Infect Dis* 30:633–638, 2000.

Limperopoulos C, Majnemer A, Shevell MI, and others: Predictors of developmental disabilities after open heart surgery in young children with congenital heart defects, *J Pediatr* 141:51–58, 2002.

Maar SP: Emergency care in pediatric septic shock, *Pediatr Emerg Care* 20(9):617–624, 2004.

Majnemer A, Limperopoulos C: Developmental progress of children with congenital heart defects requiring open heart surgery, *Semin Pediatr Neurol* 6:12–19, 1999.

Margossian R: Contemporary management of pediatric heart failure. *Expert Rev Cardiovasc Ther* 6(2):187–197, 2008.

Maron BJ: Hypertrophic cardiomyopathy. In Allen HD, Driscoll DJ, Shaddy RE, and others, editors: *Moss and Adams' heart disease in infants, children, and adolescents*, ed 6, Philadelphia, 2001, Lippincott Williams & Wilkins.

McCrindle BW, Urbina EM, Dennison BA, and others: Drug therapy of high-risk lipid abnormalities in children and adolescents: a scientific statement from the American Heart Association Atherosclerosis, Hypertension, and Obesity in Youth Committee, Council of Cardiovascular Disease in the Young, with the Council on Cardiovascular Nursing, *Circulation* 115:1948–1967, 2007.

Michelakis ED, Wilkins MR, Rabinovitch M: Emerging concepts and translational priorities in pulmonary arterial hypertension, *Circulation* 118:1486–1495, 2008.

Nakase J: Update on emerging infections from the Centers for Disease Control and Prevention, *Ann Emerg Med* 36(3):268–270, 2000.

National High Blood Pressure Education Program Working Group on High Blood Pressure in Children and Adolescents: The fourth report on the diagnosis, evaluation, and treatment of high blood pressure in children and adolescents, *Pediatrics* 114(2):555–576, 2004.

Newburger JW, Takahashi M, Gerber MA, and others: Diagnosis, treatment, and long-term management of Kawasaki disease: a statement for health professionals from the Committee on Rheumatic Fever, Endocarditis and Kawasaki Disease, Council on Cardiovascular Disease in the Young, American Heart Association, *Circulation* 110(17):2747–2771, 2004.

Park MK: *Pediatric cardiology handbook*, ed 5, Philadelphia, 2008, Mosby.

Rome JJ, Kreutzer J: Pediatric interventional catheterization: reasonable expectations and outcomes, *Pediatr Clin North Am* 51:1589–1610, 2004.

Rosenthal D, Chrisant MR, Edens E, and others: International Society for Heart and Lung Transplantation: practice guidelines for management of heart failure in children, *J Heart Lung Transplant* 23(12):1313–1333, 2004.

Schlente EA, Boramanand N, Funk MF: Supraventricular tachycardia in the pediatric primary care setting: age-related presentation, diagnosis, and management, *J Pediatr Health Care* 22 (5):289–299, 2008.

Scientific Registry of Transplant Recipients (SRTR): *OPTN/SRTR 2010 annual data report*. Rockville, Md, 2011, Department of Health and Human Services, Health Resources and Services Administration, Healthcare Systems Bureau, Division of Transplantation.

Shanmugam G, MacArthur K, Pollock J: Mechanical aortic valve replacement: long-term outcomes in children, *J Heart Valve Dis* 14(2):166–171, 2005.

Shillingford AJ, Glanzman MM, Ittenbach RF, and others: Inattention, hyperactivity, and school performance in a population of school-age children with complex congenital heart disease, *Pediatrics* 121:e759–e767, 2008.

Smith P: Primary care in children with congenital hearth disease, *J Pediatr Nurs* 16(5):308–319, 2001.

Spirito P, Autore C, Rapezzi C, and others: Syncope and risk of sudden death in hypertrophic cardiomyopathy, *Circulation* 1109:1703–1710, 2009.

Steltzer M, Rudd N, Pick B: Nutrition care for newborns with congenital heart disease, *Clin Perinatol* 32(4):1017–1030, 2005.

Tweddell JS, Hoffman GM, Mussatto KA, and others: Improved survival of patients undergoing palliation of hypoplastic left heart syndrome: lessons learned from 115 consecutive patients, *Circulation* 106(12 suppl 1):182–189, 2002.

Urbina E, Alpert B, Flynn J, and others: Ambulatory blood pressure monitoring in children and adolescents: recommendations for standard assessment: a scientific statement from the American Heart Association Atherosclerosis, Hypertension, and Obesity in Youth Committee of the Council on Cardiovascular Disease in the Young and the Council for High Blood Pressure Research, *Hypertension* 52:433, 2008.

Uzark K: Therapeutic cardiac catheterization for congenital heart disease: a new era in pediatric care, *J Pediatr Nurs* 16(5):300–307, 2001.

Wilder M, Palinkas L, Kao A, and others: Delayed diagnosis by physicians contributes to the development of coronary artery aneurysms in children with Kawasaki syndrome, *Pediatr Infect Dis* 26(3):256–260, 2007.

Wilson W, Taubert KA, Gewitz M, and others: Prevention of infective endocarditis: guidelines from the American Heart Association, *Circulation* 116(15):1736–1754, 2007.

The Child with Hematologic or Immunologic Dysfunction

Rosalind Bryant

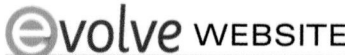 **WEBSITE**

http://evolve.elsevier.com/wong/essentials

Animations—Hemophilia A; Platelets and Blood Clotting; Sickle Cell Anemia

Case Studies—Acute Lymphoblastic Leukemia; Idiopathic Thrombocytopenic Purpura; Iron Deficiency Anemia; Sickle Cell Anemia

Key Point Summaries

NCLEX-Style Review Questions

Nursing Care Plans—The Child with Anemia; The Child with Cancer; The Child with Hemophilia; The Child with Sickle Cell Disease

CHAPTER OUTLINE

Hematologic and Immunologic Dysfunction, 869

Red Blood Cell Disorders, 869

    Anemia, 869

        Classification, 869

        Consequences of Anemia, 869

    Iron-Deficiency Anemia, 872

    Sickle Cell Anemia, 873

        Nursing Care Plan: The Child with Sickle Cell Anemia, 879

    β-Thalassemia (Cooley Anemia), 881

    Aplastic Anemia, 882

Defects in Hemostasis, 883

    Hemophilia, 883

    Immune Thrombocytopenia (Idiopathic Thrombocytopenic Purpura), 886

Disseminated Intravascular Coagulation, 887

Epistaxis (Nosebleeding), 888

Neoplastic Disorders, 888

    Leukemias, 888

    Lymphomas, 892

        Hodgkin Lymphoma, 893

        Non-Hodgkin Lymphoma, 894

Immunologic Deficiency Disorders, 894

    Human Immunodeficiency Virus Infection and Acquired Immunodeficiency Syndrome, 894

    Severe Combined Immunodeficiency Disease, 897

    Wiskott-Aldrich Syndrome, 897

Technologic Management of Hematologic and Immunologic Disorders, 897

    Blood Transfusion Therapy, 897

    Hematopoietic Stem Cell Transplantation, 899

    Apheresis, 899

LEARNING OBJECTIVES

On completion of this chapter the reader will be able to:

- Distinguish between the various categories of anemia.
- Describe the prevention of and care of the child with iron-deficiency anemia.
- Compare sickle cell anemia and β-thalassemia major in relation to pathophysiology and nursing care.
- Describe the mechanisms of inheritance and nursing care of the child with hemophilia.
- Relate the pathophysiology and clinical manifestations of leukemia.

- Demonstrate an understanding of the rationale of therapies for neoplastic disease.
- Outline a care plan for the child with neoplastic disease and the family.
- Contrast the pathophysiology and management of the immunodeficiency disorders.
- List nursing precautions and responsibilities during blood transfusion.
- Describe the types of hematopoietic stem cell transplants.

HEMATOLOGIC AND IMMUNOLOGIC DYSFUNCTION

Several tests can be performed to assess hematologic function, including additional procedures to identify the cause of the dysfunction. The following discussion is limited to a description of the most common and one of the most valuable tests, the **complete blood cell count (CBC)**. Other procedures, such as those related to iron, coagulation, and immune status, are discussed throughout the chapter as appropriate. The nurse should be familiar with the significance of the findings from the CBC (Table 26-1) and be aware of normal values for age, which are listed in Appendix B.

As with any disorder, the history and physical examination are essential to identify hematologic dysfunction, and the nurse is often the first person to suspect a problem based on information from these sources. Comments by the parent regarding the child's lack of energy, food diary of poor sources of iron, frequent infections, and bleeding that is difficult to control offer clues to the more common disorders affecting the blood. A careful physical appraisal, especially of the skin, can reveal findings (e.g., pallor, petechiae, bruising) that may indicate minor or serious hematologic conditions. Nurses need to be aware of the clinical manifestations of blood diseases to assist in recognizing symptoms and establishing a diagnosis.

> **NURSING TIP** A common term used in describing an abnormal CBC is **shift to the left**, which refers to the presence of immature neutrophils in the peripheral blood from hyperfunction of the bone marrow, as seen during a bacterial infection.

RED BLOOD CELL DISORDERS

ANEMIA

The term **anemia** describes a condition in which the number of red blood cells (RBCs) or the hemoglobin (Hgb or Hb) concentration is reduced below normal values for age. This diminishes the oxygen-carrying capacity of the blood, causing a reduction in the oxygen available to the tissues. Anemia is the most common hematologic disorder of infancy and childhood and is not a disease itself but an indication or manifestation of an underlying pathologic process.

Classification

Anemias are classified in relation to (1) etiology or physiology, manifested by erythrocyte or Hgb depletion, and (2) morphology, the characteristic changes in RBC size, shape, or color (Box 26-1). Although the morphologic classification is more useful in terms of laboratory evaluation of anemia, the etiologic approach provides direction for planning nursing care. For example, anemia with reduced Hgb concentration may be caused by a dietary depletion of iron, and the principal intervention is replenishing iron stores. The classification of anemias is found in Fig. 26-1.

Consequences of Anemia

The basic physiologic defect caused by anemia is a decrease in the oxygen-carrying capacity of blood and consequently a reduction in the amount of oxygen available to the cells. When the anemia has developed slowly, the child usually adapts to the declining Hgb level.

The effects of anemia on the circulatory system can be profound. Because the viscosity of blood depends almost entirely on the concentration of RBCs, the resulting hemodilution of severe anemia decreases

peripheral resistance, causing greater quantities of blood to return to the heart. The increased circulation and turbulence within the heart may produce a murmur. Because the cardiac workload is greatly increased, especially during exercise, infection, or emotional stress, cardiac failure may ensue.

Children seem to have a remarkable ability to function well despite low levels of Hgb. **Cyanosis** (the result of the quantity of deoxygenated Hgb in arterial blood) is typically not evident. Growth retardation, resulting from decreased cellular metabolism and coexisting anorexia, is a common finding in chronic severe anemia and is frequently accompanied by delayed sexual maturation in the older child.

Diagnostic Evaluation

In general, anemia may be suspected based on findings on the history and physical examination, such as a lack of energy, easy fatigability, and pallor, but unless the anemia is severe, the first clue to the disorder may be alterations in the CBC, such as decreased RBCs, and decreased Hgb and hematocrit (Hct) levels (see Fig. 26-1). Although anemia is sometimes defined as an Hgb level below 10 or 11 g/dl, this arbitrary cutoff is inappropriate for all children because Hgb levels normally vary with age (see Table 26-1 and Appendix B).

Other tests specific to a particular type of anemia are used to determine the underlying cause of anemia. These are discussed in relation to the particular disorder.

Therapeutic Management

The objective of medical management is to reverse the anemia by treating the underlying cause and to make up for any deficiency of blood, blood component, or substance the blood needs for normal functioning. For example, blood or blood cells are replaced after hemorrhage; in nutritional anemias, the specific deficiency is replaced.

In patients with severe anemia, supportive medical care may include oxygen therapy, bed rest, and replacement of intravascular volume with intravenous (IV) fluids. The prognosis for anemia depends on the correction of the cause.

Nursing Care Management

The assessment of anemia includes the basic techniques that are applicable to any condition. The age of the infant or child provides some clues regarding the possible etiology of the anemia. For example, iron-deficiency anemia occurs more frequently in toddlers between 12 and 36 months of age and during the growth spurt of adolescence.

Racial or ethnic background is significant. For example, the anemias related to abnormal Hgb levels are found in Southeast Asians and persons of African or Mediterranean ancestry. These same groups may be genetically deficient in the enzyme lactase after the period of infancy. Affected individuals are unable to tolerate lactose in the diet, with consequent intestinal irritation and chronic blood loss.

Special emphasis is placed on a careful history to elicit any information that might help identify the cause of the anemia. For example, a statement such as "My child drinks lots of milk" is a frequent finding in toddlers with iron-deficiency anemia. An episode of diarrhea may have precipitated temporary lactose intolerance in a young child.

Stool examination for occult (microscopic) blood (Hemoccult test) can identify chronic intestinal bleeding that results from a primary or secondary lactase deficiency. It is also important to understand the significance of various blood tests (see Table 26-1).

Prepare the Child and Family for Laboratory Tests

Usually, several blood tests are ordered, but because they are generally done sequentially rather than at one time, the child is subjected to

TABLE 26-1	TESTS PERFORMED AS PART OF A COMPLETE BLOOD COUNT
TEST (AVERAGE VALUE)*	**DESCRIPTION, COMMENTS**
RBC count (4.5–5.5 million/mm³)	Number of RBCs/mm³ of blood
	Indirectly estimates Hgb content of blood
	Reflects function of bone marrow
Hgb determination (11.5–15.5 g/dl)	Amount of Hgb (g)/dl of whole blood
	Total blood Hgb primarily depends on number of circulating RBCs but also on amount of Hgb in each cell
Hct (35%–45%)	Percent volume of packed RBCs in whole blood
	Indirectly measures Hgb content
	Is approximately three times Hgb content
RBC indices	
MCV (77–95 fl)	Average or mean volume (size) of a single RBC
	MCV values are expressed as femtoliters (fl) or cubic microns (mm³)
MCH (25–33 pg/cell)	Average or mean quantity (weight) of Hgb in a single RBC
	MCH values are expressed as picograms (pg) or micromicrograms (mmcg)
	Whereas MCV and MCH depend on accurate counts of RBCs, MCHC does not; therefore, MCHC is often more reliable
	All indices depend on average cell measurements and do not show individual RBC variations (anisocytosis)
MCHC (31%–37% Hgb [g]/dl RBC)	Average concentration of Hgb in a single RBC
	MCHC values are expressed as percent Hgb (g)/cell or Hgb (g)/dl RBC
RBC volume distribution width (13.4% ± 1.2%)	Average size of RBCs
	Differentiates some types of anemia
Reticulocyte count (0.5%–1.5% erythrocytes)	Percent reticulocytes in RBCs
	Index of production of mature RBCs by bone marrow
	Decreased count indicates depressed bone marrow function
	Increased count indicates erythrogenesis in response to some stimulus
	When reticulocyte count is extremely high, other forms of immature RBCs (normoblasts, even erythroblasts) may be present
	Indirectly estimates hypochromic anemia
	Usually elevated in patients with chronic hemolytic anemia
WBC count (4.5–13.5 × 10³ cells/mm³)	Number of WBCs/mm³ of blood
	Total number of WBCs less important than differential count
Differential WBC count	Inspection and quantification of WBC types present in peripheral blood
	Values are expressed as percentages; to obtain absolute number of any type of WBC, multiply its respective percentage by total number of WBCs
Neutrophils (polys) (54%–62%) (3–5.8 × 10³ cells/mm³)	Primary defense in bacterial infection; capable of phagocytizing and killing bacteria
Bands (3%–5%) (0.15–0.4 × 10³ cells/mm³)	Immature neutrophil
	Increased numbers in bacterial infection
	Also capable of phagocytosis and killing
Eosinophils (1%–3%) (0.05–0.25 × 10³ cells/mm³)	Named for their staining characteristics with eosin dye
	Increased in allergic disorders, parasitic diseases, certain neoplasms, and other diseases
Basophils (0.075%) (0.015–0.030 × 10³ cells/mm³)	Named for their characteristic basophilic stippling
	Contain histamine, heparin, and serotonin; believed to cause increased blood flow to injured tissues while preventing excessive clotting
Lymphocytes (25%–33%) (1.5–3.0 × 10³ cells/mm³)	Involved in development of antibody and delayed hypersensitivity
Monocytes (3%–7%)	Large phagocytic cells that are involved in early stage of inflammatory reaction
ANC (>1000/mm³)	Percent neutrophils/bands times WBC count
	Indicates body's capability to handle bacterial infections
Platelet count (150–400 × 10³/mm³)	Number of platelets/mm³ of blood
	Cellular fragments that are necessary for clotting to occur
Stained peripheral blood smear	Visual estimation of amount of Hgb in RBCs and overall size, shape, and structure of RBCs
	Various staining properties of RBC structures may be evidence of immature forms of erythrocytes
	Shows variation in size and shape of RBCs: microcytic, macrocytic, poikilocytic (variable shapes)

ANC, Absolute neutrophil count; *Hct,* hematocrit; *Hgb,* hemoglobin; *MCH,* mean corpuscular hemoglobin; *MCHC,* mean corpuscular hemoglobin concentration; *MCV,* mean corpuscular volume; *RBC,* red blood cell; *WBC,* white blood cell.
*See Appendix B for normal values according to age.

multiple finger or heel punctures or venipunctures. Laboratory technicians frequently are not aware of the trauma that repeated punctures represent to a child. However, these invasive procedures need not be painful (see Blood Specimens, Chapter 22). For example, the topical application of EMLA (an eutectic mix of lidocaine and prilocaine) or 4% lidocaine (Ela-Max or LMX) before needle punctures can eliminate pain (see Pain Management, Chapter 7). Therefore, the nurse is responsible for preparing the child and family for the tests by:

- Explaining the significance of each test, particularly why the tests are not all done at one time
- Encouraging parents or another supportive person to be with the child during the procedure

- Allowing the child to play with the equipment on a doll or participate in the actual procedure (e.g., by cleansing the finger with an alcohol swab)

Older children may appreciate the opportunity to observe the blood cells under a microscope or in photographs. This experience is especially important if a serious blood disorder, such as leukemia, is suspected because it serves as a foundation for explaining the pathophysiology of the disorder.

Bone marrow aspiration is not a routine hematologic test but is essential for definitive diagnosis of the leukemias, lymphomas, and certain anemias.

BOX 26-1 RED BLOOD CELL MORPHOLOGY

Size (Cell Size)
Variation in RBC sizes (anisocytosis)
- Normocytes (normal cell size)
- Microcytes (smaller than normal cell size)
- Macrocytes (larger than normal cell size)

Shape (Cell Shape)
Variation in RBC shapes (poikilocytosis)
- Spherocytes (globular cells)
- Drepanocytes (sickle-shaped cells)
- Numerous other irregularly shaped cells

Color (Cell Staining Characteristics)
Variation in hemoglobin concentration in the RBC
- Normochromic (sufficient or normal amount of hemoglobin per RBC)
- Hypochromic (reduced amount of hemoglobin per RBC)
- Hyperchromic (increased amount of hemoglobin per RBC)

RBC, Red blood cell.

NURSING TIP The following are suggested explanations for teaching children about blood components:
Red blood cells—Carry the oxygen you breathe from your lungs to all parts of your body
White blood cells—Help keep germs from causing infection
Platelets—Small parts of cells that help make bleeding stop by forming a clot (scab) over the hurt area
Plasma—The liquid portion of blood, which has clotting factors that help make bleeding stop

---

Decrease Tissue Oxygen Needs

Because the basic pathologic process in anemia is a decrease in oxygen-carrying capacity, an important nursing responsibility is to assess the child's energy level and minimize excess demands. The child's level of tolerance for activities of daily living and play is assessed, and adjustments are made to allow as much self-care as possible without undue exertion. During periods of rest, the nurse takes vital signs and observes behavior to establish a baseline of nonexertion energy expenditure. During periods of activity, the nurse repeats these measurements and observations to compare them with resting values.

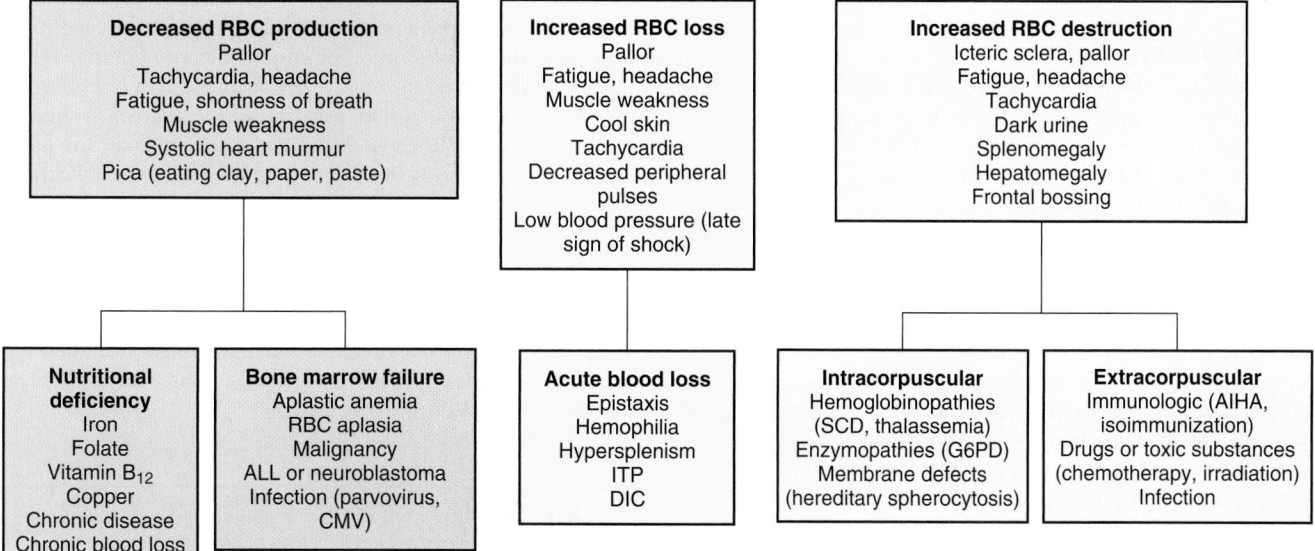

FIG 26-1 Classifications of anemias. *AIHA,* Autoimmune hemolytic anemia; *ALL,* acute lymphoid leukemia; *CMV,* cytomegalovirus; *DIC,* disseminated intravascular coagulation; *G6PD,* glucose-6-phosphate dehydrogenase; *ITP,* idiopathic thrombocytopenic purpura; *RBC,* red blood cell; *SCD,* sickle cell disease.

> **NURSING TIP** Signs of exertion include tachycardia, palpitations, tachypnea, dyspnea, shortness of breath, hyperpnea, breathlessness, dizziness, lightheadedness, diaphoresis, and change in skin color. The child looks fatigued (sagging, limp posture; slow, strained movements; inability to tolerate additional activity; difficulty sucking in infants).

Prevent Complications

Children who are so severely anemic that they are hospitalized may require oxygen to prevent or reduce tissue hypoxia. Because these children are susceptible to infection, every effort is expended to prevent exposure to infectious agents. All of the usual precautions are taken to prevent infection, such as practicing thorough hand washing, selecting an appropriate room in a noninfectious area, restricting visitors or hospital personnel with active infection, and maintaining adequate nutrition. The nurse also observes for signs of infection, particularly temperature elevation and leukocytosis.

IRON-DEFICIENCY ANEMIA

Anemia caused by an inadequate supply of dietary iron is the most prevalent nutritional disorder in the United States and the most preventable mineral disturbance. The prevalence of iron-deficiency anemia has decreased during infancy in the United States, probably in part because of families' participation in the Women, Infants, and Children (WIC) program, which provides iron-fortified formula for the first year of life and routine screening of Hgb levels during early childhood (Baker, Greer, and Committee on Nutrition American Academy of Pediatrics [AAP], 2010; Cusick, Mei, Freedman, and others, 2008). Preterm infants are especially at risk because of their reduced fetal iron supply. Children 12 to 36 months of age are at risk for anemia as a result of primarily cow milk intake and not eating an adequate amount of iron-containing food (Andrews, Ullrich, and Fleming, 2009; Baker, Greer, and Committee on Nutrition AAP, 2010; Richardson, 2007). Adolescents are also at risk because of their rapid growth rate combined with poor eating habits, menses, obesity, or strenuous activities.

Pathophysiology

Iron-deficiency anemia can be caused by any number of factors that decrease the supply of iron, impair its absorption, increase the body's need for iron, or affect the synthesis of Hgb. Although the clinical manifestations and diagnostic evaluation are similar regardless of the cause, the therapeutic and nursing care management depend on the specific reason for the iron deficiency. The following discussion is limited to iron-deficiency anemia resulting from inadequate iron in the diet.

During the last trimester of pregnancy, iron is transferred from the mother to the fetus. Most of the iron is stored in the circulating erythrocytes of the fetus, with the remainder stored in the fetal liver, spleen, and bone marrow. These iron stores are usually adequate for the first 5 to 6 months in a full-term infant but for only 2 to 3 months in preterm infants and multiple births. If dietary iron is not supplied to meet the infant's growth demands after the fetal iron stores are depleted, iron-deficiency anemia results. Physiologic anemia should not be confused with iron-deficiency anemia resulting from nutritional causes.

Although most toddlers with iron-deficiency anemia are underweight, many infants are overweight because of excessive milk ingestion (known as **milk babies**). These children become anemic for two reasons: milk, a poor source of iron, is given almost to the exclusion of solid foods, and 50% of iron-deficient infants fed cow's milk have an increased fecal loss of blood.

Therapeutic Management

After the diagnosis of iron-deficiency anemia is made, therapeutic management focuses on increasing the amount of supplemental iron the child receives. This is usually done through dietary counseling and the administration of oral iron supplements.

In formula-fed infants, the most convenient and best sources of supplemental iron are iron-fortified commercial formula and iron-fortified infant cereal. Iron-fortified formula provides a relatively constant and predictable amount of iron and is not associated with an increased incidence of gastrointestinal (GI) symptoms, such as colic, diarrhea, or constipation. Infants younger than 12 months of age should *not* be given fresh cow's milk because it may increase the risk of GI blood loss occurring from exposure to a heat-labile protein in cow's milk or cow's milk–induced GI mucosal damage resulting from a lack of cytochrome iron (heme protein) (Glader, 2007; Richardson, 2007). If GI bleeding is suspected, the child's stool should be guaiac tested on at least four or five occasions to identify any intermittent blood loss.

Dietary addition of iron-rich foods is usually inadequate as the sole treatment of iron-deficiency anemia because the iron is poorly absorbed and thus provides insufficient supplemental quantities of iron. If dietary sources of iron cannot replace body stores, oral iron supplements are prescribed for approximately 3 months. Ferrous iron, more readily absorbed than ferric iron, results in higher Hgb levels. Ascorbic acid (vitamin C) appears to facilitate absorption of iron and may be given as vitamin C–enriched foods and juices with the iron preparation.

If the Hgb level fails to rise after 1 month of oral therapy, it is important to assess for persistent bleeding, iron malabsorption, noncompliance, improper iron administration, or other causes of the anemia. Parenteral (IV or intramuscular [IM]) iron administration is safe and effective but painful, expensive, and occasionally associated with regional lymphadenopathy, transient arthralgias or serious allergic reaction (Andrews, Ullrich, and Fleming, 2009; Glader, 2007; McKenzie, 2004). Therefore, parenteral iron is reserved for children who have iron malabsorption or chronic hemoglobinuria. Transfusions are indicated for the most severe anemia and in cases of serious infection, cardiac dysfunction, or surgical emergency when anesthesia is required. Packed RBCs (2–3 ml/kg), not whole blood, are used to minimize the chance of circulatory overload. Supplemental oxygen is administered when tissue hypoxia is severe.

Prognosis

The prognosis for a child with this condition is very good. However, some evidence indicates that if the iron-deficiency anemia is severe and longstanding, cognitive, behavioral, and motor impairment may result (Andrews, Ullrich, and Fleming, 2009; Lokeshwar, Mehta, Mehta, and others, 2011; McCann and Ames, 2007).

> **QUALITY PATIENT OUTCOMES:** Iron Deficiency Anemia
> - Early recognition of signs and symptoms of iron deficiency anemia
> - Appropriate quantity of milk, use of iron-fortified infant formula, and introduction of solid foods
> - Adherence to oral iron supplement and appropriate administration
> - Hemoglobin increase within 1 month and anemia resolved within 6 months

Case Study—Iron Deficiency Anemia

Nursing Care Management

An essential nursing responsibility is instructing parents in the administration of iron. Oral iron should be given as prescribed in two divided doses between meals, when the presence of free hydrochloric acid is greatest, because more iron is absorbed in the acidic environment of the upper GI tract. A citrus fruit or juice taken with the medication aids in absorption.

 DRUG ALERT

Cow's milk contains substances that bind the iron and interfere with absorption. Iron supplements should not be administered with milk or milk products (Carley, 2003).

An adequate dosage of oral iron turns the stools a tarry green color. The nurse advises parents of this normally expected change and inquires about its occurrence on follow-up visits. Absence of the greenish black stool may be a clue to poor administration of iron, either in schedule or in dosage. Vomiting or diarrhea can occur with iron therapy. If the parents report these symptoms, the iron can be given with meals and the dosage reduced and then gradually increased until tolerated.

 DRUG ALERT

Liquid preparations of iron may temporarily stain the teeth. If possible, the medication should be taken through a straw or given through a syringe or medicine dropper placed toward the back of the mouth. Brushing the teeth after administration of the drug lessens the discoloration. Because iron ingestion in excessive quantities is toxic or even fatal, parents should be instructed to keep no more than a month's supply in the home and store it safely away from the reach of children.

If parenteral iron preparations are prescribed, iron dextran must be injected deeply into a large muscle mass using the Z-track method. The injection site is *not* massaged after injection to minimize skin staining and irritation. Because no more than 1 ml should be given in one site, the IV route should be considered to avoid multiple injections. Careful observation is required because of the risk of adverse reactions, such as anaphylaxis, with IV administration. A test dose is recommended before routine use. Recently, a new IV iron preparation (ferumoxytol) was approved in the United States that shows promise in complete replacement of iron with little toxicity (Auerbach, 2011).

Diet

A primary nursing objective is to prevent nutritional anemia through family education. Because breast milk is a low iron source, the nurse must reinforce the importance of administering iron supplementation to exclusively breastfed infants by 4 months of age (Baker, Greer, and Committee on Nutrition AAP, 2010; Lokeshwar, Mehta, Mehta, and others, 2011). The AAP recommends that preterm, marginally low and low–birth-weight infants, or infants with inadequate iron stores at birth receive iron supplements at approximately 2 months of age (Berglund, Westrup, and Domellof, 2010).

In formula-fed infants, the nurse discusses with parents the importance of using iron-fortified formula and of introducing solid foods at the appropriate age during the first year of life. Traditionally, cereals are one of the first semisolid foods to be introduced into the infant's diet at approximately 6 months of age (Baker, Greer, and Committee on Nutrition AAP, 2010; Glader, 2007; Lokeshwar, Mehta, Mehta, and others, 2011). The best solid-food source of iron is commercial iron-fortified cereals. It may be difficult at first to teach the infant to accept foods other than milk. The same principles are applied as those for introducing new foods (see Nutrition, Chapter 10), especially feeding the solid food before the milk. Predominantly milk-fed infants rebel against solid foods, and parents are cautioned about this and the need to be firm in not relinquishing control to the child. It may require intense problem solving on the part of both the family and the nurse to overcome the child's resistance.

A difficulty encountered in discouraging the parents from feeding milk to the exclusion of other foods is dispelling the popular myth that milk is a "perfect food." Many parents believe that milk is best for infants and equate weight gain with a "healthy child" and "good mothering." The nurse can also stress that overweight is not synonymous with good health.

Diet education of teenagers is especially difficult, especially because teenage girls are particularly prone to following weight-reduction diets. Emphasizing the effect of anemia on appearance (pallor) and energy level (difficulty maintaining popular activities) may be useful. (See Mineral Imbalances, Chapter 11.)

SICKLE CELL ANEMIA

Sickle cell anemia (SCA) is one of a group of diseases collectively termed hemoglobinopathies in which normal adult Hgb (Hgb A [HbA]) is partly or completely replaced by abnormal sickle Hgb (HbS). Sickle cell disease (SCD) includes all those hereditary disorders whose clinical, hematologic, and pathologic features are related to the presence of HbS. Even though the term *SCD* is sometimes used to refer to SCA, this use is incorrect. Other correct terms for SCA are SS and homozygous SCD.

The following are the most common forms of SCD in the United States:

SCA, the homozygous form of the disease (HbgSS or SS)

Sickle cell–C disease, a heterozygous variant of SCD, including both HbS and HbC (SC)

Sickle cell–hemoglobin E disease, a variant of SCD in which glutamic acid has been substituted for lysine in the number 26 position of the β-chain (SE)

Sickle thalassemia disease, a combination of sickle cell trait and β-thalassemia trait (Sβthal). β^+ refers to the ability to still produce some normal HbA. β^0 indicates that there is no ability to produce HbA.

Of the SCDs, SCA is the most common form in African Americans followed by sickle cell–C disease and sickle thalassemia. Sickle syndromes exist when the HbS is paired with other mutant globins.

Sickle cell disease is one of the most common genetic diseases worldwide. SCD affects approximately 90,000 Americans, primarily African American, followed by Hispanics, with a lower incidence in the other ethnic groups (Driscoll, 2007). The incidence of the disease varies in different geographic locations. Among African Americans, the incidence of sickle cell trait is about 9%. In West Africa, the incidence is reported to be as high as 40% among native Africans. The high incidence of sickle cell trait in West Africans is believed by some to be the result of selective protection afforded trait carriers against one type of malaria.

The gene that determines the production of HbS is situated on an autosome and, when present, is always detectable and therefore dominant. Heterozygous persons who have both normal HbA and abnormal HbS are said to have sickle cell trait. Persons who are homozygous have predominantly HbS and have SCA. The inheritance pattern is

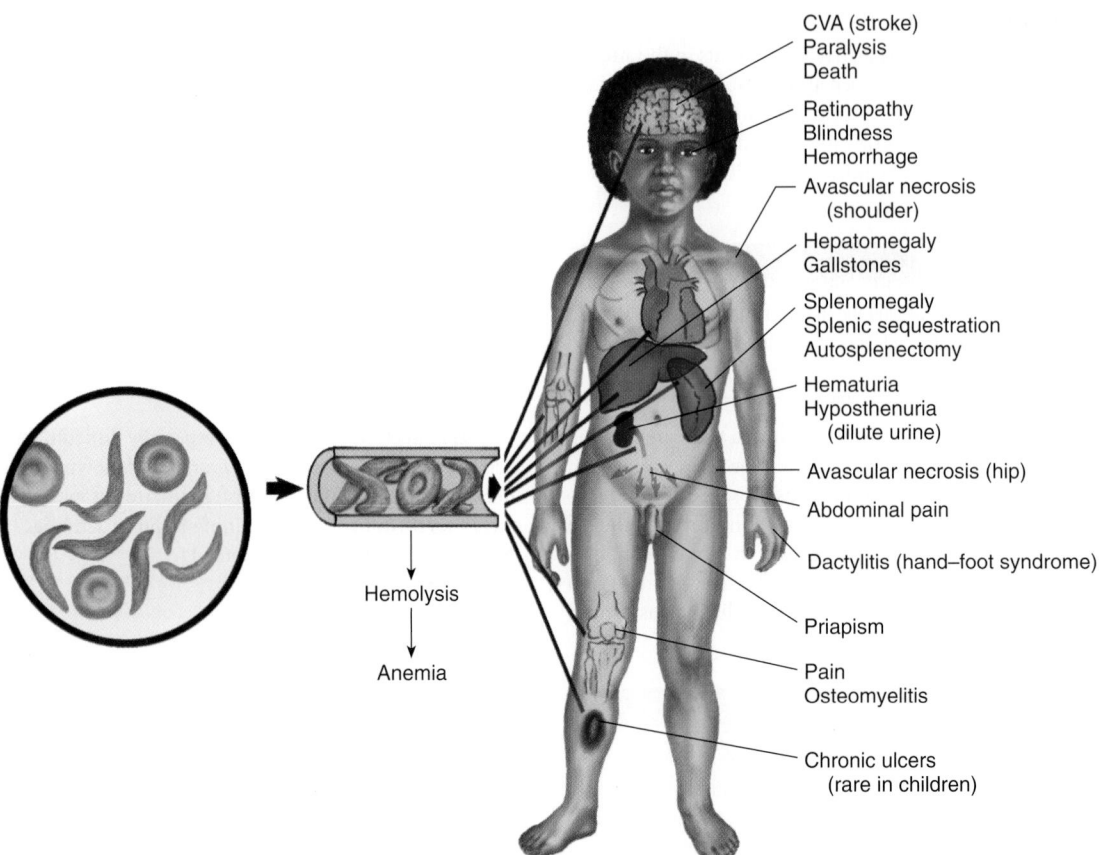

CVA (stroke)
Paralysis
Death

Retinopathy
Blindness
Hemorrhage

Avascular necrosis
(shoulder)

Hepatomegaly
Gallstones

Splenomegaly
Splenic sequestration
Autosplenectomy

Hematuria
Hyposthenuria
(dilute urine)

Avascular necrosis (hip)

Abdominal pain

Dactylitis (hand–foot syndrome)

Priapism

Pain
Osteomyelitis

Chronic ulcers
(rare in children)

Hemolysis

Anemia

FIG 26-2 Clinical features of sickle cell anemia from red blood cell obstruction and destruction. *CVA*, cerebrovascular accident.

essentially that of an autosomal recessive disorder. Therefore, when both parents have sickle cell trait, there is a 25% chance with each pregnancy of producing an offspring with SCA.

Although the defect is inherited, the sickling phenomenon is usually not apparent until later in infancy because of the presence of fetal Hbg (HbF). As long as the child has predominantly HbF, sickling does not occur because there is less HbS. Newborns with SCA are generally asymptomatic because of the protective effect of HbF (60%–80% HbF), but this rapidly decreases during the first year, so these children are at risk for sickle cell–related complications (Driscoll, 2007; Heeney and Dover, 2009).

Pathophysiology

The clinical features of SCA are primarily the result of (1) **obstruction** caused by the sickled RBCs, (2) vascular inflammation, and (3) increased RBC **destruction** (Fig. 26-2). The abnormal adhesion, entanglement, and enmeshing of rigid sickle-shaped cells accompanied by the inflammatory process intermittently blocks the microcirculation causing vasoocclusion (Fig. 26-3). The resultant absence of blood flow to adjacent tissues causes local hypoxia, leading to tissue ischemia and infarction (cellular death). Most of the complications seen in SCA can be traced to this process and its impact on various organs of the body (Box 26-2).

The clinical manifestations of SCA vary greatly in severity and frequency. The most acute symptoms of the disease occur during periods of exacerbation called **crises**. There are several types of episodic crises, including vasoocclusive, acute splenic sequestration, aplastic, hyperhemolytic, cerebrovascular accident, chest syndrome, and

infection. The crises may occur individually or concomitantly with one or more other crises. The **vasoocclusive crisis (VOC)**, preferably called a "painful episode," is characterized by ischemia causing mild to severe pain that may last from minutes to days. **Sequestration crisis** is a pooling of a large amount of blood usually in the spleen and infrequently in the liver that causes a decreased blood volume and ultimately shock. **Aplastic crisis** is diminished RBC production usually caused by viral infection that may result in profound anemia. **Hyperhemolytic crisis** is an accelerated rate of RBC destruction characterized by anemia, jaundice, and reticulocytosis.

Another serious complication is **acute chest syndrome (ACS)**, which is clinically similar to pneumonia. It is the presence of a new pulmonary infiltrate and may be associated with chest pain, fever, cough, tachypnea, wheezing, and hypoxia. A **cerebrovascular accident (CVA, stroke)** is a sudden and severe complication, often with no related illnesses. Sickled cells block the major blood vessels in the brain, resulting in cerebral infarction, which causes variable degrees of neurologic impairment. The current treatment for SCD children who have experienced a stroke is chronic transfusion therapy. Repeat CVAs causing progressively greater brain damage occur in approximately 70% of untreated children who have experienced one stroke (Heeney and Dover, 2009).

Diagnostic Evaluation

Newborn screening for SCA is mandatory in most of the United States so that infants can be identified before symptoms occur. At birth, infants have up to 80% of HbF, which does not carry the defect. Because levels of HbS are low at birth, Hgb electrophoresis or other

Normal red blood cells

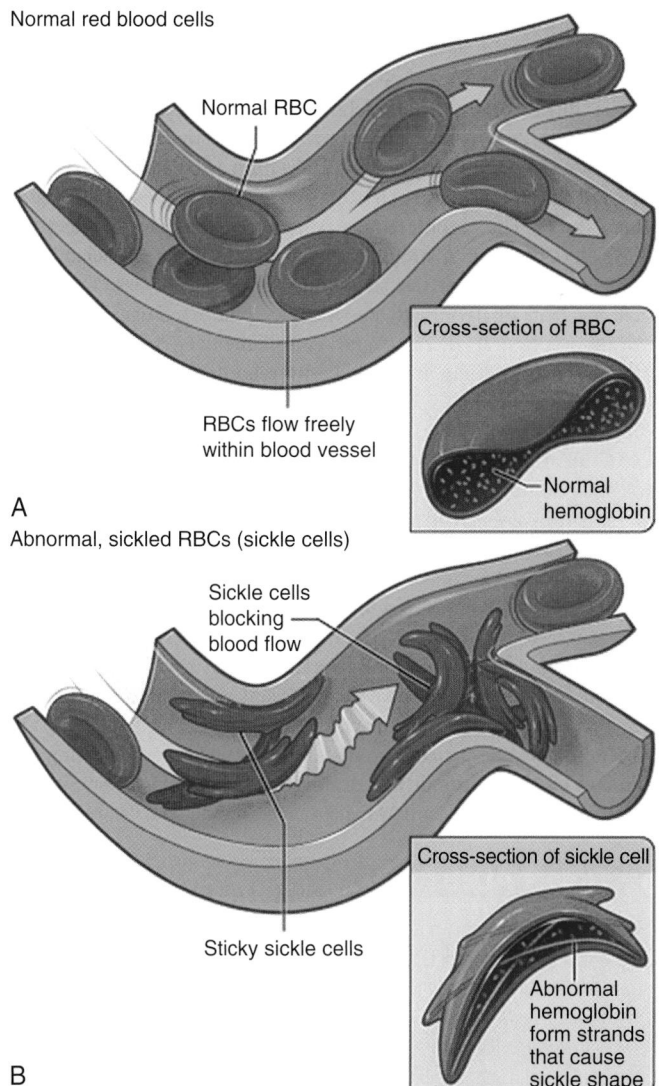

A

Abnormal, sickled RBCs (sickle cells)

Sickle cells blocking blood flow

Sticky sickle cells

Cross-section of RBC

RBCs flow freely within blood vessel

Normal hemoglobin

Cross-section of sickle cell

Abnormal hemoglobin form strands that cause sickle shape

B

Normal RBC

FIG 26-3 **A,** Normal red blood cells (RBCs) flowing freely in a blood vessel. The *inset* shows a cross-section of a normal RBC with normal hemoglobin. **B,** Abnormal, sickled RBCs clumping and blocking blood flow in a blood vessel. (Other cells also may play a role in this clumping process.) The *inset* shows a cross-section of a sickle cell with abnormal hemoglobin. (From National Heart, Lung, and Blood Institute: *What is sickle cell anemia?* Bethesda, Md, August 2008, Author.)

BOX 26-2 CLINICAL MANIFESTATIONS OF SICKLE CELL ANEMIA

General
Possible growth retardation
Chronic anemia (hemoglobin level of 6–9 g/dl)
Possible delayed sexual maturation
Marked susceptibility to sepsis

Vasoocclusive Crisis
Pain in area(s) of involvement
Manifestations related to ischemia of involved areas
  Extremities—Painful swelling of hands and feet (sickle cell dactylitis, or hand–foot syndrome), painful joints
  Abdomen—Severe pain resembling acute surgical condition
  Cerebrum—Stroke, visual disturbances
  Chest—Symptoms resembling pneumonia, protracted episodes of pulmonary disease
  Liver—Obstructive jaundice, hepatic coma
  Kidney—Hematuria
  Genitalia—Priapism (painful penile erection)

Sequestration Crisis
Pooling of large amounts of blood
  Hepatomegaly
  Splenomegaly
  Circulatory collapse

Effects of Chronic Vasoocclusive Phenomena
Heart—Cardiomegaly, systolic murmurs
Lungs—Altered pulmonary function, susceptibility to infections, pulmonary insufficiency
Kidneys—Inability to concentrate urine, enuresis, progressive renal failure
Liver—Hepatomegaly, cirrhosis, intrahepatic cholestasis
Spleen—Splenomegaly, susceptibility to infection, functional reduction in splenic activity progressing to autosplenectomy
Eyes—Intraocular abnormalities with visual disturbances; sometimes progressive retinal detachment and blindness
Extremities—Avascular necrosis of hip or shoulder; skeletal deformities, especially lordosis and kyphosis; chronic leg ulcers; susceptibility to osteomyelitis
Central nervous system—Hemiparesis, seizures

---

tests that measure Hgb concentrations are indicated. Early diagnosis (before 3 months of age) enables initiation of appropriate interventions to minimize complications. The family is taught to administer prophylactic antibiotics and identify early signs of infection to seek medical therapy as soon as possible.

If SCA is not diagnosed in early infancy, it is likely to manifest symptoms during the toddler and preschool years. SCA is occasionally first diagnosed during a crisis that follows an acute respiratory tract or GI infection. Routine hematologic tests are done to evaluate the anemia. Several specific tests detect the presence of the abnormal Hgb in the heterozygote or the homozygote. For screening purposes the sickle-turbidity test (Sickledex) is frequently used because it can be performed on blood from a fingerstick and yields accurate results in 3 minutes. However, if the test result is positive, Hgb electrophoresis

is necessary to distinguish between children with the trait and those with the disease. Hemoglobin electrophoresis ("fingerprinting" of the protein) is an accurate, rapid, and specific test for detecting the homozygous and heterozygous forms of the disease, as well as the percentages of the various types of Hgb.

Therapeutic Management

The aims of therapy are to (1) prevent the sickling phenomena, which are responsible for the pathologic sequelae, and (2) treat the medical emergencies of sickle cell crisis. The successful achievement of the aims depends on prompt nursing interventions, medical therapies, patient and family preventive measures, and use of innovative treatments.

Medical management of a crisis is usually directed toward supportive and symptomatic treatment. The main objectives are to provide (1) rest to minimize energy expenditure and to improve oxygen utilization; (2) hydration through oral and IV therapy; (3) electrolyte replacement because hypoxia results in metabolic acidosis, which also promotes sickling; (4) analgesia for the severe pain from vasoocclusion; (5) blood replacement to treat anemia and to reduce the viscosity of the sickled blood; and (6) antibiotics to treat any existing infection.

Administration of pneumococcal and meningococcal vaccines is recommended for these children because of their susceptibility to infection as a result of functional asplenia. In addition to routine immunizations, children with SCD should receive a yearly influenza vaccination (see Immunizations, Chapter 10). Oral penicillin prophylaxis is also recommended by 2 months of age to reduce the chance of pneumococcal sepsis (see Evidence-Based Practice box) (AAP, Committee on Infectious Diseases and Pickering, 2009; Hirst and Owusu-Ofori, 2010; National Institutes of Health, National Heart, Lung, and Blood Institute, 2002; Pack-Mabien and Haynes, 2009).

Oxygen therapy is of little therapeutic value unless the patient has hypoxia (Heeney and Dover, 2009). Severe hypoxia must be prevented because it causes massive systemic sickling that can be fatal. Oxygen administration is usually not effective in reversing sickling or reducing pain because the oxygen is unable to reach the enmeshed sickled erythrocytes in clogged vessels. In addition, prolonged administration of oxygen can depress bone marrow, further aggravating the anemia.

Another important component of care is the use of blood transfusions. Exchange RBC transfusion (erythrocytapheresis) is the replacement of sickle cells with normal RBCs. Exchange transfusion is a successful, rapid method of reducing the number of circulating sickle cells and therefore slowing down the vicious circle of hypoxia, thrombosis, tissue ischemia, and injury. The procedure is advocated as a possible technique in preventing reoccurrence of ACS and CVA (Velasquez, Mariscalco, Goldstein, and others, 2009). A transcranial Doppler (TCD) test identifies the child with SCD who is at high risk for developing a CVA by monitoring the intracranial vascular flow (Driscoll, 2007; Kwiatkowski, Yim, Miller, and others, 2011). The TCD is performed yearly for children from 2 to 16 years of age. The recommended treatment for children with confirmed abnormal TCD is chronic transfusion therapy (Armstrong-Wells, Grimes, Sidney, and others, 2009; Driscoll, 2007; Kwiatkowski, Yim, Miller, and others, 2011). Multiple transfusions carry the risk of transmission of viral infection, hyperviscosity, transfusion reactions, alloimmunization, and hemosiderosis (Driscoll, 2007; Heeney and Dover, 2009). After a CVA, blood transfusions are usually given every 3 to 4 weeks to help prevent a repeat stroke. To reduce iron overload from chronic transfusion therapy, chelation therapy may be started (see p. 882).

In children with recurrent life-threatening splenic sequestration, splenectomy may be a lifesaving measure. However, the spleen usually atrophies on its own through progressive fibrotic changes (**functional asplenia**) by 6 years of age in children with SCA. Prophylactic penicillin and pneumococcal vaccines have decreased the incidence of pneumococcal sepsis. Packed RBC transfusions are recommended for treatment of splenic sequestration and stroke and are used preoperatively accompanied with maintenance IV hydration for most surgical procedures in children with SCD.

The most common and debilitating symptom experienced by patients with SCD is VOC that is accompanied by increasing health care cost because of prolonged hospitalization associated with pulmonary and GI complications (Driscoll, 2007; Raphael, Mei, Mueller, and others, 2011). The chronic nature of this pain can greatly affect the child's development. A multidisciplinary team (e.g., physician, psychologist, family, nurse, social worker) approach is best for vasoocclusive pain management that includes pharmacologic treatment, hydration, physical therapy, and complementary treatment (e.g., prayer, spiritual healing, massage, herbs, relaxation, acupuncture, and biofeedback) (Brandow, Weisman, and Panepinto, 2011; Redding-Lallinger and Knoll, 2006). When mild to moderate VOC is reported, nonsteroidal anti-inflammatory medication (e.g., ibuprofen, ketorolac) or acetaminophen (Tylenol) is used initially. If these drugs are not effective alone, codeine can be added. The dosages of both drugs are titrated (adjusted) to a therapeutic level. Opioids such as immediate- and sustained-release morphine, oxycodone, hydromorphone (Dilaudid), and methadone are administered intravenously or orally for severe pain and are given around the clock. In conjunction with the opioid, IV ketorolac for a maximum of a 5-day course is commonly used to enhance the pain management effect. Patient-controlled analgesia (PCA) has been used successfully for sickle cell–related pain. PCA reinforces the patient's role and responsibility in managing the pain and provides flexibility in dealing with pain, which may vary in severity over time (see Pain Management, Chapter 7).

💊 DRUG ALERT

Meperidine (Demerol) is not recommended. Normeperidine, a metabolite of meperidine, is a central nervous system (CNS) stimulant that produces anxiety, tremors, myoclonus, and generalized seizures when it accumulates with repetitive dosing. Patients with SCD are particularly at risk for normeperidine-induced seizures (Howard and Davies, 2007; National Institutes of Health, National Heart, Lung, and Blood Institute, 2002).

Prognosis

The prognosis varies, but most patients live into the fifth decade. Most of the time, children are without symptoms and participate in normal activities without restrictions. The greatest risk is usually in children younger than 5 years of age, and the majority of deaths in these children are caused by overwhelming infection. Consequently, SCA is a chronic illness with a potentially terminal outcome. Physical and sexual maturation are delayed in adolescents with SCA. Although

---

EVIDENCE-BASED PRACTICE

Sickle Cell Anemia and Penicillin Prophylaxis

Ask the Question
Picot Question
In children with SCA, does prophylaxis with penicillin reduce the risk of pneumococcal infection?

Search for the Evidence
Search Strategies
Search selection criteria included English-language publications within the past 25 years, research-based articles (level 3 or lower), and child populations.

Databases Used
PubMed, Cochrane Collaboration, MD Consult

Critically Analyze the Evidence
- Hirst and Owusu-Ofori (2010) conducted an updated systematic Cochrane review of three trails that showed a reduced rate of infection in children with SCD receiving penicillin preventatively. Two trials looked at whether treatment was effective. The third trial followed from one of the early trials and looked at when it was safe to stop treatment. Adverse drug effects were rare

EVIDENCE-BASED PRACTICE

Sickle Cell Anemia and Penicillin Prophylaxis—cont'd

and minor. Penicillin given preventatively reduces the rate of pneumococcal infections in children with SCD younger than 5 years old.

- Researchers combined the clinical experiences of three sickle cell programs in the eastern United States in an attempt to determine the age and disease-specific risk of *Streptococcus pneumoniae* bacteremia and meningitis in children with SCD at a time when penicillin prophylaxis was routine. Forty-seven pneumococcal infections (44 bacteremia; 3 meningitis) among 40 patients with SCD were observed. Most children in whom infections developed were taking prophylactic penicillin and received Pneumovax at 24 months of age. The observed severe pneumococcal infection rate in HgbSS children younger than 5 years of age was less than that reported before penicillin prophylaxis in this specific population (Hord, Byrd, Stowe, and others, 2002).

- Administration of oral prophylactic penicillin was compared with the 14-valent pneumococcal vaccine in preventing pneumococcal infection in 242 children between the ages of 6 months and 3 years with HgbSS. In the first 5 years of the trial, there were 11 pneumococcal infections in the pneumococcal vaccine group and higher infection rates in those given the vaccine before 1 year of age. No pneumococcal isolates were found in the group receiving penicillin, although four pneumococcal isolates were found in this group within 1 year of stopping the penicillin prophylaxis at age 3 years. This study supported the use of penicillin prophylaxis to prevent pneumococcal infection in children younger than 3 years of age (John, Ramlal, Jackson, and others, 1984).

- In a multicenter, randomized, double-blind, placebo-controlled clinical trial, 105 children received penicillin twice daily; a control group of 110 children received a placebo twice daily. The trial was terminated 8 months early when an 84% reduction in the incidence of pneumococcal infections was observed in the group treated with penicillin compared with the placebo group. There were no deaths in the penicillin group, but three deaths from infection occurred in the placebo group. Researchers stressed the importance of screening children during the neonatal period and prescribing prophylactic penicillin to decrease the morbidity and mortality associated with pneumococcal infection (Gaston, Verter, Woods, and others, 1986).

- Zarkowsky, Gallagher, Gill, and others (1986) conducted a retrospective analysis of 178 episodes of bacteremia in children with sickle hemoglobinopathies that occurred during 13,771 patient-years of follow-up (*n* = 3451). The predominant pathogen in patients younger than 6 years of age was *S. pneumoniae* (66%), and gram-negative organisms were responsible for 50% of the bacteremias in patients 6 years and older. The incidence of pneumococcal bacteremia in children with SCA younger than 3 years of age was 6.1 events per 100 patient-years. The results of this study supported prophylactic administration of penicillin for prevention of pneumococcal bacteremia in children younger than 3 years of age.

- A cohort study of 315 patients with HgbSS who lived in Jamaica was conducted between June 1973 and December 1981. The patients were divided into three groups to determine whether interventions such as penicillin prophylaxis, parental education in early diagnosis of acute splenic sequestration, and close monitoring in a sickle cell clinic improved survival. A significant decline in deaths from acute splenic sequestration and pneumococcal septicemia and meningitis was found. The research indicated that early detection of SCD and prophylactic measures could significantly reduce deaths associated with HgbSS (Lee, Thomas, Cupidore, and others, 1995).

- Riddington and Owusu-Ofori (2002) conducted a systematic review of randomized controlled trials evaluating the effectiveness of prophylactic antibiotic administration in preventing pneumococcal infection in children with SCD. The review of published research found that penicillin prophylaxis significantly reduced the risk of pneumococcal infection in children with HgbSS with minimal adverse reactions.

Apply the Evidence: Nursing Implications

There is **good evidence** with a **strong recommendation** (Guyatt, Oxman, Vist, and others, 2008) that penicillin prophylaxis significantly reduces the risk of pneumococcal infection in children with SCA. The epidemiologic studies strongly suggest that all children with SCA should be started on prophylactic penicillin at 2 months of age. Parents and children with SCA should be instructed in the importance of taking the prophylactic penicillin twice daily and seeking medical attention immediately for acute illness, especially if the temperature exceeds 38.3° C (101° F), regardless of the use of prophylaxis.

QSEN Quality and Safety Competencies: Evidence-Based Practice*

Knowledge

Differentiate clinical opinion from research and evidence-based summaries.

Summarize the epidemiologic studies that strongly suggest that children with SCA should be started on prophylactic penicillin.

Skills

Base individualized care plan on patient values, clinical expertise, and evidence.

Integrate evidence into practice by making sure infants with SCD are started on penicillin at 2 months of age.

Attitudes

Value the concept of evidence-based practice as integral to determining best clinical practice.

Appreciate strengths and weakness of evidence for preventing pneumococcal infection in children with SCD.

References

Gaston MH, Verter JI, Woods G, and others: Prophylaxis with oral penicillin in children with sickle cell anemia: a randomized trial, *N Engl J Med* 314(25):1593–1599, 1986.

Guyatt GH, Oxman AD, Vist GE, and others: GRADE: an emerging consensus on rating quality of evidence and strength of recommendations, *BMJ* 336:924–926, 2008.

Hirst C, Owusu-Ofori S: Prophylactic antibiotics for preventing pneumococcal infection in children with sickle cell disease, *Cochrane Syst Rev* (11), CD003427, 2010.

Hord J, Byrd R, Stowe L, and others: *Streptococcus pneumoniae* sepsis and meningitis during the penicillin prophylaxis era in children with sickle cell disease, *J Pediatr Hematol Oncol* 24(6):470–472, 2002.

John AB, Ramlal A, Jackson H, and others: Prevention of pneumococcal infection in children with homozygous sickle cell disease, *BMJ* 288(6430):1567–1570, 1984.

Lee A, Thomas P, Cupidore L, and others: Improved survival in homozygous sickle cell disease: lessons from cohort study, *BMJ* 311(7020):1600–1602, 1995.

Riddington C, Owusu-Ofori S: Prophylactic antibiotics for preventing pneumococcal infection in children with sickle cell disease, 2002, *Cochrane Database Syst Rev* (3):CD003427, 2002.

Zarkowsky HS, Gallagher D, Gill FM, and others: Bacteremia in sickle hemoglobinopathies, *J Pediatr* 109(4):579–585, 1986.

HgbSS, Homozygous sickle cell disease; *SCA,* sickle cell anemia; *SCD,* sickle cell disease.

*Adapted from the QSEN at http://www.qsen.org.

adults achieve normal height, weight, and sexual function, the delay may present problems to adolescents (Heeney and Dover, 2009; Redding-Lallinger and Knoll, 2006).

Individuals with SCD who have higher levels of HbF tend to have a milder disease with fewer complications than those with lower levels (Anderson, 2006; Driscoll, 2007). Hydroxyurea is a U.S. Food and Drug Administration–approved medication that increases the production of HbF, reduces endothelial adhesion of sickle cells, improves the sickle cell hydration, increases nitric oxide production (a vasodilator), and lowers leukocyte and reticulocyte counts (McGann and Ware, 2011; National Institutes of Health, National Heart, Lung, and Blood Institute, 2002). Long-term follow-up of patients taking hydroxyurea alone revealed a 40% reduction in mortality and decreased frequency of VOC, ACS, hospital admissions, and need for transfusions, thus making SCD crises milder (Anderson, 2006; Strouse, Lanzkron, Beach, and others, 2008). Pediatric studies have shown that hydroxyurea can be safely used in children (Wang, Ware, Miller, and others, 2011; Zimmerman, Schultz, Davis, and others, 2004).

Hematopoietic stem cell transplantation (HSCT) offers a curative approach for some children with SCD with event-free survival of 95% (Driscoll, 2007; Haining, Duncan, and Lehmann, 2009) (see p. 899).

QUALITY PATIENT OUTCOMES: Sickle Cell Disease
- Early recognition of signs and symptoms of sickle cell anemia
- Tissue deoxygenation minimized
- Sickle cell crisis prevented or quickly managed
- Pain appropriately managed
- Stroke prevented
- Prophylactic penicillin regimen followed
- Hypoxia prevented when surgery is necessary
- Pneumococcal, *H. influenzae* type b, and meningococcal vaccines administered

---

Nursing Care Management
Educate the Family and Child

Family education begins with an explanation of the disease and its consequences (see Nursing Care Plan). After this explanation, the most important issues to teach the family are to (1) seek early intervention for problems, such as fever of 38.5° C (101.3° F) or greater; (2) give penicillin as ordered; (3) recognize signs and symptoms of splenic sequestration, as well as respiratory problems that can lead to hypoxia; and (4) treat the child normally. The nurse tells the family that the child is normal but can get sick in ways that other children cannot.

NURSING TIP One simple yet graphic way to demonstrate the effect of sickling is to roll rounded objects, such as marbles or beads, through a tube to simulate normal circulation and then roll pointed objects, such as screws or jacks, through the tube. The effect of sickling and clumping of the pointed objects is especially noticeable at a bend or slight narrowing of the tube.

The nurse emphasizes the importance of adequate hydration to prevent sickling and to delay the adhesion–stasis–thrombosis–ischemia cycle. It is not sufficient to advise parents to "force fluids" or "encourage drinking." They need specific instructions on how many daily glasses or bottles of fluid are required. Many foods are also a source of fluid, particularly soups, flavored ice pops, ice cream, sherbet, gelatin, and puddings.

Increased fluids combined with impaired kidney function result in the problem of enuresis. Parents who are unaware of this fact fre-

quently use the usual measures to discourage bedwetting, such as limiting fluids at night, and may resort to punishment and shame to force bladder control. Enuresis is treated as a complication of the disease, such as joint pain or some other symptom, to alleviate parental pressure on the child.

Promote Supportive Therapies During Crises

The success of many of the medical therapies relies heavily on nursing implementation. Management of pain is an especially difficult problem and often involves experimenting with various analgesics, including opioids, and schedules before relief is achieved. Unfortunately, these children tend to be undermedicated, resulting in their "clock watching" and demands for additional doses sooner than might be expected. Often this incorrectly raises suspicions of drug addiction, when in fact the problem is one of improper dosage (see Family-Centered Care box). In choosing and scheduling analgesics, the goal should be *prevention* of pain.

NURSING TIP Advise parents to be particularly alert to situations in which dehydration may be a possibility, such as hot weather, and to recognize early signs of reduced intake, such as decreased urinary output (e.g., fewer wet diapers) and increased thirst.

Any pain program should be combined with psychologic support to help the child deal with the depression, anxiety, and fear that may accompany the disease. This includes regular visits with the child to discuss any concerns during the hospitalization and positive reinforcement of coping skills, such as successful methods of dealing with the pain and compliance with treatment prescriptions. To reduce the negative connotation associated with the term *crisis*, it is best to say *pain episode* (see Complementary & Alternative Therapy box).

If blood transfusions or exchange transfusions are given, the nurse has the responsibility of observing for signs of transfusion reaction (see Table 26-3, p. 898). Because hypervolemia from too-rapid transfusion can increase the workload of the heart, the nurse also is alert to signs of cardiac failure.

In splenic sequestration the size of the spleen is gently measured by abdominal palpation (see Abdomen, Chapter 6). The nurse should be aware of spleen size because increasing splenomegaly is an ominous sign. A decreasing spleen size denotes response to therapy. Vital signs and blood pressure are also closely monitored for impending shock. Anemia is typically not a presenting complication in vasoocclusive crises but is a critical problem in other types of crises. The nurse monitors for evidence of increasing anemia and institutes appropriate nursing interventions (see p. 869). Oxygen is not beneficial in vaso-occlusive episodes unless hypoxemia is present (Heeney and Dover, 2009). It does not reverse sickled RBCs, and if used in a nonhypoxic patient, it will decrease erythropoiesis (Vichinsky and Styles, 1996). Because prolonged use of oxygen can aggravate the anemia, signs of lack of therapeutic benefit, such as restlessness, increased pallor, and continued pain, are reported.

Record intake, especially of IV fluids, and output. The child's weight should be taken on admission to serve as a baseline for evaluating hydration. Because diuresis can result in electrolyte loss, the nurse also observes for signs of hypokalemia and should be familiar with normal serum electrolyte values to report changes.

Recognize Other Complications

Nurses also need to be aware of the signs of ACS and CVA, both potentially fatal complications.

◎ NURSING CARE PLAN

The Child with Sickle Cell Anemia

NURSING DIAGNOSIS	PATIENT OUTCOMES	NURSING INTERVENTIONS	RATIONALE
Risk for Injury related to abnormal hemoglobin level, decreased ambient oxygen level **Child's Defining Characteristics (Subjective and Objective Data)** Shortness of breath, dyspnea Fatigue, headache, pallor Icteric sclera or jaundice Systolic murmur, cyanosis, increased pulse rate	Child will avoid situations that reduce tissue oxygenation and allow for adequate tissue oxygenation. **The Following NOC Concept Applies to This Outcome** Risk Control	Explain measures to minimize complications related to physical exertion and emotional stress. Prevent infection. Advise to avoid low-oxygen environments (e.g., high altitudes, nonpressurized airplane flights). **The Following NIC Concepts Apply to These Interventions** Health Education Behavior Modification	To avoid additional tissue oxygen needs At risk for infection because of reduced tissue oxygenation To prevent a decrease in oxygenation
Deficient Fluid Volume **Child's Defining Characteristics (Subjective and Objective Data)** Dry mucous membranes Loss of skin turgor Sunken eyes No or diminished tears Sunken fontanel Dark urine Rapid, thready pulse Rapid breathing Lethargy, weakness	Child will take adequate amounts of fluids and show no signs of dehydration. **The Following NOC Concepts Apply to This Outcome** Fluid Balance Electrolyte and Acid–Base Balance	Calculate recommended daily fluid intake (1600 ml/m^2/day) and base child's fluid requirements on this amount. Increase fluid intake above minimum requirements during physical exercise or emotional stress and during a crisis. Give parents written instructions regarding specific quantity of fluid required daily. Encourage child to drink. Stress importance of avoiding overheating. Teach family signs of dehydration. **The Following NIC Concepts Apply to These Interventions** Fluid Management Fluid/Electrolyte Management	To ensure adequate hydration To compensate for additional fluid needs To encourage compliance To ensure adequate hydration To minimize fluid loss To avoid delay in rehydration therapy
Acute Pain related to tissue anoxia (vasoocclusive crisis) **Child's Defining Characteristics (Subjective and Objective Data)** Pain can be in any location in the body; can be rapid in onset and severe; may be localized or generalized Low-grade fever may be present Localized swelling over joints with arthralgia can occur	Child will experience no or minimal pain. **The Following NOC Concepts Apply to This Outcome** Comfort Level Pain Control	Discuss preventive schedule of medication around the clock with parents. Encourage high level of fluid intake. Recognize that various analgesics, including opioids and medication schedules, may need to be tried. Reassure child and family that analgesics, including opioids, are medically indicated, that high doses may be needed, and that children rarely become addicted. Apply heat to or massage affected area. Avoid applying cold compresses. Instruct parents to seek medical attention immediately for sudden, persistent headache; weakness on one side of the body; sudden gait or speech problems; or altered mental status. **The Following NIC Concepts Apply to These Interventions** Medication Management Pain Management Patient-Controlled Analgesia Assistance	To prevent pain To ensure hydration To ensure satisfactory pain relief To avoid needless suffering because of unfounded fears To prevent vasoconstriction that may enhance sickling To prevent vasoconstriction that may enhance sickling To prevent progressive CNS damage through recognition of acute CNS events

Continued

NURSING CARE PLAN

The Child with Sickle Cell Anemia—cont'd

NURSING DIAGNOSIS	PATIENT OUTCOMES	NURSING INTERVENTIONS	RATIONALE
Risk for Infection **Child's Defining Characteristics** <u>(Subjective and Objective Data)</u> Fever, chills, pain, redness Lethargy, increased pallor, listlessness, irritability Increased pulse and respiration rates History of prior sepsis	Child will remain free of infection. **The Following NOC Concept Applies to This Outcome** Infection Severity	Stress importance of adequate nutrition; routine immunizations, including pneumococcal and meningococcal vaccinations; protection from known sources of infection; and frequent health evaluation and regularly scheduled comprehensive evaluation. Report any signs of infection immediately. Promote compliance with prophylactic antibiotic therapy Instruct parents regarding signs and symptoms of splenic sequestration and regular palpation of the spleen. **The Following NIC Concepts Apply to These Interventions** Environmental Management Communicable Disease Management Medication Prescribing Medication Administration Medication Management	To encourage preventive measures and decrease risk for infection exposure To avoid delay in treatment To prevent and treat infection To enable early recognition of splenic sequestration crisis
Deficient Knowledge related to understanding of sickle cell disease and its management **Child's/Family's Defining Characteristics** <u>(Subjective and Objective Data)</u> Lack of understanding Inability to identify signs and symptoms of painful crises Inability to follow disease management guidelines Difficulty describing treatment plan Improper medication administration	Child and family will demonstrate understanding of the disease, its cause, and its treatment. **The Following NOC Concepts Apply to This Outcome** Family Coping Knowledge: Illness Care	Teach family and children characteristics of basic genetic defect and measures to minimize complications. Stress importance of informing significant health personnel of child's disease. Explain signs of developing complications such as fever, pallor, respiratory distress, persistent headaches, and pain. Reinforce basic information regarding trait transmission and refer to genetic counseling services. Teach parents to be an advocate for their child. Educate the school and teachers regarding the cause of sickle cell disease and measures to avoid complications within the classroom. Stress with educators the need to provide tutorials and to allow child time to make up schoolwork during medical absences. **The Following NIC Concepts Apply to These Interventions** Teaching: Disease Process Teaching: Prescribed Medication	To minimize complications of sickling To provide support and prevent complications To ensure prompt and appropriate treatment To allow for informed decision making To provide support and prevent complications To provide support and prevent complications To provide support and prevent complications

CNS, Central nervous system; *NIC,* Nursing Interventions Classification; *NOC,* Nursing Outcomes Classification.

FAMILY-CENTERED CARE

Fear of Addiction

Although the pain during a sickle cell crisis is usually severe and opioids are needed, many families fear that their child will become addicted to the narcotic. Unfortunately, misinformed health professionals may foster this unfounded fear, which results in needless suffering. Extremely few children who receive opioids for severe pain become behaviorally addicted to the drug (American Pain Society, 1999; Howard and Davies, 2007; National Institutes of Health, National Heart, Lung, and Blood Institute, 2002). Families and older children, especially adolescents, need to be reassured that opioids are medically indicated, high doses may be needed, and children rarely become addicted.

COMPLEMENTARY & ALTERNATIVE THERAPY

Heat to the affected area can be soothing. Cold compresses are not applied to the area because they enhance sickling and vasoconstriction. Bed rest is usually well tolerated during a crisis, although actual rest depends greatly on pain alleviation and organized schedules of nursing care. Some activity, particularly passive range-of-motion exercises, is beneficial to promote circulation. Usually the best course of action is to let children dictate their activity tolerance.

NURSING TIP Report signs of the following immediately:

ACS:
- Severe chest, back, or abdominal pain
- Fever of 38.5° C (101.3° F) or higher
- Cough
- Dyspnea, tachypnea
- Retractions
- Declining oxygen saturation (oximetry)

CVA:
- Severe, unrelieved headaches
- Severe vomiting
- Jerking or twitching of the face, legs, or arms
- Seizures
- Strange, abnormal behavior
- Inability to move an arm or leg
- Stagger or an unsteady walk
- Stutter or slurred speech
- Weakness in the hands, feet, or legs
- Changes in vision

Support the Family

Families need the opportunity to discuss their feelings regarding transmitting a potentially fatal, chronic illness to their child. Because of the widely publicized prognosis for children with SCA, many parents express their prevalent fear of the child's death. Three manifestations of SCD that may appear in the first 2 years of life (dactylitis, severe anemia, leukocytosis) can be predictors of disease severity (DeBaun and Vichinsky, 2007; Ohls and Christensen, 2007). The nurse should care for the family as for any family with a child who has a chronic and life-threatening illness and give consideration to the siblings' reactions, the stress on the marital relationship, and the childrearing attitudes displayed toward the child (see Chapter 18). Several resources are available to families with a sickling disorder.*

---

*Sickle Cell Disease Association of America, Inc., 231 E. Baltimore St., Suite 800, Baltimore, MD 21202; 410-528-1555, 800-421-8453; fax: 410-528-1495; e-mail: scdaa@sicklecelldisease.org; http://www.sicklecelldisease.org; Sickle Cell Information Center, PO Box 109, Grady Memorial Hospital, 80 Jesse Hill Jr Drive SE, Atlanta, GA 30303; 404-616-3572; fax: 404-616-5998; e-mail: aplatt@emory.edu; http://www.scinfo.org; National Heart, Lung, and Blood Institute, PO Box 30105, Bethesda, MD 20824-0105; 301-592-8573, fax: 240-629-3246; http://www.nhlbi.nih.gov. *Sickle cell disease in newborns and infants: a guide for parents*, Pub No AHCPR 93-0564. Available from the AHCPR Publications Clearinghouse, PO Box 8547, Silver Spring, MD 20907-8547; 800-358-9295; http://www.ahcpr.gov. *Guideline for the management of acute and chronic pain in sickle-cell disease* is available from the American Pain Society, 4700 W. Lake Ave., Glenview, IL 60025-1485; 847-375-4715; fax: 866-574-2654; e-mail: info@ampainsoc.org; http://www.ampainsoc.org.

The nurse advises parents to inform all treating personnel of the child's condition. The use of medical identification, such as a bracelet, is another way of ensuring awareness of the disease.

If family members have the SCD trait or SCA, genetic counseling is necessary. A primary consideration in genetic counseling is informing parents of the 25% chance with each pregnancy of having a child with the disease when both parents carry the trait.

β-THALASSEMIA (COOLEY ANEMIA)

Worldwide, thalassemia is a common genetic disorder, affecting as many as 15 million people (Yaish, 2010). The term thalassemia, which is derived from the Greek word *thalassa*, meaning "sea," is applied to a variety of inherited blood disorders characterized by deficiencies in the rate of production of specific globin chains in Hgb. The name appropriately refers to descendants of or people living near the Mediterranean Sea, who have the highest incidence of the disease, namely Italians, Greeks, and Syrians. Evidence suggests that the high incidence of the disorders among these groups is a result of the selective advantage the trait confers in relation to malaria, as is postulated in SCD. However, the disorder has a wide geographic distribution, probably as a result of genetic migration through intermarriage or possibly as a result of spontaneous mutation.

β-Thalassemia is the most common of the thalassemias and occurs in four forms:

- Two heterozygous forms, thalassemia minor, an asymptomatic silent carrier, and thalassemia trait, which produces a mild microcytic anemia
- Thalassemia intermedia, which is manifested as splenomegaly and moderate to severe anemia
- A homozygous form, thalassemia major (also known as Cooley anemia), which results in a severe anemia that would lead to cardiac failure and death in early childhood without transfusion support

Pathophysiology

Normal postnatal Hgb is composed of two α- and two β-polypeptide chains. In β-thalassemia, there is a partial or complete deficiency in the synthesis of the β-chain of the Hgb molecule. Consequently, there is a compensatory increase in the synthesis of α-chains, and γ-chain production remains activated, resulting in defective Hgb formation. This unbalanced polypeptide unit is very unstable; when it disintegrates, it damages RBCs, causing severe anemia.

To compensate for the hemolytic process, an overabundance of erythrocytes is formed unless the bone marrow is suppressed by transfusion therapy. Excess iron from hemolysis of supplemental RBCs in transfusions and from the rapid destruction of defective cells is stored in various organs (hemosiderosis).

Diagnostic Evaluation

The onset of thalassemia major may be insidious and not recognized until the latter half of infancy. The clinical effects of thalassemia major are primarily attributable to (1) defective synthesis of HbA, (2) structurally impaired RBCs, and (3) shortened life span of erythrocytes (Box 26-3).

Hematologic studies reveal the characteristic changes in RBCs (i.e., microcytosis, hypochromia, anisocytosis, poikilocytosis, target cells, and basophilic stippling of various stages). Low Hgb and Hct levels are seen in severe anemia, although they are typically lower than the reduction in RBC count because of the proliferation of immature erythrocytes. Hgb electrophoresis confirms the diagnosis, and radiographs of involved bones reveal characteristic findings.

BOX 26-3 CLINICAL MANIFESTATIONS OF β-THALASSEMIA

Anemia (Before Diagnosis)
Pallor
Unexplained fever
Poor feeding
Enlarged spleen or liver

Progressive Anemia
Signs of chronic hypoxia
 Headache
 Precordial and bone pain
 Decreased exercise tolerance
 Listlessness
 Anorexia

Other Features
Small stature
Delayed sexual maturation
Bronzed, freckled complexion (if not receiving chelation therapy)

Bone Changes (Older Children If Untreated)
Enlarged head
Prominent frontal and parietal bossing
Prominent malar eminences
Flat or depressed bridge of the nose
Enlarged maxilla
Protrusion of the lip and upper central incisors and eventual malocclusion
Generalized osteoporosis

Therapeutic Management

The objectives of supportive therapy are to maintain sufficient Hgb levels to prevent bone marrow expansion and the resulting bony deformities and to provide sufficient RBCs to support normal growth and normal physical activity. Transfusions are the foundation of medical management with the goal of maintaining the Hgb level above 9.5 g/dl, an aim that may require transfusions as often as every 3 to 5 weeks. The advantages of this therapy include (1) improved physical and psychologic well-being because of the ability to participate in normal activities, (2) decreased cardiomegaly and hepatosplenomegaly, (3) fewer bone changes, (4) normal or near-normal growth and development until puberty, and (5) fewer infections.

One of the potential complications of frequent blood transfusions is iron overload (hemosiderosis). Because the body has no effective means of eliminating the excess iron, the mineral is deposited in body tissues. To minimize the development of hemosiderosis, the oral iron chelator deferasirox has been shown to be a safe equivalent to **deferoxamine (Desferal)**, a parenteral iron-chelating agent, and more tolerable by patients and families (Cappellini, Porter, El-Beshlawy, and others, 2010; Vichinsky, Bernaudin, Forni, and others, 2011; Vichinsky, Onyekwere, Porter, and others, 2007).

In some children with severe splenomegaly who require repeated transfusions, a splenectomy may be necessary to decrease the disabling effects of abdominal pressure and to increase the life span of supplemental RBCs. Over time, the spleen may accelerate the rate of RBC destruction and thus increase transfusion requirements. After a splenectomy, children generally require fewer transfusions, although the basic defect in Hgb synthesis remains unaffected. A major postsplenectomy complication is severe and overwhelming infection. Therefore,

these children continue to receive prophylactic antibiotics with close medical supervision for many years and should receive the pneumococcal and meningococcal vaccines in addition to the regularly scheduled immunizations (see Immunizations, Chapter 10).

> **NURSING TIP** Ensure that the family and patient understand the need to notify the health professional of all fevers of 38.5° C (101.3° F) or greater because of the risk of sepsis in a child with asplenia.

Prognosis

Most children treated with blood transfusion and early chelation therapy survive well into adulthood. The most common causes of death are heart disease, postsplenectomy sepsis, and multiple-organ failure secondary to hemochromatosis (Cunningham, Sankaran, Nathan, and others, 2009). A curative treatment for some children is HSCT. Children younger than 16 years of age who undergo allogeneic HSCT have a high rate of complication-free survival; approximately 80% of these children are cured (Lucarelli and Gaziev, 2008).

Nursing Care Management

The objectives of nursing care are to (1) promote compliance with transfusion and chelation therapy, (2) assist the child in coping with the anxiety-provoking treatments and the effects of the illness, (3) foster the child's and family's adjustment to a chronic illness, and (4) observe for complications of multiple blood transfusions. Basic to each of these goals is explaining to parents and older children the defect responsible for the disorder, its effect on RBCs, and the potential effects of untreated iron overload (e.g., diabetes and heart disease). Because the prevalence of this condition is high among families of Mediterranean descent, the nurse also inquires about the family's previous knowledge about thalassemia. All families with a child with thalassemia should be tested for the trait and referred for genetic counseling.

As with any chronic illness, the family's needs must be met for optimal adjustment to the stresses imposed by the disorder (see Chapter 18). Sources of information for the family include the Cooley's Anemia Foundation* and the Northern California Comprehensive Thalassemia Center.† Genetic counseling for the parents and fertile offspring is mandatory, and both prenatal diagnosis using amniocentesis at 20 weeks' gestation or fetal blood sampling at 10 weeks and screening for thalassemia trait are available.

APLASTIC ANEMIA

Aplastic anemia (AA) refers to a bone marrow failure condition in which the formed elements of the blood are simultaneously depressed. The peripheral blood smear demonstrates pancytopenia or the triad of profound anemia, leukopenia, and thrombocytopenia. **Hypoplastic anemia** is characterized by a profound depression of RBCs but normal or slightly decreased white blood cells (WBCs) and platelets.

Etiology

Aplastic anemia can be **primary** (**congenital**, or present at birth) or **secondary** (**acquired**). The best-known congenital disorder of which AA is an outstanding feature is **Fanconi syndrome**, a rare hereditary disorder characterized by pancytopenia, hypoplasia of the bone

*330 Seventh Ave., No. 200, New York, NY 10001; 800-522-7222; fax: 212-279-5999; http://www.cooleysanemia.org.
†747 52nd St., Oakland, CA 94609; 510-428-3885, ext. 4398; http://www.thalassemia.com.

marrow, and patchy brown discoloration of the skin resulting from the deposit of melanin and associated with multiple congenital anomalies of the musculoskeletal and genitourinary systems. The syndrome appears to be inherited as an autosomal recessive trait with varying penetrance; therefore, affected siblings may demonstrate several different combinations of defects.

Several etiologic factors contribute to the development of acquired hypoplastic anemia; however, most of the cases are considered idiopathic (Box 26-4). Acquired AA is classified as either severe acquired AA or moderate acquired AA. The following discussion focuses on severe acquired AA, which carries a poorer prognosis and follows a more rapidly fatal course than the primary types.

Diagnostic Evaluation

The onset of clinical manifestations, which include anemia, leukopenia, and decreased platelet count, is usually insidious. Definitive diagnosis is determined from bone marrow examination, which demonstrates the conversion of red bone marrow to yellow, fatty bone marrow. Severe AA is defined as less than 25% bone marrow cellularity with at least two of the following findings: absolute granulocyte count less than 500/mm³, platelet count less than 20,000/mm³, and absolute reticulocyte count less than 40,000/mm³ (Hord, 2007; Passweg and Marsh, 2010). Moderate AA is defined as more than 25% bone marrow cellularity with the presence of mild or moderate cytopenia (Shimamura and Guinan, 2009).

Therapeutic Management

The objectives of treatment are based on the recognition that the underlying disease process is failure of the bone marrow to carry out its hematopoietic functions. Therefore, therapy is directed at restoring function to the marrow and involves two main approaches: (1) immunosuppressive therapy to remove the presumed immunologic functions that prolong aplasia or (2) replacement of the bone marrow through transplantation. Bone marrow transplantation is the treatment of choice for severe AA when a suitable donor exists (see p. 889).

Antilymphocyte globulin (ALG) or antithymocyte globulin (ATG) is the principal drug treatment used for AA. The rationale for using ATG is based on the theory that AA may be a result of autoimmunity. ATG and cyclosporine suppress T cell–dependent autoimmune responses but do not cause bone marrow suppression. Cyclosporine is administered orally for several weeks to months. ATG usually is administrated intravenously over 12 to 16 hours for 4 days after a test dose to check for hypersensitivity. A course may be repeated, depending on the reduction in circulating lymphocytes and the

patient's response. Because of the hypersensitivity response associated with ATG (i.e., fever, chills, myalgias), methylprednisolone is given intravenously to prevent these side effects. Colony-stimulating factor (CSF) and granulocyte-macrophage colony-stimulating factor (GM-CSF), given parenterally, may be used to enhance bone marrow production. Androgens may be used with ATG to stimulate erythropoiesis if the AA is unresponsive to initial therapies.

Hematopoietic stem cell transplantation should be considered early in the course of the disease if a compatible donor can be found. Transplantation is more successful when performed before multiple transfusions have sensitized the child to leukocyte and human leukocyte antigens (HLA). HSCT is associated with an approximately 90% survival rate in patients who receive a bone marrow transplant from an HLA-identical sibling (Hord, 2007; Marsh, 2005; Trigg, 2004).

Nursing Care Management

The care of the child with AA is similar to that of the child with leukemia (see p. 890) and includes preparing the child and family for the diagnostic and therapeutic procedures, preventing complications from the severe pancytopenia, and emotionally supporting them in the face of a potentially fatal outcome. Information and support are available from the Aplastic Anemia and MDS International Foundation, Inc.*

Because the aspects of nursing care are discussed in the section on leukemia, only the exceptions are presented here. The drug ATG is usually administered by way of a central vein. If not, vigilant care must be directed to the IV infusion to prevent extravasation. Meticulous care of the venous access is essential because of the child's susceptibility to infection. CSFs are usually given by subcutaneous injection over several days. Chemotherapeutic agents have been reported in the treatment of relapsed patients with AA after ATG and CSF therapy. Many of the side effects associated with chemotherapy such as nausea and vomiting, alopecia, and mucositis are experienced by children receiving treatment for AA. Specialized care is required for children who have HSCT (see p. 889).

DEFECTS IN HEMOSTASIS

Hemostasis is the process that stops bleeding when a blood vessel is injured. Vascular and plasma clotting factors, as well as platelets, are required. A complex system of clotting, anticlotting, and clot breakdown (fibrinolysis) mechanisms exists in equilibrium to ensure clot formation only in the presence of blood vessel injury and to limit the clotting process to the site of vessel wall injury. Dysfunction in these systems leads to bleeding or abnormal clotting. Although the coagulation process is complex, clotting depends on three factors: (1) vascular influence, (2) platelet role, and (3) clotting factors.

HEMOPHILIA

The term hemophilia refers to a group of bleeding disorders in which there is a deficiency of one of the factors (proteins) necessary for coagulation of the blood. Although the symptomatology is similar regardless of which clotting factor is deficient, the identification of specific factor deficiencies allows definitive treatment with replacement agents.

In about 80% of all cases of hemophilia, the inheritance pattern is demonstrated as X-linked recessive. The two most common forms of

---

*100 Park Avenue, Suite 108, Rockville, MD 20850; 800-747-2820, 301-279-7202; fax: 301-279-7205; e-mail: help@aamds.org; http://www.aamds.org.

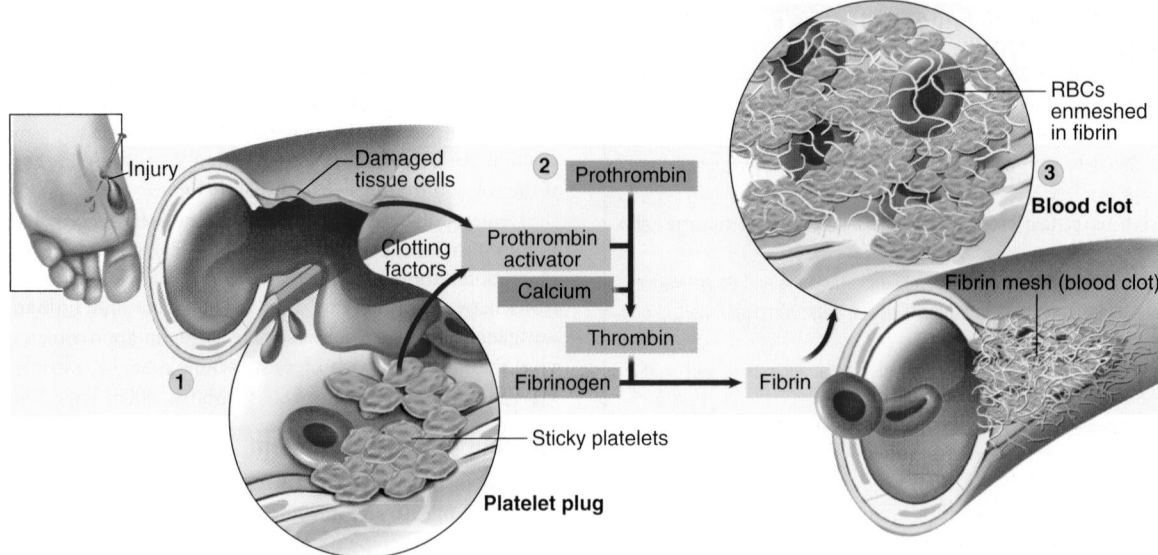

FIG 26-4 Blood clotting. The extremely complex clotting mechanism can be distilled into three basic steps: (1) release of clotting factors from both injured tissue cells and sticky platelets at the injury site (which form a temporary platelet plug); (2) a series of chemical reactions that eventually result in the formation of thrombin; and (3) formation of fibrin and trapping of red blood cells (RBCs) to form a clot. (From Thibodeau GA: *The human body in health and disease*, ed 5, St. Louis, 2010, Mosby.)

the disorder are **factor VIII deficiency (hemophilia A, or classic hemophilia)** and **factor IX deficiency (hemophilia B, or Christmas disease). Von Willebrand disease (vWD)** is another hereditary bleeding disorder characterized by a deficiency, abnormality, or absence of the protein called von Willebrand factor (vWF) and a deficiency of factor VIII. Unlike hemophilia, vWD affects both males and females. The following discussion is primarily concerned with factor VIII deficiency, which accounts for 80% of all hemophilia cases.

Pathophysiology

The basic defect of hemophilia A is a deficiency of **factor VIII (antihemophilic factor [AHF]).** AHF is produced by the liver and is necessary for the formation of thromboplastin in phase I of blood coagulation (Fig. 26-4). The less AHF found in the blood, the more severe the disease. Individuals with hemophilia have two of the three factors required for coagulation: vascular influence and platelets. Therefore, they may bleed for longer periods but not at a faster rate.

Bleeding into subcutaneous and IM tissue is common. Hemarthrosis, which is bleeding into a joint space, is the most frequent type of internal bleeding. Bony changes and crippling deformities occur after repeated bleeding episodes over several years. Signs of hemarthrosis are swelling, warmth, redness, pain, and loss of movement. Bleeding in the neck, mouth, or thorax is serious because the airway can become obstructed. Intracranial hemorrhage can have fatal consequences and is one of the major causes of death. Hemorrhage anywhere along the GI tract can lead to anemia, and bleeding into the retroperitoneal cavity is especially hazardous because of the large space for blood to accumulate. Hematomas in the spinal cord can cause paralysis.

Diagnostic Evaluation

Overt, prolonged hemorrhage is readily apparent; bleeding into tissues is less apparent (Box 26-5). The diagnosis is usually made from a history of bleeding episodes, evidence of X-linked inheritance (only one third of the cases are new mutations), and laboratory findings. The tests specific for hemophilia plasma depend on specific factors for a

BOX 26-5   CLINICAL MANIFESTATIONS OF HEMOPHILIA

- Prolonged bleeding anywhere from or in the body
- Hemorrhage from any trauma—Loss of deciduous teeth, circumcision, cuts, epistaxis, injections
- Excessive bruising, even from a slight injury, such as a fall
- Subcutaneous and intramuscular hemorrhages
- Hemarthrosis (bleeding into the joint cavities), especially the knees, ankles, and elbows
- Hematomas—Pain, swelling, and limited motion
- Spontaneous hematuria

reaction to occur, such as the partial thromboplastin time (PTT). Specific determination of factor deficiencies requires assay procedures normally performed in specialized laboratories. Carrier detection is possible in classic hemophilia using deoxyribonucleic acid (DNA) testing and is an important consideration in families in which female offspring may have inherited the trait.

Therapeutic Management

The primary therapy for hemophilia is replacement of the missing clotting factor. The products available are **factor VIII concentrates,** either produced through genetically engineering (recombinant) or derived from pooled plasma, which are reconstituted with sterile water immediately before use. A synthetic form of vasopressin, **1-deamino-8-d-arginine vasopressin (DDAVP),** increases plasma factor VIII activity and is the treatment of choice in mild hemophilia and certain types of vWD if the child shows an appropriate response. DDAVP is not effective in the treatment of severe hemophilia A, severe vWD, or any form of hemophilia B. Aggressive factor concentrate replacement therapy is initiated to prevent chronic crippling effects from joint bleeding.

Other drugs may be included in the therapy plan, depending on the source of the hemorrhage. Corticosteroids are given for hematuria, acute hemarthrosis, and chronic synovitis. Nonsteroidal anti-inflammatory drugs (NSAIDs), such as ibuprofen, are effective in relieving pain caused by synovitis; however, they are occasionally used with caution because they inhibit platelet function (Curry, 2004). Oral administration of ε-aminocaproic acid (Amicar) prevents clot destruction. Its use is limited to mouth or trauma surgery with a dose of factor concentrate given first.

A regular program of exercise and physical therapy is an important aspect of management. Physical activity within reasonable limits strengthens muscles around joints and may decrease the number of spontaneous bleeding episodes.

Treatment without delay results in more rapid recovery and a decreased likelihood of complications; therefore, most children are treated at home. The family is taught the technique of venipuncture and to administer the AHF to children older than 2 to 3 years of age. The child learns the procedure for self-administration at 8 to 12 years of age. Home treatment is highly successful, and the rewards, in addition to the immediacy, are less disruption of family life, fewer school or work days missed, and enhancement of the child's self-esteem and independence.

Primary prophylaxis in hemophilia patients has proved to be effective in preventing bleeding complications by administrating periodic factor replacement. Primary prophylaxis involves the infusion of factor VIII concentrate on a regular basis before the onset of joint damage. Secondary prophylaxis involves the infusion of factor VIII concentrate on a regular basis after the child experiences his or her first joint bleed. The infusions are given three times a week. Aggressive or on-demand factor replacement may be a cost-effective alternative to primary prophylaxis, but prophylaxis decreases the development of joint disease compared with on-demand factor replacement treatment (Manco-Johnson, Abshire, Shapiro, and others, 2007). Prompt appropriate treatment of hemorrhage and prophylactic therapy are key to excellent care and prevention of long-term morbidity in patients with hemophilia (Montgomery, Gill, and DiPaola, 2009; Sharathkumar and Pipe, 2008).

Prognosis

Although there is no cure for hemophilia, its symptoms can be controlled and its potentially crippling deformities greatly reduced or even avoided. Today many children with hemophilia function with minimal or no joint damage. They are normal children with an average life expectancy in every respect but one: they have a tendency to bleed, which is a significant inconvenience but not necessarily a life-threatening event.

Gene therapy may prove to be a treatment option in the future. This therapy involves introducing a working copy of the factor VIII gene into a patient who has a flawed copy of the gene. Problems exist with appropriate selection of the vector, identification of the cell for gene expression, and control of side effects (Matrai, Chuah, and VandenDriessche, 2010; Montgomery, Gill, and DiPaola, 2009).

QUALITY PATIENT OUTCOMES: Hemophilia
- Early recognition of signs and symptoms of hemophilia
- Bleeding episodes prevented
- Bleeding episodes treated early with factor replacement
- Adherence to prophylactic factor replacement program when indicated
- Hemarthrosis prevented when possible with limited joint damage
- Exercise program and physical therapy ongoing

Nursing Care Management

The earlier a bleeding episode is recognized, the more effectively it can be treated. Signs that indicate internal bleeding are especially important to recognize. Children are aware of internal bleeding and are reliable in telling the examiner where an internal bleed is. In addition to the manifestations described (see Box 26-5), the nurse maintains a high level of suspicion when a child with hemophilia demonstrates signs such as headache, slurred speech, loss of consciousness (from cerebral bleeding), and black tarry stools (from GI bleeding).

Prevent Bleeding

The goal of prevention of bleeding episodes is directed toward decreasing the risk of injury. Prevention of bleeding episodes is geared mostly toward appropriate exercises to strengthen muscles and joints and to allow age-appropriate activity. During infancy and toddlerhood, the normal acquisition of motor skills creates innumerable opportunities for falls, bruises, and minor wounds. Restraining the child from mastering motor development can foster more serious long-term problems than allowing the behavior. However, the environment should be made as safe as possible, with close supervision during playtime to minimize incidental injuries.

For older children, the family usually needs assistance in preparing for school. A nurse who knows the family can be instrumental in discussing the situation with the school nurse and in jointly planning an appropriate activity schedule. Because almost all persons with hemophilia are boys, the physical limitations in regard to active sports may be a difficult adjustment, and activity restrictions must be tempered with sensitivity to the child's emotional and physical needs. Use of protective equipment, such as padding and helmets, is particularly important, and noncontact sports, especially swimming, walking, jogging, tennis, golf, fishing, and bowling, are encouraged (National Hemophilia Foundation, 2006). However, the use of prophylaxis to prevent joint hemorrhage or overuse during low-impact athletic participation remains unknown (Ross, Goldenberg, Hund, and others, 2009).

To prevent oral bleeding, some readjustment in terms of dental hygiene may be needed to minimize trauma to the gums, such as use of a water irrigating device, softening the toothbrush in warm water before brushing, or using a sponge-tipped disposable toothbrush. A regular toothbrush should be soft bristled and small.

Because any trauma can lead to a bleeding episode, all persons caring for these children must be aware of their disorder. These children should wear medical identification, and older children should be encouraged to recognize situations in which disclosing their condition is important, such as during dental extraction or injections. Health personnel need to take special precautions to prevent the use of procedures that may cause bleeding, such as IM injections. The subcutaneous route is substituted for IM injections whenever possible. Venipunctures for blood samples are usually preferred for these children. There is usually less bleeding after the venipuncture than after finger or heel punctures. Neither aspirin nor any aspirin-containing compound should be used. Acetaminophen is a suitable aspirin substitute, especially for controlling pain at home.

Recognize and Control Bleeding

As noted, the earlier a bleeding episode is recognized, the more effectively it can be treated. Factor replacement therapy should be instituted according to established medical protocol, and supportive measures may be implemented, such as RICE, which stands for *rest, ice, compression,* and *elevation.* When parents and older children are taught such measures beforehand, they can be prepared to initiate immediate treatment. Plastic bags of ice or cold packs should be kept in the freezer for such emergencies. However, such measures do not take the place of factor replacement.

Prevent Crippling Effects of Bleeding

As a result of repeated episodes of hemarthrosis, incompletely absorbed blood in the joints, and limitation of motion, bone and muscle changes occur that result in flexion contractures and joint fixation. During bleeding episodes, the joint is elevated and immobilized. Active range-of-motion exercises are usually instituted after the acute episode. This allows the child to control the degree of exercise and discomfort. If an exercise program is instituted in the home, a physical therapist or public health nurse may need to supervise compliance with the regimen. Rarely, orthopedic intervention, such as casting, application of traction, or aspiration of blood, may be necessary to preserve joint function. Diet is also an important consideration because excessive body weight can increase the strain on affected joints, especially the knees, and predispose the child to hemarthrosis. Consequently, calories need to be supplied in accordance with energy requirements.

Support the Family and Prepare for Home Care

Genetic counseling is essential as soon as possible after diagnosis. Unlike many other disorders in which both parents carry the trait, the feeling of responsibility for this condition usually rests with the mother. Without an opportunity to discuss her feelings, the marital relationship can suffer. Technology is now available to identify carriers in approximately 80% of cases and may reduce the anxiety regarding childbearing in women who may be at risk of carrying the defective gene, such as sisters or maternal aunts of an affected boy. Factor concentrates have greatly changed the outlook for these children by minimizing bleeding and allowing the child to live a normal, unrestricted life. Children are taught to take responsibility for their disease at an early age. They learn their limitations, other preventive measures, and self-administration of the prophylactic AHF.

The needs of families who have children with hemophilia are best met through a comprehensive team approach of physicians (pediatrician, hematologist, orthopedist), nurse practitioner, nurse, social worker, and physical therapist. Parent-group discussions are beneficial in meeting the needs that are often best met by similarly affected families. For example, with the improved prognosis for these children, parents and adolescents with hemophilia face vocational and financial problems in addition to concern over future childbearing. After children reach 21 years of age, many insurance companies will no longer carry them. This can be disastrous in terms of the cost of treatment. Financial support is particularly important. A person with severe hemophilia may require factor replacement therapy and other medical treatments that cost in excess of $100,000 a year. The National Hemophilia Foundation* and the Canadian Hemophilia Society† provide numerous services and publications for both health providers and families.

Children who have become infected with human immunodeficiency virus (HIV) through transfusions and factor replacement products are faced with the consequences of this dreaded disease. Consequently, they need the support of health professionals, especially in the areas of safe sexual practices to avoid disease transmission and public education regarding acquired immunodeficiency syndrome (AIDS) and ways to deal with public reactions to persons who have AIDS.

IMMUNE THROMBOCYTOPENIA (IDIOPATHIC THROMBOCYTOPENIC PURPURA)

Idiopathic or immune thrombocytopenic purpura (ITP), as a formerly used term because purpura is an infrequent sign at presentation, is now referred to as immune thrombocytopenia (Rodeghiero, Stasi, Gernsheimer, and others, 2009). ITP is an acquired hemorrhagic disorder characterized by (1) thrombocytopenia, (2) absence or minimal signs of bleeding (easy bruising, mucosal bleeding, petechiae) in most childhood cases, and (3) normal bone marrow with normal or increased number of immature platelets (megakaryocytes) and eosinophils. Although all causes of ITP are not known, it is understood that ITP involves the evolution of antibodies against multiple platelet antigens, leading to reduced platelet survival and impaired platelet production (Consolini, 2011; McCrae, 2011). It is the most frequently occurring thrombocytopenia of childhood. The greatest frequency of occurrence is in children younger than 10 years of age with the peak incidence at age 2 to 5 years (Consolini, 2011; McCrae, 2011; Wilson, 2009).

The disease occurs in one of two forms: an acute, self-limiting course or a chronic condition (>12 months' duration). The acute form is most often seen after upper respiratory tract infections; after the childhood diseases measles, rubella, mumps, and chickenpox; or after infection with parvovirus B19.

Diagnostic Evaluation

The diagnosis is suspected on the basis of clinical manifestations (Box 26-6). In ITP, the platelet count is reduced to below 20,000/mm³; therefore, tests that depend on platelet function, such as the tourniquet test, bleeding time, and clot retraction, have abnormal results. Although there is no definitive test on which to establish a diagnosis of ITP, several tests are usually performed to rule out other disorders in which thrombocytopenia is a manifestation, such as systemic lupus erythematosus, lymphoma, or leukemia.

BOX 26-6 CLINICAL MANIFESTATIONS OF IMMUNE THROMBOCYTOPENIA (IDIOPATHIC THROMBOCYTOPENIC PURPURA)

Easy bruising
- Petechiae
- Ecchymoses
- Most often over bony prominences

Bleeding from mucous membranes
- Epistaxis
- Bleeding gums
- Internal hemorrhage evidenced by:
  - Hematuria
  - Hematemesis
  - Melena
  - Hemarthrosis
  - Menorrhagia
  - Hematomas over lower extremities

---

*116 W. 32nd St., 11th Floor, New York, NY 10001; 800-42-HANDI, 212-328-3700; fax: 212-328-3777; e-mail: handi@hemophilia.org; http://www.hemophilia.org.
†625 President Kennedy Ave., Suite 505, Montreal, QC H3A 1K2; 800-668-2686, 514-848-0503; fax: 514-848-9661; e-mail: chs@hemophilia.ca; http://www.hemophilia.ca.

BOX 26-7 CRITERIA FOR ANTI-D ANTIBODY THERAPY

- Age between 1 and 19 years; Rh(D)-positive blood type
- Normal WBC count and hemoglobin level for age; platelet count of 20,000/mm^3
- No active mucosal bleeding
- No history of reaction to plasma products
- No known immunoglobulin A deficiency
- No concurrent infection
- Absence of Evans syndrome (characterized by the combination of idiopathic thrombocytopenic purpura and autoimmune hemolytic anemia)
- No suspicion of lupus erythematosus or other collagen vascular disorder
- No splenectomy

WBC, White blood cell.

Therapeutic Management

Management of ITP is primarily supportive because the course of the disease is self-limited in the majority of cases. Activity is restricted at the onset while the platelet count is low and while active bleeding or progression of lesions is occurring. Treatment for acute presentation is symptomatic and has included prednisone, IV immune globulin (IVIG), and anti-D antibody. These are not curative therapies. Anti-D antibody is a relatively new therapy for ITP. Infusion of anti-D antibody causes a transient hemolytic anemia in the patient. Along with the clearance of antibody-coated RBCs, there is prolonged survival of platelets resulting from the blockade of the Fc receptors of the reticuloendothelial cells. The platelet count does not increase until 48 hours after an infusion of anti-D antibody; therefore, it is not appropriate therapy for patients who are actively bleeding. The benefits of choosing anti-D antibody therapy over prednisone or IVIG is that anti-D antibody can be given in one dose over 5 to 10 minutes and is significantly less expensive than IVIG. Historically, patients who are treated with prednisone may first undergo a bone marrow examination to rule out leukemia, which is controversial because leukemia rarely manifests with low platelet count alone (Scott and Montgomery, 2007; Wilson, 2009). Therefore, the use of anti-D antibody and IVIG alleviates the need for a bone marrow examination. Before receiving the initial dose of anti-D antibody, patients must meet certain criteria (Box 26-7). Premedication with acetaminophen 5 to 10 minutes before the infusion is recommended.

> **NURSING TIP** After administration of anti-D antibody, observe the child for a minimum of 1 hour and maintain a patent IV line. Obtain baseline vital signs before the infusion and again 5, 20, and 60 minutes after beginning the infusion. Fever, chills, and headache may occur during or shortly after the infusion. If so, diphenhydramine (Benadryl) and hydrocortisone (Solu-Cortef) should be given and the patient observed for an additional hour.

Splenectomy is for patients who have chronic ITP that is not responsive to pharmacologic management and have increased risk of severe hemorrhage. It is the useful option associated with long-term remission for the majority of these children and reduces the risk of hemorrhage (McCrae, 2011; Scott and Montgomery, 2007; Wilson, 2009). Before splenectomy is considered, waiting until the child is older than 5 years of age is generally recommended because of the increased risk of bacterial infection. Pneumococcal and meningococcal vaccines are recommended before splenectomy (see Immunizations, Chapter 10). The child also receives penicillin prophylaxis after splenectomy.

The length of prophylactic therapy is controversial, but in general, a minimum of 3 years is recommended.

Prognosis

The majority of children have a self-limited course without major complications. Some children may develop chronic ITP and require ongoing therapy. A splenectomy may modify the disease process, and the child will be asymptomatic.

> **QUALITY PATIENT OUTCOMES: ITP**
> - Serious bleeding episode prevented
> - Activities that increase risk for serious bleeding avoided
> - Treatment administered without serious side effects

Nursing Care Management

Nursing care is largely supportive and should include teaching regarding possible side effects of therapy and limitation in activities while the child's platelet count is less than 50,000/mm^3 (Consolini, 2011). Children with ITP should not participate in *any* contact sports, bike riding, skateboarding, in-line skating, gymnastics, climbing, or running. Parents are encouraged to engage their children in quiet activities and to prevent any injuries to the child's head. The harmful effects of using aspirin and NSAIDs to control pain are critical for these children; therefore, salicylate substitutes (e.g., acetaminophen) are always used. As in any condition with an uncertain outcome, the family needs emotional support.

DISSEMINATED INTRAVASCULAR COAGULATION

Disseminated intravascular coagulation (DIC), also known as consumption coagulopathy, is characterized by diffuse fibrin deposition in the microvasculature, consumption of coagulation factors, and endogenous generation of thrombin and plasmin. DIC is a secondary disorder of coagulation that occurs as a complication of a number of pathologic processes, such as hypoxia, acidosis, shock, and endothelial damage. It can result from many severe systemic diseases, such as congenital heart disease, necrotizing enterocolitis, gram-negative bacterial sepsis, rickettsial infections, and some severe viral infections.

Pathophysiology

Disseminated intravascular coagulation occurs when the first stage of the coagulation process is abnormally stimulated. Although no well-defined sequence of events occurs, two distinct phases can be identified. First, when the clotting mechanism is triggered in the circulation, thrombin is generated in greater amounts than can be neutralized by the body. Consequently, there is rapid conversion of fibrinogen to fibrin, with aggregation and destruction of platelets. If local and widespread fibrin deposition in blood vessels takes place, obstruction and eventual necrosis of tissues occur. Second, the fibrinolytic mechanism is activated, causing extensive destruction of clotting factors. With a deficiency of clotting factors, the child is vulnerable to uncontrollable hemorrhage into vital organs. An additional complication is damage and hemolysis of RBCs.

Diagnostic Evaluation

Disseminated intravascular coagulation is suspected when the patient has an increased tendency to bleed (Box 26-8). Hematologic findings include prolonged prothrombin time, PTT, and thrombin time. There is a profoundly depressed platelet count, fragmented RBCs, and depleted fibrinogen.

Case Study—Idiopathic Thrombocytopenic Purpura

BOX 26-8   **CLINICAL MANIFESTATIONS OF DISSEMINATED INTRAVASCULAR COAGULATION**

Petechiae
Purpura
Bleeding from openings in the skin
- Venipuncture site
- Surgical incision
Bleeding from umbilicus, trachea (newborn)
Evidence of gastrointestinal bleeding
Hypotension
Organ dysfunction from infarction and ischemia

Therapeutic Management

Treatment of DIC is directed toward control of the underlying or initiating cause, which in most instances stops the coagulation problem spontaneously. Platelets and fresh-frozen plasma may be needed to replace lost plasma components, especially in children whose underlying disease remains uncontrolled. Extremely ill newborn infants may require exchange transfusion with fresh blood. The IV administration of heparin to inhibit thrombin formation is most often restricted to patients who have not responded to treatment of the underlying disease or replacement of coagulation factors and platelets.

Nursing Care Management

The goals of nursing care are to be aware of the possibility of DIC in severely ill children and to recognize signs that might indicate its presence. The skills needed to monitor IV infusion and blood transfusions and to administer heparin are the same as for any child receiving these therapies. (See Chapter 18 for care of children with life-threatening illnesses.)

EPISTAXIS (NOSEBLEEDING)

Isolated and transient episodes of epistaxis, or nosebleeding, are common in childhood. The nose, especially the septum, is a highly vascular structure, and bleeding usually results from direct trauma, including blows to the nose, foreign bodies, and nose picking, or from mucosal inflammation associated with allergic rhinitis and upper respiratory tract infections. The bleeding ordinarily stops spontaneously or with minimal pressure and requires no medical evaluation or therapy.

Recurrent epistaxis and severe bleeding may indicate an underlying disease, particularly vascular abnormalities, leukemia, thrombocytopenia, and clotting factor deficiency diseases (e.g., hemophilia, vWD). Nosebleeds are sometimes associated with administration of aspirin, even in normal amounts. Persistent episodes of epistaxis require medical evaluation.

Nursing Care Management

In the event of a nosebleed, an essential intervention is to remain calm. Otherwise, the child will become more agitated, the blood pressure will increase, and the child will not cooperate. Although in most instances a nosebleed is not serious, it can be upsetting to family members as well. They need reassurance that the loss of blood is not serious and that the bleeding usually stops in less than 10 minutes with nasal pressure.

✚ EMERGENCY TREATMENT
Epistaxis

- Have child sit up and lean forward (not lie down).
- Apply continuous pressure to nose with thumb and forefinger for at least 10 minutes.
- Insert cotton or wadded tissue into each nostril and apply ice or cold cloth to bridge of nose if bleeding persists.
- Keep child calm and quiet.

To control the bleeding, the child is instructed to sit up and lean forward (not to lie down) to avoid aspiration of blood. Most of the nosebleeding originates in the anterior part of the nasal septum and can be controlled by applying pressure to the soft lower portion of the nose with the thumb and forefinger (see Emergency Treatment box). During this time, the child breathes through the mouth.

In the event that hemorrhage continues, the child should be evaluated by a practitioner, who may pack the nose with epinephrine-soaked gauze. After a nosebleed, petroleum or water-soluble jelly can be inserted into each nostril to prevent crusting of old blood and to lessen the likelihood of the child's picking at the nose and restarting the hemorrhage. If a child has numerous nosebleeds, factors believed to increase the likelihood of bleeds are eliminated, such as discouraging nose picking or altering the household humidity by placing a cool-mist humidifier in the child's room. Repeated bleeding episodes lasting longer than 30 minutes may be an indication to refer the child for evaluation for the possibility of a bleeding disorder.

NEOPLASTIC DISORDERS

Neoplastic disorders are the leading cause of death from disease in children past infancy, and almost half of all childhood cancers involve the blood or blood-forming organs. Leukemias and lymphomas are discussed here. Malignant solid tumors of childhood are discussed elsewhere in relation to the tissues or organs involved.

LEUKEMIAS

Leukemia, cancer of the blood-forming tissues, is the most common form of childhood cancer. The annual incidence is three to four cases per 100,000 white children (Jemal, Siegel, Ward, and others, 2009). It is more common in boys and whites, with the peak onset between 2 and 5 years of age (Hutter, 2010; Margolin, Rabin, Steuber, and others, 2011; Pui, Relling, and Downing, 2004). It is one of the forms of cancer that has demonstrated dramatic improvements in survival rates. Whereas current long-term disease-free survival for children with acute lymphoid leukemia approaches 80% (Margolin, Rabin, Steuber, and others, 2011; Pui, Relling, and Downing, 2004), acute nonlymphoid leukemia has a 50% to 65% survival rate (Kaspers and Creutzig, 2005; Pearce and Sills, 2005). (See also Prognosis, p. 889.)

Classification

Leukemia is a broad term given to a group of malignant diseases of the bone marrow and lymphatic system. Research has revealed that it is a complex disease of varying heterogeneity. Consequently, classification has become increasingly complex, sophisticated, and essential because identification of the subtype of leukemia has therapeutic and prognostic implications. The following is a brief overview of the major classification systems currently being used.

Morphology

Two forms are generally recognized in children, acute lymphoid leukemia (ALL) and acute nonlymphoid (myelogenous) leukemia (ANLL or AML). Synonyms for ALL include lymphatic, lymphocytic, lymphoblastic, and lymphoblastoid leukemia. Usually the terms stem cell or blast cell leukemia also refer to the lymphoid type. Synonyms for the AML type include granulocytic, myelocytic, monocytic, myelogenous, monoblastic, and monomyeloblastic.

Cytochemical markers—Several chemical stains (e.g., terminal deoxynucleotidyl transferase [TdT]) aid in differentiation between ALL and ANLL.

Chromosome studies—Chromosome analysis has become an important tool in the diagnosis of ALL. For example, children with trisomy 21 have 20 times the risk of other children for developing ALL. Children with more than 50 chromosomes on the leukemic cells (hyperdiploid) have the best prognosis (Margolin, Rabin, Steuber, and others, 2011). Translocations of chromosomes also found on the leukemic cells can denote good prognosis, as in the trisomies 4 and 10, or a poor prognosis, as in the t(9:22) or Philadelphia chromosome.

Cell-surface immunologic markers—Cell-surface antigens have permitted differentiation of ALL into three broad classes: B-cell ALL; T-cell ALL; and common ALL antigen (CALLA or CD 10+) formally known as non-T, non-B ALL, which is actually of early B-cell lineage (Margolin, Rabin, Steuber, and others, 2011). Children with the common ALL antigen on their cell surfaces have the more favorable prognosis (Margolin, Rabin, Steuber, and others, 2011).

Pathophysiology

Leukemia is an unrestricted proliferation of immature WBCs in the blood-forming tissues of the body. Although not a "tumor" as such, the leukemic cells demonstrate the same neoplastic properties as solid cancers. Therefore, the resulting pathologic condition and clinical manifestations are caused by infiltration and replacement of any tissue of the body with nonfunctional leukemic cells. Highly vascular organs, such as the spleen and liver, are the most severely affected.

To understand the pathophysiology of the leukemic process, it is important to clarify two common misconceptions. First, although leukemia is an overproduction of WBCs, most often in the acute form, the leukocyte count is low (thus the term *leukemia*). Second, these immature cells do not deliberately attack and destroy the normal blood cells or vascular tissues. Cellular destruction takes place by infiltration and subsequent competition for metabolic elements.

In all types of leukemia, the proliferating cells depress the production of formed elements of the blood in bone marrow by competing for and depriving the normal cells of the essential nutrients for metabolism. The most frequent presenting signs and symptoms of leukemia are a result of infiltration of the bone marrow. The three main consequences are (1) anemia from decreased RBCs, (2) infection from neutropenia, and (3) bleeding from decreased platelet production. The invasion of the bone marrow with leukemic cells gradually causes a weakening of the bone and a tendency toward fractures. As leukemic cells invade the periosteum, increasing pressure causes severe pain.

The spleen, liver, and lymph glands demonstrate marked infiltration, enlargement, and eventually fibrosis. Hepatosplenomegaly is typically more common than lymphadenopathy. The next most important site of involvement is the central nervous system (CNS) secondary to leukemic infiltration, which may cause increased intracranial pressure (see Box 28-1, p. 929).

Leukemic cells may also invade the testes, kidneys, prostate, ovaries, GI tract, and lungs. With long-term survivors becoming more common, such sites of leukemia invasion, especially the testes, are becoming more important clinically.

Diagnostic Evaluation

Leukemia is usually suspected based on the history and physical presentation that often includes fever, signs and symptoms of low blood counts, lymph node enlargement, and an enlarged liver and spleen. Peripheral blood smear may reveal immature forms of leukocytes, frequently combined with low blood counts. Definitive diagnosis is based on bone marrow aspiration or biopsy. Flow cytometry identifies the specific type of blast cell. Typically, the bone marrow is hypercellular, with primarily blast cells. After the diagnosis is confirmed, a lumbar puncture is performed to determine whether there is any CNS involvement. A few children will have CNS involvement at diagnosis, although most are asymptomatic.

Therapeutic Management

Treatment of leukemia involves the use of chemotherapeutic agents, with or without cranial irradiation, in four phases: (1) induction therapy, which achieves a complete remission or less than 5% leukemic cells in the bone marrow; (2) CNS prophylactic therapy, which prevents leukemic cells from invading the CNS; (3) intensification therapy (consolidation), which eradicates residual leukemia cells, followed by delayed intensification, which prevents emergence of resistant leukemic clones; and (4) maintenance therapy, which serves to maintain the remission phase.

Hematopoietic Stem Cell Transplantation

Hematopoietic stem cell transplantation has been used successfully for treating children who have ALL and AML. HSCT is *not* recommended for children with ALL during the first remission because of the excellent results possible with chemotherapy. In the United States, patients with intermediate- and high-risk AML with a suitable donor available are recommended for transplant during the first clinical remission (Bollard, Krance, and Heslop, 2011).

Hematopoietic stem cell transplantation may be not only from antigen-matched related donors but also from matched unrelated donors or mismatched donors. Peripheral blood stem cell transplants are capable of differentiating into specialized cells of the hematologic system and can be obtained from related or unrelated donors or from umbilical cord blood. Regardless of the type of transplant, it is accompanied by significant morbidity and mortality, including graft-versus-host disease (GVHD), overwhelming infection, or severe organ damage.

Prognosis

The most important prognostic factors for determining long-term survival for children with ALL (in addition to treatment) are (1) the initial WBC count, (2) the child's age at the time of diagnosis, (3) the type of cell involved, (4) the sex of the child, and (5) karyotype analysis. Children with a normal or low WBC count who are CALLA positive have a much better prognosis than those with a high count or other cell types. Children diagnosed between 2 and 9 years of age have consistently demonstrated a better outlook than those diagnosed before 2 or after 10 years of age, and girls appear to have a more favorable prognosis than boys. Children with more than 50 chromosomes indicated by a DNA index greater than 1.16 (hyperdiploid) have a better prognosis. Similarly, patients with ALL and trisomies of chromosomes 4 and 10 have a good prognosis with a low risk of treatment failure (Margolin, Rabin, Steuber, and others, 2011).

Late Effects of Treatment

Although vigorous treatment of childhood cancers has resulted in dramatically improved survival rates, increasing concern surrounds late effects—adverse changes related to treatment modalities—and recurrence of the disease process. Almost no organ is exempt, and almost every antineoplastic agent, especially irradiation, is responsible for some adverse effect.

The most devastating late effect is development of a second malignancy. Children who received cranial irradiation at age 5 years or younger are most susceptible to developing brain tumors and increase risk of developing cognitive defects that can affect school performance (Bhatia, 2004; Hutter, 2010). Treatment with an anthracycline is associated with cardiomyopathy; cranial irradiation and intrathecal chemotherapy are associated with cognitive and neuropsychologic deficits, which are just a few of the long-term sequelae. Consequently, close monitoring for late effects is essential, especially with the advent of additional clinical trials.

Nursing Care Management

Nursing care of the child with leukemia is directly related to the therapeutic regimen. General psychologic interventions during each phase of therapy are discussed in Chapter 18.

Prepare the Child and Family for Diagnostic and Therapeutic Procedures

From the time before diagnosis to cessation of therapy, children must undergo several tests; the most traumatic are bone marrow aspiration, bone marrow biopsy, and lumbar punctures. Multiple finger sticks and venipunctures for blood analysis and drug infusion are common occurrences. Therefore, the child needs an explanation of each procedure and what can be expected. In addition, effective pharmacologic measures, including conscious and unconscious sedation, and non-pharmacologic strategies are used to reduce discomfort associated with these painful procedures.

Relieve Pain

The effective use of analgesia is especially important when the malignant process is uncontrolled and causes acute pain. Dosages of opioids (narcotics) are adjusted, or *titrated,* to the child's needs and administered *around the clock* for optimal pain control. Nonpharmacologic strategies should be implemented as needed but are not substitutes for pharmacologic management. Readers are encouraged to review the principles of pain assessment and management presented in Chapter 7 and Preparation for Diagnostic and Therapeutic Procedures, Chapter 22, when caring for a child with leukemia.

Prevent Complications of Myelosuppression

The leukemic process and most of the chemotherapeutic agents cause myelosuppression. The reduced numbers of blood cells result in secondary problems of infection, bleeding tendencies, and anemia. Supportive care involves both medical and nursing management. Because these are so closely linked, they are discussed together.

Infection. A frequent complication of treatment for childhood cancer is overwhelming infection secondary to neutropenia. The child is most susceptible to overwhelming infection during three phases of the disease: (1) at the time of diagnosis and relapse when the leukemic process has replaced normal leukocytes; (2) during immunosuppressive therapy; and (3) after prolonged antibiotic therapy, which predisposes the child to the growth of resistant organisms. However, the use of granulocyte colony-stimulating factor (GCSF) has reduced the incidence and duration of infection in children receiving treatment for cancer.

The first defense against infection is prevention. When the child is hospitalized, the nurse uses all measures to control transfer of infection. These typically include the use of a private room, restriction of all visitors and health personnel with active infection, and strict hand-washing technique with an antiseptic solution. In some research centers, special germ-free environments are available during complete myelosuppression from intensive chemotherapy or for bone marrow transplant. The nurse should be aware of these guidelines and educate patients and families.

> **NURSING TIP** The child is not immunized against live viral vaccines (measles, rubella, mumps) until the immune system is capable of responding appropriately to the vaccine (AAP, Committee on Infectious Diseases and Pickering, 2009; Koh and Pizzo, 2011). Most institutions have individual guidelines regarding vaccinations in children undergoing immunosuppressive therapy.

The child is evaluated for potential sites of infection (e.g., mucosal ulceration; skin abrasion; skin tear, such as a hangnail) and observed for any elevation in temperature. To identify the source of infection, chest radiographs and blood, stool, urine, and nasopharyngeal cultures are taken. IV antibiotics are administered, and if this therapy is prolonged, a venous access device, such as a peripherally inserted central catheter or intermittent infusion device (saline lock or PRN [as-needed] adaptor), is used to maintain IV access.

Prevention of infection continues to be a priority after discharge from the hospital. Ordinarily, the child is allowed to return to school when the WBC count is at a satisfactory level, usually an absolute neutrophil count greater than $500/mm^3$ (see Nursing Care Guidelines box). At all times, family members are encouraged to practice good hand washing to prevent introducing pathogens into the home. The child may need to be isolated from school contacts in the event of an outbreak of a childhood disease, especially chickenpox.

Nutrition is another important component of infection prevention. An adequate protein-caloric intake provides the child with better host defenses against infection and increased tolerance to chemotherapy and irradiation. However, providing optimal nutrition during periods of anorexia and vomiting from chemotherapy is a tremendous challenge (see Feeding the Sick Child, Chapter 22).

Hemorrhage. Before the use of transfused platelets, hemorrhage was a leading cause of death in patients with leukemia. Now most bleeding episodes can be prevented or controlled with the administration of platelet concentrates or platelet-rich plasma.

📋 NURSING CARE GUIDELINES
Calculating the Absolute Neutrophil Count

Determine the total percent of neutrophils ("polys," or "segs," and bands). Multiply WBC count by percent of neutrophils.

Example:
WBC = 1000; neutrophils = 7%; nonsegmented neutrophils (bands) = 7%
Step 1: 7% + 7% = 14%
Step 2: 0.14 × 1000 = 140 ANC

ANC, Absolute neutrophil count; *WBC,* white blood cell.

Skin punctures are avoided whenever possible because bleeding sites can become easily infected. When finger sticks, venipunctures, IM injections, and bone marrow aspirations are performed, aseptic technique must be used along with continued observation for bleeding. Meticulous mouth care is essential because gingival bleeding with resultant mucositis is a frequent problem. Because the rectal area is prone to ulceration from various drugs, feces and urine are removed immediately, and the perianal area is washed. Using rectal temperatures is avoided to prevent trauma. Children are advised to avoid activities that might cause injury or bleeding, such as riding bicycles and skateboards, climbing trees and playground equipment, and playing contact sports.

Platelet transfusions are generally reserved for active bleeding episodes that do not respond to local treatment and that may occur during induction or relapse therapy. Epistaxis and gingival bleeding are the most common. The nurse teaches parents and older children measures to control nosebleeding (see p. 888). Pressure at the site without disturbing clot formation is the general rule.

During bleeding episodes, the parents and child need much emotional support. Often parents request a platelet transfusion, unaware of the need for trying local measures first. The nurse can be instrumental in allaying anxiety by acknowledging the feelings of the child and family and explaining the reason for delaying a platelet transfusion until absolutely necessary.

Anemia. Initially, anemia may be profound from complete replacement of the bone marrow by leukemic cells. During induction therapy, blood transfusions may be necessary. The usual precautions in caring for the child with anemia are instituted (see p. 869).

Use Precautions in Administering and Handling Chemotherapeutic Agents

In addition to the nurse's many responsibilities in regard to the child and family, nurses must also use safeguards to protect themselves. Handling chemotherapeutic agents may present risks to handlers and to their offspring, although the exact degree of risk is not known. Many chemotherapeutic agents are vesicants (sclerosing agents) that can cause severe cellular damage if even minute amounts of the drug infiltrate surrounding tissue. Only nurses experienced with chemotherapeutic agents should administer vesicants. Guidelines are available* and must be followed exactly to prevent tissue damage to patients. Interventions for extravasation vary, but each nurse should be aware of the institution's policies and implement them at once.

In addition to extravasation, a potentially fatal complication is anaphylaxis, especially from L-asparaginase, teniposide (VM-26), etoposide (VP-16), bleomycin, and cisplatin. Nursing responsibilities include prevention of, recognition of, and preparation for serious reactions. Prevention begins with a careful history for known allergies.

Most children with cancer have a venous access device, which facilitates administration of IV drugs. During treatment and remission, many drugs are taken orally at home. Compliance with the medication schedule is essential, and nurses play an important role in educating the family about the drugs and encouraging adherence to the plan.

> **NURSING TIP** Chemotherapeutic drugs must be given through a free-flowing IV line. The infusion is stopped immediately if any sign of infiltration (pain, stinging, swelling, or redness at the cannulation site) occurs. When chemotherapeutic and immunologic agents are given, the child must be observed for 20 minutes after the infusion for signs of anaphylaxis (cyanosis, hypotension, wheezing, severe urticaria). Emergency equipment (especially blood pressure monitor and bag valve mask) and emergency drugs (especially oxygen, epinephrine, antihistamine, aminophylline, corticosteroids, and vasopressors) must be available. If a reaction is suspected, the drug is discontinued, the IV line is flushed with saline, and the child's vital signs and subsequent responses are monitored.

Manage Problems of Drug Toxicity

Chemotherapy presents several nursing challenges. The complexity of the treatment protocols is often overwhelming to families. In addition, each therapy is associated with a number of predictable side effects. Nurses must be aware of these side effects and use judgment in recognizing reactions, as well as toxicities.[†]

Nausea and Vomiting. The nausea and vomiting that occur shortly after administration of several of the drugs and from cranial or abdominal radiation can be profound. The serotonin-receptor antagonists (e.g., ondansetron, granisetron, palonosetron) are effective in the control of nausea and vomiting occurring after emetogenic chemotherapy and radiotherapy. When combined with dexamethasone, these agents are the treatment of choice in the prevention of delayed emesis (Lindley, Goodin, McCune, and others, 2005; Saito, Aogi, Sekine, and others, 2009).

The most beneficial regimen for antiemetic control has been the administration of the antiemetic *before* chemotherapy begins. The goal is to prevent the child from ever experiencing nausea or vomiting, thus preventing development of anticipatory symptoms (the conditioned response of developing nausea and vomiting before receiving the drug).

Anorexia. Loss of appetite is a direct consequence of the chemotherapy or irradiation. It is a major problem for parents because it is the one area they feel responsible for, particularly when so many other facets of care are outside their control. There are no universally successful techniques for encouraging a sick child to eat. However, the guidelines in Chapter 22 can be helpful during the anorexic period and can prevent additional problems during the remission.

Some children still do not eat despite these approaches. When loss of appetite and weight persist, the nurse should investigate the family situation to determine whether any factors (e.g., conditioned aversion to food, environmental stress related to eating, controlling behavior, anger) might be contributing to the problem. Nasogastric tube feedings or total parenteral nutrition may be implemented for children with significant nutritional problems.

Mucosal Ulceration. One of the most distressing side effects of several drugs is GI mucosal cell damage, which can produce ulcers anywhere along the alimentary tract. Oral ulcers greatly compound anorexia because eating is extremely uncomfortable, but the following interventions may be helpful: (1) provide a bland, moist, soft diet appropriate for the child's age and preferences; (2) use a soft sponge toothbrush (Toothettes) or cotton-tipped applicator; (3) provide frequent mouthwashes with normal saline (using a solution of 1 tsp of table salt and

---

Cancer Chemotherapy Guidelines can be obtained from the Oncology Nursing Society, 125 Enterprise Drive, Pittsburgh, PA 15275; 866-257-4ONS, 412-859-6100; fax: 877-369-5497; e-mail: customer.service@ons.org; http://www.ons.org.

[†]Detailed chemotherapeutic agents are outlined in Wilson D, Hockenberry MJ: *Wong's clinical manual of pediatric nursing*, ed 8, St. Louis, 2008, Mosby.

1 pt of water) or sodium bicarbonate mouth rinses (using a solution of 1 tsp of baking soda in 1 qt of water); and (4) use local anesthetics (e.g., Chloraseptic lozenges) or nonprescription preparations without alcohol (e.g., hydrocortisone dental paste [Orabase], antiseptic mouth rinse [UlcerEase], diphenhydramine [Benadryl] and aluminum and magnesium hydroxide [Maalox] solution). Although local anesthetics are effective in temporarily relieving the pain, many children dislike the taste and numb feeling they produce.

> **NURSING TIP** Viscous lidocaine is not recommended for young children; if applied to the pharynx, it may depress the gag reflex, increasing the risk of aspiration. Seizures have been rarely associated with the use of oral viscous lidocaine, most likely as a result of the rapid absorption into the bloodstream via the oral lesions (Cho, Cheng, and Cheng, 2000).

Other preparations that may be used to prevent or treat mucositis include chlorhexidine gluconate (Peridex) because of its dual effectiveness against candidal and bacterial infections, antifungal troches (lozenges) or mouthwash, and lip balm (e.g., Aquaphor) to keep the lips moist. Agents that should not be used include lemon glycerin swabs (irritate eroded tissue and can decay teeth), hydrogen peroxide (delays healing by breaking down protein), and milk of magnesia (dries mucosa).

Stomatitis may cause such difficulty with eating that the child may require hospitalization for hydration, parenteral nutrition, and pain control (often with IV morphine). The child will usually choose the foods that are best tolerated, and the nurse should encourage parents to relax any eating pressures. Because the stomatitis is a temporary condition, the child can resume good food habits after the ulcers heal. Dental hygiene can become a serious problem for children with orthodontic appliances. Sometimes it may be necessary to remove the braces to allow chemotherapy to continue.

Rectal ulcers are managed by meticulous toilet hygiene, warm sitz baths after each bowel movement, and use of an occlusive ointment or dressing applied to the ulcerated area to promote epithelialization. Stool softeners are necessary to prevent further discomfort. Parents are advised to record bowel movements because the child may voluntarily avoid defecation to prevent discomfort. Rectal thermometers and suppositories are contraindicated because insertion may further traumatize the area.

Neuropathy. Vincristine and, to a lesser extent, vinblastine can cause various neurotoxic effects. Nursing interventions for management of these effects include (1) administering stool softeners or laxatives for severe constipation caused by decreased bowel innervation; (2) maintaining good body alignment and, if patient is on bed rest, using a footboard or high-top shoes to minimize or prevent footdrop; (3) carrying out safety measures during ambulation because of weakness and numbing of the extremities, which may cause difficulty in walking or fine hand movement; and (4) providing a soft or liquid diet for severe jaw pain.

Hemorrhagic Cystitis. Sterile hemorrhagic cystitis, a side effect of chemical irritation to the bladder from cyclophosphamide, can be decreased and often prevented by (1) promoting a liberal fluid intake (at least $1\frac{1}{2}$ times the recommended daily fluid requirement); (2) frequent voiding immediately after feeling the urge, before bed, and after arising; (3) administering the drug early in the day to allow for sufficient oral intake and voiding; and (4) administering mesna (an agent that provides protection to the bladder) as ordered. If oral home administration is prescribed, the family needs *specific* instructions regarding exactly how much fluid the child must have.

> **NURSING TIP** If signs of cystitis occur, such as burning or bleeding on urination, prompt medical evaluation is needed.

Alopecia. Hair loss is a common side effect of several chemotherapeutic drugs and cranial irradiation, although not all children lose their hair during drug therapy. It is better to warn children and parents of this side effect than to allow them to think that it is only a remote possibility. A soft cotton cap is the most comfortable headwear for children. Polyester increases perspiration and causes itching. Other options include scarves, hats, or a wig.

The nurse should also inform the family that hair regrows in 3 to 6 months and may be of a different color and texture. Frequently, the hair is darker, thicker, and curlier than before. If the child chooses not to wear a wig, attention to some type of head covering, especially in cold climates and during exposure to sun, and scalp hygiene are important. The scalp should be washed like any other body part.

Moon Face. Short-term steroid therapy produces no acute toxicities and produces two beneficial reactions: increased appetite and a sense of well-being. However, it does produce alterations in appearance, which, although not clinically significant, can be extremely distressing to older children. One of these is moon face, in which the child's face becomes rounded and puffy. It is helpful to reassure the child that after cessation of the drug, the facial shape will return to normal. Unlike hair loss, little can be done to camouflage this obvious change. If the child resumes activity early in the course of treatment, the change may be less noticeable to peers than after a long absence.

Mood Changes. Shortly after beginning steroid therapy, children experience a number of mood changes that range from feelings of well-being and euphoria to depression and irritability. If parents are unaware of these drug-induced changes, they may become unduly concerned. The nurse should warn them of the reactions and encourage them to discuss the behavioral changes with each other and the child.

Provide Emotional Support

An important aspect of continued emotional support involves the prognosis. Although leukemia is no longer invariably fatal, it must be remembered that survival statistics are only average estimates and apply to those children treated with the latest protocols since diagnosis. For low-risk children, the chances may be better, but for high-risk children, they may be significantly poorer. Of those who do survive after discontinuing therapy, some will relapse. Therefore, at present, only the passage of time is positive confirmation of the child's being ultimately "cured" of the disease. Remission, even in excess of 5 years, cannot be equated with a cure. With increasing concern regarding late effects of treatment, continued surveillance of the child's health status is needed. The nurse who is working with family members must individualize information regarding the "numbers" and the potential risks. An understanding of each member's emotional needs, as well as competent care of physical ones, is essential to the positive, growth-promoting support of the family. Comprehensive emotional support for the family of the child with a potentially fatal illness is discussed in Chapter 18.

LYMPHOMAS

Pediatric lymphomas are the third most common group of malignancies in children and adolescents. The lymphomas, a group of neoplastic diseases that arise from the lymphoid and hematopoietic systems, are

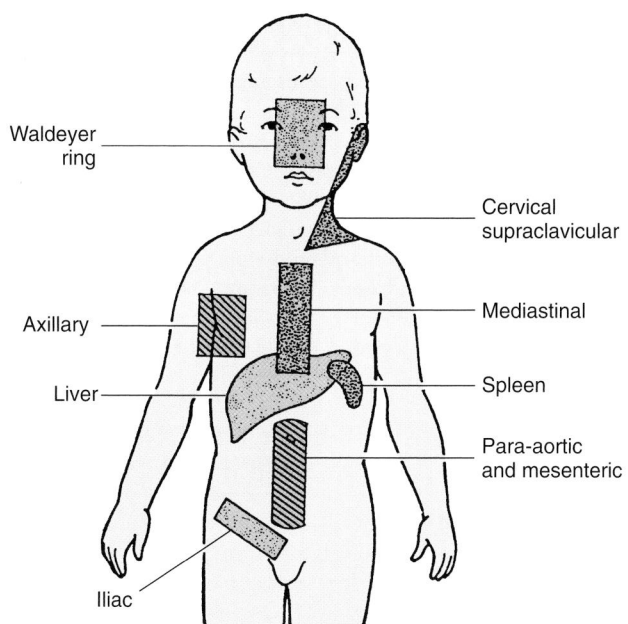

FIG 26-5 Main areas of lymphadenopathy and organ involvement in Hodgkin lymphoma.

Waldeyer ring
Cervical supraclavicular
Axillary
Mediastinal
Liver
Spleen
Para-aortic and mesenteric
Iliac

divided into Hodgkin lymphoma (HL) and non-Hodgkin lymphoma (NHL). These diseases are further subdivided according to tissue type and extent of disease. Whereas NHL is more prevalent in children younger than 14 years of age, HL is prevalent in adolescence and the young adult period, with a striking increase between ages 15 and 19 years.

Hodgkin Lymphoma

Hodgkin lymphoma is a neoplastic disease that originates in the lymphoid system and primarily involves the lymph nodes. It predictably metastasizes to nonnodal or extralymphatic sites, especially the spleen, liver, bone marrow, and lungs, although no tissue is exempt from involvement (Fig. 26-5). It is classified according to four histologic types: (1) lymphocytic predominance, (2) nodular sclerosis, (3) mixed cellularity, and (4) lymphocytic depletion. Accurate staging of the extent of disease is the basis for treatment protocols and expected prognoses.

The Ann Arbor staging system assigns a stage based on the number of sites of lymph node involvement, presence of extranodal disease, and history of any symptoms. Patients are classified as A if asymptomatic and as B if they have the following symptoms: temperature of 38° C (100.4° F) or higher for 3 consecutive days, drenching night sweats, or unexplained loss of body weight (≥10%) over the preceding 6 months. Nonspecific systemic symptoms include fatigue, anorexia, mild to severe pruritus, and slight weight loss (Metzger, Krasin, Hudson, and others, 2011).

Asymptomatic enlarged cervical or supraclavicular lymphadenopathy is the most common presentation of HL. Other systemic symptoms may be manifested, including cough, abdominal discomfort, and anorexia. Because multiple organs may be involved, diagnosis is based on several tests and the extent of metastatic disease. Tests include a CBC, erythrocyte sedimentation rate, serum copper, ferritin level, fibrinogen, immunoglobulins, uric acid level, liver function tests, T-cell function studies, and urinalysis. Radiographic tests include chest radiography and computed tomography (CT) of the neck and chest; CT and magnetic resonance imaging of the abdomen and pelvis; and

positron emission tomography (PET), which is replacing the gallium scan and bone scan to identify metastatic disease.

A lymph node biopsy is essential to establish histologic diagnosis and staging. The presence of Reed-Sternberg cells is characteristic of HL. These large cells, which are multilobed and nucleated with abundant cytoplasm and a typically halolike clear zone around the nucleolus, are often described as having an "owl's eyes" appearance (Metzger, Krasin, Hudson, and others, 2011). A bone marrow aspiration and biopsy is usually performed in patients with advanced disease, B symptoms, or disease recurrence (Metzger, Krasin, Hudson, and others, 2011). With the advent of CT and PET scans to identify metastatic disease and multiagent therapy to eradicate metastatic disease, surgical staging involving a laparotomy with splenectomy is no longer performed.

Therapeutic Management

The primary modalities of therapy are radiation and chemotherapy. Each may be used alone or in combination based on the clinical staging. Radiation may involve only the involved field (IF), an extended field (EF) (involved areas plus adjacent nodes), or total nodal irradiation (TNI), depending on the extent of involvement.

An effective combination of chemotherapy widely used is MOPP (mechlorethamine, vincristine [Oncovin], procarbazine, prednisone) or ABVD (Adriamycin, bleomycin, vinblastine, dacarbazine). However, this therapy combination has caused severe late effects, especially secondary malignancies. Other drug combinations such as COPP (cyclophosphamide, vincristine, prednisone, procarbazine) as a substitute for MOPP have minimized late effects.

Follow-up care of children no longer receiving therapy is essential to identify relapse and secondary cancers. In children with splenic irradiation, prophylactic antibiotics are administered for an indefinite period. Also, immunizations against pneumococci and meningococci are recommended.

Prognosis. Long-term survival for all stages of HL is excellent. The goal for pediatric HL's curative treatment is to provide minimal morbidity with the highest quality of life (Metzger, Krasin, Hudson, and others, 2011).

Nursing Care Management

Nursing care involves the same objectives as for patients with other types of cancer, specifically: (1) preparation for diagnostic and operative procedures, (2) explanation of treatment side effects, and (3) child and family support (see Chapter 18). Because this is most often a disease of adolescents and young adults, the nurse must have an appreciation of their psychologic needs and reactions during the diagnostic and treatment phases.

The most common side effect of irradiation is fatigue. This is particularly difficult for active, outgoing school-age children and adolescents because it prevents them from keeping up with their peers. Sometimes adolescents will push themselves to the point of physical exhaustion rather than admit and succumb to the decreased activity tolerance. The nurse cautions parents to observe for behavior such as extreme fatigue at the end of the day, falling asleep at the dinner table, inability to concentrate on homework, or an increased susceptibility to infection. A regular bedtime and scheduled rest periods are important for these children, especially during chemotherapy, when myelosuppression increases the risk of infection and debilitation. Before discharge, the nurse should discuss a feasible school schedule with the parents and child.

An area of concern for adolescents is the high risk of sterility from irradiation and chemotherapy. Both drugs, particularly procarbazine and alkylating agents, and irradiation to the gonads can lead to infertility. Adolescents should be informed of these side effects early in the course of the diagnosis and treatment. Sperm banking is now offered at many cancer centers before the initiation of treatment in adolescent boys. Sexual function is not altered, although the appearance of secondary sexual characteristics and menstruation may be delayed in pubescent children. Delayed sexual maturation may be an extremely sensitive and stressful issue for children (see Chapter 17).

Non-Hodgkin Lymphoma

Non-Hodgkin lymphoma occurs more frequently in children than HL. Histologic classification of childhood NHL is strikingly different from that of HL, as demonstrated in the following statements:
- The disease is usually diffuse rather than nodular.
- The cell type is either undifferentiated or poorly differentiated.
- Dissemination occurs early, more often, and rapidly.
- Mediastinal involvement and invasion of meninges are common.

NHL exhibits a variety of morphologic, cytochemical, and immunologic features, similar to the diversity seen in leukemia. Classification is based on the histologic pattern: (1) lymphoblastic, (2) Burkitt or non-Burkitt, or (3) large cell. Immunologically, these cells are also classified as T cells; B cells; or non-T, non-B cells (lacking immunologic properties). The clinical staging system used in HL is of little value in NHL, although it has been modified, and other systems have been developed.

Diagnostic Evaluation

Because the clinical presentation of most children with NHL is widespread disseminated disease, thorough pathologic staging is unnecessary. Clinical manifestations depend on the anatomic site and extent of involvement. These manifestations include many of those seen in Hodgkin disease and leukemia, as well as organ symptoms related to pressure from enlargement of adjacent lymph nodes, such as intestinal or airway obstruction, cranial nerve palsies, and spinal paralysis.

Recommendations for staging include a surgical biopsy of an enlarged node, histopathologic confirmation of disease with cytochemical and immunologic evaluation, bone marrow examination, radiographic studies (especially tomograms of the lungs and GI organs), and lumbar puncture.

Therapeutic Management

The treatment protocols for NHL include aggressive use of irradiation and chemotherapy. Similar to leukemic therapy, the protocols include induction, consolidation, and maintenance phases, some with intrathecal chemotherapy. Several antineoplastic agents used in the treatment of NHL include vincristine, prednisone, L-asparaginase, methotrexate, 6-mercaptopurine, cytarabine, cyclophosphamide, anthracyclines, and teniposide or etoposide. Chemotherapy is the main component of treatment for NHL in children (Gross and Perkins, 2011).

Prognosis. The prognosis is excellent for children with NHL. In developed countries, more than 80% of children with NHL are now cured with modern therapy, even patients with widely disseminated disease (Gross and Perkins, 2011).

Nursing Care Management

Nursing care of children with NHL is similar to that required for children with leukemia. Many of the same drugs are used, although the schedules differ. Because of the intense chemotherapy, nursing care is primarily directed toward managing the side effects of these agents and providing supportive care to the child and family.

IMMUNOLOGIC DEFICIENCY DISORDERS

A number of disorders can cause profound, often life-threatening alterations within the body's immune system. The most serious are those conditions that completely depress immunity, such as severe combined immunodeficiency disease (SCID). However, the one disorder that generates the most anxiety, within both the family and the community at large, is HIV infection/AIDS.

Several classifications of immune dysfunction exist. AIDS, SCID, and Wiskott-Aldrich syndrome (WAS) are syndromes wherein the body is unable to mount an immune response. The immune response can also be misdirected. In autoimmune disorders, antibodies, macrophages, and lymphocytes attack healthy cells.

HUMAN IMMUNODEFICIENCY VIRUS INFECTION AND ACQUIRED IMMUNODEFICIENCY SYNDROME

Since the first cases of AIDS were identified in the early 1980s, HIV infection has generated intense medical investigation. Research has led to early diagnosis of and improved medical treatments for HIV infection, changing this disease from a rapidly fatal one to a chronic disease.

Epidemiology

The first AIDS cases in the pediatric population in the United States were identified in children born to HIV-infected mothers and in children who received blood products. More than 90% of these children acquired the disease perinatally from their mothers. Smaller numbers of children were infected through the transfusion of contaminated blood or blood products before 1985 or were infected through sexual abuse. Currently, the principal modes of HIV transmission to the pediatric population are mother-to-child transmission and adolescent risky behaviors such as sexual activity and IV drug use (Simpkins, Siberry, and Hutton, 2009).

The estimated number of children with perinatally acquired AIDS peaked in 1992; subsequent years have seen significant declines. This trend is a result of implementation of recommended HIV counseling and voluntary testing practices and the use of highly active antiretroviral therapy (HAART) to prevent perinatal transmission. HAART, typically a combination of two nucleoside analog reverse transcriptase inhibitors and a protease inhibitor, is the current standard in the United States for the treatment of HIV-infected pregnant women, and it has significantly reduced the transmission of HIV (Perinatal HIV Guidelines Working Group, 2007; Simpkins, Siberry, and Hutton, 2009). Routine HIV counseling and voluntary testing using the opt-out approach (right of refusal) is the recommended standard of care for pregnant women in the United States (Centers for Disease Control and Prevention [CDC], 2007; AAP, Committee on Pediatric AIDS, 2008; Simpkins, Siberry, and Hutton, 2009).

Etiology

Human immunodeficiency virus is a retrovirus that is transmitted by lymphocytes and monocytes. It is found in the blood, semen, vaginal secretions, and breast milk. It has an incubation or latency period of months to years (Yogev and Chadwick, 2007). There are different strains of HIV. Whereas HIV-2 is prevalent in Africa, HIV-1 is the dominant strain in the United States and elsewhere. Horizontal transmission of HIV occurs through intimate sexual contact or parenteral exposure to blood or body fluids containing visible blood. Perinatal (vertical) transmission occurs when an HIV-infected pregnant woman passes the infection to her infant. There is no evidence that *casual* contact between infected and uninfected individuals can spread the virus.

Pathophysiology

The HIV virus primarily infects a specific subset of T lymphocytes, the CD_4^+ T cells. The virus takes over the machinery of the CD_4^+ lymphocyte, using it to replicate itself, rendering the CD_4^+ cell dysfunctional. The CD_4^+ lymphocyte count gradually decreases over time, leading to progressive immunodeficiency. The count eventually reaches a critical level below which there is substantial risk of opportunistic illnesses, followed by death.

Clinical Manifestations

Common clinical manifestations of HIV infection in children are varied (Box 26-9). The diagnosis of AIDS is associated with certain illnesses or conditions. The most common AIDS-defining conditions observed among American children are listed in Box 26-10. Other problems in these children may include short stature, malnutrition, and cardiomyopathy. CNS abnormalities resulting from HIV infection may include neuropsychologic deficits; developmental disabilities; and deficits in motor skills, communication, and behavioral functioning.

Diagnostic Evaluation

For children 18 months of age and older, the HIV enzyme-linked immunosorbent assay (ELISA) and Western blot immunoassay are performed to determine HIV infection. In infants born to HIV-infected mothers, these assays will be positive because of the presence of maternal antibodies derived transplacentally. Maternal antibodies may persist in the infant up to 18 months of age. Therefore, other diagnostic tests are used, most commonly the HIV polymerase chain reaction for detection of proviral DNA. With this technique, almost all infected infants can be diagnosed between 1 and 6 months of age (Goldschmidt and Fogler, 2006; Yogev and Chadwick, 2007).

The CDC (1994) has developed a classification system to describe the spectrum of HIV disease in children (Table 26-2). The system indicates the severity of clinical signs and symptoms and the degree of immunosuppression. Mild signs and symptoms include lymphadenopathy, parotitis, hepatosplenomegaly, and recurrent or persistent sinusitis or otitis media. Moderate signs and symptoms include lymphoid interstitial pneumonitis (LIP) and a variety of organ-specific dysfunctions or infections. Severe signs and symptoms include AIDS-defining illnesses with the exception of LIP. Children with LIP have a better prognosis than those with other AIDS-defining illnesses. In children whose HIV infection is not yet confirmed, the letter *E* (vertically exposed) is placed in front of the classification. The immune categories are based on CD_4^+ lymphocyte counts and percentages. Age adjustment of these numbers is necessary because normal counts, which are relatively high in infants, decline steadily until 6 years of age, when they reach adult norms.

Therapeutic Management

The goals of therapy for HIV infection include slowing the growth of the virus, preventing and treating opportunistic infections, and providing nutritional support and symptomatic treatment. Antiretroviral drugs work at various stages of the HIV life cycle to prevent reproduction of functional new virus particles. Although not a cure, these drugs can suppress viral replication, preventing further deterioration of the immune system, and thus delay disease progression. Classes of antiretroviral agents include nucleoside reverse transcriptase inhibitors (e.g., zidovudine, didanosine, stavudine, lamivudine, abacavir), nonnucleoside reverse transcriptase inhibitors (e.g., nevirapine, delavirdine, efavirenz), nucleotide reverse transcriptase inhibitors (e.g., adefovir),

---

BOX 26-9 COMMON CLINICAL MANIFESTATIONS OF HUMAN IMMUNODEFICIENCY VIRUS INFECTION IN CHILDREN

- Lymphadenopathy
- Hepatosplenomegaly
- Oral candidiasis
- Chronic or recurrent diarrhea
- Failure to thrive
- Developmental delay
- Parotitis

BOX 26-10 COMMON DEFINING CONDITIONS FOR ACQUIRED IMMUNODEFICIENCY SYNDROME IN CHILDREN

- *Pneumocystis carinii* pneumonia
- Lymphoid interstitial pneumonitis
- Recurrent bacterial infections
- Wasting syndrome
- Candidal esophagitis
- Human immunodeficiency virus encephalopathy
- Cytomegalovirus disease
- *Mycobacterium avium-intracellulare* complex infection
- Pulmonary candidiasis
- Herpes simplex disease
- Cryptosporidiosis

TABLE 26-2 PEDIATRIC HUMAN IMMUNODEFICIENCY VIRUS INFECTION CLASSIFICATION*

IMMUNOLOGIC CATEGORY	N: NO SIGNS OR SYMPTOMS	A: MILD SIGNS OR SYMPTOMS	B: MODERATE SIGNS OR SYMPTOMS†	C: SEVERE SIGNS OR SYMPTOMS†
No evidence of suppression	N1	A1	B1	C1
Evidence of moderate suppression	N2	A2	B2	C2
Severe suppression	N3	A3	B3	C3

From Centers for Disease Control and Prevention: 1994 Revised classification system for human immunodeficiency virus infection in children less than 13 years of age, *MMWR Recomm Rep* 43(RR-12):1–10, 1994.
*Children whose human immunodeficiency virus infection status is not confirmed are classified by using this table with the letter E (for perinatally exposed) placed before the appropriate classification code (e.g., EN2).
†Both category C and lymphoid interstitial pneumonitis in category B are reportable to state and local health departments as acquired immunodeficiency syndrome.

protease inhibitors (e.g., indinavir, saquinavir, ritonavir, nelfinavir, amprenavir), and adjunctive antiretrovirals (e.g., hydroxyurea). Combinations of antiretroviral drugs are used to stall the emergence of drug resistance. Antiretroviral therapy regimens and guidelines are continually evolving. Therapy is lifelong, making adherence difficult. Laboratory markers (CD_4^+ lymphocyte count, viral load) assist in monitoring both disease progression and response to therapy.

Pneumocystis carinii pneumonia (PCP) is the most common opportunistic infection of children infected with HIV. It occurs most frequently between 3 and 6 months of age. All infants born to HIV-infected women should receive prophylaxis until HIV infection is reasonably excluded (AAP, Committee on Pediatric AIDS, 2000a; Havens, Mofenson, and Committee on Pediatric AIDS, 2009; Simpkins, Siberry, and Hutton, 2009). Trimethoprim–sulfamethoxazole (TMP-SMZ) is the agent of choice. If adverse effects are experienced with TMP-SMZ, dapsone or pentamidine can be used.

Prophylaxis is often employed for other opportunistic infections, such as disseminated *Mycobacterium avium-intracellulare* complex, candidiasis, or herpes simplex. IV gamma globulin (IVGG) has been helpful in preventing recurrent or serious bacterial infections in some HIV-infected children.

Immunization against common childhood illnesses, including the pneumococcal and influenza vaccines, is recommended for all children exposed to and infected with HIV (AAP, Committee on Pediatric AIDS, 2000b; Simpkins, Siberry, and Hutton, 2009). Varicella (chickenpox) vaccine and measles, mumps, and rubella (MMR) vaccine can be administered if there is no evidence of severe immunocompromise. Because antibody production to vaccines may be poor or decrease over time, immediate prophylaxis after exposure to several vaccine-preventable diseases (e.g., measles, varicella) is warranted. It should be recognized that children receiving IVGG prophylaxis may not respond to the MMR vaccine if given in close proximity to the IVGG dose (Allen, 2007; CDC, 2003).

HIV infection often leads to marked failure to thrive and multiple nutritional deficiencies. Nutritional management may be difficult because of recurrent illness, diarrhea, and other physical problems. Intensive nutritional interventions should be instituted when the child's growth begins to slow or weight begins to decrease.

Prognosis

Early recognition and improved medical care have changed HIV disease from a rapidly fatal illness to a chronic disease. After the introduction of combination antiretroviral therapy, the numbers of new AIDS cases and deaths declined substantially. In the United States, the annual number of AIDS cases affecting children younger than 13 years of age had a sharp, steady decline since the early 1990s (Klause and Johnson, 2007; Simpkins, Siberry, and Hutton, 2009). In contrast, adolescents and young adults (13–24 years of age) with AIDS that represent a minority of U.S. cases (≈5%) constitute one of the fastest growing groups of newly infected persons in the country (Simpkins, Siberry, and Hutton, 2009; Yogev and Chadwick, 2007).

QUALITY PATIENT OUTCOMES: HIV
- Early recognition of signs and symptoms of HIV
- HIV infection slowed or maintained
- Growth and development promoted
- No infectious complications or cancer development
- Adherence to antiretroviral therapy
- Prolonged survival
- Quality of life supported

Nursing Care Management

Education concerning transmission and control of infectious diseases, including HIV infection, is essential for individuals with HIV infection and anyone involved in their care. The basic tenets of standard precautions should be presented in an age-appropriate manner, with careful consideration of the educational levels of the individuals (see Infection Control, Chapter 22). Safety issues, including appropriate storage of special medications and equipment (e.g., needles and syringes), are emphasized.

Unfortunately, relatives, friends, and others in the general public may be fearful of contracting HIV infection, and criticism and ostracism of the child and family may occur. In an effort to protect the child, the family may limit the child's activities outside the home. Although certain precautions are justified in limiting exposure to sources of infections, they must be tempered with concern for the child's normal developmental needs. Both the family and the community need ongoing education about HIV to dispel many of the myths that have been perpetuated by uninformed persons.*

Prevention is a key component of HIV education. Educating adolescents about HIV is essential in preventing HIV infection in this age group. Education should include the routes of transmission, the hazards of IV and other recreational drug use, and the value of sexual abstinence and safe sex practices. Such education should be a part of anticipatory guidance provided to all adolescent patients. Nurses can also encourage adolescents at risk to undergo HIV counseling and testing. In addition to identifying infected teenagers and getting them into care, such counseling affords adolescents an opportunity to learn about and possibly change their risky behaviors.

The multiple complications associated with HIV disease are potentially painful (Ezekowitz, 2009). Aggressive pain management is essential for these children to have an acceptable quality of life. Their pain may be caused by infections (e.g., otitis media, dental abscess), encephalopathy (e.g., spasticity), adverse effects of medications (e.g., peripheral neuropathy), or an unknown source (e.g., deep musculoskeletal pain). Pain is not only related to the disease processes but also to various treatments these children often undergo, including venipunctures, lumbar punctures, biopsies, and endoscopies. Ongoing assessment of pain is crucial and is most easily accomplished in older children who are able to communicate. Nonverbal and developmentally delayed children are more difficult to assess. The nurse should be alert for signs of pain such as emotional detachment, lack of interactive play, irritability, and depression. Effective pain management depends on the appropriate use of pharmacologic agents, including EMLA or LMX cream, acetaminophen, NSAIDs, muscle relaxants, and opioids. Tolerance to opioids may indicate increased dosing; monitored use ensures safety. Nonpharmacologic interventions (e.g., guided imagery, hypnosis, relaxation, and distraction techniques) are useful adjuncts.

Common psychosocial concerns include disclosing the diagnosis to the child, making custody plans when the parent is infected, and anticipating the loss of a family member. Other stressors may include financial difficulties, HIV-associated stigma, efforts to keep the diagnosis secret, other infected family members, and the multiple losses associated with HIV. Most mothers of these children are single mothers who are also HIV infected. As primary caretakers, they often attend to the needs of their child first, neglecting their own health in the process. The nurse is an integral part of the multidisciplinary team necessary

---

*Additional information is available from the National HIV/AIDS Hotline: 800-448-0440; outside the United States: 301-315-2816.

for the successful management of the complex medical and social problems of these families.

Children with HIV infection attend daycare centers and schools. It is well established that the risk of HIV transmission in these settings is minimal. These institutions are required to follow CDC and Occupational Safety and Health Administration (OSHA) guidelines for infection control measures. Standard precautions describing proper management of blood and body fluids should also be followed. It is recommended that school personnel receive current HIV information and include it in the health education curriculum for kindergarten through twelfth grade (AAP, Committee on Pediatric AIDS and Committee on Infectious Diseases, 1999; AAP, Committee on Pediatric AIDS, 2000a). School nurses play a vital role in educating the school staff, students, and parents. They are also invaluable in monitoring the needs of known affected children.

Confidentiality is another major issue in daycare or school attendance. Parents and legal guardians have the right to decide whether they inform the daycare or school of their child's HIV diagnosis. Unfortunately, myths about HIV infection continue to exist, and the family often wishes to avoid any potential criticism or ostracism of the child.

SEVERE COMBINED IMMUNODEFICIENCY DISEASE

Severe combined immunodeficiency disease is a defect characterized by absence of both humoral and cell-mediated immunity. The terms Swiss-type lymphopenic agammaglobulinemia (an autosomal recessive form of the disease) and X-linked lymphopenic agammaglobulinemia have been used to describe this disorder, which, as the names imply, can follow either mode of inheritance.

Susceptibility to infection occurs early in life, most often in the first month of life. The child has chronic infections, fails to completely recover from infections, is frequently reinfected, and is infected with unusual agents. Failure to thrive is a consequence of the persistent illnesses.

Diagnosis is usually based on a history of recurrent, severe infections from early infancy; a familial history of the disorder; and specific laboratory findings, which include lymphopenia, lack of lymphocyte response to antigens, and absence of plasma cells in the bone marrow. Documentation of immunoglobulin deficiency is difficult during infancy because of the normally delayed response of infants in producing their own immunoglobulins and material transfer of immunoglobulin G (IgG).

Therapeutic Management

The definitive treatment for SCID is HSCT from a histocompatible donor, a haplo-identical donor (usually a parent), or a matched unrelated donor. IVIG infusions and PCP prophylaxis are used to augment the humoral immunity until the transplant is performed. Several investigators are attempting gene therapy with some success, offering hope that gene therapy may eventually be the treatment of choice for cases of SCID (Bonilla and Geha, 2009; Buckley, 2007).

Nursing Care Management

Nursing care focuses on preventing infection and supporting the child and family. The care is consistent with that needed for HSCT for any condition (see p. 889). Because the prognosis for SCID is very poor if a compatible bone marrow donor is not available, nursing care is directed at supporting the family in caring for a child with a life-threatening illness (see Chapter 18). Genetic counseling is essential because of the modes of transmission in either form of the disorder.

WISKOTT-ALDRICH SYNDROME

Wiskott-Aldrich syndrome is an X-linked recessive disorder characterized by a triad of abnormalities: (1) thrombocytopenia, (2) eczema, and (3) immunodeficiency of selective functions of B lymphocytes and T lymphocytes. An abnormal gene has been identified on the proximal arm of the X chromosome and designated the WAS protein (Bonilla and Geha, 2009; Buckley, 2007). At birth, the presenting feature may be bleeding such as bloody diarrhea as a result of thrombocytopenia. As the child grows older, recurrent infection and eczema become more severe, and the bleeding becomes less frequent.

Eczema is typical of the allergic type and readily becomes superinfected. Chronic infection with herpes simplex is a frequent problem and may lead to chronic keratitis of the eye with loss of vision. Chronic pulmonary disease, sinusitis, and otitis media result from repeated infections. In children who survive the bleeding episodes and overwhelming infections, malignancy presents an additional risk to survival. Medical treatment involves:

- Counteracting the bleeding tendencies with platelet transfusions
- Administering IVIG to provide passive immunity
- Administering prophylactic antibiotics to prevent and control infection.
- Providing aggressive local therapy for the eczema

WAS can be cured with HSCT (Albert, Notarangelo, and Ochs, 2010; Buckley, 2007). Several clinical trials focused on replacing the normal WAS gene are being conducted to determine the most effective vector (Albert, Notarangelo, and Ochs, 2010).

Nursing Care Management

Because of the poor prognosis for these children, the main nursing consideration is supporting the family in the care of a fatally ill child (see Chapter 18). Physical care is directed at controlling the problems imposed by the disorder. The measures used to control bleeding are similar to those for hemophilia and vWD (see previous discussions). Another major goal is prevention or control of infection. Because eczema is a troublesome problem, nursing measures specific to this condition are especially important (see Chapter 30). The genetic implications of this X-linked recessive disorder differ little from those of any other X-linked disorder.

TECHNOLOGIC MANAGEMENT OF HEMATOLOGIC AND IMMUNOLOGIC DISORDERS

BLOOD TRANSFUSION THERAPY

Technologic advances in blood banking and transfusion medicine enable the administration of only the blood component needed by the child, such as packed RBCs in anemia or platelets for bleeding disorders. However, regardless of the blood component infused, all transfusions have some risks. Nurses need to be aware of the possible complications and the appropriate interventions. Table 26-3 summarizes the major hazards of transfusions, the signs and symptoms typically associated with each, and nursing responsibilities. General guidelines that apply to all transfusions include:

- Take vital signs, including blood pressure, *before* administering blood to establish baseline data for intratransfusion and posttransfusion comparison; 15 minutes after initiation; hourly while blood is infusing; and on completion of transfusion.
- Check the identification of the recipient with the donor's blood group and type regardless of the blood product being used.

TABLE 26-3   NURSING CARE OF THE CHILD RECEIVING BLOOD TRANSFUSIONS

COMPLICATION	SIGNS AND SYMPTOMS	PRECAUTIONS AND NURSING RESPONSIBILITIES
Immediate Reactions		

Hemolytic reactions
Most severe type but rare
Incompatible blood
Incompatibility in multiple
  transfusions
	Sudden, severe headache
	Chills
	Shaking
	Fever
	Pain at needle site and along
	  venous tract
	Nausea and vomiting
	Sensation of tightness in chest
	Red or black urine
	Flank pain
	Progressive signs of shock or
	  renal failure
		Identify donor and recipient blood types and groups before transfusion is begun; verify
		  with another nurse or practitioner.
		Transfuse blood slowly for first 15–20 min or initial 20% of blood volume; remain with
		  patient.
		Stop transfusion immediately in event signs or symptoms occur, maintain patent IV line,
		  and notify practitioner.
		Save donor blood to recrossmatch with patient's blood.
		Monitor for evidence of shock.
		Insert urinary catheter and monitor hourly outputs.
		Send samples of patient's blood and urine to laboratory for presence of hemoglobin
		  (indicates intravascular hemolysis).
		Observe for signs of hemorrhage resulting from DIC.
		Support medical therapies to reverse shock.

Febrile reactions Leukocyte or platelet antibodies Plasma protein antibodies	Fever Chills	May give acetaminophen for prophylaxis. Leukocyte-poor RBCs are less likely to cause reaction. Stop transfusion immediately; report to practitioner for evaluation.
Allergic reactions Recipient reaction to allergens in donor's blood	Urticaria Pruritus Flushing Asthmatic wheezing Laryngeal edema	Give antihistamines for prophylaxis to children with tendency to allergic reactions. Stop transfusion immediately. Administer epinephrine for wheezing or anaphylactic reaction.

Circulatory overload
Too rapid transfusion (even a
  small quantity)
Transfusion of excessive
  quantity of blood (even slowly)
	Precordial pain
	Dyspnea
	Rales
	Cyanosis
	Dry cough
	Distended neck veins
	Hypertension
		Transfuse blood slowly.
		Prevent overload by using packed RBCs or administering divided amounts of blood.
		Use infusion pump to regulate and maintain flow rate.
		Stop transfusion immediately if there are signs of overload.
		Place child upright with feet in dependent position to increase venous resistance.

Air emboli
May occur when blood is
  transfused under pressure
	Sudden difficulty in breathing
	Sharp pain in chest
	Apprehension
		Normalize pressure before container is empty when infusing blood under pressure.
		Clear tubing of air by aspirating air with syringe at nearest Y connector if air is observed
		  in tubing; disconnect tubing and allow blood to flow until air has escaped only if a Y
		  connector is not available.

Hypothermia	Chills Low temperature Irregular heart rate Possible cardiac arrest	Allow blood to warm at room temperature (<1 hr). Use approved mechanical blood warmer or electric warming coil to warm blood rapidly; never use microwave oven. Take temperature if patient complains of chills; if subnormal, stop transfusion.

Electrolyte disturbances
Hyperkalemia (in massive
  transfusions or in patients
  with renal problems)
	Nausea, diarrhea
	Muscular weakness
	Flaccid paralysis
	Paresthesia of extremities
	Bradycardia
	Apprehension
	Cardiac arrest
		Use washed RBCs or fresh blood if patient is at risk.

Delayed Reactions		

Transmission of infection
Hepatitis
HIV infection
Malaria
Syphilis
Other bacterial or viral infection
	Signs of infection (e.g., jaundice)
	Toxic reaction—High fever,
	  severe headache or substernal
	  pain, hypotension, intense
	  flushing, vomiting or diarrhea
		Blood is tested for antibodies to HIV, hepatitis C virus, and hepatitis B core antigen; in
		  addition, blood is tested for hepatitis B surface antigen and alanine aminotransferase,
		  and a serologic test is performed for syphilis. Units that test positive are destroyed.
		  Individuals at risk for carrying certain viruses are deterred from donation.
		Report any sign of infection, and if it occurs during transfusion, stop transfusion
		  immediately, send sample for culture and sensitivity testing, and notify practitioner.

Alloimmunization
Antibody formation
Occurs in patients receiving
  multiple transfusions
	Increased risk of hemolytic,
	  febrile, and allergic reactions
		Use limited number of donors.
		Observe carefully for signs of reactions.

Delayed hemolytic reaction	Destruction of RBCs and fever 5–10 days after transfusion	Observe for posttransfusion anemia and decreasing benefit from successive transfusion.

DIC, Disseminated intravascular coagulation; *HIV,* human immunodeficiency virus; *IV,* intravenous; *RBC,* red blood cell.

- Administer the first 50 ml of blood or 20% of the volume (whichever is smaller) *slowly* and stay with the child.
- Administer with normal saline on a piggyback setup or have normal saline available.
- Administer blood through an appropriate filter to eliminate particles in the blood and prevent the precipitation of formed elements; gently shake the container frequently.
- Use blood within 30 minutes of its arrival from the blood bank; if it is not used, return it to the blood bank—do not store it in the regular unit refrigerator.
- Infuse a unit of blood (or the specified amount) within 4 hours. If the infusion will exceed this time, the blood should be divided into appropriately sized quantities by the blood bank and the unused portion refrigerated under controlled conditions.
- If a reaction of any type is suspected, stop the transfusion, take vital signs, maintain a patent IV line with normal saline and new tubing, notify the practitioner, and do not restart the transfusion until the child's condition has been medically evaluated.

Although hemolytic reactions are rare, ABO incompatibility remains the most common cause of death from blood transfusion, and human error (administration of the wrong type to the patient or mislabeling of the blood product) is usually responsible (Bell, 2007; Tondon, Pandey, Mickey, and others, 2010). Hemolysis can also cause the release of large quantities of phospholipids, which are capable of stimulating DIC. Acute kidney shutdown and eventual renal failure are a result of renal vasoconstriction from antigen–antibody complexes derived from the RBC surface.

Blood is usually administered to children by infusion pump; therefore, the usual precautions and management related to pumps apply. When the blood is started with a standard transfusion set, the filter chamber is filled to allow the total filter to be used. The drip chamber is partially filled with blood to permit counting of the drops. In adjusting the flow rate, it is important to remember that blood administration sets do not use microdrops (60 drops/ml) but regular drops (usually 10–15 drops/ml). The nurse must consider this when calculating the flow rate.

HEMATOPOIETIC STEM CELL TRANSPLANTATION

Hematopoietic stem cell transplantation is used to establish healthy hematopoiesis in both malignant and nonmalignant disease. Candidates for transplantation are children who have disorders that are unlikely to be cured by other means. The most common conditioning allogenic regimens use intensive ablative therapy consisting of high-dose combination chemotherapy with or without total-body irradiation (Bollard, Krance, and Heslop, 2011). After the immune system is suppressed to prevent rejection of the transplanted marrow, the stem cells are harvested from the bone marrow, peripheral blood, or the umbilical vein of the placenta and given to the patient by IV transfusion. The newly transfused stem cells will begin to repopulate the ablative bone marrow. In essence, the recipient will accept a new blood-forming organ.

The selection process for a suitable donor and the potential complications in transplantation are related to the HLA system complex. Some of the major HLA antigens are A, B, C, D, and DR. There is a wide diversity for each of these HLA loci. There are more than 20 different HLA-A antigens that can be inherited and more than 40 different HLA-B antigens.

The genes are inherited as a single unit or haplotype. A child inherits one unit from each parent; thus, a child and each parent have one identical and one nonidentical haplotype. Because the possible haplotype combinations among siblings follow the laws of mendelian genetics, there is a one in four chance that two siblings have two identical haplotypes and are perfectly matched at the HLA loci.

The importance of HLA matching is to prevent the serious complication known as GVHD. Because the child's immune system is essentially rendered nonfunctional, there is little difficulty with bone marrow rejection by the recipient. However, the donor's marrow may contain antigens not matched to the recipient's antigens, which begin attacking body cells. The more closely the HLA systems match, the less likely GVHD is to develop. However, for patients with low-risk disease, the increase risk of chronic GVHD needs to be balanced against the risk of relapse (Bollard, Krance, and Heslop, 2011).

Different types of HSCT are now performed. Allogeneic HSCT involves matching a histocompatible donor with the recipient. However, allogeneic HSCT is limited by the presence of a suitable marrow donor.

Because of the limited numbers of patients having HLA-identical siblings, other types of allogeneic transplants have evolved. Umbilical cord blood stem cell transplantation is an established, rich source of hematopoietic stem cells. Because stem cells can be found with high frequency in the circulation of newborns, cord blood transplantation has become an alternative for some children. The benefit of using umbilical cord blood is the blood's relative immunodeficiency at birth because of naivety of cord T cells, which have a lower risk of GVHD-related problems (Bollard, Krance, and Heslop, 2011).

Autologous HSCTs use the patient's own marrow that was collected from disease-free tissue, frozen, and sometimes treated to remove malignant cells. Children with solid tumors such as neuroblastoma, lymphomas, rhabdomyosarcoma, Ewing sarcoma, and Wilms tumor have been treated with autologous HSCTs.

Peripheral stem cell transplants (PSCTs) are also used in children with cancer. PSCT, a type of autologous transplant, differs in the way stem cells are collected from the patient. CSF is first given to stimulate the production of peripheral blood stem cells (PBSCs) as an alternative to marrow as source of stem cells (Bollard, Krance, and Heslop, 2011). After the WBC count is high enough, the stem cells are collected by an apheresis machine. This machine filters out peripheral stem cells from whole blood, returning the remainder of the blood cells and plasma to the child. The peripheral stem cells are then frozen until the patient is ready for the PSCT.

Nursing Care Management

The care of children undergoing HSCT is similar to that of any child receiving chemotherapy and radiotherapy. These children are usually hospitalized for several weeks after HSCT. Because of the risk of infection, the unit may use such measures as strict handwashing, screening visitors, laminar airflow rooms, and institutional isolation policies. Throughout this long ordeal, the family is concerned with successful engraftment and fear of fatal complications (see Family-Centered Care box). Consequently, nurses need to provide sensitive care and maintain a supportive attitude during the many crises that may arise. If the procedure is not successful, the families need care consistent with that required by the family of any child with a life-threatening disorder (see Chapter 18).

APHERESIS

Apheresis is the removal of blood from an individual, separation of the blood into its components, retention of one or more of these components, and reinfusion of the remainder of the blood into the individual. Apheresis is most often used to remove large quantities of platelets from healthy adult donors. These transfusion products have greatly

FAMILY-CENTERED CARE

The Decision for a Hematopoietic Stem Cell Transplant

A family's decision for a child to undergo HSCT may be fraught with challenges. Often the child is facing certain death from the malignancy. The preparation of the child for the transplant also places the patient at great medical risk.

When the preparatory regimen is begun and the child's immune system is destroyed, there is no turning back. Unlike kidney transplantation, HSCT does not have a "rescue" procedure, such as dialysis, for supportive therapy. If the donor is a sibling, the issue of his or her marrow "saving" the brother or sister can be a concern, especially if the transplant fails. Parents often must leave the home to stay at the transplant center and encounter additional stressors such as arranging child care, taking a leave from work, and managing finances. The patient faces the greatest stress—fear of HSCT failure or life-threatening complications.

HSCT, Hematopoietic stem cell transplantation.

prolonged the survival of patients with hematologic and oncologic diseases.

This technique is used to remove PBSCs from children before they receive HSCT or high-dose chemotherapy or radiotherapy, which is severely toxic to the bone marrow. These PBSCs can then be used to restore the child's bone marrow. Apheresis is also used as a therapeutic modality. The blood component that is diseased or toxic is separated from the blood, and the remainder is returned to the individual. Therapeutic apheresis is considered part of standard therapy for many diseases. Plasma is selectively removed from individuals with hyperviscosity, life-threatening complications of myasthenia gravis, Guillain-Barré syndrome, thrombotic thrombocytopenic purpura, and certain drug overdoses. WBCs are removed from individuals with high-WBC-count leukemia.

Nursing Care Management

Difficult venous access and small blood volume can limit the ability to use this therapy in infants and young children. Education of the family and child includes the purposes of the therapy and the technology.

Specially trained individuals perform the apheresis procedure. Attention focuses on the rate of removal, blood component separation, and reinfusion of blood into the child. Vital signs are monitored, and the child is continuously observed for any adverse reactions secondary to the circulatory volume changes and the anticoagulant used.

When apheresis components are infused, nursing measures differ depending on whether the product is autologous (blood component from the child) or allogeneic (blood component from another individual). Autologous components are the child's own blood; therefore, a major precaution is proper identification to ensure the correct component. The rate of infusion should be adjusted to the child's tolerance. If the product is allogeneic, all precautions for blood transfusions apply.

KEY POINTS

- Anemia is defined as reduction of RBCs or Hgb concentration to levels below normal for age; disorders are classified by etiology and physiology or morphology.
- The nurse's role in treatment of anemia is to assist in establishing a diagnosis, prepare the child for laboratory tests, administer prescribed medications, decrease tissue oxygen needs, implement safety precautions, and observe for complications.
- The main nursing goal in prevention of nutritional anemia is parent education regarding correct feeding practices.
- SCA is a hereditary hemoglobinopathy caused by normal adult HbA being partly or completely replaced by sickle HbS.
- Nursing care of the child with SCA focuses on teaching the family how to prevent and recognize sickle cell problems; managing pain during crises; and helping the child and parents adjust to a lifelong, chronic disease.
- Nursing care of the child with β-thalassemia includes observing for complications of multiple blood transfusions, assisting the child in coping with the effects of illness, and fostering parent–child adjustment to long-term illness.
- Causes of acquired AA include irradiation, drugs, industrial and household chemicals, infections, and infiltration and replacement of myeloid elements; however, the majority of cases are idiopathic.

- Clotting depends on three processes: vascular spasm, platelet aggregation, and coagulation and clot formation.
- Nursing care of the child with hemophilia involves preventing bleeding by decreasing the risk of injury, recognizing and managing bleeding with factor replacement, preventing the crippling effects of joint degeneration, and preparing and supporting the child and family for home care.
- Goals in the care of the child with leukemia are to prepare the family for diagnostic and therapeutic procedures, prevent complications of myelosuppression, manage problems of irradiation and drug toxicity, and provide continued emotional support.
- The lymphomas include HL and NHL and are disorders involving the lymphoid system.
- Immunodeficiency disorders render the affected individual unable to fight infectious organisms.
- HIV infection is primarily acquired in infancy from a HIV-infected parent and in adolescence from engaging in high-risk behaviors.
- Blood transfusions supply needed blood components.
- HSCT replaces the diseased or malfunctioning bone marrow with viable blood stem cells.
- Apheresis is the selective removal of a blood component. It can be used to supply cellular elements needed for therapy (i.e., platelets or stem cells) or to remove diseased components.

REFERENCES

Albert MH, Notarangelo LD, Ochs HD: Clinical spectrum, pathophysiology and treatment of Wiskott-Aldrich syndrome, *Curr Opin Hematol* 18:42–48, 2010.

Allen UD: Immunizations for children with cancer, *Pediatr Blood Cancer* 49:1102–1108, 2007.

American Academy of Pediatrics, Committee on Infectious Diseases, Pickering L, editor: *Red book: report of the Committee on Infectious Diseases,* ed 28, Elk Grove Village, Ill, 2009, Author.

American Academy of Pediatrics, Committee on Pediatric AIDS: Identification and care of HIV-exposed and HIV-infected infants, children, and adolescents in foster care, *Pediatrics* 106(1):149–153, 2000a.

American Academy of Pediatrics, Committee on Pediatric AIDS: Technical report: perinatal human immunodeficiency virus testing and prevention of transmission, *Pediatrics* 106(6): 1–12, 2000b.

American Academy of Pediatrics, Committee on Pediatric AIDS: HIV testing and prophylaxis to prevent mother-to-child transmission in the United States, *Pediatrics* 122:1127–1134, 2008.

American Academy of Pediatrics, Committee on Pediatric AIDS and Committee on Infectious Diseases: Issues related to human immunodeficiency virus transmission in schools, child care, medical settings, the home, and community, *Pediatrics* 104(2):318–324, 1999.

American Pain Society: *Guidelines for the management of acute and chronic pain in sickle-cell disease*, Glenview, Ill, 1999, Author.

Anderson N: Hydroxyurea therapy: improving the lives of patients with sickle cell disease, *Pediatr Nurs* 32(6):541–543, 2006.

Andrews NC, Ullrich CK, Fleming MD: Disorders of iron metabolism and sideroblastic anemia. In Orkin SH, Nathan D, Ginsburg D, and others, editors: *Nathan and Oski's hematology of infancy and childhood*, ed 7, Philadelphia, 2009, Saunders.

Armstrong-Wells J, Grimes S, Sidney D, and others: Utilization of TCD screening for primary stroke prevention in children with sickle cell disease, *Neurology* 72:1316–1321, 2009.

Auerbach M: Should intravenous iron be upfront therapy for iron deficiency anemia? *Pediatr Blood Cancer* 56:511–512, 2011.

Baker RD, Greer FR, Committee on Nutrition American Academy of Pediatrics: Diagnosis and prevention of iron deficiency and iron-deficiency anemia in infants and young children (0–3 years of age), *Pediatrics* 126:1040–1050, 2010.

Bell MD: Red blood cell transfusions, *Pediatr Rev* 28(8):299–304, 2007.

Berglund S, Westrup B, Domellof M: Iron supplements reduce the risk of iron deficiency anemia in marginally low birth weight infants, *Pediatrics* 126:e874–e883, 2010.

Bhatia S: Epidemiology. In Wallace WHB, Green DM, editors: *Late effects of childhood cancer*, London, 2004, Arnold.

Bollard CM, Krance RA, Heslop HE: Hematopoietic stem cell transplantation in pediatric oncology. In Pizzo PA, Poplack DG, editors: *Principles and practice of pediatric oncology*, ed 6, Philadelphia, 2011, Lippincott.

Bonilla FA, Geha RS: Primary immunodeficiency diseases. In Orkin SH, Nathan D, Ginsburg D, and others, editors: *Nathan and Oski's hematology of infancy and childhood*, ed 7, Philadelphia, 2009, Saunders.

Brandow AM, Weisman SJ, Panepinto JA: The impact of a multidisciplinary pain management model on sickle cell disease pain hospitalizations, *Pediatr Blood Cancer* 56: 789–793, 2011.

Buckley RH: Evaluation of the immune system. In Behrman RE, Kliegman RM, Jenson HTS, and others, editors: *Nelson textbook of pediatrics*, ed 18, Philadelphia, 2007, Saunders.

Cappellini MD, Porter JB, El-Beshlawy A, and others: Tailoring iron chelation by iron intake and serum ferritin trends: the prospective multicenter EPIC study of desferasirox in 1744

patients with various transfusion-dependent anemias, *Haematologica* 95:557–566, 2010.

Carley A: Anemia: when is it iron deficiency? *Pediatr Nurs* 29(2):127–133, 2003.

Centers for Disease Control and Prevention: 1994 revised classified system for human immunodeficiency virus infection in children less than 13 years of age, *MMWR Recomm Rep* 43(RR-12):1–10, 1994.

Centers for Disease Control and Prevention: Advancing HIV prevention: new strategies for a changing epidemic—United States, *MMWR Morb Mortal Wkly Rep* 52(15):329–332, 2003.

Centers for Disease Control and Prevention: *Mother-to-child (perinatal) HIV transmission and prevention*, Atlanta Department of Health and Human Services, 2007, retrieved from http://www.cdc.gov/hiv/topics/perinatal/resources/factsheets/perinatal.htm#2.

Cho S, Cheng AC, Cheng MCK: Oral care for children with leukemia, *Hong Kong Med J* 6(2):203–208, 2000.

Consolini DM: Thrombocytopenia in infants and children, *Pediatr Rev* 32:135–151, 2011.

Cunningham MJ, Sankaran VG, Nathan DG, and others: The thalassemias. In Orkin SH, Nathan DG, Ginsburg D, and others, editors: *Nathan and Oski's hematology of infancy and childhood*, ed 7, Philadelphia, 2009, Saunders.

Curry H: Bleeding disorder basics, *Pediatr Nurs* 30(5):402–405, 2004.

Cusick SE, Mei Z, Freedman DS, and others: Unexplained decline in the prevalence of anemia among U.S. children and women between 1988–1994 and 1999–2002, *Am J Clin Nutr* 88:1611–1617, 2008.

DeBaun MR, Vichinsky E: Hemoglobinopathies. In Kliegman RM, Jenson HB, Behrman RE, and others, editors: *Nelson textbook of pediatrics*, ed 18, Philadelphia, 2007, Saunders.

Driscoll MC: Sickle cell disease, *Pediatr Rev* 28(7):259–267, 2007.

Ezekowitz RAB: Hematologic manifestations of systemic diseases. In Orkin SH, Nathan DG, Ginsburg D, and others, editors: *Nathan and Oski's hematology of infancy and childhood*, ed 7, Philadelphia, 2009, Saunders.

Glader B: Anemias of inadequate production. In Behrman RE, Kliegman RM, Jenson HTS, and others, editors: *Nelson textbook of pediatrics*, ed 18, Philadelphia, 2007, Saunders.

Goldschmidt RH, Fogler JA: Opportunities to prevent HIV transmission to newborns, *Pediatrics* 117(1):208–209, 2006.

Gross TG, Perkins SL: Malignant non-Hodgkin lymphomas in children. In Pizzo PA, Poplack DG, editors: *Principles and practice of pediatric oncology*, ed 6, Philadelphia, 2011, Lippincott.

Haining, WN, Duncan C, Lehmann LE: Principles of bone marrow and stem cell transplantation. In Orkin SH, Nathan DG, Ginsburg D, and others, editors: *Nathan and Oski's hematology of infancy and childhood*, ed 7, Philadelphia, 2009, Saunders.

Havens PL, Mofenson LM, Committee on Pediatric AIDS: Evaluation and management of the infant exposed to HIV-1 in the United States, *Pediatrics* 122:1127–1134, 2009.

Heeney M, Dover GJ: Sickle cell disease. In Orkin SH, Nathan DG, Ginsburg D, and others, editors: *Nathan and Oski's hematology of infancy and childhood*, ed 7, Philadelphia, 2009, Saunders.

Hirst C, Owusu-Ofori S: Prophylactic antibiotics for preventing pneumococcal infection in children with sickle cell disease, *Cochrane Syst Rev* (11): CD003427, 2010.

Hord JD: The acquired pancytopenia. In Behrman RE, Kliegman RM, Jenson HTS, and others, editors: *Nelson textbook of pediatrics*, ed 18, Philadelphia, 2007, Saunders.

Howard J, Davies SC: Sickle cell disease in North Europe, *Scand J Clin Lab Invest* 67:27–38, 2007.

Hutter JJ: Childhood leukemia, *Pediatr Rev* 31:234–241, 2010.

Jemal A, Siegel R, Ward E, and others: Cancer statistics, 2009, *CA Cancer J Clin* 59(4):225–249, 2009.

Kaspers GJ, Creutzig U: Pediatric acute myeloid leukemia: international progress and future directions, *Leukemia* 19(12):2025–2029, 2005.

Klause BD, Johnson M: Paradigm shift: new testing guidelines for HIV, *Adv Nurse Pract* 15(3):59–93, 2007.

Koh AY, Pizzo PA: Infectious complications in pediatric cancer patients. In Pizzo PA, Poplack DG, editors: *Principles and practice of pediatric oncology*, ed 6, Philadelphia, 2011, Lippincott.

Kwiatkowski JL, Yim E, Miller S, and others for the STOP 2 study investigators: Effect of transfusion therapy on transcranial Doppler ultrasonography velocities in children with sickle cell disease, *Pediatr Blood Cancer* 56:777–782, 2011.

Lindley C, Goodin S, McCune J, and others: Prevention of delayed chemotherapy-induced nausea and vomiting after moderately high to highly emetogenic chemotherapy, *Am J Clin Oncol* 28(3):270–276, 2005.

Lokeshwar HR, Mehta M, Mehta N, and others: Prevention of iron deficiency anemia (IDA): how far have we reached? *Indian J Pediatr* 78(5):593–602, 2011.

Lucarelli G, Gaziev J: Advances in the allogeneic transplantation for thalassemia, *Blood Rev* 22:53–63, 2008.

Manco-Johnson MJ, Abshire TC, Shapiro AD, and others: Prophylaxis versus episodic treatment to prevent joint disease in boys with severe hemophilia, *N Engl J Med* 357:535–544, 2007.

Margolin JF, Rabin KR, Steuber CP, and others: Acute lymphoblastic leukemia. In Pizzo PA, Poplack DG, editors: *Principles and practice of pediatric oncology*, ed 6, Philadelphia, 2011, Lippincott.

Marsh JCW: Management of acquired aplastic anemia, *Blood Rev* 19:143–151, 2005.

Matrai J, Chuah MKL, VandenDriessche T: Preclinical and clinical progress in hemophilia gene therapy, *Curr Opin Hematol* 17:387–392, 2010.

McCann JC, Ames BN: An overview of evidence for a causal relation between iron deficiency during development and deficits in cognitive or behavioral function, *Am J Clin Nurs* 85(4): 931–945, 2007.

McCrae K: Immune thrombocytopenia: no longer "idiopathic," *Cleve Clin J Med* 78(6):358–373, 2011.

McGann PT, Ware RE: Hydroxyurea for sickle cell anemia: what have we learned and what questions remain? *Curr Opin Hematol* 18:158–165, 2011.

McKenzie SB: Anemias of disordered iron metabolism and heme synthesis. In McKenzie SB, editor: *Clinical laboratory hematology*, Upper Saddle River, NJ, 2004, Pearson Prentice Hall.

Metzger M, Krasin MJ, Hudson MM, and others: Hodgkin lymphoma. In Pizzo PA, Poplack DG, editors: *Principles and practice of pediatric oncology*, ed 6, Philadelphia, 2011, Lippincott.

Montgomery RR, Gill JC, DiPaola J: Hemophilia and von Willebrand disease. In Orkin SH, Nathan D, Ginsburg D, and others, editors: *Nathan and Oski's hematology of infancy and childhood*, ed 7, Philadelphia, 2009, Saunders.

National Hemophilia Foundation, Bleeding Disorders Information Center: Newly diagnosed: parents FAQ 2006, retrieved July 11, 2011, from http://www.hemophilia.org/bdi/bdi_newly7c.htm.

National Institutes of Health; National Heart, Lung, and Blood Institute, Division of Blood Disease and Resources: *The management of sickle cell disease*, NIH Pub No 02-2117, Bethesda, Md, 2002, NHLBI Health Information Network.

Ohls R, Christensen RD: Hemoglobin disorders. In Behrman RE, Kliegman RM, Jenson HTS, and others, editors: *Nelson textbook of pediatrics*, ed 18, Philadelphia, 2007, Saunders.

Pack-Mabien A, Haynes J: A primary care provider's guide to prevention and acute care management of adults and children with sickle cell disease, *J Am Acad Nurse Pract* 21:250–257, 2009.

Passweg JR, Marsh JCW: Aplastic anemia: first-line treatment by immunosuppression and sibling marrow transplantation, *Hematol Am Soc Hematol* 36–42, 2010.

Pearce JM, Sills RH: Childhood leukemia, *Pediatr Rev* 26(3):96–104, 2005.

Perinatal HIV Guidelines Working Group, Public Health Service Task Force: Recommendations for use of antiretroviral drugs in pregnant HIV-infected women for maternal health and interventions to reduce perinatal HIV transmission in the United States, 2007, retrieved March 24, 2008, from http://www.aidsinfo.nih.gov/ContentFiles/PerinatalGL.pdf.

Pui CH, Relling MV, Downing JR: Acute lymphoblastic leukemia, *N Engl J Med* 350:1535–1548, 2004.

Raphael JL, Mei M, Mueller BU, and others: High resource hospitalizations among children with vaso-occlusive crises in sickle cell disease, *Pediatr Blood Cancer*, 2011, in press.

Redding-Lallinger R, Knoll C: Sickle cell disease-pathophysiology and treatment, *Curr Probl Pediatr Adolesc Health Care* 36(10):346–376, 2006.

Richardson M: Microcytic anemia, *Pediatr Rev* 28(1):5–13, 2007.

Rodeghiero F, Stasi R, Gernsheimer T, and others: Standardization of terminology, definitions, and outcome criteria in immune thrombocytopenic purpura of adults and children: report from an international working group, *Blood* 113:2386–2393, 2009.

Ross C, Goldenberg NA, Hund D, and others: Athletic participation in severe hemophilia: bleeding and joint outcomes in children on prophylaxis, *Pediatrics* 124:1267–1272, 2009.

Saito M, Aogi K, Sekine I, and others: Palonosetron plus dexamethasone versus granisetron plus dexamethasone for prevention of nausea and vomiting during chemotherapy: a double-blind, double-dummy, randomised, comparative phase III trial, *Lancet Oncol* 10(2):115–124, 2009.

Scott JP, Montgomery RR: Platelet and blood vessel disorder. In Behrman RE, Kliegman RM, Jenson HTS, and others, editors: *Nelson textbook of pediatrics*, ed 18, Philadelphia, 2007, Saunders.

Sharathkumar AA, Pipe SW: Post-thrombotic syndrome in children: a single center experience, *J Pediatr Hematol Oncol* 30(4):261–266, 2008.

Shimamura A, Guinan EC: Acquired aplastic anemia. In Orkin SH, Nathan D, Ginsburg D, and others, editors: *Nathan and Oski's hematology of infancy and childhood*, ed 7, Philadelphia, 2009, Saunders.

Simpkins EP, Siberry GK, Hutton N: Thinking about HIV infection, *Pediatr Rev* 30:337–349, 2009.

Strouse JJ, Lanzkron S, Beach MC, and others: Hydroxyurea for sickle cell disease: a systematic review for efficacy and toxicity in children, *Pediatrics* 122(6):1332–1342, 2008.

Tondon R, Pandey P, Mickey KB, and others: Errors reported in cross match laboratory: a prospective data analysis, *Transfus Aphers Sci* 43:309–314, 2010.

Trigg M: Hematopoietic stem cells, *Pediatrics* 113(4):1051–1057, 2004.

Velasquez MP, Mariscalco MM, Goldstein SL, and others: Erythrocytapheresis in children with sickle cell disease and acute chest syndrome, *Pediatr Blood Cancer* 53(6):1060–1063, 2009.

Vichinsky E, Bernaudin F, Forni GL, and others: Long-term safety and efficacy of deferasirox (Exjade) for up to 5 years in transfusional iron-overloaded patients with sickle cell disease, *Br J Haematol* 154(3):387–197, 2011.

Vichinsky E, Onyekwere O, Porter J, and others: A randomized comparison of deferasirox versus deferoxamine for the treatment of transfusional iron overload in sickle cell disease, *Br J Haematol* 136:501–508, 2007.

Vichinsky E, Styles L: Sickle cell disease: pulmonary complications, *Hematol Oncol Clin North Am* 10(6):1275–1286, 1996.

Wang WC, Ware RE, Miller ST, and others: Hydroxycarbamide in very young children with sickle-cell anaemia: a multicentre, randomized, controlled trial (BABY HUG), *Lancet* 377:1663–1672, 2011.

Wilson DB: Acquired platelet defects. In Orkin SH, Nathan DG, Ginsburg D, and others, editors: *Nathan and Oski's hematology of infancy and childhood*, ed 7, Philadelphia, 2009, Saunders.

Yaish HM: Pediatric thalassemia, 2010, *Medscape*, retrieved June 10, 2011, from http://emedicine.medscape.com/article/958850-overview#a0199.

Yogev R, Chadwick EG: Acquired immunodeficiency syndrome (human immunodeficiency virus). In Kliegman RM, Jenson HB, Behrman RE, and others, editors: *Nelson textbook of pediatrics*, ed 18, Philadelphia, 2007, Saunders.

Zimmerman S, Schultz W, Davis J, and others: Sustained long-term hematologic efficacy of hydroxyurea at maximum tolerated dose in children with sickle cell disease, *Blood* 103(6):2039–2045, 2004.

The Child with Genitourinary Dysfunction

Barbara A. Montagnino and Patricia A. Ring

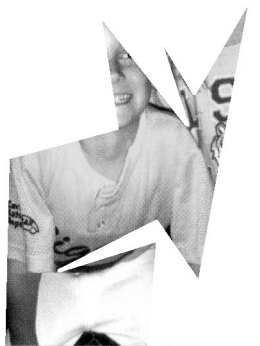

evolve WEBSITE

http://evolve.elsevier.com/wong/essentials
Animations—Bladder; Kidney Function
Case Studies—Acute Renal Failure; Urinary Tract Infection
Key Point Summaries

NCLEX-Style Review Questions
Nursing Care Plans—The Child with Acute Renal Dysfunction;
   The Child with Nephrotic Syndrome

CHAPTER OUTLINE

Genitourinary Dysfunction, 903
   Clinical Manifestations, 903
   Laboratory Tests, 904
   Nursing Care Management, 904
Genitourinary Tract Disorders and
   Defects, 904
   Urinary Tract Infection, 904
   Obstructive Uropathy, 910

External Defects, 911
   *Psychologic Problems Related to
      Genital Surgery, 911*
Glomerular Disease, 912
   Nephrotic Syndrome, 912
   Acute Glomerulonephritis, 915
Miscellaneous Renal Disorders, 916
   Hemolytic Uremic Syndrome, 916
   Wilms Tumor, 917

Renal Failure, 918
   Acute Renal Failure, 919
      *Nursing Care Plan: The Child with
      Acute Renal Dysfunction, 920*
   Chronic Renal Failure, 921
Technologic Management of Renal
   Failure, 924
   Dialysis, 924
   Transplantation, 925

LEARNING OBJECTIVES

On completion of this chapter the reader will be able to:
- Describe the various factors that contribute to urinary tract infections in infants and children.
- Discuss the preoperative preparation of the child and parents when the child has a structural defect of the genitourinary tract.
- Demonstrate an understanding of the causes and mechanisms of edema formation in nephrotic syndrome.
- Outline a nursing care plan for a child with nephrotic syndrome.

- Compare the child with minimal-change nephrotic syndrome and the child with acute glomerulonephritis in terms of clinical manifestations and nursing care.
- Contrast the causes, complications, and management of acute and chronic renal failure.
- List the types of renal dialysis.
- Recognize signs of kidney transplant rejection.

GENITOURINARY DYSFUNCTION

Assessment of kidney and urinary tract integrity and diagnosis of renal or urinary tract disease are based on several evaluative tools. Physical examination, history taking, and observation of symptoms are the initial procedures. In suspected urinary tract diseases or disorders, further assessment by laboratory, radiologic, and other evaluative methods is carried out. Figure 27-1 provides a review of the kidney and nephron structures.

CLINICAL MANIFESTATIONS

As in most disorders of childhood, the incidence and type of kidney or urinary tract dysfunction change with the age and maturation of the child. In addition, the presenting complaints and the significance of these complaints vary with maturation. For example, a complaint of enuresis has greater significance at age 8 years than at age 4 years. In newborns, urinary tract disorders are associated with a number of obvious malformations of other body systems, including the curious

Animation—Kidney Function

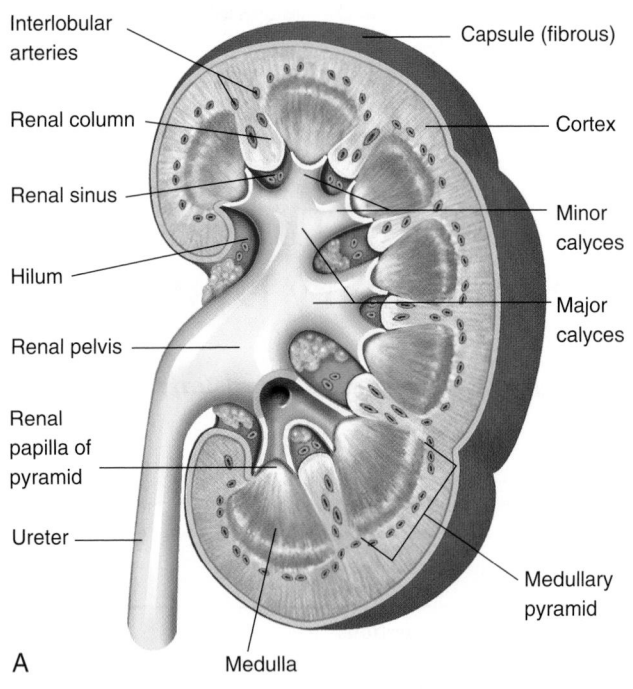

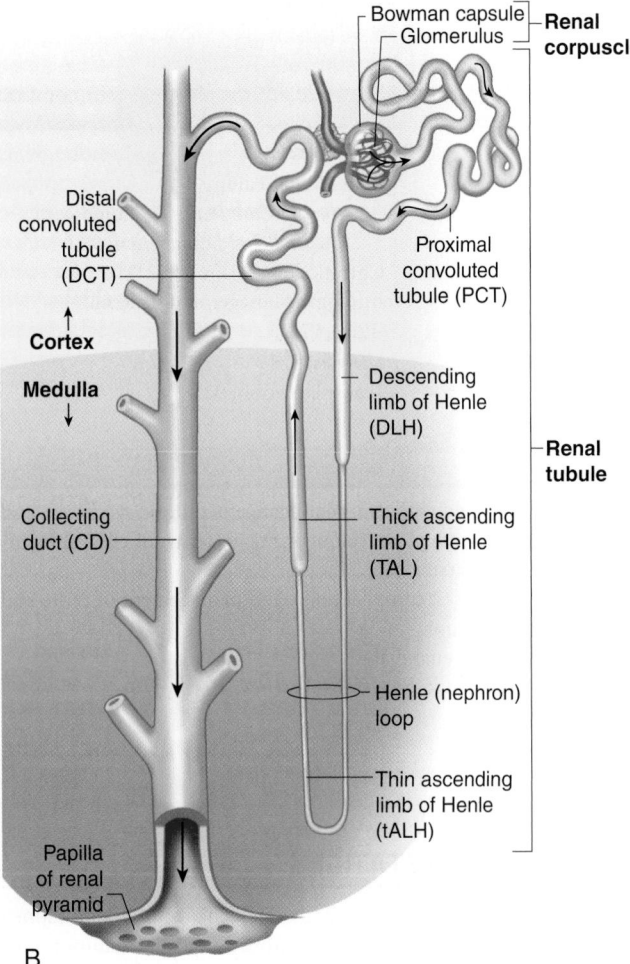

FIG 27-1 **A,** Kidney structure. **B,** Components of the nephron. (From Patton KT, Thibodeau GA: *Anatomy and physiology*, ed 7, St. Louis, 2010, Mosby.)

and unexplained but frequent association between malformed or low-set ears and urinary tract anomalies.

Many of the clinical manifestations of renal disease are common to a variety of childhood disorders, but their presence is an indication to obtain further information from the child's history, family history, and laboratory studies as part of a complete physical examination. Suspected renal disease can be further evaluated by means of radiographic studies and renal biopsy (Table 27-1).

LABORATORY TESTS

Both urine and blood studies contribute vital information for detection of renal problems. The single most important test is probably routine urinalysis. Specific urine and blood tests provide additional information. Because nurses are usually the persons who collect the specimens for examination and who often perform many of the screening tests, they should be familiar with the test, its function, and factors that can alter or distort the results of the test. The major urine and blood tests are outlined in Tables 27-2 and 27-3.

NURSING CARE MANAGEMENT

Nursing responsibilities in the assessment of genitourinary disorders or diseases begin with observation of the child for any manifestations that might indicate dysfunction. Many conditions have specific characteristics that distinguish them from other disorders. These are discussed as appropriate throughout the chapter.

The nurse is generally the one who is responsible for preparing infants, children, and parents for tests and for collection of urine and (sometimes) blood specimens for observation and laboratory analysis (see Preparation for Diagnostic and Therapeutic Procedures, and Collection of Specimens, Chapter 22). An important nursing responsibility is to maintain careful intake and output measurements and blood pressure for most children with genitourinary dysfunction and those who might be at risk for developing renal complications (e.g., children in shock, postoperative patients). For example, any significant degree of renal disease can diminish the glomerular filtration rate (GFR), a measure of the amount of plasma from which a given substance is totally cleared in 1 minute. A number of substances can be used, but the most useful clinical estimation of glomerular filtration is the clearance of creatinine, an end product of protein metabolism in muscle and a substance that is freely filtered by the glomerulus and secreted by renal tubular cells. The nurse's responsibility in this test is collection of urine, usually a 12- or 24-hour specimen.

GENITOURINARY TRACT DISORDERS AND DEFECTS

URINARY TRACT INFECTION

Infection of the genitourinary tract is one of the most common conditions of childhood. Up to 10% of children will have a febrile urinary tract infection (UTI) during the first 2 years of life (Kanellopoulos, Salakos, Spiliopoulou, and others, 2006). Among febrile boys, circumcision status is important in determining the risk for UTI. Uncircumcised male infants younger than 3 months of age had the highest prevalence of UTI (20.1%) of any group, male or female (Shaikh, Morone, Bost, and others, 2008). Circumcision status should be assessed in male infants with unexplained fever. UTI may involve the urethra and bladder (lower urinary tract) or the ureters, renal pelvis, calyces, and renal parenchyma (upper urinary tract).

TABLE 27-1	RADIOLOGIC AND OTHER TESTS OF URINARY SYSTEM FUNCTION		
TEST	**PROCEDURE**	**PURPOSE**	**COMMENTS AND NURSING RESPONSIBILITIES**
Urine culture and sensitivity	Collection of sterile specimen	Determines presence of pathogens and the drugs to which they are sensitive	Does not require specific parental permission Send specimen to laboratory immediately after collection Catheterization, clean-catch, or suprapubic specimen
Renal and bladder ultrasonography	Transmission of ultrasonic waves through renal parenchyma, along ureteral course, and over bladder	Allows visualization of renal parenchyma and renal pelvis without exposure to external-beam radiation or radioactive isotopes Visualization of dilated ureters and bladder wall also possible	Noninvasive procedure
Testicular (scrotal) ultrasonography	Transmission of ultrasonic waves through scrotal contents and testis	Allows visualization of scrotal contents, including testis Testicular ultrasonography is used to identify masses, and Doppler-enhanced ultrasonography is used to differentiate hyperemia of epididymo-orchitis from ischemia or torsion	Noninvasive procedure
Scout film	Flat plate radiograph of abdomen and pelvis for KUB	Detects and establishes renal outlines, presence of calculi, or opaque foreign bodies in bladder	Prepare as for routine x-ray film
Voiding cystourethrography	Contrast medium injected into bladder through urethral catheter until bladder is full; films taken before, during, and after voiding	Visualizes bladder outline and urethra, reveals reflux of urine into ureters, and shows complications of bladder emptying	Prepare child for catheterization
Radionuclide (nuclear) cystogram	Radionuclide-containing fluid injected through urethral catheter until bladder is full; images generated before, during, and after voiding	Alternative to voiding cystourethrography in children with allergy to intravesical contrast material Allows evaluation of reflux, although visualization of anatomic details is relatively poor	Prepare child for catheterization Reassure patient and parents that allergic response to contrast materials is avoided by use of radionuclide
Radioisotope imaging studies	Contrast medium injected intravenously; computer analysis to measure uptake or washout (excretion) for analysis of organ function	DTPA radioisotope used to measure GFR; estimate of differential renal function and renal washout to determine presence and location of upper urinary tract obstruction DMSA radioisotope used to visualize renal scars and differential renal function; does not visualize ureters and bladder MAG3 radioisotope combines features of DTPA (evaluation of upper urinary tract obstruction) with features of DMSA radioisotope (differential renal function)	Insert or assist with insertion of IV infusion Monitor IV infusion Urethral catheterization may accompany DTPA radioisotope scan; prepare child for catheterization when indicated
IVP (IV urography; excretory urography)	IV injection of a contrast medium Medium secreted and concentrated by tubules X-ray films made 5, 10, and 15 minutes after injection; delayed films (30, 60 minutes, and so on) are obtained if obstruction suspected	Defines urinary tract Provides information about integrity of kidneys, ureters, and bladder Retroperitoneal masses visualized when they shift position of ureters	Preparation for test: **Infants up to 2 years of age**—no solid food; omit one bottle on morning of examination; perform studies early to avoid withholding of fluids **Children ages 2–14 years**—give cathartic evening before examination, nothing orally after midnight, enema (soapsuds) morning of examination
CT	Narrow-beam x-rays and computer analysis provide precise reconstruction of area	Visualizes vertical or horizontal cross section of kidney Especially valuable to distinguish tumors and cysts	Noncontrast scan is noninvasive Contrast-enhanced CT scan preparation similar to that for IVP
Cystoscopy	Direct visualization of bladder and lower urinary tract through small scope inserted via urethra	Investigation of bladder and lower tract lesions; visualizes ureteral openings, bladder wall, trigone, and urethra	Give nothing orally after midnight Carry out preoperative preparations Prepare the child for cystoscopy

Continued

TABLE 27-1　RADIOLOGIC AND OTHER TESTS OF URINARY SYSTEM FUNCTION—cont'd

TEST	PROCEDURE	PURPOSE	COMMENTS AND NURSING RESPONSIBILITIES
Retrograde pyelography	Contrast medium injected through ureteral catheter	Visualizes pelvic calyces, ureters, and bladder	Give cathartic if ordered Give preoperative medication if ordered Observe for reaction to contrast medium Monitor vital signs after procedure
Renal angiography	Contrast medium injected directly into renal artery via catheter placed in femoral artery (or umbilical artery in newborn) and advanced to renal artery	Visualizes renal vascular system, especially for renal arterial stenosis	Prepare child for insertion of a spinal needle or perfusion catheter in renal pelvis (anesthetic often required)
Whitaker perfusion test	Injection of contrast material through renal pelvis and ureters Measures pressures in renal pelvis and urinary bladder	Determine presence of obstruction causing upper urinary tract dilation	
Renal biopsy	Removal of kidney tissue by open or percutaneous technique for study by light, electron, or immunofluorescent microscopy	Yields histologic and microscopic information about glomeruli and tubules; helps distinguish among types of nephritic syndromes Distinguishes other renal disorders	Nothing orally 4–6 hours before test Premedicate as ordered Prepare setup for procedure Assist with procedure Take vital signs Apply pressure to area with pressure dressing and, if feasible, a sandbag Bed rest for 24 hours Observe for abdominal pain, tenderness Monitor input and output Surgical incision may be required in infants
Urodynamics	Set of tests designed to measure bladder filling, storage, and evacuation functions **Uroflowmetry**—Test to determine efficiency of urination **Cystometrography**—Graphic comparison of bladder pressure as a function of volume **Voiding pressure study**—Comparison of detrusor contraction pressure, sphincter electromyelogram, and urinary flow	Determine characteristic of voiding dysfunction Used to identify type (cause) of incontinence or urinary retention Especially valuable for voiding dysfunction complicated by urinary infection, urinary retention, or neurogenic bladder dysfunction	Prepare child for urinary catheterization The bladder will be filled with saline solution, and filling pressures will be recorded; the child may experience fullness, coolness from the saline fluid, and urine leakage during the study Insertion of needles may be required for sphincter EMG

CT, Computed tomography; *DMSA,* dimercaptosuccinic acid; *DTPA,* diethylenetriamine pentaacetic acid; *EMG,* electromyography; *GFR,* glomerular filtration rate; *IV,* intravenous; *IVP,* intravenous pyelography; *KUB,* kidney, ureters, and bladder; *MAG3,* mercaptoacetyltriglycine.

Because it is often impossible to localize the infection, the broad designation UTI is applied to the presence of significant numbers of microorganisms anywhere within the urinary tract except the distal third of the urethra, which is usually colonized with bacteria.

Classification

Infection of the urinary tract may be present with or without clinical symptoms. As a result, the site of infection is often difficult to pinpoint with any degree of accuracy. Various terms used to describe urinary tract disorders include:

Bacteriuria—Presence of bacteria in the urine

Asymptomatic bacteriuria—Significant bacteriuria (usually defined as >100,000 colony-forming units [CFUs]) with no evidence of clinical infection

Symptomatic bacteriuria—Bacteriuria accompanied by physical signs of UTI (dysuria, suprapubic discomfort, hematuria, fever)

Recurrent UTI—Repeated episode of bacteriuria or symptomatic UTI

Persistent UTI—Persistence of bacteriuria despite antibiotic treatment

Febrile UTI—Bacteriuria accompanied by fever and other physical signs of UTI; presence of a fever typically implies pyelonephritis

Cystitis—Inflammation of the bladder

Urethritis—Inflammation of the urethra

Pyelonephritis—Inflammation of the upper urinary tract and kidneys

Urosepsis—Febrile UTI coexisting with systemic signs of bacterial illness; blood culture reveals presence of urinary pathogen

Etiology

A variety of organisms can be responsible for UTI. *Escherichia coli* (80% of cases) and other gram-negative enteric organisms are most frequently implicated; these organisms are usually found in the anal and perineal region. Other organisms associated with UTI include

TABLE 27-2 URINE TESTS OF RENAL FUNCTION

TEST	NORMAL RANGE	DEVIATIONS	SIGNIFICANCE OF DEVIATIONS
Physical Tests			
Volume	Age related	Polyuria	Osmotic factors (urinary glucose level in diabetes mellitus)
	Newborn—30–60 ml	Oliguria	Retention caused by obstructive disease
	Children—Bladder capacity (oz)		Inadequate bladder emptying caused by neurogenic bladder or obstructive disorder
	= Age (years) + 2	Anuria	Obstruction of urinary tract; ARF
Specific	With normal fluid	High	Dehydration
gravity	intake—1.016–1.022		Presence of protein or glucose
	Newborn—1.001–1.020		Presence of radiopaque contrast medium after radiologic examinations
	Others—1.001–1.030	Low	Excessive fluid intake
			Distal tubular dysfunction
			Insufficient ADH
			Diuresis
Osmolality	Newborn—50–600 mOsm/L	Fixed at 1.010	Chronic glomerular disease
	Thereafter—50–1400 mOsm/L	High or low	Same as for specific gravity
			More sensitive index than specific gravity
Appearance	Clear pale yellow to deep gold	Cloudy	Contains sediment
		Cloudy reddish pink to reddish brown	Blood from trauma or disease
			Myoglobin after severe muscle destruction
		Light	Dilute
		Dark	Concentrated
		Red	Trauma
Chemical Tests			
pH	Newborn—5–7	Weak acid or neutral	If associated with metabolic acidosis, suggests tubular acidosis
	Thereafter—4.8–7.8	Alkaline	If associated with metabolic alkalosis, suggests potassium deficiency
	Average—6		Urinary infection
			Metabolic alkalosis
Protein level	Absent	Present	Abnormal glomerular permeability (e.g., glomerular disease, changes in blood pressure)
			Most kidney disease
			Orthostatic in some individuals
Glucose level	Absent	Present	Diabetes mellitus
			Infusion of concentrated glucose-containing fluids
			Glomerulonephritis
			Impaired tubular reabsorption
Ketone levels	Absent	Present	Conditions of acute metabolic demand (stress)
			Diabetic ketoacidosis
Leukocyte esterase	Absent	Present	Can identify both lysed and intact WBCs via enzyme detection
Nitrites	Absent	Present	Most species of bacteria convert nitrates to nitrites in the urine
Microscopic Tests			
WBC count	<1 or 2	>5 polymorphonuclear leukocytes/field	Urinary tract inflammatory process
		Lymphocytes	Allograft rejection
			Malignancy
RBC count	<1 or 2	4–6/field in centrifuged specimen	Trauma
			Stones
			Glomerular injury
			Infection
			Neoplasms
Presence of bacteria	Absent to a few	>100,000 organisms/ ml in centrifuged specimen	UTI
Presence of casts	Occasional	Granular casts	Tubular or glomerular disorders
		Cellular casts	Degenerative process in advanced renal disease
		WBC	Pyelonephritis
		RBC	Glomerulonephritis
		Hyaline casts	Proteinuria; usually transient

ADH, Antidiuretic hormone; *ARF,* acute renal failure; *RBC,* red blood cell; *UTI,* urinary tract infection; *WBC,* white blood cell.

TABLE 27-3	**BLOOD TESTS OF RENAL FUNCTION**		
TEST	**NORMAL RANGE (MG/DL)**	**DEVIATIONS**	**SIGNIFICANCE OF DEVIATIONS**
BUN	Newborn—4-18 Infant, child—5-18	Elevated	Renal disease—acute or chronic (the higher the BUN, the more severe the disease) Increased protein catabolism Dehydration Hemorrhage High protein intake Corticosteroid therapy
Uric acid	Child—2.0-5.5	Increased	Severe renal disease
Creatinine	Infant—0.2-0.4 Child—0.3-0.7 Adolescent—0.5-1.0	Increased	Renal impairment

BUN, Blood urea nitrogen.

Proteus, Pseudomonas, Klebsiella, and *Haemophilus* spp.; *Staphylococcus aureus*; and coagulase-negative *Staphylococcus* organisms. Several factors contribute to the development of UTI in childhood.

Anatomic and Physical Factors

The structure of the lower urinary tract is believed to account for the increased incidence of bacteriuria in females (Rosenthal, 2004). The short urethra, which measures about 2 cm (0.75 inch) in young girls and 4 cm (1.6 inches) in mature women, provides a ready pathway for invasion of organisms. In addition, the closure of the urethra at the end of micturition may return contaminated bacteria to the bladder. The longer male urethra (as long as 20 cm [8 inches] in an adult) and the antibacterial properties of prostatic secretions inhibit the entry and growth of pathogens.

> **NURSING TIP** Considerable evidence suggests there are fewer UTIs among circumcised male infants than among uncircumcised male infants, but the difference is not significant enough to recommend routine circumcision in newborns (American Academy of Pediatrics, Task Force on Circumcision, 1999).

The single most important host factor influencing the occurrence of UTI is **urinary stasis**. Ordinarily, urine is sterile, but at 37° C (98.6° F), it provides an excellent culture medium. Under normal conditions, the act of completely and repeatedly emptying the bladder flushes away any organisms before they have an opportunity to multiply and invade surrounding tissue. However, urine that remains in the bladder allows bacteria from the urethra to rapidly become established in the rich medium. Incomplete bladder emptying (stasis) may result from **reflux** (see Vesicoureteral Reflux, p. 909), anatomic abnormalities (especially those involving the ureters), dysfunction of the voiding mechanism, or extrinsic ureteral or bladder compression that may be caused by constipation. The key to preventing UTI is to maintain adequate blood supply to the bladder wall by avoidance of overdistention and high bladder pressure.

Altered Urine and Bladder Chemistry

Several mechanical and chemical characteristics of the urine and bladder mucosa help maintain urinary sterility. Increased fluid intake promotes flushing of the normal bladder and lowers the concentration of organisms in the infected bladder. Diuresis also seems to enhance the antibacterial properties of the renal medulla.

Most pathogens favor an alkaline medium. Normally, urine is slightly acidic with a median pH of 6. A urine pH of about 5 hampers but does not eliminate bacterial multiplication. Much has been reported about the use of cranberry products to increase urine acidity in an effort to prevent UTI. Recent review of the literature in adult subjects supports the use of cranberry products in reducing the incidence of UTI in women (Jepson, Mihaljevic, and Craig, 2008). Results of one study in children suggests that daily consumption of concentrated cranberry juice can prevent recurrence of symptomatic UTIs (Ferrara, Romaniello, Vitelli, and others, 2009). Further research that controls for type of cranberry product used, dosing regimens, and patient selection based on age and underlying medical condition is required to clarify unanswered questions before recommendations can be made regarding the use of this supplement, especially in the pediatric population.

Diagnostic Evaluation

The clinical manifestations of UTI depend on the child's age (Box 27-1). Diagnosis of UTI is confirmed by detection of bacteriuria in urine culture, but urine collection is often difficult, especially in infants and very small children. Several factors may alter a urine specimen, and contamination of a specimen by organisms from sources other than the urine, such as perineal and perianal flora in bag specimens, is the most frequent cause of false-positive results. Unless the specimen is a first morning sample, a recent high fluid intake may indicate a falsely low organism count. Therefore, children should not be encouraged to drink large volumes of water in an attempt to obtain a specimen quickly.

> **! NURSING ALERT**
>
> A child who exhibits the following should be evaluated for UTI:
> - Incontinence in a toilet-trained child
> - Strong-smelling urine
> - Frequency or urgency

More accurate estimates of bacterial content are obtained from **suprapubic aspiration** (in children younger than 2 years of age) and properly performed bladder catheterization (as long as the first few milliliters are excluded from collection). The specimen should be taken directly to the laboratory for immediate culture.

Tests to detect bacteriuria are being used with increased frequency in screening for UTI. The dipstick tests for leukocyte esterase or nitrite are quick and inexpensive methods for detecting infection before obtaining final culture results.

Localization of the infection site may involve more specific tests, including percutaneous kidney taps and bladder washout procedures. Other tests, such as ultrasonography, voiding cystourethrogram (VCUG), intravenous pyelogram (IVP), and DMSA (dimercaptosuccinic acid) scan, may be performed after the infection subsides to identify anatomic abnormalities contributing to the development of infection and existing kidney changes from recurrent infection.

Therapeutic Management

The objectives of treatment of children with UTI are to (1) eliminate current infection, (2) identify contributing factors to reduce the risk

BOX 27-1 CLINICAL MANIFESTATIONS OF URINARY TRACT DISORDERS OR DISEASE

Neonatal Period (Birth–1 Month)
Poor feeding
Vomiting
Failure to gain weight
Rapid respiration (acidosis)
Respiratory distress
Spontaneous pneumothorax or pneumomediastinum
Frequent urination
Screaming on urination
Poor urine stream
Jaundice
Seizures
Dehydration
Other anomalies or stigmata
Enlarged kidneys or bladder

Infancy (1–24 Months)
Poor feeding
Vomiting
Failure to gain weight
Excessive thirst
Frequent urination
Straining or screaming on urination
Foul-smelling urine
Pallor
Fever
Persistent diaper rash
Seizures (with or without fever)
Dehydration
Enlarged kidneys or bladder

Childhood (2–14 Years)
Poor appetite
Vomiting
Growth failure
Excessive thirst
Enuresis, incontinence, frequent urination
Painful urination
Swelling of face
Seizures
Pallor
Fatigue
Blood in urine
Abdominal or back pain
Edema
Hypertension
Tetany

(including trimethoprim and sulfisoxazole in combination), the cephalosporins, and nitrofurantoin.

If anatomic defects such as primary reflux or bladder neck obstruction are present, surgical correction of these abnormalities may be necessary to prevent recurrent infection. Follow-up study is an important component of medical management because the relapse rate is high and infection tends to recur 1 to 2 months after termination of treatment. The aim of therapy and careful follow-up is to reduce the chance of renal scarring. However, recurrent infection of the urinary bladder predisposes the individual to transient episodes of vesicoureteral reflux (VUR).

Vesicoureteral Reflux

Vesicoureteral reflux refers to the abnormal retrograde flow of bladder urine into the ureters. During voiding, urine is swept up the ureters and then flows back into the empty bladder, where it acts as a reservoir for bacterial growth until the next void. **Primary reflux** results from congenitally abnormal insertion of ureters into the bladder; **secondary reflux** occurs as a result of an acquired condition.

It is not clear that reflux necessarily causes infections. What is clear is that reflux is more likely to be associated with recurring kidney infections rather than simple bladder infections (cystitis). In the presence of reflux, infected urine (bacteria) from the bladder has access to the kidney, resulting in kidney infections (pyelonephritis). These children are usually very symptomatic with high fevers, vomiting, and chills. Reflux, when associated with UTI, is the most common cause of renal scarring in children. Renal scarring may occur with the first episode of febrile UTI. Reflux in the presence of sterile urine does not cause renal damage. Therefore, the most important concept in managing VUR is preventing bacteria from reaching the kidneys. VUR is managed conservatively with daily low-dose antibiotic therapy. A urine culture should be done every 2 to 3 months and any time the child has a fever. This method of management requires a motivated, reliable, and cooperative family. Many children outgrow the reflux over a period of years. An annual VCUG is done to assess the status of the reflux.

For children with mild to moderate reflux, a minimally invasive endoscopic option (subtrigonal injection or STING) is an alternative to daily antibiotics or open surgical intervention. A bulking agent—dextranomer–hyaluronic acid polymer (Deflux)—is injected into the mucous membrane of the ureter, making retrograde flow of urine more difficult. Overall cure rates relate to degree of reflux and range from 67.4% to 88.3%, although more than one injection may be needed to achieve resolution (Chen, Yeh, and Chou, 2010).

Indications for open surgical intervention include significant anatomic abnormality at the ureterovesical junction, recurrent UTIs, severe forms of VUR, noncompliance with medical therapy, intolerance to antibiotics, and VUR after puberty in women.

Prognosis

With prompt and adequate treatment at the time of diagnosis, the long-term prognosis for UTI is usually excellent. However, the hazard of progressive renal injury is greatest when infection occurs in young children (especially those younger than 2 years of age) and is associated with congenital renal malformations and reflux. Therefore, early diagnosis of children at risk is particularly important.

QUALITY PATIENT OUTCOMES: Urinary Tract Infections
• Treatment based on culture and sensitivity
• Renal function maintained
• Appropriate diagnosis of renal abnormalities

---

of recurrence, (3) prevent systemic spread of the infection, and (4) preserve renal function. Antibiotic therapy should be initiated on the basis of identification of the pathogen, the child's history of antibiotic use, and the location of the infection. Several antimicrobial drugs are available for treating UTI, but all of them can occasionally be ineffective because of resistance of organisms. Common antiinfective agents used for UTI include the penicillins, sulfonamide

Nursing Care Management

Nurses should instruct parents to observe regularly for clues suggesting UTI. Unfortunately, the signs of UTI are not as evident as those of upper respiratory tract infection. Therefore, many cases go undetected because no one thought to investigate this very common problem.

Because infants and young children often are unable to express their feelings and sensations verbally, it is difficult to detect discomfort they may be experiencing from dysuria. A careful history regarding voiding habits, stooling pattern, and episodes of unexplained irritability may assist in detecting less obvious cases of UTI. Consequently, parents should be cautioned to observe for specific clues of UTI in suspected cases.

> **NURSING TIP**   Check the diaper every half hour. This increases the opportunity for observing the stream for such findings as straining or fretting before voiding begins, signs of discomfort before and during urinating, starting and stopping the stream intermittently, and frequent dripping of small amounts of urine.

When infection is suspected, collecting an appropriate specimen is essential. It is the nurse's responsibility to take every precaution to obtain acceptable clean-voided specimens to avoid the use of other more invasive collecting procedures except when absolutely indicated. Because of the unreliability of a specimen obtained via a urine collection bag, suprapubic aspiration of urine or sterile catheterization should be done in infants and young children who are seen with fever.

Frequently, additional tests are performed to detect anatomic defects. Children are prepared for these tests as appropriate for their age. This includes an explanation of the procedure, its purpose, and what the children will experience (see Preparation for Diagnostic and Therapeutic Procedures, Chapter 22). Sometimes a simple description of the urinary system is helpful. Especially for preschool children, the nurse must clarify that the urinary tract is separate from any sexual function and that the test is for a problem that they did not cause. Children may associate blame for perceived wrongdoing (e.g., masturbation) or unacceptable thoughts with the reason for the illness or the tests. For children younger than 3 to 4 years of age, the procedure can be explained on a doll. For those who are older, a simple drawing of the bladder, urethra, ureters, and kidneys makes the procedure more understandable.

Handling actual equipment when feasible can be helpful in allaying anxiety in children of all ages. Anticipatory instruction on distraction techniques such as deep breathing, storytelling, and imagery may help the child relax and be more cooperative during the actual procedures. If surgery is indicated, facts and understanding of the procedure will help decrease the child's fear and anxiety concerning more extensive medical-surgical intervention.

Because antibacterial drugs are indicated in UTI, the nurse advises parents of proper dosage and administration. When antiseptics such as nitrofurantoin are used for prolonged therapy to maintain urine sterility, parents need an explanation of the drug's continued necessity when no signs of infection are present. For all children, an adequate or increased fluid intake is encouraged.

Prevention

Prevention is the most important goal in both primary and recurrent infection, and most preventive measures are simple hygienic habits that should be a routine part of daily care (see Nursing Care Guidelines box). For example, parents are taught to cleanse their infant's genital areas from front to back to avoid contaminating the urethral area with fecal organisms. Girls are taught to wipe from front to back after

NURSING CARE GUIDELINES
Prevention of Urinary Tract Infection

Factors Predisposing to Development
Short female urethra close to vagina and anus
Incomplete emptying (reflux) and overdistention of bladder
Concentrated urine
Constipation

Measures of Prevention
Practice perineal hygiene: wipe from front to back.
Avoid tight clothing or diapers; wear cotton panties rather than nylon.
Check for vaginitis or pinworms, especially if child scratches between legs.
Avoid "holding" urine; encourage child to void frequently, especially before long trips or other circumstances in which toilet facilities are not available.
Empty bladder completely with each void. Have the child "double void" (void, wait a few minutes, and void again). Severe cases may require clean, intermittent catheterization or biofeedback instruction.
Avoid straining during defecation and avoid constipation.
Encourage generous fluid intake.

CRITICAL THINKING CASE STUDY
Urinary Tract Infection and Constipation

During your assessment of Lisa, a 5-year-old girl admitted to the hospital for a severe UTI, her mother tells you that Lisa has bowel movements every third or fourth day. They are usually large, hard-formed stools, and Lisa sometimes has trouble evacuating the stool.

Questions
1. Evidence—Is there sufficient evidence to draw conclusion about Lisa's UTI and constipation?
2. Assumptions—Describe an underlying assumption about each of the following:
   a. UTIs and girls
   b. Normal bowel patterns for 4-year-old children
   c. Association between UTIs and constipation
3. What priorities for nursing care should be established for Lisa?
4. Does the evidence support your nursing intervention?

UTI, Urinary tract infection.

voiding and defecating. Children should void as soon as they feel the urge (see Critical Thinking Case Study box).

Sexually active female adolescents are advised to urinate as soon as possible after they have intercourse to flush out bacteria introduced during the activity. Children who have recurrent UTIs or neurogenic bladder are frequently maintained on daily low-dose antibiotics. Giving the dose at bedtime allows the drug to remain in the bladder overnight. The nurse should reinforce the importance of compliance to parents and older children.

OBSTRUCTIVE UROPATHY

Structural or functional abnormalities of the urinary system that obstruct the normal flow of urine can produce renal disorders. When there is interference with urine flow, the backup of urine above the obstruction causes **hydronephrosis** (dilation of the renal pelvis from distention) with eventual pressure destruction of renal parenchyma,

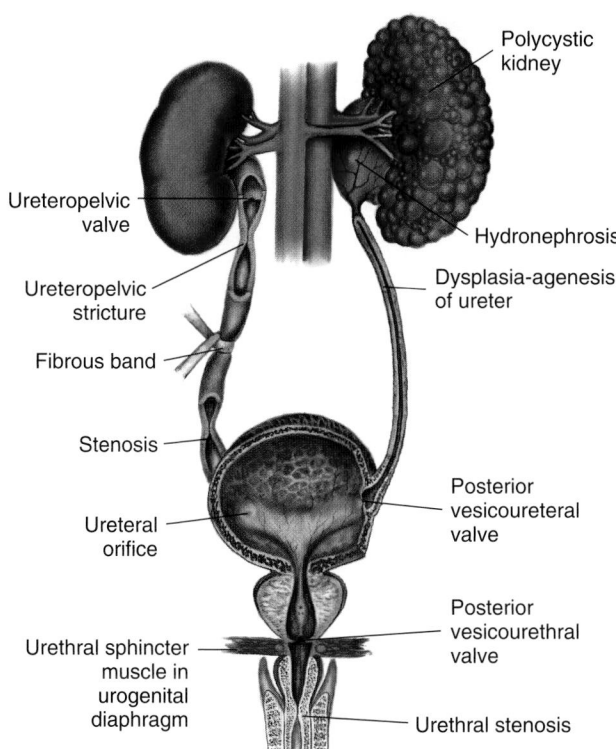

Polycystic kidney

Ureteropelvic valve

Ureteropelvic stricture

Fibrous band

Stenosis

Ureteral orifice

Urethral sphincter muscle in urogenital diaphragm

Hydronephrosis

Dysplasia-agenesis of ureter

Posterior vesicoureteral valve

Posterior vesicourethral valve

Urethral stenosis

FIG 27-2 Major sites of urinary tract obstruction.

although the dilating ureters form a reservoir that reduces the effect on the kidneys for a long time.

Obstruction may be congenital or acquired, unilateral or bilateral, and complete or incomplete with acute or chronic manifestations. The obstruction can occur at any level of the upper or lower urinary tract (Fig. 27-2). Partial obstruction may not be symptomatic unless there is a water or solute diuresis. Boys are affected more frequently than girls, and malformations should be suspected when patients have some other congenital defects (e.g., prune belly syndrome, chromosomal anomalies, anorectal malformations, defects of the pinna of the ear).

Damage to distal nephrons in chronic uropathy alters the ability to concentrate urine, contributing to increased urine flow and metabolic acidosis occurring from decreased excretion of acid secondary to impaired ability of the distal nephron to secrete hydrogen ions. Partial obstruction results in progressive loss of renal function as a result of irreversible damage to the nephrons. Pooled urine serves as a medium for bacterial growth; therefore, UTIs further increase the extent of renal damage.

Early diagnosis and surgical correction or procedures that divert the flow of urine to bypass the obstruction, such as placement of a temporary percutaneous nephrostomy tube or cutaneous ureterostomy, are essential to prevent progressive renal damage. Medical complications of acute or chronic renal failure (CRF) or infection are managed as described for those disorders.

Nursing Care Management

Nursing goals in urinary tract obstruction include helping to identify cases, assisting with diagnostic procedures, and caring for children with complications (described elsewhere). Preparing parents and children for procedures is a major nursing responsibility. Preparation for urinary diversion procedures is of special importance (see Preparation for Diagnostic and Therapeutic Procedures, Chapter 22).

Parents and children need emotional support and counseling during the lengthy management of these disorders. Many children are discharged with ureteral drainage systems in place that must be protected from damage, and the danger of infection is a constant concern. Parents are taught to care for the equipment and recognize the signs of possible obstruction or infection within the system. Maintaining adequate urine flow is imperative. Fluids should be encouraged. The tube should be observed frequently for indications of obstruction resulting from sediment, small blood clots, or kinking. The physician should inspect any drainage from around the tube.

Children with external diversional systems need psychologic support and guidance, especially as they reach adolescence and body image concerns assume more prominence. Those with progressive renal deterioration may face the prospect of dialysis or transplantation and the emotions that accompany these procedures.

EXTERNAL DEFECTS

Defects of the external genitourinary tract are serious conditions primarily because of the psychologic impact on the child. Satisfactory surgical repair is successful for the more common disorders and is carried out or initiated as early as possible. The major anomalies of the lower genitourinary tract, their description, and their management are outlined in Table 27-4.

Psychologic Problems Related to Genital Surgery

Surgery involving sexual organs can be particularly disruptive to children, especially preschoolers fearing punishment, retaliation, body mutilation, or castration. Some of the problems of hospitalization, separation, and anxiety can be eased by hospital practices that are sensitive to the child's needs (see Chapter 21).

A child's body image is largely derived as a result of feedback from the primary caregivers, and parental anxiety regarding an acceptable physical appearance and adequate future sexual competency is readily communicated to an affected child. Therefore, children with birth defects are at risk for developing a distorted body image that reflects the caregiver's subtly communicated evaluation of their bodies. The trend toward repair of visible genital defects is based in large part on these psychologic variables. The earlier a repair can be achieved, the more likely it is that the child will develop a normal body image.

During the years from 3 to 6, the phallic-oedipal period, children show a strong interest and concern about the genital area, sex differences, and genital normality or its lack. It is also a time when children are frightened of what they perceive to be threats to their body and bodily function. They also view any untoward happening as a punishment for real or imagined wrongdoing or unacceptable sexual feelings, such as masturbation, sex play, or erotic feelings. Surgical repair is recommended before these fears and anxieties develop.

After extensive review of the emotional, cognitive, and body image problems that may occur in children undergoing surgical reconstruction of a genital deformity, Kass (1996) recommended that surgery be accomplished between the ages of 6 and 15 months to minimize the psychologic effects of surgery and anesthesia.

Nursing Care Management

Preparing children and their families for diagnostic and surgical procedures (see Preparation for Diagnostic and Therapeutic Procedures, Chapter 22) and for home care is a major nursing function. Most postoperative care involves care of the surgical site. Tub baths are discouraged for 1 week after simple surgeries. The surgical site is kept clean and otherwise protected from infection and is inspected for signs

TABLE 27-4 DEFECTS OF THE GENITOURINARY TRACT

DEFECT	THERAPEUTIC MANAGEMENT
Inguinal hernia—Protrusion of abdominal contents through inguinal canal into scrotum	Detected as painless inguinal swelling of variable size Surgical closure of inguinal defect
Hydrocele—Fluid in scrotum	Surgical repair indicated if spontaneous resolution not accomplished in 1 year
Phimosis—Narrowing or stenosis of preputial opening of foreskin	**Mild cases**—Manual retraction of foreskin and proper cleansing of area **Severe cases**—Circumcision or vertical division and transverse suturing of foreskin

Hypospadias—Urethral opening located behind glans penis or anywhere along ventral surface of penile shaft	Objectives of surgical correction:
	   Enable child to void in standing position and direct stream voluntarily in usual manner
	   Improve physical appearance of genitalia
	   Produce a sexually adequate organ

Chordee—Ventral curvature of penis, often associated with hypospadias	Surgical release of fibrous band causing the deformity
Epispadias—Meatal opening located on dorsal surface of penis	Surgical correction, usually including penile and urethral lengthening and bladder neck reconstruction (if necessary)

Cryptorchidism—Failure of one or both testes to descend normally through inguinal canal	Detected by inability to palpate testes within scrotum
	Medical—Administration of human chorionic gonadotropin (older child)
	Surgical—Orchiopexy
	Objectives of therapy:
	   Prevent damage to undescended testicle
	   Decrease incidence of malignant tumor formation
	   Avoid trauma and torsion
	   Close inguinal canal
	   Prevent cosmetic and psychologic disability from empty scrotum

Exstrophy of bladder—Eversion of posterior bladder through anterior bladder wall and lower abdominal wall; associated with open pubic arch (a severe defect)	Potential objectives of surgical correction:
	   Preserve renal function
	   Attain urinary control
	   Provide adequate reconstructive repair
	   Improve sexual function (especially in males)

Disorders of Sexual Differentiation	
Masculinized female (female pseudohermaphrodite)	Assign gender as female; assign gender while avoiding irreversible surgery, realizing some children may change gender later in life; family participation essential
Incompletely masculinized male (male pseudohermaphrodite)	Assign gender while avoiding irreversible surgery, realizing some children may change gender later in life; family participation essential
True hermaphrodite (both ovaries and testes)	Assign gender while avoiding irreversible surgery, realizing some children may change gender later in life; gender assignment depends on predominant characteristics; family participation essential
Mixed gonadal dysgenesis	Assign gender while avoiding irreversible surgery, realizing some children may change gender later in life; gender assignment depends on predominant characteristics; family participation essential

of infection. Dressings, if any, are inspected regularly. More complex surgeries require additional care and observation (e.g., catheter care for urethral reconstruction and care of urinary diversion stomas and collection devices).

Some older children's activities, such as pushing, lifting, playing with straddle toys or in sandboxes, swimming, and rough activities, may be restricted after some types of surgical repairs. Precise restrictions depend on the specific type of surgery. Activities of infants and toddlers are not limited.

In most cases, the results of surgery are satisfactory. However, in some of the more severe defects, such as exstrophy and those that require stomas, additional emotional interventions may be needed. A major concern of parents and children is related to surgery affecting the genitalia directly. Concerns about penis size, appearance of the genitalia, potential ability to procreate, and rejection by peers (especially the opposite sex) are potential fears that require psychologic adjustment, particularly during adolescence.

GLOMERULAR DISEASE

NEPHROTIC SYNDROME

Nephrotic syndrome is a clinical state that includes massive proteinuria, hypoalbuminemia, hyperlipidemia, and edema. The disorder can occur as (1) a primary disease known as idiopathic nephrosis, childhood nephrosis, or minimal-change nephrotic syndrome (MCNS); (2) a secondary disorder that occurs as a clinical manifestation after or in association with glomerular damage that has a known or presumed cause; or (3) a congenital form inherited as an autosomal recessive disorder. The disorder is characterized by increased glomerular permeability to plasma protein, which results in massive urinary protein loss. The glomerulus is responsible for the initial step in the formation of urine, and the filtration rate depends on an intact glomerular membrane. This discussion is devoted to MCNS because it constitutes 80% of nephrotic syndrome cases.

Pathophysiology

The onset of MCNS can occur at any age but predominantly occurs in children between 2 and 7 years of age. It is rare in children younger than 6 months of age, uncommon in infants younger than 1 year of age, and unusual after the age of 8 years. Patients with MCNS are twice as likely to be male.

The pathogenesis of MCNS is not fully understood. There may be a metabolic, biochemical, physiochemical, or immune-mediated disturbance that causes the basement membrane of the glomeruli to become increasingly permeable to protein, but the cause and mechanisms are only speculative.

The glomerular membrane, normally impermeable to albumin and other proteins, becomes permeable to proteins, especially albumin, that leak through the membrane and are lost in urine (**hyperalbuminuria**). This reduces the serum albumin level (**hypoalbuminemia**), decreasing the colloidal osmotic pressure in the capillaries. As a result, the vascular hydrostatic pressure exceeds the pull of the colloidal osmotic pressure, causing fluid to accumulate in the interstitial spaces (**edema**) and body cavities, particularly in the abdominal cavity (**ascites**). The shift of fluid from the plasma to the interstitial spaces reduces the vascular fluid volume (**hypovolemia**), which in turn stimulates the renin–angiotensin system and the secretion of antidiuretic hormone and aldosterone. Tubular reabsorption of sodium and water is increased in an attempt to increase intravascular volume. The elevation of serum lipids is not fully understood. The sequence of events in nephrotic syndrome is diagrammed in Figure 27-3.

Diagnostic Evaluation

The disease is suspected on the basis of clinical manifestations (Box 27-2), especially when weight gain in a previously well child increases slowly over days or weeks. The generalized edema may develop rapidly or gradually but eventually prompts the family to seek medical attention. Parents usually give a history of the child being well but steadily gaining weight; appearing edematous; and then becoming anorexic, irritable, and less active.

The diagnosis of MCNS is suspected on the basis of the history and clinical manifestations (edema, proteinuria, hypoalbuminemia, and hypercholesterolemia in the absence of hematuria and hypertension) in children between the ages of 2 and 8 years. The hallmark of MCNS is massive proteinuria (higher than 2+ on urine dipstick). Hyaline casts, oval fat bodies, and a few red blood cells (RBCs) can be found in the urine of some affected children, although there is seldom gross hematuria. The GFR is usually normal or high.

Total serum protein concentration is low, with the serum albumin significantly reduced and plasma lipids elevated. Hemoglobin and hematocrit are usually normal or elevated as a result of hemoconcentration. The platelet count may be elevated. Serum sodium concentration may be low. If the patient does not respond to a 4- to 8-week course of steroids, a renal biopsy may be needed to distinguish among other types of nephrotic syndrome. The biopsy results of children with MCNS are remarkable for effacement of the foot processes of the epithelial cells lining the basement membrane, but otherwise the kidney tissue is normal.

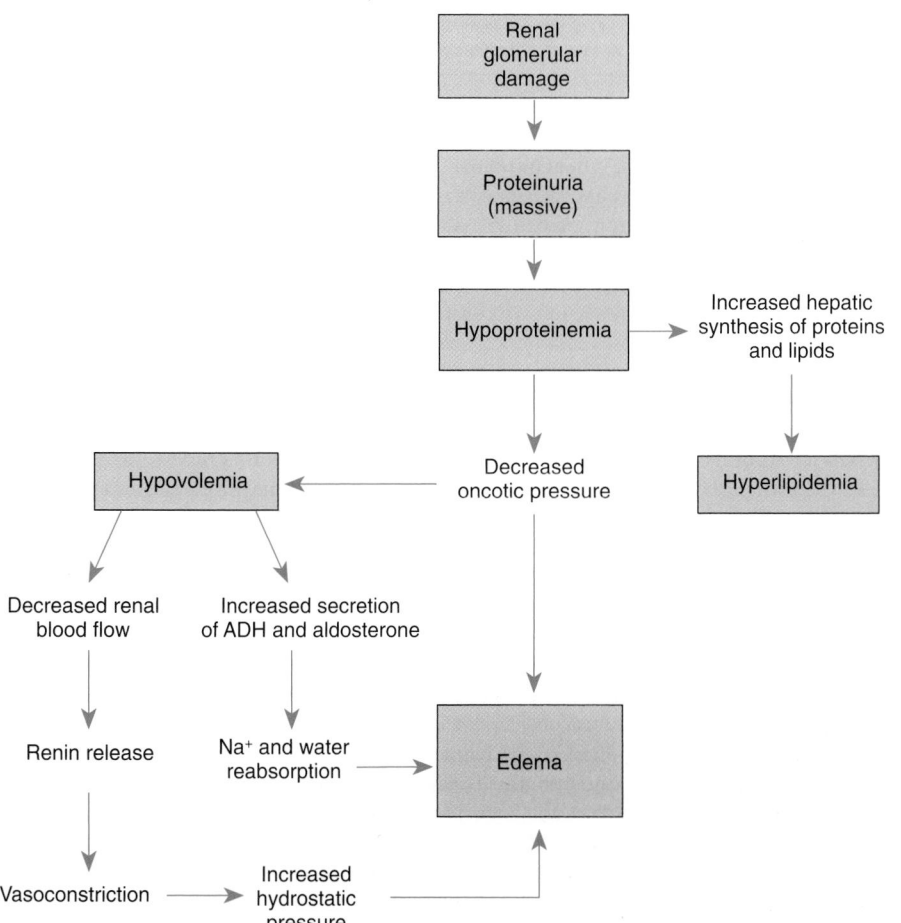

FIG 27-3 Sequence of events in nephrotic syndrome. *ADH,* Antidiuretic hormone.

BOX 27-2 CLINICAL MANIFESTATIONS OF NEPHROTIC SYNDROME

Weight gain
Puffiness of face (facial edema):
- Especially around the eyes
- Apparent on arising in the morning
- Subsides during the day

Abdominal swelling (ascites)
Pleural effusion
Labial or scrotal swelling
Edema of intestinal mucosal, possibly causing:
- Diarrhea
- Anorexia
- Poor intestinal absorption

Ankle or leg swelling
Irritability
Easily fatigued
Lethargic
Blood pressure normal or slightly decreased
Susceptibility to infection
Urine alterations:
- Decreased volume
- Frothy

Therapeutic Management

Objectives of therapeutic management include (1) reducing excretion of urinary protein, (2) reducing fluid retention in the tissues, (3) preventing infection, and (4) minimizing complications related to therapies. Dietary restrictions include a low-salt diet and, in more severe cases, fluid restriction. If complications of edema develop, diuretic therapy may be initiated to provide temporary relief from edema. Sometimes infusions of 25% albumin are used. Acute infections are treated with appropriate antibiotics.

Corticosteroids are the first line of therapy for MCNS. The starting dosage for prednisone is usually 2 mg/kg body weight/day for 6 weeks followed by 1.5 mg/kg every other day for 6 weeks (Gipson, Massengill, Yao, and others, 2009). About two thirds of children with MCNS have a relapse, heralded first by increased urine protein. Relapses can be diagnosed early if parents are taught routine home monitoring of urine protein by dipstick. Relapses are treated with a repeated, but usually shorter, course of high-dose steroid therapy. Side effects of the steroids include weight gain, rounding of the face, behavior changes, and increased appetite. Long-term therapy may result in hirsutism, growth retardation, cataracts, hypertension, gastrointestinal bleeding, bone demineralization, infection, and hyperglycemia. Children who do not respond to steroid therapy, those who have frequent relapses, and those in whom the side effects threaten their growth and general health may be considered for a course of therapy using other immunosuppressant medications (cyclophosphamide, chlorambucil, or cyclosporine).

Episodes of MCNS, both the first episode and relapse, often happen in conjunction with a viral or bacterial infection. Relapses can also be triggered by allergies and immunizations. Relapses in children with MCNS may continue over many years.

Complications of nephrotic syndrome include infection, circulatory insufficiency secondary to hypovolemia, and thromboembolism. Infections that may be seen in children with nephrotic syndrome

include peritonitis, cellulitis, and pneumonia and require prompt recognition and vigorous treatment with appropriate antibiotic therapy.

Prognosis

The prognosis for ultimate recovery in most cases is good. It is a self-limiting disease, and in children who respond to steroid therapy, the tendency to relapse decreases with time. With early detection and prompt implementation of therapy to eradicate proteinuria, progressive basement membrane damage is minimized so that when the tendency to relapse is past, renal function is usually normal or near normal. It is estimated that approximately 80% of affected children have this favorable prognosis.

QUALITY PATIENT OUTCOMES: Nephrotic Syndrome
- Protein-free urine
- Acute infections prevented
- Edema absent or minimal
- Nutrition maintained
- Metabolic abnormalities controlled

Nursing Care Management

Continuous monitoring of fluid retention or excretion is an important nursing function. Strict intake and output records are essential but may be difficult to obtain from very young children. Application of collection bags is irritating to edematous skin that is readily subject to breakdown. Applying diapers or weighing wet pads may be necessary.

NURSING TIP Another strategy for obtaining a daily urine protein is to place cotton balls in the diaper at night before bedtime and then squeeze them out in the morning.

Other methods of monitoring progress include urine examination for albumin, daily weight, and measurement of abdominal girth. Assessment of edema (e.g., increased or decreased swelling around the eyes and dependent areas), the degree of pitting, and the color and texture of skin are part of nursing care. Vital signs are monitored to detect any early signs of complications such as shock or an infective process.

Infection is a constant source of danger to edematous children and those receiving corticosteroid therapy. These children are particularly vulnerable to upper respiratory tract infection; therefore, they must be kept warm and dry, active, and protected from contact with infected individuals (e.g., roommates, visitors, and personnel). Vital signs are monitored to detect any early signs of an infective process.

Loss of appetite accompanying active nephrosis creates a perplexing problem for nurses. During this time, the combined efforts of nurse, dietitian, parents, and child are needed to formulate a nutritionally adequate and attractive diet. Salt is usually restricted (but not eliminated) during the edema phase and while the child is on steroid therapy. Fluid restriction (if prescribed) is limited to short-term use during massive edema. Every effort should be made to serve attractive meals with preferred foods and a minimum of fuss, but it usually requires considerable ingenuity to entice the child to eat (see Feeding the Sick Child, Chapter 22).

Children usually adjust activities according to their tolerance level. However, they may require guidance in selecting play activities. Suitable recreational and diversional activities are an important part of their care. Irritability and mood swings that accompany steroid therapy are not unusual in these children and may create an additional challenge for the nurse and family.

Family Support and Home Care

Continuous support of the child and family is one of the major nursing considerations. Most children are treated at home during relapses. Parents are taught to detect signs of relapse and to call for changes in treatment at the earliest indications. Unless the edema and proteinuria are severe or the parents, for some reason, are unable to care for the ill child, *home care is preferred*. Parents are instructed in testing urine for albumin, administering medications, and providing general care. Parents are also instructed regarding avoiding contact with infected playmates, but the child should attend school.

The prolonged course of the relapsing form of nephrotic syndrome is taxing to both the child and the family. The up-and-down course of remissions and exacerbations with periodic disruption of family life by hospitalization places a severe strain on the child and the family, both psychologically and financially. Reassurance regarding this characteristic of the course of the disease, with emphasis on the importance of long-term care, needs to be provided to parents and children to gain their cooperation. A satisfactory response is more likely when relapses are detected and therapy is instituted early, and remissions are prolonged when instructions are carried out faithfully. Continuous support of the child and family is one of the major nursing considerations (see Chapter 18).

ACUTE GLOMERULONEPHRITIS

Acute glomerulonephritis (AGN) may be a primary event or a manifestation of a systemic disorder that can range from minimal to severe. Common features include oliguria, edema, hypertension and circulatory congestion, hematuria, and proteinuria. Most cases are postinfectious and have been associated with pneumococcal, streptococcal, and viral infections. Acute poststreptococcal glomerulonephritis (APSGN) is the most common of the postinfectious renal diseases in childhood and the one for which a cause can be established in the majority of cases. APSGN can occur at any age but affects primarily early school-age children, with a peak age of onset of 6 to 7 years. It is uncommon in children younger than 2 years of age, and boys outnumber girls two to one.

Etiology

Acute poststreptococcal glomerulonephritis is an immune-complex disease that occurs after an antecedent streptococcal infection with certain strains of the group A β-hemolytic streptococcus. Most streptococcal infections *do not* cause APSGN. A latent period of 10 to 21 days occurs between the streptococcal infection and the onset of clinical manifestations. Disease secondary to streptococcal pharyngitis is more common in the winter or spring, but when APSGN is associated with pyoderma (principally impetigo), it may be more prevalent in later summer or early fall, especially in warmer climates. Second episodes of AGN are rare.

Pathophysiology

The pathophysiology of APSGN is still uncertain. Immune complexes are deposited in the glomerular basement membrane. The glomeruli become edematous and infiltrated with polymorphonuclear leukocytes, which occlude the capillary lumen. The resulting decrease in plasma filtration results in an excessive accumulation of water and retention of sodium that expands plasma and interstitial fluid volumes, leading to circulatory congestion and edema. The cause of the hypertension associated with AGN cannot be completely explained by fluid retention. Excess renin may also be produced.

BOX 27-3   CLINICAL MANIFESTATIONS OF ACUTE POSTSTREPTOCOCCAL GLOMERULONEPHRITIS

Edema:
- Especially periorbital
- Facial edema more prominent in the morning
- Spreads during the day to involve extremities and abdomen

Anorexia

Urine:
- Cloudy, smoky brown (resembles tea or cola)
- Severely reduced volume

Pallor

Irritability

Lethargy

Child appearing ill

Child seldom expresses specific complaints

Older children complaining of:
- Headaches
- Abdominal discomfort
- Dysuria

Vomiting possible

Mild to severely elevated blood pressure

Diagnostic Evaluation

Typically, affected children are in good health until they experience streptococcal infection. In some instances, they have a history of only a mild cold or no previous infection at all. The onset of nephritis appears after an average latency period of about 10 days (Box 27-3). Because the child appears to be well during the latency period, parents do not recognize the association. The edema is relatively moderate and may not be appreciated by someone unfamiliar with the child's normal appearance.

Urinalysis during the acute phase characteristically shows hematuria and proteinuria. Proteinuria generally parallels the hematuria and may be 3+ or 4+ in the presence of gross hematuria. Gross discoloration of the urine reflects RBC and hemoglobin content. Microscopic examination of the sediment shows many RBCs, leukocytes, epithelial cells, and granular and RBC casts. Bacteria are not seen.

Azotemia that results from impaired glomerular filtration is reflected in elevated blood urea nitrogen (BUN) and creatinine levels in at least 50% of cases. Occasionally, proteinuria is excessive, and the patient may have nephrotic syndrome (i.e., hypoproteinemia and hyperlipidemia).

Cultures of the pharynx are rarely positive for streptococci because the renal disease occurs weeks after the infection.

Some serologic tests are necessary to make the diagnosis of AGN. Circulating serum antibodies to streptococci indicate the presence of a previous infection. The antistreptolysin O (ASO) titer is the most familiar and readily available test for streptococcal infection. Other antibodies that may aid in diagnosis are elevated antihyaluronidase (AHase), antideoxyribonuclease B (ADNase-B), and streptozyme.

All patients with APSGN have reduced serum complement (C3) activity in the early stages of the disease. Rising C3 levels are used as a guide to indicate improvement of the disease and should be normal in almost all patients 8 weeks after the disease onset.

Studies that may be useful include chest x-ray examination, which generally shows cardiac enlargement, pulmonary congestion, or pleural effusion during the edematous phase of acute disease. Renal biopsy for diagnostic purposes is seldom required but may be useful in the diagnosis of atypical cases.

Therapeutic Management

Management consists of general supportive measures and early recognition and treatment of complications. Children who have normal blood pressure and a satisfactory urinary output can generally be treated at home. Those with substantial edema, hypertension, gross hematuria, or significant oliguria should be hospitalized because of the unpredictability of complications.

Dietary restrictions depend on the stage and severity of the disease, especially the extent of edema. Moderate sodium restriction and even fluid restriction may be instituted for children with hypertension and edema. Foods with substantial amounts of potassium are generally restricted during the period of oliguria.

Regular measurement of vital signs, body weight, and intake and output is essential to monitor the progress of the disease and to detect complications that may appear at any time during the course of the disease. *A record of daily weight is the most useful means for assessing fluid balance.* Rarely, children with AGN will develop acute renal failure (ARF) with oliguria that significantly alters the fluid and electrolyte balance (resulting in hyperkalemia, acidosis, hypocalcemia, or hyperphosphatemia). These children require careful management. Peritoneal dialysis or hemodialysis is seldom needed.

Acute hypertension must be anticipated and identified early. Blood pressure measurements are taken every 4 to 6 hours. A variety of antihypertensive medications and diuretics are used to control hypertension. Antibiotic therapy is indicated only for children with evidence of persistent streptococcal infections. It is used to prevent transmission of nephritogenic streptococci to other family members.

Prognosis

Almost all children correctly diagnosed as having APSGN recover completely, and specific immunity is conferred, so subsequent recurrences are uncommon. Some of these children have been reported to develop chronic disease, but most of these cases are now believed to be different glomerular diseases misdiagnosed as poststreptococcal disease.

Nursing Care Management

Nursing care of the child with glomerulonephritis involves careful assessment of the disease status, with regular monitoring of vital signs (including frequent measurement of blood pressure), fluid balance, and behavior.

Vital signs provide clues to the severity of the disease and early signs of complications. They are carefully measured, and any deviations are reported and recorded. The volume and character of urine are noted, and the child is weighed daily. Children with restricted fluid intake, especially those who are not severely edematous or those who have lost weight, are observed for signs of dehydration.

Assessment of the child's appearance for signs of cerebral complications is an important nursing function because the severity of the acute phase is variable and unpredictable. The child with edema, hypertension, and gross hematuria may be subject to complications, and anticipatory preparations such as seizure precautions and intravenous (IV) equipment are included in the nursing care plan.

For most children, a regular diet is allowed, but it should contain no added salt. Foods high in sodium and salted treats are eliminated, and parents and friends are advised not to bring snacks such as potato chips or pretzels. However, the total amount of salt ingested is usually less than prescribed because of the child's poor appetite. Fluid restriction, if prescribed, is more difficult, and the amount permitted should be evenly divided throughout the waking hours. Meal preparation and service require special attention because the child is indifferent to meals during the acute phase. Again, collaboration with parents and the dietitian and special consideration for food preferences facilitate meal planning.

During the acute phase, children are generally content to lie in bed. As they begin to feel better and their symptoms subside, they will want to be up and about. Activities should be planned to allow for frequent rest periods and avoidance of fatigue. Children who have mild edema and no hypertension, as well as convalescent children who are being treated at home, need follow-up care. Parents are instructed regarding general measures, including diet and prevention of infection.

Health supervision is continued with weekly followed by monthly visits for evaluation and urinalysis. Parent education and support in preparation for discharge and home care include education in home management and the need for follow-up care and health supervision.

MISCELLANEOUS RENAL DISORDERS

HEMOLYTIC UREMIC SYNDROME

Hemolytic uremic syndrome (HUS) is an uncommon, acute renal disease that occurs primarily in infants and small children between the ages of 6 months and 5 years. HUS is one of the most frequent causes of acquired ARF in children (Duzova, Bakkaloglu, Kalyoncu, and others, 2010). The clinical features of the disease include acquired hemolytic anemia, thrombocytopenia, renal injury, and central nervous system (CNS) symptoms. The etiology of HUS is thought to be associated with bacterial toxins, chemicals, and viruses. The appearance of the disease has been associated with *Rickettsia* organisms, viruses (especially coxsackievirus, echovirus, and adenovirus), *E. coli*, pneumococci, shigellae, and salmonellae and may represent an unusual response to these infections. Multiple cases of HUS caused by enteric infection of the *E. coli* O157:H7 serotype have been traced to undercooked meat, especially ground beef. Other sources are unpasteurized milk or fruit juice, especially apple; alfalfa sprouts; lettuce; and salami. Drinking or swimming in sewage-contaminated water can also cause infection. The clinical presentation is usually a history of a prodromal illness (most often gastroenteritis or an upper respiratory tract infection) followed by the sudden onset of hemolysis and renal failure.

Pathophysiology

The primary site of injury appears to be the endothelial lining of the small glomerular arterioles, which become swollen and occluded with deposits of platelets and fibrin clots (intravascular coagulation). RBCs are damaged as they attempt to move through the partially occluded blood vessels. These damaged cells are removed by the spleen, causing acute hemolytic anemia. The platelet aggregation within the damaged blood vessels or the damage and removal of platelets produce the characteristic thrombocytopenia.

Diagnostic Evaluation

The triad of anemia, thrombocytopenia, and renal failure is sufficient for diagnosis (Box 27-4). Renal involvement is evidenced by proteinuria, hematuria, and urinary casts; BUN and serum creatinine levels are elevated. A low hemoglobin and hematocrit and a high reticulocyte count confirm the hemolytic nature of the anemia.

Therapeutic Management

The goals of therapy are early diagnosis and aggressive, supportive care of the ARF and hemolytic anemia. The most consistently effective

BOX 27-4   CLINICAL MANIFESTATIONS OF HEMOLYTIC UREMIC SYNDROME

Vomiting
Irritability
Lethargy
Marked pallor
Hemorrhagic manifestations:
- Bruising
- Petechiae
- Jaundice
- Bloody diarrhea

Oliguria or anuria
CNS involvement:
- Seizures
- Stupor or coma

Signs of acute heart failure (sometimes)

CNS, Central nervous system.

BOX 27-5   CLINICAL MANIFESTATIONS OF WILMS TUMOR

Abdominal swelling or mass:
- Firm
- Nontender
- Confined to one side

Hematuria (less than one fourth of cases)
Fatigue and malaise
Hypertension (occasionally)
Weight loss
Fever
Manifestations resulting from compression of tumor mass
Secondary metabolic alterations from tumor or metastasis
If metastasis, symptoms of lung involvement:
- Dyspnea
- Cough
- Shortness of breath
- Chest pain (sometimes)

treatment of HUS is hemodialysis or peritoneal dialysis, which is instituted in any child who has been anuric for 24 hours or who demonstrates oliguria with uremia or hypertension and seizures. Other treatments include use of pharmacologic agents, fresh-frozen plasma, and plasmapheresis. Blood transfusions with fresh, washed packed cells are administered for severe anemia but are used with caution to prevent circulatory overload from added volume.

Prognosis

With prompt treatment, the recovery rate is about 95%, but residual renal impairment ranges from 10% to 50%. Long-term complications include CRF, hypertension, and CNS disorders. Death is usually caused by residual renal impairment or CNS injury.

Nursing Care Management

Nursing care is the same as that provided in ARF and, for children with continued impairment, includes management of chronic disease. Because of the sudden and life-threatening nature of the disorder in a previously well child, parents are often ill prepared for the impact of hospitalization and treatment. Therefore, support and understanding are especially important aspects of care.

WILMS TUMOR

Wilms tumor, or nephroblastoma, is the most common malignant renal and intraabdominal tumor of childhood. The incidence is estimated to be 8.0 cases per million children. Approximately 500 new cases are diagnosed each year in the United States, with 6% involving both kidneys (Cendren and Gomez, 2010). Wilms tumor occurs about three times more often in African Americans than in East Asians in the United States. The peak age at diagnosis is approximately 3 years, and occurrence is slightly more frequent in boys than in girls. The majority of patients with Wilms tumor are diagnosed at younger than 5 years of age, with 1% to 2.5% having a familial origin. Unfortunately, there is no method of identifying gene carriers at this time.

Etiology

Wilms tumor probably arises from a malignant, undifferentiated cluster of primordial cells capable of initiating the regeneration of an abnormal structure. Its occurrence slightly favors the left kidney, which

is advantageous because surgically this kidney is easier to manipulate and remove. In about 10% of cases, both kidneys are involved. Studies have shown that development of Wilms tumor is frequently associated with aniridia, hemihypertrophy, Beckwith-Wiedemann syndrome, or genitourinary anomalies (Cendron and Gomez, 2010; Dome, Perlman, Ritchey, and others, 2006).

Diagnostic Evaluation

In a child suspected of having Wilms tumor, special emphasis is placed on the history and physical examination for the presence of congenital anomalies, a family history of cancer, and signs of malignancy (e.g., weight loss, size of liver and spleen, indications of anemia, lymphadenopathy). Most children with Wilms tumor are brought to the practitioner because of abdominal swelling or an abdominal mass (Box 27-5). Specific tests include radiographic studies, including abdominal ultrasonography and abdominal and chest computed tomography scan; hematologic studies; biochemical studies; and urinalysis. Studies to demonstrate the relationship of the tumor to the ipsilateral kidney and the presence of a normal, functioning kidney on the contralateral side are essential. If a large tumor is present, an inferior venacavogram is necessary to demonstrate possible tumor involvement adjacent to the vena cava. A bone marrow aspiration may be performed to rule out metastasis, which is rare in children with Wilms tumor.

> **! NURSING ALERT**
>
> To reinforce the need for caution, it may be necessary to post a sign on the bed that reads "DO NOT PALPATE ABDOMEN." Careful bathing and handling are also important in preventing trauma to the tumor site.

Therapeutic Management

Combined treatment with surgery and chemotherapy with or without radiation is based on the histologic pattern and clinical stage (Box 27-6).

Surgery is scheduled as soon as possible after confirmation of a renal mass, usually within 24 to 48 hours of admission. A large transabdominal incision is performed for optimal visualization of the abdominal cavity. The tumor, affected kidney, and adjacent adrenal gland are removed. Great care is taken to keep the encapsulated tumor

BOX 27-6   STAGING OF WILMS TUMOR

Stage I—Tumor is limited to kidney and completely resected.
Stage II—Tumor extends beyond kidney but is completely resected.
Stage III—Residual nonhematogenous tumor is confined to abdomen.
Stage IV—Hematogenous metastases; deposits are beyond stage III, namely, to lung, liver, bone, and brain.
Stage V—Bilateral renal involvement is present at diagnosis.

intact because rupture can seed cancer cells throughout the abdomen, lymph channel, and bloodstream. The contralateral kidney is carefully inspected for evidence of disease or dysfunction. Regional lymph nodes are inspected, and a biopsy is performed when indicated. Any involved structures, such as part of the colon, diaphragm, or vena cava, are removed. Metal clips are placed around the tumor site for exact marking during radiotherapy.

If both kidneys are involved, the child may be treated with radiotherapy or chemotherapy before surgery to decrease the size of the tumor, allowing more conservative surgery. It may be possible to perform a partial nephrectomy on the less affected kidney, with a total nephrectomy on the opposite side. When a transplant is feasible, such as from a twin, sibling, or parent, bilateral nephrectomy is considered as a last resort.

Postoperative radiotherapy is indicated for children with large tumors, metastasis, residual postoperative disease, unfavorable histologic characteristics, or recurrence. Chemotherapy is indicated for all stages. The most effective agents for treating Wilms tumor are actinomycin D (dactinomycin), vincristine, and adriamycin, with the addition of cyclophosphamide for unfavorable histology or advanced disease (Cendron and Gomez, 2010; Dome, Perlman, Ritchey, and others, 2006). The duration of therapy ranges from 6 to 15 months.

Prognosis

Survival rates for Wilms tumor are the highest among all childhood cancers. Children with localized tumor (stages I and II) have a 90% chance of cure with multimodal therapy. Factors that favorably affect the success of further therapy include initial treatment with only vincristine and dactinomycin, relapse to the lungs only, relapse in the abdomen of a patient who received no prior abdominal irradiation, and relapse more than 12 months after diagnosis. Wilms tumor may recur, especially in the lungs. Both chemotherapy and radiotherapy can induce second malignancies, usually in areas that have been irradiated (Cendron and Gomez, 2010; Dome, Perlman, Ritchey, and others, 2006).

Nursing Care Management

Nursing care of the child with Wilms tumor is similar to that of children with other cancers treated with surgery, irradiation, and chemotherapy. However, there are some significant differences; these are discussed for each phase of nursing intervention.

Preoperative Care

The preoperative period is one of swift diagnosis. The nurse faces the challenge of preparing the child and parents for all laboratory and operative procedures within 24 to 48 hours of admission. Because of the minimal preparatory time, explanations should be simple, repetitive, and focused on the child's actual experiences. In addition to the usual preoperative observations, blood pressure is monitored because hypertension from excess renin production is a possibility.

There are several special preoperative concerns, the most important of which is that the *tumor is not palpated unless absolutely necessary* because manipulation of the mass may cause dissemination of cancer cells to adjacent and distant sites.

Because radiotherapy and chemotherapy are usually begun immediately after surgery, parents need an explanation of what to expect, such as major benefits and side effects. The timing of the information should be considered to avoid overwhelming the family. Ideally, the nurse should be present during physician–parent conferences to answer questions as they arise. It is usually better to postpone telling the child about these side effects until after surgery. Alopecia, usually of most concern to older children, does not occur until approximately 2 weeks after the initial treatment regimen. Therefore, the child can be prepared for the hair loss postoperatively.

Postoperative Care

Despite the extensive surgical intervention necessary in many children with Wilms tumor, the recovery is usually rapid. The major nursing responsibilities are the same as those after any abdominal surgery (see Surgical Procedures, Chapter 22). Because these children are at risk for intestinal obstruction from vincristine-induced ileus, radiation-induced edema, and postsurgical adhesion formation, the nurse carefully monitors gastrointestinal activity, such as bowel movements, bowel sounds, distention, vomiting, and pain. The nurse also monitors blood pressure, urinary output, and signs of infection and institutes pulmonary hygiene to prevent postoperative pulmonary complications.

Family Support

The postoperative period is frequently difficult for parents. The shock of seeing their child immediately after surgery may be the first realization of the seriousness of the diagnosis. It also marks the confirmation of the stage of the tumor. During this period, the nurse should be with the parents to assure them of the child's recovery after surgery and to assess the parents' understanding of the total experience. They need an opportunity to express their feelings and need to be provided the same emotional care discussed in Chapter 18 for families who have a child with a life-threatening disorder.

Older children need an opportunity to deal with their feelings concerning the many procedures to which they have been subjected in rapid succession. Play therapy with dolls or puppets or through drawing can be extremely beneficial in helping them adjust. It is not unusual for children to feel angry because of the extent of surgery, the need for additional therapy, or the seriousness of the disorder.

! NURSING ALERT

Prompt detection and treatment of any genitourinary signs or symptoms are mandatory. Children with a solitary kidney should be assessed and advised on the need for protective equipment before engaging in contact, collision, or limited contact activities (Rice and Council on Sports Medicine and Fitness, 2008).

RENAL FAILURE

Renal failure is the inability of the kidneys to excrete waste material, concentrate urine, and conserve electrolytes. It can occur suddenly (**acute renal failure [ARF]**) in response to inadequate perfusion, kidney disease, or urinary tract obstruction, or it can develop slowly (**chronic renal failure [CRF]**) as a result of longstanding kidney disease or an anomaly.

> ## BOX 27-7   CLINICAL MANIFESTATIONS OF ACUTE RENAL FAILURE
>
> Specific:
> - Oliguria
> - Anuria uncommon (except in obstructive disorders)
>
> Nonspecific (may develop):
> - Nausea
> - Vomiting
> - Drowsiness
> - Edema
> - Hypertension
>
> Manifestations of underlying disorder or pathologic condition

---

Azotemia and *uremia* are terms often used in relation to renal failure. **Azotemia** is the accumulation of nitrogenous waste within the blood. **Uremia** is a more advanced condition in which retention of nitrogenous products produces toxic symptoms. Whereas azotemia is not life threatening, uremia is a serious condition that often involves other body systems.

ACUTE RENAL FAILURE

Acute renal failure is said to exist when the kidneys suddenly are unable to regulate the volume and composition of urine appropriately in response to food and fluid intake and the needs of the organism. The principal feature of ARF is oliguria* associated with azotemia, metabolic acidosis, and diverse electrolyte disturbances. ARF is not common in childhood, but the outcome depends on the cause, associated findings, and prompt recognition and treatment.

The pathologic conditions that produce ARF caused by glomerulonephritis and HUS are discussed in relation to those disorders. ARF can also develop as a result of a large number of related or unrelated clinical conditions: poor renal perfusion; urinary tract obstruction; acute renal injury; or the final expression of chronic, irreversible renal disease. The most common cause in children is transient renal failure resulting from severe dehydration or other causes of poor perfusion that may respond to restoration of fluid volume.

Pathophysiology

Acute renal failure is usually reversible, but the deviations of physiologic function can be extreme, and mortality in the pediatric age group remains high. There is severe reduction in the GFR, an elevated BUN level, and a significant reduction in renal blood flow.

The clinical course is variable and depends on the cause. In reversible ARF, there is a period of severe oliguria, or a low-output phase, followed by an abrupt onset of diuresis, or a high-output phase, and then a gradual return to (or toward) normal urine volumes.

Diagnostic Evaluation

In many instances of ARF, the infant or child is already critically ill with the precipitating disorder, and the explanation for development of oliguria may or may not be readily apparent (Box 27-7). When a previously well child develops ARF without an obvious cause, a careful history is taken to reveal symptoms that may be related to glomerulonephritis, obstructive uropathy, or exposure to nephrotoxic chemicals

---

*The definition of oliguria varies extensively in the literature, from 1.8 to 4 dl/m^2/24 hr.

(e.g., ingestion of heavy metals, inhalation of carbon tetrachloride or other organic solvents, or medications such as nonsteroidal antiinflammatory drugs [Patzer, 2008] known to be toxic to the kidneys). Significant laboratory measurements during renal shutdown that serve as a guide for therapy are BUN, serum creatinine, pH, sodium, potassium, and calcium.

> ## ! NURSING ALERT
>
> Diminished urinary output and lethargy in a child who is dehydrated, is in shock, or has recently undergone surgery should be evaluated for possible ARF.

> ## ! NURSING ALERT
>
> Any of the following signs of hyperkalemia constitute an emergency and are reported immediately:
> - Serum potassium concentrations in excess of 7 mEq/L
> - Presence of electrocardiographic abnormalities, such as prolonged QRS complex, depressed ST segment, high peaked T waves, bradycardia, or heart block

Therapeutic Management

Treatment of ARF is directed toward (1) treatment of the underlying cause, (2) management of the complications of renal failure, and (3) provision of supportive therapy within the constraints imposed by the renal failure.

Treatment of poor perfusion resulting from dehydration consists of volume restoration, as described in Chapter 24 in treatment of dehydration. If oliguria persists after restoration of fluid volume or if the renal failure is caused by intrinsic renal damage, the physiologic and biochemical abnormalities that have resulted from kidney dysfunction must be corrected or controlled. Initially, a Foley catheter is inserted to rule out urine retention, to collect available urine for analysis, and to monitor results of diuretic administration. The catheter may or may not be removed during the oliguric phase.

The amount of exogenous water provided should not exceed the amount needed to maintain zero water balance. It is calculated on the basis of estimated endogenous water formation and losses from sensible (primarily gastrointestinal) and insensible sources. No allotment is calculated for urine as long as oliguria persists (see Nursing Care Plan).

When the output begins to increase, either spontaneously or in response to diuretic therapy, the intake of fluid, potassium, and sodium must be monitored and adequate replacement provided to prevent depletion and its consequences. Some patients pass enormous amounts of electrolyte-rich urine.

Complications

The child with ARF has a tendency to develop water intoxication and hyponatremia, which makes it difficult to provide calories in sufficient amounts to meet the child's needs and reduce tissue catabolism, metabolic acidosis, hyperkalemia, and uremia. If the child is able to tolerate oral foods, food sources high in concentrated carbohydrate and fat but low in protein, potassium, and sodium may be provided. However, many children have functional disturbances of the gastrointestinal tract, such as nausea and vomiting; therefore, the IV route is generally preferred and usually consists of essential amino acids or a combination of essential and nonessential amino acids administered by the central venous route.

NURSING CARE PLAN

The Child with Acute Renal Dysfunction

NURSING DIAGNOSIS	PATIENT OUTCOMES	NURSING INTERVENTIONS	RATIONALE
Risk for Injury related to accumulated electrolytes and waste products	The child will exhibit no evidence of waste product accumulation.	Assist with renal dialysis.	To maintain renal excretory function
		Administer sodium polystyrene sulfonate (Kayexalate).	To reduce serum potassium levels
Child's/Family's Defining Characteristics (Subjective and Objective Data)	**The Following NOC Concept Applies to This Outcome**	Provide diet low in potassium, sodium, and phosphorus.	To reduce excretory demand on kidneys
Excesses in potassium, sodium, and phosphorus	Risk Control	Observe for evidence of accumulated waste products.	To ensure prompt treatment
Evidence of hyperkalemia, hyperphosphatemia, uremia		**The Following NIC Concepts Apply to These Interventions**	
Excess BUN		Risk Identification	
		Medication Administration	
		Surveillance	
		Teaching: Individual	
Altered Nutrition: Less Than Body Requirements related to restricted diet	The child will consume an adequate amount of appropriate foods.	Provide dietary instructions for foods that reduce excretory demands on kidneys and provide sufficient calories and protein for growth.	To encourage appropriate diet, which can reduce kidney demands
	The child will show no evidence of deficiencies or weight loss.	Limit phosphorus, salt, and potassium as prescribed.	To prevent mineral excess
Child's/Family's Defining Characteristics (Subjective and Objective Data)		Encourage intake of carbohydrates and foods high in calcium.	To provide calories for growth and calcium to prevent bone demineralization
Weight loss, inadequate growth	**The Following NOC Concepts Apply to These Outcomes**	Arrange for renal dietitian to meet with family to review allowable foods and assist in dietary planning.	To provide family with understanding of the child's dietary needs
Poor nutritional intake	Nutritional Status: Nutrient Intake	Help hemodialysis patient to fill out menu requests for meals.	To promote appropriate food choice decisions
	Nutritional Status: Food and Fluid Intake		
	Weight Control	**The Following NIC Concepts Apply to These Interventions**	
		Teaching: Prescribed Diet	
		Vital Signs Monitoring	
		Fluid Management	
		Nutrition Management	
		Nutrition Therapy	
		Nutritional Monitoring	

BUN, Blood urea nitrogen; *NIC,* Nursing Interventions Classification; *NOC,* Nursing Outcomes Classification.

Control of water balance in these patients requires careful monitoring of feedback information, such as accurate intake and output, body weight, and electrolyte measurements. In general, during the oliguric phase, no sodium, chloride, or potassium is given unless there are other large, ongoing losses. Regular measurement of plasma electrolyte, pH, BUN, and creatinine levels is required to assess the adequacy of fluid therapy and to anticipate complications that require specific treatment.

Hyperkalemia is the most immediate threat to the life of the child with ARF. Hyperkalemia can be minimized and sometimes avoided by eliminating potassium from all food and fluid, reducing tissue catabolism, and correcting acidosis. Measures used for the reduction of serum potassium levels are oral or rectal administration of an ion-exchange resin such as sodium polystyrene sulfonate (Kayexalate) and peritoneal dialysis or hemodialysis (see p. 924). The resin produces its effect by exchange of its sodium for the potassium, thus binding potassium for removal from the body. This increased sodium concentration may contribute to fluid overload, hypertension, and cardiac failure. Dialysis removes potassium and other waste products from the serum by diffusion through a semipermeable membrane.

Hypertension is a frequent and serious complication of ARF, and to detect it early, blood pressure measurements are made every 4 to 6 hours. The most common cause of hypertension in ARF is overexpansion of extracellular fluid and plasma volume together with activation of the renin–angiotensin system. Hypertension is controlled with antihypertensive drugs. Other measures that may be used include limiting fluids and salt.

Anemia is frequently associated with ARF, but transfusion is not recommended unless the hemoglobin drops below 6 g/dl. Transfusions, if used, consist of fresh, packed RBCs given slowly to reduce the likelihood of increasing blood volume, hypertension, and hyperkalemia.

Seizures occur often when renal failure progresses to uremia and are also related to hypertension, hyponatremia, and hypocalcemia. Treatment is directed to the specific cause when known. More obscure causes are managed with antiepileptic drugs.

Cardiac failure with pulmonary edema is almost always associated with hypervolemia. Treatment is directed toward reduction of fluid volume, with water and sodium restriction and administration of diuretics.

Prognosis

The prognosis of ARF depends largely on the nature and severity of the causative factor or precipitating event and the promptness and competence of management. The outcome is least favorable in children with rapidly progressive nephritis and cortical necrosis. Children in whom ARF is a result of HUS or AGN may recover completely, but residual renal impairment or hypertension is more often the rule. Complete recovery is usually expected in children whose renal failure is a result of dehydration, nephrotoxins, or ischemia. ARF after cardiac surgery is less favorable. It is often impossible to assess the extent of recovery for several months.

> **QUALITY PATIENT OUTCOMES: Acute Renal Failure**
> - Underlying cause of ARF identified and treated
> - Water balance maintained
> - Hypertension controlled
> - Electrolyte balance maintained
> - Diet maintains calories while minimizing tissue catabolism, metabolic acidosis, hyperkalemia, and uremia

Nursing Care Management

Meticulous attention to fluid intake and output is mandatory and includes all of the physical measurements discussed previously in relation to problems of fluid balance. Monitoring fluid balance and vital signs is a continuous process, and observers are constantly on the alert for signs of complications so that appropriate interventions can be implemented. Because these children require intensive observation and often specialized treatment, such as dialysis, they are usually admitted to an intensive care unit in which needed equipment and trained personnel are available (see also Nursing Care Plan).

Limiting fluid intake requires ingenuity on the part of caregivers to cope with the child who is thirsty. Rationing the daily intake in small amounts of fluid served in containers that give the impression of larger volumes is one strategy. Older children who understand the rationale of fluid limits can help determine how their daily ration should be distributed.

Meeting nutritional needs is sometimes a problem; the child may be nauseated, and encouraging concentrated foods without fluids may be difficult. When nourishment is provided by the IV route, careful monitoring is essential to prevent fluid overload. In addition, nursing measures such as maintaining an optimal thermal environment, reducing any elevation of body temperature, and reducing restlessness and anxiety are used to decrease the rate of tissue catabolism.

The nurse must be continually alert for changes in behavior that indicate the onset of complications. Infection from reduced resistance, anemia, and general morbidity is a constant threat. Fluid overload and electrolyte disturbances can precipitate cardiovascular complications such as hypertension and cardiac failure. Fluid and electrolyte imbalances, acidosis, and accumulation of nitrogenous waste products can produce neurologic involvement manifested by coma, seizures, or alterations in sensorium.

Although children with ARF are usually quite ill and voluntarily diminish their activity, infants may become restless and irritable, and children are often anxious and frightened. Frequent, painful, and stress-producing treatments and tests must be performed. A supportive, empathetic nurse can provide comfort and stability in a threatening and unnatural environment.

Family Support

Providing support and reassurance to parents is among the major nursing responsibilities. The seriousness of ARF and its emergency nature are stressful to parents, and most feel some degree of guilt regarding the child's condition, especially when the illness is a result of ingestion of a toxic substance, dehydration, or a genetic disease. They need reassurance and a sympathetic listener. They also need to be kept informed of the child's progress and provided explanations regarding the therapeutic regimen. The equipment and the child's behavior are sometimes frightening and anxiety provoking. Nurses can do much to help parents comprehend and deal with the stresses of the situation.

CHRONIC RENAL FAILURE

The kidneys are able to maintain the chemical composition of fluids within normal limits until more than 50% of functional renal capacity is destroyed by disease or injury. Chronic renal insufficiency or failure begins when the diseased kidneys can no longer maintain the normal chemical structure of body fluids under normal conditions. Progressive deterioration over months or years produces a variety of clinical and biochemical disturbances that eventually culminate in the clinical syndrome known as uremia.

A variety of diseases and disorders can result in CRF. The most frequent causes are congenital renal and urinary tract malformations, VUR associated with recurrent UTI, chronic pyelonephritis, hereditary disorders, chronic glomerulonephritis, and glomerulonephropathy associated with systemic diseases such as anaphylactoid purpura and lupus erythematosus.

Pathophysiology

Early in the course of progressive nephrotic destruction, the child remains asymptomatic with only minimal biochemical abnormalities. Unless the presence of CRF is detected in the process of routine assessment, signs and symptoms that indicate advanced renal damage frequently emerge only late in the course of the disease. Midway in the disease process, as increasing numbers of nephrons are totally destroyed and most others are damaged to varying degrees, the few that remain intact are hypertrophied but functional. These few normal nephrons are able to make sufficient adjustments to stresses to maintain reasonable degrees of fluid and electrolyte balance. Definitive biochemical examination at this time will reveal restricted tolerance to excesses or restrictions. As the disease progresses to the end stage, because of a severe reduction in the number of functioning nephrons, the kidneys are no longer able to maintain fluid and electrolyte balance, and the features of uremic syndrome appear.

The accumulation of various biochemical substances in the blood resulting from diminished renal function produces complications such as the following:

Retention of waste products, especially BUN and creatinine

Water and sodium retention, which contributes to edema and vascular congestion

Hyperkalemia of dangerous levels

Metabolic acidosis of a sustained nature because of continual hydrogen ion retention and bicarbonate loss

Calcium and phosphorus disturbances, resulting in altered bone metabolism, which in turn causes growth arrest or retardation, bone pain, and deformities known as renal osteodystrophy

Anemia caused by hematologic dysfunction, including a shortened life span of RBCs, impaired RBC production related to decreased production of erythropoietin, prolonged bleeding time, and nutritional anemia

Growth disturbance, probably caused by such factors as renal osteodystrophy, poor nutrition associated with dietary restrictions and loss of appetite, and biochemical abnormalities

Children with CRF seem to be more susceptible to infection, especially pneumonia, UTI, and septicemia, although the reason for this is unclear. These children become extraordinarily sensitive to changes in vascular volume that may cause pulmonary overload, CNS symptoms, hypertension, and cardiac failure.

Diagnostic Evaluation

The diagnosis of CRF is usually suspected on the basis of any number of clinical manifestations, a history of prior renal disease, or biochemical findings. The onset is usually gradual, and the initial signs and symptoms are vague and nonspecific (Box 27-8).

Laboratory and other diagnostic tools and tests are of value in assessing the extent of renal damage, biochemical disturbances, and related physical dysfunction (see Tables 27-1 to 27-3). Often they can help establish the nature of the underlying disease and differentiate among other disease processes and the pathologic consequences of renal dysfunction.

Therapeutic Management

In irreversible renal failure, the goals of medical management are to (1) promote maximum renal function, (2) maintain body fluid and electrolyte balance within safe biochemical limits, (3) treat systemic complications, and (4) promote as active and normal a life as possible for the child for as long as possible. The child is allowed unrestricted activity and is allowed to set his or her own limits regarding rest and extent of exertion. School attendance is encouraged as long as the child is able. When the effort is too great, home tutoring is arranged.

Diet regulation is the most effective means, short of dialysis, of reducing the quantity of materials that require renal excretion. The goal of diet management in renal failure is to provide sufficient calories and protein for growth while limiting the excretory demands made on the kidneys, to minimize metabolic bone disease (**osteodystrophy**), and to minimize fluid and electrolyte disturbances. Dietary protein intake is limited only to the reference daily intake (RDA) for the child's age. Restriction of protein intake below the RDA is believed to negatively affect growth and neurodevelopment. Malnutrition may develop in patients with CRF even before they need dialysis (Sylvestre, Fonseca, Stinghen, and others, 2007).

Sodium and water are not usually limited unless there is evidence of edema or hypertension, and potassium is not usually restricted. However, restrictions of any or all three may be imposed in later stages or at any time that abnormal serum concentrations are evident.

Dietary phosphorus is controlled through reduction of protein and milk intake to prevent or correct the calcium–phosphorus imbalance. Phosphorus levels can be further reduced by oral administration of calcium carbonate preparations or other phosphate-binding agents that combine with the phosphorus to decrease gastrointestinal absorption and thus the serum levels of phosphate. Treatment with 25-OH vitamin D is begun to increase calcium absorption and suppress elevated parathyroid hormone levels.

Metabolic acidosis is alleviated through administration of alkalizing agents such as sodium bicarbonate or a combination of sodium and potassium citrate.

BOX 27-8   CLINICAL MANIFESTATIONS OF CHRONIC RENAL FAILURE

Early signs:
- Loss of normal energy
- Increased fatigue on exertion
- Pallor, subtle (may not be noticed)
- Elevated blood pressure (sometimes)

As the disease progresses:
- Decreased appetite (especially at breakfast)
- Less interest in normal activities
- Increased or decreased urinary output with compensatory intake of fluid
- Pallor more evident
- Sallow, muddy appearance of skin

Child may complain of:
- Headache
- Muscle cramps
- Nausea

Other signs and symptoms:
- Weight loss
- Facial edema
- Malaise
- Bone or joint pain
- Growth retardation
- Dryness or itching of the skin
- Bruised skin
- Sensory or motor loss (sometimes)
- Amenorrhea (common in adolescent girls)

Uremic syndrome (untreated):
- Gastrointestinal symptoms
  - Anorexia
  - Nausea and vomiting
- Bleeding tendencies
  - Bruises
  - Bloody diarrheal stools
  - Stomatitis
  - Bleeding from lips and mouth
- Intractable itching
- Uremic frost (deposits of urea crystals on skin)
- Unpleasant "uremic" breath odor
- Deep respirations
- Hypertension
- Congestive heart failure
- Pulmonary edema
- Neurologic involvement
  - Progressive confusion
  - Dulled sensorium
  - Coma (ultimately)
  - Tremors
  - Muscular twitching
  - Seizures

Growth failure is one major consequence of CRF, especially in preadolescents. These children grow poorly both before and after the initiation of hemodialysis. The use of recombinant human growth hormone to accelerate growth in children with growth retardation secondary to CRF has been successful (Vimalachandra, Hodson, Willis, and others, 2006). **Osseous deformities** that result from renal osteodystrophy, especially those related to ambulation, are troublesome and require correction if they occur. Dental defects are common in children with CRF, and the earlier the onset of the disease, the more severe are the dental manifestations (including hypoplasia, hypomineralization, tooth discoloration, alteration in size and shape of teeth, malocclusion, and ulcerative stomatitis). Therefore, regular dental care is important in these children.

Anemia in children with CRF is related to decreased production of erythropoietin. Recombinant human erythropoietin (rHuEPO) is being offered to these children as thrice-weekly or weekly subcutaneous injections and is replacing the need for frequent blood transfusions. The drug corrects the anemia and in turn increases appetite, activity, and general well-being in the children who receive it.

Hypertension may be managed initially by cautious use of a low-sodium diet, fluid restriction, and perhaps diuretics such as hydrochlorothiazide or furosemide. Severe hypertension requires the use of antihypertensive agents, singly or in combination.

Intercurrent infections are treated with appropriate antimicrobials at the first sign of infection; however, any drug eliminated through the kidneys is administered with caution. Other complications are treated symptomatically (e.g., central-acting antiemetics for nausea, antiepileptics for seizures, and diphenhydramine [Benadryl] for pruritus).

When evidence of end-stage renal disease (ESRD) appears in a child, the disease runs its relentless course and results in death in a few weeks unless waste products and toxins are removed from body fluids by dialysis or kidney transplantation. These techniques have been adapted for infants and small children and are implemented in most cases of renal failure after conservative management is no longer effective (see Technologic Management of Renal Failure, p. 924).

Prognosis

Dialysis and transplantation are the only treatments currently available for children with ESRD. Although children may survive on dialysis, it is not an ideal long-term modality. Complications include infection of access sites, growth failure, and disruption of normal socialization. Many pediatric centers encourage families of children with ESRD to consider kidney transplantation. The North American Pediatric Renal Trials and Collaborative Studies' annual transplant report documents graft survival of 96% at 1 year and 84% at 5 years for living donor kidneys and 95% at 1 year and 78% at 5 years for deceased donor kidneys (2010).

Posttransplant complications include infection, hypertension, steroid toxicity, hyperlipidemia, aseptic necrosis, malignancy, and growth retardation (Dharnidharka and Araya, 2009). Long-term graft survival is not guaranteed, and many children require a second or third transplant. Successful kidney transplantation does improve rehabilitation of children with CRF, both educationally and psychologically. Increasing use of primary or preemptive kidney transplants is becoming the optimal form of renal replacement therapy, leading to substantial improvement in quality of life (Goldstein, Graham, Burwinkle, and others, 2006).

QUALITY PATIENT OUTCOMES: Chronic Renal Failure
- Sufficient calories and protein for growth maintained
- Excretory demands made on the kidney are limited
- Metabolic bone disease (osteodystrophy) minimal
- Fluid and electrolyte disturbances managed
- Hypertension managed
- Growth retardation treated

Nursing Care Management

The multiple complications of ESRD are managed according to medical protocols such as the National Kidney Foundation Kidney Disease Outcomes Quality Initiative's evidence-based clinical practice guidelines (http://www.kidney.org/professionals/KDOQI). However, progressive disease places a number of stresses on the child and family, including those of a potentially fatal illness (see Chapter 18). There is a continuing need for repeated examinations that often entail painful procedures, side effects, and frequent hospitalizations. Diet therapy becomes progressively more restricted and intense, and the child is required to take a variety of medications. Ever present in all aspects of the treatment regimen is the agonizing realization that without treatment, death is inevitable.

Some specific stresses related to ESRD and its treatment are predictable. When it first becomes apparent that ESRD is inevitable, both parents and child experience depression and anxiety. Acceptance is particularly difficult if renal failure progresses rapidly after diagnosis. Denial and disbelief are usually pronounced, especially among the parents. After renal failure is established and symptoms become progressively more distressing, the initiation of dialysis is usually perceived as a positive experience, and after experiencing initial concerns regarding the treatment, the child begins to feel better, and parental anxiety is relieved for a time.

Initiating a dialysis regimen is a traumatic and anxiety-provoking experience for most children because it involves surgery for implantation of a graft, fistula, or peritoneal catheter. The initial experience with the dialysis procedure is frightening to most children. They need reassurance about the nature of the preparations for dialysis and the conduct of the treatment.

Both the graft and the fistula require needle insertions at each dialysis. The goal is to perform pain-free venipuncture. Using buffered lidocaine with a small-gauge needle (30 gauge) to anesthetize the area before venipuncture of the graft or fistula is one method. Using an anesthetizing topical preparation such as EMLA (eutectic mixture of local anesthetics [lidocaine and prilocaine]) 1 hour before venipuncture is another approach (see Pain Management, Chapter 7). External dual-lumen venous access devices eliminate the need for needles but are more prone to infection and other central line complications.

Adolescents, with their increased need for independence and their urge for rebellion, usually adapt less well than younger children. They resent the control and enforced dependence imposed by the rigorous and unrelenting therapy program. They resent being dependent on hemodialysis technology, their parents, and the professional staff. Depression or hostility is common in adolescents undergoing hemodialysis.

The availability of home peritoneal dialysis has offered a greater degree of freedom for persons undergoing long-term dialysis. The nurse is responsible for teaching the family about (1) the disease, its implications, and the therapeutic plan; (2) the possible psychologic effects of the disease and the treatment; and (3) the technical aspects of the procedure. The family learns to manage the various aspects of the dialysis procedure, how to maintain accurate records, and how to observe for signs of complications that need to be reported to the proper persons.

Body changes related to the disease process, such as pale or ashen skin color, growth retardation, and lack of sexual maturation, are stress provoking. Dietary restrictions are particularly burdensome for both children and parents. Children feel deprived when they are unable to eat foods previously enjoyed and that are unrestricted for other family members. Consequently, they may fail to cooperate. Diet restrictions may be interpreted as punishment. Some children, unable to

FAMILY-CENTERED CARE

Family Priorities

Families that have children with long-term chronic illnesses, such as end-stage renal disease, spend much time in hospitals, outpatient clinics, and primary health care facilities. When they miss appointments or respond less quickly than anticipated, sometimes they are quickly labeled "noncompliant." It is important to remember that families have to develop priorities for the unit as a whole. Sometimes the family may decide that it is more important for the parent to go to work or to attend a sibling's school performance than to attend an appointment scheduled for them by health care personnel. The chronically ill child cannot and should not always be the number one priority for the family. The professional staff who works with the family can help the parents prioritize the needs of the ill child within the needs of the family constellation.

Teresa Hall, MS, RN
Hathaway Children's Services
Sylmar, Calif.

understand fully the purpose of restrictions, will sneak forbidden food items at every opportunity. Allowing children, especially adolescents, maximum participation in and responsibility for their own treatment program is helpful.

After months or years of dialysis, the parents and child feel anxiety associated with the prognosis and continued pressures of the treatment. The relentless need for treatment interferes with family plans. The time spent in transportation to and from the dialysis unit and the time spent undergoing dialysis treatments cut into time for outside activities, including school. Graft and fistula problems, as well as peritoneal catheter exit site infections, may develop and present a common source of aggravation (see Family-Centered Care box).

The possibility of kidney transplantation often provides hope for relief from the rigors of hemodialysis and peritoneal dialysis. Most children and families respond well to a kidney transplant, and most children can be successfully rehabilitated.

The National Kidney Foundation* and other agencies provide a number of services and information for families of children with renal disease.

TECHNOLOGIC MANAGEMENT OF RENAL FAILURE

DIALYSIS

Dialysis is the process of separating colloids and crystalline substances in solution by the difference in their rate of diffusion through a semipermeable membrane. Methods of dialysis currently available for clinical management of renal failure are peritoneal dialysis, wherein the abdominal cavity acts as a semipermeable membrane through which water and solutes of small molecular size move by osmosis and diffusion according to their respective concentrations on either side of the membrane, and hemodialysis, in which blood is circulated outside the body through artificial membranes that permit a similar passage of water and solutes. A third type of dialysis is hemofiltration, in which

*30 E. 33rd St., New York, NY 10016; 212-889-2210, 800-622-9010; http://www.kidney.org. In Canada: Kidney Foundation of Canada, 300–5165 Sherbrooke St. West, Montreal, QC H4A 1T6; 514-369-4806, 800-361-7494; http://www.kidney.ca.

blood filtrate is circulated outside the body by hydrostatic pressure exerted across a semipermeable membrane with simultaneous infusion of a replacement solution. Types of hemofiltration include continuous venovenous hemofiltration, continuous venovenous hemodialysis, and continuous venovenous hemodiafiltration. These continuous renal replacement therapies are used in ARF, severe fluid overload, and inborn errors of metabolism or after bone marrow transplant.

Peritoneal dialysis is the preferred form of dialysis for infants, children and parents who wish to remain independent, families who live a long distance from the medical center, and children who prefer fewer dietary restrictions and a gentler form of dialysis. Chronic peritoneal dialysis is most often performed at home. The two types of peritoneal dialysis are continuous ambulatory peritoneal dialysis and continuous cycling peritoneal dialysis. In both methods, commercially available sterile dialysis solution is instilled into the peritoneal cavity through a surgically implanted indwelling catheter tunneled subcutaneously and sutured into place. The warmed solution is allowed to enter the peritoneal cavity by gravity and remains a variable length of time according to the rate of solute removal and glucose absorption in individual patients. The care and management of the procedure are the responsibility of the parents of young children. Some centers have initiated use of home health nurses to give parents respite from care. Older children and adolescents can carry out the procedure themselves, which provides them with some control and less dependency. This is especially important for adolescents.

! NURSING ALERT

Observe for changes in the color of the dialysate draining from the child. The spent solution should be clear. If the color is cloudy, notify the practitioner immediately (Schaefer, 2003).

Hemodialysis requires the creation of a vascular access and the use of special dialysis equipment—the hemodialyzer, or so-called artificial kidney. Vascular access may be one of three types: fistulas, grafts, or external vascular access devices. An arteriovenous fistula is an access in which a vein and artery are connected surgically. The preferred site is the radial artery and a forearm vein that produces dilation and thickening of the superficial vessels of the forearm to provide easy access for repeated venipuncture. An alternative is the creation of a subcutaneous (internal) arteriovenous graft by anastomosing artery and vein, with a synthetic prosthetic graft for circulatory access. The most commonly used material is expanded polytetrafluoroethylene (ePTFE). Both the graft and the fistula require needle insertions with each dialysis treatment.

For external vascular access devices, percutaneous catheters are inserted in the femoral, subclavian, or internal jugular veins, even in very small children. A more permanent form of external access is available via a central catheter inserted surgically into the internal jugular vein. This catheter has a dual lumen, which allows a larger volume of blood flow with minimum recirculation. Catheters eliminate the need for skin punctures but may require some home care.

Hemodialysis is best suited to children who do not have someone in the family who is able to perform home peritoneal dialysis and to those who live close to a dialysis center. The procedure is usually performed three times per week for 4 to 6 hours, depending on the child's size. Hemodialysis achieves rapid correction of fluid and electrolyte abnormalities but can cause problems in association with this rapid change, such as muscle cramping and hypotension. Disadvantages include school absence during dialysis and strict fluid and dietary restrictions between dialysis sessions. Boredom for the child and family

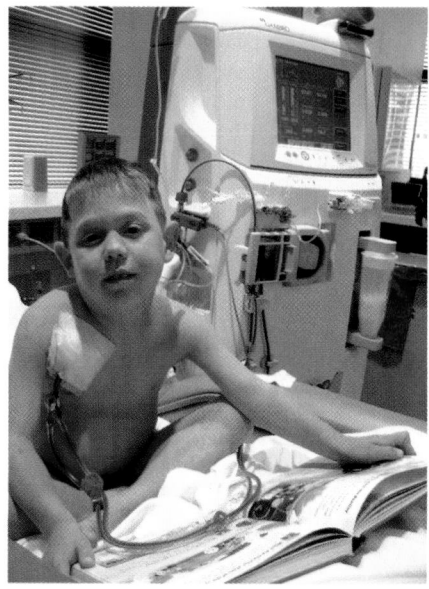

FIG 27-4 Diversional activities help lessen the boredom children can experience during hemodialysis.

is often a problem during dialysis, and planned activities should be introduced (Fig. 27-4).

Most children show rapid clinical improvement with the implementation of dialysis, although it is directly related to the duration of uremia before dialysis and good nutrition. Growth rate and skeletal maturation improve, but recovery of normal growth is infrequent. In many cases, sexual development, although delayed, progresses to completion.

TRANSPLANTATION

Kidney transplantation is an acceptable and effective means of therapy in the pediatric age group. Although peritoneal dialysis and hemodialysis are life preserving, both require major alterations in lifestyle.

Transplantation offers the opportunity for a relatively normal life and is the preferred form of treatment for children with ESRD. Primary or preemptive transplants maintain the greatest amount of normalcy in the family's life.

Kidneys for transplant are available from two sources: a living related donor, usually a parent or a sibling, or a cadaver donor, wherein the family of a dead or brain-dead patient consents to donation of a healthy kidney. Retransplantation may be required.

The primary goal in transplantation is the long-term survival of grafted tissue by securing tissue that is antigenically similar to that of the recipient and by suppressing the recipient's immune mechanism. The immunosuppressant therapy of choice has been corticosteroids (prednisone) in conjunction with cyclosporine or tacrolimus and mycophenolate mofetil. Other therapies include antilymphoblast globulin or monoclonal antibodies. New immunosuppressant medications and early withdrawal of steroids or steroid-free protocols are rapidly coming into clinical trials and use in large transplant centers (Grenda and Webb, 2010). It is important for the nurse to learn about the medications used in the antirejection protocol(s) and their side effects. Because the immunosuppressant medications are taken indefinitely, transplant patients experience many side effects of the drugs, including hypertension, growth retardation, cataracts, risk of infection, obesity, characteristics of Cushing syndrome, and hirsutism (McDonald, 2011).

> **! NURSING ALERT**
>
> The child with a kidney transplant who exhibits any of the following should be evaluated immediately for possible rejection:
> - Fever
> - Swelling and tenderness over graft area
> - Diminished urinary output
> - Elevated blood pressure
> - Elevated serum creatinine

Rejection of the transplanted kidney is the most common cause of transplant failure. Rejection is treated aggressively with immunosuppressant medications and can often be reversed. Some patients do not respond to treatment of acute rejection or develop chronic rejection and must eventually return to dialysis or undergo another kidney transplant.

■ KEY POINTS

- Common inflammatory disorders of the genitourinary tract include UTI, nephrotic syndrome, and AGN.
- Management of UTIs is directed at eliminating infection, detecting and correcting functional or anatomic abnormalities, preventing recurrences, and preserving renal function.
- VUR is the retrograde flow of bladder urine into the ureters.
- Obstructive uropathy is a result of structural or functional abnormalities of the urinary system that obstruct the normal flow of urine.
- The more common defects of the genitourinary tract include phimosis, cryptorchidism, inguinal hernia, hydrocele, and hypospadias.
- Body image concerns and castration anxiety are particularly intense in children with defects in the genital area.
- Nephrotic syndrome is characterized by increased glomerular permeability to protein, with massive urinary loss of protein resulting in hypoproteinemia and edema.

- Management of nephrotic syndrome is aimed at reducing excretion of protein, reducing or preventing fluid retention by tissues, and preventing infection and other complications.
- Common features of AGN are oliguria, edema, hypertension, circulatory congestion, hematuria, and proteinuria.
- Therapeutic management of AGN involves maintenance of fluid balance, treatment of hypertension, and antibiotic therapy.
- Management of HUS is aimed at control of complications and hematologic manifestations of renal failure.
- Wilms tumor is the most common malignant neoplasm of the kidney in infants and children.
- In ARF, management is directed at determining treatment of the underlying cause, managing complications of renal failure, and providing supportive therapy.
- Abnormalities in CRF are waste product retention, water and sodium retention, hyperkalemia, acidosis, calcium and phosphorus disturbance, anemia, and growth disturbances.

KEY POINTS—cont'd

- The types of dialysis used in ESRD are peritoneal dialysis and hemodialysis.
- When the child will need home dialysis, the nurse educates the family about the disease, its implications, the therapeutic plan, possible psychologic effects of the disease, and the treatment and technical aspects of the procedure.

- The major concerns in kidney transplantation are tissue matching and prevention of rejection; psychologic concerns involve self-image as related to possible body changes as a result of the effects of corticosteroid therapy.

REFERENCES

American Academy of Pediatrics, Task Force on Circumcision: Circumcision policy statement, *Pediatrics* 103(3):686–693, 1999.

Cendron M, Gomez P: *Wilms tumor*, retrieved December 16, 2010, from http://emedicine. medscape.com/article/453076-overview.

Chen HC, Yeh CM, Chou CM: Endoscopic treatment of vesicoureteral reflux in children with dextranomer/hyaluronic acid—a single surgeon's 6 year experience, *Diagn Ther Endosc Epub* 2010, in press.

Dharnidharka VR, Araya CE: Complications of renal transplantation. In Avner ED, Harmon WE, Niaudet P, and other, editors: *Pediatric nephrology*, ed 6, Berlin Heidelberg, 2009, Springer-Verlag.

Dome JS, Perlman EJ, Ritchey ML, and others: Renal tumors. In Pizzo PA, Poplack DP, editors: *Principles and practices of pediatric oncology*, ed 5, Philadelphia, 2006, Lippincott.

Duzova A, Bakkaloglu A, Kalyoncu M, and others: Etiology and outcome of acute kidney injury in children, *Pediatr Nephrol* 25(8):1453–1461, 2010.

Ferrara P, Romaniello L, Vitelli O, and others: Cranberry juice for the prevention of recurrent urinary tract infections: a randomized controlled trial in children, *Scan J Uro Nephrol* 43:369–372, 2009.

Gipson DS, Massengill SF, Yao L, and others: Management of childhood onset nephrotic syndrome, *Pediatrics* 124(2):747–757, 2009.

Goldstein SL, Graham N, Burwinkle T, and others: Health-related quality of life in pediatric patients with ESRD, *Pediatr Nephrol* 21(6): 846–850, 2006.

Grenda R, Webb NJ: Steroid minimization in pediatric renal transplantation: early withdrawal or avoidance? *Pediatr Transplantation* 14(8): 961–967, 2010.

Jepson RG, Mihaljevic L, Craig J: Cranberries for preventing urinary tract infections, *Cochrane Database Syst Rev* (2):CD001321, 2008.

Kanellopoulos TA, Salakos C, Spiliopoulou I, and others: First urinary tract infection in neonates, infants and young children: a comparative study, *Pediatr Nephrol* 21(8):1131–1137, 2006.

Kass E: Timing of elective surgery on the genitalia of male children with particular reference to the risks, benefits, and psychological effects of surgery and anesthesia, *Pediatrics* 97(4): 590–594, 1996.

McDonald RA: Immunosuppression in renal transplantation in children, *UpToDate* 2011, retrieved May 20, 2011, from http:// www.uptodate.com.

National Kidney Foundation: *The National Kidney Foundation kidney disease outcomes quality initiative* (NKF KDOQI™), retrieved June 6, 2011, from http://www.kidney.org/professionals/ kdoqi.

North American Pediatric Renal Trials and Collaborative Studies: *NAPRTCS 2010 annual transplant report*, retrieved May 6, 2011, from https://web.emmes.com/study/ped/annlrept/ 2010_Report.pdf.

Patzer L: Nephrotoxicity as a cause of acute kidney injury in children, *Pediatr Nephrol* 23(12):2159–2173, 2008.

Rice SG, Council on Sports Medicine and Fitness: Medical conditions affecting sports participation, *Pediatrics* 121(4):841–848, 2008.

Rosenthal M: Current concept in managing UTIs in children, *Infect Dis Child* 17(3):30–31, 2004.

Schaefer F: Management of peritonitis in children receiving chronic peritoneal dialysis, *Paediatr Drugs* 5(5):315–325, 2003.

Shaikh N, Morone NE, Bost JE, and others: Prevalence of urinary tract infection in childhood: a meta-analysis, *Pediatr Infect Dis J* 27(4):302–308, 2008.

Sylvestre LC, Fonseca K, Stinghen A, and others: The malnutrition and inflammation axis in pediatric patients with chronic kidney disease, *Pediatr Nephrol* 22(6):864–873, 2007.

Vimalachandra D, Hodson EM, Willis NS, and others: Growth hormone for children with chronic kidney disease, *Cochrane Database Syst Rev* (3):CD003264, 2006.

The Child with Cerebral Dysfunction

Cheryl C. Rodgers and Valerie J. Groben

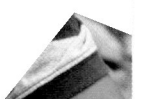

CHAPTER OUTLINE

Cerebral Dysfunction, 928
  Increased Intracranial Pressure, 928
  Altered States of Consciousness, 928
    Levels of Consciousness, 928
    Coma Assessment, 929
  General Aspects, 929
  Neurologic Examination, 930
    Vital Signs, 930
    Skin, 930
    Eyes, 930
    Motor Function, 931
    Posturing, 932
    Reflexes, 932
  Special Diagnostic Procedures, 932
Nursing Care of the Unconscious Child, 934
  Respiratory Management, 935
  Intracranial Pressure Monitoring, 935
    Nursing Activities, 936
    Suctioning, 936

Nutrition and Hydration, 937
  Altered Pituitary Secretion, 937
Medications, 937
Thermoregulation, 937
Elimination, 937
Hygienic Care, 937
Positioning and Exercise, 938
Stimulation, 938
  Regaining Consciousness, 938
Family Support, 938
Cerebral Trauma, 938
  Head Injury, 938
  Submersion Injury, 945
Nervous System Tumors, 946
  Brain Tumors, 946
  Neuroblastoma, 949
Intracranial Infections, 949
  Bacterial Meningitis, 950
  Nonbacterial (Aseptic) Meningitis, 953

Encephalitis, 954
Rabies, 955
Reye Syndrome, 956
Seizure Disorders, 956
  Etiology, 956
  Pathophysiology, 956
  Seizure Classification and Clinical Manifestations, 957
    Nursing Care Plan: The Child with Seizures, 963
  Febrile Seizures, 966
Cerebral Malformations, 966
  Cranial Deformities, 966
  Hydrocephalus, 967

LEARNING OBJECTIVES

On completion of this chapter the reader will be able to:
- Describe the various modalities for assessment of cerebral function.
- Differentiate among the stages of consciousness.
- Formulate a care plan for the unconscious child.
- Distinguish among the types of head injuries and the serious complications.
- Describe the nursing care of a child with a tumor of the central nervous system.

- Outline a care plan for the child with bacterial meningitis.
- Differentiate between the various types of seizure disorders.
- Demonstrate an understanding of the manifestations of a seizure disorder and the management of a child with such a disorder.
- Describe the preoperative and postoperative care of a child with hydrocephalus.

CEREBRAL DYSFUNCTION

Most of the information about the status of the brain is obtained by indirect measurements. Some of these measurements are discussed elsewhere in relation to numerous aspects of child care (e.g., as part of assessments of health [Chapter 6], newborn status [Chapter 8], intellectual disability [Chapter 19], hypoxic injury [cerebral palsy, Chapter 32], and attainment of developmental milestones at each stage of development). Because increased intracranial pressure (ICP) and altered states of consciousness have such prominent places in neurologic dysfunction, they are described here followed by techniques for neurologic assessment and diagnostic tests.

INCREASED INTRACRANIAL PRESSURE

The brain, tightly enclosed in the solid bony cranium, is well protected but highly vulnerable to pressure that may accumulate within the enclosure (Fig. 28-1). The cranium's total volume—brain (80%), cerebrospinal fluid (CSF) (10%), and blood (10%)—must remain approximately the same at all times. A change in the proportional volume of one of these components (e.g., increase or decrease in intracranial blood) must be accompanied by a compensatory change in another. In this way, the volume and pressure normally remain constant. Examples of compensatory changes are reduction in blood volume, decrease in CSF production, increase in CSF absorption, or shrinkage of brain mass by displacement of intracellular and extracellular fluid. Children with open fontanels compensate by skull expansion and widened sutures. However, at any age, the capacity for spatial compensation is limited. An increase in ICP may be caused by tumors or other space-occupying lesions, accumulation of fluid within the ventricular system, bleeding, or edema of cerebral tissues. When compensation is exhausted, any further increase in the cranium's volume will result in a rapid rise in ICP.

Early signs and symptoms of increased ICP are often subtle and assume many patterns (Box 28-1). As pressure increases, signs and symptoms become more pronounced, and the level of consciousness (LOC) deteriorates.

ALTERED STATES OF CONSCIOUSNESS

Consciousness implies awareness—the ability to respond to sensory stimuli and have subjective experiences. There are two components of consciousness: alertness, an arousal-waking state, including the ability to respond to stimuli, and cognitive power, including the ability to process stimuli and produce verbal and motor responses.

An altered state of consciousness usually refers to varying states of unconsciousness that may be momentary or may extend for hours, for days, or indefinitely. Unconsciousness is depressed cerebral function—the inability to respond to sensory stimuli and have subjective experiences. Coma is defined as a state of unconsciousness from which the patient cannot be aroused even with powerful stimuli.

Levels of Consciousness

Assessment of LOC remains the earliest indicator of improvement or deterioration in neurologic status. LOC is determined by observations of the child's responses to the environment. When LOC is being assessed in young children, it is often useful to have a parent present to help elicit a desired response. An infant or child may not respond in an unfamiliar environment or to unfamiliar voices. Children older than 3 years of age should be able to give their name, although they may not be cognizant of place or time. Other diagnostic tests, such as motor activity, reflexes, and vital signs, are more variable and do not

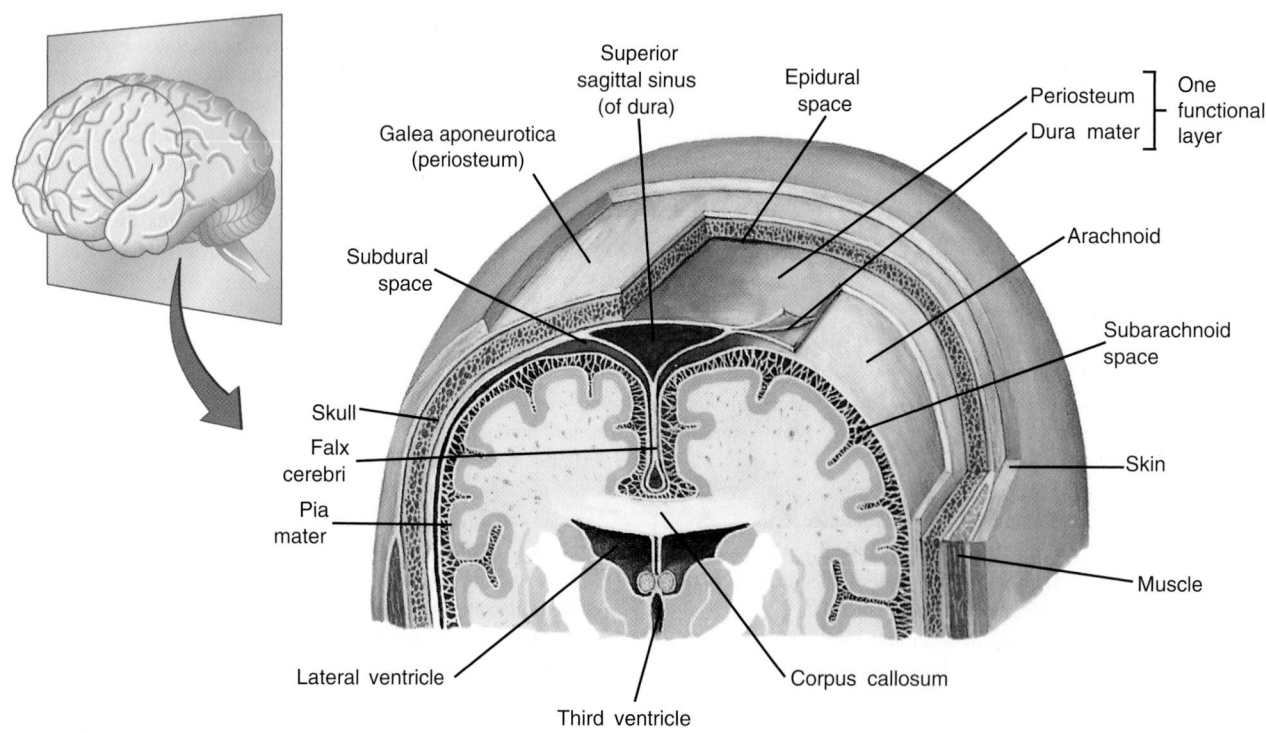

FIG 28-1 Coronal section of the top of the head showing meningeal layers. (From Patton KT, Thibodeau GA: *Anatomy and physiology*, ed 8, St. Louis, 2013, Mosby.)

Modified from Seidel HM, Ball JW, Dains JE, and others, editors: *Mosby's guide to physical examination*, ed 5, St. Louis, 2003, Mosby. LOC, Level of consciousness.

BOX 28-1 CLINICAL MANIFESTATIONS OF INCREASED INTRACRANIAL PRESSURE IN INFANTS AND CHILDREN

Infants

Tense, bulging fontanel
Separated cranial sutures
Macewen (cracked-pot) sign
Irritability and restlessness
Drowsiness
Increased sleeping
High-pitched cry
Increased frontooccipital circumference
Distended scalp veins
Poor feeding
Crying when disturbed
Setting-sun sign

Children

Headache
Nausea
Forceful vomiting
Diplopia, blurred vision
Seizures
Indifference, drowsiness
Decline in school performance
Diminished physical activity and motor performance
Increased sleeping
Inability to follow simple commands
Lethargy

Late Signs in Infants and Children

Bradycardia
Decreased motor response to command
Decreased sensory response to painful stimuli
Alterations in pupil size and reactivity
Extension or flexion posturing
Cheyne-Stokes respirations
Papilledema
Decreased consciousness
Coma

BOX 28-2 LEVELS OF CONSCIOUSNESS

Full consciousness—Awake and alert, orientated to time, place, and person; behavior appropriate for age
Confusion—Impaired decision making
Disorientation—Confusion regarding time, place; decreased LOC
Lethargy—Limited spontaneous movement, sluggish speech, drowsy, falling asleep quickly
Obtundation—Arousable with stimulation
Stupor—Remaining in a deep sleep, slow response to vigorous and repeated stimulation or moaning responses to stimuli
Coma—No motor or verbal response or extension posturing to noxious (painful) stimuli
Persistent vegetative state—Permanently lost function of the cerebral cortex. Eyes follow objects only by reflex or when attracted to the direction of loud sounds; all four limbs are spastic but can withdraw from painful stimuli; hands show reflexive grasping and groping; the face can grimace, some food may be swallowed, and the child may groan or cry but utter no words.

brain death among children of all ages (Mathur, Peterson, Stadtier, and others, 2008).

GENERAL ASPECTS

Children younger than 2 years of age require special evaluation because they are unable to respond to directions designed to elicit specific neurologic responses. Early neurologic responses in infants are primarily reflexive; these responses are gradually replaced by meaningful movement in the characteristic cephalocaudal direction of development. This evidence of progressive maturation reflects more extensive myelinization and changes in neurochemical and electrophysiologic properties.

Most information about infants and small children is gained by observing their spontaneous and elicited reflex responses as they develop increasingly complex motor skills and by eliciting progressively sophisticated communicative and adaptive behaviors. Delay or deviation from expected milestones helps identify high-risk children. Persistence or reappearance of reflexes that normally disappear indicates a pathologic condition. In evaluating an infant or young child, it is also important to obtain the pregnancy and delivery history to determine the possible impact of intrauterine environmental influences known to affect the orderly maturation of the central nervous system (CNS). These influences include maternal infections, cigarette or alcohol consumption, drug use, toxin exposure, trauma, and metabolic insults.

General aspects of assessment that provide clues to the etiology of dysfunction include:

Family history—Sometimes offers clues regarding possible genetic disorders with neurologic manifestations
Health history—May provide valuable clues regarding the cause of dysfunction. Information should include Apgar scores, age of developmental milestones, trauma or injuries, acute and chronic illnesses, encounters with animals or insects, and ingestion or inhalation of neurotoxic substances.

necessarily directly parallel the depth of the comatose state. The most consistently used terms are described in Box 28-2.

Coma Assessment

Several scales have been devised in an attempt to standardize the description and interpretation of the degree of depressed consciousness. The most popular of these is the Glasgow Coma Scale (GCS), which consists of a three-part assessment: eye opening, verbal response, and motor response (Fig. 28-2). Numeric values of 1 through 5 are assigned to the levels of response in each category. The sum of these numeric values provides an objective measure of the patient's LOC. A person with an unaltered LOC would score the highest, 15; a score of 8 or below is generally accepted as a definition of coma; and the lowest score, 3, indicates deep coma. A decrease in the GCS score indicates a deterioration of the patient's condition. In 1987, major medical and legal societies developed specific guidelines for the determination of

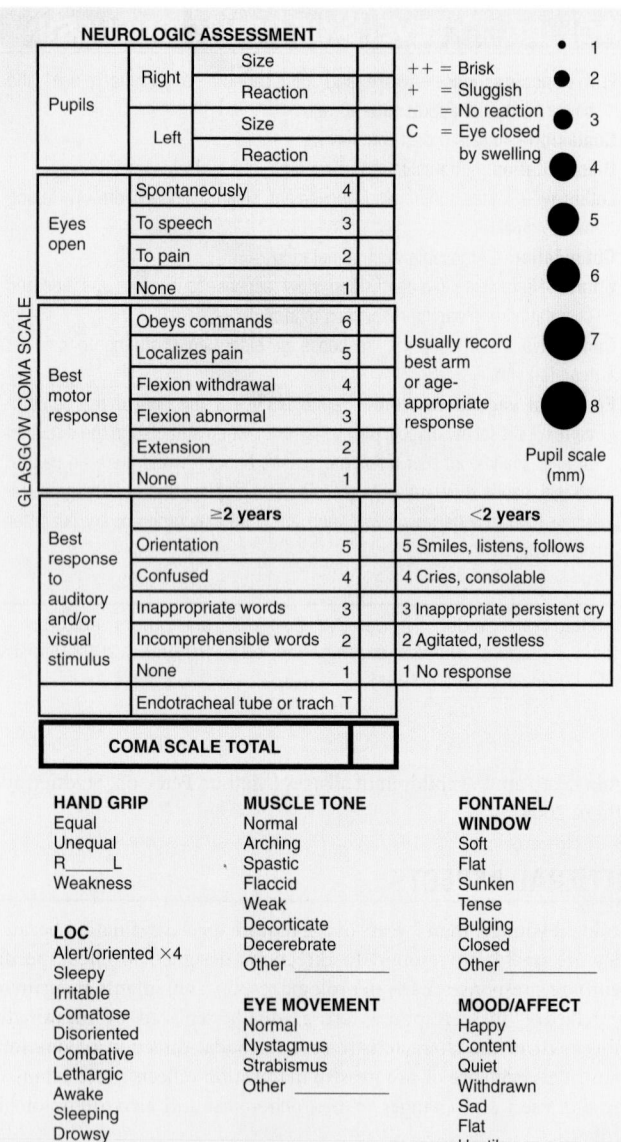

FIG 28-2 Pediatric coma scale. *LOC,* Level of consciousness.

Physical evaluation of infants—Includes assessment of:
- Level of alertness
- Size and shape of the head, including presence of fontanels
- Sensory responses
- Motor function, including posture, tone, and muscle strength
- Motility, including symmetry of movements and involuntary movements
- Respirations, including signs of prolonged apnea, ataxic breathing, paradoxic chest movement, or hyperventilation
- Dysmorphic facial features
- Behavioral cues, including consolability and habituation
- Primitive and deep tendon reflexes
- Cranial nerves

NEUROLOGIC EXAMINATION

The purpose of the neurologic examination is to establish an accurate, objective baseline of neurologic information. It is essential that the neurologic examination be documented in a fashion that can be reproduced by others. This allows for a comparison of the findings so the observer can detect subtle changes in the neurologic status that might not otherwise be evident. Descriptions of behaviors should be simple, objective, and easily interpreted: "Drowsy but awake and conversationally rational/oriented"; "Sleepy but arousable with vigorous physical stimuli. Pressure to nail base of right hand results in upper extremity flexion/lower extremity extension."

Vital Signs

Pulse, respiration, and blood pressure provide information regarding the adequacy of circulation and the possible underlying cause of altered consciousness. Autonomic activity is most intensively disturbed in cases of deep coma or brainstem lesions.

Body temperature is often elevated, and sometimes the elevation may be extreme. High temperature is most frequently a sign of an acute infectious process or heat stroke but may also be caused by ingestion of some drugs (especially salicylates, alcohol, and barbiturates) or by intracranial bleeding, especially subarachnoid hemorrhage. Hypothalamic involvement may cause elevated or decreased temperature. Coma of a toxic origin may produce hypothermia.

The **pulse** is variable and may be rapid, slow and bounding, or feeble. **Blood pressure** may be normal, elevated, or very low. The Cushing reflex, or pressor response, causes a slowing of the pulse and an increase in blood pressure and is uncommon in children; when it occurs, it is a very late sign of ICP. Medications may affect the vital signs. For assessment purposes, actual *changes* in pulse and blood pressure are more important than the direction of the change.

Respirations are often slow, deep, and irregular. Slow, deep breathing is often seen in the heavy sleep caused by sedatives, after seizures, or in cerebral infections. Slow, shallow breathing may result from sedatives or opioids (narcotics). Hyperventilation (deep and rapid respirations) is usually a result of metabolic acidosis or abnormal stimulation of the respiratory center in the medulla caused by salicylate poisoning, hepatic coma, or Reye syndrome (RS).

Breathing patterns have been described with a number of terms (e.g., apneustic, cluster, ataxic, Cheyne-Stokes). However, it is better to describe what is being observed rather than to place a label on it because the traditional terms are often used and interpreted incorrectly. Periodic or irregular breathing is an ominous sign of brainstem (especially medullary) dysfunction that often precedes complete apnea. The **odor** of the breath may provide additional clues (e.g., the fruity, acetone odor of ketosis; the foul odor of uremia; the fetid odor of hepatic failure; or the odor of alcohol).

Skin

The skin may offer clues to the cause of unconsciousness. The head should be examined for trauma such as lacerations, ecchymosis, or hematoma, and the body surface should be examined for signs of injury, needle marks, petechiae, bites, and ticks. Evidence of toxic substances may be found on the hands, face, mouth, and clothing, especially in small children.

Eyes

Pupil size and reactivity are assessed (Fig. 28-3; see also Fig. 28-2). Pinpoint pupils are commonly observed in poisoning, such as opiate or barbiturate poisoning, and in brainstem dysfunction. Widely dilated and reactive pupils are often seen after seizures and may involve only one side. Dilated pupils may also be caused by eye trauma. Widely dilated and fixed pupils suggest paralysis of cranial nerve III secondary to pressure from herniation of the brain through the tentorium. A

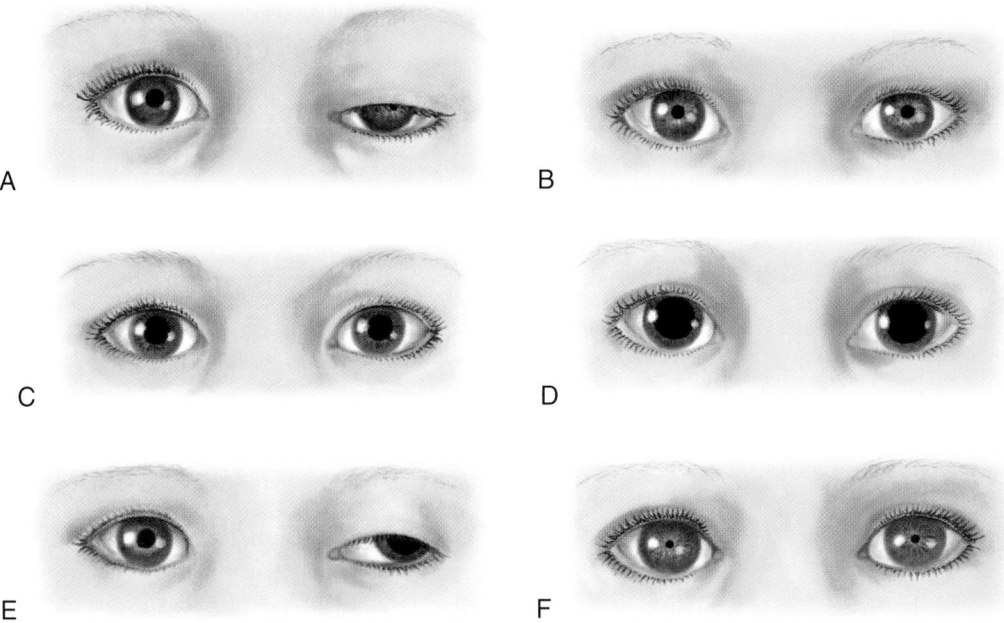

FIG 28-3 Variations in pupil size with altered states of consciousness. **A,** Ipsilateral pupillary constriction with slight ptosis. **B,** Bilateral small pupils. **C,** Midposition, light fixed to all stimuli. **D,** Bilateral dilated and fixed pupils. **E,** Dilated pupils, left eye abducted with ptosis. **F,** Pinpoint pupils.

unilateral fixed pupil usually suggests a lesion on the same side. If pupils are fixed bilaterally for more than 5 minutes, brainstem damage is usually implied. Dilated and nonreactive pupils are also seen in hypothermia, anoxia, ischemia, poisoning with atropine-like substances, or prior instillation of mydriatic drugs.

> **! NURSING ALERT**
>
> The sudden appearance of a fixed and dilated pupil(s) is a neurologic emergency.

The description of eye movements should indicate whether one or both eyes are involved and how the reaction was elicited. The parents should be asked about preexisting strabismus, which will cause the eyes to appear normal under compromise. Posttraumatic strabismus indicates cranial nerve VI damage.

Special tests, usually performed by qualified persons, include:

Doll's head maneuver—Elicited by rotating the child's head quickly to one side and then to the other. Conjugate (paired or working together) movement of the eyes in the direction opposite to the head rotation is normal. Absence of this response suggests dysfunction of the brainstem or oculomotor nerve (cranial nerve III).

> **! NURSING ALERT**
>
> Any tests that require head movement are not attempted until after cervical spine injury has been ruled out.

Caloric test, or oculovestibular response—Elicited with the child's head up (head of bed is elevated 30 degrees) by irrigating the external auditory canal with 10 ml of ice water for 20 seconds, which normally causes conjugate movement of the eyes toward the side of stimulation. This movement is lost when the pontine centers are impaired, thus providing important information in assessment of the comatose patient.

> **! NURSING ALERT**
>
> The caloric test is painful and is never performed on a child who is awake or on an individual with a ruptured tympanic membrane.

Funduscopic examination—Reveals additional clues. Papilledema will not be evident early in the course of unconsciousness because it takes 24 to 48 hours to develop, if it develops at all. Papilledema is characterized by optic disc swelling, indistinct optic disc margins, hemorrhage, tortuosity of vessels, and absence of venous pulsations. The presence of preretinal (subhyaloid) hemorrhages in children is almost invariably a result of acute trauma with intracranial bleeding, usually subarachnoid or subdural hemorrhage.

Motor Function

Observing spontaneous activity, gait, and response to painful stimuli provides clues to the location and extent of cerebral dysfunction. Even subtle movements (e.g., the outward rotation of a hip) should be noted and the child observed for other signs. Asymmetric movements of the limbs or absence of movement suggests paralysis. In hemiplegia, the affected limb lies in external rotation and will fall uncontrollably when lifted and allowed to drop. In patients with cerebellum abnormalities, heel-to-toe walking is difficult. Patients with cerebellar ataxia have an unsteady, broad-based gait. All motor functions should be described rather than labeled.

In the deeper comatose states, there is little or no spontaneous movement, and the musculature tends to be flaccid. There is considerable variability in the motor behavior in lesser degrees of coma. For example, the child may be relatively immobile or restless and hyperkinetic; muscle tone may be increased or decreased. Tremors, twitching, and spasms of muscles are common observations. The patient may display purposeless movements. Combative or negativistic behavior is common. Hyperactivity is more common in toxic states than in cases of increased ICP. Seizures are common in children and may be present

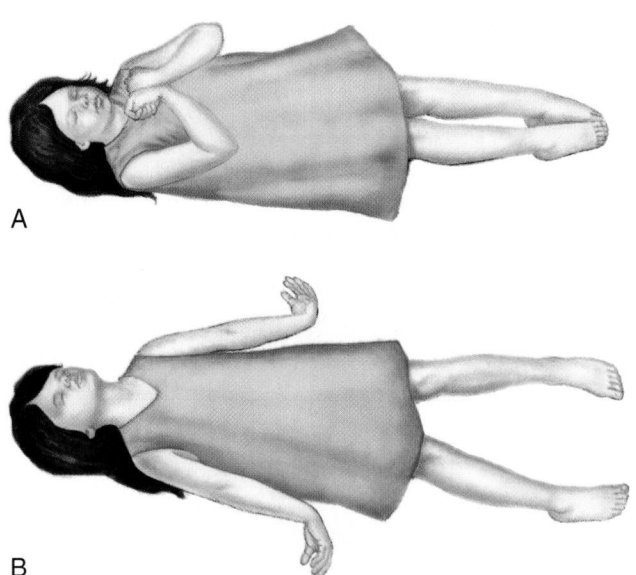

FIG 28-4 A, Flexion posturing. **B,** Extension posturing.

from any cause. Any repetitive or seizure movements should be precisely described.

Posturing

Primitive postural reflexes emerge as cortical control over motor function is lost in brain dysfunction. These reflexes are evident in posturing and motor movements directly related to the area of the brain involved. Posturing reflects a balance between the lower exciting and the higher inhibiting influences and strong muscles overcoming weaker ones. Decorticate or *flexion posturing* (Fig. 28-4, *A*) is seen with severe dysfunction of the cerebral cortex or with lesions to corticospinal tracts above the brainstem. Typical posturing includes rigid flexion with the arms held tightly to the body; flexed elbows, wrists, and fingers; plantar flexed feet; legs extended and internally rotated; and possibly the presence of fine tremors or intense stiffness. Decerebrate posture or *extension posturing* (see Fig. 28-4, *B*) is a sign of dysfunction at the level of the midbrain or lesions to the brainstem. It is characterized by rigid extension and pronation of the arms and legs, flexed wrists and fingers, a clenched jaw, an extended neck, and possibly an arched back. Unilateral decerebrate posture is often caused by tentorial herniation.

Posturing may not be evident when the child is quiet but can usually be elicited by applying painful stimuli, such as a blunt object pressed on the base of the nail. Nurses should avoid applying thumb pressure to the supraorbital region of the frontal bone (risk of orbital damage). Noxious stimuli (e.g., suctioning) will elicit a response, as may turning or touching. When the nurse is describing posturing, the stimulus needed to provoke the response is as important as the reaction.

Reflexes

Testing of some reflexes may be of limited value. In general, the corneal, pupillary, muscle-stretch, superficial, and plantar reflexes tend to be absent in deep coma. The state of reflexes is variable in lighter grades of unconsciousness and depends on the underlying pathologic process and the location of the lesion. Absence of corneal reflexes and presence of a tonic neck reflex are associated with severe brain damage. The Babinski reflex (see Extremities, Chapter 6) may be of value if it is found to be present consistently in children older than 18 months.

A positive Babinski reflex is significant in assessment of pyramidal tract lesions when it is unilateral and associated with other pyramidal signs.

> **! NURSING ALERT**
>
> Three key reflexes that demonstrate neurologic health in young infants are the Moro, tonic neck, and withdrawal reflexes.

SPECIAL DIAGNOSTIC PROCEDURES

Numerous diagnostic procedures are used for the assessment of cerebral function. Laboratory tests that may help delineate the cause of unconsciousness include blood glucose, urea nitrogen, and electrolyte (pH, sodium, potassium, chloride, calcium, and bicarbonate) tests; blood ammonia levels; clotting studies, hematocrit, and a complete blood count; liver function tests; blood cultures if there is fever; and urine toxicology screen and blood lead levels if clinically indicated.

An electroencephalogram (EEG) may provide important information. For example, generalized random, slow activity suggests suppressed cortical function, and localized slow activity suggests a space-occupying issue such as a hematoma, tumor, or infectious process. A flat tracing is one of the criteria used as evidence of brain death.

Examination of spinal fluid is performed when toxic encephalopathy or infection is suspected. Lumbar puncture is ordinarily delayed if intracranial hemorrhage is suspected and is contraindicated in the presence of ICP because of the potential for tentorial herniation.

Auditory and visual evoked potentials are sometimes used in neurologic evaluation of infants and very young children. Visual evoked potentials are useful in evaluating visual abnormalities from the retina to the visual cortex, and brainstem auditory evoked potentials are useful for assessing hearing acuity and brainstem function. Both are particularly useful for detecting demyelinating disease and neoplasms.

Highly sophisticated tests are carried out with specialized equipment. Two imaging techniques, computed tomography (CT) and magnetic resonance imaging (MRI), assist in diagnosis by scanning both soft tissues and solid matter. Most of these tests are outlined in Table 28-1. Because such tests can be threatening to children, the nurse needs to prepare patients for the tests and provide support and reassurance during the tests (see Preparation for Diagnostic and Therapeutic Procedures, Chapter 22). Children who are old enough to understand require careful explanation of the procedure, reason for the procedure, what they will experience, and how they can help. School-age children usually appreciate a more detailed description of why contrast material is injected. The importance of lying still for tests needs to be stressed. Children unfamiliar with the machines can be shown a picture beforehand.

Although radiographic examinations are not painful, the machinery is often so frightening in appearance that the child protests because of anxiety. This is especially true of CT and MRI, both of which require that the child's head be placed within a special immobilizing device. Chin and cheek pads are sometimes used to prevent the slightest head movement, and straps are applied to the body to prevent a slight change in body position. The nurse can explain these events to a frightened child by comparing them to an astronaut's preparation for a space flight. It is important to emphasize to the child that at no time is the procedure painful.

The nurse should not expect cooperation from a young child. Sedation may be required. Many different agents are currently used for

TABLE 28-1	**NEUROLOGIC DIAGNOSTIC PROCEDURES**		
TEST	**DESCRIPTION**	**PURPOSE**	**COMMENTS**
LP	Spinal needle is inserted between L3–L4 or L4–L5 vertebral spaces into subarachnoid space; CSF pressure is measured, and sample is collected.	Diagnostic—Measures spinal fluid pressure, obtains CSF for laboratory analysis Therapeutic—Injection of medication	Contraindicated in patients with increased ICP or infected skin over puncture site.
Subdural tap	Needle is inserted into anterior fontanel or coronal suture (midline to pupil).	Helps rule out subdural effusions Removes CSF to relieve pressure	Place infant in semi-erect position after subdural tap to minimize leakage from site; prevent child from crying if possible. Check site frequently for evidence of leakage.
Ventricular puncture	Needle is inserted into lateral ventricle via coronal suture (midline to pupil).	Removes CSF to relieve pressure	Risk of intracerebral or ventricular hemorrhage.
EEG	EEG records changes in electrical potential of brain. Electrodes are placed at various points to assess electrical function in a particular area. Impulses are recorded by electromagnetic pen or digitally.	Detects spikes, or bursts of electrical activity that indicate the potential for seizures Used to determine brain death	Patient should remain quiet during procedure; may require sedation. Minimize external stimuli during procedure.
Nuclear brain scan	Radioisotope is injected intravenously and then counted and recorded after fixed time intervals. Radioisotope accumulates in areas where blood–brain barrier is defective.	Identifies focal brain lesions (e.g., tumors, abscesses) Positive uptake of material with encephalitis and subdural hematoma Visualizes CSF pathways	Requires IV access; patient may require sedation. In normal children or noncommunicating hydrocephalus, no retrograde filling of ventricles occurs. Areas of concentrated uptake of material are termed *hot spots*.
Endocephalography	Pulses of ultrasonic waves are beamed through head; echoes from reflecting surfaces are recorded graphically.	Identifies shifts in midline structures from their normal positions as a result of intracranial lesions May show ventricular dilation	Simple, safe, rapid procedure. Fontanel must be patent.
RTUS	Similar to CT but uses ultrasound instead of ionizing radiation.	Allows high-resolution anatomic visualization in variety of imaging planes	Produces images similar to CT scan. Especially useful in neonatal CNS problems. Anterior fontanel must be patent.
Radiography	Skull films are taken from different views—lateral, posterolateral, axial (submentoventricular), half-axial.	Shows fractures, dislocations, spreading suture lines, craniosynostosis Shows degenerative changes, bone erosion, calcifications	Simple, noninvasive procedure.
CT scan	Pinpoint x-ray beam is directed on horizontal or vertical plane to provide series of images that are fed into computer and assembled in image displayed on video screen. CT uses ionizing radiation.	Visualizes horizontal and vertical cross section of brain in three planes (axial, coronal, sagittal) Distinguishes density of various intracranial tissues and structures—congenital abnormalities, hemorrhage, tumors, demyelinating and inflammatory processes, calcification	Requires IV access if contrast agent is used. Patient may require sedation. Rapid.
MRI	MRI produces radiofrequency emissions from elements (e.g., hydrogen, phosphorus), which are converted to visual images by computer.	Permits visualization of morphologic feature of target structures Permits tissue discrimination unavailable with many techniques	MRI is noninvasive procedure except when IV contrast agent is used. No exposure to radiation occurs. Patient may require sedation. Parent or attendant can remain in room with child. MRI does not visualize bone detail or calcifications. No metal can be present in scanner. Requires lengthy period of immobility.
PET	PET involves IV injection of positron-emitting radionucleotide; local concentrations are detected and transformed into visual display by computer.	Detects and measures blood volume and flow in brain, metabolic activity, and biochemical changes within tissue	Minimum exposure to radiation occurs. Patient may require sedation.

Continued

TABLE 28-1	NEUROLOGIC DIAGNOSTIC PROCEDURES—cont'd		
TEST	**DESCRIPTION**	**PURPOSE**	**COMMENTS**
DSA	Contrast dye is injected intravenously; computer "subtracts" all tissues without contrast medium, leaving clear image of contrast medium in vessels studied.	Visualizes vasculature of target tissue. Visualizes finite vascular abnormalities	Safe alternative to angiography. Patient must remain still during procedure; may require sedation.
SPECT	Involves IV injection of photon-emitting radionuclide; radionuclides are absorbed by healthy tissue at different rate than by diseased or necrotic tissue; data are transferred to computer that converts image to film.	Provides information regarding blood flow to tissues; analyzing blood flow to organ may help determine how well it is functioning	Requires lengthy period of immobility. Minimum exposure to radiation occurs. Patient may require sedation.

CNS, Central nervous system; *CSF,* cerebrospinal fluid; *CT,* computed tomography; *DSA,* digital subtraction angiography; *EEG,* electroencephalography; *ICP,* intracranial pressure; *IV,* intravenous; *LP,* lumbar puncture; *MRI,* magnetic resonance imaging; *PET,* positron emission tomography; *RTUS,* real-time ultrasonography; *SPECT,* single-photon emission computed tomography.

sedation of children undergoing neurologic diagnostic procedures. Chloral hydrate, pentobarbital, or benzodiazepines have been used for decades as short-term sedative agents and remain safe methods of pediatric outpatient sedation (Mason, 2008). Chloral hydrate and pentobarbital have no analgesic proprieties but can provide successful sedation for nonpainful procedures such as CT and MRI (Mason, 2008). In recent years, propofol has been used as a sedation agent for diagnostic procedures because of its short induction and recovery time, but this medication should be used with caution because it can cause respiratory depression and apnea with little warning (Machata, Willschke, Kabon, and others, 2008; Mason, 2008). (See Pain Management, Chapter 7.)

Physical preparation for the diagnostic test may involve administration of a sedative. If so, children should be helped through the preparation and administration and assured that someone will remain with them (if possible). Children need continual support and reinforcement during procedures in which they remain conscious. Vital signs and physiologic responses to the procedure are monitored throughout. Many diagnostic procedures performed on an outpatient basis require sedation, and children need recovery time and observation. The nurse should review written instructions with parents if the child is discharged after a procedure. Children who have undergone a procedure with a general anesthetic require postanesthesia care, including positioning, to prevent aspiration of secretions and frequent assessment of the vital signs and LOC. In addition, other neurologic functions such as pupillary responses, motor strength, and movement are tested at regular intervals. Any surgical wound resulting from the test is checked for bleeding, CSF leakage, and other complications. Children who undergo repeated subdural taps should have their hematocrit monitored to detect excessive blood loss from the procedure.

NURSING CARE OF THE UNCONSCIOUS CHILD

The unconscious child requires nursing attention, with observation, recording, and evaluation of changes in objective signs. These observations provide valuable information regarding the patient's progress. Often they serve as a guide to the diagnosis and treatment. Therefore, careful and detailed observations are essential for the patient's welfare. In addition, vital functions must be maintained and complications prevented through conscientious and meticulous nursing care. The outcome of unconsciousness may be early and complete recovery, death within a few hours or days, persistent and permanent unconsciousness, or recovery with varying degrees of residual mental or physical disability. The outcome and recovery of the unconscious child may depend on the level of nursing care and observational skills.

Emergency measures are directed toward ensuring a patent airway, breathing, and circulation; stabilizing the spine when indicated; treating shock; and reducing ICP if present. Delayed treatment often leads to increased damage. As soon as emergency measures have been implemented—and in many cases concurrently—therapies for specific causes are begun. Because nursing care is closely related to medical management, both are considered here.

Continual observation of LOC, pupillary reaction, and vital signs is essential to manage CNS disorders. Regular assessment of neurologic status is an essential part of nursing comatose children. The assessment frequency depends on the cause of unconsciousness, the LOC, and the progression of cerebral involvement. Intervals may be as short as every 15 minutes or as long as every 2 hours. Significant alterations must be reported immediately.

Vital signs provide important information about the status of the unconscious child. Hypothalamic and brainstem disorders may affect the patient's thermoregulation, so frequent monitoring is needed. The temperature is taken every 2 to 4 hours, depending on the patient's condition. Hypothermia is defined as a core body temperature less than 35° C (95° F). EEG slowing is noted at 30° C, and loss of pupillary light reflex is lost at 28° C (Young, 2009). Hyperthermia is defined as a core body temperature greater than 38.5° C (101.3° F) and temperatures greater than 42° C can cause EEG slowing, seizures, and encephalopathy (Young, 2009).

The neurologic examination is performed periodically and includes evaluating pupillary abnormalities, brainstem function, LOC, and motor response (Sharma, Kochar, Sankhyan, and other, 2010). Pupils are observed for their size, symmetry, and reaction to light. Signs of meningeal irritation such as nuchal rigidity are also assessed. The presence of the oculovestibular response, corneal (blink) response, and cough and gag reflexes are evaluated. Aspects of LOC assessment include response to vocal commands, resistance to care, and response to painful stimuli. Spontaneous movement, changes in muscle tone or strength, and body position are noted. Seizure activity is described according to the duration and body areas involved.

Pain management for the comatose child requires astute nursing observation and management. Responses to pain include motor reactions such as increased agitation or posturing; facial changes such as grimaces; and physiological reactions such as tachycardia, tachypnea, diaphoresis, or hypertension (Schnakers and Zasler, 2007). Because these findings may not be specific for pain, the nurse should observe for their appearance during times of induced or suspected pain and their disappearance after the end of the inciting procedure or the administration of analgesia. A pain assessment record should be used to document indications of pain and the effectiveness of interventions (see Pain Assessment, Chapter 7).

The use of opioids, such as morphine, to relieve pain is controversial because they may mask signs of altered consciousness or depress respirations. However, unrelieved pain activates the stress response, which can elevate ICP. To block the stress response, some authorities advocate the use of analgesics; sedatives; and, in some cases, paralyzing agents via continuous intravenous (IV) infusion. A frequently used combination is fentanyl, midazolam, and vecuronium (Norcuron). If there are concerns about assessing the LOC or respiratory depression, naloxone (Narcan) can be used to reverse the opioid effects. Regardless of which drugs are used, adequate dosage and regular administration are essential to provide optimal pain relief (see Pain Management, Chapter 7).

Other measures to relieve discomfort include providing a quiet, dimly lit environment; limiting visitors; preventing any sudden, jarring movement, such as banging into the bed; and preventing an increase in ICP. The last is most effectively achieved by proper positioning and prevention of straining, such as during coughing, vomiting, suctioning, and defecating.

> ## 💊 DRUG ALERT
>
> When opioids are used, bowel elimination must be closely monitored because of the potential constipating effect. Stool softeners should be given with laxatives as needed to prevent constipation.

RESPIRATORY MANAGEMENT

Respiratory effectiveness is the primary concern in the care of the unconscious child, and establishment of an adequate airway is *always* the first priority. Carbon dioxide has a potent vasodilating effect and will increase cerebral blood flow (CBF) and ICP. Cerebral hypoxia that lasts longer than 4 minutes nearly always causes irreversible brain damage.

> ## ❗ NURSING ALERT
>
> Respiratory obstruction and subsequent compromise leads to cardiac arrest. Maintaining an adequate, patent airway is of the utmost importance.

Children in lighter states of coma may be able to cough and swallow, but those in deeper states are unable to handle secretions, which tend to pool in the throat and pharynx. Dysfunction of cranial nerves IX and X places the child at risk for aspiration and cardiac arrest; therefore, the child is positioned to prevent aspiration of secretions, and the stomach is emptied to reduce the likelihood of vomiting. In infants, blockage of air passages from secretions can happen in seconds. In addition, upper airway obstruction from laryngospasm is a frequent complication in comatose children.

An oral airway can be used for children who have a temporary loss of consciousness, such as after a contusion, seizure, or anesthesia. For children who remain unconscious for a longer time, a nasotracheal or orotracheal tube is inserted to maintain the open airway and facilitate removal of secretions. Endotracheal intubation should be considered in children with a GCS score of less than 8, evidence of herniation,

apnea, or inability to maintain an airway (Sankhyan, Raju, Sharma, and other, 2010). A tracheostomy is performed in cases in which laryngoscopy for introduction of an endotracheal tube would be difficult or for a child who needs long-term ventilatory support. Suctioning is used only as needed to clear the airway, exerting care to prevent increasing ICP. Respiratory status is observed and evaluated regularly. Signs of respiratory distress may be an indication for ventilatory assistance.

When the respiratory center is involved, mechanical ventilation is usually indicated (see Chapter 22). Blood gas analysis is performed regularly, and oxygen is administered as indicated. Moderately severe hypoxia and respiratory acidosis are often present but not always evident from clinical manifestations. Hyperventilation frequently accompanies unconsciousness and may lead to respiratory alkalosis, or it may represent the body's attempt to compensate for metabolic acidosis. Therefore, blood gas and pH determinations are essential guides for therapy. Chest physiotherapy is carried out on a regular basis, and the child's position is changed at least every 2 hours to prevent pulmonary complications.

INTRACRANIAL PRESSURE MONITORING

 An acute rise in ICP can cause secondary brain injury (Singhi and Tiwari, 2009), and management of the child with increased ICP is a complex and important task. ICP monitoring is used to guide therapy to reduce ICP and provides information on intracranial compliance, cerebrovascular status, and cerebral perfusion (Sankhyan, Raju, Sharma, and other, 2010). Nonetheless, ICP monitoring is an invasive procedure that has associated risks, including infection, hemorrhage, malfunction, and obstruction (Singhi and Tiwari, 2009). Indications for inserting an ICP monitor are as follows:

- GCS evaluation of less than 8
- Traumatic brain injury with an abnormal head CT scan
- Deterioration of condition
- Subjective judgment regarding clinical appearance and response

Four major types of ICP monitors are

1. Intraventricular catheter with fibroscopic sensors attached to a monitoring system
2. Subarachnoid bolt (Richmond screw)
3. Epidural sensor
4. Anterior fontanel pressure monitor

Direct ventricular pressure measurement with an intraventricular catheter remains the gold standard of ICP monitoring (Singhi and Tiwari, 2009). Subarachnoid and epidural monitoring can be used when a catheter cannot be cannulated in the ventricle, but they often must be replaced after several days because of measurement drift (Singhi and Tiwari, 2009). Transducers for both ventricular and subarachnoid monitoring should be set up without the use of a flush device.

Placement of the intraventricular catheter and subarachnoid bolt occurs through a burr hole in the skull. The intraventricular method involves introduction of a catheter into the lateral ventricle on the nondominant side, if known. The subarachnoid bolt involves placement of a bolt in the subarachnoid space, and the epidural sensor involves placement of a sensor between the dura and the skull. The intraventricular catheter has the advantage of providing a means for recalibration when measurement drift occurs, but both the catheter and the bolt can be used for therapeutic CSF drainage to reduce pressure. A drainage bag attached to the system is kept at the level of the ventricles and can be lowered to decrease ICP (see Critical Thinking Case Study).

Animation—Cerebral Perfusion

❓ CRITICAL THINKING CASE STUDY

Hydrocephalus

Three-year-old Emma had a posterior fossa tumor removed 5 days ago. Although an EVD was placed to treat her hydrocephalus, she continues to demonstrate signs of increased ICP, including holding the back of her head, anorexia, crying when moved or when strangers enter the room, and intermittent lethargy. On examination, fluid drainage is noted on the mother's clothes, and Emma is experiencing repetitive, rapid eyelid blinking.

Questions

1. Evidence—Is there sufficient evidence to draw conclusions about Emma's behavior, physical assessment findings, and ICP?
2. Assumptions—Describe any underlying assumption about each of the following:
   a. A preschool-age child who had a posterior fossa tumor removed 5 days ago
   b. A preschool-age child who has an EVD placed to treat the hydrocephalus
   c. A preschool-age child with an EVD who continues to demonstrate physical signs associated with increased ICP after recent surgery
3. What priorities for nursing care should be established?
4. Does the evidence support your nursing intervention?

EVD, External ventricular drain; *ICP*, intracranial pressure.

❗ NURSING ALERT

If the external ventricular drain is unclamped for CSF drainage, carefully monitor the level of the collection container. If the container is too low, improper CSF decompression could lower ICP too rapidly, causing bleeding and pain.

❗ NURSING ALERT

The bolt is stabilized with dressings, and these are not changed or disturbed, even to check the site.

Placement of the subarachnoid bolt is not adjusted by anyone except the neurosurgeon who placed the device. The neurosurgeon is notified if a satisfactory waveform on the ICP monitoring is not observed.

An epidural sensor provides a readout of the ICP with a stopcock assembly and transducer. Although less invasive, ICP measurements may be inconsistent. In infants, a fontanel transducer can be used to detect impulses from a pressure sensor and convert them to electrical energy. The electrical energy is then converted to visible waves or numeric readings on an oscilloscope. ICP measurement from the anterior fontanel is noninvasive but may prove to be inaccurate if the equipment is poorly placed or inconsistently recalibrated.

Intracranial pressure can be increased by instillation of solutions; therefore, antibiotics are administered systemically if a positive CSF culture is obtained. CSF is a body fluid; therefore, standard precautions are implemented according to hospital policy (see Infection Control, Chapter 22).

Nurses caring for patients with intracranial monitoring devices must be acquainted with the system, assist with insertion, interpret the monitor readings, and be able to distinguish between danger signals and mechanical dysfunction.

For sustained ICP elevations greater than 20 to 25 mm Hg, several medical measures are available. Osmotic diuretics may provide rapid relief in emergency situations. Although their effect is transient, lasting only about 6 hours, they can be lifesaving in emergencies. These substances are rapidly excreted by the kidneys and carry with them large quantities of sodium and water. Mannitol (or sometimes urea) administered intravenously is the drug most frequently used for rapid reduction and can lower ICP in 1 to 5 minutes. The infusion is generally given slowly but may be pushed rapidly in cases of herniation or impending herniation. Hypertonic saline in concentrations of 3% to 23% have been shown to reduce ICP by its osmotic force and can be beneficial for hypovolemic and hypotensive patients by increasing intravascular volume and blood pressure (Singhi and Tiwari, 2009). Adrenocorticosteroids are not recommended for cerebral edema secondary to head trauma. $PaCO_2$ should be maintained at 25 to 30 mm Hg to produce vasoconstriction, which reduces CSF, thereby decreasing ICP, but this effect is sustained only 11 to 20 hours because the CSF equilibrates to the new $PaCO_2$ level (Singhi and Tiwari, 2009).

Nursing Activities

In cases of high levels of increased ICP, procedures tend to trigger reactive pressure waves in many patients. For example, increased intrathoracic or abdominal pressure is transmitted to the cranium. Particular care should be taken in positioning these patients to avoid neck vein compression, which may further increase ICP by interfering with venous return.

The child can be propped to one side or the other, and the use of an alternating-pressure mattress reduces the chance of prolonged pressure to vulnerable areas. Frequent clinical assessment of the child cannot be replaced by an ICP monitoring device.

❗ NURSING ALERT

The head of the bed is elevated to 30 degrees, and the child is positioned so that the head is maintained in midline to facilitate venous drainage and avoid jugular compression (Sankhyan, Raju, Sharma, and other, 2010). Turning side to side is contraindicated because of the risk of jugular compression.

It is important to avoid activities that may increase ICP by causing pain or emotional stress. Gentle range-of-motion exercises can be carried out but should not be performed vigorously. Nontherapeutic touch can cause an increase in ICP. Any disturbing procedures to be performed should be scheduled to take advantage of therapies that reduce ICP, such as osmotherapy and sedation. Efforts are taken to minimize or eliminate environmental noise. Assessment and intervention to relieve pain are important nursing functions to decrease ICP. Individualizing nursing activities and minimizing environmental stimuli by decreasing elective procedures help control ICP (Sankhyan, Raju, Sharma, and other, 2010).

Suctioning

Suctioning and percussion are poorly tolerated and are therefore contraindicated unless concurrent respiratory problems exist. Hypoxia and the Valsalva maneuver associated with cough both acutely elevate ICP. Vibration, which does not increase ICP, accomplishes excellent results and should be tried first if treatment is needed. If suctioning is necessary, it should be brief and preceded by hyperventilation with 100% oxygen, which can be monitored during suctioning with a pulse oxygen sensor reading to determine oxygen saturation.

NUTRITION AND HYDRATION

In the unconscious child, fluids and calories are supplied initially by the IV route (see Chapter 22). An IV infusion is started early, and the type of fluid administered is determined by the patient's general condition. Fluid therapy requires careful monitoring and adjustment based on neurologic signs and electrolyte determinations. The goal of fluid therapy is euvolemia. Often, comatose children are unable to cope with the same amounts of fluid they could tolerate when they are healthy, and overhydration must be avoided to prevent fatal cerebral edema. When cerebral edema is a threat, fluids may be restricted to reduce the chance of fluid overload. Skin and mucous membranes are examined for signs of dehydration. Observation for signs of altered fluid balance related to abnormal pituitary secretions is a part of nursing care.

Long-term nutrition is provided with a balanced formula via a nasogastric or gastrostomy tube. Most children have continuous feedings, but if bolus feedings are used, the tube is rinsed with water after each feeding. Avoid overfeeding to prevent vomiting and the risk of aspiration.

Altered Pituitary Secretion

An altered ability to handle fluid loads is attributed in part to the syndrome of inappropriate antidiuretic hormone secretion (SIADH) and diabetes insipidus (DI) resulting from hypothalamic dysfunction (see Chapter 29). SIADH frequently accompanies CNS diseases such as head injury, meningitis, encephalitis, brain abscess, brain tumor, and subarachnoid hemorrhage. In patients with SIADH, scant quantities of urine are excreted, electrolyte analysis reveals hyponatremia and hyposmolality, and manifestations of overhydration are evident. It is important to evaluate all parameters because the reduced urinary output might be erroneously interpreted as a sign of dehydration. The treatment of SIADH consists of restriction of fluids until serum electrolytes and osmolality return to normal levels.

Diabetes insipidus may occur after intracranial trauma. In DI, there are large amounts of diluted urine and the accompanying danger of dehydration. Adequate replacement of fluids is essential, and observation of electrolyte balance is necessary to detect signs of hypernatremia and hyperosmolality. Exogenous vasopressin may be administered.

MEDICATIONS

The cause of unconsciousness determines specific drug therapies. Children with infectious processes are given antibiotics appropriate to the disease and the infecting organism. Corticosteroids are prescribed for inflammatory conditions and edema. Cerebral edema is an indication for osmotherapy. Sedatives or antiepileptics are prescribed for seizure activity (see p. 960).

 DRUG ALERT

Sedation in the combative child provides amnesic and anxiolytic properties in conjunction with a paralytic agent. The combination decreases ICP and allows treatment of cerebral edema. Usual drugs include morphine, midazolam, and pancuronium (Pavulon). Midazolam is appealing because of its short half-life. Prolonged use of propofol should be avoided in children because of the risk of metabolic acidosis (Orliaguet, Meyer, and Baugnon, 2008).

Deep coma induced by administration of barbiturates is controversial in the management of ICP. Barbiturates are currently reserved for the reduction of increased ICP when all else has failed. Barbiturates decrease the cerebral metabolic rate for oxygen and protect the brain during times of reduced cerebral perfusion pressure. Barbiturate coma requires extensive monitoring, cardiovascular and respiratory support, and ICP monitoring to assess response to therapy. Paralyzing agents such as pancuronium also may be needed to aid in performing diagnostic tests, improving effectiveness of therapy, and reducing risks of secondary complications. Elevation of ICP or heart rate of patients who are being given paralyzing agents or are under sedation may indicate the need for another dose of either or both medications.

THERMOREGULATION

Hyperthermia often accompanies cerebral dysfunction; if it is present, measures are implemented to reduce the temperature to prevent brain damage and to reduce metabolic demands generated by the increased body temperature. Antipyretic agents are usually ineffective with hyperthermia as a result of traumatic brain injury; therefore, external cooling should be used (Badjatia, 2009). External cooling consists of evaporation (sponge baths), conduction (ice packs, cooling blankets), convection (fans), and radiation (skin exposure) (Badjatia, 2009). Laboratory tests and other methods are used in an attempt to determine the cause of the hyperthermia.

ELIMINATION

A urinary catheter is usually inserted in the acute phase, although diapers may be used and weighed to record urinary output. The child who formerly had bowel and bladder control is generally incontinent. If the child remains comatose for a long period, the indwelling catheter may be removed, and periodic bladder emptying can be accomplished by intermittent catheterization. Stool softeners are usually sufficient to maintain bowel function, but suppositories or enemas may be needed occasionally for adequate elimination and to prevent fecal impaction. The passage of liquid stool after a period of no bowel activity is usually a sign of an impaction. To avoid this preventable problem, daily recording of bowel activity is essential.

HYGIENIC CARE

Routine measures for cleansing and maintaining skin integrity are an integral part of nursing care of the unconscious child (see Maintaining Healthy Skin, Chapter 22).

Mouth care is performed at least twice daily because the mouth tends to become dry or coated with mucus. The teeth are carefully brushed with a soft toothbrush or cleaned with gauze saturated with saline. Commercially prepared cleansing devices, such as Toothettes, are convenient for cleansing the mouth and teeth. Lips are coated with ointment or other preparations to protect them from drying, cracking, or blistering.

Unconscious children are susceptible to eye irritation. The corneal reflexes are absent; therefore, the eyes are easily irritated or damaged by linen, dust, or other substances that may come in contact with them. Excessive dryness results from incomplete closure of the eyes or decreased secretions, especially if the child is undergoing osmotherapy to reduce or prevent cerebral edema.

! NURSING ALERT

The eyes should be examined regularly and carefully for early signs of irritation or inflammation. Artificial tears or a lubricating ointment is placed in the eyes every 1 to 2 hours. Eye dressings may be necessary to protect the eyes from possible damage.

POSITIONING AND EXERCISE

The unconscious child is positioned to minimize ICP and to prevent aspiration of saliva, nasogastric secretions, and vomitus. The head of the bed is elevated, and the child is placed in a side-lying or semiprone position. A small, firm pillow is placed under the head, and the uppermost limbs are flexed and supported with pillows. The weight of the body should not rest on the dependent arm. In the semiprone position, the child lies with the dependent arm at the side behind the body, the opposite side supported on pillows, and the uppermost arm and leg flexed and resting on the pillows. This position prevents undue pressure on the dependent extremities. The dependent position of the face encourages drainage of secretions and prevents the flaccid tongue from obstructing the airway.

Normal range-of-motion exercises help maintain function and prevent contractures of joints. Exercises should be performed gently and with full range of motion. A small rolled pad can be placed in the palms to help maintain proper position of fingers; footboards or high-top shoes can help prevent footdrop; and splinting may be needed to prevent severe contractures of the wrist, knee, or ankle in decerebrate children.

STIMULATION

Sensory stimulation is important in the care of the unconscious child. For a temporarily unconscious or semiconscious child, sensory stimulation helps arouse the child to the conscious state and orient the child to time and place. Auditory and tactile stimulation are especially valuable. Tactile stimulation is not appropriate for children in whom it may elicit an undesirable response. However, for other children, tactile contact often has a relaxing and calming effect. When the child's condition permits, holding or rocking has a soothing effect and provides the body contact needed by young children. Involving family members with the sensory stimulation can create a positive effect on the child and allows the family to participate in the care (Abbasi, Mohammadi, and Rezayi, 2009).

The auditory sense is often intact in a state of coma. Hearing is the last sense to be lost and the first one to be regained; therefore, the child should be spoken to as any other child. Conversation around the child should not include thoughtless or derogatory remarks. Soft music is frequently used to provide auditory stimulation. Singing the child's favorite songs or reading a favorite story is a tactic used to maintain the child's contact with a familiar world. Playing songs or stories recorded in the parents' voices can provide a continuous source of familiar stimulation.

Regaining Consciousness

Awakening from a coma is a gradual process; however, sometimes children regain consciousness within a short time. Regaining orientation involves knowing person, place, and time in that order.

Certain behaviors have been observed when children awaken from the unconscious state. The stress and anxiety they appear to feel in a strange and unfamiliar environment can be expressed in silent, withdrawn behavior. Children respond to basic questioning but usually do not display their prehospitalization personality and social behavior until they are transferred from the critical care area.

FAMILY SUPPORT

Helping the parents of an unconscious child cope with the situation is especially difficult. They may demonstrate all of the guilt, fear, hostility, and anxiety of any parent of a seriously ill child (see Chapter 18). In addition, these parents are faced with the uncertain outcome of the cerebral dysfunction. The fear of death, intellectual disability, or other permanent disability is present. Nursing intervention with parents depends on the nature of the pathologic condition, the parents' personality, and the parent–child relationship before the injury or illness. Parents need the most intensive nursing intervention during the period of crisis and uncertainty. Throughout the treatment and recovery phase, the nurse provides parents with information and encourages them to become involved in the child's care.

Probably the most difficult situations involve children who never regain consciousness. Family members often attempt to construct a representation of the child by bringing items that belong to the child, such as favorite toys or music. This is interpreted as an attempt to provide stimulation for the child in the hope of eliciting a response, to let the hospital staff know the child as the unique individual he or she was, and to reconstitute an image of the child "lost" to them and for whom they mourn. Unlike losing a child through death, these situations lack finality, which often leaves family members in a state of prolonged grief and searching for signs of hope. An awareness of these behaviors and coping mechanisms provides nurses with the understanding that helps them support the parents in their grief process.

Superimposed on the process of grieving for the "lost" child, parents may be faced with difficult decisions. When the child's brain is so severely damaged that vital functions must be maintained by artificial means, the parents along with guidance from the health care team must make the final decision of whether to remove life-support systems. Nurses continue to provide specialty care during this time that maintains the patient's physiological status while addressing informational and psychological needs of the family (Ashwal and Serna-Fonseca, 2006). This decision is difficult for parents, but having an open and honest dialog about the child's medical condition and prognosis can help make patient-centered conclusions (Young, 2009). Parents' cultural, religious, and language needs along with their intellectual level, decision-making preferences, and emotional state are considered during the discussions (Truog, Campbell, Curtis, and others, 2008). Sometimes parents may choose to refuse or not initiate treatment if they believe it to be best for the child and the family (informed dissent). At other times, parents request that "everything possible" be done for the child.

When the child has survived the cerebral insult and is not comatose, but physical or mental capacity is limited, either minimally or severely, families must cope with the long and tedious rehabilitation process and the uncertain outcome. The drain on financial, emotional, and social resources can be enormous.

For parents who choose to care for their child at home, planning for home care begins early in the recovery process. The family should become involved with the child's care as soon as they indicate an interest and ability to do so. They need education and support in learning to care for the child, regular follow-up observation and assessment of the home management, and planning for some respite care of the child. Parents need to understand that it is important to plan for periodic relief from the continual care of the child (see Preparing for Discharge and Home Care, Chapter 21, and Family-Centered Home Care, Chapter 20).

CEREBRAL TRAUMA

HEAD INJURY

Head injury is a pathologic process involving the scalp, skull, meninges, or brain as a result of trauma. According to national statistics and Safe

Kids Worldwide,* unintentional injuries are the number one health risk for children and the leading cause of death in children older than 1 year of age. Yearly, one in eight children in the United States will sustain an injury serious enough to require medical attention. Tragically, 5100 children ages 1 to 14 years are killed every year by injuries (Safe Kids, 2009). It has been estimated that 500,000 children per year sustain a traumatic brain injury and that 2170 children per year die as a result of the brain injury (Faul, Xu, Wald, and others, 2010). Evidence demonstrates that a previous head injury increases a child's risk of having a subsequent head injury (Swaine, Tremblay, Platt, and others, 2007).

Etiology

The three major causes of brain damage in childhood, in order of importance, are falls, motor vehicle injuries, and bicycle or sports-related injuries. Neurologic injury accounts for the highest mortality rate, with boys affected twice as often as girls. In motor vehicle accidents, children younger than 2 years of age are almost exclusively injured as passengers, but older children may also be injured as pedestrians or cyclists. The majority of deaths from brain trauma caused by bicycle injuries occur between the ages of 5 and 14 years. Bicycle helmet laws have been effective in reducing the risk of head injury by 85% and brain injury by 88% (Rivara and Grossman, 2011).

The exposed nature of the head renders it particularly vulnerable to trauma, and many of the physical characteristics of children predispose them to craniocerebral trauma. For example, infants can be left unattended on beds, in high chairs, and in other places from which they can fall. Because the head of an infant or toddler is proportionately larger and heavier in relation to other body parts, it is the most likely to be injured. Incomplete motor development contributes to falls at young ages, and the natural curiosity and exuberance of children also increase their risk of injury.

Pathophysiology

The pathology of brain injury is directly related to the force of impact. Intracranial contents (brain, blood, CSF) are damaged because the force is too great to be absorbed by the skull and musculoligamentous support of the head. Although nervous tissue is delicate, it usually requires a severe blow to cause significant damage.

Primary head injuries are those that occur at the time of trauma and include skull fracture, contusions, intracranial hematoma, and diffuse injury. Subsequent complications include hypoxic brain damage, increased ICP, infection, and cerebral edema. The predominant feature of a child's brain injury is the amount of diffuse swelling that occurs. Hypoxia and hypercapnia threaten the energy requirements of the brain and increase CBF. The added volume across the blood–brain barrier, along with the loss of autoregulation, exacerbates cerebral edema. Pressure inside the skull that is greater than arterial pressure results in inadequate perfusion.

A child's response to head injury is different from that of an adult. The larger head size and insufficient musculoskeletal support render the very young child particularly vulnerable to head injuries. Physical forces act on the head through acceleration, deceleration, or deformation. Acceleration or deceleration is responsible for most head injuries. When the stationary head receives a blow, the sudden acceleration causes deformation of the skull and mass movement of the brain. Continued movement of the intracranial contents allows the brain to strike parts of the skull (e.g., the sharp edges of the sphenoid or the

*1301 Pennsylvania Ave. NW, Suite 1000, Washington, DC 20004-1707; 202-662-0600; http://www.safekids.org.

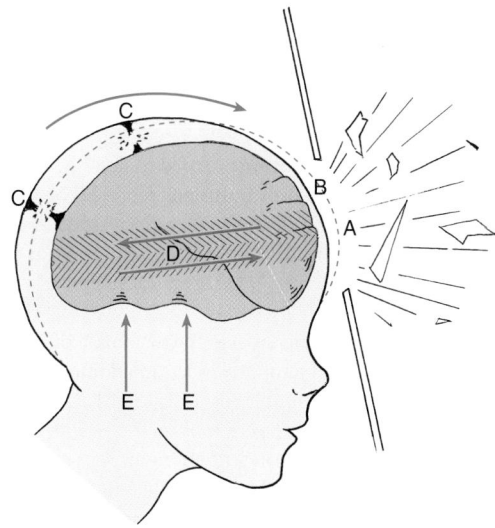

FIG 28-5 Mechanical distortion of the cranium during a closed head injury. **A,** Preinjury contour of the skull. **B,** Immediate postinjury contour of the skull. **C,** Torn subdural vessels. **D,** Shearing forces. **E,** Trauma from contact with the floor of the cranium. (Redrawn from Grubb RL, Coxe WS: Central nervous system trauma: cranial. In Eliasson SG, Presky AL, Hardin Jr WB, editors: *Neurological pathophysiology*, New York, 1974, Oxford University Press.)

irregular surface of the anterior fossa) or the edges of the tentorium. Sudden deceleration, such as takes place in a fall, causes the greatest cerebral injury at the point of impact.

Although the brain volume remains unchanged, significant distortion takes place as the brain changes shape in response to the force of impact to the skull. This movement can cause bruising at the point of impact (coup) or at a distance as the brain collides with the unyielding surfaces far removed from the point of impact (contrecoup) (Fig. 28-5). Thus, a blow to the occipital region can cause severe injury to the frontal and temporal areas of the brain. Children with an acceleration–deceleration injury demonstrate diffuse generalized cerebral swelling produced by increased blood volume or a redistribution of cerebral blood volume (cerebral hyperemia) rather than by increased water content (edema), as seen in adults.

Another effect of brain movement is shearing stresses, which may tear small arteries and cause subdural hemorrhages. Damage can also occur when severe compression of the skull causes the brain to be forced through the tentorial opening. This can produce irreparable damage to the brainstem (Fig. 28-6).

Concussion

The most common head injury is concussion, an alteration in neurologic or cognitive function with or without loss of consciousness, which occurs immediately after a head injury (Landry, 2011). Confusion and amnesia after head injury are the hallmarks of concussion; however, loss of consciousness is not an accurate indicator for the presence of a concussion (Meehan and Mannix, 2010). Concussions usually resolve in 7 to 10 days without complications; however, some individuals may require several months to recover from a concussion (Lee, 2007).

The pathogenesis of concussion is still unclear but may be a result of shearing forces that cause stretching, compression, and tearing of nerve fibers, particularly in the area of the central brainstem, the seat of the reticular activating system. It has also been suggested that the anatomic alterations of nerve fibers cause the release of large quantities of acetylcholine into the CSF and a reduction in oxygen consumption with increased lactate production.

Contusion and Laceration

The terms contusion and laceration are used to describe visible bruising and tearing of cerebral tissue. Contusions represent petechial hemorrhages or localized bruising along the superficial aspects of the brain at the site of impact (coup injury) or a lesion remote from the site of direct trauma (contrecoup injury). In serious accidents, there may be multiple sites of injury.

The major areas of the brain susceptible to contusion or laceration are the occipital, frontal, and temporal lobes. In addition, the irregular surfaces of the anterior and middle fossae at the base of the skull are capable of producing bruises or lacerations on forceful impact. Contusions may cause focal disturbances in strength, sensation, or visual awareness. The degree of brain damage in the contused areas varies according to the extent of vascular injury. Signs vary from mild, transient weakness of a limb to prolonged unconsciousness and paralysis. However, the signs and symptoms may be clinically indistinguishable from those of concussion.

The lower incidence of cerebral contusion in infancy has been attributed to infants' pliable skulls with less convolutional markings of the inner space between brain tissue and bone. However, infants who are roughly shaken (shaken baby syndrome) can sustain profound neurologic impairment, seizures, retinal hemorrhages, intracranial subarachnoid or subdural hemorrhages, high cervical spinal cord hemorrhages, and contusions (Walls, 2006).

Cerebral lacerations are generally associated with penetrating or depressed skull fractures. However, they may occur without fracture in small children. When brain tissue is actually torn, with bleeding into and around the tear, more severe and prolonged unconsciousness and paralysis occur, leaving permanent scarring and some degree of disability.

Fractures

⊝ Because of its flexibility, the immature skull is able to sustain a greater degree of deformation than the adult skull before it incurs a fracture. A great deal of force is required to produce a fracture in an infant's skull.

The types of skull fractures that occur are linear, depressed, comminuted, basilar, open, and growing fractures. As a rule, the faster the blow, the greater the likelihood of a depressed fracture; a low-velocity impact tends to produce a linear fracture.

Linear fractures are a single fracture line that starts at the point of maximum impact but does not cross suture lines. Linear fractures constitute the majority of childhood skull fractures. Most linear skull fractures are associated with an overlying hematoma or soft-tissue swelling (Erlichman, Blumfield, Rajpathak, and other, 2010).

Depressed fractures are those in which the bone is locally broken, usually into several irregular fragments that are pushed inward, causing pressure on the brain. Depressed skull fractures may be associated with direct underlying parenchymal damage and should be suspected when a child's head appears misshapen. Surgery may be needed to elevate the depressed bone fragment if there is an associated intracranial hematoma or pressure.

Comminuted fractures consist of multiple associated linear fractures. They usually result from intense impact. These types of fractures often result from repeated blows against an object and may suggest child abuse.

Basilar fractures involve the basilar portion of the frontal, ethmoid, sphenoid, temporal, or occipital bones. Because of the proximity of the fracture line to structures surrounding the brainstem, a basal skull fracture is a serious head injury. Approximately 80% of the cases may include clinical features such as subcutaneous bleeding in the posterior neck area and over the mastoid process (battle sign), bleeding around the eyes (raccoon eyes), bleeding behind the tympanic membrane (hemotympanum), or CSF leakage from the nose or ear (Perheentupa, Kinnunen, Grenman, and others, 2010).

Open fractures cause communication between the skull and the scalp or the mucosa of the upper respiratory tract. Open fractures increase the risk of CNS infection when the fracture creates an opening in the paranasal sinuses or middle ear that causes CSF leakage. They may have a skin laceration overlying the bone fracture called a *compound fracture*. Antibiotics are recommended to prevent osteomyelitis.

Growing fractures are skull fractures associated with an underlying dural tear that may be caused by a leptomeningeal cyst, dilated ventricles, or a herniated brain. Ninety percent of all growing fractures occur before the age of 3 years (Vignes, Jeelani, Jeelani, and others, 2007). Physical examination reveals a pulsatile mass or sunken skull defect, and symptoms include headaches, seizures, or both.

Complications

The major complications of trauma to the head are hemorrhage, infection, edema, and herniation through the brainstem. Infection is always a hazard in open injuries, and edema is related to tissue trauma. Vascular rupture may occur even in minor head injuries, causing hemorrhage between the skull and cerebral surfaces. Compression of the underlying brain produces effects that can be rapidly fatal or insidiously progressive.

! NURSING ALERT

Posttraumatic meningitis should be suspected in children with increasing drowsiness and fever who also have basilar skull fractures.

Epidural Hemorrhage

An epidural hemorrhage is bleeding between the dura and the skull to form a hematoma. This bleeding causes the dura to be stripped from bone, forcing the underlying brain contents downward and inward as the brain expands (see Fig. 28-6, *A*). Because bleeding is generally arterial, brain compression occurs rapidly. Most often the expanding hematoma is located in the parietal and temporal regions, although they can occur in the frontal or occipital posterior fossa (Case, 2008). The lower incidence of epidural hematoma in childhood has been attributed to the fact that the middle meningeal artery is not embedded in the bone surface of the skull until approximately 2 years of age. Therefore, a fracture of the temporal bone is less likely to lacerate the artery. Second, the dura closely adheres to the inner table of the skull, especially at the level of the sutures, making separation from bleeding less likely. However, a child's skull can be indented with sufficient force to tear the middle meningeal artery and rebound intact without causing a fracture. Hemorrhage can also derive from dural veins or the dural sinuses, especially in infants and small children, in whom fracture is less likely to occur. In 20% to 40% of children, a skull fracture is not detectable. The classic clinical picture of epidural hemorrhage (momentary unconsciousness followed by a normal period and then lethargy or coma) can be less evident in children (see Box 28-3 for clinical manifestations). The period of impaired consciousness is

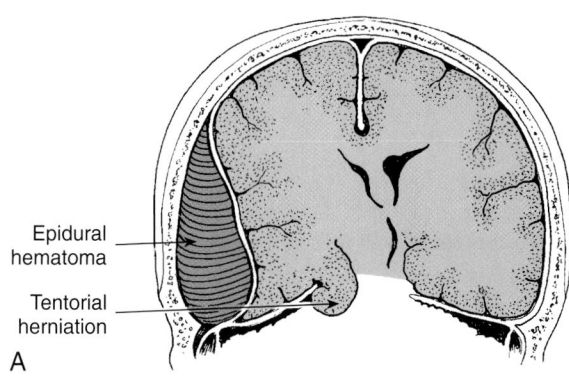

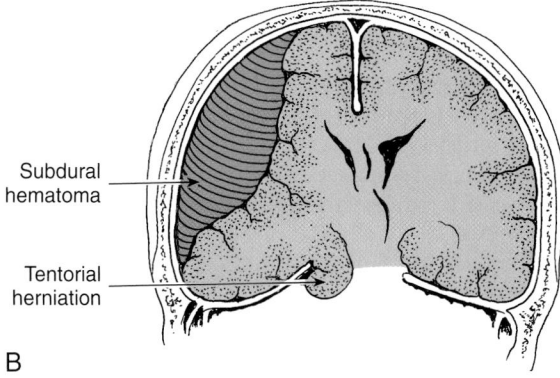

FIG 28-6 A, Epidural (extradural) hematoma and compression of temporal lobe through tentorial hiatus. **B,** Subdural hematoma.

frequently lacking, and the symptom-free period is atypical because of nonspecific symptoms such as irritability, headache, and vomiting. Physical findings can include pallor with anemia and cephalhematoma with infants exhibiting hypotonia and a bulging fontanel. If the severity of the child's signs and symptoms is not recognized, herniation and death will occur.

Subdural Hemorrhage

A subdural hemorrhage is bleeding between the dura and the arachnoid membrane, usually as a result of rupture of cortical veins that bridge the subdural space (see Fig. 28-6, *B*). Subdural hematomas are more common than epidural hematomas, occurring most often in infancy.

Unlike epidural hemorrhage, which develops inwardly against the less resistant brain tissue, subdural hemorrhage tends to develop more slowly and spreads thinly and widely until it is limited by the dural barriers—the falx and tentorium. Subdural hematomas are fairly common in infants, frequently as a result of birth trauma, falls, assaults, or violent shaking. Presenting signs can include irritability, vomiting, increased head circumference, bulging fontanels in infants, lethargy, or seizures. The small subdural space and dura firmly attached to the skull in this area are highly vulnerable to increased ICP. Hemiparesis, hemiplegia, and unequal pupils are signs of brainstem compression and increased ICP.

> ### ! NURSING ALERT
>
> Children with a subdural hematoma and retinal hemorrhages should be evaluated for the possibility of child abuse, especially shaken baby syndrome.

BOX 28-3 CLINICAL MANIFESTATIONS OF ACUTE HEAD INJURY

Minor Injury
May or may not lose consciousness
Transient period of confusion
Somnolence
Listlessness
Irritability
Pallor
Vomiting (one or more episodes)

Signs of Progression
Altered mental status (e.g., difficulty arousing child)
Mounting agitation
Development of focal lateral neurologic signs
Marked changes in vital signs

Severe Injury
Signs of increased intracranial pressure (see Box 28-1)
Bulging fontanel (infant)
Retinal hemorrhages
Extraocular palsies (especially cranial nerve III)
Hemiparesis
Quadriplegia
Elevated temperature
Unsteady gait
Papilledema

Associated Signs
Scalp trauma
Other injuries (e.g., to extremities)

Subdural taps often provide relief in the infant, as revealed by follow-up CT scans, improved neurologic status, and a flat anterior fontanel. The need for surgical evacuation of the hematoma depends on the physical examination, size of the hematoma, and CT scan abnormalities.

Cerebral Edema

Some degree of brain edema is expected, especially 24 to 72 hours after craniocerebral trauma. Cerebral edema associated with traumatic brain injury may be caused by direct cellular injury leading to intracellular swelling or vascular injury leading to increased intracellular fluid. Either mechanism can result in increased ICP as a result of the increased intracranial volume and changes in CBF.

Diagnostic Evaluation

A detailed health history, both past and present, is essential in evaluating the child with a craniocerebral trauma. Certain disorders, such as drug allergies, hemophilia, diabetes mellitus, or epilepsy, may produce similar symptoms. Even minor traumatic injury can aggravate a preexisting disease process, thereby producing neurologic signs out of proportion to the injury. It must be determined whether the infant or child exhibited alterations in consciousness, and any other signs and behaviors exhibited by the child must be noted. Because head injuries are frequently accompanied by injuries in other areas, the examination is performed with care to avoid further damage.

> ⚠ **NURSING ALERT**
>
> Stabilize a child's spine after head injury until a spinal cord injury is ruled out.

Initial Assessment

Priorities in the initial stabilization phase of a child with a head injury include assessment of the ABCs (airway, breathing, circulation); evaluation for shock; a neurologic examination focusing on mental status, pupillary responses, and motor responses; and assessment for spinal cord injury. The assessment is carried out quickly in relation to vital signs (see Emergency Treatment box).

> ⚠ **NURSING ALERT**
>
> Deep, rapid, periodic, or intermittent and gasping respirations; wide fluctuations or noticeable slowing of the pulse; and widening pulse pressure or extreme fluctuations in blood pressure are signs of brainstem involvement. Note that marked hypotension may represent internal injuries.

Ocular signs such as fixed, dilated, and unequal pupils; fixed and constricted pupils; and pupils that are poorly reactive or nonreactive to light and accommodation indicate increased ICP or brainstem involvement. It is important to remain with the child who demonstrates fixed and dilated pupils because these are ominous signs with a high probability of respiratory arrest. Dilated, nonpulsating blood vessels indicate increased ICP before the appearance of papilledema. Retinal hemorrhages are seen in acute head injuries, including shaken baby syndrome.

> ⚠ **NURSING ALERT**
>
> Observation of asymmetric pupils or one dilated, nonreactive pupil in a comatose child is a neurologic emergency.

Less urgent but important additional assessments include examination of the scalp for lacerations and palpation for other abnormalities. A significant amount of blood loss can occur from scalp lacerations. An underlying skull fracture should be ruled out by CT scan.

> ⚠ **NURSING ALERT**
>
> Bleeding from the nose or ears needs further evaluation, and a watery discharge from the nose (rhinorrhea) that is positive for glucose (as tested with Dextrostix) suggests leaking of CSF from a skull fracture.

An accurate assessment of clinical signs provides baseline information. Serial evaluations, preferably by a single observer, help to detect changes in the neurologic status. Alterations in mental status, evidenced by increased difficulty in rousing the child, mounting agitation, development of focal lateral neurologic signs, or marked changes in vital signs, usually indicate extension or progression of the basic pathologic process.

Special Tests

After a thorough clinical examination, a variety of diagnostic tests are helpful in providing a more definitive diagnosis of the type and extent of the trauma. The severity of a head injury may not be apparent on clinical examination of a child but is detectable on a CT scan. Whenever the child has a history consistent with a serious head injury (unrestrained occupant in a severe motor vehicle accident or a fall from a

> ✚ **EMERGENCY TREATMENT**
>
> ### Head Injury
>
> 1. Assess child:
>   - **A**—Airway
>   - **B**—Breathing
>   - **C**—Circulation
> 2. Stabilize neck and spine immediately. Use jaw thrust, not chin lift, to open airway.
> 3. Clean any abrasions with soap and water.
>   - Apply clean dressing.
>   - If bleeding, apply pressure and then ice to relieve pain and swelling.
> 4. Keep NPO until instructed otherwise.
> 5. Assess pain but do not give analgesics or sedatives.
> 6. Check pupil reaction every 4 hours (including twice during night) for 48 hours.
> 7. Awaken twice during the night to check LOC.
> 8. Seek medical attention if any of the following apply:
>   - Injury sustained:
>   - At high speed (e.g., automobile)
>   - In a fall from a significant distance (e.g., height greater than that of the child)
>   - From great force (e.g., baseball bat)
>   - Under suspicious circumstances
>   - Loss of consciousness
>   - Amnesia
>   - Discomfort (crying) more than 10 minutes after injury
>   - Headache that is severe, worsening, interferes with sleep, or lasts more than 24 hours
>   - Fluid leak from ears or nose; blackened eyes
>   - Vomiting three or more times, beginning after injury, or continuing 4 to 6 hours after injury
>   - Swelling in front of or above earlobe or swelling that increases in size
>   - Confusion or abnormal behaving
>   - Difficulty arousing child from sleep
>   - Difficulty speaking
>   - Blurred vision or diplopia
>   - Unsteady gait
>   - Difficulty using extremities, weakness, or incoordination
>   - Neck pain or stiffness
>   - Pupils dilated, unequal, or fixed
>   - Infant with bulging fontanel
>   - Seizures

LOC, Level of consciousness; *NPO*, nothing by mouth.

significant height), it is important to perform a diagnostic scan even if the child initially appears alert and oriented. All children with head injuries who have any alteration of consciousness, headache, vomiting, skull fracture, seizure, or a predisposing medical condition should undergo CT scanning.

After early head injury, MRI may be useful in evaluating cerebral edema or structural brain abnormalities, and neurobehavioral assessment can document any cognitive impairments. Skull radiographs are of little benefit in diagnosing skull fractures. EEG is not helpful for diagnosis of head injury but is useful for defining seizure activity. Lumbar puncture is rarely used in craniocerebral trauma and is contraindicated in the presence of increased ICP because of the possibility of herniation.

FAMILY CENTERED-CARE
Maintaining Contact

Maintaining contact with parents for continued observation and reevaluation of the child, when indicated, facilitates early diagnosis and treatment of possible complications from head injury, such as hematoma, hydrocephalus, and posttraumatic seizures. Children are generally hospitalized for 24 to 48 hours of observation if their family lives far from medical facilities or lacks transportation or a telephone that would provide access to immediate help. Other circumstances, such as language or other communication barriers, or even emotional trauma, may hinder learning and make it difficult for families to feel confident in caring for their child at home.

Posttraumatic Syndromes

Posttraumatic syndromes include postconcussion syndrome, posttraumatic seizures, and structural complications after a head injury.

Postconcussion syndrome is a common sequela to brain injury with or without loss of consciousness. Symptoms can develop within hours to days after a mild head injury but can also occur after moderate to severe head injury. The manifestations vary with the child's age and include nausea, dizziness, headache, diplopia, disorientation, and other mental status changes. The duration of manifestations can vary from several days to several months. Death from concussion is preventable unless overwhelming secondary brain injury has occurred (Blinman, Houseknecht, Synder, and others, 2009).

Posttraumatic seizures occur in a number of children who survive a head injury and are more common in children than in adults (Boran, Boran, Barut, and others, 2006). Seizures are more likely to occur within the first few days after a severe head injury.

Structural complications (e.g., hydrocephalus) may occur as a result of head injuries. Clinical sequelae include cognitive deterioration, motor deficits, optic atrophy, cranial nerve palsies, or aphasia. The type of residual effect depends on the location and nature of the trauma.

Therapeutic Management

The majority of children with mild traumatic brain injury who have not lost consciousness can be cared for and observed at home after a careful examination reveals no serious intracranial injury. Nurses should provide parents with verbal and written instructions of signs and symptoms that warrant concern and the need for medical reevaluation (see Family-Centered Care box).

Parents are instructed to check the child every 2 hours to determine any changes in responsiveness. The sleeping child should be wakened to see if he or she can be roused normally. Parents are advised to maintain contact with the health professional, who typically examines the child again in 1 or 2 days. The manifestations of epidural hematoma in children do not generally appear until 24 hours or more after injury.

Children with severe injuries, those who have lost consciousness for more than a few minutes, and those with prolonged and continued seizures or other focal or diffuse neurologic signs must be hospitalized until their condition is stable and their neurologic signs have diminished. The child is maintained on NPO status (nothing by mouth) or restricted to clear liquids until it is determined that vomiting will not occur. IV fluids are indicated in the child who is comatose, displays dulled sensorium, or is persistently vomiting. Fluid balance is closely monitored by daily weights; accurate intake and output measurements; and serum osmolality to detect early signs of water retention, excessive dehydration, and states of hypertonicity or hypotonicity.

The volume of IV fluid is carefully monitored to minimize the possibility of overhydration in cases of SIADH and cerebral edema. However, damage to the hypothalamus or pituitary gland may produce DI with its accompanying hypertonicity and dehydration.

DRUG ALERT

Sedating drugs are commonly withheld in the acute phase. Headaches are usually controlled with acetaminophen, although opioids may be needed. Antiepileptics are used for seizure control. Antibiotics may be administered if lacerations, penetrating injuries, or CSF leakage is noted. Cerebral edema is managed as described for the unconscious child. Hyperthermia is controlled with tepid sponges or a hypothermia blanket.

Surgical Therapy

Scalp lacerations are sutured after the underlying bone is carefully examined. Depressed fractures require surgical reduction and removal of bone fragments. Torn dura is sutured. Ping-pong ball skull fractures in very young infants ordinarily correct themselves within a few weeks; however, some may require surgical intervention.

Prognosis

The outcome of craniocerebral trauma depends on the extent of injury and complications. In general, the prognosis is more favorable for children than for adults. More than 90% of children with concussions or simple linear fractures recover without symptoms after the initial period. Outcomes in children with brain injuries are increasingly focused on long-term cognitive, emotional, and mental problems. The vulnerability of young children's developing brains can result in detrimental disruptions after significant brain injury (Bonnier, Marique, Van Hout, and others, 2007).

True coma (not obeying commands, eyes closed, and not speaking) usually does not last more than 2 weeks. A child's eventual outcome can range from brain death to a persistent vegetative state to complete recovery. However, even the best recovery after a coma may be associated with personality changes, including mood lability and loss of confidence, impaired short-term memory, headaches, and subtle cognitive impairments. Many children are left with significant disabilities after head injury that appear months later as learning difficulties, behavioral changes, or emotional disturbances (Bonnier, Marique, Van Hout, and others, 2007).

> **QUALITY PATIENT OUTCOMES: Acute Head Injury**
> • Early recognition of signs and symptoms of increased ICP
> • Adequate ventilation, oxygenation, and circulation maintained
> • Cerebral oxygen requirements minimized
> • Sedation and analgesia provided while allowing for neurologic assessment

Nursing Care Management

The hospitalized child requires careful neurologic assessment and evaluation that are repeated at frequent intervals to establish a correct diagnosis, identify signs and symptoms of increased ICP, determine clinical management, and prevent many complications.

The child is placed on bed rest, usually with the head of the bed elevated slightly and the head in midline position. Appropriate safety measures, such as side rails kept up and seizure precautions, are implemented. Children may be restless and irritable, but often their reaction is to fall asleep when left undisturbed. A quiet environment helps reduce restlessness and irritability. For extremely restless children, hard surfaces may need to be padded and restraint used to prevent the possibility of further injury. Care is individualized according to the child's specific needs. Shining bright lights directly into the child's face is irritating and makes assessment of ocular responses difficult.

Frequent examinations of vital signs, neurologic signs, and LOC are extremely important nursing observations. When possible, they should be performed by a single observer to better detect subtle changes that may indicate worsening neurologic status. Pupils are checked for size, equality, reaction to light, and accommodation. After the initial elevations usually seen after injury, the vital signs generally return to normal unless there is brainstem involvement.

The most important nursing observation is assessment of the child's LOC. Alterations in consciousness appear earlier in the progression of an injury than alterations of vital signs or focal neurologic signs. Some expected responses may be misinterpreted as deviations from the normal. Frequent examinations of alertness are fatiguing to the child; therefore, the child often desires to fall asleep, which may be confused with depressed consciousness. It is common to observe ocular divergence through the partially closed eyelids.

A key nursing role is to provide sedation and analgesia for the child. The conflict between the need to promote comfort and relieve anxiety in the child versus the need to assess for neurologic changes presents a dilemma. Both goals can be achieved with close observation of the child's LOC and response to analgesics, use of a pain assessment record, and effective communication with the practitioner. Decreasing restlessness after administration of an analgesic most likely reflects pain control rather than a declining LOC.

Observations of position and movement provide additional information. Any abnormal posturing is noted, as well as whether it occurs continuously or intermittently. Questions nurses might consider include:

- Are the child's handgrips strong and equal in strength?
- Are there any signs of flexion or extension posturing?
- What is the child's response to stimulation?
- Is movement purposeful, random, or absent?
- Are movement and sensation equal on both sides or restricted to one side only?

The child may complain of headache or other discomfort. A child who is too young to describe a headache may be fussy and resist being handled. A child who has vertigo will often assume a position of comfort and vigorously resist efforts to be moved. Forcible movement causes the child to vomit and display spontaneous nystagmus. Seizures are relatively common in children with head trauma and may be of any type. Carefully observe, record, and report in detail any seizure activity. Children in postictal (postseizure) states are lethargic, with sluggish pupils.

Document drainage from any orifice. Bleeding from the ear suggests the possibility of a basal skull fracture. Clear nasal drainage is suggestive of an anterior basal skull fracture. The amount and characteristics of the drainage should be observed, recorded, and reported.

> ### ! NURSING ALERT
>
> Suctioning through the nares is contraindicated because of the risk of the catheter entering the brain parenchyma through a fracture in the skull.

Head trauma is frequently accompanied by other undetected injuries; therefore, any bruises, lacerations, or evidence of internal injuries or fractures of the extremities are noted and reported. Associated injuries are evaluated and treated appropriately.

The child with normal LOC is usually allowed clear liquids unless fluid is restricted. If the child has an IV infusion, it is maintained as prescribed. The diet is advanced to that appropriate for the child's age as soon as the condition permits. Intake and output are measured and recorded, and any incontinence of bowel or bladder is noted if the child has been toilet trained.

Observe the child for any unusual behavior, but behavior should be interpreted in relation to the child's normal behavior. For example, urinary incontinence during sleep would be of no consequence in a child who routinely wets the bed but would be highly significant for one who is always dry. Parents are valuable resources in evaluating objective behavior of their child. Information obtained from parents at or shortly after admission is helpful in evaluating the child's behavior (e.g., the ease with which the child is roused normally, the usual sleeping position and patterns, motor activities [rolling over, sitting up, climbing], hearing and visual acuity, appetite, and manner of eating [spoon, bottle, cup]).

Family Support

The emotional and educational support of the family presents a challenging aspect to nursing care. Witnessing the parents' grief and helplessness on seeing their child in an altered state, connected to monitoring equipment, and in an intensive care unit evokes empathy. The nurse can encourage the family to be involved in the child's care, to bring in familiar belongings, or to make a tape recording of familiar voices and sounds. Parents may need a demonstration on how to touch or cuddle their child and may want to talk about their grief. The nurse can listen attentively, reinforce what is being done to assist the child, and direct parents toward signs and symptoms of recovery to instill hope without promises. Honesty and kindness, along with competent care, can help families through this difficult time.

When the child is discharged, the parents are advised of probable posttraumatic symptoms that may be expected. They should understand necessary monitoring and how to contact health care providers in case the child develops any unusual signs or symptoms. The importance of follow-up evaluation should be emphasized.

Rehabilitation

Rehabilitation and management of the child with permanent brain injury are essential aspects of care. Rehabilitation begins as soon as feasible and usually involves the family and a rehabilitation team. Careful assessment of the child's capabilities, limitations, and probable potential is made as early as possible, and appropriate interventions are implemented to maximize the residual capacities. The Brain Injury Association of America* provides information and listings of rehabilitation services and support groups throughout the country.

Pediatric trauma rehabilitation is a national concern. Coordinating care and services for early rehabilitation involves identifying the child's and family's response to the traumatic injury and disability, securing available resources, and recognizing the parental role in the process.

Children with disabilities resulting from head trauma require assessment on a physical, cognitive, emotional, and social level. These children have experienced separation, pain, sensory deprivation and overload, changes in circadian cycle, and fear of the unknown. Recovery and transition require new coping strategies at the same time that regressive and acting-out behavior may start. Parents and children

---

*1608 Spring Hill Road, Suite 110, Vienna, VA 22182; 703-761-0750; fax: 703-761-0755; http://www.biausa.org.

need honest communication for decision making. Rehabilitation is advocated when the child has progressed beyond what can be provided in a hospital setting. The Rancho Los Amigos Scale provides a systematic assessment of the possible progress a child may achieve after a severe head injury.

Prevention

Tremendous strides have been taken in the prevention of cerebral damage after head injury in children. New developments are directed toward the prevention of cellular injury or the primary insult. Nurses can exert a valuable influence on prevention of children's head injuries through education. Preventable head injuries occur because unnecessary risks go unchecked. Inadequate supervision combined with children's natural sense of indestructibility and exploration can lead to lethal results. Nurses are in the unique position of influencing caregivers in terms of growth and development risks. Banning the use of infant walkers is an example. This equipment does not help develop motor skills and places infants at risk for head and neck injuries from falls, especially down steps. Public education coupled with legislative support can prevent childhood injuries. (For extensive discussions of childhood injuries and prevention, see Chapters 10, 12, 13, 15, and 16. See also Childhood Mortality, Chapter 1.)

SUBMERSION INJURY

Submersion injury is a major cause of accidental death in children older than 1 year of age. The term *submersion injury* has replaced *near-drowning* to include any person who experiences distress from submersion or immersion in liquid that either results in death (drowning) or survival at least 24 hours after submersion (near-drowning) (Weiss and American Academy of Pediatrics [AAP] Committee on Injury, Violence, and Poison Prevention, 2010). Most cases of submersion are accidental, usually involving children who are helpless in water, such as inadequately attended children in or near swimming pools or infants in bathtubs; small children who fall into ponds, streams, and flooded excavations; occupants of pleasure boats who fail to wear life preservers; children who have diving accidents; and children who are able to swim but overestimate their endurance. Accidental drowning occurs more commonly in toddlers, boys, and African Americans (Nasrullah and Muazzam, 2011). Drowning can take place in any body of liquid, and sites of drowning are important to consider for preventive education. Children younger than 1 year old are most likely to drown in a bathtub, and buckets filled with fluid cause a risk of drowning to top-heavy toddlers who can fall head first into the buckets (Hon and Leung, 2010). Preschoolers are at risk for drowning in swimming pools, and drowning in school-age children and adolescents most commonly occurs in natural bodies of water such as lakes, ponds, and rivers (Shephard and Quan, 2011). The suction created at the outlet of pools, hot tubs, or whirlpool spas is strong enough to trap any child, even larger children, underwater. Drowning as a form of fatal child abuse has also been recognized as a problem.

Pathophysiology

Hypoxia is the primary cause of injury when submersion occurs and can cause damage to the brain, lungs, heart, kidneys, liver, and gastrointestinal system. Cerebral hypoxia is the major component of morbidity and mortality with submersion events. Within minutes of a submersion, a lack of oxygen leads to coma and ultimately cardiac arrest (Shephard and Quan, 2011). Recovery depends on the timeliness and effectiveness of initial resuscitation and subsequent supportive care measures.

Pathophysiologic features in submersion injuries are hypoxia, aspiration, and hypothermia.

Hypoxia is related to the duration of anoxia and asphyxia. Different cells tolerate variable lengths of anoxia, causing variations of cell damage. Neurons, especially cerebral cells, sustain irreversible damage after 4 to 6 minutes of submersion; but the heart and lungs can survive up to 30 minutes. Regardless of the amount of water aspirated, there is arterial hypoxemia (resulting from atelectasis with shunting of blood through the nonventilated alveoli) and a combined respiratory acidosis (resulting from retained carbon dioxide) and metabolic acidosis (caused by buildup of acid metabolites from anaerobic metabolism). Approximately 10% of drowning victims die without aspirating fluid but succumb from acute asphyxia as a result of prolonged reflex laryngospasm.

Aspiration of fluid is quickly absorbed in the pulmonary circulation resulting in pulmonary edema, atelectasis, and airway spasm, which aggravates the hypoxia. No clinical or physiologic difference, therapy, or outcome has been noted among human survivors in the submersion of salt water versus fresh water (Shephard and Quan, 2011).

Hypothermia is common after submersion, and children are at an increased risk of hypothermia because of their large surface area relative to body mass, decreased subcutaneous fat, and limited thermoregulation (Shephard and Quan, 2011). The temperature of the liquid plays an important role in developing hypoxemia. Cold water decreases metabolic demands and activates the diving reflex, which causes blood to be shunted away from the periphery and concentrated to the brain and heart. However, prolonged submersion in cold liquids can impair cognition, coordination, and muscle strength, ultimately resulting in a loss of consciousness, decreased cardiac output, and cardiac arrest (Shephard and Quan, 2011).

Therapeutic Management

The outcome of children after a submersion event depends on the circumstances and duration of the submersion and the speed and effectiveness of resuscitation efforts (Shephard and Quan, 2011). Resuscitative measures should begin at the scene of a drowning, and the victim should be transported to the hospital with maximal ventilatory and circulatory support. In the hospital, intensive care is implemented and continued according to the patient's needs.

In general, the management of the victims with submersion injuries is based on the degree of cerebral insult. The first priority is to restore oxygen delivery to the cells and prevent further hypoxic damage. A spontaneously breathing child will do well in an oxygen-enriched atmosphere; a more severely affected child will require endotracheal intubation and mechanical ventilation. Blood gases and pH are monitored frequently as a guide to oxygen, fluid, and electrolyte therapies.

> **! NURSING ALERT**
>
> All children who have a submersion injury should be hospitalized for observation. Almost half of asymptomatic or minimally symptomatic alert children experience complications (e.g., respiratory compromise, cerebral edema) during the first 24 hours after the incident (Shephard and Quan, 2011).

Aspiration pneumonia is a frequent complication that occurs about 48 to 72 hours after the episode. Bronchospasm, alveolocapillary membrane damage, atelectasis, abscess formation, and acute respiratory distress syndrome are other complications that occur after aspiration of fluid.

NURSING CARE GUIDELINES
Establishing Brain Death in Children

1. Coma and apnea must coexist. Child must exhibit complete loss of consciousness, vocalization, and volitional activity.
2. Brainstem function must be absent, as defined by:
   a. Midposition or fully dilated pupils that do not respond to light. Drugs may influence and invalidate pupillary assessment.
   b. Absence of spontaneous eye movements and those induced by oculocephalic and caloric (oculovestibular) testing.
   c. Absence of movement of bulbar musculature, corneal, gag, cough, sucking, and rooting reflexes.
   d. Absence of respiratory movements with standardized methods for testing apnea.
3. Child must not be hypothermic or hypotensive for age.
4. Flaccid tone and absence of spontaneous or induced movements, excluding activity mediated at the spinal cord level.
5. Examination should remain consistent with brain death throughout the observation and testing period.
6. Observation periods according to age:
   Seven days to 2 months—Two separate examinations and two EEGs separated by at least 48 hours
   Two months to 1 year—Two separate examinations and two EEGs separated by at least 24 hours
   Over 1 year—Two separate examinations separated by at least 12 hours

Modified from Ashwal S, Serna-Fonseca T: Brain death in infants and children, *Crit Care Nurse* 26:117–128, 2006.
EEG, Electroencephalogram.

Prognosis

The best predictors of a good outcome are length of submersion less than 5 minutes and the presence of sinus rhythm, reactive pupils, and neurologic responsiveness at the scene. The worst prognoses—for death or severe neurologic impairment—are children submerged for more than 10 minutes and not responding to advanced life support within 25 minutes. All children without purposeful movement and normal brainstem function 24 hours after a submersion injury have sustained severe neurologic deficits or death (Shephard and Quan, 2011). (See Nursing Care Guidelines box.)

Nursing Care Management

Nursing care depends on the child's condition. A child who survives may need intensive respiratory nursing care with attention to vital signs, mechanical ventilation, or tracheostomy, blood gas determination, chest physiotherapy, and IV infusion. Frequently, a child who has sustained a submersion injury requires the same care as an unconscious child. A difficult aspect in the care of the child victim of submersion injury is helping the parents cope with severe guilt reactions. Given the magnitude of the event, parents need repeated assurance that everything possible is being done to treat the child.

The parents of the child who is saved from death face the anxiety of not knowing the final outcome. The situation generates such intense feelings of loneliness and guilt that it is important for families to know that they are not alone. They should be reminded frequently that people are available to assist them during the crisis. Additional sources of support include psychiatric and social work consultants, community services, and religious support. Self-help groups may be beneficial if these are available in the community.

Nurses often have difficulty relating to the parents if obvious neglect has precipitated the accident and subsequent problems; therefore, it is important for those who care for these children and their families to assess their own feelings about the situation in addition to assessing the family's coping abilities and resources. Caring for victims of a submersion injury and their families requires nurses to be sensitive to the needs of the child and family and to recognize their own reactions and emotions.

Prevention

Most submersion injuries are preventable. The most common cause of submersion injury of infants and young children is inadequate adult supervision, including a momentary lapse of supervision (Weiss and AAP Committee on Injury, Violence, and Poison Prevention, 2010). Close adult supervision of infants and children around any body of water is essential and should include the adult not engaging in any distracting activities. Other strategies include environmental prevention strategies such as pool fencing; pool covers; water-entry alarms; and lifeguard and individual prevention such as swimming and survival skills, cardiopulmonary resuscitation training, and the use of personal floatation devices (Weiss and AAP Committee on Injury, Violence, and Poison Prevention, 2010). (See also Injury Prevention, Chapters 10, 12, 13, 15, and 16.)

NERVOUS SYSTEM TUMORS

Central nervous system tumors account for approximately 20% of all childhood cancers, with an estimated annual incidence of 3.1 cases per 100,000 children younger than 15 years of age (Howlader, Noone, Krapcho, and others, 2011).

BRAIN TUMORS

Brain tumors are the most common solid tumor in children and are the second most common childhood cancer. In children, the use of reference terms *benign* or *malignant* is generally avoided because any tumor, despite its nature, can be fatal or associated with significant morbidities in the developing brain of a child.

Central nervous system tumors can arise from any cell within the brain or spinal cord. The cell origin provides a histologic classification. For instance, astrocytes (cells that form the supportive tissue for neurons) may form a common glial tumor called an astrocytoma. A specific type of tumor called ependymoma typically arises within or adjacent to the ependymal lining of the ventricular system. CNS tumors in children are typically glial or neuronal in origin, located in the infratentorium, and generally sensitive to radiation and adjuvant chemotherapy (Merchant, Pollack, and Loeffler, 2010). Infratentorial brain tumors occur in the area of the brain below the tentorium cerebelli involving the cerebellum or brainstem. Types of infratentorial tumors include medulloblastoma, ependymoma, cerebellar astrocytoma, and brainstem glioma. Tumors above the tentorium are referred to as supratentorial and may include astrocytoma, primitive neuroectodermal tumor, craniopharyngioma, and optic pathway glioma. The suprasellar and pineal regions of the brain often are the location of germ cell tumors.

Diagnostic Evaluation

The signs and symptoms of brain tumors are directly related to their anatomic location and size and, to some extent, the child's age.

Supratentorial tumors can cause symptoms that include seizures, contralateral hemiparesis, memory loss, personality and behavioral changes, decline in school performance, and vision loss. Infratentorial tumors often cause the obstruction of normal CSF flow, resulting in signs and symptoms of increased ICP. Tumors involving the brainstem may cause cranial neuropathies, difficulty in micturition (if the pontine micturition center is affected), weakness, hypertonicity, and changes in respiratory pattern. Cerebellar tumors often cause ataxia, dysmetria, or nystagmus. In infants and very young children whose cranial sutures are still open, initial signs and symptoms of increased ICP (headache, vomiting, and lethargy) may not be evident, and symptoms may include irritability, failure to thrive, and loss of developmental milestones. Brain tumors involving the pineal gland or suprasellar region often present with endocrinopathies, which include growth failure, precocious puberty, DI, and adrenal insufficiency.

Diagnosis of a brain tumor is based subjectively on presenting clinical signs, objectively on neurologic tests, along with surgical confirmation of the histologic diagnosis. A number of tests may be used in the neurologic evaluation, but the most common diagnostic procedure is MRI, which determines the location and extent of the tumor. Other tests that may be used include CT, angiography, EEG, and lumbar puncture. CT or MRI is routinely performed before a lumbar puncture procedure to identify intracranial abnormalities that may cause a contraindication to the procedure (Lin and Safdieh, 2010). Lumbar puncture is dangerous in the presence of increased ICP because of the possibility of brainstem herniation after a sudden release of pressure. The definitive diagnosis of a brain tumor is based on brain tissue specimens obtained during surgery.

Therapeutic Management

Treatment may involve the use of surgery, radiotherapy, and chemotherapy or a combination of these treatment modalities. The optimum treatment is complete surgical resection of the primary tumor with preservation of adequate neurologic function. Radiation therapy is an integral part of treatment for many brain tumors but can cause significant neurocognitive side effects as well as endocrinopathies. Because rapid brain development occurs during the first 3 years of life, radiation therapy, particularly craniospinal radiation, is avoided in children younger than 3 years of age. Chemotherapy may be used as primary treatment or in an effort to delay radiation therapy until patients are older and may experience fewer neurocognitive side effects. One of the challenges in using chemotherapy for CNS tumors is the blood–brain barrier, which is a natural barrier that significantly influences the penetration of substances into the CNS. Commonly used chemotherapy agents for treatment of brain tumors in children include vincristine, cisplatin, carboplatin, cyclophosphamide, etoposide, lomustine, and temozolomide (Blaney, Haas-Kogan, Young Poussaint, and others, 2011).

Prognosis

The prognosis for a child with a brain tumor is quite variable and depends on the type of brain tumor, the size of the tumor, the extent of the disease, age, and surgical resectability. Recent advances in surgical instrumentation allowing aggressive surgical intervention, modifications in radiation, and use of chemotherapy have increased the long-term survival rates for many children with brain tumors. Currently, the overall survival rate for CNS tumors in children younger than 15 years of age is approximately 75% (Howlader, Noone, Krapcho, and others, 2011). Despite an improvement in overall survival, children with brain tumors, particularly those who are very young at diagnosis,

may have significant physical, cognitive, and endocrinologic sequelae because of their tumor and associated treatment (Shaw, 2009).

Nursing Care Management

If a brain tumor is suspected in a child admitted to the hospital for cerebral dysfunction, establishing baseline data with which to compare preoperative and postoperative changes is an essential step. It also allows the nurse to assess the degree of physical incapacity and the family's emotional reaction to the diagnosis.

Vital signs, including blood pressure and pulse pressure (the difference between systolic and diastolic pressures), are taken routinely and more often when any change is noted. Any sudden variations are reported immediately. Observation for symptoms of Cushing triad—a hallmark sign of increased ICP, which includes bradycardia, hypertension, and irregular respirations—is a crucial role of the nurse. It is also important to note a change in vital signs during or after diagnostic procedures. A routine neurologic assessment is performed at the same time as vital signs, and head circumference should be measured for infants and very young children. The child is observed for evidence of headache, vomiting, and any seizure activity. The location, severity, and duration of the headache are noted, as well as its relationship to activity, time of day, and any associated factors. Behaviors such as lying flat and facing away from light or refusing to engage in play are clues to discomfort in nonverbal children. The child's gait is observed at least once daily. Head tilt while talking or performing an activity as well as other changes in posturing should always be documented.

Prevent Postoperative Complications

Usually the surgeon will prescribe specific orders for vital signs, neurologic checks, positioning, fluid regulation, and medication. These vary somewhat, depending on the location of the craniotomy. The following are general principles of care for infratentorial or supratentorial surgery. Additional aspects of care that are discussed elsewhere may include care of the child with seizures and neurologic assessment of the unconscious child.

Vital signs are taken as frequently as every 15 to 30 minutes until the child is stable. Temperature measurement is particularly important because of hyperthermia resulting from surgical intervention in the hypothalamus or brainstem and from some types of general anesthesia. To prepare for this reaction, a cooling blanket is often placed on the bed *before* the child returns to the unit so it is ready for use when needed. The temperature is monitored carefully when any cooling measures are taken because hypothermia can occur suddenly. Recognizing signs of other complications such as increased ICP, meningitis, and respiratory tract infection is imperative.

> **! NURSING ALERT**
>
> When temperature is elevated, an infectious process must always be suspected, particularly if the febrile state occurs 1 to 2 days after surgery. It is important for the bedside nurse to remember that cultures (blood, urine, or CSF) should be obtained before the administration of any antibiotics in a febrile postoperative patient.

Neurologic checks are an essential aspect of care and include pupillary reaction to light, LOC, sleep patterns, and response to stimuli. Although children may be less responsive for a few days after surgery, when they regain full consciousness, there should be a steady increase in alertness. Regression to a lethargic, irritable state indicates increasing ICP, possibly caused by hemorrhage, cerebral edema, or meningitis.

> ⚠ **NURSING ALERT**
>
> Sluggish, dilated, or unequal pupils are reported immediately because they may indicate increased ICP and potential brainstem herniation, a medical emergency.

Observations for function are not instituted until the child regains consciousness. However, as soon as possible, the nurse should begin testing reflexes, handgrip, and functioning of the cranial nerves. Muscle strength is usually diminished as a result of general weakness after surgery but should improve daily. Ataxia may be significantly worse with cerebellar intervention but will slowly improve. Edema near the cranial nerves may depress important functions such as the gag, blink, or swallowing reflex.

Dressings are observed for evidence of drainage. If soiled, the dressing is not removed but is reinforced with dry sterile gauze. The approximate amount of drainage is estimated and recorded. A drain may be placed in the operative site.

> ⚠ **NURSING ALERT**
>
> To keep an accurate account of drainage, the soiled area is circled with a pen every hour or so. In this way, continuous bleeding is easily recognized. The presence of colorless drainage is reported immediately because it most likely is CSF from the incisional area. A foul odor from the dressing may indicate an infection. This should be reported immediately, and the nurse should anticipate cultures to be taken from the site.

Correct positioning after surgery is critical to prevent pressure against the operative site, reduce ICP, and avoid the danger of aspiration. If a large tumor was removed, the child is not placed on the operative side because the brain may suddenly shift to that cavity, causing trauma to the blood vessels, linings, and the brain itself. The nurse confers with the surgeon to be certain of the correct position, including degree of neck flexion. The first 24 to 48 hours after brain surgery are critical. If the child's position is restricted, notice of this is posted above the head of the bed. When the child is turned, every precaution is used to prevent jarring or malalignment to prevent undue strain on the sutures. Two nurses are needed—one supporting the head and the other supporting the body. The use of a turning sheet may facilitate turning a heavy child.

The child with an infratentorial procedure is usually positioned on either side with the bed flat. When a supratentorial craniotomy is performed, the head of bed is elevated 20 to 30 degrees with the child on either side or on the back. In a supratentorial craniotomy, the head elevation facilitates CSF drainage and decreases excessive blood flow to the brain to prevent hemorrhage. Pillows should be placed against the child's back, not head, to maintain the desired position. Ordinarily, the head and neck are kept in midline with the body, and the neck should not be flexed to support venous drainage (Christie, 2008).

> ⚠ **NURSING ALERT**
>
> The Trendelenburg position is contraindicated in both infratentorial and supratentorial surgeries because it increases ICP and the risk of hemorrhage. If shock is impending, the practitioner is notified immediately before the head is lowered.

With an infratentorial craniotomy, the child is kept NPO for at least 24 hours or longer if the gag and swallowing reflexes are depressed or the child is comatose. With a supratentorial operation, cranial neuropathy is less likely, and clear fluids may be resumed soon after the child is alert, sometimes within 24 hours. If the child vomits, oral liquids are stopped. Vomiting not only predisposes the child to aspiration but also increases ICP and the potential for incisional rupture.

The child should be fed to conserve energy and minimize movement. If there is any sign of cranial nerve deficits, the child is fed slowly to prevent choking and aspiration. Thickening agents can be used if the patient experiences dysphagia with thin liquids. Sometimes enteral feeding is necessary when body functions are too depressed to permit safe oral feedings or when the child refuses to eat or drink. IV fluids are continued until oral fluids are well tolerated or a method of enteral feeding is established. Because of the postoperative cerebral edema and danger of increased ICP, fluid status is carefully monitored.

Ⓔ Headache may be severe and is largely a result of cerebral edema. Measures to relieve some of the discomfort include providing a quiet, dimly lit environment; restricting visitors; preventing any sudden jarring movement, such as banging into the bed; and preventing an increase in ICP. Avoiding increased ICP is most effectively achieved by proper positioning and prevention of straining, such as during coughing, vomiting, or defecating. The use of opioids, such as morphine, to relieve pain is controversial because it is thought that they may mask signs of altered consciousness or depress respirations. However, opioids can be given safely because naloxone can be used to reverse opioid effects, such as sedation or respiratory depression. Acetaminophen and codeine are also effective analgesics for mild to moderate pain. When giving medication such as acetaminophen for pain, the nurse should be aware that this medication may also mask the presence of a fever, which could indicate postoperative infection. Regardless of the drugs used, adequate dosage and regular administration are essential to providing optimal pain relief (see also Pain Assessment; Pain Management, Chapter 7). Placing an ice bag on the forehead may also provide some headache relief, especially if facial edema is severe. Constipation is a common postoperative issue because of anesthesia and immobility. It is important to note that the use of narcotics for pain control may further contribute to constipation. Patients should be given a bowel regimen during the postoperative period until normal bowel function returns.

Support the Child and Family

The family's emotional needs are immense when the diagnosis is a brain tumor, and feelings are influenced by the extent of surgery, any neurologic deficits, the expected prognosis, and possible additional therapy. Because few definitive answers can be given before surgery, the surgeon's report after surgery is a significant finding that can vary from a low-grade, completely resected neoplasm to a highly malignant, invasive, and only partially removed tumor. Although parents often try to prepare themselves for the worst possible scenario, being given the news that their child has a potentially fatal tumor or may have significant neurologic impairment from the necessary treatment is always devastating.

Parents should be encouraged to verbalize their feelings about the diagnosis. Often they express tremendous guilt for viewing the insidious onset of symptoms, such as ataxia, visual difficulty, or headache, as "minor complaints" by the child. In retrospect, many parents feel guilt that they did not associate their child's decline in school performance with an actual medical problem. The nurse needs to exercise particular care not to make any comments that insinuate that the parents should have sought medical advice sooner because this will only compound any feelings of guilt that already exist. During this period, the nurse should also discuss with the parents what they plan to tell the child. If the child was prepared honestly, the diagnosis can be expressed in a similar age-appropriate manner. During recovery, the child will need additional explanation about the treatment and the reason for any residual neurologic effects, such as ataxia or blindness. The increasing availability of child life specialists has served as a tremendous resource in explaining diagnoses such as brain tumors to children and helping them cope with hospitalization and necessary treatment as well as understand and physical sequelae they may experience (Reynolds and Boyd, 2010).

NEUROBLASTOMA

Neuroblastomas are the most common malignant extracranial solid tumors in children, accounting for 8% to 10% of all childhood cancers (Mullassery, Dominic, Jesudason, and others, 2009). They occur in about 1 per 7000 live births, with a slightly higher incidence in boys (Brodeur, Hogarty, Mosse, and others, 2011). Approximately 95% of children with neuroblastoma manifest the disease before 10 years of age, with the median age of occurrence at 23 months (Park, Eggert, and Caron, 2010). These tumors originate from embryonic neural crest cells that normally give rise to the adrenal medulla and the sympathetic ganglia. Consequently, the majority of tumors develop in the abdomen along the adrenal gland or the retroperitoneal sympathetic chain. Other sites may be in the head, neck, chest, or pelvis.

The signs and symptoms of neuroblastoma depend on the location and stage of the disease. Neuroblastoma is commonly referred to as a "silent" tumor because about half of the patients present with localized disease and display few symptoms. However, children with advanced disease are ill appearing with symptoms of periorbital ecchymoses, proptosis, bone pain, and irritability caused by extensive tumor metastasis, usually in the lymph nodes, bone marrow, skeletal system, skin, or liver (Park, Eggert, and Caron, 2010).

Diagnostic Evaluation

The objective of diagnosis is to locate the primary site and areas of metastasis. Skeletal survey; skull, neck, chest, abdominal, and bone CT scans; and bilateral bone marrow aspirations and biopsies are used to locate a tumor mass and metastasis. A metaiodobenzylguanidine (MIBG) scan is used to determine involvement of bone, bone marrow, and soft tissue involvement.

Urinary excretion of catecholamines is detected in approximately 95% of children with adrenal or sympathetic tumors. Analyzing the breakdown products excreted in the urine, namely vanillylmandelic acid, homovanillic acid, dopamine, and norepinephrine, permits detection of suspected tumor before and after medical-surgical intervention (Mullassery, Dominic, Jesudason, and others, 2009). Amplification of proto-oncogene, known as the *MYCN* gene, and chromosomal abnormalities correlates strongly with advanced-stage disease, rapid tumor progression, and a poor prognosis (Brodeur, Hogarty, Mosse, and others, 2011).

Therapeutic Management

Accurate clinical staging is important for establishing initial treatment. Therefore, surgery is used both to remove as much of the tumor as possible and to obtain biopsies. In early stages, complete surgical removal of the tumor is the treatment of choice. If the tumor is large, partial resection is attempted, with a course of irradiation postoperatively to shrink the tumor in the hope of complete removal at a later date. Surgery is usually limited to biopsy in stages III and IV because of the extensive metastasis, although the use of additional

surgery to assess tumor regression or remove a regressed tumor is not unlikely.

Because radiotherapy can cause vertebral damage and growth arrest, it is contraindicated with intraspinal tumors; however, it can be used for emergency management of a massive neuroblastoma that is causing spinal cord compression (Mullassery, Dominic, Jesudason, and others, 2009). Radiotherapy also offers palliation for metastatic lesions in the bones, lung, liver, or brain.

Chemotherapy is the mainstay of therapy for extensive local or disseminated disease. Agents used in various combinations include cyclophosphamide, doxorubicin, cisplatin, etoposide, vincristine, ifosfamide, carboplatin, topotecan, and teniposide. In children with high-risk or recurrent disease, retinoic acid, radiotherapy, and myeloablative chemotherapy with peripheral stem cell rescue may be used to obtain a longer remission even though a poor overall survival rate is seen (Brodeur, Hogarty, Mosse, and others, 2011).

Prognosis

If all stages are grouped together, the 5-year disease-free survival rates range from 95% for children in the low-risk stage to only 30% in children in the high-risk stage (Park, Eggert, and Caron, 2010). Generally, the younger the child at diagnosis (especially younger than 1 year of age), the better the survival rate. Neuroblastoma is one of the few tumors demonstrating spontaneous regression (especially stage IV-S), possibly as a result of maturity of the embryonic cell or the development of an active immune system.

Nursing Care Management

Nursing considerations are similar to those discussed for leukemia and brain tumors, including psychologic and physical preparation for diagnostic and operative procedures; prevention of postoperative complications for abdominal, thoracic, or cranial surgery; and explanation of chemotherapy, radiotherapy, and their side effects.

Because this tumor carries a poor prognosis for many children, every consideration must be given to the family in terms of coping with a life-threatening illness (see Chapter 18). Because of the high degree of metastasis at the time of diagnosis, many parents experience substantial guilt for not having recognized signs earlier. Parents need much support in dealing with these feelings and expressing them to the appropriate people.

INTRACRANIAL INFECTIONS

The nervous system is subject to infection by the same organisms that affect other organs of the body. However, the nervous system is limited in the ways in which it responds to injury. Laboratory studies are needed to identify the causative agent. The inflammatory process can affect the meninges (meningitis) or brain (encephalitis).

Meningitis can be caused by a variety of organisms, but the three main types are (1) bacterial, or pyogenic, caused by pus-forming bacteria, especially meningococci, pneumococci, and *Haemophilus* organisms; (2) viral, or aseptic, caused by a wide variety of viral agents; and (3) tuberculous, caused by the tuberculin bacillus. The majority of children with acute febrile intracranial infections have either bacterial meningitis or viral meningitis as the underlying cause. Bacterial meningitis is considered much more serious than viral meningitis. Compared with viral meningitis, which typically is short lived, self-limiting, and followed by complete recovery, complications from bacterial meningitis can be quite severe and include shock, coma, seizures, intellectual deficits, hearing loss, vision loss, and death (Somand and Meurer, 2009).

BACTERIAL MENINGITIS

Bacterial meningitis is an acute inflammation of the meninges and CSF. Suspected bacterial meningitis is a medical emergency, and immediate action must be taken to identify the causative organism and to initiate prompt treatment.

The advent of antimicrobial therapy has had a significant effect on the overall clinical course and prognosis of children with bacterial meningitis. However, the introduction of vaccines has made the most significant impact on the incidence of this disease. After the introduction of the *Haemophilus* influenza type b (Hib) vaccine in 1990 and the pneumococcal conjugate vaccines in 2000, the incidence of bacterial meningitis declined in all age groups except children younger than 2 months of age. The incidence of bacterial meningitis caused by *Haemophilus influenzae, Streptococcus pneumoniae, Neisseria meningitidis,* group B streptococcus (GBS), and *Listeria monocytogenes* in children from 2 months of age to 17 years decreased from approximately 17 cases per 100,000 in 1998 to approximately 8 cases per 100,000 in 2007 (Thigpen, Whitney, Messonnier, and others, 2011).

Although it is encouraging to recognize the dramatic decline in the incidence of bacterial meningitis, this disease still results in death with the fatality rate of approximately 6.9% in children. The incidence is highest for patients younger than 2 months of age, and GBS is the most common causative organism in these patients. In children older than 2 months of age, *S. pneumoniae* and *N. meningitidis* are the most common etiologies for bacterial meningitis (Thigpen, Whitney, Messonnier, and others, 2011). Other causative organisms include β-hemolytic streptococci, *Staphylococcus aureus,* and *Escherichia coli.* The leading causes of neonatal meningitis are GBS, *E. coli,* and *L. monocytogenes. E. coli* infection is seldom seen beyond infancy. Meningococcal meningitis occurs in epidemic form and is the only type readily transmitted by droplet infection from nasopharyngeal secretions. Although this condition may develop at any age, the risk of meningococcal infection increases with the number of contacts; therefore, it occurs predominantly in school-age children and adolescents. College students, especially those living in dormitory residences, are at moderately increased risk for meningococcal disease compared with other persons their age. The meningococcal conjugate vaccine should be given to all people age 11 to 18 years with a booster dose administered 5 years later (Granoff and Gilsdorf, 2011).

There appear to be some seasonal variations with the organisms. Meningitis caused by *H. influenzae* primarily occurs in autumn or early winter. Pneumococcal and meningococcal infections can occur at any time but are more common in later winter and early spring.

Pathophysiology

The most common route of infection is vascular dissemination from a focus of infection elsewhere. For example, organisms from the nasopharynx invade the underlying blood vessels and enter the cerebral blood supply or form local thromboemboli that release septic emboli into the bloodstream. Invasion by direct extension from infections in the paranasal and mastoid sinuses is less common. Organisms also gain entry by direct implantation after penetrating wounds, skull fractures that provide an opening into the skin or sinuses, lumbar puncture or surgical procedures, anatomic abnormalities such as spina bifida, or foreign bodies such as an internal ventricular shunt or an external ventricular device. After implanting, the organisms spread into the CSF, by which the infection spreads throughout the subarachnoid space.

The infective process is similar to that seen in any bacterial infection and includes inflammation, exudation, white blood cell accumulation,

and varying degrees of tissue damage. The brain becomes hyperemic and edematous, and the entire surface of the brain is covered by a layer of purulent exudate that varies with the type of organism. For example, meningococcal exudate is most marked over the parietal, occipital, and cerebellar regions; the thick, fibrinous exudate of pneumococcal infection is confined chiefly to the surface of the brain, particularly the anterior lobes; and the exudate of streptococcal infections is similar to that of pneumococcal infections but thinner. As infection extends to the ventricles, thick pus, fibrin, or adhesions may occlude the narrow passages and obstruct the flow of CSF.

Clinical Manifestations

Patients with bacterial meningitis may present with fever and signs of meningeal irritation, including nausea, vomiting, irritability, anorexia, headache, photophobia, confusion, back pain, and nuchal rigidity. A history of an upper respiratory infection often precedes these symptoms. See Box 28-4 for clinical manifestations of bacterial meningitis. Nuchal rigidity is manifested by inability to flex neck and place chin on chest as well as presence of Kernig and Brudzinski signs. The Kernig sign is present if the patient, in the supine position with the hip and knee flexed at 90 degrees, cannot extend the knee more than 135 degrees and pain is felt in the hamstrings. Flexion of the opposite knee may also occur. The Brudzinski sign is present if the patient, while in the supine position, flexes the lower extremities if passive flexion of the neck is attempted (Feigin and Cutrer, 2009).

> **! NURSING ALERT**
>
> Any child who is ill and develops a purpuric or petechial rash may have (overwhelming) meningococcemia and must receive medical attention immediately.

Diagnostic Evaluation

A lumbar puncture is the definitive diagnostic test for meningitis. The fluid pressure is measured, and samples are obtained for culture, Gram stain, blood cell count, and determination of glucose and protein content. These findings are usually diagnostic. Culture and sensitivity testing are needed to identify the causative organism. Spinal fluid pressure is usually elevated, but interpretation is often difficult when the child is crying. Sedation with fentanyl and midazolam can alleviate the child's pain and fear associated with this procedure. If there is evidence or suspicion of increased ICP (papilledema, focal neurologic deficits, bulging fontanel), a CT scan of the head is warranted before the procedure. Lumbar puncture is contraindicated in any patient with imaging to suggest that the procedure is not safe (e.g., midline shift, mass effect, transependymal migration of CSF). However, a "normal" CT does not always mean a lumbar puncture is safe in the case of bacterial meningitis. It is important to take the clinical status into careful consideration. Clinical signs, including recent seizure, deteriorating LOC, or brainstem signs (posturing, pupillary changes, respiratory pattern changes), are clinical predictors of when a lumbar puncture should be delayed (Joffe, 2007).

The patient with meningitis generally has an elevated white blood cell count, often predominantly polymorphonuclear leukocytes. Typically, in bacterial meningitis, the CSF glucose level is reduced, generally in proportion to the duration and severity of the infection. It is a common misconception that the CSF glucose is low because of bacterial consumption of glucose. However, CNS infections may alter glucose transport across the blood–CSF barrier, resulting in a low CSF glucose value. The CSF glucose value in viral meningitis is usually

BOX 28-4   CLINICAL MANIFESTATIONS OF BACTERIAL MENINGITIS

Children and Adolescents
Usually abrupt onset
Fever
Chills
Headache
Vomiting
Alterations in sensorium
Seizures (often the initial sign)
Irritability
Agitation
May develop:
- Photophobia
- Delirium
- Hallucinations
- Aggressive behavior
- Drowsiness
- Stupor
- Coma

Nuchal rigidity; may progress to opisthotonos
Positive Kernig and Brudzinski signs
Hyperactivity but variable reflex responses
Signs and symptoms peculiar to individual organisms:
- Petechial or purpuric rashes (meningococcal infection), especially when associated with a shocklike state
- Joint involvement (meningococcal and *Haemophilus influenzae* infection)
- Chronically draining ear (pneumococcal meningitis)

Infants and Young Children
Classic picture (above) rarely seen in children between 3 months and 2 years of age
Fever
Poor feeding

Vomiting
Marked irritability
Frequent seizures (often accompanied by a high-pitched cry)
Bulging fontanel
Nuchal rigidity possible
Brudzinski and Kernig signs not helpful in diagnosis
Difficult to elicit and evaluate in this age group
Subdural empyema (*H. influenzae* infection)

Neonates
Specific Signs
Extremely difficult to diagnose
Manifestations vague and nonspecific
Child well at birth but within a few days begins to look and behave poorly
Refuses feedings
Poor sucking ability
Vomiting or diarrhea
Poor tone
Lack of movement
Weak cry
Full, tense, and bulging fontanel may appear late in course of illness
Neck usually supple

Nonspecific Signs That May Be Present
Hypothermia or fever (depending on the infant's maturity)
Jaundice
Irritability
Drowsiness
Seizures
Respiratory irregularities or apnea
Cyanosis
Weight loss

---

normal (Logan and MacMahon, 2008). The protein concentration is usually increased.

A blood culture is advisable for all children suspected of having meningitis and occasionally will be positive when CSF culture is negative. Nose and throat cultures may provide helpful information in some cases.

Therapeutic Management

Acute bacterial meningitis is a medical emergency that requires early recognition and immediate institution of therapy to prevent death or residual disabilities. The initial therapeutic management includes:

- Isolation precautions
- Initiation of antimicrobial therapy
- Restrict hydration
- Maintenance of ventilation
- Reduction of increased ICP
- Management of systemic shock
- Control of seizures
- Control of temperature
- Treatment of complications

The child is isolated from other children, usually in an intensive care unit for close observation. An IV infusion is started to facilitate the administration of antimicrobial agents, fluids, antiepileptic drugs, and blood, if needed. The child is placed on a cardiac monitor and in respiratory isolation.

Drugs

Until the causative organism is identified, the choice of antibiotic is based on the known sensitivity of the organism most likely to be the infective agent. After identification of the organism, antimicrobial agents are adjusted accordingly.

💊 DRUG ALERT

Dexamethasone may play a role in the initial management of increased ICP and cerebral herniation, but its ability to reduce long-term complications of bacterial meningitis remains controversial. Evidence indicates that dexamethasone therapy decreases the risk of neurologic sequelae in children with Hib meningitis, but data regarding the benefits in other types of bacterial meningitis are inconclusive (Prober and Dyner, 2011a). It is not recommended to be used if aseptic or nonbacterial meningitis is suspected (Granoff and Gilsdorf, 2011).

Signs of gastrointestinal hemorrhage or secondary infection may complicate steroid administration. Antibiotic treatment with cephalosporins demonstrates superiority for promptly sterilizing the CSF and reducing the incidence of severe hearing impairment.

Nonspecific Measures

Maintaining hydration is a prime concern, and the type and amount of IV fluids are determined by the patient's condition. Children with bacterial meningitis must be monitored closely for electrolyte and fluid abnormalities. The optimum hydration involves correction of any fluid deficits followed by fluid restriction until normal serum sodium levels and no signs of increased ICP are present. If needed, measures to decrease ICP are implemented (see p. 935). Long-term fluid restriction is not the standard of care because a lack of adequate fluid volume can reduce blood pressure and cerebral perfusion pressure, causing CNS ischemia (Prober and Dyner, 2011a).

Complications are treated appropriately, such as aspiration of subdural effusion in infants and treatment for disseminated intravascular coagulation syndrome. Shock is managed by restoration of circulating blood volume and maintenance of electrolyte balance. Seizures can occur during the first few days of treatment. These are controlled with the appropriate antiepileptic drug. Hearing loss is common. The patient should undergo auditory evaluation 6 months after the illness has resolved.

Lumbar puncture is carried out as needed to determine the effectiveness of therapy. The patient is evaluated neurologically during the convalescent period.

Prognosis

Fewer than 10% of cases of bacterial meningitis in children are fatal (Thigpen, Whitney, Messonnier, and others, 2011). The child's age, duration of illness before antibiotic therapy, rapidity of diagnosis after onset, type of organism, and adequacy of therapy are important in the prognosis of bacterial meningitis. Survivors can experience significant physical and neurologic sequelae. The most common sequelae in children include hearing loss, intellectual disability, spasticity or paresis, and seizure disorder. Approximately half of the survivors of pediatric bacterial meningitis will have at least one sequelae at a 5-year follow-up time point (Chandran, Herbert, Misurski, and other, 2011).

Clinical features that are associated with an increased risk of developing neurologic complications include young age, infection with *S. pneumoniae*, CSF with more than 10^7 colony forming units/ml or low CSF glucose content, delay in antimicrobial therapy for longer than 2 days, prolonged or complicated seizures, focal neurologic deficits, and adequacy of response to infection (Chandran, Herbert, Misurski, and other, 2011). The residual deficits in infants are primarily a result of communicating hydrocephalus and the greater effects of cerebritis on the immature brain. In older children, the residual effects are related to the inflammatory process itself or result from vasculitis associated with the disease.

QUALITY PATIENT OUTCOMES: Bacterial Meningitis
- Early recognition of signs and symptoms of meningitis
- Antibiotics administered as soon as diagnosis is established
- Cerebral edema prevented
- Exposure prevented by early isolation
- Side effects managed
- Neurologic sequelae prevented

Prevention

Vaccines are available for types A, C, Y, and W-135 meningococci and Hib. Meningococcal polysaccharide vaccination is routinely given to children 11 years of age or older; however, children 2 to 11 years may be given the vaccine if they are at increased risk for meningococcal disease (Granoff and Gilsdorf, 2011). Routine vaccinations for Hib are recommended for all children beginning at 2 months of age (see Immunizations, Chapter 10). Pneumococcal conjugate vaccine is now recommended for all children beginning at 2 months of age (Prober and Dyner, 2011a) (see Evidence-Based Practice box).

! NURSING ALERT

A major priority of nursing care of a child suspected of having meningitis is to administer antibiotics as soon as they are ordered. The child is placed on respiratory isolation for at least 24 hours after initiation of antimicrobial therapy.

Nursing Care Management

The room is kept as quiet as possible, and environmental stimuli are kept to a minimum because most children with meningitis are sensitive to noise, bright lights, and other external stimuli. Most children are more comfortable without a pillow and with the head of the bed slightly elevated. A side-lying position is more often assumed because of nuchal rigidity. The nurse should avoid actions that cause pain or increase discomfort, such as lifting the child's head. Evaluating the child for pain and implementing appropriate relief measures are important during the initial 24 to 72 hours. Acetaminophen with codeine is often used. The nurse should be cautious to evaluate if a patient is febrile before giving acetaminophen or ibuprofen because either of these medications may mask a fever, which is an important clinical indication of infection.

The nursing care of the child with meningitis is determined by the child's symptoms and treatment. Observation of vital signs, neurologic signs, LOC, urinary output, and other pertinent data is carried out at frequent intervals. The child who is unconscious is managed as described previously (see p. 934), and all children are observed carefully for signs of the complications just described, especially increased ICP, shock, or respiratory distress. Frequent assessment of the open fontanels is needed in the infant because subdural effusions and obstructive hydrocephalus can develop as a complication of meningitis.

Fluids and nourishment are determined by the child's status. The child with dulled sensorium is usually kept NPO. Other children are allowed clear liquids initially and, if these are tolerated, progress to a diet suitable for their age. Careful monitoring and recording of intake and output are needed to determine deviations that might indicate impending shock or increasing fluid accumulation, such as cerebral edema or subdural effusion.

One of the most difficult problems in the nursing care of children with meningitis is maintaining IV infusion for the length of time needed to provide adequate antimicrobial therapy (usually 10 days). Because continuous IV fluids are usually not necessary, an intermittent infusion device is used. In some cases, children who are recovering uneventfully are sent home with the device, and the parents are taught IV drug administration.

Family Support

The sudden nature of the illness makes emotional support of the child and parents extremely important. Parents are upset and concerned about their child's condition and often feel guilty for not having suspected the seriousness of the illness sooner. They need much reassurance that the natural onset of meningitis is sudden and that they acted responsibly in seeking medical assistance when they did. The nurse encourages the parents to openly discuss their feelings to minimize blame and guilt. They also are kept informed of the child's progress and of all procedures, results, and treatments. In the event that the child's condition worsens, they need the same psychologic supportive care as parents who face the possible death of their child (see Chapter 18).

EVIDENCE-BASED PRACTICE

Children with Bacterial Meningitis and Preventive Vaccines

Ask the Question
Picot Question
In children and adolescents with bacterial meningitis, has the administration of Hib, pneumococcal, and meningococcal preventive vaccines reduced the incidence and mortality associated with bacterial meningitis?

Search for Evidence
Search Strategies
Search selection criteria included English-language publications within the past 10 years, research-based articles (level 3 or lower), and children and adult populations.

Databases Used
PubMed and Cochrane Collaboration

Critically Analyze the Evidence
- Laval, Pimenta, de Andrade, and others (2003) conducted a systematic review of studies done in developed and developing countries that compared the effect of the conjugate of the Hib vaccine in the early 1990s with the more recent use of the heptavalent pneumococcal and the serogroup C meningococcal vaccines. The researchers concluded that all the vaccines mentioned have contributed directly to the decline in acute bacterial meningitis.
- Data trends on *Streptococcus pneumoniae* infections from the Bacterial Core Surveillance of the Centers for Disease Control and Prevention were evaluated during 1998 to 2001. After being licensed in early 2000, the pneumococcal conjugate vaccine significantly reduced the number of invasive pneumococcal cases, with the largest decline in children younger than 2 years of age (Whitney, Farley, Hadler, and others, 2003).
- Haddy, Perry, Chacko, and others (2005) compared the incidence of *S. pneumoniae* disease before and after the introduction of conjugated pneumococcal vaccine from 1999 to 2002. The trend in the rates of invasive pneumococcal disease cases showed significant declines during the study period for all ages after the introduction of the heptavalent *S. pneumoniae* protein conjugate vaccine.
- Children's Hospital of Pittsburgh reported the occurrence of bacterial meningitis before and after the licensure of the Hib conjugate vaccine. A total of 221 children, ages 1 month to 18 years, diagnosed with bacterial meningitis were identified from 1988 to 1998. *Haemophilus influenzae* was the organism responsible for approximately 58% of cases of bacterial meningitis. The absolute number of cases of bacterial meningitis caused by *H. influenzae* declined to 2.5 cases per year after the introduction of the Hib conjugate vaccine (Neuman and Wald, 2001).
- Watt, Wolfson, O'Brien, and others (2009) performed a literature review with studies evaluating Hib disease incidence, fatality ratios, and the effect of Hib vaccine. In 2000, there were 173,000 cases of Hib meningitis and 78,300 deaths among children younger than the age of 5 years worldwide. Expanded use of Hib vaccine can reduce the incidence and mortality of Hib-related disease.

- A recent Cochrane review determined the effect, duration of protection, and age-specific effects of polysaccharide SgAV to prevent meningococcal meningitis in children. The vaccine had a 95% protective effect during the first year in children older than 5 years of age, but its efficacy after the first year could not be determined. Children ages 1 to 5 years in low-income countries were also protected, but the exact efficacy could not be determined (Patel and Lee, 2010).

Apply the Evidence: Nursing Implications
There is **good evidence** with a **strong recommendation** (Guyatt, Oxman, Vist, and others, 2008) to suggest that all children should be immunized against the most common organisms responsible for bacterial meningitis (i.e., Hib, *S. pneumoniae*, and *Neisseria meningitidis*) as preventive vaccines to decrease the incidence of bacterial meningitis. The nurse should stress to the parents, children, adolescents, and young adults the importance of adhering to the immunization schedule to protect the child against serious childhood diseases.

QSEN Quality and Safety Competencies:
Evidence-Based Practice*
Knowledge
Differentiate clinical opinion from research and evidence-based summaries.
Describe the rationale for using vaccines to prevent bacterial meningitis.

Skills
Base individualized care plan on patient values, clinical expertise, and evidence.
Integrate evidence into practice by determining whether a patient needs Hib, pneumococcal, or meningococcal preventive vaccines.

Attitudes
Value the concept of evidence-based practice as integral to determining best clinical practice.
Appreciate the strengths and weakness of evidence for preventive vaccination in children.

References
Guyatt GH, Oxman AD, Vist GE, and others: GRADE: an emerging consensus on rating quality of evidence and strength of recommendations, *BMJ* 336:924–926, 2008.
Haddy RI, Perry K, Chacko CE, and others: Comparison of incidence in invasive *Streptococcus pneumoniae* disease among children before and after introduction of conjugated pneumococcal vaccine, *Pediatr Infect Dis J* 24(4):320–330, 2005.
Laval CA, Pimenta FC, de Andrade JG, and others: Progress towards meningitis prevention in the conjugate vaccines era, *Braz J Infect Dis* 7(5):315–324, 2003.
Neuman HB, Wald ER: Bacterial meningitis in childhood at the Children's Hospital of Pittsburgh: 1988–1998, *Clin Pediatr (Phila)* 40(11):595–600, 2001.
Patel M, Lee CK: Polysaccharide vaccines for preventing serogroup A meningococcal meningitis, *Cochrane Database Syst Rev* (1):CD001093, 2010.
Watt JP, Wolfson LJ, O'Brien KL, and others: Burden of disease caused by *Haemophilus influenzae* type b in children younger than 5 years, *Lancet* 374:903–911, 2009.
Whitney CG, Farley MM, Hadler J, and others: Decline in invasive pneumococcal disease after the introduction of protein–polysaccharide conjugate vaccine, *N Engl J Med* 348(18):1737–1746, 2003.

Hib, *Haemophilus influenzae* type b; *SgAV*, serogroup A vaccine.
*Adapted from the QSEN at http://www.qsen.org.

NONBACTERIAL (ASEPTIC) MENINGITIS

Aseptic meningitis is caused by many different viruses, including arbovirus, herpes simplex virus (HSV), cytomegalovirus, adenovirus, and human immunodeficiency virus (HIV). Enteroviruses are the most common cause of viral meningitis (Prober and Dyner, 2011b). The term *aseptic meningitis* refers to the onset of meningeal symptoms, fever, and pleocytosis without bacterial growth from CSF cultures. Viral meningitis can occur at any age but is most common in very young children. Viral meningitis has many of the same presenting signs and symptoms as bacterial meningitis, including headache, fever, photophobia, and nuchal rigidity. Viral meningitis can also be

TABLE 28-2	VARIATION OF CEREBROSPINAL FLUID ANALYSIS IN BACTERIAL AND VIRAL MENINGITIS	
MANIFESTATIONS	**BACTERIAL***	**VIRAL**
WBC count	Elevated; increased polys	Slightly elevated; increased lymphs
Protein content	Elevated	Normal or slightly increased
Glucose content	Decreased	Normal
Gram stain; bacteria culture	Positive	Negative
Color	Cloudy	Clear

WBC, White blood cell.
*Results may vary in the neonate.

accompanied by cutaneous and mucosal manifestations of enterovirus, including hand, foot, and mouth syndrome; herpangina; and maculopapular rash. The clinical course of viral meningitis is much shorter and typically without any significant complications (Logan and MacMahon, 2008).

Diagnosis is based on clinical features and CSF findings. Variations in CSF values in bacterial and viral meningitis are listed in Table 28-2. It is important to differentiate this self-limiting disorder from the more serious forms of meningitis.

Treatment is primarily symptomatic, such as acetaminophen for headache and muscle pain, maintenance of hydration, and positioning for comfort. Until a definitive diagnosis is made, antimicrobial agents may be administered and isolation enforced as a precaution against the possibility that the disease might be of bacterial origin. Nursing care is similar to the care of the child with bacterial meningitis.

ENCEPHALITIS

Encephalitis is an inflammatory process of the CNS resulting in inflammation of the brain parenchyma itself and is caused by a variety of organisms, including bacteria, spirochetes, fungi, protozoa, helminths, and viruses. Most infections are associated with viruses, and this discussion is limited to those agents.

Etiology

Encephalitis can occur as a result of (1) direct invasion of the CNS by a virus or (2) postinfectious involvement of the CNS after a viral disease. Often the specific type of encephalitis may not be identified. The cause of more than half of the cases reported in the United States is unknown. The majority of cases of known etiology are associated with the childhood diseases of measles, mumps, varicella, and rubella and, less often, with the enteroviruses, herpesviruses, and West Nile virus.

Herpes simplex encephalitis is an uncommon disease, but 30% of cases involve children. The initial clinical findings are nonspecific (fever, altered mental status), but most cases evolve to demonstrate focal neurologic signs and symptoms. Children may experience focal seizures. The CSF is abnormal in most cases. Because of a rise in the number of children with HSV encephalitis, suspected cases require prompt attention, especially because the diagnosis can be difficult. CSF polymerase chain reaction testing can confirm the clinical diagnosis rapidly. The early use of IV acyclovir reduces mortality and morbidity. Empiric therapy with acyclovir is given before precise virologic diagnosis has been established. Approximately two thirds of children with

BOX 28-5	CLINICAL MANIFESTATIONS OF ENCEPHALITIS

Onset
  Malaise
  Fever
  Headache
  Dizziness
  Apathy
  Lethargy
  Nuchal rigidity
Severe Cases
  High fever
  Stupor
  Seizures
  Disorientation
  Nausea and vomiting
  Ataxia
  Tremors
  Hyperactivity
  Speech difficulties—mutism
  Altered mental status
  Spasticity
  Coma (may proceed to death)
  Ocular palsies
  Paralysis

HSV encephalitis will have residual neurologic deficits (James, Kimberlin, and Whitley, 2009).

The multiplicity of causes of viral encephalitis makes diagnosis difficult. Most are those involved with arthropod vectors (togaviruses and bunyaviruses) and those associated with hemorrhagic fevers (arenaviruses, filoviruses, and hantaviruses). In the United States, the vector reservoir for most agents pathogenic for humans is the mosquito (St. Louis or West Nile encephalitis); therefore, most cases of encephalitis appear during the hot summer months and subside during the autumn.

The clinical features of encephalitis are similar regardless of the agent involved. Manifestations can range from a mild benign form that resembles aseptic meningitis, lasts a few days, and is followed by rapid and complete recovery to a fulminating encephalitis with severe CNS involvement. The onset may be sudden or may be gradual with malaise, fever, headache, dizziness, apathy, nuchal rigidity, nausea and vomiting, ataxia, tremors, hyperactivity, and speech difficulties (Box 28-5). In severe cases, the patient has a high fever, stupor, seizures, disorientation, spasticity, and coma that may proceed to death. Ocular palsies and paralysis also may occur.

Diagnostic Evaluation

The diagnosis is made on the basis of clinical findings and, when possible, identification of the specific virus. Early in the course of encephalitis, CT scan results may be normal. Later, hemorrhagic areas in the frontotemporal region may be seen. Togaviruses (some of which were formerly labeled arboviruses) are rarely detected in the blood or spinal fluid, but viruses of herpes, mumps, measles, and enteroviruses may be found in the CSF. Serologic testing may be required. The first blood sample should be drawn as soon as possible after onset, with the second sample drawn 2 or 3 weeks later. There are a number of characteristic EEG findings in encephalitis, particularly in HSV encephalitis, and an

EEG is often part of the diagnostic evaluation (Somand and Meurer, 2009).

Therapeutic Management

Patients suspected of having encephalitis are hospitalized promptly for observation. Only HSV encephalitis has specific treatment available. In other cases, treatment is primarily supportive and includes conscientious nursing care, control of cerebral manifestations, and adequate nutrition and hydration, with observation and management as for other cerebral disorders. Viral encephalitis can cause devastating neurologic injury. Cerebral edema, seizures, abnormal fluid and electrolyte balances, aspiration, and cardiac or respiratory arrest occur in severe viral encephalitis, and close monitoring is needed (Prober and Dyner, 2011b).

The prognosis for the child with encephalitis depends on the child's age, the type of organism, and residual neurologic damage. Long-term outcomes of HSV encephalitis in children can be serious, and deficits include visual, auditory, motor, and psychiatric (Prober and Dyner, 2011b). Very young children (younger than 2 years of age) may exhibit increased neurologic disabilities, including learning difficulties and seizure disorders. Follow-up care with periodic reevaluation is important because symptoms are often subtle, and rehabilitation is essential for patients who develop residual effects of the disease.

> **QUALITY PATIENT OUTCOMES: Encephalitis**
> - Early recognition of signs and symptoms of meningitis
> - Cerebral edema prevented
> - Side effects managed
> - Neurologic sequelae prevented

Nursing Care Management

Nursing care of the child with encephalitis is the same as for any unconscious child and for children with meningitis. Additional nursing interventions include observation for deterioration in consciousness. Isolation of the child is not necessary; however, good hand-washing technique must be followed. A main focus of nursing management is the control of rapidly rising ICP. Neurologic monitoring, administration of medications, and support of the child and parents are the major aspects of care.

RABIES

Rabies is an acute infection of the nervous system caused by a virus that is almost invariably fatal if left untreated. It is transmitted to humans by the saliva of an infected mammal and is introduced through a bite or skin abrasion. After entry into a new host, the virus multiplies in muscle cells and is spread through neural pathways without stimulating a protective host immune response.

Approximately 92% of rabies cases are transmitted by wild animals and the remainder from domestic animals (Blanton, Palmer, and Rupprecht, 2010). Wild animals such as skunks, raccoons, foxes, and bats are the animals most often infected with rabies and the cause of most indigenous cases of human rabies in the United States. The likelihood of human exposure to a rabid domestic animal has decreased greatly. In 2009, only four cases of human rabies were reported in the United States (Blanton, Palmer, and Rupprecht, 2010).

The circumstances of a biting incident are important. An unprovoked attack is more likely than a provoked attack to indicate a rabid animal. Bites inflicted on a child attempting to feed or handle an apparently healthy animal can generally be regarded as provoked. Any child bitten by a wild animal is assumed to be exposed to rabies.

> **! NURSING ALERT**
>
> Unusual behavior in an animal is cause for suspicion; children should be warned to beware of wild animals that appear to be friendly.

Although rabies is common among wildlife species, human rabies is rarely acquired. Modern-day prophylaxis is nearly 100% successful. The highest incidence occurs in children younger than age 15 years. The incubation period usually ranges from 1 to 3 months but may be as short as 5 days or as long as 8 months (Willoughby, 2011). Only 10% to 15% of persons bitten develop the disease, but when symptoms are present, rabies progresses to a fatal outcome. In the United States, human fatalities associated with rabies occur in people who fail to seek medical attention, usually because they are unaware of their exposure.

The disease is characterized by a period of nonspecific symptoms, including general malaise, fever, headache, and weakness, followed by typical symptoms of severe encephalitis, including agitation, changes in LOC, and seizures. Attempts at swallowing may cause such severe spasm of the pharynx, neck, and diaphragm muscles that apnea, cyanosis, and anoxia are produced—the characteristics from which the term *hydrophobia* was derived.

Diagnosis is made on the basis of history and clinical features. Hydrophobia is a cardinal sign of a rabies diagnosis.

Therapeutic Management

Treatment is of little avail after symptoms appear, but the long incubation period allows time for the induction of active and passive immunity before the onset of illness. Two types of immunizing products are available for use in humans: (1) the inactivated rabies vaccines, which induce an active immune response, and (2) the globulins, which contain preformed antibodies. The two types of products should be used concurrently for rabies postexposure treatment when prophylaxis is indicated; however, they are contraindicated after rabies symptoms develop (Willoughby, 2011).

The current therapy for a rabid animal bite consists of thorough cleansing of the wound with soap and water and administering antibiotics as indicated. Suturing of the wound should be avoided whenever possible. Passive immunization with human rabies immunoglobulin should be administered as soon as possible after exposure to provide rapid, short-term passive immunity (Manning, Rupprecht, Fishbein, and others, 2008).

Postexposure active immunity is conferred by administration of the human diploid cell rabies vaccine. The first intramuscular injection of the vaccine is given at the same time as the immunoglobulin (day 0) and is followed by injections at 3, 7, 14, and 28 days after the first dose (Manning, Rupprecht, Fishbein, and others, 2008). Before antirabies prophylaxis is initiated, the local or state health department should be consulted.

Nursing Care Management

Parents and children are frightened by the urgency and seriousness of the situation. They need anticipatory guidance for the therapy and support and reassurance regarding the efficacy of the preventive measures for this dreaded disease. The vaccine is well tolerated by children, although they need preparation for the series of injections. Mass immunization is unnecessary and unlikely to be implemented. In areas where rabies is rare, the schedule given is sufficient. However, certain circumstances may warrant preexposure vaccination, such as when a child is being taken to an area of the world where rabies in stray dogs is still a problem.

REYE SYNDROME

Reye syndrome is a disorder defined as acute encephalopathy associated with other characteristic organ involvement. It is characterized by fever, profoundly impaired consciousness, and disordered hepatic function.

The etiology of RS is not well understood, but most cases follow a common viral illness, typically influenza or varicella. RS is a condition characterized pathologically by cerebral edema and fatty changes of the liver. The onset of RS is notable for profuse effortless vomiting and varying degrees of neurologic impairment, including personality changes, seizures, and coma, that lead to increase ICP, herniation, and death (Carey and Balistreri, 2011). The cause of RS is abnormal mitochondrial function induced by various viruses, drugs, exogenous toxins, and genetic factors. Elevated serum ammonia levels tend to correlate with the clinical manifestations and prognosis.

Definitive diagnosis is established by liver biopsy. The staging criteria for RS are based on liver dysfunction and on neurologic signs that range from lethargy to coma. As a result of improved diagnostic techniques, children who in the past would have been diagnosed with RS are now diagnosed with other illnesses such as viral or metabolic diseases. Cases of unrecognized, drug-induced encephalopathy by antiemetics given to children during viral illnesses have symptoms similar to those of RS.

The potential association between aspirin therapy for the treatment of fever in children with varicella or influenza and the development of RS precludes its use in these patients. However, by the time the Food and Drug Administration required aspirin product labeling in 1986, most of the decline in RS incidence had already occurred.

Nursing Care Management

The most important aspect of successful management of a child with RS is early diagnosis and aggressive supportive therapy. Rapid progression to coma and high peak ammonia concentrations are associated with a more serious prognosis. Cerebral edema with increased ICP represents the most immediate threat to life.

Care and observations are implemented as for any child with an altered state of consciousness (see p. 934) and increasing ICP. Accurate and frequent monitoring of intake and output is essential for adjusting fluid volumes to prevent both dehydration and cerebral edema. Because of related liver dysfunction, laboratory studies to determine impaired coagulation, such as prolonged bleeding time, should be monitored.

Parents of children with RS need to be kept informed of the child's progress, to have diagnostic procedures and therapeutic management explained, and to be given concerned and sympathetic support. Families need to be aware that salicylate, the alleged offending ingredient in aspirin, is contained in other products (e.g., Pepto-Bismol). They should refrain from administering any product for influenza-like symptoms without first checking the label for "hidden" salicylates.

Prognosis

Recovery from RS is rapid and usually without sequelae if the diagnosis is determined early and therapy is initiated promptly. Patients who survive have full liver function recovery; however, approximately one third may have subtle neuropsychological deficits (Carey and Balistreri, 2011; Pugliese, Beltramo, and Torre, 2008).

▌SEIZURE DISORDERS

Seizures are the most common pediatric neurologic disorder. About 4% of children will have at least one seizure by the age of 15 years with half of those episodes being febrile seizures (Friedman and Ghazala, 2006). Seizures are caused by excessive and disorderly neuronal discharges in the brain. The manifestation of seizures depends on the region of the brain in which they originate and may include unconsciousness or altered consciousness; involuntary movements; and changes in perception, behaviors, sensations, and posture.

Seizures are a symptom of an underlying disease process. Causes of seizures may be infectious, neurologic, metabolic, traumatic, or related to ingestion of toxins (Friedman and Ghazala, 2006). Epilepsy is a condition characterized by two or more unprovoked seizures and can be caused by a variety of pathologic processes in the brain. A single seizure event should not be classified as epilepsy and is generally not treated with long-term antiepileptic drugs. Some seizures may result from an acute medical or neurologic illness and cease after the illness is treated. In other cases, children may have a single seizure without the cause ever being known.

After it is determined that the child has had a seizure, it is important to classify the seizure, according to the International Classification of Epileptic Seizures, and assign it to the appropriate epilepsy syndrome, according to the International Classification of Epilepsies and Epileptic Syndromes. Optimum treatment and prognosis require an accurate diagnosis and a determination of the cause whenever possible.

ETIOLOGY

Seizures in children have many different causes. Seizures are classified not only according to type but also according to etiology. Acute symptomatic seizures are associated with an acute insult such as head trauma or meningitis. Remote symptomatic seizures are those without an immediate cause but with an identifiable prior brain injury such as major head trauma, meningitis or encephalitis, hypoxia, stroke, or a static encephalopathy such as cognitive impairment or cerebral palsy. Cryptogenic seizures are those occurring with no clear cause. Idiopathic seizures are genetic in origin. A partial list of causative factors is presented in Box 28-6.

PATHOPHYSIOLOGY

Regardless of the etiologic factor or type of seizure, the basic mechanism is the same. Abnormal electrical discharges (1) may arise from central areas in the brain that affect consciousness; (2) may be restricted to one area of the cerebral cortex, producing manifestations characteristic of that particular anatomic focus; or (3) may begin in a localized area of the cortex and spread to other portions of the brain and, if sufficiently extensive, produce generalized seizure activity.

Seizure activity begins with a group of neurons in the CNS that because of excessive excitation and loss of inhibition amplify their discharge simultaneously. In response to physiologic stimuli, such as cellular dehydration, severe hypoglycemia, electrolyte imbalance, sleep deprivation, emotional stress, and endocrine changes, these hyperexcitable cells activate normal cells in surrounding areas and in distant, synaptically related cells. A generalized seizure develops when the neuronal excitation from the epileptogenic focus spreads to the brainstem, particularly the midbrain and reticular formation. These centers within the brainstem, known as the centrencephalic system, are responsible for the spread of the epileptic potentials. The discharges can originate spontaneously in the centrencephalic system or be triggered by a focal area in the cortex. On the basis of these characteristic neuronal discharges (as recorded by the EEG), seizures are designated as partial, generalized, and unclassified epileptic seizures.

BOX 28-6   ETIOLOGY OF SEIZURES IN CHILDREN

Nonrecurrent (Acute)
Febrile episodes
Intracranial infection
Intracranial hemorrhage
Space-occupying lesions (cyst, tumor)
Acute cerebral edema
Anoxia
Toxins
Drugs
Tetanus
Lead encephalopathy
Shigella or *Salmonella* organisms
Metabolic alterations:
- Hypocalcemia
- Hypoglycemia
- Hyponatremia or hypernatremia
- Hypomagnesemia
- Alkalosis
- Disorders of amino acid metabolism
- Deficiency states
- Hyperbilirubinemia

Recurrent (Chronic)
Idiopathic epilepsy
Epilepsy secondary to:
- Trauma
- Hemorrhage
- Anoxia
- Infections
- Toxins
- Degenerative phenomena
- Congenital defects
- Parasitic brain disease
- Hypoglycemia injury
Epilepsy—sensory stimulus
Epilepsy-stimulating states
- Narcolepsy and catalepsy
- Psychogenic
- Tetany from hypocalcemia, alkalosis
Hypoglycemic states
- Hyperinsulinism
- Hypopituitarism
- Adrenocortical insufficiency
- Hepatic disorders
Uremia
Allergy
Cardiovascular dysfunction or syncopal episodes
Migraine

SEIZURE CLASSIFICATION AND CLINICAL MANIFESTATIONS

There are many different types of seizures, and each has unique clinical manifestations. Seizures are classified into three major categories:

Partial seizures, which have a local onset and involve a relatively small location in the brain

Generalized seizures, which involve both hemispheres of the brain and are without local onset

Unclassified epileptic seizures

Descriptions of the different types of seizures are found in Box 28-7 and Table 28-3.

Diagnostic Evaluation

Establishing a diagnosis is critical for establishing a prognosis and planning the proper treatment. The process of diagnosis in a child suspected of having epilepsy includes (1) determining whether epilepsy or seizures exist and not an alternative diagnosis and (2) defining the underlying cause, if possible. The assessment and diagnosis rely heavily on a thorough history, skilled observation, and several diagnostic tests.

It is especially important to differentiate epilepsy from other brief alterations in consciousness or behavior. Clinical entities that mimic seizures include migraine headaches, toxic effects of drugs, syncope (fainting), breath-holding spells in infants and young children, movement disorders (tics, tremor, chorea), prolonged QT syndrome, sleep disturbances (night terrors), psychogenic seizures, rage attacks, and transient ischemic attacks (rare in children) (Friedman and Ghazala, 2006). Cocaine intoxication should be considered in the differential diagnosis of new-onset seizure activity in a newborn infant.

The history of the seizure should be detailed, including the type of seizure or description of the child's behavior during the event, the age at onset, and the time at which the seizure occurs (e.g., early morning, before meals, while awake, or during sleep). Any factors that may have precipitated the seizure are important, including fever, infection, head trauma, anxiety, fatigue, sleep deprivation, menstrual cycle, alcohol, and activity (e.g., hyperventilation or exposure to strong stimuli such as bright flashing light or loud noises). Record any sensory phenomena that the child can describe. The duration and progression of the seizure (if any) and the postictal feelings and behavior (e.g., confusion, inability to speak, amnesia, headache, and sleep) should also be recorded. It is important to determine whether more than one seizure type exists. It is often more informative to ask the parents to mime the seizure rather than relying on their oral description. Miming often reveals features, such as head turning, that would otherwise go unrecognized. Some seizures are overlooked by parents. For example, some parents may not identify brief head nods or brief single jerks as seizures unless specifically asked whether their child has these symptoms. The family history should include whether other family members have had a seizure, cognitive impairments, cerebral palsy, or other neurologic disorders. A family history can offer clues to paroxysmal disorders such as migraine headaches, breath-holding spells, febrile seizures, or neurologic diseases.

A complete physical and neurologic examination, including developmental assessment of language, learning, behavior, and motor abilities, may provide clues to the cause of the seizures. A number of laboratory and neuroimaging tests may be ordered depending on the child's age, whether it is a new-onset seizure, characteristics of the seizure, and the history. Laboratory studies that may prove to be of value include a venous lead level if the history warrants or white blood cell count (for signs of infection). Blood glucose measurements may

Hallmark early systemic clinical changes during a generalized seizure include tachycardia, hypertension, hyperglycemia, and hypoxemia. Brief seizures rarely produce significant durable side effects. In contrast, prolonged seizures can lead to lactic acidosis rhabdomyolysis, hyperkalemia, hyperthermia, and hypoglycemia. All of these changes can cause long-term neurologic damage (Friedman and Ghazala, 2006).

BOX 28-7   CLASSIFICATION AND CLINICAL MANIFESTATIONS OF SEIZURES

Partial Seizures

Simple Partial Seizures with Motor Signs

Characterized by:

- Localized motor symptoms
- Somatosensory, psychic, autonomic symptoms
- Combination of these
- Abnormal discharges remaining unilateral

Manifestations

- Aversive seizure (most common motor seizure in children)—Eye or eyes and head turn away from the side of the focus; awareness of movement or loss of consciousness
- Rolandic (Sylvan) seizure—Tonic-clonic movements involving the face, salivation, arrested speech; most common during sleep
- Jacksonian march (rare in children)—Orderly, sequential progression of clonic movements beginning in a foot, hand, or face and moving, or "marching," to adjacent body parts

Simple Partial Seizures with Sensory Signs

Uncommon in children younger than 8 years of age

Characterized by various sensations, including:

- Numbness, tingling, prickling, paresthesia, or pain originating in one area (e.g., face or extremities) and spreading to other parts of the body
- Visual sensations or formed images
- Motor phenomena such as posturing or hypertonia

Complex Partial Seizures (Psychomotor Seizures)

Observed more often in children from 3 years through adolescence

Characterized by:

- Period of altered behavior
- Amnesia for event (no recollection of behavior)
- Inability to respond to environment
- Impaired consciousness during event
- Drowsiness or sleep usually following seizure
- Confusion and amnesia possibly prolonged
- Complex sensory phenomena (aura)—Most frequent sensation is strange feeling in the pit of the stomach that rises toward the throat and is often accompanied by odd or unpleasant odors or tastes; complex auditory or visual hallucinations; ill-defined feelings of elation or strangeness (e.g., déjà vu, a feeling of familiarity in a strange environment); strong feelings of fear and anxiety; a distorted sense of time and self; and in small children, emission of a cry or attempt to run for help

Patterns of motor behavior:

- Stereotypic
- Similar with each subsequent seizure
- May suddenly cease activity, appear dazed, stare into space, become confused and apathetic, and become limp or stiff or display some form of posturing
- May be confused
- May perform purposeless, complicated activities in a repetitive manner (automatisms), such as walking, running, kicking, laughing, or speaking incoherently, most often followed by postictal confusion or sleep; may exhibit oropharyngeal activities, such as smacking, chewing, drooling, swallowing, and nausea or abdominal pain followed by stiffness, a fall, and postictal sleep; rarely manifests actions such as rage or temper tantrums; aggressive acts uncommon during seizure

Generalized Seizures

Tonic-Clonic Seizures (Formerly Known as Grand Mal)

Most common and most dramatic of all seizure manifestations

Occur without warning

Tonic phase lasts approximately 10 to 20 seconds

Manifestations:

- Eyes roll upward
- Immediate loss of consciousness
- If standing, falls to floor or ground
- Stiffens in generalized, symmetric tonic contraction of entire body musculature
- Arms usually flexed
- Legs, head, and neck extended
- May utter a peculiar piercing cry
- Apneic, may become cyanotic
- Increased salivation and loss of swallowing reflex

Clonic phase lasts about 30 seconds but can vary from only a few seconds to a half hour or longer

Manifestations:

- Violent jerking movements as the trunk and extremities undergo rhythmic contraction and relaxation
- May foam at the mouth
- May be incontinent of urine and feces

As event ends, movements less intense, occurring at longer intervals and then ceasing entirely

Status epilepticus—Series of seizures at intervals too brief to allow the child to regain consciousness between the time one event ends and the next begins

- Requires emergency intervention
- Can lead to exhaustion, respiratory failure, and death

Postictal state:

- Appears to relax
- May remain semiconscious and difficult to arouse
- May awaken in a few minutes
- Remains confused for several hours
- Poor coordination
- Mild impairment of fine motor movements
- May have visual and speech difficulties
- May vomit or complain of severe headache
- When left alone, usually sleeps for several hours
- On awakening, is fully conscious
- Usually feels tired and complains of sore muscles and headache
- No recollection of entire event

Absence Seizures (Formerly Called Petit Mal or Lapses)

Characterized by:

- Onset usually between 4 and 12 years of age
- More common in girls than boys
- Usually cease at puberty
- Brief loss of consciousness
- Minimum or no alteration in muscle tone
- May go unrecognized because of little change in child's behavior
- Abrupt onset; suddenly develops 20 or more attacks daily
- Event often mistaken for inattentiveness or daydreaming
- Events possibly precipitated by hyperventilation, hypoglycemia, stresses (emotional and physiologic), fatigue, or sleeplessness

BOX 28-7 CLASSIFICATION AND CLINICAL MANIFESTATIONS OF SEIZURES—cont'd

Manifestations:
- Brief loss of consciousness
- Appear without warning or aura
- Usually last about 5 to 10 seconds
- Slight loss of muscle tone may cause child to drop objects
- Ability to maintain postural control; seldom falls
- Minor movements such as lip smacking, twitching of eyelids or face, or slight hand movements
- Not accompanied by incontinence
- Amnesia for episode
- May need to reorient self to previous activity

Atonic and Akinetic Seizures (Also Known as Drop Attacks)
Characterized by:
- Onset usually between 2 and 5 years of age
- Sudden, momentary loss of muscle tone and postural control
- Events recurring frequently during the day, particularly in the morning hours and shortly after awakening

Manifestations:
- Loss of tone causing child to fall to the floor violently
- Unable to break fall by putting out hand
- May incur a serious injury to the face, head, or shoulder
- Loss of consciousness only momentary

Myoclonic Seizures
A variety of seizure episodes
May be isolated as benign essential myoclonus
May occur in association with other seizure forms

Characterized by:
- Sudden, brief contractures of a muscle or group of muscles
- Occur singly or repetitively
- No postictal state
- May or may not be symmetric
- May or may not include loss of consciousness

Infantile Spasms
Also called infantile myoclonus, massive spasms, hypsarrhythmia, salaam episodes, or infantile myoclonic spasms
Most commonly occur during the first 6 to 8 months of life
Twice as common in boys as girls
Numerous seizures during the day without postictal drowsiness or sleep
Poor outlook for normal intelligence
Manifestations:
- Possible series of sudden, brief, symmetric, muscular contractions
- Head flexed, arms extended, and legs drawn up
- Eyes sometimes rolling upward or inward
- May be preceded or followed by a cry or giggling
- May or may not include loss of consciousness
- Sometimes flushing, pallor, or cyanosis

Infants who are able to sit but not stand:
- Sudden dropping forward of the head and neck with trunk flexed forward and knees drawn up—the *salaam* or *jackknife* seizure

Less often: alternate clinical forms
- Extensor spasms rather than flexion of arms, legs, and trunk, and head nodding
- Lightning events involving a single, momentary, shocklike contraction of the entire body

TABLE 28-3 COMPARISON OF SIMPLE PARTIAL, COMPLEX PARTIAL, AND ABSENCE SEIZURES

CLINICAL MANIFESTATIONS	SIMPLE PARTIAL	COMPLEX PARTIAL	ABSENCE
Age of onset	Any age	Uncommon before age 3 years	Uncommon before age 3 years
Frequency (per day)	Variable	Rarely over one or two times	Multiple
Duration	Usually <30 sec	Usually >60 sec, rarely <10 sec	Usually >10 sec, rarely >30 sec
Aura	May be sole manifestation of seizure	Frequent	Never
Impaired consciousness	Never	Always	Always; brief loss of consciousness
Automatisms	Never	Frequent	Frequent
Clonic movements	Frequent	Occasional	Occasional
Postictal impairment	Rare	Frequent	Never
Mental disorientation	Rare	Common	Unusual

give evidence of hypoglycemic episodes, and serum electrolytes, blood urea nitrogen, calcium, serum amino acids, lactate, ammonia, and urine organic acids may indicate metabolic disturbances. Blood for chromosomal analysis may also be tested if a genetic etiology is suspected. A toxic screen should be performed if alcohol or drug ingestion is suspected. Lumbar puncture can confirm a suspected diagnosis of meningitis. CT may be done to detect a cerebral hemorrhage, infarctions, and gross malformations. MRI provides greater anatomic detail and is used to detect developmental malformations, tumors, and cortical dysplasias.

An EEG is obtained for most children with seizures and is the most useful tool for evaluating a seizure disorder. The EEG confirms the presence of abnormal electrical discharges and provides information on the seizure type and the focus. The EEG is carried out under varying conditions—with the child asleep, awake, awake with provocative stimulation (flashing lights, noise), and hyperventilation. Stimulation may elicit abnormal electrical activity, which is recorded on the EEG. Various seizure types produce characteristic EEG patterns: high-voltage spike discharges are seen in tonic-clonic seizures, with abnormal patterns in the intervals between seizures; a three-per-second spike and wave pattern is observed in an absence seizure; and absence of electrical activity in an area suggests a large lesion, such as an abscess or subdural collection of fluid.

A normal EEG does not rule out seizures because the EEG is only a surface recording and only represents approximately 1 hour of time and therefore may show normal interictal activity. If there is concern about whether a child has seizures or the seizure type cannot be determined, then a long-term video EEG may be done to record the child during wakefulness and sleep. The full-body image is recorded on video, with selected EEG channels displayed on the same screen for simultaneous recording and viewing. EEG monitoring is also available in digital EEG and digital video imaging, which allows for greater selection of EEG channels and is available in both routine and long-term EEGs. Although the EEG is very valuable, it should not be used alone to determine the type of seizure. Rather, the EEG interpretation along with a thorough clinical description of the patient's behavior during the seizure episode will guide to the correct classification of the seizure and the appropriate treatment choice.

Therapeutic Management

The goal of treatment of seizure disorders is to control the seizures or to reduce their frequency and severity, discover and correct the cause when possible, and help the child live as normal a life as possible. If the seizure activity is a manifestation of an infectious, traumatic, or metabolic process, the seizure therapy is instituted as part of the general therapeutic regimen and may only be necessary for a certain period of time if the underlying cause is corrected. Management of epilepsy has four treatment options: drug therapy, the ketogenic diet, vagus nerve stimulation (VNS), and epilepsy surgery.

Drug Therapy

It is known that persons predisposed to epilepsy have seizures when their basal level of neuronal excitability exceeds a critical point; no event occurs if the excitability is maintained below this threshold. The administration of antiepileptic drugs serves to raise this threshold and prevent seizures. Consequently, the primary therapy for seizure disorders is the administration of the appropriate antiepileptic drug or combination of drugs in a dosage that provides the desired effect without causing undesirable side effects or toxic reactions. Antiepileptic drugs are believed to exert their effect primarily by reducing the responsiveness of normal neurons to the sudden, high-frequency nerve impulses that arise in the epileptogenic focus. Thus, the seizure is effectively suppressed; however, the abnormal brain waves may or may not be altered. Complete control of seizures can be achieved in 70% to 80% of children (Curatolo, Moavero, Lo Castro, and Cerminara, 2009; Lozsadi, Von Oertzen, and Cock, 2010).

The initiation of anticonvulsant therapy is based on several factors, including the child's age, type of seizure, risk of recurrence, and other comorbid or predisposing medical issues. For children who develop recurrent seizures or epilepsy, treatment is begun with a single drug known to be effective and have the lowest toxicity (i.e., the safest side effect profile for the child's particular type of seizure). The dosage is gradually increased until the seizures are controlled or the child develops side effects. If the drug is effective but does not sufficiently control the seizures, a second drug is added in gradually increasing doses. When seizures are controlled, the first drug may be tapered to reduce the potential adverse effects and drug interactions of polytherapy. Monotherapy remains the treatment method of choice for epilepsy, but a combination of medications may be a viable alternative for children who cannot attain seizure control with only one medication (Mikati, 2011).

Measurement of blood levels of the drug is important if the seizures continue when the child is on a therapeutic dose of medication, to adjust the dosage and to assist in determining which medication may be causing the side effects if the child is on multiple antiepileptic medications. Some possible causes of low serum blood concentrations are noncompliance, poor absorption, and drug interactions. The

dosage needs to be increased as the child grows. Blood cell counts, urinalysis, and liver function tests are obtained at frequent intervals in children receiving particular antiepileptic medications that can affect organ function.

If complete seizure control is maintained on an anticonvulsant drug for 2 years, it is safe to discontinue the drug for patients with no risk factors. Risk factors include children older than 12 years of age at onset, history of neonatal seizures, numerous seizures before control is achieved, and the presence of a neurologic dysfunction (e.g., motor or cognitive impairment). Up to 40% of children whose medications are discontinued will experience seizure recurrence. Recurrence occurs most frequently within 6 months of discontinuation (Sillanpää and Schmidt, 2006).

When seizure medications are discontinued, the dosage is decreased gradually over several weeks. Sudden withdrawal of a drug is not recommended because it can cause an increase in the number and severity of seizures.

> ### 💊 DRUG ALERT
>
> Fosphenytoin is often used to treat seizures instead of IV phenytoin because of possible complications and drug interactions associated with IV phenytoin. If IV phenytoin is used, it should be administered via slow IV push at a rate that does not exceed 50 mg/min. Because phenytoin precipitates when mixed with glucose, only normal saline is used to flush the tubing or catheter. Fosphenytoin may be given in saline or glucose solutions at a rate of up to 150 mg PE (phenytoin equivalent)/min, and it may be given intramuscularly if necessary.

Ketogenic Diet

The ketogenic diet is a high-fat, low-carbohydrate, and adequate protein diet (Freeman, Kossoff, and Hartman, 2007). Consumption of such a diet forces the body to shift from using glucose as the primary energy source to using fat, and the individual develops a state of ketosis. The diet is rigorous. All foods and liquids the child consumes must be carefully weighed and measured. The diet is deficient in vitamins and minerals; therefore, vitamin supplements are necessary. Early side effects of the diet are diarrhea, hypoglycemia, dehydration, acidosis, and lethargy, and long-term side effects include dyslipidemia, kidney stones, and poor growth (Freeman, Kossoff, and Hartman, 2007).

The ketogenic diet has been shown to be an efficacious and tolerable treatment for medically refractory seizures (Freeman, Kossoff, and Hartman, 2007). Studies have shown that as many as 56% of children on the diet had greater than a 50% reduction in seizure episodes (Hartman and Vining, 2007).

Vagus Nerve Stimulation

Vagus nerve stimulation uses an implantable device that reduces seizures in individuals who have not had effective control with drug therapy. It is currently indicated as adjunct therapy in patients 12 years and older with partial-onset seizures (with or without secondary generalization) who are refractory to antiepileptic drugs (Elliott, Rodgers, Bassani, and others, 2011). A programmable signal generator is implanted subcutaneously in the chest. Electrodes tunneled underneath the skin deliver electrical impulses to the left vagus nerve (cranial nerve X). The device is programmed noninvasively to deliver a precise pattern of stimulation to the left vagus nerve. The patient or caregiver can activate the device using a magnet at the onset of a seizure. No long-term adverse effects have been reported with VNS, but dysphonia, throat or neck pain, and cough can occur during stimulation.

Studies show that about one third to one half of patients have a reduction in seizures after 1 year of therapy (Elliott, Rodgers, Bassani, and others, 2011).

Surgical Therapy

When seizures are determined to be caused by a hematoma, tumor, or other cerebral lesion, surgical removal is the treatment. In children with epilepsy, surgery is reserved for those who have incapacitating, refractory seizures. Refractory seizures are usually defined as the persistence of seizures despite adequate trials of three antiepileptic medications, alone or in combination (Mikati, 2011). An extensive medical (e.g., invasive EEG monitoring), psychosocial, and psychoneurologic evaluation is required before surgery. There are several types of surgical interventions. Focal resection entails removal of the epileptogenic zone, and hemispherectomy involves removing all or most of one hemisphere in patients with catastrophic hemispheric epilepsy (Mikati, 2011). Corpus callosotomy consists of the separation of the connections between the two hemispheres in the brain to prevent seizure activity by blocking epileptic discharges (Spencer and Huh, 2008). Patients undergoing surgical resection can experience a decrease in the frequency and severity of seizures, a decrease in antiepileptic medication requirements, and an improvement in their quality of life (Spencer and Huh, 2008).

Status Epilepticus

Status epilepticus is a continuous seizure that lasts more than 30 minutes or a series of seizures from which the child does not regain a premorbid LOC (Huff and Fountain, 2011). It has been suggested that the term *impending status epilepticus* be used for a continuous or series of seizures lasting between 5 and 30 minutes (Mikati, 2011). The initial treatment is directed toward support and maintenance of vital functions, that is, the ABCs of life support, administering oxygen, and gaining IV access, immediately followed by IV administration of antiepileptic agents.

> **💊 DRUG ALERT**
>
> Buccal midazolam and rectal diazepam are quick, effective, and safe treatments for home or prehospital treatment of status epilepticus (Shorvon, 2011). Cessation of seizure occurred in 8 minutes with buccal midazolam and 15 minutes with rectal diazepam (Shorvon, 2011). Respiratory depression is a potential side effect of both medications, and patients should be monitored closely after administration (Mikati, 2011).

For in-hospital management of status epilepticus, IV diazepam or lorazepam (Ativan) is the first-line drug of choice (Mikati, 2011). Lorazepam is the preferred agent because of its rapid onset (2–5 minutes) and long half-life (12–24 hours). The child must be closely monitored during administration to detect early alterations in vital signs that may indicate impending respiratory depression. When a benzodiazepine (diazepam or lorazepam) is ineffective, fosphenytoin followed by phenobarbital is given as the next line of treatment. This combination of therapy places the child at high risk for apnea; therefore, respiratory support is generally necessary. Children may also receive an antiepileptic medication, intravenous valproate, which does not cause respiratory compromise (Mikati, 2011). Children who continue to have seizures despite this drug treatment may require general anesthesia with a continuous infusion of midazolam, propofol, or pentobarbital (Shorvon, 2011). In this situation, the patient may need to be intubated and continuous EEG monitoring is typically done to monitor for and treat electrographic seizures (Friedman and Ghazala, 2006).

> **💊 DRUG ALERT**
>
> Diazepam is incompatible with many drugs. To give it intravenously, inject it slowly and directly into the vein or through tubing as close as possible to the vein insertion site.

Nursing care of a child with status epilepticus includes, in addition to the ABCs of life support, monitoring blood pressure and body temperature. During the first 30 to 45 minutes of the seizure, the blood pressure may be elevated. Thereafter, the blood pressure typically returns to normal but may be decreased depending on the medications being administered for seizure control. Hyperthermia requiring treatment may occur as a result of increased motor activity.

Prognosis

Most children who experience a second seizure will experience additional seizures with as many as 72% of children having additional seizures within 5 years after the second seizure (Berg, 2008). Therefore, a history of two seizures is sufficient to diagnose epilepsy. Epidemiologic studies using population- or community-based cohorts show that the underlying etiology of the child's epilepsy is the most important factor affecting prognosis (Nei and Bagla, 2007). Children with epilepsy and severe neurologic disorders were 22 times more likely to die than children with epilepsy and a normal neurologic status (Nei and Bagla, 2007). Mortality is also associated with the severity and frequency of the child's seizures. Mortality does not significantly increase in children who are seizure free but can be as high as 46% in patients with status epilepticus (Nei and Bagla, 2007).

> **QUALITY PATIENT OUTCOMES: Seizures**
> - Etiology of seizure determined
> - Seizures controlled or reduced in frequency and severity
> - Family and child receive education to manage seizures
> - Child adhering to treatment
> - Side effects of treatment minimized
> - No physical injury as a result of seizure activity

Nursing Care Management

An important nursing responsibility is to observe the seizure episode and accurately document the events. Any alterations in behavior preceding the seizure and the characteristics of the episode, such as sensory-hallucinatory phenomena (e.g., an aura), motor effects (e.g., eye movements, muscular contractions), alterations in consciousness, and postictal state, are noted and recorded (Box 28-8). The nurse should describe only what is observed rather than trying to label a seizure type. Note the duration of the seizure with start and stop times.

Based on a thorough assessment, several nursing diagnoses are identified. The more common diagnoses for the child with a seizure disorder are included in the Nursing Care Plan.

The child must be protected from injury during the seizure. Nursing observations made during the event provide valuable information for diagnosis and management of the disorder (see Emergency Treatment box, p. 965).

It is impossible to halt a seizure after it has begun, and no attempt should be made to do so. The nurse must remain calm, stay with the child, and prevent the child from sustaining any harm during the seizure. If possible, the child should be isolated from the view of others by closing a door or pulling screens. A seizure can be upsetting to the child, other visitors, and their families. If other persons are present, they should be assured that everything is being done for the child. After

Nursing Care Plan—The Child with a Seizure Disorder

BOX 28-8   GENERAL OBSERVATIONS: THE CHILD DURING A SEIZURE

Observations During Seizure

Describe

Order of events (before, during, and after)

Duration of seizure

- Tonic-clonic—from first signs of event until jerking stops
- Absence—from loss of consciousness until consciousness is regained
- Complex partial—from first sign of unresponsiveness, motor activity, and automatisms until there are signs of responsiveness to environment

Onset

Time of onset

Significant precipitating events—missed medication dosage, illness, stress, sleep deprivation, menses

Behavior

Change in facial expression

Cry or other sound

Stereotypic or automatous movements

Random activity (wandering)

Position of eyes, head, body, extremities

Unilateral or bilateral posturing of one or more extremities

Movement

Change of position, if any

Site of commencement—hand, thumb, mouth, generalized

Tonic phase—length, parts of body involved

Clonic phase—twitching or jerking movements, parts of body involved, sequence of parts involved, generalized, change in character of movements

Lack of movement or muscle tone of body part or entire body

Face

Color change—pallor, cyanosis, flushing

Perspiration

Mouth—position, deviating to one side, teeth clenched, tongue bitten, frothing at mouth, flecks of blood or bleeding

Lack of expression

Asymmetric expression

Eyes

Position—straight ahead, deviation upward or outward, conjugate or divergent gaze

Pupils—change in size, equality, reaction to light

Respiratory Effort

Presence and length of apnea

Other

Incontinence

Postictal Observations

Duration of postictal period

State of consciousness

Orientation

Arousability

Motor ability

- Any change in motor function
- Ability to move all extremities
- Paresis or weakness

Speech

Sensations

- Complaint of discomfort or pain
- Any sensory impairment
- Recollection of preseizure sensations or aura

---

the seizure, they can be given a simple explanation about the event as needed.

If the nurse is able to reach the child in time, a child who is standing or seated in a chair (including a wheelchair) is eased to the floor immediately. During (and sometimes after) the tonic-clonic seizure, the swallowing reflex is lost, salivation increases, and the tongue is hypotonic. Therefore, the child is at risk for aspiration and airway occlusion. Placing the child on the side facilitates drainage and helps maintain a patent airway. Suctioning the oral cavity and posterior oropharynx may be necessary. Take vital signs and allow the child to rest if at school or away from home. When feasible, the child is integrated into the environment as soon as possible. Sending a child with a chronic seizure disorder home from school is not necessary unless requested by the parents.

Seizure precautions are required for children who are known to have seizures or who are under observation for seizures. The extent of these measures depends on the type and frequency of the seizure (Box 28-9).

! NURSING ALERT

Do not move or forcefully restrain the child during a tonic-clonic seizure and do not place a solid object between the teeth.

Long-Term Care

Care of the child with a recurrent seizure disorder involves physical care and instruction regarding the importance of the drug therapy and, probably more significant, the problems related to the emotional aspects of the disorder. Few diseases generate as much anxiety among relatives as epilepsy. Fears and misconceptions about the disease and its treatment are common. For many, it represents the archetype of severe hereditary affliction. Nursing care is directed toward educating the child and family about epilepsy and helping them develop strategies to cope with the psychologic and sociologic problems related to epilepsy.

Children with epilepsy are prescribed antiepileptic medications. These medications are administered at regular intervals to maintain adequate levels in the blood. The nurse can help the parents plan the administration of the medication at convenient times to avoid disruptions of family routines as much as possible. It is important to impress on the family the necessity of giving the antiepileptic medication regularly and for as long as required. In general, antiepileptic medications are continued until the child has been seizure free for 2 years (Johnston and Smith, 2007). The medication is then slowly tapered over a period of weeks to avoid the possibility of precipitating a seizure. It is sometimes easy to skip doses or omit them for a variety of reasons, especially when the child is free of seizures most of the time. This is particularly

NURSING CARE PLAN

The Child with Seizures

NURSING DIAGNOSIS	PATIENT OUTCOMES	NURSING INTERVENTIONS	RATIONALE
Risk for Injury related to CNS dysfunction and inability to control self (motor) secondary to type of seizure	Child will not experience physical injury as a result of seizure activity.	Administer AEDs.	To prevent seizure activity
		Teach family and child, as appropriate, the purpose of AEDs, expected response and action, potential side effects, timing, dosage, route of administration, and how to monitor effects.	To promote understanding of chronic condition
Child's Defining Characteristics <u>(Subjective and Objective Data)</u>	**The Following NOC Concepts Apply to This Outcome**		To prevent seizure activity and encourage self-care
Change in LOC	Risk Control	Monitor for side effects of AEDs and therapeutic levels according to child's growth, illness factors that affect metabolism, and effects of drug.	To prevent secondary effects of AEDs and to prevent seizures from occurring because of subtherapeutic drug levels
Disorientation	Safety Behavior: Personal		
Clonic movements	Safety Behavior: Home Physical Environment	Stress importance of adherence to medication regimen even if child has no evidence of seizure activity.	To prevent seizure activity
Automatisms	Safety Status: Falls Occurrence	Teach patient and family to identify and avoid situations that are known to precipitate a seizure (e.g., blinking lights, sleep deprivation, excess activity or exercise, physical factors).	To prevent seizure activity
Aura			
Postictal impairment (dependent on the type of seizure)		Initiate seizure precautions in the hospital:	To prevent physical harm
		• Pad side rails of bed, crib, or wheelchair.	
		• Keep bed relatively free of objects.	
		• Set up suction and oxygen in room.	
		Educate family to initiate seizure precautions at home:	To prevent physical harm
		• Bathroom safety includes taking showers instead of baths to prevent drowning. Use shower seat if falls occur during typical seizure. Leave bathroom door unlocked.	
		• Kitchen safety includes cooking when someone else is nearby, using back burners of the stove to prevent accidental burns, and using shatterproof containers as much as possible.	
		• Sports safety includes wearing protective equipment, having others nearby, not climbing higher than 10 feet without special equipment.	
		Teach family seizure first aid:	To prepare the family for emergencies
		• If child is at risk of falling at beginning of episode, ease child to floor.	
		• Loosen tight or restrictive clothing.	
		• Turn the child to side-lying position.	
		• Prevent child from hitting head on objects.	
		• Time the seizure.	
		• Allow seizure to end spontaneously.	
		• Reassure the child when awakening from seizure.	
		• Do not put anything in child's mouth.	
		• Do not attempt to restrain child or use force.	
		• Call EMS (see Emergency Treatment box, p. 965) if seizure persists more than 5 minutes, for repeated seizures, or if the child does not wake up after the movements have stopped.	
		Counsel women of childbearing age about contraception and birth defects associated with AEDs.	To prevent birth defects
		The Following NIC Concepts Apply to These Interventions	
		Area Restriction	
		Surveillance Safety	
		Environmental Management: Safety	
		Medication Administration	
		Teaching: Medication Administration	
		Emergency Care	
		Oxygen Administration	
		Seizure Precautions	

Continued

⊚ NURSING CARE PLAN

The Child with Seizures—cont'd

NURSING DIAGNOSIS	PATIENT OUTCOMES	NURSING INTERVENTIONS	RATIONALE
Risk for Aspiration, and Ineffective Breathing Pattern, related to impaired motor activity, LOC, and loss of airway protection (tonic-clonic seizure) **Child's Defining Characteristics** <u>(Subjective and Objective Data)</u> Decreased LOC Depressed cough reflex Apnea Decreased inspiratory pressure	Child's airway will remain patent. Child will have effective ventilation. **The Following NOC Concepts Apply to These Outcomes** Aspiration Control Respiratory Status: Airway Patency Respiratory Status: Ventilation	In the event of a seizure, place child in a side-lying position on a flat surface such as floor or bed. Remain with patient. Remove secretions, food, and liquids from mouth when seizure subsides. In postictal state, monitor oxygenation status. Administer oxygen as necessary. Administer rescue breaths if spontaneous respirations do not resume shortly after seizure subsides. Administer medications intended to stop seizure longer than 5 minutes (rectal diazepam, IV Dilantin, IV lorazepam) **The Following NIC Concepts Apply to These Interventions** Risk Identification Aspiration Control Oxygen Administration Medication Administration	To prevent aspiration and choking To protect the airway To prevent aspiration To determine the need for oxygen To prevent hypoxia To prevent hypoxia To prevent continued seizure activity
Anxiety/Fear, Parent, related to child having life-threatening and incapacitating seizure activity* **Child's or Family's Defining Characteristics** <u>(Subjective and Objective Data)</u> Anguish Fear Feelings of inadequacy and hopelessness Worry, apprehension Report of apprehension Panic Excitement	Parent will cope with child's condition and receive adequate support. **The Following NOC Concepts Apply to This Outcome** Anxiety Control Coping Fear Control	Allow parent to remain with child during seizure. Instruct parent on proper protection interventions during child's seizure activity, including positioning, safety, airway maintenance, reassurance techniques, and emergency medication administration. Provide information regarding nature (type) of seizure, therapeutic interventions, and lifestyle modifications. Encourage family involvement in daily care of child with goal of normalization and promotion of optimum growth and development. Involve parents in discussion of fears, anxieties, and resources and support options available to family. **The Following NIC Concepts Apply to These Interventions** Support Group Coping Enhancement Anxiety Reduction Family Process Maintenance Active Listening Counseling Decision-Making Support Family Involvement Promotion	To decrease fear of unknown and allow parent to see measures taken to protect child To promote parent participation and to foster sense of control over situation To promote knowledge of condition, parental intervention, and sense of control To provide hope To promote family functioning and coping

AED, Antiepileptic drug; *CNS*, central nervous system; *EMS*, emergency medical services; *IV*, intravenous; *LOC*, level of consciousness; *NIC*, Nursing Interventions Classification; *NOC*, Nursing Outcomes Classification.

*Nursing diagnosis may also apply to child in the postictal phase, depending on the type of seizure and the child's understanding and cognition level.

✚ EMERGENCY TREATMENT

Seizures

Tonic-Clonic Seizure

During the Seizure

Remain calm.

Time seizure episode.

If child is standing or seated, ease child down to the floor.

Place pillow or folded blanket under child's head.

Loosen restrictive clothing.

Remove eyeglasses.

Clear area of any hazards or hard objects.

Allow seizure to end without interference.

If vomiting occurs, turn child to one side.

Do not:
- Attempt to restrain child or use force
- Put anything in child's mouth
- Give any food or liquids

After the Seizure

Time postictal period.

Check for breathing. Check position of head and tongue.

Reposition if head is hyperextended. If child is not breathing, give rescue breathing and call EMS.

Keep child on side.

Remain with child.

Do not give food or liquids until child is fully alert and swallowing reflex has returned.

Call EMS when necessary.

Look for medical identification and determine what factors occurred before onset of seizure that may have been triggering factors.

Check head and body for possible injuries.

Check inside of mouth to see if tongue or lips have been bitten.

Complex Partial Seizure

During the Seizure

Do not restrain.

Remove harmful objects from area.

Redirect to safe area.

Do not agitate; instead, talk in calm, reassuring manner.

Do not expect child to follow instructions.

Watch to see if seizure generalizes.

After the Seizure

Stay with child and reassure until fully conscious.

Call Emergency Medical Services If

Child stops breathing.

There is evidence of injury or child is diabetic or pregnant.

Seizure lasts for more than 5 minutes (unless duration of seizure is typically longer than 5 minutes) and written medical order is present.

Status epilepticus occurs.

Pupils are not equal after seizure.

Child vomits continuously 30 minutes after seizure has ended (sign of possible acute problem).

Child cannot be awakened and is unresponsive to pain after seizure has ended.

Seizure occurs in water.

This is child's first seizure.

Modified from *Seizure recognition and first aid*, 2001, Epilepsy Foundation, retrieved March 5, 2007, from http://www.epilepsyfoundation.org. *EMS,* Emergency medical services.

BOX 28-9   SEIZURE PRECAUTIONS

The extent of precautions depends on type, severity, and frequency of seizures. They may include:
- Side rails raised when child is sleeping or resting
- Side rails and other hard objects padded
- Waterproof mattress or pad on bed or crib

Appropriate precautions during potentially hazardous activities may include:
- Swimming with a companion
- Showers preferred; bathing only with close supervision
- Use of protective helmet and padding during bicycle riding, skateboarding, in-line skating
- Supervision during use of hazardous machinery or equipment

Have child carry or wear medical identification.

Alert other caregivers to need for any special precautions.

Child may not drive or operate hazardous machinery or equipment unless seizure free for designated period (varies by state).

---

repeated vomiting, gastrointestinal surgery, or status epilepticus. Parents can learn to administer rectal antiepileptic medication for home treatment. Buccal midazolam or rectal diazepam is a useful adjunctive home treatment for children at risk for prolonged seizures or clusters of seizures and can minimize the need for hospitalization while enhancing parental confidence.

💊 DRUG ALERT

Children taking phenobarbital or phenytoin should receive adequate vitamin D and folic acid because deficiencies of both have been associated with these drugs. Phenytoin should not be taken with milk.

Nurses should educate the child and parents about the possible adverse reactions to the medications used to treat seizures. Parents should understand the common side effects and be encouraged to report their observations to their health care provider. Parents should understand that the child needs periodic physical assessment and laboratory studies. Possible adverse effects on the hematopoietic system, liver, and kidneys may be reflected in symptoms such as fever, sore throat, enlarged lymph nodes, jaundice, and bleeding (e.g., easy bruising, petechiae, ecchymoses, epistaxis). A common factor in status epilepticus is inadequate blood levels of antiepileptic drugs.

Although children with epilepsy are at increased risk for injury, few limitations should be placed on activities. The degree to which activities are restricted is individualized for each child and depends on the

---

so when the child is older and assumes responsibility for his or her medication. The seizure threshold may be lowered during any illness but particularly with fever. Therefore, parents should be aware that if their child has an illness, he or she is at increased risk for seizures. Parents should contact their health professional if their child misses medications during an illness because of vomiting.

Rectal preparations of some antiepileptic medications are highly effective when a child is unable to take oral medications because of

type, frequency, and severity of the seizures; the child's response to therapy; and the length of time the seizures have been controlled. To prevent head injuries, children should always wear appropriate safety devices, such as helmets, and should avoid activities involving heights. Although bike riding is safe for most children, children with frequent seizures and impairment of consciousness should avoid it. Skating, in-line skating, and skateboarding should be restricted only in children with frequent seizures. Helmets must be worn while participating in these activities.

Children with epilepsy are at higher risk for submersion injury than children without epilepsy. Young children should never be left alone in the bathtub, even for a few seconds. Older children and adolescents should be encouraged to use a shower and reminded not to lock the bathroom door when showering. They should never swim unsupervised.

Because the child is encouraged to attend school, camp, and other normal activities, the school nurse and teachers should be made aware of the child's condition and therapy. They can help ensure regularity of medication administration and provision of any special care the child might need. Teachers, child care providers, camp counselors, youth organization leaders, coaches, and other adults who assume responsibility for children should be instructed regarding care of the child during a seizure so they can act calmly for the child's welfare and influence the attitude of the child's peers.

Triggering Factors

Careful and detailed documentation of seizures over time may indicate a pattern of seizures. In the general population, as many as 90% of individuals with epilepsy can recognize at least one trigger for their seizures (Haut and Lipton, 2009). When this occurs, the child, nurse, or responsible adult can intervene to make changes in the lifestyle or environment that may prevent seizures or decrease their frequency. Often the necessary changes are simple but can make an enormous difference in the lives of the child and family.

The most common factors that may trigger seizures in children include emotional stress, sleep deprivation, fatigue, fever, and illness (Nakken, Solaas, Kjeldsen, and others, 2005). Other precipitating factors include flickering lights, menstrual cycle, and alcohol (Haut and Lipton, 2009). Some individuals have pattern- or photo-sensitive epilepsy, that is, seizures precipitated by changes in dark–light patterns, such as those that occur with a flash on a camera, automobile headlights, reflections of light on snow or water, or rotating blades on a fan. Most of these individuals have absence, myoclonic, or generalized tonic-clonic seizures. Some children have seizures while playing video games. Although the actual incidence of video game–induced epilepsy is unknown, it most commonly affects children between the ages of 9 and 15 years (Shoja, Tubbs, Malekian, and others, 2007). These children are sensitive to intermittent photic stimulation, usually more than 3 flashes per second, that can trigger an epileptic episode (Shoja, Tubbs, Malekian, and others, 2007). The prognosis for pattern- or photo-epilepsy is good. Prevention techniques such as keeping a distance greater than 2 m from the television or computer screen, using a smaller screen, and taking frequent breaks can reduce the incidence (Shoja, Tubbs, Malekian, and others, 2007).

FEBRILE SEIZURES

Febrile seizures are one of the most common neurologic conditions of childhood, affecting approximately 2% to 5% of children between the ages of 6 and 60 months (Steering Committee on Quality Improvement and Management, Subcommittee on Febrile Seizures AAP, 2008).

Febrile seizures are classified as simple or complex. Simple febrile seizures occur in children between the ages of 6 months and 5 years with no preexisting neurologic abnormality and consist of a general tonic-clonic seizure that occurs with a fever (>38.0° C) and resolves within 15 minutes with a return to alert mental status after the seizure and no further seizure occurring within a 24-hour period (Hampers and Spina, 2011). On the other hand, complex febrile seizures can occur in children of any age usually with a previous neurologic impairment and consist of a prolonged seizure lasting more than 15 minutes that can reoccur within 24 hours and can result in neurologic deficits after the seizure (Fetveit, 2008). Most febrile seizures occur between 6 months and 5 years of age, with the peak incidence occurring at 18 months of age (Østergaard, 2009).

The cause of febrile seizures is still uncertain. Risk factors for simple febrile seizures include viral infections and a family history of febrile seizures (Fetveit, 2008). Associations with chromosomal mutations, premature birth, and developmental delay have been evaluated but have not demonstrated any conclusive evidence (Fetveit, 2008). Most febrile seizures have stopped by the time the child is taken to a medical facility and require no treatment. However, if the seizure continues, treatment consists of controlling the seizure with IV or rectal diazepam and reducing the temperature with acetaminophen or ibuprofen (Hampers and Spina, 2011). Antiepileptic prophylaxis is usually not indicated. Antipyretic therapy may lower the child's temperature and provide symptomatic relief but will not prevent a seizure (Steering Committee on Quality Improvement and Management, Subcommittee on Febrile Seizures AAP, 2008). Tepid sponge baths are not recommended for several reasons: they are ineffective in significantly lowering the temperature, the shivering effect further increases metabolic output, and cooling causes discomfort to the child. Parental education and emotional support are important interventions, and information may need to be repeated depending on the parents' anxiety and education level. Parents need reassurance regarding the benign nature of simple febrile seizures. Several large studies show no difference in neurologic deficits, cognitive functioning, or memory impairments in children with simple or complex febrile seizures compared with population control participants (Fetveit, 2008).

Long-term antiepileptic therapy is usually not required for children with simple febrile seizures. Whereas children with a simple febrile seizure have only a 1% risk of developing epilepsy, children with a complex febrile seizure along with a preexisting neurologic abnormality and a family history of afebrile seizure have a 10% risk of developing epilepsy (Hampers and Spina, 2011).

> **! NURSING ALERT**
>
> If a febrile seizure lasts more than 5 minutes, parents should seek medical attention right away. Parents should call for emergency assistance (911) and not place the child who is actively having a seizure in the car.

CEREBRAL MALFORMATIONS

CRANIAL DEFORMITIES

In a normal newborn, the cranial sutures are separated by membranous seams several millimeters wide. Up to 2 days after birth, the cranial bones are highly mobile, which allows them to mold and slide over one another, adjusting the circumference of the head to accommodate to the changing shape and character of the birth canal. The principal sutures in the infant's skull are the sagittal, coronal, and lambdoidal sutures, and the major soft areas at the juncture of these sutures are the anterior and posterior fontanels (see Fig. 8-6).

After birth, growth of the skull bones occurs in a direction **perpendicular** to the line of the suture, and normal closure occurs in a regular and predictable order. Although there are wide variations in the age at which closure takes place in individual children, normally all sutures and fontanels are ossified by the following ages:

Eight weeks—Posterior fontanel closed

Six months—Fibrous union of suture lines and interlocking of serrated edges

Eighteen months—Anterior fontanel closed

After 12 years—Sutures unable to be separated by increased ICP

Solid union of all sutures is not completed until late childhood. Craniosynostosis, closure of a suture before the expected time, inhibits the perpendicular growth. Because normal increase in brain volume requires expansion, the skull is forced to grow in a direction *parallel* to the fused suture. This alteration in skull growth always produces a distortion of the head shape when the underlying brain growth is normal. A small head with closed and normal shape is a result of deficient brain growth; the suture closure is secondary to this brain growth failure. Failure of brain growth is not secondary to suture closure.

Various types of cranial deformities are encountered in early infancy. These include an enlarged head with frontal protrusion (**bossing**; characteristic of hydrocephalus), parietal bossing that is seen in chronic subdural hematoma, a small head, and a variety of skull deformities. Some occur during prenatal development; in others, head circumference is usually within normal limits at birth, and the deviation from normal development becomes apparent with advancing age.

Prognosis

The majority of infants with craniosynostosis have normal brain development. The exceptions are those with genetic disorders that involve brain pathologic conditions.

Nursing Care Management

Nursing care of families in which there is a child with a cranial defect involves identifying children with deformities and referring them for evaluation. Because no therapy is available for children with microcephaly, nursing care is directed toward helping parents adjust to caring for a child with brain damage (see Chapter 19).

Infants who benefit from surgery require special emphasis on observation for signs of anemia because of the large blood loss during surgery (see Family-Centered Care box). Nursing care includes observation for signs of hemorrhage, infection, pain, and swelling, as well as parental education for suture care and safety. Surgical sutures should remain dry and intact. Parents need to observe for any signs of redness, drainage, or swelling and report any temperature greater than 38.4° C (101° F).

🏠 FAMILY-CENTERED CARE
Blood Donation

Parents may wish to provide a compatible blood donor for their infant undergoing a planned surgical correction for craniosynostosis. Nurses need to inform and guide parents through the blood bank procedure.

Early surgical management of craniosynostosis in children ages 3 to 9 months allows proper expansion of the brain and the creation of an acceptable appearance (Ursitti, Fadda, Papetti, and others, 2011). Parents require special support and education during this time, especially from the health care team.

HYDROCEPHALUS

Hydrocephalus is a condition caused by an imbalance in the production and absorption of CSF in the ventricular system. When production is greater than absorption, CSF accumulates within the ventricular system, usually under increased pressure, producing passive dilation of the ventricles.

Pathophysiology

The causes of hydrocephalus are varied, but the result is either (1) impaired absorption of CSF fluid within the subarachnoid space, obliteration of the subarachnoid cisterns, or malfunction of the arachnoid villi (**nonobstructive** or **communicating hydrocephalus**) or (2) obstruction to the flow of CSF through the ventricular system (**obstructive** or **noncommunicating hydrocephalus**) (Kinsman and Johnston, 2011). Any imbalance of secretion and absorption causes an increased accumulation of CSF in the ventricles, which become dilated (ventriculomegaly) and compress the brain substance against the surrounding rigid bony cranium. When this occurs before fusion of the cranial sutures, it causes enlargement of the skull and dilation of the ventricles (Fig. 28-7). In children younger than 10 to 12 years

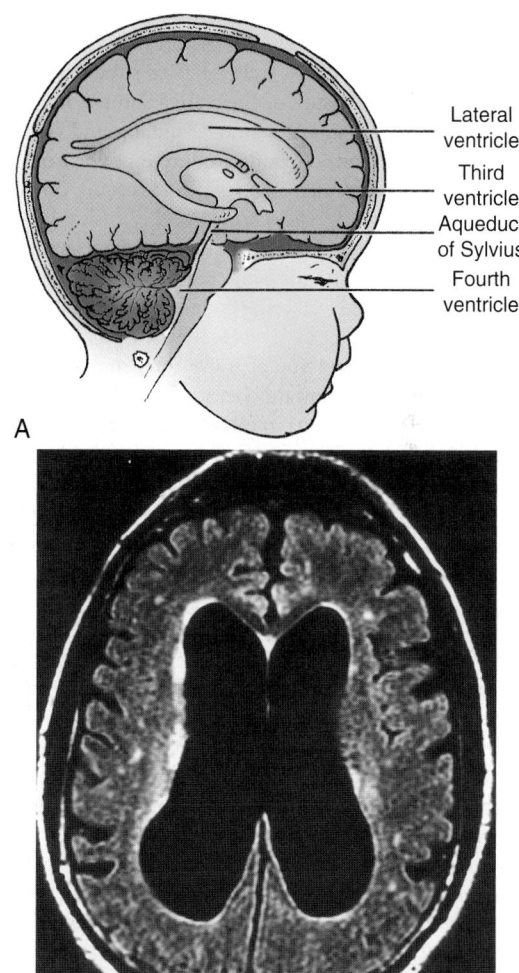

Lateral ventricle

Third ventricle

Aqueduct of Sylvius

Fourth ventricle

A

B

FIG 28-7 Hydrocephalus: a block in flow of cerebrospinal fluid (CSF). **A,** Patent CSF circulation. **B,** Normal-pressure hydrocephalus. (**B,** From Grossman RI, Yousem DM: *Neuroradiology: the requisites,* ed 3, St. Louis, 2010, Mosby.)

of age, partially closed suture lines, especially the sagittal suture, may become diastatic or opened. After 12 years of age, the sutures are fused and will not open.

Most cases of noncommunicating hydrocephalus are a result of developmental malformations. Although the defect usually is apparent in early infancy, it may become evident at any time from the prenatal period to late childhood or early adulthood. Other causes include neoplasms, infections, and trauma. An obstruction to the normal flow can occur at any point in the CSF pathway to produce increased pressure and dilation of the pathways proximal to the site of obstruction.

Developmental defects (e.g., Arnold-Chiari malformations, aqueduct stenosis, aqueduct gliosis, and atresia of the foramina of Luschka and Magendie [Dandy-Walker syndrome]) account for most cases of hydrocephalus from birth to 2 years of age. Hydrocephalus is so often associated with myelomeningocele that all such infants should be observed for its development. In the remainder of cases, there is a history of intrauterine infection, hemorrhage, and neonatal meningoencephalitis. In older children, hydrocephalus is most often a result of intracranial masses, intracranial infections, hemorrhage, preexisting developmental defects (e.g., aqueduct stenosis, Arnold-Chiari malformation), or trauma.

Clinical Manifestations

The factors that influence the clinical picture in hydrocephalus are the time of onset, acuity of onset, and associated structural malformations. In infancy, before closure of the cranial sutures, head enlargement is the predominant sign, but in older infants and children, the lesions responsible for hydrocephalus produce other neurologic signs through pressure on adjacent structures before causing CSF obstruction (Box 28-10).

In infants with hydrocephalus, the head grows at an abnormal rate; fontanels are bulging and nonpulsatile; scalp veins are dilated, especially when the infant cries; and skull bones are thin with separated sutures, causing a cracked-pot sound (Macewen sign) when palpated. In severe cases, infants display frontal protrusion (frontal bossing), eyes depressed and rotated downward (setting-sun sign), and sluggish pupils. The signs and symptoms in early to late childhood are caused by increased ICP, and specific manifestations are related to the focal lesion. Most commonly resulting from posterior fossa neoplasms and aqueduct stenosis, the clinical manifestations are primarily those associated with space-occupying lesions (e.g., headaches on awakening with improvement after emesis or being in an upright position, strabismus, ataxia).

Diagnostic Evaluation

Hydrocephalus in infants is based on head circumference that crosses at least one percentile line on the head measurement chart within 2 to 4 weeks. In evaluation of a preterm infant, specially adapted head circumference charts are consulted to distinguish abnormal head growth from normal rapid head growth. The primary diagnostic tools to detect hydrocephalus in older infants and children are CT and MRI. Diagnostic evaluation of children who have symptoms of hydrocephalus after infancy is similar to that used in those with suspected intracranial tumor. In neonates, echoencephalography is useful in comparing the ratio of lateral ventricle to cortex.

Therapeutic Management

The treatment of hydrocephalus is directed toward relief of the hydrocephalus, treatment of the cause, treatment of associated complications, and management of problems related to the effect of the disorder on psychomotor development. The treatment is, with few exceptions,

---

BOX 28-10   CLINICAL MANIFESTATIONS OF HYDROCEPHALUS

Infancy (Early)
Abnormally rapid head growth
Bulging fontanels (especially anterior) sometimes without head enlargement:
- Tense
- Nonpulsatile

Dilated scalp veins
Separated sutures
Macewen sign (cracked-pot sound on percussion)
Thinning of skull bones

Infancy (Later)
Frontal enlargement, or bossing
Depressed eyes
Setting-sun sign (sclera visible above the iris)
Pupils sluggish with unequal response to light

Infancy (General)
Irritability
Lethargy
Infant cries when picked up or rocked and quiets when allowed to lie still
Early infantile reflex acts may persist
Normally expected responses fail to appear
May display:
- Change in LOC
- Opisthotonos (often extreme)
- Lower extremity spasticity
- Vomiting

Advanced cases:
- Difficulty in sucking and feeding
- Shrill, brief, high-pitched cry
- Cardiopulmonary embarrassment

Childhood
Headache on awakening; improvement after emesis or upright posture
Papilledema
Strabismus
Extrapyramidal tract signs (e.g., ataxia)
Irritability
Lethargy
Apathy
Confusion
Incoherence
Vomiting

LOC, Level of consciousness.

---

surgical. This is accomplished by direct removal of an obstruction (e.g., a tumor) or placement of a shunt that provides primary drainage of the CSF from the ventricles to an extracranial compartment, usually the peritoneum (ventriculoperitoneal [VP] shunt) (Fig. 28-8).

Most shunt systems consist of a ventricular catheter, a flush pump, a unidirectional flow valve, and a distal catheter. In all models, the valves are designed to open at a predetermined intraventricular pressure and close when the pressure falls below that level, thus preventing backflow of secretions.

The major complications of VP shunts are malfunction and infection. All shunts are subject to mechanical difficulties, such as kinking,

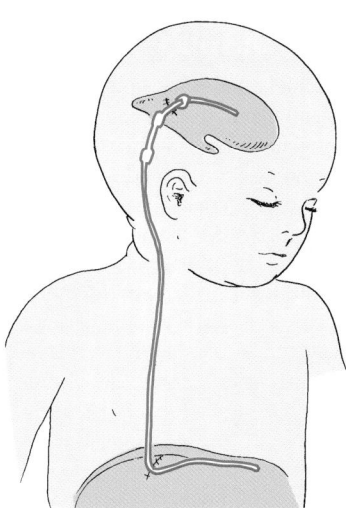

FIG 28-8 Ventriculoperitoneal shunt. The catheter is threaded beneath the skin.

plugging, or separation or migration of the tubing. Malfunction is most often caused by mechanical obstruction either within the ventricles from particulate matter (tissue or exudate) or at the distal end from thrombosis or displacement as a result of growth. Revisions are needed when signs of malfunction appear. The child with a shunt obstruction is often first seen in an emergency department with clinical manifestations of increased ICP, frequently accompanied by worsening neurologic status.

The most serious complication, shunt infection, can occur at any time, but the period of greatest risk is 1 to 2 months after placement. The infection is generally a result of intercurrent infections at the time of shunt placement. Infections include septicemia, bacterial endocarditis, wound infection, shunt nephritis, meningitis, and ventriculitis. Meningitis and ventriculitis are of greatest concern because any complicating CNS infection is a significant predictor of poor intellectual outcome. Infection is treated with antibiotics administered intravenously or intrathecally for a minimum of 7 to 10 days. A persistent infection requires removal of the shunt until the infection is controlled. External ventricular drainage (EVD) is used until CSF is sterile. The EVD allows for removal of CSF through a tube that is placed in the child's ventricle and flows by gravity into a collection device.

An alternative to shunt placement is the endoscopic third ventriculostomy in children with noncommunicating hydrocephalus. In this procedure, a small opening is made in the floor of the third ventricle that allows the CSF to flow freely through the previously blocked ventricle. Complications include CSF leak, intraventricular hemorrhage, meningitis, cranial nerve injury, obstruction, and hypothalamic injury (Hader, Walker, Myles, and others, 2008).

Prognosis

The prognosis for children with treated hydrocephalus depends largely on the rate at which hydrocephalus develops, the duration of increased ICP, the frequency of complications, and the cause of the hydrocephalus. For example, children with malignant tumors may have a high mortality rate regardless of other complicating factors.

Surgically treated hydrocephalus with continued neurosurgical and medical management has a survival rate of about 80%, with the highest incidence of mortality occurring within the first year of treatment (Paulsen, Lundar, and Lindegaard, 2010). Of the surviving children, approximately 60% were reported to have normal intellectual ability,

but only 30% had an intelligence quotient (IQ) above 90 (Gupta, Park, Solomon, and others, 2007). Although most children with a history of hydrocephalus are good-natured and friendly, some children can have aggressive or delinquent behavior and may be depressed (Gupta, Park, Solomon, and others, 2007; Kinsman and Johnson, 2011).

Nursing Care Management

An infant with diagnosed or suspected hydrocephalus is observed carefully for signs of increasing ventricular size and increasing ICP. In infants, the head is measured daily at the largest point, the occipitofrontal circumference (see Head Circumference, Chapter 6, for technique). Fontanels and suture lines are palpated for size, signs of bulging, tenseness, and separation. Irritability, lethargy, or seizure activity, as well as altered vital signs and feeding behavior, may indicate an advancing pathologic condition.

In older children, the most valuable indicators of increasing ICP are alterations in the child's LOC, headaches, and changes with environmental interactions. Changes are identified by observation and by comparison of present behavior with customary behavior, sleep patterns, developmental capabilities, and habits, obtained through a detailed history and a baseline assessment. This baseline information serves as a guide for postoperative assessment and evaluation of shunt function.

The nurse is responsible for preparing the child for diagnostic tests such as MRI or CT scan and for assisting with procedures such as a ventricular tap, which is often performed to relieve excessive pressure during the preoperative period and for CSF examination. Sedation is required because the child must remain absolutely still during diagnostic testing (see Preparation for Diagnostic and Therapeutic Procedures, Chapter 22).

> **! NURSING ALERT**
>
> If surgery is anticipated, IV lines should not be placed in a scalp vein on a child with hydrocephalus.

Postoperative Care

In addition to routine postoperative care and observation, the infant or child is positioned carefully on the unoperated side to prevent pressure on the shunt valve. The child is kept flat to avoid complications resulting from too-rapid reduction of intracranial fluid. The surgeon indicates the position to be maintained and the extent of activity allowed. Pain management can be achieved with acetaminophen with or without codeine for mild to moderate pain and opioids for severe pain (see Pain Management, Chapter 7).

Observation is continued for signs of increased ICP, which indicates obstruction of the shunt. Neurologic assessment includes evaluation of pupillary dilation (pressure causes compression or stretching of the oculomotor nerve, producing dilation on the same side as the pressure) and blood pressure (hypoxia to the brainstem causes variability in these vital signs). If there is increased ICP, the surgeon will prescribe elevation of the head of the bed and allow the child to sit up to enhance gravity flow through the shunt.

> **! NURSING ALERT**
>
> Arbitrary pumping of the shunt may cause obstruction or other problems and should not be performed unless indicated by a neurosurgeon.

Because infection is the greatest hazard of the postoperative period, nurses are continually on the alert for the usual manifestations of CSF infection, such as elevated temperature, poor feeding, vomiting, decreased responsiveness, and seizure activity. There may be signs of local inflammation at the operative sites and along the shunt tract. The child is also observed for abdominal distention because CSF may cause peritonitis or a postoperative ileus as a complication of distal catheter placement. Antibiotics are administered by the IV route as ordered, and the nurse may also need to assist with intraventricular instillation. The incision site is inspected for leakage, and any suspected drainage is tested for glucose, an indication of CSF.

Family Support

Specific needs and concerns of parents during periods of hospitalization are related to the reason for the child's hospitalization (shunt revision, infection, diagnosis) and the diagnostic and surgical procedures to which the child is subjected. Parents may have little understanding of anatomy; therefore, they need further exploration and reinforcement of information that was given to them by the physician and neurosurgeon, including information about what to expect. They are especially frightened of any procedure that involves the brain, and the fear of intellectual disability or brain damage is real and pervasive. Nurses can calm their anxiety with explanations of the rationale underlying the various nursing and medical activities, such as positioning or testing, and by simply being available and willing to listen to their concerns.

To prepare for the child's discharge and home care, the parents are instructed on how to recognize signs that indicate shunt malfunction or infection. Active children may have injuries, such as a fall, that can damage the shunt, and the tubing may pull out of the distal insertion site or become disconnected during normal growth. Contact sports should be avoided, and a helmet should be worn when outside play is vigorous.

The management of hydrocephalus in a child is a demanding task for both family and health professionals, and helping a family cope with the child's difficulties is an important nursing responsibility. Children with hydrocephalus have lifelong special health care needs and require evaluation on a regular basis. The overall aim is to establish realistic goals and an appropriate educational program that will help the child to achieve his or her optimal potential.

Families can be referred to community agencies for support and guidance. The National Hydrocephalus Foundation* and the Hydrocephalus Association† provide information on the condition for families and assist interested groups in establishing local organizations.

---

*12413 Centralia Road, Lakewood, CA 90715-1653; 562-924-6666, 888-857-3434; http://www.nhfonline.org.
†870 Market St., Suite 705, San Francisco, CA 94102; 415-732-7040, 888-598-3789; http://www.hydroassoc.org.

▌ KEY POINTS

- LOC is the most important indicator of neurologic health; altered levels include full consciousness, confusion, disorientation, lethargy, obtundation, stupor, coma, and a persistent vegetative state.
- Complete neurologic examination includes LOC; posture; motor, sensory, cranial nerve, and reflex testing; and vital signs.
- Nursing care of the unconscious child focuses on ensuring respiratory management; performing neurologic assessment; monitoring ICP; supplying adequate nutrition and hydration; providing drug therapy; promoting elimination, hygienic care, proper positioning, exercise, and stimulation; and providing family support.
- Fractures resulting from head injuries may be classified as linear, depressed, comminuted, basilar, open, and growing fractures.
- Primary head injury involves features that occur at the time of trauma, including fractured skull, contusions, intracranial hematoma, and diffuse injury. Secondary complications include hypoxic brain damage, increased ICP, infection, cerebral edema, and post-traumatic syndromes.
- The young child's response to head injury is different because of the following features: larger head size, expandable skull, larger blood volume to the brain, and small subdural spaces.
- Problems resulting from submersion injury include hypoxia, asphyxiation, aspiration, and hypothermia.
- Nursing care of the child with a brain tumor includes observing for signs and symptoms related to the tumor, preparing the child and family for diagnostic tests and operative procedures, preventing postoperative complications, planning for discharge, and promoting a return to optimal health.
- Nursing care of the child with meningitis includes administering antibiotics, taking isolation precautions, removing environmental

stimuli, ensuring correct positioning, monitoring vital signs, administering IV therapy, promoting adequate fluid and nutritional status, and providing supportive care to the family.
- Routine immunization of infants with Hib and pneumococcal conjugate vaccines has reduced the incidence of bacterial meningitis.
- Encephalitis may result from direct invasion of the CNS by a virus or from involvement of the CNS after viral disease.
- A seizure is a symptom of an underlying pathologic condition and may be manifested by sensory-hallucinatory phenomena, motor effects, sensorimotor effects, or loss of consciousness.
- Partial seizures are categorized as simple (without associated impairment of consciousness) or complex (with impaired consciousness); both types may become generalized.
- Generalized seizures are categorized as tonic, clonic, tonic-clonic, absence, atonic, and myoclonic.
- Long-term care of a child with recurrent seizure disorders includes physical care and education regarding the importance of drug therapy and problems related to emotional aspects of the disorder.
- Febrile seizures are the most common type of childhood seizure.
- Many cranial deformities are amenable to surgical correction.
- Hydrocephalus is a symptom of underlying brain pathologic condition demonstrated by impaired absorption of CSF or obstruction to the flow of CSF within the ventricles.
- Therapy for hydrocephalus involves relief of the hydrocephalus, treatment of the underlying brain disorder if possible, prevention or treatment of complications, and management of problems related to development.

REFERENCES

Abbasi M, Mohammadi E, Rezayi S: Effect of a regular family visiting program as an affective, auditory, and tactile stimulation on the consciousness level of comatose patients with a head injury, *Jpn J Nurs Sci* 6:21–26, 2009.

Ashwal S, Serna-Fonseca T: Brain deaths in infants and children, *Crit Care Nurse* 26(2):117–128, 2006.

Badjatia N: Hyperthermia and fever control in brain injury, *Crit Care Med* 37(7 suppl): S250–S255, 2009.

Berg AT: Risk of recurrence after a first unprovoked seizure, *Epilepsia* 49(suppl 1): 13–18, 2008.

Blaney SM, Haas-Kogan D, Young Poussaint T, and others: Gliomas, ependymomas, and other nonembryonal tumors of the central nervous system. In Pizzo PA, Poplack DG, editors: *Principles and practice of pediatric oncology*, ed 6, Philadelphia, 2011, Lippincott Williams & Wilkins.

Blanton JD, Palmer D, Rupprecht CE: Rabies surveillance in the United States during 2009, *J Am Vet Med Assoc* 237(6):646–657, 2010.

Blinman TA, Houseknecht E, Snyder C, and others: Postconcussive symptoms in hospitalized pediatric patients after mild traumatic brain injury, *J Pediatr Surg* 44:1223–1228, 2009.

Bonnier C, Marique P, Van Hout A, and other: Neurodevelopmental outcome after severe traumatic brain injury in very young children, *J Child Neurol* 22:519–529, 2007.

Boran BO, Boran P, Barut N, and others: Evaluation of mild head injury in a pediatric population, *Pediatr Neurosurg* 42:203–207, 2006.

Brodeur GM, Hogarty MD, Mosse YP, and other: Neuroblastoma. In Pizzo PA, Poplack DG, editors: *Principles and practice of pediatric oncology*, ed 6, Philadelphia, 2011, Lippincott Williams & Wilkins.

Carey RG, Balistreri WF: Mitochondrial hepatopathies. In Kliegman RM, Stanton BF, St. Geme JW, and others, editors: *Nelson textbook of pediatrics*, ed 19, Philadelphia, 2011, Elsevier/Saunders.

Case ME: Accidental traumatic head injury in infants and young children, *Brain Pathol* 18:583–589, 2008.

Chandran A, Herbert H, Misurski D, and other: Long-term sequelae of childhood bacterial meningitis: an underappreciated problem, *Pediatr Infect Dis J* 30(1):3–6, 2011.

Christie RJ: Therapeutic positioning of the multiply-injured trauma patient in ICU, *Br J Nurs* 17(10):638–642, 2008.

Curatolo P, Moavero R, Lo Castro A, and other: Pharmacotherapy of idiopathic generalized epilepsies, *Expert Opin Pharmacother* 10(1): 5–17, 2009.

Elliott RE, Rodgers SD, Bassani L, and others: Vagus nerve stimulation for children with treatment resistant epilepsy, *J Neurosurg Pediatr* 7:491–500, 2011.

Erlichman DB, Blumfield E, Rajpathak S, and other: Association between linear skull fractures and intracranial hemorrhage in children with minor head trauma, *Pediatr Radiol* 40:1375–1379, 2010.

Faul M, Xu L, Wald MM, and other: *Traumatic brain injury in the United States*, Atlanta, 2010, Centers for Disease Control and Prevention, retrieved July 11, 2011, from http://www.cdc.gov/traumaticbraininjury/pdf/tbi_blue_book_age.pdf.

Feigin RD, Cutrer WB: Bacterial meningitis beyond the neonatal period. In Feigin RD, Cherry JD, Demmler-Harrison GJ, and other, editors: *Textbook of pediatric infectious diseases*, ed 6, Philadelphia, 2009, Saunders.

Fetveit A: Assessment of febrile seizures in children, *Eur J Pediatr* 167:17–27, 2008.

Freeman JM, Kossoff EH, Hartman AL: The ketogenic diet: one decade later, *Pediatrics* 119(3):535–543, 2007.

Friedman MJ, Ghazala SQ: Seizures in children, *Pediatr Clin North Am* 53:257–277, 2006.

Granoff DM, Gilsdor JR: *Neisseria* meningitis. In Kliegman RM, Stanton BF, St. Geme JW, and others, editors: *Nelson textbook of pediatrics*, ed 19, Philadelphia, 2011, Elsevier/Saunders.

Gupta N, Park J, Solomon C, and others: Long-term outcomes in patients with treated childhood hydrocephalus, *J Neurosurg* 106:334–339, 2007.

Hader WJ, Walker RL, Myles ST, and other: Complications of endoscopic third ventriculostomy in previously shunted patients, *Neurosurgery* 63:168–175, 2008.

Hampers LC, Spina LA: Evaluation and management of pediatric febrile seizures in the emergency department, *Emerg Med Clin North Am* 29(1):83–93, 2011.

Hartman AL, Vining EP: Clinical aspects of the ketogenic diet, *Epilepsia* 48(1):31–42, 2007.

Haut SR, Lipton RB: Predicting seizures: a behavioral approach, *Neurol Clin* 27:925–940, 2009.

Hon KE, Leung AK: Childhood accidents: injuries and poisoning, *Adv Pediatr* 57:33–62, 2010.

Howlader N, Noone AM, Krapcho M, and others: *SEER cancer statistics review 1975–2008*, National Cancer Institute, retrieved July 28, 2011, from http://seer.cancer.gov/csr/1975_2008/.

Huff JS, Fountain NB: Pathophysiology and definitions of seizures and status epilepticus, *Emerg Med Clin North Am* 29(1):1–13, 2011.

James SH, Kimberlin DW, Whitley RJ: Antiviral therapy for herpesvirus central nervous system infections, *Antiviral Res* 83:207–213, 2009.

Joffe AR: Lumbar puncture and brain herniation in acute bacterial meningitis: a review, *J Intensive Care Med* 22(4):194–207, 2007.

Johnston A, Smith P: Sudden unexpected death in epilepsy, *Expert Rev Neurother* 7(12):1751–1761, 2007.

Kinsman SL, Johnston MV: Hydrocephalus. In Kliegman RM, Stanton BF, St. Geme JW, and others, editors: *Nelson textbook of pediatrics*, ed 19, Philadelphia, 2011, Elsevier/Saunders.

Landry GL: Head and neck injuries. In Kliegman RM, Stanton BF, St. Geme JW, and others, editors: *Nelson textbook of pediatrics*, ed 19, Philadelphia, 2011, Elsevier/Saunders.

Lee LK: Controversies in the sequelae of pediatric mild traumatic brain injury, *Pediatr Emerg Care* 23:580–583, 2007.

Lin AL, Safdieh JE: The evaluation and management of bacterial meningitis, current practice and emerging developments, *Neurologist* 16(3):143–151, 2010.

Logan SA, MacMahon E: Viral meningitis, *BMJ* 336:36–40, 2008.

Lozsadi DA, Von Oertzen J, Cock HR: Epilepsy: recent advances, *J Neurol* 257:1946–1951, 2010.

Machata AM, Willschke H, Kabon B, and others: Propofol-based sedation regimen for infants and children undergoing ambulatory magnetic resonance imaging, *Br J Anaesth* 101(2):239–243, 2008.

Manning SE, Rupprecht CE, Fishbein D, and others: Human rabies prevention—United States 2008, *MMWR* 57(No. RR-3), retrieved July 1, 2011, from http://www.cdc.gov/mmwr/preview/mmwrhtml/rr57e507a1.htm.

Mason KP: The pediatric sedation service: who is appropriate to sedate, which medications should I use, who should prescribe the drugs, how do I bill, *Pediatr Radiol* 38(suppl):S218–S224, 2008.

Mathur M, Peterson L, Stadtler M, and others: Variability in pediatric brain death determination and documentation in Southern California, *Pediatrics* 121(5):988–993, 2008.

Meehan WP, Mannix R: Pediatric concussions in United States emergency departments in the years 2002 to 2006, *J Pediatr* 157(6):889–893, 2010.

Merchant TE, Pollack IF, Loeffler JS: Brain tumors across the age spectrum: biology, therapy and late effects, *Semin Radiat Oncol* 20(1):58–66, 2010.

Mikati MA: Treatment of seizures and epilepsy. In Kliegman RM, Stanton BF, St. Geme JW, and others, editors: *Nelson textbook of pediatrics*, ed 19, Philadelphia, 2011, Elsevier/Saunders.

Mullassery D, Dominici D, Jesudason EC, and others: Neuroblastoma: contemporary management, *Arch Dis Child Educ Pract Ed* 94:177–185, 2009.

Nakken KO, Solaas MH, Kjeldsen MJ, and others: Which seizure-precipitating factors do patients with epilepsy most frequently report? *Epilepsy Behav* 6:85–89, 2005.

Nasrullah M, Muazzam S: Drowning mortality in the United States 1999–2006, *J Community Health* 36:69–75, 2011.

Nei M, Bagla R: Seizure-related injury and death, *Curr Neurol Neurosci Rep* 7:335–341, 2007.

Orliaguet G, Meyer PG, Baugnon T: Management of critically ill children with traumatic brain injury, *Pediatr Anesth* 18:455–461, 2008.

Østergaard JR: Febrile seizures, *Acta Paediatr* 98:771–773, 2009.

Park JR, Eggert A, Caron H: Neuroblastoma: biology, prognosis, and treatment, *Hematol Oncol Clin North Am* 24(1):65–86, 2010.

Paulsen AH, Lundar T, Lindegaard KF: Twenty-year outcome in young adults with childhood hydrocephalus: assessment of surgical outcome, work participation, and health-related quality of life, *J Neurosurg Pediatr* 6:527–535, 2010.

Perheentupa U, Kinnunen I, Grénman R, and others: Management and outcome of pediatric skull base fractures, *Int J Pediatr Otorhinolaryngol* 74:1245–1250, 2010.

Prober CG, Dyner L: Acute bacterial meningitis beyond the neonatal period. In Kliegman RM, Stanton BF, St. Geme JW, and others, editors: *Nelson textbook of pediatrics*, ed 19, Philadelphia, 2011a, Elsevier/Saunders.

Prober CG, Dyner L: Viral meningoencephalitis. In Kliegman RM, Stanton BF, St. Geme JW, and others, editors: *Nelson textbook of pediatrics*, ed 19, Philadelphia, 2011b, Elsevier/Saunders.

Pugliese A, Beltramo T, Torre D: Reye's and Reye's-like syndromes, *Cell Biochem Funct* 26(7):741–746, 2008.

Reynolds D, Boyd M: Child life specialists and nurses working together, *Imprint* 57(1):22–25, 2010.

Rivara FP, Grossman DC: Injury control. In Kliegman RM, Stanton BF, St. Geme JW, and others, editors: *Nelson textbook of pediatrics*, ed 19, Philadelphia, 2011, Elsevier/Saunders.

Safe Kids: *Report to the nation: trends in unintentional childhood injury mortality and parental views on child safety, 2008*, 2009, Safe Kids Worldwide, retrieved June 26, 2011, from http://www.safekids.org/assets/docs/ourwork/ research/research-report-safe-kids-week-2008. pdf.

Sankhyan N, Raju KN, Sharma S, and other: Management of raised intracranial pressure, *Indian J Pediatr* 77:1409–1416, 2010.

Sharma S, Kochar GS, Sankhyan N, and other: Approach to the child with coma, *Indian J Pediatr* 77:1279–1287, 2010.

Shaw S: Endocrine late effects in survivors of pediatric brain tumors, *J Pediatr Oncol Nurs* 26(5):295–302, 2009.

Schnakers C, Zasler ND: Pain assessment and management in disorders of consciousness, *Curr Opin Neurol* 20:620–626, 2007.

Shephard E, Quan L: Drowning and submersion injury. In Kliegman RM, Stanton BF, St. Geme JW, and others, editors: *Nelson textbook of pediatrics*, ed 19, Philadelphia, 2011, Elsevier/ Saunders.

Shoja MM, Tubbs RS, Malekian A, and others: Video game epilepsy in the twentieth century: a review, *Childs Nerv Syst* 23:265–267, 2007.

Shorvon S: The treatment of status epilepticus, *Curr Opin Neurol* 24:165–170, 2011.

Sillanpää M, Schmidt D: Prognosis of seizure recurrence after stopping antiepileptic drugs in seizure-free patients: a long term population-based study of childhood-onset epilepsy, *Epilepsy Behav* 8(4):713, 2006.

Singhi SC, Tiwari L: Management of intracranial hypertension, *Indian J Pediatr* 76:519–529, 2009.

Somand D, Meurer W: Central nervous system infections, *Emerg Med Clin North Am* 27:89–100, 2009.

Spencer S, Huh L: Outcomes of epilepsy surgery in adults and children, *Lancet Neurol* 7:525–537, 2008.

Steering Committee on Quality Improvement and Management, Subcommittee on Febrile Seizures American Academy of Pediatrics: Febrile seizures: clinical practice guideline for the long-term management of the child with simple febrile seizures, *Pediatrics* 121(6):1281–1286, 2008.

Swaine BR, Tremblay C, Platt RW, and others: Previous head injury is a risk factor for subsequent head injury in children: a longitudinal cohort study, *Pediatrics* 119(4): 749–758, 2007.

Thigpen MC, Whitney CG, Messonnier NE, and others: Bacterial meningitis in the United States 1998–2007, *N Engl J Med* 364(21):2016–2025, 2011.

Truog RD, Campbell ML, Curtis JR, and others: Recommendations for end-of-life care in the intensive care unit, *Crit Care Med* 36(3): 953–963, 2008.

Ursitti F, Fadda T, Papetti L, and others: Evaluation and management of nonsyndromic craniosynostosis, *Acta Paediatr* 100(9):1185–1194, 2011.

Vignes JR, Jeelani NU, Jeelani A, and others: Growing skull fracture after minor closed-head injury, *J Pediatr* 151:316–318, 2007.

Walls C: Shaken baby syndrome education: A role for nurse practitioners working with families of small children, *J Pediatr Health Care* 20(5):304–310, 2006.

Weiss J, American Academy of Pediatrics Committee on Injury, Violence, and Poison Prevention: Prevention of drowning, *Pediatrics* 126:e253–e262, 2010.

Willoughby RE Jr: Rabies. In Kliegman RM, Stanton BF, St. Geme JW, and others, editors: *Nelson textbook of pediatrics*, ed 19, Philadelphia, 2011, Elsevier/Saunders.

Young GB: Coma, *Ann NY Acad Sci* 1157:32–47, 2009.

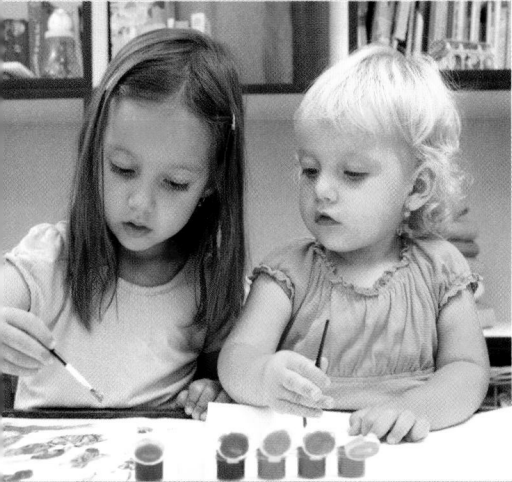

CHAPTER
29

The Child with Endocrine Dysfunction

Elizabeth Record and Linda K. Ballard

evolve WEBSITE

http://evolve.elsevier.com/wong/essentials
Animations—Adrenal Function; Insulin Injection
Case Studies—Diabetes Mellitus; Diabetes Insipidus
Key Point Summaries

NCLEX-Style Review Questions
Nursing Care Plans—The Child with Diabetes Mellitus; The Child
with Diabetic Ketoacidosis (DKA)

CHAPTER OUTLINE

The Endocrine System, 973
   Hormones, 976
Disorders of Pituitary Function, 977
   Hypopituitarism, 977
   Pituitary Hyperfunction, 979
   Precocious Puberty, 979
   Diabetes Insipidus, 980
   Syndrome of Inappropriate Antidiuretic
     Hormone, 981
Disorders of Thyroid Function, 981
   Juvenile Hypothyroidism, 982
   Goiter, 982

Lymphocytic Thyroiditis, 983
Hyperthyroidism, 983
Disorders of Parathyroid Function, 985
   Hypoparathyroidism, 985
   Hyperparathyroidism, 986
Disorders of Adrenal Function, 987
   Acute Adrenocortical Insufficiency, 987
   Chronic Adrenocortical Insufficiency
     (Addison Disease), 988
   Cushing Syndrome, 989
   Congenital Adrenal Hyperplasia, 990
   Pheochromocytoma, 991

Disorders of Pancreatic Hormone
   Secretion, 992
   Diabetes Mellitus, 992
    *Nursing Care Plan: The Child with
    Diabetes Mellitus, 1000*

LEARNING OBJECTIVES

On completion of this chapter the reader will be able to:
- Differentiate between the disorders caused by hypopituitary and hyperpituitary dysfunction.
- Describe the manifestations of thyroid hypofunction and hyperfunction and the management of children with the disorders.
- Distinguish between the manifestations of adrenal hypofunction and hyperfunction.

- Differentiate among the various categories of diabetes mellitus.
- Discuss the management and nursing care of the child with diabetes mellitus in the acute care setting.
- Distinguish between a hypoglycemic and a hyperglycemic reaction.
- Formulate a teaching plan for instructing the parents of a child with diabetes mellitus.

THE ENDOCRINE SYSTEM

The endocrine system consists of three components: (1) the cells, which send chemical messages by means of hormones; (2) the target cells, or end organs, which receive the chemical messages; and (3) the environment through which the chemicals are transported (blood, lymph, extracellular fluids) from the sites of synthesis to the sites of

cellular action. The endocrine system controls or regulates metabolic processes governing energy production, growth, fluid and electrolyte balance, response to stress, and sexual reproduction (Baxter and Ribeiro, 2004). The endocrine glands, which are distributed throughout the body, are listed in Table 29-1; also listed are several additional structures sometimes considered endocrine glands, although they are not usually included. The pathophysiology review in Figure 29-1

TABLE 29-1 HORMONES AND THEIR FUNCTION

HORMONE	EFFECT	HYPOFUNCTION	HYPERFUNCTION
Adenohypophysis (Anterior Pituitary)*			
STH or GH (somatotropin) *Target tissue*—Bones	Promotes growth of bone and soft tissues Has main effect on linear growth Maintains a normal rate of protein synthesis Conserves carbohydrate utilization and promotes fat mobilization Is essential for proliferation of cartilage cells at epiphyseal plate Is ineffective for linear growth after epiphyseal closure Has hyperglycemic effect (anti-insulin action)	Epiphyseal fusion with cessation of growth Prepubertal dwarfism Pituitary cachexia (Simmonds disease) Generalized growth retardation Hypoglycemia	Prepubertal gigantism Acromegaly (after full growth is attained) Diabetes mellitus Postpubertal hypoproteinemia
Thyrotropin (TSH) *Target tissue*—Thyroid gland	Promotes and maintains growth and development of thyroid gland Stimulates TH secretion	Hypothyroidism Marked delay of puberty Juvenile myxedema	Hyperthyroidism Thyrotoxicosis Graves disease
ACTH *Target tissue*—Adrenal cortex	Promotes and maintains growth and development of adrenal cortex Stimulates adrenal cortex to secrete glucocorticoids and androgens	Acute adrenocortical insufficiency (Addison disease) Hypoglycemia Increased skin pigmentation	Cushing syndrome
Gonadotropins *Target tissue*—Gonads FSH *Target tissue*—Ovaries, testes	Stimulate gonads to mature and produce sex hormones and germ cells *Male*—Stimulates development of seminiferous tubules; initiates spermatogenesis *Female*—Stimulates graafian follicles to mature and secrete estrogen	Absent or incomplete spontaneous puberty Hypogonadism Sterility Absence or loss of secondary sex characteristics Amenorrhea	Precocious puberty Early epiphyseal closure Precocious puberty Primary gonadal failure Hirsutism Polycystic ovary Early epiphyseal closure
Luteinizing hormone (LH)[†] *Target tissue*—Ovaries, testes	*Male*—Stimulates differentiation of Leydig cells, which secrete androgens, principally testosterone *Female*—Produces rupture of follicle with discharge of mature ovum; stimulates secretion of progesterone by corpus luteum	Hypogonadism Sterility Impotence Absence or loss of secondary sex characteristics Ovarian failure Eunuchism	Precocious puberty Primary gonadal failure Hirsutism Polycystic ovary Early epiphyseal closure
Prolactin (luteotropic hormone) *Target tissue*—Ovaries, breasts	Stimulates milk secretion Maintains corpus luteum and progesterone secretion during pregnancy	Inability to lactate Amenorrhea	Galactorrhea Functional hypogonadism
MSH *Target tissue*—Skin	Promotes pigmentation of skin	Diminished or absent skin pigmentation	Increased skin pigmentation
Neurohypophysis (Posterior Pituitary)			
ADH (vasopressin) *Target tissue*—Renal tubules	Acts on distal and collecting tubules, making them more permeable to water, thus increasing reabsorption and decreasing excretion of urine	Diabetes insipidus	SIADH Fluid retention Hyponatremia
Oxytocin *Target tissue*—Uterus, breasts	Stimulates powerful contractions of uterus Causes ejection of milk from alveoli into breast ducts (letdown reflex)		
Thyroid			
THs—T$_4$ and T$_3$	Regulate metabolic rate; control rate of growth of body cells Especially important for growth of bones, teeth, and brain Promote mobilization of fats and gluconeogenesis	Hypothyroidism Myxedema Hashimoto thyroiditis General growth greatly reduced; extent dependent on age at which deficiency occurs Intellectual disability in infant	Exophthalmic goiter (Graves disease) Accelerated linear growth Early epiphyseal closure
Thyrocalcitonin	Regulates calcium and phosphorus metabolism Influences ossification and development of bone		

TABLE 29-1	HORMONES AND THEIR FUNCTION—cont'd		
HORMONE	**EFFECT**	**HYPOFUNCTION**	**HYPERFUNCTION**
Parathyroid Glands			
PTH	Promotes calcium reabsorption from blood, bone, and intestines	Hypocalcemia (tetany)	Hypercalcemia (bone demineralization)
	Promotes excretion of phosphorus in kidney tubules		Hypophosphatemia
Adrenal Cortex			
Mineralocorticoids	Stimulate renal tubules to reabsorb sodium, thus	Adrenocortical insufficiency	Electrolyte imbalance
Aldosterone	promoting water retention but potassium loss		Hyperaldosteronism
Sex hormones—Androgens,	Influence development of bone, reproductive organs,	Male feminization	Adrenogenital syndrome
estrogens, progesterone	and secondary sex characteristics		
Glucocorticoids	Promote normal fat, protein, and carbohydrate	Addison disease	Cushing syndrome
Cortisol (hydrocortisone and	metabolism	Acute adrenocortical insufficiency	Severe impairment of growth
compound F)	Mobilize body defenses during periods of stress	Impaired growth and sexual	with slowing in skeletal
Corticosterone (compound B)	Suppress inflammatory reaction	function	maturation
			In excess, tend to accelerate gluconeogenesis and protein and fat catabolism
Adrenal Medulla			
Epinephrine (adrenaline),	Produce vasoconstriction of heart and smooth muscles		Hyperfunction caused by:
norepinephrine	(raise blood pressure)		Pheochromocytoma
(noradrenaline)	Increase blood glucose via glycolysis		Neuroblastoma
	Inhibit GI activity		Ganglioneuroma
	Activate sweat glands		
Islets of Langerhans of Pancreas			
Insulin (β cells)	Promotes glucose transport into the cells	Diabetes mellitus	Hyperinsulinism
	Increases glucose utilization, glycogenesis, and glycolysis		
	Promotes fatty acid transport into cells and lipogenesis		
	Promotes amino acid transport into cells and protein synthesis		
Glucagon (α cells)	Acts as antagonist to insulin, thereby increasing blood		Hyperglycemia
	glucose concentration by accelerating		May be instrumental in
	glycogenolysis		genesis of DKA in DM
	Able to inhibit secretion of both insulin and glycogen		
Somatostatin (δ cells)	Able to inhibit secretion of both insulin and glycogen		
Ovaries			
Estrogen	Accelerates growth of epithelial cells, especially in	Lack of or repression of sexual	Precocious puberty, early
	uterus after menses	development	epiphyseal closure
	Promotes protein anabolism		
	Promotes epiphyseal closure of bones		
	Promotes breast development during puberty and pregnancy		
	Plays role in sexual function		
	Stimulates water and sodium reabsorption in renal tubules		
	Stimulates ripening of ova		
Progesterone	Prepares uterus for nidation of fertilized ovum and aids in maintenance of pregnancy		
	Aids in development of alveolar system of breasts during pregnancy		
	Inhibits myometrial contractions		
	Has effect on protein catabolism		
	Promotes salt and water retention, especially in endometrium		

Continued

TABLE 29-1	HORMONES AND THEIR FUNCTION—cont'd		
HORMONE	**EFFECT**	**HYPOFUNCTION**	**HYPERFUNCTION**
Testes			
Testosterone	Accelerates protein anabolism for growth	Delayed sexual development or	Precocious puberty, early
	Promotes epiphyseal closure	eunuchoidism	epiphyseal closure
	Promotes development of secondary sex characteristics		
	Plays role in sexual function		
	Stimulates testes to produce spermatozoa		

ACTH, Adrenocorticotropic hormone; *ADH*, antidiuretic hormone; *DKA*, diabetic ketoacidosis; *DM*, diabetes mellitus; *FSH*, follicle-stimulating hormone; *GH*, growth hormone; *GI*, gastrointestinal; *MSH*, melanocyte-stimulating hormone; *PTH*, parathyroid hormone; *SIADH*, syndrome of inappropriate antidiuretic hormone secretion; *STH*, somatotropin hormone; T_3, triiodothyronine; T_4, thyroxine; *TH*, thyroid hormone; *TSH*, thyroid-stimulating hormone.
*For each anterior pituitary hormone there is a corresponding hypothalamic-releasing factor. A deficiency in these factors caused by inhibiting anterior pituitary hormone synthesis produces the same effects. (See text for more detailed information.)
†In males, LH is sometimes known as interstitial cell–stimulating hormone (ICSH).

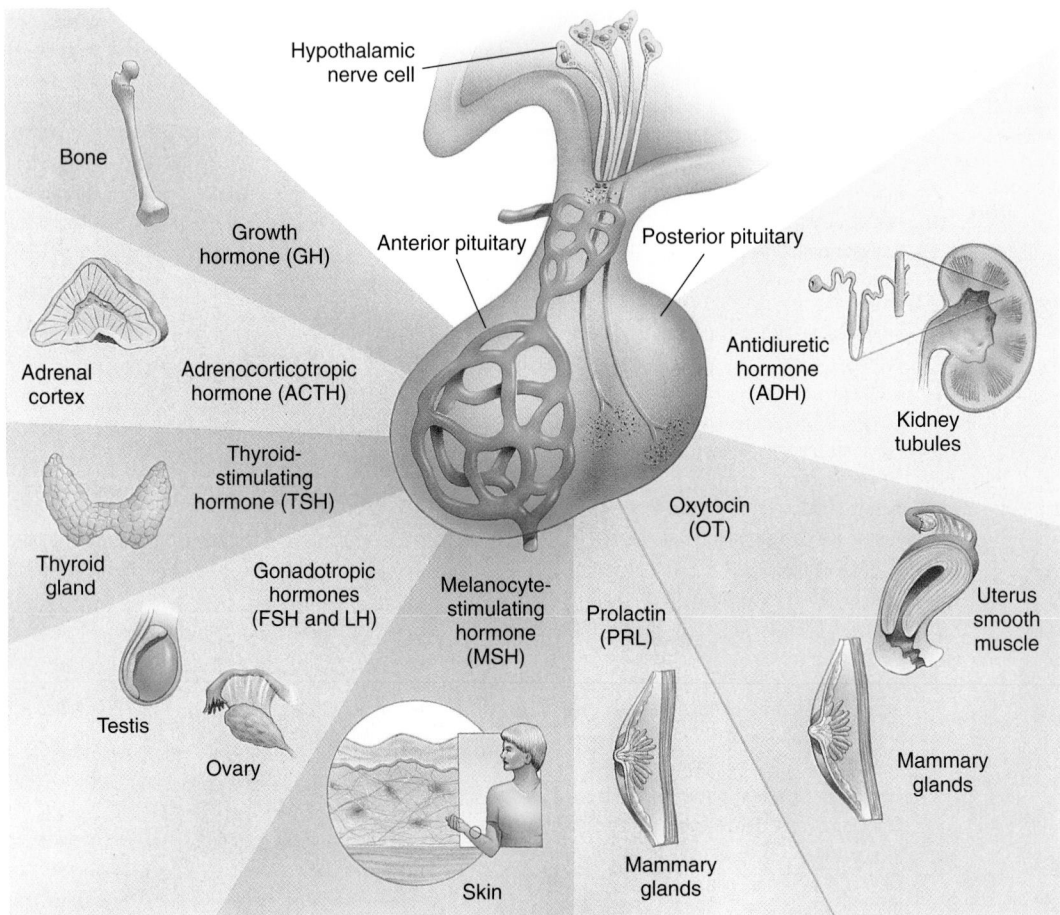

FIG 29-1 Principal anterior and posterior pituitary hormones and their target organs. *FSH,* Follicle-stimulating hormone; *LH,* luteinizing hormone. (From Patton KT, Thibodeau GA: *Anatomy and physiology,* ed 8, St. Louis, 2013, Mosby.)

provides a summary of the principle pituitary hormones and their target organs.

HORMONES

A hormone is a complex chemical substance produced and secreted into body fluids by a cell or group of cells that exerts a physiologic controlling effect on other cells (Kliegman, Stanton, St. Geme, and others, 2011). These effects may be local or distant and may affect either most cells of the body or specific "target" tissues. Hormones are released by the endocrine glands into the bloodstream, and production is regulated by a feedback mechanism (see Table 29-1). The master gland of the endocrine system is the anterior pituitary, which is in turn controlled by the hypothalamus. Some hormones, such as insulin, are regulated by other mechanisms.

DISORDERS OF PITUITARY FUNCTION

The pituitary gland is divided into two lobes, the anterior and the posterior lobes. Each lobe is responsible for different hormones. Disorders of the anterior pituitary hormones may be attributable to organic defects or have an idiopathic etiology and may occur as a single hormonal problem or in combination with other hormonal disorders. The clinical manifestations depend on the hormones involved and the age of onset. Panhypopituitarism is often defined clinically as the loss of all anterior pituitary hormones, leaving only posterior function intact (Toogood and Stewart, 2008).

> ## ❗ NURSING ALERT
>
> Children with panhypopituitarism should wear medical identification, such as a bracelet.

HYPOPITUITARISM

Hypopituitarism is diminished or deficient secretion of pituitary hormones. The consequences of the condition depend on the degree of dysfunction and can lead to gonadotropin deficiency with absence or regression of secondary sex characteristics; growth hormone (GH) deficiency, in which children display retarded somatic growth; thyroid-stimulating hormone (TSH) deficiency, which produces hypothyroidism; and corticotropin deficiency, which results in manifestations of adrenal hypofunction. Hypopituitarism can result from any of the conditions listed in Box 29-1. The most common organic cause of pituitary undersecretion is tumors in the pituitary or hypothalamic region, especially the craniopharyngiomas. Congenital hypopituitarism can be seen in newborn infants, often as a result of birth trauma. Symptoms of hypoglycemia and seizure activity often manifest within the first 24 hours after birth (Toogood and Stewart, 2008).

Idiopathic hypopituitarism, or idiopathic pituitary growth failure, is usually related to GH deficiency, which inhibits somatic growth in all cells of the body (Miller and Zimmerman, 2004). Growth failure is defined as an absolute height of less than -2 standard deviation (SD) for age or a linear growth velocity consistently less than -1 SD for age. When this occurs without the presence of hypothyroidism, systemic disease, or malnutrition, then an abnormality of the GH–insulin-like growth factor (IGF-I) axis should be considered (Richmond and Rogol, 2008). Not all children with short stature have GH deficiency. In most instances, the cause is either familial short stature or constitutional growth delay. **Familial short stature** refers to otherwise healthy children who have ancestors with adult height in the lower percentiles. **Constitutional growth delay** refers to individuals (usually boys) with delayed linear growth, generally beginning as a toddler, and skeletal and sexual maturation that is behind that of age mates (Halac and Zimmerman, 2004; Miller and Zimmerman, 2004). Typically, these children will reach normal adult height. Often there is a history of a similar pattern of growth in one of the child's parents or other family members. The untreated child will proceed through normal changes as expected on the basis of bone age. Although treatment with GH is not usually indicated, its use has become controversial, especially in relation to parental and child requests for treatment to accelerate growth.

Clinical Manifestations

Children with hypopituitarism generally grow normally during the first year and then follow a slowed growth curve that is below the third percentile. Skeletal proportions and weight are normal for the age, but

---

BOX 29-1   CLINICAL MANIFESTATIONS OF PANHYPOPITUITARISM

Growth Hormone
Short stature but proportional height and weight
Delayed epiphyseal closure
Retarded bone age proportional to height
Premature aging common in later life
Increased insulin sensitivity

Thyroid-Stimulating Hormone
Short stature with infantile proportions
Dry, coarse skin; yellow discoloration, pallor
Cold intolerance
Constipation
Somnolence
Bradycardia
Dyspnea on exertion
Delayed dentition, loss of teeth

Gonadotropins
Absence of sexual maturation or loss of secondary sexual characteristics
Atrophy of genitalia, prostate gland, breasts
Amenorrhea without menopausal symptoms
Decreased spermatogenesis

Adrenocorticotropic Hormone
Severe anorexia, weight loss
Hypoglycemia
Hypotension
Hyponatremia, hyperkalemia
Adrenal apoplexy, especially in response to stress
Circulatory collapse

Antidiuretic Hormone
Polyuria
Polydipsia
Dehydration

Melanocyte-Stimulating Hormone
Decreased pigmentation

---

these children may appear younger than their chronologic age. Dentition is delayed, and teeth may be overcrowded and malpositioned because of the undeveloped jaw. Sexual development is usually delayed but is otherwise normal unless the gonadotropin hormones are deficient. Growth may extend into the third or fourth decade of life, but permanent height is usually diminished if the disorder is left untreated. Symptoms such as headache and vision changes may indicate the presence of a tumor. Clinical manifestations of panhypopituitarism are listed in Box 29-1.

Diagnostic Evaluation

Only a small number of children with delayed growth or short stature have hypopituitary dwarfism. In the majority of instances, the cause is constitutional delay. Diagnostic evaluation is aimed at isolating organic causes, which, in addition to GH deficiency, may include hypothyroidism, oversecretion of cortisol, gonadal aplasia, chronic illness, nutritional inadequacy, Russell-Silver dwarfism, or hypochondroplasia.

A complete diagnostic evaluation should include a family history, a history of the child's growth patterns and previous health status,

Modified from Vogiatzi MG, Copeland KC: The short child, *Pediatr Rev* 19(3):92–99, 1998.

BOX 29-2 EVALUATING THE GROWTH CURVE

Ensure reliability of measurements. Accurately obtain and plot height and weight measurements.

Determine absolute height. The child's absolute height bears some relationship to the likelihood of a pathologic condition. However, the majority of children who have a height below the lowest percentile (either the third or fifth percentile on the height curve) do not have a pathologic growth problem.

Assess height velocity. The most important aspect of a growth evaluation is the observation of a child's height over time, or height velocity. Accurate determination of height velocity requires at least 4 and preferably 6 months of observation. A substantial deceleration in height velocity (crossing several percentiles) between 3 and 12 or 13 years of age indicates a pathologic condition until proven otherwise.

Determine weight-to-height relationship. Determination of the weight-to-height ratio has some diagnostic value in ascertaining the cause of growth retardation in a short child.

Project target height. The height of a child can be judged inappropriately short only in the context of his or her genetic potential. Determine the target height of the child with the formula:

[Father's height (cm) + Mother's height (cm) + 13]/2 for boys

or

[Father's height (cm) + Mother's height (cm) − 13]/2 for girls

Most children achieve an adult stature within approximately 10 cm (4 inches) of the target height.

Modified from Vogiatzi MG, Copeland KC: The short child, *Pediatr Rev* 19(3):92–99, 1998.

BOX 29-3 BONE AGE FOR EVALUATING GROWTH DISORDERS

Bone age refers to a method of assessing skeletal maturity by comparing the appearance of representative epiphyseal centers obtained on x-ray examination with age-appropriate published standards.

Most conditions that cause poor linear growth also cause a delay in skeletal maturation and a retarded bone age. Observation of even a profoundly delayed bone age is never diagnostic or even indicative of a specific diagnosis. A delayed bone age merely indicates that the associated short stature is to some extent "partially reversible" because linear growth will continue until epiphyseal fusion is complete. In comparison, a bone age that is not delayed in a short child is of much greater concern and may, in fact, be of some diagnostic value under certain circumstances.

Modified from Vogiatzi MG, Copeland KC: The short child, *Pediatr Rev* 19(3):92–99, 1998.

physical examination, psychosocial evaluation, radiographic surveys, and endocrine studies. Accurate measurement of height (using a calibrated stadiometer) and weight and comparison with standard growth charts are essential. Multiple height measures reflect a more accurate assessment of abnormal growth patterns (Box 29-2) (Hall, 2000). Parental height and familial patterns of growth are important clues to diagnosis.

A skeletal survey in children younger than 3 years of age and radiographic examination of the hand–wrist for centers of ossification (bone age) (Box 29-3) in older children are important in evaluating growth.

Definitive diagnosis is based on absent or subnormal reserves of pituitary GH. Because GH levels are variable in children, GH stimulation testing is usually required for diagnosis. Initial assessment of the serum IGF-I and IGF binding protein 3 (IGFBP3) indicates a need for further evaluation of GH dysfunction if levels are less than −1 SD below the mean for age. It is recommended that GH stimulation tests be reserved for children with low serum IGF-I and IGFBP3 levels and poor growth who do not have other causes for short stature (Richmond and Rogol, 2008). GH stimulation testing involves the use of pharmacologic agents such as levodopa, clonidine, arginine, insulin, propranolol, or glucagon to provoke the release of GH (Kliegman, Stanton, St. Geme, and others, 2011). Children with poor linear growth, delayed bone age, and abnormal GH stimulation tests are considered GH deficient.

Therapeutic Management

Treatment of GH deficiency caused by organic lesions is directed toward correction of the underlying disease process (e.g., surgical removal or irradiation of a tumor). The definitive treatment of GH deficiency is replacement of GH, which is successful in 80% of affected children. Biosynthetic GH is administered subcutaneously on a daily basis. Growth velocity increases in the first year and then declines in subsequent years. Final height is likely to remain less than normal (Bryant, Baxter, Cave, and others, 2007), and early diagnosis and intervention are essential (Leschek, Rose, Yanovski, and others, 2004).

The decision to stop GH therapy is made jointly by the child, family, and health care team. Growth rates of less than 1 inch per year and a bone age of more than 14 years in girls and more than 16 years in boys are often used as criteria to stop GH therapy (Kliegman, Stanton, St. Geme, and others, 2011). Children with other hormone deficiencies require replacement therapy to correct the specific disorders.

Nursing Care Management

The principal nursing consideration is identifying children with growth problems. Even though the majority of growth problems are not a result of organic causes, any delay in normal growth and sexual development poses special emotional adjustments for these children.

The nurse may be a key person in helping establish a diagnosis. For example, if serial height and weight records are not available, the nurse can question parents about the child's growth compared with that of siblings, peers, or relatives. Preparation of the child and family for diagnostic testing is especially important if a number of tests are being performed, and the child requires particular attention during provocative testing. Blood samples are usually taken every 30 minutes for a 3-hour period. Children also have difficulty overcoming hypoglycemia generated by tests with insulin, so they must be observed carefully for signs of hypoglycemia, but those receiving glucagon are at risk of nausea and vomiting. Clonidine may cause hypotension, requiring administration of intravenous (IV) fluids.

Child and Family Support

Children undergoing hormone replacement require additional support. The nurse should provide education for patient self-management during the school-age years. Nursing functions include family education concerning medication preparation and storage, injection sites, injection technique, and syringe disposal (see Chapter 22). Administration of GH is facilitated by family routines that include a specific time of day for the injection. Younger children may enjoy using a calendar and colorful stickers to designate received injections.

> **NURSING TIP** Optimum dosing is often achieved when GH is administered at bedtime. Physiologic release is more normally stimulated as a result of pituitary release of GH during the first 45 to 90 minutes after the onset of sleep.

Even when hormone replacement is successful, these children attain their eventual adult height at a slower rate than their peers; therefore, they need assistance in setting realistic expectations regarding improvement. Because these children appear younger than their chronologic age, others frequently relate to them in infantile or childish ways. Parents and teachers benefit from guidance directed toward setting realistic expectations for the child based on age and abilities. For example, in the home, such children should have the same age-appropriate responsibilities as their siblings. As they approach adolescence, they should be encouraged to participate in group activities with peers. If abilities and strengths are emphasized rather than physical size, such children are more likely to develop a positive self-image.

Professionals and families can find resources for research, education, support, and advocacy from the Human Growth Foundation.* The treatment is expensive, but the cost is often partially covered by insurance if the child has a documented deficiency. Children with panhypopituitarism should be advised to wear medical identification at all times.

PITUITARY HYPERFUNCTION

Excess GH before closure of the epiphyseal shafts results in proportional overgrowth of the long bones until the individual reaches a height of 2.4 m (8 ft) or more. Vertical growth is accompanied by rapid and increased development of muscles and viscera. Weight is increased but is usually in proportion to height. Proportional enlargement of head circumference also occurs and may result in delayed closure of the fontanels in young children. Children with a pituitary-secreting tumor may also demonstrate signs of increasing intracranial pressure, especially headache.

If oversecretion of GH occurs after epiphyseal closure, growth is in the transverse direction, producing a condition known as **acromegaly**. Typical facial features include overgrowth of the head, lips, nose, tongue, jaw, and paranasal and mastoid sinuses; separation and malocclusion of the teeth in the enlarged jaw; disproportion of the face to the cerebral division of the skull; increased facial hair; thickened, deeply creased skin; and an increased tendency toward hyperglycemia and diabetes mellitus (DM). Acromegaly can develop slowly, leading to delays in diagnosis and treatment.

Diagnostic Evaluation

Diagnosis is based on a history of excessive growth during childhood and evidence of increased levels of GH. Radiographic studies may reveal a tumor in an enlarged sella turcica, normal bone age, enlargement of bones (e.g., the paranasal sinuses), and evidence of joint changes. Endocrine studies to confirm excess of other hormones, specifically thyroid, cortisol, and sex hormones, should also be included in the differential diagnosis.

Therapeutic Management

If a lesion is present, surgery is performed to remove the tumor when feasible. Other therapies aimed at destroying pituitary tissue include

*997 Glen Cove Ave., Suite 5, Glen Head, NY 11545; 800-451-6434; e-mail: hgf1@hgfound.org; http://www.hgfound.org.

external irradiation and radioactive implants. New pharmacologic agents have evolved and may be use in combination with other therapies (Natchtigall, Delgado, Swearingen, and others, 2008). Depending on the extent of surgical extirpation and degree of pituitary insufficiency, hormone replacement with thyroid extract, cortisone, and sex hormones may be necessary.

Nursing Care Management

The primary nursing consideration is early identification of children with excessive growth rates. Although medical management is unable to reduce growth already attained, further growth can be retarded. The earlier the treatment, the more control there is in predetermining a normal adult height. Nurses should also observe for signs of a tumor, especially headache, and evidence of concurrent hormonal excesses, particularly the gonadotropins, which cause sexual precocity. Children with excessive growth rates require as much emotional support as those with short stature.

PRECOCIOUS PUBERTY

Manifestations of sexual development before age 9 years in boys or age 8 years in girls have traditionally been considered precocious development, and these children were recommended for further evaluation (Kempers and Otten, 2002; Midyett, Moore, and Jacobson, 2003). Recent examination of the age limit for defining when puberty is precocious reveals that the onset of puberty in girls is occurring earlier than previous studies have documented (Biro, Huang, Crawford, and others, 2006; Slyper, 2006). The mean onset of puberty was 10.2 years in white girls and 9.6 years in African-American girls. Based on these findings, precocious puberty evaluation for a pathologic cause should be performed for white girls younger than 7 years of age or for African-American girls younger than 6 years of age. No change in the guidelines for evaluation of precocious puberty in boys is recommended. However, recent data suggest that boys may be beginning maturation earlier as well (Herman-Giddens, 2006; Slyper, 2006).

Normally, the hypothalamic-releasing factors stimulate secretion of the gonadotropic hormones from the anterior pituitary at the time of puberty. In boys, interstitial cell–stimulating hormone stimulates Leydig cells of the testes to secrete testosterone; in girls, follicle-stimulating hormone (FSH) and luteinizing hormone stimulate the ovarian follicles to secrete estrogens (Nebesio and Eugster, 2007). This sequence of events is known as the **hypothalamic–pituitary–gonadal axis**. If for some reason the cycle undergoes premature activation, the child will display evidence of advanced or precocious puberty. Causes of precocious puberty are found in Box 29-4.

Isosexual precocious puberty is more common among girls than boys. Approximately 80% of children with precocious puberty have **central precocious puberty (CPP)**, in which pubertal development is activated by the hypothalamic gonadotropin-releasing hormone (GnRH) (Greiner and Kerrigan, 2006). This produces early maturation and development of the gonads with secretion of sex hormones, development of secondary sex characteristics, and sometimes production of mature sperm and ova (Lee, 2006; Root, 2000). CPP may be the result of congenital anomalies; infectious, neoplastic, or traumatic insults to the central nervous system (CNS); or treatment of longstanding sex hormone exposure (Trivin, Couto-Silva, Sainte-Rose, and others, 2006). CPP occurs more frequently in girls and is usually idiopathic, with 95% demonstrating no causative factor (Greiner and Kerrigan, 2006; Nebesio and Eugster, 2007; Root, 2000). A CNS insult or structural abnormality is found in more than 90% of boys with CPP (Root, 2000).

BOX 29-4 CAUSES OF PRECOCIOUS PUBERTY

Central Precocious Puberty

Idiopathic, with or without hypothalamic hamartoma
Secondary
- Congenital anomalies
- Postinflammatory—Encephalitis, meningitis, abscess, granulomatous disease
- Radiotherapy
- Trauma
- Neoplasms

After effective treatment of longstanding pseudososexual precocity

Peripheral Precocious Puberty

Familial male-limited precocious puberty
Albright syndrome
Gonadal or extragonadal tumors
Adrenal
- Congenital adrenal hyperplasia
- Adenoma, carcinoma
- Glucocorticoid resistance

Exogenous sex hormones
Primary hypothyroidism

Incomplete Precocious Puberty

Premature thelarche
Premature menarche
Premature pubarche or adrenarche

Modified from Root AW: Precocious puberty, *Pediatr Rev* 21(1):10–19, 2000.

Peripheral precocious puberty (PPP) includes early puberty resulting from hormone stimulation other than the hypothalamic GnRH–stimulated pituitary gonadotropin release. Isolated manifestations that are usually associated with puberty may be seen as variations in normal sexual development (Greiner and Kerrigan, 2006). They appear without other signs of pubescence and are caused by excess secretion of sex hormones through the gonads or adrenal glands and may be isosexual or contrasexual. Included are premature thelarche (development of breasts in prepubertal girls), premature pubarche (premature adrenarche, early development of sexual hair), and premature menarche (isolated menses without other evidence of sexual development).

Therapeutic Management

Treatment of precocious puberty is directed toward the specific cause when known. In 50% of cases, precocious pubertal development regresses or stops advancing without any treatment (Carel and Leger, 2008). If needed, precocious puberty of central (hypothalamic–pituitary) origin is managed with monthly injections of a synthetic analog of luteinizing hormone–releasing hormone, which regulates pituitary secretions (Greiner and Kerrigan, 2006; Muir, 2006). The available preparation, leuprolide acetate (Lupron Depot), is given in a dosage of 0.2 to 0.3 mg/kg intramuscularly once every 4 weeks. Longer acting formulations have recently been developed as well. Breast development regresses or does not advance, and growth returns to normal rates, enhancing predicted height. Studies suggest that not all patients attain adult targeted heights, and the addition of GH therapy may be warranted (Carel and Leger, 2008). Treatment is discontinued at a chronologically appropriate time, allowing pubertal changes to resume. Psychologic management of the patient and family is an important aspect of care. Both parents and the affected child should be taught the injection procedure.

Nursing Care Management

Psychologic support and guidance of the child and family are the most important aspects of management. Parents need anticipatory guidance, support and information resources, and reassurance of the benign nature of the condition (Greiner and Kerrigan, 2006; O'Sullivan and O'Sullivan, 2002). Dress and activities for the physically precocious child should be appropriate to the chronologic age. Sexual interest is not usually advanced beyond the child's chronologic age, and parents need to understand that the child's mental age is congruent with the chronologic age.

DIABETES INSIPIDUS

The principal disorder of posterior pituitary hypofunction is diabetes insipidus (DI), also known as neurogenic DI, resulting from undersecretion of antidiuretic hormone (ADH), or vasopressin (Pitressin), and producing a state of uncontrolled diuresis (Makaryus and McFarlane, 2006). This disorder is not to be confused with nephrogenic DI, a rare hereditary disorder affecting primarily males and caused by unresponsiveness of the renal tubules to the hormone.

Neurogenic DI may result from a number of different causes. Primary causes are familial or idiopathic; of the total cases, approximately 45% to 50% are idiopathic. Secondary causes include trauma (accidental or surgical), tumors, granulomatous disease, infections (meningitis or encephalitis), and vascular anomalies (aneurysm). Certain drugs, such as alcohol and phenytoin (diphenylhydantoin), can cause a transient polyuria. DI may be an early sign of an evolving cerebral process (De Buyst, Massa, Christophe, and others, 2007).

The cardinal signs of DI are polyuria and polydipsia. In older children, signs such as excessive urination accompanied by a compensatory insatiable thirst may be so intense that the child does little more than go to the toilet and drink fluids (Cheetham and Baylis, 2002). Frequently, the first sign is enuresis. In infants, the initial symptom is irritability that is relieved with feedings of water but not milk. These infants are also prone to dehydration, electrolyte imbalance, hyperthermia, azotemia, and potential circulatory collapse.

Dehydration is usually not a serious problem in older children, who are able to drink larger quantities of water. However, any period of unconsciousness, such as after trauma or anesthesia, may be life threatening because the voluntary demand for fluid is absent. During such instances, careful monitoring of urine volumes, blood concentration, and IV fluid replacement is essential to prevent dehydration.

> **! NURSING ALERT**
>
> Children with DI complicated by congenital absence of the thirst center must be encouraged to drink sufficient quantities of liquid to prevent electrolyte imbalance.

Diagnostic Evaluation

The simplest test used to diagnose this condition is restriction of oral fluids and observation of consequent changes in urine volume and concentration. Normally, reducing fluids results in concentrated urine and diminished volume. In DI, fluid restriction has little or no effect on urine formation but causes weight loss from dehydration. Accurate results from this procedure require strict monitoring of fluid intake and urinary output, measurement of urine concentration (specific gravity or osmolality), and frequent weight checks. A weight loss between 3% and 5% indicates significant dehydration and requires termination of the fluid restriction.

> ### ❗ NURSING ALERT
>
> Small children require close observation during fluid deprivation to prevent them from drinking, even from toilet bowls, flower vases, and other unlikely sources of fluid.

If this test result is positive, the child should be given a test dose of injected aqueous vasopressin, which should alleviate the polyuria and polydipsia. Unresponsiveness to exogenous vasopressin usually indicates nephrogenic DI. An important diagnostic consideration is to differentiate DI from other causes of polyuria and polydipsia, especially DM. DI may be the early sign of an evolving cerebral process (De Buyst, Massa, Christophe, and others, 2007).

Therapeutic Management

The usual treatment is hormone replacement, either with an intramuscular or subcutaneous injection of vasopressin tannate in peanut oil or with a nasal spray of aqueous lysine vasopressin (Makaryus and McFarlane, 2006; Verbalis, 2003). The injectable form has the advantage of lasting 48 to 72 hours, which affords the child a full night's sleep. However, it has the disadvantage of requiring frequent injections and proper preparation of the drug.

> **NURSING TIP** To be effective, vasopressin must be thoroughly resuspended in the oil by being held under warm running water for 10 to 15 minutes and shaken vigorously before being drawn into the syringe. If this is not done, the oil may be injected minus the ADH. Small brown particles, which indicate drug dispersion, must be seen in the suspension.

Nursing Care Management

The initial objective is identification of the disorder. Because an early sign may be sudden enuresis in a child who is toilet trained, excessive thirst with bedwetting is an indication for further investigation. Another clue is persistent irritability and crying in an infant that is relieved only by bottle feedings of water. After head trauma or certain neurosurgical procedures, the development of DI can be anticipated; therefore, these patients must be closely monitored.

Assessment includes measurement of body weight, serum electrolytes, blood urea nitrogen (BUN), hematocrit, and urine specific gravity. Fluid intake and output should be carefully measured and recorded. Alert patients are able to adjust intake to urine losses, but unconscious or very young patients require closer fluid observation. In children who are not toilet trained, collection of urine specimens may require application of a urine-collecting device.

After confirmation of the diagnosis, parents need a thorough explanation regarding the condition with specific clarification that DI is a different condition from DM. They must realize that treatment is lifelong. Caregivers should be taught the correct procedure for preparation and administration of the injectable form of the drug. When children are old enough, they should be encouraged to assume full responsibility for their care.

For emergency purposes, these children should wear medical alert identification. Older children should carry the nasal spray with them for temporary relief of symptoms. School personnel need to be aware of the problem so they can grant children unrestricted use of the lavatory.

SYNDROME OF INAPPROPRIATE ANTIDIURETIC HORMONE

The disorder that results from hypersecretion of ADH from the posterior pituitary hormone is known as syndrome of inappropriate ADH secretion (SIADH). It is observed with increased frequency in a variety of conditions, especially those involving infections, tumors, or other CNS disease or trauma, and is the most common cause of hyponatremia in the pediatric population (Lin, Liu, and Lim, 2005; Rivkees, 2008).

The manifestations are directly related to fluid retention and hypotonicity. Excess ADH causes most of the filtered water to be reabsorbed from the kidneys back into central circulation. Serum osmolality is low, and urine osmolality is inappropriately elevated. When serum sodium levels are diminished to 120 mEq/L, affected children may display anorexia, nausea (and sometimes vomiting), stomach cramps, irritability, and personality changes. With progressive reduction in sodium, other neurologic signs, stupor, and convulsions may be evident. The symptoms usually disappear when the underlying disorder is corrected.

The immediate management consists of restricting fluids. Subsequent management depends on the cause and severity. Fluids continue to be restricted to one-fourth to one-half maintenance. When there are no fluid abnormalities but SIADH can be anticipated, fluids are often restricted expectantly at two-thirds to three-fourths maintenance.

Nursing Care Management

The first goal of nursing management is recognizing the presence of SIADH from symptoms described in patients at risk.

> ### ❗ NURSING ALERT
>
> Nausea, vomiting, and malaise may precede the onset of more severe stages such as disorientation, confusion, coma, and seizures (Majzoub and Muglia, 2003).

Accurately measuring intake and output, noting daily weight, and observing for signs of fluid overload are primary nursing functions, especially in children receiving IV fluids. Seizure precautions are implemented, and the child and family need education regarding the rationale for fluid restrictions. The rare child with chronic SIADH will be placed on long-term ADH-antagonizing medication, and the child and family will require instructions for its administration.

▮ DISORDERS OF THYROID FUNCTION

The thyroid gland secretes two types of hormones: thyroid hormone (TH), which consists of the hormones thyroxine (T_4) and triiodothyronine (T_3), and calcitonin. The secretion of THs is controlled by TSH from the anterior pituitary, which in turn is regulated by thyrotropin-releasing factor (TRF) from the hypothalamus as a negative feedback response. Consequently, hypothyroidism or hyperthyroidism may result from a defect in the target gland or from a disturbance in the secretion of TSH or TRF. Because the functions of T_3 and T_4 are qualitatively the same, the term *thyroid hormone* is used throughout the discussion.

The synthesis of TH depends on available sources of dietary iodine and tyrosine. The thyroid is the only endocrine gland capable of storing excess amounts of hormones for release as needed. During circulation in the bloodstream, T_4 and T_3 are bound to carrier proteins (thyroxine-binding globulin). They must be unbound before they are able to exert their metabolic effect.

The main physiologic action of TH is to regulate the basal metabolic rate and thereby control the processes of growth and tissue differentiation. Unlike GH, TH is involved in many more diverse activities that influence the growth and development of body tissues. Therefore, a deficiency of TH exerts a more profound effect on growth than that seen in hypopituitarism.

Calcitonin helps maintain blood calcium levels by decreasing the calcium concentration. Its effect is the opposite of parathyroid hormone (PTH) in that it inhibits skeletal demineralization and promotes calcium deposition in the bone.

JUVENILE HYPOTHYROIDISM

Hypothyroidism is one of the most common endocrine problems of childhood. It may be either congenital (see Chapter 9) or acquired and represents a deficiency in secretion of TH (Foley, 2001).

Beyond infancy, primary hypothyroidism may be caused by a number of defects. For example, a congenital hypoplastic thyroid gland may provide sufficient amounts of TH during the first year or two but be inadequate when rapid body growth increases demands on the gland. A partial or complete thyroidectomy for cancer or thyrotoxicosis can leave insufficient thyroid tissue to furnish hormones for body requirements. Radiotherapy for Hodgkin disease or other malignancies may lead to hypothyroidism (Pizzo and Poplack, 2010). Infectious processes may cause hypothyroidism. It can also occur when dietary iodine is deficient, although it is now rare in the United States because iodized salt is a readily available source of the nutrient.

Clinical manifestations depend on the extent of dysfunction and the child's age at onset. Primary congenital hypothyroidism is characterized by low levels of circulating THs and raised levels of TSH at birth (Macchia, 2000). If left untreated, congenital hypothyroidism causes decreased mental capacity. Improvements in newborn screening have led to earlier detection and prevention of complications (American Academy of Pediatrics [AAP], Rose, Section on Endocrinology and Committee on Genetics of the American Thyroid Association, and others, 2006). The GnRH test and baseline measurement of gonadotropin and sex hormone serum concentrations at 3 months of age are promising options for assessment of hypothalamic–pituitary—gonadal function in infants with congenital hypothyroidism (van Tijn, Schroor, Delemarre-van de Waal, and others, 2007). The presenting symptoms are decelerated growth from chronic deprivation of TH or thyromegaly. Impaired growth and development are less severe when hypothyroidism is acquired at a later age, and because brain growth is nearly complete by 2 to 3 years of age, intellectual disability and neurologic sequelae are not associated with juvenile hypothyroidism. Other manifestations are myxedematous skin changes (dry skin, puffiness around the eyes, sparse hair), constipation, lethargy, and mental decline (Box 29-5).

Therapy is TH replacement, the same as for hypothyroidism in infants, although the prompt treatment needed in infants is not required in children. L-thyroxine is administered over a period of 4 to 8 weeks to avoid symptoms of hyperthyroidism. Researchers have found that children treated early continue to have mild delays in

---

> **BOX 29-5** **CLINICAL MANIFESTATIONS OF JUVENILE HYPOTHYROIDISM**
>
> Decelerated growth
> - Less when acquired at later age
>
> Myxedematous skin changes
> - Dry skin
> - Puffiness around eyes
> - Sparse hair
> - Constipation
> - Sleepiness
> - Mental decline

---

reading, comprehension, and arithmetic but catch up by grade six (Rovet and Ehrlich, 2000). However, adolescents may demonstrate problems with memory, attention, and visuospatial processing.

Nursing Care Management

The importance of early recognition in the infant is discussed in Chapter 9. Growth cessation or retardation in a child whose growth has previously been normal should alert the observer to the possibility of hypothyroidism. After diagnosis and implementation of thyroxine therapy, the importance of compliance and periodic monitoring of response to therapy should be stressed to parents. Children should learn to take responsibility for their own health as soon as they are old enough, at about 9 or 10 years of age.

GOITER

A goiter is an enlargement or hypertrophy of the thyroid gland. It may occur with deficient (hypothyroid), excessive (hyperthyroid), or normal (euthyroid) TH secretion. It can be congenital or acquired. Congenital disease occurs as a result of maternal administration of antithyroid drugs or iodides during pregnancy or as an inborn error of TH production. Acquired disease can result from increased secretion of pituitary TSH in response to decreased circulating levels of TH or from infiltrative neoplastic or inflammatory processes. In most children, goiter is caused by chronic autoimmune thyroiditis (deVries, Bulvik, and Phillip, 2009). In areas where dietary iodine (essential for TH production) is deficient, goiter can be endemic.

Enlargement of the thyroid gland may be mild and noticeable only when there is an increased demand for TH (e.g., during periods of rapid growth). Enlargement of the thyroid at birth can be sufficient to cause severe respiratory distress. Colloid goiters are diffuse, benign, and occur more frequently in adolescent girls. Thyroid function is normal, and the gland will gradually decrease over several years without treatment. TH replacement may be necessary to treat the hypothyroidism and reverse the TSH effect on the gland.

Nursing Care Management

Large goiters are identified by their obvious appearance. In older children, each lobe of the thyroid should be approximately the same as the terminal phalanx of the child's thumb (deVries, Bulvik, and Phillip, 2009). Smaller nodules may be evident only on palpation. Benign enlargement of the thyroid gland may occur during adolescence and should not be confused with pathologic states. Nodules rarely are caused by a cancerous tumor but always require evaluation. Questions regarding exposure to radiation should be included in the assessment.

> **! NURSING ALERT**
>
> If an infant is born with a goiter, immediate precautions are instituted for emergency ventilation, such as supplemental oxygen and a tracheostomy set nearby. Hyperextension of the neck often facilitates breathing.

Immediate surgery to remove part of the gland may be lifesaving in infants born with a goiter. When thyroid replacement is necessary, parents have the same needs regarding its administration as discussed for the parents of children who have hypothyroidism (see Chapter 9).

LYMPHOCYTIC THYROIDITIS

Lymphocytic thyroiditis (Hashimoto disease, chronic autoimmune thyroiditis) is the most common cause of thyroid disease in children and adolescents and accounts for the largest percentage of juvenile hypothyroidism (Szymborska and Staroszczyk, 2000). It accounts for many of the enlarged thyroid glands formerly designated *thyroid hyperplasia of adolescence* or *adolescent goiter*. Although it can occur during the first 3 years of life, it occurs more frequently after age 6 years. It reaches a peak incidence during adolescence, and there is evidence that the disease is self-limiting. The presence of a goiter and elevated thyroglobulin antibody with progressive increase in both thyroid peroxidase antibody and TSH may be predictive factors for future development of hypothyroidism (Radetti, Gottardi, Bona, and others, 2006).

The presence of the enlarged thyroid gland is usually detected during a routine examination, although it may be noted by parents when the child swallows. In most children, the entire gland is enlarged symmetrically (although it may be asymmetric) and is firm, freely movable, and nontender. There may be manifestations of moderate tracheal compression (sense of fullness, hoarseness, and dysphagia), but it is extremely rare for a nontoxic diffuse goiter to enlarge to the extent that it causes mechanical obstruction. Most children are euthyroid, but some display symptoms of hypothyroidism, including delayed growth, puberty, and declining school performance. Other signs suggestive of thyroiditis are found in Box 29-6.

> **BOX 29-6 CLINICAL MANIFESTATIONS OF LYMPHOCYTIC THYROIDITIS**
>
> **Enlarged Thyroid Gland**
> Usually symmetric
> Firm
> Freely movable
> Nontender
>
> **Tracheal Compression**
> Sense of fullness
> Hoarseness
> Dysphagia
>
> **Hyperthyroidism (Possible)**
> Nervousness
> Irritability
> Increased sweating
> Hyperactivity

Diagnostic Evaluation

Thyroid function test results are usually normal, although TSH levels may be slightly or moderately elevated. With progressive disease, the T_4 decreases followed by a decrease in T_3 levels and an increase in TSH. The majority of children have antithyroid antibody titers. However, levels in children are lower than in adults; therefore, repeated measurements may be needed in doubtful cases because titers may increase later in the disease.

Therapeutic Management

In many cases, the goiter is transient and asymptomatic and regresses spontaneously within a year or two. Therapy of a nontoxic diffuse goiter is usually simple, uncomplicated, and effective. Oral administration of TH decreases the size of the gland significantly and provides the feedback needed to suppress TSH stimulation, and the hyperplastic thyroid gland gradually regresses in size. TSH levels should be monitored, with the goal of restoring normal growth and development. Surgery is contraindicated in this disorder. Untreated patients should be evaluated periodically.

Nursing Care Management

Nursing care consists of identifying the child with thyroid enlargement, reassuring the child that the condition is probably only temporary, and reinforcing instructions for thyroid therapy.

HYPERTHYROIDISM

The largest percentage of hyperthyroidism in childhood is caused by Graves disease, which is usually associated with an enlarged thyroid gland and exophthalmos (Ma, Xie, Kuang, and others, 2006; Streetman and Khanderia, 2004; Thompson, 2002). Most cases of Graves disease in children occur between ages 6 and 15 years, with a peak incidence at 12 to 14 years of age, but the disease may be present at birth in children of thyrotoxic mothers. The incidence is five times higher in girls than in boys.

The hyperthyroidism of Graves disease is apparently caused by an autoimmune response to TSH receptors, but no specific etiology has been identified. There is definitive evidence for familial association, with a high concordance incidence in twins. Patients with Graves disease possess the histocompatibility antigens A1, B8, and DR3 (Dallas and Foley, 2003; Simmonds, Howson, Heward, and others, 2005). There may be an association with other autoimmune diseases such as rheumatoid arthritis and lupus.

The development of manifestations is highly variable. Signs and symptoms develop gradually, with an interval between onset and diagnosis of approximately 6 to 12 months. The principal clinical features are excessive motion, including irritability, hyperactivity, short attention span, tremors, insomnia, and emotional lability. Clinical manifestations are presented in Box 29-7.

Exophthalmos (protruding eyeballs), which is observed in many children, is accompanied by a wide-eyed staring expression, increased blinking, eyelid lag, lack of convergence, and absence of wrinkling of the forehead when looking upward. As protrusion of the eyeball increases, the child may not be able to completely cover the cornea with the eyelid. Visual disturbances may include blurred vision and loss of visual acuity. Ophthalmopathy can develop long before or after the onset of hyperthyroidism. A consistent pathogenic link between them has not been identified. It is now thought that Graves ophthalmopathy is a disorder of autoimmune origin caused by a complex interplay of endogenous and environmental factors (Bartalena, Tanda, Piantanida, and others, 2003).

BOX 29-7 CLINICAL MANIFESTATIONS OF HYPERTHYROIDISM (GRAVES DISEASE)

Cardinal Signs
Emotional lability
Physical restlessness, characteristically at rest
Decelerated school performance
Voracious appetite with weight loss in 50% of cases
Fatigue

Physical Signs
Tachycardia
Widened pulse pressure
Dyspnea on exertion
Exophthalmos (protruding eyeballs)
Wide-eyed, staring expression with eyelid lag
Tremor
Goiter (hypertrophy and hyperplasia)
Warm, moist skin
Accelerated linear growth
Heat intolerance (may be severe)
Hair fine and unable to hold a curl
Systolic murmurs

Thyroid Storm
Acute onset:
• Severe irritability and restlessness
• Vomiting
• Diarrhea
• Hyperthermia
• Hypertension
• Severe tachycardia
• Prostration
May progress rapidly to:
• Delirium
• Coma
• Death

Diagnostic Evaluation

The presence of a thyroid mass in a child requires a thorough history, including inquiry into prior irradiation to the head and neck and exposure to a goitrogen. The diagnosis is established on the basis of increased levels of T_4 and T_3. TSH is suppressed to unmeasurable levels (Ma, Xie, Kuang, and others, 2006). Graves disease is confirmed by measurement of thyroid-stimulating immunoglobulin.

Therapeutic Management

Therapy for hyperthyroidism is controversial, but all methods are directed toward retarding the rate of hormone secretion. The three acceptable modes available are antithyroid drugs (methimazole), which interferes with the biosynthesis of TH; subtotal thyroidectomy; and ablation with radioiodine (^{131}I iodide) (Rivkees and Cornelius, 2003; Streetman and Khanderia, 2004). Each is effective, but each has advantages and disadvantages. Pharmacologic therapy may induce a remission, and treatment may be discontinued. However, relapse may occur. Radioactive iodine ablation is usually effective but response may be slower, and there have been concerns about a possible link

to thyroid cancer in younger children. Surgery is often used when other treatments are not effective. These children require lifelong monitoring.

When affected children exhibit signs and symptoms of hyperthyroidism (e.g., increased weight loss, pulse, pulse pressure, and blood pressure), their activity should be limited to classwork only. Vigorous exercise is restricted until thyroid levels are decreased to normal or near-normal values.

Thyrotoxicosis (thyroid "crisis" or thyroid "storm") may occur from sudden release of the hormone. Although thyrotoxicosis is unusual in children, a crisis can be life threatening. These "storms" are evidenced by the acute onset of severe irritability and restlessness, vomiting, diarrhea, hyperthermia, hypertension, severe tachycardia, and prostration. There may be rapid progression to delirium, coma, and even death. A crisis may be precipitated by acute infection, surgical emergencies, or discontinuation of antithyroid therapy. Treatment, in addition to antithyroid drugs, is administration of β-adrenergic blocking agents (propranolol), which provide relief from the adrenergic hyperresponsiveness that produces the disturbing side effects of the reaction. Therapy is usually required for 2 to 3 weeks.

The American Thyroid Association* has an extensive website with information related to prevention, treatment, and cure of thyroid disease.

Nursing Care Management

The initial nursing objective is identification of children with hyperthyroidism. Because the clinical manifestations often appear gradually, the goiter and ophthalmic changes may not be noticed, and the excessive activity may be attributed to behavioral problems. Nurses in ambulatory settings, particularly schools, need to be alert to signs that suggest this disorder, especially weight loss despite an excellent appetite, academic difficulties resulting from a short attention span and inability to sit still, unexplained fatigue and sleeplessness, and difficulty with fine motor skills such as writing. Exophthalmos may develop long before the onset of signs and symptoms of hyperthyroidism and may be the only presenting sign (Thompson, 2002). Exophthalmos is less common in adults than children (Jospe, 2001).

Much of these children's care is related to treating physical symptoms before a response to drug therapy is achieved. A regular routine is beneficial in providing frequent rest periods, minimizing the stress of coping with unexpected demands, and meeting the children's needs promptly. Physical activity is restricted. Mood swings and irritability can disrupt interpersonal relationships, creating difficulties within and outside the home. The child and parents should be encouraged to express feelings about the behavior and its effect on others. Heat intolerance may be minimized by the use of light cotton clothing, good ventilation, air conditioning or fans, frequent baths, and adequate hydration. Dietary requirements should be adjusted to meet the child's increased metabolic rate. Rather than three large meals, the child's appetite may be better satisfied by five or six moderate meals throughout the day.

When therapy is instituted, the nurse explains the drug regimen, emphasizing the importance of observing for side effects of antithyroid drugs. These include skin rashes, arthralgias, vasculitis, liver dysfunction, and agranulocytosis. Parents should also be aware of the signs of hypothyroidism, which can occur from overdose of the drugs. The most common indications are lethargy and somnolence.

---

*6066 Leesburg Pike, Suite 550, Falls Church, VA 22041; 800-THYROID; e-mail: thyroid@thyroid.org; http://www.thyroid.org.

> **! NURSING ALERT**
>
> Children being treated with methimazole must be carefully monitored for side effects of the drug. Because sore throat and fever accompany the grave complication of leukopenia, these children should be seen by a practitioner if such symptoms occur. Parents and children should be taught to recognize and report symptoms immediately.

> **! NURSING ALERT**
>
> The earliest indication of hypoparathyroidism may be anxiety and mental depression followed by paresthesia and evidence of heightened neuromuscular excitability, such as:
>
> **Chvostek sign**—Facial muscle spasm elicited by tapping the facial nerve in the region of the parotid gland
>
> **Trousseau sign**—Carpal spasm elicited by pressure applied to nerves of the upper arm
>
> **Tetany**—Carpopedal spasm (sharp flexion of wrist and ankle joints), muscle twitching, cramps, seizures, and stridor

DISORDERS OF PARATHYROID FUNCTION

The parathyroid glands secrete PTH, the main function of which, along with vitamin D and calcitonin, is homeostasis of serum calcium concentration (Perheentupa, 2003). The effect of PTH on calcium is opposite that of calcitonin. The net result of the integrated action of PTH and vitamin D is maintenance of serum calcium levels within a narrow normal range and the mineralization of bone. Secretion of PTH is controlled by a negative feedback system involving the serum calcium ion concentration. Low ionized calcium levels stimulate PTH secretion, causing absorption of calcium by the target tissues; high ionized calcium concentrations suppress PTH.

HYPOPARATHYROIDISM

Hypoparathyroidism is a spectrum of disorders that result in deficient PTH. Congenital hypoparathyroidism may be caused by a specific defect in the synthesis or cellular processing of PTH or by aplasia or hypoplasia of the gland (Perheentupa, 2003).

Hypoparathyroidism can also occur secondary to other causes, including infection and autoimmune syndromes. Postoperative hypoparathyroidism may follow thyroidectomy with acute or gradual onset and be transient or permanent. Two forms of transient hypoparathyroidism may be present in newborns, both of which are the result of a relative PTH deficiency. One type is caused by maternal hyperparathyroidism or maternal DM. A more common, later form appears almost exclusively in infants fed a milk formula with a high phosphate-to-calcium ratio.

Pseudohypoparathyroidism occurs when there is a genetic defect in the cellular receptors to PTH. The result is normal parathyroid gland and PTH levels. Abnormal calcium and phosphorus levels are not affected by administration of PTH. These children typically have a short, stocky build; a round face; and abnormally shaped hands and fingers. Other endocrine dysfunction may be found concurrently (Shoback, 2008).

Clinical signs of hypoparathyroidism are found in Box 29-8. Muscle cramps are an early symptom, progressing to numbness, stiffness, and tingling in the hands and feet. A positive Chvostek or Trousseau sign or laryngeal spasms may be present. Convulsions with loss of

> **BOX 29-8   CLINICAL MANIFESTATIONS OF HYPOPARATHYROIDISM**
>
> **Pseudohypoparathyroidism**
> Short stature
> Round face
> Short, thick neck
> Short, stubby fingers and toes
> Dimpling of skin over knuckles
> Subcutaneous soft tissue calcifications
> Intellectual disability a prominent feature
>
> **Idiopathic Hypoparathyroidism**
> None of the above physical characteristics observed
> May include papilledema
> May have intellectual disability
>
> **Both Types**
> Dry, scaly, coarse skin with eruptions
> Hair often brittle
> Nails thin and brittle with characteristic transverse grooves
> Dental and enamel hypoplasia
> Muscle contractions:
> - Tetany
> - Carpopedal spasm
> - Laryngospasm (laryngeal stridor)
> - Muscle cramps and twitching
> - Positive Chvostek sign or Trousseau sign (see Nursing Alert, this page)
> - Paresthesias, tingling
>
> Neurologic:
> - Headache
> - Seizures (generalized, absence, or focal)
> - Swings of emotion
> - Loss of memory
> - Depression
> - Confusion possible
>
> Gastrointestinal:
> - Muscle cramps
> - Diarrhea
> - Vomiting
> - Retarded skeletal growth

consciousness may occur. These episodes may be preceded by abdominal discomfort, tonic rigidity, head retraction, and cyanosis. Headaches and vomiting with increased intracranial pressure and papilledema may occur and may suggest a brain tumor (Kliegman, Stanton, St. Geme, and others, 2011).

Diagnostic Evaluation

The diagnosis of hypoparathyroidism is made on the basis of clinical manifestations associated with decreased serum calcium and increased serum phosphorus. Levels of plasma PTH are low in idiopathic hypoparathyroidism but high in pseudohypoparathyroidism. End-organ responsiveness is tested by the administration of PTH with measurement of urinary cyclic adenosine monophosphate (cAMP). Kidney function tests are included in the differential diagnosis to rule out renal insufficiency. Magnesium levels should also be tested. Although bone radiograph findings are usually normal, they may demonstrate increased bone density and suppressed growth.

Therapeutic Management

The objective of treatment is to maintain normal serum calcium and phosphate levels with minimum complications. Acute or severe tetany is corrected immediately by IV and oral administration of calcium gluconate and follow-up daily doses to achieve normal levels. Twice-daily serum calcium measurements are taken to monitor the efficacy of therapy and prevent hypercalcemia. When diagnosis is confirmed, vitamin D therapy is begun. Vitamin D therapy is somewhat difficult to regulate because the drug has a prolonged onset and a long half-life. Some authorities advocate beginning with a lower dose with stepwise increases and careful monitoring of serum calcium until stable levels are achieved. Others prefer rapid induction with higher doses and rapid reduction to lower maintenance levels (Cooper and Gittoes, 2008; Kliegman, Stanton, St. Geme, and others, 2011).

Long-term management usually consists of vitamin D and oral calcium supplementation. Blood calcium and phosphorus are monitored frequently until the levels have stabilized and then routinely thereafter. Renal function, blood pressure, and serum vitamin D levels are measured every 6 months. Serum magnesium levels are measured to permit detection of hypomagnesemia, which may raise the requirement for vitamin D.

Nursing Care Management

The initial objective is recognition of hypocalcemia. Unexplained convulsions, irritability (especially to external stimuli), gastrointestinal symptoms (diarrhea, vomiting, cramping), and positive signs of tetany should lead the nurse to suspect this disorder. Much of the initial nursing care is related to the physical manifestations and includes institution of seizure and safety precautions; reduction of environmental stimuli; and observation for signs of laryngospasm such as stridor, hoarseness, and a feeling of tightness in the throat. A tracheostomy set and injectable calcium gluconate should be available for emergency use. The administration of calcium gluconate requires precautions against extravasation of the drug and tissue destruction.

After initiating treatment, the nurse discusses with the parents the need for continuous daily administration of calcium salts and vitamin D. Because vitamin D toxicity can be a serious consequence of therapy, parents are advised to watch for signs that include weakness, fatigue, lassitude, headache, nausea, vomiting, and diarrhea. Early renal impairment is manifested by polyuria, polydipsia, and nocturia.

HYPERPARATHYROIDISM

Hyperparathyroidism is rare in childhood but can be primary or secondary. The most common cause of primary hyperparathyroidism is adenoma of the gland (Kliegman, Stanton, St. Geme, and others, 2011). The most common causes of secondary hyperparathyroidism are chronic renal disease, renal osteodystrophy, and congenital anomalies of the urinary tract. The common factor is hypercalcemia. The clinical signs of hyperparathyroidism are listed in Box 29-9.

Diagnostic Evaluation

Blood studies to identify elevated calcium and decreased phosphorus levels are routinely performed. Measurement of PTH, as well as several tests to isolate the cause of the hypercalcemia, such as renal function studies, should be included. Other procedures used to substantiate the physiologic consequences of the disorder include electrocardiography and radiographic bone surveys.

> **BOX 29-9 CLINICAL MANIFESTATIONS OF HYPERPARATHYROIDISM**
>
> **Gastrointestinal**
> Nausea
> Vomiting
> Abdominal discomfort
> Constipation
>
> **Central Nervous System**
> Delusions
> Confusion
> Hallucinations
> Impaired memory
> Lack of interest and initiative
> Depression
> Varying levels of consciousness
>
> **Neuromuscular**
> Weakness
> Easy fatigability
> Muscle atrophy (especially proximal muscles of lower limbs)
> Tongue twitching
> Paresthesias in extremities
>
> **Skeletal**
> Vague bone pain
> Subperiosteal resorption of phalanges
> Spontaneous fractures
> Absence of lamina dura around teeth
>
> **Renal**
> Polyuria
> Polydipsia
> Renal colic
> Hypertension

Therapeutic Management

Treatment depends on the cause of hyperparathyroidism. The treatment of primary hyperparathyroidism is surgical removal of the tumor or hyperplastic tissue. Treatment of secondary hyperparathyroidism is directed at the underlying contributing cause, which subsequently restores the serum calcium balance. However, in some instances, such as in chronic renal failure, the underlying disorder is irreversible. In this case, treatment is aimed at raising serum calcium levels to inhibit the stimulatory effect of low levels on the parathyroids. This includes oral administration of calcium salts, high doses of vitamin D to enhance calcium absorption, a low-phosphorus diet, and administration of a phosphorus-mobilizing aluminum hydroxide to reduce phosphate absorption.

Nursing Care Management

The initial nursing objective is recognition of the disorder. Because secondary hyperparathyroidism is a consequence of chronic renal failure, the nurse is always alert to signs that suggest this complication, especially bone pain and fractures. Because urinary symptoms are the earliest indication, assessment of other body systems for evidence of high calcium levels is indicated when polyuria and polydipsia coexist. Clues to the possibility of hyperparathyroidism include change in behavior, especially inactivity; unexplained gastrointestinal symptoms; and cardiac irregularities.

DISORDERS OF ADRENAL FUNCTION

The adrenal cortex secretes three main groups of hormones collectively called steroids and classified according to their biologic activity: (1) glucocorticoids (cortisol, corticosterone), (2) mineralocorticoids (aldosterone), and (3) sex steroids (androgens, estrogens, and progestins). Alterations in the levels of these hormones produce significant dysfunction in a variety of body tissues and organs. Because the adrenocortical cells are capable of producing any of the steroids, pathologic conditions may result in a deficiency or an excess of more than one type of hormone. However, most are rare in children.

The adrenal medulla secretes the catecholamines epinephrine and norepinephrine. Both hormones have essentially the same effects on various organs as those caused by direct sympathetic stimulation except that the hormonal effects last several times longer. Catecholamine-secreting tumors are the primary cause of adrenal medullary hyperfunction.

ACUTE ADRENOCORTICAL INSUFFICIENCY

The acute form of adrenocortical insufficiency (adrenal crisis) may have a number of causes during childhood. Although a rare disorder, some of the more common etiologic factors include hemorrhage into the gland from trauma, which may be caused by a prolonged, difficult labor; fulminating infections, such as meningococcemia, which result in hemorrhage and necrosis (Waterhouse-Friderichsen syndrome); abrupt withdrawal of exogenous sources of cortisone or failure to increase exogenous supplies during stress; or congenital adrenogenital hyperplasia of the salt-losing type.

Early symptoms of adrenocortical insufficiency include increased irritability, headache, diffuse abdominal pain, weakness, nausea and vomiting, and diarrhea. Other clinical signs are found in Box 29-10. In newborns, adrenal crisis is accompanied by extreme hyperpyrexia (high temperature), tachypnea, cyanosis, and seizures. Usually there is no evidence of infection or purpura. However, hemorrhage into the adrenal gland may be evident as a palpable retroperitoneal mass.

Diagnostic Evaluation

There is no rapid, definitive test for confirmation of acute adrenocortical insufficiency. Routine procedures such as measurement of plasma cortisol levels are too time consuming to be practical. Therefore, diagnosis is usually made based on clinical presentation, especially when a fulminating sepsis is accompanied by hemorrhagic manifestations and signs of circulatory collapse despite adequate antibiotic therapy. Because there is no real danger in administering a cortisol preparation for a short period, treatment should be instituted immediately. Improvement with cortisol therapy confirms the diagnosis.

Therapeutic Management

Treatment involves replacement of cortisol, replacement of body fluids to combat dehydration and hypovolemia, administration of glucose solutions to correct hypoglycemia, and specific antibiotic therapy in the presence of infection. Initially, IV hydrocortisone (Solu-Cortef) is administered. Normal saline containing 5% glucose is given parenterally to replace lost fluid, electrolytes, and glucose. If hemorrhage has been severe, whole blood may be replaced. In the event that these

---

BOX 29-10   CLINICAL MANIFESTATIONS OF ACUTE ADRENOCORTICAL INSUFFICIENCY

Early Symptoms
Increased irritability
Headache
Diffuse abdominal pain
Weakness
Nausea and vomiting
Diarrhea

Generalized Hemorrhagic Manifestations (Waterhouse-Friderichsen Syndrome)
Fever (increases as condition worsens)
Central nervous system signs:
- Nuchal rigidity
- Seizures
- Stupor
- Coma

Shocklike State
Weak, rapid pulse
Decreased blood pressure
Shallow respirations
Cold, clammy skin
Cyanosis
Circulatory collapse (terminal event)

Newborn
Hyperpyrexia
Tachypnea
Cyanosis
Seizures
Gland evident as palpable retroperitoneal mass (hemorrhagic)

---

measures do not reverse the circulatory collapse, vasopressors are used for immediate vasoconstriction and elevation of blood pressure.

After the child's condition has been stabilized, oral doses of cortisone, fluids, and salt are given, similar to the regimen used for chronic adrenal insufficiency. To maintain sodium retention, aldosterone is replaced by synthetic salt-retaining steroids.

Nursing Care Management

Because of the abrupt onset and potentially fatal outcome of this condition, prompt recognition is essential. Vital signs and blood pressure are taken every 15 minutes to monitor the hyperpyrexia and shocklike state. Seizure precautions are instituted because convulsions from the elevated temperature are not uncommon. As soon as therapy is instituted, the nurse should monitor the child's response to fluid and cortisol replacement. Whereas too rapid administration of fluids can precipitate cardiac failure, overdosage with cortisol produces hypotension and a sudden fall in temperature.

When the acute phase is over and the hypovolemia has been corrected, the child is given oral fluids, such as small quantities of ginger ale, fruit juice, or salted broth. Too rapid ingestion of oral fluids may induce vomiting, which increases dehydration. Therefore, the nurse should plan a gradual schedule for reintroducing liquids.

The sudden, severe nature of this disorder necessitates a great deal of emotional support for the child and family. The child may be placed in an intensive care unit where the surroundings are strange and frightening. Despite the need for emergency intervention, the nurse must be sensitive to the family's psychologic needs and prepare them for each procedure even if this is a brief statement such as "The IV infusion is necessary to replace fluid that the child is losing." Because recovery within 24 hours is often dramatic, the nurse should keep the parents apprised of the child's condition, emphasizing signs of improvement, such as a lowered temperature and elevated blood pressure.

CHRONIC ADRENOCORTICAL INSUFFICIENCY (ADDISON DISEASE)

Chronic adrenocortical insufficiency is rare in children. Causes include infections, destructive lesion of the adrenal gland or neoplasms, autoimmune processes, or idiopathic. At one time, generalized tuberculosis was the leading cause of adrenal gland destruction.

Evidence of this disorder is usually gradual in onset because 90% of adrenal tissue must be nonfunctional before signs of insufficiency are manifested. However, during periods of stress, when demands for additional cortisol are increased, symptoms of acute insufficiency may appear in a previously well child (Box 29-11).

Definitive diagnosis is based on measurements of functional cortisol reserve. The fasting serum cortisol and urinary 17-hydroxy-corticosteroid levels are low and fail to rise, and plasma **adrenocorticotropic hormone (ACTH)** levels are elevated with corticotropin (ACTH) stimulation, the definitive test for the disease.

Therapeutic Management

Treatment involves replacement of **glucocorticoids (cortisol)** and **mineralocorticoids (aldosterone)**. Some children are able to be maintained solely on oral supplements of cortisol (cortisone or hydrocortisone preparations) with a liberal intake of salt. During stressful situations, such as fever, infection, emotional upset, or surgery, the dosage must be tripled to accommodate the body's increased need for glucocorticoids. Failure to meet this requirement will precipitate an acute crisis. Overdosage produces appearance of cushingoid signs.

Children with more severe states of chronic adrenal insufficiency require mineralocorticoid replacement to maintain fluid and electrolyte balance. Other forms of therapy include monthly injections of desoxycorticosterone acetate or implantation of desoxycorticosterone acetate pellets subcutaneously every 9 to 12 months.

Nursing Care Management

After the disorder is diagnosed, parents need guidance concerning drug therapy. They must be aware of the continuous need for cortisol replacement. Sudden termination of the drug because of inadequate

BOX 29-11   CLINICAL MANIFESTATIONS OF CHRONIC ADRENOCORTICAL INSUFFICIENCY

Neurologic Symptoms
Muscular weakness
Mental fatigue
Irritability, apathy, and negativism
Increased sleeping, listlessness

Pigmentary Changes
Previous scars
Palmar creases
Mucous membranes
Hair
Hyperpigmentation over pressure points (elbows, knees, or waist)
Less frequently, vitiligo (loss of pigmentation)

Gastrointestinal Symptoms
Dehydration
Anorexia
Weight loss

Circulatory Symptoms
Hypotension
Small heart size
Dizziness
Syncopal (fainting) attacks

Hypoglycemia
Headache
Hunger
Weakness
Trembling
Sweating

Other Signs (Seen in Some Children)
Recurrent, unexplained seizures
Intense craving for salt
Acute abdominal pain
Electrolyte imbalances

supplies or inability to ingest the oral form because of vomiting places the child in danger of an acute adrenal crisis. Therefore, parents should always have a spare supply of the medication in the home. Ideally, they will have a prefilled syringe of hydrocortisone and be instructed in proper technique for intramuscular administration of the drug in case of crisis. Unnecessary administration of cortisone will not harm the child, but if it is needed, it may be lifesaving. Any evidence of acute insufficiency should be reported to the practitioner immediately.

Parents also need to be aware of side effects of the drugs. Undesirable side effects of cortisone include gastric irritation, which is minimized by ingestion with food or the use of an antacid; increased excitability and sleeplessness; weight gain, which may require dietary management to prevent obesity; and, rarely, behavioral changes, including depression or euphoria. Parents should be aware of signs of overdose and report these to the practitioner. In addition, the drug has a bitter taste, which creates a challenge for nurses and parents in its administration.

Adapted from Magiakou MA, Mastorakos G, Oldfield EH, and others: Cushing's syndrome in children and adolescents: presentation, diagnosis, and therapy, *N Engl J Med* 331(10):629–636, 1994. *ACTH,* Adrenocorticotropic hormone.

Because the body cannot supply endogenous sources of cortical hormones during times of stress, the home environment should be stable and relatively unstressful. Parents need to be aware that during periods of emotional or physical crisis, the child requires additional hormone replacement. The child should wear medical identification, such as a bracelet, to permit medical personnel to adjust requirements during emergency care.

CUSHING SYNDROME

Cushing syndrome is a characteristic group of manifestations caused by excessive circulating free cortisol. It can result from a variety of causes, which generally fall into one of five categories (Box 29-12). Cushing syndrome in young children may be caused by an adrenal tumor (Moshang, 2003).

Cushing syndrome is uncommon in children. When seen, it is often caused by excessive or prolonged steroid therapy that produces a cushingoid appearance (Fig. 29-2). This condition is reversible after the steroids are gradually discontinued. Abrupt withdrawal will precipitate acute adrenal insufficiency. Gradual withdrawal of exogenous supplies is necessary to allow the anterior pituitary an opportunity to secrete increasing amounts of ACTH to stimulate the adrenals to produce cortisol.

Clinical Manifestations

Because the actions of cortisol are widespread, clinical manifestations are equally profound and diverse. The symptoms that produce changes in physical appearance occur early in the disorder and are of considerable concern to school-age and older children. The physiologic disturbances, such as hyperglycemia, susceptibility to infection, hypertension, and hypokalemia, may have life-threatening consequences unless recognized early and treated successfully. Children with short stature may be responding to increased cortisol levels, resulting in Cushing syndrome. Cortisol inhibits the action of GH.

Diagnostic Evaluation

Several tests are helpful in confirming excess Cushing syndrome. Serum cortisol levels should be measured at midnight and in the morning along with corticotropin hormone, urinary free cortisol, fasting blood glucose levels for hyperglycemia, serum electrolyte levels for hypokalemia and alkalosis, and 24-hour urinary levels of elevated 17-hydroxycorticoids and 17-ketosteroids. Imaging of the pituitary

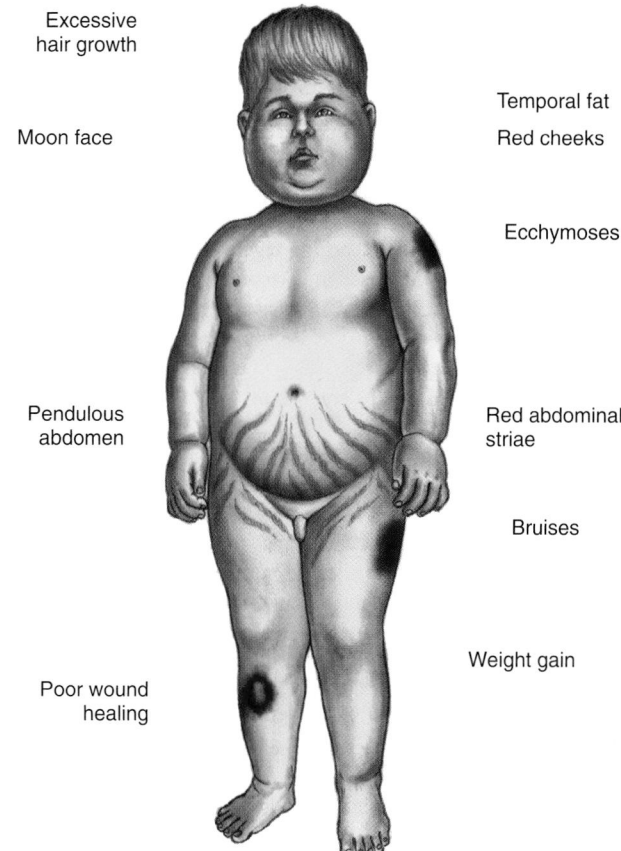

Excessive hair growth

Moon face

Temporal fat
Red cheeks

Ecchymoses

Pendulous abdomen

Red abdominal striae

Bruises

Weight gain

Poor wound healing

FIG 29-2 Characteristics of Cushing syndrome.

and adrenal glands to assess for tumors, bone density studies for evidence of osteoporosis, and skull radiographs to determine enlargement of the sella turcica may also aid in the diagnosis. Another procedure used to establish a more definitive diagnosis is the dexamethasone (cortisone) suppression test (Nieman and Ilias, 2005). Administration of an exogenous supply of cortisone normally suppresses ACTH production. However, in individuals with Cushing syndrome, cortisol levels remain elevated. This test is helpful in differentiating between children who are obese and those who appear to have cushingoid features.

Therapeutic Management

Treatment depends on the cause. In most cases, surgical intervention involves bilateral adrenalectomy and postoperative replacement of the cortical hormones (the therapy for this is the same as that outlined for chronic adrenocortical insufficiency). If a pituitary tumor is found, surgical extirpation or irradiation may be chosen. In either of these instances, treatment of panhypopituitarism with replacement of GH, thyroid extract, ADH, gonadotropins, and steroids may be necessary for an indefinite period (Nieman and Ilias, 2005).

Nursing Care Management

Nursing care also depends on the cause. When cushingoid features are caused by steroid therapy, the effects may be lessened with administration of the drug early in the morning and on an alternate-day basis. Giving the drug early in the day maintains the normal diurnal pattern of cortisol secretion. If given during the evening, it is more likely to produce symptoms because endogenous cortisol levels are already low, and the additional supply exerts more pronounced effects. An alternate-day schedule allows the anterior pituitary an opportunity to maintain more normal hypothalamic–pituitary–adrenal control mechanisms.

If an organic cause is found, nursing care is related to the treatment regimen. Although a bilateral adrenalectomy permanently solves one condition, it reciprocally produces another syndrome. Before surgery, parents need to be adequately informed of the operative benefits and disadvantages. Postoperative teaching regarding drug replacement is the same as discussed in the previous section.

> **! NURSING ALERT**
>
> Postoperative complications of adrenalectomy are related to the sudden withdrawal of cortisol. Observe for shocklike symptoms (e.g., hypotension, hyperpyrexia).

Anorexia and nausea and vomiting are common and may be improved with the use of nasogastric decompression. Muscle and joint pain may be severe, requiring use of analgesics. The psychologic depression can be profound and may not improve for months. Parents should be aware of the physiologic reasons behind these symptoms in order to be supportive of the child.

CONGENITAL ADRENAL HYPERPLASIA

Congenital adrenal hyperplasia (CAH) is a family of disorders caused by decreased enzyme activity required for cortisol production in the adrenal cortex. The adrenal gland produces excessive amounts of cortisol precursors and androgens to compensate. The most common defect is 21-hydroxylase deficiency, which constitutes more than 90% of all cases of CAH (AAP, Section on Endocrinology and Committee on Genetics, 2000, reaffirmed 2005). This deficiency is an autosomal recessive disorder that results in improper steroid hormone synthesis. It occurs in approximately 1 per 12,000 to 15,000 births and can be life threatening in its most severe form (Glatt, Garzon, and Popovic, 2005).

Excessive androgens cause masculinization of the urogenital system at approximately the tenth week of fetal development. The most pronounced abnormalities occur in girls, who are born with varying degrees of ambiguous genitalia. Masculinization of external genitalia causes the clitoris to enlarge so that it appears as a small phallus. Fusion of the labia produces a saclike structure resembling the scrotum without testes. However, no abnormal changes occur in the internal sexual organs, although the vaginal orifice is usually closed by the fused labia. The label *ambiguous genitalia* should be applied to any infant with hypospadias or micropenis and no palpable gonads, and a diagnostic evaluation for CAH should be contemplated. Males do not display genital abnormalities at birth (New and Ghizzoni, 2003).

Increased pigmentation of skin creases and genitalia caused by increased ACTH may be a subtle sign of adrenal insufficiency. A saltwasting crisis frequently occurs, usually within the first few weeks of life (Kliegman, Stanton, St. Geme, and others, 2011). Infants fail to gain weight, and hyponatremia and hyperkalemia may be significant. Cardiac arrest can occur.

Untreated CAH results in early sexual maturation, with enlargement of the external sexual organs; development of axillary, pubic, and facial hair; deepening of the voice; acne; and a marked increase in musculature with changes toward an adult male physique. However, in contrast to precocious puberty, breasts do not develop in girls, and

they remain amenorrheic and infertile. In boys, the testes remain small, and spermatogenesis does not occur. In both sexes, linear growth is accelerated, and epiphyseal closure is premature, resulting in short stature by the end of puberty.

Diagnostic Evaluation

Clinical diagnosis is initially based on congenital abnormalities that lead to difficulty in assigning sex to the newborn and on signs and symptoms of adrenal insufficiency. Newborn screening is currently done in all 50 U.S. states by measurement of the cortisol precursor 17-hydroxyprogesterone. Definitive diagnosis is confirmed by evidence of increased 17-ketosteroid levels in most types of CAH (AAP, Section on Endocrinology and Committee on Genetics, 2000, reaffirmed 2005). In complete 21-hydroxylase deficiency, blood electrolytes demonstrate loss of sodium and chloride and elevation of potassium. In older children, bone age is advanced, and linear growth is increased. DNA analysis for positive sex determination and to rule out any other genetic abnormality (e.g., Turner syndrome) is always done in any case of ambiguous genitalia.

Another test that can be used to visualize the presence of pelvic structures is ultrasonography, a noninvasive, painless imaging technique that does not require anesthesia or sedation. It is especially useful in CAH because it readily identifies the absence or presence of female reproductive organs or male testes in a newborn or child with ambiguous genitalia. Because ultrasonography yields immediate results, it has the advantage of determining the child's gender long before the more complex laboratory results for chromosome analysis or steroid levels are available.

Therapeutic Management

After diagnosis is confirmed, medical management includes administration of glucocorticoids to suppress the abnormally high secretions of ACTH and adrenal androgens (Glatt, Garzon, and Popovic, 2005). If cortisone is begun early enough, it is very effective. Cortisone depresses the secretion of ACTH by the adenohypophysis, which in turn inhibits the secretion of adrenocorticosteroids, which stems the progressive virilization. The signs and symptoms of masculinization in girls gradually disappear, and excessive early linear growth is slowed. Puberty occurs normally at the appropriate age.

The recommended oral dosage is divided to simulate the normal diurnal pattern of ACTH secretion. Because these children are unable to produce cortisol in response to stress, it is necessary to increase the dosage during episodes of infection, fever, surgery, or other stresses. Acute emergencies require immediate IV or intramuscular administration. Children with the salt-losing type of CAH require aldosterone replacement, as outlined under chronic adrenal insufficiency, and supplementary dietary salt. Frequent laboratory tests are conducted to assess the effects on electrolytes, hormonal profiles, and renin levels. The frequency of testing is individualized to the child.

Gender assignment and surgical intervention in the newborn with ambiguous genitalia is complex and controversial. It is a significant stress for families, who need support from a multidisciplinary team of experienced specialists. Factors that influence gender assignment include genetic diagnosis, genital appearance, surgical options, fertility, and family and cultural preferences. Generally, genetically female (46XX) infants should be raised as girls. Early reconstructive surgery should be considered only in the case of severe virilization (Lee, Houk, Ahmed, and others, 2006). Emphasis is on functional rather than cosmetic outcomes, and surgery can often be delayed. Reports concerning sexual satisfaction after partial clitoridectomy indicate that the capacity for orgasm and sexual gratification is not necessarily impaired. Male infants may require phallic reconstruction by an experienced surgeon.

Unfortunately, not all children with CAH are diagnosed at birth and raised in accordance with their genetic sex. Particularly in the case of affected females, masculinization of the external genitalia may have led to sex assignment as a male. In males, diagnosis is usually delayed until early childhood, when signs of virilism appear. In these situations, it is advisable to continue rearing the child as a male in accordance with assigned sex and phenotype. Hormone replacement may be required to permit linear growth and to initiate male pubertal changes. Surgery is usually indicated to remove the female organs and reconstruct the phallus for satisfactory sexual relations. These individuals are not fertile.

Nursing Care Management

Of major importance is recognition of ambiguous genitalia and diagnostic confirmation in newborns. Parents need assistance in understanding and accepting the condition and time to grieve for the loss of perfection in their newborn child. As soon as the sex is determined, parents should be informed of the findings and encouraged to choose an appropriate name, and the child should be identified as a male or female with no reference to ambiguous sex.

In general, rearing a genetically female child as a girl is preferred because of the success of surgical intervention and the satisfactory results with hormones in reversing virilism and providing a prospect of normal puberty and the ability to conceive. This is in contrast to the choice of rearing the child as a boy, in which case the child is sterile and may never be able to function satisfactorily in heterosexual relationships. If the parents persist in their decision to assign a male sex to a genetically female child, a psychologic consultation should be requested to explore their motivations and ensure their understanding of the future consequences for the child.

Nursing care management regarding cortisol and aldosterone replacement are the same as those discussed for chronic adrenocortical insufficiency. Because infants are especially prone to dehydration and salt-losing crises, parents need to be aware of signs of dehydration and the urgency of immediate medical intervention to stabilize the child's condition. Parents should have injectable hydrocortisone available and know how to prepare and administer the intramuscular injection (see Chapter 22).

In the unfortunate situation in which the sex is erroneously assigned and the correct sex determined later, parents need a great deal of help in understanding the reason for the incorrect sex identification and the options for sex reassignment or medical-surgical intervention.

Parents should be referred for genetic counseling before they conceive another child because CAH is an autosomal recessive disorder. Prenatal diagnosis and treatment are available.

> ### ⚠ NURSING ALERT
>
> The parents should be advised that there is no physical harm in treating for suspected adrenal insufficiency that is not present, but the consequence of not treating acute adrenal insufficiency can be fatal.

PHEOCHROMOCYTOMA

Pheochromocytoma is a rare tumor characterized by secretion of catecholamines. The tumor most commonly arises from the chromaffin cells of the adrenal medulla but may occur wherever these cells are found, such as along the paraganglia of the aorta or thoracolumbar sympathetic chain (Pacak, Eisenhofer, Ahlman, and others, 2007).

Approximately 10% of these tumors are located in extraadrenal sites. In children, they are frequently bilateral or multiple and are generally benign. Often there is a familial transmission of the condition as an autosomal dominant trait (Kliegman, Stanton, St. Geme, and others, 2011).

The clinical manifestations of pheochromocytoma are caused by an increased production of catecholamines, producing hypertension, tachycardia, headache, decreased gastrointestinal activity with resultant constipation, increased metabolism with anorexia, weight loss, hyperglycemia, polyuria, polydipsia, hyperventilation, nervousness, heat intolerance, and diaphoresis. In severe cases, signs of congestive heart failure are evident.

Diagnostic Evaluation

The clinical manifestations mimic those of other disorders, such as hyperthyroidism or DM. Usually the tumor is identified by computed tomography (CT) scan or magnetic resonance imaging (MRI). Definitive tests include 24-hour measurement of urinary levels of the catecholamine metabolites, histamine stimulation, and α-adrenergic blocking agents.

Therapeutic Management

Definitive treatment consists of surgical removal of the tumor. In children, the tumors may be bilateral, requiring a bilateral adrenalectomy and lifelong glucocorticoid and mineralocorticoid therapy. The major complications that can occur during surgery are severe hypertension, tachyarrhythmias, and hypotension. The first two are caused by excessive release of catecholamines during manipulation of the tumor, and the latter results from catecholamine withdrawal and hypovolemic shock.

Preoperative medication to inhibit the effects of catecholamines is begun 1 to 3 weeks before surgery to prevent these complications. The major group of drugs used is the α-adrenergic blocking agents with or without β-adrenergic blocking agents. The most commonly used β-adrenergic blocker is phenoxybenzamine (Dibenzyline), a long-acting medication given orally every 12 hours. The shorter acting phentolamine (Regitine) is equally effective but less satisfactory for long-term use, although it is useful for acute hypertension. To control catecholamine release when β-adrenergic blocking agents are inadequate, the child is given β-adrenergic blocking agents.

Success of therapy is judged by lowering of blood pressure to normal, absence of hypertensive attacks (flushing or blanching, fainting, headache, palpitations, tachycardia, nausea and vomiting, profuse sweating), heat tolerance, a decrease in perspiration, and disappearance of hyperglycemia. A disadvantage of these drugs is their inability to block the effects of catecholamines on β receptors.

Nursing Care Management

An initial nursing objective is identification of children with this disorder. Outstanding clues are hypertension and hypertensive attacks. Because of behavioral changes (nervousness, excitability, overactivity, and even psychosis), increased cardiac and respiratory activity may appear to be related to an acute anxiety attack. Therefore, a careful history of the onset of symptoms and association with stressful events is helpful in distinguishing between an organic and a psychologic cause for the symptoms.

Preoperative nursing care involves frequent monitoring of vital signs and observation for evidence of hypertensive attacks and congestive heart failure. Therapeutic effects are evidenced by normal vital signs and absence of glycosuria. Daily blood glucose levels, urine acetone, and any signs of hyperglycemia are noted and reported immediately.

> **! NURSING ALERT**
>
> Do not palpate the mass. Preoperative palpation of the mass releases catecholamines, which can stimulate severe hypertension and tachyarrhythmias.

The environment is made conducive to rest and free of emotional stress. This requires adequate preparation during hospital admission and before surgery. Parents are encouraged to room-in with their child and to participate in care. Play activities need to be tailored to the child's energy level without being overly strenuous or challenging because these can increase metabolic rate and promote frustration and anxiety.

After surgery, the child is observed for signs of shock from removal of excess catecholamines. If a bilateral adrenalectomy was performed, the nursing interventions are those discussed for chronic adrenocortical insufficiency.

DISORDERS OF PANCREATIC HORMONE SECRETION

DIABETES MELLITUS

Diabetes mellitus is a chronic disorder of metabolism characterized by a partial or complete deficiency of the hormone **insulin**. It is the most common metabolic disease, resulting in metabolic adjustment or physiologic change in almost all areas of the body. The most recent statistics (2010) indicate that in the United States, approximately 215,000 children younger than age 20 years have either type 1 or type 2 diabetes (Centers for Disease Control and Prevention [CDC], 2010). The odds are higher for African-American and Hispanic children: nearly 50% of them will develop diabetes (Urrutia-Rojas and Menchaca, 2006). DM in children can occur at any age but has a peak incidence between ages 10 and 15 years, with 75% diagnosed before 18 years of age. The incidence in boys is slightly higher than in girls (1 : 1 to 1.2 : 1).

Traditionally, DM had been classified according to the type of treatment needed. The old categories were insulin-dependent diabetes mellitus (IDDM), or type I, and non–insulin-dependent diabetes mellitus (NIDDM), or type II. In 1997, these terms were eliminated because treatment can vary (some people with NIDDM require insulin) and because the terms do not indicate the underlying problem. The new terms are type 1 and type 2, using Arabic symbols to avoid confusion (e.g., type II could be read as type eleven) (American Diabetes Association, 2001). The characteristics of type 1 DM and type 2 DM are outlined in Table 29-2.

In the age group younger than 10 years, most diabetes cases are type 1 and occur most frequently in non-Hispanic whites. In the age group 10 to 19 years, type 1 diabetes is more prominent in non-Hispanic whites followed by African Americans and then Hispanics; the lowest prevalence is among American Indians. In type 2 diabetes, American Indians have the highest incidence followed by African Americans, Asian Pacific individuals, and Hispanics; the lowest prevalence is in non-Hispanic whites (CDC, 2011). The Pima Indian tribe reports a greater than 51% incidence of type 2 DM.

Type 1 diabetes is characterized by destruction of the pancreatic β cells, which produce insulin; this usually leads to absolute insulin deficiency. Type 1 diabetes has two forms. Immune-mediated DM results from an autoimmune destruction of the β cells; it typically starts in children or young adults who are slim, but it can arise in adults of any age. **Idiopathic type 1** refers to rare forms of the disease that have no known cause.

TABLE 29-2	CHARACTERISTICS OF TYPE 1 AND TYPE 2 DIABETES MELLITUS	
CHARACTERISTIC	**TYPE 1**	**TYPE 2**
Age at onset	<20 years	Increasingly occurring in younger children
Type of onset	Abrupt	Gradual
Sex ratio	Affects males slightly more than females	Females outnumber males
Percentage of diabetic population	5%–8%	85%–90%
Heredity:		
Family history	Sometimes	Frequently
Human leukocyte antigen	Associations	No association
Twin concordance	25%–50%	90%–100%
Ethnic distribution	Primarily whites	Increased incidence in American Indians, Hispanics, African Americans
Presenting symptoms	3 Ps common: polyuria, polydipsia, polyphagia	May be related to long-term complications
Nutritional status	Underweight	Overweight
Insulin (natural):		
Pancreatic content	Usually none	>50% normal
Serum insulin	Low to absent	High or low
Primary resistance	Minimum	Marked
Islet cell antibodies	80%–85%	<5%
Therapy:		
Insulin	Always	20%–30% of patients
Oral agents	Ineffective	Often effective
Diet only	Ineffective	Often effective
Chronic complications	>80%	Variable
Ketoacidosis	Common	Infrequent

Type 2 diabetes usually arises because of insulin resistance in which the body fails to use insulin properly combined with relative (rather than absolute) insulin deficiency. People with type 2 can range from predominantly insulin resistant with relative insulin deficiency to predominantly deficient in insulin secretion with some insulin resistance. It typically occurs in those who are older than 45 years of age, are overweight and sedentary, and have a family history of diabetes.

The symptomatology of diabetes is more readily recognizable in children than in adults, so it is surprising that the diagnosis may sometimes be missed or delayed. Diabetes is a great imitator; influenza, gastroenteritis, and appendicitis are the conditions most often diagnosed when it turns out that the disease is really diabetes (Box 29-13).

Pathophysiology

Insulin is needed to support the metabolism of carbohydrates, fats, and proteins, primarily by facilitating the entry of these substances into the cells. Insulin is needed for the entry of glucose into the muscle and fat cells, prevention of mobilization of fats from fat cells, and storage of glucose as glycogen in the cells of liver and muscle. Insulin is not needed for the entry of glucose into nerve cells or vascular tissue. The chemical composition and molecular structure of insulin are such that it fits into receptor sites on the cell membrane. Here it initiates a

BOX 29-13 CLINICAL MANIFESTATIONS OF TYPE 1 DIABETES MELLITUS

Polyphagia
Polyuria
Polydipsia
Weight loss
Enuresis or nocturia
Irritability; "not himself" or "herself"
Shortened attention span
Lowered frustration tolerance
Dry skin
Blurred vision
Poor wound healing
Fatigue
Flushed skin
Headache
Frequent infections
Hyperglycemia
- Elevated blood glucose levels
- Glucosuria
Diabetic ketosis
- Ketones and glucose in urine
- Dehydration in some cases
Diabetic ketoacidosis
- Dehydration
- Electrolyte imbalance
- Acidosis
- Deep, rapid breathing (Kussmaul respirations)

Ketoacidosis

When insulin is absent or insulin sensitivity is altered, glucose is unavailable for cellular metabolism, and the body chooses alternate sources of energy, principally fat. Consequently, fats break down into fatty acids, and glycerol in the fat cells is converted by the liver to ketone bodies (β-hydroxybutyric acid, acetoacetic acid, acetone). Any excess is eliminated in the urine (ketonuria) or the lungs (acetone breath). The ketone bodies in the blood (ketonemia) are strong acids that lower serum pH, producing ketoacidosis.

Ketones are organic acids that readily produce excessive quantities of free hydrogen ions, causing a fall in plasma pH. Then chemical buffers in the plasma, principally bicarbonate, combine with the hydrogen ions to form carbonic acid, which readily dissociates into water and carbon dioxide. The respiratory system attempts to eliminate the excess carbon dioxide by increased depth and rate (Kussmaul respirations, or the hyperventilation characteristic of metabolic acidosis). The ketones are buffered by sodium and potassium in the plasma. The kidneys attempt to compensate for the increased pH by increasing tubular secretion of hydrogen and ammonium ions in exchange for fixed base, thus depleting the base buffer concentration.

With cellular death, potassium is released from the cells (intracellular fluid) into the bloodstream (extracellular fluid) and excreted by the kidneys, where the loss is accelerated by osmotic diuresis. The total body potassium is then decreased even though the serum potassium level may be elevated as a result of the decreased fluid volume in which it circulates. Alteration in serum and tissue potassium can lead to cardiac arrest.

If these conditions are not reversed by insulin therapy in combination with correction of the fluid deficiency and electrolyte imbalance, progressive deterioration occurs, with dehydration, electrolyte imbalance, acidosis, coma, and death. Diabetic ketoacidosis (DKA) should be diagnosed promptly in a seriously ill patient and therapy instituted in an intensive care unit.

Long-Term Complications

Long-term complications of diabetes involve both the microvasculature and the macrovasculature. The principal microvascular complications are nephropathy, retinopathy, and neuropathy. Microvascular disease develops during the first 30 years of diabetes, beginning in the first 10 to 15 years after puberty, with renal involvement evidenced by proteinuria and clinically apparent retinopathy. Macrovascular disease develops after 25 years of diabetes and creates the predominant problems in patients with type 2 DM. The process appears to be one of glycosylation, wherein proteins from the blood become deposited in the walls of small vessels (e.g., glomeruli), where they become trapped by "sticky" glucose compounds (glycosyl radicals). The buildup of these substances over time causes narrowing of the vessels, with subsequent interference with microcirculation to the affected areas (Rosenson and Herman, 2008).

With poor diabetic control, vascular changes can appear as early as 2½ to 3 years after diagnosis; however, with good to excellent control, changes can be postponed for 20 or more years. Intensive insulin therapy appears to delay the onset and slow the progression of retinopathy, nephropathy, and neuropathy. Hypertension and atherosclerotic cardiovascular disease are also major causes of morbidity and mortality in patients with DM (Karnik, Fields, and Shannon, 2007).

Other complications have been observed in children with type 1 DM. Hyperglycemia appears to influence thyroid function, and altered function is frequently observed at the time of diagnosis and in poorly controlled diabetes. Limited mobility of small joints of the hand occurs

sequence of poorly defined chemical reactions that alter the cell membrane to facilitate the entry of glucose into the cell and stimulate enzymatic systems outside the cell that metabolize the glucose for energy production.

With a deficiency of insulin, glucose is unable to enter the cells, and its concentration in the bloodstream increases. The increased concentration of glucose (hyperglycemia) produces an osmotic gradient that causes the movement of body fluid from the intracellular space to the interstitial space and then to the extracellular space and into the glomerular filtrate to "dilute" the hyperosmolar filtrate. Normally, the renal tubular capacity to transport glucose is adequate to reabsorb all the glucose in the glomerular filtrate. When the glucose concentration in the glomerular filtrate exceeds the renal threshold (6180 mg/dl), glucose spills into the urine (glycosuria) along with an osmotic diversion of water (polyuria), a cardinal sign of diabetes. The urinary fluid losses cause the excessive thirst (polydipsia) observed in diabetes. This water "washout" results in a depletion of other essential chemicals, especially potassium.

Protein is also wasted during insulin deficiency. Because glucose is unable to enter the cells, protein is broken down and converted to glucose by the liver (glucogenesis); this glucose then contributes to the hyperglycemia. These mechanisms are similar to those seen in starvation when substrate (glucose) is absent. The body is actually in a state of starvation during insulin deficiency. Without the use of carbohydrates for energy, fat and protein stores are depleted as the body attempts to meet its energy needs. The hunger mechanism is triggered, but increased food intake (polyphagia) enhances the problem by further elevating blood glucose.

Nursing Care Plan—The Child with Diabetic Ketoacidosis (DKA)

in 30% of 7- to 18-year-old children with type 1 DM and appears to be related to changes in the skin and soft tissues surrounding the joint as a result of glycosylation.

> ! **NURSING ALERT**
>
> Recurrent vaginal and urinary tract infections, especially with *Candida albicans*, are often an early sign of type 2 DM, especially in adolescents.

Diagnostic Evaluation

Three groups of children who should be considered as candidates for diabetes are (1) children who have glycosuria, polyuria, and a history of weight loss or failure to gain despite a voracious appetite; (2) those with transient or persistent glycosuria; and (3) those who display manifestations of metabolic acidosis, with or without stupor or coma. In every case, diabetes must be considered if there is glycosuria, with or without ketonuria, and unexplained hyperglycemia.

Glycosuria by itself is not diagnostic of diabetes. Other sugars, such as galactose, can produce a positive result with certain test strips, and a mild degree of glycosuria can be caused by other conditions, such as infection, trauma, emotional or physical stress, hyperalimentation, and some renal or endocrine diseases.

An 8-hour fasting blood glucose level of 126 mg/dl or more, a random blood glucose value of 200 mg/dl or more accompanied by classic signs of diabetes, or an oral glucose tolerance test (OGTT) finding of 200 mg/dl or more in the 2-hour sample is almost certain to indicate diabetes (American Diabetes Association, 2005). Postprandial blood glucose determinations and the traditional OGTTs have yielded low detection rates in children and are not usually necessary for establishing a diagnosis. Serum insulin levels may be normal or moderately elevated at the onset of diabetes; delayed insulin response to glucose indicates impaired glucose tolerance.

Ketoacidosis must be differentiated from other causes of acidosis or coma, including hypoglycemia, uremia, gastroenteritis with metabolic acidosis, salicylate intoxication encephalitis, and other intracranial lesions. DKA is a state of relative insulin insufficiency and may include the presence of hyperglycemia (blood glucose level ≥200 mg/dl), ketonemia (strongly positive), acidosis (pH <7.30 and bicarbonate <15 mmol/L), glycosuria, and ketonuria (Wolsdorf, Craig, Daneman, and others, 2009). Tests used to determine glycosuria and ketonuria are the glucose oxidase tapes (Keto-Diastix).

Therapeutic Management

The management of the child with type 1 DM consists of a multidisciplinary approach involving the family; the child (when appropriate); and professionals, including a pediatric endocrinologist, diabetes nurse educator, nutritionist, and exercise physiologist. Often psychological support from a mental health professional is also needed. Communication among the team members is essential and extends to other individuals in the child's life, such as teachers, school nurse, school guidance counselor, and coach.

The definitive treatment is replacement of insulin that the child is unable to produce. However, insulin needs are also affected by emotions, nutritional intake, activity, and other life events such as illnesses and puberty. The complexity of the disease and its management requires that the child and family incorporate diabetes needs into their lifestyle. Medical and nutritional guidance are primary, but management also includes continuing diabetes education, family guidance, and emotional support.

Insulin Therapy

Insulin replacement is the cornerstone of management of type 1 DM. Insulin dosage is tailored to each child based on home blood glucose monitoring. The goal of insulin therapy is maintaining near-normal blood glucose values while avoiding too frequent episodes of hypoglycemia. The goals of treatment are to maintain near-normal glucose levels of less than 126 mg/dl and glycosylated hemoglobin (hemoglobin A1c) of 7% or less (Hannon, Gungor, and Arslanian, 2006). Glycemic control decreases the likelihood of long-term complications in patients with DM (Petitti, Imperatore, Palla, and others, 2007). Insulin is administered as two or more injections per day or as continuous subcutaneous infusion using a portable insulin pump.

Healthy pancreatic cells secrete insulin at a low but steady basal rate with superimposed bursts of increased secretion that coincide with intake of nutrients. Consequently, insulin levels in the blood increase and decrease coincidentally with rises and falls in blood glucose levels. In addition, insulin is secreted directly into the portal circulation; therefore, the liver, which is the major site of glucose disposal, receives the largest concentration of insulin. No matter which method of insulin replacement is used, this normal pattern cannot be duplicated. Subcutaneous injection results in absorption of the drug into the general circulation, thus reducing the concentrations of insulin to which the liver is exposed.

Insulin Preparations. Insulin is available in highly purified pork preparations and in human insulin biosynthesized by and extracted from bacterial or yeast cultures. Most clinicians suggest human insulin as the treatment of choice. Insulin is available in rapid-, intermediate-, and long-acting preparations, and all are packaged in the strength of 100 units/ml. Some insulins are available as premixed insulins, such as 70/30 and 50/50 ratios, the first number indicating the percentage of intermediate-acting insulin and the second number the percentage of rapid-acting insulin. The different types of insulin are found in Box 29-14.

> ! **NURSING ALERT**
>
> The human insulins from various manufacturers may be interchangeable, but human insulin and pork insulin or pure pork insulin should never be substituted for one another.

Dosage. Conventional management has consisted of a **twice-daily insulin** regimen of a combination of **rapid-acting** and **intermediate-acting** insulin drawn up into the same syringe and injected before breakfast and before the evening meal. The amount of morning regular insulin is determined by patterns in the late morning and lunchtime blood glucose values. The morning intermediate-acting dosage is determined by patterns in the late afternoon and supper blood glucose values. Fasting blood glucose patterns at breakfast help determine the evening dose of intermediate insulin, and the blood glucose patterns at bedtime help determine the evening dose of rapid-acting (regular) insulin. For some children, better morning glucose control is achieved by a later (bedtime) injection of intermediate-acting insulin.

Regular insulin is best administered at least 30 minutes before meals. This allows sufficient time for absorption and results in a significantly greater reduction in the postprandial rise in blood glucose than if the meal were eaten immediately after the insulin injection. Intensive therapy consists of multiple injections throughout the day with a once- or twice-daily dose of long-acting (Ultralente) insulin to simulate the basal insulin secretion and injections of rapid-acting insulin before each meal. A multiple daily injection program reduces microvascular complications of diabetes in young, healthy patients who have type 1 DM.

The precise dose of insulin needed cannot be predicted. Therefore, the total dosage and percentage of regular- to intermediate-acting insulin should be determined empirically for each child. Usually 60% to 75% of the total daily dose is given before breakfast, and the remainder is given before the evening meal. Furthermore, insulin requirements do not remain constant but change continuously during growth and development; the need varies according to the child's activity level and pubertal status. For example, less insulin is required during spring and summer months when children are more active. Illness also alters insulin requirements. Some children require more frequent insulin administration. This includes children with difficult-to-control diabetes and children during the adolescent growth spurt.

Methods of Administration. Daily insulin is administered subcutaneously by twice-daily injections, by multiple-dose injections, or by means of an insulin infusion pump. The insulin pump is an electromechanical device designed to deliver fixed amounts of regular or lispro insulin continuously (basal rate), thereby more closely imitating the release of the hormone by the islet cells (Phillip, Battelino, Rodriguez, and others, 2007). Although the pump delivers a programmed amount of basal insulin, the child or parent must program a dose for the pump to deliver before each meal.

The system consists of a syringe to hold the insulin, a plunger, and a computerized mechanism to drive the plunger. The insulin flows from the syringe through a catheter to a needle inserted into subcutaneous tissue (the abdomen or thigh), and the lightweight device is worn on a belt or a shoulder holster. The needle and catheter are changed every 48 to 72 hours by the child or parent using aseptic technique and then taped in place.

Although the pump provides more consistent insulin delivery, it has certain disadvantages. Pump therapy is expensive and requires commitment from the parent and child. A certain level of math skills is required to calculate infusion rates. It should also not be removed for more than 1 hour at a time, which may limit some activities. Skin infections are common, and as with any other mechanical device, it is subject to malfunction. However, the pumps are equipped with alarms that signal problems, such as a depleted battery, an occluded needle or tubing, or a microprocessor malfunction.

Monitoring

Daily monitoring of blood glucose levels is an essential aspect of appropriate DM management. Plasma blood glucose and hemoglobin A1c goal ranges are found in Table 29-3.

Blood Glucose. Self-monitoring of blood glucose (SMBG) has improved diabetes management and is used successfully by children from the onset of their diabetes. By testing their own blood, children are able to change their insulin regimen to maintain their glucose level in the euglycemic (normal) range of 80 to 120 mg/dl. Diabetes management depends to a great extent on SMBG. In general, children tolerate the testing well.

Glycosylated Hemoglobin. The measurement of glycosylated hemoglobin (hemoglobin A1c) levels is a satisfactory method for assessing control of the diabetes. As red blood cells circulate in the bloodstream, glucose molecules gradually attach to the hemoglobin A molecules and remain there for the lifetime of the red blood cell, approximately 120 days. The attachment is not reversible; therefore, this glycosylated hemoglobin reflects the average blood glucose levels over the previous 2 to 3 months. The test is a satisfactory method for assessing control, detecting incorrect testing, monitoring the effectiveness of changes in treatment, defining patients' goals, and detecting nonadherence. Nondiabetic hemoglobin A1c values are generally between 4% and 6% but can vary by laboratory. Diabetes control for

---

BOX 29-14   TYPES OF INSULIN

There are four types of insulin, based on the following criteria:
- How soon the insulin starts working (onset)
- When the insulin works the hardest (peak time)
- How long the insulin lasts in the body (duration)

However, each person responds to insulin in his or her own way. That is why onset, peak time, and duration are given as ranges.

Rapid-acting insulin (e.g., NovoLog) reaches the blood within 15 minutes after injection. The insulin peaks 30 to 90 minutes later and may last as long as 5 hours.

Short-acting (regular) insulin (e.g., Novolin R) usually reaches the blood within 30 minutes after injection. The insulin peaks 2 to 4 hours later and stays in the blood for about 4 to 8 hours.

Intermediate-acting insulins (e.g., Novolin N) reach the blood 2 to 6 hours after injection. The insulins peak 4 to 14 hours later and stay in the blood for about 14 to 20 hours.

Long-acting insulin (e.g., Lantus) takes 6 to 14 hours to start working. It has no peak or a very small peak 10 to 16 hours after injection. The insulin stays in the blood between 20 and 24 hours.

Some insulins come mixed together (e.g., Novolin 70/30). For example, you can buy regular insulin and NPH insulins already mixed in one bottle, which makes it easier to inject two kinds of insulin at the same time. However, you cannot adjust the amount of one insulin without also changing how much you get of the other insulin.

Adapted from American Diabetes Association: *Resource guide 2005,* retrieved April 10, 2008, from http://www.diabetes.org/rg2005/insulin.jsp.
NPH, Neutral protamine Hagedorn.

TABLE 29-3   PLASMA BLOOD GLUCOSE AND HEMOGLOBIN A1C GOALS FOR TYPE 1 DIABETES MELLITUS BY AGE GROUP

AGE	VALUE* BEFORE MEALS (mg/dl)	VALUE* AT BEDTIME/ OVERNIGHT (mg/dl)	HEMOGLOBIN A1C (%)	IMPLICATIONS
Toddlers and preschoolers (<6 years)	100–180	110–200	≤8.5% (but ≥7.5%)	High risk and vulnerability to hypoglycemia
School age (6–12 years)	90–180	100–180	<8%	Risks of hypoglycemia and relatively low risk of complications before puberty
Adolescents (>12 years) and young adults	90–130	90–150	<7.5%	Risk of hypoglycemia Developmental and psychologic issues

Modified from American Diabetes Association: Standards of medical care in diabetes, *Diabetes Care* 28(suppl):S4–36, 2005.
*Plasma blood glucose goal range.

children depends on age, with hemoglobin A1c levels of 6.5% to 8% indicating a slightly elevated but acceptable range (American Diabetes Association, 2005). Hemoglobin A1c levels of less than 7% are a well-established goal at most care centers.

Urine. Urine testing for glucose is no longer used for diabetes management; there is poor correlation between simultaneous glycosuria and blood glucose concentrations. However, urine testing can be carried out to detect evidence of ketonuria.

> **! NURSING ALERT**
>
> It is recommended that urine be tested for ketones every 3 hours during an illness or whenever the blood glucose level is over 240 mg/dl when illness is not present.

Nutrition

Essentially, the nutritional needs of children with diabetes are no different from those of healthy children. Children with diabetes need no special foods or supplements. They need sufficient calories to balance daily expenditure for energy and to satisfy the requirement for growth and development. Unlike children without diabetes, whose insulin is secreted in response to food intake, insulin injected subcutaneously has a relatively predictable time of onset, peak effect, duration of action, and absorption rate depending on the type of insulin used. Consequently, the timing of food consumption must be regulated to correspond to the timing and action of the insulin prescribed.

Meals and snacks must be eaten according to peak insulin action, and the total number of calories and proportions of basic nutrients must be consistent from day to day. The constant release of insulin into the circulation makes the child prone to hypoglycemia between the three daily meals unless a snack is provided between meals and at bedtime. The distribution of calories should be calculated to fit the activity pattern of each child. For example, a child who is more active in the afternoon will need a larger snack at that time. This larger snack might also be split to allow some food at school and some food after school. Food intake should be altered to balance food, insulin, and exercise. Extra food is needed for increased activity.

Concentrated sweets are discouraged, and because of the increased risk of atherosclerosis in persons with DM, fat is reduced to 30% or less of the total caloric requirement. Dietary fiber has become increasingly important in dietary planning because of its influence on digestion, absorption, and metabolism of many nutrients. It has been found to diminish the rise in blood glucose after meals.

For growing children, food restriction should never be used for diabetes control, although caloric restrictions may be imposed for weight control if the child is overweight. In general, the child's appetite should be the guide for the amount of calories needed, with the total caloric intake adjusted to appetite and activity.

Exercise

Exercise is encouraged and never restricted unless indicated by other health conditions. Exercise lowers blood glucose levels, depending on the intensity and duration of the activity. Consequently, exercise should be included as part of diabetes management, and the type and amount of exercise should be planned around the child's interests and capabilities. However, in most instances, children's activities are unplanned, and the resulting decrease in blood glucose can be compensated for by providing extra snacks before (and if the exercise is prolonged, during) the activity. In addition to a feeling of well-being,

regular exercise aids in utilization of food and often results in a reduction of insulin requirements.

Hypoglycemia

Occasional episodes of hypoglycemia are an integral part of insulin therapy, and an objective of diabetes management is to achieve the best possible glycemic control while minimizing the frequency and severity of hypoglycemia. Even with good control, a child may frequently experience mild symptoms of hypoglycemia. If the signs and symptoms are recognized early and promptly relieved by appropriate therapy, the child's activity should be interrupted for no more than a few minutes.

> **! NURSING ALERT**
>
> Hypoglycemic episodes most commonly occur before meals or when the insulin effect is peaking.

The signs and symptoms of hypoglycemia are caused by both increased adrenergic activity and impaired brain function. The increased adrenergic nervous system activity plus increased secretion of catecholamines produces nervousness, pallor, tremulousness, palpitations, sweating, and hunger (Cryer, 2008). Weakness, dizziness, headache, drowsiness, irritability, loss of coordination, seizures, and coma are more severe responses and reflect CNS glucose deprivation and the body's attempts to elevate the serum glucose levels.

It is often difficult to distinguish between hyperglycemia and a hypoglycemic reaction (Table 29-4). Because the symptoms are similar and usually begin with changes in behavior, the simplest way to differentiate between the two is to test the blood glucose level. The blood glucose level is low in hypoglycemia, but in hyperglycemia, the glucose level is significantly elevated. Urinary ketones may be present after hypoglycemia as a result of starvation ketone production. In doubtful situations it is safer to give the child some simple carbohydrate. This will help alleviate the symptoms in the case of hypoglycemia but will do little harm if the child is hyperglycemic.

Children are usually able to detect the onset of hypoglycemia, but some are too young to implement treatment. Parents should become adept at recognizing the onset of symptoms—for example, a change in a child's behavior, such as tearfulness or euphoria. In the majority of cases, 10 to 15 g of simple carbohydrate, such as 1 Tbsp of table sugar, will elevate the blood glucose level and alleviate the symptoms. The simpler the carbohydrate, the more rapidly it will be absorbed (8 oz of milk equals 15 g of carbohydrate). The rapidly releasing sugar is followed by a complex carbohydrate such as a slice of bread or a cracker and by a protein such as peanut butter or milk.

For a mild reaction, milk or fruit juice is a good food to use in children. Milk supplies them with lactose or milk sugar, as well as a more prolonged action from the protein and fat (aids in decreased absorption). Other glucose sources include Insta-Glucose (cherry-flavored glucose), carbonated drinks (not sugarless), sherbet, gelatin, or cake icing. All children with diabetes should carry with them glucose tabs, Insta-Glucose, sugar cubes, or sugar-containing candy such as LifeSavers or Charms. A difficulty with candies or icing is that the child may learn to fake a reaction to get the sweets; therefore, commercial treatment products such as Insta-Glucose or glucose tabs may be preferred.

Glucagon is sometimes prescribed for home treatment of hypoglycemia. It is available as an emergency kit that must be mixed at the time of use and is administered intramuscularly or subcutaneously. Glucagon functions by releasing stored glycogen from the liver and requires about 15 to 20 minutes to elevate the blood glucose level.

TABLE 29-4	COMPARISON OF MANIFESTATIONS OF HYPOGLYCEMIA AND HYPERGLYCEMIA	
VARIABLE	**HYPOGLYCEMIA**	**HYPERGLYCEMIA**
Onset	Rapid (minutes)	Gradual (days)
Mood	Labile, irritable, nervous, weepy	Lethargic
Mental status	Difficulty concentrating, speaking, focusing, coordinating Nightmares	Dulled sensorium Confusion
Inward feeling	Shaky feeling Hunger Headache Dizziness	Thirst Weakness Nausea and vomiting Abdominal pain
Skin	Pallor Sweating	Flushed Signs of dehydration
Mucous membranes	Normal	Dry, crusty
Respirations	Shallow, normal	Deep, rapid (Kussmaul)
Pulse	Tachycardia, palpitations	Less rapid, weak
Breath odor	Normal	Fruity, acetone
Neurologic	Tremors	Diminished reflexes Paresthesia
Ominous signs	Late—Hyperreflexia, dilated pupils, seizure Shock, coma	Acidosis, coma
Blood:		
Glucose	Low: <60 mg/dl	High: ≥250 mg/dl
Ketones	Negative	High, large
Osmolarity	Normal	High
pH	Normal	Low (≤7.25)
Hematocrit	Normal	High
Bicarbonate	Normal	<20 mEq/L
Urine:		
Output	Normal	Polyuria (early) to oliguria (late)
Glucose	Negative	Enuresis, nocturia
Ketones	Negative or trace	High
Visual	Diplopia	Blurred vision

! NURSING ALERT

Vomiting may occur after administration of glucagon; therefore, precautions against aspiration must be taken (e.g., placing the child on the side) because the child often becomes unconscious.

When the child is responsive, the lost glycogen stores are replaced by small amounts of sugar-containing fluid administered frequently until the child feels comfortable trying solid foods.

Morning Hyperglycemia. The management of elevated morning blood glucose levels depends on whether the increase is a true dawn phenomenon, insulin waning, or a rebound hyperglycemia (the Somogyi effect). Insulin waning is a progressive rise in blood glucose levels from bedtime to morning. It is treated by increasing the nocturnal insulin dose. The true dawn phenomenon shows relatively normal blood glucose level until about 3 AM, when the level begins to rise. The Somogyi effect may occur at any time but often entails an elevated blood glucose level at bedtime and a drop at 2 AM with a rebound rise following. The treatment for this phenomenon is decreasing the nocturnal insulin dose to prevent the 2 AM hypoglycemia. The rebound rise in the blood glucose level is a result of counterregulatory hormones (epinephrine, GH, and corticosteroids), which are stimulated by hypoglycemia. More frequent blood monitoring (especially at times of anticipated peak insulin action) will usually identify these conditions. Trace amounts of urinary ketones aid in identifying undetected hypoglycemia.

Illness Management

Illness alters diabetes management, and maintaining control is usually related to the seriousness of the illness. In a well-controlled child, an illness will run its course as it does in unaffected children. The goals during an illness are to restore euglycemia, treat urinary ketones, and maintain hydration. Blood glucose levels and urinary ketones should be monitored every 3 hours. Some hyperglycemia and ketonuria are expected in most illnesses, even with diminished food intake, and are an indication for increased insulin. Insulin should never be omitted during an illness, although dosage requirements may increase, decrease, or remain unchanged, depending on the severity of the illness and the child's appetite. Often the child will need supplemental insulin between usual dose times. If the child vomits more than once, if blood glucose levels remain above 240 mg/dl, or if urinary ketones remain high, the health care practitioner should be notified. Simple carbohydrates may be substituted for carbohydrate-containing exchanges in the meal plan. Although insulin and diet are important tools in sick-day care, fluids are the most important intervention. Fluids must be encouraged to prevent dehydration and to flush out ketones.

Therapeutic Management of Diabetic Ketoacidosis

Diabetic ketoacidosis, the most complete state of insulin deficiency, is a life-threatening situation. Management consists of rapid assessment, adequate insulin to reduce the elevated blood glucose level, fluids to overcome dehydration, and electrolyte replacement (especially potassium).

Because DKA constitutes an emergency situation, the child should be admitted to an intensive care facility for management. The priority is to obtain a venous access for administration of fluids, electrolytes, and insulin. The child should be weighed, measured, and placed on a cardiac monitor. Blood glucose and ketone levels are determined at the bedside, and samples are obtained for laboratory measurement of glucose, electrolytes, BUN, arterial pH, PO_2, PCO_2, hemoglobin, hematocrit, white blood cell count and differential, calcium, and phosphorus.

Oxygen may be administered to patients who are cyanotic and in whom arterial oxygen is less than 80%. Gastric suction is applied to unconscious children to avoid the possibility of pulmonary aspiration. Antibiotics may be administered to febrile children after appropriate specimens are obtained for culture. A Foley catheter may or may not be inserted for urine samples and measurement. Unless the child is unconscious, a collection bag is usually sufficient for accurate assessments.

Fluid and Electrolyte Therapy

All patients with DKA experience dehydration (10% of total body weight in severe ketoacidosis) because of the osmotic diuresis, accompanied by depletion of electrolytes, sodium, potassium, chloride, phosphate, and magnesium. Serum pH and bicarbonate reflect the degree of acidosis. Prompt and adequate fluid therapy restores tissue perfusion and suppresses the elevated levels of stress hormones.

The initial hydrating solution is 0.9% saline solution. Traditionally, deficits have been replaced at a rate of 50% over the first 8 to 12 hours and the remaining 50% over the next 16 to 24 hours. Current trends suggest more cautious fluid management to reduce the risk of cerebral edema. The fluid deficit is replaced evenly over a period of 36 to 48 hours (Cooke and Plotnick, 2008).

> ### ! NURSING ALERT
>
> Potassium must never be given until the serum potassium level is known to be normal or low and urinary voiding is observed. All maintenance IV fluids should include 20 to 40 mEq/L of potassium. Never give potassium as a rapid IV bolus, or cardiac arrest may result.

Serum potassium levels may be normal on admission, but after fluid and insulin administration, the rapid return of potassium to the cells can seriously deplete serum levels, with the attendant risk of cardiac arrhythmias. As soon as the child has established renal function (is voiding at least 25 ml/hr) and insulin has been given, vigorous potassium replacement is implemented. The cardiac monitor is used as a guide to therapy, and configuration of T waves should be observed every 30 to 60 minutes to determine changes that might indicate alterations in potassium concentration (widening of the QT interval and the appearance of a U wave following a flattened T wave indicate hypokalemia; an elevated and spreading T wave and shortening of the QT interval indicate hyperkalemia).

Insulin should not be given until urinary ketones and a blood glucose level have been obtained. Continuous IV regular insulin is given at a dosage of 0.1 units/kg/hr. Insulin therapy should be started after the initial rehydration bolus because serum glucose levels fall rapidly after volume expansion. Blood glucose levels should decrease by 50 to 100 mg/dl/hr. When blood glucose levels fall to 250 to 300 mg/dl, dextrose is added to the IV solution. The goal is to maintain blood glucose levels between 120 and 240 mg/dl by adding 5% to 10% dextrose. Sodium bicarbonate is used conservatively; it is used for pH less than 7.0, severe hyperkalemia, or cardiac instability. Because sodium bicarbonate has been associated with an increased risk for cerebral edema, children receiving this substance must be carefully monitored for changes in level of consciousness (Brown, 2004).

When the critical period is over, the task of regulating the insulin dosage in relation to diet and activity is started. Children should be actively involved in their own care and are given responsibility according to their ability and the guidance of the nurse.

> ### ! NURSING ALERT
>
> Because insulin can chemically bind to plastic tubing and in-line filters, thereby reducing the amount of medication reaching the systemic circulation, an insulin mixture is run through the tubing to saturate the insulin-binding sites before the infusion is started.

Nursing Care Management

Children with DM may be admitted to the hospital at the time of their initial diagnosis; during illness or surgery; or for episodes of ketoacidosis, which may be precipitated by any of a variety of factors (see the Evidence-Based Practice box evaluating hospitalization compared with outpatient care for children newly diagnosed with type 1

DM). Many children are able to keep the disease under control with periodic assessment and adjustment of insulin, diet, and activity as needed under the supervision of a practitioner. Under most circumstances, these children can be managed well at home and require hospitalization only for serious illnesses or upsets.

However, a small number of children with diabetes exhibit a degree of metabolic lability and have repeated episodes of DKA that require hospitalization, which interferes with their education and social development. These children appear to display a characteristic personality structure. They tend to be unusually passive and nonassertive and to come from families that are inclined to smooth over conflicts without resolution. Children in this type of setting experience emotional arousal with little, if any, opportunity or ability to resolve it. Other children from psychosocially dysfunctional families display behavioral and personality problems. This emotional stress causes an increased production of endogenous catecholamines, which stimulate fat breakdown, leading to ketonemia and ketonuria.

Hospital Management

Children with DKA require intensive nursing care. Vital signs should be observed and recorded frequently. Hypotension caused by the contracted blood volume of the dehydrated state may cause decreased peripheral blood flow, which can be particularly hazardous to the heart, lungs, and kidneys. An elevated temperature may indicate infection and should be reported so that treatment can be implemented immediately.

Careful and accurate records should be maintained, including vital signs (pulse, respiration, temperature, blood pressure), weight, IV fluids, electrolytes, insulin, blood glucose level, and intake and output. A urine collection device or retention catheter is used to obtain the urine measurements, which include volume, specific gravity, and glucose and ketone values. The volume relative to the glucose content is important because 5% glucose in a 300-ml sample is a significantly greater amount than a similar reading from a 75-ml sample. A diabetic flow sheet maintained at the bedside provides an ongoing record of the vital signs, urine and blood tests, amount of insulin given, and intake and output. The level of consciousness is assessed and recorded at frequent intervals. The comatose child generally regains consciousness fairly soon after initiation of therapy but is managed like any unconscious child until then.

When the critical period is over, the task of regulating insulin dosage to diet and activity is begun. The same meticulous records of intake and output, urine glucose and acetone levels, and insulin administration are maintained. Capable children should be actively involved in their own care and are given responsibility for keeping the intake and output record; testing the blood and urine; and, when appropriate, administering their own insulin—all under the supervision and guidance of the nurse (see Nursing Care Plan).

Child and Family Education

Several organizations are prepared to assist with education and dissemination of knowledge about diabetes. The American Diabetes Association,* Canadian Diabetes Association,† Juvenile Diabetes Research Foundation International,‡ and American Association

---

*1701 N. Beauregard St., Alexandria, VA 22311; 800-342-2383; http://www.diabetes.org.

†1400–522 University Ave., Toronto, ON M5G 2R5; 800-226-8464; http://www.diabetes.ca.

‡26 Broadway, 14th Floor, New York, NY 10004; 800-533-CURE; http://www.jdrf.org.

EVIDENCE-BASED PRACTICE

Hospital Admission or Outpatient Care for Children Newly Diagnosed with Type 1 Diabetes Mellitus

Ask the Question
Picot Question

Is hospitalization necessary for children newly diagnosed with type 1 DM who are not acutely ill?

Search for the Evidence
Search Strategies

Searched the literature to obtain clinical research studies related to this issue. Selection criteria included English-language publications within the past 10 years; research-based articles; infant, child, and adolescent populations.

Databases Used

PubMed, CINAHL, Cochrane Collaboration, AHRQ

Critically Analyze the Evidence

In a Cochrane Review, seven studies were found evaluating routine hospital admission compared with outpatient or home care for children newly diagnosed with type 1 DM (Clar, Waugh, and Thomas, 2009). The overall quality of the six studies was low, making results of the review inconclusive. Overall, it appears that outpatient home management of type 1 DM in children at diagnosis does not lead to any disadvantages in terms of metabolic control, acute diabetic complications and hospitalizations, adjustment to the disease, or total financial costs (Chase, Crews, Garg, and others, 1992; Dougherty, Schiffrin, White, and others, 1998; Galatzer, Schoshana, Gil, and others, 1982; Simell, Putto-Laurila, Nanto-Salonen, and others, 1995; Spaulding and Spaulding, 1976). However, high-quality RCTs are needed.

One RCT found that home-based management of children newly diagnosed with type 1 DM may lead to slight improvement in long-term metabolic control (Dougherty, Schiffrin, White, and others, 1998). No differences were found in any psychosocial or behavioral parameters evaluated or the rate of complications within 2 years of the diagnosis.

Apply the Evidence: Nursing Implications

There is **low-quality evidence** with a **weak recommendation** (Guyatt, Oxman, Vist, and others, 2008) that hospitalization is not necessary for children newly diagnosed with type 1 DM. The main tasks after diagnosis of type 1 DM in children are to achieve metabolic stabilization and prevent complications, to provide support to the child and family, and to educate them on how to manage the disease. No definitive conclusion can be made from the research found on this issue. However, the few studies that exist suggest that there are no adverse effects associated with outpatient home management of a child newly diagnosed with type 1 DM.

QSEN **Quality and Safety Competencies:**
Evidence-Based Practice*
Knowledge

Differentiate clinical opinion from research and evidence-based summaries.

Identify the pros and cons of hospital admission for newly diagnosed children with type 1 DM.

Skills

Base individualized care plan on patient values, clinical expertise, and evidence.

Integrate evidence into teaching newly diagnosed children and their families the principles of DM management.

Attitudes

Value the concept of evidence-based practice as integral to determining best clinical practice.

Appreciate strengths and weakness of evidence for hospitalization for newly diagnosed children with type 1 DM.

References

Chase PH, Crews KR, Garg S, and others: Outpatient management vs in-hospital management of children with new-onset diabetes, *Clin Pediatr* 31(8):450–456, 1992.
Clar C, Waugh N, Thomas S: Routine hospital admission versus out-patient or home care in children at diagnosis of type 1 diabetes mellitus, *Cochrane Database Syst Rev* (3):CD004099, 2009.
Dougherty G, Schiffrin A, White D, and others: Home-based management can achieve intensification cost-effectively in type 1 diabetes, *Pediatrics* 103(1):122–128, 1998.
Galatzer A, Schoshana A, Gil R, and others: Crisis intervention programme in newly diagnosed diabetic children, *Diabetes Care* 5(4):414–419, 1982.
Guyatt GH, Oxman AD, Vist GE, and others: GRADE: an emerging consensus on rating quality of evidence and strength of recommendations, *BMJ* 336:924–926, 2008.
Simell T, Putto-Laurila A, Nanto-Salonen K, and others: Randomized prospective trial of ambulatory treatment and one-week hospitalisation of children with newly diagnosed IDDM, *Diabetes* 44(suppl 1):162A, 1995.
Spaulding R, Spaulding W: The diabetic daycare unit: comparison of patients and costs of initiating insulin therapy in the unit and a hospital, *Can Med Assoc J* 114:780–783, 1976.

DM, Diabetes mellitus; *RCT,* randomized controlled trial.
*Adapted from the QSEN at http://www.qsen.org.

---

of Diabetes Educators* are valuable resources for a wide variety of educational materials. The National Institute of Diabetes and Digestive and Kidney Diseases† publishes a number of comprehensive annotated bibliographies, including "Educational Materials for and About Young People with Diabetes," a compilation of resource materials for children, siblings, parents, teachers, and health professionals, and "Sports and Exercise for People with Diabetes."

Medical Identification

One of the first things the nurse should call to the parents' attention is the need for the child to wear some means of medical identification.

Usually recommended is the Medic-Alert identification, a stainless steel or silver- or gold-plated identification bracelet that is visible and immediately recognizable. It contains a collect telephone number that medical personnel can call around the clock for medical records and personal information.

Nature of Diabetes

The better the parents understand the pathophysiology of diabetes and the function and action of insulin and glucagon in relation to caloric intake and exercise, the better they will understand the disease and its effects on the child. Parents need answers to a number of questions (voiced or unvoiced) to increase their confidence in coping with the disease. For example, they may want to know about the various procedures performed on their child and treatment rationale, such as what is being put in the IV bottle and the expected effect.

*200 W. Madison St., Suite 800, Chicago, IL 60606; 800-338-3633; e-mail: education@aadenet.org; http://www.diabeteseducator.org.
†Office of Communications and Public Liaison, NIDDK, NIH, Building 31, Room 9A06, 31 Center Drive, MSC 2560, Bethesda, MD 20892-2560; 301-496-3583; http://www.niddk.nih.gov.

Meal Planning

Normal nutrition is a major aspect of the family education program. Diet instruction is usually conducted by the nutritionist, with reinforcement and guidance from the nurse. The emphasis is on adequate intake for age, consistent menus, complex carbohydrates, and consistent eating times. The family is taught how the meal plan relates to the requirements of growth and development, the disease process, and the insulin regimen. Meals and snacks are modified based on the child's preferences and current menu, preserving cultural patterns and preferences as much as possible. Extensive exchange lists are available that include foods compatible with most lifestyles.

Learning about foods within specific food groups helps in making choices. Weights and measures of foods are used as eye-training devices for defining serving sizes and should be practiced for about 3 months, with gradual progression to estimation of food portions. Even when the child and family become competent in estimating portion sizes, reassessment should take place weekly or monthly and when there is any change of brands.

Family members should also be guided in reading labels for the nutritional value of foods and food content. They need to become familiar with the carbohydrate content of food groups. Substitution with foods of equal carbohydrate content is the skill needed for

---

◎ NURSING CARE PLAN

The Child with Diabetes Mellitus

NURSING DIAGNOSIS	PATIENT OUTCOMES	NURSING INTERVENTIONS	RATIONALE
Risk for Injury related to insulin deficiency	Child will demonstrate normal blood glucose levels.	Obtain blood glucose level.	To determine most appropriate dosage of insulin
		Administer insulin as prescribed.	To maintain normal blood glucose level
Child's Defining Characteristics (Subjective and Objective Data)	**The Following NOC Concepts Apply to This Outcome**	Understand the action of insulin, including differences in composition, time of onset, and duration of action for the various preparations.	To ensure accurate insulin administration
Polyphagia			
Polydipsia	Blood Glucose Control		
Polyuria	Nutritional Status: Nutrient Intake	Use aseptic techniques when preparing and administering insulin.	To prevent infection
Weight loss			
Enuresis or nocturia		Rotate sites.	To enhance absorption of insulin
Abnormal blood profile—glucose, insulin			
Irritability			
Shortened attention span		**The Following NIC Concepts Apply to These Interventions**	
Fatigue		Health Education	
Dry skin		Hyperglycemia Management	
Blurred vision		Hypoglycemia Management	
Headache		Nutritional Management	
Frequent infections		Medication Administration	
Hyperglycemia			
Flushed skin			
Risk for Injury related to hypoglycemia	Child will exhibit no evidence of hypoglycemia.	Recognize signs of hypoglycemia early. Be alert at times when blood glucose levels are lowest (before meals and snacks; 2–4 AM; after bursts of physical activity without additional food; or with a delayed, omitted, or incompletely consumed meal or snack).	To prevent hypoglycemia
Child's Defining Characteristics (Subjective and Objective Data)	**The Following NOC Concept Applies to This Outcome**	Test blood glucose.	To evaluate glucose level
Shaky feeling		Offer 10–15 g of readily absorbed carbohydrates, such as orange juice, hard candy, or milk.	To elevate blood glucose level and alleviate symptoms of hypoglycemia
Hunger	Blood Glucose Control		
Headache			
Dizziness			
Difficulty concentrating, speaking, or focusing		Follow with complex carbohydrate and protein, such as bread or cracker spread with peanut butter or cheese.	To maintain blood glucose level
Tremors		Administer glucagons to unconscious or combative child; position child to minimize risk of aspiration because vomiting may occur.	To elevate blood glucose level
Tachycardia			
Shallow respirations			
Can lead to convulsion, shock, and coma		**The Following NIC Concepts Apply to These Interventions**	
		Health Education	
		Hypoglycemia Management	

◎ NURSING CARE PLAN

The Child with Diabetes Mellitus—cont'd

NURSING DIAGNOSIS	PATIENT OUTCOMES	NURSING INTERVENTIONS	RATIONALE
Knowledge Deficit (Diabetes Management) related to care of a child with newly diagnosed diabetes mellitus	Child and family will have attitude conducive to learning.	Select methods, vocabulary, and content appropriate to learner's level.	To maximize learning
		Allow time for family and child to begin to adjust to initial impact of the diagnosis.	To allow child and family to set pace
		Select an environment conducive to learning.	To promote learning
Child's or Family's Defining Characteristics		Involve all senses and use a variety of teaching strategies, especially participation.	To promote effective learning
(Subjective and Objective Data)		Provide pamphlets or other supplementary materials.	To promote learning
Lack of understanding	Child and family will demonstrate understanding of meal planning.	Emphasize relationship between normal nutritional needs and the disease.	To encourage sense of normalcy
Inability to prepare and administer insulin		Become familiar with family's culture and food preferences.	To include culture preferences in meal planning
Inability to follow meal planning guidelines		Teach or reinforce learners' understanding of the basic food groups and the prescribed meal plan.	To reinforce existing knowledge base
Difficulty describing treatment plan		Help child and family estimate portion sizes by volume.	To provide a more practical method than weighing food
		Suggest low-carbohydrate snack items.	To promote appropriate food choices
		Guide family in assessing labels of food products for carbohydrate content.	To reinforce that consistency in carbohydrate portions is essential
	Child and family will demonstrate knowledge of and ability to administer insulin.	Teach child and family the characteristics of the insulins prescribed.	To increase understanding that there are several insulin preparations
		Teach proper mixing of insulins.	To prevent contaminating the vials
		Teach injection procedure.	To promote appropriate administration
		Teach basic techniques using an orange or similar item.	To build confidence
		Use demonstration and return demonstration techniques on another adult before injecting child.	To minimize stress for the child
		Help families and child work out a set rotational pattern.	To ensure maximum absorption of insulin and prevent hypertrophy at injection site
		Teach proper care of insulin and equipment.	To prevent contamination and minimize complications
	Child and family will demonstrate ability to test blood glucose level.	Teach family and child, if old enough, blood glucose monitoring or use of equipment, interpretation of results, and care and maintenance of equipment.	To ensure that child and family learn how to adjust insulin based on blood glucose level
	Child and family will demonstrate knowledge of management of hyperglycemia and hypoglycemia.	Instruct learners in how to recognize signs of hyperglycemia and hypoglycemia.	To prevent delay of treatment
		Explain relationship of insulin needs to illness, activity, and intense emotion.	To ensure appropriate treatment
		Teach how to adjust food, activity, and insulin at times of illness and during other situations that alter blood glucose levels.	To ensure appropriate treatment
		Suggest carrying source of carbohydrate, such as sugar cubes or hard candy, in pocket.	To prevent delay in treatment
		Instruct parents and child in how to treat hypoglycemia with food, simple sugars, or glucagons.	To establish health practices that last a lifetime
	Child and family will demonstrate understanding of proper hygiene.	Emphasize importance of personal hygiene.	To promote child's general health
		Encourage regular dental care and yearly ophthalmologic examinations.	To minimize risk of infection
		Teach proper care of cuts and scratches; teach proper foot care.	To prevent infection

Continued

NURSING CARE PLAN

The Child with Diabetes Mellitus—cont'd

NURSING DIAGNOSIS	PATIENT OUTCOMES	NURSING INTERVENTIONS	RATIONALE
	The Following NOC Concepts Apply to These Outcomes Blood Glucose Control Knowledge: Medication Knowledge: Treatment Regimen	The Following NIC Concepts Apply to These Interventions Health Education Hyperglycemia Management Hypoglycemia Management	

NIC, Nursing Interventions Classification; *NOC,* Nursing Outcomes Classification.

successful carbohydrate counting. Substitution might be necessary if a food is not available in sufficient quantity or for the teenager who wishes to eat fast food with peers. The use of a multiple daily injection program lends flexibility to the timing of meals.

Lists of popular fast-food items and items served at the major fast-food chains can be obtained from the restaurants to help guide food selections. It is important that the child know the nutritional value of these items (the major chains are remarkably uniform), but the child should be cautioned to avoid high-fat and high-sugar/high-carbohydrate items; for example, the child could choose a plain hamburger instead of a double cheeseburger.

Children should use sugar substitutes in moderation in items such as soft drinks. Artificial sweeteners have been shown to be safe, but if there is any question about amounts, the physician, dietitian, or nurse specialist can provide guidelines based on body weight. Sugar-free chewing gum and candies made with sorbitol may be used in moderation by children with DM. Although sorbitol is less cariogenic than other varieties of sugar substitutes, it is an alcohol sugar that is metabolized to fructose and then to glucose. Furthermore, large amounts can cause osmotic diarrhea. Most dietetic foods contain sorbitol. They are more expensive than regular foods. Also, although a product may be sugar free, it is not necessarily carbohydrate free.

Traveling

Traveling requires planning, especially when a trip involves crossing time zones. A number of tips are included in pamphlets available free of charge. Suggestions for traveling encompass what will be needed from the practitioner before leaving, what and how much to take along, needs in transit, what to consider at the destination, and planning for when the child returns home. Planning is needed no matter what type of travel is considered—automobile, plane, bus, or train.

Insulin

Families need to understand the treatment method and the insulin prescribed, including the effective duration, onset, and peak action. They also need to know the characteristics of the various types of insulins, the proper mixing and dilution of insulins, and how to substitute another type when their usual brand is not available (insulin is a nonprescription drug). Insulin need not be refrigerated but should be maintained at a temperature between 15° and 29.4° C (59° and 85° F). Freezing renders insulin inactive.

Insulin bottles that have been "opened" (i.e., the stopper has been punctured) should be stored at room temperature or refrigerated for up to 28 to 30 days. After 1 month, these vials should be discarded. Unopened vials should be refrigerated and are good until the expiration date on the label. Diabetic supplies should not be left in a hot environment.

Injection Procedure

Learning to give insulin injections is a source of anxiety for both parents and children. It is helpful for the learner to know that this important aspect of care will become as routine as brushing the teeth. First, the basic injection technique is taught using an orange or similar item and sterile normal saline for practice. To gain children's confidence, the nurse can demonstrate the technique by giving a skillful injection to the parent and then having the parent return the demonstration by giving the nurse an injection. With practice and confidence, the parents will soon be able to give the insulin injection to their children, and their children will trust them. Another effective strategy is to instruct the children and then have them teach the technique to the parents while the nurse observes. Both parents should participate, and as little time as possible should elapse between instruction and the actual injection, especially with parents and teenage learners.

Insulin can be injected into any area in which there is adipose (fat) tissue over muscle; the drug is injected at a 90-degree angle. Newly diagnosed children may have lost adipose tissue, and care should be exerted not to inject intramuscularly. The pinch technique is the most effective method for tenting the skin to allow easy entrance of the needle to subcutaneous tissues in children. The site selected will sometimes depend on whether children or parents administer the insulin. The arms, thighs, hips, and abdomen are usual injection sites for insulin. The children can reach the thighs, abdomen, and part of the hip and arm easily but may require help to inject other sites. For example, a parent can pinch a loose fold of skin of the arm while the child injects the insulin.

The parents and child are helped to work out a rotation pattern to various areas of the body to enhance absorption because insulin absorption is slowed by fat pads that develop in overused injection areas. The most efficient rotation plan involves giving about four to six injections in one area (each injection about 2.5 cm [1 inch] apart, or the diameter of the insulin vial from the previous injection) and then moving to another area.

It is important to remember that the absorption rate varies in different parts of the body (Table 29-5). The methodical use of one anatomic area and then movement to another (as described in the previous paragraph) minimizes variations in absorption

TABLE 29-5	ONSET AND DURATION OF ACTION RELATED TO INJECTION SITE			
	SITE OF INJECTION			
	ABDOMEN	ARM	LEG	BUTTOCK
Rate	Very fast	Fast	Slow	Very slow
Duration	Very short	Short	Long	Very long

From Albisser AM, Sperlich M: Adjusting insulins, *Diabetes Educ* 18(3):211–218, 1992.

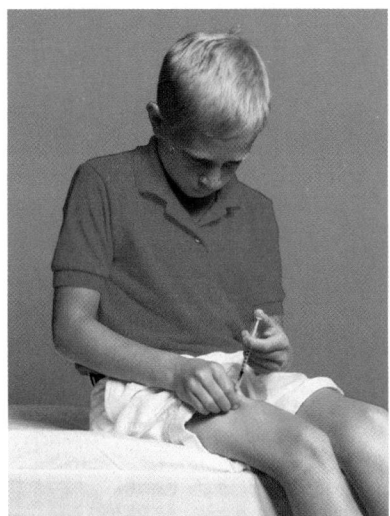

FIG 29-3 School-age children are able to administer their own insulin.

rates. However, absorption is also altered by vigorous exercise, which enhances absorption from exercised muscles; therefore, it is recommended that a site be chosen other than the exercising extremity (e.g., avoiding legs and arms when playing in a tennis tournament).

Injection sites for an entire month can be determined in advance on a simple chart. For example, a "paper doll" (body outline) can be constructed and insulin sites marked by the child. After injection, the child places the date on the appropriate site. To keep in practice, it is a good idea for the parent to give two or three injections a week in areas that are difficult for the child to reach. The same basic methodology is used when teaching children to give their own insulin injections (Fig. 29-3). They should practice first on an orange or a doll, building courage gradually. Other devices are available for insulin injection and may offer advantages to some children. Children who do not wish to give themselves injections can be taught to use a syringe-loaded injector (Inject-Ease). With the device, puncture is always automatic. Adolescents respond well to a self-contained and compact device resembling a fountain pen (NovoPen), which eliminates conventional vials and syringes. Preloaded pens may also cause less pain because the needle is not blunted by piercing the rubber top of the insulin vial (Rex, Jensen, and Lawton, 2006).

Continuous Subcutaneous Insulin Infusion. Some children are considered candidates for use of a portable insulin pump, and even some young children with unsatisfactory metabolic control can benefit from its use. The child and the parents are taught to operate the device, including the mechanics of the pump, battery changes, and alarm systems. A number of devices are on the market that vary in the basal

ATRAUMATIC CARE
Minimizing Pain of Blood Glucose Monitoring

To enhance blood flow to the finger, hold it under warm water for a few seconds before the puncture.

When obtaining blood samples, use the ring finger or thumb (blood flows more easily to these areas) and puncture the finger just to the side of the finger pad (more blood vessels and fewer nerve endings).

To prevent a deep puncture, press the platform of the lancet device lightly against the skin and avoid steadying the finger against a hard surface.

Use lancet devices with adjustable-depth tips. Begin with the shallowest setting.

Use glucose monitors that require small blood samples (e.g., Ascensia Elite) to avoid repeated punctures.

rates they are able to deliver and in the cost of the equipment. Families can investigate the various devices and select the model that best suits their needs. Product information is available from pump manufacturers and distributors.*

Parents and children learn (1) the technical aspects of the pump and self-monitoring of blood glucose; (2) prevention and treatment for hyperglycemia, sick-day management, and meal planning; (3) the effects of exercise, stress, and diet on blood glucose levels; and (4) decision-making strategies to evaluate blood glucose patterns and make adjustments in all aspects of the regimen.

Numerous blood glucose measurements (at least four times per day) are an essential part of infusion pump use. Intensive education and supervision are critical to obtaining maximum efficiency and control. This is particularly important if the family has been accustomed to a conventional insulin regimen. They must realize that simply wearing the pump will not normalize blood glucose. The pump is merely an insulin delivery device, and frequent, routine blood glucose determinations are necessary to adjust the insulin delivery rate.

The major problems with use of the insulin pump are inflammation from irritation and infection at the insertion site. The site should be cleaned thoroughly before the needle is inserted and then covered with a transparent dressing. The site is changed and rotated every 48 to 72 hours (this may vary) or at the first sign of inflammation. Nurses working where pumps are part of the therapeutic regimen should become familiar with the operation of the specific device being used and the protocol of disease management. Others should be aware of this management technique and be prepared to assist patients using the pump.

Monitoring

Nurses should also be prepared to teach and supervise blood glucose monitoring. SMBG is associated with few complications, and although it does not necessarily lead to improved metabolic control, it provides a more accurate assessment of blood glucose levels than can be obtained with the historical urine testing. Blood glucose monitoring has the added advantage that it can be performed anywhere (see Atraumatic Care box).

Blood for testing can be obtained by two different methods: manually or with a mechanical bloodletting device. A mechanical device is recommended for children, although the child and family should learn

---

*Medtronic MiniMed, http://www.minimed.com; Disetronic, http://www.disetronic-usa.com; Animas, http://www.animascorp.com.

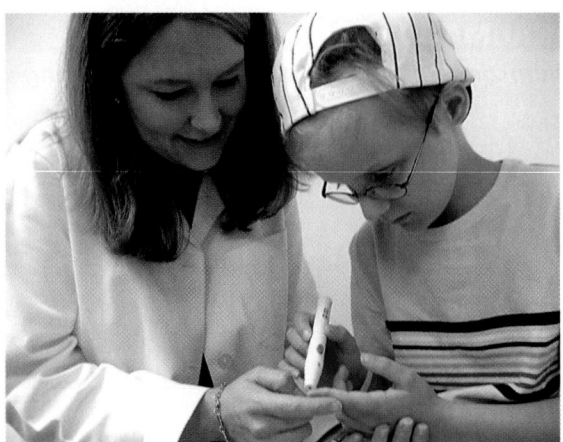

FIG 29-4 Child using a finger-stick device to obtain a blood sample.

to use both methods in the event of mechanical failure. Several lancet devices are available, and each provides a means for obtaining a large drop of blood for testing (Fig. 29-4).

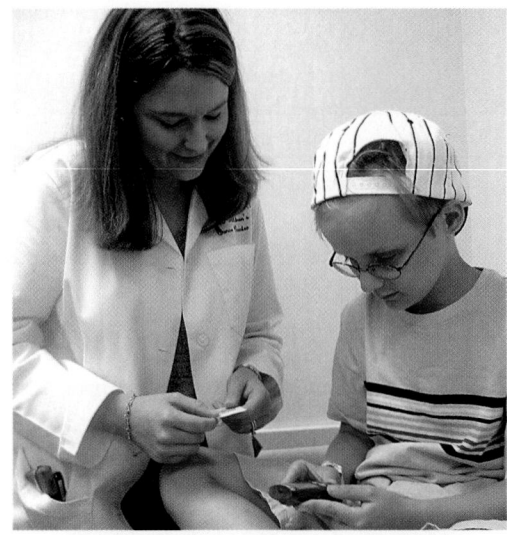

FIG 29-5 Child using a blood glucose monitor and reagent strips to test his blood for glucose.

> **⚠ NURSING ALERT**
>
> Caution children not to allow anyone else to use their lancet because of the risk of contracting hepatitis B virus or human immunodeficiency virus infection.

The blood sample may be obtained from fingertips or alternate sites such as the forearm. Alternate site testing requires a meter that can test a small volume of blood. Not all meters are capable of this.

Signs of redness and soreness at the site of finger puncture should be examined by the practitioner. It may be evidence of poor technique, poor hygiene, or poor skin healing relative to poor control. Many types of blood-testing meters are available for home use. Newer technology has brought about improvements in meter size and ease of use. The family should be shown features of several meters, including advantages and disadvantages, and allowed to choose equipment that best meets their needs.

The least expensive testing method uses a reagent strip to which blood is applied (Fig. 29-5). After blotting, the color change is compared against a color scale for an estimation of the blood glucose level. The strips can be cut in half (although not all professionals recommend this) to obtain two readings per strip. This method is not accepted practice but may be necessary for some families or situations.

Urine Testing. Testing for urinary ketones is recommended during times of illness and when blood glucose values are elevated. Information on a specific ketone-testing product should include correct procedure, storage, and product expiration. Families need a clear understanding of home management of ketones (fluids and additional insulin as directed by the health care team).

Signs of Hyperglycemia

Severe hyperglycemia is most often caused by illness, growth, emotional upset, or missed insulin doses. Emotional stress from school finals or examinations or physical response to immunizations are examples of causes of hyperglycemia. With careful glucose monitoring, any elevation can be managed by adjustment of insulin or food intake. Parents should understand how to adjust food, activity, and insulin at the time of illness or when the child is treated for an illness with a medication known to raise the blood glucose level (e.g., steroids). The hyperglycemia is managed by increasing insulin soon after the increased glucose level is noted. Health care professionals should be aware that adolescent girls often become hyperglycemic around the time of their menses and should be advised to increase insulin dosages if necessary.

Signs of Hypoglycemia

Hypoglycemia is caused by imbalances of food intake, insulin, and activity. Ideally, hypoglycemia should be prevented, and parents need to be prepared to prevent, recognize, and treat the problem. They should be familiar with the signs of hypoglycemia and instructed in treatment, including care of the child with seizures. Early signs are adrenergic, including sweating and trembling, which help raise the blood glucose level, similar to the reaction when an individual is startled or anxious. The second set of symptoms that follow an untreated adrenergic reaction is neuroglycopenic (also called brain hypoglycemia). These symptoms typically include difficulty with balance, memory, attention, or concentration; dizziness or lightheadedness; and slurred speech. Severe and prolonged hypoglycemia leads to seizures, coma, and possible death (Cryer, 2008). Hypoglycemia can be managed effectively as outlined in the Emergency Treatment box.

It is advisable for parents to plan for anticipated excitement or exercise. In addition, gastroenteritis may decrease insulin needs slightly as a result of poor appetite, vomiting, or diarrhea. If the blood glucose level is low but urinary ketones are present, the family should be aware of the increased need for simple carbohydrates and liquids.

Hygiene

All aspects of personal hygiene should be emphasized for children with diabetes. Children should be cautioned against wearing shoes without socks, wearing sandals, and walking barefoot. Correct nail and extremity care tailored to the individual child (with the guidance of a podiatrist) can begin health practices that last a lifetime. These children's eyes should be checked once a year unless the child wears glasses and then as directed by the ophthalmologist. Regular dental care is emphasized, and cuts and scratches should be treated with plain soap and water unless otherwise indicated. Diaper rash in infants and candidal infections in teens may indicate poor diabetes control.

✚ EMERGENCY TREATMENT

Hypoglycemia

Mild Reaction—Adrenergic Symptoms

Give child 10 to 15 g of a simple, high-carbohydrate substance (preferably liquid, e.g., 3–6 oz of orange juice).
Follow with starch-protein snack.

Moderate Reaction—Neuroglycopenic Symptoms

Give child 10 to 15 g of a simple carbohydrate as above.
Repeat in 10 to 15 minutes if symptoms persist.
Follow with larger snack.
Watch child closely.

Severe Reaction—Unresponsive, Unconscious, or Seizures

Administer glucagon as prescribed.
Follow with planned meal or snack when child is able to eat or add a snack of 10% of daily calories.

Nocturnal Reaction

Give child 10 to 15 g of a simple carbohydrate.
Follow with snack of 10% of daily calories.

Exercise

Exercise is an important component of the treatment plan. If the child is more active at one time of the day than at another time, food or insulin can be altered to meet that activity pattern. Food should be increased in the summer, when children tend to be more active. Decreased activity on return to school may require a decrease in food intake or increase in insulin dosage. Children who are active in team sports will need a snack about a half hour before the anticipated activity. Races or other competition may call for a slightly higher food intake than at practice times.

Food intake will usually need to be repeated for prolonged activity periods, often as frequently as every 45 minutes to 1 hour. Families should be informed that if increased food is not tolerated, decreased insulin is the next course of action. If the timing of the exercise is changed so that the supper meal is delayed, the insulin in the second or third dose of the day may be moved back to precede the mealtime. Sugar may sometimes be needed during exercise periods for quick response. Elevated blood glucose levels after extreme activity may represent the body's adrenergic response to exercise. If the blood glucose level is elevated (>240 mg/dl) before planned exercise, urinary ketones should be checked, and the activity may need to be postponed until the blood glucose is controlled.

❗ NURSING ALERT

Ketonuria in the presence of hyperglycemia is an early sign of ketoacidosis and a contraindication to exercise.

Record Keeping

Home records are an invaluable aid to diabetes self-management. The nurse and family devise a method to chart insulin administered, blood glucose values, urine ketone results, and other factors and events that affect diabetes control. The child and family are encouraged to observe for patterns of blood glucose responses to events such as exercise. If lapses in management occur (e.g., eating a candy bar), the child should be encouraged to note this and not be criticized for the transgression.

Self-Management

Self-management is the key to close control. Being able to make changes when they are needed rather than waiting until the next contact with health care professionals is important for self-management and gives the individual and family the feeling that they have control over the disease. Psychologically, this helps family members believe they are useful and participating members of the team. Allowing the child to learn to look at records objectively promotes independence in self-management support. As children grow and assume more responsibility for self-management, they develop confidence in their ability to manage their disease and confidence in themselves as persons. They learn to respond to the disease and to make more accurate interpretations and changes in treatment when they become adults.

Puberty is associated with decreased sensitivity to insulin that normally would be compensated for by an increased insulin secretion. Health care professionals should anticipate that pubertal patients will have more difficulty maintaining glycemic control. Insulin doses commonly need to be increased, often dramatically (Tfayli and Arsianian, 2007). Patients should be taught to give themselves additional doses of rapid-acting insulin (5%–10% of their daily dose) when their blood glucose levels are increased. The use of supplemental rapid-acting insulin is preferred to withholding food in adolescents.

Child or Adolescent and Family Support

Just as the physiologic responses affect the child, the parents and other family members of the child with newly diagnosed DM experience various emotional responses to the crisis. Care in the acute setting is short but may create fears and frustrations. The prospect of a chronic illness in their child engenders all the feelings and concerns that are faced by parents of children with other chronic illnesses (see Chapter 18). The threat of complications and death is always present, as well as the continuing drain on emotional and financial resources.

Certain fears may develop as a result of past experiences with the disease. A severe insulin reaction with seizures can contribute to fear of repetition. If parents observe a seizure or the adolescent has one in a public place, the desire to maintain better control is reinforced. They must understand how to prevent problems and how to handle problems calmly and coolly if they occur, and they must understand the complexities of the body, the disease, and its complications. Young children usually adjust well to problems related to the disease. With toddlers and preschoolers, insulin injections and glucose testing may be difficult at first. However, they usually accept the procedures when the parents use a matter-of-fact approach, without calling attention to a "hurt," and treat the procedure like any other routine part of the child's life. After the injection, time with some special and positive attention, such as reading or talking, or another pleasant activity, is one way to convert children who initially refuse injections to those who accept them.

In the years before adolescence, children probably accept their condition most easily. They are able to understand the basic concepts related to their disease and its treatment. They are able to test blood glucose and urine, recognize food groups, give injections, keep records, and distinguish fear or excitement from hypoglycemia. They understand how to recognize, prevent, and treat hypoglycemia. However, they still need considerable parental involvement.

NURSING TIP Ongoing motivation to adhere to a regimen is difficult. An older child and parent (or another caregiver) may enjoy negotiating a day off when the responsibility for testing and recording blood glucose is delegated from the child to the caregiver (or vice versa).

Adolescents appear to have the most difficulty adjusting. Adolescence is a time of stress in trying to be perfect and similar to one's peers, and no matter what others say, having diabetes is being different. Some adolescents are more upset about not being able to have a candy bar than about injections, diet, and other aspects of management. If children can accept the difference as a part of life—in other words, that each person is different in some way—then, with adequate parental support, they should be able to adjust well (see Critical Thinking Case Study).

Camping and other special group activities are useful. At diabetes camp, children learn that they are not alone. As a result, they become more independent and resourceful in other settings. Useful information about such camps and organizations can be obtained from the American Diabetes Association. A list of accredited camps specifically for children and teenagers with diabetes is also available from the American Camping Association.*

---

*5000 State Road 67 N., Martinsville, IN 46151; 765-342-8456; http://www.acacamps.org.

? CRITICAL THINKING CASE STUDY

Type 1 Diabetes Mellitus

Shelly, a 14-year-old adolescent with a 3-year history of type 1 DM, has been admitted to the pediatric intensive care unit for treatment of DKA. This is her fifth hospital admission for DKA in the past year. Shelly's parents are divorced, and she has four younger siblings, none of whom has diabetes. Shelly's mother has maintained two jobs for the past 5 years and frequently leaves Shelly in charge of the household. In anticipation of her discharge, you are planning a patient education program for Shelly and her mother. What important issues regarding Shelly's unstable diabetes management must you consider to plan the education program?

Questions

1. Evidence—Is there sufficient evidence to draw conclusions about Shelly's recurrent episodes of DKA?
2. Assumptions—Describe an underlying assumption about each of the following:
   a. Type 1 DM in adolescence
   b. Type 1 DM and menses
   c. Emotional stress and elevated blood glucose levels
   d. Blood glucose monitoring for insulin management
3. What priorities for nursing care should be established for Shelly?
4. Does the evidence support your nursing intervention?

DKA, Diabetic ketoacidosis; *DM,* diabetes mellitus.

▮ KEY POINTS

- The endocrine system has three components: the cells, which send chemicals message via hormones; target cells, which receive the message; and the environment through which the chemical is transported from the site of synthesis to the sites of cellular action.
- Pituitary dysfunction is manifested primarily by growth disturbance.
- The main physiologic action of TH is to regulate the basal metabolic rate and control the processes of growth and tissue differentiation.
- Disorders of thyroid function include hypothyroidism, autoimmune thyroiditis, goiter, and hyperthyroidism.
- Therapy for hyperthyroidism is directed at retarding the rate of hormone secretion and may include drug therapy, thyroidectomy, or radioiodine therapy.
- Classic forms of hypoparathyroidism in childhood are idiopathic (deficient production of PTH) and pseudohypoparathyroidism (increased PTH production with end-organ unresponsiveness to PTH).

- The adrenal cortex secretes three important groups of hormones: glucocorticoids, mineralocorticoids, and sex steroids.
- Disorders of adrenal function include acute adrenocortical insufficiency, chronic adrenocortical insufficiency, Cushing syndrome, and CAH.
- Five categories of Cushing syndrome are pituitary, adrenal, ectopic, iatrogenic, and food dependent.
- Management of CAH includes assignment of a sex according to genotype; administration of cortisone; and, possibly, reconstructive surgery.
- DM is categorized as type 1 diabetes and type 2 diabetes.
- The focus of type 1 DM is insulin replacement, diet, and exercise.
- Education of families includes explanation of diabetes, meal planning, administering insulin injections, monitoring general hygienic practices, promoting exercise, record keeping, and observing for complications.

REFERENCES

American Academy of Pediatrics, Rose SR, Section on Endocrinology and Committee on Genetics of the American Thyroid Association, and others: Update of newborn screening and therapy for congenital hypothyroidism, *Pediatrics* 7(6):2290–2303, 2006.

American Academy of Pediatrics, Section on Endocrinology and Committee on Genetics: Technical report: congenital adrenal hyperplasia, *Pediatrics* 106(6):1511–1518, 2000. Reaffirmation statement published 2005.

American Diabetes Association: Report of the Expert Committee on the Diagnosis and Classification of Diabetes Mellitus, *Diabetes Care* 24(suppl 1):S5–S20, 2001.

American Diabetes Association: Care of children and adolescents with type 1 diabetes, *Diabetes Care* 28:186–212, 2005.

Bartalena L, Tanda ML, Piantanida E, and others: Oxidative stress and Graves' ophthalmopathy: in vitro studies and therapeutic implications, *Biofactors* 19(3–4):155–163, 2003.

Baxter JD, Ribeiro RCJ: Introduction to endocrinology. In Greenspan FS, Gardner DG, editors: *Basic and clinical endocrinology,* ed 7, New York, 2004, Lange Medical Books/McGraw-Hill.

Biro FM, Huang B, Crawford PB, and others: Pubertal correlates in black and white girls, *J Pediatr* 148(2):234–240, 2006.

Brown TB: Cerebral edema in childhood diabetic ketoacidosis: is treatment a factor? *Emerg Med J* 21:141–144, 2004.

Bryant J, Cave C, Milne R: Recombinant growth hormone for idiopathic short stature in children and adolescents, *Cochrane Database Syst Rev* (3):CD004440, 2007.

Carell C, Leger J: Precocious puberty, *N Engl J Med* 358:2366–2377, 2008.

Centers for Disease Control and Prevention: *Children and diabetes: more information*, Atlanta, March 2010, Author.

Centers for Disease Control and Prevention: *National Diabetes Fact Sheet 2011: national estimates and general information on diabetes and prediabetes in the U.S.*, Atlanta, 2011, Author.

Cheetham T, Baylis PH: Diabetes insipidus in children: pathophysiology, diagnoses and management, *Paediatr Drugs* 4(12):785–796, 2002.

Cooke D, Plotnick L: Management of diabetic ketoacidosis in children and adolescents, *Pediatr Rev* 29:431–436, 2008.

Cooper MS, Gittoes NJ: Diagnosis and management of hypocalcemia, *BMJ* 336:1298–1302, 2008.

Cryer PE: The barriers of hypoglycemia in diabetes, *Diabetes* 57(12):3169–3176, 2008.

Dallas JS, Foley TP: Hyperthyroidism. In Lifshitz F, editor: *Pediatric endocrinology*, ed 4, New York, 2003, Marcel Dekker.

De Buyst J, Massa G, Christophe C, and others: Clinical, hormonal and imaging findings in 27 children with central diabetes insipidus, *Eur J Pediatr* 166(1):43–49, 2007.

DeVries L, Bulvik S, Phillip M: Chronic autoimmune thyroiditis in children and adolescents: at presentation and during long term follow up, *Arch Dis Child* 94(1):33–37, 2009.

Foley TP: Hypothyroidism. In Hoekelman RA, Adam HM, Nelson NM, and others, editors: *Primary pediatric care*, ed 4, St. Louis, 2001, Mosby.

Glatt K, Garzon D, Popovic J: Congenital adrenal hyperplasia due to 21-hydroxylase deficiency, *Soc Pediatr Nurs* 10(3):104–114, 2005.

Greiner MV, Kerrigan JR: Puberty: timing is everything, *Pediatr Ann* 35(12):916–922, 2006.

Halac I, Zimmerman D: Evaluating short stature in children, *Pediatr Ann* 33(3):171–176, 2004.

Hall DMB: Growth monitoring, *Arch Dis Child* 82(1):10–15, 2000.

Hannon TS, Gungor N, Arslanian SA: Type 2 diabetes in children and adolescents: a review for the primary care provider, *Pediatr Ann* 35(12):880–887, 2006.

Herman-Giddens ME: Recent data on pubertal milestones in United States children: the secular trend toward earlier development, *Int J Androl* 29(1):241–246, 2006.

Jospe N: Hyperthyroidism. In Hoekelman RA, Adam HM, Nelson NM, and others, editors: *Primary pediatric care*, ed 4, St. Louis, 2001, Mosby.

Karnik AA, Fields AV, Shannon RP: Diabetic cardiomyopathy, *Curr Hypertens Rep* 9(6):467–473, 2007.

Kempers MJ, Otten BJ: Idiopathic precocious puberty versus puberty in adopted children: auxological response to gonadotrophin-releasing

hormone agonist treatment and final height, *Eur J Endocrinol* 147(5):609–616, 2002.

Kliegman RM, Stanton B, St. Geme J, and others: *Nelson textbook of pediatrics*, ed 19, Philadelphia, 2011, Saunders.

Lee PA, Houk CP, Ahmed SF, and others: Consensus statement on management of intersex disorders, *Pediatrics* 118:e488, 2006.

Leschek EW, Rose SR, Yanovski FA, and others: Effect of growth hormone treatment on adult height in peripubertal children with idiopathic short stature: a randomized, double blind, placebo-controlled trial, *J Clin Endocrino Metab* 89(7):3140–3148, 2004.

Lin M, Liu SJ, Lim IT: Disorders of water imbalance, *Emerg Med Clin North Am* 23(3):749–770, 2005.

Ma C, Xie JW, Kuang AR, and others: Radioiodine treatment for pediatric Grave's disease (protocol), *Cochrane Database Syst Rev* (4):CD006294, 2006.

Macchia PE: Recent advances in understanding the molecular basis of primary congenital hypothyroidism, *Mol Med Today* 6(1):36–42, 2000.

Majzoub JA, Muglia LJ: Disorders of water homeostasis. In Lifshitz F, editor: *Pediatric endocrinology*, ed 4, New York, 2003, Marcel Dekker.

Makaryus AN, McFarlane SI: Diabetes insipidus: diagnosis and treatment of a complex disease, *Cleve Clin J Med* 73(1):65–71, 2006.

Midyett LK, Moore WV, Jacobson JD: Are pubertal changes in girls before age 8 benign? *Pediatrics* 111(1):47–51, 2003.

Miller BS, Zimmerman D: Idiopathic short stature in children, *Pediatr Ann* 33(3):177–181, 2004.

Moshang T: Cushing's disease, 70 years later … and the beat goes on (editorial), *J Clin Endocrinol Metab* 88(1):31–33, 2003.

Muir A: Precocious puberty, *Pediatr Rev* 27(10):373–381, 2006.

Natchtigall L, Delgado A, Swearingen B, and others: Extensive clinical experience: changing patterns in diagnosis and therapy of acromegaly over two decades, *J Clin Endocrinol Metab* 93(6):2035–2041, 2008.

Nebesio TD, Eugster EA: Current concepts in normal and abnormal puberty, *Curr Prob Pediatr Adolesc Health Care* 37(2):50–72, 2007.

New MI, Ghizzoni L: Update on congenital adrenal hyperplasia. In Lifshitz F, editor: *Pediatric endocrinology*, ed 4, New York, 2003, Marcel Dekker.

Nieman LK, Ilias I: Evaluation and treatment of Cushing's syndrome, *Am J Med* 118(12):1340–1346, 2005.

O'Sullivan E, O'Sullivan M: Precocious puberty: a parent's perspective, *Arch Dis Childhood* 86:320–321, 2002.

Pacak K, Eisenhofer G, Ahlman H, and others: Pheochromocytoma: recommendations for clinical practice from the First International Symposium, *Nat Clin Pract Endocrinol Metab* 3(2):92–102, 2007.

Perheentupa J: Hypoparathyroidism and mineral homeostasis. In Lifshitz F, editor: *Pediatric*

endocrinology, ed 4, New York, 2003, Marcel Dekker.

Petitti BD, Imperatore G, Palla SL, and others: Serum lipids and glucose control: the SEARCH for Diabetes in Youth study, *Arch Pediatr Adolesc Med* 161(2):159–165, 2007.

Phillip M, Battelino T, Rodriguez H, and others: Use of insulin pump therapy in the pediatric age group, *Diabetes Care* 30:1653–1662, 2007.

Pizzo PA, Poplack DG: *Principles and theories of pediatric oncology*, Philadelphia, 2010, Lippincott Williams & Wilkins.

Radetti G, Gottardi E, Bona G, and others: The natural history of euthyroid Hashimoto's thyroiditis in children, *J Pediatr* 149(6):827–832, 2006.

Rex J, Jensen KH, Lawton SA: A review of 20 years of experience with the Novopen family of insulin injection devices, *Clin Drug Invest* 26(7):367–401, 2006.

Richmond EJ, Rogol AD: Growth hormone deficiency in children, *Pituitary* 71:115–120, 2008.

Rivkees SA: Differentiating appropriate antidiuretic hormone secretion, inappropriate antidiuretic hormone secretion and cerebral salt wasting: the common, uncommon and misnamed, *Curr Opin Pediatr* 20:448–452, 2008.

Rivkees SA, Cornelius EA: Influence of iodine-131 dose on the outcome of hyperthyroidism in children, *Pediatrics* 111(4):745–748, 2003.

Root AW: Precocious puberty, *Pediatr Rev* 21(1):10–19, 2000.

Rosenson RS, Herman WH: Glycated proteins and cardiovascular disease in glucose intolerance and type 11 diabetes, *Curr Cardiovascular Risk Rep* 2(1):43–46, 2008.

Rovet JF, Ehrlich R: Psychoeducational outcome in children with early-treated congenital hypothyroidism, *Pediatrics* 105(3):515–522, 2000.

Shoback D: Clinical practice: hypoparathyroidism, *N Engl J Med* 359(4):391–403, 2008.

Simmonds MJ, Howson JM, Heward JM, and others: Regression mapping of association between the human leukocyte antigen region and Graves disease, *Am J Hum Genet* 76(1):157–163, 2005.

Slyper AH: The pubertal timing controversy in the USA, and a review of possible causative factors for the advance in timing of onset of puberty, *Clin Endocrinol (Oxf)* 65(1):1–8, 2006.

Streetman DD, Khanderia U: Diagnosis and treatment of Graves disease, *Am J Nurse Pract* 8(1):27–36, 2004.

Szymborska M, Staroszczyk B: Thyroiditis in children, *Med Wieku Rozwoj* IV(4):383–391, 2000.

Tfayli H, Arsianian S: The challenge of adolescence: hormonal changes and sensitivity to insulin, *Diabetic Voice* 52:28–30, 2007.

Thompson GB: Surgical management in Graves' disease, *Panminerva Med* 44(4):287–293, 2002.

Toogood M, Stewart PM: Hypopituitarism: clinical features, diagnosis, and management, *Endocrino Metab Clin North Am* 37:235–261, 2008.

Trivin C, Couto-Silva AC, Sainte-Rose Z, and others: Presentation and evolution of organic central precocious puberty according to the type of CNS lesion, *Clin Endocrinol (Oxf)* 65(2):239–245, 2006.

Urrutia-Rojas X, Menchaca J: Prevalence of risk for type 2 diabetes in school children, *J Sch Health* 76(5):189–194, 2006.

Van Tijn DA, Schroor EJ, Delemarre-van de Waal HA, and others: Early assessment of hypothalamic-pituitary-gonadal function in patients with congenital hypothyroidism of central origin, *J Clin Endocrinol Metab* 92(1):104–109, 2007.

Verbalis JG: Diabetes insipidus, *Rev Endocr Metab Disord* 4(2):177–185, 2003.

Wolsdorf J, Craig ME, Daneman D, and others: Diabetic ketoacidosis in children and adolescents with diabetes: ISPAD Clinical Practice Consensus Guidelines 2009 Compendium, *Pediatric Diabetes* 10(suppl 12):118–133, 2009.

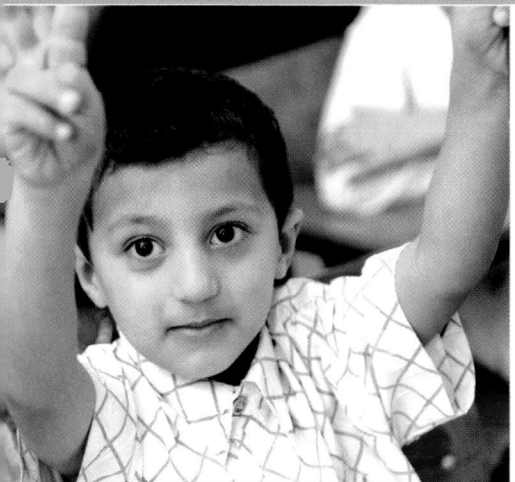

The Child with Integumentary Dysfunction

*Marilyn J. Hockenberry, Rose U. Baker,
and Mary A. Mondozzi*

evolve WEBSITE

http://evolve.elsevier.com/wong/essentials

Animations—Burns in Children; Tick Paralysis

Case Studies—Acne Vulgaris; Burns; Impetigo; Poison Ivy; Tinea
   Capitis

Key Point Summaries

NCLEX-Style Review Questions

Nursing Care Plan—The Child with Burns: Management and
   Rehabilitative Stages

CHAPTER OUTLINE

Integumentary Dysfunction, 1010
   Skin Lesions, 1010
      Skin of Younger Children, 1010
   Wounds, 1010
      Epidermal Injuries, 1013
      Injury to Deeper Tissues, 1013
      Process of Wound Healing, 1013
      Factors That Influence Healing, 1013
   General Therapeutic
      Management, 1013
      Dressings, 1013
      Topical Therapy, 1014
      Systemic Therapy, 1015
   Nursing Care Management, 1015
      Wound Care, 1015
      Relief of Symptoms, 1016
      Topical Therapy, 1016
   Home Care and Family Support, 1016

Infections of the Skin, 1017
   Bacterial Infections, 1017
   Viral Infections, 1017
   Dermatophytoses (Fungal
      Infections), 1017
   Systemic Mycotic (Fungal)
      Infections, 1020
Skin Disorders Related to Chemical or
   Physical Contacts, 1022
   Contact Dermatitis, 1022
   Poison Ivy, Oak, and Sumac, 1022
   Drug Reactions, 1022
   Foreign Bodies, 1024
Skin Disorders Related to Animal
   Contacts, 1024
   Arthropod Bites and Stings, 1024
   Scabies, 1024
   Pediculosis Capitis, 1027

Rickettsial Diseases, 1028
   Lyme Disease, 1029
   Pet and Wild Animal Bites, 1029
   Human Bites, 1030
   Cat Scratch Disease, 1030
Miscellaneous Skin Disorders, 1030
Skin Disorders Associated with Specific
   Age Groups, 1030
   Diaper Dermatitis, 1030
   Atopic Dermatitis (Eczema), 1032
   Seborrheic Dermatitis, 1035
   Acne, 1035
Thermal Injury, 1037
   Burns, 1037
      Characteristics of Burn Injury, 1037
   Sunburn, 1047
   Cold Injury, 1048

LEARNING OBJECTIVES

On completion of this chapter the reader will be able to:
- Describe the distribution and configuration of various skin lesions.
- List the benefits of a moist environment for wound healing.
- Discuss the nursing care related to therapies for skin disorders.
- Contrast the manifestations of and therapies for bacterial, viral, and
  fungal infections of the skin.
- Compare the skin manifestations related to age in children.
- Outline a care plan to prevent and treat diaper dermatitis.
- Outline a care plan for a child with atopic dermatitis.
- Formulate a teaching plan for an adolescent with acne.
- Describe the methods for assessing a burn wound.
- Discuss the physical and emotional care of a child with a severe
  burn wound.

INTEGUMENTARY DYSFUNCTION

SKIN LESIONS

Lesions of the skin result from a variety of etiologic factors. Skin lesions originate from (1) contact with injurious agents (infective organisms, toxic chemicals, and physical trauma), (2) hereditary factors, (3) external factors (e.g., allergens), or (4) systemic diseases (e.g., measles, lupus erythematosus, nutritional deficiency diseases). Responses to these agents or factors are highly individualized. An agent that is harmless to one individual may be damaging to another, and a single agent may produce varying degrees of response

An important factor in the etiology of skin manifestations is the child's age. Infants are subject to "birthmark" malformations and atopic dermatitis (AD) that appear early in life, school-age children are susceptible to ringworm of the scalp, and acne is a characteristic skin disorder of puberty. Contact dermatitis, such as poison ivy, is seen only when the noxious agent is found in the environment. Tension and anxiety may produce, modify, or prolong skin conditions.

Skin of Younger Children

The major skin layers arise from different embryologic origins. Early in the embryonic period, a single layer of epithelium forms from the ectoderm while simultaneously the corium develops from the mesenchyme. In infants and small children, the epidermis is loosely bound to the dermis. This poor adherence causes the layers to separate easily during an inflammatory process to form blisters. This is especially true in preterm infants, who have a propensity to blister formation and separation of the skin with minor trauma such as the removal of adhesive tape. In contrast, the skin of older children is thinner, and the cells of all the strata are more compressed.

Pathophysiology of Dermatitis

More than half of the dermatologic problems in children are forms of dermatitis. This implies a sequence of inflammatory changes in the skin that are grossly and microscopically similar but diverse in course and causation. Acute responses produce intercellular and intracellular edema, the formation of intradermal vesicles, and an initial infiltration of inflammatory cells into the epidermis. In the dermis, there is edema, vascular dilation, and early perivascular cellular infiltration. The location and manner of these reactions produce the lesions characteristic of each disorder. The changes are usually reversible, and the skin ordinarily recovers without blemish unless complicating factors such as ulceration from the primary irritant, scratching, and infection are introduced or underlying vascular disease develops. In chronic conditions, permanent effects are seen that vary according to the disorder, the general condition of the affected individual, and the available therapy.

Diagnostic Evaluation

Although the history and subjective symptoms of skin lesions are explored first, the obvious objective characteristics of the lesions are often noted simultaneously. Many skin lesions are easily diagnosed after careful inspection.

History and Subjective Symptoms

Many cutaneous lesions are associated with local symptoms. The most common local symptom is itching (pruritus), which varies in intensity. Pain or tenderness often accompanies some skin lesions. Other skin sensations such as burning, prickling, stinging, or crawling are also described. Alterations in local feeling include absence of sensation (anesthesia); excessive sensitivity (hyperesthesia); diminished sensation (hypesthesia or hypoesthesia); or abnormal sensation, such as burning or prickling (paresthesia). These symptoms may remain localized or migrate; may be constant or intermittent; and may be aggravated by a specific activity, such as exposure to sunlight.

It is important to determine whether the child has an allergic condition such as asthma or hay fever or history of a previous skin disease. AD, often associated with allergies, frequently begins in infancy. Important questions for the parent include when the lesion or symptom first appeared; whether it occurred with ingestion of a food or other substance, including any medication; and whether the condition was related to activity such as contact with plants, insects, or chemicals.

Objective Findings

The distribution, size, morphology, and arrangement of skin lesions provide significant information. Extrinsic causes usually result from physical, chemical, or allergic irritants or from an infectious agent such as bacteria, fungi, viruses, or animal parasites. Skin manifestations are also produced by intrinsic causes such as an infection (measles or chickenpox), drug sensitization, or other allergic phenomena.

Types of Lesions

Skin lesions assume distinct characteristics that are related to the pathologic process. Nurses should become familiar with the common terms that are applied to skin lesions because these terms are used in the processes of record keeping and communication. These terms include:

Erythema—A reddened area caused by increased amounts of oxygenated blood in the dermal vasculature

Ecchymoses (bruises)—Localized red or purple discolorations caused by extravasation of blood into dermis and subcutaneous tissues

Petechiae—Pinpoint, tiny, and sharp circumscribed spots in the superficial layers of the epidermis

Primary lesions—Skin changes produced by a causative factor; common primary lesions in pediatric skin disorders are macules, papules, and vesicles (Fig. 30-1)

Secondary lesions—Changes that result from alteration in the primary lesions, such as those caused by rubbing, scratching, medication, or involution and healing (Fig. 30-2)

Distribution pattern—The pattern in which lesions are distributed over the body, whether local or generalized, and the specific areas associated with the lesions

Configuration and arrangement—The size, shape, and arrangement of a lesion or groups of lesions (e.g., discrete, clustered, diffuse, or confluent)

Laboratory Studies

If a skin problem is related to a systemic disease (e.g., collagen or immunodeficiency disease), laboratory studies are performed to identify these conditions. Diagnostic techniques include microscopic examination, cultures, skin scrapings or biopsy, cytodiagnosis, patch testing, Wood light examination, allergic skin testing, and other laboratory tests such as blood count and sedimentation rate.

WOUNDS

Wounds are structural or physiologic disruptions of the skin that activate normal or abnormal tissue repair responses. Wounds are classified as acute or chronic. Acute wounds are those that heal uneventfully within 2 to 3 weeks. Chronic wounds are those that do not heal in the expected time frame or are associated with complications. Cofactors

Macule—flat; nonpalpable; circumscribed; <1 cm in diameter; brown, red, purple, white, or tan in color
Examples: Freckles, flat moles, rubella, rubeola

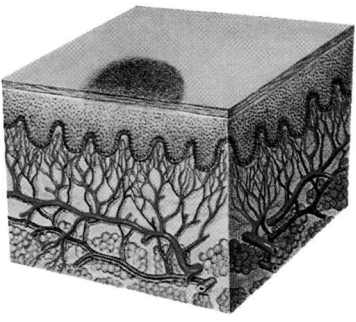

Plaque—elevated; flat topped; firm; rough; superficial papule >1 cm in diameter; may be coalesced papules
Examples: Psoriasis, seborrheic and actinic keratoses

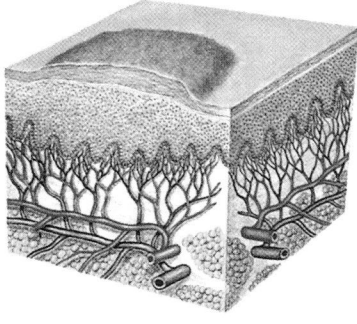

Patch—flat; nonpalpable; irregular in shape; macule that is >1 cm in diameter
Examples: Vitiligo, port-wine marks

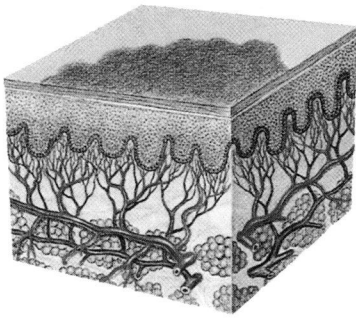

Wheal—elevated, irregularly shaped area of cutaneous edema; solid, transient, changing, variable diameter; pale pink with lighter center
Examples: Urticaria, insect bites

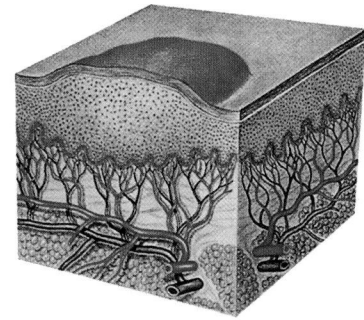

Papule—elevated; palpable; firm; circumscribed; <1 cm in diameter; brown, red, pink, tan, or bluish red in color
Examples: Warts; drug-related eruptions; pigmented nevi

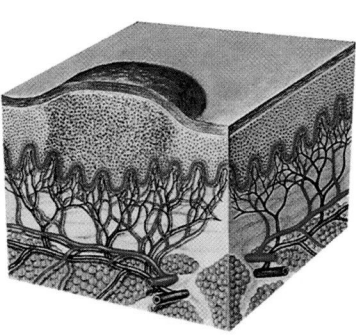

Nodule—elevated; firm; circumscribed; palpable; deeper in dermis than papule; 1 to 2 cm in diameter
Examples: Erythema nodosum, lipomas

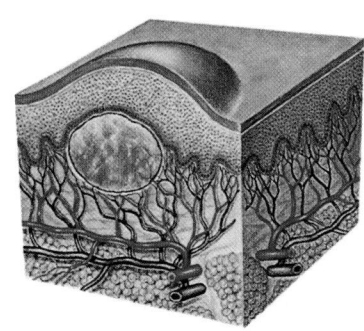

Vesicle—elevated; circumscribed; superficial; filled with serous fluid; <1 cm in diameter
Examples: Blister, varicella

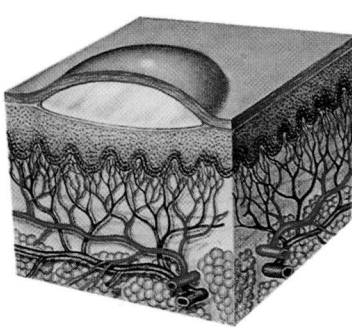

Pustule—elevated; superficial; similar to vesicle but filled with purulent fluid
Examples: Impetigo, acne, variola

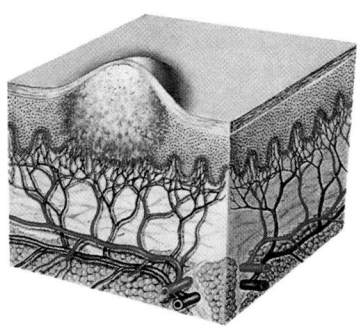

Bulla—vesicle >1 cm in diameter
Examples: Blister, pemphigus vulgaris

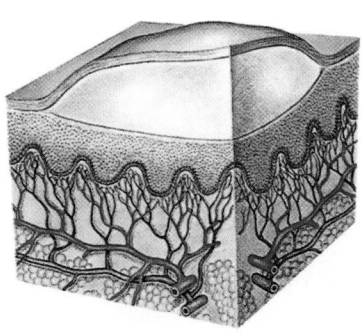

Cyst—elevated; circumscribed; palpable; encapsulated; filled with liquid or semisolid material
Example: Sebaceous cyst

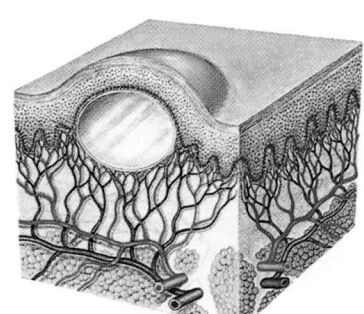

FIG 30-1 Primary skin lesions. (From Seidel HM, Ball JW, Dains JE, and others: *Mosby's guide to physical examination*, ed 6, St. Louis, 2006, Mosby.)

Scale—heaped-up keratinized cells; flaky exfoliation; irregular; thick or thin; dry or oily; varied size; silver, white, or tan in color
Examples: Psoriasis, exfoliative dermatitis

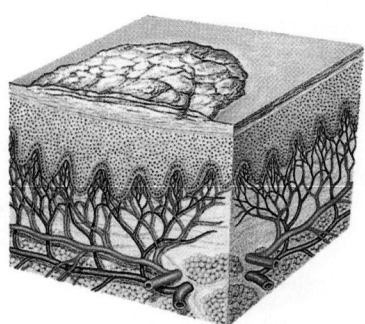

Crust—dried serum, blood, or purulent exudate; slightly elevated; size varies; brown, red, black, tan, or straw in color
Examples: Scab on abrasion, eczema

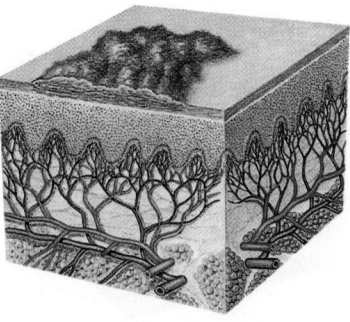

Lichenification—rough, thickened epidermis; accentuated skin markings caused by rubbing or irritation; often involves flexor aspect of extremity
Example: Chronic dermatitis

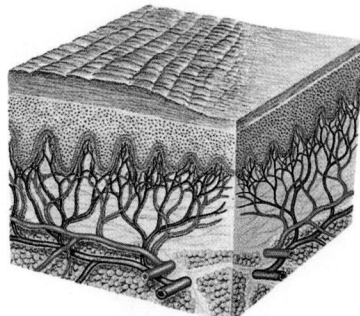

Scar—thin to thick fibrous tissue replacing injured dermis; irregular; pink, red, or white in color; may be atrophic or hypertrophic
Example: Healed wound or surgical incision

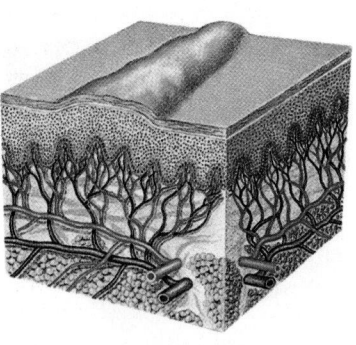

Keloid— irregularly shaped, elevated, progressively enlarging scar; grows beyond boundaries of wound; caused by excessive collagen formation during healing
Example: Keloid from ear piercing or burn scar

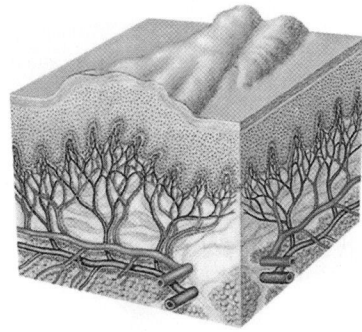

Excoriation—loss of epidermis; linear or hollowed-out crusted area; dermis exposed
Examples: Abrasion, scratch

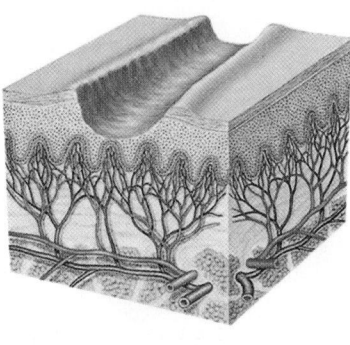

Fissure—linear crack or break from epidermis to dermis; small; deep; red
Examples: Athlete's foot, cheilosis

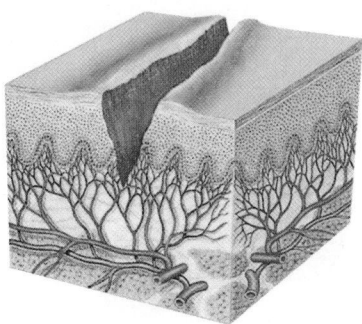

Erosion—loss of all or part of epidermis; depressed; moist; glistening; follows rupture of vesicle or bulla; larger than fissure
Examples: Varicella, variola following rupture

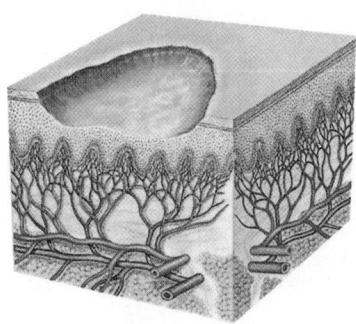

Ulcer—loss of epidermis and dermis; concave; varies in size; exudative; red or reddish blue
Examples: Decubiti, stasis ulcers

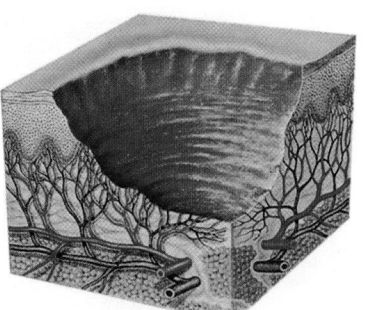

FIG 30-2 Secondary skin lesions. (From Seidel HM, Ball JW, Dains JE, and others: *Mosby's guide to physical examination,* ed 6, St. Louis, 2006, Mosby.)

that disrupt or delay wound healing include compromised perfusion, malnutrition, and infection. In children, most wounds are acute and can be prevented from becoming chronic wounds through appropriate nursing care. Wounds are also classified as surgical and nonsurgical and then further classified in the same manner as burns: superficial, partial thickness, or full thickness (complex wounds that include muscle or bone).

Epidermal Injuries

Abrasions are the most common epidermal wounds in children, usually in the form of a skinned knee or elbow. In most injuries, the margins of the abraded area are superficial, involving only the outer layers of epidermis, although the central portion may extend into the dermis. Epithelial tissue is composed of labile cells, which are constantly destroyed and replaced throughout the life span. Therefore, epidermal injuries usually result in rapid, uneventful healing and recovery.

Injury to Deeper Tissues

Tissues composed of permanent cells such as muscle and nerve cells are unable to regenerate. These tissues repair themselves by substituting fibrous connective tissue for the injured tissue. This fibrous tissue, or scar, serves as a patch to preserve or restore the continuity of the tissue. Wounds involving permanent cells include surgical incisions, lacerations, ulcers, evulsions, and full-thickness burns.

Process of Wound Healing

When the skin is injured, its normal protective barrier function is broken. In a healthy immunocompetent individual, acute traumatic abrasions, lacerations, and superficial skin and soft tissue injuries heal spontaneously without complications. The process of tissue healing involves complex cellular interactions and biochemical reactions. The healing process is segregated into four phases that are characterized by the particular cells involved and the chemicals produced. The four stages of wound healing are hemostasis, inflammation, proliferation, and remodeling (Krasner, Rodeheaver, and Sibbald, 2007). Some authorities combine the first two phases.

In the hemostasis phase, platelets act to seal off the damaged blood vessels and to form a stable clot. Hemostasis occurs within minutes of the initial injury to the skin unless there is an underlying clotting disorder.

Inflammation, the second stage of wound healing, presents a clinical picture that involves erythema, swelling, and warmth, often associated with pain at the wound site. This stage usually lasts up to 4 days after injury. The inflammation phase involves white blood cells such as the neutrophils, monocytes, and macrophages. These cells mount an initial defense against microbial invasion and secrete proteolytic enzymes that destroy nonviable tissue and microorganisms in the wound area.

The proliferative phase, which includes granulation and contracture, is the third stage of healing. This phase lasts from 4 to 21 days in acute wounds, depending on the size of the wound. The phase involves the replacement of dermal tissues and subdermal tissues in deep wounds, as well as the contraction of the wound. The phase is characterized clinically by the presence of granulation tissue, the "beefy," pebbled red tissue in the wound base. Fibroblasts, or immature connective tissue cells, secrete collagen, which provides the foundation for dermal regeneration. Angiocytes regenerate the outer layers of capillaries, and endothelial cells produce the lining in a process called angiogenesis. The formation of granulation tissue, which provides the foundation for the wound, depends on angiogenesis. The keratinocytes

are responsible for epithelialization. In the final stage of epithelialization, contracture occurs as the keratinocytes differentiate and form the protective outer layer, or stratum corneum, of the skin.

Remodeling, or maturation, is the final phase of the healing process. This phase occurs in the dermis as fibroblasts increase the tissue tensile strength and gradually replace type 3 collagen in the scar tissue with type 1 collagen, thicken the collagen fibers, and reorient the collagen fibers along the lines of tissue tension. Fibroblasts disappear as the wound becomes stronger. The wound edges are brought closer together, and a mature scar is formed. Children heal aggressively with abundant scar tissue, especially during growth spurts. The highly elastic quality of children's skin pulls on the wound, and the wound defends against this pull by forming scar tissue. Remodeling and maturation occur over several months and can take up to 2 years. Thus, some wounds that appear to be completely healed can break down suddenly if attention is not paid to the initial causative factors.

The phases of wound healing are complex and may be interrupted by disease conditions, medications, and other systemic and local factors that influence the healing process. When a wound does not follow the "normal wound healing trajectory," it may become stuck in one of the stages and become a chronic wound. It is important that health care providers understand and address the factors that influence wound healing and prevent the development of chronic wounds.

Factors That Influence Healing

Wound care management has shifted from interventions aimed at maintaining a dry environment to those that promote a moist, crust-free environment that enhances the migration of epithelial cells across the wound and facilitates remodeling. Whereas an acute full-thickness wound kept in a moist environment usually reepithelializes in 12 to 15 days, the same wound when kept open to the air heals in about 25 to 30 days.

Numerous factors can delay healing (Table 30-1). For example, traditional practices, such as the use of antiseptics (hydrogen peroxide and povidone–iodine [Betadine] solutions), which were once thought to prevent infection, are now known to have a cytotoxic effect on healthy cells and minimal effect on controlling infections. Povidone–iodine may also be absorbed through the skin in neonates and young children.

GENERAL THERAPEUTIC MANAGEMENT

Some skin disorders demand aggressive therapy, but by and large, the major aim of treatment is to prevent further damage, eliminate the cause, prevent complications, and provide relief from discomfort while tissues undergo healing (McCord and Levy, 2006). Factors that contribute to the development of dermatitis and that prolong the course of the disease should be eliminated when possible. The most common causative agents of dermatitis in infants, children, and adolescents are environmental factors (soaps, bubble baths, shampoos, rough or tight clothing, wet diapers, blankets, and toys) and the natural elements (e.g., dirt, sand, heat, cold, moisture, and wind). Dermatitis may also result from home remedies and medications.

Dressings

No one dressing meets the needs of all wounds. The traditional dry gauze dressing should not be used on open wounds because it allows the wound surface to dry, does little to prevent bacterial invasion, and adheres to the dried scab so that removal disturbs the newly regenerating epithelial cells. In most instances, traditional gauze dressings have been replaced by dressings that promote moist wound healing. Moist

TABLE 30-1   FACTORS THAT DELAY WOUND HEALING

FACTOR	EFFECT ON HEALING
Dry wound environment	Allows epithelial cells to dry out and die; impairs migration of epithelial cells across wound surface
Nutritional deficiencies	
Vitamin A	Results in inadequate inflammatory response
Vitamin B$_1$	Results in decreased collagen formation
Vitamin C	Inhibits formation of collagen fibers and capillary development
Protein	Reduces supply of amino acids for tissue repair
Zinc	Impairs epithelialization
Immunocompromise	Results in inadequate or delayed inflammatory response
Impaired circulation	Inhibits inflammatory response and removal of debris from wound area
	Reduces supply of nutrients to wound area
Stress (pain, poor sleep)	Releases catecholamines that cause vasoconstriction
Antiseptics	
Hydrogen peroxide	Toxic to fibroblasts; can cause subcutaneous gas formation (mimics gas-forming infection)
Povidone–iodine	Toxic to WBCs, RBCs, and fibroblasts
Chlorhexidine	Toxic to WBCs
Medications	
Corticosteroids	Impair phagocytosis
	Inhibit fibroblast proliferation
	Depress formation of granulation tissue
	Inhibit wound contraction
Chemotherapy	Interrupts the cell cycle; damages DNA or prevents DNA repair
Antiinflammatory drugs	Decrease the inflammatory phase
Foreign bodies	Increase inflammatory response
	Inhibit wound closure
Infection	Increases inflammatory response
	Increases tissue destruction
Mechanical friction	Damages or destroys granulation tissue
Fluid accumulation	Accumulation in area inhibits tissues from approximating
Radiation	Inhibits fibroblastic activity and capillary formation
	May cause tissue necrosis
Diseases	
Diabetes mellitus	Inhibits collagen synthesis
	Impairs circulation and capillary growth
	Hyperglycemia impairs phagocytosis
Anemia	Reduces oxygen supply to tissues
Peripheral vascular disease	Reduces oxygen supply to wounds
Uremia	Decreases collagen and granulation tissue

DNA, Deoxyribonucleic acid; *RBC*, red blood cell; *WBC*, white blood cell.

wound healing increases the rate of collagen synthesis and reepithelialization and decreases pain and inflammation. It also creates an environment for autolytic débridement of necrotic tissue, which creates a clean wound bed and enhances granulation. However, a balance must be achieved between creating a moist wound bed and maintaining a dry periwound area that protects the skin and wound from maceration. The dressing type and frequency of dressing changes help to achieve this balance. The frequency of dressing changes is based on the presence of infection, the type of dressing, the location of the wound, and the amount of drainage. Dressings should always be changed when they are loose or soiled. They should be changed more frequently in areas where contamination is likely (e.g., the sacral area, the buttocks, the tracheal area) or when wound infection is suspected or present.

Topical Therapy

Several agents and methods are available for treatment. In selecting a therapeutic regimen, the practitioner considers (1) the choice of active ingredient, (2) the proper vehicle or base, (3) the cosmetic effect, (4) the cost, and (5) instructions for use. Several basic concepts must also be considered. Overtreatment is avoided. For example, when dermatitis is acute, topical applications should be mild and bland to avoid further irritation. Broken or inflamed skin, especially in children, is more absorbent than intact skin, and chemicals that are nonirritating to intact skin may be quite irritating to inflamed skin.

Topical applications may be applied to treat the disorder, reduce itching, decrease external stimuli, or apply external heat or cold. The emollient action of soaks, baths, and lotions provides a soothing film over the skin surface that reduces external stimuli. Ordinarily, lukewarm, tepid, or cool applications offer the greatest relief.

> **! NURSING ALERT**
>
> Application of heat tends to aggravate most conditions, and its use is usually reserved for reducing specific inflammatory processes, such as folliculitis and cellulitis.

Ointments in a petrolatum base provide protection from moisture. Therefore, this type of ointment is indicated around gastrostomy tubes, in skinfolds, and in the diaper area. Creams are absorbed by the skin and are used for areas where a nongreasy "feel" is desired (e.g., face, hands).

Topical Corticosteroid Therapy

Glucocorticoids are the therapeutic agents used most frequently for skin disorders. Their local antiinflammatory effects are merely palliative, so the medication must be applied until the condition undergoes a remission or the causative agent is eliminated. Corticosteroids are applied directly to the affected area, are essentially nonsensitizing, and have only minor side effects. As with the use of any steroids, their use in large amounts may mask signs of infection, and symptoms may be exacerbated after termination of the drug. Families are cautioned that the medication cannot be used for all skin disorders. The concentrations available without prescription are not adequate for stubborn skin conditions (e.g., psoriasis) and may further aggravate inflammation caused by fungus or bacteria. Most parents and children apply too much topical hydrocortisone; therefore, they should be counseled that it is both effective and economical to apply only a thin film and to massage it into the skin. Parents and children should also be advised to use the application for no more than 5 to 7 days because these agents may cause depigmentation and other changes in the skin.

Other Topical Therapies

Other topical treatments include chemical cautery (especially useful for warts), cryosurgery, electrodesiccation (chiefly used for warts, granulomas, and nevi), ultraviolet (UV) therapy (primarily used in psoriasis and acne), laser therapy (especially for birthmarks), and acne therapies such as dermabrasion and chemical peels. New drugs called topical immunomodulators are effective in reducing the itching of AD (eczema) and preventing the recurrence of "flares."

Systemic Therapy

Systemic drugs may be used as an adjunct to topical therapy in some dermatologic disorders. The drugs most frequently used are corticosteroids, antibiotics, and antifungal agents. Corticosteroids are valuable because of their capacity to inhibit inflammatory and allergic reactions. The dosage is carefully adjusted and gradually tapered to the minimum dosage that is effective and tolerated. In infants and children, the dosage is larger than is usually calculated from body weight ratios. However, prolonged use may temporarily suppress growth.

Antibiotics are used in severe or widespread skin infections. However, because these drugs tend to produce hypersensitivity in some patients, they are used with caution. Antifungal agents are the only means for treating systemic fungal infections.

NURSING CARE MANAGEMENT

The child's subjective symptoms and the parent's history provide valuable information to help establish a diagnosis. Older children often describe the condition as painful, itching, or tingling or in other descriptive terms. However, much can be determined by also observing the younger child's behavior. Does the child scratch? Is the child restless or irritable? Does the child favor or avoid using a body part? A careful history provides important clues. Has the child had access to chemicals or been in the woods or around a woodpile? Has the child eaten a new food? Is the child taking medication? Has the child any known allergy? Do siblings or playmates have similar lesions? What soap or bubble bath is used for bathing?

It is important for nurses to not only describe but also assess skin lesions and wounds. The color, shape, and distribution of lesions and wounds are important. Individual lesions are described according to standard terminology. Sometimes two descriptors are used for a particular characteristic (e.g., maculopapular rash). To confirm or amplify the findings made by inspection, the nurse may gently palpate the skin to detect characteristics such as temperature, moisture, texture, elasticity, and edema. Wounds are assessed for depth of tissue damage, evidence of healing, and signs of infection.

> **! NURSING ALERT**
>
> Signs of wound infection are:
> - Increased erythema, especially beyond the wound margin
> - Edema
> - Purulent exudate
> - Pain
> - Increased temperature

The frequency of wound assessment depends on the severity and complexity of the wound. For example, simple or chronic wounds are assessed weekly; infected or complex wounds are assessed daily. Wounds are measured at least weekly (height, width, and depth). The wound bed is assessed for color, drainage, odor, necrosis, granulation tissue, fibrin slough, undermining and condition of the wound edges, and the color and condition of the surrounding skin (Butler, 2007).

Therapeutic programs are designed to include general measures such as rest, protection, and relief of discomfort and specific treatments such as medication and physical techniques. Only a few skin diseases are contagious; therefore, it is usually not necessary to isolate the affected child except from persons in danger of acquiring a secondary infection (e.g., a child receiving large doses of corticosteroids or other immunosuppressant drugs or a child with an immunologic deficiency disorder). However, if the skin manifestation is caused by a viral exanthema, such as measles or chickenpox, the child is prevented from exposing other susceptible children.

Wound Care

Parents can generally manage small skin lesions or wounds at home. The parents are instructed to wash their hands and then wash the wound gently with mild soap and water or normal saline. They are cautioned to avoid povidone–iodine, alcohol, and hydrogen peroxide because these products are toxic to wounds.

> **! NURSING ALERT**
>
> Do not put anything in a wound that you would not put in the eye. The safest solution is normal saline.

Open wounds are covered with a dressing, such as a commercial adhesive bandage, although larger wounds may benefit from the use of occlusive dressings. If occlusive dressings are applied, parents should learn how to apply and remove the dressings correctly. For example, hydrocolloid dressings adhere best if a wide margin is left around the wound and the dressing is pressed against intact skin until it adheres. If a dressing needs to be secured, a nonalcohol skin barrier can be applied to protect the skin, or the wound can be "picture framed" with hydrocolloid dressing and dressing tape can be secured to the hydrocolloid. This method of securing the dressing protects the skin when the tape is removed. Montgomery straps or stretch netting can also be used to secure dressings and to avoid the use of tape.

> **! NURSING ALERT**
>
> Advise parents that the yellow gel forming under hydrocolloid dressings may look like pus and has a distinct odor (somewhat fruity) but is normal leakage.

Dressings are removed carefully to protect intact skin and the epithelial surface of the wound. When removing transparent or hydrocolloid dressings, the nurse or parent should raise one edge of the dressing and pull *parallel* to the skin to loosen the adhesive. The longer the dressings are left on, the easier they are to remove. Less frequent dressing changes decrease wound contamination.

Lacerations present a special challenge. The injured child and family are usually distressed by the bleeding. In particular, scalp lacerations tend to bleed profusely. Parental guilt and shock usually accompany the injury. The initial nursing intervention is to apply pressure to the area and to attempt to calm the child before further examination. Unless there is bleeding from a severed artery, the wound is cleansed with a forced jet of sterile tepid water or saline (via syringe) and examined for extent; depth; and presence of foreign material such as dirt, glass, or fabric fragments.

The location of the wound facilitates assessment. Wounds over bony areas may contain bone chips, and clear fluid seeping from severe head wounds may indicate cerebrospinal fluid. A pressure dressing is applied for transfer to medical care. After the child is in a medical facility, he or she is prepared for suturing.

Puncture wounds that do not require a tetanus booster are soaked in warm water and soap for several minutes. Causing the wound to rebleed may be helpful. An adhesive bandage can be applied if desired. Puncture wounds of the head, chest, or abdomen or those that could still contain a portion of the puncturing object must be evaluated carefully.

Parents are cautioned against opening blisters or kissing a wound "to make it better." The wound can easily become contaminated from germs in the human mouth. If scabs form, they are allowed to slough off without assistance; picking or early removal may cause scarring and secondary infection. Parents are advised to seek medical help if there is evidence of infection.

Relief of Symptoms

Most therapeutic regimens for skin lesions are directed toward relief of pruritus, the most common subjective complaint. Cooling the affected area and increasing the skin pH with cool baths or compresses and alkaline applications (e.g., baking soda baths) are helpful in reducing the itching. Clothing and bed linens should be soft and lightweight to decrease the irritation from friction and stimulation.

During treatment, both the affected and the unaffected skin is protected from damage and secondary infection. Preventing scratching is important. Older children can cooperate, although they may need to be reminded to stop scratching or rubbing. However, small or uncooperative children may require the use of devices such as mittens (especially during sleep) or special coverings. Keeping fingernails clean, short, and trimmed reduces the risk of secondary infection.

Antipruritic medications, such as diphenhydramine (Benadryl) or hydroxyzine (Atarax), may be prescribed for severe itching, especially if it disturbs the child's rest. Pain and discomfort are usually managed with nonpharmacologic measures and mild analgesia. Severe pain requires more potent medication. Occlusive dressings over wounds reduce pain. For suturing wounds a topical anesthetic or intradermal buffered lidocaine should be used (see Pain Management, Chapter 7).

Topical Therapy

The specific type of topical therapy and the mode of application depend on the nature and location of the lesion. It is especially important to wash the hands before and after application of any topical therapy. The skin is assessed before the application and reassessed after treatment. Any observed changes are noted and described.

Wet compresses or dressings cool the skin by evaporation, relieve itching and inflammation, and cleanse the area by loosening and removing crusts and debris. A variety of ingredients, such as plain water or Burow solution (available without a prescription), can be applied on Kerlix gauze; plain gauze; or (preferably) soft cotton cloths such as freshly laundered handkerchiefs or strips from diaper, sheeting, or pillowcase material.

Dressings immersed in the desired solution are wrung out slightly and applied to the affected area wet but not dripping. They are applied flat and smooth in such a way that motion is not totally restricted—fingers are wrapped separately, and arms and legs are wrapped so that elbows and knees can bend. Dressings are held in place by Kerlix or other cotton wrap, tubular stockinette, mittens, and socks (two pairs—one to hold the dressings in place and the other to protect from movement). When evaporation begins to dry them, the dressings are removed, rewet in the solution, and reapplied using aseptic technique. The solution is *not* poured or applied with a syringe directly over the dressings. As fluid evaporates, the solution becomes more concentrated, and this could damage sensitive lesions.

Fresh solution at room temperature is applied at 2-, 3-, or 4-hour intervals and allowed to remain on the lesion for 20 to 90 minutes. Wet dressings are seldom continued after about 48 hours. The child is protected against chilling during treatment, and no more than 20% of the body is covered with a dressing at one time to avoid the risk of hypothermia. After treatment, the skin is dried thoroughly by patting with a towel. Lotion or other medication (if prescribed) is applied at this time.

When children are uncooperative in the use of wet dressings, soaks are often used for removal of crusts and for their mild astringent action. The same solutions are used as for wet compresses. Gaining young children's cooperation for hand or foot soaks is difficult unless the procedure is accompanied by play. Older infants and toddlers delight in playing with brightly colored objects or poker chips scattered over the bottom of the receptacle, and preschoolers can be challenged to hold a floating item beneath the water's surface. However, these activities require supervision; infants and small children place items in their mouths, and children easily lose control with water play. Washing dishes, cars, dolls, or doll clothes will also occupy time during soaks.

Although older children can cooperate, they, too, need something to do during the procedure, such as listening to music or a story or watching television. Placing the solution and the extremity in a plastic sealable bag is an effective method to soak a hand or foot.

Baths are useful in the treatment of widespread dermatitis by evenly distributing the soothing antipruritic and antiinflammatory effects of the solution, usually oatmeal or mineral oil preparations. The solution is added to a tub of lukewarm water. The temperature of the bath is tepid, and the treatment usually lasts 15 to 30 minutes. Therapeutic baths are more interesting when toy boats or other items for water play accompany the procedure.

Topical applications are applied to skin lesions to ease discomfort, prevent further injury, and facilitate healing. A thin application of the ointment or cream may be covered with a plastic film and anchored with adhesive, covered with a commercial transparent dressing, or wrapped in Kerlix gauze and held in place by a stretchy net dressing. Topical preparations are applied systematically with the contour of the body surface (not simply up and down). Children love to be "painted," and lotion applications can be fun when an ordinary paintbrush is used. Regardless of the type of preparation used, parents need detailed information on how to apply it and how long the preparation should remain on the skin.

> **! NURSING ALERT**
>
> Provide written instructions and demonstrate to parents the correct amount of topical medication to apply (e.g., size of a pea, thin film to cover). If more than one preparation is applied, mark the containers with numbers so the parents remember the correct order of application. Stress that more is not necessarily better with some medications, such as steroids.

HOME CARE AND FAMILY SUPPORT

Dermatologic conditions always involve the family, but few situations require hospitalization, and most care is delivered at home. Because the family members must carry out the treatment plan, their cooperation is essential. Regimens that are simple to accomplish in the clinic, hospital, or primary care provider's office may be frustrating and baffling at home. The family may also need assistance in adapting equipment available for home therapy.

It is important that the child and family be given as detailed explanations as possible about both the expected and the unexpected results of treatment, including any ill effects that might occur. If unexplained reactions develop, the family is directed to discontinue treatment and report the reactions to the appropriate person. The use of over-the-counter medicines is discouraged unless the preparations have been discussed with the health care provider and have received approval.

Because the skin is the most visible portion of the body, defects in its surface alter its appearance and cause distress for the child. Skin problems may also result in rejection by others. Parents of other children may fear that their children will "catch" the disorder. Occasionally, the affected child's own family members reduce their interaction or physical contact with the child. This is seldom a problem with dermatitis of short duration, but chronic conditions can frequently create problems and affect the child's self-esteem.

INFECTIONS OF THE SKIN

BACTERIAL INFECTIONS

Normally, the skin harbors a variety of bacterial flora, including the major pathogenic varieties of staphylococci and streptococci. The degree of pathogenicity of the organism depends on its invasiveness and toxicity, the integrity of the skin, and the immune and cellular defenses of the host. Children with congenital or acquired immunodeficiency disorders (e.g., acquired immunodeficiency syndrome [AIDS]), those in a debilitated condition, those receiving immunosuppressant therapy, and those with a generalized malignancy such as leukemia or lymphoma are at risk for developing bacterial infections.

Because of the characteristic "walling-off" process of the inflammatory reaction (abscess formation), staphylococci are more difficult to treat, and the local infected area is associated with an increase in bacteria all over the skin surface that serves as a source of continuing infection. In previous years, methicillin-resistant *Staphylococcus aureus* (MRSA) infections were primarily seen in nursing homes and hospitals. In recent years, the number of MRSA community-acquired infections has risen (Kaplan, 2006). All of these factors underline the importance of careful hand washing and cleanliness when caring for infected children and their lesions to prevent the spread of infection and as an essential prophylactic measure when caring for infants and small children. Common bacterial skin disorders are outlined in Table 30-2.

Nursing Care Management

The major nursing functions related to bacterial skin infections are to prevent the spread of infection and to prevent complications. Impetigo contagiosa and MRSA infection can easily spread by self-inoculation; therefore, caution the child against touching the involved area. Hand washing is mandatory before and after contact with an affected child. Also emphasize hand washing to both the child and the family. Many children with AD are colonized with MRSA in the nares and under the fingernails (Rosenthal, 2004). For many bacterial infections and for MRSA infection in particular, the child should be provided with washcloths and towels separate from those of other family members. The child's pajamas, underwear, and other clothes should be changed daily and washed in hot water. Razors used for shaving should be discarded after each use and not shared. To prevent recurrence, some infectious disease specialists recommend bathing in a chlorine bath once or twice weekly. A 5-minute soak of 2.5 ml of bleach diluted in 13 gallons of water or ½ cup of bleach diluted in a standard 50-gallon tub one fourth filled with water could decrease community-acquired MRSA colonies by more than 99.9% (Fisher, Chain, Hair, and others, 2008; Kaplan, 2008). In addition, mupirocin can be applied to the nares of patients and families twice daily for 2 to 4 weeks to prevent reinfection (Dohil and Eichenfield, 2005).

Children and parents are often tempted to squeeze follicular lesions. They must be warned that squeezing will not hasten the resolution of the infection and that there is a risk of making the lesion worse or spreading the infection. No attempt should be made to puncture the surface of the pustule with a needle or sharp instrument. A child with a sty may waken with the eyelids of the affected eye sealed shut with exudate. The child or the parents are instructed to gently wipe the eyelid from the inner to the outer edge with warm water and a clean washcloth until the exudate is removed.

The child with limited cellulitis of an extremity is usually managed at home on a regimen of oral antibiotics and warm compresses. The parents are taught the procedures and instructed in administration of the medication. Children with more extensive cellulitis, especially around a joint with lymphadenitis or on the face, are usually admitted to the hospital for parenteral antibiotics with continued treatment at home. Nurses are responsible for teaching the family to administer the medication and apply compresses.

VIRAL INFECTIONS

Viruses are intracellular parasites that produce their effect by using the intracellular substances of the host cells. Composed of only a deoxyribonucleic acid (DNA) or ribonucleic acid (RNA) core enclosed in an antigenic protein shell, viruses are unable to provide for their own metabolic needs or to reproduce themselves. After a virus penetrates a cell of the host organism, it sheds the outer shell and disappears within the cell, where the nucleic acid core stimulates the host cell to form more virus material from its intracellular substance. In a viral infection, the epidermal cells react with inflammation and vesiculation (as in herpes simplex) or by proliferating to form growths (warts).

Many of the communicable viral diseases of childhood are associated with rashes, and each rash is characteristic. The type of lesion and the configuration of rubeola, rubella, and chickenpox are described in Table 14-1. Other common viral disorders of the skin are outlined in Table 30-3.

DERMATOPHYTOSES (FUNGAL INFECTIONS)

The dermatophytoses (ringworm) are infections caused by a group of closely related filamentous fungi that invade primarily the stratum corneum, hair, and nails. These are superficial infections that live on, not in, the skin. They are confined to the dead keratin layers and are unable to survive in the deeper layers. Because the keratin is desquamated constantly, the fungus must multiply at a rate that equals the rate of keratin production to maintain itself; otherwise, the infection would be shed with the discarded skin cells. Common dermatophytoses are outlined in Table 30-4.

Dermatophytoses are designated by the Latin word *tinea*, with further designation related to the area of the body where they are found (e.g., tinea capitis [ringworm of the scalp]). Dermatophyte infections are most often transmitted from one person to another or from infected animals to humans. Diagnosis is made from microscopic examination of scrapings taken from the advancing periphery of the lesion, which almost always produces a scale.

TABLE 30-2	BACTERIAL INFECTIONS		
DISORDER AND ORGANISM	**MANIFESTATIONS**	**MANAGEMENT**	**COMMENTS**
Impetigo contagiosa (Fig. 30-3)— *Staphylococcus*	Begins as a reddish macule Becomes vesicular Ruptures easily, leaving superficial, moist erosion Tends to spread peripherally in sharply marginated irregular outlines Exudate dries to form heavy, honey-colored crusts Pruritus common *Systemic effects*—Minimal or asymptomatic	Careful removal of undermined skin, crusts, and debris by softening with 1:20 Burow solution compresses Topical application of bactericidal ointment Systemic administration of oral or parenteral antibiotics (penicillin) in severe or extensive lesions	Tends to heal without scarring unless secondary infection Autoinoculable and contagious Common in toddlers and preschoolers May be superimposed on eczema
Pyoderma— *Staphylococcus*, *Streptococcus*	Deeper extension of infection into dermis Tissue reaction more severe *Systemic effects*—Fever, lymphangitis	Soap and water cleansing Wet compresses Bathing with antibacterial soap as prescribed Do not share washcloths or towels Mupirocin to nares and lesions as prescribed Systemic antibiotics	Autoinoculable and contagious May heal with or without scarring
Folliculitis (pimple), furuncle (boil), carbuncle (multiple boils)— *Staphylococcus aureus*	Folliculitis—Infection of hair follicle Furuncle—Larger lesion with more redness and swelling at a single follicle Carbuncle—More extensive lesion with widespread inflammation and "pointing" at several follicular orifices *Systemic effects*—Malaise if severe	Skin cleanliness Local warm, moist compresses Topical application of antibiotic agents Systemic antibiotics in severe cases Incision and drainage of severe lesions followed by wound irrigations with antibiotics or suitable drain implantation	Autoinoculable and contagious Furuncle and carbuncle tend to heal with scar formation Never squeeze a lesion
Cellulitis— *Streptococcus*, *Staphylococcus*, *Haemophilus influenzae* (Fig. 30-4)	Inflammation of skin and subcutaneous tissues with intense redness, swelling, and firm infiltration Lymphangitis "streaking" frequently seen Involvement of regional lymph nodes common May progress to abscess formation *Systemic effects*—Fever, malaise	Oral or parenteral antibiotics Rest and immobilization of both affected area and child Hot, moist compresses to area	Hospitalization may be necessary for child with systemic symptoms Otitis media may be associated with facial cellulites
Staphylococcal scalded skin syndrome— *S. aureus*	Macular erythema with "sandpaper" texture of involved skin Epidermis becoming wrinkled (in ≤2 days), and large bullae appearing	Systemic administration of antibiotics Gentle cleansing with saline, Burow solution, or 0.25% silver nitrate compresses	Infants subject to fluid loss; impaired body temperature regulation; and secondary infection, such as pneumonia, cellulitis, and septicemia Heals without scarring

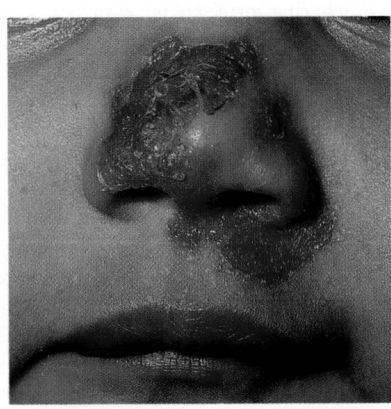

FIG 30-3 Impetigo contagiosa. (From Weston WL, Lane AT: *Color textbook of pediatric dermatology*, ed 4, St. Louis, 2007, Mosby.)

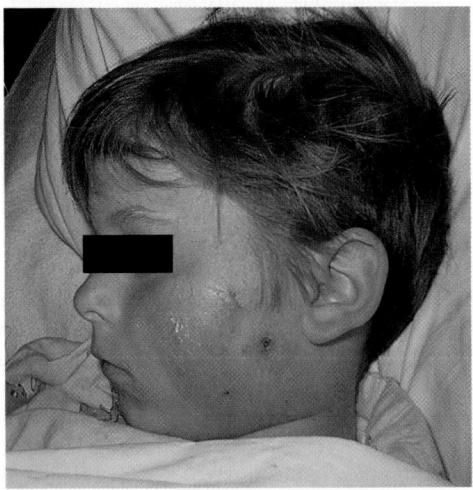

FIG 30-4 Cellulitis of cheek from a puncture wound. (From Weston WL, Lane AT: *Color textbook of pediatric dermatology*, ed 4, St. Louis, 2007, Mosby.)

TABLE 30-3	**VIRAL INFECTIONS**		
INFECTION	**MANIFESTATIONS**	**MANAGEMENT**	**COMMENTS**
Verruca (warts) *Cause*—Human papillomavirus (various types)	Usually well-circumscribed, gray or brown, elevated, firm papules with a roughened, finely papillomatous texture Occur anywhere but usually appear on exposed areas such as fingers, hands, face, and soles May be single or multiple Asymptomatic	Not uniformly successful Local destructive therapy, individualized according to location, type, and number—surgical removal, electrocautery, curettage, cryotherapy (liquid nitrogen), caustic solutions (lactic acid and salicylic acid in flexible collodion, retinoic acid, salicylic acid plasters), x-ray treatment, laser	Common in children Tend to disappear spontaneously Course unpredictable Most destructive techniques tend to leave scars Autoinoculable Repeated irritation will cause to enlarge Apply topical anesthetic EMLA
Verruca plantaris (plantar wart)	Located on plantar surface of feet and, because of pressure, are practically flat; may be surrounded by a collar of hyperkeratosis	Apply caustic solution to wart and wear foam insole with hole cut to relieve pressure on wart; soak 20 minutes after 2–3 days; repeat until wart comes out	Destructive techniques tend to leave scars, which may cause problems with walking Apply topical anesthetic EMLA
Herpes simplex virus Type I (cold sore, fever blister) Type II (genital)	Grouped, burning, and itching vesicles on inflammatory base, usually on or near mucocutaneous junctions (lips, nose, genitalia, buttocks) Vesicles dry, forming a crust followed by exfoliation and spontaneous healing in 8–10 days May be accompanied by regional lymphadenopathy	Avoidance of secondary infection Burow solution compresses during weeping stages Topical therapy (penciclovir) to shorten duration of cold sores Oral antiviral (acyclovir) for initial infection or to reduce severity in recurrence Valacyclovir (Valtrex), an oral antiviral, used for episodic treatment of recurrent genital herpes; reduces pain, stops viral shedding, and has a more convenient administration schedule than acyclovir	Heal without scarring unless secondary infection Type I cold sores prevented by using sunscreens protecting against UVA and UVB light to prevent lip blisters Aggravated by corticosteroids Positive psychologic effect from treatment May be fatal in children with depressed immunity
Varicella-zoster virus (herpes zoster; shingles)	Caused by same virus that causes varicella (chickenpox) Virus has affinity for posterior root ganglia, posterior horn of spinal cord, and skin; crops of vesicles usually confined to dermatome following along course of affected nerve Usually preceded by neuralgic pain, hyperesthesias, or itching May be accompanied by constitutional symptoms	Symptomatic Analgesics for pain Mild sedation sometimes helpful Local moist compresses Drying lotions sometimes helpful Ophthalmic variety: use systemic corticotropin (ACTH) or corticosteroids Acyclovir Lidocaine (Lidoderm) topical anesthetic	Pain in children usually minimal Postherpetic pain does not occur in children Chickenpox may follow exposure; isolate affected child from other children in a hospital or school May occur in children with depressed immunity; can be fatal
Molluscum contagiosum *Cause*—Pox virus Small, benign tumors	Flesh-colored papules with a central caseous plug (umbilicated) Usually asymptomatic	Cases in well children resolve spontaneously in about 18 months Treatment reserved for troublesome cases Apply topical anesthetic EMLA and remove with curette Use tretinoin gel 0.01% or cantharidin (Cantharone) liquid* Curettage or cryotherapy	Common in school-age children Spread by skin-to-skin contact, including autoinoculation and fomite-to-skin contact

ACTH, Adrenocorticotropic hormone; *EMLA*, eutectic mix of lidocaine and prilocaine; *UVA*, ultraviolet A; *UVB*, ultraviolet B.
*Not available in the United States but can be purchased in Canada.

Nursing Care Management

When teaching families how to care for ringworm, the nurse should emphasize good health and hygiene. Because of the infectious nature of the disease, affected children should not exchange grooming items, headgear, scarves, or other articles of apparel that have been in proximity to the infected area with other children. Affected children are provided with their own towels and directed to wear a protective cap at night to avoid transmitting the fungus to bedding, especially if they sleep with another person. Because the infection can be acquired by animal-to-human transmission, all household pets should be examined for the disorder. Other sources of infection are seats with headrests (theater seats), seats in public transportation vehicles, helmets, and gymnasium mats.

Both 2% ketoconazole and 1% selenium sulfide shampoos may reduce colony counts of dermatophytes. These shampoos can be used in combination with oral therapy to reduce the transmission of disease to others. The shampoo should be applied to the scalp for 5 to 10 minutes at least three times per week. The child may return to school after the therapy is initiated.

Alternately, if the child is treated with the drug griseofulvin, the therapy frequently continues for weeks or months, and because subjective symptoms subside, children or parents may be tempted to decrease

TABLE 30-4 DERMATOPHYTOSES (FUNGAL INFECTIONS)

DISEASE AND ORGANISM	MANIFESTATIONS	MANAGEMENT	COMMENTS
Tinea capitis—*Trichophyton tonsurans, Microsporum audouinii, Microsporum canis* (Fig. 30-5, *A*)	Lesions in scalp but may extend to hairline or neck Characteristic configuration of scaly, circumscribed patches or patchy, scaling areas of alopecia Generally asymptomatic but severe, deep inflammatory reaction may occur that manifests as boggy, encrusted lesions (kerions) Pruritic Microscopic examination of scales is diagnostic	Oral griseofulvin Oral ketoconazole for difficult cases Selenium sulfide shampoos Topical antifungal agents (e.g., clotrimazole, haloprogin, miconazole)	Person-to-person transmission Animal-to-person transmission Rarely, permanent loss of hair *M. audouinii* transmitted from one human being to another directly or from personal items; *M. canis* usually contracted from household pets, especially cats Atopic individuals more susceptible
Tinea corporis—*Trichophyton rubrum, Trichophyton mentagrophytes, M. canis,* Epidermophyton (see Fig. 30-4, *B*)	Generally round or oval, erythematous scaling patch that spreads peripherally and clears centrally; may involve nails (tinea unguium) *Diagnosis*—Direct microscopic examination of scales Usually unilateral	Oral griseofulvin Local application of antifungal preparation such as tolnaftate, haloprogin, miconazole, clotrimazole; apply 1 inch beyond periphery of lesion; continual application 1–2 weeks after no sign of lesion	Usually of animal origin from infected pets Majority of infections in children caused by *M. canis* and *M. audouinii*
Tinea cruris ("jock itch")—*Epidermophyton floccosum, T. rubrum, T. mentagrophytes*	Skin response similar to tinea corporis Localized to medial proximal aspect of thigh and crural fold; may involve scrotum in boys Pruritic *Diagnosis*—Same as for tinea corporis	Local application of tolnaftate liquid Wet compresses or sitz baths may be soothing	Rare in preadolescent children Health education regarding personal hygiene
Tinea pedis ("athlete's foot")—*T. rubrum, Trichophyton interdigitale, E. floccosum*	On intertriginous areas between toes or on plantar surface of feet Lesions vary: Maceration and fissuring between toes Patches with pinhead-sized vesicles on plantar surface Pruritic *Diagnosis*—Direct microscopic examination of scrapings	Oral griseofulvin Local applications of tolnaftate liquid and antifungal powder containing tolnaftate *Acute infections*—Compresses or soaks followed by application of glucocorticoid cream Elimination of conditions of heat and perspiration by clean, light socks and well-ventilated shoes; avoidance of occlusive shoes	Most frequent in adolescents and adults; rare in children, but occurrence increases with wearing of plastic shoes Transmission to other individuals rare despite general opinion to contrary Ointments not successful
Candidiasis (moniliasis)—*Candida albicans*	Grows in chronically moist areas Inflamed areas with white exudate, peeling, and easy bleeding Pruritic *Diagnosis*—Characteristic appearance	Amphotericin B, nystatin ointment, or other antifungal preparations to affected areas	Common form of diaper dermatitis (see Fig. 30-11, p. 1032) Oral form common in infants (see Chapter 9) Vaginal form in older girls May be disseminated in immunosuppressed children

or discontinue the drug. The nurse should emphasize to family members the importance of maintaining the prescribed dosage schedule and of taking the medication with high-fat foods for best absorption. They are also instructed regarding possible drug side effects, such as headache, gastrointestinal upset, fatigue, insomnia, and photosensitivity. For children who take the drug over many months, periodic testing is required to monitor leukopenia and assess liver and renal function. Newer antifungal medications such as terbinafine, itraconazole, and fluconazole may be used when there are adverse reactions to griseofulvin. Currently, these drugs are being studied to determine their efficacy and safety in treating tinea capitis in children but are not approved by the U.S. Food and Drug Administration (FDA) for this indication at this time.

SYSTEMIC MYCOTIC (FUNGAL) INFECTIONS

Mycotic (systemic or deep fungal) infections have the capacity to invade the viscera, as well as the skin. The most common infections are the lung diseases, which are usually acquired by inhalation of fungal spores. These fungi produce a variable spectrum of disease, and some are common in certain geographic areas. They are not transmitted from person to person but appear to reside in the soil, from which their spores are airborne. The cutaneous lesions caused by deep fungal infections are granulomatous and appear as ulcers, plaques, nodules, fungating masses, and abscesses. The course of deep fungal diseases is chronic with slow progression that favors sensitization (Table 30-5).

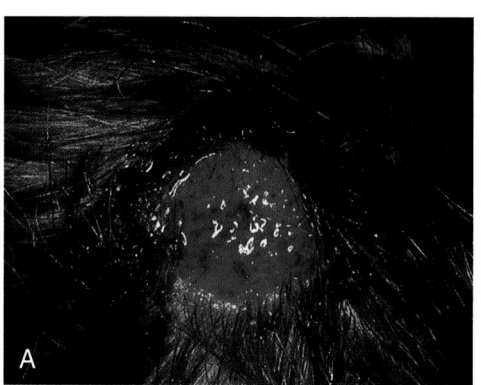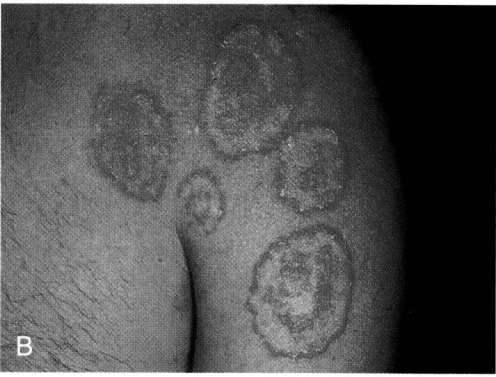

FIG 30-5 A, Tinea capitis. **B,** Tinea corporis. Both infections are caused by *Microsporum canis*, the "kitten" or "puppy" fungus. (From Habif TP: *Clinical dermatology: a color guide to diagnosis and therapy*, ed 4, St. Louis, 2004, Mosby.)

TABLE 30-5	**SYSTEMIC MYCOSES**			
DISORDER AND ORGANISM	**SKIN MANIFESTATIONS**	**SYSTEMIC MANIFESTATIONS**	**MANAGEMENT**	**COMMENTS**
North American blastomycosis— *Blastomyces dermatitidis*	Chronic granulomatous lesions and microabscesses in any part of body Initial lesion is a papule; undergoes ulceration and peripheral spread	Pulmonary symptoms, such as cough, chest pain, weakness, and weight loss May have skeletal involvement, with bone destruction and formation of cutaneous abscesses	IV administration of amphotericin B	Usual portal of entry is lungs Source of infection unknown Noninfectious Pulmonary infections may be mild and self-limiting and require no treatment Progressive disease often fatal
Cryptococcosis— *Cryptococcus neoformans* (*Torula histolytica*)	Usually on face; acneiform, firm, nodular, painless eruption	*CNS manifestations*— Headache, dizziness, stiff neck, and signs of increased intracranial pressure Low-grade fever, mild cough, lung infiltration	IV amphotericin B; may be administered intrathecally for CNS involvement 5-Fluorocytosine for meningitis Excision and drainage of local lesions	Acquired by inhalation of dust but may enter through skin Prognosis serious Noninfectious Increased incidence in persons receiving corticosteroids with lymphoreticular malignancies or type 2 diabetes
Histoplasmosis— *Histoplasma capsulatum*	Not distinctive or uniform but most appear as punched-out or granulomatous ulcers	General systemic symptoms may include pallor, diarrhea, vomiting, irregular spiking temperature, hepatosplenomegaly, and pulmonary symptoms Any tissue of body may be involved with related symptoms	IV amphotericin B for severe cases Oral ketoconazole	Organism cultured from soil, especially where contaminated with fowl droppings Fungus enters through skin or mucous membranes of mouth and respiratory tract Endemic in Mississippi and Ohio River valleys Disseminated diseases most common in infants and children
Coccidioidomycosis (valley fever)— *Coccidioides immitis*	Erythema nodosum Erythema multiforme Erythematous maculopapular rash	Primary lung disease usually asymptomatic May be sign of acute febrile illness Disseminated disease is serious	IV amphotericin B IV miconazole (synthetic imidazole) Intraventricular miconazole plus oral ketoconazole for CNS involvement Surgical resection of persistent pulmonary cavities	Inhalation of aerospores from soil Endemic in southwestern United States Usually resolves spontaneously Increased incidence in dark-skinned races (Filipino, African American, Hispanic, Asian)

CNS, Central nervous system; *IV,* intravenous.

SKIN DISORDERS RELATED TO CHEMICAL OR PHYSICAL CONTACTS

CONTACT DERMATITIS

Contact dermatitis is an inflammatory reaction of the skin to chemical substances, natural or synthetic, that evoke a hypersensitivity response or direct irritation. The initial reaction occurs in an exposed region, most commonly the face and neck, backs of the hands, forearms, male genitalia, and lower legs. Early in the reaction, there is usually a sharp delineation between inflamed and normal skin that ranges from a faint, transient erythema to massive bullae on an erythematous swollen base. Itching is a constant symptom.

The cause may be a primary irritant or a sensitizing agent. A primary irritant is one that irritates any skin. A sensitizing agent produces an irritation on those individuals who have met the irritant or something chemically related to it, have undergone an immunologic change, and have become sensitized. Prior exposure is not necessarily a factor in the reaction. A sensitizer irritates in relatively low concentrations only persons who are allergic to it.

In infants, contact dermatitis occurs on the convex surfaces of the diaper area. Other agents that produce contact dermatitis include plants (poison ivy, oak, or sumac), animal irritants (wool, feathers, and furs), metal (nickel found in jewelry and the snaps on sleepers and denim), vegetable irritants (oleoresins, oils, and turpentine), synthetic fabrics (e.g., shoe components), dyes, cosmetics, perfumes, and soaps (including bubble baths). The list is endless.

The major goal in treatment is to prevent further exposure of the skin to the offending substance. Provided there is no further irritation, the skin's normal recuperative powers will often produce healing without treatment. Otherwise, treatment of contact dermatitis is based on severity. Mild cases are treated with topical steroids. Mild to moderately severe cases may require a 2-week course of strong topical corticosteroids. Very severe cases require systemic corticosteroids.

Nursing Care Management

Nurses frequently detect evidence of contact dermatitis during routine physical assessments. Skin manifestations in specific areas suggest limited contact, such as around the eyes (mascara), areas of the body covered by clothing but not protected by undergarments (wool), or areas of the body not covered by clothing (UV injury). Generalized involvement is more likely to be caused by bubble bath or soap. Often nurses can determine the offending agent and counsel families regarding management. However, if the lesions persist, are extensive, or show evidence of infection, medical evaluation is indicated.

POISON IVY, OAK, AND SUMAC

Contact with the dry or succulent portions of any of three poisonous plants (ivy, oak, and sumac) produces localized, streaked or spotty, oozing, and painful impetiginous lesions. The offending substance in these plants is an oil, urushiol, that is extremely potent. Sensitivity to urushiol is not inborn but is developed after one or two exposures and may change over a lifetime. All parts of the plants contain the oil, including dried leaves and stems (Fig. 30-6). Even smoke from burning brush piles can produce a reaction.

Animals do not seem to be affected by the oil; however, dogs or other animals that have run or played in the plants may carry the sap on their fur, and animals that eat the plants can transfer the oil in their saliva. Shoes, tools, and toys can transfer the oil. Golf balls that have been in the rough are another source of contact.

Urushiol takes effect as soon as it touches the skin. It penetrates through the epidermis and bonds with the dermal layer, where it initiates an immune response. The full-blown reaction is evident after about 2 days, with redness, swelling, and itching at the site of contact. Several days later, streaked or spotty blisters oozing serum from damaged cells produce the characteristic impetiginous lesions (see Fig. 30-6, B). The lesions dry and heal spontaneously, and itching stops by 10 to 14 days.

Therapeutic Management

As soon as an exposure is realized, there is no time to waste. The earlier the skin is cleansed, the greater the chance of removing the urushiol before it attaches to the skin. The exposed skin can be cleansed with isopropyl alcohol followed by water. A shower with soap and warm water should follow. Clothes, tools, shoes, and any other objects that had contact with the plants should be cleaned with alcohol and then water.

Treatment of the lesions includes calamine lotion, soothing Burow solution compresses, or Aveeno baths to relieve discomfort. Topical corticosteroid gel is effective for prevention or relief of inflammation, especially when applied before blisters form. Oral corticosteroids may be needed for severe reactions, and a sedative such as diphenhydramine may be ordered.

Nursing Care Management

When it is known that the child has made contact with the plant, the area is immediately flushed (preferably within 15 minutes) with *cold* running water to neutralize the urushiol not yet bonded to the skin. If there is a stream nearby, an effective method is to have the child enter the water (clothes and all) and allow the water to rinse the oil from both skin and clothing. Harsh soap is contraindicated because it removes protective skin oils and dilutes the urushiol, allowing it to spread; hard scrubbing irritates the skin. All clothing that has come in contact with the plant is removed with care and thoroughly laundered in hot water and detergent. Every effort is made to prevent the child from scratching the lesions. Although the lesions do not spread by contact with the blister serum or from scratching, they can become secondarily infected.

Prevention

Prevention is best accomplished by avoiding contact and removing the plant from the environment. All children, especially those known to be sensitive, should be taught to recognize the plant. Information regarding means for destroying plants can be obtained from the U.S. Department of Agriculture or U.S. Forestry Service. Home garden sprays that kill broad-leaf plants or all vegetation (e.g., Roundup or Spectracide) are ineffective. If poisonous plants are growing in public community area, the local authorities should be contacted to remove the plants. A cream that protects exposed skin from poison oak and ivy is Ivy Block.

DRUG REACTIONS

Adverse reactions to drugs are seen more often in the skin than in any other organ, although any organ of the body can be affected. The reaction may be a result of toxicity related to drug concentration, individual intolerance to the average dosage of the drug, or an allergic or idiosyncratic response. The manifestations may be associated with side effects or secondary effects of a drug, either of which are unrelated to its primary pharmacologic actions.

Although any drug is capable of producing a reaction in the susceptible individual, some drugs have a tendency to produce a particular

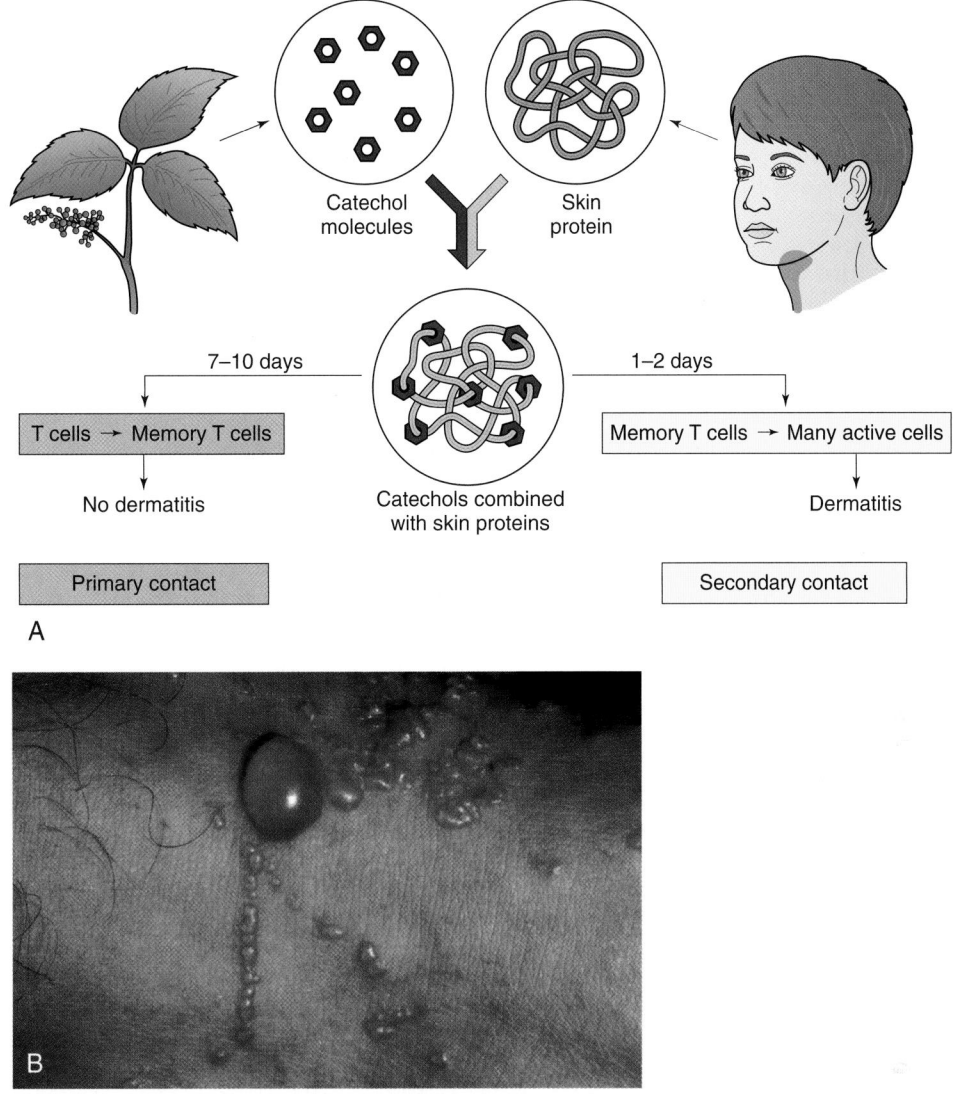

FIG 30-6 A, Development of allergic contact dermatitis. **B,** Poison ivy lesions; note the "streaked" blisters surrounding one large blister. (**A,** From McCance K, Huether S: *Pathophysiology: the biological basis for disease in adults and children,* ed 6, St. Louis, 2010, Mosby. **B,** From Habif TP: *Clinical dermatology: a color guide to diagnosis and therapy,* ed 5, St. Louis, 2010, Mosby.)

reaction consistently, and others are more likely to produce an untoward effect. Many are allergenic responses that occur after a previous administration of the drug, even a topical application. Other factors influence a drug response in a particular individual. For example, the incidence increases with the amount and number of drugs given.

> **! NURSING ALERT**
>
> IV drugs are more likely to cause a reaction than oral drugs. Stop the drug but maintain the infusion with normal saline.

Manifestations of drug reactions may be delayed or immediate. A period of 7 days is usually required for a child to develop sensitivity to a drug that has never been administered previously. With prior sensitivity, the manifestations appear almost immediately. Rashes are the most common manifestation of adverse drug reactions in children. However, individual drug reactions may vary from a single lesion to extensive, generalized epidermal necrosis such as that seen in

Stevens-Johnson syndrome (see Table 30-8). Cutaneous manifestations can resemble almost any skin disease and can be seen in almost any degree of severity. With few exceptions, the distribution of a drug eruption is widespread because it results from a circulating agent; appears as an inflammatory response with itching; is sudden in onset; and may be associated with constitutional symptoms such as fever, malaise, gastrointestinal upsets, anemia, or liver and kidney damage.

In most cases, treatment for simple cutaneous reactions consists of discontinuing the drug. Sometimes a decision is made to continue the drug (e.g., an antibiotic in an infant or small child) until the cause of the rash is clearly indicated. In urticarial-type eruptions, antihistamines may be ordered, and for widespread and severe lesions, corticosteroids are beneficial. Severe anaphylactic reactions are a medical emergency (see Anaphylaxis, Chapter 25).

Nursing Care Management

The most effective means of management is prevention. Parents always remember a severe reaction. A careful history will elicit evidence of a previous drug reaction. The history should include the name of the drug, nature of the reaction, drug dosage, and how soon after administration the reaction occurred (see Chapter 6).

Nurses who suspect that a rash is caused by a medication should withhold any further dose and report the eruption to the practitioner. Frequent offenders in drug reactions are penicillin and sulfonamides, and nurses must be alert to this possibility. However, even common drugs, including aspirin, barbiturates, chemical agents in some foods, flavoring agents, and preservatives, are capable of producing an undesired response. Persons who have severe reactions should wear a medical identification bracelet or necklace in case of emergency or inadvertent administration of the offending drug.

FOREIGN BODIES

Parents can remove small wooden splinters with a needle and tweezers that have been sterilized with alcohol or a flame. The area around the sliver is washed with soap and water before removal is attempted. The sliver is exposed with the needle and then grasped firmly by the tweezers and pulled out. Some foreign bodies, such as a fishhook, pieces of glass, a difficult-to-see object, or a deeply embedded object (e.g., a needle in a foot or near a joint), require medical evaluation.

Small cactus prickles or spines are troublesome to remove, but the following methods may prove helpful:

- Apply a thin layer of water-soluble household glue and cover it with gauze; when the glue dries, peel off the gauze.
- Apply hair removal wax or body sugar, let it dry, and remove.
- Place cellophane tape, sticky side down, over the spines and lift it off.

SKIN DISORDERS RELATED TO ANIMAL CONTACTS

ARTHROPOD BITES AND STINGS

Bites and stings account for a significant amount of mild to moderate discomfort in children. Most bites and stings are managed by simple symptomatic measures, such as compresses, calamine lotion, and prevention of secondary infection. Arthropods include insects and arachnids, such as mites, ticks, spiders, and scorpions. Most arthropods in the United States, including tarantulas, are relatively harmless. Although all spiders produce venom that is injected via fangs, some are unable to pierce the skin, and others produce venom that is insufficiently toxic to be harmful. Only scorpions and two spiders—the brown recluse and the black widow—inject venom deadly enough to require immediate attention. Children bitten by these arachnids must receive medical attention as soon as possible. Major offending creatures, their manifestations, and management are outlined in Table 30-6. A brown recluse spider bite is shown in Fig. 30-7.

When a hymenopteran (bees in particular) stings, its barbed stinger penetrates the skin. As long as the stinger remains in the skin, the muscles push the stinger deeper, and the venom is pumped into the wound. The best approach is to remove the stinger as quickly as possible and to get away from the vicinity of other insects to prevent further injury. Children who have become sensitized to hymenopteran bites may demonstrate a severe systemic response that can be life threatening. One sting can produce generalized urticaria, respiratory difficulty (from laryngeal edema), hypotension, and death. Intramuscular administration of epinephrine provides immediate relief and must be available for emergency use.

Hypersensitive children should wear a medical identification bracelet. They should also have a kit that contains epinephrine and a

hypodermic syringe. Families are reminded to check the expiration date on the kit and to replace an outdated one. They should determine whether a nurse is available at the school and find out what the school policy is regarding administration of drugs. If a school nurse is not present, someone at the school should be designated to inject the epinephrine in case of an emergency.

SCABIES

Scabies is an endemic infestation caused by the scabies mite, *Sarcoptes scabiei*. Lesions are created as the impregnated female burrows into the stratum corneum of the epidermis (never into living tissue) to deposit her eggs and feces. The inflammatory response and intense itching occur after the host becomes sensitized to the mite, approximately 30 to 60 days after initial contact. If the person has been previously sensitized to the mite, the response occurs within 48 hours after exposure. After this time, the areas over which the mite has traveled will begin to itch and develop the characteristic eruption (Box 30-1). Consequently, mites will not necessarily be located at all sites of eruption.

There is great variability in the type of lesions. Infants often develop an eczematous eruption; therefore, the observer must look for discrete papules, burrows, or vesicles.

Nursing Care Management

The treatment of scabies is the application of a scabicide. The drug of choice in children and infants older than 2 months is permethrin 5% cream (Elimite). Alternative drugs are 10% crotamiton, ivermectin, or 1% lindane cream or lotion. Lindane can be neurotoxic and is contraindicated in several age groups. Lindane should be reserved for treatment of patients who fail to respond to other preparations (American Academy of Pediatrics [AAP], Committee on Infectious Diseases and Pickering, 2009).

Ivermectin, an oral medication, may be used to treat scabies in patients with secondary excoriations for whom topical scabicides are irritating and not well tolerated or whose infestation is refractory (AAP, Committee on Infectious Diseases and Pickering, 2009). However, the safety and efficacy of ivermectin for children younger than 5 years of age or children weighing less than 15 kg (33 lb) has not been established.

Because of the length of time between infestation and physical symptoms (30–60 days), all persons who were in close contact with the affected child need treatment. This may include boyfriends or girlfriends, babysitters, grandparents, and immediate family members. The objective is to treat as thoroughly as possible the first time. Enough medication for the entire family should be prescribed, with 2 oz allowed for each adult and 1 oz for each child.

PEDICULOSIS CAPITIS

Pediculosis capitis (head lice) is an infestation of the scalp by *Pediculus humanus capitis,* a common parasite in school-age children. The adult louse lives only about 48 hours when away from a human host, and the life span of the average female is 1 month. The female lays her eggs at night at the junction of a hair shaft and close to the skin because the eggs need a warm environment. The nits, or eggs, hatch in approximately 7 to 10 days. Itching is usually the only symptom. Common areas involved are the occipital area, behind the ears, and the nape of the neck (Box 30-2).

Diagnostic Evaluation

Diagnosis is made by observation of the white eggs (nits) firmly attached to the hair shafts (Fig. 30-8). Because of their brief life span

TABLE 30-6	**SKIN LESIONS CAUSED BY ARTHROPODS**	
MECHANISM AND CHARACTERISTIC	**MANIFESTATIONS**	**MANAGEMENT**

Insect Bites—Flies, Gnats, Mosquitoes, Fleas

Mechanism—Foreign protein in insects' saliva introduced when skin is penetrated for a blood-sucking meal
Distribution:
  Almost everywhere—Fleas, mosquitoes, ants
  Suburbs and rural areas—Bees
  Urban areas—Hornets, wasps, yellow jackets
	Hypersensitivity reaction
	Papular urticaria
	Firm papules; may be capped by vesicles or excoriated
	Little or no reaction in nonsensitized person
		Treatment:
		  Use antipruritic agents and baths.
		  Administer antihistamines.
		  Prevent secondary infection.
		Prevention:
		  Avoid contact.
		  Remove focus, such as treating furniture, mattresses, carpets, and pets, where insects may live.
		  Apply insect repellent when exposure is anticipated.

Chiggers—Harvest Mites

Mechanism—Attach with claws and secrete a digestive substance that liquefies the host's epidermis
Manifestations:
  Erythematous papules
  Intense itching
	Same as insect bites
	Favor warm areas of body, especially intertriginous areas and areas covered with clothing
		Avoid contact, especially in areas of tall grass and underbrush.
		Apply insect repellant when exposure is anticipated.
		Administer systemic steroids for extensive bites.

Hymenopterans—Bees, Wasps, Hornets, Yellow Jackets, Fire Ants

Mechanism:
  Injection of venom through stinging apparatus
  Venom contains histamine; allergenic proteins; and often a spreading factor, hyaluronidase
  Severe reactions caused by hypersensitivity or multiple stings
	Local reaction—Small red area, wheal, itching, and heat
	Systemic reactions—May be mild to severe, including generalized edema, pain, nausea and vomiting, confusion, respiratory embarrassment, and shock
		Treatment:
		  Carefully scrape off stinger or pull out stinger as quickly as possible.
		  Cleanse with soap and water.
		  Apply cool compresses.
		  Apply common household product (e.g., lemon juice, paste made with aspirin or baking soda).
		  Administer antihistamines.
		Severe reactions—Administer epinephrine, corticosteroids; treat for shock.
		Prevention:
		  Teach child to wear shoes; to avoid wearing bright clothing, flowery prints, shiny jewelry, or perfumed grooming products (cologne, scented hairspray), which might attract the insect; and to avoid places where the insect may be contacted.
		  Hypersensitive children should wear medical identification to indicate allergy and therapy needed; family should keep emergency medication and be taught its administration.

Black Widow Spider

Mechanism—Venom injected through a clawlike appendage; has neurotoxic action
Characteristics:
  Shiny black spider, with a body about 1.25 cm (0.5 inch) long and a red or orange hourglass-shaped marking on underside
  Avoids light and bites in self-defense
	Mild sting at time of bite
	Area becomes swollen, painful, and erythematous
	Dizziness, weakness, and abdominal pain
	May produce delirium, paralysis, seizures, and (if large amount of venom absorbed) death
		Treatment:
		  Cleanse wound with antiseptic.
		  Apply cool compresses.
		  Administer antivenin.
		  Administer muscle relaxant, such as calcium gluconate; analgesics or sedatives; hydrocortisone or diazepam intravenously.
		Prevention—Teach children to avoid places that harbor the spider (e.g., woodpiles).

Continued

TABLE 30-6 SKIN LESIONS CAUSED BY ARTHROPODS—cont'd

MECHANISM AND CHARACTERISTIC	MANIFESTATIONS	MANAGEMENT
Brown Recluse Spider		
Mechanism:	Mild sting at time of bite	*Treatment:*
Venom injected via fangs	Transient erythema followed by bleb or blister;	Apply cool compresses locally.
Venom contains powerful necrotoxin	mild to severe pain in 2–8 hours; purple,	Administer antibiotics, corticosteroids.
Characteristics:	star-shaped area in 3–4 days; necrotic	Relieve pain.
Slender spider, with long legs and body length	ulceration in 7–14 days (see Fig. 30-7)	Wound may require skin graft.
of 1–2 cm; color is fawn to dark brown;	Systemic reactions may include fever, malaise,	*Prevention*—Teach children to avoid possible nesting
recognized by fiddle-shaped mark on head	restlessness, nausea, vomiting, and joint pain	sites.
Shy; bites only when annoyed or surprised	Generalized petechial eruption	
Prefers dark areas where seldom disturbed	Wounds heal with scar formation	
Scorpions		
Mechanism:	Intense local pain, erythema, numbness,	*Treatment:*
Sting by means of a hooked caudal stinger	burning, restlessness, vomiting	Delay absorption of venom by keeping child quiet;
that discharges venom	Ascending motor paralysis with seizures,	place involved area in dependent position.
Venom of more venomous species contains	weakness, rapid pulse, excessive salivation,	Administer antivenin.
hemolysins, endotheliolysins, and	thirst, dysuria, pulmonary edema, coma, and	Relieve pain.
neurotoxins	death	Admit to pediatric intensive care unit for surveillance.
Characteristics—Usual habitat southwestern	Some species produce only local tissue reaction	*Prevention*—Teach children to avoid possible nesting
United States	with swelling at puncture site (distinctive)	sites.
	Symptoms subside in a few hours	
	Deaths occur among children younger than	
	4 years of age, usually in first 24 hours	
⊖ Ticks		
Mechanism—In process of sucking blood, head	Tick usually attached to skin, head embedded	*Treatment:*
and mouth parts are buried in skin	Produce firm, discrete, intensely pruritic nodules	Grasp tick with tweezers (forceps) as close as possible
Characteristics:	at site of attachment	to point of attachment.
Feed on blood of mammals	May cause urticaria or persistent localized	Pull straight up with steady, even pressure; if using
Significant in humans because of pathologic	edema	bare hands, use a tissue to touch tick during removal;
organism carried		wash hands thoroughly with soap and water.
May be vectors of various infectious diseases,		Remove any remaining part (e.g., head) with sterile
such as Rocky Mountain spotted fever,		needle.
Q fever, tularemia, relapsing fever, Lyme		Cleanse wounds with soap and disinfectant.
disease, tick paralysis		*Prevention*—Teach children to avoid areas where
Must attach and feed for 1–2 hours to		prevalent.
transmit disease		Inspect skin (especially scalp) after being in wooded
Usual habitat is wooded area		areas.
		(See discussion on p. 1029.)

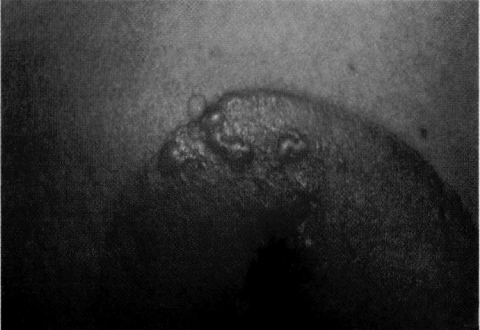

FIG 30-7 Brown recluse spider bite. Note central necrosis surrounded by purplish area and blisters. (From Weston WL, Lane AT: *Color textbook of pediatric dermatology*, ed 4, St. Louis, 2007, Mosby.)

BOX 30-1 CLINICAL MANIFESTATIONS OF SCABIES

Lesion

Children—Minute grayish brown, threadlike (mite burrows), pruritic
- Black dot at end of burrow (mite)

Infants—Eczematous eruption, pruritic

Distribution

Generally in intertriginous areas—Interdigital, axillary-cubital, popliteal, inguinal

Children older than 2 years of age—Primarily hands and wrists

Children younger than 2 years—Primarily feet and ankles

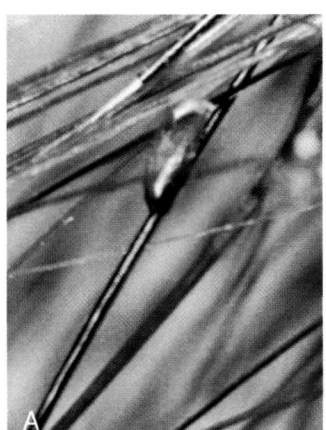 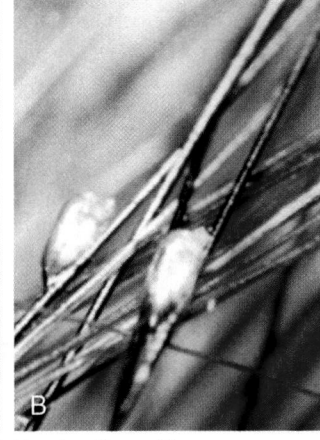

FIG 30-8 A, Empty nit case. **B,** Viable nits. (From *The contemporary approach to the control of head lice in schools and communities,* Pittsburgh, 1991, SmithKline Beecham.)

and mobility, adult lice are more difficult to locate. Nits must be differentiated from dandruff, lint, hair spray, and other items of similar size and shape. Scratch marks or inflammatory papules, caused by secondary infection, may also be found on the scalp in the vulnerable areas.

Therapeutic Management

Treatment consists of the application of pediculicides and manual removal of nit cases. The drug of choice for infants and children is permethrin 1% cream rinse (Nix), which kills adult lice and nits. This product and preparations of pyrethrin with piperonyl butoxide (RID or A-200 Pyrinate) can be obtained without a prescription and are more effective and safer than lindane (Strong and Johnstone, 2008). Most experts advise a second treatment at 7 to 10 days to ensure a cure (AAP, Committee on Infectious Diseases and Pickering, 2009). However, pyrethrin products are contraindicated for individuals with contact allergy to ragweed or turpentine. If neither permethrin nor pyrethrin products are effective, the prescription drug 0.5% malathion, which has been approved for treatment of head lice, can be used. However, malathion contains flammable alcohol, must remain in contact with the scalp for 8 to 12 hours, and is not recommended for children younger than 2 years of age.

Because of concerns that head lice may be developing resistance to chemical shampoos and that repeated exposure of children to strong chemicals on the scalp may be unwise, effective nonchemical control measures are essential. Daily removal of nits from the child's hair with a metal nit comb at least every 2 or 3 days is a control measure

following treatment with a pediculicide (Mumcuoglu, Barker, Burgess, and others, 2007).

Nursing Care Management

An important nursing role is educating the parents about pediculosis. Nurses should emphasize that *anyone* can get pediculosis; it has no respect for age, socioeconomic level, or cleanliness. Lice do not jump or fly, but they can be transmitted from one person to another on personal items. Lice are more likely to infest white children, those with straight hair, and girls. Children are cautioned against sharing combs, hair ornaments, hats, caps, scarves, coats, and other items used on or near the hair. Children who share lockers are more likely to become infested, and slumber parties place children at risk. Lice are not carried or transmitted by pets.

Nurses or parents should carefully inspect children who scratch their heads more than usual for bite marks, redness, and nits. The hair is systematically spread with two flat-sided sticks or tongue depressors, and the scalp is observed for any movement that indicates a louse. Nurses should wear gloves when examining the hair. Lice are small and grayish tan, have no wings, and are visible to the naked eye. The nits, or eggs, appear as tiny whitish oval specks adhering to the hair shaft about 6 mm (0.25 inch) from the scalp. The adherent nature of the nits distinguishes them from dandruff, which falls off readily. **Empty nit cases**, indicating hatched lice, are translucent rather than white and are located more than 6 mm from the scalp (see Fig. 30-8).

If evidence of infestation is found, it is important to treat the child according to the directions on the label of the pediculicide. Parents are advised to read the directions carefully before beginning treatment. The child is made as comfortable as possible during the application process because the pediculicide must remain on the scalp and hair for several minutes. Playing "beauty parlor" while shampooing is a useful strategy. The child lies supine with the head over a sink or basin and covers the eyes with a dry towel or washcloth. This prevents medication, which can cause chemical conjunctivitis, from splashing into the eyes. If eye irritation occurs, the eyes must be flushed well with tepid water. It is not necessary to remove the nits after treatment because only live lice cause infestation. However, because none of the pediculicides is 100% effective in killing all the eggs, the makers of some pediculicides recommend manual removal of the nits after treatment. An extra-fine-tooth comb that is included in many commercial pediculicides or is available at community pharmacies facilitates manual removal. If the comb is ineffective in removing the nit cases, the examiner should remove them by scraping them off the strands of hair with his or her fingernails.

Live lice survive for up to 48 hours away from the host, but nits are shed into the environment and are capable of hatching in 7 to 10 days; retreatment may be required. Therefore, measures must be taken to prevent further infestation (see Community Focus box). Spraying with insecticide is not recommended because of the danger to children and animals. Families should also be advised that the pediculicide is relatively expensive, especially when several members of the household require treatment. Families may be inclined to try home remedies to treat the lice. A recent study by Lee, Rios, Aten, and others (2004) showed that home remedies such as petroleum jelly, oils, vinegar, butter, alcohol, and mayonnaise did little to kill louse eggs but increased the risk for skin infection with *S. aureus*. Another study by Pearlman (2004) showed that dry-on pediculicide lotions may effectively treat lice without the use of current shampoos with neurotoxins, nit removal, or extensive housecleaning. Another study (Goates, Atkin, Wilding, and others, 2006) demonstrated that one 3-minute application of hot air has the potential to eliminate lice infestations.

Preventing the Spread and Recurrence of Pediculosis

- Machine wash all washable clothing, towels, and bed linens in hot water and dry them in a hot dryer for at least 20 minutes. Dry clean nonwashable items.
- Thoroughly vacuum carpets, car seats, pillows, stuffed animals, rugs, mattresses, and upholstered furniture.
- Seal nonwashable items in plastic bags for 14 days if unable to dry clean or vacuum.
- Soak combs, brushes, and hair accessories in lice-killing products for 1 hour or in boiling water for 10 minutes.
- In daycare centers, store children's clothing items such as hats and scarves and other headgear in separate cubicles.
- Discourage the sharing of items such as hats, scarves, hair accessories, combs, and brushes among children in group settings such as daycare centers.
- Avoid physical contact with infested individuals and their belongings, especially clothing and bedding.
- Inspect children in a group setting regularly for head lice.
- Provide educational programs on the transmission of pediculosis, its detection, and treatment.

Modified from Chin J, editor: *Control of communicable diseases manual*, Washington, DC, 2000, American Public Health Association.

Prevention

The increasing incidence of pediculosis in schoolchildren is a serious concern for school nurses, parents, and community health agencies. However, school head lice screening programs have not proven to have a significant effect on the incidence of head lice in the school setting; parent education programs may be more helpful in the management of head lice. Children with head lice should be allowed to return to school after proper treatment. Both the AAP and the National Association of School Nurses discourage a "no nit" policy for schools.

RICKETTSIAL DISEASES

The organisms responsible for a number of disorders are transmitted to human beings via arthropods (Table 30-7). Mammals become infected only through the bites of infected lice, fleas, ticks, and mites, all of which serve as both infectors and reservoirs. Rickettsiae are intracellular parasites, similar in size to bacteria that inhabit the alimentary tract of a wide range of natural hosts. Rickettsial diseases are more common in temperate and tropical climates where humans live in association with arthropods. Infection in humans is incidental (except epidemic typhus) and not necessary for the survival of the rickettsial species. However, after the organism invades a human, it causes a disease that varies in intensity from a benign, self-limiting illness to a disease that is fulminating and fatal.

LYME DISEASE

Lyme disease is the most common tickborne disorder in the United States. It is caused by the spirochete *Borrelia burgdorferi*, which enters the skin and bloodstream through the saliva and feces of ticks, especially the deer tick (Moreno, 2011). Most cases of Lyme disease are

TABLE 30-7	ERUPTIONS CAUSED BY RICKETTSIAE		
DISORDER, ORGANISM, AND HOST	**MANIFESTATIONS**	**MANAGEMENT**	**COMMENTS**
Rocky Mountain spotted fever—*Rickettsia rickettsii* Arthropod—Tick Transmission—Tick Mammal source—Wild rodents, dogs	*Gradual onset*—Fever, malaise, anorexia, myalgia *Abrupt onset*—Rapid temperature elevation, chills, vomiting, myalgia, severe headache Maculopapular or petechial rash primarily on extremities (ankles and wrists) but may spread to other areas, characteristically on palms and soles	*Control*—Protection from tick bite by wearing proper apparel, tick repellent Tetracycline or chloramphenicol Vigorous supportive therapy	Usually self-limiting in children Onset in children may resemble any infectious disease Severe disease rare in children Inspect children and dogs regularly if they play in wooded areas See Table 30-6 for management of ticks
Epidemic typhus—*R. prowazekii* Arthropod—Body louse Transmission—Infected feces into broken skin Mammal source—Humans	Abrupt onset of chills, fever, diffuse myalgia, headache, malaise Maculopapular rash becoming petechial 4–7 days later, spreading from trunk outward	*Control*—Immediate destruction of vectors Tetracycline or chloramphenicol Supportive treatment	Patient should be isolated until deloused See discussion on p. 1027 for management of pediculosis Excreta from infected lice also in dust; disinfect patient's clothing, bedding, and possessions and wash in hot water
Endemic typhus—*R. typhi* Arthropod—Rat fleas or lice Transmission—Flea bite; inhaling or ingesting flea excreta Mammal source—Rats	Headache, arthralgia, backache followed by fever; may last 9–14 days Maculopapular rash after 1–8 days of fever; begins in trunk and spreads to periphery; rarely involves face, palms, soles	*Control*—Eliminate rat reservoir, insect vectors, or both Tetracycline or chloramphenicol Supportive treatment	Fairly common in United States Shorter duration than epidemic typhus Mild, seldom fatal illness Difficult to distinguish from epidemic typhus
Rickettsialpox—*R. akari* Arthropod—Mouse mite Transmission—Mite Mammal source—House mouse	Maculopapular rash after primary lesion; eschar at site of bite; fever, chills, headache	*Control*—Eradication of rodent reservoir and mite vector Tetracycline or chloramphenicol Supportive treatment	Self-limiting nonfatal disease Endemic in New York City Found in many cities in United States

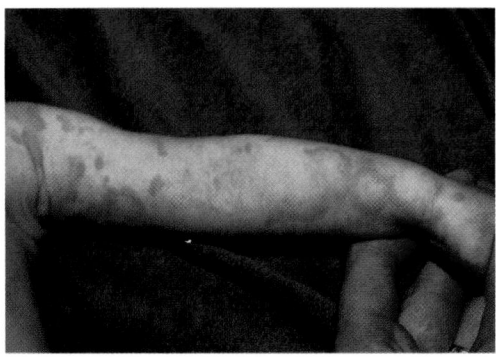

FIG 30-9 Lyme disease. Note annular red rings in erythema chronicum migrans. (From Weston WL, Lane AT: *Color textbook of pediatric dermatology,* ed 4, St. Louis, 2007, Mosby.)

reported in the Northeast from southern Maine to northern Virginia. The disease may initially appear in any of three stages:

Stage 1 consists of the tick bite at the time of inoculation, followed in 3 to 31 days by the development of erythema migrans at the site of the bite (Fig. 30-9).

Stage 2, the most serious stage of the disease, is characterized by systemic involvement of neurologic, cardiac, and musculoskeletal systems that appears several weeks after the cutaneous phase is completed.

Stage 3, or the late stage, includes musculoskeletal pain that involves the tendons, bursae, muscles, and synovia. Arthritis may occur, and late neurologic problems include deafness and chronic encephalopathy.

Diagnostic Evaluation

Diagnosis is best made clinically during the early stages by recognizing the characteristic rash, erythema migrans. Serologic testing may be used to establish the diagnosis in later stages of the disease.

Therapeutic Management

Early and appropriate treatment is essential to prevent complications. Children older than 8 years of age are treated with oral doxycycline; amoxicillin is recommended for children younger than 8 years of age (Centers for Disease Control and Prevention [CDC], 2009). For patients who are allergic to penicillin, alternative drugs include cefuroxime or erythromycin. Most experts treat individuals with early Lyme disease for 14 to 21 days. Persons who have removed ticks from themselves should be monitored closely for signs and symptoms of tickborne diseases for 30 days; in particular, they should be monitored for erythema migrans, a red expanding skin lesion at the site of the tick bite that may suggest Lyme disease. People who develop a skin lesion or viral infection–like illness within 1 month of an attached tick should seek prompt medical attention (Wormser, Dattwyler, Shapiro, and others, 2006). Treatment of erythema migrans most often prevents development of later stages of Lyme disease.

Nursing Care Management

The major thrust of nursing care should be educating parents to protect their children from exposure to ticks. Children should avoid tick-infested areas or wear light-colored clothing so that ticks can be spotted easily, tuck pant legs into socks, and wear a long-sleeved shirt tucked into pants when in wooded areas. Parents and children need to perform regular tick checks when they are in infested areas (with special attention to the scalp, neck, armpits, and groin areas) (Network

to Reduce Lyme Disease in School-Aged Children, 2010). Parents should also be alert for signs of the skin lesion, especially if their children have been in tick-infested areas. Insect repellents containing diethyltoluamide (DEET) and permethrin can protect against ticks, but parents should use these chemicals cautiously. Although there have been reports of serious neurologic complications in children resulting from frequent and excessive application of DEET repellants, the risk is low when they are used properly. Products with DEET should be applied sparingly according to label instructions and not applied to a child's face, hands, or any areas of irritated skin. After the child returns indoors, treated skin should be washed with soap and water. Information about Lyme disease can be obtained from the American Lyme Disease Foundation, Inc.*

PET AND WILD ANIMAL BITES

Animal bites are common in childhood. However, children are bitten more often by animals belonging to the family or to neighbors than by stray animals. The majority of victims of dog bites are boys between the ages of 5 and 9 years (CDC, 2003). Most dog or cat injuries are to the upper extremities. Small children are likely to be bitten or scratched on the head, face, and neck because they tend to put their heads near the animal's head and flail their arms rather than protecting their heads (Kaye, Belz, and Kirschner, 2009). Animal bites are potentially serious because of the likelihood of significant infection. Injuries vary in intensity from small puncture wounds to complete evulsion of tissue that is associated with significant crush injury.

Therapeutic Management

General wound care consists of rinsing the wound with copious amounts of saline or lactated Ringer solution under pressure via a large syringe and of washing the surrounding skin with mild soap. A clean pressure dressing is applied, and the extremity is elevated if the wound is bleeding. Medical evaluation is advised because of the danger of tetanus and rabies, although dogs in most urban areas must be immunized against rabies. Bites from wild animals, such as squirrels, bats, raccoons, foxes, and skunks, are also dangerous.

Prophylactic antibiotics are indicated for puncture wounds and wounds in areas that may prove to be cosmetically or functionally impaired if infected. Extensive lacerations are débrided and loosely sutured to allow drainage in the event of infection. Tetanus toxoid is administered according to standard guidelines (see Immunizations, Chapter 10), and rabies protocol is followed (see Rabies, Chapter 28). Injuries to poorly vascularized areas, such as the hands, are more likely to become infected than those in more vascularized areas, such as the face; puncture wounds are more likely to become infected than lacerations.

Nursing Care Management

The most important aspect related to animal bites is prevention. Children should understand animal behavior and develop respect for animals (see Community Focus box). Parents should monitor their children's behavior with dogs and instruct them not to tease or surprise dogs, invade their territory, interfere with their feeding or sleeping, take their toys, or interact with sick or injured dogs or dogs with pups. Parents who are considering getting a pet, especially a dog, for themselves or their children should select a dog that has a high level of sociability with, and is unlikely to be a danger to, children.

---

*PO Box 466, Lyme, CT 06371; e-mail: inquire@aldf.com; http://www.aldf.com.

Animal Safety

- Teach children to avoid all strange animals, especially wild, sick, or injured ones, that may be carriers of rabies (use the same techniques used in teaching children not to talk to strangers).
- Teach children to avoid dangerous and nervous animals in the neighborhood.
- Vaccinate your own dog against rabies.
- Never permit children to break up an animal fight even when their own pet is involved. Use a rake, broom, or garden hose to separate animals.
- Teach children the danger of mistreating or teasing pets (animals will bite if mauled, annoyed, or frightened).
- Spay or neuter your pets (spaying or neutering reduces aggression, not protectiveness).
- Avoid direct eye contact with a threatening dog and remain motionless until a threatening dog leaves the area.
- Never hold your face close to an animal.
- Teach children not to disturb an animal that is eating; sleeping; or caring for young puppies, kittens, and so on.
- Never tease; pull the tail; or take away food, a bone, or a toy with which an animal is playing.
- Never approach a strange dog that is confined or restrained; do not keep animals confined with short ropes or chains (this can make them aggressive or vicious, especially when teased).
- Do not run, ride a bicycle, or skate in front of a dog (it will startle the dog); teach children the importance of avoiding bike routes where dogs are known to chase vehicles.
- Do not allow an inexperienced child or adult to feed a dog (if the person pulls back when the animal moves to take the food, this can frighten and startle the animal).
- If a dog is asleep or unaware of your presence or has not seen you approach, speak to the animal to make it aware of your presence to avoid startling the animal.
- Allow a dog to see and sniff a child before the child attempts to pet the animal.
- Do not permit a child to lead a large dog.
- Train or socialize a dog for appropriate behavior; avoid aggressive play with pets.
- Do not adopt pets for children until children demonstrate their maturity and ability to handle and care for pets.

From Humane Society of the United States: *Preventing and avoiding dog bites*, Washington, DC, 1998, Author.

HUMAN BITES

Children often acquire lacerations from the teeth of other humans in rough play, during fights, or as victims of child abuse. Many preschool children bite others out of frustration or anger. Because human dental plaque and gingiva harbor pathogenic organisms, all human bites should receive attention. Delayed treatment increases the risk of infection.

If the laceration is less than 6 mm (0.25 inch) in length, the wound can be treated at home. The wound is washed vigorously with soap and water, and a pressure dressing is applied to stop bleeding. Ice applications minimize discomfort and swelling. Increased pain or redness at the wound site is an indication that the child should receive medical attention for antibiotic therapy. Tetanus toxoid is needed if the child is insufficiently immunized. Wounds larger than 6 mm should receive medical attention.

CAT SCRATCH DISEASE

Cat scratch disease is the most common cause of regional lymphadenitis in children and adolescents. It usually follows the scratch or bite of an animal (a cat or kitten in 99% of cases). The disease is usually a benign, self-limiting illness that resolves spontaneously in about 2 to 4 months. Diagnosis is made on the basis of (1) history of contact with a cat or kitten, (2) the presence of regional lymphadenopathy for several days, and (3) serologic identification of the causative organism by indirect fluorescent antibody assay or polymerase chain reaction test. The disease may persist for several months before gradual resolution. In some children, especially those who are immunocompromised, the adenitis may progress to suppuration and serious complications. Treatment is primarily supportive, but antibiotic therapy may hasten the resolution of adenopathy in the disease (CDC, 2002).

MISCELLANEOUS SKIN DISORDERS

A number of miscellaneous skin lesions occur in children. Some occur as a result of congenital disorders and are inherited as an autosomal dominant trait (Table 30-8). **Ichthyoses** are a heterogeneous group of disorders characterized by scaling that create challenging problems in treatment. These disorders are not discussed in detail here because of their wide variability.

SKIN DISORDERS ASSOCIATED WITH SPECIFIC AGE GROUPS

Several common dermatologic conditions are confined to children in specific age groups. These conditions include diaper, atopic, and seborrheic dermatitis, which occurs predominantly in infants, and acne, which is most common in adolescence.

DIAPER DERMATITIS

Diaper dermatitis is common in infants and one of several acute inflammatory skin disorders caused either directly or indirectly by wearing diapers. The peak age of occurrence is 9 to 12 months of age, and the incidence is greater in bottle-fed infants than in breastfed infants.

Pathophysiology and Clinical Manifestations

Diaper dermatitis is caused by prolonged and repetitive contact with an irritant (e.g., urine, feces, soaps, detergents, ointments, friction). Although the irritant in the majority of cases is urine and feces, a combination of factors contributes to irritation.

Prolonged contact of the skin with diaper wetness produces higher friction, greater abrasion damage, increased transepidermal permeability, and increased microbial counts. Healthy skin is less resistant to potential irritants.

Although ammonia was once thought to cause diaper rash because of the association between the strong odor on diapers and dermatitis, ammonia alone is not sufficient. The irritant quality of urine is related to an increase in pH from the breakdown of urea in the presence of fecal urease. The increased pH promotes the activity of fecal enzymes, principally the proteases and lipases, which act as irritants. Fecal enzymes also increase the permeability of skin to bile salts, another potential irritant in feces.

The eruption of diaper dermatitis is manifested primarily on convex surfaces or in folds. The lesions represent a variety of types and configurations. Eruptions involving the skin in most intimate contact

TABLE 30-8   MISCELLANEOUS SKIN DISORDERS

DISEASE AND CAUSATIVE AGENT	LOCAL MANIFESTATIONS	MANAGEMENT	COMMENTS
Urticaria—Usually allergic response to drugs or infection	Development of wheals Vary in size and configuration and tend to appear quickly, spread irregularly, and fade within a few hours May be constant or intermittent, sparse or profuse, small or large, discrete or confluent May be acute, chronic, or recurrent in acute attacks	Local soothing and antipruritic applications Antihistamines Epinephrine or ephedrine Cortisone in severe cases Severe upper respiratory tract involvement may require tracheostomy	Known etiologic agents should be avoided May be accompanied by malaise, fever, lymphadenopathy Severe cases may involve mucous membranes, internal organs, and joints Obstruction to air passages constitutes medical emergency (see Chapter 25)
Intertrigo—Mechanical trauma and aggravating factors of excessive heat, moisture, and sweat retention	Red, inflamed, moist, partially denuded, marginated areas, the shape of which is determined by location Appears where opposing skin surfaces rub together, such as intergluteal folds, groin, neck, and axilla Excessive moisture and obesity are often factors	Affected areas kept clean and dry Skinfolds kept separated with a generous supply of nonmedicated powder Expose to air and light Remove excess clothing	A form of diaper irritation Prevent recurrence by keeping susceptible areas clean and dry Frequently associated with overheating from too much clothing; common in tracheostomy patients with short necks and copious secretions
Psoriasis—Unknown; hereditary predisposition; may be triggered by stress	Round, thick, dry, reddish patches covered with coarse, silvery scales over trunk and extremities; first lesions commonly appear in scalp; facial lesions more common in children than in adults Affected cells proliferate at a much more rapid rate than normal cells	Tar preparations in combination with UVB light or natural sunlight Topical corticosteroids Topical vitamin D analog calcipotriene Phenol and saline solutions followed by a tar shampoo to remove scales Keratolytic agents (salicylic acid) Acitretin Emollients may provide relief	Uncommon in children younger than 6 years old Patients are otherwise healthy Coal tar acts synergistically with UVB light Keratolytic agents enhance absorption of corticosteroids Humidifiers may help in winter
Alopecia*			
Alopecia areata	Sudden onset of asymptomatic, noninflammatory, round, bald patches in hairy parts of body	Psychologic support Inducement of allergic contact dermatitis to stimulate growth of hair Minoxidil (peripheral vasodilator)	Family history in 10%–26% of cases Some concern regarding drug therapy safety Refer to support groups*
Traumatic alopecia	Traction alopecia around scalp margins from tight hair styles (e.g., braids, pony tails, corn rows)	Counseling regarding hair styling, use of hair cosmetics, hot combs, rollers	More prevalent in African-American children and adolescents Prolonged traction can produce fibrosis of hair root and permanent loss
Trichotillomania	Compulsive hair pulling	Determine and treat cause	Chronic hair pulling may require psychologic therapy
Tinea capitis	See Table 30-4	See Table 30-4	See Table 30-4
Erythema multiforme (Stevens-Johnson syndrome)—Unknown; associated with ingestion of some drugs; often follows upper respiratory tract infection	Erythematous papular rash Lesions enlarge by peripheral expansion, develop central vesicle Involves most skin surfaces except scalp May extend to mucous membranes, especially oral, ocular, and urethral	Symptomatic and supportive Maintain adequate intake of fluids (oral or intravenous), calories, and protein Moist wound care, hydrogels such as CarraGauze, Vaseline, or Aquaphor Appropriate treatment of complications Diligent monitoring of urine volume and specific gravity, hemoglobin and hematocrit, serum electrolyte levels, total body weight	Rash often preceded by fever and malaise Complications include renal failure and severe eye disease Respiratory involvement in a number of cases Self-limiting, but recovery may extend for weeks; skin lesions may subside without scarring; mucous membrane lesions may persist for months Recurrence rate, 20%; mortality rate as high as 10% High mutation rate
Neurofibromatosis—Inherited disorder; autosomal dominant inheritance pattern	Café-au-lait spots, pigmented nevi, axillary freckling Slow-growing cutaneous and subcutaneous neurofibromas	Symptomatic treatment of associated manifestations (e.g., speech defects, seizures, skeletal defects [scoliosis, kyphosis], learning disabilities) Surgical removal of troublesome tumors	Refer to support groups† Family needs to know about genetic implications

UVB, Ultraviolet B.

*National Alopecia Areata Foundation, 14 Mitchell Blvd., San Rafael, CA 94903; 415-472-3780; fax: 415-472-5343; e-mail: info@naaf.org; http://www.naaf.org.

†Children's Tumor Foundation, 95 Pine St., 16th Floor, New York, NY 10005; 800-323-7938 or 212-344-6633; fax: 212-747-0004; e-mail: info@ctf.org; http://www.ctf.org.

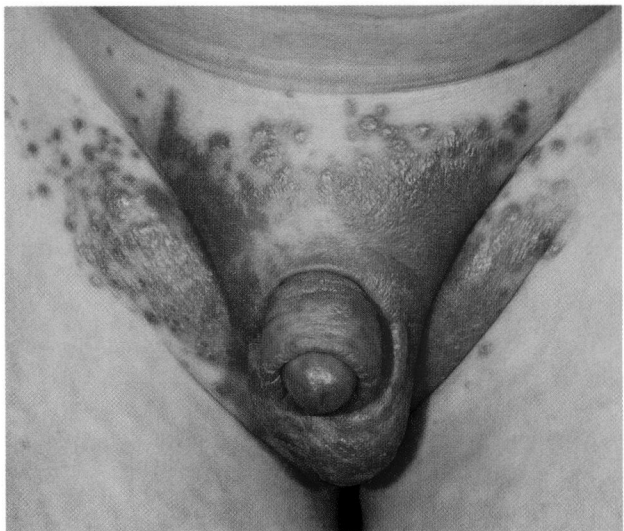

FIG 30-10 Irritant diaper dermatitis. Note the sharply demarcated edges. (From Habif TP: *Clinical dermatology: a color guide to diagnosis and therapy*, ed 5, St. Louis, 2010, Mosby.)

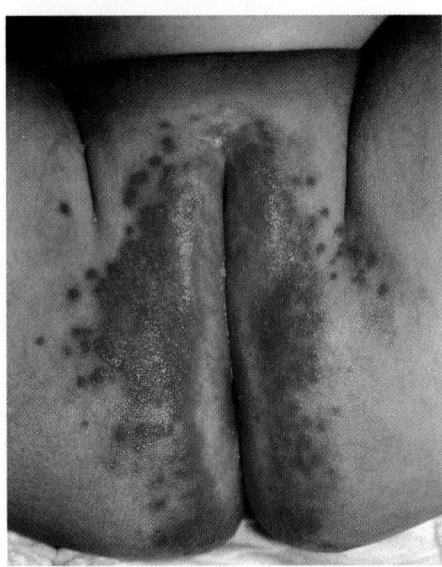

FIG 30-11 Candidiasis of diaper area. Note the beefy red central erythema with satellite pustules. (From Paller AS, Mancini AJ: *Hurwitz clinical pediatric dermatology*, ed 4, St. Louis, 2011, Saunders Elsevier.)

with the diaper (e.g., the convex surfaces of buttocks, inner thighs, mons pubis, scrotum) but sparing the folds are likely to be caused by chemical irritants, especially from urine and feces (Fig. 30-10). Other causes are detergents or soaps from inadequately rinsed cloth diapers or the chemicals in disposable wipes. Perianal involvement is usually the result of chemical irritation from feces, especially diarrheal stools. *Candida albicans* infection produces perianal inflammation and a maculopapular rash with satellite lesions that may cross the inguinal fold (Fig. 30-11). It is seen in up to 90% of infants with chronic diaper dermatitis and should be considered in diaper rashes that are recalcitrant to treatment.

Nursing Care Management

Nursing interventions are aimed at altering the three factors that produce dermatitis: wetness, pH, and fecal irritants. The most

<table>
<tr><td colspan="2">

FAMILY-CENTERED CARE
Controlling Diaper Rash

Keep skin dry.*
- Use superabsorbent disposable diapers to reduce skin wetness.
- If using cloth diapers, use only overwraps that allow air to circulate; avoid rubber pants.
- Change diapers as soon as soiled—especially with stool—whenever possible, preferably once during the night.
- Expose healthy or only slightly irritated skin to air, not heat, to dry completely.

Apply ointment, such as zinc oxide or petrolatum, to protect skin, especially if skin is very red or has moist, open areas.
- Avoid removing skin barrier cream with each diaper change; remove waste material and reapply skin barrier cream.
- To completely remove ointment, especially zinc oxide, use mineral oil; do not wash vigorously.

Avoid overwashing the skin, especially with perfumed soaps or commercial wipes, which may be irritating.
- May use a moisturizer or nonsoap cleanser, such as cold cream or Cetaphil, to wipe urine from skin.
- Gently wipe stool from skin using water and mild soap, such as Dove.
- When traveling, fill an old baby wipe container with soft paper towels and warm water.

</td></tr>
</table>

*Powder helps keep the skin dry, but talc is dangerous if breathed into the lungs. Plain cornstarch or cornstarch-based powder is safer. When using any powder product, first shake it into your hand and then apply it to the diaper area. Store the container away from the infant's reach; keep the container closed when not in use.

significant factor amenable to intervention is the moist environment created in the diaper area. Changing the diaper as soon as it becomes wet eliminates a large part of the problem, and removing the diaper to expose healthy skin to air facilitates drying. The use of a hair dryer or heat lamp is not recommended because these devices can cause burns.

Diaper construction has a significant impact on the incidence and severity of diaper dermatitis. Superabsorbent disposable paper diapers reduce diaper dermatitis. They contain an absorbent gelling material that binds water tightly to decrease skin wetness, maintains pH control by providing a buffering capacity, and decreases skin irritation by preventing mixing of urine and feces in the diaper. Another advance in diapers is the addition of an inner layer or top sheet that is impregnated with petrolatum (as in Pampers Swaddler with Absorb Away Liner).

Guidelines for controlling diaper rash are presented in the Family-Centered Care box. A common misconception about using cornstarch on skin is that it promotes the growth of *C. albicans*. Neither cornstarch nor talc promotes the growth of fungi under conditions normally found in the diaper area. Cornstarch is more effective in reducing friction and tends to cake less than talc when the skin is wet. On the basis of these properties and its safety in terms of inhalation injury, cornstarch is the preferred product. Talc should not be used.

ATOPIC DERMATITIS (ECZEMA)

Eczema or eczematous inflammation of the skin refers to a descriptive category of dermatologic diseases and not to a specific etiology. AD is a type of pruritic eczema that usually begins during infancy and is associated with an allergic contact dermatitis with a hereditary tendency (atopy) (Jacob, Yang, Herro, and others, 2010). AD manifests in three forms based on the child's age and the distribution of lesions:

BOX 30-3   CLINICAL MANIFESTATIONS OF ATOPIC DERMATITIS

Distribution of Lesions

Infantile form—Generalized, especially cheeks, scalp, trunk, and extensor surfaces of extremities (Fig. 30-12)

Childhood form—Flexural areas (antecubital and popliteal fossae, neck), wrists, ankles, and feet

Preadolescent and adolescent form—Face, sides of neck, hands, feet, face, and antecubital and popliteal fossae (to a lesser extent)

Appearance of Lesions

Infantile Form

Erythema

Vesicles

Papules

Weeping

Oozing

Crusting

Scaling

Often symmetric

Childhood Form

Symmetric involvement

Clusters of small erythematous or flesh-colored papules or minimally scaling patches

Dry and may be hyperpigmented

Lichenification (thickened skin with accentuation of creases)

Keratosis pilaris (follicular hyperkeratosis) common

Adolescent or Adult Form

Same as childhood manifestations

Dry, thick lesions (lichenified plaques) common

Confluent papules

Other Physical Manifestations

Intense itching

Unaffected skin dry and rough

African-American children likely to exhibit more papular or follicular lesions than are white children

May exhibit one or more of the following:

• Lymphadenopathy, especially near affected sites

• Increased palmar creases (many cases)

• Atopic pleats (extra line or groove of lower eyelid)

• Prone to cold hands

• Pityriasis alba (small, poorly defined areas of hypopigmentation)

• Facial pallor (especially around nose, mouth, and ears)

• Bluish discoloration beneath eyes ("allergic shiners")

• Increased susceptibility to unusual cutaneous infections (especially viral)

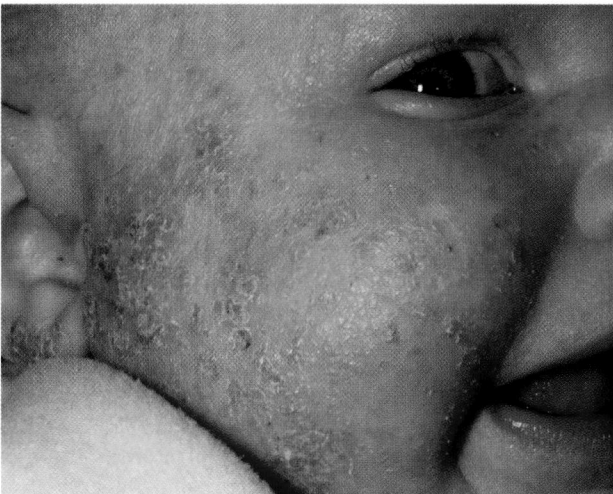

FIG 30-12 Atopic dermatitis. (From Habif TP: *Clinical dermatology: a color guide to diagnosis and therapy*, ed 5, St. Louis, 2010, Mosby.)

threshold compared with children who do not have AD for cutaneous itching, and many authorities believe the dermatologic manifestations appear subsequent to scratching from the intense pruritus (Alanne, Nermes, Soderlund, and others, 2011). For example, infants rub their faces against bed linen, and their crawling (a form of scratching) results in irritation of knees and elbows. Lesions disappear if the scratching is stopped.

The majority of children with infantile AD have a family history of eczema, asthma, food allergies, or allergic rhinitis, which strongly supports a genetic predisposition. The cause is unknown but appears to be related to abnormal function of the skin, including alterations in perspiration, peripheral vascular function, and heat tolerance. Manifestations of the chronic disease improve in humid climates and get worse in the fall and winter, when homes are heated and environmental humidity is lower. The disorder can be controlled but not cured. A recent study of 134 infants with AD showed that itching and scratching and sleep disturbance were specific features detracting from quality of life in these young children (Alanne, Nermes, Soderlund, and others, 2011).

Therapeutic Management

The major goals of management are to (1) hydrate the skin, (2) relieve pruritus, (3) reduce flare-ups or inflammation, and (4) prevent and control secondary infection. The general measures for managing AD focus on reducing pruritus and other aspects of the disease. Management strategies include avoiding exposure to skin irritants or allergens; avoiding overheating; and administering medications such as antihistamines, topical immunomodulators, topical steroids, and (sometimes) mild sedatives as indicated.

Enhancing skin hydration and preventing dry, flaky skin are accomplished in a number of ways, depending on the child's skin characteristics and individual needs. A tepid bath with a mild soap (Dove or Neutrogena), no soap, or an emulsifying oil followed immediately by application of an emollient (within 3 minutes) assists in trapping moisture and preventing its loss. Bubble baths and harsh soaps should be avoided. The bath may need to be repeated once or twice daily, depending on the child's status; excessive bathing without emollient application only dries out the skin. Some lotions are not effective, and emollients should be chosen carefully to prevent excessive skin

1. **Infantile** (infantile eczema)—Usually begins at 2 to 6 months of age; generally undergoes spontaneous remission by 3 years of age

2. **Childhood**—May follow the infantile form; occurs at 2 to 3 years of age; 90% of children have manifestations by age 5 years

3. **Preadolescent and adolescent**—Begins at about 12 years of age; may continue into the early adult years or indefinitely

The diagnosis of AD is based on a combination of history and morphologic findings (Box 30-3). Children with AD have a lower

drying. Aquaphor, Cetaphil, and Eucerin are acceptable lotions for skin hydration. A nighttime bath followed by emollient application and dressing in soft cotton pajamas may help alleviate most nighttime pruritus.

Sometimes colloid baths, such as the addition of 2 cups of cornstarch to a tub of warm water, provide temporary relief of itching and may help the child sleep if given before bedtime. Cool wet compresses are soothing to the skin and provide antiseptic protection.

Oral antihistamine drugs such as hydroxyzine or diphenhydramine usually relieve moderate or severe pruritus. Nonsedating antihistamines such as loratadine (Claritin) or fexofenadine (Allegra) may be preferred for daytime pruritus relief. Because pruritus increases at night, a mildly sedating antihistamine may be needed.

Occasional flare-ups require the use of topical steroids to diminish inflammation. Low-, moderate-, or high-potency topical corticosteroids are prescribed, depending on the degree of involvement, the area of the body to be treated, the child's age, the potential for local side effects (striae, skin atrophy, and pigment changes), and the type of vehicle to be used (e.g., cream, lotion, ointment). Patients receiving topical corticosteroid therapy for chronic conditions should be evaluated for risk factors for suboptimal linear growth and reduced bone density. Topical immunomodulators, a new nonsteroidal treatment for AD, are best used at the beginning of a "flare-up" just as the skin becomes red and itches. Two newer immunomodulator medications used in children with AD are tacrolimus and pimecrolimus (Walling and Swick, 2010). Tacrolimus is available in two ointment strengths (0.03% and 0.1%); the 0.03% concentration has been approved for use in children 2 years of age and older (Doss, Kamoun, Dubertret, and others, 2010). Pimecrolimus is available in a 1% cream that has no systemic accumulation or effects. This drug is approved for use in children with mild to moderate AD. Both drugs can be used freely on the face without worrying about steroid side effects.

If secondary skin infections occur in children with AD, these infections are managed with appropriate systemic antibiotics. In a subgroup of patients with moderate to severe AD, the disease may require systemic treatment (Ricci, Dondi, Patrizi, and others, 2009).

Nursing Care Management

Assessment of the child with AD includes a family history for evidence of atopy, a history of previous involvement, and any environmental or dietary factors associated with the present and previous exacerbations. The skin lesions are examined for type, distribution, and evidence of secondary infection. Parents are interviewed regarding the child's behavior, especially in relation to scratching, irritability, and sleeping patterns. Exploration of the family's feelings and methods of coping is also important.

The nursing care of the child with AD is challenging. Controlling the intense pruritus is imperative if the disorder is to be successfully managed because scratching leads to new lesions and may cause secondary infection. In addition to the medical regimen, other measures can be taken to prevent or minimize the scratching. Fingernails and toenails are cut short, kept clean, and filed frequently to prevent sharp edges. Gloves or cotton stockings can be placed over the hands and pinned to shirtsleeves. One-piece outfits with long sleeves and long pants also decrease direct contact with the skin. If gloves or socks are used, the child needs time to be free from such restrictions. An excellent time to remove gloves, socks, or other protective devices is during the bath or after receiving sedative or antipruritic medication.

Conditions that increase itching are eliminated when possible. Woolen clothes or blankets, rough fabrics, and furry stuffed animals are removed from the child's environment. Because heat and humidity cause perspiration (which intensifies itching), proper dress for climatic conditions is essential. Pruritus is often precipitated by exposure to the irritant effects of certain components of common products such as soaps, detergents, fabric softeners, perfumes, and powders. Most children experience less itching when soft cotton fabrics are worn next to the skin. During cold months, synthetic fabrics (not wool) should be used for overcoats, hats, gloves, and snowsuits. Exposure to latex products, such as gloves and balloons, should also be avoided.

Clothes and sheets are laundered in a mild detergent and rinsed thoroughly in clear water (without fabric softeners or antistatic chemicals). Putting the clothes through a second complete wash cycle without using detergent reduces the amount of residue remaining in the fabric.

Preventing infection is usually accomplished by preventing scratching. Baths are given as prescribed; the water is kept tepid; and soaps (except as indicated), bubble baths, oils, and powders are avoided. Skinfolds and diaper areas need frequent cleansing with plain water. A room humidifier or vaporizer may benefit children with extremely dry skin. The skin lesions are examined for signs of infection—usually honey-colored crusts or pustules with surrounding erythema. Any signs of infection are reported to the practitioner.

> **! NURSING ALERT**
>
> If the child is being treated with baths for hydration, it is imperative that the emollient preparation be applied immediately after bathing (while the skin is still slightly moist) to prevent drying.

Wet soaks and compresses are applied and medications for pruritus or infection are administered as directed. The family is given explicit instructions on the preparation and use of soaks, special baths, and topical medications, including the order of application if more than one is prescribed. It is important to emphasize that one thick application of topical medication is *not* equivalent to several thin applications and that excessive use of an agent (particularly steroids) can be hazardous. If children have difficulty remaining still for a 10- or 15-minute soak, bath, or dressing application, these can be carried out at naptime or when the child is engrossed in watching television, listening to a story, or playing with tub toys.

Diet modification is another source of frustration to parents. When a hypoallergenic diet is prescribed, parents need help to understand the reason for the diet and the guidelines for avoiding hyperallergenic foods (see Nursing Care Guidelines box). Because hypoallergenic diets take time before visible effects are apparent, parents need reassurance that results may not be seen immediately. If airborne allergens make eczema worse, the family is counseled about "allergy proofing" the home (see Asthma, Chapter 23).

Family Support

Parents are assured that the lesions will not produce scarring (unless secondarily infected) and that the disease is not contagious. However, the child may have repeated exacerbations and remissions. Spontaneous and permanent remission takes place at approximately 2 to 3 years of age in most children with the infantile disorder.

During acute phases, emotional stress can become intense for the family. They need time to discuss negative feelings and to be reassured that these feelings are normal. Stress tends to aggravate the severity of the condition. Therefore, efforts to relieve as much anxiety as possible in both the parents and the child have a beneficial emotional and physical effect.

NURSING CARE GUIDELINES
Preventing Atopy in Children

Identify Children at Risk
Family history of allergy
Increased immunoglobulin E in cord blood and postnatal serum
Dry, flaky skin

Prenatal Precautions (Last Trimester)
Avoid any known food allergens
Avoid milk and other dairy products, peanuts, and eggs
Minimize ingestion of other hyperallergenic foods

Postnatal Precautions
Breast milk or casein-whey hydrolysate formula (e.g., Nutramigen, Pregestimil, Alimentum) exclusively for at least 6 months
No solid food for first 6 months
No cow's milk or soy formula for 12 months
No eggs, fish, corn, citrus, peanuts, nuts, or chocolate for 12 to 18 months
One new food added at 5- to 7-day intervals to identify possible reaction

Environmental Control
Limited exposure to dust, molds, furry animals, and cigarette smoke

Data from Johnstone D: Strategy for intervention of food allergy in infants, *Int Pediatr* 4(4):319–325, 1989; Zeiger R, Heller S, Mellon M, and others: Effectiveness of dietary manipulation in the prevention of food allergy in infants, part II, *J Allergy Clin Immunol* 78(1 Pt 2): 224–238, 1986; Wood RA: Prospects for the prevention of allergy in children, *Curr Opin Pediatr* 8(6):601–605, 1995.

SEBORRHEIC DERMATITIS

Seborrheic dermatitis is a chronic, recurrent, inflammatory reaction of the skin. It occurs most commonly on the scalp (cradle cap) but may involve the eyelids (blepharitis), external ear canal (otitis externa), nasolabial folds, and inguinal region. The cause is unknown, although it is more common in early infancy, when sebum production is increased. The lesions are characteristically thick, adherent, yellowish, scaly, oily patches that may or may not be mildly pruritic. Unlike AD, seborrheic dermatitis is not associated with a positive family history for allergy and is common in infants shortly after birth and in adolescents after puberty. Diagnosis is made primarily on the basis of the appearance and the location of the crusts or scales.

Nursing Care Management

Cradle cap may be prevented with adequate scalp hygiene. Frequently, parents omit shampooing the infant's hair for fear of damaging the "soft spots," or fontanels. The nurse should discuss how to shampoo the infant's hair and emphasize that the fontanel is similar to skin anywhere else on the body—it does not puncture or tear with mild pressure.

When seborrheic lesions are present, the treatment is directed at removing the crusts. Parents are taught the appropriate procedure to clean the scalp. Education may need to include a demonstration. Shampooing should be done daily with a mild soap or commercial baby shampoo; medicated shampoos are not necessary, but an antiseborrheic shampoo containing sulfur and salicylic acid may be used. Shampoo is applied to the scalp and allowed to remain on the scalp until the crusts soften. Then the scalp is thoroughly rinsed. A fine-tooth comb or a soft facial brush helps remove the loosened crusts from the strands of hair after shampooing.

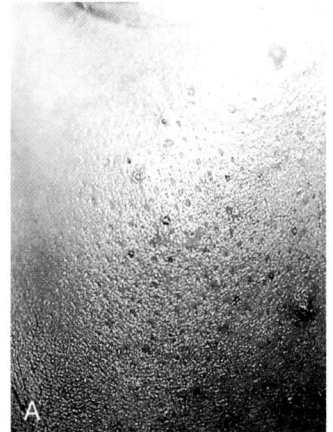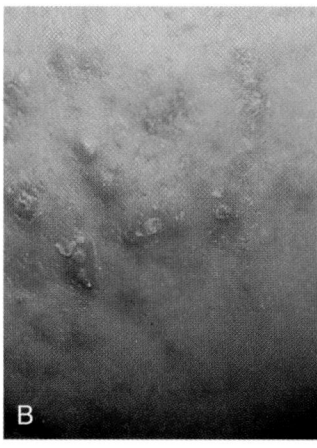

FIG 30-13 Acne vulgaris. **A,** Acne vulgaris. **B,** Comedones with a few inflammatory pustules. (From Zitelli BJ, McIntire SC, Nowalk AJ: *Zitelli and Davis' atlas of pediatric physical diagnosis*, ed 6, St. Louis, 2012, Saunders.)

ACNE

Acne vulgaris is the most common skin problem treated by physicians during patients' adolescence. Acne is not caused by dirt but by testosterone, a hormone present in boys and girls that increases during puberty. It stimulates the sebaceous glands of the skin to enlarge, or produce oil, and plug the pores. Whiteheads, blackheads, and pimples are present in teenage acne.

Half of the adolescent population experiences acne by the end of the teenage years. Although the disorder can appear before the age of 10 years, the peak incidence occurs in middle to late adolescence (age 16–17 years in girls and 17–18 years in boys). It is more common in boys than in girls. The degree to which an individual is affected may range from nothing more than a few isolated comedones to a severe inflammatory reaction. Although the disease is self-limiting and not life threatening, it has great significance to adolescents. Health professionals should not underestimate the impact that acne has on teens.

Numerous factors affect the development and course of acne. Its distribution in families and a high degree of concordance in identical twins suggest hereditary factors. Premenstrual flare-ups of acne occur in nearly 70% of adolescent girls, suggesting a hormonal cause. Studies do not indicate a clear association between stress and acne, but adolescents commonly cite stress as a cause for acne outbreaks. Cosmetics containing lanolin, petrolatum, vegetable oils, lauryl alcohol, butyl stearate, and oleic acid can increase comedone production. Exposure to oils in cooking grease can be a precursor in adolescents who work over fast-food restaurant hot oils. There is no known link between dietary intake and the development or worsening of acne.

Pathophysiology

Contributors to acne development include sebum secretion, abnormal desquamation of follicles, bacterial growth, and inflammation (Kim and Armstrong, 2011). **Comedogenesis** (formation of comedones) results in a noninflammatory lesion that may be either an **open comedone** ("blackhead") or a **closed comedone** ("whitehead"). Inflammation occurs with the proliferation of *Propionibacterium acnes*, which draws in neutrophils, causing inflammatory papules, pustules, nodules, and cysts (Fig. 30-13).

Therapeutic Management

Successful management of acne depends on a cooperative effort among the health care provider, the adolescent, and the parents. Unlike many other dermatologic conditions, acne lesions resolve slowly, and improvement may not be apparent for at least 6 weeks. Individual comedones can take several weeks to months to resolve, and papules and pustules usually resolve in about 1 week. The multifactorial causes of acne necessitate a combined approach for successful treatment. Treatment consists of general measures of care and specific treatments determined by the type of lesions involved.

General Measures

Improvement of the adolescent's overall health status is part of the general management. Adequate rest, moderate exercise, a well-balanced diet, reduction of emotional stress, and elimination of any foci of infection are all part of general health promotion.

Cleansing

Dirt or oil on the surface of the skin does not cause acne. Gentle cleansing with a mild cleanser once or twice daily is usually sufficient. Antibacterial soaps are ineffective and may be too drying when used in combination with topical acne medications. For some adolescents, hygiene of the hair and scalp appears to be related to the clinical activity of the acne. Acne on the forehead may improve with brushing the hair away from the forehead and more frequent shampooing.

Medications

Treatment success depends on commitment from the adolescent. Before prescribing treatment, the practitioner should determine the adolescent's level of comfort and readiness to begin treatment.

Tretinoin (Retin-A) is the only drug that effectively interrupts the abnormal follicular keratinization that produces microcomedones, the invisible precursors of the visible comedones. Tretinoin alone is usually sufficient for management of comedonal acne (Kim and Armstrong, 2011). Tretinoin is available as a cream, gel, or liquid. This drug can be extremely irritating to the skin and requires careful patient education for optimal usage. The patient should be instructed to begin with a pea-sized dot of medication, which is divided into the three main areas of the face and then gently rubbed into each area. The medication should not be applied for at least 20 to 30 minutes after washing to decrease the burning sensation. The avoidance of the sun and the daily use of sunscreen must be emphasized because sun exposure can result in severe sunburn. Adolescents should be advised to apply the medication at night and to use a sunscreen with a sun protection factor (SPF) of at least 15 in the daytime.

Topical benzoyl peroxide is an antibacterial agent that inhibits the growth of *P. acnes* organisms. It is effective against both inflammatory and noninflammatory acne and is an effective first-line agent. This medication is available as a cream, lotion, gel, or wash. The patient should be informed that the medication may have a bleaching effect on sheets, bedclothes, and towels. The adolescent can be reassured that skin bleaching will not occur. Accommodation to the medication can be gained with a gradual increase in the strength and frequency of application.

When inflammatory lesions accompany the comedones, a topical antibacterial agent may be prescribed. These agents are used to prevent new lesions and to treat preexisting acne. Clindamycin, erythromycin, metronidazole, azelaic acid, and the combination of either benzoyl peroxide and erythromycin (Benzamycin) or benzoyl peroxide and glycolic acid are all choices for topical antibacterial therapy. The combination of 5% benzoyl peroxide and 3% erythromycin is especially beneficial, although the exact mechanism of action is not understood (Kim and Armstrong, 2011).

Systemic antibiotic therapy is used when moderate to severe acne does not respond to topical treatments. Oral antibiotics such as tetracycline, erythromycin, minocycline, and doxycycline are considered safe to use (Fanelli, Kupperman, Lautenbach, and others, 2011; Leyden and Del Rosso, 2011).

Young women with mild to moderate acne may respond well to topical treatment and the addition of an oral contraceptive pill (OCP). OCPs reduce the endogenous androgen production and decrease the bioavailability of the woman's circulating androgens. Both of these actions result in decreased acne.

Isotretinoin, 13-*cis*-retinoic acid (Accutane), is a potent and effective oral agent that is reserved for severe cystic acne that has not responded to other treatments. Isotretinoin is the only agent available that affects factors involved in the development of acne. However, treatment with isotretinoin should be managed *only* by a dermatologist. Adolescents with multiple, active, deep dermal or subcutaneous cystic and nodular acne lesions are treated for 20 weeks. Multiple side effects can occur, including dry skin and mucous membranes, nasal irritation, dry eyes, decreased night vision, photosensitivity, arthralgia, headaches, mood changes, aggressive or violent behaviors, depression, and suicidal ideation. Adolescents taking this drug should be monitored for depression, depressive symptoms, and suicidal ideation (Misery, 2011). The drug should be given only at the recommended doses for no longer than the recommended duration. The most significant side effects of this drug are the teratogenic effects. Isotretinoin is absolutely contraindicated in pregnant women. Sexually active young women must use an effective contraceptive method during treatment and for 1 month after treatment. Patients receiving isotretinoin should also be monitored for elevated cholesterol and triglyceride levels. Significant elevation may require discontinuation of the medication.

Nursing Care Management

Because acne is so common and its appearance may seem so mild, the health care provider may underestimate the relative importance of the disease to the adolescent. The nurse should assess the individual adolescent's level of distress, current management, and perceived success of any regimen before initiating a referral. If adolescents do not perceive the acne to be a problem, they may lack motivation to follow the treatment plan.

The nurse can provide ongoing support for the adolescent when a treatment plan is initiated. The family is also encouraged to support the adolescent in his or her efforts. Use of medications and basic skin care information should be discussed in detail with the adolescent. Written instructions should accompany the verbal discussion. Information to dispel myths regarding the use of abrasive cleansing products can prevent unnecessary costs and trauma to the skin.

Teenagers need education about the factors that aggravate and damage the skin, such as too vigorous scrubbing. In addition, picking, squeezing, and manual expression with fingernails break down the ductal walls of lesions and cause the acne to worsen. Mechanical irritation, such as vinyl helmet straps that rub areas predisposed to acne, can also cause the development of lesions.

THERMAL INJURY

BURNS

Burn injuries are usually attributed to extreme heat sources but may also result from exposure to cold, chemicals, electricity, or radiation. Most burns are relatively minor and do not require definitive medical treatment. However, burns involving a large body surface area, critical body parts, or the geriatric or pediatric population often benefit from treatment in specialized burn centers. The American Burn Association has established criteria to guide decisions regarding the severity of injury and the need for transfer for specialized care.* Burn prevention is also discussed in Chapters 10, 12, 15, and 16.

When burns are categorized according to the patient's age and type of injury, the following patterns become apparent: (1) hot-water scalds are most frequent in toddlers, (2) flame-related burns are more common in older children, (3) 10% to 20% of documented cases of child abuse include burn injuries (Herndon, 2007), and (4) children playing with matches or lighters account for 1 in 10 house fires.

The extent of tissue destruction is determined by the intensity of the heat source, the duration of contact or exposure, the conductivity of the tissue involved, and the rate at which the heat energy is dissipated by the skin. A brief exposure to high-intensity heat from a flame can produce burn injuries similar to those induced by long exposure to less intense heat in hot water.

Characteristics of Burn Injury

The physiologic responses, treatment modalities, prognosis, and disposition of the injured child are all directly related to the *amount of tissue destroyed*. Therefore, the severity of the burn injury is assessed on the basis of the percentage of **total body surface area (TBSA)** burned and depth of the burn. Among children in the school-age group or younger age groups, a burn that is 10% TBSA can be life threatening if not treated correctly. Other important factors in determining the seriousness of the injury are the location of the wounds, the child's age and general health, the causative agent, the presence of respiratory involvement, and any associated injury or condition.

Type of Injury

The majority of burns result from contact with thermal agents such as a flame, hot surfaces, or hot liquids. Electrical injuries caused by household current have the greatest incidence in young children, who insert conductive objects into electrical outlets and bite or suck on connected electrical cords (Herndon, 2007). These burns occur most commonly during the spring and summer months and are also associated with risk-taking behaviors in boys. Direct contact with high- or low-voltage current, as well as lightning strikes, is the most frequent mechanism of injury. The resistance of the tissue and the path of the electric current are responsible for the damage incurred. Electric current travels through the body following the path of least resistance, which involves the tissues, fluid, blood vessels, and nerves. A more localized burn is produced if skin resistance is high at the area of contact, and a more systemic pattern of injury is produced if skin resistance is low. Often compared with a crush injury, serious electrical trauma results from current passing through vital organs, muscle compartments, and nerve or vascular pathways. Loss of limbs, cardiac fibrillation, respiratory collapse, and burns are common occurrences after exposure to electrical energy. Criteria for admission, as derived from evidence-based practice for electrical burn injuries, includes a history of loss of consciousness, electrocardiographic (ECG) changes, 10% TBSA affected, or the need for monitoring an affected extremity. Cardiac monitoring is therefore included in standard burn care when ECG changes are identified on admission (Arnoldo, Klein, and Gibran, 2006).

Chemical burns are seen in the pediatric population and can cause extensive injury. The severity of injury is related to the chemical agent (acid, alkali, or organic compound) and the duration of contact. The mechanism of injury differs from that in other burns in that there is a chemical disruption and alteration of the physical properties of the exposed body area. Noxious agents exist in many cleaning products commonly found in the home. In addition to concern for localized damage, the potential for systemic toxicity must be addressed. Of particular concern is the exposure of the eyes to chemical agents, the ingestion of caustic substances, and inhalation of toxic gases produced from chemicals.

Extent of Injury

The extent of a burn is expressed as a percentage of the TBSA. This is most accurately estimated by using specially designed age-related charts (Fig. 30-14). It is more efficient to use a chart designed to assign body proportions to children of different ages.

Depth of Injury

A thermal injury is a three-dimensional wound that is also assessed in relation to depth of injury. Traditionally, the terms *first*, *second*, and *third degree* have been used to describe the depth of tissue injury. However, with the current emphasis on wound healing, these have been replaced by more descriptive terms based on the extent of destruction to the epithelializing elements of the skin (Fig. 30-15).

Superficial (first-degree) burns are usually of minor significance. This type of injury involves the epidermal layer only. There is often a latent period followed by erythema. Tissue damage is minimal, and there is no blistering. The protective functions of the skin remain intact and systemic effects are rare. Pain is the predominant symptom, and the burn heals in 5 to 10 days without scarring. A mild sunburn is an example of a superficial burn.

Partial-thickness (second-degree) burns involve the epidermis and varying degrees of the dermal layer. These wounds are painful, moist, red, and blistered. With superficial partial-thickness burns, dermal elements are intact, and the wound should heal in approximately 14 to 21 days with variable amounts of scarring (Fig. 30-16). The wound is extremely sensitive to temperature changes, exposure to air, and light touch. Although classified as second-degree or partial-thickness burn, deep dermal burns resemble full-thickness injuries in many respects except that sweat glands and hair follicles remain intact. The burn may appear mottled, with pink, red, or waxy white areas exhibiting blisters and edema formation. Systemic effects are similar to those encountered with full-thickness burns. Although many of these wounds heal spontaneously, healing time may be extended beyond 21 days. These burn wounds often heal with extensive scarring.

Full-thickness (third-degree) burns are serious injuries that involve the entire epidermis and dermis and extend into subcutaneous tissue (see Fig. 30-15). Nerve endings, sweat glands, and hair follicles are destroyed. The burn varies in color from red to tan, waxy white, brown, or black and is distinguished by a dry, leathery appearance (Fig. 30-17). Normally, full-thickness burns lack sensation in the area of injury because of the destruction of nerve endings. However, most full-thickness burns have superficial and partial-thickness burned areas at the periphery of the burn, where nerve endings are intact and exposed. As the peripheral fibers regenerate, painful sensations return. Consequently, children often experience severe pain related to the size and depth of the burn. Full-thickness wounds are not capable of reepithelialization and require surgical excision and grafting to close the wound.

---

*The American Burn Association offers an Advanced Burn Life Support Program; http://www.ameriburn.org/ablsnow.php.

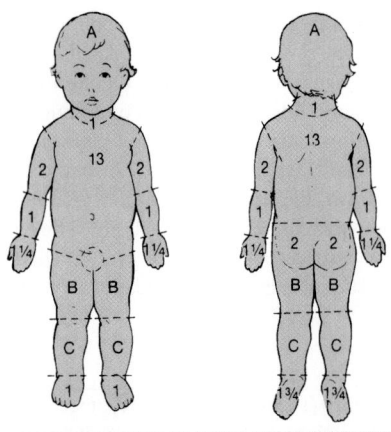

RELATIVE PERCENTAGES OF AREAS AFFECTED BY GROWTH

A

AREA	BIRTH	AGE 1 YR	AGE 5 YR
A = ½ of head	9½	8½	6½
B = ½ of one thigh	2¾	3¼	4
C = ½ of one leg	2½	2½	2¾

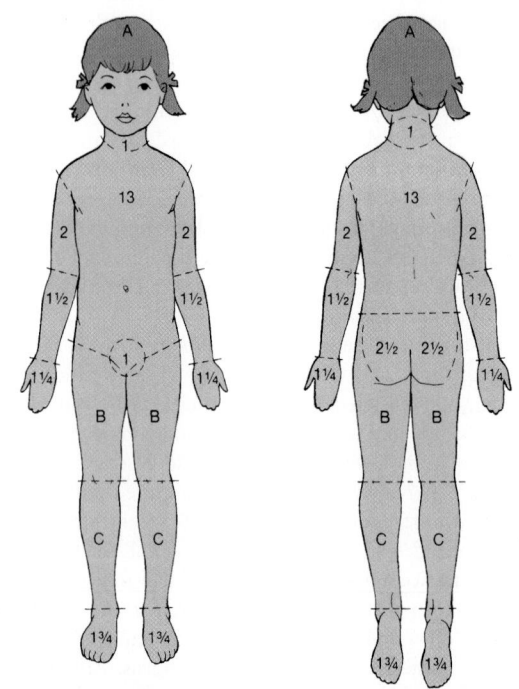

RELATIVE PERCENTAGES OF AREAS AFFECTED BY GROWTH

B

AREA	AGE 10 YR	AGE 15 YR	ADULT
A = ½ of head	5½	4½	3½
B = ½ of one thigh	4½	4½	4¾
C = ½ of one leg	3	3¼	3½

FIG 30-14 Estimation of distribution of burns in children. **A,** Children from birth to age 5 years. **B,** Older children.

Fourth-degree burns are full-thickness burns that involve underlying structures such as muscle, fascia, and bone. The wound appears dull and dry, and ligaments, tendons, and bone may be exposed (Fig. 30-18).

Severity of Injury

Burns are classified as minor, moderate, or major, which is useful in determining the disposition of the patient for treatment. Burn patients are categorized as (1) those with a **major burn injury,** who require the services and facilities of a specialized burn center; (2) those with a **moderate burn,** who may be treated in a hospital with expertise in burn care; and (3) those with **minor injuries,** who may be treated on an outpatient basis. The extent and depth of the burn (Table 30-9), the causative agent, the body area involved, the patient's age, and concomitant injuries and illnesses determine the severity of the injury.

Because the skin of infants is so thin, they are likely to sustain deeper injuries compared with older children. Children younger than 2 years of age, especially 6 months or younger, have a significantly higher mortality rate than older children with burns of similar magnitude. Acute or chronic illnesses or superimposed injuries also complicate burn care and response to treatment.

Inhalation Injury

Trauma to the tracheobronchial tree often follows inhalation of heated gases and toxic chemicals produced during combustion. Although direct thermal injury to the upper airway may occur, heat damage below the vocal cords is rare. Inspired heated air is cooled in the upper airway before reaching the trachea. Reflex closure of the cords and laryngospasm also prevent full inhalation. However, evidence of direct thermal injury to the upper airway includes burns of the face and lips, singed nasal hairs, and laryngeal edema. Clinical manifestations may be delayed as long as 24 to 48 hours. Wheezing, increasing secretions, hoarseness, wet rales, and carbonaceous secretions are signs of respiratory tract involvement. Upper airway obstruction is often associated with burn shock and fluid resuscitation. In such situations, endotracheal intubation may also be necessary to preserve a patent airway.

Inhalation of carbon monoxide is suspected when the injury has occurred in an enclosed space. Mucosal erythema and edema followed by sloughing of the mucosa are manifestations of respiratory tract injury. A mucopurulent membrane replaces the mucosal lining and seriously compromises respiration and ventilation. A significant increase in mortality has been observed when inhalation injury and pneumonia are both present. Deep burns, especially those encircling the thorax, may cause restriction of chest excursion as a result of edema and inelastic eschar formation. Young children are particularly at risk because of the pliability of the skeletal structure.

Pathophysiology

Thermal injuries produce both local and systemic effects that are related to the extent of tissue destruction. In superficial burns, the tissue damage is minimal. In partial-thickness burns, there is considerable edema and more severe capillary damage. With a major burn greater than 30% TBSA, there is a systemic response involving an increase in capillary permeability, allowing plasma proteins, fluids, and electrolytes to be lost. Maximum edema formation in a small wound occurs about 8 to 12 hours after injury. After a larger injury, hypovolemia, associated with this phenomenon, will slow the rate of edema formation, with maximum effect at 18 to 24 hours.

Another systemic response is anemia, caused by direct heat destruction of red blood cells (RBCs), hemolysis of injured RBCs, and trapping of RBCs in the microvascular thrombi of damaged cells. A long-term decrease in the number of RBCs may occur as a result of increased RBC fragility. Initially, there is an increased blood flow to the heart, brain, and kidneys, with decreased blood flow to the gastrointestinal tract. There is an increase in metabolism to maintain body heat, providing for the increased energy needs of the body.

Complications

Thermally injured children are subject to a number of serious complications, both from the wound and from systemic alterations resulting

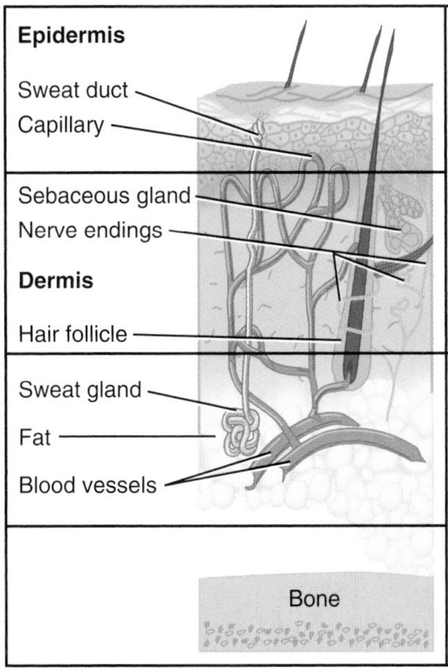

	Wound Appearance	Wound Sensation	Course of Healing
Partial-Thickness Burn — 1st Degree	Epidermis remains intact and without blisters Erythema; skin blanches with pressure	Painful	Discomfort lasts 48–72 hours. Desquamation occurs in 3–7 days.
Partial-Thickness Burn — 2nd Degree	Wet, shiny, weeping surface Blisters Wound blanches with pressure	Painful Very sensitive to touch, air currents	Superficial partial-thickness burn heals in <21 days. Deep partial-thickness burn requires >21 days for healing. Healing rates vary with burn depth and presence or absence of infection.
Full-Thickness Burn — 3rd Degree	Color variable (i.e., deep red, white, black, brown) Surface dry Thrombosed vessels visible No blanching	Insensate (↓ pinprick sensation)	Autografting is required for healing.
Full-Thickness Burn — 4th Degree	Color variable Charring visible in deepest areas Extremity movement limited	Insensate	Amputation of extremities is likely. Autografting is required for healing.

Diagram labels: Epidermis — Sweat duct, Capillary; Sebaceous gland, Nerve endings; **Dermis** — Hair follicle; Sweat gland, Fat, Blood vessels; Bone

FIG 30-15 Classification of burn depth according to depth of injury. (From Black JM: *Medical-surgical nursing: clinical management for positive outcomes*, ed 8, Philadelphia, 2008, Saunders.)

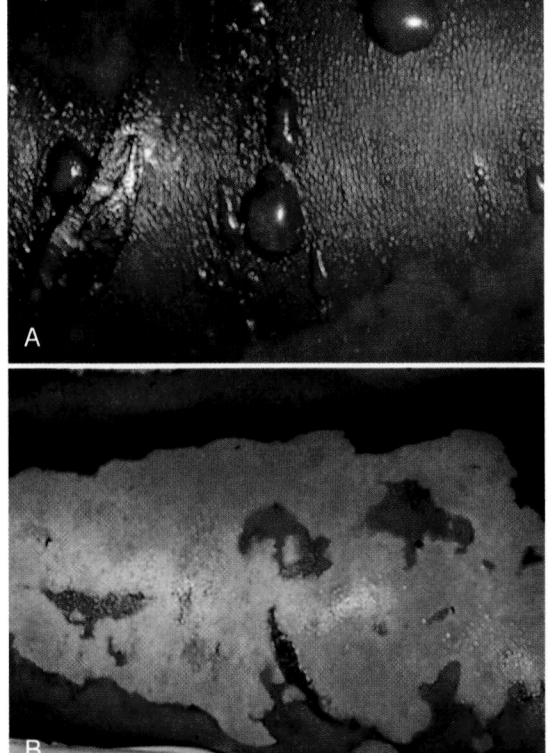

FIG 30-16 Superficial partial-thickness burns on an African-American child. **A,** Blisters intact. **B,** Blisters removed. (Courtesy Hillcrest Medical Center, Tulsa, Okla.)

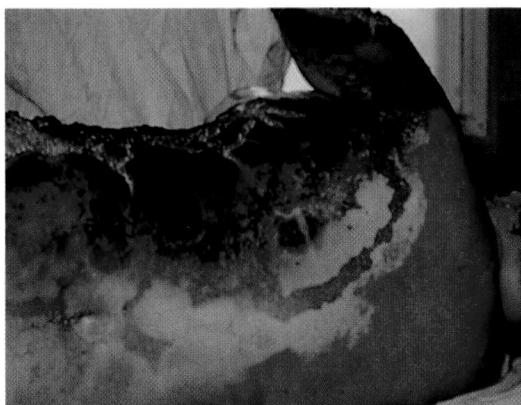

FIG 30-17 *Bottom* to *top:* Deep partial-thickness burn (*red area*), full-thickness burn (*white area*), and full-thickness burn with eschar (*brown area*). (Courtesy Hillcrest Medical Center, Tulsa, Okla.)

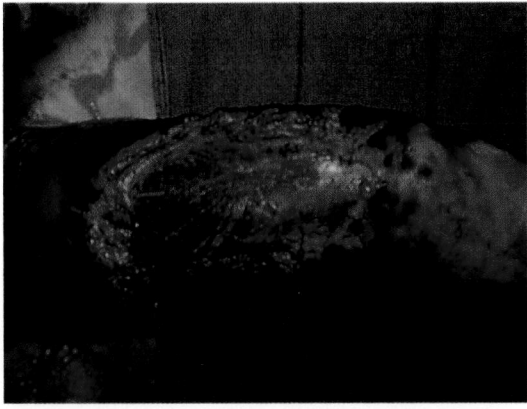

FIG 30-18 Full-thickness burn with muscle and fascia involved. (Courtesy Hillcrest Medical Center, Tulsa, Okla.)

TABLE 30-9	SEVERITY GRADING SYSTEM ADOPTED BY THE AMERICAN BURN ASSOCIATION		
	MINOR*	**MODERATE**	**MAJOR**
Partial-thickness burns (% TBSA)	<10	10–20	>20
Full-thickness burns			All
Treatment	Usually outpatient; may require 1- to 2-day admission	Admission to hospital, preferably one with expertise in burn care	Admission to a burn center

From Vaccaro P, Trofino RB: Care of the patient with minor to moderate burns. In Trofino RB, editor: *Nursing care of the burn-injured patient*, Philadelphia, 1991, FA Davis.
TBSA, Total body surface area.
*Minor burns exclude any burn involving the face, hands, feet, perineum or crossing joints; electrical burns; any injury complicated by the presence of inhalation injury or concomitant trauma; and children with psychosocial factors affecting the injury.

from the injury. The immediate threat to life is related to airway compromise and profound shock. During healing, infection—both local and systemic sepsis—is the primary complication. Mortality associated with thermal trauma in children increases with the severity of injury and decreases as age advances. In children older than 3 years, the mortality rate is similar to that of adults. Below this age, the survival rate with burns and their associated complications lessens considerably.

A less apparent respiratory tract injury is inhalation of carbon monoxide. Carbon monoxide has a greater affinity for hemoglobin than does oxygen, thereby depriving peripheral tissues and oxygen-dependent organs (e.g., the heart and brain) of the oxygen needed for survival. Treatment for either of these two problems is 100% oxygen, which reverses the situation rapidly.

Pulmonary problems are a major cause of fatality in children with either thermal burns or complications in the respiratory tract. Early in the postburn period, most pulmonary infections result from nosocomial exposure, immobility, and abdominal distention. The hematogenous variety occurs later and is related to the septic burn wound or other foci, such as phlebitis at the site of an invasive intravenous (IV) line. Respiratory problems include inhalation injuries, aspiration in unconscious patients, bacterial pneumonia, pulmonary edema, pulmonary embolus, posttraumatic pulmonary insufficiency, and atelectasis. The most common cause of respiratory failure in the pediatric age group is bacterial pneumonia, which requires prolonged intubation and sometimes a tracheostomy. Tracheostomies increase the incidence of serious complications and are performed only in extreme cases.

A less common complication is pulmonary edema resulting from fluid overload or acute respiratory distress syndrome (ARDS) in association with gram-negative sepsis. ARDS results from pulmonary capillary damage and leakage of fluid into the interstitial spaces of the lung. A loss of compliance and interference with oxygenation are the consequences of pulmonary insufficiency in conjunction with systemic sepsis.

✚ EMERGENCY TREATMENT
Burns

Minor Burns
Stop the burning process:
- Apply cool water to the burn or hold the burned area under cool running water.
- Do not use ice.

Do not disturb any blisters that form unless the injury is from a chemical substance.
Do not apply anything to the wound.
Cover with a clean cloth if risk of damage or contamination.
Remove burned clothing and jewelry.

Major Burns
Stop the burning process:
- Flame burns—smother the fire.
- Place victim in the horizontal position.
- Roll victim in a blanket or similar object; avoid covering the head.

Assess for an adequate airway and breathing.
If child is not breathing, begin mouth-to-mouth resuscitation.
Remove burned clothing and jewelry.
Cover wound with a clean cloth.
Keep victim warm.
Transport to medical aid.
Begin intravenous and oxygen therapy as prescribed.

Wound Sepsis

Sepsis is a critical problem in the treatment of burns and an ever-present threat after the shock phase. Decreased level of consciousness and lethargy are early signs of sepsis. Initially, burn wounds are relatively pathogen free unless they are contaminated with potentially infectious material, such as dirt or polluted water. However, dead tissue and exudate provide a fertile field for bacterial growth. On approximately the third postburn day, early colonization of the wound surface by a preponderance of gram-positive organisms (primarily staphylococci) changes to predominantly gram-negative opportunistic organisms, particularly *Pseudomonas aeruginosa*. By the fifth postburn day, bacterial invasion is well under way beneath the surface of the burn wound. Early surgical excision of eschar together with placement of autograft reduces the incidence of sepsis.

Therapeutic Management
Emergency Care
The initial management of the burn patient begins at the scene of injury. The first priority is to stop the burning process (see Emergency Treatment box). The child should then be transported immediately to the nearest medical facility for treatment and evaluation. The child and the family are usually extremely frightened and anxious; sensitivity to their emotional state and reassurance should be provided during the transport process.

Stop the Burning Process. The chief aim of rescue in flame burns is to smother the fire, not fan it. Children tend to panic and run, which spreads the flames and makes assistance more difficult. The injured child should be placed in a horizontal position and rolled in a blanket, rug, or similar article, with care taken not to cover the head and face because of the danger of inhalation of toxic fumes. If nothing is available, the victim should lie down and roll over slowly to extinguish the flames. Remaining in the vertical position may cause the hair to ignite or the inhalation of flames, heat, or smoke.

Major burns with large amounts of denuded skin should not be cooled. Heat is rapidly lost from burned areas, and additional cooling leads to a drop in core body temperature and potential circulatory collapse. Wet dressings also promote vasoconstriction because of cooling, resulting in impaired circulation to the burned area and increased tissue damage. Chemical burns require continuous flushing with large amounts of water before transport to a medical facility. The use of neutralizing agents on the skin is contraindicated because a chemical reaction is initiated and further injury may result. If the chemical is in powder form, the addition of water may spread the caustic agent. The powder should be brushed off if possible before flushing the area.

Burned clothing is removed to prevent further damage from smoldering fabric and hot beads of melted synthetic materials. Jewelry is removed to eliminate the transfer of heat from the metal and constriction resulting from edema formation. This also provides access to the wound and prevents painful removal later.

Assess the Victim's Condition. As soon as the flames are extinguished, the child is assessed. Airway, breathing, and circulation are the primary concerns. Cardiopulmonary complications may result from exposure to electric current, inhalation of toxic fumes and smoke, hypovolemia, and shock. Emergency measures are instituted as appropriate.

Cover the Burn. The burn wound should be covered with a clean dry cloth to prevent contamination, decrease pain by eliminating air contact, and prevent hypothermia. No attempt should be made to treat the burn. Application of topical ointments, oils, or other home remedies is contraindicated.

Transport the Child to Medical Aid. The child with an extensive burn is not given anything by mouth to avoid aspiration in the presence of paralytic ileus and upper airway edema and to prevent water intoxication. The child is transported to the nearest medical facility. If this cannot be accomplished within a relatively short period, IV access should be established, if possible, with a large-bore catheter. Oxygen is administered, if available, at 100%. A report of the initial assessment, associated trauma, and any interventions implemented is given to the medical facility assuming care of the child.

Provide Reassurance. Providing reassurance and psychological support to both the family and the child helps immeasurably during the period of postinjury crisis. Reducing anxiety conserves energy the family and child will need to cope with the physiologic and emotional stress of injury.

Minor Burns

Treatment of burns classified as minor can usually be managed adequately on an outpatient basis when it is determined that the parent can be relied on to carry out instructions for care and observation. Patients with less than optimum circumstances may require close follow-up to ensure adherence with treatment.

The wound is cleansed with a mild soap and tepid water. Débridement of the wound includes removal of any embedded debris, chemicals, and devitalized tissue. Removal of intact blisters remains controversial. Some authorities argue that blisters provide a barrier against infection; others maintain that blister fluid is an effective medium for the growth of microorganisms. However, blisters should be broken if the injury is from a chemical agent to control absorption. Most practitioners favor covering the wound with an antimicrobial ointment to reduce the risk of infection and to provide some form of pain relief. The dressing consists of nonadherent fine-mesh gauze placed over the ointment and a light wrap of gauze dressing that avoids interference with movement. This helps keep the wound clean and protect it from trauma. The caregiver is instructed to wash the wound, reapply the dressing, and return the child to the office or clinic as directed for wound observation. The frequency of dressing changes may vary from every other day to once a day.

Some practitioners prefer an occlusive dressing, such as a hydrocolloid, which is placed over the wound after cleansing. Hydrogel dressings, which are soothing and nonadherent, may also be used. The dressing is changed when leakage occurs—at regular intervals or at least weekly. This method eliminates the discomfort associated with frequent dressing changes but limits visualization of the wound surface.

If there is a high probability of infection or other complications or if there is doubt about the ability to carry out instructions, the caregiver may be directed to bring the patient in daily for dressing changes and inspection. Another option is have a nurse make a home visit to inspect the wound and perform the dressing change. Frequent removal of the dressing is an effective mode of débridement. Soaking the dressing in tepid water or normal saline before removal helps loosen the dressing and debris and reduce discomfort. Burns of the face are usually treated by an open method. The wound is washed and débrided in the same manner, and a thin film of antimicrobial ointment is applied.

A tetanus history is obtained on admission. If there is no history of immunization or if more than 5 years have passed since the last immunization, tetanus prophylaxis is administered. A mild analgesic such as acetaminophen is usually sufficient to relieve discomfort; the antipyretic effect of the drug also alleviates the sensation of heat.

Most minor burns heal without difficulty, but if the wound margin becomes erythematous; gross purulence is noted; or the child develops evidence of systemic reaction, such as fever or tachycardia, hospitalization is indicated. The child should also be evaluated for functional impairment, and the caregiver should be instructed in the exercise and ambulation program. After wound healing, an evaluation of scar maturation and range of motion will indicate any need for further therapy.

Major Burns

The first priority is airway maintenance. The inhalation of noxious agents or respiratory burns is suggested when there is a history of injury in an enclosed space; edema of the oral and nasal membranes; thermal injury to the face, nares, and upper torso; hyperemia; and blisters or evidence of trauma to the upper respiratory passages. When respiratory involvement is suspected or evident, 100% oxygen is administered and blood gas values, including carbon monoxide levels, are determined.

If the child exhibits changes in sensorium, air hunger, or other signs of respiratory distress, an endotracheal tube is inserted to maintain the airway. When severe edema of the face and neck is anticipated, intubation is performed before swelling makes intubation difficult or impossible. Controlled intubation is preferred to an emergency intubation. Intubation allows for the delivery of humidified oxygen, the removal of secretions from respiratory passages, and the provision of ventilatory support. When full-thickness burns encircle the chest, constricting eschar may limit chest wall excursion, and ventilation of the child becomes more difficult. Escharotomy of the chest relieves this constriction and improves ventilation.

Fluid Replacement Therapy. The objectives of fluid therapy are to (1) compensate for water and sodium lost to traumatized areas and interstitial spaces, (2) reestablish sodium balance, (3) restore circulating volume, (4) provide adequate perfusion, (5) correct acidosis, and (6) improve renal function.

Fluid replacement is required during the first 24 hours because of fluid shifts that occur after the injury. Various formulas are used to calculate fluid needs, and the one adopted depends on practitioner preference. Crystalloid solutions are used during this initial phase of therapy. Parameters such as vital signs (especially heart rate), urinary output volume, adequacy of capillary filling, and state of sensorium determine adequacy of fluid resuscitation.

After the initial 24-hour period, theoretically there is a capillary seal, and capillary permeability is restored. Colloid solutions such as albumin, Plasma-Lyte, or fresh-frozen plasma are useful in maintaining plasma volume. However, children with burn injuries usually require fluids in excess of their calculated maintenance and replacement volume. Reasons for this may include underestimation of burn size (particularly in pediatric patients), pulmonary injury that sequesters resuscitation fluid in the lung, electrical injury with greater tissue destruction than that which is visible, and a delay in the initiation of fluid resuscitation. Irreversible burn shock that persists despite aggressive fluid resuscitation remains a significant cause of death in the immediate postburn period. Fluid balance may continue to be a problem throughout the course of treatment, especially during periods in which there may be considerable evaporative loss from the wound.

Nutrition. The enhanced metabolic requirements and catabolism in severe burns make nutritional needs of paramount importance and often difficult to satisfy. To avoid protein breakdown, the diet must provide sufficient calories to meet the increased metabolic needs and enough protein. Hypoglycemia can result from the stress of the burn injury because the liver glycogen stores are rapidly depleted.

A high-protein, high-calorie diet is encouraged. Many children have poor appetites and are unable to meet energy requirements solely by oral feeding. Oral feedings are encouraged unless the child is intubated or paralytic ileus persists. Most children with burns in excess of 25% TBSA require supplementation with tube feeding. Early and continued nutritional support is an important part of therapy for seriously burned patients. Enteral feeding provides direct nourishment to the gastrointestinal tract and helps reverse the defective gut barrier that accompanies burn shock (Purdue, 2007). Children who require enteral supplementation must be monitored for feeding intolerance and tube malposition. The nurse should also monitor and report any abdominal distention, diarrhea, or electrolyte and metabolic deviations. If nutritional requirements cannot be met entirely by the enteral route, parenteral hyperalimentation is used to supplement intake. However, enteral feeding increases blood flow in the intestinal tract, preserves gastrointestinal function, and minimizes bacterial translocation by decreasing mucosal atrophy of the intestines. These factors make enteral feeding the preferred route of nutritional support (Herndon, 2007).

To facilitate growth and proliferation of epithelial cells, administration of vitamins A and C is begun early in the postburn period. Zinc is also supplemented because of its important role in wound healing and epithelialization.

Medication. Antibiotics are usually not administered prophylactically. The administration of systemic antibiotics to control wound colonization is not indicated because decreased circulation to the injured area prevents delivery of the medication to areas of deepest injury. Surveillance cultures and monitoring of the clinical course provide the most reliable indicators of developing infection. Appropriate antibiotics are instituted to treat the specific identified organism Otitis media should not be overlooked as a source of fever in the pediatric population (Herndon, 2007).

Some form of sedation and analgesia is required in the care of burned children. Morphine sulfate is the drug of choice for severe burn injuries. Morphine has extensive distribution but is metabolized rapidly; continuous infusion or frequent administration is needed for pain management in burns. Morphine is administered intravenously and titrated to individual needs. The unstable circulatory status and edema formation preclude intramuscular or subcutaneous administration. When combined, midazolam (Versed) and fentanyl (Sublimaze) also provide excellent IV sedation and analgesia to control procedural pain in children with burns (Herndon, 2007). The oral form of fentanyl, Oralet, provides effective analgesia in a convenient form that children can suck. Dosage monitoring is important because tolerance to opioids may develop. IV analgesics are most effective when they are administered just before the onset of procedural pain.

The use of short-acting anesthetic agents, such as propofol (Diprivan) and nitrous oxide, has proved beneficial in eliminating procedural pain. Pharyngeal reflexes remain intact, thus ensuring a patent airway. Propofol is an IV sedative hypnotic agent that produces sedation in less than 1 minute and lasts only a few minutes. Nitrous oxide is a useful short-term analgesic when given in a mixture of gases on a fixed ratio of 50% nitrous oxide and 50% oxygen (Annequin, Carbajal, Chauvin, and others, 2000). Initiation of action is approximately 1 minute, with peak effect reached in 3 to 5 minutes. Nitrous oxide is useful to alleviate anxiety and raise the threshold of pain during procedures. The child may self-administer the nitrous oxide mixture with assistance. For any conscious or unconscious sedation, the child must be monitored continuously during the procedure (see Preoperative Care, Chapter 22; and Pain Assessment and Pain Management, Chapter 7).

Management of the Burn Wound. After the initial period of shock and the restoration of fluid balance, the primary concern is the burn wound. The objectives of wound management include prevention of infection, removal of devitalized tissue, and closure of the wound. The application of dressings and topical antimicrobial therapy reduce pain by minimizing the exposure to air.

Primary Excision. In children with large, full-thickness burn wounds, excision is performed as soon as the patient is hemodynamically stable after initial resuscitation. Because the burn wound precipitates an exaggerated physiologic response, many complications do not resolve until the eschar is excised and the wound is closed. Early excision of deep partial- and full-thickness burns reduces the incidence of infection and the threat of sepsis.

Débridement. Partial-thickness wounds require débridement of devitalized tissue to promote healing. Débridement is painful and requires analgesia and a sedative before the procedure. Medications given for pain need to be readily available during this procedure and may need to be titrated up during the procedure. Hydroxyzine and diphenhydramine are often needed for itching that occurs after whirlpool and débridement. The itching becomes particularly bothersome as the burns heal.

Hydrotherapy is used to cleanse the wound and involves soaking in a tub or showering at least once a day for no more than 20 minutes. The water acts to loosen and remove sloughing tissue, exudate, and topical medications. Hydrotherapy helps to cleanse not only the wound but also the entire body and aids in maintenance of range of motion. Mesh gauze serves to entrap the exudative slough and is readily removed during hydrotherapy. Any loose tissue is carefully trimmed away before the wound is redressed.

Topical Antimicrobial Agents. Methods used for managing the burn wound include:

Exposure—Wounds are left open to air; crust forms on partial-thickness wounds, and eschar forms on full-thickness burns.

Open—Topical antimicrobial agent is applied directly to the wound surface, and the wound is left uncovered.

Modified—Antimicrobial agent is applied directly or impregnated into thin gauze and applied to the wound; gauze or net secures the area.

Occlusive—Antimicrobial agent is impregnated in gauze or applied directly to the wound; multiple layers of bulky gauze are placed over the primary layer and secured with gauze or net.

All of these methods provide wound coverage and use some type of topical agent. Topical agents do not eliminate organisms from the wound but can effectively inhibit bacterial growth. To be effective, a topical application must be nontoxic, capable of diffusing through eschar, harmless to viable tissue, inexpensive, and easy to apply. A topical ointment should not encourage the development of resistant strains of bacteria and should produce minimal electrolyte derangement. A variety of specific agents are available; examples include Bacitracin, Silver Sulfadiazine (Thermazine), Santyl (Collagenase), and Mafenide Acetate (Sulfamylon). Some topical agents are packaged and prepared on a fine-meshed gauze that allows ease of application. The gauze provides necessary protection for the wound, maximizes patient comfort, increases rate of healing, decreases the necessity for frequent dressing changes, and is cost effective. Examples include a nanocrystalline film of pure silver (Acticoat), a hydrofiber with ionic silver (Aquacel Ag), a flexible nylon mesh matrix with oat-beta glucan and silver (Glucan Silver Matrix), and a silicone foam dressing with silver (Mepilex Ag).

Biologic Skin Coverings. Permanent coverage of extensive burns is a prolonged process that requires repeated operative procedures using general anesthesia for atraumatic care in débridement and grafting. Early closure shortens the period of metabolic stress and decreases the likelihood of burn wound sepsis. In the acute phase, biologic dressings cover and protect the wound from contamination, reduce fluid and protein loss, increase the rate of epithelialization, reduce pain, and facilitate movement of joints to retain range of motion.

Allograft (homograft) skin is obtained from human cadavers that are screened for communicable diseases. Allograft is particularly useful in the coverage of surgically excised deep partial- and full-thickness wounds in extensive burns when available donor sites are limited. Severe immunosuppression occurs in massively burned children, and the allograft becomes adherent. The allograft can remain in place until suitable donor sites become available. Typically, rejection is seen approximately 3 to 4 weeks after application (Herndon, 2007). The availability of tissue banks and a supply of suitable donors limit the use of allografts.

Xenograft from a variety of species, most notably pigs, is commercially available. In large burns, the porcine xenograft is commonly applied when extensive early débridement is indicated to cover a partial-thickness burn; this provides a temporary covering for the wound until an available autograft can be applied to the full-thickness areas (Herndon, 2007). Pigskin dressings are replaced every 1 to 3 days. They are particularly effective in children with partial-thickness scald burns of the hands and face because they allow relatively pain-free movement, which reduces contracture formation and has the added benefit of improving appetite and morale.

When applied early to a superficial partial-thickness injury, biologic dressings stimulate epithelial growth and faster wound healing. However, biologic dressings must be applied to clean wounds. If the dressing covers areas of heavy microbial contamination, infection occurs beneath the dressing. In the case of partial-thickness burns, such infection may convert the wound to a full-thickness injury.

Synthetic skin coverings are available for the management of partial-thickness burn wounds. Ideally, the dressing should provide the properties of human skin, including adherence, elasticity, durability, and hemostasis. Synthetic skin substitutes are readily available, have an indefinite shelf life, and are relatively inexpensive.

Synthetic dressings are composed of a variety of materials and can be used successfully in the management of superficial partial-thickness burns and donor sites. Examples include adherent elastic films; hydro-active materials; or colloidal suspensions that are usually permeable to air, vapor, and fluids.

Biobrane is a flexible silicone–nylon membrane bonded to collagenous peptides of porcine skin. Calcium alginate is another treatment for donor sites. As with biologic dressings, it is important that the wound be free of debris before the dressing is applied. Body temperature elevation or evidence of purulence, erythema, or cellulitis around the wound edges may indicate that the wound has become infected beneath the dressing. If this occurs, prompt discontinuance of the synthetic dressing is indicated. All synthetic dressings are reputed to hasten wound healing and reduce discomfort.

Permanent Skin Coverings. Permanent coverage of deep partial- and full-thickness burns is usually accomplished with a split-thickness skin graft. This graft consists of the epidermis and a portion of the dermis removed from an intact area of skin by a special instrument, the **dermatome** (Fig. 30-19). With extensive burns, it is often difficult to find enough viable skin to cover the wounds; therefore, available donor sites and special techniques are used. Split-thickness skin grafts may be sheet graft or mesh graft.

Sheet Graft. A sheet of skin removed from the donor site is placed intact over the recipient site and sutured in place; this is used in areas where cosmetic results are most visible (Fig. 30-20).

Mesh Graft. A sheet of skin is removed from the donor site and passed through a mesher, which produces tiny slits in the skin that allow the skin to cover 1.5 to 9 times the area of the sheet graft; this results in a less desirable cosmetic and functional outcome (Fig. 30-21).

The donor site is dressed with synthetic wound coverings or fine-mesh gauze until the dressing separates at 10 to 14 days when the wound is healed. Dressings are not changed on donor sites to avoid damage to newly healed, delicate epithelium. Healed donor sites are available for reharvesting in patients with extensive burns and limited undamaged skin, but the quality of skin is decreased when multiple grafts are taken.

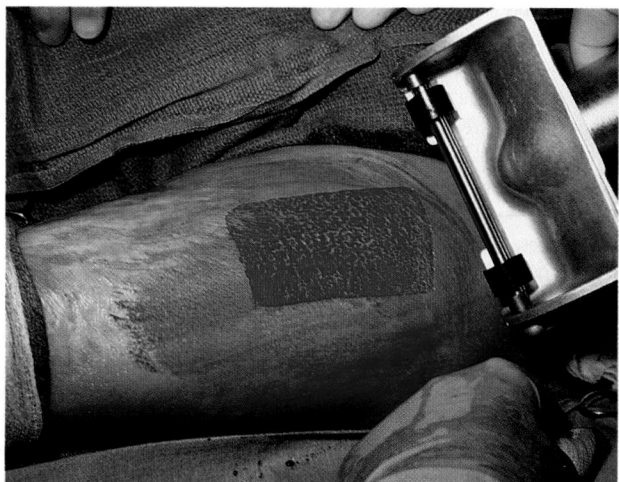

FIG   30-19 Removal of split-thickness skin graft with a dermatome.

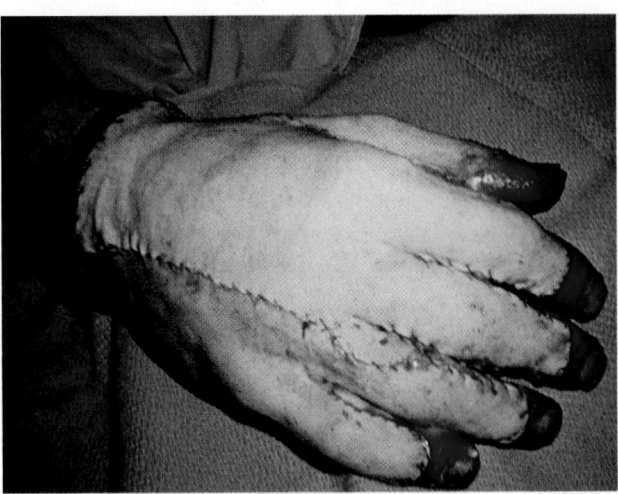

FIG 30-20 Sheet graft.

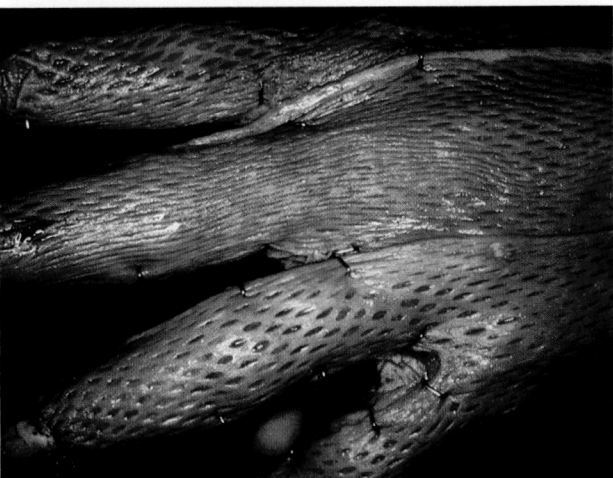

FIG 30-21 Mesh graft.

Artificial Skin. The development of Integra, a product that allows the dermis to regenerate, has produced significant improvement in burn wound healing and decreased scar formation. It is applied to partial- and full-thickness burns. The two-layer membrane is made of collagen (a fibrous protein from animal tendons and cartilage) and silicone rubber (i.e., Silastic). The Silastic layer is peeled off after the dermis is formed. The application of artificial skin does not replace the grafting procedure, but it prepares the burn wound to accept an ultrathin autograft. Advantages include faster healing of the burn wound when integrity of the dermis is restored, faster healing of donor sites with the use of ultrathin grafts, and restoration of sweat glands and hair follicles. A disadvantage is its high cost.

Cultured Epithelium. When burns are extensive and donor sites for split-thickness skin grafting are limited, it is possible to culture cells from a full-thickness skin biopsy and produce coherent sheets that can be applied to clean, excised full-thickness wounds. Epithelial cell culture grafts offer the possibility of an unlimited source of autografts in patients with extensive burns. Cultured epithelial autografts are effective in early wound closure. The child's own skin is fractionated and cultured in a porcine media to form a thin epithelial layer that is applied to the burn wound. This technique offers an improved rate of survival in patients with extensive burns and limited donor sites.

Prognosis

Children differ from adults in their responses to thermal injury, and the mortality rates in young children are significantly higher than those in older children and adults. Mortality is greatest for children younger than 48 months of age. Many children who do survive have long-term functional and cosmetic impairments.

Nursing Care Management

Because the care of burned children encompasses a broad range of skills, nursing care has been divided into segments that correspond with the major phases of burn treatment. The acute phase, also referred to as the *emergent* or *resuscitative phase*, involves the first 24 to 48 hours. The management phase extends from the completion of adequate resuscitation through wound coverage. The rehabilitative phase begins when the majority of the wounds have healed and rehabilitation has become the predominant focus of the care plan. This phase continues until all reconstructive procedures and corrective measures are accomplished (often a period of months or years).

Acute Phase

The primary emphasis during the emergent phase is the treatment of burn shock and the management of pulmonary status. Monitoring vital signs, output, fluid infusion, and respiratory parameters are ongoing activities in the hours immediately after injury. IV infusion is begun immediately and is regulated to maintain a urinary output of at least 1 to 2 ml/kg in children weighing less than 30 kg (66 pounds); an output of 30 to 50 ml/hr is expected in children weighing more than 30 kg. Urinary output and specific gravity, vital signs, laboratory data, and objective signs of adequate hydration guide the rate of fluid administration.

Children who are hospitalized with burns require constant observation and assessment for complications. Alterations in electrolyte balance produce clinical symptoms of confusion, weakness, cardiac irregularities, and seizures. Changes in respiratory function and gas exchange are reflected clinically by restlessness, irritability, increased work of breathing, and alterations in blood gas values. The loss of protective function of the skin exposes burned children to increased risk of hypothermia. Edema formation and circulatory impairment result in the loss of sensation and deep, throbbing pain.

> ### ! NURSING ALERT
>
> Evaluate the burned extremity and check the pulse every hour. If unable to palpate, use Doppler to ascertain loss of circulation and pulse. If the pulse is lost, escharotomy may be necessary to relieve the edema causing pressure on blood vessels to restore adequate circulation.

Burn centers maintain a pictorial record of wounds to record progress and for legal purposes (if child abuse is suspected). Burn wounds are treated according to the protocol of the specific burn center. The burn team monitors infection control procedures and ensures that staff and visitors comply with established protocols to prevent cross-contamination in the burn unit.

Throughout the acute phase of care, the psychosocial needs of the children and their families should not be overlooked. The child is frightened, uncomfortable, and often confused. Children may be isolated from familiar persons and surroundings; the overwhelming physical needs at this time are the primary focus of the staff and parents. In addition to feeling concern for their child, the family experiences guilt, which may be related to the fact that the parents did not or could not protect their child from injury. Consistency in the information presented and in the attitude of the staff creates a sense of familiarity and stability during the acute phase of care. Consistent caregivers can also help decrease the patient's and family's anxiety and provide coordination of care. For example, when many teams of consultants and specialists are involved in the child's care, appointing a burn team "spokesperson" decreases the confusion and enhances communication regarding the child's care.

Management and Rehabilitative Phases

After the patient's condition is stabilized, the management phase begins. The multidisciplinary team concentrates on preventing wound infections, closing the wound as quickly as possible, and managing the numerous complications. Although the rehabilitative phase begins when permanent wound closure has been achieved, rehabilitation issues are identified on admission and are included in the care plan throughout the hospital course.

> **⚠ NURSING ALERT**
>
> In a pediatric burn patient, a decreased level of consciousness, increased restlessness, and lethargy are some of the first signs of overwhelming sepsis and may indicate inadequate hydration. Assessment of capillary refill and pulses are another important indicator of the adequacy of hydration. With inadequate hydration, a spiking fever and diminished bowel sounds accompanied by paralytic ileus are noted and progressively increase over 48 to 72 hours, after which the temperature falls to subnormal limits. At this time, the wound deteriorates, the white blood cell count is depressed, and septic shock becomes manifest.

Comfort Management

The severe pain of the wound and resultant therapies, the anxiety generated by these experiences, sleep deprivation, itching related to wound healing, and the conscious and unconscious interpretations of traumatic events contribute to the psychologic behaviors commonly observed in children with burns. It is always difficult to deal with a child in pain, and inflicting pain on a helpless child is contrary to the empathic nature of nursing. Interventions to promote comfort may include medications (including IV morphine, fentanyl, or midazolam and short-term anesthetics such as propofol), relaxation techniques, distraction therapy, behavioral techniques, operant conditioning (e.g., tokens, star chart), and family participation.

Children need age-appropriate explanations before all procedures. When children appear to accept pain with little or no response, psychologic consultation may be needed. Consistency in caregivers is important. If this is not possible, a carefully developed, multidisciplinary care plan is necessary to provide consistency.

Care of the Burn Wound

The nurse has a major responsibility for cleansing, débriding, and applying topical medications and dressings to the burn wound. Pain medication should be administered so that the peak effect of the drug coincides with the procedure. Children who have an understanding of the procedure to be performed and some perceived control demonstrate less maladaptive behavior. Children also respond well to participating in decisions (see Atraumatic Care box).

Outer dressings are removed. Any dressings that have adhered to the wound can be more easily removed by applying tepid water or normal saline. Loose or easily detached tissue is débrided during the cleansing process. In dressing the wound, it is important that all areas be clean, that medication is amply applied, and that no two burned surfaces touch each other (e.g., fingers or toes; ears touching the side

> **ATRAUMATIC CARE**
> ### *Reducing the Stress of Burn Care Procedures*
>
> - Have all materials ready before beginning.
> - Administer appropriate analgesics and sedatives.
> - Remind the child of the impending procedure to allow sufficient time to prepare.
> - Allow the child to test and approve the temperature of the water.
> - Allow the child to select the area of the body on which to begin.
> - Allow the child to request a short rest period during the procedure.
> - Allow the child to remove the dressings if desired.
> - Provide something constructive for the child to do during the procedure (e.g., holding a package of dressings or a roll of gauze).
> - Inform the child when the procedure is near completion.
> - Praise the child for cooperation.

of the head). If they are touching, the burned surfaces will heal together, causing deformity or dysfunction.

Topical medications may be applied directly to the wound with a tongue blade or gloved hand as well as using impregnated fine-mesh gauze. Dressings are then applied to assist in exudate absorption, wound débridement, and increased patient comfort. All dressings applied circumferentially should be wrapped in a distal-to-proximal manner. The dressing is applied with sufficient tension to remain in place but not so tightly as to impair circulation or limit motion. An elastic net is then applied to secure the dressing in place. A stable dressing is especially important when the child is ambulatory.

Standard precautions, including the use of protective garb and barrier techniques, should be followed when caring for patients with burns. Frequent hand and forearm washing is the single most important element of the infection control program. Strict policies for cleaning the environment and patient care equipment should be implemented to minimize the risk of cross-contamination. All visitors and members of other departments should be oriented to the infection control policies, including the importance of hand and forearm washing and use of protective garb. Visitors should be screened for infection and contagious diseases before patient contact.

Prevention of Complications
Acute Care

The maintenance of body temperature is important to children with burns. Core body temperature is supported when energy is conserved with an environmental temperature of 28° to 33° C (82.4° to 91.4° F). Large areas of the body should not be exposed simultaneously during dressing changes. Warmed solutions, linens, occlusive dressings, heat shields, a radiant warmer, and warming blankets assist in preventing hypothermia.

The chief danger during acute care is infection—wound infection, generalized sepsis, or bacterial pneumonia. Accurate and ongoing assessments of all parameters that provide clues to the early diagnosis and treatment of infection are essential. Symptoms of sepsis include a decreased level of consciousness, a rising or falling white blood cell count, hyperthermia progressing to hypothermia, increasing fluid requirements, hypoactive or absent bowel sounds, a rising or falling blood glucose level, tachycardia, tachypnea, and thrombocytopenia. Infection delays the progress of wound healing.

Children are reluctant to move if movement causes pain, and they are likely to assume a position of comfort. Unfortunately, the most comfortable position often encourages the formation of contractures and loss of function. Ongoing efforts to prevent contractures include

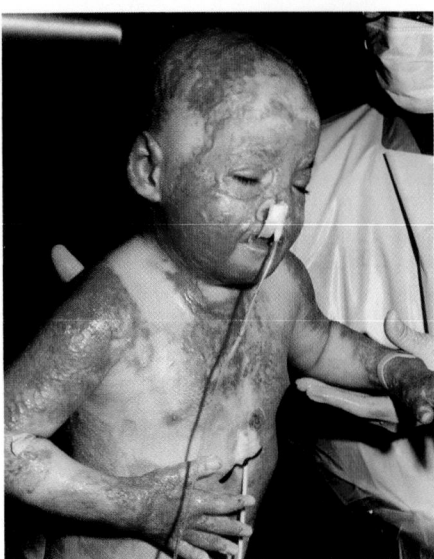

FIG 30-22 Extensive scars from a flame burn. (Courtesy The Paul and Carol David Foundation Burn Institute, Akron, Ohio.)

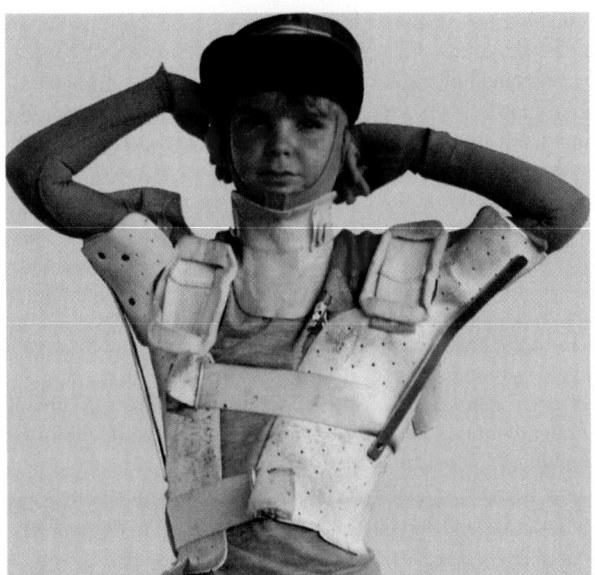

FIG 30-23 Child in an elasticized (Jobst) garment and "airplane" splints.

maintaining proper body alignment, positioning and splinting involved extremities in extension, providing active and passive physical therapy, and encouraging spontaneous movement when feasible. Frequent position changes are important to promote adequate bronchopulmonary hygiene and capillary perfusion to common pressure areas. Low–air loss beds are beneficial for morbidly obese children or children with posterior grafts. Special attention should be given to areas at risk for increased pressure, such as the posterior scalp, heels, sacrum, and areas exposed to mechanical irritation from splints and dressings.

Long-Term Care

When the burn heals, the rehabilitative phase of care begins. Scar formation becomes a major problem as burn wounds heal (Fig. 30-22). Contractile properties of the scar tissue can result in disabling contractures, deformity, and disfigurement.

Uniform pressure applied to the scar decreases the blood supply. When pressure is removed, blood supply to the scar is immediately increased; therefore, periods without pressure should be brief to avoid nourishment of the hypertrophic tissue. Continuous pressure to areas of scarring can be achieved by elastic bandages or commercially available pressure garments. Because these custom-made garments are often worn for months, revisions may be required as the child grows. It is much easier to prevent scarring and contracture of the wound than to resolve an existing problem. Splints and appliances may also be needed until wound maturation is achieved (Fig. 30-23).

Scar tissue has certain significant properties, particularly for growing children. Intense itching occurs in healing burn wounds and scar tissue until the scar is no longer active. Itching is usually treated with a combination of H_1 and H_2 antagonists such as cetirizine (Zyrtec) and cimetidine (Tagamet) (Baker, Zeller, Klein, and others, 2001); an H_1 antagonist alone; and frequent applications of a moisturizer, such as Vaseline Intensive Care Rescue, Aveeno Baby, Alpha Keri, or Eucerin. Massage therapy during the application of moisturizers is also beneficial to stretch scar tissue and aid in contracture prevention. Scar tissue has no sweat glands, and children with extensive scarring may experience difficulty during hot weather. Caregivers should be alerted to this possibility and be prepared to institute alternate methods of cooling when necessary.

Scar tissue does not grow and expand as does normal tissue, which may create difficulties, especially in functional areas such as on the hands and over joints. Additional surgery is sometimes required to allow independent functioning in daily activities, to improve cosmetic appearance, or to restore anatomic integrity.

The nursing activities in the rehabilitative phase of treatment focus on the child's and family's adaptation to the burn injury and their ability to reintegrate into the community. The psychologic pain and sequelae of severe burn injury are as intense as the physical trauma. The impact of severe burns taxes the coping mechanisms at all ages. Very young children, who suffer acutely from separation anxiety, and adolescents, who are developing an identity, are probably the most affected psychologically. Toddlers cannot understand why the parents they love and who have protected them can leave them in such a frightening and unfamiliar place. Adolescents, in the process of achieving independence from the family, find themselves in a dependent role with a damaged body. Being different from others at a time when conformity with peers is so important is difficult to accept.

Anticipation of the return to school can be overwhelming and frightening. It is essential that health care professionals recognize the importance of preparing teachers and classmates for the child's return. Teachers need to be provided with information to assist the child and family and to promote the child's optimal adjustment. Hospital-sponsored school reentry programs use a variety of methods to provide education and information about the implications of the injury, the garments and appliances, and the need for support and acceptance. Telephone calls, videotapes, information packets, and visits by members of the health care team offer opportunities to help with reintegration into the school environment—a focal point of the child's life.

Psychosocial Support of the Child

Children should begin early to do as much for themselves as possible and to be active participants in their care. Loss of control and perceived helplessness may result in acting-out behaviors. During illness, children can regress to a previous developmental level that allows them to deal with stress. As children begin to participate in their care, they gain confidence and self-esteem. Fears and anxieties diminish with accomplishment and self-confidence. If the child demonstrates nonadherence in the rehabilitative phase, a behavior modification program can be initiated to promote or reward the child's accomplishment in care.

Children need to know that their injury and the treatments are not punishment for real or imagined transgressions and that the nurse understands their fear, anger, and discomfort. They also need body contact. This is often difficult to arrange for the child with massive burns. Stroking areas of unburned skin is comforting. Even older children enjoy sitting on the parent's lap and being cuddled and hugged. This can be a reward or a comfort in times of stress, but most of all it should be kept in mind that it is a natural part of childhood.

Psychosocial Support of the Family

Recognizing and respecting each family's strengths, differences, and methods of coping allow the nurse to respond to their unique needs by implementing a family-centered approach to care. In the acute phase, all attention is focused on the child, and the parents feel powerless and ineffectual. Most parents feel overwhelming guilt, whether or not the guilt is justified. They feel responsible for the injury. These feelings may impede the child's rehabilitation. Parents may indulge the child and allow nonadherent behaviors that affect physical and emotional recovery. Parents need to be informed of the child's progress and helped to cope with their feelings while providing support to their child. The nurse can help them understand that it is not selfish to look after themselves and their own needs to meet their child's needs. It is important to recognize the parents' need to grieve the change in their child's normal appearance as part of the grieving process. Definitive professional help may be needed for parents whose response to the injury is severe or whose response to stress is manifested in destructive behavior.

The parents are members of the multidisciplinary team and participate in the development of the care plan. It is important to facilitate their input; to consider all aspects of the physical, emotional, social, and cultural factors affecting the child and family; and to establish a realistic home therapy program. The family's willingness to assume responsibility for care and their ability to implement the therapeutic regimen are assessed. Home, school, and other environmental factors are explored; financial concerns and available community resources are discussed; and a specific care plan for the child, with an anticipated follow-up program, is developed.

Prevention of Burn Injury

The best intervention is to prevent burns from occurring. Hot liquids in the kitchen and bathroom most commonly injure infants and toddlers. Hot liquids should be kept out of reach; tablecloths and dangling appliance cords are often pulled by toddlers, who spill hot grease and liquids on themselves. Electrical cords and outlets represent a potential risk to small children, who may chew on accessible cords and insert objects into outlets.

The Consumer Product Safety Commission recommends a reduction of water heater thermostats to a maximum of 48.9° C (120° F). The "dial-down" recommendation has been suggested by utility companies, burn treatment centers, medical personnel, and others interested in public safety. However, many water heaters continue to remain set at levels well above the safe level. Small children are especially at risk for scald injuries from hot tap water because of their decreased reaction time and agility, their curiosity, and the thermal sensitivity of their skin. Caregivers should never leave a child unattended in a bath and without adult supervision. Water should always be tested before a child is placed in the tub or shower.

The increased use of microwave ovens has resulted in burn injuries from the extremely hot internal temperatures generated in heated items. Baby formula, jelly-filled pastries, and hot liquids and dishes may result in cutaneous scalds or the ingestion of overheated liquids. Parents should use caution when removing items from the microwave oven and should always test the food before giving it to children.

As children mature, risk-taking behaviors increase. Matches and lighters are dangerous in the hands of children. Adults must remember to keep potentially hazardous items out of the reach of children; a lighter, like a match, is a tool for adult use.

Education related to fire safety and survival should begin with very young children. They can practice "stop, drop, and roll" to extinguish a fire. The fire escape route, including a safe meeting place away from the home in case of fire, also should be practiced. Additional information on burn care and prevention can be obtained from the American Burn Association* and the National Safety Council†.

Community activities are also helpful in supporting burn survivors and preventing burns. The Aluminum Cans for Burned Children (ACBC) is an exemplary effort based at the Paul and Carol David Foundation Burn Institute in Akron, Ohio‡. Activities funded by ACBC include a Burn Survivors Support Group, Burn Camp, and meetings of Juvenile Firestoppers (for children with fire-setting behavior). Adult weekend retreats and school and family education sessions are a part of this program. The burn center and fire department provide the personnel to present programs.

SUNBURN

Sunburn is a common skin injury caused by overexposure to ultraviolet radiation (UVR). The sun emits a continuous spectrum of visible and nonvisible light rays that range in length from very short to very long. The shorter, higher frequency waves are more damaging than longer wavelengths, but much of the light is filtered out as it travels through the atmosphere. Of the light that does filter through, ultraviolet A (UVA) waves are the longest and cause only minimum burning, but they play a significant role in photosensitive and photoallergic reactions. They are also responsible for premature aging of the skin and potentiate the effects of ultraviolet B (UVB) waves. UVB waves are shorter and are responsible for tanning, burning, and most of the harmful effects attributed to sunlight, especially skin cancer.

Numerous factors influence the amount of UVR exposure. Maximum exposure occurs at midday (10 AM–4 PM), when the distance from the sun to a given spot on the earth is shortest. There is more exposure at higher altitudes and near the equator and less when the sky is hazy (although the amount of UVR that does penetrate is easily underestimated). Window glass effectively screens out UVB but not UVA rays. Fresh snow, water, and sand reflect UVR, especially when the sun is directly overhead.

Sunburn is usually an epidermal burn, although severe sunburn can be a partial-thickness burn with blister formation. Treatment of sunburn involves stopping the burning process, decreasing the inflammatory response, and rehydrating the skin. Local application of cool tap water soaks or immersion in a tepid-water bath (temperature slightly below 36.7° C [98° F]) for 20 minutes or until the skin is cool limits tissue destruction and relieves the discomfort. After the cool applications, a bland oil-in-water moisturizing lotion can be applied.

---

*625 North Michigan Ave., Suite 2550, Chicago, IL 60611; 312-642-9260; fax: 312-642-9130; e-mail: info@ameriburn.org; http://www.ameriburn.org.
†1121 Spring Lake Drive, Itasca, IL 60143-3201; 630-285-1121, e-mail: info@nsc.org; http://www.nsc.org.
‡Akron Children's Hospital, One Perkins Square, Akron, OH 44308-1062; 330-543-1000; fax: 330-543-9998; http://www.akronchildrens.org.

Partial-thickness burns are treated the same as those from any heat source (see earlier discussion on burns).

Nursing Care Management

Protection from sunburn is the major goal of management, and the harmful effects of the sun on the delicate skin of infants and children are currently receiving increased attention. To protect skin exposed to the sun for extended periods, skin should be covered with clothing, and FDA-approved sun protection agents should be applied.

Two types of products are available for sun protection: topical sunscreens, which partially absorb UVR, and sun blockers, which block out UVR by reflecting sunlight. The most frequently recommended sun blockers are zinc oxide and titanium dioxide ointments. Sunscreens are products containing a sun protection factor (SPF) based on evaluation of effectiveness against UVR. For example, if individuals normally burn in 10 minutes without a sunscreen, use of a sunscreen with SPF 15 allows them to remain in the sun 15 times 10, or 150 minutes (2½ hours) before acquiring the same degree of burns. The most effective sunscreens against UVB are *p*-aminobenzoic acid (PABA) and PABA-esters. However, many individuals are allergic to PABA, and sunscreens without PABA are encouraged to prevent these reactions in children.

Sunscreens are applied evenly to all exposed areas, with special attention to skin folds and areas that might become exposed as clothing shifts. Avoid eye contact. Parents are directed to read labels of sunscreen products carefully for the SPF and follow the manufacturer's directions for application.

> **! NURSING ALERT**
>
> Sunscreens are not recommended for infants younger than 6 months of age. However, infants younger than 6 months of age may have sunscreen applied over small areas of skin such as the back of hands that may not be adequately covered by clothing when they are in the sun. Infants should be kept out of the sun or physically shaded from it. Fabric with a tight weave, such as cotton, offers good protection.

Individuals who work in the community, such as teachers, daycare workers, coaches, and youth group leaders, as well as relatives, should all be made aware of sun safety for children. Sunscreens must be applied *liberally and frequently*.

COLD INJURY

In cold injuries the nature of the heat-regulating mechanisms of the body are such that the inner portion of the body, or core, produces heat, and the periphery, or outer area, conserves or dissipates heat. When the body attempts to conserve heat, the outer tissues are subjected to low temperatures, and local trauma may result.

Chilblain, redness and swelling of the skin, occurs when extremities, usually the hands, are exposed intermittently to temperatures of 1.1° to 15.5° C (30° to 60° F). The response may vary but is characterized by intense vasodilation that increases the temperature of involved tissues above that of unaffected tissue and produces edematous, reddish blue patches that itch and burn. As warming takes place, the sensations become more intense, but ordinarily they subside in a few days.

Frostbite is the term used to describe tissue damage caused when excessive heat loss to local tissues allows ice crystals to form in tissues. The frostbitten part appears white or blanched, feels solid, and is without sensation. Rapid rewarming is associated with less tissue necrosis than slow thawing. It restores blood flow and shortens the period of cellular damage. Rewarming produces a flush (sometimes deep purple) and a return of sensation, which is extremely painful. Large blisters may appear in 24 to 48 hours after rewarming and begin to reabsorb within 5 to 10 days followed by the formation of a hard black eschar. Superficial injury often heals without incident. Rewarming is accomplished by immersing the part in well-agitated water at 37.8° to 42.2° C (100° to 108° F). Discomfort is managed with analgesics and sedatives. Care of blistered skin is similar to that described for burns. It is seldom possible to estimate the extent of tissue loss until new skin layers are revealed after the eschar layer separates.

■ KEY POINTS

- A variety of factors can produce lesions of the skin.
- It is important for nurses to be able to describe skin lesions accurately.
- The process of wound healing consists of hemostasis, inflammation, proliferation, and remodeling.
- A moist environment promotes wound healing.
- Bacterial, viral, and fungal infections are common in childhood.
- Some skin diseases are transmitted by arthropod vectors, especially ticks.
- The most common skin infestations of childhood—scabies and pediculosis capitis—affect children of any age and from any social class.
- Contact dermatitis may involve a primary irritant or a sensitizing agent.
- Adverse reactions to drugs are manifested more often in the skin than in any other body organ.
- The most common skin disorders of infancy are diaper dermatitis, seborrheic dermatitis, and AD.
- Acne, a disorder affecting many adolescents, is related to hormonal fluctuation, stimulation of the sebaceous glands, excessive sebum production, the formation of comedones, and the overgrowth of the *P. acnes* organism.
- Medication and gentle facial cleansing are the treatments of choice for acne.
- Burns are caused by thermal, chemical, electric, or radioactive agents.
- Burns are assessed on the extent, depth, and severity of the wound.
- Essentials of emergency care of burn injury include stopping the burning process, covering the burn, transporting the injured child to medical aid, and providing reassurance to the child and family.
- Management of minor burns consists of facilitating wound healing, relieving discomfort, and preventing complications.
- Management of major burns consists of facilitating wound healing, relieving discomfort, replacing destroyed skin, preventing or treating complications, and providing rehabilitation.
- Sunscreen is recommended for use when the skin is exposed to the damaging effects of the sun's rays.
- Thermal injuries to the skin can result from exposure to extreme cold.

REFERENCES

Alanne S, Nermes M, Soderlund R, and others: Quality of life in infants with atopic dermatitis and healthy infants: a follow-up from birth to 24 months, *Acta Pediatr* 100(8):e65–e70, 2011.

American Academy of Pediatrics, Committee on Infectious Diseases, Pickering LK, editor: *Red book: report of the Committee on Infectious Diseases*, ed 28, Elk Grove Village, Ill, 2009, Author.

Annequin D, Carbajal R, Chauvin P, and others: Fixed 50% nitrous oxide oxygen mixture for painful procedures: a French survey, *Pediatrics* 105(4):E47, 2000.

Arnoldo B, Klein M, Gibran NS: Practice guidelines for the management of electrical injuries, *J Burn Care Res* 27(4):439–447, 2006.

Baker RAU, Zeller RA, Klein RL, and others: Burn wound itch control using H$_1$ and H$_2$ antagonists, *J Burn Care Rehabil* 22(4):263–268, 2001.

Butler C: Pediatric skin care: guidelines for assessment, prevention, and treatment, *Dermatol Nurs* 19(5):471–485, 2007.

Centers for Disease Control and Prevention: Cat-scratch disease in children—Texas, September 2000–August 2001, *MMWR Morb Mortal Wkly Rep* 51(10):212–214, 2002.

Centers for Disease Control and Prevention: Nonfatal dog bite–related injuries treated in hospital emergency departments—United States, 2001, *MMWR Morb Mortal Wkly Rep* 52(26):605–610, 2003.

Centers for Disease Control and Prevention: Lyme disease, 2009, retrieved February 11, 2010, from http://www.cdc.gov/ncidod/dvbid/lyme/index.htm.

Dohil MA, Eichenfield LF: A treatment approach for atopic dermatitis, *Pediatr Ann* 34(3):201–210, 2005.

Doss N, Kamoun MR, Dubertret L, and others: Efficacy of tacrolimus 0.03% ointment as second-line treatment for children with moderate-to-severe atopic dermatitis, *Pediatr Allergy Immunol* 21:321–329, 2010.

Fanelli M, Kupperman E, Lautenbach E, and others: Antibiotics, acne and *Staphylococcus aureus* colonization, *Arch Dermatol* 147(8):917–921, 2011.

Fisher RG, Chan RL, Hair PS, and others: Hypochlorite killing of community-acquired methicillin-resistant *Staphylococcus aureus*, *Pediatr Infect Dis J* 27(10):934–935, 2008.

Goates BM, Atkin JS, Wilding KG, and others: An effective nonchemical treatment for head lice: a lot of hot air, *Pediatrics* 118(5):1962–1970, 2006.

Herndon DN, editor: *Total burn care*, ed 3, London, 2007, Saunders.

Jacob SE, Yang A, Herro E, and others: Contact allergens in a pediatric population, *J Clin Aesthet Derm* 3(101):29–35, 2010.

Kaplan SL: Community-acquired methicillin-resistant *Staphylococcus aureus* infections in children, *Semin Pediatr Infect Dis* 17(3):113–119, 2006.

Kaplan SL: Commentary: prevention of recurrent staphylococcal infections, *Pediatr Infect Dis J* 27(10):935–937, 2008.

Kaye AE, Belz JM, Kirschner RE: Pediatric dog bites injuries: a 4-year review of experience at the Children's Hospital of Philadelphia, *Plast Reconstr Surg* 124:551–558, 2009.

Kim RH, Armstrong AQ: Current state of acne treatment: highlighting lasers, photodynamic therapy, and chemical peels, *Dermatol Online J* 17(3):1–13, 2011.

Krasner DL, Rodeheaver GT, Sibbald RG: *Chronic wound care: a clinical source book for healthcare professionals*, ed 4, Wayne, Pa, 2007, HMP Communications.

Leyden JJ, Del Rosso JQ: Oral antibiotic therapy for acne vulgaris, *Clin Aesthet Derm* 4(2):40–47, 2011.

McCord SS, Levy ML: Practical guide to pediatric wound care, *Semin Plast Surg* 20(3):92–199, 2006.

Misery L: Consequences of psychological distress in adolescents with acne, *J Invest Derm* 131:290–292, 2011.

Moreno MA: Lyme disease in children and adolescents, *Arch Pediatr Adolesc Med* 165(1):96, 2011.

Mumcuoglu KY, Barker SC, Burgess IE, and others: International guidelines for effective control of head louse infestations, *J Drugs Dermatol* 6(4):409–414, 2007.

Network to Reduce Lyme Disease in School-Aged Children: You can make a difference to a child by reducing risk of Lyme disease, *NASN School Nurse* 25:110–113, 2010.

Pearlman DL: A simple treatment for head lice: dry on, suffocation based pediculicide, *Pediatrics* 114(3):e275–e279, 2004.

Purdue GF: American Burn Association presidential address 2006 on nutrition: yesterday, today, and tomorrow, *J Burn Care Res* 28(1):1–5, 2007.

Ricci G, Dondi A, Patrizi A, and others: Systemic therapy of atopic dermatitis in children, *Drugs* 69(3):297–306, 2009.

Rosenthal M: Bacterial colonization, hyperresponsive immune systems conspire in eczema: diagnosing dermatological disorders, *Infect Dis Child* 17(3):47–48, 2004.

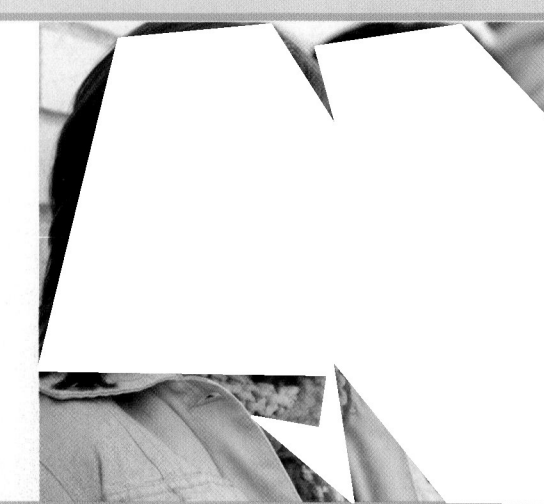

CHAPTER OUTLINE

The Immobilized Child, 1051
  Immobilization, 1051
    Physiologic Effects of
      Immobilization, 1051
    Psychologic Effects of
      Immobilization, 1051
    Effect on Families, 1054
Traumatic Injury, 1055
  Soft-Tissue Injury, 1055
    Contusions, 1055
    Dislocations, 1055
    Sprains, 1056
    Strains, 1056
  Fractures, 1057
    Types of Fractures, 1057
    Growth Plate (Physeal)
      Injuries, 1057
    Bone Healing and Remodeling, 1058
  The Child in a Cast, 1059
    The Cast, 1060

The Child in Traction, 1062
  Purposes of Traction, 1062
  Types of Traction, 1063
  Distraction, 1065
    External Fixation, 1065
  Amputation, 1066
Sports Participation and Injury, 1066
  Overuse Syndromes, 1067
    Stress Fractures, 1067
  Nurse's Role in Sports for Children and
    Adolescents, 1067
Birth and Developmental Defects, 1068
  Developmental Dysplasia of the Hip, 1068
  Clubfoot, 1071
  Metatarsus Adductus (Varus), 1072
  Skeletal Limb Deficiency, 1072
  Osteogenesis Imperfecta, 1073
Acquired Defects, 1074
  Legg-Calvé-Perthes Disease, 1074
  Slipped Capital Femoral Epiphysis, 1075

  Kyphosis and Lordosis, 1076
  Idiopathic Scoliosis, 1076
Infections of Bones and Joints, 1079
  Osteomyelitis, 1079
  Septic Arthritis, 1080
  Skeletal Tuberculosis, 1081
Bone and Soft-Tissue Tumors, 1081
  General Concepts: Bone Tumors, 1081
  Osteosarcoma, 1081
  Ewing Sarcoma (Primitive
    Neuroectodermal Tumor), 1082
  Rhabdomyosarcoma, 1083
Disorders of Joints, 1084
  Juvenile Idiopathic Arthritis (Juvenile
    Rheumatoid Arthritis), 1084
    Classification of Juvenile Idiopathic
      Arthritis, 1084
  Systemic Lupus Erythematosus, 1086

LEARNING OBJECTIVES

On completion of this chapter the reader will be able to:

- Outline a plan of care for a child immobilized with an injury or a degenerative disease.
- Develop a teaching plan for the parents of a child in a cast.
- Explain the functions of the various types of traction.
- Devise a nursing care plan for a child in traction.
- Differentiate among the various congenital skeletal defects.
- Design a teaching plan for the parents of a child with a congenital skeletal deformity.

- Describe the therapies and nursing care of a child with idiopathic scoliosis.
- Outline a care plan for a child with osteomyelitis.
- Differentiate between osteosarcoma and Ewing sarcoma.
- Describe the nursing care of a child with juvenile idiopathic arthritis.
- Demonstrate an understanding of the management of a child with systemic lupus erythematosus.

THE IMMOBILIZED CHILD

IMMOBILIZATION

One of the most difficult aspects of illness in children is the immobility it often imposes on a child. Children's natural tendency to be active influences all aspects of their growth and development. Impaired mobility presents a challenge to children, their families, and their caregivers.

Physiologic Effects of Immobilization

Many clinical studies, including space program research, have documented predictable consequences that occur after immobilization and the absence of gravitational force. Functional and metabolic responses to restricted movement can be noted in most of the body systems. Each has a direct influence on the child's growth and development because of homeostatic mechanisms that thrive on normal use and feedback to maintain dynamic equilibrium. Inactivity leads to a decrease in the functional capabilities of the whole body as dramatically as the lack of physical exercise leads to muscle weakness.

Disuse from illness, injury, or a sedentary lifestyle can limit function and potentially delay age-appropriate milestones. Most of the pathologic changes that occur during immobilization arise from decreased muscle strength and mass, decreased metabolism, and bone demineralization, which are closely interrelated, with one change leading to or affecting the others.

The major effects of immobilization are outlined briefly in Table 31-1 and are related directly or indirectly to decreased muscle activity, which produces numerous primary changes in the musculoskeletal system with secondary alterations in the cardiovascular, respiratory, skeletal, metabolic, and renal systems. The musculoskeletal changes that occur during disuse are a result of alterations in the effect of gravity and stress on the muscles, joints, and bones. Muscle disuse leads to tissue breakdown and loss of muscle mass (**atrophy**). Muscle atrophy causes decreased strength and endurance, which may take weeks or months to restore.

During immobilization, a **joint contracture** begins when the arrangement of collagen, the main structural protein of connective tissues, is altered, resulting in a denser tissue that does not glide as easily. Eventually, muscles, tendons, and ligaments can shorten and reduce joint movement, ultimately producing contractures that restrict function. The daily stresses on bone created by motion and weight bearing maintain the balance between bone formation (osteoblastic activity) and bone resorption (osteoclastic activity). During immobilization, increased calcium leaves the bone, causing osteopenia (demineralization of the bones), which may predispose bone to pathologic fractures.

The major musculoskeletal consequences of immobilization are:
- Significant decrease in muscle size, strength, and endurance
- Bone demineralization leading to osteoporosis
- Contractures and decreased joint mobility

Circulatory stasis combined with hypercoagulability of the blood, which results from factors such as damage to the endothelium of blood vessels (Virchow triad), can lead to thrombus and embolus formation. **Deep venous thrombosis (DVT)** involves the formation of a thrombus in a deep vein such as the iliac and femoral veins and can cause significant morbidity if it remains undetected and untreated. The larger the portion of the body immobilized and the longer the immobilization, the greater the risks of immobility.

Psychologic Effects of Immobilization

For children, one of the most difficult aspects of illness is immobilization. Throughout childhood, physical activity is an integral part of daily life and is essential for physical growth and development. It also serves children as an instrument for communication and expression and as a means for learning about and understanding their world. Activity helps them deal with a variety of feelings and impulses and provides a mechanism by which they can exert control over inner tensions. Children respond to anxiety with increased activity. Removal of this power deprives them of necessary input and a natural outlet for their feelings and fantasies. Through movement, children also gain sensory input, which provides an essential element for developing and maintaining body image.

When children are immobilized by disease or as part of a treatment regimen, they experience diminished environmental stimuli with a loss of tactile input and an altered perception of themselves and their environment. Sudden or gradual immobilization narrows the amount and variety of environmental stimuli children receive by means of all their senses: touch, sight, hearing, taste, smell, and proprioception (a feeling of where they are in their environment). This sensory

TABLE 31-1	SUMMARY OF PHYSICAL EFFECTS OF IMMOBILIZATION WITH NURSING INTERVENTIONS*	
PRIMARY EFFECTS	**SECONDARY EFFECTS**	**NURSING CONSIDERATIONS**
Muscular System		
Decreased muscle strength, tone, and endurance	Decreased venous return and decreased cardiac output	Use antiembolism stockings or intermittent compression devices to promote venous return (monitor circulatory and neurovascular status of extremities when such devices are used).
	Decreased metabolism and need for oxygen	
	Decreased exercise tolerance	Plan play activities to use uninvolved extremities.
	Bone demineralization	Place in upright posture when possible.
Disuse atrophy and loss of muscle mass	Catabolism	Have patient perform range-of-motion, active, passive, and stretching exercises.
	Loss of strength	
Loss of joint mobility	Contractures, ankylosis of joints	Maintain correct body alignment.
		Use joint splints as indicated to prevent further deformity.
		Maintain range of motion.
Weak back muscles	Secondary spinal deformities	Maintain body alignment.
Weak abdominal muscles	Impaired respiration	See nursing considerations for respiratory system.

Continued

TABLE 31-1	SUMMARY OF PHYSICAL EFFECTS OF IMMOBILIZATION WITH NURSING INTERVENTIONS—cont'd	
PRIMARY EFFECTS	**SECONDARY EFFECTS**	**NURSING CONSIDERATIONS**
Skeletal System		
Bone demineralization— osteoporosis, hypercalcemia	Negative bone calcium uptake	With paralysis, use upright posture on tilt table.
	Pathologic fractures	Handle extremities carefully when turning and positioning.
	Calcium deposits	Administer calcium-mobilizing drugs (diphosphonates) and normal saline infusions if ordered.
	Extraosseous bone formation, especially at hip, knee, elbow, and shoulder	Ensure adequate intake of fluid; monitor output.
	Renal calculi	Acidify urine.
		Promptly treat urinary tract infections.
Negative bone calcium uptake	Life-threatening electrolyte imbalance	Monitor serum calcium levels.
		Provide electrolyte replacement as indicated.
Metabolism		
Decreased metabolic rate	Slowing of all systems	Mobilize as soon as possible.
	Decreased food intake	Have patient perform active and passive resistance exercises and deep-breathing exercises.
		Ensure adequate food intake.
		Provide a high-protein, high fiber diet.
Negative nitrogen balance	Decline in nutritional state	Encourage small, frequent feedings with protein and preferred foods.
	Impaired healing	Prevent pressure areas.
Hypercalcemia	Electrolyte imbalance	See nursing consideration for skeletal system.
Decreased production of stress hormones	Decreased physical and emotional coping capacity	Identify causes of stress.
		Implement appropriate interventions to lower physical and psychosocial stresses.
Cardiovascular System		
Decreased efficiency of orthostatic neurovascular reflexes	Inability to adapt readily to upright position (orthostatic intolerance)	Monitor peripheral pulses and skin temperature changes.
	Pooling of blood in extremities in upright posture	Use antiembolism stockings or intermittent compression devices to decrease pooling when upright.
Diminished vasopressor mechanism	Orthostatic intolerance with syncope, hypertension, deceased cerebral blood flow, tachycardia	Provide abdominal support.
		In severe cases, use antigravitational pants.
		Position horizontally.
Altered distribution of blood volume	Increased cardiac workload	Monitor hydration, blood pressure, and urinary output.
	Decreased exercise tolerance	
Venous stasis	Pulmonary emboli or thrombi	Encourage and assist with frequent position changes.
		Elevate extremities without knee flexion.
		Ensure adequate fluid intake.
		Have patient perform active or passive exercises or movement as needed.
		Prescribe routine wearing of antiembolism stockings or intermittent compression devices.
		Monitor for signs of pulmonary embolism—sudden dyspnea, chest pain, respiratory arrest.
		Promptly intervene to maintain adequate oxygenation if signs and symptoms of pulmonary emboli are noted.
		Measure circumference of extremities periodically.
		Give anticoagulant drugs as prescribed.
Dependent edema	Tissue breakdown and susceptibility to infection	Administer skin care.
		Turn every 2–4 hr.
		Monitor skin color, temperature, and integrity.
		Use pressure-reduction surface as necessary to prevent skin breakdown. (See Chapter 22.)

TABLE 31-1	SUMMARY OF PHYSICAL EFFECTS OF IMMOBILIZATION WITH NURSING INTERVENTIONS—cont'd		
PRIMARY EFFECTS	**SECONDARY EFFECTS**	**NURSING CONSIDERATIONS**
Respiratory System		
Decreased need for oxygen	Altered oxygen–carbon dioxide exchange and metabolism	Promote exercise as tolerated.
Decreased chest expansion and diminished vital capacity	Diminished oxygen intake	Encourage deep-breathing exercises.
	Dyspnea and inadequate arterial oxygen saturation; acidosis	Position for optimum chest expansion. Semi-Fowler position may assist in lung expansion if patient can tolerate.
		Use prone positioning without pressure on abdomen to allow gravity to aid in diaphragmatic excursion.
		Ensure that patient maintains proper alignment when sitting to prevent pressure on respiratory mechanism.
Poor abdominal tone and distention	Interference with diaphragmatic excursion	Avoid restriction of chest and abdominal musculature.
		Supply torso support to promote chest expansion.
Mechanical or biochemical secretion retention	Hypostatic pneumonia	Change position frequently.
	Bacterial and viral pneumonia	Carry out chest percussion, vibration, and drainage (or suctioning) as necessary.
	Atelectasis	Use incentive spirometer
		Monitor breath sounds.
Loss of respiratory muscle strength	Poor cough	Encourage coughing and deep breathing.
		Support chest wall by splinting with pillow when patient coughs.
		Use incentive spirometer.
		Observe for signs of respiratory distress with pulse oximetry or blood gas measurement as necessary.
	Upper respiratory tract infection	Prevent contact with infected persons.
		Provide adequate hydration.
		Administer immunizations as necessary (pneumococcal, meningococcal).
Gastrointestinal System		
Distention caused by poor abdominal muscle tone	Interference with respiratory movements	Monitor bowel sounds.
	Difficulty in feeding in prone position	Encourage small, frequent feedings.
		Have patient sit in upright position in bedside chair if possible.
No specific primary effect	Possible constipation caused by gravitational effect on feces through ascending colon or weakened smooth muscle tone	Carry out bowel training program with hydration, stool softeners, increased fiber intake, and mild laxatives if necessary.
	Anorexia	Stimulate appetite with favored foods.
Urinary System		
Alteration of gravitational force	Difficulty in voiding in prone position	Position as upright as possible to void.
Impaired ureteral peristalsis	Urinary retention in calyces and bladder	Hydrate to ensure adequate urinary output for age.
	Infection	Stimulate bladder emptying with warm running water, as necessary.
	Renal calculi	Catheterize only for severe urinary retention.
		Administer antibiotics as indicated.
Integumentary System		
Altered tissue integrity	Decreased circulation and pressure leading to tissue injury	Turn and reposition at least every 2–4 hr.
		Frequently inspect total skin surface.
		Eliminate mechanical factors causing pressure, friction, moisture, or irritation.
		Place on pressure-reduction mattress.
	Difficulty with personal hygiene	Assess ability to perform self-care and assist with bathing, grooming, and toileting as needed.
		Encourage self-care to potential ability.
		Ensure adequate intake of protein, vitamins, and minerals.

*Individualize care according to child's needs; interventions may vary in different institutions.

deprivation frequently leads to feelings of isolation and boredom and of being forgotten, especially by peers.

Physical interference with the activity of infants and young children gives them a feeling of helplessness. Even speech and language skills require sensorimotor activity and experience. For toddlers, exploration and imitative behaviors are essential to developing a sense of autonomy. Preschoolers' expression of initiative is evidenced by the need for vigorous physical activity. School-age children's development is strongly influenced by physical achievement and competition. Adolescents rely on mobility to achieve independence. The quest for mastery at every stage of development is related to mobility.

The monotony of immobilization may lead to sluggish intellectual and psychomotor responses; decreased communication skills; increased fantasizing; and rarely, hallucinations and disorientation. Children are likely to become depressed over loss of ability to function or the marked changes in body image. They may regress to earlier developmental behaviors, such as wanting to be fed, bedwetting, and baby talk.

Children may react to immobility by active protest, anger, and aggressive behavior, or they may become quiet, passive, and submissive. They may believe the immobilization is a justified punishment for misbehavior. Children should be allowed to display their anger, but it should be within the limits of safety to their self-esteem and not damaging to the integrity of others (see Providing Opportunities for Play and Expressive Activities, Chapter 21). When children are unable to express anger, aggression is often displayed inappropriately through regressive behavior and outbursts of crying or temper tantrums.

Effect on Families

Even brief periods of immobilization may disrupt family function, and catastrophic illness or disability may severely tax a family's resources and coping abilities. The family's needs often must be met by the services of a multidisciplinary team, and nurses play a key role in anticipating the services they will need and in coordinating conferences to plan care. In preparation for discharge, home management is frequently planned before discharge, including special considerations for addressing cultural, economic, physical, and psychological needs. A child with a severe disability is very dependent, and caregivers need respite to revitalize themselves. Individual and group counseling is beneficial for solving problems in advance and provides an emotional support system. Parent groups are also helpful and often allow nonthreatening social contact. The families of children with permanent disabilities need long-term resources because some of the most difficult problems arise as they try to sustain high-quality care for many years (see Chapter 20).

Nursing Care Management

Physical assessment of the child who is immobilized for any number of reasons (e.g., injury or illness) includes a focus not only on the injured part (e.g., fracture) but also on the functioning of other systems that may be affected secondarily—the circulatory, renal, respiratory, muscular, and gastrointestinal systems. With long-term immobilization, there may also be neurologic impairment and changes in electrolytes (especially calcium), nitrogen balance, and the general metabolic rate. The psychological impact of immobilization should also be assessed.

Children who require prolonged total immobility and are unable to move themselves in bed should be placed on a pressure-reduction mattress to prevent skin breakdown. Frequent position changes also help prevent dependent edema and stimulate circulation, respiratory

function, gastrointestinal motility, and neurologic sensation. Children at greater risk for skin breakdown include those with prolonged immobilization; mechanical ventilation; orthotic and prosthetic devices, including wheelchairs; and casts. Additional risk factors include poor nutrition, friction (from bed linen with traction), and moist skin (from urine or perspiration). Nursing care of children at risk includes strategies for preventing skin breakdown when such conditions are present. The Braden Q Scale is a reliable, objective tool that may be used in the assessment for pressure ulcer development in children who are acutely ill or who are at risk for skin breakdown from neurologic conditions and immobilization (Noonan, Quigley, and Curley, 2011).

The use of antiembolism stockings or intermittent compression devices prevents circulatory stasis and dependent edema in the lower extremities and the development of DVT. Anticoagulant therapy may also be implemented with low-molecular-weight heparin, vitamin K antagonists, or unfractionated heparin. The child should be allowed as much activity as possible within the limitations of the illness or treatment. Any functional mobility, however minimal, is preferred to total immobility. High-protein, high-calorie foods are encouraged to prevent negative nitrogen balance, which may be difficult to correct by diet, especially if there is anorexia as a result of immobility and decreased gastrointestinal function (decreased motility and possibly constipation). Stimulating the appetite with small servings of attractively arranged, preferred foods may be sufficient. Sometimes supplementary nasogastric or gastrostomy feedings or intravenous (IV) fluids may be needed, but these are reserved for serious disability in which oral intake is impossible.

Adequate hydration and, when possible, an upright position and remobilization promote bowel and kidney function and help prevent complications in these systems. Children are encouraged to be as active as their condition and restrictive devices allow. This poses few problems for children, whose innate ingenuity and natural inclination toward mobility provide them with the impetus for physical activity. They need the opportunity, the materials or objects to stimulate activity, and the encouragement and participation of others. Those who are unable to move benefit from passive exercise and movement in consultation with a physical therapist.

Whenever possible, transporting the child outside the confines of the room increases environmental stimuli and allows social contact with others. Specially designed wheelchairs for increased mobility and independence are available. While hospitalized, children benefit from same-age visitors, computers, books, interactive video games, and other items brought from their own room at home, all of which help them to function in a more normal way. While hospitalized, they also benefit from frequent visitors, accessibility of clocks and calendars, and a program of diversional therapy to help them function more normally. A child life specialist should be consulted for recreational planning. An activity center or slanting tray can be helpful for the child with limited mobility to use for drawing, coloring, writing, and playing with small toys such as trucks and cars. Children are able to express frustration, displeasure, and anger through play activities (see Chapter 21), which is helpful in the child's recovery. Hospitalized children should be allowed to wear their own clothes (street clothes, especially for preadolescent and adolescent girls) and resume school and preinjury activities. A parent or siblings should be allowed to stay overnight and room in with the hospitalized child to prevent the effects of family disruption from hospitalization. All efforts should be made to minimize family disruption resulting from the hospitalization. Although most of the suggestions discussed relate to hospital care, the same consultations (physical therapist, occupational therapist, child life specialist, speech therapist) and environment may be considered in the home as well to help the child and family achieve independence and normalization (see Chapter 20).

Using dolls, stuffed animals, or puppets to illustrate and explain the immobilization method (e.g., traction, cast) is a valuable tool for small children. Placing a cast, tubing, or other restraining equipment on the doll offers the child a nonthreatening opportunity to express, through the doll, feelings concerning the restrictions and feelings toward the nurse and other health care providers. The doll or puppet may also be used for teaching the child and family procedures such as IV therapy, procedural sedation, and general anesthesia.

One of the most useful interventions to help children cope with immobility is participation in their own care. Self-care to the maximum extent is usually well received by children. They can help plan their daily routine; select their diet; and choose "street clothes," including innovative adornment, such as a baseball cap or brightly colored stockings to express their autonomy and individuality. They are encouraged to do as much for themselves as they are able to keep their muscles active and their interest alive.

Visits from significant persons, such as family members and friends, offer occasions for emotional support and also provide opportunities for learning how to care for the child. Privacy is necessary, especially for adolescents.

For a child with greatly restricted movement (e.g., child with a large bilateral hip spica cast), nursing care is often a challenge. These situations require long-term care either in the hospital or at home, but wherever the care occurs, consistent planning and coordination of activities with other health care workers and significant others are vital nursing functions.

With the increased trend toward early mobilization, early discharge, and home health care, many children are discharged home within a few days of hospitalization. Follow-up treatment may take place in the home setting or an outpatient ambulatory facility.

Family Support and Home Care

The needs of a child with severe disabilities can be complex, and family members require time to assimilate the teachings and demonstrations needed to understand the child's situation and care. Even a child who is confined on a short-term basis can be a challenge for the family, which is usually unprepared for the problems imposed by the child's special needs. Home modification is usually needed for facilitating care, especially when it involves traction, a large cast, or extended confinement. Suitable child care may be needed for times when all family members work.

Just as in the hospital, the child at home is encouraged to be as independent as possible and to follow a schedule that approximates his or her normal lifestyle as nearly as possible, such as continuing school lessons, regular bedtime, and suitable recreational activities.

TRAUMATIC INJURY

SOFT-TISSUE INJURY

Injuries to the muscles, ligaments, and tendons are common in children (Fig. 31-1). In young children, soft-tissue injury usually results from mishaps during play. In older children and adolescents, participation in sports is a common cause of such injuries.

Contusions

A contusion (bruise) is damage to the soft tissue, subcutaneous structures, and muscle. The tearing of these tissues and small blood vessels

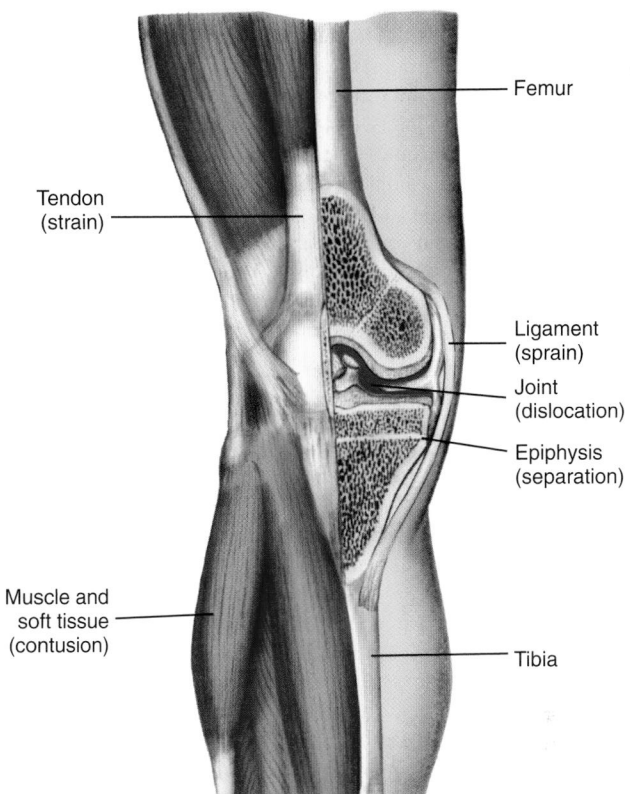

FIG 31-1 Sites of injuries to bones, joints, and soft tissues.

and the inflammatory response lead to hemorrhage, edema, and associated pain when the child attempts to move the injured part. The escape of blood into the tissues is observed as **ecchymosis**, a black-and-blue discoloration.

Large contusions cause gross swelling, pain, and disability and usually receive immediate attention from health personnel. Smaller injuries may go unnoticed, allowing continued participation. However, they can become disabling after rest because of pain and muscle spasm. Immediate treatment consists of cold application, as in the treatment of sprains described below. Return to participation is allowed when the strength and range of motion of the affected extremity are equal to those of the opposite extremity or are demonstrated under conditions such as sport-specific tests. **Myositis ossificans** may occur from deep contusions to the biceps or quadriceps muscles; this condition may result in a restriction of flexibility of the affected limb.

Crush injuries occur when children's extremities or digits are crushed (e.g., fingers slammed in doors, folding chairs, or equipment) or hit (as when hammering a nail). A severe crush injury involves the bone, with swelling and bleeding beneath the nail (subungual) and sometimes laceration of the pulp of the nail. The **subungual hematoma** can be released by creating a hole at the proximal end of the nail with a special cautery device or a heated sterile 18-gauge needle.

Dislocations

Long bones are held in approximation to one another at the joint by ligaments. A dislocation occurs when the force of stress on the ligament is so great as to displace the normal position of the opposing bone ends or the bone end to its socket. The predominant symptom is pain that increases with attempted passive or active movement of the extremity. In dislocations, there may be an obvious deformity and inability to move the joint. Children with naturally lax joints are more prone to dislocation of joints. Dislocation of the phalanges is the most common type seen in children, followed by elbow dislocation. In the adolescent population, shoulder dislocations are more common and dislocation unaccompanied by fracture is rare.

A common injury in young children is subluxation, or partial dislocation, of the radial head, also called *pulled elbow* or **nursemaid's elbow**. In the majority of cases, the injury occurs in a child younger than 5 years of age who receives a sudden longitudinal pull or traction at the wrist while the arm is fully extended and the forearm pronated. It usually occurs when an individual who is holding the child by the hand or wrist gives a sudden pull or jerk to prevent a fall or attempts to lift the child by pulling the wrist or when the child pulls away by dropping to the floor or ground. The child often cries, appears anxious, complains of pain in the elbow or wrist, and refuses to use the affected limb. The practitioner manipulates the arm by applying firm finger pressure to the head of the radius and then supinates and flexes the forearm to return the bone structure to normal alignment. A click may be heard or felt, and functional use of the arm returns within minutes. Immobilization is not required. However, the longer the subluxation is present, the longer it takes for the child to recover mobility after treatment. No anesthetic is usually required, but a mild pain reliever such as acetaminophen or ibuprofen may be administered. In an older child, severe elbow injury or dislocation should be immediately evaluated by a practitioner. If a traumatic elbow injury in a younger child is not a subluxation or if attempts at reduction are unsuccessful, the child should be carefully evaluated, with the consideration of radiographs.

In children younger than 5 years of age, the hip can be dislocated by a fall. The greatest risk after this injury is the potential loss of blood supply to the head of the femur. Relocation of the hip within 60 minutes after the injury provides the best chance for prevention of damage to the femoral head.

Shoulder dislocations and separations occur most often in older adolescents and are often sports related. Temporary restriction of the joint, with a sling or bandage that secures the arm to the chest in a shoulder dislocation, can provide sufficient comfort and immobilization until medical attention is received.

Simple dislocations should be reduced as soon as possible with the child under procedural sedation combined with local anesthesia. An unreduced dislocation may be complicated by increased swelling, making reduction difficult and increasing the risk of neurovascular problems. Treatment is determined by the severity of the injury.

Sprains

A sprain occurs when trauma to a joint is so severe that a ligament is partially or completely torn or stretched by the force created as a joint is twisted or wrenched, often accompanied by damage to associated blood vessels, muscles, tendons, and nerves. Common sprain sites include ankles and knees.

The presence of joint laxity is the most valid indicator of the severity of a sprain. In a severe injury, the child complains of the joint "feeling loose" or as if "something is coming apart" and may describe hearing a "snap," "pop," or "tearing." Pain may or may not be the principal subjective symptom, and in some children, it may prevent optimal examination of ligamentous instability. There is a rapid onset of swelling, often diffuse, accompanied by immediate disability and appreciable reluctance to use the injured joint.

Strains

A strain is a microscopic tear to the musculotendinous unit and has features in common with sprains. The area is painful to touch and swollen. Most strains are incurred over time rather than suddenly, and the rapidity of the appearance provides clues regarding severity. In general, the more rapidly the strain occurs, the more severe the injury. When the strain involves the muscular portion, there is more bleeding, often palpable soon after injury and before edema obscures the hematoma.

Therapeutic Management

The first 12 to 24 hours are the most critical period for virtually all soft-tissue injuries. Basic principles of managing sprains and other soft-tissue injuries are summarized in the acronyms RICE and ICES.

Rest	**I**ce
Ice	**C**ompression
Compression	**E**levation
Elevation	**S**upport

Soft-tissue injuries should be iced immediately. This is best accomplished with crushed ice wrapped in a towel, a screw-top ice bag, or a resealable plastic storage bag. Chemical-activated ice packs are also effective for immediate treatment but are not reusable and must be closely monitored for leakage. A wet elastic wrap, which transfers cold better than dry wrap, is applied to provide compression and to keep the ice pack in place. A cloth barrier should be used between the ice container and the skin to prevent trauma to the tissues. Ice has a rapid cooling effect on tissues that reduces edema and pain. Ice should never be applied for more than 30 minutes at a time.

> **NURSING TIP** A plastic bag of frozen vegetables, such as peas, serves as a convenient ice pack for soft-tissue injuries. It is clean, watertight, and easily molded to the injured part. When available, snow placed in a plastic bag may serve as an ice bag.

Elevating the extremity uses gravity to facilitate venous return and reduce edema formation in the damaged area. The point of injury should be kept several inches above the level of the heart for therapy to be effective. Several pillows can be used for elevation. Allowing the extremity to be dependent causes excessive fluid accumulation in the area of injury, delaying healing and causing painful swelling.

Torn ligaments, especially those in the knee, are usually treated by immobilization with a knee immobilizer or a knee brace that allows flexion and extension until the child is able to walk without a limp. Crutches are used for mobility to rest the affected extremity. Passive leg exercises, gradually increased to active ones, are begun as soon as sufficient healing has taken place. Parents and children are cautioned against using any form of liniment or other heat-producing preparation before examination. If the injury requires casting or splinting, the heat generated in the enclosed space can cause extreme discomfort and even tissue damage. In some cases, torn knee ligaments are managed with arthroscopy and ligament repair or reconstruction as necessary depending on the extent of the tear, ligaments involved, and child's age. Surgical reconstruction of the anterior cruciate ligament may be performed in young athletes who wish to continue in active sports (Sarwark, 2010).

FRACTURES

⊖ Bone fractures occur when the resistance of bone against the stress being exerted yields to the stress force. Fractures are a common injury at any age but are more likely to occur in children and older adults. Because childhood is a time of rapid bone growth, the pattern of fractures, problems of diagnosis, and methods of treatment differ in children compared with adults. In children, fractures heal much faster than in adults. Consequently, children may not require as long a period of immobilization of the affected extremity as an adult with a fracture.

Fracture injuries in children are most often a result of traumatic incidents at home, at school, in a motor vehicle, or in association with recreational activities. Children's everyday activities include vigorous play that predisposes them to injury, including climbing, falling down, running into immovable objects, skateboarding, trampolines, skiing, playground activities, and receiving blows to any part of their bodies by a solid, immovable object.

Aside from automobile accidents or falls from heights, true injuries that cause fractures rarely occur in infancy. Bone injury in children of this age group warrants further investigation. In any small child, radiographic evidence of fractures at various stages of healing is, with few exceptions, a result of nonaccidental trauma (child abuse). Any investigation of fractures in infants, particularly multiple fractures, should include consideration of osteogenesis imperfecta (OI) after nonaccidental trauma has been ruled out.

Fractures in school-age children are often a result of playground falls or bicycle–automobile or skateboard injuries. Adolescents are vulnerable to multiple and severe trauma because they are mobile on bicycles, all-terrain vehicles, skateboards, skis, snowboards, trampolines, and motorcycles and are active in sports.

A distal forearm (radius, ulna, or both) fracture is the most common fracture in children. The clavicle is also a common fracture sustained in childhood, with approximately half of clavicle fractures occurring in children younger than 10 years of age. Common mechanisms of injury include a fall with an outstretched hand or direct trauma to the bone. In neonates, a fractured clavicle may occur with a large newborn and a small maternal pelvis. This may be noted in the first few days after birth by a unilateral Moro reflex or at the 2-week well-child check, when a fracture callus is palpated on the infant's healing clavicle.

Types of Fractures

A fractured bone consists of fragments—the fragment closer to the midline, or the proximal fragment, and the fragment farther from the midline, or the distal fragment. When fracture fragments are separated, the fracture is complete; when fragments remain attached, the fracture is incomplete. The fracture line can be any of the following:

Transverse—Crosswise at right angles to the long axis of the bone
Oblique—Slanting but straight between a horizontal and a perpendicular direction
Spiral—Slanting and circular, twisting around the bone shaft

The twisting of an extremity while the bone is breaking results in a spiral break. If the fracture does not produce a break in the skin, it is a simple, or closed, fracture. Open, or compound, fractures are those with an open wound through which the bone protrudes. If the bone fragments cause damage to other organs or tissues (e.g., lung, liver), the injury is said to be a complicated fracture. When small fragments of bone are broken from the fractured shaft and lie in the surrounding tissue, the injury is a comminuted fracture. This type of fracture is rare in children. The types of fractures that are seen most often in children are described in Box 31-1 and in Figure 31-2.

BOX 31-1   TYPES OF FRACTURES IN CHILDREN

Plastic deformation—Occurs when the bone is bent but not broken. A child's flexible bone can be bent 45 degrees or more before breaking. However, if bent, the bone will straighten slowly but not completely, producing some deformity but without the angulation seen when the bone breaks. Bends occur most commonly in the ulna and fibula, often in association with fractures of the radius and tibia.

Buckle, or **torus**, **fracture**—Produced by compression of the porous bone; appears as a raised or bulging projection at the fracture site. These fractures occur in the most porous portion of the bone near the metaphysis (the portion of the bone shaft adjacent to the epiphysis) and are more common in young children.

Greenstick fracture—Occurs when a bone is angulated beyond the limits of bending. The compressed side bends, and the tension side fails, causing an incomplete fracture similar to the break observed when a green stick is broken.

Complete fracture—Divides the bone fragments. These fragments often remain attached by a **periosteal hinge,** which can aid or hinder reduction.

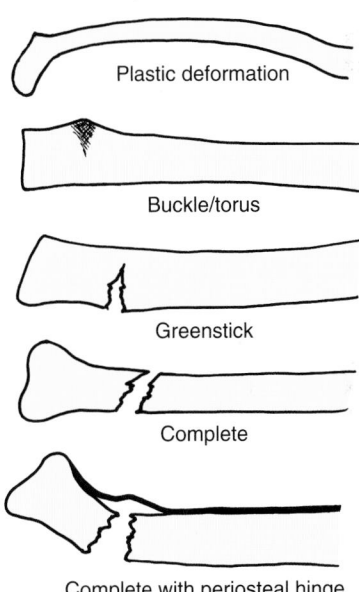

Plastic deformation

Buckle/torus

Greenstick

Complete

Complete with periosteal hinge

FIG 31-2 Types of fractures in children.

Growth Plate (Physeal) Injuries

The weakest point of long bones is the cartilage growth plate, or the physis. Consequently, this is a frequent site of damage of childhood trauma. Growth plate fractures are classified with the Salter-Harris classification system (Fig. 31-3). Detection of physeal injuries is sometimes difficult but critical. Close monitoring and early treatment, if indicated, is essential to prevent longitudinal or angular growth deformities (or both). Treatment of these fractures may include surgical open reduction and internal fixation to prevent or reduce growth disturbances.

Immediately after a fracture occurs, the muscles contract and physiologically splint the injured area. This phenomenon accounts for the muscle tightness observed over a fracture site and the deformity that is produced as the muscles pull the bone ends out of alignment. This

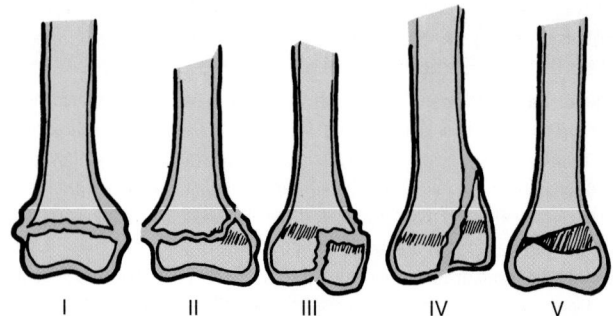

FIG 31-3 Salter-Harris fracture classification. Types of epiphyseal injury in order of increasing risk. The injuries are classified as follows: type I, separation or slip of growth plate without fracture of the bone; type II, separation of growth plate and breaking off of section of metaphysis; type III, fracture of epiphysis extending through joint surface; type IV, fracture of growth plate, epiphysis, and metaphysis; and type V, crushing injury of epiphysis (can be diagnosed only in retrospect). This classification of epiphyseal injuries was developed by orthopedists RB Salter and WR Harris. (First published in Salter RB, Harris WR: Injuries involving the physeal plate, *J Bone Joint Surg Am* 45[3]:587–622, 1963.)

muscle response must be overcome by traction or complete muscle relaxation (e.g., anesthesia) to realign the distal bone fragment to the proximal bone fragment.

Bone Healing and Remodeling

Bone healing is rapid in growing children because of the thickened periosteum and generous blood supply. When there is a break in the continuity of bone, the osteoblasts are stimulated to maximal activity. New bone cells are formed in immense numbers almost immediately after the injury and, in time, are evidenced by a bulging growth of new bone tissue between the fractured bone fragments. This is followed by deposition of calcium salts to form a callus. Remodeling is a process that occurs in the healing of long bone fractures in growing children. The irregularities produced by the fracture become indistinct as the angles and bone overgrowth are smoothed out, giving the bone a straighter appearance. A general rule of thumb is that an angulated fracture in a growing child will remodel by one degree per month (Green and Swiontkowski, 2008).

Fractures heal in less time in children than in adults. The approximate healing times for a femoral shaft are as follows:

Neonatal period—2 to 3 weeks
Early childhood—4 weeks
Later childhood—6 to 8 weeks
Adolescence—8 to 12 weeks

Diagnostic Evaluation

A history of the injury may be lacking in childhood injuries. Infants and toddlers are unable to communicate, and older children may not volunteer information (even under direct questioning) when the injury occurred during questionable activities. Whenever possible, it is helpful to obtain information from someone who witnessed the injury. In cases of nonaccidental trauma, providers may give false information to protect themselves or family members.

The child may exhibit the same manifestations seen in adults (Box 31-2). However, often a fracture is remarkably stable because of intact periosteum. The child may even be able to use an affected arm or walk on a fractured leg. Because bones are highly vascular, a soft, pliable hematoma may be felt around the fracture site.

Signs of injury:
- Generalized swelling
- Pain or tenderness
- Deformity
- Diminished functional use of affected limb or digit

May also demonstrate:
- Bruising
- Severe muscular rigidity
- Crepitus (grating sensation at fracture site)

> **! NURSING ALERT**
>
> A fracture should be strongly suspected in a small child who refuses to walk or crawl.

Radiographic examination is the most useful diagnostic tool for assessing skeletal trauma. The calcium deposits in bone make the entire structure radiopaque. Radiographic films are taken after fracture reduction and, in some cases, may be taken during the healing process to determine satisfactory progress.

Therapeutic Management

The goals of fracture management are:
- To regain alignment and length of the bony fragments (reduction)
- To retain alignment and length (immobilization)
- To restore function to the injured parts
- To prevent further injury and deformity

The majority of children's fractures heal well, and nonunion is rare. Fractures are splinted or casted to immobilize and protect the injured extremity. Children with displaced fractures may have immediate surgical reduction and fixation (internal or external) rather than being immobilized by traction (Fig. 31-4). This practice is more common and holds true for all types of fractures, including femur fractures, although there is variation based on provider preference and institutional practice. Some conditions require immediate medical attention, including open fractures, compartment syndrome, fractures associated with vascular or nerve injury, and joint dislocations that are unresponsive to reduction maneuvers.

In children, immobilization is used until adequate callus is formed. The position of the bone fragments in relation to one another influences the rapidity of healing and residual deformity. Weight bearing and active movement for the purpose of regaining function may begin after the fracture site is determined to be stable by the medical provider. The child's natural tendency to be active is usually sufficient to restore normal mobility, and physical or occupational therapy is rarely indicated.

Children are most frequently hospitalized for fractures of the femur and supracondylar area of the distal humerus. If simple reduction cannot be achieved or a neurovascular problem is detected after the injury, observation in a hospital setting may be indicated. The trend is to avoid hospitalization. The major methods for immobilizing a fracture, casting and traction, are described later.

Nursing Care Management

Nurses are frequently the persons who make the initial assessment of a child with a suspected fracture (see Emergency Treatment box).

The child and parents may be frightened and upset, and the child is often in pain. Therefore, if the child is alert and there is no evidence of hemorrhage, the initial nursing interventions are directed toward calming and reassuring the child and parents so that a more extensive assessment can be more easily accomplished.

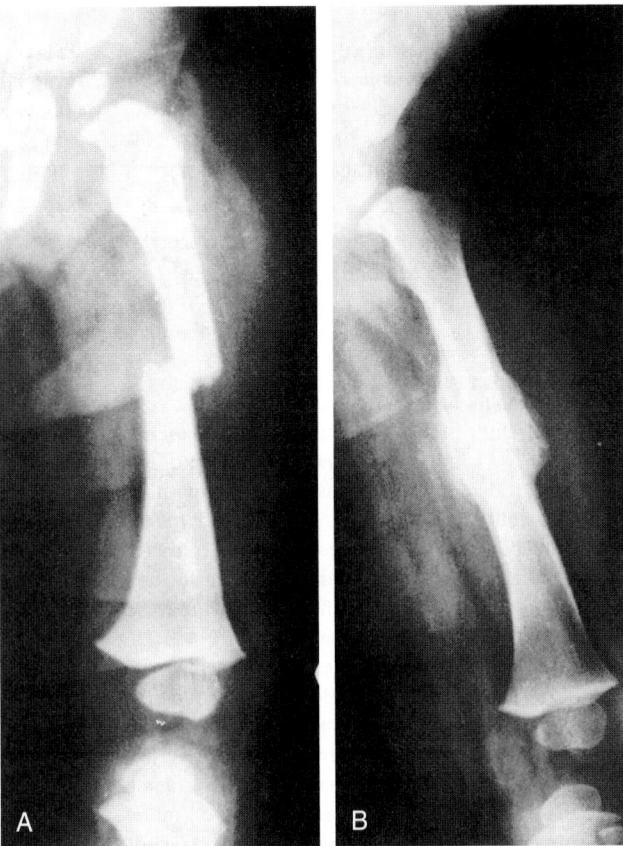

FIG 31-4 Fractured femur. Most fractured femurs in childhood are of the spiral type shown here. Note comparison of **A,** original radiography, with **B,** 6-month postfracture radiography showing callus formation. (Courtesy Henrietta Egleston Hospital for Children, Atlanta. From Hilt NE, Schmitt EW: *Pediatric orthopedic nursing,* St. Louis, 1975, Mosby.)

✚ EMERGENCY TREATMENT

Fracture

Determine the mechanism of injury.
Assess the 6 Ps.
Move the injured part as little as possible.
Cover open wounds with a sterile or clean dressing.
Immobilize the limb, including joints above and below the fracture site; do not attempt to reduce the fracture or push protruding bone under the skin.
Use a soft splint (pillow or folded towel) or rigid splint (rolled newspaper or magazine).
Uninjured leg can serve as a splint for a leg fracture if no splint is available.
Reassess neurovascular status.
Apply traction if circulatory compromise is present.
Elevate the injured limb if possible.
Apply cold to the injured area.
Call emergency medical services or transport to medical facility.

While remaining calm and speaking in a quiet voice, the nurse can ask the parents and older child to describe what happened. The child may arrive with the limb supported in some manner; if not, careful support or immobilization may be provided to the affected site. In the event that the limb is supported or immobilized, it may be best not to touch the child but to ask him or her to point to the painful area and to wiggle the fingers or toes. By this time the child may feel relatively safe and will allow someone to gently touch the area just enough to feel the pulses and test for sensation. A child's anxiety is greatly influenced by previous experiences with injury and with health personnel. However, he or she needs to be told what will happen and what to do to help. The affected limb need not be palpated, and it should not be moved unless properly splinted. If the child is at home or if the practitioner is not present to examine the child, some type of splint is applied carefully for transport to the medical facility. Parental anxiety may be heightened by the child's pain reaction and fear and possibly by other events surrounding the accident. It is important to communicate to the parent that the child will receive the necessary care, including pain management.

❗ NURSING ALERT

Compartment syndrome is a serious complication that results from compression of nerves, blood vessels, and muscle inside a closed space. This injury may be devastating, resulting in tissue death, and thus requires emergency treatment (fasciotomy). The six Ps of ischemia from a vascular, soft-tissue, nerve, or bone injury should be included in an assessment of any injury:
1. Pain
2. Pulselessness
3. Pallor
4. Paresthesia
5. Paralysis
6. Pressure (Box 31-3)

THE CHILD IN A CAST

The completeness of the fracture, the type of bone involved, and the amount of weight bearing influence how much of the extremity must be included in the cast to immobilize the fracture site completely. In most cases, the joints above and below the fracture are immobilized to eliminate the possibility of movement that might cause displacement at the fracture site. Four major categories of casts are used for fractures: upper extremity to immobilize the wrist or elbow, lower extremity to immobilize the ankle or knee, spinal and cervical to immobilize the spine, and spica casts to immobilize the hip and knee (Fig. 31-5).

BOX 31-3   **COMPARTMENT SYNDROME EVALUATION**

Assess the extent of injury—6 *P*s:
1. **Pain:** Severe pain that is not relieved by analgesics or elevation of the limb, movement that increases pain
2. **Pulselessness:** Inability to palpate a pulse distal to the fracture or compartment
3. **Pallor:** Pale appearing skin, poor perfusion, capillary refill greater than 3 seconds
4. **Paresthesia:** Tingling or burning sensations
5. **Paralysis:** Inability to move extremity or digits
6. **Pressure:** Involved limb or digits may feel tense and warm; skin is tight, shiny; pressure within the compartment is elevated

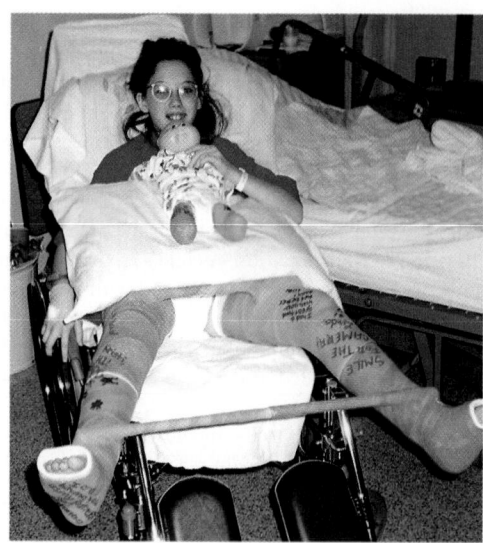

FIG 31-5 Spica cast with hip abductor. Note the casts on the doll as well.

The Cast

Casts are constructed from gauze strips and bandages impregnated with plaster of Paris or, more commonly, from synthetic lighter weight and water-resistant materials (e.g., waterproof liners, fiberglass and polyurethane resin).

Both types of casting produce heat from chemical reaction activated by water immediately after application. Plaster casts mold closely to the body part, take 10 to 72 hours to dry, have a smooth exterior, and are inexpensive. The newer synthetic casting material is lightweight, dries in 5 to 20 minutes, permits earlier weight bearing, and is water resistant when applied with a waterproof liner. It is always desirable to give children choices, and synthetic casting materials come in a variety of colors. The disadvantages of synthetic casting are its inability to mold closely to body parts and its rough exterior, which may scratch surfaces. Synthetic casts are also difficult to write on; a waterproof marker or color markers may be used.

Cast Application

The child's developmental age should be considered before the cast is applied. For preschoolers who fear bodily harm and fantasize about the loss of an extremity, it may be helpful to use a plastic doll or stuffed animal to explain the procedure beforehand. Toddlers and preschoolers do not have easily defined body boundaries; if an extremity is wrapped in a bandage, cast, or splint, to the young child the extremity ceases to function or exist. It is also helpful to explain that some synthetic cast material will become warm during application but will not burn. During the application of the cast, various distraction methods can be used, including discussing favorite pets or activities at school, blowing bubbles, and so forth. In this age group, explanations such as "This will help your arm get better" are futile because the child has no concept of causality.

Before the cast is applied, the extremities are checked for any abrasions, cuts, or other alterations in the skin surface and for the presence of rings or other items that might cause constriction from swelling; such objects are removed. A tube of cloth stockinette or Gore-Tex liner is stretched over the area to be casted, and bony prominences are padded with soft cotton sheeting. Dry rolls of casting material are immersed in a pail of water. The wet rolls are put on in a bandage

fashion and molded to the extremity. During application of the cast, the underlying stockinette is pulled over the rough edges of the cast and secured with casting material to form a padded edge to protect the skin.

Nursing Care Management

The complete evaporation of the water from a hip spica cast can take 24 to 48 hours when older types of plaster materials are used. Drying occurs within minutes with fiberglass cast material. The cast must remain uncovered to allow it to dry from the inside out. Turning the child in a plaster cast at least every 2 hours will help to dry a body cast evenly and prevent complications related to immobility. A regular fan or cool-air hair dryer to circulate air may be helpful when the humidity is high.

> **! NURSING ALERT**
>
> Heated fans or dryers are not used because they cause the cast to dry on the outside and remain wet beneath or cause burns from heat conduction by way of the cast to the underlying tissue.

A wet plaster cast should be supported by a pillow that is covered with plastic and handled by the palms of the hands to prevent indenting the cast, which can create pressure areas. A dry plaster-of-Paris cast produces a hollow sound when it is tapped with the finger. After it has dried, "hot spots" felt on the cast surface or a foul-smelling odor may indicate an infection. This should be reported for further evaluation, and if concern continues, an opening, or a "window," may be exposed over the area of concern to evaluate the site.

During the first few hours after a cast is applied, the chief concern is that the extremity may continue to swell to the extent that the cast becomes a tourniquet, shutting off circulation and producing neurovascular complications (compartment syndrome) (see Box 31-3). To reduce the likelihood of this potential problem, the body part can be elevated, thereby increasing venous return. If edema is excessive, casts are bivalved (i.e., cut to make anterior and posterior halves that are held together with an elastic bandage). The cast and the involved extremity are observed frequently for neurovascular integrity and any signs of compromise. Permanent muscle and tissue damage can occur within a few hours.

> **! NURSING ALERT**
>
> Observations such as pain (unrelieved by pain medication 1 hour after administration, especially with passive range of motion), swelling, discoloration (pallor or cyanosis) of the exposed portions, decreased pulses, decreased temperature, paresthesia, or the inability to move the distal exposed part(s) should be reported immediately. Pallor, paralysis, and pulselessness are late signs (see Box 31-3).

When an extremity that has sustained an open fracture is casted, a window is often left over the wound area to allow for observation and dressing of the wound. For the first few hours after surgery, substantial bleeding may soak through the cast. Periodically, the circumscribed bloodstained area should be outlined with a waterproof marker and the time indicated to provide a guide for assessing the amount of bleeding.

Appropriate cast care guidelines for the child's caregiver are necessary before discharge. Instructions are also given for checking for signs and symptoms that indicate that the cast is too tight (see Family-Centered Care box). Parents should also be told to take the child to the

⚕ FAMILY-CENTERED CARE

Cast Care

Keep the casted extremity elevated on pillows or similar support for the first day or as directed by the health professional.

Avoid denting the plaster cast with fingertips (use palms of hand to handle) while it is still wet to avoid creating pressure points.

Expose the plaster cast to air until dry.

Observe the extremities (fingers or toes) for any evidence of swelling or discoloration (darker or lighter than a comparable extremity) and contact the health professional if noted.

Check movement and sensation of the visible extremities frequently.

Follow health professional's orders regarding any restriction of activities.

Restrict strenuous activities for the first few days.
- Engage in quiet activities but encourage use of muscles.
- Move the joints above and below the cast on the affected extremity.

Encourage frequent rest for a few days, keeping the injured extremity elevated while resting.

Avoid allowing the affected limb to hang in a dependent position for any length of time.
- Keep an injured upper extremity elevated (e.g., in a sling) while upright.
- Elevate a lower limb when sitting and avoid standing for too long.

Do not allow the child to put anything inside the cast. Keep small items that might be placed inside the cast away from small children.

Keep a clear path for ambulation. Remove toys, hazardous floor rugs, pets, and other items over which the child might stumble.

Use crutches appropriately if lower limb fracture requires non–weight bearing on affected extremity.

The crutches should fit properly, have a soft rubber tip to prevent slipping, and be well padded at the axilla.

With crutch walking, the child's body weight is supported on the hand grips, not the axilla.

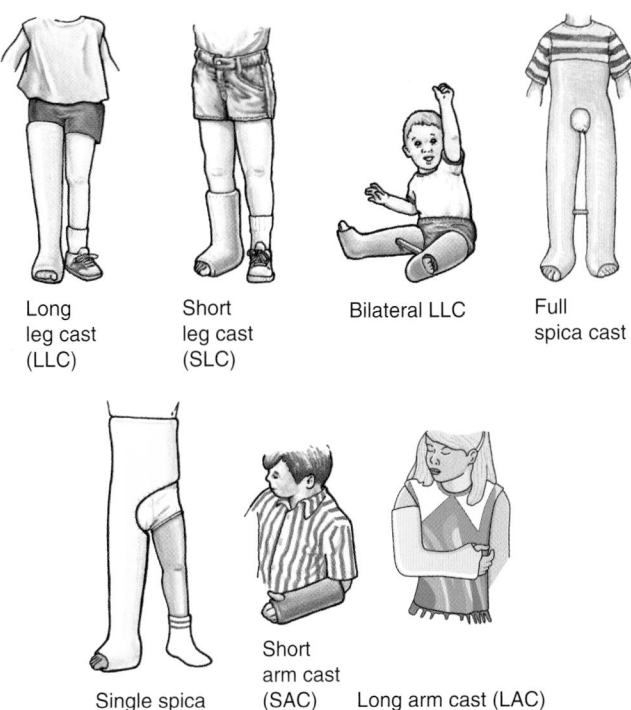

Long leg cast (LLC)   Short leg cast (SLC)   Bilateral LLC   Full spica cast

Single spica   Short arm cast (SAC)   Long arm cast (LAC)

FIG 31-6 Types of casts.

health professional for attention if the cast becomes too loose because a loose cast no longer serves its purpose.

Nurses can help families adapt the child's home environment to meet the temporary encumbrance of a large cast or one that restricts the child's mobility (e.g., a long-leg or spica cast [Fig. 31-6]). Commonplace situations become problematic (e.g., transporting a child safely and comfortably in a car). Standard seat belts and car seats may not be readily adapted for use by children in some casts. Specially designed car seats and restraints are available that meet safety requirements.* Alterations to standard car seats to accommodate the cast are not recommended because the structure may be adversely altered and fail to properly restrain the child. A bedside commode or rental wheelchair maybe be necessary equipment for a child who is nonambulatory.

Parents are taught the proper care of the cast or brace and are helped to devise means for maintaining cleanliness. A superabsorbent disposable diaper is tucked beneath the entire perineal opening of the cast. A larger diaper can be applied and fastened over the small diaper

and cast to hold the smaller diaper in place. In the event that the larger diaper becomes wet or soiled, it is likely the cast is as well.

For tightly fitting casts, transparent film dressings can be cut into strips as for petaling with one edge applied to the cast edge and the other directly to the perineum; this forms a continuous, waterproof bridge between the perineum and the cast to prevent leakage. An additional advantage to the use of this transparent dressing is that it keeps both the skin and the cast dry while allowing for observation of skin beneath the dressing.

Older infants and small children may stuff bits of food, small toys, or other items under the cast; parents should be alerted to this possibility so they can initiate suitable preventive measures.

Feeding an infant in a hip spica cast offers problems in positioning. Very young infants can be fed in the supine position with the head elevated. With the infant's hips and legs supported on a pillow at the side, the parent can cuddle the infant in his or her arms during feeding. A somewhat similar position can be used for breastfeeding (i.e., with the infant supported on pillows or held in a "football" hold facing the mother with the legs behind her). An alternate position is to hold the infant upright on the caregiver's lap with the legs of the infant astride the adult's leg.

Children in spica casts usually find the prone position easier for self-feeding from a small table placed next to the dining table; alternatively, they may manage a semisitting position in bed or in a wheelchair (see Fig. 31-5). The use of a conventional toilet is almost impossible. A bedside toilet can be adapted for use. Small bedpans or other containers offer alternatives for elimination. The nurse may suggest waterproofing methods by devising plastic wraps for elimination and showers. Baths are possible only if the plaster cast is kept out of the water and covered to prevent it from becoming wet.

Cast Removal

Cutting the cast to remove it or to relieve tightness is frequently a frightening experience for children. They fear the sound of the cast

---

*For information on specially adapted molded-plastic chairs for children who have spica casts, contact Snug Seat at 800-336-7684; http://www.snugseat.com/en-US/Welcome-to-Snug-Seat.aspx. The E-Z-On vest is a special safety harness for larger children with poor trunk control. Additional safety restraints and a listing of distributors are available from SafetyBeltSafe U.S.A., http://www.carseat.org. Another resource is the National Center for the Safe Transportation of Children with Special Health Care Needs; 800-543-6227; http://www.preventinjury.org/specNeeds.asp.

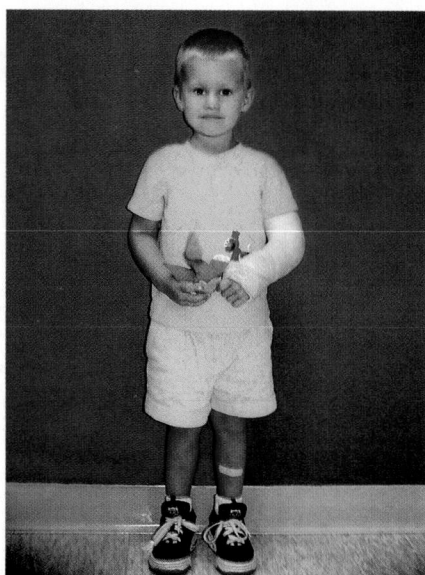

FIG 31-7 Young children usually adapt well to a cast but often fear removal of the cast.

cutter and are terrified that their flesh, as well as the cast, will be cut. The oscillating blade vibrates rapidly back and forth and will not cut when placed *lightly* on the skin. Children have described it as producing a "tickly" sensation. The vibration also generates heat that may be felt by the child. Both of these feelings should be explained.

Preparation for the procedure will help reduce anxiety, especially if a trusting relationship has been established between the child and the nurse. Many young children come to regard the cast as part of themselves, which intensifies their fear of removal (Fig. 31-7). They need continual reassurance that all is going well and that their behavior is accepted. After the cast is removed, the parents and child should be given the option of keeping the cast. If the cast has been in place for a lengthy period, decreased muscle mass will be noted. The child should be reassured that resuming exercise and routine activities will return function and appearance (provided there was no significant trauma beforehand).

After the cast is removed, the skin surface will be caked with desquamated skin and sebaceous secretions. Application of mineral oil (e.g., baby oil) or lotion may remove the particles as well as provide comfort. Soaking the extremity in a bathtub is usually sufficient for their removal, but it may take several days to eliminate the accumulation completely. The parents and child should be instructed not to pull or forcibly remove this material with vigorous scrubbing because it may cause excoriation and bleeding.

THE CHILD IN TRACTION

The ever-changing health care arena has witnessed the demise of many long-term treatments involving lengthy hospitalization; one such change is in the area of traction. Most balanced skeletal traction is applied in children after a severe or complex injury to allow physiologic stability, align bone fragments, and permit closer evaluation of the injured site. Newer technology has produced orthopedic fixation devices that allow partial or full mobility, thus preventing long-term immobilization and its consequences. In many situations, surgical intervention may be carried out within a matter of days; therefore, skeletal traction devices described herein may be used infrequently in pediatrics.

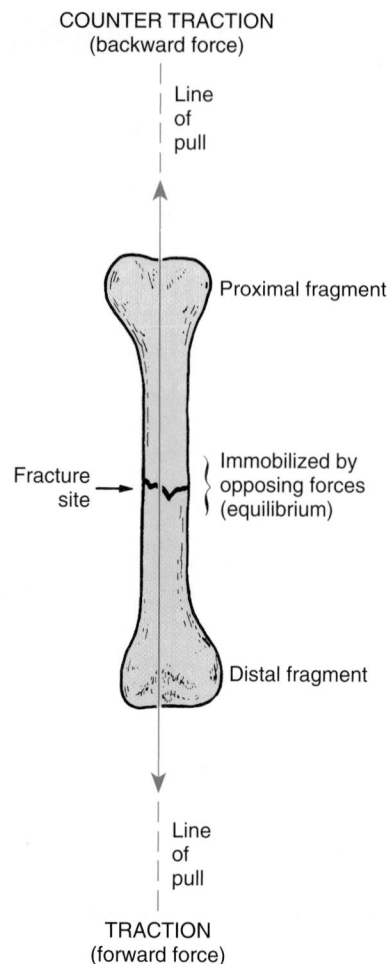

FIG 31-8 Application of traction to maintain bone alignment.

Purposes of Traction

The six primary purposes of traction are:
1. To fatigue the involved muscles and reduce muscle spasm so that bones can be realigned
2. To position the distal and proximal bone ends in desired realignment to promote satisfactory bone healing
3. To immobilize the fracture site until realignment has been achieved and sufficient healing has taken place to permit casting or splinting
4. To help prevent or improve contracture deformity
5. To provide immobilization of specific areas of the body
6. To reduce muscle spasms (rare in children)

The three essential components of traction management are traction, counter traction, and friction (Fig. 31-8). To reduce or realign a fracture site, **traction** (forward force) is produced by attaching weight to the distal bone fragment. Body weight provides **counter traction** (backward force), and the patient's contact with the bed constitutes the **frictional** force. These forces are used to align the distal and proximal bone fragments by adjusting the line of pull upward or downward and adducting or abducting the extremity.

To attain equilibrium, the amount of forward force is adjusted by adding weight to or subtracting weight from the traction, or counter traction can be increased by elevating the foot of the bed to create a greater gravitational pull to the backward force.

BOX 31-4   TYPES OF TRACTION

Manual traction—Applied to the body part by the hand placed distal to the fracture site. Manual traction may be provided during application of a cast but more commonly when a closed reduction is performed.

Skin traction—Applied directly to the skin surface and indirectly to the skeletal structures. The pulling mechanism is attached to the skin with adhesive material or an elastic bandage. Both types are applied over soft, foam-backed traction straps to distribute the traction pull.

Skeletal traction—Applied directly to the skeletal structure by a pin, wire, or tongs inserted into or through the diameter of the bone distal to the fracture.

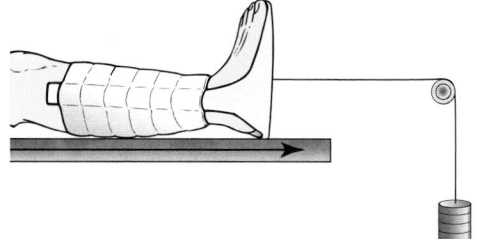

FIG 31-9 Buck extension traction. (From Lewis SL, Heitkemper MM, Dirksen S, and others, editors: *Medical-surgical nursing: assessment and management of clinical problems*, ed 8, St. Louis, 2011, Mosby.)

The **all-or-none law**, characteristic of muscle contractility, influences the complete relaxation. When muscles are stretched, muscle spasm ceases, which permits the realignment of the bone ends. The continuous maintenance of traction is important during this phase because releasing the traction allows the muscle's normal contracting ability to again cause a malpositioning of the bone ends.

The realignment of the fragments is a gradual process that is achieved more rapidly in infants, who have limited muscle tone, than in muscular teenagers. The desired vector force and callus formation are checked periodically by radiographic examination. The traction pull to some degree immobilizes the fracture site; however, adjunctive immobilizing devices such as splints or casts are sometimes used with skeletal traction. Immobilization with traction is maintained until the bone ends are in satisfactory realignment after which a less confining type of immobilization—a cast, pins, or external stabilization device—is applied.

Types of Traction

The pull needed for traction can be applied to the distal bone fragment in several ways (Box 31-4). The type of traction applied is determined primarily by the child's age, the condition of the soft tissues, and the type and degree of displacement of the fracture. Fractures most commonly treated by application of traction are those involving the femur and vertebrae. The major types of traction for specific fractures are briefly discussed below.

The use of upper extremity traction in children is uncommon. Newer surgical techniques allow for early mobilization and optimal results without traction. Nursing care of the child with upper extremity traction is the same as that for lower extremity traction, which is discussed below.

The frequent site for a femoral fracture is in the middle third of the shaft. With this fracture, there may be significant overriding but minimal displacement. In a fracture in the lower third of the shaft, the pull of the gastrocnemius muscle causes the distal fragment to become downwardly displaced.

Fractures of the femur can often be reduced with immediate application of a hip spica cast in young children. When traction is required, several types may be used based on the initial assessment.

Bryant traction is a type of running traction in which the pull is in only one direction. Skin traction is applied to the legs, which are flexed at a 90-degree angle at the hips. The child's trunk (with the buttocks raised slightly off the bed) provides counter traction.

Buck extension traction (Fig. 31-9) is a type of traction with the legs in an extended position. Except for fracture cases, turning from side to side with care is permitted to maintain the involved leg in alignment. Buck extension traction is used primarily for short-term immobilization, such as preoperative management of a child with a dislocated hip, or for correction of contractures or bone deformities, such as in Legg-Calvé-Perthes disease. Buck traction may be accomplished with either skin straps or a special foam boot designed for traction.

Russell traction uses skin traction on the lower leg and a padded sling under the knee. Two lines of pull, one along the longitudinal line of the lower leg and one perpendicular to the leg, are produced. This combination of pulls allows realignment of the lower extremity and immobilizes the hip and knee in a flexed position. The hip flexion must be kept at the prescribed angle to prevent fracture malalignment because there is no direct support under the fracture and the skin traction may slip. Special nursing measures include carefully checking the position of the traction so that the amount of desired hip flexion is maintained and damage to the common peroneal nerve under the knee does not produce footdrop.

A common skeletal traction is **90-degree–90-degree traction** (90-90 traction). The lower leg is supported by a boot cast or a calf sling, and a skeletal Steinmann pin or Kirschner wire is placed in the distal fragment of the femur, resulting in a 90-degree angle at both the hip and the knee. From a nursing standpoint, this traction facilitates position changes, toileting, and prevention of complications related to traction.

Balanced suspension traction may be used with or without skin or skeletal traction. Unless used with another traction, the balanced suspension merely suspends the leg in a desired flexed position to relax the hip and hamstring muscles and does not exert any traction directly on a body part. A **Thomas splint** extends from the groin to midair above the foot, and a **Pearson attachment** supports the lower leg. Towels or pieces of felt covered with stockinette are clipped or pinned to the splints for leg support. When the child is lifted off the bed, the traction lifts with the child without loss of alignment. This traction requires careful checking of splints and ropes to make certain that no slippage or fraying has occurred. The traction is of great value in an older and heavier child when it is essential to lift the patient for care.

The cervical area is a vulnerable site for flexion or extension injuries to muscle, vertebrae, or the spinal cord. Cervical muscle trauma without other complications is treated with a cervical hard collar to relieve the weight of the head from the fracture site. When a child displaces or fractures a cervical vertebra, it may be necessary to reduce and immobilize the site with cervical skeletal traction. The spinal cord runs through the intravertebral canal, and dislocation or fracture of the vertebrae can also cause spinal cord injury. Nursing assessment of neurologic function is essential to prevent further injury during the application and use of cervical skeletal traction.

Most cervical traction is accomplished with the use of a **halo brace** or **halo vest** (Fig. 31-10, *A*) This device consists of a steel halo attached

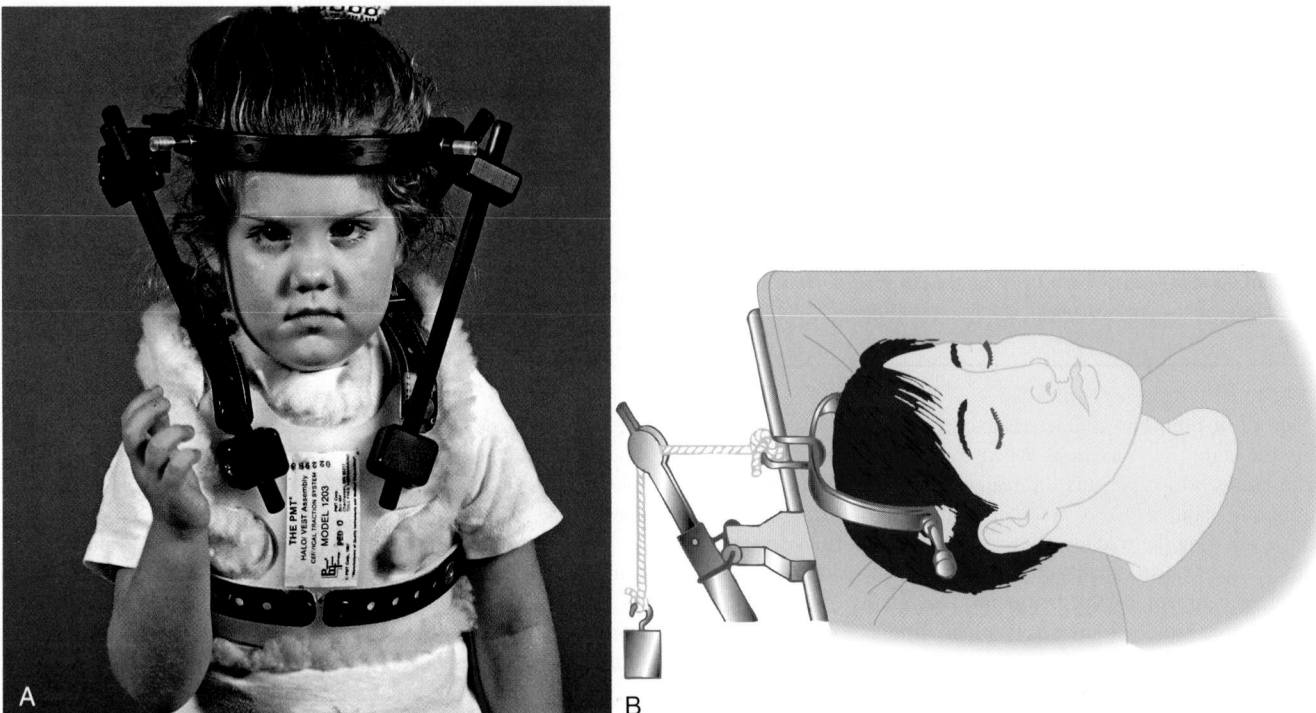

FIG 31-10 A, Halo vest. **B,** Crutchfield tong traction. (**A,** from Herring JA: *Tachdjian's pediatric orthopaedics,* ed 4, Philadelphia, 2008, Saunders; **B,** from Black JM, Hawks JH: *Medical-surgical nursing: clinical management for positive outcomes,* ed 8, Philadelphia, 2009, Saunders Elsevier.)

to the head by four screws inserted into the outer skull; several rigid bars connect the halo to a vest that is worn around the chest, thus providing greater mobility of the rest of the body while avoiding cervical spinal motion altogether. If the injury has been limited to a vertebral fracture without neurologic deficit, a halo brace can be applied to permit earlier ambulation. Gardner-Wells tongs may be used with cervical traction to immobilize the cervical spine (Fig. 31-10, *B*) (Fisher, Williams, and Levine, 2008). Gardner-Wells tongs are spring loaded, so making burr holes and shaving hair are not required; a local anesthetic may be used during application. As the neck muscles fatigue with constant traction pull, the vertebral bodies gradually separate so that the cord is no longer pinched between the vertebrae. Immobilization until fracture healing or surgical fixation can occur is an essential goal of cervical traction. If immobilization is required in an infant or young child, a special cervical spine cast (Minerva cast) is applied.

Nursing Care Management

To assess the child in traction, it is essential to know the purpose for which the traction is applied and to understand the basic principles of traction. Regular assessment of both the child and the traction apparatus is required (see Nursing Care Guidelines box). Many of the nursing problems associated with a child in traction are related to immobility. Modifying the child's diet, encouraging fluids, increasing fiber, and offering a mild stool softener may be necessary to prevent constipation.

When indicated by the attending practitioner, the nurse may remove nonadhesive skin traction. In these cases, intermittent traction is periodically released and reapplied as ordered. A child may have several types of traction at one time, and each one must be assessed separately to avoid problems.

> **! NURSING ALERT**
>
> Skeletal traction is never released by the nurse (except under direct supervision by the practitioner). This precaution includes not lifting the weights that are applying traction (e.g., for moving the child in bed, for repositioning).

In addition to routine skin observation and care, the child in skeletal traction will need special skin care at the pin sites according to hospital policy or practitioner preference. Pin sites should be frequently assessed and cleaned to prevent infection; after the first 48 to 72 hours, pin site care may be performed once daily or weekly for mechanically stable pins (Holmes, Brown, and Pin Site Care Expert Panel, 2005). Use of a 2-mg/ml chlorhexidine solution has been proposed as best practice care for skeletal pin sites by the National Association of Orthopaedic Nurses (Holmes, Brown, and Pin Site Care Expert Panel, 2005). A pressure-reduction device, such as a pressure-reduction mattress, decreases the chance of skin breakdown.

> **NURSING TIP** A small hand mirror facilitates visualization of inaccessible skin areas.

When the child is first placed in traction, increased discomfort is common as a result of the traction pull fatiguing the muscle. It has been determined that orthopedic conditions are associated with a higher-than-average number of painful events and a higher percentage of bodily symptoms than other common conditions. Analgesics, including IV opioids, and muscle relaxants, help during this phase of care and should be administered liberally.

NURSING CARE GUIDELINES

Traction Care

Understand Therapy
Understand purpose of traction.
Understand function of traction in each specific situation.

Maintain Traction
Check desired line of pull and relationship of distal fragment to proximal fragment. Check whether fragment is being directed upward, adducted, or abducted.
Check function of each component:
- Position of bandages, frames, splints, specialized boot
- Ropes—In center track of pulley, taut, no fraying, knots tied securely
- Pulleys—In original position on attachment bar; have not slid from original site; wheels freely movable
- Weights—Correct amount of weight, hanging freely, in safe location

Check bed position—Head or foot elevated as directed for desired amount of pull and counter traction.
Do not remove skeletal traction or adhesive traction straps on skin traction.

Maintain Alignment
Observe for correct body alignment with emphasis on alignment of shoulder, hip, and leg.
Check after child has moved.
Maintain correct angles at joints.

Skin Traction
Replace nonadhesive straps or elastic bandage on skin traction *when permitted* or absolutely necessary but make certain that traction on limb is maintained by someone during procedure.
Assess straps or bandages to ascertain if they are correctly applied (diagonal or spiral) and not too loose or too tight, which could cause slippage and malalignment of traction.
Assess traction boot to ensure it has not slipped and is not causing compression of the foot, thus impairing the circulation.

Skeletal Traction
Check pin sites frequently for signs of bleeding, inflammation, or infection.
Cleanse and dress pin sites per institution protocol or as ordered.
Apply topical antiseptic or antibiotic to pin sites daily as ordered.

Cover ends of pins with protective rubber or padding to prevent child being scratched by pin.
Note pull of traction on pin; pull should be even.
Check pin screws to be certain that screws are tight in metal clamp that attaches traction apparatus to pin.

Prevent Skin Breakdown
Provide alternating-pressure mattress underneath hips and back.
Make total-body skin checks for redness or breakdown, especially over areas that receive greatest pressure.
Wash and dry skin at least daily.
Inspect pressure points daily or more often if risk for breakdown is observed.
Use a skin breakdown assessment scale such as Braden Q.
Stimulate circulation with gentle massage over pressure areas.
Change position at least every 2 hours to relieve pressure.
Encourage increase in intake of oral fluids.
Provide and encourage patient to eat a balanced diet, including vegetables and fruits.

Prevent Complications
Check pulses in affected area and compare with pulses in contralateral site.
Assess circular dressings for excessive tightness.
Assess restrictive bandages or devices used to maintain traction on affected limb.
- Make certain that they are not too loose or too tight.
- Remove periodically and check for skin breakdown or pressure areas.

Encourage deep breathing or use of incentive spirometry.
- Monitor the 6 Ps (see p. 1059).

Take immediate action to correct problem or report to practitioner if neurovascular changes are present.
Record findings of neurovascular changes.
Carry out passive, active, or active-with-resistance exercises of uninvolved joints.
Note if any tightness, weakness, edema, or contractures are developing in uninvolved joints and muscles.
Take measures to correct or prevent further development of weakness, such as applying footboard or foot orthoses to prevent footdrop.

! NURSING ALERT

For skeletal traction to be effective, ensure that the weights are hanging freely at all times.

The specific nursing responsibilities for the patient in traction are outlined in the Nursing Care Guidelines box above.

DISTRACTION

Unlike traction, which helps bones realign and fuse properly, **distraction** is the process of separating opposing bone to encourage regeneration of new bone in the created space. Distraction can also be used when limbs are of unequal lengths and new bone is needed to elongate the shorter limb.

External Fixation

Monolateral, Taylor Spatial Frame, and **Ilizarov external fixators (IEFs)** are common external fixation devices. The IEF uses a system of wires, rings, and telescoping rods that permits limb lengthening to occur by manual distraction (Fig. 31-11). In addition to lengthening bones, the device can be used to correct angular or rotational defects or to immobilize fractures. The device is attached surgically by securing a series of external full or half rings to the bone with wires. External telescoping rods connect the rings to each other. Manual distraction is accomplished by manipulating the rods to increase the distance between the rings. A percutaneous osteotomy is performed when the device is applied to create a "false" growth plate. A special osteotomy or corticotomy involves cutting only the cortex of the bone while preserving its blood supply, bone marrow, endosteum, and periosteum.

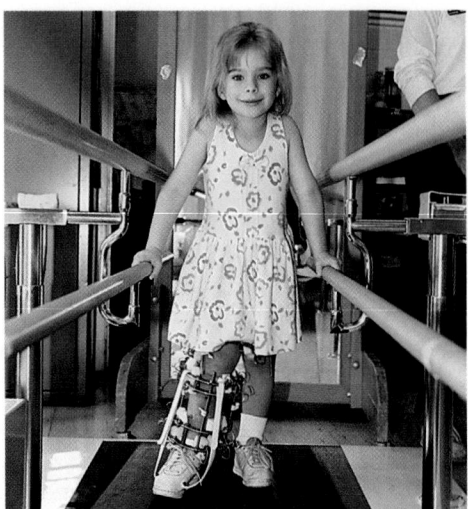

FIG 31-11 Child with Ilizarov external fixator during physical therapy on parallel bars.

Capillary blood flow to the transected area is essential for proper bone growth. Cut bone ends typically grow at a rate of 1 cm (0.4 inches) per month. The IEF can result in up to a 15-cm (6-inch) gain in length.

Nursing Care Management

Success of the fixation devices depends on the child's and family's cooperation; therefore, before surgery, they must be fully informed of the appearance of the device, how it accomplishes bone growth and limits bone mobility, alterations in activities, and home and follow-up care. Children are involved in learning to adjust the device to accomplish distraction. Children and parents should be instructed in pin care, including observation for infection and loosening of the pins. Cleaning routines for the pin sites vary among practitioners but should not traumatize the skin.

Children who participate actively in their care report less discomfort. Because the device is external, the child and family need to be prepared for the reactions of others and assisted in camouflaging the device with appropriate apparel, such as wide-legged pants that close with self-adhering fasteners around the device. A loose sock or stockinette may also be used over the device to decrease public awareness. Partial weight bearing is allowed, and the child learns to walk with crutches. Alterations in activity include modifications at school and in physical education. Full weight bearing is not allowed until the distraction is completed and bone consolidation has occurred. Follow-up care is essential to maintain appropriate distraction until the desired limb length is achieved. The device is removed surgically after the bone has consolidated, and the child may need to use crutches or have a cast for 4 to 6 weeks after removal to reduce the risk of fracture.

AMPUTATION

A child may be born with the congenital absence of an extremity, have a traumatic loss of an extremity, or need a surgical amputation for a pathologic condition such as osteosarcoma (see p. 1081). With today's surgical technology and the quick thinking of bystanders who save a traumatically amputated body part, some children have had fingers and arms sewn back on with variable degrees of functional use regained.

> ### ! NURSING ALERT
>
> For an amputated limb or body part that may be reattached, do the following:
> 1. Rinse limb gently with normal saline.
> 2. Loosely wrap limb in sterile gauze.
> 3. Place wrapped limb in a watertight bag.
> 4. Cool (without freezing) bag in ice water (do not pack in ice because this may harm tissue).
> 5. Label with child's name, date, and time, and transport with the child to the hospital.

Surgical amputation or the surgical repair of a permanently severed limb focuses on constructing an adequately nourished residual limb. A smooth, healthy, padded stump, free of nerve endings, is important in prosthesis fitting and subsequent ambulation. In some situations in which there is no vascular or neurologic deficit, a cast is applied to the stump immediately after the procedure, and a pylon, metal extension, and artificial foot are attached so the patient can walk on the temporary prosthesis within a few hours.

Nursing Care Management

Stump shaping is done postoperatively with special elastic bandaging using a figure-eight bandage, which applies pressure in a cone-shaped fashion. This technique decreases stump edema, controls hemorrhage, and aids in developing desired contours so the child will bear weight on the posterior aspect of the skin flap rather than on the end of the stump. Stump elevation may be used during the first 24 hours, but after this time, the extremity should not be left in this position because contractures in the proximal joint will develop and seriously hamper ambulation. Monitoring proper body alignment will further decrease the risk of flexion contractures.

For older children and adolescents, arm exercises, bed pushups, and prosthesis-training programs using parallel bars help build up the arm muscles necessary for walking with crutches. Full range-of-motion exercises of joints above the amputation must be performed several times daily using active and isotonic exercises. Young children are often spontaneously active and require little encouragement.

Depending on the child's age, children or their parents will need to learn hygiene, including carefully washing with soap and water every day and checking for skin irritation, breakdown, and infection. A tube of stockinette or powder is used to slide the prosthesis on more easily. Skin must be checked carefully every time the prosthesis is removed, and prosthesis tolerance time must be adjusted to prevent skin breakdown.

For children who have had an amputation, phantom limb sensation is an expected experience because the nerve–brain connections are still present. Gradually, these sensations fade, although in many people who have had amputations, they persist for years. Preoperative discussion of this phenomenon will aid a child in understanding these "unusual feelings" and not hiding the experiences from others. Limb pain, especially pain that increases with ambulation, should be evaluated for the possibility of a neuroma at the free nerve endings in the stump or other problems such as a poorly fitting prosthesis or joint instability.

SPORTS PARTICIPATION AND INJURY

Every sport has the potential for injury to participants—whether an adolescent engages in serious competition or participates for

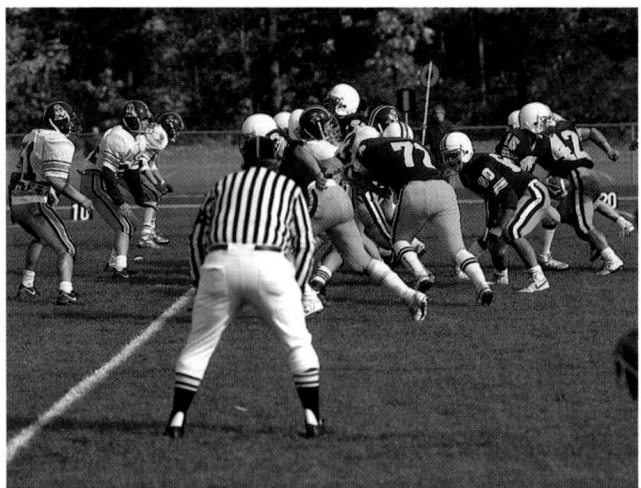

FIG 31-12 A number of injuries may occur with sports participation.

enjoyment. Serious injury occurs most often during rough contact sports or to persons who are not physically prepared for the activity. Injuries also occur when the children's or adolescents' bodies are not suited to the sport, when their muscles and body systems (respiratory and cardiovascular) are not conditioned to endure physical stress, or when they lack the insight and judgment to recognize that an activity exceeds their physical abilities. Rapidly growing bones, muscles, joints, and tendons are especially vulnerable to unusual strain. In general, more injuries occur during recreational sports participation than during organized athletic competition.

The environment and the sports or recreational equipment can also present risks (Fig. 31-12). Children and adolescents who participate in physical activity or sports do so in many different environments, including indoors and outdoors, on floors, on the ground and snow, on or beneath water surfaces, and sometimes in free air space. Most of these activities also involve equipment, which children and adolescents may not be physically mature enough to manage safely. A common example is skateboarding when the child or adolescent does not take safety precautions and perceives increased risk taking as a part of the sport.

Acute overload injuries are those that occur suddenly during an activity and produce immediate symptoms. A blow or overstretching, twisting, or sudden stress to tissues can cause these injuries. For descriptions and management of traumatic injuries see pp. 1055-1056.

OVERUSE SYNDROMES

To excel in sports, young athletes are forced to train longer, harder, and earlier in life than previously. The rewards are an increased level of fitness, better performance, faster times, and the satisfaction of attaining a personal goal. However, risks are associated when young people overtrain; these risks include recurrent upper respiratory infections, sleep and mood disturbances, loss of appetite, decreased interest in training and competition, and inability to concentrate (Winsley and Matos, 2011). Growing numbers of young people participate in organized sports, resulting in an increase in overuse injuries. Nearly half of all injuries evaluated in pediatric sports medicine are overuse injuries (Biber and Gregory, 2010).

The risk of overuse injury is always present and can be related to several factors, including training errors, muscle–tendon imbalance, anatomic malalignment (e.g., femoral anteversion, excessive lumbar lordosis, tibial torsion), incorrect footwear or playing surface, an associated disease state, and growth (growth cartilage is less resistant to microtrauma). Chronic pain in athletes is often associated with overuse injury, which can occur at any level of athletic participation. The common feature in overuse injuries is the **repetitive microtrauma** that occurs to a particular anatomic structure Performing the same movements repeatedly can cause several types of injury:

- **Frictional**, or rubbing of one structure against another
- **Tractional**, or repeated pull on a ligament or tendon
- **Cyclic**, or repetitive loading of impact forces (stress fractures)

The end result is inflammation of the involved structure with complaints of pain, tenderness, swelling, and disability.

Stress Fractures

Stress fractures are a consequence of repetitive, excessive stress on the bone that causes microfractures within the bone. Continued stress to the bone can lead to spread of the microfracture and eventual macrofracture. The pathogenesis of stress injury to the bone is multifactorial and includes everything from the footwear to the fitness level of the athlete. Stress fractures occur most commonly in the lower extremities, particularly the tibia. Track and field athletes have the highest incidence of stress fractures (Patel, 2010).

The most common symptom of stress fracture is a sharp, persistent, progressive pain or a deep, persistent dull ache located over the bone. Sometimes there is pain on impact (heel strike), but the most important clinical sign is pain over the involved bony surface. Diagnosis is based on clinical observation and history. Plain radiographs are rarely diagnostic of stress fractures during the initial few weeks because callus formation is not yet evident. Magnetic resonance imaging (MRI) is used when other causes of pain must be ruled out.

Therapeutic Management

Development of inflammation is common to all overuse syndromes; therefore, management involves rest or alteration of activities, physical therapy, and medication. Rest is the primary therapy, usually interpreted as reduced activity and the use of alternative exercise—not bed rest or immobilization with an orthosis. The main purpose is to alleviate the repetitive stress that initiated the symptoms. It is important to keep the adolescent mobile, and training can be continued. Alternative exercise is selected that maintains conditioning without aggravating the injury. For example, pool running (treading water in the deep end of a pool) can use the same movements as running but without the weight bearing; bicycling, swimming, and rowing are viable alternatives.

Other modalities include cryotherapy and cold whirlpool baths. Sometimes taping, bracing, splinting, and other orthoses are used, depending on the injury. **Nonsteroidal antiinflammatory drugs (NSAIDs)** are often prescribed to reduce inflammation and pain. Topical medications are of questionable value.

NURSE'S ROLE IN SPORTS FOR CHILDREN AND ADOLESCENTS

Nurses are often involved in sports activities in the areas of preparation and evaluation for activities, prevention of injury, treatment of injuries, and rehabilitation after injury. Selecting an appropriate sport for both recreation and competition is a joint effort of the adolescent, parents, and health professionals. The best approach to counseling children, adolescents, and parents regarding sports participation is to encourage activities that are most likely to provide pleasure and physical benefits throughout childhood and into adulthood. Exposure to a variety of activities is better for young children than limiting them to one sport. Parents should be cautioned against overcommitting children to sports activities so they have time for other activities.

When children sustain athletic injuries, nurses are often responsible for instructions regarding care. Instructions (e.g., schedule for appointments, application of ice, any restrictions in activity) should be clear and accompanied by written directions. The importance of taking medications as prescribed is emphasized, especially if medications are needed for an extended period and if adherence is an issue. Antiinflammatory medications given an hour before practice or competition may help children continue their activities.

Prevention of sports injuries is the most important aspect of athletic programs. Children should be suited to the activity, and the environment and the equipment must be safe. Children should be prepared for the sport, especially if it requires strenuous or continuous physical exertion. Nurses, coaches, and athletic trainers must collaborate to ensure that safety measures are implemented. Stretching exercises, warm-up and cool-down activities, and appropriate training are requirements for safe participation. Protective measures such as pads, taping, and wrapping are also important to prevent injury. Finally, nurses must be aware of environmental safety risks (see Head Injury, Chapter 28).

BIRTH AND DEVELOPMENTAL DEFECTS

Some skeletal defects may be diagnosed at birth or within days, weeks, or months after birth. In other cases, the deviation may be difficult to detect without careful inspection. Therefore, it is imperative that nurses become acquainted with signs of these defects and understand the principles of therapy in order to direct others in the care and management of these children.

DEVELOPMENTAL DYSPLASIA OF THE HIP

The broad term developmental dysplasia of the hip (DDH) describes a spectrum of disorders related to abnormal development of the hip that may occur at any time during fetal life, infancy, or childhood. A change in terminology from *congenital hip dysplasia* and *congenital dislocation of the hip* to DDH more properly reflects a variety of hip abnormalities in which there is a shallow acetabulum, subluxation, or dislocation.

The incidence of hip instability is approximately 1.5 per 1000 live births, and approximately 15% to 50% of infants with DDH are born breech. Girls are affected more commonly (80%) and there is a positive family history in approximately 12% to 33% of affected individuals (Sankar, Horn, Wells, and others, 2011a).

Pathophysiology

The cause of DDH is unknown, but certain factors such as gender, birth order, family history, intrauterine position, delivery type, joint laxity, and postnatal positioning are believed to affect the risk of DDH. Predisposing factors associated with DDH may be divided into three broad categories: (1) physiologic factors, which include maternal hormone secretion and intrauterine positioning; (2) mechanical factors, which involve breech presentation, multiple fetus, oligohydramnios, and large infant size (other mechanical factors may include continued maintenance of the hips in adduction and extension that will in time cause a dislocation); and (3) genetic factors, which entail a higher incidence of DDH in siblings of affected infants and an even greater incidence of recurrence if a sibling and one parent were affected.

Some experts categorize DDH into two major groups: (1) idiopathic, in which the infant is neurologically intact, and (2) teratologic, which involves a neuromuscular defect such as arthrogryposis or myelodysplasia. The teratologic forms usually occur in utero and are much less common.

Three degrees of DDH are illustrated in Figure 31-13:

1. **Acetabular dysplasia**—This is the mildest form of DDH, in which there is neither subluxation nor dislocation. There is a delay in acetabular development evidenced by osseous hypoplasia of the acetabular roof that is oblique and shallow, although the cartilaginous roof is comparatively intact. The femoral head remains in the acetabulum.

2. **Subluxation**—The largest percentage of DDH, subluxation, implies incomplete dislocation of the hip and is sometimes regarded as an intermediate state in the development from primary dysplasia to complete dislocation. The femoral head remains in contact with the acetabulum, but a stretched capsule and ligamentum teres cause the head of the femur to be partially displaced. Pressure on the cartilaginous roof inhibits ossification and produces a flattening of the socket.

3. **Dislocation**—The femoral head loses contact with the acetabulum and is displaced posteriorly and superiorly over the fibrocartilaginous rim. The ligamentum teres is elongated and taut.

Factors related to infant handling are indicated in the Cultural Considerations box.

Recently, several prominent orthopedic specialty organizations recommended that infants' hips be placed in slight flexion and abduction during swaddling. It was further recommended that infants' knees be maintained in slight flexion and that forced or sustained passive hip extension in the first few months should be avoided (Price and Schwend, 2011). These recommendations were supported by evidence that demonstrated a significant relationship between tight swaddling

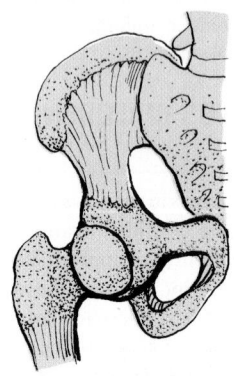 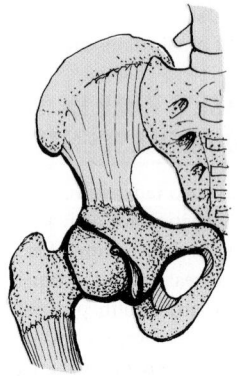 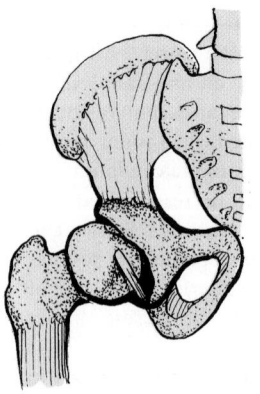 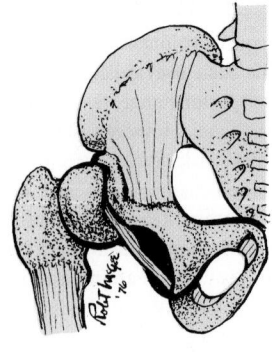

Normal   Dysplasia   Subluxation   Dislocation

FIG 31-13 Configuration and relationship of structures in developmental dysplasia of the hip.

and hip dysplasia and are aimed at decreasing the incidence of hip dysplasia in infants.

Diagnostic Evaluation

Developmental dysplasia of the hip is often not detected at the initial examination after birth; thus, all infants should be carefully monitored for hip dysplasia at follow-up visits throughout the first year of life at routine well-child checks. In the newborn period, hip dysplasia usually appears as hip joint laxity rather than as outright dislocation (Fig. 31-14). Subluxation and the tendency to dislocate can be demonstrated by the Ortolani or Barlow tests (see Fig. 31-14, *B*, *C*, and *D*). The Ortolani and Barlow tests are most reliable from birth to 4 weeks of age. With the Barlow test, the thighs are adducted; the Ortolani test involves abducting the thighs to test for hip subluxation or dislocation (Seidel, Ball, Dains, and others, 2006). Other signs of

🌐 CULTURAL CONSIDERATIONS
Developmental Dysplasia of the Hip

A striking relationship exists between the development of hip dislocation and methods of swaddling the hips. Among the cultures with the highest incidence of dislocation, newly born infants are tightly wrapped with the hips adducted and extended in blankets or other swaddling material or are strapped to cradle boards. In cultures such as those in Central and South America and Asia, where mothers traditionally carry infants on their backs with the infants' hips in the abducted and flexed hip position, hip dysplasia is much less common.

DDH are shortening of the limb on the affected side (see Fig. 31-14, *C*), asymmetric thigh and gluteal folds (see Fig 31-14, *A*), broadening of the perineum (in bilateral dislocation) (Box 31-5), and decreased hip abduction on the affected side.

❗ NURSING ALERT

These tests must be performed by an experienced clinician to prevent an injury to the infant's hip.

Radiographic examination in early infancy is not reliable because ossification of the femoral head does not normally take place until the fourth to sixth month of life. However, the cartilaginous head can be visualized directly by ultrasonography. Universal newborn screening with ultrasonography has been proposed; however, numerous studies reveal that this approach has a high rate of false-positive results and subsequent overtreatment. Therefore, ultrasonography is recommended as an adjunct to other diagnostic procedures (American Academy of Pediatrics [AAP], 2000; Sankar, Horn, Wells, and others, 2011a). In infants older than age 4 months and in children, radiographic examination is useful in confirming the diagnosis. An upward slope in the roof of the acetabulum (the acetabular angle) greater than 30 degrees with upward and outward displacement of the femoral head is a frequent finding in older children. Computed tomography (CT) may be useful to assess the position of the femoral head relative to the acetabulum after closed reduction and casting. The AAP (2000) has

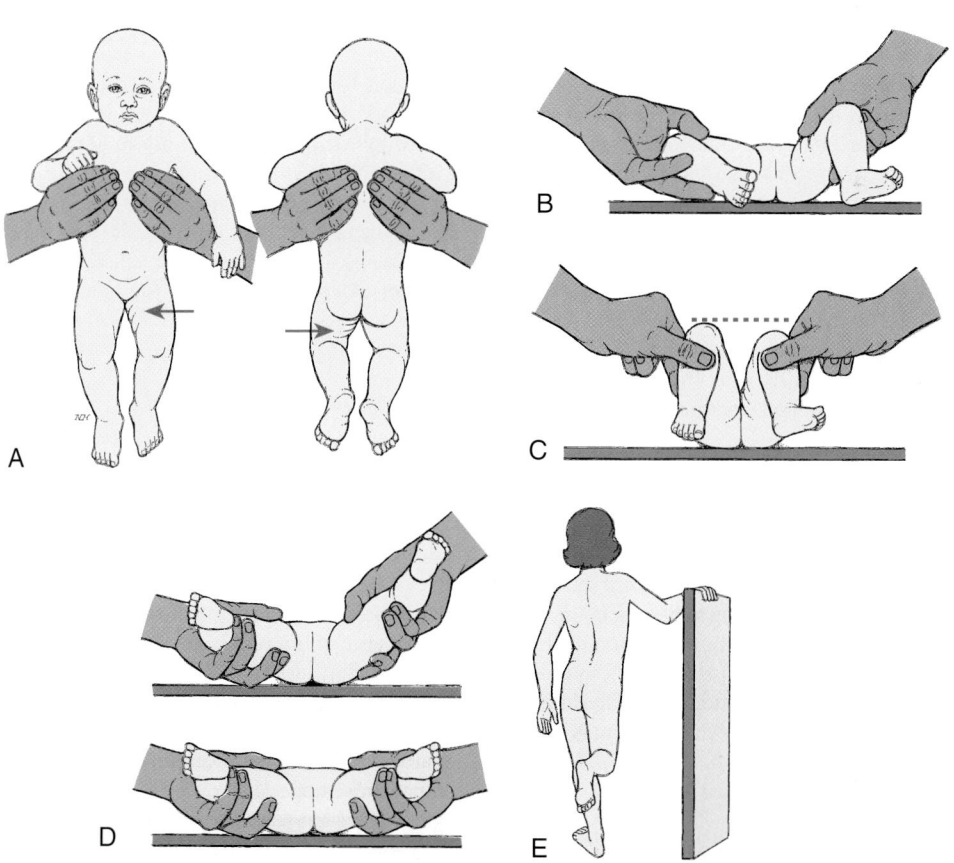

FIG 31-14 Signs of developmental dysplasia of the hip. **A,** Asymmetry of gluteal and thigh folds. **B,** Limited hip abduction, as seen in flexion. **C,** Apparent shortening of the femur, as indicated by the level of the knees in flexion. **D,** Ortolani maneuver with clunk elicited (in infants <4 weeks of age). **E,** Positive Trendelenburg sign with lordosis (if child is weight bearing).

BOX 31-5 CLINICAL MANIFESTATIONS OF DEVELOPMENTAL DYSPLASIA OF THE HIP

Infants

Shortening of limb on affected side (Galeazzi sign)

Restricted abduction of hip on affected side

Unequal gluteal folds (best visualized with infant prone)

Positive Ortolani test (hip is reduced by abduction)

Positive Barlow test (hip is dislocated by adduction)

Older Infants and Children

Affected leg appears shorter than the other

Telescoping or piston mobility of joint—Head of femur felt to move up and down in buttock when extended thigh is pushed first toward child's head and then pulled distally

Trendelenburg sign—When child stands first on one foot and then on the other (holding onto a chair, rail, or someone's hands) bearing weight on affected hip, pelvis tilts downward on normal side instead of upward, as it would with normal stability

Greater trochanter prominent and appearing above a line from anterosuperior iliac spine to tuberosity of ischium

Marked lordosis and waddling gait (bilateral hip dislocation)

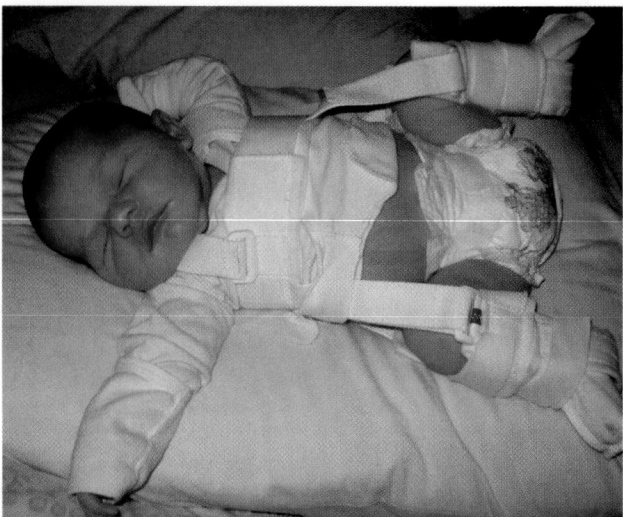

FIG 31-15 Child in Pavlik harness. (Courtesy Amanda Politte, St. Louis)

published extensive clinical guidelines for screening and early detection of DDH.

Therapeutic Management

Treatment is begun as soon as the condition is recognized because early intervention is more favorable to the restoration of normal bony architecture and function. The longer treatment is delayed, the more severe the deformity, the more difficult the treatment, and the less favorable the prognosis. The treatment varies with the child's age and the extent of the dysplasia. The goal of treatment is to obtain and maintain a safe, congruent position of the hip joint to promote normal hip joint development.

Newborns to Age 6 Months

The hip joint is maintained by dynamic splinting in a safe position with the proximal femur centered in the acetabulum in an attitude of flexion. Of the numerous devices available, the **Pavlik harness** is the most widely used, and with time, motion, and gravity, the hip works into a more abducted, reduced position (Fig. 31-15). The harness is worn continuously until the hip is proved stable on clinical and ultrasound examination, usually in 6 to 12 weeks.

When adduction contracture is present, other devices (e.g., Bryant traction [p. 1063]) are used to slowly and gently stretch the hip to full abduction, after which wide abduction is maintained until stability is attained. When there is difficulty in maintaining stable reduction, a hip spica cast is applied and changed periodically to accommodate the child's growth. After 3 to 6 months, sufficient stability is acquired to allow transfer to a removable protective abduction brace. The duration of treatment depends on development of the acetabulum but is usually accomplished within the first year.

Ages 6 to 24 Months

In this age group, the dislocation is often not recognized until the child begins to stand and walk, when attendant shortening of the limb and contractures of hip adductor and flexor muscles become apparent (DDH hip radiograph). A surgical closed reduction is performed, and

the child is placed in a spica cast for approximately 12 weeks. An abduction orthosis may be used instead of a hip spica cast. In the event that the hip remains unstable, an open reduction is performed (Sankar, Horn, Wells, and others, 2011a).

Older Children

Correction of the hip deformity in older children is inherently more difficult than in the preceding age groups because secondary adaptive changes and other etiologic factors (e.g., juvenile arthritis or nonambulatory cerebral palsy) complicate the condition. Operative reduction, which may involve preoperative traction, tenotomy of contracted muscles, and any one of several innominate osteotomy procedures designed to construct an acetabular roof, often combined with proximal femoral osteotomy, are usually required. After cast removal, range-of-motion exercises help restore movement. Successful reduction and reconstruction become increasingly difficult after the age of 4 years and are usually impossible or inadvisable in children older than 6 years of age because of severe shortening and contracture of muscles and deformity of the femoral and acetabular structures.

Nursing Care Management

Nurses are in a unique position to detect DDH in early infancy. During the infant assessment process and routine nurturing activities, the hips and extremities are inspected for any deviations from normal. These observations are reported to the attending practitioner, and an ambulatory child who displays a limp or an unusual gait should be referred for evaluation. This may indicate an orthopedic or neurologic problem. Nonambulatory children with cerebral palsy should also be assessed for evidence of hip problems.

The major nursing problems in the care of an infant or child in a cast or other device are related to maintenance of the device and adaptation of nurturing activities to meet the patient's needs. Generally, treatment and follow-up care of these children are carried out in an outpatient setting.

! NURSING ALERT

The former practice of double or triple diapering for DDH is not recommended because there is no evidence to support its efficacy.

The primary nursing goal is teaching parents to apply and maintain the reduction device. The Pavlik harness allows for easy handling of the infant and usually produces less apprehension in the parent than heavy braces and casts. Because of infants' rapid growth, the straps should be checked in the beginning of therapy and every 1 to 2 weeks for adjustments (Hart, Albright, Rebello, and others, 2006). It is important that parents understand the correct use of the appliance, which may or may not allow for its removal during bathing. Removing the harness is determined individually on the basis of the provider's recommendation, the family's level of understanding, and the degree of hip deformity. Parents are instructed to not adjust the harness. The child should be examined by the practitioner before any adjustment is attempted to make certain the hips are in correct placement.

Skin care is an important aspect of the care of an infant in a harness. The following instructions for preventing skin breakdown are stressed:

- Always put an undershirt (or a shirt with extensions that close at the crotch) under the chest straps and put knee socks under the foot and leg pieces to prevent the straps from rubbing the skin.
- Check frequently (at least two or three times a day) for red areas under the straps and the clothing.
- Gently massage healthy skin under the straps once a day to stimulate circulation. In general, avoid lotions and powders because they can cake and irritate the skin.
- Always place the diaper under the straps.

Parents are encouraged to hold the infant with a harness and continue care and nurturing activities. The nurse can assist by being available for parents' questions about the necessary adaptations to daily care to decrease the parents' anxiety and possible feelings about the child being hurt by routine caring.

Casts and orthotic devices (braces) offer more challenging nursing and caregiver problems because they cannot be removed for routine care, although sometimes a brace may be removed for bathing. Care of an infant or small child with a cast requires nursing innovation to reduce irritation and to maintain cleanliness of both the child and the cast, particularly in the diaper area. (See p. 1060 for care of the child in a cast.)

It is important for nurses, parents, and other caregivers to understand that children in corrective devices need to be involved in all of the activities of any child in the same age group. Confinement in a cast or appliance should not exclude children from family (or unit) activities. They can be held astride the lap for comfort and transported to areas of activity. The child may be allowed to walk in a cast or orthotic device. An adapted wheelchair, stroller, or scooter can offer mobility to an older infant or child.

CLUBFOOT

Clubfoot is a complex deformity of the ankle and foot that includes forefoot adduction, midfoot supination, hindfoot varus, and ankle equinus. Deformities of the foot and ankle are described according to the position of the ankle and foot. The more common positions involve the following variations:

Talipes varus—An inversion, or bending inward

Talipes valgus—An eversion, or bending outward

Talipes equinus—Plantar flexion, in which the toes are lower than the heel

Talipes calcaneus—Dorsiflexion, in which the toes are higher than the heel

Talipes equinovarus—Toes lower than the heel and facing inward

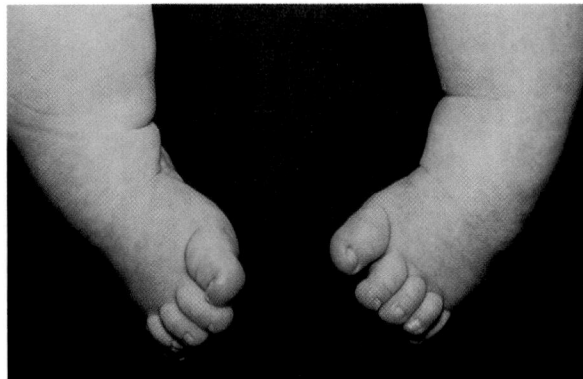

FIG 31-16 Bilateral congenital talipes equinovarus (congenital clubfoot) in a 2-month-old infant. (From Zitelli BJ, McIntire SC, Nowalk AJ: *Zitelli and Davis' atlas of pediatric physical diagnosis*, ed 6, St. Louis, 2012, Saunders.)

Most cases of clubfoot are a combination of these positions, and the most frequently occurring type of clubfoot (≈95% of cases) is the composite deformity talipes equinovarus (TEV), in which the foot is pointed downward (plantar flexed) and inward in varying degrees of severity (Fig. 31-16). Clubfoot may occur as an isolated deformity or in association with other disorders or syndromes, such as chromosomal abnormalities, arthrogryposis, cerebral palsy, or spina bifida.

The incidence of clubfoot in the general population is approximately 1 per 1000 live births, with boys affected twice as often as girls. Bilateral clubfeet occur in 50% of the cases (Hosalkar, Spiegel, and Davidson, 2011). The precise cause of clubfoot is unknown. Some authorities attribute the defect to abnormal positioning and restricted movement in utero, although the evidence is not conclusive. Other experts implicate arrested or abnormal embryonic development. Whereas arrested development during this early stage tends to result in a rigid deformity, mechanical pressures from intrauterine positioning are likely causes of more flexible deformities (Shyy, Wang, Sheffield, and others, 2010).

Classification

Clubfoot may be further divided into three categories: (1) positional clubfoot (also called transitional, mild, or postural clubfoot), which is believed to occur primarily from intrauterine crowding and responds to simple stretching and casting; (2) syndromic (or teratologic) clubfoot, which is associated with other congenital anomalies such as myelomeningocele or arthrogryposis and is a more severe form of clubfoot that is often resistant to treatment; and (3) congenital clubfoot, also referred to as idiopathic, which may occur in an otherwise normal child and has a wide range of rigidity and prognosis.

The mild, or postural, clubfoot may correct spontaneously or may require passive exercise or serial casting. There is no bony abnormality, but there may be tightness and shortening of the soft tissues medially and posteriorly. The teratologic clubfoot usually requires surgical correction and has a high incidence of recurrence. The congenital idiopathic clubfoot, or "true clubfoot," almost always requires surgical intervention because there is bony abnormality.

Diagnostic Evaluation

The deformity is readily apparent and easily detected prenatally through ultrasonography or at birth. However, it must be differentiated from some positional deformities that can be passively corrected or overcorrected. Paralytic changes in the lower extremity of children

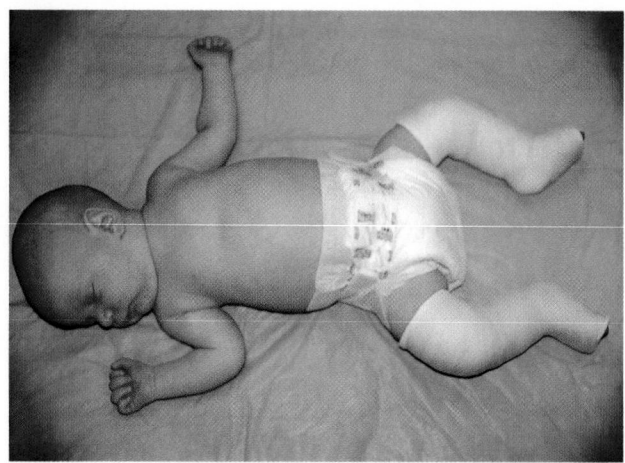

FIG 31-17 Feet casted for correction of bilateral talipes equinovarus.

with neuromuscular involvement often produce equinovarus deformity. An increased risk of hip dysplasia is associated with clubfoot deformities.

Therapeutic Management

The goal of treatment for clubfoot is to achieve a painless, plantigrade, and stable foot. Treatment of clubfoot involves three stages: (1) correction of the deformity, (2) maintenance of the correction until normal muscle balance is regained, and (3) follow-up observation to avert possible recurrence of the deformity. Some feet respond to treatment readily; some respond only to prolonged, vigorous, and sustained efforts; and the improvement in others remains disappointing even with maximal effort on the part of all concerned.

A common approach to clubfoot management is the Ponseti method (Ponseti, 1996). Serial casting is begun shortly after birth. Weekly gentle manipulation and serial long-leg casts allow for gradual repositioning of the foot (Fig. 31-17). The extremity or extremities are casted until maximum correction is achieved, usually within 6 to 10 weeks. The majority of the time, a percutaneous heel cord tenotomy is performed at the end of the serial casting to correct the equinus. After the tenotomy, a long-leg cast is applied and left in place for 3 weeks. A Denis Browne bar with Ponseti sandals or straight-laced shoes placed in abduction are then fitted to prevent recurrence. Inability to achieve normal foot alignment after casting and tenotomy indicates the need for surgical intervention.

Nursing Care Management

Nursing care of the child with clubfoot is the same as for any child who has a cast (see p. 1060). Because the child will spend considerable time in a corrective device, nursing care plans include both long- and short-term goals. Conscientious observation of the skin and circulation is particularly important in young infants because of their rapid growth rate. Because treatment and follow-up care are handled in the orthopedist's office, clinic, or outpatient department, parent education and support are important in nursing care of these children.

It is important for parents to understand the overall treatment program, the importance of regular cast changes, and the role they play in the long-term effectiveness of the therapy. Reinforcing and clarifying the orthopedist's explanations and instructions, teaching parents about care of the cast or appliance (including vigilant observation for potential problems), and encouraging parents to facilitate

normal development within the limitations imposed by the deformity or therapy are all part of nursing responsibilities.

METATARSUS ADDUCTUS (VARUS)

Metatarsus adductus, or metatarsus varus, is probably the most common congenital foot deformity. In most instances, it is a result of abnormal intrauterine positioning, particularly in a firstborn child, and is usually detected at birth. The deformity is characterized by medial adduction of the toes and forefoot, frequently in association with inversion, and by convexity of the lateral border of the foot. Metatarsus adductus may be divided into three categories: type I, in which the forefoot is flexible and corrects easily with manipulation; type II, in which there is only partial flexibility in the forefoot and it corrects passively past neutral position but only to neutral position with active manipulation; and type III, in which the forefoot is rigid and will not stretch to neutral position with manipulation. Unlike TEV, with which it is often confused, the angulation occurs at the tarsometatarsal joint, but the heel and ankle remain in a neutral position. Ankle range of motion is normal. This deformity often causes a pigeon-toed gait in the child.

Management depends on the rigidity and type of the deformity. With types I and II, correction can usually be accomplished by gentle manipulation and passive stretching of the foot, which the parent is taught to perform. Repeated and consistent stretching is continued for the first 6 weeks, after which the treatment is based on the flexibility of the foot. With type III, the child usually requires serial manipulation and casting to correct the defect. Casting is performed every 1 to 2 weeks for 6 to 8 weeks, after which a corrective shoe or orthosis may be used. Surgical correction is rarely required for the condition but may be performed in children 4 to 6 years of age who have considerable pain on ambulation or an inability to wear certain kinds of shoes as a result of the defect (Hosalkar, Spiegel, and Davidson, 2011).

Nursing Care Management

The nursing role primarily involves identifying the defect so that early therapy and instruction of the parents can be initiated. The nurse teaches the parents how to hold the heel firmly and to stretch only the forefoot; otherwise, undue force on the heel may produce a valgus deformity. If casting or an orthosis is required, the nurse instructs the parents in cast care and observation of the corrective device (see p. 1060).

SKELETAL LIMB DEFICIENCY

Congenital limb deficiencies, or reduction malformations, are manifested by a variety of degrees of loss of functional capacity. They are characterized by underdevelopment of skeletal elements of the extremities. The range of malformation can extend from minor defects of the digits to serious abnormalities, such as amelia, absence of an entire extremity; or meromelia, partial absence of an extremity, which includes phocomelia (seal limbs), the interposed deficiency of long bones with relatively good development of hands and feet attached at or near the shoulder or the hips. Most reduction defects are primary defects of development of the limb, but prenatal destruction of the limb can occur, such as full or partial amputation of a limb in utero from constriction of an amniotic band (amniotic band syndrome). Neonates with congenital limb deficiencies often have associated malformations and should be thoroughly investigated for cardiovascular, central nervous system (CNS), renal, and digestive abnormalities (Stoll, Alembik, Dott, and others, 2010).

Pathophysiology

Limb deficiencies can be attributed to both heredity and environment and can originate at any stage of limb development. Formation of limbs may be suppressed at the time of limb bud formation, or there may be interference in later stages of differentiation and growth. Heredity appears to play a prominent role, and prenatal environmental insults have been implicated in a number of cases, such as the well-publicized thalidomide tragedy of the 1950s and early 1960s, which demonstrated a clear relationship between the time of exposure of the pregnant woman to the antiemetic drug and the presence and type of limb deformity in the newborn. There still are many drugs that may have similar teratogenic effects in the first trimester of pregnancy; therefore, medication administration during this period should be carefully evaluated by the practitioner. Deletion or shortening of digits or limbs may also be associated with chorionic villus sampling, especially before 10 to 12 weeks of gestation; however, the incidence and relationship remain uncertain.

Therapeutic Management

Children with congenital limb deficiencies should be fitted with prosthetic devices, and the devices should be applied at the earliest possible stage of development in an attempt to match the infant's motor readiness. This favors natural progression of prosthetic use. For example, an infant with an upper extremity deficiency is fitted with a simple passive device, such as a mitten prosthesis, to encourage limb exploration, sitting (with the extremities needed for support), and bilateral hand activities.

Lower limb prostheses are applied when the infant begins sitting up and can maintain balance. In preparation for prosthetic devices, surgical modification may be necessary to ensure the most favorable use of the device because severe deformity can interfere with its effective use. Phocomelic digits are preserved for controlling switches of externally powered appliances in the upper extremities. Digits (in both the upper and lower extremities) provide the child with surfaces for tactile exploration and stimulation. Prostheses are replaced to accommodate the child's growth and increasing capabilities.

Nursing Care Management

Prosthetic application training and habilitation are most successfully carried out in a center that specializes in meeting the special needs of these children, especially very young children and those with amputations or missing limbs. Management involves a prosthetist, who specializes in the development, fitting, and maintenance of prosthetic limbs, and other health care workers such as physical and occupational therapists. Parents need special attention and support and are encouraged to assist the child in making age-commensurate adjustments to the environment. Although these children need assistance, overprotection may produce overdependence, with later maladjustment to school and other situations.

OSTEOGENESIS IMPERFECTA

Osteogenesis imperfecta is the most common osteoporosis syndrome in childhood. However, it is very rare. OI is a heterogeneous, autosomal dominant disorder characterized by fractures and bone deformity. There are at least eight described types of OI, which accounts for significant disease variability. Clinical features may include varying degrees of bone fragility, deformity, and fracture; blue sclerae; hearing loss; and dentinogenesis imperfecta (hypoplastic discolored teeth). Although inheritance follows an autosomal dominant pattern in most cases, rare autosomal recessive inheritance exists primarily

---

BOX 31-6   CLASSIFICATION OF OSTEOGENESIS IMPERFECTA

Type I*
  A—Mild bone fragility; blue sclerae; normal teeth; hearing loss (occurs between ages 20 and 30 years); autosomal dominant inheritance
  B—Same as A except dentinogenesis imperfecta instead of normal teeth
  C—Same as B but no bone fragility
Type II—Lethal; stillborn or die in early infancy; severe bone fragility, multiple fractures at birth; 10% of cases of OI; autosomal recessive inheritance
Type III—Severe bone fragility leading to severe progressive deformities; normal sclerae; marked growth failure; most autosomal recessive inheritance; few autosomal dominant inheritance
Type IV
  A—Mild to moderate bone fragility; normal sclerae; normal teeth; short stature; variable deformity; autosomal dominant inheritance
  B—Same as A except dentinogenesis imperfecta instead of normal teeth; approximately 6% of cases of OI
Type V—Clinically similar to type IV; hyperplastic callus; collagen mutation is negative
Type VI—Sclerae and dentition normal; moderate to severe bone fragility; diagnosis by bone biopsy because of similarities to other types; only identified in eight persons to date (Land, Rauch, Travers, and others, 2007)
Types VII and VIII (recessive form)—Clinically overlap types II and III but have white sclerae, rhizomelia, and small to normal head circumference; severe osteochondroplasia and short stature in survivors (Marini, 2011)

OI, Osteogenesis imperfecta.
*Two thirds of cases are type I.

---

in populations with consanguineous marriages (Marini, 2011) (Box 31-6).

Most types of OI have defects in the *COL1A1* or *COL1A2* genes, which code for polypeptide chains in type 1 procollagen, a precursor of type 1 collagen, a major structural component of bone. The error results in faulty bone mineralization, abnormal bone architecture, and increased susceptibility to fracture.

Osteogenesis imperfecta has several classifications based on clinical features and patterns of inheritance (see Box 31-6). Clinically, type I is the most common, with wide variability of bone fragility; some affected family members have significant deformity and disability, but others lead agile, active lives. Type II variants are the most severe and are considered lethal in infancy. Type III OI is characterized by multiple fractures, bone deformity, and severe disability, including scoliosis and vertebral compression; affected individuals rarely live to 30 years of age. Growth failure and short stature are common. Type IV is similar to type I with blue or white sclerae. Another variant, or type V, has been described in which those affected have a hyperplastic callus, a radiodense metaphyseal band, and calcification of the interosseous membrane of the forearm; no collagen mutations are noted in this group (Marini, 2011). A type VI has been described with a characteristic mineralization defect, which does not respond to pamidronate therapy as do types I to V (Land, Rauch, Travers, and others, 2007). Children affected with this type have no dental involvement and normal sclerae; a bone biopsy is the only way to establish a diagnosis because of the similarities to other types. Types VII and VIII overlap types II and III in relation to clinical features, but those types who survive have white sclerae, a normal to small head circumference, short stature, and rhizomelia (Marini, 2011).

Therapeutic Management

The treatment for OI is primarily supportive, although patients and families are optimistic about new research advances. The use of bisphosphonate therapy with IV pamidronate to promote increased bone density and prevent fractures has become standard therapy for many children with OI; however, long bones are weakened by prolonged treatment. One of the advantages of bisphosphonate therapy is the decrease in vertebral compression and scoliosis (Marini, 2011).

The goals of a rehabilitative approach to management are directed toward preventing (1) positional contractures and deformities, (2) muscle weakness and osteoporosis, and (3) malalignment of lower extremity joints prohibiting weight bearing.

Lightweight braces and splints help support limbs, prevent fractures, and aid in ambulation. Physical therapy helps prevent disuse osteoporosis and strengthens muscles, which in turn improves bone density.

Surgery is sometimes used to help treat the manifestations of the disease. Surgical techniques are used to correct deformities that interfere with bracing, standing, or walking. For a child with recurrent fractures, inserting an intramedullary rod provides stability to bones.

Nursing Care Management

Infants and children with this disorder require careful handling to prevent fractures. They must be supported when they are being turned, positioned, moved, and held. Even changing a diaper may cause a fracture in severely affected infants. These children should never be held by the ankles when being diapered but should be gently lifted by the buttocks or supported with pillows.

Both parents and the affected child need education regarding the child's limitations and guidelines in planning suitable activities that promote optimal development and protect the child from harm. Realistic occupational planning and genetic counseling are part of the long-term goals of care. Educational materials and information can be obtained from the Osteogenesis Imperfecta Foundation,* which also has a network that can put a family in contact with other families with a similar problem.

Osteogenesis imperfecta is a differential diagnosis that must be ruled out in the event of multiple fractures that could be attributed to nonaccidental injury (child abuse). A detailed history, no evidence of associated soft-tissue injury, and the presence of other symptoms related to OI help to determine the diagnosis.

> **! NURSING ALERT**
>
> Children with multiple fractures should be screened for OI. The possibility that nonaccidental trauma is the cause of fractures in children must be carefully evaluated by a multidisciplinary team.

ACQUIRED DEFECTS

LEGG-CALVÉ-PERTHES DISEASE

Legg-Calvé-Perthes disease, sometimes called *coxa plana* or *osteochondritis deformans juvenilis*, is a self-limiting disorder in which there is aseptic necrosis of the femoral head. The disease affects children ages 2 to 12 years, but most cases occur in boys between 4 and 8 years of age as an isolated event. In approximately 10% of cases, the involvement is bilateral; most of the affected children have a skeletal age

*804 W. Diamond Ave., Suite 210, Gaithersburg, MD 20878; 800-981-2663; http://www.oif.org.

> **BOX 31-7 RADIOGRAPHIC STAGES OF LEGG-CALVÉ-PERTHES DISEASE**
>
> **Stage I: Initial,** or **avascular, stage**—Aseptic necrosis or infarction of the femoral capital epiphysis with degenerative changes producing flattening of the upper surface of the femoral head
>
> **Stage II: Fragmentation,** or **revascularization, stage**—Capital bone resorption and revascularization with fragmentation (vascular resorption of the epiphysis) that gives a mottled appearance on radiographs
>
> **Stage III: Reossification,** or **reparative, stage**—New bone formation, which is represented on radiographs as calcification and ossification or increased density in the areas of radiolucency; this filling-in process appears to take place from the periphery of the head centrally
>
> **Stage IV: Residual,** or **regenerative, stage**—Gradual reformation of the head of the femur without radiolucency and, it is hoped, to a spherical form

significantly below their chronologic age (Sankar, Horn, Wells, and others, 2011b). The male-to-female ratio is 4:1 or 5:1. White children are affected 10 times more frequently than African-American children.

Pathophysiology

The cause of the disease is unknown, but a disturbance of circulation to the femoral capital epiphysis produces an ischemic aseptic necrosis of the femoral head. During middle childhood, circulation to the femoral epiphysis is more tenuous than at other ages and can become obstructed by trauma, inflammation, coagulation defects, and a variety of other causes. The pathologic events seem to take place in four stages (Box 31-7). The entire process may encompass as little as 18 months or continue for several years. The reformed femoral head may be severely altered or appear entirely normal.

Clinical Manifestations and Diagnostic Evaluation

The onset of Legg-Calvé-Perthes disease is usually insidious, and the history may reveal only intermittent appearance of a limp on the affected side or a symptom complex, including hip soreness, ache, or stiffness, which can be constant or intermittent. The parents may report seeing the child limping, and the limp becomes more pronounced with increased activity. The pain may be experienced in the hip, along the entire thigh, or in the vicinity of the knee joint. The pain and limp are usually most evident on arising and at the end of a long day of activities. The pain is usually accompanied by joint dysfunction and limited range of motion. There may be a vague history of trauma. The diagnosis is established by history, examination, radiographs, and rarely, MRI.

Therapeutic Management

Because deformity occurs early in the disease process, the aims of treatment are to eliminate hip instability; restore and maintain adequate range of hip motion; prevent capital femoral epiphyseal collapse, extrusion, or subluxation; and ensure a well-rounded femoral head at the time of healing. Treatment varies according to the child's age at the time of diagnosis and the appearance of the femoral head vasculature and position within the acetabulum. Nonsurgical containment of the femoral head may be accomplished with abduction casts, immobilization, and NSAIDs, and a pelvic or proximal femoral osteotomy may be used to contain the femoral head. Activity causes microfractures of the soft ischemic epiphysis, which tend to induce synovitis, stiffness, and adductor contracture. The initial therapy is rest and non–weight bearing, which helps reduce inflammation and restore motion. Later, active motion is encouraged. In some cases, traction is applied to stretch tight adductor muscles.

Containment can be accomplished in several ways. One is the use of non–weight-bearing devices, such as an abduction brace (e.g., Atlanta Scottish Rite orthosis), leg casts, or a leather harness sling, which prevent weight bearing on the affected limb. Another includes the use of various weight-bearing appliances, such as abduction-ambulation braces or casts after a period of bed rest and traction. A third option consists of surgical reconstruction and containment procedures. Conservative therapy must be continued for 2 to 4 years, although braces constructed from lightweight materials allow the child to maintain a nearly normal activity level. Surgical correction, although subjecting the child to additional risks (e.g., from anesthesia, infection, blood transfusion), returns the child to normal activities in 3 to 4 months. The use of home traction has also been explored.

Another surgical option is total hip resurfacing; in this procedure the hip joint is replaced with a metal cup in the acetabulum that interfaces with a capped bearing located on the femoral head. Hip resurfacing decreases the risk of dislocation and is more bone conserving than hip arthroplasty (Costa, Johnson, Naziri, and others, 2011).

The disease is self-limiting, but the ultimate outcome of therapy depends on early and efficient treatment and the child's age at the onset of the disorder. Younger children (5 years and younger), whose epiphyses are more cartilaginous, have the best prognosis for complete recovery. Children 10 years and older have a significant risk for degenerative arthritis, especially with femoral head deformity at the time of diagnosis. The later the diagnosis is made, the more femoral damage will have occurred before treatment is implemented. In most cases, with good patient compliance with the prescribed regimen, the prognosis is excellent.

Nursing Care Management

Nurses may be the first health professionals to identify affected children and to refer them for medical evaluation. They are also persons on whom the child and the family can rely to help them understand and adjust to the therapeutic measures. Because most of the child's care is conducted on an outpatient basis, the major emphasis of nursing care is teaching the family the care and management of the corrective appliance selected for therapy. The family needs to learn the purpose, function, application, and care of the corrective device and the importance of compliance to achieve the desired outcome (see Family-Centered Care box).

One of the most difficult aspects associated with the disorder is coping with a normally active child who feels well but must remain relatively inactive during periods when non–weight bearing is required. Suitable activities must be devised to meet the needs of a child in the process of developing a sense of initiative or industry. Activities that meet the creative urges are well received.

SLIPPED CAPITAL FEMORAL EPIPHYSIS

Slipped capital femoral epiphysis (SCFE) refers to the spontaneous displacement of the proximal femoral epiphysis in a posterior and inferior direction. It develops most frequently shortly before or during accelerated growth and the onset of puberty (children between the ages of 9 and 16 years; median age, 13 years for boys and 12 years for girls) and is most frequently observed in boys and obese children. The incidence is 11 cases per 100,000 children. Bilateral involvement occurs in up to 60% of cases (Lehmann, Aarons, Loder, and others, 2006; Sankar, Horn, Wells, and others, 2011c).

FAMILY-CENTERED CARE
Legg-Calvé-Perthes Disease

A family with five healthy children was one day startled to learn that their 2-year-old son could no longer walk. He was diagnosed with Legg-Calvé-Perthes disease. Through several years of prosthetic devices and numerous physician visits, hospitalizations, and surgeries, this family turned a potentially devastating experience into one with cherished memories.

Today, the parents reflect on how their family coped with the reality of a debilitating disease. It was difficult for the parents to observe an eager, energetic child watch other children riding bicycles, running, or playing outdoor games. They are warmed by memories of watching their other children make the difference for their sibling. They all developed a strong bond through caring and sharing with one another. Coping as a family was an easy adjustment and, most of all, therapeutic. Today, more than 20 years later, the parents believe that each family member has grown with feelings of faith and trust. The experience proved to them that life will go on and that life is what you make it!

Shona Swenson Lenss, MS, RN, FNP
Cheyenne, Wyo.

BOX 31-8   CLINICAL MANIFESTATIONS OF SLIPPED CAPITAL FEMORAL EPIPHYSIS

Very often obese (body mass index >95%)
Limp on affected side
Possible inability to bear weight because of severe pain
Pain in groin, thigh, or knee
 • May be acute, chronic, or acute-on-chronic
 • Continuous or intermittent
Affected leg is externally rotated
Loss of abduction and internal rotation as severity increases
Shortening of lower extremity

Pathophysiology

Most cases of SCFE are idiopathic, although it can be associated with endocrine disorders, growth hormone therapy, renal osteodystrophy, and radiotherapy. The cause of idiopathic SCFE is multifactorial and includes obesity, physeal architecture and orientation, and pubertal hormone changes that affect physeal strength. Although obesity stresses the physeal plate, SCFE can also occur in children who are not obese. Radiographs show medial displacement of the epiphysis and uncovered upper portion of the femoral neck adjacent to the physis. There is a widened growth plate and irregular metaphysis. The capital femoral epiphysis remains in the acetabulum, but the femoral neck slips, deforming the femoral head and stretching blood vessels to the epiphysis.

Diagnostic Evaluation

The disorder is suspected when an adolescent or preadolescent displays clinical signs or complains of hip, groin, thigh, or knee pain (Box 31-8). The diagnosis is confirmed by anteroposterior and frog-leg radiographic examination that reflects a change in position of the proximal femoral epiphysis.

Therapeutic Management

The treatment goals of SCFE are to (1) prevent further slipping until physeal closure, (2) avoid further complication such as avascular necrosis, and (3) maintain adequate hip function (Loder, 2006; Sankar, Horn, Wells, and others, 2011c). After the diagnosis has been established, the child should be non–weight bearing to prevent further slippage. Some surgeons prefer to take the child to surgery within 24 hours of the onset of acute symptoms and avoid further risk for avascular necrosis (Loder, 2006). Surgical treatment varies with the degree of displacement. Surgical pinning in situ involves the placement of a single pin or multiple pins and screws through the femoral neck into the proximal femoral epiphysis to prevent further slippage. An osteotomy for deformity is seldom needed in the acute setting. Hip arthroscopy performed before in situ pinning has been shown to be effective in decreasing hip pain and allowing early hip movement in some children with SCFE (Jayakumar, Ramachandran, Youm, and others, 2012). Postsurgical care includes non–weight bearing with crutch ambulation until acceptable, painless range of motion is achieved. SCFE is an emergency and requires early diagnosis and treatment to increase the likelihood of an acceptable outcome.

Nursing Care Management

Nursing care is the same as that for a child in a cast or in traction, as discussed earlier in this chapter. Postoperative care involves hemodynamic stabilization and assessment for complications.

> **! NURSING ALERT**
>
> Children with hip issues such as Legg-Calvé-Perthes or SCFE often present with groin, thigh, or knee pain. This is often because of referred pain and is anatomically related to the obturator nerve. Any time a child presents with groin, thigh, or knee pain, a complete hip examination is paramount to rule out underlying hip pathology.

KYPHOSIS AND LORDOSIS

The spine, consisting of numerous segments, can acquire deformity curves of three types: kyphosis, lordosis, and scoliosis (Fig. 31-18). Kyphosis is an abnormally increased lateral angulation in the convex curvature of the spine (see Fig. 31-18, *B*). It can occur secondary to disease processes such as tuberculosis (TB), chronic arthritis, osteodystrophy, or compression fractures of the thoracic spine. The most common form of kyphosis is postural. Children, especially during the time when skeletal growth outpaces growth of muscle, are prone to exaggeration of a normal kyphosis. They assume abnormal sitting and standing positions. Scheuermann kyphosis is a thoracic curve greater than 45 degrees with wedging greater than 5 degrees of at least three adjacent vertebral bodies and vertebral irregularity.

Postural (flexible) kyphosis is almost always accompanied by a compensatory postural lordosis, an abnormally exaggerated concave lumbar curvature. Treatment of kyphosis consists of exercises to strengthen shoulder and abdominal muscles and bracing for more marked deformity. With adolescents, who are self-conscious about their appearance, the best approach is to emphasize the cosmetic value of corrective therapy and to place the responsibility on the adolescent for carrying out an exercise program at home with regular visits to and assessments by a therapist. Treatment with a brace may be indicated until skeletal maturity, and surgical fusion may be considered for severe, painful, or progressive thoracic curves such as Scheuermann kyphosis.

Lordosis is an accentuation of the cervical or lumbar curvature beyond physiologic limits (see Fig. 31-18, *C*). It may be a secondary complication of a disease process, a result of trauma, or idiopathic. It is often seen in association with flexion contractures of the hip, scoliosis, obesity, DDH, and SCFE. During the pubertal growth spurt, lordosis of varying degrees is observed in teenagers, especially girls. In obese children, the weight of the abdominal fat alters the center of gravity, causing a compensatory lordosis. Unlike kyphosis, severe lordosis is usually accompanied by pain.

Treatment involves management of the predisposing cause when possible, such as weight loss and correction of deformities. Postural exercises or support garments are helpful in relieving symptoms in some cases; however, these do not usually effect a permanent cure.

IDIOPATHIC SCOLIOSIS

Idiopathic scoliosis is a complex spinal deformity in three planes, usually involving lateral curvature, spinal rotation causing rib

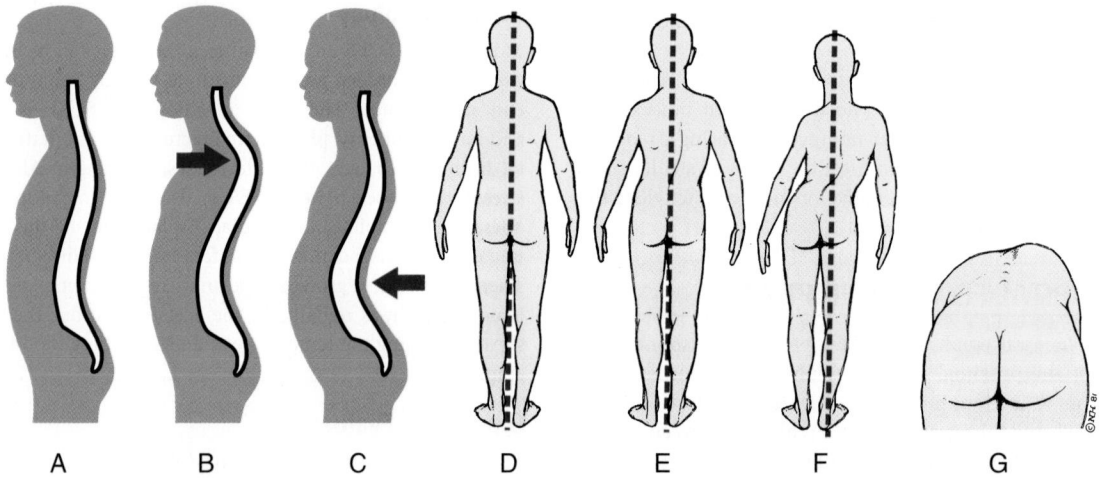

FIG 31-18 Defects of spinal column. **A,** Normal spine. **B,** Kyphosis. **C,** Lordosis. **D,** Normal spine in balance. **E,** Mild scoliosis in balance. **F,** Severe scoliosis not in balance. **G,** Rib hump and flank asymmetry seen in flexion caused by rotary component. (Redrawn from Hilt NE, Schmitt EW: *Pediatric orthopedic nursing*, St. Louis, 1975, Mosby.)

Animation—Spine Structure

asymmetry, and thoracic hypokyphosis. It is the most common spinal deformity and can be further classified according to age of onset: infantile, at birth or up to 3 years of age; childhood or juvenile, which develops during childhood (4–10 years); or, most commonly, adolescent (diagnosed at age 10 years or later), which develops during the growth spurt of early adolescence.

Scoliosis can be caused by a number of conditions and may occur alone or in association with other diseases, particularly neuromuscular conditions. In most cases, however, there is no apparent cause, hence the name idiopathic scoliosis. There appears to be a genetic component to the etiology of idiopathic scoliosis; however, the exact relationship has yet to be established. The following section is limited to a discussion of adolescent idiopathic scoliosis.

Idiopathic scoliosis is most noticeable during the preadolescent growth spurt. Parents frequently bring a child for follow-up on an abnormal school scoliosis screening or because of ill-fitting clothes, such as poorly fitting slacks. School screening is somewhat controversial because no controlled studies have demonstrated improved outcomes, and a reported number of false-positive results leads to referrals. The American Academy of Orthopaedic Surgeons and the AAP published a joint statement favoring scoliosis screening for preadolescents and adolescents either in the school, physician's office, or nurses' clinic (Richards and Vitale, 2008). According to the American Academy of Orthopaedic Surgeons (Richards and Vitale, 2008), girls should be screened at ages 10 and 12 years, and boys should be screened once either at age 13 or 14 years. The benefits of early detection, referral, and medical treatment are considered to be significant, but the persons performing the screenings must be educated in the detection of spinal deformity.

Diagnostic Evaluation

Observation is performed behind an undressed (in undergarments), standing child, noting shoulder height, scapular or flank shape, and hip height and alignment. When the child bends forward at the waist (the Adams forward bend test) with hanging arms, asymmetry of the ribs and flanks may be noted. A scoliometer is also used in the initial screening to measure the angle of truncal rotation. Often a primary curve and a compensatory curve will place the head in alignment with the gluteal cleft. However, in the uncompensated curve, the head and hips are not aligned (see Fig. 31-18, E and F). (See Spine, Chapter 6, for additional information.) Definitive diagnosis is made by radiographs of the child in the standing position and use of the Cobb technique that establishes the degree of curvature. The Risser

scale is used to evaluate skeletal maturity on the radiographs; the scale assists in making a determination of the likely progression of the spinal angulature based on growth potential. Radiographic curves need to be measured at least 10 degrees for diagnosis. Curves of less than 25 degrees are mild and require observation during growth (Newton and Wenger, 2005).

> ## ! NURSING ALERT
>
> Intraspinal conditions or other disease processes that can cause scoliosis must be ruled out. The presence of pain, sacral dimpling or hairy patches, cutaneous vascular changes, absent or abnormal reflexes, bowel or bladder incontinence, or left thoracic curve may indicate an intraspinal abnormality such as syringomyelia, diastematomyelia, or tethered cord syndrome. An MRI scan should be obtained for evaluation.

Therapeutic Management

Current management options include observation with regular clinical and radiographic evaluation, orthotic intervention (bracing), and surgical spinal fusion. Treatment decisions are based on the magnitude, location, and type of curve; the child's age and skeletal maturity; and any underlying or contributing disease process.

Bracing and Exercise

For many curves in growing children and adolescents, bracing may be the treatment of choice. It is important to understand that bracing is not curative but that it may slow the progression of the curvature to allow skeletal growth and maturity. The two most common types of bracing are (1) the Boston and Wilmington braces, which are underarm orthoses customized from prefabricated plastic shells, with corrective forces for each patient using lateral pads and decreasing lumbar lordosis, and (2) a TLSO (thoracolumbosacral orthosis), which is an underarm orthosis made of plastic that is custom molded to the body and then shaped to correct or hold the deformity (Fig. 31-19). The Milwaukee brace, or CTLSO, which is an individually adapted brace that includes a neck ring, is rarely used in scoliosis but is sometimes used in the treatment of kyphosis. The Charleston nighttime bending brace is worn only when the child is in bed because it prevents walking because of the severity of the trunk bend. Compliance in wearing the brace is difficult because of the child's age and preoccupation with body image and appearance. Bracing is the standard treatment for moderate curvatures in growing children (Sponseller, 2011).

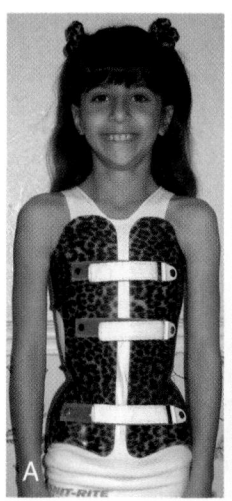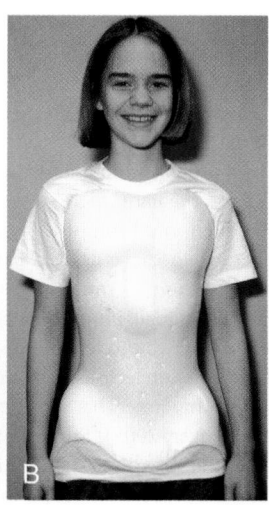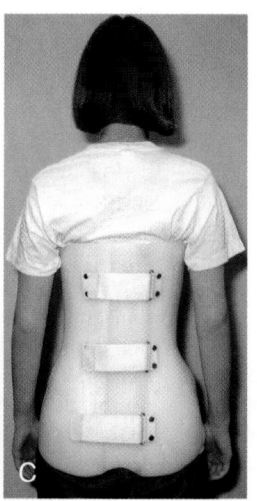

FIG 31-19 A, Standard thoracolumbosacral orthotic (TLSO) brace for idiopathic scoliosis. The brace may be decorated to make it more acceptable to adolescents. **B,** Variation of a standard TLSO brace that fastens in the back to provide needed support. **C,** Posterior view of the same brace.

Exercises, transcutaneous electrical stimulation, and chiropractic treatment are rarely of value for managing scoliosis. Exercises are of benefit when used in conjunction with bracing to maintain and strengthen spinal and abdominal muscles during treatment.

Surgical Management

Surgical intervention may be required for treatment of severe curves, which are typically greater than 45 degrees. The degree of curvature, its behavior, the etiology, and symptoms guide the decision for surgery. Bracing is ineffective in managing curves greater than 45 degrees. Progressive curves that do not respond to bracing and progressive congenital and neuromuscular curves require surgical intervention.

The surgical technique of a spinal fusion consists of realignment with internal fixation and instrumentation combined with bony fusion (arthrodesis) of the realigned spine. Bone from the iliac crest or donor bone is used to fuse the spine. The goals of surgical intervention are to improve the curvatures on the sagittal and coronal planes and to have a solid, pain-free fusion in a well-balanced torso, with maximum mobility of the remaining spinal segments. Surgical approaches may be posterior, anterior, or both.

Many instrumentation systems are available, including Dwyer, Zielke, Luque, Cotrel-Dubousset, Isola, TSRH (Texas Scottish Rite Hospital), and Moss Miami. Selection of the system is individualized according to the patient's needs and surgeon's preference. Combinations of rods, hooks, wires, and pedicle screws may be used.

The Luque-rod segmental spinal instrumentation provides segmental stability with the use of wires and L-shaped rods. By way of a posterior approach, the wires are threaded beneath the lamina of each vertebra and tightened around the rods resting along the transverse processes to stabilize the spine. The advantage of this method is that the patient can be mobile within a few days and requires no postoperative immobilization. A higher risk of nerve damage has been reported.

The Cotrel-Dubousset instrumentation is a newer generation of spinal instrumentation and implements bilateral rods and hooks at many sites. Anterior approaches using the Dwyer or Zielke instrumentation involve screws into the vertebral bodies connected by a cable or rod. These systems require postoperative immobilization with a custom-fitted plastic jacket.

Nursing Care Management

Treatment for scoliosis extends over a significant portion of the affected child's period of growth. In adolescents, this period is the one in which their identity, both physical and psychologic, is formed. The identification of scoliosis as a "deformity," in combination with unattractive appliances and a significant surgical procedure, can have a negative effect on the already fragile adolescent body image. The adolescent and family require excellent nursing care not only for physical needs to be met but also for psychologic needs associated with the diagnosis, surgery, postoperative recovery, and eventual rehabilitation. Although adolescents with scoliosis are encouraged to participate in most peer activities, necessary therapeutic modifications are likely to make them feel different and apart. Nursing care of the adolescent who is facing scoliosis surgery, potential social isolation, pain, and uncertainty, in addition to misunderstood emotions and body image issues, must be evaluated from the adolescent's perspective to be successful in meeting the individual's needs (Napierkowski, 2007).

When a child or adolescent first faces the prospect of a prolonged period in a brace or other device, the therapy program and the nature of the device must be explained thoroughly to both the child and the parents so they will understand the anticipated results, how the appliance corrects the defect, the freedoms and constraints imposed by the device, and what they can do to help achieve the desired goal.

Management involves the skills and services of a team of specialists, including the orthopedist, neurosurgeon, physical therapist, orthotist (a specialist in fitting orthopedic braces), nurse, social worker, and sometimes a thoracic or pulmonary specialist.

It is difficult for a child or adolescent to be restricted at any phase of development, but adolescents need continual positive reinforcement, encouragement, and as much independence as can be safely assumed during this time. Adolescents appreciate guidance and assistance regarding anticipated problems, such as selection of clothing and participation in social activities. Socialization with peers is strongly encouraged, and every effort is expended to help the adolescent feel attractive and worthwhile.

Preoperative Care

The preoperative workup usually involves a radiographic series, including bending and traction films, pulmonary function studies, and laboratory studies (including prothrombin, partial thromboplastin, and platelet function test; blood count; electrolyte levels; urinalysis and urine culture; and blood levels of any medications). Because spinal surgery usually involves considerable blood loss, several options are considered preoperatively to maintain or replace blood volume. These options include autologous blood donations obtained from the patient before the surgery; intraoperative blood salvage; intraoperative hemodilution; erythropoietin administration; and controlled induced hypotension, which must be carefully monitored at all times to prevent physiologic instability (Newton and Wenger, 2005).

Surgery for spinal fusion is complex, and often adolescents who require the procedure because of idiopathic scoliosis are not familiar with medical terms, procedures, or experiences. Preoperative teaching is critical for the adolescent to be able to cooperate and participate in his or her treatment and recovery. Because the surgery is extensive, the patient is taught how to manage his or her own patient-controlled analgesia (PCA) pump; how to log roll; and the use and function of other equipment, such as a chest tube (for anterior repair) and Foley catheter. It is recommended that the child or adolescent bring a favorite toy (age dependent) or personal items such as a favorite stuffed animal, laptop computer (with Internet access), cell phone or iPod, or movie player, for postoperative use. Meeting with a peer who has undergone a similar surgery may also be valuable. Parents should be informed that the child's appearance after surgery may be quite different; prone positioning for the length of the surgery and fluid shifting may cause considerable edema.

Postoperative Care

After surgery, patients are monitored in an acute care setting and log rolled when changing position to prevent damage to the fusion and instrumentation. Skin care is important, and pressure-relieving mattresses or beds may be needed to prevent pressure wounds (see Maintaining Healthy Skin, Chapter 22).

In addition to the usual postoperative assessments of wound, circulation, and vital signs, the neurologic status of the patient's extremities requires special attention. Prompt recognition of any neurologic impairment is imperative because delayed paralysis may develop that requires surgical intervention. Common postoperative problems after spinal fusion include neurologic injury or spinal cord injury, hypotension from acute blood loss, wound infection, syndrome of inappropriate antidiuretic hormone, atelectasis, pneumothorax, ileus, delayed neurologic injury, and implanted hardware complications (Freeman, 2007; Newton and Wenger, 2005). Superior mesenteric artery syndrome may occur several days after spinal surgery; this involves duodenal compression by the aorta and superior mesenteric artery and may result in acute partial or complete duodenal obstruction. Clinical manifestations include epigastric pain, nausea, copious vomiting, and eructation; symptoms are aggravated in the supine position and often relieved with the patient in a left lateral decubitus or prone position.

The child usually has considerable pain for the first few days after surgery and requires frequent administration of pain medication, preferably IV opioids administered on a regular schedule. For children able to understand the concept, PCA is recommended (see Pain Assessment; Pain Management, Chapter 7).

In most cases, the patient begins ambulation as soon as possible, depending on the instrumentation used—generally by the second or third postoperative day. The patient is discharged by 1 week, depending on the surgical approach. In addition to pain management, the patient is evaluated for skin integrity, adequate urinary output, fluid and electrolyte balance, and ileus. Discharge planning should include a timetable for follow-up with the practitioner and resumption of regular activities.

The patient may start physical therapy as soon as he or she is able, beginning with range-of-motion exercises on the first postoperative day and many of the activities of daily living in the following days. Self-care, such as washing and eating, is always encouraged. Throughout the hospitalization, age-appropriate activities and contact with family and friends are important parts of nursing care and planning (see Immobilization, p. 1051).

The family is encouraged to become involved in the patient's care to facilitate the transition from hospital to home management. An organization that provides education and services to both families and professionals is the National Scoliosis Foundation.* The American Academy of Orthopaedic Surgeons† and Scoliosis Research Society,‡ an organization of physicians and scientists, have published an excellent book, *Scoliosis*, and the Scoliosis Research Society has educational information available on its website.

INFECTIONS OF BONES AND JOINTS

OSTEOMYELITIS

Osteomyelitis, an infectious process in the bone, can occur at any age but most frequently is seen in children 10 years of age or younger. Boys are more commonly affected than girls, and the median age of diagnosis is 5 to 6 years of age. The limbs most commonly affected include the foot, femur, tibia, and pelvis. It is estimated that 1 in 5000 children younger than the age of 13 years is diagnosed each year with this condition (Zaoutis, Localio, Leckerman, and others, 2009). *Staphylococcus aureus* is the most common causative organism. Neonates are also likely to have osteomyelitis caused by group B streptococci. Children with sickle cell disease may develop osteomyelitis from *Salmonella* organisms as well as *S. aureus*. *Neisseria gonorrhoeae* is a potential causative organism in sexually active adolescents. *Kingella kingae* has been reported as one of the most causative organisms in children younger than age 5 years (Kaplan, 2011a).

Acute hematogenous osteomyelitis results when a bloodborne bacterium causes an infection in the bone. Common foci include infected lesions, upper respiratory tract infections, otitis media, tonsillitis, abscessed teeth, pyelonephritis, and infected burns. **Exogenous osteomyelitis** is acquired from direct inoculation of the bone from a puncture wound, open fracture, surgical contamination, or adjacent

---

*5 Cabot Place, Stoughton, MA 02072; 800-673-6922; http://www.scoliosis.org.
†6300 N. River Road, Rosemont, IL 60018-4262; 847-823-7186; http://www.aaos.org.
‡555 E. Wells St., Suite 1100, Milwaukee, WI 53202; 414-289-9107; http://www.srs.org/about/contact.

BOX 31-9   CLINICAL MANIFESTATIONS OF ACUTE OSTEOMYELITIS

General Manifestations
Possible history of trauma to affected bone
Child appears very ill
Irritability
Restlessness
Elevated temperature
Rapid pulse
Dehydration

Local Manifestations
Tenderness
Increased warmth
Diffuse swelling over involved bone
Involved extremity painful, especially on movement
Involved extremity held in semiflexion
Surrounding muscles tense and resistant to passive movement

---

tissue infection. **Subacute osteomyelitis** has a longer course and may be caused by less virulent microbes with a walled-off abscess or **Brodie abscess,** typically in the proximal or distal tibia. **Chronic osteomyelitis** is a progression of acute osteomyelitis and is characterized by dead bone, bone loss, and drainage and sinus tracts.

Generally, healthy bone is not likely to become infected. Factors that contribute to infection include inoculation with a large number of organisms, presence of a foreign body, bone injury, high virulence of an organism, immunosuppression, and malnutrition; certain types and locations of bone are also more vulnerable to infection.

Typically, children with acute hematogenous osteomyelitis are seen with a 2- to 7-day history of pain, warmth, tenderness, and decreased range of motion in the affected limb along with systemic symptoms of fever, irritability, and lethargy (Box 31-9). Infants may have an adjacent joint effusion as well. Symptoms often resemble those observed in other conditions involving bones such as arthritis, leukemia, or sarcoma.

Pathophysiology

In acute osteomyelitis, bacteria adhere to bone, causing a suppurative infection with inflammatory cells, edema, vascular congestion, and small-vessel thrombosis; the result is bone destruction, abscess formation, and dead bone (sequestra). Infection within the bone can rupture through the cortex into the subperiosteal space, stripping loose periosteum and forming an abscess. As dead bone is resorbed, new bone is formed along the live bone and infection borders. This surrounding sheath of live bone is called an **involucrum**. Sinus tracts from perforations in the involucrum may drain pus through soft tissue to the skin.

The pathology of osteomyelitis is different in infants, children older than 1 year of age, and adults. In infants, blood vessels cross the growth plate into the epiphysis and joint space, which allows infection to spread into the joint. In children, the infection is contained by the growth plate, and joint infection is less likely (unless the infection is intracapsular). In older adolescents (with a closed growth plate), the infection is poorly contained and the joint is compromised. Adult periosteum is attached to bone; consequently, rupture through the periosteum and sinus drainage is more common in adults.

Diagnostic Evaluation

Organism identification and antibiotic susceptibility testing are essential for effective therapy. Cultures of aspirated purulent drainage

Animation—Osteomyelitis

Case Study—Osteomyelitis

along with cultures of blood, joint fluid, and infected skin samples should be obtained. Bone biopsy is indicated if blood culture results and radiographic findings are not consistent with osteomyelitis. Supporting evidence for osteomyelitis includes leukocytosis and elevated erythrocyte sedimentation rate (ESR) and C-reactive protein (CRP). Radiographic signs, except for soft-tissue swelling, are evident only after 2 to 3 weeks. A three-phase technetium bone scan can show areas of increased blood flow, such as occurs in early stages in infected bone, and is useful in locating multiple sites; however, it is not a diagnostic test. CT can detect bone destruction, and MRI provides anatomic details useful in delineating the area of involvement, especially if surgical intervention is planned. MRI is reported to be the most sensitive diagnostic radiologic tool for diagnosing osteomyelitis (Kaplan, 2011a). Sometimes the osteomyelitis may be unrecognized if it occurs as a complication of a severe toxic and debilitating disease. Neonates may not present with clinical manifestations other than limited mobility of the affected extremity; fever may or may not be present, and the neonate may not appear to be sick (Kaplan, 2011a).

Therapeutic Management

After culture specimens are obtained, empiric therapy is started with IV antibiotics covering the mostly likely organisms. For *S. aureus*, nafcillin or clindamycin is generally used. Consideration should be given to the increased rates of community-acquired methicillin-resistant *S. aureus* (MRSA) in the selection of first-line antibiotic therapy; MRSA may require vancomycin, or in some cases, clindamycin may be appropriate. In one study, children with MRSA osteomyelitis had an increased length of hospitalization, longer antibiotic course, and a greater number of complications (Saavedra-Lozano, Mejías, Ahmad, and others, 2008). When the infectious agent is identified, administration of the appropriate antibiotic is initiated and continued for at least 3 to 4 weeks, but the length of therapy is determined by the duration of the symptoms, the response to treatment, and the sensitivity of the organism; 6 weeks to 4 months may be required in some cases (Kaplan, 2011a). In selected cases, oral antibiotic therapy may follow the IV treatment. Because of the prolonged duration of high-dose antibiotic therapy, it is important to monitor for hematologic, renal, hepatic, ototoxic, and other potential side effects. To prevent antibiotic-associated diarrhea in some children, administration of a probiotic may be considered.

Surgery may be indicated if there is no response to specific antibiotic therapy, a penetrating injury, persistent soft-tissue abscess is seen, or the infection spreads to the joint. Opinions differ regarding surgical intervention, but many advocate sequestrectomy and surgical drainage to decompress the metaphyseal space before purulent fluid erupts and spreads to the subperiosteal space, forming abscesses that strip the periosteum from bone or form draining sinuses. When these complications occur, a chronic infection usually persists, which may require antibiotic therapy for several months.

Nursing Care Management

During the acute phase of illness, movement of the affected limb will cause discomfort; therefore, the child is positioned comfortably with the affected limb supported. A temporary splint or cast may be applied. Weight bearing is avoided in the acute phase, and moving and turning are carried out carefully to minimize pain. The child may require long-term pain medication to deal with the bone pain. Postoperatively, pain medication should be considered as with any other surgical procedure.

Antibiotic therapy requires careful observation and monitoring of the IV equipment and site. A peripherally inserted central catheter (PICC) may be inserted for long-term antibiotic therapy. Antibiotic therapy is often continued at home or through an outpatient infusion clinic.

Standard precautions are implemented for all children with osteomyelitis. If there is an open wound, it is managed according to standard wound care precautions. If a PICC line or central venous catheter (CVC) is inserted, meticulous care should be taken to prevent catheter-related infection. One study reported a high number of catheter-related complications in children discharged on IV antibiotics and a CVC (Ruebner, Keren, Coffin, and others, 2006).

Provision of diversional and constructive activities becomes an important nursing intervention. Children are usually confined to bed for some time during the acute phase but may be allowed to move about on a stretcher or in a wheelchair if isolation is not necessary.

As the infection subsides, physical therapy is instituted to ensure restoration of optimum function. The child may eventually be transitioned to a regimen of oral antibiotics, and progress is followed closely for some time.

SEPTIC ARTHRITIS

Septic arthritis is a bacterial infection in the joint. It usually results from hematogenous spread or from direct extension of an adjacent cellulitis or osteomyelitis. Direct inoculation from trauma accounts for 15% to 20% of septic arthritis cases. The most common causative organism is *S. aureus*. Community-acquired MRSA is commonly a cause of septic arthritis. In addition to *S. aureus*, pathogens seen in neonates include group B streptococci, *Escherichia coli*, and *Candida albicans*. In children 2 months to 5 years of age, *S. aureus*, *Streptococcus pyogenes*, *Streptococcus pneumoniae*, and *K. kingae* are the primary organisms causing infection. Children older than 5 years are more likely to be infected by *S. aureus* and *S. pyogenes*, and sexually active adolescents may be infected by *N. gonorrhoeae* (Gutierrez, 2005; Kaplan, 2011b).

The knees, hips, ankles, and elbows are the most common joints affected. Clinical manifestations include severe joint pain, swelling, warmth of overlying tissue, and occasionally erythema. An infection involving the hip, however, is considered a surgical emergency to prevent compromised blood supply to the head of the femur (Kaplan, 2011b).

The child is resistant to any joint movement. Features of systemic illness such as fever, malaise, headache, nausea, vomiting, and irritability may also be present.

Therapeutic Management and Nursing Care Management

The affected joint is aspirated and the specimen evaluated by Gram stain, cultures (including separate cultures for *H. influenzae* and *N. gonorrhoeae*), and determination of leukocyte count. In addition, perform blood cultures and obtain complete blood count with differential and ESR or CRP level. Early radiographic findings are limited to soft-tissue swelling but may reveal a foreign body, and such films always provide a baseline for comparison. Technetium scans reveal areas of increased blood flow but will not differentiate between sites. MRI and CT scans provide more detailed images of cartilage loss, joint narrowing, erosions, and ankylosis of progressive disease. Ultrasonography is helpful in the detection of joint effusions and fluid in the soft tissue and subperiosteum (Kaplan, 2011b).

Treatment is IV antibiotic therapy based on Gram stain results and the clinical presentation. The benefits of serial aspirations to demonstrate sterility of synovium fluid and reduce pressure or pain are controversial. Pain management is an important aspect of nursing care, particularly with involvement of a large joint such as the hip. Surgical intervention may also be required if there was a penetrating wound or a foreign object was possibly involved. Physical therapy may be initiated for the child who is immobilized to prevent flexion contractures. Additional nursing care is the same as for osteomyelitis.

SKELETAL TUBERCULOSIS

In children, tubercular infection of the bones and joints is acquired by lymphohematogenous spread at the time of primary infection. Occasionally, it is from chronic pulmonary tuberculosis. Skeletal tubercular infection is not common in the United States but should be considered in communities with high TB case rates. The condition is a late manifestation of TB and is most likely to involve the vertebrae, causing tubercular spondylitis. If the infection is progressive, it causes Pott disease with destruction of the vertebral bodies and results in kyphosis and spinal malalignment. Symptoms are insidious. The child may report persistent or intermittent pain. Other findings include joint swelling and stiffness; fever and weight loss are not common. Tubercular arthritis can also affect single joints such as a knee or hip and tends to cause severe destruction of adjacent bone. Infection in the fingers causes spina ventosa, a tuberculous dactylitis.

As with pulmonary tuberculosis, the index case should be located. A family and environmental history needs to be obtained and tuberculin skin tests (TSTs) performed. Results of TSTs are positive for the majority of children with tuberculous arthritis; however, the results are not diagnostic, and the clinical and laboratory features do not differentiate tubercular arthritis from a nontubercular septic arthritis. Diagnosis requires isolation of *Mycobacterium tuberculosis* from the site. Patients with the susceptible organism start treatment with combined antituberculosis chemotherapy (isoniazid, rifampin, and pyrazinamide); directly observed therapy (DOT) is preferred. (See also Chapter 23.)

Nursing Care Management

Nursing care depends on the site and extent of infection. Tuberculous spondylitis and hip infection may require immobilization, casting, and surgical fusion. Nursing care is individualized but is generally the same as for osteomyelitis and septic arthritis.

▎ BONE AND SOFT-TISSUE TUMORS

GENERAL CONCEPTS: BONE TUMORS

Bone tumors account for about 6% of all malignant neoplasms in children. Approximately 90% of all primary malignant bone tumors in children are either osteogenic sarcoma or Ewing sarcoma; osteosarcoma, the most common, occurs in 56% of all cases. The peak age for pediatric bone tumors is 15 years, and they occur more often in boys.

Most malignant bone tumors produce localized pain in the affected site, which may be severe or dull and may be attributed to trauma or the vague complaint of "growing pains." The pain is often relieved by a flexed position, which relaxes the muscles overlying the stretched periosteum. Frequently, it draws attention when the child limps, curtails physical activity, or is unable to hold heavy objects (Box 31-10). A palpable mass is also a common manifestation of bone tumors, but systemic symptoms such as fever and other clinical symptoms such as spinal cord compression and respiratory distress are more frequent in patients with Ewing sarcoma.

BOX 31-10   CLINICAL MANIFESTATIONS OF BONE TUMORS

Pain localized at affected site
- May be severe or dull
- Often relieved by position of flexion

Frequently brought to attention when child:
- Limps
- Curtails own physical activity
- Is unable to hold heavy objects

Diagnostic Evaluation

Diagnosis begins with a thorough history and physical examination. A primary objective is to rule out causes such as trauma or infection. Careful questioning regarding pain is essential in attempting to determine the duration and rate of tumor growth. Physical assessment focuses on functional status of the affected area; signs of inflammation; size of the mass; and any systemic indication of generalized malignancy, such as anemia, weight loss, and frequent infection.

Definitive diagnosis is based on radiologic studies, such as plain films and CT or MRI of the primary site, CT of the chest, and radioisotope bone scans to evaluate metastasis and bone marrow examination in patients with Ewing sarcoma. A needle or surgical biopsy is necessary to establish the diagnosis. Ewing sarcoma most commonly involves the pelvis, long bones of the lower extremities, and chest wall, and radiographically involves the diaphysis with detachment of the periosteum from the bone (Codman triangle). In osteosarcoma, lesions are most commonly located in the metaphyseal region of the bone, often involving the long bones. Radial ossification in the soft tissue gives the tumor a "sunburst" appearance on plain radiograph.

OSTEOSARCOMA

Osteosarcoma (osteogenic sarcoma) is the most common bone cancer in children and most commonly affects patients in the second decade of life during their growth spurt. It presumably arises from bone-forming mesenchyme, which gives rise to malignant osteoid tissue. Most primary tumor sites are in the diametaphyseal region (wider part of the shaft, adjacent to the epiphyseal growth plate) of long bones, especially in the lower extremities. More than half occur in the femur, particularly the distal portion, with the rest involving the humerus, tibia, pelvis, jaw, and phalanges.

Therapeutic Management

Optimum treatment of osteosarcoma includes surgery and chemotherapy. The surgical approach consists of surgical biopsy followed by either limb salvage or amputation. To ensure local control, all gross and microscopic tumors must be resected. A limb salvage procedure involves en bloc resection of the primary tumor with prosthetic replacement of the involved bone. For example, with osteosarcoma of the distal femur, a total femur and joint replacement is performed. Frequently, children undergoing a limb salvage procedure receive preoperative chemotherapy in an attempt to decrease the tumor size and make surgery more manageable (Gorlick, Bielack, Teot, and others, 2011; Lanzkowsky, 2005).

Chemotherapy plays a vital role in treatment of osteosarcoma. Antineoplastic drugs, such as high-dose methotrexate with citrovorum factor rescue, doxorubicin, cisplatin, ifosfamide, and etoposide, may be administered singly or in combination and may be used both before or after surgical resection of the tumor. The use of postoperative chemotherapy after amputation has comparable results to trials using preoperative chemotherapy followed by limb salvage surgery. Preoperative chemotherapy allows for examination of the surgical specimen at the time of definitive surgery, which predicts clinical outcome. When pulmonary metastases are found, thoracotomy and chemotherapy have resulted in prolonged survival and potential cure. These combined-modality approaches have significantly improved the prognosis in osteosarcoma to approximately 78% for nonmetastatic patients (Lanzkowsky, 2005). Ongoing trials are evaluating the use of biologic agents such as muramyl tripeptide phosphatidylethanolamine to eradicate micrometastases by stimulating macrophages to kill tumor cells not eliminated by chemotherapy (Lanzkowsky, 2005).

Nursing Care Management

Nursing care depends on the type of surgical approach. Obviously, the family may have more difficulty adjusting to an amputation than a limb salvage procedure. In either instance, preparation of the child and family is critical. Straightforward honesty is essential in gaining the child's cooperation and trust. The diagnosis of cancer should not be disguised with falsehoods such as "infection." To accept the need for radical surgery, the child must be aware of the lack of alternatives for treatment. Although the responsibility of telling the child is generally left to the physician, the nurse should be present at the discussion or be aware of exactly what is said. The child should be told a few days before surgery to allow him or her time to think about the diagnosis and consequent treatment and to ask questions. (See Nursing Care Plan: The Child with a Bone Tumor.*)

Sometimes children have many questions about the prosthesis, limitations on physical ability, and prognosis in terms of cure. At other times they react with silence or with a calm manner that belies their concern and fear. Either response must be accepted because it is part of the grieving process of a loss. For those who desire information, it may be helpful to introduce them to another person who has had an amputation before surgery or to show them pictures of the prosthesis.[†] However, the nurse must be careful not to overwhelm children with information. A sound approach is to answer questions without offering additional information. For those who do not pursue additional information, the nurse expresses a willingness to talk.

The child is also informed of the need for chemotherapy and its side effects before surgery. Exercise caution about offering too much information at one time. When discussing hair loss, emphasize positive aspects, such as wearing a wig or hats that are unique. Because bone tumors affect adolescents and young adults, it is not unusual for them to become angry over all of the radical body alterations.

If an amputation is performed, the child is usually fitted with a temporary prosthesis immediately after surgery, which permits early functioning and fosters psychologic adjustment. If this is not done, the child requires stump care, which is the same as for any person with an amputation. A permanent prosthesis is usually fitted within 6 to 8 weeks. During hospitalization, the child begins physical therapy to become proficient in the use and care of the device.

Phantom limb pain may develop after amputation. This symptom is characterized by sensations such as tingling; itching; and, more frequently, pain felt in the amputated limb. The child and family need to know that the sensations are real, not imagined. Amitriptyline (Elavil) has been used successfully in children to decrease the pain. In addition, an epidural is often used preoperatively as a nerve block in an effort to decrease or eliminate the occurrence of phantom limb pain. Much research is needed to further delineate the best care for these patients (Ong, Arneja, and Ong, 2006).

Discharge planning must begin early in the postoperative period. After the child has begun physical therapy, the nurse should consult with the therapist and practitioner to evaluate the child's physical and emotional readiness to reenter school. It is an opportune time to involve a community nurse in the child's home care. Every effort is made to promote normalcy and gradual resumption of realistic preamputation activities.* Role-playing in anticipation of such experiences is beneficial in preparing the child for the inevitable confrontation by others. Environmental barriers, such as stairs, are assessed in terms of the accessibility in the school and home, especially because the child may need to use crutches or a wheelchair before complete healing and prosthetic competency are achieved.

The nurse encourages the child to select clothing that best camouflages the prosthesis, such as pants or long-sleeved shirts. Well-fitted prostheses are so natural looking that girls can usually wear sheer stockings without revealing the device. Emphasizing feminine or masculine apparel helps the child regain a feeling of self-identity. Even during the postoperative period, encouraging the child to wear blue jeans and a T-shirt may distract attention from the deformity and focus it on familiar aspects of appearance.

The family and child need much support in adjusting not only to a life-threatening diagnosis but also to alteration in body form and function. Because loss of a limb entails a grieving process, those caring for the child need to recognize that the reactions of anger and depression are normal and necessary. Often parents view the anger as a direct affront to them for allowing the amputation to occur, or they see the depression as rejection. These are not personal attacks but the child's attempts to cope with a loss.

EWING SARCOMA (PRIMITIVE NEUROECTODERMAL TUMOR)

Ewing sarcomas, or the Ewing sarcoma family of tumors, which includes primitive neuroectodermal tumor of the bone, are the second most common malignant bone tumor (after osteosarcoma) in childhood (Lanzkowsky, 2005). Ewing sarcoma arises in the marrow spaces of the bone rather than from osseous tissue. The tumor originates in the shaft of long and trunk bones, most often affecting the pelvis, femur, tibia, fibula, humerus, ulna, vertebra, scapula, ribs, and skull. It occurs almost exclusively in individuals younger than age 30 years and affects whites much more often than other races.

Therapeutic Management

Limb salvage procedures might be feasible in extremity lesions, and amputation may be considered if the results of radiotherapy render the extremity useless or deformed (e.g., from restricted growth in young children). The treatment of choice for the majority of lesions is involved field radiotherapy and chemotherapy. A widely used drug regimen includes vincristine, doxorubicin, cyclophosphamide alternating with ifosfamide, and etoposide. The addition of ifosfamide and

---

*In Wilson D, Hockenberry MJ: *Wong's clinical manual of pediatric nursing,* ed 8, St. Louis, 2012, Mosby.
[†]Information about prostheses can be obtained from the National Amputation Foundation, 40 Church St., Malverne, NY 11565; 516-887-3600; http://www.nationalamputation.org.

---

*Information about special programs for children with amputations is available from the Candlelighters Childhood Cancer Foundation, 8323 Southwest Freeway, Suite 435, Houston, TX 77074 ; 713-270-4700; http://www.candle.org.

etoposide has increased the 3-year survival rate to 78% for patients with localized disease (Lanzkowsky, 2005).

Nursing Care Management

The psychologic adjustment to Ewing sarcoma is typically less traumatic than it is to osteosarcoma because of the preservation of the affected limb. Many families accept the diagnosis with a sense of relief in knowing that this type of bone cancer does not necessitate amputation, and initially they may not be aware of the damaging effects on the irradiated site. Consequently, they need preparation for the various diagnostic tests, including bone marrow aspiration and surgical biopsy, and adequate explanation of the treatment regimen. High-dose radiotherapy often causes a skin reaction of dry or moist desquamation followed by hyperpigmentation. The child should wear loose-fitting clothes over the irradiated area to minimize additional skin irritation. Because of increased sensitivity, the area should be protected from sunlight and sudden changes in temperature, such as from heating pads or ice packs. Encourage the child to use the extremity as tolerated. Occasionally, the physical therapist may plan an active exercise program to preserve maximum function.

The child needs the same considerations for adjusting to the effects of chemotherapy as any other patient with cancer. The drug regimen usually results in hair loss, severe nausea and vomiting, peripheral neuropathy, and possibly cardiotoxicity. Make every effort to outline a treatment plan that allows the child maximum resumption of a normal lifestyle and activities. (See Nursing Care Plan: The Child with Cancer.*)

RHABDOMYOSARCOMA

Rhabdomyosarcoma (*rhabdo*, striated) is the most common soft-tissue sarcoma in children. Striated (skeletal) muscle is found almost anywhere in the body, so these tumors occur in many sites, the most common of which are the head and neck, especially the orbit. The disease occurs in children in all age groups but is most common in children younger than 5 years of age. Its incidence is approximately 8.5 per 1 million for white children but only 4.0 per 1 million for African-American children in the age group from 2 to 19 years (Lanzkowsky, 2005).

Rhabdomyosarcoma arises from embryonic mesenchyme. Three subtypes are recognized, embryonal, alveolar, and pleomorphic. Soft-tissue sarcomas are the fourth most common type of solid tumors in children. These malignant neoplasms originate from undifferentiated mesenchymal cells in muscles, tendons, bursae, and fascia or in fibrous, connective, lymphatic, or vascular tissue. They derive their name from the specific tissue(s) of origin, such as myosarcoma (*myo*, muscle).

The initial signs and symptoms are related to the site of the tumor and compression of adjacent organs (Table 31-2). Some tumor locations, such as the orbit, manifest early in the course of the illness. Other tumors, such as those of the retroperitoneal area, only produce symptoms when they are relatively large and compress adjacent organs. Unfortunately, many of the signs and symptoms attributable to rhabdomyosarcoma are vague and frequently suggest a common childhood illness, such as "earache" or "runny nose." Rarely, the site of the primary tumor site is never identified.

Diagnostic Evaluation

Diagnosis begins with a careful history and physical examination. Radiographic studies to delineate the primary tumor site should

*In Wilson D, Hockenberry MJ: *Wong's clinical manual of pediatric nursing,* ed 8, St. Louis, 2012, Mosby.

TABLE 31-2	**CLINICAL MANIFESTATIONS OF RHABDOMYOSARCOMA ACCORDING TO TUMOR SITE**
LOCATION	**SIGNS AND SYMPTOMS**
Central nervous system	Headaches
	Morning vomiting
	Diplopia
Orbit	Rapidly developing unilateral proptosis
	Ecchymosis of conjunctiva
	Loss of extraocular movements (strabismus)
Nasopharynx	Stuffy nose (earliest sign)
	Nasal obstruction—dysphagia, nasal voice (obstruction of posterior nasal conches), serous otitis media (obstruction of eustachian tube)
	Pain (sore throat and ear)
	Epistaxis
	Palpable neck nodes
	Visible mass in oropharynx (late sign)
Paranasal sinuses	Nasal obstruction
	Local pain
	Discharge
	Sinusitis
	Swelling
Middle ear	Signs of chronic serous otitis media
	Pain
	Sanguinopurulent drainage
	Facial nerve palsy
Retroperitoneal area (usually a "silent" tumor)	Abdominal mass
	Pain
	Signs of intestinal or genitourinary obstruction
Perineum	Visible superficial mass
	Bowel or bladder dysfunction (from tumor compression)
Extremity	Pain
	Palpable fixed mass
	Regional lymph node enlargement

BOX 31-11	**STAGING OF RHABDOMYOSARCOMA**

Group I—Localized disease; tumor completely resected, and regional nodes not involved
Group II—Localized disease with microscopic residual, or regional disease with no residual or with microscopic residual
Group III—Incomplete resection or biopsy with gross residual disease
Group IV—Metastatic disease present at diagnosis

include CT or MRI. Metastatic evaluation should include a CT of the chest, bone scan, and bilateral bone marrow aspirates and biopsies. For patients with tumors in the parameningeal area, a lumbar puncture should be done to examine the spinal fluid. An excisional biopsy or surgical resection of the tumor, when possible, is done to confirm the diagnosis.

Careful staging is extremely important for planning treatment and determining the prognosis. The Intergroup Rhabdomyosarcoma Study has developed a surgicopathologic staging system, shown in Box 31-11 (Helman, 2011; Lanzkowsky, 2005).

With the use of contemporary multimodal therapy, more than 80% of patients with nonmetastatic disease are expected to survive (Helman, 2011; Lanzkowsky, 2005). If relapse occurs, the prognosis for long-term survival is poor.

Therapeutic Management

All rhabdomyosarcomas are high-grade tumors with the potential for metastases. Therefore, multimodal therapy is recommended for all patients. Complete removal of the primary tumor is advocated whenever possible. However, because the tumor is chemosensitive, radical procedures with high morbidity should be avoided. In the majority of cases, a biopsy is followed by chemotherapy, irradiation, or both. Patients with embryonal tumors and group I disease can be treated with chemotherapy alone, but all others require chemotherapy and radiotherapy. Drugs that are used most often for the treatment of rhabdomyosarcoma include vincristine, actinomycin D, cyclophosphamide (VAC), ifosfamide, topotecan, irinotecan, and doxorubicin, which are administered for about 1 year (Lanzkowsky, 2005).

Nursing Care Management

The nursing responsibilities are similar to those for other types of cancer, especially the solid tumors when surgery is used. Specific objectives include (1) careful assessment for signs of the tumor, especially during well-child examinations; (2) preparation of the child and family for the multiple diagnostic tests; and (3) supportive care during each stage of multimodal therapy.

DISORDERS OF JOINTS

JUVENILE IDIOPATHIC ARTHRITIS (JUVENILE RHEUMATOID ARTHRITIS)

Juvenile idiopathic arthritis (JIA) is the name replacing *juvenile rheumatoid arthritis (JRA)* in the research literature and now in clinical practice. The JRA nomenclature revision to JIA was partly attributable to the minimally applicable reference to "rheumatoid" in JRA. Only a small percentage of children have a positive rheumatoid factor, yet the name burdens the family with images of adult disfiguring rheumatoid arthritis, a distinctly different disease. Furthermore, the JRA classification system focused more on disease at onset versus disease progression, which is more important.

Semantics aside, JIA is a chronic autoimmune inflammatory disease causing inflammation of joints and other tissue with an unknown cause. JIA starts before age 16 years with a peak onset between 1 and 3 years of age. Twice as many girls as boys are affected. The reported incidence of chronic childhood arthritis varies from 1 to 20 cases per 100,000 children with a prevalence of 10 to 400 per 100,000 (Cassidy and Petty, 2011). The cause is unknown, but two factors are hypothesized: immunogenic susceptibility and an environmental or external trigger such as a virus (e.g., rubella, Epstein-Barr virus, parvovirus B19). There are a few known genetic risk factors, including HLA class I and class II genes, the *PTPN22* gene, and the *IL2RA/CD 25* gene; however, the genetic contribution is complicated and still not well understood.

Pathophysiology

The disease process is characterized by chronic inflammation of the synovium with joint effusion and eventual erosion, destruction, and fibrosis of the articular cartilage. Adhesions between joint surfaces and ankylosis of joints occur if the inflammatory process persists.

Clinical Manifestations

The outcome of JIA is variable and unpredictable. The disease, even in severe forms, is rarely life threatening but can cause significant disability. The arthritis tends to wax and wane; however, patterns of clinical remission indicate approximately 25% will obtain clinical remission off medication for a follow-up duration of at least 4 years. Children with arthritis in four or fewer joints had the greatest likelihood for a sustained remission. Children with extensive arthritis and a positive rheumatoid factor were less likely to have a sustained remission (Wallace, Huang, and Bandeira, 2005). Their arthritis can cause significant joint deformity and functional disability, requiring medication, physical therapy, and perhaps future joint replacement. Chronic and acute uveitis can cause permanent vision loss if undiagnosed and not aggressively treated.

Classification of Juvenile Idiopathic Arthritis

Juvenile idiopathic arthritis is not a single disease but a heterogeneous group of diseases. The universal Durban classification of JIA, revised and published in 1998, lists several disease categories, each with its own set of criteria and exclusions, which continue to be revised (Petty, Southwood, Manners, and others, 2004):

Systemic arthritis is arthritis in one or more joints associated with at least 2 weeks of quotidian fever, rash, lymphadenopathy, hepatosplenomegaly, and serositis.

Oligoarthritis is arthritis in one to four joints for the first 6 months of disease. It is subdivided to *persistent oligoarthritis* if it remains in four joints or fewer or becomes *extended oligoarthritis* if it involves more than four joints after 6 months.

Polyarthritis rheumatoid factor negative affects five or more joints in the first 6 months with a negative rheumatoid factor.

Polyarthritis rheumatoid factor positive also affects five or more joints in first 6 months, but these children have a positive rheumatoid factor.

Psoriatic arthritis is arthritis with psoriasis or an associated dactylitis, nail pitting, or onycholysis or psoriasis in a first-degree relative.

Enthesitis-related arthritis is arthritis or enthesitis associated with at least two of the following: sacroiliac or lumbosacral pain, HLA-B27 antigen, arthritis in a boy older than 6 years, acute anterior uveitis, inflammatory bowel disease, Reiter syndrome, or acute anterior uveitis in a first-degree relative.

Undifferentiated arthritis fits no other category above or fits more than one category.

Diagnostic Evaluation

Juvenile idiopathic arthritis is a diagnosis of exclusion; there are no definitive tests. Classifications are based on the clinical criteria of age of onset before age 16 years, arthritis in one or more joints for 6 weeks or longer, and exclusion of other causes. Laboratory tests may provide supporting evidence of disease. The ESR may or may not be elevated. Leukocytosis is frequently present during exacerbations of systemic JIA. Antinuclear antibodies are common in JIA but are not specific for arthritis; however, they help identify children who are at greater risk for uveitis. Plain radiographs are the best initial imaging studies and may show soft-tissue swelling and joint space widening from increased synovial fluid in the joint. Later films can reveal osteoporosis, narrow joint space, erosions, subluxation, and ankylosis. A slit lamp eye examination is necessary to diagnose uveitis, inflammation in the anterior chamber of the eye, which is most common in antinuclear antibody–positive young girls with oligoarthritis. Routine examinations are necessary for early diagnosis and treatment to avoid or minimize sight-threatening disease (Qian and Acharya, 2010).

Therapeutic Management

There is no cure for JIA. The major goals of therapy are to control pain, preserve joint range of motion and function, minimize effects of inflammation such as joint deformity, and promote normal growth and development. Outpatient care is the mainstay of therapy; lengthy hospitalizations are infrequent in this era of managed care. The treatment plan can be exhaustive and intrusive for the child and family, including medications, physical and occupational therapy, ophthalmologic slit lamp examinations, splints, comfort measures, dietary management, school modifications, and psychosocial support.

Medications

Many arthritis medications are available, and most are effective in suppressing the inflammatory process and relieving pain. These drugs may be given alone or in combination and are prescribed in a stepwise manner dependent on arthritis severity.

Nonsteroidal antiinflammatory drugs are the first drugs used. Naproxen, ibuprofen, tolmetin, indomethacin, celecoxib, meloxicam, and aspirin are approved for use in children. They are effective with few common side effects other than gastrointestinal irritation and bruising; with naproxen, skin fragility is a possible side effect. NSAIDs must be taken with food. Aspirin, once the drug of choice, has been replaced by other NSAIDs because they have fewer side effects and easier administration schedules.

Methotrexate is the second-line medication used in children who have failed with NSAIDs alone. It is started in combination with an NSAID. It is effective, with acceptable toxicity, which requires monitoring of complete blood cell counts and liver functions. Patient education about possible side effects, including discussions with teens about birth defects and avoiding alcohol, is essential.

Corticosteroids are potent immunosuppressives used for life-threatening complications, incapacitating arthritis, and uveitis. They are administered at the lowest effective dosage for the briefest period and discontinued on a tapering schedule. They may be administered orally, as intraarticular joint injections, as IV infusions, or in eye drop form for uveitis. A single intraarticular injection may provide effective relief for children with pauciarticular disease unresponsive to NSAIDs. Prolonged use of systemic steroids is associated with significant side effects, including Cushing syndrome, osteoporosis, increased infection risk, glucose intolerance, cataracts, and growth suppression.

Biologic agents that work by several mechanisms to interrupt and minimize the inflammatory process are used in children with severe or progressive arthritis. Biologic agents may be used in combination with methotrexate. The Food and Drug Administration (FDA) has approved etanercept, adalimumab and abatacept use in children with JIA. Etanercept is a tumor necrosis factor-α (TNF-α) receptor blocker and an effective drug for children with JIA unresponsive to methotrexate (Lovell, Giannini, Reiff, and others, 2003). It is given once or twice a week via subcutaneous injections. The long-term safety and efficacy of etanercept have been confirmed (Giannini, Ilowite, Lovell, and others, 2009). Adalimumab is a monoclonal antibody that also inhibits TNF, thereby reducing inflammation; it is a subcutaneous injection given every 2 weeks (Lovell, Ruperto, and Goodman, 2008). Abatacept reduces inflammation by inhibiting T cells and is given intravenously every 4 weeks. Possible side effects of biologics include an increased infection risk, rare reports of demyelinating disease and pancytopenia, and allergic reactions. Because of the infection risk, children should be evaluated for TB exposure before starting these medications. Live vaccines should be avoided while taking these agents. There is a reported potential increased risk of malignancy with anti-TNF agents etanercept, adalimumab, and infliximab (FDA, 2009). Parents and patients should be informed that biologic drugs are new therapies, and more will be learned about potential side effects in the postmarketing period.

Physical and Occupational Therapy

Programs of physical management are individualized for each child and designed to reach the ultimate goal: preserving function or preventing deformity. Physical therapy is directed toward specific joints, focusing on strengthening muscles, mobilizing restricted joint motion, and preventing or correcting deformities. Occupational therapy assumes responsibility for generalized mobility and performance of activities of daily living.

General treatment or maintenance programs vary; physical therapists may be involved several times weekly to monthly in management of a home program, or their visits may be limited to infrequent review of the home program for compliance, effectiveness, and need. Normal activities of daily living and the child's natural tendency to be active are usually sufficient to maintain muscle strength and joint mobility.

Exercising in a pool is excellent therapy because it allows freedom of movement with support and minimal gravitational pull. If there is pain on motion, a hot pack or warm bath before therapy may help.

Practitioners may recommend nighttime splinting to help minimize pain and reduce flexion deformity. Joints most frequently splinted are the knees, wrists, and hands. Loss of extension in the knee, hip, and wrist causes special problems and requires vigilance to detect the earliest signs of involvement and vigorous attention to prevent deformity with specialized passive stretching, positioning, and resting splints.

Nursing Care Management

⊝ Nursing the child with JIA involves assessment of the child's general health, the status of involved joints, and the child's emotional response to all ramifications of the disease—discomfort, physical restrictions, therapies, and self-concept.

The effects of JIA are manifest in every aspect of the child's life, including physical activities, social experiences, and personality development. Nursing interventions to support the parents may foster successful adaptation for the entire family. Parental concerns about the disease prognosis, financial and insurance issues, spouse and sibling relationships, and job and schedule conflicts must all be addressed. Referral to social workers, counselors, or support groups may be needed.

Relieve Pain

The pain of JIA is related to several aspects of the disease, including disease severity, functional status, individual pain threshold, family variables, and psychologic adjustment. The aim is to provide as much relief as possible with medication and other therapies to help children tolerate the pain and cope as effectively as possible. Nonpharmacologic modalities such as behavioral therapy and relaxation techniques have proved effective in modifying pain perception (see Pain Management, Chapter 7) and activities that aggravate pain. Opioid analgesics are typically avoided in juvenile arthritis; however, for children immobilized with refractory pain, short-term opioid analgesics can be part of a comprehensive plan that uses multiple pain relief techniques (Connelly and Schanberg, 2006).

Promote General Health

The child's general health must be considered. A well-balanced diet with sufficient calories to maintain growth is essential. If the child is relatively inactive, caloric intake needs to match energy needs to avoid excessive weight gain, which places additional stress on affected joints.

Sleep and rest are essential for children with JIA. Some children require rest during the day; however, daytime napping that interferes with nighttime sleepiness should be avoided. A bedtime routine that involves comfort measures can help induce sleep. A firm mattress, electric blanket, or sleeping bag helps provide warmth, comfort, and rest. Nighttime splints needed to maintain range of motion might initially be a source of bedtime conflict. The family needs to be instructed on how to use the splint appropriately; the splint should not be painful or impede sleep. Behavior modification programs that reward splint and exercise compliance may be helpful in reducing adherence barriers. Well-child care to assess growth, development, and immunization requirements needs to be coordinated between the primary care provider and the rheumatologist. Common childhood illnesses, such as upper respiratory tract infections, may cause arthritis to worsen; consequently, medical attention must be sought quickly for relatively minor illness to prevent arthritis flares. Effective communication among the family, the primary care provider, and the rheumatology team is essential for care coordination.

Children are encouraged to attend school even on days when they have some pain or discomfort. The school nurse's assistance is enlisted so that a child is permitted to take the prescribed medication at school and to arrange for rest in the nurse's office during the day. Split days or half days may help a child remain involved in school. Permitting the child to come to school late allows time to gain joint movement and reduces the time at school to avoid exhaustion. It is important that the child attend school to learn skills and engage in social interaction, especially if the JIA continues to limit physical skills. Arranging for two sets of textbooks eliminates the need to carry books to and from school, thus reducing discomfort and difficulty walking. A formal school hearing may be necessary to obtain an Individualized Education Program, ensured by public law, which includes intensive school modifications.

Facilitate Adherence

The child and family are involved in the therapeutic plan. They need to know the purpose and correct use of any splints and appliances and the medication regimen. The family is instructed regarding administration of medications and the value of a regular schedule of administration to maintain a satisfactory drug level in the body. They need to know that NSAIDs should not be given on an empty stomach and to be alert for signs of medication toxicity. If evidence of drug toxicity is noted, the family is instructed to notify the health professional and follow that person's instructions.

Encourage Heat and Exercise

Heat has been shown to be beneficial to children with arthritis. Moist heat is best for relieving pain and stiffness, and the most efficient and practical method is in the bathtub with warm water. In some cases, a daily whirlpool bath, paraffin bath, or hot packs may be used as needed for temporary relief of acute swelling and pain. Hot packs are easily applied using a bath towel wrung out after being immersed in hot water or heated in a microwave oven, applied to the area, and covered with plastic for 20 minutes. Commercial pads that warm in only a few minutes in the microwave are also available. Painful hands or feet can be immersed in a pan of warm water for 10 minutes two or three times daily in addition to tub baths.

Pool therapy is the easiest method for exercising a large number of joints. Swimming activities strengthen muscles and maintain mobility in larger joints. Very small children who are frightened of the water can carry out their exercises in the bathtub. Small children love to splash, kick, and throw things in the water. Remember, adult supervision is necessary for all water activities.

Activities of daily living provide satisfactory exercise for older children to maintain maximal mobility with minimal pain. These children are encouraged in their efforts to be independent and patiently allowed to dress and groom themselves, to assume daily tasks, and to care for their belongings. It is often difficult for children to manipulate buttons, comb or brush their hair, and turn faucets, but unless there is an acute flare, parents and other caregivers should not offer assistance. In addition, children should learn and understand why others do not help them. Many helpful devices, such as self-adhering fasteners, tongs for manipulating difficult items, and grab bars installed in bathrooms for safety, can be used to facilitate tasks. A raised (higher) toilet seat often makes the difference between dependent and independent toileting because weak quadriceps muscles and sore knees inhibit the ability to raise the body from a low sitting position.

A child's natural affinity for play offers many opportunities for incorporating therapeutic exercises. Throwing or kicking a ball and riding a tricycle (with the seat raised to achieve maximum leg extension) are excellent moving and stretching exercises for a very young child whose daily living activities are physically limited.

An effective approach to beginning the day's activities is to awaken children early to give them their medication and then to allow them to sleep for an hour. On arising, children take a hot bath (or shower) and perform a simple ritual of limbering-up exercises, after which they commence the activities of the day, such as going to school. Exercise, heat, and rest are spaced throughout the remainder of the day according to the child's individual needs and schedules. Parents are instructed in exercises that meet the child's needs.

The Arthritis Foundation and the American Juvenile Arthritis Alliance* (an organization within the Arthritis Foundation) provide information and services for both parents and professionals, and nurses can refer families to these agencies as an added resource.

Support Child and Family

Juvenile idiopathic arthritis affects every aspect of life for the child and family. Physical limitations may interfere with self-care, school participation, and recreational activities. The intensive treatment plan, including multiple medications, physical therapy, comfort measures, and medical appointments, is intrusive and disruptive to the parents' work schedule and the family routine. To prevent isolation and foster independence, the family is encouraged to pursue their normal activities. Unfortunately, the adaptations necessary to make that occur take resourcefulness and commitment from all family members. At diagnosis and throughout the span of JIA, it is essential to recognize signs of stress and counterproductive coping and provide the necessary support to maximize adaptation. The problems and needs of these families are discussed in Chapter 18, and readers are directed to that chapter for guidance in planning care.

SYSTEMIC LUPUS ERYTHEMATOSUS

Systemic lupus erythematosus (SLE) is a chronic, multisystem, autoimmune disease of the connective tissues and blood vessels characterized by inflammation in potentially any body tissue. Its course and symptoms are variable and unpredictable, with mild to life-threatening complications. In addition to SLE, there are other forms of lupus, such as neonatal lupus, which occurs when maternal autoantibodies cross the placenta and cause transient lupus-like symptoms in a newborn,

---

*PO Box 7669, Atlanta, GA 30357; 800-283-7800; http://www.arthritis.org. In Canada: The Arthritis Society, 393 University Ave., Suite 1700, Toronto, ON M5G 1E6; 416-979-7228; fax: 416-979-8366; http://www.arthritis.ca.

BOX 31-12   CLINICAL MANIFESTATIONS OF SYSTEMIC LUPUS ERYTHEMATOSUS RELATED TO TISSUES INVOLVED

Constitutional—Fever, fatigue, weight loss, anorexia

Cutaneous—Erythematous butterfly rash over bridge of nose and across cheeks, discoid rash, photosensitivity, mucocutaneous ulceration, alopecia, periungual telangiectasias

Musculoskeletal—Arthritis, arthralgia, myositis, myalgia, tenosynovitis

Neurologic—Headache, seizure, forgetfulness, behavior change, change in school performance, psychosis, chorea, stroke, cranial and peripheral neuropathy, pseudotumor cerebri

Pulmonary and cardiac—Pleuritis, basilar pneumonitis, atelectasis, pericarditis, myocarditis, endocarditis

Renal—Glomerulonephritis, nephrotic syndrome, hypertension

Gastrointestinal—Abdominal pain, nausea, vomiting, blood in stool, abdominal crisis, esophageal dysfunction, colitis

Hepatic, splenic, and nodal—Hepatomegaly, splenomegaly, lymphadenopathy

Hematologic—Anemia, cytopenia

Ophthalmologic—Cotton wool spots, papilledema, retinopathy

Vascular—Raynaud phenomenon, thrombophlebitis, livedo reticularis

BOX 31-13   DIAGNOSTIC CRITERIA FOR SYSTEMIC LUPUS ERYTHEMATOSUS

Four of the following criteria must be met for diagnosis:
1. Malar rash—fixed malar erythema
2. Discoid rash—patchy erythematous lesions
3. Photosensitivity—rash with sun exposure
4. Oronasal ulcers—painless ulcers in mouth or nose
5. Arthritis—swelling, tenderness, or effusion in two or more peripheral joints (nonerosive)
6. Serositis—pleuritis, pericarditis
7. Renal disorder—proteinuria, casts
8. Neurologic disorder—psychosis, seizures
9. Hematologic disorder—hemolytic anemia, thrombocytopenia, leukopenia, lymphopenia
10. Immunologic disorder—anti–double-stranded DNA, anti-Sm, antiphospholipid antibodies; lupus anticoagulant; false-positive syphilis test (rapid plasma reagin [RPR])
11. Antinuclear antibodies

DNA, Deoxyribonucleic acid; *Sm,* Smith.

with the potential serious complication of heart block. The remaining discussion focuses on SLE.

Evidence suggests that survival rates in children with SLE have significantly improved; 5-year survival rates are said to be almost 100%, and 10-year survival rates are close to 90% (Ravelli, Ruperto, and Martini, 2005). SLE is more common in girls, with an approximate 5:1 female-to-male ratio, and typically occurs between the ages of 10 and 19 years. There is a familial tendency, although many newly diagnosed patients are unaware of other affected family members. SLE has been reported in all cultures, but within the United States, there has been a disproportionately higher incidence in African-American, Asian, and Hispanic children.

The cause of SLE is not known. It appears to result from a complex interaction of genetics with an unidentified trigger that activates the disease. Suspected triggers include exposure to ultraviolet light, estrogen, pregnancy, infections, and drugs. Genetic predisposition to SLE is evidenced in an increased concordance rate in twins (10-fold), increased incidence within family members (10%–16%), and increased frequency of certain gene alleles in population-based studies.

Clinical Manifestations and Diagnostic Evaluation

The child with SLE may have any clinical manifestation with mild to life-threatening severity (Box 31-12). The diagnosis is established when 4 of the 11 diagnostic criteria are met (Box 31-13). Kidney involvement heralds progressive disease and the need for rigorous therapeutic management.

Therapeutic Management

The goal of treatment is to ensure the child's health by balancing the medications necessary to avoid exacerbation and complications while preventing or minimizing treatment-associated morbidity. Therapy involves the use of specific medications and general supportive care. The drugs used to control inflammation are corticosteroids administered in doses sufficient to control inflammation and then tapered to the lowest suppressive dose. Other drugs include antimalarial preparations, which are useful for rash and arthritis; NSAIDs, which relieve muscle and joint inflammation; and immunosuppressive agents, such as cyclophosphamide, for renal and CNS disease. Mycophenolate, azathioprine, and methotrexate are effective immunosuppressive drugs that may be use to control SLE and allow steroids to be reduced. Antihypertensives, aspirin, and antibiotics are just a few of the additional drugs that may be necessary to treat or avoid complications.

General supportive care includes sufficient nutrition, sleep and rest, and exercise. Exposure to the sun and ultraviolet B (UVB) light is limited because of its association with SLE exacerbation.

Nursing Care Management

The principal nursing goal is to help the child and family positively adjust to the disease and therapy. The child and family must learn to recognize subtle signs of disease exacerbation and potential complications of medication therapy and to communicate these concerns to their care provider. Consequently, patient and family education is an ongoing process initiated at diagnosis and tailored to the patient's individual needs. Referral to a social worker, psychologist, or support group may help the child and family make a successful adjustment. Support groups are associated with the Lupus Foundation of America* and the Arthritis Foundation.†

Key issues include therapy compliance; body-image problems associated with rash, hair loss, and steroid therapy; school attendance; vocational activities; social relationships; sexual activity; and pregnancy. (See Chapter 18 for a discussion on adjusting to a chronic illness.) Specific instructions for avoiding exposure to the sun and UVB light, such as using sunscreens, wearing sun-resistant clothing, and altering outdoor activities, must be provided with great sensitivity to ensure compliance while minimizing the associated feeling of being different from peers (see Sunburn, Chapter 30). Patients need to be instructed to maintain regular medical supervision and seek attention quickly during illness or before elective surgical procedures, such as dental extraction, because of potential needs for increased steroids or prophylactic antibiotics. People with SLE should carry medical identification for their disease and steroid dependence.

---

*2000 L St. NW, Suite 710, Washington, DC 20036; 202-349-1155, 800-558-0121; http://www.lupus.org/newsite.
†PO Box 7669, Atlanta, GA 30357-0669; 800-283-7800; http://www.arthritis.org/index.php. In Canada, the Arthritis Society may be contacted for locations of all local Canadian province offices: http://www.arthritis.ca.

KEY POINTS

- Immobility has a profound effect on all aspects of growth and development.
- The major physical consequences of immobilization are loss of muscle strength, endurance, and muscle mass; bone demineralization; loss of joint mobility; and potential contractures.
- Features of children's fractures not observed in adults include the presence of growth plate, thicker and stronger periosteum, bone porosity, more rapid healing, and less joint stiffness.
- The goals of fracture management are to regain alignment and length of fractured bones, retain alignment and length, and restore function.
- The method of fracture reduction is determined by the child's age, degree of displacement, amount of overriding, amount of edema, condition of the skin and soft tissues, sensation, and circulation distal to the fracture.
- The primary purposes of traction are to fatigue involved muscles and reduce muscle spasm (comfort), position bone ends in desired alignment, and immobilize the fracture site until realignment has been achieved to permit casting or splinting.
- The development of DDH is related to gender, birth order, intrauterine positioning, and genetic and postnatal factors.
- Tight swaddling of infants' hips and lower extremities is not recommended in the first several months of life to prevent or decrease the incidence of hip dysplasia.
- Treatment of clubfoot consists of manipulation and casting to correct the deformity, maintenance of the correction, possible heel cord tenotomy, and prevention of recurrence.
- Acquired hip deformities are managed with alteration in activities, physical therapy, immobilization devices, or surgical stabilization with or without casting.
- Observation for scoliosis via the Adams forward bend test is an important part of a routine physical assessment.
- Scoliosis is managed by observation, bracing, or surgical intervention.
- Bone infections are managed with vigorous antibiotic therapy, immobilization of the affected limb, and sometimes surgical irrigation and debridement.
- Osteosarcoma is a neoplasm of bone-forming tissues; Ewing sarcoma is a neoplasm that arises from bone marrow spaces.
- Rhabdomyosarcoma may occur almost anywhere in the body, but the most common sites are the head and neck.
- Nursing care of a child with arthritis consists of promoting general health, relieving discomfort, preventing deformity, and preserving function.
- SLE is a chronic autoimmune disorder that affects the collagen tissues of the body.

REFERENCES

American Academy of Pediatrics: Clinical practice guideline: early detection of developmental dysplasia of the hip, *Pediatrics* 105(4):896–905, 2000.

Biber R, Gregory A: Overuse injuries in youth sports: is there such a thing as too much sports? *Pediatr Ann* 39(5):286–292, 2010.

Cassidy JT, Petty RE. Chronic arthritis in childhood. In Cassidy JT, Petty RE, Laxer RM, Lindsley CB, editors: *Textbook of pediatric rheumatology*, ed 6, Philadelphia, 2011, Elsevier Saunders.

Connelly M, Schanberg L: Opioid therapy for the treatment of refractory pain in children with juvenile rheumatoid arthritis, *Nat Clin Pract Rheumatol* 2(12):636–637, 2006.

Costa CR, Johnson AJ, Naziri Q, and others: Review of total hip resurfacing and total hip arthroplasty in young patients who had Legg-Calvé-Perthes disease, *Orthop Clin N Am* 42(3):419–422, 2011.

Fisher TJ, Williams SL, Levine AM. Spinal orthosis. In Browner BD, Jupiter JB, Levine AM, and others, editors, *Skeletal trauma: basic science, management, and reconstruction*, ed 4, Philadelphia, 2008, Saunders.

Food and Drug Administration: Postmarket drug safety information for patients and providers/ drug safety information for health professionals, Silver Spring, Md, 2009, Food and Drug Administration, retrieved August 5, 2009, from http://www.fda.gov/NewsEvents/Newsroom/ PressAnnouncements/ucm175803.htm.

Freeman BL III: Scoliosis and kyphosis. In Canale ST, Beaty JH, editors: *Campbell's operative orthopaedics*, ed 11, Philadelphia, 2007, Mosby.

Giannini EH, Ilowite NT, Lovell DJ, and others: Long-term safety and effectiveness of etanercept in children with selected categories of juvenile idiopathic arthritis, *Arthritis Rheum* 60(9): 2794–2804, 2009.

Gorlick R, Bielack S, Teot L, and others: Osteosarcoma: biology, diagnosis, treatment and remaining challenges. In Pizzo PA, Poplack DG, editors: *Principles and practices of pediatric oncology*, ed 6, Philadelphia, 2011, Lippincott.

Green NE, Swiontkowski MF: *Skeletal trauma in children*, ed 4, Philadelphia, 2008, WB Saunders Company.

Gutierrez K: Bone and joint infections in children, *Pediatr Clin North Am* 52(3):779–794, 2005.

Hart ES, Albright MB, Rebello GN, and others: Developmental dysplasia of the hip: nursing implications and anticipatory guidance for parents, *Orthop Nurs* 25(2):100–109, 2006.

Helman LJ: Rhabdomyosarcoma and the undifferentiated sarcomas of childhood. In Pizzo PA, Poplack DG, editors: *Principles and practices of pediatric oncology*, ed 6, Philadelphia, 2011, Lippincott.

Holmes SB, Brown SJ, Pin Site Care Expert Panel: Skeletal pin site care: National Association of Orthopaedic Nurses guidelines for orthopaedic nursing, *Orthop Nurs* 24(2):99–107, 2005.

Hosalkar HS, Spiegel DA, Davidson RS: Talipes equinovarus (clubfoot). In Kliegman RM, Stanton BF, St. Geme JW, and others: *Nelson textbook of pediatrics*, ed 19, Philadelphia, 2011, Saunders.

Jayakumar P, Ramachandran M, Youm T, and others: Arthroscopy of the hip for paediatric and adolescent disorders, *J Bone Joint Surg* 94(3):290–296, 2012.

Kaplan SL: Osteomyelitis. In Kliegman RM, Stanton BF, St. Geme JW, and others: *Nelson textbook of pediatrics*, ed 19, Philadelphia, 2011a, Saunders.

Kaplan SL: Septic arthritis. In Kliegman RM, Stanton BF, St. Geme JW, and others: *Nelson textbook of pediatrics*, ed 19, Philadelphia, 2011b, Saunders.

Land C, Rauch F, Travers R, and others: Osteogenesis imperfecta type VI in childhood and adolescence: effects of cyclical intravenous pamidronate treatment, *Bone* 40(3):638–644, 2007.

Lanzkowsky P: *Manual of pediatric hematology and oncology*, ed 4, San Diego, 2005, Academic Press.

Lehmann CL, Aarons RR, Loder RT, and others: The epidemiology of slipped capital femoral epiphysis: an update, *J Pediatr Orthop* 26(3): 286–290, 2006.

Loder RT: Controversies in slipped capital femoral epiphysis, *Orthop Clin North Am* 37(2):211–221, 2006.

Lovell DJ, Giannini EH, Reiff A, and others: Long-term efficacy and safety of etanercept in children with polyarticular-course juvenile rheumatoid arthritis: interim results from an ongoing multicenter, open-label, extended-treatment trial, *Arthritis Rheum* 48(1):218–226, 2003.

Lovell DJ, Ruperto N, Goodman S, and others: Adalimumab with or without methotrexate in juvenile rheumatoid arthritis, *N Engl J Med* 359(8):810–820, 2008.

Marini JC: Osteogenesis imperfect. In Kliegman RM, Stanton BF, St. Geme JW, and others: *Nelson textbook of pediatrics*, ed 19, Philadelphia, 2011, Saunders.

Napierkowski DB: Scoliosis: a case study in an adolescent boy, *Orthop Nurs* 26(3):147–153, 2007.

Newton PO, Wenger DR: Idiopathic scoliosis. In Morrissy RT, Weinstein SL, editors: *Lovell and Winter's pediatric orthopaedics*, Philadelphia, 2005, Williams & Wilkins.

Noonan C, Quigley S, Curley MA: Using the Braden Q Scale to predict pressure ulcer risk in pediatric patients, *J Pediatr Nurs* 26(6):566–575, 2011.

Ong BY, Arneja A, Ong EW: Effects of anesthesia on pain after lower-limb amputation, *J Clin Anesth* 18(8):600–604, 2006.

Patel DR: Stress fractures: diagnosis and management in the primary care setting. *Pediatr Clin North Am* 57(3):819–827, 2010.

Petty RE, Southwood TR, Manners P, and others: International League of Associations for Rheumatology classification of juvenile idiopathic arthritis, second revision, Edmonton, 2001, *J Rheumatol* 31(2):390–392, 2004.

Ponseti IV: *Congenital clubfoot: fundamentals of treatment*, Oxford, 1996, Oxford University Press.

Price CT, Schwend RM: Improper swaddling a risk factor for developmental dysplasia of hip, *AAP News* 32(9):11–12, 2011.

Qian Y, Acharya NR: Juvenile idiopathic arthritis-associated uveitis, *Curr Opin Ophthalmol* 21(6):468–472, 2010.

Ravelli A, Ruperto N, Martini A: Outcome in juvenile onset lupus erythematosus, *Curr Opin Rheumatol* 17(5):568–573, 2005.

Richards BS, Vitale MG: Screening for idiopathic scoliosis in adolescents: an information statement, *J Bone Joint Surg* 90(1):195–198, 2008.

Ruebner R, Keren R, Coffin S, and others: Complications of central venous catheters used for the treatment of acute hematogenous osteomyelitis, *Pediatrics* 117(4):1210–1215, 2006.

Saavedra-Lozano J, Mejías A, Ahmad N, and others: Changing trends in acute osteomyelitis in children: impact of methicillin-resistant *Staphylococcus aureus* infections, *J Pediatr Orthop* 28(5):569–575, 2008.

Sankar WN, Horn D, Wells L, and others: Developmental dysplasia of the hip. In Kliegman RM, Stanton BF, St. Geme JW, and others: *Nelson textbook of pediatrics*, ed 19, Philadelphia, 2011a, Saunders.

Sankar WN, Horn D, Wells L, and others: Legg-Calvé-Perthes disease. In Kliegman RM, Stanton BF, St. Geme JW, and others: *Nelson textbook of pediatrics*, ed 19, Philadelphia, 2011b, Saunders.

Sankar WN, Horn D, Wells L, and others: Slipped capital femoral epiphysis. In Kliegman RM, Stanton BF, St. Geme JW, and others: *Nelson textbook of pediatrics*, ed 19, Philadelphia, 2011c, Saunders.

Sarwark JF, editor: *Essentials of musculoskeletal care*, ed 4, Rosemont, Ill, 2010, American Academy of Orthopaedic Surgeons.

Seidel HM, Ball JW, Dains JE, and others: *Mosby's guide to physical examination*, ed 5, St. Louis, 2006, Mosby.

Shyy W, Wang K, Sheffield VC, and others: Evaluation of embryonic and perinatal myosin gene mutations and the etiology of congenital idiopathic clubfoot, *J Pediatr Orthop* 30(3):231–234, 2010.

Sponseller PD: Bracing for adolescent idiopathic scoliosis in practice today, *J Pediatr Orthop* 31(suppl 1):S53–S60, 2011.

Stoll C, Alembik Y, Dott B, and others: Associated malformations in patients with limb reduction deficiencies, *Eur J Med Genet* 53(5):286–290, 2010.

Wallace C, Huang B, Bandeira M, and others: Patterns of clinical remission in select categories of juvenile idiopathic arthritis, *Arthritis Rheum* 52(11):3554–3562, 2005.

Winsley R, Matos N: Overtraining and elite young athletes, *Med Sport Sci* 56:97–105, 2011.

Zaoutis T, Localio AR, Leckerman K, and others: Prolonged intravenous therapy versus early transition to oral antimicrobial therapy for acute osteomyelitis in children, *Pediatrics* 123(2):636–642, 2009.

The Child with Neuromuscular or Muscular Dysfunction

Jean Stansbury, Barbara Montagnino, and David Wilson

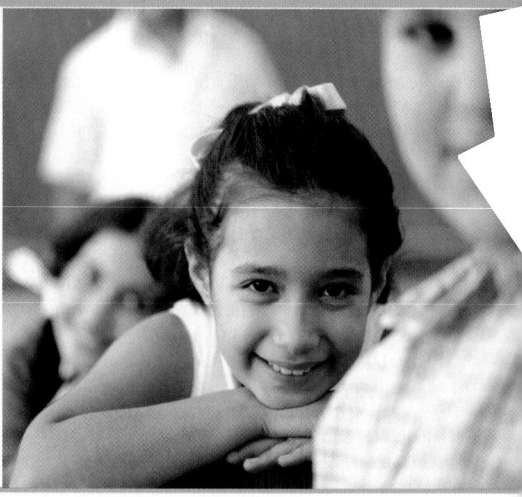

evolve WEBSITE

http://evolve.elsevier.com/wong/essentials
Animation—Guillain-Barré Syndrome
Case Study—Cerebral Palsy
Key Point Summaries

NCLEX-Style Review Questions
Nursing Care Plans—The Child with Cerebral Palsy; The Child with Myelomeningocele (Spina Bifida)

CHAPTER OUTLINE

Congenital Neuromuscular or Muscular Disorders, 1090
  Cerebral Palsy, 1090
  Neural Tube Defects (Myelomeningocele), 1098
    Latex Allergy, 1104
  Spinal Muscular Atrophy, Type 1 (Werdnig-Hoffmann Disease), 1105

Spinal Muscular Atrophy, Type 3 (Kugelberg-Welander Disease), 1106
Muscular Dystrophies, 1106
  Duchenne (Pseudohypertrophic) Muscular Dystrophy, 1106
Acquired Neuromuscular Disorders, 1109
  Guillain-Barré Syndrome (Infectious Polyneuritis), 1109

Tetanus, 1111
Botulism, 1113
  Infant Botulism, 1113
Spinal Cord Injuries, 1114

LEARNING OBJECTIVES

On completion of this chapter the reader will be able to:
- Discuss the nursing role in helping parents care for the child who has cerebral palsy.
- Formulate a nursing care plan for the preoperative and postoperative care of a child with myelomeningocele.
- Outline a care plan for a child with Guillain-Barré syndrome.

- Discuss the home care management of the child with a neuromuscular disease such as spinal muscular atrophy.
- Discuss the prevention and treatment of tetanus.
- Identify the causes of botulism in infants and children.
- List three causes of spinal cord injury in children.

CONGENITAL NEUROMUSCULAR OR MUSCULAR DISORDERS

CEREBRAL PALSY

A new definition proposed in 2006 describes cerebral palsy (CP) as a "group of permanent disorders of the development of movement and posture, causing activity limitation, that are attributed to nonprogressive disturbances that occurred in the developing fetal or infant brain" (Rosenbaum, Paneth, Leviton, and others, 2007). In addition to motor disorders, the condition often involves disturbances of sensation, perception, communication, cognition, and behavior; secondary musculoskeletal problems; and epilepsy (Rosenbaum, Paneth, Leviton, and others, 2007). The etiology, clinical features, and course vary and are characterized by abnormal muscle tone and coordination as the primary disturbances. CP is the most common permanent physical disability of childhood, and the incidence is reported to be between 2.4 to 3.6 per every 1000 live births in the United States (Hirtz, Thurman, Gwinn-Hardy, and others, 2007; Yeargin-Allsopp, Van Naarden Braun, Doernberg, and others, 2008). Since the 1960s, the prevalence of CP has risen approximately 20%, which most likely reflects the improved survival of extremely low–birth-weight and very low–birth-weight infants.

Although the prevalent traditional hypothesis has been that CP results from perinatal problems, especially birth asphyxia, it is now believed that CP results more often from existing prenatal brain abnormalities; the exact cause of these abnormalities remains elusive but may include genetic factors, including clotting disorders as well as brain malformations. It has been estimated that as many as 80% of CP cases are attributable to unidentified prenatal factors (Krigger, 2006). Intrauterine exposure to maternal chorioamnionitis is associated with an increased risk of CP in infants of normal birth weight and preterm infants (Hermansen and Hermansen, 2006); however, not all term infants exposed to chorioamnionitis develop CP (Grether, Nelson, Walsh, and others, 2003; Wu, Escobar, Grether, and others, 2003). Perinatal ischemic stroke is also associated with a later diagnosis of CP (Golomb, Saha, Garg, and others, 2007). Additional factors that may contribute to the development of CP postnatally include bacterial meningitis, multiple births, viral encephalitis, motor vehicle crashes, and child abuse (shaken baby syndrome [traumatic brain injury]) (Krigger, 2006). One study found a higher risk of CP occurring among infants born at 42 weeks or later than among those born at 37 or 38 weeks' gestation (Moster, Wilcox, Vollset, and others, 2010). A significant percentage (15% to 60%) of children with CP also have epilepsy. In summary, as many as 80% of the total cases of CP may be linked to a perinatal or neonatal brain lesion or brain maldevelopment, regardless of the cause (Krageloh-Mann and Cans, 2009).

Pathophysiology

It is difficult to establish a precise location of neurologic lesions on the basis of etiology or clinical signs because there is no characteristic pathologic picture. In some cases, there are gross malformations of the brain. In others, there may be evidence of vascular occlusion, atrophy, loss of neurons, and laminar degeneration that produce narrower gyri, wider sulci, and low brain weight. Anoxia appears to play the most significant role in the pathologic state of brain damage, which is often secondary to other causative mechanisms.

There are a few exceptions. In some cases, the manifestations or etiology are related to anatomic areas. For example, CP associated with preterm birth is usually spastic diplegia caused by hypoxic infarction or hemorrhage with periventricular leukomalacia in the area adjacent to the lateral ventricles. The athetoid (extrapyramidal) type of CP is most likely to be associated with birth asphyxia but can also be caused by kernicterus and metabolic genetic disorders such as mitochondrial disorders and glutaricaciduria (Johnston, 2011). Hemiplegic (hemiparetic) CP is often associated with a focal cerebral infarction (stroke) secondary to an intrauterine or perinatal thromboembolism, usually a result of maternal thrombosis or hereditary clotting disorder (Johnston, 2011). Cerebral hypoplasia and sometimes severe neonatal hypoglycemia are related to ataxic CP. Generalized cortical and cerebral atrophy often cause severe quadriparesis with cognitive impairment and microcephaly.

Clinical Classification

A revision of the Winter classification was proposed in 2005 to reflect the child's actual clinical problems and their severity, an assessment of the child's physical and quality-of-life status across time, and long-term support needs (Bax, Goldstein, Rosenbaum, and others, 2005; Nehring, 2010). The proposed new definition has four major dimensions of classification (Bax, Goldstein, Rosenbaum, and others, 2005):

Motor abnormalities—Nature and typology of the motor disorder; functional motor abilities

Associated impairments—Seizures; hearing or vision impairment; attentional, behavioral, communicative, or cognitive deficits; oral motor and speech function

Anatomic and radiologic findings—Anatomic distribution or parts of the body affected by motor impairments or limitations; radiologic findings sometimes including white matter lesions or brain anomaly noted on computed tomography (CT) or magnetic resonance imaging (MRI)

Causation and timing—Identification of a clearly identified cause such as a postnatal event (e.g., meningitis, traumatic brain injury)

Cerebral palsy has four primary types of movement disorders: spastic, dyskinetic, ataxic, and mixed (Nehring, 2010). The most common clinical type, spastic CP, represents an upper motor neuron muscular weakness (Box 32-1). The reflex arc is intact, and the characteristic physical signs are increased stretch reflexes, increased muscle tone, and (often) weakness. Early neurologic manifestations are usually generalized hypotonia or decreased tone that lasts for a few weeks or may extend for months or even as long as 1 year.

Diagnostic Evaluation

Infants at risk according to known etiologic factors associated with CP warrant careful assessment during early infancy to identify the signs of neuromotor dysfunction as soon as possible. The neurologic examination and history are the primary means for diagnosis. Neuroimaging of the child with suspected brain abnormality and CP is now recommended for diagnostic assessment, with MRI preferred to CT scan. Metabolic and genetic testing is recommended if no structural abnormality is identified by neuroimaging; laboratory tests are no longer recommended in the diagnostic process for CP.

Early recognition is made more difficult by the lack of reliable neonatal neurologic signs. However, nurses should monitor infants with known etiologic risk factors and evaluate them closely in the first 2 years of life. Because cortical control of movement does not occur until later in infancy, motor impairment associated with voluntary control is usually not apparent until after 2 to 4 months of age at the earliest. More often the diagnosis cannot be confirmed until the age of 2 years because motor tone abnormalities may be indicative of another neuromuscular illness. In addition, some children who show signs consistent with CP before 2 years do not demonstrate such signs after 2 years (Nehring, 2010). However, there is no consensus regarding an age cut-off for the onset of symptoms. Clinical manifestations of CP at the time of diagnosis are listed in Box 32-2; early warning signs are listed in Box 32-3, but these are not considered diagnostic.

Establishing a diagnosis may be easier with the persistence of primitive reflexes: (1) either the asymmetric tonic neck reflex or the persistent Moro reflex (beyond 4 months of age) and (2) the crossed extensor reflex. The tonic neck reflex normally disappears between 4 and 6 months of age. An obligatory response is considered abnormal. This is elicited by turning the infant's head to one side and holding it there for 20 seconds. When a crying infant is unable to move from the asymmetric posturing of the tonic neck reflex when crying, it is considered obligatory and an abnormal response. The crossed extensor reflex, which normally disappears by 4 months, is elicited by applying a noxious stimulus to the sole of one foot with the knee extended. Normally, the contralateral foot responds with extensor, abduction, and then adduction movements. The possibility of CP is suggested if these reflexes occur after 4 months.

A number of assessment instruments are now available to evaluate muscle spasticity; functional independence in self-care, mobility, and cognition; self-initiated movements over time; and capability and

BOX 32-1 CLINICAL CLASSIFICATION OF CEREBRAL PALSY

Spastic (Pyramidal)

Characterized by persistent primitive reflexes, positive Babinski reflex, ankle clonus, exaggerated stretch reflexes, eventual development of contractures

- Seventy percent to 80% of all cases of CP
- Diplegia—All extremities affected; lower more than upper (30%–40% of spastic CP)
- Tetraplegia—All four extremities involved: legs and trunk, mouth, pharynx, and tongue (10%–15% of spastic CP)
- Triplegia—Three limbs involved
- Monoplegia—Only one limb involved
- Hemiplegia—Motor dysfunction on one side of the body; upper extremity more affected than lower (20%–30% of spastic CP)

Other features:

- Hypertonicity with poor control of posture, balance, and coordinated motion
- Impairment of fine and gross motor skills

Dyskinetic (Nonspastic, Extrapyramidal)

Athetoid—Chorea (involuntary, irregular, jerking movements); characterized by slow, wormlike, writhing movements that usually involve the extremities, trunk, neck, facial muscles, and tongue

Dystonic—Slow, twisting movements of the trunk or extremities; abnormal posture

Involvement of the pharyngeal, laryngeal, and oral muscles causing drooling and dysarthria (imperfect speech articulation)

Ataxic (Nonspastic, Extrapyramidal)

Wide-based gait

Rapid, repetitive movements performed poorly

Disintegration of movements of the upper extremities when the child reaches for objects

Mixed Type

Combination of spastic CP and dyskinetic CP

May be labeled *mixed* when no specific motor pattern is dominant; however, this term is losing favor to more precise descriptions of motor function and affected area of brain involved (Rosenbaum, Paneth, Leviton, and others, 2007)

Data from Nehring W: Cerebral palsy. In Allen PJ, Vessey JA, Schapiro NA, editors: *Primary care of the child with a chronic condition*, ed 5, St. Louis, 2010, Mosby; Jones MW, Morgan E, Shelton JE, and others: Cerebral palsy: introduction and diagnosis, part 1, *J Pediatr Health Care* 21(3):146–152, 2007; and National Institute of Neurologic Disorders and Stroke: *Cerebral palsy: hope through research*, 2006, retrieved July 9, 2007, from http://www.ninds.nih.gov/disorders/cerebral_palsy/detail_cerebral_palsy.htm. *CP*, Cerebral palsy.

performance of functional activities in self-care, mobility, and social function (Krigger, 2006).

Therapeutic Management

The goals of therapy for children with CP are early recognition and promotion of optimal development to enable affected children to attain normalization and their potential within the limits of their existing health problems. The disorder is permanent, and therapy is primarily preventive and symptomatic.

Therapy has five broad goals:

BOX 32-2 CLINICAL MANIFESTATIONS OF CEREBRAL PALSY (AT TIME OF DIAGNOSIS)

Delayed Gross Motor Development

- A universal manifestation
- Delay in all motor accomplishments
- Increases as growth advances
- Delays more obvious as growth advances

Abnormal Motor Performance

- Very early preferential unilateral hand preference
- Abnormal and asymmetric crawl
- Standing or walking on toes
- Uncoordinated or involuntary movements
- Poor sucking
- Feeding difficulties
- Persistent tongue thrust

Alterations of Muscle Tone

- Increased or decreased resistance to passive movements
- Opisthotonic posturing (arching of back)
- Feels stiff on handling or dressing
- Difficulty in diapering
- Rigid and unbending at the hip and knee joints when pulled to sitting position (early sign)

Abnormal Postures

- Maintains hips higher than trunk in prone position with legs and arms flexed or drawn under the body
- Scissoring and extension of legs with feet plantar flexed in supine position
- Persistent infantile resting and sleeping position
- Arms abducted at shoulders
- Elbows flexed
- Hands fisted

Reflex Abnormalities

- Persistence of primitive infantile reflexes
- Obligatory tonic neck reflex at any age
- Nonpersistence beyond 6 months of age
- Persistence or hyperactivity of the Moro, plantar, and palmar grasp reflexes
- Hyperreflexia, ankle clonus, and stretch reflexes elicited in many muscle groups on fast, passive movements

Associated Disabilities*

- Altered learning and reasoning
- Seizures
- Impaired behavioral and interpersonal relationships
- Sensory impairment (vision, hearing)

From Nehring WM: Cerebral palsy. In Allen PJ, Vessey JA, Schapiro NA, editors, *Primary care of the child with a chronic condition*, ed 5, St. Louis, 2010, Mosby/Elsevier. Adapted from Jones MW, Morgan E, Shelton JE: Primary care of the child with cerebral palsy: a review of systems (part II), *J Pediatr Health Care* 21, 226–237, 2007.
*May or may not be present.

1. To establish locomotion, communication, and self-help skills
2. To gain optimal appearance and integration of motor functions
3. To correct associated defects as effectively as possible
4. To provide educational opportunities adapted to the child's needs and capabilities

BOX 32-3 EARLY SIGNS OF CEREBRAL PALSY

- Failure to meet any developmental milestones such as rolling over, raising head, sitting up, crawling
- Persistent primitive reflexes such as Moro, atonic neck
- Poor head control (head lag) and clenched fists after 3 months of age
- Stiff or rigid arms or legs; scissoring legs
- Pushing away or arching back; stiff posture
- Floppy or limp body posture, especially while sleeping
- Inability to sit up without support by 8 months
- Using only one side of the body or only the arms to crawl
- Feeding difficulties
- Persistent gagging or choking when fed
- After 6 months of age, tongue pushing soft food out of the mouth
- Extreme irritability or crying
- Failure to smile by 3 months
- Lack of interest in surroundings

Data from Pathways Awareness Foundation: *Parents . . . if you see any of these warning signs . . . don't delay,* Chicago, 1991, Author; Nehring W: Cerebral palsy. In Allen PJ, Vessey JA, editors: *Primary care of the child with a chronic condition*, St. Louis, 2004, Mosby; and Jones MW, Morgan E, Shelton JE, and others: Cerebral palsy: introduction and diagnosis, part 1, *J Pediatr Health Care* 21(3):146–152, 2007.

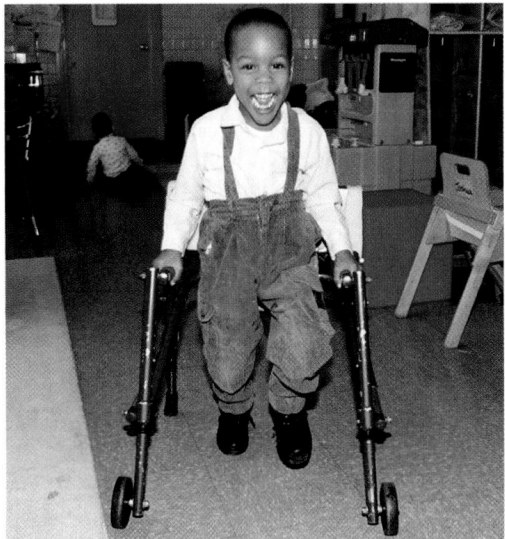

FIG 32-1 Mobilization device for a child.

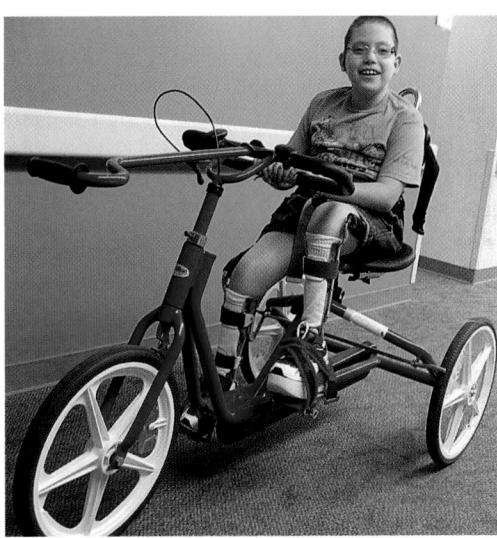

FIG 32-2 Bike walker used to provide mobility and to enhance leg muscle strength. (Courtesy Texas Children's Hospital, Houston.)

5. To promote socialization experiences with other affected and unaffected children

Each child is evaluated and managed on an individual basis. The scope of the child's needs requires multidisciplinary planning and care coordination among professionals and the child's family. The outcome for the child and family with CP is normalization and promotion of self-care activities that empower the child and family to achieve maximum potential.

Ankle–foot orthoses (AFOs, braces) are worn by many of these children and are used to help prevent or reduce deformity, increase the energy efficiency of gait, and control alignment. Wheeled go-carts that provide sitting balance may serve as early "wheelchair" experience for young children. Manual or powered wheelchairs allow for more independent mobility (Figs. 32-1 and 32-2). Strollers can be equipped with custom seats for dependent mobilization.

Orthopedic surgery may be required to correct contracture or spastic deformities, to provide stability for an uncontrollable joint, and to provide balanced muscle power. This includes tendon-lengthening procedures, release of spastic muscles, and correction of hip and adductor muscle spasticity or contracture to improve locomotion. Hip dislocation often occurs in children with CP. Spinal fusion may be required for scoliosis. Computerized motion analysis, radiographs, and clinical findings are used to make decisions about orthopedic surgery. Selective dorsal rhizotomy provides marked improvement in some children with CP. The procedure involves selectively cutting dorsal column sensory rootlets that have an abnormal response to electrical stimulation. Achieving the benefits from the surgery requires intensive physical therapy and family commitment. Because the procedure results in flaccid muscles, the child must be retaught to sit, stand, and walk.

Surgical intervention is usually reserved for children who do not respond to the more conservative measures, but it is also indicated for children whose spasticity causes progressive deformities. Surgery is primarily used to improve function rather than for cosmetic purposes and is followed by physical therapy.

Intense pain may occur with muscle spasms in patients with CP. Pharmacologic agents given orally (dantrolene sodium, baclofen [Lioresal], and diazepam [Valium]) have had little effectiveness in improving muscle coordination in children with CP; however, they are effective in decreasing overall spasticity. The most common side effects of these agents include hepatotoxicity (dantrolene), drowsiness, fatigue, and muscle weakness; less commonly, diaphoresis and constipation may be seen with baclofen. Diazepam is used frequently but should be restricted to older children and adolescents.

Botulinum toxin A (Botox) is also used to reduce spasticity in targeted muscles. Botulinum toxin A is injected into a selected muscle (commonly the quadriceps, gastrocnemius, or medial hamstrings) after a topical anesthetic is applied. The drug acts to inhibit the release of acetylcholine into a specific muscle group, thereby preventing muscle movement. When it is administered early in the course of the condition, affected muscle contractures may be minimized, particularly in lower extremities, thus avoiding surgical procedures with possible adverse effects. The goal is to allow stretching of the muscle as it relaxes and permit ambulation with an AFO. The major reported adverse effects of botulinum toxin A injection are pain at the injection site and temporary weakness (Lukban, Rosales, and Dressler, 2009). Prime candidates for botulinum toxin A injections are children with spasticity confined to the lower extremities; the drug weakens spasticity so the muscles can be stretched and the child may walk with or without orthoses. The onset of action occurs within 24 to 72 hours, with a peak effect observed at 2 weeks and a duration of action of 3 to 6 months.

Children with CP may also experience pain as a result of surgical procedures intended to reduce contracture deformities, body position, gastroesophageal reflux, and physical therapy (McKearnan, Kieckhefer, Engel, and others, 2004). Therefore, pain management is an important aspect of care of children with CP.

The neurosurgical and pharmacologic approach to managing the spasticity associated with CP involves the implantation of a pump to infuse baclofen directly into the intrathecal space surrounding the spinal cord to provide relief of spasticity. Intrathecal baclofen therapy is best suited for children with severe spasticity that interferes with activities of daily living (ADLs) and ambulation. Patients may be screened before pump placement by the infusion of a "test dose" of intrathecal baclofen delivered via a lumbar puncture. Close monitoring for side effects (hypotonia, somnolence, seizures, nausea, vomiting, headache) occurs. Relief of spasticity occurs for several hours after the infusion. If a positive effect is noted, the patient is considered a candidate for pump placement. The implantation procedure is done in the operating room by a neurosurgeon. The pump, which is approximately the size of a hockey puck, is placed in the subcutaneous space of the midabdomen. An intrathecal catheter is tunneled from the lumbar area to the abdomen and connected to the pump. The pump is filled with baclofen and programmed to provide a set dose using a telemetry wand and a computer. Benefits of intrathecal baclofen include fewer systemic side effects than oral baclofen, dosage titration for maximizing effects, and reversibility of therapy with removal of the pump if so desired. The patient may remain hospitalized for 3 to 7 days to adjust the dosage and ensure proper healing. Outpatient visits to refill the pump and make dosage adjustments occur about every 3 to 6 months, depending on the patient's response to the treatment. This procedure is most suited for a multidisciplinary setting where rehabilitation specialists are readily available and consistently involved in the patient's ongoing care. Abrupt withdrawal of intrathecal baclofen may result in adverse effects such as rebound spasticity, pruritus, hyperthermia, rhabdomyolysis, disseminated intravascular coagulation, multiorgan failure, and death; in some cases, intrathecal baclofen withdrawal may mimic sepsis.

Antiepileptic drugs (AEDs) such as carbamazepine (Tegretol) and divalproex (valproate sodium and valproic acid; Depakote) are prescribed routinely for children who have seizures. Other medications include levodopa to treat dystonia; Artane for treating dystonia, and for increasing the use of upper extremities and vocalizations; and reserpine for hyperkinetic movement disorders such as chorea or athetosis (Johnston, 2011). All medications should be monitored for maintenance of therapeutic levels and avoidance of subtherapeutic or toxic levels.

Dental hygiene is essential in the care of children with CP. Regular visits to the dentist and prophylaxis, including brushing, fluoride, and flossing, should be started as soon as the teeth erupt. Dental care is especially important for children being given phenytoin because they often develop gum hyperplasia. Decreased oral intake can lead to more tartar buildup. Additional problems common among children with CP include constipation caused by neurologic deficits and lack of exercise, poor bladder control and urinary retention, chronic respiratory tract infections, problems with airway clearance, and aspiration

pneumonia. These occur as a result of gastroesophageal reflux, abnormal muscle tone, immobility, and altered positioning, and skin problems may occur as a result of altered positioning, poor nutrition, and immobility.

A wide variety of technical aids are available to improve the functioning of children with CP. Airway clearance devices help mobilize secretions. Eye–hand coordination can also be enhanced by computerized toys and games. Toys may be operated by a head or hand switch. Microcomputers combined with voice synthesizers aid children with speech difficulties to "speak." Smart phones with speech applications are appropriate for some children.

Many other electronic devices allow independent functioning. Sensors can be activated and deactivated by using a head stick or tongue or other voluntary muscle movement over which the child has control. Voice-activated computer technology may also allow increased mobility and ambulation with specially designed devices such as wheelchairs. The application of this technology makes it possible for persons with CP to function in their own residences and can be extended into the workplace.

There is some evidence that **neuromuscular electrical stimulation (NMES)** in addition to dynamic splinting may result in increased muscle strength, range of motion, and function of upper limbs in children with CP. Further studies are needed in children with CP to support the use of botulinum toxin A in conjuction with NMES to decrease muscle spasticity and improve function (Wright, Durham, Ewins, and others, 2012).

Behavior problems may occur and often interfere with the child's development. Attention-deficit/hyperactivity disorder and other learning problems require professional attention. In addition, children with CP may have vision difficulties such as strabismus, nystagmus, and optic atrophy (Johnston, 2011). Speech-language therapy involves the services of a speech-language pathologist who may also assist with feeding problems.

Physical therapy is one of the most frequently used conservative treatment modalities. It requires the specialized skills of a qualified therapist with an extensive repertoire of exercise methods who can design a program to stimulate each child to achieve his or her functional goals.

An active therapy program involves the family; the physical therapist; and often other members of the health team, including the nurse. The most common approach uses traditional types of therapeutic exercises that consist of stretching, passive, active, and resistive movements applied to specific muscle groups or joints to maintain or increase range of motion, strength, or endurance.

Prognosis

The prognosis for the child with CP depends largely on the type and severity of the condition. Children with mild to moderate involvement (85%) have the capability of achieving ambulation between the ages of 2 and 7 years (Berker and Yalçin, 2008). If the child does not achieve independent ambulation by this time, chances are poor for ambulation and independence. Approximately 30% to 50% of individuals with CP have significant cognitive impairments, and an even higher percentage have mild cognitive and learning deficits. However, many children with severe spastic tetraplegic CP have normal intelligence. Growth is affected in children with spastic tetraplegia, and many children remain below the 5th percentile for age and sex.

As children with CP become adults, about 30% remain in the home and are cared for by a parent or caregiver; 50% of individuals with spastic tetraplegia live in independent settings and function at appropriate social levels considering their disability (Green, Greenberg, and

Hurwitz, 2003). Vocational rehabilitation and higher education are possible for adults with CP. Children with severe CP mobility impairment and feeding problems often succumb to respiratory tract infection in childhood. The few survival rate studies on children or adults with CP show that survival is influenced by existing comorbidities (Nehring, 2010).

Prevention of some cases of CP may become a reality in the near future. Studies indicate that early neuroprotection in term infants with the use of therapeutic hypothermia (head cooling or whole-body cooling) within 6 hours of birth improved survival without CP by approximately 40% (Johnston, Fatemi, Wilson, and others, 2011).

! NURSING ALERT

The use of mobile infant walkers is discouraged in children with CP. They pose a risk of injury to normal children and are especially hazardous for children with CP. Also, jumping seats, such as those that hang in doorways, should not be used.

Nursing Care Management

Because children with CP are being identified and treated at an earlier age, parents are participating earlier in treatment programs for their children with disabilities. They are taught the proper handling and home care of young children with CP and need a carefully planned program so that their change of role from parent to caregiver can be melded into the already established relationship. Close work with other multidisciplinary team members is essential. Nurses reinforce the therapeutic plan and assist the family in devising and modifying equipment and activities to continue the therapy program in the home. The nursing process in the care of the child with CP is outlined in the Nursing Care Plan.

Because children with CP expend so much energy in their efforts to accomplish ADLs, more frequent rest periods should be arranged to avoid fatigue. The diet should be tailored to the child's activity and metabolic needs. Gastrostomy feedings may be necessary to supplement regular feedings and ensure adequate weight gain, particularly in children at risk for growth failure and chronic malnutrition, those with severe CP and subsequent oral feeding difficulties, and children whose

---

◎ NURSING CARE PLAN

The Child with Cerebral Palsy

NURSING DIAGNOSIS	PATIENT OUTCOMES	NURSING INTERVENTIONS	RATIONALE
Impaired Physical Mobility related to neuromuscular impairment	The child will demonstrate active muscle movement.	Carry out and teach family to perform stretching exercises on affected muscles.	To prevent muscle contractures
	The child will have adequate mobility to perform ADLs to maximum potential.	Use assistive devices such as wheelchair, AFOs, and wrist splints.	To increase mobility and prevent contractures
Child's Defining Characteristics (Subjective and Objective Data)		Administer medications (specify) intended to decrease muscle spasticity.	To minimize pain and decrease spasticity
Postural instability during performance of routine ADLs	**The Following NOC Concepts Apply to These Outcomes**	Encourage and teach parent(s) to use jaw control during feedings.	To facilitate eating
Limited ability to perform gross motor skills	Body Mechanics Performance	Position child semiupright during feedings.	To decrease chance of aspiration and facilitate mobilization of food and fluids through esophagus
Limited range of motion	Ambulation: Wheelchair		
Limited ability to perform fine motor skills	Joint Movement: Elbow, Wrist, Neck, Knee, Hip, Ankle	Encourage play exercises that involve joint movement and promote fine and gross motor skill acquisition and repetition.	To promote joint movement
Gait changes	Mobility		To promote achievement of developmental milestones
Movement-induced tremor			
Persistence of primitive reflexes		**The Following NIC Concepts Apply to These Interventions**	
		Exercise Therapy: Joint Mobility	
		Exercise Promotion: Stretching	
		Self-Care Assistance	
Risk for Injury (Falls, Aspiration) related to mobility limitation, neuromuscular impairment, and perception and cognitive impairment	Child will remain injury free. Home physical environment will be safe.	Educate family regarding child's physical limitations that place him or her at greater risk for injury.	To prevent accidental injury during mobilization
		Instruct family in steps to avoid injury, including padded furniture, lowered bed or side rails as appropriate, gates on stairs, avoidance of throw rugs, thick carpeting.	To promote family involvement in injury prevention
Child's Defining Characteristics (Subjective and Objective Data)	**The Following NOC Concepts Apply to These Outcomes**		
Physical factors: altered mobility	Personal Safety Behavior	Position child in semiupright position after feedings.	To prevent aspiration
Limited ability to chew food and swallow food particles	Falls Occurrence	Assess child's ability to manage (chewing and swallowing) oral feedings.	To determine appropriate feeding method and prevent aspiration
Neuromuscular factors:		Use jaw support as needed during feedings.	To prevent choking and possible aspiration
• Limited perception of danger			
• Uncontrollable muscular movements		Use appropriate mobilization devices and ensure they are safe for child's age.	To prevent muscle contractures

Continued

◎ NURSING CARE PLAN

The Child with Cerebral Palsy—cont'd

NURSING DIAGNOSIS	PATIENT OUTCOMES	NURSING INTERVENTIONS	RATIONALE
		Encourage mobilization and play activities that stretch muscles.	To promote personal safety
		Teach child which ADLs are safe and appropriate to perform without assistance of another person.	To promote self-care
		The Following NIC Concepts Apply to These Interventions Risk Identification Environmental Management: Safety Surveillance: Safety Physical Restraint Parent Education: Childrearing, Family	
Pain (chronic) related to involuntary muscle movements (spasticity) and treatments for muscle spasticity **Child's Defining Characteristics (Subjective and Objective Data)** Observed evidence of guarded behavior, grimace, crying, restlessness, irritability Atrophy of involved muscle group Altered ability to continue previous ADLs	Child's optimum comfort level will be maintained. **The Following NOC Concepts Apply to This Outcome** Comfort Level Pain: Disruptive Effects Depression Level	Administer medications to control spasticity (specify).	To prevent muscle spasm pain
		Perform stretching exercises after pain medication has been administered (60 minutes for oral medications).	To manage pain impulses during exercises
		Administer pain medications (specify) such as NSAIDs.	To minimize pain
		For treatments such as botulinum toxin A (Botox) injections, assist with administration of appropriate pain medications and monitoring child for pain sensation (specify).	To decrease pain of injection at site
		For postoperative pain, administer pain medications on an around-the-clock schedule for 48 to 72 hours; use PCA pump as child's cognitive and motor skills allow.	To promote personal physical comfort
		Use objective pain scale to assess pain level.	To provide objective measure of pain for intervention
		Encourage child to verbalize effects of pain on ADLs.	To provide outlet for frustration related to chronic pain experience
		Use assistive devices such as AFOs or KAFOs.	To decrease muscle spasticity and contractures.
		Teach parent(s) and child appropriate positions to assume while sitting and recumbent to minimize effects of muscle spasticity.	To promote self-care
		The Following NIC Concepts Apply to These Interventions Medication Administration Analgesic Administration Emotional Support Splinting Environmental Management: Comfort Exercise Promotion	

ADLs, Activities of daily living; *AFO,* ankle–foot orthosis; *KAFO,* knee–ankle–foot orthoses; *NIC,* Nursing Interventions Classification; *NOC,* Nursing Outcomes Classification; *NSAID,* nonsteroidal antiinflammatory drug; *PCA,* patient-controlled analgesia.

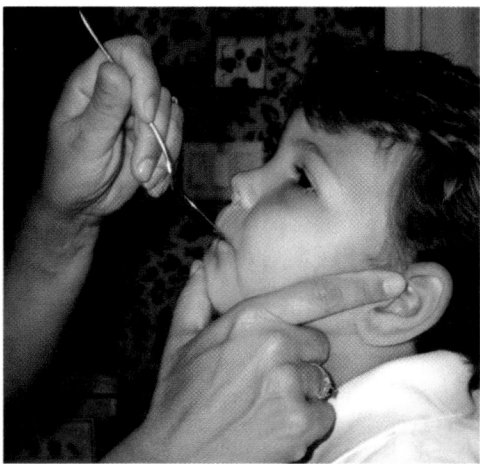

FIG 32-3 Manual jaw control provided anteriorly.

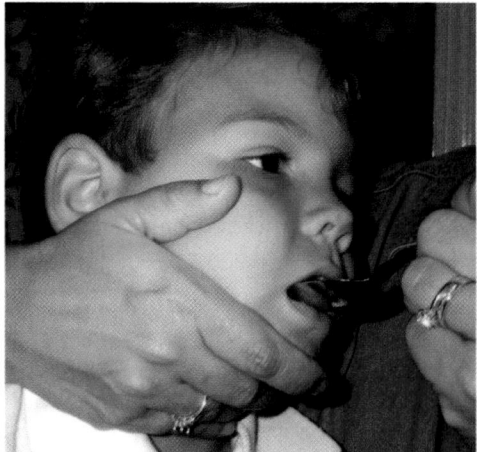

FIG 32-4 Manual jaw control provided from the side.

well-being is affected by illness and decreased fluid or medication intake (Rogers, 2004). Oral feedings may be continued to maintain oral motor skills. Weight gain is perceived as an important measure of adequate oral feeding efficiency.

Parents may need assistance and advice with medication administration through a gastrostomy tube to prevent clogging. A skin-level gastrostomy is particularly suited for children with CP. Because jaw control is often compromised, more normal control can be achieved if the feeder provides stability of the oral mechanism from the side or front of the face. When directed from the front, the middle finger of the nonfeeding hand is placed posterior to the body portion of the chin, the thumb is placed below the bottom lip, and the index finger is placed parallel to the child's mandible (Fig. 32-3). Manual jaw control from the side assists with head control, correction of neck and trunk hyperextension, and jaw stabilization. The middle finger of the nonfeeding hand is placed posterior to the bony portion of the chin, the index finger is placed on the chin below the lower lip, and the thumb is placed obliquely across the cheek to provide lateral jaw stability (Fig. 32-4).

Safety precautions are implemented, such as having children wear protective helmets if they are subject to falls or capable of injuring their heads on hard objects. Because children with CP are at risk for altered proprioception and subsequent falls, the home and play environments should be adapted to their needs to prevent bodily harm. Appropriate

immunizations should be administered to prevent childhood illnesses and protect against respiratory tract infections such as influenza or pneumonia. Dental problems may be more common in children with CP, which creates a need for meticulous attention to all aspects of dental care. Transportation of the child with motor problems and restricted mobility may be especially challenging for the family and child. Attention must be given to the child's safety when riding in a motor vehicle; a federally approved safety restraint should be used at all times. It is recommended that children with CP ride in a rear-facing position as long as possible because of their poor head, neck, and trunk control (Lovette, 2008). Car restraints especially designated for children with poor head and neck control are available and should be used.*

The involvement of physical therapy, speech therapy, and occupational therapy is particularly important in establishment and maintenance of muscle function, development of adequate speech and phonation, and identification of modifications necessary for the child's environment so that ADLs can be performed to the child's satisfaction.

As in all aspects of care, educational requirements are determined by the child's needs and potential. Children with mild to moderate cognitive involvement are generally able to participate in regular classes. Resource rooms are available in most schools to provide more individualized attention. Integration of children with CP into regular classrooms should be the initial goal. For those who are unable to benefit from formal education, a vocational training program may be appropriate. At adolescence, prevocational and vocational counseling and guidance are arranged. At any phase or in any setting, education is geared toward the child's assets.

Recreation and after-school activities should be considered for children who are unable to participate in the regular athletic programs and other peer activities. Some children can compete in athletic and artistic endeavors, and many games and pastimes are suited to their capabilities. Competitive sports are also becoming increasingly available to children with disabilities and offer an added dimension to physical activities. Recreational activities serve to stimulate children's interest and curiosity, help them adjust to their disability, improve their functional abilities, and build self-esteem. Any accomplishment that helps children approach a normal way of life enhances their self-concept.

Support the Family

Probably the nursing interventions most valuable to the family are support and help in coping with the emotional aspects of the disorder, many of which are discussed in relation to the child with a disability (see Chapter 18). Initially, the parents need supportive counseling directed toward understanding the meaning of the diagnosis and all of the feelings that it engenders. Later they need clarification regarding what they can expect from the child and from health professionals. Educating families in the principles of family-centered care and parent–professional collaboration is essential. The family may require help in modifying the home environment for care of the child (see also Chapter 20). Transportation to the practitioner's office and other health care agencies often requires special arrangements.

---

*For information on specially adapted molded-plastic chairs for children with CP, contact Snug Seat at 800-336-7684; http://www.snugseat.com/en-US/Welcome-to-Snug-Seat.aspx. The E-Z-On vest is a special safety harness for larger children with poor trunk control. Additional safety restraints and a listing of distributors are available from SafetyBeltSafe U.S.A., http://www.carseat.org. Another resource is National Center for the Safe Transportation of Children with Special Health Care Needs; 800-543-6227; http://www.preventinjury.org/specNeeds.asp.

The Reality of Acceptance of Cerebral Palsy

Acceptance is rarely achieved in the length of time implied in the literature.

In the first place, what is acceptance? To me, it is the end of comparing my son with every other child I see. I focus on *his* gains, not society's expectations.

It is also being able to laugh periodically *at* his "clumsiness." It is "gallows humor" as he achieves adulthood; jokes about CP can be funny now.

The bitterness is gone; I am now happy for people who have children without CP.

I no longer feel sorry for my son but rather for the people who cannot see him for the great person he is; the CP does *not* come first.

He is now a young man of 25 years, and I am learning to accept his independence.

It is a "never-ending story."

Elaine A. Dunham, RN
Shriners Hospitals for Children
Springfield, Mass.

Care coordination for the child and family with CP is an important nursing role. The home health nurse or care manager has an important role in the support and encouragement for families who assume the primary care of a child with CP. Having a child with CP implies numerous problems of daily management and changes in family life, and the nurse can help with education, assessment, and mobilization of resources.

The nurse needs to support the parents in their frustration, problem solving, concerns, approaches to helping the child, and the positive approaches they use. Parents and other family members may need support and counseling. Siblings of a child with a disability are affected and may respond to the child's presence with overt or less evident behavioral problems. The family needs a relationship with nurses who can provide continued contact, support, and encouragement through the long process of habilitation.

Parents may also find help and comfort from parent groups, with whom they can share problems and concerns and from whom they can derive comfort and practical information. Parent support groups are most helpful through sharing experiences and accomplishments. For example, parents can learn from others what it is like to have a child with CP, which is generally not possible from professionals (see Family-Centered Care box). The national organization United Cerebral Palsy* has branches in most communities. The association provides a variety of services for children and families. A number of excellent books also are available to guide parents and nurses who work with children with CP.

Support Hospitalized Child

Cerebral palsy is not a disorder that requires ongoing hospitalization; therefore, when children with CP are hospitalized, they are usually admitted for illness or corrective surgery. Nursing care of the child with CP similar to that of any child with a disability, and children with CP should be approached as would any child in the hospital. Speech impairment is common in children with CP, but this may not correlate with their ability to understand. Therapy programs should be

*1660 L St. NW, Suite 700, Washington, DC 20036; 800-872-5827; fax: 202-776-0414; e-mail: info@ucp.org; http://www.ucp.org. The website also has links to each state's United Cerebral Palsy organization.

continued, when appropriate, during the time they are hospitalized. Encouraging the parent to room-in and actively participate in the child's care helps promote family-centered care. However, it is also important to remember that hospitalization may be the first time a parent can defer care to a nurse and not be the primary caregiver. Discuss this with the family to find the right level of involvement for them.

NEURAL TUBE DEFECTS (MYELOMENINGOCELE)

Abnormalities that derive from the embryonic neural tube (neural tube defects [NTDs]) constitute the largest group of congenital anomalies that are consistent with multifactorial inheritance. Normally, the spinal cord and cauda equina are encased in a protective sheath of bone and meninges (Fig. 32-5, *A*). Failure of neural tube closure produces defects of varying degrees (Box 32-4). They may involve the entire length of the neural tube or may be restricted to a small area.

In the United States, rates of NTDs have declined from 1.3 per 1000 births in 1970 to 0.3 per 1000 births after the introduction of mandatory food fortification with folic acid in 1998. One concern is that NTD rates have not decreased among Hispanic and non-Hispanic white mothers since 1999 (Centers for Disease Control and Prevention [CDC], 2009). In 2005, the rates for spina bifida (SB) were estimated by the CDC to be 17.96 per 100,000 live births, thus making this one of the most common birth defects in the United States (Matthews, 2009; Wolff, Witkop, Miller, and others, 2009). Increased use of prenatal diagnostic techniques and termination of pregnancies have also affected the overall incidence of NTDs. (see also Prevention, p. 1102).

Anencephaly, the most serious NTD, is a congenital malformation in which both cerebral hemispheres are absent. The condition is usually incompatible with life, and many affected infants are stillborn. For those who survive, no specific treatment is available. The infants have a portion of the brainstem and are able to maintain vital functions (e.g., temperature regulation and cardiac and respiratory function) for a few hours to several weeks but eventually die of respiratory failure.

Myelodysplasia refers broadly to any malformation of the spinal canal and cord. Midline defects involving failure of the osseous (bony) spine to close are called spina bifida (SB), the most common defect of the central nervous system (CNS). SB is categorized into two types, SB occulta and SB cystica.

Spina bifida occulta refers to a defect that is not visible externally. It occurs most frequently in the lumbosacral area (L5 and S1) (Fig. 32-5, *B*). SB occulta may not be apparent unless there are associated cutaneous manifestations or neuromuscular disturbances.

Spina bifida cystica refers to a visible defect with an external saclike protrusion. The two major forms of SB cystica are meningocele, which encases meninges and spinal fluid but no neural elements (Fig. 32-5, *C*), and myelomeningocele (or meningomyelocele), which contains meninges, spinal fluid, and nerves (Fig. 32-5, *D*). Meningocele is not associated with neurologic deficit, which occurs in varying, often serious, degrees in myelomeningocele. Clinically, the term *spina bifida* is used to refer to myelomeningocele.

Pathophysiology

The pathophysiology of SB is best understood when related to the normal formative stages of the nervous system. At approximately 20 days of gestation, a decided depression, the neural groove, appears in the dorsal ectoderm of the embryo. During the fourth week of gestation, the groove deepens rapidly, and its elevated margins develop laterally and fuse dorsally to form the neural tube. Neural tube formation begins in the cervical region near the center of the embryo and

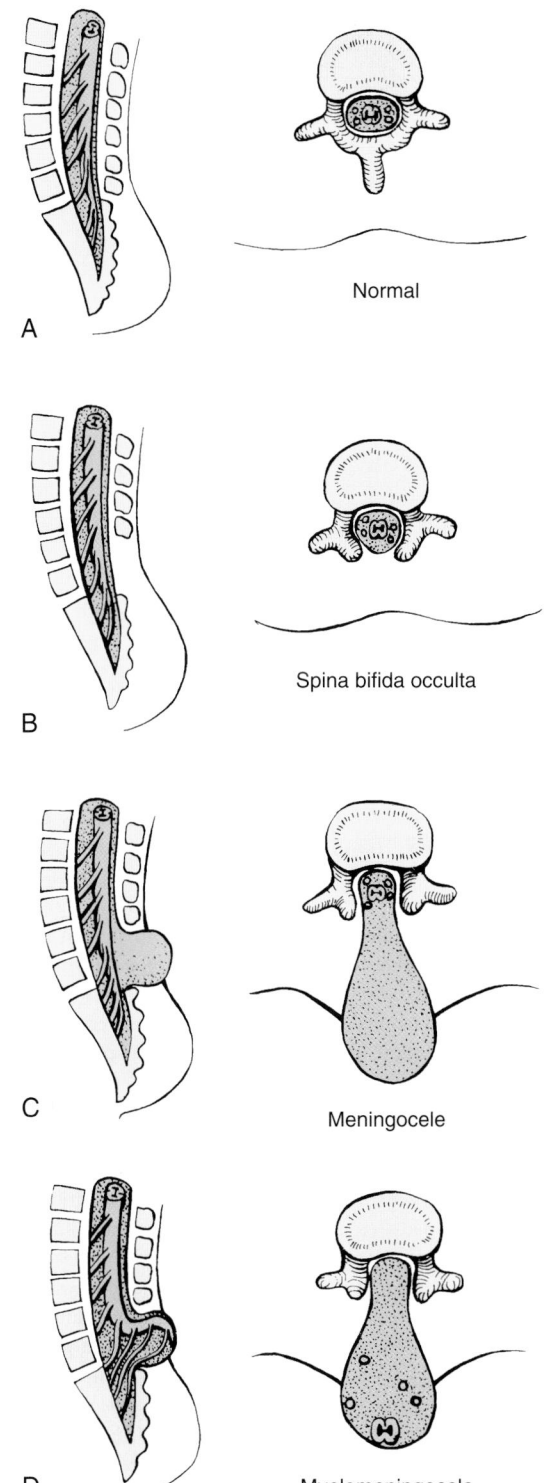

A

Normal

B

Spina bifida occulta

C

Meningocele

D

Myelomeningocele

FIG 32-5 Midline defects of the osseous spine with varying degrees of neural herniations.

BOX 32-4 SIGNIFICANT NEURAL TUBE DEFECTS

Cranioschisis—A skull defect through which various tissues protrude

Exencephaly—Brain totally exposed or extruded through an associated skull defect; fetus usually aborted

Anencephaly—If fetus with exencephaly survives, degeneration of the brain to a spongiform mass with no bony covering; incompatible with life usually beyond a few days to weeks

Encephalocele—Herniation of brain and meninges through a defect in the skull, producing a fluid-filled sac; can be frontal or posterior

Rachischisis or **spina bifida**—Fissure in the spinal column that leaves the meninges and spinal cord exposed

Meningocele—Hernial protrusion of a saclike cyst of meninges filled with spinal fluid (see Fig. 32-5, *C*)

Myelomeningocele (meningomyelocele)—Hernial protrusion of a saclike cyst containing meninges, spinal fluid, and a portion of the spinal cord with its nerves (see Fig. 32-5, *D*)

neural tube as a result of an abnormal increase in cerebrospinal fluid (CSF) pressure during the first trimester.

Etiology

There is evidence of a multifactorial etiology, including drugs, radiation, maternal malnutrition, chemicals, and possibly a genetic mutation in folate pathways in some cases, which may result in abnormal development. There is also evidence of a genetic component in the development of SB; myelomeningocele may occur in association with syndromes such as trisomy 18, PHAVER (limb pterygia, congenital heart anomalies, vertebral defects, ear anomalies, and radial defects) syndrome, and Meckel-Gruber syndrome (Shaer, Chescheir, and Schulkin, 2007). Additional factors predisposing children to an increased risk of NTDs include prepregnancy maternal obesity, maternal diabetes mellitus, low maternal vitamin B_{12} status, maternal hyperthermia, and the use of AEDs in pregnancy. The genetic predisposition is supported by evidence of the risk of recurrence after one affected child (3%–4%) and a 10% risk of recurrence with two previously affected children (Kinsman and Johnston, 2011).

The degree of neurologic dysfunction depends on where the sac protrudes through the vertebrae, the anatomic level of the defect, and the amount of nerve tissue involved. The majority of myelomeningoceles (75%) involve the lumbar or lumbosacral area (Fig. 32-6). Hydrocephalus is a frequently associated anomaly in 80% to 90% of the children. About 80% of patients with myelomeningocele develop a type II Chiari malformation (Kinsman and Johnston, 2011).

Diagnostic Evaluation

The diagnosis of SB is made on the basis of clinical manifestations (Box 32-5) and examination of the meningeal sac. Diagnostic measures used to evaluate the brain and spinal cord include MRI, ultrasonography, and CT. A neurologic evaluation will determine the extent of involvement of bowel and bladder function as well as lower extremity neuromuscular involvement. Flaccid paralysis of the lower extremities is a common finding with absent deep tendon reflexes.

Prenatal Detection

It is possible to determine the presence of some major open NTDs prenatally. Ultrasonographic scanning of the uterus and elevated maternal concentrations of α-fetoprotein (AFP, or MS-AFP), a fetal-specific γ-₁-globulin, in amniotic fluid may indicate anencephaly or

advances in both directions—caudally and cephalically—until by the end of the fourth week of gestation, the ends of the neural tube, the anterior and posterior neuropores, close.

Most authorities believe the primary defect in neural tube malformations is a failure of neural tube closure. However, some evidence indicates that the defects are a result of splitting of the already closed

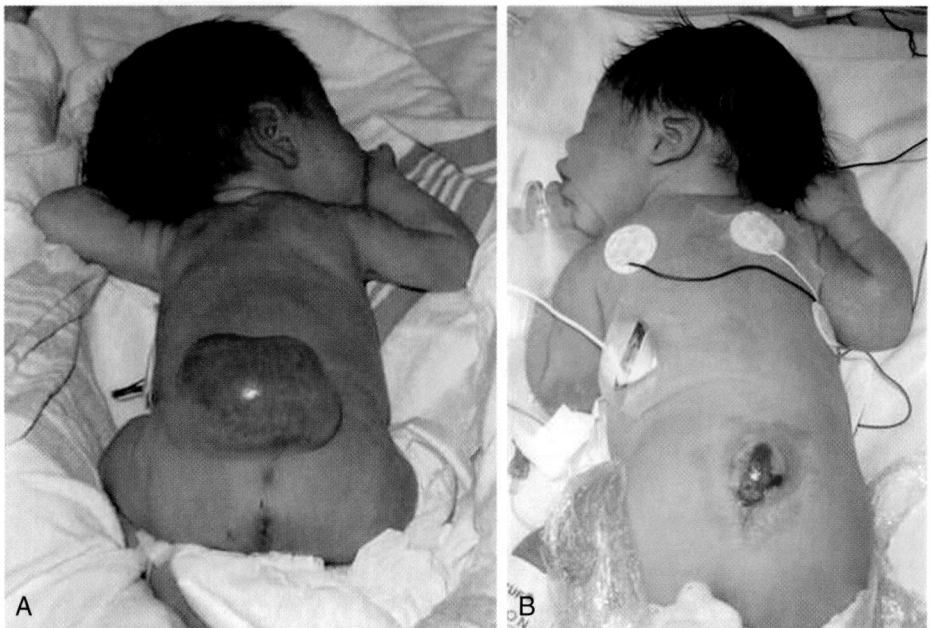

FIG 32-6 A, Myelomeningocele with an intact sac. **B,** Myelomeningocele with a ruptured sac. (Courtesy Dr. Robert C. Dauser, Neurosurgery, Baylor College of Medicine, Houston.)

BOX 32-5   CLINICAL MANIFESTATIONS OF SPINA BIFIDA

Spina Bifida Cystica
Sensory disturbances usually parallel to motor dysfunction
- Below second lumbar vertebra:
  - Flaccid, partial paralysis of lower extremities
  - Varying degrees of sensory deficit
  - Overflow incontinence with constant dribbling of urine
  - Lack of bowel control
  - Rectal prolapse (sometimes)
- Below third sacral vertebra:
  - No motor impairment
  - May have saddle anesthesia with bladder and anal sphincter paralysis
Joint deformities (sometimes produced in utero):
- Talipes valgus or varus contractures
- Kyphosis
- Lumbosacral scoliosis
- Hip dislocation or subluxation

Spina Bifida Occulta
Frequently no observable manifestations
May be associated with one or more cutaneous manifestations:
- Skin depression or dimple
- Port-wine angiomatous nevi
- Dark tufts of hair
- Soft, subcutaneous lipomas
May have neuromuscular disturbances:
- Progressive disturbance of gait with foot weakness
- Bowel and bladder sphincter disturbances

myelomeningocele. The optimum time for performing these diagnostic tests is between 16 and 18 weeks of gestation before AFP concentrations normally diminish and in sufficient time to permit a therapeutic abortion. It is recommended that such diagnostic procedures and genetic counseling be considered for all mothers who have borne an affected child, and testing is offered to all pregnant women (Kirkham, Harris, and Grzybowski, 2005). Chorionic villus sampling is also a method for prenatal diagnosis of NTDs; however, it carries certain risks (skeletal limb depletion) and is not recommended before 10 weeks of gestation.

Therapeutic Management

Management of the child who has a myelomeningocele requires a multidisciplinary team approach involving the specialties of neurology, neurosurgery, pediatrics, urology, orthopedics, rehabilitation, physical therapy, occupational therapy, and social services, as well as intensive nursing care in a variety of specialty areas. The collaborative efforts of these specialists focus on (1) the myelomeningocele and the problems associated with the defect—hydrocephalus, paralysis, orthopedic deformities (e.g., developmental dysplasia of the hip, clubfoot; scoliosis), and genitourinary abnormalities; (2) possible acquired problems that may or may not be associated, such as Chiari II malformation, meningitis, seizures, hypoxia, and hemorrhage; and (3) other abnormalities, such as cardiac or gastrointestinal (GI) malformations. Many hospitals have routine outpatient care by multidisciplinary teams to provide the complex follow-up care needed for children with myelodysplasia.

Many authorities believe that early closure, within the first 24 to 72 hours, offers the most favorable outcome. Surgical closure within the first 24 hours is recommended if the sac is leaking CSF (Kinsman and Johnston, 2011).

A variety of neurosurgical and plastic surgical procedures are used for skin closure without disturbing the neural elements or removing any portion of the sac. The objective is satisfactory skin coverage of

the lesion and meticulous closure. Wide excision of the large membranous covering may damage functioning neural tissue.

Associated problems are assessed and managed by appropriate surgical and supportive measures. Shunt procedures provide relief from imminent or progressive hydrocephalus (see Chapter 28). When diagnosed, ventriculitis, meningitis, urinary tract infection, and pneumonia are treated with vigorous antibiotic therapy and supportive measures. Surgical intervention for Chiari II malformation is indicated only when the child is symptomatic (i.e., high-pitched crowing cry, stridor, respiratory difficulties, oral-motor difficulties, upper extremity spasticity).

Early surgical closure of the myelomeningocele sac through fetal surgery has been evaluated in relation to prevention of injury to the exposed spinal cord tissue and the improvement of neurologic and urologic outcomes in the affected child. The Management of Myelomeningocele Study, a clinical trial supported by the National Institute of Health, found that prenatal surgery for myelomeningocele reduced the need for shunting (for hydrocephalus), evaluated at 12 months, and there was an improvement in mental and motor function scores at 30 months in the children who had prenatal surgery (compared with children who had postnatal surgery) (Adzick, Thom, Spong, and others, 2011). Outcome data for urologic and bowel function are not available at this time.

Infancy

Initial care of the newborn involves preventing infection; performing a neurologic assessment, including observing for associated anomalies; and dealing with the impact of the anomaly on the family. Although meningoceles are repaired early, especially if there is danger of rupture of the sac, the philosophy regarding skin closure of myelomeningocele varies. Most authorities believe that early closure, within the first 24 to 72 hours, offers the most favorable outcome. Early closure, preferably in the first 12 to 18 hours, not only prevents local infection and trauma to the exposed tissues but also avoids stretching of other nerve roots (which may occur as the meningeal sac expands during the first hours after birth), thus preventing further motor impairment. Broad-spectrum antibiotics are initiated, and neurotoxic substances such as povidone–iodine are avoided at the malformation.

Improved surgical techniques do not alter the major physical disability and deformity or chronic urinary tract and pulmonary infections that affect the quality of life for these children. Superimposed on these physical problems are the disorder's effects on family life and finances and on school and hospital services.

Orthopedic Considerations

According to most orthopedists, musculoskeletal problems that will affect later locomotion should be evaluated early, and treatment, when indicated, should be instituted without delay. Neurologic assessment will determine the neurosegmental level of the lesion and enable recognition of spasticity and progressive paralysis, potential for deformity, and functional expectations. Orthopedic management includes prevention of joint contractures, correction of any existing deformities, prevention or minimization of the effects of motor and sensory deficits, prevention of skin breakdown, and acquisition of the best possible function of affected lower extremities. Common orthopedic problems requiring attention in SB include deformities of the knees, hips, feet, and spine; fractures and insensate skin further complicate orthopedic care. Other problems that may occur later include kyphosis and scoliosis (Lazzaretti and Pearson, 2010). Because children with this condition often have decreased sensitivity in their lower extremities, preventive skin care is important. A high percentage (60%) of children seen in a wound clinic for skin breakdown had myelomeningocele (Samaniego, 2003). The status of the neurologic deficit remains the most important factor in determining the child's ultimate functional abilities.

With technologic advances, a variety of lightweight orthoses, including braces, special "walking" devices, and custom-built wheelchairs, are available to provide mobility to children with spinal cord lesions (see also Chapter 31). Early in infancy, intervention with passive range-of-motion exercises, positioning, and stretching exercises may help decrease the incidence of muscle contractures. Corrective surgical procedures, when indicated, are best initiated at an early age so the child will not lag significantly behind age mates in developmental progress. When there is little hope for lower extremity functioning, surgery is seldom recommended unless it will improve sitting position in a wheelchair and function for ADLs and mobility.

Management of Genitourinary Function

Myelomeningocele is one of the most common causes of neuropathic (neurogenic) bladder dysfunction among children. In infants, the goal of treatment is to preserve renal function. In older children, the goal is to preserve renal function and achieve optimal urinary continence. Urinary incontinence is a chronic, often debilitating problem for the child. In addition, the neuropathic bladder may produce urinary system distress, characterized by symptomatic urinary tract infections, ureterohydronephrosis, and vesicoureteral reflux or renal insufficiency. The characteristics of bladder dysfunction in children vary according to the level of the neurologic lesion and the influence of bony growth and development on the spine. Therefore, ongoing urologic monitoring is essential. Evidence is growing that early intervention, based on evaluation during the neonatal period and before complications occur, improves bladder function, reduces the risk of subsequent urinary system distress, and decreases the need for reconstructive surgery of the lower urinary tract (Snodgrass and Gorgollo, 2010; Tarcan, Onol, Ilker, and others, 2006).

Treatment of renal problems includes (1) regular urologic care with prompt and vigorous treatment of infections; (2) a method of regular emptying of the bladder, such as clean intermittent catheterization (CIC) taught to and performed by parents and self-catheterization taught to children; (3) medications to improve bladder storage and continence, such as oxybutynin chloride (Ditropan) and tolterodine (Detrol); and (4) surgical procedures such as vesicostomy (bladder surgically brought out to the abdominal wall, allowing continuous urinary drainage) and augmentation enterocystoplasty (using a segment of bowel or stomach to increase bladder capacity, thereby reducing high bladder pressures).

However, despite the combined efforts of CIC, medication, and surgical intervention, some children with myelodysplasia may continue to experience debilitating urinary incontinence. Many of these children are able to attain social continence with a continent urinary diversion commonly referred to as a Mitrofanoff procedure. In this procedure, a catheterizable channel is surgically created from appendix, ureter, or tapered bowel. The proximal end of the channel is connected to the bladder with the distal end brought out as a small stoma on the abdominal wall, usually near the umbilicus. The bladder neck may be sutured to prevent urinary leakage from the urethra. CIC through the easily accessible abdominal route fosters greater independence in children, especially in those unable to transfer from wheelchair to toilet to perform CIC.

Bowel Control

Some degree of fecal continence can be achieved in most children with myelomeningocele with diet modification, regular toilet habits, and prevention of constipation and impaction. It is frequently a lengthy process. Dietary fiber supplements (recommended 10 g/day), laxatives, suppositories, or enemas aid in producing regular evacuation. Older children and adolescents seeking more independence may attain bowel continence and higher quality of life after undergoing an antegrade continence enema (ACE) procedure (Doolin, 2006). In a procedure similar to the Mitrofanoff, the appendix or ileum is used to create a catheterizable channel with attachment of the proximal end to the colon. The distal end of the channel exits through a small abdominal stoma. Every 1 or 2 days, a catheter is passed through the stoma, allowing enema solution to be instilled directly into the colon. After administration of the enema solution, the child sits on the toilet for 30 to 60 minutes as stool is flushed out through the rectum. The frequency of enemas and volume of solution used to completely evacuate the bowel vary among individuals.

Prognosis

The early prognosis for the child with myelomeningocele depends on the neurologic deficit present at birth, including motor ability, bladder innervation, and associated neurologic anomalies. Early surgical repair of the spinal defect, antibiotic therapy to reduce the incidence of meningitis and ventriculitis, prevention of urinary system dysfunction, and early detection and correction of hydrocephalus have significantly increased the survival rate and quality of life in such children. Children with spina bifida have normal intelligence. Many children with SB achieve partial independent living and gainful employment. Reports of survival rates vary, and many include adults who were born before medical advances and surgical techniques seen in the past 25 years. Coordinated care for adults with SB is essential; however, multidisciplinary adult care is often inadequate (Lazzaretti and Pearson, 2010). In children and adolescents with SB, the achievement of urinary continence is associated with improved self-concept and esteem, especially among girls (Moore, Kogan, and Parekh, 2004). This chronic condition has an array of associated complications, including hydrocephalus and shunt malfunctions, scoliosis, bowel and bladder management issues, latex allergy, and epilepsy. However, based on current medical knowledge and ethical considerations, aggressive, early management is favored for the child with myelomeningocele.

Prevention

The CDC (2009) continues to affirm that 50% to 70% of NTDs can be prevented by daily consumption of 0.4 mg of folic acid among women of childbearing age. The data indicate that serum folate concentrations among women of childbearing age decreased 16% from 2003 to 2004 in all ethnic groups studied. Lowest serum folate levels were seen in non-Hispanic whites in 2003 to 2004; however, overall serum folate levels remained below recommended levels in non-Hispanic African Americans during all three periods studied (CDC, 2007). These results indicate that nurses and other health care workers have an important task in disseminating information that may decrease the incidence of birth defects in children by promoting maternal consumption of folic acid.*

To ensure adequate daily intake of the recommended amount of folic acid, women must take a folic acid supplement, eat a fortified

breakfast cereal containing 100% of the Recommended Dietary Allowance of folic acid (e.g., Kellogg's Product 19, General Mills Total, Multigrain Cheerios Plus), or increase their consumption of fortified foods (cereal, bread, rice, grits, pasta) and foods naturally rich in folate (green, leafy vegetables and citrus fruits). For women who have had a previous pregnancy affected by NTDs, folic acid intake is increased to 4 mg under the supervision of a practitioner beginning 1 month before a planned pregnancy and continuing through the first trimester. Supplementation of 4 mg of folate should not be given solely in multivitamin preparations because of the risk of overdose of other vitamins. Drugs that affect folic acid metabolism and increase the risk of myelomeningocele should be avoided before pregnancy (if plans are to become pregnant in the near future) and during pregnancy; these include trimethoprim and the AEDs carbamazepine, phenytoin, phenobarbital, valproic acid, and primidone (Kinsman and Johnston, 2011).

Nursing Care Management

At birth, an examination is performed to assess the intactness of the membranous cyst. During transport to the nursery, every effort is made to prevent trauma to this protective covering. In addition to the routine assessment of the newborn (see Chapter 8), the infant is assessed for the level of neurologic involvement. Movement of extremities or skin response, especially an anal reflex that might provide clues to the degree of motor or sensory impairment, is noted. It is important to observe the infant's behavior in conjunction with the stimulus because limb movements can be induced in response to spinal cord reflex activity that has no connection with the higher centers. Observation of urinary output, especially if a diaper remains dry, may indicate urinary retention. Abdominal assessment revealing bladder distention, even with a wet diaper, may indicate urinary overflow in a retentive bladder. The head circumference is measured daily (see Chapter 6), and the fontanels are examined for signs of tension or bulging.

Care of the Myelomeningocele Sac

The infant is usually placed in an incubator or warmer so temperature can be maintained without clothing or covers that might irritate the spinal lesion. When an overhead warmer is used, the dressings over the defect require more frequent moistening because of the dehydrating effect of the radiant heat.

Before surgical closure, the myelomeningocele is prevented from drying by the application of a sterile, moist, nonadherent dressing over the defect. The moistening solution is usually sterile normal saline. Dressings are changed frequently (every 2–4 hours), and the sac is closely inspected for leaks, abrasions, irritation, and any signs of infection. The sac must be carefully cleansed if it becomes soiled or contaminated. Sometimes the sac ruptures during delivery or transport, and any opening in the sac greatly increases the risk of infection to the CNS.

> **NURSING TIP** To prevent stool contamination of the SB defect preoperatively, obtain a surgical drape (e.g., Steri-Drape). Cut a portion of the drape to fit the infant's sacrum and secure the drape using nonlatex tape. Place the rest of the drape loosely over the dressing, covering the defect and thus preventing exposure to stool.

> **! NURSING ALERT**
>
> Observe for early signs of infection, such as temperature instability (axillary), irritability, and lethargy, and for signs of increased intracranial pressure, which might indicate developing hydrocephalus.

*Information is available from CDC, National Center on Birth Defects and Developmental Disabilities, Division of Birth Defects and Developmental Disabilities, 1600 Clifton Road NE, MS E-86, Atlanta, GA 30333; 800-CDC-INFO; e-mail: cdcinfo@cdc.gov; http://www.cdc.gov/ncbddd/folicacid and from the March of Dimes Resource Center, 1275 Mamaroneck Ave., White Plains, NY 10605; http://www.marchofdimes.com.

One of the most important and challenging aspects in the early care of the infant with myelomeningocele is positioning. Before surgery, the infant is kept in the prone position to minimize tension on the sac and the risk of trauma. The prone position allows for optimal positioning of the legs, especially in cases of associated hip dysplasia. The infant is placed prone with the hips slightly flexed and supported to reduce tension on the defect. The legs are maintained in abduction with a pad between the knees to counteract hip subluxation, and a small roll is placed under the ankles to maintain a neutral foot position. A variety of aids, including diaper rolls, pads, small foam pads, or specially designed frames and appliances, can be used to maintain the desired position.

Prevent Complications

The prone position affects other aspects of the infant's care. For example, in this position, the infant is more difficult to keep clean, pressure areas are a constant threat, and feeding becomes a problem. The infant's head is turned to one side for feeding. Fortunately, most defects are repaired early, and the infant can be held for feeding soon after surgery. Special care must be taken to avoid pressure on the operative site.

Diapering the infant may be contraindicated until the defect has been repaired and healing is well advanced or epithelialization has taken place. The padding beneath the diaper area is changed as needed to keep the skin dry and free of irritation. When urinary retention is detected, CIC is used. Because the bowel sphincter is frequently affected, there is continual passage of stool, often misinterpreted as diarrhea, which is a constant irritant to the skin and a source of infection to the spinal lesion.

Areas of sensory and motor impairment are subject to skin breakdown and therefore require meticulous care. Placing the infant on a special mattress or mattress overlay reduces pressure on the knees and ankles. Periodic cleansing, application of lotion, and gentle massage aid circulation.

Gentle range-of-motion exercises are carried out to prevent contractures, and stretching of contractures is performed when indicated. However, these exercises may be restricted to the foot, ankle, and knee joint. When the hip joints are unstable, stretching against tight hip flexors or adductor muscles, which act much like bowstrings, may aggravate a tendency toward subluxation. Consultation with a physical therapist is an important aspect of the short- and long-term management of infants with myelomeningocele.

Cuddling infants with unrepaired myelomeningocele is contraindicated. Their need for tactile stimulation is met by caressing, stroking, and other comfort measures. Individualized developmental care with age-appropriate stimulation is provided (see Developmental Outcome, Chapter 9).

Provide Postoperative Care

Postoperative care of the infant with myelomeningocele involves the same basic care as that of any postsurgical infant and includes monitoring vital signs, monitoring intake and output, providing nourishment, observing for signs of infection, and managing pain. Care of the operative site is carried out under the direction of the surgeon and includes close observation for signs of leakage of CSF. General care is continued as preoperatively.

The prone position is maintained after surgical closure, although many neurosurgeons allow a side-lying or partial side-lying position unless it aggravates a coexisting hip dysplasia or permits undesirable hip flexion. This offers an opportunity for position changes, which reduces the risk of pressure sores and facilitates feeding. If permitted, the infant can be held upright against the body, with care taken to avoid pressure on the operative site. After the effects of anesthesia have subsided and the infant is alert, feedings may be resumed unless there are other anomalies or associated complications.

Support Family and Educate about Home Care

As soon as the parents are able to cope with the infant's condition, they are encouraged to become involved in care. They need to learn how to continue at home the care that has been initiated in the hospital, including positioning, feeding, skin care, and range-of-motion exercises when appropriate. They are taught CIC technique when it is prescribed. Parents also need to know the signs of complications (urinary, neurologic, orthopedic) and how to obtain assistance when needed.

The mother who wishes to breastfeed the infant is encouraged to do so because this will be beneficial. Shortly after delivery, the mother is started on a program of pumping to initiate and maintain milk supply until the infant is stable enough to begin breastfeeding (Hurtekant and Spatz, 2007). This process may require considerable support from nurses, physicians, and family members because of separation from the infant for surgical care and recovery.

The long-range planning with and support of the parents and newborn begin in the hospital continuing throughout childhood and even into young adulthood. The life expectancy of children with SB extends well into adulthood; therefore, planning should involve long-term goals and plans for optimum function as an adult. Discussion about aspects of adulthood such as receiving educational or vocational training and education, living independently, having a mate, having sexual relationships, and bearing and rearing children is important and should not be overlooked. The unique service needs of adolescents with SB as they attempt to gain independence from family and establish lives of their own have not been adequately addressed in the literature (Sawyer and Macnee, 2010). Betz, Linroth, Butler, and others (2010) interviewed young people with SB making the transition to adulthood. Some common themes that emerged among these young people were as follows: (1) challenges in preparation for self-management, (2) limited social relationships, (3) awareness of their cognitive challenges, and (4) the cost of independence. Nurses assume an important role as central members of the health team. As a care manager and coordinator, nurses review information with the family, take responsibility for family teaching, and act as a liaison between inpatient and outpatient services. The child will need numerous hospitalizations over the years, and each one will be a source of stress to which the younger child is especially vulnerable (see Chapter 18 for a discussion of care of the child with a disability).

Habilitation involves not only solving problems of self-help and locomotion but also solving the most distressing problem of urinary or bowel incontinence, which threatens the child's social acceptability. Assistance in preparing the child and the school regarding the child's special needs helps provide a better initial adjustment to this broader social experience.

A Life Course Model has been developed for patients, families, caregivers, teachers, and clinicians to facilitate, through a developmental approach, the care of the child and young person with SB; this

---

BOX 32-6 MEDICAL CONDITIONS ASSOCIATED WITH RISK OF LATEX ALLERGY

- Spina bifida
- Urogenital anomalies
- Imperforate anus
- Tracheoesophageal fistula
- VATER association
- Preterm infants
- Ventriculoperitoneal shunt
- Cognitive impairment
- Cerebral palsy
- Spinal cord injuries
- Multiple surgeries
- Atopy

VATER, Vertebral defects, imperforate anus, tracheoesophageal fistula, and radial and renal dysplasia.

NURSING CARE GUIDELINES
Identifying Latex Allergy

- Does your child have any symptoms, such as sneezing, coughing, rashes, or wheezing, when handling rubber products (e.g., balloons, tennis or Koosh balls, adhesive bandage strips) or when in contact with rubber hospital products (e.g., gloves, catheters)?
- Has your child ever had an allergic reaction during surgery?
- Does your child have a history of rashes; asthma; or allergic reactions to medication or foods, especially milk, kiwi, bananas, or chestnuts?
- How would you identify or recognize an allergic reaction in your child?
- What would you do if an allergic reaction occurred?
- Has anyone ever discussed latex or rubber allergy or sensitivity with you?
- Has your child had any allergy testing?
- When did your child last come in contact with any type of rubber product? Were you present?

Modified from Romanczuk A: Latex use with infants and children: it can cause problems, *MCN Am J Matern Child Nurs* 18(4):208–212, 1993.

---

program has been made into a web-based tool that can be used to assist in the transition to adulthood (Dicianno, Fairman, Juengst, and others, 2010). Additional information regarding this program is available through the Spina Bifida Association's website at http://www.sbpreparations.org.

The Spina Bifida Association of America* is organized to provide services and support for families of children with spinal lesions.

Latex Allergy

Latex allergy, or latex hypersensitivity, was identified as being a serious health hazard when a report linked intraoperative anaphylaxis with latex in children with SB. Latex, a natural product derived from the rubber tree, is used in combination with other chemicals to give elasticity, strength, and durability to many products. Children with SB are at high risk for developing latex allergy because of repeated exposure to latex products during surgery and procedures. Therefore, such children should not be exposed to latex products from birth onward to minimize the occurrence of latex hypersensitivity. Allergic reactions range from urticaria, wheezing, watery eyes, and rashes, to anaphylactic shock. More severe reactions tend to occur when latex comes in contact with mucous membranes, wet skin, the bloodstream, or an airway. There also can be cross-reactions to a number of foods (e.g., banana, avocado, kiwi, chestnut).

Allergic reactions to latex protein can also occur when the substance is transferred to food by food handlers wearing latex gloves, prompting several states to pass legislation that prohibits the use of latex gloves in food service. In addition to patients with SB, high-risk populations include patients with urogenital anomalies or multiple surgeries as well as health care workers. Box 32-6 lists medical conditions associated with the risk of latex allergy.

The most important goals are prevention of latex sensitivity and identification of children with a known hypersensitivity (see Nursing Care Guidelines box). High-risk and latex-allergic individuals must be managed in a latex-free environment. Take care that they do not come in direct or secondary contact with products or equipment containing latex at *any time* during medical treatment. Allergy testing can identify

latex sensitivity with varying success. Skin prick testing and provocation testing carry the risk of allergic reaction or anaphylaxis. Several commercially available assays can be useful in confirming latex sensitivity. To date, none of these tests demonstrates complete diagnostic reliability, and they should not be the sole determinant of the presence or absence of an allergic response to latex.

Because children who have SB are prone to develop sensitivity to latex, reducing exposure from birth onward may decrease the chance of allergy development. Nonlatex products lists are available to parents and health care workers; these products may be substituted for those containing latex. In the health care arena, it is important to use products with the lowest potential risk of sensitizing patients and staff members.*

The identification of those sensitive to latex is best accomplished through careful screening of all patients. During the health interview with the parent or child, ask *all* patients, not only those at risk, about sensitivity to latex. Be certain this is a routine part of all preoperative and preprocedural histories. Stress the importance of the allergy history to all personnel (e.g., phlebotomists). (See Nursing Care Guidelines box for questions related to latex allergy.) Children with latex hypersensitivity should carry some form of allergy identification, such as a Medic-Alert bracelet. Education programs regarding latex hypersensitivity are aimed at those who care for high-risk groups, such as children with SB, and may include relatives, school nurses, teachers, child care workers, and babysitters. In addition to educating caregivers about the child's exposure to medical products that contain latex, nurses need to inform them of common nonmedical latex objects such as water toys, pacifiers, and plastic storage bags.[†] Items brought to the hospital, such as floral bouquets, should also be screened for latex toys and balloons. Parents should also receive literature explaining signs and symptoms of latex hypersensitivity and appropriate emergency treatment. (See Anaphylaxis, Chapter 25.)

---

*4590 McArthur Blvd. NW, Suite 250, Washington, DC 20007-4226; 202-944-3285, 800-621-3141; fax: 202-944-3295; http://www.sbaa.org.

*For a list of latex products and alternative products, see the SBAA National Resource Center and then Latex List on the Spina Bifida Association's home page, http://www.spinabifidaassociation.org.
[†]Latex-free product lists are available from the American Latex Allergy Association's online resource manual, available at http://www.latexallergyresources.org/ResourceManual/section1/index.cfm. American Latex Allergy Association, PO Box 198, Slinger, WI 53086; 888-972-5378; http://www.latexallergyresources.org.

SPINAL MUSCULAR ATROPHY, TYPE 1 (WERDNIG-HOFFMANN DISEASE)

Spinal muscular atrophy (SMA) type 1 (Werdnig-Hoffmann disease) is a disorder characterized by progressive weakness and wasting of skeletal muscles caused by degeneration of anterior horn cells. It is inherited as an autosomal recessive trait and is the most common paralytic form of the floppy infant syndrome (congenital hypotonia). The sites of the pathologic condition are the anterior horn cells of the spinal cord and the motor nuclei of the brainstem, but the primary effect is atrophy of skeletal muscles. The age of onset is variable, but the earlier the onset, the more disseminated and severe the motor weakness. The disorder may be manifested early—often at birth—and almost always before 2 years of age; death may occur as a result of respiratory failure by age 2 years (Iannaccone and Burghes, 2002; Lunn and Wang, 2008). The manifestations (Box 32-7) and prognosis are categorized according to the age of onset, severity of weakness, and clinical course; some children may fluctuate between exhibiting symptoms of types 1 and 2 or types 2 and 3 in regard to clinical function (Sarnat, 2011a). Some experts also categorize SMA according to the highest level of motor function (Lunn and Wang, 2008); type 1 includes "nonsitters," type 2 includes "sitters," and type 3 includes "walkers" (Iannaccone, 2007). A severe rare fetal form of SMA, classified as type 0, is reported to be quite lethal in the perinatal period; motor neuron degeneration may be noted as early as midgestation in type 0 (Sarnat, 2011a). Type 4 may present between 20 and 30 years of age and may be referred to as proximal adult type SMA (Prior, 2010).

Diagnostic Evaluation and Therapeutic Management

The diagnosis is based on the molecular genetic marker for the *SMN* (survival motor neuron) gene, which is located on chromosome 5q13. Prenatal diagnosis may be made by genetic analysis of circulating fetal cells in maternal blood (Beroud, Karliova, Bonnefont, and others, 2003) or circulating fetal cells in amniotic fluid. The risk of subsequent affected offspring in carriers of the mutant gene or in families with known cases of SMA may also be evaluated genetically. Further diagnostic studies include muscle electromyography (EMG), which demonstrates a denervation pattern, and muscle biopsy; however, the genetic analysis has become the gold standard for diagnosis of the condition.

There is no cure for the disease, and treatment is symptomatic and preventive, primarily preventing joint contractures and treating orthopedic problems, the most serious of which is scoliosis. Hip subluxation and dislocation may also occur. Many children benefit from powered wheelchairs, lifts, special pressure-adjustable mattresses, and accessible environmental controls. Muscle and joint contractures require careful attention and care to prevent further complications. Nutritional growth failure may occur in infants and toddlers as a result of poor feeding; supplemental gastrostomy feedings may be required to maintain adequate nutritional status and maintain weight gain. The use of lower extremity orthoses may assist with ambulation, but eventually, the child may be confined to a wheelchair as muscle atrophy progresses. Restrictive lung disease is the most serious complication of SMA (Iannaccone, 2007). Upper respiratory tract infections often occur and are treated with antibiotic therapy; they are the cause of death in many children. Rapid eye movement (REM)–related sleep-disordered breathing is common in children with SMA type 1; this progresses to sleep-disordered breathing during REM and non-REM sleep followed by respiratory failure, which often requires nocturnal noninvasive mechanical ventilation (Schroth, 2009). Noninvasive ventilation methods such as bilevel positive airway pressure (BiPAP) have decreased the morbidity and increased the survival rate of children

with SMA types 1 and 2. A decreased ability to cough and clear secretions may be managed with airway clearance therapies such as the cough-assist machine and manual cough assistance. Guidelines for the standardization of respiratory care for patients with SMA have been published elsewhere (Schroth, 2009).

BOX 32-7   CLINICAL MANIFESTATIONS OF SPINAL MUSCULAR ATROPHY*

Type 1 (Werdnig-Hoffmann Disease)
Clinical manifestations within first few weeks or months of life
Onset within 6 months of life
Inactivity the most prominent feature
Infant lying in a frog-leg position with legs externally rotated, abducted, and flexed at knees
Generalized weakness
Absent deep tendon reflexes
Limited movements of shoulder and arm muscles
Active movement usually limited to fingers and toes
Diaphragmatic breathing with sternal retractions (diaphragmatic paralysis may occur)
Abnormal tongue movements (at rest)
Weak cry and cough
Poor suck reflex
Tiring quickly during feedings (if breastfed, may lose weight before noticeable)
Growth failure (nutritional)
Alert facies
Normal sensation and intellect
Affected infants not able to sit alone, roll over, or walk
Early death possible from respiratory failure or infection

Type 2 (Intermediate Spinal Muscular Atrophy)
Onset before age 18 months
    Early—Weakness confined to arms and legs
    Later—Becomes generalized
Legs usually involved to greater extent than arms
Prominent pectus excavatum
Movements absent during complete relaxation or sleep
Some infants able to sit if placed in position, but few can ambulate
Life span from 7 months to 7 years, although many have normal life expectancy

Type 3 (Kugelberg-Welander Disease; Mild Spinal Muscular Atrophy)
Onset of symptoms after 18 months of age
Normal head control and ability to sit unassisted by 6 to 8 months of age
Thigh and hip muscles weak
Scoliosis common
Failure to walk a common presentation
In those who manage to walk:
- Waddling gait
- Genu recurvatum
- Protuberant abdomen
- Ambulation becoming increasingly difficult
- Confinement to a wheelchair by second decade
- Deep tendon reflexes possibly present early but disappear

*These classifications are general, but some research suggests there may be variations in life span and other characteristics (Iannaccone and Burghes, 2002; Russman, 1996; Russman, Iannaccone, Buncher, and others, 1992).

Prognosis

Prognosis varies according to the age of onset or group as described in Box 32-7. Individuals with SMA type 1 may succumb to respiratory infections or failure between 1 and 24 months of age (Iannaccone and Burghes, 2002; Sarnat, 2011a); however, some may live into their third or fourth decade of life. A significant number of infants with SMA require a tracheotomy, and associated medical conditions in survivors include gastroesophageal reflux, scoliosis, early onset puberty, hip dysplasia, and recurrent oral candidiasis (Bach, 2007). Drug therapy with riluzole, valproic acid, gabapentin, and oral phenylbutyrate has been shown to slow the progression of the condition, but none has demonstrated significant overall benefits (Bosboom, Vrancken, van den Berg, and others, 2009; Sarnat, 2011a).

Nursing Care Management

An infant or small child with progressive muscle weakness requires nursing care similar to that of an immobilized patient (see Chapter 31). However, the underlying goal of treatment should be to assist the child and family in dealing with the illness while progressing toward a life of normalization within the child's capabilities. Special attention should be directed to preventing muscle and joint contractures, promoting independence in performance of ADLs, and becoming incorporated into the mainstream of school when possible. In addition, parents need support and resources to be able to provide for the child and remain an intact family. Because children with neuromuscular disease have abnormal breathing patterns that often contribute to early death, it is important to assess adequate oxygenation, especially during the sleep phase when shallow breathing occurs and hypoxemia may develop. Home pulse oximetry may be used to assess the child during sleep and provide noninvasive mechanical ventilation as necessary (Bush, Fraser, Jardine, and others, 2005; Young, Lowe, Fitzgerald, and others, 2007) (see Duchenne [Pseudohypertrophic] Muscular Dystrophy, below, for respiratory management). Supportive care also includes management of orthoses and other orthopedic equipment as required. Because children with SMA are intellectually normal, verbal, tactile, and auditory stimulation are important aspects of developmental care. Supporting them so they can see the activities around them and transporting them in appropriate conveyances (e.g., wagon, power wheelchair) for a change of environment provide stimulation and a broader scope of contacts.

Children who are able to sit require proper support and attention to alignment to prevent deformities and other complications. Children who survive beyond infancy need attention to educational needs and opportunities for social interaction with other children. The parents of a child who is chronically ill require much support and encouragement* (see Chapter 18). Parents who have not sought genetic counseling should be encouraged to do so to evaluate further risk potential.

SPINAL MUSCULAR ATROPHY, TYPE 3 (KUGELBERG-WELANDER DISEASE)

Spinal muscular atrophy type 3 (Kugelberg-Welander disease) is a result of anterior horn cell and motor nerve degeneration. The disease is characterized by a pattern of muscular weakness similar to that of type 1 SMA (see Box 32-7). Several modes of inheritance have been

*Family resources include Families of SMA, 925 Busse Road, Elk Grove Village, IL 60007; 800-886-1762; http://www.fsma.org. In Canada: Families of Spinal Muscular Atrophy Canada, 103–7134 Vedder Rd., Chilliwack, BC V2R 4G4; toll free 855-824-1266; http://www.curesma.ca. Muscular Dystrophy Association–USA, 3300 E. Sunrise Drive, Tucson, AZ 85718; 800-572-1717; http://www.mda.org.

reported for the disease: autosomal recessive, autosomal dominant, and X-linked recessive.

The onset occurs from younger than 1 year of age into adulthood, with symptoms resembling type 3 SMA. Proximal muscle weakness (especially of the lower limbs) and muscular atrophy are the predominant features. The disease runs a slowly progressive course. Some children lose the ability to walk 8 to 9 years after the onset of symptoms, but many can still walk after 30 years or more. Many affected persons have a normal life expectancy (Lunn and Wang, 2008).

Therapeutic Management and Nursing Care Management

The management is primarily symptomatic and supportive and is related to maintaining mobility as long as possible, preventing complications such as skin breakdown, optimizing and maintaining respiratory function, and providing support to the child and family. The discussion of family support in the section for Duchenne muscular dystrophy is also applicable to families of children with SMA.

MUSCULAR DYSTROPHIES

Muscular dystrophies (MDs) constitute the largest and most important single group of muscle diseases of childhood. The MDs have a genetic origin in which there is gradual degeneration of muscle fibers, and they are characterized by progressive weakness and wasting of symmetric groups of skeletal muscles, with increasing disability and deformity. In all forms of MD, there is an insidious loss of strength, but each type differs in regard to the muscle groups affected (Fig. 32-7), age of onset, rate of progression, and inheritance pattern. The most common form, Duchenne muscular dystrophy (DMD), is discussed separately in the next section.

Facioscapulohumeral (Landouzy-Dejerine) muscular dystrophy is inherited as an autosomal dominant disorder with onset in early adolescence. It is characterized by difficulty in raising the arms over the head, lack of facial mobility, and a forward slope of the shoulders. The progression is slow, and the life span is usually unaffected.

Limb-girdle muscular dystrophy (LGMD) is a heterogenous group of disorders with autosomal dominant and recessive inheritance whose clinical manifestations often appear in later childhood, adolescence, or early adulthood with variable but usually slow progression (Quan, 2011). All types of LGMD are characterized by weakness of proximal muscles of the pelvic and shoulder girdles. Other forms of MD include myotonic dystrophy, scapulohumeral MD (Emery-Dreifuss MD), fascioscapulohumeral MD (Landouzy-Dejerine disease), and congenital MD; these forms consist of subtypes of MD and are discussed at length elsewhere (see Sarnat, 2011b).

Treatment of the MDs consists mainly of supportive measures, including physical therapy, orthopedic procedures to minimize deformity, ventilation support, and assistance for the affected child in meeting the demands of daily living.

DUCHENNE (PSEUDOHYPERTROPHIC) MUSCULAR DYSTROPHY

Duchenne muscular dystrophy is the most severe and the most common MD of childhood. It is inherited as an X-linked recessive trait, and the single-gene defect is located on the short arm of the X chromosome. DMD has a high mutation rate, with a positive family history in about 65% of cases. Genetic counseling is an important aspect of the care of the family. In about 30% of cases, it is a new mutation, and the mother is *not* the carrier (Sarnat, 2011b).

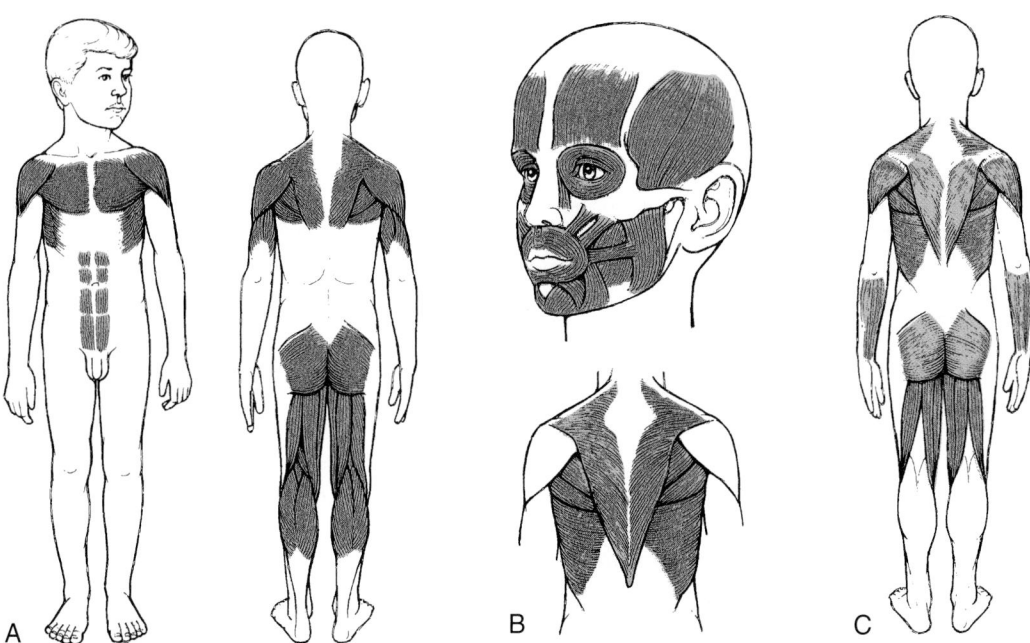

FIG 32-7 Initial muscle groups involved in muscular dystrophies. **A,** Pseudohypertrophic. **B,** Fascioscapulohumeral. **C,** Limb girdle.

BOX 32-8   CHARACTERISTICS OF DUCHENNE MUSCULAR DYSTROPHY

- Early onset, usually between 3 and 7 years of age
- Progressive muscular weakness, wasting, and contractures
- Calf muscle hypertrophy in most patients
- Loss of independent ambulation by 9 to 12 years of age
- Slowly progressive, generalized weakness during teenage years

---

As in all X-linked disorders, males are affected almost exclusively. The female carrier may have an elevated serum creatine kinase, but muscle weakness is usually not a problem; however, about 10% of female carriers develop cardiomyopathy (Manzur, Kinali, and Muntoni, 2008). In rare instances, a female may be identified with DMD disease yet with muscular weakness that is milder than in boys (Sarnat, 2011b). At the genetic level, both DMD and Becker MD (a milder variant) result from mutations of the gene that encodes dystrophin, a protein product in skeletal muscle. Dystrophin is absent from the muscles of children with DMD and is reduced or abnormal in children with Becker MD. Children with Becker MD have a later onset of symptoms, which are usually not as severe as those seen in DMD. The incidence is approximately 1 in 3600 male births for the Duchenne form and approximately 1 in 30,000 live births for the Becker type (Sarnat, 2007, 2011). Box 32-8 describes the characteristics of DMD.

Most children with DMD reach the appropriate developmental milestones early in life, although they may have mild, subtle delays. Evidence of muscle weakness usually appears during the third to seventh year, although there may have been a history of delay in motor development, particularly walking. Difficulties in running, riding a bicycle, and climbing stairs are usually the first symptoms noted. Typically, affected boys have a waddling gait and lordosis, fall frequently, and develop a characteristic manner of rising from a squatting or sitting position on the floor (**Gower sign**) (Fig. 32-8). Lordosis occurs

as a result of weakened pelvic muscles, and the waddling gait is a result of weakness in the gluteus medius and maximus muscles (Battista, 2010). In the early years, rapid developmental gains may mask the progression of the disease.

Muscles, especially in the calves, thighs, and upper arms, become enlarged from fatty infiltration and feel unusually firm or woody on palpation (Box 32-9). The term **pseudohypertrophy** is derived from this muscular enlargement. Profound muscular atrophy occurs in the later stages; contractures and deformities involving large and small joints are common complications as the disease progresses. Ambulation usually becomes impossible by 12 years of age. The loss of mobilization further increases the spectrum of complications, which may include osteoporosis, fractures, constipation, skin breakdown, and psychosocial and behavioral problems. Atrophy of facial, oropharyngeal, and respiratory muscles does not occur until the advanced stage of the disease. Ultimately, the disease process involves the diaphragm and auxiliary muscles of respiration, and cardiomyopathy is seen in approximately 50% to 80% of patients with DMD (Sarnat, 2011b).

Obesity is a common complication that contributes to premature loss of ambulation. Children who have restricted opportunities for physical activity and who are bored easily consume calories in excess of their needs. This may be compounded by overfeeding by well-meaning family and friends. Proper dietary intake and a diversified recreational program help reduce the likelihood of obesity and enable children to maintain ambulation and functional independence for a longer time.

Mild to moderate cognitive impairment is commonly associated with MD. A deficiency of dystrophin isoforms in brain tissue causes cognitive and intellectual impairment (Manzur, Kinali, and Muntoni, 2008). The mean intelligence quotient (IQ) is approximately 20 points below normal, and frank mental deficit is present in 20% to 30% of these children. Verbal IQ is markedly low in boys with DMD, and emotional disturbance is more common than in other children with disabilities; however, children with DMD should be involved in early learning programs and eventually moved into regular classrooms as much as possible. Patients with Becker MD present later in life than

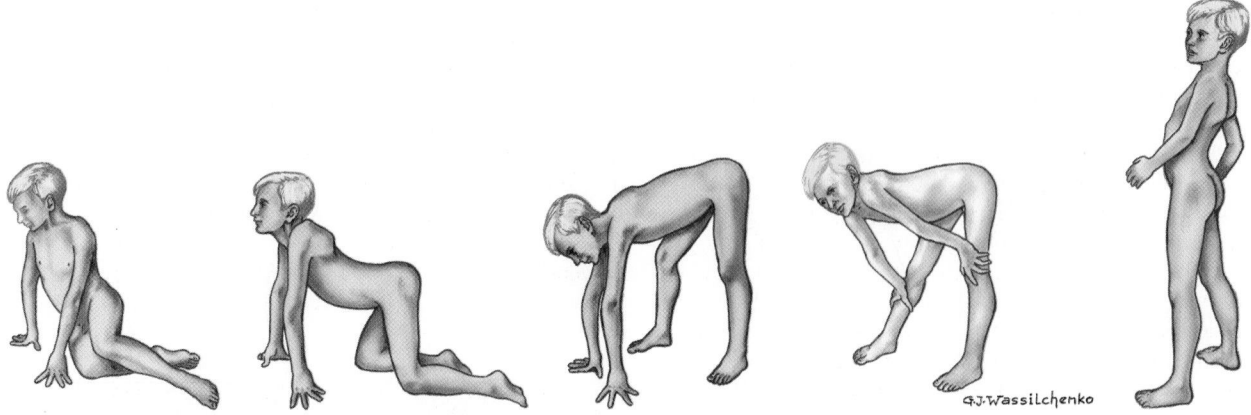

FIG 32-8 A child with Duchenne muscular dystrophy attains standing posture by kneeling and then gradually pushing his torso upright (with knees straight) by "walking" his hands up his legs (Gower sign). Note the marked lordosis in an upright position.

BOX 32-9 CLINICAL MANIFESTATIONS OF DUCHENNE MUSCULAR DYSTROPHY

Relentless progression of muscle weakness; possible death from respiratory or cardiac failure
Waddling gait
Lordosis
Frequent falls
Gower sign (child turns onto side or abdomen; flexes knees to assume a kneeling position; and then with knees extended, gradually pushes torso to an upright position by "walking" the hands up the legs)
Enlarged (hypertrophied) muscles (especially calves, thighs, and upper arms); feel unusually firm or woody on palpation
Later stages—profound muscular atrophy
Mental deficiency (common)
- Mild (≈20 IQ points below normal)
- Mental deficit present in 25% to 30% of patients
Complications:
- Contracture deformities of hips, knees, and ankles
- Disuse atrophy
- Cardiomyopathy
- Obesity and at times undernutrition
- Respiratory compromise and cardiac failure

---

those with DMD, but they often do not survive past the middle of the second decade, with few patients living into their 40s (Sarnat, 2011b).

Diagnostic Evaluation

The diagnosis of DMD is primarily established by blood polymerase chain reaction (PCR) for the dystrophin gene mutation (Sarnat, 2011b). Prenatal diagnosis is also possible as early as 12 weeks of gestation. Serum enzyme measurement, muscle biopsy, and EMG may also be used in establishing the diagnosis. Serum creatine kinase (CK) levels are extremely high in the first 2 years of life before the onset of clinical weakness. If the child demonstrates the usual characteristics, has a positive family history for DMD, and the PCR result is positive, the muscle biopsy may be deferred.

Therapeutic Management

No effective treatment exists for childhood MD. The use of the corticosteroids prednisone and deflazacort has been evaluated as a treatment for DMD. Several clinical trials demonstrated increased muscle strength and improved performance and pulmonary function, with significant decrease in the progression of weakness, when prednisone was administered for 6 months to 2 years (Manzur, Kuntzer, Pike, and others, 2008). The American Academy of Neurology has published a practice parameter for the administration of corticosteroids in the treatment of DMD (Moxley, Ashwal, Pandya, and others, 2005). Major side effects in these studies included weight gain and a cushingoid facial appearance.

Maintaining optimal function in all muscles for as long as possible is the primary goal; secondary is the prevention of contractures. Children with DMD who remain as active as possible are able to avoid wheelchair confinement for a longer time. Maintenance of function often involves stretching exercises, strength and muscle training, breathing exercises to increase and maintain vital lung capacity, range-of-motion exercises, surgery to release contracture deformities, bracing, and performance of ADLs.

Parents should always be involved in making decisions about the child's care, and teaching regarding home safety and prevention of falls is important as well. Parents should also be encouraged to have the child keep follow-up appointments for medical care and physical and occupational therapy. Because respiratory tract infections are most troublesome in these children, influenza and pneumococcal vaccines are encouraged, and contact with persons with respiratory tract infections should be avoided. Action plans for prompt treatment of respiratory illness are important.

Eventually, respiratory and cardiac problems become the central focus of the debilitating illness. Children with neuromuscular disease develop abnormal breathing patterns, and hypoxia may occur as a result of inadequate oxygenation. The child and parents should be involved in a discussion of long-term ventilation options. Cardiac and respiratory assessment during wake–sleep cycles is imperative. Respiratory care for children with neuromuscular conditions such as SMA and DMD may involve the use of noninvasive ventilation with BiPAP on a temporary or full-time basis, mechanically assisted coughing (MAC), or tracheotomy and relief of airway obstruction with coughing and suctioning devices; the tracheotomy, however, is associated with more complications (Simonds, 2006; Young, Lowe, Fitzgerald, and others, 2007). Home pulse oximetry may be used to monitor oxygenation during sleep or to aid in decision making regarding the use of MAC to clear the airways.

Several devices are available for children with neuromuscular disease to assist in clearing the airway when the cough reflex is ineffective or diminished. The mechanical cough in-exsufflator (MIE; also referred to as cough assist) has been found to be safe and effective in the daily management of respiratory function (Kravitz, 2009; Miske, Hickey, Kolb, and others, 2004). The MIE delivers positive inspiratory pressures at a set rate followed by negative pressure exsufflation coordinated with the patient's own breathing rhythm. The exsufflation is designed to mimic a cough reflex so mucus can be effectively cleared. Airway suctioning after exsufflation is accomplished as necessary to clear the airways. In children, the MIE device may be connected directly to a tracheostomy or used with a mouthpiece or face mask. The Boitano (2009) reference contains a variety of equipment options, including various masks that can be used to deliver noninvasive positive pressure.

Manual cough-assisting techniques include glossopharyngeal breathing or air stacking (frog breathing); the abdominal thrust, which is similar to the Heimlich maneuver (Kravitz, 2009); and manual hyperinflation with a self-inflating resuscitation bag (without oxygen) and a mouthpiece. Hyperinflation may be used in conjunction with abdominal thrusts to improve peak cough flows (Boitano, 2009).

The use of routine chest physiotherapy (postural drainage) for DMD has not been adequately evaluated for its effectiveness in clearing the airway of mucus except when there is focal atelectasis and mucus plugging the airways (Kravitz, 2009).

Survival in individuals with DMD may be prolonged several years with the use of noninvasive ventilation and MAC as alternatives to tracheotomy and airway suctioning (Bach and Martinez, 2011; Simonds, 2006). The American Thoracic Society (2004) has published extensive guidelines for respiratory monitoring and care of children and adults with DMD.

The American Academy of Pediatrics (AAP) Section on Cardiology and Cardiac Surgery (2005) recommends an extensive cardiac evaluation of the child diagnosed with either DMD or Becker MD. Patients with neuromuscular conditions may not be seen with the typical signs and symptoms of cardiac dysfunction. Therefore, symptoms such as weight loss, nausea and vomiting, cough, increased fatigue on performance of ADLs, and orthopnea should be carefully evaluated to detect early signs of cardiomyopathy.

Genetic counseling is recommended for parents, sisters, and maternal aunts and their daughters. Long-term care, end-of-life care, and palliative care options are issues that the health care team must discuss with the child and family affected by MD (Finder, 2009). Professional counseling is necessary in some cases to allow frank discussion of these issues, and referrals should be made as appropriate.

Nursing Care Management

The care and management of a child with MD involve the combined efforts of a multidisciplinary health care team. Nurses can help clarify the roles of these health care professionals to family and others. The major emphasis of nursing care is to help the child and family cope with a chronic, progressive, incapacitating disease; to help design a program that will afford maximal independence and reduce the predictable and preventable disabilities associated with the disorder; and to help the child and family deal constructively with the limitations the disease imposes on their daily lives. Because of advances in technology, children with MD may live into early adulthood; therefore, the goals of care should also involve decisions regarding quality of life, achievement of independence, and transition to adulthood.

Working closely with other team members, nurses assist the family in developing the child's self-help skills to give the child the satisfaction of being as independent as possible for as long as possible. This requires continual evaluation of the child's capabilities, which are often difficult to assess. Fortunately, most children with MD instinctively recognize the need to become as independent as possible and strive to do so.

Practical difficulties faced by families are physical limitations of housing and mobility. Some families live in houses or apartments that are unsuited to wheelchairs. Transportation may also be a barrier for families of children with MD. Assisting with these challenges requires team problem solving. Diet, nutritional needs, and nutrition modification are discussed according to the needs of the individual child and family.

Children with MD tend to become socially isolated as their physical condition deteriorates to the point that they can no longer keep up with their friends and classmates. Their physical capabilities diminish, and their dependency increases at the age at which most children are expanding their range of interests and relationships. To gain peer associations, they often learn and use behaviors that bring them the rewards of other children's company. These friends are often children who have been rejected by more able-bodied classmates.

The parents' social activities are also restricted, and the family's activities must be continually modified to accommodate the needs of the affected child. When the child becomes increasingly incapacitated, the family may consider home-based care, an assisted living facility, or respite care. Unless the child is severely incapacitated, he should also be involved in the decisions regarding such care. Nurses can assist with decision making by exploring all available options and resources and support the child and family in the decision. Older boys with MD may also need psychiatric or psychologic counseling to deal with issues such as depression, anger, and quality of life. Parents also need to be encouraged to become involved in support groups because evidence indicates that adequate social support from family, community, and other parents is crucial to appropriate coping in families with children with chronic illness.

Regardless of how successful the program or how well the family adapts to the disorder, superimposed on the physical and emotional problems associated with a child with a long-term disability is the constant knowledge of the ultimate outcome of the disease. All of the manifestations seen in the child with a chronic fatal illness are encountered in these families (see Chapter 18).

Nurses are especially valuable health professionals as they come to know the family and the family's problems. Nurses can be alert to the family's problems and needs and make necessary referrals when supplementary services are indicated. The Muscular Dystrophy Association–USA* has branches in most communities to assist families that have a member with MD.

ACQUIRED NEUROMUSCULAR DISORDERS

GUILLAIN-BARRÉ SYNDROME (INFECTIOUS POLYNEURITIS)

Guillain-Barré syndrome (GBS), also known as infectious polyneuritis, is an uncommon acute demyelinating polyneuropathy with a progressive, usually ascending flaccid paralysis. The hallmark of GBS

---

*3300 E. Sunrise Drive, Tucson, AZ 85718; 800-572-1717; e-mail: mda@mdausa.org; http://www.mda.org. In Canada: Muscular Dystrophy Canada, 2345 Yonge St., Suite 900, Toronto, ON M4P 2E5; 866-MUSCLE-8; fax: 416-488-7523; http://www.muscle.ca/national/home.html.

Animation—Guillain-Barré Syndrome

is acute peripheral motor weakness. The paralysis usually occurs approximately 10 days after a nonspecific viral infection; GBS has also been reported after administration of certain vaccines (rabies, influenza, polio, and meningococcal) (Sarnat, 2011c). Several subtypes of GBS include acute inflammatory demyelinating neuropathy, acute motor axonal neuropathy, acute motor sensory axonal neuropathy, and Miller Fisher syndrome. Children are less often affected than adults; among children, those between ages 4 and 10 years have higher susceptibility. The male-to-female ratio is reported to be 1.5:1. Two peak periods with an increased incidence of GBS have been identified: late adolescence and young adulthood.

Chronic inflammatory demyelinating polyradiculoneuropathies (CIDP) are chronic types of GBS that recur intermittently or do not improve over a period of months to years (Sarnat, 2011c). The following discussion focuses on GBS.

Congenital GBS is rare yet may occur in the neonatal period and consists of hypotonia, weakness, and decreased or absent reflexes. Maternal neuromuscular disease may or may not be present. Diagnosis is established by the same criteria as in older children, but the symptoms gradually subside over the first few months of life and disappear by 12 months (Sarnat, 2011c).

Pathophysiology

Guillain-Barré syndrome is an immune-mediated disease often associated with a number of viral or bacterial infections or the administration of certain vaccines. It has been associated with infectious mononucleosis, measles, mumps, *Campylobacter jejuni* (gastroenteritis), cytomegalovirus, *Borrelia burgdorferi* (Lyme disease), Epstein-Barr virus, *Helicobacter pylori*, and *Mycoplasma* and *Pneumocystis* infections. Onset of GBS symptoms usually occurs within 10 days of the primary infection. Pathologic changes in spinal and cranial nerves consist of inflammation and edema with rapid, segmented demyelination and compression of nerve roots within the dural sheath. Nerve conduction is impaired, producing ascending partial or complete paralysis of muscles innervated by the involved nerves. GBS has three phases:

1. **Acute**—Phase starts when symptoms begin and continues until new symptoms stop appearing or deterioration ceases; it may last as long as 4 weeks.
2. **Plateau**—Symptoms remain constant without further deterioration; it may last from days to weeks.
3. **Recovery**—Patient begins to improve and progress to optimal recovery; it usually lasts a few weeks to months depending on the deficits incurred by the illness.

Diagnostic Evaluation

The diagnosis of GBS is based on clinical manifestations (Box 32-10), CSF analysis, and EMG findings. CSF analysis reveals an abnormally elevated protein concentration, normal glucose, and fewer than 10 white blood cells (WBCs)/mm^3 (Sarnat, 2011c). EMG shows evidence of acute muscle denervation, but other laboratory studies are usually noncontributory. The symmetric nature of the paralysis helps differentiate this disorder from spinal paralytic poliomyelitis, which usually affects sporadic muscles.

Therapeutic Management

Treatment of GBS is primarily supportive. In the acute phase, patients are hospitalized because respiratory and pharyngeal involvement may require assisted ventilation, sometimes with a temporary tracheostomy. Treatment modalities include aggressive ventilatory support in the event of respiratory compromise, intravenous (IV) administration

---

BOX 32-10   CLINICAL MANIFESTATIONS OF GUILLAIN-BARRÉ SYNDROME

Initial Symptoms

Muscle tenderness

Paresthesia and cramps (sometimes)

Proximal symmetric muscle weakness

Ascending paralysis from lower extremities

Frequently involves muscles of trunk and upper extremities and those supplied by cranial nerves (especially facial)

Flaccid paralysis with loss of reflexes

May involve facial, extraocular, labial, lingual, pharyngeal, and laryngeal muscles

Intercostal and phrenic nerve involvement:
- Breathlessness in vocalizations
- Shallow, irregular respirations

Other Manifestations

Tendon reflexes depressed or absent

Variable degrees of sensory impairment

Muscle tenderness or sensitivity to slight pressure

Urinary incontinence or retention and constipation

---

of immunoglobulin (IVIG), and sometimes steroids; plasmapheresis and immunosuppressive drugs may also be used. Plasmapheresis has been shown to decrease the length of recovery in patients with severe GBS yet is expensive, and side effects include hypotension, fever, bleeding disorders, chills, urticaria, and bradycardia. Some evidence reports equal benefits to treatment of GBS with IVIG administration or plasmapheresis; both sped up recovery time in studies reviewed (Hughes and Cornblath, 2005). There is evidence, however, of significant improvement in children with high-dose IVIG therapy (vs. supportive treatment alone) (Hughes, Swan, and van Doorn, 2010). IVIG is now recommended as the primary treatment of GBS when administered within 2 weeks of disease onset (Hughes, 2008). Corticosteroids alone do not decrease the symptoms or shorten the duration of the disease.

Medications that may be administered during the acute phase include a low-molecular-weight heparin to prevent deep vein thrombosis (DVT), a mild laxative or stool softener to prevent constipation, pain medication such as acetaminophen, and a histamine-antagonist to prevent stress ulcer formation. Chronic neuropathic pain after GBS may be treated with gabapentin, which is reported to be more effective than carbamazepine (Sarnat, 2011c).

Rehabilitation after the acute phase may involve physical therapy, occupational therapy, and speech therapy. Additional consideration should be given to problems of general weakness and retraining for toileting and feeding (Lyons, 2008).

Course and Prognosis

Better outcomes are associated with younger age, no requirement for mechanical respiratory assistance, slower progression of disease, normal peripheral nerve function on EMG, and treatment with either IVIG or plasmapheresis. Recovery usually begins within 2 to 3 weeks, and most patients regain full muscle strength. The recovery of muscle strength progresses in the reverse order of onset of paralysis, with lower extremity strength being the last to recover. Poor prognosis with subsequent residual effects in children is reportedly associated with cranial nerve involvement, extensive disability at time of presentation, and intubation.

Most deaths associated with GBS are caused by respiratory failure; therefore, early diagnosis and access to respiratory support are especially important. The rate of recovery is usually related to the degree of involvement and may extend from a few weeks to months. The greater the degree of paralysis, the longer the recovery phase.

Nursing Care Management

Nursing care is primarily supportive and is the same as that required for children with immobilization and respiratory compromise. The emphasis of care is on close observation to assess the extent of paralysis and on prevention of complications, including aspiration, ventilator-associated pneumonia (VAP), atelectasis, DVT, pressure ulcer, fear and anxiety, autonomic dysfunction, and pain.

During the acute phase of the disease, the nurse should carefully observe the child's condition for possible difficulty in swallowing and respiratory involvement. Closely monitor the child's respiratory function and keep the oxygen source, appropriate-sized insufflation bag and mask, endotracheal intubation and suctioning equipment, tracheotomy tray, and vasoconstrictor drugs available. Monitor vital signs frequently, including neurologic signs and level of consciousness. For children who develop respiratory impairment, the care is the same as that for any child with respiratory distress requiring mechanical ventilation.

Respiratory care, if intubation is required, requires close monitoring of oxygenation status (usually by pulse oximetry and sometimes arterial blood gases), maintenance of an open airway with suctioning, and postural changes to prevent pneumonia. Consideration should be given to preventing opportunistic infections such as VAP; meticulous oral care and hypopharynx suctioning, elevation of the head of bed 30 degrees, and strict asepsis with suctioning equipment (including catheters, a Yankauer device, or both) should be implemented to prevent VAP. Children with oral and pharyngeal involvement may be fed via a nasogastric or gastrostomy tube to ensure adequate feeding. It is also important to consider the possibility of stress ulcers in such patients and administer a proton pump inhibitor. Immobilization, which occurs with GBS, decreases GI function; therefore, attention to problems such as decreased gastric emptying, constipation, and feeding residuals requires nursing assessment and appropriate collaborative interventions. Temporary urinary catheterization may be required; urinary retention is common, and appropriate assessment of urinary output is vital. Sensory impairment and paralysis in the lower extremities make the child susceptible to skin breakdown; therefore, attention should be given to meticulous skin care. Passive range-of-motion exercises and application of orthoses to prevent muscle contracture are important when paralysis is present. Prevention of DVT is accomplished with pneumatic compression (antiembolism) devices, administration of a low-molecular-weight heparin, and early mobilization and ambulation. Autonomic dysfunction may be life threatening; thus, close monitoring of vital signs in the acute phase is essential.

A key to recovery in the child with GBS is the prevention of muscle and joint contractures, so passive range-of-motion exercises must be carried out routinely to maintain vital function. Although the child may have a generalized paralysis, cognitive function remains intact; therefore, it is important for nursing care to involve communication with the child or adolescent regarding procedures and treatments that may be frightening, especially if mechanical ventilation is required. Encourage parents to talk to the child and make eye and physical contact and to reassure the child during this phase of the illness.

Pain management is crucial in the care of children with GBS. Although neuromuscular impairment may make pain perception more difficult to accurately evaluate, objective pain scales should be used. Gabapentin and carbamazepine may be used to manage neuropathic pain in patients with GBS.

Physical therapy may be limited to passive range-of-motion exercises during the evolving phase of the disease. Later, as the disease stabilizes and recovery begins, an active physical therapy program is implemented to prevent contracture deformities and facilitate muscle recovery. This may include active exercise, gait training, and bracing.

Throughout the course of the illness, child and parent support is paramount. The usual rapidity of the paralysis and the long recovery period greatly tax the emotional reserves of all family members. The parents and child benefit from repeated reassurance that recovery is occurring and from realistic information regarding the possibility of permanent disability. In the event of a residual disability, the family needs assistance in accepting and adjusting to the loss of function. (See Chapter 18.) The GBS/CIDP Foundation International* is a nonprofit organization devoted to support, education, and research. It provides families with support from recovered persons, publishes informational literature and a newsletter, and maintains a list of practitioners experienced with the disease.

TETANUS

Tetanus, or lockjaw, is an acute, preventable, but often fatal disease caused by an exotoxin produced by the anaerobic spore-forming, gram-positive bacillus *Clostridium tetani*. It is characterized by painful muscular rigidity primarily involving the masseter and neck muscles. There are four requirements for the development of tetanus: (1) presence of tetanus spores or vegetative forms of the bacillus, (2) injury to the tissues, (3) wound conditions that encourage multiplication of the organism, and (4) a susceptible host.

Tetanus spores are found in soil; dust; and the intestinal tracts of humans and animals, especially herbivorous animals. The organisms are more prevalent in rural areas but are readily carried to urban areas by the wind. The organisms are not invasive but enter the body by way of wounds, particularly a puncture wound, burn, or crushed area. They may enter through a minor, unnoticed break in the skin, such as a thorn or needle prick, bee sting, or scratch. In newborns, infection may occur through the umbilical cord, usually in situations in which infants are delivered in severely contaminated surroundings or the mother is not adequately immunized. The disease has the greatest incidence in months when persons are more involved in outdoor activities.

Pathophysiology

When prevention efforts are not effective and conditions are favorable, the organisms proliferate and form potent exotoxins, one of which is tetanospasmin. Tetanospasmin affects the CNS to produce the clinical manifestations of the disease. The ideal conditions for the organisms' growth are devitalized tissues without access to air, such as wounds that have not been washed or kept clean and those that have crusted over, trapping pus beneath. The exotoxin appears to reach the CNS by way of either the neuron axons or the vascular system. The toxin becomes fixed on nerve cells of the anterior horn of the spinal cord and the brainstem. The toxin acts at the myoneural junction to produce muscular stiffness and lower the threshold for reflex excitability.

---

*The Holly Building, 104½ Forrest Ave., Narberth, PA 19072; 610-667-0131, 866-224-3301; http://www.gbs-cidp.org.

BOX 32-11 CLINICAL MANIFESTATIONS OF TETANUS

Initial Symptoms

Progressive stiffness and tenderness of muscles in neck and jaw

Characteristic difficulty in opening the mouth (**trismus**)

Risus sardonicus (sardonic smile) caused by facial muscle spasm

Progressive Involvement

Opisthotonic positioning

Boardlike rigidity of abdominal and limb muscles

Difficulty swallowing

Extreme sensitivity to external stimuli (slight noise, gentle touch, or bright light):

- Trigger paroxysmal muscle contractions that last seconds to minutes
- Contractions recur with increased frequency until almost continuous (sustained, tetanic)

Laryngospasm and tetany of respiratory muscles:

- Accumulated secretions
- Respiratory arrest
- Atelectasis
- Pneumonia

Other Aspects

Mentation unaffected; patient alert

Pain, anxiety, and distress reflected in:

- Rapid pulse
- Sweating
- Anxious facial expression
- Fever usually absent or only mild

The incubation period for tetanus varies from 2 days to months and averages 8 days; most cases occur within 14 days. In neonates, it is usually 5 to 14 days. Shorter incubation periods have been associated with more heavily contaminated wounds, more severe disease, and a worse prognosis (AAP, Committee on Infectious Diseases and Pickering, 2009).

The manner of onset varies, but the initial symptoms are usually a progressive stiffness and tenderness of the muscles in the neck and jaw. Eventually, all voluntary muscles are affected (Box 32-11). As the child recovers from the disease, the paroxysms become less frequent and gradually subside. Survival beyond 4 days usually indicates recovery, but complete recovery may require weeks.

Therapeutic Management

Primary prevention is key and occurs through immunization and boosters (AAP, Committee on Infectious Diseases and Pickering, 2009). After an injury has occurred, further preventive measures are based on the child's immune status and the nature of the injury. Specific prophylactic therapy after trauma is administration of **tetanus toxoid** (note that **equine tetanus antitoxin [TAT]** is not available in the United States) (see Immunizations, Chapter 10, for age-specific recommendations).

An unprotected or inadequately immunized child who sustains a "tetanus-prone" wound (including wounds contaminated with dirt, feces, soil, and saliva; puncture wounds; avulsions; and wounds resulting from missiles, crushing, burns, and frostbite) should receive **tetanus immunoglobulin (TIG)**. Concurrent administration of both TIG and tetanus toxoid at separate sites is recommended both to provide protection and to initiate the active immune process.

After the individual has received primary tetanus immunization, antitoxin is believed to provide protection for at least 10 years and for a longer period after booster immunization (AAP, Committee on Infectious Diseases and Pickering, 2009). Recently, the Advisory Committee on Immunization Practices (CDC, 2011) recommended no specific time intervals between the administration of a tetanus- or diphtheria-toxoid containing vaccine and Tdap (tetanus, diphtheria, and pertussis) to provide protection against pertussis; other than a localized pain reaction, no other side effects were noted in persons who received the Td and Tdap at intervals as short as 18 months. Completion of active immunization is carried out according to the usual pattern. Antibiotic treatment with penicillin G (or erythromycin or tetracycline in older children with allergy to penicillin) is important in the management of tetanus as an adjunct against clostridia; metronidazole is a viable alternative (Arnon, 2011a).

> ## ⚡ SAFETY ALERT
>
> TIG and tetanus toxoid are always administered via the intramuscular route in separate syringes and at separate sites; they are never administered by the intravenous route.

Aggressive supportive care is necessary to treat tetanus in the acute phase. Acutely ill children are best treated in an intensive care facility where close and constant observation and equipment for monitoring and respiratory support are readily available. A quiet environment is preferred to reduce external stimuli.

General supportive care is indicated, including maintaining an adequate airway and fluid and electrolyte balance, managing pain, and ensuring adequate caloric intake. Indwelling oral or nasogastric feedings may be required to maintain adequate fluid and caloric intake; continued laryngospasm may necessitate total parenteral nutrition or gastrostomy feeding. Severe or recurrent laryngospasm or excessive secretions may require advanced airway management such as endotracheal intubation or tracheotomy.

Tetanus immunoglobulin therapy to neutralize toxins is the most specific therapy for tetanus. Local care of the wound by surgical débridement and cleansing helps reduce the numbers of proliferating organisms at the site of injury. The cleansing should be repeated several times during the first 48 hours, and deep, infected lacerations are usually exposed and débrided. Infiltration of the wound with TIG is no longer considered necessary (AAP, Committee on Infectious Diseases and Pickering, 2009).

Diazepam is the drug of choice for seizure control and muscle relaxation (Arnon, 2011a), but lorazepam (Ativan) may be used in some cases. Intrathecal baclofen, IV magnesium sulfate, dantrolene sodium, and midazolam may also be used in the management of muscle spasticity associated with tetanus. Patients with severe tetanus and those who do not respond to other muscle relaxants may require the administration of a neuromuscular blocking agent, such as rocuronium or vecuronium; intrathecal baclofen may be used as a muscle relaxant but only in the intensive care unit because it often induces apnea. Because of their paralytic effect on respiratory muscles, use of these drugs requires mechanical ventilation with endotracheal intubation or tracheotomy and constant cardiopulmonary monitoring. Endotracheal tube insertion or tracheotomy is often indicated and should be performed before severe respiratory distress develops. Despite the absence of pain manifestation with these drugs, it is important to administer adequate analgesia. The administration of corticosteroids has met with success in some cases.

Nursing Care Management

The care of the child with tetanus requires supportive management with particular attention to airway and breathing. Respiratory status is carefully evaluated for any signs of distress, and appropriate emergency equipment is kept available at all times. The location, extent, and severity of muscle spasms are important nursing observations. Muscle relaxants, opioids, and sedatives that may be prescribed can also cause respiratory depression; therefore, the child should be assessed for excessive CNS depression. Attention to hydration and nutrition involves monitoring an IV infusion, monitoring nasogastric or gastrostomy feedings, and suctioning oropharyngeal secretions when indicated.

In caring for a child with tetanus during the acute phase, every effort should be made to control or eliminate stimulation from sound, light, and touch. Although a darkened room is ideal, sufficient light is essential so that the child can be carefully observed; light appears to be less irritating than vibratory or auditory stimuli. The infant or child is handled as little as possible, and extra effort is expended to avoid any sudden or loud noise to prevent seizures.

If a potent muscle relaxant such as vecuronium is used, the total paralysis makes oral communication impossible. The drug is not a sedative, however, and anxiety should be considered in children who are intubated. Therefore, all the child's needs must be anticipated and procedures carefully explained beforehand. Additional care is focused on preventing the complications associated with prolonged immobility, including decreased bowel and bladder tone and subsequent constipation, anorexia, DVT, pneumonia, and skin breakdown.

Because their mental status is clear, children are aware of what is happening to them and are often extremely anxious. They should not be left alone, and all efforts should be made to reduce anxiety, which can contribute to muscle spasms. Parents are encouraged to stay with the child to offer security and support. They also need support, information, and reassurance from the nurse.

BOTULISM

Botulism is an acute flaccid paralysis caused by the preformed toxin produced by the anaerobic bacillus *Clostridium botulinum.* In classic, or foodborne botulism, the most common source of the toxin is a contaminated food source. The disease has a wide variation in severity, from constipation to progressive sequential loss of neurologic function and respiratory failure. The most common source of the toxin is improperly sterilized home-canned foods. CNS symptoms appear abruptly approximately 12 to 36 hours after ingestion of contaminated food and may or may not be preceded by acute digestive disturbance (Box 32-12).

Human botulism is caused by neurotoxins A, B, E, and rarely F (AAP, Committee on Infectious Diseases and Pickering, 2009). Types A and B are the most common causes of infant botulism. In addition to foodborne botulism, other forms include wound botulism; infant botulism; and artificial botulism, usually a result of bioterrorism.

Treatment consists of IV administration of botulism antitoxin and general supportive measures, primarily respiratory and nutritional. Toxins vary in protein-binding capacity. Some have a relatively short half-life and do not bind to tissues firmly; therefore, therapy is continued until paralysis subsides. Other toxins appear to bind irreversibly to nerve endings and are therefore not amenable to neutralization.

Infant Botulism

Infant botulism, unlike foodborne botulism in older persons, is caused by ingestion of spores or vegetative cells of *C. botulinum* and the subsequent release of the toxin from organisms colonizing the GI tract.

BOX 32-12   CLINICAL MANIFESTATIONS OF BOTULISM

General Signs

Weakness
Dizziness
Headache
Difficulty talking and speaking
Diplopia
Vomiting
Progressive, life-threatening respiratory paralysis

Infant Botulism*

Constipation (a common symptom)
Generalized weakness
Decrease in spontaneous movements
Diminished or absent deep tendon reflexes
Loss of head control
Poor feeding
Weak cry
Reduced gag reflex
Progressive respiratory paralysis

*Most commonly diagnosed as "rule out sepsis" in the acute phase because of clinical presentation. Sometimes may be misdiagnosed as spinal muscular atrophy or metabolic disease.

C. botulinum types A and B are the most common causative strains of infant botulism. This form of botulism has become more prevalent than any other form. Many cases of infant botulism occur in breastfed infants who are being introduced to nonhuman milk substances (AAP, Committee on Infectious Diseases and Pickering, 2009). There appears to be no common food or drug source of the organisms; however, the *C. botulinum* organisms have been found in honey. Botulism may occur in infants as young as 1 week of age up to 12 months of age with peak incidence between 2 and 4 months of age.

The severity of the disease varies widely, from mild constipation to progressive sequential loss of neurologic function and respiratory failure (see Box 32-12). The affected infant is usually well before the onset of symptoms. Constipation is a common presenting symptom, and almost all infants exhibit generalized weakness and a decrease in spontaneous movements. Deep tendon reflexes are usually diminished or absent. Cranial nerve deficits are common, as evidenced by loss of head control, difficulty in feeding, weak cry, and reduced gag reflex. Type 1 SMA and metabolic disorders are often mistaken for infant botulism in the initial diagnostic phase because of the similarities in clinical manifestations of hypotonia, lethargy, and poor feeding (Arnon, 2011b). Presenting clinical signs also often mimic those of sepsis in young infants. Botulism toxin exerts its effect by inhibiting the release of acetylcholine at the myoneural junction, thereby impairing motor activity of muscles innervated by affected nerves.

Diagnosis is made on the basis of the clinical history, physical examination, and laboratory detection of the organism in the patient's stool and, less commonly, blood. However, isolation of the organism may take several days; therefore, suspicion of botulism by clinical presentation should require emergent treatment (Arnon, 2011b). EMG may be helpful in establishing the diagnosis; however, results may be normal early in the course of the illness.

Treatment consists of immediate administration of botulism immune globulin intravenously (BIG-IV) (Arnon, 2011b) without delaying for laboratory diagnosis. Early administration of BIG-IV neutralizes the toxin and stops the progression of the disease. The human-derived botulism antitoxin (BIG-IV) has been evaluated and is now available nationwide for use only in infant botulism. Infants treated with BIG-IV usually have a shortened hospital stay from approximately 6 weeks to 2 weeks, reportedly as a result of decreased requirements for mechanical ventilation and intensive care (Arnon, 2011b). Approximately 50% of affected infants require intubation and mechanical ventilation; therefore, respiratory support is crucial, as is nutritional support because theses infants are unable to feed. Trivalent equine botulinum antitoxin and bivalent antitoxin, used in adults and older children, are not administered to infants. Antibiotic therapy is not part of the management because the botulinum toxin is an intracellular molecule, and antibiotics would not be effective; aminoglycosides in particular should not be administered because they may potentiate the blocking effects of the neurotoxin (Arnon, 2011b).

The prognosis is generally good if the patient is adequately treated, although recovery may be slow, requiring a few weeks after severe illness. Untreated patients may require a longer hospitalization.

> ### ! NURSING ALERT
>
> Although the precise source of *C. botulinum* spores has not been identified as originating from honey in many cases of infant botulism, it is still recommended that honey not be given to infants younger than 12 months of age because the spores have been found in honey (CDC, 2010).

Nursing Care Management

Nursing responsibilities include observing, recognizing, and reporting signs of poor feeding, constipation, and muscle impairment in the infant with botulism and providing intensive nursing care when an infant is hospitalized. (See Nursing Care Management for the infant with SMA, p. 1106, and Nursing Care of the High-Risk Newborn and Family, Chapter 9.) Parental support and reassurance are important. Most infants recover when the disorder is recognized and BIG-IV therapy is implemented. Nursing care of the infant on mechanical ventilation requires observation of oxygenation status and vigilance for any complications. Parents should be aware that during recovery, infants fatigue easily when muscular action is sustained. This has important implications for timing the resumption of feedings because of the risk of aspiration. Parents should also be advised that normal bowel activity may not return for several weeks. Therefore, a stool softener can be beneficial.

SPINAL CORD INJURIES

Spinal cord injuries (SCIs) with major neurologic involvement traditionally have not been a common cause of physical disability in children. However, a sufficient number of children with these injuries are admitted to major medical centers, and because of the increased survival rate as a result of improved management, nurses are often involved in the care and rehabilitation of children with SCI.

Mechanisms of Injury

The most common cause of serious spinal cord damage in children is trauma involving motor vehicle crashes (MVCs) (including automobile-bicycle, all-terrain vehicles, and snowmobiles), sports injuries (especially from diving, trampoline activities, gymnastics, and football), birth trauma, and nonaccidental trauma. MVCs accounted for 56% of SCI in children and adolescents and falls and firearm injury caused 14% and 9% of SCIs, respectively. The children injured (SCI) in MVCs were not properly restrained in 67.7% of the cases (Vitale,

Goss, Matsumoto, and others, 2006). The increased use of recreational activities involving motorized vehicles such as jet water skis, all-terrain vehicles, and motorcycles has also increased the incidence of SCIs in children. Congenital defects of the spine such as myelomeningocele also may in some cases produce the effects of SCI.

Transverse myelitis (inflammation of the spinal cord) may be caused by illness and has also been reported to develop from inadvertent intraarterial administration of long-acting penicillin injected into the buttocks. Damage can be extensive enough to result in paraplegia or even lower limb amputation.

In MVCs, most SCIs in children are a result of indirect trauma caused by sudden hyperflexion or hyperextension of the neck, often combined with a rotational force. Trauma to the spinal cord without evidence of vertebral fracture or dislocation (SCI without radiographic abnormality, or SCIWORA) is particularly likely to occur in an MVC when proper safety restraints are not used. An unrestrained child becomes a projectile during sudden deceleration and is subject to injury from contact with a variety of objects inside and outside the vehicle. Individuals who use only a lap seat belt restraint are at greater risk of SCI than those who use a combination lap and shoulder restraint. High cervical spine injuries have been reported in children younger than 2 years of age who are improperly restrained in forward-facing car seats. Infants who are improperly restrained in an infant car seat may experience cervical trauma in a car crash. Small children may also be severely injured by deploying front seat air bags.

Falling from heights occurs less often in children than in adults, but vertebral compression from blows to the head or buttocks can occur in water sports (diving and surfing), falls from horses, or other athletic activities. Birth injuries may occur in breech deliveries from traction force on the spinal cord during delivery of the head and shoulders. When shaken, infants commonly sustain cervical cord damage, as well as subdural hematoma and retinal hemorrhage; cognitive impairment and death may occur subsequent to the traumatic event. Infants have weak neck muscles, and during vigorous shaking, their large and heavy heads rapidly wobble back and forth. A significant number of adolescents receive SCIs secondary to gunshot wounds, stabbings, and other violent inflicted injury.

Because of the marked mobility of the neck, fracture or subluxation (partial dislocation) is the most common immediate cause of SCI, particularly in the lower cervical region. Although unusual in adults, SCI without fracture is common in children, whose spines are suppler, weaker, and more mobile than those of adults. Therefore, the force is more easily dissipated over a larger number of segments. In infants and small children younger than the age of 5 years, upper cervical spine fractures and spinal compression are more common, but adolescents tend to have lower cervical and thoracolumbar fracture dislocations (Retake, 2011).

The severity of the force, the mechanisms of the injury, and the degree of the individual's muscular relaxation at the time of the injury greatly influence the extent of the trauma. SCIs are classified as either complete or incomplete. In a complete injury, there is no motor or sensory function more than three segments below the neurologic level of the injury (Mathison, Kadom, and Krug, 2008). Incomplete lesions have several typical characteristics (Mathison, Kadom, and Krug, 2008):

Central cord syndrome—Central gray matter destruction and preservation of peripheral tracts; tetraplegia with sacral sparing common; some motor recovery gained

Anterior cord syndrome—Complete motor and sensory loss with trunk and lower extremity proprioception and sensation of pressure

Posterior cord syndrome—Loss of sensation, pain, and proprioception with normal cord function, including motor function; able to move extremities but have difficulty controlling such movements

Brown-Séquard syndrome—Unilateral cord lesion with a motor deficit on the opposite side of the body from the primary insult; absence of pain and temperature sensation on the opposite side from the injury

Spinal cord concussion—Transient loss of neural function below the level of the acute spinal cord lesion, resulting in flaccid paralysis and loss of tendon, autonomic, and cutaneous reflex activity; may last hours to weeks

The American Spinal Injury Association (ASIA) (2009) Standards for neurologic classification of SCI worksheet is available online at http://www.asia-spinalinjury.org/publications/2006_Classif_worksheet.pdf. The ASIA Impairment Scale (Box 32-13) combines motor and sensory function and is used to determine the severity of impairment from the injury (complete or incomplete). It may also be used to measure neurologic changes and functional goals for rehabilitation (Mathison, Kadom, and Krug, 2008).

The injury sustained can affect any of the spinal nerves, and the higher the injury, the more extensive the damage. The child can be left with complete or partial paralysis of the lower extremities (**paraplegia**) or with damage at a higher level and without functional use of any of the four extremities (**tetraplegia**). A high cervical cord injury that affects the phrenic nerve paralyzes the diaphragm and leaves the child dependent on mechanical ventilation.

A mild but equally frightening form of cord trauma is **spinal cord compression**, a temporary neural dysfunction without visible damage to the cord. Complete tetraplegia can result but initially may not be differentiated from serious cord injury.

Clinical Manifestations

It is often difficult to determine the extent and severity of damage at first. Immediate loss of function is caused by both anatomic and impaired physiologic function, and improved function may not be evident for weeks or even months. Manifestation of the initial response to acute SCI is flaccid paralysis below the level of the damage. This stage is often referred to as **spinal shock syndrome** and is caused by the sudden disruption of central and autonomic pathways. Local effects of cord edema and ischemia produce a physiologic transection with or without an anatomic severance. Most children with an SCI experience some spinal shock. Manifestations include the absence of reflexes at or below the cord lesion, with flaccidity or limpness of the involved muscles, loss of sensation and motor function, and autonomic dysfunction (symptoms of hypotension, low or high body temperature, loss of bladder and bowel control, and autonomic dysreflexia).

Autonomic paralysis also affects thermoregulatory functions. Afferent impulses from temperature receptors in the skin are not integrated; therefore, the patient is subject to temperature increases or decreases in response to alterations in environmental temperature. Hyperthermia can result from excessive ambient temperature, such as too many covers.

Except in the situations previously mentioned, flaccid paralysis is replaced by spinal reflex activity and increasing spasticity or, in incomplete lesions, greater or lesser degree of neurologic recovery.

The paralytic nature of autonomic function is replaced by **autonomic dysreflexia**, especially when the lesions are above the midthoracic level. This autonomic phenomenon is caused by visceral distention or irritation, particularly of the bowel or bladder. Sensory impulses are triggered and travel to the cord lesion, where they are

---

BOX 32-13   AMERICAN SPINAL INJURY ASSOCIATION IMPAIRMENT SCALE

A—Complete: No motor or sensory function is preserved in the sacral segments S4–S5.

B—Incomplete: Sensory but not motor function is preserved below the neurologic level and includes the sacral segments S4–S5.

C—Incomplete: Motor function is preserved below the neurologic level, and more than half of key muscles below the neurologic level have a muscle grade less than 3.

D—Incomplete: Motor function is preserved below the neurologic level, and at least half of key muscles below the neurologic level have a muscle grade of 3 or more.

E—Normal: Motor and sensory function are normal.

Clinical Syndromes (Optional)
Central cord
Brown-Séquard
Anterior cord
Conus medullaris
Cauda equina

Used with permission, American Spinal Injury Association, 2006.

---

blocked, which causes activation of sympathetic reflex action with disturbed central inhibitory control. Excessive sympathetic activity is manifested by a flushing face, sweating forehead, pupillary constriction, marked hypertension, headache, and bradycardia. The precipitating stimulus may be merely a full bladder or rectum or other internal or external sensory input. It can be a catastrophic event unless the irritation is relieved.

Additional clinical findings of SCI may include numbness, tingling, or burning; priapism; weakness; and loss of bowel and bladder control (Hayes and Arriola, 2005).

Neurogenic shock occurs as a result of a disruption in the descending sympathetic pathways with loss of vasomotor tone and sympathetic innervations to the cardiovascular system (Hayes and Arriola, 2005). Hypotension, bradycardia, and peripheral vasodilation occur as a result of neurogenic shock.

Children with suspected SCI may have suffered multiple injuries (e.g., head injury); therefore, multiple clinical manifestations may occur that may mask those of an SCI.

Therapeutic Management

Initial care begins at the scene of the accident with proper immobilization of the cervical, thoracic, and lumbar spine. Because of the complexity of these injuries, it is usually recommended that these persons be transported to a spinal injury center for care by specially trained health care personnel as soon as possible after the injury for appropriate diagnostic evaluation and intervention.

The initial management of the child with a suspected SCI should begin with an assessment of the ABCs: airway, breathing, and circulation. Guidelines for the child who is found unconscious with an unknown cause are discussed in Chapter 23 (Cardiopulmonary Resuscitation). The airway should be opened using the jaw-thrust technique to minimize damage to the cervical spine. The child is monitored for cardiovascular instability, and measures are taken to support systemic blood pressure and maintain optimal cardiac output. Because MVC and other trauma in children may involve internal organ damage and potential bleeding, abdominal distention and other signs are acted on immediately to prevent further systemic shock. After the child is stabilized and transported to a regional trauma center, a thorough evaluation of neurologic status and any other associated trauma is carried out by the multidisciplinary team. In the emergency department, spinal immobilization should be maintained until a thorough neurologic assessment is completed; in children, this typically involves a CT scan and possibly an MRI. Additional interventions are discussed in the Nursing Care Management section.

Spinal cord injury management guidelines and standards of care have been published for adult and pediatric patients with SCIs by the American Association of Neurological Surgeons and the Congress of Neurological Surgeons. However, there are no evidence-based guidelines for the management of SCI in children (Mathison, Kadom, and Krug, 2008).

Intravenous methylprednisone may be started within the first 8 hours after the injury to decrease inflammation and minimize further injury. Therapy is continued for 23 to 48 hours; however, there is controversy about its use in small children.

A number of progressive rehabilitation modalities have been developed in recent years that have the potential for increasing the quality of life for children with SCI. One treatment is functional electrical stimulation (FES), also referred to as functional neuromuscular stimulation, or neuromuscular electrical stimulation. With this treatment, an electrical stimulator is surgically implanted under the skin in the abdomen, and electrode leads are tunneled to paralyzed leg muscles, enabling the child to sit, stand, and walk with the aid of crutches, a walker, or other orthoses. The stimulator can also be used to elicit a voluntary grasp and release with the hand. Before the latter can be accomplished, a number of surgical tendon transfers may be required for elbow extension, wrist extension, and finger and thumb flexion. In addition, FES has therapeutic benefits, which include increased muscle strength, improved gait function, and increased cardiovascular fitness (Thrasher and Popovic, 2008). Tendon transfers have been shown to be successful in enhancing hand and arm function, increasing pinch force, and facilitating independence in ADLs (Hosalkar, Pandya, Hsu, and others, 2009). Restoration of hand and arm function enables children with SCI to perform self-catheterization and achieve greater independence in personal hygiene.

Exercise is considered an integral part of SCI rehabilitation; exercise may enhance neuroplasticity and decrease further muscle atrophy. Examples of exercise modalities in SCI patients include upper body strength training and hand cycling (Hosalkar, Pandya, Hsu, and others, 2009).

Administration of pharmacologic agents such as clonidine hydrochloride may improve ambulation in patients with partial SCIs, and exercise therapy through interactive locomotor training has helped some individuals with SCI regain ambulatory function.

A number of orthoses or ambulation aids such as crutches may still be necessary to achieve upright mobility, yet as robotic technology advances, so do the chances for improved mobilization in children with SCI. Mechanical or robotic orthoses may be used in conjunction with FES to enable ambulation in persons with SCI (To, Kirsch, Kobetic, and others, 2005). Gait training may be achieved with a number of different modalities, including a stationary cycle; however, no specific method has proved superior to the others. FES has also been effective in reducing complications from bladder and bowel incontinence and in assisting males in achieving penile erection.

Surgical interventions for SCI include early cord decompression (decompression laminectomy) and cervical or thoracic fusion. Crutchfield, Vinke, or Gardner-Wells tongs and skeletal traction may be used for early cervical vertebral stabilization. A halo vest may be suited for ambulation after the acute phase. (See also discussion of cervical traction in Chapter 31.) After cervical spinal fusion, a hard cervical collar or sterno-occipital-mandibular immobilizer brace may be worn until the fusion is solidified.

Nursing Care Management

The nursing care of the child affected by SCI is complex and challenging. A multidisciplinary SCI team is equipped to manage the acute phase of the injury, and some members, including the nurse, may follow the patient to eventual recovery. Nursing management is concerned with ensuring adequate initial stabilization of the entire spinal column with a rigid cervical collar with supportive blocks on a rigid backboard. The traumatic event causing the injury may or may not be recalled if the child lost consciousness; such events are extremely frightening to the child. The young child may also be frightened by the immobilization process and the inability to move the extremities; therefore, it is important to reassure and comfort the child during this process.

During the acute phase of the injury, it is imperative that airway patency be ensured, complications prevented, and function maintained. Evaluate the extent of the neurologic damage early to establish a baseline for neurologic function. Continual assessment of sensory and motor function should occur to prevent further deterioration of neurologic status as a result of spinal cord edema. The ASIA Impairment Scale can be used to assess neurologic function on a routine basis during the patient's recovery. After the patient is admitted, further evaluation of his or her ability to perform ADLs and need for assistance during recovery can be made with the Functional Independence Measure scale.

Nursing care during the acute phase should also focus on frequent monitoring of neurologic signs to determine any changes in neurologic function that require further intervention (e.g., level of consciousness using the Glasgow Coma Scale). In addition to airway maintenance, the nurse should monitor for changes in hemodynamic status that may require immediate medical attention. Neurogenic shock consists of hypotension, bradycardia, and vasodilation. Inotropic medications may be required to maintain adequate perfusion. Renal function is closely monitored by measuring urinary output and fluids administered. The child with a head injury may experience elevated intracranial pressure; therefore, changes in neurologic status are reported to the practitioner. Fluid restriction may be required if intracranial pressure is elevated, so fluid intake should be closely monitored.

The nursing care of the child with an SCI is, in most respects, the same as that of any immobilized child (see The Immobilized Child, Chapter 31). Additional aspects of care that should be addressed on an individual basis include hypercalcemia in adolescent boys, DVT, latex sensitization, autonomic dysreflexia, and sleep-disordered breathing (Vogel, Hickey, Klaas, and others, 2004).

Respiratory care often focuses on maintaining an adequate airway and effective ventilation. The child with a high-level cervical injury (C3 and above) requires continuous ventilatory assistance. In most instances, a tracheostomy is the method of choice for greater ease in clearing secretions and for less trauma to tissues during long-term ventilatory dependence. In some children, breathing pacemaker devices (phrenic nerve stimulators) are implanted to stimulate the phrenic nerve and produce diaphragmatic contractions and lung expansion without assisted ventilation. In the child who does not require mechanical ventilation, special attention to clearance of secretions is vital because of decreased pulmonary function. In addition to percussion and postural drainage, the child may require a cough-assist device to clear secretions effectively (see Duchenne [Pseudohypertrophic] Muscular Dystrophy: Therapeutic Management).

Temperature is often poorly regulated in children with SCI; therefore, body temperature must be monitored closely for fluctuations. Response to environmental temperature changes may be slow or absent, and the ability to dissipate heat through the process of shivering may be compromised.

Children with SCI have unique needs in relation to skin care. Because of decreased sensation and impaired mobility, they depend on others to assess and assist in the management of intact skin. Skin care practices are the same as those for any child who is immobilized. A skin score scale such as the Braden Q Scale should be used to objectively evaluate risks for skin breakdown and skin conditions (Noonan, Quigley, and Curley, 2011). An alternating-pressure mattress or other pressure relief or reduction device is kept underneath the child, and the skin is thoroughly inspected at least once a day (or more often if there is increased risk) for signs of pressure and breakdown, especially over bony prominences.

Bowel and bladder function is often affected in the child with SCI. CIC may be required to regularly empty the neurogenic bladder and prevent urinary tract infections. A regular bowel management program is tailored to the child's needs.

Pain management is vital in children and adolescents with SCI. In children with upper motor neuron involvement, the spasticity that develops may require administration of an antispasmodic medication such as diazepam. Baclofen is considered the drug of choice for reducing muscle spasticity. Gabapentin may be used to treat neuropathic pain. Botulinum toxin type A and α_2-adrenergic agonists may be used in older children with SCI to decrease muscle spasticity.

All adaptive devices help children increase their mobility, function, and endurance. Children with some lower extremity function progress to parallel bars and then to a walker; children with tetraplegia learn to use a wheelchair—among the most valuable aids available to children with SCIs (Fig. 32-9). The wheelchair should be selected carefully in relation to where it will be used, the architectural barriers, and the child's functional capacity. For children with severe upper extremity paralysis, a variety of motorized wheelchairs are used; however, the more complex they are, the greater their cost, weight, and tendency to break down. Wheelchair tolerance is gained over time and is accompanied by measures to prevent orthostatic hypotension and pressure ulcers.

A variety of orthoses and other appliances can be adapted for use by many children. The primary purpose of lower extremity bracing in children with SCIs is for ambulation.

During the recovery and rehabilitation phase, patients with SCI must be carefully monitored for complications of immobility such as

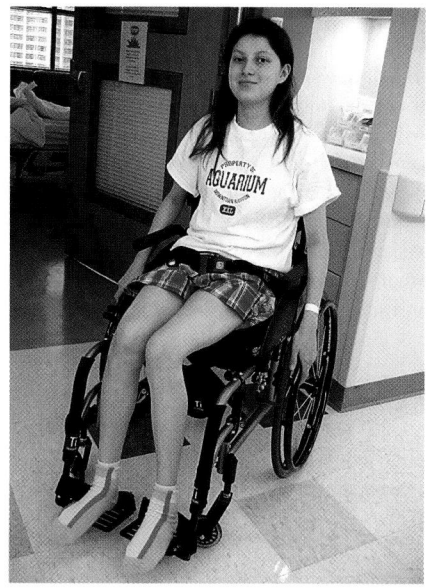

FIG 32-9 A wheelchair allows an adolescent mobility and independence. (Courtesy Texas Children's Hospital, Houston.)

DVT and pulmonary embolus. Children with high-level lesions are susceptible to the development of autonomic dysreflexia, which requires prompt action to prevent encephalopathy and shock. Clinical manifestations of autonomic dysreflexia include a drastic increase in systemic blood pressure, headache, bradycardia, profuse diaphoresis, cardiac arrhythmias, flushing, piloerection, blurred vision, nasal congestion, anxiety, spots on the visual field, or absent or minimum symptoms (Vogel, Hickey, Klaas, and others, 2004).

The child and family with SCI are prepared for the eventual discharge from the acute care facility to a rehabilitation center. The major aims of physical rehabilitation are to prepare the child and family to achieve normalization and resume life at home and in the community. Additional goals of rehabilitation in children with SCI are to promote independence in mobility and self-care skills, academic achievement, independent living, and employment.

The nurse is a crucial member of the health care team in relation to helping the family cope with the magnitude of the injury and disability, understand the extent of the disability, verbalize expected outcomes, and move toward eventual rehabilitation and normalization within the child's capabilities. The goals of rehabilitation include preparing the child and family to live at home and function as independently as possible.

KEY POINTS

- Clinical manifestations of CP include delayed gross motor development, altered motor performance, alterations of muscle tone and subsequent muscle contractures, abnormal posture, and associated disabilities such as seizures and sensory impairment.
- Therapy for CP takes into account the nature of the physical disability, defects associated with the disorder, and interpersonal and social influences encountered by the affected child.
- Care of the infant and child with myelomeningocele is directed toward protecting the meningeal sac, preventing infection and skin breakdown, observing for signs of urologic and bowel complications, promoting early parent–infant interaction, and planning appropriate interventions to optimize the child's development.
- SMA type 1 (Werdnig-Hoffmann disease) is characterized by progressive weakness and wasting of skeletal muscles caused by degeneration of anterior horn cells of the spinal cord.
- MDs are the most prevalent cause of neuromuscular dysfunction of childhood.
- Children with neuromuscular disease require careful monitoring of respiratory function and prompt interventions to prevent hypoxia and hypercarbia.

■ **KEY POINTS—cont'd**

- Major complications of DMD include joint contractures, disuse atrophy, obesity, cardiomyopathy, sleep-disordered breathing, and respiratory failure as the condition progresses.
- Nursing care of the child with GBS consists of maintaining a patent airway; monitoring vital signs and neurologic signs; maintaining adequate nutritional status; and providing physical therapy, reassurance, and support to the child and family.
- Tetanus occurs when tetanus spores or vegetative bacilli enter a wound and multiply in a susceptible host.
- Clinical manifestations of infant botulism include constipation, decreased activity, poor feeding, and lethargy.
- Therapeutic management of SCI is directed toward immobilizing the entire spinal column at the scene of the traumatic event, transporting safely by health care personnel trained to transport possible spinal trauma victims, evaluating neurologic damage, preventing further neurologic damage, and implementing an aggressive rehabilitation program designed to help achieve independence and movement.

REFERENCES

Adzick NS, Thom EA, Spong CY, and others: A randomized trial of prenatal versus postnatal repair of myelomeningocele, *N Engl J Med* 364(11):993–1104, 2011.

American Academy of Pediatrics, Committee on Infectious Diseases, Pickering L, editor: *Red book: 2009 report of the Committee on Infectious Diseases*, ed 28, Elk Grove Village, Ill, 2009, Author.

American Academy of Pediatrics Section on Cardiology and Cardiac Surgery: Cardiovascular health supervision for individuals affected by Duchenne or Becker muscular dystrophy, *Pediatrics* 116(6):1569–1573, 2005.

American Spinal Injury Association: *Standard neurological classification of spinal cord injury*, Atlanta, 2009, Author, retrieved July 2, 2011, from http://www.asia-spinalinjury.org/publications/2006_Classif_worksheet.pdf.

American Thoracic Society: Respiratory care of the patient with Duchenne muscular dystrophy, *Am J Respir Crit Care Med* 170(4):456–465, 2004.

Arnon SS: Tetanus (*Clostridium tetani*). In Kliegman RM, Stanton BF, St. Geme JW, and others, editors: *Nelson textbook of pediatrics*, ed 19, Philadelphia, 2011a, Saunders.

Arnon SS: Anaerobic bacterial infections: botulism (*Clostridium botulinum*). In Kliegman RM, Stanton BF, St. Geme JW, and others, editors: *Nelson textbook of pediatrics*, ed 19, Philadelphia, 2011b, Saunders.

Bach JR: Medical considerations of long-term survival of Werdnig-Hoffmann disease, *Am J Phys Med Rehabil* 86(5):349–355, 2007.

Bach JR, Martinez D: Duchenne muscular dystrophy: continuous noninvasive ventilatory support prolongs survival, *Respir Care* 56(6):744–750, 2011.

Battista V: Muscular dystrophy, Duchenne. In Jackson PL, Vessey JA, Schapiro NA, editors: *Primary care of the child with a chronic illness*, ed 5, St. Louis, 2010, Mosby.

Bax M, Goldstein M, Rosenbaum P, and others: Proposed definition and classification of cerebral palsy, *Dev Med Child Neurol* 47(8):571–576, 2005.

Berker AN, Yalçin MS: Cerebral palsy: orthopedic aspects and rehabilitation, *Pediatr Clin North Am* 55(5):1209–1225, 2008.

Beroud C, Karliova M, Bonnefont JP, and others: Prenatal diagnosis of spinal muscular atrophy by genetic analysis of circulating fetal cells, *Lancet* 361(9362):1013–1014, 2003.

Betz C, Linroth R, Butler C, and others: Spina bifida: what we learned from consumers, *Pediatr Clin NA* 57(4):935–944, 2010.

Boitano LJ: Equipment options for cough augmentation, ventilation, and noninvasive interfaces in neuromuscular respiratory management, *Pediatrics* 123(suppl 4):S226–S230, 2009.

Bosboom WM, Vrancken AF, van den Berg LH, and others: Drug treatment for spinal muscular atrophy type I, *Cochrane Database Syst Rev* (1):CD006281, 2009.

Bush A, Fraser J, Jardine E, and others: Respiratory management of the infant with type 1 spinal muscular atrophy, *Arch Dis Child* 90(7):709–711, 2005.

Centers for Disease Control and Prevention: Folate status in women of childbearing age, by race/ethnicity—United States, 1999–2000, 2001–2002, and 2003–2004, *MMWR Morb Mortal Wkly Rep* 55(51):1377–1380, 2007.

Centers for Disease Control and Prevention: Racial/ethnic differences in the birth prevalence of spina bifida—United States, 1995–2005, *MMWR Morb Mortal Wkly Rep* 57(53):1409–1413, 2009.

Centers for Disease Control and Prevention: *Botulism: general information: frequently asked questions*, 2010, retrieved July 2, 2011, from http://www.cdc.gov/nczved/divisions/dfbmd/diseases/botulism.

Centers for Disease Control and Prevention: Updated recommendation for use of tetanus toxoid, reduced diphtheria toxoid and acellular pertussis (Tdap) vaccine form the Advisory Committee on Immunization Practices, 2010, *MMWR Morb Mortal Wkly Rep* 60(01):13–15, 2011.

Dicianno BE, Fairman AD, Juengst SB, and others: Using the spina bifida Life Course Model in clinical practice: an interdisciplinary approach, *Pediatr Clin North Am* 57(4):945–957, 2010.

Doolin E: Bowel management for patients with myelodysplasia, *Surg Clin North Am* 86(2):505–514, 2006.

Finder JD: A 2009 perspective on the 2004 American Thoracic Society statement, "Respiratory care of the patient with Duchenne muscular dystrophy," *Pediatrics* 123(suppl 4):S239–S241, 2009.

Golomb MR, Saha C, Garg BP, and others: Association of cerebral palsy with other disabilities in children with perinatal arterial ischemic stroke, *Pediatr Neurol* 37(4):245–249, 2007.

Green L, Greenberg GM, Hurwitz E: Primary care of children with cerebral palsy, *Clin Fam Pract* 5(2):1–21, 2003.

Grether JK, Nelson KB, Walsh E, and others: Intrauterine exposure to infection and risk of cerebral palsy in very preterm infants, *Arch Pediatr Adolesc Med* 157(1):26–32, 2003.

Hayes JS, Arriola T: Pediatric spinal injuries, *Pediatr Nurs* 31(6):464–467, 2005.

Hermansen MC, Hermansen MG: Perinatal infections and cerebral palsy, *Clin Perinatol* 33(2):315–333, 2006.

Hirtz D, Thurman DJ, Gwinn-Hardy K, and others: How common are the "common" neurological disorders? *Neurology* 68(5):326–337, 2007.

Hosalkar H, Pandya NK, Hsu J, and others: Specialty update: what's new in orthopaedic rehabilitation, *J Bone Joint Surg Am* 91(9):2296–2310, 2009.

Hughes R: The role of IVIG in autoimmune neuropathies: the latest evidence, *J Neuro* 255(suppl 3):7–11, 2008.

Hughes RA, Cornblath DR: Guillain-Barré syndrome, *Lancet* 366(9497):1653–1666, 2005.

Hughes RA, Swan AV, van Doorn PA: Intravenous immunoglobulin for Guillain-Barré syndrome, *Cochrane Database Syst Rev* (6):CD002063, 2010.

Hurtekant KM, Spatz DL: Special considerations for breastfeeding the infant with spina bifida, *J Perinat Neonatal Nurs* 21(1):69–75, 2007.

Iannaccone ST: Modern management of spinal muscular atrophy, *J Child Neurol* 22(8):974–978, 2007.

Iannaccone ST, Burghes A: Spinal muscular atrophies, *Adv Neurol* 88:83–98, 2002.

Johnston MV: Cerebral palsy. In Kliegman RM, Stanton BF, St. Geme JW, and others, editors: *Nelson textbook of pediatrics*, ed 19, Philadelphia, 2011, Saunders.

Johnston MV, Fatemi A, Wilson MA, and others: Treatment advances in neonatal neuroprotection and neurointensive care, *Lancet Neurol* 10(4):372–382, 2011.

Kinsman SL, Johnston MV: Myelomeningocele. In Kliegman RM, Stanton BF, St. Geme JW, and others, editors: *Nelson textbook of pediatrics*, ed 19, Philadelphia, 2011, Saunders

Kirkham C, Harris S, Grzybowski S: Evidence-based prenatal care, part I, general prenatal care and counseling issues, *Am Fam Physician* 71(7):1307–1316, 2005.

Krageloh-Mann I, Cans C: Cerebral palsy update, *Brain Dev* 31(7):537–544, 2009.

Kravitz RM: Airway clearance in Duchenne muscular dystrophy, *Pediatrics* 123(suppl 4): S231–S235, 2009.

Krigger KW: Cerebral palsy: an overview, *Am Fam Physician* 73(1):91–100, 101–102, 2006.

Lazzaretti CC, Pearson C: Myelodysplasia. In Allen PJ, Vessey JA, editors: *Primary care of the child with a chronic condition*, ed 5, St. Louis, 2010, Mosby.

Lovette B: Safe transportation for children with special needs, *J Pediatr Health Care* 22(5): 323–328, 2008.

Lukban MB, Rosales RL, Dressler D: Effectiveness of botulinum toxin A for upper and lower limb spasticity in children with cerebral palsy: a summary of evidence, *J Neural Transm* 116(3): 319–331, 2009.

Lunn MR, Wang CH: Spina muscular atrophy, *Lancet* 371(9630):2120–2133, 2008.

Lyons R: Elusive belly pain and Guillain-Barré syndrome, *J Pediatr Health Care* 22(5):310–314, 2008.

Manzur AY, Kinali M, Muntoni F: Update on the management of Duchenne muscular dystrophy, *Arch Dis Child* 93(11):986–990, 2008.

Manzur AY, Kuntzer T, Pike M, and others: Glucocorticoid corticosteroids for Duchenne muscular dystrophy, *Cochrane Database Syst Rev* (1):CD003725, 2008.

Mathison DJ, Kadom N, Krug SE: Spinal cord injury in the pediatric patient, *Clin Pediatr Emerg Med* 9(2):106–123, 2008.

Matthews TJ: *Trends in spina bifida and anencephalus in the United States, 1991–2006*, Hyatsville, Md, 2009, National Center on Health Statistics, retrieved June 1, 2009, from http://www.cdc.gov/nchs/products/pubs/pubd/hestats/spine_anen.pdf.

McKearnan KA, Kieckhefer GM, Engel JM, and others: Pain in children with cerebral palsy: a review, *J Neurosci Nurs* 36(5):252–259, 2004.

Miske LJ, Hickey EM, Kolb SM, and others: Use of the mechanical in-exsufflator in pediatric patients with neuromuscular disease and impaired cough, *Chest* 125(4):1406–1412, 2004.

Moore C, Kogan BA, Parekh A: Impact of urinary incontinence on self-concept in children with spina bifida, *J Urol* 171(4):1659–1662, 2004.

Moster D, Wilcox AJ, Vollset SE, and others: Cerebral palsy among term and postterm births, *JAMA* 304(9):976–982, 2010.

Moxley RT, Ashwal S, Pandya S, and others: Practice parameter: corticosteroid treatment of Duchenne dystrophy, *Neurology* 64(1):13–20, 2005.

Nehring WM: Cerebral palsy. In Jackson PL, Vessey JA, Schapiro NA, editors: *Primary care of the child with a chronic illness*, ed 5, St. Louis, 2010, Mosby.

Noonan C, Quigley S, Curley MA: Using the Braden Q Scale to predict pressure ulcer risk in pediatric patients, *J Pediatr Nurs* 26(6): 566–575, 2011.

Prior TW: Spinal muscular atrophy: newborn and carrier screening, *Obstet Gynecol Clin North Am* 37(1):23–26, 2010.

Quan D: Muscular dystrophies and neurologic diseases that present as myopathy, *Rheum Dis Clin North Am* 37(2):233–244, 2011.

Retake HL: Spinal cord injuries in children. In Kliegman RM, Stanton BF, St. Geme JW, and others, editors: *Nelson textbook of pediatrics*, ed 19, Philadelphia, 2011, Saunders.

Rogers B: Feeding method and health outcomes of children with cerebral palsy, *J Pediatr* 145(2 suppl):S28–S32, 2004.

Rosenbaum P, Paneth N, Leviton A, and others: A report: the definition and classification of cerebral palsy April 2006, *Dev Med Child Neurol* 49(S109):1–44, 2007.

Russman BS: Function changes in spinal muscular atrophy II and III: the DCN/SMA Group, *Neurology* 47(4):973–976, 1996.

Russman BS, Iannaccone ST, Buncher CR, and others: Spinal muscular atrophy: new thoughts on the pathogenesis and classification schema, *J Child Neurol* 7(4):347–353, 1992.

Samaniego IA: A sore spot in pediatrics: risk factors for pressure ulcers, *Pediatr Nurs* 29(4): 278–282, 2003.

Sarnat HB: Spinal muscular atrophies. In Kliegman RM, Stanton BF, St. Geme JW, and others, editors: *Nelson textbook of pediatrics*, ed 19, Philadelphia, 2011a, Saunders.

Sarnat HB: Guillain-Barré syndrome. In Kliegman RM, Stanton BF, St. Geme JW, and others, editors: *Nelson textbook of pediatrics*, ed 19, Philadelphia, 2011b, Saunders.

Sarnat HB: Muscular dystrophies. In Kliegman RM, Stanton BF, St. Geme JW, and others, editors: *Nelson textbook of pediatrics*, ed 19, Philadelphia, 2011c, Saunders.

Sarnat HB: Neuromuscular disorders. In Kliegman RM, Behrman RE, Jenson HB and others, editors: *Nelson textbook of pediatrics*, ed 18, Philadelphia, 2007, Saunders.

Sawyer SM, Macnee S: Transition to adult health care for adolescents with spina bifida: research issues, *Dev Disabil Res Rev* 16(1):60–65, 2010.

Schroth MK: Special considerations in the respiratory management of spinal muscular atrophy, *Pediatrics* 123(suppl 4):S245–S249, 2009.

Shaer CM, Chescheir N, Schulkin J: Myelomeningocele: a review of the epidemiology, genetics, risk factors for conception, prenatal diagnosis, and prognosis for affected individuals, *Obstet Gynecol Surv* 62(7):471–479, 2007.

Simonds AK: Recent advances in respiratory care for neuromuscular disease, *Chest* 130(6):1879–1886, 2006.

Snodgrass WT, Gargollo PC: Urologic care of the neurogenic bladder in children, *Urol Clin North Am* 37(2):207–214, 2010.

Tarcan T, Onol FF, Ilker Y, and others: The timing of primary neurosurgical repair significantly affects neurogenic bladder prognosis in children with myelomeningocele, *J Urol* 176(3):1161–1165, 2006.

Thrasher TA, Popovic MR: Functional electrical stimulation of walking: function, exercise and rehabilitation, *Ann Readapt Med Phys* 51(6): 452–460, 2008.

To CS, Kirsch RF, Kobetic R, and others: Simulation of a functional neuromuscular stimulation powered mechanical gait orthosis with coordinated joint locking, *IEEE Trans Neural Syst Rehabil Eng* 13(2):227–235, 2005.

Vitale MG, Goss JM, Matsumoto H, and others: Epidemiology of pediatric spinal cord injury in the United States: years 1997 and 2000, *J Pediatr Orthop* 26(6):745–749, 2006.

Vogel LC, Hickey KJ, Klaas SJ, and others: Unique issues in pediatric spinal cord injury, *Orthop Nurs* 23(5):300–308, 2004.

Wolff T, Witkop CT, Miller T, and others: Folic acid supplementation for the prevention of neural tube defects: an update of the evidence for the U.S. Preventive Services Task Force, *Ann Intern Med* 150(9):632–639, W112–W115, 2009.

Wright PA, Durham S, Ewins DJ, and others: Neuromuscular electrical stimulation for children with cerebral palsy: a review, *Arch Dis Child* 97(4):364–371, 2012.

Wu YW, Escobar GJ, Grether JK, and others: Chorioamnionitis and cerebral palsy in term and near-term infants, *JAMA* 290(20): 2677–2684, 2003.

Yeargin-Allsopp M, Van Naarden Braun K, Doernberg NS, and others: Prevalence of cerebral palsy in 8-year-old children in three areas of the United States in 2002: a multisite collaboration, *Pediatrics* 121(3):547–554, 2008.

Young HK, Lowe A, Fitzgerald DA, and others: Outcome of noninvasive ventilation in children with neuromuscular disease, *Neurology* 68(3): 198–201, 2007.

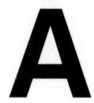

A

Growth Measurements

BODY MASS INDEX FORMULA

English Formula

$$BMI = [\text{Weight in pounds} \div \text{Height in inches} \div \text{Height in inches}] \times 703$$

Fractions and ounces must be entered as decimal values.

FRACTION	OUNCES	DECIMAL
$\frac{1}{8}$	2	0.125
$\frac{1}{4}$	4	0.25
$\frac{3}{8}$	6	0.375
$\frac{1}{2}$	8	0.5
$\frac{5}{8}$	10	0.625
$\frac{3}{4}$	12	0.75
$\frac{7}{8}$	14	0.875

Example: A 33-lb, 4-oz child is 37 $\frac{5}{8}$ inches tall.

$$[(33.25\,\text{lb} \div 37.625\,\text{in}) \div 37.625\,\text{in}] \times 703 = 16.5$$

Metric Formula

$$BMI = \text{Weight in kilograms} \div [\text{Height in meters}]^2$$

or

$$BMI = [(\text{Weight in kilograms} \div \text{Height in cm}) \div \text{Height in cm}] \times 10,000$$

Example: A 16.9-kg child is 105.2 cm tall.

$$[(16.9\,\text{kg} \div 105.2\,\text{cm}) \div 105.2\,\text{cm}] \times 10,000 = 15.3$$

From Kuczmarski RJ, Ogden CL, Grummer-Strawn LM, and others: *CDC growth charts: United States: advance data from vital and health statistics,* no 314, Hyattsville, Md, June 8, 2000, National Center for Health Statistics; retrieved from www.cdc.gov/nchs/about/major/nhanes/growthcharts/fullreport.htm.

HEIGHT AND WEIGHT MEASUREMENTS FOR BOYS

AGE*	HEIGHT BY PERCENTILES						WEIGHT BY PERCENTILES					
	5		50		95		5		50		95	
	cm	inches	cm	inches	cm	inches	kg	lb	kg	lb	kg	lb
Birth	46.4	18¼	50.5	20	54.4	21½	2.54	5½	3.27	7¼	4.15	9¼
3 mo	56.7	22¼	61.1	24	65.4	25¾	4.43	9¾	5.98	13¼	7.37	16¼
6 mo	63.4	25	67.8	26¾	72.3	28½	6.20	13¾	7.85	17¼	9.46	20¾
9 mo	68.0	26¾	72.3	28½	77.1	30¼	7.52	16½	9.18	20¼	10.93	24
1	71.7	28¼	76.1	30	81.2	32	8.43	18½	10.15	22½	11.99	26½
1½	77.5	30½	82.4	32½	88.1	34¾	9.59	21¼	11.47	25¼	13.44	29½
2†	82.5	32½	86.8	34¼	94.4	37¼	10.49	23¼	12.34	27¼	15.50	34¼
2½†	85.4	33½	90.4	35½	97.8	38½	11.27	24¾	13.52	29¾	16.61	36½
3	89.0	35	94.9	37¼	102.0	40¼	12.05	26½	14.62	32¼	17.77	39¼
3½	92.5	36½	99.1	39	106.1	41¾	12.84	28¼	15.68	34½	18.98	41¾
4	95.8	37¾	102.9	40½	109.9	43¼	13.64	30	16.69	36¾	20.27	44¾
4½	98.9	39	106.6	42	113.5	44¾	14.45	31¾	17.69	39	21.63	47¾
5	102.0	40¼	109.9	43¼	117.0	46	15.27	33¾	18.67	41¼	23.09	51
6	107.7	42½	116.1	45¾	123.5	48½	16.93	37¼	20.69	45½	26.34	58
7	113.0	44½	121.7	48	129.7	51	18.64	41	22.85	50¼	30.12	66½
8	118.1	46½	127.0	50	135.7	53½	20.40	45	25.30	55¾	34.51	76
9	122.9	48½	132.2	52	141.8	55¾	22.25	49	28.13	62	39.58	87¼
10	127.7	50¼	137.5	54¼	148.1	58¼	24.33	53¾	31.44	69¼	45.27	99¾
11	132.6	52¼	143.3	56½	154.9	61	26.80	59	35.30	77¾	51.47	113½
12	137.6	54¼	149.7	59	162.3	64	29.85	65¾	39.78	87¾	58.09	128
13	142.9	56¼	156.5	61½	169.8	66¾	33.64	74¼	44.95	99	65.02	143¼
14	148.8	58½	163.1	64¼	176.7	69½	38.22	84¼	50.77	112	72.13	159
15	155.2	61	169.0	66½	181.9	71½	43.11	95	56.71	125	79.12	174½
16	161.1	63½	173.5	68¼	185.4	73	47.74	105¼	62.10	137	85.62	188¾
17	164.9	65	176.2	69¼	187.3	73¾	51.50	113½	66.31	146¼	91.31	201¼
18	165.7	65¼	176.8	69½	187.6	73¾	53.97	119	68.88	151¾	95.76	211

Modified from National Center for Health Statistics, Health Resources Administration, Department of Health, Education and Welfare, Hyattsville, Md.

Conversion of metric data to approximate inches and pounds by Ross Laboratories.

*Years unless otherwise indicated.

†Height data include some recumbent length measurements, which make values slightly higher than if all measurements had been of stature (standing height).

Birth to 24 months: Boys
Length-for-age and Weight-for-age percentiles

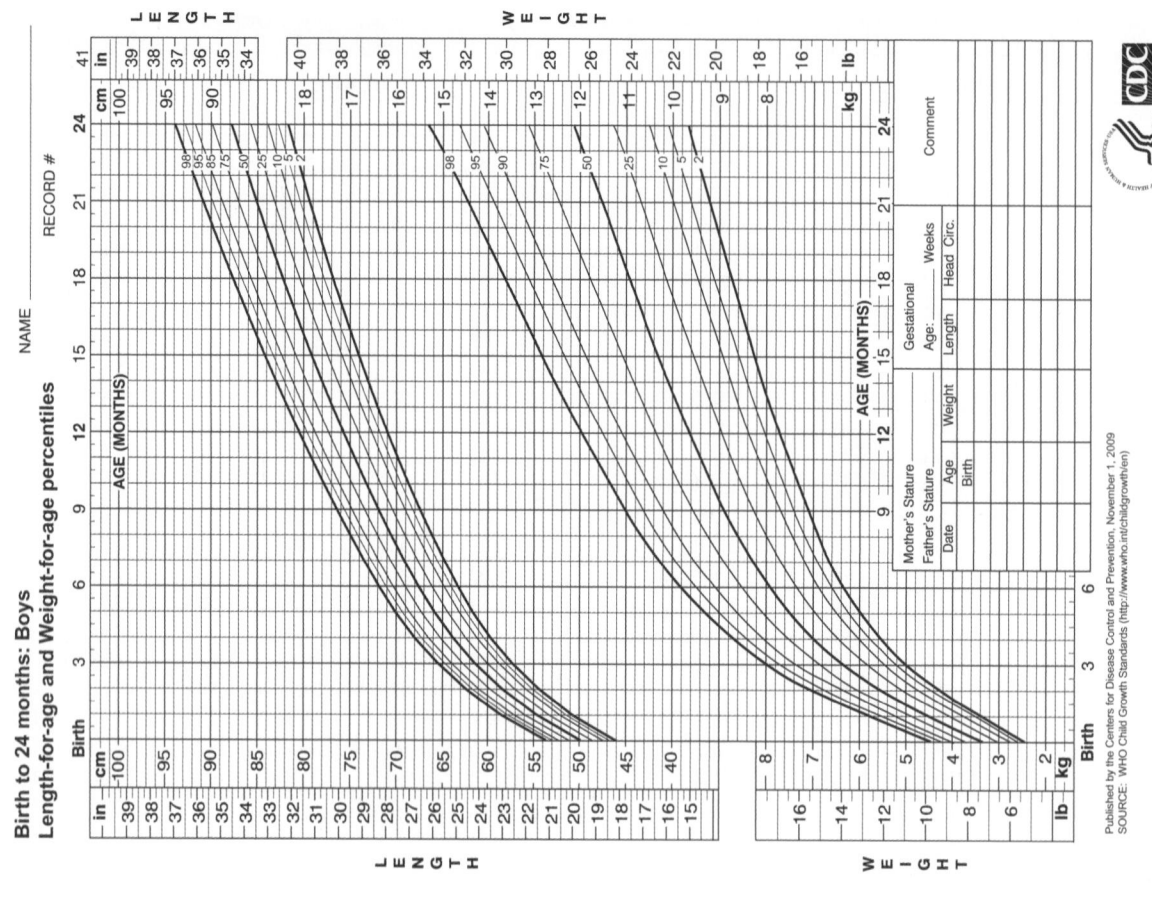

FIG A-2 Birth to 24 months: boys. Length-for-age and weight-for-age percentiles. Published by the Centers for Disease Control and Prevention, November 1, 2009. Source: WHO Child Growth Standards (http://www.who.int/childgrowth/en).

Birth to 24 months: Boys
Head circumference-for-age and
Weight-for-length percentiles

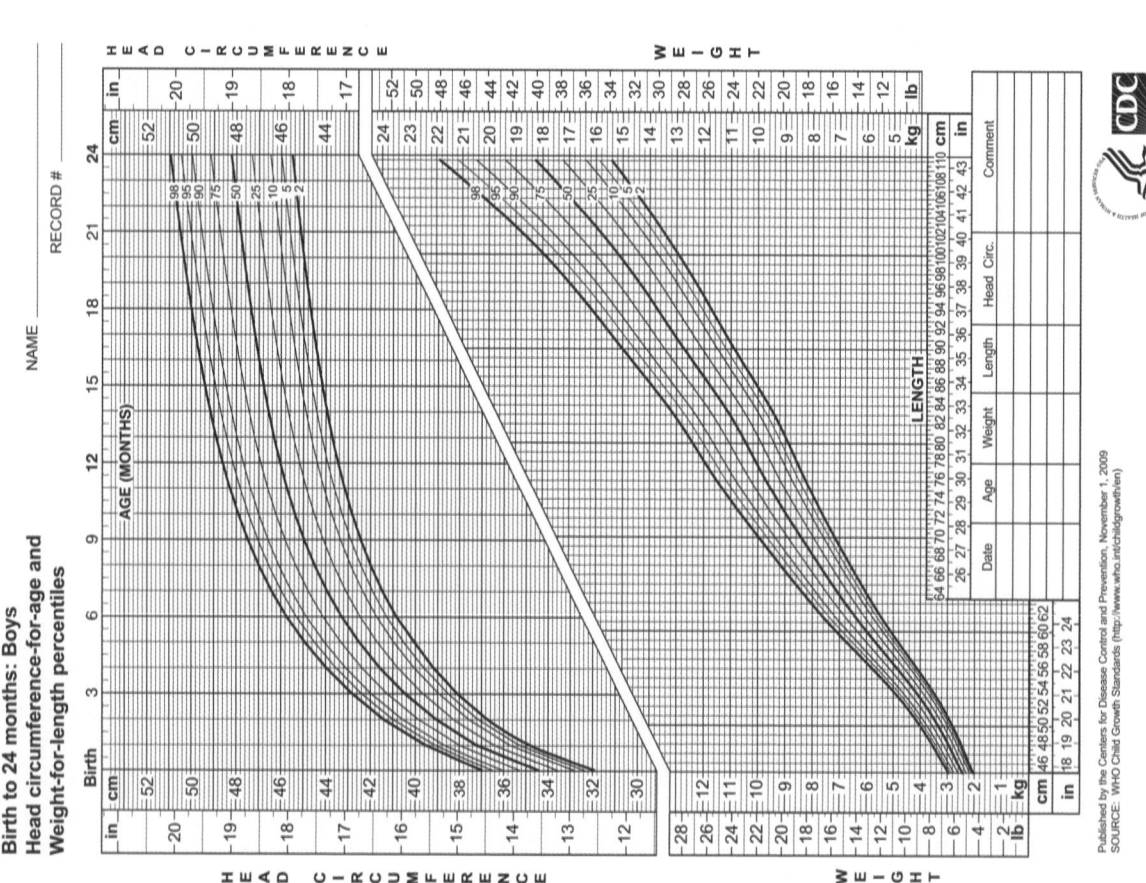

FIG A-1 Birth to 24 months: boys. Head circumference–for-age and weight-for-length percentiles. Published by the Centers for Disease Control and Prevention, November 1, 2009. Source: WHO Child Growth Standards (http://www.who.int/childgrowth/en).

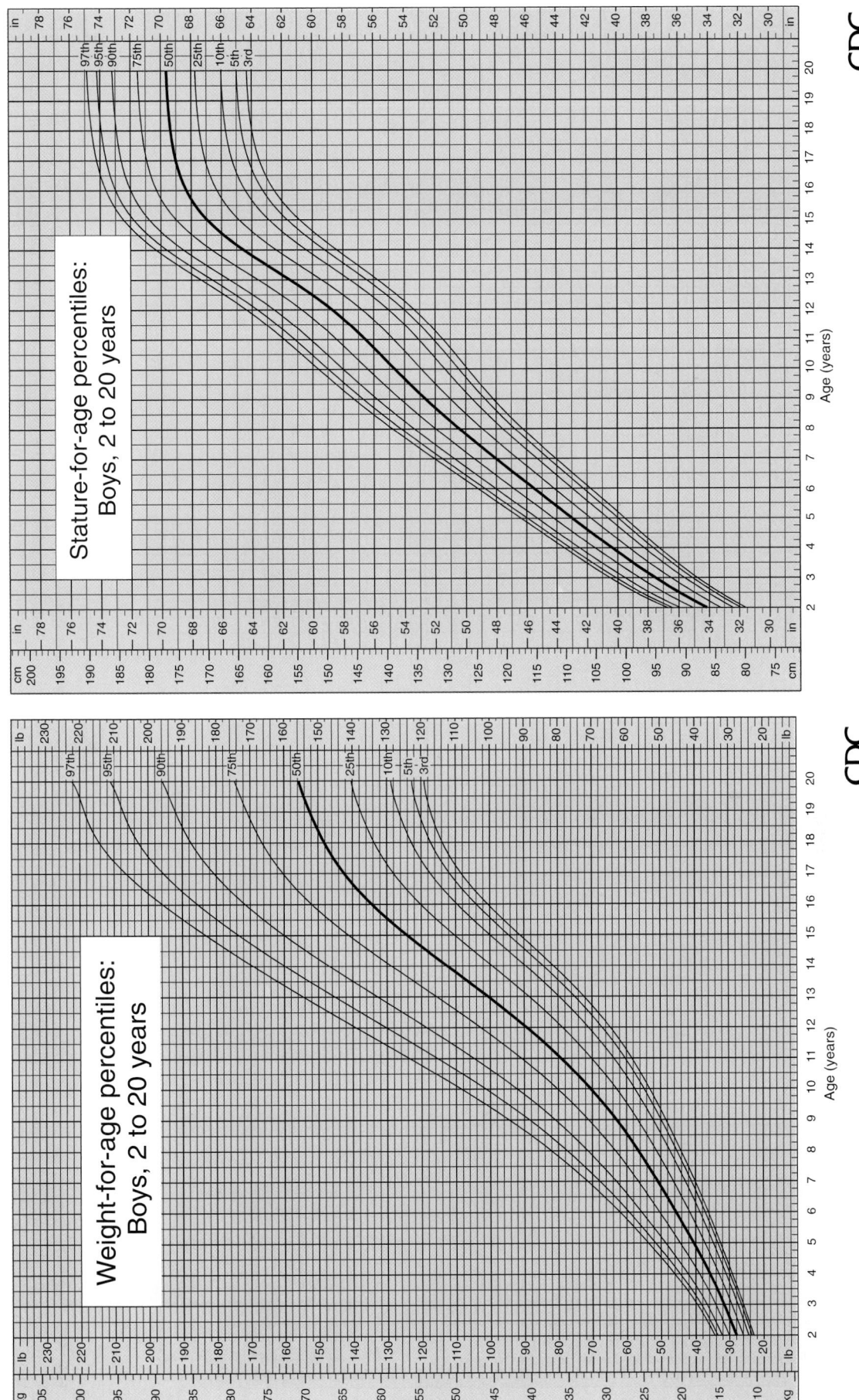

FIG A-4 Stature-for-age percentiles, boys, 2 to 20 years, CDC growth charts: United States. (Developed by the National Center for Health Statistics in collaboration with the National Center for Chronic Disease Prevention and Health Promotion, 2000.)

FIG A-3 Weight-for-age percentiles, boys, 2 to 20 years, CDC growth charts: United States. (Developed by the National Center for Health Statistics in collaboration with the National Center for Chronic Disease Prevention and Health Promotion, 2000.)

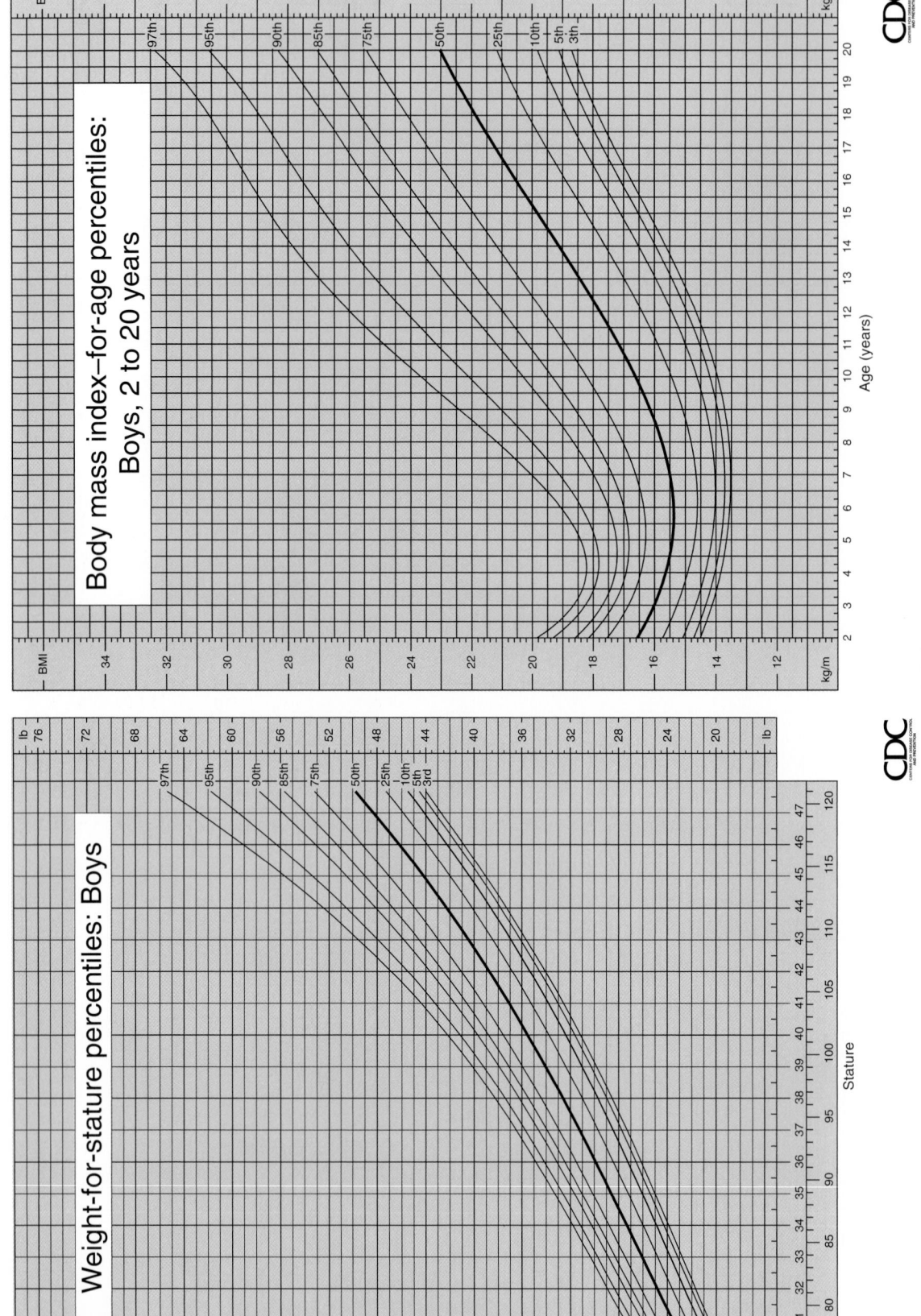

FIG A-5 Weight-for-stature percentiles, boys, CDC growth charts: United States. (Developed by the National Center for Health Statistics in collaboration with the National Center for Chronic Disease Prevention and Health Promotion, 2000.)

FIG A-6 Body mass index-for-age percentiles, boys, 2 to 20 years, CDC growth charts: United States (Developed by the National Center for Health Statistics in collaboration with the National Center for Chronic Disease Prevention and Health Promotion, 2000.)

HEIGHT AND WEIGHT MEASUREMENTS FOR GIRLS

	HEIGHT BY PERCENTILES						WEIGHT BY PERCENTILES					
	5		50		95		5		50		95	
AGE*	cm	inches	cm	inches	cm	inches	kg	lb	kg	lb	kg	lb
Birth	45.4	17¾	49.9	19¾	52.9	20¾	2.36	5¼	3.23	7	3.81	8½
3 mo	55.4	21¾	59.5	23½	63.4	25	4.18	9¼	5.4	12	6.74	14¾
6 mo	61.8	24¼	65.9	26	70.2	27¾	5.79	12¾	7.21	16	8.73	19¼
9 mo	66.1	26	70.4	27¾	75.0	29½	7.0	15½	8.56	18¾	10.17	22½
1	69.8	27½	74.3	29¼	79.1	31¼	7.84	17¼	9.53	21	11.24	24¾
1½	76.0	30	80.9	31¾	86.1	34	8.92	19¾	10.82	23¾	12.76	28¼
2†	81.6	32¼	86.8	34¼	93.6	36¾	9.95	22	11.8	26	14.15	31¼
2½†	84.6	33¼	90.0	35½	96.6	38	10.8	23¾	13.03	28¾	15.76	34¾
3	88.3	34¾	94.1	37	100.6	39½	11.61	25½	14.1	31	17.22	38
3½	91.7	36	97.9	38½	104.5	41¼	12.37	27¼	15.07	33¼	18.59	41
4	95.0	37½	101.6	40	108.3	42¾	13.11	29	15.96	35¼	19.91	44
4½	98.1	38½	105.0	41¼	112.0	44	13.83	30½	16.81	37	21.24	46¾
5	101.1	39¾	108.4	42¾	115.6	45½	14.55	32	17.66	39	22.62	49¾
6	106.6	42	114.6	45	122.7	48¼	16.05	35½	19.52	43	25.75	56¾
7	111.8	44	120.6	47½	129.5	51	17.71	39	21.84	48¼	29.68	65½
8	116.9	46	126.4	49¾	136.2	53½	19.62	43¼	24.84	54¾	34.71	76½
9	122.1	48	132.2	52	142.9	56¼	21.82	48	28.46	62¾	40.64	89½
10	127.5	50¼	138.3	54½	149.5	58¾	24.36	53¾	32.55	71¾	47.17	104
11	133.5	52½	144.8	57	156.2	61½	27.24	60	36.95	81½	54.0	119
12	139.8	55	151.5	59¾	162.7	64	30.52	67¼	41.53	91½	60.81	134
13	145.2	57¼	157.1	61¾	168.1	66¼	34.14	75¼	46.1	101¾	67.3	148¼
14	148.7	58½	160.4	63¼	171.3	67½	37.76	83¼	50.28	110¾	73.08	161
15	150.5	59¼	161.8	63¾	172.8	68	40.99	90¼	53.68	118¼	77.78	171½
16	151.6	59¾	162.4	64	173.3	68¼	43.41	95¾	55.89	123¼	80.99	178½
17	152.7	60	163.1	64¼	173.5	68¼	44.74	98¾	56.69	125	82.46	181¾
18	153.6	60½	163.7	64½	173.6	68¼	45.26	99¾	56.62	124¾	82.47	181¾

Modified from National Center for Health Statistics, Health Resources Administration, Department of Health, Education and Welfare, Hyattsville, Md.

Conversion of metric data to approximate inches and pounds by Ross Laboratories.

*Years unless otherwise indicated.

†Height data include some recumbent length measurements, which make values slightly higher than if all measurements had been of stature.

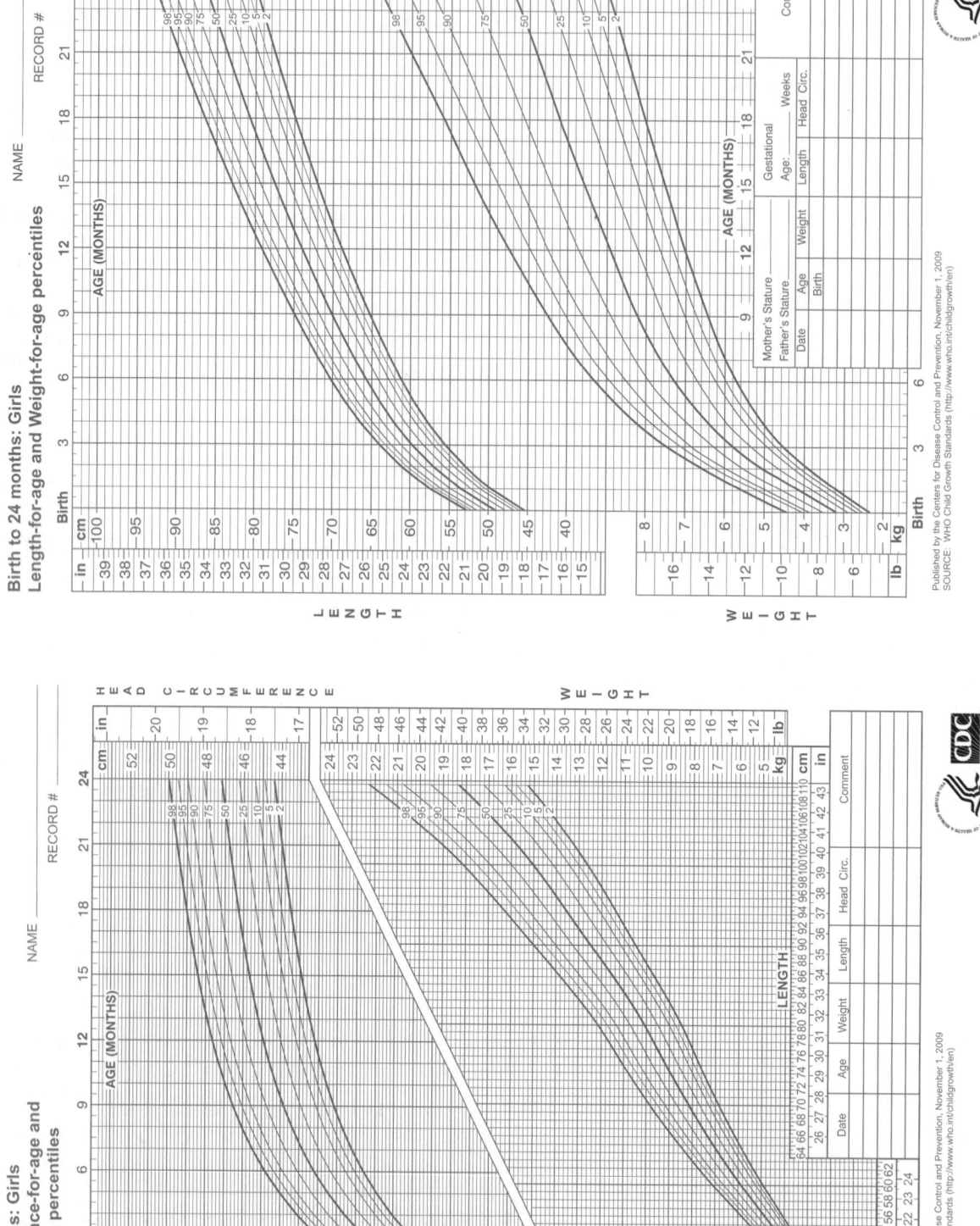

Birth to 24 months: Girls
Length-for-age and Weight-for-age percentiles

NAME _____

RECORD # _____

Published by the Centers for Disease Control and Prevention, November 1, 2009
SOURCE: WHO Child Growth Standards (http://www.who.int/childgrowth/en)

FIG A-8 Birth to 24 months: girls. Length-for-age and weight-for-age percentiles. Published by the Centers for Disease Control and Prevention, November 1, 2009. Source: WHO Child Growth Standards (http://www.who.int/childgrowth/en).

Birth to 24 months: Girls
Head circumference-for-age and
Weight-for-length percentiles

NAME _____

RECORD # _____

Published by the Centers for Disease Control and Prevention, November 1, 2009
SOURCE: WHO Child Growth Standards (http://www.who.int/childgrowth/en)

FIG A-7 Birth to 24 months: girls. Head circumference-for-age and weight-for-length percentiles. Published by the Centers for Disease Control and Prevention, November 1, 2009. Source: WHO Child Growth Standards (http://www.who.int/childgrowth/en).

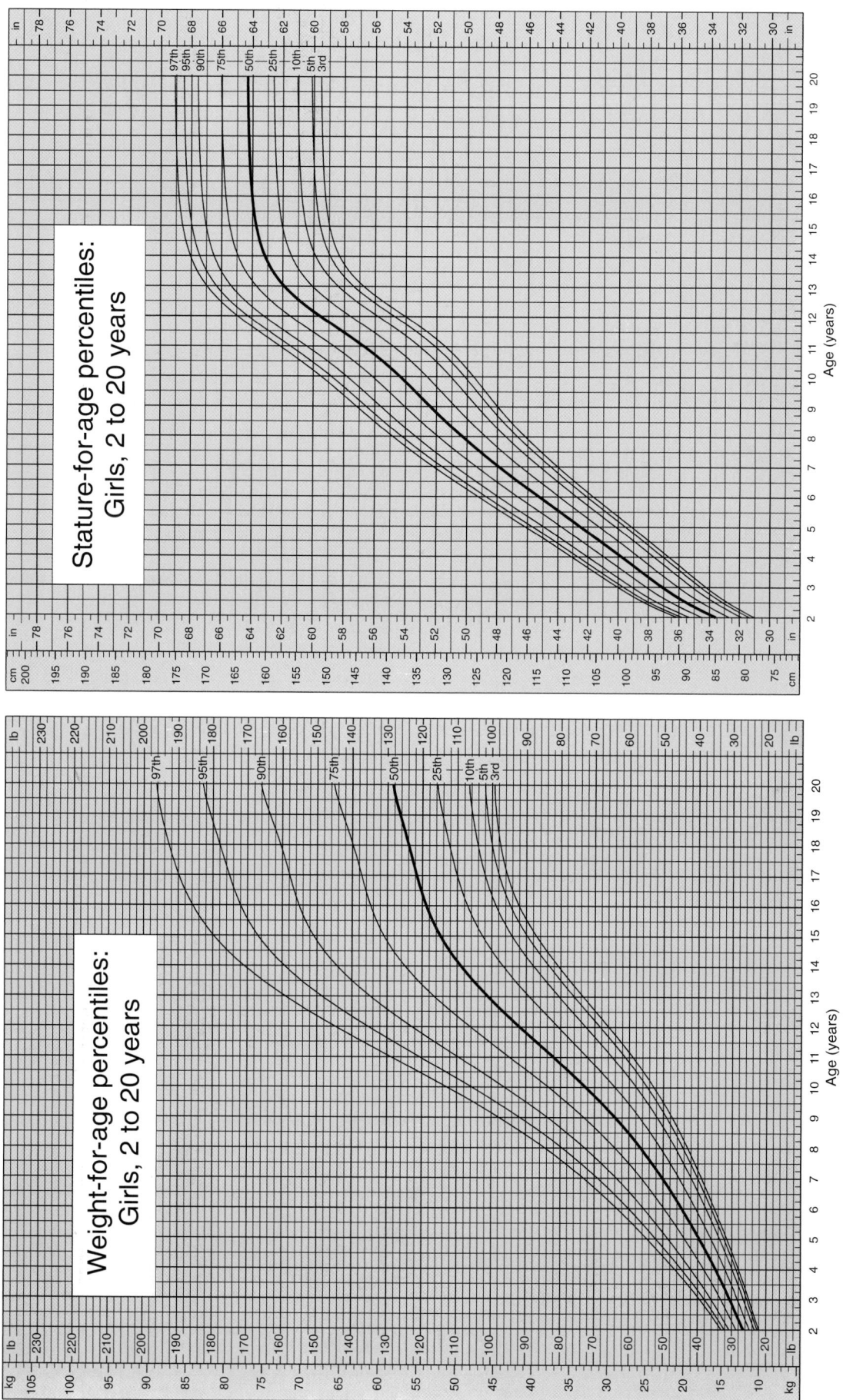

FIG A-9 Weight-for-age percentiles, girls, 2 to 20 years, CDC growth charts: United States. (Developed by the National Center for Health Statistics in collaboration with the National Center for Chronic Disease Prevention and Health Promotion, 2000.)

FIG A-10 Stature-for-age percentiles, girls, 2 to 20 years, CDC growth charts: United States. (Developed by the National Center for Health Statistics in collaboration with the National Center for Chronic Disease Prevention and Health Promotion, 2000.)

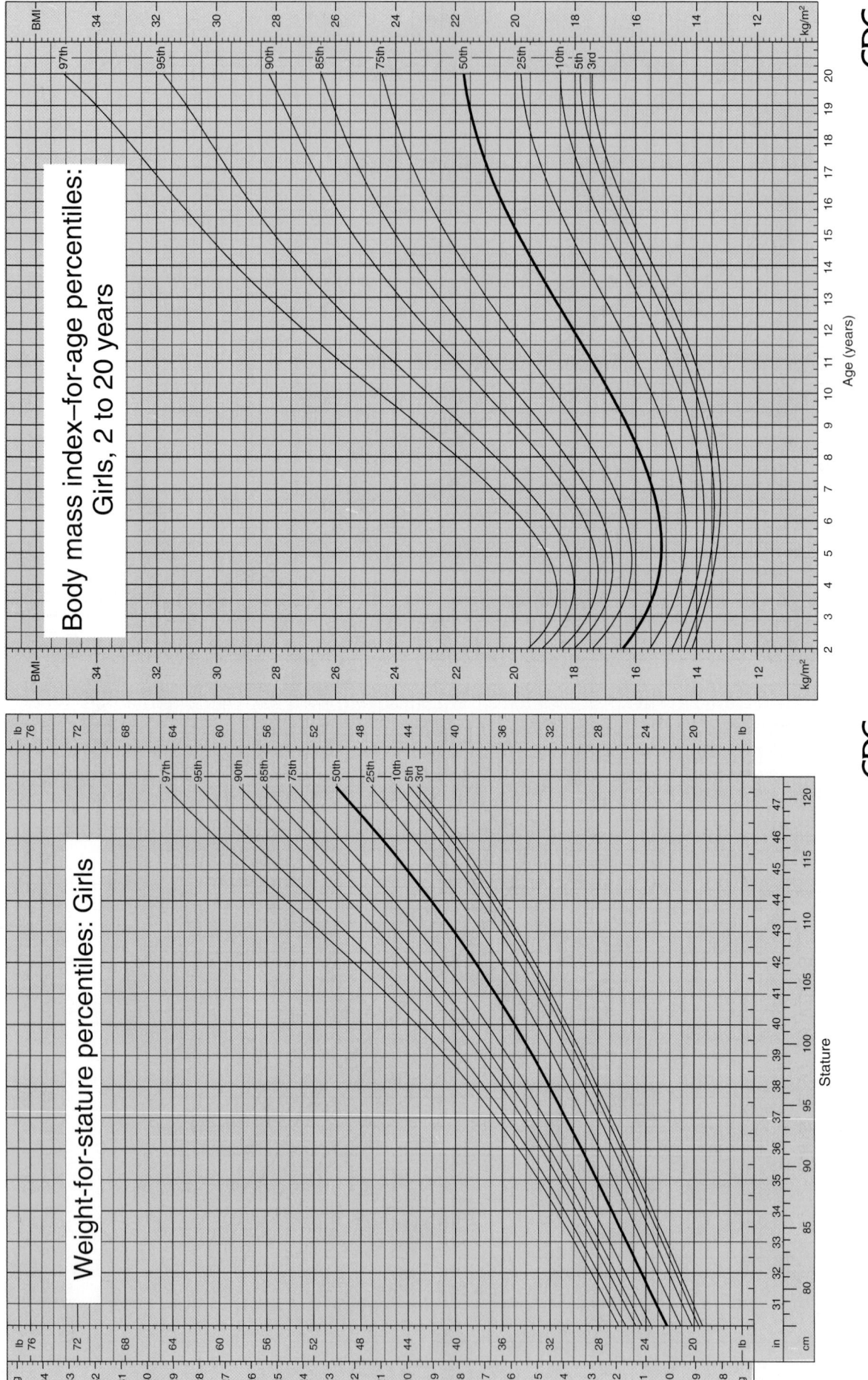

FIG A-11 Weight-for-stature percentiles, girls, CDC growth charts: United States. (Developed by the National Center for Health Statistics in collaboration with the National Center for Chronic Disease Prevention and Health Promotion, 2000.)

FIG A-12 Body mass index–for-age percentiles, girls, 2 to 20 years, CDC growth charts: United States. (Developed by the National Center for Health Statistics in collaboration with the National Center for Chronic Disease Prevention and Health Promotion, 2000.)

Common Laboratory Tests

COMMON LABORATORY TESTS AND TESTS RESULTS*

| TEST/SPECIMEN | AGE/GENDER/REFERENCE | NORMAL RANGES | | | |
		CONVENTIONAL UNITS		INTERNATIONAL UNITS (SI)	
Acetaminophen					
Serum or plasma	Therap. conc.	10–30 mcg/ml		66–200 µmol/L	
	Toxic conc.	>200 mcg/ml		>1300 µmol/L	
Ammonia nitrogen					
Plasma or serum	Newborn	90–150 mcg/dl		64–107 µmol/L	
	0–2 wk	79–129 mcg/dl		56–92 µmol/L	
	>1 mo	29–70 mcg/dl		21–50 µmol/L	
	Thereafter	0–50 mcg/dl		0–35.7 µmol/L	
Antistreptolysin O titer (ASO)					
Serum	2–4 yr	<160 Todd units			
	School-age children	170–330 Todd units			
Base excess					
Whole blood	Newborn	(–10)–(–2) mEq/L		(–10)–(–2) mmol/L	
	Infant	(–7)–(–1) mEq/L		(–7)–(–1) mmol/L	
	Child	(–4)–(+2) mEq/L		(–4)–(+2) mmol/L	
	Thereafter	(–3)–(+3) mEq/L		(–3)–(+3) mmol/L	
Bicarbonate (HCO₃)					
Serum	Arterial	21–28 mEq/L		21–28 mmol/L	
	Venous	22–29 mEq/L		22–29 mmol/L	
Bilirubin, total		**Premature** (mg/dl)	**Full term** (mg/dl)	**Premature** (µmol/L)	**Full term** (µmol/L)
Serum	Cord	<2.0	<2.0	<34	<34
	0–1 d	<8.0	<6.0	<137	<103
	1–2 d	<12.0	<8.0	<205	<137
	2–5 d	<16.0	<12.0	<274	<205
	Thereafter	<20.0	<10.0	<340	<171
Bilirubin, direct (conjugated)					
Serum		0.0–0.2 mg/dl		0–3.4 µmol/L	
Bleeding time					
Blood from skin puncture					
Ivy	Normal	2–7 min		2–7 min	
	Borderline	7–11 min		7–11 min	
Simplate (G-D)		2.75–8 min		2.75–8 min	
Blood volume					
Whole blood	Male	52–83 ml/kg		0.052–0.083 L/kg	
	Female	50–75 ml/kg		0.050–0.075 L/kg	
C-reactive protein (CRP)					
Serum	Cord	52–1330 ng/ml		52–1330 mcg/L	
	2–12 yr	67–1800 ng/ml		67–1800 mcg/L	

*For a description of abbreviations, see p. 1139.

Continued

TEST/SPECIMEN	AGE/GENDER/REFERENCE	NORMAL RANGES	
		CONVENTIONAL UNITS	INTERNATIONAL UNITS (SI)
Calcium, ionized			
Serum, plasma, or	Cord	5.0–6.0 mg/dl	1.25–1.50 mmol/L
whole blood	Newborn, 3–24 hr	4.3–5.1 mg/dl	1.07–1.27 mmol/L
	24–48 hr	4.0–4.7 mg/dl	1.00–1.17 mmol/L
	Thereafter	4.8–4.92 mg/dl or 2.24–2.46 mEq/L	1.12–1.23 mmol/L
Calcium, total			
Serum	Cord	9.0–11.5 mg/dl	2.25–2.88 mmol/L
	Newborn, 3–24 hr	9.0–10.6 mg/dl	2.3–2.65 mmol/L
	24–48 hr	7.0–12.0 mg/dl	1.75–3.0 mmol/L
	4–7 d	9.0–10.9 mg/dl	2.25–2.73 mmol/L
	Child	8.8–10.8 mg/dl	2.2–2.70 mmol/L
	Thereafter	8.4–10.2 mg/dl	2.1–2.55 mmol/L
Carbon dioxide, partial pressure (PCO_2)			
Whole blood,	Newborn	27–40 mm Hg	3.6–5.3 kPa
arterial	Infant	27–41 mm Hg	3.6–5.5 kPa
	Thereafter: Male	35–48 mm Hg	4.7–6.4 kPa
	Female	32–45 mm Hg	4.3–6.0 kPa
Carbon dioxide, total (tCO_2)			
Serum or plasma	Cord	14–22 mEq/L	14–22 mmol/L
	Premature (1 wk)	14–27 mEq/L	14–27 mmol/L
	Newborn	13–22 mEq/L	13–22 mmol/L
	Infant, child	20–28 mEq/L	20–28 mmol/L
	Thereafter	23–30 mEq/L	23–30 mmol/L
Cerebrospinal fluid (CSF)			
Pressure		70–180 mm H_2O	70–180 mm H_2O
Volume	Child	60–100 ml	0.06–0.10 L
	Adult	100–160 ml	0.10–0.16 L
Chloride			
Serum or plasma	Cord	96–104 mEq/L	96–104 mmol/L
	Newborn	97–110 mEq/L	97–110 mmol/L
	Thereafter	98–106 mEq/L	98–106 mmol/L
Sweat	Normal (homozygote)	<40 mEq/L	<40 mmol/L
	Marginal (e.g., asthma, Addison disease, malnutrition)	45–60 mEq/L	45–60 mmol/L
	Cystic fibrosis	>60 mEq/L	>60 mmol/L
Cholesterol, total			
Serum or plasma†	Acceptable	<170 mg/dl	<4.4 mmol/L
	Borderline	170–199 mg/dl	4.4–5.1 mmol/L
	High	≥200 mg/dl	≥5.2 mmol/L
Clotting time (Lee-White)			
Whole blood		5–8 min (glass tubes)	5–8 min
		5–15 min (room temp)	5–15 min
		30 min (silicone tube)	30 min
Creatine kinase (CK, CPK)			
Serum	Cord	70–380 U/L	70–380 U/L
	5–8 hr	214–1175 U/L	214–1175 U/L
	24–33 hr	130–1200 U/L	130–1200 U/L
	72–100 hr	87–725 U/L	87–725 U/L
	Adult	5–130 U/L	5–130 U/L
Creatinine			
Serum	Cord	0.6–1.2 mg/dl	53–106 μmol/L
	Newborn	0.3–1.0 mg/dl	27–88 μmol/L
	Infant	0.2–0.4 mg/d	18–35 μmol/L
	Child	0.3–0.7 mg/dl	27–62 μmol/L
	Adolescent	0.5–1.0 mg/dl	44–88 μmol/L
	Adult: Male	0.6–1.2 mg/dl	53–106 μmol/L
	Female	0.5–1.1 mg/dl	44–97 μmol/L

†From National Cholesterol Education Program: Report of the expert panel on blood cholesterol levels in children and adolescents, *Pediatrics* 89(3 pt 2):527, 1992.

TEST/SPECIMEN	AGE/GENDER/REFERENCE	NORMAL RANGES	
		CONVENTIONAL UNITS	INTERNATIONAL UNITS (SI)
Urine, 24 hr	Premature	8.1–15.0 mg/kg/24 hr	72–133 μmol/kg/24 hr
	Full term	10.4–19.7 mg/kg/24 hr	92–174 μmol/kg/24 hr
	1.5–7 yr	10–15 mg/kg/24 hr	88–133 μmol/kg/24 hr
	7–15 yr	5.2–41 mg/kg/24 hr	46–362 μmol/kg/24 hr
Creatinine clearance (endogenous)			
Serum or plasma	Newborn	40–65 ml/min/1.73 m²	
and urine	<40 yr: Male	97–137 ml/min/1.73 m²	
	Female	88–128 ml/min/1.73 m²	
Digoxin			
Serum, plasma;	Therap. conc.		
collect at least	CHF	0.8–1.5 ng/ml	1.0–1.9 nmol/L
12 hr after dose	Arrhythmias	1.5–2.0 ng/ml	1.9–2.6 nmol/L
	Toxic conc.		
	Child	>2.5 ng/ml	>3.2 nmol/L
	Adult	>3.0 ng/ml	>3.8 nmol/L
Eosinophil count			
Whole blood,		50–250 cells/mm³ (μl)	50–250 × 10⁶ cells/L
capillary blood			
Erythrocyte (RBC) count			
Whole blood	Cord	3.9–5.5 million/mm³	3.9–5.5 × 10¹² cells/L
	1–3 d	4.0–6.6 million/mm³	4.0–6.6 × 10¹² cells/L
	1 wk	3.9–6.3 million/mm³	3.9–6.3 × 10¹² cells/L
	2 wk	3.6–6.2 million/mm³	3.6–6.2 × 10¹² cells/L
	1 mo	3.0–5.4 million/mm³	3.0–5.4 × 10¹² cells/L
	2 mo	2.7–4.9 million/mm³	2.7–4.9 × 10¹² cells/L
	3–6 mo	3.1–4.5 million/mm³	3.1–4.5 × 10¹² cells/L
	0.5–2 yr	3.7–5.3 million/mm³	3.7–5.3 × 10¹² cells/L
	2–6 yr	3.9–5.3 million/mm³	3.9–5.3 × 10¹² cells/L
	6–12 yr	4.0–5.2 million/mm³	4.0–5.2 × 10¹² cells/L
	12–18 yr: Male	4.5–5.3 million/mm³	4.5–5.3 × 10¹² cells/L
	Female	4.1–5.1 million/mm³	4.1–5.1 × 10¹² cells/L
Erythrocyte sedimentation rate (ESR)			
Whole blood			
Westergren	Child	0–10 mm/hr	0–10 mm/hr
(modified)	<50 yr: Male	0–15 mm/hr	0–15 mm/hr
	Female	0–20 mm/hr	0–20 mm/hr
Wintrobe	Child	0–13 mm/hr	0–13 mm/hr
	Adult: Male	0–9 mm/hr	0–9 mm/hr
	Female	0–20 mm/hr	0–20 mm/hr
Fibrinogen			
Plasma	Newborn	125–300 mg/dl	1.25–3.00 g/L
	Thereafter	200–400 mg/dl	2.00–4.00 g/L
Galactose			
Serum	Newborn	0–20 mg/dl	0–1.11 mmol/L
	Thereafter	<5 mg/dl	<0.28 mmol/L
Urine	Newborn	≤60 mg/dl	≤3.33 mmol/L
	Thereafter	<14 mg/24 hr	<0.08 mmol/d
Glucose			
Serum	Cord	45–96 mg/dl	2.5–5.3 mmol/L
	Newborn, 1 d	40–60 mg/dl	2.2–3.3 mmol/L
	Newborn, >1 d	50–90 mg/dl	2.8–5.0 mmol/L
	Child	60–100 mg/dl	3.3–5.5 mmol/L
	Thereafter	70–105 mg/dl	3.9–5.8 mmol/L
Whole blood	Adult	65–95 mg/dl	3.6–5.3 mmol/L
CSF	Adult	40–70 mg/dl	2.2–3.9 mmol/L
Urine (quantitative)		<0.5 g/d	<2.8 mmol/d
Urine (qualitative)		Negative	Negative

Continued

TEST/SPECIMEN	AGE/GENDER/REFERENCE	NORMAL RANGES			
		CONVENTIONAL UNITS		INTERNATIONAL UNITS (SI)	
Glucose tolerance test (GTT), oral					
Serum					
Dosages		**Normal**	**Diabetic**	**Normal**	**Diabetic**
Adult: 75 g	Fasting	70–105 mg/dl	≥126 mg/dl	3.9–5.8 mmol/L	≥7.0 mmol/L
Child: 1.75 g/kg of	60 min	120–170 mg/dl	≥200 mg/dl	6.7–9.4 mmol/L	≥11 mmol/L
ideal weight up	90 min	100–140 mg/dl	≥200 mg/dl	5.6–7.8 mmol/L	≥11 mmol/L
to maximum of	120 min	70–120 mg/dl	≥200 mg/dl	3.9–6.7 mmol/L	≥11 mmol/L
75 g					
Growth hormone (GH, somatotropin)					
Plasma	1 d	5–53 ng/ml		5–53 mcg/L	
	1 wk	5–27 ng/ml		5–27 mcg/L	
	1–12 mo	2–10 ng/ml		2–10 mcg/L	
	Fasting child/adult	<0.7–6.0 ng/ml		<0.7–6.0 mcg/L	
Hematocrit (HCT, Hct)					
Whole blood	1 d (cap)	48%–69%		0.48–0.69 vol fraction	
	2 d	48%–75%		0.48–0.75 vol fraction	
	3 d	44%–72%		0.44–0.72 vol fraction	
	2 mo	28%–42%		0.28–0.42 vol fraction	
	6–12 yr	35%–45%		0.35–0.45 vol fraction	
	12–18 yr: Male	37%–49%		0.37–0.49 vol fraction	
	Female	36%–46%		0.36–0.46 vol fraction	
Hemoglobin (Hb)					
Whole blood	1–3 d (cap)	14.5–22.5 g/dl		2.25–3.49 mmol/L	
	2 mo	9.0–14.0 g/dl		1.40–2.17 mmol/L	
	6–12 yr	11.5–15.5 g/dl		1.78–2.40 mmol/L	
	12–18 yr: Male	13.0–16.0 g/dl		2.02–2.48 mmol/L	
	Female	12.0–16.0 g/dl		1.86–2.48 mmol/L	
Hemoglobin A					
Whole blood		>95% of total		>0.95 fraction of Hb	
Hemoglobin F					
Whole blood	1 d	63%–92% HbF		0.63–0.92 mass fraction HbF	
	5 d	65%–88% HbF		0.65–0.88 mass fraction HbF	
	3 wk	55%–85% HbF		0.55–0.85 mass fraction HbF	
	6–9 wk	31%–75% HbF		0.31–0.75 mass fraction HbF	
	3–4 mo	<2%–59% HbF		<0.02–0.59 mass fraction HbF	
	6 mo	<2%–9% HbF		<0.02–0.09 mass fraction HbF	
	Adult	<2.0% HbF		<0.02 mass fraction HbF	
Immunoglobulin A (IgA)					
Serum	Cord	1.4–3.6 mg/dl		14–36 mg/L	
	1–3 mo	1.3–53 mg/dl		13–530 mg/L	
	4–6 mo	4.4–84 mg/dl		44–840 mg/L	
	7–12 mo	11–106 mg/dl		110–1060 mg/L	
	2–5 yr	14–159 mg/dl		140–1590 mg/L	
	6–10 yr	33–236 mg/dl		330–2360 mg/L	
	Adult	70–312 mg/dl		700–3120 mg/L	
Immunoglobulin D (IgD)					
Serum	Newborn	None detected		None detected	
	Thereafter	0–8 mg/dl		0–80 mg/L	
Immunoglobulin E (IgE)					
Serum	Male	0–230 IU/ml		0–230 kIU/L	
	Female	0–170 IU/ml		0–170 kIU/L	
Immunoglobulin G (IgG)					
Serum	Cord	636–1606 mg/dl		6.36–16.06 g/L	
	1 mo	251–906 mg/dl		2.51–9.06 g/L	
	2–4 mo	176–601 mg/dl		1.76–6.01 g/L	
	5–12 mo	172–1069 mg/dl		1.72–10.69 g/L	
	1–5 yr	345–1236 mg/dl		3.45–12.36 g/L	
	6–10 yr	608–1572 mg/dl		6.08–15.72 g/L	
	Adult	639–1349 mg/dl		6.39–13.49 g/L	

TEST/SPECIMEN	AGE/GENDER/REFERENCE	NORMAL RANGES		
		CONVENTIONAL UNITS		INTERNATIONAL UNITS (SI)
Immunoglobulin M (IgM)				
Serum	Cord	6.3–25 mg/dl		63–250 mg/L
	1–4 mo	17–105 mg/dl		170–1050 mg/L
	5–9 mo	33–126 mg/dl		330–1260 mg/L
	10–12 mo	41–173 mg/dl		410–1730 mg/L
	2–8 yr	43–207 mg/dl		430–2070 mg/L
	9–10 yr	52–242 mg/dl		520–2420 mg/L
	Adult	56–352 mg/dl		560–3520 mg/L
Iron				
Serum	Newborn	100–250 mcg/dl		18–45 µmol/L
	Infant	40–100 mcg/dl		7–18 µmol/L
	Child	50–120 mcg/dl		9–22 µmol/L
	Thereafter: Male	65–170 mcg/dl		12–30 µmol/L
	Female	50–170 mcg/dl		9–30 µmol/L
	Intoxicated child	280–2550 mcg/dl		50.12–456.5 µmol/L
	Fatally poisoned child	>1800 mcg/dl		>322.2 µmol/L
Iron-binding capacity, total (TIBC)				
Serum	Infant	100–400 mcg/dl		17.90–71.60 µmol/L
	Thereafter	250–400 mcg/dl		44.75–71.60 µmol/L
Lead				
Whole blood	Child	<10 mcg/dl		<0.48 µmol/L
Urine, 24 hr		<80 mcg/L		<0.39 µmol/L
Leukocyte count (WBC count)		×1000 cells/mm³ (µl)		×10⁹ cells/L
Whole blood	Birth	9.0–30.0		9.0–30.0
	24 hr	9.4–34.0		9.4–34.0
	1 mo	5.0–19.5		5.0–19.5
	1–3 yr	6.0–17.5		6.0–17.5
	4–7 yr	5.5–15.5		5.5–15.5
	8–13 yr	4.5–13.5		4.5–13.5
	Adult	4.5–11.0		4.5–11.0
		×1000 cells/mm³ (µl)		×10⁶ cells/L
CSF (cell count)	Premature	0–25 mononuclear		0–25
		0–10 polymorphonuclear		0–10
		0–1000 RBC		0–1000
	Newborn	0–20 mononuclear		0–20
		0–10 polymorphonuclear		0–10
		0–800 RBC		0–800
	Neonate	0–5 mononuclear		0–5
		0–10 polymorphonuclear		0–10
		0–50 RBC		0–50
	Thereafter	0–5 mononuclear		0–5
Leukocyte differential count				
Whole blood	Myelocytes	0%	0 cells/mm³ (µl)	Number fraction 0
	Neutrophils—"bands"	3%–5%	150–400 cells/mm³ (µl)	Number fraction 0.03–0.05
	Neutrophils—"segs"	54%–62%	3000–5800 cells/mm³ (µl)	Number fraction 0.54–0.62
	Lymphocytes	25%–33%	1500–3000 cells/mm³ (µl)	Number fraction 0.25–0.33
	Monocytes	3%–7%	285–500 cells/mm³ (µl)	Number fraction 0.03–0.07
	Eosinophils	1%–3%	50–250 cells/mm³ (µl)	Number fraction 0.01–0.03
	Basophils	0%–0.75%	15–50 cells/mm³ (µl)	Number fraction 0–0.0075
Mean corpuscular hemoglobin (MCH)				
Whole blood	Birth	31–37 pg/cell		0.48–0.57 fmol/cell
	1–3 d (cap)	31–37 pg/cell		0.48–0.57 fmol/cell
	1 wk–1 mo	28–40 pg/cell		0.43–0.62 fmol/cell
	2 mo	26–34 pg/cell		0.40–0.53 fmol/cell
	3–6 mo	25–35 pg/cell		0.39–0.54 fmol/cell
	0.5–2 yr	23–31 pg/cell		0.36–0.48 fmol/cell
	2–6 yr	24–30 pg/cell		0.37–0.47 fmol/cell
	6–12 yr	25–33 pg/cell		0.39–0.51 fmol/cell
	12–18 yr	25–35 pg/cell		0.39–0.54 fmol/cell
	18–49 yr	26–34 pg/cell		0.40–0.53 fmol/cell

Continued

TEST/SPECIMEN	AGE/GENDER/REFERENCE	NORMAL RANGES	
		CONVENTIONAL UNITS	INTERNATIONAL UNITS (SI)
Mean corpuscular hemoglobin concentration (MCHC)			
Whole blood	Birth	30%–36% Hb/cell or g Hb/dl RBC	4.65–5.58 mmol Hb/L RBC
	1–3 d (cap)	29%–37% Hb/cell or g Hb/dl RBC	4.50–5.74 mmol Hb/L RBC
	1–2 wk	28%–38% Hb/cell or g Hb/dl RBC	4.34–5.89 mmol Hb/L RBC
	1–2 mo	29%–37% Hb/cell or g Hb/dl RBC	4.50–5.74 mmol Hb/L RBC
	3 mo–2 yr	30%–36% Hb/cell or g Hb/dl RBC	4.65–5.58 mmol Hb/L RBC
	2–18 yr	31%–37% Hb/cell or g Hb/dl RBC	4.81–5.74 mmol Hb/L RBC
	>18 yr	31%–37% Hb/cell or g Hb/dl RBC	4.81–5.74 mmol Hb/L RBC
Mean corpuscular volume (MCV)			
Whole blood	1–3 d (cap)	95–121 μm^3	95–121 fl
	0.5–2 yr	70–86 μm^3	70–86 fl
	6–12 yr	77–95 μm^3	77–95 fl
	12–18 yr: Male	78–98 μm^3	78–98 fl
	Female	78–102 μm^3	78–102 fl
Osmolality			
Serum	Child, adult	275–295 mOsm/kg H_2O	
Urine, random		50–1400 mOsm/kg H_2O, depending on fluid intake; after 12-hr fluid restriction: >850 mOsm/kg H_2O	
Urine, 24 hr		≅300–900 mOsm/kg H_2O	
Oxygen, partial pressure (PO_2)			
Whole blood, arterial	Birth	8–24 mm Hg	1.1–3.2 kPa
	5–10 min	33–75 mm Hg	4.4–10.0 kPa
	30 min	31–85 mm Hg	4.1–11.3 kPa
	>1 hr	55–80 mm Hg	7.3–10.6 kPa
	1 d	54–95 mm Hg	7.2–12.6 kPa
	Thereafter (decreased with age)	83–108 mm Hg	11–14.4 kPa
Oxygen saturation (SaO_2)			
Whole blood, arterial	Newborn	85%–90%	Fraction saturated 0.85–0.90
	Thereafter	95%–99%	Fraction saturated 0.95–0.99
Partial thromboplastin time (PTT)			
Whole blood (Na citrate)			
Nonactivated		60–85 s (Platelin)	60–85 s
Activated		25–35 s (differs with method)	25–35 s
pH			H^+ concentration
Whole blood, arterial (must be corrected for body temperature)	Premature (48 hr)	7.35–7.50	31–44 nmol/L
	Birth, full term	7.11–7.36	43–77 nmol/L
	5–10 min	7.09–7.30	50–81 nmol/L
	30 min	7.21–7.38	41–61 nmol/L
	>1 hr	7.26–7.49	32–54 nmol/L
	1 d	7.29–7.45	35–51 nmol/L
	Thereafter	7.35–7.45	35–44 nmol/L
Urine, random	Newborn/neonate	5–7	0.1–10 μmol/L
	Thereafter	4.5–8 (average ≅6)	0.01–32 μmol/L (average ≅1.0 μmol/L)
Stool		7.0–7.5	31–100 nmol/L
Phenylalanine			
Serum	Premature	2.0–7.5 mg/dl	120–450 μmol/L
	Newborn	1.2–3.4 mg/dl	70–210 μmol/L
	Thereafter	0.8–1.8 mg/dl	50–110 μmol/L
Urine, 24 hr	10 d–2 wk	1–2 mg/d	6–12 μmol/d
	3–12 yr	4–18 mg/d	24–110 μmol/d
	Thereafter	Trace—17 mg/d	Trace—103 μmol/d
Plasma volume			
Plasma	Male	25–43 ml/kg	0.025–0.043 L/kg
	Female	28–45 ml/kg	0.028–0.045 L/kg
Platelet count (thrombocyte count)			
Whole blood (EDTA)	Newborn (after 1 wk, same as adult)	84–478 × 10^3/mm³ (μl)	84–478 × 10^9/L
	Adult	150–400 × 10^3/mm³ (μl)	150–400 × 10^9/L

		NORMAL RANGES	
TEST/SPECIMEN	**AGE/GENDER/REFERENCE**	**CONVENTIONAL UNITS**	**INTERNATIONAL UNITS (SI)**
Potassium			
Serum	Newborn	3.0–6.0 mEq/L	3.0–6.0 mmol/L
	Thereafter	3.5–5.0 mEq/L	3.5–5.0 mmol/L
Plasma (heparin)		3.4–4.5 mEq/L	3.4–4.5 mmol/L
Urine, 24 hr		2.5–125 mEq/d (varies with diet)	2.5–125 mmol/L
Protein			
Serum, total	Premature	4.3–7.6 g/dl	43–76 g/L
	Newborn	4.6–7.4 g/dl	46–74 g/L
	1–7 yr	6.1–7.9 g/dl	61–79 g/L
	8–12 yr	6.4–8.1 g/dl	64–81 g/L
	13–19 yr	6.6–8.2 g/dl	66–82 g/L
Total			
Urine, 24 hr		1–14 mg/dl	10–140 mg/L
		50–80 mg/d (at rest)	50–80 mg/d
		<250 mg/d (after intense exercise)	<250 mg/d (after intense exercise)
CSF		Lumbar: 8–32 mg/dl	80–320 mg/L
Prothrombin time (PT)			
One-stage (Quick)			
Whole blood (Na	In general	11–15 s (varies with type of thromboplastin)	11–15 s
citrate)	Newborn	Prolonged by 2–3 s	Prolonged by 2–3 s
Two-stage modified (Ware and Seegers)			
Whole blood (sodium citrate)		18–22 s	18–22 s
RBC count: see Erythrocyte (RBC) count			
Red blood cell volume			
Whole blood	Male	20–36 ml/kg	0.020–0.036 L/kg
	Female	19–31 ml/kg	0.019–0.031 L/kg
Reticulocyte count			
Whole blood	Adults	0.5%–1.5% of erythrocytes or 25,000–75,000/mm^3 (μl)	0.005–0.015 (number fraction) or 25,000–75,000 × 10^6/L
Capillary	1 d	0.4%–6.0%	0.004–0.060 (number fraction)
	7 d	<0.1%–1.3%	<0.001–0.013 (number fraction)
	1–4 wk	<0.1%–1.2%	<0.001–0.012 (number fraction)
	5–6 wk	<0.1%–2.4%	<0.001–0.024 (number fraction)
	7–8 wk	0.1%–2.9%	0.001–0.029 (number fraction)
	9–10 wk	<0.1%–2.6%	<0.001–0.026 (number fraction)
	11–12 wk	0.1%–1.3%	0.001–0.013 (number fraction)
Salicylates			
Serum, plasma	Therap. conc.	15–30 mg/dl	1.1–2.2 mmol/L
	Toxic conc.	>30 mg/dl	>18.5 mmol/L
Sedimentation rate: see Erythrocyte sedimentation rate (ESR)			
Sodium			
Serum or plasma	Newborn	134–146 mEq/L	134–146 mmol/L
	Infant	139–146 mEq/L	139–146 mmol/L
	Child	138–145 mEq/L	138–145 mmol/L
	Thereafter	136–146 mEq/L	136–146 mmol/L
Urine, 24 hr		40–220 mEq/L (diet dependent)	40–220 mmol/L
Sweat	Normal	<40 mEq/L	<40 mmol/L
	Indeterminate	45–60 mEq/L	45–60 mmol/L
	Cystic fibrosis	>60 mEq/L	>60 mmol/L
Specific gravity			
Urine, random	Adult	1.002–1.030	1.002–1.030
	After 12-hr fluid restriction	>1.025	>1.025
Urine, 24 hr		1.015–1.025	

Continued

TEST/SPECIMEN	AGE/GENDER/REFERENCE	NORMAL RANGES			
		CONVENTIONAL UNITS		INTERNATIONAL UNITS (SI)	
Theophylline					
Serum, plasma	Therap. conc.				
	Bronchodilator	10–20 mcg/ml		56–110 μmol/L	
	Premature apnea	5–10 mcg/ml		28–56 μmol/L	
	Toxic conc.	>20 mcg/ml		>110 μmol/L	
Thrombin time					
Whole blood (Na citrate)		Control time ±2 s when control is 9–13 s		Control time ±2 s when control is 9–13 s	
Thyroxine, total (T_4)					
Serum	Cord	8–13 mcg/dl		103–168 nmol/L	
	Newborn	11.5–24 mcg/dl (lower in low-birth-weight infants)		148–310 nmol/L	
	Neonate	9–18 mcg/dl		116–232 nmol/L	
	Infant	7–15 mcg/dl		90–194 nmol/L	
	1–5 yr	7.3–15 mcg/dl		94–194 nmol/L	
	5–10 yr	6.4–13.3 mcg/dl		83–172 nmol/L	
	Thereafter	5–12 mcg/dl		65–155 nmol/L	
	Newborn screen (filter paper)	6.2–22 mcg/dl		80–284 nmol/L	
Triglycerides (TG)		**Male** (mg/dl)	**Female** (mg/dl)	**Male** (g/L)	**Female** (g/L)
Serum, after ≥2-hr fast	Cord	10–98	10–98	0.10–0.98	0.10–0.98
	0–5 yr	30–86	32–99	0.30–0.86	0.32–0.99
	6–11 yr	31–108	35–114	0.31–1.08	0.35–1.14
	12–15 yr	36–138	41–138	0.36–1.38	0.41–1.38
	16–19 yr	40–163	40–128	0.40–1.63	0.40–1.28
Triiodothyronine (T_3), free					
Serum	Cord	20–240 pg/dl		0.3–3.7 pmol/L	
	1–3 d	200–610 pg/dl		3.1–9.4 pmol/L	
	6 wk	240–560 pg/dl		3.7–8.6 pmol/L	
	Adults (20–50 yr)	230–660 pg/dl		3.5–10.0 pmol/L	
Triiodothyronine, total (T_3–RIA)					
Serum	Cord	30–70 ng/dl		0.46–1.08 nmol/L	
	Newborn	72–260 ng/dl		1.16–4 nmol/L	
	1–5 yr	100–260 ng/dl		1.54–4 nmol/L	
	5–10 yr	90–240 ng/dl		1.39–3.70 nmol/L	
	10–15 yr	80–210 ng/dl		1.23–3.23 nmol/L	
	Thereafter	115–190 ng/dl		1.77–2.93 nmol/L	
Urea nitrogen					
Serum or plasma	Cord	21–40 mg/dl		7.5–14.3 mmol/L	
	Premature (1 wk)	3–25 mg/dl		1.1–9 mmol/L	
	Newborn	3–12 mg/dl		1.1–4.3 mmol/L	
	Infant/child	5–18 mg/dl		1.8–6.4 mmol/L	
	Thereafter	7–18 mg/dl		2.5–6.4 mmol/L	
Urine volume					
Urine, 24 hr	Newborn	50–300 ml/d		0.05–0.3 L/d	
	Infant	350–550 ml/d		0.35–0.5 L/d	
	Child	500–1000 ml/d		0.5–1 L/d	
	Adolescent	700–1400 ml/d		0.7–1.4 L/d	
	Thereafter: Male	800–1800 ml/d		0.8–1.8 L/d	
	Female	600–1600 ml/d (varies with intake and other factors)		0.6–1.6 L/d	

WBC: see Leukocyte count (WBC count)

ABBREVIATIONS USED IN LABORATORY TESTS

ABBREVIATION	TERM
cap	capillary
CHF	congestive heart failure
conc.	concentration
CSF	cerebrospinal fluid
d	day; diem
EDTA	ethylenediaminetetraacetate
g	gram
H^+	hydrogen ion
H_2O	water
Hb	hemoglobin
HbF	fetal hemoglobin
hr	hour
IU	International unit
L	liter
m	meter
mEq	milliequivalent
min	minute
mm	millimeter
mm Hg	millimeters of mercury
mm H_2O	millimeters of water
mm^3	cubic millimeter
mo	month
mol	mole
mOsm	milliosmole
Na	sodium
Pa	pascal
RBC	red blood cells
s	second
temp	temperature
therap.	therapeutic
U	international unit of enzyme activity
vol	volume
WBC	white blood cells
wk	week
yr	year
>	greater than
≥	greater than or equal to
<	less than
≤	less than or equal to
±	plus/minus
≅	approximately equal to

PREFIXES DENOTING DECIMAL FACTORS

PREFIX	SYMBOL	AMOUNT
kilo	k	one thousand (10^3)
deci	d	one tenth (10^{-1})
centi	c	one hundredth (10^{-2})
milli	m	one thousandth (10^{-3})
micro	mc, μ	one millionth (10^{-6})
nano	n	one billionth (10^{-9})
pico	p	one trillionth (10^{-12})
femto	f	one quadrillionth (10^{-15})

Translations of Wong-Baker FACES
Pain Rating Scale*

	0	1	2	3	4	5
0-5 coding	0	1	2	3	4	5
0-10 coding	0	2	4	6	8	10
English	No Hurt	Hurts Little Bit	Hurts Little More	Hurts Even More	Hurts Whole Lot	Hurts Worst
Spanish	No duele	Duele un poco	Duele un poco más	Duele mucho	Duele mucho más	Duele el máximo
French	Pas mal	Un petit peu mal	Un peri plus mal	Encore plus mal	Très mal	Très mal
Italian	Non fa male	Fa male un poco	Fa male un po di piu	Fa male ancora di piu	Fa molto male	Fa maggior-mente male
Portuguese	Não doi	Doi um pouco	Doi um pouco mais	Doi muito	Doi muito mais	Doi o máximo
Bosnian	Ne boli	Boli samo malo	Boli malo više	Boli još više	Boli puno	Boli najviše
Vietnamese	Không dau	Hồi dau	Dau hòn chút	Dau nhiêu hòn	Dau thât nhiêu	Dau qúa dô
Chinese	無痛	微痛	較痛	更痛	很痛	劇痛
Greek	Δεν Πονάϊ	Πονάϊ Λιγο	Πονάϊ Λιγο Πιο Πολν	Πονάϊ Πολν	Πονάϊ Πιο Πολν	Πονάϊ Παρα Πολν
Romanian	No doare	Doare puțin	Doare un pic mai mult	Doare și mai mult	Doare foarte tare	Doare cel mai mult

*Wong-Baker FACES Pain Rating Scale: Available at no charge from The Purdue Frederick Company, 100 Connecticut Ave., Norwalk, CT 06850-3590; http://www.partnersagainstpain.com. Spanish and Portuguese translations by Ellen Johnsen; French translation from Wong DL: *Soins infirmiers pediatrie*, Laval, Que, 2002, Editions Etudes Vivantes, Groupe Educalivres, Inc.; Italian translation by Madeline Mitchko; Bosnian translation by Barbara Bogomolov; Vietnamese translation by Yen B. Isle; Chinese translation by Hung-Shen Lin; Greek translation by Nicholas Mamalis; Romanian translation by Bogdan R. Dinu.

Brief Word Instructions (Above)

Point to each face using the words to describe the pain intensity. Ask person to choose face that best describes own pain and record the appropriate number. Rating scale can be used with people ages 3 years and older.

Note: In a study of 148 children ages 4 to 5 years, there were no differences in pain scores when children used the original or brief word instructions. (In Wong D, Baker C: *Reference manual for the Wong-Baker FACES Pain Rating Scale,* Duarte, Calif, 1998, City of Hope Mayday Pain Resource Center; retrieved from http://evolve.elsevier.com/Wong/essentials.)

Original Instructions

English. Explain to the person that each face is for a person who feels happy because he has no pain (hurt) or sad because he has some or a lot of pain. **Face 0** is very happy because he doesn't hurt at all. **Face 1** hurts just a little bit. **Face 2** hurts a little more. **Face 3** hurts even more. **Face 4** hurts a whole lot. **Face 5** hurts as much as you can imagine, although you don't have to be crying to feel this bad. Ask the person to choose the face that best describes how he or she is feeling.

Rating scale is recommended for persons ages 3 years and older.

Spanish. Expliquele a la persona que cada cara representa una persona que se siente feliz porque no tiene dolor o triste porque siente un poco o mucho dolor. **Cara 0** se siente muy feliz porque no tiene dolor. **Cara 1** tiene un poco de dolor. **Cara 2** tiene un poquito más de dolor. **Cara 3** tiene más dolor. **Cara 4** tiene mucho dolor. **Cara 5** tiene el dolor más fuerte que usted pueda imaginar, aunque usted no tiene que estar llorando para sentirse asi de mal. Pidale a la persona que escoja la cara que mejor describe su proprio dolor.

Esta escala se puede usar con personas de tres años de edad o más.

French. Expliquez à la personne que chaque visage représent une personne qui est heureux parce qu'elle n'a pas point du mal ou triste parce qu'elle a un peu ou beaucoup du mal. **Visage 0** est trés heureux parce qu'elle n'a pas point du mal. **Visage 1** a un petit peu de mal. **Visage 2** a plus du mal. **Visage 3** a encore plus du mal. **Visage 4** a beaucoup du mal. **Visage 5** a autant mal que vous pouvez imaginer, bien que ces mauvais sentiments ne finissent pas nécessaira a vous faire pleurer. Demandez à la personne de choisir le visage qui convient le mieux avec ses sentiments.

Ces evaluations sont recommendés pour des personnes de trois ans et davantage.

Italian. Spiegare a la persona che ogni facien è per una persona che si sente felice perchè non tiene dolore oppure triste perchè ha poco o molto dolore. **Faccia 0** è molto felice perchè non tiene dolore. **Faccia 1** tiene poco dolore. **Faccia 2** tiene un po più di dolore. **Faccia 3** tiene più dolore. **Faccia 4** tiene molto dolore. **Faccia 5** tiene molto dolore che non puoi immaginare però non devi piangere per tenere dolore. Domandi ala persona di scegliere quale faccia meglio descrive come si sente.

Grado scale è raccomandata a la persona di tre anni in sù.

Portuguese. Explique a pessoa que cada face representa uma pessoa que está feliz porque não têm dor, ou triste por ter um pouco ou muita dor. **Face 0** está muito feliz porque não têm nenhuma dor. **Face 1** têm apenas um pouco de dor. **Face 2** têm um pouco mais de dor. **Face 3** têm ainda mais dor. **Face 4** têm muita dor. **Face 5** têm uma dor máxima, apesar de que nem sempre provoca o choro. Peça a pessoa que escolhe a face que melhor descreve como ele se sente.

Esta escala é aplicável a pessoas de tres anos de idade ou mais.

Romanian. Explicati copilului că fiecare desen (figură) corespunde unei persoane care este veselă, pentru ca nu are nici o durere, sau unei persoane care este tristă, pentru că are dureri. **Figura 0** este foarte fericită pentru că nu are nici o durere. **Figura 1** arată că doare doar un

pic. **Figura 2** arată că doare ceva mai mult. **Figura 3** arată că doare s,i mai mult. **Figura 4** arată că doare foarte tare. **Figura 5** arată că doare atât de tare cât se poate imagina, chiar dacă nu este însotita neapărat de lacrimi. Cereti copilului (persoanei) să indice figura care exprimă cel mai bine cum se simte el.

Scala de evaluare a durerii este recomandată pentru copiii în vârstùă de trei ani s,i peste.

Bosnian. Objasnite osobi da je svako lice namjenjeno za osobu koja se osjec´a sretnom jer ne osjec´a bol ili tužnom jer osjec´a malo ili puno boli. **Lice 0** je sretno jer ne osjec´a nikakvu bol. **Lice 1** osjec´a samo malu bol. **Lice 2** osjec´a malo više boli. **Lice 3** osjec´a još vec´u bol. **Lice 4** osjec´a puno boli. **Lice 5** osjec´a onoliku bol koju je moguc´e zamisliti, što ne znac´i da osoba koja osjec´a tu bol mora plakati. Upitajte osobu da izabere lice koje najbolje opisuju kako se osjec´a. Skala procijene bola se preporu c´uje za osobe starosti 3 godine ili više.

Upirati prstom na svako lice objašnjavajuc´i rijec´ima intensitet boli. Pitajte dijete da izabere lice koje najbolje opisuje njihovu bol i zabiljezue odgovarajuc´i broj.

German. Erläutern Sie dem Kind, daß jedes Gesicht zu einer Person gehört, die froh darüber ist, keine Schmerzen zu haben, oder die sehr traurig ist, weil sie mäßige bis starke Schmerzen hat. **Gesicht 0** ist sehr froh, weil es keine Schmerzen hat. **Gesicht 1** sagt, es tut ein bißchen weh. **Gesicht 2** hat ein bißchen mehr Schmerzen. **Gesicht 3** sagt, es tut noch mehr weh, und **Gesicht 4,** es tut ziemlich weh. **Gesicht 5** leidet unter so starken Schmerzen, wie Du Dir nur vorstellen kannst, auch wenn dabei nicht unbedingt Tränen fließen müssen. Bitten Sie das Kind, das Gesicht auszuwählen, das seinem Empfinden am besten entspricht.

Empfohlen für Kinder ab drei Jahren.

Vietnamese

Xin cắt nghĩa cho mỗi người, từng khuôn mặt của một người cãm thấy vui vẽ tại vì không có sự đau đớn hoặc, buồn vì có chút ít hay rất nhiều sự đau đớn.

Cái mặt với **số 0** thì rất là vui tại vì mặt ấy không có sự đau đớn. **Mặt số 1** chỉ đau một chút thôi. **Mặt số 2** hơi đau hơn một chút nữa. **Mặt số 3** đau hơn chút nữa. **Mặt số 4** đau thật nhiều. **Mặt số 5** đau không thể tưởng tượng, mặc dù người ta không cần phải khóc mới cảm thấy được sự buồn khổ như thế.

Bạn hỏi từng người tự chọn khuôn mặt nào diễn tả được sự đau đớn của chính mình.

Japanese

3歳以上の患者に望ましい。それぞれの顔は、患者の痛み (pain, hurt) がないのでご機嫌な感じ、または、ある程度の痛み・沢山の痛みがあるので悲しい感じを表現していることを説明して下さい。0＝痛みがまったくないから、とても幸せな顔をしている、1＝ほんの少し痛い、2＝もう少し痛い、3＝もっと痛い、4＝とっても痛い、5＝痛くて涙を流す必要はないけれども、これ以上の痛みは考えられないほど痛い。今、どのように感じているか最もよく表わしている顔を選ぶよう、患者に求めて下さい。

Chinese

解釋給人聽用每張臉譜來代表著一個人的感覺是因為沒有疼痛〔傷痛〕而感快樂或是因為些許疼痛或者是許多疼痛而感傷心。第零張臉是很快樂的因為他一點也不覺得疼痛。第一張臉只痛一丁點兒。第二張臉又痛多了一些。第三張臉痛得更多了。第四張臉是非常痛了。第五張臉是為人們所能想像到的劇痛即使感到這樣難過，卻不一定哭出來。請這人選擇出最能代表他現在感覺的一張臉譜。此量表適用於三歲以上的人。

Spanish–English Translations

ENGLISH PHRASE	SPANISH PHRASE
PHYSICAL EXAMINATION	
Open your mouth	Abre la boca
Breathe deeply	Respira profundo
Turn over	Voltéate
Hoarse	Ronco
Rash or skin lesion produced by insect bite	Rozadura o una lesión en la piel producida por una picadura de insecto
Rash	Roncha, salpullido, rozadura
Ringworm	Tiña
To tighten (grip)	Apretar
To loosen	Relajar, aflojar
Bruise	Moretón
Skin "spot" (like a blanching)	Mancha
Snore, stertor	Roncar
Snoring sound	Ronquido
Swollen	Hinchado
SYMPTOMS	
I would like to know if you have (or have had):	Quisiera saber si tienes (o has tenido):
Cough	Tos
Runny nose	Moquera
Fever	Fiebre o calentura
Vomiting or nausea	Vómito o náusea
Diarrhea	Diarrea
Constipation	Estreñimiento
Pain	Dolor
Allergic reaction	Reacción alérgica
Seizure	Convulsión
Sore throat	Dolor de garganta
Diaper dermatitis	Dermatitis por el pañal
Dizzy	Mareado(a)
HISTORY	
Are you sleeping well?	¿Estás durmiendo bien?
Have you had any trauma?	¿Has tenido algún trastorno o algún trauma?
Have you had any hemorrhage or loss of blood?	¿Has tenido una hemorragia o pérdida de sangre?
Problems during pregnancy or delivery?	¿Problemas en el embarazo o parto?

ENGLISH PHRASE	SPANISH PHRASE
Born at term or premature?	¿Nació a tiempo o fue prematuro?
Did he get better after the treatment or the medicine given?	¿Mejoró después del tratamiento o después de haberle dado la medicina?
How many times did (he/she) urinate today?	¿Cuántas veces orinó hoy?
How many wet diapers has (he/she) had?	¿Cuántos pañales ha mojado?
How many dirty diapers?	¿Cuántos pañales sucios?
Where does it hurt?	¿Dónde te duele?
When did it start?	¿Cuándo empezó?
Does (he/she) have any allergies to medicine or food?	¿Él (ella) tiene alergia a alguna medicina o comida?
Up-to-date	Al día
Contagious	Contagioso
Stool (various terms)	Excremento, heces, popo
Has (she/he) had any chronic illnesses?	¿Él (ella) ha tenido alguna enfermedad crónica?
How many times did he/she vomit today?	¿Cuántas veces vomitó hoy?
Wheezing or adventitious sounds (in lungs)	Pillido o ruidos en los pulmones
Nasal secretions	Secreción nasal
Stuffy nose	Bloqueo nasal
Breathing problems	Dificultad para respirar
Thick discharge	Flujo grueso
Wound	Herida
Blood pressure	Presión arterial
Temperature	Temperatura
Fever	Calentura, fiebre
Pulse	Pulso
Heartbeat	Latido del corazón
Airway	Vía respiratoria
Vital signs	Signos vitals
SPECIFIC CONDITIONS	
Flu	Gripa
Croup	Crup
Bronchitis	Bronquitis
Burn	Quemadura
Rash or dermatitis	Erupción o rozadura
Pneumonia	Neumonía

ENGLISH PHRASE	SPANISH PHRASE
Pertussis	Tos ferina
Measles	Sarampión
Mumps	Paperas
Chickenpox	Varicela
Rubella	Rubéola
Polio	Polio
Tetanus	Tétano
Vomiting	Vómito
Diarrhea	Diarrea
Asthma	Asma
Mucous	Moco
Seizures	Convulsións
Drainage	Drenaje
Immunization	Vacuna
Poison ivy	Hiedra venenosa
Bacterial infection	Infección bacterial
Viral infection	Infección viral
Diaper dermatitis	Dermatitis por causa del pañal
Rash or skin lesion produced by insect bite	Rozadura o lesión de la piel hecha por una picadura de insecto
Ulcer (as in mouth ulcers or chancre sores)	Úlceras o llagas en la boca
Gastritis	Gastritis, agruras
Constipation	Estreñimiento
Home remedies	Tratamientos caseros
Fracture	Fractura
Intensive care	Cuidado intensivo
Immunizations	Vacunas
Animal bite	Mordida de animal
Menstrual period	Menstruación, período
Birth control	Anticonceptivo

EQUIPMENT

ENGLISH PHRASE	SPANISH PHRASE
Tube; can also mean nasogastric tube or urinary catheter or any tube that has to be inserted into body (MicKey button, gastrostomy)	Sonda, catéter urinario, tubo que se introduce en el cuerpo
Gown	Bata
Suction	Succión
Sheet	Sábana
Diaper	Pañal
Bulb syringe	Saca mocos
Clothes, clothing	Ropa
Splint or cast	Férula o yeso
Dressing, bandage	Bendaje, gaza
Infusion pump	Máquina para infusion
Tape	Cinta
Teaspoon	Cucharadita
Cup (as in small medicine cup or drinking cup)	Taza
Syringe	Jeringa
Pill	Pastilla, píldora
Needle	Aguja
Antibiotic	Antibiótico
Cotton swab	Algodón
Pacifier	Chupón
Bottle, as in baby bottle or medicine bottle	Biberón

ENGLISH PHRASE	SPANISH PHRASE
Juice	Jugo
Milk	Leche

BODY PARTS

ENGLISH PHRASE	SPANISH PHRASE
Bone	Hueso
Blood	Sangre
Tongue	Lengua
Head	Cabeza
Arm	Brazo
Finger	Dedo
Leg	Pierna
Neck	Cuello
Elbow	Codo
Foot	Pie
Ear	Oreja
Nose	Nariz
Mouth	Boca
Bladder	Vejiga
Back	Espalda
Chest	Pecho
Spleen	Bazo
Gallbladder	Vesícula

PAIN MANAGEMENT

ENGLISH PHRASE	SPANISH PHRASE
Do you have any pain…?	¿Tienes dolor…?
Headache	De cabeza
Stomachache	De estómago
Backache	De espalda
Chest pain	En el pecho
In the arm	En el brazo
In the legs	En las piernas
In the mouth	En la boca
In the eyes	En los ojos
In the bladder	En la vejiga
How many hours, days, months, years have you had pain…?	¿Por cuántos (cuántas) horas, días, meses, años has tenido dolor…?
Please show me where it hurts	Muéstreme dónde te duele, por favor.
What medicine are you taking for pain?	¿Qué medicina estás tomando para el dolor?
What medicine have you taken for pain?	¿Qué medicina has tomado para el dolor?
Calm down	Cálmate
This won't hurt	Esto no te va a doler

PROCEDURES

ENGLISH PHRASE	SPANISH PHRASE
Injection	Inyección
Lumbar puncture	Punción lumbar
Oral hydration solution (e.g., Pedialyte)	Suero oral o por la boca
Intravenous fluids	Suero intravenoso o por la vena
Start an intravenous line	Vamos a ponerle suero intravenoso o por la vena
Normal saline drops	Gotas de solución salina
Humidity	Humedad
Vaporizer	Vaporizador de aire
Breathing treatment	Tratamiento para la respiración
Humidity in the bathroom with a hot shower running	El vapor en el baño de la regadera o ducha de agua caliente
Stool sample	Muestra de heces (popo) excremento

Continued

ENGLISH PHRASE	SPANISH PHRASE
We need to take some blood to see what exactly (illness) (he/she) has	Tenemos que tomar una muestra de sangre para saber con seguridad lo que el o ella tiene o padece
The results of your blood test show…	Los resultados de la sangre muestran…
The most important thing is to decrease the fever with Tylenol or Motrin	Lo más importante es reducir la fiebre con Tylenol o Motrin
We will have to catheterize (him/her)	Tendremos que ponerle una sonda en la vejiga
Topical treatment	Tratamiento tópico
To suture	Suturar
A suture	Sutura
To swab (as in "swab the mouth" or "to place a cream on…")	Untar
He/she should take lots of clear liquids	Debe tomar bastantes líquidos claros

ENGLISH PHRASE	SPANISH PHRASE
To nurse, breastfeed	Amamantar
To burp	Eructar
X-ray	Radiografía
Computed tomography scan	Tomografía
Nasal drops	Gotas nasales
Put ice on it	Póngale hielo

MISCELLANEOUS PHRASES

He/she will need to be hospitalized for treatment (observation)	Tendrá que ser hospitalizado(a) para darle tratamiento (ser observado[a])
We need a urine specimen in this cup	Necesitamos su muestra de orina en esta taza
Take him/her to the primary doctor tomorrow	Llévelo mañana a su doctor principal o de cabecera
He/she's very sick	Está muy enfermo(a)

Blood Pressure Levels

		SYSTOLIC BP (mm Hg)							DIASTOLIC BP (mm Hg)						
		PERCENTILE OF HEIGHT							PERCENTILE OF HEIGHT						
AGE (yr)	BP PERCENTILE*	5th	10th	25th	50th	75th	90th	95th	5th	10th	25th	50th	75th	90th	95th
1	50th	80	81	83	85	87	88	89	34	35	36	37	38	39	39
	90th	94	95	97	99	100	102	103	49	50	51	52	53	53	54
	95th	98	99	101	103	104	106	106	54	54	55	56	57	58	58
	99th	105	106	108	110	112	113	114	61	62	63	64	65	66	66
2	50th	84	85	87	88	90	92	92	39	40	41	42	43	44	44
	90th	97	99	100	102	104	105	106	54	55	56	57	58	58	59
	95th	101	102	104	106	108	109	110	59	59	60	61	62	63	63
	99th	109	110	111	113	115	117	117	66	67	68	69	70	71	71
3	50th	86	87	89	91	93	94	95	44	44	45	46	47	48	48
	90th	100	101	103	105	107	108	109	59	59	60	61	62	63	63
	95th	104	105	107	109	110	112	113	63	63	64	65	66	67	67
	99th	111	112	114	116	118	119	120	71	71	72	73	74	75	75
4	50th	88	89	91	93	95	96	97	47	48	49	50	51	51	52
	90th	102	103	105	107	109	110	111	62	63	64	65	66	66	67
	95th	106	107	109	111	112	114	115	66	67	68	69	70	71	71
	99th	113	114	116	118	120	121	122	74	75	76	77	78	78	79
5	50th	90	91	93	95	96	98	98	50	51	52	53	54	55	55
	90th	104	105	106	108	110	111	112	65	66	67	68	69	69	70
	95th	108	109	110	112	114	115	116	69	70	71	72	73	74	74
	99th	115	116	118	120	121	123	123	77	78	79	80	81	81	82
6	50th	91	92	94	96	98	99	100	53	53	54	55	56	57	57
	90th	105	106	108	110	111	113	113	68	68	69	70	71	72	72
	95th	109	110	112	114	115	117	117	72	72	73	74	75	76	76
	99th	116	117	119	121	123	124	125	80	80	81	82	83	84	84
7	50th	92	94	95	97	99	100	101	55	55	56	57	58	59	59
	90th	106	107	109	111	113	114	115	70	70	71	72	73	74	74
	95th	110	111	113	115	117	118	119	74	74	75	76	77	78	78
	99th	117	118	120	122	124	125	126	82	82	83	84	85	86	86
8	50th	94	95	97	99	100	102	102	56	57	58	59	60	60	61
	90th	107	109	110	112	114	115	116	71	72	72	73	74	75	76
	95th	111	112	114	116	118	119	120	75	76	77	78	79	79	80
	99th	119	120	122	123	125	127	127	83	84	85	86	87	87	88
9	50th	95	96	98	100	102	103	104	57	58	59	60	61	61	62
	90th	109	110	112	114	115	117	118	72	73	74	75	76	76	77
	95th	113	114	116	118	119	121	121	76	77	78	79	80	81	81
	99th	120	121	123	125	127	128	129	84	85	86	87	88	88	89
10	50th	97	98	100	102	103	105	106	58	59	60	61	61	62	63
	90th	111	112	114	115	117	119	119	73	73	74	75	76	77	78
	95th	115	116	117	119	121	122	123	77	78	79	80	81	81	82
	99th	122	123	125	127	128	130	130	85	86	86	88	88	89	90
11	50th	99	100	102	104	105	107	107	59	59	60	61	62	63	63
	90th	113	114	115	117	119	120	121	74	74	75	76	77	78	78
	95th	117	118	119	121	123	124	125	78	78	79	80	81	82	82
	99th	124	125	127	129	130	132	132	86	86	87	88	89	90	90

BLOOD PRESSURE (BP) LEVELS FOR BOYS BY AGE AND HEIGHT PERCENTILE

Continued

BLOOD PRESSURE (BP) LEVELS FOR BOYS BY AGE AND HEIGHT PERCENTILE—cont'd

AGE (yr)	BP PERCENTILE*	SYSTOLIC BP (mm Hg) PERCENTILE OF HEIGHT							DIASTOLIC BP (mm Hg) PERCENTILE OF HEIGHT						
		5th	10th	25th	50th	75th	90th	95th	5th	10th	25th	50th	75th	90th	95th
12	50th	101	102	104	106	108	109	110	59	60	61	62	63	63	64
	90th	115	116	118	120	121	123	123	74	75	75	76	77	78	79
	95th	119	120	122	123	125	127	127	78	79	80	81	82	82	83
	99th	126	127	129	131	133	134	135	86	87	88	89	90	90	91
13	50th	104	105	106	108	110	111	112	60	60	61	62	63	64	64
	90th	117	118	120	122	124	125	126	75	75	76	77	78	79	79
	95th	121	122	124	126	128	129	130	79	79	80	81	82	83	83
	99th	128	130	131	133	135	136	137	87	87	88	89	90	91	91
14	50th	106	107	109	111	113	114	115	60	61	62	63	64	65	65
	90th	120	121	123	125	126	128	128	75	76	77	78	79	79	80
	95th	124	125	127	128	130	132	132	80	80	81	82	83	84	84
	99th	131	132	134	136	138	139	140	87	88	89	90	91	92	92
15	50th	109	110	112	113	115	117	117	61	62	63	64	65	66	66
	90th	122	124	125	127	129	130	131	76	77	78	79	80	80	81
	95th	126	127	129	131	133	134	135	81	81	82	83	84	85	85
	99th	134	135	136	138	140	142	142	88	89	90	91	92	93	93
16	50th	111	112	114	116	118	119	120	63	63	64	65	66	67	67
	90th	125	126	128	130	131	133	134	78	78	79	80	81	82	82
	95th	129	130	132	134	135	137	137	82	83	83	84	85	86	87
	99th	136	137	139	141	143	144	145	90	90	91	92	93	94	94
17	50th	114	115	116	118	120	121	122	65	66	66	67	68	69	70
	90th	127	128	130	132	134	135	136	80	80	81	82	83	84	84
	95th	131	132	134	136	138	139	140	84	85	86	87	87	88	89
	99th	139	140	141	143	145	146	147	92	93	93	94	95	96	97

Retrieved November 22, 2011, from http://www.nhlbi.nih.gov/health/prof/heart/hbp/hbp_ped.pdf.
*The 90th percentile is 1.28 standard deviation (SD), the 95th percentile is 1.645 SD, and the 99th percentile is 2.326 SD over the mean.

BLOOD PRESSURE (BP) LEVELS FOR GIRLS BY AGE AND HEIGHT PERCENTILE

AGE (yr)	BP PERCENTILE*	SYSTOLIC BP (mm Hg) PERCENTILE OF HEIGHT							DIASTOLIC BP (mm Hg) PERCENTILE OF HEIGHT						
		5th	10th	25th	50th	75th	90th	95th	5th	10th	25th	50th	75th	90th	95th
1	50th	83	84	85	86	88	89	90	38	39	39	40	41	41	42
	90th	97	97	98	100	101	102	103	52	53	53	54	55	55	56
	95th	100	101	102	104	105	106	107	56	57	57	58	59	59	60
	99th	108	108	109	111	112	113	114	64	64	65	65	66	67	67
2	50th	85	85	87	88	89	91	91	43	44	44	45	46	46	47
	90th	98	99	100	101	103	104	105	57	58	58	59	60	61	61
	95th	102	103	104	105	107	108	109	61	62	62	63	64	65	65
	99th	109	110	111	112	114	115	116	69	69	70	70	71	72	72
3	50th	86	87	88	89	91	92	93	47	48	48	49	50	50	51
	90th	100	100	102	103	104	106	106	61	62	62	63	64	64	65
	95th	104	104	105	107	108	109	110	65	66	66	67	68	68	69
	99th	111	111	113	114	115	116	117	73	73	74	74	75	76	76
4	50th	88	88	90	91	92	94	94	50	50	51	52	52	53	54
	90th	101	102	103	104	106	107	108	64	64	65	66	67	67	68
	95th	105	106	107	108	110	111	112	68	68	69	70	71	71	72
	99th	112	113	114	115	117	118	119	76	76	76	77	78	79	79
5	50th	89	90	91	93	94	95	96	52	53	53	54	55	55	56
	90th	103	103	105	106	107	109	109	66	67	67	68	69	69	70
	95th	107	107	108	110	111	112	113	70	71	71	72	73	73	74
	99th	114	114	116	117	118	120	120	78	78	79	79	80	81	81

BLOOD PRESSURE (BP) LEVELS FOR GIRLS BY AGE AND HEIGHT PERCENTILE—cont'd

AGE (yr)	BP PERCENTILE*	SYSTOLIC BP (mm Hg) PERCENTILE OF HEIGHT							DIASTOLIC BP (mm Hg) PERCENTILE OF HEIGHT						
		5th	10th	25th	50th	75th	90th	95th	5th	10th	25th	50th	75th	90th	95th
6	50th	91	92	93	94	96	97	98	54	54	55	56	56	57	58
	90th	104	105	106	108	109	110	111	68	68	69	70	70	71	72
	95th	108	109	110	111	113	114	115	72	72	73	74	74	75	76
	99th	115	116	117	119	120	121	122	80	80	80	81	82	83	83
7	50th	93	93	95	96	97	99	99	55	56	56	57	58	58	59
	90th	106	107	108	109	111	112	113	69	70	70	71	72	72	73
	95th	110	111	112	113	115	116	116	73	74	74	75	76	76	77
	99th	117	118	119	120	122	123	124	81	81	82	82	83	84	84
8	50th	95	95	96	98	99	100	101	57	57	57	58	59	60	60
	90th	108	109	110	111	113	114	114	71	71	71	72	73	74	74
	95th	112	112	114	115	116	118	118	75	75	75	76	77	78	78
	99th	119	120	121	122	123	125	125	82	82	83	83	84	85	86
9	50th	96	97	98	100	101	102	103	58	58	58	59	60	61	61
	90th	110	110	112	113	114	116	116	72	72	72	73	74	75	75
	95th	114	114	115	117	118	119	120	76	76	76	77	78	79	79
	99th	121	121	123	124	125	127	127	83	83	84	84	85	86	87
10	50th	98	99	100	102	103	104	105	59	59	59	60	61	62	62
	90th	112	112	114	115	116	118	118	73	73	73	74	75	76	76
	95th	116	116	117	119	120	121	122	77	77	77	78	79	80	80
	99th	123	123	125	126	127	129	129	84	84	85	86	86	87	88
11	50th	100	101	102	103	105	106	107	60	60	60	61	62	63	63
	90th	114	114	116	117	118	119	120	74	74	74	75	76	77	77
	95th	118	118	119	121	122	123	124	78	78	78	79	80	81	81
	99th	125	125	126	128	129	130	131	85	85	86	87	87	88	89
12	50th	102	103	104	105	107	108	109	61	61	61	62	63	64	64
	90th	116	116	117	119	120	121	122	75	75	75	76	77	78	78
	95th	119	120	121	123	124	125	126	79	79	79	80	81	82	82
	99th	127	127	128	130	131	132	133	86	86	87	88	88	89	90
13	50th	104	105	106	107	109	110	110	62	62	62	63	64	65	65
	90th	117	118	119	121	122	123	124	76	76	76	77	78	79	79
	95th	121	122	123	124	126	127	128	80	80	80	81	82	83	83
	99th	128	129	130	132	133	134	135	87	87	88	89	89	90	91
14	50th	106	106	107	109	110	111	112	63	63	63	64	65	66	66
	90th	119	120	121	122	124	125	125	77	77	77	78	79	80	80
	95th	123	123	125	126	127	129	129	81	81	81	82	83	84	84
	99th	130	131	132	133	135	136	136	88	88	89	90	90	91	92
15	50th	107	108	109	110	111	113	113	64	64	64	65	66	67	67
	90th	120	121	122	123	125	126	127	78	78	78	79	80	81	81
	95th	124	125	126	127	129	130	131	82	82	82	83	84	85	85
	99th	131	132	133	134	136	137	138	89	89	90	91	91	92	93
16	50th	108	108	110	111	112	114	114	64	64	65	66	66	67	68
	90th	121	122	123	124	126	127	128	78	78	79	80	81	81	82
	95th	125	126	127	128	130	131	132	82	82	83	84	85	85	86
	99th	132	133	134	135	137	138	139	90	90	90	91	92	93	93
17	50th	108	109	110	111	113	114	115	64	65	65	66	67	67	68
	90th	122	122	123	125	126	127	128	78	79	79	80	81	81	82
	95th	125	126	127	129	130	131	132	82	83	83	84	85	85	86
	99th	133	133	134	136	137	138	139	90	90	91	91	92	93	93

Retrieved November 22, 2011, from http://www.nhlbi.nih.gov/health/prof/heart/hbp/hbp_ped.pdf.

*The 90th percentile is 1.28 standard deviation (SD), the 95th percentile is 1.645 SD, and the 99th percentile is 2.326 SD over the mean.

Answers to Case Studies

CHAPTER 3

Parenting the Adopted Child

1. Yes. Although there is no one best time to tell children they are adopted, most authorities believe that children should be informed before they enter school to avoid learning about it from third parties. In addition, authorities agree that children should be told at an age young enough so that, as they grow older, they do not remember a time when they did not know they were adopted.
2. a. The best time is highly individualized and based on the child's readiness. For some children, this may be when they ask about where babies come from. Children have a more difficult adjustment if disclosure occurs when they are older, and waiting until adolescence is too late.
   b. Parents should be completely honest with the child and provide information about the adoption in a matter-of-fact way. Sharing the story of adoption is an important parental responsibility and can be handled much like a parent shares birth experiences with a biologic child.
   c. Parents should anticipate that children may act out after being told that they are adopted. Some children use the fact of their adoption as a weapon to manipulate and threaten their parents. Allowing children to express their feelings and emotions after they have been told about their adoption is important.
3. Because Justin's parents have requested guidance, it is appropriate for you, as the nurse, to provide information about how and when they should tell Justin he is adopted. However, the nurse's first priority is to be certain that Justin's parents are comfortable with this information and that they feel free to ask any further questions and to obtain additional information. Because Justin is only 12 months old, his parents have time to think about how they will present this information to Justin and to prepare for the disclosure. They also have time to discuss how they will react to the feelings, emotions, and behaviors that Justin may demonstrate after he learns he is adopted.
4. Yes, at the present time, most authorities agree that children should be told about the fact that they are adopted and that disclosure of this information should occur before the school-age years.

CHAPTER 4

Reducing Cultural Shock

1. An understanding of the Arab culture provides insight into the woman's hesitancy to make decisions in her husband's absence.
2. a. Typically, in the Arab culture men make the decisions, and women are expected to support these decisions.

b. The need for an interpreter is evident to make certain the mother understands the seriousness of the situation.
   c. Knowledge of the process for obtaining approval for emergency procedures without informed consent will facilitate the best care for the child.
   d. Appropriate documentation of how approval was obtained without parental consent is essential.
3. The first priority is to make certain the child is receiving the best care possible and that the necessary procedure is performed as soon as possible. The next priority is to ensure that the mother understands the urgency of the situation by using an interpreter.
4. The child's health status is most important at this time.

CHAPTER 9

Jaundice

1. Yes, there are sufficient data to arrive at some possible conclusions.
2. a. See text, pp. 256–263.
   b. Serum bilirubin levels are within acceptable limits, and based on the available data, the infant is within the low-intermediate risk zone. Based on the available data, ABO incompatibility–related hemolysis is not evident but may warrant further investigation.
   c. Oral intake is adequate; urine and stool output is appropriate (based on urine output of 1 wet diaper per each day of life = 5 wets).
   d. The assessment of behavior and reflexes indicates no particular concerns; the newborn appears to be healthy.
3. No immediate intervention to reduce bilirubin is warranted at this time, although the treatment is a medical decision. Nursing care should focus on alleviating parents' concerns regarding condition of infant, who appears to be healthy, and addressing their concerns about the misinformation on the potential for brain damage (which is a nonexistent problem at this point). Encourage the mother to continue breastfeeding on demand and observe the infant's activity levels, intake, and urinary and stool output. Emphasize that jaundice and hyperbilirubinemia are transient conditions of the newborn. At this point, a follow-up appointment should be scheduled with the primary practitioner in 24 hours to monitor the bilirubin level, address the parents' concerns, and monitor the infant's weight.
4. Yes, the infant's laboratory data and physical assessment data support these conclusions. Additionally, knowledge about physiologic hyperbilirubinemia of the newborn supports these conclusions. Phototherapy does not seem warranted at this time based on the available data.

CHAPTER 10

Childhood Immunizations and Autism

1. There is sufficient evidence to arrive at some possible conclusions regarding Monica's concerns about immunizing her children.
2. See text, pp. 335 and 340.
   a. To date, objective and retrospective studies in the United States and Europe do not support a correlation between any childhood vaccines such as MMR (measles, mumps, and rubella) and the rate of autism or any other pervasive disorders. Schechter and Grether (2008) found that rates of autism continued to rise in California even after the removal of thimerosal from childhood vaccines.
   b. It is not uncommon for parents who have not lived in an era during which childhood communicable diseases were not commonplace to state that communicable diseases have been eradicated from developed countries and do not pose a threat. This is partially true; however, with ever-increasing population mobility, children in the suburban United States may accidentally come in contact with an individual who was recently exposed (unknowingly) to a communicable disease in another country. This occurred recently in the case of the measles outbreak in Hennepin County, Minnesota (Centers for Disease Control and Prevention, 2011).
   c. Herd immunity, or community immunity, implies that individuals who are immunized against certain illnesses build an immunity to those and prevent the transmission of that particular communicable disease to others who are not immunized. Herd immunity is less effective as the number of immunized persons decreases and vice versa. Population-based surveys in the United States are often conducted to identify the number of children being vaccinated to compare with the communicable disease occurrence rates; recommendations from state or local public health agencies may be made to increase the number of immunizations if the vaccination rate is low. Such was the case recently when pertussis vaccination rates were found to be low in adolescents ages 13 to 18 years; the Advisory Committee on Immunization Practices (Centers for Disease Control and Prevention) recommended a booster of the Tdap (diphtheria, tetanus, and pertussis) vaccine for adolescents age 16 years who had received the DTaP (diphtheria, tetanus, and pertussis) series and 1 Tdap at age 12 or 13 years.
3. Here are some suggestions about talking to parents who have concerns about vaccines.
   * Provide accurate and user-friendly information on vaccines (the necessity for each one, the disease each prevents, potential adverse effects).
   * Realize that the parent is expressing concern for the child's health.
   * Acknowledge the parent's concerns in a genuine, empathetic manner.
   * Respect the parent's ultimate wishes.
   * Be knowledgeable about the benefits of individual vaccines, the common adverse effects, and how to minimize those effects.
   * Help the parent make an informed decision regarding the administration of each vaccine.
   * Be flexible and provide parents options regarding the administration of multiple vaccines, especially in infants, who must receive multiple injections at 2, 4, and 6 months (i.e., allow parents to space the vaccinations at different visits to decrease the total number of injections at each visit; make provisions for office visits for immunization purposes only [does not incur a practitioner fee except for administration of vaccine], provided the child is healthy).
   * Provide parents with a copy of the VIS (Vaccine Information Statement) for each of the childhood vaccines even if they decide not to have the children vaccinated.
   * Avoid the use of guilt-laden statements to "convince" the parents what is best for their children.
   * Remain neutral while providing objective information.
   * Listen attentively to the parents' concerns. If you cannot remain objective and caring during the discussion, suggest that another person discuss the parents' concerns with them (identify such a person beforehand in the department for such occasions).
4. The evidence has been supported by the available literature.

   Centers for Disease Control and Prevention: Notes from the field: measles outbreak—Hennepin County, Minnesota, February–March 2011, *MMWR Weekly* 60(13):421, 2011.

   Schechter R, Grether JK: Continuing increases in autism reported to California's developmental services system: mercury in retrograde, *Arch Gen Psychiatry* 65(1):19–24, 2008.

CHAPTER 11

Food Allergy Anaphylaxis

1. There is sufficient evidence to indicate that Jason is having an anaphylactic reaction to an ingested food (peanuts in this case). Peanuts are the most common food allergen in children in the United States.
2. See p. 359.
   a. Clinical manifestations of anaphylaxis include itching, hoarseness, wheezing, difficulty swallowing, cyanosis, hypotension, and respiratory arrest.
   b. The emergency treatment is to administer an intramuscular (IM) dose of epinephrine.
   c. In this scenario, it would be most appropriate to administer a dose of IM epinephrine.
   d. It just so happens that the school nurse has two EpiPens—one is an EpiPen Jr. of 0.15 mg and the other is of 0.3 mg. Which one would you administer? It is estimated that Jason weighs 45 lb. (See p. 360.)
3. Implications for nursing care.
   * The immediate priority is to administer the epinephrine. Jason should be closely monitored, including vital signs, work of breathing, comfort, and anxiety. Several reports in the literature indicate that children often die from food allergy anaphylaxis because of the fear of administering epinephrine for its potential side effects.
   * The second and third priorities would be to call 911 and then call Jason's parents and notify them of Jason's reaction, the intervention taken, and Jason's status.
   * Meanwhile, Jason should continue to be observed by the nursing students and school nurse (until emergency medical services arrives)
4. The results could be lethal as discussed above. It is within the scope of practice of the school nurse to administer the IM epinephrine when the signs and symptoms of anaphylaxis are observed.
5. Yes, there is sufficient evidence for these interventions based on the literature on food allergy anaphylaxis in children.

CHAPTER 16

Discussing the Future

1. Yes, there is sufficient information to arrive at a conclusion about what advice to give Jeremy's mother.
2. a. During adolescence, teens consider all of their past relationships as they attempt to form their own personal identity. They attempt to formulate a satisfactory identity from a multiplicity of roles, aspirations, and identifications. The process of developing this identity is time consuming and can be associated with confusion and discouragement.
   b. If significant others are too persistent and demand that adolescents make specific decisions or behave in definite ways, adolescents often make premature decisions and accept roles that do not incorporate their own personal goals or aspirations.
   c. Parents who communicate well with their teens have an open, nonjudgmental, nondictatorial manner. They demonstrate that they are available and willing to listen to their teenagers. However, they also wait until the teenager opens the discussion, and then they listen attentively and allow the teen to explore issues.
3. The nursing priority in this situation is to have the mother become more aware that Jeremy is not likely to discuss his concerns on a timetable and that it is important for her to respect his point of view. Although Jeremy wants his mother's guidance and support, he does not want to be told what to do, and he needs an opportunity to express his own feelings and views. An example of appropriate advice to give Jeremy's mother might be: "Be open and available to Jeremy. Tell him what you think but *not what to do.*"
4. Yes, the information about how teens formulate a personal identity and the principles of effective parent communication allow the nurse to formulate this response.

Discussing Sexual Orientation with Adolescents

1. No, there are insufficient data to arrive at a conclusion about John's sexual orientation. Further discussion with him is necessary before making any assumptions.
2. a. Studies of gay men and lesbians indicate that adolescence is the time when individuals become aware of same-sex attraction. Homosexual and bisexual youths are at risk for health-damaging behaviors such as early initiation of sexual behavior, substance abuse, suicide, and running away from home.
   b. Homosexual and bisexual youths are often confronted with the antihomosexual attitudes and values of society. This reaction of society makes it difficult for homosexual and bisexual youths to grow up and become healthy physically and mentally.
   c. Health care professionals who work with adolescents should consider the adolescent's increasing independence and responsibility while ensuring confidentiality.
3. The nurse's first priority in this situation is to give John permission to discuss his feelings about this topic. He has come to the nurse practitioner to discuss this matter, and he probably feels comfortable sharing this information with the nurse practitioner. The nurse practitioner needs to be open and nonjudgmental in interactions with John. He needs to know that the nurse practitioner will maintain confidentiality, appreciate his feelings, and remain sensitive to his need to talk about this topic. An example of an appropriate response for the nurse practitioner might be: "John, tell me more about how you came to this conclusion."

4. Yes, the information about sexual orientation in adolescence and the role of the health care professional support this conclusion.

Respecting Privacy

1. Yes, there is sufficient evidence for the nurse to formulate a response to Jamie's mother.
2. a. As teenagers progress through adolescence, they are able to assume more responsibility for their own health. They can take prescribed medications, keep health care appointments, and discuss their care with health care professionals.
   b. Parents of adolescents should respect their teenagers' independence while maintaining some level of involvement with their children. However, in matters of health care, they should gradually assume the role of a consultant and allow their children to take an increasingly active role in relating to health professionals.
   c. Health professionals who work with adolescents must consider adolescents' increasing independence and responsibility while also maintaining privacy and ensuring confidentiality. In most adolescent clinics, health care professionals meet with the adolescent and the parent together followed by individual time with both the adolescent and the parent.
3. The first priority for nursing care at this point is to reassure both Jamie and her mother that they will each have an opportunity to express their concerns to the nurse practitioner. Because Jamie is the nurse practitioner's patient and the setting is an adolescent clinic, the nurse practitioner should speak with Jamie first after meeting briefly with Jamie and her mother together. An appropriate response by the nurse practitioner might be: "I would like to begin by speaking with both of you together and then spend some time with just you, Jamie, and then with just you, Mrs. S." Knowing that her mother will also have an opportunity to express her concerns, Jamie will likely be more open and may even say, "I know what my mother will tell you," and address the issue herself. This response will also demonstrate to Jamie that the nurse practitioner respects her privacy and will maintain confidentiality. If the nurse speaks with Jamie first, Jamie might think that her privacy is being violated and become distrustful of both the nurse practitioner and her mother. In addition, if the nurse practitioner speaks with Mrs. S. first, Jamie is likely to become defensive and spend her time trying to draw from the nurse practitioner what her mother said.
4. Yes, the information about adolescent growth and development and the roles of adolescents, their parents, and the health care professional support this conclusion.

CHAPTER 17

Attention-Deficit/Hyperactivity Disorder

1. Yes, there are sufficient data to arrive at a possible conclusion.
2. a. Methylphenidate is a stimulant that increases dopamine and norepinephrine levels that lead to stimulation of the inhibitory system of the central nervous system.
   b. Common side effects of methylphenidate include nausea, anorexia, decreased appetite, and insomnia.
   c. Although the absorption rate of methylphenidate is increased when the drug is taken with meals, side effects such as decreased appetite may become more pronounced with this schedule of administration. Side effects can be alleviated by changing the times that the drug is administered or by switching to a sustained time-release form of the drug that is taken once per day in the morning.

3. Although Johnnie seems to have responded favorably to his medication and has demonstrated several positive effects of methylphenidate (improvement in math class and increasing self-confidence in social skills), the nurse should be concerned about the fact that Johnnie has not eaten his lunch for the past week and that he is not hungry. Decreased appetite is a negative side effect of methylphenidate.

4. Yes, the data indicate that Johnnie is currently experiencing a decrease in his appetite. Because decreased appetite is a common side effect of methylphenidate, there is a high probability that this symptom is related to Johnnie's medication. However, adjusting or changing the times the medication is administered can often alleviate this side effect. Another option is to ask Johnnie's physician to switch his medication to a sustained time-release form of methylphenidate that can be given once per day in the morning.

Testicular Self-Examination

1. Yes. Although testicular cancer is not common in adolescence, when it does occur, it is generally malignant. Testicular cancer is very curable if detected early.

2. a. The best way to detect testicular tumors is by performing testicular self-examination every month.

    b. The usual presenting symptom for testicular cancer is a heavy, hard painless mass (either smooth or nodular) that is palpated on the testis.

    c. Adolescent boys are self-conscious about their genital anatomy. However, as a pediatric nurse practitioner at the school-based clinic, Paul is in an excellent position to teach young men how to perform this examination. It is highly probable that he has already won their trust and confidence through his routine daily nursing activities, such as providing sports physical examinations and treating their episodic illnesses. Paul will be able to present the class in a manner that is respectful of the young boys while allaying their anxieties and providing them with an important health skill.

    d. The class should be presented in a matter-of-fact way with an explanation of both the characteristics of normal testicles as well as a description of abnormal findings.

3. The first priority is to make certain that all adolescent boys with health problems feel comfortable visiting the health suite and sharing their concerns with the nurse practitioner. The ultimate goal is to be certain that no adolescent boy with a potential testicular tumor fails to get an immediate assessment and referral for treatment.

4. Yes, the information about testicular cancer, and the importance of detecting it early, provides a definite rationale for the class.

Anorexia Nervosa

1. Using the clinical manifestations of anorexia nervosa (AN) (see Box 17-8), there is sufficient evidence to support the conclusion that Jane has AN.

2. a. Young adolescent girls with AN are often high achievers or excellent students. They have an abundance of energy, a distorted body image, and a fear of gaining weight.

    b. A family crisis can influence AN. Jane's parents are currently in the middle of a divorce, and in this type of situation, some teens feel they have no control over events in their life. Consequently, some adolescents take control by refusing to eat and developing AN.

    c. Jane is engaging in increased physical activity and is skipping lunch several days each week. On physical examination, she has a decreased body temperature (36° C [96.8° F]) and she has lost 9 kg (20 lb) in the past year (she is at <85% of her expected weight). She also told the nurse practitioner that she has not had her menstrual period for 3 months. These manifestations are all congruent with AN.

    d. AN is treated by a team of health professionals who address the abnormal eating patterns and altered body image of the patient and the dysfunctional family dynamics that accompany this disorder.

3. Jane should be referred to a specialist who deals with adolescents with AN.

4. Yes, the evidence supports the conclusion.

Prescription Medication Abuse in Adolescence

1. Yes. It is apparent that the adolescent needs further evaluation and should not be returned to class at this time. The slurred speech, short-term memory lapse, and elevated heart rate indicate further evaluation should be sought.

2. Legally, the nurse must call the girl's parents and inform them that she appears to need medical attention. It is up to the parents or guardians to take the next step (i.e., take her to the nearest emergency department [ED] or to her primary care practitioner). As a school nurse, Sally must decide if the girl's life is in immediate danger (e.g., vital signs and neurologic signs unstable); it does not appear to be at this time. Sally does not have the authority to call emergency medical services (EMS) or to take the girl to the ED at this time.

3. a. The assessment findings of memory lapse, slurred speech, decreased respirations, sluggish pupil reactivity, and tachycardia indicate a need for further medical evaluation and observation.

    b. See pp. 526–530.

4. Nursing implications include close observation for any signs of deterioration in vital signs or respiratory status. Sally must notify the girl's parents or guardians. In the event they cannot be reached, the nurse should call EMS and ask that the girl be transported to an acute care facility for observation. In the ED, the girl will be triaged, and vital signs will be taken. Urine drug screen will be obtained to determine what she has in her system, and frequent neurologic signs will be monitored. She will also probably have a peripheral intravenous line started and some blood tests drawn for baseline (chemistry and electrolytes, possibly a liver panel). If it is determined that an opioid was taken, naloxone may be administered, depending on her status at the time.

CHAPTER 19

Diagnosis of Down Syndrome

1. Yes. Shocked parents with three children are notified that their newborn has Down syndrome.

2. a. Melissa is a developmentally delayed newborn who requires time-consuming care.

    b. Melissa will develop a variety of medical problems, causing a huge financial expense.

    c. Melissa will always require parent and sibling supervision and care.

3. The first priority is to allow the parents to express their feelings of grief, anger, sadness, and guilt regarding the birth of a children with an intellectual disability.

    • The nurse should not take anything for granted or give definite suggestions regarding children with disabilities.

- The nurse should demonstrate acceptance of the child because parents are sensitive to the professional's attitude.
4. Yes. The parents' response suggests unexpressed feelings of anger, loss, sadness, and confusion.

Hearing Impairment

1. Yes. Jason is severely hearing impaired and awakening in an unfamiliar environment after a surgical procedure. Jason recovers in an unfamiliar environment with monitors, an intravenous line, and other equipment that may create fear, anxiety, and agitation.
2. a. Jason's inability to hear and communicate promotes frustration and fear.
   b. Jason's increasing agitation may be because of not having his hearing aids.
   c. Jason, who is recovering from regional block for herniorrhaphy, is unable to clearly verbalize or use sign language to express his needs.
3. The first priority is to establish communication with Jason by directly facing him to facilitate lip reading, touching him to get his attention, and correctly placing his hearing aids if available.
   - Determine his usual means of communicating and encourage expression of feelings and questions regarding environment, equipment, and procedures.
   - Explain procedures before performing them, using gestures, objects, or pictures; speak slowly and clearly.
   - Allow ample time for child to show understanding of explanations.
   - Decrease environmental noise.
   - Listen closely as the child speaks and focus on his pronunciation of words.
4. Yes. Jason's behavior does not suggest the transitory confusion associated with the initial emergence from anesthesia. Rather, it suggests that he became increasingly frustrated as he became aware of his environment with the inability to communicate his desires and feelings. Although pain is a possibility and needs to be evaluated, regional blocks are typically given during surgery to keep children comfortable until after they are discharged.

CHAPTER 20

Family-Centered Home Care and Conflicts

1. Yes. There is sufficient evidence to arrive at some possible conclusions (see p. 604).
2. a. Sarah demonstrates tongue thrusting, which is common in healthy children from birth to 4 or 5 months and in children who have little experience with oral feedings and oral stimulation. This indicates she may not be ready for oral feedings; an assessment by a speech-language pathologist (SLP) would be helpful. (See Feeding Resistance, Chapter 9.)
   b. Given Sarah's history and assessment data, there are risks, primarily choking and aspiration, involved in starting oral feedings.
   c. The mother's request is not unusual. Parents want the best for their children despite disabilities that often set them apart from other peers. Although it may seem complicated to engage in communication, negotiation, and consultation over the seemingly simple issue of giving baby food to a 3-year-old child, many issues must be considered. The family appears to have legitimate reasons for wanting their daughter started on baby foods. The nurse should further explore reasons for wanting the child to be fed orally. They may believe that health care

providers have overlooked this aspect of normal development. They may be attempting to assist their daughter in achieving age-appropriate skills and may also want their daughter to participate in family mealtimes. These are legitimate, commendable goals, and the family should be supported in making such choices for their child.
3. A child who is 3 years old and has not been fed orally will benefit from an oral-motor assessment by an occupational therapist (OT)/SLP to explore the possibility of starting minimum oral feedings. Specific plans with incremental steps to reduce oral-motor defensiveness and improve the ability to accept foods orally should precede feeding. Nutritional consultation may also be important as feeding plans shift from gastrostomy to oral feedings. The nurse and the family should continue to discuss the issue, plan for consultations and evaluations related to the child's oral-motor progress, and thereby arrange to meet the family's goals of oral feeding in safer incremental steps. Communication between the nurse and the family may also lead to other approaches to normalizing mealtimes for Sarah and her family. After the OT/SLP has completed the assessment, specific short- and long-term goals for modified oral feedings may be developed, involving the family in such discussions. In addition, the family should be made aware of potential problems with oral feedings, including aspiration pneumonia or airway obstruction with further respiratory compromise.
4. Yes. The evidence supports implementing this care plan. The nurse should not dismiss the parents' request for oral feedings yet should not acquiesce to their request without assessing the situation, developing conclusions based on the assessment, and implementing an appropriate care plan that may be evaluated by the outcomes. It would not be appropriate to begin oral feedings without first consulting an OT/SLP regarding Sarah's oral-motor abilities.

Maintaining Therapeutic Boundaries

1. Yes. There is sufficient evidence to arrive at some conclusions regarding the situation.
2. a. Home care of any person, especially a child with a chronic debilitating condition, is stressful on any family, regardless of its stability and resources. The seeming lack of coping skills and decreased financial resources make the stress worse. It is not unusual for stress and conflict to surround the child's care, especially if one parent seems to be less involved in the daily care. The needs of the primary caretaker, Mrs. Jones in this instance, are not being met, and she is expressing that frustration to the nurse, who perhaps is perceived as an ally in the situation.
   b. The impact of a chronic condition on parents can be devastating and lead to misunderstandings, competition over the child's care, and neglect of the feelings of one's partner. Because the child's prognosis is poor, this can exacerbate feelings of frustration, anger, helplessness, fatigue, and conflict between the parents. The parents may feel guilty about their feelings toward the child. On one hand, they may love and care for the child; on the other hand, the presence of a child with a chronic condition with a poor prognosis who requires constant physical care may engender a desire to see an end to the situation with the child's death. These ambivalent feelings are not unusual in parents, and there may also be gender differences in how feelings over such conditions are expressed. Unmet expectations are a source of conflict among parents with a child who is sick; expectations of each other's role in the family setting may have suffered with the

loss of the "perfect" child. These feelings may last for months or even years without an appropriate resolution if adequate resources for resolution are not provided.

c. The status of the marriage appears to be strained at this time; however, there is not sufficient evidence to draw a simple conclusion without further exploration (assessment). This may be the way each parent deals with crisis situations—the mother fusses and complains, and the father withdraws by going to work and being less involved. Some anticipatory grieving may be occurring, but this needs to be explored by health care persons who can be objective and properly evaluate the marriage status.

3. The concept of therapeutic boundaries supports the idea that they are not rigid and fixed. The home care nurse must be responsive to the relationship preferred by the family and the style with which the family operates. Individual roles change according to the expectations that person has about her or his role and the particular situation. In this case, it would be appropriate for the nurse to mention that home care can be stressful for a family, indicate that referrals for counseling may be provided if desired by the parents, and listen and reflect with Mrs. Jones about her feelings. Exploring issues such as an additional home care aide to help take care of Derek might be appropriate; this would enable Mrs. Jones to take a break from his care and have time to herself. Additional financial aid may be explored by a qualified case manager or social worker so Mr. Jones would not have to work as much away from home. It is important to explore the couple's feelings regarding Derek's condition and care and their role in providing for him, as well as their relationship with each other. It is not unusual for families in crisis to become so involved in the care of the child that they forget what their marriage and relationship is about. If one or both parties do not desire counseling by another professional, perhaps other avenues such as family support groups could be explored as an option. No matter what your opinion, it would be inappropriate to agree with Mrs. Jones that her husband is not helping enough with the child's care. Such an action implies a judgment that is outside the nurse's role and undermines rather than supports the family system. Families in crisis often require professional assistance in the form of counseling to explore coping skills and help involve appropriate community resources.

4. Some preliminary evidence supports the argument that professional help is warranted in this situation. In addition, as the feelings of Mr. and Mrs. Jones are explored, additional evidence may arise that alters the course of action proposed.

CHAPTER 21

Complementary and Alternative Medicine

1. There is limited evidence to draw certain conclusions without obtaining more data from the parents. It would be appropriate to gather more information before jumping to any major conclusions at this time.

2. a. Complementary and alternative medicine (CAM) is more common in U.S. households than previously reported. Much of the concern surrounding complementary therapies, especially in children, is the lack of sufficient data regarding their effectiveness, benefit, and the potential harm that may occur as a result of such treatments. In some cases, CAM therapies may counteract certain medications or the effects of prescribed therapies. It has become more common for practitioners in emergency medicine to encounter patients who are taking CAM therapy in addition to prescription medications or treatments for

conditions such as eczema, asthma, colds, and upper respiratory tract problems.

b. Folk remedies are common among certain ethnic groups and subgroups within the United States. Many are based on traditional family remedies that have been proven to be neither effective nor entirely harmful in most cases. However, a few remedies could be potentially harmful, especially to children, if these remedies counteract the effects of prescribed treatments that are known to be effective.

c. The nurse's role in such cases is to gather sufficient data from the family about the practice, discuss the treatment (CAM) in a nonjudgmental manner, and be cognizant of the effects of the treatment on the child's current health status and potential effects on other medical treatment regimens.

3. Give the family their penny and open a dialog about the traditional practice they are using. Additional information should be gathered in a nonjudgmental manner, and the discussion should center on the family's traditional beliefs regarding the practices, the prescribed medical regimen, and whether there is a conflict or potential for harm. There is no need to stop the treatment unless potential harm to the child may occur. A discussion with the primary practitioner regarding the use of CAM for Maria should ensue followed by a discussion with the entire family, if necessary. The contents of the bottle will more than likely be revealed during the discussion with the family. It is important to respect the family's wishes regarding traditional folk or CAM rituals yet remain mindful of potential harmful effects on the child. It is not likely that telling the family to stop the ritual will be successful because these beliefs are deeply ingrained into cultural, religious, and medical practice; the family is more likely to continue the ritual at home on discharge and further disregard other instructions for care if a confrontational approach is adopted by the nursing and medical staff. The important concept for the staff and family to focus on is the ultimate well-being of the child. What you have probably observed is Santeria, the African-Caribbean religion that was brought to the New World by slaves from West Africa. It is common among immigrants from Cuba, Puerto Rico, Brazil, and Santo Domingo, and it is believed that a majority of Latin American immigrants will have contact with Santeria sometime in their lives.

4. As yet, there is insufficient evidence to indicate that harm is being done by the CAM ritual. Further data need to be gathered, and then a decision about further discussion of the CAM practice may occur.

Playroom and Hospital Procedures

1. There is sufficient evidence regarding this incident to draw some conclusions.

2. a. Regardless of how minor a procedure such as a venipuncture may seem to an adult health care worker, it represents a major threat to a child. One must consider the child's age, illness, developmental level, and previous experiences with venipunctures.

b. Play is an important function of childhood whether the child is sick or well. Through play, children may act out fears, concerns, anger, and other behaviors they may not feel comfortable expressing to adults in a confrontational manner. Play is an important part of the hospitalized child's life, and it is a vehicle for promoting optimal development.

c. It is important to have the blood drawn so that Dr. Lung may plan a therapeutic regimen; however, one must consider another issue: there appears to have been no advance preparation of the child's skin to minimize or prevent pain from the procedure. Regardless of the phlebotomist's skill in performing the procedure, it is also important to consider the fact that the negative repercussions for performing the procedure at this point may outweigh the positive benefits.

d. All staff on the pediatric floor must be in agreement about respecting the child's personal space in the playroom and about adhering to unit policies or rules so that respect is maintained. Failure to respect the child's space may engender fear in other children who perceive that the playroom is not a safe place after all. The fear of having other procedures performed in the playroom may prevent children from going there to participate in therapeutic and interactive play.

3. It is important to maintain a fair balance between what constitutes therapeutic management of illness and childhood recreation. It would be appropriate in this situation to intervene and ask the phlebotomist to return in 30 minutes to an hour and indicate that the child will be ready for the venipuncture in the treatment room at that time. It is important to stress that the playroom is off limits for procedures. It would be appropriate to discuss this plan with Joel, indicating that the procedure will be performed at the designated time. It is also important to explore pain management issues with Joel—does he usually use local anesthetic or other topical remedies to prevent pain at the site? If so, it will be necessary to make such arrangements in advance, possibly now, so his pain is managed appropriately. As the nurse, it is appropriate to discuss a delay in obtaining the laboratory results with Dr. Lung and the reasons for the delay. As workers on the pediatric floor, it is important for medical and nursing staff to communicate effectively. If this arrangement does not suit Dr. Lung's time frame for accomplishing certain tasks, one might suggest a trade-off. The nurse may draw the blood in the treatment room after preparations are made and Joel agrees on a time. Remember, however, that school-age children are prone to "bargain" for more time to delay or prevent the event because it is painful. One must be gently firm about the agreed-on time of the procedure and not allow further delays to accommodate the child who just does not want the procedure performed—ever, in most cases.

4. Yes, there is sufficient evidence to support these decisions and the plan of action.

CHAPTER 23

Croup Syndrome

1. Yes, there are sufficient data to arrive at a possible conclusion in this situation.
2. a. Epiglottitis is a serious obstructive inflammatory process that occurs in children 2 to 8 years of age.
   b. Symptoms of epiglottitis include throat pain, restlessness, and drooling, and the child usually prefers to sit upright rather than lie down.
   c. Because epiglottitis can quickly progress to severe respiratory distress, the nurse should never examine the child's throat with a tongue depressor or take a throat culture.
   d. Nursing interventions for the child with epiglottitis include monitoring the child's respiratory status, allowing the child to remain in the position that is most comfortable, preparing to administer a racemic epinephrine (nebulized) aerosol treatment, having emergency airway equipment available, and assisting with insertion of an intravenous line and administration of antibiotics.

3. The suspicion of epiglottitis constitutes an emergency. The priorities for nursing care at this time are to maintain the child's airway, keep the child comfortable, and reassure the child and parent. An antipyretic may be administered for the fever as per standing practitioner's orders.
4. Yes, the evidence supports the conclusion.

CHAPTER 24

Diarrhea

1. Yes, there are sufficient data for the nurse practitioner to arrive at some conclusions.
2. a. See Table 24-3, Evaluating Extent of Dehydration, and note the criteria for mild dehydration.
   b. Infants or children with mild dehydration are managed with oral rehydration therapy (ORT) and early reintroduction of an adequate diet. In cases of severe dehydration or when infants and children have uncontrollable vomiting, intravenous fluids are used in the management of acute diarrhea.
   c. Breastfeeding generally can be continued in mild dehydration.
   d. Antidiarrheal medications are not recommended for the treatment of acute infectious diarrhea. These medications have adverse effects such as slowed motility and can prolong the illness.
3. At present, Mary meets all the criteria for mild dehydration. It is highly probable that she has acute infectious diarrhea because her mother noted that she has had a "cold" for several days, she is vomiting and having diarrhea, and she has an elevated temperature. The priority for nursing care at this time is to provide rehydration via ORT. ORT is an effective, safe, and cost-effective way to treat mild dehydration. The nurse practitioner should provide the mother with instructions to give Mary oral rehydration solution at frequent intervals and in small amounts. The mother should also be instructed to continue with breastfeeding and normal feedings. Early reintroduction of normal nutrients is desirable in cases of mild dehydration; delayed introduction of food may be harmful and can prolong the illness. Mary's mother should also be told to avoid the use of antidiarrheal medications.
4. Yes, the evidence supports this initial plan of management.

Constipation

1. Yes, there are sufficient data to arrive at some conclusions for an initial plan of management.
2. a. Constipation in infancy can be caused by medical conditions such as Hirschsprung disease, hypothyroidism, or strictures, or it can be simple functional constipation.
   b. In infancy, changes in dietary practices such as a change from human milk to formula may precipitate functional constipation.
   c. Functional constipation is usually treated by dietary modifications such as increasing the amount of carbohydrate, fruit, or vegetables in the infant's diet.
3. Initially, the nurse practitioner can tell Harry's mother that functional constipation may occur with changes in the diet (e.g., the change from breastfeeding 6 weeks ago to bottle-formula feeding). The nurse practitioner can recommend that Harry's mother slowly introduce cereal and prune juice into Harry's diet. Cereal and one or two offerings of fruit juice each day may help to prevent further constipation. Often, simple measures such as the introduction of solid foods or other dietary modifications help to remedy functional constipation.

4. The initial data seem to point to the conclusion that Harry has functional constipation. However, the one episode of diarrhea and the two episodes of passage of ribbonlike stools do not usually occur with functional constipation.

Inflammatory Bowel Disease

1. Yes, there is sufficient evidence to arrive at some conclusions about what to include in Susan's discharge planning.
2. a. The goals of nutritional support for a patient with Crohn disease (CD) include (1) correction of nutrient deficits and replacement of ongoing losses, (2) provision of adequate energy and protein for healing, and (3) provision of adequate nutrients to support normal growth.
   b. See Gavage Feeding, Chapter 22 (pp. 695–698).
   c. Adolescents who are diagnosed with CD must adjust to the fact that they have a chronic illness that is characterized by remissions and exacerbations. CD may affect their activities of daily living, their social interactions with peers, and their ability to attend school. An important goal of therapy for adolescents with CD is to allow them to have as normal a lifestyle as possible.
3. The most immediate priority for discharge is to teach Susan and her family how to insert the nasogastric (NG) tube, how to administer the feedings, how to obtain the supplies needed for the tube feedings at home, and how to observe for any untoward effects of the NG feedings. As Susan's discharge nurse, you should have Susan and another family member insert the NG tube and demonstrate how to check the placement of the NG tube and how to start and stop the feedings while Susan is in the hospital. As Susan's nurse, you will also need to arrange before discharge for the appropriate vendors to deliver the feeding tube supplies and feeding pump to Susan's home so the supplies will be in place when Susan is discharged. While doing all this teaching, you should also be alert to any questions, worries, or anxieties that Susan or her family members may express.
4. Yes, Susan is to receive nighttime NG tube infusions at home, and her family has expressed a desire to perform this procedure at home. Therefore, this discharge teaching is needed and required.

CHAPTER 25

Cardiac Catheterization

1. Yes. This patient has just undergone an invasive diagnostic procedure. Bleeding is a potential risk after cardiac catheterization.
2. a. Complications after cardiac catheterization can include acute hemorrhage from the catheterization entry site, low-grade fever, nausea and vomiting, loss of pulses in the catheterized extremity, and transient dysrhythmias.
   b. Nausea and vomiting can occur after heart catheterization but are not directly related to acute blood loss. However, if the child had significant vomiting immediately after the procedure and was not able to keep his leg straight, the vomiting might have increased the chance of bleeding at the catheterization entry site.
   c. Significant blood loss can occur in a short time after the use of an artery for cardiac catheterization.
3. The first priority is to prevent bleeding. Pressure is applied above the visible catheterization site where the vessel was accessed. Place the child flat in bed to decrease the effect of gravity on the rate of bleeding. Notify the practitioner immediately. Replacement fluids may need to be administered, and pharmacologic control of emesis is important.

4. This may be an arterial bleed, and Tommy is at risk for losing a large amount of blood in a short time. Your first priority should be to control the bleeding. Appropriate measures are to treat the patient like a shock patient by immediately laying the child flat to help control bleeding.

Supraventricular Tachycardia

1. Yes. The infant has a history of poor feeding and irritability and has an abnormally fast heart rate that is nonvariable consistent with supraventricular tachycardia.
2. a. Clinical manifestations of congestive heart failure include irritability, tachypnea, poor feeding, and pallor.
   b. Because the infant is younger than 3 months old, an accurate temperature should be taken because of infants' increased risk for infection, which can also correlate with poor feeding and irritability. Newborns are at increased risk for meningitis and other community-acquired infections (both viral and bacterial) and have not been immunized against common organisms that could otherwise be tolerated in an older child.
   c. Supraventricular tachycardia (SVT) is the most common arrhythmia in the pediatric population and is characterized by a consistent heart rate greater than 200 beats/min. The QRS complex is narrow, and there is no variation in the rate.
3. The nurse should immediately assure that respiratory status is closely observed and that the infant maintains stable oxygen saturations above 95%. Oxygen therapy should be administered if there is any compromise in perfusion (as in this case). Blood pressure should be monitored closely. A practitioner should immediately be notified because infants can tolerate SVT for 6 hours but then may rapidly deteriorate. If no intravenous (IV) access is readily accessible, a bag of ice may be placed on the infant's face or on the diaper region (femoral area) for 15 to 20 seconds to stimulate the vagal-dive reflex. Continuous cardiorespiratory monitoring should be in place. The practitioner, after IV access is obtained, may order adenosine if the infant remains in SVT.
4. Yes, the infant is in SVT, and following basic life support protocol, airway and respiratory management are the priority. In the case of stable SVT, vagal maneuvers and adenosine are the first line in management. If those interventions are unsuccessful, electrical cardioversion may be performed only in the presence of an experienced practitioner.

CHAPTER 27

Urinary Tract Infection and Constipation

1. Yes. Lisa's mother reports a history of constipation with large, hard-formed stools occurring only every 3 or 4 days. Lisa was diagnosed with a urinary tract infection (UTI) severe enough to be admitted to the hospital.
2. a. The structure of the lower urinary tract is believed to account for the increased incidence of bacteriuria in females.
   b. A history of hard, large stools occurring every 3 or 4 days is not a normal elimination pattern for 4-year-old children.
   c. A large stool mass within the colon is likely to cause pressure on the bladder and urethra and not allow the bladder to empty completely. Stasis of the urine can lead to infection.
3. The first priority at this time is to begin treatment for the UTI. Lisa's diet and fluid intake should be evaluated and a plan developed to prevent constipation in the future.
4. Yes. Lisa's history reflects chronic problems with constipation that must be addressed.

CHAPTER 28

Hydrocephalus

1. Yes. Emma's fussiness, holding the back of her head, intermittent periods of lethargy, and repetitive, rapid eye blinking are signs of increased intracranial pressure (ICP).
2. a. Emma's posterior fossa tumor removal places her at risk for cerebral edema with associated increased ICP.
   b. Emma's external ventricular drainage (EVD) may be occluded and should be assessed. Positioning of the EVD is important to evaluate because the cerebrospinal fluid (CSF) drains by gravity; repositioning may be necessary to promote adequate drainage and decrease ICP.
   c. The physical signs and behavior are indicative of increased ICP, which may occur if Emma's EVD is obstructed or is draining improperly. There is evidence that CSF is draining on the mother's clothing, which is an abnormal finding with an EVD; the EVD is a closed system, and breakage or malfunction may cause the child further harm if bacteria colonize the reservoir.
3. The nurse should inspect the EVD site, assess Emma's neurologic status, and notify the medical provider of the findings. A transparent dressing should be placed over the EVD site to observe for CSF drainage, an abnormal finding. The EVD should remain positioned so that gravity drainage of CSF is enhanced (at the level of the external auditory meatus with the head at a 20- to 30-degree elevation); rapid CSF drainage is undesirable because it may result in subdural complications. A computed tomography scan may be useful in determining the status of the drainage device.
4. Yes. Emma's signs of increased ICP and CSF drainage on her mother's clothes support the nurse's actions.

CHAPTER 29

Type 1 Diabetes Mellitus

1. Yes. Shelly has had five hospital admissions for diabetic ketoacidosis (DKA) in the past year. Numerous factors must be involved with her unstable disease.
2. a. The normal tasks of adolescence can play a significant role in blood glucose instability.
   b. Adolescent girls with diabetes have frequent fluctuations of blood glucose levels immediately before, during, or after their menses.
   c. Shelly's personal loss from the divorce, her mother's absence because of a heavy work schedule, and the added responsibilities of the household may cause significant stress, resulting in elevated blood glucose levels.
   d. Careful, frequent, consistent monitoring of blood glucose levels is essential for effective insulin management during adolescence.
3. The first priority would be to focus directly on the issues of hyperglycemia. Determination of Shelly's practice of monitoring and managing her diabetes at home is essential. Areas of diabetes management that should be emphasized include careful dietary management, an appropriate exercise program, conscientious self-testing of blood glucose, appropriate administration of daily insulin, and adherence to sliding-scaling insulin therapy. Discussion of the emotional stressors she identifies at this time is appropriate.
4. Yes, Shelly's history of DKA over the past year supports her inability to monitor and manage her diabetes.

A

Abdomen
  auscultation of, 136
  contour of, 135
  distention of, 808b
  examination of, 134–136, 135f–136f
  in Down syndrome, 577b
  movement of, 135
  of neonate, 199, 203t–206t
    circumference of, 192
    contour of, 199
  palpation of, 136, 136b, 137f
Abdominal migraine, 784
Abdominal pain
  colicky, 808b
  paroxysmal, in infant, 367–368, 368b, 368f
  recurrent (functional), 178, 784–785
    management of, 784
Abdominal thrusts, subdiaphragmatic, 759, 759f
Abdominal wall, defects of, 807t
Abducens nerve, assessment of, 141f, 142t
Ablation, radiofrequency, for supraventricular
    tachycardia, 854
ABO incompatibility, 264, 265t
Abrasion(s), 1013
  in maltreated child, 450b
Abscess, Brodie, 1079
Absence seizures, 958b–959b, 959t. See also
    Seizure(s).
Absolute neutrophil count, 870t
  calculation of, 890b
Absorption, defects of, 813
Abstinence, sexual, 512t–514t
Abuse
  child characteristics and, 447
  emotional, 446, 449, 450b, 451
  environmental characteristics and, 447
  parental characteristics and, 447
  physical, 446–447, 449, 450b, 451, 452b
    factors predisposing to, 446
  prevention of, 453–454
  sexual. See Sexual abuse.
  substance. See Substance abuse.
  suspected, assessment data in, 453b
  warning signs of, 449b
Abusers, characteristics of, 447–448
ABVD regimen, for Hodgkin lymphoma, 893
Acceptance, in chronic illness/disability, 544
Accessory nerve, assessment of, 141f, 142t
Accessory skin structures, examination of,
    119–120
Accidental decannulation, in tracheostomy, 693
Accommodation, pupillary, 121
Accomplishment, sense of, in school-age child,
    459
Acetabular dysplasia, in developmental dysplasia
    of hip, 1068, 1068f

Acetaminophen
  for fever, 651
  for pain, 162, 163t
  poisoning with, 438b–439b
Acetone breath, 993
Achilles reflex, 141f
Achondroplasia, 507
Acid mantle, of neonatal skin, 210, 244
Acid-base imbalance, in neonate, 277–279, 277t,
    279t
Acid-base ratio, altered, 279
Acid-base status, assessment of, 277t
Acidosis, 277
  metabolic, in chronic renal failure, 921
Acne, 1035–1036
Acne vulgaris, 1035
Acoustic feedback, of hearing aid, 580–581
Acoustic nerve, assessment of, 141f, 142t
Acquaintance rape, definition of, 516b
Acquired immunodeficiency syndrome (AIDS),
    894–897. See also Human immunodeficiency
    virus (HIV) infection.
Acrodynia, 441
Acromegaly, 979
Activated charcoal, for poisoning, 440
Activities of daily living (ADL)
  in chronic illness/disability, 552
  in juvenile rheumatoid arthritis, 1086
Activity and exercise
  for adolescent, 490–491, 491f
  for infant, 330
  for neonate, 201, 202t
  for obesity, 522–523
  for preschooler, 418–419, 419t
  for school-age child, 468–469, 469f
  for toddler, 393–394
  in cognitive impairment, 573–574, 573f–574f
  progressive, after congenital heart disease
    surgery, 847
Acute chest syndrome, in sickle cell anemia, 874
Acute lung injury, 733–734
Acute lymphoid leukemia, 889
Acute myelogenous leukemia, 889
Acute pain. See also Pain entries.
  assessment of, 145–151, 145f, 146t–150t
Acute poststreptococcal glomerulonephritis, 915,
    915b
Acute renal failure, 919–921
  complications of, 919–921
  diagnosis of, 919, 919b
  nursing care management for, 920b, 921
  pathophysiology of, 919
  prognosis of, 921
  treatment of, 919–921
Acute respiratory distress syndrome, 733–734
Acyclovir
  for herpes simplex infection, 233–234
  for immunocompromised child, 423–431
Addiction
  fear of, 880b
  to opioids, 175b, 563
Addison disease, 988–989, 988b
Adenohypophysis (anterior pituitary), 974t–976t

Adenoidectomy, 715–716
Adequate Intake (AI), of nutrients, 99, 103b
Adherence, 646–647
Adhesives, in neonatal skin care, 244b–245b
Adipose brown tissue, in neonate, 186
Admission
  assessment for, 618, 619b–620b
  emergency, 631, 632b
  guidelines for, 621b
  preparation for, 618–621, 621f
  to intensive care unit, 631–633, 631f, 633b
Adolescent(s)
  adoptive parents of, 36
  biologic development of, 477–481, 477b–478b,
    479f–480f
  body art and, 492
  body image of, self-concept and, 486–487, 488t
  chronic illness/disability in, developmental
    effects of, 546t–547t
  cognitive development of, 482, 488t
  communication with, 92, 483b
  concepts of and reactions to death in,
    558t–559t
  contraception for, 511–514, 512t–514t
  definition of, 477
  dental health of, 491
  eating disorders in, 517–527. See also specific
    disorder.
  eating habits and behavior of, 489–490, 490f
  eczema in, 1033, 1033b
  family rules for, 495b
  family-centered care for, 495, 495b
  firearms and, 494–495
  goiter in, 983
  growth and development of, 477–487
    altered, 507–508, 508t
  growth patterns of, 478–481, 488t
    sex differences in, 478–481
  health promotion for, 487–495
  hearing in, 491
  hyperlipidemia in, 490
  hypertension in, 490
  immunizations for, 488–489
  informed consent of, 637
  injury prevention in, 493–495, 494b
  interests and activities of, 484–485, 484f
  interviewing of, 487b
  loss of control in, 616
  moral development of, 482
  nutrition for, 489–490, 490f
  obesity in, 490, 517–523, 518f, 520b–522b
  pelvic inflammatory disease in, 514–516
  personal care of, 491–492
  physical examination of, 107t
  physiologic changes in, 481
  posture of, 491–492
  pregnant, 511
  preparation of, for procedures, 639b–640b
  privacy for, 487b
  psychosocial development of, 481–482, 488t
  relationships of
    with parents, 483, 488t
    with peers, 483–484, 484f, 488t

Page numbers followed by *f* indicate figures;
t, tables; *b*, boxes.

Adolescent(s) (Continued)
reproductive disorders in, 508–510
rest for, 490–491
safety promotion for, 493–495
separation anxiety in, 615
sexual assault (rape) of, 516–517, 516b–517b
sexual maturation of, 477–478, 477b–478b. See also Puberty.
in boys, 478, 480f
in girls, 477–478, 479f–480f
sexuality of, 485–486, 485f, 488t
cognitive impairment and, 575
education and guidance in, 493
problems related to, 510–517
sexually transmitted disease in, 514, 515t
sleep and activity in, 490–491, 491f
social development of, 483–485, 484f
spiritual development of, 482–483
sports injuries in, 495
stress reduction for, 492, 492b, 492f
substance abuse by, 527–531
suicide by, 531–533, 531b–532b
tanning by, 492
vehicular injuries and, 493–494
vision in, 491
Adolescent Pediatric Pain Tool (APPT), 156
Adoption, 35–37, 36f
adolescence and, 36
cross-racial and international, 36–37
issues of origin in, 36
Adrenal cortex, hormones of, 974t–976t, 987
Adrenal crisis, 987
Adrenal disorder(s), 987–992
acute adrenocortical insufficiency, 987–988, 987b
chronic adrenocortical insufficiency, 988–989, 988b
congenital adrenal hyperplasia, 990–991
Cushing syndrome, 989–990, 989b, 989f
pheochromocytoma, 991–992
Adrenal hyperplasia, congenital, 990–991
Adrenal medulla, hormones of, 974t–976t, 987
Adrenarche, 477–478
Adrenocortical insufficiency
acute, 987–988, 987b
chronic (Addison disease), 988–989, 988b
Adrenocorticotropic hormone (ACTH), 974t–976t, 977b
Adult(s), cognitive impairment in, 572t
Advanced life support (ALS), 755
Adventitious sounds, 132
Advocacy, family, 9, 9b
Aerosol therapy, 680
Affect, in cognitive development, 319–320
African-American families
and relationship with health care providers, 52
health beliefs and practices of, 58t–59t
Aganglionic megacolon, congenital, 779
Age
bone, 68
developmental, 65b
gestational
clinical assessment of, 189–201, 190b, 190f–191f
weight related to, 189–192
parental, 32
Agglutinogens, 263

Aggression, in preschooler, 416–417
Agnosia, 580
Air bags, death from, 348
Airborne precautions, in infection control, 653, 654b
Airway, in cardiopulmonary resuscitation, 757–758, 758f
Airway clearance therapy, for cystic fibrosis, 749–750, 750f
Airway obstruction, 758–759
by foreign body, 731–732
in asthma, 737, 737f
in children, 759, 759f
in infants, 758–759, 759f
Airway patency, in neonate, 206–207
Akinetic seizures, 958b–959b. See also Seizure(s).
Alcohol
adolescent use of, 528–529, 528b
intrauterine exposure to, 289, 296t
Alertness, definition of, 928
Alkalosis, 277
Allele, 80
Allergens
exposure to, 359
food, definition of, 358
in asthma
avoidance of, 744
control of, 739
Allergic reaction(s)
as contraindication to immunization, 341
history of, 97, 97b
to food, 358, 359b–361b. See also specific food.
to latex, in spina bifida, 1104, 1104b
Allografts (homografts), for burns, 1043
All-terrain vehicle injuries, prevention of, 472
Alopecia, 1031t
chemotherapy-induced, 892
Alternate cover test, 123, 123f
Alveolar unit, prenatal development of, 262–263, 268f
Ambiguous genitalia, 990
gender assignment in, 990–991
Amblyopia, 122, 584b–585b
photoscreening for, 123
Ambulation aids, for spinal cord injuries, 1116
Ambulatory blood pressure monitoring, 115, 115t
Ambulatory care, 629–630
discharge from, 630b
Amelia, 1072
Amenorrhea, 508–509
American Nurses Association Code of Ethics for Nurses (2001), 556
American Sign Language, 582
American Spinal Injury Association Impairment Scale, 1115b
5-Aminosalicylates, for inflammatory bowel disease, 790
Amish families, and relationship with health care providers, 53
Amnesia, in head trauma, 939
Amniocentesis, 265
Amniotic band syndrome, 1072
Amoxicillin, for otitis media, 718
Amputation, 1066
Amylase, 309–314
Anaclitic depression, 613
Anal patency, in neonate, 199

Anal reflex, 138
Anal stage, in psychosexual development, 71, 71t
Analgesia
adjuvant, 162–163
administration of, routes and methods of, 166b–167b
effectiveness of, 172–173
epidural, 168
for circumcision, 212
for leukemia, 890
for postoperative headache, 948
patient-controlled, 163–164, 168f
mode of administration of, 163
preemptive, 177
transdermal, 168, 168f
transmucosal, 168
Analgesic patches, in pain management, 169b
Anaphylaxis, 862–863
emergency management of, 360b
food allergy, 360b
Androgens, in puberty, 477
Anemia, 869–872
aplastic, 882–883, 883b
classification of, 869, 871b, 871f
consequences of, 869
Cooley (β-thalassemia), 881–882, 882b
definition of, 869
diagnosis of, 869, 870t, 871b
in acute renal failure, 920
in chronic renal failure, 922–923
in leukemia, 889
prevention of, 891
iron-deficiency, 872–873
nursing care management for, 869–872
physiologic, in infancy, 309
sickle cell, 873–881. See also Sickle cell anemia.
treatment of, 869
Anencephaly, 1098, 1099b
Anesthesia
for circumcision, 212
induction of, parental presence during, 644, 644f
Anesthetic cream, 168
Anger, in chronic illness/disability, 544
Angiography
digital subtraction, of cerebral function, 933t–934t
renal, 905t–906t
Angiotensin-converting enzyme (ACE) inhibitors, for congestive heart failure, 835
Animal bites, 1024–1030
in infancy, 347t–348t
Animal safety, 1030b
Animism, 416
Anisometropia, 584b–585b
Ankle-foot orthosis, in cerebral palsy, 1093
Ann Arbor staging system, for Hodgkin lymphoma, 893
Anoplasty, for anorectal malformations, 812
Anorectal malformations, 810–812, 811b, 811f
Anorexia
chemotherapy-induced, 891
physiologic, in toddler, 390
Anorexia nervosa, 523
case study of, 525b
characteristics of, 524t
clinical manifestations of, 524b

Antacids, for peptic ulcer disease, 793
Antegrade continence enema, 1101–1102
Anterior cord syndrome, 1114
Anthropometry, 102
Antibiotics
    for acne, 1036
    for conjunctivitis, 208
    for inflammatory bowel disease, 790
    for otitis media, 718
    for sepsis, 283
    intravenous, for cystic fibrosis, 750
    prophylactic
        for infective bacterial endocarditis, 848–849,
            849b
        for ophthalmia neonatorum, 208
        for puncture wounds, 1029
        for rheumatic fever, 849–850
    topical, for burns, 1042–1043
Antibodies, in neonate, 188
Anticholinergics, for asthma, 740
Anticipatory grief, 249, 565
Anticipatory guidance
    in care of families, 350
    in communication, 89
Anticonvulsants, for seizures, 960
Anti-D antibody therapy, for idiopathic
        thrombocytopenic purpura, 887, 887b
Antidepressants, tricyclic, for cancer pain, 180
Antidiuretic hormone (ADH). See Vasopressin
        (antidiuretic hormone).
Antidotes, for poisoning, 440
Antiemetics, 782
Antiepileptic agents
    for cerebral palsy, 1094
    rectal preparations of, 965
Antigens, 263
Antihemophilic factor, 884
Antihistamines, for atopic dermatitis, 1034
Antilymphocyte globulin, for aplastic anemia,
        883
Antipyretics, for fever, 651
Antiretroviral agents, for human
        immunodeficiency virus infection, 895–896
Antiseptic agents, in neonatal skin care,
        244b–245b
Antistreptolysin O titer, in rheumatic fever, 849
Antithymocyte globulin, for aplastic anemia, 883
Anus. See also Anal entries.
    examination of, 138
    imperforate, 811, 811f
Anxiety
    in school-age child, 505
    separation
        in hospitalization, 613–615, 613b, 613f–614f
            prevention or minimization of, 621
        in infant, 321
Aortic coarctation, 827, 828b–829b
Aortic stenosis, 828b–829b
    subvalvular, 828b–829b
    valvular, 828b–829b
Aortic valves, 133
Apgar scoring system, in neonatal assessment,
        189, 189t
Aphasia, 580
Apheresis, 899–900
Aphthous stomatitis, 433
Apical impulse (AI), 132

Aplastic anemia, 882–883, 883b
Aplastic crisis, 874
Apnea, 754
    of prematurity, 273t–274t
    sleep, 369–370
        obstructive, 754
Apnea monitors, 373, 373b
    electrode placement for, 373–374, 374f
Apparent life-threatening event (ALTE), in
        infant, 372–374
    diagnosis of, 372–373
    family support for, 374
    nursing care management for, 373–374, 374f
    treatment of, 373, 373b
Appendectomy, 786
Appendicitis, 785–786, 785b
    nursing care plan for, 787b–788b
Appendix
    ruptured, 786
    vermiform, 785
Approach behaviors, 542, 543b
Appropriate for gestational age (AGA), 191, 191f
Arab families, and relationship with health care
        providers, 52
Arm circumference, measurement of, 111
Arm restraints, 656, 657f
Arm strength, 140
Arrhythmia(s), 134, 853–854, 854b. See also
        specific type.
    classification of, 853
Arterial blood sampling, 662
Arteriovenous fistula, in dialysis, 924
Arteriovenous graft, in dialysis, 924
Arthritis
    in Kawasaki disease, 859–860
    rheumatoid, juvenile, 1084–1086
    septic, 1080–1081
Arthrodesis, 1078
Arthropod bites, 1024–1028, 1025t–1026t, 1026f
Ascariasis (roundworm), 434t
Ascites, 913
    management of, 798
Aseptic (nonbacterial) meningitis, 953–954,
        954t
Asian-American families, and relationship with
        health care providers, 52
Asphyxia, in infancy, 347t–348t
Aspiration
    bone marrow, positioning for, 658
    child safety home checklist for, 349b
    foreign body, 731–732
        in toddler, 397t–398t, 403
    in infancy, 345b–346b
    in submersion injury, 945
    pneumonia due to, 732–733, 945
    suprapubic, 661–662, 662b, 908
Aspirin
    for Kawasaki disease, 859
    poisoning with, 438b–439b
Assisted suicide, 555–556
Associative play, 76, 77f
Asthma, 724t, 736–747
    allergens in, avoidance of, 744
    bronchospasm in, relief of, 744–747, 746f
    clinical manifestations of, 738b
    diagnosis of, 738–739
    etiology of, 736–737, 737b

Asthma (Continued)
    exercise-induced, 740
    management of
        acute care plan in, 742b, 743–744, 743f
        allergen control in, 739
        breathing exercises in, 740–741, 747
        drug therapy in, 739–740
        hyposensitization in, 741
    nursing care plan for, 743–747, 745b
    prognosis of, 741–743
    self-care in, 747
    severity of, classification of, 736, 736b
    status asthmaticus in, 741
    triggers for, 737b
Astigmatism, 584b–585b
Astrocytoma, 946
Ataxic movement, in cerebral palsy, 1091, 1092b
Athlete's foot, 1020t
Atonic seizures, 958b–959b. See also Seizure(s).
Atopic dermatitis (eczema), 1032–1034, 1033b,
        1033f
    in Wiskott-Aldrich syndrome, 897
Atopy, 359
Atraumatic care, 8–9
Atresia
    biliary, 798–800, 799b
    esophageal, 803–805, 803f
        long-gap, 804
    tricuspid, 830b–831b
Atrial septal defect, 826b–827b
Atrioventricular canal defect, 826b–827b
Atrioventricular valves, 133
Attachment, development of, in infancy, 320–321,
        320f
Attachment behaviors, of neonate, 202, 202b
Attention-deficit/hyperactivity disorder, 501–504,
        503b
    definition of, 501
    diagnosis of, 501–502, 502b
    nursing care management for, 504
    treatment of, 502–504, 504b
Atypical pneumonia, 726. See also Pneumonia.
Auditory acuity
    in infant, 315
    in neonate, 188
Auditory imperception, central, 580
Auditory nerve, assessment of, 141f, 142t
Auditory sense, in coma, 938
Auditory tests, 127, 128t
Augmentation enterocystoplasty, 1101
Aural temperature, measurement of, 113t
Auricle, inspection of, 125
Auscultation
    effective, 131b
    in cardiovascular dysfunction, 821
    of abdomen, 136
    of breath sounds, in neonate, 197–198
    of heart, 133–134
        sequence of sounds in, 134t
    of lungs, 131–132, 131b
Autism, immunization and, 335b
Autism spectrum disorders, 590–593
    clinical manifestations of, 592
    diagnosis of, 591b, 592
    etiology of, 590–591
    family support in, 593
    nursing care management for, 593

Autism spectrum disorders (Continued)
  prognosis of, 592–593
  thimerosal-containing vaccines and, 592b
Automatic implantable cardioverter defibrillator, 856
Automobile safety
  for infant, 344–348, 344f, 345b–346b, 347t–348t
    high-risk, 251–252
  for toddler, 396–401
  in chronic illness/disability, 552
Automobile-related injuries, 3, 5f
  of adolescent, 493–494, 494b
  of school-age child, 472t–473t
  of toddler, 397t–398t, 400–401
  to spinal cord, 1114–1115
Autonomic dysreflexia, 1115, 1117
Autonomic system, of neonate, 188
Autonomy, 11
  of special needs adolescent, 554
  of special needs child, 553
  sense of, in toddler, 380
  vs. shame and doubt, in psychosocial development, 71t, 72
Autopsy, 565
Avoidance behaviors, 542, 543b
Avulsion, tooth, 470
  emergency treatment for, 471b
Axillary sensor thermometer, 116b
Axillary temperature
  measurement of, 113t
  of neonate, 192, 192f
Axillary thermometer, infrared, 193
Azotemia, 919
Azotorrhea, in cystic fibrosis, 747

B
Babinski reflex, 139, 200, 200f, 932
Baby bottle tooth decay, 395–396, 396f
Baby food, commercially prepared, 328
Baby-Friendly Hospital Initiative (BFHI), 215
Bacille Calmette-Guérin (BCG) vaccine, 731
Back blows, for airway obstructions, 758–759, 759f
Baclofen pump, for cerebral palsy, 1094
Bacterial endocarditis, infective, 848–849, 848b–849b
Bacterial infections, cutaneous, 1017, 1018f, 1018t
Bacterial meningitis, 950–952
  cerebrospinal fluid analysis in, 954t
  clinical manifestations of, 950, 951b
  diagnosis of, 950–951
  nursing care management for, 952
  pathophysiology of, 950
  prevention of, 952, 953b
  prognosis of, 952
  treatment of, 951–952
Bacterial overgrowth, in short-bowel syndrome, 815
Bacterial pneumonia, 726. See also pneumonia.
Bacterial tracheitis, 721t, 723
Bacteriuria
  asymptomatic, 906
  symptomatic, 906
Bad breath, assessment of, in respiratory function, 709b

Balance, cerebellar control of, 140
Balances suspension traction, 1063
Baptism, of high-risk neonate, 253
Barbiturates, coma caused by, 937
Bariatric surgery, for obesity, 521
Barrel chest, 129
Barrier methods, of contraception, 512t–514t
Basal metabolic rate (BMR), 763–764
Basilar fracture, of skull, 940
Bathing, 648–649
  of neonate, 209–210, 211f
    at high risk, 244b–245b
Bathing trunk nevus, 234
Baths, in dermatitis, 1016
Bed wetting (enuresis), 499, 500b. See also Urinary incontinence.
Bedding, soft, sudden infant death syndrome and, 370
Bee stings, 1024, 1025t–1026t
Behavior(s)
  approach, 542, 543b
  avoidance, 542, 543b
  examination of, 119
  of neonate, 194, 219
    assessment of, 201–202, 201b
    attachment, 202, 202b
    in Brazelton Neonatal Behavioral Assessment Scale, 201, 201b
    stressed/fatigued, 280t
  of school-age child
    dishonest, 466–467
    disorders of, 501–507, 502b
  parental, in chronic illness/disability, responses to, 547
  personal-social, 384
    of preschooler, 410–411, 411f
  posthospital, 616b
  related to divorce, 38b
Behavior modification theory, positive and negative reinforcement in, 34
Behavior problems, in cerebral palsy, 1094
Behavioral contract
  in eating disorders, 526
  in pain management, 160b
Behavioral methods, of contraception, 512t–514t
Behavioral Pain Assessment Scales, 146t–147t
Behavioral Pain Score (BPS), 146t–147t
Behavioral restraints, 656
Behavioral signs, in cognitive impairment, 571b
Behavioral strategies, in compliance, 647
Behavioral therapy
  cognitive, for eating disorders, 525
  for attention-deficit/hyperactivity disorder, 503
  for obesity, 522
Beneficence, 11
Benzoyl peroxide, for acne, 1036
Beta-adrenergic agonists, for asthma, 740
Beta-blockers, for congestive heart failure, 835
Bibliotherapy, in communication with children, 93
Biculture, 49. See also Culture.
Bicycle injuries, 4
  prevention of, 472, 472f
Bicycle safety, 474b
Bike walker, in cerebral palsy, 1093, 1093f
Biliary atresia, 798–800, 799b
Bilingual education, 49

Bilirubin, 257
  conjugated, 257
  excessive. See Hyperbilirubinemia.
  neurotoxicity of, 260
  unconjugated, 257, 259–260
Bilirubin encephalopathy, 260
Bilirubinometry, transcutaneous, 258
Bill of Rights, for children and teens, 623b
Binocularity, 315
Binuclear family, 27
Bioavailability, of micronutrients, in human milk, 214
Biochemical tests, in nutritional assessment, 102
Biologic agents, for juvenile rheumatoid arthritis, 1085
Biologic development, 309–317
  of adolescent, 477–481, 477b–478b, 479f–480f
  of infant
    fine motor skills in, 315, 315f
    gross motor skills in, 315–317
    head control in, 315, 316f
    locomotion in, 317, 318f
    maturation of systems in, 309–315
    proportional changes in, 309, 310t–314t
    rolling over in, 315–316, 317f
    sitting in, 316, 317f
  of preschooler, 408, 408f
  of school-age child, 458–459, 458f
  of toddler, 379–380
    gross and fine motor development in, 379–380
    maturation of systems in, 379
    proportional changes in, 379
    sensory changes in, 379
Biologic skin coverings, for burns, 1043
Biologic therapies, for inflammatory bowel disease, 790
Biopsy, renal, 905t–906t
Birth(s)
  circulatory changes at, 823–824, 824f
  multiple, 30–31, 30f, 31t. See also Twins.
  and subsequent children, 221–222, 222f
  parental adjustment to, 31
Birth defects, 1068–1074. See also specific defect.
Birth history, 96
Birth injury(ies), 229–232, 230f–232f
Birth order, 29–30
Birth weight, assessment of, 189–192, 191f
Birthmarks, 234–235, 234f
Bisexual family, 27–28
Bismuth compounds, for peptic ulcer disease, 793
Bites
  animal, 1024–1030
    in infancy, 347t–348t
  arthropod, 1024–1028, 1025t–1026t, 1026f
  human, 1030
    by infant, 319
Bitterness, in chronic illness/disability, 544
Black eye (hematoma), 586b
Black widow spider bites, 1025t–1026t
Blackhead (open comedone), 1035
Bladder capacity, in school-age child, 458
Bladder catheterization, in urine collection, 660–662, 660t, 661b–662b
Bladder chemistry, in urinary tract infections, 908

Bladder control
  in spina bifida, 1101
  in spinal cord injuries, 1117
  nighttime, 387
Bladder dysfunction, neuropathic, 1101
Bladder exstrophy, 912t
Bladder temperature, measurement of, 112b
Bladder ultrasonography, 905t–906t
Blanket swaddling, 246
Bleeding. See Hemorrhage.
Blended (reconstituted) family, 27, 39
Blepharitis, 1035
Blindness, legal, 584
Blisters, fever, 433, 1019t
Blood glucose testing
  in diabetes mellitus, 995–996, 995t, 1003–1004,
    1004f
  minimizing pain of, 1003b
Blood group incompatibility, hemolytic disease
    of newborn and, 263–264
Blood lead levels, 434t
  reduction of, 445b
Blood pressure. See also Hypertension;
    Hypotension.
  in neonate, at high risk, 235–236
  in neurologic examination, 930
  measurement of, 115–118, 115t
    cuff selection in, 116–117, 116t, 117f
    in neonate, 193, 193f
    interpretation in, 117–118
    sites for, 116–117, 117f, 117t
  postoperative, 645t
Blood pressure cuff, selection of, 116–117, 116t,
    117f
Blood pressure tables, 118b
Blood sampling, 662–664
  arterial, 662
  capillary, 662
  from central venous catheters, 663b
  heel lance for, 662–664, 664b, 664f
  venous, 662. See also Venipuncture.
Blood test(s)
  Guthrie, 298–299
  of renal function, 908t
Blood transfusions. See Transfusion(s).
Blood volume, of neonate, 186–187
Blue spells, 841
Bodily injury
  child safety home checklist for, 349b
  fear of, in hospitalization, 623–624
  of adolescent, 494b
  of infant, 345b–346b
  of school-age child, prevention of, 472t–473t
  of toddler, 397t–398t, 403
Body art, in adolescence, 492
Body fluids, distribution of, 763–771
Body image, development of, 74–75
  in adolescent, 486–487, 488t
  in infant, 320, 320f
  in preschooler, 409–410
  in school-age child, 464, 465t–466t
  in toddler, 383
Body mass index (BMI), 517–518
  calculation of, 520
  in adolescent girls vs. boys, 479
Body surface area (BSA), 764
  in drug dosage determination, 665

Body systems, maturation of, 309–315
Body temperature. See Temperature.
Bone(s)
  formation of, 68
  healing of, 1058
  in school-age child, 458
  infection of, 1079–1081
  long, birth-related fracture of, 231
  ossification of, 68
  shape of, 139
Bone age, 68
  growth disorders and, 978, 978b
Bone marrow aspiration, positioning for, 658
Bone remodeling, 1058
Bone tumors, 1081, 1081b
Books, for hospitalized child, 625
Booster seats, 398–399, 399f
Bossing, 967
  frontal, 968
Boston brace, 1077
Bottle feeding. See Formula feeding.
Botulinum toxin A, for cerebral palsy, 1093–1094
Botulism, 1113–1114, 1113b
  infant, 1113–1114
Botulism immune globulin, intravenous,
    1113–1114
Bowel control
  in spina bifida, 1101–1102
  in spinal cord injuries, 1117
Bowel elimination
  in home care, 702
  ostomies in, 702
  problems of, 499–501, 500b
Bowel training, 387
Bowen's family systems theory, 24
Bowleg (genu varum), 139, 139f
Brace
  Boston, 1077
  Charleston nighttime bending, 1077
  for scoliosis, 1077–1078, 1077f
  halo, 1063–1064
  Wilmington, 1077
Brachial palsy, in neonate, 231–232, 232f
Bradydysrhythmias, 853–854
Braille, 587
Brain. See also Cerebral entries; specific part.
  nuclear scan of, 933t–934t
Brain death, establishing, 946b
Brain injury
  hypoxic-ischemic, 281t
  neuroinflicted, 446
Brain tumors, 946–949
Brainstem glioma, 946
Brazelton Neonatal Behavioral Assessment Scale,
    clusters of neonatal behaviors in, 201,
    201b
Breast(s)
  development of, 130, 477–478, 479f
  male, enlarged, 510
  neonatal, 197
  pubertal, 130
Breast milk, 214–215. See also Breastfeeding.
  donor, 241
  expressed, 241
  for infant, 326
Breast milk jaundice, 257t, 258
Breast pumping, 326–327

Breastfeeding, 215–216
  alternative to, 327. See also Formula(s);
    Formula feeding.
  atopy avoidance with, 360
  contraindications to, 215
  criteria promoting successful, 216, 216f
  growth patterns and, 108
  in first 6 months, 326–328
  in second 6 months, 328
  jaundice associated with, 257t, 258
  of high-risk neonate, 241
  successful, steps to, 215b
  with twins, 216, 216f
Breath
  acetone, 993
  odor of, 930
Breath sounds, 130
  classification of, 131b
  diminished or absent, 131–132
Breathing. See also Respiration(s).
  assessment of, in respiratory function, 709b
  deep, encouragement of, 131b
  obstructive sleep-disordered, 754
  patterns of, 132b
    in neurologic examination, 930
  periodic, in neonate, 197
Breathing exercises, for asthma, 740–741, 747
British antilewisite, as chelating agent, 444
British Sign Language, 582
Brodie abscess, 1079
Bronchial (postural) drainage, 689
Bronchiolitis, 723–725, 724t
Bronchitis, 723, 724t
Bronchodilators, for cystic fibrosis, 750
Bronchoprovocation test, in asthma, 738
Bronchopulmonary dysplasia, 273–277, 273t–274t
Bronchospasm
  exercise-induced, 740
  relief of, 744–747, 746f
Bronchus(i), conditions affecting, 724t
Broviac catheter, 675t
Brown fat, in neonate, 186
Brown recluse spider bites, 1025t–1026t, 1026f
Brown-Séquard syndrome, 1115
Brudzinski sign, 950
Bruises (ecchymoses), 450b, 1010
Bryant traction, 1063
Buck extension traction, 1063, 1063f
Buckle fracture, 1057b, 1057f
Buddhism, 61t–62t
Bulb syringe, for oropharyngeal suctioning, in
    neonate, 206–207
Bulimia, 523
  characteristics of, 524t
Bulla, 1011f
Bullying, 462, 505–506
  long-term consequences of, 462–463
Bupivacaine, for procedural pain, 176
Burns, 5, 5f, 1036–1047
  acute care for, 1045–1046
  allografts (homografts) for, 1043
  artificial skin for, 1044
  biologic skin coverings for, 1043
  characteristics of, 1037–1038
  chemical, 734, 1037
    to eye, 586b
  child safety home checklist for, 349b

Burns *(Continued)*
  complications of, 1038–1040
    prevention of, 1045–1047, 1046f
  cultured epithelium for, 1044
  débridement of, 1042
  depth of, 1037–1038, 1039f
    characteristics of, 1037–1038, 1039f
    classification of, 1039f
  distribution of, 1038f
  drug therapy for, 1042
  electrical, 1037
    in infancy, 347t–348t
    in toddler, 401
  emergency care for, 1040–1041, 1040b
  excision in, 1042
  extent of, 1037, 1039f
  fluid management in, 1041–1042
  fourth-degree, 1038
  full-thickness (third-degree), 1037, 1039f
  grading of, 1040t
  hydrotherapy for, 1042
  in adolescence, 494b
  in infancy, 345b–346b, 347t–348t
  in maltreated child, 450b
  in school-age child, prevention of, 472t–473t
  in toddler, 397t–398t, 401–402, 402f
  inhalation, 734–735, 1038
  long-term care for, 1046, 1046f
  major, 1038, 1040t
    treatment of, 1041–1044
  mesh graft for, 1043, 1044f
  minor, 1038, 1040t
    treatment of, 1041
  moderate, 1038, 1040t
  nursing care management for, 1044–1045
  nutritional support in, 1042
  ocular, 586b
  pain associated with, 177
  partial-thickness (second-degree), 1037, 1039f
  pathophysiology of, 1038–1040
  prevention of, 1047
  prognosis of, 1044
  psychologic interventions for, 177
  psychosocial support of child with, 1046–1047
  psychosocial support of family in, 1047
  sepsis in, 1040
  severity grading system of, 1040t
  severity of, 1038, 1040t
  sheet graft for, 1043, 1044f
  skin coverings for
    permanent, 1043, 1043f
    synthetic, 1043
  superficial (first-degree), 1037, 1039f
  topical antibiotics for, 1042–1043
  total body surface area of, 1037, 1038f
  treatment of, 1040–1044
  type of, 1037
  wound care for, 1045
  xenografts for, 1043

C

Cadaver kidney donor, 925
Café au lait spots, 234
Calcitonin, 981–982
Calcium imbalance
  in chronic renal failure, 921
  in infant, 356

Calcium intake
  for preschooler, 417
  for toddler, 392
Calendar method, of contraception, 512t–514t
Caloric test, 931
Campylobacter jejuni, diarrhea due to, 772t–774t
Cancer. *See* Neoplastic disease; *specific neoplasm.*
Candidiasis, 1020t
  in neonate, 232–233, 233f
  of diaper area, 1030–1032, 1032f
Capillary blood sampling, 662
Capillary (strawberry) hemangioma, 234, 234f
Capillary refill time test, 133
Capnometry, 689
Caput succedaneum, 229, 230f
Car seat/restraint
  for child with disabilities, 399–400
  for neonate, at high risk, 251–252, 252b
  for toddler, 396–400, 399f
Carbohydrate(s), in human milk, 214
Carbon dioxide monitoring, end-tidal, 689
Carbon dioxide narcosis, oxygen-induced, 688
Cardiac catheterization, in cardiovascular
      dysfunction, 821t–822t, 822, 823b
Cardiac demands, decreased, for congestive heart
      failure, 836, 839
Cardiac involvement, in Kawasaki disease,
      859
Cardiac resynchronization therapy, for congestive
      heart failure, 835
Cardiogenic shock, 860b
Cardiomyopathy, 855–856
  dilated, 855
  hypertrophic, 855
  restrictive, 855
Cardiopulmonary resuscitation (CPR), 755–758
  breaths in, 758, 758f
  chest compressions in, 757, 757f
  medications in, 758
  open airway in, 757–758, 758f
  pulse check in, 757, 757f
  resuscitation procedure in, 755–758, 756f
Cardiovascular dysfunction, 819–865. *See also*
      Heart disease.
  acquired, 848–856
  auscultation in, 821
  cardiac catheterization in, 821t–822t, 822,
      823b
  congenital, 823–830. *See also* Congenital heart
      disease.
  diagnosis of, 821–822, 821t
  echocardiography in, 821, 821t
  electrocardiography in, 821, 821t
  history of, 820–823
  inspection in, 820–821
  nursing care management for, 822–823
  palpation and percussion in, 821
  physical examination of, 820–823
Cardiovascular support, for shock, 861–862
Cardiovascular system
  effect of immobilization on, 1051t–1053t
  in neonate, complications of, 279, 280t
Cardioversion, synchronized, for supraventricular
      tachycardia, 854
Cardioverter defibrillator, automatic implantable,
      856
Carditis, in rheumatic fever, 850b

Caregiver-child interaction, maltreatment and,
      448–449
Caries. *See* Dental caries.
Casein (curds), 309–314
  in human milk, 214
Casts, 1059–1062
  application of, 1060
  care of, 1060–1062, 1061b
  construction of, 1060
  for clubfoot, 1072, 1072f
  for developmental dysplasia of hip, 1070,
      1070f
  for fractures, 1059b, 1060, 1060f
  removal of, 1061–1062, 1062f
  types of, 1061f
Cat scratch disease, 1030
Cataracts, 584b–585b
Catheter
  central, peripherally inserted, 674
  central venous, blood sampling from, 663b
  Foley, 660t
  Groshong, 675t
  nontunneled, 673
  safety, for parenteral fluid therapy, 682, 684f
  tracheostomy suction, 691, 691f
  tunneled (Hickman or Broviac), 675t
Catheter toes, 240
Catheterization
  bladder, in urine collection, 660–662, 660t,
      661b–662b
  cardiac, in cardiovascular dysfunction,
      821t–822t, 822, 823b
  clean intermittent, 1101
Causal relationship, in cognitive development,
      381, 409
Cavernous venous hemangioma, 234
CCR5 gene, 80–81
CD_4+ T cells, in human immunodeficiency virus
      infection, 895
Celiac disease (gluten-sensitive enteropathy),
      812–815, 813f, 814b
Cell phones, 50, 484, 484f
Cell-surface immunologic markers, in leukemia,
      889
Cellulitis, 1017, 1018f, 1018t
Centers for Disease Control and Prevention
      (CDC) classification, of human
      immunodeficiency virus infection, 895,
      895t
Central auditory imperception, 580
Central cord syndrome, 1114
Central nervous system depressants, adolescent
      use of, 529
Central nervous system prophylactic therapy, for
      leukemia, 889
Central nervous system stimulants, adolescent
      use of, 529
Central precocious puberty, 979, 980b
Central venous access device (CVAD), 673–676,
      675t
  long-term, 675, 675t, 676f
  short-term, 673
  site care for, 677b–678b
Central venous catheter, blood sampling from,
      663b
Cephalhematoma, 229, 230f
Cephalopelvic disproportion, 229

Cereal
  infant, 328
  iron-fortified, for toddler, 392
Cerebellum, function of, 140, 140b
Cerebral contusion, 940
Cerebral dysfunction, 927–970
  altered states of consciousness in, 928–929,
    929b, 930f
  assessment of
    diagnostic procedures in, 932–934,
      933t–934t
    neurologic examination in, 930–932,
      931f–932f
  general aspects of, 929–930
  in aseptic meningitis, 953–954, 954t
  in bacterial meningitis, 950–952, 951b, 953b
  in brain tumors, 946–949
  in cranial deformities, 966–967
  in encephalitis, 954–955, 954b
  in head trauma, 938–945
  in hydrocephalus, 936b, 967–970, 967f, 968b,
    969f
  in neuroblastoma, 949
  in rabies, 955
  in Reye syndrome, 956
  in seizures, 956–966, 957b–959b, 959t,
    962b–965b
    febrile, 966
  in submersion injury, 945–946
  increased intracranial pressure in, 928, 928f,
    929b
  nursing care in, 934–938
Cerebral edema, 941
Cerebral lacerations, 940
Cerebral malformation(s), 966–970
  cranial defects, 966–967
  hydrocephalus, 936b, 967–970, 967f, 968b,
    969f
Cerebral palsy, 1090–1098
  acceptance of, 1098b
  care plan for, 1095b–1096b
  clinical classification of, 1091, 1092b
  definition of, 1090
  diagnosis of, 1091–1092, 1092b
  early signs of, 1093b
  family support for, 1097–1098
  hospitalization in, 1098
  nursing care management for, 1095–1098,
    1097f
  pathophysiology of, 1091
  prevention of, 1095
  prognosis of, 1094–1095
  treatment of, 1092–1095, 1093f
Cerebral trauma, 938–945. See also Head trauma.
Cerebrospinal fluid, analysis of, in bacterial and
  viral meningitis, 954t
Cerebrovascular accident, in sickle cell anemia,
  874
Cerumen, 125
Cervical cap, 512t–514t
Charcoal, activated, for poisoning, 440
Charleston nighttime bending brace, 1077
Cheating, by school-age child, 467
Chelating agents, 444
Chelation therapy
  for heavy metal poisoning, 441
  for lead poisoning, 444, 445b

Chemical(s)
  defects caused by, 294–295, 296t
  use of, in health history, 97–98
Chemical burns, 734, 1037. See also Burns.
  to eye, 586b
Chemical irritants, skin lesions caused by,
  1022–1024
Chemical methods, of contraception,
  512t–514t
Chemically induced defects, in neonate, 294–295,
  296t
Chemotherapy
  for Hodgkin lymphoma, 893
  for leukemia, 891
  for neuroblastoma, 949
  for non-Hodgkin lymphoma, 894
  for osteosarcoma, 1081–1082
  for retinoblastoma, 590
  for Wilms tumor, 918
  lumbar puncture for, 179
Chest
  examination of, 129–130, 130f–131f
  of infant, 309
  of neonate, 197, 203t–206t
Chest circumference
  of neonate, 192
  of toddler, 379
Chest compressions, in cardiopulmonary
  resuscitation, 757, 757f
Chest pain, assessment of, in respiratory
  function, 709b
Chest physiotherapy, 689–690
  for cystic fibrosis, 749–750
  in Duchenne muscular dystrophy, 1109
Chest radiography, in cystic fibrosis, 749
Chest thrusts, for airway obstructions, 758–759,
  759f
Chest tube drainage, 693–694, 694f, 695b
Chest wall, movement of, 130, 131f
Cheyne-Stokes respiration, 564, 564b
Chickenpox (varicella), 424f, 424t–430t
  immunization against, 332f–333f, 337–338
  maternal infection with, 291t–292t
Chigger bites, 1025t–1026t
Chilblains, 1048
Child care facilities, alternate, for infants,
  323–324
Child center–based care, 323
Child health promotion, social, cultural, and
  religious influences on, 43–63. See also
  Cultural entries; Culture; Religious beliefs;
  Social entries; Socialization.
Child pornography, 447
Child prostitution, 447
Child safety home checklist, 349b
Childhood
  hearing impairment in, 581–584, 582b
  visual impairment in, 586–587
Childhood eczema, 1033, 1033b
Childhood morbidity, 8
Childhood mortality, 7–8, 7t
Childrearing practices, temperament related to,
  310t–314t, 323
Children's Hospital of Eastern Ontario Pain Scale
  (CHOOPS), 146t–147t, 147
Chinese families, health beliefs and practices of,
  58t–59t

Chlamydia infection, 514
  maternal, 291t–292t
Chloride concentration, in cystic fibrosis, 749
Chlorothiazide, for congestive heart failure, 836t
Choking, during toddler years, 397t–398t, 403
Cholesterol, serum levels of, 851t
Cholesterol screening, 852b
Cholestyramine, for hyperlipidemia, 851
Choline magnesium trisalicylate, for pain, 163t
Chordee, 912t
Chorea, in rheumatic fever, 850, 850b
Chorionic villous sampling, 265
Christian Scientists, 61t–62t
Chromosomal abnormalities, 294, 295t
  in congenital heart disease, 823
  sex, 508, 508t
Chromosomal deletion, 294
Chromosomal translocation, 294
Chromosome analysis, in leukemia, 889
Chronic illness/disability, 536–567
  acknowledgment of, 544
  activities of daily living in, 552
  assessment of, 548, 548t
  coping mechanisms in, 542, 545–547, 545b,
    545f
    of child, 551
    of parents, 549–551
    of parent-to-parent, 551
    of siblings, 551–552
  developmental aspects of, 538
  end-of-life in, 555–560. See also Death and
    dying.
    decision making at, 555–560
  family feelings in, management of, 543–544
  family of child with, 540–544, 540b, 542b
  family stresses with, 542
  family support system in
    at time of diagnosis, 548–549, 549f
    coping methods in, 549–552
    establishment of, 544
  family-centered care in, 538
    cultural role in, 538–539
  family–health care provider communication
    in, 538
  family's adjustment to, 543–544
  functional burden in, 544, 544b
  health care education in, 547, 552
  home care in, 539
  hopefulness in, 547
  impact of, 540–541
    on parents, 540–541, 540b
    on siblings, 541, 542b
  mainstreaming in, 539
  managed care in, 540
  nature and severity of, 537, 537t
  normal development in, 546t–547t, 552–554
    in adolescence, 554
    in early childhood, 553, 553b, 553f
    in school-age child, 553–554, 554f
  normalization in, 539–540
    promotion of, 551b
  nursing care guidelines for, 550b
  pain assessment in, 156
  parental behavior in, responses to, 547
  parental empowerment and, 542–543
    advocate for, 551
  primary health care in, 552

Chronic illness/disability (Continued)
  realistic goals in, 554–555
  reintegration of family life in, 544
  safe transportation in, 552
  scope of problem in, 537
  self-care in, 547
  shared decision making in, 539, 539b
  shock and denial in, 543
  special considerations in, 550b
  stress and periodic crisis in, 542–543
  therapeutic relationships in, 538
  trends in care for, 538–540
  type of, 547
Chronic immune thyroiditis, 983
Chronic pain. See also Pain entries.
  assessment of, 151
  definition of, 151
Chronic pain syndromes, 175
Chronic renal failure, 921–924
  diagnosis of, 922, 922b
  nursing care management for, 923–924
  pathophysiology of, 921–922
  prognosis of, 923
  treatment of, 922–923
Church of Christ, Scientist, 61t–62t
Church of Jesus Christ of Latter-day Saints, 61t–62t
Chvostek sign, 985b
Cigarette smoking. See Smoking.
Circular reactions, in cognitive development, 319
Circulation
  neonatal, 186
  prenatal and postnatal, 823–824, 824f
Circumcision, 211–214
  anesthesia and analgesia for, 212
  cultural considerations in, 214b
  female, 214b
  pain management during, 212b–213b
  proper positioning for, 212, 212f
  risks and benefits of, 211–212, 211b
Cirrhosis, 797–798
Classroom placement, appropriate, attention-deficit hyperactivity disorder and, 503
Clavicle fracture, birth-related, 230
Clean intermittent catheterization, 1101
Clean-catch urine specimen, 659
Cleft lip/cleft palate, 800–803, 800f, 802b
Clinical reasoning, 12
Clitoris, in neonate, 199
Cloaca, 811
  persistent, 811, 811f
Closed comedone (whitehead), 1035
Closed (simple) fracture, 1057
Clostridium botulinum, diarrhea due to, 772t–774t
Clostridium difficile, diarrhea due to, 772t–774t, 775
Clostridium perfringens, diarrhea due to, 772t–774t
Clubbing of fingers, 841, 841f
Clubfoot, 1071–1072, 1071f
  correction of, 1072, 1072f
Clubs, for school-age child, 462–463
Coagulopathy, consumption, 887–888, 888b
Coanalgesics, for pain, 162–163
Coarctation of aorta, 827, 828b–829b

Cobedding
  of twins, 221, 222f
  sudden infant death syndrome and, 370
Cocaine
  adolescent use of, 529
  intrauterine exposure to, 289
Coccidioidomycosis, 1021t
Codeine, for pain, 164t
Cognition, definition of, 72, 319
Cognitive behavioral therapy, for eating disorders, 525
Cognitive development, 71t, 72–73
  definition of, 571
  of adolescent, 482, 488t
  of infant, 319–320, 319f
  of preschooler, 408–409, 413t–414t
  of school-age child, 460, 461f
  of toddler, 380–382, 381f, 382b
Cognitive impairment, 571–579
  care plan for, 575
  child/family teaching in, 572–573, 573f
  classification of, 571, 572t
  communication in, 574, 574f
  developmental delay and, 571
  diagnosis of, 571, 571b
  discipline in, 574–575
  education in, 572–573, 573f
  etiology of, 571–572
  hospitalization in, 575–576
  in Down syndrome, 576–578, 576f, 577b
  in fragile X syndrome, 578–579, 579b
  nursing care for, 550b, 572–576
  optimal development in, 573
  pain assessment in, 153–156
  play and exercise in, 573–574, 573f–574f
  prevention of, 576
  self-care skills in, 573
  sexuality in, 575
  socialization in, 575
Cognitive power, definition of, 928
Coitus interruptus, 512t–514t
COL1A genes, in osteogenesis imperfecta, 1073
Cold, common, 710–714, 711b–714b
Cold injury, 1048
Cold packs, for respiratory infections, 709–710
Cold sore (fever blister), 433, 1019t
Cold stress, in high-risk neonate, consequences of, 237–238
Colectomy, subtotal, for inflammatory bowel disease, 790–791
Colestipol, for hyperlipidemia, 851
Colic, in infant, 367–368, 368b, 368f
Colitis, ulcerative, 789, 789t
Collaboration, in pediatric nursing, 11
Collar bone fracture, birth-related, 230
Color Tool, in pain assessment, 148t–150t
Color vision, 125
Color vision deficit, 125
Colostomy, 702
  for anorectal malformations, 812
Coma, 929b
  assessment of, 929, 930f
  awakening from, 938
  barbiturate-induced, 937
  definition of, 928
  diabetes insipidus in, 937

Coma (Continued)
  drug therapy in, 937
  elimination in, 937
  exercise in, 938
  family support in, 938
  hydration in, 937
  hygiene in, 937
  intracranial pressure monitoring in, 935–936
  nursing care in, 934–938
  nutrition in, 937
  pain management in, 934–935
  positioning in, 938
  respiratory management in, 935
  stimulation in, 938
  suctioning in, 936
  syndrome of inappropriate antidiuretic hormone secretion in, 937
  thermoregulation in, 937
Comedogenesis, 1035
Comedone
  closed (whitehead), 1035
  open (blackhead), 1035
Comfort
  of burn patients, 1045, 1045b
  promotion of, for respiratory infections, 708–710
COMFORT Scale, in pain assessment, 145
Comminuted fracture, 1057
  of skull, 940
Common cold, 710–714, 711b–714b
Communal family, 27
Communicable disease(s), 423–432, 423b, 424t–430t. See also specific disease.
Communication. See also Interview.
  anticipatory guidance in, 89
  blocks to, avoidance of, 89, 89b
  cultural aspects of, 47–48, 53–54
  empathy on, 89
  guidelines for, 87–88
  impaired, pain assessment in, 153–156, 157f–158f
  in cognitive impairment, 574, 574f
  in home care, 604
  listening skills in, 89
  nonverbal, 53–54, 574, 574f
  privacy and confidentiality in, 87–88, 87f
  setting for, 87–88
  silence in, 89
  with children, 90–92, 91b
    in adolescence, 92, 483b
    in early childhood, 91, 92f
    in infancy, 91
    in school-age years, 91–92
    related to thought process development, 91–92, 91b
    techniques of, 92–95, 93b–94b
  with families, 88–95
    through interpreter, 89–90, 90b
  with parents, 88–90
Community
  definition of, 16–17
  nursing in, 16
  support of, 48
Community evaluation, 20
Community factors, obesity and, 519
Community health diagnosis, 19–20

Community health nursing, 17
Community implementation, 20
Community needs assessment, 19–20
Community planning, 20, 21b
Community-based nursing care, 16–22
    concepts in, 16–19
    demographics in, 18
    economics in, 19
    epidemiology in, 18–19, 18b, 18f
    evaluation in, 20
    implementation in, 20
    nurse's roles and function in, 17, 17b
    nursing process in, 19–20, 19b
    planning in, 20, 21b
Compartment syndrome, evaluation of, 1059b
Compensated shock, 861, 861b
Complementary and alternative medicine
    classes of, 162
    cultural health influences in, 55b
    definition of, 159–162
    for sickle cell anemia, 881b
    for toddler, 393
    in home care, 604b
    safety topics in, 56b
    spiritual practices in, 55b
Complete atrioventricular block, 853–854
Complete blood count (CBC), 868, 870t
Complete fracture, 1057b, 1057f
Complete heart block, 853–854
Complex pain. See also Pain entries.
    assessment of, 156
Complex partial seizures, 958b–959b, 959t.
        See also Seizure(s).
Compliance, 646–647
Compound fracture, of skull, 940
Computed tomography (CT)
    of cerebral function, 933t–934t
    of urinary function, 905t–906t
Computer(s)
    in home care, 606–607
    privacy issues in, 88
Concept of conservation, in school-age child,
        460, 461f
Conceptual thinking, in school-age child, 460
Concrete operational thought, in cognitive
        development, 71t, 73
Concussion
    in head trauma, 939–940
    spinal cord, 1115
Condoms, 512t–514t
Conduction, heat loss through, 207
Conductive hearing loss, 580–581, 581f. See also
        Hearing impairment.
Conductive-sensorineural hearing loss, 580.
        See also Hearing impairment.
Confidentiality
    in interview, 87–88
    informed consent and, 637
Confusion, 929b
    in head trauma, 939
    opioid-induced, 165t–166t
Congenital adrenal hyperplasia, 990–991
Congenital aganglionic megacolon, 779
Congenital anomalies, 81, 293–295, 293b. See also
        specific anomaly.
    genetic etiology of, 294, 295t
    nursing care guidelines for, 550b

Congenital heart disease, 820, 823–830
    acyanotic, 824
    aortic coarctation in, 828b–829b
    aortic stenosis in, 828b–829b
    atrial septal defect in, 826b–827b
    atrioventricular canal defect in, 826b–827b
    chromosomal anomalies associated with,
        823
    circulatory changes in, 823–824, 824f
    classification of, 824–830, 825f, 826b–827b
    clinical consequences of, 830–843
    congestive heart failure in, 830–843. See also
        Congestive heart failure.
    cyanotic, 824
    decreased pulmonary blood flow in, defects
        with, 827–830, 830b–831b, 830f
    family adjustment in, 843
    family education in, 843–844
    family help in, 844–845
    hemodynamic defects in, 824
    hypoplastic left heart syndrome in,
        831b–834b
    hypoxemia in, 840–843
    incidence of, 823
    increased pulmonary blood flow in, defects
        with, 825, 825f, 826b–827b
    invasive procedures for
        comfort and emotional support after, 847
        complications of, 846b
        discharge and home care planning in,
            847–848, 848b
        fluid monitoring in, 846–847
        patient/family preparation in, 845
        postoperative care in, 845–847, 846b
        respiratory status in, 846
        rest and progressive activity after, 847
        vital signs observation in, 845–846
    mixed defects in, 830, 831b–834b
    nursing care in, 843–848
    obstructive defects in, 825–827, 825f,
        828b–829b
    patent ductus arteriosus in, 826b–827b
    pulmonic stenosis in, 828b–829b
    shunts in, 824
    tetralogy of Fallot in, 830b–831b
    total anomalous pulmonary venous
        connection in, 831b–834b
    transposition of great arteries in, 831b–834b
    tricuspid atresia in, 830b–831b
    truncus arteriosus in, 831b–834b
    valvular aortic stenosis in, 828b–829b
    ventricular septal defect in, 826b–827b
Congestive heart failure, 830–843
    clinical manifestations of, 835, 835b
    left-sided, 834
    nursing care management for, 836–840,
        837b–838b
    pathophysiology of, 834, 834f
    right-sided, 834
    treatment of, 835–836, 836t
Conjunctiva, examination of, 121
Conjunctivitis
    in neonates, treatment of, 208
    in toddler/preschooler, 432, 432b
Consanguineous relationships, in families, 24
Conscience, 380
    in preschooler, 408

Consciousness
    altered states of, 928–929. See also Coma.
    assessment of, 929, 930f
    definition of, 928
    full, 929b
    levels of, 928–929, 929b
    regaining, 938
Consent, informed. See Informed consent.
Conservation, concept of, in school-age child,
        460, 461f
Conservative Judaism, 61t–62t
Constipation, 778–779, 779b–780b
    in cystic fibrosis, 751
    opioid-induced, 165t–166t, 169–171
    urinary tract infections and, 910b
Consummatory behavior, of neonate, 218–219
Consumption coagulopathy, 887–888, 888b
Contact dermatitis, 1022, 1023f
Contact lenses, 589
Contact precautions, in infection control, 654,
        654b
Containment, in pain management, 159
Continuous ambulatory peritoneal dialysis
        (CAPD), 924
Continuous cycling peritoneal dialysis (CCPD),
        924
Contraception, 511–514, 512t–514t
Contracture
    in wound healing, 1013
    joint, 1051
Contusions
    cerebral, 940
    soft tissue, 1055
Convection, heat loss through, 207
Conversion reaction (hysteria), in school-age
        child, 506
Cool mist
    for laryngotracheobronchitis, 722
    for respiratory infections, 708
Cooley (β-thalassemia) anemia, 881–882, 882b
Cooling procedures
    for fever, 651
    for hyperthermia, 651
Coombs test
    direct, 265
    indirect, 265
Cooperation, social relationships and, 462–463,
        462f
Cooperative play, 77, 77f
Coordination
    cerebellar control of, 140
    in pediatric nursing, 11
Coordination of secondary schemas, in cognitive
        development, 320
Coping behaviors, in chronic illness/disability,
        542, 543b
Coping mechanisms
    in chronic illness/disability, 542, 545–547,
        545b, 545f
    of child, 551
    of parents, 549–551
    of parent-to-parent, 551
    of siblings, 551–552
    in posttraumatic stress disorder, 505
Cornea, examination of, 121
    in neonate, 197
Corneal light reflex test, 122–123, 122f

Corneal reflex, 197
Corporal (physical) punishment, 35
Corrosives, poisoning with, 438b–439b
Corticosteroids
for asthma, 739–740
for juvenile rheumatoid arthritis, 1085
for minimal-change nephrotic syndrome, 914
Costal angle, 129
Cotrel-Dubousset instrumentation, 1078
Cough, assessment of, in respiratory function, 709b
Cough-assisting techniques, manual, in Duchenne muscular dystrophy, 1109
Counseling, 10–11
for attention-deficit/hyperactivity disorder, 503
telephone triage and, 88, 88b
Countercoup injury, 939
Coup injury, 939
Couplet care (dyad), 222
Cover test, 123
alternate, 123, 123f
Cow's milk allergy, 360–361, 361b
Cow's milk–based formula, 217
Coxa plana, 1074–1075, 1074b
Coxsackievirus, maternal infection with, 291t–292t
Crackles, 132
neonatal, 197
Cradle cap, 1035
Cranial deformities, 966–967
Cranial nerves, assessment of, 140, 141f, 142t
Cranial sutures, 195, 196f
Cranioschisis, 1099b
Craniosynostosis, 192, 967
Craniotabes, physiologic, 195–196
Craniotomy, infratentorial, 948
Crawl reflex, 200f
Crawling, 317
Creative activities, in hospitalization, 625–626, 625f
Creativity, in play, 77
Creeping, 317
Cremasteric reflex, 137, 138f
Crepitus, 230
Crib, falls from, 402–403
CRIES, 148t–150t, 153
Crohn disease, 789, 789t
Cromolyn sodium, for asthma, 740
Cross-racial adoption, 36–37
Croup, 720
spasmodic, 723
Croup syndromes, 720–723, 721t, 722b
Croup tent, 688
Crown-to-rump measurements, of neonate, 192
Crush injury, 1055
Crust, 1012f
Crutchfield tong traction, 1063–1064, 1064f
Cry (crying)
nighttime, 365t
graduated extinction method for, 365
of neonate, 202, 202t
vocalization during, 322
Cryptococcosis, 1021t
Cryptorchidism, 912t
Cued speech, 582
Cultural awareness, 56b, 57–62, 58t–59t, 60b
listening and, 89

Cultural competence, importance of, to nurses, 56–57, 57b
Cultural customs, 52–54
Cultural factors
in chronic illness/disability, 538–539
in circumcision, 214b
in communication, 47–48, 53–54
in complementary and alternative medicine, 55b–56b
in health beliefs and practices, 43, 56b
in pain assessment, 156
in schools, 48
Cultural health influences, 55b
Cultural humility, 44
Cultural relativity, 52
Cultural sensitivity, 46
Cultural shock, 46, 46b
Culturally diverse families, developing relationship with, 603–604, 603b
Culture, 43–46
communities and, 48
definitions of, 44b
dominant, practices considered abusive by, 56, 56b
ethnicity and, 47, 47f. See also Race/ethnicity.
North American, 45
peer-group, 48–49, 48f
religion and, 60, 60b, 60f, 61t–62t
self-esteem and, 45–46
subcultures and, 44
Curds (casein), 309–314
in human milk, 214
Cushing syndrome, 989–990, 989b, 989f
Customs, food, 54
Cyanosis, 119t, 840–841, 869
assessment of, in respiratory function, 709b
Cyst, 1011f
pilonidal, 199
Cystic fibrosis, 747–754
clinical manifestations of, 749b
diagnosis of, 748–749
endocrine complications in, 747–748
management of, 751
family support in, 753
gastrointestinal complications in, 748
management of, 751
home care in, 752–753
hospital care in, 752
nursing care in, 752–754
pathophysiology of, 747–748, 748f
prognosis of, 751–752
pulmonary complications in, 748
management of, 749–751, 750f
reproductive complications in, 748
screening for, 749
transition to adulthood in, 753–754
treatment of, 749–752
Cystic fibrosis transmembrane regulator (CFTR), 747
Cystitis, 906
hemorrhagic, chemotherapy-induced, 892
Cystometrography, 905t–906t
Cystoscopy, 905t–906t
Cytochemical markers, in leukemia, 889
Cytomegalovirus (CMV)
in hepatitis, 794–795
maternal infection with, 291t–292t

D

Dance reflex, 200f
Date rape, definition of, 516b
Daycare, for preschooler, 40, 40b
Dead space, in drug administration, 667
1-Deamino-8-d-arginine vasopressin (DDAVP), for hemophilia, 884
Death and dying. See also Mortality.
at home, 564, 564b
autopsy and, 565
children's understanding of and reactions to, 558t–559t
decision making in
by parents, 557
by physician and health care team, 557
dying child in, 557–558, 558t–559t
ethical considerations in, 555–556
family needs and support in, 563
fear of actual death in, 564, 564b
fear of dying in, 563, 563f
fear of pain and suffering in, 560–563
grief and mourning and, 565–566
home care in, 558
hospice care in, 559–560
hospital care in, 558
in hospital, 564
nurses' reactions to, 566–567
nursing care guidelines in, 550b
nursing care plan for, 560b–562b
of high-risk neonate, 252–253
organ or tissue donation and, 565
pain and symptom management in, 556b, 562–563, 563b
palliative care in, 555
Death rattle, 564, 564b
Débridement, of burns, 1042
Decannulation, accidental, in tracheostomy, 693
Decibels, sound intensity expressed in, 580t
Decompensated shock, 861, 861b
Decongestants, for respiratory infections, 709
Deep palpation, of abdomen, 136
Deep tendon reflex, 140
Deep vein thrombosis, 1051
Defense mechanisms, in toddler, 379
Deferoxamine, for Cooley anemia, 882
Dehydration, 764–771
clinical manifestations of, 767, 768t
degrees of, 767–768, 767t
diagnosis of, 768
hypertonic, 767
hypotonic, 767
in intestinal obstruction, 808b
isotonic, 767
nursing care management for, 769–771
treatment of, 768–769, 769t
types of, 766–767
Delivery room, stabilization and resuscitation in, 278b
Deltoid muscle, drug administration into, 667–671, 670f
Demand feeding, of neonate, 218
Demographics, in community-based nursing care, 18
Denial, 613, 613b
in chronic illness/disability, 543–544
Dental. See also Teeth.

Dental caries, 2–3
early childhood, 330, 395–396, 396f
in school-age child, 470
Dental defects, in chronic renal failure, 922–923
Dental examinations, 129
regular, 394
Dental health
of adolescent, 491
of preschooler, 419
of school-age child, 469–470, 470f, 471b
of toddler, 394–396, 394f, 395t, 396f
Dental hygiene. *See also* Oral hygiene.
in cerebral palsy, 1094
Dental injury, 470
Dental plaque, removal of, 394–395
Dental sealants, pit and fissure, 491
Denver Development Screening Test (DDST), 78–79
Denver Development Screening Test–Revised (Denver II), 78–80, 79b
Denver II Prescreening Developmental Questionnaire, 80
Depressants, CNS, adolescent use of, 529
Depressed fracture, of skull, 940
Depression
anaclitic, 613
childhood, 506–507, 506b
Deprivation dwarfism, 507
Depth perception (stereopsis), 315
Dermatitis
atopic, 1032–1034, 1033b, 1033f
in Wiskott-Aldrich syndrome, 897
baths for, 1016
contact, 1022, 1023f
diaper, 232, 1030–1036, 1032f
control of, 1032b
treatment of, 244b–245b
flea-bite, 232
pathophysiology of, 1010
seborrheic, 1035
Dermatome, 423–431
removal of split-thickness skin graft with, 1043, 1043f
Dermatophytosis (ringworm), 1017–1020, 1020t, 1021f
Desensitization, in preschooler, 416
Despair, 613, 613b
Detachment, 613, 613b
Development, 64–85
assessment of, 78–80, 79b
biologic, 309–317. *See also* Biologic development.
cognitive, 71t, 72–73. *See also* Cognitive development.
definition of, 65
family, 24b, 25, 25t
fetal, 81
genetic factors influencing, 80–84, 82b. *See also* Genetic *entries.*
growth and, 65–70. *See also* Growth and development.
home care and, 607–608, 607b, 607f
in chronic illness/disability, 538, 545, 545f, 546t–547t, 552–554
in adolescence, 554
in early childhood, 553, 553b, 553f
in school-age child, 553–554, 554f

Development (*Continued*)
in cognitive impairment, optimal, 573
intellectual, 77
theoretic foundations of, 72–74
language, 73
moral, 71t, 73–74. *See also* Moral development.
of body image, 74–75. *See also under body image.*
of personality, 71–75, 71t
theoretic foundations of, 71–72
of self-concept, 74–75
of temperament, 322–323
pace of, 66
play in, 75–78. *See also* Play.
psychologic, 66
psychosexual, 71, 71t, 318–319
psychosocial, 71–72, 71t, 72f, 318–319. *See also* Psychosocial development.
sensorimotor, 77
social. *See* Social development.
spiritual, 71t, 74. *See also* Spiritual development.
stages of, 65b, 74–75
Developmental delay, cognitive impairment and, 571
Developmental dysplasia of hip, 1068–1071
clinical manifestations of, 1070b
diagnosis of, 1069–1070, 1069f
nursing care management for, 1070–1071
pathophysiology of, 1068–1069, 1068f
treatment of, 1070, 1070f
Developmentally appropriate activities, in hospitalization, 624
Dextrocardia, 198
Diabetes insipidus, 980–981
in coma, 937
neurogenic, 980
Diabetes mellitus, 992–1006
blood glucose testing in, 995–996, 995t, 1003–1004, 1003b, 1004f
child/family education in, 998–999
child/family support in, 1005–1006
cystic fibrosis–related, 747–748
diagnosis of, 994
exercise in, 996, 1005
glucogenesis in, 993
glycosuria in, 993
glycosylated hemoglobin measurement in, 995–996, 995t
hospitalization in, 998, 999b
hygiene in, 1005
hyperglycemia in, 993, 997, 1004
hypoglycemia in, 996–997, 997t, 1004, 1005b
illness management in, 997
insulin for, 994–995
administration of, 995
dosage of, 994–995
duration of, 1002
injection of, 1002–1003, 1003f, 1003t
preparation of, 994
types of, 995b
ketoacidosis in, 993
management of, 997–998
long-term complications of, 993–994
maternal, 285–286, 286b, 286f
meal planning in, 1000–1002
Medic-Alert identification in, 999

Diabetes mellitus (*Continued*)
nature of, 999
nephropathy in, 993
neuropathy in, 993
nursing care management for, 998–1006, 1000b–1002b
nutrition in, 996
pathophysiology of, 992–994
polydipsia in, 993
polyuria in, 993
record keeping in, 1005
retinopathy in, 993
self-management in, 1005
Somogyi effect in, 997
travel and, 1002
treatment of, 994–997
type 1, 992, 992t, 993b, 1006b
type 2, 3, 992, 992t
urine glucose testing in, 996, 1004
Diabetic ketoacidosis, 993
management of, 997–998
Diagnostic procedures. *See* Procedures.
Dialysis, 924–925, 925f
Diaper dermatitis, 232, 1030–1036, 1032f
control of, 1032b
treatment of, 244b–245b
Diapering, in spina bifida, 1103
Diaphragm, contraceptive, 512t–514t
Diarrhea, 771–778
acute, 772
infectious causes of, 772t–774t
chronic, 772
chronic nonspecific, 772
diagnosis of, 775
etiology of, 772–775, 772t–774t
in kwashiorkor, 357
intractable, 772
nursing care management for, 777
pathophysiology of, 775
prevention of, 776–778
treatment of, 775–776, 776t
Diastasis recti, 199
Diazepam, for seizures, 1112
Diet. *See also* Nutrition.
constipation and, 779, 780b
dental health and
in infant, 330
in toddler, 395–396, 396f
for toddler, 391–392
gluten-free, 814
high-fiber, for abdominal pain, 784–785
in chronic renal failure, 922
in cystic fibrosis, 751
in glomerulonephritis, 916
in health history, 96
iron sources in, 873
ketogenic, for seizures, 960
Mediterranean-type, for hyperlipidemia, 851
modification of, obesity and, 520, 520b
phenylalanine restriction in, 299
vegetarian, 392–393
Dietary fiber supplements, in spina bifida, 1101–1102
Dietary intake, 99–101, 102f, 103b
Dietary Reference Intakes (DRIs), 99, 103b
Differentiation, definition of, 65

Digestive processes
 defects in, 812
 in toddler, 379
Digital sensor, 116b
Digital subtraction angiography (DSA), of
 cerebral function, 933t–934t
Digital thermometers, infrared, 193
Digoxin
 administration of, 839b
 for congestive heart failure, 835
 toxicity of, 838, 839b
Dilated cardiomyopathy, 855
Diphtheria, 424t–430t
 immunization against, 332f–333f, 335–336
Disability. *See* Chronic illness/disability.
Discharge checklist, for neonate, 223b
Discharge criteria, for neonate, 222b
Discharge planning, 629
 after congenital heart disease surgery, 847–848,
  848b
 for neonate, 222–223, 222b–223b
  at high risk, 251–252, 252b
Discipline
 in cognitive impairment, 574–575
 of infant, 324
 of school-age child, 466
 of special needs child, 553
Disease
 distribution of, 18, 18b
 prevention of, 9
 screening for, in neonate, 209
Dishonest behavior, of school-age child, 466–467
Dislocation(s), 1055–1056
 in developmental dysplasia of hip, 1068, 1068f
 in maltreated child, 450b
Disorientation, 929b
Disseminated intravascular coagulation (DIC),
 887–888, 888b
Distraction
 during procedures, 641
 in pain management, 160b
 osseous, 1065–1066, 1066f
Distributive shock, 860b
Diuretics, for congestive heart failure, 835–836,
 836t, 840
Diversional activities, in hospitalization, 624–625,
 625f
Diverticulum, Meckel, 786–789, 788b
Divorce
 custody and parenting partnerships after, 39
 impact of, 37–38, 38b
 parenting and, 37–39
 stages of, 37, 37b
 telling children of, 38
Do not resuscitate (DNR) orders, 557
Documentation, of nursing process, 13
Dog guide, 587
Doll's head maneuver, 931
Donor milk banks, 241
Doppler ultrasonography, blood pressure
 monitoring with, 115
Double effect principle, 563, 563b
Double-walled incubator, 238–239
Down syndrome (trisomy 21), 81–82, 295t
 diagnosis of, 576, 576f, 577b–578b
  prenatal, 578
 etiology of, 576

Down syndrome (trisomy 21) *(Continued)*
 nursing care management for, 577–578
 prognosis of, 577
 treatment of, 576–577
Dramatic play, 76. *See also* Play.
 during hospitalization, 626
 of preschooler, 411
Drawing
 during hospitalization, 625–626, 625f
 in communication with children, 94
Dreams, in communication with children, 93
Dressings, in wound care, 1013–1014
Drop attacks, 958b–959b
Droplet precautions, in infection control,
 653–654, 654b
Drowning, 5, 5f. *See also* Submersion injury.
 of adolescent, 494b
 of infant, 345b–346b, 347t–348t
 of school-age child, prevention of, 472t–473t
 of toddler, 397t–398t, 401
Drug abuse/misuse, 527. *See also* Substance
 abuse.
Drug dosage, determination of, 665
Drug reactions, adverse, 1022–1024, 1031t
Drug therapy. *See also named drug or drug group.*
 administration of, 665–681
  aerosol, 680
  dosage in, 665
  in high-risk neonate, 244–246
  in home care, 680–681
  intradermal, 671
  intramuscular, 667–671, 668b–669b,
   669t–670t, 671f, 672b
  intravenous, 671–676, 673b–674b, 673t,
   675t, 676f, 677b–678b
  nasal, 679, 680f
  nasogastric, 676, 678b
  optic, 679, 679f
  oral, 665–667, 666b, 667f
  orogastric, 676, 678b
  otic, 679
  rectal, 678–679
  subcutaneous, 671
  via gastrostomy, 676, 678b
 for attention-deficit/hyperactivity disorder,
  502, 504b
 for burns, 1042
 for coma, 937
 for eating disorders, 525
 for obesity, 520
 for pain, 162–175, 163t–166t, 166b–167b
 for seizures, 960
 intrauterine exposure to, 286–290, 287b
 medication history of, 97
 subcutaneous administration of, 671
 teratogenic effects of, 294
Drug tolerance, 527
Drug toxicity, management of, 891–892
DTaP/DTP vaccine, 336
Dual-earner family, 39–40
Dubowitz Scale, 189
Duchenne muscular dystrophy, 1106–1109,
 1107b–1108b, 1107f–1108f
Ducher Scale, in pain assessment, 148t–150t
Ductus arteriosus, 823–824, 824f
Duodenal ulcer, 792
Duvall's Developmental Stages of Family, 26b

Dwarfism
 psychosocial (deprivation), 507
 Russell-Silver, 977
Dyad (couplet care), 222
Dysacousis, 580
Dysgraphia, 503
Dyskinetic movement, in cerebral palsy, 1091,
 1092b
Dyslipidemia, 851
Dysmenorrhea, 509
Dysphoria, opioid-induced, 165t–166t
Dysreflexia, autonomic, 1115, 1117
Dysrhythmia(s), 134, 853–854, 854b. *See also*
 specific type.
Dyssomnias, 364

E

Ear(s)
 examination of, 125–127
  external structures in, 125, 125f
  internal structures in, 125–127
  positioning of child for, 125–127, 126f
 foreign bodies in, 127
 in Down syndrome, 577b
 of neonate, 197, 203t–206t
Ear drops, 679
Ear sensor thermometer, 116b
Eardrum, bony landmarks of, 127
Early intervention program, in cognitive
 impairment, 572–573
Eating disorder(s), 517–527. *See also specific
 disorder.*
 diagnosis of, 524, 524t
 etiology and pathophysiology of, 523–524
 nursing care management for, 525–526
 screening for, 525
 treatment of, 524–525
Eating disorder not otherwise specified
 (EDNOS), 523
Eating habits, of adolescent, 489–490, 490f
Ecchymoses (bruises), 119t, 1010
Eccrine glands, of neonate, 187
Echocardiography (ECHO), in cardiovascular
 dysfunction, 821, 821t
Economics, in community-based nursing care, 19
Eczema (atopic dermatitis), 1032–1034, 1033b,
 1033f
 in Wiskott-Aldrich syndrome, 897
Edema, 913
 cerebral, 941
 pulmonary, 733
Education
 bilingual, 49
 client/family. *See* Health/family education.
 during hospitalization, 626–627
 in chronic illness/disability, 547, 552
 in cognitive impairment, 572–573, 573f
 in home care, 607–608
 in human immunodeficiency virus infection,
  896
 in visual impairment, 587–588
 of special needs child, 539
  supplemental programs in, 539–540
 parenting, 32, 32f
 safety, 403
 sexuality, 493
Edward syndrome (trisomy 18), 295t

Ego mastery, in school-age child, 463–464
Elbow, nursemaid's (pulled), 1056
Elbow restraint, 656–657, 657f
Electrical burns, 1037. *See also* Burns.
    in infancy, 347t–348t
    in toddler, 401
Electrical equipment, safety of, 652
Electrocardiography (ECG), in cardiovascular
        dysfunction, 821, 821t
Electrode(s), placement of, for apnea monitors,
        373–374, 374f
Electroencephalography (EEG), 933t–934t
Electrolyte balance
    disturbances of, 764–771, 765t–766t
    in neonate, 187
Electrolyte therapy, for diabetic ketoacidosis,
        997–998
Electronic continuous thermometer, 112, 116b
Electronic intermittent thermometer, 112, 116b
Electrophoresis, hemoglobin, in sickle cell
        anemia, 875
Elimination. *See* Bowel elimination.
E-mail, in home care, 606–607
Emancipated minors, informed consent of, 637
Embryogenesis, 81
Emergency admission, 631, 632b
Emergency care, socioeconomic influences on,
        51
Emergency medical service (EMS), 755
Emergency protocol review, 608
Emergency treatment
    of eye injuries, 586b
    of poisoning, 437–441, 437b
EMLA cream, 168
Emollients, in neonatal skin care, 244, 244b–245b
Emotion, expression of, 551b
Emotional abuse, 446, 449, 450b, 451
Emotional neglect, 446, 452b
Emotional support
    after congenital heart disease surgery, 847
    for leukemia patients, 892
Emotionality, in adolescence, 482
Empathy, in communication, 89
En face position, in maternal attachment, 219,
        219f
Encephalitis, 954–955, 954b
Encephalocele, 1099b
Encephalopathy, bilirubin, 260
Encopresis, 500–501, 501b, 778
Endocarditis, bacterial, 848–849, 848b–849b
Endocephalography, 933t–934t
Endocrine system
    of neonate, 188
    structure and function of, 973–976, 974t–976t,
        976f
End-of-life. *See also* Death and dying.
    decision making at, 555–560
    perspectives on, 555–560
End-of-life care, 597
    pain management in, 180, 556b
Endotracheal tube
    intubation with, 690
    suctioning of, saline installation before,
        271b–272b
End-stage liver disease, 798b
End-stage renal disease, 923
End-tidal carbon dioxide monitoring, 689

Enema, 701–702, 701t
    antegrade continence, 1101–1102
Energy expenditure, 518
Energy intake, 518
Energy needs, of high-risk neonate, 243–244,
        243f
Enteral nutrition. *See also* Nutrition; Nutritional
        entries.
    for high-risk neonate, 237
    for necrotizing enterocolitis, 284
    gavage feeding in, 242–243, 695–698,
        696b–697b, 698f
Enterobiasis (pinworm), 435–436, 436b
Enterocolitis, necrotizing, 284–285, 285b
Enterocystoplasty, augmentation, 1101
Enthnocentrism, 47
Enucleation, 590
Enuresis (bed wetting), 499, 500b. *See also*
        Urinary incontinence.
Environmental influences
    in abusive situations, 447
    obesity and, 519
    primary- and secondary-group, 45
Environmental manipulation, for attention-
        deficit/hyperactivity disorder, 503
Environmental noise, 580
Environmental safety issues, 652–653, 652f
Environmental stressors, in intensive care unit,
        633b
Eosinophils, 188
Ependymoma, 946
Epicanthal folds, 122–123
Epidemiologic triangle, 18–19, 18f
Epidermal injuries, 1013
Epidermal stripping, 648
Epidural analgesia, 168
Epidural hemorrhage, 940–941, 941f
Epiglottitis, acute, 721t
Epileptic seizures. *See also* Seizure(s).
    unclassified, 957
Epinephrine, 974t–976t
    for anaphylaxis, 360b, 862
    for laryngotracheobronchitis, 722
EpiPen, 360b
Epispadias, 912t
Epistaxis (nosebleed), 888
Epithelial pearls, 199
Epithelium, cultured, for burns, 1044
Epstein pearls, 197, 210
Epstein-Barr virus (EBV)
    in hepatitis, 794–795
    in mononucleosis, 719–720
Equine tetanus antitoxin, 1112
Erb-Duchenne palsy, 200
    in neonate, 231–232, 232f
Erikson theory, of psychosocial development,
        71–72, 71t, 72f
    in adolescent, 481–482
    in infant, 318–319
    in preschooler, 408
    in school-age child, 459, 459f
    in toddler, 380, 381f
Erosion, skin, 1012f
Erythema, 119t, 1010
Erythema infectiosum (fifth disease), 424t–430t,
        425f
    maternal infection with, 291t–292t

Erythema marginatum, in rheumatic fever, 850b
Erythema migrans, in Lyme disease, 1029, 1029f
Erythema multiforme, 1023, 1031t
Erythema toxicum neonatorum, 232
Erythroblastosis fetalis (fetal hydrops), 264
Erythroblasts, 264
Escherichia coli, diarrhea due to, 772t–774t
Esophageal atresia, 803–805, 803f
    long-gap, 804
Esophageal temperature, measurement of, 112b
Esophageal varices, 798
Estimated Average Requirement (EAR), of
        nutrients, 99, 103b
Estrogen(s), 974t–976t
    for dysmenorrhea, 509
    in puberty, 477
Ethical decision making, 11
Ethical issues, in end-of-life care, 555–556
Ethnic pride, 46
Ethnicity. *See* Race/ethnicity.
Euthanasia, 555–556
Evaporated milk formula, 218
Evaporation, heat loss through, 207, 239
Evidence-based practice, 11–12, 12t
Evil eye, 56
Ewing sarcoma, 1082–1083
Exanthem subitum (roseola infantum),
        424t–430t, 426f
Exchange transfusion
    for hemolytic disease of newborn, 266
    for sickle cell anemia, 876
Excision, of burns, 1042
Excoriation, 1012f
Exencephaly, 1099b
Exercise(s). *See also* Activity and exercise.
    breathing, for asthma, 740–741, 747
    in coma, 938
    in diabetes mellitus, 996, 1005
    in juvenile rheumatoid arthritis, 1086
    in scoliosis, 1077–1078
Exercise-induced bronchospasm, 740
Exhibitionism, 447
Exophalmos (protruding eyeballs), 983
Expressive skills, in cognitive impairment, 574
Exstrophy, bladder, 912t
Extended family, 27, 27f
Extension posturing, 932, 932f
External fixation, for fractures, 1065–1066, 1066f
Extracorporeal membrane oxygenation (ECMO),
        for respiratory distress syndrome, 277
Extrauterine life, adjustment to, 186–189. *See also*
        Neonate(s).
    immediate, 186
    physiologic, 186, 187b
Extravasation, definition of, 687
Extremity(ies)
    examination of, 139, 139f
    of neonate, 198t, 199–200, 203t–206t
Extremity venipuncture, positioning for, 657,
        658f
Eye(s). *See also* Vision; Visual *entries; specific part*.
    examination of, 121–125
        external structures in, 121, 121f
        fundoscopic, 122, 122f, 931
        guidelines in, 124t
        internal structures in, 121–122
        neurologic, 930–931, 931f

Eye(s) (Continued)
    preparation of child for, 121–122
    vision testing in, 122–125, 122f–123f
  in Down syndrome, 577b
  in neonate, 196–197, 198t, 203t–206t
    ophthalmia neonatorum prophylaxis
      and, 208
  injuries to, 586b
  irritation of, in coma, 937
  lazy, 122
Eye drops, administration of, 679, 679f
Eyeballs, protruding (exophthalmos), 983
Eyelids, examination of, 119
E-Z-On vest, 399–400

F
Face, moon, chemotherapy-induced, 892
Facebook, 484
Faces Pain Rating Scale, 148t–150t, 150
Facial nerve, assessment of, 141f, 142t
Facial paralysis, in neonate, 231, 231f
Facioscapulohumeral muscular dystrophy, 1106
Factor VIII concentrate, for hemophilia, 884
  prophylactic, 885
Factor VIII deficiency, 884. See also Hemophilia.
Failure to thrive, 362–364
  classification of, 362
  diagnosis of, 362
  feeding child with, 364b
  nursing care management for, 363–364, 363b, 364f
  prognosis of, 363
  psychosocial, 507
  treatment of, 362
  zinc deficiency and, 355–356
Faith healing, 56
Falls
  child safety home checklist for, 349b
  in adolescence, 494b
  in infancy, 345b–346b, 347t–348t
  in toddler years, 397t–398t, 402–403
  prevention of, 653
Familial short stature, 977
Family(ies)
  binuclear, 27
  bisexual, 27–28
  blended (reconstituted), 27, 39
  communal, 27
  communication with, 88–95
    through interpreter, 89–90, 90b
  consanguineous relationships in, 24
  culturally diverse, developing relationships
    with, 603–604, 603b
  definition of, 24
  developmental theory of, 24b, 25, 25t
  dual-earner, 39–40
  effect of immobilization on, 1054
  extended, 27, 27f
  foster, 41
  functioning style of, 28
  gay/lesbian, 27–28
  general concepts of, 24–26
  grieving, support for, 566b
  influence of, obesity and, 518, 522
  migrant, 51–52
  North American, 45

Family(ies) (Continued)
  nuclear, 26
    traditional, 26
  nursing interventions for, 26, 26b
  of ALTE infant, support of, 374
  of dying child, 557–558, 557b, 558t–559t
  of SIDS infant, care of, 371–372
  of special needs child, 540–544, 540b, 542b
    stresses within, 542
  polygamous, 27
  preparation of, for procedures, 642, 643b
  roles and relationships of, 28–31. See also
    Parent(s); Sibling(s).
  school-age child's relationship with, 463
  single-parent, 27, 39
  size and configuration of, 28, 29f
  strengths of, 26b, 28
  stressors on, 24–25
  structure of, 26–28, 98–99, 100b–101b
  transgender, 27–28
Family advocacy, 9, 9b
Family assessment interview, 100b–101b
Family life, reintegration of, in chronic illness/
  disability, 544
Family medical history, 98
Family planning services, 511–514, 512t–514t
Family rules, for adolescent, 495b
Family stress theory, 24–25, 25t
Family support system
  during hospitalization, 627–628
  in acute renal failure, 921
  in bacterial meningitis, 952
  in brain tumor, 950
  in cerebral palsy, 1097–1098
  in chronic illness/disability
    at time of diagnosis, 548–549, 549f
    coping methods in, 549–552
    establishment of, 544
  in coma, 938
  in congestive heart failure, 840
  in cystic fibrosis, 753
  in diabetes mellitus, 1005–1006
  in head trauma, 944
  in hemophilia, 886
  in hydrocephalus, 970
  in inflammatory bowel disease, 791–792
  in juvenile rheumatoid arthritis, 1086
  in nephrotic syndrome, 915
  in sickle cell anemia, 881
  in skin disorders, 1016–1017
  in spina bifida, 1103–1104
  in Wilms tumor, 918
Family system theory, 24, 25t
Family-based therapy, for eating disorders, 526
Family-centered care, 8, 8b, 13b, 603–610
  conflicts in, 605b
  diversity in, 603–604
  fever and, 652–653, 652b
  guidance during adolescence in, 495, 495b
  guidance during infancy in, 350, 350b
  guidance during preschool years in, 420, 420b
  guidance during school-age years in, 472, 474b
  guidance during toddler years in, 403, 404b
  hyperbilirubinemia and, 262–263
  in chronic illness/disability, 538
    cultural role in, 538–539
  in hospitalization, 628, 628b

Family-centered care (Continued)
  of high-risk neonate, 248–249, 249b
  parent-professional collaboration in, 604–605
  sibling visitation in, 221, 221f
Family-to-family support, in home care, 609–610
Fanconi syndrome, 882–883
Fasting, preoperative, 642–644, 644t
Fat(s)
  brown, in neonate, 186
  in human milk, 214
Father
  engrossment of, with neonate, 220–221, 220f
  of special needs child, 541
  single, 39
Fatigue, signs of, in neonate, 280t
Fear
  in preschooler, 416
  in school-age child, 467–468
  nighttime, 365t
  of actual death, 564, 564b
  of dying alone, 563, 563f
  of pain and suffering, 560–563
  stranger, in infant, 321
    coping with, 323
Febrile seizures, 651, 966. See also Seizure(s).
Fecal incontinence, 500–501, 501b
Feeding. See also Food.
  alternative techniques of, 694–701
  gastrostomy, 698–700, 698f, 699b–700b, 700f
  gavage, 242–243, 695–698, 696b–697b, 698f.
    See also Enteral nutrition.
  of high-risk neonate, 242–243
  in cleft lip/cleft palate infant, 801–802
  infant. See also Breastfeeding; Formula feeding.
    in first 6 months, 326–328
    in first year, 329b
    in second 6 months, 328
    nighttime, 365t
    solid foods in
      introduction of, 329
      preparation of, 328
  neonatal
    behavioral stages in, 218–219
    schedules for, 218
  of sick child, 649–650, 650b
  resistance to, in high-risk neonate, 243
Feeding readiness, 241–242
Feelings, expression of, during procedures,
  641–642, 642f
Feet, in Down syndrome, 577b
Femoral epiphysis, slipped capital, 1075–1076,
  1075b
Femoral fracture, 1058, 1059f
Femoral hernia, 136, 136f
Femoral pulses
  of neonate, 203t–206t
  palpation of, 136, 137f
Femoral venipuncture, positioning for, 657, 657f
Fentanyl, for pain, 162, 164t
Fetal alcohol spectrum disorder (FASD), 289,
  296t
Fetal alcohol syndrome (FAS), 289
Fetal development, 81
Fetal hydrops (erythroblastosis fetalis), 264
Fever, 650–651
  as contraindication to immunization, 341
  in respiratory infections, 710

Fever (Continued)
  in urinary tract infections, 906
  management of, 651, 652b
  seizures and, 651
Fever blister (cold sore), 433, 1019t
Fibrinolysis, 883
Fibrosis, pancreatic, in cystic fibrosis, 747
Fifth disease (erythema infectiosum), 424t–430t, 425f
  maternal infection with, 291t–292t
Filipino families, and relationship with health care providers, 52
Fingers, clubbing of, 841, 841f
Finger-stick device, for blood glucose testing, 1003–1004, 1004f
Fire ant bites, 1025t–1026t
Firearms
  adolescent and, 494–495
  improper use of, 5, 5f
Fissure, 1012f
Fistula
  arteriovenous, in dialysis, 924
  omphalomesenteric, 786
  perineal, 811b, 812
  rectovaginal, 811, 811f
  tracheoesophageal, 803–805, 803b, 803f
Five-point harness restraint, 398
FLACC Postoperative Pain Tool, 146t–147t
FLACC Scale, 146t–147t, 147
Flame burns. See also Burns.
  in toddler, 401
Flea-bite dermatitis, 232
Flexion posturing, 932, 932f
Flies, biting, 1025t–1026t
Floppy infant syndrome, 1105
Fluid(s). See also Water entries.
  extracellular, 763
  intracellular, 763
  monitoring of, during congenital heart disease surgery, 846–847
Fluid balance
  basal metabolic rate and, 764
  body surface area and, 764
  daily requirements for, 764, 764t
  disturbances of, 764–771, 765t–766t
  in infant, 345–346, 763–764
  in neonate, 187
    hydration and, 239–240
  insensible losses and, 763
  intake and output measurements in, 681
  maintenance of, 681–687
  renal function and, 764
Fluid intake, measurement of, 681
Fluid intoxication, 764
Fluid management
  in bacterial meningitis, 951–952
  in burns, 1041–1042
  in coma, 937
  in diabetic ketoacidosis, 997–998
  in high-risk neonate, 239–240
  promotion of, for respiratory infections, 710
Fluid output, measurement of, 681
Fluid requirements
  altered, 763
  daily maintenance, 764, 764t
Fluid therapy, parenteral. See Parenteral fluid therapy.

Fluid volume, changes in, growth and, 763–764
Fluoride
  in dental care, 330
  in dental health, 395, 395t
  supplemental, 326
Fluorosis, 129
Flush lines, intravenous, 673t
Flutter mucus clearance device, 750, 750f
Foley catheter, 660t
Folic acid, supplemental, 355
Folk healers, 55–56
Folk medicine, 55–56
Folliculitis, 1018t
Fontanel(s), 195, 196f
  anterior and posterior, 195
Food. See also Diet; Feeding; Nutrition.
  allergies to, 358. See also specific food.
    clinical manifestations of, 359, 359b
    definition of, 358
    diagnosis of, 360
    nursing care management for, 360
    treatment of, 360
  fiber content of, 780b
  hot-cold classification of, 55
  iron-rich
    for iron-deficiency anemia, 872
    for toddler, 392
  solid, for infants
    introduction of, 329
    selection and preparation of, 328
Food allergens, definition of, 358
Food customs, 54
Food diary, 101
  analysis of, 102
Food intolerance, 358
Food practices, 102b
Foreign body(ies)
  aspiration of, 731–732
    in toddler, 403
  in ear, 127
  in eye, 586b
  in skin, 1024
Formal operational thought, in cognitive development, 71t, 73
Formula(s)
  alternate milk products in, 218
  caloric density of, 840
  commercially prepared, 217–218
  iron-fortified, 327, 872
  phenylalanine-free, 300
  preparation of, 218
Formula feeding, 217
  commercially prepared formulas for, 217–218
  growth patterns and, 108
  in first 6 months, 326–328
  in second 6 months, 328
  of high-risk neonate, 242
Foster care, definition of, 41
Foster homes, 41
Foster parents, 41
Fowler's spiritual development theory, 71t, 74
Fracture(s), 1057–1059. See also specific type of fracture.
  birth-related, 230–231
  casts for, 1059–1062, 1060f–1062f, 1061b
  diagnosis of, 1058, 1058b
  external fixation of, 1065–1066, 1066f

Fracture(s) (Continued)
  healing of, 1058
  in maltreated child, 450b
  nursing care management for, 1058–1059
  Salter-Harris classification of, 1057, 1058f
  skull, 940
  treatment of, 1058, 1059f
    emergency, 1059b
  types of, 1057, 1057b, 1057f
Fragile X syndrome, 81–82, 578–579, 579b
Frenotomy, 197
Frenulum, 197
Freudian theory, of psychosexual development, 71, 71t
Friction, pressure ulcers and, 648
Friends, best, 484
Frostbite, 1048
Fruit juice, for infants, 328
Frustration, in preschooler, 416
Functional burden, in chronic illness/disability, 544, 544b
Functional Disability Inventory, 151
Functional electrical stimulation, for spinal cord injuries, 1116
Fundus, examination of, 122, 122f, 931
Funeral arrangements, for deceased infant, 253
Fungal infections, cutaneous, 1017–1020, 1020t, 1021f
  systemic, 1020, 1021t
Furlow double-opposing Z-plasty, for cleft palate, 801
Furniture, safety of, 652
Furosemide, for congestive heart failure, 836t

G
Gag reflex, 241–242
Gait training, for spinal cord injuries, 1116
Galactose-1-phosphate uridyltransferase (GALT), 300–301
Galactosemia, 300–301
Games, 76. See also Play.
  for hospitalized child, 625
  quiet, for school-age child, 463, 464f
Gamma globulin, intravenous, for Kawasaki disease, 859
Gang violence, 463
Gardner-Wells tongs, 1063–1064
Gas(es), noxious, injury from, 734–735
Gastric decontamination, for poisoning, 440
Gastric lavage, for poisoning, 440
Gastric ulcer, 792
Gastric varices, 798
Gastroesophageal reflux, 782–784
  clinical manifestations and complications of, 782b
  diagnosis of, 783
  in cystic fibrosis, 751
  nursing care management for, 783–784
  pathophysiology of, 782–783
  treatment of, 783, 783f
  vs. gastroesophageal reflux disease, 782
Gastrointestinal disorders, 771–785. See also specific disorder.
  hepatic, 794–800
  inflammatory, 785–793
  obstructive, 805–812, 808b
  of malabsorption, 812–816

Gastrointestinal disorders *(Continued)*
    of motility, 771–784
    parasitic, 433–436, 434t
    structural, 800–805
Gastrointestinal hypersensitivity, immediate, 359
Gastrointestinal system
    effect of immobilization on, 1051t–1053t
    of infant, 309–314
    of neonate, 187, 187b
Gastroschisis, 807t
Gastrostomy feedings, in cerebral palsy, 1095–1097
Gastrostomy tube
    drug administration via, 676, 678b
    feeding via, 698–700, 698f, 699b–700b, 700f
Gavage feeding, 242–243, 695–698, 696b–697b, 698f. *See also* Enteral nutrition.
    of high-risk neonate, 242–243
Gay/lesbian family, 27–28
Gaze, cardinal positions of, 140, 142f
Gel mattress, heated, 238–239
Gender assignment, in ambiguous genitalia, 990–991
Gender identity, of toddler, 383
Gene(s), 80–81
    mutation of, 80
    single defect of, 294
    substitution or alteration of, 293
Gene therapy, for hemophilia, 885
Generalized seizures, 957, 958b–959b. *See also* Seizure(s).
Genetic counseling
    in Down syndrome, 578
    in Duchenne muscular dystrophy, 1109
Genetic disorders, 81–82. *See also specific disorder.*
    assessment of, 293b
    counseling and testing for, 301–302, 302t
    education, care, and support for, 83–84
    identification and referral for, 83
    psychologic aspects of, 302
Genetic factors, influencing development, 80–84
Genetic knowledge, application and integration of, 82–83
Genetic testing, types of, 302t
Genetics
    overview of, 80–84
    role of nurses in, 82, 82b
Genital stage, in psychosexual development, 71, 71t
Genitalia
    ambiguous, 990
        gender assignment in, 990–991
    examination of, 136–138
        in female, 137–138, 138f
        in male, 137, 137f–138f
    in Down syndrome, 577b
    of neonate
        female, 199, 203t–206t
        male, 199, 203t–206t
Genitourinary disorder(s), 903–925
    acute glomerulonephritis, 915–916, 915b
    clinical manifestations of, 903–904, 905t–906t
    external, 911–912, 912t
    glomerular, 912–916

Genitourinary disorder(s) *(Continued)*
    hemolytic-uremic syndrome, 916–917, 917b
    in spina bifida, management of, 1101
    laboratory findings in, 904, 907t–908t
    nephrotic syndrome, 912–915, 913f, 914b
    nursing care management for, 904
    obstructive, 910–911, 911f
    renal failure
        acute, 919–921, 919b–920b
        chronic, 921–924, 922b
        technical management of, 924–925
    surgery for
        nursing care in, 911–912
        psychologic problems related to, 911
    urinary tract infections, 904–910
    Wilms tumor, 917–918, 917b–918b
Genomic knowledge, application and integration of, 82–83
Genomics, overview of, 80–84
Genu valgum (knock knee), 139, 139f
Genu varum (bowleg), 139, 139f
Germ cell tumors, 946
German measles (rubella), 424t–430t, 429f
    immunization against, 332f–333f, 337
    maternal infection with, 291t–292t
Gestational age
    clinical assessment of, 189–201, 190b, 190f–191f
    weight related to, 189–192
Giant pigmented nevus, 234
Giardiasis, 434–435, 435b, 435f
Gingiva (gums), examination of, 129
Gingivitis, in school-age child, 470
Gingivostomatitis, herpetic, pain in, 176
Glans penis, examination of, 137
Glasgow Coma Scale (GCS), 929
Glasses, for visual impairment, 589
Glaucoma, 584b–585b
Glioma, brainstem, 946
Glomerulonephritis
    acute, 714, 915–916, 915b
    poststreptococcal, 915
Glossopharyngeal nerve, assessment of, 141f, 142t
Glucagon, 974t–976t
Glucocorticoids, 974t–976t
    for Addison disease, 988
Glucogenesis, in diabetes mellitus, 993
Glucose testing, in diabetes mellitus
    blood, 995–996, 995t, 1003–1004, 1003b, 1004f
    urine, 996, 1004
Glucuronyl transferase, 257
    neonatal live function and, 187
Gluteal fields, 138
Gluten free diet, 814
Gluten-sensitive enteropathy (celiac disease), 812–815, 813f, 814b
Glycosuria, in diabetes mellitus, 993
Glycosylated hemoglobin A1c, in diabetes mellitus, 995–996, 995t
Gnat bites, 1025t–1026t
Goat's milk, 218
Goiter, 982–983
    adolescent, 983
Gomco clamp, for circumcision, 212
Gonadotropins, 974t–976t, 977b

Gonorrhea, 514
    maternal infection with, 291t–292t
Gower sign, 1107, 1108f
Graduated extinction method, for nighttime crying, 365
Graft(s)
    arteriovenous, in dialysis, 924
    for burns
        allograft (homograft), 1043
        mesh graft, 1043, 1044f
        sheet graft, 1043, 1044f
        xenograft, 1043
Graft-versus-host disease, in transplant patient, 899
Grand mal seizures, 958b–959b. *See also* Seizure(s).
Granulation, in wound healing, 1013
Grasp, 319
    palmar, 315
    pincer, 315, 315f
Grasp (plantar) reflex, 139, 200, 200f
Gratification, delayed, 318
Graves disease, 983, 984b
Great arteries, transposition of, 831b–834b
Greenstick fracture, 1057b, 1057f
Grief, 565–566
    anticipatory, 249, 565
    nurses experiencing, 253
    parental, 565
    sibling, 565–566
Grief reactions, complicated, 565
Grieving families, support for, 566b
Griseofulvin, for dermatophytoses, 1019–1020
Groshong catheter, 675t
Group A β-hemolytic streptococci, pharyngitis due to, 714–715, 849
Group identity
    in adolescence, 481
    vs. alienation, 481
Group therapy, for obesity, 522
Growing fracture, of skull, 940
Growth
    changes in fluid volume and, 763–764
    definition of, 65
    in adolescence
        constitutional delay of, 507
        patterns of, 478–481, 488t
            sex differences in, 478–481
    in infancy, 309
    measurements of, 106–111
    skeletal, 68
Growth and development, 65–70. *See also* Development.
    biologic determinants of, 67–68, 67f, 68t
    directional trends in, 65–66, 66f
    external proportions in, 67
    foundations of, 65–66, 65b
    history taking of, 97
    individual differences in, 66
    metabolism in, 69
    nutrition in, 69–70
    of adolescent, 477–487
        altered, 507–508, 508t
    of infant, 309–325, 310t–314t
        concerns related to, 323–325
    of lymphoid tissues, 68–69
    of organ systems, 69

Growth and development *(Continued)*
  of preschooler, 408–417, 413t–414t
    concerns related to, 412–417, 415f
  of school-age child, 458–468
    concerns related to, 464–468
  of toddler, 379–390, 386t–387t
    concerns related to, 385–390, 388f–389f
  pace of, 66
  patterns of, 65–66
  physiologic changes in, 69
  rates of, 67, 67f
  sensitive periods in, 66
  sequential trends in, 66
  sleep/rest and, 69
  temperament and, 70, 70b
  temperature and, 69
Growth charts, 107–109
  different versions of, 109, 109f
Growth curve
  evaluation of, 977–978, 978b
  intrauterine, 190f–191f, 191
Growth delay, constitutional, 977
Growth disorders, bone age and, 978, 978b
Growth failure, in chronic renal failure, 922–923
Growth hormone (GH), 974t–976t, 977b
Growth hormone deficiency, treatment of, 978
Growth plate injuries, 1057–1058, 1058f
Growth spurt, pubertal, 68t
Guided imagery, in pain management, 160b
Guillain-Barré syndrome, 1109–1111, 1110b
  meningococcal conjugate vaccine-4 and, 339
  vaccine-induced, 717
Guilt, in chronic illness/disability, 543
Guns, adolescent and, 494–495
Guthrie blood test, 298–299
Gynecomastia, 130, 510

H
H₂-receptor antagonists
  for gastroesophageal reflux, 782
  for peptic ulcer disease, 793
Habits, history taking of, 97–98, 97b
Haemophilus influenzae type B infection,
    immunization against, 332f–333f, 337
Hair, inspection of, 119
Hair care, 649
Hair follicles, growth phases of, in neonate,
    187–188
Hair loss, chemotherapy-induced, 892
Haitian families, health beliefs and practices of,
    58t–59t
Hallucinations, opioid-induced, 165t–166t
Hallucinogens, adolescent use of, 530
Halo brace, 1063–1064
Halo vest, 1063–1064, 1064f
Hand, foot, and mouth disease, stomatitis in,
    433
Hand(s), in Down syndrome, 577b
Hand strength, 140
Hard palate, examination of, 129
Hardy-Rand-Rittler test, 125
Harness systems, types of, 398
Hashimoto disease, 983
Head
  coronal section of, 928f
  examination of, 120–121
  in Down syndrome, 577b

Head circumference
  measurement of, 111
  of neonate, 192
  of toddler, 379
Head contour, of neonate, 194–196
Head control
  of infant, 121, 315, 316f
  of neonate, 196, 196f
Head growth, in infant, 309
Head lag, in neonate, 196
Head lice, 1024–1028, 1027b–1028b, 1027f
Head posture, 121
Head trauma, 938–945
  abusive, 446
  birth-related, 229–230, 230f
  cerebral edema in, 941
  clinical manifestations of, 941b
  complications of, 940–941
  concussion in, 939–940
  coup/countercoup injury in, 939
  epidural hemorrhage in, 940–941, 941f
  etiology of, 939
  evaluation of, 941–943
    initial assessment in, 942
    posttraumatic syndromes in, 943
    special tests in, 942
  family support in, 944
  fractures in, 940
  inflicted, 446
  nursing care management for, 943–945
  pathophysiology of, 939–940, 939f
  prevention of, 945
  prognosis of, 943
  rehabilitation after, 944–945
  subdural hemorrhage in, 941, 941f
  treatment of, 942b, 943
Headache, recurrent, 177–178
Head-to-heel length, of neonate, 192, 192f
Health beliefs, 55
Health care
  for children, 2–8, 2b
  in chronic illness/disability, 552
Health care providers, relationships with, 52–54,
    53f
Health education, in chronic illness/disability,
    547, 552
Health history, 95–99. *See also* History taking.
Health Insurance Portability and Accountability
    Act (1996), 637
Health maintenance, in school-age child,
    471–472
Health practices, 55–56, 56b
Health problems. *See* Illness.
Health promotion, 2–3, 9. *See also* Pediatric
    nursing.
  developmental influences on, 64–85. *See also*
    Development.
  during adolescence, 487–495
  during preschool years, 417–420
  during school years, 468–472
Health teaching, 10
Health/family education
  in chronic illness/disability, 547, 552
  in congenital heart disease, 843–844
  in diabetes mellitus, 998–999
  in sickle cell anemia, 878
Healthy People 2020, 2b

Hearing
  in adolescent, 491
  in coma, 938
  in neonate, 188, 197, 198t
    screening for, 209
  in toddler, 379
Hearing aid(s), 580–581, 581f
Hearing impairment, 579–584
  case study in, 583b
  classification of, 579–580, 580t
  clinical manifestations of, 582b
  conductive, 580–581, 581f
  definition of, 579–580
  etiology of, 579–580
  hospitalization in, 583
  mixed, 580
  noise-induced, 580
  nursing care management for, 581–584, 582b
  pathology of, 580
  prevention of, 583–584
  profound, 579
  sensorineural, 580–581
  slight to moderate, 579
  socialization and, 582–583
  symptom severity in, 580, 580t
  treatment of, 580–581, 581f
  with visual impairment, 589
Heart. *See also* Cardiac; Cardio- *entries*.
  blood flow through, 820f
  examination of, 132–134, 133f–134f,
    134t–135t
  in infant, 309
  in neonate, 198–199, 203t–206t
Heart block, complete, 853–854
Heart disease
  acquired, 820, 848–856
    bacterial endocarditis in, 848–849,
      848b–849b
    cardiomyopathy in, 855–856
    dysrhythmias in, 853–854, 854b
    hyperlipidemia in, 850–853, 851t, 852b
    pulmonary artery hypertension in, 854–855
    rheumatic fever in, 849–850, 850b
  cardiac catheterization in, 822, 822t, 823b
  congenital. *See* Congenital heart disease.
  diagnosis of, 821–822, 821t
  echocardiography in, 821
  electrocardiography in, 821
  history in, 820–823
  nursing care management for, 822–823
  physical examination in, 820–823
  transplantation for, 856–857
Heart failure
  congestive, 830–843. *See also* Congestive heart
    failure.
  in acute renal failure, 921
Heart murmurs, 134
  grading of, 135t
  in neonate, 198–199
Heart rate
  in infancy, 309
  in neonate, 198
  postoperative, 645t
Heart sounds
  auscultation of, 134t
  evaluation of, 134
  in neonate, 198–199

Heart sounds (Continued)
  normal, differentiation of, 133–134, 134f, 134t
  origin of, 133–134
Heart transplantation, 856–857
  heterotopic, 856
  orthotopic, 856
Heat injury, 734. See also Burns.
Heat loss, evaporative, 207, 239
Heat therapy, for juvenile rheumatoid arthritis, 1086
Heavy metal poisoning, 441
Heel lance, 662, 664b
  complications of, 662–664, 664f
Heel puncture
  for hypothyroidism, 297
  in neonate, 210b
Height
  general trends in, 67, 68t
  measurement of, 110, 110f
  of infant, 309
Heimlich maneuver, 759, 759f
Helicobacter pylori, and ulcers, 792
Helmet, customized, for positional plagiocephaly, 366, 366f
Hemangioma
  capillary (strawberry), 234, 234f
  cavernous venous, 234
Hematocrit, 870t
Hematologic disorder(s), 869
  anemia, 869–872
  complete blood count in, 870t
  hemostatic, 883–888
  neoplastic, 888–894
  technologic management of, 897–900
Hematoma, ocular (black eye), 586b
Hematopoietic stem cell transplantation, 899, 900b
  allogeneic, 899
  autologous, 899
  for aplastic anemia, 883
  for leukemia, 889
  for severe combined immunodeficiency disease, 897
  peripheral, 899
Hematopoietic system
  of infant, 309
  of neonate, 186
Hemodialysis, 924
Hemodynamic defects, in congenital heart disease, 824
Hemofiltration, 924
Hemoglobin, determination of, 870t
Hemoglobin A1c, glycosylated, in diabetes mellitus, 995–996, 995t
Hemoglobin electrophoresis, for sickle cell anemia, 875
Hemolytic disease of newborn, 263–266, 264f, 265t
  clinical manifestations of, 264–265
  diagnosis of, 265
  nursing care management for, 266
  prognosis of, 266
  treatment of, 265–266
Hemolytic-uremic syndrome, 916–917, 917b
Hemophilia, 883–886
  diagnosis of, 884, 884b
  nursing care management for, 885–886

Hemophilia (Continued)
  pathophysiology of, 884
  prognosis of, 885
  treatment of, 884–885
Hemophilia A, 884
Hemorrhage
  after throat surgery, 716
  epidural, 940–941, 941f
  in hemophilia
    control of, 885–886
    crippling effects of, 886
    prevention of, 885
  in leukemia, 889
    prevention of, 890–891
  intracranial, 281t
  intraventricular, 281t
  subdural, 941, 941f
  subgaleal, 229–230, 230f
Hemorrhagic cystitis, chemotherapy-induced, 892
Hemostasis, 883
  in wound healing, 1013
Hemostatic disorder(s), 883–888
  disseminated intravascular coagulation, 887–888
  epistaxis, 888
  hemophilia, 883–886
  idiopathic thrombocytopenic purpura, 886–887
Heparin flush, for intravenous lines, 673b–674b
Heparin lock, 672–673
Hepatic portoenterostomy, for biliary atresia, 799
Hepatitis, 794–797
  clinical manifestations of, 796
  diagnosis of, 796–797
  etiology of, 794–795
  management of, 797
  nursing care management for, 797
  pathophysiology of, 796
  prevention of, 797
  prognosis of, 797
  types of, 794t
Hepatitis A, 794t, 795
  immunization against, 331, 797
Hepatitis B, 794t, 795
  immunization against, 331–335, 332f–333f, 797
  in neonate, 209
Hepatitis B immune globulin (HBIG), 797
Hepatitis B vaccine, for adolescent, 489
Hepatitis B virus, maternal infection with, 291t–292t
Hepatitis C, 794t, 795
Hepatitis D, 795
Hepatitis E, 795
Hepatitis G, 795
Herbs, 393
  for lactating mothers, 327
Hernia(s), 805, 806t–807t
  femoral, 136, 136f
  hiatal, 806t
  incarcerated, 805
  inguinal, 135–136, 136f, 912t
    in neonate, 199
    strangulated, 805
  umbilical, 135, 136f, 806t
Herpangina, stomatitis in, 433

Herpangina ulcers, pain in, 176
Herpes labialis, recurrent, 433
Herpes simplex encephalitis, 954
Herpes simplex virus (HSV)
  type I, 1019t
  type II, 1019t
Herpes simplex virus (HSV) infection, 433, 433f
  in neonate, 233–234
Herpes zoster (shingles), 423–431, 1019t
Herpetic gingivostomatitis, 433, 433f
  pain in, 176
Heterophil antibody tests, for mononucleosis, 720
Heterosexual relationships, 485, 485f
Hiatal hernia, 806t
Hickman catheter, 675t
High-density lipoproteins (HDLs), 851
Highly active antiretroviral therapy, for human immunodeficiency virus infection, 894
High-risk infant. See Neonate(s), high-risk.
Hinduism, 61t–62t
Hip, developmental dysplasia of, 1068–1071
  clinical manifestations of, 1070b
  diagnosis of, 1069–1070, 1069f
  nursing care management for, 1070–1071
  pathophysiology of, 1068–1069, 1068f
  treatment of, 1070, 1070f
Hirschberg test, 122–123, 122f
Hirschsprung's disease, 779–781, 780b, 780f
Hispanic families, and relationship with health care providers, 52
Histoplasmosis, 1021t
History taking, 95–99
  birth history in, 96
  chief complaint in, 95–96
  family medical history in, 98
  family structure in, 98–99, 100b–101b
  geographic location in, 98
  health history in, 95–99
  identifying information in, 95
  informant in, 95
  of allergies, 97, 97b
  of diet, 96
  of growth and development, 97
  of habits, 97–98, 97b
  of immunization record, 97
  of present illness, 96
  of previous illnesses, injuries, and operations, 96
  psychosocial history in, 99
  sexual history in, 98, 98b
  symptom analysis in, 96, 101b
  system review in, 99
Hodgkin lymphoma, 893–894, 893f
Home care
  after congenital heart disease surgery, 847–848
  alternative feeding techniques in, 701
  benchmarking in, 602–603
  bowel elimination in, 702
  case management in, 600–601, 601b
  communication in, 604
  concepts of, 596–603, 597f
  cost of care in, 597–598
  developmental aspects of, 607–608, 607b, 607f
  discharge planning for, 598–600, 599b
    emergency protocol review in, 608
    individualized care plan in, 599, 600b

Home care *(Continued)*
neonate and, 222–223, 223b
predischarge assessment in, 599, 600b
diversity in, 603–604
drug administration in, 680–681
education and, 607–608
effective, 598, 599b
evidence-based practice in, 602–603
family-centered, 603–610. *See also* Family-centered care.
family-to-family support in, 609–610
for infant, 323
house rules for, 605b
in chronic illness/disability, 539
in cystic fibrosis, 752–753
in death and dying, 558
in hemophilia, 886
in nephrotic syndrome, 915
in skin disorders, 1016–1017
in spina bifida, 1103–1104
intermittent skilled nursing in, 598, 599b
nursing care standards in, 601–603, 602b
nursing process in, 605–607, 606b
parent-professional collaboration in, 604–605
permanency planning and, 598
primary caregiver responsibilities in, 598
private-duty nursing in, 598
quality improvement program in, 602–603
resources for, 602b
respite care and, 598
safety issues in, 608–609, 609b, 609f
self-care in, 607–608
therapeutic boundaries in, 606b
training in, 601–603, 601f
transition to, after hospitalization, 629
trends in, 597–598
technologic, 606–607
vs. hospice care, 597
Home care agency, 598, 599b
public or private, 602, 602b
Home deaths, 564, 564b
Homelessness, 51
Honey, avoidance of, 327
Hookworm disease, 434t
Hopefulness, in chronic illness/disability, 547
Hormonal methods, of contraception, 512t–514t
Hormone(s), 976. *See also specific hormone.*
function of, 974t–976t
in puberty
changes of, 477
influences of, 479–481
Hormone replacement therapy, for hypopituitarism, 978–979
Hornet stings, 1025t–1026t
Hospice care, 559–560
concepts of, 559–560
for terminal neonate, 253
vs. home care, 597
Hospice philosophy, 559
Hospital deaths, 564
Hospitalization, 612–633
activities in
creative, 625–626, 625f
developmentally appropriate, 624
diversional, 624–625, 625f
expressive, 624–626

Hospitalization *(Continued)*
admission in
assessment for, 618, 619b–620b
emergency, 631, 632b
guidelines for, 621b
preparation for, 618–621, 621f
ambulatory or outpatient care in, 629–630
discharge from, 630b
beneficial effects of, 617, 625–627
child's routine in, 622–623, 622f
discharge planning in, 629
for neonate, 222–223, 222b–223b
educational opportunities in, 626–627
effects of, on child, 616–617, 616b
encouraging independence in, 623
family support during, 627–628
family-centered care in, 628, 628b
fear of injury in, 623–624
freedom of movement in, 622
in cerebral palsy, 1098
in cognitive impairment, 575–576
in cystic fibrosis, 752
in death and dying, 558
in diabetes mellitus, 998, 999b
in hearing impairment, 583
in intensive care unit, 631–633, 631f, 633b
in visual impairment, 588
information in, 628
isolation precaution in, 628–629
loss of control in, 615–616
minimization of, 622–623, 622f, 623b
nursing interventions in, 621–627
parental absence during, 621–622, 622f
parental participation during, 628–629
parental response to, 617, 617b
parent-child relationships in, 626
play in, 624–626, 624b
dramatic, 626
therapeutic, 625
preparation for, 617–621
promoting understanding in, 623, 623b
self-mastery in, promotion of, 627
separation anxiety in, 613–615, 613b, 613f–614f
prevention or minimization of, 621
sibling response to, 617
socialization in, 627, 627f
stressors in, 613–617, 633b
risk factors for, 616–617, 616b
toys in, 625
transition to home care after, 629
Hot or cold remedies, 55
Hot packs, for respiratory infections, 709–710
Hot-cold food classification, 55
HOTV test, 123, 124t
House dust mites, asthma due to, 739
Household safety, 403
Huffing, in cystic fibrosis, 750
Human bites, 1030
by infant, 319
Human diploid cell rabies vaccine, 955
Human immunodeficiency virus (HIV), 794–795
maternal infection with, 291t–292t
Human immunodeficiency virus (HIV) infection, 894–897
clinical manifestations of, 895, 895b
diagnosis of, 895, 895t

Human immunodeficiency virus (HIV) infection *(Continued)*
epidemiology of, 894
etiology of, 894–895
nursing care management for, 896–897
pathophysiology of, 895
prognosis of, 896
treatment of, 895–896
Human leukocyte antigen (HLA), 883
Human leukocyte antigen (HLA) complex, 899
Human milk. *See* Breast milk.
Human papillomavirus (HPV) infection, 514
immunization against, 339
Human papillomavirus (HPV) vaccine, for adolescent, 489
Human parvovirus B19, infections caused by, 423
Hyaline membrane disease, 267. *See also* Respiratory distress syndrome.
Hydration. *See* Fluid management.
Hydrocarbons, poisoning with, 438b–439b
Hydrocele, 912t
noncommunicating, 199
Hydrocephalus, 967–970
clinical manifestations of, 968, 968b
communicating, 967–968
diagnosis of, 968
noncommunicating, 967–968
nursing care management for, 969–970
pathophysiology of, 967–968, 967f
prognosis of, 969
treatment of, 968–969, 969f
Hydrocodone with acetaminophen, for pain, 164t
Hydromorphone
for pain, 162, 164t
in patient-controlled analgesia, 164
Hydronephrosis, 910–911
Hydrophobia, 955
Hydrotherapy, for burns, 1042
21-Hydroxylase deficiency, 990
Hygiene
dental, in cerebral palsy, 1094
in coma, 937
in diabetes mellitus, 1005
oral, 649
Hymenal tag, 199
Hymenopteran stings, 1024, 1025t–1026t
Hyperalbuminemia, 913
Hyperbilirubinemia, 256–263
complications of, 259–260
diagnosis of, 258–259, 259f
discharge planning and, 263
nursing care management for, 261, 263b
pathophysiology of, 257–258
prognosis of, 261
treatment of, 260–261, 260f
types of, 256, 257t
Hypercholesterolemia, 850–853, 851t, 852b
Hypercyanotic spells, 841
treatment of, 841, 842b, 842f, 842t
Hyperemia, reactive, 647
Hyperfunction, pituitary, 979
Hyperglycemia
in diabetes mellitus, 993, 997, 1004
morning, 997
vs. hypoglycemia, 997t

Hyperhemolytic crisis, 874
Hyperkalemia, 765t–766t
  in acute renal failure, 920
  in chronic renal failure, 921
Hyperlipidemia, 850–853, 851t, 852b
  in adolescent, 490
Hypernatremia, 765t–766t
Hyperopia, 584, 584b–585b
Hyperparathyroidism, 986–987, 986b
Hyperphenylalaninemia, 298
Hypertension
  in acute renal failure, 920
  in adolescent, 490
  in chronic renal failure, 923
  pulmonary artery, 854–855
  systemic, 857–858
    clinical manifestations of, 857b
    diagnosis of, 857
    essential, 857
    nursing care management for, 858
    secondary, 857
    treatment of, 858
Hyperthermia, 650. *See also* Fever.
  automobile-related, 401
  definition of, 934
  in coma, 937
  management of, 651
Hyperthyroidism, 983–984, 984b
  of Graves disease, 983, 984b
Hypertrophic cardiomyopathy, 855
Hypertrophic pyloric stenosis, 805–809, 808b, 808f
Hypervitaminosis A, 355
Hypervitaminosis D, 355
Hypoalbuminemia, 913
Hypocalcemia, characteristics of, 267t
Hypochondroplasia, 977
Hypoglossal nerve, assessment of, 141f, 142t
Hypoglycemia
  characteristics of, 267t
  in diabetes mellitus, 996–997, 1004, 1005b
  in infants of diabetic mothers, 285
  vs. hyperglycemia, 996–997, 1005b
Hypokalemia, 765t–766t
Hyponatremia, 765t–766t
Hypoparathyroidism, 985–986, 985b
  congenital, 985
Hypopituitarism, 977–979, 977b–978b
  congenital, 977
  idiopathic, 977
Hypoplastic left heart syndrome, 831b–834b
Hyposensitization, for asthma, 741
Hypospadias, 912t
Hypotension, orthostatic, 118
Hypothalamic-pituitary-gonadal axis, 979
Hypothermia
  definition of, 934
  in submersion injury, 945
  therapeutic, 280, 1095
Hypothyroidism, juvenile, 982, 982b
Hypotonia, 200
  congenital, 1105
Hypovolemia, 913
Hypovolemic shock, 860b
Hypoxemia, 840–843
  clinical manifestations of, 841, 841f
  diagnosis of, 841

Hypoxemia (*Continued*)
  nursing care management for, 841–843
  treatment of, 841, 842f, 842t
Hypoxia, 840–841
  in submersion injury, 945
Hysteria (conversion reaction), in school-age child, 506

I

Ibuprofen
  for fever, 651
  for pain, 163t
Ice, compression, elevation, support (ICES), for soft tissue injuries, 1056, 1056t
Ichthyoses, 1030
Icterus neonatorum, 257–258, 257t
Identity
  development of, in adolescence, 481–482
  vs. role confusion, in psychosocial development, 71t, 72
Idiopathic thrombocytopenic purpura, 886–887, 886b–887b
Ileostomy, for inflammatory bowel disease, 790–791
Ileus, meconium, 778
  in cystic fibrosis, 747
Ilizarov external fixator, 1065–1066, 1066f
Illness
  chronic. *See* Chronic illness/disability.
  distribution of, 18
  in childhood, 3–6
  present, history taking of, 96
  previous, history taking of, 96
  susceptibility to, 51
  terminal. *See* Death and dying.
Imaginary playmates, 412
Imaginative play, of preschooler, 411, 411f
Imbalance of forces, in health beliefs and practices, 43
Imitation, in cognitive development, 319–320
Imitative play, of preschooler, 411, 411f
Immobilization, 1051–1055
  effect of, on families, 1054
  nursing care management for, 1054–1055
  physiologic effects of, 1051, 1051t–1053t
  psychologic effects of, 1051–1054
Immune system
  in infant, 314
  in school-age child, 458
Immune thyroiditis, chronic, 983
Immunization(s), 3
  administration of, 341–344, 342b–343b
  against bacterial meningitis, 952, 953b
  against diphtheria, 332f–333f, 335–336
  against *Haemophilus influenzae* type B, 332f–333f, 337
  against hepatitis A, 331
  against hepatitis B, 331–335, 332f–333f, 489
    in neonate, 209
  against human papillomavirus infection, 339, 489
  against influenza, 332f–333f, 338–339, 717
  against measles, 332f–333f, 337
  against meningococcal infection, 332f–333f, 339
  against mumps, 332f–333f, 337
  against pertussis, 332f–333f, 336

Immunization(s) (*Continued*)
  against pneumococcal infection, 332f–333f, 338
  against poliomyelitis, 336–337
  against rubella, 332f–333f, 337
  against tetanus, 332f–333f, 336
    booster, 431, 488–489
  against varicella, 332f–333f, 337–338
  autism and, 335b
  communicating with parents about, 341b
  contraindications to, 340–341
  for adolescent, 488–489
  for infants, 330–344
    schedule of, 330–331
  history taking of, 97
  order of, 342b
  pain associated with, 176
  precautions for, 340–341
  reactions to, 339–340
  routine, recommendations for, 331–339, 331b, 332f–333f
  selected, recommendations for, 339
  with pneumococcal conjugate vaccine, 719
Immunocompromised patient, as contraindication to immunization, 341
Immunoglobulin(s)
  intravenous
    for hyperbilirubinemia, 260
    for Kawasaki disease, 859
  tetanus, 1112
Immunoglobulin A (IgA)
  in breast milk, 241
  secretory, 314
Immunoglobulin D (IgD), 314
Immunoglobulin E (IgE), 314
Immunoglobulin G (IgG), 314
Immunoglobulin M (IgM), 314
Immunologic deficiency disorder(s), 894–897
  human immunodeficiency virus infection, 894–897
  severe combined immunodeficiency disease, 897
  technologic management of, 897–900
  Wiskott-Aldrich syndrome, 897
Immunologic markers, cell-surface, in leukemia, 889
Immunomodulators, for inflammatory bowel disease, 790
Immunosuppression, after heart transplantation, 856
Imperforate anus, 811, 811f
Impetigo, poststreptococcal glomerulonephritis and, 915
Impetigo contagiosa, 1018f, 1018t
Inborn errors of metabolism, 295–301
Incest, 447
Income, poverty, and health insurance coverage in U.S., 51b
Incomplete precocious puberty, 980b
Incontinence
  fecal, 500–501, 501b
  urinary. *See* Urinary incontinence.
Increased intracranial pressure, 928
  clinical manifestations of, 929b
  monitoring of, in coma, 935–936

Incubator
  double-walled, 238–239
  servo-controlled, 238–239
Independence
  in visual impairment, 587
  of special needs adolescent, 554
  of special needs child, 553
Individual identity, in adolescence, 481–482
Individuals with Disabilities Education Act
    (IDEA), 572–573
Individuating-reflexive stage, of spiritual
    development, 71t, 74
Induction therapy, for leukemia, 889
Industry, of special needs child, 553
Industry vs. inferiority, in psychosocial
    development, 71t, 72
Infant(s)
  airway obstruction in, 758–759, 759f
  apparent life-threatening event in, 372–374
  biologic development of, 309–317
    fine motor skills in, 315, 315f
    gross motor skills in, 315–317
    head control in, 315, 316f
    locomotion in, 317, 318f
    maturation of systems in, 309–315
    proportional changes in, 309, 310t–314t
    rolling over in, 315–316, 317f
    sitting in, 316, 317f
  body image development in, 320, 320f
  breast- and formula-fed, growth patterns in,
    108
  child care arrangements for, 323–324
  chronic illness/disability in, developmental
    effects of, 546t–547t
  cognitive development of, 319–320, 319f
  colic in, 367–368, 368b, 368f
  communication with, 91
  concepts of and reactions to death in,
    558t–559t
  constipation in, 778–779
  dental health in, 330
  discipline for, 324
  growth and development of, 309–325,
    310t–314t
    concerns related to, 323–325
  hearing impairment in, 581–584, 582b
  height and weight gain of, 68t
  immunizations in, 330–344. See also
    Immunization(s).
  injury prevention in, 344–350
    nurse's role in, 348–350
  intramuscular injections in, 671, 671f
  loss of control in, 615
  newborn. See Neonate(s).
  nutrition for, 326–330, 326b, 329b. See also
    Nutrition; Nutritional entries.
  pacifier for, 324–325, 324b
  peptic ulcers in, 792b
  physical examination of, 107t
  pneumonia in, 725
  preparation of, for procedures, 639b–640b
  psychosocial development of, 318–319
  separation and stranger fear in, 323
  setting limits for, 324
  sleep and activity in, 330
  sleep disturbances in, 364–366, 365t
  social development of, 320–322, 320f

Infant(s) (Continued)
  sudden death of, 368–372. See also Sudden
    infant death syndrome (SIDS).
  teething in, 325, 325f
  temperament of, 322–323
  thumb sucking by, 324–325
  transportation of, 654–655, 655f
  visual acuity testing in, 123–124
  visual impairment in, 586
  water balance in, 763–764
Infant mortality, 6–7, 7t
Infant restraints, 344–346, 344f
  anchoring of, 344–346
Infantile eczema, 1033, 1033b
Infantile spasms, 958b–959b
Infants of diabetic mothers (IDMs), 285–286,
    286b, 286f
Infection(s). See also specific infection.
  communicable, 423–432, 423b, 424t–430t
  in chronic renal failure, recurrent, 923
  in leukemia, 889
  in neonate
    defenses against, 188
    identification of, 208
    maternal infections and, 290, 291t–292t
  intracranial, 949–956
  of bones and joints, 1079–1081
  skin
    bacterial, 1017, 1018f, 1018t
    fungal, 1017–1020, 1020t, 1021f
      systemic, 1020, 1021t
    viral, 1017, 1019t
  visual impairment and, 586
Infection control, 653–654, 654b, 655f
  for neonate
    at high risk, 239
    prevention of, 208–214
  in home setting, 608
  in leukemia, 890
Infectious mononucleosis, 719–720, 720b
Infective bacterial endocarditis, 848–849,
    848b–849b
Inferiority, sense of, in school-age child, 459
Inflammation, in wound healing, 1013
Inflammatory bowel disease, 789–792, 789t
  diagnosis of, 789–790
  etiology of, 789
  family support in, 791
  nursing care management for, 791–792
  pathophysiology of, 789
  prognosis of, 791
  treatment of
    drug therapy in, 790
    nutritional support in, 790
    surgical, 790–791
Influenza, 716–717
  immunization against, 332f–333f, 338–339,
    717
Influenza A, H1N1 subtype of, 716–717
Influenza vaccine, 717
Informant, in history taking, 95
Information, identification of, in history
    taking, 95
Informed consent, 636–637
  and confidentiality, 637
  and parental right to child's medial chart, 637
  eligibility for giving, 637

Informed consent (Continued)
  evidence of, 637
  for hyperbilirubin treatment, 262
  of mature and emancipated minors, 637
  of parents or guardians, 637
  requirements for, 636–637
  treatment without, 637
Infrared thermometer, 112, 116b
  axillary and digital, 193
Infusion device, peripheral intermittent, 672–673
Infusion pumps
  in parenteral fluid therapy, 683
  in patient-controlled analgesia, 163
Inguinal hernia, 135–136, 136f, 912t
  in neonate, 199
  strangulated, 805
Inhalation injury, 1038. See also Burns.
  smoke-induced, 734–735
Inhalation therapy, 687–689, 688f
  monitoring of, 688–689, 688f
Inhaled nitric oxide, for respiratory distress
    syndrome, 277
Inheritance, multifactorial, 294
Initiative vs. guilt, in psychosocial development,
    71t, 72, 72f
Injection(s)
  intradermal, 671
  intramuscular, 667–671, 668b–669b, 669t–670t,
    671f, 672b
  intravenous, 671–676, 673b–674b, 673t, 675t,
    676f, 677b–678b
  needle-free, 170b
  subcutaneous, 671
Injury. See Traumatic injury; specific type of
    injury.
In-line skate safety, 474b
Insect bites, 1025t–1026t
Institutional factors, obesity and, 519
Insulin, 974t–976t, 994–995, 1002
  administration of, 995
  dosage of, 994–995
  duration of, 1002
  injection of, 1002–1003, 1003f, 1003t
  intermediate-acting, 994, 995b
  long-acting, 994, 995b
  preparation of, 994
  rapid-acting, 994, 995b
  regular, 994, 995b
  types of, 995b
Insulin infusion, continuous subcutaneous,
    1003
Insulin pump, 995
  portable, 1003
Integumentary system. See Skin entries.
Intellectual development
  theoretic foundations of, 72–74
  through play, 77
Intellectual disability, 571, 571b. See also
    Cognitive impairment.
  definition of, 571
Intelligence quotient, 571
Intensification therapy, for leukemia, 889
Intensive care unit, 631–633, 631f, 633b
Intercostal retraction, in neonate, 197
Intercostal spaces, 129
Interests and activities, of adolescent, 484–485,
    484f

Intermittent infusion device, peripheral, 672–673. *See also* Intravenous administration.

Intermittent skilled nursing, in home care, 598, 599b

International adoption, 36–37

Internet, 50

Internet chatrooms, 484

Internet services, in home care, 606–607

Interpreter, communicating with families through, 89–90, 90b

Intertrigo, 1031t

Interview
directing focus in, 88–89
encouraging parents to talk in, 88
family assessment, 100b–101b
introductions in, 87
of adolescent, 92, 487b
privacy and confidentiality in, 87–88, 87f
without judgment, 89b

Intestinal obstruction. *See also specific type.*
clinical manifestations of, 808b
distal, in cystic fibrosis, 748

Intestines
malrotation of, 810
of neonate, 187, 187b

Intracranial hemorrhage, 281t

Intracranial infection(s), 949–956

Intracranial pressure, increased, 928
clinical manifestations of, 929b
monitoring of, in coma, 935–936

Intradermal drug administration, 671

Intramuscular drug administration, 667–671, 668b–669b, 671f, 672b
site determination in, 667–671, 669t–670t
syringe and needle selection in, 667

Intraosseous infusion, 681–682

Intrauterine device, copper-releasing, 512t–514t

Intrauterine disorders, 81

Intrauterine growth curves, 190f–191f, 191

Intrauterine transfusion, Rh isoimmunization and, 265–266

Intravenous drug administration, 671–676, 676f
central venous access device for, 673–676, 675t
heparin flush for, 673b–674b
peripheral intermittent infusion device for, 672–673
saline flush for, 673b–674b

Intravenous flush lines, 673t

Intravenous pyelography (IVP), 905t–906t

Intraventricular hemorrhage, 281t

Introductions, in interview, 87

Intubation, rapid sequence, 690

Intuitive-projective stage, of spiritual development, 71t, 74

Intussusception, 809–810, 809f, 810b

Invasive procedures, pain management of, 176–177

Invisible poverty, 50

Involucrum, 1079

Iris, examination of, 121

Iron
absorption of, 392, 393b
poisoning with, 438b–439b
supplemental, administration of, 326, 326b

Iron-deficiency anemia, 872–873

Iron-rich diet, 873
for toddler, 392

Irradiation. *See* Radiation therapy.

Irreversible (terminal) shock, 861, 861b

Islam, 61t–62t

Islet of Langerhans, 974t–976t

Isoimmunization (Rh incompatibility), prevention of, 265

Isolation precautions, 628–629

Isoniazid (INH), for tuberculosis, 730–731

Isosexual precocious puberty, 979

Isotretinoin, for acne, 1036

Ivermectin, for scabies, 1024

Ivy, poison, 1022, 1023f

J

Jacket restraints, 656

Japanese families
and relationship with health care providers, 52
health beliefs and practices of, 58t–59t

Jaundice, 119t, 256, 263b. *See also* Hyperbilirubinemia.
breast milk, 257t, 258
breastfeeding-associated, 257t, 258
in biliary atresia, 798–799, 799b
neonatal, 261b
physiologic, 257–258, 257t

Jaw control, manual, in cerebral palsy, 1097, 1097f

Jehovah's Witnesses, 61t–62t

Jitteriness, 279

Joint(s)
contracture of, 1051
examination of, 139

Joint disorder(s)
infectious, 1079–1081
rheumatoid, 1084–1086

J-tip administration, of lidocaine, 170b

Judaism, 61t–62t

Judgment, interviewing without, 89b

Junctional (compound) nevus, 234

Juvenile hypothyroidism, 982, 982b

Juvenile melanoma, 234

Juvenile rheumatoid arthritis, 1084–1086
child/family support in, 1086
classification of, 1084
heat and exercise for, 1086
pain relief for, 1085
treatment of, 1085
drug therapy in, 1085
physical and occupational therapy in, 1085

K

Kangaroo (skin-to-skin) holding
for high-risk neonate, 239, 246–247, 246f
in pain management, 159, 162f

Kasabach-Merritt syndrome, 234

Kasai procedure, for biliary atresia, 799

Kawasaki disease, 858–860, 859b
acute phase in, 858–859
subacute phase in, 858–859

Keloid, 1012f

Kernicterus, 259–260, 262

Ketamine, for cancer pain, 180

Ketoacidosis, diabetic, 993
management of, 997–998

Ketogenic diet, for seizures, 960

Ketones, 993

Ketonuria, 993

Kidney(s). *See also* Nephro-; Renal *entries.*
for transplant, 925
of neonate, 203t–206t
structure of, 904f
transplantation of, 925

Kindergarten experience, 412–415, 415f

Klinefelter syndrome, 295t, 508, 508t

Klippel-Trenaunay-Weber syndrome, 234

Klumpke palsy, 200

Knee jerk (patellar) reflex, 140, 141f

Knock knee (genu valgum), 139, 139f

Kohlberg's moral development theory, 71t, 73–74
in adolescent, 482
in preschooler, 409
in school-age child, 460

Korean families, and relationship with health care providers, 53

Kugelberg-Walander syndrome, 1105b, 1106

Kwashiorkor, 357
marasmic, 357

Kyphosis, 1076, 1076f

L

Labia majora
examination of, 138, 138f
in neonate, 199

Labia minora
examination of, 138, 138f
in neonate, 199

Laceration(s)
cerebral, 940
in maltreated child, 450b
nursing care management for, 1015

Lactase, 526

Lactase deficiency
developmental, 526
primary, 526
secondary, 526
symptoms of, 527b

Lactation. *See* Breastfeeding.

Lacto-ovo vegetarians, 392

Lactose intolerance, 526–527

Lactovegetarians, 392

Lancets, safe disposal of, 609b

Landouzy-Dejerine muscular dystrophy, 1106

Language
development of, 73
in infant, 321–322
in toddler, 384, 386t–387t
in preschooler, 409–410, 410f, 413t–414t
sign, 582

Language disorders, in autism, 591–592

Laptop computers, in home care, 606–607

Large family child care home, 323

Large-for-gestational age (LGA) infant, 286, 286f

Laryngitis, spasmodic, 721t, 723

Laryngotracheobronchitis, acute, 721t, 722–723

LATCH safety seat system, 399, 400f

Latchkey children, 466

Latency period, in psychosexual development, 71, 71t

Latex allergy, in spina bifida, 1104, 1104b

Latex-free environment, 1104

Lead, sources of, 442b

Lead poisoning, 441–445
anticipatory guidance in, 443
blood lead levels in, 434t

Lead poisoning *(Continued)*
  causes of, 441–442, 441b
  chelation therapy for, 444, 445b
  diagnosis of, 442–443
  nursing care management for, 444–445
  pathophysiology and clinical manifestations of, 442, 443f
  prognosis of, 444
  screening for, 443
  treatment of, 443–444
Learning disability
  attention-deficit/hyperactivity disorder and, 501
  definition of, 501
Lea's shield, 512t–514t
Leg restraints, 656
Leg strength, 140
Legal blindness, 584
Legal guardians, informed consent of, 637
Legg-Calvé-Perthes disease, 1074–1075, 1074b
Length. *See also* Growth; Height.
  recumbent, measurement of, 109, 110f
Lethargy, 929b
Letonogestrel implant (Implanon), 512t–514t
Letonogestrel intrauterine system (Mirena), 512t–514t
Leukemia, 888–892
  acute lymphoid, 889
  acute myelogenous, 889
  classification of, 888–889
  diagnosis of, 889
  morphology in, 889
  nursing care management for, 890–892, 890b
  pathophysiology of, 889
  prognosis of, 889
  treatment of, 889
    chemotherapy in, 891
    drug toxicity in, 891–892
    late effects of, 890
Leukorrhea, 509
Leukotrienes, for asthma, 740
Levorphanol, for pain, 164t
Levothyroxine, for hypothyroidism, 298
Lice, head, 1024–1028, 1027b–1028b, 1027f
Lichenification, 1012f
Lidocaine
  for pain, during peripheral intravenous access, 171b
  for urethral catheterization, 661b
  needle-free injection of, 170b
Ligaments, torn, treatment of, 1056
Limb deficiency, congenital, 1072–1073
Limb salvage procedure, for osteosarcoma, 1081
Limb-girdle muscular dystrophy, 1106
Limit setting
  for infant, 324
  for school-age child, 466
Linear fracture, of skull, 940
Lingual frenulum, 197
Lingual tonsil, 715, 715f
Lip(s)
  cleft, 800–803, 800f, 802b
  examination of, 128
Lipase, 314
Lipoproteins, 851
Lip-reading, 581–582, 583b
Liquid crystal skin contact thermometer, 116b

Listening skills, in communication, 89
Listeriosis, maternal infection with, 291t–292t
Live attenuated influenza vaccine (LAIV), 338
Liver
  of infant, 314
  of neonate, 187, 203t–206t
Liver disease. *See also* Cirrhosis; Hepatitis.
  end-stage, 798b
Liver transplantation, for cirrhosis, 798
Living related kidney donor, 925
Lockjaw (tetanus), 1111–1113, 1112b
  immunization against, 332f–333f, 336
Locomotion, development of, 317, 318f
Long bone fracture, birth-related, 231
Lordosis, 1076, 1076f
  in Duchenne muscular dystrophy, 1107
Loss of control, in hospitalization, 615–616
  minimization of, 622–623, 622f, 623b
Low-density lipoproteins (LDLs), 851
Lumbar puncture, 933t–934t
  for chemotherapy, 179
  in bacterial meningitis, 950
  positioning for, 657–658, 658f
Lumirubin, 260
Lung(s). *See also* Pulmonary; Respiratory *entries*.
  examination of, 130–132, 131b–132b, 132f
  of neonate, 197–198, 203t–206t
Lupus, neonatal, 1086–1087
Luque-rod instrumentation, 1078
Luteinizing hormone (LH), 974t–976t
Luteinizing hormone–releasing hormone (LHRH), for precocious puberty, 980
Lying, by school-age child, 467
Lyme disease, 1028–1029, 1029f
Lymph nodes
  examination of, 120, 120f
  in neonate, 199
Lymphocytes, 188
Lymphocytic thyroiditis, 983, 983b
Lymphoid tissue, growth and development of, 68–69
Lymphoma, 892–894
  Hodgkin, 893–894, 893f
  non-Hodgkin, 894
Lysozyme(s), in human milk, 214

M
Macewen sign, 968
Macrobiotic diet, 392
Macrominerals, 355–356
Macrophage system, in neonate, 188
Macula, examination of, 122
Macular stain, transient, 234
Macule, 1011f
Magic tricks, in communication with children, 94
Magical thinking, of preschooler, 409
Magnetic resonance imaging (MRI), of cerebral function, 933t–934t
Mainstreaming. *See also* Education; School.
  of special needs child, 539
Maintenance therapy, for leukemia, 889
Malabsorption syndromes, 812–816
Malnutrition, protein-energy, 356–358
  nursing care management for, 358
  treatment of, 357–358
Malocclusion, 470

Malrotation, of intestine, 810
Maltreatment, 445–454. *See also* Abuse; Neglect.
  caregiver-child interaction and, 448–449
  clinical manifestations of, 450b
  discharge planning and, 453
  history and interview of, 449–451
  nursing care for, 448–454, 449b, 452b
  physical assessment of, 451
  prevention of, 453–454, 454b
  support for child and, 453
  support for family and, 453
Manual cough-assisting techniques, in Duchenne muscular dystrophy, 1109
Manual jaw control, in cerebral palsy, 1097, 1097f
Manual traction, 1063b
Manubrium, examination of, 129
Marasmus, 357
Marfan syndrome, 294
Marijuana, intrauterine exposure to, 290
Mass media, influences of, 49–50
Masturbation, in preschooler, 416
Maternal attachment, to neonate, 219–220, 219f
Maternal diabetes, 285–286, 286b, 286f
Maternal infections, 290, 291t–292t
Maternal smoking, sudden infant death syndrome and, 370
Maturation
  definition of, 65
  neurologic, 68
  skeletal, 68
Meal planning, in diabetes mellitus, 1000–1002
Mean arterial pressures (MAPs), 115, 115t
Measles (rubeola), 424t–430t, 427f
  immunization against, 332f–333f, 337
Measles-mumps-rubella-varicella (MMRV) vaccine, 337
Meatus, nasal, 128
Mechanical ventilation, 690
Meckel diverticulum, 786–789, 788b
Meconium aspiration syndrome, 273t–274t
Meconium ileus, 778
  in cystic fibrosis, 747
Medic-Alert identification, 999
Medical-surgical restraints, 655–656
Medication(s). *See* Drug therapy; *specific drug*.
Mediterranean-type diet, for hyperlipidemia, 851
Medroxyprogesterone acetate (Depo-Provera), 512t–514t
Medulloblastoma, 946
Megacolon, congenital aganglionic, 779
Megavitamin(s), 393. *See also* Vitamin(s).
Meibomian glands, 121
Melanin, in neonate, 188
Melanocyte-stimulating hormone (MSH), 974t–976t, 977b
Melanoma, juvenile, 234
Memory, eating behaviors and, 519
Meningitis
  aseptic (nonbacterial), 953–954, 954t
  bacterial, 950–952, 951b, 953b, 954t
Meningocele, 1099b, 1099f
Meningococcal conjugate vaccine (MCV), 339
Meningococcal infection, immunization against, 332f–333f, 339
Meningococcal vaccine, sickle cell anemia and, 876
Mental health problems, 6

Mental representation, in cognitive development, 319, 381, 381f
Mental retardation, definition of, 571
Meperidine
  for pain, 164t
  in patient-controlled analgesia, 164
Mercury poisoning, 441
Mercy killing, 555–556
Meromelia, 1072
Mesh graft, for burns, 1043, 1044f
Metabolic acidosis, in chronic renal failure, 921
Metabolism
  effect of immobilization on, 1051t–1053t
  low, obesity and, 519
  neonatal, 187
    complications of, 266, 267t
    inborn errors of, 295–301
Metalloporphyrins, for hyperbilirubinemia, 260
Metatarsus adductus, 1072
Metatarsus varus, 1072
Metered-dose inhaler (MDI)
  for asthma, 739
  use of, 744, 746b, 746f
Methadone, for pain, 164t
Methamphetamine
  adolescent use of, 529
  intrauterine exposure to, 289–290
Methicillin-resistant *Staphylococcus aureus* (MRSA) infection, 1017
Methotrexate, for juvenile rheumatoid arthritis, 1085
Mexican American families, health beliefs and practices of, 58t–59t
Microcephaly, 192
Microminerals (trace elements), 355–356
  bioavailability of, in human milk, 214
Midstream urine specimen, 659
Migraine, abdominal, 784
Migrant families, 51–52
Milk
  evaporated, 218
  for toddler, 392
  goat's, 218
  human, 214–215. *See also* Breastfeeding.
  witch's, 197
Milk babies, 872
Milk products, alternate, 218
Millard procedure, for cleft lip, 801
Mind-altering drugs, adolescent use of, 530
Mineral imbalances, in infant, 355–356
Mineral supplements, for protein-energy malnutrition, 357
Mineralocorticoids, 974t–976t
  for Addison disease, 988
Minimal-change nephrotic syndrome, 912
Minorities, 47. *See also* Race/ethnicity.
Minors, emancipated, informed consent of, 637
Misbehavior
  consequences of, 35
  minimizing, 33, 34b
Mitral valves, 133
Mixed defects, in congenital heart disease, 830, 831b–834b
Mixed movement, in cerebral palsy, 1091, 1092b
Mobility, spinal, 139
Mobilization device, in cerebral palsy, 1093, 1093f

Modeling, of aggression, 416–417
Modified Behavioral Pain Score (MBPS), 146t–147t
Mogen clamp, for circumcision, 212
Molestation, 447
Molluscum contagiosum, 1019t
Mongolian spots, 210
Moniliasis. *See* Candidiasis.
Monoclonal antibodies, for asthma, 740
Monocytes, 188
Mononucleosis, infectious, 719–720, 720b
Monosomy, 294
Monospot test, for mononucleosis, 720
Monotropy, 221
Mons pubis, examination of, 138, 138f
Mood changes, chemotherapy-induced, 892
Moon face, chemotherapy-induced, 892
MOPP regimen, for Hodgkin lymphoma, 893
Moral development, 71t, 73–74
  of adolescent, 482
  of preschooler, 409
  of school-age child, 460
Morality, play and, 78, 78f
Morbidity
  childhood, 8
  rates of, 18, 18b
Mormonism, 61t–62t
Moro reflex, 200, 200f
Morphine
  for cancer pain, 179–180
  for pain, 162, 164t
  in patient-controlled analgesia, 163–164
Mortality. *See also* Death and dying.
  childhood, 7–8, 7t
  infant, 6–7, 7t
  rates of, 18, 18b
Mosquito bites, 1025t–1026t
Mother
  attachment of, to neonate, 219–220, 219f
  of special needs child, 541
  working, 40, 40b
Mother-infant care (dyad), 222
Mother's milk. *See* Breast milk.
Mother-twin bonding, 221
Motility disorders, 771–784
Motivation
  activities promoting, 70b
  in substance abuse, 527
Motor development
  fine
    in infant, 310t–314t, 315, 315f
    in preschooler, 408, 413t–414t
    in toddler, 380, 386t–387t
  gross
    in infant, 310t–314t, 315–317
    in preschooler, 408, 408f, 413t–414t
    in toddler, 379, 386t–387t
Motor function, in neurologic examination, 931–932
Motor vehicle. *See* Automobile *entries.*
Mourning, 565–566
Mouth. *See also* Oral *entries.*
  examination of, 128–129, 129f
  in Down syndrome, 577b
  of neonate, 197, 198t, 203t–206t
Movement, freedom of, in hospitalization, 622

Movement disorder(s), in cerebral palsy, 1091, 1092b
Mucocutaneous lymph node syndrome, 858–860, 859b
Mucosa
  gastrointestinal, in neonate, 187
  ulceration of, chemotherapy-induced, 891–892
Mucosal protective agents, for peptic ulcer disease, 793
Mucositis, oral, in cancer patients, 179
Mucous membranes
  in neonate, 188
  nasal, 128
  oral, 128–129
Mucus, in respiratory tract, 271
Multifactorial inheritance, 294
Multimodal therapy, for attention-deficit/hyperactivity disorder, 503
Multiple births, 30–31, 30f, 31t. *See also* Twins.
  and subsequent children, 221–222, 222f
  parental adjustment to, 31
Multiple disabilities. *See also* Chronic illness/disability.
  nursing care guidelines for, 550b
Mummy restraints, 656, 657f
Mumps, 424t–430t
  immunization against, 332f–333f, 337
Munchausen syndrome by proxy, 446
Muscle(s), examination of, 139–140
Muscle tone, in neonate, 200
Muscular dystrophy, 1106, 1107f
  Duchenne, 1106–1109, 1107b–1108b, 1107f–1108f
  Landouzy-Dejerine, 1106
  limb-girdle, 1106
Muscular system
  effect of immobilization on, 1051t–1053t
  in neonates, 188
Musculoskeletal disorder(s). *See also specific disorder.*
  acquired, 1074–1079
  amputation for, 1066
  casts for, 1059–1062
  congenital, 1068–1074
  distraction therapy for, 1065–1066
  infectious, 1079–1081
  neoplastic, 1081–1084
  traction for, 1062–1064
  traumatic, 1055–1066
Musculoskeletal system
  in Down syndrome, 577b
  in neonate, 188
Muslims, 61t–62t
Mutations
  genetic, 80
  in fragile X syndrome, 578–579
Mutilation, female, 214b
Mutual affection and equality, between parent and adolescent, 483
Mutual play, of preschooler, 412
Mutual storytelling, in communication with children, 93
Mycotic infections. *See* Fungal infections.
Myelination, in neonate, 188
Myelitis, transverse, 1114
Myelodysplasia, 1098

Myelomeningocele, 1098–1104, 1099b, 1099f. *See also* Spina bifida.
Myelomeningocele sac, 1099, 1100f
  care of, 1102–1103
Myelosuppression, in leukemia, 890–891
Myoclonic seizures, 958b–959b. *See also* Seizure(s).
Myopia, 584, 584b–585b
Myositis ossificans, 1055
MyPlate, 99, 102f
MyPyramid for Preschoolers, 417–418
Myringotomy, for otitis media, 718–719
Mythical-literal stage, of spiritual development, 71t, 74

N

Nails, examination of, 119–120
Naming, of deceased infant, 253
Narcissism, 318–319
Narcotics, adolescent use of, 529
Nasal canal, patency of, in neonate, 197
Nasal cannula, oxygen delivery via, 688
Nasal meatus, 128
Nasal mucus, assessment of, in respiratory function, 709b
Nasal septum, 128
Nasal turbinates, 128
Nasal vestibule, anterior, 128
Nasal washing, 665
Nasoduodenal tube, feeding via, 700–701
Nasogastric tube
  drug administration via, 676, 678b
  feedings via, 635
  placement of, 696b–697b
Nasojejunal tube, feeding via, 700–701
Nasopharyngeal temperature, measurement of, 112b
Nasopharyngitis, viral, 710–714, 711b–712b
  clinical manifestations of, 713b
  complications of, 714b
Nasotracheal intubation, for epiglottitis, 721
Natal teeth, vs. neonatal teeth, 197
National Childhood Vaccine Injury Act (1986), 344
National Children's Study, 2b
Native American families, health beliefs and practices of, 58t–59t
Natural forces, in health beliefs and practices, 43
Nausea
  chemotherapy-induced, 891
  opioid-induced, 165t–166t
Near-drowning. *See* Submersion injury.
Neck
  examination of, 120–121
  in Down syndrome, 577b
  of neonate, 197, 203t–206t
Necrotizing enterocolitis, 284–285, 285b
Needle(s)
  safe disposal of, 609b
  selection of, in intramuscular drug administration, 667, 668b–669b
Needleless system
  in lidocaine injections, 170b
  in parenteral fluid therapy, 682, 684f
Negativism, during toddler years, 380, 390

Neglect, 445–446
  definition of, 445
  history and interview in, 449
  physical assessment of, 450b, 451
  types of, 446
Neonatal Abstinence Scoring System, 288
Neonatal abstinence syndrome, 200, 287
Neonatal Infant Pain Scale (NIPS), 148t–150t
Neonatal Intensive Care Unit Network Neurobehavioral Scale (NNNS), 288
Neonatal lupus, 1086–1087
Neonatal Pain, Agitation, and Sedation Scale (NPASS), 148t–150t, 153
Neonate(s)
  abdomen in, 199, 203t–206t
    circumference of, 192
    contour of, 199
  acid-base imbalance in, 277–279, 277t, 279t
  adjustment of, to extrauterine life, 186–189
  alcohol-exposed, 289
  anal patency in, 199
  assessment of, 189–202
    Apgar scoring in, 189, 189t
    attachment behaviors in, 202, 202b
    behavioral, 201–202, 201b
    birth weight in, 189–192, 191f
    clinical, 189–201, 190b, 190f–191f
    general appearance in, 194
    general measurements in, 192–194, 192f–193f
    gestational age in, 189–201, 190b, 190f–191f
    initial, 189, 189t
    physical, 202, 203t–206t
    reflexes in, 198t
    transitional, 201
  auditory acuity in, 188
  axillary temperature in, 192, 192f
  bathing of, 209–210, 211f
  behavior of, 194, 219
  birth injuries in, 229–232, 230f–232f
  birthmarks in, 234–235, 234f
  blood pressure measurement in, 193, 193f
  blood volume in, 186–187
  brown fat in, 186
  candidiasis in, 232–233, 233f
  cardiovascular complications in, 279, 280t
  chemically induced defects in, 294–295, 296t
  chest in, 197, 203t–206t
    circumference of, 192
  circulatory system in, 186
  circumcision in, 211–214, 211b, 212f
    cultural considerations in, 214b
    pain management during, 212b–213b
  cocaine-exposed, 289
  congenital anomalies in, 293–295, 293b
    genetic etiology of, 294, 295t
  congenital hypothyroidism in, 297–298, 297b
  constipation in, 778
  crackles in, 197
  cry of, 202, 202t
  discharge planning for, 222–223, 222b–223b
  drug-exposed, 286–290, 287b
  ears in, 197, 203t–206t
  eccrine glands in, 187
  endocrine system in, 188
  erythema toxicum neonatorum in, 232
  extremities in, 198t, 199–200, 203t–206t

Neonate(s) *(Continued)*
  eyes in, 196–197, 198t, 203t–206t
    ophthalmia neonatorum prophylaxis and, 208
  feeding behavior of, 218–219
  feeding schedules for, 218
  femoral pulses in, 203t–206t
  fluid and electrolyte balance in, 187
  galactosemia in, 300–301
  gastrointestinal system in, 187, 187b
  genetic disease in
    counseling and testing for, 301–302, 302t
    psychologic aspects of, 302
  genitalia in
    female, 199, 203t–206t
    male, 199, 203t–206t
  gestational age of, 189–201, 190b, 190f–191f
  hair follicle growth phases in, 187–188
  head circumference of, 192
  head contour of, 194–196
  head control in, 196, 196f
  head-to-heel length of, 192, 192f
  hearing in, 188, 197, 198t
    screening for, 209
  heart in, 198–199, 203t–206t
  heart rate in, 198
  heart sounds in, 198–199
  heat loss in, 207
  heel punctures in, 210b
  hematopoietic system in, 186
  hemolytic disease of, 263–266, 264f, 265t
  herpes simplex infection in, 233–234
  high-risk, 235–253
    baptism of, 253
    breastfeeding of, 241
    care of, 235–253
    classification of, 235, 236b
    definition of, 235
    developmental outcome in, 246–248, 246f, 248b, 280t
    discharge planning for, 251–252, 252b
    energy conservation in, 243–244, 243f
    family support for, 248–249, 249b
    feeding resistance in, 243
    gavage feeding of, 242–243
    hydration in, 239–240
    hyperbilirubinemia in, 256–263, 257t, 259f–260f
    identification of, 235
    infection prevention in, 239
    loss of, 252–253
    nipple feeding of, 241–242, 242f
    nutrition for, 240–243
    parent-infant relationships and, 249–251, 250f
    physical assessment of, 237b
    physiologic monitoring of, 237
    postterm, 256
    preterm, 253–256, 254b, 255f–256f
    respiratory support for, 236
    siblings of, 251, 251f
    skin care in, 244, 244b–245b
    support groups and, 251
    systematic assessment of, 235
    thermoregulation in, 236–239, 239f
  home care after discharge and, 222–223, 223b
  immunization of, hepatitis B, 209

Neonate(s) *(Continued)*
infection in
defenses against, 188
identification of, 208
maternal infections and, 290, 291t–292t
necrotizing enterocolitis, 284–285, 285b
prevention of, 208–214
sepsis, 282–284, 283b
intestines in, 187, 187b
kidneys in, 203t–206t
liver in, 187, 203t–206t
lungs in, 197–198, 203t–206t
marijuana-exposed, 290
maternal attachment to, 219–220, 219f
maternal diabetes and, 285–286, 286b, 286f
melanin in, 188
metabolic rate in, 187
metabolism in
complications of, 266, 267t
inborn errors of, 295–301
methamphetamine-exposed, 289–290
mouth in, 197, 198t, 203t–206t
multiple births and subsequent children and,
221–222, 222f
musculoskeletal system in, 188
myelination in, 188
neck in, 197, 203t–206t
neurologic system in, 188, 198t, 200–201, 200f
complications of, 279, 281t
nose in, 197, 198t, 203t–206t
nursing care of, 189–223
nutrition for, 214–219
alternate milk products in, 218
bottle feeding and, 217
breastfeeding and, 215–216, 215b, 216f
commercially prepared formulas in, 217–218
human milk in, 214–215
pain assessment in, 152–153, 153b, 154t–155t
parental bonding with, 219–222, 219f
patent airway in, maintenance of, 206–207
paternal engrossment with, 220–221, 220f
peptic ulcers in, 792b
phenylketonuria in, 298–300, 299f
physical examination of, 206b
pneumonia in, 725
posture of, 194, 203t–206t
pseudomenstruation in, 188
pulse in, 193
pulse oximetry in, 193, 194b–195b
rectum in, 199, 203t–206t
reflexes in, 198t. *See also specific reflexes.*
renal system in, 187
respirations in, 193, 197
respiratory distress syndrome in, 267–273,
268f–269f, 269b, 270t
respiratory system in, 186
complications of, 273–279, 273t–274t
salivary glands in, 187
screening for disease in, 209
sebaceous glands in, 187
seizures in, 279–282, 281b, 282t
selective serotonin reuptake inhibitor–exposed,
290
sensory functions of, 188–189
siblings of, 221, 221f
skin of, 187–188, 194, 203t–206t
sleep/activity patterns in, 201, 202t

Neonate(s) *(Continued)*
smell in, 188–189
spine in, 199, 203t–206t
spleen in, 203t–206t
stomach capacity in, 187
tactile stimulation in, 186
taste in, 189
thermoregulation in, 186–189
axillary temperature in, 192, 192f
maintenance of stable temperature and, 207
throat in, 197, 198t, 203t–206t
touch in, 189
umbilical cord in, 203t–206t
umbilicus in, care of, 211
vision in, 188
vitamin K administration in, 208–209
weight loss in, 192
Neoplastic disease, 888–894
genetic-environment interplay in, 80
leukemias, 888–892
lymphomas, 892–894
pain associated with, 179–180
testicular, 510
Nephroblastoma (Wilms tumor), 917–918,
917b–918b
Nephropathy, diabetic, 993
Nephrosis
childhood, 912
idiopathic, 912
Nephrotic syndrome, 912–915
diagnosis of, 913, 914b
nursing care management for, 914–915
pathophysiology of, 913, 913f
prognosis of, 914
treatment of, 914
Nervous system tumors, 946–949
Nesting, 246
Neural tube defects, 1098–1104, 1099b, 1099f.
See also Spina bifida.
Neurobehavioral organization, in toddler, 379
Neuroblastoma, 949
Neuroectodermal tumor, primitive, 1082–1083
Neurofibromatosis, 1031t
Neurogenic shock, 1115
Neurohypophysis (posterior pituitary), 974t–976t
Neurologic system
examination of, 140, 140b, 140f–142f, 142t,
930–932
in infant, 309, 310t–314t
in neonate, 188, 198t, 200–201, 200f
complications of, 279, 281t
maturation of, 68
Neuromuscular disorder(s). *See also specific
disorder.*
acquired, 1109–1117
congenital, 1090–1109
Neuromuscular electrical stimulation, in cerebral
palsy, 1094
Neuropathic pain, opioid infusion for, 180
Neuropathy
chemotherapy-induced, 892
diabetic, 993
Neutrophils, 188
Nevus
bathing trunk, 234
giant pigmented, 234
junctional (compound), 234

Nevus flammeus, 234, 234f
New Ballard Scale, 189, 190f–191f
Newborn Assessment of Pain Inventory (NAPI),
146t–147t
Nightmares, vs. sleep terrors, 418, 419t
90-degree–90-degree traction, 1063
Nipple(s)
position of, 130
supernumerary, 197
Nipple feeding, of high-risk neonate, 241–242,
242f
Nissen fundoplication, for gastroesophageal
reflux, 782, 783f
Nitric oxide, inhaled, for respiratory distress
syndrome, 277
Nitrous oxide, for procedural pain, 176–177
Nits, 1024, 1027b, 1027f
Nocturnal enuresis, 499, 500b. *See also* Urinary
incontinence.
Nodule, 1011f
Noise, environmental, 580
Noise pollution, excessive, 584
Non-commuicating Children's Pain Checklist,
156, 157f–158f
Non-Hodgkin lymphoma, 894
Nonmaleficence, 11
Nonnutritive sucking, 243
in pain management, 159, 159f
Nonpenetrating wounds, to eye, 586
Nonpharmacologic strategies, in pain
management, 159–162, 159f, 160b, 162f
Nonpoisonous plants, 437b
Nonsmoking strategies, 529b
Nonsteroidal antiinflammatory drugs
(NSAIDs)
for dysmenorrhea, 509
for juvenile rheumatoid arthritis, 1085
for pain, 162, 163t
Nontunneled catheter, 673
Nonverbal communication, 53–54, 574, 574f
techniques of, with children, 94
Norepinephrine, 974t–976t
Normalization
concept of, 597
in chronic illness/disability, 539–540
promotion of, 551b
North American blastomycosis, 1021t
North American family, 45
Norwalk-like organisms, diarrhea due to,
772t–774t
Nose. *See also* Nasal; Naso- *entries.*
examination of, 127–128, 128f, 128t
in Down syndrome, 577b
in neonate, 197, 198t, 203t–206t
Nose drops, 679, 680f
Nosebleed (epistaxis), 888
Noxious irritants, inhalation of, 734
Nuclear brain scan, 933t–934t
Nuclear family, 26
traditional, 26
Numeric Scale, in pain assessment, 148t–150t
Nursemaid's elbow, 1056
Nursing care, of neonate, 189–223
Nursing care guidelines, 10b, 14b
Nursing caries, 395–396, 396f
Nursing diagnosis, 12–13, 13b
Nursing informatics, 88

Nursing practice, evidence-based practice in, 11–12, 12t
Nursing process, 12–13
  assessment in, 12
  documentation in, 13
  evaluation in, 13
  implementation in, 13
  in community-based nursing care, 19–20, 19b
  in home care, 605–607, 606b
  nursing diagnosis in, 12–13, 13b
  planning in, 13
Nursing research, 11–12
Nutrition, 2. *See also* Diet.
  assessment of, 99–102
    biochemical tests in, 102
    clinical examination in, 102, 104t–105t
    evaluation of, 102, 102f
  enteral
    for high-risk neonate, 237
    for necrotizing enterocolitis, 284
    gavage feeding in, 242–243, 695–698, 696b–697b, 698f
  for adolescent, 489–490, 490f
  for infant, 326–330, 326b, 329b
    in first 6 months, 326–328
    in second 6 months, 328
    solid foods in
      introduction of, 329
      preparation of, 328
    weaning in, 329–330
  for neonate, 214–219
    alternate milk products in, 218
    at high risk, 240–243
    bottle feeding and, 217
    breastfeeding and, 215–216, 215b, 216f
    commercially prepared formulas in, 217–218
    human milk in, 214–215
  for preschooler, 417–418, 418f
  for school-age child, 468–472
  for toddler, 391, 393b
    counseling in, 391
    dietary guidelines in, 391–392
  socioeconomic aspects of, 51
  total parenteral
    in inflammatory bowel disease, 790
    in short-bowel syndrome, 815
Nutritional counseling, for obesity, 521–522
Nutritional disorders. *See also* Malnutrition; *specific disorder or nutrient.*
  in infant, 354–366
  nursing care management for, 356
Nutritional support
  in burns, 1042
  in cirrhosis, 798
  in coma, 937
  in congestive heart failure, 840
  in diabetes mellitus, 996
  in growth and development, 69–70
  in inflammatory bowel disease, 790
  in respiratory infections, 710
  in short-bowel syndrome, 815
Nutritional therapy, for eating disorders, 525
NuvaRing, 512t–514t
Nystagmus, in neonate, 197
Nystatin, for oral candidiasis, 233

O
Oak, poison, 1022
Obesity, 3, 3f
  adolescent, 490, 517–523
  diagnosis of, 519–520
  etiology and pathophysiology of, 518–519, 518f
  nursing care management for, 521–523, 521b–522b
  prevention of, 520b, 522b
  treatment of, 520–521
Object permanence
  in infant, 319, 319f
  in toddler, 381
Objective Pain Score (OPS), 146t–147t
Obstructive defects, in congenital heart disease, 825–827, 825f, 828b–829b
Obstructive sleep apnea syndrome, 754
Obstructive uropathy, 910–911, 911f
Obtundation, 929b
Occupational therapy, for juvenile rheumatoid arthritis, 1085
Ocular alignment, 122–125, 122f–123f
Oculomotor nerve, assessment of, 141f, 142t
Oculovestibular response, 931
Odor of breath, 930
Olfactory nerve, assessment of, 141f, 142t
Omphalocele, 807t
Omphalomesenteric fistula, 786
Onlooker play, 76
Only child, 30
Open comedone (blackhead), 1035
Open fracture, of skull, 940
Open (compound) fracture, 1057
Ophthalmia neonatorum, prophylaxis for, 208
Opioid(s)
  addiction to, 175b, 563
  dosages of, 164t
  for neuropathic pain, 180
  for pain, 162, 164t
  physical dependence on, 175b
  side effects of, 165t–166t, 168–172, 172b
  tolerance to, 171–172, 173f–174f, 175b, 563
  weaning flowsheet for, 171–172, 173f–174f
Optic disc, examination of, 122
Optic nerve, assessment of, 141f, 142t
Oral administration, of drugs, 665–667, 666b, 667f
Oral candidiasis (thrush), in neonate, 232–233, 233f
Oral care, in coma, 937
Oral contraceptives, 512t–514t
  for dysmenorrhea, 509
Oral hygiene, 649. *See also* Dental health; Dental hygiene.
  in infant, 330
Oral rehydration solutions
  for dehydration, 768, 769t
  for diarrhea, 775, 775b, 776t
  for respiratory infections, 710
Oral stage, in psychosexual development, 71, 71t
Oral temperature, measurement of, 113t
Organ donation, 565
Organ systems
  growth and development of, 69
  review of, in history taking, 99
Organizational strategies, in compliance, 647

Orogastric administration, of drugs, 676, 678b
Oropharynx, examination of, 129
Ortho Evra transdermal system, 512t–514t
Orthodox Judaism, 61t–62t
Orthophoric eyes, 122–123, 122f
Orthostatic hypotension, 118
Osseous deformities, in chronic renal failure, 922–923
Ossification centers, 68
Osteochondritis deformans juvenilis, 1074–1075, 1074b
Osteodystrophy, renal, 921
Osteogenesis imperfecta, 1073–1074
  classification of, 1073b
Osteomyelitis, 1079–1080, 1079b
  acute hematogenous, 1079
  chronic, 1079
  subacute, 1079
Osteosarcoma, 1081–1082
  amputation for, 1066
Ostomies, 702
Otitis externa, 1035
Otitis media, 717–719, 718b
  clinical manifestations of, 718, 718b
  nursing care management for, 719
  pain in, 176
  prevention of, 719
  treatment of, 718–719
Otitis media with effusion, 718b, 719
Otoscopy, 127
  reducing distress from, 125b
Oucher Pain Scale, 150, 156
Outcome and Assessment Information Set (OASIS), 602–603
Outpatient care, 629–630
Ovarian hormones, 974t–976t
Overeating, during adolescence, 490
Overprotection, in chronic illness/disability, 544, 553b
Overuse syndrome, 1067
Owl eyes appearance, in Hodgkin lymphoma, 893
Oximetry, pulse, 688, 688f
Oxycodone, for pain, 162, 164t
Oxygen mask, 688
Oxygen tent, 688
Oxygen therapy, 687–689, 688f
  for respiratory distress syndrome, 270, 270t
  for sickle cell anemia, 876
  in delivery room, 278b
  monitoring of, 688–689, 688f
Oxymetazoline, for respiratory infections, 709
Oxytocin, 974t–976t

P
Pacemakers, permanent, 854
Pacifier, 324–325, 324b
  in pain management, 159
  sudden infant death syndrome and, 370
Padded overhead shield restraint, 398
PAH gene, 298
Pain
  abdominal. *See* Abdominal pain.
  burn, 177
  cancer, 179–180
  emotional response to, 151

Pain (Continued)
fear of, 560–563
in primary care, 175–176
in sickle cell disease, 178–179
intensity of, 145–150, 145f, 146t–150t
of recurrent headaches, 177–178
physical recovery after, 150–151
postoperative, 177
responses to, 145b
untreated, consequences of, 175
Pain assessment, 144–152, 145b
cultural differences in, 156
in acute conditions, 145–151, 145f, 146t–150t
in chronic illness, 156
in chronic or recurrent conditions, 151
in communication and cognitive impaired child, 153–156, 157f–158f
in complex pain, 156
in neonate, 152–153, 153b, 154t–155t
multidimensional measures in, 151–152, 152f
Pain Assessment Tool (PAT), 148t–150t
Pain diaries, 151
Pain Indicator for Communicatively Impaired Children (PICIC), 156
Pain management, 156–175
adverse events and symptoms in, 150
during circumcision, 212b–213b
effectiveness of, 172–175
for comatose child, 934–935
for invasive procedural pain, 176–177
for minor procedures, 161b–162b
improvement and satisfaction with, judgment of, 150
in end-of-life care, 180, 562–563, 563b
in human immunodeficiency virus infection, 896
in juvenile rheumatoid arthritis, 1085
in leukemia, 890
in spinal cord injuries, 1117
nonpharmacologic, 159–162, 159f, 160b, 162f
pharmacologic, 162–175, 163t–166t, 166b–167b
analgesic patches in, 169b
buffered lidocaine in, 171b
epidural analgesia in, 168
needle-free injection system in, 170b
patient-controlled analgesia in, 163–164, 168f
side effects of, 168–172, 172b, 173f–174f
transmucosal and transdermal analgesia in, 168, 168f
proper positioning in, 159
Pain Rating Scales, 148t–150t
Painting, during hospitalization, 625–626, 625f
Palate
cleft, 800–803, 802b
hard and soft, examination of, 129
in neonate, 197
Palatine (faucial) tonsil, 715, 715f
Palliative care, 555. See also Death and dying.
Pallor, 119t
Palm, examination of, 120, 120f
Palmar grasp, 315
Palpation
in cardiovascular dysfunction, 821
of abdomen, 136, 136b, 137f

Palpation (Continued)
of femoral pulses, 136, 137f
of joints, 139
of scrotum, 137
of skull, 121, 195
Palpebral fissures, examination of, 121
Pancreatic enzymes, replacement of, in cystic fibrosis, 751
Pancreatic fibrosis, in cystic fibrosis, 747
Pancreatic hormones, 974t–976t
disorders of, 992–1006
Pandemic, WHO definition of, 716–717
Papule, 1011f
Parachute reflex, 315–316, 317f
Parallel play, 76, 76f
Paralysis, in neonate
brachial, 231–232, 232f
facial, 231, 231f
phrenic nerve, 232
Parasitic disease(s), 433–436, 434t
enterobiasis, 435–436, 436b
giardiasis, 434–435, 435b, 435f
nursing care management for, 433–434
prevention of, 434b
Parasomnias, 364
Parasuicide, 531. See also Suicide.
Parathyroid disorder(s), 985–987
hyperparathyroidism, 986–987, 986b
hypoparathyroidism, 985–986, 985b
Parathyroid hormone (PTH), 974t–976t, 985
Parent(s), 31–35. See also Family(ies); Father; Mother.
abusive, 447
accommodating contemporary parenting situations of, 41
adolescent relationships with, 483, 488t
age of, 32
authoritarian (dictorial), 33
authoritative (democratic), 33
behaviors of, 33
communication with, 88–90. See also Communication.
about immunizations, 341b
discipline by
guidelines for implementing, 33–34, 34b
types of, 34–35, 35b, 35f
divorced, 37–39, 37b–38b
education of, 32, 32f
father involvement as, 32, 32f, 53, 53f
foster, 41
grieving, 565
informed consent of, 637
limit setting by, 33–35, 34b–35b, 35f
minimizing misbehavior by, 33, 34b
motivation for parenthood and, 31
of adoptive child, 25, 36f
of high-risk neonate, psychologic tasks of, 249, 249b
of hospitalized child
absence of, 621–622, 622f
participation of, 628–629
reactions of, 617, 617b
of school-age child, 466
of special needs child, 540–541, 540b
empowerment of, 542–543, 551
response to behavior of, 547
support for, 549–551

Parent(s) (Continued)
of twins, 30–31, 30f, 31t
adjustment of, 31
parenting styles of, 33
permissive, 33
preparation for parenthood and, 31
presence and support of
for induction of anesthesia, 644, 644f
for procedures, 638–640
rape victim's, support for, 517b
roles of, 28
single, 27, 39
support systems for, 32–33, 33f
transition to parenthood and, 31–33, 32f–33f
Parental consent, treatment without, 637
Parental right to child's medical chart, informed consent and, 637
Parent-child attachment, in visual impairment, 587
Parent-child interactions, 99
Parent-child relationships, during hospitalization, 626
Parenteral fluid therapy, 681–687
complications of, 687
for dehydration, 769
for high-risk neonate, 239–240
infusion pumps for, 683
intravenous care in, 685b–686b
intravenous set changes in, 686b
line removal in, 684–687
line securement in, 684, 684f
safety catheters and needleless systems in, 682, 684f
site for, 681–682, 682f
Parent-infant bonding, promotion of, 219–222, 219f
Parent-infant relationships, of high-risk neonate, 249–251, 250f
Parent-professional collaboration
in home care, 604–605
successful, 31–35
Parent's Postoperative Pain Measure (PPPM), 147
Parent's Postoperative Pain Rating Scale (PPPRS), 147
Partial seizures, 957, 958b–959b, 959t. See also Seizure(s).
Parvovirus B19 (erythema infectiosum), maternal infection with, 291t–292t
Patau syndrome (trisomy 13), 295t
Patch, 1011f
Patent ductus arteriosus (PDA), 826b–827b
Paternal engrossment, with neonate, 220–221, 220f
Patient-Centered Outcome Measures, 1
Patient-controlled analgesia, 163–164, 168f
mode of administration of, 163
Paun-Brunell test, for mononucleosis, 720
Pavlik harness, 1070, 1070f
PCV (pneumococcal conjugate vaccine), 338
Peak expiratory flow meter (PEFM), 738, 744b
Peak expiratory flow rate (PEFR), 738
Pearson attachment, 1063
Pediatric coma scale, 930f
Pediatric nurse, role of, 9–11, 17b
Pediatric nursing, 1–14
atraumatic care in, 8–9
clinical reasoning in, 12

Pediatric nursing *(Continued)*
  coordination and collaboration in, 11
  dental care in, 2–3
  disease prevention in, 9
  ethical decision making in, 11
  evidence-based practice in, 11–12, 12t
  family advocacy and caring in, 9, 9b
  family-centered care in, 8, 8b
  goal of, 2
  health problems in, 3–6, 3f–6f, 4b, 4t
  health promotion in, 2–3, 9
  health teaching in, 10
  immunizations in, 3
  injury prevention in, 10
  morbidity in, 8
  mortality in
    childhood, 7–8, 7t
    infant, 6–7, 7t
  nutrition in, 2
  philosophy of care in, 8–9
  process in, 12–13
  quality outcome measures in, 13–14, 14b
  support and counseling in, 10–11
  therapeutic relationship in, 9
Pediatric obesity prevention protocol, 522b
Pediatric shock, 437
Pediculosis capitis, 1024–1028, 1027b–1028b,
    1027f
Pedophilia, 447
Peer(s), adolescent relationships with, 483–484,
    484f, 488t
Peer groups
  culture of, 48–49, 48f
  school-age child and, 462–463
Penetrating wounds, to eye, 586, 586b
Penicillin, prophylactic
  for rheumatic fever, 849–850
  for sickle cell anemia, 876, 876b–877b
Penicillin G, for streptococcal pharyngitis, 714
Penis
  circumcised, care of, 212
  examination of, 137
  in neonate, 199
Peptic ulcer disease, 792–793, 792b
Perceptual thinking, in school-age child, 460
Percussion
  in cardiovascular dysfunction, 821
  in coma, 936
Perinatal ischemic stroke, 1091
Perineal fistula, 811b, 812
Periodic breathing, in neonate, 197
Periodontal disease, in school-age child, 470
Periodontitis, in school-age child, 470
Peripheral blood smear, 870t
Peripheral intermittent infusion device, 672–673
Peripheral intravenous access
  frequency of set changes in, 686b
  lidocaine for pain during, 171b
Peripheral intravenous line
  care of, 685b–686b
  removal of, 684–687
  securement of, 684, 684f
Peripheral lock, 672–673
Peripheral precocious puberty, 980, 980b
Peripheral stem cell transplantation, 899
Peripheral vision, 124–125
Peripherally inserted central catheter, 674

Peristalsis, 136
Peristaltic waves, 135
Peritoneal dialysis, 924
Peritonitis, 785
Periungual desquamation, in Kawasaki disease,
    859–860
PERRLA, 121
Persistent pulmonary hypertension of newborn,
    273t–274t
Persistent vegetative state, 929b
Personal care, in adolescence, 491–492
Personal identity, vs. role diffusion, 481
Personal relationships, in adolescence, 484
Personality, development of, 71–75, 71t
  theoretic foundations of, 71–72
Personal-social behavior
  of preschooler, 410–411, 411f
  of toddler, 384
Personnel, in atraumatic care, 8–9
Pertussis (whooping cough), 424t–430t, 728–729
  immunization against, 332f–333f, 336
Petechiae, 119t, 1010
Petit mal seizures, 958b–959b, 959t. *See also*
    Seizure(s).
PH, compensated and uncompensated, 279
PHACE syndrome, 234
Phallix stage, in psychosexual development, 71, 71t
Phantom limb sensation, 1066
Pharyngeal tonsil, 715, 715f
Pharyngitis
  pain in, 176
  streptococcal, 714–715, 714f
Phenylalanine, 298
Phenylalanine hydroxylase, 298
Phenylephrine, for respiratory infections, 709
Phenylketonuria (PKU), 298–300, 299f
  neonatal screening for, 209
Phenylpyruvic acid, 298
Pheochromocytoma, 991–992
Phimosis, 912t
Phobia, school, 505
Phocomelia, 1072
Phosphorus, dietary, 922
Phosphorus imbalance
  in chronic renal failure, 921
  in infant, 356
Photograph, of deceased infant, 253
Photoisomerization, 260
Photoscreening, for amblyopia, 123
Phototherapy
  and parent-child interaction, 263b
  commercial delivery of, 260–261
  for hyperbilirubinemia, 250f, 260, 262
  home, 263
Phrenic nerve paralysis, in neonate, 232
Physeal injuries, 1057–1058, 1058f
Physical abuse, 446–447, 449, 450b, 451, 452b
  factors predisposing to, 446
Physical activity. *See* Activity and exercise.
Physical dependence, on opioids, 175b
Physical disability. *See also* Chronic illness/
    disability.
  nursing care guidelines for, 550b
Physical distress, 8–9
Physical examination, 106–140, 108f
  general appearance in, 118–119
  growth measurements in, 106–111, 109f–111f

Physical examination *(Continued)*
  of abdomen, 134–136, 135f–137f
    in neonate, 199
  of anus, 138
    in neonate, 199
  of chest, 129–130, 130f–131f
    in neonate, 197, 203t–206t
  of ears, 125–127, 125f–127f
    in neonate, 197, 203t–206t
  of extremities, 139, 139f
    in neonate, 198t, 199–200, 203t–206t
  of eyes, 121–125, 121f–123f, 124t
    in neonate, 196–197, 198t, 203t–206t
  of genitalia, 136–138
    female, 137–138, 138f
      in neonate, 199, 203t–206t
    male, 137, 137f–138f
      in neonate, 199, 203t–206t
  of head and neck, 120–121
    in neonate, 194–197
  of heart, 132–134, 133f–134f, 134t–135t
    in neonate, 198–199, 203t–206t
  of joints, 139
  of lungs, 130–132, 131b–132b, 132f
    in neonate, 197–198, 203t–206t
  of lymph nodes, 120, 120f
  of mouth and throat, 128–129, 129f
    in neonate, 197, 198t, 203t–206t
  of muscles, 139–140
  of neonate, 206b
  of neurologic system, 140, 140b, 140f–142f,
    142t
    in neonate, 188, 198t, 200–201, 200f
  of nose, 127–128, 128f, 128t
    in neonate, 197, 198t, 203t–206t
  of skin, 119–120, 119t, 120f
    in neonate, 187–188, 195, 203t–206t
  of spine, 138–140
    in neonate, 199, 203t–206t
  physiologic measurements in, 111–118. *See
    also* Vital signs.
  preparation of child for, 102–103, 103f, 106f,
    107t
  sequence of examination in, 102
Physical inactivity, obesity and, 519
Physical irritants, skin lesions caused by,
    1022–1024
Physical neglect, 446, 452b
Physical stressors, in intensive care unit, 633b
Physical therapy
  chest, 689–690
  in cerebral palsy, 1094
  in juvenile rheumatoid arthritis, 1085
Physiologic anorexia, in toddler, 390
Physiologic jaundice, 257–258, 257t
Piaget cognitive theory, 71t, 72–73
  in adolescent, 482, 488t
  in infant, 319–320, 319f
  in preschooler, 409
  in school-age child, 460
  in toddler, 380–382, 381f, 382b
Piercing, in adolescence, 492
Pigeon chest, 129
Pigeon toe, 139
Pilonidal cyst, 199
Pincer grasp, 315, 315f
Pinna, inspection of, 125, 125f

Pinworm (enterobiasis), 435–436, 436b
Pit and fissure sealants, 491
Pituitary
　anterior (adenohypophysis), 974t–976t
　posterior (neurohypophysis), 974t–976t
Pituitary disorder(s), 977–981
　diabetes insipidus, 980–981
　hyperfunction, 979
　hypopituitarism, 977–979, 977b–978b
　precocious puberty, 979–980, 980b
　syndrome of inappropriate antidiuretic
　　hormone secretion, 981
Pituitary hormones, 974t–976t
Pituitary secretion, altered, 937
Plagiocephaly, positional, 366–367, 366f
Plantar (grasp) reflex, 139, 200, 200f
Plantar wart, 1019t
Plants
　nonpoisonous, 437b
　poisonous, 437b, 1022, 1023f
Plaque, cutaneous, 1011f
Plastibell procedure, in circumcision, 212
Plastic deformation fracture, 1057b, 1057f
Plastic hood, oxygen delivery via, 688, 688f
Platelet count, 870t
Play, 75–78
　classification of, 75
　content of, 75–76, 75f–76f
　during hospitalization, 624–626, 624b
　　dramatic, 626
　　therapeutic, 625
　during procedures, 642, 643b
　functions of, 77–78, 78f
　in cognitive development, 319–320
　in cognitive impairment, 573–574, 573f–574f
　in communication with children, 93b–94b,
　　94–95
　in social development
　　of infant, 320, 322
　　of preschooler, 411–412, 411f
　　of school-age child, 463–464
　　of toddler, 384–385, 385f
　in visual impairment, 587
　rules of, 463
　social character of, 76–77, 76f–77f
　team, 463
　therapeutic value of, 77–78, 78f
　toys in, 78
Play rituals, of school-age child, 463
Pneumococcal conjugate vaccine PCV7
　(Prevnar), 719
Pneumococcal conjugate vaccine PCV13, 726
Pneumococcal infection, immunization against,
　332f–333f, 338
Pneumococcal polysaccharide vaccine (PPV), 338
Pneumococcal vaccine, sickle cell anemia and,
　876
Pneumocystis jiroveci (carinii) pneumonia, in
　human immunodeficiency virus infection,
　896
Pneumonia, 725–728
　aspiration, 732–733, 945
　atypical, 726
　bacterial, 726
　complications of, 726, 728b
　nursing care management for, 590, 728f
　Pneumocystis jiroveci (carinii), 896

Pneumonia *(Continued)*
　prevention of, 726
　ventilator-associated, 690
　　prevention of, 727b
　viral, 726, 726b
Pneumonitis, 725
Pneumothorax, 273–277, 273t–274t, 728b
Point of maximum intensity (PMI)
　in neonate, 198
　of pulse, 133
Poison(s), ingestion of, 436–445
Poison control center (PCC), 437
Poison ivy, 1022, 1023f
Poison oak, 1022
Poison sumac, 1022
Poisoning, 5, 6f
　child safety home checklist for, 349b
　digoxin, 838, 839b
　drug, management of, 891–892
　emergency treatment of, 437–441, 437b
　gastric decontamination for, 440
　heavy metal, 441
　lead, 441–445. *See also* Lead poisoning.
　mercury, 441
　of adolescent, 494b
　of infant, 345b–346b, 347t–348t
　of preschooler, 436–445, 437b–439b
　of school-age child, prevention of, 472t–473t
　of toddler, 397t–398t, 402, 402f, 436–445,
　　437b–439b
　prevention of, 440–441, 441b
Poisonous plants, 437b, 1022, 1023f
Poker Chip Tool, in pain assessment, 148t–150t
Poliomyelitis
　immunization against, 336–337
　paralysis of, vaccine-associated, 336–337
Polyandry, 27
Polyarthritis, in rheumatic fever, 850b
Polycythemia, 841
Polydactyly, 139, 199
Polydipsia, in diabetes mellitus, 993
Polygamous family, 27
Polygamy, 27
Polygyny, 27
Polyneuritis, infectious, 1109–1111, 1110b
Polyuria, in diabetes mellitus, 993
Pool therapy, for juvenile rheumatoid arthritis,
　1086
Pornography, child, 447
Port(s), implanted, 675t
Port wine stain, 234, 234f
Positioning
　in coma, 938
　proper, in pain management, 159
Positive self-talk, in pain management, 160b
Positron emission tomography (PET), of cerebral
　function, 933t–934t
Postconcussion syndrome, 943
Posterior cord syndrome, 1115
Posterior sagittal anorectoplasty (PSARP), for
　anorectal malformations, 812
Posthospital behaviors, 616b
Postoperative Pain Score, 148t–150t
Post-pubescence, definition of, 477
Poststreptococcal glomerulonephritis, 915, 915b
Postterm infant(s), 256. *See also* Neonate(s).
Posttraumatic seizures, 943. *See also* Seizure(s).

Posttraumatic stress disorder, 504–505
　definition of, 504
Posttraumatic syndromes, 943
Posture
　of adolescent, 491–492
　of neonate, 194, 203t–206t
Posturing, in neurologic examination, 932, 932f
Potassium depletion, 765t–766t
Potassium excess, 765t–766t
Pouchitis, 790–791
Poverty, 50–51
Preadolescence, 459
Precocious puberty, 979–980, 980b
Prefeeding behavior, of neonate, 218–219
Pregnancy
　adolescent, 511
　as contraindication to MMR immunization,
　　341
　drug use during, 286–290, 287b
Prehension, 315
Premature Infant Pain Profile (PIPP), 148t–150t,
　153
Prematurity. *See* Preterm infant(s).
Prenatal testing, in Down syndrome, 578
Preoperational thought, in cognitive
　development, 71t, 73, 381–382, 382b
Prepubescence, 459
　definition of, 477
Prepuce, 199
　examination of, 138, 138f
Preschool experience, 412–415, 415f
Preschooler(s)
　aggression in, 416–417
　biologic development of, 408, 408f
　body image of, 409–410
　cognitive development of, 408–409
　cognitive impairment in, 572t
　communication with, 91, 92f
　concepts of and reactions to death in,
　　558t–559t
　constipation in, 779
　daycare for, 40, 40b
　dental health of, 419
　developmental effects of chronic illness/
　　disability in, 546t–547t
　fears of, 416
　growth and development of, 408–417,
　　413t–414t
　　concerns related to, 412–417, 415f
　infectious diseases in, 423–433, 424t–430t
　injury prevention in, 419–420
　intestinal parasitic diseases in, 433–436, 434t
　loss of control in, 615
　maltreatment of, 445–454, 450b, 452b
　moral development of, 409
　nutrition for, 417–418, 418f
　peptic ulcers in, 792b
　physical examination of, 107t
　pneumonia in, 725
　poisonous ingestions by, 436–445, 437b–439b
　preparation of, for procedures, 639b–640b
　preschool/kindergarten experience of,
　　412–415, 415f
　psychosocial development of, 408
　separation anxiety in, 614
　sex education for, 415–416
　sexual development of, 410

Preschooler(s) (Continued)
    sleep and activity in, 418–419, 419t
    social development of, 410–412, 410f–411f,
        413t–414t
    speech problems in, 417
    spiritual development of, 409
    stress in, 416
Prescription medication abuse, adolescent, 530b
Presence, definition of, 621
Pressure ulcers, 648
Preterm infant(s), 253–256. See also Neonate(s).
    breastfeeding of, 241
    car seat for, 251–252
    diagnosis of, 254–256, 255f–256f
    late, 235, 254
    treatment of, 256
Primary care, pain in, 175–176
Primary prevention, of disease, 19
Privacy
    computer, 88
    for adolescent, 487b
    in interview, 87, 87f
Private-duty nursing, in home care, 598
Procedures
    child involvement in, 641
    distraction during, 641
    explanation for, 640–641, 641t
    expression of feelings during, 641–642, 642f
    for alternative feeding techniques, 694–701
    for drug administration, 665–681
    for elimination problems, 701–702
    for fluid management, 681–687
    for hygiene and skin care, 647–651
    for respiratory disorders, 687–694
    for specimen collection, 658–665
    guidelines for, 638b
    informed consent for, 636–637
    neurologic, 932–934, 933t–934t
    parental presence and support for, 638–640
    performance of, 641
    play activities for, 642, 643b
    positioning for, 657–658, 657f–658f
    positive reinforcement during, 642
    postprocedural support for, 642
    preparation for
        age-specific, 639b–640b
        family, 642, 643b
        physical, 641
        psychologic, 637–641
    restraint, 655–657, 656t, 657f
    safety, 652–657
    success of, 641
    surgical, 642–646. See also Surgery.
    trust and support for, 638
Progesterone, 974t–976t
Progestin-only pill, 512t–514t
Prolactin, 974t–976t
Prone sleeping, sudden infant death syndrome
    and, 370
Prostacyclin, for pulmonary artery hypertension,
    855
Prostitution, child, 447
Protein(s), in human milk, 214
Protein-energy malnutrition, 356–358
    nursing care management for, 358
    treatment of, 357–358
Protest, stages of, 613b

Pruritus
    control of, 1034
    opioid-induced, 165t–166t
Pseudohypoparathyroidism, 985, 985b
Pseudomenstruation, in neonate, 188
Pseudostrabismus, 122–123, 122f
Psoriasis, 1031t
Psychologic distress, 8–9
Psychologic factors, affecting eating patterns, 519
Psychologic stressors, in intensive care unit, 633b
Psychomotor seizures, 958b–959b, 959t. See also
    Seizure(s).
Psychosexual development, 71, 71t, 318–319
Psychosocial concerns, in human
    immunodeficiency virus infection, 896–897
Psychosocial development, 71–72, 72f, 318–319
    of adolescent, 481–482, 488t
    of preschooler, 408
    of school-age child, 459, 459f
    of toddler, 380, 381f
Psychosocial dwarfism, 507
Psychosocial history, 99
Psychosocial support
    for family of burn patient, 1047
    of burn patient, 1046–1047
Psychostimulants
    for attention-deficit/hyperactivity disorder, 528
    side effects of, 504
Ptyalin, 309–314
Puberty
    body hair changes in, 480f, 481
    constitutional delay of, 507
    definition of, 477
    growth spurt in, 68t
    hormonal changes in, 477
    hormonal influences in, 479–481
    precocious, 979–980, 980b
    responses to, 487, 488t
Pubic hair, 480f, 481
Pudendum, examination of, 138, 138f
Puerto Rican families, health beliefs and practices
    of, 58t–59t
Pulled elbow, 1056
Pulmonary artery hypertension, 854–855
Pulmonary artery temperature, measurement of,
    112b
Pulmonary blood flow
    decreased, defects with, 827–830, 830b–831b,
        830f
    increased, defects with, 825, 825f, 826b–827b
Pulmonary edema, 733
Pulmonary function tests, in asthma, 738
Pulmonic stenosis, 828b–829b
Pulse, 100
    femoral, palpation of, 136, 137f
    grading of, 115t
    in neonate, 193
    location of, 132, 133f
    variable, 930
Pulse check, in cardiopulmonary resuscitation,
    757, 757f
Pulse oximetry, 688, 688f
    in neonate, 193, 194b–195b
Pupils
    examination of, 121
    in neonate, 188
    size variation of, 930–931, 931f

Puppets, for hospitalized child, 626
Purging, 523
Pustule, 1011f
Pyelonephritis, 906
Pyloric stenosis, hypertrophic, 805–809,
    808b, 808f
Pyloromyotomy, for pyloric stenosis, 808
Pyoderma, 1018t

Q
Q-T interval, prolonged, sudden infant death
    syndrome and, 370
Quality outcome measures, in pediatric nursing,
    13–14, 14b

R
Rabies, 955
Race/ethnicity
    culture and, 47, 47f. See also Cultural entries;
        Culture.
    relationship with health care providers and,
        52–54, 53f
    skin color and, 119, 119t
Rachischisis, 1099b
Radiation, heat loss through, 207
Radiation therapy
    for Hodgkin lymphoma, 893
    for retinoblastoma, 589
    for Wilms tumor, 918
    side effects of, 893
Radiofrequency ablation, for supraventricular
    tachycardia, 854
Radiography, of cerebral function, 933t–934t
Radioisotope imaging studies, of urinary
    function, 905t–906t
Radionuclide cystography, 905t–906t
Range of motion
    of extremities, 200
    of head and neck, 121
    of joints, 139
Range-of-motion exercises
    in coma, 938
    in spina bifida, 1103
Rape. See also Sexual assault.
    clinical manifestations of, 516, 517b
    definition of, 516b
Rape victim's parents, support for, 517b
Rapid sequence intubation, 690
Rapprochement, in social development, 383
Rash, neonatal, 232
Rating game, in communication with children,
    93
Reactive attachment disorder, 321
Reactive hyperemia, 647
Reading ability, in school-age child, 460
Reading materials, developmental effects of, 43
Ready-to-use therapeutic food (RTUF), for
    protein-energy malnutrition, 358
Reagents strips, for blood glucose testing, 1004,
    1004f
Rebound effect, after phototherapy, 262
Receptive skills, in cognitive impairment, 574
Recommended Daily Allowance (RDA), 99,
    103b
Record keeping, in diabetes mellitus, 1005
Recreational activities, in cerebral palsy, 1097
Rectal administration, of drugs, 678–679

Rectal prolapse, in cystic fibrosis, 748, 751
Rectal temperature, measurement of, 113t
Rectal ulcers, chemotherapy-induced, 892
Rectovaginal fistula, 811, 811f
Rectum, of neonate, 199, 203t–206t
Recurrent pain, assessment of, 151
Red blood cell(s)
  packed, for iron-deficiency anemia, 872
  sickled, 874, 874f
Red blood cell count, 870t
Red blood cell disorders, 869–883. *See also specific disorder.*
Red blood cell indices, 870t
Red blood cell morphology, 871b
Red blood cell transfusion
  for Cooley anemia, 882
  for sickle cell anemia, 876
Red reflex, 122, 197
Reed-Sternberg cells, in Hodgkin lymphoma, 893
Refeeding syndrome, 357
Reflex(es)
  Achilles, 141f
  anal, 138
  Babinski, 139, 200, 200f, 932
  corneal, 197
  crawl, 200f
  cremasteric, 137, 138f
  dance, 200f
  deep tendon, 140
  gag, 241–242
  in cerebral palsy, 1091
  infants use of, 319
  knee jerk (patellar), 140, 141f
  Moro, 200, 200f
  neonatal, 198t
  parachute, 315–316, 317f
  plantar (grasp), 139, 200, 200f
  primitive, 188
  red, 122, 197
  rooting, 197, 218–219
  startle, 197, 198t
  sucking, 197
  testing of, 140, 141f, 932
  tonic neck, 200f
Reflux
  gastroesophageal. *See* Gastroesophageal reflux.
  vesicoureteral, 909
Refraction, 584
Refrigerant sprays, analgesic, 168
Regression, during toddler years, 390
Rehabilitation
  for burn patients, management of, 1045
  for head trauma patients, 944–945
Reinforcement
  in aggression, 417
  positive, during procedures, 642
Rejection
  after heart transplantation, 856
  after renal transplantation, 925
  in chronic illness/disability, 544
Relaxation
  during abdominal palpation, 136b
  in pain management, 160b
Religion, 60
Religious beliefs, 60–62
  affecting nursing care, 61t–62t, 62

Religious rituals, 56
Remodeling (maturation), in wound healing, 1013
Renal angiography, 905t–906t
Renal biopsy, 905t–906t
Renal disease, end-stage, 923
Renal failure, 918–924
  acute, 919–921, 919b–920b
  chronic, 921–924, 922b
  dialysis for, 924–925, 925f
  transplantation for, 925
Renal function
  blood tests of, 908t
  fluid balance and, 764
  urine tests of, 907t
Renal osteodystrophy, 921
Renal system
  of infant, 345
  of neonate, 187
Renal ultrasonography, 905t–906t
Reproductive system, disorders of, 508–510. *See also specific disorder.*
Resources, for home care, 602b
Respiration(s). *See also* Breathing.
  Cheyne-Stokes, 564, 564b
  evaluation of, 130
  in cardiopulmonary resuscitation, 758, 758f
  in neonate, 193, 197
  in neurologic examination, 930
Respiratory arrest, 754
Respiratory care, in spinal cord injuries, 1116–1117
Respiratory depression, opioid-induced, 165t–166t, 168–169
  management of, 172b
Respiratory disorders. *See also specific disorder.*
  asthma causing, 736–747. *See also* Asthma.
  bronchial (postural) drainage for, 689
  chest physical therapy for, 689–690
  chest tube drainage for, 693–694, 694f, 695b
  foreign body aspiration causing, 731–732
  infectious. *See* Respiratory infection.
  inhalation therapy for, 687–689, 688f
    monitoring of, 688–689, 688f
  long-term, 736–754
  mechanical ventilation for, 690
  rapid sequence intubation for, 690
  tracheostomy for, 690–693, 691f
    routine care and, 693, 693f
    suctioning during, 691–693, 691f, 692b
    tube occlusion and accidental decannulation and, 693
Respiratory distress, 267
  evaluation of, 269, 269f
  in intestinal obstruction, 808b
Respiratory distress syndrome, 267–273
  acute, 733–734
  diagnosis of, 269, 269b, 269f
  in neonate, 267–273, 268f–269f, 269b, 270t
  nursing care management for, 271–273, 273b–274b
  pathophysiology of, 268–269, 268f
  prevention of, 271
  prognosis of, 271
  treatment of, 269–271, 270t
Respiratory emergencies, 754–759
  recovery position after, 759, 759f

Respiratory failure, 754–755, 755b
  definition of, 754
Respiratory infections, 707–710. *See also specific infection.*
  acute, 709b
  age and, 707
  clinical manifestations of, 707, 708b
  etiology of, 707
  lower tract, 723–728, 724t
  nursing care plan for, 707–710, 709b
  organisms causing, 707
  resistance to, 707
  seasonal variations in, 707
  spread of, prevention of, 710
  upper tract, 710–720, 711b–713b
Respiratory movements, evaluation of, 130
Respiratory rate
  in infancy, 309
  measurement of, 115
  postoperative, 645t
Respiratory secretions, collection of, 271, 664–665
Respiratory status, during congenital heart disease surgery, 846
Respiratory support, for high-risk neonate, 236
Respiratory syncytial virus (RSV) infection, 723–725
  clinical manifestations of, 724, 724b
  nursing care management for, 725
  prevention of, 725
  treatment of, 724–725
Respiratory system, effect of immobilization on, 1051t–1053t
Respiratory tract
  lower, 707
  mucus collection in, 271, 664–665
  of neonate, 186
    complications of, 273–279, 273t–274t
  upper, 707
Respite care, 598
Rest
  after congenital heart disease surgery, 847
  for adolescent, 490–491
  for school-age child, 468
  need for, 69
  promotion of, for respiratory infections, 708
Rest, *ice, compression, elevation* (RICE)
  for hemophilia, 885–886
  for soft tissue injuries, 1056, 1056t
Restraints, methods of, 655–657, 656t, 657f
Restrictive cardiomyopathy, 855
Resuscitation
  cardiopulmonary, 755–758. *See also* Cardiopulmonary resuscitation (CPR).
  in delivery room, 278b
RET protooncogene, in Hirschsprung's disease, 779
Rete pegs, 244
Reticulocyte count, 870t
Retinoblastoma, 589–590
  diagnosis of, 589, 589b, 590f
  nursing care management for, 590
  prognosis of, 590
  treatment of, 589–590
Retinopathy, diabetic, 993
Retinopathy of prematurity, 273–277, 273t–274t
Retrograde pyelography, 905t–906t

Revised Infant Temperament Questionnaire (RITQ), 322–323
Reye syndrome, 956
Rh antigens, maternal sensitization to, 264, 264f
Rh incompatibility, 263–264, 264f
  prevention of, 265
Rh negative, 263–264
Rh positive, 263–264
Rhabdomyosarcoma, 1083–1084, 1083b, 1083t
Rheumatic fever, 714, 849–850, 850b
Rheumatoid arthritis, juvenile, 1084–1086
Rib cage, 129, 130f
Rickets, vitamin D–deficient, 214
Rickettsial disease, 1028–1030, 1028t
Rickettsialpox, 1028t
Riley Infant Pain Scale (RIPS), 146t–147t
Rimantadine, for influenza, 717
Ringworm (dermatophytosis), 1017–1020, 1020t, 1021f
Ritalin, for attention-deficit/hyperactivity disorder, 504b
Rituals, in play, of school-age child, 463
Rocky Mountain spotted fever, 1028t
Role confusion, vs. identity, in psychosocial development, 71t, 72
Rolling over, in infancy, 315–316, 317f
Roman Catholicism, 61t–62t
Romberg's test, 140
Rooting reflex, 197, 218–219
Roseola infantum (exanthem subitum), 424t–430t, 426f
Rotavirus, diarrhea due to, 772, 772t–774t
Rotavirus vaccine, 776
Roundworm (ascariasis), 434t
Rubella (German measles), 424t–430t, 429f
  immunization against, 332f–333f, 337
  maternal infection with, 291t–292t
Rubeola (measles), 424t–430t, 427f
  immunization against, 332f–333f, 337
Rules, in play, 463
Russell traction, 1063
Russell-Silver dwarfism, 977

S
S₁ heart sound, 133–134
S₂ heart sound, 133
S₃ heart sound, 133
S₄ heart sound, 133
Safety belts, shoulder-hip, 399
Safety catheters, for parenteral fluid therapy, 682, 684f
Safety concerns, 652–657
  environmental factors in, 652–653, 652f
  for falls, 653
  for toys, 652–653
  in complementary and alternative medicine, 56b
  in infancy, 344–350, 345b–346b, 347t–348t
  in motor vehicle injuries, 344–348, 344f, 345b–346b
  in toddler years, 396–403
Safety education, 403
Safety issues, in home care, 608–609, 609b, 609f
Safety precautions, 1097
Safety promotion, in adolescence, 493–495
Saline, installation of, before endotracheal or tracheostomy suctioning, 271b–272b, 692b

Saline flush, for intravenous lines, 673b–674b
Saline flush solutions, in intravenous lines, 770b–771b
Salivary glands, of neonate, 187
Salmeterol, for asthma, 740
Salmonella organisms, diarrhea due to, 772–775, 772t–774t
Salter-Harris classification, of fractures, 1057, 1058f
Satiety behavior, of neonate, 218–219
Scabies, 1024, 1026b
Scald burns. See also Burns.
  in toddler, 401
Scale, 1012f
Scale for use in Newborns (SUN), 148t–150t
Scalp, examination of, 119
Scalp vein, for parenteral fluid therapy, 681, 682f
Scar(s), 1012f
  extensive, from flame burns, 1045, 1046f
Scarlet fever, 424t–430t, 430f
Scheduled feeding, of neonate, 218
Scheuermann kyphosis, 1076
Schizophrenia, childhood, 507
School, as cultural influence, 48
School experience, 464–466, 467b
School health, 471–472
School phobia, 505
School-age child
  airway obstruction in, 759, 759f
  attention-deficit/hyperactivity disorder in, 501–504, 502b–503b
  behavioral disorders in, 501–507, 502b
  biologic development of, 458–459, 458f
  bullying of, 505–506
  cognitive impairment in, 572t
  communication with, 91–92
  concepts of and reactions to death in, 558t–559t
  constipation in, 779
  conversion reaction in, 506
  dental health of, 469–470, 470f, 471b
  depression in, 506–507, 506b
  developmental effects of chronic illness/disability in, 546t–547t
  discipline of, 466
  dishonest behavior of, 466–467
  elimination problems in, 499–501, 500b
  exercise and activity for, 468–469, 469f
  family-centered care for, 472, 474b
  fear in, 467–468
  growth and development of, 458–468
    concerns related to, 464–468
  health maintenance in, 471–472
  injury prevention in, 472, 472f, 472t–473t
  latchkey, 466
  loss of control in, 615–616
  moral development of, 460
  nutrition for, 468–472
  parents of, 466
  peptic ulcers in, 792b
  physical examination of, 107t
  pneumonia in, 725
  posttraumatic stress disorder in, 504–505
  preparation of, for procedures, 639b–640b
  psychosocial development of, 459, 459f
  rest for, 468

School-age child (Continued)
  schizophrenia in, 507
  school experience for, 464–466, 467b
  school phobia in, 505
  self-concept development in, 464, 465t–466t
  separation anxiety in, 614–615
  setting limits for, 466
  sex education for, 470–471
  sleep in, 468
  social development of, 460–464, 462f, 464f
  spiritual development of, 460
  stress in, 467–468
  teachers and, 464–466
Sclerosing agent, 687
Scoliometer, 1077
Scoliosis, 139
  idiopathic, 1076–1079, 1077f
Scooter safety, 474b
Scorpion bites, 1025t–1026t
Scout film, 905t–906t
Screening
  cholesterol, 852b
  for cystic fibrosis, 749
  for disease, 209
  for eating disorders, 525
  for hearing, 209
  for lead poisoning, 443
  for phenylketonuria, 209
  in community-base nursing care, 19
Scrotum
  examination of, 137
  of neonate, 199
Sebaceous glands, of neonate, 187
Seborrheic dermatitis, 1035
Secondary prevention, of disease, 19
Sedation
  in end-of-life care, 180
  opioid-induced, 165t–166t
  preoperative, 644–645
Seeing Eye Dog, 587
Seizure(s), 956–966
  classification of, 957–966, 958b–959b, 959t
  clinical manifestations of, 957–966, 958b–959b, 959t
  diagnosis of, 957–960
  etiology of, 956, 957b
  febrile, 651, 966
  in acute renal failure, 920
  in status epilepticus, 961
  long-term care for, 962–966
  neonatal, 279–282, 281b
    classification of, 279, 282t
  nursing care management for, 961–966, 962b–964b
  observations during, 962b
  pathophysiology of, 957
  posttraumatic, 943
  precautions in, 965b
  prognosis of, 961
  treatment of, 960–961
    drug therapy in, 960
    emergency, 965b
    for status epilepticus, 961
    ketogenic diet in, 960
    surgical, 961
    vagus nerve stimulation in, 960–961
  triggering factors in, 966

Selective serotonin reuptake inhibitors (SSRIs), intrauterine exposure to, 290
Self-accusation, in chronic illness/disability, 543
Self-awareness, through play, 77
Self-care, 623
  in chronic illness/disability, 547
  in home care, 607–608
Self-care skills, in cognitive impairment, 573
Self-concept, development of, 74–75
  in adolescent, 486–487, 488t
  in school-age child, 464, 465t–466t
Self-esteem
  and culture, 45–46
  development of, 75
Self-mastery, in hospitalization, 627
Self-talk, positive, in pain management, 160b
Semilunar valves, 133
Semimotor stage, of cognitive development, 71t, 73
Semi-vegetarians, 392
Sense of identity, in adolescent, 481–482
Sense of industry, in school-age child, 459
Sense-pleasure play, 75, 75f
Sensitivity, cultural, 46
Sensitization, 359
Sensorimotor development, 77, 319–320
Sensorineural hearing loss, 580–581. See also Hearing impairment.
Sensory functions, of neonate, 188–189
Sensory stimulation, in coma, 938
Sentence completion, in communication with children, 93–94
Separation, coping with, 323
Separation anxiety
  in hospitalization, 613–615, 613b, 613f–614f
    prevention or minimization of, 621
  in infant, 321
Separation-individuation, 321
Sepsis, 863–864, 863b, 864t
  in intestinal obstruction, 808b
  neonatal, 282–284, 283b
  wound, 1040
Septal defect(s)
  atrial, 826b–827b
  ventricular, 826b–827b, 827–830
Septic arthritis, 1080–1081
Septic shock, 863–864, 863b, 864t
  definition of, 863
Septum, nasal, 128
Sequence, definition of, 293
Serologic tests, for celiac disease, 814
Servo-controlled incubator, 238–239
Setting-sun sign, 968
Severe combined immunodeficiency disease, 897
Sex characteristics
  primary, 477
  secondary, 477, 479f–480f
Sex chromosome abnormalities, 508, 508t
Sex differences, in adolescent growth patterns, 478–481
Sex education
  for preschooler, 415–416
  for school-age child, 470–471
Sex hormones, 974t–976t
  maternal, 188
Sex typing, 410
Sex-role identity, in adolescence, 481

Sex-role imitation, 410
Sexual abuse, 447–448, 448b
  clinical manifestations of, 450b
  history and interview in, 449–451
  initiation and perpetuation of, 448, 448b
  physical assessment of, 451
  preventing and dealing with, 454b
  protection of child from further, 451–454
  victims of, 447–448
Sexual activity, children pressured into, 448b
Sexual assault, 516–517
  definitions of, 516b
  diagnosis of, 516–517, 517b
  nursing care management for, 517, 517b
  treatment of, 517
Sexual assault nurse examiners (SANEs), 517
Sexual development, of preschooler, 410
Sexual differentiation, disorders of, 912t
Sexual history, 98, 98b
Sexual identity, 531b
  development of, 485
Sexual maturation
  early, 528b
  of adolescent, 477–478, 477b–478b. See also Puberty.
    in boys, 478, 480f
    in girls, 477–478, 479f–480f
Sexual orientation, 485–486, 486b, 531b
  development of, 486
Sexuality
  adolescent, 485–486, 485f, 488t
    education and guidance in, 493
  in cognitive impairment, 575
Sexually transmitted disease(s), 511–514, 512t–514t
Shaken baby syndrome, 446
Shampoos
  for dermatophytes, 1019
  for head lice, 1027
Shear, pressure ulcers and, 648
Sheet graft, for burns, 1043, 1044f
Shigella organisms, diarrhea due to, 772–775, 772t–774t
Shingles (herpes zoster), 423–431, 1019t
Shock, 860–862
  anaphylactic, 862
  cardiogenic, 860b
  clinical manifestations of, 861b
  compensated, 861, 861b
  cultural, 46, 46b
  decompensated, 861, 861b
  distributive, 860b
  emergency treatment of, 863b
  hypovolemic, 860b
  in chronic illness/disability, 543
  in dehydration, 768
  in intestinal obstruction, 808b
  irreversible (terminal), 861, 861b
  neurogenic, 1115
  pediatric, 437
  septic, 863–864, 863b, 864t
Short stature, familial, 977
Short-bowel syndrome, 815–816
Shoulder-hip safety belts, 399
Shunt(s)
  left-to-right, 824
  right-to-left, 824

Shunt(s) *(Continued)*
  surgical, 842t
  ventriculoperitoneal, for hydrocephalus, 968, 969f
Sibling(s)
  active relationships of, 29
  functions of, 29
  grieving, 565–566
  interactions of, 29
  of neonate, 221, 221f
    at high risk, 251, 251f
  of special needs child, 541, 542b, 551–552
  older, in large families, 28
  ordinal position of, 29–30, 30b
  reactions of, to hospitalization, 617
  rivalry of, toddler and, 389
  spacing of, 29, 29f
  support of, during hospitalization, 628b
Sick-child care, 323
Sickle cell anemia, 873–881
  acute chest syndrome in, 874
  cerebrovascular accident in, 874
  clinical manifestations of, 875b
  crisis in, 874, 876
    supportive therapies during, 878
  diagnosis of, 874–875
  nursing care management for, 878–881
  nursing care plan in, 879b–880b
  pathophysiology of, 874, 874f–875f, 875b
  prognosis of, 876–878
  treatment of, 875–878
    complementary and alternative, 881b
Sickle cell crisis, 874, 876
  supportive therapies during, 878
Sickle cell disease, 873
  pain in, 178–179
  vitamin deficiencies in, 355
Sickle cell trait, 873–874
Sickle cell–C disease, 873
Sickle cell–hemoglobin B disease, 873
Sickle thalassemia disease, 873
Sickle-turbidity test (Sickledex), 875
Sight, partial, 584. See also Visual impairment.
Sighted human guide, 587
Sign language, 582
Silence, in communication, 89
Simple partial seizures. See also Seizure(s).
  with motor signs, 958b–959b, 959t
  with sensory signs, 958b–959b, 959t
Single father, 39
Single-gene defects, 294
Single-parent family, 27, 39
  special needs child in, 541
Single-photon emission computed tomography (SPECT), of cerebral function, 933t–934t
Sinus arrhythmia, 134
  in infancy, 309
Sinus bradycardia, 853
Sinus tachycardia, 854
Site selection, in intramuscular drug administration, 667–671, 668b–669b, 669t–670t
Sitting ability, development of, 316, 317f
Skateboard safety, 474b
Skeletal system. See also Musculoskeletal system.
  effect of immobilization on, 1051t–1053t
  growth and maturation of, 68
  in neonate, 188

Skeletal traction, 1063b
Skill play, 76, 76f
Skilled nursing, intermittent, in home care, 598, 599b
Skills, acquisition of, in school-age child, 469
Skin
  abdominal, 135
  artificial, for burns, 1044
  effect of immobilization on, 1051t–1053t
  examination of, 119–120, 119t, 120f
  healthy, maintenance of, 647–648
  in Down syndrome, 577b
  in neurologic examination, 930
  of neonate, 187–188, 194, 203t–206t
Skin breakdown, treatment of, 244b–245b
Skin care, 647–651, 648b
  in neonate, at high risk, 244, 244b–245b
  in spinal cord injuries, 1117
Skin color, in neonate, 194
Skin coverings, for burns
  permanent, 1043, 1043f
  synthetic, 1043
Skin disorder(s), 1009–1048. See also specific disorder.
  age-specific, 1030–1036
  animal-related, 1024–1030, 1025t–1026t, 1028t
  burns, 1036–1047. See also Burns.
  family support in, 1016–1017
  from chemical or physical irritants, 1022–1024, 1023f, 1026f
  home care for, 1016–1017
  infectious
    bacterial, 1017, 1018f, 1018t
    fungal, 1017–1020, 1020t, 1021f
      systemic, 1020, 1021t
    viral, 1017, 1019t
  lesions in, 1010, 1011f–1012f
  miscellaneous, 1030, 1031t
  nursing care management for, 1015–1016
  treatment of, 1013–1015
    systemic therapy in, 1015
    topical therapy in, 1014–1015
  wounds in, 1010–1013, 1014t. See also Wound entries.
Skin lesions, 1010, 1011f–1012f
Skin prick test, in asthma, 738
Skin temperature, measurement of, 112b
Skin traction, 1063b
Skinfold thickness, 102
  measurement of, 111
Skin-to-skin (kangaroo) holding
  for high-risk neonate, 239, 246–247, 246f
  in pain management, 159, 162f
Skull
  fracture of, 940
    birth-related, 231
  palpation of, 121, 195
Sleep
  in adolescent, 490–491, 491f
  in infant, 330
  in neonate, 201, 202t
  in preschooler, 418–419, 419t
  in school-age child, 468
  in toddler, 393–394
  need for, 69
Sleep apnea, 369–370
  obstructive, 754

Sleep disorders
  in chronic and recurrent pain, 151
  in infancy and early childhood, 364–366, 365t
Sleep habits, in health history, 97
Sleep terrors, vs. nightmares, 418, 419t
Sleeping position, supine, sudden infant death syndrome and, 370
Sleep-wake cycles, in toddler, 379
Slipped capital femoral epiphysis, 1075–1076, 1075b
Small family child care home, 323
Small-for-gestational age (SGA), 191, 191f
Smegma, 199
Smell
  in neonate, 188–189
  in toddler, 379
Smoke, tobacco, environmental exposure to, 735–736, 736b
Smoke inhalation injury, 734–735
Smokeless tobacco, 528
Smoking
  adolescent, 527–528, 528b
  maternal
    intrauterine exposure to, 296t
    sudden infant death syndrome and, 370
Snellen letter chart, 123
Soave endorectal pull-through procedure, for Hirschsprung's disease, 781
Social affective play, 75
Social development
  of adolescent, 483–485, 484f
  of infant, 320–322
    attachment in, 320–321, 320f
    language in, 321–322
    play in, 322
    separation anxiety in, 321
    stranger fear in, 321
  of preschooler, 410–412, 410f–411f, 413t–414t
  of school-age child, 460–464, 462f, 464f
  of toddler, 383–385, 384f–385f, 386t–387t
Social media
  influences of, 50
  role of, in adolescence, 484
Social networking sites, 50, 484
Social relationships, and cooperation, 462–463, 462f
Social roles, 45–46
Social stressors, in intensive care unit, 633b
Socialization, 48. See also Cultural entries; Culture.
  in cognitive impairment, 575
  in hearing impairment, 582–583
  in hospitalization, 627, 627f
  in visual impairment, 587
  peer groups and, 48–49, 48f
  through play, 77
Socioeconomic status
  class and, 47–48
  homelessness and, 51
  influences of, 50–52
  of migrant families, 51–52
  poverty and, 50–51, 51b
Sodium concentration, in cystic fibrosis, 749
Sodium depletion, 765t–766t
Sodium excess, 765t–766t
Sodium retention, in chronic renal failure, 921

Soft bedding, sudden infant death syndrome and, 370
Soft palate, examination of, 129
Soft tissue injuries, 1055–1056, 1055f
  birth-related, 229
  treatment of, 1056, 1056t
Soft tissue tumors, 1070b, 1083–1084, 1083t
Solid food. See also Food.
  for infants
    introduction of, 329
    selection and preparation of, 328
Solitary play, 76
Somatostatin, 974t–976t
Somogyi effect, 997
Sorrow, in chronic illness/disability, 544
Sound intensity, expressed in decibels, 580t
Soy protein–based formulas, 217
Spasmodic laryngitis, 721t, 723
Spasms, infantile, 958b–959b
Spasticity, in cerebral palsy, 1091, 1092b
Spatial relationship, in cognitive development, 381
Special needs children. See Chronic illness/disability; Cognitive impairment.
Specimen collection, 658–665
  of blood, 662–664, 663b–664b, 664f. See also Blood sampling; Venipuncture.
  of respiratory secretions, 664–665
  of stool samples, 662
  of urine, 658–662, 659f, 660t, 661b–662b
  steps common in, 658
Speech, 73
  cued, 582
  delayed, in autism, 591–592
  in preschooler, 417
  rate of development of, 73
  telegraphic, 410
Speech language therapy, 582
Spermicides, 512t–514t
Spica casts, 1059, 1060f–1061f
Spina bifida, 199, 1098–1104
  bladder control in, 1101
  bowel control in, 1101–1102
  complications of, prevention of, 1103
  diagnosis of, 1099–1100, 1100b
  etiology of, 1099, 1100f
  family support in, 1103–1104
  home care in, 1103–1104
  latex allergy in, 1104, 1104b
  myelomeningocele sac care in, 1102–1103
  nursing care management for, 1102–1104
  pathophysiology of, 1098–1099
  postoperative care in, 1103
  prevention of, 1102
  prognosis of, 1102
  treatment of, 1100–1102
    in infancy, 1101
    orthopedic considerations in, 1101
Spina bifida cystica, 1098, 1100b
Spina bifida occulta, 1098, 1099f, 1100b
Spinal cord compression, 1115
Spinal cord concussion, 1115
Spinal cord injuries, 1114–1117, 1115b
  clinical manifestations of, 1115
  mechanisms of, 1114–1115
  nursing care management for, 1116–1117, 1117f
  treatment of, 1115–1116

Spinal muscular atrophy
type 1 (Werdnig-Hoffmann disease), 1105–1106, 1105b
type 2 (intermediate), 1105b
type 3 (Kugelberg-Walander syndrome), 1105b, 1106
Spinal shock syndrome, 1115
Spine
curvature of, 138–139
examination of, 138–140
of neonate, 199, 203t–206t
Spiritual beliefs, 74
Spiritual development, 71t, 74
of adolescent, 482–483
of preschooler, 409
of school-age child, 460
of toddler, 382–383
Spiritual practices, 55b
integration of, into pediatric nursing practice, 60b
Spirituality, 60
assessment of, 603b
Spironolactone, for congestive heart failure, 836t
Spleen, of neonate, 203t–206t
Splenectomy
for Cooley anemia, 882
for idiopathic thrombocytopenic purpura, 887
for sickle cell anemia, 876
Splint, Thomas, 1063
Sports
nurse's role in, 1067–1068
participation in, 1066–1068
Sports injuries, 1066–1068, 1067f
in adolescence, 495
overuse, 1067
prevention of, 1068
Sports participation, of school-age child, 469, 469f
Spot test, for hypothyroidism, 297
Sprains, 1056
Sputum
blood-streaked, in cystic fibrosis, 750
collection of, 664–665
Standard precautions, in infection control, 653, 654b
Staphylococcal scalded skin syndrome, 1018t
Staphylococcus organisms, diarrhea due to, 772t–774t
Startle reflex, 197, 198t
Stasis, urinary, 908
Statins, for hyperlipidemia, 851–853
Status asthmaticus, 741. *See also* Asthma.
Status epilepticus, 961. *See also* Seizure(s).
Statutory rape, definition of, 516b
Statutory rape laws, 516
Stealing, by school-age child, 467
Steatorrhea, in cystic fibrosis, 747
Stem cell transplantation
hematopoietic. *See* Hematopoietic stem cell transplantation.
umbilical cord, 899
Stenosis, 825. *See also at anatomic site.*
Stereopsis (depth perception), 315
Sternal angle (angle of Inuis), 129
Sternum, examination of, 129
Steroids
oral, for laryngotracheobronchitis, 722
topical, for atopic dermatitis, 1034

Stevens-Johnson syndrome, 1023, 1031t
Stimulants, CNS, adolescent use of, 529
Stimulation
in coma, 938
in psychosocial growth, 322
tactile
of infant, 319
of neonate, 186
Stings, arthropod, 1024–1028, 1025t–1026t
Stoma, tracheostomy, care of, 693
Stomach capacity, of neonate, 187
Stomatitis
chemotherapy-induced, 892
in toddler/preschooler, 432–433, 433f
Stool specimens, collection of, 662
Stool-softening agents, 779
Stork bites, 210
Strabismus, 122, 584, 584b–585b
in neonate, 197
Strains, 1056
"Stranger danger" concept, 403
Stranger fear, in infant, 321
coping with, 323
Stranger rape, 516
Strawberry hemangioma, 234, 234f
Strep throat, 714
Streptococcal pharyngitis, 714–715, 714f
Stress
cold, in high-risk neonate, consequences of, 237–238
family, 24–25
in adolescence, reduction of, 492, 492b, 492f
in chronic illness/disability, coping with, 542–543
in hospitalization, 613–617, 633b
risk factors for, 616–617, 616b
in neonate, 280t
in preschooler, 416
in school-age child, 467–468
reduction of, in burn care procedures, 1045b
Stress fractures, 1067
Stress responses, to pain, 173–175
Stress ulcer, 792
Stressors, 613
in intensive care unit, 633b
Stroke
in sickle cell anemia, 874
perinatal ischemic, 1091
Strong families, qualities of, 28b
Strongyloidiasis, 434t
Stump shaping, postoperative, 1066
Stupor, 929b
Sturge-Weber syndrome, 234
Stuttering, 417
Subcultures, 44. *See also* Cultural *entries*; Culture.
influences on, 46–50
Subcutaneous administration, of drugs, 671
Subdiaphragmatic abdominal thrusts, 759, 759f
Subdural hemorrhage, 941, 941f
Subdural tap, 933t–934t
Subgaleal compartment, 229–230
Subgaleal hemorrhage, 229–230, 230f
Subluxation, 1056
in developmental dysplasia of hip, 1068, 1068f
Submersion injury
aspiration in, 945
cerebral dysfunction in, 945–946

Submersion injury *(Continued)*
hypothermia in, 945
hypoxia in, 945
Substance abuse, 6
acute care for, 530
adolescent, 527–531
prescription medication abuse in, 530b
dependence in, 527
family support in, 530–531
intrauterine
alcohol in, 289, 296t
cocaine in, 289
marijuana in, 290
methamphetamine in, 289–290
selective serotonin reuptake inhibitors in, 290
long-term management for, 530
motivation in, 527
prevention of, 531
types of drugs in, 527–530
Subvalvular aortic stenosis, 828b–829b
Succimer, as chelating agent, 444
Sucking, nonnutritive, 243
in pain management, 159, 159f
Sucking reflex, 197
Suctioning, in coma, 936
Sudden infant death syndrome (SIDS), 368–372
aborted (near-miss). *See* Apparent life-threatening event (ALTE).
care of family with, 371–372
definition of, 368–369
epidemiology of, 369t
etiology of, 369–370
nursing care management for, 371–372
protective factors for, 370–371
risk factors for, 370
infant, 371
Suffering, fear of, 560–563
Suffocation, 5, 5f
child safety home checklist for, 349b
in infancy, 345b–346b, 347t–348t
of toddler, 397t–398t, 403
safety home checklist for, 349b
Suicidal ideation, 531
Suicide, 531–533
assisted, 555–556
attempted, 531
copycat, 532
definition of, 6, 531
high risk for, 531–532
methods of, 532
motivation for, 532
warning signs of, 532b
Sumac, poison, 1022
Sunburns, 1047–1048. *See also* Burns.
in toddler, 401–402
Superego, 380
in preschooler, 408
Superficial palpation, of abdomen, 136
Superior mesenteric artery syndrome, 1078–1079
Supernatural forces, in health beliefs and practices, 43
Supernumerary nipples, 197
Supine sleeping position, sudden infant death syndrome and, 370
Supplemental feeding, of neonate, 218

Support groups. *See also* Family support system.
 for parents of high-risk neonate, 251
 for parents of special needs child, 544, 544b
Supraglottitis, acute, 721–722, 721t
Suprapubic aspiration, 661–662, 662b, 908
Suprasternal notch, examination of, 129
Supraventricular tachycardia, 854, 854b
Surfactant, 268
 complications of, 270
 for respiratory distress syndrome, 270
Surgery. *See also specific procedure.*
 bariatric, 521
 for congenital heart disease, 845. *See also*
  Congenital heart disease, invasive
  procedures for.
 for Wilms tumor, 917–918
 orthopedic, for cerebral palsy, 1093
 postoperative care in, 645–646, 645t, 646b
 preoperative care in, 642–645, 644f, 644t
Sutures, cranial, 191f, 195
Swaddle restraints, 656, 657f
Swaddling, blanket, 246
Sweat, in cystic fibrosis patients, 749
Symbols, in cognitive development, 319
Symptom analysis, in history taking, 96, 101b
Syndactyly, 139, 199
Syndrome, definition of, 293
Syndrome of inappropriate antidiuretic hormone
 secretion, 937, 981
Synthetic-convention stage, of spiritual
 development, 71t, 74
Syphilis, maternal infection with, 291t–292t
Syringe selection, in intramuscular drug
 administration, 667
Syrup of ipecac, for poisoning, 440
Systemic inflammatory response syndrome, 863,
 863b
Systemic injury, from gases, 734–735
Systemic lupus erythematosus, 1086–1087, 1087b

T
Tablet computers, in home care, 606–607
Tachydysrhythmias, 854
Tactile play, of toddler, 385
Tactile stimulation
 of infant, 319
 of neonate, 186
Talipes calcaneus, 1071
Talipes equinovarus, 1071, 1071f
Talipes equinus, 1071
Talipes valgus, 1071
Talipes varus, 1071
Talk, encouraging parents to, 88
Tanner stages, of sexual maturation, 477, 477b
Tanning, by adolescent, 492
Tantrums, during toddler years, 389–390
Taping, 648
Tapping method, visual impairment and, 587
Task analysis, in cognitive impairment, 572
Taste
 in neonate, 189
 in toddler, 379
Taste preferences, in toddler, 379
Tattooing, in adolescence, 492
Teachers, 464–466
Team play, 463
Technology, developmental effects of, 50

Teenager(s). *See* Adolescent(s).
Teeth. *See also* Dental *entries.*
 avulsed, 470, 471b
 care of, 2–3
  deficient, 51
  in infant, 330
 eruption of, 314
  in infancy, 325, 325f
  sequence of, 325, 325f
 method of brushing of, 470
 natal, vs. neonatal teeth, 197
 permanent, eruption of, 469, 470f
Telecommunication devices for deaf (TDD), 582
Telegraphic speech, 410
Telephone triage, 88, 88b
Teletypewriters, 582
Television, developmental effects of, 43, 50f
Television viewing, during preschool years, 412
Temper tantrums, during toddler years, 389–390
Temperament, 69–70, 322–323
 attributes of, 70b
 childrearing practices related to, 310t–314t,
  323
 definition of, 70
 significance of, 70, 70b
Temperature
 axillary, in neonate, 192, 192f
 elevated. *See* Fever.
 in neurologic examination, 930
 in toddler, 379
 measurement of, 112, 112b, 114b–116b
 postoperative, 645t
 skin, in neonate, 192
 stable, maintenance of, in neonate, 207
Temporal artery temperature, measurement of,
 113t
Temporal artery thermometers, 193
Tennison-Randall procedure, for cleft lip, 801
Teratogenic agents, 81
Terminally ill. *See also* Death and dying.
 treatment options for, 558–560
Tertiary circular reactions, in cognitive
 development, 380–381
Tertiary prevention, of disease, 19
Testes
 of neonate, 199
 palpation of, 137
 self-examination of, 510, 510b
Testicular cancer, 510
Testicular hormones, 974t–976t
Testicular ultrasonography, 905t–906t
Testosterone, 974t–976t
Tet spells, 841
Tetanus (lockjaw), 1111–1113, 1112b
 immunization against, 332f–333f, 336
Tetanus and acellular pertussis (Tdap) vaccine,
 booster, 431, 488–489
Tetanus immunoglobulin, 1112
Tetanus toxin, 1112
Tetany, 985b
Tetralogy of Fallot, 830b–831b
Text messaging, 485
β-Thalassemia (Cooley) anemia, 881–882, 882b
Thalassemia intermedia, 881
Thalassemia major, 881
Thalassemia minor, 881
Thalassemia trait, 881

Thalidomide, teratogenic effects of, 1073
Thelarche, 477–478
Theophylline, for asthma, 740
Therapeutic care, 8–9
Therapeutic holding, 655–657, 656t, 657f
Therapeutic play. *See also* Play.
 during hospitalization, 625
Therapeutic procedures. *See* Procedures.
Therapeutic relationship, 9
Thermal devices, use of, 244b–245b
Thermal environment, neutral, 237
 maintenance of, 238–239, 239f
Thermal injuries. *See* Burns.
Thermal stability, in high-risk neonate, 237
Thermogenesis (shivering), 315
Thermometers
 axillary and digital, infrared, 193
 temporal artery, 193
 types of, 112, 116b
Thermoregulation, 69
 in coma, 937
 in infant, 315
 in neonate, 186–189
  at high risk, 236–239, 239f
  axillary temperature in, 192, 192f
  maintenance of stable temperature and, 207
Thimerosal-containing vaccines, and autism
 spectrum disorders, 592b
Third-person technique, of communication with
 children, 93
Thomas splint, 1063
Thoracic cavity, 129
Thoracolumbosacral orthosis, 1077, 1077f
Thoracotomy, for tracheoesophageal fistula, 804
Thought, preoperational, in cognitive
 development, 381–382, 382b
Thought process, development of,
 communication related to, 91–92, 91b
Thought stopping, in pain management, 160b
Throat. *See also* Oropharyngeal; Pharyngeal
 entries.
 examination of, 128–129, 129f
 of neonate, 197, 198t, 203t–206t
Thrombosis, deep vein, 1051
Thrush (oral candidiasis), in neonate, 232–233,
 233f
Thumb sucking, in infancy, 324–325
Thyrocalcitonin, 974t–976t
Thyroid crisis, 984, 984b
Thyroid disorder(s), 981–984
 goiter, 982–983
 hyperthyroidism, 983–984, 984b
 juvenile hypothyroidism, 982, 982b
 lymphocytic thyroiditis, 983, 983b
Thyroid hormones, 974t–976t
Thyroid hyperplasia of adolescence, 983
Thyroid storm, 984, 984b
Thyroiditis, lymphocytic, 983, 983b
Thyroid-stimulating hormone (TSH), 977b
Thyrotoxicosis, 984, 984b
Thyrotropin, 974t–976t
Thyrotropin-releasing factor, 981–982
Thyroxine (T$_4$), 974t–976t, 981–982
Tick bites, 1025t–1026t
Time-out, disciplinary, 35, 35b, 35f
Tinea capitis, 1020t, 1021f
Tinea corporis, 1020t, 1021f

Tinea cruris, 1020t
Tinea pedis, 1020t
Tissue donation, 565
Tissue oxygenation, improved, for congestive heart failure, 836
Tobacco. *See also* Smoking.
  adolescent use of, 527–528
  smokeless, 528
Tobacco smoke, environmental exposure to, 735–736, 736b
Toddler(s)
  automobile safety for, 396–401
  biologic development of, 379–380
  body image of, 383
  burns in, 397t–398t, 401–402, 402f
  car restraints for, 396–400, 399f
  care of families with, 403, 404b
  choking in, 397t–398t, 403
  cognitive development of, 380–382, 381f, 382b
  complementary and alternative medicine for, 393
  concepts of and reactions to death in, 558t–559t
  dental health of, 394–396, 394f, 395t, 396f
  developmental effects of chronic illness/ disability in, 546t–547t
  drowning of, 397t–398t, 401
  falls in, 397t–398t, 402–403
  gender identity of, 383
  growth and development of, 379–390, 386t–387t
    concerns related to, 385–390, 388f–389f
  infectious diseases in, 423–433, 424t–430t
  injury to
    automobile-related, 397t–398t, 400–401
    bodily, 397t–398t, 403
    prevention of, 396–403, 397t–398t
  intestinal parasitic diseases in, 433–436, 434t
  loss of control in, 615
  maltreatment of, 445–454, 450b, 452b
  negativism in, 380, 390
  nutrition for, 391, 393b
  physical examination of, 107t
  poisoning in, 397t–398t, 402, 402f
  poisonous ingestions by, 436–445, 437b–439b
  preparation of, for procedures, 639b–640b
  psychosocial development of, 380, 381f
  regression in, 390
  separation anxiety in, 614
  sibling rivalry and, 389
  sleep and activity in, 393–394
  social development of, 383–385, 384f–385f, 386t–387t
  spiritual development of, 382–383
  suffocation in, 397t–398t, 403
  temper tantrums in, 389–390
  toilet training of, 385–389, 387b, 388f
Toddler-Preschooler Postoperative Pain Scale (TPPS), 147
Toe(s)
  catheter, 240
  pigeon, 139
Toilet training, 385–389, 387b, 388f
  readiness phase of, 388, 388f
Tolerable Upper Intake Level, of nutrients, 99, 103b

Tolerance, to opioids, 171–172, 173f–174f, 175b, 563
Tolmetin, for pain, 163t
Tone, muscle, 139
Tongue, examination of, 129
Tonic neck reflex, 200f
Tonic-clonic seizures, 958b–959b. *See also* Seizure(s).
Tonsillectomy, 715
Tonsillitis, 715–716, 715f
Tonsils, 715, 715f
Topical therapy, anesthetic, 168
TORCH complex, 290
Torticollis (wryneck), 121
Torus fracture, 1057b, 1057f
Total anomalous pulmonary venous connection (TAPVC), 831b–834b
Total parenteral nutrition (TPN). *See also* Nutrition; Nutritional *entries.*
  in inflammatory bowel disease, 790
  in short-bowel syndrome, 815
Touch
  in neonate, 189
  in toddler, 379
Toxic shock syndrome, 864–865, 865b
Toxicity. *See* Poisoning.
Toxocariasis, 434t
Toxoplasmosis, maternal infection with, 291t–292t
Toys, 78. *See also* Play.
  appropriate, for toddler, 385
  in hospitalization, 625
  safety concerns for, 652–653
  selection of, 574
Tracheitis, bacterial, 721t, 723
Tracheobronchitis, 723, 724t
Tracheoesophageal fistula, 803–805, 803b, 803f
Tracheomalacia, 804
Tracheostomy, 690–693, 691f
  for epiglottitis, 721
  routine care for, 693, 693f
  suctioning during, 691–693, 691f
    saline installation before, 271b–272b, 692b
  tube occlusion and accidental decannulation in, 693
Tracheostomy tube, occlusion of, 693
Traction, 1062–1064
  counter, 1062
  nursing care guidelines for, 1064, 1065b
  purpose of, 1062–1063, 1062f
  types of, 1063–1064, 1063b
Traditional nuclear family, 26
Transcutaneous oxygen monitoring, 688
Transdermal analgesia, 168, 168f
Transfusion(s)
  blood, 897–899
    nursing care in, 898t
  exchange, for hemolytic disease of newborn, 266
  intrauterine, Rh isoimmunization and, 265–266
  red blood cell
    for Cooley anemia, 882
    for sickle cell anemia, 876
Transgender family, 27–28
Transilluminators, 681, 682f
  in vascular access, 683b

Translators, children as, 90b
Transmission-based precautions, in infection control, 653, 654b
Transmucosal analgesia, 168
Transplantation
  heart, 856–857
  hematopoietic stem cell. *See* Hematopoietic stem cell transplantation.
  kidney, 925
  liver, for cirrhosis, 798
Transportation, of infants and children, 654–655, 655f
Transposition of great arteries, 831b–834b
Traumatic injury, 3–5, 5f–6f, 1055–1066. *See also at anatomic site; specific type of injury.*
  automobile-related
    in adolescence, 493–494, 494b
    in toddler years, 397t–398t, 400–401
  birth-related, 1068–1074
  distribution of, 18
  in visual impairment, 586
  mortality due to, 3, 4t
  nonaccidental, 396
  prevention of, 10
    in adolescence, 493–495, 494b
    in infancy, 344–350, 345b–346b, 347t–348t
      nurse's role in, 348–350
    in preschooler, 419–420
    in school-age child, 472, 472f, 472t–473t
    in toddler, 396–403, 397t–398t
  risk factors for, 3, 4b
  soft tissue, 1055–1056
  sports-related, 1066–1068
Travel, diabetes mellitus and, 1002
Treatment strategies, in compliance, 647
Tremor, definition of, 279
Tremulousness, 279
Tretinoin (Retin-A), for acne, 1036
Trichuriasis, 434t
Tricuspid atresia, 830b–831b
Tricuspid valves, 133
Tricyclic antidepressants, for cancer pain, 180
Trigeminal nerve, assessment of, 141f, 142t
Triiodothyronine (T$_3$), 974t–976t, 981–982
Triple-drug therapy, for *Helicobacter pylori* infection, 793
Trisomy, 294
Trisomy 13 (Patau syndrome), 295t
Trisomy 18 (Edward syndrome), 295t
Trisomy 21 (Down syndrome), 81–82, 295t
Trochlear nerve, assessment of, 141f, 142t
Trousseau sign, 985b
Truncus arteriosus, 831b–834b
Trust
  development of, 318–319
  vs. mistrust, 318
    in psychosocial development, 71t, 72
Trypsin, 314
T-shield restraint, 398
Tubal tonsil, 715, 715f
Tuberculin skin test, 729, 730b
  positive, definition of, 729, 730b
Tuberculosis, 729–731, 729b
  clinical active, 729–730
  latent, 729–730
  skeletal, 1081

Tumors. *See also specific tumor.*
bone, 1081, 1081b
nervous system, 946–949
soft tissue, 1070b, 1083–1084, 1083t
Tunneled catheter, 675t
Turbinates, nasal, 128
Turner syndrome, 81–82, 295t, 508, 508t
Twenty-four hour urine collection, 659–660
Twins, 30–31, 30f
breastfeeding with, 216, 216f
characteristics of, 31t
Twitter, 484
Tympanic membrane
landmarks of, 126, 126f
otoscopic examination of, 127
Tympanostomy tube placement, for otitis media, 719
Typhus
endemic, 1028t
epidemic, 1028t
Tyrosine, 298

U

Ugly duckling stage, 458
Ulcer(s)
duodenal, 792
gastric, 792
herpangina, pain in, 176
mucosal, chemotherapy-induced, 891–892
peptic, 792–793, 792b
pressure, 648
primary, 792
rectal, chemotherapy-induced, 892
skin, 1012f
stress, 792
Ulcerative colitis, 789, 789t
Ultrasonography (US)
bladder, 905t–906t
of cerebral function, 933t–934t
renal, 905t–906t
testicular, 905t–906t
Ultraviolet A waves, 1047
Ultraviolet B waves, 1047
Ultraviolet burns. *See also* Burns.
to eye, 586b
Umbilical cord, 203t–206t
Umbilical cord stem cell transplantation, 899
Umbilical hernia, 806t
Umbilicus
care of, 211
inspection of, 135
Unconsciousness. *See also* Coma.
definition of, 928
nursing care in, 934–938
Undereating, during adolescence, 490
Undifferentiated stage, of spiritual development, 71t, 74
United Nations' Declaration of Rights of Child, 9b
Unoccupied behavior, play and, 76
Uremia, 919, 921
Urethral meatus, examination of
in female, 138
in male, 137
Urethritis, 906
Urinary retention, opioid-induced, 165t–166t
Urinary stasis, 908

Urinary system, effect of immobilization on, 1051t–1053t
Urinary tract infections, 904–910
altered urine and bladder chemistry in, 908
anatomic factors in, 908
classification of, 906
constipation and, 910b
diagnosis of, 908, 909b
etiology of, 906–908
febrile, 906
nursing care management for, 910
physical factors in, 908
prevention of, 910, 910b
prognosis of, 909
treatment of, 908–909
vesicoureteral reflux in, 909
Urine chemistry, in urinary tract infections, 908
Urine collection, techniques of, 660–662, 660t, 661b–662b
Urine culture, 905t–906t
Urine glucose testing, in diabetes mellitus, 996, 1004
Urine specimen
clean-catch, 659
midstream, 659
twenty-four hour, 659–660
Urine tests, of renal function, 907t
Uroflowmetry, 905t–906t
Uropathy, obstructive, 910–911, 911f
Urosepsis, 906
Urticaria, 1031t
Uvula
examination of, 129
of neonate, 197

V

Vaccine(s). *See also* Immunization(s); *specific vaccine.*
and autism, 335b
thimerosal-containing, and autism spectrum disorders, 592b
Vaccine Adverse Events Reporting System, 344
Vaccine Compensation Amendments (1987), 344
Vaccine information statement (VIS), 344
Vaccine-associated poliomyelitis paralysis (VAPP), 336–337
VACTERL association, 803
Vaginal discharge, in neonate, 199
Vaginal orifice, examination of, 138
Vaginitis, 509–510
Vagus nerve, assessment of, 141f, 142t
Vagus nerve stimulation, for seizures, 960–961
Valsalva maneuver, for supraventricular tachycardia, 854
Valvular aortic stenosis, 828b–829b
Varicella (chickenpox), 424f, 424t–430t
immunization against, 332f–333f, 337–338
maternal infection with, 291t–292t
Varicella-zoster immune globulin (VariZIG), for immunocompromised child, 423–431
Varicella-zoster virus (VZV), 423–431, 1019t
Varices
esophageal, 798
gastric, 798
Vascular access, transilluminator devices in, 683b

Vascular dysfunction, 857–865
anaphylaxis in, 862–863
hypertension in, 857–858, 857b
Kawasaki disease in, 858–860, 859b
septic shock in, 863–864, 863b, 864t
shock in, 860–862, 860b–861b, 863b
toxic shock syndrome in, 864–865, 865b
Vascular malformations, 234, 234f
Vasodilator therapy, for pulmonary artery hypertension, 855
Vasoocclusive crisis, in sickle cell anemia, 874, 876
Vasopressin (antidiuretic hormone), 974t–976t, 977b
for diabetes insipidus, 981
in neonate, 188
Vastus lateralis muscle, drug administration into, 667–671, 669f, 672b
VATER association, 803
Veau-Wardill-Kilner V-Y pushback procedure, for cleft palate, 801
Vegans, 392
Vegetarian diet, 392–393
Venipuncture, 662. *See also* Blood sampling.
extremity, positioning for, 657, 658f
femoral, positioning for, 657, 657f
Venous hemangioma, cavernous, 234
Ventilation
for shock, 861, 863b
mechanical, 690
Ventilator-associated pneumonia, 690. *See also* Pneumonia.
prevention of, 727b
Ventricular puncture, 933t–934t
Ventricular septal defect, 826b–827b, 827–830
Ventriculoperitoneal shunt, for hydrocephalus, 968, 969f
Ventrogluteal site, drug administration into, 667, 670f, 672b
Verbal skills, in cognitive impairment, 574
Verbal techniques, of communication with children, 93–94
Vernix caseosa, 194, 315
Verrucae (warts), 1019t
Very low–birth-weight infant(s), growth patterns in, 108
Vesicant, 687
Vesicle, 1011f
Vesicoureteral reflux, 909
Vest, halo, 1063–1064, 1064f
Vestibulocochlear nerve, assessment of, 141f, 142t
Vibrio cholerae, diarrhea due to, 772t–774t
Vietnamese families
and relationship with health care providers, 52–53
health beliefs and practices of, 58t–59t
Violence, 5–6
gang, 463
Viral infections. *See also specific viral infection.*
cutaneous, 1017, 1019t
oral, pain in, 176
Viral meningitis, 953–954, 954t
Viral nasopharyngitis, 710–714, 711b–712b
clinical manifestations of, 713b
complications of, 714b
Viral pneumonia, 726, 726b. *See also* Pneumonia.
Virchow triad, 1051

Visible poverty, 50
Vision. *See also* Eye(s).
  color, 125
  in adolescent, 491
  in neonate, 188
  peripheral, 124–125
Vision testing, 122–125, 122f–123f
Visual acuity
  in neonate, 188
  in toddler, 379
Visual acuity testing, 123, 124t
Visual Analog Scale, in pain assessment,
    148t–150t
Visual impairment, 584–589
  classification of, 584
  definition of, 584
  education in, 587–588
  etiology of, 584–586, 584b–585b
  hospitalization in, 588
  in hyperthyroidism, 983
  independence in, 587
  infections and, 586
  nursing care management for, 586–589
  optimal development in, 587
  parent-child attachment in, 587
  partial, 584
  permanent, 584
  play and socialization in, 587
  prevention of, 588–589
  trauma and, 586
  types of, 584b–585b
  with hearing impairment, 589
Visually evoked potentials (VEPs), 124
Vital signs
  age-specific, in septic shock, 864t
  brain tumors and, 947
  in neurologic examination, 930
  observation of, during congenital heart disease
      surgery, 845–846
  postoperative, 645t
Vitamin(s)
  excessive doses of, definition of, 355
  misuse of, 393
  supplemental, for protein-energy
      malnutrition, 357
Vitamin A
  deficiency of, 355
  supplemental, 431
Vitamin C, for toddler, 392
Vitamin D
  for hypoparathyroidism, 986
  for toddler, 392
  supplemental, 326, 355
Vitamin D–deficient rickets, 214
Vitamin imbalances, in infant, 355
Vitamin K administration, of neonate, 208–209
Vocalization
  during crying, 322
  during infancy, 310t–314t

Voiding cystourethrography, 905t–906t
Voiding pressure study, 905t–906t
Volvulus, 810
Vomiting, 781–782
  bilious, 781
  chemotherapy-induced, 891
  cyclic, 782
  in pyloric stenosis, 807, 808b
  opioid-induced, 165t–166t
Vulnerable child syndrome, 262–263
Vulva, examination of, 138, 138f

W

Waldeyer tonsillar ring, 715
Warm mist, for respiratory infections, 708
Warts (verrucae), 1019t
Wasp stings, 1025t–1026t
Waste products, in chronic renal failure,
    retention of, 921
Water. *See also* Fluid *entries.*
  depletion of, 765t–766t
  excess of, 765t–766t
Water balance, in infants, 763–764
Water intoxication, 764, 765t–766t
Water losses
  insensible, 239, 763
  transepidermal, 244b–245b
Water retention, in chronic renal failure, 921
Waterson-Friderichsen syndrome, 987, 987b
Weaning, 329–330
  definition of, 329
Weaning flowsheet, for opioids, 171–172,
    173f–174f
Weight
  general trends in, 67, 68t
  measurement of, 110–111, 111f
    in neonate, 192
  related to gestational age, 189–192
Weight loss
  in adolescent, 523
  in neonate, 192
Weight loss programs, 523
Welts, 450b
Werdnig-Hoffmann disease, 1105–1106, 1105b
Wet compresses, in wound care, 1016
Wheal, 1011f
Wheelchair, 552, 1117, 1117f
  in cerebral palsy, 1093
Wheeze, 132
  assessment of, in respiratory
      function, 709b
Whey (lactalbumin), in human milk, 214
Whey-hydrolysate formulas, 217
Whey-to-casein ratio, in prepared
    formulas, 217
Whitaker perfusion test, 905t–906t
White blood cell count, 870t
  differential, 870t
Whitehead (closed comedone), 1035

Whooping cough (pertussis), 424t–430t,
    728–729
  immunization against, 332f–333f, 336
Wilmington brace, 1077
Wilms tumor (nephroblastoma), 917–918,
    917b–918b
Winter classification, modified, of cerebral
    palsy, 1091
Wiskott-Aldrich syndrome, 897
Witch's milk, 197
Withdrawal, drug, in neonates, 287b
Withdrawal Assessment Tool-1 (WAT-1),
    171–172, 173f–174f
Wong-Baker Faces Pain Rating Scale, 150
Word association game, in communication with
    children, 93
Word-Graphic Rating Scale, in pain assessment,
    148t–150t
Work-based group care, 323
Working mother, 40, 40b
Wound(s), 1010–1013, 1014t
  acute, 1010–1013
  burn. *See* Burns.
  chronic, 1010–1013
  deep tissue, 1013
  epidermal, 1013
  open, 1015
  puncture, 1016
  to eye, 586
Wound care
  corticosteroid therapy in, 1014
  dressings in, 1013–1014
  for animal bites, 1029
  for burns, 1045
  nursing care in, 1015–1016
  relief of symptoms in, 1016
  systemic therapy in, 1015
  topical therapy in, 1014–1016
Wound healing
  factors influencing, 1013, 1014t
  process of, 1013
Wound sepsis, 1040
Wrist restraint, 656, 657f
Writing, in communication with children, 94
Wryneck (torticollis), 121

X

Xenografts, for burns, 1043

Y

Yellow jacket stings, 1025t–1026t
Yersinia enterocolitis, diarrhea due to, 772t–774t

Z

Zanamivir, for influenza, 717
Zinc deficiency
  in failure to thrive, 355–356
  in neonate, 244
Zollinger-Ellison syndrome, 792